BRUNNER AND SUDDARTH'S

Textbook of Medical-Surgical Nursing

Lippincot

Philadelphia • New Yo

BRUNNER AND SUDDARTH'S

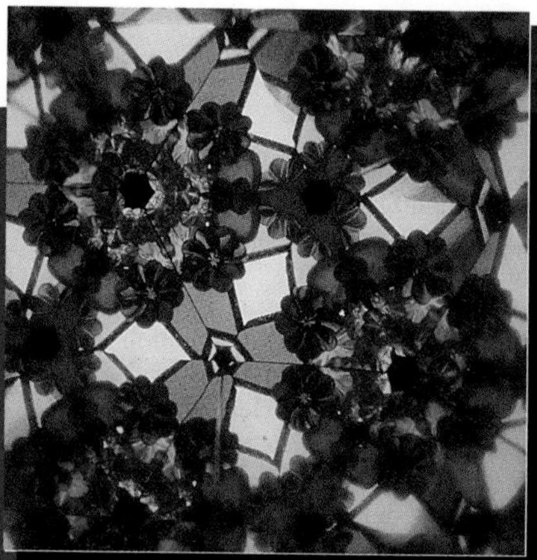

Textbook of Medical-Surgical Nursing

EIGHTH EDITION

Suzanne C. Smeltzer, RN, EdD, FAAN

Associate Professor and Nurse Researcher
Thomas Jefferson University
Philadelphia, Pennsylvania

Brenda G. Bare, RN, MSN

Assistant Vice President for Nursing
The Alexandria Hospital
Alexandria, Virginia

With 41 Contributors

Sponsoring Editor: Lisa Stead
Coordinating Editorial Assistants: Sarah Andrus and Brian MacDonald
Project Editor: Tom Gibbons
Indexer: Ann Cassar
Art Director: Susan Hermansen
Interior Designer: Anne O'Donnell
Cover Designer: Jerry Cable
Production Manager: Helen Ewan
Production Coordinator: Kathryn Rule
Compositor: Compset Inc.
Printer/Binder: R.R. Donnelly & Sons Company/Willard
Cover Printer: The Lehigh Press, Inc.

8th Edition

6 5 4

Library of Congress Cataloging-in-Publication Data

Brunner and Suddarth's textbook of medical-surgical nursing.—8th ed./ [edited by] Suzanne C. Smeltzer, Brenda G. Bare ; with 41 contributors.
p. cm.
Includes bibliographical references and index.
ISBN 0-397-55073-1
ISBN 0-397-55480-X (unbound version)
1. Nursing. 2. Surgical nursing. I. Brunner, Lillian Sholtis. II. Suddarth, Doris Smith. III. Smeltzer, Suzanne C. O'Connell. IV. Bare, Brenda G. V. Title: Textbook of medical-surgical nursing.
[DNLM: 1. Nursing Care. 2. Surgical Nursing. WY 150 B8972 1995]
RT41.T46 1995
610.73–dc20
DNLM/DLC
for Library of Congress 95-2835
CIP

The material contained in this volume was submitted as previously unpublished material, except in the instances in which credit has been given to the source from which some of the illustrative material was derived.

Any procedure or practice described in this book should be applied by the health-care practitioner under appropriate supervision in accordance with professional standards of care used with regard to the unique circumstances that apply in each practice situation. Care has been taken to confirm the accuracy of information presented and to describe generally accepted practices. However, the authors, editors, and publisher cannot accept any responsibility for errors or omissions or for any consequences from application of the information in this book and make no warranty, express or implied, with respect to the contents of the book.

The authors and publisher have exerted every effort to ensure that drug selection and dosage set forth in this text are in accordance with current recommendations and practice at the time of publication. However, in view of ongoing research, changes in government regulations, and the constant flow of information relating to drug therapy and drug reactions, the reader is urged to check the package insert for each drug for any change in indications and dosage and for added warnings and precautions. This is particularly important when the recommended agent is a new or infrequently employed drug.

To Lillian Sholtis Brunner and Doris Smith Suddarth

With appreciation for the many years you have helped
countless nursing students and practitioners in the art and science of nursing

Contributors

Margaret Ahearn-Spera, R.N., C., M.S.N.
Director, Medical Patient Care Services
Danbury Hospital
Danbury, Connecticut
Assistant Clinical Professor
Yale University School of Nursing
New Haven, Connecticut
Chapter 60: Management of Patients With Neurologic Disorders

Daleen Aragon, R.N., M.S.N., C.C.R.N.
Education Specialist, ICU
Orlando Regional Health Care System
Orlando, Florida
Chapter 56: Assessment and Management of Patients With Vision Problems and Eye Disorders

Debra A. Bancroft, R.N., B.S.N.
Speciality Coordinator, Rheumatology
Columbia Hospital
Milwaukee, Wisconsin
Chapter 52: Management of Patients With Rheumatic Disorders

Linda J. Burns, Ph.D., R.N.
Assistant Professor, College of Nursing
Seton Hall University
South Orange, New Jersey
Chapter 19: Preoperative Nursing Management
Chapter 20: Intraoperative Nursing and Anesthesia
Chapter 21: Postoperative Nursing Management

Jacqueline Fowler Byers, R.N., M.S.N., C.C.R.N.
Director of Nursing Research
Orlando Regional Health Care System
Orlando, Florida
Chapter 55: Management of Patients With Burn Injury

Patricia Ann Cady, Ph.D., R.N., C.C.R.N.
Clinical Nurse III, Surgical Intensive Care Unit
Beth Israel Hospital
Boston, Massachusetts
Chapter 5: Ethical Issues in Medical-Surgical Nursing

Corinne Lewis Conlon, M.S.N., R.N., C.S.
Assistant Professor
Piedmont Virginia Community College
Charlottesville, Virginia
Chapter 32: Assessment and Management of Patients With Hematologic Disorders

Juliet Corbin, R.N., D.N.S.
Lecturer, School of Nursing
San Jose State University
San Jose, California
Chapter 17: Chronic Illness

Ann Dellaira, Ph.D., R.N., C.
Assistant Professor, Department of Nursing
Faculty of Arts and Sciences, Rutgers University
Camden, New Jersey
Chapter 48: Assessment of Immune Function
Chapter 49: Management of Patients With Immunodeficiency Disorders
Chapter 50: Acquired Immunodeficiency Syndrome
Chapter 51: Management of Patients With Allergic Disorders

Gladys E. Deters, R.N., M.S.N., O.C.N.
Associate Professor
University of Virginia School of Nursing
Charlottesville, Virginia
Chapter 53: Assessment of Integumentary Function
Chapter 54: Management of Patients With Dermatologic Problems

Nancy Donegan, R.N., M.P.H., C.I.C.
Director, Infection Control
Washington Hospital Center
Washington, D.C.
Chapter 65: Management of Patients With Infectious Diseases

Karen Hassey Dow, R.N., Ph.D., F.A.A.N.
Associate Professor
University of Central Florida
Orlando, Florida
Chapter 46: Assessment and Management of Patients With Breast Disorders

Barbara Springer Edwards, R.N., C.C.R.N., M.T.S.
Acting Director, Cardiac Surgical Unit
The Alexandria Hospital
Alexandria, Virginia
Ethical Issues Displays

Kathleen Keller Furniss, R.N., C., M.S.N.
Women's Health Care Nurse Practitioner
University of Medicine and Dentistry of New Jersey
Newark, New Jersey
Chapter 44: Assessment and Management of Patients With Problems Related to Female Physiologic Processes
Chapter 45: Management of Patients With Disorders of the Female Reproductive System
Chapter 46: Assessment and Management of Patients With Breast Disorders

Maureen Giuffre, R.N., Ph.D.
Clinical Research Consultant
Salisbury, Maryland
Chapter 13: Pain Management

Janet Goshorn, R.N., M.S.N.
Clinical Educator
Florida Hospital
Orlando, Florida
Chapter 43: Management of Patients With Urinary and Renal Disorders

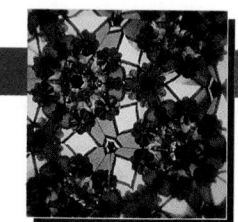

Doreen Chaffinch Grzelak, M.S.N., R.N., O.C.N.
Director Medical/Oncology Nursing
Reston Hospital Center
Reston, Virginia
Chapter 34: Management of Patients With Ingestive Problems and Upper Gastrointestinal Disorders
Chapter 36: Management of Patients With Gastric and Duodenal Disorders

Gail P. Hamilton, R.N., C., D.S.W.
Associate Professor
Department of Nursing, College of Allied Health Professions
Temple University
Philadelphia, Pennsylvania
Chapter 12: Health Care of the Older Adult

Lois M. Hoskins, Ph.D., R.N., F.A.A.N.
Associate Professor
The Catholic University of America
Washington, D.C.
Chapter 8: Homeostasis and Pathophysiologic Processes
Chapter 9: Stress and Adaptation

Ann N. Hotter, R.N., M.S.N., C.C.R.N.
Clinical Nurse Specialist—Critical Care
Mayo Foundation Hospitals
Assistant Professor of Nursing
Mayo Medical School
Rochester, Minnesota
Chapter 25: Respiratory Care Modalities

Ryan Iwamoto, R.N., C.S., M.N.
Clinical Nurse Specialist—Radiation Oncology
Virginia Mason Medical Center
Seattle, Washington
Chapter 47: Assessment and Management of Patients With Disorders of the Male Reproductive System

Ann Robicheau Kaisen, R.N., B.S.N., M.P.A.
Nursing Education Specialist
Yale–New Haven Hospital
New Haven, Connecticut
Chapter 26: Assessment of Cardiovascular Function

Dorothy B. Liddel, M.S.N., R.N., O.N.C.
Assistant Professor
Columbia Union College
Takoma Park, Maryland
Chapter 18: Principles and Practices of Rehabilitation
Chapter 61: Assessment of Musculoskeletal Function
Chapter 62: Management Modalities for Patients With Musculoskeletal Dysfunction
Chapter 63: Management of Patients With Musculoskeletal Disorders
Chapter 64: Management of Patients With Musculoskeletal Trauma

Martha V. Manning, R.N., M.S.N.
Milieu Nurse Specialist
Commonwealth Day Treatment Program
Fairfax, Virginia
Chapter 33: Assessment of Digestive and Gastrointestinal Function
Chapter 37: Management of Patients With Intestinal and Rectal Disorders

Barbara J. Maschak-Carey, R.N., C.S., M.S.N., C.D.E.
Diabetes Clinical Nurse Specialist
Hospital of the University of Pennsylvania
Philadelphia, Pennsylvania
Chapter 39: Assessment and Management of Patients With Diabetes Mellitus

Shawn M. McCabe, R.N., M.S.N., C.C.R.N.
Clinical Nurse Specialist, Trauma
University of Medicine and Dentistry of New Jersey
Newark, New Jersey
Chapter 58: Assessment of Neurologic Function
Chapter 59: Management of Patients With Neurologic Dysfunction

Kathleen Miller, R.N., M.B.A., M.S.N.
Assistant Vice President Nursing and Support Services
The Alexandria Hospital
Alexandria, Virginia
Chapter 66: Emergency Nursing

Kathleen Collins Monahan, R.N., M.S.N.
Nursing Consultant
Formerly of Yale–New Haven Hospital
New Haven, Connecticut
Chapter 26: Assessment of Cardiovascular Function

Nancy A. Morrissey, Ph.D., R.N., C.
Director, Surgical Unit
The Alexandria Hospital
Alexandria, Virginia
Chapter 35: Gastrointestinal Intubation and Special Nutritional Management

Martha Mulvey, R.N., M.S., C.N.S.
Clinical Nurse Specialist—Surgery
University Hospital, University of Medicine and Dentistry of New Jersey
Newark, New Jersey
Chapter 14: Fluids and Electrolytes: Balance and Disturbances

Catherine Paradiso, R.N., C.C.R.N., M.S.N.
Clinical Nurse Specialist
Mobile Health Unit Coordinator
The Visiting Nurse Association
Home Care of Staten Island
Staten Island, New York
Chapter 41: Assessment of Urinary and Renal Function
Chapter 42: Management of Patients With Urinary and Renal Dysfunction

Anne G. Peach, R.N., M.S.N., C.N.A.
Site Administrator, Sand Lake Hospital
Orlando Regional Health Care System
Orlando, Florida
Chapter 22: Assessment of Respiratory Function
Chapter 23: Management of Patients With Conditions of the Upper Respiratory Tract
Chapter 24: Management of Patients With Conditions of the Chest and Lower Respiratory Tract

Janice Smith Pigg, B.S.N., R.N., M.S.
Nurse Consultant, Rheumatology
Columbia Musculoskeletal Center, Columbia Hospital
Milwaukee, Wisconsin
Chapter 52: Management of Patients With Rheumatic Disorders

Kimberly J. Pollock, R.N., B.S.N., M.B.A., C.O.R.L.N.
Administrator, Department of Otorhinolaryngology
University of Texas Southwest Medical Center
Dallas, Texas
Chapter 57: Assessment and Management of Patients With Hearing Problems and Ear Disorders

Kathryn A. Pollon, R.N., M.S.N., C.S.
Mental Health Therapist
Northwest Center for Community Mental Health
Chantilly, Virginia
Chapter 10: Human Response to Illness

Linda Robinson, M.S.N., R.N., C.S.
Doctoral Candidate
University of Pennsylvania School of Nursing
Philadelphia, Pennsylvania
Chapter 15: Shock and Multisystem Failure

Susan Rokita, R.N., M.S.
Clinical Nurse Specialist—Adult Oncology
University Hospital, Pennsylvania State University
Hershey, Pennsylvania
Chapter 16: Oncology: Nursing the Patient With Cancer

Linda H. Schakenbach, M.S.N., R.N., C.C.R.N., C.E.T.N., C.S.
Clinical Nurse Specialist, Surgical Nursing
Fairfax Hospital
Fairfax, Virginia
Chapter 28: Management of Patients With Cardiac Disorders and Related Complications
Chapter 29: Management of Patients With Structural, Infectious, or Inflammatory Cardiac Disorders
Chapter 30: Management of the Cardiac Surgery Patient

Loretta Spittle, R.N., M.S., C.C.R.N.
Staff Nurse, MICU
Georgetown University Hospital
Washington, D.C.
Chapter 27: Management of Patients With Dysrhythmias and Conduction Problems
Chapter 28: Management of Patients With Cardiac Disorders and Related Complications
Chapter 29: Management of Patients With Structural, Infectious, or Inflammatory Cardiac Disorders

Cindy Stern, R.N., M.S.N.
Clinical Research Associate
Thomas Jefferson University Hospital
Philadelphia, Pennsylvania
Chapter 16: Oncology: Nursing the Patient With Cancer

Marshelle Thobaben, M.S., P.H.N, R.N., F.N.P.
Professor
Humboldt State University
Arcata, California

Judith Troyer-Caudle, R.N., M.S.N.
Vascular and Wound Clinical Nurse Specialist
Veterans' Affairs Medical Center
Kansas City, Missouri
Chapter 31: Assessment and Management of Patients With Vascular Disorders and Problems of Peripheral Circulation

Reviewers

Kathy M. Howard, R.N., C., M.S.N.
Standard Maintenance Representative
Medical-Surgical Adult Health Division
Newark Beth Israel Medical Center
Newark, New Jersey

Joan Klemballa, R.N., M.A., Ph.D.
Professor of Nursing
The College of West Virginia
Beckley, West Virginia

Cathy Mallone, R.N., B.S.N., M.S.N.
Assistant Professor
University of North Alabama
Florence, Alabama

Dorothy Obester, Ph.D., M.S.N., B.S.N.E., R.N.
Professor of Nursing
Saint Francis College
Loretta, Pennsylvania

Katherine Dentoni Ricossa, B.S.N., R.N., C., Ph.N.
Associate Faculty
Mission Community College
Santa Clara, California
Staff Nurse III, Surgical Orthopedic Neurosurgical Department
Good Samaritan Hospital
San Jose, California

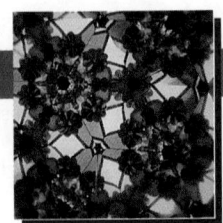

Preface

As the end of the 20th century approaches, the health care system and nursing, as an integral part of that system, are entering a new era characterized by heretofore unknown challenges. With health care shifting from the acute care hospital to community-based settings and the home in an effort to reduce costs of health care, the profession of nursing and nurses are faced with the need to respond to an array of demands and changes.

The "graying of America" reflects the aging of the population and an increasing incidence of chronic illnesses among the patients in our care. The ethnic and cultural characteristics of patients, clients, and health care providers alike are becoming more diverse. The beliefs and values of nurses that health and health care are important and that people have a vital role in maintaining their own health may conflict with the beliefs and values of other cultures. The problem of homelessness in individuals and whole families creates a challenge and dilemma to the nurse whose goal for patients is optimal health and well-being. It creates a dilemma for nurses who take for granted the availability of shelter, food, and clothing.

Acute care hospitals promote discharge of patients as early as possible because of financial losses incurred if patients are hospitalized beyond the number of days for which the hospital receives reimbursement. At the same time, nurses must consider the well-being of patients as their families reorganize their lives so they can assume care for the patient who is discharged within days of major surgery or acute illness. The need to discharge patients from the hospital while they are in the very early stages of recovery creates challenges for the nurse who must teach the patient and family about detection, prevention, and management of complications that previously were attended to during hospitalization. The need to begin discharge planning often before the patient is hospitalized for surgery requires new approaches to planning and implementing interventions to ensure the patient's recovery and well-being.

As nurses deal with these changes in the health care system, they are also called upon to respond to changes related to technologic and scientific advances in health care. Examples of these changes include the discovery of new genetic markers that provide information about a patient's likelihood of developing potentially fatal or disabling diseases in the future and advanced technologies and therapeutic regimens that enable the survival of those who previously would have succumbed to their illness or injury. As these changes are occurring, patients are taking on an increasingly active role in decision making about their own health care. Patients are urged to consider advanced directives and to make known their opinions and wishes about their own care.

Although the value of nurses' contributions to patient care has been acknowledged in the past, the need for nurses to take an active, more visible role in influencing health-related social policy at the local and national levels is becoming increasingly important because of the relationship between social issues, such as violence and drug abuse, and health. The proliferation of other categories of health care providers makes it imperative that nurses effectively articulate the contributions of nursing to health promotion and maintenance, disease prevention, and patient and family well-being. A voice at the table of decision-making about health policy and health-related social issues is critical if nursing as a profession is to thrive.

The changes and challenges described above make it essential that the nurse is knowledgeable about the problems faced by patients and their families during and following hospitalization and has well-developed critical-thinking skills that will allow examination of issues encountered in the course of providing care in the hospital, outpatient clinic, nursing center, community setting, and home. An understanding of the influences of culture and ethnicity on the patient and an ability to identify and analyze ethical issues in nursing practice are essential if the nurse is to provide the high-quality care that the public expects.

This edition of *Brunner and Suddarth's Textbook of Medical-Surgical Nursing* was written with today's changing health care system as a key focus.

Organization

The book is divided into 17 units, dealing with various aspects of health care and the physiologic disorders that constitute the essence of medical-surgical nursing.

Unit 1 addresses broad general issues in the current health care scene and in nursing education. Chapters in this unit deal with such topics as Health Care Delivery and Nursing Practice; Community-Based Nursing Practice; Critical Thinking and the Nursing Process; Health Teaching and Health Promotion; and Ethical Issues in Medical-Surgical Nursing.

Unit 2 describes the components of health assessment, including approaches to Clinical Interviewing and Physical Examination and Nutritional Assessment.

Unit 3 examines a range of biophysical and psychosocial concepts and includes chapters on Homeostasis and Pathophysiology; Stress and Adaptation; Human Response to Illness; Transcultural Perspectives in Nursing; and Health Care of the Older Adult.

Unit 4, Concepts and Challenges in Patient Management, addresses the topics of Pain Management; Fluids and Electrolytes; Shock and Multisystem Failure; Oncology; Chronic Illness; and Rehabilitation.

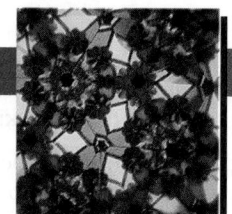

Unit 5 on Perioperative Concepts and Management provides the student with the general principles involved in preoperative, intraoperative, and postoperative management. Individual chapters address each of these stages of perioperative nursing.

Units 6 to 16 focus on specific areas of human physiologic function and the dysfunctions associated with each of the major body systems. The areas covered include Oxygen–Carbon Dioxide Exchange and Respiratory Function; Cardiovascular, Circulatory, and Hematologic Function; Digestive and Gastrointestinal Function; Metabolic and Endocrine Function; Urinary and Renal Function; Reproductive Function; Immunologic Function; Integumentary Function; Sensorineural Function; Neurologic Function; and Musculoskeletal Function. Each body system unit includes chapters on assessment, general management and therapeutic interventions, and specific physiologic disorders and problems.

Unit 17, the last unit, deals with the acute problems of Infectious Diseases and Emergency Nursing.

New to This Edition

As expected with a new edition, the chapters throughout the book have been thoroughly reviewed and updated to ensure that the material reflects current information and developments.

- *New chapters* have been added to address the pressing issues and new concepts mentioned earlier in the Preface:
  Chapter 2: Community-Based Nursing Practice
  Chapter 3: Critical Thinking and the Nursing Process
  Chapter 11: Transcultural Perspectives in Nursing
  Chapter 15: Shock and Multisystem Failure
  Chapter 17: Chronic Illness
  Chapter 50: Acquired Immunodeficiency Syndrome
- *New elements* to this edition include collaborative problems; examples of critical pathways; special charts and boxed displays on patient education, prevention, and health promotion guidelines; ethical decision-making situations; procedural guidelines; and critical thinking exercises at the end of each chapter. Each of these elements and other features are described in more detail in the following paragraphs.
- *Full color* has been introduced into this edition to provide a richer visual impact and to highlight the illustrations as well as the various display elements, charts, and tables.
- *A clinical handbook,* covering the major disorders encountered in medical-surgical nursing practice, accompanies this edition. The information is presented in outline format and offers the student a portable, easy-to-use clinical reference.

Critical Thinking Emphasis

Nurses have traditionally drawn on their critical thinking skills in providing nursing care. However, with the changing health care scene, nurses are working in more diverse settings and with more independence; thus, the need to develop critical thinking skills early in the education process has become even more important. The text and its accompanying learning package provide several means for helping students develop and refine these essential thinking skills:

- Chapter 3, "Critical Thinking and the Nursing Process," offers a general discussion of critical thinking along with specific guidelines for developing these skills. The student can thus obtain a solid overview of methods for applying critical thinking in the clinical setting.
- *Critical Thinking Exercises* at the end of each chapter provide the student with specific situations in which to apply thinking skills. Classroom discussion of students' responses to these exercises can provide a forum for exploring the different thinking processes involved in dealing with these situations.
- *The Study Guide* that accompanies the text contains additional critical thinking exercises and situations to further help students develop and refine their cognitive skills.
- *A computer disc* enclosed at the back of the book provides a self-testing medium for the student and offers the rationale for decision-making responses. Continued use of this computer program will enhance the student's ability to think critically.

Transcultural Awareness

The rich and varied cultural texture of our society requires a sensitive and open-minded approach in the delivery of health care. The text has attempted to increase an awareness of methods for caring for people from varied ethnic and cultural backgrounds:

- Chapter 11, "Transcultural Perspectives in Nursing," is devoted to this subject and offers specific guidelines and considerations in dealing with ethnic and cultural diversity in the health care setting.
- The *Critical Thinking Exercises* at the end of each chapter contain numerous instances of cultural diversity to reinforce this important consideration in nursing practice.

Special Features

- *Nursing Process:* The nursing process continues to be the focus for discussing the delivery of nursing care. As in previous editions, it is presented in a consistent format for most of the major disorders covered in the text. Assessment, Diagnosis (Nursing Diagnoses and Collaborative Problems), Planning and Implementation, Nursing Interventions, and Evaluation with Expected Outcomes represent the major framework for discussing the nursing process.
- *Collaborative Problems:* Since working collaboratively with other members of the health care team represents an essential nursing responsibility, collaborative problems have been incorporated into the nursing process framework as part of assessment and monitoring activities and as an important component of nursing interventions.
- *Critical Pathways:* Selected examples of critical pathways are included. These depict the manner in which

cost containment goals based on DRGs have prompted hospitals to construct clinical management tools that delineate the daily collaborative activities that must be carried out within a set time frame to achieve identifiable patient outcomes.

- *Care Plans:* As in past editions, numerous care plans abound throughout the text and are based on the nursing process. Whereas critical pathways present broad-based collaborative activity involved in patient care, the nursing care plans delineate the specific nursing interventions to be carried out in delivering effective nursing care to achieve the desired patient outcomes.
- *Patient Education Charts and Prevention and Health Promotion Guidelines:* These charts and boxed displays underscore the importance of health promotion and preventive care as a key component of nursing practice. They highlight specific points related to guiding patients in promoting their health, preventing illness and carrying out self-care activity while recovering from specific illnesses.
- *Procedure Guidelines:* In selected instances when nursing care is based on procedural activity in a medical-surgical setting, the steps involved in carrying out the procedure are presented in chart form for easy access.
- *Home Care Considerations:* With so many patients being discharged early in the course of their recovery, home care and patient teaching have gained increasing importance in the delivery of health care. The activities involved in carrying out or overseeing care in the home, either through home care visits by the nurse or through family and patient teaching, are delineated for a wide range of disorders and are clearly highlighted under specific headings in the text. This specific information augments the general guidelines for home care delivery discussed in Chapter 2, "Community-Based Nursing Practice."
- *Gerontologic Considerations:* The increasing number of elderly people in our society requires that special attention be directed to the care of this segment of the population. Therefore, the text continues to include a special heading for discussing gerontologic considerations throughout the clinical chapters and devotes a full chapter to this topic: Chapter 12, "Health Care of the Older Adult."
- *Research Profiles:* The results of nursing research continue to influence nursing care. This edition retains the extremely popular Nursing Research Profile feature that appears at the end of the clinical units. These profiles contain a collection of key current research studies related to selected main topics covered in the unit. The student is thus given an overview of the diverse nature of the research that has been conducted and can gain an awareness and appreciation of the importance of such research to nursing practice.
- *Chapter Outlines and Learning Objectives:* The outlines and objectives that appear at the beginning of each chapter help orient the reader to the content of the chapter. The outlines identify the organizational elements within the chapter. The learning objectives alert the reader to the key concepts and points to be gained from studying the chapter.
- *Bold-Face Type:* Key terms are presented in bold face when first introduced in the chapter to highlight the words and definitions and alert the reader to their importance.

Teaching/Learning Package

The teaching/learning package that accompanies this edition of *Brunner and Suddarth's Textbook of Medical-Surgical Nursing* contains items for both the student and the instructor. For the student there is a study guide, a computer program for self-evaluation, and a clinical handbook. For the instructor there is a computerized testbank, a printed testbank, an instructor's manual, and a set of overhead transparencies.

For the Student

- *The Study Guide* is structured to follow the chapter sequence of the text and offers a variety of different types of questions to help students evaluate their grasp of the contents of the text. Critical thinking questions and case studies provide an opportunity to apply higher-level cognitive skills.
- *A Computer Disc* inserted at the back of the text offers further practice in evaluating knowledge and thinking skills. Students are offered different modes for self-evaluation and are provided with rationale to explain the appropriateness of their responses.
- *A Clinical Handbook* to cover the most frequent disorders encountered in medical-surgical nursing accompanies this edition. An alphabetical organization and an outline format provide an easy-to-use reference for the clinical setting.

For the Instructor

- *A Computerized Testbank,* based on the ParTEST program, consists of 1000 new questions for this edition and is available free to instructors upon adoption of the text. ParTEST is a sophisticated program that allows instructors to edit the questions in the testbank or add new questions, if so desired.
- *A Printed Testbank,* consisting of the questions in the computerized testbank, is available to enable instructors to see the questions for a particular chapter or unit at a glance.
- *Instructor's Manual*
- *Overhead Transparencies*

The eighth edition of *Brunner and Suddarth's Textbook of Medical-Surgical Nursing* is designed to address current issues and to promote the skills necessary in today's changing health care system. Chronicity, home care, and gerontologic considerations have received special emphasis because of their increasing importance in our society. This textbook, which retains the focus on the caring values that have characterized previous editions and prepares the nurse for the beginning of the 21st century, and the educational materials that have been developed to accompany it are designed to assist students and their faculty to respond to the changing health care environment.

Suzanne C. O'Connell Smeltzer
Brenda G. Bare

Acknowledgments

The authors and publisher wish to thank the following people for their hard work and dedication to this project:

Diane M. Billings, R.N., B.S.N., M.S.Ed.
Associate Professor
Indiana University School of Nursing
Indianapolis, Indiana

Mary Jo Boyer, R.N., D.N.Sc.
Associate Dean
Allied Health and Nursing
Delaware County Community College
Media, Pennsylvania

Curtis Buck, C.R.N.A., R.R.T.
Director, Respiratory Therapy
Mayo Foundation Hospitals
Rochester, Minnesota

Kathleen M. Bury, R.N.
Coordinator, IV Services
The Alexandria Hospital
Alexandria, Virginia

Randi Cardonick, M.S., R.D.
Out-Patient Dietician
Hospital of the University of Pennsylvania
Philadelphia, Pennsylvania

Dolly Daniel, R.N.C., B.S.N., C.D.E.
Diabetes Nurse Specialist
The Alexandria Hospital
Alexandria, Virginia

Douglas Gracey, M.D.
Consultant in Pulmonary and Critical Care Medicine
Mayo Clinic
Rochester, Minnesota

Tracey B. Hopkins, R.N., A.D.N.
The Graduate Hospital
Philadelphia, Pennsylvania

Diana Intenzo
Editor

Gary Koenig, R.N.
Nurse Coordinator for Pulmonary Ventilator Respiratory Unit
Mayo Foundation Hospitals
Rochester, Minnesota

Nina S. McClesky, M.L.S.
Director, Medical Library
The Alexandria Hospital
Alexandria, Virginia

Norma M. Metheny, Ph.D., R.N., F.A.A.N.
Professor of Nursing
St. Louis University School of Nursing
St. Louis, Missouri

William L. Meyerhoff, M.D., Ph.D.
Professor and Chairman
Department of Otorhinolaryngology
University of Texas Southwest Medical Center
Dallas, Texas

Margaret Rafferty, R.N., M.A., M.P.H.C.S., N.P.
Associate Professor
Long Island College Hospital School of Nursing
Brooklyn, New York

Carol S. Rosenberg, M.S.N., R.N., C.D.E.
Diabetes Clinical Nurse Specialist
Bay Shores Medical Group
Torrence, California

Ronald K. Smeltzer, Ph.D.

P. Dee G. Stephenson, M.D.
Stephenson Eye Association
Venice, Florida

Elizabeth Sullivan
Manager of Clinical Outcomes
Hahnemann University Hospital
Philadelphia, Pennsylvania

Betty Temples-Mill, R.N., Ph.D.

Rose Wilcox, R.N., M.S.
Instruction Coordinator
Columbus Public Schools
Columbus, Ohio

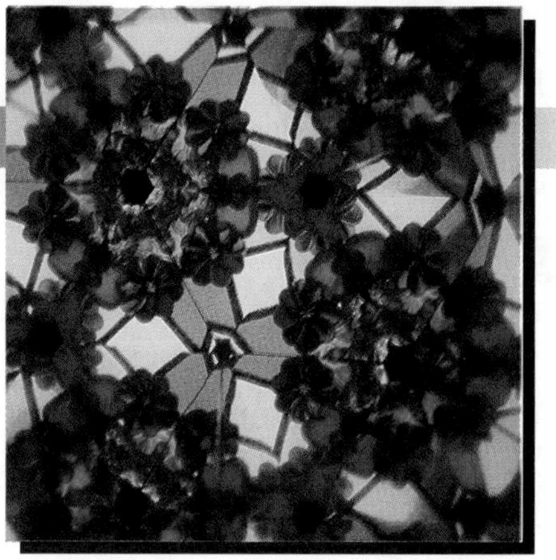

Contents

11 ■ Transcultural Perspectives in Nursing 133

12 ■ Health Care of the Older Adult 141

UNIT 4
Concepts and Challenges in Patient Management 177

13 ■ Pain Management 179

14 ■ Fluids and Electrolytes: Balance and Disturbances 205

37 ■ Management of Patients With Intestinal and Rectal Disorders 909

UNIT 9
Metabolic and Endocrine Function 959

38 ■ Assessment and Management of Patients With Hepatic and Biliary Disorders 961

39 ■ Assessment and Management of Patients With Diabetes Mellitus 1017

40 ■ Assessment and Management of Patients With Endocrine Disorders 1069

UNIT 11
Reproductive Function 1231

44 ■ Assessment and Management of Patients With Problems Related to Female Physiologic Processes 1233

45 ■ Management of Patients With Disorders of the Female Reproductive System 1269

46 ■ Assessment and Management of Patients With Breast Disorders 1301

63 ■ Management of Patients With Musculoskeletal Disorders 1879

64 ■ Management of Patients With Musculoskeletal Trauma 1907

UNIT 17
Other Acute Problems 1951

65 ■ Management of Patients With Infectious Diseases 1953

66 ■ Emergency Nursing 1999

UNIT 1

Health Maintenance and Health Needs

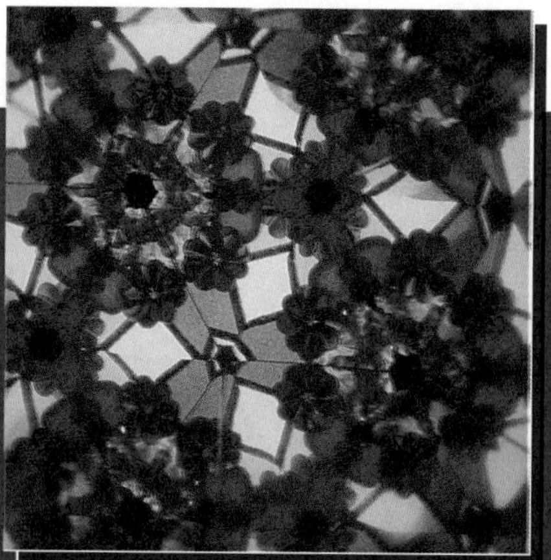

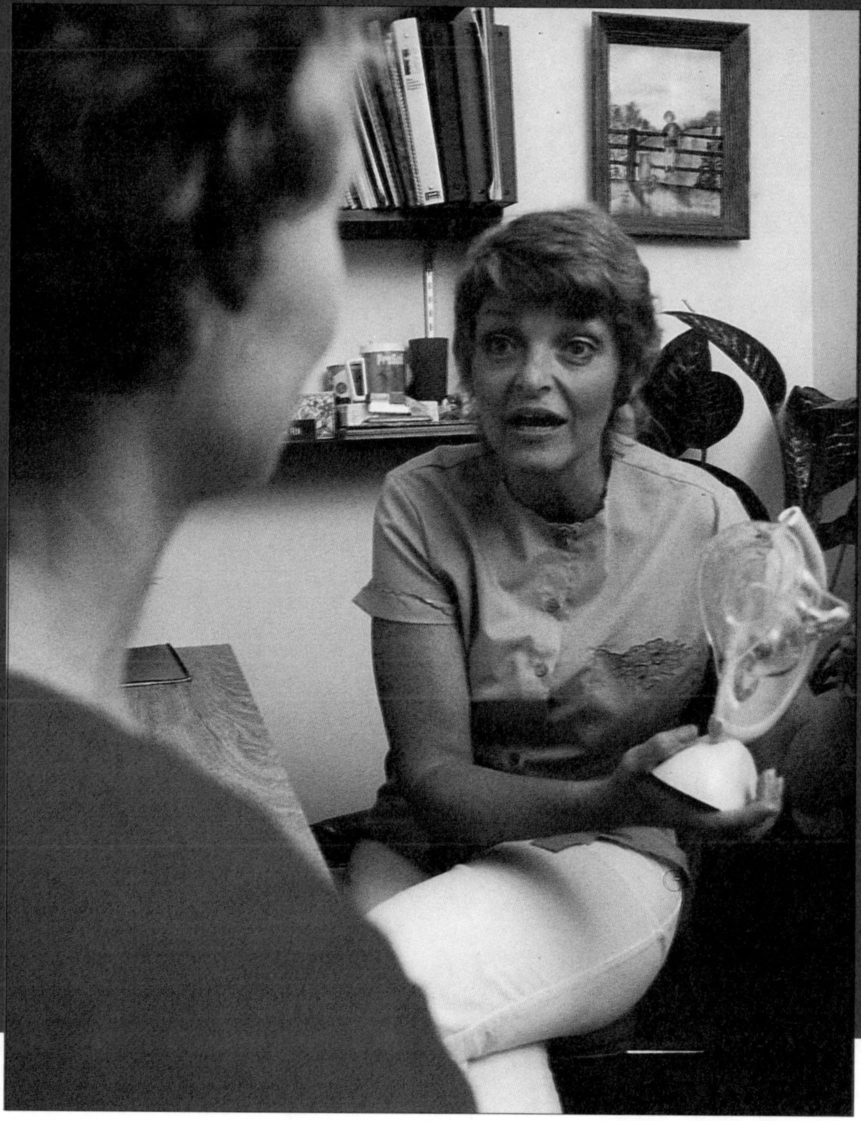

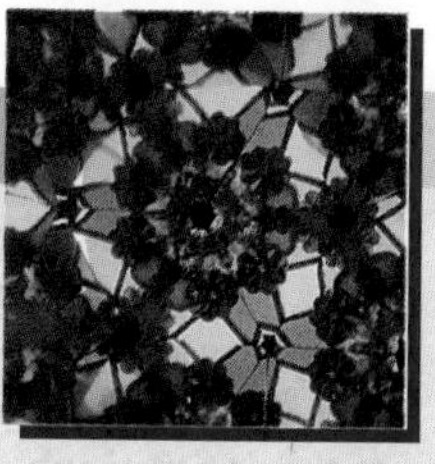

1 Health Care Delivery and Nursing Practice

CHAPTER OUTLINE

The Health Care Delivery System
Health and Health Promotion
The Changing Health Care Scene
Measures for Cost-Effective, Quality Care
Managed Health Care
Nursing and the Nursing Delivery System
Nursing Defined
Nursing Delivery Systems
Community-Based Nursing
The Patient/Client: Consumer and Recipient of Health Care
The Patient's Basic Needs
Cultural Diversity
Roles of the Nurse
Practitioner Role
Leadership Role
Research Role
Advanced Practice Nursing
Collaborative Practice
Critical Thinking Exercises

LEARNING OBJECTIVES

On completion of the chapter, the learner will be able to:

1. Define **health** within the context of the current health care delivery system
2. Describe factors that are causing significant changes in the health care delivery system
3. Specify the expanded roles of the nurse
4. Describe the practitioner, leadership, and research roles of the nurse
5. Describe primary nursing, case management, and collaborative practice

The health care industry, like other industries in American society, has experienced numerous changes during the past several decades. These changes are a culmination of societal, technologic, scientific, economic, and political changes that have occurred throughout the 20th century.

All these changes have a significant impact on nursing, not the least of which are the increase in the aging population, the changing pattern of diseases, the cultural diversity of the population, and the rising cost of health care, which is being addressed through health care reform efforts.

In addition, nursing is significantly affected by changes that have led to increased outpatient care services, decreased length of hospital stays, and more and more care provided in the community and in the home. These changes are having a dramatic influence on where nurses practice, with an increasing trend for nurses to provide health care in community and home settings.

As an increasing proportion of the population reaches age 65 and older and as disease patterns shift from acute illnesses to chronic illnesses, the focus of the health care professions is shifting from disease treatment and cure to prevention, health promotion, and management of chronic conditions. This shift in focus coincides with a nationwide emphasis on cost control and resource management, directed toward providing cost-efficient and cost-effective health care services to the population as a whole.

The changes occurring in the health care system make change in nursing inevitable. Likewise, nursing, as a health care profession and a major component of the health care delivery system, has been and will continue to be an important force in shaping the future of that system.

The Health Care Delivery System

Health and Health Promotion

Our health care system has traditionally been disease-oriented. However, current trends place greater emphasis on health and its promotion.

Health. How health is perceived depends on how health is defined. The World Health Organization (WHO) defines health as a "state of complete physical, mental, and social well being and not merely the absence of disease and infirmity."* Such a definition of health does not allow for any variation in the degrees of wellness or illness. On the other hand, the concept of a health–illness continuum allows for a greater range in describing a person's health status. By viewing health and illness on a continuum, it is possible to consider a person as having neither complete health nor complete illness. Instead, a person's state of health is ever-changing and has the potential for ranging from high-level wellness to extremely poor health and imminent death. The model of the health–illness continuum makes it possible to view a person as simultaneously possessing degrees of both health and illness.

The limitations of the WHO definition of health are clear in relation to chronic illness. A chronically ill person cannot meet the standards of health as established by the WHO definition. However, when viewed from the perspective of the health–illness continuum, people with chronic illness can be understood as having the potential to attain a high level of wellness, if they are successful in meeting their health potential within the limits of their chronic illness.

Wellness. Wellness has been defined as being equivalent to health. Leddy and Pepper (1993, p. 222) acknowledge that wellness is difficult to quantify, but they contend that it may be indicated by "(1) the capacity of the person to perform to the best of his ability, (2) the ability to adjust and adapt to varying situations, (3) a reported feeling of well-being, and (4) a feeling that 'everything is together' and 'harmonious.' " With this in mind, it becomes evident that the goal of health care providers is to promote positive changes that are directed toward health and well-being.

Health Promotion. Today increasing emphasis is placed on health, health promotion, wellness, and self-care. Health is seen as resulting from a lifestyle that is oriented toward wellness. The result has been the evolution of a wide range of health promotion strategies, including multiphasic screening, lifetime health monitoring programs, environmental and mental health programs, risk reduction, and nutrition and health education. A growing interest in self-care skills is evidenced by the large number of health-related publications, conferences, and workshops designed for the lay public. Organized self-care education programs emphasize health promotion, disease prevention, management of illness, self-medication, and use of the professional health care system. In addition, well over 500,000 self-help groups exist for the purpose of sharing experiences and information about self-care with peers who have similar chronic diseases or disability problems.

Special efforts are being made by health care professionals to reach and motivate members of various cultural and socioeconomic groups concerning lifestyle and health practices. Stress, improper diet, lack of exercise, smoking, drugs, high-risk behaviors and sexual practices, and poor hygiene are all related to the concept that lifestyle affects health. Health care professionals, then, should be concerned with encouraging behavior that promotes health. The goal is to motivate people so that they will make improvements in the way they live, modify risky behaviors, and adopt healthy behaviors.

The Changing Health Care Scene

The health care delivery system is rapidly changing as society's health needs and expectations change.

During the past 50 years, the health problems of the American people have changed significantly. Many infectious diseases have been controlled or eradicated; others (*e.g.*, tuberculosis, AIDS, sexually transmitted diseases) are on the rise. The majority of health problems seen today are chronic in nature. Almost 50% of the U.S. population have one or more chronic conditions.

The elderly population has increased significantly and will continue to grow in future years. In 1991, the nation's 32 million elderly constituted 12% of the population; it is predicted that the number will reach 22% of the population by the year 2030. Those 85 and older constitute one of the fastest-growing segments of the population. By the year 2000, half of the older population will be age 75 and older. Many of the elderly suffer from multiple chronic conditions

*Preamble of the Constitution of the World Health Organization.

that are exacerbated by acute episodes. Their health care needs are complex and demand significant investments, both professional and financial, by the health care industry.

Societal and legislative factors are significant in the changing patterns of health care. Changes in the population in general are affecting the need for and the delivery of health care. It is estimated that by the year 2000, there will be close to 300 million people in the United States (U.S. Department of Health and Human Services, 1990). This population expansion has in part been attributed to improved public health services and improved nutrition.

Not only is the population increasing, but the composition of the population is also changing. The decline in birth rate and the increase in life span due to improved health care have resulted in fewer school-age children and more senior citizens. The majority of the population reside in highly congested urban areas, with a steady migration of minority groups to the inner cities and a migration of middle-class persons to suburban areas. The number of homeless people, including entire families, has increased significantly. The population has become more culturally diverse as increasing numbers of people from different national backgrounds enter the country.

Because of such population changes, the need for health care for specific age groups and for persons within specific geographic localities is altering the effectiveness of the traditional means of providing health care and is necessitating far-reaching changes in the overall health care delivery system.

Technologic advances have occurred in greater numbers during the past several decades than in all other time periods of human civilization. This is an era of sophisticated electronic machines, which have revolutionized the way surgery and diagnostic tests are performed. This is also an era of sophisticated communication systems, connecting most parts of the world. A variety of systems have been devised for storing, retrieving, and disseminating information. Such scientific and technologic advances are themselves precipitating rapid change as well as rapid obsolescence.

Measures for Cost-Effective, Quality Care

The general public has become increasingly interested in and knowledgeable about health care and health promotion. This awareness has been stimulated by television, newspapers, magazines, and other communications media and by political debate. The public has become more health conscious and has in general begun to subscribe strongly to the belief that health and health care constitute a basic right, rather than a privilege for a chosen few.

Health care providers have become increasingly aware of the public's beliefs about health and health care. One indication of such awareness is the time-honored Patient's Bill of Rights prepared by the American Hospital Association, which is directed toward the promotion of more effective patient care and patient satisfaction (Chart 1-1).

The National League for Nursing (NLN) has also issued a statement on patients' rights, which "specifies ways in which a respect for patients' rights and a commitment to safeguarding them can be incorporated into nursing education programs and upheld and reinforced by those in nursing service. In many cases, nurses can directly involve themselves in assuring specific rights; in others, they can make their influence felt indirectly" (Chart 1-2).

Awareness of the public's beliefs and concerns about health and health care has also been acknowledged by Congress. The National Health Planning and Resources Act of 1974 emphasized the need for planning and providing quality health care for all Americans by means of coordinated health services, manpower, and facilities at the national, state, and local levels. Medically underserved populations were the target for the primary care services that were provided for by this act. However, growing adherence to the philosophy that comprehensive, quality health care should be provided for all citizens has prompted governmental concern about spiraling health care costs and wide variations in costs among providers. These concerns led to the Medicare prospective payment system and to the continuing debate about health care reform that has received so much Congressional attention in the last few years.

Diagnosis-Related Groups (DRGs)

In 1983, Congress enacted the most significant health legislation since the Medicare program in 1965. The government was no longer able to afford to reimburse hospitals for patient care that was delivered without any defined limits or costs. Thus, it approved a prospective payment system for hospital inpatient services. This system of reimbursement, referred to as diagnosis-related groups (DRGs), set the rates for Medicare payments for hospital services. Hospitals receive payment at a fixed rate for patients in specific DRGs. A fixed payment has been predetermined for over 470 possible diagnostic categories, which cover the majority of medical diagnoses of all patients admitted to the hospital. Thus, hospitals receive the same payment for every patient with a given diagnosis or DRG. If the cost of the patient's care is lower than the payment, the hospital gains a profit; if the cost is higher, the hospital incurs a loss. In order to qualify for Medicare reimbursement, hospitals must contract with peer review organizations (PROs) to perform quality and utilization review. The PROs monitor admission patterns, lengths of stay, transfers, and the quality of services, and validate DRG coding. The burden is now on hospitals to reduce costs, utilization, and lengths of patient stay.

The DRG system provides hospitals with an incentive to cut unnecessary costs and to discharge patients as quickly as possible. The importance of an effective discharge planning program along with utilization review and quality assurance programs is unquestionable.

The impact of these initiatives on nurses is that they must assume responsibility with other health care team members for maintaining quality care while facing pressures to discharge patients and decrease staffing costs. Consequently, nurses in hospitals are caring for patients who are older and sicker and require more nursing services, and nurses in the community are caring for patients who have been discharged earlier and need acute care services and high technology and long-term care.

Quality Assurance Programs

At the same time that hospitals are dealing with shorter hospital stays, health care agencies are implementing ongoing quality assurance programs. These programs were required

CHART 1-1
AHA's Patient's Bill of Rights

1. The patient has the right to considerate and respectful care.
2. The patient has the right to obtain from his physician complete current information concerning his diagnosis, treatment, and prognosis in terms the patient can be reasonably expected to understand. When it is not medically advisable to give such information to the patient, the information should be made available to an appropriate person in his behalf. He has the right to know, by name, the physician responsible for coordinating his care.
3. The patient has the right to receive from his physician information necessary to give informed consent prior to the start of any procedure and/or treatment. Except in emergencies, such information for informed consent should include but not necessarily be limited to the specific procedure and/or treatment, the medically significant risks involved, and the probable duration of incapacitation. Where medically significant alternatives for care or treatment exist, or when the patient requests information concerning medical alternatives, the patient has the right to such information. The patient also has the right to know the name of the person responsible for the procedures and/or treatment.
4. The patient has the right to refuse treatment to the extent permitted by law and to be informed of the medical consequences of his action.
5. The patient has the right to every consideration of his privacy concerning his own medical care program. Case discussion, consultation, examination, and treatment are confidential and should be conducted discreetly. Those not directly involved in his care must have the permission of the patient to be present.
6. The patient has the right to expect that all communications and records pertaining to his care should be treated as confidential.
7. The patient has the right to expect that within its capacity a hospital must make reasonable response to the request of a patient for services. The hospital must provide evaluation, service, and/or referral as indicated by the urgency of the case. When medically permissible, a patient may be transferred to another facility only after he has received complete information and explanation concerning the needs for and alternatives to such a transfer. The institution to which the patient is to be transferred must first have accepted the patient for transfer.
8. The patient has the right to obtain information as to any relationship of his hospital to other health care and educational institutions insofar as his care is concerned. The patient has the right to obtain information as to the existence of any professional relationships among individuals, by name, who are treating him.
9. The patient has the right to be advised if the hospital proposes to engage in or perform human experimentation affecting his care or treatment. The patient has the right to refuse to participate in such research projects.
10. The patient has the right to expect reasonable continuity of care. He has the right to know in advance what appointment times and physicians are available and where. The patient has the right to expect that the hospital will provide a mechanism whereby he is informed by his physician or a delegate of the physician of the patient's continuing health care requirements following discharge.
11. The patient has the right to examine and receive an explanation of his bill regardless of source of payment.
12. The patient has the right to know what hospital rules and regulations apply to his conduct as a patient.

(Reprinted with the permission of the American Hospital Association.)

for reimbursement for services and for accreditation by the Joint Commission on Accreditation of Healthcare Organizations (JCAHO). The concept of quality assurance establishes a sense of accountability on the part of the health professions to society for the quality, appropriateness, and cost of health services provided.

JCAHO developed a generic model that required monitoring and evaluation of quality and appropriateness of care. The model was implemented in health care institutions and agencies through organization-wide quality assurance (QA) programs and reporting systems. Many aspects of the programs were centralized in a quality assurance department. In addition, each patient care and patient services department was responsible for developing its own plan for monitoring and evaluation. Objective and measurable indicators were used to monitor, evaluate, and communicate the quality and appropriateness of care delivered.

In the early 1990s quality assurance received intense scrutiny. It was recognized that quality of care as defined by regulatory agencies continues to be difficult to measure. Quality assurance criteria were identified as measures to ensure minimal expectations only; they did not provide mechanisms for identifying causes of problems or for determining systems or processes that need improvement.

Continuous Quality Improvement

Continuous quality improvement (CQI) has been identified as a more effective mechanism for improving the quality of health care. In 1992 the revised standards of JCAHO initiated a mandate that health care organizations move toward implementation of continuous quality improvement.

Unlike quality assurance, which focuses on individual incidents or errors and minimal expectations, CQI focuses on the processes used to provide care, with the aim of improving quality by assessing and improving those interrelated processes between different departments and health care professionals that most affect patient care outcomes and patient satisfaction. CQI involves analyzing, understanding, and improving clinical, financial, or operational

CHART 1-2

NLN's Statement on Patient's Rights

According to the NLN statement, nurses have a responsibility to uphold the following rights of patients:

- To health care that is accessible and that meets professional standards, regardless of the setting.
- To courteous and individualized health care that is equitable, humane and given without discrimination as to race, color, creed, sex, national origin, source of payment, or ethical or political beliefs.
- To information about their diagnosis, prognosis, and treatment—including alternatives to care and risks involved—in terms they and their families can readily understand, so that they can give their informed consent.
- To informed participation in all decisions concerning their health care.
- To information about the qualifications, names, and titles of personnel responsible for providing their health care.
- To refuse observation by those not directly involved in their care.
- To privacy during interview, examination, and treatment.
- To privacy in communicating and visiting with persons of their choice.
- To refuse treatment, medications, or participation in research and experimentation, without punitive action being taken against them.
- To coordination and continuity of health care.
- To appropriate instruction or education from health care personnel so that they can achieve an optimal level of wellness and an understanding of their basic health needs.
- To confidentiality of all records (except as otherwise provided for by law or third party payer contracts) and all communications, written or oral, between patients and health care providers.
- To access to all health records pertaining to them, and the right to challenge and correct their records for accuracy, and the right to transfer all such records in the case of continuing care.
- To information on the charges for services, including the right to challenge these.
- To be fully informed as to all their rights in all health care settings.

(National League for Nursing. Nursing's Role in Patient's Rights. New York, The League, 1977. Used with permission.)

processes. Problems that are identified as more than isolated events are analyzed and all of the issues that may affect the outcome are studied. The main focus is on the processes that surround the quality issue.

As health care agencies move toward implementation of CQI, nurses are provided with many opportunities to be involved in quality improvement. Nurse managers as well as nurses directly involved in delivery of care are involved in analyzing the processes that are being evaluated. Their knowledge of the processes and conditions that affect patient care is critical in designing changes that will improve the quality of the care provided.

Managed Health Care

The steady rise of health care costs over the last few decades has led to alternative health care delivery systems, including health maintenance organizations, preferred provider organizations, and managed health care.

Health Maintenance Organizations

Health maintenance organizations (HMOs) are prepaid, group health practice systems designed to deliver comprehensive health care services to a defined group of voluntarily enrolled individuals. HMOs are based on the holistic concept of care—providing outpatient (ambulatory) and inpatient care that meets the health care needs of the whole person. The goal of HMOs is to give comprehensive health care that is of the best quality and quantity for the money available, while eliminating fragmentation and duplication of services. As HMOs have grown, they have expanded to include specialist services and programs for Medicare and Medicaid populations.

Studies have shown that HMOs are cost-effective and that the quality of care provided by these health care delivery systems is comparable to the care provided elsewhere in the same communities.

Preferred Provider Organizations

HMOs paved the way and served as the model for **preferred provider organizations** (PPOs). In contrast to the HMO, the PPO is not a distinct entity. Rather, it is a business arrangement between a group of providers, usually hospitals and physicians, who contract to provide health care to subscribers, usually businesses, for a negotiated fee that usually is discounted. PPOs allow businesses to decrease their expenses for employee health care benefits, and they allow hospitals and physicians to market their services to employers.

Managed Care

HMOs and PPOs have given rise to a much broader pattern of reimbursement and cost control—**managed health care.** Managed care is considered a most important trend in health care and the dominant theme of the current decade. The failure of the regulatory efforts of the past decades to cut costs and the resulting escalation of health care costs that are predicted to reach from 15% to 22% of the gross domestic product (GDP) by the year 2000 prompted business, labor, and government to assume greater control over financing and delivery of health care. The result is significant expansion of managed health care to the point that distinctions between HMOs, PPOs, exclusive provider arrangements (EPAs), managed indemnity plans, and self-insured managed care are blurring. The common features which characterize them as managed care include prenegotiated payment rates, mandatory precertification, utilization review, limited choice of provider, and fixed-price reimbursement. The scope of managed care has broadened from in-hospital services to ambulatory, long-term, and home care services as well as related diagnostic and therapeutic services.

The results of managed care are already evident: dramatic reduction in in-patient hospital days, continuing expansion of ambulatory care, fierce competition, and marketing strategies that appeal to consumers as well as to insurers and regulators. Hospitals are faced with a declining number of patients, more severely ill patients, and shorter lengths of stay. As patients return to the community, they have more health care needs than ever before, and many of these needs are complex. The demand for home care and community-based services is escalating by leaps and bounds.

Despite their successes, managed care organizations are faced with the challenge of providing quality services under even greater resource constraints. They are meeting this challenge. Efforts toward health care reform encourage the use of managed care options to control costs and to improve access to health care.

Nursing and the Nursing Delivery System

The delivery of nursing care has obviously been affected by the changes that have occurred in the health care system. However, the purpose and aim of nursing care have continued to be directed at the goals inherent in the definition of nursing.

Nursing Defined

The definition of nursing has evolved over time. Since the time of Florence Nightingale, who wrote in 1858 that the real goal of nursing was "to put the patient in the best condition for nurture to act upon him," nursing leaders have defined nursing as both an art and a science. The American Nurses Association (ANA), in its *Social Policy Statement* of 1995, defines nursing as "the diagnosis and treatment of human responses to health and illness" and provides the following illustrative list of phenomena that are the focus for nursing care and research:

- Self-care processes
- Physiologic and pathophysiologic processes in areas such as rest, sleep, respiration, circulation, reproduction, activity, nutrition, elimination, skin, sexuality, communication
- Comfort, pain and discomfort
- Emotions related to experiences of health and illness
- Meanings ascribed to health and illnesses
- Decision making and ability to make choices
- Perceptual orientations such as self-image and control over one's body and environments
- Transitions across the life span, such as birth, growth, development, and death
- Affiliative relationships, including freedom from oppression and abuse
- Environmental systems

Nurses have a responsibility to carry out their role as defined in the social policy statement and to comply with the nurse practice act of the state in which they practice, as well as the code for nurses as spelled out by the International Council of Nurses (ICN) and the ANA.

Nursing Delivery Systems

Nursing care can be carried out through a variety of organizational methods such as team nursing, which had its origins in the 1950s and 1960s, to more recent forms of care delivery such as primary nursing and case management. In team nursing, care is given by a variety of nursing personnel under the supervision of a single nurse who has minimal involvement in giving care. Primary nursing, on the other hand, has been shown to increase significantly the quality of patient care and to be more cost-effective. However, more research is needed to substantiate these findings.

Primary Nursing

Primary nursing (not to be confused with primary health care, which deals with first-contact general health care) refers to comprehensive, individualized care that is provided by the same nurse throughout the period of care. This type of nursing care allows the nurse to give direct patient care rather than manage and supervise the functions of others who care for the patient. In essence, it allows the nurse the opportunity to implement the practitioner and leadership roles within the framework of rendering direct patient care.

The focus of primary nursing is the patient. The primary nurse accepts total 24-hour responsibility for quality nursing care for the patient. Thus, nursing care is directed toward meeting total, individualized patient needs. The primary nurse is responsible and accountable for involving the patient and family directly in all facets of care and has autonomy in making decisions in this regard. The nurse is thus a facilitator of family-centered as well as patient-centered nursing care. Communications with other members of the health team regarding the patient's health care are made by the primary nurse, thereby providing continuity of care and promoting collaborative efforts directed toward quality patient care. It provides the other health care professionals with the opportunity to communicate directly with the nurse who is responsible for the patient's care.

Prior to the patient's discharge to another health care facility or to his or her home, the primary nurse assumes the responsibility for making the appropriate referrals and for ensuring that all relevant information is provided to those persons who will be involved in his or her care, including the family.

During the times when the primary nurse is not scheduled to work, an associate nurse or co-nurse assists in overseeing the delivery of care. The associate nurse implements the nursing care plan and provides feedback to the primary nurse for evaluating the plan of care. However, the primary nurse has the responsibility to make sure that the patient's needs are met and that continuity of care is maintained.

The long-term survival of primary nursing as it is currently implemented is uncertain. As cost-containment measures accelerate and patient acuity increases, staffing ratios of patients to nurses are increasing. Many nursing service departments and agencies are meeting the increased workload demands by making modifications in their approach to primary nursing or by reverting to team or functional systems for delivering care. Others are changing their staffing mixes and redesigning their models of practice to accommodate nurse extender roles. Still others are changing to more innovative systems such as case management.

Case Management

Case management has become a prominent method for coordinating health care services to assure cost-effectiveness, accountability, and quality care. The case management process dates back to the public health programs of the early 1900s, and it has always been the dominant role of public health nursing. Over the years, the process has varied in form and function, but the basic theme has remained: responsibility for meeting patient needs rests with one individual or team whose purpose is to provide the patient and family with access to required services, to assure coordination of these services, and to evaluate how effectively these services are delivered.

The reasons case management has gained such prominence can be traced to the decrease in length of hospital stay coupled with rapid and frequent interunit transfers from specialty to standard care units.

The case manager role, instead of focusing on direct patient care, focuses on managing the care of an entire caseload of patients and collaborating with the nurses and other health care personnel who care for the patients. In most instances, the caseload is limited in scope to patients with similar diagnoses, needs, and therapies, and the case managers function across units. They are experts in their specialty areas and function to coordinate the inpatient and outpatient services needed by patients. The goals of this coordination include quality, appropriateness, and timeliness of services as well as cost reduction. The case manager follows the patient after discharge in an effort to access and promote coordination of health care services that will avert or delay rehospitalization.

Critical Pathways. With the expansion of managed care nationwide, a new dimension is being added to case management—critical pathways. **Critical pathways** serve as the interdisciplinary care plan and the tool for tracking a patient's progress toward achieving positive outcomes within a specified time frame. Critical paths have been developed for certain DRGs (*e.g.*, open heart surgery, pneumonia with comorbidity, fractured hip), for high-risk patients (*e.g.*, patients receiving chemotherapy), and for patients with certain common health problems (*e.g.*, patients with chronic pain). They identify certain key events such as diagnostic tests, treatments, activities, medications, consultation, and education that must occur within specified times for the patient to achieve the desired and timely outcomes (Fig. 1-1). The nurse case manager facilitates and coordinates interventions to assure that the patient progresses through the key events and achieves the desired outcomes.

Through case management and the use of critical paths, patients and the care they receive are continually assessed from preadmission to discharge and in many cases post-discharge, and in the home care and community setting. The resultant continuity of care, effective utilization of services, and cost-containment are expected to be major benefits for society and for the health care system.

Community-Based Nursing

As trends continue toward shortened hospital stays and increased utilization of outpatient health care services, the need for nursing care in the home and community setting has increased tremendously.

Because nursing services are being provided outside as well as within the hospital, nurses have a choice of practicing in a variety of health care delivery settings: acute medical centers, ambulatory care settings, clinics, urgent care centers, outpatient departments, neighborhood health centers, home health care agencies, independent or group nursing centers, and managed care agencies.

Home health care and community nursing, which have traditionally focused on maternal and child health, chronic care, and health promotion, now are expanding to meet the needs of many other groups of patients with a variety of problems and needs. In addition to health departments and visiting nurse associations, home and community services are provided by community-based programs for specific populations, such as the elderly, as well as by hospital-based home health care agencies, hospices, independent professional nursing practices, and large and small free-standing health care agencies.

Community nursing centers, which have emerged over the past two decades with the advent of nurse practitioners, are nurse-managed and provide primary care services including ambulatory and outpatient care, immunizations, health assessment and screening services, and patient and family education and counseling. The populations that these centers serve are varied, but most typically include a high proportion of patients who are very young, very old, poor, and of racial minorities—groups that are generally underserved.

As the numbers and kinds of agencies that provide care in the home and community have expanded, the needs of patients requiring care have also expanded. Patients are discharged from acute care institutions to their homes and communities at much earlier stages of recovery and at more acute levels of illness. Many are elderly and many have multiple medical and nursing diagnoses and multisystem health problems that require acute and intensive nursing care. Medical technologies, such as ventilators and intravenous and total parenteral nutrition therapy, once limited to acute care settings, have been adapted to the home care setting.

As a result, the home health care setting is becoming one of the largest practice areas for nursing, and home care nursing is becoming a specialty area that requires advanced knowledge and skills in general nursing practice, with emphasis on community health and acute medical-surgical nursing. Also required are high-level assessment skills and

CRITICAL PATHWAY

Mastectomy **LOS 3.6** **DRG 258**

	DAY 1	O	C	DAY 2	O	C	DAY 3	O	C	DAY 4	O	C
Special Orders Tests (Consults)	PAT: CBC, SMA6, urinalysis, CXR, ECG (> 40 year OR H/O cardiac disease).						Liver scan, CBC if increase blood loss during OR. Post for bone scan as outpatient.					
Nutrition	Clear liquids/advance as tolerated.			Increase diet as tolerated.								
Treatment	VS q 4h. IM pain med q 4h prn. Assess dressing and reinforce prn. No Rx or needlesticks affected arm (post sign). Empty & measure J.P. drain q 8h. I&O. Respiratory care – q 2h while awake q 4h at night (turn, cough, and deep breathe, use incentive spirometry).			VS q shift. PO pain meds if tolerating food and fluids. Change dressing, assess incision. Measure J.P. outputs. Respiratory care q 4h while awake q 8h at night. Liver scan if indicated. Schedule for outpatient bone scan before discharge (if indicated). Demonstrate or begin post mastectomy exercises (per surgeon request).			Change dressing, assess incision measure J.P. output. Mastectomy exercises (per surgeon).					
Activity	OOB with assistance.			OOB ambulating with assistance. Encourage "normal" use of arm.			OOB ambulating in hall. Increase use of arm affected side as tolerated, i.e. abduction. Reinforce walking fully erect and not guarding on affected side.					
Teaching	Instruct incentive spirometry and pulmonary toilet. Verbalizes understanding of rationale for pulmonary toilet.			Verbalizes how to care for affected arm, prevent infection, manage lymphedema. Verbalizes rationale for exercises. Demonstrate post mastectomy exercises (per surgeon request). Views incision and verbalizes feelings.			Demonstrate how to empty & care for J.P. drain. Demonstrate mastectomy exercises correctly. Verbalize S&S infection, when to contact MD. Acknowledge change in body image.			Importance of mammography.		
Discharge Planning	Explain Reach for Recovery Organization; contact per patient's request. Explain Arm in Arm Support Group at HHC – give pamphlet.						Give pamphlet or literature for Reach for Recovery, Arm in Arm and Mastectomy Exercises and Arm Care.					
Variance												

EXPECTED OUTCOMES

1. The patient will ______________________________ date
2. The patient will ______________________________ date
3. The patient will ______________________________ date

O = Ordered
C = Completed

FIGURE 1-1. An example of a clinical or critical pathway. This pathway indicates the type of clinical treatment or patient care activities to be carried out for each day of hospitalization expected for a patient undergoing a mastectomy. The DRG category for a mastectomy is listed as 258; the length of stay (LOS) is identified as 3.6 days. Hospitals are developing pathways such as this based on their experiences in treating patients with specific disorders. (Courtesy of Harbor Hospital Center, Baltimore, MD.)

decision-making skills in a setting where other health care professionals are not available to validate observations, conclusions, and decisions.

Community health nurses are functioning as acute care nurses in the home, providing high-tech, high-touch services to patients with acute health care needs. In addition, they are responsible for patient and family teaching and for accessing community resources and coordinating the continuing care of the patient and family. For these reasons, the scope of medical-surgical nursing encompasses not only the acute care setting within hospitals, but also the acute care setting as it expands into the community and the home. Throughout this textbook, emphasis is placed on the home health care needs of patients, with particular attention given to the teaching and health maintenance needs of patients and their families.

The Patient/Client: Consumer and Recipient of Health Care

The term **patient,** which is derived from the Latin verb meaning "to suffer," has traditionally been used to describe those persons who are recipients of care. The connotation commonly attached to the word is one of dependence. For this reason, many nurses prefer to use the term **client,** which is derived from the Latin verb meaning "to lean" and which connotes alliance and interdependence. For the purposes of this book, the term **patient** will be used throughout but with the understanding that either term is acceptable.

The central figure in health care services is, of course, the patient. The patient who comes to the hospital or health care facility with a health problem or problems (increasing numbers of people have multiple health problems) also comes as an individual, a member of a family, and a citizen of the community. Depending upon the problem, associated circumstances, and past experiences, patients' needs will vary. One of the nurse's important functions is to identify the patient's immediate needs and take measures to alleviate them.

The Patient's Basic Needs

Certain needs are basic to all persons and demand satisfaction accordingly. Such needs are dealt with on the basis of priority, meaning that certain needs are more pressing than others. However, once an essential need is met, a person moves to a need on a higher level. Approaching needs according to priority reflects Maslow's hierarchy of needs (Fig. 1-2), which are ranked as follows: physiologic needs; safety and security; belongingness and affection; esteem and self-respect; and self-actualization, which includes self-fulfillment, desire to know and understand, and aesthetic needs. Lower-level needs always remain, but because there is a reduction in need tension, the person is able to move to higher-level needs. A person's pursuit of higher-level needs indicates that he or she is moving toward psychologic health and well-being. Such a hierarchy of needs is a useful organizational framework that can be applied to the various

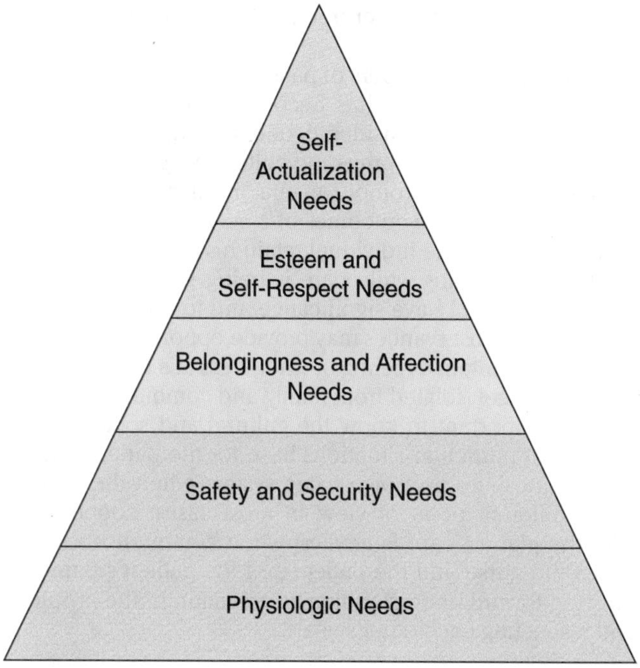

FIGURE 1-2. This scheme of Maslow's hierarchy of human needs shows how a person moves from basic need fulfillment to higher levels of needs, with the ultimate goal of integrated human functioning and health.

nursing models for assessment of patients' strengths, limitations, and need for nursing interventions.

Cultural Diversity

It is predicted that by the second decade of the 21st century, minority populations in the United States will outnumber the rest of the population. As the cultural composition of the population changes, it becomes increasingly important to address cultural considerations in the delivery of health care. Patients from diverse sociocultural groups bring to the health care setting different health care beliefs, values, and practices. These factors significantly affect the way an individual responds to health care problems or illness, to those who provide the care, and to the care itself. Unless these factors are understood and respected by the health care providers, the care provided may be ineffective and health care outcomes may be negatively affected.

Culture is defined as learned patterns of behavior, beliefs, and values that are characteristic of a particular group of people. Included among the many characteristics that distinguish cultural groups are "mode of dress, language, values, rules or norms for behavior, economics, politics, law and social control, artifacts, technology, dietary practices, and health care. Health preservation, sickness prevention, causes of sickness, treatment, coping, caring, dying, and death are part of the health component of every culture" (Germain, 1992, p. 1).

Every person has a unique belief and value system that has been shaped at least in part by his or her cultural environment. This belief and value system is very important and guides the individual's thinking, decisions, and actions. It provides direction for interpreting and responding to illness and to health care.

As increasing numbers of patients come from culturally diverse backgrounds, it has become evident that cultural differences must be considered, understood, and respected and that the care given must be culturally appropriate and sensitive in order to promote an effective nurse–patient relationship and positive outcomes of care. All attempts should be made to help the individual retain his or her unique cultural characteristics while care is being given. To provide special foods that have significance and to arrange for special religious observances may provide opportunities for the patient to maintain a feeling of wholeness at a time when he or she may feel isolated from family and community.

It is important to know the cultural and social significance that particular situations have for the patient and to avoid imposing one's own value system when the patient has a different point of view. In most cases, cooperation with the plan of care is greatest when communication between the nurse and the patient and the patient's family is directed toward understanding the situation or the problem and respecting each other's goals.

Roles of the Nurse

The professional nurse in both institutional and community health care settings assumes three roles: the practitioner role, the leadership role, and the research role. Although each role carries specific responsibilities, these roles relate to one another and are found in all nursing positions. These roles are designed to meet the immediate and future health care and nursing needs of the health care consumers who are the recipients of nursing care.

Practitioner Role

The **practitioner role** of the nurse involves those actions that the nurse takes when assuming responsibility that is directed toward meeting the health care and nursing needs of individual patients, their families, and significant others. This role is the dominant role of nurses in primary, secondary, and tertiary health care settings and in home care and community nursing. It is a role that can be achieved only through utilization of the nursing process, the basis for all nursing practice.

Leadership Role

The **leadership role** of the nurse has traditionally been perceived as a specialized role assumed only by those nurses who have titles that suggest leadership and who are the leaders of large groups of nurses or related health care professionals. However, the definition of nursing leadership developed by Yura, Ozimek, and Walsh (1981) gives a broader scope to the concept and identifies leadership as a role that is inherent within all nursing positions. The leadership role of the nurse involves those actions that the nurse accomplishes when assuming responsibility for affecting the actions of others that are directed toward determining and achieving goals.

Nursing leadership is a process that involves four components: decision-making, relating, influencing, and facilitating. Each of these components is directed toward change and the ultimate outcome of goal achievement. Basic to the entire process is communication, the effectiveness of which determines the accomplishment of the process.

Thus, the leadership process in nursing can be said to be an interpersonal process in which the nurse, as a leader, uses interpersonal skills to effect change in the behavior of others. The components of the leadership process are appropriate during all phases of the nursing process.

Research Role

The **research role** of the nurse was traditionally viewed as being carried out only by academicians, nurse scientists, and graduate nursing students. Today, participation in the research process is considered to be the responsibility of nurses in clinical practice.

The primary task of nursing research is to contribute to the scientific base of nursing practice. Studies are needed to determine the effectiveness of nursing interventions and nursing care. Through such research efforts, the science of nursing will grow and a scientifically based rationale for making changes in nursing practice will be generated.

Nurses who have preparation in research methodology can use their research knowledge and skills to initiate and implement timely studies of nursing. This is not to say that nurses who do not initiate and implement nursing research studies do not play a significant role in nursing research. Every nurse has valuable contributions to make to nursing research and a responsibility to make these contributions. All nurses must constantly be alert for nursing problems and important questions about the practice of nursing, which can serve as the basis for the identification of researchable questions.

Those nurses directly involved in patient care are often in the best position to identify potential research problems and questions. Their clinical insights are invaluable. Nurses also have a responsibility to become actively involved in ongoing research studies. This participation may involve facilitating the data collection process, or it may involve the actual collection of data. Explaining the study to other health care professionals or to patients and their families is often of invaluable assistance to the nurse who is conducting the study.

Above all, nurses must use research findings in their nursing practice. Research for the sake of research is meaningless. Only with the use of research findings in nursing practice will the science of nursing be furthered. Research findings can be substantiated only through utilization, validation, and dissemination. Nurses must continually be aware of studies that are directly related to their own area of clinical practice.

Advanced Practice Nursing

Professional nursing is adapting to meet changing health needs and expectations. One such adaptation is through the **expanded role of the nurse**, which has developed in response to the need to improve the distribution of health care services and to decrease the cost of health care. The nurse who functions in advanced practice provides direct care to patients through independent practice, or practice within a health care agency or with a physician. Specialization has evolved within the expanded roles of nursing, a result of the recent explosion of technology.

Nurses receive advanced education in such specialties as intensive care, coronary care, respiratory care, oncologic care, neonatal intensive care, rehabilitation, trauma, and gerontologic nursing, to name just a few. With the expanded role of the nurse, various titles have emerged that attempt to specify the functions as well as the educational preparation of nurses. Two of these titles are nurse practitioner and clinical nurse specialist, as well as the more recent title of advanced practice nursing that encompasses both nurse practitioners and clinical specialists.

Although initially the educational preparation for nurse practitioners was in certificate programs, both nurse practitioners and clinical nurse specialists require graduate level education. The two programs, which originally differed significantly in scope and in the definition of the role component, now have many similarities and areas of overlap. Nurse practitioners and clinical nurse specialists (along with certified nurse midwives and certified registered nurse anesthetists) are identified as advanced practice nurses.

Nurse practitioners are, for the most part, prepared as generalists (*e.g.*, pediatric nurse practitioner, geriatric nurse practitioner). They define their role in terms of the direct provision of a broad range of primary health care services to patients and families. The focus is on providing direct patient care in an environment that promotes a significant degree of autonomy and collaboration with other health professionals. They practice in both acute and nonacute care settings.

Clinical nurse specialists, on the other hand, are prepared as specialists who practice within a circumscribed area of care (*e.g.*, cardiovascular clinical nurse specialist, oncology clinical nurse specialist). They define their role as having four major components: clinical practice, education, consultation, and research. Studies have shown that in reality the focus is often on the education and consultation roles: education and counseling of patients and families, and education, counseling, and consultation with nursing staff. Although they may practice in a variety of settings, most often their practice is within the acute care hospital setting. Most recently, clinical nurse specialists have been identified by many nursing leaders as ideal case managers. They have the educational background and the clinical expertise to organize and coordinate services and resources to meet the patient's health care needs in a cost-effective and efficient manner.

With advanced practice roles has come a continuing effort by state nursing associations to define more clearly the practice of nursing. Nurse practice acts have been amended to give nurses the authority to perform functions that were previously restricted to the practice of medicine. These functions include nursing diagnosis, treatment, performance of invasive procedures, and prescription of medications and treatments. Regulations regarding these functions are stipulated by the board of nursing in each state, which defines the education and experience required and the clinical situations in which a nurse may perform these functions.

In general, initial care, ambulatory health care, and anticipatory guidance are all becoming increasingly important in nursing practice. The advanced practice roles enable the nurse to function interdependently with other health care professionals and to establish a more collegial relationship between physician and nurse. With changes in health care, the role of advanced practice nurses, especially in primary care, is expected to increase in terms of scope, responsibility, and recognition.

Collaborative Practice

Throughout this chapter, we have explored the changing role of nursing. Many references have been made to the significance of nurses as members of the health care team. As the unique competencies of nurses are becoming more clearly articulated, there is increasing evidence that nursing provides certain health care services that are unique to the profession. However, nursing continues to recognize the importance of collaboration with other health care disciplines in meeting all of the health care needs of patients.

In some institutions the **nurse–physician collaborative practice model** is used. Within a decentralized organizational structure, nurses and physicians function collaboratively in making clinical decisions. A joint practice committee, with equal representation from both professions, may function at the unit level to monitor, support, and foster collaboration. Collaborative practice is further enhanced with integration of the clinical record and with joint patient care record reviews. Figure 1-3 compares the traditional model with the collaborative practice model.

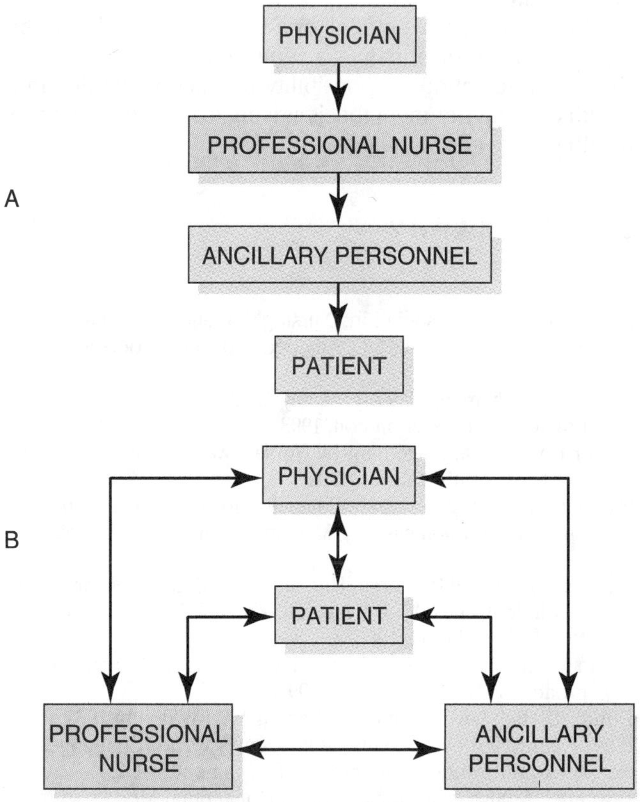

FIGURE 1-3. Comparison of traditional practice model (**A**) and collaborative practice model (**B**).

CRITICAL THINKING EXERCISES

1. Your clinical assignment is on a medical-surgical unit in an acute care hospital. Identify a patient care issue, *e.g.*, patient education, that could be improved. Describe the mechanism that is available within the hospital to address such quality improvement issues.
2. You are caring for an elderly patient who has several chronic medical conditions and who is soon to be discharged. A case manager has been assigned to this patient. How would you explain the role of the case manager to the patient and her daughter?
3. You are assigned to care for a patient whose health care is covered by a managed health care plan. How have managed health care plans affected nursing care delivery in acute care hospitals and outpatient settings? How might this specific patient's care be affected?

The Secretary of Health and Human Services Commission on Nursing, in its report in 1988, recognized the essential nature of collaborative practice to health care delivery by recommending that employers of nurses and the medical profession foster collaboration between members of the health care team.

The collaborative model, or a variation of it, should be a primary goal for nursing—a venture that would promote shared participation, responsibility, and accountability in a health care environment that is striving to meet the complex health care needs of the public.

BIBLIOGRAPHY

Books

American Nurses Association. Nursing's Agenda for Health Care Reform. Kansas City, MO, American Nurses Association, June 1991.

Barnum BS. Nursing Theory: Analysis, Application, Evaluation. Philadelphia, JB Lippincott, 1993.

Bower KA. Case Management by Nurses. Washington, DC, American Nurses Publications, 1992.

Cabinet on Nursing Research. Education for Participation in Nursing Research. Kansas City, MO, American Nurses Association, 1989.

Cabinet on Nursing Research. Human Rights Guidelines for Nurses in Clinical and Other Research. Kansas City, MO, American Nurses Association, 1985.

Chinn P and Jacobs MK. Theory and Nursing: A Systematic Approach. St. Louis, CV Mosby, 1991.

Dunn HL. High-Level Wellness. Arlington, VA, RW Beatty, 1961.

Ellis JR and Hartley CL. Nursing in Today's World: Challenges, Issues, and Trends. Philadelphia, JB Lippincott, 1992.

Fawcett J. Analysis and Evaluation of Conceptual Models of Nursing. Philadelphia, FA Davis, 1989.

Fitzpatrick JJ and Whall AL. Conceptual Models of Nursing: Analysis and Application. Norwalk, CT, Appleton and Lange, 1989.

George JB. Nursing Theories. The Base for Professional Nursing Practice. Norwalk, CT, Appleton and Lange, 1990.

Hamric AB and Spross JA (eds). The Clinical Nurse Specialist in Theory and Practice. Philadelphia, WB Saunders, 1989.

Henderson V. The Nature of Nursing. New York, Macmillan, 1966.

Johnson DE. The behavioral system model for nursing. In Parker ME. Nursing Theories in Practice. New York, National League for Nursing, 1990.

Johnson DE. The behavioral system model in nursing. In Riehl JP and Roy C (eds). Conceptual Models for Nursing Practice. New York, Appleton-Century-Crofts, 1980.

King IM. A Theory for Nursing: Systems, Concepts, Process. New York, John Wiley & Sons, 1981.

King IM. King's general systems framework and theory. In Riehl-Sisca JP. Conceptual Models for Nursing Practice. Norwalk, CT, Appleton and Lange, 1989.

King IM. King's theory of goal attainment. In Parse RR. Nursing Science: Major Paradigms, Theories, and Critiques. Philadelphia, WB Saunders, 1989.

Leddy S and Pepper JM. Conceptual Bases of Professional Nursing. Philadelphia, JB Lippincott, 1989.

Maslow AH. Motivation and Personality. New York, Harper & Brothers, 1970.

Mayer GG and Madden MJ. Patient Care Delivery Models. Rockville, MD, Aspen Systems Corporation, 1990.

Meleis AI. Theoretical Nursing: Development and Progress. Philadelphia, JB Lippincott, 1991.

Mitchell PR and Grippando GM. Nursing Perspectives & Issues. Albany, NY, Delmar Publishers, 1993.

Moloney MM. Professionalization of Nursing: Current Issues and Trends. Philadelphia, JB Lippincott, 1992.

Neuman B. The Neuman Systems Model: Application to Nursing Education and Practice. Norwalk, CT, Appleton and Lange, 1982, 1989.

Newman MA. Health as Expanding Consciousness. St. Louis, CV Mosby, 1986.

Nightingale F. Notes on Nursing: What It Is, and What It Is Not. New York, D Appleton, 1860.

Nursing: A Social Policy Statement. Washington, DC, American Nurses Association, 1995.

Orem DE. Nursing: Concepts of Practice. St Louis, CV Mosby–Year Book, 1980, 1985, 1991.

Parse RR. Man-living-health: A theory of nursing. In Riehl-Sisca JP. Conceptual Models for Nursing Practice. Norwalk, CT, Appleton and Lange, 1989.

Parse RR. Nursing Science: Major Paradigms, Theories, and Critiques. Philadelphia, WB Saunders, 1987.

Peplau HE. Interpersonal Relations in Nursing. New York, GP Putnam's Sons, 1952.

Rogers ME. Nursing: A science of unitary man. In Riehl JP and Roy C (eds). Conceptual Models for Nursing Practice. New York, Appleton-Century-Crofts, 1980.

Rogers ME. Nursing: Science of unitary irreducible human beings: Update 1990. In Barrett EAM. Visions of Roger's Based Nursing. New York, National League for Nursing, 1990.

Roy C. Roy's adaptation model. In Parse R. Nursing Science: Major Paradigms, Theories, and Critiques. Philadelphia, WB Saunders, 1987.

Roy C and Roberts SL. Theory Construction in Nursing: An Adaptation Model. Englewood Cliffs, NJ, Prentice-Hall, 1981.

U.S. Department of Health and Human Services. Public Health Service. Healthy People 2000: National Health Promotion and Disease Prevention Objectives. Washington, DC, U.S. Government Printing Office, 1990.

Watson J. Nursing: Human Science and Human Care. Norwalk, CT Appleton-Century-Crofts, 1985.

Watson J. Watson's philosophy and theory of human caring in nursing. In Riehl-Sisca JP. Conceptual Models for Nursing Practice. Norwalk, CT, Appleton and Lange, 1989.

Yura H, Ozimek D, and Walsh MB. Nursing Leadership: Theory and Process. New York, Appleton-Century-Crofts, 1981.

Journals

Asterisks indicate nursing research articles.

Theories and Concepts of Nursing

Barger S and Rosenfeld P. Models in community health care: Findings from a national study of community nursing centers. Nurs Health Care 1993 Oct; 14(8): 426–431.

Bernal EW. The nurse as patient advocate. Hastings Center Report 1992 Jul-Aug; 22(4): 18–23.

*Bostrom J and Mitchell M. Relationship of direct nursing care hours to DRG and severity of illness. Nurs Economics 1991 Mar-April; 9(2): 105–111.

Brent NJ. Delegation and supervision of patient care. Home Healthcare Nurse 1993 July-Aug; 11(4): 7–8.

Cesta TG. The link between continuous quality improvement and case management. J Nurs Admin 1993 June; 23(6): 55–61.

Corbin JM and Strauss A. A nursing model for chronic illness management based upon the trajectory framework. Scholar Inq Nurs Pract 1991 Feb; 5(3): 155–174.

Deming QB. A prescription for national health care reform. Hospital Practice 1993 April 15; 28(4): 21, 25–28.

Drew JC. Health maintenance organizations: History, evolution, and survival. Nurs Health Care 1990 March; 11(3): 145–149.

Dunn JL. What high-level wellness means. Health Values 1977 Jan-Feb; 1: 9–16.

Dunston J. How managed care can work for you. Nursing 1990 Oct; 20(10): 56–59.

Fagin CM. Collaboration between nurses and physicians: No longer a choice. Academic Medicine 1992 May; 67(5): 295–303.

*Geissler EM. Nursing diagnoses: A study of cultural relevance. J Professional Nurs 1992 Sept-Oct; 8(5): 301–307.

Germain CP. Cultural care: A bridge between sickness, illness, and disease. Holistic Nurse Pract 1992 April; 6(3): 1–9.

Giger JN and Davidhizar R. Transcultural nursing assessment: A method for advancing nursing practice. Int Nurs Rev 1990 Jan-Feb; 37(1): 199–202.

Hampton DC. Implementing a managed care framework through care maps. J Nurs Admin 1993 May; 23(5): 21–27.

Hicks L et al. Nursing challenges in managed care. Nurs Econ 1992 Jul-Aug; 10(4): 265–276.

Hodes JR and Crombrugghe PV. Nurse-physician relationships. Nurs Manage 1990 July; 21(7): 73–75.

*Hoesen NS and Eriksen LR. The impact of diagnosis-related groups in patient acuity, quality of care, and length of stay. J Nurs Admin 1990 Sept; 20(9): 20–23.

Hoffman CA. The house of medicine. JAMA 1972 July 31; 221(5): 483–485.

*Hughes K and Marcantonio R. Practice patterns among home health, public health and hospital nurses. Nurs Health Care 1992 Oct; 13(10): 532–536.

Jensen L and Allen M. Wellness: The dialectic of illness. Image: Journal of Nursing Scholarship 1993 Fall; 25(3): 220–223.

Keane A and Richmond T. Tertiary Nurse Practitioners. Image: Journal of Nursing Scholarship 1993 Winter; 25(4).

Klessig J. Cross-cultural medicine. A decade later. West J Med 1992 Sep; 157: 316–322.

Leininger MM. Transcultural diversity and universality: A theory of nursing. Nurs Health Care 1985 June; 6(6): 209–212.

Leininger MM. Transcultural nursing: The study and practice field. Imprint 1991 April/May; 38(2): 55, 57, 59.

*Mark B. Characteristics of nursing practice models. J Nurs Admin 1992 Nov; 22(11): 57–63.

Mayhew PA. Evaluating research for use in practice. MEDSURG Nursing 1993 Dec; 2(6): 496–498.

Mayhew PA. The importance of the practicing nurse in nursing research. MEDSURG Nursing 1993 Jun; 2(3): 210–211, 246.

Mosher C et al. Upgrading practice with critical pathways. Am J Nurs 1992 Jan; 92(1): 41–44.

Naylor MD and Brooten D. The roles and functions of clinical nurse specialists. Image: Journal of Nursing Scholarship 1993 Spring; 25(1): 73–78.

Newman MA. Newman's theory of health as praxis. Nurs Sci Quart 1990 Spring 3(1): 37–41.

Papenhausen JL. Case management: A model of advanced practice? Clinical Nurse Specialist 1990 April; 4(4): 169–170.

Peplau HE. The art and science of nursing: Similarities, differences and relations. Nurs Sci Quart 1988 Feb; 1(1): 8–15.

Phillips CY et al. Case manager/nurse manager: A blending of roles. Nurs Manage 1993 Oct; 24(10): 26–28.

Redford LJ. Case management. The wave of the future. J Case Management 1992 Spring; 1(1): 5–8.

Rothenburger RL. Transcultural nursing. Overcoming obstacles to effective communication. AORN J 1990 May; 51(5): 1349–1354, 1357–1363.

Scholz J. Cultural expressions affecting patient care. Dimens Oncol Nurs 1990 Spring; 4(1): 16–26.

Schroer K. Case management: Clinical nurse specialist and nurse practitioner, converging roles. Clinical Nurse Specialist 1991 Winter; 5(4): 189–194.

Sharp N. Recognizing APN's: It's now or never! Nurs Manage 1994 Feb; 25(2): 14–16.

Sherer JL. Health care reform: Nursing's vision of change. Hospitals 1993 April 20; 67(8): 20–26.

Smith MC. Case management and nursing theory-based practice. Nurs Sci Quart 1993 Spring; 6(1): 8–9.

Stulginsky MM. Nurses' home health experience. Part I: The practice setting. Nurs Health Care 1993 Oct; 14(8): 402–407.

Stulginsky MM. Nurses' home health experience. Part II: The unique demands of home visits. Nurs Health Care 1993 Nov; 14(9): 476–485.

Thobaben M and Mattingly HJ. Cultural sensitivity. Educating home healthcare nurses to be transcultural nurses. Home Healthcare Nurs 1993 July/August; 11(4): 61–63.

Woods RG et al. Managed care: The missing link in quality improvement. J Nurs Care Qual 1992 July; 6(4): 55–65.

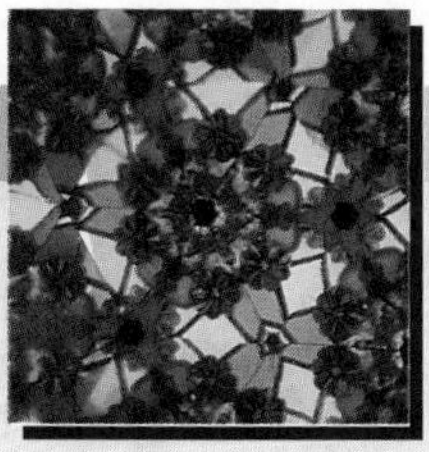

2 Community-Based Nursing Practice

CHAPTER OUTLINE

The Growing Need for Community-Based Health Care

Home Health Care

Hospital Versus Community-Based Nursing Care
Discharge Planning for Home Care
Community Resources and Referrals
Preparing for a Home Visit
Personal Safety Precautions
Conducting a Home Visit
Determining the Need for Future Visits
Closing the Visit

Other Community-Based Health Care Settings

Ambulatory Settings
Occupational Health Programs
School Health Programs
Care for the Homeless

Critical Thinking Exercises

LEARNING OBJECTIVES

On completion of the chapter, the learner will be able to:

1. Discuss the changes in the health care system that have increased the need for medical-surgical nurses to practice in community-based settings
2. Compare the differences and similarities between community-based and hospital nursing
3. Describe the discharge planning process in relation to home care preparation
4. Explain methods for identifying community resources and making referrals
5. Discuss how to prepare for a home health care visit and how to conduct the visit
6. Identify personal safety precautions a home health nurse should take when making home visits
7. Describe the various types of nursing functions carried out in ambulatory care facilities, school nursing programs, and primary care clinics
8. Explain the difficulties involved in providing health care services to the homeless

The Growing Need for Community-Based Health Care

As described in Chapter 1, the changes that have occurred in the health care system in the past decade or so have led to an increase in the amount of care being provided in ambulatory health care settings and in the home. These changes have increased the need for nurses to provide nursing care in the community and the home setting.

The shift in health care delivery is a result of changes in federal legislation, tighter insurance regulations, and the development of alternative health care delivery systems. As a result of federal legislation passed in 1983, hospitals are now reimbursed at a fixed rate for patients with the same diagnosis as defined by Diagnostic Related Groups (DRGs). Under this system, hospitals can cut costs and even earn income by carefully monitoring the types of services they provide and by discharging patients as soon as possible. Consequently, patients are being discharged from acute care facilities to their homes or to residential or long-term facilities at much earlier stages of recovery than in the past. High-level technical equipment, such as IV lines and ventilators, have become part of home health care.

Alternative health care delivery systems, such as health maintenance organizations (HMOs), preferred provider organizations (PPOs), and managed health care systems, have contributed to the drive to control costs and the type of health care services available to patients. These regulations have dramatically reduced the length of hospital stays and led to patients being treated more frequently in ambulatory care settings and at home. Chapter 1 provides a more thorough discussion of alternative health care delivery systems.

As more health care delivery shifts into the community, more nurses are finding employment outside the hospital and are working in a variety of settings and sites, such as ambulatory health clinics, prenatal and well-baby clinics, hospice agencies, industrial settings (as occupational nurses), homeless shelters, nursing centers, and patients' homes.

Nurses working in these settings deliver care without direct on-site supervision or back-up by other hospital staff personnel. They must be self-directed, flexible, adaptable, and tolerant of various types of lifestyles and living conditions. Expertise in independent decision-making, critical thinking, physical assessment, health education, and competence in basic nursing care are essential abilities and skills necessary to function effectively in the evolving health care system.

Home Health Care

As a result of the changes in the health care industry, home health care is becoming one of the biggest practice areas for nurses. Because of the acuity level of patients, nurses with acute care and high-technology experience are in demand in this field. Many home health care patients are acutely ill and many have chronic health problems. Health and social services are provided to the patient by a multidisciplinary team that includes professional nurses, home health aides, social workers, and physical, speech, and occupational therapists. The care is under the direction of a physician and provided on an intermittent or part-time basis.

Health care services are provided by official, publicly funded agencies, nonprofit agencies, proprietary chains, and hospital-based agencies. Some agencies specialize in high-technology services. Most agencies are reimbursed from a variety of sources, including Medicare and Medicaid programs, private insurance, and direct payments by patients. Each funding source has its own requirements for services rendered, the number of visits allowed, and the amount of reimbursement the agency will receive. However, over one half the home health care expenditures are funded by Medicare.

The elderly are the most frequent users of home health services. To be eligible for service, the patient must be acutely ill, homebound, and in need of skilled nursing services. Nursing care includes skilled assessment of the patient's physical, psychological, social, and environmental status. Nursing interventions include giving the patient intravenous therapy and injections, total parenteral nutrition feedings, or performing venipunctures; inserting catheters; treating pressure sores; changing dressings; and providing ostomy care. The nurse instructs the patient and family in skills and self-care strategies as well as in health maintenance and promotion activities, such as nutritional counseling, exercise programs, and stress management techniques (Fig. 2-1).

Medicare allows nurses to manage and evaluate (MAE) patient care for seriously ill patients who have complex, labile conditions and are at high risk for rehospitalization. The nurse serves as a case manager and monitors the delivery of care provided to patients in their homes.

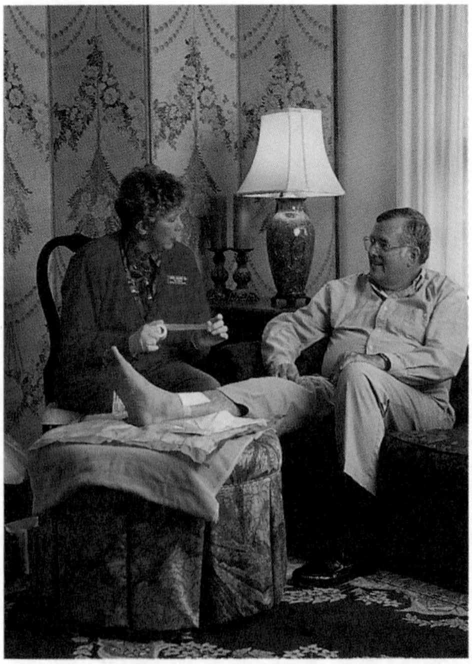

FIGURE 2-1. Home care nurses perform different types of care, including changing dressings and providing patient education. (Courtesy Horizons Home Care, Raleigh, NC.)

Hospital Versus Community-Based Nursing Care

Home health visits are a unique aspect of community-based nursing. These visits are made by nurses who work for home health and public health agencies and visiting nurse associations or by hospital-employed nurses. Such visits can also be part of the responsibilities of school nurses, clinic nurses, or occupational nurses. The type of nursing services provided to patients in their homes varies from agency to agency. Nurses working for home health or hospice agencies make home visits to provide skilled nursing care to patients discharged from the hospital and to prevent hospitalization or rehospitalization. Clinic nurses conduct home visits as part of patient follow-up. Public health and school nurses may make visits to provide anticipatory guidance to high-risk families and follow-up care to patients with communicable diseases.

Giving nursing care in a patient's home is different from providing care in a hospital. Patients must sign a release form to stay and receive treatment. They have little control over what happens to them, and they are expected to comply with the hospital's rules, regulations, and schedule of activities. They sleep in the hospital's beds and wear hospital gowns or similar-looking sleeping clothes. They are given their treatments, care, baths, and medications at a time that is usually determined by institutional schedules rather than at a time that is convenient for them. Although they may select meals from a daily menu, there is a limited choice in the type of food they are offered. Family members and friends are allowed to visit at the hospital's discretion.

Home care nurses are considered to be guests in the patient's home and need permission to visit and give care. They will have minimal control over the lifestyle, living situations, and health practices of the patients they visit. The lack of full decision-making authority can create a conflict for the nurse and lead to problems in the nurse–patient relationship. To work successfully with patients, no matter what the setting, it is important for a nurse to be nonjudgmental and to convey respect for the patient's beliefs, even when they differ sharply from the nurse's. This can be difficult for a nurse when a patient's lifestyle involves activities that the nurse considers harmful or unacceptable, such as alcohol or drug abuse.

The cleanliness of a patient's home may not meet the standards of a hospital. Although the nurse can provide teaching points about maintaining clean surroundings, the patient and family determine whether or not to implement the nurse's suggestions. The nurse must accept the reality of the situation and deliver the care required regardless of the sanitary conditions of the surroundings.

The kind of equipment and supplies or resources usually available in acute care settings are often unavailable in the patient's home. The nurse has to learn to improvise when providing care, such as when changing a dressing or catheterizing a patient in a regular bed that is not adjustable and lacks a bedside stand.

Infection control is as important in the home as it is in the hospital, but can be more challenging and requires more creative approaches. As in any situation, it is important to wash one's hands before and after giving direct patient care, even in a home that does not have running water. If aseptic technique is called for in a patient's home, it is essential to plan for implementing this before going to the home. This applies to using universal precautions, instituting isolation precautions if warranted, and disposing of bodily secretions and excretions. If injections are part of the care given, the nurse should use a closed container to dispose of syringes. Injectable and other medications need to be kept out of the reach of children during visits and stored in a safe place if they are to remain in the house. Nurses performing invasive procedures need to be up to date with their immunizations, including hepatitis B and tetanus.

The home environment often has more distractions than a hospital. The home can be filled with background noise and crowded with people and objects. A nurse may have to request that the television be turned down during the visit or that the patient move to a more private place to be interviewed.

Friends, neighbors, or family members may ask the nurse about the patient's condition. A patient has a right to confidentiality, and information should be shared only with the patient's permission. If the nurse carries the patient's chart into the house, it must be put in a secure place to avoid it being picked up by others or misplaced.

Discharge Planning for Home Care

Discharge planning begins when a patient is admitted in order to prepare for early discharge and the possible need for follow-up care in the home. Several different personnel or agencies may be involved in the planning process. In hospitals, social workers or nurses may serve as the discharge planners. Some home health agencies have liaison nurses who work with the discharge planners to ensure that the patient's needs are met when released from the hospital. Professionals in ambulatory health care settings may refer sick patients for home care services to prevent hospitalization. Public health nurses have patients referred for anticipatory guidance for high-risk families, for case finding, and follow-up treatment for patients with communicable diseases.

The development of a comprehensive discharge plan requires collaboration with professionals both at the referring agency and the home health or public health agency. The process involves identifying the patient's needs and developing a thorough plan to meet them. Communication with and cooperation of the patient and family are essential.

Community Resources and Referrals

Home health nurses and public health nurses act as case managers. After assessing the patient's needs, they might make referrals to other team members, such as home health aides and social workers. They work collaboratively with the health team and the agency or person who referred the patient for service.

Continuous coordinated care among all health care providers involved in the patient's care is essential to avoid duplication of effort by the various personnel caring for the patient.

Home health and public health nurses have the responsibility of providing the patient and family with information regarding other types of community resources available to meet their needs. During the initial and subsequent visits they help patients identify these community services and encourage the patient and family to contact the appropriate agencies. On occasion the nurse may need to make the initial contact if the patient and family are unable to do so themselves.

A community-based nurse needs to be knowledgeable about community resources available to patients and the services the agencies provide, eligibility requirements, and any possible charges for the services. Most communities have directories of health and social service agencies that the nurse can consult. These directories need to be continually updated as resources change. If a community does not have a resource booklet, the agency may develop one for the staff. It should include the commonly used community resources that patients need, the cost of the services, and eligibility requirements. The telephone book is also a good resource for helping patients identify the locations of grocery and drug stores, banks, health care facilities, ambulances, physicians, dentists, pharmacists, folk healers, social service agencies, and senior citizen programs.

Preparing for a Home Visit

Most agencies have a policy manual that states their philosophy and procedures and defines the services they provide. Becoming familiar with these policies is an essential step before initiating a home visit. It is also important to know the agency's policies and the state law regarding what action to take if the nurse finds a patient dead, encounters an abusive situation in the family, or determines that a patient cannot remain safely at home.

Before making a home visit, the nurse should review the patient's referral form and other pertinent data concerning the patient. It may be necessary to contact the referring agency if the purpose for the referral is unclear or if important information is missing.

The first step is to call the patient to obtain permission to visit, schedule a time for the visit, and verify the address. This initial phone conversation provides an opportunity to introduce oneself, identify the agency, and explain the reason for the visit.

If a patient does not have a telephone, the nurse should see if those who made the referral have a number where a phone message can be left for the patient. If an unannounced visit must be made to a patient's home, the nurse should ask permission to come in before entering the house. Explaining the purpose of the referral at the outset and setting up the time for future visits before leaving are also recommended approaches.

Most agencies supply nurses with bags that contain standard supplies and equipment needed during home visits. It is important to keep the bag properly supplied and to bring any additional items that might be needed for the visit. Patients usually do not have medical supplies that are needed for treatment.

Personal Safety Precautions

Whenever a nurse makes a home visit, the agency should know the nurse's schedule and the locations of the visits. The nurse should learn about the neighborhood and obtain directions for reaching the expected destination. A plan of action should always be established in case of emergencies.

Nurses are not expected to disregard their personal safety in an effort to make or complete home visits. If nurses encounter dangerous situations during visits, they should return to their agencies and contact their supervisors and/or law enforcement officials.

A list of suggested precautions to take when making a home visit is presented in Chart 2-1.

Conducting a Home Visit

The first visit sets the tone for subsequent visits and is a crucial step in establishing the nurse–patient relationship. The situations encountered can vary depending on numerous factors. Patients may be in pain and unable to care for themselves. Families may be overwhelmed and doubt their ability to care for their loved one. They may not understand why the patient was sent home from the hospital before being totally rehabilitated. They may not comprehend what home care is or why they cannot have 24-hour nursing services. It is critical that the nurse try to convey an understanding of what the patient and family are experiencing and how the illness is affecting their lives.

During the initial home visit, which usually lasts less than an hour, the patient is evaluated and a plan of care established that is followed or modified on subsequent visits. The nurse informs the patient of the agency's practices and policies and hours of operation. If the agency is to be reimbursed for the visit, the patient will have to provide evidence of insurance information, such as a Medicare card or Medicaid stickers.

The initial assessment includes evaluating the patient, the home environment, the patient's self-care abilities or the family's ability to provide care, and the patient's need for additional resources (Fig. 2-2). Identifying any possible hazards such as cluttered walk areas, potential fire risks, pollution (air, water), or inadequate sanitation facilities is also part of the initial assessment.

Documentation considerations for home visits follow fairly specific regulations. The patient's needs and the nursing care given are documented accurately to assure that the agency will qualify for payment for the visit. Medicare, Medicaid, and third-party payers require documentation of the patient's homebound status and the need for skilled professional nursing care. The medical diagnosis and specific detailed information on the functional limitations of the patient are usually part of the documentation. The goals and the actions appropriate for attaining them need to be identified. Expected outcomes of the nursing interventions must be stated in terms of the patient's behaviors and must be realistic and measurable. They must reflect the nursing diagnosis or the patient's problems and specify those actions that are expected to solve the patient's problems. If the doc-

CHART 2-1
Safety Precautions in Home Health Care

1. Know the phone number of the agency, police, and emergency services.
2. Let the agency know your daily schedules and the phone numbers of your patients so that you can be located if you do not return when expected.
3. Know where the patient lives before leaving to make the visit and carry a map for quick referral.
4. Keep your car in good working order and have sufficient gas in the tank.
5. Park the car near the patient's home and lock it during the visit.
6. Do not drive an expensive car or wear expensive jewelry when making visits.
7. Know the routes when using public transportation or walking to the patient's house.
8. Carry agency identification and have enough change to make phone calls in case you get lost or have problems. (Some agencies provide cellular phones for their nurses to enable them to contact the agency in case of an emergency or if unexpected situations arise.)
9. When making visits in high-crime areas, visit with another nurse rather than alone.
10. Schedule visits only during daylight hours.
11. Never walk into a patient's home uninvited.
12. If you do not feel safe entering a patient's home, leave the area.
13. Become familiar with the layout of the house, including exits from the house.
14. If a patient or family member is intoxicated, hostile, or obnoxious, reschedule the visit and leave.
15. If a family is having a serious argument or abusing the patient, reschedule the visit and contact your supervisor and report the abuse to the appropriate authorities.

umentation is not done correctly, the agency may not be paid for the visit.

Determining the Need for Future Visits

In the process of conducting an assessment of the patient's situation, the nurse evaluates the need for future visits and the frequency with which those visits may need to be made.

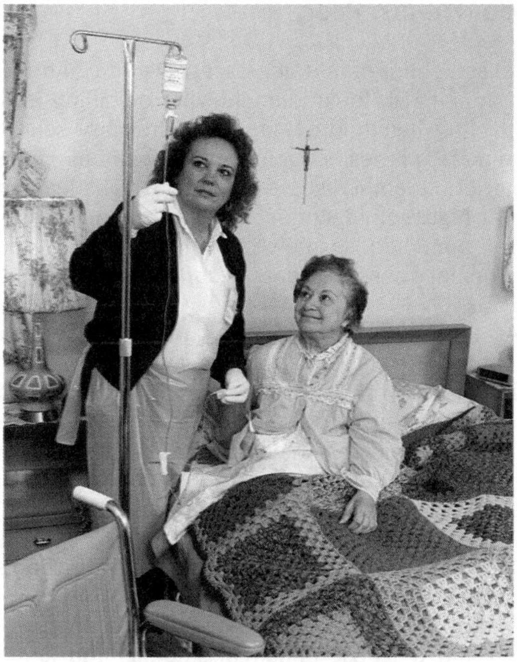

FIGURE 2-2. Intravenous therapy is one of the types of skilled nursing care that may be provided in the home. (Courtesy Good Samaritan Certified Home Health Agency, Babylon, NY.)

To make these judgments, the nurse may find it helpful to consider the following factors:

- *The patient's current health status:* How well is the patient progressing? How serious are the present signs and symptoms? Has the patient shown signs of progressing as expected or does it seem that recovery will be delayed?
- *The level of self-care abilities:* Is the patient capable of self-care? What is the patient's level of independence? Is the patient ambulatory or bedridden? Does the patient have sufficient energy or is he or she frail and easily fatigued?
- *The level of nursing care needed:* What level of nursing care does the patient require? Is the care related to basic skills or does it require more complex interventions?
- *The prognosis:* What is the expectation of recovery in this particular instance? What are the chances that complications may develop if nursing care is not provided?
- *Patient education needs:* How well has the patient or family grasped the teaching points made? Is there a need for further follow-up and retraining? What level of proficiency does the patient or family show in carrying out the necessary care?
- *Mental status:* How alert is the patient? Are there signs of confusion or thinking difficulties? Does the patient tend to be forgetful or have a limited attention span?
- *The home environment:* Are there worrisome safety factors apparent? Are family or friends available to provide care or is the patient alone?
- *Level of adherence:* Is the patient following the instructions provided? Does the patient seem capable of doing so? Are the family members helpful in this regard or are they unwilling or unable to assist in caring for the patient as expected?

With each subsequent visit, these factors are evaluated to determine the continuing health needs of the patient. As progress is made and the patient becomes more capable of self-care and more independent, the need for home visits may decline.

Closing the Visit

As the visit comes to a close, it is important to summarize the main points of the visit for the patient and family and identify expectations for future visits or patient achievements.

The following points should be considered at the end of each visit:

- What are the main points the patient or family should remember from the visit?
- What positive attributes have been noted about the patient and the family that will give them a sense of accomplishment?
- What were the main points of the teaching plan or the treatments needed to assure that the patient and family understand what they must do? A written set of instructions should be left with the patient or family, provided they can read.
- Who should the patient or family call in case they need to contact someone immediately? Are current emergency phone numbers readily available?
- What signs of complications should be reported immediately?
- What is the day and time of the next visit? Will a different nurse make the visit? How frequently will visits be made and for how long, if discernible at this time?

Other Community-Based Health Care Settings

Ambulatory Settings

Ambulatory health care is provided for patients in community- or hospital-based settings. The types of agencies that provide ambulatory health care are medical clinics, ambulatory care units, urgent care centers, cardiac rehabilitation programs, mental health centers, student health centers, community outreach programs, and nursing centers. Some ambulatory centers provide care to a specific population, such as migrant workers or Native Americans. Neighborhood health centers provide services to patients who live in a geographically defined area. The centers may operate in free-standing buildings, storefronts, or mobile units. Agencies can provide ambulatory health care in addition to other services, such as offering an adult day care or health program. The kinds of services offered and the patients served depend on the agency's mission.

Nursing responsibilities in ambulatory health care settings include providing direct patient care, conducting patient intake screenings, treating patients with acute or chronic illnesses or emergency conditions, referring patients to other agencies for additional services, teaching patients self-care activities, and offering health education programs that promote health maintenance. Nurses also work as the clinic managers and direct the operation of the clinic and supervise other health team members.

Nurse practitioners, educated in primary care, often practice in ambulatory care settings with a focus on gerontology, pediatrics, family or adult health, or family planning.

Occupational Health Programs

Federal legislation, especially the Occupational Safety and Health Act, has had a major impact on health conditions in the workplace. The intent of the law is directed at creating safer and healthier work conditions. It is in an employer's interest to try to provide a safe working environment because the result is reduced costs associated with employee absenteeism, hospitalization, and disability.

Occupational nurses can work in solo units in an industrial setting, may serve as consultants on a limited or part-time basis, or may be members of an interdisciplinary team composed of a variety of health care workers such as nurses, physicians, exercise physiologists, health educators, counselors, nutritionists, safety engineers, and industrial hygienists.

The occupational health nurse functions in several ways and may provide direct care to employees who become ill, conduct health education programs for company staff members, or set up health programs aimed at establishing specific health behaviors, such as eating properly and getting enough exercise. The nurse must also be knowledgeable about federal regulations pertaining to occupational health and be familiar with other pertinent legislation, such as the Americans with Disabilities Act.

School Health Programs

School-age children and adolescents with health problems are at major risk for underachieving or failing in school. The leading health problems of elementary school—age children are injuries, influenza and pneumonia, infections, malnutrition, dental disease, and cancer. The leading problems for high school students are alcohol and drug abuse, injuries, homicide, sexually transmitted disease, sports injuries, dental disease, pregnancy, and mental and emotional problems.

An ideal school health program would have an interdisciplinary health team consisting of physicians, nurses, dentists, social workers, counselors and the school administrators, and parents and students. The school would serve as the site for a family health clinic, which would offer primary health and mental health services to children and adolescents as well as to all family members in the community.

Nurse practitioners are ideally suited to provide the primary care in these settings, and several schools have established school nurse programs to provide care in the community. The nurse practitioners perform physical examinations and diagnose and treat students and families for acute and chronic illnesses. These clinics are cost effective and are especially beneficial for students from low-income families who lack access to health care or have no health insurance.

The roles of the school nurse are care provider, health educator, consultant, and counselor. The school nurse collaborates with the students, their parents, administrators, and other health and social service professionals regarding a student's health problems. Nurses perform health screenings, give basic care for minor injuries and complaints, administer medications, monitor students' and families' immunizations status, and identify children with health problems. They need to be knowledgeable about state and local regulations affecting school-age children, such as ordinances for excluding students from school because of communicable diseases, lice, scabies, or other parasites.

The school nurse is a health education consultant for teachers. In addition to providing information on health practices, teaching health classes, or helping with the development of the health education curriculum, the school nurse educates the teacher and class when one of the students has a special problem, a disability, or a disease such as hemophilia or AIDS.

The school nurse can train volunteers to perform basic health screenings, interpret the results to the parents, make referrals, and follow-up to ensure that the student has received adequate care.

Care for the Homeless

No exact figures exist on the number of homeless people in the United States. It is a growing problem and includes increasing numbers of women, children, and elderly. The homeless are a heterogeneous group that includes the chronically mentally ill, people who abuse alcohol and other drugs, members of dysfunctional families, the unemployed, and those who cannot find affordable housing. Some are temporarily homeless as a result of catastrophic natural disasters.

The homeless often have difficulty affording or gaining access to health care. Because of numerous obstacles, they seek health care late in the course of the disease and deteriorate more quickly than other patients. Many of the health problems they experience are related in large part to their living situations. Street life exposes the homeless to the extremes of hot and cold environments and compounds the health risks these people face.

The homeless have high rates of trauma, tuberculosis, upper respiratory infection, poor nutrition and anemia, lice, scabies, peripheral vascular problems, sexually transmitted diseases, dental problems, arthritis, hypothermia, and foot problems. Common chronic health problems of the homeless include diabetes, hypertension, and heart disease. The management of these problems is made more difficult by the patient living on the street and being discharged to a homeless situation. The homeless who live in shelters frequently encounter overcrowded, unventilated quarters that provide an ideal environment for the spread of communicable diseases such as tuberculosis.

Community-based nurses who work with the homeless must be nonjudgmental, patient, and understanding. They must be proficient in dealing with many different kinds of people with a wide variety of health problems and needs. Nursing interventions will be aimed at attempting to obtain health care services for the homeless and evaluate the health care needs of those who reside in the shelters. However, unless the social problems that underlie homelessness are resolved, the plight of the homeless will continue to be a major problem in this country.

CRITICAL THINKING EXERCISES

1. A patient who will require long-term intravenous antibiotic therapy has been referred to a home health care agency for care following discharge from the hospital. How would you explain to this patient the kind of care that will be provided by the home health care nurse?
2. You are exploring employment opportunities in community-based health care facilities. What criteria would you use to determine if a particular agency is one in which you would be interested in working?
3. A homeless patient has sought medical care in the Emergency Department. How does the assessment of this patient differ from that of a patient who is not homeless?

BIBLIOGRAPHY

Books

Clark MJ. Nursing in the Community. Norwalk, CT, Appleton & Lange, 1992

Rice R. Home Health Nursing Practice: Concepts and Application. St Louis, MO, Mosby-Year Book, 1992.

Spradley BW. Readings in Community Health Nursing, 4th ed. Philadelphia, JB Lippincott, 1991.

Stanhope M and Lancaster J. Community Health Nursing: Process and Practice for Promoting Health, 3rd ed. St Louis, MO, Mosby-Year Book, 1992.

Swanson JM and Albrecht M. Community Health Nursing: Promoting the Health of Aggregates. Philadelphia, WB Saunders, 1993.

Journals

Allen SA. Medicare case management. Home Healthcare Nurse 1994; 12(3):21–27.

Burgel BJ. Occupational health: Nursing in the workplace. Nurs Clin North Am 1994 Sept; 29(3):431–441.

Carter KF et al. Health needs of homeless clients: Accessing nursing care at a free clinic. J Community Health Nurs 1994; 11(3): 139–147.

Dee-Kelly PA, Heller S, and Sibley M. Managed care: An opportunity for home care agencies. Nurs Clin North Am 1994 Sept; 29(3):471–481.

Ellenbecker CA and Shea K. Documenting in home health care practice: Evidence of quality care. Nurs Clin North Am 1994 Sept; 29(3):495–506.

Gurfolina V. Hospice nursing. The concept of palliative care. Nurs Clin North Am 1994 Sept; 29(3):533–546.

Hodnicki DR. Homelessness: Health-care implications. Journal of Community Health Nursing 1990; 7(2):59–67.

Hootman J. Nursing our most valuable natural resource: School age children. Nurs Forum 1994 July–Sept; 29(3):5–17.

Igoe JB. School nursing. Nurs Clin North Am 1994 Sept; 29(3): 443–457.

Stulginsky MM. Nurses' home health experience. Part I: The practice setting. Nursing and Health Care 1993 Oct; 14(8):402–407.

Stulginsky MM. Nurses' home health experience. Part II: The unique demands of home visits. Nursing and Health Care 1993 Nov; 14(9):476–485.

Uphold CR and Graham MV. Schools as centers for collaborative services for families: A vision for change. Nurs Outlook 1993 Sept/Oct; 41(5):204–211.

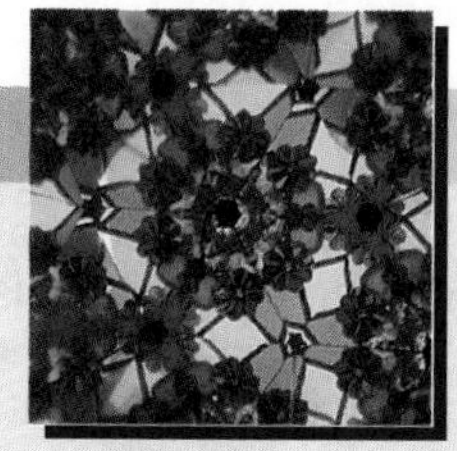

3 Critical Thinking and the Nursing Process

CHAPTER OUTLINE

Critical Thinking
Aspects of Critical Thinking
Steps of the Nursing Process
Assessment
Health History
The Health Assessment
Other Components of the Data Base
Recording the Data Base
Diagnosis
Nursing Diagnosis
Collaborative Problems
Planning
Setting Priorities
Establishing Goals for Nursing Action
Establishing Expected Outcomes
Implementation
Recording Outcomes
Evaluation
Critical Thinking Exercises

LEARNING OBJECTIVES

On completion of the chapter, the learner will be able to:

1. Describe the skills of critical thinking and the components of the nursing process
2. Identify the variables involved in effectively conducting a nursing history and a health assessment
3. Describe the process of developing nursing diagnoses, collaborative problems, goals, and expected outcomes
4. Identify the purposes and essential components of the nursing care plan
5. Develop a nursing care plan for a patient

Critical Thinking

In today's health care arena the nurse is faced with increasingly complex issues and situations resulting from advanced technology, a greater acuity of patients in hospital and community settings, the aging population, complex disease processes, and continually changing ethical and cultural factors. Traditionally, nurses have used a problem-solving approach in planning and providing nursing care. Today the decision-making part of problem solving has become increasingly more complex and requires critical thinking.

Critical thinking is a cognitive or mental process that involves rational examination and analysis of all available information and ideas and the formulation of conclusions and decisions. Independent judgments and decisions evolve from a sound knowledge base and the ability to synthesize information within the context in which it presents. Nursing skills related to the use of the scientific method, application of the nursing process, and clinical decision making are essential components of critical thinking.

Aspects of Critical Thinking

Thinking is a continuous, ongoing process that involves the interaction of a series of thoughts and perceptions. Critical thinking, as a type of thinking, is also a continuous process. However, certain cognitive or mental activities can be identified as key components of critical thinking.

A person who has developed the skill of critical thinking will generally engage in the following mental activity while thinking critically:

- Ask questions to determine the reason and cause of why certain developments have occurred and to see if more information is needed.
- Gather as much relevant information as possible to consider all factors involved.
- Validate the information presented to make sure that it is accurate, not just supposition or opinion, and that it makes sense and is based on fact and evidence.
- Analyze the information to determine what it means and to see if it forms clusters or patterns that point to certain conclusions.
- Draw upon past clinical experience and knowledge to explain what is happening and to anticipate what might happen next.
- Maintain a flexible attitude that allows the facts to guide the thinking and takes into account all possibilities.
- Consider available options and examine each in terms of their advantages and disadvantages.
- Formulate decisions that reflect creativity and independent decision making.

Developing the skill of critical thinking takes time and practice. Throughout this text, critical thinking exercises are offered as a means of practicing one's ability to think critically. Additional exercises can be found in the Study Guide that accompanies the text. The questions listed in Chart 3-1 can serve as a guide in working through the exercises, although it is important to remember that each situation is unique and calls for an approach that fits the particular circumstances being described.

Nurses must use critical thinking skills in all practice settings: acute care, ambulatory, and extended care settings as well as in the home and community. Each patient situa-

CHART 3-1

The Inquiring Mind: Critical Thinking in Action

Throughout the critical thinking process, a continuous flow of questions evolves in the thinker's mind. While the questions will vary according to the particular clinical situation, certain general inquiries can serve as a basis for reaching conclusions and determining a course of action.

When faced with a patient situation, it is often helpful to seek answers to some or all of the following questions in an attempt to determine those actions that are most appropriate:

- What relevant assessment information do I need and how do I interpret this information? What does this information tell me?
- What problems does this information point to? Have I identified the most important ones? Does the information point to any other problems that I should consider?
- Have I gathered all the information I need? (signs/symptoms, lab values, medication history, emotional factors, mental status)? Is anything missing?
- Is there anything that needs to be reported immediately? Do I need to seek additional assistance?
- Does this patient have any special risk factors? Which ones are most significant? What must I do to minimize these risks?
- What possible complications must I watch for?
- What are the most important problems that we are facing in this situation? Do the patient and the patient's family see the same problems?
- What are the desired outcomes for this patient? Which have the highest priority? Do the patient and I see eye to eye on these points?
- What is going to be my first action in this situation?
- How can I construct a plan of care to achieve the goals?
- Are there any age-related factors involved and will they require some special approach? Will I need to make some change in the plan of care to take these factors into account?
- How do the family dynamics affect this situation, and will this have an impact on my actions or plan of care?
- Are there cultural factors that I must address and consider?
- Am I dealing with an ethical problem here? If so, how am I going to resolve it?
- Has any nursing research been conducted on this subject?

tion, regardless of the setting, is viewed as unique and dynamic. The unique factors that the patient brings to the health care situation are considered, studied, analyzed, and interpreted. Interpretation of the information presented then allows the nurse to focus on those factors that are most relevant and that are most significant to the clinical situation. Decisions about what to do and how to do it are then developed into a plan of action. The critical thinking skills that are necessary to make such decisions are used in all the steps of the nursing process.

Steps of the Nursing Process

The nursing process has been accepted as the essence of nursing. It is a deliberate system for identifying and solving health problems in order to meet a person's health care and nursing needs. Although the steps of the nursing process have been delineated in various ways by different writers, the common components cited include assessment, diagnosis, planning, implementation, and evaluation. The 1991 American Nurses Association Standards of Clinical Nursing Practice includes an additional component entitled outcome identification and establishes the sequence of steps in the following order: assessment, diagnosis, outcome identification, planning, implementation, and evaluation. For the purposes of this text, the nursing process will be based on the traditional five steps and will delineate two components in the diagnosis step: nursing diagnoses and collaborative problems. The steps are defined as follows:

1. *Assessment*—the systematic collection of data to determine the patient's health status and to identify any actual or potential health problems. (Analysis of data is included as part of the assessment. For those who wish to emphasize its importance, analysis may be identified as a separate step of the nursing process.)
2. *Diagnosis*—identification of the following two types of patient problems:
   a. *Nursing diagnoses*—actual or potential health problems that can be managed by independent nursing interventions
   b. *Collaborative problems*—certain physiologic complications that nurses monitor to detect onset or changes in status. Nurses manage collaborative problems using physician-prescribed and nursing-prescribed interventions to minimize the complications of the events (Carpenito, 1993, p. 30).
3. *Planning*—development of goals and a plan of care designed to assist the patient in resolving the diagnosed problems
4. *Implementation*—actualization of the plan of care through nursing interventions
5. *Evaluation*—determination of the patient's responses to the nursing interventions and the extent to which the goals have been achieved

Dividing the nursing process into five distinct components or steps serves to emphasize the essential nursing actions that must be taken to resolve the patient's nursing diagnoses and manage any collaborative problems or complications. However, we must remember that the divisions of the process into separate steps is artificial and that the process functions as an integrated whole, with the steps being interrelated, interdependent, and recurrent (Fig. 3-1). Chart 3-2 presents an overview of the nursing activities involved in applying the nursing process.

Assessment

The gathering of assessment data is carried out by means of the health history and the health assessment and by ongoing monitoring to remain aware of the patient's needs and the effectiveness of the nursing care that he or she receives.

Health History

The health history is conducted for the purpose of determining the individual's state of wellness or illness and is best accomplished as part of a planned interview. The interview is a dialogue between the patient and the nurse and involves the sensitive direction of a conversation in order to obtain information. The nurse's approach to the person will largely determine the amount and quality of information that is received. Achieving a relationship of mutual trust and respect requires the ability to communicate a sincere interest in the person. Examples of effective therapeutic

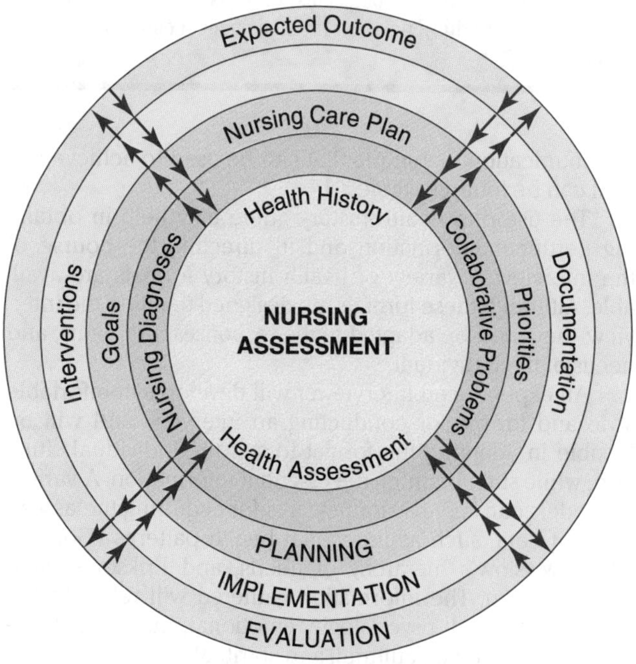

FIGURE 3-1. The nursing process is depicted schematically in this circle. Starting from the innermost circle, nursing assessment, the process moves outward through the formulation of nursing diagnoses and collaborative problems, planning, the setting of goals and priorities, establishing the nursing care plan, and actual implementations and documentation, and arrives at the ongoing process of evaluation and expected outcomes.

CHART 3-2
Steps of the Nursing Process

Assessment

1. Conduct the health history.
2. Perform the health assessment.
3. Interview the patient's family or significant others.
4. Study the health record.
5. Organize, analyze, synthesize, and summarize the collected data.

Diagnosis

Nursing Diagnosis

1. Identify the patient's nursing problems.
2. Identify the defining characteristics of the nursing problems.
3. Identify the etiology of the nursing problems.
4. State nursing diagnoses concisely and precisely.

Collaborative Problems

1. Identify potential problems or complications that require collaborative interventions.
2. Identify health team members with whom collaboration is essential.

Planning

1. Assign priority to the nursing diagnoses.
2. Specify the goals.
   a. Develop immediate, intermediate, and long-term goals.
   b. State the goals in realistic and measurable terms.
3. Identify nursing interventions appropriate for goal attainment.
4. Establish expected outcomes.
   a. Make sure that the outcomes are realistic and measurable.
   b. Identify critical times for the attainment of outcomes.
5. Develop the written nursing care plan.
   a. Include nursing diagnoses, goals, nursing interventions, expected outcomes, and critical times.
   b. Write all entries precisely, concisely, and systematically.
   c. Keep the plan current and flexible to meet the patient's changing problems and needs.
6. Involve the patient, his family or significant others, nursing team members, and other health team members in all aspects of planning.

Implementation

1. Put the nursing care plan into action.
2. Coordinate the activities of the patient, family or significant others, nursing team members, and other health team members.
3. Record the patient's responses to the nursing actions.

Evaluation

1. Collect objective data.
2. Compare the patient's behavioral outcomes with the expected outcomes. Determine the extent to which the goals were achieved.
3. Include the patient, family or significant others, nursing team members, and other health care team members in the evaluation.
4. Identify alterations that need to be made in the nursing diagnoses, collaborative problems, goals, nursing interventions, and expected outcomes.
5. Continue all steps of the nursing process: assessment, diagnosis, planning, implementation, and evaluation.

communication technique that can be used to achieve this goal can be found in Table 3-1.

The use of a health history guide may help in obtaining pertinent information and in directing the course of the interview. A variety of health history formats are available. Although these formats are designed to guide the interview, they must be adapted to the responses, problems, and needs of the individual.

An experienced interviewer will develop a comfortable style and format for conducting an interview and will be flexible in adapting the format to suit the individual situation, while still obtaining the essential information. A variety of models can serve as frameworks for acquiring the assessment of data, such as functional health patterns (Gordon, 1993), Maslow's hierarchy of needs, and Erikson's eight stages of man. The information gathered will relate to the person's physical, psychologic, emotional, intellectual, developmental, social, cultural, and spiritual needs.

The questions in Chart 3-3 are offered as guidelines for interviewing, but the questions actually asked are determined by the reaction of the individual.

In some instances it may be appropriate for the patient to fill out a health history form. When a form is used, it is the responsibility of the nurse to verify and clarify the information provided by the patient and to seek any additional information that is necessary to identify the individual's nursing needs.

The Health Assessment

A health assessment or physical assessment may be carried out prior to, during, or following the health history, depending on the patient's physical and emotional state and the immediate priorities of his or her illness situation.

The purpose of the health assessment is to identify those aspects of the person's physical, psychologic, and emotional state that indicate the existence of a nursing need. It requires the use of the senses of sight, hearing, touch, and smell as well as the appropriate interview skills and techniques. Physical examination techniques as well as techniques and strategies for assessing behaviors and role changes are discussed in Chapters 6 and 7.

Other Components of the Data Base

Additional relevant information should be obtained from the person's family or significant others, from other members of the health team, and from the person's health rec-

TABLE 3-1 Summary of Therapeutic Communication Techniques

Technique	Definition	Therapeutic Value
Listening	An active process of receiving information and examining one's reaction to the messages received	Nonverbally communicates nurse's interest in patient.
Silence	Periods of no verbal communication among participants	Nonverbally communicates nurse's acceptance of patient
Establishing guidelines	Statements regarding roles, purpose, and limitations for a particular interaction	Helps patient to know what is expected of him
Open-ended comments	General comments asking the patient to determine the direction the interaction should take	Allows patient to decide what material is most relevant and encourages him to continue
Reducing distance	Diminishing physical space between the nurse and patient	Nonverbally communicates that nurse wants to be involved with patient
Acknowledgment	Recognition given to a patient for contribution to an interaction	Demonstrates the importance of the patient's role within the relationship
Restating	Repeating to the patient what the nurse believes is the main thought or idea expressed	Asks for validation of nurse's interpretation of the message
Reflecting	Directing back to the patient his ideas, feelings, questions, or content	Attempts to show patient the importance of his own ideas, feelings, and interpretations
Seeking clarification	Asking for additional inputs to understand the message received	Demonstrates nurse's desire to understand patient's communication
Seeking consensual validation	Attempts to reach a mutual denotative and connotative meaning of specific words	Demonstrates nurse's desire to understand patient's communication
Focusing	Questions or statements to help the patient develop or expand an idea	Directs conversation toward topics of importance
Summarizing	Statement of main areas discussed during interaction	Helps patient to separate relevant from irrelevant material: serves as a review and closing for the interaction
Planning	Mutual decision making regarding the goals, direction, and so on, of future interactions	Reiterates patient's role within relationship

(Reprinted with permission from Sundeen SJ et al. Nurse–Client Interaction: Interpreting the Nursing Process. St. Louis, Mosby-Year Book, 1994.)

ord or chart. Depending on the person's immediate illness needs, this information may have been obtained prior to the health history and the health assessment. Whatever the sequence of events, it is important to use all available sources of pertinent data to complete the nursing assessment.

Recording the Data Base

After the health history and health assessment are completed, the information obtained is recorded in the patient's permanent record. The record provides a means of communication between the members of the health care team and facilitates coordinated planning and continuity of care. The record fulfills other functions as well:

- It serves as the business and legal record for the health care agency and for the professional staff responsible for the person's care.
- It serves as a basis for evaluating the quality and appropriateness of care as well as for reviewing the effective use of patient care services.
- It provides data useful in research, education, and short- and long-range planning.

There are a variety of systems used for documenting patient care. Each health care agency selects the system that

CHART 3-3
Suggestions for Interviewing Patients

Current Health Status

Nursing Focus: At the beginning of the interview, focus on what is most troublesome to the patient.

Suggested Initial Statement: "Please tell me why you are seeking health care."

- What is causing you the most discomfort?
- When did the symptoms appear?
- What did you do when you noticed these symptoms?
- Does anything seem to relieve these symptoms?
- Do you believe you are getting better or worse? (the directional trend: improvement or deterioration)
- How do you feel now?
- What do you know about your illness or condition?
- What do you do for yourself at home when you are sick?
- How has the illness affected your way of life? For how long?
- What factors aggravate or help your condition?
- Are you taking any medications?
- Do you have any allergies? (food, drugs)
- What is your greatest concern?
- What have you been told about the treatment or tests that have been planned for you?
- Who or what has been your chief source of information?

Past Health History

Nursing Focus: Learn about the patient's background and experience in order to determine his or her needs.*

Suggested Initial Statement: "It will be helpful if you will tell me about your past health history."†

- Would you tell me a little about yourself, your family, your way of life?
- What types of things do you do to try to stay healthy?
- How do you usually react to being ill?
- Whom do you usually turn to for help?
- What type of work do you do?
- Has your illness interfered with your work?
- How do you like to be treated when you are ill?
- What activities, hobbies, and forms of recreation do you enjoy?

Nursing Needs

Nursing Focus: Ascertain what can be done to support the patient and help the individual to make the best use of his or her resources.

Suggested Initial Statement: "Please tell me what you think your needs are, your strengths, and your limitations."*

- What would you like to be able to do to help yourself get better?
- What kinds of help do you need?
- Who do you think could provide this help?
- What aspects of your life are being disrupted by your illness?
- How do you think your illness will affect your family?
- What do you think will be the hardest part of the situation?
- What are your food preferences? Dislikes?
- What are your sleeping habits?
  Regular retiring time?
  Do you like a night light?
  How many pillows do you use?
- What are your elimination habits (bowel and urinary)?
- Do you have any limitations of seeing? hearing? walking?
- Would it be helpful to have a family member or friend stay with you?

If the interview is being conducted in the hospital:

- What concerns you most about being in the hospital?
- What do you miss the most in the hospital?
- How long do you think you will stay?
- What do you not understand as well as you would like to?
- What could the nursing staff do that would be most helpful for you?

*Social, cultural, developmental, and educational levels and the patient's readiness to learn are assessed throughout the interview.

†General requests for information often prompt the patient to discuss his or her health status, problems, and needs openly and fully; if such requests result in complete and appropriate sharing of information, more specific questions are often unnecessary.

best meets its needs. The types of systems available include the problem-oriented health record system or more simplified charting processes such as Focus Charting, Patient Outcome Charting, Problem Intervention Evaluation (PIE) Charting, and Charting by Exception (CBE). In addition, many health care agencies have moved toward computerized documentation systems which appear to save time, improve the monitoring of quality improvement issues, and make it easier to gain access to patient information.

Diagnosis

The assessment component of the nursing process serves as the basis for identifying nursing diagnoses and collaborative problems. Soon after the completion of the health history and the health assessment, the nurse organizes, analyzes, synthesizes, and summarizes the data collected and determines the patient's need for nursing care.

Nursing Diagnosis

Nursing, unlike medicine, does not yet have a complete taxonomy of diagnostic labels that convey the same meaning to all nurses. The purpose for establishing a formal list of nursing diagnoses was to identify those nursing functions for which nurses are held legally responsible and accountable. Nursing diagnoses have fostered the development of autonomy and accountability in nursing and have helped to delineate the scope of practice. Standards of practice have become increasingly more definitive, and collaboration of nursing with other disciplines has been facilitated.

Many state nurse practice acts include nursing diagnosis as a nursing function, and nursing diagnosis is included in the American Nurses Association Standards of Nursing Practice and in the standards developed by many nursing specialty organizations.

The official organization that has assumed formal responsibility for formulating acceptable nursing diagnoses is the North American Nursing Diagnosis Association (NANDA). NANDA has approved a taxonomy for classification of nursing diagnoses and continues to develop it further. Efforts have been made to include the taxonomy in the World Health Organization's tenth revision of the International Classification of Diseases (ICD-10).

The diagnostic categories identified by NANDA (Chart 3-4) have been generally accepted by nurses but require further validation and expansion. They are not yet complete or mutually exclusive. More research is needed to determine the predictive and prognostic attributes of the diagnostic labels. Only through clinical use and research of nursing diagnostic labels can these labels be validated and expanded.

Formulating a Nursing Diagnosis

When developing the nursing diagnoses for a particular patient, the nurse must first identify the commonalities among the assessment data collected. These common features lead to the categorization of related data that reveal the existence of a problem and the need for nursing intervention. *The patient's nursing problem is then defined as the nursing diagnosis.*

It must be remembered that nursing diagnoses are *not* medical diagnoses; they are *not* medical treatments prescribed by the physician; they are *not* diagnostic studies; they are *not* the equipment used to implement medical therapy; and they are *not* the problems that the nurse experiences while caring for the patient. They *are* the patient's actual or potential health problems that are amenable to resolution by independent nursing actions. Nursing diagnoses that are succinctly stated in terms of the specific problems of the patient will guide the nurse in the development of the nursing care plan.

In order to give additional meaning to the diagnosis, the characteristics and the etiology of the problem must be identified and included as part of the diagnosis. For example, the nursing diagnoses and their defining characteristics and etiology for a patient who has rheumatoid arthritis may include:

- Impaired physical mobility related to restricted joint movement
- Self-care deficits (feeding, bathing, dressing, toileting) related to fatigue and joint stiffness
- Self-esteem disturbance related to loss of independence
- Altered nutrition (less than body requirements) related to fatigue and inadequate food intake

Collaborative Problems

In addition to nursing diagnoses and their related nursing interventions, nursing practice encompasses certain situations and interventions that do not fall within the definition of nursing diagnoses. These activities pertain to potential problems or complications that are medical in origin and require collaborative interventions with the physician and other members of the health care team. The term **collaborative problem** is used to identify these situations.

- Collaborative problems are certain physiologic complications that nurses monitor to detect onset or changes in status. Nurses manage collaborative problems using physician-prescribed and nursing-prescribed interventions to minimize the complications of the events (Carpenito, 1993, p. 30).

Thus, a primary focus of the nurse in dealing with collaborative problems is to monitor the patient for onset of complications or changes in the status of existing complications. The complications are usually related to the patient's disease process or to treatments, medications, or diagnostic studies. In addition, the nurse prescribes nursing interventions that are appropriate for managing the complications and implements the treatments prescribed by the physician. Figure 3-2 depicts the differences between nursing diagnoses and collaborative problems.

After the nursing diagnoses and collaborative problems have been identified, they are recorded on the nursing care plan.

Planning

Once the nursing diagnoses have been identified, the planning component of the nursing process is developed. This phase involves the following:

1. Assigning priorities to the nursing diagnoses and collaborative problems
2. Specifying immediate, intermediate, and long-term goals of nursing action
3. Identifying specific nursing interventions appropriate for attaining the goals
4. Identifying interdependent interventions
5. Specifying expected outcomes
6. Documenting the nursing diagnoses, collaborative problems, goals, nursing interventions, and expected outcomes on the nursing care plan
7. Communicating to appropriate personnel any assessment data that point to health needs that can best be met by other members of the health care team

Setting Priorities

Assigning priorities to the nursing diagnoses and to the collaborative problems is a joint effort by the nurse and the patient or the family members. Any disagreement about the priorities is resolved in a way that is mutually acceptable. Consideration must be given to the urgency of the problems, the most critical problems receiving the highest priorities. Maslow's hierarchy of needs provides a useful framework for determining priority problems, with high priority being given to physical needs, followed by lower-level needs.

CHART 3-4
NANDA Approved Nursing Diagnoses—1994

Activity Intolerance
Activity Intolerance, Risk for
Adjustment, Impaired
Airway Clearance, Ineffective
Altered Family Processes: Alcoholism
Anxiety
Aspiration, Risk for
Body Image Disturbance
Body Temperature, Risk for Altered
Breastfeeding, Effective
Breastfeeding, Ineffective
Breastfeeding, Interrupted
Breathing Pattern, Ineffective
Caregiver Role Strain
Caregiver Role Strain, Risk for
Commuication, Impaired Verbal
Community Coping, Potential for Enhanced
Community Coping, Ineffective
Confusion, Acute
Confusion, Chronic
Constipation
Constipation, Colonic
Constipation, Perceived
Decisional Conflict (Specify)
Decreased Cardiac Output
Defensive Coping
Denial, Ineffective
Diarrhea
Disuse Syndrome, Risk for
Diversional Activity Deficit
Dysreflexia
Energy Field Disturbance
Environmental Interpretation Syndrome, Impaired
Family Coping, Compromised, Ineffective
Family Coping, Disabling, Ineffective
Family Coping: Potential for Growth
Family Processes, Altered
Fatigue
Fear
Fluid Volume Deficit
Fluid Volume Deficit, Risk for
Fluid Volume Excess
Gas Exchange, Impaired
Grieving, Anticipatory
Grieving, Dysfunctional
Growth and Development, Altered
Health Maintenance, Altered
Health-Seeking Behaviors (Specify)
Home Maintenance Management, Impaired
Hopelessness
Hyperthermia
Hypothermia
Incontinence, Bowel
Incontinence, Functional
Incontinence, Reflex
Incontinence, Stress
Incontinence, Total
Incontinence, Urge
Individual Coping, Ineffective
Infant Feeding Pattern, Ineffective
Infant Behavior, Risk for Disorganized
Infant Behavior, Disorganized
Infant Behavior, Potential for Enhanced Organized
Infection, Risk for
Injury, Risk for
Intracranial: Decreased Adaptive Capacity
Knowledge Deficit (Specify)
Loneliness, Risk for
Memory, Impaired
Noncompliance (Specify)
Nutrition: Less Than Body Requirements, Altered
Nutrition: More Than Body Requirements, Altered
Nutrition: Potential for More Than Body Requirements, Altered
Oral Mucuous Membrane, Altered
Pain
Pain, Chronic
Parental Role Conflict
Parenting, Altered
Parenting, Risk for Altered
Parent/Infant/Child Attachment, Risk for Altered
Personal Identity Disturbance
Peripheral Neurovascular Dysfunction, Risk for
Perioperative Positioning Injury, Risk for
Physical Mobility, Impaired
Poisoning, Risk for
Post-Trauma Response
Powerlessness
Protection, Altered
Rape-Trauma Syndrome
Rape-Trauma Syndrome: Compound Reaction
Rape-Trauma Syndrome: Silent Reaction
Relocation Stress Syndrome
Role Performance, Altered
Self-Care Deficit, Bathing/Hygiene
Self-Care Deficit, Feeding
Self-Care Deficit, Dressing/Grooming
Self-Care Deficit, Toileting
Self-Esteem, Chronic Low
Self-Esteem, Situational Low
Self-Esteem Disturbance
Self-Mutilation, Risk for
Sensory/Perceptual Alterations (Specify) (Visual, auditory, kinesthetic, gustatory, tactile, olfactory)
Sexual Dysfunction
Sexuality Patterns, Altered
Skin Integrity, Impaired
Skin Integrity, Risk for Impaired
Sleep Pattern Disturbance

(continued)

CHART 3-4 *(continued)*

NANDA Approved Nursing Diagnoses—1994

Social Interaction, Impaired
Social Isolation
Spiritual Distress (Distress of the Human Spirit)
Spiritual Well-Being, Potential for Enhanced
Suffocation, Risk for
Swallowing, Impaired
Therapeutic Regimen: Families, Ineffective Management of
Therapeutic Regimen: Community, Ineffective Management of
Therapeutic Regimen: Individual, Ineffective Management of
Thermoregulation, Ineffective
Thought Processes, Altered
Tissue Integrity, Impaired
Tissue Perfusion, Altered (Specify Type) (Renal, cerebral, cardiopulmonary, gastrointestinal, peripheral)
Trauma, Risk for
Unilateral Neglect
Urinary Elimination, Altered
Urinary Retention
Ventilation, Inability to Sustain Spontaneous
Ventilatory Weaning Response, Dysfunctional
Violence, Risk for: Self-directed or directed at others

Establishing Goals for Nursing Action

After the priorities of the nursing diagnoses have been established, the immediate, intermediate, and long-term goals and the nursing actions appropriate for attaining the goals are identified. The patient and his or her family are included in the establishment of the goals for the nursing actions. The immediate goals are those that can be reached in a short period of time. The intermediate and long-term goals require a longer period of time to be achieved, and they usually involve preventing complications and other health problems and promoting health education and rehabilitation. For example, goals for a diabetic patient with a nursing diagnosis of "knowledge deficit relative to the prescribed diet" may be stated as follows:

Immediate goal: Oral intake and tolerance of 1500-calorie diabetic diet spaced in three meals and one snack
Intermediate goal: Planning of meals for 1 week based on diabetic exchange system
Long-term goal: Adherence to prescribed diabetic diet

Establishing Expected Outcomes

Expected outcomes of the nursing interventions are stated in terms of the patient's behaviors and the time period in which they are to be achieved. These outcomes must be realistic and measurable. Standard outcome criteria for people with specific health problems have been established by health care agencies. These outcomes should be used whenever possible, although they may need to be adapted to establish realistic criteria for the specific person involved.

- The outcomes that define the expected behavior of the patient will indicate that the problem is being resolved or that progress toward resolving the problem is being made. The outcomes also serve as the basis for evaluating the effectiveness of the nursing interventions.
- The critical time periods provide a time frame for determining the effectiveness of the nursing interventions and whether additional nursing care is needed or whether the care plan needs to be adjusted.

The information incorporated into the nursing care plan is written in a concise, systematic manner that facilitates its use by all nursing personnel. Space must be provided in the care plan for documenting the patient's response to the nursing interventions—the outcomes. It must be remembered that the care plan is subject to change as the patient's problems change, as the priorities of the problems shift, as problems are resolved, and as additional information about the patient's state of health is collected. As the nursing interventions are implemented, the patient's responses are evaluated and documented, and the care plan is modified accordingly. A well-developed, continuously updated plan of care is the greatest assurance that the patient's nursing diagnoses and collaborative problems will be addressed and his or her basic needs will be met. (An example of a care plan can be found on page 35.)

Implementation

The implementation phase of the nursing process follows the formulation of the nursing care plan. Implementation refers to carrying out the proposed plan of care. The nurse assumes responsibility for the implementation but includes the patient and the family and other members of the nursing team and the health care team as appropriate. The activities of all persons involved in implementation are coordinated by the nurse.

- The nursing care plan serves as the basis for implementation.
- The immediate, intermediate, and long-term goals are used as a focus for the implementation of the designed nursing interventions.
- While implementing nursing care, the nurse continually assesses the patient and his or her response to the nursing care.
- Alterations are made in the care plan as the patient's condition, problems, and responses change and as a reassignment of priorities is required.

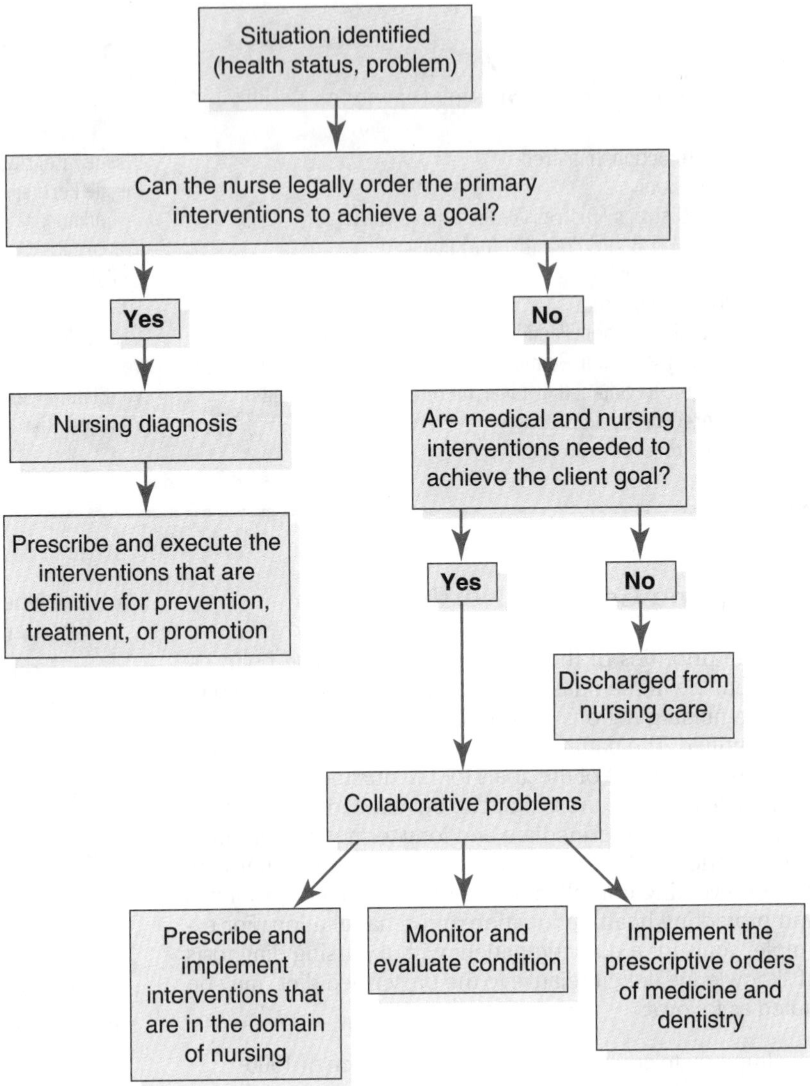

FIGURE 3-2. Differentiating nursing diagnoses from collaborative problems. (Carpenito LJ. Nursing Diagnosis: Application to Clinical Practice [6th ed]. Philadelphia, JB Lippincott, 1995; © 1990, 1988, 1985, Lynda Juall Carpenito.)

Implementation includes carrying out the nursing interventions that are directed toward resolving the patient's nursing diagnoses and collaborative problems and meeting his or her health needs.

Included among nursing interventions are assisting with hygienic care; promoting physical and psychologic comfort; supporting respiratory and elimination functions; facilitating the ingestion of food, fluids, and nutrients; managing the patient's immediate surroundings; offering health teaching; promoting a therapeutic relationship; and carrying out a host of therapeutic nursing activities. Judgment, critical thinking, and decision-making skills are essential in the selection of appropriate nursing interventions that are based on scientific principles.

- All nursing interventions are patient-focused and goal-directed. They are based on scientific principles and are implemented with compassion, confidence, and a willingness to accept and understand the patient's responses.

Many nursing actions are independent. Others are interdependent, such as carrying out prescribed treatment for medications and therapies and collaborating with other health care team members to accomplish specific expected outcomes and to monitor and manage potential complications. Such interdependent functioning is just that—interdependent. Requests from other health care team members should not be followed blindly but should be assessed critically and questioned as necessary.

Recording Outcomes

The implementation phase of the nursing process is concluded when the nursing interventions have been completed and the patient's responses to them have been recorded. Recordings are made concisely, precisely, and objectively and satisfy the following criteria:

- They relate to the nursing diagnoses and collaborative problems.
- They describe the nursing interventions and the patient's responses to the interventions.
- They include any additional pertinent data.

NURSING CARE PLAN 3–1
Example of an Individualized Nursing Care Plan

Mr. John Lee, a 50-year-old management consultant, was admitted to the nursing unit from his physician's office. A routine physical examination 3 months previously had revealed essential hypertension with BP 170/110 and decreased urine creatinine clearance. During the subsequent 3 months the blood pressure elevation did not respond to diet therapy. Mr. Lee admitted that he had not been successful in adhering to the low-sodium, low-cholesterol, weight-reduction diet that had been prescribed for him. He stated "my life is just too busy—I work all hours of the day and night." He indicated that in addition to his work he and his wife share the responsibility for raising their two teenage daughters. He drinks five to seven cups of coffee daily and drinks alcohol only at social occasions. Admission physical examination revealed BP 162/112, P 96, R 20, T 37°C, height 5'10", weight 210 lbs, and slight edema of the ankles and feet. Mr. Lee stated that his feet are "always puffy at night." There were several darkened areas (2 cm in diameter) on the anterior lower legs bilaterally. A brief hospitalization was planned for thorough evaluation and initiation of therapy. The physician's orders on admission included: activity as desired; Lasix, 40 mg bid; monitor vital signs every 4 hours while awake; 1500 calorie, 1 g sodium, low cholesterol diet.

NURSING DIAGNOSIS

1. Altered health maintenance related to hypertension, stress, obesity, and caffeine
2. Ineffective individual coping relative to role responsibilities at work and home
3. Noncompliance with dietary regimen related to knowledge deficit and life-style

COLLABORATIVE PROBLEMS

1. Ischemic ulcers of lower legs

GOALS

Immediate: Gradual decrease in blood pressure
Intermediate: Initiation of life-style alterations to decrease stress
Long-term: Alteration of life-style to reduce emotional and environmental stressors
Compliance with dietary regimen
Absence of ischemic leg ulcers

Nursing Interventions	Expected Outcomes	Outcomes
Monitor BP lying, sitting, and standing every 4 hr	Experiences no further increase in BP	BP range of 162/112–138/98 since admission No variation greater than 5 mm Hg in systolic or diastolic pressures with position changes No variation between right and left arms Maximum BP from 24 hr after admission to time of discharge: 138/98
Monitor fluid status:		
I&O	Urinary output adequate in relation to oral intake	Intake: 1850 ml Output: 1685 ml
Peripheral edema	No evidence of peripheral edema	Minimal edema of feet late in evening
Promote atmosphere conducive to physical and mental rest:		
Encourage alternation of rest and activity	Alternates periods of rest and activity	Rests in bed 1 hr in morning and 2 hr in afternoon; disconnects phone during rest periods Awake at intervals during night: 8 hr of uninterrupted sleep at night after initiation of 30 mg Dalmane at bedtime
Encourage limitation of visitors and interactions that are stress-producing	Limits visitors to family in the evenings	Wife and daughters visit 2 hr in evening; patient calm and relaxed after visits

(*continued*)

NURSING CARE PLAN 3–1 *(continued)*
Example of an Individualized Nursing Care Plan

Nursing Interventions	Expected Outcomes	Outcomes
	Avoids stress-producing interactions	Wife and daughters aware of need to decrease stress: they consult with patient about regular family activities
Assist patient to alter life-style to decrease stress:		
Discuss relationship between emotional stress and physiologic functioning	Describes stress as a precursor to alteration in physiologic functioning	Accurately described relationship between stress and hypertension
Encourage patient to identify stress-producing stimuli	Identifies life-style factors that produce stress	Identified the following stressors: Self-imposed demands of job; unwillingness to refer clients; Excessive involvement in daughters' school and recreational activities
Encourage patient to identify adjustments necessary to reduce stress	Identifies life-style adjustments necessary to reduce stress	Verbalized plans to make more referrals; Identified need to decrease work hours to maximum of 8 hr per day
	Discusses life-style adjustments with family	Consulted with wife and daughters; will alternate with wife in attending daughters' activities; all family members supportive
Encourage patient to identify obesity and caffeine as stressors and aggravators of hypertension; request consultation with dietitian and reinforce instructions given.	Identifies harmful effects of obesity and caffeine	Accurately described effects of obesity and caffeine on blood pressure
	Makes plans for losing weight	Plans to go to Weight Watchers; has had success with this program in the past
	Makes plans for decreasing caffeine intake	Drinks 1 cup of coffee for breakfast; uses decaffeinated coffee at mid morning, lunch, and dinner, expressed satisfaction with this plan
Assess for ischemic leg ulcers; report changes in darkened spots on legs to physician	Absence of changes in skin integrity on lower extremities	No changes noted in characteristics of skin of lower legs on days 2 and 3
Teach foot care: daily inspection and washing, nail care, avoidance of caustic solutions, lubrication of dry skin, avoidance of heat to feet, well-fitting shoes and socks, avoidance of crossing legs	Describes principles and techniques of proper foot care	Discussed importance of proper foot care; demonstrated proper technique of foot care; shoes and socks fit well; does not cross legs when sitting

Evaluation

Evaluation is the final step of the nursing process and is directed toward determining the patient's response to the nursing interventions and the extent to which the goals have been achieved. The nursing care plan provides the basis for evaluation; the nursing diagnoses, collaborative problems, goals, nursing interventions, and expected outcomes provide the specific guidelines that dictate the focus of the evaluation.

Evaluation will answer the following questions:

- Were the nursing diagnoses and collaborative problems accurate?
- Did the patient reach the expected outcomes?
- Did the patient attain the expected outcomes within the critical time periods?
- Have the patient's nursing diagnoses been resolved?
- Have the collaborative problems been resolved?
- Have the patient's nursing needs been met?
- Should the nursing interventions be retained, altered, or discontinued?
- Have new problems evolved for which nursing interventions have not been planned or implemented?
- What factors influenced the achievement or lack of achievement of the goals?
- Do priorities need to be reassigned?
- Should changes be made in the goals and expected outcomes?

Objective data that answer these questions must be collected from all available sources (*i.e.*, patient, family or significant others, nursing and other health care team members). These data should be available in the patient's record and must be substantiated by direct observation of the patient.

CRITICAL THINKING EXERCISES

1. How does the approach to critical thinking differ among nursing practice settings, *i.e.*, acute care, ambulatory, extended care, home, and community settings?
2. You have just completed the physical assessment of your assigned patient. How would you develop the patient's nursing diagnoses? Describe the kind of resources that are available to help you with identifying these diagnoses.
3. You have developed a nursing care plan for your assigned patient. Describe how you used critical thinking skills to develop this care plan. How did you integrate your critical thinking into the nursing process?

An example of a care plan based on a case study is presented on pages 35-36.

BIBLIOGRAPHY

Books

American Nurses Association. Standards of Clinical Nursing Practice. Kansas City, MO, ANA, 1991.

Alfaro R. Applying Nursing Diagnoses and Nursing Process: A Step-by-Step Guide. Philadelphia, JB Lippincott, 1994.

Bates B. A Guide to Physical Examination and History Taking. Philadelphia, JB Lippincott, 1995.

Bowers AC and Thompson JM. Clinical Manual of Health Assessment. St Louis, CV Mosby, 1992.

Carnevali DL and Thomas MD. Diagnostic Reasoning and Treatment Decision Making in Nursing. Philadelphia, JB Lippincott, 1993.

Carpenito LJ. Handbook of Nursing Diagnosis (6th ed). Philadelphia, JB Lippincott, 1995.

Carpenito LJ. Nursing Diagnosis: Application to Clinical Practice (5th ed). Philadelphia, JB Lippincott, 1993.

Carroll–Johnson RM and Paquette M (eds). Classification of Nursing Diagnoses. Proceedings of the Tenth Conference, North American Nursing Diagnosis Association. Philadelphia, JB Lippincott, 1994.

Gordon M. Nursing Diagnosis: Process and Application. St Louis, Mosby-Year Book, 1993.

Guzzeta CE et al. Clinical Assessment Tools for Use With Nursing Diagnoses. St Louis, CV Mosby, 1989.

Maas M, Buckwalter KC, and Hardy M. Nursing Diagnoses and Interventions for the Elderly. Menlo Park, CA, Addison–Wesley Nursing, 1991.

Malasanos L et al. Health Assessment. St Louis, CV Mosby, 1990.

McFarland GK and McFarlane EA. Nursing Diagnosis and Intervention. Planning for Patient Care. St Louis, CV Mosby, 1993.

Sundeen SJ et al. Nurse–Client Interaction: Implementing the Nursing Process. St Louis, Mosby Year-Book, 1994.

Tucker SM. Patient Care Standards: Nursing Process, Diagnosis, and Outcome. St Louis, CV Mosby, 1992.

Yura H and Walsh MB. The Nursing Process: Assessing, Planning, Implementing, Evaluating. Norwalk, CT, Appleton and Lange, 1988.

Journals

Asterisks indicate nursing research articles.

Braverman BG. Eliciting assessment data from the patient who is difficult to interview. Nurs Clin North Am 1990 Dec; 25(4): 743–750.

Briody ME, Jones DA, and Fitzpatrick JJ. Toward further understanding of nursing diagnosis. Nursing Diagnosis 1992 July-Sep; 3(3): 124–128.

Edelstein J. A study of nursing documentation. Nurs Manage 1990 Nov; 21(11): 40–46.

*Etheridge S, Bos S, and Bos N. Staff nurse identification of nursing diagnosis from a written case study. Nursing Diagnosis 1992 Jan-Mar; 3(1): 30–35.

Frisch N. How nursing diagnosis helps to direct and inform practice. Home Healthcare Nurse 1993 Mar-Apr; 11(2): 64–65, 70.

Geissler EM. Transcultural nursing and nursing diagnosis. Nurs Health Care 1991 April; 12(4): 190–192, 203.

Germain CP. Cultural care: A bridge between sickness, illness, and disease. Holistic Nurse Pract 1992 April; 6(3): 1–9.

Grant JS and Kinney MR. The need for operational definitions for defining characteristics. Nursing Diagnosis 1991 Oct-Dec; 2(4): 181–185.

Gryfinski JJ. Implementing focus charting: Process and critique. Clinical Nurse Spec 1990 Winter; 4(4): 200–205.

Guido GW. Legal aspects of documentation. Med-Surg Nursing Quarterly 1993 Spring; 1(4): 97–105.

Guido GW. Trends in documentation. Med-Surg Nursing Quarterly 1993 Spring; 1(4): 87–95.

Gwozdz DT and Togno-Armanasco VD. Streamlining patient care documentation. J Nurs Adm 1992 May; 22(5): 35–39.

Holmes SB, Fuhrmann M, and Ivancin L. Development of a nursing documentation system. Orthop Nurs 1992 Jan-Feb; 11(1): 55–70.

Hoskins LM. Axes: Focus of Taxonomy II. Nursing Diagnosis 1992 July-Sept; 3(3): 117–123.

Lekander BJ, Lehmann S, and Lindquist R. Therapeutic listening: key intervention for several nursing diagnoses. Dimens Crit Care Nurs 1993 Jan-Feb; 12(1): 24–29.

*Loomis ME and Conco D. Patients' perceptions of health, chronic illness, and nursing diagnosis. Nursing Diagnosis 1991 Oct-Dec; 2(4): 162–170.

Lucatorto M et al. Documentation. A focus for cost savings. J Nurs Adm 1991 Mar; 21(3): 32–36.

*Lutjens LRJ. The nature and use of nursing diagnosis in hospitals. Nursing Diagnosis 1993 July-Sept; 4(3): 107–113.

Murphy J and Burke LJ. Charting by Exception. Nursing 1990 May; 20(5): 65–67.

Rosenbaum JN. A cultural assessment guide. Can Nurse 1991 April; 87(4): 32–33.

Scholz J. Cultural expressions affecting patient care. Dimens Oncol Nurs 1990 Spring; 4(1): 16–26.

Seifert PC and Grandusky RJ. Nursing diagnoses. Their use in developing care plans. AORN J 1990 April; 51(4): 1008–1021.

Steck AM and Sangermano C. Documentation: Incorporating the nursing process. Semin Perioper Nurs 1992 Oct; 1(4): 240–248.

Thompson C. Evaluating the patient's response to care: Outcomes documentation. Med-Surg Nursing Quarterly 1993 Spring; 1(4): 79–86.

Turner SJ. Nursing process, nursing diagnoses, and care plans in a clinical setting. J Nurs Staff Dev 1991 Sep-Oct; 7(5): 239–243.

Weber G. Making nursing diagnosis work for you and your client. Nurs Health Care 1991 Oct; 12(8): 424–430.

Wooldridge JB, Brown OF, and Herman J. Nursing diagnosis: The central theme in nursing knowledge. Nursing Diagnosis 1993 April-June; 4(2): 50–55.

Wright K. An overview of nursing process. Gastroenterol Nurse 1992 Aug; 15(1): 14–17.

Journals

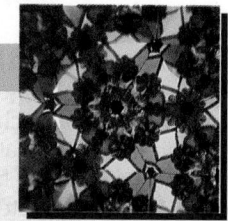

4

Health Education and Health Promotion

CHAPTER OUTLINE

Health Education Today
The Purpose of Health Education
Adherence to the Therapeutic Regimen
Gerontologic Considerations
The Nature of Teaching and Learning
Learning Readiness
The Learning Atmosphere
Teaching Techniques
Gerontologic Considerations
The Nursing Process in Patient Teaching
Assessment
Nursing Diagnosis
Planning
Implementation
Evaluation
Health Promotion
Health and Wellness
Definition of Health Promotion
Health Promotion Principles
Health Promotion Throughout the Life Span
Children and Adolescents
Young and Middle-Aged Adults
Elderly Adults
Implications for Nursing
Critical Thinking Exercises

LEARNING OBJECTIVES

On completion of this chapter, the learner will be able to:

1. Describe the purposes and significance of health education
2. Describe the concept of adherence to a therapeutic regimen
3. Identify variables that influence the elderly person's adherence to a therapeutic regimen
4. Describe the variables that affect learning readiness
5. Describe strategies that facilitate elderly people's learning abilities
6. Describe the relationship of the teaching–learning process to the nursing process
7. Develop a teaching plan for a patient
8. Define the concepts of health, wellness, and health promotion
9. Describe the health promotion principles of self-responsibility, nutrition, stress management, and exercise
10. Specify the variables that affect health promotion activities for children, young and middle-aged adults, and elderly adults
11. Describe the role of the nurse in health promotion

Health Education Today

One of the greatest challenges facing nursing today is meeting the health education needs of the American public. In this respect, nursing has placed increasing emphasis on the role of the nurse as teacher. Teaching, as a function of nursing, is included in many state nurse practice acts and in the American Nurses Association Standards of Nursing Practice. Thus, health education is considered to be an independent function of nursing practice and a primary responsibility of the nursing profession.

Health education is an essential component of nursing care and is directed toward promoting, maintaining, and restoring health; preventing illness; and assisting people to deal with the residual effects of illness.

Teaching activities by nurses take place in many settings including prenatal clinics, well baby clinics, neighborhood health centers, physicians' offices, schools, hospitals, home health settings, and other community-based locales.

Every contact a nurse has with a health care consumer, whether that person is ill or not, should be considered an opportunity for health teaching. While the person has a right to decide whether or not to learn, the nurse has the responsibility to present information that will motivate the person to appreciate the need for learning.

The Purpose of Health Education

The emphasis on health education stems in part from the belief of many health care leaders that the public has the right to expect and receive comprehensive health care, including health education. It also reflects the emergence of a better-informed public that is asking more significant questions about health and the health care services it receives. Because of the emphasis that American society places on health and the responsibility that each of us has to maintain and promote our own health, it is the obligation of the members of the health care system and, specifically, nurses to make health education available to the American public.

One of the largest groups of people in need of health education today are those with chronic illnesses. As the life span of our population continues to increase, the number of people with such illnesses will also increase. Many health care leaders believe that persons with chronic illness are entitled to health care information to enable them to participate actively in and assume responsibility for much of their own care. Health education can aid these individuals to adapt to illness, prevent complications, cooperate with prescribed therapy, and learn to solve problems when confronted with new situations. It can also prevent rehospitalization; people with chronic conditions are frequently readmitted because they do not know how to care for themselves.

- The goal of health education is to teach people to live life to its healthiest—that is, to strive toward achieving one's maximum health potential.

The changes that have occurred in the health care system as a result of cost reduction and cost containment have placed greater significance on patient education. It is viewed as a strategy for reducing cost by preventing illness and avoiding expensive medical treatment and by decreasing lengthy hospital stays and facilitating earlier discharge. For hospitals it is also viewed as a public relations tool for increasing patient satisfaction. It is also viewed as a cost-avoidance strategy for those who believe that positive staff-patient relationships avert malpractice suits.

Adherence to the Therapeutic Regimen

One of the aims of patient education is to encourage people to adhere to their therapeutic regimen. The term **compliance** is often used to describe this behavior—implying that patients will change their behavior or "comply" because they have been told to do so. However, this term suggests that the learner's role is passive.

Noncompliance has been accepted as a nursing diagnosis by NANDA. However, many nursing authors contend that, from historical, philosophical, ethical, and theoretical perspectives, noncompliance as a nursing diagnosis runs counter to the basic nursing principle of respect for the individual. According to Keeling et al., "It negates the client's value system and personal interpretation of the illness experience" (1993, p. 96).

Several alternative nursing diagnosis terms have been suggested, such as nonadherence to the therapeutic regimen, need for commitment to treatment, and inability to adapt to the treatment regimen. These, and perhaps other terms, will need to be tested and validated to support their use as appropriate and clinically useful.

For the purposes of this discussion, the term **adherence** to a therapeutic regimen will be used to describe the patient's role and behaviors in achieving positive health care practices. This term more clearly implies active, voluntary collaborative efforts between the patient and the health care provider.

Adherence to a therapeutic regimen requires that the person make one or more lifestyle changes to carry out specific activities such as taking medications, maintaining a diet, restricting activities, self-monitoring for signs and symptoms of illness, practicing specific hygienic measures, seeking periodic health evaluation, and attending to a host of other therapeutic and preventive measures. The fact that many people do not adhere to their prescribed regimens cannot be ignored or minimized; rates of adherence are generally very low, especially when the regimens are complex or of long duration.

The characteristics of people who do not adhere to their prescribed therapy have been the subject of many studies. For the most part, the findings have been inconclusive. No one factor has been found to be the predominant cause of nonadherence. Instead, it seems that a wide range of variables influence the degree of adherence:

- Demographic variables, such as age, gender, race, socioeconomic status, and education
- Illness variables, such as the severity of the illness and the relief of symptoms afforded by the therapy
- Therapeutic regimen variables, such as the complexity of the regimen and uncomfortable side effects
- Psychosocial variables, such as intelligence, attitudes toward health professionals, acceptance or denial of ill-

ness, religious or cultural beliefs, and the financial and other costs involved in following the regimen

Teaching programs are more likely to succeed if variables that have an effect on the person's adherence are identified and incorporated into the teaching plan.

The problem of nonadherence to therapeutic regimens is a substantial one that needs to be remedied to assist people to participate in self-care and to achieve their maximum health potential.

Although knowledge alone has not been found to be a sufficient stimulus to motivate total adherence, studies indicate that some degree of adherence is obtained through teaching programs and other methods directed toward stimulating motivation. For example, sometimes establishing a written contract between the nurse and the learner will help promote motivation toward adherence. In this system, a series of goals is established, beginning with small, easily attainable objectives and moving to more advanced goals so that frequent positive reinforcement is provided as the person makes progress from one goal to the next. A weight reduction program, for example, based on a progression of small attainable goals has a better chance of succeeding than one which merely identifies a general goal of losing 30 pounds.

Gerontologic Considerations

Nonadherence to therapeutic regimens is a significant problem with elderly people, because it can lead to increased morbidity and mortality and increased cost of treatment (U.S. Department of Health and Human Services, 1990). In addition, a significant number of nursing home admissions and hospital admissions have been linked to nonadherence.

Elderly persons frequently have one or more chronic illnesses that are managed with numerous medications and are periodically complicated by acute episodes. Elderly people also have other problems that affect adherence to therapeutic regimens, such as increased sensitivity to medications and their side effects, difficulty in adjusting to change and stress, financial constraints, forgetfulness, inadequate support systems, lifetime habits of self-medication with over-the-counter medications, visual impairments, hearing impairments, and mobility limitations (Fig. 4-1).

To promote adherence among the elderly, time and effort must be taken to assess all variables that may affect health behavior. In addition, the person's strengths and limitations must be assessed so that the strengths can be used to compensate for limitations. Above all, health care professionals must work together to provide continuous, coordinated care; otherwise, the efforts of one health care professional may be negated by the efforts of another.

The Nature of Teaching and Learning

Learning can be defined as acquiring knowledge, attitudes, or skills. Teaching is defined as helping another person to learn. These definitions indicate that the teaching–learning process is an active one, requiring the involvement of both teacher and learner in the effort to reach the desired outcome: change in behavior. The teacher does not give knowledge to the learner, but instead serves as a facilitator of learning.

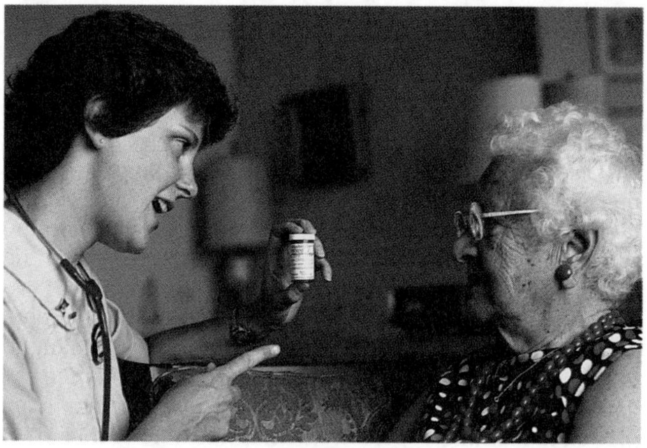

FIGURE 4-1. Instruction on pharmocologic use and interaction is extremely important in the elderly population.

In general, there is no definitive theory about how learning occurs and how it is affected by teaching. No single theory of learning explains how learning occurs. However, studies indicate that learning can be affected by certain factors such as readiness to learn, the learning environment, and the teaching techniques employed.

Learning Readiness

One of the most significant factors influencing learning is the learner's readiness to learn—including physical and emotional status and past experiences in learning.

Physical readiness is of vital importance because until a person is physically capable of learning, attempts at teaching and learning may be both futile and frustrating. Someone who is experiencing acute pain will be unable to focus attention away from the pain long enough to concentrate on learning. Likewise, a person who is short of breath will concentrate on breathing rather than on learning.

Emotional readiness involves the motivation to learn. A person who has not accepted an existing illness, or the fact that illness is a possible threat, will not be motivated to learn. A person who does not accept a therapeutic regimen, or views it as conflicting with his or her lifestyle, may consciously avoid learning. Until a person recognizes the need to learn and acknowledges an ability to learn, teaching efforts may be thwarted. However, it is not always wise to wait for a patient to become emotionally ready to learn—this time may never come unless efforts are made by the nurse to stimulate the individual's motivation.

Illness and the threat of illness are usually accompanied by anxiety and stress. The nurse who recognizes such reactions to illness or threatened illness can use simple explanations and instructions to alleviate these anxieties and to provide further motivations to learn. It must be remembered that because learning involves changes in behavior, it normally produces mild anxiety. Such anxiety is often a useful motivating factor.

Emotional readiness can be promoted by creating a warm, accepting, positive atmosphere and by establishing realistic learning goals with the person so that he or she can realize success and a feeling of accomplishment, which in themselves are motivators of learning.

Feedback about progress also serves to motivate learning. Such feedback should be presented in the form of positive reinforcement when the learner is successful and in the form of constructive suggestions for improvement when he or she is unsuccessful.

Experiential readiness to learn refers to past experiences that enable a person to learn what is being taught. Previous educational experiences and life experiences in general are significant determinants of an individual's approach to learning. A person who has had little or no formal education may not be able to understand the instructional materials presented. The person who has experienced difficulty in learning in the past may be hesitant to make new attempts to learn. Many behaviors required for meeting one's maximum health potential demand a rather extensive background of knowledge, physical skills, and attitudes. If the person does not have this background on which to build, learning may be very difficult and very slow. For example, someone who does not understand the basics of normal nutrition may not be able to understand the restrictions of a special diet. Also, a person who is not future-oriented will be unable to appreciate many aspects of preventive health teaching. And a person who does not view the desired learning as personally meaningful will reject teaching efforts.

Thus, experiential readiness is closely related to emotional readiness, because motivation tends to be stimulated by one's appreciation for the need to learn and by those learning tasks that are familiar, interesting, and meaningful.

- Prior to initiating a teaching–learning program, it is important to assess the learner's physical and emotional readiness to learn as well as his or her ability to learn what is being taught. This information then becomes the basis for the goals to be established—goals that in themselves can motivate the person to learn.
- Involving the learner in the establishment of goals that are mutually acceptable serves the purpose of encouraging active involvement in the learning process and a willingness to share responsibility for learning.

The Learning Atmosphere

Although learning can take place without a teacher, most people who are attempting to learn new or altered health behaviors will need the services of a nurse-teacher at least part of the time. The interpersonal interaction between the learner and the nurse who is attempting to meet the individual's learning needs may be formal or informal, depending on the method and techniques of teaching that are found to be most appropriate.

Learning can be encouraged by manipulating those external variables that affect learning. For example, the physical setting of the teaching session should be such that it is conducive to learning. That is, the room temperature, lighting, noise levels, and so on, should be appropriate to the learning situation. Also, the time selected for teaching should be suited to the individual's needs. Scheduling a teaching session at a time of day when the person is fatigued or anxious about a pending diagnostic or therapeutic procedure or when visitors are present does not provide an atmosphere conducive to learning. On the other hand, if family members are to participate in providing care, the sessions should be timed to take place when the family is present so they can learn any necessary skills or techniques.

Teaching Techniques

The teaching techniques and methods selected will also enhance learning if they are appropriate to the individual's needs. Numerous techniques are available including lectures, group teaching, and demonstrations, all of which can be enhanced with specially prepared teaching materials.

The **lecture or explanation** method of teaching is commonly used but should always be accompanied by discussion. The discussion is important because it affords the learner an opportunity to express personal feelings and concerns, to ask questions, and to receive clarification of any possible misinformation or misunderstandings.

Group teaching is appropriate for some people because it allows them not only to receive the information that is needed but also to feel secure as a member of a group. Those with similar problems or learning needs have the opportunity to identify with each other and thus to gain moral support and encouragement. However, it must be remembered that not everyone relates well in groups and therefore may not benefit from such experiences. It must also be remembered that if group teaching is used, assessment and follow-up of each individual are imperative to ensure that each has gained the knowledge and skills needed.

Demonstration and practice are often essential ingredients of a teaching program, especially when skills are to be learned. It is best to demonstrate the skill and then allow the learner ample opportunity to practice the skill. When the skill involves special equipment such as insulin syringes, colostomy bags, or dressings, it is important to teach with the same equipment that will be used in the home setting. Learning to perform a skill with one kind of equipment and then having to change to a different kind can lead to confusion and mistakes.

Teaching aids are available to enhance learning and include materials such as books, pamphlets, pictures, films, slides, audio and video tapes, models, programmed instruction, and computer-assisted learning modules (Fig. 4-2). Such teaching aids are invaluable when used appropriately, and they can save a significant amount of personnel time and related cost. However, all such aids should be reviewed before they are used to be sure that they are designed to meet the individual person's learning needs.

Reinforcement and follow-up are important because learning takes time. Allowing ample time to learn and reinforcing what is learned are successful teaching strategies. A single teaching session is never adequate. Follow-up sessions are imperative to promote the learner's confidence in his or her ability to follow through with what has been learned. Such sessions also provide an opportunity to evaluate the person's progress and to plan for additional teaching

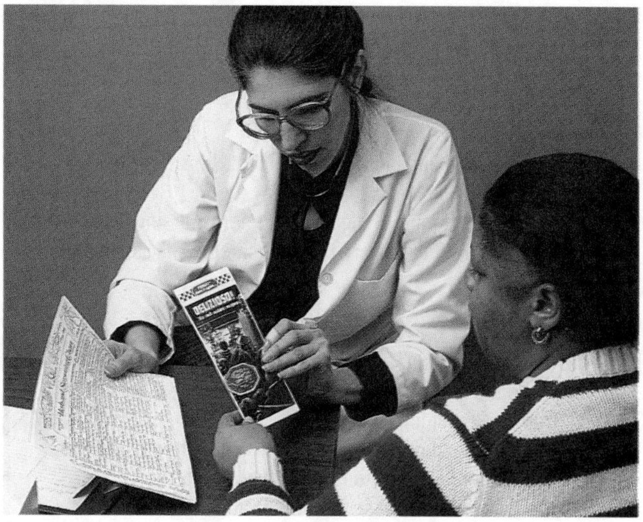

FIGURE 4-2. Teaching aids enhance learning.

sessions as required. It is also important to realize that a hospitalized patient may not be able to transfer what has been learned in the hospital to the home setting. Thus, arrangements for follow-up after discharge are often essential to ensure that the full benefits of the previous teaching program have been realized.

Gerontologic Considerations

Nurses caring for elderly people must be aware of how the normal changes that occur with aging affect learning abilities and how an elderly person can be assisted to adjust to these changes. Above all, it is most important to recognize that just because a person is elderly does not mean that he or she cannot learn. Many studies have shown that older adults can learn and remember if the information to be learned is paced appropriately, is relevant, and is followed by appropriate feedback strategies that apply to all learners. It is also important to be aware that the changes associated with aging vary significantly among elderly persons. Therefore, it is essential that thorough assessment of each person's level of physiologic and psychologic functioning be conducted before teaching begins.

Changes in cognition resulting from age include slowed mental functioning; decreases in short-term memory, abstract thinking, and concentration abilities; and an increase in reaction time. These changes are often accentuated by the host of disease conditions that cause the elderly to seek health care in the first place. Teaching strategies that are often effective include a slowly paced presentation of small amounts of material at a time, frequent repetition of information, and the use of reinforcement techniques such as audiovisual and written materials and repeated practice sessions. The teaching environment must be one in which distracting stimuli are minimized as much as possible.

Sensory changes associated with aging also affect teaching and learning. Teaching strategies to accommodate decreased visual acuity include large-print and easy-to-read materials that are printed on nonglare paper. Because color discrimination is often impaired, the use of color-coded or highlighted teaching materials may not be effective. To maximize hearing, the teacher speaks distinctly in a normal or lowered pitch voice, facing the person so he or she can lip read. Visual cues are often helpful to reinforce verbal teaching.

Family members are involved in teaching sessions when possible. They provide another source for reinforcement of material and can help the learner to recall instructions later. They can also provide valuable information about the person's living situation and related learning needs.

When the nurse, the family, and other involved health care professionals work collaboratively to facilitate an elderly person's learning, the chances of success will be maximized. Successful learning for the elderly should result in improved self-care abilities, enhanced self-esteem, and a willingness to learn in future sessions.

The Nursing Process in Patient Teaching

The steps of the nursing process—assessment, diagnosis, planning, implementation, and evaluation—are used when constructing a teaching plan to meet an individual's teaching and learning needs (Chart 4-1).

Assessment

Assessment in the teaching–learning process is directed toward the systematic collection of data about the person's learning needs and readiness to learn and about the family's learning needs. All internal and external variables that affect the patient's readiness to learn are assessed. A learning assessment guide may be used for this purpose. Some of the learning assessment guides available are very general and are directed toward the assessment of general health information. Others are specific to common medication regimens or disease processes. Such guides serve to facilitate the assessment but must be adapted to the individual's responses, problems, and needs.

As soon as possible after completing the assessment, the nurse organizes, analyzes, synthesizes, and summarizes the data collected and determines the patient's need for teaching.

Nursing Diagnosis

Nursing diagnoses that specifically relate to the patient's and the family's learning needs are then succinctly stated and serve as a guide in the development of the teaching plan.

Planning

Once the nursing diagnoses have been identified, the planning component of the teaching–learning process is estab-

CHART 4-1
A Guide to Patient Education

Assessment

1. Assess the person's readiness for health education.
   a. What are the person's health beliefs and behaviors?
   b. What psychosocial adaptation is the person making?
   c. Is the learner ready to learn?
      Is he or she able to learn these behaviors?
      What additional information about the person is needed?
      What are the person's expectations?
      What does he or she want to learn?
2. Organize, analyze, synthesize, and summarize the collected data.

Nursing Diagnosis

Formulate the nursing diagnoses that relate to the person's learning needs.

1. Identify the learning needs, their characteristics, and etiology.
2. State nursing diagnoses concisely and precisely.

Planning

1. Assign priority to the nursing diagnoses that relate to the individual's learning needs.
2. Specify the immediate, intermediate, and long-term teacher–learner-established learning goals.
3. Identify teaching strategies appropriate for goal attainment.
4. Establish expected outcomes.
5. Develop the written teaching plan.
   a. Include diagnoses, goals, teaching strategies, and expected outcomes.
   b. Put the information to be taught in logical sequence.
   c. Write down the key points.
   d. Select appropriate teaching aids.
   e. Keep the plan current and flexible to meet the person's changing learning needs.
6. Involve the learner, family or significant others, nursing team members, and other health care team members in all aspects of planning.

Implementation

1. Put the teaching plan into action.
2. Use language the person can understand.
3. Use appropriate teaching aids.
4. Use the same equipment that the person will use after discharge.
5. Encourage the person to participate actively in learning.
6. Record the learner's responses to the teaching actions.
7. Give feedback.

Evaluation

1. Collect objective data.
   a. Observe the person.
   b. Ask questions to determine if the person understands.
   c. Use rating scales, checklists, anecdotal notes, and written tests when appropriate.
2. Compare the person's behavioral responses with the expected outcomes. Determine the extent to which the goals were achieved.
3. Include the person, family or significant others, nursing team members, and other health care team members in the evaluation.
4. Identify alterations that need to be made in the teaching plan.
5. Make referrals to appropriate sources or agencies for reinforcement of learning after discharge.
6. Continue all steps of the teaching process: assessment, diagnosis, planning, implementation, and evaluation.

lished in accordance with general criteria followed in the nursing process:

1. Assigning priorities to the diagnoses
2. Specifying the immediate, intermediate, and long-term goals of learning
3. Identifying specific teaching strategies appropriate for attaining goals
4. Specifying the expected outcomes
5. Documenting the diagnoses, goals, teaching strategies, and expected outcomes on the teaching plan

As in the nursing process, the assignment of priorities to the diagnoses should be a joint effort by the nurse and the learner or family members. Consideration must be given to the urgency of the individual's learning needs, with the most critical needs receiving the highest priority.

After the priorities of the diagnoses have been established, the immediate, intermediate, and long-term goals and the teaching strategies appropriate for attaining the goals are identified. Studies have indicated that teaching is most effective when the learner's goals and the nurse's goals are in agreement. Goal-directed learning begins with the establishment of goals that are appropriate to the situation and that are realistic in terms of the individual's ability and desire to achieve them. Involving the patient and family in establishing goals and the subsequent planning of teaching strategies promotes their cooperation in the implementation of the teaching plan.

Expected outcomes of the teaching strategies are stated in terms of the person's behaviors and the family's behaviors, when appropriate. Every effort is made to develop outcomes that are realistic and measurable. The critical time periods within which the outcomes should be demonstrated by the person are also identified. The outcomes and the critical time periods will serve as a basis for evaluating the effectiveness of the teaching strategies.

During the planning phase, the nurse gives consideration to the sequence in which the subject matter will be presented in each of the teaching strategies. Critical information (such as survival skills for the person with diabetes) and information that the person or family has identified as of particular importance or interest to them generally receives high priority in the sequence of material to be presented. An outline is often helpful for arranging subject matter and for ensuring that all necessary information is included. Also during this time, appropriate teaching aids to be used in implementing the teaching strategies are prepared or selected.

The entire planning phase of the teaching–learning process is concluded with the formulation of the teaching plan. This teaching plan communicates the following information to all members of the nursing team:

1. The nursing diagnoses that specifically relate to the individual's learning needs and the priorities of these diagnoses
2. The goals of the teaching strategies
3. The teaching strategies, which are expressed in the form of teaching orders
4. The expected outcomes, which identify the expected behavioral responses of the learner
5. The critical time period within which each outcome is expected to be met
6. The individual's behavioral responses (which must be documented on the teaching plan)

The same rules that apply to writing and revising the nursing care plan apply to the teaching plan.

Implementation

In the implementation phase of the teaching–learning process, the patient, the family, and other members of the nursing team and the health care team carry out the activities outlined in the teaching plan. The activities of all of these persons are coordinated by the nurse.

It is important to remain flexible during the implementation phase of the teaching–learning process and to assess the individual's responses to the teaching strategies continuously, making alterations in the teaching plan as necessary. Creativity in promoting and sustaining the learner's motivation to learn is essential; and it is important to anticipate new learning needs that may arise following discharge from the hospital or after home care visits have ended.

The implementation phase is concluded when the teaching strategies have been completed and when the individual's responses to the actions have been recorded. This record serves as the basis for evaluating how well the defined goals and expected outcomes have been achieved.

Evaluation

Evaluation of the teaching–learning process is directed toward determining how effectively the person has responded to the teaching strategies and to what extent the goals have been achieved. An important part of the evaluation phase addresses the question: "What should be done to improve the teaching?" Answers to this question will dictate changes that must be made in the teaching plan.

It should never be assumed that an individual has learned because he or she has been taught. Learning does not automatically follow teaching. A variety of measurement techniques can be used to determine changes in behavior as evidence that learning has taken place. These techniques include directly observing the behavior; using rating scales, checklists, or anecdotal notes to document the behaviors; and indirectly measuring results through oral questioning and written tests. Measurement of actual behavior (direct measurement) is the most accurate and appropriate technique in many patient-teaching situations. However, it should be supplemented with indirect measurements whenever possible. When more than one measurement technique is employed, the reliability of the resultant data is enhanced because each individual measurement technique carries with it a potential source of error.

Using measurement techniques is only the beginning of evaluation. It is followed by interpreting the data and making value judgments about the learning and teaching. Such evaluation should be done periodically throughout the teaching–learning program, at its conclusion, and at varying periods after the program has ended.

Evaluation of learning after hospitalization is highly desirable and extends into home care. With shortened lengths of hospital stay and with short-stay and same-day surgical procedures, there is a particular need for follow-up evaluation in the home. Coordination of efforts and sharing of information between hospital-based and community-based nursing personnel serve to facilitate such post-teaching evaluation.

- It should always be remembered that evaluation is not the end step in the teaching–learning process. The information gathered during evaluation should be used to redirect teaching actions with the goal of improving the learner's responses and outcomes.

Health Promotion

Health teaching and health promotion are linked by a major common goal—to encourage people to achieve as high a level of wellness as possible so that they can live maximally healthy lives and avoid preventable illnesses.

The call for health promotion has become a major cornerstone in health policy today because of the need to control health care costs and reduce unnecessary sickness and death.

The nation's first public health agenda was established in 1979 and set goals for improving the health of all Americans. Additional goals were defined in 1980 by a list of objectives referred to as "the 1990 health objectives." These goals identified improvements that needed to be made in health status, reduction of risks, public awareness, health services, and protective measures.

The most recent national health goals have been specified in "Healthy People 2000." The priorities identified include health promotion, health protection, and preventive services (Chart 4-2). Increased emphasis has been placed on the following objectives: prevention of disability and morbidity; greater attention to improvements in the health status of specific groups that are at highest risk for premature death; and increased provision for early detection of asymptomatic disease conditions in an attempt to prevent disability and early death. These objectives are directed toward meeting the World Health Organization's goal of "health for all by the year 2000" (Healthy People 2000, 1990).

Health and Wellness

The concept of health promotion has evolved from a changing definition of health and from an awareness that wellness

CHART 4-2
Healthy People 2000 Priority Areas

Health Promotion
1. Physical Activity and Fitness
2. Nutrition
3. Tobacco
4. Alcohol and Other Drugs
5. Family Planning
6. Mental Health and Mental Disorders
7. Violent and Abusive Behavior
8. Educational and Community-Based Programs

Health Protection
9. Unintentional Injuries
10. Occupational Safety and Health
11. Environmental Health
12. Food and Drug Safety
13. Oral Health

Preventive Services
14. Maternal and Infant Health
15. Heart Disease and Stroke
16. Cancer
17. Diabetes and Chronic Disabling Conditions
18. HIV Infection
19. Sexually Transmitted Diseases
20. Immunization and Infectious Diseases
21. Clinical Preventive Services

Surveillance and Data Systems
22. Surveillance and Data Systems

Age-Related Objectives
Children
Adolescents and Young Adults
Adults
Older Adults

(From U.S. Department of Health and Human Services. Healthy People 2000: National Health Promotion and Disease Prevention Objectives. DHHS Publication No. (PHS) 91-50213. Washington, DC, U.S. Government Printing Office, 1990.)

exists at many levels of functioning. The definition of health as the mere absence of disease is no longer accepted. Today, health is viewed as a dynamic, ever-changing condition that enables a person to function at an optimum potential at any given point in time. The ideal health status is one in which people are successful in achieving their full potential regardless of any disabilities they might have.

Wellness, as a reflection of health, involves a conscious and deliberate attempt to maximize one's health. Wellness does not just happen—it requires planning and conscious commitment. It is the result of lifestyle behaviors that are designed for the purpose of attaining one's highest potential for well-being. Wellness is not the same for every person. The person with a chronic illness or disability can reach a level of wellness equivalent to someone without illness or disability. The key to wellness is whether or not the person is functioning at this highest potential within the limitations over which he or she has no control.

A significant amount of research has shown that people, by virtue of what they do or fail to do, influence their own health. Today, many of the major causes of illnesses are chronic diseases that have been closely related to lifestyle behaviors (*e.g.*, heart disease, lung and colon cancer, chronic obstructive pulmonary diseases, hypertension, cirrhosis, peptic ulcers, traumatic injury, human immunodeficiency virus [HIV] infection, and AIDS). Thus, a person's health status to a large extent reflects his or her style of living.

Definition of Health Promotion

Health promotion can be defined as activities that, by accentuating the positive, assist a person to develop those resources that will maintain or enhance well-being and improve the quality of life. It refers to the activities that a person does personally in the absence of symptoms in an attempt to remain healthy; these activities do not need the assistance of a member of the health care team.

The purpose of health promotion is to focus on the person's potential for wellness and to encourage him or her to alter personal habits, lifestyle, and environment in ways that will reduce risks and enhance health and well-being. Health promotion is an active process, that is, it is not something that can be prescribed or dictated. It is up to the individual to decide whether or not to make the changes that will help promote a higher level of wellness. Choices must be made, and only the individual can make these choices.

Health Promotion Programs

The concepts of health, wellness, health promotion, and disease prevention have been extensively addressed in the lay literature and news media as well as in professional journals. The result has been a public demand for health information and a tremendous response by health care professionals and agencies to provide this information. Health promotion programs that were once limited to hospital settings have now moved into the community in settings such as clinics, schools, churches, businesses, and industry. The workplace is quickly becoming an important site for health promotion programs, as employers strive to reduce costs associated with absenteeism, hospitalization, disability, excessive turnover of personnel, and early death.

Health Promotion Principles

Certain principles underlie the concept of health promotion as an active process: self-responsibility, nutritional awareness, stress reduction and management, and physical fitness.

Self-Responsibility

Taking responsibility for oneself is the key to successful health promotion. It recognizes that the individual, and only the individual, has control over his or her life. Each of us, alone, can make those choices that determine whether our individual lifestyle is one that promotes health. As more people recognize the significant effect that lifestyle and behavior have on health, they assume responsibility for avoiding high-risk behaviors such as smoking, alcohol and drug abuse, overeating, driving while intoxicated, risky sexual practices, and other unhealthy practices. They also assume responsibility for developing practices that have been found to be positive influences in promoting health, such as engaging in regular exercise, wearing a seat belt, and following a balanced diet.

A variety of different techniques have been used to try to encourage people to accept responsibility for promoting their health. These methods have ranged from extensive educational programs to reward systems. Studies have not shown any one technique to be superior to any other. Instead, it seems that self-responsibility for health promotion is very individualized and depends on the person's desires and inner motivations. Health promotion programs are important tools for offering encouragement to individuals to assume responsibility for their health and to develop behaviors that positively affect health.

Nutrition

Nutrition as a component of health promotion has become the focus of considerable attention and publicity. A vast array of books and magazine articles exist that address the topics of special diets, natural foods, and the hazards of certain substances such as sugar, salt, cholesterol, and food additives. Good nutrition has been suggested as the single most significant factor in determining health status and longevity.

Nutritional awareness involves an understanding of the importance of a properly balanced diet that supplies all of the essential nutrients and an awareness of the relationship between diet and disease. A diet that promotes health is thought to be one that substitutes natural foods for processed and refined ones and that reduces the intake of sugar, salt, fat, caffeine, alcohol, and food additives and preservatives.

Chapter 7, Physical Assessment and Nutritional Assessment, contains detailed information on the assessment of the individual's nutritional status. Physical signs indicating nutritional status, anthropometric measurements, assessment of food intake (food record, 24-hour recall), comparison of food intake to the dietary guidelines outlined in the Food Guide Pyramid, and calculation of ideal body weight are covered in that chapter.

Stress Management

Stress management and stress reduction have become important aspects of health promotion. Studies have shown the negative effects of stress on health and a cause-and-effect relationship between stress and infectious diseases, traumatic injuries including motor vehicle crashes, and some chronic illnesses. Stress, as a part of the modern way of life, has become inevitable in "high-tech," urban societies in which self-imposed demands for productivity have become excessive. To counter the negative impact of stress, more and more emphasis is placed on encouraging people to manage their stress appropriately and to reduce stress that is counterproductive. Techniques such as relaxation training, exercise, and modification of stress-producing situations are often included in health promotion programs that deal with stress. Further information on stress management, including health risk appraisal and stress reduction methods such as biofeedback and the relaxation response, can be found in Chapter 9, Stress and Adaptation.

Exercise

Physical fitness is another important component of health promotion. Studies that have examined the relationship between health and physical fitness have found that a regular exercise program can promote health by improving the function of the circulatory system and the lungs, decreasing cholesterol and low-density lipoproteins, lowering body weight by increasing calorie expenditure, delaying degenerative changes such as osteoporosis, and improving flexibility and overall muscle strength and endurance. On the other hand, exercise can be harmful if it is not started gradually and increased slowly in accordance with the individual's response. An exercise program should be designed specifically for the individual, with consideration given to age, physical condition, and any known cardiovascular risk factors. An appropriate exercise program can have a significant positive effect on the individual's performance capacity, appearance, and general state of health.

Health Promotion Throughout the Life Span

Health promotion as a concept and a process extends throughout the life span. Studies have shown that the health of a child can be affected, either positively or negatively, by the health practices of the mother during the prenatal period. Thus, health promotion starts before birth and extends through childhood, adulthood, and old age.

Children and Adolescents

Health screening has traditionally been an important aspect of childhood health care. The goal has been to detect health problems at an early age so that they can be treated early in the child's life. Today, health promotion goes beyond the mere screening of children for disabilities. Extensive efforts are made to promote positive health practices at a very young age. Because health habits and practices are formed early in life, children should be encouraged to develop positive health attitudes. For this reason, more and more programs are being offered to school-age children and to adolescents to help them develop good health habits. While the negative results of such practices as smoking, risky sexual activities, alcohol and drug abuse, and poor nutrition are explained, emphasis is also placed on values training, self-esteem, and healthy lifestyle practices. The programs are designed to appeal to the particular age-group, with emphasis on learning experiences that are fun, interesting, and relevant.

Young and Middle-Aged Adults

Young and middle-aged adults represent an age group that not only expresses an interest in health and health promotion but responds enthusiastically to suggestions that show how lifestyle practices can improve health. Thus, they are highly motivated in changing their lifestyles in ways that are believed to enhance health and wellness. Many adults who wish to improve their health turn to health-promotion programs to assist them in making the desired changes in their lifestyles. They respond in overwhelming numbers to programs that focus on such topics as general wellness, smoking cessation, exercise, physical conditioning, weight control, and stress management. Because of the nationwide emphasis on health during the reproductive years, young adults actively seek out programs that address prenatal health, parenting, family planning, and women's health issues.

Programs that provide health screening, such as those that screen for cancer, hypertension, diabetes, and hearing impairments, are quite popular with this age group. Programs that deal with health promotion for persons with specific chronic illnesses such as cancer, diabetes, heart disease, and pulmonary disease are also popular. It is becoming more and more evident that chronic disease does not preclude health and wellness; rather, positive health attitudes and practices can promote optimal health for persons who must live with the limitations imposed by the chronic nature of their illnesses.

Health promotion programs are offered in a variety of settings, including the community and neighborhood. Common sites include local clinics, elementary schools, high schools, community colleges, recreation centers, and churches. Health fairs are held in civic centers and shopping malls. The outreach idea for health promotion programs has served to meet the needs of many adults who otherwise would not avail themselves of opportunities to strive toward a healthier lifestyle.

The workplace has also become a center for health promotion activity. Employers are increasingly concerned about the rising costs of health care insurance to treat illnesses that are related to lifestyle behaviors. They are also concerned about increased absenteeism and lost productivity. For these reasons, many businesses have instituted health promotion programs in the workplace. Some employ health promotion specialists to develop and implement the program; others purchase packaged programs that have already been developed by health care agencies or private health promotion corporations.

The programs that are offered at the workplace usually include employee health screening and counseling, physical fitness, nutritional awareness, work safety, and stress management and reduction. In addition, efforts are made to promote a safe and healthy work environment. Many large businesses provide exercise facilities for their employees and offer their health promotion programs to retirees. If employers can show cost containment benefits from such programs, their dollars will be considered well spent, and more businesses will provide health promotion programs as a benefit of employment.

Elderly Adults

Health promotion is as important for the elderly as it is for other age groups. Despite the fact that 80% of people over the age of 65 have one or more chronic illnesses and about 50% of the aged population are limited in their activity, the elderly as a group experience significant gains from health promotion. Studies have shown that the elderly are very health-conscious and that most view their health positively and are willing to adopt practices that will improve their health and well-being. Although their chronic illnesses and disabilities cannot be eliminated, these adults can benefit from activities that help them maintain independence and achieve an optimal level of health.

Many health promotion programs have been developed to meet the needs of older Americans. Many of these began within the Department of Health and Human Services. Both public and private organizations have been responsive to this initiative, and more programs that serve the elderly are emerging. Many of these are offered by health care agencies, churches, recreational centers, senior citizen residences, and a variety of other organizations.

Activities directed toward health promotion for the elderly are the same as those for other age groups: physical fitness and exercise, nutrition, safety, and stress management and stress reduction.

CRITICAL THINKING EXERCISES

1. You are developing a patient teaching plan for a patient with diabetes mellitus. Describe the strategies you would develop for promoting adherence to the therapeutic regimen. Indicate the possible variables that could influence the patient's willingness or ability to follow the instructions.
2. You are assigned to teach an elderly patient about the medications that she will be taking at home. How would you assess this patient's condition and psychosocial situation to determine how best to instruct her about her medications?
3. A neighbor tells you that he has heard about a health fair that is being offered at a nearby civic center. He asks you if you think that he should attend. Describe the reasons you might give for why he should attend.

Implications for Nursing

Nurses, by virtue of their expertise in health and health care and their long-established credibility with consumers, play a vital role in health promotion. In many instances they have initiated health promotion programs or have participated with other health care personnel in developing and providing wellness services in a variety of settings.

As health care professionals, nurses have a responsibility to promote activities that foster well-being, self-actualization, and personal fulfillment. Every interaction with consumers of health care must be viewed as an opportunity to promote positive health attitudes and behaviors.

REFERENCES AND BIBLIOGRAPHY

Books

Edelman C and Mandle CL. Health Promotion Throughout the Lifespan. St. Louis, CV Mosby, 1990.

Haggard A. Handbook of Patient Education. Rockville, MD, Aspen Publishers, 1989.

Knollmueller RN. Prevention Across the Life Span: Healthy People For the Twenty-First Century. Washington, DC, American Nurses Publishing, 1993.

Murray RB and Zentner JP. Nursing Assessment and Health Promotion Through the Life Span. Englewood Cliffs, NJ, Prentice-Hall, 1989.

Pender NJ. Health Promotion in Nursing Practice. Norwalk, CT, Appleton and Lange, 1987.

Rankin SH and Stallings KD. Patient Education: Issues, Principles, Practices. Philadelphia, JB Lippincott, 1990.

Redman B. The Process of Patient Education. St. Louis, Mosby-Year Book, 1993.

U.S. Department of Health and Human Services, Office of the Inspector General. Medication Regimens: Causes of Noncompliance. Washington, DC, U.S. Department of Health and Human Services, 1990.

U.S. Department of Health and Human Services, Public Health Service. Healthy People 2000: National Health Promotion and Disease Prevention Objectives. Washington, DC, U.S. Government Printing Office, 1990.

Journals

Asterisks indicate nursing research articles.

Bigbee JL and Jansa N. Strategies for promoting health protection. Nurs Clin North Am 1991 Dec; 26(4): 895–912.

Carethers M. Health promotion in the elderly. Am Fam Physician 1992 May; 45(5): 2253–2259.

*Conn VS, Taylor SG, and Kelley S. Medication regimen complexity and adherence among older adults. Image: Journal of Nursing Scholarship 1991 Winter; 23(4): 231–236.

Hickey T and Stilwell DL. Health promotion for older people: All is not well. Gerontologist 1991 Dec; 31(6): 822–829.

Homedes N. Do you know how to influence patients' behavior? Tips to improve patient's adherence. Fam Pract 1991 Dec; 8(4): 412–423.

Keeling A et al. Noncompliance revisited: A disciplinary perspective on a nursing diagnosis. Nursing Diagnosis 1993 July-Sept; 4(3): 91–98.

Morris LS and Schulz RM. Patient compliance—an overview. J Clin Pharm Ther 1992 Oct; 17(5): 283–295.

Padilla GV and Bulcavage LM. Theories used in patient/health education. Semin Oncol Nurs 1991 May; 7(2): 87–96.

Pencak M. Workplace health promotion programs. An overview. Nurs Clin North Am 1991 March; 26(4): 233–240.

Rakel BA. Interventions related to patient teaching. Nurs Clin North Am 1992 June; 27(2): 397–405.

Redland AR and Stuifbergen AK. Strategies for maintenance of health-promoting behaviors. Nurs Clin North Am 1993 June; 28(2): 427–442.

Rega MD. A model approach for patient education. MEDSURG Nursing 1993 Dec; 2(6): 477–479.

*Simons MR. Interventions related to compliance. Nurs Clin North Am 1992 June; 27(2): 477–484.

Spellbring AM. Nursing's role in health promotion. An overview. Nurs Clin North Am 1991 Dec; 26(4): 805–814.

Tanner EKW. Assessment of a health-promotive lifestyle. Nurs Clin North Am 1991 Dec; 26(4): 845–854.

Tripp SL and Stachowick B. Health maintenance, health promotion: Is there a difference? Public Health Nurs 1992 Sept; 9(3): 155–161.

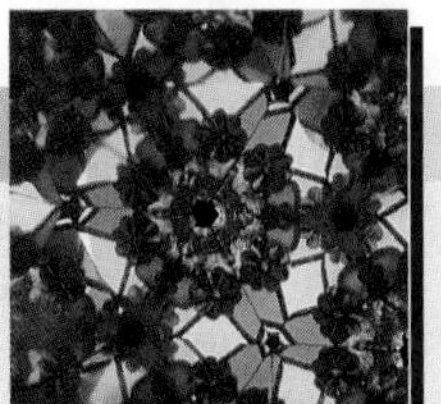

5 Ethical Issues in Medical-Surgical Nursing

CHAPTER OUTLINE

Definition of Ethical Terms
Ethics Versus Morality
Approaches to Ethics
Moral Situations

Classic Ethical Theories
Teleological Theory
Deontological Theory
Virtue Ethics
Ethical Pluralism

Domain of Nursing Ethics
Types of Ethical Problems in Nursing
Ethical Decision Making

Preventive Ethics
Advance Directives

Critical Thinking Exercises

LEARNING OBJECTIVES

On completion of the chapter, the learner will be able to:

1. Define ethics and nursing ethics
2. Identify several ethical dilemmas common to the medical-surgical area of nursing practice
3. Specify strategies that can be helpful to nurses in ethical decision making

In the complex world in which we live, we are surrounded by ethical issues in all facets of our lives. Consequently, there has been a heightened interest in the field of ethics in an attempt to gain a better understanding of how these issues influence us. Specifically, in health care, the focus on ethics has intensified in response to controversial developments including increased technologic advances and diminished resources. Both of these areas have an impact on the role of the professional nurse.

In the past, medicine had few ways to combat disease; thus, the nurse's role was primarily one of support and comfort. Today, sophisticated technology can frequently prolong life indefinitely. Questions have been raised about whether it is always appropriate to use this technology, and if not, why not.

The development of technologic support has had an influence on all stages of life. For example, the prenatal period has been influenced by genetic screening, *in vitro* fertilization, the harvesting and freezing of embryos, and prenatal surgery. In the early stages of life, premature infants are given a chance for survival as a result of technical support. And children and adults who would have died as a result of organ failure are living longer because of organ transplants. Technologic advances have also contributed to an increase in the average life expectancy. However, these advances in technology have been a "mixed blessing." While many individuals are afforded a better quality of life, others face extended suffering as a result of efforts to prolong life, usually at a great expense.

The cost of health care has generated much controversy in the discussion of ethical issues. Presently, approximately 14% of the gross domestic product (GDP) is spent on health care. Issues surrounding the way this money is spent abound. Utilizing advanced technology because it is available may not always be appropriate and may escalate cost of care when the outcomes are questionable. Some may argue that the money spent on these futile efforts might be better used providing health care for the many people who lack adequate health insurance or access to care. Another factor affecting health care costs is the vast number of people diagnosed with AIDS. Some people insist that more research dollars should be spent to develop better treatment for AIDS patients and to find a cure for this dread disease. There are also the ethical issues that surround those practices or policies that seem to allocate health care resources unjustly on the basis of age, race, gender, or social mores.

These ethical issues have had an impact on the role of the professional nurse. The accepted definition of professional nursing has inspired a new advocacy role for nurses. The American Nurses Association, in the publication *Nursing: A Social Policy Statement* (1995), defines nursing as "the diagnosis and treatment of human responses to health and illness." This definition supports the claim that nurses must be actively involved in the decision-making process regarding ethical concerns surrounding health care and human responses. However, this belief may come into conflict in health care settings in which the traditional roles of the nurse are delineated within a bureaucratic structure. Health care settings in which nurses are valued members of the health care team promote multidisciplinary communication and may enhance patient care. To practice effectively in these settings, nurses must be aware of ethical issues and assist patients in voicing their moral concerns.

The focus of this chapter will be on providing an overview of ethical theory. A review of common terminology and ethical theories will be included to provide a background for more advanced investigation. Understanding the role of the professional nurse in ethical decision making will assist nurses in identifying the steps used in the analytic decision-making model and in articulating their ethical positions. Initially, the subject of ethical decision making may appear overwhelming because the terminology or "language" is different from everyday language. However, one must remember that the language can be learned, as can the skill to make ethical decisions.

Definition of Ethical Terms

Ethics Versus Morality

The terms **ethics** and **morality** are used in relation to beliefs about right and wrong and to appropriate guidelines for action. The two terms, while referring to similar concepts, differ slightly in meaning. **Ethics** refers to the philosophic study of morality, in which one relies on formal theory, rules, principles, or codes of conduct to determine the "right" course of action. In contrast, **morality** describes one's personal commitment to values that are frequently influenced by societal norms and expectations. For example, children learn from their parents that it is wrong to steal. Society has fostered the belief that stealing is wrong; thus, an individual may incorporate these social mores into his or her own value system. In an ethical inquiry, individuals would analyze why it is wrong to steal and may base their arguments on the fact that stealing violates fundamental moral principles such as respect for persons, justice, and fidelity (promise keeping).

In essence ethics is the more formal, systematic study of moral beliefs, whereas morality is the adherence to informal personal values. Because the distinction between the two is slight, they are used interchangeably. For our purposes ethics and morality will be used synonymously in this chapter.

Approaches to Ethics

There are two broad approaches to ethics—non-normative and normative. The non-normative approach is further divided into metaethics and descriptive ethics, whereas the normative approach is divided into general normative ethics and applied ethics.

Non-normative Ethics

Metaethics is concerned with understanding the concepts and linguistic terminology used in ethics, such as what it means to be "good," "virtuous," or "right." An example of metaethics in the health care environment would be analysis of the concept of "informed consent." Nurses are aware that patients must give consent prior to surgery, but sometimes a question arises as to whether the patient is truly informed. Thus, delving deeper into the whole concept of informed consent would be a metaethical inquiry.

In **descriptive ethics**, the goal is to identify various ethical behaviors and beliefs. There is no attempt to place a judgment on the practices; thus, it may be described as being ethically neutral. This type of approach is frequently used by historians, anthropologists, and sociologists as they study the behavior of different groups of individuals. For example, studies of American Eskimos revealed the common practice of placing the elderly on ice rafts and letting them float away and die since they were no longer productive members of society. With this type of descriptive research, there is no attempt to judge if this practice is morally acceptable; rather, it is merely stating "the way it is." As the field of nursing ethics develops, nurse researchers may employ descriptive ethics to gain a better perspective of the ethical beliefs held by practicing nurses.

Normative Ethics

Normative ethics is the branch of moral philosophy one usually associates with ethics. When one hears the words "ought" or "should," it is in reference to identifying the morally correct course of behavior in answering the question, "What should I (we) do in this situation?" When this approach is used to identify global problems that transcend all fields, it is referred to as **general normative ethics.** For example, how should governments interact to obtain world peace? When questions are asked within a specific discipline it is referred to as **applied ethics**.

Various disciplines utilize the frameworks of general ethical theories and moral principles and apply them to specific problems within their domain. For example, bioethics is the study of ethical problems in biology and medicine, although it may also be referred to as medical, clinical, or health care ethics. Nursing ethics may be considered a distinct form of applied ethics because it addresses many moral situations that are specific to the nursing profession. Some ethical problems that affect nursing may also apply to the broader area of health care ethics. However, because the nursing profession is a "caring" rather than a predominantly "curing" profession, with its own professional code of ethics, it is *imperative* that one not equate nursing ethics solely with medical ethics.

Moral Situations

Many different words are used to describe a moral situation, including moral dilemma, moral uncertainty, and moral distress. The most common word used is **dilemma**. It is important to clarify the precise meaning of this word so as not to confuse a moral dilemma with a moral problem: what may appear to be a dilemma may actually be a moral problem.

With a moral dilemma, a clear conflict exists between two or more moral principles or competing moral claims. The choice of one action over another may lead to an unpleasant outcome, and the person must choose "the lesser of two evils." For example, for a severely ill patient, adhering to the principle of sanctity of life may require the use of prolonged life-sustaining treatment. On the other hand, one may feel that the life-sustaining measures only prolong the person's suffering. In this case, both alternatives are unpleasant: continuing treatment and possibly prolonging suffering, versus discontinuing treatment, resulting in the patient's probable death.

This example poses a true moral dilemma if the patient is incompetent (not able to make his or her own decisions). However, if the patient is competent and voices personal views, making such statements as, "I want to live . . . do everything you can," then even if the nurse feels it is morally wrong to continue treatment, it should be continued. A competent adult has the right to make these decisions, and the person's wishes take precedence. This example depicts a **moral problem** rather than a moral dilemma because there is no conflict of moral principles. By adhering to the principle of respect for autonomy, there is only one morally correct choice of action—continuing treatment.

Moral Uncertainty and Moral Distress

Two other possible moral situations nurses may encounter in practice are moral uncertainty and moral distress (Jameton, 1984). In **moral uncertainty**, one cannot accurately define what the moral situation is or what moral principles may apply, but there is a strong feeling that something is not right. Consider the example of an elderly person who undergoes surgery and does not progress well postoperatively. One may hear the comment, "The surgery was a success, but because the patient has so many other problems he is not getting better." Frequently, this type of patient requires significant nursing care. Prolonged bedrest may have resulted in the patient becoming dependent on others for ambulation, skin care, or other activities of daily living. There may be minimal medical intervention needed at this time, but the patient is not ready to be discharged. Gradually, this patient receives less attention than the other, sicker patients. Nurses may be aware that this particular patient is not receiving the necessary attention, but the precise moral situation is difficult to identify.

The second moral situation identified by Jameton is **moral distress**. In this situation, the nurse is aware of the correct action, but institutional constraints stand in the way of pursuing the correct action. For example, a patient asks a nurse if he has cancer. The surgeon and family have made the decision not to tell the patient the diagnosis. From an ethical perspective, patients should be told their diagnoses if they specifically ask. Ideally, this information should come from the physician, with the nurse present to assist the patient in understanding the terminology and to provide further support if necessary. The nurse could experience moral distress if the hospital threatens disciplinary action or job termination if the information is disclosed without the agreement of the physician and/or the family.

It is essential that nurses freely engage in dialogue concerning moral situations, even though such dialogue is difficult for everyone involved. Improved interdisciplinary communication is supported when all members of the health care team can voice their concerns and come to an understanding of the moral situation.

Classic Ethical Theories

The goal of ethical theory is to justify the question "What should be done?" in terms of a specific ethical framework. Ethical theories are broad frameworks consisting of moral rules and principles. Thus, ethical theories serve as the foundation for normative judgments or courses of action.

While there are a variety of ethical frameworks, two ethical theories predominate: teleological theory and deontological theory. Two other frameworks are virtue ethics and ethical pluralism.

Teleological Theory

Teleological comes from the Greek word *telos,* meaning "ends." According to this theory, one is predominantly concerned with the end results or consequences of actions. This theory is also commonly referred to as **consequentialism**.

The most famous formulation of consequentialism is called **utilitarian theory**. The saying "the greatest good for the greatest number" is the basis of utilitarian theory. Therefore, one's moral choice is to choose that action that maximizes the good consequences over the bad.

A strong supporter of utilitarianism was the philosopher John Stuart Mill. In his work, Mill (1871/1977) proposed that the foundation of moral judgments is the principle of utility, which is also referred to as the "greatest happiness principle." For Mill, "actions are right in proportion as they tend to promote happiness, wrong as they tend to produce the reverse of happiness." The desirable end points are freedom and absence of pain. This utilitarian perspective may apply to specific moral acts or rules. When using moral rules, one should apply the principle of utility to the specific moral rules that lead to the greatest possible happiness for all people. Although Mill's theory may be classified as **hedonistic**, the principle of utility, or pleasure, probably means more than pleasure in the common usage of the term. Nonetheless, other utilitarian philosophers favor other intrinsic values in addition to pleasure, such as knowledge, health, or friendship, as the goal for the attainment of the aggregate good.

There are many criticisms of a teleological moral framework based on consequences. The most obvious flaw in this type of approach is the uncertainty and difficulty in measuring various intrinsic values. How can one accurately measure and compare happiness or pleasure, or values such as health and friendship? In addition, basing one's moral actions on "the greatest good for the greatest number" may be problematic in certain situations. How can one morally justify decisions that may adversely affect individuals who do not belong to the majority? And, finally, teleological theory has been criticized because of its reliance on consequences. If the overall consequences are morally good, does this justify attaining these goals by nonmoral actions or behavioral means? These questions certainly raise some issues within a teleological framework. An alternative approach, the deontological approach, attempts to address these issues.

Deontological Theory

The word **deontology** comes from the Greek word *deon,* which means duty or obligation. A deontological or **formalist** theory, in contrast to utilitarian theory (which focuses on the consequences of the act) argues that there are moral standards that exist independent of the ends. These moral standards refer to the various universal moral principles (Chart 5-1). The distinguishing feature among formalist thinkers is that one's justification of moral actions is more important than the specific consequences or results of the actions.

As with teleological theory, significant differences exist among followers of the formalist tradition. One difference concerns whether there is only one moral principle that takes precedence (a monistic perspective) or several moral principles (a pluralistic perspective).

An example of monistic reasoning is found in the writings of Immanual Kant, an 18th-century German philosopher. Kant (1785/1983) held that morality must ultimately be founded on principles of reason that all rational people possess. It is essential that individuals possess a "good will" that chooses actions *for the sake of duty,* not merely *in accordance with duty.* Therefore, the motives that compel one to act must be identified. To use an example in nursing: if a nurse makes a medication error and reports it only from fear of punitive action if the error is later discovered, rather than from concern for the potential harmful effects to the patient, then this nurse is not acting within a moral perspective. Although the action of revealing the medication error is correct, the motives behind the action are different.

Kant's perspective is considered **monistic** (an adherence to one moral principle or imperative) because he calls for one essential test of rationality called the **categorical imperative**, which is absolute and universal without exception. Although the categorical imperative does not espouse a single moral principle *per se,* it provides the logical test for any acceptable moral principle.

Within the categorical imperative, Kant espoused various formulations. For example: "Act only according to that maxim whereby you can at the same time will that it should become a universal law." This formulation is similar to "the Golden Rule" espoused in theologic beliefs and is also similar to the moral principle of respect for others. Another formulation of his categorical imperative is "Act in such a way that you treat humanity, whether in your own person or in that of another, always at the same time as an end and never simply as a means." This perspective may be sharply contrasted to the utilitarian approach, where the consequences of the action are of primary importance.

This distinction is important to clarify in the area of health care research. For example, even though the goal of patient participation in a research study is to advance scientific knowledge, patients are not being used merely as a means to obtain this goal provided they are truly informed and participate freely in the research.

A major criticism of Kant's theory is that it does not specify which moral principles take precedence or what to do when two or more actions (duties) are in conflict. Other formalist philosophers have attempted to resolve this issue.

For a **pluralistic** view, which stresses the existence of several moral principles, we can use the example of W. D. Ross, a 20th century British philosopher. Ross (1930) identified two types of duties: *prima facie* and actual. The term *prima facie* may be roughly translated as conditional or all other things being equal. A *prima facie* duty must be acted upon unless it comes in conflict with another equal or

CHART 5-1
Common Ethical Principles

Common ethical principles one may use to validate moral claims.

Autonomy

Derived from the Greek words *autos* ("self") and *nomos* ("rule" or "law"), thus refers to self-rule. In contemporary discourse it has broad meanings, including individual rights, privacy, and choice. Autonomy entails the ability to make a choice free from external constraints.

Beneficence

The duty to do good and the active promotion of benevolent acts (for example, goodness, kindness, and charity). May also include the injunction not to inflict harm (see *Nonmaleficence*).

Confidentiality

This principle relates to the concept of privacy. Information obtained from an individual will not be disclosed to another unless it will benefit the person or there is a direct threat to the social good.

Double Effect

A principle that may morally justify some actions that may produce both good and evil effects. All four of the following criteria must be fulfilled:

1. The action itself is good or morally neutral.
2. The agent sincerely intends the good and not the evil effect (the evil effect may be foreseen but not intended).
3. The good effect is not achieved by means of the evil effect.
4. There is proportionate or favorable balance of good over evil.

Fidelity

Promise keeping. The duty to be faithful to one's commitments. It includes both explicit and implicit promises to another.

Justice

From a broad perspective, justice states that like cases should be treated alike. A more restricted version of justice is distributive justice, which refers to the distribution of social benefits and burdens. Various theories of distributive justice may include the following notions: That each person receive

A. Equally
B. According to need
C. According to effort
D. According to societal contribution
E. According to merit or
F. According to legal entitlement.

Retributive justice is concerned with the distribution of punishment.

Nonmaleficence

The duty not to inflict as well as to prevent and remove harm. May be included within the principle of beneficence, in which case nonmaleficence would be more binding.

Paternalism

The intentional limitation of another's autonomy justified by an appeal to beneficence or the welfare or needs of another. Thus, the prevention of any evils or harm is greater than any potential evils caused by the interference of the individual's autonomy or liberty.

Respect for Persons

Frequently used synonymously with autonomy. However, it goes beyond accepting the notion or attitude that people have autonomous choice to treat others in such a way that enables them to make the choice.

Sanctity of Life

The perspective that life is the highest good. Thus, all forms of life, including mere biological existence, should take precedence over external criteria for judging quality of life.

Veracity

The obligation to tell the truth and not to lie or deceive others.

stronger duty. For example, it is a moral wrong to tell a lie; however, one may on occasion justify this action if there is a more compelling duty (for example, avoiding harm to another). The major criticism of Ross's theory, along with other formalist approaches, is that it does not specify which moral principles are the most important and/or take precedence.

Virtue Ethics

In contrast to the teleological and deontological theories which focus on specific principles, actions, and the consequences of one's actions, ethics based on virtues focuses on the character traits of the individual. This approach is consistent with the writings of Aristotle and Plato, which espoused that moral conduct was directly related to the cultivation of virtuous character behaviors. Virtues are seen as specific habits or dispositions that a person possesses or aspires to possess. Thus, for Aristotle the moral question was "What shall I be?" rather than "What shall I do?" However, virtues may take many forms. For example, faith, hope, love, and charity are frequently expressed as virtues within religious writings. The question must then be asked, "Which virtues are moral?" One response may be that moral virtues are those specific traits that enable one to act morally and responsibly.

Because this response is vague, some philosophers are reluctant to classify virtue ethics as a primary specific moral theory. Rather, they view virtue ethics as fundamental corollaries to the other normative ethical theories. Their reasoning is that many of the virtues inherently correspond to the various moral principles. For example, the virtues of benevolence and fairness correspond to the principles of beneficence and justice, respectively. However, it is helpful to have a basic understanding of the ethics of virtue because this focus has been addressed as the nursing profession attempts to delineate its own philosophic basis.

Ethical Pluralism

The aim of delineating moral theory into contrasting frameworks is to illustrate how moral philosophy has evolved within the philosophic domain. While some philosophers would advocate that one's ethical reasoning should be consistent with one particular framework, in actual practice this is difficult to uphold. In the applied discipline of health care ethics, one frequently hears comments that reflect this notion of diversity. The ethical problem of allocation of scarce resources may serve as an illustration. Consider the situation in which a hospital is questioning whether to allocate funds to initiate a heart–lung transplant program. The hospital anticipates that in the first year there will be five candidates for this surgical procedure. However, the costs for implementing this program are substantial; therefore, to subsidize the program the hospital will close four community health clinics. The board of directors decides to vote against the transplant program. Their reasoning is that more people will benefit from the community health centers. In this example, a utilitarian framework based on the consequences of "the greatest good for the greatest number" was the moral basis for the claim to maintain the health clinics. Thus, on the "macro" level, utilitarian theory has substantial merit.

But consider another example. One of the patients in the intensive care unit is an 87-year-old woman with congestive heart failure. The physician in charge of the unit would like to transfer this patient to the general unit so that a younger, "more viable" patient may be admitted. Because the elderly woman continues to require the intensive care resources, her immediate caretakers argue that she should remain in the intensive care unit. The moral basis for their claim rests on the principles of respect for persons and nonmaleficence (do no harm). In this case, a formalist approach based on universal moral principles was the foundation of the moral decision.

It is clear, then, that one's moral reasoning may depend on the context of the moral problem. It should not be presupposed that one moral framework is inherently "better" than another. One general rule of thumb is that on the "macro" level (broad policy decisions), utilitarian theory is very useful, and on the "micro" level, where one particular patient is the focus of decision making, a formalist approach has particular merit.

It is essential to highlight the perspective of moral pluralism to clarify some misconceptions frequently held by students of ethics. Initially, students may become frustrated in their attempts to strictly adhere to a particular moral framework. They may find it more effective to take into consideration various frameworks. This may entail understanding the moral principles and applying them to specific moral situations as well as questioning what virtues or behaviors the student as a member of society wants to espouse. For nurses, one approach in assessing the ethical issues in the discipline of nursing may be taking into consideration a variety of perspectives.

Domain of Nursing Ethics

A reciprocal relationship exists between the nursing profession and society: nurses provide continuing care to all people regardless of disease or social status, and society recognizes the profession's expectation that its members act responsibly and according to a code of ethics.

As a profession, nursing is accountable to society. This accountability is spelled out in the American Hospital Association's Patient's Bill of Rights (see Chart 1-1), which reflects social beliefs about health and health care. In addition to accepting this document as one measure of accountability, nursing has further defined its standards of accountability through a formal Code of Ethics that explicitly states nursing's values and goals. The Code (Chart 5-2), which was established by the American Nurses Association, consists of ethical standards, each with its own interpretive statements. In the most recent revision of the Code of Ethics, the interpretive statements were amplified to incorporate universal moral principles. The Code could be considered a pluralistic framework because it espouses a variety of universal principles and the virtues of professional behavior. The Code is an excellent framework for nurses to use to help in ethical decision making.

The ethical dilemmas a nurse may encounter in the medical-surgical arena are numerous and diverse. However, in order to reason through these dilemmas, nurses must be aware of the underlying philosophic concepts. Because ethical reasoning can be enhanced through a basic understanding of moral philosophy, a significant portion of this chapter has been devoted to these philosophic concepts.

Common ethical principles that apply in nursing include the following: autonomy, beneficence, confidentiality, double effect, fidelity, justice, nonmaleficence, paternalism, respect for persons, sanctity of life, and veracity. The definitions of each of these terms can be found in Chart 5-1. Because these principles are so important in understanding ethical situations in nursing, the reader is advised to refer to the chart before reading further.

Types of Ethical Problems in Nursing

The factors mentioned in the introduction to this chapter—technologic advances and diminished resources—have been instrumental in raising numerous ethical questions and controversies. These factors have provoked discussion about many facets of health care practice, including "life and death" issues. However, to focus only on the sensational issues of life and death is to ignore the many situations that involve ethical considerations. Levine (1977) states:

> *There are overlooked ethical challenges in the mundane, everyday routine activities of professional practice, and these have largely gone unexamined. Ethical behavior is not the display of one's moral*

CHART 5-2

American Nurses Association Code for Nurses

1. The nurse provides services with respect for human dignity and the uniqueness of the client, unrestricted by considerations of social or economic status, personal attributes, or the nature of the health problems.
2. The nurse safeguards the client's right to privacy by judiciously protecting information of a confidential nature.
3. The nurse acts to safeguard the client and the public when health care and safety are affected by the incompetent, unethical, or illegal practice of any person.
4. The nurse assumes responsibility and accountability for individual nursing judgments and actions.
5. The nurse maintains competence in nursing.
6. The nurse exercises informed judgment and uses individual competence and qualifications as criteria in seeking consultation, accepting responsibilities, and delegating nursing activities to others.
7. The nurse participates in activities that contribute to the ongoing development of the profession's body of knowledge.
8. The nurse participates in the profession's efforts to implement and improve standards of nursing.
9. The nurse participates in the profession's efforts to establish and maintain conditions of employment conducive to high-quality nursing care.
10. The nurse participates in the profession's effort to protect the public from misinformation and misrepresentation and to maintain the integrity of nursing.
11. The nurse collaborates with members of the health professions and other citizens in promoting community and national efforts to meet the health needs of the public.

(Reprinted with permission from American Nurses Association. Code for Nurses with Interpretive Statements. Kansas City, MO, American Nurses Association, 1985.)

rectitude in times of crises. It is the day-by-day expression of one's commitment to other persons and the ways in which human beings relate to one another in their daily interactions.

This perspective underscores the basic ethical framework of the nursing profession, the phenomenon of human caring. Nursing theories that incorporate the bio-psycho-social-spiritual dimensions portray a holistic framework with humanism or caring as the core. As the nursing profession strives to delineate its own theory of ethics, *caring* is often cited as the *moral* foundation. For nurses to embrace this professional ethos, it is necessary to be aware not only of major ethical dilemmas but also of those daily interactions with health care consumers that frequently give rise to ethical challenges that are not as easily identified.

Confidentiality

We all need to be aware of the confidential nature of the information dealt with in daily practice. When nursing assessments are performed, patients should be informed of the purpose of the assessment and told that information will be recorded in their health record. Occasionally, patients will provide information that is extraneous to either the medical or nursing diagnosis, or they will request that certain information not be included in the record. If the information is not pertinent to the case, the nurse should question if it is prudent to record it in the chart. In the practice setting, discussion of the patient with other members of the health care team is often necessary. However, these discussions should occur in a private area, not in the cafeteria or an elevator, where there is a strong possibility that the conversation could be overheard.

Another threat to keeping information confidential is the widespread use of computers and the easy access people have to them. This can increase the potential for misuse of information that may have negative social consequences. For example, laboratory results regarding AIDS testing or genetic screening may lead to loss of employment or insurance if the information is leaked. Because of these possibilities, sensitivity to the principle of confidentiality is essential.

Restraints

The use of restraints is another area that carries ethical overtones. It is important to weigh carefully the risks of limiting a person's autonomy by using restraints (both physical and pharmacologic measures) against the safety risks involved in not using restraints. Restraints often can have an unexpected effect, by making the person more agitated or confused. Before restraints are used, other strategies should be tried such as asking family members or volunteers to sit with a confused patient or by engaging the person in diversionary activities.

Trust Issues

Telling the truth is one of the basic principles in our cultural mores. Two ethical dilemmas in clinical practice that can come in direct conflict with this principle of veracity are the use of placebos and revealing a diagnosis to the patient. Both involve the issue of trust, which is an essential element in the nurse–patient relationship. To foster trust, there must be the understanding that both the patient and the nurse will be truthful to one another. Use of placebos in clinical studies (in which some patients are given a nonacting drug while others are given the actual drug being tested) may carry overtones of deception and may severely undermine the nurse–patient relationship. Consequently, the use of placebos should be considered only when the patient is involved in the decision-making process and is aware that placebos are one approach used in the treatment regimen.

Informing patients of their diagnoses represents a common ethical situation in nursing practice. Frequently, physicians and families withhold such information from patients for fear of causing additional distress. Patients often are aware of their diagnosis and ask specific questions that indicate that they are ready to hear the information. However, evasive comments by the nursing staff often are used as a means to maintain professional relationships with other health practitioners. This area is indeed complex because it challenges the nurse's integrity. Some strategies the nurse could consider in this situation include:

1. Not lying to the patient
2. Providing all information related to nursing procedures and diagnoses
3. Communicating to the family and physician the patient's requests for information

Families often are unaware of the patient's repeated questions to the nurse. With a better understanding of the situation, families may change their perspective. Finally, although providing the information may be the morally appropriate behavior, the manner in which the patient is told is important. Nurses must remember to be compassionate and caring while informing patients; disclosure of information merely for the sake of patient autonomy does not convey respect for others.

Death and Dying Issues

Dilemmas that revolve around death and dying are prevalent in medical-surgical practice and frequently initiate moral discussion. The dilemmas are compounded by the fact that the idea of curing is paramount in health care. With advanced technology, it may be difficult to accept the fact that "nothing more can be done" or that technology may prolong life, but at the expense of comfort. Focusing on the caring as well as the curing role may assist nurses in dealing with these difficult moral situations.

DNR Orders. The "do not resuscitate" (DNR) order is frequently a controversial issue. When a patient is competent to make decisions, his or her choice for a DNR order should be honored, according to the principles of autonomy or respect for the individual. However, it should be clear to nurses that a DNR order does not mean "do not treat." Frequently, these patients have significant medical and nursing needs, all of which demand attention. Unfortunately, a DNR order is at times interpreted to mean that the patient requires less nursing time. All patients deserve appropriate nursing interventions, regardless of their resuscitation status.

Life Support. In contrast to the previous situations are those situations in which the decision not to resuscitate has not been made for a dying patient. The nurse may be put in the uncomfortable position of initiating life supportive measures when the patient's status appears futile. This frequently occurs when the patient is not competent to make the decision and the family (or surrogate decision maker) refuses DNR as an option. The nurse may be told to perform "a slow code" (*i.e.*, not to rush to resuscitate the patient). This is an unacceptable order.

Probably the best recourse for nurses in these situations is to open up the channels of communication. Discussing the matter with the physician may lead to further communication with the family and to a reconsideration of their decision, especially when they are afraid to make the decision to let a loved one die with no further efforts to resuscitate. Finally, when working with colleagues who are dealing with such difficult situations, it helps to talk and listen to their concerns as a way of providing support.

Food and Fluid. In addition to requesting that no heroic measures be taken to prolong life, a dying patient may request that no more food or fluid be administered. Many individuals feel that food and hydration are basic human needs and are not considered "invasive measures"; thus, they should always be maintained. However, some consider food and hydration as a means of prolonging suffering. In evaluating this issue, nurses must take into consideration the potential harm as well as the benefit to the patient of either administering or withdrawing sustenance. Evaluation of harm necessitates a careful review of the reasons the person has requested the withdrawal of food and hydration. Although the principle of autonomy has considerable merit and is supported by the Code for Nurses, there may be situations when the request for withdrawal of food and hydration cannot be upheld. For patients who are not competent, the issues are more complex. Some of these cases have actually reached law courts. Different states have different case-law precedents for these matters.

At present, there are no firm guidelines to assist nurses in this area. In general, the provision of food and hydration is usually in the patient's best interest. However, there may be situations where food and hydration are futile attempts to maintain life. This issue is one of the most perplexing dilemmas confronting health care professionals and needs careful scrutiny. As professionals, nurses must provide care while balancing the inherent rights of individuals.

Pain Control. The use of narcotics to alleviate a patient's pain is another dilemma for nurses. Patients with excruciating pain may require large dosages of pain medication, which at times can lead to a decrease in respiratory function. Fear of respiratory depression should not prevent nurses from attempting to alleviate pain for the dying patient. In this situation, the actions may be justified by the principle of double effect (see definition in Chart 5-1). The intent or goal of nursing interventions is to alleviate pain and suffering while promoting comfort. The risk of respiratory depression is not the intent of the actions and should not be used as an excuse for withholding pain medication. However, the patient's respiratory status should be carefully monitored; any signs of respiratory depression are reported to the physician.

Underutilization of pain medication represents an area of ethical debate. While a pain assessment may appear to be a clinical judgment, it may also be considered a moral judgment as well, in that one is making a value judgment concerning another person's pain. For example, the nurse in assessing a patient's complaint of pain may determine that the pain is not as severe as described by the patient since medication was given only 1 hour ago. Rather than dispute the patient's claim, the nurse indicates that more medication will be administered, but then waits until the next dose is due. The nurse's rationale is based on the principles of beneficence and nonmaleficence, because the reason for not immediately administering more medication is an unfounded fear of the patient becoming addicted to narcotics. While appearing to "do no harm" the nurse is violating the principle of veracity by stating that more pain medication will be administered and then waiting for the prescribed length of time before doing so.

Refusing Care

Any nurse who feels compelled to refuse to provide care for a particular type of patient faces an ethical dilemma. The reasons given for refusal range from a conflict of personal values to fear of personal risk of injury. Such instances have increased with the advent of AIDS as a major health problem.

The ethical obligation to care for all patients is clearly identified in Statement One of the Nursing Code of Ethics. However, to avoid facing these moral situations, a nurse can follow certain strategies. For example, when applying for a job, one should ask questions regarding the patient population. If one is uncomfortable with a particular situation, then the choice would be not to accept the position. On the other hand, while the nurse has a moral obligation to serve, the health care institution has some obligations to its employees, by providing current information regarding safe practice and the necessary supplies and equipment needed to follow universal precautions, as well as adequate disability and workers' compensation. The denial of care or providing substandard nursing care to some members of our society is not acceptable nursing practice.

Ethical Decision Making

As indicated in the preceding discussions, ethical situations are common and diverse in nursing practice. Although the moral situations can vary, the fundamental philosophic principles remain. Experience indicates there are no clear solutions to these dilemmas. The process of moral reflection will help nurses to justify their actions.

The approach to ethical decision making can follow the steps of the nursing process: **assessment**, in which the ethical situation is examined and analyzed; **planning**, in which information is gathered and validated; **implementation**, in which alternative actions are identified; and **evaluation**, in which the choice of action is determined and evaluated. Chart 5-3 outlines the steps of an ethical analysis. A case study applying these steps is depicted in Chart 5-4.

CHART 5-3
Steps of an Ethical Analysis

The following are guidelines to assist nurses in ethical decision making. These guidelines reflect an active process in decision making, similar to the nursing process detailed in Chapter 2.

Assessment

1. Assess the ethical/moral situations of the problem.
   This step entails the recognition of the ethical, legal, and professional dimensions of the situation.
   A. Does the situation entail *substantive* moral problems? (Conflicts among ethical principles or professional obligations?)
   B. Are there *procedural* conflicts? (For example, who should make the decisions? Any conflicts among the health care providers, family, guardians, and patient?)
   C. Identify the significant people involved and those affected by the decision.

Planning

2. Collect information.
   A. Include the following information: the medical facts, treatment options, nursing diagnoses, legal data, and the values, beliefs, and religious components.
   B. Make a distinction between the factual and the values/beliefs.
   C. Validate the patient's capacity, or lack of capacity, to make decisions.
   D. Identify any other relevant information that shoud be elicited.
   E. Identify the ethical/moral issues and the competing claims.

Implementation

3. List the alternatives.
   Compare alternatives with applicable ethical principles and professional code of ethics. May choose either framework below, or follow both and compare outcomes.

   Utilitarian Approach
   A. Predict the consequences of the alternatives.
   B. Assign a positive or negative value to each consequence.
   C. Choose the consequence that predicts the highest positive value or "the greatest good for the greatest number."

   Deontological Approach
   A. Identify the relevant moral principles.
   B. Compare alternatives with moral principles.
   C. Appeal to the "higher level" moral principle if there is a conflict.

Evaluation

4. Decide and evaluate decision.
   A. What is the best or morally correct action?
   B. Give the ethical reasons for your decision.
   C. What are the ethical reasons against your decision?
   D. How do you respond to the reasons against your decision?

CHART 5-4

Case Analysis

Guidelines that can be used in ethical decision making are outlined in Chart 5–3 and illustrated in the example that follows.

Mr. G. is a 68-year-old male admitted to the medical-surgical unit with a 1-month history of abdominal pain and a recent history of nausea, vomiting, and blood in his stools for the last 48 hours. Mr. G. is a retired manager who lives with his wife; his three children are all grown and living on their own. He states he has kept busy in his retirement years by playing golf, volunteering at the church, and "tinkering around the house."

A complete GI workup revealed a colon mass and possible perforation. He is scheduled for immediate exploratory surgery. Prior to the surgery he appears quite anxious and states to the nurse that he is scared. In addition he states that "I hope they don't find anything bad, even though there is a good probability that they may. I don't know what I would do. My brother died in the hospital two years ago and that was horrible. I never want to die the way he did, with all those machines and tubes hooked up to him. And my wife, I do not want her to be alone, but I'm reluctant to talk to her about this and get her all nervous and upset. I'll just pray that everything will go okay. Luckily, I've always had faith in the church."

The surgery revealed advanced carcinoma with metastasis. The surgery was palliative to remove the obstruction with a transverse colostomy, but there is a high probability of sepsis from the perforation. Mr. G. returns to the unit from the recovery room with intravenous fluids, antibiotics, and narcotic orders, along with a do not resuscitate (DNR) order. The nurse questioned the DNR order but was told "there is nothing more we can do for him."

Assessment

1. Are there substantive moral problems?
   Yes. In this case there appears to be a conflict among the moral principles of autonomy, respect for persons, beneficence, and paternalism.
2. Are there procedural conflicts?
   Yes. Between the physician and the nurse. The concern is that the patient was not included in the decision-making process.

Planning

Facts: Advanced cancer with metastases. Physician feels that chemotherapy is not an option because of the advanced stage of the disease. States he is ordering the other treatments because "this would be the best for this patient."

Legally, the patient is competent to make the decisions.

Although the nurse agrees with the intent of the DNR order, her concern is that the patient was not consulted. She feels that the comment by the physician that "this would be the best for this patient" is a value judgment that needs to be clarified. The nurse feels that it is essential to assess Mr. G.'s perspectives of his health situation and his personal values and beliefs. Although she feels Mr. G. would agree to the DNR order, she also thinks that including Mr. G. will allow him to determine how much pain medication he needs, which in turn will allow him to be alert enough to discuss the situation with his family and clergy.

Moral Claims

Physician: Maintain the DNR order, it would be in the patient's best interests not to cause him additional distress. (*Alternative 1*)

Nurse: Include the patient and family in the decision-making process. (*Alternative 2*)

Implementation

The two alternatives to the moral problem are delineated above under the moral claims. In assessing the interventions, it is essential to evaluate the alternatives in light of the universal moral principles.

(continued)

Preventive Ethics

As previously mentioned, a dilemma refers to a conflict between two unpleasant alternatives. In such instances, one's moral decision is to choose the "lesser evil" of the two. However, there are various strategies available to assist nurses in ethical decision making. These strategies may be referred to as "preventive" because they may be helpful in anticipating and avoiding certain kinds of ethical dilemmas.

Frequently, dilemmas occur when the health care practitioners are unsure of the patient's wishes, because the person is unconscious or too cognitively impaired to communicate directly. One famous court case in this area of clinical ethics is that of Nancy Cruzan. Nancy Cruzan was a young woman involved in a single car crash after which she remained in a persistent vegetative state. Her family endured a 3-year legal battle to have her feeding tube removed so that she could be allowed to die. The U.S. Supreme Court decided that a state may require "clear and convincing evidence" of the patient's wishes before withdrawing life support. This ruling and the public response to it served as an impetus to legislation on advance directives, entitled the Patient Self-Determination Act (PSDA), effective December 1991. The intent of this legislation is to encourage people to prepare advance directives in which they indicate their wishes concerning the degree of supportive care to be provided if they become incapacitated. The regulatory language is quite broad and allows for different institutions to have latitude in implementing the person's directives. It should be noted that this legislation does not require a patient to have an advance directive, but that the patient be informed about them. Subsequently it is one area where nursing can play a significant role in patient education.

CHART 5-4 *(continued)*

Case Analysis

Alternative 1: This is based on the principles of paternalism and beneficence. In essence, limiting Mr. G.'s autonomy is justified by the benevolent acts of doing good and not inflicting additional harm. In this case, the ratio of benefit/harm is such that greater harm could result with the additional distress of allowing Mr. G. to make this difficult decision when there is no more medical treatment available to benefit him.

Alternative 2: This claim is based on the principles of autonomy, respect for persons, and beneficence. The nurse feels that because Mr. G. is a competent adult, he has the individual right to make this personal decision. The principle of respect for persons goes beyond admitting that the person has the choice, but also enables the person to make the choice free from external constraints. In addition, the nurse feels that the benefit/burden ratio is weighted in the opposite direction. It would be more beneficial to allow Mr. G. to participate in the decision-making process because he could solicit the support from his clergy and family. Finally, the nurse substantiates her claim with Statement 1 of the Code of Ethics, which states, "The nurse provides services with respect for human dignity and the uniqueness of the client, unrestricted by considerations of social or economic status, personal attributes, or the nature of the health problems." Because each patient is unique, health providers cannot assume that all patients will respond in the same manner of distress with the additional information. Thus, patients should be given the information and the choice to make their own decisions. The nursing interventions would be to evaluate the patient's *responses* to the information and provide supportive services.

Evaluation

This case poses a difficult moral dilemma. Some may argue that there is only one valid claim (including the patient in the decision making) because the patient is a competent adult. However, the physician's claim not to inflict additional harm is valid and based on universal principles. If the physician had not included these principles but had relied on his previous comments that "it would be the best for this patient," then the claim would not be valid because it would be based on his personal values and beliefs.

However, when the two alternatives or moral claims are valid, one must appeal to the "higher order" principle. In this case, the principles of autonomy and respect for persons are more influential than paternalism. Although the principle of beneficence is considered a strong moral principle, in this case it would hold less weight than autonomy or respect for persons because Mr. G. continues to have the mental capacity to make decisions. Consequently, Alternative 2 would be the morally correct decision.

Because the morally correct course of action is not always apparent, this case underscores how moral decision making must occur among all the health care providers actively involved in the case. Moral decisions are typically difficult decisions for everyone involved, and it is essential that all members of the health care team listen and respect the views of others. Through an open, nonjudgmental dialogue, the course of action that reflects the "best interests" of the patient will usually emerge.

Advance Directives

Advance directives provide valuable information and may assist health care providers in decision making. Advance directives are legal documents that specify the patient's wishes prior to hospitalization. A **living will** is one type of advance directive. In most situations, living wills are limited to situations where the patient's medical condition is deemed terminal. Because it is difficult to define "terminal" accurately, the living will is not always honored. Another potential drawback to the living will is that these documents are frequently written when the person is in good health. It is not unusual for people to change their minds as their illness progresses. Therefore, the patient maintains the option to nullify the document.

Another type of advance directive is the **durable power of attorney** (PA). With the PA, the patient has identified another individual to make decisions on his or her behalf. In this type of decision making, the patient may have clarified his or her wishes concerning a variety of medical situations. As such, the power of attorney is a less restrictive type of advanced directive. These advance directives vary among state jurisdictions. However, even in states where these documents are not legally binding, they provide helpful information. They assist health care practitioners in determining the patient's prior expressed wishes in situations where this information can no longer be obtained directly.

Another type of preventive ethics is available through **institutional ethics committees**, which exist in many hospitals to assist practitioners with ethical dilemmas. The purpose of these multidisciplinary committees may vary among institutions. In some hospitals, the committee exists solely for the purpose of developing policies; others may have a strong educative or consultative focus. Because these committees usually are comprised of individuals with some advanced background in ethical decision making, nurses can consult with the committee members. Nurses with particular interest or expertise in the area of ethics are valuable members of ethics committees.

The heightened interest in ethical decision making has resulted in many continuing education programs, ranging from small seminars or workshops to full-semester courses offered by local colleges or professional organizations.

Finally, an increasing number of nursing and medical journals contain articles on ethical issues, and numerous textbooks on clinical ethics or nursing ethics are available. These books are valuable resources because they cover the ethical theory and dilemmas of practice in greater depth. The American Nurses Association also has publications available to assist nurses in this emergent field of inquiry.

CRITICAL THINKING EXERCISES

1. A family member of your patient tells you information about the patient that the patient has not revealed. How would you determine if you should communicate this information to the patient's primary nurse?
2. The physician is discussing the prognosis of a terminally ill patient with the patient's family. The family members are adamant that they want everything possible done for the patient. From a nursing perspective, describe the information that you might provide to help the family. How might your approach differ if the family seems uncertain of what to do?
3. You have identified what you believe to be an ethical dilemma with a hospitalized patient. How would you determine if the situation is indeed an ethical dilemma that requires intervention and resolution? What resources are available to you within the hospital that would be helpful in making this determination?

REFERENCES AND BIBLIOGRAPHY

Books

Philosophical and Clinical Ethics

Beauchamp T and Childress J. Principles of Biomedical Ethics, 3rd ed. New York, Oxford University Press, 1989.

Beauchamp T and Walters LR (eds). Contemporary Issues in Bioethics, 3rd ed. Belmont, CA, Wadsworth Publishing, 1989.

Cranford R and Doudera AE (eds). Institutional Ethics Committees and Health Care Decision Making. Ann Arbor, MI, Health Administration Press, 1984.

Fletcher J, Quist N, and Jonsen A. Ethics Consultation in Health Care. Ann Arbor, MI, Health Administration Press, 1989.

Garrett T, Baillie H, and Garrett R. Health Care Ethics: Principles and Problems. Englewood Cliffs, NJ, Prentice Hall, 1989.

Kant I. Grounding for the metaphysics of morals. In Ellington JW (trans). Kant's Ethical Philosophy. Indianapolis, IN, Hackett Publishing, 1983 (original work published 1785).

Lynn J (ed). By No Extraordinary Means: The Choice to Forego Life Sustaining Food and Water. Bloomington, IN, Indiana University Press, 1986.

Mill JS. Utilitarianism. In Reiser S, Dyck A, and Curran W (eds). Ethics in Medicine: Historical Perspectives and Contemporary Concerns. Cambridge, MA, MIT Press, 1871/1977.

President's Commission for the Study of Ethical Problems in Medicine and Biomedical and Behavioral Research. Deciding to Forego Life Sustaining Treatment. Washington, DC, U.S. Government Printing Office, 1983.

President's Commission for the Study of Ethical Problems in Medicine and Biomedical and Behavioral Research. Making Health Care Decisions, Vol 1: Report. Washington, DC, U.S. Government Printing Office, 1983.

Reich W. Encyclopedia of Bioethics. New York, Free Press, 1978.

Ross WD. The Right and the Good. Oxford, Clarendon Press, 1930.

The Hastings Center. Guidelines on the Termination of Life-Sustaining Treatment and the Care of the Dying. New York, The Hastings Center, 1987.

Veatch R. A Theory of Medical Ethics. New York, Basic Books, 1981.

Nursing Ethics

American Nurses Association. Code for Nurses with Interpretive Statements. Kansas City, MO, American Nurses Association, 1985.

American Nurses Association. Ethical Dilemmas Confronting Nurses. Kansas City, MO, American Nurses Association, 1985.

American Nurses Association. Ethics in Nursing Practice and Education. Kansas City, MO, American Nurses Association, 1980.

American Nurses Association. Ethics in Nursing: Position Statements and Guidelines. Kansas City, MO, American Nurses Association, 1988.

American Nurses Association. Nursing: A Social Policy Statement. Washington, DC, American Nurses Association, 1995.

Bandman E and Bandman B. Nursing Ethics Through the Life Span, 2nd ed. Norwalk, CT, Appleton & Lange, 1990.

Benjamin M and Curtis J. Ethics in Nursing, 3rd ed. New York, Oxford University Press, 1992.

Benner P and Wrubel J. The Primacy of Caring: Stress and Coping in Health and Illness. Menlo Park, CA, Addison-Wesley Publishing, 1989.

Davis A and Aroskar M. Ethical Dilemmas and Nursing Practice, 3rd ed. Norwalk, CT, Appleton & Lange, 1991.

Fowler M and Levine-Ariff J. Ethics at the Bedside. Philadelphia, JB Lippincott, 1987.

Jameton A. Nursing Practice: The Ethical Issues. Englewood Cliffs, NJ, Prentice-Hall, 1984.

Thompson J and Thompson H. Professional Ethics in Nursing. Malabar, FL, Robert E. Krieger, 1990.

Watson J. Nursing: Human Science and Human Care. New York, National League for Nursing, 1988.

Journals

Asterisks indicate nursing research articles.

Aroskar M. Anatomy of an ethical dilemma: The theory. Am J Nurs 1980 April; 80(4): 658–660.

Aroskar M. Incompetent, unethical, or illegal practice—teaching students to cope. Journal of Professional Nursing 1993 May-June; 9(3): 130.

Aroskar M. Ethics in nursing and health care reform: Back to the future? Hastings Center Report 1994 May–June; 24(3): 11–12.

Boyle L. Legal implications of the patient self-determination act. Nurse Practitioner Forum 1992 March; 3(1): 12–15.

Brody H. Ethics, technology, and the human genome project. Journal of Clinical Ethics 1991 Winter; 2(4): 278–281.

Buchanan S and Cook L. Nursing ethics committees: The time is now. Nursing Management 1992 August; 23(8): 40–41.

Campbell M. Terminal weaning: It's not simply "pulling the plug." Nursing94 1994 Sep; 24(9): 34–39.

Catalano J. Systems of ethics: A perspective. Critical Care Nurse 1992 December; 12(8): 91–96.

Childress J. Ethics, public policy, and human fetal tissue transplantation. Kennedy Institute of Ethics Journal 1991 June; 1(2): 93–121.

Copp L. An ethical responsibility for pain management. Journal of Advanced Nursing 1993 Jan; 18(1): 1–3.

*Corley M and Raines D. An ethical practice environment as a caring environment. Nursing Administration Quarterly 1993 Winter; 17(2): 68–74.

Davis A. Ethics rounds with intensive care nurses. Nurs Clin North Am 1979 Mar; 14(1): 45–55.

Davis A. Helping your staff address ethical dilemmas. J Nurs Adm 1982 Feb; 12(2): 9–13.

*Davis A. Clinical nurses' ethical decision making in situations of informed consent. Adv Nurs Sci 1989 April; 11(3): 63–69.

Downes J. Acquired immunodeficiency syndrome: The nurse's legal duty to serve. Journal of Professional Nursing 1991 Nov–Dec; 7(6): 333–340.

Edwards B. When the physician won't give up. Am J Nurs 1993 Sep; 93(9): 34–37.

Flarey D. Legal and ethical issues in HIV testing: Part 1. J Nurs Adm 1992 Oct; 22(10): 14–20.

Flarey D. Legal and ethical issues in HIV testing: Part 2. J Nurs Adm 1992 Nov; 22(11): 27–32.

Flarey D. Organ donation and transplantation: An ethical analysis. Health Care Supervisor 1991 Sept; 10(1): 14–22.

Forrow L, Arnold R, and Parker L. Preventive ethics: Expanding the horizons of clinical ethics. J Clin Ethics 1993 Winter; 4(4): 287–294.

Fox A. Confronting the use of placebos for pain. Am J Nurs 1994 Sep; 94(9): 42–46.

Fry S (ed). Ethics, part I: Issues in nursing. Nurs Clin North Am 1989 June; 24(2): 461–577. (Note: half this issue devoted to articles on ethics.)

Fry S (ed). Ethics, part II: Applications in nursing practice. Nurs Clin North Am 1989 Dec; 24(4): 951–1057. (Note: half this issue devoted to articles on ethics.)

Fry S (ed). Nursing ethics. Journal of Medicine and Philosophy 1991 June; 16(3): 231–367. (Note: entire issue devoted to articles on ethics.)

Grady C, Jacob J, and Romano C. Confidentiality: A survey in a research hospital. Journal of Clinical Ethics 1991 Spring; 2(1): 25–30.

Greco P, Schulman K, Lavizzo-Mourey R, Hansen-Flaschen J. The patient self-determination act and the future of advance directives. Annals of Internal Medicine 1991; 115(8): 639–643.

Hassmiller S. Bringing the patient self-determination act into practice. Nursing Management 1991; 22(12): 29–32.

*Henneman E, Baird B, Bellamy P, Faber L, and Oye R. Effect of do-not-resuscitate orders on the nursing care of critically ill patients. Am J Crit Care 1994 Nov; 3(6): 467–475.

*Holly C. The ethical quandaries of acute care nursing practice. Journal of Professional Nursing 1993 Mar–April; 9(2): 110–115.

Huerta S and Oddi L. Refusal to care for patients with human immunodeficiency virus/acquired immunodeficiency syndrome: Issues and responses. Journal of Professional Nursing 1992 July–Aug: 8(4): 221–230.

Kass N. Insurance for the insurers: The use of genetic tests. Hastings Center Report 1992 Nov–Dec; 22(6): 6–12.

Levine M. Nursing ethics and the ethical nurse. Am J Nurs 1977 May; 77(5): 845–847.

Lumpp Sister F. The role of the nurse in the bioethical decision-making process. Nurs Clin North Am 1979 Mar; 14(1): 13–21.

Maltz A. When the patient doesn't want to be resuscitated. RN 1991; 54(2): 65–69.

McCloskey E. The patient self-determination act. Kennedy Institute of Ethics Journal 1991 June; 1(2): 163–169.

Meyer C. "End of life" care patients. Am J Nurs 1993 Feb; 93(2): 40–47.

Miedema F. Withdrawing treatment from the hopelessly ill . . . the ethical case. Dimensions of Critical Care Nursing 1993 Jan–Feb; 12(1): 40–45.

Mitchell C. Code gray: Ethical dilemmas in nursing. Nurs Life 1986 Jan/Feb; 6(1): 18–23.

Mitchell C. Ethical dilemmas in nursing: Part 2. Nurs Life 1986 Mar/Apr; 6(2): 26–30.

Moss R and La Puma J. The ethics of mechanical restraints. Hastings Center Report 1991 Jan–Feb; 21(1): 22–25.

Murphy P. 'ACT': Taking a positive approach to end-of-life care. Am J Nurs 1995 Mar; 95(3): 42–43.

*Nursing '93 editors. To tell or not to tell: A special survey report on HIV and ethics. Nursing 1993 March; 23(3): 50–53.

Obade C. Whisper down the lane: AIDS, privacy and the hospital "grapevine." Journal of Clinical Ethics 1991 Summer; 2(2): 133–137.

RN editors. It's your decision: A practical guide to modern nursing ethics. RN 1988 Oct; 51(10): 26–88. (Note: entire issue devoted to articles on ethics.)

*Rosenblum R and Deatrick J. Role of the nurse in ethically ambiguous situation. Dimensions of Critical Care Nursing 1992 Nov–Dec; 11(6): 318–325.

Rouse F. Patients, providers, and the PSDA. In "Practicing the PSDA," Special Supplement, Hastings Center Report 1991 Sept–Oct; 21(5): S2–S3.

Schneiderman L, Jecker N, and Jonsen A. Medical futility: Its meaning and ethical implications. Annals of Internal Medicine 1990 June 15; 112(12): 949–954.

Schwartz J. Living wills and health care proxies. Nursing and Health Care 1992; 13: 92–96.

Silverman H, Fry S, and Armistead N. Nurses' perspectives on implementation of the patient self-determination act. J Clin Ethics 1994 Spring; 5(1): 30–37.

Smith S. When ethics and orders conflict. RN 1991 Sept; 54(9): 61–68.

Stolley J. Freeing your patients from restraints. Am J Nurs 1995 Feb; 95(2): 27–31.

Strother A. Drawing the line between life and death. Am J Nurs 1991 April; 91(4): 24–25.

*Tucker D. Working with the patient designated "Do not resuscitate:" How the nurse copes. Focus on Critical Care 1992 Feb; 19(1): 35–40.

Twomey J. Analysis of the claim to distinct nursing ethics: Normative and nonnormative approaches. Adv Nurs Sci 1989 Apr; 11(3): 25–32.

Uustal D (ed). Ethics. Critical Care Nursing Clinics of North America 1990 September; 2(3): 421–520. (Note: half this issue devoted to articles on ethics.)

Walters L. Ethical issues in human gene therapy. Journal of Clinical Ethics 1991 Winter; 2(4): 267–274.

Weber G. The patient self-determination act: The nurse's proactive role. Journal of Professional Nursing 1992 Jan–Feb; 8(1): 6.

Wegmann J and Jassak P. Ethical issues in cancer care. Seminars in Oncology Nursing 1989 May; 5(2): 75–131. (Note: entire issue devoted to articles on ethics.)

Wicclair M. Differentiating ethical decisions from clinical standards. Dimensions of Critical Care Nursing 1991 Sept–Oct; 10(5): 280–288.

Wise CT. Understanding advance directives. Virginia Nurse 1991 Spring; 59(1): 8–11.

Wurzbach ME. The dilemma of withholding or withdrawing nutrition. Image: Journal of Nursing Scholarship 1990 Winter; 22(4): 226–230.

UNIT 2
Health Assessment of the Client/Patient

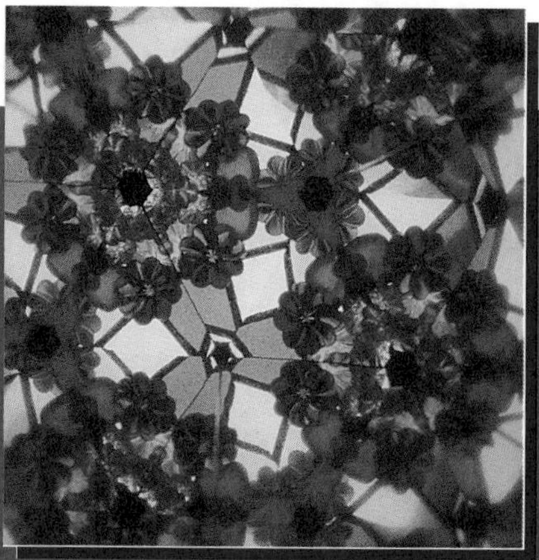

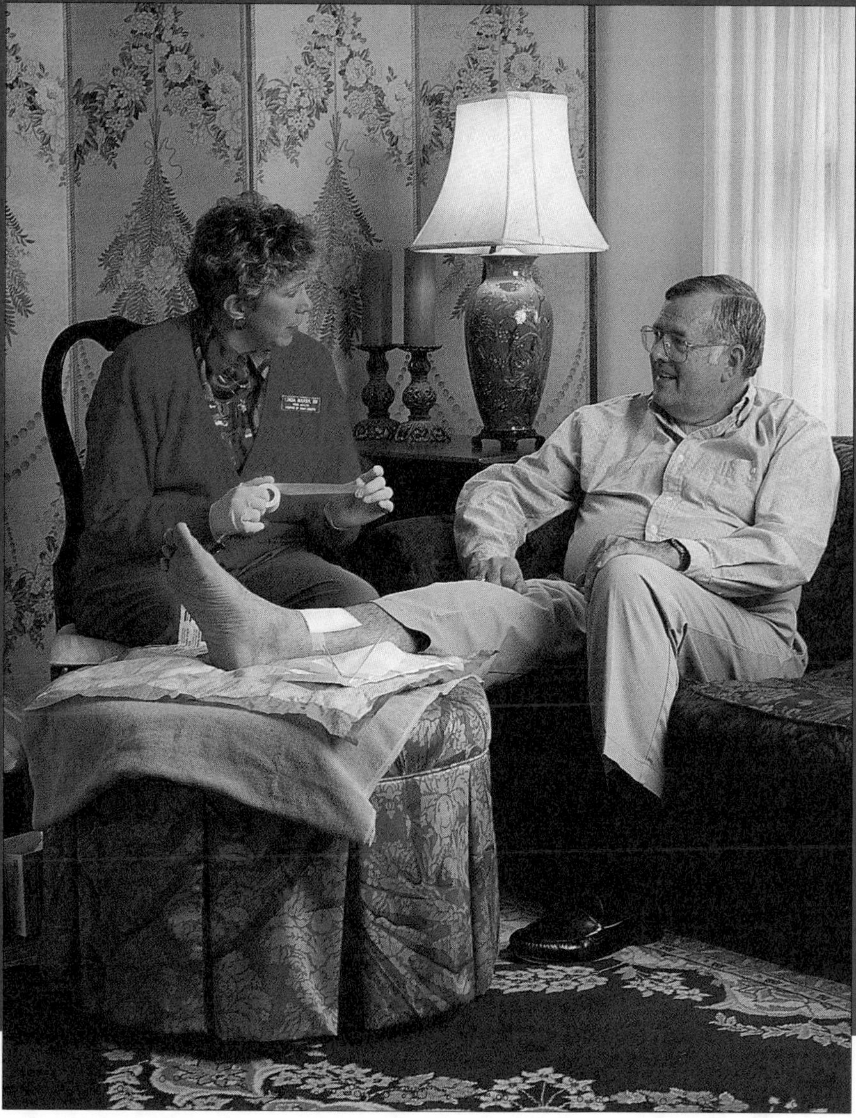

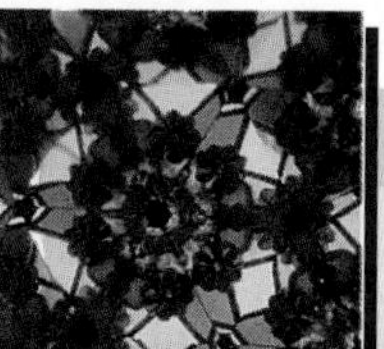

6 Clinical Interviewing: The Health History

CHAPTER OUTLINE

The Role of the Nurse
The Health History
Ethical Considerations in Data Collection
Basic Guidelines for the Interviewer
Reducing Anxiety
Encouraging Communication
Remaining Flexible
Conveying Empathy
Personal Awareness
Nonverbal Communication
Level of Understanding
Cultural Considerations
Summarizing the Interview
Content of the Interview
Biographical Data
The Informant
Chief Complaint
History of Present Illness
Health History
Family History
Review of Systems
Patient Profile
Gerontologic Considerations
Other Health History Formats
Critical Thinking Exercises

LEARNING OBJECTIVES

On completion of the chapter, the learner will be able to:

1. Describe the components of the health history
2. Identify ethical considerations necessary for protection of the individual's rights related to data collected for health assessment
3. Identify the interviewing skills and techniques used to conduct a successful interview
4. Describe effective use of the health history form
5. Specify the essential components of the data base
6. Discuss cultural, ethnic, religious, socioeconomic, and educational backgrounds as significant variables in the interview process
7. Describe specific modifications that may be necessary in obtaining a health history from an elderly patient
8. Conduct a patient interview for the purpose of obtaining a data base

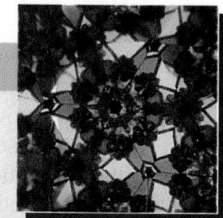

The clinical interview is one of the most important facets of the nurse–patient relationship. It establishes the quality of the relationship, provides the information needed to conduct a thorough assessment of the person's health status, and identifies the foundation for making nursing diagnoses. Behaviors appropriate to the interview and the techniques required to elicit appropriate information are not part of our everyday social lives. These behaviors and techniques must be learned. Interviewing skills require careful development and are refined through practice and experience.

The Role of the Nurse

The role of the nurse in the provision of health care is an ever-changing one. The scope of nursing practice includes not only those functions for which the nurse has traditionally been prepared but also many activities once reserved for physicians and other members of the health care team. To facilitate the nursing process, nurses obtain the patient's history and frequently perform a physical examination. The concept that only the physician diagnoses patient problems and plans appropriate interventions has also changed. A growing list of nursing diagnoses is used by nurses to identify and categorize patient problems that nurses have the knowledge, skills, and responsibility to treat.

Intrinsic to the concept of the health care team is the interdependence of health professionals, including physicians, nurses, nutritionists, social workers, and others, each using his or her unique skills and knowledge to contribute to the resolution of patient problems. A variety of formats for the nursing assessment and health history have been developed. Regardless of the format, the data base obtained by the nurse is complementary to the data bases obtained by other members of the health care team, focusing on nursing's unique concern for the patient.

The Health History

Throughout the nursing assessment, and particularly in the history, attention is focused on the impact of psychosocial, ethnic, and cultural patterns on the person's health, illness, and health promotion behaviors. The interpersonal and physical environments, as well as the person's lifestyle and activities of daily living, are explored in depth. Many nurses are also responsible for obtaining a detailed history of the person's current health problems, past medical history, family history, and a review of functional status or body systems. Including this information within the context of the history obtained by the nurse has resulted in a total health profile that focuses on health as well as illness and is more appropriately called a health history rather than a medical or a nursing history.

The format of the health history has traditionally been a combination of the medical history and the nursing assessment, although formats based on nursing frameworks such as functional health patterns have also become a current standard. Both the review of systems and patient profile are expanded to include individual and family relationships, lifestyle patterns, health practices, and coping strategies. These components of the health history are the backbone of the nursing assessment and can easily be adapted so that they are consistent with the philosophy of nursing at a particular institution or agency and meet the needs of a particular patient population.

The consolidation of the information obtained by the physician or primary care provider and by the nurse within one health history avoids a duplication of information, minimizes efforts on the part of the person to provide this information, and encourages collaboration between the nurse and physician who share in the collection and interpretation of the data base.

In order to contribute significantly to the health history, the nurse must be cognizant of (1) ethical considerations in data collection; (2) basic guidelines, skills, and techniques for conducting the interview; and (3) the content of the health history.

Ethical Considerations in Data Collection

Whenever information is elicited from a person, that person has the right to know why the information is sought and how it will be used. For this reason, it is most important to explain in detail what a health history is, how the information is elicited, and how it will be used.

It is also important that the individual be fully informed about the process of data collection and that the decision to participate be freely made. A private setting for the interview promotes trust and encourages open, honest communication.

Following the interview, the nurse selectively records on the health history form information that is pertinent to the health status. Isolated personal facts and highly sensitive information (arrest record, illegal drug use) are not initially entered in the health record but are discussed first with the primary health care provider.

When the interview is completed and the data recorded, the written record is maintained in a secure place and made available only to those health professionals directly involved in the care of the patient. This is another method of ensuring confidentiality and maintaining a high standard of nursing care and professional conduct.

Basic Guidelines for the Interviewer

Reducing Anxiety

- The interviewer approaches the person as a unique individual, puts him or her at ease, and provides for his or her comfort.

People who seek health care for a specific problem are often anxious because of uncertainty about the significance of their symptoms. Anxiety is compounded by fears related to potential disruption of lifestyle and, perhaps, by apprehension about the costs of health care. Given this set of circumstances, the person feels helpless and not in control of his or her health and economic well-being.

To minimize the patient's anxieties, it is important to introduce oneself, identify one's role, and describe the purpose of the health history. The next step is to explain that the health history will be used to identify areas of concern regarding the person's health status. The patient is reassured that all the information shared is confidential and that only health professionals directly involved in the care will have access to that information.

A private setting should be used for the interview. If visitors are present, they are asked to leave, because the patient may find it difficult to communicate when others are present. However, if the person expresses a desire to have a family member present during the interview, this request is acceptable and may generate additional information that the patient might otherwise forget or be unable to share. Distractions, such as those caused by radios or television sets, are reduced or eliminated.

The interview is conducted with consideration for the person's comfort and self-respect. Before beginning, the nurse makes sure that the person is comfortable. The patient who is short of breath may be more comfortable in a sitting position than in a supine position. If the patient is in pain or needs to go to the bathroom, these discomforts are attended to before the interview begins.

Encouraging Communication

- The interviewer permits the individual to express himself or herself fully.

The goal of the clinical interview is to obtain all of the facts that will ultimately influence both the nursing diagnoses and the plan of care. This is best achieved in an atmosphere that encourages spontaneous responses. Such spontaneity is influenced by the physical setting and by the behavior of the interviewer. Even the simple act of the interviewer sitting during the interview conveys an important message of having time and interest in what is being said (Fig. 6-1).

It is important to put the person at ease and to encourage an open and honest description of the problem. Nonverbal communication on the part of the interviewer is a critical element in encouraging open discussion. Nodding one's head or repeating the last few words may prompt the person to elaborate or continue. A puzzled look will encourage the person to clarify what is being said.

Questions posed should be open-ended. "How can we help you?" "Tell me about it," "How did it feel?" are all appropriate questions. Examples of inappropriate questions are: "Was it a sharp pain?" "Did it happen only on weekdays?" Such questions suggest the answer and "lead" the person to respond accordingly. Although one certainly wishes to obtain this information, it is best sought in a more open-ended way; otherwise, the person may attempt to provide the answer he or she thinks the interviewer wants to hear.

The use of open-ended questions is not a technique to be employed throughout the entire interview. In order to refine the details that are important to the analysis of symptoms, some degree of direct questioning is necessary. Such questions offer options. For example, the question "Does the pain have any relationship to meals?" gives the person the option of answering yes or no. Similarly, the question "Does the pain come before the meal, during the meal, or after the meal?" provides an opportunity to select from among several options.

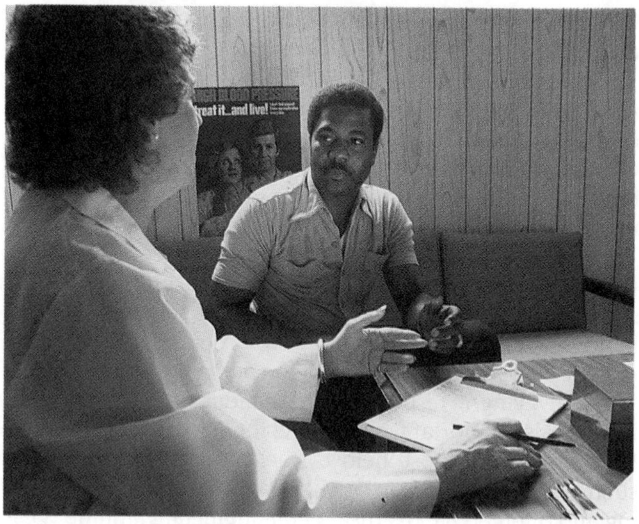

FIGURE 6-1. A comfortable, relaxed atmosphere is essential for a successful clinical interview.

Not every interview will follow the same pattern. In some instances a more direct approach to the questioning will be necessary. An experienced interviewer will develop the sophistication to modify interview techniques as needed.

Remaining Flexible

- The interviewer usually uses a health history form to guide the interview and adjusts the sequence of questions to coincide with the flow of conversation.

The health history form is a tool designed to assist in the collection of data relevant to the person's health status. For this reason, the form is not memorized or rigidly adhered to at the expense of what the individual wants to say. For example, if the person is sharing information about a particular problem and the interviewer interrupts to ask direct questions about occupation, education, or family relationships, the flow of information may be broken and important facts overlooked.

It is also essential to *listen* when the person answers the questions. Brief note-taking during the interview is acceptable, but when overdone it is highly distracting to the person being interviewed. It also limits eye contact and conveys an impersonal message.

Conveying Empathy

- The interviewer demonstrates an understanding of the nature and intensity of the person's problem.

The interviewing process does not consist entirely of questions and answers. The manner in which the interviewer responds nonverbally demonstrates an ability to listen and conveys a genuine interest in the person's concerns. Such behavior is often reassuring and helps enhance the therapeutic effects of the interview.

Extended pauses or silent moments during the interview may indicate that the person is emotionally overcome or may be attempting to formulate an accurate description of events. Such silences need not be interrupted by the interviewer. Tearful episodes are also not interrupted, and the urge to say that everything is going to be all right is resisted. Things may not be all right, and the reassurance may appear false. Moreover, much can be learned by exploring the person's fears and anxieties. Sometimes, open-ended statements such as "You look sad" or "You seem frightened" will convey empathy and encourage the person to elaborate.

Conveying a respect for the patient's beliefs and attitudes is also important, even if such beliefs and attitudes differ sharply from those held by the interviewer. Statements such as "You don't really believe that, do you?" are demeaning and often create distrust. A nonjudgmental attitude is especially important when dealing with matters related to sexuality, drug and alcohol use, and cultural patterns.

Personal Awareness

- The interviewer is aware of his or her own feelings and attitudes.

Behaviors and beliefs that the nurse might find personally offensive may arouse hostility, anger, anxiety, or even, at times, revulsion. An ethical or moral sense may make it difficult to develop relationships with patients who have different lifestyles, sexual practices, or health practices. However, it is inappropriate to convey negative reactions or judgments. Sometimes a personal fear about a certain illness may lead to a feeling of discomfort when dealing with people who have that particular disorder. The first step in dealing effectively with patients with such health problems is to understand the underlying factors that contribute to these behaviors and one's own reactions to them.

Nonverbal Communication

- The interviewer is attuned to nonverbal communication and learns to recognize gestures that convey defensiveness, hostility, confidence, impatience, and similar feelings.

Body language can provide as much information as the spoken word, especially when body language contradicts verbal expression and raises questions about the person's real feelings. In such instances it often helps to mention the apparent inconsistency in order to elicit further information.

Level of Understanding

- The interviewer communicates in a manner that is consistent with the individual's level of understanding.

It is important to take into consideration the individual's educational background and language. People who are not proficient in English and those who have had little contact with the health care system may be unfamiliar with terms commonly used by health care professionals. Therefore, questions should be phrased in a way that is easily understandable, and technical terms should be avoided. A person who does not understand what is being said is unlikely to ask questions for fear of appearing ignorant. Careful questioning on the part of the interviewer may reveal if anything was misunderstood.

Cultural Considerations

- The interviewer takes into account the person's cultural background.

Cultural attitudes and belief about family relationships, the role of women in the culture, and the meaning of health must be accepted at face value, in the same way as attitudes toward pain, illness, and hospitalization are viewed. These beliefs and attitudes are derived from each person's experiences, which vary according to the person's ethnic and cultural background. A person from another culture may have a different view of personal health practices from someone born and raised in an American suburb. For example, women from certain cultures do not view pregnancy as requiring care until labor begins. Such women do not understand the need for prenatal care as advocated by health professionals and therefore do not seek health care until they begin labor. Similarly, people from some ethnic backgrounds will not complain of pain, even when it is severe, because their culture does not condone outward expressions of pain. In some instances they may refuse to take analgesics. Other cultures have their own folklore for the treatment of illnesses.

All such differences in outlook must be taken into account and accepted when dealing with members of other cultures. Trying to force one's own point of view on people who have other beliefs and customs leads to conflict and mistrust and may have a negative effect on the nurse–patient relationship and the care given.

Summarizing the Interview

- The interviewer terminates the interview in an appropriate manner that summarizes the information obtained and ensures that the person has understood major points discussed.

At the end of the interview, the examiner asks if the person has any questions. One method for identifying any possible misunderstanding is to summarize briefly the person's responses, thereby providing the person with an opportunity to correct misinformation and add facts that may have been omitted.

Content of the Interview

When the patient is seen for the first time by a member of the health team (except in the emergency care situation), the first requisite is to obtain a **data base**. The framework for organizing the information may vary, but the content, regardless of format, covers the same general topics. A traditional approach includes the following parts:

1. Biographical data
2. Informant
3. Chief complaint
4. History of present illness (or present health concern)
5. Past medical history
6. Review of systems
7. Family history
8. Patient profile
9. Physical examination
10. Radiologic and laboratory information
11. Problem formulation (medical and nursing diagnoses)

Biographical Data

Biographical or introductory information helps to put much of the history in context. This information includes the person's name, address, age, sex, marital status, occupation, and ethnic origins. Some interviewers prefer to ask more personal questions at this juncture to obtain a full patient profile. Others prefer to wait until more trust and confidence have been established. Moreover, someone in pain or with an equally urgent problem is unlikely to put a great deal of confidence in an interviewer who is more concerned about marital or occupational status than with quickly addressing the problem at hand.

The Informant

The informant, or the person providing the information, may not always be the patient, as in the case of a child or a disoriented or confused person or someone who is unconscious, in a coma, or suffering a severe psychiatric disturbance. The interviewer assesses the reliability of the informant and the usefulness of the information provided. For example, hysterical or depressed patients are unlikely to provide a reliable data base, while those who abuse drugs and alcohol are likely to deny using these substances. It is reasonable for the interviewer to make a judgment about the reliability of the information (based on the context of the entire interview) and to include this evaluation in the record.

Chief Complaint

The chief complaint is the issue that brings the person to seek help. Questions such as "Why have you come to the health center today?" or "Why have you been admitted to the hospital?" usually elicit the chief complaint. Frequently, there is no specific complaint, as in the instance of someone getting a "checkup." This reason would be recorded instead of a chief complaint. When a complaint is voiced, the person's exact words are recorded in quotation marks. However, a statement such as "My doctor sent me" should not be recorded as a chief complaint. Although such information can be included as part of the introductory patient profile, the person should be asked the reason for seeking health care, and this reason should be entered as the chief complaint.

When more than one problem exists, the problems are listed in order of the priority in which they are reported.

History of Present Illness

The history of any illness is the single most important factor in assisting the health professional in arriving at a diagnosis or determining the person's needs. The physical examination is helpful but usually reveals manifestations that are expected consequences of the story that has unfolded. Occasionally, diagnostic test results can be helpful; only rarely do they establish the diagnosis. On the other hand, a careful history assists in correct selection of appropriate diagnostic tests.

If the present illness is only the latest episode in a series of episodes, the entire sequence of events is recorded. For example, an episode of insulin shock is only one event in a series of occurrences that define a history of diabetes. In such an instance, the entire course of the diabetic illness is described in order to put the current complaint in context. Although the episode of insulin shock is highlighted in the history, the course of the illness is described and documented in the record. After all the facts have been obtained, the details of the present illness or health concern, from onset until the time of contact with the health care team, are constructed. These facts are recorded in *chronologic order*, beginning with, for example, "The patient was in good health until . . ." or "The patient first experienced abdominal pain 2 months prior to seeking help."

The history of the present illness includes such information as the date and manner (sudden, gradual) in which the problem occurred, the setting in which the problem developed (at home, at work, after an argument, after exercise), manifestations of the problem, and the course of the illness or problem. The course of the illness or problem includes self-treatment, medical interventions, progress and effects of treatment, and the patient's perceptions of the cause or meaning of the problem.

Specific symptoms (pain, headache, fever, change in bowel habits) are delineated in detail, along with location and radiation (if pain), quality, severity, and duration. The interviewer also inquires if the chief complaint is persistent or intermittent, what factors aggravate or alleviate it, and if any associated manifestations exist.

Associated manifestations are symptoms that occur simultaneously with the chief complaint. The presence or absence of associated symptoms may shed light on the origin or extent of the problem, as well as on the diagnosis. These symptoms are referred to as significant positive or negative findings and are derived from a review of systems directly related to the chief complaint. For instance, if the person reports a vague symptom, such as fatigue or weight loss, all body systems are reviewed and included in the history of the present illness. If, on the other hand, the person's chief complaint is chest pain, only the cardiopulmonary and gastrointestinal systems may be included in the history of the present illness. In either situation, both positive and negative findings are recorded in order to define the problem further.

Health History

A detailed summary of the person's health history is a valuable component of the data base. After the general health status is determined, inquiries are made about immunization status and any known allergies to drugs or other substances. The dates of immunization, along with the type of allergy and adverse reactions, are recorded. The person is asked to provide information, if known, about his or her last physical examination, chest x-ray, electrocardiogram (ECG), eye examination, hearing tests, dental checkup, and Papanicolaou (Pap) smear (if female). Previous illnesses are then discussed. Negative as well as positive responses to a list of specific diseases are recorded. Dates, or the age of the patient at the time of illness, as well as the names of the primary care provider and hospital, the diagnosis, and the treatment are also recorded. A history of the following areas is elicited.

- Childhood illness—rubeola, rubella, polio, whooping cough, mumps, chickenpox, scarlet fever, rheumatic fever, strep throat
- Adult illnesses
- Psychiatric illnesses
- Injuries—burns, fractures, head injuries
- Hospitalizations
- Surgical and diagnostic procedures
- Current medications—prescription, over-the-counter, home remedies
- Use of alcohol and other drugs

If a particular hospitalization or major medical intervention is related to the present illness, it need not be repeated; rather, a reference is made to the appropriate part of the report, such as "see history of present illness" or "see HPI" on the data sheet.

Family History

The age and health status, or the age and cause of death, of first-order relatives (parents, siblings, spouse, children) and second-order relatives (grandparents, cousins) are elicited to identify diseases that may be hereditary, communicable, or possibly environmental in cause. The following diseases are generally covered: cancer, hypertension, heart disease, diabetes, epilepsy, mental illness, tuberculosis, kidney disease, arthritis, allergies, asthma, alcoholism, and obesity. One of the easiest methods of recording such data is by using the family tree or genogram (Fig. 6-2).

Review of Systems

The system review includes an overview of general health as well as symptoms related to each body system. Questions are asked about each of the major body systems in terms of past or present symptoms. Reviewing each body system helps reveal any relevant data. Negative as well as positive answers are recorded. If the patient responds positively to

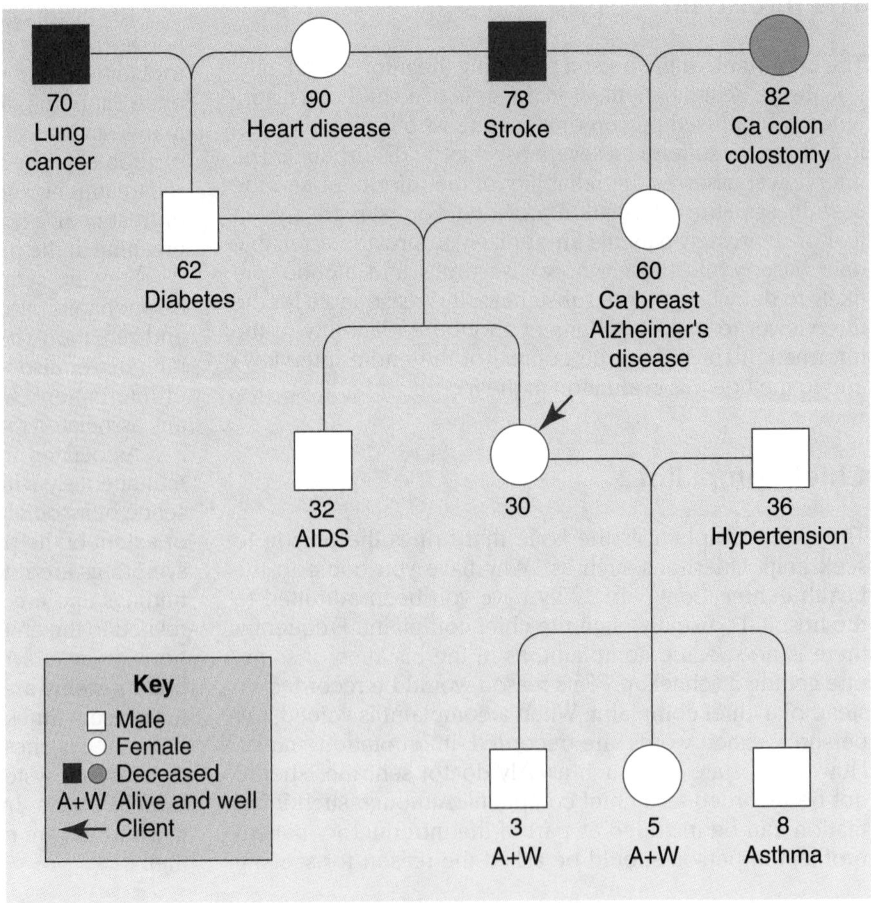

FIGURE 6-2. Sample recording of family history as a "family tree." Grandparents, parents, siblings, spouse, and children are identified.

questions about a particular system, the information is analyzed carefully. If any illnesses were previously mentioned or recorded, it is not necessary to repeat them in this part of the history. Instead, reference is made to the appropriate place in the history where the information can be found.

A review of systems can be organized in a formal checklist, which becomes a part of the health history. One advantage of a checklist is that it can be easily audited and is less subject to error than a system that relies heavily on the interviewer's memory.

Patient Profile

In the patient profile, more biographical information is gathered. A complete composite, or profile, of the patient is critical to an analysis of the chief complaint and of the person's ability to deal with the problem.

The information elicited at this point in the interview is highly personal and subjective. During this stage, the person is encouraged to express feelings in an uninhibited manner and to discuss personal experiences. It is best to begin with general, open-ended questions and to move to direct questioning when specific facts are needed. The patient is often less anxious when the interview progresses from information that is less personal (birthplace, occupation, education) to information that is more personal (sexuality, body image, coping abilities).

A general patient profile consists of the following content areas:

1. Past life events related to health
2. Education and occupation
3. Environment (physical, spiritual, cultural, interpersonal)
4. Lifestyle (patterns and habits)
5. Self-concept
6. Sexuality
7. Risk for abuse
8. Stress and coping response

The patient profile is outlined in Chart 6-1.

CHART 6-1
Patient Profile

Past Events Related to Health

Place of birth
Places lived
Significant childhood/adolescent experiences

Education and Occupation

Jobs held in past
Current position/job
Length of time at position
Educational preparation
Work satisfaction and career goals
Financial resources
Insurance coverage

Environment

Physical
Living arrangements (type of housing, neighborhood, presence of hazards)

Spiritual
Extent to which religion is a part of individual's life
Religious beliefs related to perception of health and illness
Religious practices

Interpersonal
Ethnic background (language spoken, customs and values held, folk practices used to maintain health or to cure illness)
Family relationships (family structure, roles, communication patterns, support system)
Friendships (quality of relationship)

Lifestyle

Patterns
Sleep (time individual retires, hours per night, comfort measures, awakens rested)
Exercise (type, frequency, time spent)
Nutrition (24-hour diet recall, idiosyncrasies, restrictions)
Recreation (type of activity, time spent)
Caffeine (coffee, tea, cola, chocolate)—kind, amount
Smoking (cigarette, pipe, cigar, marijuana)—kind, amount per day, number of years, desire to quit
Alcohol—kind, amount, pattern over past year
Drugs—kind, amount, route of administration

Self-Concept

View of self in present
View of self in future
Body image (level of satisfaction, concerns)

Sexuality

Perception of self as a man or woman
Quality of sexual relationships
Concerns related to sexuality or sexual functioning

Risk for Abuse

Physical injury in past
Afraid of partner, caregiver, family

Stress and Coping Response

Major concerns or problems at present
Daily "hassles"
Past experiences with similar problems
Past coping patterns and outcomes
Present coping strategies and anticipated outcomes
Individual's expectations of family/friends and health care team in problem resolution

Past Life Events Related to Health

The patient profile begins with a brief life history. Questions about place of birth and past places of residence help focus attention on the earlier years of life. Personal experiences during childhood or adolescence that have special significance may be elicited by asking, "Was there anything that you experienced as a child or adolescent that would be helpful for me to know about?" The interviewer's intent is to encourage the person to make a quick review of his or her earlier life, highlighting an event or circumstance of particular significance. Sometimes the person will not be able to recall anything that was meaningful. On the other hand, he or she may take the opportunity to share information such as a personal achievement, a failure, a developmental crisis, or an instance of physical or emotional abuse.

Education and Occupation

Inquiring about current occupation can reveal much about a person's economic status and educational preparation. A statement such as "Tell me about your job" often elicits information about role, job tasks, and satisfaction with the position. It may be necessary to ask direct questions about past employment and career goals if the person does not initially provide this information.

Asking the person what kind of educational requirements were necessary to attain his or her present job is a more sensitive approach to educational background than asking whether he or she graduated from high school. It is rarely necessary to know the actual numerical value of the person's salary; the information needed is whether income is sufficient to meet expenses and support the lifestyle to which he or she is accustomed. Questions such as "Do you have any financial concerns at this time?" or "Sometimes there just doesn't seem to be enough money to make ends meet. Are you finding this true?" may be helpful. Inquiry about the person's insurance coverage and plans for health care payment are also appropriate.

Environment

The person's physical environment and its potential hazards, spiritual awareness, cultural background, interpersonal relationships, and support system are included in the concept of environment.

Physical Environment. The type of housing (apartment, duplex, single family) in which the person lives, its location, and information related to safety and comfort within the person's home and neighborhood are elicited. The nurse attempts to identify environmental hazards, such as isolation, inadequate protection, potential fire risks, pollution (noise, air, water), and inadequate sanitation facilities.

Spiritual Environment. One's spiritual environment refers to the degree to which one is thoughtful or contemplative about one's existence, accepts challenges in one's life, and seeks and finds answers to personal questions. For many people, this spirituality is expressed through identification with a particular religion. Like cultural influences, spiritual values and beliefs direct a person's behavior and approach to health problems and can influence how he or she reacts to sickness. Illness can be a time of spiritual crisis and can place considerable stress on a person's internal resources and beliefs. Including this facet of a person's being in the health history can help identify possible support systems as well as beliefs and customs that need to be considered in planning care. Thus, information should be gathered in the following three areas:

1. The extent to which religion is a part of the person's life
2. Religious beliefs related to the person's perception of health and illness
3. Religious practices

The following questions can be used in a spiritual assessment:

- Is religion or God important to you?
- If *yes,* in what way?
- If *no,* what is the most important thing in your life?
- Are there any religious practices that are important to you?
- Do you have any spiritual concerns because of your present health problem?

Interpersonal and Cultural Environment. Cultural influences, relationships with family and friends, and the presence or absence of a support system are all a part of one's interpersonal environment.

The beliefs and practices that have been shared from generation to generation are known as cultural or ethnic patterns. They are expressed through language, dress, dietary choices, and role behaviors, in perceptions of health and illness, and in health-related behaviors. The influence of these beliefs and customs on how a person reacts to health problems and interacts with health care providers cannot be underestimated. For this reason, the health history includes information on ethnic identity (cultural and social) and racial identity (biologic). The following questions may assist in obtaining relevant information:

- Where did your parents or ancestors come from? When?
- What language do you speak at home?
- Are there certain customs or values that are important to you?
- Is there anything special you do to keep in good health?
- Do you have any specific practices for treating illness?

Family Relationships and Support System. An assessment of family structure (members, ages, roles), patterns of communication, and the presence or absence of a support system is an integral part of the patient profile. Although the traditional "family" is recognized as a mother, a father, and children, many different types of living arrangements exist within our society. "Family" may mean two or more people bound by emotional ties or commitments. Live-in companions, roommates, and close friends can all play a significant role in an individual's support system.

Lifestyle

The lifestyle section of the patient profile provides an opportunity to gain information about health-related behaviors.

These behaviors include patterns of sleep, exercise, nutrition, and recreation, as well as personal habits of smoking and the use of drugs, alcohol, and caffeine. Most people have little difficulty sharing particulars about their sleeping patterns or recreational choices. On the other hand, many are quite sensitive when asked about smoking, alcohol use, and drug use, and they may deny or understate the degree to which they use such substances. Questions can be worded so as to elicit more information, such as "What kind of alcohol do you enjoy drinking at a party" rather than "Do you drink?" Describing the person as a "social drinker" is vague and not recommended. Instead, the specific type of alcohol (*e.g.*, wine, liquor, beer) and the amount ingested per day or per week (*e.g.*, 1 pint of whiskey daily for 2 years) are described.

When alcohol abuse is suspected, additional information may be obtained by asking, "Has anyone ever said that drinking might be causing a problem for you?" or "Have you ever considered cutting down your alcohol intake?" The same approach can be used to elicit information about smoking and caffeine consumption.

Questions about drug use follow naturally after questions about smoking, caffeine consumption, and alcohol use. A nonjudgmental approach will make it easier for the person to respond truthfully and factually. It is often helpful to ask questions that require responses other than a simple "yes" or "no." If "street names" or unfamiliar terms are used to describe drugs, ask the person to define the terms used.

Self-Concept

Self-concept refers to the impression one has of oneself; an image that has developed over many years. Sometimes the interviewer can assess self-concept by asking how the person views life: "How do you feel about your life in general?", "What will your life be like in the future?" or "How do you see yourself in a few years?"

A person's self concept can be threatened very easily. For example, body image, or the mental picture one has of oneself, can be affected by normal developmental crises such as may occur with adolescence, pregnancy, or aging. The impact of certain medical conditions or surgical interventions, such as a colostomy or a mastectomy, can pose an even greater threat to body image. The following question may elicit useful information concerning self image:

- Do you have any particular concerns about your body?

Sexuality

No area of assessment is more personal than the sexual history. Interviewers are frequently uncomfortable with such questions and ignore this area of the patient profile or conduct a very cursory interview at this point. A lack of knowledge about sexuality, combined with anxiety about one's own sexuality, may hamper the interviewer's effectiveness in dealing with this subject.

Sexual assessment can be approached at the end of the interview at the time interpersonal or lifestyle factors are assessed, or it can be a part of the genitourinary history within the review of systems. For instance, it may be easier to approach a discussion of sexuality following a discussion of menstruation. A similar discussion with the male patient would follow questions related to the urinary system.

Obtaining the sexual history provides an opportunity to discuss sexual matters openly and gives the person permission to express sexual concerns to an informed professional. The interviewing style should be nonjudgmental and the language used should be appropriate to the person's age and background. It is advisable to begin the assessment with a general question concerning the person's developmental stage and the presence or absence of intimate relationships.

Such questions may lead to a discussion of concerns related to sexual expression, to the quality of a relationship, or to questions about contraception, risky sexual behaviors, and safer sex practices.

Finding out whether a person is sexually active should precede any attempts to explore issues related to sexual identity, contraception, or the quality of the sexual relationship. Avoid making assumptions related to fidelity, heterosexuality, or sexual practices. Questions are worded in such a way that the person feels free to discuss his or her sexuality regardless of marital status or sexual preference. Direct questions are usually less threatening when prefaced with such statements as "Most people feel that . . ." or "Many people worry about. . . ." This suggests the normalcy of such feelings or behavior and encourages the person to share information that might otherwise be omitted from fear of seeming different.

If the person answers abruptly or does not wish to carry the discussion any further, then the interviewer should move to the next topic. However, introducing the subject of sexuality indicates to the person that a discussion of sexual concerns is acceptable and can be approached again in the future if so desired. Further discussion of the sexual history is presented in Chapter 44.

Risk for Abuse

A topic of growing importance in today's society is physical, sexual, and psychological abuse. Such abuse occurs at all ages, to men and women from all socioeconomic, ethnic, and cultural groups. Few patients, however, will discuss this topic unless they are asked specifically about it. Therefore, it is important to ask the appropriate questions, such as:

- Is anyone physically hurting you?
- Has anyone ever hurt you physically?
- Are you ever afraid of anyone close to you (your partner, caretaker, or other family members)?

If the person's response indicates that abuse is a risk, further assessment is called for and efforts are made to assure the person's safety and provide access to appropriate community and professional resources and support systems.

Stress and Coping Responses

Each of us handles stress in our own way. How well we adapt depends on our ability to cope. When conducting a health history, it helps to explore past coping patterns, as well as perceptions of current stresses and anticipated outcomes, to identify the person's overall ability to handle stress. It is especially important to identify expectations that the person may have of family, friends, and care givers in providing support.

Gerontologic Considerations

A health history obtained from the elderly patient should be carried out in a calm, unrushed manner. Because of the increased incidence of impaired hearing and sight in the elderly, lighting should be adequate but not glaring and distracting noises should be kept to a minimum. The interviewer should assume a position that enables the person to read lips and facial expressions. If the person normally relies on a hearing aid, he or she should be asked to use it during the interview.

Elderly people often assume that new physical problems are a result of age rather than a treatable illness. In addition, the signs and symptoms of illness in the elderly are often more subtle than those in younger people and may go unreported. Therefore, the interviewer inquires about subtle physical symptoms and recent changes in function and well-being. Particular care is taken in obtaining a complete history of medications used because elderly people frequently take many different kinds of medications. Although elderly people sometimes suffer from a decrease in mental function, it should not be assumed that an elderly person is unable to provide an adequate history. However, including a member of the family in the interview process (*i.e.*, spouse, adult child, sibling, or caretaker) will help validate information and provide missing details. Further details about assessment of the elderly are provided in Chapter 12.

Other Health History Formats

The health history format presented and discussed in this chapter is only one possible format that is useful in obtaining and organizing information about a person's current and past health status. Some nurses believe that this traditional format is appropriate for physicians but inappropriate for nurses because it does not focus exclusively on the assessment of human responses to actual or potential health problems. Several attempts have been made to create an assessment format and data base with this focus in mind. One example is the nursing data base prototype based on the North American Nursing Diagnosis Association's (NANDA) Unitary Person Framework and its nine human response patterns: exchanging, communicating, relating, valuing, choosing, moving, perceiving, knowing, and feeling. Although there is some support in nursing for using this approach to obtaining the data base, a consensus for its use has not yet been established.

The National Center for Health Services Research of the U.S. Department of Health and Human Services and other groups from the public and private sectors have focused on assessing not only biological health but other dimensions of health as well. These dimensions include physical, functional, emotional, mental, and social.

Modern efforts to assess health status have focused on the manner in which disease or disability affects the patient's **functional status**, the ability of the person to function normally and perform his or her usual physical, mental, and social activities. An emphasis on functional assessment is viewed as more holistic than the traditional health or medical history. Instruments to assess health status in these ways may be of considerable assistance to nurses who use them along with their own clinical assessment skills in determining the impact of illness, disease, disability, and health problems on functional status.

Health concerns that usually are not complex (earache, tonsillectomy) and can be resolved in a short period of time usually do not require the depth or detail that is required when one is confronted with a person who is experiencing a major illness or health concern. Additional assessments that go beyond the general patient profile may be employed when the patient's health problems are acute and complex or when the illness is chronic.

Regardless of the format used, the nurse's focus during collection of data about the patient's health is different from that of the physician and other health team members; however, it complements these approaches and encourages collaboration among the health care providers, as each member brings his or her own expertise and focus to the situation.

CRITICAL THINKING EXERCISES

1. While you are conducting a health assessment of an elderly patient, she tells you that she has been abused by her family but pleads with you not to report this information to anyone. Describe the legal and ethical issues that are involved, and explain the actions you feel would be most appropriate for you to take.
2. You are conducting an assessment interview when the patient expresses annoyance at being asked questions about his health history. He claims that problems he had in the past have nothing to do with his current health concerns. Explain how you would respond or react in a way to gain his support in providing this information.
3. You need to obtain a health history from an elderly Asian patient who nods in agreement to your questions, even when the questions are open ended. How would you proceed if the patient is accompanied by her daughter? If she is alone? Can speak some English? Cannot speak English?

BIBLIOGRAPHY

Books

Clinical Interviewing

Barkauskas V. Health and Physical Assessment St. Louis, Mosby Year Book, 1994.

Bates B. A Guide to Physical Examination and History Taking, 5th ed. Philadelphia, JB Lippincott, 1995.

DeGowin RL. DeGowin and DeGowin's Diagnostic Examination, 6th ed. New York, McGraw-Hill, 1994.

Fuller J and Schaller-Ayers J. Health Assessment: A Nursing Approach. Philadelphia, JB Lippincott, 1994.

Gordon M. Nursing Diagnosis: Process and Application. St. Louis, CV Mosby, 1994.

Guzzetta CE et al. Clinical Assessment Tools for Use with Nursing Diagnosis. St. Louis, CV Mosby, 1989.

Morton PG. Health Assessment in Nursing, 2nd ed. Springhouse, PA, Springhouse, 1994.

Seidel H et al. Mosby's Guide to Physical Examination. St. Louis, CV Mosby, 1995.

Journals

Catherman A. Biopsychosocial nursing assessment: A way to enhance care plans. J Psychosocial Nursing 1990 June; 28(6): 31–33.

Feldstein MA and Rait D. Family assessment in an oncology setting. Cancer Nursing 1992 June; 15(3): 161–172.

Fields SD. History-taking in the elderly: Obtaining useful information. Geriatrics 1991 Aug; 46(8): 26–28, 34–35.

Furniss KK. Screening for abuse in the clinical setting. AWHONN's Clinical Issues 1993; 4(3): 402–406.

Gehring PE. Physical assessment begins with a history. RN 1991 Nov; 54(11): 27–32.

Hartman D and Knudson J. A nursing data base for initial patient assessment. Oncology Nursing Forum 1991 Jan–Feb; 18(1): 125–130.

Van Ruiswyk J et al. Nursing assessments: Patient severity of illness. Nursing Management 1992 Sep; 23(9): 44–46, 48.

Weiler K. Functional assessment in the determination of the need for a substitute decision maker. J Professional Nursing 1991 Nov–Dec; 7(6): 328.

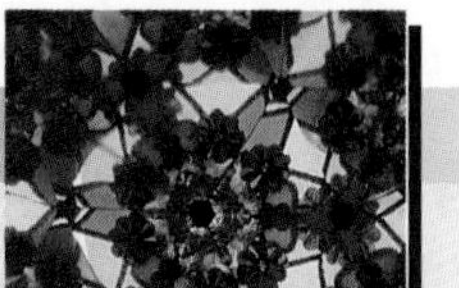

7 Physical Assessment and Nutritional Assessment

CHAPTER OUTLINE

LEARNING OBJECTIVES

On completion of this chapter, the learner will be able to:

1. Describe the physical examination processes of inspection, palpation, percussion, and auscultation
2. Use inspection, palpation, percussion, and auscultation to perform physical assessment of the major body systems
3. Describe the importance of proper physical, emotional, and educational preparation of the patient for physical assessment
4. Use clinical examination, anthropometric measurements, biochemical assessment, and assessment of food intake to assess a person's nutritional status
5. Describe factors that may contribute to altered nutritional status in the elderly

Suzanne C. Smeltzer and Brenda G. Bare: Brunner and Suddarth's Textbook of Medical-Surgical Nursing, 8th Edition. © 1996 Lippincott-Raven Publishers.

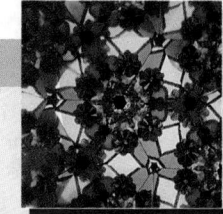

Physical assessment, or the physical examination, is an integral part of nursing assessment. The basic techniques and tools typically used in performing a physical examination are described in general in this chapter. The detailed discussion required for the thorough examination of specific systems, including special maneuvers, is found in appropriate chapters throughout the book. Because the patient's nutritional status is an important element of the total health profile, a section on nutritional assessment is included in this chapter.

The Physical Assessment

The physical examination is usually performed after the health history is taken. To facilitate this portion of the data collection process, the examination is carried out in a well-lighted, warm area. The patient is undressed and draped appropriately so that only the area to be examined is exposed. The person's physical and psychologic comfort is considered at all times; procedures and their rationale are fully explained. An explanation of what to expect precedes each part of the examination. The examiner's hands are washed prior to and immediately following the examination. Fingernails are kept short to avoid injuring the patient. Gloves are worn by the examiner when there is a possibility of coming in contact with blood or other body secretions during the physical examination.

The key to obtaining appropriate data in the least possible amount of time is an organized and systematic examination. Such an approach refines physical assessment skills and encourages cooperation and trust on the part of the patient.

The individual's health history provides the examiner with a complete health profile that guides all aspects of the physical examination. It begins with questions that focus on problems or symptoms of concern to the patient.

The complete physical examination usually proceeds in a logical head-to-toe sequence, as follows:

- Skin
- Head and neck
- Thorax and lungs
- Breasts
- Cardiovascular system
- Abdomen
- Rectum
- Genitalia
- Neurologic system
- Musculoskeletal system

In actual practice, all relevant body systems are tested throughout the physical examination, not necessarily in the sequence described. For example, when the face is examined, it is appropriate at the same time to check for facial asymmetry and, thus, for the integrity of the seventh cranial nerve; one does not return to this point later, as part of a neurologic examination. When systems are combined in this manner, the person is spared the sequence of sitting up, lying down, sitting up, and so forth, which can be exhausting and time consuming.

A "complete" physical examination is not a "routine." Many of the elements are selectively addressed as a function of the individual's particular problem. If, for example, a healthy 20-year-old college student reports for an examination in order to satisfy a requirement to play basketball and reports no history of neurologic abnormality, the requirements for an adequate survey of the neurologic system are minimal. Conversely, a complaint of transient numbness and diplopia (double vision) usually necessitates a complete neurologic investigation. Similarly, a person with pleuritic chest pain receives a much more intensive examination of the chest than the person with a headache.

The process of physical examination is a thoughtful one. Attempts to elicit physical findings are based on all the information available at the time the examination is conducted. In general, it is the individual's health history that directs the examiner in efforts to obtain additional data for a complete patient profile.

The process of learning physical examination requires memorization, repetition, and reinforcement in a clinical setting. Only after basic physical assessment techniques are mastered can the examiner tailor the routine screening examination to include thorough assessments of a particular system, including special maneuvers.

The basic tools of the physical examination are the human senses of vision, hearing, touch, and smell. These human senses may be augmented by special instruments or tools (*e.g.*, stethoscope, ophthalmoscope) to permit a better definition of what is seen or heard, but these tools should be recognized only as extensions of the human senses; they are simple instruments that anyone can learn to use well. Expertise comes with practice, and sophistication comes with the interpretation of what is seen and heard.

Assessment in the Home

Assessment of the person in the home consists of collecting information specific to any existing health problem—including physiologic and emotional status, the home environment, the adequacy of support systems or care given by family and other care providers, and the availability of needed resources. In addition, the ability of the individual and family to cope with and address their respective needs is evaluated.

The physical assessment in the home consists of the same techniques used in the hospital, clinic, or office setting. Privacy is provided and efforts are made to make the person as comfortable as possible.

The Process of Physical Examination

Four fundamental processes are employed in the physical examination: *inspection, palpation, percussion,* and *auscultation.*

Inspection

The first fundamental process is inspection or observation. The power to observe is one that must be cultivated. General inspection begins at the first moment of contact with the patient. Introducing oneself to the patient, shaking hands, and exchanging the first words set the stage. Many impressions register in this exchange, and numerous valuable observations can be made. The person is old or young (how old? how young? does the person's appearance correspond to his or her stated age?); the person is thin or obese; the person is anxious or depressed; the person's body structure is normal or perhaps deformed in some way (what way? how different from normal?).

It is essential to pay attention to the details in observation. Vague, general statements are an inadequate substitute for specific descriptions based on careful observation:

1. *The person looks sick.* In what way does he or she look sick? Is the skin clammy, pale, jaundiced, or cyanotic; is the person grimacing in pain; is breathing difficult; does he or she have edema? What specific physical features or behavioral manifestations convey that the person is "sick?"
2. *The person appears chronically ill.* In what way does he or she appear chronically ill? Does the person appear to have lost weight? People who lose weight secondary to AIDS, malignancy, or other muscle-wasting diseases have a different appearance than those who are merely thin. The distribution of their weight loss takes a different form. Does the skin have the appearance of chronic illness? That is, is it pale, or does it give the appearance of dehydration or loss of subcutaneous tissue? These important observations are documented in the chart or medical record.

Among general observations that should be noted in the initial examination of the patient are posture and stature, body movements, nutrition, speech pattern, and body temperature.

Posture and Stature. The posture that a person assumes often provides valuable information about the illness. Patients who have breathing difficulties (dyspnea) secondary to cardiac disease prefer to sit and may complain of feeling "smothered" if forced to lie flat for even brief periods of time. Persons with emphysema not only sit upright but also assume a posture that is quite characteristic. They thrust their arms forward and laterally onto the edge of the bed (tripod position) in order to place accessory muscles of respiration at an optimum mechanical advantage for respiratory assistance. Those with abdominal pain due to peritonitis prefer to lie perfectly still. Even slight jarring of the bed by the examiner will incite agonizing pain. On the other hand, patients with abdominal pain due to renal or biliary colic are very restless. They may writhe in bed or even get up and pace the room. Patients with meningeal irritation associated with headache cannot bend the head or flex the knees without aggravating their pain.

Body Movements. Abnormalities of body movement may be of two general kinds: generalized disruption of voluntary or involuntary movement and asymmetry of movement. The first category includes tremors of a wide variety; some tremor may occur at rest (Parkinson's disease), whereas others occur only on voluntary movement (cerebellar ataxia). Other tremors may exist during both rest and activity (alcohol withdrawal delirium, thyrotoxicosis). Some voluntary or involuntary movements are fine, others quite coarse. At the extreme are the convulsive movements of epilepsy or tetanus and the gross choreiform (involuntary and irregular) movements of patients with rheumatic fever or Huntington's disease.

Asymmetry of movement, in which only one side of the body is affected, is seen in patients with disease of the central nervous system (CNS), principally in those who have had cerebral vascular accidents (strokes). The patient may manifest drooping of one side of the face or be incapable of normal movement of the right or left upper and lower extremities. Strength is impaired on the involved side, and the person walks with a foot-dragging gait.

Nutrition. Nutritional status is important to note. Obesity may be generalized as a function of excessive intake of calories or may be specifically localized to the trunk in those with endocrine disorders (Cushing's disease) or those who have been taking steroids for long periods of time. Loss of weight may be generalized as a function of caloric deprivation or may be reflected more strikingly in loss of muscle mass in people whose diseases interfere with protein synthesis. A more detailed discussion of nutritional assessment is presented later in this chapter.

Speech Pattern. Speech may be slurred because of CNS disease or because of incapacity to articulate as a result of damage to cranial nerves. Damage to the recurrent laryngeal nerve will produce hoarseness, as will those diseases that produce edema or swelling of the vocal cords. Speech may be halting, slurred, or interrupted in flow in some CNS disorders (multiple sclerosis).

Body Temperature. The recording of body temperature is a part of every physical examination. Fever is an increase in body temperature above normal. A normal oral temperature for most persons is an average of 37.0°C (98.6°F). It should be recognized that there is some variation that is still within the range of normal. Some people's temperatures are quite normal at 36.6°C (98°F) and others at 37.3°C (99°F). Children playing hard during summer months quite regularly run temperatures as high as 37.7°C (100°F) and occasionally higher, but this should decrease quickly with rest. Moreover, it should be recognized that there is a normal diurnal variation of a degree or two in body temperature throughout the day. Most persons achieve their low temperature early in the morning. Body temperature rises during the day to 37.3° to 37.5°C (99° to 99.5°F) and then subsides through the night.

Palpation

Palpation is a vital part of the physical examination. Many structures of the body, although not visible, are accessible by the hand and may be assessed through touch (Fig. 7-1). Examples include superficial blood vessels, lymph nodes, the thyroid, the organs of the abdomen and pelvis, and the rectum. It should be noted that when the abdomen is examined, auscultation is performed *before* palpation and percussion to avoid altering bowel sounds.

Sounds generated within the body, if within specified frequency ranges, also may be detected through touch. Thus, certain murmurs generated in the heart or within blood vessels (thrills) may be detected. Thrills cause a sensation to the hand much like the purring of a cat. Voice sounds are transmitted along the bronchi to the periphery of the lung. These may be perceived by touch and will be

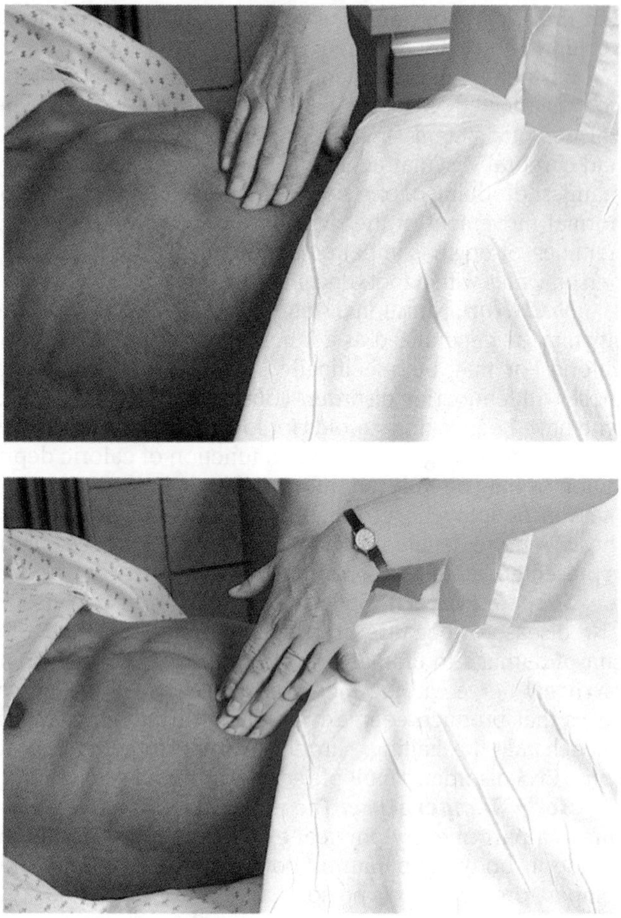

FIGURE 7-1. Palpation technique showing light palpation (**top**) and deep palpation (**bottom**). (Photo © Ken Kasper.)

altered by certain disease states within the lung. The phenomenon is called **tactile fremitus** and is useful in assessing diseases of the chest. The significance of these findings is discussed in the relevant chapters of this book.

Percussion

The technique of percussion translates the application of physical force into sound. It is a difficult skill to perfect but one capable of yielding much information about disease processes in the chest and abdomen. The principle is to set the chest wall or abdominal wall into vibration by striking it with a firm object. The sound produced is reflective of the density of the underlying structure. Certain densities produce sounds that can be identified as percussion notes. These sounds, listed in a sequence that proceeds from the least to the most dense, are called **tympany, hyperresonance, resonance, dullness,** and **flatness.**

Tympany is the drumlike sound produced by percussing the air-filled stomach. **Resonance** is the sound elicited over air-filled lungs. **Hyperresonance** is audible when one percusses over inflated lung tissue in someone with emphysema. Percussion of the liver produces a **dull sound**, whereas percussion of the thigh results in **flatness.**

The procedure for percussing for right-handed persons (hands should be reversed if the examiner is left-handed) is conducted as follows (Fig. 7-2). The distal phalanx (distal portion) of the left middle finger is placed firmly against the chest wall. The other fingers should be held away from the chest wall, because any pressure they might exert against the thorax would tend to mute or dampen the sound produced. The right hand now becomes the striking object. The middle finger of the right hand is used to strike the terminal phalanx of the middle finger of the left hand just behind the nail bed. If the action is performed sharply, a brief resonant tone will be produced. The motion of the right hand should be predominantly a wrist action. The forearm itself should be held steady. The clarity of the sound produced is dependent on the brevity of the action. The intensity is a function of the force used.

Percussion gives one the capacity to assess such normal anatomic details as the degree to which the diaphragm descends during inspiration. The sound over lung tissue is normally resonant; the sound over the diaphragm is dull. One may percuss the border of the heart. One may determine the level of pleural effusion (fluid in the pleural cavity) or the location of a consolidated area caused by pneumonia or atelectasis (collapse) of a lobe of the lung. Further application of the technique is discussed under examination of the thorax and abdomen.

Auscultation

Sound is produced within the body either by the movement of air through hollow structures or by the forces set up by the movement of columns of fluid that set solid structures in motion. Examples include the movement of air through the trachea and bronchi (breath sounds), the movement of air past functioning vocal cords (spoken voice), the movement of air through the intestines (bowel sounds), the movement of blood through vascular structures that provide critical resistance to flow (murmurs), and the impedance to flowing blood provided by closed valves and the heart wall (heart sounds). Physiologic sounds may be normal (*e.g.*, first and second heart sounds) or pathologic (*e.g.*, murmurs in diastole produced in the heart, or crackles in the lung). Some normal sounds may be distorted by pathology of structures

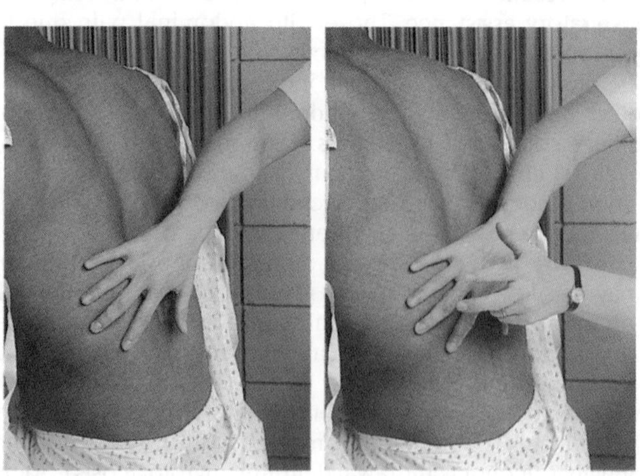

FIGURE 7-2. Percussion technique. The middle finger of one hand strikes the terminal phalanx of the middle finger of the other hand. (Photo © Ken Kasper.)

through which the sound must travel (*e.g.*, changes in the character of breath sounds as they travel through the consolidated lung of the patient with lobar pneumonia).

Sound produced within the body, if of sufficient amplitude, will set in vibration all structures between the origin of the sound and the body surface. Sound vibrations emanating from the body surface may be captured directly by the examiner's ear or, more appropriately, by the stethoscope, an instrument that functions as an extension of the human ear.

Although the **stethoscope** does not have the capacity to amplify sound, it does channel sound, thereby making physiologic sound more readily available for critical evaluation. Two end-pieces are available for the stethoscope: the **bell** and the **diaphragm** (Fig. 7-3). Many stethoscopes come with both pieces built into a single head. Alternating between the two pieces becomes a matter of turning the head of the stethoscope or flipping a switch. The bell is a small disc mounted on a conical base; it is attached to a larger disc, the diaphragm. The bell is better suited for the transmission of very low-frequency sounds. It is important to place the bell so that the entire surface of the disc rests lightly on the skin surface, to avoid flattening the skin and reducing audible vibratory sensations. The diaphragm, the larger disc, is constructed for the reception of high-frequency sounds. It is placed firmly against the skin for optimal transmission of sound.

The head of the stethoscope is held between the index and middle fingers to provide a firm contact with the skin surface (Fig. 7-4). Care is taken to avoid touching the tubing or rubbing other surfaces (hair, clothing) during auscultation to minimize extraneous noises. The earpieces of the stethoscope should fit snugly into the ear canals, and the tubing should not be more than 20 cm in length. Dual tubing transmits sound more faithfully than single tubing.

Sound produced by the body, like any other sound, is characterized by intensity, frequency, and quality. The **intensity**, or loudness, associated with physiologic sound is low. Rarely may sounds of the body, except for speech, be heard without direct application of the ear or the stethoscope to the body surface. With respect to **frequency,** or pitch, it may be said that physiologic sound is in reality "noise," in that most sounds consist of a frequency spectrum as opposed to single-frequency sounds that we associate with music or the tuning fork. The frequency spectrum may be quite low, yielding a rumbling noise, or comparatively high, producing a harsh or blowing sound. The third feature of sound is **quality**. This relates to overtones and is the characteristic of sound that allows one to differentiate sound produced by the piano from that produced by the violin. Sound quality enables the examiner to distinguish between the musical quality of high-pitched wheezing and the low-pitched rumbling of a diastolic murmur.

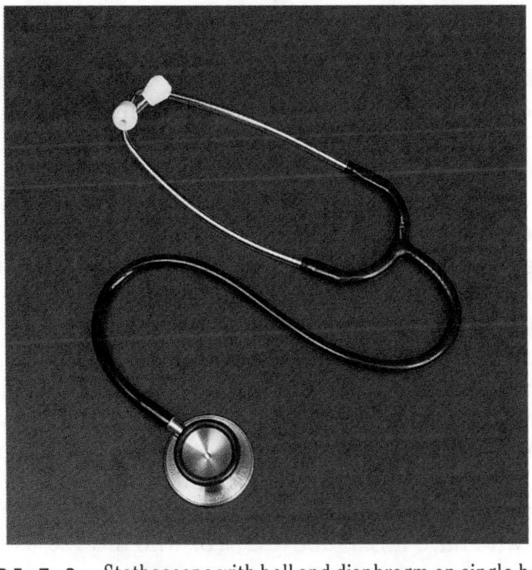

FIGURE 7-3. Stethoscope with bell and diaphragm on single head.

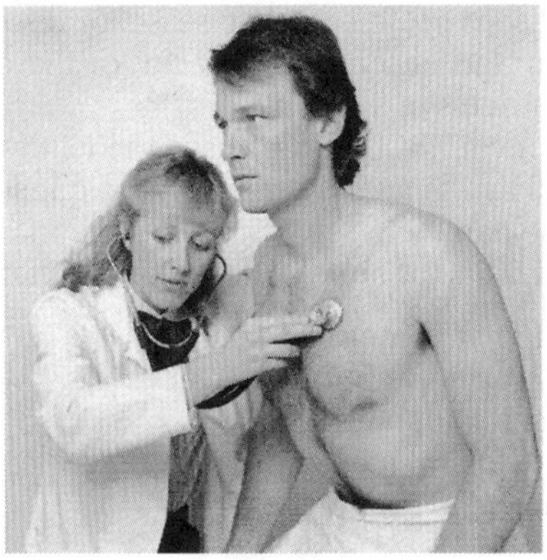

FIGURE 7-4. Auscultation technique for examining heart. (From Fuller J and Schaller-Ayers J. Health Assessment: A Nursing Approach, 2nd ed. Philadelphia, JB Lippincott, 1994.)

The Nutritional Assessment

Nutrition plays an important role in maintaining health and preventing disease. Although diseases caused by nutritional deficiency are less frequent than they once were, they have been replaced in frequency by diseases caused by overeating or eating poorly balanced meals, which contribute to the leading causes of illness and death in the United States today. Examples of health problems associated with dietary excess, imbalance, or inadequate consumption of specific nutrients include obesity, coronary artery disease, osteoporosis, cirrhosis, diverticulitis, and eating disorders. When illness or injury occurs, nutrition is an essential factor in promoting healing and resisting infection. Assessment of the person's nutritional status provides information on obesity, undernutrition, weight loss, malnutrition, deficiencies in specific nutrients, metabolic abnormalities, the effects of medications on nutrition, and special problems of the hospitalized patient and the person who is cared for in the home and in community settings.

Certain signs and symptoms that suggest possible nutritional deficiency are easy to note because they are specific. However, other physical signs may have no relation to poor diet and must be carefully distinguished from nutritional deficiencies. A physical sign that suggests a nutritional abnormality should be considered a clue rather than a diagnosis and as such should be pursued further. For example, certain signs that may appear to indicate nutritional deficiency may actually reflect other systemic conditions, such as endocrine disorders, infectious disease, or disorders affecting digestion and absorption capacity or the excretion or storage of nutrients in the body.

The acronym ABCD may be used to identify parameters of nutritional assessment. Although the sequence of assessment of these parameters may vary, evaluation of nutritional status includes one or more of the following methods:

1. **A**nthropometric measurement
   Weight/height and body mass index
   Triceps skinfold thickness
   Midarm and arm muscle circumferences
2. **B**iochemical measurements
   Albumin
   Transferrin
   Total lymphocyte count
   Electrolyte levels
   Creatinine/height index
3. **C**linical examination findings
4. **D**ietary data

Anthropometric Measurements

The most common anthropometric measurements include height, weight, and the circumferences of the upper arm and arm muscle. When anthropometric measurements are gathered as part of data collection, standardized equipment and procedures are used, as well as standard measurement guides. Although such measurements focus on undernutrition, they also detect obesity. Chart 7-1 provides guidelines for calculating ideal body weight. Chart 7-2 provides a guide to determine frame size.

CHART 7-1
Guidelines for Calculating Ideal Body Weight

Women

- Allow 100 lbs for 5 ft of height
- Add 5 lbs for each additional inch over 5 feet
- Subtract 10% for small frame; add 10% for large frame

Men

- Allow 106 lbs for each 5 feet of height
- Add 6 lbs for each additional inch over 5 feet
- Subtract 10% for small frame, add 10% for large frame

Example: IBW for a 5'6" adult is

	Female	**Male**
5' of height	100 lbs	106 lbs
Per additional inch	6" × 5 lbs/inch = 30 lb	6" × 6 lbs/inch = 36 lb
Ideal body weight	130 lbs ± 13 lb depending on frame size	142 lbs ± 14 lb depending on frame size

(Dudek SG. Nutrition Handbook for Nursing Practice, 2nd ed. Philadelphia, JB Lippincott, 1993.)

CHART 7-2
Guidelines for Calculating Frame Size

- Measure height in centimeters
- Measure wrist circumference in centimeters by placing a tape measure around the wrist where it bends at the styloid process
- Calculate the ratio of height to wrist circumference to estimate frame size

Height (cm)/Wrist circumference (cm)

	Female	**Male**
Small frame	>11	>10.4
Medium frame	10.1 – 11	9.6 – 10.4
Large frame	<10.1	<9.6

Example: Height = 5'10"(178 cm) adult

Wrist circumference = 6.2"(15.4 cm)
178/15.4 = 11.6
Result: A ratio of 11.6 indicates a small frame for females and males

(Based on Fuller J and Schaller-Ayers J. Health Assessment: A Nursing Approach. Philadelphia, JB Lippincott, 1994.)

Weight loss is an extremely important measurement because it reflects inadequate calorie intake. In someone who is semistarved, weight loss indicates an increased loss of protein from the body cell mass. Decreased height may be considered an indication of osteoporosis, an important problem related to nutrition, especially in older women. A loss of 2 or 3 inches of height may indicate osteoporosis.

Measurement of skinfold thickness and arm and muscle circumference is described in Figures 7-5 and 7-6. **Triceps skinfold thickness** (TSF) indicates fat stores. **Midarm muscle circumference** (MAMC), calculated from midarm circumference (MAC) and TSF, indicates the state of muscle protein. Thus, these measures provide information about protein–calorie malnutrition. The calculation for midarm muscle circumference is as follows:

$$\text{MAMC (cm)} = \text{MAC (cm)} - [0.314 \times \text{TSF(mm)}]$$

The TSF, MAC, and MAMC values obtained from these procedures (Table 7-1) are compared with the standards for anthropometric measurements to assess the person's nutritional status.

Body mass index (BMI) is a weight-to-height ratio composed of the body weight (in kilograms) divided by the square of the height (in meters). The obtained value is then compared to the established standards; however, trends or changes in values over time are considered more useful than isolated or one-time measurements. The BMI is highly correlated with body fat, but increased lean body mass or a large body frame can also increase the BMI. Individuals who have a BMI below 24 (or who are 80% or less of their desirable body weight for height) are at increased risk for poor nutritional status and the problems associated with it. Those who have a BMI above 27 (or who are 120% or more

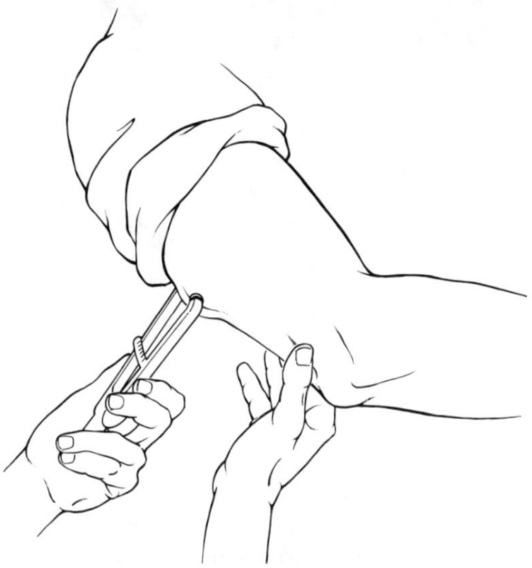

FIGURE 7-5. Measurement of triceps skinfold thickness. The nondominant arm is used for measurement. The midpoint of the arm is located; this is the midpoint between the acromial process of the scapula (at the top of the humerus) and the olecranon process of the ulna (elbow). With the arm hanging loosely at the side, a double fold of skin (not muscle) is grasped by the calipers. The measurement is recorded in millimeters.

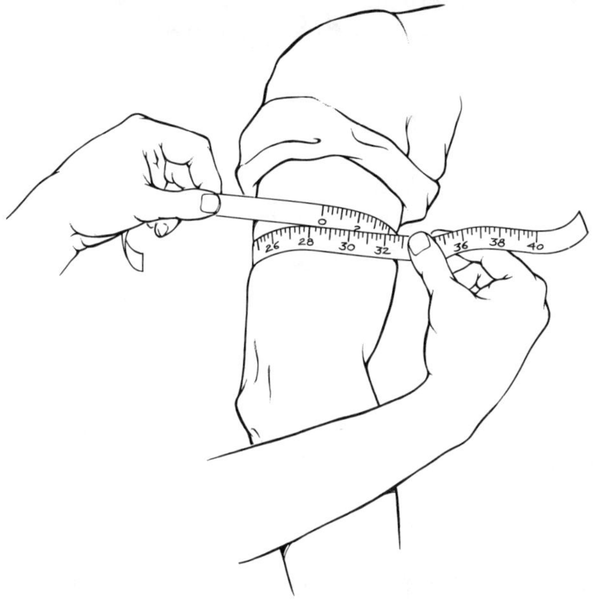

FIGURE 7-6. Measurement of midarm circumference. A flexible tape is placed midway between the top of the acromial process of the scapula and the olecranon process of the ulna; the tape is held firmly but gently to avoid compressing the soft tissue. The measurement is recorded in centimeters.

of their desirable body weight) are considered obese and are at high risk for problems associated with obesity (hypertension, diabetes, osteoarthritis.)

Biochemical Assessment

Biochemical assessment reflects both the tissue level of a given nutrient and any abnormality of metabolism in the utilization of nutrients. These determinations are made from studies of serum (serum protein, serum albumin and globulin, transferrin hemoglobin, serum vitamin A, carotene, and vitamin C) and from urine (creatinine, thiamine, riboflavin, niacin, and iodine). Some of these tests, while reflecting recent intake of the elements detected, can also identify below-normal levels when there are no clinical symptoms of deficiency. (See Table 7-2 for a guide for the interpretation of laboratory data.)

Low serum **albumin** and **transferrin** levels are often used as measures of protein deficits in adults and are expressed as percentages of normal values. Albumin synthesis depends on normal liver function and an adequate supply of amino acids. Because the body stores a large amount of albumin, albumin serum level may not decrease until

TABLE 7-1 Standard and Decreased Values for Anthropometric Measurements for Adults

	Standard	90% of Standard	70% Reference
Triceps Skinfold Thickness (mm)			
Men	12.5	11.3	8.8
Women	16.5	14.9	11.6
Midarm Circumference (cm)			
Men	29.3	26.3	20.5
Women	28.5	25.7	20.0
Midarm Muscle Circumference (cm)			
Men	25.3	22.8	17.7
Women	23.2	20.9	16.2

(Based on Dudek SG. Nutrition Handbook for Nursing Practice, 2nd ed. Philadelphia, JB Lippincott, 1993.)

TABLE 7-2 Standards for Laboratory Indices

Serum Values	Normal Ranges	Percent Deficiency		
		Mild	Moderate	Severe
Albumin (g/dl)	3.5–5	3.2–3.5	2.8–3.2	< 2.8
Transferrin (mg/dl)	230–400	180–200	160–180	< 160
Total lymphocyte count (number/mm^3)	1500–4000	1800–5000	900–1500	< 900

(Adapted from Steffee WP. Nutritional support of elderly patients. Clin Consult Nutr Support 1982; 2(5), by Nelson R. Nutrition and aging. Med Clin North Am 1989; 73(6):1541.)

malnutrition is severe; thus, its usefulness in detecting recent protein depletion is limited. Decreased albumin levels may also occur with liver or renal disease, congestive heart failure, and excessive protein loss because of burns, major surgery, infection, and cancer. Transferrin is a protein that binds and carries iron from the intestine through the serum. Because of its short half-life, decreased transferrin levels respond more quickly to protein depletion than albumin. Serial measurements of these, as well as **prealbumin** levels, are used to assess the results of nutritional therapy.

Reduced numbers of **lymphocytes** in people who become acutely malnourished as a result of stress and low-calorie feeding are associated with impairment of cellular immunity. Anergy, the absence of an immune response to injection of small concentrations of recall antigen under the skin, may also indicate malnutrition because of delayed antibody synthesis and response.

Information about **electrolyte balance** provides an assessment of kidney function as a metabolic response to infused electrolytes. The **creatinine/height index** calculated over a 24-hour period assesses the metabolically active tissue and indicates the degree of protein depletion, comparing expected body mass for height and actual body cell mass. A 24-hour urine sample is obtained and the amount of creatinine is measured and compared to normal ranges based on the patient's height and gender. Values less than normal may indicate loss of lean body mass and protein malnutrition.

Clinical Examination

The state of nutrition is often reflected in a person's appearance. Although the most obvious physical sign of good nutrition is a normal body weight with respect to height, body frame, and age, other tissues can serve as indicators of general nutritional status and adequate intake of specific nutrients; these include the hair, skin, teeth, gums, mucous membranes, mouth and tongue, skeletal muscles, abdomen, lower extremities, and thyroid gland (Table 7-3). Specific clinical examination parameters useful in identifying a person with nutritional deficits include oral examination and assessment of skin for turgor, edema, elasticity, dryness, subcutaneous tone, poorly healing wounds and ulcers, purpura, and bruises. Additionally, the musculoskeletal examination will provide information about muscle-wasting and weakness.

Dietary Intake

The appraisal of food intake considers the quantity and quality of the diet and also the frequency in which certain food items are consumed in order to determine current or customary intake of nutrients. Commonly used methods of determining individual eating patterns include the food record and the 24-hour food recall, which can help estimate if the food intake is adequate and appropriate. If these tools are used, instructions for keeping the records are given when the patient's diet history is obtained.

Food Record. The food record is used most often in nutritional status studies. The person is asked to keep a record of food actually consumed over a period of time, varying from 3 to 7 days. Some instructions are given for accurately estimating and describing the specific foods consumed. This method appears to be fairly accurate, depending on the subject's willingness to provide factual information and ability to estimate quantity of food.

24-Hour Recall. The 24-hour recall method is, as the name implies, a recall of food intake over a 24-hour period. The person is asked by the interviewer to recall all food eaten during the previous day and to estimate the quantities of the food consumed. Information obtained by this method does not always represent usual intake. For this reason, at the end of the interview the patient is asked if the previous day's food intake was a typical one. To obtain supplementary information about the typical diet, the interviewer should also ask how frequently foods from the major food groups are eaten.

Conducting the Interview

As was indicated in the chapter on interviewing techniques, it is important that the interviewer establish rapport with the person in order to promote respect and trust. The success of the interviewer in eliciting pertinent information for dietary assessment depends on the quality of communication established at the outset.

In the initial stages, the interviewer introduces and explains the purpose of the interview. The rest of the session is conducted in a nondirective and exploratory way, allowing the respondent to express his or her feelings and thoughts. At the same time, the respondent is encouraged to answer specific questions.

TABLE 7-3 Physical Signs Indicative of Nutritional Status

	Signs of Good Nutrition	Signs of Poor Nutrition
General appearance	Alert, responsive	Listless, appears acutely or chronically ill
Hair	Shiny, lustrous; firm, healthy scalp	Dull and dry, brittle, depigmented, easily plucked; thin and sparse
Face	Skin color uniform; healthy appearance	Skin dark over cheeks and under eyes, skin flaky, face swollen or hollow/sunken cheeks
Eyes	Bright, clear, moist	Eye membranes pale, dry (xerophthalmia); increased vascularity, cornea soft (keratomalacia)
Lips	Good color (pink), smooth	Swollen and puffy; angular lesion at corners of mouth (cheilosis)
Tongue	Deep red in appearance; surface papillae present	Smooth appearance, swollen, beefy red, sores, atrophic papillae
Teeth	Straight, no crowding, no dental caries, bright	Dental caries, mottled appearance (fluorosis), malpositioned
Gums	Firm, good color (pink)	Spongy, bleed easily, marginal redness, recession
Glands	No enlargement of the thyroid	Thyroid enlargement (simple goiter)
Skin	Smooth, good color, moist	Rough, dry, flaky, swollen, pale, pigmented; lack of fat under skin
Nails	Firm, pink	Spoon-shaped, ridged, brittle
Skeleton	Good posture, no malformation	Poor posture, beading of ribs, bowed legs or knock knees
Muscles	Well developed, firm	Flaccid, poor tone, wasted, underdeveloped
Extremities	No tenderness	Weak and tender; edematous
Abdomen	Flat	Swollen
Nervous system	Normal reflexes	Decreased or absent ankle and knee reflexes
Weight	Normal for height, age, and body build	Overweight or underweight

The manner in which a question is asked will influence the extent to which the respondent will cooperate. To this end, the interviewer should be nonjudgmental and must avoid expressing disapproval, either directly by comment or indirectly by facial expression.

Sometimes several questions are necessary to elicit the information needed. Consider the following exchange:

Interviewer: "What time did you get out of bed yesterday?"
Respondent: "I got up at 6 o'clock in the morning and I had a cup of coffee."
Interviewer: "Did you put anything in your coffee?"
Respondent: "Only a teaspoon of sugar, nothing else."
Interviewer: "Did you have anything else with your coffee?"
Respondent: "No, not at that time. I had breakfast later, around 8 o'clock in the morning."

When attempting to elicit information about the type and quantity of food eaten at a particular time, the interviewer should not ask a leading question, such as "Did you put sugar or cream in your coffee?" Also, assumptions should not be made about the size of servings. Instead, questions should be phrased so that quantities are more clearly determined. For example, to help determine the size of one hamburger eaten, the following question may be asked: "How many hamburgers were prepared out of the pound of ground meat you bought?" Another approach to determining quantities is to use food models of known sizes in estimating portions of meat, cake, or pie or to record quantities in common measurements, such as cups or spoonfuls (or according to the size of containers, when discussing intake of bottled beverages).

In recording a particular combination dish, such as a casserole, it is useful to ask for the ingredients in the recipe, recording the largest quantities first. When recording quantities of ingredients, one notes if the quantity of the food item was raw or cooked and the number of servings provided by the recipe. When the client has finished listing the foods for the recall questionnaire, it may be helpful to read the list of foods back and ask if anything was forgotten, such as fruit, cake, candy, between-meal snacks, or cocktails.

Additional information obtained during the interview should include methods of preparing food, sources available for food (donated foods, food stamps), food-buying practices, vitamin and mineral supplements, and income range.

Cultural Considerations

An individual's culture determines to a large extent what foods are eaten and how they are prepared and served. Culture and religion together often determine if certain foods are prohibited and if certain foods and spices are eaten on certain holidays or at specific family gatherings. Because of the importance of culture and religious beliefs to many individuals, it is important to be sensitive to these factors when obtaining a dietary history. It is, however, equally important not to stereotype individuals and assume that because they are from a certain culture or religion that they adhere to specific dietary customs.

Evaluating the Dietary Information

Once the dietary information has been obtained, the diet must be evaluated for its nutritive value. The choice of a method for dietary evaluation depends on the purpose of the assessment. If the goal is to determine if the person generally eats a healthful diet, the food intake is compared to the Dietary Guidelines outlined in the Food Guide Pyramid (Fig. 7-7). The Food Guide Pyramid was released by the U.S Department of Agriculture and the Department of Health and Human Services. The pyramid divides foods into five major groups and offers recommendations for variety in the diet, proportion of food from each food group, and moderation in eating fats, oils, and sweets. The person's food intake is compared with recommendations based on various food groups for various age levels.

If the nurse or dietitian is interested in knowing about the intake of specific nutrients, such as vitamin A, iron, or calcium, then the patient's food intake would be analyzed by consulting an official publication listing foods according to composition and nutrient content. The diet is then calculated in terms of grams and milligrams of specific nutrients. The total nutritive value is then compared with the Recommended Dietary Allowances, or RDAs (Table 7-4), and the nutritional evaluation is expressed in terms of percentage of adequacy for each nutrient.

The nurse frequently participates in the nutrition screening of patients and communicates the information to the dietitian and the rest of the team for more detailed assessment and for clinical nutrition intervention.

Factors Influencing Nutritional Status in Varied Settings

Many disease conditions produce metabolic alterations that result in **negative nitrogen balance** (when nitrogen output exceeds nitrogen intake). When these conditions are coupled with anorexia (loss of appetite), they can lead to malnutrition. It is known that malnutrition interferes with wound healing, increases susceptibility to infection, and contributes to an increased incidence of complications, lengthier hospital stay, and prolonged confinement of the patient to bed.

Although home-cooked meals are generally considered more appealing than hospital food, an advantage of being hospitalized is that food is provided even if the patient is unable to obtain and prepare the food. The person who is at home may feel too sick or fatigued to shop and prepare food or may be unable to eat because of other physical problems or limitations. In addition, people with limited or fixed incomes or those who must buy several kinds of medications may not have enough money to purchase nutritious foods.

Because complex treatments (such as those requiring ventilators, intravenous infusions, etc.) that were once used only in the hospital setting and are now being provided in the home, nutritional assessment of the patient cared for in the home is as important as that of the hospitalized patient. Many of the factors that contribute to poor nutritional status are identified in Chart 7-3.

Many medications also influence nutritional status by depressing the appetite, irritating the mucosa, or causing nausea and vomiting. Others may influence bacterial flora in the intestine or directly affect nutrient absorption so that secondary malnutrition results. Because of the effects of medications on nutritional status, it is important to assess the person's use of prescription and over-the-counter medications.

The body in starvation may convert protein to glucose for energy; the result is persistent loss of muscle tissue. One sensitive indicator of the body's gain or loss of protein is its **nitrogen balance**. An adult is said to be in **nitrogen equilibrium** when the nitrogen intake (from food) equals the nitrogen output (in urine, feces, and perspiration); it is a sign of health. A **positive nitrogen balance** exists when nitrogen intake exceeds nitrogen output and indicates tissue growth, such as occurs during pregnancy, childhood, recovery from surgery, and rebuilding of wasted tissue. **Negative nitrogen balance** indicates that tissue is breaking down faster than it is being replaced. It can be brought about by fever, surgery, burns, and other debilitating diseases, as well as by starvation. For instance, each gram of nitrogen loss in excess of intake represents the depletion of 6.25 g of protein or 25 g of muscle tissue. Therefore, a negative nitrogen balance of 10 g/day for 10 days could mean the wasting of 2.5 kg (5.5 pounds) of muscle tissue.

Analysis of Nutritional Status

Anthropometric, biochemical, clinical, and dietary data are used together to determine the patient's nutritional status. Often the anthropometric and biochemical measures and dietary data provide more information about the patient's nutritional status than the clinical examination because the clinical examination may not detect subclinical deficiencies unless such deficiencies become so advanced that overt signs develop. A low dietary intake of nutrients over a period of time may lead to low biochemical levels and, without nutritional intervention, may result in characteristic and observable signs and symptoms (see Table 7-3). A plan of action for nutritional intervention is based on the results of the dietary assessment and the client's profile. Objectives derived from the nutritional assessment and evaluation are:

- Appropriate food selection for a balanced diet
- Appropriate food intake for weight control

Gerontologic Considerations

It has been estimated that one in four elderly persons is malnourished. Elderly people who are malnourished tend to have longer and more expensive hospital stays than those who are adequately fed; the risk of costly complications is also increased in those who are malnourished. As the proportion of elderly persons in the population increases, the

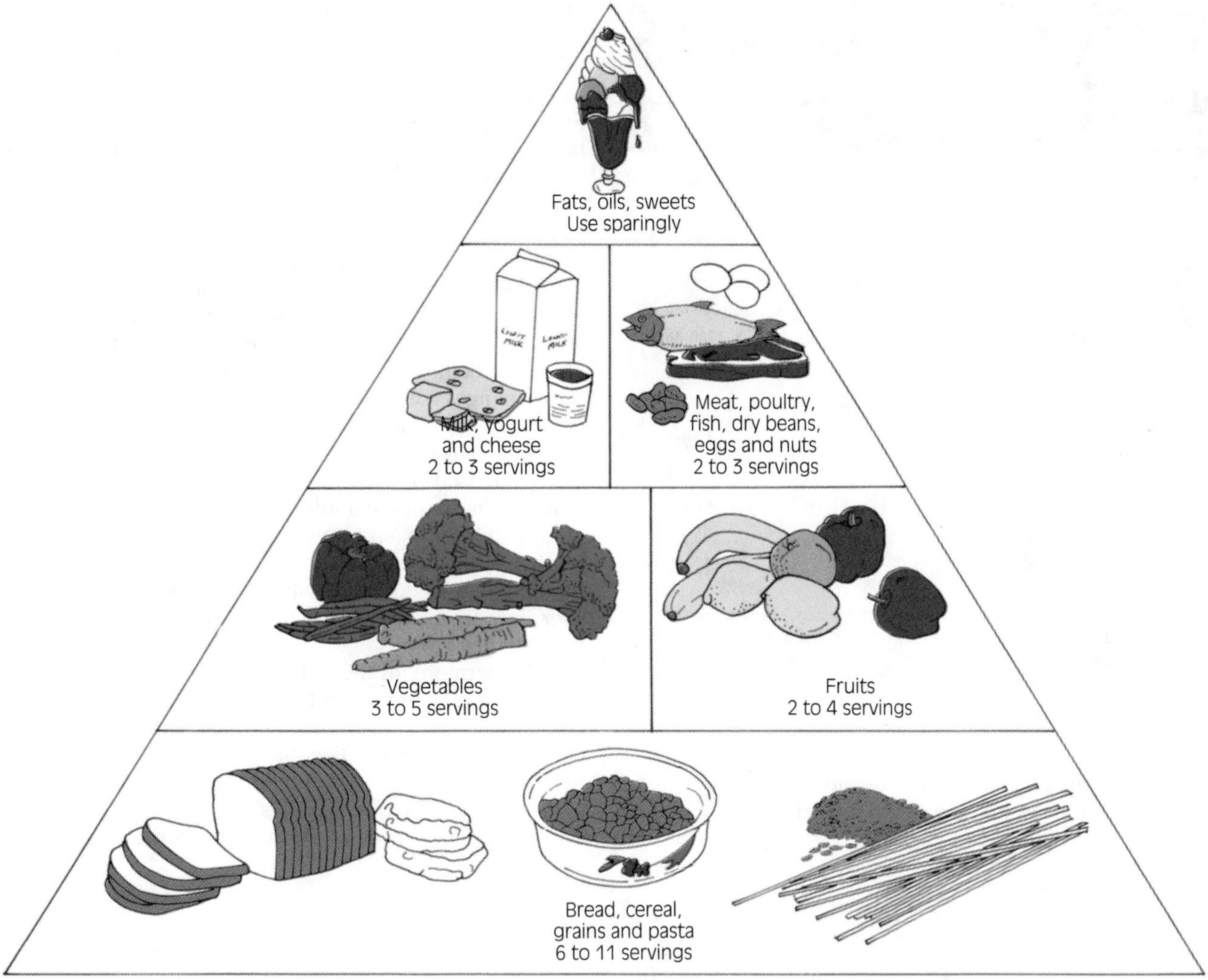

What Counts as 1 Serving?

The amount of food that counts as 1 serving is listed below. If you eat a larger portion, count it as more than 1 serving. For example, a dinner portion of spaghetti would count as 2 or 3 servings of pasta.

Be sure to eat at least the lowest number of servings from the five major food groups listed below. You need them for the vitamins, minerals, carbohydrates, and protein they provide. Just try to pick the lowest fat choices from the food groups. No specific serving size is given for the fats, oils, and sweets group because the message is USE SPARINGLY.

Food Groups

Milk, Yogurt, and Cheese

1 cup of milk or yogurt	1½ ounces of natural cheese	2 ounces of process cheese

Meat, Poultry, Fish, Dry Beans, Eggs, and Nuts

2–3 ounces of cooked lean meat, poultry, or fish	½ cup of cooked dry beans, 1 egg, or 2 tablespoons of peanut butter count as 1 ounce of lean meat

Vegetable

1 cup of raw leafy vegetables	½ cup of other vegetables, cooked or chopped raw	¾ cup of vegetable juice

Fruit

1 medium apple, banana, orange	½ cup of chopped or cooked, or canned fruit	¾ cup of fruit juice

Bread, Cereal, Rice, and Pasta

1 slice of bread	1 ounce of ready-to-eat cereal	½ cup of cooked cereal, rice, or pasta

FIGURE 7-7. The Food Guide Pyramid emphasizes foods from the five major food groups shown in the three lower sections of the Pyramid. Each of these food groups provides some, but not all, of the nutrients you need. Foods in one group cannot replace those in another. No one of these major food groups is more important than another. (Source: U.S. Department of Agriculture/U.S. Department of Health and Human Services.)

TABLE 7-4 Food and Nutrition Board, National Academy of Sciences: National Research Council Recommended Daily Dietary Allowances for Adults, Revised 1989

Nutrient	Male	Female
Vitamin B_6	2.0 mg	1.6 mg
Vitamin B_{12}	2.0 μg	2.0 μg
Calcium (age 25 and older)	800 mg	800 mg
Calcium (11–24 years of age)	1200 mg	1200mg
Vitamin C	60 mg	60 mg
Folate	200 μg	180 μg
Vitamin K	80 μg	65 μg
Iron	10 mg	15 mg
Magnesium	350 mg	280 mg
Selenium	70 μg	55 μg
Zinc	15 mg	12 mg

(Data from National Research Council. Recommended Dietary Allowances, 10th ed. Washington, DC, National Academy Press, 1989. Copyright 1989 by the National Academy of Sciences.)

importance of assessing the nutritional status of the elderly will increase.

Inadequate dietary intake in the elderly may result from physiologic changes in the gastrointestinal tract, social and economic factors, drug interactions, disease, excessive use of alcohol, and poor dentition or missing teeth. Malnutrition is a common consequence of these factors and in turn leads to illness and frailty of the elderly. Important aspects of care of the elderly in the hospital, home, or extended care facility include recognizing risk factors and identifying those at risk for inadequate nutrition. The goal of diet therapy in the elderly is to maintain nutrition and replace nutrient losses in order to maintain the individual's health and well-being.

Elderly persons may take excessive and inappropriate medications; this is referred to as **"polypharmacy."** The number of adverse reactions increases proportionately with the number of prescribed and over-the-counter medications taken. Age-related physiologic and pathophysiologic changes may alter the metabolism and elimination of many agents. Consequently, medications can influence food intake by producing side effects such as nausea, vomiting, decreased appetite, and changes in sensorium. They may alter nutrient metabolism by interfering with the distribution, utilization, and storage of nutrients. Disorders affecting any part of the gastrointestinal tract can alter nutritional requirements and health status in people of any age; however, they are likely to occur quickly and more frequently in the elderly.

Furthermore, in the elderly, nutritional problems often occur or are precipitated by such illnesses as pneumonia and urinary tract infections. Like malnutrition, acute and chronic diseases may affect the metabolism and utilization of nutrients, which already are altered because of the aging process. Use of antibiotics, appropriate vaccines, and other preventive measures (Meals on Wheels) may reduce

CHART 7-3

Factors Associated With Potential Nutritional Deficits in Hospitalized and Home Care Patients

Factors	Possible Consequences
Dental and oral problems	Inadequate intake of high-fiber foods
NPO for diagnostic testing	Inadequate caloric and protein intake; dehydration
Prolonged use of glucose and saline IV fluids	Inadequate caloric and protein intake
Nausea and vomiting	Inadequate caloric and protein intake; loss of fluid, electrolytes and minerals
Stress of illness, surgery and/or hospitalization	Increased protein and caloric requirement; increased catabolism
Wound drainage	Loss of protein, fluid, electrolytes, and minerals
Pain	Loss of appetite; inability to shop, cook, eat
Fever	Increased caloric and fluid requirement; increased catabolism
Gastrointestinal intubation	Loss of protein, fluid, and minerals
Tube feedings	Inadequate amounts; various nutrients in each formula
Gastrointestinal disease	Inadequate intake and malabsorption of nutrients
Alcoholism	Inadequate intake of nutrients; increased consumption of calories without other nutrients; vitamin deficiencies
Depression	Loss of appetite; inability to shop, cook, eat
Eating disorders (anorexia, bulimia)	Inadequate caloric and protein intake; loss of fluid, electrolytes, and minerals
Medications	Inadequate intake due to dry mouth, loss of appetite, decreased taste perception, difficulty swallowing, nausea and vomiting, physical problems that limit shopping, cooking, eating; malabsorption of nutrients

CRITICAL THINKING EXERCISES

1. Compare the approaches you would use in assessing a patient who is experiencing severe acute pain; is blind or hard of hearing; is mentally retarded; is from a culture with very different values from yours.
2. Your nutritional assessment reveals that your patient has an inadequate protein intake. How would you develop dietary instructions for the patient who is a vegetarian? For the elderly patient with a fixed income? For the patient who has an intolerance for dairy foods?
3. The findings of your physical and nutritional assessment of an 18-year-old college student suggests to you that she may have an eating disorder. How would you further assess this patient and develop a plan of management for her?

the incidence of infection and minimize the risk of illness-associated malnutrition.

Even the well elderly may be nutritionally at risk because of limited ability to shop and cook, financial hardship, and the fact that they often eat alone. Additionally, reduction in exercise with age without concomitant changes in carbohydrate intake places the elderly at risk for obesity.

The American Nurses Association has participated in a national, multidisciplinary effort to promote routine nutrition screening for older Americans through the Nutrition Screening Initiative. Easy-to-use screening tools have been developed to assist in identifying older individuals at risk for poor nutrition and in responding to poor nutrition in the elderly. Information about the Nutrition Screening Initiative can be found at the end of this chapter.

BIBLIOGRAPHY

Books

Bates B. A Guide to Physical Examination and History Taking, 5th ed. Philadelphia, JB Lippincott, 1995.

Bowers AC and Thompson JM. Clinical Manual of Health Assessment. St. Louis, CV Mosby, 1988.

DeGowin RL. DeGowin and DeGowin's Diagnostic Examination, 6th ed. New York, McGraw-Hill, 1994.

Dudek SG. Nutrition Handbook for Nursing Practice, 2nd ed. Philadelphia, JB Lippincott, 1993.

Fuller J and Schaller-Ayers J. Health Assessment: A Nursing Approach, 2nd ed. Philadelphia, JB Lippincott, 1994.

Gordon M. Manual of Nursing Diagnosis 1988–1989. St. Louis, CV Mosby, 1989.

Gordon M. Nursing Diagnosis: Process and Application. St. Louis, CV Mosby, 1994.

Midwest Nursing Research Society. Individual, Family and Community Interventions to Improve Exercise and Nutrition Behaviors. Sigma Theta Tau, Indianapolis, 1989.

National Research Council. Recommended Dietary Allowances, 10th ed. Washington, DC, National Academy Press, 1989.

Nutrition Screening Initiative. Nutrition Interventions Manual for Professionals Caring for Older Americans. Executive Summary, 1992.

Nutrition Screening Initiative. Nutrition Screening Manual for Professionals Caring for Older Americans. 1991.

Seidel H et al. Mosby's Guide to Physical Examination. St. Louis, CV Mosby, 1995.

Summers S and Ebbert DW. Ambulatory Surgical Nursing: A Nursing Approach. Philadelphia, JB Lippincott, 1992.

U.S. Department of Health and Human Services, Public Health Service. Surgeon General's Report on Nutrition and Health. Washington, DC, U.S. Government Printing Office, 1988.

Journals

General Assessment

Bishop BS. Pathologic pupillary signs: Self-learning module, Part I. Critical Care Nurse 1991 June; 11(6): 58–63; Part II July-Aug; 11(7): 58–67; Part III Sep; 11(8): 30.

Brown M. How do you spell assessment? Am J Nurs 1991 Sept; 91(9): 55–56.

Finesilver C. Respiratory assessment. RN 1992 Feb; 55(2): 22–29.

Fitzgerald MA. The physical exam. RN 1991 Sept; 54(11): 34–39.

Hartman D and Knudson J. A nursing data base for initial patient assessment. Oncology Nursing Forum 1991 Jan–Feb; 18(1): 125–130.

Holmgren C. Abdominal assessment. RN 1992 Mar; 55(3): 28–33.

Krach P. Discovering the secret: Nursing assessment of elderly alcoholics in the home. J Gerontological Nursing 1990 Nov; 16(11): 32–38.

Larson EB and Ramsbottom-Lucier M. Talking to patients [editorial]. J Gen Internal Med 1992 July–Aug; 7(4): 464–465.

Lipp-Ziff EL et al. Guidelines for use of critical care assessment tool. Critical Care Nurse 1991 June; 11(6): 32.

Lutner RE et al. The automated interview versus the personal interview. Anesthesiology 1991 Sept; 75(3): 394–400.

McConnell EA. Clinical do's and don'ts: Assessing the skin. Nursing '92 1992 April; 22(4): 86.

Nardone DA et al. A model for the diagnostic medical interview: Nonverbal, verbal, and cognitive assessments. J Gen Internal Med 1992 July–Aug; 7(4): 437–442.

National Institutes of Health. National Institutes of Health Consensus Development Conference Statement: Geriatric assessment methods for clinical decision-making. J Am Geriatr Soc 1988 April; 36(4): 342–347.

Pousada L and Leipzig RM. Rapid bedside assessment of postoperative confusion in older patients. Geriatrics 1990 May 45(5): 59–66.

Sackett DL. A primer on the precision and accuracy of the clinical examination. JAMA 1992 May; 267(19): 2638–2644.

Sackett DL. The science of the art of the clinical examination. JAMA 1992 May; 267(19): 2650–2652.

Smith M and Martin F. Domestic violence: Recognition, intervention, and prevention. Med-Surg Nurs 1995 Feb; 4(1): 21–25.

Smith RC and Hoppe RB. The patient's story: Integrating the patient- and physician-centered approaches to interviewing. Annals of Internal Medicine 1991 Sept 15; 115(6): 470–477.

Stiesmeyer JK. A four-step approach to pulmonary assessment. Am J Nurs 1993 Aug; 93(8): 22–28.

Volker DL. Needs assessment and resource identification. Oncology Nursing Forum 1991 Jan–Feb; 18(1): 119–123.

Nutritional Assessment

Blaylock B. Factors contributing to protein-calorie malnutrition in older adults. Medsurg Nursing 1993 Oct; 2(5): 397–401.

Cerrato PL. Assessing your patient's diet. RN 1991 Jan; 54(1): 60–63.

Cerrato PL. Surgery, stress, and metabolism. RN 1991 Aug; 54(8): 63–65.
Cerrato PL. Your elderly patient needs special attention. RN 1990 Sep; 53(9): 77–78, 80, 82.
Chandra RK et al. Nutrition of the elderly. Can Med Assoc J 1991 Dec 1; 145(11): 1475–1487.
Constans T et al. Protein-energy malnutrition in elderly medical patients. J Am Geriatr Soc 1992 Mar; 40(3): 263–268.
Dwyer JT, Gallo JJ and Reichel W. Assessing nutritional status in elderly patients. Am Fam Physician 1993 Feb 15; 47(3): 613–620.
Gizis FC. Nutrition in women across the life span. Nurs Clin North Amer 1992 Dec; 27(4): 971–982.
Grindel CG. Fatigue and nutrition. Med-Surg Nurs 1994 Dec; 3(6): 475–481, 499.
Ham RJ. Indicators of poor nutritional status in older Americans. Am Fam Physician 1992 Jan; 45(1): 219–228.
Herron DG. Strategies for promoting a healthy dietary intake. Nurs Clin North Amer 1991 Dec 26(4): 875–884.
Jeejeebhoy KN, Detsky AS and Baker JP. Assessment of nutritional status. J Parenteral and Enteral Nutrition 1990 Sept–Oct; 14(5 Suppl): 193S–196S.
Johnson K and Kligman EW. Preventive nutrition: An "optimal" diet for older adults. Geriatrics 1992 Oct; 47(10): 56–60.
Kelly KG. Advances in perioperative nutritional support. Med Clinics North America 1993 Mar; 77(2): 465–475.
Kondrup J, Nielsen K, and Hamberg O. Nutritional therapy in patients with liver cirrhosis. European Journal of Clinical Nutrition 1992 Apr; 46(4): 239–246.
Lacy JA. Albumin overview: Use as a nutritional marker and as a therapeutic intervention. Critical Care Nurse Jan; 11(1): 46–49.
Lin EM. Nutrition support: Making the difficult decisions. Cancer Nursing 1991; 14(5): 261–269.
Lipschitz DA, Ham RJ and White JV. An approach to nutrition screening for older Americans. Am Fam Physician 1992 Feb: 45(2): 601–608.
Nelson KJ et al. Prevalence of malnutrition in the elderly admitted to long-term-care facilities. J Am Dietetic Assoc 1993 April; 93(4): 459–461.
Nixon DW. Nutrition and cancer: American Cancer Society guidelines, programs, and initiatives. CA 1990 Mar/April; 40(2): 71–75.
Roe DA. Medications and nutrition in the elderly. Prim Care 1994 Mar; 21(1): 135–147.
Roe DA. Drug and food interactions as they affect the nutrition of older individuals. Aging 1993 Apr; 5(2 Suppl 1): 51–53.
Saffel-Shrier S and Athas BM. Effective provision of comprehensive nutrition case management for the elderly. Am Dietetic Assoc 1993 April; 93(4): 439–444.
Trujillo EB et al. Assessment of nutritional status, nutrient intake, and nutrition support in AIDS patients. Am Dietetic Assoc 1992 April; 92(4): 477–478.
U.S. Department of Health and Human Services. Diet, nutrition, and cancer prevention: The good news. (NIH Publication No. 87–2878) Bethesda, MD, National Institutes of Health, 1986.
Utley R. Mid-arm circumference. Estimating patients' weight. Dimens Crit Care Nurs 1990 Mar/April; 9(2): 75–81.
Young VR, Marchini JS and Cortiella J. Assessment of protein nutritional status. J Nutr 1990 Nov; 120(Suppl 11): 1496–1502.

RESOURCES

American Dietetic Association
216 West Jackson Blvd, Suite 800
Chicago, IL 60606
Consumer Nutrition Hotline: 800-366-1655

American Heart Association
7320 Greenville Avenue
Dallas, TX 75231
National Center: 214-373-6300
Nutrition Information: 214-706-1179

National Cancer Institute
Cancer Information Service
9000 Rockville Pike
Building 31, Room 10A-24
Bethesda, MD 20892
800-4-CANCER

Nutrition Screening Initiative
2626 Pennsylvania Avenue, N.W.
Suite 301
Washington, DC 20037
202-625-1662

Pennsylvania State Nutrition Center
The Pennsylvania State University
Ruth Building, 417 East Calder Way
University Park, PA 16802
814-865-6323

UNIT 3

Biophysical and Psychosocial Concepts

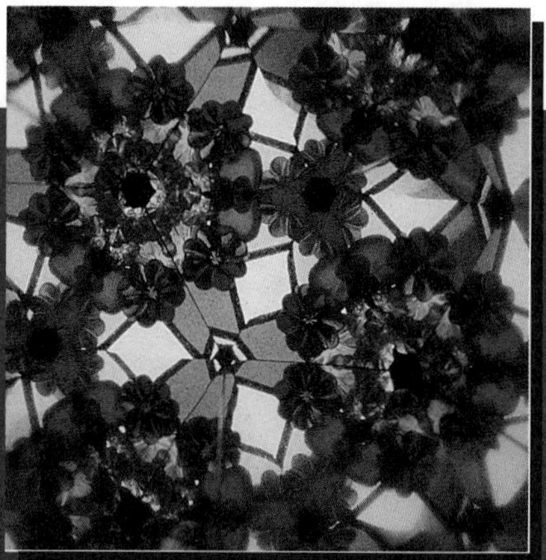

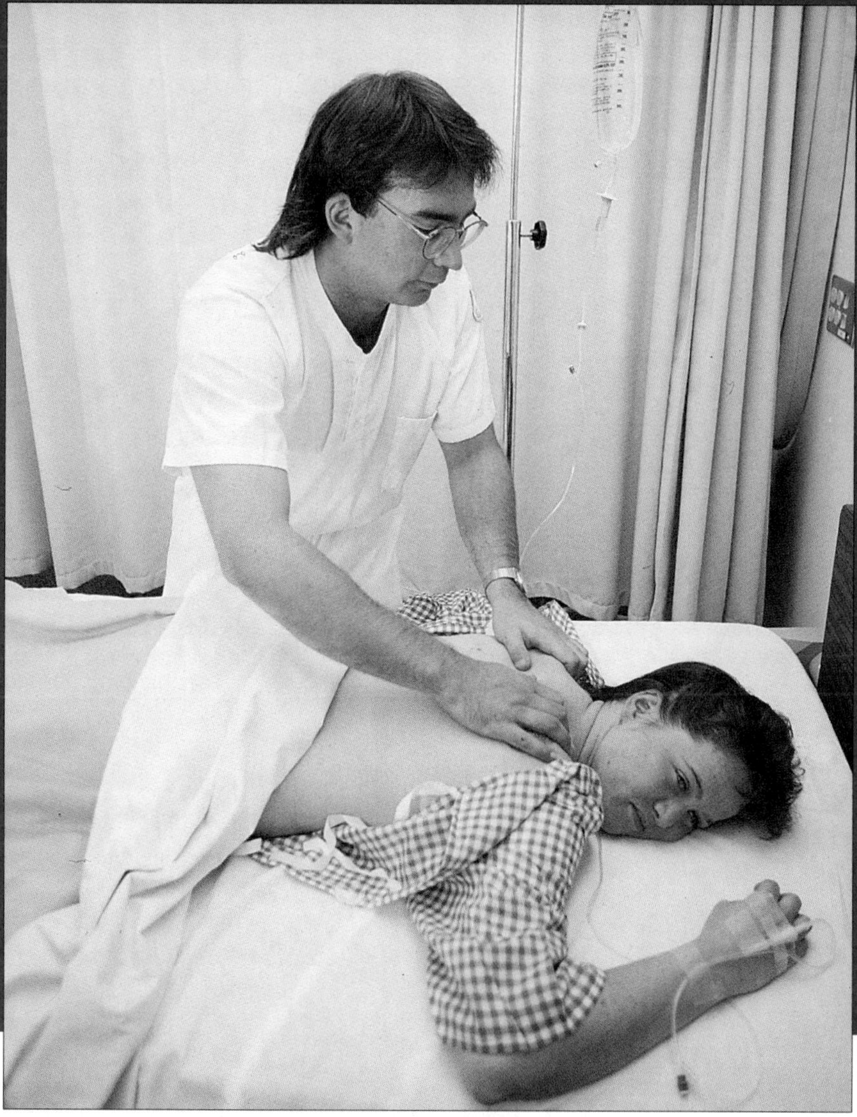

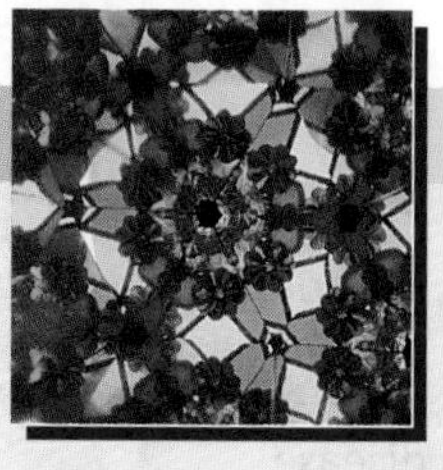

8

Homeostasis and Pathophysiologic Processes

CHAPTER OUTLINE

LEARNING OBJECTIVES

On completion of the chapter, the learner will be able to:

1. Relate the principles of internal constancy, homeostasis, and adaptation to the concept of steady state
2. Identify the significance of the body's compensatory mechanisms in the promotion of adaptation and the maintenance of the steady state
3. Describe the relationship of the process of negative feedback to the maintenance of the steady state
4. Compare the adaptive processes of hypertrophy, atrophy, hyperplasia, and metaplasia
5. Identify external and internal environmental factors that can cause cellular injury and cellular death
6. Describe the inflammatory and reparative processes
7. Compare healing by regeneration to healing by replacement
8. Assess the health patterns of an individual and their effects on maintenance of the steady state

When the body is threatened or suffers an injury, its response may involve functional and structural changes; these changes may be adaptive (having a positive effect) or maladaptive (having a negative effect). The defense mechanisms that the body can mount will determine the difference between adaptation and maladaptation—health and disease.

Physiology is the study of the functional activities of the living organism and its parts. **Pathophysiology** is the study of disordered function of the body. **Mechanisms** are patterns of action performed by different parts of the body to serve a common goal. These mechanisms may be **compensatory** to restore a lost balance, such as breathing rapidly (hyperpnea) to correct an oxygen deficit and lactic acid excess following running. Or, they may be pathophysiologic, as in failure of the heart, when the body reacts by retaining sodium and water and increasing venous pressure, which contributes to further disorder. These physiologic mechanisms give rise to **signs** that may be observed by the nurse or **symptoms** that may be reported by the patient. These observations and a knowledge of the physiologic processes involved can help determine the existence of a problem and can guide the nurse in planning the appropriate course of action.

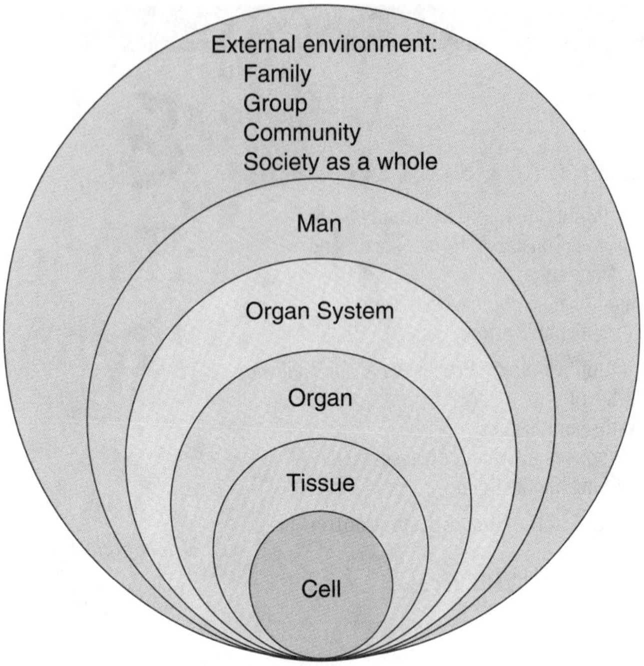

FIGURE 8-1. Constellation of systems. Each system is a subsystem of the larger system (suprasystem) of which it is a part. In this figure the cell is the smallest system, being a subsystem of all other systems.

Dynamic Balance: The Steady State

Physiologic mechanisms must be understood in the context of the body as a whole. The person, as a living system, has both an internal and an external environment. Information and matter are continuously exchanged between one environment and the other. Within the body itself, each organ, tissue, and cell is also a system or subsystem of the whole, each with its own internal and external environment, each exchanging information and matter (Fig. 8-1). The goal of the interaction of the body's subsystems is to produce a dynamic balance or **steady state** (even in the presence of change), so that all subsystems are in harmony with each other, just as an individual seeks harmony with those with whom he or she interacts.

A better understanding of the concept of steady state can be gained by examining the development of the principles of internal constancy, homeostasis, and adaptation.

Internal Constancy, Homeostasis, and Adaptation

Claude Bernard, a French physiologist in the 19th century, developed the biologic principle that for a "free life" there must be a **constancy** or "fixity of the internal milieu," despite changes in the external environment. The internal milieu he addressed was the fluid that bathes the cells, and the constancy was the balanced internal state maintained by physiologic and biochemical processes; his principle implied a static process.

Later, Walter B. Cannon coined the term **homeostasis** to describe the stability of the internal environment, which he said was coordinated by homeostatic or compensatory processes that responded to changes in the internal environment. Any change within the internal environment initiated a "righting" response or a response to minimize the change. These processes sought physiochemical balance and were under involuntary control.

Dubos (1965) provided further insight into the dynamic nature of responses. He stated that there are two complementary concepts: homeostasis and **adaptation**. Homeostasis refers to the necessary adjustments that the body can make *rapidly* to maintain its internal composition within an acceptable range, while adaptation refers to the adjustments that develop *over time*. Dubos also emphasized that there are acceptable ranges of response to stimuli and that these responses will vary for different individuals; "absolute constancy is only a concept of the ideal." Homeostasis and adaptation are both necessary for survival in a changing world.

Maintenance of the Steady State

Homeostasis, then, refers to a steady state within the body. When a change or stress occurs that causes a body function to deviate from its stable range (the change disrupts the constancy), adjustment processes are initiated to restore and maintain the dynamic balance. When these adjustment processes, or **compensatory mechanisms**, are not adequate, the steady state is threatened, function will become disordered, and pathophysiologic mechanisms will occur. The pathophysiologic mechanisms can lead to disease and may be active during disease. **Disease** is a threat to the steady state. It is an abnormal variation in the structure or function of any part of the body. Disease disrupts function and therefore limits the person's freedom of action.

An analogy can be made to the pendulum of a clock. As it swings to and fro, maintaining correct time, it is in dynamic balance, or a steady state. Someone tips the clock, and the pendulum swings a bit to one side but is still able to maintain reasonably accurate time. The clock is tipped more; now the pendulum swings more to one side than the other, and with each swing the pendulum's own weight increases the erratic movement. The clock's functional ability to provide accurate time is damaged and, if nothing intervenes, the clock may be destroyed altogether.

Nursing Implications

It is important for the nurse to realize that the optimal point of intervention to promote health is during the stage when the individual's own compensatory processes are still functioning. It is therefore imperative to be able to relate the presenting signs and symptoms to the physiology they represent. This makes it possible to identify the individual's position on the continuum of function, from health and compensation to pathophysiology and disease. Thus, if a middle-aged woman presented for a checkup and was found to be overweight, with a blood pressure of 130/85 mm Hg, the nurse would most likely counsel her with respect to diet and activity. The nurse would encourage weight loss; question the woman's intake of salt, which affects fluid balance, and her intake of caffeine, for its stimulant effect; and discuss ways to decrease the stress in her life. The ultimate goal would be to control the woman's blood pressure and prevent hypertension.

Another reason for relating symptomatology to physiology is the vast number of diseases that exist—too many to memorize. However, the number of physiologic processes is limited. Having a knowledge of these processes makes it possible to detect the abnormalities or the degree of risk involved and to intervene effectively.

Pathophysiologic Processes at the Cellular Level

The processes described may occur at all levels of the biologic organism. (They also occur in society and populations, but in this chapter we will focus on the physiology of the individual.) If the cell is considered the smallest unit or subsystem (tissues being aggregates of cells, organs aggregates of tissues, etc.), the processes of health and disease or adaptation and maladaptation may all occur at the cellular level. Indeed, pathologic processes are described at the subcellular or molecular level. The cell may then be described as existing on a continuum of function and structure, ranging from the normal cell, to the adapted cell, to the injured or diseased cell, to the dead cell (Fig. 8-2).

Nature of Changes

Changes from one state to another may occur rapidly and may not be readily detectable, because each state does not have distinct or discrete boundaries, and disease represents an extension and distortion of normal processes. For example, tanning of the skin is an adaptive, morphologic response to exposure to the rays of the sun. If the exposure is continued, however, sunburn and injury may occur, and some cells may die, as is evidenced by desquamation or "peeling."

The earliest changes occur at the molecular or subcellular level and are not easily detectable. Not until steady-state functions or structures are altered do changes become apparent. With cell injury some changes may be reversible, whereas others are lethal and lead to death.

Responses to Stimuli/Stressors

Different cells and tissues respond to stimuli with different patterns and rates of response, some being more vulnerable to one type of stimulus or stressor than another. Thus, cardiac muscle cells respond to hypoxia (inadequate oxygenation) more quickly than smooth muscle cells. The cell involved, its ability to adapt, and its physiologic state are determinants of the response.

Other determinants of the response are the type or nature of the stressor, its duration, and its severity. For example, the body can develop a tolerance to regular small amounts of a barbiturate but one large dose may result in unconsciousness and death.

Nursing Implications

Organs are capable of a wide range of activity, for example, the normal heart rate and the normal respiratory rate and volume can vary markedly; thus, the ability of the body to compensate and adapt to different situations and environmental conditions is remarkable. When injury does occur, it may be reversible up to a point; the earliest morphologic or structural changes may be regarded as "fingerprints of

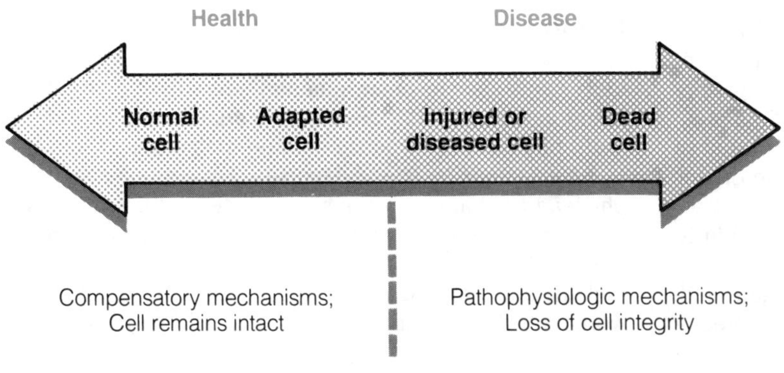

FIGURE 8-2. The cell on a continuum of function and structure. Changes in the cell are not as easily discerned as the diagram depicts. The point at which compensation is lost and pathophysiology begins is not clearly defined.

disease; when the damage is slight the prints can be erased" (Sheldon, 1992). To assure the person's health, it is imperative to detect these early changes.

Control of the Steady State: Control Systems

The concept of the cell on a continuum of function and structure (Fig. 8-2) includes the relationship of the "normal cell" and the "adapted cell" to compensatory mechanisms. These mechanisms include the adjustment processes that are continuously occurring in the body to maintain the dynamic balance, or steady state. These processes are primarily regulated by the autonomic nervous system and the endocrine system, with control achieved through negative feedback.

Negative Feedback Process

Through the process of negative feedback, deviations from a predetermined set point or range of adaptability are detected, and these changes trigger a response aimed at offsetting the deviation. Blood pressure, acid–base balance, blood glucose level, body temperature, and fluid and electrolyte balance are examples of parameters regulated through such compensatory mechanisms. Each of these parameters has a range for optimal function. If there is either an excess or a deficiency, negative feedback will trigger activity to cause a return to the optimal level.

A familiar illustration of the negative feedback process in a simple control system is the control of room temperature. The door is opened and a cold draft reduces room temperature, which is detected by a thermometer and relayed to a thermostat. The thermostat compares this temperature with a preset reference point. Detecting that the room is cooler, it sends a message to the furnace to fire up, with the effect of heating the room air. The new temperature is fed into the thermostat, and if it is equal to the reference point, the furnace is signaled to shut off. This is **negative feedback**, which is a series of actions in which the goal is to counter the influence of an initiating stimulus or disturbance. It does not change the disturbance, only its effect. In this case, the door was not closed, but its cooling effect was offset by the heating action of the furnace.

Organs of Homeostasis or Adjustment. Most of the human body's control systems are integrated at the level of the brain and are affected through the nervous and endocrine systems. Control activities involve detecting deviations from the predetermined reference point and stimulating compensatory responses in the muscles and glands of the body. The major organs affected are the heart, lungs, kidneys, liver, gastrointestinal tract, and skin. When stimulated, these organs alter the rate of their activity or the amount of secretions they produce. They have been called the organs of homeostasis or adjustment.

Local Responses: Feedback Loops. In addition to the responses controlled by the nervous and endocrine systems, there are local responses that consist of small feedback loops in a group of cells or tissues. The cells detect a change in their immediate environment and initiate an action to counteract its effect. For example, the accumulation of lactic acid in an exercised muscle will stimulate dilation of blood vessels in the area to increase blood flow and improve the delivery of oxygen and removal of waste products.

The net result of the activities of the control system through feedback loops is homeostasis—a steady state achieved by the continuous, variable action of the organs that are involved in making the adjustment, along with continuous small exchanges of chemical substances between cells, interstitial fluid, and blood throughout the body. For example, an increase in the carbon dioxide concentration of the extracellular fluid leads to increased pulmonary ventilation, which in turn decreases the carbon dioxide level. On a cellular level, the increased carbon dioxide raises the hydrogen ion concentration of the blood. This is detected by chemosensitive receptors in the respiratory control center of the medulla. This in turn stimulates an increase in the rate of discharge of the neurons, which innervates the diaphragm and intercostal muscles, and increases the rate of respiration. Excess carbon dioxide is exhaled, the hydrogen ion concentration returns to normal, and the chemically sensitive neurons are no longer stimulated.

Positive Feedback

Before concluding this discussion, another type of feedback, positive feedback, should be mentioned. Positive feedback perpetuates the chain of events set in motion by the original disturbance. Compensation does not occur, and the system becomes more imbalanced; disorder and disintegration occur. (There are some exceptions to this: blood clotting in humans, for example, is an important positive feedback mechanism.)

Cellular Adaptation and Injury

Cells are complex units dynamically responding to the changing demands and stresses of daily life. They possess a maintenance function and a specialized function: the maintenance function refers to the activities that the cell must perform with respect to itself; specialized functions are those that the cell performs in relation to the tissues and organs of which it is a part. Individual cells may cease to function without posing a threat to the organism; however, as the dead cells multiply, the specialized functions are altered and the individual's health is threatened.

Common Adaptations

Cells can adapt to environmental stress by structural and functional changes. Some of these adaptations include hypertrophy, atrophy, hyperplasia, and metaplasia (Table 8-1).

Hypertrophy and Atrophy. Hypertrophy and atrophy lead to changes in the size of cells and hence the size of the organs they form. **Compensatory hypertrophy** resulting in an enlarged muscle mass commonly occurs in skeletal and cardiac muscle under prolonged, increased workloads. The bulging muscles of the athlete who engages

TABLE 8-1 Cellular Adaptation

	Stimulus	Example
Hypertrophy		
Increase in cell size, leading to increase in organ size	Increased workload	Leg muscles of runner Arm muscles of tennis player Cardiac muscle in person with hypertension
Atrophy		
Shrinkage in size of cell, leading to decrease in organ size	Decrease in: 1. Use 2. Blood supply 3. Nutrition 4. Hormonal stimulation 5. Innervation	Secondary sex organs in aging person Extremity immobilized in plaster cast
Hyperplasia		
Increase in number of new cells (increase in mitosis)	Hormonal influence Tissue removal or destruction	Breast changes of a girl in puberty or of a pregnant woman Regeneration of liver cells New red blood cells in blood loss
Metaplasia		
Transformation of one adult cell type to another (reversible)	Stress applied to highly specialized cell	Changes in epithelial cells lining bronchi in response to smoke irritation (cells become less specialized)

in body building is one example. **Atrophy** can be the consequence of a disease or of disuse but is more readily associated with aging. There is a decrease in cell and organ size that affects, principally, skeletal muscle, secondary sex organs, the heart, and the brain.

Hyperplasia. **Hyperplasia** is an increase in the number of new cells in an organ or tissue; as cells multiply, volume increases. It is a mitotic response (a change occurring with mitosis), but it is reversible when the stimulus is removed. This distinguishes it from neoplasia or malignant growth, which continues after the stimulus is removed. Hyperplasia may be hormonally induced.

Metaplasia. **Metaplasia** is a cell transformation in which a highly specialized cell changes to a less specialized cell. This serves a protective function, because the less specialized cell is more resistant to the stress that stimulated the change. In smokers, the ciliated columnar epithelium lining the bronchi is replaced by squamous epithelium. The squamous cells can survive; however, loss of the cilia and protective mucus can have damaging consequences.

Thus, the adaptations allow the survival of the organism. They reflect changes in the normal cell in response to stress. If the stress continues, the function of the adapted cell may succumb and cell injury will occur.

Injury

Injury is defined as a disorder in steady-state regulation; any stressor that alters the ability of the cell or system to maintain optimal balance of its adjustment processes will lead to injury. Structural and functional damage then occurs, which may be reversible, permitting recovery; or it may be irreversible, leading to disability or death. Homeostatic adjustments are concerned with the small, minute-by-minute changes within the body's systems. With adaptive changes, compensation occurs and a steady state is achieved, although it may be at new levels; with injury, steady-state regulation is lost and changes in functioning ensue.

Causes of disorder and injury in the system (cell, tissue, organ, body) may arise from the external or internal environment of the system (Fig. 8-3). Causes may include the following: hypoxia, nutritional imbalance, physical agents, chemical agents, infectious agents, immune mechanisms, genetic defects, and psychogenic factors.

The most common causes are hypoxia (oxygen deficiency), chemical injury, and infectious agents. In addition, the presence of one injury makes the system more susceptible to another; for example, inadequate oxygenation and nutritional deficiencies make the system vulnerable to infection. These agents act at the cellular level by damaging or destroying the following:

- The integrity of the cell membrane, necessary for ionic balance
- The ability of the cell to transform energy (aerobic respiration, production of adenosine triphosphate [ATP])
- The ability of the cell to synthesize enzymes and other necessary proteins

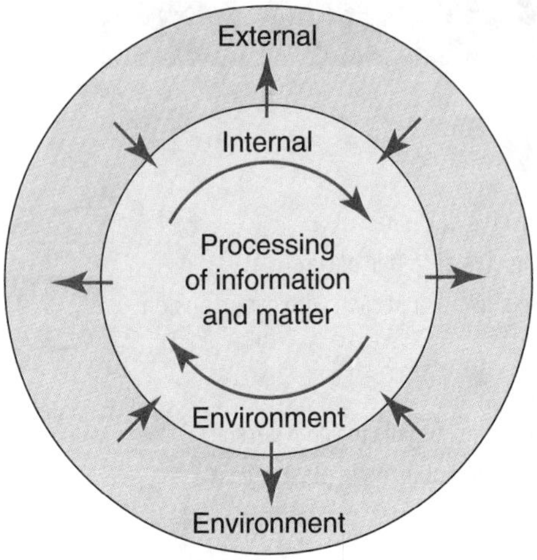

FIGURE 8-3. Influences leading to disorder may arise from the internal environment and the external environment of the system. Excesses or deficits of information and matter may occur or there may be faulty regulation of processing.

- The ability of the cell to grow and reproduce (genetic integrity)

Hypoxia

Inadequate cellular oxygenation **(hypoxia)** interferes with the cell's ability to transform energy. Hypoxia may be caused by:

- A decrease in blood supply to an area
- A decrease in the oxygen-carrying capacity of the blood (decreased hemoglobin)
- A ventilation–perfusion or respiratory problem, reducing the amount of oxygen available in the blood
- A problem in the cell's enzyme system, making it unable to use the oxygen delivered to it

The usual cause is **ischemia**, or deficient blood supply. Ischemia is commonly seen in myocardial cell injury in which arterial blood flow is decreased because of atherosclerotic narrowing of blood vessels. Ischemia also results from intravascular clots (thrombi, emboli) that may form and interfere with blood supply; they are a common cause of strokes or cerebrovascular accidents. The length of time different tissues can survive without oxygen varies; for example, brain cells may succumb in 3 to 6 minutes (sources vary). If the condition leading to hypoxia is slowly progressive, collateral circulation may develop, whereby blood is supplied by other blood vessels in the area. However, this mechanism is not highly reliable.

Nutritional Imbalance

Nutritional imbalance refers to a relative or absolute deficiency or excess of one or more essential nutrients. This may be manifested as undernutrition, in which there is an inadequate consumption of food or calories, or as overnutrition, in which there is a caloric excess. Caloric excess to the point of obesity, in which the person is 20% or more above the ideal weight, overloads cells in the body with lipids. By requiring more energy to maintain the extra tissue, obesity places a strain on the body and has been associated with the development of disease, especially pulmonary and cardiovascular disease.

Specific deficiencies arise when an essential nutrient is deficient or when there is a disproportion of nutrients. Protein deficiencies and avitaminosis (deficiency of vitamins) are examples.

An energy deficit leading to cell injury can occur when there is insufficient glucose or insufficient oxygen to transform the glucose into energy. A lack of insulin, or the inability to utilize insulin, may also prevent glucose from entering the cell from the blood. This is the problem in diabetes mellitus, which represents a metabolic disorder, leading to nutritional deficiency.

Physical Agents

Physical agents, including extremes of temperature, radiation, electrical shock, and mechanical trauma, may cause injury to the cells or the entire body. The duration of exposure and the intensity of the stressor determine the severity of damage.

Extremes of High Temperature. When a person's temperature is elevated, irrespective of cause, hypermetabolism occurs: the respiratory rate, heart rate, and basal metabolic rate increase. With fever induced by infections, the hypothalamic thermostat may be reset at a higher temperature. Thus, the person responds to external heat and cold with a new setpoint of perhaps 40°C (104°F), just as he or she did with the normal setpoint of 37°C (98.6°F). When the fever breaks, the thermostat returns to normal. The increase in body temperature is achieved through physiologic mechanisms. Body temperatures above 41°C (105.8°F) suggest **hyperthermia**; the physiologic function of the thermoregulatory center breaks down, and temperature soars. This occurs in persons with heat stroke. Eventually, the high temperature causes coagulation of cell proteins, and the cells die. It is imperative that the body be cooled rapidly to prevent brain damage.

The local response to **thermal** or **burn injury** is similar. There is an increase in metabolic activity, and as heat increases, protein is coagulated, enzyme systems are destroyed, and, in the extreme, charring or carbonization occurs. Burns of the epithelium are classified as partial-thickness burns if epithelializing elements remain to support healing; full-thickness burns lack such elements and must be grafted for healing. The amount of body surface involved determines the prognosis for the patient. If the injury is severe, the entire body system becomes involved, and hypermetabolism will develop as a pathophysiologic response.

Extremes of Low Temperature. Extremes of low temperature or cold cause vasoconstriction; blood flow becomes sluggish, and clots may form, leading to ischemic damage in the involved tissues. With still lower temperatures, ice crystals may form, and the cells may burst.

Radiation and Electrical Shock. Radiation may be used for diagnosis and treatment of diseases. Ionizing forms of radiation may cause injury by their ionizing action. Electrical shock may produce burns as a result of the heat generated when electric current travels through the body. It may also stimulate nerves abnormally; for example, fibrillation of the heart may occur.

Mechanical Trauma. Mechanical trauma can result in wounds that disrupt the cells and tissues of the body. The severity of the wound, the amount of blood loss, and the extent of nerve damage are significant factors in the outcome.

Chemical Agents

Chemical injuries may be caused by known poisons, such as lye, which has a corrosive action on epithelial tissue, or by heavy metals, such as mercury, arsenic, and lead, each with its own specific destructive action. Many other chemicals may be toxic in certain amounts, in certain people, and in certain tissues; these include compounds of extrinsic and intrinsic origin. Too much hydrochloric acid can damage the stomach lining; large amounts of glucose can cause osmotic shifts, affecting the fluid and electrolyte balance; and too much insulin can cause less than normal levels of sugar in the blood (hypoglycemia) and lead to coma.

Drugs, including medications prescribed by the physician, may cause chemical poisoning. Some individuals are less tolerant of drugs than others and manifest toxic reactions at customary dosages. Aging tends to decrease tolerance to medications. Polypharmacy (taking many medications at one time) also often occurs in the aging population. It is a problem because of the unpredictable effects of the resulting drug interactions.

Alcohol (ethanol) is a chemical irritant. In the body, alcohol is broken down into acetaldehyde, which has a direct toxic effect on liver cells that leads to a variety of liver abnormalities, including cirrhosis in susceptible individuals. Disordered liver cell function leads to complications in other organs of the body.

Infectious Agents

Biologic agents known to cause disease in humans are viruses, bacteria, rickettsiae, mycoplasmas, fungi, protozoa, and nematodes. The severity of the infectious disease depends on the number of microorganisms entering the body, their virulence, and the host's defenses, such as health, age, and immune defenses.

Some **bacteria**, such as those in tetanus and diphtheria, produce exotoxins that circulate and create cell damage. Some, such as the gram negative bacteria, produce endotoxins when they are killed; and others, such as the tubercle bacillus, induce an immune reaction.

Viruses, as the smallest living organisms, survive as parasites of the living cells they invade. Viruses infect specific cells; through a complex mechanism, they replicate within the cells they invade and then burst out to invade other cells and continue to replicate. An immune response is mounted by the body to eliminate the viruses, and the cells harboring the viruses can be injured in the process.

Typically, an inflammatory response and immune reaction are the physiologic responses of the body to the presence of infection.

Immune Mechanisms

The immune system is an exceedingly complex system; its purpose is to defend the body from invasion by any foreign object or foreign cell type, such as cancerous cells. This is a steady-state mechanism, but like other adjustment processes it can become disordered, and cell injury will occur. Basically, the immune response detects foreign bodies by distinguishing nonself substances from self substances and destroying the nonself entities. The entrance of an antigen (foreign body) into the body evokes the production of antibodies that attack and destroy the antigen (antigen–antibody reaction).

The immune system can be hypoactive or hyperactive. When it is hypoactive, immunodeficiency diseases occur; when it is hyperactive, hypersensitivity disorders arise. A disorder of the immune system itself can result in damage to the body's own tissues. Such disorders are labelled **autoimmune diseases** (see Unit 12).

Genetic Disorders

Genetic defects as causes of disease are of intense interest as more environmental pollutants are identified and their effects on genetic structure are studied. Many of these produce mutations that have no recognizable effect, such as lack of a single enzyme; others contribute to more obvious congenital abnormalities, such as Down's syndrome. Sickle cell disease, the hemophilias, and phenylketonuria are examples of diseases arising from genetic defects.

Psychogenic Factors

Mental conflict and stress may give rise to organic illness or disease (see also Chapter 9). MacSween and Whaley (1992) list three overlapping groups of such diseases: (1) acquired mental disease such as depression, (2) diseases of addiction, particularly to alcohol, tobacco, and some drugs, and (3) psychosomatic disorders. The exact means by which psychosomatic disorders (sometimes called diseases of maladaptation) are caused is uncertain but they are associated with chronic stress, anxiety, and frustration.

Response to Injury: Inflammation

Cells or tissues of the body may be injured or killed by any of the agents (physical, chemical, infectious) just described. When this happens there is a naturally occurring response in the healthy tissues adjacent to the site of injury. This is called the **inflammatory response,** or **inflammation**. It is a defensive reaction the intent of which is to neutralize, control, and/or eliminate the offending agent and to prepare the site for repair. It is a nonspecific response (not dependent on a particular cause) meant to serve a protective function. For example, inflammation may be observed at the site of a bee sting, in a sore throat, in a surgical incision, and in a burn. Inflammation also occurs in cell injury events such as strokes and myocardial infarctions.

It is important to distinguish between inflammation and infection. An infectious agent is only one of several agents that may trigger an inflammatory response. An infection exists when the infectious agent is living, growing, and multiplying in the tissues and is able to overcome the body's normal defenses.

Regardless of the cause, there is a general sequence of events that can be described as the local inflammatory response. This sequence involves changes in the microcirculation in the area of the injury that include vasodilation, increased vascular permeability, and leukocytic cellular infiltration. As these changes take place, **five cardinal signs**

of inflammation are produced: redness, heat, swelling, pain, and loss of function.

A transient vasoconstriction that occurs immediately after injury is followed by vasodilation and an increased rate of blood flow through the microcirculation. **Local heat** and **redness** result. Next, vascular permeability increases, and plasma fluids (including proteins and solutes) leak into the inflamed tissues, producing **swelling**. The **pain** produced is attributed to the pressure of fluids (swelling) on nerve endings and to direct irritation of nerve endings by chemical mediators released at the site. Bradykinin is one of the chemical mediators suspected of causing pain. **Loss of function** is most likely related to the pain and swelling, but the exact mechanism has not been explained.

As the blood flow increases and fluid leaks into the surrounding tissues, the formed elements (red blood cells, white blood cells, and platelets) remain in the blood and the blood becomes more viscous and sluggish. Leukocytes (white blood cells) collect in the vessels, exit, and migrate to the site of injury to engulf offending organisms and to remove cellular debris in a process called **phagocytosis**. Fibrinogen in the leaked plasma fluid coagulates, forming fibrin for clot formation that serves to wall off the injured area and prevent the spread of infection.

Chemical Mediators

Injury initiates the inflammatory response, but chemical substances released at the site induce the vascular changes. Foremost among these are histamine and the kinins. **Histamine** is present in many tissues of the body but is concentrated in mast cells. It is released when injury occurs and is responsible for the early changes in vasodilation and vascular permeability. **Kinins** increase vasodilation and vascular permeability; they also attract neutrophils to the area. **Prostaglandins**, another group of chemical substances, are also suspected of causing increased permeability.

The process described is complex. Although it has phases, once started they may all occur at the same time. The process may be modified by different variables, the most important of which are (1) the nature and intensity of the injury, (2) the site and tissue affected, and (3) the resistance of the host.

The inflammatory response may be confined to the site, and only local signs may appear. On the other hand, systemic responses throughout the body may also occur. **Fever** is the most common sign of a systemic response to injury. It is most likely caused by endogenous pyrogens (internal substances that cause fever) released from neutrophils and macrophages (specialized forms of leukocytes). These substances reset the hypothalamic thermostat controlling body temperature and produce fever. **Leukocytosis**, an increase in the synthesis and release of neutrophils from bone marrow, may occur to provide the body with greater ability to fight infection. Constitutional symptoms may develop, including malaise, loss of appetite, aching, and weakness.

Types of Inflammation

Inflammation is categorized primarily by its duration and the type of exudate produced. It may be acute, subacute, or chronic. A typical case of **acute inflammation** is characterized by the local vascular and exudative changes described above and usually lasts for less than 2 weeks. An acute inflammatory response is immediate, and it serves a protective function. When the injurious agent is removed, the inflammation subsides, and healing takes place with the return of normal or near-normal structure and function.

Chronic inflammation develops when the injurious agent persists and the acute response is perpetuated. Symptoms may appear for many months or years. Chronic inflammation may also begin insidiously and never have an acute phase. The chronic response does not serve a beneficial and protective function but, on the contrary, is debilitating and may produce long-lasting effects. As the inflammation becomes chronic, changes occur at the site of injury and the nature of the exudate becomes proliferative. There is a continuing cycle of cellular infiltration, necrosis, and fibrosis (repair and breakdown occur simultaneously). Considerable scarring may occur, resulting in permanent tissue damage.

Subacute inflammation falls between acute and chronic inflammation. There are elements of the active exudative phase of the acute response, and simultaneously there is some repair occurring, as in the chronic response. The term is not widely used.

Repair

The reparative process begins at approximately the same time as the injury and is interwoven with inflammation. Healing proceeds after the inflammatory debris is removed. Healing may be by **regeneration**, in which there is gradual repair of the defect by proliferation of cells of the same type as those destroyed, or it may be by **replacement** with cells of another type, usually connective tissue, resulting in scar formation.

Healing by Regeneration. The ability of cells to regenerate depends on whether they are labile, permanent, or stable. **Labile cells** include those that multiply constantly to replace cells worn out by normal physiologic processes; these include epithelial cells of the skin and those lining the gastrointestinal tract. **Permanent cells** include neurons—the nerve cell bodies, not their axons. Destruction of a neuron is a permanent loss, but axons may regenerate. If normal activity is to return, tissue regeneration must occur in a functional pattern, especially in the growth of several axons. **Stable cells** have a latent ability to regenerate. Under normal physiologic processes, they are not shed and do not need replacement, but if they are damaged or destroyed, they are able to regenerate. These include functional cells of the kidney, liver, pancreas, and other organs of the body.

Healing by Replacement. Healing may be by primary intention or secondary intention. In **primary intention healing**, the wound is clean and dry and the edges are approximated, such as may occur in a surgical wound. Little scar formation occurs, and the wound is usually healed in a week. In **secondary intention healing**, the wound or defect is larger and gaping and has more necrotic or dead material. The wound fills from the bottom upward with granulation tissue. The process of repair takes longer and results in more scar formation with loss of specialized function. Persons who have recovered from myocardial infarctions will have abnormal electrocardiographic (ECG) tracings because the electrical signal cannot be conducted through the connective tissue that replaces the defect.

As this chapter has already emphasized, the condition of the host, the environment, and the nature and severity of the injury affect the processes and outcomes—in this case, the processes of inflammation and repair.

Cell Death

Any of the injuries discussed in the preceding pages can lead to death of the cell. Essentially, the cell membrane becomes impaired, resulting in a nonrestricted flow of ions. Sodium and calcium enter the cell, followed by water, which leads to edema, and energy transformation ceases. Nerve impulses are no longer transmitted; muscles no longer contract. As the cells rupture, lysosomal enzymes that destroy tissues escape; cell death and necrosis occur.

A Representative Pathophysiologic Process: Hypertensive Heart Disease

Hypertensive heart disease is presented here as a representative pathophysiologic process. Unfortunately, words and figures can only partly portray the person's condition moment by moment or day by day in acute illness, or week by week in chronic illness. The influence of physiologic changes, of social adjustments between patient and health care personnel or family, of unknown or expressed concern and anxiety, and of the person's total life experience in the development and course of disease is well recognized by the health care team. These variables cannot be inserted into a flow diagram, yet they may be major factors governing the course of the disease.

Mechanisms of Blood Pressure Regulation

A brief summary of selected mechanisms for regulating blood pressure will facilitate the understanding of hypertensive heart disease. The regulation of arterial pressure involves complex nervous system and hormonal controls that interrelate to affect the cardiac output and peripheral vascular resistance. This relationship is expressed in the following equation:

$$\text{mean arterial pressure} = \text{cardiac output} \times \text{total peripheral resistance}$$

Cardiac output is determined by the stroke volume and the heart rate. Peripheral resistance is determined by the diameter of the arterioles. If the diameter is decreased (vasoconstriction), peripheral resistance increases; if the diameter is increased (vasodilation), peripheral resistance decreases.

Primary regulation of arterial pressure is effected by the baroreceptors in the carotid sinus and aortic arch which relay impulses to the sympathetic nervous centers in the medulla. These impulses act to inhibit the stimulation of the sympathetic nervous system. When the arterial pressure is increased, the baroreceptor endings are stretched. They fire, inhibiting the sympathetic center. This reduces the discharge of the sympathetic center, with the result that the heart rate decreases, the arterioles dilate, and the arterial pressure returns to its former level. The reverse happens with a fall in arterial pressure. The baroreceptors control only temporary changes in blood pressure.

One other mechanism, which has a longer-term effect, will be described. Renin, produced by the kidneys when their blood flow is decreased, leads to the formation of angiotensin I, which converts to angiotensin II. Angiotensin II elevates the blood pressure by direct constriction of arterioles. It also indirectly stimulates the release of aldosterone, which leads to renal retention of sodium and water. This response increases the extracellular fluid volume, which in turn increases the flow of blood returned to the heart, thereby raising the stroke volume and cardiac output. The kidneys also have an intrinsic mechanism to increase sodium and water retention.

When a *persistent* disturbance that causes arteriolar constriction occurs, total peripheral resistance is increased and the mean arterial pressure rises. In the face of the persistent disturbance, cardiac output must increase to maintain balance in the system (see equation). This is necessary to overcome the peripheral resistance, so that delivery of oxygen and nutrients to the cells and removal of cellular waste products will be maintained. To increase the cardiac output, the sympathetic nervous system stimulates the heart to beat faster; it also increases the stroke volume by causing a selective vasoconstriction in peripheral organs, thus returning more blood to the heart. With chronic hypertension, the baroreceptors are reset at a higher level, and they respond as though the new level were normal.

Initially, this mechanism is compensatory. This adaptive mechanism, however, exacts a toll by increasing the workload on the heart. At the same time, degenerative changes take place in the arterioles that are subjected to continuous high pressure. These changes occur in organs throughout the body, including the heart, which may contribute to a depleted blood supply in the myocardium. To eject blood, the heart must exert enough force to overcome the pressure reflected back to the aortic inlet. In response to this workload, the muscle of the left ventricle hypertrophies or enlarges. Eventually, it dilates, and the heart becomes enlarged. These two structural changes are adaptive; they improve the stroke volume delivered by the heart. At rest, these compensatory mechanisms may be effective, but on exertion, the heart cannot meet the demands of the body; the person is easily fatigued and becomes short of breath.

The point at which compensation ends and injury and failure begin is not continuous or separate. With the increased demands, there are changes in the distribution of blood flow that result in a reduced flow to the kidneys. This stimulates the renin–angiotensin–aldosterone mechanism. This mechanism, once compensatory, now aggravates the failing heart by increasing the extracellular fluid volume and the peripheral resistance. The heart becomes engorged with blood that it cannot pump out, and left ventricular heart failure occurs. Failure of the left ventricle has both forward and backward effects. The forward effects are due to low output, which decreases the perfusion of tissues of the body. The decreased perfusion activates sodium and water retention mechanisms in the kidneys and glands, giving positive feedback to the failing heart. The backward effects are due to the decreased emptying of the left ventricle, which raises the end-diastolic pressure. This rise in pressure is reflected back into the left atrium and the pulmonary veins, and congestion occurs in the pulmonary capillaries. Gas exchange is disrupted, and fluid exudes from the capillaries into the alveolar spaces, leading to pulmonary edema. Crackles will be heard upon auscultation of the lungs; severe dyspnea (difficult breathing) and orthopnea (inability to breath when lying down) will be present; coughing will occur; and, with pulmonary edema, pink, frothy sputum may be present. Eventually, this backward progression will affect the right side of the heart and lead to right-sided heart failure accompanied by congestion in the veins and organs drained by the vena cavae. The system is in total failure, and death is imminent.

The initial disturbance that caused the increased peripheral resistance may be unknown, as is the case in primary or essential hypertension, although a number of agents have been postulated as being contributory. The pathologic mechanism was hypoxia due to failure of the blood transportation system. In the latter stages, oxygen saturation of the blood was also decreased because of the pulmonary edema.

Nursing Implications

In the assessment of the person who seeks health care, objective signs will be the primary indicators of the physiologic processes that are occurring. The following questions are addressed during the assessment: Are the heart rate, respiratory rate, and temperature normal? If not, is any change only a temporary one? Are there other indicators of steady-state deviation? What is the person's blood pressure, height, and weight? Are there any problems in movement or sensation? Does the person demonstrate any problems in orientation or memory? Are there obvious lesions or deformities? Further signs of change are indicated in laboratory data, including electrolytes, blood urea nitrogen (BUN), blood glucose, and urinalysis. In making a nursing diagnosis, the nurse must relate the symptoms or complaints expressed by the patient to the physical signs that are present.

As previously noted, the state of the person and the environment are predictors of the health outcome in all situations. These are directly related to the health patterns of the individual. The nurse has a significant role and responsibility in identifying the health patterns of the person receiving care. If those patterns are not achieving physiologic, psychological, and social balance, the nurse is obligated—with the assistance and agreement of the patient—to seek ways to promote balance.

While this chapter has analyzed such patterns as nutrition–metabolism, elimination, activity–exercise, and sleep–rest from a physiologic perspective, the way that one copes with stress, the way one relates to others, and the values and goals held are interwoven in those physiologic patterns. To evaluate the patient's health patterns and to intervene if a problem exists requires a total assessment of the patient. Specific problems and their nursing management are addressed in greater depth in other chapters.

CRITICAL THINKING EXERCISES

1. Think back to a time when you had an acute illness or injury. How was homeostasis maintained or disrupted, and what compensatory mechanisms were evident?
2. Select a patient to whom you are assigned who has an acute illness or injury. Describe the manner in which homeostasis has been maintained or disrupted and the compensatory mechanisms that are evident. How does the patient's medical treatment support the compensatory mechanisms? How do you determine the nursing interventions that are appropriate for promoting the healing process?

REFERENCES AND BIBLIOGRAPHY

Books

Andreoli TE et al. Cecil Essentials of Medicine, 3rd ed. Philadelphia, WB Saunders, 1993.

Bullock BL and Rosendahl PP. Pathophysiology: Adaptations and Alterations in Function, 3rd ed. Philadelphia, JB Lippincott, 1992.

Carrieri VK, Lindsey AM, and West CM. Pathophysiological Phenomena in Nursing. Philadelphia, WB Saunders, 1993.

Cotran RS, Kumar V, and Robbins SL. Pathologic Basis of Disease, 4th ed. Philadelphia, WB Saunders, 1989.

Dubos R. Man Adapting. New Haven, CT, Yale University Press, 1965.

Groer MW and Shekleton ME. Basic Pathophysiology, A Conceptual Approach, 3rd ed. St. Louis, CV Mosby, 1989.

Guyton AC. Textbook of Medical Physiology. Philadelphia, WB Saunders, 1991.

Harrison TR et al. Harrison's Principles of Internal Medicine, 11th ed. New York, McGraw–Hill, 1991.

MacSween RNM and Whaley K. Muir's Textbook of Pathology, 13th ed. London, Edward Arnold, 1992.

Marieb EN. Human Anatomy and Physiology. Redwood City, CA, Benjamin/Cummings Publishing Company, 1992.

Price SA and Wilson LM. Pathophysiology, Clinical Concepts of Disease Processes. New York, McGraw–Hill, 1992.

Purtilo DT and Purtilo RB. A Survey of Human Diseases, 2nd ed. Boston, Little, Brown and Company, 1989.

Sheldon H. Boyd's Introduction to the Study of Disease, 11th ed. Philadelphia, Lea & Febiger, 1992.

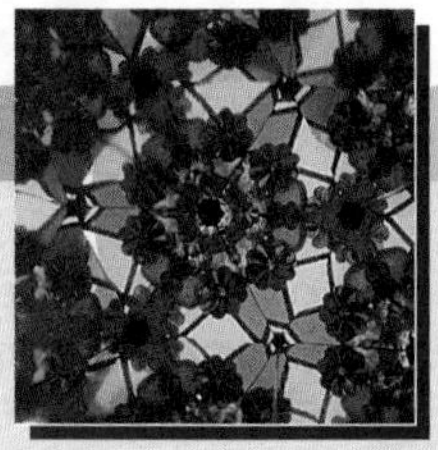

9 Stress and Adaptation

CHAPTER OUTLINE

LEARNING OBJECTIVES

On completion of the chapter, the learner will be able to:

1. Define stress and adaptation
2. Identify physiologic and psychosocial stressors
3. Compare the sympathetic–adrenal–medullary response to stress to the hypothalamic–pituitary response to stress
4. Describe the influence of social support on coping with stress
5. Describe the General Adaptation Syndrome as a theory of adaptation to biologic stress
6. Identify ways in which maladaptive responses to stress can increase the risk of illness and cause disease
7. Describe the nursing implications of health risk appraisal
8. Identify measures that are useful for reduction of stress
9. Specify the functions of social networks and support groups in the reduction of stress

"Between 1980 and 1990, the number of stress disability claims made by California state workers increased by more than 800 percent!" (Pelletier, 1992, p. xxi). Job stress, burnout, environmental stress, marital stress, and examination stress are examples that abound in everyday life. Talk of stress surrounds us, yet the ability to define and predict stress remains elusive. Scientists in the fields of physiology, psychology, and sociology have developed bodies of knowledge on the subject of stress, but they have not focused on the possible connections that might exist among these various bodies of knowledge. Recent discoveries and knowledge from studies in the field of psychoneuroimmunology are providing insight into the complex relationship of the domains of psychology (the mind and emotions), neurology (the brain and central nervous system), and immunology (the body's cellular defenses against internal and external invaders). These studies demonstrate ways that the mind and emotions can affect physical health. The findings deepen our understanding of the effects of stress on the body.

The focus of this chapter is on the process of stress and associated nursing implications.

Stress and Adaptation Defined

Three theoretical approaches (reflective of the disciplines of physiology, psychology, and sociology) have been used to define stress in nursing research (Barnfather, 1993; Lyon & Werner, 1987). One approach defines stress as a **response**. The predominant theory in this context is that of Hans Selye (1956, 1976). Selye defined stress as the nonspecific response of the body to any demand, regardless of its nature. This response included a series of physiologic reactions that he labelled the General Adaptation Syndrome (GAS).

Another theoretical approach defines stress as a **stimulus**, or the cause of the response. In this context stress is viewed as external to the individual. In this psychosocial model, life events are measured as predictors of illness. Stress is considered as a predisposing or precipitating factor increasing the individual's vulnerability to illness (Rahe, 1975).

The third approach defines stress as a transaction. In the transactive model there is an exchange or transaction, between the person and the environment, which provides feedback to the person-environment relationship. The transactional model most frequently cited is that of Richard Lazarus. Lazarus and Folkman (1984, p. 19) defined psychologic stress as a "particular *relationship* between the person and the environment that is appraised by the person as taxing his or her resources and endangering his or her well-being." Nursing research studies have used the transaction model more than the stimulus or response models.

Stress

Stress is a state produced by a change in the environment that is perceived as challenging, threatening, or damaging to the person's dynamic balance or equilibrium. There is an actual or perceived imbalance in the person's ability to meet the demands of the new situation. The change or stimulus that evokes this state is the **stressor**. The nature of the stressor is variable: an event or change that will produce stress in one person will be neutral for another, and an event that may produce stress at one time and place for one person may not do so for the same person at another time and place. A person appraises and copes with changing situations. The desired goal is adaptation, or adjustment to the change so that the person is again in equilibrium and has the energy and ability to meet new demands. This is the stress-coping process, a compensatory process with physiologic and psychologic components.

Adaptation

Adaptation is a constant, ongoing process that requires a change in structure, function, or behavior so that the person is better suited to the environment. The process involves an interaction between the person and the environment. The outcome depends upon the degree of fit between the skills and capacities of the person and his or her sources of social support on the one hand, and the types of challenges or stressors being confronted on the other. As such, adaptation is an individual process with each individual having different levels of ability to cope or respond. As new challenges are met, this ability to cope and adapt can change, thereby providing the individual with a wide range of adaptation ability from which to draw. Adaptation goes on throughout the life span and during that process many developmental and situational challenges will be encountered, especially in situations of health and illness. The goal of these encounters is to promote adaptation. In situations of health and illness this goal is realized by optimal wellness.

Because both stress and adaptation may exist at different levels of a system, it is possible to study these reactions at cell, tissue, and organ levels. The biologist's study is mainly concerned with subcellular components or with subsystems of the total body. Sociologists study stress and adaptation in individuals, families, groups, and societies, and thus, they speak of the adaptation of groups, in the sense that a group's organizational features are modified to meet the requirements of the social and physical environment in which they exist. Adaptation is a continuous process of seeking harmony in an environment. The desired end goals of adaptation for any system are survival, growth, and reproduction.

Stressors: The Sources of Stress

Each person operates at a certain level of adaptation and regularly encounters a certain amount of change. Such change is expected: it contributes to growth, and it enhances life. Stressors, however, can upset this equilibrium. A stressor may be defined as, "an internal or external event, condition, situation, and/or cue, that has the potential to bring about or actually activates significant physical or psychosocial reactions" (Werner, 1993, p. 15).

Types of Stressors

Stressors exist in many forms and categories. They may be described as physical, physiologic, or psychosocial. Physical stressors might include cold, heat, or chemical agents; physiologic stressors might include pain or fatigue; and psychosocial stressors might result from emotional reactions, such as fear of failing an exam or not getting a job. Stressors can also occur as normal life transitions that require some adjustment, such as going from childhood into puberty, giving birth, or entering marriage.

Stressors have also been classified as: (1) day-to-day stressors, or commonly occurring frustrations or hassles; (2) major complex occurrences, which may involve large groups, even entire nations; and (3) stressors that occur less frequently and involve fewer people. The first group, the day-to-day stressors, includes such common occurrences as getting caught in a traffic jam, experiencing computer downtime, and having an argument with a spouse or roommate. These experiences vary in effect; for example, encountering a rainstorm while one is vacationing at the beach will most likely evoke a more negative response than it might at another time. These less dramatic, frustrating, and irritating events, called "daily hassles," have been shown to have a greater health impact than major life events because of the cumulative effect they have over time. They can lead to high blood pressure, palpitations, or similar physiologic problems.

Some stressors influence larger groups of people, possibly even entire nations. These include events of history such as terrorism and war, which are threatening situations when experienced either directly, in the war zone, or indirectly through live news coverage. The demographic, economic, and technologic changes occurring in society also serve as stressors. The stress produced by any stressor is sometimes a result not only of the change itself but also of the speed with which the change occurs.

Life Event Stressors

The third group of stressors has been studied most extensively and deals with relatively infrequently occurring situations that directly affect the individual. This category includes the influence of life events, such as death, birth, marriage, divorce, and retirement. It includes the psychosocial crises described by Erikson as occurring in the life-cycle stages of the human experience. More enduring chronic stressors have also been placed in this category and may include such things as having a permanent functional disability or dealing with the burden associated with providing long-term care to a frail elderly parent.

Relating life events to illness (the theoretical approach which defines stress as a stimulus) has been a major focus of psychosocial studies. This can be traced to Adolph Meyer, who in the 1930s observed in "life charts" of his patients a linkage between illnesses and critical life events. Harold Wolff, following this line of research, concluded that people under constant stress had a high incidence of psychosomatic disease (reported in Dohrenwend et al., 1993). Holmes and Rahe (1967) developed life events scales that assign numerical values, called **life-change units**, to typical life events. Stress is defined as an accumulation of changes in one's life that require psychologic adaptation.

Using a life events scale, checking off the number of recent events, and deriving a total score, one can predict the likelihood of illness. The items reflect events that require a change in the person's life pattern; the variable of change is important because it requires adjustment. The Recent Life Changes Questionnaire (RLCQ) (Tausig, 1982) contains 118 items related to events such as death, birth, marriage, divorce, promotions, serious arguments, and vacations. The events listed include both desirable and undesirable happenings. Research findings in nursing and other disciplines have demonstrated only weak to moderate associations between stressful life events and outcomes (Werner, 1993).

Time-Related Stressors

Stressors can also be categorized according to their duration. They may be **acute**, time-limited stressors, such as awaiting surgery or a final examination. They may be **stressor sequences** consisting of a series of events over a period of time that result from some initiating event such as job loss or divorce. They may be **chronic intermittent** (hassles fall into this category), or they may be **chronic enduring** sources of stress that persist over time.

Ballard (1981) identified immobilization, isolation, orientation, and sensory deprivation as stressful conditions in a study of patients in the surgical intensive care unit. She observed that nurses could alter many of the stressors in the intensive care unit. She also observed that not only are illness and major surgery stressors, but the role changes and financial demands occasioned by the illness are additional stressors. This is an example of the stressor sequence: over time, one event may lead to others or may have an impact on existing situations.

Mediating Processes

Following the recognition of a stressor, the person will consciously or unconsciously react to manage the situation. This is called the **mediating process**. The theory developed by Lazarus emphasizes cognitive appraisal and coping. Appraisal and coping will be influenced by antecedent variables which include the internal and external resources of the person.

Appraisal and Coping

Cognitive appraisal (Lazarus, 1991a; Lazarus & Folkman, 1984) is a process through which an event is evaluated with respect to what is at stake (primary appraisal) and what might and can be done (secondary appraisal).

What is at stake, or **primary appraisal**, is influenced by the personal goals and commitments or motivation of the individual. For example, How important or how relevant is what is happening? Is it in conflict with what the person wants or desires? Does the situation threaten the person's own sense of strength and ego-identity?

As an outcome of primary appraisal, the situation will be identified as either nonstressful or stressful. If *nonstressful*, the situation is **irrelevant or benign-positive**. A *stressful* situation may be one of three kinds: (1) those in which **harm or loss** has occurred; (2) those that are **threatening**, in that harm or loss is anticipated; and (3) those that are **challenging**, in that some opportunity or gain is anticipated.

Secondary appraisal is an evaluation of what might and can be done. This includes assigning blame or credit to those responsible for a frustrating event, thinking about whether or not one can do something about the situation (one's coping potential), and determining future expectancy, or whether things are likely to change for better or worse (Lazarus, 1991a, 1991c). The degree of stress is determined by a comparison of what is at stake and what can be done about it (a sort of risk–benefit analysis).

Reappraisal also occurs and refers to a changed appraisal based on new information. The appraisal process is not necessarily sequential; primary and secondary appraisal and reappraisal may occur simultaneously. Information learned from an adaptational encounter can be stored so that when a similar situation is encountered again the whole process does not need to be repeated.

The appraisal process contributes to the development of an **emotion**. Negative emotions such as fear and anger accompany harm/loss appraisals, while positive emotions such as happiness and joy accompany challenge. Besides the subjective component or feeling which accompanies a particular emotion, each emotion also includes a tendency to act in a certain way. To illustrate this concept, an unexpected quiz in the classroom might be judged as threatening by the unprepared student, and fear, anger, and resentment might be felt. These emotions might be expressed by outwardly hostile behavior or comments.

Lazarus (1991a) has expanded his former ideas about stress, appraisal, and coping into a more complex model relating emotion to adaptation. He calls this a cognitive–motivational–relational theory with **relational** "standing for a focus on negotiation with a physical and social world" (p. 13). A theory of emotion is proposed as the bridge to connect psychology, physiology, and sociology. "More than any other arena of psychological thought, emotion is an integrative, organismic concept that subsumes psychological stress and coping within itself and unites motivation, cognition, and adaptation in a complex configuration" (p. 40).

Coping, according to Lazarus, consists of the cognitive and behavioral efforts made to manage the specific external or internal demands that tax a person's resources. Coping can be **emotion-focused** or **problem-focused**. Coping that is emotion-focused seeks to make the person feel better by lessening the emotional distress felt. Problem-focused coping aims to make direct changes in the environment so that the situation can be dealt with more effectively. Both types of coping usually occur in a stressful situation. Even when the situation is viewed as challenging or beneficial, coping efforts may be required to develop and sustain the challenge, that is, to maintain the positive benefits of the challenge and to ward off any threats. In harmful or threatening situations successful coping will reduce or eliminate the source of stress and relieve the emotion it generated.

Personal Resources

Appraisal and coping are affected by the internal characteristics of the person. These include health and energy, as well as the person's belief system including existential beliefs (faith, religious beliefs), commitments or life goals (motivational properties), and the person's own sense of self including self-esteem, control, and mastery. They also include knowledge, problem-solving skills, and social skills (ability to communicate and interact with others).

Those characteristics that have been studied the most in nursing research include health-promoting lifestyle and hardiness (Ruiz-Bueno, 1993). A health-promoting lifestyle buffers the effect of stressors. From a nursing practice standpoint this outcome supports nursing's goal of promoting health. In many circumstances, promoting a healthy lifestyle is more achievable than reducing and altering the stressors.

Hardiness is the name given to a general quality that comes from rich, varied, and rewarding childhood experiences. It is a personality characteristic composed of control, commitment, and challenge. Hardy persons perceive stressors as something they can change and therefore control. Potential stressful situations are interesting and meaningful (commitment); change and new situations are viewed as an opportunity for growth (challenge). Some positive support has been found for hardiness as a mediator of the psychosocial stress associated with chronic illness (Ruiz-Bueno, 1993).

External Resources

Social Support. Social support is a major external resource. The nature of social support and its influence on coping have been studied extensively, and it has been demonstrated to be an effective moderator of life stress. Cobb (1976) defined social support as information belonging to one or more of three categories. The first category of information leads the individual to believe that he or she is cared for and loved. This appears most often in a relationship between two people in which mutual trust and attachment are expressed by helping one another meet their needs. Such expressions, sometimes called **emotional support**, are most commonly thought of in the marital relationship.

The second category of information leads the individual to believe that he or she is esteemed and valued. This is most effective when there is a public announcement that demonstrates the favorable position the individual has in the group. It elevates the person's sense of self-worth. This is called **esteem support**.

The third category of information leads the individual to believe that he or she belongs to a **network of communication and mutual obligation**. Information is shared by the members of the network, they all know what it is, and they are all aware that it is shared. This information is of two types. One is communications, which are "the essence of history"—what is going on, who is affected, and so forth. Another type of communication in this category is the knowledge that goods and services are available to the members on demand; for example, a person can call on a close friend in an emergency. Cobb emphasized that social support encourages independent behavior; it does not lead to dependency.

Social support begins *in utero;* it is fostered through maternal and paternal attachment behavior and develops through family, peer, and community relationships as the person grows. A number of sociologic and family theories attest to increased stress and illness when the family structure is disrupted.

Social support facilitates the coping behaviors of a person; however, this is conditional on the nature of the social support. People can have extensive relationships and interact frequently, but the necessary support comes only when there is a deep level of involvement and concern, not when people merely touch the surface of each other's lives. The critical qualities within the network are the exchange of intimate communications and the presence of solidarity and trust.

Material Resources. Material resources are another source of external support, and include the goods and services that can be purchased. Coping with constraints in the environment is much easier for individuals with adequate financial resources because their sense of vulnerability to threat is decreased.

Coping with Illness

The five predominant ways of coping with illness identified in a review of 57 nursing research studies were: "(1) trying to be optimistic about the outcome, (2) using social support, (3) using spiritual resources, (4) trying to maintain control either over the situation or over feelings, and (5) trying to accept the situation" (Jalowiec, 1993, p. 80).

Both patients and family members in the studies used a combination of emotion-focused and problem-focused coping in dealing with illness-related stressors. Other ways of coping found in the studies included information-seeking, reprioritizing needs and roles, lowering expectations, making compromises, comparison to others, activity planning to conserve energy, taking things one step at a time, listening to their body, and using self-talk for encouragement.

Physiologic Response

Interpretation of Stimuli by the Brain

The physiologic response to a stressor is a protective and adaptive mechanism to maintain the homeostatic balance of the body. As described by McEwen and Mendelson (1993), the stress response is a "cascade of neural and hormonal events that have short- and long-lasting consequences for both brain and body . . . a stressor is an event that challenges homeostasis, with a disease outcome being looked upon as a failure of the normal process of adaptation to the stress" (p. 101).

Neural and hormonal actions to maintain homeostatic balance are integrated by the hypothalamus. The hypothalamus is located in the center of the brain, surrounded by the limbic system and the cerebral hemispheres. It integrates autonomic nervous system mechanisms that maintain the chemical constancy of the internal environment of the body. The hypothalamus and the limbic system regulate emotions and many visceral behaviors necessary for survival (*e.g.*, eating, drinking, temperature control, reproduction, defense, and aggression). The hypothalamus is made up of a number of nuclei; the limbic system contains the amygdala, hippocampus, and septal nuclei, along with other structures.

Research supports the concept that each of these structures responds differently to stimuli, and each has its characteristic response. The cerebral hemispheres are concerned with cognitive functions: thought processes, learning, and memory. The limbic system has connections with both the cerebral hemispheres and the brain stem. In addition, the reticular activating system (RAS), which is a network of cells that forms a two-way communication system, extends from the brainstem into the midbrain and limbic system. This network controls the alert or "waking" state of the body; it sends signals that are relayed up to the cortex and relays signals from the cortex downward.

In the stress response, afferent impulses are carried from sensory organs (eye, ear, nose, skin) and internal sensors (baroreceptors, chemoreceptors) to nerve centers in the brain. Stress may be perceived by different centers ranging from the cortex down to the brainstem, which in turn relay information to the hypothalamus. The response to the perception of stress is integrated in the hypothalamus, which coordinates the adjustments necessary to return to homeostatic balance. The degree and duration of the response will vary; major stress evokes both sympathetic and pituitary adrenal responses.

Neuroendocrine Response

Neural and neuroendocrine pathways under the control of the hypothalamus are activated in the stress response. First, there is a sympathetic nervous system discharge followed by a sympathetic–adrenal–medullary discharge, and finally, if the stress persists, the hypothalamic–pituitary system is activated (Fig. 9-1).

Sympathetic Nervous System Response. The sympathetic nervous system response is rapid and short-lived. Norepinephrine is released at nerve endings in direct contact with their respective end organs to cause an increase in function of the vital organs and a state of general body arousal. The heart rate is increased. Peripheral vasoconstriction occurs, raising the blood pressure. Blood is also shunted away from abdominal organs. The purpose of these activities is to provide better perfusion of vital organs (brain, heart, skeletal muscles). Blood glucose is increased and supplies more readily available energy. The pupils are dilated, and mental activity is increased; a greater sense of awareness exists. Constriction of the blood vessels of the skin limits bleeding in the event of trauma. Subjectively, the person is likely to experience cold feet, clammy skin and hands, chills, palpitations, and a "knot" in the stomach. Typically, the person appears tense, with the muscles of the neck, upper back, and shoulders tightened; respirations may be rapid and shallow, with the diaphragm tense.

Sympathetic–Adrenal–Medullary Response. In addition to its direct effect on major end organs, the sympathetic nervous system (SNS) stimulates the medulla of the adrenal gland to release the hormones epinephrine and norepinephrine into the bloodstream. The action of these hormones is similar to that of the SNS and has the effect of sustaining and prolonging its actions. Epinephrine and norepinephrine both also stimulate the nervous system

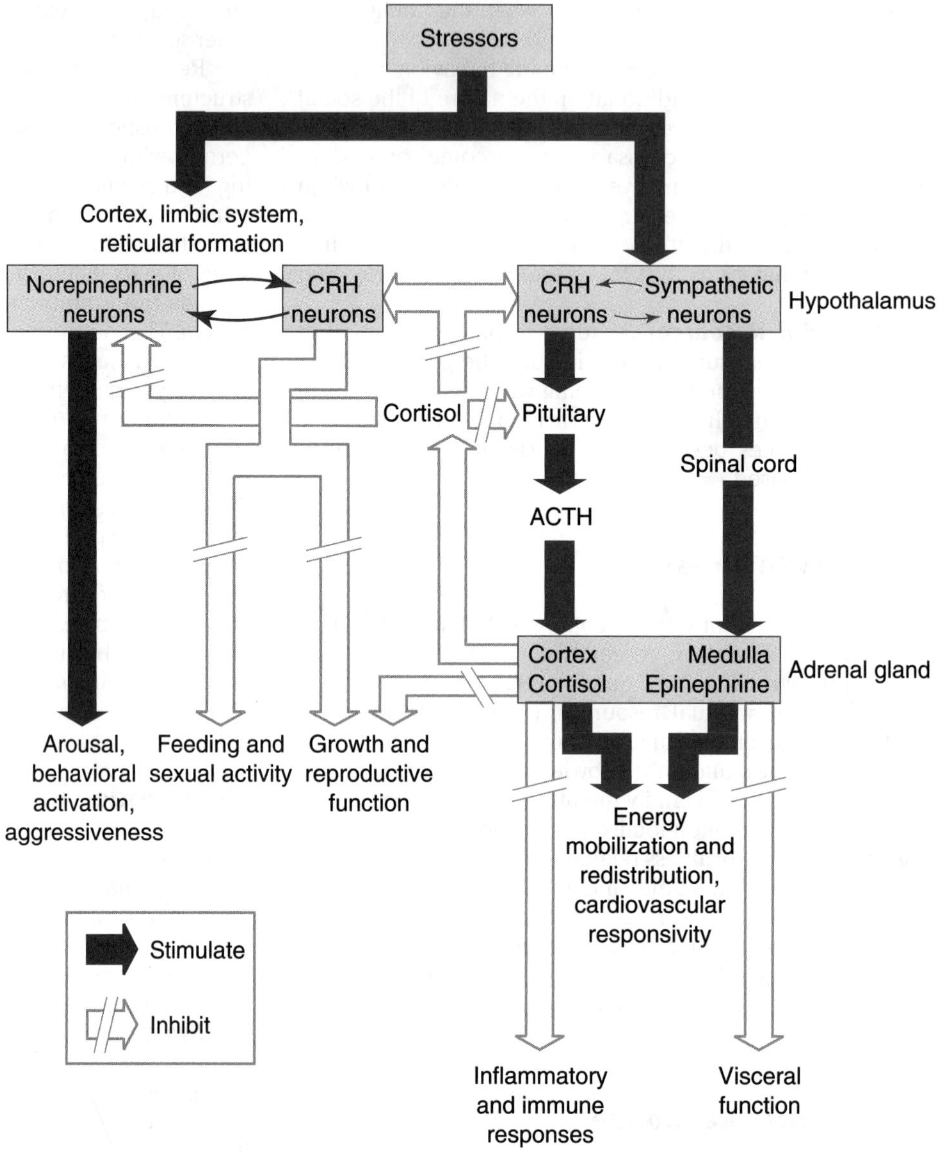

FIGURE 9-1. Integrated responses to stress mediated by the sympathetic nervous system and the hypothalamic–pituitary–adrenocortical axis. The responses are mutually reinforcing, both at the central and peripheral levels. Negative feedback by cortisol also can limit an overresponse that might be harmful to the individual. *Colored arrows,* stimulation; *open arrows,* inhibition; CRH, corticotropin-releasing hormone; ACTH, adreno-corticotropic hormone. (Reproduced with permission from Berne RM and Levy MN. Physiology. St. Louis, Mosby-Year Book, 1993.)

and produce metabolic effects that increase the blood glucose level and increase the metabolic rate. The effect of the sympathetic and adrenal–medullary responses is summarized in Table 9-1. This effect is called the "fight or flight" reaction.

Hypothalamic–Pituitary Response. The longest-acting phase of the physiologic response, which is more likely to occur in persistent stress, involves the hypothalamic–pituitary pathway. The hypothalamus secretes corticotropin-releasing factor, which stimulates the anterior pituitary to produce adrenocorticotropic hormone (ACTH). ACTH in turn stimulates the adrenal cortex to produce glucocorticoids, primarily cortisol. Cortisol stimulates protein catabolism, releasing amino acids; stimulates liver uptake of amino acids and their conversion to glucose (gluconeogenesis); and inhibits glucose uptake (anti-insulin action) by many body cells but not those of the brain and heart. These cortisol-induced metabolic effects provide the body with a ready source of energy during a stressful situation. There are some important implications to this effect: a person with diabetes who is under stress, such as that caused by an infection, will need more insulin than usual. Any patient who is under stress (illness, surgery, prolonged psychologic stress) will catabolize body protein and need supplements. Children subjected to severe stress will have retarded growth.

The actions of the catecholamines (epinephrine and norepinephrine) and cortisol are most important in the general response to stress. Other hormones that are released are antidiuretic hormone (ADH) from the posterior pituitary and aldosterone from the adrenal cortex. ADH and aldosterone promote sodium and water retention, which is an adaptive mechanism in the event of hemorrhage or loss of fluids through excessive perspiration. ADH has also been shown to influence learning and so may facilitate coping in new and threatening situations. Growth hormone and glucagon are secreted and stimulate the uptake of amino acids by cells, helping to mobilize energy resources. The secretion of other hormones is also affected, but their adaptive function is less clear.

The production of endorphin, an endogenous opiate, is also increased during stress and enhances the threshold for tolerance of painful stimuli. It may also affect mood. It has been implicated in the so-called "high" that long-distance runners experience.

TABLE 9-1 Sympathetic–Adrenal–Medullary Response

Effect	Purpose	Mechanism
↑ Heart rate ↑ Blood pressure	Better perfusion of vital organs	Increased cardiac output due to increased myocardial contractility and heart rate; also, increased venous return (peripheral vasoconstriction)
↑ Blood glucose	Increased available energy	Increased liver and muscle glycogen breakdown; also, increased breakdown of adipose tissue triglycerides
↑ Mental activity	Alert state	
Dilated pupils	Increased awareness	
↑ Tension of skeletal muscles	Preparedness for activity, decreased fatigue	Excitation of muscles; also, increase in amount of blood shunted to the muscles from the abdominal viscera
↑ Ventilation (may be rapid and shallow)	Provision of oxygen for energy	
↑ Coagulability of blood	Prevention of hemorrhage in event of trauma	Vasoconstriction of surface vessels

Stress and the Immune System

Glucocorticoids depress the immune system. When they are present in high concentrations, there is a reduction in the inflammatory response to injury or infection. The steps of the inflammatory process are inhibited, lymphocytes are destroyed in lymphoid tissues, and antibody production is decreased. As a result, the ability of the person to resist infections is reduced. The inhibition of the inflammatory response can be used to advantage pharmacologically in the prescription of cortisol to treat the inflammatory and immune responses in arthritis, asthma, and transplant rejection.

The relationship of stress to the immune response is a subject of new fields of study called behavioral immunology, psychoneuroimmunology, and neuroimmunomodulation. Studies of animals have shown that extreme psychologic stress can have a profound effect on immune competence. Studies in humans have not been as conclusive (partially because of problems in experimental design and control), but investigators believe that the mind influences immune responses with consequences that can be harmful to the host (Kiecolt-Glaser & Glaser, 1992).

Selye and the General Adaptation Syndrome

Because of his profound influence on the scientific development of the study of stress and the manner in which he popularized the concept, it is important to understand Hans Selye's theory. In 1936, Selye, experimenting with animals, first described a syndrome consisting of enlargement of the adrenal cortex; shrinkage of the thymus, spleen, lymph nodes, and other lymphatic structures; and the appearance of deep, bleeding ulcers in the stomach and duodenum. He identified this as a nonspecific response to diverse, noxious stimuli. From this beginning, he developed a theory of adaptation to biologic stress, which he named the **general adaptation syndrome** (GAS).

Phases of the GAS

The GAS has three phases: **alarm, resistance,** and **exhaustion**. During the acute phase, or alarm reaction, the sympathetic fight or flight response is activated with release of adrenal medullary hormones, and the ACTH–adrenal cortical response begins. The alarm reaction is defensive and anti-inflammatory but self-limited. Because it is impossible to live in a continuous state of alarm (death would ensue), the person moves into the second stage, resistance. During this stage, adaptation to the noxious stressor occurs. Cortisol activity is still increased. If exposure to the stressor is prolonged, exhaustion sets in and endocrine activity increases, producing deleterious effects on the body systems (especially circulatory, digestive, and immune) that can lead to death. Stages one and two of this syndrome are repeated, in different degrees, throughout life as the person encounters stressors.

Selye also compared the GAS with the life process. During childhood, there are few encounters with stress to promote the development of adaptive functioning, and the child is vulnerable. During adulthood, the person encounters a number of life's stressful events and develops a resistance or adaptation. During the later years, the accumulation of life's stressors and the wear and tear on the organism again deplete the person's ability to adapt, resistance falls, and eventually death ensues.

Local Adaptation Syndrome

According to Selye's theory, there is also a local adaptation syndrome (LAS). This syndrome includes the inflammatory response and repair processes that occur at the local site of tissue injury. The LAS occurs in small, topical injuries, such as in contact dermatitis. If the local injury were severe enough the general adaptation syndrome would be activated also.

Selye emphasized that stress is the nonspecific response common to all stressors, regardless of whether they are physiologic, psychologic, or social. The fact that different demands are interpreted by different people as stressors is explained by the many conditioning factors in each person's environment. Conditioning factors also account for differences in the tolerance of different persons for stress. Some may develop diseases of adaptation, such as hypertension and migraine headaches, while others appear to be unaffected.

Additional Views

In his early research, Selye used extremes of physical stressors to study the stress response. With better techniques for detecting hormones, a variety of stressors of differing intensities have been used, and multihormonal patterns of response have been detected. These studies indicate that there are different patterns of response to different stimuli, **stimulus specificity**, and that each person develops a characteristic pattern of autonomic response that carries over from one type of stress to another, **individual response specificity**. It has been suggested that the nonspecific response is not elicited by a diverse number of stimuli but rather by one factor, emotional arousal, and that it is the degree of the arousal that affects the intensity of the hormonal response and thus the manifestations displayed by the individual (Mason, 1975).

Indicators of Stress

Indicators of stress and stress response include subjective and objective measures. Chart 9-1 lists signs and symptoms that may be observed directly or reported by the person. Some are psychologic, some physiologic, some behavioral, and some reflect social behaviors and thought processes. Some of these reactions may be coping behaviors. Over time, each person tends to develop a characteristic pattern of behavior in stress that is a warning that the system is out of balance.

Laboratory measurements of indicators of stress have helped in understanding this complex process. Among the measures, blood and urine analyses can be used to demonstrate changes in hormonal levels and hormonal breakdown products. Reliable measures of stress include blood levels of catecholamines, corticoids, ACTH, and eosinophils. The serum creatine/creatinine ratio and elevations of cholesterol and free fatty acids can also be measured. Immunoglobulin assays may be determined. With the growth of neuroimmunology, improved laboratory measures are likely to follow.

Galvanic skin resistance, which measures the electrical conductivity of the skin, may be assessed. This is primarily a measure of sweat excretion, which rises in stress, and is typically used in lie detector tests. Rises in blood pressure and heart rate can also be measured.

In addition to using laboratory tests, researchers have developed questionnaires to identify and assess stressors, stress, and coping. Many of these are discussed in the research monograph developed by Barnfather and Lyon (1993) based on a synthesis conference held by nurse scientists on the state of the science in stress and coping nursing research. Miller and Smith (1993) provide a stress audit and a stress profile measurement that is available in the popular literature.

Maladaptive Responses

As indicated earlier, the stress response serves as an adaptation to meet threatening situations. It has been retained

CHART 9-1
Indices of Stress

- General irritability, hyperexcitation, or depression
- Dryness of the throat and mouth
- Overpowering urge to cry or run and hide
- Easily fatigued, loss of interest
- "Floating anxiety"—do not know exactly why or what
- Easily startled
- Stuttering or other speech difficulties
- Hypermotility: pacing, moving about, cannot sit still
- Gastrointestinal signs and symptoms: "butterflies" in the stomach, diarrhea, vomiting
- Change in menstrual cycle
- Loss of or excessive appetite
- Increased use of legally prescribed drugs, such as tranquilizers or psychic energizers
- Accident proneness
- Disturbed behavior
- Pounding of the heart
- Impulsive behavior, emotional instability
- Inability to concentrate
- Feelings of unreality, weakness, or dizziness
- Tension, alertness
- Trembling, nervous tics
- Nervous laughter
- Grinding of teeth
- Insomnia
- Perspiring
- Increased frequency of urination
- Muscle tension and migraine headaches
- Pain in the neck or lower back
- Increased smoking
- Alcohol and drug addiction
- Nightmares

(Based on Selye H. Stress in Health and Disease. Stoneham, MA, Butterworths, 1976. Reprinted by permission of the publisher.)

from the human evolutionary past and it is questionable whether it fits the needs of life in civilized societies. The fight or flight response, for example, is an anticipatory response that mobilized the bodily resources of our ancestors to deal with predators and other harsh factors in their environment. This same mobilization comes into play in response to emotional stimuli unrelated to danger. For example, a person may get an "adrenaline rush" when competing over a decisive point in a ball game, or when excited about attending a party.

The stress response can be both beneficial and harmful. When the body has been prepared physiologically to act and does not do so, the result is likely to be frustrating and injurious to the person's health.

When the responses to stress are ineffective, they are referred to as maladaptive. **Maladaptive responses** are chronic, recurrent responses or patterns of response over time that do not promote the goals of adaptation. The goals of adaptation can be categorized into three areas. One is somatic or physical health, the goal being optimal wellness. Another is psychologic health or having a sense of well-being (happiness, satisfaction with life, morale). The other area is that of social functioning, which includes work, social, and family relationships, with the goal being positive relationships. Maladaptive responses that threaten these goals include faulty appraisals and inappropriate coping (Lazarus, 1991a).The focus of this discussion is on somatic health.

The frequency, intensity, and duration of stressful situations contribute to the development of negative emotions and subsequent patterns of neurochemical discharge. By appraising situations more adequately and by coping more appropriately it is possible to anticipate and defuse some of these situations. For example, frequent potentially stressful encounters (marital discord) might be avoided with better communication and problem solving; or a pattern of procrastination (delaying work on tasks) can contribute to stress when the deadline of the task approaches.

Coping processes that include the use of alcohol, drugs, or abusive substances to reduce stress increase the risk of illness. Other inappropriate coping patterns may increase the risk of illness more indirectly. As an example, people with type-A behaviors are driving, competitive, and achievement-oriented. The pattern they have developed reflects a socialization process that emphasizes the work ethic. Mobilization of type-A behavior increases the output of catecholamines, the adrenal-medullary hormones, with their attendant effects on the body. One might say the life of a type-A person is a series of fight or flight responses.

Other forms of inappropriate coping include denial, avoidance, and distancing. Denial may be illustrated by the woman who feels a lump in her breast but denies its seriousness and delays seeking medical attention. The intent of the denial is to control the threat, but it may endanger life.

Ego defenses are called "defensive reappraisals" by Lazarus (1991a, p. 113). They are a learned and automatic (unconscious) strategy to deal with conflicts over a particular emotion. In this case the emotion itself, anger for example, is the threat. The individual "learns" to appraise situations that would or should provoke anger as being benign or irrelevant. Subsequently, when provoking situations arise, the anger is "short-circuited," repressed, or suppressed.

Models of Illness

A **general model of illness**, based on Selye's theory, basically suggests that any stressor elicits a state of disturbed physiologic equilibrium. If this state is prolonged or the response excessive, it will increase the susceptibility of the person to illness. This susceptibility, coupled with a predisposition in the person (genetic traits, health, age), leads to illness.

In instances in which the sympathetic adrenal–medullary response is prolonged or excessive, a state of chronic arousal develops, which may lead to high blood pressure, arteriosclerotic changes, and cardiovascular disease. When the production of the adrenal cortical hormone is prolonged or excessive, behavior patterns of withdrawal and depression are seen. In addition, the immune response is decreased, and infections and tumors may develop.

Selye (1976, pp. 169–170) proposed a list of disorders which he called diseases of maladaptation. These include the following:

> *High blood pressure, diseases of the heart and blood vessels, diseases of the kidney, eclampsia, rheumatic and rheumatoid arthritis, inflammatory diseases of the skin and eyes, infections, allergic and hypersensitivity diseases, nervous and mental diseases, sexual derangements, digestive diseases, metabolic diseases, cancer, and diseases of resistance in general.*

The **specificity model of illness** has developed in contrast to the general model. This model flows from the work of Mason and others cited earlier in this chapter indicating that there are specific patterns of physiologic response to specific emotions. Specific illnesses can flow from these patterned disturbances.

Stress Management: Nursing Interventions

Stress or the potential for stress is ubiquitous; that is, it can be everywhere and anywhere at once. Throughout this book, health problems will be identified that carry with them the potential for stress. Anxiety is the usual emotion associated with stress. In the presence of anxiety, the customary activities of daily living may be disrupted; for example, sleep disturbance may be present, and eating and activity patterns may be altered.

The usual nursing diagnosis related to stress is anxiety, which is defined as a vague, uneasy feeling whose source may be nonspecific or not known to the person. Coping patterns may be ineffective, thought processes may be impaired, and role relationships may suffer. These are reflected in the nursing diagnoses of impaired adjustment, ineffective individual coping, defensive coping, and ineffective denial, all of which indicate poor adaptive responses (NANDA, 1992).

Methods for stress management aim to reduce and control stress and to improve coping. Nurses might use these methods not only with their patients but also in their own lives. The need to prevent illness, improve the quality of life, and decrease the cost of health care makes efforts to promote health crucial. Stress control is a significant health promotion goal. The selected stress reduction methods and coping enhancements that will be described in the next section are divided into two groups: those using the person's internal resources and those using external resources.

Internal Resources

Health-Promoting Lifestyles

An individual's personal resources that aid in coping include health and energy. A health-promoting lifestyle provides these resources and buffers or cushions the impact of stressors. Lifestyles or habits that contribute to the risk of developing illness can be reduced or eliminated.

Health Risk Appraisal. Health risk appraisal is an assessment method designed to promote health by examining the individual's personal habits and recommending changes where health risk is identified. Health risk questionnaires estimate the likelihood that a person with a given set of characteristics will become ill, often within a given time span. It is reasoned that if people are provided with this information, they will alter their activities (*e.g.,* stop smoking, have periodic screening examinations) to improve their health status. Questionnaires typically identify the following types of information:

1. Demographic data: age, sex, race, ethnic background
2. Personal and family history of certain diseases and health problems
3. Lifestyle factors
   a. Eating, sleeping, exercise, smoking, drinking, and driving habits
   b. Stressors on the job
   c. Role relationships and associated stressors
4. Physical measurements
   a. Blood pressure
   b. Height, weight
   c. Laboratory analyses of blood and urine
5. Membership or nonmembership in a high-risk group, such as a family with a history of cancer

The personal information is compared with average population risk data, and the risk factors are identified and weighted. From this analysis the person's risks and major health hazards are identified. If the person makes suggested changes, further comparisons with population data can estimate how many years will be added to his or her life span. Research so far has not demonstrated that providing people with such information ensures that they will change their habits (Doerr & Hutchins, 1981; Kaman, Licciardone, & Hoffman, 1991).

Although the collection of data bases like the one just described is a common part of taking a health history, the analysis of risk is not customary. A national *nursing* data base that supplies the essential information for making decisions about patient care has not yet been developed.

Health risk appraisal and patient education to improve health behavior are activities that nurses can perform to prevent health problems and reduce stress. In those who *already* have health problems, there will be some degree of stress, and the nurse can anticipate changes based on the stress response. For example, the postsurgical patient will have fluid and electrolyte changes resulting from the general neuroendocrine response. This response has a snowballing effect. Although it does not primarily affect the kidney, the vasoconstriction induced as part of the stress response may decrease the flow of blood to the kidney, which stimulates the renin–angiotensin mechanism, leading to an increase in aldosterone with extracellular fluid retention.

Coping Enhancement. McCloskey and Bulechek (1992) identify "coping enhancement" as a nursing intervention and define it as "assisting a patient to adapt to perceived stressors, changes, or threats which interfere with meeting life demands and roles" (Chart 9-2). After completing a health risk appraisal the nurse could use "coping enhancement" to assist the patient in an analysis of the appraisal and to explore methods to improve the person's coping abilities, including appraisal of his or her own personal resources.

Relaxation Training

In reviewing the research on nursing interventions for stress that was conducted from 1980 to 1990, Snyder (1993) and Egan (1993) identified relaxation techniques as the major method used to relieve stress. Commonly used techniques cited were progressive muscle relaxation, relaxation with guided imagery, and Benson's relaxation response (described in the next section). The goal of relaxation training is to produce a response that counters the stress response. When this goal is achieved, the action of the hypothalamus adjusts and decreases the activity of the sympathetic and parasympathetic nervous systems. The sequence of physiologic effects and their signs and symptoms are interrupted, and psychologic stress is reduced. This is a learned response and requires practice to achieve.

The different relaxation techniques share four similar elements: (1) a quiet environment, (2) a comfortable position, (3) a passive attitude, and (4) a mental device (something on which to focus the attention, such as a word, phrase, or sound).

Progressive Muscle Relaxation. Progressive muscle relaxation involves tensing and releasing the muscles of the body in sequence, and sensing the difference in feeling. It is best if the person lies on a soft cushion on the floor, in a quiet room, breathing easily. Someone usually reads the instructions in a low tone and a slow and relaxed manner, or a tape of the instructions can be played. The person tenses the muscles in the whole body, holds, senses the tension, and then relaxes. Then he or she begins tensing individual muscle groups, keeping the rest of the body relaxed—hands, then arms, then shoulders, etc.—each time feeling the tension and relaxation. When completed, the whole body should be relaxed (Benson, 1993; Scandrett-Hibdon & Uecker, 1992).

Benson's Relaxation Response. Benson and Proctor (1984) describe the following steps of the Benson Relaxation Response (pp. 106–117):

CHART 9-2
Coping Enhancement

Definition: Assisting a patient to adapt to perceived stressors, changes, or threats which interfere with meeting life demands and roles

Activities

Appraise a patient's adjustment to changes in body image as indicated
Appraise the impact of the patient's life situation on roles and relationships
Encourage patient to identify a realistic description of change in role
Appraise the patient's understanding of the disease process
Appraise and discuss alternative responses to situation
Use a calm, reassuring approach
Provide an atmosphere of acceptance
Assist the patient in developing an objective appraisal of the event
Help the patient to identify the information he/she is most interested in obtaining
Provide factual information concerning diagnosis, treatment, and prognosis
Provide the patient with realistic choices about certain aspects of care
Encourage an attitude of realistic hope as a way of dealing with feelings of helplessness
Evaluate the patient's decision-making ability
Seek to understand the patient's perspective of a stressful situation
Discourage decision-making when the patient is under severe stress
Encourage gradual mastery of the situation
Encourage patience in developing relationships
Encourage relationships with persons who have common interests and goals
Encourage social and community activities
Encourage the acceptance of limitations of others
Acknowledge the patient's spiritual/cultural background
Encourage the use of spiritual resources if desired
Explore patient's previous achievements of success
Explore patient's reasons for self-criticism
Confront patient's ambivalent (angry or depressed) feelings
Foster constructive outlets for anger and hostility
Arrange situations that encourage patient's autonomy
Assist patient in identifying positive responses from others
Encourage the identification of specific life values
Explore with the patient previous methods of dealing with life problems
Introduce patient to persons (or groups) who have successfully undergone the same experience
Support the use of appropriate defense mechanisms
Encourage verbalization of feelings, perceptions, and fears
Discuss consequences of not dealing with guilt and shame
Encourage the patient to identify own strengths and abilities
Assist the patient in identifying appropriate short- and long-term goals
Assist the patient in breaking down complex goals into small, manageable steps
Assist the patient in examining available resources to meet the goals
Reduce stimuli in the environment that could be misinterpreted as threatening
Appraise patient needs/desires for social support
Assist the patient to identify available support systems
Determine the risk of the patient's inflicting self-harm
Encourage family involvement as appropriate
Encourage the family to verbalize feelings about ill family member
Provide appropriate social skills training
Assist the patient to identify positive strategies to deal with limitations and manage needed lifestyle or role changes
Assist the patient to problem-solve in a constructive manner
Instruct the patient on the use of relaxation techniques as needed
Assist the patient to grieve, and work through the losses of chronic illness and/or disability if appropriate
Assist the patient to clarify misconceptions
Encourage the patient to evaluate his/her own behavior

(Reproduced with permission from McCloskey JC and Bulechek GM. Nursing Intervention Classification (NIC). St. Louis, Mosby-Yearbook, 1992.)

Step One: Pick a brief phrase or word that reflects your basic belief system.
Step Two: Choose a comfortable position.
Step Three: Close your eyes.
Step Four: Relax your muscles.
Step Five: Become aware of your breathing, and start using your selected focus word.
Step Six: Maintain a passive attitude.
Step Seven: Continue for a set period of time.
Step Eight: Practice the technique twice daily.

This response combines meditation with relaxation. Along with the repeated word or phrase, a passive attitude is essential. Other thoughts or distractions (noises, the pain of an ailment) may occur; however, Benson recommends not fighting the distraction but simply continuing to repeat the focus phrase. The time of day is not important, but the exercise works best on an empty stomach.

Relaxation With Guided Imagery. Simple guided imagery is the "purposeful use of imagination to achieve relaxation and/or direct attention away from undesirable sensations" (McCloskey & Bulechek, 1992, p. 77). The nurse helps the person to select a pleasant scene or experience from his or her past, such as watching the ocean, dabbling the feet in a cool stream. This image serves as the mental device in this technique. As the person sits comfortably and quietly, the nurse guides him or her to review the scene, trying to feel and relive the imagery with all of the senses. A tape recording may be made of his or her description of the image, or commercial tape recordings for guided imagery and relaxation can be used.

Other Relaxation Techniques. Other relaxation techniques include meditation, breathing techniques, therapeutic touch, massage, music therapy, biofeedback, and the use of humor.

Providing Sensory and Procedural Information

Two commonly prescribed nursing interventions, the provision of sensory information and procedural information (such as preoperative teaching) have the goal of improving the patient's coping ability. Major nursing research using these interventions has been conducted by Leventhal and Johnson (1983). They have tested the theory that people acquire a sense of control over events when they are given information that makes it possible for them to form a mental image of the event. For example, if people were provided with a description of the sensations they could expect to feel (*e.g.*, pulling, burning, pressure), if the routine of the procedure were described to them, and if they were given instructions in coping behaviors (deep breathing, coughing, turning, exercises), they would experience less distress and have better outcomes (less pain, better mood, fewer analgesics needed, more rapid recovery). In their work, the researchers have tested these techniques alone and in combination in different short-term and long-term threatening situations (diagnostic examinations and surgery). The outcomes have been complex and illustrate that individual differences in the perception of stress and its management must be taken into consideration.

Among their findings, Leventhal and Johnson discovered that the combination of sensory information and postoperative exercise instruction was not consistently effective. If the instruction provided the patient with a way of coping when he or she previously had none, it was more likely to be effective. If he or she already had an effective coping strategy, any new ones could be considered conflicting. In some instances, attempting to use the new strategy rather than relying on existing strategies was thought to delay recovery, particularly after the patient went home. Specific coping strategies were usually more effective in short-term than in long-term events. Individual differences were found to be significant.

This research can help the nurse to decide who will benefit from the information provided, the goal to be achieved, and the specific outcome criteria to be used in evaluating the information.

Preparatory Education

Preparatory education includes giving structured content, such as a lesson in childbirth preparation to expectant parents, or cardiovascular content to the cardiac patient. Studies using these techniques purport to alter the person–environment relationship such that something that might have been viewed as a harm or threat is now appraised more positively. This also reduces the emotional response so that patients are able to concentrate more effectively, and their problem-solving skills are enhanced.

External Resources

Social Support

The function of social networks in dealing with stress includes the following:

- The maintenance of positive social identity
- The provision of emotional support
- The provision of material aid and tangible services
- Access to information
- Access to new social contacts and new social roles

The emotions—anxiety, fear, guilt—that accompany stress are unpleasant and often increase in a spiraling fashion if relief is not provided. Emotional support from family and significant others provides a person with love and a sense of sharing the burden. Being able to talk with someone and express one's feelings openly may help to gain mastery of the situation. Nurses can provide this source of support; however, it is important to identify the person's social support system and encourage its use. People who are "loners" or isolated, or who withdraw in times of stress have a high risk of coping failure.

Anxiety may also distort a person's ability to process information. Perception is narrowed, thoughts may be unclear, and reality may be distorted. For a time, this cognitive blurring is adaptive and allows the person to tolerate a threat, perhaps some bad news. However, reality must be faced for the longer run. It helps to seek information and advice from others who can assist with analyzing the threat and developing a strategy to manage it. Again, this use of others helps the person to maintain mastery of a situation and to retain self-esteem.

Support Groups and Therapy Groups. Support groups exist especially for groups of people with similar stressful situations. Groups have been formed by parents of children with leukemia, people with ostomies, mastectomy

CRITICAL THINKING EXERCISES

1. Think back to a time when you had an acute illness or injury. Describe the illness-related or injury-related stressors you experienced. How did you cope with these stressors? What evidence was there that your coping ability was successful or unsuccessful?
2. You are caring for a patient in the home care setting. Describe how you would assess the patient's health status and life-style to determine health promotion activities that should be explored with the patient and his family. How would your plans vary if the patient is weak and debilitated versus a patient who is recuperating according to schedule; has failing eyesight; is alone most of the day?

patients (Reach to Recovery) and those with other kinds of cancer or other serious diseases. There are groups for single parents, Alcoholics Anonymous and spouses of alcoholics, drug addiction groups, and groups for victims of child abuse. Professional, civic, and religious support groups are active in the community. There are also encounter groups, assertiveness training programs, and consciousness-raising groups to help people modify their usual behavior in person–environment transactions. Being a member of a group with similar problems or goals has a releasing effect on the person that promotes freedom of expression and exchange of ideas.

REFERENCES AND BIBLIOGRAPHY

Books

Aldwin CM. Stress, Coping, and Development. New York, Guilford Press, 1994.

Barnfather JS. History, overview and project methodology. In Barnfather JS and Lyon BL (eds). Stress and Coping: State of the Science and Implications for Nursing Theory, Research and Practice. Indianapolis, Indiana, Sigma Theta Tau International Inc., 1993.

Barnfather JS and Lyon BL (eds). Stress and Coping: State of the Science and Implications for Nursing Theory, Research and Practice. Indianapolis, Indiana, Sigma Theta Tau International Inc., 1993.

Benson H. The relaxation response. In Goleman D and Gurin J (eds). Mind Body Medicine: How to Use Your Mind for Better Health. Yonkers, NY Consumer Reports Books, 1993.

Benson H and Proctor W. Beyond the Relaxation Response. New York, Berkley Books, 1984.

Berne RM and Levy MN. Physiology. St. Louis, Mosby Year Book, 1993.

Bulechek GM and McCloskey JC. Nursing Interventions: Essential Nursing Treatments. Philadelphia, WB Saunders, 1992.

Bullock BL and Rosendahl PB. Pathophysiology: Adaptations and Alterations in Function, 3rd ed. Philadelphia, JB Lippincott, 1992.

Carrieri VK, Lindsey AM, and West CM. Pathophysiological Phenomena in Nursing. Philadelphia, WB Saunders, 1993.

Dohrenwend BP et al. The structured event probe and narrative rating method for measuring stressful life events. In Goldberger L and Breznitz S (eds). Handbook of Stress, 2nd ed. New York, The Free Press, 1993.

Egan EC. Intervention and the stress-related health outcome linkage: Theoretical orientations. In Barnfather JS and Lyon BL (eds). Stress and Coping: State of the Science and Implications for Nursing Theory, Research and Practice. Indianapolis, Indiana, Sigma Theta Tau International Inc., 1993.

Elliott G. Stress and illness. In Cheren S (ed). Psychosomatic Medicine: Theory, Physiology, and Practice (2 vols). Madison, CT, International Universities Press, 1989.

Goldberger L and Breznitz S (eds). Handbook of Stress, 2nd ed. New York, The Free Press, 1993.

Goleman D and Gurin J. Mind Body Medicine: How to Use Your Mind for Better Health. Yonkers, NY, Consumer Reports Books, 1993.

Guyton AC. Textbook of Medical Physiology. Philadelphia, WB Saunders, 1991.

Jalowiec A. Coping with illness: Synthesis and critique of the nursing literature from 1980-1990. In Barnfather JS and Lyon BL (eds). Stress and Coping: State of the Science and Implications for Nursing Theory, Research and Practice. Indianapolis, Indiana, Sigma Theta Tau International Inc., 1993.

Jasmin G. Stress Revisited. Basel, Switzerland, Karger, 1991.

Joneja JV and Bielory L. Understanding Allergy, Sensitivity, and Immunity. New Brunswick, Rutgers University Press, 1990.

Lazarus RS. Why we should think of stress as a subset of emotion. In Goldberger L and Breznitz S (eds). Handbook of Stress, 2nd ed. New York, The Free Press, 1993.

Lazarus RS. Emotion and Adaptation. New York, Oxford University Press, 1991a.

Lazarus RS and Folkman S. Stress, Appraisal, and Coping. New York, Springer Publishing Company, 1984.

Leventhal H and Johnson JE. Laboratory and field experimentation: Development of a theory of self-regulation. In Wooldridge PJ et al (eds). Behavioral Science and Nursing Theory. St. Louis, CV Mosby, 1983.

Lyon BL and Werner JS. Stress. In Fitzpatrick J and Taunton R (eds). Annual Review of Nursing Research. New York, Springer Publishing Company, 1987.

McCloskey JC and Bulechek GM (eds). Nursing Interventions Classification (NIC). St. Louis, Mosby Year Book, 1992.

McEwen BS and Mendelson S. Effects of stress on the neurochemistry and morphology of the brain: Counterregulation versus damage. In Goldberger L and Breznitz S (eds). Handbook of Stress, 2nd ed. New York, The Free Press, 1993.

Miller JF. Coping with Chronic Illness, 2nd ed. Philadelphia, FA Davis, 1992.

Miller LH and Smith AD. The Stress Solution. New York, Pocket Books, 1993.

Moyers B. Healing and the Mind. New York, Doubleday, 1993.

North American Nursing Diagnosis Association. NANDA Nursing Diagnoses: Definitions and Classifications 1992-1993. Philadelphia, Nursecom, 1992.

Pelletier KR. Mind as Healer, Mind as Slayer, 2nd ed. New York, Dell Publishing Company. Text copyright, 1977. Preface copyright 1992.

Plotnikoff N, Murgo A, Faith R, and Wybran J. Stress and Immunity. Boca Raton, CRC Press, 1991.

Ruiz-Bueno JB. Commentary on resources as mediators of the stress-health outcome linkage. In Barnfather JS and Lyon BL (eds). Stress and Coping: State of the Science and Implications for Nursing Theory, Research and Practice. Indianapolis, Indiana, Sigma Theta Tau International Inc., 1993.

Scandrett-Hibdon S and Uecker S. Relaxation Training. In Bulechek GM and McCloskey JC. Nursing Interventions: Essential Nursing Treatments. Philadelphia, WB Saunders, 1992.

Selye H. The Stress of Life, rev ed. New York, McGraw Hill, 1976.

Selye H. The Stress of Life. New York, McGraw Hill, 1956.

Snyder M. The influence of interventions on the stress-health outcome linkage. In Barnfather JS and Lyon BL (eds). Stress and Coping: State of the Science and Implications for Nursing Theory, Research and Practice. Indianapolis, Indiana, Sigma Theta Tau International Inc., 1993.

Werner JS. Stressors and health outcomes: Synthesis of nursing research, 1980-1990. In Barnfather JS and Lyon BL (eds). Stress and Coping: State of the Science and Implications for Nursing Theory, Research and Practice. Indianapolis, Indiana, Sigma Theta Tau International Inc., 1993.

Journals

Ballard KS. Identification of environmental stressors for patients in a surgical intensive care unit. Issues Mental Health Nurs 1981 Jan–Jun; 3: 89–108.

Brandt P and Weinert C. The PRQ—A social support measure. Nurs Res 1981 Sept/Oct; 30(5): 277–280.

Cobb S. Social support as a moderator of life stress. Psychosom Med 1976 Sept/Oct; 38(5): 300–314.

Doerr BT and Hutchins EB. Health risk appraisal: Process, problems, and prospects for nursing practice and research. Nurs Res 1981 Sept/Oct; 30(5): 277–280.

Funk SC. Hardiness: A review of theory and research. Health Psychology 1992; 11(5): 335–345.

Harbuz MS and Lightman SL. Stress and the hypothalamo-pituitary-adrenal axis: Acute, chronic and immunological activation. J Endocrinology 1992; 134: 327–339.

Holmes TH and Rahe RH. The social readjustment rating scale. J Psychosom Res 1967 Aug; 11: 213–218.

Kaman RL, Licciardone JC, and Hoffman MA. Comparison of health risk prevalence reported in a health risk appraisal and predicted through demographic analysis. Am J Health Promot 1991; 5(5): 378–383.

Kiecolt-Glaser JK and Glaser R. Psychoneuroimmunology: Can psychological interventions modulate immunity. J Consulting and Clinical Psychology 1992 Aug; 60(4): 569–575.

Lazarus RS. Cognition and motivation in emotion. Am Psychologist 1991b April; 46(4): 352–367.

Lazarus RS. Progress on a cognitive-motivational-relational theory of emotion. Am Psychologist 1991c Aug; 46(8): 819–834.

Mason JW. A historical view of the stress field, Part II. J Hum Stress 1975 June; 1(2): 22–36.

Norbeck JS, Lindsey AM, and Carrieri VL. The development of an instrument to measure social support. Nurs Res 1981 Sept/Oct; 30(5): 264–269.

Rahe RH. Editorial. J Hum Stress 1975 June; 1(2): 3.

Tausig M. Measuring life events. J Health Soc Behav 1982 March; 23(1): 52–64.

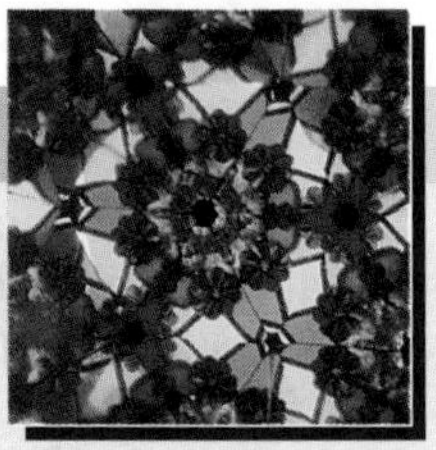

10

Human Response to Illness

CHAPTER OUTLINE

LEARNING OBJECTIVES

On completion of this chapter, the reader will be able to:

1. Identify the stages of illness and the role of the nurse during each of these stages
2. Describe the significance of the patient's need for inclusion, control, and affection during his or her adaptation to illness
3. Specify nursing strategies that are appropriate for assisting patients to develop and maintain a positive self-image and body image
4. Explain the emotions of anxiety, anger, hostility, grief, mourning, and hope as related to illness adaptation
5. Use the nursing process as a framework for care of patients with emotional reactions to illness and treatment: anxiety, anger and hostility, grief, mourning, and hope
6. Assess the significance of role changes that result from illness
7. Identify nursing actions that promote effective coping strategies

The experience of illness generates many stressful feelings and reactions, including frustration, anxiety, anger, denial, shame, grief, and uncertainty. Those who become ill, along with their families, have to adapt to the demands of the different stages of illness. Painful and disturbing symptoms lead to diagnostic tests and medical treatment. Dreaded questions arise about the prognosis, possible body changes, and the reactions of others. If hospitalization becomes necessary, it creates stress by placing the person in an unfamiliar and often frightening environment that stirs feelings of vulnerability and loss of control. Acute illness calls for immediate action; chronic illness involves intricate changes in lifestyle with an uncertain future.

People who are ill are often sensitive and vulnerable. Their whole lives are changed, at least temporarily. They struggle with the memories of past experiences as they cope with the present reality and an uncertain future. Issues of mortality, dependency, trust, and identity come to the fore.

Serious illness or injury is always more than just physical pain and inconvenience. Life goals, family, work and income, mobility, body image, and lifestyle may be drastically altered. Whether the changes are temporary or permanent, the situation may develop into a crisis—a crisis that affects family, friends, and professional helpers.

In the midst of this uncertainty, the nurse stands as a central figure who, through understanding and intelligent action, assists the individual in maintaining basic security, self-esteem, and integrity and in coping with the crisis of illness.

Providing optimal help to patients and families depends on an understanding of the following:

- The usual stages of illness and accompanying emotional responses
- The major tasks of adapting to significant illness or injury
- The typical coping strategies used by individuals and families
- The psychologic, social, and cultural factors that help or hinder coping

Stages of Illness

The transition from health to illness is a complex and highly individualized experience. Dealing with this situation not only involves attempting to restore physiologic balance but also includes making the following two adjustments: (1) modifying body image, self concept, and relations to other people and work, and (2) readjusting realistically to the limitations imposed by the condition. These two adjustments begin in the setting in which the person is being treated for the health problem.

In the cycle of health and illness, most people go through three stages: (1) the transition from health to illness, (2) the period of "accepted" illness, and (3) convalescence. The duration and quality of the experience vary with differences in personality, the specific disorder, and the changes made in the person's life.

First Stage

The transition from health to illness usually begins with the development of symptoms which are generally accompanied by unpleasant sensations, loss of vigor and stamina, and a decrease in the ability to function. Certain symptoms, such as chest pain, indigestion, and headache, may increase in frequency and intensity. Anxiety often is present and is handled with the person's usual coping mechanisms. To avoid the prospect of illness, one person may continue with everyday activity. Another may become passive and withdrawn, hoping that the vague symptoms will go away. A person may put off seeking medical care for fear of the diagnosis, especially if something serious is suspected, such as cancer. Anxiety, guilt, shame, and denial are prominent during this initial period.

If the symptoms persist, the person will generally seek medical help, although fear of undergoing examination and diagnostic tests may lead to procrastination or to canceled or missed appointments. A feeling of resistance may lead the person to ignore initial recommendations or not take prescribed medication. Some people go from caregiver to caregiver, hoping to learn "what's really the matter" or that a previous diagnosis was inaccurate.

A person who experiences a sudden catastrophe, such as heart attack or stroke, is suddenly cast into a state of illness. Fear in this instance may center around concern that help will not arrive in time. Apprehension may be expressed through excessive demands, denial that the problem exists, refusal to cooperate or accept the proposed treatment, withdrawal, and suspicion of the motives and methods of those trying to help. In such instances it helps to contact the patient's close relatives, significant others, and primary care provider, if possible. Calmly explaining the necessary procedures and demonstrating professional skill will convey a sense of competency and reduce the anxiety and fear.

When patients and families are experiencing shock, disbelief, and denial of the condition, it is often helpful for them to verbalize their feelings. In a noncritical way, the nurse does not support the denial but accepts their need to cope with the situation in this way. Orienting patients to the immediate environment, answering questions, and addressing concerns will also have a calming effect.

Second Stage

The second stage in the transition from health to illness includes accepting the illness. The person recognizes and acknowledges the illness and the need for assistance from others, especially from the medical and nursing staffs. Frequently there is a tendency to adopt the patient role, which is evident by an abdication from usual responsibilities and cooperation in the task of getting well. In this stage, patients may become preoccupied with themselves, their symptoms, and their treatment. Increased dependency accompanies preoccupation with somatic concerns. This behavior is often described as regressive, because it is a return to earlier forms of behaving, feeling, and relating to others.

A certain amount of regression is necessary so that patients can allow themselves to rest in bed, eat specified diets, sleep, and let their bodies heal. People who normally resist being dependent may find this very difficult and may continue to deny their condition in part or refuse prescribed treatment. The other extreme of dependency problems is seen in those who receive so much gratification from dependency that they attempt to continue it indefinitely.

A frequent reaction to dependency includes anger, guilt, and resentment, which may be expressed as criticism of the care being given and of the caregivers as well. The most helpful nursing approach is to view this reaction as the person's attempt to deal with the situation and to encourage the expression of feelings without passing judgment, moralizing, or arguing. Expressing an understanding of the person's feelings (*i.e.*, "This must be difficult to deal with" or "You must be feeling a loss of control") will encourage the person to verbalize fears.

When people become sick, they often feel helpless and hopeless. While nurses assume responsibility for providing care, they recognize individual differences and needs, and they provide opportunities, whenever possible, for the person to make decisions and assume personal responsibility. A person who feels assured of the nurse's availability, interest, and competence will become less anxious and will be able to relinquish dependency.

Third Stage

The third stage of illness is the convalescent or restitution period. Health and physical strength often return before the person feels or acts "well." Just as a lag usually occurs in the initial stage between the appearance of physical symptoms and the emotional acceptance of illness, a reverse lag occurs in recovery. Getting well implies giving up a dependent, regressive position and resuming adult responsibilities and normal relationships with others. Although some people are reluctant to give up the dependent role, most are motivated toward health but may be afraid or hesitant to try new skills. This is particularly true if the illness and treatment require major changes in work and family relations.

People in this stage can be helped through guidance, advice, and encouragement to progress. They are encouraged to experiment with new skills that may be needed for self-care, for coping, or for enhancing relationships with others. And they are guided to renew interest in the world, communicate better with family, and make plans for the future.

If the assistance of a support group is needed, such as for those who have had strokes, mastectomies, and other conditions, a member of the group may be asked to visit to talk to the person to convey hope and to give realistic, first-hand information on useful coping strategies. While the person may at first be too overwhelmed by anxiety or grief to use these services, it may help to offer a reminder of these support services at a later time. If, on the other hand, the person does not want to affiliate with such groups, then these preferences should be acknowledged and accepted as the individual's right to choose.

Adapting to Illness

Just what is it that patients and families have to cope with when they or a loved one become sick? The major tasks involved have been identified by Moos (1984) as follows:

- Dealing with the discomfort, incapacitation, and symptoms of the illness or injury
- Managing the stress of treatment, procedures, and possible hospitalization
- Developing and maintaining adequate relationships with caregivers who may include nurses, physicians, family members, and community-based and home health care personnel
- Preserving a satisfactory self-image and maintaining a sense of competence and mastery
- Balancing the disturbing feelings aroused by illness and treatment
- Maintaining relationships with family and friends despite a change in role identity
- Preparing for an uncertain future in which further loss, death, or recovery are possibilities

These adaptive tasks often occur simultaneously or recur at different stages of the illness.

Basic Emotional Needs

Everyone has the same basic emotional needs, including the need for love, trust, autonomy, identity, self-esteem, recognition, and security. Schultz (1966) summarized these needs as the interpersonal needs for inclusion, control, and affection. If these needs are not fulfilled, the result may be undesired feelings and behaviors, such as anxiety, anger, loneliness, and self-doubt.

The interpersonal needs for inclusion, control, and affection are overlapping and continuous. Inclusion is primarily related to the formation of a relationship, whereas control and affection are demonstrated within the relationship. Inclusion is feeling "in" or "out"; control is "top" or "bottom"; and affection is "remote" or "close." Generally, people establish equilibrium between themselves and others in these three areas. Illness disturbs this balance, giving rise to a wide variety of new stresses.

Need for Inclusion

The need for inclusion is defined behaviorally as the need to establish and maintain satisfactory relationships with people. It refers to establishing and maintaining a feeling of mutual interest in others. The need for inclusion is the need to feel that the self is significant and worthwhile. Inclusion behavior refers to association between individuals and is indicated by such words as *associate, interact, belong, join,* and *communicate.* Lack of inclusion is connoted by words such as *excluded, ignored, withdrawn, aloof,* and *isolated.* The need to be included is shown by the desire to attract attention and interest. Sometimes illness brings out a strong need for inclusion, as in the patient who seems overly "demanding" in seeking attention.

The desire for prestige and status is a part of inclusion needs; each of us needs people to pay attention to us, know who we are, and distinguish us from others. Identity is closely related to inclusion. One is known as a distinct individual, who therefore deserves attention. The height of inclusion is to be understood, which implies that someone is interested enough to seek and discover our particular characteristics, likes, and dislikes.

In a health care setting inclusion needs can be met by providing information and answering questions, explaining one's own responsibilities in providing care, and acknowledging the individual's needs and preferences.

Need for Control

The need for control is associated with the need to establish and maintain a satisfactory relationship with others with regard to power, decision making, and authority. It has to do with the feeling of mutual respect for the competence and responsibility of oneself and others. Control needs are suggested by such words as *dominance, influence, boss, rebellion, submission, leader, noncooperation,* and *follower.* Control represents assumption of power over others and therefore over one's own future, whereas *being* controlled means giving up responsibility for oneself.

The need for control becomes an issue for a person entering the health care system because many basic decisions which the individual is used to making, such as when to get up, what to eat, and when to go to the bathroom, are now determined to some degree by others. Different people react in different ways to this situation. At one extreme is the person who completely gives up or abdicates personal responsibility and becomes a clinging, helpless patient who seeks direction from everyone about what to do and how to do it. Behind this behavior often lie anxiety, hostility, and a lack of trust in others as well as oneself. Nursing interventions that assist the person to assume responsibility for making decisions about personal care contribute to restoring control.

The other extreme in control behavior is reflected in the actions of a patient who constantly rebels against any limitations and tries to dominate the situation. Such a person may have difficulty accepting the need for dependency in such matters as bed rest or following "doctor's orders." Allowing this kind of person some say in selective decisions will help promote a sense of control. Nurses also need to examine their own needs for power and control in relation to patients, co-workers, and physicians.

Need for Affection

The third major need is that of affection, in which individuals establish a give-and-take relationship based on mutual liking. Affection is suggested by such words as *love, like, emotionally close, personal, friendship,* and *intimacy.* Lack of affection is connoted by *hate, dislike,* and *emotionally distant.* The need for affection usually is met by family members, spouses, and close friends. Illness or hospitalization may disrupt sources of support. Being emotionally close to another generally results in confiding one's innermost anxieties, wishes, and feelings. Patients may turn to the nurse to share these thoughts, especially if a family member is unavailable or too anxious to listen.

Self-Image and Body Image

Body image represents the picture that each of us has of ourself. Serious illness and injury can abruptly interfere with that self-concept. Adapting to the changes imposed by illness can affect one's sense of identity. A major disability can be viewed as a limitation to be challenged. On the other hand it may lead to a feeling of being "crippled."

Threats to Body Image. Threats to body image, and hence to self-esteem, are often accompanied by feelings of shame, inadequacy, and guilt. In the health care setting, people deal with numerous situations that threaten their self-esteem. Violation of modesty and invasion of privacy cause anxiety and embarrassment. Exposure of the body during physical examinations and such treatments as enemas and catheterizations may be upsetting, even though expected as part of the therapeutic regimen. The need for using a bedpan or talking about bowel and bladder habits can also threaten self-esteem. Severe threats to body image can result from drastic changes brought about by a colostomy or ileostomy, an amputation, mastectomy, or similar type of surgical procedure. Treatments such as those involving radiation or chemotherapy can also affect appearance and thus one's perception of oneself.

Changes in body image may result from side effects of medication, such as development of a moon face from taking steroids or changes in secondary sex characteristics and growth of facial hair. Besides the sudden changes in body structure and functioning that occur through injury or surgical intervention, subtle changes occur in progressive conditions such as arthritis, obesity, and multiple sclerosis. Even normal changes in the body, such as occur in puberty and pregnancy, pose a problem of altering the body image. During adolescence there is a sensitive, often painful awareness of the body and its many changes. Complexion, weight, and development of primary and secondary sexual characteristics are closely linked to feelings of worth and sexual desirability.

Nursing Implications. The first step in understanding the concept of body image is to become more aware of one's own attitude toward health, illness, disfigurement, and changes in body functioning. Anxiety, revulsion, and pity are common responses to abnormal body appearance and functioning. To care for patients who have these conditions, nurses must come to terms with their own feelings. A nurse reacting adversely to a patient's appearance can have a damaging effect on that person's ability to adjust in a positive manner.

The nurse needs to learn what the body change means to the individual and what adjustments will be required. In formulating the nursing care plan it is important to assess the ability of the family to help the patient cope with changes, to determine how realistic the person is about the body change, and to identify specific problems in coping and methods of coping. The nurse needs to determine ways of supporting the family and the methods for responding to the patient's reactions. Frequent reactions include grief, mourning, and anger. Yet hope is essential and must be supported and encouraged, as must efforts at rehabilitation.

Social Adjustments. Even after the person has begun to accept the change in body image and feels worthwhile and accepted by caregivers, he or she must adjust to dealing with the outside world. Because nurses are familiar with illness and injury, they may lose sight of the fact that many people respond negatively when they encounter someone who is disfigured or incapacitated. They may stare or ask intrusive questions about the person's condition or treat the person as if he or she were completely helpless. Patients may need help in learning how to handle such situations. They also need to be cautioned about dwelling on their problem. Talking about one's health status, body functioning, and difficulties in adjustment is appropriate with health care personnel and close family and friends. With other people, excessive dwelling on these topics may lead to rejection and ostracism.'

Emotional Reactions to Illness

Many disturbing feelings are aroused by acute and chronic illnesses and the treatment they require. Some emotional reactions commonly experienced by patients and their families are anxiety, anger, grief, hope, shame, guilt, courage, pride, despair, love, depression, helplessness, envy, loneliness, and faith. How they are experienced and expressed depends on the person's basic personality, the perception of the situation, and the extent of support from others. There is no right or wrong way to feel about serious illness. Nurses can anticipate different reactions and can encourage patients and families to express feelings in a constructive way.

Anxiety

Anxiety is a normal reaction to stress and threat of harm. It is an emotional reaction to the perception of danger, real or imagined. Anxiety and fear are often used synonymously; however, fear generally refers to a specific threat; anxiety to a nonspecific threat. A person experiencing anxiety may feel uneasy and apprehensive and may have a vague sense of dread. Feelings of helplessness and inadequacy may be present, along with a sense of alienation and insecurity. The intensity of these feelings may be mild or severe enough to cause panic, and the intensity may increase or diminish depending upon the person's coping abilities and resources at any particular point in time.

Anxiety is a common reaction to illness because illness is perceived as posing the following threats: a general threat to life, health, and body integrity; exposure and embarrassment; discomfort from pain and fatigue; changes in diet; deprivation of sexual satisfaction; restriction of movement; isolation; interruption or loss of one's means of livelihood; precipitation of a financial crisis; rejection or ridicule from others as the result of the condition; inconsistent and unpredictable behavior of the authority figures on whom one's welfare depends; frustration of goals and expectations; confusion and uncertainty about the present and the future; and separation from family and friends if hospitalization is necessary.

Physiologic reactions to anxiety are primarily reactions of the autonomic nervous system. They include increases in pulse and respiratory rates; shifts in blood pressure and temperature; relaxation of the smooth muscles in the bladder and bowel; cold, clammy skin; increased perspiration; dilated pupils; and dry mouth. The bodily responses to mild anxiety initially promote learning and the ability to function, but as the reaction increases in severity, learning decreases, perception is reduced or distorted, and the ability to concentrate is greatly diminished.

Nurses must be able to evaluate the level of anxiety in a patient so that it can be effectively reduced. An extremely anxious person is very uncomfortable; has difficulty giving or receiving information of any kind, and learns little about health matters; and magnifies or distorts what is heard.

Characteristic manifestations of anxiety depend on the individual and may include withdrawal, silence, hyperactivity, swearing, talking and joking excessively, striking out verbally or physically, fantasizing, complaining, and crying. The specific means of coping with anxiety, whether successful or not, vary with individuals and with the situation.

Nursing Interventions. Nursing intervention directed toward reducing anxiety has four aspects:

1. Recognizing that the person is anxious and being aware of situations that can potentially precipitate anxiety, as evidenced by physiologic, emotional, and behavioral clues
2. Encouraging the person to recognize and express any feelings of anxiety
3. Assisting the person to understand and cope with the anxiety by asking open-ended questions such as "Tell me what happened," "What was going on?" or "What did you expect to happen?"
4. Extending a sense of caring through the appropriate use of touch, physical care, and tone of voice

Nursing Care Plan 10-1 provides an example of a care plan for a person with anxiety.

Anger and Hostility

In addition to anxiety, expressions of anger are a common reaction to illness. The outward expression is often demonstrated as aggression, a complex reaction of feelings and behavior that varies in intensity, duration, and expression. Words such as *irritated, sullen, unfriendly, hostile, assertive, belligerent, defiant, uncooperative, resentful, enraged, furious,* and *indignant* describe various forms of aggressiveness.

Anger, the general term for this emotion, is one way of handling anxiety, particularly in response to real or perceived threat, insult, or injury. To be sick often means being helpless, controlled by others, and assaulted—however therapeutically—by needles, catheters, enemas, and surgical procedures. Being told to wait for medication angers many patients who are in pain. Being awakened in the middle of the night to cough and take deep breaths can tax one's patience. Being confined to one's home or forced to limit one's activities may arouse feelings of anger. Being uncertain of the prognosis or the future can lead to angry outbursts or sullen behavior.

Such expressions of anger may decrease markedly as the element of the unknown is reduced and the person learns more about what to expect. On the other hand, anger may increase if the threat grows and the person's needs are not met adequately. Allowing the person choices provides some measure of personal control and often helps reduce feelings of anger and frustration.

A person who is angry as a result of illness may behave in a variety of ways: by being argumentative, demanding, unappreciative, sarcastic, and unwilling to cooperate. A person may exhibit nonverbal expressions of anger—glaring eyes, clenched fist, or a sneer. Occasionally, a person is aggressive to the point of violence—shouting, cursing, doing or threatening to do physical harm.

The expression of anger in the clinical situation may reflect the person's best manner of coping with perceived threats and may be an attempt to relieve feelings of helpless-

NURSING CARE PLAN 10–1
Care of the Patient With Anxiety

Mr. Vernon Hughes, a 40-year-old, married father of two, is brought to the emergency department on the insistence of his wife. He complains of pressure in his chest and is having some difficulty breathing. Mr. Hughes' skin is pale and moist and he is very anxious. Ms. Daniel, the primary nurse introduces herself and takes his blood pressure, pulse and respiration—BP 150/100, P 100, R 24. She then applies a 12-lead EKG, which reveals ST elevation leads II, III, and AVF. Mr. Hughes is admitted to CCU with the diagnosis of acute inferior myocardial infarction. Upon arrival to CCU he is given a tissue plasminogen activator (TPA). He experiences some reperfusion ectopy. Ms. Daniel begins explaining procedures and monitors to Mr. Hughes. His speech is rapid. He complains of a dry mouth, excessive perspiration, and increased restlessness and he frequently requests the urinal. He had difficulty focusing on the information presented by Ms. Daniel as evidenced by his repeatedly asking, "What are you saying—I don't understand."

NURSING DIAGNOSIS

1. Pain related to myocardial infarction
2. Anxiety related to crisis situation particularly fear of dying

GOALS

1. Relief of pain
2. Use of effective methods to cope with and lessen anxiety

Nursing Interventions	Expected Outcomes	Outcomes
1. Relieve pain and discomfort. To minimize myocardial damage, pain control takes priority. Once pain has been relieved, nursing measures directed toward alleviating Mr. Hughes' anxiety will be appropriate and meaningful.		
a. Administer nitroglycerin IV drip as prescribed for pain control.	a. Experiences relief from pain	• Reported less discomfort after nitroglycerin administered
b. Observe for side effects of analgesic.	b. Absence of side effects	• No evidence of side effects; BP within acceptable range
c. Assess TPR BP, q1h and more frequently if necessary.	c. Vital signs normal	• Elevation of vital signs continues 24 hr after admission: T 37.4° C, P 90–100, R 22–26, BP 130/86–146/90
d. Monitor for return of chest pain.	d. Absence of chest pain	• No evidence of chest pain
e. Monitor heart rhythm continuously.	e. Absence of dysrhythmias	• No dysrhythmias noted
2. Establish relationship built on trust.		
a. Introduce self.	a. Acknowledges presence of nurse	• Called primary nurse by name
b. Obtain patient's perceptions of problem.	b. Verbalizes events leading to hospitalization and feelings about possible death	• On admission, reconstructed events leading to hospitalization and events that followed; described feelings as "I don't know what will happen now"; unable to identify fears
c. Provide consistency in care and in approach to patient. d. Accept patient as an individual.	c–d. Exhibits behavior indicative of trust	• One day after admission, expressed fears of unknown and anger at the situation; fearful about death, dependence, recovery
e. Provide instructions in clear, simple manner.	e. Focuses on instructions related to procedures	• Verbalized that talking is helpful; asked when nurse will return; body posture relaxed. Provided accurate feedback of instructions

(continued)

NURSING CARE PLAN 10–1 *(continued)*
Care of the Patient With Anxiety

Nursing Interventions	Expected Outcomes	Outcomes
3. Assist patient to identify anxious feelings.		
a. Encourage patient to verbalize feelings of anxiety.	a. Verbalizes feelings of anxiety	• Expressed anxiety about fear of dying
b. Remain with patient.	b. Anxiety decreases	• Physiologic reactions to anxiety decreased (*i.e.,* mouth less dry, decreased perspiration, less urinary frequency, decreased restlessness)
c. Assist in identifying events that increase anxiety.	c. Identifies events that increase anxiety	• Identified the following as increasing anxiety: hurried atmosphere, pain when analgesic wears off, alarms sounding
d. Discuss relationship between increased anxiety and physiologic functioning.	d. Identifies increased anxiety as a precursor to altered physiologic function	• Accurately described relationship between anxiety and altered physiologic functions; reported increased salivation, decreased perspiration, decreased urinary frequency
e. Discuss relationship between increased anxiety and behavior patterns.	e. Identifies increased anxiety as a precursor to alterations in behavior	• Identified increased motor activity as a consequence of increased anxiety
f. Note time and occasion of increased restlessness.	f. Decrease in restlessness	• Restlessness decreased; less adjustment of bed covers; able to process instructions; speech remained rapid at times
g. Promote use of effective coping measures to decrease anxiety.	g. Identifies effective coping mechanisms	• Identified the following as effective in decreasing anxiety: listening to music, visiting with family, reading magazines
h. Teach relaxation techniques.	h. Uses relaxation techniques to decrease anxiety	• Practiced relaxation techniques when feeling anxious; stated that relaxation techniques decreased feelings of anxiety
i. Encourage patient to use support systems.	i. Uses support of family	• Discussed fears about dying and the future with family

ness and dependency or to cope with the grief process. A patient's anger may vanish when someone helps him or her to identify what is frustrating or threatening and to take steps to successfully deal with the threat.

Nursing Interventions. Therapeutic responses to angry patients are based on the attempt to understand the person and the particular situation. Avoiding the patient is not acceptable. Instead, attempts should be made to help the person sort out the issues involved in a way that preserves the individual's dignity, pride, and self-esteem. At the same time, limits should be set on the person's behavior to avoid harm to anyone, and more appropriate means of expressing these feelings should be explored.

A plan of care can be devised based on the following questions: When does the person get angry and how does he or she show it? Does this anger interfere with the patient's receiving the care he or she needs? Why does his or her behavior bother me? How do I react? Does he or she get angry with other people too? Is there someone who does get along with him or her? What does that person do that is different? Does the patient's hostility serve a useful purpose? How much of this behavior reflects the person's usual way of reacting to people? How much is he or she willing to change? What realistic goals shall we work toward? Are there any other resources—physician, family, psychiatric nursing consultant, psychiatrist, occupational therapist, or other patients—that we could consult? If the patient stops expressing anger, will he or she develop more destructive patterns?

Learning to work therapeutically with angry, hostile patients is a challenging and rewarding part of nursing. Patients who disguise temporary fear and shame with anger appreciate the nurse who stands by them in the crisis without condemnation, rejection, or retaliation. Patients who have made a lifelong adjustment by means of hostile attack are also grateful (although they may never express it directly) to the nurse who refuses to be alienated and who attempts to understand and be supportive. Nursing Care Plan 10-2 is an example of a nursing care plan for the patient with anger and hostility.

Grief and Mourning

Grief is an emotional response to the anticipated or actual loss of someone or something valued. The loss may be that

NURSING CARE PLAN 10–2
Care of the Patient With Anger and Hostility

Mr. Hughes is transferred to PCU on day 3. He has no further complaints of chest pain. His ECG shows that he is in normal sinus rhythm with no recurrent ectopy. Mr. Hughes is angry and not interested in attending to cardiac teaching/learning offered by Ms. Daniel. Mr. Hughes becomes sarcastic and demanding. He complains that "no one has been in to check on me and I could have died—then all you nurses would be in trouble." He demands that Ms. Daniel "take care of me just like the doctor said" and then he tells her to leave the room and "send someone else who knows what they're doing."

NURSING DIAGNOSIS

1. Ineffective coping
   a. Verbal abuse related to feelings of helplessness
   b. Uncooperative behavior related to feelings of loss of control

GOALS

1. Restoration of appropriate communication
2. Verbalization of feelings
3. Participation in therapeutic regimen

Nursing Interventions	Expected Outcomes	Outcomes
1. Promote appropriate communications.		
a. Establish relationship built on trust (see Nursing Care Plan 10-1).		
b. Remain calm; do not take verbal abuse personally.	b. Communicates within normal limits of volume	• Voice raised only occasionally at 24 hr
c. Set and keep limits; withdraw attention as needed.	c. Communicates appropriately	• Requests, observations, questions expressed verbally in an appropriate manner
d. Encourage patient to express feelings.	d. Verbalizes how anger affects his verbal communication	• Apologized for shouting and belittling behavior; verbalized ways in which he used anger to avoid dealing with loss of control, loss of independence, and fear of dying
2. Promote verbalization of feelings.		
a. Encourage patient to express feelings about dependency.	a. Verbalizes feelings about dependency	• Described feeling dependent on nursing staff for satisfaction of basic needs
b. Allow patient to make as many choices as possible.	b. Maintains as much control as possible	• Established own schedule for ADL
c. Involve patient in goal establishment.	c. Verbalizes goals and expectations	• Identified realistic expectations for therapy, discharge, and rehabilitation; established goals for changes in lifestyle. Identified changes that had occurred since hospital admission; expressed his perception of the effect of these changes on lifestyle; identified need to regain control and to learn to care for self
3. Promote participation in therapeutic regimen.		
a. Emphasize strengths and potential.	a. Identifies own strengths and potentials	• Identified social supports, age, physical condition, lifestyle, and stamina; expressed desire to talk with discharge planner to facilitate interim plan for outpatient cardiac rehabilitation.
b. Encourage involvement in self-care.	b. Accomplishes self-care activities	• After establishing schedule for ADL, began active participation in own care; self-sufficient in ADL by 72 hr

of a relative or friend, a part of the body, a job, health, or life. Feelings of anxiety, helplessness, hopelessness, guilt, anger, depression, remorse, sadness, and loneliness are part of grief. Grieving refers to the process that follows the loss and ultimately results in the grief being overcome.

The intensity of grief and mourning depends on the significance and extent of the loss to the person. It is generally greater if the loss, especially through death, comes suddenly. If the survivor has been particularly dependent on the deceased person or in any way feels responsible for the death, grief is intensified. Ambivalence (mixed feelings) is present in all significant relationships. If the ambivalence is marked, grief may be particularly intense. Guilt and irrational ideas about the causation of the death may prevent a person from mourning effectively.

The stages of grieving are similar to the stages of adaptation to illness—shock and disbelief, awareness, and restitution. The initial response to loss includes a sinking feeling, tightness in the throat, loss of appetite, fatigue, tension, and acute anxiety. Perceptions are altered, and there is a feeling of unreality and distance from others. There is a preoccupation with the deceased or lost object and a hope that it will return. Feelings of guilt may be present, accompanied by soul-searching and remorse about things that could have been done differently. The grieving person may withdraw from others and from normal activities or become purposely busy. Often the shock of the loss is accepted and the person goes through the motions of making arrangements and caring for others. Emotional reactions may be muted as a protective mechanism.

In the stage of developing awareness, the person experiences pain, anguish, emptiness, and acute sadness. Crying or the desire to cry is common and often elicits support from others. Many people cannot allow themselves to cry in public and need privacy to handle their grief.

In the stage of restitution, the reality of the loss is accepted. In the case of death, the funeral makes this fact unavoidable. In the case of amputation, the sight of the stump and the first attempt at using a prosthesis underline the reality. The mourner begins a long process of coping with the loss. The process includes talking repetitively about the person or object, with a tendency to idealize, so that only pleasant memories are reinforced. Gradually, emotional attachment subsides and new interests develop with energy invested in other people. The relationship is remembered more realistically, with its good and bad aspects.

Nursing Interventions. Nursing interventions to help patients and families with the experience of grief and mourning include anticipating reactions to loss, supporting the usual coping mechanisms, and allowing the expression of feelings. If a death has occurred in an institutional setting, the family is given time to mourn in private. When a body part or function is lost, specific nursing care is designed and steps are taken to prevent additional loss of self esteem. By listening and empathizing, the nurse provides a sense of caring and offers comfort and support. By being aware of the usual patterns of grief and mourning, the nurse can recognize maladaptive patterns and help evaluate the need for other types of therapeutic intervention, such as psychotherapy. Nursing Care Plan 10-3 is an example of a nursing care plan for the patient experiencing grief and mourning.

Hope

Hope is a mixture of feelings and thoughts that center on the fundamental belief that there are solutions to significant human needs and problems. Most people have hoped for and expected a long and healthy life for themselves and their significant others. Serious illness and injury can jeopardize that expectation and undermine hope.

The purpose of hope is to ward off despair, which is characterized by mental anguish, disorganization, helplessness, and hopelessness. Loss of hope leads to giving up, which results in physical and emotional disequilibrium and even death if the person gives up the will to live.

Nursing Interventions. Hope is reinforced by other people who give support and encouragement to continue the struggle. When patients see "the light at the end of the tunnel," they can persist in moving toward future goals of improved functioning. Even with patients who are dying, hope for relief of suffering and meaningful living in the present are important aspects that can be reinforced with nursing care.

Nursing Care Plan 10-4 is an example of a nursing care plan to assist the patient in restoring hope.

Cultural Considerations

There are many cultural factors involved in the specific ways that people react to illness and treatment. Some people will be stoic, exhibiting few behaviors that indicate their true emotions. When questioned about their feelings they may deny that they have any concerns about their illness or its treatment, even when the illness is serious and has the potential for significantly affecting their well-being or their way of life. In contrast, others will display their emotions in elaborate ways, such as ritualistic weeping and public display.

These extremes of behaviors as well as less extreme reactions are learned and can best be understood if the person's sociocultural background is understood. This is possible only through exchange of information between the nurse and the patient and family with the goal of building mutual trust and understanding. It is often critical to explore the meaning of the behavior for the patient. Only by understanding the cultural and social meanings of particular behaviors and particular situations for patients can the nurse begin to assist the patient to cope with the situation and to acquire health behaviors that are compatible with his or her beliefs and values.

Role Changes

People frequently undergo role changes when they become ill or injured. These changes can affect the ways others interact and relate to them; relationships with family and friends may frequently be altered and adjusted.

Some of the most important role changes affecting a family are those in which parents are no longer able to carry out their usual activities. In some instances the children end up caring for their parents. In the usual life cycle, aging parents become increasingly dependent on their middle-aged children for help and direction; serious illness makes this role reversal even more pressing.

NURSING CARE PLAN 10-3
Care of the Patient Experiencing Grief and Mourning

As time progresses, Mr. Hughes is noticeably more quiet and withdrawn. He verbalizes fear of dying before his children are on their own and leaving his wife to raise them alone. He is often observed staring at a blank wall. He also verbalizes concerns about sexual relationships with his wife. He tells his family and friends that he is not sure he can adapt to the lifestyle changes needed as a result of the MI.

NURSING DIAGNOSIS

1. Anticipatory grieving related to life changes caused by MI
2. Knowledge deficit related to cardiac procedures

GOALS

1. Acceptance of losses
2. Alteration of lifestyle to accommodate loss
3. Acceptance and cooperation during cardiac testing procedures

Nursing Interventions	Expected Outcomes	Outcomes
1. Encourage patient to identify meaning of loss.		
a. Establish relationship built on trust (see Nursing Care Plan 10-1).		
b. Encourage expression of feelings about loss.	b. Identifies feelings about loss	• Cried and talked about loss of independence
c. Encourage to identify effects of loss.	c. Identifies effects of loss on lifestyle	• Talked about decreased mobility and need to go to outpatient cardiac rehabilitation
d. Assist in decreasing depressive symptoms.	d. Experiences decrease in symptoms of depression	• Reported increase in appetite and extended periods of uninterrupted sleep; increased ability to concentrate while reading a book; participating in ADL and exhibited more spontaneous conversation
e. Facilitate movement through the stages of grieving and loss.	e. Resolves loss	• Talked positively about rehabilitation; expressed interest in actively participating in rehabilitative program; described family support system
2. Teach patient about procedures:		
a. Instruct about cardiac catheterization procedure.	a. Understands need for cardiac catheterization	• Complies with requests and cooperates with procedure
b. Instruct about percutaneous transluminal coronary angioplasty (PTCA).	b. Understands need for PTCA	

Role changes affecting occupational functioning also can have an impact. Many people base their sense of self-worth on the ability to work and be productive. If forced to retire or go into a long period of convalescence, a person may feel lost and bereft of important links with others. Vocational rehabilitation is an important part of health planning for patients who must make major alterations in this area of life.

Coping Strategies

Adapting to illness involves numerous strategies, depending on the coping skills the person has used in other difficult, stressful situations. Moos (1984) described seven categories of coping skills: denial, seeking information, requesting emotional support, learning self care, setting concrete limited goals, rehearsing alternative outcomes, and finding meaning in illness. At different stages of illness, one or more of the coping skills may predominate.

Denial

Denial involves refusing to accept or acknowledge the seriousness of the illness. This approach downplays the symptoms as evidence of illness or disregards the serious-

NURSING CARE PLAN 10–4
Assisting the Patient in Restoring Hope

Mr. Hughes has made progress. He speaks to Ms. Daniel about his plans after discharge: "Of course I'll have to go to outpatient cardiac rehabilitation for a while and I don't think it will be long before I'm stronger. My family is supportive of the lifestyle changes I'll have to make. My wife and I are talking about my fears about sexual function and other things. Things really do look hopeful."

NURSING DIAGNOSIS

1. Disturbance in self-concepts: self-esteem, independence/dependence, role performance
2. Potential noncompliance with therapeutic regimen

GOALS

1. Improvement in self-concept
2. Resumption of independent lifestyle
3. Compliance with therapeutic regimen

Nursing Interventions	Expected Outcomes	Outcomes
1. Increase self-esteem.		
a. Give positive feedback for progress made in self-care and lifestyle changes.	a. Describes feelings about changes made in self-care and lifestyle	• Verbalized fears related to self-care and changes in lifestyle
b. Help patient identify strengths and potentials.	b. Identifies strengths and potentials	• Made a list of physical activities he will be able to continue; identified supports within family and community; verbalized self-determination as an inner strength
c. Give positive feedback for progress made in accepting lifestyle changes.	c. Describes feelings about how lifestyle has changed	• Verbalized sadness related to loss of independence and put into perspective the effect of this loss on self and family; stated he was looking forward to returning to his apartment
2. Encourage efforts toward successfully altering lifestyle.	2. Makes necessary arrangement for promoting cardiac rehabilitation	• Adheres to arrangements promoting cardiac rehabilitation
3. Encourage adherence to therapeutic regimen.		
a. Encourage participation in discharge planning.	a. Participates in making plans for discharge	• Attended discharge planning conference; consulted with cardiac rehab. team
b. Provide patient with discharge instructions.	b. Exercises according to plan; keeps appointments with physician and cardiac rehabilitation team	

ness of the diagnosis. The first reaction to loss is shock and disbelief. Denial or numbing of feelings gives one time to absorb the meaning and protects one from being overwhelmed by emotions. Denial and isolation are ego defense mechanisms that protect against anxiety. In time, the increase or persistence of symptoms generally forces the person to abandon denial and face the reality of the situation.

As a coping skill, denying or minimizing the problem helps to maintain psychologic equilibrium. It can be harmful when it leads to avoidance behavior such as missing appointments or refusing to follow the prescribed treatment. Inappropriate cheerfulness and lack of concern about symptoms may indicate denial. If anxiety, depression, and anger are not expressed in situations where they are expected, the person may be using denial for self-protection or protection of others. The latter occurs when patients are aware that they are dying but believe that the family would be more comfortable not knowing this fact. In such instances, it may help to provide the person with an opportunity to talk about fears and feelings in the face of impending death.

Nursing Interventions. Dealing with denial of illness involves assessing the extent to which the denial is harmful or beneficial. Since denial is a defense mechanism, it is best not to challenge it directly. Neither is it encouraged. Showing a willingness to discuss matters can help provide an opportunity to talk things through. Using nonthreatening exploratory questions may help lead the person to accept reality. When this point is reached, further support may be necessary to help deal with the emotional reactions that result from giving up the denial and facing reality.

Seeking Information

The coping skill of seeking information involves (1) seeking relevant information that can relieve anxiety caused by misconceptions and uncertainty, and (2) using one's intellectual resources effectively. Patients and families are often relieved by information about the illness, its treatment, and the course the illness is expected to take. This awareness provides a framework for making plans and taking effective action. Learning that other people with the same condition have been treated successfully provides encouragement and hope. Misconceptions are clarified and correct facts provided. Giving a time range in which treatment will be effective helps to decrease feelings of helplessness. People who are informed are better able to participate in their own treatment.

Requesting Emotional Support

Being able to elicit emotional support from family, friends, and health care providers while maintaining a sense of personal competence is important. Illness frequently causes fear and anxiety and a sense of isolation. A valuable coping skill is being able to reach out for help from others, thereby maintaining hope through encouragement. Whether illness imposes temporary or permanent limitations, people often need to have a sense of mastery over their lives. Encouragement can be gained by talking with other people who have the same condition. Support groups are helpful in encouraging the expression of feelings, sharing practical problems, and passing along effective ways of coping.

Learning Self-Care

Learning to take care of oneself confirms one's personal ability and effectiveness. People can learn to care for themselves even in the aftermath of catastrophic illness and injury. Helplessness is decreased because the sense of pride in accomplishments helps to restore or maintain self-esteem. Patient teaching is thus an essential element in promoting self care. Since family members play an increasingly important role in caregiving during acute as well as chronic illness, they should be included in the teaching sessions and shown how to carry out appropriate procedures and provide effective care.

Setting Concrete, Limited Goals

The overall tasks of adapting to serious illness seem overwhelming at first, yet they can be mastered. Breaking tasks into small, manageable goals will eventually lead to success. In this way motivation is maintained and feelings of helplessness are decreased. Instead of worrying, the person takes effective action. Principles of learning are important in accomplishing the eventual long-term goals.

Rehearsing Alternative Outcomes

There are often several alternatives in every situation. Recognizing these options helps a person to feel less helpless. Exploring options with the nurse and one's family helps to expand the reality base on which to make decisions. Anticipatory planning reduces helplessness by asking "What will happen if . . . ?"

This coping skill is often used in conjunction with information seeking. It helps to decrease anxiety by preparing for the future. Recalling how one has been able to manage past difficulties bolsters confidence.

When there is a choice of several treatment modalities, discussing the alternatives is a vital part of self-determination. Health professionals do not always know what is best. They can give information based on knowledge and past experience; the final decision belongs to the patient and family. Skill in rehearsing alternatives is very important for those who have lost a body part or function. They may need to rehearse what to do in a variety of social situations. Groups of people with the same condition may be helped by role-playing situations.

Finding Meaning in Illness

Illness is a human experience. Many people have found serious illness to be a turning point in their lives, both spiritually and philosophically. Sometimes people find solace in the belief that their suffering may have some meaning or be helpful to others. They may participate in research projects or training programs to this end.

Families may be brought together by illness in a painful but very meaningful way. People experience a sense of their basic worth as well as that of others. Many survivors of serious illness report that they experienced a change in values and priorities, greater concern for others, and a heightened appreciation for the beauty of nature. After serious illness, some people may find meaning in helping others through support groups or as volunteers for health-related organizations or political action groups.

Dying and Death

Stages of Dying

Death is a natural part of life and comes to all beings. Some societies treat death as a naturally occurring phenomenon and accept it in an open and nonthreatening manner. In our culture, however, death is often treated as taboo. Children are "protected" from the reality of death and grow to adulthood with very little exposure to it. For most people, the thought of death is frightening and impossible to comprehend. Regardless of religious beliefs, it is difficult to imagine oneself not existing in the world.

People face death in many ways. According to Kübler-Ross (1969), the emotional responses of a person facing death can be traced through five stages: denial and isolation, anger, bargaining, depression, and acceptance. These five stages do not always occur in sequence, and they may overlap one another. Patients and their families move back and forth through the experience and may be at different stages at a given time.

Denial and isolation occur as a first reaction to the possibility of impending death. The person cannot accept the fact that death is near. Denial permits hope to exist.

The next emotion expressed is anger. The question "Why me?" is frequently on the person's mind. Although it is impossible to answer this question, allowing the person to express feelings and listening to concerns can help him or her move through this stage to the next.

Bargaining is a phase of coping during which the dying person attempts to negotiate a trade. Usually it involves a deal with God or fate: "If I can live long enough to attend my son's wedding, I'll be ready to die." If possible, everything should be done to grant patients their requests.

Depression is evident when the person realizes the full impact of the inevitable. Defense mechanisms are no longer effective; sadness and anguish are felt and expressed. The resolution of this phase leads quietly into the final stage.

Acceptance is a time of relative peace. The person seems to want to review the past and contemplate the unknown future. Often, the person does not talk a great deal but wants others nearby. If pain is relieved, the person who has accepted death often wants to be comforted by having contact with those who are meaningful.

Tasks of Mourning

Worden (1991) describes the four tasks of mourning or adapting to loss. Like developmental tasks that are necessary for a child's growth and development, tasks of mourning must be completed if growth and development are to continue.

The first task of mourning is to accept the reality of the loss both intellectually and emotionally. Fluctuating from belief to disbelief is evident as the bereaved negotiate this task.

Working through the pain of grief is the second task. The pain of grief takes many forms, *i.e.* physical pain, emotional pain, and behavioral pain. Denial and avoidance of this pain only result in other symptoms such as depression or unhealthy behaviors. The only way through this task is through feeling and acknowledging the pain of grief.

The third task deals with adjusting to the environment in which the deceased is missing. The bereaved must adjust by developing new skills, assuming new roles, and changing their sense of the world, as in finding new meaning and directions in one's life.

The fourth and final task is that of emotional relocation of the deceased and moving on with life. The idea is that one's energy and attachments do not remain with the deceased, but are actively invested in forming new relationships.

The resolution of grief work comes when the bereaved become future oriented, derive pleasure from life, and are able to adapt to new roles. It is important to remember that this is a process that takes time and work.

In our society, dying and death can occur in a variety of settings. The nurse in these settings must not only be available to the dying patient, but to friends and family who need to be supported as they support the dying person. Care must be provided in a sensitive manner. When aggressive measures are instituted in a critical care setting, the needs of the family must be considered and communication lines between the patient, staff, and family maintained. The family is often waiting vigilantly for limited, scheduled visiting times only to see their loved one attached to various machines, tubes, and monitors.

CRITICAL THINKING EXERCISES

1. You are caring for two patients, both of whom have cancer. One patient has only recently been told of her diagnosis. The other patient has been receiving treatment for the cancer for almost a year. How might the coping needs of these two patients differ? How might your plan of care differ for each?
2. The daughter of a patient approaches you and expresses her frustration that her father, who has hypertension, denies that his illness is serious and refuses to adhere to his prescribed diet. Based on your knowledge of the various ways that people cope with illness, how might you explain the patient's reaction to his daughter? Describe the strategies you might suggest to get the patient to adhere to the prescribed treatment.
3. The husband of a patient who is dying indicates his concern that his wife will not talk to him or to his children about the fact that she is dying; whenever he raises the subject with her, she says that she is too tired to talk. Considering what you have learned about emotional responses to dying, how would you explain his wife's behavior? If the husband were the one in denial, how would you proceed?

When a person dies at home, the family or friends are usually responsible for the physical needs of the dying person. The nurse's role in this instance is to teach the family how to carry out certain procedures and to provide comfort and support for all concerned.

Frequently, the family will arrange for hospice care. Hospice care can be provided in a freestanding hospice facility, in a part of the general hospital set aside for hospice care, or in the home. The goal of hospice care is to maintain the dying person in as pain-free a state as possible in the final phases of life. The nurse working in the hospice setting provides psychosocial and spiritual support to the dying patient and his or her family.

Nursing homes, convalescent homes, and extended care facilities are alternative settings when the family is unable to care for the dying person. In these settings, the family and friends often provide whatever limited care they are able to provide, such as cooking favorite foods and feeding the dying person. As death is often expected in these facilities, care is usually aimed toward a peaceful and dignified death.

REFERENCES AND BIBLIOGRAPHY

Books

Benner P and Wurbel J. The Primacy of Caring: Stress and Coping in Health and Illness. Menlo Park, CA, Addison-Wesley, 1989.

Brown GW and Harris TO. Life Events and Illness. New York, Guilford Press, 1989.

Derogatis LR and Wise TN. Anxiety and Depressive Disorders in the Medical Patient. Washington, DC, American Psychiatric Press, 1989.

Kennerley H. Managing Anxiety. New York, Oxford University Press, 1990.

Kübler-Ross E. On Death and Dying. New York, Macmillan, 1969.

Lerner H. The Dance of Anger. New York, Harper and Row, 1985.

Moos R (ed). Coping With Physical Illness, vol. 2. New York, Plenum Medical Book Co., 1984.

Schultz W. The Interpersonal Underworld. Palo Alto, CA, Science and Behavior Books, 1966.

Strauss A and Corbin J. Chronic Illness and the Quality of Life. St. Louis, CV Mosby, 1984.

Sundeen SJ et al. Nurse-Client Interaction: Implementing the Nursing Process. St. Louis, Mosby Year-Book, 1994.

Wilson HS and Kneisl CR. Psychiatric Nursing, 3rd ed. Menlo Park, CA, Addison-Wesley, 1988.

Worden JW. Grief Counseling and Grief Therapy, 2nd ed. New York, Springer, 1991.

Journals

Asterisks indicate nursing research articles.

Badger JM. Calming the anxious patient. Am J Nurs 1994 May; 94(5); 46–50.

*Cowles KV and Rodgers BL. The concept of grief: A foundation for nursing research and practice. Res in Nurs and Health 1991; 14: 119–127.

*Davis T et al. Identifying depression in medical patients. Image: J Nurs Sch 1988 Winter; 20(4): 191–195.

Frisch N. Home care nursing and psychosocial-emotional needs of clients. Home Healthcare Nurs 1993 Mar-April; 11(2): 64–70.

*Fryback P and Reinert B. Facilitating health in people with terminal diagnoses by encouraging a sense of control. Medsurg Nurs 1993 June 2(3): 197–201.

Groves C et al. Nursing ground rounds: ICU psychosis. Helping your patient return to reality. Nursing 1982 Jan; 12(1): 58–63.

*Gurklis JA et al. Identification of stressors and use of coping methods in chronic hemodialysis patients. Nurs Res 1988 July–Aug; 37(4): 236–239.

*Harrison TM et al. Assessing nurses' communication: A cross- sectional study. West J Nurs Res 1989 Feb; 11(1): 75–91.

*Kaempf G et al. The effect of music on anxiety: A research study. AORN J 1989 July; 50(1): 112, 114–118.

Kelly JH and Lehman L. Assessment of anxiety, depression, and suspiciousness in the home care setting. Home Healthcare Nur 1993 Mar–April; 11(2): 16–20.

Kelly JH and Lehman L. Nursing interventions for anxiety, depression and suspiciousness in the home care setting. Home Healthcare Nur 1993 May–June; 11(3): 35–40.

*Leja AM. Using guided imagery to combat post-surgical depression. J Gerontol Nurs 1989 April; 15(4): 6–11, 40–41.

*McGinnis S. How can nurses improve the quality of life of the hospice client and family? Hospice J 1986; 2: 23–36.

Perrin K. Psychoneuroimmunology and nursing practice. Nurs Spectrum 1993 Aug; 3(16): 5.

Ufema J. Mrs. Murphy's strange behavior . . . "dying" talk. Nursing 1989 May; 19(5): 84–85.

Ufema J. Facing death: Look to the past. Nursing 1988 Nov; 18(11): 93–94.

Ufema J. Insights on death and dying. Nursing 1988 Oct; 18(10): 93–94.

Zerwekh J. The truth tellers. How hospice nurses help patients confront death. Am J Nurs 1994 Feb; 94(2): 31–34.

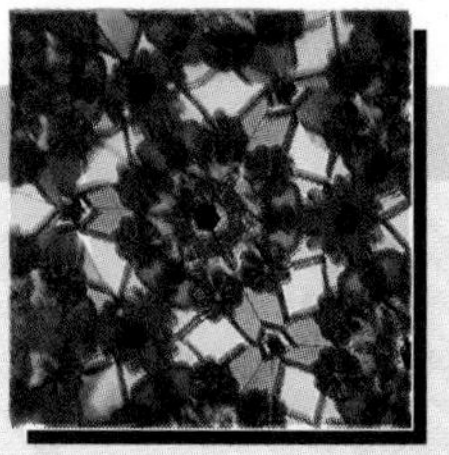

11 Transcultural Perspectives in Nursing

CHAPTER OUTLINE

LEARNING OBJECTIVES

On completion of this chapter, the learner will be able to:

1. Apply transcultural nursing principles, concepts, and theories when providing nursing care for patients (individuals, families, groups, and communities)
2. Identify key components of cultural assessment for self and clients
3. Critically analyze the influence of culture on nursing care decisions and actions for patients
4. Develop strategies for planning, providing, and evaluating culturally competent nursing care for patients from diverse backgrounds

Definitions of Culture

The concept of culture and its relationship to the health care beliefs and practices of patients and their family and friends provides the foundation for transcultural nursing. This awareness of culture in the delivery of nursing care has been described in different ways including culturally competent nursing care (American Academy of Nursing, 1993; Andrews & Boyle, 1995; Campinha-Bacote, 1994; Cross et al, 1989) or culturally congruent nursing care (Leininger, 1991).

The term culture was initially defined by the British anthropologist Sir Edward Tylor in 1871 as including the knowledge, belief, art, morals, laws, customs, and any other capabilities and habits acquired by humans as members of society. Today, culture can be defined in 200 different ways. According to Dr. Madeleine Leininger, founder of the specialty called transcultural nursing, culture is the "learned and transmitted knowledge about a particular culture with its values, beliefs, rules of behavior, and lifestyle practices that guides a designated group in their thinking and actions in patterned ways" (Leininger, 1978, p. 491).

Culture has four basic characteristics:

1. It is learned from birth through language and socialization.
2. It is shared by all members of the same cultural group.
3. It is influenced by specific conditions related to environmental and technical factors and to the availability of resources,
4. It is dynamic and ever-changing.

Subcultures and Minorities

Although culture is a universal phenomenon, it takes on specific and distinctive features for a particular group, encompassing all of the knowledge, beliefs, customs, and skills acquired by the members of that group. When such groups function within a large cultural group, they are referred to as **subcultures**.

The term **subculture** is used for relatively large groups of people who share characteristics that are not common to all members of the culture and that enable them to be identified as a distinct entity. Examples of subcultures based on ethnicity (*i.e.*, subcultures with common traits such as physical characteristics, language, or ancestry) include African Americans, Hispanics, and Native Americans. It should be noted that each of the aforementioned subcultures may be further divided. For example, Native Americans consist of American Indians and Alaska Natives, who represent more than 500 federally and state-recognized tribes in addition to an unknown number of tribes that receive no official recognition.

Subcultures also may be based on religion (more than 1200 exist in the United States); occupation (including nurse, physician, and other members of the health care team); age (infants, children, adolescents, older adults); gender (man or woman); sexual orientation (gays, lesbians, or bisexuals); or geographic location (such as Texans, Southerners, Appalachians).

The term *minority* refers to a group of people whose physical or cultural characteristics differ from the majority of people in a society. At times minorities may be singled out or isolated from others in society or treated in different or unequal ways. Although there are four federally identified minority groups (Blacks, Hispanics, Asian/Pacific Islanders, and Native Americans), the concept of minority varies widely and must be understood in a cultural context. For example, men may be considered minorities within the nursing profession, but they comprise a majority within the field of medicine. Because at times the term minority connotes inferiority, members of many racial and ethnic groups object to being identified as minorities.

Transcultural Nursing

Transcultural nursing, a term sometimes used interchangeably with cross-cultural, intercultural, or multicultural nursing, refers to a formal area of study and practice that focuses on the cultural care (caring) values, beliefs, and practices of individuals and groups from a particular culture. The underlying focus of transcultural nursing is to provide culture-specific and culture-universal care that promotes the well-being or health for individuals, families, groups, communities, and institutions (Leininger, 1978, 1991). When the care is delivered beyond the nurse's national boundaries, the terms international or transnational nursing are often used.

Although many nurses, anthropologists, and others have written about the cultural aspects of nursing and health care, Dr. Madeleine Leininger has developed a comprehensive research-based theory called "Culture Care Diversity and Universality." The goal of the theory is to provide culturally congruent nursing care to improve care to people of different or similar cultures. This means helping clients, through culturally based care, to recover from illness, to prevent conditions that would limit the client's health or well-being, or to facilitate a peaceful death in ways that are culturally meaningful and appropriate. Nursing care needs to be tailored or fit to the client's cultural values, beliefs, and lifeways.

Some of the terms described in Leininger's theory include culture care accommodation, culture care repatterning or restructuring, and the basic definition of culturally congruent care:

- Culture care accommodation refers to those professional actions and decisions that help people of a designated culture adapt to achieve a beneficial or satisfying health outcome.
- Culture care repatterning or restructuring refers to those professional actions and decisions that help clients reorder, change, or modify their lifestyles for new, different, or more beneficial health care patterns. At the same time the client's cultural values and beliefs are respected and a better (or healthier) lifestyle is provided.
- Culturally congruent nursing care refers to those cognitively based acts or decisions that are tailor-made to fit with an individual, group, or institution's cultural val-

ues, beliefs, and lifestyles to provide meaningful, beneficial, and satisfying health care.

Other terms and definitions that provide further insight into culture and health care include:

- *Acculturation*, the process by which members of a cultural group adapt to or learn how to take on the behaviors of another group.
- *Cultural blindness*, the inability of an individual to recognize his or her own values, beliefs, and practices and those of others because of strong ethnocentric tendencies.
- *Cultural imposition*, the tendency to impose one's cultural beliefs, values, and patterns of behavior on a person or persons from a different culture.
- *Cultural taboos*, those activities governed by rules of behavior that are avoided, forbidden, or prohibited by a particular cultural group.

Culturally Competent Nursing Care

Culturally competent or congruent nursing care refers to a complex integration of attitudes, knowledge, and skills (including assessment, decision making, judgments, critical thinking, and evaluation) that enables the nurse to provide care in a culturally sensitive manner.

This concept also applies to health care institutions which must develop culturally sensitive policies and provide an atmosphere that fosters the provision of culturally congruent and competent care by nurses, a group whose members frequently reflect the multicultural complexion of our society. For example, it is estimated that 9%, or 207,000 registered nurses in the United States, come from racial or ethnic minority backgrounds.

Policies that promote culturally congruent care establish flexible regulations pertaining to visitors (number, frequency, and length of visits); consider the role of folk healers in the planning, implementation, and evaluation of care; provide interpretation services for non-English speaking patients; recognize special dietary needs of patients from selected cultural groups; and create an environment in which the spiritual and religious practices of patients are encouraged.

Cultural Assessment

Cultural nursing assessment refers to a systematic appraisal or examination of individuals, families, groups, and communities in terms of their cultural beliefs, values, and practices. The purpose of such an assessment is to provide culturally congruent care. Because the nurse-client interaction is the focal point of nursing, nurses should consider their own cultural orientation when conducting assessment of the patient and the patient's family and friends.

In an effort to establish a database for determining a patient's cultural background, nurses have developed cultural assessment tools or have modified existing assessment tools (Andrews & Boyle, 1995; Leininger, 1991) to assure that transcultural considerations are included in the plan of care. Regardless of the particular cultural assessment instrument that is used, the following principles can be used to guide the assessment.

- Know your own cultural attitudes, values, beliefs, and practices.
- Regardless of "good intention," everyone has cultural "baggage" that ultimately results in ethnocentrism (the tendency to view one's own culture as superior to others).
- In general, it is easier to understand those whose cultural heritage is similar to our own, while viewing those who are unlike us as strange and different.
- Maintain a broad, open attitude. Expect the unexpected. Enjoy surprises.
- Avoid seeing all people as alike, *i.e.*, avoid cultural stereotypes such as "all Chinese like rice" or "all Italians eat spaghetti."
- Try to understand the reason(s) for any behavior by discussing commonalities and differences.
- If a client has said or done something that you do not understand, ask for clarification. Be a good listener. Most clients will respond positively to questions that arise from a genuine concern for and interest in them.
- If at all possible, speak the client's language (even simple greetings and social courtesies will be appreciated). Avoid feigning an accent or using words that are ordinarily not part of your vocabulary.
- Be yourself. There are no right or wrong ways to learn about cultural diversity.

Cross-Cultural Communication

Communication occurs through words, body language, and other linguistically related cues such as voice, tone, and loudness. These principles apply to nurse-client interactions, as well as to communications among members of a multicultural health care team.

Verbal Communication

Approximately 150 different languages are spoken in the United States with Spanish accounting for the largest percentage among minority groups. Obviously, nurses cannot become fluent in all languages, but certain strategies for fostering effective cross-cultural communication are necessary when providing care for patients who are not fluent in English. It should be noted that during illness, clients of all ages tend to regress, and the regression often involves language skills. Chart 11-1 summarizes suggested strategies for overcoming language barriers. The nurse also will want to assess how well the patient and family have understood what has been said. The following may signal lack of effective communication:

- *Efforts to change the subject.* This could indicate that the patient does not understand what you are saying and is attempting to talk about something more familiar.

CHART 11-1
Overcoming Language Barriers

- Greet the patient using the last or complete name. Avoid being too casual or familiar. Gesture to yourself and say your name. Smile.
- Proceed in an unhurried manner. Pay attention to any effort by the patient or family to communicate.
- Speak in a low, moderate voice. Avoid talking loudly. Remember that there is a tendency to raise the volume and pitch of your voice when the listener appears not to understand. The listener may perceive that you are shouting and/or angry.
- Organize your thoughts. Repeat and summarize frequently. Use audiovisual aids when feasible.
- Use short, simple sentence structure and speak in the active voice.
- Use simple words, such as "pain" instead of "discomfort." Avoid medical jargon, idioms, and slang. Avoid using contractions, *e.g.*, don't, can't, won't, etc.
  Use nouns repeatedly instead of pronouns.
  Example:
  Do not say: "He has been taking his medicine, hasn't he?"
  Do say: "Does Juan take medicine?"
- Pantomime words and simple actions while verbalizing them.
- Give instructions in the proper sequence.
  Example:
  Do not say: "Before you rinse the bottle, sterilize it."
  Do say: "First wash the bottle. Second, rinse the bottle."
- Discuss one topic at a time and avoid giving too much information in a single conversation. Avoid using conjunctions.
  Example:
  Do not say: "Are you cold and in pain?"
  Do say: "Are you cold?" (while pantomiming) "Are you in pain?"
- Validate if the person understands by having him or her repeat instructions, demonstrate the procedure, or act out the meaning.
- Use any words you know in the person's language. This indicates that you are aware of and respect the patient's primary means of communicating.
- Try a third language. Many Indo-Chinese speak French. Europeans often know three or four languages. Try Latin words or phrases, if you are familiar with the language.
- Ask who among the patient's family and friends could serve as an interpreter. Be aware of culturally based gender and age differences and diverse socioeconomic, educational and tribal/regional differences when choosing an interpreter.
- Obtain phrase books from a library or bookstore, make or purchase flash cards, contact hospitals for a list of interpreters, and use both formal and informal networking to locate a suitable interpreter. Although costly, some telecommunication companies provide translation services.

- *Absence of questions.* Paradoxically, this often means that the listener is not grasping the message and therefore has difficulty formulating questions to ask.
- *Inappropriate laughter.* A self-conscious giggle may signal poor comprehension and may be an attempt to disguise embarrassment.
- *Nonverbal cues.* Although a blank expression may signal poor understanding, among some Asian-Americans it may reflect a desire to avoid overt expression of emotion. Similarly, avoidance of eye contact may be a cultural expression of respect for the speaker (*e.g.*, some Native Americans and Asian-Americans).

Cultural Awareness

Because so many human behaviors and attitudes are shaped by cultural influences, nurses should be aware that patients act and behave in a variety of ways, based on their cultural background. However, although certain attributes and attitudes are frequently associated with particular cultural groups, as described in the following pages, it is important to realize that not all people from the same cultural background share the same behaviors and views. Although failing to consider a patient's cultural preferences and beliefs is considered insensitive and possibly indifferent, assuming that all members of any one culture act and behave in the same way runs the risk of stereotyping people. The best way to avoid stereotyping is to view each patient as an individual and to find out which cultural preference, if any, the patient has.

Space and Distance

People tend to regard the space in their immediate vicinity as an extension of themselves. How much space they need between themselves and others to feel comfortable is a culturally determined phenomenon.

Because nurses and patients usually are not consciously aware of their personal space requirements, they frequently have difficulty understanding different behaviors in this regard. For example, positioning oneself close to another may be perceived as an expression of warmth and care by one person but as a threatening invasion of personal space by another. Research reveals that individuals from the United States, Canada, and Great Britain require the most personal space between themselves and others, whereas those from Latin America, Japan, and the Middle East need the least amount of space and feel comfortable standing close to others.

If patients seem to position themselves too close or too far away, the nurse should consider cultural preferences for space and distance. Ideally, patients should be permitted to assume a position that is comfortable to them in terms of personal space and distance. Because a significant amount of communication during nursing care requires close physical contact, the nurse should be aware of these important cultural differences and consider them when delivering care.

Eye Contact

Eye contact is also a culturally determined behavior. Although most nurses have been taught to maintain eye contact when speaking with clients, some people from culturally diverse backgrounds may interpret this behavior differently. Some Asians, Native Americans, Indo-Chinese, Arabs, and Appalachians may consider direct eye contact impolite or aggressive, and they may avert their own eyes when talking with nurses and others they perceive to be in positions of authority. Some Native Americans will stare at the floor during conversations, a cultural behavior conveying respect and indicating that the listener is paying close attention to the speaker. Some Hispanic clients maintain down-cast eyes as a sign of appropriate deferential behavior toward others on the basis of age, gender, social position, economic status, and position of authority. Being aware that eye contact carries certain meanings in such circumstances will help the nurse understand a patient's behavior and will provide an atmosphere in which the patient can feel comfortable.

Time

Attitudes about time vary widely among cultures and can be a common barrier to effective communication between nurses and patients. Views about punctuality and the use of time are culturally determined, as is the concept of waiting. Symbols of time such as watches, sunrises, and sunsets represent methods for measuring the duration and passage of time.

For most health care providers, time is extremely important, as is promptness. For example, nurses frequently expect patients to arrive at an exact time for an appointment, despite the fact that the patient is often kept waiting by health care providers who are running late. Health care providers are likely to function according to an appointment system in which there are short intervals of perhaps only a few minutes. For clients from some cultures time is a relative phenomenon, with little attention paid to the *exact* hour or minute. Some Hispanic clients, for example, consider time in a wider frame of reference and make the primary distinction between day and night. Time also may be determined according to traditional times for meals, sleep, and other activities or events. For people from some cultures, the present is of the greatest importance and time is viewed in broad ranges rather than in terms of a fixed hour. Being flexible in regard to schedules is the norm.

Value differences also may influence a person's sense of priority when it comes to time. For example, responding to a family matter may be more important to a client than a scheduled health care appointment. Allowing for these different views is essential in maintaining an effective nurse-patient relationship. Scolding a client for being late or acting annoyed undermines the patient's confidence in the health care system and might result in further missed appointments or indifference to health care suggestions.

Touch

The meaning people associate with touching is culturally determined to a great degree. In some cultures (*e.g.*, Hispanic and Arab), male health care providers may be prohibited from touching or examining certain parts of the female body. Similarly, it may be inappropriate for females to care for males. Among many Asian-Americans, it is impolite to touch a person's head because the spirit is believed to reside there. Thus, assessment of the head or evaluation of head injury requires alternate approaches. The client's culturally defined sense of modesty also must be considered when providing nursing care (*e.g.*, some Jewish and Muslim women believe that modesty requires covering their head, arms, and legs with clothing).

Observance of Holidays

All cultures celebrate civil and religious holidays. Nurses should familiarize themselves with major holidays for members of the cultural groups they serve. Information about these important celebrations is available from various sources including religious organizations, hospital chaplains, and patients themselves. Routine health appointments, diagnostic tests, surgery, and other major procedures should be scheduled to avoid those holidays a patient identifies as significant.

Culture and Diet

The cultural meanings associated with food vary widely, but usually include one or more of the following: relief of hunger; promotion of health and healing; prevention of disease or illness; expression of caring for another; promotion of interpersonal closeness among individuals, families, groups, communities or nations; promotion of kinship and family alliances; solidification of social ties; celebration of life events (*e.g.*, birthdays, marriages, funerals); expression of gratitude or appreciation; recognition of achievement or accomplishment; validation of social, cultural, or religious ceremonial functions; facilitation of business negotiations; and expression of affluence, wealth, or social status.

Culture determines what foods are served and when they are served; the number and frequency of meals; who eats with whom; who is given the choicest portions; how foods are prepared, served, and eaten (*e.g.*, chop sticks, hands, fork-knife-spoon); and where people shop for their favorite food items (*e.g.*, ethnic grocery stores and specialty food markets).

Religious practice may include fasting (*e.g.*, Mormons, Catholics, Buddhists, Jews, Muslims, and others), abstaining from selected foods at particular times (*e.g.*, Catholics abstain from meat on Ash Wednesday and the Fridays of Lent), and the ritualistic use of food and beverages (*e.g.*, Passover dinner, consumption of bread and wine during religious ceremonies). Table 11-1 summarizes some dietary practices of selected religious groups.

Many groups tend to feast, often in the company of family and friends, on selected holidays. For example, many

TABLE 11-1 Dietary Practices of Selected Religious Groups

Prohibited Foods and Beverages

Hinduism
All meats
Animal shortenings

Islam
Pork
Alcoholic products and beverages (including extracts such as vanilla or lemon)
Animal shortenings
Gelatin made with pork, marshmallow, and other confections made with gelatin

Judaism
Pork
Predatory fowl
Shellfish and scavenger fish (*e.g.*, shrimp, crab, lobster, escargot, catfish). Fish with fins and scales are permissible.
Mixing milk and meat dishes at same meal
Blood by ingestion (*e.g.*, blood sausage, raw meat). Blood by transfusion is acceptable.
Note: Packaged foods will contain labels identifying *kosher* ("properly preserved" or "fitting") and *parve* (made without meat or milk) items.

Mormonism (Church of Jesus Christ of Latter-Day Saints)
Alcohol
Tobacco
Beverages containing stimulants (coffee, tea, colas, and selected carbonated soft drinks)

Seventh-Day Adventism
Pork
Certain seafood including shellfish
Fermented beverages
Note: Optional vegetarianism is encouraged.

Christians eat large dinners on Christmas and Easter, and consume other traditional high-calorie, high-fat foods such as seasonal cookies, pastries, and candies.

These culturally based dietary practices are especially significant in the care of patients with diabetes, hypertension, gastrointestinal disorders, and other conditions in which diet plays a key role.

Causes of Illness

There are three major views or paradigms that attempt to explain the causes of disease and illness: the biomedical or scientific view, the naturalistic or holistic perspective, and the magico-religious view.

The biomedical or scientific world view prevails in most health care settings and is embraced by most nurses and other health care providers. The basic assumptions underlying the biomedical perspective are that all events in life have a cause and effect, that the human body functions much like a machine, and that all of reality can be observed and measured (*e.g.*, intelligence tests). Among the biomedical explanations for disease is germ theory, which identifies microscopic organisms as the cause of communicable diseases.

The second way that some cultures attempt to explain the cause of illness is through the naturalistic or holistic perspective, a viewpoint that is found among many Native Americans, Asians, and others who believe that human life is only one aspect of nature. According to this view, the forces of nature must be kept in natural balance or harmony.

Many Asian-Americans hold a belief in the yin/yang theory, in which health is believed to exist when all aspects of a person are in perfect balance or harmony. Rooted in the ancient Chinese philosophy of Tao (The Way), the yin/yang theory proposes that all organisms and objects in the universe consist of yin and yang energy. The seat of the energy forces are within the autonomic nervous system where balance between the opposing forces is maintained during health. Yin energy represents the female and negative forces, such as emptiness, darkness, and cold, whereas the yang forces are male and positive, emitting warmth and fullness. Foods are classified as hot and cold in this theory and are transformed into yin and yang energy when metabolized by the body. Yin foods are cold and yang foods are hot. Cold foods are eaten with a hot illness, and hot foods are eaten with a cold illness. The yin/yang theory is the basis for Eastern or Chinese medicine and is embraced by some Asian-Americans.

According to the naturalistic world view, breaking the laws of nature creates imbalances, chaos, and disease. Individuals embracing the naturalistic paradigm use metaphors such as "the healing power of Nature." From the perspective of the Chinese, for example, illness is not seen as an intruding agent, but as a part of life's rhythmic course and as an outward sign of disharmony within.

Many Hispanic, African-American, and Arab groups embrace the *hot/cold theory* of health and illness. The four humors of the body—blood, phlegm, black bile, and yellow bile—regulate basic bodily functions and are described in terms of temperature, dryness, and moisture. The treatment of disease consists of adding or subtracting cold, heat, dryness, or wetness to restore the balance of the humors. Beverages, foods, herbs, medicines, and diseases are classified as hot or cold according to their perceived effects on the body, not on their physical characteristics. According to the hot/cold theory, the individual as a whole, not just a particular ailment, is significant. Those who embrace the hot/cold theory maintain that health consists of a positive state of total well-being, including physical, psychological, spiritual, and social aspects of the person.

The third major way in which people view the world and explain the causes of illness is the *magico-religious* world view. The basic premise is that the world is seen as an arena in which supernatural forces dominate. The fate of the world and those in it depend on the action of supernatural forces for good or evil. Examples of magical causes of illness include belief in voodoo or witchcraft among some African-Americans and others from Caribbean countries. *Faith healing* is based on religious beliefs and is most prevalent among selected Christian religions including Christian Scientism, whereas various healing rituals may be found in many other religions such as Roman Catholicism, Mormonism (Church of Jesus Christ of Latter-day Saints), and others.

Of course it is possible to hold a combination of world views, and many patients are likely to offer more than one explanation for the cause of their illness. As a profession, nursing largely embraces the scientific/biomedical world view, but some aspects of holism have begun to gain popularity, including a wide variety of techniques for managing chronic pain such as hypnosis, therapeutic touch, and biofeedback. Belief in spiritual power also is held by many nurses who credit supernatural forces with various unexplained phenomena related to patients' health and illness states.

Regardless of the view held and whether or not the nurse agrees with the patient's beliefs in this regard, it is important to be aware of how people view their illness and their health and to work within this framework to promote the individual's care and well-being.

Folk Healers

Several cultures believe in folk or indigenous healers. The nurse may find some Hispanic patients turning to a *curandero/a*, *espiritualista* (spiritualist), *yerbo* (herbalist), or *sabador* (healer who manipulates bones and muscles). Some African-American patients may seek assistance from a *hougan* (voodoo priest or priestess), *spiritualist*, or *root doctor* (usually a woman who uses magic rituals to treat diseases), "*old lady*" (an older woman who has successfully raised a family and who specializes in child care and folk remedies). Native American patients may seek assistance from a *shaman* or *medicine man* or *woman*. Clients of Asian descent may mention that they have visited *herbalists*, *acupuncturists*, or *bone setters*. Several cultures have their own healers, most of whom speak the native tongue of the client, make house calls, and cost significantly less than healers practicing in the biomedical/scientific health care system.

It is best not to ridicule a patient's belief in a folk healer or try to undermine trust in the healer. To do so may alienate and drive the patient away from receiving the care prescribed. Efforts should be made to accommodate one set of beliefs while advocating the treatment proposed by modern health science.

CRITICAL THINKING EXERCISES

1. You are assigned to care for a hospitalized young adult whose cultural background is different from yours. Describe how you would assess his cultural beliefs and practices in developing a nursing care plan. Explain why it is important to examine your own feelings about his cultural background.
2. An elderly patient who does not speak English is hospitalized following elective surgery. Even though he is progressing well and his discharge has been planned, his family insists on staying with him for as many hours as possible, refusing to leave when visiting hours are over. How can you help the nursing staff to explore the meaning of the family's behavior and understand their own feelings about this behavior? Devise a strategy that you think will help resolve this situation.
3. You are preparing for a home visit to provide care for an elderly patient who is of foreign origin. The record indicates that she does not speak English and lives in a neighborhood where most of the residents are from the same ethnic background as the patient. Describe how you would plan for this visit in order to ensure that you can communicate with the patient and family while providing the necessary nursing care. Explore other aspects of the patient's and family's background that you would want to assess before making the visit and while you are at the home.

The Future of Transcultural Nursing Care

By the middle of the 21st century, the average patient will trace his or her ancestry to Africa, Asia, the Pacific Islands, or the Hispanic or Arab worlds, rather than to Europe. With increasing frequency, nurses will be expected to provide culturally congruent and competent care for patients and to work effectively with other health care team members whose ancestry also reflects the multicultural complexion of contemporary society.

REFERENCES AND BIBLIOGRAPHY

American Academy of Nursing. Promoting cultural competence in and through nursing education. Subpanel on Cultural competence in Nursing Education. New York, American Academy of Nursing, 1995.

Andrews MM, and Boyle JS. Transcultural Concepts in Nursing Care, 2nd ed. Philadelphia, JB Lippincott, 1995.

Campinha-Bacote J. The Process of Cultural Competence in Health Care. Wyoming, OH, Transcultural CARE Associates, 1994.

Cross TL et al. Towards a culturally competent system of care. Monograph produced by the CASSP Technical Assistance Center at Georgetown University Child Development Center, 1989.

Leininger MM. Culture Care Diversity and Universality: A Theory of Nursing. New York, National League for Nursing Press, 1991.

Leininger MM. Transcultural Nursing: Concepts, Theories, and Practices. New York, John Wiley & Sons, 1978.

RESOURCES

Organizations

Asian-Pacific Islander Nurses Association
c/o College of Mount Saint Vincent
6301 Riverdale Avenue, Riverdale NY 10471
(718) 405-3354

Council on Nursing and Anthropology
c/o Dr. Mildred Roberson
Nursing and Health Sciences, Salisbury State University
Salisbury, MD 21801

Native American Indian Association
927 Treadale Lane, Cloquet MN 55720
(218) 879-1227

National Association of Hispanic Nurses
1501 16th Street, NW, Washington DC 20036
(202) 387-2477

National Black Nurses Association
P.O. Box 1823, Washington DC 20012-1823
(202) 393-6870

Office of Minority Health
U.S. Department of Health and Human Services
P.O. Box 37337, Washington DC 20013-7337
(800) 444-6472
No cost for accessing database, information specialists, resource network, and publications on major health problems affecting African-Americans, Hispanics, Native Americans, and Asian/Pacific Islanders.

Transcultural Nursing Society
c/o Madonna University
College of Nursing and Health
36600 Schoolcraft Road, Livonia MI 48150-1173
(800) TCN-9995

Journals

Journal of Transcultural Nursing
Journal of Cultural Diversity
Multicultural Nursing Journal

Databases

Med-Line
Cumulative Index of Nursing and Allied Health Literature (CINAHL)
PsychLit
Native American Resource and Information Service (NARIS)

Translation Services

AT & T Language Line Services
(800) 752-6096
Provides written and oral translation in 140 languages

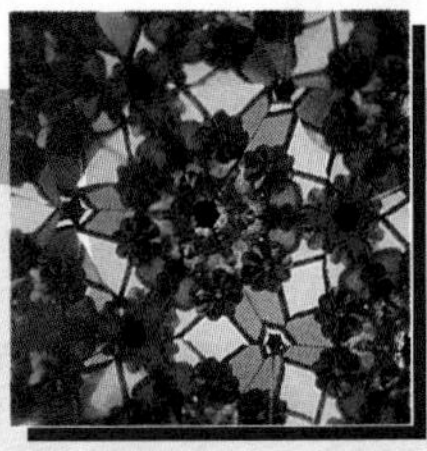

12
Health Care of the Older Adult

CHAPTER OUTLINE

LEARNING OBJECTIVES

On completion of this chapter, the learner will be able to:

1. Develop a definition of aging based on developmental and sociologic theories of aging
2. Describe the aging American population based on demographic trends and statistical data
3. Discuss the physiologic aspects of aging that occur as a result of both normal and pathologic changes
4. Describe the significance of preventive health care and health promotion for the elderly
5. Identify the important physical and mental health problems of aging and their impact upon the functioning of older persons and their families
6. Use the nursing process as a framework for care of patients with Alzheimer's disease
7. Specify nursing implications relative to medication therapy in older persons
8. Examine the concerns of older people and their families in the home and community, the acute care setting, and in a protected environment
9. Identify major legal and ethical issues that are of consideration in the care of older persons

Suzanne C. Smeltzer and Brenda G. Bare: Brunner and Suddarth's Textbook of Medical-Surgical Nursing, 8th Edition. © 1996 Lippincott-Raven Publishers.

Aging, the normal process of time-related change, begins with birth and continues throughout life. Old age is the final phase of the life span.

The older segment of the total American population is growing more rapidly than the rest of the population. U.S. Census Bureau projections indicate that by the year 2030 there will be more people over age 65 years (22%) than people under age 18 years (21%). With an increased older population, more people are living to be "very old." Health professionals are challenged to deal with the higher prevalence of illness occurring within this aging population. Many chronic conditions commonly found among older people can be managed, limited, and even prevented. Older people will be more likely to maintain good health and functional independence if appropriate, community-based support services are available.

Definitions

Geriatrics, the study of old age, includes the physiology, pathology, diagnosis, and management of the diseases of older adults. The broader field of **gerontology** is the study of the aging process and includes the biologic, psychologic, and sociologic sciences. Because old age is a normal occurrence within the life span that encompasses all experiences of life, care and concern for the elderly cannot be limited to one discipline. Optimal care of elderly persons can best be provided through a cooperative effort. The **interdisciplinary team,** made up of specialists from many fields, can combine expertise and resources in contributing knowledge and research to provide insight into all aspects of the aging process.

Gerontologic or **gerontic nursing** is the field of nursing that specializes in care of the elderly. Standards and Scope of Gerontological Nursing Practice were originally developed in 1969 and revised in 1976 and 1987 by the American Nurses Association. The nurse gerontologist can be either a specialist or a generalist offering comprehensive nursing care to the older person. The basic nursing process of assessment, diagnosis, planning, implementation, and evaluation is used in combination with a specialized knowledge of aging.

Gerontologic nursing can be provided in acute, chronic, or community settings. Emphasis of care is placed on promoting, maintaining, and restoring health and independence. Strengths of older adults are identified and used to help them achieve optimal independence. The nurse helps the older person to maintain dignity and maximum autonomy despite physical, social, and psychologic losses. The role of patient advocate calls for collaboration with the interdisciplinary team to provide non-nursing services and a holistic approach to care. In addition, creativity in instituting nursing interventions can help the older person achieve positive physical and mental health.

Old Age Defined

The definition of old age varies depending upon the individual's frame of reference. Thirty-five-year-old parents may be considered old by their children and young by their parents. The active, healthy person of age 65 may consider 75 years as the beginning of old age.

When the retirement age was set at 65 years through Social Security legislation in the 1930s, American society accepted 65 years as the beginning of old age. This represents the chronologic definition of old age that is used most often by society. However, functional and physiologic age differ with the individual and therefore cannot be standardized. Functionally, a professional basketball player is old at the age of 35, although he may be in superb physical health and physiologically young. Gerontologists have attempted to allow for individual differences by using the classification of young–old for 65 to 74 years, and old–old for 75 years and beyond.

Life Span Versus Life Expectancy

Life span is the maximum number of years a person can live under the best of conditions in the absence of disease. The longest verified time that anyone has lived is 120 years. A Japanese man reached this age in 1986 and later that year died of pneumonia (National Institute on Aging, 1993). There has been little change in the life span in recorded history.

Life expectancy is the average number of years that a person can be expected to live. In the 20th century, life expectancy from birth has risen dramatically from an average of 47.3 years (1900) to 75.4 years (1990), with women (79.0 years) living about 7 years longer than men (72.1 years). Early in this century, increased life expectancy was attributed to the decreased death rates of infants and young people. Since 1970, however, increases in life expectancy have been due to decreased mortality among the middle-aged and elderly populations. In 1990, life expectancy differences between men and women were 6.9 years at birth and 4.4 years at 65 years (Table 12-1) (National Center for Health Statistics, 1992; U.S. Senate Committee on Aging, 1991).

TABLE 12-1 Projected Life Expectancy at Birth and Age 65, by Sex: 1990–2050

Year	At Birth		At Age 65	
	Men	Women	Men	Women
1990	72.1	79.0	15.0	19.4
2000	73.5	80.4	15.7	20.3
2010	74.4	81.3	16.2	21.0
2020	74.9	81.8	16.6	21.4
2030	75.4	82.3	17.0	21.8
2040	75.9	82.8	17.3	22.3
2050	76.4	83.3	17.7	22.7

SOURCE: Projections of the population of the United States, by age, sex, and race: 1988 to 2080, Spencer G. Current Population Reports Series P-25, No. 1018 January 1989.

It is predicted that in future years, more people will live longer. Therefore, health professions will be challenged to make these added years healthy and productive ones.

Profile of an Aging America

The older population of 20th-century America has multiplied dramatically in proportion and numbers (4.1% in 1900 to 12.7% in 1993; 3.1 million in 1900 to 32.8 million in 1991). The high birth rate prior to 1920 is evident in the present generation of older people. The baby boom generation, accounting for notable population growth between 1946 and 1964, has been followed by a dramatic decline in the birth rate. These birth rate variations in combination with the rise in longevity have resulted in an ever-increasing proportion of older persons. The median age of the population has expanded from 28 in 1970 to 33 in 1990. It will rise to 36 years by 2000 and to 42 years by 2030. Between 2010 and 2030, when the baby boom generation reaches age 65, the aged population will increase rapidly. In 1993 there were 32.8 million Americans over age 65; presently, one in eight persons is over 65 years (Fig. 12-1). Those 85 and older constitute one of the fastest-growing segments of the population. By the turn of the century, half of the older population will be age 75 and older. This will place greater demands for care upon the health care system (U.S. Senate Committee on Aging, 1991).

In retirement years, older persons become financially dependent upon Social Security benefits in combination with asset income and earnings, pensions, and savings. Social Security is the major source of income for many older families and individuals. Although there is a growing perception that the elderly are well off financially, they are economically vulnerable because of inflation and an increased threat to loss of independence and health. Economic status varies considerably within the older age group, with some older people holding substantial resources. However, approximately one fifth (20%) of the older population was either below or barely above the poverty level in 1993 (defined as $8740 for an older couple or $6930 for a single person in 1993). Older consumers spent proportionately more of their incomes on housing, food, and health care than their younger counterparts (U.S. Bureau of the Census, 1992).

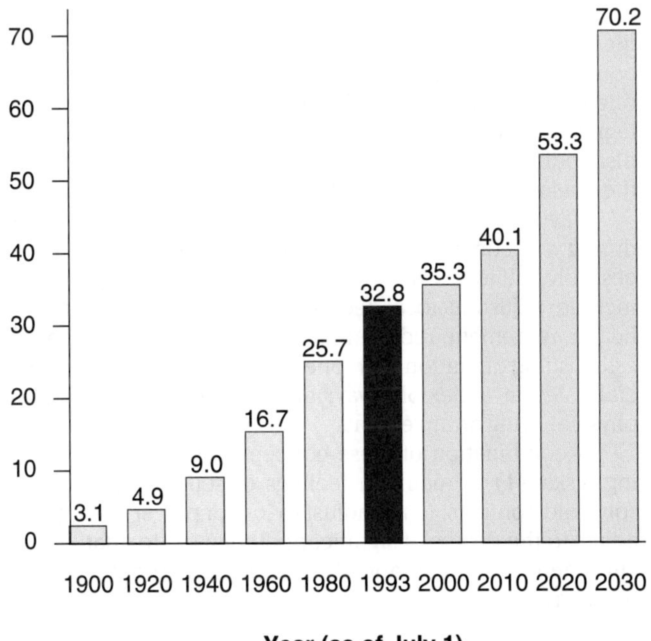

FIGURE 12-1. Increase in 65+ population (in millions 1900–2030). Figures through 1993 are actual figures. Those after 1993 are projected. Note that increments in years on horizontal scale are uneven. (Based on data from U.S. Bureau of the Census.)

Health Status of the Elderly

Although most older persons consider themselves to be in good health, 4 out of 5 suffer from at least one chronic illness (Fig. 12-2). In later life acute conditions occur with less frequency, while chronic illnesses are more common. Progression of the disease process threatens independence and quality of life by impeding ability to perform personal care and everyday tasks. Of the 30 million older persons living in the community in 1990, 4.4 million (14.5%) had difficulty with at least one of five activities of daily living (eating, bathing, dressing, transferring, toileting) (U.S. Senate Committee on Aging, 1991).

Heart disease followed by cancer and stroke account for more than 75% of elderly deaths (Table 12-2). The use of health care resources is greater among older people, particularly in the last year of life. On the average, older people are hospitalized three times more frequently and remain in the hospital 50% longer than people under age 65 (Schick and Schick, 1994; U.S. Senate Committee on Aging, 1991).

Psychosocial Aspects of Aging

Successful psychologic aging is reflected in the older person's ability to adapt to physical, social, and emotional losses and achieve contentment, serenity, and life satisfactions. Because changes in life patterns are inevitable over a lifetime, the person must show resiliency and coping skills when confronting stresses and change. The nurse can encourage participation in decision making, optimal independence, social activities, and involvement in productive, fulfilling activities. Flexibility, humor, and curiosity all contribute to the older person's social and psychologic adjustment. A positive self-image enhances risk taking and participation in new, untested roles.

Although attitudes toward old people differ in ethnic subcultures, a subtle theme of ageism predominates. **Ageism** is a prejudice against or dislike of older people. It is often based upon **stereotypes,** simplified and often untrue beliefs, that reinforce society's negative image of the aged person. Elderly people make up an extremely heterogeneous group, yet negative stereotypes are attributed to all of them.

Fear of aging and the inability for many to confront their own aging process may trigger ageist beliefs. Retire-

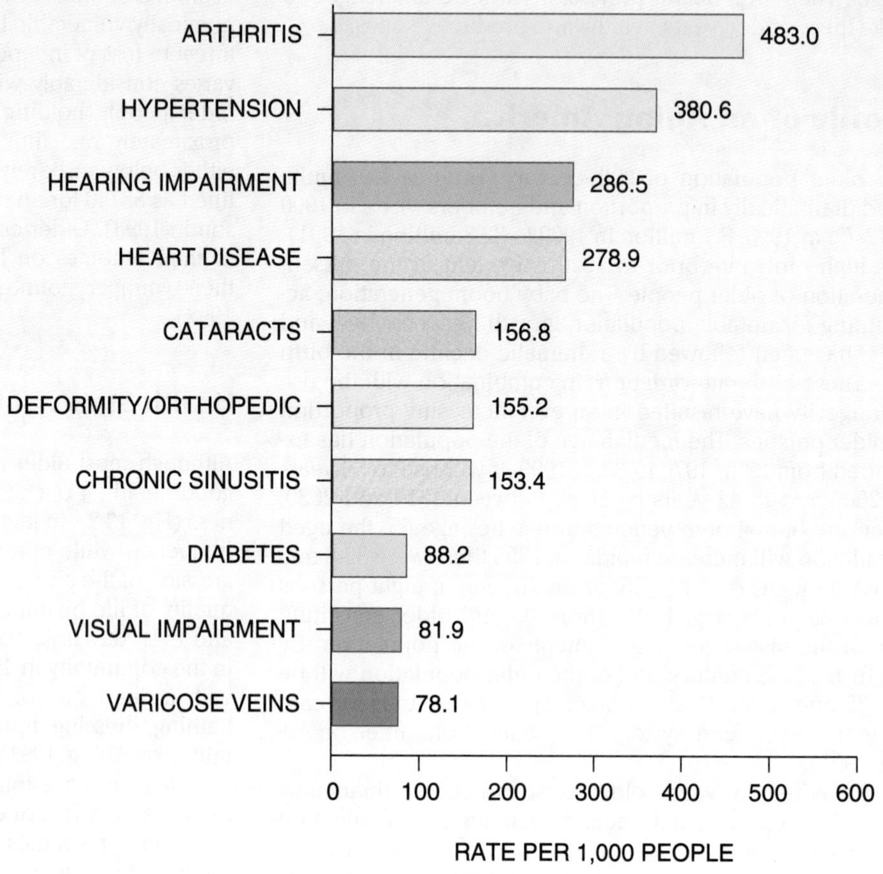

FIGURE 12-2. The top ten chronic conditions for persons 65+: 1990. (National Center for Health Statistics, National Health Interview Survey, 1990.)

ment and perceived nonproductivity are also responsible for negative feelings. The younger working person may see the older person as one who is not contributing to society and is draining economic resources. This negative image is so common in American society that the elderly themselves often believe it. Stereotypes call for certain behaviors, and the elderly may adopt these expected roles. Thus, negative stereotypes are reinforced.

Health professionals may be instrumental in perpetuating a negative image. Nurses who care for sick old people see many problems that they may generalize to the entire elderly community. Only through an understanding of the aging process and respect for each person as an individual can the myths of aging be dispelled. If aged persons are treated with dignity and encouraged to make decisions and maintain autonomy, the quality of their lives should improve.

Developmental Theories

Erikson (1963) developed the concept of eight stages of man, each stage representing crucial turning points in the life span stretching from birth to death. He delineated the major developmental task of old age as ego integrity versus despair. **Ego integrity** suggests an acceptance of one's lifestyle and a belief that choices made were the best that could be made at a particular time. One is still in control of one's life, a life of dignity. **Despair,** the opposite of ego integrity, implies that the older person feels dissatisfied and disappointed with his or her life. If given another chance, the person would live life differently.

Havighurst (1972) lists developmental tasks that occur during a lifetime. A person who completes the tasks successfully will feel contentment. These tasks of aging persons include adjusting to a decrease in physical strength and health, retirement, reduced income, and death of a spouse; establishing affiliation with one's age group; adapting to social roles in a flexible way; and establishing satisfactory physical living arrangements.

A combination of these concepts results in the following tasks: (1) to maintain feelings of self-worth; (2) to resolve old conflicts; (3) to adjust to loss of power roles; (4) to adjust to the deaths of significant others; (5) to adapt to environmental changes; and (6) to maintain an optimal level of wellness.

Sociologic Theories of Aging

Three major theories of aging have emerged from the early scientific studies of aging conducted four and five decades

TABLE 12-2 Death Rates for Ten Leading Causes of Death Among Older People, by Age: 1988 (rates per 100,000 population in age group)

Cause of Death	65+	65 to 74	75 to 84	85+
ALL CAUSES	5,105	2,730	6,321	15,594
Diseases of the heart	2,066	984	2,543	7,098
Malignant neoplasms	1,068	843	1,313	1,639
Cerebrovascular diseases	431	155	554	1,707
Chronic obstructive pulmonary disease	226	152	313	394
Pneumonia and influenza	225	60	257	1,125
Diabetes	97	62	125	222
Accidents	89	50	107	267
Atherosclerosis	69	15	70	396
Nephritis, nephrotic syndrome, nephrosis	61	26	78	217
Septicemia	56	24	71	199

SOURCE: National Center for Health Statistics. Advanced report of final mortality statistics, 1988. Monthly Vital Statistics Report 1990 Nov 28; 39(7) Supplement.

ago: disengagement, activity, and continuity. These theories attempt to predict and explain the social interactions and roles that contribute to a successful life adjustment of a person in old age.

The **disengagement theory** (Cummings & Henry, 1961) suggests that an elderly person, by withdrawing from society at the same time that society is withdrawing its support from his or her age group, achieves high morale and life satisfaction. This theory has been refuted by research findings showing that engaged, active persons achieve higher life satisfaction than disengaged, more passive people.

The **activity theory** (Havighurst, 1968) proposes that life satisfaction in normal aging involves maintaining the active lifestyle of middle age. This theory reflects the thinking of the majority of middle-class America. It assumes that the older person will find satisfying replacements for activities.

The **continuity theory** (Atchley, 1989; Neugarten, 1964) proposes that successful adjustment to old age rests with the ability of the person to continue life patterns across a lifetime. It is important to retain a continuity or connection to the past. Old habits, values, and interests are integral to a person's present life.

Cognitive Aspects of Aging

Intelligence

Stereotypes suggest that older people have slow thinking processes, forgetfulness, confusion, and senility. Many people erroneously believe that it is difficult, if not impossible, to introduce new learning to an older adult.

Intelligence tests measure the ability to accomplish intellectual tasks such as forming concepts, solving problems, acquiring information, and reasoning. When intelligence test scores from people of all ages are compared (cross-sectional testing), test scores for older adults show a progressive decline beginning in midlife. However, studies show that environment and health have a considerable influence on scores. Interpretation of research findings is controversial. Good cardiovascular health, a stimulating environment, high levels of education, occupational status, and income all seem to have a positive effect upon intelligence scores in later life.

Research studies, as well as demonstrations of creativity by older adults, show that creativity is found in all persons regardless of age. Creative performance in older adults is best manifested within a society that will provide stimulating opportunities and reward risk taking.

Learning and Memory

The ability to learn and acquire new skills and information decreases in the older adult, especially past the age of 70. Despite this, many older persons continue to learn and participate in varied educational experiences. Motivation, performance speed, ill health, and physical status all are important factors that influence learning.

Memory, an integral part of learning, has components that include short-term memory (5 to 30 seconds), recent memory (1 hour to several days), and long-term memory (lifetime). Acquisition of information, registration (recording), retention (storing), and recall (retrieval) are essential components of the memory process. Sensory losses, distractions, and disinterest interfere with acquiring and recording information. Age-related loss occurs more frequently with short-term and recent memory. In the absence of a pathologic process it is called benign senescent forgetfulness. The process by which older adults learn is facilitated when the nurse:

- Supplies mnemonics to enhance recall of related data
- Encourages ongoing use of the intellect
- Links new information with familiar information

- Uses visual, auditory, and other sensory cues
- Encourages the learners to wear their glasses and hearing aids
- Provides glare-free lighting
- Provides a quiet, nondistracting environment
- Sets short-term goals with input from the learning group
- Keeps teaching periods short
- Paces learning tasks according to the stamina of the group
- Encourages verbal participation by the learners
- Reinforces successful learning in a positive manner

Normal Biologic Aging

Intrinsic Versus Extrinsic Aging

Intrinsic aging (from within the person) refers to those changes caused by the normal aging process that are genetically programmed and essentially universal within a species. Universality is the major criterion to use in distinguishing normal from abnormal aging. **Extrinsic changes** of aging result from influences outside the person. Illness and disease, air pollution, and sunlight are examples of extrinsic factors that may hasten the aging process. These abnormal aging processes can be eliminated or reduced through effective health care interventions.

Age-Related Cellular, Tissue, and Organ Changes

Cellular and extracellular changes of old age cause a deterioration of physical appearance and function. Measurable changes in the shape and body make-up occur. The aged person is shorter, with diminished shoulder width and increased circumference of the chest and abdomen, and diameter of the pelvis. Skin appears thin and wrinkled. Lean body mass diminishes and fat mass increases. The adipose tissue (fat) is redistributed from subcutaneous tissues and the extremities to the trunk.

The body's ability to maintain homeostasis or constancy becomes increasingly diminished with cellular aging. Organ systems cannot function at full efficiency because of cellular and tissue deficits. Cells become less able to replace themselves. They accumulate a pigment known as lipofuscin. Within the connective tissue, a degradation of elastin and collagen causes tissues to become stiffer and less elastic.

Age-Related Body System Changes: Health Promotion

The well-being of an aged person depends on physical, mental, social, and environmental factors. A total assessment includes an evaluation of all major body systems, social and mental status, and the ability of the person to function independently despite the presence of a chronic illness. (See Table 12-3 for nursing assessment and interventions for age-related changes in body systems.)

Cardiovascular Changes

Heart disease is a leading cause of death for all age groups including the aged (see Table 12-2). The mortality rate from cardiovascular disease also increases with age. The normal structural changes of aging that occur in the heart and vascular system reduce their ability to function efficiently. The heart valves become thicker and stiffer, and the heart and arteries lose their elasticity. Calcium and fat deposits accumulate within arterial walls. Veins become increasingly tortuous.

Although function is maintained under normal circumstances, the cardiovascular system has less reserve, and its ability to respond to stress is reduced. The resting cardiac output (heart rate [HR] × stroke volume) decreases about 1% annually after age 20. Under conditions of stress, both the maximum cardiac output and the maximum heart rate diminish annually. The relationship between maximum heart rate and age is:

$$\text{maximum HR} = 220 - \text{age in years}$$

Systolic hypertension was once believed to be part of the normal aging process. Hypertension, commonly referred to as high blood pressure, although not universal, is a common problem in the older population. Hypertension has been shown to be a prominent risk factor at all ages for cardiovascular disease and stroke. Older people with a blood pressure reading of less than 140/90 mm Hg live longer than persons with higher readings. A diagnosis of hypertension should be made only after it has been confirmed by at least two subsequent readings.

In older persons, the diagnosis of hypertension is classified as:

1. Isolated systolic hypertension in which the systolic reading exceeds 160 mm Hg, with the diastolic measurement normal or near normal (below 90 mm Hg)
2. Essential hypertension in which the diastolic pressure is greater than or equal to 90 regardless of the systolic pressure
3. Secondary hypertension or hypertension that can be attributed to an underlying cause

Cardiovascular dysfunction may become exaggerated and interfere with normal activities of daily living. The normal changes of aging, genetic factors, and lifestyle may contribute to major disorders that include cardiac dysrhythmias, congestive heart failure, coronary artery disease, arteriosclerosis, hypertension, intermittent claudication (leg pain caused by walking), myocardial infarction, peripheral vascular disease, and cerebrovascular accidents (strokes).

Promotion of Cardiovascular Health

Cardiovascular health in the elderly can be promoted by advocating regular exercise, proper diet, weight control, regular blood pressure check ups, avoidance of stress, and no smoking (see Table 12-3 for details). Additional assessment parameters include being alert for adverse responses to medication, including orthostatic hypotension, electrolyte imbalance, confusion, and depression. To avoid lightheadedness, fainting, and possible falls caused by orthostatic hy-

TABLE 12-3 Body Systems: Changes in Functional Status With Nursing Recommendations

Changes	Subjective and Objective Findings	Health Promotion/Nursing Recommendations
Cardiovascular System		
Decreased cardiac output; diminished ability to respond to stress; heart rate and stroke volume do not increase with maximum demand; slower heart recovery rate; increased blood pressure	Complaints of fatigue with increased activity Increased heart rate recovery time Normal BP ≤140/90 mm Hg	Exercise regularly; pace activities; avoid smoking; eat a low fat, low salt diet; participate in stress reduction activities; check blood pressure regularly, medication compliance, weight control.
Respiratory System		
Increase in residual lung volume; decrease in vital capacity; decreased gas exchange and diffusing capacity; decreased cough efficiency	Fatigue and breathlessness with sustained activity; impaired healing of tissues due to decreased oxygenation; difficulty coughing up secretions	Exercise regularly; avoid smoking; take adequate fluids to liquify secretions; receive yearly influenza immunization; avoid exposure to upper respiratory tract infections.
Integumentary System		
Decreased protection against trauma and solar exposure; decreased protection against temperature extremes; diminished secretion of natural oils and perspiration	Skin appears thin and wrinkled; complaints of injuries, bruises, and sunburn; complaints of intolerance to heat; bone structure is prominent; dry skin	Avoid solar exposure (clothing, sunscreen, stay indoors); dress appropriately for temperature; maintain a safe indoor temperature; bathe only 1–2 times weekly; lubricate skin.
Reproductive System		
Female: Vaginal narrowing and decreased elasticity; decreased vaginal secretions Male: Decreased size of penis and testes Male and female: Slower sexual response	*Female:* Painful intercourse; vaginal bleeding following intercourse; vaginal itching and irritation; delayed orgasm. *Male:* Delayed erection and achievement of orgasm.	May require a prescription for estrogen/antibiotic cream; use a lubricant with intercourse; seek health/sexual counseling if needed.
Musculoskeletal System		
Loss of bone density; loss of muscle strength and size; degenerated joint cartilage	Height loss; prone to fractures; kyphosis; complaints of back pain. Loss of strength, flexibility, and endurance. Complaints of joint pain.	Exercise regularly; eat a high-calcium diet; limit phosphorus intake. Hormones and calcium supplements may be prescribed.
Genitourinary System		
Male and female: Bladder capacity decreases; delayed sensation to void Male: Benign prostatic hyperplasia Female: Relaxed perineal muscles	Urinary retention Difficulty voiding Urgency, frequency, and incontinence of urine	Seek regular medical supervision; have ready access to toilet; wear easily manipulated clothing; drink adequate fluids; maintain an acid urine; avoid bladder irritants (*e.g.* caffeinated beverages, alcohol, sweeteners); practice pelvic floor muscle exercises. Maintain perineal hygiene: skin clean and dry; absorbent pads; water resistant skin cream; clean underclothes.
Gastrointestinal System		
Decreased salivation; difficulty swallowing food; delayed esophageal and gastric emptying; reduced gastrointestinal motility	Complaints of dry mouth Complaints of fullness, heartburn, and indigestion Complaints of constipation, flatulence, and abdominal discomfort	Use ice chips, mouthwash; brush, floss, and massage gums daily; receive regular dental care. Eat small, frequent meals; sit up and avoid heavy activity after eating; limit antacids. Eat a high fiber, low fat diet; limit laxatives; toilet regularly; drink adequate fluids.

(continued)

TABLE 12-3 (continued)

Changes	Subjective and Objective Findings	Health Promotion/Nursing Recommendations
Nervous System		
Reduced speed in nerve conduction; increased confusion with physical illness and loss of environmental cues; reduced cerebral circulation (becomes faint, loses balance)	Slower to respond and react; learning takes longer; becomes confused with hospital admission; complaints of faintness; frequent falls	Pace teaching. With hospitalization, encourage visitors; enhance sensory stimulation; with sudden confusion, look for cause. Encourage slow rising from a resting position; encourage use of a cane.
Special Senses		
Vision: Diminished ability to focus on close objects; inability to tolerate glare; difficulty adjusting to changes of light intensity; decreased ability to distinguish colors	Holds objects far away from face; complaints of glare; complaints of poor night vision; confuses colors	Wear eyeglasses; use sunglasses outdoors; avoid abrupt changes from dark to light; use adequate indoor lighting with area lights and nightlights. Use large printed books; use magnifier for reading; avoid night driving; use contrasting colors for color coding; avoid glare of shiny surfaces and direct sunlight.
Hearing: Decreased ability to hear high frequency sounds	Gives inappropriate responses; asks people to repeat words; strains forward to hear	Recommend a hearing examination; reduce background noise; face person; enunciate clearly; speak with a low-pitched voice; use nonverbal cues.
Taste and smell: Decreased ability to taste and smell	Uses excessive sugar and salt	Encourage use of lemon, spices, herbs.

potension, the older person should be counseled to rise slowly from a lying, to a sitting, to a standing position.

Respiratory Changes

Age-related changes in the respiratory system that affect lung capacity and function include the following: an increase in the anteroposterior chest diameter, osteoporotic collapse of vertebrae resulting in kyphosis (increased convex curvature of the spine), calcification of the costal cartilages and reduced mobility of the ribs, diminished efficiency of the respiratory muscles, an increase in lung rigidity, and a decrease in alveolar surface area. The increased rigidity or loss of elastic recoil in the lung results in an increase in residual lung volume and a decrease in vital capacity. Gas exchange and diffusing capacity are diminished.

Decreased cough efficiency, reduced ciliary activity, and increased respiratory dead space make the older person more vulnerable to respiratory infections. Although older adults have sufficient respiratory function to carry out activities of daily living, there is a diminished ventilatory capacity. This results in a decreased tolerance for sustained exercise and a need for short rest periods during prolonged activity.

Promotion of Respiratory Health

Health promotion activities that will help the elderly maintain adequate respiratory function include regular exercise, appropriate fluid intake, yearly influenza immunizations, and avoidance of smoking and respiratory infections.

Integumentary Changes

The functions of the skin include protection, temperature regulation, sensation, and excretion. With advanced age, intrinsic and extrinsic changes occur that affect the function and appearance of the skin. The epidermis and dermis become thinner. Elastic fibers are reduced in number; collagen becomes stiffer. Subcutaneous fat diminishes, particularly in the extremities. A loss of capillaries in the skin results in a decreased blood supply. These changes result in a loss of resiliency and a wrinkling and sagging of the skin. Hair pigmentation decreases and hair becomes gray. The skin becomes drier and susceptible to irritations because of decreased activities of the sebaceous and sweat glands. Spotty and irregular distribution of pigment occurs, particularly in areas that have been exposed previously to sunlight. These changes in the integument reduce tolerance to extremes of temperature and solar exposure. Skin dryness makes the person susceptible to itching and skin irritation.

Promotion of Integumentary Health

Health teaching points to promote healthy skin function include avoiding exposure to the sun, wearing appropriate clothes to protect the skin, maintaining a suitable temperature indoors, using a lubricating skin cream, and avoiding long soaks in the tub.

Reproductive Changes

Ovarian production of estrogen and progesterone ceases with menopause. Changes occurring in the female reproductive system include thinning of the vaginal wall with a narrowing in size and a loss of elasticity; decreased vaginal secretions, resulting in vaginal dryness, itching, and decreased acidity; involution (atrophy) of the uterus and ovaries; and decreased pubococcygeal muscle tone, resulting in a relaxed vagina and perineum. These changes contribute to vaginal bleeding and painful intercourse. In older men, the penis and testes decrease in size and levels of androgens diminish.

Promotion of Sexual Health

Sexual desire and activity decline but do not disappear, nor should sexual activity be discouraged. Society often views older people erroneously as asexual. The nurse can explain that sexual activity varies individually but is related to sexual behavior at an earlier age. If further counseling is needed, a referral to a trained professional can be suggested. Additional suggestions include using a vaginal lubricant or inquiring about estrogen replacement therapy.

Genitourinary Changes

The genitourinary system continues to function adequately in older people, although there is a loss in kidney mass due primarily to loss of nephrons. Changes in kidney function include decreased filtration rate, diminished tubular function with less efficiency in resorbing and concentrating the urine, and a slower restoration of acid–base balance in response to stress. The ureters, bladder, and urethra lose muscle tone. The bladder capacity decreases, and the older person may be unable to empty the bladder completely. Retention of urine increases the risk of infections. Frequency, urgency, and incontinence are also common problems. Older women may have decreased perineal muscle tone resulting in stress incontinence and urgency. Benign prostatic hyperplasia (enlarged prostate gland) is a common finding in older men. Enlargement of the prostate causes chronic urinary retention, frequency, and incontinence.

Health Promotion of the Genitourinary System

Adequate consumption of fluids is necessary to prevent bladder infections and to maintain fluid balance. Problems of urinary incontinence and frequency can be reduced if the older person follows these guidelines:

- Having ready access to toilet facilities
- Voiding regularly
- Practicing pelvic floor exercises

Pelvic floor exercises, first described by Kegel (1948), can be highly useful in reducing the symptoms of stress and urge incontinence. Because achieving better muscle control takes at least several weeks to accomplish, the elderly person is encouraged to persist regularly with the exercises. Teaching the patient how to do the exercises begins with identifying the pubococcygeus muscle. Point out that this muscle is the same one that is used to hold back flatus or to voluntarily stop the flow of urine. The abdomen, thighs, and buttocks are to remain relaxed. The pubococcygeus muscle is first tightened and then relaxed, each for 10 seconds. These two exercises should be alternated and repeated ten times, four to six times a day. The person can practice them when standing, sitting, or lying down. The nurse can suggest incorporating the exercises into other daily activities because they are undetectable by others. These exercises are also recommended for men with dribbling incontinence related to prostatic surgery. The nurse instructs the patient to tighten the rectal sphincter until the penis retracts. Frequent repetition produces the desired muscle tone.

Constipation can be a major factor contributing to urinary incontinence. Encourage the person to eat a high-fiber diet, drink adequate fluids, and increase mobility to promote regular bowel function. Additional health maintenance practices can be found in Table 12-3.

Gastrointestinal Changes

The function of the gastrointestinal tract usually remains adequate throughout life. Nevertheless, many older people suffer from discomforts that are related to the sluggish passage of food or delayed motility. About half of the population have lost all their teeth by the age of 60. Although it is not an inevitable consequence of aging, periodontal disease leading to tooth decay and loss of teeth is common. Salivary flow diminishes, and the older person may experience a dry mouth.

Peristalsis in the esophagus is less efficient in the elderly. In addition, the gastroesophageal sphincter may fail to relax, leading to delayed esophageal emptying and dilation of the lower esophagus. Major complaints often center upon feelings of fullness, heartburn, and indigestion. Gastric motility may decrease, resulting in delayed emptying of stomach contents. Diminished secretion of acid and pepsin reduces the absorption of iron, calcium, and vitamin B_{12}.

Absorption of nutrients in the small intestine appears to be diminished with age but is adequate. The function of the liver, gallbladder, and pancreas is generally maintained, although some inefficiencies exist in absorption and tolerance to fat. The incidence of gallstones and common bile duct stones increases progressively with advanced years. Abdominal surgery in persons 60 years and older is performed more frequently for gallbladder disease than for any other disorder.

Constipation is high on the list of complaints of aged persons. When mild, the symptoms involve abdominal discomfort and flatulence. However, more serious consequences include fecal impaction that contributes to diarrhea around the impaction, fecal incontinence, and obstruction. Predisposing factors for constipation include lack of dietary bulk, prolonged use of laxatives, ignoring the urge to defecate, side effects of medications, emotional problems, inactivity, insufficient fluid intake, and excessive dietary fat.

Health Promotion for the Gastrointestinal System

Older people may be guided to promote gastrointestinal function by following certain health promotion practices such as brushing and flossing their teeth on a daily basis; receiving regular dental care; eating small, frequent meals; avoiding heavy activity after eating; eating a high-fiber, low-fat diet; ingesting an adequate amount of fluids; establishing regular bowel habits; and avoiding the use of laxatives and antacids.

Nutritional Health

The social, psychologic, and physiologic functions of eating influence the dietary habits of the aged person. Decreased physical activity and a slower metabolic rate reduce the number of calories needed by the older adult to maintain an ideal weight. Although fewer calories are desirable, the older person continues to require the same nutrients. Apathy, immobility, depression, loneliness, poverty, inadequate knowledge, lack of oral health, and lack of taste discrimination contribute to undesirable eating habits. Wasted, empty calories are found primarily in foods that are high in fats, cholesterol, and sugar.

Health promotion teaching includes encouraging a diet low in sodium and saturated fats, with an emphasis on vegetables, fruits, and fish. The older adult requires a variety of foods to maintain balanced nutrition. Fats, particularly saturated fats, should be avoided because they are high in calories and contribute to atherosclerosis. No more than 20% to 25% of dietary calories should be consumed as fat intake. Reducing salt intake is also advocated because sodium reduction has been shown to reduce levels of hypertension.

Protein intake should remain the same in later adulthood. Dried beans and peas are inexpensive and excellent sources of protein and fiber. Red meats, whole milk, eggs, and cheese should be replaced by chicken, fish, and low-fat dairy products to provide adequate protein and reduce fat intake.

Carbohydrates, a major source of energy, should supply the diet with 55% to 60% of the daily calories. Simple sugars should be avoided and complex carbohydrates encouraged. Potatoes, whole grains, brown rice, and fruit provide the person with minerals, vitamins, and fiber; eating these foods should be encouraged, even though they are more difficult to prepare and chew. Commercially processed foods often have a low nutritional and high-sodium content in proportion to the number of calories they contain.

Insufficient consumption of water leads to dehydration and constipation, common problems for older people. Adequate fluid balance is necessary to maintain peristalsis and urinary function. Eight glasses of water are recommended daily unless contraindicated by a medical condition.

Musculoskeletal Changes

A gradual, progressive decrease in bone mass begins before the age of 40 years. Excessive loss of bone density results in osteoporosis (see Chapter 63). This condition is most apparent in postmenopausal women and is associated with inactivity, inadequate calcium intake, and loss of estrogens. Its incidence is higher in northern Europeans and other whites and in the Chinese and Japanese. The danger of fracture due to bone resorption is especially high for the dorsal vertebra, humerus, radius, femur, and tibia. A loss of height occurs in later life. This shortening of the trunk is due to osteoporotic changes of the spine, kyphosis (excessive convex curvature of the spine), and flexion of the hips and knees. These changes negatively affect mobility, balance, and internal organ function.

The muscles diminish in size and lose strength, flexibility, and endurance with decreased activity and advanced age. Back pain is common. Beginning in middle age, the cartilage of joints progressively deteriorates. Degenerative joint disease is found in all older persons past the age of 70.

Health Promotion for Bones

Osteoporosis is a common problem in older women. The demineralization that occurs in osteoporosis is accelerated by the loss of estrogens, inactivity, and a low-calcium, high-phosphorus diet. The nurse can recommend:

- A high calcium intake (dairy products and dark green vegetables are excellent sources, as are soups and broths made with a soup bone and cooked with added vinegar to leach calcium from the bone)
- A low-phosphorus diet (a calcium:phosphorus ratio of 1:1 is ideal; red meats, cola drinks, and processed foods that are low in calcium and high in phosphorus are avoided)
- Exercise (the pull of muscle insertions on the long bones strengthens them and retards calcium resorption)

Calcium supplements, vitamin D, fluoride, and estrogens are often prescribed for the person who is at high risk or who already has osteoporosis. Although osteoporosis cannot be reversed, the disease process can be prevented or arrested.

Health Promotion for Musculoskeletal Function

A program of regular exercise can be lifelong or begun in later life. The axiom "use it or lose it" is very relevant when considering the physical capacity of aged persons. A major barrier to exercise is societal attitudes in general and a negative attitude of older people themselves. Old people are considered to be frail and physically unfit. Many elderly believe that they need less exercise, that vigorous exercise has many risks, and that they have limited ability to perform exercise. They tend to stay indoors and often lack motivation to initiate or maintain physical activity.

The nurse plays an important role by encouraging and challenging older adults to participate in a regular exercise program. Research shows that exercise enhances cardiovascular and respiratory efficiency. Regular exercise increases the strength and efficiency of heart contractions and improves oxygen uptake by cardiac and skeletal muscles. Exercise has been shown to reduce fatigue, increase energy, and reduce cardiovascular risk factors. Muscle endurance, strength, and flexibility—all outcomes of regular exercise—help to promote independence and psychologic well-being. Aerobic exercises are the foundation of programs of cardiovascular endurance conditioning. A physical examination by a physician or nurse practitioner is necessary prior to initiating an exercise program. The program is based on current health status and past activity, with a warm-up and cool-down period before and after exercise. The older person should perform exercises in moderation and use short rests to avoid undue fatigue. Swimming and brisk walking are often recommended because they are managed easily and usually enjoyed by the older person.

Nervous System Changes

The structure and function of the nervous system change with advanced age. A progressive loss in brain mass is attributed to a loss of nerve cells that are not replaced. There is a reduction in the synthesis and metabolism of the major neurotransmitters. Nerve impulses are conducted more slowly, and therefore older persons take a longer time to respond and react. The autonomic nervous system performs less efficiently, and postural hypotension, which causes the person to feel lightheaded upon standing up quickly, may occur. Cerebral ischemia with related lightheadedness may interfere with mobility and safety. Homeostasis is more difficult to maintain, but in the absence of pathologic changes the older person functions adequately and retains cognitive and intellectual abilities. Accompanying the nervous system changes is a reduction of cerebral blood flow. However, under ordinary circumstances, oxygen and glucose supply are adequate.

Health Promotion for the Nervous System

A slowed reaction time places the older person at risk for accidents and injury. Loss of consciousness or a feeling of faintness may occur when the person rises too rapidly from a lying or sitting position. The nurse advises the person to allow a longer time to respond to a stimulus and to move more deliberately. Mental function is threatened by physical or emotional stresses. A sudden onset of confusion may be the first symptom of an infection or change in physical condition (pneumonia, urinary tract infection, drug interactions, dehydration, and others).

Sensory Changes

The sensory organs of sight, hearing, taste, touch, and smell allow each of us to communicate with the environment. Messages received from our surroundings keep us oriented, interested, and contented. Sensory losses with old age affect all sensory organs and threaten this interaction. This is a time of life when the older person is less able to perform physically and is sedentary. Sensory losses can be devastating to the person who cannot see to read or watch television, who cannot hear conversation well enough to communicate, or who cannot discriminate taste well enough to enjoy food.

Sensory Losses Versus Sensory Deprivation

The diminishing function of the sensory organs results in sensory losses that can often be helped by assistive devices such as glasses or hearing aids. Sensory deprivation is the absence of stimuli in the environment, or the inability to interpret existing stimuli (perhaps as a result of a sensory loss). This deprivation can lead to boredom, confusion, irritability, disorientation, and anxiety. Meaningful sensory stimulation offered to the older person is often helpful in correcting this problem. Although all old people have sensory losses and as a result are at high risk for sensory deprivation, all do not suffer from sensory deprivation. One sense can substitute for another in observing and interpreting stimuli. The nurse can enhance sensory stimulation in the environment with colors, pictures, textures, tastes, smells, sounds, and so forth. The stimuli are most meaningful when they are interpreted to the older person and if they are changed often. The confused person responds well to touching and to familiar songs.

Vision

As new cells form on the outside surface of the lens of the eye, the older central cells accumulate and become yellow, rigid, dense and cloudy. Thus, only the outer portion of the lens is elastic enough to change shape (accommodate) and focus at near and far distances. As the lens become less flexible, the near point of focus gets farther away. This condition, **presbyopia**, usually begins in the 40s. Reading glasses to magnify objects are required. In addition, the yellowing, cloudy lens causes light to scatter and therefore makes the older person susceptible to glare. The ability to discern blue from green declines. The pupil dilates slowly and less completely because of increased stiffness of the muscles of the iris. The older person takes longer to adjust when going to and from dark and light environments/settings and needs brighter light for close vision. Although pathologic visual conditions are not a part of normal aging, there is an increased incidence of eye disease in older persons. Those most commonly occurring include cataracts, glaucoma, senile macular degeneration, and diabetic retinopathy.

Hearing

Loss of the ability to hear high-frequency tones occurs in midlife. This age-related hearing loss, called **presbycusis**, is attributed to irreversible inner ear changes. Older persons are often unable to follow conversation because tones of high-frequency consonants (letters *f, s, th; ch, sh; b, t, p*) all sound alike. Unable to communicate, they feel isolated and withdraw from social events. When hearing difficulties are suspected, the ears and hearing should be assessed. Wax buildup or other correctable problems may be responsible for major hearing difficulties. A properly prescribed and fitted hearing aid may be useful in reducing hearing deficits.

Hearing loss may cause the older person to respond inappropriately, to misunderstand conversation, and to avoid social interaction. This behavior may be erroneously interpreted as confused or "senile."

Touching

The sense of touch offers the most intimate of messages and is easiest to interpret. When other senses diminish, touching can reduce feelings of isolation and give a sense of well-being. Although sensory receptors dull with age, they do not disappear. Older persons are eager to touch and be touched. Reduced mobility and fewer social contacts often diminish such opportunities. The nurse can enhance touching contact by offering back rubs, foot massages, and gentle touch. Companion animals may also be used to focus emotions. These pets offer many older persons love, warmth, and touching stimulation that vastly improve their quality of life.

Taste and Smell

The four basic tastes are sweet, sour, salty, and bitter. Of these, sweet tastes are particularly dulled in older persons. This explains why they tend to use sweets excessively. Blunted taste may contribute to the preference for salty, highly seasoned foods. Herbs, onions, garlic, and lemon are encouraged as substitutes for salt to flavor food.

Health Promotion for Sensory Disorders

Health promotion strategies for maintaining sensory function consist of those strategies discussed under each of the aforementioned senses. Additional suggestions can be found in Table 12-3.

Mental Health Disorders

Mental health disorders constitute a major problem and threat to older adults and their families. It is estimated that 15% to 25% of all persons over age 65 have serious symptoms due to a mental or psychiatric disorder (U.S. Senate Committee on Aging, 1991). Within nursing homes this percentage is higher than in the community. Several studies document that in a majority of nursing home residents, psychiatric problems are given as a primary or secondary diagnosis. As many as 75% of persons in nursing homes display signs of dementia. Depressive illness in institutionalized older people is second only to organic mental disorders. Of the nonorganic disorders of older adults that include depression, schizophrenia, and anxiety, depression is most likely to have its onset in later life (Cohen, 1990; Koenig & Blazer, 1992).

Organic mental disorders or syndromes, called degenerative and cerebrovascular disorders, are associated with abnormal cognitive, physical, or behavioral functioning that accompany pathologic changes in the brain. Although not a normal occurrence of old age, organic mental disorders occur in an estimated 10% of persons over 65 and nearly half (47%) of persons over 85 years. They can be chronic or acute, reversible or irreversible. At least half are due to Alzheimer's disease. The remainder can be categorized as (1) delirium or confusional states, (2) amnesia states, and (3) non-Alzheimer dementias.

Older adults are less likely than younger persons to seek treatment for mental health symptoms. Health professionals are challenged to recognize, assess, refer, collaborate, treat, and support those older adults who exhibit noticeable changes in intellect or affect. In a community setting, the nurse may be the only health provider who has contact with the person. Symptoms should not be dismissed as age-related changes. A thorough assessment may reveal a treatable, reversible physical or mental condition. Related concerns include family involvement, access and quality of care, treatment costs and compliance, and ethical issues.

Age-Related Stress and Coping Mechanisms

Coping patterns and the ability to adapt to stress are developed over the course of a lifetime and remain consistent with earlier life. Knowledge of successes and competence in younger adulthood helps the person develop a positive self-image that remains solid even with adversities of old age. The person's abilities to adapt to changes, make decisions, and respond predictably are all determined by the past. Continuity of self provides the older person with defense against erosion of self-esteem. A flexible, well-functioning individual will probably continue as such. However, losses may accumulate within a short period of time and be overwhelming. The older person will have fewer choices and diminished resources to deal with stress. Common stressors of old age include normal aging changes that impair physical function, activities, and appearance; disabilities of chronic illness; social and environmental losses of income, roles, and activities; and the death of significant others.

Affective Disorders

Depression is the most common affective or mood disorder of old age and is often responsive to treatment. Its classification and diagnosis vary according to the number, severity, and duration of symptoms. Depression disrupts quality of life, increases the risk of suicide, and becomes self-perpetuating. A person with depression is not in control of this illness and benefits from interventions by health professionals. Contrary to the beliefs of many, data from recent epidemiologic studies have shown that depressive disorders and even depressive symptoms are less prevalent among older people than they are among the younger population (George, 1993; Koenig & Blazer, 1992). Rates of occurrence are higher for those older adults who are hospitalized (as high as 40% when all depressive disorders are included) (Finch, Ramsey, & Katona, 1992). Within the nursing home setting it is estimated that 12% to 16% of the residents are suffering with a major depression and as many as 30% to 35% of the remainder have a depressive disorder (Koenig & Blazer, 1992).

Depressive disorders vary and are classified according to the number, cause, severity, and duration of symptoms. A major, or clinical, depression presents with symptoms of greater severity and duration. A lesser depression, although not considered a clinical depression, can, nonetheless, have a negative impact upon quality of life. Signs of depression include feelings of sadness, fatigue, diminished memory and concentration, feelings of guilt or worthlessness, sleep disturbances, appetite disturbances with excessive weight loss or gain, restlessness, impaired attention span, and suicidal ideation. Suicide attempts are a potential risk when depression exists. The suicide rate in older white males is higher than in any other age group. A suicidal attempt in an older person is less often a "gesture" and more often "successful" (Valente, 1994).

Geriatric depression is difficult to diagnose. Symptoms of dementia and depression often overlap and cognitive impairment may be due to depression rather than organic mental disease. At times, depression accompanies dementia and successful treatment of the depression may resolve confusion otherwise attributed to the dementia. When depression and medical illnesses coexist, and they often do, neglect of the depression can retard physical recovery. Symptoms might be secondary to a medication interaction or an undiagnosed physical condition. The mental status and depression examinations are vital components of physical assessment and must not be overlooked (see Tables 12-4 and 12-5).

For mild or moderate depression, a psychotherapeutic approach that uses cognitive and behavioral therapies is the treatment of choice. This is often in combination with antidepressant medications. For the more severe depression, medications are of primary importance. The serotonin reuptake inhibitors such as fluoxetine (Prozac) or paroxetine (Paxil) are clinically useful and exhibit rapid action with low occurrence of adverse effects. CNS overstimulation, including such symptoms as anxiety and tremor, can occur. The tricyclic antidepressants, specifically nortriptyline, desipramine, and doxepine, are also clinically therapeutic for depression. Anticholinergic, cardiac, and orthostatic side effects, as well as interactions with other medications, require that these agents be used with care. Accordingly, the dosage must be managed carefully to relieve symptoms and at the same time avoid drug toxicity. It may take 4 to 6 weeks for symptoms to recede, so the nurse should offer explanations and encouragement during this period of time. Electroconvulsive therapy may be indicated for severe depression that is nonresponsive to pharmacologic treatment.

TABLE 12-4 Items of Mini-Mental State Examination

Maximum Score	
	Orientation
5	What is the (year) (season) (date) (day) (month)?
5	Where are we (state) (county) (city) (hospital) (floor)?
	Registration
3	Name three objects: One second to say each. Then ask the patient all three after you have said them. Give one point for each correct answer. Repeat them until he learns all three. Count trials and record number. Number of trials
	Attention and calculation
5	Begin with 100 and count backwards by 7 (stop after five answers). Alternatively, spell "world" backwards.
	Recall
3	Ask for the three objects repeated above. Give one point for each correct answer.
	Language
2	Show a pencil and a watch and ask subject to name them.
1	Repeat the following: "No 'if's,' 'and's,' or 'but's.' "
3	A three-stage command, "Take a paper in your right hand; fold it in half and put it on the floor."
1	Read and obey the following: (show subject the written item). CLOSE YOUR EYES
1	Write a sentence.
1	Copy a design (complex polygon as in Bender-Gestalt).
30	Total score possible

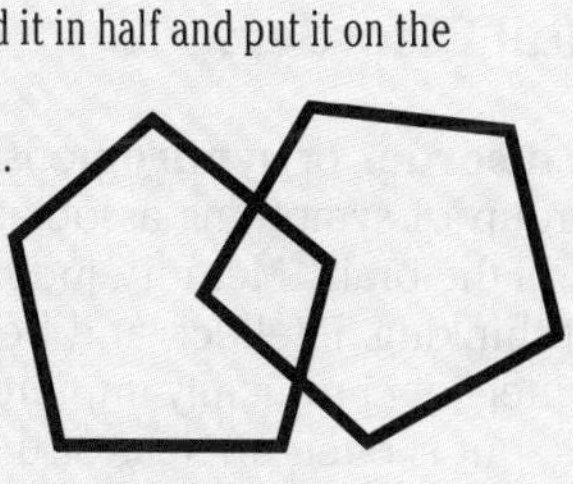

Reprinted from Folstein MF, Folstein S, and McHugh PR. Mini-mental state: A practical method for grading the cognitive state of patients for the clinician. Journal of Psychiatric Research 1975; 12:189–198 with permission from Pergamon Press Ltd, Headington Hill Hall, Oxford OX3 OBW, UK.

TABLE 12-5 Geriatric Depression Scale (GDS).

Choose the best answer for how you felt this past week.

*1.	Are you basically satisfied with your life?	YES	NO
2.	Have you dropped many of your activities and interests?	YES	NO
3.	Do you feel that your life is empty?	YES	NO
4.	Do you often get bored?	YES	NO
*5.	Are you hopeful about the future?	YES	NO
6.	Are you bothered by thoughts you can't get out of your head?	YES	NO
*7.	Are you in good spirits most of the time?	YES	NO
8.	Are you afraid that something bad is going to happen to you?	YES	NO
*9.	Do you feel happy most of the time?	YES	NO
10.	Do you often feel helpless?	YES	NO
11.	Do you often get restless and fidgety?	YES	NO
12.	Do you prefer to stay at home, rather than going out and doing new things?	YES	NO
13.	Do you frequently worry about the future?	YES	NO
14.	Do you feel you have more problems with memory than most?	YES	NO
*15.	Do you think it is wonderful to be alive now?	YES	NO
16.	Do you often feel downhearted and blue?	YES	NO
17.	Do you feel pretty worthless the way you are now?	YES	NO
18.	Do you worry a lot about the past?	YES	NO
*19.	Do you find life very exciting?	YES	NO
20.	Is it hard for you to get started on new projects?	YES	NO
*21.	Do you feel full of energy?	YES	NO
22.	Do you feel that your situation is hopeless?	YES	NO
23.	Do you think that most people are better off than you are?	YES	NO
24.	Do you frequently get upset over little things?	YES	NO
25.	Do you frequently feel like crying?	YES	NO
26.	Do you have trouble concentrating?	YES	NO
*27.	Do you enjoy getting up in the morning?	YES	NO
28.	Do you prefer to avoid social gatherings?	YES	NO
*29.	Is it easy for you to make decisions?	YES	NO
*30.	Is your mind as clear as it used to be?	YES	NO

* Appropriate (nondepressed) answers = yes, all others = no

Score: ☐ (Number of "depressed" answers)

Norms

Normal	5 ± 4
Mildly depressed	15 ± 6
Very depressed	23 ± 5

Yesavage J et al. Development and validation of a geriatric screening scale: A preliminary report. Journal of Psychiatric Research 1983; 17. (Reprinted with permission from Pergamon Press PLC, Headington Hill Hall, Oxford OX3 OBW, UK.)

Organic Mental Disorders

Organic mental disorder or **syndrome** is a general term that refers to a group of symptoms associated with pathologic dysfunction of the brain. Memory, judgment, cognitive function, abstract thinking, intellect, and behavior patterns commonly are acutely or chronically impaired. The etiology may be presumed, but is often unclear or unknown. Two of the most commonly occurring syndromes that will be discussed in this chapter are delirium (usually acute) and dementia (usually chronic) (Table 12-6).

Delirium

Delirium, often called acute confusional state, begins with confusion and progresses to disorientation and change in the level of consciousness which may range from stupor to excessive activity. Thinking is disorganized, and the attention span is characteristically short. Hallucinations, delusions, fear, anxiety, and paranoia may be evident. Because of the acute and unexpected onset of symptoms and the unknown underlying cause, this situation represents a medical emergency. The nurse must recognize the grave implications

TABLE 12-6 Summary of Differences Between Dementia and Delirium

	Dementia		Delirium
	Alzheimer's Disease (AD)	**Multi-Infarct Dementia**	
Etiology	Familial (Genetic). [Chromosomes 14, 19, 21] Sporadic	Cardiovascular disease Cerebrovascular disease Hypertension	Drug toxicity and interactions. Acute disease. Trauma. Chronic disease exacerbation. Fluid and electrolyte disorder.
Risk Factors	Advanced age; genetic factor	Preexisting CV disease	Preexisting cognitive impairment
Occurrence	50–60% of dementias	20% of dementias	20% of hospitalized older people
Onset	Slow	Often abrupt Follows a stroke or TIA	Rapid, acute onset A harbinger of acute medical illness
Age of Onset	Early onset AD: 30s–65 Late onset AD: 65 + Most commonly: 85 +	Most commonly 50–70 years	Any age, but predominately in older persons
Sex	Males and females equally	Predominantly males	Males and females equally
Course	Chronic, irreversible. Progressive, regular, downhill	Chronic, irreversible Fluctuating, stepwise progression	Acute
Duration	2–20 years	Variable. Years.	Lasts 1 day to 1 month
Symptom Progress	Onset insidious. *Early*—Mild and subtle. *Middle and Late*—Intensified. Progression to death (infection or malnutrition).	Depends upon location of infarct and success of treatment. Death due to underlying CV disease.	Symptoms are fully reversible with adequate treatment. Can progress to chronicity or death if underlying condition is ignored.
Mood	Early depression (30%)	Labile. Mood swings.	Variable
Speech/Language	Speech remains intact until late in disease. *Early*—Mild anomia (cannot name objects). Deficits progress until speech lacks meaning. Echoes and repeats words and sounds. Mutism.	May have speech deficit /aphasia depending upon location of lesion	Fluctuating. Often cannot concentrate long enough to speak.
Physical Signs	*Early*—No motor deficits. *Middle*—Apraxia [70%] (cannot perform purposeful movement). *Late*—Dysarthria (impaired articulation). Mutism. *End stage*—Loss of all voluntary activity—positive neurologic signs.	According to location of lesion: Focal neurologic signs, seizures Commonly exhibits motor deficits	Secondary to underlying disease
Orientation	Becomes lost in familiar places (topographic disorientation) Has difficulty drawing 3-dimensional objects (visual and spatial disorientation) Disorientation to time, place, and person—with disease progression		May fluctuate between lucidity and complete disorientation to time, place, and person
Memory	Loss is an early sign of dementia. Loss of recent memory is soon followed by progressive decline in recent and remote memory.		Impaired recent and remote memory. May fluctuate between lucidity and confusion.
Personality	Apathy, indifference, irritability *Early disease*—Social behavior intact. Hides cognitive deficits. *Advanced disease*—Disengages from activity and relationships. Suspicious. Paranoid delusions caused by memory loss. Aggressive. Catastrophic reactions.		Fluctuating. Cannot focus attention to converse. Alarmed by symptoms (when lucid). Hallucinations. Paranoid.
Functional Status/ADLs	Poor judgment in everyday activities. Has progressive decline in ability to handle money, use telephone, function in home and workplace.		Impaired

(continued)

TABLE 12-6 *(continued)*

	Dementia		Delirium
	Alzheimer's Disease (AD)	Multi-Infarct Dementia	
Attention Span	Distractable. Short attention span.		Highly impaired. Cannot maintain or shift attention.
Psychomotor Activity	Wandering, hyperactivity, pacing, restlessness, agitation		Variable. Alternates between high agitation, hyperactivity, restlessness, and lethargy.
Sleep–Wake Cycle	Often is impaired. Wandering and agitation at nighttime.		Takes brief naps throughout day and night

of the acute symptoms and report them immediately. If the delirium goes unrecognized and the underlying cause is not treated, permanent, irreversible brain damage or death can follow.

Delirium is secondary to any number of causes, including physical illness, drug or alcohol toxicity, dehydration, fecal impaction, malnutrition, infection, head trauma, lack of environmental cues, and sensory deprivation or overload. Older adults are particularly vulnerable to acute confusion because of their marginal biologic reserve and the high number of medications that they take. The course of this syndrome is short, usually lasting less than a week and no more than a month.

Therapeutic interventions vary, depending on the reason for the symptoms. Because drug interactions and toxicity are often implicated, it is desirable that nonessential medications be withdrawn. Nutritional and fluid intake should be supervised and monitored. The environment should be quiet and calm. To increase orientation and provide familiar environmental cues, the nurse encourages family members or friends to touch and talk to the patient. With a newly admitted patient, it is important to question the family carefully about his or her prior cognitive state. Ongoing mental status assessments using this baseline will be helpful in evaluating responses to treatment.

Dementia

Dementia (senile dementia, chronic brain syndrome) is a syndrome rather than a distinct disease entity. It is usually progressive and irreversible and is not a part of normal aging. It is characterized by a general decline in intellectual functioning that may include losses of memory, abstract reasoning ability, judgment, and language. Personality changes occur and abilities to perform activities of daily living deteriorate over time. Symptoms are usually subtle in onset and often progress slowly until they are very obvious and profoundly devastating. The three most common nonreversible dementias are Alzheimer's disease (AD), multi-infarct dementia (MID), and mixed Alzheimer's disease and multi-infarct dementia (MIX).

Alzheimer's Disease

Alzheimer's disease (AD) is sometimes called primary degenerative dementia or senile dementia of the Alzheimer's type (SDAT). It accounts for at least 50% of all the dementias suffered by the elderly (Lamy, 1992). It is a progressive, irreversible, degenerative neurologic disease that begins insidiously and is characterized by gradual losses of cognitive function and disturbances in behavior and affect. Alzheimer's disease is not found exclusively in old people. In 1% to 10% of the cases, its onset may be in middle age and it is then called **early-onset dementia**. However, both early-onset and late-onset (onset after 65 years) dementias are considered to be clinically and pathologically identical.

Prevalence rates are strongly associated with age. About 10% of the population over 65 years has Alzheimer's disease. For those persons older than 85 years, this rate increases to 47.2% (Evans, Funkenstein, & Albert, 1990; U.S. Committee on Aging, 1991). With an expanding older population, Alzheimer's disease presents an ever-increasing problem. Approximately 4 million Americans are presently afflicted with it. The course of the disease ranges from 3 to 20 years, until the death of the patient (Lamy, 1992).

Pathophysiology

There are specific neuropathologic and biochemical changes found with Alzheimer's disease. These include neurofibrillary tangles (a tangled mass of nonfunctioning neurons) and senile or neuritic plaques (deposits of beta-amyloid protein, part of a larger protein, amyloid precursor protein [APP]). This neuronal damage occurs primarily in the cerebral cortex and results in decreased brain size. Similar changes are found to a lesser extent in normal brain tissue of older adults. Cells principally affected by this disease are the ones that use the neurotransmitter acetylcholine. Biochemically, the enzyme active in producing acetylcholine is decreased. Acetylcholine is specifically involved in memory processing.

In the fall of 1993, the FDA approved the first Alzheimer's medication, Tacrine hydrochloride, for the treatment of the symptoms of Alzheimer's disease. This agent enhances acetylcholine in the brain and has been shown on two clinical trials to benefit memory in patients with mild to moderate Alzheimer's disease. Because use of this medication causes liver toxicity, patients must be closely monitored (FDA Medical Bulletin, 1993).

Etiology

Age and family history are the two established risk factors for Alzheimer's disease. If family members have at least one other relative with this disease, they are classified as "familial." A familial component nonspecifically includes environmental triggers and genetic determinants. Alzheimer's disease that occurs with no known family history is called "sporadic." Intense research effort is presently being made to identify the chromosomes and specific genes that predispose persons to developing this disease.

In 1987, chromosome 21 was first implicated in some families with early-onset familial Alzheimer's disease (FAD). Soon after, the gene coding for amyloid precursor protein (APP) was also found to be on chromosome 21. However, it took until 1991 for an actual mutation in association with FAD to be found in the APP gene of chromosome 21. For these cases, onset of Alzheimer's disease began in their 50s. Only a few of the cases of FAD have been found to have this genetic mutation. Then, in 1992, chromosome 14 was found to contain an unidentified mutation also linked to FAD. For these persons, the onset age of Alzheimer's disease is in their 40s. Researchers speculate that more genetic factors are to be discovered because there remain some cases of FAD that cannot be linked to either of these chromosomes (Breteler et al.,1992).

As discussed previously, most persons who develop AD do so after the age of 65. These patients with late-onset AD show no chromosome 14 or 21 disturbances. In 1991, a genetic linkage was made between chromosome 19 and late-onset AD. The gene that produces a protein called ApoE is located on chromosome 19. One of the three forms of ApoE, ApoE4, is associated with an increased risk of late-onset AD. A connection between AD and ApoE4 has been discovered even in those with no family history of AD. Therefore, it is thought that the ApoE gene may be a factor in many AD cases previously thought to be sporadic. Many now believe that genetics is a more important factor than was previously suspected. It is also believed that biochemical processes are responsible for modifying or controlling the brain changes of AD. Research continues. Known now is the fact that similar clinical and pathological findings of AD have been correlated with chromosomes 14, 19, and 21 (Alzheimer's Association, 1993; Hodes, 1994; National Institute on Aging, 1994).

Diagnostic Evaluation

History, clinical symptoms, physical examination, and laboratory tests including electroencephalography (EEG), computed tomography (CT scan), magnetic resonance imaging (MRI), and examination of the blood and cerebrospinal fluid (CSF) may all refute or support a diagnosis of Alzheimer's disease. Depression can closely mimic early-stage AD and coexists in many AD cases. A depression scale and a cognitive function test such as the Mini-Mental State Examination (MMSE) should be used for screening (see Tables 12-4 and 12-5). A clinical presentation of cognitive impairment may be due to depression and must be considered. The EEG changes are not always specific. The CT and MRI scans are very useful for excluding hematoma, brain tumor, stroke, normal pressure hydrocephalus, and atrophy but are not reliable in making a definitive diagnosis of Alzheimer's disease. Infections, physiologic disturbances, and biochemical abnormalities can be excluded by examination of the blood and cerebrospinal fluid, but findings are not specific enough to make the diagnosis. A diagnosis of "probable AD" is made when medical history, physical examination, and laboratory tests have excluded all known causes of other dementias. It can be confirmed only by cerebral biopsy or autopsy.

Clinical Manifestations

In the early stages of Alzheimer's disease, forgetfulness and subtle memory loss occur. There may be small difficulties in work or social activities, but the patient has adequate cognitive function to hide the loss and can function independently. Depression may occur at this time. With further progression of the disease the deficits can no longer be concealed. Forgetfulness is manifested in many daily actions. These patients may lose their ability to recognize familiar faces, places, and objects and get lost in a familiar environment. They may repeat the same stories because they forget that they told them. Trying to reason with the person and use reality orientation only increase the patient's anxiety without increasing function, because this is also forgotten.

Conversation becomes difficult because the patient forgets what he or she was about to say or may not be able to remember words. The ability to formulate concepts and think abstractly disappears. The patient can interpret a proverb only in concrete terms. The patient is often unable to appreciate the consequences of his or her actions and will therefore exhibit impulsive behavior. For example, on a hot day he or she may decide to wade in the city fountain fully clothed. He or she will have difficulty with everyday activities such as operating simple appliances and handling money.

Personality changes are usually negative. The patient may become depressed, suspicious, paranoid, hostile, and even combative. Progression of the disease intensifies the symptoms. Speaking skills deteriorate to nonsense syllables; agitation and physical activity increase. A voracious appetite often develops because of the high activity level. The patient may wander at night for hours. Eventually he or she will need help in all areas of personal care, including eating and toileting; dysphagia (an inability or difficulty in swallowing) occurs and incontinence develops. The terminal stage may last for months. The patient is usually immobile and requires total care. Occasionally the patient may recognize family or caretakers. Death occurs as a result of a complicating condition such as pneumonia, malnutrition, or dehydration.

Nursing Interventions

Interventions by the nurse are aimed at helping the person in maintaining optimal cognitive function, promoting physical safety, reducing anxiety and agitation, improving communication, promoting independence in self-care activities, providing for the patient's needs for socialization and intimacy, maintaining adequate nutrition, managing sleep pattern disturbances, and supporting and educating family caregivers.

Supporting Cognitive Function

As the patient's cognitive ability declines, the nurse provides a calm, predictable environment that helps the person interpret his or her surroundings and activities. Environmental stimuli are limited and a regular routine is followed. A quiet, pleasant manner of speaking and offering clear and simple explanations, along with using memory aids and cues help to minimize confusion and disorientation and give the patient a sense of security. A prominently displayed clock and calendar will enhance orientation to time. Color-coding the doorway will help the patient who has difficulty locating his or her room.

Promoting Physical Safety

A safe environment will allow the person to move about as freely as possible and relieve the family of constant worry about safety. To prevent falls and other accidents, all obvious hazards are removed. Night lights, a call light, and a low bed with half bed rails are used at bedtime. The patient's intake of medications and food is monitored. Smoking is allowed only with supervision. A hazard-free environment allows the patient maximum independence and a sense of autonomy. Because of a short attention span and forgetfulness, wandering behavior can often be reduced by gently persuading or distracting the person. Restraints are avoided because they may increase agitation. Doors leading from the house must be secured. Outside the home all activities must be supervised to protect the person. The person should wear an identification bracelet or neck chain in case he or she becomes separated from the caregiver.

Reducing Anxiety and Agitation

Despite profound cognitive losses, there will be times when the patient is aware of his or her rapidly diminishing abilities. The patient will need constant emotional support that will reinforce a positive self-image. When losses of skills occur, goals are adjusted to fit the patient's declining ability.

Because recreation is important, the person is encouraged to enjoy simple activities. Realistic goals that provide satisfaction are appropriate. Hobbies and activities (walking, exercise, socializing) can improve the quality of life.

The environment should be kept simple, familiar, and noise-free. Excitement and confusion can be upsetting and may precipitate a combative, agitated state known as a **catastrophic reaction** (overreaction to excessive stimulation). During such a reaction, the patient responds by screaming, crying, or becoming abusive (physical or verbal assault). This is his or her way of expressing an inability to deal with the environment. When this occurs, it is important to remain calm and unhurried. Measures such as listening to music, stroking, rocking, or distraction may quiet the patient. Frequently he or she forgets what triggered the reaction. Structuring activities is also helpful. Being familiar with the person's predicted responses to certain stressors will help caregivers avoid similar situations.

Improving Communication

To promote the patient's interpretation of messages, the nurse remains unhurried and reduces noises and distractions. Clear, easy-to-understand sentences are used to convey messages because the meaning of words is frequently forgotten or there is difficulty with organizing and expressing a thought. Lists and simple written instructions can serve as reminders to the patient and are often helpful.

Sometimes the patient can point to an object or use nonverbal language to communicate. Tactile stimuli such as a hug or a hand pat are usually interpreted as signs of affection, concern, and security.

Promoting Independence in Self-Care Activities

Pathophysiologic changes in the cerebral cortex make it difficult for a person with a self-care deficit to achieve physical independence. Efforts are directed toward helping the person maintain independent functioning for as long as possible. One suggestion is to simplify daily activities by organizing them into short, achievable steps so that the patient can experience a sense of accomplishment. Frequently the occupational therapist is able to suggest ways to simplify tasks or recommend adaptive equipment. Direct patient supervision is sometimes necessary.

Maintaining personal dignity and autonomy is important for the person with Alzheimer's disease. He or she is encouraged to make choices when appropriate and to participate in self-care activities as much as possible.

Providing for Socialization and Intimacy Needs

Because socialization with old friends can be comforting, visits, letters, and phone calls are encouraged. Visits should be brief and nonstressful; limiting visitors to one or two at a time is recommended.

The confused, lonely person may find stimulation, comfort, and contentment in the soft fur, melodious purr, or warm, wet tongue of a pet. The nonjudgmental friendliness of an animal can be helpful. Care of the pet by the patient can provide satisfying activity and an outlet for energy.

Alzheimer's disease does not eliminate the need for intimacy. The patient and his or her spouse may or may not continue to enjoy sexual activity. The spouse should be encouraged to talk about any sexual concerns, and sexual counseling may be suggested if necessary. Simple expressions of love, such as touching and holding, are often meaningful for this couple.

Inappropriate sexual behaviors seldom occur, but when they do they can cause extreme embarrassment to family members. For example, the person may undress in a public place on a hot day or may masturbate publicly. The use of gentle distraction is recommended.

Promoting Adequate Nutrition

Mealtime can be a pleasant, social occasion, or it can become a time of upset and distress. Mealtime should be kept simple and calm, without confrontations. The patient will prefer familiar foods that look appetizing and taste good. To avoid "playing" with the food, one dish is offered at a time. Food is cut into small pieces to prevent choking. Liquids may be easier to swallow if they are converted to gelatin. Hot food and beverages are served warm. The temperature of the foods should be checked to prevent burns.

When lack of coordination interferes with self-feeding, adaptive equipment is helpful. Some patients may do well eating with their fingers. If this is the case, an apron or a smock, rather than a bib, is used to protect clothing. As deficits progress, it may be necessary to feed the patient. Forgetfulness, disinterest, dental problems, incoordination, overstimulation, and choking can all provide barriers to good nutrition.

Promoting Balanced Activity and Rest

Many patients with Alzheimer's disease exhibit sleep disturbances and wandering behavior. These behaviors are most likely to occur when the patient is bored, restless, agitated, or disoriented, particularly in a new setting and frequently at night. The patient who wanders outside of the house is often unable to find his or her way home and is at risk for accident and injury. Family members and neighbors must frequently search for the patient.

All Alzheimer's patients should wear some form of visible identification (bracelet or neck chain) at all times. Although the patient is allowed to walk around in a protected environment, access to the outdoors should be blocked. If sleep is disturbed or he or she is unable to go to sleep, music, warm milk, or a back rub may help the person relax. During the day the patient should be given sufficient opportunity to participate in exercise activities, because a regular pattern of activity and rest will enhance nighttime sleep. Long periods of daytime sleeping are discouraged.

Supporting and Educating Family Caregivers

The emotional burden placed upon the family of a patient with Alzheimer's disease is enormous. The physical health of the patient is often excellent, and the mental degeneration is gradual. Because the diagnosis is not specific, the family may cling to the hope that the diagnosis is incorrect and that the person will improve if he or she tries harder. Aggression and hostility exhibited by the patient are often misunderstood by the caregiver or family, who feel unappreciated, frustrated, and angry. Feelings of guilt, nervousness, and worry contribute to caregiver fatigue, depression, and family dysfunction.

The multiple needs of family caregivers have been addressed by the Alzheimer's Association (formerly known as ADRDA). This national organization with more than 100 local chapters is a coalition of family members and professionals sharing the goals of family support and service, education, research, and advocacy. Family support groups, respite care, and adult day care are available through the Alzheimer's Association. Concerned volunteers are trained to provide structure to caregiver support groups. Through the use of respite care, a service commonly provided, the caregiver can get away from the home for short periods of time while someone else is tending to the patient's needs.

The nurse must be sensitive to the highly emotional issues that the family is confronting. Support and education of the caregivers are essential components of care. The family can contact the Alzheimer's Association or a comparable group that provides the opportunity to meet with others experiencing similar problems. (See Nursing Care Plan 12-1: Care of the Patient With Alzheimer's Disease.)

Multi-infarct Dementia

Multi-infarct dementia (MID) is an organic mental disorder second only to Alzheimer's disease in incidence. About 20% of the cases of dementia are attributed to this disease. It is characterized by an uneven, downward decline in mental function. Multi-infarct dementia is sometimes confused with Alzheimer's disease, paranoia, or delirium because of its unpredictable clinical course. The diagnosis can sometimes be even more difficult because the patient may be suffering from both Alzheimer's disease and multi-infarct dementia.

Cerebral damage occurs when blood supply to the brain is disrupted. Infarction, the death of brain tissue, occurs with striking rapidity. Multiple small cerebral infarctions, clinically manifested as small strokes, result in multi-infarct dementia. Instead of displaying the progressively downhill course of Alzheimer's disease, the progress of multi-infarct dementia is uneven. Every small infarct is followed by some recovery and a plateau until the next infarction occurs. Often the patient has a history of cardiovascular and cerebrovascular disease. The age of onset is between 50 and 70 years, and the condition occurs more frequently in men than in women.

Dizziness, headaches, and decreased mental and physical vigor are early signs of the disease. In more than half the cases, the disease appears acutely as sudden confusion. This is followed by gradual, spotty memory loss. The patient may hallucinate and display symptoms of delirium. Speech disturbances may be present. Early treatment of hypertension and vascular disease may prevent progression of the disease. In later stages, manifestations of the decline are similar to the signs discussed with Alzheimer's disease, and often they cannot be distinguished.

text continues on page 165

NURSING CARE PLAN 12–1
Care of the Patient with Alzheimer's Disease

Nursing Interventions	Rationale	Expected Outcomes
NURSING DIAGNOSIS: Alterations in thought processes (altered cognition, perception, confusion, and disorientation) related to neuronal degeneration and progressive dementia		
GOAL: Maintenance of optimal cognitive functions		
1. Reduce environmental confusion. a. Approach patient in a pleasant, calm way. b. Be predictable in your manner and conversation. c. Keep the environment simple and pleasing. d. Maintain a regular daily schedule. e. Devise memory aids as needed (lists, reminding notes, labels on items, pictures, diagrams).	1. Simple and limited stimuli will facilitate interpretation and reduce distortion of input; predictable behavior is less threatening than unpredictable behavior; memory aids will assist the patient to remember.	• Maintains optimal memory function • Shows a reduction in confused behavior • Demonstrates an appropriate response to tactile, visual, and auditory stimuli • Verbalizes a sense of security and protection • Demonstrates optimal orientation to time, place, and person
2. Increase environmental cues. a. Identify yourself when interacting with the patient. b. Address patient by name. c. Offer environmental cues for orientation to time, place, and person (pictures, photos, clock, calendar with crossed-off days, color-coded halls and doors). d. Provide hourglass timer if unable to tell time on clock. e. Interpret environmental stimulation as part of the conversation.	2. Environmental cues will enhance orientation to time, place, and person by filling memory gaps and serving as reminders; as memory loss increases, it may be necessary to identify yourself at the beginning of every interaction with the patient.	
NURSING DIAGNOSIS: High risk for injury related to impulsive behavior, impaired judgement, lack of insight, and dysfunctional behaviors		
GOAL: Maintenance of physical safety		
1. Control the environment. a. Remove obvious hazards. b. Reduce injury potential from bedtime falls. (1) Use only half bedrails. (2) Keep bed in low position. (3) Use night lights. (4) Have accessible call light. c. Monitor medication regimen. d. Permit smoking only with supervision. e. Monitor food temperature. f. Supervise all activities outside of the home.	1. A hazard-free environment will reduce the risk of injury and free the family from constant worry. Outside the home, everything is assumed to be a hazard.	• Complies with safety procedures • Moves freely and independently around the home • Verbalizes a sense of security and contentment
2. Permit maximum independence and freedom. a. Allow freedom in the "safe" environment. b. Avoid use of restraints. c. When wandering, distract rather than force. d. Keep identification tag on patient.	a. This will give the patient a sense of autonomy. b. Restraints may increae agitation. c. Force will increase anxiety. Distraction is facilitated by immediate memory loss. d. A name and phone number will facilitate a safe return when the patient wanders away.	

(continued)

NURSING CARE PLAN 12–1 *(continued)*
Care of the Patient with Alzheimer's Disease

Nursing Interventions	Rationale	Expected Outcomes
NURSING DIAGNOSIS: Anxiety related to cognitive losses and reduction in self concept		
GOAL: Maintenance of an optimal level of psychological functioning		
1. Reduce anxiety-provoking situations in daily routine. a. Keep reality orientation nonthreatening. b. Be patient with forgetfulness. c. Accept harmless eccentric behavior. d. Maintain a daily, regular routine. e. Keep stimuli simple. f. Distract rather than confront unacceptable behavior. g. When the patient demonstrates a negative attitude in interacting, leave patient and return in a short time. h. Avoid situations that have upset patient in the past. i. Reassure following a catastrophic reaction. j. Do not try to reason with the patient.	a–c. Constant corrections will increase anxiety and may result in a highly agitated, angry, and combative state known as a catastrophic reaction. d–e. Simple, structured stimuli are easiest to interpret. f–g. Often forgets immediately and becomes involved in new activity. j. Unable to conduct abstract thinking.	• Shows fewer episodes of catastrophic reactions, angry outbursts, and crying • Demonstrates less restlessness, irritability, and agitation • Verbalizes feelings of calmness and contentment • Seeks out the companionship of others • Participates in activities willingly • Shows a greater level of self assurance in difficult situations
2. Enhance the quality of life. a. Offer multiple opportunities for fulfillment (music, pets, walks, exercise, old hobbies, simple chores). b. Provide comfort and security.	2. Goals are minute-by-minute. The patient has the capacity to enjoy and experience happiness.	
3. Encourage positive feelings of self. a. Treat the patient as a person with feelings. b. Openly discuss feelings of anxiety and offer encouragement. c. Praise appropriately. d. Do not infantilize (treat as a child) by using baby talk or child terms. e. When skills are lost, do not try to retrain.	3. Acceptance will give support. This person is in the process of grieving over profound losses; infantilization increases the anxiety. Deterioration of the cognitive processes makes loss of skills inevitable.	
NURSING DIAGNOSIS: Impaired verbal communication related to cognitive losses		
GOAL: Attainment of an optimal exchange of ideas between the patient and others		
1. Implement strategies to promote the patient's interpretation of messages. a. Be calm, pleasant, and unhurried. b. Keep verbal messages short and simple. c. Avoid decision-making situations. d. Use nonverbal messages along with words. e. Be consistent in conversation. f. Avoid competing noises and distractions.	a–g. Simple, short messages are easiest to interpret.	• Shows an improved ability to understand messages • Shows an improved ability to express self verbally • Uses alternate methods of communication (writing, nonverbal) • Shows fewer frustrations when communicating

(continued)

NURSING CARE PLAN 12–1 *(continued)*
Care of the Patient with Alzheimer's Disease

Nursing Interventions	Rationale	Expected Outcomes
g. Avoid complex issues.		
h. Write down simple instructions and lists.	h. Alternate methods for communication often are successful.	
i. Observe patient's expression for signs that he or she understands.	i. A good listener must be responsive to feedback.	
j. Talk to the patient even if he or she gives little response.	j. The patient's response may not reflect how much he or she understands of the conversation.	
2. Develop strategies to improve the patient's ability to express messages.	2. This will allow the patient to express needs and feelings. Feelings of isolation are reduced.	
a. Supply forgotten words when possible. b. Guess the message and confirm with the patient. c. Ignore mistakes.	a–c. Active, helpful listening can minimize frustrations when the patient needs help communicating.	
d. Allow adequate time for conversation. e. Encourage short, simple sentences. f. Ask "yes/no" questions.	d–f. An unhurried attitude will enhance communication.	
g. Provide alternative methods for communication (pointing, describing, pictures).	g. Certain methods may be more successful than others.	
h. Acknowledge the frustration that the patient is experiencing.	h. Acknowledging the patient's frustration communicates acceptance.	

NURSING DIAGNOSIS: Self-care deficits related to confusion, cognitive losses, and dysfunctional behaviors

GOAL: Maintenance of maximum independence in activities of daily living

Nursing Interventions	Rationale	Expected Outcomes
1. Develop strategies to facilitate daily performance of activities.		
a. Provide adaptive devices. b. Maintain a regular daily schedule at a time convenient with the patient. c. Keep the environment simple and pleasant. d. Keep instructions simple and divide tasks into small parts.	a–d. A regular schedule, adaptive equipment, and simple tasks will reduce confusion, enhance ability to care for self, and assure safety.	• Performs activities of daily living at expected optimal level • Demonstrates the ability to use adaptive equipment • Uses safety measures to prevent injury • Verbalizes an awareness of dignity and autonomy
e. Monitor function of body systems.	e. Supervision will promote optimal function and detect early problems.	• Has fewer episodes of incontinence
2. Provide specific safeguards of safety in bathing.		
a. Monitor bath water temperature.	a. The patient is unreliable in adjusting bath temperature.	
b. Encourage use of safety devices (*e.g.* handrails, rubber mats).	b. Impulsive behavior increases the risk of accidents.	
3. Allow patient autonomy and dignity while providing needed care.	3. Encouraging autonomy will enhance a sense of dignity and well-being.	
a. Encourage patient to make choices (*e.g.* clothing, foods, schedule). b. Provide adequate privacy.		

(continued)

NURSING CARE PLAN 12–1 *(continued)*
Care of the Patient with Alzheimer's Disease

Nursing Interventions	Rationale	Expected Outcomes
4. Provide specific measures to encourage continence.		
a. Provide accessibility to the bathroom. If needed, color code the door of bathroom.	a. Visual stimuli can reinforce recognition.	
b. Use clothing that opens easily.	b. This facilitates continence when haste is necessary.	
c. Maintain toileting schedule (every 2 hours, after meals).	c–d. These help to maintain normal elimination.	
d. Encourage adequate fluids, fiber, and activity for regular bowel elimination.		
e. Recommend restricting fluids in evening hours.	e. Excessive fluids in the evening may interfere with the sleep-activity routine.	

NURSING DIAGNOSIS: Alterations in family process related to care of a dysfunctional family member

GOAL: Attainment of family adaptation and harmony

Nursing Interventions	Rationale	Expected Outcomes
1. Initiate and enhance family knowledge of disease. a. Teach family about Alzheimer's disease. b. Encourage family members to read "The 36 Hour Day" and ask questions.	1. If the family understands the disease, they will be better prepared to help the patient and adjust their style of living to his or her needs.	The family will: • Provide appropriate care and support of the patient • Discuss feelings and frustrations with the nurse • Seek appropriate help from community agencies • Join a self-help group
2. Acknowledge the emotional impact of the disease upon the family system. a. Elicit family reaction to patient's illness. b. Encourage family to talk about their worry, guilt, anger, and frustrations. c. Encourage use of stress reduction techniques. d. Encourage family to share concerns and feelings with patient if appropriate.	2. This illness has profound effects upon the family. They will be frightened, frustrated, angry, and guilty, and feel helpless.	
3. Initiate referrals to obtain community help.		
a. Assist family to contact community agencies to receive such support services as respite care, adult day care, visiting nurse services, and social work services.	a. Community services will provide respite care, suggestions for home management, financial advice, and nursing. These will help the family cope and manage this family crisis in the best possible way.	
b. Encourage the family to contact Alzheimer's Association and participate in a self-help group.	b. A support group will help the family better understand how others are dealing with similar problems.	

(continued)

NURSING CARE PLAN 12–1 *(continued)*
Care of the Patient with Alzheimer's Disease

Nursing Interventions	Rationale	Expected Outcomes
NURSING DIAGNOSIS: Impaired social interaction related to cognitive impairment and dysfunctional behaviors		
GOAL: Enhancement of socialization and fulfillment of intimacy needs		
1. Encourage social encounters with family and friends. Encourage family and friends to:		• Participates in social events with family and friends • Increases touching behavior • Verbalizes or demonstrates contentment when socializing and interacting with others • Engages in sexual activity or intimate behavior with spouse • Meets sexual needs privately in an acceptable manner
a. Use touching to maintain contact with patient.	a. Tactile stimulation is easiest to interpret.	
b. Touch, hug, and demonstrate affection. c. Share feelings honestly and openly with patient.	b–c. The patient continues to need love and affection.	
d. React objectively to negative responses. e. Accept patient despite negative interactions.	d–e. Positive interactions are best maintained if the family overlooks negative encounters.	
f. Limit numbers of visitors to 1 or 2 at a time.	f. Fewer visitors will help maintain simple stimuli and avoid a catastrophic reaction.	
g. Provide a companion animal if possible and appropriate.	g. Pets provide loving acceptance, opportunities for touching, and are a catalyst to socialization.	
2. Provide opportunities for meeting intimacy needs and sexual expression. a. Encourage expressions of intimacy and tenderness with spouse. b. Encourage a sexual relationship with spouse if interest exists. c. Provide privacy if patient masturbates or exposes self.	2. Intimacy and sexual expression will provide a sense of contentment and fulfillment to the patient.	
NURSING DIAGNOSIS: Alterations in nutrition related to confusion and imbalance of intake / activity		
GOAL: Maintenance of an optimal level of nutrition		
1. Monitor food intake and observe food habits. a. Note weight loss or gain. b. Encourage adequate fluid intake. c. Provide regular mealtime schedule.	1. Encouragement and reminders to eat will help this patient eat adequately and regularly.	• Eats a balanced diet and drinks needed fluids • Demonstrates enjoyment and maximum independence at mealtime • Teeth and gums are brushed regularly
2. Maintain a favorable environment for eating. a. Allow patient optimal independence.	a. Finger foods, adaptive equipment, and a large apron will facilitate independence if lack of coordination interferes with the patient's ability to use utensils.	
b. Maintain a calm, pleasant environment. c. Offer a menu choice. d. Offer familiar foods.	b–d. If mealtime is pleasant, with favorite and familiar foods, the patient will eat well with enjoyment.	
3. Promote regular mouthcare. a. Encourage care of gums and teeth after meals. b. Encourage the patient's participation in care.	3. Healthy teeth and properly fitted dentures are important for maintaining nutritional health. A reminder may be necessary if patient forgets.	

(continued)

NURSING CARE PLAN 12-1 *(continued)*
Care of the Patient with Alzheimer's Disease

NURSING DIAGNOSIS: Sleep pattern disturbance related to anxiety, confusion, and activity/rest imbalance

GOAL: Maintenance of a balance of sleep and activity

Nursing Interventions	Rationale	Expected Outcomes
1. Reduce night-time distractions. a. Identify and reduce noise and anxiety. b. Avoid disturbing patient during the night for procedures or medications.	1. A nonstimulating environment will decrease confusion and minimize hyperactive behavior.	• Establishes rest and sleep patterns on a regular schedule • Reduces wandering behaviors at night • Verbalizes a feeling of safety and comfort at bedtime • Establishes activity patterns on a regular schedule
2. Take measures to increase safety. a. Provide nightlights. b. Block accessibility to the outdoors. c. Confine patient to a safe area. d. Provide patient with identification bracelet.	2. These will enhance the patient's safety if he or she wanders at night.	
3. Enhance comfort if awake at night. a. Avoid the use of restraints. b. Provide comfort measures when awake at night (warm milk, bath, backrub, soft music, rocking, caressing pet).	3. A pleasant, nonrestrictive environment will enhance return to sleep, minimize anxiety, and increase the patient's sense of well-being.	
4. Design a balanced schedule of activity/sleep. a. Increase daytime wakefulness and encourage short rests rather than long naps. b. Encourage regular exercise and activity programs.	4. Daily activity and regular exercise reduce agitation and produce a calming effect.	

Medications and the Elderly

Older people use more medications than any other age group. Representing 12.6% of the total population, they use 30% of the prescribed medications and 40% of all over-the-counter medications. Studies show that those persons who have symptoms of disease are the persons most likely to be taking medications. Medications have improved the health and well-being of older persons by alleviating symptoms of discomfort, treating chronic illnesses, and curing infectious processes. However, problems commonly occur because of drug interactions, multiple drug effects, multiple drug use (polypharmacy), and noncompliance. Those medications that are most frequently overprescribed and misprescribed are mind-affecting agents (tranquilizers, sedatives, hypnotics, and antipsychotics), cardiovascular agents, and gastrointestinal agents (U.S. Committee on Aging, 1991).

In any medication regimen for the elderly, one must bear in mind that medications are capable of altering the person's nutritional status, which may already be compromised by a marginal diet and chronic disease and its treatment. Medications can depress the appetite, cause nausea and vomiting, irritate the stomach, cause constipation and diarrhea, and decrease absorption of nutrients. In addition, they can alter the electrolyte balance and carbohydrate and fat metabolism. A few examples of medications that are capable of altering the nutritional status are antacids (produce thiamine deficiency), cathartics (diminish absorption), antibiotics and phenytoin (Dilantin) (reduce use of folic acid), and phenothiazines, estrogens, and steroid hormones (increase food intake and weight gain).

Physiologic Considerations

There is great variability in the absorption, distribution, metabolism, and excretion of medications in older persons (Table 12-7). In part, this is due to a reduced capacity of the liver and kidneys to metabolize and excrete the medications and to lowered levels of circulatory and nervous system efficiency in coping with the effect of certain drugs. Many medications and their metabolites are excreted by the kidney. With advanced age there are decreases in body weight, total body water, lean body mass, and plasma albumin (protein) and an increase in body fat. Consequently, highly protein-binding agents will have fewer binding sites and higher pharmacologic activity. Fat-soluble agents will have more binding sites, thus enhancing storage and delaying elimination.

TABLE 12-7 Altered Drug Responses in Older People

Age-Related Changes	Impact of Age-Related Change	Applicable Drugs
Absorption		
Reduced gastric acid; increased *p*H (less acid)	Rate of drug absorption—possibly delayed	
Reduced GI motility; prolonged gastric emptying	Extent of drug absorption—not affected	
Distribution		
Decreaed albumin sites	Serious alterations in drug binding to plasma proteins. (The unbound drug gives the pharmacologic response.) Highly protein-bound drugs will have fewer binding sites, leading to increased effects and accelerated metabolism and excretion.	*Selected highly protein binding drugs:* Oral anticoagulants (warfarin) Oral hypoglycemic agents (sulfonylureas) Barbiturates Calcium channel blockers Furosemide (Lasix) Nonsteroidal anti-inflammatory drugs (NSAIDs) Sulfonamides Quinidine Phenytoin (Dilantin)
Reduced cardiac output	Decreased perfusion of many bodily organs	
Impaired peripheral blood flow	Decreased perfusion	
Increased percentage of body fat	Proportion of body fat increases with age and thus gives the body an increased ability to store fat-soluble drugs. This causes drug accumulation, prolonged storage, and delayed excretion.	*Selected fat-soluble drugs* Barbiturates Diazepam (Valium) Lidocaine Phenothiazines (antipsychotics)
Decreased lean body mass	Decreased body volume allows higher peak levels of drugs.	Ethanol Morphine
Metabolism		
Decreased cardiac output and decreased perfusion of the liver	Decreased metabolism and delay of breakdown of drugs, resulting in prolonged duration of action, accumulation, and drug toxicity	All drugs metabolized by the liver
Excretion		
Decreased renal blood flow; loss of functioning nephrons; decreased renal efficiency	Decreased rates of elimination and increased duration of action Danger of accumulation and drug toxicity	*Selected drugs with prolonged action:* Aminoglycoside antibiotics Cimetidine (Tagamet) Chlorpropamide (Diabinase) Digoxin Lithium Procainamide

Nursing Implications

The nurse administering medications to older persons must be aware of the following:

- Those commonly used medications that are removed from the body primarily by renal excretion remain in the body for a longer time in persons with decreased renal function. Dosages often must be reduced. Overdosage and drug toxicity at usual therapeutic dosages commonly occur.
- Medications with a narrow safety margin (*e.g.*, digitalis glycosides) must be administered cautiously.
- A decline in cardiac output may decrease the delivery rate to the target organ or storage tissue.
- The circulatory and central nervous systems of older persons are less able to cope with the effect of certain medications even when blood levels are "normal."
- Medication dosages often must be reduced because overdosage and drug toxicity at usual therapeutic dosages may result.
- Paradoxical or unusual responses to medications may be manifested in the form of toxic reactions and complications.
- As a result of a slowing metabolism medication levels may increase in the tissues and plasma, leading to prolonged drug action.
- Many elderly persons have multiple medical problems that require treatment with one or more medications. The possibility of interactions between medications is

further magnified if the older person is also taking one or more over-the-counter medications.
- A high-fiber diet, use of psyllium (Metamucil), or other laxatives may accelerate transport of medications taken concurrently and reduce absorption.
- If for any reason the person is not dependable about taking medication, the nurse must be sure that the pill or capsule is actually swallowed and not retained between the cheeks and the gums or teeth.

Self-Administered Medications

Teaching self-administration of medication involves asking questions of the patient and requesting return demonstrations to be sure learning has occurred. It is important to consider possible sensory and memory losses as well as decreased manual dexterity. The following steps can be instituted to help the person manage his or her medications and improve compliance:

- Explain the action, side effects, and dosage of each medication.
- Write out the drug schedule.
- Encourage the use of standard containers rather than safety lids (if there are no children in the household).
- Destroy old, unused medications.
- Review the medication schedule periodically.
- Discourage the use of over-the-counter drugs without consulting a health professional.
- Encourage sips of water first, followed by several more swallows of water with the pill to help it go down more easily.
- Explain that capsules will dissolve better if the water is at room temperature rather than iced.

Chronic Illness and Common Disturbances of Well-Being

Urinary Incontinence

The older person often does not report this very common problem unless specifically asked about it. It can be acute and develop during an illness, or it can develop chronically over a period of years. Using the acronym DRIP, transient causes can be attributed to delirium, dehydration (D), restricted mobility (R), inflammation, infection, impaction (I), and pharmaceuticals or polyuria (P). Established incontinence may be due to neurologic or structural pathologies. Often these can be helped or corrected with nonsurgical interventions such as Kegel exercises or environmental manipulation (see Health Promotion of the Genitourinary System in Table 12-3). The patient with this problem should be urged to seek help from appropriate health personnel.

Fatigue

There is a well-circulated myth that older people should "take it easy" and avoid vigorous activity. Many of the elderly, therefore, may expect to feel tired and adopt an inactive role. Activity, however, is a desired state in older adults. Normal fatigue following strenuous or sustained exercise is expected with the aging process. A short rest usually restores vigor.

General chronic fatigue is not normal and may be a consequence of oversedation. Fatigue may be an indicator of depression or a symptom of physical illness such as anemia or heart disease.

Headaches

Most headaches are caused by incorrect posture and muscle strain around the head and neck. Heat, ice, massage, and exercise are used to relieve the symptoms. Serious organic disease such as brain tumor or hematoma may be the underlying cause and needs to be excluded. The patient should be encouraged to seek medical advice if headaches persist.

Back Pain

The common complaint of back pain can accompany a number of chronic problems requiring medical attention. Back pain may be a sign of osteoporosis; accompanying vertebral fractures may press on the spinal nerves, causing severe pain that radiates to the legs (sciatica). Other, less common causes of back pain include metastatic cancer and infection. Muscle spasms responsible for much of the discomfort can be relieved by heat, ice, and rest. When acute back pain subsides, recurrence can be prevented by initiating a low back muscle exercise program.

Sleep Disturbances

Drowsiness is often due to boredom, habit, depression, or organic disease. Sleep patterns change with advanced age. Stages 3 and 4 of the sleep cycle are the stages of deepest sleep when arousal is most difficult. These levels of deepest sleep occur with less frequency in later life. Many brief arousals are predominant in the sleep of older persons. This increased wakefulness, although brief, may create an impression of sleeplessness or insomnia. Daytime napping and inactivity contribute to reduced sleep at night. Arthritis, muscle aches, nocturia, and sleep apnea may cause interruption in sleep.

A positive and reassuring attitude is necessary when counseling older adults about sleep. Daytime physical activity is encouraged. Quiet activity and reading are alternatives if sleep does not come. Symptoms are dealt with individually and sedatives discouraged. Some people find a warm bath and a glass of milk at bedtime helpful.

Heartburn and Indigestion

Heartburn and indigestion occur as a result of a reflux of stomach acid into the esophagus. Common causes include overeating, an incompetent lower esophageal sphincter, hiatal hernia, side effects of medications, and organic disease.

Advise the older person to chew food carefully, eat small meals, avoid heavy spices, and sit rather than recline after eating. Medical evaluation is necessary if symptoms persist.

Dyspnea

A normal decline in pulmonary function may be responsible for shortness of breath following physical exertion. Obesity, anemia, smoking, lung disease, respiratory infections, and heart disease are all causes of increased breathlessness. Because fever may not occur with respiratory infection in the older adult, increased respirations followed by increased pulse rate often are the first observable signs of acute illness.

Foot Problems

The feet of the older person should be given particular attention. Diminished subcutaneous fat reduces the protective padding and makes the skin more vulnerable to injury. Diminished blood supply as a result of circulatory impairment puts the older person at high risk for foot infections and subsequent complications. Ingrown toenails, corns, and calluses all cause discomfort and may lead to infection and tissue necrosis. Toenails often are thick and difficult to cut.

If the older person is unable to care for his or her toenails, the nurse can provide nail care. The feet are soaked in warm water and dried thoroughly. Debris around the cuticles and between the toes is removed with a soft towel. The nails are cut straight across beyond the nail grooves. Sharp edges are blunted with an emery board. Lotion is applied regularly. For the diabetic, only a podiatrist or other specially trained person should cut the nails.

The Older Person in the Community

Ninety-five percent of the elderly live in the community; 75% own their homes. In 1991, 31% were living alone (79% women). In the 65 and older age group, half as many women as men were married and living with their spouses (40% of women, 74% of men). Half of the women over age 65 (48%), but only 15% of the men, were widowed (Fowles, 1992). This difference in marital status is due to several factors: women have a longer life expectancy than men, women tend to marry older men, and women remain widowed whereas men often remarry.

Family

Planning for care and understanding the psychosocial aspects of the older person must be accomplished within the context of the family. When dependency needs occur, the spouse assumes the role of primary caregiver. In the absence of the surviving spouse, an adult child usually assumes caregiver responsibilities and eventually may need help in providing care and support. A widely held myth within American society is that adult children and their aged parents are socially alienated. Furthermore, many believe that adult children abandon their parents when health and other dependency problems arise. Extensive research refutes these beliefs. The family is an important source of support for older persons. Eighty-one percent of the elderly have living children. Of those living alone, two-thirds have at least one child living within 30 minutes of their home, and 62% see at least one adult child weekly (Fowles, 1992).

Illness presents special problems for persons who are alone. If community resources and/or adult children are unable to provide care, the elderly are at high risk for institutionalization. Social attitudes and cultural values often dictate that adult children should provide services and financial support, and assume the burden of care if their aged parents are unable to care for themselves. Regardless of the amount of responsibility and love the adult child exhibits toward the dependent aged parents, strains will develop if care continues over a period of time. Research exploring the relationship between aged parents and their adult children shows that with poor health of the parent, the quality of the parent–child relationship declines. Under certain circumstances of high risk, strains in intergenerational relationships can result in elder abuse.

Elder abuse is an active or passive act or behavior that is harmful to the elderly person. Such behavior includes physical violence, personal neglect, financial exploitation, violation of rights, denial of health care, and self-inflicted abuse. Before elder abuse occurs, when strains are evident, preventive action should be taken. Interdisciplinary team members can be enlisted to help the caregiver develop self-awareness, increased insight, and understanding of the aging process. At the same time, community resources may be useful for both the aged person and the caregiver.

The Home Environment

Safety and Comfort

Accidents rank seventh as a cause of death for older people. Falls, the major cause of accidents in the elderly, are not often fatal but threaten health and the quality of life. Normal and pathologic consequences of aging that contribute to increased falls include visual changes, such as loss of depth perception, susceptibility to glare, loss of visual acuity, and difficulty in light accommodation; neurologic changes, including loss of balance, loss of position sense, and delayed reaction time; cardiovascular changes resulting in cerebral hypoxia and postural hypotension; cognitive changes, including confusion, loss of judgment, and impulsive behavior; and musculoskeletal changes, including altered posture and decreased muscle strength. Many medications, drug interactions, and alcohol use precipitate falls by causing drowsiness, incoordination, and postural hypotension.

There are lifestyle and environmental changes that the nurse can encourage the older adult and his family to adopt. Adequate lighting with minimal glare and shadow calls for small area lamps, indirect lighting, sheer curtains to diffuse direct sunlight, dull rather than shiny surfaces, and night lights. Sharply contrasting colors can be used to mark the edges of stairs. Grab bars by the tub and toilet are useful. Canes are excellent deterrents to falls, particularly outdoors where many hazards exist. Loose clothing, improperly fitting shoes, scatter rugs, small objects, and pets create hazards and increase the risk of accidents. A person will function best in familiar settings if furniture and objects remain unchanged. When the older person enters a new environment, he or she should be watched carefully, assisted often, and urged to use a cane because the potential for accidents is greater in unfamiliar spaces.

Personal Space

The older person needs a place of his or her own, a very special location that can offer security, comfort, and privacy. This important "charted territory" can be a house, a room, or part of a room. It will contain treasures and mementos from a lifetime. The nurse can help the older person to maintain his or her own space. If the patient is moved, he or she will adjust more easily if he or she can establish a new area of privacy. Clutter is understandable if the space is small and the items are many. These articles can be touched, thought about, and enjoyed regularly to enhance the quality of life. Within the nursing home, hoarding and collecting behavior may be viewed negatively. If hoarding becomes a problem, the nurse and patient should constructively work out a solution. Personal items should *never* be removed without consent. Even if dementia is evident, it is preferable to clean up the area through a cooperative approach.

Community Programs and Health Services

Hospital and health services are used more by the elderly than by other age groups in the population. They are hospitalized three times more often than younger people, stay 50% longer, and use more prescription medications (U.S. Senate Committee on Aging, 1991). Chronic rather than acute disease is the major cause of illness, but hospital admissions are often required for acute exacerbations of chronic conditions. Over 80% of people 65 and older have at least one chronic condition; multiple conditions are common. With advancing age, disabilities resulting from these chronic illnesses create the need for help with basic activities of daily living. Twenty-two percent of the elderly are limited to a point where they can no longer carry on regular daily activities. Community programs provide help beyond the capabilities of informal supports. Such valuable services as health care at home or in an adult day care center, opportunities for socialization, transportation, and home-delivered meals often keep the older person in the community and postpone or possibly eliminate the need for a nursing home.

Medicare and Medicaid

Medicare is a federal social insurance program designed to provide health care for older persons who are entitled to Social Security benefits. It has two parts: part A is hospital insurance and part B is medical insurance. All entitled persons receive part A, which provides limited coverage for hospital and posthospital nursing home care and unlimited visits for home health care. Part B is a voluntary program that costs a small additional monthly premium. Part B pays for limited outpatient medical services and doctor's visits. Major items not covered by either part include nonskilled home nursing care, ongoing nursing home care, prescription drugs, eyeglasses, and dental care. Medicare pays about 45% of the health costs of older people (U.S. Senate Committee on Aging, 1991).

Medicaid is a health assistance program financed by state funds and matching federal grants. This program varies from state to state and is available only to the poor. It is the major source of public funding that provides nursing home care for the poor elderly. This program covers all the basic medical services and often covers such items as medications, eyeglasses, and dental care. Eligibility requirements prevent many low-income people from receiving financial support for health care.

Home Care

The older adult usually prefers to live independently, even if he or she has difficulty getting around the home. This may be against the wishes of the person's adult children. If the older person is capable of accepting responsibility for the personal risk involved and other persons are not endangered, the adult children should not interfere with this decision. There are many community supports that help the older person maintain independence. Informal sources of help such as family, friends, the mail carrier, church members, and neighbors can all keep an informal watch. Area agencies on aging (AAAs) perform many community services, including telephone reassurance, friendly visitors, home repair services, and home-delivered meals. Homemaker and chore services can be obtained at an hourly rate through AAAs or the local community nursing services. If the person is financially unable to pay, these services are subsidized through local and state funds. Nursing care and rehabilitation services requiring the expertise of a registered nurse and appropriate health professionals are paid by Medicare.

There are other community support services available to help the older person outside of the home. Senior centers have social and health promotion activities; some provide a nutritious noontime meal. Adult day care facilities offer daily nursing care and social opportunities. Family members can carry on daily activities while the older person is at the day care center.

Ethical and Legal Issues

Loss of rights, victimization, and other grave consequences face the person who has made no plans for personal and property management in the event of disability or death. The advice and services of a competent attorney regarding financial and personal issues can preserve future autonomy and self-determination. The nurse as an advocate can encourage the older person to give advance directives for future decision making in the event of incapacitation.

Power of attorney is a legal agreement that authorizes a person who is designated by the older person to act in specific, outlined purposes on behalf of the signer. This is a form of voluntary guardianship; permission is freely granted when the older person is competent. Unless stated otherwise, this power of attorney is invalidated upon the incapacity of the signer. A **durable power of attorney** is a similar agreement that continues even if the older person is disabled or incapacitated. This power can include financial and/or personal decisions depending upon the desires of the older person.

A **trust** is another option that the competent older person can consider. With a trust, the person designates someone to manage his or her property, stipulates how and under what circumstances the property will be managed, and designates a beneficiary. If incompetency or disability occurs, management of the property will be according to the person's wishes.

If no advance arrangement has been made, and the older person seems unable to make decisions, anyone can petition the court for an incompetency hearing. If the court rules that the person is incompetent, the judge will appoint a **guardian,** a third party who is given powers by the court to assume responsibility for making financial and/or personal decisions for that person. There are two kinds of guardians—guardian of the person and guardian of the estate. Because such a court action strips the civil liberties and constitutional rights from the older person, there is potential for great harm. Safeguards include (1) the older person must be given notice, (2) he or she must be given an opportunity to be legally represented, and (3) medical testimony can be cross-examined. A less restrictive form of guardianship called the **limited guardianship** transfers to the appointed guardian only those powers or duties that the older person cannot exercise. Although this alternative is not widely used, it remains an option.

In the event of severe illness with no reasonable expectation of recovery, the older person may not want to have his or her life extended by heroic measures. Those who want to avoid technologic interventions can give an **advance directive** regarding medical treatment through the use of a **living will.** This written document must be signed by the individual and have two witnesses. It should be given to the physician and incorporated into the medical record. Many states have enacted legislation to accept such a document. The nurse can help the person keep this document current and encourage discussion with the physician. The doctor must write and sign a no-code or do not resuscitate (DNR) order. Otherwise, resuscitative measures are taken if a medical emergency occurs.

The Older Adult in an Acute Care Setting: Altered Responses to Illness

Host Defenses: Susceptibility to Infectious Disease

Infectious diseases present a significant threat of morbidity and mortality to older people. In part, this is due to a blunted response of host defenses caused by a reduction both in cell-mediated and humoral immunity (see Chapters 48 and 49). Also, age-related loss of physiologic reserve and chronic illnesses contribute to an increased susceptibility. Pneumonia, urinary tract infections, tuberculosis, gastrointestinal infections, and skin infections are some of the commonly occurring infectious diseases in older people.

The impact of influenza and pneumococcal infections upon older people is significant. Estimates place the number of deaths from influenza at 10,000 to 40,000, while pneumococcal infections are responsible for 40,000 deaths annually. Of these deaths, at least 85% are older people. Safe and effective vaccines with very few systemic reactions are available. Clinical studies show that the influenza vaccine is about 50% to 60% effective in preventing pneumonia and hospitalization and 60% to 70% effective in preventing death. It is estimated that the pneumococcal vaccine is about 60% to 70% effective in older persons. The only contraindication is a history of anaphylactic hypersensitivity to eggs or a previous severe reaction (Centers for Disease Control, 1992).

The influenza vaccine is prepared yearly to adjust for the specific immunologic characteristics that are present in the influenza viruses at that time. It is an inactivated preparation that should be taken annually in the fall, preferably November. The pneumococcal vaccine has 23 type-specific capsular polysaccharides. Protection lasts 4 years or more. Revaccination is rarely recommended due to the higher incidence of local reaction on subsequent immunizations. Both of these injections can be received at the same time in separate injection sites. The nurse should urge older persons to receive these vaccines. All health providers working with older people or high-risk chronically ill persons should also be immunized (Centers for Disease Control, 1991c).

Tuberculosis (TB) incidence dropped from a peak of 84,000 cases in 1953 to a low of 22,000 cases in 1984. Since then, newly reported cases have increased to an incidence of 26,673 cases in 1992. Other than in HIV-infected persons, case rates for TB are highest among the 65+ population. Nursing home residents account for the majority of the cases in the older population. Much of the infection rate is attributed to reactivation of old infection. Pulmonary and extrapulmonary TB often have subtle, nonspecific symptoms. This is of particular concern in the nursing home, because an active case of TB places patients and staff in jeopardy of infection (Centers for Disease Control, 1993; Dutt & Stead, 1992).

Centers for Disease Control and Prevention (CDC) Guidelines suggest that all new admissions to nursing homes receive a Mantoux test (PPD test) unless there is a history of TB or a previous positive response. All patients whose tests are not positive (positive = induration >10mm at 48–72 hours) should receive a second test in 1 week. The first PPD serves to boost the suppressed immune response that may occur with an older person. Chest x-rays and possibly sputum studies should be used to follow up on PPD positive responders and converters. For positive converters, a course of preventive therapy for 6 to 12 months with Isoniazid (INH) reduces the risk of active disease by 70%. All negative testers should be periodically retested. The nurse can facilitate this process within the care facility (Centers for Disease Control, 1991b; Dutt & Stead, 1992).

Pain and Fever

Many altered physical, emotional, and systemic reactions to disease are attributed to age-related changes in the older person. Useful and reliable physical indicators of illness in the young and middle-aged person cannot be relied upon for the diagnosis of potential life-threatening problems in the older adult. The response to pain in the older person may be lessened because of reduced acuity of touch, alterations in neural pathways, and diminished processing of sensory data. Research has demonstrated the absence of chest pain in 81% of older adults experiencing a myocardial infarction. Hiatal hernia or upper gastrointestinal distress is often responsible for chest pain in the elderly. Acute abdominal conditions such as mesenteric infarction and appendicitis often go unrecognized in elders because of atypical signs and absence of pain.

In the older person, the baseline body temperature is approximately one degree Fahrenheit below that of a younger person. Therefore, in the event of illness, the body temperature of an older person may not reach a sufficient elevation to qualify as the traditionally defined "fever." A temperature of 37.8°C (100°F) in combination with systemic symptoms may signal infection. A temperature of 38.3°C (101°F) is almost certainly a serious infection that needs prompt attention. A blunted fever in the face of an infection often indicates a poor prognosis. Elevations in temperature rarely exceed 39.5°C (103°F). The nurse must be alert to other subtle signs of infection: mental confusion, increased respirations, tachycardia, and changed facial appearance and color.

Emotional Impact

The emotional component of illness in older persons may differ from that of younger people. Many elderly equate good health with the absence of old age. "You are as old as you feel" is a belief of many. An illness that requires hospitalization or a change in lifestyle is an imminent threat to well-being. Admission to the hospital is often feared and actively avoided. Economic concerns and fear of becoming a burden to the family often lead to high anxiety in an older person. The nurse must recognize the implications of fear, anxiety, and dependency in the elderly patient. Autonomy and independent decision making are encouraged. A positive and confident demeanor from the nurse and the family help lift the mental outlook of an elderly person. In addition to anxiety and fear, older persons are at high risk for disorientation, confusion, change in levels of consciousness, and other symptoms of delirium if they are admitted to the hospital.

Systemic Impact

The systemic impact of illness upon the aged person has far-reaching effects. The decline in organ function that occurs in every system of the aging body eventually forces one or more body systems to function at full capacity. Illness places new demands upon body systems that have little or no reserve to meet this crisis. Homeostasis, the ability of the body to maintain an internal balance of function and chemical composition, is jeopardized. The older person may be unable to respond effectively to an acute illness or, if he or she has a chronic health condition, unable to sustain appropriate responses over a long period of time. Furthermore, the older person's ability to respond to definitive treatment is impaired.

The Older Adult in a Protected Environment

Many housing communities for older people will perform routine maintenance and provide opportunities for socialization and recreation. Easier access to shopping and health care may convince the person that a new location will solve many residential problems. When preparation time is sufficient and money, energy, and health are adequate, a move to a new home can be a positive life experience.

Retirement communities have living quarters of apartments, condominiums, and houses that are developed specifically for the older person. An independent lifestyle is enhanced with social and recreational events. Health services are not provided. **Life care (continuing care) communities** offer all the features of retirement communities plus health care and skilled nursing care units. When entering such a community, the resident must be capable of independent living.

Although only 5% of the elderly population live in nursing homes at any given time, an estimated 43% of people who were 65 years old in 1990 will use a nursing home at some time in their remaining life. Nursing homes offer a variety of health and personal services that include skilled

CRITICAL THINKING EXERCISES

1. Your clinical assignment is in an adult day care center. Based on your knowledge of the aging process and theories about aging, describe the strategies and goals you would devise to enhance communication with the elderly clients.
2. You are assigned to care for two hospitalized patients. One is a young adult and the other is elderly; both are recovering from abdominal surgery. How will the nursing assessment of these two patients differ? How will their care differ? What will be the differences in their discharge planning needs?
3. A neighbor whose wife has recently been diagnosed as having Alzheimer's disease approaches you expressing concern about his wife. He appears quite distraught and expresses anxiety about how he will be able to continue to care for her. Drawing upon your knowledge about the course of this condition and the problems it presents to both the afflicted person and the caregiver, describe the guidance you would offer.
4. You are caring for an elderly patient in the home setting. Describe the focus of your assessment to determine if any changes need to be made in the patient's home environment and support systems to better meet his physical and psychosocial needs.

nursing care and rehabilitation. They do not provide acute care. Medicare will not pay for personal care and will only pay skilled nursing home costs for a limited number of days. The cost of nursing home care comes out of the patient's and family's funds. When money and all assets are totally depleted, the costs will be paid by Medicaid.

Often, a decision for a nursing home placement is made by the family without consulting the older person. Research indicates that successful adjustment to the nursing home is enhanced if the older person participates in the decision-making process. The nurse and social worker as advocates can emphasize this point and encourage a family decision that includes the patient. When this occurs, the patient selects the home of his or her choice and will enter with a positive mental attitude and a feeling of control. If the patient wants to remain at home, he or she might be able to manage with the help of community supports. Decisions made "for your own good" by the family may, in fact, not be. Placement in a nursing home against the wishes of the patient should be made only as a last resort when no other alternative is available.

REFERENCES AND BIBLIOGRAPHY

Books

Carnevali DL and Patrick M. Nursing Management for the Elderly, 3rd ed. Philadelphia, JB Lippincott, 1993.

Christiansen JL and Grzybowski JM. Biology of Aging. St. Louis, CV Mosby, 1993.

Cohen GD. Psychopathology and mental health in the mature and elderly adult. In Binstock RH and George LK (eds). Handbook of Aging and the Social Sciences, 3rd ed (pp 359–371). New York, Academic Press, 1990.

Cummings E and Henry WE. Growing Old: The Process of Disengagement. New York, Basic Books, 1961.

Erikson EH. Childhood and Society, 2nd ed. New York, WW Norton, 1963.

Fowles DG. A Profile of Older Americans: 1994. American Association of Retired Persons and the Administration on Aging. Washington, DC, U.S. Department of Health and Human Services, 1994.

Havighurst RJ. Developmental Tasks and Education, 3rd ed. New York, McKay, 1972.

Kane RL, Ouslander JG, and Abrass IB. Essentials of Clinical Geriatrics, 3rd ed. New York, McGraw-Hill, 1994.

National Center for Health Statistics. Vital Statistics of the United States, 1989: Volume II, section 6 life tables. Washington, DC, Public Health Service, 1992.

National Institute on Aging. Discoveries in health for aging Americans: Progress report on Alzheimer's disease. US Department of Health and Human Services, National Institutes of Health, Washington, DC, 1994.

National Institute on Aging. In Search of the Secrets of Aging (NIH Publication No. 93-2756). Bethesda MD, National Institutes of Health, 1993.

Neugarten BL. Personality in Middle and Late Life. New York, Atherton Press, 1964.

Schick FL and Schick R (eds). Statistical Handbook on Aging Americans, 1994 Edition. Phoenix AZ, Oryx Press, 1994.

Schlenker ED. Nutrition in Aging, 2nd ed. St. Louis, CV Mosby, 1993.

U.S. Bureau of the Census. Current Population Reports, Special Studies, P23-178RV; Sixty-five plus in America. U.S. Government Printing Office, Washington, DC, 1992.

U.S. Senate Committee on Aging, American Association of Retired Persons, Federal Council on Aging, and U.S. Administration on Aging. Aging America: Trends and Projections. DHHS Publication No. (FCoA)91-28001. Washington, DC, U.S. Department of Health and Human Services, 1991.

Journals

Asterisks indicate nursing research articles.

Alzheimer's Association. Revolutionizing the genetics of Alzheimer's disease. Research and Practice 1993 Spring; 2(2): 1–2.

Atchley RC. Continuity theory of normal aging. Gerontologist 1989 April; 29(2): 183–190.

Brady R et al. Geriatric falls: Prevention strategies for the staff. J Gerontol Nurs 1993 Sept; 19(9): 26–32.

Breteler MMB et al. Epidemiology of Alzheimer's disease. Epidemiologic Reviews 1992 Jan; 14: 59–82.

*Brockapp DY et al. Nursing knowledge: Acute postoperative pain management in the elderly. J Gerontol Nurs 1993 Nov; 19(11): 31–37.

*Burgener SC and Shimer R. Variables related to caregiver behaviors with cognitively impaired elders in institutional settings. Res in Nurs and Health 1993 June; 16: 193–202.

Centers for Disease Control. Prevention and control of influenza: Recommendations of the Immunization Practices Advisory Committee (ACIP). MMWR 1991a; 40(RR-6): 1–15.

Centers for Disease Control. Prevention and control of influenza: Recommendations of the Immunization Practices Advisory Committee (ACIP). MMWR 1992; 41(RR-9): 1–10.

Centers for Disease Control. Purified protein derivative (PPD)–tuberculin anergy and HIV infection: Guidelines for anergy testing and management of anergic persons at risk of tuberculosis. MMWR 1991b; 40(RR-5): 27–32.

Centers for Disease Control. Tuberculosis morbidity—United States, 1992. MMWR 1993; 42: 363.

Centers for Disease Control. Update on adult immunization: Recommendations of the Immunization Practices Advisory Committee (ACIP). MMWR 1991c; 40(RR-12): 33–36, 43, 44.

*Conn VS. Self-management of over-the-counter medications by older adults. Public Health Nurs 1992 Sept; 9(1): 29–36.

Drugay M and Gallagher G. Patient self-determination act: Implementing an information program in a nursing facility. J Gerontol Nurs 1993 Dec; 19(12): 29–34.

Dutt AK and Stead WW. Tuberculosis. Clin Geriatr Med 1992 Nov; 8(4): 761–775.

Evans DA, Funkenstein H and Albert MS. Prevalence of Alzheimer's disease in a community population of older persons: Higher than earlier reported. JAMA 1990; 263: 2551–2556.

Finch EJL, Ramsey R and Katona CLE. Depression and physical fitness in the elderly. Clin Geriatr Med 1992 May; 8(2): 275–298.

Fraser D. Patient assessment: Infection in the elderly. J Gerontol Nurs 1993 July; 19(7): 5–11.

George LK. Depressive disorders and symptoms in later life. Generations 1993 Winter/Spring; XVII(1): 35–38.

Gerdner LA and Buckwalter KC. A nursing challenge: Assessment and management of agitation in Alzheimer's patients. J Gerontol Nurs 1994 Apr; 20(4): 11–20.

Havighurst RJ. Personality and patterns of aging. Gerontologist 1968; 8(3): 20–23.

Hodes RJ. Alzheimer's disease: Treatment research finds new targets. JAGS 1994 June; 42(6): 679–681.

Holt J. How to help confused patients. Am J Nurs 1993 Aug; 93(8): 32–36.

*Houston KA. An investigation of rocking as relaxation for the elderly. Geriatr Nurs 1993 July/Aug; 14(4): 186–189.

Kegel AH. Progressive resistance exercise in the functional restoration of the perineal muscles. Am J Obstet Gynecol 1948; 56: 238–248.

Koenig HG and Blazer DG. Epidemiology of geriatric affective disorders. Clin Geriatr Med 1992 May; 8(2): 235–251.

Lamy PP. Alzheimer's disease 1906–1991: Yesterday's future—tomorrow's reality? Elder Care News 1992 Fall; 8(4): 26–37.

Lancaster E. Tuberculosis comeback: Impact on long-term care facilities. J Gerontol Nurs 1993 July; 19(7): 16–21.
Liaw YS et al. Clinical spectrum of tuberculosis in older patients. JAGS 1995 March; 43(3): 256–260.
Lipowski ZJ. Update on delirium. Psychiatr Clin North Am 1992 June; 15(2): 335–346.
MacKay S. Durable power of attorney for health care. Geriatr Nurs 1992 Mar/Apr; 13(2): 99–108.
Madson SK. Patient self-determination act: Implications for long-term care. J Gerontol Nurs 1992 Feb; 19(2): 15–18.
Morgan S. Effects of age on cardiovascular functioning. Geriatr Nurs 1993 Sept/Oct; 14(5): 249–251.
*Munchiando JF and Kendall K. Comparison of the effectiveness of two bowel programs for CVA patients. Rehab Nurs 1993 May/June; 18(3): 168–172.
New product approvals: First Alzheimer's drug. FDA Medical Bulletin 1993 Dec; 23(3): 5.
*Pascucci MA. Measuring incentives to health promotion in older adults. J Gerontol Nurs 1992 Mar; 18(3): 16–23.
Pfister-Minogue K. Enhancing patient compliance: A guide for nurses. Geriatr Nurs 1993; 14(3): 124–132.
Schilke JM. Slowing the aging process with physical activity. J Gerontol Nurs 1991 June; 17(6): 4–8.
Stevenson C and Capezuti E. Guardianship: Protection vs. peril. Geriatr Nurs 1991 Jan/Feb; 12(1): 10–14.
Valente S. Recognizing depression in elderly patients. Am J Nurs 1994 Dec; 94(12): 19–25.

INFORMATION/RESOURCES

Agencies

Administration on Aging
330 Independence Avenue SW, Suite 4760, Washington, DC 20201, (202) 619-0556

Aging Network Services
Suite 907, 4400 East-West Highway, Bethesda, MD 20814, (301) 657-4329

Alzheimer's Association
919 Suite 1000, N. Michigan Avenue, Chicago, IL 60610, (312) 335-8700

Alzheimer's Disease Education and Referral Center (ADEAR)
P.O. Box 8250, Silver Spring, MD 20907-8250, (301) 495-3311, (800) 438-4380

American Association of Homes for the Aging
901 E Street NW, Suite 500, Washington, DC 20004-2837, (202) 783-2242

The American Association for International Aging
1133 20th Street NW, Suite 330, Washington, DC 20036, (202) 833-8893

American Association of Retired Persons
601 E Street NW, Washington, DC 20049, (202) 434-2277

American College of Health Care Administrators
325 S Patrick St, Alexandria, VA 22314, (703) 549-5822

American Federation for Aging Research (AFAR)
1414 Avenue of the Americas, 18th Floor, New York, NY 10019, (212) 572-2327

American Foundation for the Blind
15 West 16th Street, New York, NY 10011, (212) 620-2000

American Geriatrics Society, Inc.
770 Lexington Avenue, Suite 300, New York, NY 10021, (212) 308-1414

American Health Care Association
1201 L Street NW, Washington, DC 20005, (202) 842-8444

American Society on Aging
833 Market Street, Suite 516, San Francisco, CA 94130, (415) 974-9600

American Society for Geriatric Dentistry
211 East Chicago Avenue, 17th Floor, Chicago, IL 60611, (312) 440-2660

Association for Gerontology in Higher Education (AGHE)
1001 Connecticut Avenue NW, Suite 410, Washington, DC 20036, (202) 429-9277

Children of Aging Parents (CAPS)
Suite 302-A, 16098 Woodbourne Road, Levittown, PA 19057, (215) 945-6900

Elderhostel
75 Federal Street, Boston, MA 02110-1941, (617) 426-7788

Gerontological Society of America
1275 K Street NW, Suite 350, Washington, DC 20005-4006, (202) 842-1275

Gray Panthers
2025 Pennsylvania Avenue NW, Suite 821, Washington, DC 20006, (202) 466-3132

Help for Incontinent People (HIP)
P.O. Box 544, Union, SC 29379, (803) 579-7900

Legal Services for the Elderly
17th Floor, 130 West 42nd Street, New York, NY 10036, (212) 391-0120

National Aging Resource Center on Elder Abuse (NARCEA)
c/o American Public Welfare Association, Suite 500, 810 First Street NE, Washington, DC 20042-4205, (202) 682-2470

National Caucus and Center on Black Aged, Inc.
Suite 500, 1424 K Street NW, Washington, DC 20005, (202) 637-8400

National Council on the Aging, Inc.
Suite 200, 409 Third Street SW, Washington, DC 20024, (202) 479-1200

National Gerontological Nursing Association
7250 Parkway Drive, Suite 510, Hanover, MD 21076, (800) 723-0560

Nursing Research Profile for Unit 3

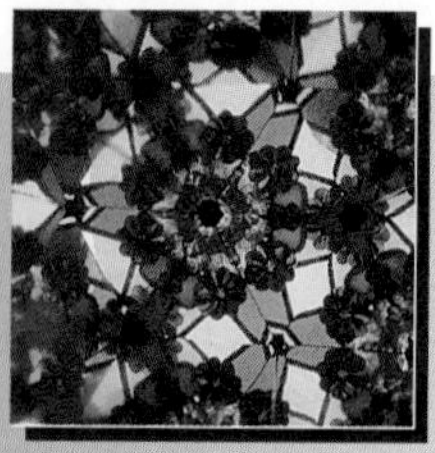

Biophysical and Psychosocial Concepts Related to Health and Illness

Overview

Nursing research in the area of biophysical and psychosocial concepts related to health and illness covers a variety of concepts. The following studies are presented as examples of the nursing research that has been conducted in the areas of stress and anxiety and gerontology. The nursing implications warrant consideration and further study.

Response to Illness

Meek SS. Effects of slow stroke back massage on relaxation in hospice clients. Image: J Nurs Scholarship 1993 Spring; 25(1):17–21.

This study used slow stroke back massage (SSBM) as a method of promoting relaxation in a sample of 30 adult hospice clients. The purpose of the study was to identify the effects of SSBM on systolic and diastolic blood pressure, cardiac rate, and skin temperature—indirect indicators of relaxation. A quasi-experimental repeated measures design was used with SSBM administered to each subject on 2 consecutive days with two pre-intervention and two post-intervention measurements of the physiologic variables.

The predicted hypotheses were supported: there were statistically significant decreases ($p < 0.001$) in systolic and diastolic blood pressures and heart rate and significant increases ($p < 0.002$) in temperature. The magnitude of these clinical changes was sufficient to demonstrate relaxation but was not great enough to place the subjects in danger of hypotension, bradycardia, or hyperthermia.

Nursing Implications. Slow stroke back massage is a simple, cost-effective measure for promotion of relaxation that does not require formal preparation in massage therapy. This technique can be used by nurses and can be taught to family caregivers of hospice patients. Caregivers may welcome this tangible means of showing care and support of their terminally ill loved one.

The physiologic changes that were used to indicate relaxation were found to be maintained 5 minutes post-intervention; effects longer than 5 minutes were not measured. Therefore, long-term effects of SSBM require further study.

Ali NS and Bennett SJ. Postmenopausal women: Factors in osteoporosis preventive behaviors. J Gerontol Nurs 1992 Dec; 18(12):23–32.

Osteoporosis-preventive health behaviors are identified as promoting behaviors such as improved nutrition and exercise and preventive behaviors such as adequate calcium intake, exercise adherence, maintenance of healthy life-style patterns, and compliance with hormone replacement therapy (HRT). This correlational study investigated the relationship of knowledge of osteoporosis prevention, perceptions of benefits of and barriers to milk intake, and health-promoting behaviors and osteoporosis-preventive behaviors among postmenopausal women.

The sample included 91 postmenopausal women, 54 to 83 years of age, recruited from residents of a senior citizen apartment complex and hospital volunteers in the Midwest. Ninety-five percent of the sample was Caucasian. The subjects completed four questionnaires. Knowledge of osteoporosis (KOP) was measured by a 10-item tool, and perception of barriers to and benefits of milk intake was measured by a 19-item Milk Barriers/Benefit Scale developed for this study. The 48-item Health Promotion Lifestyle Profile (HPLP) measured health-promoting behaviors. Osteoporosis-preventive behaviors (OPB) were measured by a 5-item questionnaire developed for this study.

Correlation coefficients and stepwise multiple regressions were used to analyze the data. Osteoporosis-preventive behaviors were significantly correlated with calcium intake, knowledge of osteoporosis prevention, total benefits of and barriers to milk intake, and health-promoting behaviors. Age was negatively correlated with knowledge of osteoporosis-preventive behaviors. Higher education levels were associated with greater knowledge of osteoporosis prevention. The KOP and the HPLP were significant predictors of osteoporosis-preventive behaviors. Also, the findings indicated that the postmenopausal women were not practicing adequate osteoporosis-preventive behaviors.

Nursing Implications. Nurses need to focus on health promotion and osteoporosis prevention in their health education efforts with older adults. In the clinical setting, nurses need to routinely assess women for risk factors for osteoporosis and provide education and/or referrals based on assessment findings. The benefit of milk as a source of calcium to prevent osteoporosis in the older adult needs to be promoted. Additional research identifying osteoporosis-preventive behaviors among other age groups and focusing on other variables such as exercise is recommended.

Kaakinen JR. Living with silence. Gerontologist 1992 Apr; 32(2):258–264.

This qualitative study used a role-play interview technique to encourage residents of nursing homes to identify how they communicate with other nursing home residents and to identify perceptions and beliefs that nursing home residents have about rules that govern their communication with other residents. The study participants consisted of 72 residents from eight nursing homes. These subjects were identified by the Directors of Nursing as meeting the inclusion criteria for the study: 65 years of age or older; fluent in English; capable of participating in a sustained conversation of 30 to 45 minutes; and no diagnosis of organic brain syndrome, Alzheimer's disease, primary psychotic disorder or acute withdrawal from alcohol or drugs, profound hearing loss, or extensive speech disorder.

Study results indicated that certain self-regulatory beliefs and rules governed verbal communication patterns and kept residents from freely interacting with other residents. Commonly occurring themes emerged: (1) more than 50% of the residents ignored persons whom they perceived to be "senile"; (2) residents would only talk to people who talked to them; (3) many did not initiate conversation with "hard of hearing" persons; (4) many did not talk with others because they feared social consequences (*e.g.*, gossip) or to avoid a social confrontation. Over 50% of the residents indicated that they believed that there were rules that prohibited complaining and talking about loneliness and dying.

Nursing Implications. Nurses can be instrumental in preventing feelings of isolation among nursing home residents. In assigning rooms to non-demented residents, the nurse should pair those who are capable of interacting verbally. Activities can be designed to stimulate conversations. Recreational events such as reminiscence groups, current events groups, and theater groups all foster verbal exchanges. Small discussion groups could be used to address topics that residents perceive as taboo. Memorial services should be held for those who die, thus addressing this often avoided topic of conversation.

Health Care of the Elderly

Abraham IL, Neundorfer MM, and Currie LJ. Effects of group interventions on cognition and depression in nursing home residents. Nurs Research 1992 Jul/Aug; 41(4):196–202.

Symptoms of depression may cause cognitive dysfunction in the absence of dementia. Although 15% of nursing home residents exhibit cognitive impairment and depressive symptoms attributable to external events, no controlled studies of interventions for depression have been reported. The purpose of this study was to identify the effects of cognitive-behavioral group therapy and focused visual imagery group therapy on cognitive functioning, depression, hopelessness, and dissatisfaction with life among depressed nursing home residents.

Seventy-six nursing home residents suffering from mild to severe depression and mild to moderate cognition decline were divided into three groups and given a 24-week course of therapy. Two intervention groups received either cognitive-behavioral or visual imagery therapy. The third group, the control group, was enrolled in an education-discussion group. Four validated instruments were used to measure cognitive status, depression, hopelessness, and life satisfaction at periodic intervals.

At completion of the study, the cognitive performance of those subjects who received either of the group therapy interventions was significantly ($p < 0.04$) improved. Depressive symptomatology was not decreased for subjects in any of the three groups.

Nursing Implications. Nurses in long-term care settings should recognize that interventions such as group therapy can reduce cognitive impairment in depressed elderly patients who do not have accompanying dementia. Not all cognitive impairment should be attributed to dementia. Further research needs to be conducted to study the influence of varied group interventions on depression and to identify the factors that are responsible for symptom improvement.

Badger TA. Physical health impairment and depression among older adults. Image: J Nurs Scholarship 1993 Winter; 25(4): 325–330.

In about 30% of the older population, depression is found concurrently with chronic physical illnesses and may contribute to decreased self-esteem, diminished quality of life, and poor social functioning. Past research has shown that depression can exert a negative effect on the physical health of older adults.

This descriptive study examined the relationship between physical health, mastery, social support, and depression in 80 community-residing older people with one or more chronic illnesses. The Older Americans Resources and Services Multidimensional Functional Assessment Questionnaire was used to measure physical health impairment, social resources, economic resources, mental health functioning, and self-care capacity. Based on their physical health impairment scores, participants were divided into two groups: Group 1 comprised 41 participants with mild physical health impairments; group 2 comprised 39 participants with moderate to severe physical health impairments.

The group with the greater physical health impairments demonstrated decreased sense of mastery, decreased social support, increased depression, and increased self-reported problem drinking when compared with the group with mild physical health impairments. Lack of social resources, economic resources, and mastery were found to be significant predictors of depression in the participants.

Nursing Implications. To prevent or alleviate depression in elderly adults with physical health impairments, nurses can initiate strategies to help these patients learn specific techniques that will assist them to improve their ability to perform those activities that they consider important. It is suggested that increased mastery of such activities allows for increased mobilization of social support. Further research is indicated to identify how best to enhance the personal and environmental resources and prevent or alleviate depression in older adults who have chronic illnesses that result in physical impairments.

Osborn CL and Marshall MJ. Self-feeding performance in nursing home residents. J Gerontol Nurs 1993 Mar; 19(3):7–14.

The incidence of feeding dependencies in nursing homes is as high as 50%. For those lacking skills or desire to feed themselves, full feeding assistance fosters dependency and promotes increased disability. This descriptive study was conducted to compare the self-feeding capabilities of cognitively impaired elderly nursing home residents with their actual self-feeding performance at mealtime.

The study sample consisted of 23 cognitively impaired nursing home residents who were identified by staff as partially dependent in feeding. At mealtime the researchers used a continuum of five helping interventions, ranging from non-verbal cues to some physical guidance to full support to assist the subjects with feeding. When less than full support was offered, some participants demonstrated hidden capabilities for self-sufficiency that were not evident in their usual performance. Using the specific tasks of drinking from a cup and eating a pureed diet, capability scores were significantly greater than total performance. Very few of the residents required full assistance when less assistance was offered. In contrast, the staff used an "all-or-nothing" approach and gave full assistance to most persons who were unable to be fully independent at mealtime.

Nursing Implications. Assistance at mealtimes should promote self-care and foster independence. Although it is important that nutritional needs be met, partially dependent older adults can be encouraged through the use of verbal cues and limited physical assistance as needed to feed themselves. Assignment of a single staff member to assist a group of partially dependent residents to eat is suggested. The professional nurse should provide suggestions and problem solving to nursing assistants in encouraging self-feeding skills of older adult nursing home residents.

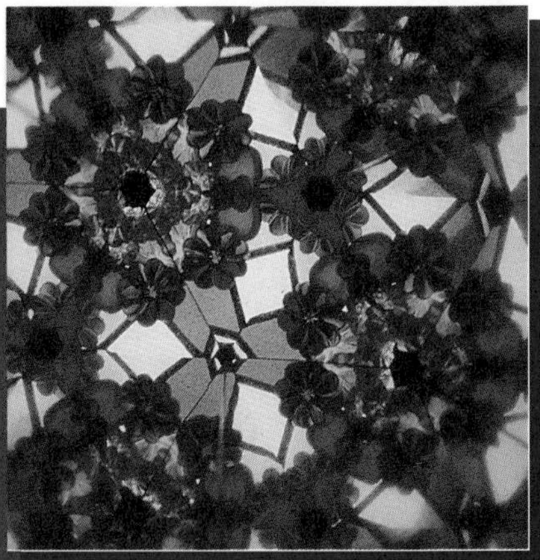

UNIT 4
Concepts and Challenges in Patient Management

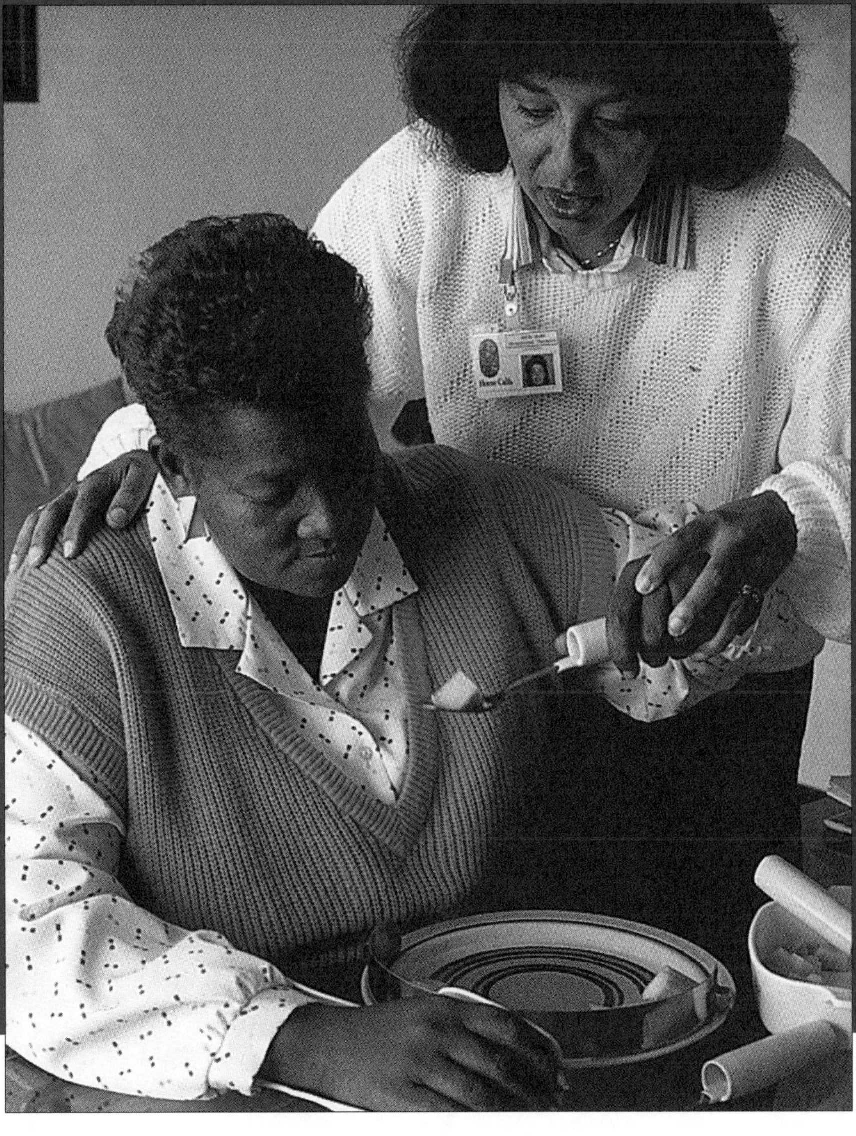

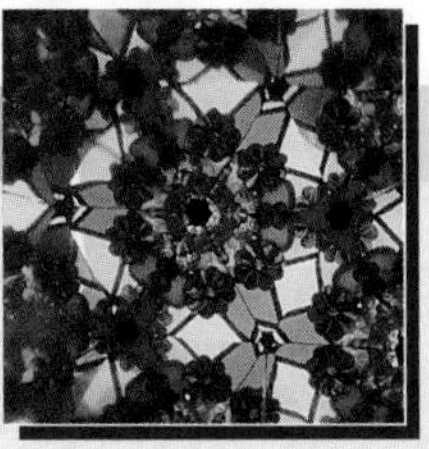

13

Pain Management

CHAPTER OUTLINE

Definition of Pain
Acute Versus Chronic Pain
Harmful Effects of Pain

Pain Perception
Neurophysiologic Mechanisms of Pain

Nursing Assessment of Pain
Assessing Perception of Pain
Assessing Physiologic and Behavioral Responses to Pain
Factors Influencing the Pain Response

Nursing Interventions
Identifying Goals for Pain Management
Nurse–Patient Relationship and Patient Teaching
Providing Physical Care
Managing Anxiety Related to Pain

Pain Management Strategies
Pharmacologic Interventions
Nonpharmacologic Measures

Patient Teaching: Care in the Home and Community

Evaluation of Effectiveness of Pain Intervention Strategies

Critical Thinking Exercises

LEARNING OBJECTIVES

On completion of this chapter, the learner will be able to:

1. Differentiate between acute and chronic pain
2. Describe the neurophysiology of pain
3. Describe physiologic and environmental factors that can alter the perception of pain
4. Explain the difference in opioid dependency, tolerance, and addiction; discuss when opioid tolerance may be a problem
5. Explain the impact of aging on pain
6. Describe the negative consequences of pain
7. Demonstrate use of appropriate pain measurement instruments
8. Identify appropriate pain-relief interventions for selected populations
9. Develop a plan to avoid adverse effects of opioids
10. Use the nursing process as a framework for care of patients with pain

Definition of Pain

Pain is an unpleasant sensory and emotional experience resulting from actual or potential tissue damage. It is the most common reason a person seeks health care. Pain occurs with many disease processes or with some diagnostic tests or treatments. Pain disables and distresses more people than any single disease. (As a preliminary to this discussion, see Chart 13-1 for a glossary of terms.)

The nurse spends more time with the patient in pain than any other health care professional and has the opportunity to help relieve pain and its harmful effects. The primary care provider's role is to identify and treat the cause of the pain and prescribe medications to relieve it. The nurse not only collaborates with other health care professionals but also administers most pain relief interventions, evaluates the effectiveness of the interventions, and serves as patient advocate when the intervention is ineffective. In addition, the nurse serves as educator to the patient and family, teaching them to manage the analgesia or pain relief regimen themselves when appropriate.

The nursing definition of pain is *whatever bodily hurt the patient says he has, existing whenever he says it does.* The cardinal rule in the care of patients with pain is that *all pain is real*, even if its cause is unknown. Therefore, the existence of pain is based simply on the patient's report that it exists. This definition is based on two important points.

First, the nurse believes patients when they indicate that they have pain. Pain is considered real even if no physical cause or origin can be identified. Although some painful sensations are associated with mental or psychological states, the patient actually feels a sensation of pain in such instances and does not merely imagine it. Most painful sensations are the result of physical stimuli *and* mental or emotional stimuli. Therefore, assessing a person's pain involves obtaining information about the physical causes of pain as well as the mental or emotional factors that influence the individual's perception of pain. Nursing intervention addresses both components.

The second point to keep in mind is what the patient "says" about pain is not limited to verbal statements. Some patients cannot or will not verbally report that they have pain. Therefore, the nurse is also responsible for observing nonverbal behaviors that *may* occur with pain.

Although it is important to believe the patient who reports pain, it is equally important to be alert to patients who deny pain when they have pain. A nurse who suspects pain in a patient who denies it should explore with the patient the reason for suspecting pain, such as the fact that the disorder or procedure is usually painful, or that the patient grimaces when moving or avoids any movement. Exploring the possible reasons why the patient is denying the pain is also helpful. Some people deny pain because they fear the treatment that may ensue if they complain of pain or they fear becoming addicted to opioids (narcotics) if these drugs are prescribed for the pain.

CHART 13-1
Glossary

Addiction A behavioral pattern of substance use characterized by a compulsion to take the drug primarily in order to experience its psychic effects.

Dermatome The region of the body that is supplied by a single pair of dorsal root ganglia.

Nociceptor Nerve fiber that transmits pain

Non-nociceptor Nerve fiber that usually does not transmit pain

Nociceptive system The system involved in transmission and perception of pain

Opioid A morphine-like compound that produces bodily effects including pain relief, sedation, constipation, and respiratory depression

Pain An unpleasant sensory and emotional experience resulting from actual or potential tissue damage.

Pain threshold The least intense stimulus that will cause pain

Pain tolerance The maximum intensity or duration of pain that a person is willing to endure

Patient-controlled analgesia (PCA) Self-administered analgesics by a patient instructed about the procedure

Acute Versus Chronic Pain

Two basic categories of pain are generally recognized: acute pain and chronic pain. Table 13-1 compares the characteristics of acute and chronic pain.

Acute Pain

Acute pain is usually of recent onset and is most commonly associated with a specific injury. Acute pain indicates that damage or injury has occurred. It draws attention to the fact that it is occurring and teaches us to avoid similar potentially painful situations. If no lasting damage occurs and no systemic disease exists, acute pain usually decreases as healing occurs; this generally occurs in less than 6 months and usually less than 1 month. For purposes of definition, acute pain can be described as lasting from a few seconds to 6 months.

Injuries or diseases that cause acute pain may heal spontaneously or may require treatment. For example, a prick of the finger usually heals rapidly, with the pain subsiding quickly, perhaps within a few seconds or minutes. In the case of a more severe condition, such as a fracture of an extremity, treatment is required with the pain decreasing in time as the bone heals.

Chronic Pain

Chronic pain is constant or intermittent pain that persists over a period of time. It lasts beyond the expected healing time and often cannot be attributed to a specific cause or injury. It may not have a well-defined onset and often is difficult to treat as it usually does not respond to treatment

TABLE 13-1 Comparison of Acute and Chronic Pain

Characteristic	Acute Pain	Chronic Pain
Purpose/benefit	Warns of injury or problem	None
Onset	Recent	Continuous or intermittent
Intensity	Mild to severe	Mild to severe
Duration	Short duration (from a few seconds to 6 months)	Long duration (6 months or more)
Autonomic response	Consistent with sympathetic stress response Increased heart rate Increased stroke volume Increased blood pressure Increased pupillary dilation Increased muscle tension Decreased gastrointestinal motility Decreased salivary flow (dry mouth)	Absence of autonomic responses
Psychologic component	Anxiety	Depression Irritability Withdrawal from outside interests Withdrawal from relationships
Others types of response		Disturbed sleep Decreased libido Decreased appetite
Examples	Surgical pain, trauma	Cancer pain, arthritis, trigeminal neuralgia

(Adapted from Porth CM. Pathophysiology: Concepts of Altered Health States, 4th ed. Philadelphia, JB Lippincott, 1994.)

directed at its cause. Although acute pain may be a useful signal that something is wrong, chronic pain usually becomes a problem in its own right.

Chronic pain is often defined as pain that lasts for 6 months or longer, although 6 months is an arbitrary period for differentiating between acute and chronic pain. An episode of pain may assume the characteristics of chronic pain before 6 months have elapsed, or some types of pain may remain primarily acute in nature for longer than 6 months. Nevertheless, after 6 months most pain experiences are accompanied by problems related to the pain itself. Chronic pain serves no useful purpose, and if it persists it may become the major disorder.

Although it is unknown why some people develop chronic pain after an injury or disease process, it is suspected that nerve endings that normally do not transmit pain develop the ability to evoke painful sensations, or those nerve endings that normally transmit only noxious (painful) stimuli transmit previously non-noxious (nonpainful) stimuli as painful stimuli.

Chronic pain may occur with cancer but this type of pain generally has an identifiable cause. Cancer pain often results from compression of a peripheral nerve or the meninges or from damage to these structures following surgery, chemotherapy, or radiation treatments, or by tumor growth and infiltration.

The nurse may come in contact with patients with chronic pain when they are admitted to the hospital for treatment or when they are seen in the home for home care. Frequently the nurse is called on in community-based settings to assist in managing the patient's pain.

Harmful Effects of Pain

Acute Pain. Regardless of the nature, pattern, or cause of pain, pain that is inadequately treated has harmful effects beyond the discomfort it causes. In addition to being uncomfortable and disturbing, unrelieved acute pain can affect the pulmonary, cardiovascular, gastrointestinal, endocrine, and immunologic systems (Yeager et al., 1987; Benedetti et al., 1984). The stress response ("neuroendocrine response to stress") that occurs with trauma also occurs with other causes of severe pain. The widespread endocrine, immunologic, and inflammatory changes that occur with stress can have significant negative effects. This is particularly true in patients compromised because of age, illness, or injury.

The stress response generally consists of increased metabolic rate and cardiac output, impaired insulin response, increased production of cortisol, and increased retention of fluids (see Chapter 9 for details about the stress response).

The stress response may increase the patient's risk for physiologic disorders (*i.e.*, myocardial infarction, pulmonary infection, thromboembolism, and prolonged paralytic ileus). The patient with severe pain and the stress associated with it may be unable to take a deep breath and experiences increased fatigue and decreased mobility. Although these effects may be tolerated by a young healthy person, they may hamper recovery of an elderly, debilitated, or critically ill person. Effective pain relief may result in a more rapid recovery and early return to previous activities, including work.

Chronic Pain. Just as acute pain has negative effects, chronic pain also has adverse effects. Suppression of immune function associated with chronic pain may promote tumor growth. Additionally, a chronic pain often results in depression and disability. Although health care providers have been concerned about the large quantities of opioid (narcotic) medications required to relieve chronic pain in some patients, it is safe to use large doses of these medications for controlling progressive chronic pain (*e.g.*, cancer pain); in fact, it may be unsafe not to do so because of the consequences of unrelieved pain (Liebeskind, 1991).

Regardless of how the patient copes with chronic pain, pain over an extended period often results in disability. The patient may be unable to continue the activities and interpersonal relationships engaged in before pain began. This may range from curtailing participation in physical activities to being unable to take care of personal needs, such as dressing or eating. The nurse needs to understand the effects of chronic pain on the patient and family and be knowledgeable about pain relief strategies and appropriate resources to assist with pain management.

Pain Perception

Many theories attempt to explain the neurologic basis of pain. However, no single theory fully explains how pain is transmitted or perceived, nor explains the complexity of the pathways that affect transmission of pain impulses, the sensation of pain, and individual differences in pain sensation. Effective management of a patient's pain requires an understanding of pain perception, also referred to as *nociception*. In addition, it is necessary to understand pain assessment strategies and the interventions used to relieve a person's pain, as well as the advantages, disadvantages, and limitations of each of those interventions.

Neurophysiologic Mechanisms of Pain

Specific structures in the nervous system are involved in transforming a stimulus into a sensation of pain. The system involved in the transmission and perception of pain is referred to as the **nociceptive system**. The sensitivity of the components of the nociceptive system can be affected by a number of factors and may differ among individuals. Not all persons exposed to the same stimulus (appendicitis, for example) experience the same intensity of pain. Sensation that is very painful to one person may be barely noticeable to another person. Further, a stimulus may result in pain at one time but not at another time. For example, pain due to chronic arthritis and postoperative pain is often worse at night. Those factors that can increase or decrease the sensitivity of the different components of the nociceptive system are described in the following discussion.

Pain Transmission

Pain Receptors (Nociceptors). Pain receptors (nociceptors) are free nerve endings in the skin that respond only to intense, potentially damaging stimuli. Such stimuli may be mechanical, thermal, or chemical in nature. The joints, skeletal muscle, fascia, tendons, and the cornea also have pain receptors that have the potential to transmit stimuli that produce pain. However, the large internal organs (viscera) do not contain nerve endings that respond only to painful stimuli. Pain originating in these organs results from intense stimulation of receptors that have other purposes. For example, inflammation, stretching, ischemia, dilation, and spasm of the internal organs all cause intense response in these multipurpose fibers and potentially cause severe pain.

The pain receptors are complex multidirectional pathways. These nerve fibers branch very near their origin in the skin and send fibers to local blood vessels, mast cells, hair follicles, and sweat glands. Stimulation of these fibers results in release of histamine from the mast cells and in vasodilation. The cutaneous fibers located more centrally further branch and communicate with the paravertebral sympathetic chain of the nervous system and with large internal organs. As a result of the connections between these nerve fibers, pain is often accompanied by vasomotor, autonomic, and visceral effects. For example, a patient with severe acute pain is likely to experience decreased or absent peristalsis of the gastrointestinal tract.

Although intense activation of the pain receptor fibers in the skin will cause a response in the visceral connections of that same fiber, the converse is also true. Intense stimulation of the visceral branch of a fiber may result in vasodilation and pain in the area of the body associated with that fiber. The result is **referred pain** (Fig. 13-1). The most widely recognized example of referred pain is pain in the left arm or jaw associated with cardiac ischemia or heart attack (myocardial infarction).

Chemical Mediators of Pain. A number of chemical substances that affect the sensitivity of the nerve endings or pain receptors are released into the extracellular tissue as a result of tissue damage. Chemicals that increase the transmission or perception of pain include *histamine, bradykinin, acetylcholine,* and *substance P. Prostaglandins* are chemical substances thought to increase the sensitivity of pain receptors by enhancing the pain-provoking effect of bradykinin.

Endorphins and Enkephalins. Other substances in the body serve as inhibitors of pain transmission. **Endorphins** and **enkephalins**, morphine-like substances produced by the body, are examples of substances that inhibit the transmission of painful impulses. The term endorphin is a combination of two words: *endogenous* and *morphine*. When the body releases these substances, one effect is pain relief.

Endorphins and enkephalins are found in heavy concentrations in the central nervous system. They are endogenous chemicals (produced by the body) similar in structure to opioids (also referred to as opiates or narcotics). Morphine and other opioid medications inhibit the transmission of noxious stimuli by mimicking enkephalin and endorphins.

Inhibitory interneuronal fibers that contain enkephalin are primarily activated through activity of (1) non-nocicep-

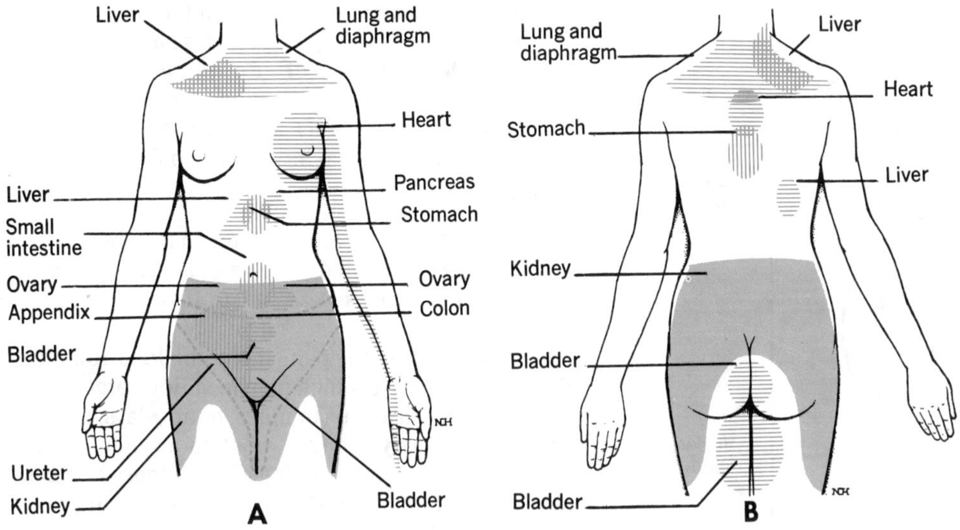

FIGURE 13-1. Referred pain. (**A**) Anterior view. (**B**) Posterior view. (From Chaffee EE and Lytle IM. Basic Physiology and Anatomy, 4th ed. Philadelphia, JB Lippincott.)

tor peripheral fibers (fibers that normally do not transmit painful or noxious stimuli) in the same receptor field as the pain receptor or nociceptor, and (2) descending fibers, grouped together in a system called "descending control" (discussed below). The enkephalins and endorphins are thought to inhibit pain impulses by blocking the transmission of these impulses in the brain and spinal cord.

The existence of enkephalins and endorphins helps explain why different people feel different amounts of pain from similar stimuli. Endorphin levels vary among individuals, as do factors, such as anxiety, that influence endorphin levels. People with more endorphins feel less pain, and those with less endorphins feel more pain.

Several techniques may be effective in relieving pain at least in part because they cause the release of endorphins. Transcutaneous electric nerve stimulation (TENS) may stimulate the release of endorphins, as may the use of placebos (inert substances) in which the patient thinks the treatment is working even though it has no value. Other methods of pain relief, such as guided imagery, may help a patient release endorphins.

Dorsal Horn and Ascending Pathways

The dorsal horn of the spinal cord can be thought of as a sensory processing area. Peripheral fibers (*e.g.*, pain receptors) terminate here and the fibers of ascending sensory tracts begin here. There are also interconnections between descending neuronal systems and the ascending sensory tracts. The ascending tracts terminate on the lower and midportions of the brain and their impulses are relayed to the cortex of the brain.

For pain to be consciously perceived, neurons in the ascending systems must be activated. Activation occurs as a result of input from the pain receptors located in the skin and internal organs. There are interconnecting neurons in the dorsal horn which, when activated, inhibit or turn off the transmission of noxious or pain-stimulating information in the ascending pathway. Frequently this area is referred to as "the gate." The gate's natural tendency is to allow all noxious input from the periphery to activate the ascending pathways and result in pain. However, if this tendency went unopposed many activities of daily living would be painful. Consequently a system exists to close the "gate." Stimulation of inhibitory interneurons of the ascending system closes the gate to pain input and prevents the transmission of pain sensations (Fig. 13-2).

The gate control theory of pain (Wall, 1978) proposes that there is interaction between pain stimuli and other sensations and that stimulation of fibers that transmit nonpainful sensations blocks or decreases the transmission of pain impulses through an inhibitory gating circuit. Inhibitory cells in the dorsal horn of the spinal cord contain enkephalin, which inhibits the transmission of pain.

This theory explains how certain activities decrease pain perception. The first response of a person who strikes the thumb with a hammer is to put the thumb in the mouth or in cold water. This action stimulates nonpain (non-nociceptive) fibers in the same receptor field as the pain-sensing fiber (nociceptors) just activated. Stimulation of large numbers of non-nociceptive fibers, which synapse on inhibitory fibers in the dorsal horn, inhibit (to some extent) transmission of painful sensation in the ascending pathways.

Descending Control System

The descending control system is a system of fibers that originate in the lower and midportion of the brain (specifically the periaqueductal gray matter) and terminate on the inhibitory interneuronal fibers in the dorsal horn of the spinal cord. This system is probably always somewhat active; it prevents continuous transmission of stimuli as painful, partly through the action of the endorphins.

Cognitive processes may stimulate endorphin production in the descending control system. The effectiveness of this system is illustrated by the effects of **distraction**. For example, individuals escaping a fire are often unaware that they have sustained burns until reaching safety. For a person to reach safety, the brain shuts off the relatively less important pain perception by stimulating the descending control system. Similarly, intense physical activity is thought to increase endorphin production in the descending control system. In addition, the distractions of visitors or a favorite TV show may increase activity in the descending

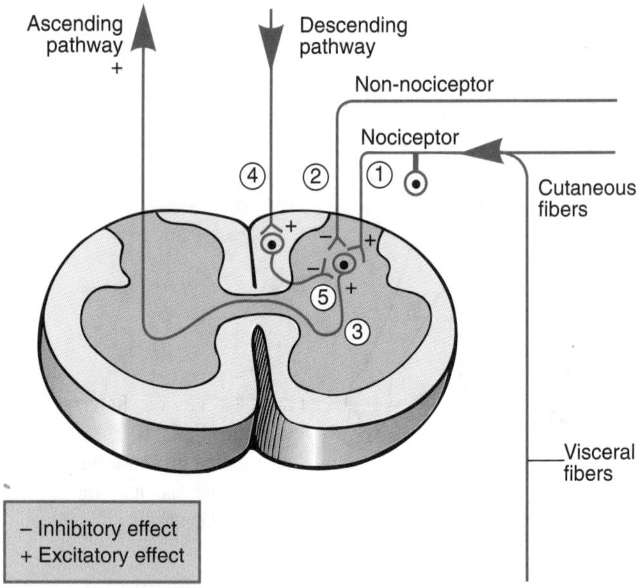

FIGURE 13-2. Schematic representation of nociception system, showing the dorsal horn with ascending and descending sensory pathways.

control system. Therefore, the person who has visitors may not report pain because activation of the descending control system results in less noxious or painful information being transmitted to consciousness. Once the distraction of the visitors ends, activity in the descending control system decreases resulting in increased transmission of painful stimuli.

Depression can have the opposite effect of distraction. People with depression often report chronic pain. Unrelenting chronic pain can cause depression; depression in turn can lead to decreased activity in the descending control system and increased perception of pain. The difference in pain perception among individuals is probably a function of unconscious yet persistent activity in the descending control system.

Nursing Assessment of Pain

Nursing assessment of a person with pain includes a description of the pain itself as well as possible other factors that may influence pain (*i.e.*, previous experience with pain, anxiety, and age) and the person's response to pain-relief strategies.

Assessing Perception of Pain

Pain assessment tools may be used to assess a patient's perception of pain. For a pain assessment tool to be useful, it must satisfy the following criteria: (1) be easy to understand and use, (2) require little effort on the part of the patient, (3) be easily scored, and (4) be sensitive to small changes in the intensity of pain. Pain assessment tools may be used to document the need for intervention, to evaluate the effectiveness of the intervention, and to identify the need for alternative or additional interventions if the initial intervention is ineffective in relieving the person's pain.

Verbal Description of Pain. The individual is the best judge of personal pain and therefore should be asked to describe and rate its severity. The information requested should describe the individual's pain in the following ways:

- The **intensity** of the pain. The person may be asked to rate the pain on a verbal scale (*e.g.*, none, slight, moderate, severe, or very severe; or 0 to 10: 0 = no pain, 10 = worst pain).
- **Characteristics** of the pain, including **location** (see Fig. 13-1 for areas to which pain in various organs may be referred), **duration** (minutes, hours, days, months, and so forth.), **rhythm** (*e.g.*, continuous, intermittent, periods of waxing and waning of the intensity or existence of pain), and **quality** (*e.g.*, pricking, burning, aching, viselike).
- **Factors that relieve pain** (*e.g.*, movement, lack of movement, exertion, rest, over-the-counter medication, and so forth) and what the person believes will help with the pain. Many people have definite ideas about what will relieve their pain. This attitude is often based on experience or trial and error.
- **Effects of pain on activities of daily living** (*e.g.*, sleep, appetite, concentration, interactions with others, physical movement, work, and leisure activities). Acute pain is often associated with anxiety, and chronic pain with depression.
- **The person's concern about the pain.** This may include a wide variety of concerns, such as financial burdens, prognosis, interference with roles, and body image changes.

Visual Analogue Scales (VAS). Visual analogue scales (Fig. 13-3) are useful in assessing the intensity of pain. The scale is comprised of a horizontal 10-cm line, and anchors (ends) indicating the extremes of pain. The person is asked to place a mark on the line indicating where the current pain lies along that continuum. The left anchor usually represents "none" or "no pain," whereas the right anchor usually represents "severe" or "worst possible pain." To score the results, a ruler is placed along the line and the distance the person marked the line from the "no pain" extreme is measured and reported in centimeters.

Guidelines for Using Pain Assessment Scales

Using a written scale to assess pain may not be possible if the person is seriously ill or in severe pain or has just returned from surgery. In these cases the patient can be asked: "On a scale of zero to ten, zero being 'no pain' and ten being 'pain as bad as it can be,' how bad is your pain now?" Patients usually can respond without difficulty. If possible, the nurse can show the patient how the pain scale works before the pain occurs (*i.e.*, preoperatively). The individual's numerical rating is documented and used to assess the effectiveness of the pain-relief interventions.

If the person does not speak English or is unable to communicate clearly information needed to manage pain,

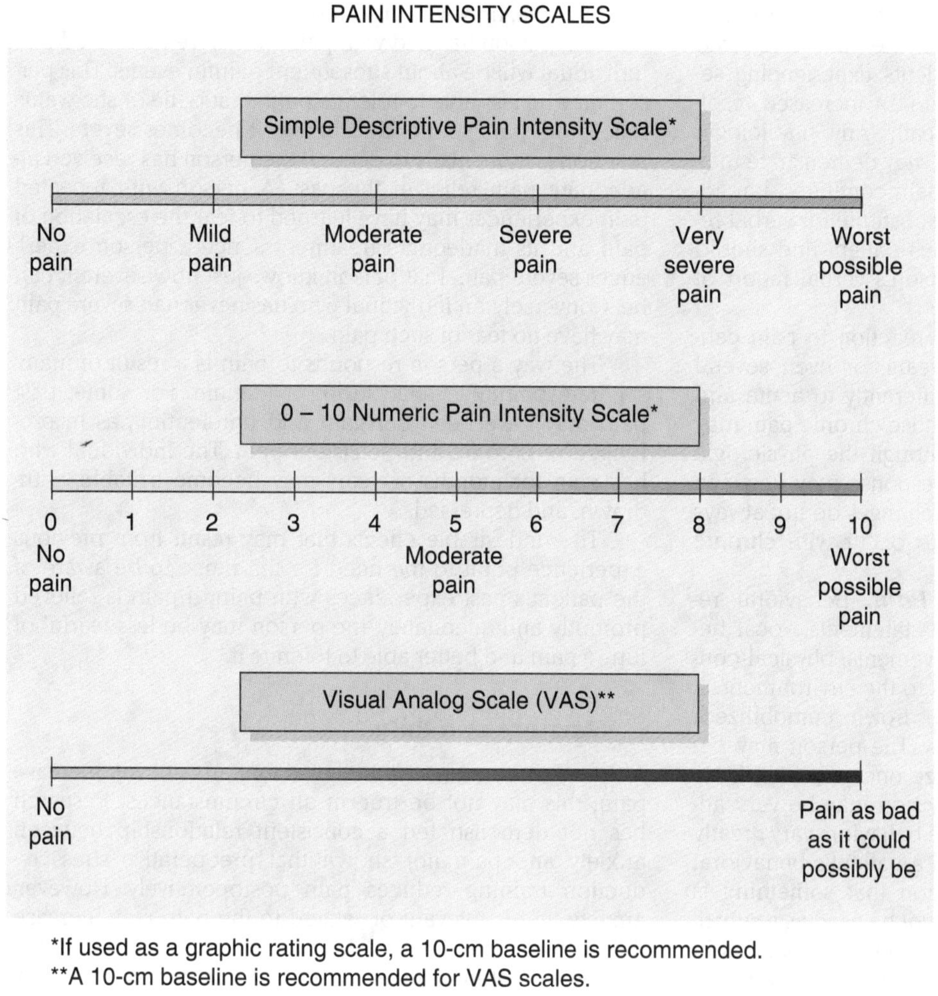

FIGURE 13-3. Examples of pain intensity scales. (Agency for Health Care Policy and Research [AHCPR]. Acute Pain Management: Operative or Medical Procedures and Trauma. Clinical Practice Guidelines. Rockville, MD; Agency for Health Care Policy and Research, Public Health Service, U.S. Department of Health and Human Services, Feb 1992.)

an interpreter, translator, or family member familiar with the person's method of communication should be consulted and a method established for pain assessment.

When a person with pain is cared for at home by family caregivers or the home care nurse, a pain scale may be helpful in assessing the effectiveness of the interventions implemented, if the scale is used before and after the interventions are administered. Scales that address the location and pattern of pain may be useful to the home care nurse in identifying new sources or sites of pain in the chronically or terminally ill patient and in monitoring changes in the patient's level of pain. The patient and family caregivers can be taught how to use a pain assessment scale to assess and manage the patient's pain. The home care nurse who sees the patient only at intervals may thus benefit from a written record of the pain scores in evaluating how effective the pain management strategies have been over time.

On occasion, a person will deny having pain when most people in similar circumstances would report significant pain. For example, it is not uncommon for a patient recovering from a total joint replacement to deny feeling "pain" but on further questioning will readily admit to having a "terrible ache, but I wouldn't call it pain." From then on, when evaluating this person's pain, the nurse would use the patient's words rather than the word "pain."

Assessing Physiologic and Behavioral Responses to Pain

Assessing physiologic and behavioral indications of pain is sometimes difficult, if not impossible. Observable physiologic and behavioral indicators of pain may be minimal or absent; however, this does not mean that the patient does not have pain.

Many health care providers are more familiar with acute pain than chronic pain. Consequently, a health care provider unfamiliar with physiologic and behavioral pain responses may question the existence of pain in a patient who calmly reports severe pain or in someone who sleeps soundly immediately before or after reporting severe pain. However, not all patients with severe pain exhibit physiologic or behavioral signs of pain. The absence of these signs should not lead the nurse to conclude that pain is absent; the presence of these signs does not always mean that a patient has pain.

Physiologic Indicators of Pain. Involuntary physiologic changes were once considered more accurate indicators of pain than the patient's verbal report. However, these involuntary responses—increased pulse and respiratory rates, pallor and perspiration—are indicators of autonomic nervous system arousal, not pain.

Some patients' heart rates may decrease in response to acute pain and increase only after the pain is relieved (Moltner, Holzl & Strain, 1990). Patients experiencing severe acute pain may not demonstrate an increased respiratory rate, but may hold their breath. Any physiologic response to acute pain that a patient *may* demonstrate may only last a few minutes, even if the pain continues. Physiologic responses should be used as a substitute for verbal reports of pain only in the unconscious patient and should not be used to try to validate a person's verbal report of pain.

Because an intense physiologic reaction to pain cannot be maintained for weeks or years, or even several hours, a patient usually responds differently to acute and chronic pain. A patient with very intense chronic pain may exhibit no physiologic changes. Although the physiologic changes associated with the stress response may occur in some persons with acute pain, such changes do not always occur; further, they are less likely to occur with chronic pain.

Behavioral Responses to Pain. Behavioral responses to pain may include verbal statements, vocal behaviors, facial expressions, body movements, physical contact with others, or altered responses to the environment. A person in acute pain may cry, moan, frown, immobilize a body part, clench a fist, or withdraw. The person may become angry or irritable and apologize once the pain is relieved. Sounds from a radio or television may be very annoying to the person with pain. These behaviors vary greatly from one time to the next. Although a patient's behavioral responses may be the first indication that something is wrong, behavioral responses should *not* be used as a substitute for pain measurement except in unusual situations in which pain measurement is not possible (*e.g.*, the person is severely mentally retarded or is unconscious).

A person with pain of sudden onset may react very differently to pain that lasts more than a few minutes or becomes chronic. Pain may cause fatigue and leave the person too exhausted to moan or cry if such behavior is the normal response to pain. The patient may sleep, even with severe pain. The patient may appear relaxed and involved in activities because of becoming a master at distraction from pain. The person who has succeeded in minimizing the effect of chronic pain on life should be encouraged rather than discouraged from coping in this way.

Factors Influencing the Pain Response

A person's pain experience is influenced by a number of factors, including past experiences with pain; anxiety; age; and expectations about pain relief (placebo effect). These factors may increase or decrease the person's perception of pain, increase or decrease tolerance for pain, and affect the manner of responses to pain.

Past Experience With Pain

It is tempting to expect that a person who has had multiple or prolonged experiences with pain will be less anxious and more tolerant of pain than one who has had little pain. For most people, however, this is not true. Often, the more experience a person has had with pain, the more frightened that individual will be about subsequent painful events. This person may be less able to tolerate pain; that is, he or she wants relief from pain sooner and before it becomes severe. This reaction is more likely to occur if the person has received inadequate pain relief in the past. A person with repeated pain experiences may have learned to fear the escalation of pain and its inadequate treatment. Once a person experiences severe pain, that person knows just how severe it can be. Conversely, an individual who has never had severe pain may have no fear of such pain.

The way a person responds to pain is a result of many separate painful events during a lifetime. For some, past pain may have been constant and unrelenting, as in prolonged or chronic and persistent pain. The individual who has pain for months or years may become irritable, withdrawn, and depressed.

The undesirable effects that may result from previous experience point to the need for the nurse to be aware of the patient's past experiences with pain. If pain is relieved promptly and adequately, the person may be less fearful of future pain and better able to tolerate it.

Anxiety and Pain

Although it is commonly believed that anxiety will increase pain, this may not be true in all circumstances. Research has not demonstrated a consistent relationship between anxiety and pain nor shown that preoperative stress reduction training reduces pain postoperatively. However, anxiety that is relevant or related to the pain may increase the patient's perception of pain. For example, a patient who was treated 2 years ago for breast cancer and now has hip pain may fear that the pain indicates metastases. In this case the anxiety may result in increased pain. Anxiety that is unrelated to the pain may distract the patient and may actually decrease the perception of pain. For example, a mother who is hospitalized with complications from a cholecystectomy and is anxious about her children may perceive less pain as her anxiety about her children increases.

The routine use of antianxiety medications to treat anxiety in someone with pain may prevent the person from reporting pain because of excessive sedation and may impair the patient's ability to take deep breaths, get out of bed, and cooperate with the recovery plan. In general, the most effective way to relieve pain is by directing the treatment at the pain rather than at the anxiety.

Culture and Pain

Culture and ethnicity have an influence on how a person responds to pain (how the pain is described or the way one behaves in response to pain). However, culture and ethnicity do not affect pain perception (Zatzick & Dimsdale, 1990).

Early in childhood individuals learn from those around them what responses to pain are acceptable or unacceptable. For example, a child may learn that a sports injury is not expected to hurt as much as a comparable injury caused by a motor vehicle crash. Others teach the child what stimuli are expected to be painful and what behavioral responses are acceptable. These beliefs vary from one culture to another; therefore, people from different cultures who experience the same intensity of pain may not report it or respond to it in the same ways.

The cultural expectations about pain that a person learns throughout life rarely are altered by exposure to the opposing values of other cultures. Consequently, individuals believe that their perceptions of and reactions to pain are normal and acceptable.

The nurse's cultural values may differ from those of a patient from another culture. The nurse's cultural expectations and values may include avoiding exaggerated expressions of pain, such as excessive crying and moaning; seeking immediate relief from pain and giving complete descriptions of the pain. A patient's cultural expectations may be to moan and complain about pain, to refuse pain-relief measures that do not cure the cause of the pain, and to use adjectives like "unbearable" in describing the pain. A patient from another cultural background may behave differently, in a very quiet stoic manner rather than expressing the pain loudly. The nurse must react to the person's pain perception and not to the pain behavior because the behavior is different from that of the nurse.

Many other attitudes and behaviors—such as a patient's preference for having visitors or being alone or an attitude toward diagnosis—may vary from one culture to another.

Recognizing the values of one's own culture and learning how these values differ from those of other cultures help to avoid evaluating the patient's behavior on the basis of one's own cultural expectations and values. It is equally important, however, to avoid stereotyping patients by culture. A nurse who recognizes cultural differences will have a greater understanding of the patient's pain and will be more accurate in assessing pain and behavioral responses to pain as well as more effective in relieving the patient's pain.

Age and Pain

The influence of age on pain perception and pain tolerance is largely unknown. Assessment of pain in the elderly may be difficult because of physiologic and psychosocial changes that accompany aging. The way an older person responds to pain may differ from the way younger people respond. Or the pain in an elderly person may be referred far from the site of injury or disease. Pain perception in the elderly may be diminished as a result of pathologic changes associated with some disorders (*e.g.*, diabetes), but in a healthy elderly person pain perception may be unchanged. Because elderly people have slower metabolism and greater ratios of body fat to muscle mass than younger people, small doses of analgesics may be sufficient to relieve the pain. When given the opportunity to self-administer postoperative analgesia, the elderly have been shown to obtain pain relief from smaller doses of opioids (Giuffre et al., 1991).

Although many elderly people seek health care because of pain, others are reluctant to seek help even when in severe pain because they consider pain to be part of normal aging. It has been estimated that more than 85% of older adults have at least one chronic health problem that could cause pain. The elderly tend to under report pain and endure greater pain for longer periods before reporting it or seeking health care. Others fail to seek care because they fear that the pain may indicate serious illness or they fear loss of control. An elderly person may respond to pain by using over-the-counter medications or medications prescribed for other illnesses. The elderly deal with pain according to their lifestyle, personality, and cultural background. Many elderly people are very fearful of addiction and as a result will not report that they are in pain or ask for pain medication.

It is essential that the elderly receive adequate pain relief after surgery or trauma. When an elderly person becomes confused following surgery or trauma, the confusion is often attributed to medications, which are then discontinued. However, confusion in the elderly may be a result of untreated and unrelieved pain. In some cases, postoperative confusion in the elderly clears once the pain is relieved. Judgments about pain and the adequacy of treatment should be based on the patient's report of pain and pain relief rather than on the basis of age.

Placebo Effect

A **placebo effect** occurs when a person responds to the medication or other treatment because of an expectation that it will work rather than because it actually works. Simply receiving a medication or treatment may produce positive effects.

The placebo effect results from the natural (endogenous) production of endorphins in the descending control system. It is a true physiologic response that can be reversed by naloxone, a narcotic antagonist.

A patient's positive expectations about treatment may increase the effectiveness of a medication or other intervention. Often the more cues the patient receives about the intervention's effectiveness, the more effective it will be. A person who is informed that a medication is expected to relieve pain is more likely to experience pain relief than one who is told that a medication is unlikely to have any effect. A positive nurse–patient relationship may also serve a very important role in enhancing the placebo effect.

Because of misperceptions about placebos and the placebo effect, the following principles and guidelines should be kept in mind:

- The placebo effect is *not* an indication that the person does not have pain; rather, it is a *true* physiologic response.
- Placebos *should never* be used to test the person's truthfulness about pain or as the first line of treatment.
- A positive response to a placebo, that is reduction in pain, *should never* be interpreted as an indication that the person's pain is not real.
- A patient *should never* be given a placebo ("sugar pill") as a substitute for analgesia. Although a placebo can

produce analgesia, patients receiving a placebo may report pain relief or that they feel better simply to avoid disappointing the nurse.

Nursing Interventions

Before discussing what the nurse can do to intervene in the patient's pain, the nurse's role in pain management is reviewed. The nurse helps relieve pain by administering pain-relieving interventions (including both pharmacologic and nonpharmacologic approaches), assessing the effectiveness of those interventions, monitoring for adverse effects, and serving as advocate for the patient when the prescribed intervention is ineffective in relieving pain. In addition, the nurse serves as educator to the patient and family to enable them to manage the prescribed intervention themselves when appropriate.

Identifying Goals for Pain Management

The information the nurse obtains by assessing the patient is used to identify goals for managing the pain. The goals identified are shared or validated with the patient. For a few patients, the goal may be total elimination of the pain. For many, however, this expectation is unrealistic. Other goals may include a decrease in the intensity, duration, or frequency of pain and a decrease in the negative effects the pain has on the patient. For example, pain may have a negative effect by decreasing appetite or interfering with sleep and thereby hampering recovery from an acute illness. In such instances the goals might be to sleep soundly and to take adequate nutrition. Chronic pain may decrease the person's quality of life by interfering with work or interpersonal relationships. Thus, a goal may be to decrease time lost from work or increase the quality of interpersonal relationships.

To determine the goal, a number of factors are considered. The first is the severity of the pain, as judged by the patient. The second factor is the anticipated harmful effects of pain. A "high-risk" patient is at much greater risk for the harmful effects of pain than a young healthy patient. The third factor is the anticipated duration of the pain. In patients with pain from a disease such as cancer, the pain may be prolonged, possibly for the remainder of the patient's life. In these cases interventions will be needed for some time and should not detract from the quality of life. A different set of interventions is available to those likely to have pain for only a few days or weeks.

The goals for the patient may be accomplished by pharmacologic or nonpharmacologic, noninvasive means. In the acute stages of illness, the patient may be unable to participate actively in relief measures, but when sufficient mental and physical energy is present, the patient may learn self-management techniques to relieve the pain. Thus, as the patient progresses through the stages of recovery, a goal may be to increase the patient's use of self-management pain-relief measures.

Nurse–Patient Relationship and Patient Teaching

Two nursing measures basic to all others in pain management are: (1) the nurse–patient relationship and (2) patient teaching about pain and how to relieve it. These activities may reduce pain in the absence of other pain-relief measures. Each may also enhance the effectiveness of other pain-relief measures used.

A positive nurse–patient relationship is essential to effective communication and teaching. Trust is an important element in this relationship. Conveying to the patient the nurse's belief that the patient has pain often helps reduce anxiety. To say to the patient, "I know that you have pain," often will set the patient's mind at rest. Occasionally, a patient who fears that no one believes his or her reports of pain is relieved when he or she knows that the nurse can be trusted and believes the pain exists.

The nurse also provides information through patient teaching about how pain can be controlled. The patient is informed, for example, that pain should be reported in the early stages. When the patient waits too long to report pain, the pain may become so intense that it is difficult to relieve.

A positive nurse–patient relationship and teaching are key to the management of analgesia in the patient with pain because open communication and patient cooperation are essential to success. Teaching is equally important because the patient or family may be responsible for managing the pain at home and preventing and managing side effects.

Providing Physical Care

The patient in pain may be unable to participate in usual activities of daily living or to perform usual self-care. Therefore, it is important to assist the person whose pain interferes with self-care to carry out these activities. The patient is often more comfortable when physical and self-care needs have been met and effort has been made to assure as comfortable a position as possible. A fresh gown and change of bed linens along with efforts to make the person feel refreshed (*e.g.*, brushing teeth, combing hair) often increase the level of comfort and improve the effectiveness of the pain-relief measures.

Providing physical care to the patient also gives the nurse the opportunity to perform a complete assessment and to identify problems that may contribute to the patient's discomfort and pain. Appropriate and gentle physical touch during care may be reassuring and comforting.

Managing Anxiety Related to Pain

Anxiety may affect a patient's response to pain. The patient who anticipates pain may become increasingly anxious. Teaching the patient about the nature of the impending painful experience and the ways available to reduce pain often decreases anxiety. A person who is experiencing pain will use previously learned strategies to reduce pain. Learning about measures to relieve pain may lessen the threat of pain and give the person a sense of control.

What the nurse explains about the available pain-relief measures and their effectiveness may also affect anxiety. The patient's anxiety may be reduced by explanations that point out the degree of pain relief that can be expected from each measure. For example, the patient who is informed beforehand that an intervention may not eliminate pain completely is less likely to become anxious when a certain amount of pain persists. Anxiety resulting from anticipation of pain or the pain experience itself may often be managed effectively by establishing a relationship with the patient and by patient teaching (see Nurse–Patient Relationship and Patient Teaching, p. 188).

A patient who is anxious about pain, may be less tolerant of the pain. This in turn may increase the level of anxiety further. It is important to interrupt this process to prevent the pain and anxiety from escalating. Low levels of pain are easier to reduce or control than are more intense levels. Consequently, pain-relief measures should be used before pain becomes severe. Many patients believe that they should not request pain-relief measures until they are unable to tolerate the pain, making it difficult for medications to provide relief. Therefore, it is important to explain to all patients that pain relief or control is more successful if pain-relief measures are used *before* pain becomes unbearable.

Pain Management Strategies

Reducing pain to a "tolerable" level was once considered the goal of pain management. However, even patients who have described pain relief as adequate often report disturbed sleep and marked distress because of pain. In view of the harmful effects of pain and inadequate pain management, the goal of merely making the pain tolerable has been replaced by the goal of relieving the pain. Pain management strategies include both pharmacologic and nonpharmacologic approaches. These approaches are selected on the basis of the individual patient's requirements and goals. Appropriate analgesics are used as prescribed and should *not* be considered only as a last resort when other pain relief measures fail. Any intervention will be most successful if initiated before the pain becomes severe, and the greatest success is often achieved if several interventions are applied simultaneously.

Pharmacologic Interventions

Managing a patient's pain through pharmacologic interventions is accomplished in collaboration with the physician or other primary care provider and the patient. Specific medications for pain management may be prescribed or an epidural catheter may be inserted to administer the initial dose. However, it is the nurse who maintains the analgesia, assesses its effectiveness, and reports if the intervention is ineffective or produces side effects. Management of pain requires close collaboration and effective communication among health care providers.

Assessment Prior to Administering Analgesia

Prior to administration of any medication, the patient is asked about allergies to medications and the nature of any previous allergic responses. True allergic or anaphylactic responses to opioids are uncommon. The patient's description of responses or reactions should be documented and reported before the medication is administered.

The patient's medication history (*i.e.*, current, usual, or recent use of prescription and over-the-counter medications) is obtained along with a history of health problems. Certain drugs or conditions may affect the analgesia's effectiveness or the metabolism and excretion of analgesic medications.

Prior to administering analgesic agents for pain relief, the nurse should assess the patient's current status, including the intensity of the pain, changes in intensity of pain following the previous dose of medication, and side effects of the medication.

Approaches for Using Analgesic Agents

Medications are most effective when the dose and interval between doses is individualized to meet the patient's needs. The only safe and effective way to administer analgesic medications is by asking the patient to rate the pain and by observing the response to medications.

Preventive Approach

A preventive approach to administering analgesics is considered the most effective strategy for relieving pain because it maintains a therapeutic level of the medication in the patient's serum. With the preventive approach, analgesics are administered at set intervals so that the medication is given before the pain becomes intensely severe; when the pain becomes intense, the serum level has fallen to a sub-therapeutic level. The lower the serum opioid level has fallen, the more difficult it will be to achieve the therapeutic level with the next dose.

Administering analgesic medication on a time basis, rather than on the basis of the patient's complaint or report of pain prevents the serum level from falling to subtherapeutic levels. If the patient's pain is likely to occur around the clock or for a great portion of a 24-hour period, a regular around-the-clock schedule of administering analgesia may be indicated. Even if the analgesic is prescribed "as-needed" or "prn," it can be administered on a preventive basis before it is needed as long as the prescribed interval between doses is observed. The preventive approach reduces the peaks and troughs in the serum level and provides more pain relief for the patient with fewer adverse effects.

Smaller doses of medication are needed with the preventive approach because the pain does not escalate to a level of severe intensity. Thus, a preventive approach may result in less medication over a 24-hour period, thereby helping prevent tolerance to analgesics and decreasing the severity of side effects (*e.g.*, sedation and constipation). Better pain control can be achieved with a preventive approach, reducing the amount of time the patient spends in pain. In addition, there is low risk of the patient craving analgesia because of pain.

With the "as-needed" or "prn" approach, the patient usually experiences pain, obtains the analgesic, and waits for it to take effect. This may result in the person spending several hours within a 24-hour period in pain. A person who receives inadequate analgesia for pain is more likely to crave the medication than one whose pain is relieved before it becomes distressing.

Individualized Doses

The dose and the interval between doses should be based on the individual patient's requirements rather than on an inflexible standard or routine. People metabolize and absorb medications at different rates and experience different levels of pain. Therefore, one dosage of an opioid (narcotic) medication given at specified intervals may be effective for one patient but ineffective for another.

Because of the fear of promoting addiction or causing respiratory depression, health care providers tend to prescribe or administer inadequate doses of opioid agents to treat acute pain or chronic pain in the terminally ill patient. However, even prolonged administration of opioid agents is associated with an extremely low incidence of addiction. Furthermore, small doses are not necessarily safe doses. For example, some patients receiving 25 mg to 50 mg of meperidine intramuscularly (IM) have been reported to suffer life-threatening respiratory depression, whereas other patients have not exhibited any sedation or respiratory depression after 200 mg of meperidine IM.

Therefore, it is essential that the effects of opioids be monitored, especially when the first dose is given or when the dose is changed or given more frequently. The time, date, the patient's pain rating (scale of 0 to 10), the analgesic agent, other pain-relief measures, side effects, and patient activity are recorded.

When the first dose of an analgesic is administered it is important to record a pain rating score, blood pressure, and respiratory and pulse rates. If the pain has not decreased 1 hour later and the patient is reasonably alert and has a satisfactory respiratory status, blood pressure, and pulse rate, then some change in analgesia is indicated. Although the analgesia dose is safe for this patient, it is ineffective in relieving the pain. Therefore, another dose of analgesia may be indicated. In such instances, the nurse consults with the physician to determine what further action is warranted.

Patient-Controlled Analgesia

Patient-controlled analgesia (PCA) has been used effectively to manage postoperative pain as well as chronic pain. PCA allows patients to control the administration of their own medication within predetermined safety limits. This approach can be used with oral analgesics as well as with continuous infusions of opioid analgesics by intravenous, subcutaneous, or epidural routes. Additionally, PCA can be used in the hospital or home setting.

PCA pumps (Fig. 13-4) permit patients to self-administer continuous infusions of medication within limits of safety, thus enabling them to administer extra medication with episodes of increased pain or painful activities. A PCA pump is an electronically controlled infusion pump with a timing device. Patients experiencing pain can administer small amounts of medication directly into their intravenous, subcutaneous, or epidural catheter by pressing a button. The pump then delivers a preset amount of analgesic medication.

The timer can be programmed to prevent additional doses from being administered until a specified time period has elapsed. This safety measure prevents the patient from administering a second dose until the first dose has had time to exert its maximal effect. Even if the patient pushes the button multiple times in rapid succession, no additional doses are released. If another dose is required at the end of the delay period, the button must be pushed again to receive the dose. Patients who are controlling their own opioid administration usually become sedated and stop pushing the button before any significant respiratory depression occurs. Nevertheless, assessing respiratory status remains a major role for the nurse caring for the patient receiving PCA.

The PCA pump can be programmed to deliver a constant, background infusion of medication and still allow the patient to administer additional doses as needed. A background infusion plus PCA may be effective with cancer patients who require large doses of analgesia. This may allow more uninterrupted sleep, but carries with it an increased risk of sedation, especially when the patient is using small doses.

Patients who use these pumps for pain control achieve better pain relief and require less pain medication than those who are treated in the standard "prn" fashion. Because the patient is able to maintain a near-constant level of medication, periods of severe pain and sedation that occur with the traditional prn regimen are avoided.

When PCA or any analgesia is used at home or in the hospital it is important to avoid playing "catch-up." The pain should be brought under control before the pump is started. PCA pumps deliver minute amounts of medication at a time with a delay period between doses. If the patient with severe pain has a low serum level of opioid, it is very difficult to regain control with the small doses available by pump. Prior to the PCA pump being used, small doses of intravenous (IV) opioid may be administered as prescribed over a short period of time until the pain is relieved; the patient is then placed on the PCA pump. If pain control is not achieved with the maximal dose of medication prescribed, further prescriptions are obtained. The goal is to achieve a serum level of opioid that will control the pain and allow the patient to maintain that level with the PCA pump. The patient who is receiving PCA is instructed *not* to wait until the pain is severe

Home Care Considerations. If PCA is to be used in the patient's home, the patient and family are taught about the actions and side effects of the medication and the operation of the pump. Family members are cautioned not to push the button for the patient, especially if the patient is asleep, because this overrides some of the safety features of the system.

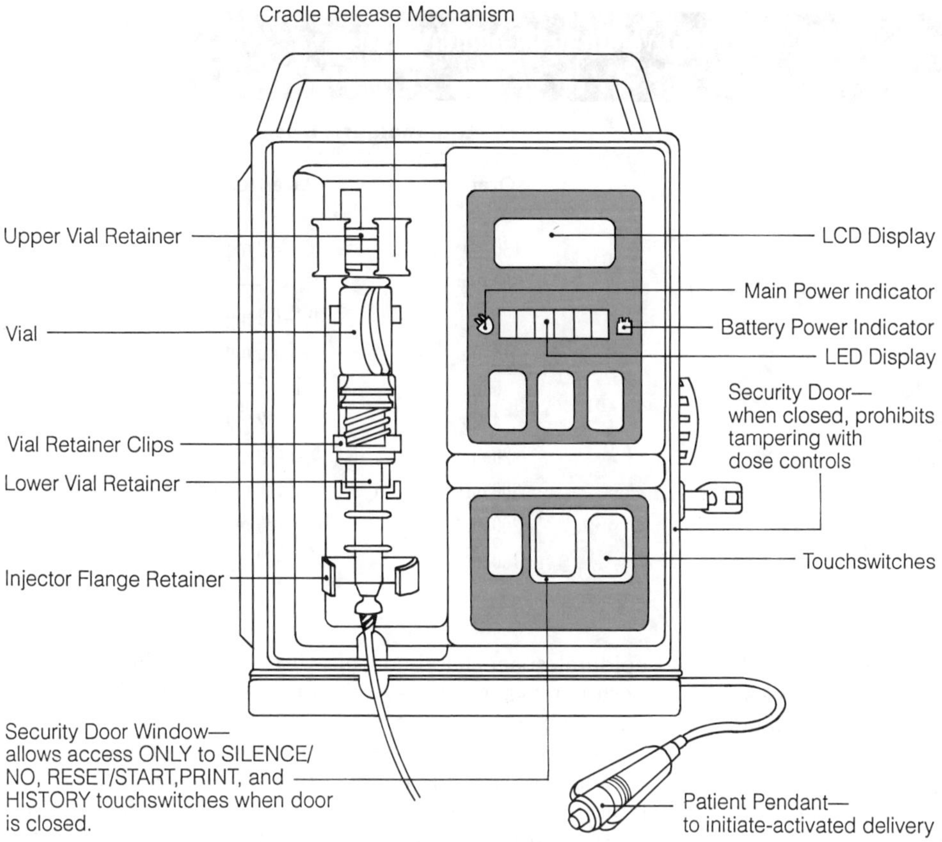

FIGURE 13-4. Patient-controlled analgesia pump.

Routes of Administration of Analgesic Agents

The route for administering analgesics is based on the patient's condition and the desired effect of the drug. Analgesics can be administered through parenteral (intravenous, intramuscular, or subcutaneous) routes, oral, rectal, and transdermal (through the skin) routes, and through epidural or intraspinal catheters. Each of these methods of administration has advantages and disadvantages; the route chosen should be based on the requirements of the individual patient.

Parenteral Administration

Parenteral administration (intramuscular, intravenous, or subcutaneous routes) of the analgesic produces more rapid effects than oral administration, but these effects are of shorter duration. Parenteral administration may also be indicated if the patient is not permitted any oral intake or is vomiting. When medication is administered by the **intramuscular route,** it enters the blood stream slowly and is metabolized slowly.

The **IV route** is an alternative to intramuscular (IM) injection of opioid analgesia. The IV route is the preferred parenteral route of administration of analgesic medications. It is much more comfortable for the patient and peak serum levels and pain relief occur much more rapidly. Because it peaks rapidly (usually within minutes) and is metabolized quickly, an appropriate IV dose will be smaller and prescribed at shorter intervals than an IM dose.

IV opioids (narcotics) may be administered by IV "push" (or "slow push," *e.g.*, over a 5- to 10-minute period) or by continuous infusion with a pump. The continuous method provides a steady level of analgesia and is indicated when pain occurs over a 24-hour period, such as postoperatively for the first day or so or in a patient with prolonged cancer pain who cannot take medication by other routes. The dose of analgesic is calculated carefully to relieve pain without producing respiratory depression and other side effects.

The **subcutaneous route** for infusion of opioid analgesics is used for patients with severe pain such as cancer pain; it is particularly useful for patients with limited intravenous access who are unable to take oral medications and patients who are managing their pain at home. The dose of opioid that can be infused through this route is limited because of the small volume that can be administered at one time into the subcutaneous tissue. However, this route is often an effective and convenient way to manage pain.

Oral Route

The oral route is preferred over parenteral administration if the patient is able to take medication by mouth, because it is easy, noninvasive, and not painful, as are injections. Severe pain can be relieved with oral narcotics *if* the doses are high enough. To be effective, however, dosage must be altered because drugs are absorbed at different rates depending on the route of administration. See Table 13-2 for a list of selected analgesics equivalent to 10 mg of morphine.

TABLE 13-2 Doses of Analgesic Equivalent to IM Administration of 10 mg of Morphine

	Equianalgesic Doses	
	Oral	Parenteral
Morphine	30 mg	10 mg
Controlled release morphine (MSContin, Roxanol)	60 mg	—
Fentanyl (Sublimaze)	—	0.1–0.2 mg
Hyromorphone (Dilaudid)	8 mg	1.5 mg
Oxymorphone (Numorphan)	6 mg	1–1.5 mg
Levophanol (Levo-Dromoran)	4 mg	2 mg
Methadone (Dolophine)	20 mg	7–10 mg
Meperidine (Demerol)	300 mg	100 mg
Codeine (with aspirin or acetaminophen)	200 mg	130 mg
Pentazocaine (Talwin)	150 mg	30–60 mg

In terminally ill patients with prolonged pain, doses may gradually be increased as the disease progresses and causes more pain or as the person builds up a tolerance to the medication. If these higher doses are increased gradually, they usually provide additional pain relief without producing respiratory depression or sedation. If the route of administration is changed from a parenteral route to the oral route at a dose that is not equivalent in strength (equianalgesic), the smaller oral dose may result in a withdrawal reaction and recurrence of pain.

Rectal Route

The rectal route of administration may be indicated in patients who are unable to take medications by any other route. Rectal suppositories of 10 mg of oxymorphone (Numorphan; two suppositories, totaling 10 mg) provide pain relief equivalent to that of 10 mg of morphine IM or 100 mg of meperidine IM. The rectal route may also be indicated for patients with bleeding problems, such as hemophilia.

Transdermal Route

The transdermal route has been used to achieve a consistent level of opioids in the serum through absorption of the medication through the skin. Commercially available transdermal systems consist of a reservoir containing the medication and a membrane. The size of the surface area of the membrane regulates the rate of drug delivery. When the transdermal system is first applied to the skin, the medication is absorbed, the opioid-binding sites in the skin slowly become saturated, and the serum level of opioid slowly rises. The slow absorption from these binding sites after the system is removed accounts for a slow decline in the serum level. This method has been used to manage postoperative pain as well as cancer pain.

Intraspinal Routes

Infusion of opioids or local anesthetic agents into the subarachnoid space (intrathecal space or spinal canal) or epidural space has been effective in controlling pain in postoperative patients as well as those with chronic pain unrelieved by other methods.

A catheter is inserted into the subarachnoid or the epidural space at the thoracic or lumbar level for administration of opioid or anesthetic agents (Fig. 13-5). With *intrathecal* administration, the medication is infused directly into the subarachnoid space and cerebrospinal fluid, which surrounds the spinal cord; with *epidural* administration, it is deposited in the dura of the spinal canal and diffuses into the subarachnoid space. Pain relief from intraspinal administration of opioids is based on the existence of opioid receptors in the spinal cord.

Repeated infusion of opioids and local anesthetics through an intrathecal or epidural catheter results in pain relief without many of the side effects of systemic analgesia, including sedation. Adverse effects associated with intraspinal administration include spinal headache because of loss of spinal fluid when the dura is punctured. The dura must be punctured with the intrathecal route and may occur inadvertently with the epidural route. Only medications without preservatives should be administered into the subarachnoid or epidural space because of potential neurotoxic effects of preservative agents.

If analgesics are required for a longer period or if the patient has persistent, severe pain secondary to a terminal disease (*e.g.*, cancer), the catheter may be tunneled through the subcutaneous tissue and the inlet or port placed under the skin. The opioid analgesic is injected through the skin into the outlet or port and catheter, which delivers the medication directly into the subarachnoid or epidural space. The analgesic may need to be injected several times a day to maintain an adequate level of pain relief.

In those patients who require more frequent doses or continuous infusions of opioids to relieve the pain, an implantable infusion device or pump may be used to administer the opioid continuously. The medication is administered at a small, constant dose at a preset rate into the epidural or subarachnoid space. The reservoir of the infusion device

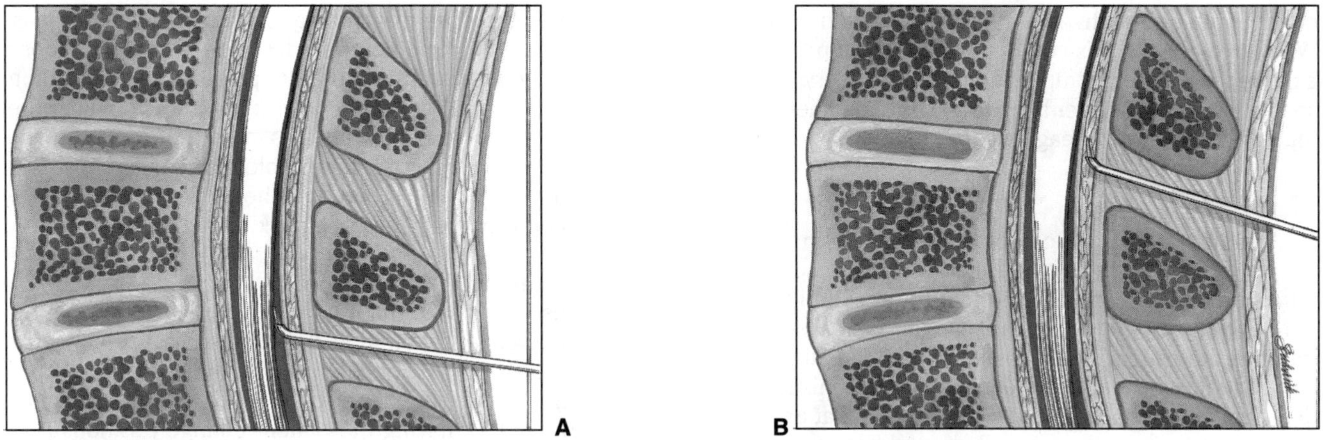

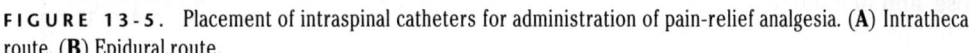

FIGURE 13-5. Placement of intraspinal catheters for administration of pain-relief analgesia. (**A**) Intrathecal route. (**B**) Epidural route.

stores the medication for slow release and needs to be refilled once every 1 or 2 months, depending on the patient's needs. This eliminates the need for repeated injections through the skin.

Very small doses of opioid analgesics can be administered by intraspinal routes to treat pain with little effect on pulse, respiration, or blood pressure. Risk of side effects such as respiratory depression and sedation is reduced because of the small doses given. However, the patient must be monitored for delayed respiratory depression. Opioid antagonists such as naloxone (Narcan) must be available to reverse respiratory depression if it occurs.

Although respiratory depression generally peaks 6 to 12 hours after epidural opioids are administered, it can occur earlier or up to 24 hours after the first injection. Therefore the patient is monitored very closely for at least the first 24 hours after the first injection and longer if changes in respiratory status or level of consciousness occur. The patient is also observed for urinary retention, pruritus, nausea, vomiting, and dizziness. Precautions must be taken to minimize the risk of infection at the catheter site and displacement of the catheter.

Nursing Considerations. When an epidural catheter is inserted for pain control it is usually the nurse who is responsible for the pain management regimen. Baseline information must be obtained to provide safe and effective pain control: (1) at what level or site has the catheter been inserted, (2) what medications (*i.e.*, local anesthetics or opioids) have been administered, and (3) what medications are anticipated in the future?

Spinal headache with loss of spinal fluid if the dura has been punctured and cardiovascular effects (hypotension and decreased heart rate) may occur owing to relaxation of the vasculature in the lower extremities. Therefore, the patient is assessed frequently for headache, decreased blood pressure, pulse rate, and urinary output.

Home Care Considerations. Both the patient who will receive analgesic at home through an epidural system and the family must be taught the correct procedure to administer the prescribed medication using sterile technique and how to assess for infection.

Specific Anesthetic and Analgesic Agents

Local Anesthetic Agents

Local anesthetics work by blocking nerve conduction when applied directly to the nerve fibers. They can be applied directly to the site of injury (*e.g.*, topical anesthetic spray for sunburn) or directly to nerve fibers through injection or at the time of surgery. Additionally, they can be administered through an epidural catheter.

Topical Application of Local Anesthetic Agents. The use of local anesthetic has been successful in reducing pain associated with thoracic or upper abdominal surgery when injected by the surgeon intercostally. Local anesthetics are rapidly absorbed into the blood stream resulting in decreased availability at the surgical or injury site and an increased anesthetic level in the blood, increasing the risk of toxicity. Therefore, a vasoconstrictive agent (*e.g.*, epinephrine or phenylephrine) is added to the anesthetic to decrease systemic absorption of the anesthetic and maintain its concentration at the surgical or injury site.

A new topical anesthetic agent has been introduced in the United States recently and is expected to be used more often. EMLA (eutectic mixture or emulsion of local anesthetics) has been used effectively for preventing pain associated with invasive procedures such as lumbar puncture. Although EMLA has been used primarily with children thus far, it is likely to be used with other age groups. To be effective, it must be applied to the site 60 to 90 minutes before the procedure is performed.

Intraspinal Administration of Local Anesthetic Agents. Intermittent or continuous administration of local anesthetics through an epidural or spinal catheter has been used for many years to produce anesthesia during surgery. Although administration of local anesthetics in the spinal canal is still largely confined to the operating room and labor and delivery suite, epidural administration of local anesthetics for pain management is increasing.

A local anesthetic administered through an epidural catheter is applied directly to the nerve root. It can be administered continuously in low doses, intermittently on a schedule, or on demand as the patient requires it, and is often combined with epidural administration of opioids. When treated with this combination, surgical patients have experienced fewer complications after surgery, ambulate sooner, and have shorter hospital stays than patients receiving standard therapy (Yeager et al, 1987).

Opioids

Opioids (narcotics) can be administered through a variety of routes, including oral, intravenous, subcutaneous, intraspinal, rectal, and transdermal routes. The goal of administration of opioids is to relieve the patient's pain and improve the patient's quality of life; therefore, the route of administration, dose, and frequency of administration are determined on an individual basis. Factors that are considered in determining the route, dose, and frequency of medication include characteristics of the patient's pain (*i.e.*, its expected duration and severity), the overall status of the patient, the patient's response to analgesics, and his or her report of pain. Although the oral route is usually preferred for the administration of opioids, oral opioids must be given frequently enough and in large enough doses to be effective.

If the patient is expected to require opioid analgesia at home, the ability of the patient and family to administer opioids as prescribed is considered in planning. Steps must be taken to ensure that the medication will be available to the patient. Many pharmacies, especially those in smaller rural areas or inner cities, may be reluctant to stock large amounts of opioids. Therefore, arrangements for obtaining these prescriptions must be made ahead of time.

With administration of opioids by any route, side effects must be considered and anticipated. Anticipating and taking steps to minimize side effects will increase the likelihood that the patient will receive adequate pain relief without interrupting their use to treat these effects.

Side Effects of Opioids (Narcotics)

Respiratory Depression and Sedation

Respiratory depression is the most serious adverse effect when opioids are administered by IV, subcutaneous, or epidural routes, yet its occurrence is relatively rare because of the small doses of opioid administered through these routes and increasing tolerance if the dose is increased slowly. The risk of respiratory depression increases with advancing age and concomitant use of other opioids or other central nervous system depressants. With the epidural route, risk of respiratory depression also increases with placement of the catheter in the thoracic area and with increased intra-abdominal or intrathoracic pressure.

The patient who is receiving opioids by any route must be assessed frequently for changes in respiratory status. Specific changes that must be noted are decreasing respiratory rate or shallow respirations. Despite the risks associated with their use, intravenous and epidural opioids are considered safe, with risks of epidural administration no greater than those of intravenous or other systemic routes of administration.

Sedation may occur with any method of administering opioids. Although it is likely to occur when opioid doses are increased, the patient often develops tolerance quickly. That is, in a short period of time, the patient no longer becomes sedated by the dose that initially caused sedation. Increasing the period of time between doses or reducing the dose temporarily, as prescribed, usually prevents deep sedation from occurring. The patient at risk for sedation must be monitored very closely for changes in respiratory status. The patient is also at risk for other problems associated with sedation and immobility. Therefore, the nurse must take measures to prevent problems such as skin breakdown.

Nausea and Vomiting

Nausea and vomiting may occur with use of opioids. When nausea and vomiting do occur it is usually some hours after the initial injection. Opioid-induced nausea and vomiting are often triggered by position change and may be prevented by having the patient change positions *very* slowly. Adequate hydration may also decrease the incidence.

Constipation

Constipation is a common side effect of opioids or narcotics. Unless prevented, constipation may become so severe that the patient is forced to choose between pain and relief of constipation. This situation can occur in the postoperative patient and in the patient who is receiving large doses to treat chronic pain due to cancer. Prevention of constipation must be a high priority in all patients receiving opioids.

A number of strategies have been used to prevent and treat opioid-related constipation. High intake of fluid and fiber and the use of mild laxatives are often effective in managing mild constipation. Unless contraindicated, a mild laxative should be administered on a regular schedule for those patients receiving opioids for pain relief. Severe constipation often requires use of a stimulating cathartic agent (*e.g.*, senna derivatives [Senokot] or bisacodyl [Dulcolax]). Using laxatives at bedtime and rectal suppositories in the morning may prevent constipation (AHCPR, 1994).

Inadequate Pain Relief

One factor commonly associated with ineffective pain relief is administration of an inadequate dose of opioid. This is most likely to occur when the route of administration of opioids is changed and the differences in absorption and action are not considered. Consequently, the patient receives doses too small to be effective and may receive them too infrequently to relieve pain adequately. For example, if an opioid is changed from the intravenous or epidural route to the oral route, the oral dose must be approximately three times greater than that given parenterally to provide relief. Because of differences in absorption of oral opioids among individuals, the patient must be assessed carefully to assure that the pain is adequately relieved. Refer to Table 13-2 for a list of opioids and dosages equivalent to morphine.

Addiction and Tolerance

Addiction is a behavioral pattern of substance use characterized by a compulsion to take the drug primarily to experience its psychic effects. Fear of patients becoming addicted or dependent on opioids has contributed to inadequate treatment of pain. This fear is common in health care providers as well as patients and results from lack of knowledge about the low risk of addiction. Research has shown that even prolonged administration of an opioid is associated with a less than 0.2% incidence of addiction (Schug et al, 1992).

Tolerance is the need for increasing doses of opioids to achieve the same effect. Patients requiring long-term use of opioids, especially cancer patients, will develop a tolerance to opioids. That is, they will need increasing doses to relieve pain; however, they are *not* addicted. Physical tolerance usually occurs in the *absence of addiction*. Tolerance to opioids is common and becomes a problem primarily in terms of delivering or administering the medication (*e.g.*, how to administer thousands of milligrams of morphine a day to a patient). On the other hand, addiction is *rare* and should rarely if ever be the primary concern of the nurse caring for a patient in pain.

Other Concerns

Pruritus (itching) is a common problem seen with opioids administered through any route. It can be relieved by administration of antihistamines or small doses of naloxone. Epidural opioids may also cause urinary retention which may necessitate urinary catheterization.

A number of factors may influence the safety and effectiveness of opioids. Opioid analgesics are primarily metabolized by the liver and excreted by the kidney. Therefore, metabolism and excretion of analgesic medications will be impaired in patients with *liver or kidney disease*, increasing the risk of cumulative or toxic effects. In addition, normeperidine, a metabolite of meperidine (Demerol) may accumulate to toxic levels in patients with impaired kidney function and can produce seizures in susceptible patients.

Patients with untreated *hypothyroidism* are more susceptible to analgesic effects and side effects of opioids. On the other hand, patients with *hyperthyroidism* may require larger doses for relief of pain. Patients with *decreased respiratory reserve* from disease or aging may be more susceptible to the depressant effects of opioids and must be carefully monitored for respiratory depression.

Dehydrated patients are at increased risk for the hypotensive effects of opioids. Patients who become *hypotensive* following administration of an opioid should be kept recumbent and rehydrated unless contraindicated. Patients who are dehydrated are also more likely to experience nausea and vomiting with opiod use. Rehydration usually relieves these symptoms.

Patients who have been receiving certain *other medications*, such as monoamine oxidase (MAO) inhibitors, phenothiazines, or tricyclic antidepressants, may have an exaggerated response to the depressant effects of opioids. Patients on these medications should receive small doses of opioids and must be monitored closely. Continued pain in these patients indicates that a therapeutic level of the analgesic has not been achieved. The patient must be monitored for sedation even if an analgesic effect has not been obtained.

Nonsteroidal Anti-inflammatory Drugs (NSAIDs)

Nonsteroidal anti-inflammatory drug (NSAIDs) are thought to decrease pain by inhibiting the production of prostaglandin from traumatized or inflamed tissues, which prevents pain receptors from becoming sensitive to previously non-noxious stimuli. In addition to the antiprostaglandin activity of NSAIDs, these agents may also have a central action.

Aspirin is the most common nonsteroidal anti-inflammatory drug. However, because it causes frequent and severe side effects, it is infrequently used to treat significant acute or chronic pain. Ibuprofen is used now to relieve mild to moderate pain, because it is effective and has a low incidence of adverse effects.

NSAIDs are very effective in the treatment of arthritic diseases and have been used with opioids to treat postoperative and other severe pain (Parker et al., 1994; Ready et al., 1994). The use of an NSAID with an opioid relieves pain more effectively than the opioid alone. The patient is often able to obtain pain relief with less opioid and fewer side effects.

NSAIDs may be useful in patients who are susceptible to the respiratory depressing effects of opioids or have built up a tolerance to opioids because of long-term use. In these cases use of NSAID decreases the amount of opioids needed. For NSAIDs to be effective, a therapeutic level must be maintained. Therefore, they should be administered around the clock (a preventive approach).

NSAIDs are well tolerated by most patients. However, those with impaired kidney function may require a smaller dose and must be monitored closely for side effects. NSAIDs may displace other medications (*e.g.*, warfarin) from serum proteins and increase their effects.

Gerontologic Considerations

Physiologic changes in the elderly make it imperative that analgesics be administered with caution. Drug interactions are more likely to occur in the elderly because of the higher incidence of chronic illness and increased use of prescription and over-the-counter drugs. Before administering opioid and non-opioid analgesics to the elderly, it is important to obtain a careful medication history to identify potential drug interactions.

Absorption and metabolism of drugs are altered in the elderly patient because of decreased liver, renal, and gastrointestinal function. In addition, changes in body weight, protein stores, and distribution of body fluid alter the distribution of drugs in the body. As a result, drugs are not metabolized as quickly and blood levels of the drug remain higher for a longer period. The elderly patient is more sensitive to medications and is at increased risk of drug toxicity.

Opioid and non-opioid analgesics can be given effectively to the elderly, but must be used cautiously because of increased susceptibility to depression of both the nervous and the respiratory systems. Meperidine must be used with particular caution because decreased binding of the drug by plasma proteins results in blood concentrations of the drug twice those found in younger patients. Because the elderly are generally more sensitive to analgesics, it is advisable to begin with a smaller dose of a non-opioid analgesic, increase the dose slowly, and add additional medications carefully. Frequent monitoring is necessary for safe, effective pain relief.

In many cases, the initial dose of analgesia prescribed for an elderly patient may be the same as that for a younger person or slightly smaller than the normal dose, but because of slowed metabolism and excretion due to aging, the safe interval for subsequent doses may need to be lengthened. As always, the best guide to pain management and administration of analgesia in all patients regardless of age is what the patient says. The elderly may obtain more pain relief for a longer period of time than a younger patient; as a result, smaller, less frequent doses may be required.

Nonpharmacologic Measures

Many patients and health team members tend to regard medication as the only method for relieving pain. However, many nonpharmacologic nursing activities can assist in relieving pain. Although there are many anecdotal reports about the effectiveness of these measures, few of them have yet been evaluated through systematic research studies. Nonpharmacologic methods of pain relief usually have very low risks. Although such measures are not a substitute for medication, they may be all that is necessary or appropriate for brief episodes of pain lasting only seconds or minutes. In other instances, especially when there is severe pain that lasts for hours or days, combining nonpharmacologic techniques with medications may be the most effective way to relieve pain.

Cutaneous Stimulation and Massage

The gate control theory of pain as described earlier, proposes that the stimulation of fibers that transmit nonpainful sensations blocks or decreases the transmission of pain impulses. Several nonpharmacologic pain relief strategies, including rubbing the skin and using heat and cold, are based on this mechanism.

Massage is generalized cutaneous stimulation of the body, often concentrating on the back and shoulders. A massage does not specifically stimulate the nonpain receptors in the same receptor field as the pain receptors but it may have an impact through the descending control system (see earlier discussion). Massage may make the patient more comfortable because it produces muscle relaxation.

Ice and Heat Therapies

Ice and heat therapies may be effective pain relief strategies in some circumstances; however, their effectiveness and mechanism of action need further study. It is thought that ice and heat therapy work by stimulating the nonpain receptors (non-nociceptors) in the same receptor field as the injury.

Ice therapy may decrease prostaglandins, which intensify the sensitivity of pain receptors, and other substances at the site of injury by inhibiting the inflammatory process. To be effective, ice should be placed on the injury site *immediately* after injury. Cohn et al. (1989) showed that when ice was placed around the knee immediately after surgery and for 4 days postoperatively, analgesic requirements decreased by about 50%.

Application of heat has the advantage of increasing blood flow to an area and could possibly contribute to pain reduction by speeding healing. However, dry heat supplied by a heating lamp does not appear to be as effective as ice (Nam & Park, 1991). Both dry and moist heat therapies probably provide some analgesia but additional research is required to understand their mechanisms of action and the appropriate indications for their use. Both ice and heat therapy must be applied carefully and monitored to avoid injury to the skin.

Transcutaneous Electrical Nerve Stimulation

Transcutaneous electrical nerve stimulation (TENS) uses a battery-operated unit with electrodes applied to the skin to produce a tingling, vibrating, or buzzing sensation in the area of pain (Fig. 13-6). It has been used in both acute and chronic pain relief. TENS is believed to decrease pain by stimulating the nonpain receptors (non-nociceptors) in the same area as the fibers that transmit the pain. This mechanism is consistent with the gate control theory of pain. The nonpain receptors are thought to block the transmission of pain signals to the brain on the ascending pathways of the central nervous system. This would explain the effectiveness of cutaneous stimulation when applied in the same area as an injury. For example, when TENS is used in a postoperative patient, the electrodes are placed around the surgical wound. Other explanations for the effectiveness of TENS are the placebo effect (the patient expects it to be effective) and the production of endorphins, which also block pain transmission.

Research has shown that patients receiving either real or sham (placebo) TENS treatment in addition to standard care, will report a similar amount of pain relief that is greater than the pain relief obtained with standard treatment alone (Conn, et al, 1986). Some patients, especially those with chronic pain, will report as much as a 50% reduction in their pain when using TENS. Other patients will receive no benefit. Which ones will be helped is unpredictable. When patients do experience pain relief it is usually of rapid onset but quickly diminishes when the stimulator is turned off.

Distraction

Distraction, which involves focusing the patient's attention on something other than the pain, can be a very successful strategy and may be the mechanism responsible for other effective cognitive techniques (Arntz et al., 1991; Devine et al., 1990). A person, who is less aware of pain or pays less attention to it, will be less bothered by pain and more tolerant of it. Distraction is thought to reduce the perception of pain by stimulating the descending control system, resulting in fewer painful stimuli being transmitted to the brain. The effectiveness of distraction depends on the patient's ability to receive and create sensory input other than pain. Pain relief is generally increased in direct relation to the person's active participation, the number of sensory modalities used, and the person's interest in the stimuli. Therefore, the stimulation of sight, sound, and touch is likely to be more effective in reducing pain than stimulation of a single sense.

Distraction may range from simply preventing monotony to using highly complex physical and mental activities.

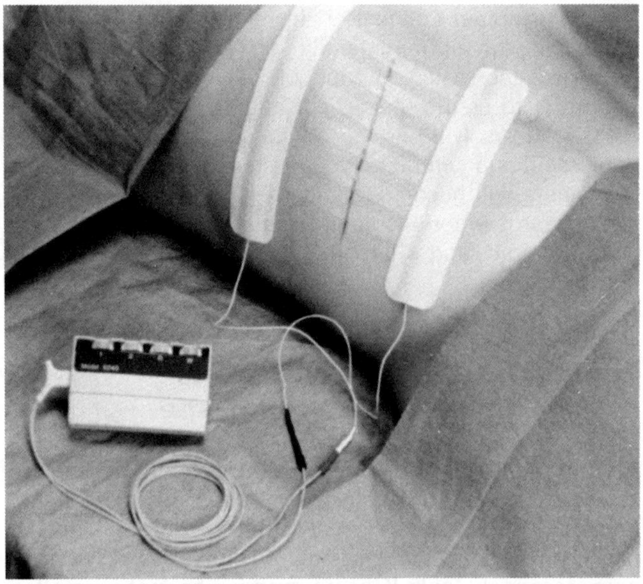

FIGURE 13-6. Transcutaneous electrical nerve stimulation (TENS) being used for relief of incisional pain postoperatively. (Courtesy of Health Care Specialties Division/3M, St. Paul, MN.)

Visits from family and friends are very effective in relieving pain. Watching an action-packed movie on a large screen with "surround sound" through headphones may be effective (provided the person finds it acceptable). Others may benefit from games and activities (*e.g.*, chess) that require concentration. Not all patients obtain pain relief with distraction, especially those in severe pain. With severe pain, the patient may be unable to concentrate well enough to participate in complex physical or mental activities.

One drawback to distraction must be considered. A patient who is using a PCA pump, during the time of effective distraction may not self-administer any analgesia. Distraction techniques usually end suddenly (*i.e.*, the activity ends or the movie ends) and the patient is left with a subtherapeutic opioid level in the serum. When intermittent distraction is used for pain relief, a continuous low level background infusion of opioid through the PCA pump may be prescribed, so that when the distraction ends it will not be necessary to try to catch up.

Relaxation Techniques

Skeletal muscle relaxation is believed to reduce pain by relaxing tense muscles that contribute to the pain. There is considerable evidence that relaxation is effective in relieving chronic low back pain (Turner & Jensen, 1993; Altmaier et al., 1992). Few studies, however, have demonstrated it to be effective in reducing postoperative pain (Lorenzi, 1991; Miller & Perry, 1990). This may be due to the relatively small role skeletal muscles play in postoperative pain or to the need for the patient to practice the relaxation technique for it to be effective. Practicing the technique may not be possible when it is taught only once, immediately before surgery. A patient who already knows a technique for relaxing may only need to be reminded to use it to reduce or prevent increased pain.

A simple relaxation technique consists of abdominal breathing at a slow, rhythmic rate. The patient may close his or her eyes and breathe slowly and comfortably. A constant rhythm can be maintained by counting silently and slowly with each inhalation ("in, two, three") and exhalation ("out, two, three"). When the nurse is teaching this technique, it is helpful to count out loud with the patient at first. Slow, rhythmic breathing may also be used as a distraction technique. Relaxation techniques, as well as other noninvasive pain relief measures, may require practice before the patient becomes skillful in using them.

Almost all people with chronic pain can benefit from some method of relaxation. Regular periods of relaxation may help to combat the fatigue and muscle tension that occur with chronic pain and which increase the pain.

Guided Imagery

Guided imagery is using one's imagination in an especially designed manner to achieve a specific positive effect. For example, guided imagery for relaxation and pain relief may consist of combining slow rhythmic breathing with a mental image of relaxation and comfort. With eyes closed, the person is instructed to imagine that with each slowly exhaled breath muscle tension and discomfort are being breathed out, leaving behind a relaxed and comfortable body. With each inhaled breath, the patient should imagine healing energy is being sent to the area of discomfort. Each time a breath is exhaled, the patient is to imagine that the exhaled air carries away the pain and tension.

If guided imagery is to be effective it requires a considerable amount of time to explain the technique and time for the patient to practice it. Usually, the patient is asked to practice guided imagery for about 5 minutes, three times a day. Several days of practice may be needed before the intensity of pain is reduced. Many patients begin to experience the relaxing effects of guided imagery the first time they try it. Pain relief can continue for hours after the imagery is used. The patient needs to be informed that guided imagery may work only for some people. Guided imagery should be used only as an adjunct to some other proven form of treatment, until research has demonstrated if and when it is effective.

Hypnosis

Hypnosis has been effective in relieving pain or decreasing the amount of analgesics required in both acute and chronic pain. It may be especially helpful in providing pain relief in particularly difficult situations (*e.g.*, burns). The mechanism by which hypnosis acts is unclear but it does not appear to be mediated by the endorphin system (Moret et al., 1991). The effectiveness of hypnosis depends on the hypnotic susceptibility of the individual. In some cases hypnosis may be effective on the first treatment; its effectiveness may increase with additional hypnotic sessions (Lewis, 1992). However, in some cases it will not work. In most situations hypnosis must be induced by a specially trained person (often a psychologist or a nurse with specialized training in hypnosis) and can be an effective addition to the use of standard analgesics.

Neurosurgical Methods of Pain Management

Several neurosurgical approaches are available and have been used successfully for patients whose pain cannot be relieved or controlled satisfactorily with medications and other nonsurgical approaches. These procedures, including those that interrupt neurologic tracts that conduct pain sensation, are discussed in Chapter 59.

Patient Teaching: Care in the Home and Community

In preparing for pain management at home, the patient and family members need to be taught and guided about what type of pain or discomfort to expect, how long that discomfort is expected to last, and when the pain or discomfort indicates a problem that should be reported. The person who has experienced acute pain as a result of injury, illness, procedures, or surgery will probably receive one or more prescriptions for analgesic medication. The patient and family need to understand the purpose of each medication, the appropriate time to use it, the side effects associated with each, and the strategies that can be used to prevent problems associated with each. The patient and family often need reassurance that pain can be successfully managed at home.

Inadequate control of pain at home is a common reason people seek health care or are readmitted to the hospital. When chronic pain exists, anxiety and fear are multiplied at the time the patient is about to return home. The patient and family are instructed about the techniques for assessing pain and administering pain medications. These instructions are given verbally and in writing as shown in Chart 13-2, which represents a sample plan for managing pain.

Opportunities are provided for the patient and family members to practice administering the medication until they are comfortable and confident with the procedure. They are instructed about the risks of respiratory and central nervous system depression associated with opioid drugs and ways to assess for these complications. If the medications cause other predictable effects, such as constipation, the instructions include measures for preventing and treating this problem as described earlier.

If the patient is to receive analgesia at home by intramuscular or subcutaneous injection or intravenous or epidural infusions, a referral to a home care nurse is indicated. The home care or community health nurse makes a home visit to assess the patient and to determine if the pain management program is being implemented and if the technique for injecting or infusing the analgesia is being carried out safely and effectively. If the patient has an implanted infusion pump in place, the nurse examines the condition of the pump or injection site and may refill the reservoir with medication as prescribed or may supervise family members in the procedure. Any change in the patient's need for analgesic medications is assessed. The nurse then assists the patient and family in modifying the medication dose in collaboration with the physician. These efforts enable the patient to obtain adequate pain relief while remaining at home and with his or her family.

If ever-increasing amounts of opioids are needed, it is important to assure the patient and family that slowly increasing doses will not cause increased risk of respiratory depression and central nervous system depression because the patient will become tolerant to these effects. However, the patient will not become tolerant to the constipating effects of opioids and will require increased efforts to prevent constipation.

Evaluating the Effectiveness of Pain Intervention Strategies

An important aspect of caring for the patient in pain is reassessing the pain after the intervention has been implemented. Evaluating how effective the measure has been is based on the patient's assessment of pain, as reflected in pain assessment tools. If the intervention has not been effective, the nurse needs to consider other measures. If these are ineffective, the goals for relieving the pain need to be reassessed in consultation with the physician. The nurse serves as a patient advocate in obtaining additional pain relief.

After interventions have had a chance to work, the patient is asked to rate the intensity of pain. This assessment is repeated at appropriate intervals after the intervention and compared to the previous rating. These assessments indicate the effectiveness of the pain relief measures and provide a basis for continuing or modifying the plan of care (Nursing Care Plan 13-1). The following expected outcomes are used to assess the effectiveness of pain relief measures:

Expected Outcomes

1. Achieves pain relief
   a. Rates pain at a lower intensity (on a scale of 0 to 10) after intervention
   b. Rates pain at a lower intensity for longer periods
2. Patient or family administers prescribed analgesic medications correctly
   a. States correct dose of medication
   b. Administers correct dose of medication using correct procedure
   c. Identifies side effects of medication
   d. Describes actions taken to prevent or correct side effects
3. Uses nonpharmacologic pain strategies as recommended
   a. Reports practice of nonpharmacologic strategies
   b. Describes expected outcome of nonpharmacologic strategies
4. Reports minimal effects of pain and minimal side effects of interventions
   a. Participates in activities important to recovery (*e.g.*, drinking fluids, coughing, ambulating)
   b. Participates in activities important to self and to family (*e.g.*, family activities, interpersonal relationships, parenting, social interaction, recreation, work)
   c. Reports adequate sleep and absence of fatigue

CHART 13-2
Pain Management Plan

Pain control plan for

____

At home, I will take the following medicines for pain control:

Medicine	How to take	How many	How often	Comments

Medicines that you may take to help treat side effects:

Side effect	Medicine	How to take	How many	How often	Comments

Constipation is a very common problem when taking opioid medications. When this occurs, do the following:

- Increase fluid intake (8 to 10 glasses of fluid)
- Exercise regularly
- Increase fiber in the diet (bran, fresh fruits, vegetables)
- Use a mild laxative, such as milk of magnesia, if no bowel movement in 3 days
- Take ____________________ every day at __________ (time) with a full glass of water
- Use a glycerin suppository every morning (this may help make a bowel movement less painful)

Non-drug pain control methods:

____

____

Additional instructions:

____

____

____

Important phone numbers:

Your doctor ____________________ Your nurse ____________________

Your pharmacy ____________________ Emergencies ____________________

Call your doctor or nurse immediately if your pain increases or if you have a new pain. Also call your doctor early for refill of pain medicines. Do not let your medicines get below 3 or 4 days' supply.

Agency for Health Care Policy and Research (AHCPR). Management of Cancer Pain. Clinical Practice Guidelines. Rockville, MD: Agency for Health Care Policy and Research, Public Health Service, U.S. Department of Health and Human Services, March 1994.

NURSING CARE PLAN 13–1
Care of the Patient With Pain

Nursing Interventions	Rationale	Expected Outcomes
NURSING DIAGNOSIS: Pain and discomfort		
GOAL: Relief of pain and discomfort or decrease in intensity of pain and discomfort		
1. Assure patient that you know pain is real and will assist him or her in dealing with it	1. Fear that pain will not be accepted as real increases tension and anxiety and decreases pain tolerance	• Reports relief that pain is accepted as real and that he will receive assistance in pain relief
2. Use pain assessment scale to identify intensity of pain and discomfort	2. Provides baseline for assessing changes in pain level and evaluating interventions	• Reports lower intensity of pain and discomfort after interventions used
3. Assess and record pain and its characteristics: location, quality, frequency, and duration	3. Data assist in evaluation of pain and pain relief and identifying multiple sources and types of pain	• Reports less disruption from pain and discomfort after use of intervention • Accepts pain medication as prescribed
4. Administer analgesics as prescribed to promote optimal pain relief	4. Analgesics are more effective if administered early in pain cycle	• Exhibits decreased physical and behavioral signs of pain and discomfort in *acute pain* (no grimacing, crying, is aware of surroundings, participates in events and activities)
5. Readminister pain assessment scale	5. Permits assessment of effectiveness of analgesia and identifies need for further action if ineffective	
6. Document severity of patient's pain on chart	6. Assists in demonstrating need for additional analgesic or alternative approach to pain management	• Identifies effective pain relief strategies • Demonstrates use of new strategies to relieve pain and reports their effectiveness
7. Identify and encourage patient to use strategies that have been successful with previous pain	7. Encourages use of pain relief strategies familiar to and accepted by patient	• Experiences minimal side effects of analgesia without interruption to treat side effects
8. Teach patient additional strategies to relieve pain and discomfort: distraction, guided imagery, relaxation, cutaneous stimulation	8. Use of these strategies along with analgesia may produce more effective pain relief	
9. Instruct patient and family about potential side effects of analgesics and their prevention and management	9. Anticipating and preventing side effects enables the patient to continue analgesia without interruption because of side effects	
NURSING DIAGNOSIS: Potential ineffective coping related to anticipation and stress of pain		
GOAL: Increased effectiveness of coping		
1. Assess patient's coping strategies and factors that produce ineffective coping	1. Provides baseline for assessing interventions and allows patient and health care provider to identify factors that have hampered effective coping	• Identifies effective and ineffective coping strategies • Demonstrates use of effective strategies • Avoids destructive coping strategies (smoking, aggression, abuse of alcohol and drugs)
2. Teach patient appropriate and safe ways to use analgesics	2. Teaches patient to use analgesics safely	• Explains safe and appropriate use of analgesics • Uses analgesics safely and appropriately • States side effects of analgesics and adequate pain relief • Exhibits absence of side effects of analgesics and adequate pain relief • Reports pain relief without side effects

(*continued*)

NURSING CARE PLAN 13–1 *(continued)*
Care of the Patient With Pain

Nursing Interventions	Rationale	Expected Outcomes
3. Assist patient to identify and use effective coping strategies	3. Previous reliance on ineffective or less effective coping strategies indicates the need for assistance in identifying effective ones	• Verbally acknowledges need for new, more effective coping strategies
4. Assist patient to plan and participate in activities	4. Provides distraction for patient and assists patient, who may have decreased all participation in activities, to become involved	• Participates in family, social, and work activities • Exhibits awareness of events and environment • Reports ability to sleep and rest • Reports less preoccupation with pain • Converses about topics other than own pain experience. • Reports that life style is appropriate and acceptable to him or her

CRITICAL THINKING EXERCISES

1. Your patient has severe cancer pain requiring increasing doses of opioids to keep her comfortable. Her family is concerned about her escalating need for pain medication and has warned her that increasing doses may be dangerous. Describe the strategies you would implement to ensure that your patient receives pain relief without dangerous side effects while reducing the family's fears about dangers of increasing doses of opioids.
2. Your patient has had a major surgical procedure that usually produces severe pain, yet he refuses all pain medication because of his fear of becoming addicted. How would you deal with this situation? What nonpharmacologic methods of pain relief would you consider for this patient? Which methods do you feel would be inappropriate?
3. A patient with a terminal disease is to receive intravenous morphine via patient-controlled analgesia (PCA) at home to control his pain. Describe the planning you would do to ensure patient safety and adequate pain control.

REFERENCES AND BIBLIOGRAPHY

Books

Agency for Health Care Policy and Research. Public Health Service. Department of Health and Human Services. Acute Pain Management: Operative or Medical Procedures and Trauma. Clinical Practice Guideline. (AHCPR 92-0032). Washington, DC, US Government Printing Office, 1992.

Agency for Health Care Policy and Research. Public Health Service. Department of Health and Human Services. Management of Cancer Pain: Adults. Clinical Practice Guidelines (AHCPR 94-0592). Washington, DC, US Government Printing Office, 1994.

American Pain Society. Principles of Analgesic Use in the Treatment of Acute Pain and Chronic Cancer Pain, 3rd ed. Skokie, IL, American Pain Society, 1992.

Benedetti C et al. Pathophysiology and therapy of postoperative pain. In: Benedetti C et al (eds.), Recent Advances in the Management of Pain. New York, Raven Press, 1984.

Ferrante FM and VadeBoncouer TR. Postoperative Pain Management. New York, Churchill Livingstone, 1993.

Patt RB. Cancer Pain. Philadelphia, JB Lippincott, 1993.

Rowlingston JC (ed). Handbook of Critical Care Pain Management. New York, McGraw-Hill, 1994.

Sevarino FB and Preble LM. A Manual for Acute Postoperative Pain Management. New York, Raven Press, 1992.

Tollison CD (ed). Handbook of Pain Management. Baltimore, Williams & Wilkins, 1994.

Wall PD et al. (eds). Textbook of Pain. New York, Churchill Livingstone, 1994.

Journals

Asterisks indicate nursing research articles.

Absi MA and Rokke PD. Can anxiety help us tolerate pain? Pain 1991 July; 46(1):43-51.

Alspach G. Pain management: Dispelling some myths [editorial]. Critical Care Nurse 1994 Oct; 14(5):13-15.

Altmaier EM et al. The effectiveness of psychological interventions for the rehabilitation of low back pain: A randomized controlled trial evaluation. Pain 1992 Jun; 49(3):329-335.

Arntz A et al. Attention, not anxiety, influences pain. Behav Res Ther 1991; 29(1):41-50.
Bostrom J and Batina M. Managing pain in a diverse medical-surgical patient population. Medsurg Nurs 1994 Dec; 3(6): 469–474.
Brofeldt BT et al. Topical lidocaine in the treatment of partial-thickness burns. J Burn Care Rehabil 1989 Jan-Feb; 10(1): 63-68.
Buchanan JM et al. Postoperative pain relief; a new approach: Narcotics compared with non-steroidal anti-inflammatory drugs. Ann R Coll Sur Engl 1988; 70:332-335.
Cameron JC. Constipation related to narcotic therapy: A protocol for nurses and patients. Cancer Nurs 1992 Oct; 15(5):372-377.
Cassuto J et al. Amide local anesthetics reduce albumin extravasation in burn injuries. Anesthesiology 1990 Feb; 72(2):302-307.
Choiniere M et al. Patient-controlled analgesia: A double-blind study in burn patients. Anaesthesia 1992 June; 47(6):467-472.
Choiniere M et al. Comparisons between patients' and nurses' assessment of pain and medication efficacy in severe burn injury. Pain 1990 Feb; 40(2):143-152.
Classification of chronic pain. Descriptions of chronic pain syndromes and definitions of pain terms. Prepared by the International Association for the Study of Pain, Subcommittee on Taxonomy. Pain Suppl 1986; 3:S1-226.
Closs SJ. Pain in elderly patients: A neglected phenomenon? J Adv Nurs 1994 Jun; 19(6):1072-1081.
Cohn BT et al. The effects of cold therapy in the postoperative management of pain in patients undergoing anterior cruciate ligament reconstruction. Am J Sports Med 1989 May-Jun; 17(3): 344-349.
Conn IG et al. Transcutaneous electrical nerve stimulation following appendicectomy: The placebo effect. Ann R Coll Surg Engl 1986 July; 68(4):191-192.
Devine DP and Spanos NP. Effectiveness of maximally different cognitive strategies and expectancy in attenuation of reported pain. J Pers Soc Psychol 1990 Apr; 58(4):672-678.
*Donovan M et al. Incidence and characteristics of pain in a sample of medical-surgical inpatients. Pain 1987 Jul;30(1):69-78.
Duggleby W and Lander J. Patient-controlled analgesia for older adults. Clinical Nursing Research 1992 Feb; 1(1):107-113.
Ennis JH. Opioid analgesics and the burning pain of Guillain-Barré syndrome. Anesthesiology 1991 Nov; 75(5):913-914.
Ferrell-Torry AT and Glick OJ. The use of therapeutic massage as a nursing intervention to modify anxiety and the perception of cancer pain. Cancer Nurs 1993 Apr; 16(2):93-101.
Fox AE. Confronting the use of placebos for pain. Am J Nurs 1994 Sep; 94(9):42-45.
Giuffre M et al. Postoperative joint replacement pain. Description and opioid requirement. Journal of Post Anesthesia Nursing 1991 Aug; 6(4): 239-245.
Gobel H and Cordes P. Circadian variation of pain sensitivity in pericranial musculature. Headache 1990 June; 30(7):418-422.
Greenwald HP. Interethnic differences in pain perception. Pain 1991 Feb; 44(2):157-163.
Guyton-Simmons J and Ehrmin J. Problem solving in pain management by expert intensive care nurses. Crit Care Nurse 1994 Oct; 14(5):37-44.
Johnson B. Analgesics for the oncology patient. Home Healthcare Nurse 1993 Nov/Dec; 11(6):52-54.
Jurna I and Brune K. Central effect of the common non-steroid anti-inflammatory agents, indomethacin, ibuprofen, and diclofenac, determined in C fibre-evoked activity in single neurones of the rat thalamus. Pain 1990 Apr; 41(1):71-80.
Kehlet H. The surgical stress response: Should it be prevented? Can J Surg 1991 Dec; 34(6):565-567.
King RB. Concerning the management of pain associated with herpes zoster and of post herpetic neuralgia. Pain 1988 April; 33(1):73-78.
Lavies N et al. Identification of patient, medical and nursing staff attitudes to postoperative opioid analgesia. Pain 1992 Mar; 48(3):313-319.
Levy MH et al. Transdermal fentanyl: Seeding trial in patients with chronic cancer pain. Journal of Pain and Symptom Management 1992 April; 7(3 Suppl):S48-50.
Levy MH et al. Supportive care in oncology. Curr Probl Cancer 1992 Nov-Dec; 16(6):329-418.
Lewis DO. Hypnoanalgesia for chronic pain: The response to multiple inductions at one session and to separate single inductions. J R Soc Med 1992 Oct; 85(10):620-624.
Liebeskind JC. Pain *can* kill. Pain 1991; 44(1):3-4.
*Lorenzi EA. Relaxation. Episiotomy incisional pain and overall discomfort. J Adv Nurs 1991 Jun; 16(6):701-709.
Maixner W and Humphrey C. Gender differences in pain and cardiovascular responses to forearm ischemia. Clin J Pain 1993 March; 9(1):16-25.
Marchand S et al. Modulation of heat pain perception by high frequency transcutaneous electrical nerve stimulation (TENS). Clin J Pain 1991 June; 7(2):122-129.
Martic B and Meherg D. Interpleural analgesia: A new technique. Critical Care Nurse 1994 Oct; 14(5):31-35.
McCaffery M and Ferrell BR. How to use the new AHCPR cancer pain guidelines. Am J Nurs 1994 Jul; 94(7):42-46.
Melzack R et al. Pain on a surgical ward: A survey of the duration and intensity of pain and the effectiveness of medication. Pain 1987 April; 29(1):67-72.
*Miller KM and Perry PA. Relaxation technique and postoperative pain in patients undergoing cardiac surgery. Heart Lung 1990 Mar; 19(2):136-146.
Miller ME and Bowers KS. Hypnotic analgesia: Dissociated experience or dissociated control? J Abnorm Psychol 1993 Feb; 102(1): 29-38.
Moller IW et al. Effect of patient-controlled analgesia on plasma catecholamine, cortisol and glucose concentrations after cholecystectomy. Br J Anaesth 1988 Aug; 61(2):160-164.
Moltner A et al. Heart rate changes as an autonomic component of the pain response. Pain 1990 Oct; 43(1):81-89
Moret V et al. Mechanism of analgesia induced by hypnosis and acupuncture: Is there a difference? Pain 1991 May; 45(2):135-140.
Naber L et al. Epidural analgesia for effective pain control. Crit Care Nurse 1994 Oct; 14(5):69-72,79-83.
*Nam HK and Park YS. A study on comparisons of ice bag and heat lamp for the relief of perineal discomfort. Kanho Hakhoe Chi Journal of Nurses Academic Society 1991 Apr; 21(1):27-40.
Nicholas MK et al. Comparison of cognitive-behavioral group treatment and an alternative non-psychological treatment for chronic low back pain. Pain 1992 Mar; 48(3):339-347.
Parker RK et al. Use of ketorolac after lower abdominal surgery. Anesthesiology 1994 Jan; 80(1);6-12.
Pasero CL and McCaffery M. Avoiding opioid-induced respiratory depression. Am J Nurs 1994 Apr; 94(4):25-30.
Pasero CL and Vanderveer BL. Epidural infusions: Not just for labor anymore. Am J Nurs 1994 Dec; 94(12):51.
Patterson DR et al. Hypnosis for the treatment of burn pain. J Consult Clin Psychol 1992 Oct; 60(5):713-717.
*Puntillo K and Weiss SJ. Pain: Its mediators and associated morbidity in critically ill cardiovascular surgical patients. Nurs Res 1994 Jan /Feb; 43(1):31–36.
Ready LB et al. Evaluation of intravenous ketorolac administered by bolus or infusion for treatment of postoperative pain. Anesthesiology 1994 Jun; 80(6):1277-1286.
*Redeker NS. Symptoms reported by older and middle-aged adults after coronary bypass surgery. Clin Nurs Res 1993 May; 2(2): 148-159.

Schug SA et al. A long term survey of morphine in cancer pain patients. Journal of Pain and Symptom Management 1992 July; 7(5):259-266.
Syrjala KL et al. Hypnosis or cognitive behavioral training for the reduction of pain and nausea during cancer treatment: A controlled clinical trial. Pain 1992 Feb; 48(2):137-146.
*Timmons ME and Bower FL. The effect of structured preoperative teaching on patients' use of patient-controlled analgesia (PCA) and their management of pain. Orthop Nurs 1993 Jan/Feb; 12(1):23-31.
Turner JA and Jensen MP. Efficacy of cognitive therapy for chronic low back pain. Pain 1993 Feb; 52(2):169-177.
Van der Does AJW. Patients' and nurses' ratings of pain and anxiety during burn wound care. Pain 1989 Oct; 39(1):95-101.
*Wall PD. The gate control theory of pain mechanisms: A re-examination and re-statement. Brain 1978; 101:1-18.
Wallace, M. Assessment and management of pain in the elderly. Medsurg Nursing. 1994 Aug; 3(4):293-298.
Weisenberg M et al. Relevant and irrelevant anxiety in the reaction to pain. Pain 1984 Dec; 20(4):371-383.
Willens JS. Giving fentanyl for pain outside the OR. Am J Nurs 1994 Feb; 94(2):24-28.
Wotring RA. Cancer pain management. Home Healthcare Nurse 1993 Sep/Oct; 11(5):40-44.
Yeager MP et al. Epidural anesthesia and analgesia in high-risk surgical patients. Anesthesiology 1987 Jun; 66(6):729-736.
Zatzick DF and Dimsdale JE. Cultural variations in response to painful stimuli. Psychosom Med 1990 Sep-Oct; 52(5):544-557.
Zylicz Z and Twycross RG. Oral opioids in the treatment of cancer pain. Neth J Med 1991 Aug; 39(1-2):108-114.

AGENCIES

American Pain Society
PO Box 186, Skokie, IL 60076

International Pain Foundation
909 NE 43rd St, Room 306, Seattle, WA 98105

Commission on Accreditation of Rehabilitation Facilities (CARF)
101 N Wilmot Rd, Suite 500, Tucson, AZ 85711, (602) 748- 1212

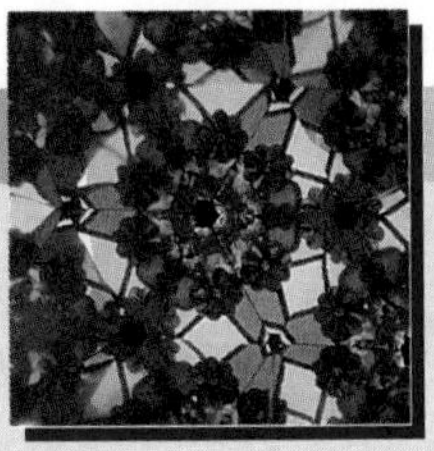

14

CHAPTER OUTLINE

Fundamental Concepts
Amount and Composition of Body Fluids
Electrolytes
Regulation of Body Fluid Compartments
Routes of Gains and Losses
Laboratory Tests to Evaluate Fluid Status
Homeostatic Mechanisms
Gerontologic Considerations

Fluid Volume Disturbances
Fluid Volume Deficit (Hypovolemia)
Fluid Volume Excess (Hypervolemia)
Gerontologic Considerations

Sodium Imbalances
Sodium Deficit (Hyponatremia)
Sodium Excess (Hypernatremia)

Potassium Imbalances
Potassium Deficit (Hypokalemia)
Potassium Excess (Hyperkalemia)

Calcium Imbalances
Calcium Deficit (Hypocalcemia)
Calcium Excess (Hypercalcemia)

Magnesium Imbalances
Magnesium Deficit (Hypomagnesemia)
Magnesium Excess (Hypermagnesemia)

Phosphorus Imbalances
Phosphorus Deficit (Hypophosphatemia)
Phosphorus Excess (Hyperphosphatemia)

Acid–Base Disturbances
Regulation of Acid–Base Balance
Metabolic Acidosis (Base Bicarbonate Deficit)
Metabolic Alkalosis (Base Bicarbonate Excess)
Respiratory Acidosis (Carbonic Acid Excess)
Respiratory Alkalosis (Carbonic Acid Deficit)
Mixed Acid–Base Disorders
Blood Gas Analysis

Parenteral Fluid Therapy
Purpose
Types of Intravenous Solutions

Nursing Management of the Patient Receiving Intravenous Therapy
Venipuncture
Monitoring Intravenous Therapy
Discontinuing an Infusion
Complications Associated With Parenteral Fluid Therapy

Critical Thinking Exercises

Fluids and Electrolytes: Balance and Disturbances

LEARNING OBJECTIVES

On completion of this chapter, the learner will be able to:

1. Differentiate between osmosis, diffusion, filtration, and active transport
2. Describe the role of the kidneys, lungs, and endocrine glands in regulation of the body's fluid composition and volume
3. Identify the effects of aging on fluid and electrolyte regulation
4. Plan effective care of patients with the following imbalances: fluid volume deficit and fluid volume excess; sodium deficit (hyponatremia) and sodium excess (hypernatremia); potassium deficit (hypokalemia) and potassium excess (hyperkalemia)
5. Describe the etiology, clinical manifestations, management, and nursing interventions for the following imbalances: calcium deficit (hypocalcemia) and calcium excess (hypercalcemia); magnesium deficit (hypomagnesemia) and magnesium excess (hypermagnesemia); phosphorus deficit (hypophosphatemia) and phosphorus excess (hyperphosphatemia)
6. Explain the role of the lungs, kidneys, and chemical buffers in maintenance of acid–base balance
7. Compare metabolic acidosis and alkalosis with regard to causes, clinical manifestations, diagnosis, and management
8. Compare respiratory acidosis and alkalosis with regard to causes, clinical manifestations, diagnosis, and management
9. Interpret arterial blood gases
10. Assess patients for evidence of acid–base imbalance
11. Demonstrate a safe and effective procedure of venipuncture
12. Describe measures used for prevention of complications of intravenous therapy

Fundamental Concepts

Amount and Composition of Body Fluids

Approximately 60% of weight in a typical adult is composed of fluid (water and electrolytes). Factors that influence the amount of body fluid are age, gender, and body fat content. As a general rule, younger people have a higher percentage of body fluid than do older people, and men have proportionately more body fluid than do women. Obese people have less fluid than thin people, because fat cells contain little water.

Body fluid is located in two fluid compartments: the intracellular space (fluid in the cells) and the extracellular space (fluid outside the cells). Approximately two-thirds of body fluid is in the **intracellular fluid compartment**, and is located primarily in the skeletal muscle mass. In a male weighing 70 kg (154 pounds), the intracellular fluid amounts to about 25 L. Approximately one-third of body fluid is extracellular and amounts to about 15 L in a 70-kg (154-pound) male.

The **extracellular fluid compartment** is further divided into the intravascular, interstitial, and transcellular fluid spaces. The *intravascular space* (the fluid within the blood vessels) contains plasma. Approximately 3 L of the average 6 L of blood volume is made up of plasma. The remaining 3 L is made up of erythrocytes, leukocytes, and thrombocytes. The *interstitial space* contains the fluid that surrounds the cell and is about 8 L in an adult. Lymph is an example of interstitial fluid. The *transcellular space* is the smallest division of the extracellular fluid and contains approximately 1 L of fluid at any given time. Examples of transcellular fluid are cerebrospinal, pericardial, synovial, intraocular, and pleural fluids; sweat; and digestive secretions.

Terms that will be useful in understanding subsequent discussion are defined in Chart 14-1.

Body fluid normally shifts between the two major compartments or spaces in an effort to maintain an equilibrium between the spaces. Loss of fluid from the body can disrupt this equilibrium. Sometimes fluid is not lost from the body, but is unavailable for use by either the intracellular fluid or extracellular fluid spaces. Loss of extracellular fluid (ECF) into a space that does not contribute to equilibrium between the intracellular fluid (ICF) and ECF is referred to as a *third space fluid shift.*

An early clue of a third space fluid shift is a decrease in urine output despite adequate fluid therapy. Urine output decreases because fluid shifts out of the intravascular space; the kidneys then receive less blood flow and attempt to compensate by decreasing urine output. Other signs and symptoms of "third spacing" that indicate an intravascular fluid volume deficit include increased heart rate, decreased blood pressure, decreased central venous pressure (CVP), edema, increased body weight, and imbalances in fluid intake and output. Examples of third space shifts occur in ascites, burns, and massive bleeding into a joint or body cavity.

Electrolytes

Electrolytes in body fluids are active chemicals (**cations**, which carry positive charges, and **anions**, which carry negative charges). The major cations in body fluid are sodium, potassium, calcium, and magnesium. The major anions are chloride, bicarbonate, phosphate, sulfate, and proteinate.

These chemicals unite in varying combinations. Therefore, electrolyte concentration in the body is expressed in

CHART 14-1
Glossary of Terms

Acidosis represents an increase in H^+ concentration (decreased blood *p*H). A low arterial *p*H due to reduced bicarbonate concentration is called metabolic acidosis. A low arterial *p*H due to increased pCO_2 is respiratory acidosis.

Alkalosis represents a reduction in H^+ concentration (increased blood *p*H). A high arterial *p*H with increased bicarbonate concentration is called metabolic alkalosis. A high arterial *p*H due to reduced pCO_2 is respiratory alkalosis.

Diffusion solutes move from an area of higher concentration to one of lower concentration. Diffusion does not require energy.

Osmosis movement of fluid across a semipermeable membrane from an area of low solute concentration to an area of high solute concentration. This process stops when the solute concentrations are equal on both sides of the membrane.

Hydrostatic pressure the pressure created by the weight of fluid against the wall of the container. In the body, this pressure in blood vessels results from the weight of fluid itself and the force resulting from cardiac contraction.

Active transport physiologic pump that moves fluid from an area of lower concentration to one of higher concentration. Active transport requires adenosine triphosphate (ATP) for energy. The production of energy depends on oxygen and glucose availability.

Osmolality number of osmoles per kilogram of solution. Expressed as mOsm/kg. Used more often in clinical practice than osmolarity to evaluate serum and urine. In addition to urea and glucose, sodium contributes the largest number of particles to osmolality.

Osmolarity number of osmoles, the standard unit of osmotic pressure per liter of solution. It is expressed as milliosmoles per liter (mOsm/L). Used to describe the concentration of solutes or dissolved particles.

Isotonic solution possesses same osmolality as serum and other body fluids. Osmolality falls within normal range for serum (280–295 mOsm/L).

Hypotonic solution possesses an osmolality lower than that of serum.

Hypertonic solution possesses an osmolality higher than that of serum.

terms of milliequivalents (mEq) per liter, a measure of chemical activity, rather than in terms of milligrams (mg), a unit of weight. More specifically, a milliequivalent is defined as being equivalent to the electrochemical activity of 1 mg of hydrogen. In a solution, cations and anions are equal in mEq/L.

Electrolyte concentrations in ICF differ from those in ECF, as reflected in Table 14-1. Because special techniques are required to measure electrolyte concentrations in the ICF, it is customary to measure the electrolytes in the most accessible portion of extracellular body fluid, namely, the plasma.

Sodium ions, which are positively charged, far outnumber the other cations in the extracellular fluid (Table 14-1). Because sodium concentration affects the overall concentration of ECF, sodium is important in the regulation of body fluid volume. Retention of sodium is associated with fluid retention; conversely, excessive loss of sodium is usually associated with decreased body fluid volume.

As shown in Table 14-1, the major electrolytes in the ICF are potassium and phosphate. The ECF has a low concentration of potassium and can tolerate only small changes in potassium concentrations. Therefore, release of large stores of intracellular potassium into the ECF by trauma to cells and tissues can be extremely dangerous.

The body expends a great deal of energy maintaining the high extracellular concentration of sodium and the high intracellular concentration of potassium. It does so by means of cell membrane pumps, which exchange sodium and potassium ions. Normal movement of fluids through the capillary wall into the tissues depends on the force of the **hydrostatic pressure** (the pressure exerted by the fluid on the walls of the blood vessel) at both the arterial and the venous ends of the vessel and the **osmotic pressure** exerted by the protein of plasma. Direction of fluid movement depends on the differences in these two opposing forces (hydrostatic vs. osmotic pressure).

In addition to electrolytes the ECF transports other substances, such as enzymes and hormones. It also carries blood components, such as red and white blood cells, throughout the body.

TABLE 14-1 Approximate Major Electrolyte Content in Body Fluid

Electrolytes	mEq/L
Extracellular Fluid (Plasma)	
Cations	
Sodium (Na^+)	142
Potassium (K^+)	5
Calcium (Ca^{2+})	5
Magnesium (Mg^{2+})	2
Total cations	154
Anions	
Chloride (Cl^-)	103
Bicarbonate (HCO_3^-)	26
Phosphate (HPO_4^{2-})	2
Sulfate (SO_4^{2-})	1
Organic acids	5
Proteinate	17
Total anions	154
Intracellular Fluid	
Cations	
Potassium (K^+)	150
Magnesium (Mg^{2+})	40
Sodium (Na^+)	10
Total cations	200
Anions	
Phosphates, Sulfates	150
Bicarbonate (HCO_3^-)	10
Proteinate	40
Total anions	200

(Metheny N. Fluid and Electrolyte Balance: Nursing Considerations. Philadelphia, JB Lippincott, 1992.)

Regulation of Body Fluid Compartments

Osmosis and Osmolality

When two different solutions are separated by a membrane impermeable to the dissolved substances, a shift of water occurs through the membrane from the region of low solute concentration to the region of high solute concentration until the solutions are of equal concentration; this diffusion of water caused by a water concentration gradient is known as **osmosis** (Fig. 14-1). The magnitude of this force depends on the *number* of particles dissolved in the solutions and not on their weights. The number of dissolved particles contained in a unit of water determines the **osmolality** or concentration of a solution, which influences the movement of water between the fluid compartments.

There are three other terms which are associated with osmosis: osmotic pressure, oncotic pressure, and osmotic diuresis.

- *Osmotic pressure* is the amount of pressure needed to stop the flow of water by osmosis.
- *Oncotic pressure* is the osmotic pressure exerted by proteins (*i.e.*, albumin).
- *Osmotic diuresis* occurs when there is increased urine output due to excretion of substances such as glucose, mannitol, or contrast agents in the urine.

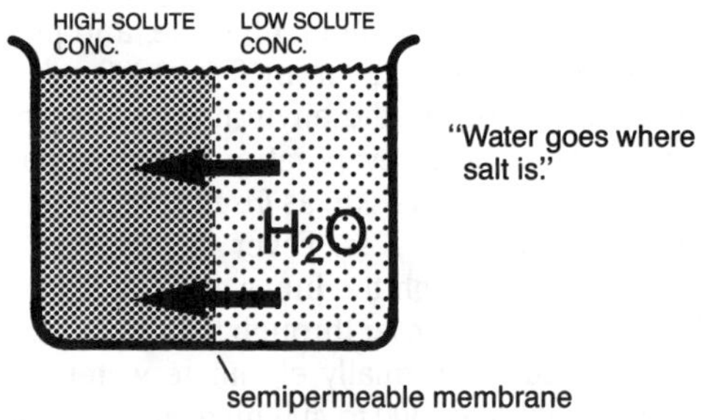

FIGURE 14-1. Osmosis. ("Water goes where salt is.") (Metheny N. Fluid and Electrolyte Balance: Nursing Considerations. Philadelphia, JB Lippincott, 1992.)

Diffusion

Diffusion is defined as the natural tendency of a substance to move from an area of higher concentration to one of lower concentration. It occurs through the random movement of ions and molecules. An example of diffusion is the exchange of oxygen and carbon dioxide between the pulmonary capillaries and alveoli.

Filtration

Hydrostatic pressure in the capillaries tends to filter fluid out of the vascular compartment into the interstitial fluid. An example of filtration is the passage of water and electrolytes from the arterial capillary bed to the interstitial fluid; in this instance, the hydrostatic pressure is furnished by the pumping action of the heart.

Sodium–Potassium Pump

As stated earlier, sodium concentration is greater in ECF than in ICF; because of this, there is a tendency for sodium to enter the cell by diffusion. This tendency is offset by the sodium–potassium pump, which is located in the cell membrane and actively moves sodium from the cell into the ECF. Conversely, the high intracellular potassium concentration is maintained by pumping of potassium into the cell. By definition, *active transport* implies that energy expenditure must take place for the movement to occur against a concentration gradient.

Routes of Gains and Losses

Water and electrolytes are gained in various ways. In health, one gains fluids by drinking and eating. In some types of illnesses, fluids may be provided by the parenteral route (intravenously or subcutaneously) or by means of an enteral feeding tube in the stomach or intestine. When fluid balance is critical, all routes of gain and all routes of loss must be recorded and the volumes compared. Organs of fluid loss include the kidneys, skin, lungs, and gastrointestinal tract.

Kidneys. The usual urine volume in the adult is between 1 and 2 liters each day. A general rule is that the output is approximately 1 ml of urine per kilogram of body weight per hour (1 ml/kg/hr) in all age groups.

Skin. *Sensible perspiration* refers to visible water and electrolyte loss through the skin by way of sweating. The chief solutes in sweat are sodium, chloride, and potassium. Actual sweat losses can vary from 0 to 1000 ml or more every hour, depending on the environmental temperature. Continuous water loss by evaporation (approximately 600 ml/day) occurs through the skin as *insensible perspiration*, a nonvisible form of water loss. Fever greatly increases insensible water loss through the lungs and the skin, as does loss of the natural skin barrier through major burns.

Lungs. The lungs normally eliminate water vapor (insensible loss) at a rate of 300 to 400 ml every day. The loss is much greater with increased respiratory rate or depth, or both.

Gastrointestinal Tract. The usual loss through the gastrointestinal tract is only 100 to 200 ml every day, even though approximately 8 liters of fluid circulate through the gastrointestinal system every 24 hours (called the "gastrointestinal circulation"). Because the bulk of fluids is reabsorbed in the small intestine, it is obvious that large losses can be incurred from the gastrointestinal tract if diarrhea or fistulas occur.

In healthy persons, the 24-hour average intake and output of water are approximately equal (Table 14-2).

Laboratory Tests to Evaluate Fluid Status

Osmolality reflects the concentration of fluid that affects the movement of water between fluid compartments by osmosis. Osmolality measures the solute concentration per *kilogram* in blood and urine. It is also a measure of a solution's ability to create osmotic pressure and affect the movement of water. Serum osmolality reflects the concentration of sodium and its anions. Urine osmolality is determined by urea, creatinine, and uric acid. It is the most reliable indicator of urine concentration. Osmolality is reported as milliosmoles per kg of water (mOsm/kg).

Osmolarity is another term which describes the concentration of solutions and is measured in milliosmoles per *liter* (mOsm/L). Osmolality, however, is used most often in clinical practice. Normal serum osmolality is 280 to 300 mOsm/kg and normal urine osmolality is 50 to 1400 mOsm/kg. Sodium predominates in extracellular fluid osmolality and holds water in this compartment.

Factors that increase and decrease serum and urine osmolality are presented in Table 14-3. Serum osmolality may be measured directly through laboratory tests or estimated at the bedside by doubling the serum sodium level or by utilizing the following formula:

$$Na^{+} \times 2 + \frac{\text{glucose}}{18} + \frac{\text{BUN}}{3} = \begin{array}{l}\text{Approximate Value}\\ \text{of Serum Osmolality}\end{array}$$

The calculated value usually is within 10 mOsm of the measured osmolality.

Urine specific gravity measures the kidney's ability to excrete or conserve water. The specific gravity of urine is

TABLE 14-2 Average Intake and Output in an Adult for a 24-Hour Period

Intake		Output	
Oral liquids	1300 ml	Urine	1500 ml
Water in food	1000 ml	Stool	200 ml
Water produced by metabolism	300 ml	Insensible	
Total	2600 ml	Lungs	300 ml
		Skin	600 ml
		Total	2600 ml

(Metheny N. Fluid and Electrolyte Balance: Nursing Considerations. Philadelphia, JB Lippincott, 1992.)

TABLE 14-3 Comparison of Serum and Urine Osmolality

	Factors Increasing Osmolality	Factors Decreasing Osmolality
Serum	Free water loss	SIADH*
	Diabetes insipidus	Renal failure
	Sodium overload	Diuretic use
	Hyperglycemia	Adrenal insufficiency
	Uremia	
Urine	Fluid volume deficit	Fluid volume excess
	SIADH*	Diabetes insipidus

*Syndrome of inappropriate antidiuretic hormone

compared to the weight of distilled water, which has a specific gravity of 1.000. The normal range of specific gravity is 1.001 to 1.040. Urine specific gravity can be measured at the bedside by placing a calibrated hydrometer or urinometer in a cylinder of approximately 20 ml of urine. Specific gravity can also be assessed with a refractometer or dipstick with reagent for this purpose. Specific gravity varies inversely with urine volume; normally, the larger the volume of urine, the lower the specific gravity. Specific gravity is a less reliable indicator of concentration than urine osmolality; increased glucose or protein in urine can cause a false high specific gravity. Factors which increase or decrease urine osmolality are the same for urine specific gravity.

Blood urea nitrogen (BUN) is made up of urea, which is an end product of protein metabolism (both from muscle and dietary intake). Amino acid breakdown produces large amounts of ammonia, which is absorbed into the bloodstream. Ammonia molecules are converted to urea and excreted in the urine. The normal BUN is 10 to 20 mg/dl (SI: 3.5–7 mmol/L). The level of BUN varies with urine output. Factors which increase BUN include GI bleeding, dehydration, increased protein intake, fever, and sepsis. Factors that decrease BUN include end-stage liver disease, a low-protein diet, starvation, and any condition that results in expanded fluid volume (*e.g.*, pregnancy).

Creatinine is the end product of muscle metabolism. It is a better indicator of renal function than BUN because it does not vary with protein intake and metabolic state. The normal serum creatinine is approximately 0.6 to 1.5 mg/dl (SI: 53–133 mmol/L); however, its concentration is dependent on lean body mass and varies from person to person.

Hematocrit measures the volume percentage of red blood cells (erythrocytes) in whole blood and normally ranges from 40% to 54% for males and 37% to 47% for females. Conditions that increase hematocrit are dehydration and polycythemia; those that decrease hematocrit are overhydration and anemia.

Urine sodium values change with sodium intake and the status of fluid volume (as sodium intake increases it results in increased excretion and as the circulating fluid volume decreases, sodium is conserved). Normal urine sodium ranges from 50 to 130 mEq/L (SI: 50–130 mmol/L). Urine sodium will be less than 20 mEq/L during periods of volume depletion and greater than 40 mEq/L as the kidneys lose the ability to conserve sodium and concentrate urine.

Homeostatic Mechanisms

Body Organs

The body is equipped with remarkable homeostatic mechanisms to keep the composition and volume of body fluid within narrow limits of normal. Organs involved in homeostasis include the kidneys, lungs, heart, adrenal glands, parathyroid glands, and pituitary gland.

Kidneys. Vital to the regulation of fluid and electrolyte balance, the kidneys normally filter 170 liters of plasma every day in the adult, while excreting only 1.5 liters of urine. They act both autonomously and in response to bloodborne messengers, such as aldosterone and antidiuretic hormone (ADH). Major functions of the kidneys in maintaining normal fluid balance include the following:

- Regulation of ECF volume and osmolality by selective retention and excretion of body fluids
- Regulation of electrolyte levels in the ECF by selective retention of needed substances and excretion of unneeded substances
- Regulation of *p*H of ECF by retention of hydrogen ions
- Excretion of metabolic wastes and toxic substances

Given the above facts, it is readily apparent that renal failure will result in multiple fluid and electrolyte problems. Renal function declines with advanced age, as do muscle mass and daily exogenous creatinine production. Thus, high-normal and minimally elevated serum creatinine values may indicate substantially reduced renal function in the elderly.

Heart and Blood Vessels. The pumping action of the heart circulates blood through the kidneys under sufficient pressure for urine to form. Failure of this pumping action interferes with renal perfusion and thus with water and electrolyte regulation.

Lungs. The lungs are also vital in maintaining homeostasis. Through exhalation, the lungs remove approximately 300 ml of water daily in the normal adult. Abnormal conditions such as hyperpnea (abnormally deep respiration) or continuous coughing increase this loss; mechanical ventilation with excessive moisture decreases it. The lungs also have a major role in maintaining acid–base balance, as will be discussed later in this chapter. Changes due to normal aging result in decreased respiratory function, causing increased difficulty in the regulation of *p*H in elderly individuals experiencing major illness or trauma.

Pituitary Gland. The hypothalamus manufactures a substance known as antidiuretic hormone (ADH), which is stored in the posterior pituitary gland and released as needed. Sometimes referred to as the "water-conserving hormone," ADH causes the body to retain water. Functions of ADH include maintaining the osmotic pressure of the cells by controlling the retention or excretion of water by the kidneys and by regulating blood volume (Fig. 14-2).

Adrenal Glands. *Aldosterone*, a mineralocorticoid secreted by the zona glomerulosa (outer zone) of the adrenal

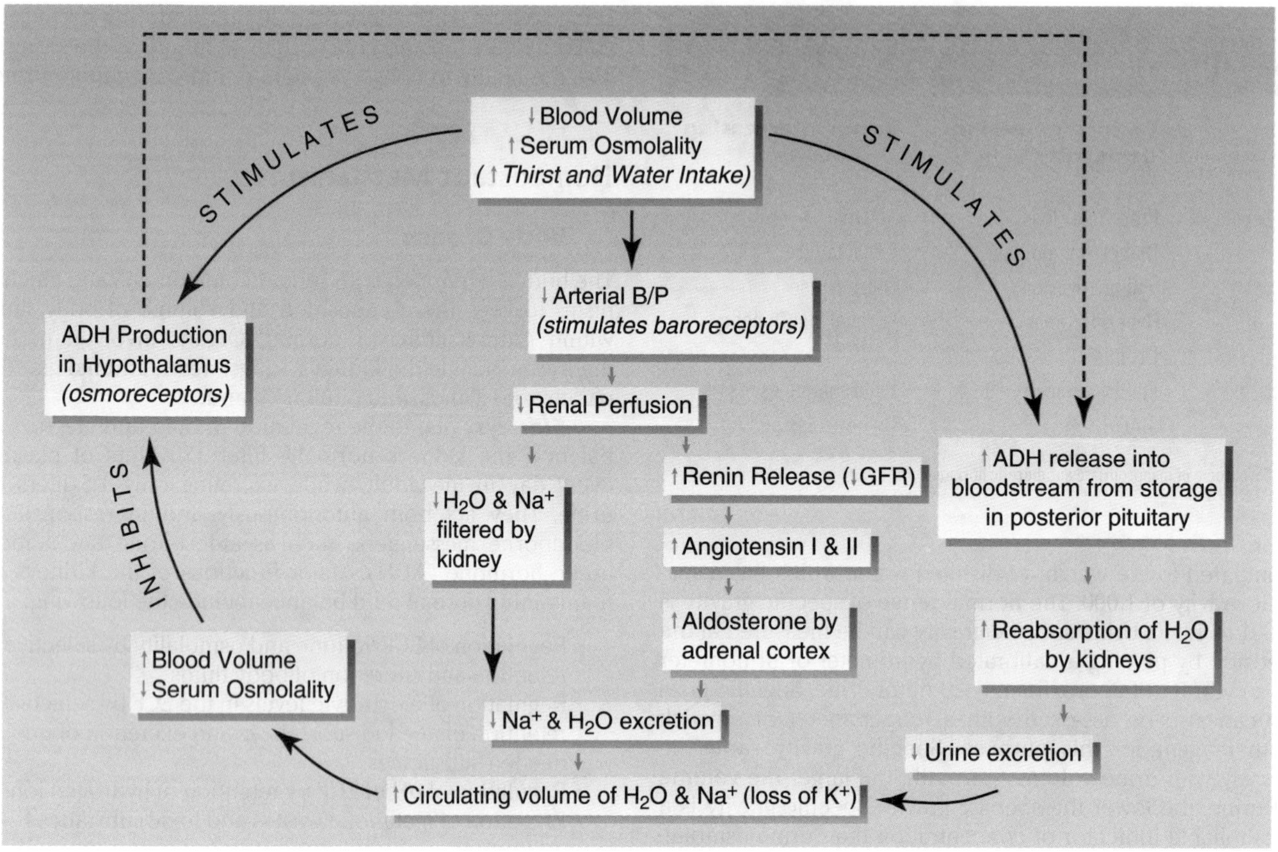

FIGURE 14-2. Fluid regulation cycle.

cortex, has a profound effect on fluid balance. Increased secretion of aldosterone causes sodium retention (and thus water retention) and potassium loss. Conversely, a decreased secretion of aldosterone causes sodium and water loss and potassium retention. *Cortisol,* another adrenocortical hormone, has only a fraction of the mineralocorticoid potency of aldosterone. When secreted in large quantities, however, it can also produce sodium and fluid retention and potassium deficit.

Parathyroid Glands. The parathyroid glands, embedded in the corners of the thyroid gland, regulate calcium and phosphate balance by means of parathyroid hormone (PTH). PTH influences bone resorption, calcium absorption from the intestines, and calcium reabsorption from the renal tubules.

Other Homeostatic Mechanisms

Changes in the volume of the interstitial compartment within the extracellular fluid space can occur without affecting body function. The vascular compartment, however, cannot tolerate change as readily and must be carefully maintained to ensure that tissues receive adequate nutrients.

Baroreceptors, which are small nerve receptors, detect changes in pressure within blood vessels and transmit this information to the central nervous system. They are responsible for monitoring the circulating volume and they regulate sympathetic and parasympathetic neural activity as well as endocrine activities. They are categorized as low pressure and high pressure baroreceptor systems. Low pressure baroreceptors are located in the cardiac atria, particularly the left atrium. The high pressure baroreceptors are nerve endings in the aortic arch and in the cardiac sinus. Additionally, another high pressure baroreceptor resides in the afferent arteriole of the juxtaglomerular apparatus of the nephron.

As arterial pressure decreases, baroreceptors transmit fewer impulses from the carotid sinuses and the aortic arch to the vasomotor center. A decrease in impulses stimulates the sympathetic nervous system and inhibits the parasympathetic nervous system. The outcome of this process is an increase in cardiac rate, conduction, and contractility and in circulating blood volume. Sympathetic stimulation constricts renal arterioles; this increases the release of aldosterone, decreases glomerular filtration, and increases sodium and water reabsorption.

Renin is an enzyme that converts angiotensinogen, an inactive substance formed by the liver, into angiotensin I and angiotensin II. An enzyme released within the lung capillaries converts angiotensin I to angiotensin II. Angiotensin II, with its vasoconstrictor properties, increases arterial perfusion pressure and stimulates thirst. As the sympathetic nervous system is stimulated, aldosterone is released in response to an increased release of renin. Aldosterone is a volume regulator and will also be released as serum potassium increases, serum sodium decreases, or ACTH levels increase.

Antidiuretic hormone (ADH) and the **thirst mechanism** have important roles in maintaining sodium concentration and oral intake of fluids. Oral intake is controlled by the thirst center located in the hypothalamus. As serum concentration or osmolality increases or blood volume decreases, neurons in the hypothalamus are stimulated by intracellular dehydration; thirst then occurs and the person increases oral intake of fluids. Water excretion is controlled by ADH, aldosterone, and baroreceptors as mentioned previously.

Osmoreceptors, located on the surface of the hypothalamus, sense changes in sodium concentration. As osmotic pressure increases, the neurons become dehydrated and quickly release impulses to the posterior pituitary which increase the release of ADH. ADH travels in the blood to the kidneys where it alters permeability to water, causing an increased reabsorption of water and a decreased urine output. The retained water dilutes the ECF and returns its concentration to normal. Restoration of normal osmotic pressure provides feedback to the osmoreceptors to inhibit future ADH release (see Fig. 14-2).

Gerontologic Considerations

Normal physiologic changes of aging, including reduced renal and respiratory function and reserve and alterations in the ratio of body fluids to muscle mass, may alter the responses of an elderly person to fluid and electrolyte changes and acid–base disturbances. In addition, the frequent use of medications in the elderly can affect renal and cardiac function and fluid balance, thereby increasing the likelihood of fluid and electrolyte disturbances. Routine procedures, such as the vigorous administration of laxatives before colon x-rays, may produce serious fluid volume deficit in the elderly, necessitating use of intravenous fluids to prevent hypotension and other effects of hypovolemia.

Alterations in fluid and electrolyte balance that may initially produce minor changes in the young and middle-aged adult have the potential to produce profound changes in the elderly, accompanied by a rapid onset of signs and symptoms. In other elderly patients, the clinical manifestations of fluid and electrolyte disturbances may be subtle or atypical. For example, fluid deficit or reduced sodium levels (hyponatremia) may cause confusion in the elderly patient, whereas in young and middle-aged people the first sign commonly is increased thirst. Rapid infusion of an excessive volume of intravenous fluids may produce fluid overload and cardiac failure in the elderly. These reactions are likely to occur more quickly and with the administration of a smaller volume of fluid than in healthy young and middle-aged adults because of the decreased cardiac reserve and reduction of renal function that accompany aging.

Increased sensitivity to fluid and electrolyte changes in the elderly requires careful assessment with attention to intake and output of fluids from all sources and changes in daily weight, careful monitoring of side effects and interactions of medications, and prompt reporting and management of disturbances. Additional gerontologic considerations relating to specific fluid and electrolyte disturbances are discussed later in this chapter.

Fluid Volume Disturbances

Fluid Volume Deficit (Hypovolemia)

Fluid volume deficit (FVD) results when water and electrolytes are lost in the same proportion as they exist in normal body fluids, so that the ratio of serum electrolytes to water remains the same. It should not be confused with the term *dehydration,* which refers to loss of water alone with increased serum sodium levels. FVD may occur alone or in combination with other imbalances. Unless other imbalances are present concurrently, serum electrolyte concentrations remain essentially unchanged.

Fluid volume deficit results from loss of body fluids and occurs more rapidly when coupled with decreased fluid intake. It is possible to develop FVD on the basis of inadequate intake alone if the decreased intake is prolonged.

Causes of FVD include abnormal fluid losses, such as those resulting from vomiting, diarrhea, gastrointestinal suction, and sweating, and decreased intake, as in the presence of nausea or inability to gain access to fluids.

Additional risk factors include diabetes insipidus, adrenal insufficiency, osmotic diuresis, hemorrhage, and coma. Third-space fluid shifts, or the movement of fluid from the vascular system to other body spaces (*i.e.,* with edema formation in burns or ascites with liver dysfunction), also produce FVD.

Clinical Manifestations

Fluid volume deficit can develop rapidly and can be mild, moderate, or severe, depending on the degree of fluid loss. Important characteristics of FVD include acute weight loss; decreased skin turgor; oliguria; concentrated urine; postural hypotension; a weak, rapid heart rate; flattened neck veins; increased temperature; decreased CVP; cool, clammy skin related to peripheral vasoconstriction; thirst; anorexia; nausea; lassitude; muscle weakness; and cramps.

Diagnostic Evaluation

Laboratory data useful in evaluating fluid volume status include the blood urea nitrogen (BUN) level and its relationship with the serum creatinine concentration. A volume-depleted patient has a BUN elevated out of proportion to the serum creatinine level (>10:1). The cause of hypovolemia may be determined by evaluating the history and physical exam. The BUN can be elevated due to dehydration or decreased renal perfusion and function. Also, the hematocrit level is greater than normal as the red blood cells become suspended in a decreased plasma volume.

Serum electrolyte changes may also exist. Potassium and sodium levels can be reduced (hypokalemia, hyponatremia) or elevated (hyperkalemia, hypernatremia).

- *Hypokalemia* can occur with gastrointestinal and renal losses.
- *Hyperkalemia* can occur with adrenal insufficiency.
- *Hypernatremia* will be seen with increased insensible losses and diabetes insipidus.
- *Hyponatremia* may exist due to increased thirst and ADH release.

Urine specific gravity is increased related to the kidneys' attempt to save water and decreased with diabetes insipidus. Normal values for these tests are listed in Table 14-4.

Management

In planning how to correct fluid loss for the patient with FVD, one must consider the usual maintenance requirements of the patient and other factors (such as fever) that can influence fluid needs. When the deficit is not severe, the oral route is preferred, provided the patient is able to drink. When fluid losses are acute or severe, however, the intravenous route is required. Isotonic electrolyte solutions (such as lactated Ringer's or 0.9% sodium chloride) are frequently used to treat the hypotensive patient with FVD, because such fluids expand plasma volume. As soon as the patient becomes normotensive, a hypotonic electrolyte solution (such as 0.45% sodium chloride) is often used to provide both electrolytes and free water for renal excretion of metabolic wastes. These and additional fluids are summarized in Table 14-5.

Accurate and frequent assessments of intake and output, weight, vital signs, central venous pressure, level of consciousness, breath sounds, and skin color should be performed to determine when therapy should be slowed to avoid volume overload. The rate of fluid administration is based on the severity of loss and the patient's hemodynamic response to volume replacement.

If the patient with severe FVD is not excreting enough urine and is therefore oliguric, it must be determined whether the depressed renal function is the result of reduced renal blood flow secondary to FVD (prerenal azotemia) or, more seriously, to acute tubular necrosis due to prolonged FVD. The test used in this situation is referred to as a *fluid challenge test.* During a fluid challenge test, volumes of fluid are administered at specific rates and intervals while the patient's hemodynamic response to this treatment is monitored (*i.e.*, vital signs, breath sounds, sensorium, central venous pressure, urine output). A typical example of

TABLE 14-4 Laboratory Tests Used to Evaluate Fluid and Electrolyte Status

Test	Usual Reference Range	SI Units
Serum sodium	135–145 mEq/L	135–145 mmol/L
Serum potassium	3.5–5.5 mEq/L	3.5–5.5 mmol/L
Total serum calcium	8.5–10.5 mg/dl (approximately 50% in ionized form)	2.1–2.6 mmol/L
Serum magnesium	1.5–2.5 mEq/L	0.80–1.2 mmol/L
Serum phosphorus	2.5–4.5 mEq/L	0.80–1.5 mmol/L
Serum chloride	100–106 mEq/L	100–106 mmol/L
Carbon dioxide content	24–30 mEq/L	24–30 mmol/L
Serum osmolality	280–295 mOsm/kg	280–295 mmol/L
Blood urea nitrogen (BUN)	10–20 mg/dl	3.5–7 mmol/L of urea
Serum creatinine	0.7–1.5 mg/dl	60–130 umol/L
BUN to creatinine ratio	10:1	
Hematocrit	Male: 44–52%	Volume fraction: 0.44–0.52
	Female: 39–47%	Volume fraction: 0.39–0.47
Serum glucose	70–110 mg/dl	3.9–6.1 mmol/L
Serum albumin	3.5–5.5 g/dl	3.5–5.5 g/L
Urinary sodium	80–180 mEq/day	80–180 mmol/day
Urinary potassium	40–80 mEq/day	40–80 mmol/day
Urinary chloride	110–250 mEq/day	110–250 mmol/day
Urinary specific gravity	1.025–1.035 = physiologic range after fluid restriction	1.025–1.035
	1.010–1.020 = random specimen with normal fluid intake.	
Urine osmolality		
Extreme range	50–1400 mOsm/L	40–1400 mmol/kg
Typical urine	500–800 mOsm/L	500–800 mmol/kg
Urinary *p*H	4.5–8.0	4.5–8.0
Typical urine	<6.6	<6.6

TABLE 14-5 Selected Water and Electrolyte Solutions

Solution	Comments
Isotonic Solutions	
0.9% NaCl (Isotonic saline) Na^+ 154 mEq/L Cl^- 154 mEq/L (308 mOsm/kg) Also available with varying concentrations of dextrose (the most frequently used is a 5% dextrose concentration)	· An isotonic solution that expands the extracellular fluid volume, used in hypovolemic states · Supplies an excess of Na^+ and Cl^-; can cause fluid volume excess and hyperchloremic acidosis if used in excessive volumes, particularly in patients with compromised renal function · Not desirable as a routine maintenance solution, as it provides only Na^+ and Cl^- (and these are provided in excessive amounts) · Sometimes used to correct mild Na^+ deficit · When mixed with 5% dextrose, the resulting solution becomes hypertonic in relation to plasma and, in addition to the above described electrolytes, provides 170 calories per liter · Only solution that may be administered with blood products
Lactated Ringer's solution (Hartmann's solution) Na^+ 130 mEq/L K^+ 4 mEq/L Ca^{2+} 3 mEq/L Cl^- 109 mEq/L Lactate (metabolized to bicarbonate) 28 mEq/L (274 mOsm/L) Also available with varying concentrations of dextrose (the most common is 5% dextrose)	· An isotonic solution that contains multiple electrolytes in roughly the same concentration as found in plasma (note that solution is lacking in Mg^{2+}) · Used in the treatment of hypovolemia, burns, and fluid lost as bile or diarrhea · Lactate is rapidly metabolized into HCO_3^- in the body. Lactated Ringer's solution should not be used in lactic acidosis because the ability to convert lactate into HCO_3^- is impaired in this disorder. · Not to be given with a $pH>7.5$, as bicarbonate is formed as lactate breaks down, causing alkalosis.
5% dextrose in water (D_5W) No electrolytes 50 g of dextrose	· An isotonic solution that supplies 170 calories per liter and free water to aid in renal excretion of solutes · Should not be used in excessive volumes in the early postoperative period (when ADH secretion is increased due to stress reaction) · Should not be used solely in treatment of fluid volume deficit, because it dilutes plasma electrolyte concentrations.
Hypotonic Solutions	
0.45% NaCl (half-strength saline) Na^+ 77 mEq/L Cl^- 77 mEq/L (154 mOsm/L) Also avilable with varying concentrations of dextrose (the most common is a 5% concentration)	· Provides Na^+, Cl^-, and free water · Free water is desirable to aid the kidneys in elimination of solute · Lacking in electrolytes other than Na^+ and Cl^- · When mixed with 5% dextrose, the solution becomes slightly hypertonic to plasma and in addition to the above-described electrolytes provides 170 calories
Hypertonic Solutions	
3% NaCl (hypertonic saline) Na^+ 513 mEq/L Cl^- 513 mEq/L (1026 mOsm/L)	· Highly hypertonic solution used only in critical situations to treat hyponatremia · Must be administered slowly and cautiously as it can cause intravascular volume overload and pulmonary edema.
5% NaCL (Hypertonic solution) Na^+ 855 mEq/L CL^- 855 mEq/L (1710 mOsm/L)	· Highly hypertonic solution used to treat symptomatic hyponatremia. · Administered slowly and cautiously as it can cause intravascular volume overload and pulmonary edema.

(Adapted from Metheny N. Fluid and Electrolyte Balance: Nursing Considerations. Philadelphia, JB Lippincott, 1992.)

a fluid challenge is 100 to 200 ml normal saline over 10 minutes. The response by a patient with FVD but normal renal function would be increased urine output and an increase in blood pressure and central venous pressure.

Shock can occur when the volume of fluid lost exceeds 25% of the intravascular volume or when fluid loss is rapid. Shock, its causes, and treatment are discussed in detail in Chapter 15.

Nursing Assessment

To assess for the presence of FVD, *fluid intake and output* are measured and evaluated at least at 8-hour intervals; sometimes, hourly measurements are indicated. As FVD is developing, body fluid losses exceed fluid intake. This loss may be in the form of excessive urination (polyuria), diarrhea, vomiting, and so on. Later, after FVD has fully developed, the kidneys attempt to conserve needed body fluids, leading to a urinary output less than 30 ml/hr in an adult; urine in this instance is concentrated and represents a healthy renal response. Daily body weight measurements are monitored; an acute weight loss of 0.5 kg (1 pound) represents a fluid loss of approximately 500 ml. (One liter of fluid weighs approximately 1 kg, or 2.2 pounds.)

The *vital signs* are closely monitored. The nurse should be particularly alert for a weak, rapid pulse and postural hypotension (*i.e.*, a drop in the systolic pressure greater than 15 mm Hg when the patient goes from a lying to a sitting position). A decrease in body temperature often accompanies fluid volume deficit, unless there is a concurrent infection.

Skin and tongue turgor are monitored on a regular basis. In a healthy person, pinched skin will immediately return to its normal position when released. This elastic property, referred to as turgor, is partially dependent on interstitial fluid volume. In a person with FVD, the skin flattens more slowly after the pinch is released; when the FVD is severe, the skin may remain elevated for many seconds. Tissue turgor is best measured by pinching the skin over the sternum, inner aspects of the thighs, or forehead. The skin turgor test is not as valid in elderly people as in younger people because skin elasticity decreases with age.

Evaluating tongue turgor, which is not affected by age, may be more valid than evaluating skin turgor. In a normal person, the tongue has one longitudinal furrow. In the person with FVD, there are additional longitudinal furrows and the tongue is smaller, because of fluid loss. The degree of oral mucous membrane moisture is also assessed; a dry mouth may indicate either FVD or mouth breathing.

Urinary concentration is monitored by measuring the urine specific gravity. In a volume-depleted patient, the urinary specific gravity should be above 1.020, indicating healthy renal conservation of fluid.

Mental function is eventually affected in severe volume depletion as a result of decreasing cerebral perfusion. Decreased peripheral perfusion can result in *cold extremities*. In patients with relatively normal cardiopulmonary function, a *low central venous pressure* is indicative of hypovolemia. Patients with acute cardiopulmonary decompensation require more extensive hemodynamic monitoring to monitor pressures in both sides of the heart.

Nursing Interventions

Preventing FVD. To prevent FVD, one must be aware of patients at risk and take measures to minimize fluid losses. For example, if the patient has diarrhea, measures should be implemented to control the diarrhea while replacing fluids. These measures may include administering antidiarrheal medications and small volumes of oral fluids at frequent intervals.

Correcting FVD. When possible, oral fluids are administered to help correct FVD, with consideration given to the patient's likes and dislikes. Also, the type of fluid the patient has lost is considered and attempts are made to select fluids most likely to replace the lost electrolytes. If the patient is reluctant to drink because of oral discomfort, frequent mouth care is given and fluids that are nonirritating to the mucosa are provided. The patient may be offered small volumes of fluids at frequent intervals rather than a large volume all at once. If nausea is present, antiemetics may be needed before oral fluid replacement can be tolerated.

If the patient is unable to eat and drink, the physician may consider an alternative route (enteral or parenteral administration) for fluid intake. This intervention is important to prevent renal damage related to prolonged FVD.

Fluid Volume Excess (Hypervolemia)

Fluid volume excess (FVE) refers to an isotonic expansion of the ECF caused by the abnormal retention of water and sodium in approximately the same proportions in which they normally exist in the ECF. It is always secondary to an increase in the total body sodium content, which, in turn, leads to an increase in total body water. Because there is isotonic retention of body substances, the serum sodium concentration remains essentially normal.

Causes of fluid volume excess may be related to simple fluid overloading or diminished function of the homeostatic mechanisms responsible for regulating fluid balance. Causative factors can include congestive heart failure, renal failure, and cirrhosis of the liver. Overzealous administration of sodium-containing fluids to someone with impaired regulatory mechanisms particularly predisposes the person to serious fluid volume excess. Excessive ingestion of table salt (sodium chloride) or other sodium salts also predisposes to fluid overload.

Clinical Manifestations

The clinical manifestations of FVE stem from expansion of the ECF compartment and include edema, distended neck veins, and crackles (abnormal lung sounds). Other manifestations of fluid volume excess include tachycardia; increased blood pressure, pulse pressure, and central venous pressure; increased weight; increased urine output; and shortness of breath and wheezing.

Diagnostic Evaluation

Laboratory data useful in the diagnosis of FVE include the BUN and hematocrit levels. In the presence of FVE, both of these values may be decreased because of plasma dilution. Other causes for abnormalities in these values include low protein intake and anemia. In chronic renal failure, both serum osmolality and sodium will be decreased due to an excessive retention of water. Urine sodium will be increased if the kidneys are attempting to excrete excess volume. Chest x-ray may indicate pulmonary congestion. Hypervolemia occurs when aldosterone is chronically stimulated (*i.e.*, cirrhosis, congestive heart failure, and nephrotic syndrome); urine sodium, therefore, will not be increased in these conditions.

Management

Management of FVE is directed at the causative factors. The treatment of edema includes measures to mobilize fluid (*i.e.*, supine positioning and supportive stockings). When the fluid excess is related to excessive administration of sodium-containing fluids, discontinuing the infusion may be all that is needed. Symptomatic treatment consists of administering diuretics and restricting fluids and sodium.

Diuretics. Diuretics are prescribed when dietary restriction of sodium alone is insufficient to reduce edema by inhibiting the reabsorption of sodium and water by the kidneys. Choices of diuretics are based on the severity of the hypervolemic state, degree of impairment of renal function, and potency of the diuretic. Generally, thiazide diuretics are prescribed for mild to moderate hypervolemia and loop diuretics for severe hypervolemia.

Electrolyte imbalances may result from the effect of the diuretic. Hypokalemia can occur with all diuretics except those (*e.g.*, spironolactone) that work in the last distal tubule of the nephrons. Potassium supplements can be prescribed to avoid this complication. Hyperkalemia can occur with diuretics that work in the last distal tubule, especially when administered to patients with decreased renal function. Hyponatremia occurs with diuresis due to increased release of ADH secondary to reduction in circulating volume. Decreased magnesium occurs with administration of loop and thiazide diuretics due to a decreased reabsorption and increased excretion of magnesium by the kidney.

Azotemia (increased nitrogen levels in the blood) can occur with FVE when urea and creatinine are not excreted due to decreased perfusion by the kidneys and decreased excretion of wastes. High uric acid levels (*hyperuricemia*) can also occur due to increased reabsorption and decreased excretion of uric acid by the kidneys.

Other Treatment Modalities. When renal function is severely impaired so that pharmacologic agents cannot act efficiently, other modalities are considered to remove sodium and fluid from the body. Hemodialysis or peritoneal dialysis may be used to remove nitrogenous wastes and control potassium and acid–base balance, and to remove sodium and fluid. Continuous arteriovenous hemofiltration (CAVH) may also be considered. See Chapter 42 for discussion of these treatment modalities.

Sodium-Restricted Diets. Treatment of FVE usually involves dietary restriction of sodium. An average daily diet not restricted in sodium contains 6 to 15 g of salt, whereas low-sodium diets can range from a mild restriction to as low as 250 mg of sodium per day, depending on the patient's needs. A mild sodium-restricted diet allows only light salting of food (about half the amount as usual) in cooking and at the table, and no addition of salt to commercially prepared foods that are already seasoned. Of course, foods high in sodium must be avoided. It is the sodium salt, sodium chloride, rather than sodium that contributes to edema formation. Therefore, patients need to read food labels carefully to determine their salt content.

Because about half of ingested sodium is in the form of seasoning, using seasoning substitutes plays a major role in decreasing sodium intake. Lemon juice, onion, and garlic are excellent substitute flavoring agents; however, some patients prefer salt substitutes. Most salt substitutes contain potassium and should be used cautiously by patients taking potassium-sparing diuretics (*e.g.*, spironolactone, triamterene, and amiloride). They should not be used at all in patients with conditions associated with potassium retention, such as advanced renal disease. Salt substitutes containing ammonium chloride can be harmful to patients with liver damage.

In some communities, the drinking water may contain too much sodium for a sodium-restricted diet. Depending on its source, water may contain as little as 1 mg or more than 1500 mg per quart. It may be necessary for patients to use distilled water when the local water supply is very high in sodium. Also, patients on sodium-restricted diets should be cautioned to avoid "water softeners" that add sodium to water in exchange for other ions, such as calcium.

Nursing Assessment

To assess for FVE, the fluid intake and output are measured at regular intervals for indication of excessive fluid retention. The patient is weighed daily, and acute weight gain is noted. (An acute weight gain of 0.9 kg [2 pounds] represents a gain of approximately 1 liter of fluid.)

It is important to assess breath sounds at regular intervals in at-risk patients, particularly when parenteral fluids are being administered. The nurse monitors the degree of edema in the most dependent parts of the body, such as the feet and ankles in ambulatory patients and the sacral region in bedridden patients. The degree of pitting edema is assessed and the extent of peripheral edema is monitored by measuring the circumference of the extremity with a tape marked in millimeters.

Nursing Interventions

Preventing FVE. Specific interventions vary somewhat with the underlying pathologic condition and the degree of FVE. Most patients, however, require sodium-restricted diets in some form. Therefore, adherence to the prescribed diet is encouraged. The patient is instructed to avoid over-the-counter medications without first checking with a health care provider, as these substances may contain sodium. When fluid retention persists despite adherence to a prescribed diet, hidden sources of sodium, such as the water supply or use of water softeners, should be considered.

Detecting and Controlling FVE. Detecting FVE is of primary importance before the condition becomes critical. Interventions include providing rest, restricting sodium, monitoring parenteral fluid therapy, and administering appropriate medications.

Some patients benefit from regular rest periods, as bed rest favors diuresis of edema fluid. The mechanism is probably related to diminished venous pooling and subsequent increase in effective circulating blood volume and renal perfusion. Sodium and fluid restriction should be instituted as indicated. Because most patients with FVE require diuretics, the patient's response to these agents is monitored. The rate of parenteral fluids and the patient's response to these fluids are also closely monitored. If dyspnea or orthopnea is present, the patient is placed in a semi-Fowler's position to promote lung expansion. The patient is turned and positioned at regular intervals, because edematous tissue is more prone to skin breakdown than normal tissue.

Because conditions predisposing to FVE are likely to be chronic, the patient is taught to monitor his or her own response to therapy by recording and evaluating fluid intake and output and body weight changes. The importance of adhering to the medical regimen is emphasized.

Edema

Edema is a common manifestation of fluid volume excess that deserves special attention. Edema formation, the result of expansion of the fluid in the interstitial fluid compartment, can be localized, for example, in the ankle; can be related to rheumatoid arthritis; or can be generalized, as in cardiac and renal failure. Severe generalized edema is called *anasarca.*

Edema will occur when there is a change in the capillary membrane, increasing the formation of interstitial fluid or decreasing removal of interstitial fluid. Burns and infection are examples of conditions associated with increasing interstitial fluid volume. Obstruction to lymphatic outflow or a decrease in plasma oncotic pressure contributes to increased interstitial fluid volume. The kidneys retain sodium and water when there is a decreased extracellular volume as a result of a decreased cardiac output from heart failure.

Ascites is a form of edema observed in the peritoneal cavity due to nephrotic syndrome or cirrhosis. Patients commonly report shortness of breath and a sense of pressure because of pressure on the diaphragm.

Edema is usually seen in dependent areas. It can be found in the ankles, sacrum, scrotum, or the periorbital region of the face. *Pitting edema* is so named because of a pit formed after one presses a finger into edematous tissue. *Pulmonary edema* is yet another form of edema in which an increase in fluid in the pulmonary interstitium and the alveoli occurs. Manifestations include shortness of breath, increased respiratory rate, diaphoresis, and crackles and wheezing on auscultation of the lungs.

Decreased hematocrit due to hemodilution, arterial blood gas results indicative of respiratory alkalosis and hypoxemia, and decreased serum sodium and osmolality due to retention of fluid may occur with edema. BUN and creatinine will increase, urine specific gravity will decrease as the kidneys attempt to excrete excess water, and urine sodium will be decreased due to increased production of aldosterone.

The *treatment* goal in edema is to preserve or restore the circulating intravascular fluid volume. In addition to treating the cause, other treatment choices may include diuretic therapy, restriction of fluids and sodium, elevation of the extremities, application of supportive stockings, paracentesis, dialysis, or continuous arterial venous hemofiltration (CAVH).

Gerontologic Considerations

The aged have special nursing care needs because of their propensity for developing fluid and electrolyte problems. Fluid balance in the elderly is often marginal at best because of certain physiologic changes associated with the aging process. Some of these changes include reduction in total body water (associated with increased body fat content and decreased muscle mass), reduction in renal function resulting in decreased ability to concentrate urine, decreased cardiovascular and respiratory function, and disturbances in hormonal regulatory functions. Although these changes are viewed as normal in the aging process, they must be considered when the elderly person becomes ill, because they predispose to fluid and electrolyte imbalances.

Assessment of the elderly patient should be modified somewhat from that of younger adults. For example, skin turgor is less valid as an assessment tool in the elderly because their skin has lost some of its elasticity; therefore, other assessment measures, such as slowness in filling of veins of the hands and feet, become more important in detecting fluid volume deficit. When skin turgor is tested in the elderly, it is best tested over the forehead or the sternum, because alterations in skin elasticity are less marked in these areas. As in any patient, skin turgor should be monitored serially to detect subtle changes.

The nurse should perform a functional assessment of the aged person's ability to determine fluid and food needs and to obtain adequate intake. For example, is the patient mentally clear? Is he able to ambulate and use his arms and hands to reach fluids and foods? Is he able to swallow? All of these questions have direct bearing on how the patient will be able to manage his own need for fluids and foods. The nurse must, of course, provide for any patient who is unable to carry out self-care activities. Another concern is that some elderly patients deliberately restrict their fluid intake to avoid embarrassing episodes of incontinence. In this situation, the nurse also implements interventions to deal with the incontinence, such as encouraging the patient to wear protective devices, carry a urinal in the car, or pace fluid intake to allow access to toilet facilities during the day.

Sodium Imbalances

Disturbances in sodium balance occur frequently in clinical practice and can develop under simple and complex circumstances.

Functions of Sodium. Sodium is the most abundant electrolyte in the ECF; its concentration ranges from 135 to 145 mEq/L (SI: 135–145 mmol/L) and consequently, it is the primary determinant of ECF osmolality. Decreased sodium is associated with parallel changes in osmolality. The fact that sodium does not easily cross the cell-wall membrane, plus its abundance or high concentration, accounts for its primary role in controlling water distribution throughout the body. In addition, sodium is the primary regulator of ECF volume. A loss or gain of sodium is usually accompanied by a loss or gain of water. Sodium also functions in establishing the electrochemical state necessary for muscle contraction and the transmission of nerve impulses.

Sodium Deficit (Hyponatremia)

Hyponatremia refers to a serum sodium level that is below normal (less than 135 mEq/L; SI: 135 mmol/L). Plasma sodium concentration represents the ratio of total body sodium to total body water. A decrease in this ratio can occur from a low quantity of total body sodium with a lesser reduction in total body water, normal total body sodium content with excess total body water, and an excess of total body sodium with an even greater excess of total body water. A hyponatremic state can, however, be superimposed on an existing fluid volume deficit (FVD) or fluid volume excess (FVE).

Sodium may be lost by way of vomiting, diarrhea, fistulas, or sweating, or it may be associated with diuretics, particularly in combination with a low-salt diet. A deficiency of aldosterone, as occurs in adrenal insufficiency, also predisposes the patient to sodium deficiency.

Dilutional Hyponatremia. In water intoxication (dilutional hyponatremia) the patient's serum sodium is diluted by an increase in the ratio of water to sodium. This causes water to move into the cell, so that the patient develops an ECF volume excess and an ICF volume excess. Predisposing conditions for this type of hyponatremia include syndrome of inappropriate antidiuretic hormone (SIADH), hyperglycemia, and increased water intake through the administration of electrolyte-poor parenteral fluids, the use of tap water enemas or irrigation of gastric tubes with water instead of normal saline.

Water may be gained abnormally by the excessive parenteral administration of dextrose and water solutions, particularly during periods of stress. It may also be gained by compulsive water drinking (psychogenic polydipsia).

SIADH. A special type of hyponatremia associated with excessive antidiuretic hormone (ADH) activity is referred to as the syndrome of inappropriate ADH secretion (SIADH). The basic physiologic disturbances in SIADH are excessive ADH activity, with water retention and dilutional hyponatremia, and inappropriate urinary excretion of sodium in the presence of hyponatremia. SIADH can be the result of either sustained secretion of ADH by the hypothalamus or production of an ADH-like substance from a tumor (aberrant ADH production). Conditions associated with SIADH include oat-cell lung tumors, head injuries, endocrine and pulmonary disorders, and use of medications such as pitocin, cyclophosphamide, vincristine, thioridazine, and amitriptyline.

Clinical Manifestations

Clinical manifestations of hyponatremia depend on the cause, magnitude, and speed with which the deficit occurs. Although nausea and abdominal cramping occur, most of the symptoms are neuropsychiatric and are probably related to the cellular swelling and cerebral edema associated with hyponatremia. As the extracellular sodium level decreases, the cellular fluid becomes relatively more concentrated and "pulls" water into the cells (Fig. 14-3). In general, those patients having acute decrease in serum sodium levels have more severe symptoms and higher mortality rates than do those with more slowly developing hyponatremia.

Features of hyponatremia associated with sodium loss and water gain include anorexia, muscle cramps, and a feeling of exhaustion. When the serum sodium level drops below 115 mEq/L (SI: 115 mmol/L), signs of increasing intracranial pressure, such as lethargy, confusion, muscular twitching, focal weakness, hemiparesis, papilledema, and seizures may occur.

Diagnostic Evaluation

Regardless of the cause of hyponatremia, the serum sodium level is less than 135 mEq/L; in SIADH it may be quite low, such as 100 mEq/L (SI: 100 mmol/L) or less. Serum osmolality is also decreased except in azotemia or ingestion of toxins. When hyponatremia is due primarily to sodium loss, the urinary sodium content is less than 10 mEq/L (SI: 10 mmol/L) and the specific gravity is low, such as 1.002 to 1.004. When hyponatremia is due to SIADH, however, the urinary sodium content is greater than 20 mEq/L and the urinary specific gravity is usually greater than 1.012. Although the patient with SIADH retains water abnormally and thus gains body weight, there is no peripheral edema; instead, the edema is inside the cells. This phenomenon is sometimes manifested as "fingerprinting" when the finger is pressed over a bony prominence, such as the sternum.

Management

Sodium Replacement. The obvious treatment for hyponatremia is careful administration of sodium. This may be accomplished orally, by nasogastric tube, or parenterally.

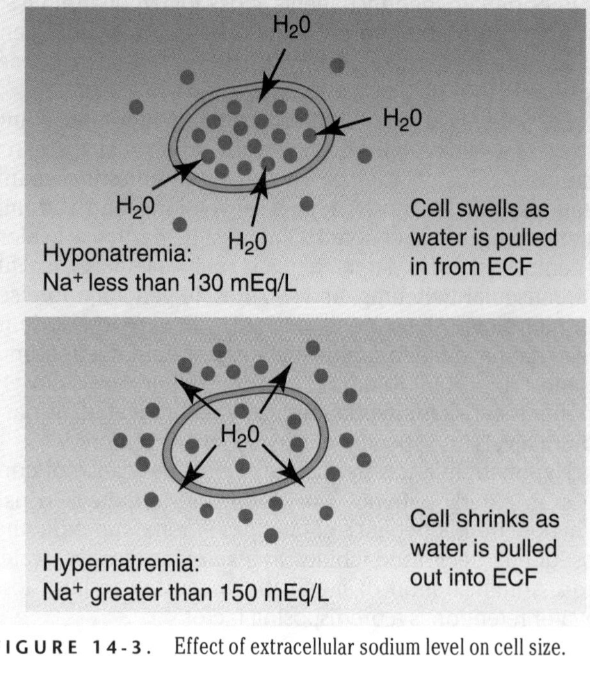

FIGURE 14-3. Effect of extracellular sodium level on cell size.

For patients who are able to eat and drink, sodium replacement is easily accomplished, because sodium is plentiful in a normal diet. For those unable to take sodium orally, lactated Ringer's solution or isotonic saline (0.9% sodium chloride) may be prescribed (Table 14-5 describes the components of selected water and electrolyte solutions). The usual daily sodium requirement in adults is approximately 100 mEq, provided there are no abnormal losses.

In SIADH, hypertonic saline alone cannot change the plasma sodium concentration. Excess sodium would be rapidly excreted in a highly concentrated urine. With the addition of furosemide (Lasix), urine is not concentrated and isotonic urine is excreted achieving a change in water balance. Additionally, in patients with SIADH, in whom water restriction is difficult, lithium or democlocycline can antagonize the osmotic effect of ADH on the medullary collecting tubule.

Water Restriction. When hyponatremia is present in a patient with normal or excess fluid volume, the treatment of choice is water restriction. This is far safer than sodium administration and is usually quite effective. When neurologic symptoms are present, however, it may be necessary to administer small volumes of a hypertonic sodium solution, such as 3% or 5% sodium chloride. Incorrect use of these fluids is *extremely dangerous;* this is understandable when one considers that a liter of 3% sodium chloride solution contains 513 mEq of sodium and a liter of 5% sodium chloride solution contains 855 mEq of sodium.

- Highly hypertonic sodium solutions (3% and 5% sodium chloride) should be administered only in intensive care settings under close observation, because only small volumes are needed to elevate the serum sodium level from a dangerously low value. These fluids are administered slowly, in small volumes, while the patient is monitored closely for fluid overload.

Nursing Assessment

It is important to identify patients at risk for hyponatremia so that they can be monitored. Early detection and treatment of this disorder are necessary to prevent serious consequences.

For patients at risk, the nurse monitors fluid intake and output as well as daily body weight. Abnormal losses of sodium or gains of water are noted. Gastrointestinal manifestations, such as anorexia, nausea, vomiting, and abdominal cramping, are also noted. One must be particularly alert for central nervous system changes, such as lethargy, confusion, muscular twitching, and seizures. In general, more severe neurologic signs are associated with very low sodium levels that have fallen rapidly because of fluid overloading. It is most important to monitor serum sodium levels closely in patients at risk for hyponatremia. When indicated, urinary sodium levels and specific gravity are also monitored.

Hyponatremia is a frequently overlooked cause of confusion in elderly patients. The elderly are at increased risk for hyponatremia because of changes in renal function and subsequent decreased ability to excrete excessive water loads. Administration of medications causing sodium loss or water retention is a predisposing factor.

Nursing Interventions

Detecting and Controlling Hyponatremia. One should be aware of patients at risk for hyponatremia and initiate measures to detect the disturbance before it becomes severe. For patients suffering abnormal losses of sodium, yet able to consume a general diet, foods and fluids with a high sodium content are encouraged and provided. For example, broth made with one beef cube contains approximately 900 mg of sodium, and 8 ounces of tomato juice contains approximately 700 mg of sodium.

It is important to be familiar with the sodium content of parenteral fluids (see Table 14-5).

Cautions. When administering fluids to patients with *cardiovascular disease,* one should monitor the patient for signs of circulatory overload, such as crackles, with auscultation of the lungs. As was stated earlier, extreme care is essential when administering highly hypertonic sodium fluids (such as 3% or 5% sodium chloride), because these fluids can be lethal if they are infused carelessly.

For patients taking *lithium,* one should be alert for lithium toxicity when sodium is lost by an abnormal route. In such instances, supplemental salt and fluid are administered. Because diuretics promote sodium loss, patients taking lithium are instructed not to use diuretics unless under close medical supervision. For all patients on lithium therapy, an adequate salt intake should be ensured.

Excess water supplements are avoided in patients receiving isotonic or hypotonic *tube feedings,* particularly if abnormal sodium loss occurs or water is being abnormally retained (as in SIADH). Actual fluid needs are determined by evaluating the intake and output, urinary specific gravity, and serum sodium levels.

Returning Sodium Level to Normal. When the primary problem is water retention, it is safer to restrict fluid intake than to administer sodium. Administering sodium to a patient with normovolemia or hypervolemia predisposes to fluid volume overload. As was stated previously, patients with cardiovascular disease receiving fluids containing sodium should be monitored very closely for signs of circulatory overload, such as crackles.

In severe hyponatremia, the aim of therapy is to elevate the serum sodium level only enough to alleviate neurologic signs. For example, it has been recommended that the serum sodium concentration be raised to a level no higher than 125 mEq/L (SI: 125 mmol/L) with hypertonic saline.

Sodium Excess (Hypernatremia)

Hypernatremia refers to a greater than normal serum sodium level, that is, a serum level greater than 145 mEq/L (SI: 145 mmol/L). It can be caused by a gain of sodium in excess of water or by a loss of water in excess of sodium. It can occur in patients with normal fluid volume or in those with FVD or FVE. Hypernatremia can occur from a disproportionate water loss or a sodium excess. With a water loss, the patient loses more water than sodium and as a result serum sodium concentration increases and the increased concentration pulls fluid out of the cell. This is both an extracellular and intracellular fluid volume deficit. In sodium excess, the patient ingests or retains more sodium than water.

Causes. A common cause of hypernatremia is deprivation of water in unconscious patients who are unable to perceive or respond to thirst. Most often affected are very old, very young, and cognitively impaired patients who are unable to communicate their thirst. Administration of hypertonic tube feedings without adequate water supplements leads to hypernatremia, as does watery diarrhea and greatly increased insensible water loss (as in hyperventilation or denuding effects of burns). Diabetes insipidus leads to hypernatremia if the patient does not experience, or cannot respond to, thirst or if fluids are excessively restricted. Less common causes are heatstroke, near drowning in sea water (which contains a sodium concentration of approximately 500 mEq/L), and malfunction of either hemodialysis or peritoneal dialysis proportioning systems. Intravenous administration of hypertonic saline or excessive use of sodium bicarbonate will also cause hypernatremia.

Clinical Manifestations

The clinical manifestations of hypernatremia are primarily neurologic and are presumably the consequence of cellular dehydration. Hypernatremia results in a relatively concentrated ECF, causing water to be pulled from the cells (see Fig. 14-3). Clinically, these changes may be manifested by restlessness and weakness in moderate hypernatremia and by disorientation, delusions, and hallucinations in severe hypernatremia. Dehydration (resulting in hypernatremia) is often overlooked as the primary reason for behavioral changes in the elderly. If hypernatremia is severe, permanent brain damage can occur (especially in children). Brain damage is apparently due to subarachnoid hemorrhages that result from brain contraction.

A primary characteristic of hypernatremia is thirst. Thirst is so strong a defender of serum sodium levels in normal people that hypernatremia never occurs unless the person is unconscious or is denied access to water; unfortunately, ill people may have an impaired thirst mechanism. Other signs include dry, swollen tongue and sticky mucous membranes. Flushed skin, peripheral and pulmonary edema, postural hypotension, and increased muscle tone and deep tendon reflexes are additional signs and symptoms which can occur with hypernatremia. A mild elevation in body temperature may occur, but when the hypernatremia is corrected, the body temperature should return to normal.

Diagnostic Evaluation

In hypernatremia the serum sodium level is greater than 145 mEq/L (SI: 145 mmol/L) and the serum osmolality is greater than 295 mOsm/kg (SI: 295 mmol/L). The urinary specific gravity and urine osmolality are increased as the kidneys attempt to conserve water (provided the water loss is from a route other than the kidneys).

Management

Treatment of hypernatremia consists of a *gradual* lowering of the serum sodium level by the infusion of a hypotonic electrolyte solution (such as 0.3% sodium chloride) or an isotonic solution (such as D_5W). A hypotonic sodium solution is considered safer than 5% dextrose in water by many clinicians because it allows a gradual reduction in the serum sodium level and thus decreases the risk of cerebral edema. A rapid reduction in the serum sodium level temporarily decreases the plasma osmolality below that of the fluid in the brain tissue, causing dangerous cerebral edema. Diuretics may also be prescribed to treat the sodium gain.

There is not consensus about the exact rate at which serum sodium levels should be reduced. As a general rule, the serum sodium level is reduced at a rate no faster than 2 mEq/L/hr to allow sufficient time for readjustment through diffusion across fluid compartments.

Desmopressin (DDAVP) can be prescribed to treat diabetes insipidus if it is the cause of hypernatremia.

Nursing Assessment

Fluid losses and gains are carefully monitored in patients at risk for hypernatremia. One should assess for abnormal losses of water or low water intake and for large gains of sodium, as might occur with ingestion of over-the-counter medications with a high sodium content (such as Alka-Seltzer). Also, it is important to obtain a medication history, as some prescription medications may have a high sodium content.

The presence of thirst or an elevated body temperature is noted and evaluated in relation to other clinical signs. The patient is monitored for changes in behavior, such as restlessness, disorientation, and lethargy.

Nursing Interventions

Preventing Hypernatremia. The nurse attempts to prevent hypernatremia by offering fluids at regular intervals, particularly in debilitated patients unable to perceive or respond to thirst. If fluid intake remains inadequate, the nurse consults with the physician to plan an alternate route for intake, either by tube feedings or by the parenteral route. If tube feedings are used, sufficient water should be administered to keep the serum sodium and blood urea nitrogen levels within normal limits. As a general rule, the higher the osmolality of the tube feeding, the greater is the need for water supplementation.

For patients with *diabetes insipidus,* it is important to ensure adequate water intake. If the patient is alert and has an intact thirst mechanism, merely providing access to water may be sufficient. If the patient has a decreased level of consciousness, or other disability interfering with adequate fluid intake, parenteral fluid replacement may be prescribed. This therapy in patients with neurologic disorders, particularly in the early postoperative period, can be anticipated.

Correcting Hypernatremia. When hypernatremia is present and parenteral fluids are necessary for its management, the nurse monitors the patient's response to the fluids by reviewing serial serum sodium levels and by observing for changes in neurologic signs. With a gradual decrease in the serum sodium level, the neurologic signs should improve. As stated in the discussion on management, too rapid reduction in the serum sodium level renders the plasma temporarily hypo-osmotic to the fluid in the brain tissue, causing dangerous cerebral edema.

Potassium Imbalances

Disturbances in potassium balance are common, as they are associated with a number of disease and injury states. They may also be induced by medications such as diuretics, laxatives, and certain antibiotics, as well as by therapies such as total parenteral nutrition (TPN) and chemotherapy. It is helpful to review some pertinent facts about potassium before proceeding to a discussion of hypokalemia and hyperkalemia.

Functions of Potassium. Potassium is the major intracellular electrolyte; in fact, 98% of the body's potassium is inside the cells. The remaining 2% is in the ECF; it is this 2% that is important in neuromuscular function. Potassium influences both skeletal and cardiac muscle activity. For example, alterations in its concentration change myocardial irritability and rhythm. Potassium is constantly moving in and out of cells according to the body's needs, under the influence of the sodium–potassium pump. The normal serum potassium concentration ranges from 3.5 to 5.5 mEq/L (SI: 3.5–5.5 mmol/L), and even minor variations are significant.

Normal renal function is necessary to maintain potassium balance because 80% of the potassium is excreted daily from the body by way of the kidneys. The other 20% is lost through the bowel and sweat glands. The kidneys are the primary regulators of potassium balance and accomplish this by adjusting the amount of potassium that is excreted in the urine. As serum potassium levels increase, so does the level in the renal tubular cell. A concentration gradient occurs favoring the movement of potassium into the renal tubule with the loss of potassium in the urine. Aldosterone will also increase the excretion of potassium by the kidney. The kidneys cannot conserve potassium as well as they can conserve sodium; therefore, potassium may still be lost in urine in the presence of potassium depletion.

Potassium Deficit (Hypokalemia)

Hypokalemia refers to a below-normal serum potassium concentration. It usually indicates a real deficit in total potassium stores; however, it may occur in patients with normal potassium stores when alkalosis is present, as alkalosis causes a temporary shift of serum potassium into the cells. (See pp. 233–234 for a discussion of alkalosis.)

As stated earlier, hypokalemia is a common imbalance. *Gastrointestinal* loss of potassium is probably the most common cause of potassium depletion. Vomiting and gastric suction frequently lead to hypokalemia, partly because potassium is actually lost when gastric fluid is lost, but more so because potassium is lost through the kidneys in association with metabolic alkalosis. Relatively large amounts of potassium are contained in intestinal fluids; for example, diarrheal fluid may contain as much as 30 mEq/L. Therefore, potassium deficit occurs frequently with diarrhea, prolonged intestinal suctioning, recent ileostomy, and villous adenoma (a tumor of the intestinal tract characterized by excretion of potassium-rich mucus).

Alterations in acid–base balance have a significant effect on potassium distribution. The mechanism involves shifts of hydrogen ions and potassium ions between the cells and extracellular fluid. Hypokalemia can cause alkalosis and, in turn, alkalosis can cause hypokalemia. For example, hydrogen ions move out of the cells in alkalotic states to help correct the high *p*H, and potassium ions move in to maintain an electrically neutral state. (See pp. 230–236 for a discussion of acid–base balance.)

Hyperaldosteronism increases renal potassium wasting and can lead to severe potassium depletion. Primary hyperaldosteronism is seen in patients with adrenal adenomas. Secondary hyperaldosteronism occurs in patients with cirrhosis, nephrotic syndrome, congestive heart failure, and malignant hypertension.

Potassium-losing diuretics, such as furosemide, the thiazides, and ethacrynic acid, can certainly induce hypokalemia, particularly when administered in large doses to patients with poor potassium intake. Other medications that can lead to hypokalemia include corticosteroids, sodium penicillin, carbenicillin, and amphotericin B.

Entry of potassium into skeletal muscle and hepatic cells is promoted by insulin. Thus, patients with persistent *insulin hypersecretion* may experience hypokalemia; this is often seen in patients receiving high-carbohydrate parenteral fluids (as in total parenteral nutrition).

Patients unable or unwilling to eat a normal diet for a prolonged period are at risk for hypokalemia. This may occur in debilitated elderly people, alcoholics, and patients with anorexia nervosa. In addition to poor intake, people with bulimia frequently suffer increased potassium loss through self-induced vomiting and laxative and diuretic abuse.

Clinical Manifestations

Potassium deficiency can result in widespread derangements in physiologic function. Most important, severe hypokalemia can result in death through cardiac or respiratory arrest. Clinical signs rarely develop before the serum potassium level has fallen below 3 mEq/L (SI: 3 mmol/L) unless the rate of fall has been rapid. Manifestations of hypokalemia include fatigue, anorexia, nausea, vomiting, muscle weakness, leg cramps, decreased bowel motility, paresthesias, dysrhythmias, and increased sensitivity to digitalis. If prolonged, hypokalemia can lead to an inability of the kidneys to concentrate urine, causing dilute urine (excessive urination [polyuria], nocturia) and excessive thirst. Potassium depletion depresses the release of insulin and results in glucose intolerance.

Diagnostic Evaluation

In hypokalemia, the serum potassium concentration is less than the lower limit of normal. Electrocardiographic changes can include flat T waves and depressed ST segments (Fig. 14-4). The presence of a U wave will also be seen on ECG. Hypokalemia increases sensitivity to digitalis, predisposing to digitalis toxicity at lower digitalis levels. Meta-

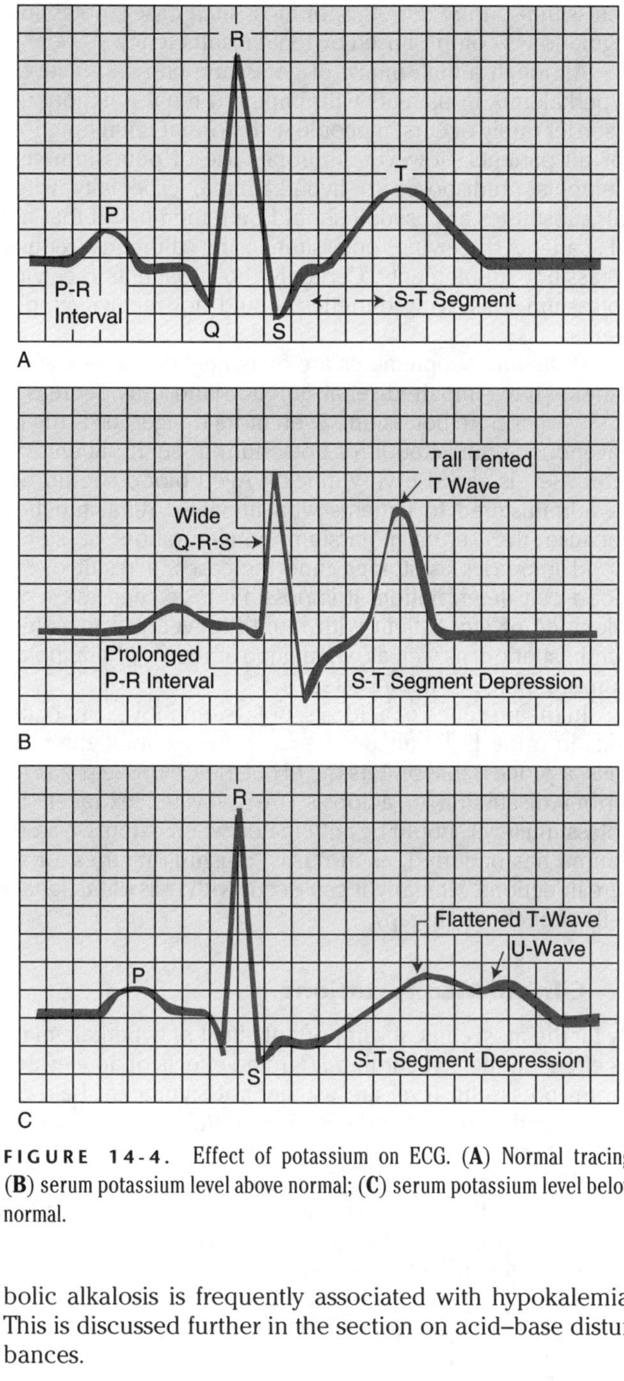

FIGURE 14-4. Effect of potassium on ECG. (**A**) Normal tracing; (**B**) serum potassium level above normal; (**C**) serum potassium level below normal.

bolic alkalosis is frequently associated with hypokalemia. This is discussed further in the section on acid–base disturbances.

Management

The best treatment of hypokalemia is prevention. Potassium loss must be corrected daily; administration of 40 to 80 mEq/day of potassium is adequate in the adult if there are no abnormal losses of potassium.

For patients at risk, a *diet* containing sufficient potassium should be provided; dietary intake of potassium in the average adult is 50 to 100 mEq/day. Foods high in potassium include raisins, bananas, apricots, oranges, avocados, beans, and potatoes.

When dietary intake is inadequate for any reason, the physician may prescribe *potassium supplements.* Many salt substitutes contain 50 to 60 mEq of potassium per teaspoon and may be all the patient needs to supplement potassium intake. Oral potassium supplements can produce small bowel lesions; therefore, the patient must be assessed for and cautioned about abdominal distention, pain, or GI bleeding.

When oral administration of potassium is not feasible, the *intravenous* route is indicated. In fact, the intravenous route is mandatory for patients with severe hypokalemia (such as a serum level of 2 mEq/L). Although potassium chloride is usually used to correct potassium deficits, the physician may prescribe potassium acetate or potassium phosphate. Intravenous potassium must be administered through an IV pump to avoid replacing potassium too quickly. When potassium is administered through a peripheral vein, the rate of administration must be decreased to avoid irritating the vein and causing a burning sensation during administration. Each hospital has its own standard of care which should be consulted; however, IV potassium should not be administered at rates faster than 20 mEq/hr or in concentrations greater than 30 to 40 mEq/L unless hypokalemia is severe, because this can cause life-threatening dysrhythmias.

- Potassium is *never* administered IV push or IM; when prepared for IV infusions, it should be agitated well to prevent bolus doses resulting from the potassium concentrating at the bottom of the IV container.

In general, concentrations greater than 60 mEq/L are not administered in peripheral veins, because venous pain and sclerosis may occur. For routine maintenance needs, potassium is administered at a rate no faster than 10 mEq/hr, suitably diluted.

In critical situations, more concentrated solutions (such as 20 mEq/dl) may be administered through a central line. Even in extreme hypokalemia, it is recommended that potassium be administered no faster than 20 to 40 mEq/hr (suitably diluted); in such a situation, the patient must be monitored by electrocardiogram (ECG) and observed closely for other signs, such as changes in muscle strength.

Nursing Assessment

Because hypokalemia can be life threatening, it is important to monitor for its early presence in patients at risk. The presence of fatigue, anorexia, muscle weakness, decreased bowel motility, paresthesias, or dysrhythmias should prompt one to examine the serum potassium concentration. When available, electrocardiograms may provide useful information. Patients receiving digitalis who are at risk for potassium deficiency should be monitored closely for signs of digitalis toxicity, because hypokalemia potentiates the action of digitalis. In fact, physicians usually prefer to keep the serum potassium level greater than 3.5 mEq/L (SI: 3.5 mmol/L) in digitalized patients.

Nursing Interventions

Preventing Hypokalemia. Measures are taken to prevent hypokalemia when possible. Prevention may take the form of encouraging intake of foods rich in potassium for the patient at risk (when the diet allows). Sources of potassium include fruit and fruit juices (bananas, melon, citrus fruit), fresh and frozen vegetables, fresh meats, and processed foods. When hypokalemia is due to abuse of laxatives or diuretics, patient education may help alleviate the problem. Part of the health history and assessment should be directed at identifying problems amenable to prevention through education.

Correcting Hypokalemia. Great care should be exercised when administering potassium intravenously. Potassium should be administered only after adequate urine flow has been established. A decrease in urine volume to less than 20 ml/hr for 2 consecutive hours is an indication to stop potassium infusion until the situation is evaluated. Potassium is primarily excreted by the kidneys; therefore, when oliguria is present, administration of potassium can cause the serum potassium concentration to rise to dangerous levels.

Potassium replacement must be administered cautiously to the elderly because they have a lower lean body mass and total body potassium level and therefore lower potassium requirements. Additionally, with the physiologic loss of renal function with advancing years, administered potassium may be retained more readily than in younger persons.

Potassium Excess (Hyperkalemia)

Hyperkalemia refers to a greater than normal serum potassium concentration. It seldom occurs in patients with normal renal function. Like hypokalemia, it is often due to iatrogenic (treatment-induced) causes. Although less common than hypokalemia, it is usually more dangerous because cardiac arrest is more frequently associated with high serum potassium levels.

Before considering true causes of hyperkalemia, one must be aware that there are a number of causes of factitious *("pseudo") hyperkalemia.* The most common are the use of a tight tourniquet around an exercising extremity while drawing a blood sample and hemolysis of the sample before analysis. Other causes include marked leukocytosis or thrombocytosis and drawing blood above a site where potassium is infusing. Failure to be aware of factitious causes of hyperkalemia can result in aggressive treatment of nonexistent hyperkalemia, resulting in serious lowering of serum potassium levels. Thus, measurements of grossly elevated levels should be verified.

The major cause of hyperkalemia is decreased renal excretion of potassium. Thus, significant hyperkalemia is commonly seen in untreated patients with renal failure, particularly when potassium is being liberated from cells during infectious processes or exogenous sources of potassium are excessive, as in diet or medications. A deficiency of adrenal corticosteroids causes sodium loss and potassium retention; thus, hypoaldosteronism and Addison's disease predispose to hyperkalemia.

Medications have been implicated as a probable contributing factor in more than 60% of the hyperkalemic episodes identified through retrospective studies. Medications commonly implicated are potassium chloride, captopril, nonsteroidal anti-inflammatory drugs (NSAIDs), and potassium-sparing diuretics. In most such cases, potassium regulation is compromised by renal insufficiency.

Although a high intake of potassium can cause severe hyperkalemia in patients with impaired renal function, the disorder rarely occurs in people with normal renal function. For all patients, however, improper use of potassium supplements predisposes to hyperkalemia, especially when salt substitutes are used. It should be remembered that not all patients receiving potassium-losing diuretics require potassium supplements. Certainly those patients receiving potassium-conserving diuretics should not receive supplements.

Potassium supplements are extremely dangerous when patients have impaired renal function and thus decreased ability to excrete potassium. Even more dangerous is the intravenous administration of potassium to such patients, as serum levels can rise very quickly. Aged blood should not be administered to patients with impaired renal function because the serum potassium concentration of stored blood increases as storage time increases, a result of red blood cell deterioration. It is possible to exceed the renal tolerance of *any* patient with rapid intravenous potassium administration, as well as when large amounts of oral potassium supplements are ingested.

In the presence of acidosis, potassium moves out of the cells into the ECF. This occurs as hydrogen ions enter the cells, a process that buffers the *p*H of the ECF. (See p. 233 for further discussion of acidosis.) An elevated extracellular potassium level should be anticipated when extensive tissue trauma has occurred, as in burns, crushing injuries, or severe infections. Similarly, it can occur with lysis of malignant cells after chemotherapy.

Clinical Manifestations

By far the most clinically important effect of hyperkalemia is its effect on the myocardium. Cardiac effects of an elevated serum potassium level are usually not significant below a concentration of 7 mEq/L (SI: 7 mmol/L), but they are almost always present when the level is 8 mEq/L (SI: 8 mmol/L) or greater. As the plasma potassium concentration is increased, disturbances in cardiac conduction occur. The earliest changes, often occurring at a serum potassium level greater than 6 mEq/L (SI: 6 mmol/L), are peaked, narrow T waves, ST depression, and a shortened QT interval. If the serum potassium level continues to rise, the PR interval becomes prolonged and is followed by disappearance of the P waves. Finally, there is decomposition and prolongation of the QRS complex (Fig. 14-4). Ventricular dysrhythmias and cardiac arrest may occur at any point in this progression.

Severe hyperkalemia causes skeletal muscle weakness and even paralysis, related to a depolarization block in muscle. Similarly, ventricular conduction is slowed. Although hyperkalemia has marked effects on the peripheral neuromuscular system, it has little effect on the central nervous system. Rapidly ascending muscular weakness leading to flaccid quadriplegia has been reported in patients with very high serum potassium levels. Paralysis of respiratory muscles and those required for speaking can also occur.

Gastrointestinal manifestations, such as nausea, intermittent intestinal colic, and diarrhea, may occur in hyperkalemic patients.

Diagnostic Evaluation

Serum potassium levels and ECG changes are crucial to the diagnosis of hyperkalemia, as discussed above under Clinical Manifestations. Arterial blood gases may show metabolic acidosis since hyperkalemia often occurs with acidosis.

Management

An immediate ECG should be performed to detect changes. Shortened repolarization and peaked T waves are seen initially. It is prudent as well to obtain a repeat serum potassium level to verify results.

In nonacute situations, restriction of dietary potassium and potassium-containing medications may suffice. For example, eliminating the use of potassium-containing salt substitutes in the patient taking a potassium-conserving diuretic may be all that is needed to deal with mild hyperkalemia.

Prevention of serious hyperkalemia by the administration, either orally or by retention enema, of cation-exchange resins (such as Kayexalate) may be necessary in patients with renal impairment. Cation exchange resins cannot be used if the patient has a paralytic ileus because intestinal perforation can occur.

Emergency Measures

In emergency situations, it may be necessary to administer calcium gluconate intravenously. Within minutes after administration, calcium antagonizes the action of hyperkalemia on the heart. Infusion of calcium does not reduce the serum potassium concentration but immediately antagonizes the adverse cardiac conduction abnormalities. Calcium chloride and calcium gluconate are not interchangeable. Calcium gluconate contains 4.5 mEq of calcium and calcium chloride contains 13.6 mEq of calcium. Monitoring the patient's blood pressure is essential as rapid administration can cause hypotension. The ECG should be continuously monitored during administration; the appearance of bradycardia is an indication to stop the infusion. The myocardial protective effects of calcium are transient, lasting about 30 minutes. Extra caution is required if the patient has been digitalized, because parenteral administration of calcium sensitizes the heart to digitalis and may precipitate digitalis toxicity.

Intravenous administration of sodium bicarbonate may be necessary to alkalinize the plasma and cause a temporary shift of potassium into the cells. Also, sodium bicarbonate furnishes sodium to antagonize the cardiac effects of potassium. Effects of this therapy begin within 30 to 60 minutes and may persist for hours; however, they are only temporary.

Intravenous administration of regular insulin and hypertonic dextrose causes a temporary shift of potassium into the cells. Glucose and insulin therapy has an onset of action within 30 minutes and lasts for several hours.

The above stopgap measures only temporarily protect the patient from hyperkalemia. If the hyperkalemic condition is not transient, actual removal of potassium from the body is required; this may be accomplished by way of cation-exchange resins, peritoneal dialysis, or hemodialysis.

Nursing Assessment

Patients at risk for potassium excess should be identified so they can be monitored closely for signs of hyperkalemia. (See the section dealing with etiologic factors.) The nurse observes for signs of muscular weakness and dysrhythmias. The presence of paresthesias is noted, as are gastrointestinal symptoms such as nausea and intestinal colic. For patients at risk, serum potassium levels are measured periodically.

It is important to remember that elevated serum potassium levels may be erroneous; thus, highly abnormal levels should always be verified. To avoid false reports of hyperkalemia, prolonged use of a tourniquet while drawing the blood sample is avoided and the patient is cautioned not to exercise the extremity immediately before the blood sample is obtained. The blood sample is taken to the laboratory as soon as possible, because hemolysis of the sample results in a falsely elevated serum potassium level.

Nursing Interventions

Preventing Hyperkalemia. Measures are taken to prevent hyperkalemia in patients at risk, when possible, by encouraging the patient to adhere to the prescribed potassium restriction. Foods high in potassium to be avoided include coffee, cocoa, tea, dried fruits, dried beans, and whole grain breads. Milk and eggs also contain substantial amounts of potassium. Conversely, foods with minimal potassium content include butter, margarine, cranberry juice or sauce, ginger ale, gumdrops or jellybeans, hard candy, root beer, sugar, and honey.

Restoring Potassium Balance. As stated earlier, it is possible to exceed the tolerance for potassium in any person if the substance is administered rapidly by the intravenous route. Therefore, great care should be taken to monitor potassium solutions closely, paying careful attention to the solution's concentration and rate of administration. When potassium is added to parenteral solutions, the potassium is mixed with the fluid by inverting the bottle several times. Potassium chloride should *never* be added to a hanging bottle because it might result in the potassium being administered as a bolus (potassium chloride is heavy and settles to the bottom of the container).

It is important to caution patients to use salt substitutes sparingly if they are taking other supplementary forms of potassium or potassium-conserving diuretics. Also, potassium-conserving diuretics (such as spironolactone, triamterene, and amiloride), potassium supplements, and salt substitutes should not be administered to patients with renal dysfunction. Most salt substitutes contain approximately 60 mEq of potassium per teaspoon.

Calcium Imbalances

Because many factors affect calcium regulation, both hypocalcemia and hypercalcemia are relatively common disturbances. To facilitate understanding of calcium disturbances, it is helpful to review factors affecting calcium balance.

Functions of Calcium. Over 99% of the body's calcium is concentrated in the skeletal system, where it is a major component of strong, durable bones and teeth. About 1% of skeletal calcium is rapidly exchangeable with blood calcium; the rest is more stable and only slowly exchanged. The small amount of calcium located outside the bone circulates in the serum, partly bound to protein and partly ionized. Calcium helps hold body cells together. In addition, calcium exerts a sedative action on nerve cells and thus plays a major role in the transmission of nerve impulses. It helps regulate muscle contraction and relaxation, including normal heartbeat. Calcium is instrumental in activating enzymes that stimulate many essential chemical reactions in the body and also plays a role in blood coagulation.

The normal total serum calcium level is 8.5 to 10.5 mg/dl (SI: 2.1–2.6 mmol/L). About 50% of the serum calcium exists in an ionized form that is physiologically active and important for neuromuscular activity and blood coagulation. The remainder of serum calcium exists bound to serum proteins, primarily albumin. Calcium is absorbed from foods in the presence of normal gastric acidity and vitamin D. Most of calcium excretion is via the feces and the remainder is in urine. Serum calcium is controlled by parathyroid hormone and calcitonin. As ionized serum calcium decreases, the parathyroid glands secrete parathyroid hormone. This event then increases calcium absorption from the GI tract, increases calcium reabsorption from the renal tubule, and releases calcium from the bone. The increase in calcium ion concentration suppresses parathyroid hormone secretion. When calcium increases excessively, the thyroid gland will secrete calcitonin. It will briefly inhibit calcium reabsorption from bone and decrease serum calcium concentration.

Calcium Deficit (Hypocalcemia)

Hypocalcemia refers to a lower than normal serum concentration of calcium, which occurs in a variety of clinical situations. A patient, however, may have a total body calcium deficit (as in osteoporosis) and maintain a normal serum calcium level. Bed rest in the elderly person with osteoporosis is hazardous because impaired calcium metabolism with increased bone resorption is associated with immobilization.

A number of factors can cause hypocalcemia. Primary hypoparathyroidism results in this disturbance, as does surgical hypoparathyroidism. The latter is far more common. Not only is it associated with thyroid and parathyroid surgery, but it can also occur after radical neck dissection and is most likely in the first 24 to 48 hours after surgery. Transient hypocalcemia can occur with massive administration of citrated blood (as in exchange transfusions in newborns), because citrate can combine with ionized calcium and temporarily remove it from the circulation.

Inflammation of the pancreas causes the breakdown of proteins and lipids. It is thought that calcium ions combine with the fatty acids released by lipolysis, forming soaps. As a result of this process, hypocalcemia occurs and is common in pancreatitis. It has also been suggested that hypocalcemia might be related to excessive secretion of glucagon from the inflamed pancreas, resulting in increased secretion of calcitonin (a hormone that lowers serum calcium).

Hypocalcemia is common in patients with renal failure because these patients frequently have elevated serum phosphate levels. Hyperphosphatemia usually causes a reciprocal drop in the serum calcium level. Other causes of hypocalcemia can include inadequate vitamin D consumption, magnesium deficiency, medullary thyroid carcinoma, low serum albumin levels, and alkalosis. Medications predisposing to hypocalcemia can include aluminum-containing antacids, aminoglycosides, caffeine, cisplatin, corticosteroids, mithramycin, phosphates, isoniazid, and loop diuretics.

Osteoporosis is associated with prolonged low intake of calcium and represents a total body calcium deficit, even though serum calcium levels are usually normal. This disorder strikes millions of Americans, mostly post-menopausal women. It is characterized by loss of bone mass, causing bones to become porous and brittle, and therefore susceptible to fracture (see Chapter 63).

Clinical Manifestations

Tetany is the most characteristic manifestation of hypocalcemia. Tetany refers to the entire symptom complex induced by increased neural excitability. These symptoms are due to spontaneous discharges of both sensory and motor fibers in peripheral nerves. Sensations of tingling may occur in the tips of the fingers, around the mouth, and, less commonly, in the feet. Spasms of the muscles of the extremities and face may occur. Pain may develop as a result of these spasms.

Trousseau's sign (Fig. 14-5) can be elicited by inflating a blood pressure cuff on the upper arm to about 20 mm Hg above systolic pressure; within 2 to 5 minutes carpopedal spasm will occur as ischemia of the ulnar nerve develops. *Chvostek's sign* consists of twitching of muscles supplied by the facial nerve when the nerve is tapped about 2 cm anterior to the earlobe, just below the zygomatic arch.

Seizures may occur because hypocalcemia increases irritability of the central nervous system as well as of the peripheral nerves. Other changes associated with hypocalcemia include mental changes such as emotional depression, impairment of memory, confusion, delirium, and even hallucinations. Prolonged QT interval is seen on the ECG due

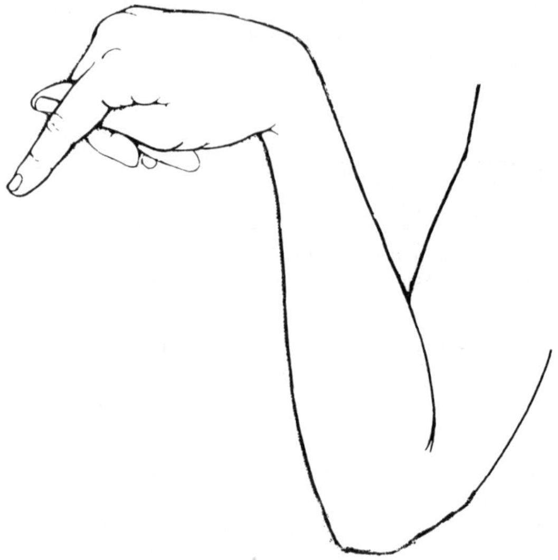

FIGURE 14-5. Trousseau's sign. Carpopedal spasm with hypocalcemia.

to an elongation of the ST segment; a form of ventricular tachycardia called Torsades de Pointes may occur.

Diagnostic Evaluation

When evaluating serum calcium levels, one must consider several other variables, such as the patient's serum albumin level and arterial *p*H. Because abnormalities in serum albumin levels may affect interpretation of the serum calcium level, it may be necessary to calculate the corrected serum calcium if the serum albumin level is abnormal. For every decrease in serum albumin of 1 g/dl below 4 g/dl, the total serum calcium level is underestimated by approximately 0.8 mg/dl. The following is a quick method to calculate the corrected serum calcium level:

$$\text{Measured total serum } Ca^{2+} \text{ level (mg/dl)} + 0.8 \times [4.0 - \text{measured albumin level (g/dl)}] = \text{corrected total calcium concentration (mg/dl)}$$

An example to demonstrate the calculations needed to obtain the corrected total serum calcium level is as follows: A patient's reported serum albumin level is 2.5 g/dl; the reported serum calcium level is 10.5 mg/dl.

- The decrease in serum albumin level from normal level (difference from normal albumin of 4 g/dl) is calculated: 4 g/dl – 2.5 g/dl = 1.5 g/dl
- The following ratio is calculated: 0.8 mg/dl : 1 g/dl = **?** mg/dl : 1.5 mg/dl **?** = 0.8 mg × 1.5 or 1.2 mg/dl calcium
- Add 1.2 to 10.5 mg (reported serum calcium level) to obtain the corrected total serum calcium level of 11.7 mg/dl.

Clinicians will often ignore a low serum calcium level in the presence of a similarly low serum albumin level. The ionized calcium level is usually normal in patients with reduced total serum calcium levels and concomitant hypoalbuminemia. When the arterial *p*H increases (alkalosis), more calcium becomes bound to protein. As a result, the ionized portion decreases. Symptoms of hypocalcemia may occur in the presence of alkalosis. Acidosis (low *p*H) has the opposite effect; that is, less calcium is bound to protein and thus more exists in the ionized form. However, relatively small changes in serum calcium levels occur during these acid-base abnormalities.

Ideally, the laboratory should measure the ionized level of calcium. In most laboratories, however, only the total calcium level is reported; thus, concentration of the ionized fraction must be estimated by simultaneous measurement of serum albumin level. Parathyroid hormone levels will be decreased in hypoparathyroidism. Magnesium and phosphorus levels need to be assessed to identify possible causes of decreased calcium.

Management

Acute symptomatic hypocalcemia is a medical emergency, requiring prompt intravenous administration of calcium. Parenteral calcium salts include calcium gluconate, calcium chloride, and calcium gluceptate. Although calcium chloride produces a significantly higher ionized calcium than an equimolar amount of calcium gluconate, it is not used as often because it is more irritating and can cause sloughing of tissue if allowed to infiltrate. Too rapid intravenous administration of calcium can induce cardiac arrest, preceded by bradycardia. Intravenous calcium administration is particularly dangerous in digitalized patients because calcium ions exert an effect similar to that of digitalis and can cause digitalis toxicity with adverse cardiac effects.

Vitamin D therapy may be instituted to increase calcium absorption from the GI tract. Aluminum hydroxide antacids may be prescribed to decrease elevated phosphorus levels prior to treating hypocalcemia. Lastly, increasing the dietary intake of calcium to at least 1000 to 1500 mg/day in the adult is recommended (milk products; green, leafy vegetables; canned salmon, sardines, and fresh oysters). If tetany does respond to IV calcium then a low magnesium level is explored as a possible cause of tetany.

Nursing Interventions

It is important to observe for hypocalcemia in patients at risk. One should be prepared to take seizure precautions when hypocalcemia is severe. The status of the airway is closely monitored because laryngeal stridor can occur. Safety precautions are taken, as indicated, if confusion is present.

Persons at high risk for osteoporosis are instructed about the need for adequate dietary calcium intake; if not consumed in the diet, calcium supplements should be considered. Also, the value of regular exercise in decreasing bone loss should be emphasized, as should the effect of medications on calcium balance. For example, alcohol and caffeine in high doses inhibit calcium absorption; and moderate cigarette smoking increases urinary calcium excretion.

Calcium Excess (Hypercalcemia)

Hypercalcemia refers to an excess of calcium in the plasma. It is a dangerous imbalance when severe; in fact, hypercalcemic crisis has a mortality rate as high as 50% if not treated promptly.

The most common causes of hypercalcemia are malignant neoplastic diseases and hyperparathyroidism. Malignant tumors can produce hypercalcemia by a variety of mechanisms. The excessive parathyroid hormone secretion associated with hyperparathyroidism causes increased release of calcium from the bones and increased intestinal and renal absorption of calcium.

Bone mineral is lost during immobilization, sometimes causing elevation of total (and especially ionized) calcium in the bloodstream. Symptomatic hypercalcemia from immobilization, however, is rare; when it does occur it is virtually limited to persons with high calcium turnover rates (such as adolescents during a growth spurt). Most cases of hypercalcemia secondary to immobility occur after severe or multiple fractures or after extensive traumatic paralysis.

Thiazide diuretics may cause a slight elevation in serum calcium levels because they potentiate the action of parathyroid hormone on the kidneys, reducing urinary calcium excretion. The milk-alkali syndrome can occur in patients with peptic ulcer treated for a prolonged period with milk and alkaline antacids, particularly calcium carbonate. Vitamin A and D intoxication, as well as the use of lithium, can cause calcium excess.

Clinical Manifestations

As a rule, the symptoms of hypercalcemia are proportional to the degree of elevation of the serum calcium level. Hypercalcemia reduces neuromuscular excitability because it suppresses activity at the myoneural junction. Symptoms such as muscular weakness, incoordination, anorexia, and constipation may be due to decreased tone in smooth and striated muscle.

Anorexia, nausea, vomiting, and constipation are common symptoms of hypercalcemia. Dehydration occurs with nausea, vomiting, anorexia, and sodium-linked calcium reabsorbtion at the proximal renal tubule. Abdominal and bone pain may also be present. Abdominal distention and paralytic ileus may complicate severe hypercalcemic crisis. Severe thirst may occur secondary to the polyuria caused by the high solute (calcium) load. Patients with chronic hypercalcemia may develop symptoms similar to those of peptic ulcer because hypercalcemia increases the secretion of acid and pepsin by the stomach.

Mental confusion, impairment of memory, slurred speech, lethargy, acute psychotic behavior, or coma may occur. The more severe symptoms tend to appear when the serum calcium level is approximately 16 mg/dl or above. However, some patients may become profoundly disturbed with serum calcium levels of only 12 mg/dl. These symptoms resolve as serum calcium levels return to normal after treatment.

Excessive urination due to disturbed renal tubular function produced by hypercalcemia may be present. Cardiac standstill can occur when the serum calcium is about 18 mg/dl. The inotropic effect of digitalis is enhanced by calcium; therefore, digitalis toxicity is aggravated by hypercalcemia.

Hypercalcemic crisis refers to an acute rise in the serum calcium level to 17 mg/dl or higher. Severe thirst and polyuria are characteristically present. Other findings may include muscular weakness, intractable nausea, abdominal cramps, obstipation (very severe constipation) or diarrhea, peptic ulcer symptoms, and bone pain. Lethargy, mental confusion, and coma may also occur. This condition is very dangerous and may result in cardiac arrest.

Diagnostic Evaluation

The serum calcium level is greater than 10.5 mg/dl (SI: 2.6 mmol/L). Cardiovascular changes may include a variety of dysrhythmias and shortening of the QT interval and ST segment. The PR interval is sometimes prolonged. The double antibody parathyroid hormone test may be used to differentiate between primary hyperparathyroidism and malignancy as a cause of hypercalcemia. Parathyroid hormone levels are increased in primary or secondary hyperparathyroidism and suppressed in malignancy. X-ray findings may indicate the presence of osteoporosis, bone cavitation, or urinary calculi.

Management

Therapeutic aims in hypercalcemia include decreasing the serum calcium level and reversing the process causing hypercalcemia. Treating the underlying cause (*i.e.*, chemotherapy for a malignancy or partial parathyroidectomy for hyperparathyroidism) is essential.

General measures include administering fluids to dilute serum calcium and promote its excretion by the kidneys, mobilizing the patient, and restricting dietary calcium intake. Administering 0.9% sodium chloride solution intravenously temporarily dilutes the serum calcium level and increases urinary calcium excretion by inhibiting tubular reabsorption of calcium. Administering intravenous phosphate can cause a reciprocal drop in serum calcium. Furosemide (Lasix) is often used in conjunction with saline administration; in addition to causing diuresis, furosemide increases calcium excretion.

Calcitonin can be used to lower the serum calcium level and is particularly useful for patients with heart disease or renal failure who cannot tolerate large sodium loads. Calcitonin reduces bone resorption, increases the deposit of calcium and phosphorus in the bones, and increases urinary excretion of calcium and phosphorus. Although available in several forms, calcitonin derived from salmon is commonly used. Skin testing for allergy to salmon calcitonin is necessary before calcitonin is administered. Systemic allergic reactions are possible since this hormone is a protein; resistance to the medication may develop later because of antibody formation. Calcitonin is administered by IM injection rather than subcutaneously because patients with hypercalcemia have poor perfusion of subcutaneous tissue.

For patients with malignant disease, treatment is directed at controlling the condition by surgery, chemotherapy, or radiation therapy. Corticosteroids may be used to decrease bone turnover and tubular reabsorption for patients with sarcoidosis, myelomas, lymphomas, and leukemias; patients with solid tumors are less responsive. The biphosphonates inhibit osteoclast activity. Pamidronate (Aredia) is the most potent of these agents and is given intravenously; it causes a transient, mild pyrexia, decreased WBC count, and myralgia. Etidronate (Didronel) is another biphosphonate that is given intravenously, but its action is slower. Mithramycin, a cytotoxic antibiotic, inhibits bone resorption and thus lowers the serum calcium levels. This agent must be used cautiously because it has significant side effects, including thrombocytopenia, nephrotoxicity, and hepatotoxicity. Inorganic phosphate salts can be administered orally or by nasogastric tube (in the form of Phospho-Soda or Neutra-Phos), rectally (as retention enemas), or intravenously. Intravenous phosphate therapy is used with extreme caution in the treatment of hypercalcemia because it can cause severe calcification in various tissues, hypotension, tetany, and acute renal failure.

Nursing Interventions

It is important to monitor for the occurrence of hypercalcemia in patients at risk for this disorder. Initiation of interventions, such as increasing patient mobility and encouraging fluids, can help prevent hypercalcemia, or at least minimize its severity. Hospitalized patients at risk for hypercalcemia are encouraged to ambulate as soon as possible; outpatients and those cared for in their homes are informed of the importance of frequent ambulation.

When encouraging oral fluids, the nurse considers the patient's likes and dislikes. Fluids containing sodium should be administered, unless contraindicated by other conditions, because sodium favors calcium excretion. Patients at home are encouraged to drink 3 to 4 quarts of fluid daily, if possible. Adequate bulk should be provided in the diet to offset the tendency for constipation. Safety precautions are taken, as necessary, when mental symptoms of hypercalcemia are present. The patient and family are informed that these mental changes are reversible with treatment. Increased calcium potentiates the effects of digitalis; therefore, the patient is assessed for signs and symptoms of digitalis toxicity. ECG changes can occur (PVCs, PATs, and heart block); therefore, the patient's pulse is monitored for any abnormalities.

Magnesium Imbalances

Functions of Magnesium. Next to potassium, magnesium is the most abundant intracellular cation. It acts as an activator for many intracellular enzyme systems and plays a role in both carbohydrate and protein metabolism. Magnesium balance is important in neuromuscular function. Because magnesium acts directly on the myoneural junction, variations in serum concentration of magnesium affect neuromuscular irritability and contractility. For example, an excess of magnesium diminishes excitability of the muscle cells, whereas a deficit increases neuromuscular irritability and contractility. Magnesium produces its sedative effect at the neuromuscular junction, probably by inhibiting the release of the neurotransmitter acetylcholine. It also increases the stimulus threshold in nerve fibers.

Magnesium exerts effects on the cardiovascular system, acting peripherally to produce vasodilation. Magnesium is thought to have a direct effect on peripheral arteries and arterioles, which results in a decreased total peripheral resistance.

Magnesium Deficit (Hypomagnesemia)

Hypomagnesemia refers to a below normal serum magnesium concentration. The normal serum magnesium level is 1.5 to 2.5 mEq/L (or 1.8–3.0 mg/dl; SI: 0.75–1.25 mmol/L). Approximately one-third of serum magnesium is bound to protein; the remaining two-thirds exist as free cations (Mg^{2+}). Like calcium, it is the ionized fraction that is primarily involved in neuromuscular activity and other physiologic processes. As with calcium levels, magnesium levels should be evaluated in combination with albumin levels. Low serum albumin levels will decrease total magnesium.

Hypomagnesemia is a common imbalance in critically ill patients, yet it is frequently overlooked. Magnesium deficit also occurs in other acutely ill patients, such as those experiencing withdrawal from alcohol and those receiving nourishment after a period of starvation, as in tube feedings or total parenteral nutrition.

An important route for magnesium loss is the gastrointestinal tract. Losses may take the form of drainage from nasogastric suction, diarrhea, or fistulas. Because fluid from the lower gastrointestinal tract is richer in magnesium (10–14 mEq/L) than is fluid from the upper tract (1–2 mEq/L), losses from diarrhea and intestinal fistulas are more likely to induce magnesium deficit than are those from gastric suction. Although magnesium losses are relatively small in nasogastric suction, hypomagnesemia will occur if losses are prolonged and parenteral fluids do not contain magnesium. Because the distal small bowel is the major site of magnesium absorption, any disruption in small bowel function, as in intestinal resection or inflammatory bowel disease, can lead to hypomagnesemia.

Alcoholism is currently the most common cause of symptomatic hypomagnesemia in the United States. It is particularly troublesome during treatment of alcohol withdrawal. Because of this, it is recommended that the serum magnesium level be measured every 2 or 3 days in patients going through withdrawal from alcohol. Although the serum magnesium level may be normal on admission, it can fall as a result of metabolic changes associated with therapy, such as the intracellular shift of magnesium associated with intravenous glucose administration.

During nutritional repletion, the major cellular electrolytes are taken from the serum and deposited in newly synthesized cells. Thus, if the enteral or parenteral feeding formula is deficient in magnesium content, serious hypomagnesemia will occur. Because of this, serum levels of these primarily intracellular ions should be measured at regular intervals during the administration of total parenteral nutrition and even during enteral feedings, especially to patients who have undergone a period of starvation.

Other causes of hypomagnesemia include the administration of aminoglycosides, cyclosporine, cisplatin, diuretics, digitalis, and amphotericin and the rapid administration of citrated blood, especially to patients with renal or hepatic disease. Magnesium deficiency is often seen in patients with diabetic ketoacidosis; it is primarily the result of increased renal excretion of magnesium during osmotic diuresis and shifting of magnesium into the cells with insulin therapy.

Clinical Manifestations

Clinical manifestations of hypomagnesemia are largely confined to the neuromuscular system. Some of the effects are due directly to the low serum magnesium level; others are due to secondary changes in potassium and calcium metabolism. Symptoms do not usually occur until the serum magnesium level is less than 1 mEq/L (SI: 0.5 mmol/L).

Among the neuromuscular changes are hyperexcitability with muscular weakness, tremors, and athetoid movements (slow, involuntary twisting and writhing movements). Others include tetany, generalized tonic-clonic or focal seizures, laryngeal stridor, and positive Chvostek's and Trousseau's signs (see discussion on p. 224), which occur, in part, because of accompanying hypocalcemia.

Magnesium deficiency predisposes to cardiac dysrhythmias, such as PVCs, supraventricular tachycardia, and ventricular fibrillation. Increased susceptibility to digitalis toxicity is associated with low serum magnesium levels. This is an important consideration because patients receiving digoxin are also likely to be on diuretic therapy, predisposing to renal loss of magnesium.

Hypomagnesemia may be accompanied by marked alterations in mood. Apathy, depression, apprehension, or extreme agitation have been noted, as well as ataxia, dizziness, insomnia, and confusion. At times, delirium and frank psychoses may occur, as may auditory or visual hallucinations.

Diagnostic Evaluation

On laboratory analysis, the serum magnesium level is less than 1.5 mEq/L or 1.8 mg/dl (SI: 0.75 mmol/L). Hypomagnesemia is frequently associated with hypokalemia and hypocalcemia. About 25% of magnesium is protein bound; principally to albumin. A decreased serum albumin can, therefore, reduce the measured total magnesium concentration; however, it does not reduce the ionized plasma magnesium concentration. ECG evaluations reflect magnesium, calcium, and potassium deficiencies, tachyarrhythmias, prolonged PR and QT intervals, widening QRS, ST depression, and flattened T waves. Torsades de Pointes, a form of ventricular tachycardia, is associated with alterations of all three electrolytes. PVCs, PATs, and heart block may also occur. Urinary magnesium levels may be helpful in identifying causes of magnesium depletion and are performed after a loading dose of magnesium sulfate.

Management

Mild magnesium deficiency can be corrected by diet alone. Principal dietary sources of magnesium are green vegetables, nuts and legumes, and fruits such as bananas, grapefruits, and oranges. Magnesium is also plentiful in peanut butter and chocolate. When necessary, magnesium salts can be administered orally to replace continuous excessive losses. Diarrhea is a common complication of oral forms of magnesium. Patients receiving total parenteral nutrition require magnesium in the intravenous solution to prevent the development of hypomagnesemia. Intravenous administration of magnesium sulfate must be given via IV pump, and calcium gluconate must be readily available in case of hypocalcemic tetany or hypermagnesiemia.

Overt symptoms of hypomagnesemia are treated with parenteral administration of magnesium. Magnesium sulfate is the most commonly used magnesium salt. Serial magnesium concentrations can be used to regulate the dosage.

Nursing Interventions

The nurse should be aware of patients at risk for hypomagnesemia and observe for its presence. Patients on digitalis are monitored closely because a deficit of magnesium predisposes to digitalis toxicity. When hypomagnesemia is severe, one should be prepared to take seizure precautions. Other safety precautions are instituted, as indicated, if confusion is present.

Because difficulty in swallowing (dysphagia) may occur in magnesium-depleted patients, the ability to swallow should be tested with water before oral medications or foods are offered. Dysphagia is probably related to the athetoid or choreiform (rapid, involuntary, and irregular jerking) movements associated with magnesium deficit.

When magnesium deficit is due to misuse of diuretics or laxatives, patient education may help alleviate the problem. For patients on a general diet who are experiencing abnormal magnesium losses, the intake of magnesium-rich foods (*e.g.*, green vegetables, nuts and legumes, bananas and oranges) is encouraged. If the deficit is due to alcohol abuse, referral to a social worker or Alcoholics Anonymous is indicated.

Magnesium Excess (Hypermagnesemia)

Hypermagnesemia refers to a greater than normal serum concentration of magnesium. A serum magnesium level can appear falsely elevated when blood specimens are allowed to hemolyze or are drawn from an extremity with an excessively tight tourniquet.

By far the most common cause of hypermagnesemia is renal failure. In fact, most patients with advanced renal failure have at least a slight elevation in serum magnesium levels. This condition is aggravated when such patients are administered magnesium to control seizures or inadvertently receive one of the many commercial antacids that contain magnesium salts.

Hypermagnesemia can occur in a patient with untreated diabetic ketoacidosis when catabolism causes release of cellular magnesium that cannot be excreted because of profound fluid volume depletion and resulting oliguria. An excess of magnesium can also result from excessive magnesium administration. Increased serum magnesium levels can also occur in adrenocortical insufficiency, Addison's disease, or hypothermia.

Clinical Manifestations

Acute elevation of the serum magnesium level depresses the central nervous system as well as the peripheral neuromuscular junction. At mildly elevated levels, there is a tendency for lowered blood pressure because of peripheral vasodilation. Nausea, vomiting, soft-tissue calcifications, facial flushing, and sensations of warmth may also occur. At higher magnesium concentrations, lethargy, difficulty speaking (dysarthria), and drowsiness can occur. Deep tendon reflexes are lost and muscular weakness and paralysis may develop. The respiratory center is depressed when serum magnesium levels exceed 10 mEq/L. Coma and cardiac arrest can occur when the serum magnesium level is greatly elevated.

Diagnostic Evaluation

On laboratory analysis, the serum magnesium level is greater than 2.5 mEq/L or 3.0 mg/dl (SI: 1.25 mmol/L). ECG findings demonstrate prolonged QT interval and AV blocks.

Management

The best treatment for hypermagnesemia is prevention. This can be accomplished by not administering magnesium to patients with renal failure and by carefully monitoring seriously ill patients who are receiving magnesium salts. In the presence of severe hypermagnesemia, all parenteral and oral magnesium salts are discontinued. When respiratory depression or defective cardiac conduction is present, emergency measures such as ventilatory support and intravenous administration of calcium are indicated. Hemodialysis with a magnesium-free dialysate is an effective treatment that should produce a safe serum magnesium level within hours. Diuretics and 0.45% sodium chloride solution enhance magnesium excretion in patients with adequate renal function. Intravenous calcium gluconate (10 ml of a 10% solution) antagonizes the neuromuscular effects of magnesium.

Nursing Interventions

Patients at risk for hypermagnesemia are identified and assessed. When hypermagnesemia is suspected, the nurse should monitor the vital signs, noting the presence of hypotension and shallow respirations, and observe for decreased patellar reflexes and changes in the level of consciousness. Care is taken to avoid giving medications that contain magnesium to patients with renal failure or compromised renal function. Similarly, one should caution patients with renal failure to check with their health care providers before they take over-the-counter medications. Caution is essential when magnesium fluids are prepared and administered parenterally because parenteral magnesium solutions are packaged in containers of various sizes (such as 2-ml ampules and 50-ml vials), all of which are sometimes loosely referred to as "amps."

Phosphorus Imbalances

Functions of Phosphorus. Phosphorus is a critical constituent of all the body's tissues. It is essential to the function of muscle and red blood cells, the formation of adenosine triphosphate (ATP) and 2,3-diphosphoglycerate (DPG), and the maintenance of acid–base balance, as well as to the nervous system and the intermediary metabolism of carbohydrate, protein, and fat. The normal serum phosphorus level ranges between 2.5 and 4.5 mg/dl (SI: 0.8–1.5 mmol/L) and may be as high as 6 mg/dl (SI: 1.94 mmol/L) in infants and children. Serum phosphorus levels are presumably greater in children because of the high rate of skeletal growth. Phosphorus is the primary anion of intracellular fluid. About 85% of phosphorus is located in bones and teeth, 14% in soft tissue, and less than 1% in extracellular fluid. Phosphorus is critical to nerve and muscle function and provides structural support to bones and teeth. Phosphorus levels decrease with age.

Phosphorus Deficit (Hypophosphatemia)

Hypophosphatemia is defined as a below normal serum concentration of inorganic phosphorus. Although it often indicates phosphorus deficiency, it may occur under a variety of circumstances in which total body phosphorus stores are normal. Conversely, phosphorus deficiency refers to an abnormally low content of phosphorus in lean tissues and may exist in the absence of hypophosphatemia.

Hypophosphatemia may occur during the administration of calories to patients with severe protein-calorie malnutrition. It is most likely to occur with overzealous intake or administration of simple carbohydrates. This syndrome can be induced in anyone with severe protein-calorie malnutrition (such as patients with anorexia nervosa or alcoholism, or elderly debilitated patients unable to eat). Some sources indicate that as many as 50% of patients hospitalized because of chronic alcoholism suffer from hypophosphatemia.

Marked hypophosphatemia may develop in malnourished patients receiving total parenteral nutrition (TPN) if the phosphorus loss is not adequately corrected. Other causes of hypophosphatemia include prolonged intense hyperventilation, alcohol withdrawal, poor dietary intake, diabetic ketoacidosis, and major thermal burns. Low magnesium, low potassium, and hyperparathyroidism related to increased urinary losses of phosphorus contribute to hypophosphatemia. Respiratory alkalosis can cause a decrease in phosphorus because of an intracellular shift of phosphorus.

Excess phosphorus binding by antacids containing magnesium, calcium, or albumin may decrease the phosphorus available from the diet to amounts below that required to maintain serum phosphorus balance. The degree of hypophosphatemia depends on the amount of phosphorus in the diet compared to the dose of antacid. Vitamin D regulates intestinal ion absorption; and, therefore, a deficiency of vitamin D may cause decreased calcium and phosphorus leading to osteomalacia.

Clinical Manifestations

Most of the signs and symptoms of phosphorus deficiency appear to result from a deficiency of adenosine triphosphate (ATP), or of 2,3-diphosphoglycerate (DPG), or of both. The former impairs cellular energy resources, and the latter impairs oxygen delivery to tissues.

A wide range of neurologic symptoms may occur, such as irritability, apprehension, weakness, numbness, paresthesias, confusion, seizures, and coma. Low levels of 2,3-DPG may reduce the delivery of oxygen to peripheral tissues, resulting in tissue anoxia. Hypoxia then leads to an increase in respiratory rate and respiratory alkalosis, causing phosphorus to move into the cells and potentiating hypophosphatemia.

It is thought that hypophosphatemia predisposes to infection. In laboratory animals, hypophosphatemia has been noted to produce depression of the chemotactic, phagocytic, and bacterial activity of granulocytes.

Muscle damage may develop as the ATP level in the muscle tissue declines. This is manifested clinically by muscle weakness, muscle pain, and, at times, acute rhabdomyolysis (disintegration of striated muscle). Weakness of respiratory muscles may greatly impair ventilation. Also, hypophosphatemia may predispose to insulin-resistance, and thus hyperglycemia. Chronic loss of phosphorus can cause bruising and bleeding due to platelet dysfunction.

Diagnostic Evaluation

On laboratory analysis, the serum phosphorus level will be less than 2.5 mg/dl (SI: 0.80 mmol/L) in adults. It is important to remember that glucose or insulin administration causes a slight decrease in the serum phosphorus level. Parathyroid hormone levels will be increased in hyperparathyroidism. Serum magnesium may be decreased due to increased excretion of magnesium in the urine. Alkaline phosphatase is increased with osteoblastic activity. X-ray studies may show skeletal changes of osteomalacia or rickets.

Management

As in any electrolyte imbalance, the best treatment is prevention. In patients at risk for hypophosphatemia, serum phosphate levels should be closely monitored and correction initiated before deficits become severe. Adequate amounts of phosphorus should be added to parenteral solutions, and attention should also be paid to phosphorus levels in enteral feeding solutions.

Severe hypophosphatemia is dangerous and requires prompt attention. Aggressive intravenous phosphorus correction is usually limited to patients with serum phosphorus levels below 1 mg/dl (SI: 0.3 mmol/L) and whose gastrointestinal tract is not functioning. Possible dangers of intravenous administration of phosphorus include hypocalcemia and metastatic calcification from hyperphosphatemia. In less acute situations, oral phosphorus replacement is usually adequate.

Nursing Interventions

The nurse should identify patients at risk for hypophosphatemia and monitor for its presence. Because malnourished patients receiving total parenteral nutrition are at risk when calories are introduced too aggressively, prevention can take the form of gradually introducing the feeding solution to avoid rapid shifts of phosphorus into the cells.

For patients with documented hypophosphatemia, careful attention should be paid to preventing infection because hypophosphatemia may produce changes in the granulocytes. For patients requiring correction of phosphorus losses, frequent monitoring of the serum phosphorus levels is indicated to augment clinical assessment. Early signs of hypophosphatemia (apprehension, confusion, change in level of consciousness) are documented and reported.

Phosphorus Excess (Hyperphosphatemia)

Hyperphosphatemia refers to a serum phosphorus level greater than normal. A variety of conditions can lead to this imbalance.

The most common cause of hyperphosphatemia is decreased excretion of phosphorus in renal failure. Other causes include chemotherapy for neoplastic disease, high phosphate intake, profound muscle necrosis, and increased phosphorus absorption. The primary complication of increased phosphorus is metastatic calcifications (soft tissue, joints, and arteries). These are seen when calcium X magnesium exceeds 70 mg/dl.

Clinical Manifestations

An elevated serum phosphorus level causes little in the way of symptoms. The most important long-term consequence is soft tissue calcification, which occurs mainly in patients with reduced glomerular filtration rates; the most important short-term consequence is tetany. High levels of serum inorganic phosphorus are harmful because they promote precipitation of calcium phosphate in nonosseous sites. Because of the reciprocal relationship between phosphorus and calcium, a high serum phosphorus level tends to cause a low calcium concentration in the serum. Tetany can result and can present as sensations of tingling in the tips of the fingers and around the mouth. Anorexia, nausea, vomiting, muscle weakness, hyperreflexia, and tachycardia may occur. Signs and symptoms are usually few and are caused by the development of decreased calcium or soft tissue calcifications.

Diagnostic Evaluation

On laboratory analysis, the serum phosphorus level is greater than 4.5 mg/dl (SI: 1.5 mmol/L) in adults. Serum phosphorus levels are normally higher in children, presumably because of the high rate of skeletal growth. Serum calcium levels are useful in assessing complications from treatments and diagnosing the primary problem. X-ray studies may show skeletal changes with abnormal bone development. Parathyroid hormone levels will be decreased in hypoparathyroidism. BUN and creatinine levels are used to assess renal function.

Management

When possible, treatment is directed at the underlying disorder. For example, hyperphosphatemia related to tumor cell lysis might be lessened by prior administration of allopurinol to prevent urate nephropathy. For patients with renal failure, measures to decrease the serum phosphate level are indicated; these include the administration of phosphate-binding gels, restriction of dietary phosphate, and dialysis.

Nursing Interventions

The nurse should be aware of patients at risk for hyperphosphatemia and monitor for its presence. When a low-phosphorus diet is prescribed, the patient is instructed to avoid foods high in phosphorus content. Such foods include hard cheese; cream; nuts; whole grain cereals, dried fruits; dried vegetables; special meats, such as kidneys, sardines, and sweetbreads; and foods made with milk. When appropriate, the nurse instructs the patient to avoid phosphate-containing substances, such as laxatives and enemas that contain phosphate. The patient is also taught the signs of impending hypocalcemia and instructed to monitor for changes in urine output.

Major fluid and electrolyte imbalances are summarized in Table 14-6.

Acid–Base Disturbances

Regulation of Acid–Base Balance

There are four types of acid–base imbalances: metabolic acidosis and alkalosis and respiratory acidosis and alkalosis. The causes, characteristics, and management of each of these disorders are discussed here.

TABLE 14-6 Summary of Major Fluid and Electrolyte Imbalances

Imbalance	Contributing Factors	Signs/Symptoms and Laboratory Findings
Fluid volume deficit (hypovolemia)	Loss of water and electrolytes, as in vomiting, diarrhea, fistulas, fever, excess sweating, burns, blood loss, gastrointestinal suction, and third-space fluid shifts; and decreased intake, as in anorexia, nausea, and inability to gain access to fluid. Diabetes insipidus and uncontrolled diabetes mellitus also contribute to a depletion of extracellular fluid volume.	Acute weight loss, decreased skin turgor, oliguria, concentrated urine, weak rapid pulse, capillary filling time prolonged, low central venous pressure, ↓ blood pressure, flattened neck veins, dizziness, weakness, thirst and confusion, ↑ pulse, muscle cramps. *Labs indicate:* ↑ hemoglobin and hematocrit, ↑ serum and urine osmolality and specific gravity, ↓ urine sodium, ↑ BUN and creatinine
Fluid volume excess (hypervolemia)	Compromised regulatory mechanisms, such as renal failure, congestive heart failure, and cirrhosis; and overzealous administration of sodium-containing fluids. Prolonged corticosteroid therapy, severe stress and hyperaldosteronism augment fluid volume excess.	Acute weight gain, edema, distended jugular veins, crackles, and elevated central venous pressure, shortness of breath, ↑ blood pressure, bounding pulse and cough. *Labs indicate:* ↓ hemoglobin and hematocrit, ↓ serum and urine osmolality, ↓ urine sodium and specific gravity.
Sodium deficit (hyponatremia) **Serum sodium < 135 mEq/L**	Loss of sodium, as in use of diuretics, loss of gastrointestinal fluids, renal disease and adrenal insufficiency. Gain of water, as in excessive administration of D_5W and excessive water supplements for patients receiving hypotonic tube feedings; disease states associated with SIADH such as head trauma and oat cell lung tumor; and pharmacologic agents associated with water retention such as oxytocin and certain tranquilizers. Hyperglycemia and congestive heart failure cause a loss of sodium.	Anorexia, nausea and vomiting, headache, lethargy, confusion, muscle cramps, muscular twitching, seizures, papilledema. *Labs indicate:* ↓ serum and urine sodium, ↓ urine specific gravity and osmolality.
Sodium excess (hypernatremia) **Serum sodium > 145 mEq/L**	Water deprivation in patients unable to drink at will, hypertonic tube feedings without adequate water supplements, diabetes insipidus, heatstroke, hyperventilation, and watery diarrhea. Excess corticosteroid, sodium bicarbonate and sodium chloride administration, and salt water near-drowning victims.	Thirst, elevated body temperature, swollen dry tongue and sticky mucous membranes, hallucinations, lethargy, restless, irritability, focal or grand mal seizures, pulmonary edema. *Labs indicate:* ↑ serum sodium, ↓ urine sodium, ↑ urine specific gravity and osmolality.
Potassium deficit (hypokalemia) **Serum potassium < 3.5 mEq/L**	Diarrhea, vomiting, gastric suction, corticosteroid administration, hyperaldosteronism, carbenicillin, amphotericin B, bulemia, osmotic diuresis, alkalosis, starvation, and digoxin toxicity.	Fatigue, anorexia, nausea and vomiting, muscle weakness, decreased bowel motility, ventricular asystole or fibrillation, paresthesias, leg cramps, ↓ blood pressure, ileus, abdominal distension, hypoactive reflexes. *ECG:* flattened T waves, prominent U waves, ST depression, and prolonged PR interval.
Potassium excess (hyperkalemia) **Serum potassium > 5.0 mEq/L**	Pseudohyperkalemia (as in hemolysis of blood sample), oliguric renal failure, use of potassium-conserving diuretics in patients with renal insufficiency, acidosis, Addison's disease, crush injury, burns, stored bank blood transfusions, and rapid intravenous administration of potassium.	Vague muscular weakness, bradycardia, dysrhythmias, flaccid paralysis, paresthesias, intestinal colic, cramps, irritability, anxiety. *ECG:* tall tented T waves, prolonged PR interval and QRS duration, absent P waves, ST depression.
Calcium deficit (hypocalcemia) **Serum calcium < 8.5 mg/dl**	Hypoparathyroidism (may follow thyroid surgery or radical neck dissection), malabsorption, pancreatitis, alkalosis, vitamin D deficiency, massive subcutaneous infection, generalized peritonitis, massive transfusion of citrated blood, and diuretic phase of renal failure.	Numbness, tingling of fingers, toes, and circumoral region; positive Trousseau's sign and Chvostek's sign; seizures, carpopedal spasms, hyperactive deep tendon reflexes, irritability, bronchospasm. *ECG:* prolonged QT interval.

(continued)

TABLE 14-6 *(continued)*

Imbalance	Contributing Factors	Signs/Symptoms and Laboratory Findings
Calcium excess (hypercalcemia) **Serum calcium > 10.5 mg/dl**	Hyperparathyroidism, malignant neoplastic disease, prolonged immobilization, overuse of calcium supplements, vitamin D excess, oliguric phase of renal failure, acidosis, and digoxin toxicity.	Muscular weakness, constipation, anorexia, nausea and vomiting, polyuria and polydipsia, hypoactive deep tendon reflexes, lethargy, deep bone pain, and pathologic features. *ECG:* shortened QT interval, bradycardia, heart blocks.
Magnesium deficit (hypomagnesemia) **Serum magnesium < 1.8 mg/dl**	Chronic alcoholism, hyperparathyroidism, hyperaldosteronism, diuretic phase of renal failure, malabsorptive disorders, diabetic ketoacidosis, refeeding after starvation, and certain pharmacologic agents (such as gentamycin, cisplatin, and cyclosporine).	Neuromuscular irritability, positive Chvostek's and Trousseau's sign, insomnia, mood changes, and anorexia and vomiting.
Magnesium excess (hypermagnesemia) **Serum magnesium > 2.7 mg/dl**	Oliguric phase of renal failure (particularly when magnesium-containing medications are administered), adrenal insufficiency, excessive intravenous magnesium administration.	Flushing, hypotension, drowsiness, hypoactive reflexes, depressed respirations, cardiac arrest and coma, diaphoresis. *ECG:* tachycardia→bradycardia, prolonged PR interval and QRS.
Phosphorus deficit (hypophosphatemia) **Serum phosphorus < 2.5 mg/dl**	Refeeding after starvation, alcohol withdrawal, diabetic ketoacidosis, respiratory alkalosis, ↓ magnesium, ↓ potassium, hyperparathyroidism, vomiting, diarrhea, hyperventilation, vitamin D deficiency associated with malabsorptive disorders.	Paresthesias, muscle weakness, bone pain and tenderness, chest pain, confusion, cardiomyopathy, respiratory failure, increased susceptibility to infection.
Phosphorus excess (hyperphosphatemia) **Serum phosphorus > 4.5 mg/dl**	Acute and chronic renal failure, excessive intake of phosphorus, vitamin D excess, respiratory acidosis, hypoparathyroidism, volume depletion, leukemia/lymphoma treated with cytotoxic agents, increased tissue breakdown, rhabdomyolysis.	Tetany, tachycardia, anorexia, nausea and vomiting, muscle weakness, and signs and symptoms of hypocalcemia.

Remarkable homeostatic mechanisms maintain plasma *p*H, an indicator of hydrogen ion (H+) concentration, within the narrow normal range of 7.35 to 7.45. These mechanisms consist of chemical buffering activity, the kidneys, and the lungs. In review, *p*H is defined as H+ concentration; the more hydrogen ions, the more acidic is the solution and the lower the pH. The *p*H range compatible with life (6.8–7.8) represents a tenfold difference in hydrogen ion concentration in plasma.

Chemical Buffers

Chemical buffers are substances that prevent major changes in the *p*H of body fluids by removing or releasing hydrogen ions; they can act quickly to prevent excessive changes in hydrogen ion concentration.

The body's major buffer system is the *bicarbonate-carbonic acid buffer system*. Normally, there are 20 parts of bicarbonate (HCO_3^-) to one part of carbonic acid (H_2CO_3). If this ratio is altered, the *p*H will change. It is the *ratio* that is important in maintaining *p*H, not absolute values. One must remember that carbon dioxide (CO_2) is a potential acid; when CO_2 is dissolved in water, it becomes carbonic acid ($CO_2 + H_2O = H_2CO_3$). Thus, when carbon dioxide is increased, the carbonic acid content is also increased and vice versa. If either bicarbonate or carbonic acid is increased or decreased so that the 20:1 ratio is no longer maintained, acid–base imbalance results.

Other less important buffer systems in the extracellular fluid include the inorganic phosphates and the plasma proteins. Intracellular buffers include proteins, organic and inorganic phosphates, and, in red blood cells, hemoglobin.

Kidneys

The kidneys regulate the bicarbonate level in extracellular fluid; they are able to regenerate bicarbonate ions as well as reabsorb them from the renal tubular cells. In the presence of respiratory acidosis, and most cases of metabolic acidosis, the kidneys excrete hydrogen ions and conserve bicarbonate ions to help restore balance. In the presence of respiratory and metabolic alkalosis, the kidneys retain hydrogen ions and excrete bicarbonate ions to help restore balance. The kidneys obviously cannot compensate for the metabolic acidosis created by renal failure. Renal compensation for imbalances is relatively slow (a matter of hours or days).

Lungs

The lungs, under the control of the brain's medulla, control the carbon dioxide, and thus carbonic acid content of extracellular fluid. They do so by adjusting ventilation in response to the amount of carbon dioxide in the blood. A rise in the partial pressure of carbon dioxide in arterial blood ($PaCO_2$) is a powerful stimulant to respiration. Of course, the partial pressure of oxygen in arterial blood (PaO_2) also influences respiration. Its effect, however, is not as marked as that produced by the $PaCO_2$.

In the presence of metabolic acidosis, the respiratory rate is increased, causing greater elimination of carbon dioxide (to reduce the acid load). In the presence of metabolic alkalosis, the respiratory rate is decreased, causing carbon dioxide to be retained (to increase the acid load).

Metabolic Acidosis (Base Bicarbonate Deficit)

Metabolic acidosis is a clinical disturbance characterized by a low *p*H (increased hydrogen concentration) and a low plasma bicarbonate concentration. It can be produced by a gain of hydrogen ion or a loss of bicarbonate. It can be divided clinically into two forms according to the values of the serum anion gap (AG): high anion gap acidosis and normal anion gap acidosis. Anion gap reflects normally unmeasured anions (phosphates, sulfates, and proteins) in plasma. Measuring the anion gap is helpful in the differential diagnosis of metabolic acidosis. The anion gap can be calculated by subtracting the sum of the serum chloride and bicarbonate concentrations (anions, or negatively charged electrolytes) from the serum sodium level (a cation, or positively charged electrolyte):

$$\text{Anion gap} = Na^+ - (Cl^- + HCO_3^-)$$

The normal value for an anion gap is 8 to 16 mEq/L. The unmeasured anions in the serum normally account for less than 16 mEq/L of the anion production. An anion gap greater than 16 mEq suggests excessive accumulation of unmeasured anions.

High anion gap acidosis results from excessive accumulation of fixed acid. It occurs in ketoacidosis, lactic acidosis, late phase of salicylate poisoning, uremia, methanol or ethylene glycol toxicity, and ketoacidosis with starvation. In all of these instances, abnormally high levels of anions flood the system, increasing the anion gap above normal limits.

Normal anion gap acidosis results from direct loss of bicarbonate, as in diarrhea, intestinal fistulas, and ureterostomies; excessive administration of chloride; and administration of parenteral nutrition without bicarbonate or bicarbonate-producing solutes (*i.e.*, lactate).

Clinical Manifestations

Signs and symptoms of metabolic acidosis vary with the severity of the acidosis. They may include headache, confusion, drowsiness, increased respiratory rate and depth, nausea, and vomiting. Peripheral vasodilation and decreased cardiac output occur when the *p*H falls below 7. Additional physical assessment findings include decreased blood pressure, cold and clammy skin, presence of dysrhythmias, and manifestations of shock.

Diagnostic Evaluation

Arterial blood gas measurements are valuable in the diagnosis of metabolic acidosis. Expected blood gas changes include a low bicarbonate level (less than 22 mEq/L) and a low *p*H (less than 7.35). Hyperkalemia may accompany metabolic acidosis, as a result of shift of potassium out of the cells. Later, as the acidosis is corrected, potassium moves back into the cells and hypokalemia may occur. Hyperventilation decreases the carbon dioxide level as a compensatory action. As stated previously, calculation of the anion gap is helpful in determining the cause of metabolic acidosis. An electrocardiogram will detect dysrhythmias caused by the increased potassium.

Management

Treatment is directed at correcting the metabolic defect. If the cause of the problem is excessive intake of chloride, treatment is aimed at eliminating the source of the chloride. When necessary, bicarbonate is administered. Although hyperkalemia occurs with acidosis, hypokalemia may occur with reversal of the acidosis and subsequent movement of potassium back into the cells. Therefore, the serum potassium level is monitored closely and hypokalemia is corrected as acidosis is reversed.

Chronic Metabolic Acidosis

Chronic metabolic acidosis is usually seen with chronic renal failure. The bicarbonate and *p*H decrease slowly, thus, the patient is asymptomatic until the bicarbonate is approximately 15 meq/L or less. Low serum calcium levels are treated prior to treatment for chronic metabolic acidosis to avoid tetany resulting from an increase in pH and decrease in ionized calcium level. Treatment of chronic metabolic acidosis may include use of alkalizing agents and hemodialysis or peritoneal dialysis.

Metabolic Alkalosis (Base Bicarbonate Excess)

Metabolic alkalosis is a clinical disturbance characterized by a high *p*H (decreased hydrogen ion concentration) and a high plasma bicarbonate concentration. It can be produced by a gain of bicarbonate or a loss of hydrogen ions.

Probably the most common cause of metabolic alkalosis is vomiting or gastric suction with loss of hydrogen and chloride ions; it also occurs in pyloric stenosis because only gastric fluid is lost in this disorder. Gastric fluid has an acid *p*H (usually 1 to 3); therefore, loss of this highly acidic fluid increases alkalinity of body fluids. Other situations predisposing to metabolic alkalosis include those associated with loss of potassium, such as the use of diuretics that lead to the excretion of potassium (*e.g.*, thiazides, furosemide, and ethacrynic acid) and the presence of excessive adrenalcorticoid hormones (as in hyperaldosteronism and Cushing's syndrome). Hypokalemia produces alkalosis in two ways: (1) in the presence of hypokalemia, the kidneys conserve potassium and thus hydrogen ion excretion is increased, and (2) cellular potassium moves out of the cells into the ECF in an attempt to maintain near-normal serum levels (as potassium ions [K+] leave the cells, hydrogen ions must enter to maintain electroneutrality). Excessive alkali ingestion through the use of antacids containing bicarbonate or the use of sodium bicarbonate during cardiopulmonary resuscitation can also cause metabolic alkalosis.

Clinical Manifestations

Alkalosis is primarily manifested by symptoms related to decreased calcium ionization, such as tingling of the fingers and toes, dizziness, and hypertonic muscles. The ionized fraction of serum calcium decreases in the presence of alkalosis as more calcium combines with serum proteins. Because it is the ionized fraction of calcium that influences neuromuscular activity, symptoms of hypocalcemia are often the predominant symptoms of alkalosis. Respirations are depressed as a compensatory action by the lungs. Atrial tachycardias may occur. As the *p*H increases above 7.6 and hypokalemia develops, ventricular disturbances may occur. Decreased motility and paralytic ileus may also occur.

Diagnostic Evaluation

Evaluating arterial blood gases reveals a *p*H greater than 7.45 and a serum bicarbonate concentration greater than 26 mEq/L. The partial pressure of carbon dioxide will increase as the lungs attempt to compensate for the excess bicarbonate by retaining carbon dioxide. This hypoventilation is more pronounced in semiconscious, unconscious, or debilitated patients than in alert patients. The former may develop marked hypoxemia as a result of hypoventilation. Hypokalemia may accompany metabolic alkalosis.

Urinary chloride levels can assist in identifying the cause of metabolic alkalosis if the patient's history does not provide adequate information. Metabolic alkalosis is the setting in which urine chloride concentration may be a more accurate estimate of volume than is the urine sodium concentration. Urine chloride concentrations help to differentiate between vomiting or diuretic ingestion or one of the causes of mineralcorticoid excess. Hypovolemia and hypochloremia in patients with vomiting or cystic fibrosis, refeeding patients, or those taking diuretics produce urine chloride concentrations less than 25 mEq/L. Signs of hypovolemia are not present and urine chloride concentration exceeds 40 mEq/L in patients with mineralcorticoid excess or alkali loading; these patients usually have expanded fluid volume. Urine chloride concentration should be less than 15 mEq/L when decreased chloride levels and hypovolemia are present.

Management

Treatment is aimed at reversing the underlying disorder. Sufficient chloride must be supplied for the kidney to absorb sodium with chloride (allowing the excretion of excess bicarbonate). Treatment also includes restoring normal fluid volume by administering sodium chloride fluids (because continued volume depletion serves to maintain the alkalosis). If hypokalemia is present, potassium is administered as KCl to replace both K^+ and Cl^- losses. Histamine H_2 receptor antagonists reduce the production of gastric HCl, thus decreasing the metabolic alkalosis associated with gastric suction. Carbonic anhydrase inhibitors are useful in treating metabolic alkalosis in those patients unable to tolerate rapid volume expansion (*i.e.*, patients with congestive heart failure). Because of volume depletion from GI loss, it is necessary to monitor intake and output carefully.

Chronic Metabolic Alkalosis

Chronic metabolic alkalosis can occur with long-term diuretic therapy (thiazides or furosemide), villous adenoma, external drainage of gastric fluids, significant potassium depletion, cystic fibrosis, and the chronic ingestion of milk and calcium carbonate. Symptoms are the same as for acute metabolic alkalosis, and as potassium decreases, frequent PVCs or U waves are seen. Management is aimed at correcting the underlying acid–base disorder.

Respiratory Acidosis (Carbonic Acid Excess)

Respiratory acidosis is a clinical disorder in which the *p*H is less than 7.35 and the partial pressure of arterial carbon dioxide ($PaCO_2$) is greater than 42 mm Hg. It may be either acute or chronic.

Respiratory acidosis is always due to inadequate excretion of carbon dioxide with inadequate ventilation, resulting in elevated plasma carbon dioxide levels and thus elevated carbonic acid levels. In addition to an elevated $PaCO_2$, hypoventilation usually causes a decrease in PaO_2. Acute respiratory acidosis occurs in emergency situations, such as acute pulmonary edema, aspiration of a foreign object, atelectasis, pneumothorax, overdosage of sedatives, sleep apnea syndrome, administration of oxygen to a patient with chronic hypercapnia (excessive levels of carbon dioxide in the blood), severe pneumonia, and ARDS (adult respiratory distress syndrome). Respiratory acidosis can also occur in diseases that impair respiratory muscles, *i.e.*, muscular dystrophy, myasthenia gravis, and Guillian-Barré syndrome. Mechanical ventilation can be associated with hypercapnia if the rate of effective alveolar ventilation is inadequate. Ventilation is fixed in these patients and CO_2 may be retained if the rate of CO_2 production is increased.

Clinical Manifestations

Clinical signs are variable in acute and chronic respiratory acidosis. Sudden hypercapnia (elevated $PaCO_2$) can cause increased pulse and respiratory rate, increased blood pressure, mental cloudiness, and feeling of fullness in the head. An elevated $PaCO_2$ causes cerebrovascular vasodilation and increased cerebral blood flow, particularly when it is higher than 60 mm Hg. Ventricular fibrillation may be the first sign of respiratory acidosis in anesthetized patients.

The patient with chronic respiratory acidosis may complain of weakness, dull headache, and symptoms of the underlying disease process. Patients with chronic obstructive pulmonary disease who gradually accumulate carbon dioxide over a prolonged period (days to months) may not develop symptoms of hypercapnia because compensatory renal changes have had time to occur. If respiratory acidosis is severe, intracranial pressure (ICP) may increase, resulting in papilledema and dilated conjunctival blood vessels. Hyperkalemia may result as hydrogen concentration overwhelms the compensatory mechanisms and moves into cells, causing a shift of potassium out of the cell.

- When the $PaCO_2$ is chronically above 50 mm Hg, the respiratory center becomes relatively insensitive to carbon dioxide as a respiratory stimulant, leaving hypoxemia as the major drive for respiration. Oxygen administration may remove the stimulus of hypoxemia, and the patient develops "carbon dioxide narcosis" unless the situation is quickly reversed. Therefore, oxygen must be administered with *extreme caution*.

Diagnostic Evaluation

Arterial blood gas evaluation reveals a *p*H less than 7.35 and a $PaCO_2$ greater than 42 mm Hg in acute respiratory acidosis. When compensation (renal retention of bicarbonate) has fully occurred, the arterial *p*H may be within the lower limits of normal. Depending on the etiology of respiratory acidosis, other diagnostic measures would include serum electrolyte evaluation, chest x-ray for determining any respiratory disease, and a drug screen if an overdose is suspected. An ECG to identify any cardiac involvement as a result of COPD (chronic obstructive pulmonary disease) may be indicated as well.

Management

Treatment is directed at improving ventilation; exact measures vary with the cause of inadequate ventilation. Pharmacologic agents are used as indicated. For example, bronchodilators help reduce bronchial spasm, and antibiotics are used for respiratory infections. Pulmonary hygiene measures are initiated, when necessary, to clear the respiratory tract of mucus and purulent drainage. Adequate hydration (2–3 L/day) is indicated to keep the mucous membranes moist and thereby facilitate removal of secretions. Supplemental oxygen is used as necessary. A mechanical ventilator, used cautiously, may improve pulmonary ventilation. Overzealous use of a mechanical ventilator may cause such rapid excretion of carbon dioxide that the kidneys will be unable to eliminate excess bicarbonate quickly enough to prevent alkalosis and seizures. For this reason, the elevated $PaCO_2$ must be decreased slowly. Placing the patient in a semi-Fowler's position facilitates expansion of the chest wall.

Chronic Respiratory Acidosis

Chronic respiratory acidosis occurs with pulmonary diseases such as chronic emphysema and bronchitis, obstructive sleep apnea, and obesity. As long as the $PaCO_2$ does not exceed the body's ability to compensate, the patient will be asymptomatic. If the $PaCO_2$ rises rapidly, cerebral vasodilation will increase ICP; cyanosis and tachypnea will develop. Treatment is the same as for acute respiratory acidosis.

- Oxygen administration must be used with *extreme caution* in those patients with chronic CO_2 retention where hypoxia rather than hypercapnia stimulates ventilation.

Respiratory Alkalosis (Carbonic Acid Deficit)

Respiratory alkalosis is a clinical condition in which the arterial *p*H is greater than 7.45 and the $PaCO_2$ is less than 38 mm Hg. As with respiratory acidosis, acute and chronic conditions can occur in respiratory alkalosis.

Respiratory alkalosis is always due to hyperventilation, which causes excessive "blowing off" of carbon dioxide and, hence, a decrease in plasma carbonic acid concentration. Causes can include extreme anxiety, hypoxemia, the early phase of salicylate intoxication, gram-negative bacteremia, and excessive ventilation by mechanical ventilators.

Diagnostic Evaluation

Analysis of arterial blood gases assists in diagnosis of respiratory alkalosis. In the acute state, the *p*H is elevated above normal as a result of a low $PaCO_2$ and a normal bicarbonate level. (The kidneys cannot alter the bicarbonate level quickly.) In the compensated state, the kidneys have had sufficient time to lower the bicarbonate level to a near normal level. Evaluation of serum electrolytes is indicated to identify any decrease in potassium as hydrogen is pulled out of the cell in exchange for potassium; decreased calcium, as severe alkalosis inhibits calcium ionization resulting in carpopedal spasms and tetany; or decreased phosphate due to alkalosis, causing an increased uptake of phosphate by the cells.

Clinical Manifestations

Clinical signs consist of lightheadedness due to vasoconstriction and decreased cerebral blood flow, inability to concentrate, numbness and tingling due to decreased calcium ionization, tinnitus, and, at times, loss of consciousness.

Management

Treatment depends on the underlying cause of respiratory alkalosis. If the cause is anxiety, the patient is instructed to breathe more slowly to cause accumulation of CO_2 or to breathe into a closed system (such as a paper bag). A sedative may be required to relieve hyperventilation in very anxious patients. Treatment for other causes of respiratory alkalosis is directed at correcting the underlying problem.

Chronic Respiratory Alkalosis

This state occurs as a result of chronic hypocapnia, resulting in decreased serum bicarbonate. Chronic hepatic insufficiency and cerebral tumors are risk factors. Patients are usually asymptomatic and the diagnostic evaluation and plan of care are the same as for acute respiratory alkalosis.

Mixed Acid–Base Disorders

At times the patient can simultaneously have both a respiratory and a metabolic imbalance. A normal *p*H in the presence of changes in the PCO_2 and plasma HCO_3^- concentration immediately suggests a mixed disorder. The only mixed disorder that cannot occur is a mixed respiratory acidosis and alkalosis, because it is impossible to have alveolar

TABLE 14-7 Acid–Base Disturbances and Compensation

Disorder	Initial Event	Compensation
Respiratory acidosis	↑ $PaCO_2$, ↑ or normal HCO_3^-, ↓ *p*H	Kidneys eliminate H^+ and retain HCO_3^-
Respiratory alkalosis	↓ $PaCO_2$, ↓ or normal HCO_3^-, ↑ *p*H	Kidneys conserve H^+ and excrete HCO_3^-
Metabolic acidosis	↓ or normal $PaCO_2$, ↓ HCO_3^-, ↓ *p*H	Lungs eliminate CO_2, conserve HCO_3^-
Metabolic alkalosis	↑ or normal $PaCO_2$, ↑ HCO_3^-, ↑ *p*H	Lungs ↓ ventilation to ↑ PCO_2, kidneys conserve H^+ to excrete HCO_3^-

hypoventilation and hyperventilation at the same time. An example of a mixed disorder is the simultaneous occurrence of metabolic acidosis and respiratory acidosis during respiratory and cardiac arrest.

Compensation

Generally, the pulmonary and renal systems will compensate for each other to return the *p*H to normal. In a single acid–base disorder, the system not causing the problem will try to compensate by returning the ratio of bicarbonate/carbonic acid to the normal 20:1. The lungs compensate for metabolic disturbances by changing CO_2 excretion. The kidneys compensate for respiratory disturbances by altering bicarbonate retention and hydrogen ion secretion. In respiratory acidosis, excess hydrogen is excreted in the urine in exchange for bicarbonate ions. In respiratory alkalosis, the renal excretion of bicarbonate is increased and hydrogen ions are retained. In metabolic acidosis, the compensatory mechanisms increase ventilation rate and the renal retention of bicarbonate. In metabolic alkalosis, the respiratory system compensates by decreasing ventilation to conserve CO_2 and raise the $PaCO_2$. Since the lungs respond to acid–base disorders within minutes, compensation for metabolic imbalances occurs faster than compensation for respiratory imbalances (Table 14-7 provides a summary of compensation effects).

Blood Gas Analysis

Blood gas analysis is often used to identify the specific acid–base disturbance and the degree of compensation that has occurred. Although it is usually based on arterial sampling, when an arterial sample cannot be obtained a mixed venous sample may be utilized. Table 14-8 compares normal ranges of venous and arterial blood gases. Chart 14-2 provides guidelines for a systematic approach to the analysis of acid–base disturbances.

Parenteral Fluid Therapy

Intravenous fluid administration is not only common in the hospital, it is also increasingly common in the home for the replacement of fluids, administration of medications, and provision of nutrients when no other route is available.

Purpose

The choice of an intravenous solution depends on the specific purpose for which it is intended. Generally, intravenous fluids are administered to achieve one or more of the following goals:

- To provide water, electrolytes, and nutrients to meet daily requirements
- To replace water and correct electrolyte deficits
- To provide a medium for intravenous administration of medications

Intravenous solutions contain dextrose or electrolytes mixed in various proportions with water. Pure or "free" water can *never* be administered intravenously because it rapidly enters red blood cells and causes them to rupture.

Types of Intravenous Solutions

Solutions are often categorized as isotonic, hypotonic, or hypertonic, according to whether their total osmolality is the same as, less than, or greater than that of blood (see p. 207 for a discussion of osmolality).

Some common water and electrolyte solutions are listed in Table 14-5, with comments about their use. Electrolyte solutions are considered *isotonic* if the total electrolyte content (anions plus cations) approximates 310 mEq/L. They are considered *hypotonic* if the total electrolyte content is less than 250 mEq/L and *hypertonic* if the total electrolyte content exceeds 375 mEq/L. The nurse must also consider a solution's osmolality, keeping in mind that the os-

TABLE 14-8 Normal Arterial and Mixed Venous Sample Blood Gases

Parameter	Arterial Sample	Venous Sample
*p*H	7.35–7.45	7.32–7.38
$PaCO_2$	35–45 mmHg	pCO_2 42–50 mmHg
PaO_2	80–100 mmHg	pO_2 40 mmHg
Oxygen saturation	95%–100%	75%
Base excess or deficit	+ or −2	+ or −2
HCO_3^-	22–26 mEq/L	23–27 Eq/L

CHART 14-2
Systematic Assessment of Arterial Blood Gases

The following steps are recommended to evaluate arterial blood gas values. They are based on the assumption that the average values are

$$pH = 7.4$$
$$PaCO_2 = 40 \text{ mm Hg}$$
$$HCO_3^- = 24 \text{ mEq/L}$$

I. *First, look at the* pH. It can be high, low, or normal as follows:

$pH > 7.4$ (alkalosis)
$pH < 7.4$ (acidosis)
$pH = 7.4$ (normal)

A normal *p*H may indicate perfectly normal blood gases, *or* it may be an indication of a *compensated* imbalance. A compensated imbalance is one in which the body has been able to correct the *p*H by either respiratory or metabolic changes (depending on the primary problem). For example, a patient with primary metabolic acidosis starts out with a low bicarbonate level but a normal carbon dioxide level. Soon afterward, the lungs try to compensate for the imbalance by exhaling large amounts of carbon dioxide (hyperventilation). Another example, a patient with primary respiratory acidosis starts out with a high carbon dioxide level; soon afterward, the kidneys attempt to compensate by retaining bicarbonate. If the compensatory maneuver is able to restore the bicarbonate to carbonic acid ratio back to 20:1, full compensation (and thus normal *p*H) will be achieved.

II. *The next step is to determine the primary cause of the disturbance. This is done by evaluating the $PaCO_2$ and HCO_3^- in relation to the* pH.

$pH > 7.4$ (alkalosis)

1. *If the $PaCO_2$ is <40 mm Hg,* the primary disturbance is respiratory alkalosis. (This situation occurs when a patient hyperventilates and "blows off" too much carbon dioxide. Recall that carbon dioxide dissolved in water becomes carbonic acid, the acid side of the "carbonic acid–bicarbonate buffer system.")
2. *If the HCO_3 is >24 mEq/L,* the primary disturbance is metabolic alkalosis. (This situation occurs when the body gains too much bicarbonate, an alkaline substance. Bicarbonate is the basic, or alkaline side of the "carbonic acid–bicarbonate buffer system.")

$pH < 7.4$ (acidosis)

1. *If the $PaCO_2$ is >40 mm Hg,* the primary disturbance is respiratory acidosis. (This situation occurs when a patient hypoventilates and thus retains too much carbon dioxide, an acidic substance.)
2. *If the HCO_3^- is <24 mEq/L,* the primary disturbance is metabolic acidosis. (This situation occurs when the body's bicarbonate level drops, either because of direct bicarbonate loss or because of gains of acids such as lactic acid or ketones).

III. *The next step involves determining if compensation has begun.*

This is done by looking at the value other than the primary disorder. If it is moving in the same direction as the primary value, compensation is underway. Consider the following gases:

*p*H	$PaCO_2$	HCO_3
(1) 7.20	60 mm Hg	24 mEq/L
(2) 7.40	60 mm Hg	37 mEq/L

The first set (1) indicates acute respiratory acidosis without compensation (the $PaCO_2$ is high, the HCO_3^- is normal). The second set (2) indicates chronic respiratory acidosis. Note that compensation has taken place; that is, the HCO_3^- has elevated to an appropriate level to balance the high $PaCO_2$ and produce a normal *p*H.

(Metheny NM. Fluid and electrolyte balance: Nursing Considerations. Philadelphia, JB Lippincott, 1992.)

molality of plasma is approximately 300 mOsm/L (SI: 300 mmol/L). For example, a 10% dextrose solution has an approximate osmolality of 505 mOsm/L.

When administering parenteral fluids, it is important to monitor the patient's response to the fluids. One should consider the fluid volume, the content of the fluid, and the patient's clinical status.

Isotonic Fluids

Fluids that are classified as isotonic have a total osmolality close to that of extracellular fluid and do not cause red blood cells to shrink or swell. The composition of these fluids may or may not approximate that of ECF. Isotonic fluids expand the extracellular fluid volume. One liter of isotonic fluid expands the extracellular fluid by 1 liter; however, it expands the plasma by only ¼ liter because it is a crystalloid fluid and diffuses quickly into the ECF compartment. For the same reason, 3 liters of isotonic fluid are needed to replace 1 liter of blood loss.

A solution of *5% dextrose in water* has a serum osmolality of 252 mOsm/L. Once administered, the glucose is rapidly metabolized, and this initially isotonic solution then disperses as a hypotonic fluid, one-third extracellular and two-thirds intracellular. Therefore, 5% dextrose in water is mainly used to supply water and to correct an increased serum osmolality. One liter of 5% dextrose in water provides less than 200 kcal and is a minor source of calories for the body's daily requirements.

Normal saline (0.9% sodium chloride) has a total osmolality of 308 mOsm/L. Because the osmolality is entirely contributed by electrolytes, the solution remains within the extracellular compartment. For this reason, normal saline is often used to treat an extracellular volume deficit. Although referred to as "normal," it contains only sodium and chloride and does not actually simulate ECF.

Several other solutions contain ions in addition to sodium and chloride and are somewhat similar to ECF in composition. *Ringer's solution* contains potassium and calcium in addition to sodium chloride. *Lactated Ringer's solution* contains bicarbonate precursors as well. These solutions are marketed, with slight variations, under a variety of different trade names.

Hypotonic Fluids

One purpose of hypotonic solutions is to replace cellular fluid, because it is hypotonic as compared with plasma. Another is to provide free water for excretion of body wastes. At times, hypotonic sodium solutions are used to treat hypernatremia and other hyperosmolar conditions. Half-strength saline (0.45% sodium chloride) is frequently used. Multiple-electrolyte solutions are also available. Excessive infusions of hypotonic solutions can lead to intravascular fluid depletion, decreased blood pressure, cellular edema, and cell damage. These solutions exert less osmotic pressure than the extracellular fluid.

Hypertonic Fluids

When *5% dextrose* is added to normal saline or Ringer's solution, the total osmolality exceeds that of ECF. The dextrose is quickly metabolized, however, and only the isotonic solution remains. Therefore, any effect on the intracellular compartment is temporary. Similarly, 5% dextrose is usually added to hypotonic multiple-electrolyte solutions. Once the dextrose is metabolized, these solutions disperse as hypotonic fluids.

Higher concentrations of dextrose, such as *50% dextrose* in water, are administered to help meet calorie requirements. These solutions are strongly hypertonic and must be administered into central veins so that they can be diluted by rapid blood flow.

Saline solutions are also available in osmolar concentrations greater than that of ECF. These solutions draw water from the intracellular compartment to the extracellular compartment and cause cells to shrink. If administered rapidly or in large quantity, they may cause an extracellular volume excess and precipitate circulatory overload and dehydration. As a result, these solutions are administered cautiously and usually only when the serum osmolality has decreased to dangerously low levels. Hypertonic solutions exert an osmotic pressure greater than that of extracellular fluid.

Other Substances Administered Intravenously

When the patient's gastrointestinal tract cannot accept food, nutritional requirements are often met intravenously. Parenteral administration may include high concentrations of glucose, protein, or fat to meet nutritional requirements.

Many medications are also delivered intravenously, either by infusion or directly into the vein. Because intravenous medications circulate rapidly, administration by this route is potentially very hazardous. Administration rates and recommended dilutions for individual medications are available in specialized texts pertaining to intravenous medications and in manufacturers' package inserts; these should be consulted to assure safe intravenous administration of medications.

Nursing Management of the Patient Receiving Intravenous Therapy

Venipuncture

The ability to gain access to the venous system for administering fluids and medications is an expected nursing skill in many settings. This responsibility includes selecting the appropriate venipuncture site and type of cannula, and being proficient in the technique of vein entry.

Before proceeding with venipuncture, it is important to select the most appropriate location and type of cannula for a particular patient. Factors influencing these choices include the type of solution to be administered, the expected duration of intravenous therapy, the patient's general condition, and the availability of veins. The skill of the person initiating the infusion is also an important consideration.

Choice of Site

Many sites can be used for intravenous therapy, but ease of access and potential hazards vary among them. Veins of the extremities are designated as peripheral locations and are ordinarily the only sites used by nurses. Because they are relatively safe and easy to enter, upper extremity veins are most commonly used. Veins of the arm and hand are shown in Figure 14-6. Leg veins should rarely, if ever, be used because of the high risk of thromboembolism; this is a last resort and can be done only with a physician's order. Additional sites to avoid include veins below a previous IV infiltration or phlebitic area; sclerosed or thrombosed veins; an arm with an arteriovenous shunt or fistula; or an arm affected by edema, infection, blood clot, or skin breakdown. Additionally, the arm on the side of a mastectomy is avoided because of impaired venous return.

Central veins frequently used by physicians include the subclavian and internal jugular veins. It is possible to access (or cannulate) these larger vessels even when peripheral sites have collapsed, and they allow administration of high-osmolar solutions. Hazards are much greater, however, and may include inadvertent entry into an artery or the pleural space.

Ideally, both arms and hands should be carefully inspected before a specific venipuncture site is chosen. A location should be selected that does not interfere with mobility. For this reason, the antecubital fossa is avoided, except as a last resort. The most distal site of the arm or hand is generally used first so that subsequent IVs can be moved progressively upward. The following are considered when selecting a site for venipuncture:

- Condition of the vein
- Type of fluid/medication to be infused
- Duration of therapy
- Patient's age and size
- Patient's medical history and current health status
- Skill of the health provider

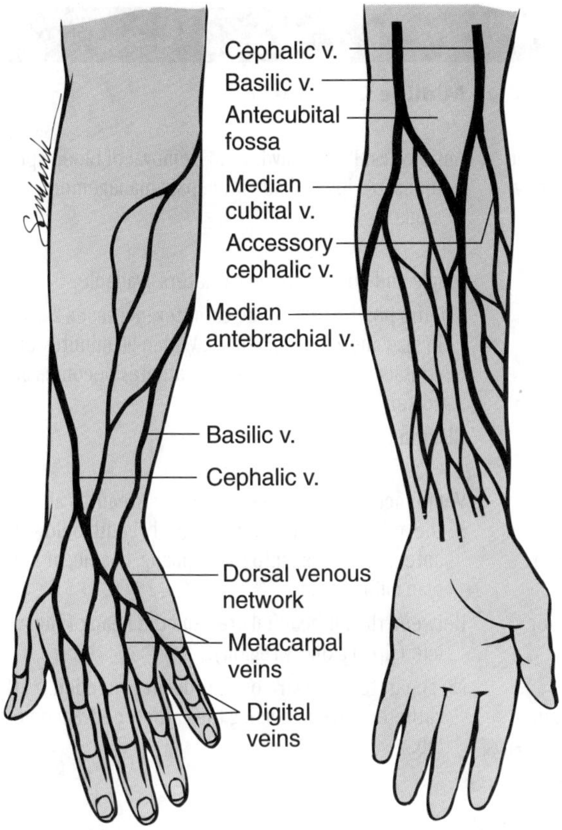

FIGURE 14-6. Sites of selection for the insertion of intravenous needles or catheters for the parenteral administration of fluids, medications, or blood products.

A vein should be assessed by palpation and inspection. It should feel firm, elastic, engorged, and round; not hard, flat, or bumpy. Because arteries lie close to veins in the antecubital fossa, the vessel should be palpated for arterial pulsation (even with a tourniquet on) and cannulation of pulsating vessels avoided. General guidelines for selecting a cannula include:

- ¾ inch–1¼ inch in length
- A small diameter of the catheter to occupy minimal space within the vein
- A 20–22 gauge for most IV fluids; a larger gauge for caustic or viscous solutions; an 18 gauge for blood administration

Hand veins are easiest to cannulate. Catheter tips should not rest in a flexion area, *e.g.*, antecubital fossa, as this would inhibit the IV flow.

Venipuncture Devices

The main types of cannulas available include steel scalp vein needles, indwelling plastic catheters inserted over a steel needle, and indwelling plastic catheters inserted through a steel needle. Scalp vein or butterfly needles are short steel needles with plastic wing handles. These are easy to insert, but because they are small and nonpliable, infiltrate easily (Fig. 14-7). The use of these needles should be limited to bolus injections or infusions lasting only a few hours, as they increase the risk of vein injury and infiltration. Insertion of an over-the-needle catheter requires the additional step of advancing the catheter into the vein after venipuncture. Because they are less likely to infiltrate, these devices are frequently preferred over scalp vein needles. Plastic catheters inserted through a hollow needle are usually called intracatheters. They are available in long lengths and are well suited for placement in central locations. Because insertion requires threading the catheter through the vein for a relatively long distance, these are difficult catheters to place.

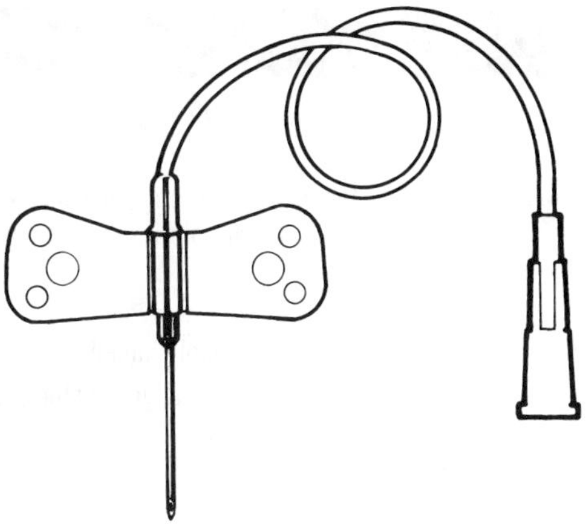

FIGURE 14-7. Scalp-vein needle: Winged infusion set. (Metheny N. Fluid and Electrolyte Balance: Nursing Considerations. Philadelphia, JB Lippincott, 1992.)

PICC and MLC Access Lines. Patients receiving home health care who need moderate to long-term parenteral therapy often have peripherally inserted central catheters (PICC) or midline catheters (MLC) inserted. These catheters are used for patients who do not have any peripheral access but who require IV antibiotics, blood, and parenteral nutrition. To utilize these catheters, the median cephalic, basilic, and cephalic veins must not be sclerosed or have been repeatedly punctured. If these veins are damaged, then central venous access via the subclavian or internal jugular vein or a venous access device must be considered as an alternative. PICC and MLC lines are compared in Table 14-9.

The principles for inserting PICC and MLC lines are much the same as those for inserting peripheral catheters; however, their insertion should be undertaken only by those who are experienced in inserting intravenous lines and have received specialized training. (See sources of information about such training at the end of this chapter.)

The physician prescribes PICC or MLC line insertion and the solution to be infused. The procedure for inserting either line requires sterile technique. The size of the catheter lumen chosen is based on the type of solution, the size of the patient, and the vein to be used. The patient's consent is obtained prior to use of these catheters. Use of the dominant arm is recommended as the site for inserting the catheter into the superior vena cava to assure adequate arm movement, which encourages blood flow and reduces the risk of dependent edema.

Needleless IV Delivery Systems. In an effort to decrease needlestick injuries and exposure to HIV, hepatitis, and other blood-borne pathogens, many hospitals are

TABLE 14-9 Comparison of PICC and MLC Lines

	Peripherally Inserted Central Catheter (PICC)	Midline Catheter (MLC)
Indications	Hyperalimentation, pain management, chemotherapeutic agents, antibiotics, intravenous hydration, blood drawing.	Antibiotics, IV fluid hydration, removal of blood specimens, peripheral nutrition, pain management infusions.
Features	Single and double lumen catheters available. 40–60 cm long; gauge variable (16–24g)	Single and double lumen catheters available. 2 hours postinsertion, the catheter increases 2 gauges in size and 2.5 cm in length. Within 90 minutes of contact with body fluids the catheter becomes 50 × softer.
Material	Radiopaque, polymer (polyurethane), silastic or aquavene materials.	Elastomeric hydrogel
Insertion Sites	Venipuncture performed in the antecubital fossa, above or below it into the basilic, cephalic, or axillary veins of the dominant arm. The median basilic is the ideal insertion site.	Venipuncture performed 2–3 finger breadths above the antecubital fossa or 1 finger breadth below the antecubital fossa into the cephalic, basilic, or median cubital vein.
Catheter Placement	The tip of the catheter lies in the superior vena cava or the brachiocephalic veins.	Between the antecubital area and the head of the clavicle (tip in axillary region).
Insertion Method	Through the needle technique, with or without a guidewire, breakaway needle with introducer or cannula with introducer (peel away sheath). (A peripherally inserted central catheter can also be used as a midline catheter.) Insertion can be accomplished at the bedside; surgery not needed for placement. Consent is required. Catheter may stay in place for up to 6 months or as long as required without complications.	No separate guidewire or introducer is needed. Stiff catheter is passed using the catheter advancement tab. Insertion can be accomlished at the bedside; surgery not needed for placement. Consent is required. Catheter may stay in place for 1–8 weeks.
Potential Complications	Malposition, pneumothorax, hemothorax, hydrothorax, dysrhythmias, nerve or tendon damage, respiratory distress, catheter embolism, thrombophlebitis or catheter occlusion. Compared with centrally placed catheters, venipuncture in the antecubital space with PICC line reduces risk of insertion complications.	Thrombosis, phlebitis, air embolism, infection, vascular perforation, bleeding, and catheter transection.
Contraindications	Dermititis, cellulitis, burns, high fluid volume infusions, rapid bolus injections, hemodialysis, and venous thrombosis.	Dermatitis, cellulitis, burns, high fluid volume infusions, rapid bolus injection, hemodialysis, and venous thrombosis.
Catheter Maintenance	Dressing changes according to agency policy and procedure. Generally, dressing changes should be done 2–3 ×/week or when wet, soiled, or nonocclusive. PICC line is flushed with 2 cc normal saline followed by heparin 1 cc (11u/ml) per lumen.	Dressing changes according to policy and procedures. Generally the dressing should be changed 2–3 ×/week, when wet, soiled, or non-occlusive. Line is flushed after each infusion or every 12 hours with 5–10 ml normal saline followed by 1 ml of heparin (100 u/ml). Catheter must be anchored securely, as the line may fall out.
Post Placement	Chest x-ray needed to confirm placement if inserted beyond axillary vein.	
Advantages	Placement of this catheter reduces cost and avoids repeated venipunctures as compared with centrally placed catheters.	Placement of this catheter reduces cost and avoids repeated venipunctures as compared with centrally placed catheters.

implementing needleless intravenous delivery systems. These systems have built-in protection against accidental needlesticks and provide a safe means of using and disposing of an IV administration set. Numerous companies are currently marketing needleless components. Collaboration with institutions and medical suppliers is helpful in developing a comprehensive and specific program.

Informing the Patient

Except in emergency situations, a patient should be prepared in advance for an intravenous infusion. A brief description of the venipuncture process, information about the expected length of infusion, and restrictions on activities are important topics. An opportunity should be given for the patient to verbalize concerns. For example, some patients believe they will die if small bubbles in the tubing enter their veins. After acknowledging this fear, the nurse can explain that usually only relatively large quantities of air administered rapidly are dangerous.

Preparation of Site

Because infection can be a major complication of intravenous therapy, the intravenous device must be sterile, as must the parenteral container and tubing. The insertion site is scrubbed with a povidone-iodine pad for 2 to 3 minutes, working from the center of the area to the periphery. This is followed with a 70% alcohol pledget. (Only alcohol pledgets are used if the patient is allergic to iodine.) The nurse must wear nonsterile disposable gloves during the venipuncture procedure because the likelihood of coming into contact with the patient's blood is high.

Vein Entry

Guidelines and a suggested sequence for venipuncture are presented in Guideline 14-1. For veins that are very small or particularly fragile, modifications in this technique may be necessary. Alternative methods can be found in journal articles or in specialized textbooks of intravenous therapy. The hospital's policy indicates if successful completion of a certification course is necessary to perform this skill.

Monitoring Intravenous Therapy

Maintaining an existing intravenous infusion is a nursing responsibility that demands knowledge of the solutions being administered and principles of flow. In addition, patients must be assessed carefully for both local and systemic complications.

Factors Affecting IV Gravity Flow

The flow of an intravenous infusion is subject to the same principles that govern fluid movement in general.

- *Flow is directly proportional to the height of the liquid column.* Raising the height of the infusion container may improve a sluggish flow.
- *Flow is directly proportional to the diameter of the tubing.* The clamp on IV tubing regulates the flow by changing the tubing diameter. In addition, the flow will be faster through cannulas of large gauge, as opposed to those of small gauge.
- *Flow is inversely proportional to the length of the tubing.* Adding extension tubing to an IV line will decrease the flow.
- *Flow is inversely proportional to the viscosity of a fluid.* Viscous intravenous solutions, like blood, require a larger cannula than do water or saline solutions.

Monitoring the Flow

Because so many factors influence the gravity flow, a solution does not necessarily continue to run at the speed originally set. Therefore, intravenous infusions must be monitored frequently to assure that the fluid is flowing at the intended rate. The IV container should be marked with tape to indicate at a glance whether the correct amount has infused. The flow rate should be calculated when the solution is originally hung, then monitored at least hourly. To calculate the flow rate, the number of drops delivered per ml must be determined; this varies with equipment and is usually printed on the solution set packaging. A formula that can be used to calculate the drop rate follows:

$$\text{gtt/ml of given set}/60 \text{ (min in hour)} \times \text{total hourly volume} = \text{gtt/min}$$

A variety of infusion pumps are available to assist in intravenous fluid delivery. These devices allow more accurate administration of fluids and medications than is possible with routine gravity-flow setups. Some pumps have flow rates calibrated in terms of milliliters/hour and are referred to as volumetric pumps. Others are calibrated in drops/minute and are referred to as infusion controllers. It is important to read the manufacturer's directions carefully before using any infusion pump or controller because there are many variations in available models. Use of these devices does not eliminate the need for frequent monitoring of the infusion and the patient.

Discontinuing an Infusion

The removal of an intravenous catheter is associated with two possible dangers: hemorrhage and catheter embolism. To prevent excessive bleeding, a dry, sterile sponge should be held over the site as the cannula is removed. Firm pressure should then be applied until all bleeding has stopped.

If a plastic IV catheter is severed, it can travel to the right ventricle and block the blood flow. To detect this complication when the catheter is removed, the expected length of the catheter is compared with its actual length. Plastic catheters should be withdrawn carefully and their length measured to make certain that no fragment has broken off. Great care must be exercised when using scissors around the dressing site. If it becomes apparent immediately that the catheter has been severed, an attempt can be made to occlude the vein above the site by applying a tourniquet to prevent the catheter from entering the central circulation (until such time as surgical removal is possible).

As always, however, it is better to *prevent* a potentially fatal problem than to deal with it after it has occurred. Fortunately, catheter embolism can easily be prevented by following simple rules, such as not using scissors near the catheter, and not withdrawing the catheter through the insertion needle. Manufacturer's guidelines should be followed carefully, such as covering the needle point with the bevel shield to prevent the catheter from being severed. Careful anchoring of the catheter will help prevent it from entering the general circulation should it accidentally separate from the adapter.

Complications Associated With Parenteral Fluid Therapy

Unfortunately, intravenous therapy predisposes to numerous hazards, including both local and systemic complications.

GUIDELINE 14–1
Starting an Intravenous Infusion

Nursing Action	Rationale
Preparation	
1. Verify order for IV therapy, check solution label, and identify patient.	1. Serious errors can be avoided by careful checking.
2. Explain procedure to patient.	2. Knowledge increases both patient comfort and cooperation.
3. Wash hands and put on disposable gloves.	3. Asepsis is essential to prevent infection. Prevents exposure of nurse to patient's blood.
4. Apply a tourniquet and identify a suitable vein.	4. This will distend the veins and allow them to be visualized.
5. Choose site.	5. Careful site selection will increase likelihood of successful venipuncture and preservation of vein.
6. Choose IV cannula.	6. Length and gauge of cannula should be appropriate for both site and purpose of infusion.
7. Connect infusion bag and tubing, and run solution through tubing to displace air; cover end of tubing.	7. Prevents delay; equipment must be attached immediately after successful venipuncture to prevent clotting.
8. Raise bed to comfortable working height and position for patient; adjust lighting. Position patient's arm below heart level to encourage capillary filling. Place protective pad on bed under the patient's arm.	8. Proper positioning will increase likelihood of success and provide comfort for patient.
Procedure	
1. Depending on hospital policy and procedure, lidocaine 1% (without epinephrine) 0.1–0.2 cc may be injected locally to the IV site.	1. Reduces pain locally from procedure.
2. Apply a new tourniquet for each patient or a blood pressure cuff 15 to 20 cm (6–8 inches) above injection site. Palpate for a pulse distal to the tourniquet. Ask patient to open and close fist several times or *hang* patient's arm down to enlarge a vein.	2. The tourniquet distends the vein and makes it easier to enter; it should never be tight enough to occlude arterial flow. If a pulse cannot be palpated distal to the tourniquet, then it is too tight. A new and separate tourniquet should be used for each patient to prevent the transmission of organisms. A blood pressure cuff may be used for elderly patients to avoid rupture of the veins. A clenched fist encourages the vein to become round and turgid.
3. Ascertain if the patient is allergic to iodine. Prepare site by scrubbing with three betadine swabs for 2–3 min. in circular motion, moving outward from injection site. Allow to dry, then cleanse site with 70% alcohol pledget to clearly view deep veins. a. If the site elected is excessively hairy, clip hair. (Check agency's policy and procedure about this practice.) b. If the patient is allergic to povidone-iodine, then 70% alcohol alone may be used.	3. Strict asepsis and careful site preparation are essential to prevent infection.
4. With hand not holding the venous access device, steady patient's arm and use finger or thumb to pull skin taut over vessel.	4. Applying traction to the vein helps to stabilize it.
5. Holding needle bevel up and at 25–45 degree angle, depending on the depth of the vein, pierce skin to reach but not penetrate vein.	5. Bevel-up position usually produces less trauma to skin and vein.
6. Decrease angle of needle to 10–20 degrees or until nearly parallel with skin, then enter vein either directly above or from the side in one quick motion.	6. Two-stage procedure decreases chance of thrusting needle through posterior wall of vein as skin is entered.
7. If backflow of blood is visible, straighten angle and advance needle. Additional steps for catheter inserted over needle:	7. Backflow may not occur if vein is small; this position decreases chance of puncturing posterior wall of vein.
a. Advance needle 0.6 cm (¼ inch) after successful venipuncture.	a. Advancing the needle slightly makes certain the plastic catheter has entered the vein.
b. Hold needle hub, and slide catheter over the needle into the vein. Never reinsert needle into a plastic catheter or pull the catheter back into the needle.	b. Reinsertion of the needle or pulling the catheter back can sever the catheter, causing catheter embolism.

(continued)

GUIDELINE 14–1 *(continued)*
Starting an Intravenous Infusion

Nursing Action	Rationale
Procedure	
c. Remove needle, while pressing lightly on the skin over the catheter tip; hold catheter hub in place.	c. Slight pressure prevents bleeding before tubing is attached.
8. Release tourniquet, and attach infusion tubing; open clamp enough to allow drip.	8. Infusion must be attached promptly to prevent clotting of blood in cannula. After 2 unsuccessful attempts at venipuncture, assistance by another nurse is suggested.
9. Slip a sterile 2 × 2 inch gauze pad under the catheter hub.	9. The gauze acts as a sterile field.
10. Anchor needle firmly in place with a tape.	10. A stable needle is less likely to become dislodged or to irritate the vein.
11. The insertion site is then covered with a Bandaid or sterile gauze; tape in place with nonallergenic tape but do not encircle extremity.	11. Tape encircling extremity can act as a tourniquet.
12. Tape a small loop of IV tubing onto dressing.	12. The loop decreases the chance of inadvertent cannula removal if the tubing is pulled.
13. Cover the insertion site with a dressing according to hospital policy and procedure. A gauze or transparent dressing may be used.	13. Transparent dressings allow assessment of the insertion site for phlebitis, infiltration and infection without removing the dressing.
14. Label dressing with type and length of cannula, date, and initials.	14. Labelling facilitates assessment and safe discontinuation.
15. Calculate infusion rate, and regulate flow of infusion.	15. Infusion must be regulated carefully to prevent overinfusion or underinfusion.
16. Document site, cannula size and type, time, solution, IV rate, and patient response to procedure.	16. Documentation is essential to facilitate care and for legal purposes.

Systemic complications occur less frequently but are often more serious than local complications and include circulatory overload, air embolism, febrile reaction, and infection.

Systemic Complications

Fluid Overload. Overloading the circulatory system with excessive intravenous fluids will cause increased blood pressure and central venous pressure, severe dyspnea, and cyanosis. Additional signs and symptoms include cough and puffy eyelids. The possible causes include rapid infusion of an IV solution or liver, cardiac, or renal disease. This is particularly likely to occur in patients with cardiac disease and is referred to as *circulatory overload.*

The treatment for circulatory overload is to decrease the IV rate, monitor vital signs frequently, assess breath sounds, and place the patient in a high Fowler's position. The physician is contacted immediately. This complication can be avoided by using an IV pump for infusions and by carefully monitoring all infusions. Complications of circulatory overload include congestive heart failure and pulmonary edema.

Air Embolism. The danger of *air embolism* is always present even though it does not occur frequently. It is most often associated with cannulation of central veins. The presence of air embolism may be manifested by dyspnea and cyanosis; hypotension; weak, rapid pulse; loss of consciousness; and chest, shoulder, and low back pain. Treatment of this complication is to immediately clamp the catheter, place the patient on his or her left side in Trendelenburg position, assess vital signs and breath sounds, and administer oxygen. Air embolism can be prevented by using a Luer-Lok adapter on all lines. Complications of air embolism include shock and death. The amount of air necessary to induce death in humans is not known; however, the rate of entry is probably as important as the actual volume of air.

Septicemia. The presence of pyrogenic substances in either the infusion solution or the administration setup can induce a febrile reaction and *septicemia.* With such a reaction, one might observe an abrupt temperature elevation shortly after the infusion is started, backache, headache, increased pulse and respiratory rate, nausea and vomiting, diarrhea, chills and shaking, general malaise, and, if severe, vascular collapse. Causes of septicemia include contamination of the IV product or a break in aseptic technique, especially in immunocompromised patients. Treatment is symptomatic and includes culturing of the IV catheter, tubing, or solution if suspect and establishing a new IV site for medication and or fluid administration.

Infection. Infection ranges in severity from local involvement of the insertion site to systemic dissemination of organisms through the bloodstream, as in septicemia. Measures to prevent infection are essential at the time the IV line is inserted and throughout the entire period of infusion. Some of these include the following:

- Carefully washing one's hands before every contact with any part of the infusion system or patient

- Examining the IV containers for cracks, leaks, or cloudiness, which may indicate a contaminated solution
- Using strict aseptic technique
- Firmly anchoring the IV cannula to prevent to-and-fro motion
- Inspecting the IV site daily and replacing sterile dressing
- Removing the IV catheter at the first sign of local inflammation, contamination, or complication
- Replacing the peripheral IV cannula every 48 to 72 hours, or as indicated
- Replacing the IV cannula inserted during emergency conditions (with questionable asepsis) as soon as possible
- Replacing the bag every 24 hours and the entire administration set at least every 48 to 72 hours, and every 24 hours when blood or lipid products are being infused

Local Complications

Local complications of intravenous therapy include infiltration, phlebitis, thrombophlebitis, hematoma, and clotting of the needle.

Infiltration. Dislodging of a needle and local infiltration of the solution into subcutaneous tissues is not uncommon. Infiltration is characterized by edema around the insertion site, discomfort, and coolness in the area of infiltration, and significant decrease in the flow rate. When the solution is particularly irritating, sloughing of tissue may result. Closely monitoring the insertion site is necessary to detect infiltration before it becomes severe.

Infiltration is easily recognized if the insertion area is larger than an identical region in the opposite extremity. Infiltration, however, is not always so obvious. A common misconception is that a backflow of blood into the tubing proves that the cannula is properly placed within the vein. If the catheter tip has pierced the wall of the vessel, however, intravenous fluid will seep into tissues as well as flow into the vein. A more reliable means of confirming infiltration is to apply a tourniquet above or proximal to the infusion site and tighten it enough to restrict venous flow. If the infusion continues to drip despite the venous obstruction, infiltration is present.

As soon as the infiltration is noticed, the infusion should be stopped and the IV discontinued. A sterile dressing is applied to the site after careful inspection. The IV infusion should be started in a new site or proximal to the infiltration if the same extremity is used. A warm compress to the affected limb may be prescribed with elevation of the arm to promote absorption of fluid. Infiltration can be detected and treated early by inspecting the site every hour for redness, edema, blood return, or coolness at the site. Using the appropriate size and type of cannula for the vein avoids this complication.

Phlebitis. Phlebitis is defined as inflammation of a vein related to both a chemical and mechanical irritation. It is characterized by a reddened, warm area around the insertion site or along the path of the vein, pain or tenderness at the site or along the vein, and swelling. The incidence of phlebitis increases with the length of time the intravenous line is in place, the composition of the fluid or medication infused (especially its *p*H and tonicity), the size and site of the cannula inserted, improper anchoring of the line, and the introduction of microorganisms at the time of insertion.

Treatment consists of discontinuing the IV and restarting it in another site, and applying a warm, moist compress to the affected site. Phlebitis can be prevented by using aseptic technique during insertion, using the appropriate size catheter and needle size for the vein, considering the composition of fluids and medications when selecting a site, observing the site for any complications every hour, and anchoring the catheter or needle well.

Thrombophlebitis. Thrombophlebitis refers to the presence of a clot plus inflammation in the vein. It is evidenced by localized pain, redness, warmth, and swelling around the insertion site or along the path of the vein, immobility of the extremity because of discomfort and swelling, sluggish flow rate, fever, malaise, and leukocytosis.

Treatment includes discontinuing the IV, applying a warm compress, elevating the extremity, and restarting the line in the opposite extremity. In the presence of signs and symptoms of thrombophlebitis, one should *not* attempt to irrigate the line. Thrombophlebitis can be prevented by avoiding trauma to the vein at the time the IV is inserted, observing the site every hour, and checking medication additives for compatibility.

Hematoma. Hematoma occurs as a result of leakage of blood into tissues surrounding the insertion site. It can be caused by perforating the opposite vein wall during venipuncture, the needle slipping out of the vein, and insufficient pressure applied to the site after the needle or catheter is removed. The signs and symptoms of a hematoma include ecchymosis, immediate swelling at the site, and the leakage of blood at the site.

Treatment includes removing the needle or catheter and applying pressure with a sterile dressing; applying an ice bag for 24 hours to the site and then a warm compress to increase absorption of blood; assessing the site; and restarting the line in another extremity if indicated. A hematoma can be prevented by carefully inserting the needle and using diligent care when a patient has a bleeding disorder, is on anticoagulants, or has advanced liver disease.

Clotting. Clotting of the needle is another local complication. It is caused by kinked IV tubing, a very slow rate, an empty IV bag, or not flushing after intermittent medications or solution administration. The signs and symptoms are decreased flow rate and blood flow back into the IV tubing.

If clotted, the IV line must be discontinued. Treatment consists of *not* irrigating or milking the tubing, *not* restoring flow by increasing the rate or hanging the solution higher, and *not* aspirating the clot from the cannula. Clotting of the needle may be prevented by not permitting the IV bag to run dry, taping the tubing to prevent kinking, maintaining an adequate flow rate and flushing the line after intermittent medication or solution administration. In some cases, urokinase (Abbokinase) is injected into the catheter to clear an occlusion resulting from fibrin or clotted blood.

Home Care Considerations

At times, IV therapy must be administered in the home setting. Home infusion therapies cover a wide range of treatments including antibiotics, analgesic medications, antineoplastics, blood or blood component therapy, and total parenteral nutrition.

Since much of the daily management of some of these therapies will rest at times with the patient and family, patient education becomes essential to teach the patient or family caregiver how to manage the fluid properly, regulate the flow rate, and be alert for possible complications. Written instructions will help reinforce the key points for all these functions.

When direct nursing care is necessary, arrangements can be made to have an infusion nurse visit the home and deliver the IV therapy as prescribed. In addition to implementing and monitoring the IV therapy, the nurse carries out a comprehensive assessment of the patient's condition and continues to teach the patient and family about the skills involved in overseeing the IV therapy setup. Any diet changes that may be necessary because of fluid or electrolyte imbalances are reinforced during such sessions. Periodic laboratory testing may be necessary to assess the effects of intravenous therapy and the patient's recovery or progress. Blood specimens may be obtained in a laboratory near the patient's home, or a home visit to obtain blood specimens may be arranged.

The nurse collaborates with the case manager in assessing the patient, family, and home environment; developing a plan of care in accordance with the patient's plan of treatment and level of ability; and arranging for appropriate referral and follow-up if necessary. Any necessary equipment may either be provided by the agency or purchased by the patient depending on the terms of the home care arrangements. Appropriate documentation is provided as needed to assure third-party payment for the service rendered.

CRITICAL THINKING EXERCISES

1. A patient is to receive intravenous antibiotics at home to treat osteomyelitis. Describe the instructions you would provide to the patient and his family to assure correct and safe administration of the prescribed antibiotic. How might your teaching strategies differ if the patient lives alone? Is unable to read? Has a faulty memory?
2. A patient expresses concern about his intravenous infusion running out; he fears that air will enter the tubing and cause an air embolism. What explanation would you give the patient about this risk?
3. Your patient is experiencing palpitations, shortness of breath, and a decrease in blood pressure. You notify the physician; she instructs you to start an intravenous infusion and tells you that she is on her way to see the patient and will arrive in approximately an hour. She does not specify what intravenous fluid should be infused. How would you proceed?

BIBLIOGRAPHY

Books

Cogan M. Fluid and Electrolytes—Physiology and Pathophysiology. Norwalk, CT, Appleton and Lange, 1991.

Fluid and Electrolytes: Video and Workbook. Springhouse, PA, Springhouse Corporation, 1994.

Gahart B. Intravenous Medications, 6th ed. St. Louis, CV Mosby, 1990.

Halperin ML and Goldstein MB. Fluid, Electrolyte and Acid–Base Physiology: A Problem-Based Approach. Philadelphia, WB Saunders, 1994.

Hartshorn J et al. Introduction to Critical Care Nursing. Philadelphia, WB Saunders, 1993.

Horne M, Easterday-Heitz U, and Swearingen P. Fluid, Electrolyte, and Acid–Base Balance. A Case Study Approach. St. Louis, Mosby–Year Book, 1991.

Horne MM and Swearingen PL. Pocket Guide. Fluid, Electrolytes, and Acid–Base Balance, 2nd ed. St. Louis, Mosby–Year Book, 1993.

Intravenous Nursing Society. Revised Intravenous Nursing Standards of Practice. Belmont, MA. Intravenous Nursing Society, 1990.

IV Therapy. Clinical Skillbuilders. Springhouse, PA, Springhouse Corporation, 1990.

Kee JL and Paulanka B. Fluids and Electrolytes With Clinical Applications, 5th ed. Albany, NY, Delmar Publishers, Inc., 1994.

Kokko J and Tannen R. Fluids and Electrolytes, 2nd ed. Philadelphia, WB Saunders, 1990.

Marino P. The ICU Book. Philadelphia, Lea & Febiger, 1991.

McFarland MR and Grant-Moeller M. Nursing Implications of Laboratory Tests, 3rd ed. Albany, NY, Delmar Publishers, Inc., 1994.

Metheny NM. Fluid and Electrolyte Balance: Nursing Considerations, 2nd ed. Philadelphia, JB Lippincott, 1992.

Pestano C. Fluids and Electrolytes in the Surgical Patient, 4th ed. Baltimore, Williams & Wilkins, 1989.

Rose B. Clinical Physiology of Acid–Base & Electrolyte Disorders, 4th ed. New York, McGraw-Hill, 1994.

Weinstein S. Plumer's Principles and Practice of Intravenous Therapy, 5th ed. JB Lippincott, 1993.

Windmer AF. IV-related infections. In Wenzel RP. Prevention and Control of Nosocomial Infections. Baltimore, Williams & Wilkins, 1993.

Journals

Asterisks indicate nursing research articles.

AARC Clinical Practice Guideline. Sampling for arterial blood gas analysis. Respiratory Care 1992 Aug; 37(8):913–917.

*Adams F. Fluid intake: How much do elders drink? Geriatr Nurs (New York) 1988 July/Aug; 9(4):218–221.

Anderson S. ABG's. Six easy steps to interpreting blood gases. Am J Nurs 1990 Aug; 90(8):42–45.

Bohony J. Fighting the needlestick battle without needles. Medsurg Nurs 1993 Dec; 2(6):469–476.

Bohony J. Nine IV complications and what to do about them. Am J Nurs 1993 Oct; 93(10):45–50.

*Bowman M et al. Effect of tube-feeding osmolality on serum sodium levels. Crit Care Nurse 1989 Jan; 9(1):22–28.

Cullen L. Interventions related to fluid and electrolyte balance. Nurs Clin North Am 1992 June; 27(2):569–576.

Cushing M. Hazards of the infiltrated IV. Am J Nurs 1990 Sept; 90(9):31–32.

Davis KD and Attie MF. Management of severe hypercalcemia. Crit Care Clin 1991 Jan; 7(1):175–190.

Dennison R and Blevins BN. Myths and facts . . . about fluid imbalance. Nursing 92 1992 Jan; 22(1):22.

Dennison R and Blevins BN. Myths and facts . . . about electrolytes. Nursing 92 1992 Feb; 22(2):26.

Dennison R and Blevins BN. Myths and facts . . . about acid–base imbalance. Nursing 92 1992 Mar; 22(3):69.

Dick M, Maree S, and Gray J. How to boost the odds of a painless IV start. Am J Nurs 1992 June; 92(6):49–50.

Freedman BI and Burkart JM. Hypokalemia. Crit Care Clin 1991 Jan; 7(1):143–153.

*Gershan J et al. Fluid volume deficit: Validating the indicators. Heart and Lung 1990 Mar; 19(2):152–156.

Guidelines for Cardiopulmonary Resuscitation and Emergency Cardiac Care. Recommendations of the 1992 National Conference. Journal of the American Medical Association 1992 Oct 28; 268(16):2172–2302.

Hedges C and Karas B. Peripherally inserted central catheters: Challenges for hospital management. Medsurg Nurs 1993 Dec; (2)6:443–451.

Hennessey B, Fitzgerald A, and Graham D. Venous air embolism. Keeping your patient out of danger. Am J Nurs 1993 Nov; 93(11):54–56.

Holder C and Alexander J. A new and improved guide to IV therapy. Am J Nurs 1990 Feb; 90(2):43–47.

*Jordan L. Effects of fluid manipulation on the incidence of vomiting during outpatient cisplatin infusion. Oncol Nurs Forum 1989 Mar/Apr; 16(2):213–218.

Jurf JB. Evaluating needleless products. Medsurg Nurs 1994 Jun; 3(3):176–180.

Lundgren A, Jorfeldt L, and Ek A. The care and handling of peripheral intravenous cannulae on 60 surgery and internal medicine patients: An observation study. J Adv Nurs 1993 Jun; 18(6):963–971.

*Maki DG et al. A prospective, randomized trial of gauze and two polyurethane dressings for site care of pulmonary artery catheters: Implications for catheter management. Crit Care Med 1994 Nov; 22(11):1729–1737.

*Maki DG. Yes, Virginia, aseptic technique is very important: Maximal barrier precautions during insertion reduce the risk of central venous catheter–related bacteremia. Infec Control Hosp Epidemiol 1994 Apr; 15(4 pt 1):227–230.

Meares C. P.I.C.C. and M.L.C. lines. Options worth exploring. Nursing 92 1992 Oct; 22(10):52–55.

*Metheny N et al. Electrolyte disturbances in tube-fed patients (abstr). Thirteenth Annual Midwest Nursing Research Society Conference (Cincinnati, OH) 1989 Apr 2: 220.

Metheny N. Why worry about IV fluids? Am J Nurs 1990 June; 90(6):50–57.

Millam D. How to teach good venipuncture technique. Am J Nurs 1993 July; 90(7):38–41.

Millam D. Starting IV's. How to develop your venipuncture expertise. Nursing 92 1992 Sep; 22(9):33–46.

Peppers MP, Geheb M; and Desai T. Hypophosphatemia and hyperphosphatemia. Crit Care Clin 1991 Jan; 7(1):201–214.

*Peters K et al. Increasing clinical use of pulse oximetry. Dimensions in Critical Care Nursing 1990 Mar/Apr; 9(2):107–111.

Ryder M. Peripherally inserted central catheters. Nurs Clin North Am 1993 Dec; 28(4):937–973.

Rountree D. The P.I.C. catheter. Am J Nurs 1991 August; 91(8):22–28.

Salem M, Munoz R, and Chernow B. Hypomagnesimia in critical illness. Crit Care Clin 1991; Jan 7(1):225–249.

Stringfield Y. Back to basics. Acidosis, alkalosis and ABG's. Am J Nurs 1993 Nov; 93(11):43–44.

*Strumpfer A. Lower incidence of peripheral catheter complications by the use of elastomeric hydrogel catheters in home intravenous therapy patients. J Intravenous Nurs 1991 July/Aug; 14(4):261–267.

*Thompson D et al. A trial of povidone-iodine antiseptic solution for the prevention of cannula-related thrombophlebitis. J Intravenous Nurs 1989; 12(2):99–102.

Van Hook JW. Hypermagnesemia. Crit Care Clin 1991 Jan; 7(1): 215–223.

Williams ME. Hyperkalemia. Crit Care Clin 1991 Jan; 7(1):155–174.

Wood L. IV vesicants: How to avoid extravasation. Am J Nurs 1993 Apr; 93(4):42–46.

Yarnell R and Craig M. Detecting hypomagnesemia. Nursing 91 1991 July; 21(7):55–57.

Zaloga GP. Hypocalcemic crisis. Crit Care Clin 1991 Jan; 7(1): 191–200.

RESOURCES

Applied Biotech Products, Inc. Instructional Manual. 1989. Landry Vein Light. P.O. Box 52703, Lafayette, LA 70505-2703.

Assessing Fluids and Electrolytes. Video Skill Series. 1989. Springhouse Corporation. 1111 Bethlehem Pike, Springhouse, PA 19477.

Detecting and Managing IV Problems. Video Skill Series. 1988. Springhouse Corporation. 1111 Bethlehem Pike, Springhouse PA, 19477.

Intravenous Nurses Society (National Chapter). Brighton St., Belmont, MA 02178. (617) 489-5205.

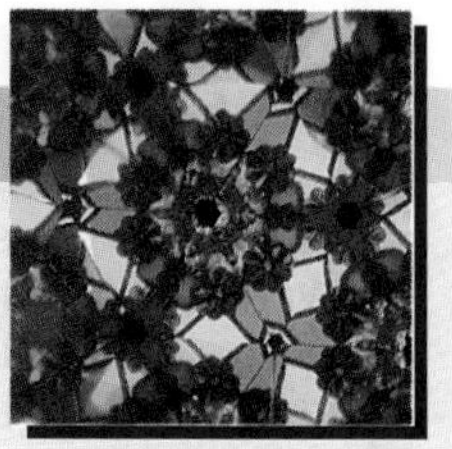

15 Shock and Multisystem Failure

CHAPTER OUTLINE

Definition of Shock
Classification of Shock

Pathophysiology of Shock
Cellular Effects of Shock
Vascular Responses
Blood Pressure Regulation

Overview of the Stages of Shock
Compensatory Stage
Progressive Stage
Irreversible Stage

Overview of Medical Management of Shock
Fluid Replacement in Shock
Vasoactive Medication Therapy in Shock
Nutritional Support in Shock

Classifications of Shock

Management of Different Types of Shock
Hypovolemic Shock
Cardiogenic Shock
Distributive Shock

Multiple Organ Failure
Clinical Manifestations
Management

Critical Thinking Exercises

LEARNING OBJECTIVES

On completion of this chapter, the learner will be able to:

1. Define shock and its underlying pathophysiology
2. Compare clinical findings of the compensatory and progressive stages of shock
3. Describe organ damage that may occur with shock
4. Compare hypovolemic, cardiogenic, and distributive shock in terms of causes, pathophysiologic effects, medical and nursing management
5. Describe indications for varying types of fluid replacement
6. Identify vasoactive medications used in the treatment of shock and describe nursing implications associated with their use
7. Discuss the importance of nutritional support in all forms of shock
8. Discuss the role of the nurse in psychosocial support of both the patient experiencing shock and the family
9. Discuss the syndrome of multiple organ failure

Suzanne C. Smeltzer and Brenda G. Bare: Brunner and Suddarth's Textbook of Medical-Surgical Nursing, 8th Edition. © 1996 Lippincott-Raven Publishers.

Definition of Shock

Shock is defined as a complex, life-threatening condition (or syndrome) characterized by inadequate blood flow to the tissues and cells of the body (Rice, 1991a). Adequate blood flow to the tissues and cells requires the following components: (1) an adequate cardiac pump, (2) an effective vasculature or circulatory system, and (3) adequate blood volume. If one of these components is impaired, blood flow to the tissues will be threatened or compromised. Inadequate blood flow to the tissues results in inadequate oxygen and nutrients to the cells, cellular starvation, cell death, organ failure, and eventual death if not treated.

Shock affects all body systems. It may develop rapidly or slowly depending on the underlying cause. During shock the body struggles to survive, calling on all its homeostatic mechanisms to restore blood flow and tissue perfusion. Shock may occur as a complication of many disorders and therefore all patients have the potential to develop shock (Rice, 1991a).

Nursing care of the patient with shock requires ongoing systematic assessment of the patient. Many of the interventions required in caring for the patient with shock call for close collaboration with other members of the health care team and a physician's order. The nurse must anticipate such orders as they need to be executed with speed and accuracy.

Before discussing the systemic impact of shock and the medical and nursing management involved, this chapter will examine the pathophysiology of shock at the cellular and circulatory system levels.

Classification of Shock

Shock can be classified according to etiology and may be described as (1) hypovolemic, (2) cardiogenic, and (3) distributive or vasogenic. Some authors identify a fourth category, obstructive shock, which is shock resulting from disorders that cause mechanical obstruction to blood flow through the central circulatory system despite normal myocardial function and intravascular volume. Examples include pulmonary embolism, cardiac tamponade, dissecting aortic aneurysm, and tension pneumothorax. In this discussion obstructive disorders will be discussed as examples of noncoronary cardiogenic shock.

Hypovolemic shock occurs when there is a decrease in the intravascular volume. Cardiogenic shock occurs when the heart has an impaired pumping ability; it may be of coronary or noncoronary origin. Distributive or vasogenic shock occurs when there is a maldistribution of the blood volume in the vasculature (Rice, 1991a). Although the treatment plan and nursing care will differ for the different types of shock (as discussed later), the ultimate dysfunction is the same for all three classifications of shock—decreased tissue perfusion.

Pathophysiology of Shock

Cellular Effects of Shock

When body cells lack an adequate blood supply and an adequate supply of oxygen, their ability to metabolize energy is impaired. Energy metabolism occurs within the cell where nutrients are chemically broken down and stored in the form of adenosine triphosphate (ATP). Cells use this stored energy to perform necessary functions such as active transport, muscular contraction, and biochemical synthesis as well as specialized cellular functions such as the conduction of electrical impulses. ATP can be synthesized aerobically (in the presence of oxygen) or anaerobically (in the absence of oxygen). However, aerobic metabolism yields far greater amounts of ATP per mole of glucose than anaerobic metabolism and therefore is a more efficient and effective means of producing energy. Additionally, anaerobic metabolism results in the accumulation of the toxic end product, lactic acid, which must be removed from the cell and transported to the liver for conversion into glucose and glycogen.

In shock, the cells lack an adequate blood supply and are deprived of oxygen and nutrients; therefore, they must produce energy through anaerobic metabolism. This results in low energy yields from nutrients, and an acidotic intracellular environment. Because of these changes, normal cell function ceases (Fig. 15-1). The cell swells and its membrane becomes more permeable, allowing electrolytes and fluids to seep from and into the cell. The sodium-potassium pump becomes impaired. Cell structures (mitochondria and lysosomes) are damaged and death of the cell results (Hardaway, 1988).

Vascular Responses

Oxygen attaches to the hemoglobin molecule in red blood cells and is carried to body cells through the blood. The amount of oxygen that is delivered to cells depends both on blood *flow* to a specific area and on blood *oxygen concentration* (Gould et al, 1993). Blood is continuously recycled back through the lungs to be reoxygenated and to eliminate end products of cellular metabolism such as carbon dioxide. The heart muscle provides the pump needed to propel the freshly oxygenated blood out to the body tissues. This process of circulation is facilitated through an elaborate and dynamic vasculature consisting of arteries, veins, arterioles, capillaries, and venules. The vasculature can dilate or constrict based on both central and local regulatory mechanisms. Central regulatory mechanisms cause dilation or constriction of the vasculature to maintain an adequate blood pressure. Local regulatory mechanisms, referred to as autoregulation, cause vasodilation or vasoconstriction in response to chemicals released by the cell communicating its need for oxygen and nutrients (Niedringhaus, Smith-Collins, & Myers, 1983).

Blood Pressure Regulation

Three major components of the circulatory system, *blood volume*, the *cardiac pump*, and the *vasculature* must respond effectively to complex neural, chemical, and hormonal feedback systems to maintain an adequate blood pressure and ultimately perfuse body tissues.

Blood pressure is regulated through a complex interaction of neural, chemical, and hormonal feedback systems

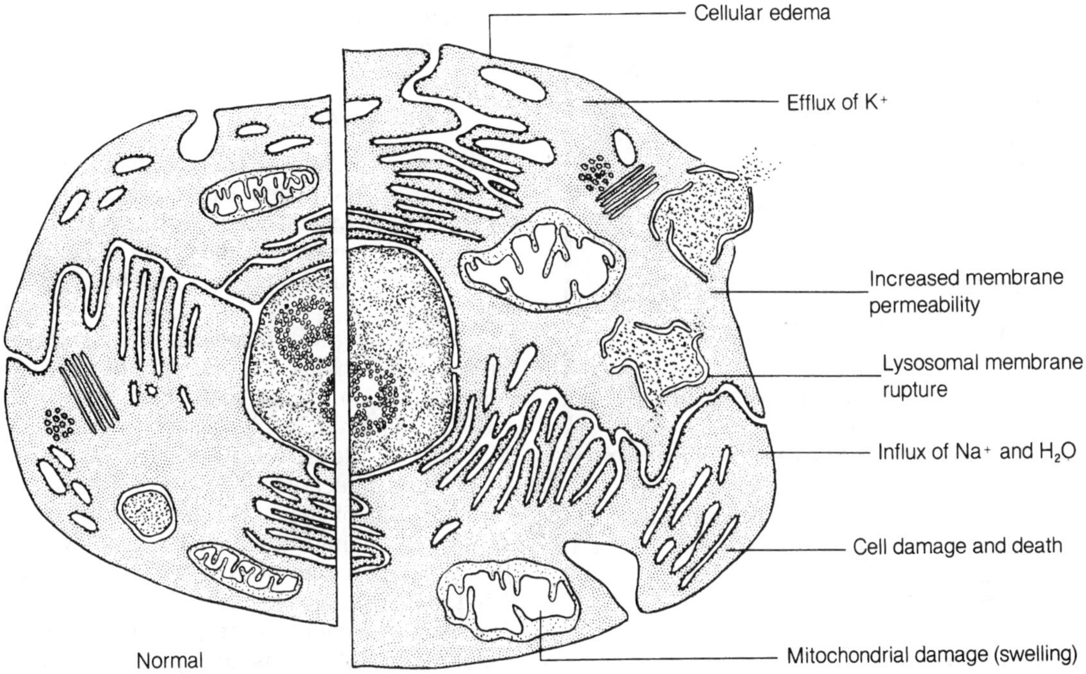

FIGURE 15-1. Cellular effects of shock. The cell swells and the cell membrane becomes more permeable, and fluids and electrolytes seep from and into the cell. Mitochondria and lysosomes are damaged and the cell dies. (From Porth CM. Pathophysiology: Concepts of Altered Health States, 3rd ed. Philadelphia, JB Lippincott, 1990.)

affecting both cardiac output and peripheral resistance. This relationship is expressed in the following equation:

$$\text{Mean arterial blood pressure} = \text{cardiac output} \times \text{peripheral resistance}$$

Cardiac output is determined by stroke volume (the amount of blood ejected at systole) and heart rate. Peripheral resistance is determined by the diameter of the arterioles.

Tissue and organ perfusion depend on mean arterial pressure (MAP). The MAP is the average pressure at which blood moves through the vasculature. True mean arterial pressure can only be calculated by complex methods. A convenient formula for clinical use in estimating MAP is provided in Chart 15-1. An average MAP of 80 to 120 mm Hg is necessary for cells to receive the oxygen and nutrients needed to metabolize energy in amounts sufficient to sustain life (Carolan, 1984).

The primary mechanism that regulates blood pressure is through the baroreceptors (pressure receptors) located in the carotid sinus and aortic arch. These pressure receptors convey impulses to the sympathetic nervous center in the medulla of the brain. In the event of a drop in blood pressure, catecholamines (epinephrine and norepinephrine) are released from the adrenal medulla of the adrenal glands, which causes an increase in heart rate and vasoconstriction, thus restoring blood pressure. Chemoreceptors, also located in the aortic arch and carotid arteries, regulate blood pressure and respiratory rate using much the same mechanism in response to changes in oxygen and carbon dioxide concentrations in the blood. These primary regulatory mechanisms can respond to changes in blood pressure on a moment-to-moment basis.

The kidneys also play an important role in blood pressure regulation. Their mechanism of blood pressure regulation is caused by the release of renin, which leads to the conversion of angiotensin I to angiotensin II, a potent vasoconstrictor. This effect indirectly leads to the release of aldosterone from the adrenal cortex, which results in the retention of sodium and water. The resultant increased blood sodium level stimulates the release of antidiuretic hormone (ADH) by the pituitary gland. ADH causes the kidneys to retain water further in an effort to raise blood volume and blood pressure. These secondary regulatory mechanisms may take hours or days to respond to changes in blood pressure.

To summarize, adequate blood volume, an effective cardiac pump, and an effective vasculature are necessary to maintain blood pressure and tissue perfusion. When one of the three components of this system begins to fail, the body is able to compensate through increased work by the other two. However, when compensatory mechanisms are no longer able to compensate for the failed system, body tissues are inadequately perfused and the syndrome of shock begins. Unless prompt intervention is initiated, shock will progress resulting in organ failure and death.

Overview of the Stages of Shock

The syndrome of shock can be conceptualized as a continuum along which the patient struggles to survive. For convenience it is useful to divide this continuum into separate stages to understand the physiologic response and subsequent clinical signs and symptoms at different points on the continuum. In this discussion, shock has been divided into three stages: compensatory, progressive, and irreversible. (Although some authors identify an *initial stage* of shock, changes attributed to this stage occur at the cellular level and are generally not detectable clinically.) The earlier

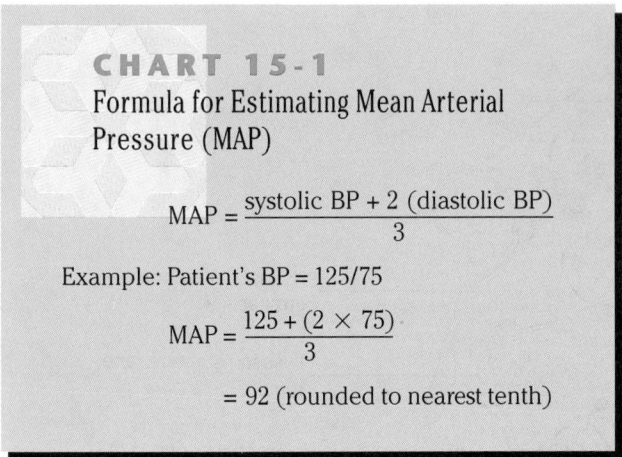

CHART 15-1
Formula for Estimating Mean Arterial Pressure (MAP)

$$MAP = \frac{\text{systolic BP} + 2\ (\text{diastolic BP})}{3}$$

Example: Patient's BP = 125/75

$$MAP = \frac{125 + (2 \times 75)}{3}$$

$$= 92 \text{ (rounded to nearest tenth)}$$

that medical management and nursing interventions can be initiated along this continuum, the greater the chance of survival for the patient.

Compensatory Stage

In the *compensatory stage* of shock the patient's blood pressure remains within normal limits. Vasoconstriction, increased heart rate, and increased contractility of the heart all contribute to maintaining adequate cardiac output. This results from stimulation of the sympathetic nervous system and subsequent release of catecholamines (epinephrine and norepinephrine). The patient is in the often-described "fight or flight" response. A redistribution of blood flow occurs to assure adequate blood supply to the brain and heart. Blood is shunted away from "nonessential" organs such as the skin, lungs, kidneys, and gastrointestinal tract (Rice, 1991b). As a result of this shunting, the patient's skin is cold and clammy, bowel sounds are hypoactive, and urine output decreases in response to the release of aldosterone and ADH.

Despite a normal blood pressure the patient shows numerous clinical signs indicating that organs are not being adequately perfused. The result of inadequate perfusion is anaerobic metabolism and buildup of lactic acid, producing *metabolic acidosis*. The respiratory rate increases from baseline in response to metabolic acidosis. This rapid respiratory rate facilitates removal of excess CO_2, but results in raising the blood *p*H and often causing a compensatory respiratory alkalosis. The alkalotic state causes mental status changes such as confusion or combativeness. If treatment is initiated in this stage of shock, the prognosis for the patient is good.

Medical Management

At this stage of shock, medical treatment is directed toward identifying the cause of the shock, correcting the underlying disorder so that shock does not progress, and supporting those physiologic mechanisms that thus far have responded successfully to the threat. Because compensation cannot be effectively maintained indefinitely, measures such as fluid replacement and use of medications must be initiated to maintain an adequate blood pressure and reestablish and maintain adequate tissue perfusion. An overview of fluid replacement and vasoactive drug therapy in shock is presented on pp. 253–254.

Nursing Management

Early intervention along the continuum of shock is the key to improving the patient's prognosis. Therefore it is necessary to assess systematically those patients at risk for developing shock to recognize the subtle clinical signs described in the compensatory stage of shock before there is a drop in blood pressure.

In assessing for inadequate tissue perfusion, the nurse monitors for changes in level of consciousness, skin, urinary output, and vital signs. Laboratory results are also closely monitored; in this stage of shock, serum sodium and blood glucose levels are elevated in response to the release of ADH and catecholamines.

The role of the nurse at the compensatory stage of shock is to monitor the patient's hemodynamic status and *promptly* report deviations to the physician, assist in identifying and treating the underlying disorder by continuous in-depth assessment of the patient, administer prescribed fluids and medications, and promote patient safety. Vital signs are key indicators of the patient's hemodynamic status; however, blood pressure is an indirect method of monitoring tissue hypoxia.

- By the time there is a drop in blood pressure, damage has already been occurring on the cellular and tissue levels. Therefore, it is imperative that the patient at risk for shock be assessed and monitored closely *before* there is a drop in blood pressure.

Although the treatment modalities are prescribed and initiated by the physician, it is often the nurse who implements them, troubleshoots equipment used in treatment, monitors the patient's status during treatment, and assesses the immediate effects of treatment. Additionally, the nurse assesses the response of the patient and the family to the crisis and to the treatment.

Because of experiencing a major threat to health and well-being and being the focus of attention of many health care providers, the patient often becomes anxious and apprehensive. Providing the patient with brief explanations about the diagnostic and treatment procedures that are being performed, supporting the patient during those procedures, and providing information about their outcomes, are often effective strategies for reducing stress and anxiety level, thus contributing to the patient's physical and mental well-being.

The nurse also monitors for threats to the patient's safety because a high anxiety level and altered mental status often impair an individual's judgment. In this stage, patients who were previously cooperative and followed instructions may now disrupt intravenous lines and catheters and further complicate their condition. Therefore, close supervision is essential.

Progressive Stage

In the progressive stage of shock, the mechanisms that regulate blood pressure are unable to continue to compensate and the mean arterial pressure (MAP) falls below normal limits with an average systolic blood pressure of less than 80 to 90 mm Hg (Rice, 1991b). Although all organ systems suffer from hypoperfusion at this stage, two events occur that further perpetuate the shock syndrome. First, the overworked heart becomes ischemic, which leads to failure of the cardiac pump even if the underlying cause of the shock is not of cardiac origin.

Second, the autoregulatory function of the microcirculation fails in response to numerous chemical mediators that are released by cells, resulting in increased capillary permeability. At this stage the prognosis for the patient worsens. A relaxation of precapillary sphincters causes fluid to leak from the capillaries, and less fluid is then returned to the heart. Even if the underlying cause of the shock is reversed, the breakdown of the circulatory system itself perpetuates the shock state and a vicious circle ensues.

Systemic Impact

Chances of survival depend on the general health of the patient prior to the shock syndrome as well as the amount of time it takes to restore tissue perfusion. As the shock syndrome progresses, organ systems decompensate.

Lungs. The lungs, which begin to be compromised early in shock, are affected at this stage. This development increases the likelihood that mechanical ventilation may be needed if shock progresses. Respirations are rapid and shallow. Crackles are heard over lung fields. Decreased pulmonary blood flow causes arterial oxygen levels to decrease and carbon dioxide levels to increase. The hypoperfused alveoli stop producing surfactant and subsequently collapse. Pulmonary capillaries begin to leak their contents, causing severe pulmonary edema (Vaughn & Brooks, 1990). This condition is sometimes referred to as *adult respiratory distress syndrome* (ARDS), *shock lung*, or *noncardiogenic pulmonary edema*. Further explanation of ARDS as well as its nursing management can be found in Chapter 24 of this text.

Heart. A lack of adequate blood supply leads to dysrhythmias and ischemia. The patient has a rapid heart rate, sometimes exceeding 150 beats per minute. The patient may complain of chest pain and even suffer a myocardial infarction. Cardiac enzymes (*e.g.*, LDH and CPK) are elevated.

Brain. As blood flow to the brain becomes impaired, the patient's mental status deteriorates. Changes in mental status occur as a result of decreased cerebral perfusion and hypoxia; the patient may initially exhibit a subtle change in behavior or confusion. Subsequently, lethargy increases and the patient begins to lose consciousness. The patient's pupils are often dilated and only sluggishly reactive to light.

Kidneys. When MAP falls below 75 mm Hg, the glomerular filtration rate of the kidneys cannot be maintained and drastic changes in renal function occur. Acute renal failure (ARF) can occur, which is characterized by an increase in blood urea nitrogen (BUN) and serum creatinine levels, fluid and electrolyte shifts, acid-base imbalances, and a loss of the renal-hormonal regulation of blood pressure. Urinary output is usually decreased to below 20 ml/hr, but can be variable depending on the phase of ARF. For a further discussion of ARF, review Chapter 43 of this text.

Liver. Decreased blood flow to the liver impairs the liver cells' ability to perform their critical metabolic and phagocytic functions. Consequently the patient is less able to metabolize drugs and metabolic waste products such as ammonia and lactic acid. The patient becomes more susceptible to infection as the liver is no longer able to filter bacteria out of the blood. Liver enzymes (SGOT [AST], SGPT [ALT], LDH) are elevated and the patient appears jaundiced.

Gastrointestinal Tract. Gastrointestinal ischemia can cause stress ulceration in the stomach placing the patient at risk for gastrointestinal bleeding. In the small intestine, the mucosa can become necrotic and slough off, causing bloody diarrhea. Beyond the local effects of impaired perfusion, ischemia of the gastrointestinal system leads to the release of toxins which enter the blood stream through the lymph system. In addition to causing infection, these toxins can cause cardiac depression and vasodilatation and interfere with healthy cells, resulting in their inability to metabolize nutrients (Collins, 1990).

Hematologic System. The combination of hypotension, sluggish blood flow, metabolic acidosis, and generalized hypoxemia can interfere with normal hemostatic mechanisms. Disseminated intravascular coagulation (DIC) can occur either as a cause or as a complication of shock. In this condition widespread clotting and bleeding occur simultaneously. Bruises (ecchymoses) and bleeding (petechiae) may appear in the skin. Coagulation times (PT, PTT) are prolonged. Clotting factors and platelets are consumed and require replacement therapy to achieve hemostasis. Further discussion on DIC appears in Chapter 16 of this text.

Medical Management

The specific medical management in the progressive stage of shock depends on the type of shock and its underlying cause. It is also based on the degree of decompensation that has occurred in the organ systems. Medical management specific to each type of shock is discussed in later sections of this chapter. Although there are a number of differences in medical management by type of shock, there are some medical interventions that are common to all types. These include use of appropriate intravenous fluids and medications to restore tissue perfusion by (1) optimizing intravascular volume, (2) supporting the pumping action of the heart, and (3) improving the competence of the vascular system. Other aspects of management may include nutritional support and use of H_2-blockers such as cimetidine and ranitidine to reduce risk of gastrointestinal (GI) bleeding. An overview of use of fluids and medications to accomplish these goals is presented on pp. 253–254.

Nursing Management

Nursing care of the patient in the progressive stage of shock requires expertise in assessing and understanding shock and the significance of changes in assessment data. The patient in the progressive stage of shock is often cared for in the intensive care setting because of the close monitoring (hemodynamic monitoring, electrocardiographic [ECG] monitoring, arterial blood gases, serum electrolyte levels, and physical and mental changes) that is essential, the rapid and frequent changes in medications and fluids that are prescribed, and the possible need to use supportive technologies such as mechanical ventilation, dialysis, and intra-aortic balloon pump.

Working closely with other members of the health care team, the nurse carefully documents treatments, medications, and fluids that are administered by all members of the team, noting the time, dosage or volume, and the patient's response. Additionally, the nurse coordinates both the scheduling of diagnostic procedures that are often carried out at the patient's bedside and the flow of health care personnel involved in the patient's care. If supportive technologies are used, the nurse attempts to reduce the risk of complications that may develop from their use and monitors the patient for early signs of complications (*e.g.*, monitors blood levels of medications, monitors neurovascular status if arterial lines are inserted, especially in the lower extremities).

Simultaneously, the nurse assures the patient's safety and comfort by ensuring that all procedures, including invasive procedures, are carried out using correct techniques and that venous and arterial puncture sites and infusion sites are managed with the goal of preventing infection. Positioning and repositioning the patient for comfort, to prevent pulmonary complications and to maintain skin integrity, are part of the nurse's role in the care of the patient in shock.

Efforts are made to minimize the cardiac workload by reducing the patient's physical activity and any fear or anxiety. Promoting rest and comfort is a priority in the patient's care. To make sure the patient gets as much uninterrupted rest as possible, care is planned so that all nonessential activities are avoided. The patient is prevented from becoming excessively warm or cold with shivering because such temperature extremes can increase the patient's metabolic rate and subsequently the cardiac workload. The patient should not be warmed too quickly, and warming blankets should not be applied because they can cause vasodilation and a subsequent drop in blood pressure.

Because the patient in shock is the object of intense attention by the health care team, the family often feels neglected; but they are often reluctant to ask questions or seek information for fear that they will be in the way or will interfere with the attention given to the patient. The nurse should assure that the family is comfortably situated and is kept informed about the patient's status. Often the family needs advice from the health care team to get some rest; they are more likely to take this advice if they feel that the patient is being well cared for and that they will be notified of any significant changes in the patient's status. A visit from the hospital chaplain may be comforting to the family and provides some attention to the family while the nurse concentrates on the patient.

Irreversible Stage

The irreversible (or refractory) stage of shock represents the point along the shock continuum where organ damage is so severe that the patient does not respond to treatment and is unable to survive. Despite treatment, blood pressure remains low. Complete renal and liver failure, compounded by the release of necrotic tissue toxins, creates an overwhelming metabolic acidosis. Anaerobic metabolism contributes to a worsening lactic acidosis. Reserves of ATP are almost totally depleted and mechanisms for storing new supplies of energy have been destroyed. Multiple organ failure has occurred and death is imminent. Multiple organ failure can occur as a progression along the shock continuum or as a syndrome unto itself and is further described later in this chapter.

Table 15-1 compares the clinical findings of the three stages of shock.

Medical Management

The medical management during this phase of shock is usually the same as for the progressive stage. Although the patient's shock may have progressed from the progressive to the irreversible stage, the judgment that the shock is irreversible can be made only retrospectively on the basis of failure of the patient to respond to treatment. Strategies that may be experimental (*i.e.*, investigational drugs) may be used in an attempt to reduce or reverse the severity of the patient's shock.

TABLE 15-1 Clinical Findings by Stages of Shock

	Compensatory Stage	Progressive Stage	Irreversible Stage
Heart rate	> 100 bpm	> 150 bpm	Erratic or asystole
Blood pressure	Normal	SBP < 80–90 mm Hg	Requires mechanical or pharmacological support
Respiratory status	> 20	Rapid, shallow respirations; crackles	Requires intubation
Skin	Cold, clammy	Mottled, petechiae	Jaundice
Urinary output	Decreased	< 20 ml/hr	Anuric, requires dialysis
Mentation	Confusion	Lethargy	Unconscious
Acid–base balance	Respiratory alkalosis	Metabolic acidosis	Profound acidosis

(Based on Rice V. Shock, a clinical syndrome: An update. Part I. Critical Care Nurse 1991; 11[4]:20–27.)

Nursing Management

As in the progressive stage of shock, the nurse's attention continues to be directed toward carrying out prescribed treatment modalities, monitoring the patient, preventing complications, protecting the patient from injury, and providing comfort. Offering brief explanations to the patient about what is happening is essential even if there is no certainty that the patient hears or understands what is being said.

As it becomes obvious that the patient is unlikely to survive, the patient's family needs to be informed about the prognosis and likely outcomes. Opportunities should be provided, throughout the patient's care, for the family to see, touch, and talk to the patient. A close family friend or clergy may be of comfort to the family in dealing with the inevitable death of the patient.

During this stage of shock, families may misinterpret the actions of the health care team. They have been told that nothing has been effective in reversing the shock and that the patient's survival is very unlikely; yet, the health care team continues to work feverishly on the patient. A distraught, grieving family may interpret this as a chance for recovery when none exists. As a result, family members may become angry when the patient dies. If different members of the health care team confer with the family, family members will have an opportunity to understand the patient's prognosis and the purpose for the measures being taken. During these conferences, it is essential to explain that the equipment and treatments being provided are for the patient's comfort and do not suggest that the patient will recover. Families should be encouraged to express their wishes concerning the use of life support measures.

Overview of Medical Management of Shock

As described above and in the discussion of types of shock to follow, medical management in all types and all phases of shock includes fluid replacement to restore intravascular volume, vasoactive medications to restore vasomotor tone and improve cardiac function, and nutritional support to address the metabolic requirements that are often dramatically increased in shock. Medical therapies described in this section require collaboration among all members of the health care team to assure that the manifestations of shock are quickly identified and that adequate and timely treatment is instituted to achieve the best outcome possible.

Fluid Replacement in Shock

Fluid replacement is given in all types of shock. The selection of fluids and the speed of delivery will vary, but fluids are given to enhance oxygenation, which is in part dependent on *flow.* The fluids administered may include crystalloids, colloids, or blood components. Selection of the best fluid to treat shock remains controversial as reflected in the literature. In emergency situations, the "best" fluid is often the fluid that is readily available. Both crystalloids and colloids, as described below, can be given to restore intravascular volume. Blood component therapy is used most frequently in hypovolemic shock and is discussed on pp. 255–256.

Crystalloids. Crystalloids are electrolyte solutions that move freely between the intravascular compartment and the interstitial spaces. Isotonic solutions are often selected because they contain the same concentration of electrolytes as the extracellular fluid and therefore can be given without altering concentrations of electrolytes in the plasma (Gould et al., 1993). Ringer's lactate solution and 0.9% sodium chloride are the two fluids of first choice used in treating hypovolemic shock (Imm & Carlson, 1993). Ringer's lactate is an electrolyte solution containing the lactate ion, which should not be confused with lactic acid. The lactate ion is converted to bicarbonate, which helps to buffer the overall acidosis that occurs in shock.

A disadvantage in using isotonic crystalloid solutions is that three parts of the volume are lost to the interstitial compartment for every one part that remains in the intravascular compartment. This occurs in response to mechanisms that store extracellular body fluid. Therefore large amounts of fluid must be given to restore intravascular volume (Gould et al., 1993).

Care must be taken when rapidly administering isotonic crytalloids to avoid causing excessive edema, particularly pulmonary edema. For this reason, and depending on the cause of the hypovolemia, a hypertonic crystalloid solution, such as 3% sodium chloride, is sometimes administered in hypovolemic shock. Hypertonic solutions have the effect of pulling fluid from the interstitial and intracellular compartments into the intravascular compartment. Therefore less volume of fluid is given to the patient with the same net effect of increasing intravascular volume (Imm & Carlson, 1993).

Colloids. Intravenous colloidal solutions contain molecules that are too large to pass through capillary membranes. Colloids expand intravascular volume by pulling fluid into the intravascular space by means of their oncotic pressure (Imm & Carlson, 1993). Colloidal solutions have the same effect as hypertonic solutions in increasing intravascular volume, but they allow less volume of fluid to be administered than is required with crystalloids. Additionally, colloids have a longer duration of action than crystalloids because the molecules remain within the intravascular compartment longer.

Five percent albumin is one of the most commonly used colloidal solutions to treat hypovolemic shock. Albumin is a plasma protein; 5% albumin solution is prepared from human plasma and is heated to reduce its potential to transmit disease. The disadvantages in using albumin are its high cost and limited availability as it is dependent on blood donors. Synthetic colloid preparations such as 6% hetastarch and 6% dextran solution are now widely used. However, dextran may interfere with platelet aggregation and therefore is not indicated if hemorrhage is the cause of the hypovolemic shock.

With all colloidal solutions, side effects include the rare occurrence of anaphylactic reactions for which the nurse must monitor.

Complications of Fluid Administration

Close monitoring of the patient during fluid replacement is necessary to identify side effects and complications. The most common and serious side effects of fluid replacement are *cardiovascular overload* and *pulmonary edema*.

Patients receiving fluid replacement should be monitored frequently for adequate urinary output, changes in mental status, skin perfusion, and changes in vital signs. The patient's lung sounds are auscultated frequently to detect any accumulation of fluid in the lungs.

Often a central venous pressure (CVP) line is inserted. In addition to physical assessment, the CVP value helps in monitoring the patient's progress with fluid replacement. A normal CVP value is 4 to 12 cm of water. Several readings are obtained to determine a range, and fluid replacement is continued within these parameters as long as the patient's overall status is improving. Hemodynamic monitoring with arterial and pulmonary artery lines may be implemented to allow close monitoring of the patient's cardiac status and to evaluate the response to therapy.

Vasoactive Medication Therapy in Shock

Vasoactive medications are given in all forms of shock to improve the patient's hemodynamic stability when fluid therapy alone will not maintain adequate mean arterial pressure. Specific drugs are selected to correct the particular hemodynamic alteration that is impeding cardiac output. Vasoactive medications increase cardiac output by strengthening contractility of the heart, reducing the workload of the heart muscle, causing vasoconstriction or regulating the heart rate (Burns, 1990).

Vasoactive drugs are selected for their action on receptors of the sympathetic nervous system. These receptors are known as alpha and beta receptors; beta receptors are further divided into $beta_1$ and $beta_2$ receptors. When alpha receptors are stimulated, constriction of the blood vessels occurs in the cardiorespiratory and gastrointestinal systems, skin, and kidneys. When $beta_1$ receptors are stimulated, the result is an increase in heart rate and myocardial contraction. Vasodilation of the heart and skeletal muscles and relaxation of the bronchioles occur with stimulation of the $beta_2$ receptors. The medications used in the treatment of shock consist of various combinations of vasoactive drugs to maximize tissue perfusion by stimulating the alpha and beta receptors.

When vasoactive drugs are administered, vital signs must be monitored frequently (at least every 15 minutes or more often if indicated). Vasoactive medications should be administered through a central intravenous line because infiltration of some vasoactive medications can cause tissue necrosis and sloughing. An intravenous pump or controller should be used to assure that the medications are delivered safely and accurately.

Individual drug dosages are often titrated by the nurse who adjusts the intravenous drip rates based on the physician's prescription and the patient's response. Dosages are changed in order to maintain the patient's mean arterial pressure (usually above 80 mm Hg) within set parameters as prescribed in relation to the patient's perfusion requirements (Burns, 1990).

- When vasoactive medications are discontinued, they should never be stopped abruptly as this could cause severe hemodynamic instability perpetuating the shock syndrome.

The dosages of vasoactive medications should be tapered and the patient weaned from the drug with frequent monitoring (every 15 minutes) of the blood pressure. Table 15-2 presents some of the commonly prescribed vasoactive medications used in the treatment of shock.

Nutritional Support in Shock

Nutritional support is an important aspect of care for the patient with shock. Increased metabolic rates during shock increase energy requirements and therefore caloric requirements. The patient in shock requires over 3000 calories per day.

The release of catecholamines early in the shock continuum causes glycogen stores to be depleted in about 8 to 10 hours. Nutritional energy requirements are then met by breaking down lean body mass. In this catabolic process skeletal muscle mass is broken down even when the patient has large stores of fat or adipose tissue. Loss of skeletal muscle can greatly prolong the recovery time for the shock patient. Parenteral or enteral nutritional support should be initiated within 3 to 4 days of the onset of shock (Kuhn, 1990).

TABLE 15-2 Vasoactive Drugs Used in Treating Shock

	Desired Action in Shock	Disadvantages
Sympathomimetics Dopamine (Intropin) Dobutamine (Dobutrex) Epinephrine (Adrenaline)	Improve contractility, increase stroke volume, increase cardiac output	Increase oxygen demand of the heart
Vasodilators Nitroprusside (Nipride) Nitroglycerine (Tridil)	Reduce preload and after load, reduce oxygen demand of heart	Cause hypotension
Vasoconstrictors Phenylephrine (Neo-Synephrine) Methoxamine (Vasoxyl)	Increase blood pressure by vasoconstriction	Increase afterload, thereby increasing cardiac work load; compromise perfusion to skin, kidneys, lungs, GI tract

Stress ulcers occur frequently in acutely ill patients because of the compromised blood supply to the gastrointestinal tract. Therefore, H_2 blockers such as cimetidine and ranitidine are prescribed to prevent ulcer formation by inhibiting gastric acid secretion.

Management of Different Types of Shock

Hypovolemic Shock

Hypovolemic shock—the most common type of shock—is characterized by a decreased intravascular volume. Body fluid is contained in intracellular and extracellular compartments. Intracellular fluid comprises approximately two thirds of the total body water. The extracellular body fluid is found in one of two compartments: intravascular (inside blood vessels) and interstitial (surrounding tissues). The volume of interstitial fluid is *approximately* three to four times that of intravascular fluid. Hypovolemic shock occurs when there is a reduction in *intravascular* volume of 15% to 25%. This would represent a loss of 750 ml to 1300 ml of blood in a 70-kg (154-lb) man.

Hypovolemic shock can be caused by external fluid losses as in hemorrhage, or internal fluid shifts as in severe dehydration, severe edema, or ascites. Intravascular volume can be reduced both by fluid loss and fluid shifting between intravascular and interstitial compartments. Table 15-3 lists conditions that place patients at risk for hypovolemic shock (Rice, 1991a).

The sequence of events in hypovolemic shock begins with a decrease in the intravascular volume. This results in decreased venous return of blood to the heart and subsequent decreased ventricular filling. Decreased ventricular filling results in decreased stroke volume (amount of blood ejected from the heart) and decreased cardiac output. When cardiac output drops, blood pressure drops, and tissues cannot be adequately perfused (Fig. 15-2).

Medical Management of Hypovolemic Shock

Major goals in treating hypovolemic shock are to (1) *restore intravascular volume* to reverse the sequence of events leading to inadequate tissue perfusion, (2) *redistribute fluid volume*, and (3) *correct the underlying cause* of the fluid loss as

TABLE 15-3 Conditions Placing Patients at Risk for Hypovolemic Shock

External fluid losses	Trauma Surgery Vomiting Diarrhea Diuresis Diabetes insipidus
Internal fluid shifts	Internal hemorrhage Burns Ascites Peritonitis

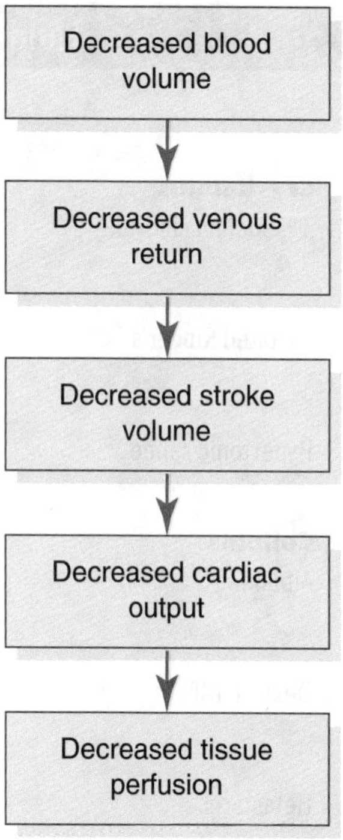

FIGURE 15-2. Pathophysiologic sequence of events in hypovolemic shock.

quickly as possible. Depending on the severity of shock and the patient's condition, it is likely that efforts will be made to address all three goals simultaneously.

Treatment of Underlying Cause. If the patient is hemorrhaging, efforts are made to stop the bleeding. This may involve application of pressure to the bleeding site or surgery may be necessary to stop internal bleeding. If the cause of the hypovolemia is diarrhea or vomiting, medications to treat diarrhea and vomiting are administered.

Fluid and Blood Replacement. Beyond reversing the primary cause for the decreased intravascular volume, fluid replacement (also referred to as fluid resuscitation) is of primary concern. At least two large-gauge intravenous lines are inserted to establish intravenous access for fluid administration. Two intravenous accesses allow simultaneous administration of fluid and blood component therapy if required. Because the goal of the fluid replacement is to restore *intravascular volume*, it is necessary to administer fluids that will remain in the intravascular compartment and thus avoid creating fluid shifts from the intravascular compartment into the intracellular compartment. Table 15-4 presents a summary of fluids commonly used in treating shock.

Ringer's lactate and 0.9% sodium chloride, both crystalloid fluids, are two isotonic fluids commonly used in treating hypovolemic shock (Imm & Carlson, 1993). Large amounts of fluid must be administered to restore intravascular volume because isotonic crystalloid solutions move freely between the fluid compartments of the body and do not remain in the vascular system.

Colloids (i.e., albumin, hetastarch, and 6% dextran) are now widely used. Dextran is not indicated if the cause of the hypovolemic shock is hemorrhage because it interferes with platelet aggregation.

Blood products, also colloids, may need to be administered, particularly when the cause of the hypovolemic shock

TABLE 15-4 Fluid Replacement in Shock

	Advantages	Disadvantages
Crystalloids		
.9% sodium chloride	Widely available, inexpensive	Requires large volume of infusion; can cause pulmonary edema
Lactated Ringer's	Lactate ion helps buffer metabolic acidosis	Requires large volume of infusion; can cause pulmonary edema
Hypertonic saline (3%, 5%, 7.5%)	Small volume needed to restore intravascular volume	Danger of hypernatremia
Colloids		
Albumin (5%, 25%)	Rapidly expands plasma volume	Expensive; requires human donors; limited supply; can cause CHF
Dextran (40, 70)	Synthetic plasma expander	Interferes with platelet aggregation; not recommended for hemorrhagic shock
Hetastarch	Synthetic; less expensive than albumin; effect lasts up to 36 hours	

is hemorrhage. However, because of the risk of transmitting blood-borne viruses and the scarcity of blood products, these products are used only if other alternatives are unavailable or blood loss is extensive and rapid. Packed red blood cells are administered to replenish the patient's oxygen-carrying capacity in conjunction with other fluids that will expand volume. Current recommendations are to base the need for transfusions on the patient's individual oxygenation needs, which are determined by vital signs, blood gases, and clinical appearance rather than an arbitrary laboratory value (Gould et al., 1993). Synthetic forms of blood (*i.e.*, compounds capable of carrying oxygen in the same way that blood does) are currently being tested.

Autotransfusion, the collection and retransfusion of the patient's own blood, may be initiated. This reduces the risk of transmitting a communicable disease or of a transfusion reaction, and eliminates the prolonged time needed for typing and cross matching blood. Autotransfusion can be performed when the patient is bleeding within a closed cavity such as the chest or abdominal cavity (Blansfield, 1990). A chest tube is inserted and blood is collected through a filter in a specifically designed collection device often attached to routine chest tube drainage systems. The blood obtained must be transfused back to the patient within 4 hours of its collection. Disadvantages of autotransfusion include damage to red blood cells during the process of collection and transfusion and the risk of microembolism (Blansfield, 1990).

Additional details about fluid replacement are presented on page 253.

Redistribution of Fluid. In addition to administering fluids to restore intravascular volume, *positioning* the patient properly assists fluid redistribution. A modified Trendelenburg position (Fig. 15-3) is recommended in hypovolemic shock. By elevating the patient's legs, the return of venous blood is enhanced by gravity. Positioning patients in a full Trendelenburg position makes breathing difficult and therefore is not recommended.

Military antishock trousers (MAST) may be used in extreme emergency situations where bleeding cannot be controlled such as in trauma or retroperitoneal bleeding (Fig. 15-4). This device is a three-chambered tourniquet that is wrapped around each of the patient's legs and torso and then inflated to force blood from the lower extremities into the upper circulation. The "suit" helps to control hemorrhage by applying pressure over the bleeding site. MAST can also be used to stabilize fractures while transporting a patient to the operating room.

Once inflated, the MAST should not be deflated to assess wound sites or to check peripheral pulses because of the risk of a rapid and severe drop in blood pressure. When

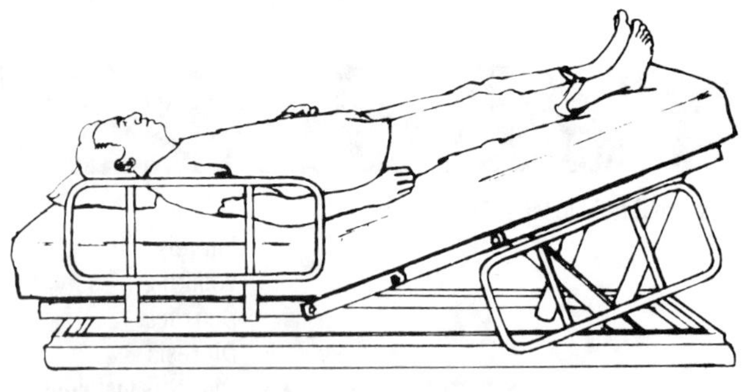

FIGURE 15-3. Proper positioning of the patient who shows signs of shock. The lower extremities are elevated to an angle of approximately 20 degrees; the knees are straight, the trunk is horizontal, and the head is slightly elevated.

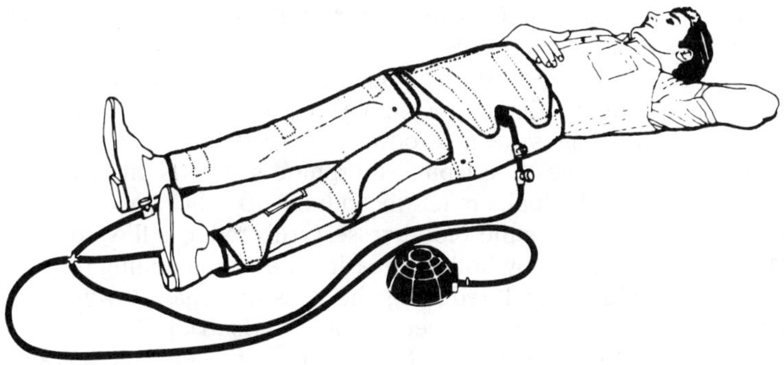

FIGURE 15-4. The military antishock trousers (MAST) is a garment designed to correct internal bleeding and hypovolemia by the application of counterpressure around the legs and abdomen. This creates an artificial peripheral resistance and helps sustain coronary perfusion. It should be applied as soon as possible after injury, preferably before the patient is transferred to the emergency department. (Courtesy of David Clark Co., Inc., Worcester, MA.)

the patient is in the operating room and ready for surgical intervention, the MAST should be deflated slowly (over 30 to 60 minutes) while administering fluids. Use of the MAST can result in circulatory compromise to the lower extremities and therefore should be used only as a last resort in maintaining blood pressure.

Medications

If fluid administration fails to reverse the shock, then the same medications given in cardiogenic shock (see p. 258) are used because unreversed hypovolemic shock progresses to cardiogenic shock (the "vicious circle").

If the underlying cause of the hypovolemia was dehydration, medications will be prescribed to reverse the cause of the dehydration. For example, insulin will be administered to patients with dehydration secondary to hyperglycemia; desmopressin (DDVP) for diabetes insipidus, antidiarrheal agents for diarrhea, and antiemetics for vomiting.

Nursing Management of the Patient With Hypovolemic Shock

Primary prevention of shock is an essential focus of nursing intervention. Hypovolemic shock can be prevented in some instances by closely monitoring patients who are at risk for fluid deficits and assisting with fluid replacement before intravascular volume is depleted. In other circumstances, hypovolemic shock cannot be prevented and nursing care focuses on assisting with treatment targeted at treating its cause and restoring intravascular volume.

General nursing measures include assuring safe administration of prescribed fluids and medications and documenting their administration and effects. Another important nursing role is monitoring for signs of complications and side effects of treatment and reporting these signs *early* in the course of treatment.

Administering blood transfusions safely is a vital nursing role. In emergency situations it is important to quickly obtain blood specimens for a baseline complete blood count (CBC) and to type and cross match the patient's blood in anticipation of blood transfusions. The patient who receives transfusion of blood products must be monitored closely for adverse effects (see Chapter 32).

Fluid replacement complications are possible, often when large volumes are administered rapidly. Therefore the nurse monitors the patient closely for cardiovascular overload and pulmonary edema. The risks of these complications are increased in the elderly and in patients with pre-existing cardiac disease. Monitoring includes: hemodynamic pressure monitoring, vital signs, arterial blood gases, hemoglobin and hematocrit levels, and fluid intake and output. Physical assessment focuses on observing the patient's jugular veins for distension and monitoring jugular venous pressure (JVP). JVP will be low in hypovolemic shock; it will increase with effective treatment and will be significantly increased with fluid overload and congestive heart failure. The patient's cardiac and respiratory status are monitored closely; changes in heart rate and rhythm and lung sounds are reported by the nurse to the physician.

Oxygen is administered to increase the amount of oxygen carried by available hemoglobin in the blood. A patient who is confused may feel apprehensive with an oxygen mask or cannula in place. Frequent explanations about the need for the mask may reduce some of the patient's fear and anxiety. Simultaneously, the nurse must direct efforts to the safety and comfort of the patient.

Cardiogenic Shock

Cardiogenic shock occurs when the heart's ability to pump blood is impaired. Cardiac output is a function of both stroke volume and heart rate. When stroke volume and heart rate decrease or become erratic, blood pressure drops and tissue perfusion is compromised. Along with other tissues and organs being deprived of adequate blood supply, the heart muscle itself receives inadequate blood and experiences impaired tissue perfusion. Patients in cardiogenic shock may experience angina and develop dysrhythmias.

Causes of cardiogenic shock are either of a coronary or noncoronary etiology (see Table 15-5 for conditions that place patients at risk for developing cardiogenic shock). Coronary cardiogenic shock is more common than noncoronary cardiogenic shock and is seen most often in

TABLE 15-5 Conditions Placing Patients at Risk for Cardiogenic shock

Coronary	Myocardial infarction
Non-coronary	Cardiomyopathies Valvular damage Cardiac tamponade Dysrhythmias

patients with myocardial infarctions where extensive ventricular damage (>40%) has occurred, particularly to the anterior wall of the myocardium (Summers, 1990).

When the heart's ability to pump blood forward is impaired, two pathologic events occur. First, because of the decreased stroke volume, there is decreased cardiac output. This results in decreased blood pressure and subsequently decreased tissue perfusion. Second, because the weakened ventricle does not fully eject its volume of blood at systole, there is an accumulation of fluid in the lungs. This sequence of events can occur rapidly, or over a period of days. Figure 15-5 depicts the sequence of events in cardiogenic shock.

Medical Management

The goals of medical management of the patient in cardiogenic shock are to (1) limit further myocardial damage, (2) preserve the healthy myocardium, and (3) improve the heart's ability to pump effectively (Rice, 1991c). In general, these goals are achieved by increasing oxygen supply to the heart muscle, while reducing oxygen demands.

As with all forms of shock, the underlying cause of cardiogenic shock must be corrected. It is necessary first to treat the oxygenation needs of the heart muscle to ensure its continued ability to pump blood to other organs. In the case of coronary cardiogenic shock, this may require thrombolytic therapy, angioplasty, or coronary artery bypass graft surgery. In the case of noncoronary cardiogenic shock the patient may require a cardiac valve replacement or correction of a dysrhythmia. For further explanation of these procedures refer to Chapters 27 and 29.

First-line treatment of cardiogenic shock involves:

- Supplying supplemental oxygen
- Controlling chest pain
- Administering vasoactive drugs
- Selective fluid support (Rice, 1991c)

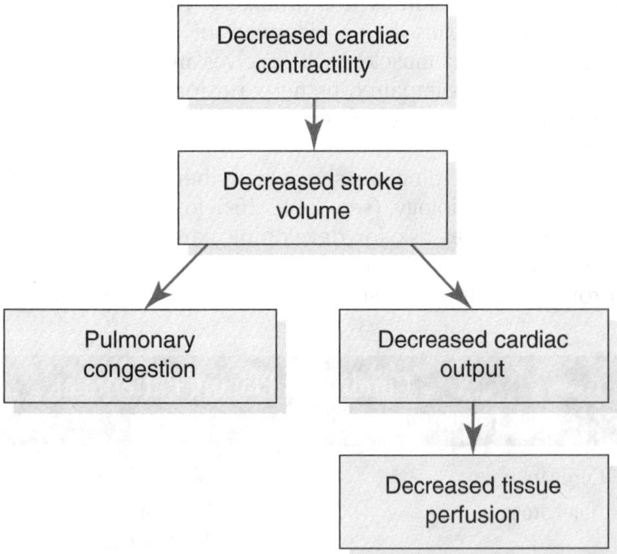

FIGURE 15-5. Pathophysiologic sequence of events in cardiogenic shock.

General Management. In the early stages of shock, supplemental oxygen is given through a nasal cannula at 3 to 5 L/minute. Arterial blood gases and pulse oximetry monitoring will indicate whether or not the patient requires a more aggressive method of oxygen delivery. If the patient experiences chest pain, morphine sulfate is given intravenously for pain relief. In addition to relieving pain, morphine dilates the blood vessels. This reduces the workload of the heart by both decreasing the cardiac filling pressure (preload) and reducing the pressure against which the heart muscle has to eject blood (afterload).

Morphine is also of benefit in treating the patient's anxiety. Cardiac enzymes are measured and 12-lead electrocardiograms (ECG) are obtained daily to assess the degree of myocardial damage.

Hemodynamic monitoring will be initiated to accurately assess the patient's response to treatment. In many institutions this will require transferring the patient to the intensive care unit. An arterial line will be inserted for accurate and continuous monitoring of blood pressure as well as for providing a port from which to obtain frequent arterial blood gas samplings without having to perform repeated arterial punctures. A multilumen pulmonary artery catheter will be inserted to measure the patient's pulmonary artery pressures and cardiac output. Further information about this topic is presented in Chapters 26 and 28.

Drug Therapy. Vasoactive drug therapy consists of multiple pharmacologic strategies to restore and maintain adequate cardiac output. In coronary cardiogenic shock, vasoactive drug therapy is aimed at improving cardiac contractility, decreasing preload and afterload, or stabilizing the heart rate.

Because improving contractility and decreasing cardiac workload are opposing pharmacologic actions, two classifications of medications are often given in combination: sympathomimetics and vasodilators. *Sympathomimetic* medications increase cardiac output by mimicking the action of the sympathetic nervous system through vasoconstriction, increasing myocardial contractility, or increasing the heart rate. *Vasodilators* are used to decrease preload and afterload, thus reducing the workload of the heart and the oxygen demand. Two medications commonly used in combination in the treatment of cardiogenic shock are dopamine and nitroglycerin.

Dopamine (Intropin) has varying vasoactive effects depending on the dose at which it is administered. Low-dose dopamine (0.5 to 3.0 μg/kg/min) increases renal and mesenteric blood flow, thereby preventing ischemia of these organs because shock causes blood to be shunted away from the kidneys and the mesentery. However, this dosage does not improve cardiac output. Medium-dose dopamine (4 to 8 μg/kg/min) has the effect of improving contractility and slightly increasing the heart rate. At this dosage, dopamine increases cardiac output and therefore is desirable. High-dose dopamine (8 to 10 μg/kg/min) causes vasoconstriction. Vasoconstriction increases afterload and thus increases cardiac workload. This effect is not desired and therefore emphasizes the importance of carefully titrating dosages. Once the patient's blood pressure has stabilized, low-dose dopamine may be continued for its effect of promoting renal perfusion in particular. In severe metabolic acidosis seen in the later stages of shock, dopamine's effectiveness is diminished. The acidosis must first be corrected with intravenous sodium bicarbonate (Rice, 1991c).

Intravenous *nitroglycerin* (Tridil) in low doses acts as a venous vasodilator and therefore reduces preload. At higher doses, nitroglycerine causes arterial vasodilation and therefore reduces afterload as well. These actions in combination with medium-dose dopamine increase cardiac output while minimizing cardiac workload. Additionally, vasodilation enhances blood flow to the myocardium improving oxygen delivery to the weakened heart muscle.

Other vasoactive medications that may be used in the management of cardiogenic shock include dobutamine (Dobutrex), norepinephrine (Levophed), epinephrine (Adrenaline), isoproterenol (Isuprel), and amrinone (Inocor). Each of these drugs stimulates different receptors of the sympathetic nervous system. A combination of these medications may be prescribed and is based on the patient's response to treatment. All vasoactive medications have adverse side effects making specific medications more useful than others at different phases of shock. Diuretics, such as furosemide (Lasix), may be administered to reduce the workload of the heart by reducing fluid accumulation.

Antidysrhythmic medication is also part of the drug regimen in cardiogenic shock. Multiple factors such as hypoxemia, electrolyte imbalances, and acid–base imbalances contribute to serious cardiac dysrhythmias in all patients with shock. Additionally, as a compensatory response to decreased cardiac output and blood pressure, the heart rate increases beyond normal limits. This impedes cardiac output further by shortening diastole and thereby decreasing time for ventricular filling. Consequently antidysrhythmic medications are required to stabilize the heart rate. For a full discussion of cardiac dysrhythmias as well as commonly prescribed medications, see Chapter 27. General principles regarding the administration of vasoactive medications are discussed on page 254.

Fluid Therapy. In addition to medications, fluids are administered in the treatment of cardiogenic shock (Alpert & Becker, 1993). Administration of fluids must be monitored closely by the nurse to detect signs of fluid overload. Incremental intravenous fluid boluses are cautiously administered starting in amounts of 50 ml to determine optimal filling pressures to improve cardiac output (Alpert & Becker, 1993).

Mechanical Support. In cases in which the patient's cardiac output does not improve despite supplemental oxygen, vasoactive medications, and fluid boluses, mechanical assistive devices are used as a temporary means of improving the heart's ability to pump. Intra-aortic balloon counterpulsation (IABC) is one means of providing temporary circulatory assistance. A polyurethane balloon catheter is inserted percutaneously through the common femoral artery and advanced into the descending thoracic aorta. The balloon catheter is connected to a console containing a gas-filled pump. The timing of the balloon inflation is synchronized electrocardiographically with the beginning of diastole, and the balloon deflation occurs just prior to systole. By augmenting the propulsion of blood volume, IABC:

- Increases stroke volume
- Improves coronary circulation
- Decreases preload
- Decreases cardiac work
- Decreases myocardial oxygen demand (Schott, 1990)

See Chapter 28 for a further discussion of IABC.

Other means of mechanical assistance include left and right ventricular assist devices and total artificial hearts. These devices consist of electrical pumps or pumps that are driven by pneumatic air and assist or replace the ventricular pumping action of the heart. Human heart transplantation may be indicated when the patient cannot be weaned from mechanical assistive devices (Rice, 1991c). Mechanical assist devices and heart transplantation are discussed in Chapter 30.

Another short-term means of providing cardiac or pulmonary support to the patient in cardiogenic shock is through an extracorporeal device similar to cardiopulmonary bypass used in open heart surgery. The cardiopulmonary bypass (CPB) system requires systemic anticoagulation, arterial and venous cannulation of the femoral artery and vein, and connection to a centrifugal, oxygenated pump. The catheter tip is advanced into the patient's right atrium. This system lowers left and right ventricular pressures, reducing the workload and oxygen needs of the heart. One of the most significant complications of CPB is thromboembolism (Cone, et al, 1992). This procedure is used only in emergency situations until definitive treatment such as a heart transplant can be initiated.

Nursing Management of the Patient with Cardiogenic Shock

Prevention. In some circumstances, cardiogenic shock can be prevented by identifying patients at risk early and promoting adequate oxygenation of the heart muscle and decreasing cardiac workload. This can be accomplished by conserving the patient's energy, promptly relieving angina, and administering supplemental oxygen. Often, however, cardiogenic shock cannot be prevented. In such instances, nursing management includes working with other members of the management team to prevent the shock from progressing and to restore adequate cardiac function and tissue perfusion.

Hemodynamic Monitoring. A major role of the nurse is monitoring the patient's hemodynamic and cardiac status. Arterial lines and ECG monitoring equipment must be maintained and functioning properly. The nurse anticipates the medications, intravenous fluids, and equipment that might be used and must be ready to assist in implementing these measures. Changes in hemodynamic, cardiac, and pulmonary status are documented and reported promptly. Additionally, the appearance of adventitious breath sounds, changes in cardiac rhythm, and other physical assessment findings are reported immediately.

Fluid Administration. The nurse has a critical role in safe and accurate administration of intravenous fluids and medications. Fluid overload and pulmonary edema are risks because of ineffective cardiac function and accumulation of blood and fluid in the pulmonary tissues. The nurse documents and records medications and treatments that are administered as well as the patient's response to treatment.

The nurse needs to be knowledgeable about the desired effects as well as side effects of medications. For example, it is important to monitor the patient for decreased blood pressure when morphine or nitroglycerin is administered. The patient receiving thrombolytic therapy must be monitored for bleeding. Arterial and venous puncture sites must be observed for bleeding and pressure applied at the sites. Intravenous infusions must be observed closely as tissue necrosis and sloughing may occur if vasopressor medications infiltrate the tissues. Urine output, BUN, and serum creatinine levels are monitored because of the possibility of decreased renal function secondary to the effects of cardiogenic shock or its treatment.

IABC. The nurse plays a critical role in the care of the patient receiving IABC. The nurse makes ongoing timing adjustments of the balloon pump to maximize its effectiveness by synchronizing it with the cardiac cycle. The patient is at great risk of circulatory compromise to the leg on the side where the catheter has been placed. Therefore, frequent neurovascular checks of the lower extremities must be made.

Safety and Comfort. While assisting with these measures, the nurse also must take an active role in assuring the patient's safety and physical comfort and in reducing the patient's anxiety. This includes administering medication to relieve chest pain, preventing infection at the multiple arterial and venous line insertion sites, protecting the patient's skin, and monitoring respiratory function. Proper positioning of the patient promotes effective breathing without decreasing blood pressure and may also increase the patient's comfort while reducing anxiety.

Brief explanations about procedures that are being performed and the use of comforting touch often provide reassurance to the patient. The patient's family is often anxious and benefits from opportunities to see and talk to the patient. Explanations of treatments and the patient's response to them are often of comfort to family members.

Distributive Shock

Distributive or vasogenic shock occurs when blood volume is abnormally displaced in the vasculature such as when blood volume pools in peripheral blood vessels. This displacement of blood volume causes a *relative* hypovolemia because not enough blood is returned to the heart, which leads to subsequent inadequate tissue perfusion. The ability of the blood vessels to constrict helps return the blood to the heart. Thus, the vascular tone is determined both by central regulatory mechanisms, as in blood pressure regulation, and by local regulatory mechanisms, as in tissue demands for oxygen and nutrients. Therefore, distributive shock can be caused either by a loss of sympathetic tone or by release of chemical mediators from cells.

The varied mechanisms leading to the initial vasodilation in distributive shock further subdivide this classification of shock into three types: (1) *neurogenic*, (2) *anaphylactic*, and (3) *septic* shock. Table 15-6 provides examples of conditions placing patients at risk for distributive shock.

TABLE 15-6 Conditions Placing Patients at Risk for Distributive Shock

Neurogenic shock	Spinal cord injury
	Spinal anesthesia
Anaphylactic shock	Penicillin sensitivity
	Transfusion reaction
	Bee sting allergy
Septic shock	Immunosuppression
	Extremes of age (<1 yr and >65 yrs)
	Malnourishment
	Chronic illness
	Invasive procedures

The different types of distributive shock cause variations in the pathophysiologic chain of events and will be explained separately. In all types of distributive shock, massive arterial and venous dilation allows blood volume to pool peripherally. Arterial dilation reduces systemic vascular resistance (SVR). Initially cardiac output can be high in distributive shock, both from the reduction in afterload (SVR) and from the heart muscle's increased effort to maintain perfusion despite the incompetent vasculature secondary to arterial dilation. Pooling of blood in the periphery results in decreased venous return. Decreased venous return results in decreased stroke volume and decreased cardiac output. Decreased cardiac output, in turn, causes decreased blood pressure and ultimately decreased tissue perfusion. Figure 15-6 presents the pathophysiologic sequence of events in distributive shock.

Neurogenic Shock

In neurogenic shock, vasodilation occurs as a result of a loss of sympathetic tone. This can be caused by spinal cord injury, spinal anesthesia, and nervous system damage. It can also occur as a result of depressant action of medications or by lack of glucose (*e.g.*, insulin reaction or shock). Neurogenic shock may have a prolonged course (spinal cord injury) or a short one (syncope or fainting).

Spinal neurogenic shock is characterized by dry, warm skin rather than the cool, moist skin seen in hypovolemic shock. Another characteristic is bradycardia rather than the tachycardia observed in other forms of shock.

Medical Management. Treatment of neurogenic shock involves restoring sympathetic tone either through the stabilization of a spinal cord injury or, in the instance of spinal anesthesia, by positioning the patient properly. Specific treatment of neurogenic shock depends on its cause. Further discussion on the management of the patient with a spinal cord injury is presented in Chapter 60. If hypoglycemia (insulin shock) is the cause, rapid administration of glucose is initiated. (Hypoglycemia and insulin reaction are described further in Chapter 39).

Nursing Management. Neurogenic shock can be prevented in the patient receiving spinal or epidural anesthesia by raising the head of the bed 15 to 20 degrees to prevent the spread of the anesthetic up the spinal cord (Rice, 1991d). In suspected spinal cord injury, neurogenic shock may be prevented by carefully immobilizing the patient to prevent further damage to the spinal cord.

In the patient with neurogenic shock, nursing interventions are directed toward supporting the patient's cardiovascular and neurologic functions until the usually transient episode of neurogenic shock resolves. Elastic stockings and

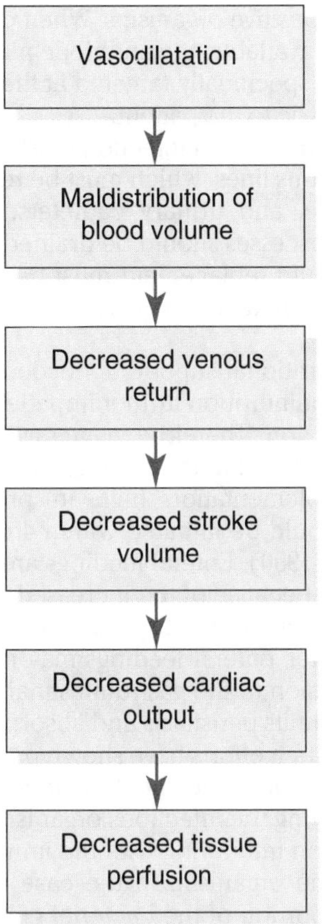

FIGURE 15-6. Pathophysiologic sequence of events in distributive shock.

elevating the foot of the bed may minimize pooling of blood in the legs.

Patients who have experienced a spinal cord injury may not report pain caused by internal injuries. Therefore, in the immediate post-injury period, the nurse must monitor the patient closely for signs of internal bleeding that could lead to hypovolemic shock.

The pooling of blood in the lower extremities places the patient at increased risk for thrombus formation. Therefore, it is important for the nurse to check the patient daily for a positive Homans' sign as well as any redness of the calves. Homans' sign is elicited by lifting the patient's leg, flexing the leg at the knee, and dorsiflexing the foot. A Homans' sign is positive and suggestive of deep vein thrombosis if pain in the calf occurs.

Administration of heparin, application of elastic compression stockings, and pneumatic compression of the legs may prevent thrombus formation. Passive range of motion of the immobile extremities also promotes circulation.

Anaphylactic Shock

Anaphylactic shock is caused by a severe allergic reaction when a patient who has already produced antibodies to a foreign substance (antigen) develops a systemic antigen–antibody reaction. This process requires that the patient has previously been exposed to the substance. An antigen–antibody reaction provokes mast cells to release potent vasoactive substances such as histamine or bradykinin, which cause widespread vasodilation and capillary permeability. Anaphylactic shock occurs rapidly and is life threatening. Because anaphylactic shock occurs in patients already exposed to an antigen and who have developed antibodies to it, it can often be prevented. Therefore, patients with known allergies must understand the significance of their subsequent exposure to the antigen and should be instructed to wear identification that identifies their sensitivities. This could prevent emergency administration of a medication that would lead to anaphylactic shock. Additionally, the patient and family need instruction about emergency use of medications to treat anaphylaxis.

Medical Management. Treatment of anaphylactic shock requires removal of the causative antigen (such as discontinuing administration of an antibiotic), administration of medications that will restore vascular tone, and emergency support of basic life functions. Epinephrine is given intravenously for its vasoconstrictive action. Diphenhydramine (Benadryl) is administered intravenously to reverse the effects of histamine, thereby reducing capillary permeability. Aminophylline is given intravenously to reverse the histamine-induced bronchospasm.

If cardiac arrest and respiratory arrest are imminent or have occurred, cardiopulmonary resuscitation (CPR) is performed. Endotracheal intubation or tracheotomy may be necessary to establish an airway. Intravenous lines are inserted to provide access for infusions of fluids and medications. Further explanation of anaphylaxis and specific chemical mediators is presented in Chapter 51.

Nursing Management. The nurse has an important role in the prevention of anaphylactic shock: assessing all patients for allergies or previous reactions to antigens (*e.g.*, medications, blood products, foods, contrast media) and communicating the existence of these allergies or reactions to others. Additionally, the patient's understanding of previous reactions and steps taken by the patient and family to prevent further exposure to antigens are assessed. When new allergies are identified, the patient is instructed to wear or carry identification that identifies the specific allergen or antigen.

When any new medication is administered, the patient must be observed for an allergic reaction. This is especially important with medications that are administered intravenously. Allergy to penicillin is one of the most common causes of anaphylactic shock.

In the hospital setting it is important to identify patients who are at risk for anaphylactic reactions to contrast media used for diagnostic studies: those with a well-known allergy to iodine or fish or those who have had previous allergic reactions to contrast media. This information must be conveyed to x-ray personnel.

The nurse must be knowledgeable about the clinical manifestations of anaphylaxis, take immediate action if signs and symptoms occur, and be prepared to begin CPR if cardiac and respiratory arrest occur. In addition to monitoring the patient's response to treatment, the nurse assists with intubation if needed, monitors the patient's hemodynamic status, ensures intravenous access for administration of medications, administers prescribed medications and fluids, and documents treatments and their effects.

Community health and home care nurses whose role includes administering antibiotics in the patient's home or other setting should also be prepared to administer epinephrine subcutaneously or intramuscularly in the event of an anaphylactic reaction.

Following recovery from anaphylaxis, the patient and family require explanation of the event. Further, the nurse provides teaching to the patient about avoiding future exposure to antigens and administering emergency medication to treat anaphylaxis.

Septic Shock

Septic shock is the most common type of distributive shock and is caused by widespread infection. Despite increased sophistication of antibiotic therapy, the incidence of septic shock has continued to rise over the past 50 years, with mortality rates ranging between 40% and 90% (Rice, 1991a). Septic shock is the most common cause of death in noncoronary intensive care units (Bone et al, 1992). (Toxic shock syndrome, a specific form of septic shock, is described in Chapter 45.)

The rate of nosocomial infection (infections occurring in the hospital) in critically ill patients has been reported to range from 15% to 25% (Hoyt, 1990.) The incidence of septic shock could be reduced by instituting infection control practices, carrying out meticulous aseptic technique, debriding wounds to remove necrotic tissue, properly cleaning and maintaining equipment, and thorough handwashing.

The most common causative microorganisms of septic shock are the gram-negative bacteria. However, other infectious agents such as gram-positive bacteria and viruses also can cause septic shock. When a microorganism invades body tissues the patient exhibits an immune response. This immune response provokes the activation of chemical mediators that have a variety of effects leading to shock. Increased capillary permeability, which leads to fluid seeping from the capillaries, and vasodilation are two such effects.

Septic shock occurs in two distinct phases. The first phase, referred to as the *hyperdynamic* or "warm" phase, is characterized by a high cardiac output with vasodilation. The patient becomes overheated or hyperthermic with warm flushed skin. Heart and respiratory rates are elevated. Urinary output may increase or may remain at normal levels. Gastrointestinal status may be compromised as evidenced by nausea, vomiting, or diarrhea.

The later phase, referred to as the *hypodynamic* or "cold" phase, is characterized by a low cardiac output with vasoconstriction reflecting the body's effort to compensate for the hypovolemia caused by the loss of intravascular volume through the capillaries. In this phase the patient's blood pressure drops, and the skin is cool and pale. Temperature may be normal or below normal. Heart and respiratory rates remain rapid. The patient no longer produces urine and multiple organ failure may occur.

Medical Management. Current treatment of septic shock involves identifying and eliminating the cause of infection. Specimens of urine, blood, sputum, and wound drainage are collected using aseptic technique. Broad-spectrum antibiotics are started prior to receiving culture and sensitivity reports to improve the patient's chances for survival (Roach, 1990). A cephalosporin agent plus an aminoglycoside may be prescribed initially. This combination will provide antibiotic coverage of most gram-negative and some gram-positive organisms. When culture and sensitivity reports are available, the antibiotic may be changed to one that is more specifically targeted at the infecting organism and is less toxic to the patient.

Any potential routes of infection must be eliminated, including intravenous lines, which must be removed and reinserted elsewhere, and urinary catheters, which must be removed. Any abscesses should be drained and necrotic areas debrided. Fluid replacement must be instituted to correct the hypovolemia that results from the incompetent vasculature.

Whereas nutritional support is needed in all classifications of shock, malnutrition further impedes the patient's resistance to infection. Therefore, aggressive nutritional supplementation is critical in the management of septic shock. Nutritional supplementation high in protein is recommended and should be initiated within 4 days of the onset of shock (Kuhn, 1990). Enteral feedings are preferred to the parenteral route because of the increased risk of iatrogenic infection resulting from the insertion of intravenous catheters; however, enteral feedings may not be possible if decreased perfusion to the gastrointestinal tract in the later stages of shock limits peristalsis and absorption.

Recent research efforts have shown promise for improving the outcomes of septic shock. Whereas past efforts focused on destroying the infectious organism, emphasis now is being placed on interfering with the immune response of the patient to the organism. In the case of gram-negative septic shock, a portion of the bacterial cell wall, called endotoxin, is released during phagocytosis (Klein & Witek-Janusek, 1992). Endotoxin is believed to be a trigger that causes the release of the chemical mediators whose effects lead to shock. Monoclonal antibodies that counter the endotoxin have been developed and are currently being studied in clinical trials. Although early evidence demonstrates the effectiveness of these anti-endotoxin monoclonal antibodies in enhancing immune function, their cost is prohibitive (Nash et al., 1991). Regardless, the shift in focus toward immunotherapy in the treatment of septic shock will continue to shed light on how the cellular response to infection can lead to shock.

Nursing Management. The nurse caring for *any* patient requires keeping in mind the risks of sepsis and the high mortality associated with septic shock. All invasive procedures must be carried out with correct aseptic technique after careful handwashing. Additionally, intravenous lines, arterial and venous puncture sites, surgical incisions, trauma wounds, urinary catheters, and pressure ulcers are monitored for signs of infection in all patients. The nurse identifies those patients at particular risk for sepsis and septic shock (*i.e.*, elderly and immunosuppressed patients; those with extensive trauma or burns; persons with diabetes). Consideration, however, must be given to the fact that these high-risk patients may not develop typical or classic signs of infection and sepsis. Confusion, for example, may be the first sign of infection and sepsis in the elderly.

When caring for the patient with septic shock, the nurse collaborates with other members of the health care team to identify the site and source of sepsis and the specific organisms involved. Appropriate specimens for culture and sensitivity are often obtained by the nurse.

Elevated body temperature (hyperthermia) is common with sepsis and raises the patient's metabolic rate and oxygen consumption. Therefore, efforts are made to reduce the patient's temperature by administering salicylates and using ice bags and hypothermia blankets. During these therapies, the nurse monitors the patient closely for shivering which further increases oxygen consumption. Efforts to increase the patient's comfort are important if the patient experiences chills, fever, or shivering. The nurse administers prescribed intravenous fluids and medications including antibiotics and vasoactive medications to restore vascular volume. Because of decreased perfusion to the kidneys and liver, serum concentrations of antibiotics that are normally cleared by these organs may increase and produce toxic effects. Therefore, the nurse monitors blood levels (antibiotic levels, BUN, creatinine, white blood count) and reports increased levels to the physician.

As with other types of shock, the nurse monitors the patient's hemodynamic status, fluid intake and output, and nutritional status. Daily weights and close monitoring of serum albumin levels aid in determining the patient's protein requirements.

Multiple Organ Failure

Multiple organ failure (MOF) or multiple organ dysfunction syndrome (MODS) can occur as a complication of all forms of shock (Cipolle et al., 1993). As previously described, in shock, all organ systems singularly suffer damage from a lack of adequate perfusion that can result in organ failure. However a syndrome of *sequential* organ failure has been further observed in patients. The exact mechanism that triggers this syndrome is unknown.

Although various causes of MOF have been identified, such as dead or injured tissue, infection, and perfusion deficits, it is not yet possible to predict which patients will develop MOF (Cipolle et al., 1993). This is partly because much of the organ damage occurs at the cellular level and therefore cannot be directly observed or measured. The sequence of organ failure usually begins in the lungs and is followed by failure of the liver and kidneys (Lekander & Cerra, 1990).

Clinical Manifestations

The clinical course of MOF follows one of two patterns. In both patterns there is an initial event that results in low blood pressure. The cause of the drop in blood pressure is treated and seemingly the patient responds. In the first pattern of MOF, occurring most often when the initiating event is a pulmonary one such as lung injury, the patient experiences respiratory compromise that necessitates intubation. This usually occurs within 24 to 72 hours of the initiating event. Respiratory failure leads rapidly to MOF and the patient survives only 2 to 4 days (Lekander & Cerra, 1990)

The second pattern of MOF occurs more insidiously. This pattern occurs most often in the patient with septic shock and progressively unfolds over the course of about 1 month. The patient also experiences respiratory failure and requires intubation. The patient remains hemodynamically stable for about 7 to 14 days. Despite this apparent stability, the patient exhibits a hypermetabolic state characterized by hyperglycemia, hyperlactatemia, and polyuria. The patient's metabolic rate is 1.5 to 2 times basal metabolic rate. Infection is usually present and skin breakdown begins to occur. During this stage there is a severe loss of skeletal muscle mass, a process referred to as *auto-catabolism*. If the hypermetabolic phase can be reversed, the mortality rate at this stage is between 25% and 40% (Lekander & Cerra, 1990).

In patients for whom the hypermetabolic phase cannot be reversed, MOF progresses and is characterized by jaundice, hyperbilirubinemia, and renal failure often requiring dialysis. The patient becomes less hemodynamically stable and begins to require vasoactive medications and fluid therapy support. This phase is prognostically significant in that the mortality rate increases from 40% to 60% in the early stage, to 90% to 100% in the late stage of MOF. The patient usually dies within about 28 days (Lekander & Cerra, 1990).

Management

Treatment measures to reverse MOF are aimed at (1) controlling the initiating event, (2) promoting adequate organ perfusion, and (3) providing nutritional support. The general plan of nursing care for the MOF patient is the same as that for the patient in septic shock. Providing information and support to family members is a critical role of the nurse in caring for patients with MOF. For those patients who sur-

CRITICAL THINKING EXERCISES

1. A patient has been brought to the emergency department in septic shock. How would you explain septic shock to the patient's family? How might your approach differ if the family members are distraught and crying? If they do not speak English well?
2. While driving home from work, you encounter a motor vehicle crash. One of the individuals in the crash is bleeding profusely. Describe the measures you would take at the scene to prevent or reduce the severity of shock and your reasons for doing so.
3. A patient has experienced second- and third-degree burns over 50% of his body. You know you must be alert for different types of shock that can occur during various phases of burn management. How would you assess for the various types of shock at different management stages, and how would the management of the different types of shock differ?
4. How would you distinguish anaphylactic shock from other forms of shock?

vive MOF, the massive loss of skeletal muscle mass makes rehabilitation a long, slow process.

REFERENCES AND BIBLIOGRAPHY

Books

Carolan JM (ed). Shock: A Nursing Guide. Oradell, NJ, Medical Economics Books, 1984.

Dolan JT. Critical Care Nursing. Philadelphia, FA Davis, 1991.

Guthrie M (ed). Contemporary Issues in Critical Care Nursing: Shock, Vol II. New York, Churchill Livingstone, 1982.

Hardaway RM (ed). Shock: The Reversible Stage of Dying. Littleton, MA, PSG Publishing, 1988.

Perry AG and Potter PA (eds). Shock: Comprehensive Nursing Management. St Louis, CV Mosby, 1983.

Spencer RT et al. Clinical Pharmacology and Nursing Management. Philadelphia, JB Lippincott, 1993.

Strange JM. Shock Trauma Care Plans. Springhouse, PA, Springhouse, 1987.

Journals

Ackerman GS, Fallon WF. Pharmacotherapeutics of hemorrhagic shock. Trauma Q 1992 Jul; 8(4):54–61.

Alpert JS and Becker RC. Mechanisms and management of cardiogenic shock. Crit Care Clin 1993; 9(2):205–218.

Baily PM. The metabolic response to injury: Overview and introduction to multiple system organ failure. Trauma Q 1991 Jan; 7(2):1–11.

Barone JE and Snyder AB. Treatment strategies in shock: Use of oxygen transport measurements. Heart Lung 1991; 20(1):81–86.

Barriere SL et al. Septic shock: Beyond antibiotics. Patient Care 1991; 25(10):95–98, 101–104, 107–109.

Bell TN. Disseminated intravascular coagulation and shock. Crit Care Nurs Clin North Am 1990; 2(2):255–268.

Blansfield J. Emergency autotransfusion in hypovolemia. Crit Care Nurs Clin North Am 1990; 2(2):195–199.

Bone RC. Let's agree on terminology: Definitions of sepsis. Crit Care Med 1991; 19(7):973–976.

Bone RC et al. Definitions for sepsis and organ failure and guidelines for the use of innovative therapies in sepsis. Chest 1992; 101(6):1644–1655.

Bonilla J et al. Hemorrhagic shock: Contemporary and future therapy. Trauma Q 1992 Jul; 8(4):38–53.

Brown KK. Septic shock: How to stop the deadly cascade. Part 1. Am J Nurs 1994 Sept; 94(9):20–26.

Brown KK. Critical interventions in septic shock, Part 2. Am J Nurs 1994 Oct; 94(10):20–25.

Buckman RF, Badellino MM, and Goldberg A. Pathophysiology of hemorrhagic hypovolemia and shock. Trauma Q 1992 Jul; 8(4):12–27.

Burns KM. Vasoactive drug therapy in shock. Crit Care Nurs Clin North Am 1990; 2(2):167–178.

Cipolle MD et al. Secondary organ dysfunction. Crit Care Clin 1993; 9(2):261–298.

Collins AS. Gastrointestinal complications in shock. Crit Care Nurs Clin North Am 1990; 2(2):269–277.

Cone M et al. Cardiopulmonary support in the intensive care unit. American Journal of Critical Care 1992; 1(1):98–108.

Dennis JW. Blood replacement, massive transfusion, and hemostasis in hemorrhagic shock. Trauma Q 1992 Jul; 8(4): 62–68.

Fallon WF. Complications of hemorrhagic shock. Trauma Q 1992 Jul; 8(4):78–90.

Gould SA et al. Hypovolemic shock. Crit Care Clin 1993; 9(2):239–259.

Hazinski MF et al. Epidemiology, pathophysiology and clinical presentation of gram-negative sepsis. American Journal of Critical Care 1993; 2(3):224–235.

Houston MC. Pathophysiology of shock. Crit Care Nurs Clin North Am 1990; 2(2):143–149.

Hoyt NJ. Preventing septic shock. Infection control in the intensive care unit. Crit Care Nurs Clin North Am 1990; 2(2):287–297.

Imm A and Carlson RW. Fluid resuscitation in circulatory shock. Crit Care Clin 1993; 9(2):313–333.

Jillings CR. Shock. Psychosocial needs of the patient and family. Crit Care Nurs Clin North Am 1990; 2(2):325–330.

Klein DM and Witek-Janusek L. Advances in immunotherapy of sepsis. Dimensions Crit Care Nurs 1992; 11(2):75–89.

Knaus WA, et al. Evaluation of definitions for sepsis. Chest 1992; 101(6):1656–1662.

Kuhn MM. Nutritional support for the shock patient. Crit Care Nurs Clin North Am 1990; 2(2):201–220.

Lancaster LE. Renal response to shock. Crit Care Nurs Clin North Am 1990; 2(2):221–233.

Lancaster LE and Rice V. Nursing care planning. Overview and application to the patient in shock. Crit Care Nurs Clin North Am 1990; 2(2):279–286.

Lekander BJ and Cerra FB. The syndrome of multiple organ failure. Crit Care Nurs Clin North Am 1990; 2(2):331–342.

Littleton MT. Trends in agents used for the management of sepsis. Crit Care Nurs Q 1993; 15(4):33–46.

Littleton MT. Prostaglandins and leukotrienes as mediators of shock and trauma. Crit Care Nurs Q 1988; 11(2):11–20.

Martin K. Oxygen delivery and consumption in septic shock. Intensive Care Nurs 1991; 7:193–199.

McMorrow ME and Cooney-Daniello M. When to suspect septic shock. RN 1991; 54(10):32–37.

Mostow SR. Management of gram-negative septic shock. Hosp Pract 1991; 25(10):121–123, 128–130.

Nash DB et al. Monoclonal antibodies for septic shock: In or out the barn door? Qual Rev Bull 1991; 17(10):310–313.

O'Neal PV. How to spot early signs of cardiogenic shock. Am J Nurs 1994 May; 94(5):36–41.

Rice V. Shock, a clinical syndrome: An update. Part I. Crit Care Nurse 1991a; 11(4):20–27.

Rice V. Shock, a clinical syndrome: An update. Part 2. Crit Care Nurse 1991b; 11(5):74–85.

Rice V. Shock, a clinical syndrome: An update. Part 3. Crit Care Nurse 1991c; 11(6):34–39.

Rice V. Shock, a clinical syndrome: An update. Part 4. Crit Care Nurse 1991d; 11(7):28–40.

Roach AC. Antibiotic therapy in septic shock. Crit Care Nurs Clin North Am 1990; 2(2):179–186.

Robins EV. Burn shock. Crit Care Nurs Clin North Am 1990; 2(2): 299–309.

Schott KE. Intra-aortic balloon counterpulsation as a therapy for shock. Crit Care Nurs Clin North Am 1990; 2(2):187–193.

Schumann LL and Remington MA. The use of Naloxone in treating endotoxic shock. Crit Care Nurse 1990; 10(2):63–73.

Shoemaker WC. Monitoring and management of acute circulatory problems: The expanded role of the physiologically oriented critical care nurse. Am J Crit Care 1992; 1(1):38–53.

Stroud M et al. Cellular and humoral mediators of sepsis syndrome. Crit Care Nurs Clin North Am 1990; 2(2):151–160.

Summers G. The clinical and hemodynamic presentation of the shock patient. Crit Care Nurs Clin North Am 1990; 2(2):161–165.

Vaughan P and Brooks C. Adult respiratory distress syndrome. A complication of shock. Crit Care Nurs Clin North Am 1990; 2(2):235–253.

Vinsant GO and Fallon WF. General principles in the management of hemorrhagic shock: Lessons learned in the early care of the trauma patient. Trauma Q 1992 Jul; 8(4):28–37.

Waters LM et al. Hetastarch: An alternative colloid in burn shock management. J Burn Care Rehabil 1989; 10(1):11–16.

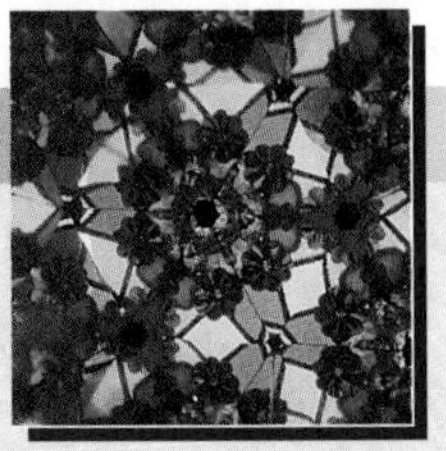

16

Oncology: Nursing the Patient With Cancer

CHAPTER OUTLINE

LEARNING OBJECTIVES

On completion of this chapter, the learner will be able to:

Cancer nursing is an area of practice that covers all age groups and nursing specialties and is carried out in a variety of health care settings, including the home, community, acute care institutions, and rehabilitation centers. The field or specialty of cancer nursing, or **oncology nursing**, has paralleled the development of medical oncology and the major therapeutic advances that have occurred in the care of the person with cancer.

The scope, responsibilities, and goals of cancer nursing are as diverse and complex as those of any nursing specialty. There is a special challenge inherent in caring for people with cancer because in our society the word *cancer* has often been equated with pain and death. Identifying one's own reactions to cancer and setting realistic goals that can be attained enables the nurse to meet this challenge.

The nurse must be equipped to support the patient and family through a wide range of physical, emotional, social, cultural, and spiritual crises. Accomplishing the desired outcomes involves providing realistic support to those receiving nursing care and using standards of practice and the nursing process as the basis of care. The major areas of responsibility for the nurse caring for the patient with cancer are listed in Chart 16-1.

Incidence

Although cancer affects every age group, most cancers occur in people over 65 years of age. Overall, men experience a higher incidence of cancer than do women.

At least 1,170,000 Americans are diagnosed each year with a cancer affecting one of various body sites (Fig. 16-1). Cancer incidence is higher in the industrialized nations of the world and in the industrial sectors of more developed countries.

Mortality Rates

Cancers are second only to cardiovascular disease as a leading cause of death in the United States. Each year, more than 496,000 Americans die of a malignant process. In order of frequency, the leading causes of cancer deaths in the United States include cancers of the lung, prostate, and colorectal area in men and cancers of the lung, breast, and colorectal area in women. Relative 5-year survival rates in 1991 are 38% for African Americans and 54% for white Americans. Cancer mortality in African Americans is higher than in any other race living in the United States. This finding is related to the higher incidence rates and later stage of diagnosis of cancer found among African Americans. The increased cancer morbidity and mortality for this group may be related more to economic factors, education, and barriers to health care than to racial characteristics.

Pathophysiology of the Malignant Process

Cancer is a disease process that begins when an abnormal cell is transformed by the genetic mutation of the cellular DNA. This abnormal cell forms a clone and begins to proliferate abnormally, ignoring growth-regulating signals in the environment surrounding the cell.

A stage is then reached in which the cells acquire invasive characteristics, and changes occur in surrounding tissues. The cells infiltrate these tissues and gain access to lymph and blood vessels, by which they can be carried to other areas of the body to form **metastases** (cancer spread) in other parts of the body.

Although the disease can be described in the general terms just used, cancer is not a single disease with a single cause; rather it is a group of distinct diseases with different causes, manifestations, treatments, and prognoses.

Benign Versus Malignant Proliferative Patterns

During a person's life span, various body tissues normally experience periods of rapid or proliferative growth that must

CHART 16-1

Responsibilities of the Nurse Caring for the Oncology Patient and Family

- Support the idea that cancer is a chronic illness that has acute exacerbations rather than one that is synonymous with death and suffering.
- Assess own level of knowledge relative to the pathophysiology of the disease process.
- Make use of current research findings and practices in the care of the patient with cancer and his or her family.
- Identify persons at high risk for the development of cancer.
- Participate in primary and secondary prevention efforts.
- Assess the nursing care needs of the person with cancer.
- Assess the learning needs, desires, and capabilities of the person with cancer.
- Identify nursing problems of the person and his or her family.
- Assess the social support networks available to the person.
- Plan appropriate interventions with the person and his or her family.
- Assist the person to identify own strengths and limitations.
- Assist the person to design short-term and long-term goals for care.
- Implement a nursing care plan that interfaces with the medical care regimen and that is consistent with the established goals.
- Collaborate with members of a multidisciplinary team to foster continuity of care.
- Evaluate the goals and resultant outcomes of care with the patient, his or her family, and the members of the multidisciplinary team.
- Reassess and redesign the direction of the care as determined by the evaluation.

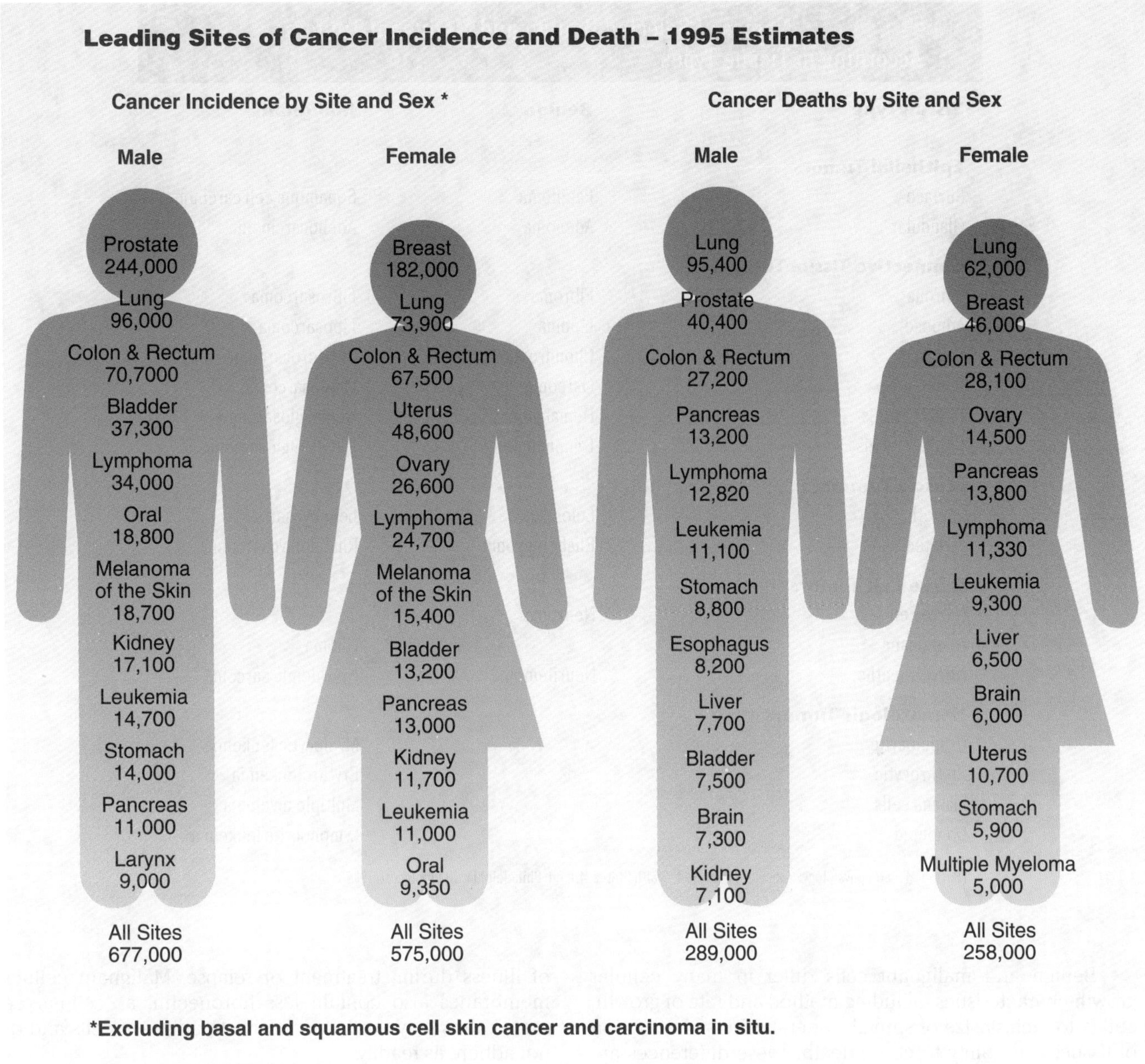

FIGURE 16-1. Leading sites of cancer incidences and deaths—1995 estimates. (From: Cancer Facts and Figures 1995.)

be distinguished from malignant growth activity. Several patterns of cell growth exist and are designated by the terms *hyperplasia, metaplasia, dysplasia, anaplasia*, and *neoplasia*.

Hyperplasia. Hyperplasia, an increase in the number of cells of a tissue, is a common proliferative process during periods of rapid body growth (*e.g.*, fetal and adolescent growth and development) and during regeneration of skin and bone marrow. It is a normal cellular response when a physiologic demand exists; it becomes an abnormal response when growth exceeds the physiologic demand such as may occur with chronic irritation.

Metaplasia. Metaplasia occurs when one type of mature cell is converted to another type by means of a stimulus that affects the parent stem cell. Chronic irritation or inflammation, vitamin deficiency, and chemical exposure may be factors leading to metaplasia. Metaplastic changes may be reversible or may progress to dysplasia.

Dysplasia. Dysplasia is bizarre cell growth resulting in cells that differ in size, shape, or arrangement from other cells of the same type of tissue. Dysplasia can occur from chemicals, radiation, or chronic inflammation or irritation. It can be reversible or can precede irreversible neoplastic change.

Anaplasia. Anaplasia is a lower degree of differentiation of dysplastic cells. (**Differentiation** refers to the extent to which the cells differ from their cells of origin and to their degree of maturity.) Anaplastic cells are poorly differentiated and irregularly shaped or disorganized with respect to growth and arrangement. Anaplastic cells lack normal cellular characteristics and are nearly always malignant.

Neoplasia. Neoplasia, described as uncontrolled cell growth that follows no physiologic demand, can be either benign or malignant. Benign and malignant neoplastic growths are classified and named by tissue of origin as described in Table 16-1.

TABLE 16-1 Names of Selected Benign and Malignant Tumors According to Tissue Types

Tissue Type	Benign	Malignant
Epithelial Tumors		
Surface	Papilloma	Squamous cell carcinoma
Glandular	Adenoma	Adenocarcinoma
Connective Tissue Tumors		
Fibrous	Fibroma	Fibrosarcoma
Adipose	Lipoma	Liposarcoma
Cartilage	Chondroma	Chondrosarcoma
Bone	Osteoma	Osteosarcoma
Blood vessels	Hemangioma	Hemangiosarcoma
Lymph vessels	Lymphangioma	Lymphangiosarcoma
Muscle Tumors		
Smooth	Leiomyoma	Leiomyosarcoma
Striated	Rhabdomyoma	Rhabdomyosarcoma
Nerve Cell Tumors		
Nerve cell	Neuroma	
Glial tissue		Glioma
Nerve sheaths	Neurilemoma	Neurilemic sarcoma
Hematologic Tumors		
Granulocytic		Myelocytic leukemia
Erythrocytic		Erythroleukemia
Plasma cells		Multiple myeloma
Lymphoid		Lymphocytic leukemia

(Porth CM. Pathophysiology: Concepts of Altered Health States. 4th ed. Philadelphia, JB Lippincott, 1994.)

Benign and malignant cells differ in many cellular growth characteristics including method and rate of growth, ability to metastasize or spread, general effects, destruction of tissue, and ability to cause death. These differences are summarized in Table 16-2. The degree of anaplasia (lack of differentiation of cells) ultimately determines the malignant potential.

Characteristics of Malignant Cells

Despite their individual differences, all cancer cells share some common cellular characteristics in relation to the cell membrane, the presence of special proteins, the nuclei, chromosomal abnormalities, and the rate of mitosis and growth. The cell membranes are altered in cancer cells, which affects fluid movement in and out of the cell. The cell membrane of malignant cells also contains proteins called *tumor-specific antigens* (such as carcinoembryonic antigen [CEA] and prostate specific antigen [PSA]), which develop as they become less differentiated (mature) over time. These proteins distinguish the malignant cell from a benign cell of the same tissue type and may be useful in measuring the extent of disease in a person and in tracking the course of illness during treatment or relapse. Malignant cellular membranes also contain less fibronectin, a "cellular cement"; thus they are less cohesive to adjacent cells and do not adhere as readily.

Nuclei of cancer cells are often large and irregularly shaped (pleomorphism). Nucleoli, structures within the nucleus that house ribonucleic acid (RNA), are larger and more numerous in malignant cells, perhaps because of increased RNA synthesis. Chromosomal abnormalities (translocations, deletions, additions) and fragility of chromosomes are commonly found on analysis of cancer cells.

Mitosis (cell division) occurs more frequently in malignant cells than in normal cells, thus increasing the growth fraction of the tumor cell population. Additionally, cancer cells have altered amounts of cyclic adenosine monophosphate (AMP) and cyclic guanosine monophosphate (GMP). These substances, which are the building blocks of nucleic acids, facilitate the use of nutrients and the synthesis of RNA. As a result, cell growth and division are promoted, requiring high levels of glucose and oxygen. If these glucose and oxygen stores are unavailable, malignant cells will use anaerobic metabolic channels to produce energy. Anaerobic means of energy production make the cell less dependent on the availability of a constant oxygen supply.

TABLE 16-2 Characteristics of Benign and Malignant Neoplasms

Characteristics	Benign	Malignant
Cell characteristics	Well-differentiated cells that resemble normal cells of the tissue from which the tumor originated	Cells often bear little resemblance to the normal cells of the tissue from which they arose; there is both anaplasia and pleomorphism
Mode of growth	Tumor grows by expansion and does not infiltrate the surrounding tissues; usually encapsulated	Grows at the periphery and sends out processes that infiltrate and destroy the surrounding tissues
Rate of growth	Rate of growth is usually slow	Rate of growth is variable and is dependent on level of differentiation; the more anaplastic the tumor, the more rapid the rate of growth
Metastasis	Does not spread by metastasis	Gains access to the blood and lymph channels and metastasizes to other areas of the body
General effects	Is usually a localized phenomenon that does not cause generalized effects unless, by its location, it interferes with vital functions	Often causes generalized effects such as anemia, weakness, and weight loss
Destruction of tissue	Does not usually cause tissue damage unless its location interferes with blood flow	Often causes extensive tissue damage as the tumor outgrows its blood supply or encroaches on blood flow to the area; may also produce substances that cause cell damage
Ability to cause death	Does not usually cause death unless by its location it interferes with vital functions	Will usually cause death unless growth can be controlled

(Porth CM. Pathophysiology: Concepts of Altered Health States. 4th ed. Philadelphia, JB Lippincott, 1994.)

Invasion and Metastasis

Malignancies have the ability to spread or transfer cancerous cells from one organ or body part to another by invasion and metastasis.

Invasion. Invasion involves the growth of the primary tumor into the surrounding host tissues. The process of invasion occurs in several ways. Mechanical pressure exerted by rapidly proliferating neoplasms may force fingerlike projections of tumor cells into surrounding tissue and interstitial spaces. Malignant cells may break off from the primary tumor and invade adjacent structures. Malignant cells are thought to possess or produce specific destructive enzymes—such as collagenases (specific to collagen), plasminogen activators (specific to plasma), and lysosomal hydrolyses that destroy surrounding tissue, including the structural tissues of the vascular basement membrane—which facilitate invasion of malignant cells. The mechanical pressure of a rapidly growing tumor may enhance this process.

Metastasis. Metastasis is the dissemination or spread of malignant cells from the primary tumor to distant sites by direct spread of tumor cells to body cavities or through lymphatic and blood circulation. Tumors growing in or penetrating body cavities may shed cells or emboli that travel within the body cavity and "seed" the surfaces of other organs. This can occur in ovarian cancer when malignant cells enter the peritoneal cavity and seed peritoneal surfaces of abdominal organs such as the liver or pancreas.

Lymphatic Spread. The most common mechanism of metastasis is transport of tumor cells through the lymphatic circulation. Tumor emboli enter the lymph channels by way of the interstitial fluid that communicates with lymphatic fluid. In addition, malignant cells may penetrate lymphatic vessels by invasion. After entering the lymphatic circulation, malignant cells either become lodged in the lymph nodes or pass between lymphatic and venous circulation. Tumors arising in areas of the body with rapid and extensive lymphatic circulation have a high risk of metastasis through lymphatic channels. Breast tumors frequently metastasize in this manner through axillary, clavicular, and thoracic lymph channels.

Hematogenous Spread. Dissemination of malignant cells through the bloodstream (hematogenous spread), is directly related to the vascularity of the tumor. Few malignant cells are able to survive the turbulent nature of arterial circulation, insufficient oxygenation, or destruction by the body's immune system. In addition, the structure of most arteries and arterioles is far too secure to permit malignant invasion. Those malignant cells that do survive this hostile environment are able to attach to endothelium and attract fibrin, platelets, and clotting factors to seal themselves from immune surveillance. The endothelium will retract, allowing the malignant cells to enter the basement membrane and secrete lysosomal enzymes to destroy surrounding body tissues, thus leading to implantation.

Angiogenesis. Malignant cells also have the ability to induce the growth of new capillaries from the host tissue to meet their needs for nutrients and oxygen. This process is referred to as *angiogenesis*. It is through this vascular network that tumor emboli can enter the systemic circulation and travel to distant sites. Large tumor emboli that become trapped in the microcirculation of distant sites may further metastasize to other sites.

In summary, metastasis from the primary tumor to other sites is not a random process. It is a complex process achieved by few malignant cells; it is estimated that only 0.01% of all cancer cells go on to produce a metastatic focus. The host provides a hostile environment that destroys most circulating tumor cells. Those successful cells that achieve metastasis are able to survive because of their virulence and adaptive abilities.

Since the late 1800s, investigators have recognized that the malignancies of specific cell classifications have a tendency to metastasize to specific organs.

Currently, investigators are focusing their attention on the following factors in metastasis: organ vascularity, immune defenses at the tissue level, surface recognition factors on tumor cells, and differing behavioral characteristics among cells within one tumor.

Carcinogenesis

Malignant transformation is thought to be at least a three-step cellular process: initiation, promotion, and progression.

Initiation is the first step, in which initiators such as chemicals, physical factors, and biologic agents escape normal enzymatic mechanisms and cause alterations in the genetic structure of the cellular deoxyribonucleic acid (DNA). These alterations may be reversed by DNA repair mechanisms or may result in permanent cellular mutations. These mutations usually are not of significance to cells until the second step of carcinogenesis occurs.

During **promotion**, repeated exposure to promoting agents causes the expression of abnormal or mutant genetic information even after long latency periods. Latency periods for the promotion of cellular mutations vary with the type of agent and the dosage of the promoter, as well as the innate characteristics of the target cell.

Cellular oncogenes, present in all mammalian systems, are responsible for the vital cellular functions of growth and differentiation. Cellular proto-oncogenes are present in cells and act as an "on switch" for cellular growth. Similarly, cancer suppressor genes act to "turn off" or regulate unneeded cellular proliferation. When these genes become mutated, rearranged, amplified, or lose regulatory capabilities, malignant transformation is allowed to occur. Once this genetic expression occurs in cells, they begin to produce mutant cell populations that are different from their original cellular ancestors.

Progression is the third step of cellular carcinogenesis. The cellular changes formed during initiation and promotion now assume increased malignant behavior. These cells now display a propensity to invade adjacent tissues and to metastasize. Those agents that initiate or promote cellular transformation are referred to as **carcinogens**.

Etiology

Certain categories of agents or factors have been implicated in the carcinogenic process. These include viruses, physical agents, chemical agents, genetic or familial factors, dietary factors, and hormonal agents.

Viruses

Viruses as a cause of human cancers are hard to ascertain because viruses are difficult to isolate. Infectious causes are considered or suspected when specific cancers appear in clusters. Viruses are thought to incorporate themselves in the genetic structure of cells, thus altering future generations of that cell population—perhaps leading to a cancer. For example, the Epstein–Barr virus is highly suspect as a causative agent in Burkitt's lymphoma and nasopharyngeal cancers. Herpes simplex type II virus, cytomegalovirus, and human papillomavirus (HPV), types 16 and 18, all have been associated with dysplasia and malignancy of the uterine cervix; the hepatitis B virus has been implicated in hepatocellular carcinoma. Similarly, the human T-cell lymphotropic virus (HTLV-I) has been associated with some lymphocytic leukemias and lymphomas, especially among individuals in southern Japan; and the HIV virus is associated with Kaposi's sarcoma.

Physical Agents

Physical factors associated with carcinogenesis include exposure to sunlight or to radiation, chronic irritation or inflammation, and tobacco use.

Excessive exposure to the ultraviolet radiation of the sun, especially in people who are fair-skinned and have blue or green eyes, increases the risk of skin cancers. Factors such as clothing styles (sleeveless dresses or shorts), use of sunscreens, occupation, recreational habits, as well as environmental variables such as humidity, altitude, and latitude all play a role in the exposure risk of ultraviolet light.

Exposure to ionizing radiation can occur with repeated diagnostic radiographic procedures or when radiation therapy is used to treat disease. Improved radiographic equipment presents a minimal risk of extensive radiation exposure when used appropriately. Radiation therapy used in disease treatment or exposure to radioactive materials at nuclear weapon sites or nuclear power plants is associated with higher incidences of leukemias, multiple myeloma, and cancers of the lung, bone, breast, thyroid, and other tissues. Natural background radiation (radon) occurring from the natural decay of the earth has also been associated with increased lung cancer. Homes displaying high levels of trapped radon should be ventilated to allow the radon gas to disperse into the atmosphere.

Exposure to electromagnetic fields (EMF) from power lines, microwaves, and cellular phones, may also increase cancer risk. Currently, findings of epidemiologic studies related to EMF that suggest an increase in leukemias, central nervous system tumors, skin malignancies, and testicular cancers remain controversial.

Chronic irritation or inflammation is thought to damage cells, leading to abnormal cell differentiation. Cell mutations secondary to chronic irritation or inflammation are associated with lip cancers among pipe smokers. Oral cancers are associated with prolonged tobacco use or ill-fitting dentures. Melanomas are associated with chronically irritated moles; colorectal cancers with ulcerative colitis; and liver cancers with cirrhosis.

Chemical Agents

Eighty-five percent of all cancers are thought to be related to the environment. Tobacco smoke is a potent chemical carcinogen that accounts for at least 35% of cancer deaths. Smoking is strongly associated with cancers of the lung, head and neck, esophagus, pancreas, cervix, and bladder. Tobacco may also act synergistically with other substances such as alcohol, asbestos, uranium, and viruses to promote cancer development. Chewing tobacco is associated with cancers of the oral activity and primarily occurs in men under 40 years of age.

Many chemical substances found in the workplace have proved to be carcinogens or co-carcinogens in the cancer process. The extensive list of suspected chemical substances continues to grow. Chemical carcinogens include aromatic amines and aniline dyes; arsenic, soots, and tars; asbestos; benzene; betel nut and lime; cadmium; chromium compounds; nickel and zinc ores; wood dust; beryllium compounds; and polyvinyl chloride.

Most hazardous chemicals produce their toxic effects by altering DNA structure in body sites distant from chemical exposure. The liver, lungs, and kidneys are the organ systems most often affected, presumably because of their roles in detoxifying chemicals.

Genetic and Familial Factors

Genetic factors also play a role in cancer cell development. If DNA damage occurs in cells where chromosomal patterns are abnormal, mutant cells may develop. Abnormal chromosomal patterns and cancer have been associated with extra chromosomes, too few chromosomes, or translocated chromosomes. Specific cancers with underlying genetic abnormalities include Burkitt's lymphoma, chronic myelogenous leukemia, meningiomas, acute leukemias, retinoblastomas, Wilms' tumor, and skin cancers.

Some cancers of adulthood and childhood display familial predisposition. These cancers tend to occur at an early age and at multiple sites in one organ or pair of organs. In cancers with a hereditary predisposition, commonly two or more first-degree relatives share the same cancer type. Cancers associated with familial inheritance include retinoblastomas, nephroblastomas, pheochromocytomas, malignant neurofibromatosis, leukemias, and breast, endometrial, colorectal, stomach, prostate, and lung cancers.

Dietary Factors

Dietary factors are thought to be related to 40% to 60% of all environmental cancers. Dietary substances can be proactive (protective), carcinogenic, or co-carcinogenic. The risk of cancer increases with long-term ingestion of carcinogens or co-carcinogens or chronic absence of proactive substances in the diet.

Dietary substances associated with an increased cancer risk include fats, alcohol, salt-cured or smoked meats, food containing nitrates and nitrites, and a high caloric dietary intake. Food substances that appear to reduce cancer risk include high-fiber foods, cruciferous vegetables (cabbage, broccoli, cauliflower, brussel sprouts, kohlrabi), carotenoids (carrots, tomatoes, spinach, apricots, peaches, dark green and deep yellow vegetables), and possibly vitamins E and C and selenium.

Hormonal Agents

Tumor growth may be promoted by disturbances in hormonal balance by either the body's own (endogenous) hormone production or administration of exogenous hormones. Cancers of the breast, prostate, and uterus are considered to be dependent on endogenous hormonal levels for growth. Oral contraceptives, diethylstilbestrol (DES), and prolonged estrogen replacement therapy have been associated with hepatocellular carcinomas, vaginal carcinomas, and breast cancer, respectively.

The Role of the Immune System

In human beings, malignant cells are capable of developing on a regular basis. There is evidence that the surveillance function of the immune system is most often able to detect the development of malignant cells and destroy them before cell growth becomes uncontrolled. When the immune system fails to identify and stop the growth of malignant cells, clinical cancer develops.

Patients who for various reasons are immunoincompetent have been shown to have an increased incidence of cancer. Organ transplant recipients who receive immunosuppressive therapy to prevent rejection of the transplanted organ have an increased incidence of lymphoma, Kaposi's sarcoma (KS), squamous cell cancer of the skin, and cervical and anogenital cancers. Patients with immunodeficiency diseases such as acquired immunodeficiency disease syndrome (AIDS) have an increased incidence of KS, lymphoma, and rectal and head and neck cancers. Some patients who have received alkylating chemotherapy agents to treat Hodgkin's disease have shown an increased incidence of secondary malignancies. Autoimmune diseases such as rheumatoid arthritis and Sjögren's syndrome are associated with increased cancer development. Finally, changes related to the aging process, such as declining organ function, increased incidence of chronic diseases, and diminished immunocompetence may contribute to an increased incidence of cancer in older people.

Normal Immune Responses

Normally, an intact immune system is able to combat cancer cells in several ways. Antigens on the cell membranes of cancer cells, known as *tumor-associated antigens*, are usually recognized by the immune system as foreign. These antigens are capable of stimulating the cellular and humoral immune responses. The T lymphocyte, the soldier of the cellular immune response, along with the macrophage is responsible for recognizing tumor cell antigens. When tumor antigens are recognized by T lymphocytes, other T lymphocytes toxic to the tumor cells are stimulated, proliferate, and are released into the circulation. In addition to possessing cytotoxic properties, T lymphocytes are capable of stimulating other components of the immune system to rid the body of malignant cells.

Certain **lymphokines**, which are substances produced by lymphocytes, are capable of killing or damaging various types of malignant cells. Other lymphokines can mobilize other cells, such as macrophages, that disrupt cancer cells. **Interferon**, a substance produced by the body in response to viral infection, also possesses some antitumor characteristics. Antibodies produced by B lymphocytes of the humoral immune response, either alone or in combination with the complement system, also defend against malignant cells. Natural killer (NK) cells, have recently been identified as a major component of the body's defense against cancer. NK cells are a subpopulation of lymphocytes that act by directly destroying cancer cells or by producing lymphokines that assist in cell destruction.

Immune System Failure

How is it, then, that malignant cells can survive and proliferate despite the immune system defense mechanisms? There are several theories about how tumor cells can overcome an apparently intact immune system. If the body fails to recognize the malignant cell as different from "self," the immune response may fail to be stimulated. The failure of the immune system to respond promptly to the malignant cells allows the tumor to grow to a size that is too large to be managed by normal immune mechanisms.

The tumor cells may actually suppress the patient's immune defenses. Tumor antigens may combine with the antibodies produced by the person and hide or mask themselves from normal immune defense mechanisms. These tumor antigen–antibody complexes can also depress further production of antibodies. Tumors are also capable of changing their appearance or producing substances that impair usual immune defenses. These substances not only promote growth of the tumor, but also increase the patient's susceptibility to infection by a variety of pathogenic organisms. As a result of prolonged contact with a tumor antigen, the patient's body may be depleted of the specific lymphocytes and no longer be able to mount an appropriate immune response.

Abnormal concentrations of host suppressor T lymphocytes may play a role in the development of malignancies. Suppressor T lymphocytes normally assist in the regulation of antibody production and diminish immune responses when they are no longer required. Studies have demonstrated that low levels of serum antibodies and high levels of suppressor cells have been found in patients with multiple myeloma, a malignancy associated with hypogammaglobulinemia (low amounts of serum antibodies). Carcinogens such as viruses or certain chemicals, including chemotherapeutic agents, may weaken the immune system and ultimately enhance tumor growth.

Detection and Prevention of Cancer

Nurses as well as physicians have traditionally been involved with *tertiary prevention,* the care and rehabilitation of the patient after cancer has been diagnosed and treated. In recent years, however, the American Cancer Society, the National Cancer Institute, clinicians, and researchers have placed greater emphasis on primary and secondary prevention of cancer. *Primary prevention* is concerned with reducing the risk or preventing the development of cancer in healthy people. *Secondary prevention* involves detection and screening efforts to achieve early diagnosis and prompt intervention to halt the cancerous process.

Nurses in all settings have an important role in cancer prevention, by acquiring the knowledge and skills necessary to educate the community about health-related behaviors, risk factors associated with the development of cancer, and screening and detection methods. Epidemiologic and laboratory studies have shown that dietary habits, exposure to the sun, tobacco use, and alcohol consumption can greatly influence the risk of developing cancer. Nurses also need teaching and counseling skills to facilitate client participation in cancer prevention programs and to promote healthy lifestyles.

Several studies have demonstrated that numerous factors such as race, cultural influences, level of education, income, and age influence the degree of knowledge people have about cancer risk factors and the type of health-promoting behaviors they practice. For example, Underwood (1991) examined perceptions of African American men concerning health maintenance behavior, cancer screening, cancer risk factors, and cancer prevention. The findings suggested that attitudes of fatalism, pessimism, and fear of cancer influenced the degree to which these men were willing to seek medical advice or follow-health promotion behaviors aimed at reducing the risk of cancer.

In planning prevention and screening programs, nurses utilize information about specific populations to improve the success of the programs. For example, Coleman et al (1991) found that the most beneficial method of teaching breast self-examination (BSE) in older women combined the use of individual instruction, role modeling, and a breast model.

Public awareness about health promotion can be increased in a variety of ways. Health education and health maintenance programs are sponsored by community organizations such as churches, senior citizen groups, and parent-teacher associations. Primary prevention programs may focus on the hazards of tobacco or the importance of nutrition. Secondary prevention programs may promote breast and testicular self-examination and Papanicolaou tests. The American Cancer Society has developed a public education program, "Taking Control," that integrates diet, exercise, and general health habit tips that people can follow to reduce their risk of developing cancer (Chart 16-2). Nurses in acute care settings can identify risks for patients and families and incorporate teaching and counseling in discharge planning.

Nurses also develop educational and counseling programs targeting patients and families with high incidences of cancer. Malignant melanoma and breast cancer are examples of malignancies often seen in more than one person in a family.

Screening efforts to detect the early occurrence of cancer usually focus on cancers with the highest incidence rates or those that have improved survival rates if diagnosed early. Examples of these types of cancer include breast, col-

CHART 16-2
Ten Steps of Cancer Prevention

Action	Rationale
Protective Factors	
1. Increase consumption of fresh vegetables (especially those of the cabbage family).	1. Increase fiber intake; increase intake of vitamins.
2. Increase fiber intake.	2. High-fiber diets reduce risk of developing certain cancers (cancer of breast, prostate, and colon).
3. Increase intake of vitamin A.	3. Reduces risk of cancers (esophagus, larynx, and lung).
4. Increase intake of foods rich in vitamin C.	4. Citrus fruits and vegetables rich in vitamin C may protect against cancer of the stomach and esophagus.
5. Practice weight control.	5. Obesity is linked to cancers of the uterus, gallbladder, breast, and colon.
Risk Factors	
6. Reduce the amount of dietary fat.	6. A high-fat diet increases risk of developing breast, colon, and prostate cancers.
7. Reduce intake of salt-cured, smoked, and nitrate-cured foods.	7. Moderation in consumption of these foods is recommended, as they have been linked to cancers of the esophagus and stomach.
8. Stop cigarette smoking.	8. Smokers are at risk for lung cancer.
9. Reduce alcohol intake.	9. Drinking large amounts of alcohol increases the risk of liver cancer. Heavy drinkers who smoke are at greater risk for cancers of the mouth, throat, larynx, and esophagus.
10. Avoid overexposure to the sun.	10. Overexposure to the sun increases the risk of skin cancer. Protective clothing or use of a sunscreen reduces the risk.

(Modified from the Taking Control Program of the American Cancer Society.)

orectal, cervical, endometrial, testicular, skin, and oropharyngeal cancers. Nurses and physicians can encourage individuals to comply with detection efforts as suggested by the American Cancer Society (Table 16-3).

Diagnosis of Cancer

The diagnosis of cancer is based on the assessment of physiologic and functional changes as well as on the results of the diagnostic evaluation. Patients with suspected cancer undergo extensive diagnostic testing to (1) determine the presence of tumor and the extent of disease; (2) identify possible spread (metastasis) or invasion of other body tissues; (3) evaluate the function of both involved and uninvolved body systems and organs; and (4) obtain tissue and cells for analysis of the cancer, including its stage and grade. Extensive testing most often includes a complete history and physical examination and radiologic, serologic, and other diagnostic and surgical procedures (Table 16-4).

Nursing Considerations. A patient undergoing extensive testing is usually fearful of the procedures themselves and anxious about the possible results of the testing. The patient and family require information about the tests to be performed, the sensations likely to be experienced and the patient's role in the testing procedures. The nurse provides opportunities for the patient and family to verbalize their fears about the test results, supports the patient and family throughout the period of diagnostic testing, and reinforces and clarifies information conveyed to them by the physician. The nurse also encourages the patient and family members to communicate and share their concerns and to discuss their questions with each other.

Staging and Grading

A complete diagnostic evaluation includes identifying the stage and grade of the malignancy. This process must be accomplished before the initiation of treatment to provide for and maintain a systematic and consistent approach to diagnosis, treatment, and evaluation of outcomes. Treatment options and prognosis are determined on the basis of staging and grading. **Staging** determines the size of the tumor and the existence of metastasis. Several systems exist for classifying the anatomic extent of disease. The **TNM system**, developed from the work of the International Union Against Cancer (IUCC) and the American Joint Committee for Cancer Staging and End Stage Reporting (AJCCS), is frequently used in describing malignancies such as breast, lung, or head and neck cancers. In this system, the *T* refers to the extent of the primary tumor, *N* refers to lymph node involvement, and *M* refers to the extent of metastasis (Table 16-5). A variety of other staging systems are available for cancers that do not lend themselves to the TNM system.

Grading refers to the classification of the tumor cells. Grading systems seek to define the type of tissue from which the tumor originated and the degree to which the tumor

TABLE 16-3 Recommendations of the American Cancer Society for Early Detection of Common Cancers

Test or Procedure	Population: Sex	Age	Frequency
Sigmoidoscopy, preferably flexible	M & F	50 and over	Every 3 to 5 years
Fecal occult blood test	M & F	50 and over	Every year
Digital rectal examination	M & F	40 and over	Every year
Pap test	F	All women who are or who have been sexually active, or have reached age 18, should have an annual Pap test and pelvic examination. After a woman has had three or more consecutive satisfactory normal annual examinations, the Pap test may be performed less frequently at the discretion of her physician.	
Pelvic examination	F	18–40 Over 40	Every 1–3 years with Pap test Every year
Endometrial tissue sample	F	At menopause, women at high risk*	At menopause
Breast self-examination	F	20 and over	Every month
Clinical breast examination	F	20–40 Over 40	Every 3 years Every year
Mammography**	F	40–49 50 and over	Every 1–2 years Every year
Health counseling and cancer checkup***	M & F M & F	Over 20 Over 40	Every 3 years Every year

*History of infertility, obesity, failure to ovulate, abnormal uterine bleeding, or estrogen therapy.
**Screening mammography should begin by age 40.
***To include examination for cancers of the thyroid, testicles, prostate, ovaries, lymph nodes, oral region, and skin.
(Levin B and Murphy GP, Revision of American Cancer Society recommendations for early detection of colorectal cancer. CA 1992 Sept/Oct; 42(5):296–299.)

cells retain the functional and histologic characteristics of the tissue of origin.

This information assists in predicting the behavior and prognosis of various tumors. Grading is assigned a numeric value ranging from I to IV. Grade I tumors, also known as *well-differentiated* tumors, closely resemble the tissue of origin in structure and function. Tumors that do not clearly resemble the tissue of origin in structure or function are described as *poorly differentiated* or *undifferentiated* and are assigned grade IV. These tumors tend to be more aggressive and less responsive to treatment than well-differentiated tumors.

Management of Cancer

Treatment options offered to cancer patients should be based on realistic and achievable goals for each specific type of cancer. The range of possible treatment goals may include complete eradication of malignant disease (**cure**), prolonged survival and containment of the growth of cancer cells (**control**), or relief of symptoms associated with the cancerous disease process (**palliation**).

It is imperative that the health care team, the patient, and the patient's family have a clear understanding of the treatment options and goals. Open communication and support are vital as the patient and family periodically reassess treatment plans and goals when complications of therapy develop or disease progresses.

Multiple modalities are often employed in cancer treatment. A variety of therapies, including surgery, radiation therapy, chemotherapy, and biologic response modifier therapy may be used at various times during the course of treatment. An understanding of the principles of each and how they interrelate is important in understanding the rationale and goals of treatment.

Surgery

Surgical removal of the entire cancer remains the best and most frequently used modality of treatment. The specific surgical approach, however, may be selected for a variety of reasons. Surgery may be selected as the primary method of treatment or it may be diagnostic, prophylactic, palliative, or reconstructive.

TABLE 16-4 Examples of Diagnostic Procedures Used in Evaluating Malignancies

Procedure	Description	Potential Uses
Tumor markers	Substances found in blood or other body fluids that are made by the tumor or by the body in response to the tumor	Breast, colon, lung, ovarian, testicular cancers
Magnetic resonance imaging (MRI)	Use of magnetic fields and radiofrequency signals to create sectional images of various body structures	Neurologic, pelvic, abdominal, thoracic cancers
Computed tomography scanning (CT scan)	Use of narrow beam x-ray to scan successive layers of tissue to provide cross-sectional views	Neurologic, pelvic, skeletal, abdominal, thoracic cancers
Fluoroscopy	Use of x-rays that show contrasts between body tissue densities; may involve the use of contrast materials	Skeletal, lung, gastrointestinal cancers
Ultrasound	Echoes of high-frequency sound waves are recorded on an imaging screen; used to assess tissues deep within the body	Abdominal and pelvic cancers
Endoscopy	Direct visualization of a body cavity or passageway by insertion of an endoscope into a body cavity or opening; allows tissue biopsy, fluid aspiration and excision of small tumors	Bronchial, gastrointestinal cancers
Nuclear medicine imaging	Uses intravenous injection or ingestion of radioisotope substances followed by imaging of tissues that have concentrated the radioisotopes	Bone, liver, kidney, spleen, brain, thyroid cancers

Surgery as Primary Treatment

When surgery is used as the primary approach in the treatment of cancer, the goal is to remove the entire tumor (or as much as is feasible, a procedure often called **debulking**) and any involved surrounding tissue, including regional lymph nodes.

Two common surgical approaches used for the treatment of primary tumors are local and wide excisions. **Local excision** is warranted when the mass is small. It includes removal of the mass and a small margin of normal tissue that is easily accessible. **Wide** or **radical excisions** include removal of the primary tumor, lymph nodes, adjacent involved structures, and surrounding structures that may be at high risk for tumor spread. This surgical method can result in disfigurement and altered functioning. Wide excisions are considered, however, if the tumor can be completely removed and the chances of cure or control are optimal.

Salvage surgery is an additional treatment option that utilizes an extensive surgical approach to treat the local recurrence of the cancer after a less extensive primary approach is used. A mastectomy to treat recurrent breast cancer following primary lumpectomy and radiation is an example of salvage surgery.

In addition to the use of surgical blades or scalpels to excise the mass and surrounding tissues, several other types of surgical interventions are available. **Electrosurgery** involves the use of electrical current to achieve tumor cell destruction. **Cryosurgery** uses liquid nitrogen to freeze tissue to cause cell destruction. **Chemosurgery** uses combined topical chemotherapy and layer-by-layer surgical removal of abnormal tissue. **Laser surgery** (light amplification by stimulated emission of radiation) involves the use of a contact tip or "laser scalpel" to focus a form of energy at an exact location and depth of tissue to destroy cancer cells.

A multidisciplinary approach is essential during and after any type of surgery. The effects of surgery on body image, self-esteem, and functional abilities are addressed. If necessary, a plan for postoperative rehabilitation is made before the surgical intervention.

It is now recognized that the growth and dissemination of cancer cells have often produced distant micrometastases by the time the patient seeks treatment. Therefore, attempting to remove wide margins of tissue in the hope of "getting all the cancer cells" is often not realistic. This reality substantiates the need for a coordinated multidisciplinary approach to cancer therapy. Once the surgery has been completed, one or more additional modalities may be chosen to increase the likelihood of destroying the cancer cells. There are, however, cancers that when treated surgically in the very early stages are considered to be curable (*e.g.*, skin cancers, testicular cancers).

Diagnostic Surgery

Diagnostic surgery is usually performed to obtain a **biopsy** (excision of a piece of tissue from a suspicious growth) to analyze the tissues and cells of the suspected malignancy. The three most common biopsy methods are the excisional, incisional, and needle methods. The **excisional method** for obtaining a biopsy is most frequently used for easily

TABLE 16-5 TNM Classification System

T* subclasses	**M‡ subclasses**
Tx—tumor cannot be adequately assessed	Mx—not assessed
T0—no evidence of primary tumor	M0—no (known) distant metastasis
TIS—carcinoma *in situ*	M1—distant metastasis present, specify site(s)
T1, T2, T3, T4—progressive increase in tumor size and involvement	**Histopathology**
N† subclasses	G1—well-differentiated grade
Nx—regional lymph nodes cannot be assessed clinically	G2—moderately well-differentiated grade
N0—regional lymph nodes demonstrably normal	G3, G4—poorly to very poorly differentiated grade
N1, N2, N3, N4—increasing degrees of demonstrable abnormalities of regional lymph nodes	

*T = Primary tumor.
†N = Regional lymph nodes.
‡M = Distant metastasis.
(American Joint Committee on Cancer. Manual for Staging of Cancer. Chicago, American Joint Committee.)

accessible tumors of the skin, breast, upper and lower gastrointestinal tract, and the upper respiratory tract. Often, removal of the entire tumor as well as surrounding normal tissue margins is possible. Removal of normal tissue beyond the area of the tumor decreases the possibility of residual microscopic disease that may lead to recurrence of the tumor. This approach not only provides the pathologist with the entire specimen but also decreases the chance of cellular seeding of the tumor. The **incisional method** is used if the tumor mass is too large to be removed.

It is imperative that the biopsy be representative of the tumor mass so that the pathologist can provide an accurate diagnosis. Negative biopsy results do not guarantee absence of malignancy. Excisional and incisional approaches are often performed through endoscopy. However, surgical incision may be required to determine the anatomic extent or stage of the tumor. For example, a diagnostic laparotomy involves the surgical opening of the abdomen to assess abdominal malignancies such as gastric cancers.

Needle biopsy is used to sample suspicious masses that are easily accessible, such as some growths in the breasts, thyroid, lung, liver, and kidney. The procedure is fast, relatively inexpensive, easy to perform, and generally requires only local anesthesia. In general, the patient experiences minimal and temporary physical discomfort. In addition, the degree to which the surrounding tissue is disturbed is kept to a minimum, thus decreasing the likelihood of disseminating cancer cells (seeding). There is, however, a chance that even the most skilled physician will obtain such a small biopsy specimen that a full description of the cellular types is not possible.

The method of biopsy chosen is based on many factors. Of greatest importance is the type of treatment anticipated if a diagnosis of cancer is confirmed. Definitive surgical approaches include the original biopsy site so that any cells dislodged during the biopsy are excised at the time of surgery. Nutrition, and hematologic, respiratory, renal, and hepatic function are considered in determining the method of treatment. If the biopsy requires general anesthesia, and subsequent surgery is likely, the effects of prolonged anesthesia on the patient are considered.

The patient and family are given an opportunity to discuss the available options before definitive plans are made. The nurse, as the patient's advocate, serves as a liaison between the patient and the physician to facilitate this process. Time should be set aside to minimize interruptions. Time for questions and for thinking through all that has been discussed should be provided.

Prophylactic Surgery

Prophylactic surgery involves the removal of nonvital tissues or organs that are likely to develop cancer. Colectomy and mastectomy are the two most common surgical procedures performed prophylactically in persons who are at a significantly high risk because of personal and family history. Some controversy, however, exists about adequate justification for prophylactic surgical procedures. For example, a strong family history of breast cancer, an abnormal physical finding on breast examination such as progressive nodularity and cystic disease, a proven history of breast cancer in the opposite breast, abnormal mammogram findings, and abnormal biopsy results may be necessary to justify prophylactic mastectomy.

Because the long-term physiologic and psychologic effects are not known, prophylactic surgery is offered selectively to patients and discussed thoroughly with the patient and family. Preoperative information and counseling, as well as long-term follow-up, should be provided.

Palliative Surgery

When cure of the cancer is not possible, the goal of treatment is to make the patient as comfortable as possible and promote a satisfying and productive life for as long as is possible. Whether the period is extremely short or lengthy, the major goal is a high quality of life—with quality defined by the patient and family. Honest and informative communication with the patient and family about the goal of surgery is essential to avoid false hope and disappointment.

Palliative surgery is performed in an attempt to relieve complications of cancer, such as ulcerations, obstructions, hemorrhage, pain, or infection. This type of surgery includes nerve block and cordotomy designed to relieve intractable pain; tumor resection to relieve obstruction that may occur if a segment of bowel is obstructed (this may result in creation of an ostomy, depending on the extent of invasion); and simple mastectomy for ulcerative breast disease.

Finally, surgical removal of hormone-producing glands that might enhance tumor growth may be performed. These glands include the pituitary, adrenals, ovaries, and testes.

Reconstructive Surgery

Reconstructive surgery may follow curative or radical surgery and is carried out in an attempt to improve function or obtain a more desirable cosmetic effect. It may be performed in one operation or in stages. Presurgery consultation and evaluation by the surgeon who is to perform later reconstructive surgery may take place preoperatively.

For example, the woman who is to have breast reconstruction performed may be seen by the surgeon before being hospitalized for a mastectomy. This approach provides the woman with something positive to focus on at a time when thoughts of disfigurement and death may be paramount. The physician performing the reconstructive surgery also benefits from seeing the way the woman's breasts appear normally and from establishing rapport with her. The nurse must be cognizant of the woman's sexuality needs and the impact that an altered body image may have on her sexuality. Providing the woman and her family with opportunities to discuss these issues is imperative. The needs of the individual must be accurately assessed and validated in each situation for any type of reconstructive surgery.

Nursing Considerations

The patient undergoing surgery for cancer requires general perioperative nursing care as described in Unit 5, along with specific care related to possible organ impairment, nutritional deficits, disorders of coagulation, and altered immunity that may increase the risk for postoperative complications. The use of combined treatment methods such as radiation and chemotherapy also contribute to postoperative complications such as infection, impaired wound healing, altered pulmonary or renal function, and the development of deep vein thrombosis. The nurse completes a thorough preoperative assessment for all factors that may affect patients undergoing surgical procedures.

The patient undergoing surgery for the diagnosis or treatment of cancer is often anxious about the surgical procedure, possible findings, postoperative limitations, changes in normal body functions, and prognosis. The patient and family require time and assistance to deal with the possible changes and outcomes resulting from the surgery.

The nurse provides education and emotional support by assessing patient and family needs and explores with them their fears and coping mechanisms, encouraging them to participate in decision-making whenever possible.

When the patient or family asks about the results of diagnostic testing and surgical procedures, the nurse's response is guided by the information the physician previously conveyed to them. The patient and family may also ask the nurse to explain and clarify information that the physician initially provided but which they did not grasp because they were so anxious at the time. It is important for the nurse to communicate frequently with the physician and other health care team members to be certain that the information provided is consistent.

After surgery, the nurse assesses the patient's responses to the surgery and monitors for possible complications such as infection, bleeding, thrombophlebitis, wound dehiscence, and organ dysfunction. The nurse also provides for patient comfort. Postoperative teaching includes wound care, activity, nutrition, and medication information.

Plans for discharge and follow-up care and treatment are initiated as early as possible to ensure continuity of care from hospital to home or from a cancer referral center to the patient's local hospital and health care provider. Patients and families are also encouraged to utilize community resources such as the American Cancer Society or Make Today Count for support and information.

Radiation Therapy

In radiation therapy, ionizing radiation is used to interrupt cellular growth. About half of patients with cancer receive a form of irradiation at some point in their course of treatment. Radiation may be used as a means of curing the cancer, such as in Hodgkin's disease, testicular seminomas, localized cancers of the head and neck, and cancers of the uterine cervix. Radiation therapy may also be used to control malignant disease when a tumor cannot be removed surgically or when local nodal metastasis is present, or it can be used prophylactically to prevent leukemic infiltration to the brain or spinal cord. Palliative irradiation is frequently used to relieve the symptoms of metastatic disease, especially when the cancer has spread to brain, bone, or soft tissue, or to treat oncologic emergencies such as superior vena cava syndrome or spinal cord compression.

Two types of ionizing radiation exist: electromagnetic rays (x-rays and gamma rays) and heavier particulate radiation (electrons [beta particles], protons, neutrons, and alpha particles). Either type of ionization can lead to tissue disruption. The most harmful tissue disruption is the alteration of the DNA molecule within the cells of the tissue. Ionizing radiation causes breakage among the strands of the DNA helix leading to cell death. Ionizing radiation can also ionize body fluids, especially water, leading to the formation of free radicals, which also cause irreversible damage to DNA. If the DNA is not repaired, the cell will die immediately, or it will die when it attempts to divide in mitosis. A tumor cell may also die if it has become sterile as a result of radiation; it dies a natural death because it cannot reproduce.

Cells are most vulnerable to the disruptive effects of radiation during DNA synthesis and mitosis (early S, G_2, and M phases of the cell cycle). Therefore, those body tissues that undergo frequent cell division are most sensitive to radiation therapy. These tissues include bone marrow, lymphatic tissue, epithelium of the gastrointestinal tract, and gonads. Slower growing tissues or tissues at rest are relatively radioresistant. Such tissues include muscle, cartilage, and connective tissues.

A *radiosensitive tumor* is one that can be destroyed by a dose of radiation that still allows for normal cell regeneration in the normal tissue. Tumors that are well oxygenated also seem to be more sensitive to radiation; therefore, radiation therapy might be enhanced if more oxygen concentrations can be delivered to tumors. In addition, if the radiation could be delivered at a time when most tumor cells are in either the S or M phases, the number of cancer cells destroyed ("cell kill") would be increased. Certain chemicals also act as radiosensitizers and sensitize more hypoxic tumors to the effects of radiation therapy.

Radiation is delivered to tumor sites by either external or internal mechanisms.

External Radiation

If external radiation therapy is used, one of several methods of delivery may be chosen, depending on the depth of the tumor to be radiated (Table 16-6). Kilovoltage therapy devices deliver the maximal radiation dose to superficial lesions such as lesions of the skin and breast, whereas gamma ray sources (cobalt-60 units) deliver the radiation dose to deeper body structures and spare the skin from possible adverse effects. Other radiation therapy machines, *linear accelerators* (Fig. 16-2) deliver their dosage to deeper structures without harming the skin and also create less scattering of radiation within the body tissues. A minimal number of centers nationwide treat more hypoxic, radioresistant tumors with cyclotrons that deliver neutron-beam therapy to the tumor.

Some centers are also testing the use of **intraoperative radiation therapy** (IORT), which involves delivering a high fraction, single dose of radiation therapy to the exposed tumor bed while the body cavity is open during surgery. Cancers in which IORT is being tested include gastric, pancreatic, colorectal, bladder, and cervical cancers and sarcomas. Toxicity with IORT is minimized because the radiation therapy is so precisely targeted to the diseased areas and exposure to overlying skin and structures is avoided. No increase in wound infection has been seen. Increases in nausea, vomiting, and postoperative ileus have been reported in some patients receiving IORT.

Internal Radiation

Internal radiation implants, or **brachytherapy**, are used to deliver a high dose of radiation to a localized area. The specific radioisotope for implantation is selected on the basis of its *half-life*, which is the time it takes for half of its radioactivity to decay. This internal radiation can be implanted by way of needles, seeds, beads, or catheters into body cavities (vagina, abdomen, pleura) or interstitial compartments (breast).

Intracavitary radioisotopes are frequently used to treat gynecologic malignancies. In these malignancies, the radioisotopes are placed into specially positioned applicators after their position is verified by x-ray as corresponding to the location of the tumor. These isotopes remain in place for a prescribed period of time and then are removed.

Patients are maintained on bedrest and logrolled to prevent displacement; an indwelling urinary catheter is inserted to ensure that the bladder is emptied. Low-residue diets and antidiarrheal agents, such as Lomotil, are provided to prevent bowel movement during therapy, again to prevent the isotopes from being dislodged.

TABLE 16-6 External Beam Radiation Therapy Equipment

Type of Radiation	Area of Maximum Dose	Indications
Kilovoltage		
Superficial radiation (10–125 Kv)	Skin surface	Superficial skin lesions
Orthovoltage radiation (125–400 Kv)	Skin surface (higher bone absorption)	Bony metastases
Gamma ray therapy		
Isotope source (cobalt or cesium)	0.5 cm below skin surface	Most malignant conditions
Megavoltage therapy		
Linear accelerators (x-rays or electrons)		
6-MV machines	1.5 cm below skin surface	Most malignant conditions; especially if deeply seated in the body
15-MV machines	3.0 cm below skin surface	
Particle beam therapy		
Cyclotrons (neutron beam therapy)	Increased uptake in fatty tissue	Late stage malignant disease; tumors that are large, anoxic, necrotic, and resistant to treatment

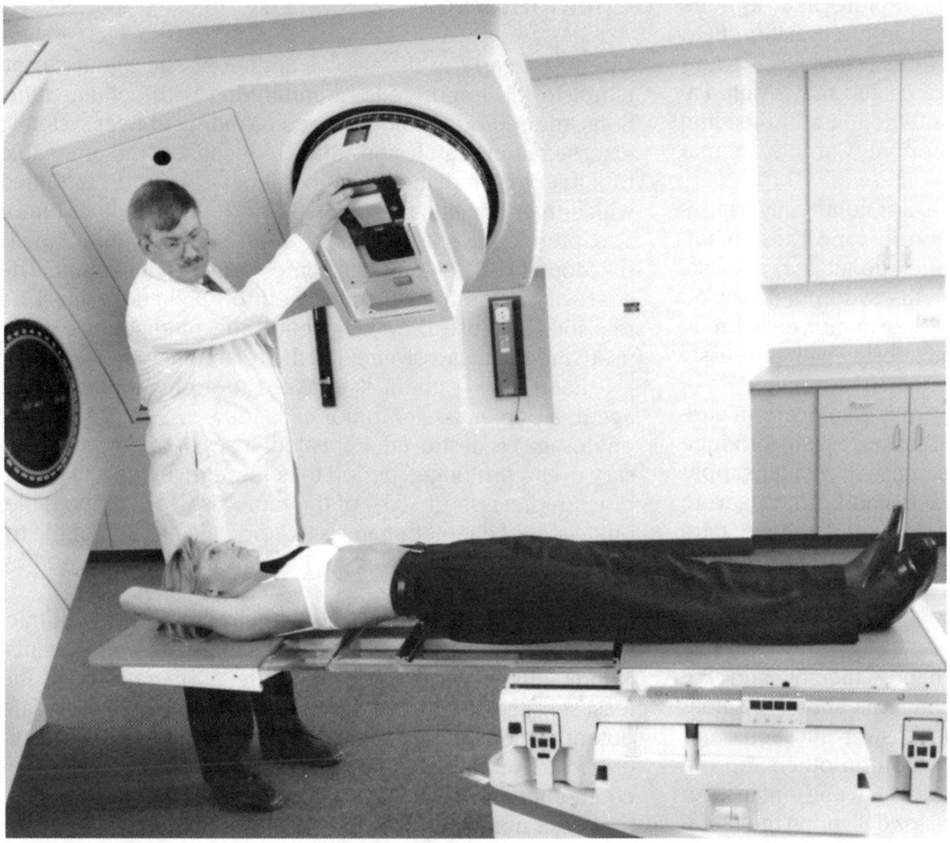

FIGURE 16-2. Mevatron, a linear electron accelerator used for radiotherapy. (Courtesy of Siemens Medical Laboratories, Inc.)

Interstitial implants may be temporary or permanent depending on the radioisotopes used.These implants usually consist of seeds, needles, wires, or small catheters positioned to provide a local radium source and are less frequently dislodged.

With internal radiation therapy, the further the tissue is from the radiation source, the less the dosage. This spares the noncancerous tissue from the radiation dose.

Patients receiving internal radiation emit radiation while the implant is in place. Principles of time, distance, and shielding must be used in planning care for these patients to minimize exposure of personnel to radiation. Safety precautions often used in caring for the patient receiving brachytherapy include assigning the person to a private room, providing appropriate notices about radiation safety precautions, having staff members wear dosimeter badges, making sure that pregnant staff members are not assigned to this patient's care, prohibiting visits by children or pregnant visitors, limiting visits from others to 30 minutes/day, and seeing that visitors maintain a 6-foot distance from the isotope source.

Radiation Dosage

The radiation dosage is dependent on the sensitivity of the target tissues to radiation and on the tumor size. The **lethal tumor dose** is defined as that dose that will eradicate 95% of the tumor yet preserve normal tissue.

The total radiation dose is delivered over several weeks to allow healthy tissue to repair and to achieve a greater cell kill by exposing more cells in the early S, G_2, or M phases of the cell cycle. Repeated radiation treatments over time (fractioned doses) also allow time for the periphery of the tumor to be reoxygenated repeatedly, as tumors shrink from the outside inward. This increases the radiosensitivity of the tumor, thus increasing tumor cell death.

Toxicity

Toxicity of radiation therapy is usually localized to the region being irradiated. Acute local reactions occur when normal cells in the treatment area are also destroyed and cellular death exceeds cellular regeneration. Body tissues most frequently affected are those that normally proliferate rapidly, such as the skin, the epithelial lining of the gastrointestinal tract including the oral cavity, and the bone marrow.

Alteration in skin integrity is a common effect and can include hair loss (alopecia), erythema, and shedding of skin (desquamation). Once treatments have been completed, reepithelialization occurs. Alterations in oral mucosal membranes secondary to radiation therapy include stomatitis, dryness of the mouth (xerostomia), change and loss of taste, and decreased salivation.

The entire gastrointestinal mucosa may be involved, and esophageal irritation with chest pain and dysphagia may result. Anorexia, nausea, vomiting, and diarrhea may occur if the stomach or colon is in the irradiated field. Symptoms subside and gastrointestinal reepithelialization occurs once treatments are complete.

Bone marrow cells proliferate rapidly, and if bone marrow–producing sites are included in the radiation field anemia, leukopenia (decreased white blood cells), and thrombocytopenia (a decrease in platelets) may result. Patients are then at increased risk for infection and bleeding until blood cell counts return to normal. Chronic anemia may occur.

Certain systemic side effects are also commonly experienced by patients receiving radiation therapy. These manifestations, which are generalized, include fatigue, malaise, headache, nausea, and vomiting. This syndrome may be secondary to substances released when tumor cells break down. The effects are temporary and subside with the cessation of treatments.

Late effects of radiation therapy may also occur in various body tissues. These effects are chronic, usually produce fibrotic changes secondary to a decreased vascular supply, and are irreversible. These late effects can be most severe when they involve vital organs such as the lungs, heart, central nervous system, and bladder.

Nursing Considerations

The patient who is receiving radiation therapy and the family often have questions and concerns about its safety. The nurse is often in a position to answer questions and allay fears about the effects of radiation on others, on the tumor, and on the patient's normal tissues and organs. An explanation of the actual procedure for delivering the radiation is provided to the patient and family, along with a description of the equipment to be used, the duration of the procedure (often minutes only), the possible need for immobilizing the patient during the procedure, and the absence of new sensations including pain during the procedure. If a radioactive implant is used, the patient is informed about the restrictions placed on visitors and health care personnel and other radiation precautions. Patients also need to understand their own role before, during, and after the procedure.

The nurse assesses the patient's skin, nutritional status, and general feeling of well-being. The skin and oral mucosa are assessed frequently for changes (particularly if radiation therapy is directed to these areas). The skin is protected from irritation, and the patient is advised to avoid using ointments, lotions, or powders on the area. Gentle oral hygiene is essential to remove debris, prevent irritation, and promote healing. If systemic changes such as weakness and fatigue occur, the patient may need assistance with activities of daily living and personal hygiene. Additionally, the nurse offers reassurance by explaining that these symptoms are a result of the treatment and do not represent deterioration or progression of the disease.

When a patient has a radioactive implant in place, it is important to take precautions to protect oneself and other personnel as well as the patient from the effects of radiation. Specific instructions are frequently provided by the radiation safety officer from the radiology department and usually include the maximal amount of time to be spent in the patient's room, shielding equipment to be used, and special precautions and actions to be taken if the implant is dislodged. Explaining the rationale for these precautions can keep the patient from feeling unduly isolated.

Chemotherapy

Chemotherapy is the use of antineoplastic agents to attempt to kill tumor cells by interfering with cellular functions and reproduction. It is used primarily to treat systemic disease rather than lesions that are localized and amenable to surgery or radiation. Chemotherapy may be combined with surgery or radiation therapy, or both, to reduce tumor size preoperatively, to destroy any remaining tumor cells postoperatively, or to treat some forms of leukemia. The goals of chemotherapy (cure, control, palliation) must be realistic, because they will define the medications to be used and the aggressiveness of the treatment plan.

Each time a tumor is exposed to a chemotherapeutic agent, a percentage of tumor cells (20% to 99%, depending on dosage) is destroyed. Repeated doses of drugs are necessary over a prolonged period to achieve regression of the tumor. Eradication of 100% of the tumor is nearly impossible, but a goal of chemotherapy is to eradicate enough of the tumor so that the remaining tumor cells can be destroyed by the body's immune system.

Actively proliferating cells within a tumor (growth fraction) are the most sensitive to chemotherapeutic agents. Nondividing cells capable of future proliferation are the least sensitive to antineoplastic drugs and consequently are potentially dangerous. They must be destroyed, however, to eradicate a malignancy completely. Repeated cycles of chemotherapy are used to kill more tumor cells by destroying these nondividing cells as they are signaled into active proliferation. These effects are related to the phases of the reproductive cycle of the cell—the cell cycle.

Reproduction of both healthy and malignant cells follows the cell cycle pattern (Fig. 16-3). The **cell cycle time** is the time required for one tissue cell to divide and reproduce into two identical daughter cells. The cell cycle of any cell has four distinct phases, each with a vital underlying function:

1. G_1 phase—RNA and protein synthesis occurs.
2. S phase—DNA synthesis occurs.
3. G_2 phase—premitotic phase; DNA synthesis is complete, mitotic spindle forms.
4. Mitosis—cell division occurs.

The G_0 phase, the resting or dormant phase of cells, can occur after mitosis and during the G_1 phase. In the G_0 phase are those dangerous cells that are not actively dividing but have the future potential for replication. The administration of certain chemotherapeutic agents (as well as administration of some other forms of therapy) is coordinated with the cell cycle.

Classification of Chemotherapeutic Agents

Certain chemotherapeutic agents (**cell cycle–specific drugs**) destroy cells in specific phases of the cell cycle. Most affect cells in the S phase by interfering with DNA and RNA synthesis. Others, such as the *vinca* or plant alkaloids, are specific to the M phase, where they halt mitotic spindle formation.

Those chemotherapeutic agents that act independently of the cell cycle phases are termed **cell cycle–nonspecific drugs**. These agents usually have a prolonged effect on cells,

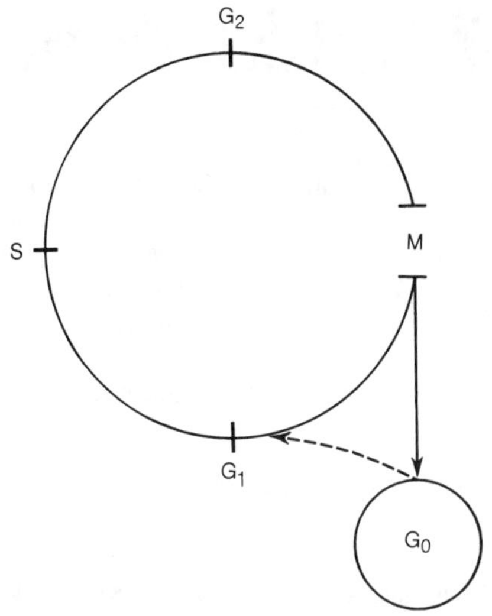

FIGURE 16-3. Phases of the cell cycle. The cycle represents the interval between the midpoint of mitosis to the subsequent end point in mitosis in a daughter cell. G_1 is the postmitotic phase during which RNA and protein synthesis is increased and cell growth occurs. G_0 is the resting or dormant phase of the cell cycle. The S phase represents synthesis of nucleic acids with chromosome replication in preparation for cell mitosis. During G_2, RNA and protein synthesis occurs as in G_1. (Porth CM. Pathophysiology: Concepts of Altered Health States, 4th ed. Philadelphia, JB Lippincott, 1994.)

leading to cellular damage or death. Many treatment plans combine cell cycle–specific and cell cycle–nonspecific drugs to increase the number of vulnerable tumor cells killed during a treatment period.

Chemotherapeutic agents are also classified according to various chemical groups, each with a different mechanism of action. These include the alkylating agents, nitrosoureas, antimetabolites, antitumor antibiotics, plant alkaloids, hormonal agents, and miscellaneous agents. The classification, mechanism of action, common drugs, cell-cycle specificity, and common side effects of antineoplastic agents are listed in Table 16-7. Chemotherapeutic agents from each category may be used to enhance the tumor cell kill during therapy by creating multiple cellular lesions. Combined drug therapy used must also include drugs of differing toxicities and with synergistic actions. Use of combination drug therapy also prevents development of drug-resistant mechanisms.

Research is continuing in an effort to find ways to combat the resistance of tumor cells to chemotherapeutic agents. Combining older drugs with other agents such as calcium channel blockers, leukovorin, hormones, or interferon has shown some benefit. Newer investigational agents are being studied for effectiveness in resistant tumor lines.

Investigational Drugs and Clinical Trials. Investigational antineoplastic drugs undergo thorough trials to test their toxicities and effectiveness. Before new chemotherapeutic agents are approved for clinical use in the treatment of cancer, they are subjected to rigorous and often lengthy evaluation to identify beneficial effects, side effects, and safety. Phase I clinical trials determine optimal drug dosing, scheduling, and toxicity. Phase II trials determine drug effectiveness with specific tumor types, and phase III clinical trials establish the effectiveness of new drug therapies as compared with conventional, established therapy.

Administration of Chemotherapeutic Agents

Routes of Administration. Chemotherapeutic drugs may be administered by topical, oral, intravenous, intramuscular, subcutaneous, arterial, intracavitary, and intrathecal routes. The route of administration is usually dependent on the type of drug, the required dose, and the type, location, and extent of tumor being treated.

Dosage. Dosage of antineoplastic agents is based primarily on the patient's total body surface area, previous response to chemotherapy or radiation therapy, major organ function, and physical performance status.

Extravasation. Special care must be taken whenever intravenous vesicant agents are administered. **Vesicant drugs** are those agents that, if deposited into the subcutaneous tissue (extravasated), cause tissue necrosis and damage to underlying tendons, nerves, and blood vessels. Although the complete mechanism of tissue destruction is unclear, it is known that the *p*H of many antineoplastic drugs is responsible for the severe inflammatory reaction as well as the binding ability of drugs to tissue DNA. Sloughing and ulceration of tissue may be so severe that skin grafting may be necessary. The full extent of tissue damage may take several weeks to become apparent. Drugs classified as vesicant agents include dactinomycin, daunorubicin, doxorubicin (Adriamycin), nitrogen mustard, mitomycin, vinblastine, vincristine, and vindesine.

Only specially trained physicians and nurses are to be involved in the administration of vesicants. Careful selection of peripheral veins, skilled venipuncture, and careful drug administration are essential. Indications of extravasation during drug administration include absence of blood return from the intravenous (IV) catheter; resistance to flow of intravenous fluid; and swelling, pain, or redness at the site. If extravasation is suspected, the drug administration is stopped immediately and ice is applied to the site (except for *vinca* alkaloid extravasation). The physician may aspirate any infiltrated drug from the tissues and inject a neutralizing solution into the area to reduce tissue damage. Selection of the neutralizing solution depends on the drug that is extravasated; examples of neutralizing solutions include sodium thiosulfate, hyaluronidase, and sodium bicarbonate. Recommendations and guidelines for management of vesicant extravasation have been issued by individual drug manufacturers, pharmacies, and the Oncology Nursing Society, and differ from one drug to the next.

When frequent, prolonged administration of vesicant antineoplastic agents is anticipated, right atrial Silastic catheters or venous access devices may be inserted. These devices promote safety during drug administration and reduce problems with access to the circulatory system (Figs. 16-4 and 16-5).

Toxicity

Toxicity associated with chemotherapy can be acute or chronic. Cells with rapid growth rates (*e.g.*, epithelium, bone marrow, hair follicles, sperm) are very susceptible to

TABLE 16-7 Classification, Actions, and Side Effects of Antineoplastic Agents

Category	Mechanism of Action	Common Drugs	Cell Cycle Specificity	Common Side Effects
Alkylating agents	Alter DNA structure by · Misreading of DNA code · Breaks in DNA molecule · Cross-linking of DNA strands	Amsacrine Nitrogen mustard Cyclophosphamide Ifosfamide Melphalan Chlorambucil Thiotepa Carboplatin Cisplatin Busulfan	Cell cycle nonspecific	Bone marrow suppression, nausea, vomiting, cystitis (cyclophosphamide and ifosfamide) stomatitis, alopecia, gonadal suppression; renal toxicity (Cisplatin)
Nitrosoureas	Similar to alkylating agents; cross blood–brain barrier	Carmustine (BCNU) Lomustine (CCNU) Semustine (methyl CCNU) Streptozocin	Cell cycle nonspecific	Delayed and cumulative myelosuppression, especially thrombocytopenia; nausea, vomiting
Antimetabolites	Interfere with the biosynthesis of metabolites/ nucleic acids necessary for RNA and DNA synthesis	Cytarabine 5-fluorouracil FUDR Methotrexate (MTX) Hydroxyurea 6-Mercaptopurine 6-Thioguanine 5-Azacytadine Pentostatin Leustatin Edatrexate	Cell cycle specific (S phase)	Nausea, vomiting, diarrhea, myelosuppression, proctitis, stomatitis, renal toxicity (MTX), hepatotoxicity.
Antitumor antibiotics	Interfere with DNA synthesis by binding DNA; prevent RNA synthesis	Dactinomycin Bleomycin Daunorubicin Idarubicin Plicamycin Mitomycin Mitoxantrone Doxorubicin (Adriamycin)	Cell cycle nonspecific	Bone marrow suppression, nausea, vomiting, alopecia, anorexia, cardiac toxicity (Daunorubicin, Doxorubicin)
Plant alkaloids/natural products	Cause metaphase arrest by inhibiting mitotic tubular formation (spindle); inhibit DNA and protein synthesis	Vincristine (VCR) Vinblastine Vindesine VP-16 VM-26 Taxol	Cell cycle specific (M phase)	Bone marrow suppression (mild with VCR), neuropathies (VCR), stomatitis Bradycardia, hypersensitivity reactions (taxol)
Hormonal agents	Bind to hormone receptor sites that alter cellular growth; block binding of estrogens to receptor sites (anti-estrogens); inhibit RNA synthesis	Androgens Estrogens Anti-estrogens Progesterone Steroids	Cell cycle nonspecific	Hypercalcemia, jaundice, increased appetite, masculinization, feminization, sodium and fluid retention, nausea, vomiting, hot flashes

(continued)

TABLE 16-7 *(continued)*

Category	Mechanism of Action	Common Drugs	Cell Cycle Specificity	Common Side Effects
Miscellaneous agents	Unknown; too complex to categorize	Asparaginase Procarbazine M-AMSA Hexamethylmelamine Dacarbazine (DTIC) Mitoxantrone Methyl-GAG	?	Anorexia, nausea, vomiting, myelosuppression, hepatotoxicity, anaphylaxis, hypotension, altered glucose metabolism

damage from these agents. Various body systems may also be affected by these drugs.

Gastrointestinal System. Nausea and vomiting are the most common side effects of chemotherapy and may persist for up to 24 hours after drug administration. The vomiting centers of the brain are stimulated by (1) stimulation of the receptors found in the chemoreceptor trigger zone (CTZ) of the medulla; (2) stimulation of peripheral autonomic pathways (gastrointestinal [GI] tract and pharynx); (3) stimulation of the vestibular pathways (inner-ear imbalances, labyrinth input); (4) cognitive stimulation (central nervous system disease, anticipatory nausea and vomiting); and (5) a combination of factors.

Drugs that can help minimize nausea and vomiting include serotonin blockers such as ondansetron (which block serotonin receptors of the CTZ), dopominergic blockers such as metoclopramide (Reglan) (which block dopamine receptors of the CTZ), phenothiazines, sedatives, steroids, and histamines, alone or in combination. Delayed nausea and vomiting which occur later than 48 to 72 hours after chemotherapy are troublesome for some patients. Antiemetic medications are often necessary for the first week at

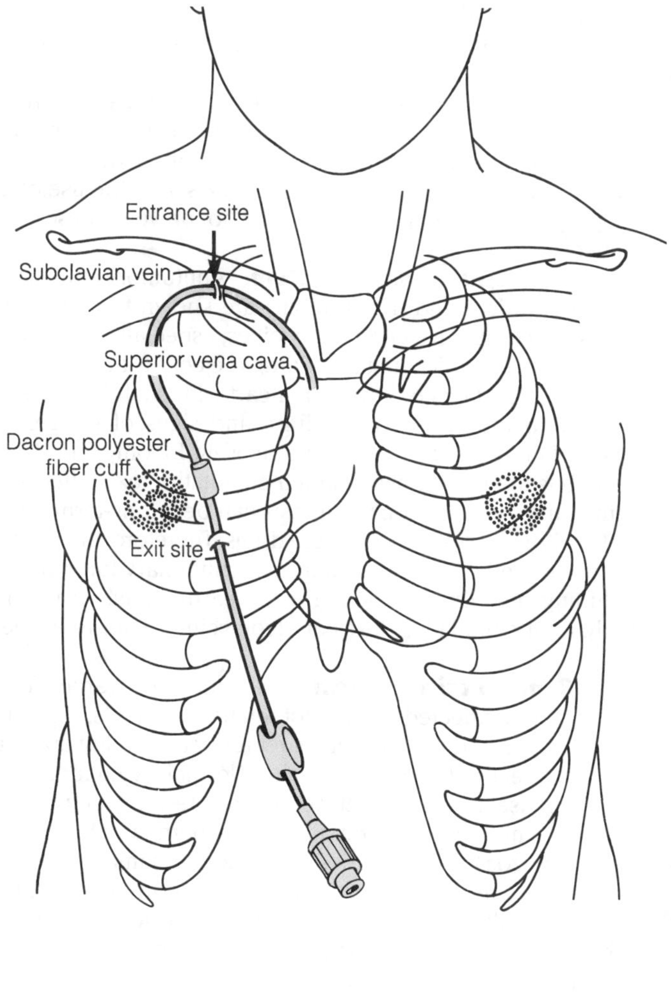

FIGURE 16-4. Right atrial catheter. The right atrial catheter is inserted into the subclavian vein and advanced until its tip is in the superior vena cava just above the right atrium. The proximal end is then tunneled from the entry site through the subcutaneous tissue of the chest wall and brought out through an exit site on the chest. The Dacron cuff helps to anchor the catheter in place and serves as a barrier to infection. (Redrawn from Viall CD. Your complete guide to central venous catheters. Nursing 1990 Feb; 20[2]:37.)

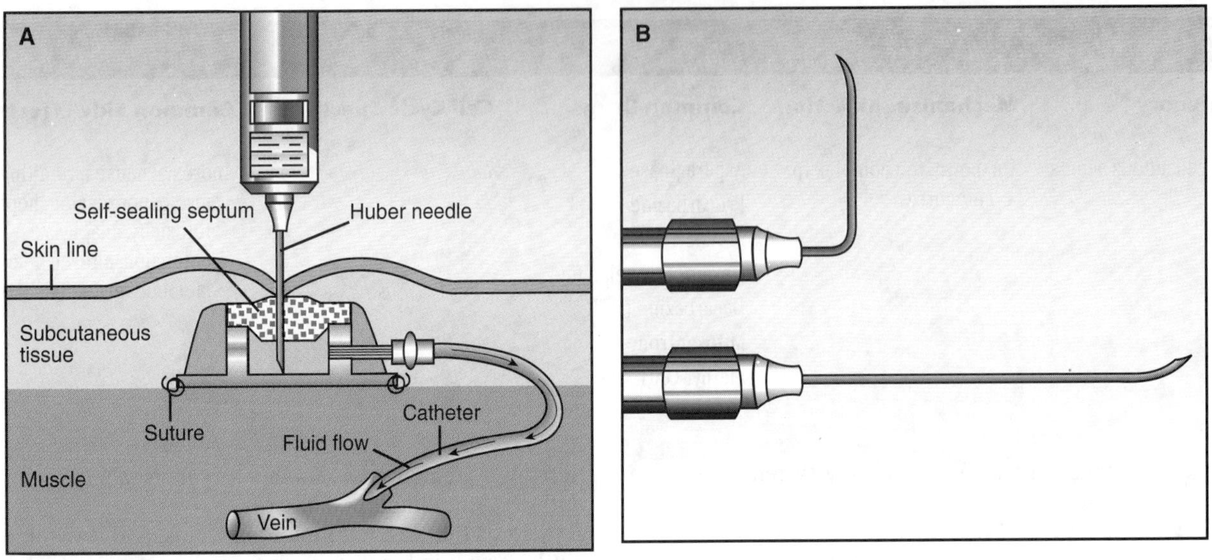

FIGURE 16-5. Implanted vascular access device. (**A**) A schematic diagram of an implanted vascular access device used for administration of medication, fluids, blood products and nutrition. The self-sealing septum permits repeated puncture by Huber needles without damage or leakage. (**B**) Two Huber needles used to enter the implanted vascular port. The 90-degree needle is used for top-entry ports for continuous infusions.

home following chemotherapy to minimize discomfort. Relaxation techniques and imagery can also help to decrease stimuli contributing to symptoms. Altering the patient's diet may reduce the frequency or severity of these symptoms.

Although the epithelium that lines the oral cavity quickly renews itself, its rapid rate of proliferation makes it susceptible to the effects of chemotherapy. As a result, stomatitis and anorexia are common. The entire gastrointestinal tract is susceptible to mucositis (inflammation of the mucosal lining), with diarrhea a common result. Antimetabolites and antitumor antibiotics are the major culprits in mucositis and other gastrointestinal symptoms.

Hematopoietic System. Most chemotherapeutic agents depress bone marrow function (myelosuppression), resulting in decreased production of blood cells. Myelosuppression decreases the number of white blood cells or leukocytes (leukopenia), red blood cells (anemia), and platelets or thrombocytes (thrombocytopenia) and increases the risk of infection and bleeding. Depression of these cells is the usual reason for limiting the dose of the chemotherapeutic drugs. Monitoring blood cell counts frequently is essential, as is protecting the patient from infection and injury, particularly while the blood cell counts are depressed.

Other agents called *colony-stimulating factors* (G-CSF, GM-CSF) are given following chemotherapy. These agents stimulate the bone marrow to produce white blood cells, especially neutrophils, at an accelerated rate, thus decreasing the duration of neutropenia. The colony-stimulating factors decrease the episodes of infection and the need for antibiotics and allow for more timely cycling of chemotherapy with less need to reduce the dosage.

Renal System. Chemotherapeutic agents can damage the kidneys because of their direct effects during excretion and the accumulation of end products after cell lysis. Cisplatin, methotrexate, and mitomycin are particularly toxic to the kidneys. Rapid tumor cell lysis after chemotherapy results in increased urinary excretion of uric acid, which can cause renal damage. In addition, intracellular contents are released into the circulation resulting in excessive levels of potassium and phosphates (hyperkalemia and hyperphosphatemia) and diminished levels of calcium (hypocalcemia). (Refer to page 313 for further discussion of tumor lysis syndrome.)

Monitoring blood urea nitrogen (BUN), serum creatinine, creatinine clearance, and serum electrolyte levels is essential. Adequate hydration, alkalinization of the urine to prevent formation of uric acid crystals, and the use of allopurinol are frequently indicated to prevent these side effects.

Cardiopulmonary System. Antitumor antibiotics (daunorubicin and doxorubicin) are known to cause irreversible cumulative cardiac toxicities, especially when total dosage reaches 550 mg/m^2. Cardiac ejection fraction (volume of blood ejected from the heart with each beat), electrocardiographic (ECG) tracings, and signs of congestive heart failure must be monitored closely. Bleomycin, BCNU, and busulfan are known for their cumulative toxic effects on lung function. Pulmonary fibrosis can be a long-term effect of prolonged dosage with these drugs. Therefore, the patient is monitored closely for changes in pulmonary function, including pulmonary function test measurements. Additionally, total cumulative doses of bleomycin are not to exceed 400 units.

Reproductive System. Testicular and ovarian function can be affected by chemotherapeutic agents, resulting in possible sterility. A woman's reproductive ability appears to be directly dependent on age. Normal ovulation, early menopause, or permanent sterility may result. Men may develop temporary or permanent azoospermia (absence of spermatozoa). Reproductive cells may be damaged during treatment and result in chromosomal abnormalities in offspring. Banking of sperm is recommended for men before treatments are initiated to protect against sterility or any mutagenic damage to sperm.

Patients and their partners need to be informed about potential changes in reproduction resulting from chemotherapy. However, patients and their partners are advised to use reliable methods of birth control while receiving chemotherapy and not to assume that sterility has resulted.

Neurologic System. The plant alkaloids, especially vincristine, can cause neurologic damage with repeated doses. Peripheral neuropathies, loss of deep tendon reflexes, and paralytic ileus may occur. These side effects are usually reversible and disappear after completion of chemotherapy. Cisplatin is also responsible for peripheral neuropathies and hearing loss due to damage to the acoustic nerve.

Nursing Considerations

The nurse has an important role in assessing and managing many of the problems experienced by the patient undergoing chemotherapy. Because of the systemic effects on normal as well as malignant cells, these problems are often widespread, affecting many body systems.

Fluid and Electrolytes. Anorexia, nausea, vomiting, altered taste, and diarrhea put the patient at risk for nutritional and fluid and electrolyte disturbances. Changes in the mucosa of the gastrointestinal tract may lead to irritation of the oral cavity and intestinal tract, further threatening the patient's nutritional status. Therefore, it is important for the nurse to assess the patient's nutritional and fluid and electrolyte status frequently and to use creative ways to encourage an adequate fluid and dietary intake.

Infection and Bleeding. Suppression of the bone marrow and immune system is an expected consequence of chemotherapy and frequently serves as a guide in determining appropriate chemotherapy dosage. However, this effect also increases the risk of anemia, infection, and bleeding disorders. Therefore, nursing assessment and care focus on identifying and modifying factors that further increase the patient's risk. Asepsis and gentle handling are indicated to prevent infection and trauma. Laboratory test results, particularly blood cell counts, are monitored closely. Untoward changes in blood test results and the occurrence of signs of infection and bleeding are reported promptly. The patient and family members are instructed about measures to prevent these problems at home. (See Nursing Care Plan 16-1 for detailed nursing care.)

Chemotherapy Administration. Local effects of the chemotherapeutic agent are also of concern. The patient is observed closely during its administration because of the risk and consequences of extravasation (particularly of vesicant agents or those that may produce tissue necrosis if deposited in the subcutaneous tissues). Local difficulties or problems with administration of chemotherapeutic agents are brought to the attention of the physician promptly so that corrective measures can be taken immediately to minimize local tissue damage.

Self Protection. Nurses involved in handling chemotherapeutic agents may be exposed to low doses of the drugs by direct contact, inhalation, and ingestion. Personnel repeatedly exposed to cytotoxic drugs have demonstrated mutagenic activity in their urine. Although not all mutagens are carcinogenic, they do have the ability to produce permanent inheritable changes in the genetic material of cells.

Although long-term studies of nurses handling chemotherapeutic agents have not been conducted, it is known that chemotherapeutic agents are associated with secondary formation of cancers and chromosome abnormalities. Nausea, vomiting, dizziness, alopecia, and nasal mucosal ulcerations have been reported in health care personnel who have handled chemotherapeutic agents.

Because of known and potential hazards associated with handling chemotherapy, the Occupational Safety and Health Administration (OSHA), Oncology Nursing Society (ONS), hospitals, and other health care agencies have developed specific precautions for those involved in the preparation and administration of chemotherapy.

The guidelines from these organizations regarding the preparation and handling of antineoplastic agents recommend the following:

1. Using a biologic safety cabinet for the preparation of all chemotherapy drugs
2. Using surgical latex gloves when handling drugs and the excretions of patients who received chemotherapy
3. Using disposable, long-sleeved gowns when preparing and administering chemotherapy drugs
4. Using Luer-Lok fittings on all intravenous tubing used to deliver chemotherapy
5. Disposing all equipment used in chemotherapy preparation and administration in appropriate, leak-proof, puncture-proof containers
6. Disposing all chemotherapy wastes as hazardous materials

When followed, these precautions greatly minimize the risk of exposure.

Bone Marrow Transplantation

Surgery, radiation therapy, and chemotherapy have greatly improved survival of cancer patients. Yet, many malignancies that originally respond to therapy continue to recur. This is true of both hematologic malignancies with disease of the bone marrow and also solid tumor malignancies treated with lower doses of anti-neoplastics to spare the bone marrow from larger, ablative doses of chemotherapy or radiation therapy. The role of bone marrow transplantation (BMT) for malignant as well as some nonmalignant diseases continues to grow. The long-term survival rate following BMT for malignant diseases is approximately 40% to 50%.

There are three types of BMT based on the source of donor tissue: (1) allogeneic (from an unrelated donor), (2) autologous (from self), and (3) syngeneic (from an identical twin).

Allogeneic BMT is used primarily for disease of the bone marrow and depends on the availability of a human leukocyte antigen (cell marker) matched donor, which greatly limits the number of transplants possible. If an allogeneic donor is found, approximately 1 to 2 liters of bone marrow must be harvested under general anesthesia. The recipient must undergo ablative doses of chemotherapy and possibly total body irradiation (TBI) to destroy all existing bone marrow and malignant disease. The harvested donor marrow is infused intravenously into the recipient and travels to sites in the body that produce bone marrow and establishes itself. This establishment of the new bone marrow is known as *engraftment*. Once engraftment is complete (2 to 4 weeks, sometimes longer), the new bone marrow becomes functional and begins producing red blood cells, white blood cells, and platelets.

Prior to engraftment, patients are at a high risk for infection, sepsis, and bleeding. Side effects of the high-dose chemotherapy and total body irradiation can be both acute and chronic. With acute side effects, patients experience nausea, vomiting, diarrhea, and severe stomatitis. With chronic side effects, patients may develop sterility, pulmonary dysfunction, cardiac dysfunction, and liver disease.

Patients are placed on immunosuppressant drugs such as cyclosporine or azathioprine (Imuran) to prevent graft-versus-host disease (GVHD). In allogenic transplants GVHD occurs when the T lymphocytes from the transplanted donor marrow mount an immune response against the recipient's tissues (skin, GI tract, liver). T lymphocytes respond in this manner because they view the recipient's tissue as being "foreign," immunologically differing from what they recognize as "self" in the donor. GVHD may occur acutely or chronically. The first 100 days following allogeneic transplant are critical days for bone marrow transplant patients until the immune system and blood making capacity (hematopoiesis) have recovered sufficiently to prevent infection and hemorrhage. Most acute side effects such as nausea, vomiting, and mucositis also resolve in the initial 100 days following transplantation.

Autologous BMT is considered for patients with disease of the bone marrow who do not have a suitable donor for allogeneic BMT and for those patients who have healthy bone marrow but require bone marrow ablative doses of chemotherapy to cure their aggressive malignancy.

Bone marrow is harvested from the patient for autologous BMT and preserved for reinfusion and, if necessary, treated to kill any malignant cells within the marrow. The patient is treated with ablative chemotherapy and possible total body irradiation to eradicate any remaining tumor. The patient's harvested bone marrow is reinfused following ablative treatment and engrafts. Until engraftment occurs in the bone marrow sites of the body, the patient is at high risk for infection, sepsis, and bleeding. Acute and chronic toxicities from chemotherapy and radiation therapy may be severe. No immunosuppressants are necessary following autologous BMT, because the patient did not receive foreign tissue.

Syngeneic BMT is the least common type of transplant because it requires an identical sibling for harvest. Obviously syngeneic transplants result in no marrow rejection because the donor is an identical tissue match to the recipient. The transplant and harvest process are the same with syngeneic transplants as with allogeneic transplants.

Nursing Considerations

Nursing care of the bone marrow transplant patient is very complex and demands a high level of skill. The success of BMT is greatly influenced by nursing care in the pre-transplant, transplant, and post-transplant periods.

Pre-transplant Care. All patients must undergo extensive pre-transplant evaluations to assess the current clinical status of the disease. Nutritional assessments, extensive physical examinations and organ function tests, as well as psychological evaluations are carried out. Blood work includes assessing past antigen exposure, such as with hepatitis virus, cytomegalovirus (CMV), herpes simplex virus (HSV), human immunodeficiency virus (HIV), and syphilis. The patient's social support systems and financial and insurance resources are also evaluated. Informed consent and patient education are vital.

Care During Treatment. Skilled nursing care is required during the treatment phase of BMT when high-dose chemotherapy and whole-body radiation is being administered. The acute toxicities of nausea, diarrhea, mucositis, and hemorrhagic cystitis will require constant nursing attention.

Through the period of bone marrow aplasia until engraftment of the new marrow occurs, patients are at high risk of dying from sepsis and bleeding. Infection may be bacterial, viral, fungal, or from protozoan sources. Renal complications arise from nephrotoxic chemotherapy drugs used in the conditioning regimen or to treat infection (amphotericin B, aminoglycosides). Tumor lysis syndrome or acute tubular necrosis also threatens patients following bone marrow transplant.

Graft-versus-host disease (GVHD) requires skillful nursing assessment to detect early GVHD effects to the spleen, liver, and gut. Veno-occlusive disease of the liver due to conditioning regimens used in BMT occurs in approximately 40% of patients and results in fluid retention, jaundice, abdominal pain, hepatomegaly, and encephalopathy. Pulmonary complications such as pulmonary edema, interstitial pneumonia, and other pneumonias often complicate the recovery after BMT.

Post-treatment Care. Ongoing nursing assessments in follow-up visits are essential to detect late effects of therapy in BMT patients. Late complications occur 100 days or later following BMT. Late effects include infections, such as varicella zoster infections. Restrictive pulmonary abnormalities and recurrent pneumonias may develop. Sterility often results. Chronic GVHD occurs involving the skin, liver, gut, esophagus, eye, lungs, joints, and vaginal mucosa. Cataracts often develop following total body irradiation.

Psychosocial assessments by nursing staff must be ongoing in this highly complex patient population. In addition to the stressors affecting patients at each phase of the transplant experience, marrow donors and family members also have unique psychosocial needs that must be addressed.

Other Nursing Concerns. Donors often experience mood alterations, decreased self-esteem, and guilt from feelings of failure. Family members must be educated and supported sufficiently to reduce anxiety and aid coping during this difficult time. Family members must also be assisted throughout this experience to maintain realistic expectations of themselves as well as those of the patient.

As BMT becomes more prevalent, many moral and ethical issues become apparent, including issues of informed consent, allocation of resources, and cost. Monitoring the quality of life in BMT patients is required to assist in prioritizing treatment options and decision-making about this option.

Hyperthermia

Hyperthermia (thermal therapy), the generation of temperatures greater than physiologic fever range (above 106.7°F or 41.5°C), has been used for many years to destroy tumors in human cancers. Research suggests that malignant cells are more sensitive than normal cells to the harmful effects of high temperatures for several reasons. Malignant cells lack the enzymes necessary to repair DNA and cell membranes damaged by elevated temperatures. These cells are deficient in enzymes that generate adenosine triphosphate (ATP), which are necessary for a normal cellular response to the increased metabolic demands that occur with hyperthermia. Most tumor cells lack an adequate blood supply to provide needed oxygen during periods of increased cellular demand, such as during hyperthermia. Cancerous tumors lack blood vessels of adequate size for dissipation of heat. Research also suggests that the body's immune system may be indirectly stimulated when hyperthermia is used.

Hyperthermia is most effective when used in combination with radiation therapy or chemotherapy. Hyperthermia and radiation therapy are thought to work well together because hypoxic tumor cells and cells in the S phase of the cell cycle are more heat-sensitive than radiosensitive; the addition of heat damages tumor cells so that they are unable to repair themselves after being damaged by radiation therapy. Hyperthermia is thought to alter cellular membrane permeability when used with chemotherapy, allowing for an increased uptake of the chemotherapeutic drug. Also, hyperthermia is thought to inhibit cellular repair processes, enhancing tumor death.

Heat can be produced by using radiowaves, ultrasound, microwaves, magnetic waves, hot water baths, or even hot wax immersions. Hyperthermia may be local or regional, or it may include the whole body.

Local or regional hyperthermia may be delivered to a cancerous extremity (for malignant melanoma) by regional perfusion, in which the affected extremity is isolated by a tourniquet and an extracorporeal circulator heats the blood flowing through the affected part. Hyperthermia probes may also be inserted around a tumor in a local area and attached to a heat source during the actual treatment period. Chemotherapeutic agents such as melphalan may also be heated and instilled into the regionally circulating blood. Local or regional hyperthermia may also include infusion of heated solutions into cancerous body organs. Whole-body hyperthermia to treat disseminated disease may be achieved by extracorporeal circulation, immersion of patients in heated water or paraffin, or enclosure in heated suits.

Side effects of hyperthermia treatments include skin burns and tissue damage, fatigue, hypotension, peripheral neuropathies, thrombophlebitis, nausea, vomiting, diarrhea, and electrolyte imbalances. Resistance to hyperthermia may develop during the treatment because cells adapt to repeated thermal insult. Research into the effectiveness of hyperthermia, methods of delivery, and side effects is ongoing.

Nursing Considerations

Although hyperthermia has been used for many years, many patients and their families are unfamiliar with this treatment for cancer. Consequently, they need explanations about the procedure, its goals, and its effects. The patient is assessed for side effects, and efforts are made to reduce their occurrence and severity. Local skin care at the site of the implanted hyperthermia probes is also required.

Photodynamic Therapy

Photodynamic therapy or phototherapy is an investigational cancer treatment that uses photosensitizing compounds such as Photofrin. When administered intravenously, this compound is retained in higher concentrations in malignant tissue than in normal tissue. This sensitizing compound is then activated by a light source, usually laser light, which penetrates body tissue. The light-activated compound then creates activated singlet oxygen molecules which are cytotoxic or harmful to body tissue cells. Because most Photofrin has been retained in malignant tissue, a more selective cytotoxicity can be achieved with minimal destruction to normal tissues.

Malignancies treated with phototherapy include endobronchial tumors, skin cancers, breast cancers, intraperitoneal tumors, and central nervous system malignancies. The major side effect of therapy is photosensitivity for 4 to 6 weeks after Photofrin administration. Patients must protect themselves from direct and indirect sunlight to prevent skin burns. Often local reactions in the area being treated are also noted. Liver and renal function should also be monitored for transient abnormalities. As with any investigational treatment, emotional support and education are vital to assist the patient and family through the treatment period.

Biologic Response Modifiers

Biologic response modifiers (BRMs) are agents or methods of treatment that can alter the immunologic relationship between the tumor and the cancer patient (host) to provide a therapeutic benefit. Although the mechanisms of action vary with each type of BRM, the goal is to destroy or stop the malignant growth. Over the years we have come to understand the role of the body's natural immune defenses against cancer. The basis of BRM treatment lies in the restoration, modification, stimulation, or augmentation of those natural immune defenses.

Nonspecific Agents

Some of the early investigations of the stimulation of the immune system involved nonspecific agents such as bacille Calmette–Guérin (**BCG**) and *Corynebacterium parvum.* These agents serve as antigens that stimulate an immune response when injected into the patient with the hope that the stimulated immune system will then eradicate malignant growths. Extensive animal and human investigations with BCG have yielded some promising results, especially in the treatment of malignant melanoma and colorectal cancer. It is considered to be a standard form of treatment for localized bladder cancer. The exact role of these agents, however, requires further investigation.

Monoclonal Antibodies

Monoclonal antibodies are another type of BRM that became available through recent technologic advances that enabled investigators to grow and produce specific antibodies for specific malignant cells. The production of monoclonal antibodies involves injecting tumor cells into mice and harvesting the antibodies produced by the immune systems of the mice. The antibodies are then infused into the cancer patient.

Preliminary investigations of monoclonal antibodies in the treatment of hematologic malignancies and solid tumors have had limited success. Currently, no monoclonal antibodies have Food and Drug Administration (FDA) approval for the treatment of cancer. Researchers are exploring the feasibility of conjugating or combining monoclonal antibodies with other substances such as radioactive materials, chemotherapy, hormones, lymphokines, and interferons. Immunoconjugate therapy combines multiple agents to enhance tumor destruction.

Monoclonal antibodies also are being used as aids in diagnostic evaluations. By attaching a radioactive substance to the monoclonal antibody, physicians are able to detect both primary and metastatic tumors through radiologic techniques.

Cytokines

Cytokines, substances produced by cells of the immune system to enhance the production and functioning of components of the immune system, are also the focus of cancer treatment research. Cytokines are grouped into families such as interferons, interleukins, colony-stimulating factors, and tumor necrosis factors.

Interferons (IFN) are examples of cytokines with both antiviral and antitumor properties. When stimulated, all nucleated cells are capable of producing these glycoproteins, which are classified according to their biologic and chemical properties: alpha-interferons are produced by leukocytes, beta-interferons are produced by fibroblasts, and gamma-interferons are produced by lymphocytes. The majority of clinical investigations have focused on the use of α-interferons. IFNs were first noted for their ability to inhibit viral infections.

Although the exact antitumor effects of IFNs have not been thoroughly established, it is thought that they either stimulate the immune system or assist in preventing tumor growth. IFNs enhance both lymphocyte and antibody production. They also facilitate the cytolytic or cell destruction role of macrophages and natural killer cells. Additionally, IFNs can inhibit cell multiplication by increasing the duration of various phases of the cell cycle.

The effects of IFN have been demonstrated in a variety of malignancies. Alpha-interferon is approved by the FDA for the treatment of hairy cell leukemia and Kaposi's sarcoma. Other positive responses have been seen in the treatment of hematologic malignancies, renal carcinomas, bladder cancer, and malignant melanoma. IFN is administered in several ways including subcutaneous, intramuscular, intravenous, and intracavitary routes. Further efforts are underway to establish the effectiveness of IFN as compared with other standard treatment regimens. The roles of beta and gamma IFN are also being explored.

Interleukins are a subgroup of cytokines known as *lymphokines* because they are produced by lymphocytes. Interleukin-2 (IL-2), is known to stimulate the production and activation of several different types of T-cell lymphocytes. In addition, IL-2 enhances the production of other types of cytokines. When combined with IL-2, the null lymphocyte (lymphocyte lacking T or B markers on the surface membrane) becomes a lymphokine-activated killer (LAK) cell capable of destroying cancer cells.

Clinical trials have combined infusions of both IL-2 and LAK cells in patients with cancers such as melanoma, sarcoma, and renal cell carcinoma. These trials are considered to be controversial by some clinicians because of the potential toxic effects of IL-2. The FDA has approved IL-2 as a treatment option for renal cell cancer in adults over the age of 18. Future trials will examine optimal dosing regimens, antitumor effects, and management of toxicities for IL-2. In addition, other interleukins such as IL-1, IL-3, IL-4, and IL-6 are being investigated for their potential roles in cancer treatment.

Colony-stimulating factors (CSFs) are hormone-like substances naturally produced by many cells within the immune system. CSFs of different types stimulate the production of all cells in the blood, including neutrophils, macrophages, monocytes, red blood cells, and platelets. Recent FDA approval of granulocyte-macrophage colony-stimulating factor (GM-CSF), granuloctye-colony stimulating factor (G-CSF), and erythropoietin has contributed significantly to the supportive care of patients with cancer.

These agents do not treat the underlying malignancy, but rather the negative effects of cancer therapies that adversely affect the bone marrow (myelotoxic), such as radiation and chemotherapy. Previously, the myelotoxic or bone marrow suppressive effects of chemotherapy have limited the doses of some chemotherapy agents and have contributed to the development of life-threatening infections.

GM-CSF is used in the treatment of neutropenia (limited number of neutrophils in the blood) associated with bone marrow transplantation. G-CSF is used to treat neutropenia associated with chemotherapy for solid tumor malignancies. Erythropoietin is used to treat anemia in cancer patients as well as anemia in dialysis patients with end-stage renal disease. Other growth factors such as macrophage colony-stimulating factor (M-CSF) and interleukin-3 (IL-3) are currently being investigated.

Tumor necrosis factor (TNF) is a cytokine naturally produced by macrophages. The exact role of TNF is still under investigation. *In vitro* studies have shown TNF to stimulate other cells of the immune response. In addition, it has demonstrated direct tumor killing activity in animal studies. Clinical trials with TNF for the treatment of melanoma, lung cancer, and renal cancer are currently underway.

Nursing Considerations

Patients receiving biologic response modifier (BRM) therapy have many of the same needs as other cancer patients undergoing more conventional therapies. However, for many patients who have failed to respond to standard treatment modalities and BRM therapy may be viewed as a last chance effort. Consequently, it is essential that the nurse assess the need for education, support, and guidance for both the patient and family and assist in planning and evaluating patient care. Some BRMs such as interferons (IFN) and granulocyte-colony stimulating factor (G-CSF) can be self administered by the patient or family in the home. Nurses teach patients and families, as needed, how to administer these agents through subcutaneous injections. Community and home health nurses are instrumental in helping with patient education and continued care in the home.

Nurses need to be familiar with each agent given and the potential adverse effects. Adverse effects, such as fever, myalgia, nausea, and vomiting as seen with interferon therapy, may not be life-threatening. However, nurses must be aware of the potential influences of these effects on the patient's quality of life. Other adverse effects may be life-threatening such as capillary leak syndrome, pulmonary edema, and hypotension, which are associated with IL-2 therapy. Nurses work very closely with physicians in assessing and managing potential toxicities of BRM therapy. Because of the investigational nature of many of these agents, the nurse will be administering them in a research setting. Accurate observations and careful documentation are essential components of the data collection process.

Gene Therapy

Gene therapy is a revolutionary approach to cancer treatment that is currently under investigation. This proposed therapy is based on the knowledge that many cancers may be the result of alterations in specific genes. Several different strategies for treating defective genes include replacing the dysfunctional genes with competent genes, inhibiting faulty genes, and introducing substances that will cause genes or cancer cells to self-destruct. Current clinical trials are investigating the potential role of gene therapy in the treatment of melanoma, renal, colon, breast, and brain cancers. Although currently gene therapy is investigational, researchers predict it will have a profound impact on medical and health care in the 21st century.

Clinical trials with gene therapy are similar to other investigational trials with chemotherapy or biologic response modifiers (BRMs) because patients participating are most often those who have not responded to standard forms of treatment. Gene therapy may be viewed as a last chance effort by the patient and family. Patients participating in preliminary clinical trials are fully informed about the experimental nature of the drugs that they receive. Although every hope is maintained that the investigational agents will effectively treat the disease, the primary purpose of early phase trials is to gather information concerning maximal tolerated doses, adverse side effects, and effects of the drugs on tumor growth. The physical and emotional needs of patients in clinical trials are addressed as with other patients who receive standard forms of cancer treatment.

Mental Imagery Techniques

Attitude and stress levels are thought to play a role in improving one's physiologic responses to fighting cancer. Mental imagery, relaxation techniques, and stress reduction measures are advocated often in conjunction with conventional treatment to assist in treating cancer.

Unproven/Unconventional Methods

A diagnosis of cancer evokes many emotions in patients and families including feelings of fear, frustration, and loss of control. Despite increasing 5-year survival rates, at least 20% to 50% of patients use or seriously consider using some form of unconventional treatment. Hopelessness, desperation, unmet needs, ignorance, and family or social pressures are major factors that motivate patients to seek unconventional methods of treatment and allow them to fall prey to deceptive practices and quackery.

Caring for patients who choose unconventional methods may place members of the health care team in difficult situations professionally, legally, and ethically. Nurses must keep in mind those ethical principles that help guide professional practice such as autonomy, beneficence, non-maleficence, and justice.

Unconventional treatments have not demonstrated scientifically, in an objective, reproducible method, the ability to cure or control cancer. In addition to being ineffective, some unconventional treatments may also be toxic to patients and incur costs to patients and families in thousands of dollars.

Most unproven cancer treatments can be categorized as machines and devices, drugs and biologicals, metabolic and dietary regimens, or mystical and spiritual approaches.

Machines and Devices. Electrical gadgets and devices are commonly reputed to cure cancers. Most are operated by persons with questionable training who report incredulous success stories. Such machines are often decorated with elaborate lights and dials and produce vibrations or other sensations of currents or energy.

Drugs and Biologicals. Medicinal agents, herbs, proteins, megavitamins, immune therapy, vaccines, enzymes, and sera have been frequent components of fraudulent cancer therapy. These agents have included oral and external medications derived from weeds, flowers, and herbs and the blood and urine of patients and animals.

Metabolic and Dietary Regimens. Metabolic and dietary regimens emphasize the ingestion of only natural substances to purify the body and retard cancerous growth. These regimens include the grape diet, the carrot juice diet, coffee enemas, and raw liver intake. Laetrile (vitamin B_{17}, amygdalin), one of the best-known forms of cancer quackery, was advocated as an agent to kill tumor cells by releasing cyanide, which is especially toxic to malignant cells. The National Cancer Institute, in response to public demand, investigated the effects of laetrile and reported no therapeutic benefits with its use. Many toxic effects (cyanide poisoning, fever, rash, headache, vomiting, diarrhea, and hypotension) were reported. Macrobiotic diets also have been advocated as a cancer treatment to reestablish balance between the major forces in the universe, yin and yang. Persons adhering to macrobiotic diets tend to develop vitamin, mineral, and protein deficiencies; experience additional weight loss due to decreased calorie intake; and achieve no therapeutic benefits from the dietary manipulation.

Mystical and Spiritual Approaches. Mystical or spiritual approaches to cancer therapy include such techniques as psychic surgery, faith healing, "laying on of hands," and invocation of mystical universal powers to kill cancerous growths. These techniques are difficult to disclaim because they are based on faith.

Nursing Considerations

A trusting relationship, supportive care, and promotion of hope in the patient and family are the most effective means of protecting them from fraudulent therapy and questionable claims of cancer cures. Truthful responses given in a nonjudgmental manner to questions and inquiries about unproven methods of cancer treatments may alleviate the fear and guilt on the part of the patient and family that they are not "doing everything" to obtain a cure. Characteristics common to fraudulent therapy may be shared with patients and their families so that they are informed and cautious in evaluating other forms of "therapy."

Nursing Care of the Patient With Cancer

The outlook for patients with cancer has greatly improved because of scientific and technological advances. However, as a result of the underlying malignancy or various treatment modalities, the patient with cancer may experience a variety of secondary problems, such as infection, reduced white cell counts, bleeding, skin problems, nutritional problems, pain, fatigue, and psychological stress. Regardless of the type of cancer treatment used, or prognosis, many patients with cancer are susceptible to these problems and complications. An important role of the nurse on the oncology team is to assess the patient for these problems and complications.

❑ *NURSING PROCESS*
The Patient With Cancer

Assessment

Infection. At all stages of cancer, the patient is assessed for those factors that can promote infection. Infection is the leading cause of death in the oncology population. Factors predisposing patients to infection are summarized in Table 16-8. The nurse monitors laboratory studies, particularly the complete blood cell count, to detect early changes in white blood cells. Common sites of infection, such as the pharynx, skin, perianal area, urinary tract, and respiratory tract, are assessed frequently. However, it is important to keep in mind that the typical signs of infection (fever, swelling, redness, drainage, and pain) may be absent in the immunosuppressed patient. The patient is monitored for sepsis, particularly if invasive catheters or infusion lines are in place.

White Blood Count. The functions of the white blood cells are often impaired in cancer patients. A decrease in circulating white blood cells (WBCs) is referred to as **leukopenia** or **granulocytopenia**.

There are three types of WBCs: neutrophils, basophils, and eosinophils. The neutrophils, totaling 60% to 70% of all the body's WBCs, play a major role in combating infection by engulfing and destroying infective agents, a process called *phagocytosis*. Both the total WBC count and concentration of neutrophils are important in determining the patient's ability to fight infection.

A differential count supplies the relative numbers of the various types of WBCs and permits tabulation of polymorphonuclear neutrophils (mature neutrophils, reported as "polys," PMNs, or "segs") and immature forms of neutrophils (reported as bands, metamyelocytes, and "stabs"). These numbers are compiled and reported as the absolute neutrophil count. **Neutropenia**, an abnormally low absolute neutrophil count, is associated with an increased risk of infection. The risk of infection rises as the absolute neutrophil count decreases and persists.

Bleeding. The cancer patient is also monitored for factors that may contribute to bleeding. These include bone marrow suppression from radiation, chemotherapy, and other drugs that interfere with coagulation and platelet functioning such as aspirin, dipyridamole (Persantine), heparin, or warfarin. Common sites assessed for bleeding include skin and mucous membranes; the intestinal, urinary, and respiratory tracts; and the brain. Gross hemorrhage as well as blood in the stools, urine, sputum or vomitus (melena, hematuria, hemoptysis, hematemesis), oozing at injection sites, bruising (ecchymosis), petechiae, and changes in mental status are monitored and reported.

Skin Problems. Skin and tissue integrity is at risk in cancer patients because of the effects of chemotherapy, radiation therapy, surgery, and invasive procedures carried out for diagnosis and therapy. As part of the assessment, the nurse identifies which of these predisposing factors are present and assesses the patient for other risk factors, including nutritional deficits, bowel and bladder incontinence, immobility, immunosuppression, and changes related to aging. Skin lesions or ulceration secondary to the tumor is noted. Alterations in tissue integrity throughout the GI tract are particularly bothersome to the patient. The oral mucous membranes and the appearance of lesions are noted, as is their effect on the patient's nutritional status and level of comfort.

Hair loss (alopecia) is another form of tissue disruption common to cancer patients who receive radiation therapy or chemotherapy. In addition to noting hair loss, the nurse also assesses the psychological impact of this side effect on the patient and the family.

Nutritional Concerns. Assessment of the patient's *nutritional concerns* is an important part of the nurse's role. Impaired nutritional status may contribute to the progression of the disease, immune incompetence, increased incidence of infection, delayed tissue repair, diminished functional ability, and decreased capacity to continue antineoplastic treatments. Alterations in nutritional status and **weight loss** may be secondary to decreased protein and calorie intake, the effect of a local tumor, systemic disease, side effects of the treatment, or the emotional status of the patient.

The patient's weight and caloric intake are monitored daily. Other information obtained through assessment includes diet history, any episodes of anorexia, changes in appetite, situations and foods that aggravate or relieve the anorexia, and medication history. Difficulty in chewing or swallowing is determined and the occurrence of nausea, vomiting, or diarrhea is noted.

Clinical and laboratory data useful in assessing the patient's nutritional status include anthropometric measurements (triceps skin fold and mid upper arm circumference), serum protein levels (albumin and transferrin), lymphocyte count, skin response to intradermal injection of antigens, hemoglobin levels, hematocrit, urinary creatinine levels, and serum iron levels.

TABLE 16-8 Factors Predisposing Cancer Patients to Infection

Factors	Underlying Mechanisms
1. Impaired skin and mucous membrane integrity	• Loss of body's first line of defense against invading organisms.
2. Chemotherapy	• Many agents cause suppression of bone marrow, resulting in decreased production and function of white blood cells. Chemotherapy agents that cause mucositis impair skin and mucous membrane integrity. Organ damage associated with certain agents may also predispose patients to infection. Organ damage such as pulmonary fibrosis or cardiomyopathy that is associated with certain agents may also predispose patients to infection.
3. Radiation therapy	• Radiation involving sites of bone marrow production may result in bone marrow suppression. May also lead to impaired tissue integrity.
4. Biologic response modifiers	• Some BRMs may cause bone marrow suppression and organ dysfunction.
5. Malignancy	• Malignant cells may infiltrate the bone marrow and interfere with production of white blood cells and lymphocytes. Hematologic malignancies (leukemias and lymphomas) are associated with impaired function and production of blood cells
6. Malnutrition	• Results in impaired function and production of cells of the immune response. May contribute to impaired skin integrity.
7. Medications	• Antibiotics disturb the balance of normal flora, allowing them to become pathogenic. This process occurs most commonly in the gastrointestinal tract. Corticosteroids and nonsteroidal anti-inflammatory drugs mask the inflammatory response.
8. Urinary catheter	• Creates port and mechanism of entry for organisms.
9. Intravenous catheter	• Results in impaired skin integrity and site of entry for organisms.
10. Other invasive procedures (surgery, paracentesis, thoracentesis, drainage tubes, endoscopies, mechanical ventilation)	• Creates port of entry and possible introduction of exogenous organisms into the system.
11. Contaminated equipment	• Environmental objects such as stagnant water in oxygen equipment are associated with growth of microorganisms.
12. Age	• Increasing age associated with declining organ function. Also associated with decreased production and functioning of the cells of the immune system.
13. Chronic illness	• Associated with impaired organ function and altered immune responses.
14. Prolonged hospitalization	• Allows increased exposure to nosocomial infection and colonization of new organisms.

Pain. Pain and discomfort in cancer may be related to the underlying malignancy, to pressure exerted by the tumor, to diagnostic testing procedures, or to many of the cancer treatments that may be used. As in any other situation involving pain, cancer pain is affected by both physical and psychosocial influences.

In addition to assessing the source and site of pain, the nurse also assesses those factors that increase the patient's perception of pain, such as fear and apprehension, fatigue, anger, and social isolation. Assessment scales for pain (see Chapter 13) are useful in assessing the patient's pain level before pain-relieving interventions are instituted and in evaluating their effectiveness in relieving pain.

Fatigue. Fatigue is often a chronic problem for individuals with cancer. The nurse assesses for feelings of weariness, weakness, lack of energy, and inability to carry out necessary and valued daily functions. Chronic fatigue may be characterized by lack of interest in usual activities, lack of motivation, and inability to concentrate. In addition, patients often do not say much and respond slowly when spoken to and appear pale with relaxed facial musculature. The nurse assesses physiologic and psychological stressors that can contribute to fatigue. Pain, nausea, dyspnea, constipation, fear, and anxiety may be associated with fatigue.

Psychosocial Status. Assessment of the cancer patient is not limited to the physiologic changes that may occur in the course of the disease. It also focuses on the patient's *psychologic and mental status* as the patient and the family face this life-threatening experience, unpleasant diagnostic tests and treatment modalities, and progression of disease. The patient's mood and emotional reaction to the results of diagnostic testing and prognosis are assessed, along with evidence that the patient is progressing through the stages of grief, and is able to talk about the diagnosis and prognosis with the family.

Body Image. Cancer patients are forced to cope with many *assaults to body image* throughout the course of disease and treatment. Entry into the health care system is often accompanied by depersonalization. Threats to self-concept are enormous as patients face the realization of illness, possible disability, and death. Many cancer patients are forced to alter their lifestyles to accommodate treatments or because of the disease pathology. Priorities and value systems are often forced to change when body image is threatened and physical characteristics become less important. Disfiguring surgery, hair loss, cachexia (emaciation), skin changes, altered communication patterns, and sexual dysfunction are some of the devastating results of cancer and its treatment that may threaten the patient's self-esteem and body image. During assessment, these potential threats are identified, as is the patient's ability to cope with these changes.

Diagnosis

Nursing Diagnoses

Based on the assessment data, nursing diagnoses of the patient with cancer may include the following:

- Impaired tissue integrity related to the effects of treatment and the disease
- Alterations in nutrition: less than body requirements related to anorexia and gastrointestinal changes
- Pain and discomfort related to disease and treatment effects
- Fatigue related to physical and psychological stressors
- Grieving related to anticipated loss and altered role function
- Body image disturbance related to changes in appearance and role functions

Collaborative Problems/Potential Complications

Based on the assessment data, potential complications that may develop include:

- Infection and sepsis
- Hemorrhage

(See pages 309–313, Oncologic Emergencies, for discussion of additional potential complications.)

Planning and Implementation

Goals. The major goals of the patient may include maintenance of tissue integrity, maintenance of nutrition, relief of pain, relief of fatigue, effective progression through the grieving process, improved body image, and absence of complications.

Nursing Interventions

Maintaining Tissue Integrity. The person with cancer is at risk for developing a variety of skin and mucous membrane impairments. The nurse in all health care settings is in an ideal position to assess and assist the patient and family in the management of these problems. Some of the most frequently encountered disturbances include skin and tissue reactions to radiation therapy, stomatitis, alopecia, and metastatic skin lesions.

The patient who is experiencing skin and tissue reactions to radiation therapy requires careful skin care to prevent further skin irritation, drying, and damage. The skin over the affected area is handled gently; rubbing and use of hot or cold water, soaps, powders, lotions, and cosmetics are avoided. Trauma to the area is prevented by using loosely fitting clothes that do not constrict, irritate, or rub the affected area. If blistering occurs, care is taken not to disrupt the blisters, thus, reducing the risk of introducing bacteria. Aseptic wound care is indicated to minimize the risk of infection and sepsis.

Stomatitis. Stomatitis is an inflammatory response of the oral tissues that most often develops within 5 to 14 days following the administration of certain chemotherapeutic agents such as doxorubicin and 5-fluorouracil. It may also occur with irradiation to the head and neck area. Stomatitis may be characterized by mild redness (erythema) and edema or, if severe, by painful ulcerations, bleeding, and secondary infection. In very severe cases of stomatitis, chemotherapy or radiation may be temporarily halted until the inflammation decreases.

As a result of normal everyday wear and tear, the epithelial cells that line the oral cavity undergo rapid turnover and slough off routinely. Chemotherapy and irradiation interfere with the body's ability to replace those cells. An inflammatory response develops as denuded areas appear in the oral cavity. Myelosuppression (bone marrow depression) as a result of the underlying malignancy or its treatment predisposes the patient to oral bleeding and infection. Pain associated with ulcerated oral tissues can significantly interfere with nutritional intake, communication, and a willingness to maintain oral hygiene. Soft-bristled toothbrushes and nonabrasive toothpaste prevent or reduce the trauma to the oral mucosa. Oral rinses with saline may be necessary for patients who cannot tolerate a toothbrush. Foods that are difficult to chew or too hot or too spicy are avoided to reduce further trauma. The patient's lips are lubricated to keep the tissues from becoming dry and cracked. Topical antifungal agents and anesthetics may be prescribed to promote healing and minimize discomfort. The patient who experiences severe pain and discomfort with stomatitis requires systemic analgesics and is encouraged and helped to use these prescribed agents and to maintain an adequate fluid and food intake. In some instances parenteral hydration and nutrition are needed.

Alopecia. The temporary or permanent thinning or complete loss of hair, referred to as *alopecia*, is a potential adverse effect of certain forms of radiation therapy and several chemotherapeutic agents. The extent of alopecia depends on the dose and duration of therapy. These treatment modalities cause alopecia by damaging stem cells and hair follicles. As a result, the hair is brittle and may fall out or break off at the surface of the scalp. Loss of other body hair is less frequent.

Many health professionals view hair loss as a minor problem when compared with the potential life-threatening consequences of the underlying malignancy. For many patients, however, hair loss poses a major threat to body image, arousing feelings of anxiety, sadness, anger, rejection, ridicule, and isolation. To patients and families, hair loss can serve as a constant reminder of cancer interference with coping abilities, interpersonal relationships, and sexuality.

The nurse's role is to provide information about alopecia and to assist the patient and family in coping with hair loss and changes in body image. The patient is encouraged to acquire a wig or hairpiece before hair loss occurs so that the replacement matches the patient's own hair. Use of attractive scarves and hats may make the patient feel less conspicuous. It is frequently of some comfort to patients that the hair usually begins to grow again after completion of the chemotherapy; however, the color and texture of the new hair may have changed.

Malignant Skin Lesions. Skin lesions may occur with local extension of the tumor or embolization of the tumor into the epithelium and its surrounding lymph and blood vessels. Secondary growth of cancer cells into the skin may result in redness (erythematous areas) or can progress to wounds involving tissue necrosis and infection. The most extensive lesions tend to disintegrate and are purulent and malodorous. In addition, these lesions are a source of considerable pain and discomfort. Although this type of wound is most often associated with breast cancer and head and neck cancers, it can also accompany lymphoma, leukemia, melanoma, and cancers of the lung, uterus, kidney, colon, and bladder. The development of severe skin lesions is usually considered to be a poor prognostic sign for expected length of survival.

Ulcerating skin lesions usually indicate the presence of widely disseminated disease. Therefore, eradicating the problem is usually not possible. The management of these lesions becomes a nursing priority. Nursing care includes carefully assessing and cleansing the skin, reducing superficial bacterial flora, controlling bleeding, reducing odor, and protecting against pain and further trauma to the skin. The patient and family require assistance and guidance to care for these skin lesions at home. Referral to a community health nurse is indicated to provide assistance and evaluation of wound care at home.

Maintaining Nutritional Status. Most cancer patients experience some degree of weight loss during their illness. Anorexia, malabsorption, and cachexia are examples of nutritional problems commonly seen in cancer patients.

Anorexia. There are many theories about the cause of anorexia in the cancer patient. Alterations in taste, manifested by increased salty, sour, and metallic taste and altered responses to sweet and bitter tastes lead to decreased appetite, decreased nutritional intake, and protein-calorie malnutrition in the cancer patient. Taste alterations may be caused by deficiencies of minerals such as zinc, increases in circulating amino acids and cellular metabolites, or the administration of chemotherapeutic agents. Patients undergoing radiation therapy to the head and neck may experience "mouth blindness," which is a severe impairment of taste. Alterations in the sense of smell also alter taste, which is a common experience of patients with head and neck cancers. Anorexia may occur because the person feels full after eating only a small amount of food. This sense of fullness occurs secondary to a decrease in digestive enzymes, abnormalities in the metabolism of glucose and triglycerides, and prolonged stimulation of gastric volume receptors which convey the feelings of being full. Psychologic distress such as fear, pain, depression, and isolation throughout illness may also have a negative impact on appetite. The person may also have developed an aversion to food because of nausea and vomiting following treatment.

Malabsorption. Many cancer patients are unable to absorb nutrients from the gastrointestinal system as a result of tumor activity and cancer treatment. Tumors can affect the gastrointestinal activity in several ways. They may impair enzyme production or create fistulas. They secrete hormones and enzymes such as gastrin, which leads to increased gastrointestinal irritation, peptic ulcer disease, and decreased fat digestion. They also interfere with protein digestion. Chemotherapy and radiation can irritate and damage mucosal cells of the bowel, inhibiting absorption. Radiation therapy can cause sclerosis of the blood vessels in the bowel and fibrotic changes in the gastrointestinal tissue. Surgical intervention may change peristaltic patterns, alter gastrointestinal secretions, and reduce the absorptive surfaces of the gastrointestinal mucosa, all leading to malabsorption.

Cachexia. Cachexia (wasting syndrome) is common in the cancer patient, especially in advanced disease states. Cancer cachexia is related to inadequate nutritional intake along with increasing metabolic demand, increased energy expenditure due to anaerobic metabolism of the tumor, impaired glucose metabolism, competition of the tumor cells for nutrients, altered lipid metabolism, and a suppressed appetite. It is characterized by loss of body weight, adipose tissue, visceral protein, and skeletal muscle.

Food should be prepared in ways to make it look and taste appealing. Unpleasant smells and unappetizing looking food are avoided. Family members are included in the dietary plan of care to encourage adequate food intake. The patient's preferences as well as physiologic and metabolic requirements are considered in selecting foods. Small, frequent meals are provided with additional supplements between meals. Oral hygiene and pain relief measures are offered before mealtime to make meals more pleasant.

If malabsorption is a problem, enzyme and vitamin replacement may be instituted, along with changing the feeding schedule, using simple diets, and relieving diarrhea. If malabsorption is severe, total parenteral nutrition (TPN) may be necessary.

TPN can be administered in several ways. A long-term venous access device, such as a right atrial Silastic catheter, may be used as shown in Figure 16-4. Another route is through an implanted venous port (Fig. 16-5) or through a peripherally inserted central catheter (PICC) (Fig. 16-6). The nurse teaches the patient and family how to care for venous access devices and how to administer TPN. Community health nurses are often called on to assist patients in administering TPN in the home.

Interventions to reduce cachexia usually do not prolong survival but may improve the patient's quality of life. Before invasive nutritional strategies are instituted, the nurse should assess the patient carefully and discuss the options with the family. Creative dietary therapies, enteral (tube) feedings, or TPN may be chosen to deliver nourishment. Nursing care is also directed toward preventing trauma, infection, and other complications that increase metabolic demands.

Relieving Pain. It is estimated that 60% to 96% of all individuals with progressive malignant disease experience pain.

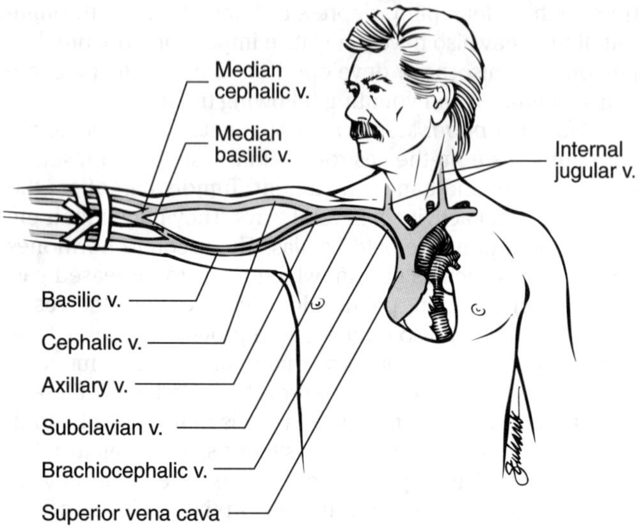

FIGURE 16-6. The venous anatomy of the upper extremity and thorax. Peripherally inserted central catheter (PICC) lines are inserted into the cephalic or basilic veins and advanced to the axillary, subclavian, or brachiocephalic veins or the superior vena cava.

Although patients with cancer may have acute pain, their pain is more frequently characterized as chronic. (For a more detailed discussion of pain, see Chapter 13.) As in other situations involving pain, the experience of cancer pain is influenced by both physical and psychosocial factors.

Malignancies can cause pain in a variety of ways. Bone destruction as a result of tumor invasion is one of the most devastating sources of pain. Bone involvement is seen commonly in multiple myeloma and cancers of the breast and prostate. Infiltration or compression of nerves can cause pain that is described as sharp and burning. Vertebral metastasis involving spinal nerves may occur with breast and lung cancer. Tumors causing lymphatic or venous obstruction may lead to a dull, throbbing type of pain. This is often associated with lymphoma or Kaposi's sarcoma. Ischemic pain results from any tumor that occludes arterial circulation. Obstruction is often associated with colon cancer. Patients with intestinal obstruction often complain of pain that is dull and poorly localized. Finally, tumors invading skin or mucous membranes may cause pain associated with inflammation, ulceration, infection, and tissue necrosis; this is common in patients with progressive head and neck malignancies and Kaposi's sarcoma.

Pain is also associated with various cancer treatment modalities. Acute pain is linked with trauma that results from surgical procedures. Some chemotherapeutic agents cause tissue necrosis, peripheral neuropathies, and stomatitis that are potential sources of pain. Radiation therapy can cause inflammation of the skin or irradiated organs.

In today's society, most people expect pain to disappear or resolve quickly, and in fact it usually does. Although it is controllable, cancer pain is often irreversible and not quickly resolved. For many patients, pain is a signal that the tumor is growing and that death is pending. As the patient anticipates the pain and becomes more anxious, pain perception is heightened, producing fear and additional pain. Chronic cancer pain, then, can be best described as a cycle progressing from pain to anxiety to fear and back to pain again.

Pain tolerance, the point past which pain can no longer be tolerated, varies among people. Pain tolerance is decreased by fatigue, anxiety, fear of death, anger, powerlessness, social isolation, changes in role identity, loss of independence, and past experiences. Tolerance to pain is enhanced by adequate rest and sleep, diversion, mood elevation, empathy, and medications such as antidepressants, antianxiety agents, and analgesics.

Inadequate pain management, which occurs all too frequently, is most often the result of misconceptions about pain assessment and pharmacologic interventions on the part of patients, families, and health care providers. Successful management of cancer pain is based on a thorough and objective pain assessment that examines physical, psychosocial, environmental, and spiritual factors. A multidisciplinary team effort is essential to determine the optimal approach for managing the patient's pain. Unlike instances of chronic nonmalignant pain, systemic analgesics play a central role in managing cancer pain.

The World Health Organization advocates a "3-Step Ladder" approach for treating cancer pain (Fig. 16-7). Analgesics are administered based on the patient's level of pain. Non-opioids (*e.g.*, acetaminophen) are used for mild pain; weak opioids (*e.g.*, codeine) are used for moderate pain, and strong opioids (*e.g.*, morphine) are used for severe pain. If the patient's pain escalates, the strength of analgesics is increased until the pain is controlled. Adjuvant medications are also administered to enhance the effectiveness of analgesics and to manage other symptoms that may contribute to the pain experience. Examples of adjuvant medications include antiemetics, antidepressants, anxiolytics, and glucocorticoids. Preventing and reducing pain help to lessen anxiety and break the previously described pain cycle. This can be accomplished best by administering analgesics on a regularly scheduled basis as prescribed (the preventive approach to pain management), with additional analgesics administered for break-through pain as needed and as prescribed.

A variety of pharmacologic and nonpharmacologic approaches offer the best methods for managing cancer pain. No reasonable approaches, even those that may be somewhat invasive, should be overlooked because of a poor or terminal prognosis. Nurses help patients and families to play an active role in managing pain. Nurses provide education and support to correct fears and misconceptions about opioid use. Inadequate pain control will lead to suffering, anxiety, fear, immobility, isolation, and depression. Improving a patient's quality of life is as important as preventing a painful death.

Decreasing Fatigue. Nurses help the patient and family to understand that fatigue is often an expected and temporary side effect of the cancer process and the treatments employed and also stems from the stress of coping with the cancer experience. It does not always signify that the cancer is advancing or that the treatment is failing. Many of the potential sources of fatigue are summarized in Chart 16-3.

Nursing strategies are designed to minimize fatigue or assist the patient to cope with existing fatigue. Helping the patient to identify sources of fatigue aid in selecting appropriate and individualized interventions. Ways to conserve energy are used to help patients plan daily activities. Alternating periods of rest and activity is beneficial. Regular, light exercise has been suggested to decrease fatigue and fa-

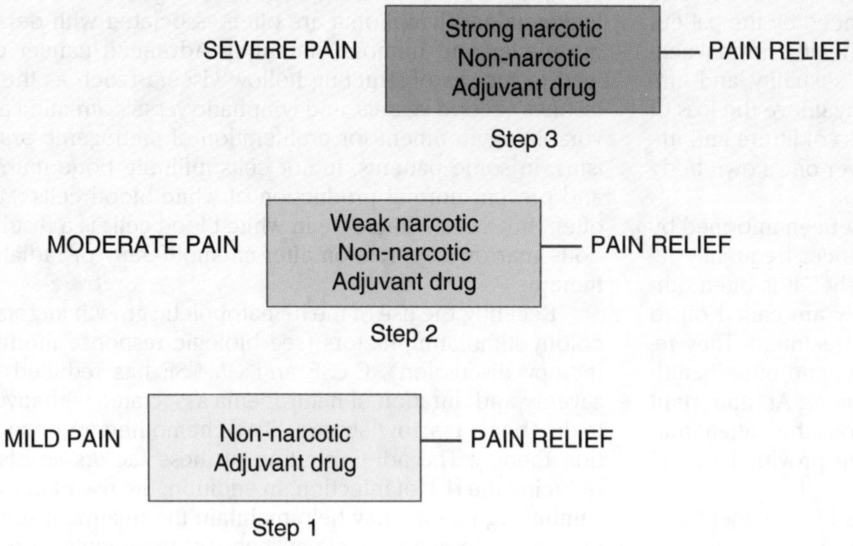

FIGURE 16-7. The World Health Organization 3-Step Ladder approach to cancer pain relief. Analgesic regimens are based on the assessment of pain ranging from mild to moderate to severe. Combinations of non-opioid and opioid drugs may be used with adjuvant drugs to control pain. (Adapted from Haviley C et al. Pharmacologic management of cancer pain: A guide for the health care professional. Cancer Nursing 1992 Oct; 15(5):331–346.)

cilitate coping in a patient with cancer. Patients are encouraged to maintain as normal a lifestyle as possible by continuing with those activities they value and enjoy. Prioritizing necessary and valued activities can assist patients in planning for each day. Both patients and families are encouraged to plan to reallocate responsibilities such as attending to child care, cleaning, and preparing meals. Patients who are employed full time may need to reduce the number of hours worked each week. The nurse assists the patient and family in coping with these changing roles and responsibilities.

Nurses also address factors that contribute to fatigue and implement pharmacologic and nonpharmacologic strategies to manage pain. Nutritional counseling is provided to patients who are not eating enough calories or protein. Serum hemoglobin and hematocrit levels are monitored for deficiencies, and blood products are administered as prescribed. Patients are monitored for alterations in oxygenation and electrolyte balances. Physical therapy and assistive devices are beneficial for patients with impaired mobility.

Improving Body Image and Self-Esteem. A positive approach is essential when caring for the patient with an altered body image. To help the patient retain control and gain a sense of self-worth, it is important to encourage independence and continued participation in self-care and decision-making. And the patient should be assisted to assume those tasks and participate in those activities that are personally of most value. Any negative feelings that the patient has about threats to body image should be expressed and aired. The nurse serves as a good listener and counselor to both the patient and the family. Referral to a support group often provides additional assistance in coping with the changes resulting from cancer or its treatment. Frequently, a cosmetologist can provide ideas about hair or wig styling, make-up, and the use of scarves and turbans to help with body image concerns. The American Cancer Society also sponsors a Look Good, Feel Better Program, which can assist patients struggling with these concerns.

Patients who are experiencing alterations in sexuality and sexual function are encouraged to share and discuss concerns openly with their partner. Alternative forms of sexual expression are explored with the patient and partner to promote positive self-worth and acceptance. The nurse who identifies serious physiologic, psychological, or communication difficulties related to sexuality or sexual function is in a key position to assist the patient and partner seek further counseling if necessary.

Progressing Through the Grieving Process. The diagnosis of cancer need not indicate a fatal outcome. Many forms of cancer are curable; many others achieve "cure" status if they are treated early. Despite these facts, many patients and their families view cancer as a fatal disease that is

CHART 16-3
Potential Sources of Fatigue in Cancer Patients

Pain, pruritus
Altered nutrition related to anorexia, nausea, vomiting, cachexia
Electrolyte imbalance related to vomiting, diarrhea
Altered protection related to neutropenia, thrombocytopenia, anemia
Impaired tissue integrity related to stomatitis, mucositis
Impaired physical mobility related to neurologic impairments, surgery, bone metastasis, pain and analgesic use
Knowledge deficit related to disease process, treatment
Anxiety related to fear, diagnosis, role changes, uncertainty of future
Ineffective breathing patterns related to cough, shortness of breath and dyspnea
Sleep pattern disturbance

inevitably accompanied by pain, suffering, debility, and emaciation. Grieving is a normal response to these fears and to the losses anticipated or experienced by the patient with cancer. These may include loss of health, normal sensations, body image, social interaction, sexuality, and intimacy. The patient, family, and friends may grieve the loss of quality time to spend with others, the loss of future and unfulfilled plans, and the loss of control over one's own body and emotional reactions.

The patient and family who have just been informed by the physician about the diagnosis of cancer frequently respond with shock, numbness, and disbelief. It is often during this stage that the patient and family are called on to make important initial decisions about treatment. They require the support of the physician, nurse, and other health care team members to make these decisions. An important role of the nurse is to answer any questions the patient and family may have and clarify information provided by the physician.

In addition to assessing the response of the patient and family to the diagnosis and planned treatment, the nurse assists them in framing their questions and concerns, identifying resources and support persons (*e.g.*, clergy, counselor), and communicating and sharing their concerns with each other. Support groups for patients and families are available through hospitals and various community organizations. These groups provide direct assistance, advice, and emotional support.

As the patient and family progress through the grieving process, they may express feelings of anger, frustration, and depression. During this time, the nurse encourages the patient and family to verbalize their feelings in an atmosphere of trust and support. The nurse continues to assess their reactions and provides assistance and support as they confront and learn to deal with new problems.

If the patient enters the terminal phase of disease, it may become obvious that the patient and family members are at different stages of the grieving process. Therefore, the nurse assists the patient and family at these different stages to come to grips with their reactions and feelings. Physical support, including holding the patient's hand or just being present at the bedside, frequently contributes to feelings of trust and peace of mind. Maintaining contact with the surviving family members after death of the cancer patient may help them to progress through the process of grieving and to work through their feelings of loss.

Monitoring and Managing Potential Complications

Infection and Sepsis. Despite advances in the care of patients with cancer, infection remains the leading cause of death. Defense against infection is compromised in many different ways. The integrity of the skin and mucous membrane, the body's first line of defense, is challenged by multiple invasive diagnostic and therapeutic procedures, by adverse effects of irradiation and chemotherapy, and by the detrimental effects of immobility. Impaired nutrition resulting from anorexia, nausea, vomiting, diarrhea, and the underlying malignant process can alter the body's ability to combat invading organisms. Medications such as antibiotics disturb the balance of normal flora, allowing the overgrowth of pathogenic organisms. Other medications can also alter the immune response (see Chapter 48). Cancer itself may be immunosuppressive. Malignancies such as leukemia and lymphoma are often associated with defects in cellular and humoral immunity. Advanced cancer can lead to tumors obstructing hollow viscera (such as the intestines), blood vessels, and lymphatic vessels, creating a favorable environment for proliferation of pathogenic organisms. In some patients, tumor cells infiltrate bone marrow and prevent normal production of white blood cells. Most often, however, a decrease in white blood cells is a result of bone marrow suppression after chemotherapy or radiation therapy.

Recently, the use of the hematopoietic growth factors or colony-stimulating factors (see biologic response modifier therapy discussion), G-CSF and GM-CSF, has reduced the severity and duration of neutropenia associated with myelotoxic (bone marrow suppressive) chemotherapy or radiation therapy. The administration of these factors assists in reducing the risk of infection. In addition, the use of colony-stimulating factors may help maintain the treatment schedules, drug dosages, the effectiveness of treatments, and the quality of life.

Infections in the myelosuppressed or immunosuppressed patient are most often nosocomial (acquired from the hospital environment). If the patient is hospitalized for courses of treatment or for management of complications, the most threatening pathogens are the gram-negative bacilli such as *Pseudomonas aeruginosa* and *Escherichia coli.* Gram-positive bacilli such as *Staphylococcus aureus* and fungal organisms such as *Candida albicans* can also contribute to serious infection.

Fever. Fever is probably the most important sign of infection in the immunocompromised patient. Although fever may be related to a variety of noninfectious conditions, including the underlying malignancy, any temperature elevation of 101°F (38.3°C) or above is reported and dealt with promptly.

Medications. Antibiotics may be prescribed to treat infections after cultures are done of wound drainage, exudate, sputum, urine, stool, or blood specimens. Individuals who are neutropenic are most often treated with broad-spectrum antibiotics before the cause of infection is identified. This course of action is necessary because of the high incidence of mortality associated with untreated infection in this group of patients. Broad-spectrum antibiotic coverage or empiric therapy includes a combination of drugs that provides defense against the major pathogenic organisms. An important component of the nurse's role is to administer these medications promptly according to the prescribed schedule to achieve adequate blood levels of the medications.

Prevention. Strict asepsis is essential when handling intravenous lines, catheters, and other invasive equipment. The patient should not be exposed to anyone with an active infection and is strongly advised to avoid crowds. A patient who is profoundly immunosuppressed, such as a recipient of bone marrow transplants, may need to be placed in a protective environment whereby the room and its contents are sterilized and the air filtered. These patients may also receive low bacterial diets avoiding fresh fruits and vegetables. Handwashing and appropriate hygiene are necessary to reduce exposure to potentially harmful bacteria and to eliminate environmental sources of contamination. Invasive procedures such as injections, vaginal or rectal examinations, rectal temperatures, and surgery are avoided. The patient is also encouraged to cough and take deep breaths frequently to prevent atelectasis and other potential respiratory problems.

Septic Shock. Assessment of the patient for infection and inflammation is frequent and continues throughout the course of the disease. Septicemia and septic shock are life-threatening complications that must be prevented or detected and treated early in their course. Patients with signs and symptoms of impending sepsis and septic shock require immediate hospitalization and aggressive treatment.

Signs and symptoms of **septic shock** (see Chapter 15) include altered mental status, either subnormal or elevated temperature, cool and clammy skin, decreased urine output, hypotension, dysrhythmias, electrolyte imbalances, and impaired arterial blood gases. The patient and family members are instructed about signs of septicemia, methods for preventing infection, and actions to take if infection or septicemia occurs.

Septic shock is most often associated with overwhelming gram-negative bacterial infections. The nurse monitors the patient's blood pressure, pulse, respirations, and temperature every 15 to 30 minutes. Neurologic assessments are carried out to assess for changes in orientation and responsiveness. Fluid and electrolyte status is monitored by measuring fluid intake and output and serum electrolytes. Arterial blood gases are obtained to determine tissue oxygenation. The nurse administers intravenous fluids, blood products, and vasopressor drugs as prescribed to maintain the patient's blood pressure and tissue perfusion. Supplemental oxygen is often necessary. Broad-spectrum antibiotics are administered as ordered to combat the underlying infection. (See Chapter 15 for a detailed discussion of management of the patient with shock.)

Bleeding and Hemorrhage. A decrease in the number of circulating platelets (thrombocytopenia) is the most common cause of bleeding in the patient with cancer. Thrombocytopenia is often a result of bone marrow depression after certain types of chemotherapy and radiation therapy. Tumor infiltration of bone marrow can also impair the normal production of platelets. In some cases, platelet destruction is associated with an enlarged spleen (hypersplenism) and abnormal antibody function that occur with leukemia and lymphoma.

Platelets are essential for normal blood clotting and coagulation (hemostasis). **Thrombocytopenia** is defined as a platelet count less than $100{,}000/mm^3$ (SI: $0.1 \times 10^{12}/L$). When the count falls to 20,000 to $50{,}000/mm^3$ (SI: 0.02 to $0.05 \times 10^{12}/L$), the risk for bleeding increases. Counts less than $20{,}000/mm^3$ (SI: $0.02 \times 10^{12}/L$) are associated with an increased risk for spontaneous bleeding and often require transfusion of platelets.

In addition to monitoring laboratory values, the nurse continues to assess the patient for evidence of bleeding. The nurse also takes steps to prevent trauma and minimize the risk of bleeding by replacing the patient's hard-bristled toothbrush with a soft-bristled one, by using an electric razor rather than a safety or straight-edge razor, and by avoiding unnecessary invasive procedures (*e.g.*, rectal temperatures, intramuscular injections, and catheterization). The patient and family are assisted in identifying and removing environmental hazards that may lead to falls or other trauma. Soft foods, increased fluid intake, and stool softeners, if prescribed, may be indicated to reduce trauma to the gastrointestinal tract. The joints and extremities are handled and moved gently to minimize the risk of spontaneous bleeding.

Hemorrhage may be related to a variety of underlying abnormalities such as thrombocytopenia and disorders of coagulation. These clinical situations are most often associated with the cancer process or the adverse effects of cancer treatments. Sites of hemorrhage may include the gastrointestinal, respiratory and genitourinary tracts, and the brain. Blood pressure, pulse, and respirations are monitored every 15 to 30 minutes when hospitalized patients experience bleeding. The serum hemoglobin and hematocrit are monitored carefully and compared with previous laboratory data for changes indicating blood loss. The nurse tests all urine, stool, and emesis for the presence of occult blood. Neurologic assessments are performed to detect changes in orientation and behavior. The nurse administers fluids and blood products as prescribed to replace any losses. Vasopressor drugs are administered as prescribed to maintain blood pressure and ensure tissue oxygenation. Supplemental oxygen is used as necessary.

Evaluation

Expected Outcomes

(See Nursing Care Plan 16-1 for specific outcomes.)

1. Maintains adequate tissue (skin and mucous membrane) integrity
2. Maintains adequate nutritional status
3. Achieves relief of pain and discomfort
4. Demonstrates increased activity tolerance and decreased fatigue
5. Progresses through the grieving process
6. Exhibits improved body image and self-esteem
7. Experiences absence of complications
   No inflammation, infection or sepsis
   No episodes of bleeding or hemorrhage

Rehabilitation

Cancer is a chronic disease that affects the physical, psychological, social, and economic dimensions of an individual's life. The diagnosis of cancer may be accompanied by emotional turmoil and changes in lifestyle or daily habits. With advances in diagnosis and treatment, however, survival rates are improving. Many patients, including those who receive primary surgical treatment and adjuvant chemotherapy or irradiation, are returning to work and their usual activities of daily living. These patients may encounter a variety of problems, including coping with changes in functional abilities and attitudes of employers, co-workers, and families who still view cancer as a terminal, debilitating disease.

Nurses play an important role in the rehabilitation of the cancer patient. Cancer rehabilitation needs to begin early in the treatment of the disease to maximize outcome. Assessment of body image changes as a result of disfiguring

Text continues on page 307

NURSING CARE PLAN 16–1
Care of the Patient With Cancer

NURSING DIAGNOSIS: Risk for infection related to altered immunologic response

GOAL: Prevention of infection

Nursing Interventions	Rationale	Expected Outcomes
1. Assess patient for evidence of infection: a. Check vital signs every 4 hours. b. Monitor WBC count and differential each day. c. Inspect all sites that may serve as entry ports for pathogens (intravenous sites, wounds, skin folds, bony prominences, perineum, and oral cavity).	1. Signs and symptoms of infection may be diminished in the immunocompromised host. Prompt recognition of infection and subsequent initiation of therapy will reduce morbidity and mortality associated with infection.	• Demonstrates normal temperature and vital signs. • Exhibits absence of signs of inflammation: local edema, erythema, pain, and warmth. • Exhibits normal breath sounds on auscultation. • Takes deep breaths and coughs every 2 hours to prevent respiratory dysfunction and infection.
2. Report fever $\geq$101°F (38.3°C), chills, diaphoresis, swelling, heat, pain, erythema, exudate on any body surfaces.		
3. Report change in respiratory or mental status, urinary frequency or burning, malaise, myalgias, arthralgias, rash, or diarrhea.		
4. Obtain cultures and sensitivities as indicated before initiation of antimicrobial treatment (wound exudate, sputum, urine, stool, blood).	4. These tests will identify organism and indicate most appropriate antimicrobial therapy. Use of inappropriate antibiotics will enhance proliferation of additional flora and encourage growth of antibiotic-resistant organisms.	• Exhibits absence of pathologic bacteria on cultures.
5. Initiate measures to minimize infection. a. Discuss with patient and family (1) Placing patient in private room if absolute WBC count $<1000/\text{mm}^3$ (2) Importance of patient avoiding contact with persons having known or recent infection or recent vaccination	5. Exposure to infection is reduced.	• Patient avoids contact with others with infections. • Patient avoids crowds. • All personnel wash hands after each voiding and bowel movement. • Excoriation and trauma of skin is avoided. • Trauma to mucous membranes is avoided (avoidance of rectal temperatures, suppositories, vaginal tampons, perianal area trauma).
b. Instruct all personnel in careful handwashing before and after entering room.	b. Hands are significant source of contamination.	• Patient uses recommended procedures and techniques if participating in management of invasive lines or catheters.
c. Avoid rectal or vaginal procedures (rectal temperatures, examinations, suppositories; vaginal tampons). d. Use stool softeners to prevent constipation and straining. e. Assist patient in practice of meticulous personal hygiene.	c. Incidence of rectal, perianal abscesses and subsequent systemic infection is high. Manipulation may cause disruption of membrane integrity and enhance progression of infection.	• Patient uses electric razor. • Patient is without skin breakdown and stasis of secretions. • Adheres to dietary and environmental restrictions.
f. Instruct patient to use electric razor.	f. Minimizes skin trauma.	
g. Encourage patient to ambulate in room unless contraindicated.	g. Minimizes chance of skin breakdown and stasis of pulmonary secretions.	
h. Avoid fresh fruits, raw meat, fish, and vegetables if absolute WBC count $<1000/\text{mm}^3$, also remove fresh flowers and potted plants.	h. Fresh fruits and vegetables harbor bacteria not removed by ordinary washing. Flowers and potted plants are also sources of organisms.	

(continued)

NURSING CARE PLAN 16–1 *(continued)*
Care of the Patient With Cancer

Nursing Interventions	Rationale	Expected Outcomes
i. Each day: change drinking water, denture cleaning fluids, and respiratory equipment containing water.	i. Stagnant water is a source of infection.	
6. Assess intravenous sites every day for evidence of infection:	6. Nosocomial staphylococcal septicemia is closely associated with intravenous catheters.	• Exhibits no signs of septicemia or septic shock. • Exhibits normal vital signs, cardiac output, and arterial pressures when monitored.
a. Change intravenous sites every other day.	a. Incidence of infection is increased when catheter is in place >72 hr.	
b. Cleanse skin with povidone-iodine before arterial puncture or venipuncture.	b. Povidone-iodine is effective against many gram-positive and gram-negative pathogens.	
c. Change central venous catheter dressings every other day.		
d. Change all solutions and infusion sets every 48 hours.	d. Once introduced into the system, microorganisms are capable of growing in infusion sets despite replacement of container and high flow rates.	
7. Avoid intramuscular injections.	7. Risk of skin abcesses is reduced.	
8. Avoid insertion of urinary catheters; if catheters are necessary, use strict aseptic technique.	8. Rates of infection *greatly* increase after urinary catheterization.	

NURSING DIAGNOSIS: Impaired skin integrity: erythematous/wet desquamation skin reactions to radiation therapy

GOAL: Maintenance of skin integrity

Nursing Interventions	Rationale	Expected Outcomes
1. In erythematous areas, a. Avoid the use of soaps, cosmetics, perfumes, powders, lotions and ointments, deodorants. b. Use only lukewarm water to bathe the area. c. Avoid rubbing or scratching the area. d. Avoid shaving the area with a straight-edge razor. e. Avoid applying hot water bottles, heating pads, ice, and adhesive tape to the area. f. Avoid exposing the area to sunlight or cold weather.	1. Care to the affected areas must focus on preventing further skin irritation, drying, and damage	• Avoids use of soaps, powders, and other cosmetics on site of radiation therapy. • States rationale for special care of skin. • Exhibits minimal change in skin. • Avoids trauma to affected skin region (avoids shaving, constricting and irritating clothing, extremes of temperature, and use of adhesive tape). • Reports change in skin promptly.
g. Avoid tight clothing in the area. Use cotton clothing.	g. Allows air circulation to affected area.	
h. Apply vitamin A&D ointment to the area.	h. Aids healing.	
2. If wet desquamation occurs. a. Do not disrupt any blisters that have formed. b. Avoid frequent washing of the area. c. Report any blistering.	2. Open weeping areas are susceptible to bacterial infection. Care must be taken to prevent introduction of pathogens.	• Demonstrates proper care of blistered or open areas. • Exhibits absence of infection of blistered and opened areas.
d. Use *prescribed* creams or ointments.	d. Decreases irritation and inflammation of the area.	
e. If area weeps, apply a thin layer of gauze dressing.	e. Enhances drying.	

(continued)

NURSING CARE PLAN 16–1 *(continued)*
Care of the Patient With Cancer

NURSING DIAGNOSIS: Alteration of oral mucous membranes: stomatitis

GOAL: Maintenance of intact oral mucous membranes

Nursing Interventions	Rationale
1. Assess oral cavity daily.	1. Provides baseline for later evaluation
2. Instruct patient to report oral burning, pain, areas of redness, open lesions on the lips, pain associated with swallowing or decreased tolerance to temperature extremes of food.	2. Identification of initial stages of stomatitis will facilitate prompt interventions, including modification of treatment as prescribed by physician.
3. Encourage and assist in oral hygiene regimens.	
Preventive	
a. Avoid commercial mouthwashes.	a. Alcohol content of mouthwashes will dry oral tissues and potentiate breakdown.
b. Brush with soft toothbrush; use nonabrasive toothpaste after meals and bedtime; floss every 24 hr.	b. Limits trauma and removes debris.
Mild stomatitis (generalized erythema, limited ulcerations, small white patches: *Candida*)	
c. Use normal saline mouth rinses every 2 hr while awake; every 6 hr at night.	c. Oxidizing action assists in removing debris, thick secretions, and bacteria.
d. Use soft toothbrush or toothette.	d. Minimizes trauma.
e. Remove dentures except for meals, be certain dentures fit well.	e. Minimizes friction and discomfort.
f. Apply lip lubricant.	f. Promotes comfort.
g. Avoid foods that are spicy or hard to chew and those with extremes of temperature.	g. Prevents local trauma.
Severe stomatitis (confluent ulcerations with bleeding and white patches covering more than 25% of oral mucosa)	
h. Obtain cultures and sensitivities of areas of infection.	h. Assists in identifying need for antimicrobial therapy.
i. Assess ability to chew and swallow; assess gag reflex.	i. Patient may be in danger of aspiration.
j. Oral rinses as prescribed or place patient on side and irrigate mouth; have suction available (may combine in solution saline, anti-*Candida* agent such as Mycostatin and topical anesthetic agent as described below).	j. Facilitates cleansing, provides for safety and comfort.
k. Remove dentures.	
l. Use toothette or gauze soaked with solution for cleansing.	l. Limits trauma, promotes comfort.
m. Use lip lubricant.	m. Promotes comfort.
n. Provide liquid or pureed diet.	n. Assures dietary intake.
o. Monitor for dehydration.	o. Decreased oral intake and ulcerations potentiate fluid deficits.

Expected Outcomes

- States rationale for frequent oral assessment and hygiene.
- Identifies signs and symptoms of stomatitis to report to nurse or physician.
- Participates in recommended oral hygiene regimen:
- Avoids mouthwashes with alcohol.
- Brushes teeth and mouth with soft bristle toothbrush.
- Uses lubricant to keep lips soft and nonirritated.
- Avoids hard to chew, spicy, and hot foods.
- Exhibits clean, intact oral mucosa.
- Exhibits no ulcerations or infections of oral cavity.
- Reports absent or decreased oral pain.
- Reports no difficulty swallowing.
- Exhibits healing (re-epithelialization) of oral mucosa within 5 to 7 days if mild stomatitis has developed.
- Exhibits healing of oral tissues within 10 to 14 days if severe stomatitis has developed.
- Exhibits no bleeding or ulcerations of oral mucosa.
- Consumes adequate fluid and food intake.
- Exhibits absence of dehydration and weight loss.

(continued)

NURSING CARE PLAN 16–1 *(continued)*
Care of the Patient With Cancer

Nursing Interventions	Rationale	Expected Outcomes
4. Minimize discomfort.		
a. Consult physician for use of topical anesthetic such as dyclonine and diphenhydramine or viscous lidocaine.	a. Alleviates pain and increases sense of well-being; promotes participation in oral hygiene and nutritional intake.	
b. Administer systemic analgesics as prescribed.		
c. Perform mouth care as described.	c. Promotes removal of debris, healing, and comfort.	
NURSING DIAGNOSIS: Impaired tissue integrity: alopecia		
GOAL: Maintenance of tissue integrity; coping with hair loss		
1. Discuss potential hair loss and regrowth with patient and family.	1. Provides information so patient and family can begin to prepare cognitively and emotionally for loss.	• Identifies alopecia as potential side effect of treatment. • Identifies positive and negative feelings and threats to self-image. • Verbalizes meaning that hair and possible hair loss have for him or her. • States rationale for modifications in hair care and treatment. • Uses mild shampoo and conditioner and shampoos hair only when necessary. • Avoids hair dryer, curlers, sprays, and other stresses on hair and scalp.
2. Explore potential impact of hair loss on self-image, interpersonal relationships, and sexuality.	2. Facilitates coping.	
3. Prevent or minimize hair loss through the following:		
a. Scalp hypothermia/scalp tourniquets.	a. Decreases hair follicle uptake of chemotherapy (not used for patients with leukemia or lymphoma because tumors cells may be present in blood vessels or scalp tissue).	
b. Cutting long hair before treatment.	b–f. Minimizes hair loss due to the weight and pulling on hair.	
c. Avoiding excessive shampooing.		
d. Using mild shampoo and conditioner, gently pat dry.		
e. Avoiding use of electric curlers, curling irons, dryers, clips, barrettes, hair sprays, hair dyes, and permanent waves.		
f. Avoiding excessive combing or brushing; use of wide-toothed comb.		
4. Prevent trauma to scalp.		
a. Lubricate scalp with vitamin A&D ointment to decrease itching.	a. Assists in maintaining skin integrity.	• Wears hat or scarf over hair when exposed to sun.
b. Have patient use sunscreen or wear hat when in the sun.	b. Prevents ultraviolet light exposure.	• Takes steps to deal with possible hair loss before it occurs; purchases wig or hair piece. • Maintains hygiene and grooming.
5. Suggest ways to assist in coping with hair loss:		
a. Purchase wig before hair loss.	a. Wig that closely resembles hair color and style is more easily selected if hair loss has not begun.	• Interacts and socializes with others.
b. If hair loss is present, take photograph to wig shop to assist in selection.	b. Facilitates adjustment.	
c. Begin to wear wig before hair loss.		
d. Contact the American Cancer Society for donated wigs, or store that specializes in this product.		
e. Wear hat, scarf, or turban.	e. Conceals loss.	

(continued)

NURSING CARE PLAN 16–1 *(continued)*
Care of the Patient With Cancer

Nursing Interventions	Rationale	Expected Outcomes
6. Encourage patient to wear own clothes and retain social contacts. 7. Explain that hair growth usually begins again once therapy is completed.	6. Assists in maintaining personal identity. 7. Reassures patient that hair loss is usually temporary.	• States that hair loss and necessity of wig are temporary.

NURSING DIAGNOSIS: Alteration in nutrition, less than body requirements, related to nausea/vomiting

GOAL: Fewer episodes of nausea/vomiting before, during, and after chemotherapy administration

Nursing Interventions	Rationale	Expected Outcomes
1. Adjust diet before and after drug administration according to patient preference and tolerance. 2. Prevent unpleasant sights, odors, and sounds in the environment. 3. Use distraction, relaxation techniques, and imagery before, during, and after chemotherapy. 4. Administer prescribed antiemetics, sedatives, and corticosteroids as prescribed. 5. Ensure adequate fluid hydration before, during, and after drug administration; assess intake and output. 6. Encourage frequent oral hygiene. 7. Provide pain relief measures, if necessary.	1. Each patient responds differently to food after chemotherapy. A diet containing foods that relieve the patient's nausea or vomiting is most helpful. 2. Unpleasant sensations can stimulate the nausea/vomiting center. 3. Decreases anxiety, which can contribute to nausea/vomiting. Psychologic conditioning may also be decreased. 4. Combination drug therapy attempts to reduce nausea/vomiting through control of the various triggering pathways. 5. Adequate fluid volume will dilute drug levels, decreasing stimulation of vomiting receptors. 6. Reduces unpleasant taste. 7. Increased comfort will increase physical tolerance of symptoms.	• Reports decrease in nausea. • Reports decrease in incidence of vomiting. • Consumes adequate fluid and food when nausea subsides. • Demonstrates use of distraction, relaxation, and imagery when indicated. • Exhibits normal skin turgor and moist mucous membranes. • Reports no additional weight loss.

NURSING DIAGNOSIS: Altered nutrition: less than body requirements, related to anorexia/cachexia/malabsorption

GOAL: Maintenance of nutritional status and of weight within 10% of pretreatment weight

Nursing Interventions	Rationale	Expected Outcomes
1. Teach patient as follows: Avoid unpleasant sights, odors, sounds in the environment during mealtime. 2. Suggest foods that are preferred and well tolerated by the patient, preferably high-calorie/high protein foods. Respect ethnic food preferences. 3. Encourage adequate fluid intake, but limit fluids at mealtime. 4. Suggest smaller, more frequent meals. 5. Promote relaxed, quiet environment during mealtime with increased social interaction as desired. 6. If possible, serve wine at mealtime with foods.	1. Anorexia can be stimulated or increased with noxious stimuli. 2. Foods preferred, well tolerated, and high in calories and protein will maintain nutritional status during periods of increased metabolic demand. 3. Fluid levels are necessary to eliminate waste products and prevent dehydration. Increased fluid levels with meals can lead to early satiety. 4. Smaller feedings given more frequently are more easily tolerated because early satiety does not occur. 5. A quiet environment promotes relaxation. Social interaction at mealtime increases appetite. 6. Wine often stimulates appetite and adds calories.	• Exhibits weight loss no greater than 10% of pretreatment weight. • Reports decreasing anorexia and increased interest in eating. • Demonstrates normal skin turgor. • Identifies rationale for dietary modifications. • Participates in calorie counts and diet histories. • Uses appropriate relaxation and imagery before meals. • Exhibits laboratory and clinical findings indicative of adequate nutritional intake: normal serum protein and transferrin levels, normal serum iron levels, normal hemoglobin, hematocrit, and lymphocyte levels, normal urinary creatinine levels.

(continued)

NURSING CARE PLAN 16–1 *(continued)*
Care of the Patient With Cancer

Nursing Interventions	Rationale	Expected Outcomes
7. Consider cold foods, if desired.	7. Cold, high-protein foods are often more tolerable and less odorous than hot foods.	• Consumes diet high in required nutrients. • Carries out oral hygiene before meals.
8. Advocate nutritional supplements, high-protein foods between meals.	8. Supplements/snacks add protein and calories to meet nutritional requirements.	• Reports that pain does not interfere with meals. • Reports decreasing episodes of nausea and vomiting.
9. Encourage frequent oral hygiene.	9. Oral hygiene measures stimulate appetite and increase saliva production.	• Participates in increasing levels of activity.
10. Provide pain relief measures.	10. Pain impairs appetite.	• States rationale for use of tube feedings or hyperalimentation.
11. Provide control of nausea/vomiting.	11. Nausea/vomiting increases anorexia.	
12. Increase activity level as tolerated.	12. Increased activity promotes appetite.	• Participates in management of tube feedings or total parenteral nutrition.
13. Decrease anxiety by encouraging verbalization of fears, concerns; use of relaxation techniques; imagery at mealtime.	13. Relief of anxiety may increase appetite.	
14. Position patient properly at mealtime.	14. Proper body position and alignment are necessary to aid chewing and swallowing.	
15. For collaborative management, provide enteral tube feedings of commercial liquid diets, elemental diets or blenderized foods through Silastic feeding tubes as prescribed.	15. Tube feedings may be necessary in the severely debilitated patient who has a functioning gastrointestinal system.	
16. Provide total parenteral nutrition with lipid supplements as prescribed.	16. Total parenteral nutrition with supplemental fats supplies needed calories and proteins to meet nutritional demands, especially in the nonfunctional gastrointestinal system.	

NURSING DIAGNOSIS: Fatigue and activity intolerance

GOAL: Increased activity tolerance and decreased fatigue level

Nursing Interventions	Rationale	Expected Outcomes
1. Encourage several rest periods during the day, especially before and after physical exertion.	1. During rest, energy is conserved and levels are replenished. Several shorter rest periods may be more beneficial than one longer rest period.	• Reports decreasing levels of fatigue. • Increases participation in activities gradually. • Rests when fatigued. • Reports restful sleep.
2. Increase total hours of nighttime sleep.	2. Sleep helps to restore energy levels.	• Requests assistance with activities appropriately.
3. Rearrange daily schedule and organize activities to conserve energy expenditure.	3. Reorganization of activities can reduce energy losses and reduce stressors.	• Reports adequate energy to participate in activities important to him (visiting with family, hobbies, etc.)
4. Allow/ask for others' assistance with necessary chores such as housework, child care, shopping, cooking.	4. Conserves energy.	• Consumes diet with recommended protein and caloric intake. • Uses relaxation exercises and imagery to decrease anxiety and promote rest.
5. Encourage reduced job workload, if possible, by reducing number of hours worked per week.	5. Reducing workload will decrease physical and psychologic stress and increase periods of rest/relaxation.	
6. Encourage adequate protein and calorie intake.	6. Protein and calorie depletion decreases activity tolerance.	
7. Encourage use of relaxation techniques, mental imagery.	7. Promotion of relaxation and psychological rest will decrease physical fatigue.	

(continued)

NURSING CARE PLAN 16–1 *(continued)*
Care of the Patient With Cancer

Nursing Interventions	Rationale	Expected Outcomes
8. Encourage participation in planned exercise programs.	8. Proper exercise programs will increase endurance and stamina.	• Participates in planned exercise program gradually. • Reports no breathlessness during activities.
9. For collaborative management, administer blood products as prescribed.	9. Lowered hemoglobin and hematocrit will predispose patient to fatigue due to decreased oxygen availability.	• Exhibits acceptable hemoglobin and hematocrit levels. • Exhibits normal fluid and electrolyte balance.
10. Assess for fluid and electrolyte disturbances.	10. May contribute to altered nerve transmission and muscle function.	• Reports decreased discomfort.
11. Assess for sources of discomfort.	11. Coping with discomfort requires energy expenditure.	• Exhibits improved mobility.
12. Provide strategies to facilitate mobility.	12. Impaired mobility requires increased energy expenditure.	

NURSING DIAGNOSIS: Pain and discomfort

GOAL: Relief of pain and discomfort

Nursing Interventions	Rationale	Expected Outcomes
1. Assess pain and discomfort characteristics: location, quality, frequency, duration, etc.	1. Provides baseline for assessing changes in pain level and evaluation of interventions.	• Reports decreased level of pain and discomfort. • Reports less disruption from pain and discomfort.
2. Assure patient that you know that pain is real and will assist him or her in reducing it.	2. Fear that pain will not be considered real increases anxiety and reduces pain tolerance.	• Explains how fatigue, fear, etc., contribute to severity of his pain and discomfort.
3. Assess other factors contributing to patient's pain: fear, fatigue, anger, etc.	3. Provides data about factors that decrease patient's ability to tolerate pain and increase pain level.	• Accepts pain medication as prescribed. • Exhibits decreased physical and behavioral signs of pain and discomfort in *acute pain* (no grimacing, crying, moaning; displays interest in surroundings and activities around him).
4. Administer analgesics to promote optimum pain relief within limits of physician's prescription.	4. Analgesics tend to be more effective when administered early in pain cycle.	
5. Assess patient's behavioral responses to pain and pain experience.	5. Provides additional information about patient's pain.	• Takes an active role in administration of analgesia. • Identifies additional effective pain relief strategies.
6. Collaborate with patient, physician, and other health care team members when changes in pain management are necessary.	6. New methods of administration of analgesia must be acceptable to patient, physician, and health care team to be effective; patient's participation decreases his or her sense of powerlessness.	• Uses alternative pain relief strategies appropriately. • Reports effective use of new pain relief strategies and decrease in pain intensity. • Reports that decreased level of pain permits participation in other activities and events.
7. Encourage strategies of pain relief that patient has used successfully in previous pain experience.	7. Encourages success of pain relief strategies accepted by patient and family.	
8. Teach patient new strategies to relieve pain and discomfort; distraction, imagery, relaxation, cutaneous stimulation, etc.	8. Increases number of options and strategies available to patient.	

(continued)

NURSING CARE PLAN 16–1 *(continued)*
Care of the Patient With Cancer

NURSING DIAGNOSIS: Grieving related to anticipatory loss; altered role functioning

GOAL: Progression through grieving process appropriately

Nursing Interventions	Rationale	Expected Outcomes
1. Encourage verbalization of fears, concerns and questions regarding disease, treatment, and future implications.	1. An increased and accurate knowledge base will decrease anxiety and dispel misconceptions.	• The patient and family will progress through the phases of grief as evidenced by increased verbalization and expression of grief. • The patient and family will identify resources available to aid coping strategies during grieving. • The patient and family use resources and supports appropriately. • The patient and family discuss the future openly with each other. • The patient and family discuss concerns and feelings openly with each other. • The patient and family use nonverbal expressions of concern for each other.
2. Encourage active participation of patient or family in care and treatment decisions.	2. Active participation will maintain patient independence and control.	
3. Visit family frequently to establish and maintain relationships and physical closeness.	3. Frequent contacts will promote trust and security and reduce feelings of fear and isolation.	
4. Encourage ventilation of negative feelings, including projected anger and hostility, within acceptable limits.	4. This allows for emotional expression without loss of self-esteem.	
5. Allow for periods of crying and expression of sadness.	5. These feelings are necessary for separation and detachment to occur.	
6. Involve clergy as desired by the patient and family.	6. This facilitates the grief process and spiritual care.	
7. Advise professional counseling as indicated for patient or family to alleviate pathologic grieving.	7. This facilitates the grief process.	
8. Allow for progression through the grieving process at the individual pace of the patient and family.	8. Grief work is variable. Not every person uses every phase of the grief process, and the time spent in dealing with each phase varies with every person. To complete grief work, this variability must be allowed.	

NURSING DIAGNOSIS: Altered body image and self-esteem related to changes in appearance, function, and roles

GOAL: Improved body image and self-esteem

Nursing Interventions	Rationale	Expected Outcomes
1. Assess patient's feelings about body image and level of self-esteem.	1. Provides baseline assessment for evaluating changes and assessing effectiveness of interventions.	• Identifies concerns of importance. • Takes active role in activities. • Maintains previous role in decision making. • Verbalizes feelings and reactions to losses or threatened losses. • Participates in self-care activities. • Permits others to assist in care when he is unable to be independent.
2. Identify potential threats to patient's self-esteem (*e.g.,* altered appearance, decreased sexual function, hair loss, decreased energy, role changes). Validate concerns with patient.	2. Anticipates changes and permits patient to identify importance of these areas to him or her.	
3. Encourage continued participation in activities and decision making.	3. Encourages/permits continued control of events and self.	
4. Encourage patient to verbalize concerns.	4. Identifying concerns is an important step in coping with them.	
5. Individualize care for the patient	5. Prevents or reduces depersonalization and emphasizes patient's self-worth.	
6. Assist patient in self-care when fatigue, lethargy, nausea, vomiting, and other symptoms prevent independence.	6. Physical well-being improves self-esteem.	

(continued)

NURSING CARE PLAN 16–1 *(continued)*
Care of the Patient With Cancer

Nursing Interventions	Rationale	Expected Outcomes
7. Assist patient in selecting and using cosmetics, scarves, hair pieces, and clothing that increase his or her sense of attractiveness.	7. Promotes positive body image.	• Exhibits interest in appearance and uses aids (cosmetics, scarves, etc.) appropriately. • Participates with others in conversations and social events and activities. • Verbalizes concern about sexual partner. • Explores alternative ways of expressing concern and affection.
8. Encourage patient and partner to share concerns about altered sexuality/sexual function and to explore alternatives to their usual sexual expression.	8. Provides opportunity for expressing concern, affection, and acceptance.	

COLLABORATIVE PROBLEM: Potential Complication: Risk for bleeding problems

GOAL: Prevention of bleeding

Nursing Interventions	Rationale	Expected Outcomes
1. Assess for potential for bleeding: monitor platelet count.	1. Mild risk: 50,000–100,000/mm^3 (SI: 0.05–0.1 × 10^{12}/L) Moderate risk: 20,000–50,000/mm^3 (SI: 0.02–0.05 × 10^{12}/L) Severe risk: less than 20,000/mm^3 (SI: 0.02 × 10^{12}/L)	• Signs and symptoms of bleeding are identified. • Exhibits no blood in feces, urine, or emesis. • Exhibits no bleeding of gums or of injection or venipuncture sites. • Exhibits no ecchymosis (bruising). • Patient and family identify ways to prevent bleeding. • Uses recommended measures to reduce risk of bleeding (uses soft toothbrush, shaves with electric razor only). • Exhibits normal vital signs. • Reports that environmental hazards have been reduced or removed. • Consumes adequate fluid. • Reports absence of constipation. • Avoids substances interfering with clotting. • Absence of tissue destruction. • Exhibits normal mental status and absence of signs of intracranial bleeding.
2. Assess for bleeding:		
a. Petechiae or ecchymosis	a. Indicates injury to microcirculation and larger vessels.	
b. Decrease in Hbg or Hct	b. Indicates blood loss.	
c. Prolonged bleeding from invasive procedures, venipunctures, minor cuts or scratches		
d. Frank or occult blood in any body excretion, emesis, sputum		
e. Bleeding from any body orifice		
f. Altered mental status	f. Indicates neurologic involvement.	
3. Instruct patient and family about ways to minimize bleeding:		
a. Use soft toothbrush or toothette for mouth care.	a. Prevents trauma to oral tissues.	
b. Avoid commercial mouthwashes.	b. Contains high alcohol content that will dry oral tissues.	
c. Use electric razor for shaving.	c. Prevents trauma to skin.	
d. Use emery board for nail care.		
e. Avoid foods that are difficult to chew.	e. Prevents oral tissue trauma.	
4. Initiate measures to minimize bleeding.		
a. Draw all blood for lab work with one daily venipuncture.	a. Minimizes trauma and blood loss.	
b. Avoid taking temperature rectally or administering suppositories and enemas.	b. Prevents trauma to rectal mucosa.	
c. Avoid intramuscular injections; use smallest needle possible.	c. Prevents intramuscular bleeding.	
d. Apply direct pressure to injections and venipuncture sites for at least 5 minutes.	d. Minimizes blood loss.	
e. Lubricate lips with petrolatum.	e. Prevents skin from drying.	

(continued)

NURSING CARE PLAN 16–1 *(continued)*
Care of the Patient With Cancer

Nursing Interventions	Rationale	Expected Outcomes
f. Avoid bladder catheterizations; use smallest catheter if necessary.	f. Prevents trauma to urethra.	• Avoids medications that interfere with clotting (aspirin).
g. Maintain fluid intake of at least 3 L/24 hr unless contraindicated.	g. Hydration helps to prevent skin drying.	• Absence of epistaxis and cerebral bleeding.
h. Use stool softeners or increase bulk in diet.	h. Prevents constipation and straining that may injure rectal tissue.	
i. Avoid medications that will interfere with clotting (*e.g.*, aspirin).	i. Minimizes risk of bleeding.	
j. Recommend use of water-based lubricant before sexual intercourse.	j. Prevents friction and tissue trauma.	
5. When platelet count is less than 20,000/mm³, institute the following:	5. Platelet count of less than 20,000/mm³ is associated with increased risk of spontaneous bleeding.	
a. Bed rest with padded side rails.	a. Reduces risk of injury	
b. Avoidance of strenuous activity.	b. Increases intracranial pressure and risk of cerebral hemorrhage.	
c. Platelet transfusions as prescribed; administer prescribed diphenhydramine hydrochloride (Benadryl) or hydrocortisone sodium succinate (Solu-Cortef) to prevent reaction to platelet transfusion.	c. Allergic reactions to blood products are associated with antigen-antibody reaction that causes platelet destruction.	
d. Supervise activity when out of bed.		
e. Caution against forceful nose-blowing.	e. Prevents trauma to nasal mucosa and increased intracranial pressure.	

treatments is necessary to facilitate the patient's adjustment to changes in appearance or functional abilities. The nurse can refer the patient and family to a variety of support groups sponsored by the American Cancer Society, such as those for people who have had laryngectomies or mastectomies. Nurses also collaborate with physical and occupational therapists in improving the patient's abilities and use of prosthetic devices.

Some patients return to work and continue to receive either chemotherapy or radiation therapy for extended periods. These people may experience transient problems such as lethargy, easy fatigue, anorexia, nausea, or vomiting. Nurses assess for the existence of these problems and assist the patient in identifying strategies for coping with them. For patients with gastrointestinal disturbances after chemotherapy, altering work hours or receiving treatments in the evenings may prove to be helpful. Nurses collaborate with dietitians to help patients plan meals that will be acceptable and meet nutritional requirements. Nurses are also involved in the ongoing assessment of patients over time to detect any long-term sequelae of cancer treatment.

Discrimination against recovering cancer patients has been demonstrated in several forms. Often employers do not understand that different kinds of cancers have different prognoses and different impact on functional ability. As a result, employers may be hesitant to hire or continue to employ people with cancer, especially if ongoing treatment regimens require adjustments in work schedules. Attitudes of co-workers can become a problem when the patient has a communication impairment such as may occur in some head and neck cancers. Finally, employers, co-workers, and families may continue to view the person as being "sick" despite ongoing recovery or completion of treatment.

Nurses can participate in efforts to educate employers and the public in general to ensure that the rights of patients with cancer are maintained. Whenever possible, nurses assist patients and families to resume preexisting roles. Nurses can encourage patients to regain the highest level of independence possible. In addition, the patient may be directed to vocational rehabilitation services of the American Cancer Society or other agencies. The diagnosis of cancer need not be a death sentence. Many people can and do resume active roles in life.

Gerontologic Considerations

As a result of the growing number of people over the age of 65, nurses are providing care for increasing numbers of elderly patients. The risk of cancer rises steadily with age. More than 57% of all cancers occur in people over the age of 65. Both cancer incidence and mortality rise with increased age. The most common sites of cancer in the elderly include lung, colon, breast, and prostate.

It is important for oncology nurses working with the elderly population to understand the normal physiologic changes that occur with aging. These changes include decreased skin elasticity; decreased skeletal mass, structure, and strength; decreased organ function and structure; impaired immune system mechanisms; alterations in neurologic function; and altered drug absorption, distribution, metabolism, and elimination. These changes ultimately influence the elderly patient's ability to tolerate treatment for cancer. In addition, many elderly patients have other chronic diseases that may also limit tolerance to treatment.

Potential toxicities associated with chemotherapeutic agents such as renal impairment, myelosuppression, and cardiomyopathy may be increased as a result of declining organ function and diminished physiologic reserves. The elderly patient receiving radiation therapy may have delayed recovery of normal tissues and may experience more severe adverse effects such as mucositis, nausea and vomiting, and myelosuppression. The older patient is slower to recover from surgery as a result of decreased tissue healing capacity and declining pulmonary and cardiovascular functioning. Elderly patients also are at increased risk for developing complications such as atelectasis, pneumonia, and wound infections.

In addition to the physical challenges encountered by the elderly with cancer, psychosocial issues such as gradual loss of supportive resources also have an impact. The declining health or loss of a spouse as well as the unavailability of relatives or friends may result in unmet needs for assistance with activities of daily living. In addition, the economic impact of health care may be difficult for those living on fixed incomes.

The nurse must be aware of the special needs of the aging population. Cancer prevention, detection, and screening efforts are directed toward the elderly as well as the younger population. Nurses carefully monitor elderly patients receiving cancer treatments for signs and symptoms of adverse effects. In addition, the elderly patient is instructed to report all symptoms to the physician. It is not uncommon for the elderly patient to delay reporting symptoms, attributing them to "old age." Many elderly persons do not want to report illness for fear of losing their independence or financial security. The nurse acts as a patient advocate, encouraging independence and identifying resources for support when indicated.

Patient Education and Home Care Considerations

In recent years a transition in the delivery of health care has occurred as patients have been discharged from acute care facilities to the home setting where families and friends are assuming increasing responsibility for continued patient care. Technological advances now make it possible to provide special care in the home related to administering chemotherapy, TPN, blood product transfusions, parenteral antibiotics, and parenteral pain management; managing symptoms; and attending to vascular access devises. Home care nurses provide support and education for patients and caregivers as they make the transition from hospital to home.

Teaching initially focuses on providing information needed by the patient and family to address the most immediate care needs they are likely to encounter at home. Side effects of treatments and changes in the patient's status that should be reported are clearly spelled out. Other learning needs are identified and are based on the priorities identified by the patient and family as well as on the complexity of treatments that will be provided in the home. Follow-up visits and phone calls from the nurse are often reassuring to the patient and family and increase their comfort in dealing with aspects of care that may be complex and new to them.

The nurse's responsibilities in the home and community also include assessing the home environment, suggesting modifications that would assist the patient and family in addressing the physical needs of the patient, assisting with the patient's physical care, and assessing the psychological and emotional impact of the illness on the patient and the family. Assessing changes in the patient's physical status and reporting relevant changes to the physician help to assure that appropriate and timely modifications in therapy are made. The nurse often facilitates the coordination of patient care by maintaining close communication with all health care providers involved in each patient's care. Informing the patient and family about the resources available (*e.g.*, local office of the American Cancer Society, home aides, church groups, and support groups) and assisting them to initiate contact with those resources often assist in reducing the stress experienced by both the patient and the family.

Care of the Patient With Advanced Cancer

The patient with advanced cancer is likely to experience many of the problems previously described, but all to a greater degree. Symptoms of gastrointestinal disturbances, nutritional problems, weight loss, and cachexia make the person more susceptible to skin breakdown, fluid and electrolyte problems, and infection.

Although not all cancer patients experience pain, those who do often fear that it will not be adequately treated. Although treatment at this stage of illness is likely to be palliative rather than curative, prevention and appropriate management of problems can improve the quality of the patient's life considerably. For example, use of analgesia on a regular basis at set intervals rather than on an "as needed" basis usually breaks the cycle of tension and anxiety associated with waiting until pain becomes so severe that pain relief is inadequate once the analgesic is given. Working with the patient and family as well as with other health care providers on a pain management program based on the patient's specific requirements frequently increases the individual's comfort and sense of control. In addition, the dose of opioid (narcotic) analgesic required is often reduced as pain becomes more manageable and other medications (*e.g.*, sedatives, tranquilizers, muscle relaxants) are added to assist in relieving pain.

The patient may be a candidate for radiation therapy or surgical intervention to relieve severe pain. The consequences of these procedures (*e.g.*, percutaneous nerve block, cordotomy) are explained to the patient and family, and measures are taken to prevent complications resulting from altered sensation, immobility, and changes in bowel and bladder function.

With the appearance of each new symptom, the patient often experiences dread and fear that the disease is progressing. However, one cannot assume that all symptoms are related to the cancer. The new symptoms and problems are evaluated and treated aggressively if possible to increase the patient's comfort and improve the quality of life.

Weakness, immobility, fatigue, and inactivity often occur in the advanced stages of cancer as a result of the tumor itself, treatment, inadequate nutritional intake, or difficulty breathing (dyspnea). The nurse works with the patient to set realistic goals and to provide rest balanced with planned activities and exercise. Other measures include assisting the patient in identifying less energy-consuming methods for accomplishing tasks and promoting activities that the patient values the most.

Efforts are made throughout the course of the disease to provide the patient with as much control and independence as desired, but with assurance that support and assistance are available when needed. Additionally, the health care team works with the patient and family to ascertain and comply with the patient's wishes about treatment methods and care as the terminal phase of illness and death approach.

Hospice

For many years, society was unable to cope appropriately with patients in the most advanced stages of cancer, and patients died in acute care settings rather than at home or in facilities specifically designed to manage the needs of patients with terminal disease. The needs of these persons often do not require advanced technology or sophisticated equipment, but are best managed by a comprehensive multidisciplinary program that focuses on relieving symptoms and providing psychosocial and spiritual support for the patient and family when cure and remission are no longer possible. The concept of hospice, which originated in Great Britain, best addresses these needs. Most importantly, the focus of care is the family, not just the patient. Hospice may take several forms: free-standing hospices, hospital-based programs, and community or home-based programs.

Because of high costs associated with maintaining free-standing hospices, care is often delivered by coordinating services provided by both the hospital and community. Although physicians, social workers, clergy, dietitians, physical therapists, and volunteers are involved in patient care, nurses are most often the coordinators of all hospice activities. It is essential that community-based nurses possess advanced skills in assessing and managing pain, nutrition, bowel dysfunction, and skin impairments.

In addition, hospice programs facilitate clear communication among family members and among health care providers. Most patients and families are informed of the prognoses and are encouraged to participate in decisions regarding pursuing or terminating treatment.

Community health nurses also are actively involved in bereavement counseling. Through collaboration with other support disciplines, nurses often assist patients and families to cope with changes in role identity, family structure, grief, and loss. In many instances, family support for survivors continues for a period of about 1 year.

Oncologic Emergencies

In addition to assessing and managing the previously described problems of the patient with cancer, the nurse also has an important role in the prompt detection and management of complications that are considered oncologic emergencies. As a result of the underlying malignancy, its metastasis, or the effects of treatment, the cancer patient is at risk for developing a unique group of acute conditions requiring immediate medical or surgical intervention. Common oncologic emergencies that require collaboration among all members of the health care team include superior vena cava syndrome, spinal cord compression, hypercalcemia, pericardial effusion, disseminated intravascular coagulation, and the syndromes of inappropriate secretion of antidiuretic hormone and tumor lysis.

Superior Vena Cava Syndrome

The superior vena cava is the major site of venous drainage from the head, neck, arms, and upper thorax. Positioned within the rigid compartment of the mediastinum, this thin-walled, low intravascular pressure vessel is closely surrounded by major structures, including the heart, lungs, vertebral bodies, and esophagus. Compression of the superior vena cava by tumor or enlarged lymph nodes can result in markedly impaired venous drainage of the head, neck, arms, and thorax. Intraluminal thrombosis that obstructs venous circulation will also impair venous drainage. In most patients, the superior vena cava syndrome (SVCS) occurs with lung cancer, but it can also occur with lymphoma and metastasis from other sites.

Clinical Manifestations. The clinical manifestations of impaired venous drainage usually develop gradually over a period of 3 to 4 weeks, but they may also appear suddenly. Progressive shortness of breath, dyspnea, cough, and facial swelling are common. Edema of the neck, arms, hands, and thorax may develop with associated sensations of skin tightness and difficulty swallowing. The jugular, temporal, and arm veins may be engorged and distended. Dilated thoracic vessels often cause prominent venous patterns visible on the chest wall. Continued venous obstruction may lead to increased intracranial pressure, associated visual disturbances, headache, and altered mental status. If untreated, SVCS may lead to cerebral anoxia (because not enough oxygen reaches the brain), laryngeal edema, bronchial obstruction, and death.

Management. Prompt diagnosis and treatment are essential in managing this syndrome. Radiation therapy is the treatment of choice to decrease the tumor size and alleviate symptoms. Chemotherapy is used when the tumor is known to be responsive to such treatment (lymphoma or small cell lung cancer). Anticoagulant or thrombolytic therapy may be used to treat SVCS related to intraluminal thrombosis. Other supportive measures such as oxygen therapy and diuretics may be used.

Nursing Interventions. Nursing care includes identifying patients at risk for developing superior vena cava syndrome. Clinical manifestations detected by the nursing assessment are reported to the physician and investigated promptly. Continued assessment of the patient's cardiopulmonary and neurologic status is essential. As a result of increasing difficulty in breathing and progressive edema, many patients become anxious and fearful of suffocating. Nursing care is directed toward facilitating breathing by positioning the patient properly, promoting comfort, and reducing anxiety. The patient's energy is conserved in an attempt to minimize shortness of breath. In addition, the patient's fluid volume status is monitored and fluids are administered cautiously to minimize edema. Patients who receive thoracic radiation are assessed for adverse effects such as dysphagia (difficulty swallowing) and esophagitis.

Spinal Cord Compression

Malignancies such as breast, lung, kidney, and prostate cancers, myeloma, and lymphoma that metastasize to the spine may cause spinal cord compression. Most lesions develop in the space between the periosteum of the vertebrae and the dura of the spinal cord (extradural), leading to compression of the cord and surrounding tissues. Vertebral collapse is another common cause of compression. Less commonly, tumors may develop in the spinal cord, meninges, ligaments, or nerve roots within the dura.

Clinical Manifestations. Spinal cord compression is compounded by local inflammation, edema, venous stasis, and impaired blood supply to the involved nervous tissues. Spinal cord compression is characterized by pain that may be constant and exacerbated by movement, coughing, sneezing, or the Valsalva maneuver (the act of bearing down). The location and characteristics of the pain depend on the area of involvement of the spinal cord.

Neurologic dysfunction develops when cord compression is prolonged or severe and may include motor and sensory deficit. Sensory deficits generally begin as loss of pinprick sensation, progressing to loss of ability to detect vibration, and finally to loss of position sense. The sense of touch usually remains intact even when motor dysfunction is advanced. Motor loss (weakness and ataxia) may be present at the time of diagnosis. If the compression progresses, flaccid paralysis ultimately occurs. The occurrence of other dysfunctions such as urinary and fecal incontinence is dependent on the level of the lesion compressing the cord. Compression of upper motor neurons above S2 can lead to incontinence owing to overflow of a full, distended bladder. Cord compression at levels S3, S4, and S5 can result in flaccid sphincter tone and bowel incontinence.

Diagnostic Evaluation. Prompt neurologic assessment is essential if sensory and motor function is to be maintained or restored. Although the myelogram has long been considered the standard diagnostic tool for spinal cord compression, magnetic resonance imaging (MRI) is being used with increasing frequency. Other diagnostic procedures such as x-rays, bone scans, and computerized tomography (CT) scans may assist in patient evaluation. Once the diagnosis is established, medical intervention is quickly initiated because symptoms can progress within a relatively short period of time.

Management. Radiation therapy is most commonly used to reduce the size of the tumor and to halt the progression of the disease. In most cases, surgical decompression is not used unless the symptoms progress despite irradiation or unless the patient has previously received a maximal amount of radiation to the area of the cord involved. Surgery may be indicated when the tumor involved is known to be nonresponsive to radiation therapy. Steroids are given in addition to radiation therapy to decrease the edema and inflammation at the site of compression. Recovery of neurologic function is influenced by how quickly the problem is diagnosed and treated. Despite treatment, patients who develop complete paralysis usually do not regain all of their neurologic function.

Nursing Interventions. Nursing interventions include ongoing assessment of neurologic function to identify existing and progressing dysfunction. Most patients will require both pharmacologic and nonpharmacologic measures to control pain. Because of pain and decreased functional abilities associated with spinal cord compression, patients are often at risk for the hazards of immobility such as skin breakdown, urinary stasis, thrombophlebitis, and decreased clearance of pulmonary secretions. Nursing measures are directed toward preventing these problems and maintaining muscle tone through range of motion exercises. For patients with bladder or bowel incontinence, intermittent urinary catheterization and bowel training programs are essential. Additionally, the patient and family require assistance in coping with the patient's pain and alterations in body functioning, lifestyles, roles, and level of independence.

Hypercalcemia

Hypercalcemia is a potentially life-threatening complication that is characterized by abnormal calcium metabolism, resulting in serum calcium levels in excess of 11 mg/dl (SI: 2.74 mmol/L) of blood. The skeletal system serves as the storage site for approximately 99% of all the calcium in the body. Hypercalcemia associated with cancer occurs when the release of calcium from the bones is more than the kidneys can excrete or the bones can reabsorb (see Chapter 14 for a discussion of normal calcium metabolism). Hypercalcemia is commonly seen in patients with multiple myeloma and cancers of the breast, lung, and head and neck. Less commonly, it develops in patients with leukemia, lymphoma, or renal cancer.

The underlying cause of hypercalcemia in the cancer patient varies. Approximately 70% of all cancer patients with hypercalcemia have metastatic bone disease. In this situation, direct invasion of the bone by tumor cells causes bone destruction and subsequent release of calcium. Hypercalcemia may also be caused by the production of *osteoclast-activating factor* and prostaglandins. These substances, produced by cancer cells, stimulate the breakdown of bone and the release of calcium. Hypercalcemia may also be caused by tumors that produce parathyroid-like substances and promote release of calcium from bones.

Factors unrelated to the underlying malignancy may contribute to hypercalcemia. These include immobility, dehydration, renal impairment, and medications such as thiazide diuretics. In addition, hormonal medications used in the treatment of breast cancer may contribute to the development of hypercalcemia.

Management. The manifestations of hypercalcemia and its medical management are discussed in Chapter 14.

Nursing Interventions. Nursing care begins with identifying those patients at risk for hypercalcemia. Careful nursing assessment will assist in identifying the signs and symptoms of hypercalcemia. These include fatigue, weakness, confusion, decreased level of responsiveness, hyporeflexia, nausea, vomiting, constipation, polyuria (exessive urination), polydipsia (excessive thirst), dehydration, and dysrhythmias.

Assessment of the patient's and family's knowledge of hypercalcemia is essential because prevention and early detection can prevent potential fatality.

Patients at risk for developing hypercalcemia receive instructions alerting them to the signs and symptoms of hypercalcemia, which they are to report. They are encouraged to maintain adequate fluid intake of 2 to 3 L of fluid per day unless contraindicated by existing renal or cardiac disease. The importance of mobility must be emphasized to prevent demineralization and breakdown of bones. Patients with alterations in mental status and mobility as a result of hypercalcemia require additional nursing measures to prevent the hazards of immobility and to promote safety.

Pericardial Effusion and Cardiac Tamponade

Cardiac tamponade is a cardiovascular disorder that occurs when fluid accumulates in the pericardial space and compresses the heart, thereby impeding cardiac filling during diastole. Neoplastic disease or its treatment is the most common cause of cardiac tamponade. Pericardial disease secondary to neoplastic growth usually occurs by direct invasion from adjacent thoracic tumors (lung, esophagus, and breast cancers) or metastasis to the pericardium (lymphomas, leukemias, sarcomas, melanomas, and carcinomas of the GI tract).

Fluid produced by the invasive tumor, metastatic lesion, or pericardial tissue in response to the malignant processes accumulates in the pericardial space, increases pressure on the myocardium, and impedes expansion of the ventricles. As ventricular volume and cardiac output fall, the cardiac pump fails and circulatory collapse develops. Radiation therapy of 4000 rad or more to the mediastinal area has also been implicated in pericardial fibrosis, pericarditis, and resultant cardiac tamponade, which may occur months or even years after the completion of radiation therapy.

Pericardial disease and cardiac tamponade may occur gradually or very rapidly. If fluid accumulates gradually, the parietal (outer) layer of the pericardial space will stretch and compensate for the increased pressure. Therefore, large amounts of fluid may accumulate before symptoms appear. When fluid accumulates rapidly, however, the pericardial pressures rise quickly and stretching cannot occur to compensate for the increase in fluid. As a result central venous pressures (CVP) increase and the jugular veins become distended.

Clinical Manifestations. Distention of neck veins during inspiration (Kussmaul's sign) is suggestive of pericardial disease. Pulsus paradoxus (a decrease in systolic blood pressure of more than 10 mm Hg during inspiration with strengthening of the pulse on expiration) may be detected in moderate cardiac tamponade. Heart sounds become distant, and increased areas of cardiac dullness may be percussed. As cardiac output decreases, the heart will begin to beat faster (compensatory tachycardia) and venous and vascular pressures increase.

As tamponade progresses, the systolic blood pressure continues to fall and the diastolic pressure rises in compensatory effort, creating a narrow pulse pressure. Shortness of breath and tachypnea may also develop. Weakness, chest pain, orthopnea, anxiety, diaphoresis, lethargy, and altered consciousness due to decreased amounts of oxygen reaching the brain (cerebral perfusion) may result. Circulatory collapse with cardiac arrest is imminent if untreated.

Diagnostic Evaluation. Electrocardiographic tracings will help in diagnosing pericardial effusion. The chest x-ray film does not usually confirm the diagnosis but shows small amounts of fluid in the pericardium (pericardial effusions). With larger effusions, however, the x-ray film will reveal a "water-bottle" heart (obliteration of vessel contour and cardiac chambers). Echocardiography and computed tomography are valuable both in diagnosing cardiac tamponade and in evaluating the effectiveness of treatment.

Management. The usual treatment of cardiac tamponade is **pericardiocentesis** (the aspiration or withdrawal of the pericardial fluid by a large-bore needle inserted into the pericardial space). Unfortunately, in malignant effusions pericardiocentesis provides only temporary relief; fluid will frequently reaccumulate. Pericardial windows or openings in the pericardium are often created surgically as a palliative measure to drain pericardial effusions into the pleural space. Catheters may also be placed in the pericardial space and sclerosing agents (such as tetracycline, bleomycin, 5-FU, or thiotepa) may be injected to prevent fluid from reaccumulating.

Other therapeutic options such as radiation therapy or antineoplastic drugs are dependent on how sensitive the primary tumor is to these treatments. In mild effusions, prednisone and diuretics may be prescribed with careful monitoring of patient status.

Nursing Interventions. Nursing assessment includes (1) frequent monitoring of vital signs; (2) assessment for pulsus paradoxus; (3) monitoring of ECG tracings; (4) assessment of heart and lung sounds, neck vein filling, level of consciousness, respiratory status, and skin color and temperature; (5) accurate monitoring of intake and output; and (6) review of laboratory study findings such as arterial blood gases and electrolytes.

Appropriate nursing actions may include elevating the head of the patient's bed; minimizing the patient's physical activity to reduce oxygen requirements; administering supplemental oxygen as prescribed; providing frequent oral hygiene; turning, and encouraging the patient to cough and take deep breaths every 2 hours; reorienting the patient, if needed; providing supportive measures; maintaining a patent intravenous access; and providing appropriate patient education.

Disseminated Intravascular Coagulopathy

Disseminated intravascular coagulopathy (DIC, consumption coagulopathy) is a disorder in which coagulation or fibrinolysis (destruction of clots) occurs, resulting in bleeding and thrombosis. DIC can occur with any malignancy, but is most commonly associated with hematologic malignancies such as leukemia and cancers of the prostate, GI tract, and lungs. Certain chemotherapeutic agents such as methotrexate, prednisone, L-asparaginase, vincristine, and 6-mercaptopurine have been associated with DIC. Certain disease processes commonly seen in the cancer patient may also initiate DIC, including sepsis, hepatic failure, and anaphylaxis.

Clot formation is initiated when the intrinsic or extrinsic mechanisms of normal coagulation are triggered. Injury to the lining of veins and arteries caused by metastatic cancer cells can stimulate coagulation through the intrinsic pathway. Some malignant cells have been shown to release thromboplastin or thromboplastin-like substances activating the extrinsic pathway of coagulation. Cell lysis induced by chemotherapy can also cause the release of thromboplastin from damaged cells. The release of endotoxins from bacterial cells during gram-negative sepsis is another mechanism by which the clotting cascade is stimulated.

Once activated, the clotting cascade continues to consume clotting factors and platelets at a rate faster than the body can replace them. Clots are deposited in the microvasculature placing the patient at great risk for impaired circulation, tissue hypoxia, and infarction. In addition, fibrinolysis occurs, breaking down clots and increasing the levels of anticoagulant substances, thereby placing the patient at risk for hemorrhage.

Laboratory results indicative of DIC include prolonged prothrombin time (PT or protime) and partial thromboplastin time (PTT), decreased platelet counts and fibrinogen levels, and increased fibrin split products. Circulating levels of clotting factors are also diminished.

Chronic DIC may produce few or no observable symptoms. Patients may exhibit easy bruising, prolonged bleeding from venipuncture sites, bleeding of the gums, and slow gastrointestinal bleeding. Acute DIC is associated with life-threatening hemorrhage and infarction. Clinical symptoms of this syndrome are varied and depend on the organ system involved in thrombus/infarction or bleeding episodes.

Management. Treatment of DIC centers on controlling the underlying disease process. Chemotherapy is given to treat the underlying malignancy. Antibiotics are used in the treatment of sepsis. Anticoagulant agents such as heparin or antithrombin III may be employed to decrease the stimulation of the coagulation pathways. Transfusion with fresh frozen plasma or cryoprecipitates (which contain clotting factors and fibrinogen) and platelets may be used as replacement therapy to prevent or control bleeding. Use of antifibrinolytic agents such as aminocaproic acid (Amicar) is controversial as it is associated with increased incidence of thrombus formation.

Nursing Interventions. Nursing assessments for the patient with DIC include monitoring vital signs; maintaining accurate intake and output measurements; assessing skin color and temperature; lung, heart, and bowel sounds; level of consciousness; headache, visual disturbances, chest pain, decreased urinary output, and abdominal tenderness; all body orifices, tube insertion sites, incisions, and bodily excretions for bleeding; and monitoring laboratory test results.

Appropriate nursing interventions involve minimizing physical activity to decrease risk of injury and oxygen requirements; applying pressure to all venipuncture sites; avoiding nonessential invasive procedures; maintaining adequate oral hygiene; assisting the patient to turn, cough, and take deep breaths every 2 hours; reorienting the patient, if needed; maintaining a safe environment; and providing appropriate patient education and supportive measures.

Syndrome of Inappropriate Secretion of Antidiuretic Hormone

The syndrome of inappropriate secretion of antidiuretic hormone (SIADH) is characterized by continuous, uncontrolled release of antidiuretic hormone (ADH), produced by the tumor cells or by the abnormal stimulation of the hypothalmic-pituitary network. Increased ADH leads to increased extracellular fluid volume with decreased osmolality,* water intoxication, hyponatremia, increased urine osmolality, and increased excretion of urinary sodium.

The most common cause of SIADH is malignancy, especially small cell cancers of the lung. It can also occur in patients with cancers of the pancreas, duodenum, brain, esophagus, colon, ovary, larynx, prostate, and nasopharynx and in those with Hodgkin's disease, thymomas, and lymphosarcomas. Antineoplastic drugs, vincristine, vinblastine, cisplatin, and cyclophosphamide, as well as the narcotic morphine, also stimulate ADH secretion and can lead to SIADH. Certain processes commonly seen in the cancer patient such as pain, stress, nausea, trauma, and hemorrhage are also associated with SIADH.

When ADH is produced, the distal renal tubules and collecting ducts of the kidney conserve and reabsorb water. In SIADH, the posterior pituitary becomes unresponsive to the normal feedback mechanisms and water conservation continues despite decreasing serum osmolality and increasing urine osmolality. As more fluid is absorbed, the circulatory volume increases, and sodium is actively excreted by the kidneys in compensation.

If the serum sodium levels fall below 120 mEq/L (SI: 120 mmol/L), patients usually display symptoms of hyponatremia, which include personality changes, irritability, nausea, anorexia, vomiting, weight gain, fatigue, muscular pain (myalgia), headache, lethargy, and confusion. If serum sodium levels continue to fall below 110 mEq/L, seizure, abnormal reflexes, papilledema, coma, and death may result. Edema is rarely seen with SIADH.

Laboratory findings indicative of SIADH include (1) decreased serum sodium, (2) increased urine osmolality, and (3) increased urinary sodium. Decreased BUN, creatinine, and serum albumin levels secondary to dilution may also occur. Abnormal results of water load tests would also indicate the presence of SIADH.

Management. Treatment of SIADH depends on the severity of symptoms. With mild symptoms, fluids are limited to 500 to 1000 ml/day to increase the serum sodium level and decrease fluid overload. If water restriction alone

*Osmolality = number of osmols per kilogram of solution. Its values change with changes in fluid and electrolyte balance.

is not effective in correcting or controlling serum sodium levels, demeclocycline or lithium carbonate is often prescribed to interfere with the antidiuretic action of ADH. When neurologic symptoms are severe, parenteral sodium replacement and diuretic therapy are indicated. Electrolytes are monitored carefully during treatment because secondary magnesium, potassium, and calcium imbalances may occur.

After the symptoms of SIADH are brought under control, the underlying malignancy is treated. If water excess continues despite treatment of the underlying cancer, pharmacologic intervention (urea and furosemide) may be indicated to control symptoms.

Nursing Interventions. Nursing assessment of the patient with SIADH includes maintaining accurate measurement of intake and output and assessing the level of consciousness, lung and heart sounds, vital signs, daily weight, and urine-specific gravity. The patient is also assessed for nausea, vomiting, anorexia, edema, fatigue, and lethargy. The nurse monitors laboratory test results, including serum electrolytes, osmolality, BUN, creatinine, and urinary sodium and osmolality.

Nursing interventions include minimizing activity, providing appropriate oral hygiene measures, maintaining environmental safety measures, and restricting fluid intake if necessary. Reorienting the patient and providing appropriate patient education and supportive measures also are indicated.

Tumor Lysis Syndrome

Tumor lysis syndrome (TLS) is a potentially fatal complication associated with radiation or chemotherapy-induced cell destruction of large or rapidly growing cancers such as leukemia, lymphoma, and small cell lung cancer. The release of intracellular contents from the tumor cells, leads to hyperkalemia, hypocalcemia, hyperphosphotemia, and hyperuricemia. These electrolyte imbalances occur when the kidneys are unable to excrete large volumes of the released intracellular metabolites. Metabolic disturbances are associated with potentially serious cardiac, neurologic, gastrointestinal, and renal manifestations such as dysrhythmias, laryngospasm, seizures, diminished mental status, vomiting, and renal failure. The clinical manifestations are dependent on the extent of the metabolic abnormalities that occur.

Management. Preventing renal failure and electrolyte imbalances are the goals of medical management of tumor lysis syndrome. Aggressive fluid hydration at a rate of 3 L/m^2 over 24 hours is initiated 48 hours before and after the initiation of cytotoxic therapy. Hydration is necessary to increase urine volume and the excretion of uric acid and electrolytes. Alkalinization of the urine increases the solubility of uric acid and prevents renal failure from uric acid precipitation in the kidneys. Alkalinization may be accomplished by administering sodium bicarbonate in each liter of intravenous fluid to maintain a urine *p*H greater than or equal to 7. Other drugs such as carbonic anhydrase inhibitor or acetazolamide may be used to alkalinize the urine. Allopurinol is administered orally to prevent the formation of uric acid by inhibiting the conversion of nucleic acids to uric acids.

CRITICAL THINKING EXERCISES

1. One of the cancer patients in your care is a 76-year-old woman who is independent, lives by herself, and insists on taking care of herself. She has decided to have outpatient chemotherapy as recommended by her physician. Describe the planning that is necessary to assure that she receives chemotherapy as prescribed and is able to manage side effects and maintain her independence.
2. A patient with advanced cancer has been advised by his physician to undergo an extensive surgical procedure followed by radiation therapy. The patient is considering herbal treatments instead and asks your opinion about what he should do. Explain what legal and ethical issues may be involved in this situation. On what basis would you decide your course of action?
3. A patient has advanced cancer, yet his physician has not informed him of his diagnosis and the patient's family has specifically stated that they do not want him informed about his diagnosis or prognosis. The patient has been asking you about his diagnosis and the cause of his symptoms. Explain the pros and cons of answering his questions directly. Which course of action would you take and why? How would you resolve the situation to the satisfaction of all involved?

Severe hyperkalemia is treated by administering a cation-exchange resin such as sodium polystyrene sulfonate (Kayexalate) that binds and eliminates potassium through the bowel. Administering hypertonic dextrose and regular insulin temporarily shifts potassium into cells and lowers serum potassium levels. Hyperphosphatemia is treated by administering phosphate-binding gels such as aluminum hydroxide that allow phosphate to be excreted in the feces. Hypocalcemia is managed by correcting elevated phosphorus levels. This is possible because of the inverse relationship that occurs between calcium and phosphorus levels. Hemodialysis is indicated when patients are unresponsive to the standard approaches for managing uric acid and electrolyte abnormalities.

Nursing Interventions. Nursing interventions for TLS begin with recognizing patients who are at risk for developing this complication. Preventive measures such as administering fluid hydration and allopurinol are essential. Nurses assess the following systems for signs and symptoms of uric acid and electrolyte imbalances: cardiac, neurologic, gastrointestinal, and renal. Serum electrolyte and uric acid levels are monitored. Patients are also assessed for evidence of fluid volume overload secondary to aggressive hydration.

Patients are instructed to report symptoms indicating electrolyte disturbances.

SELECTED REFERENCES AND READINGS

Books

Agency for Health Care Policy and Research. Public Health Service. Department of Health and Human Services. Acute Pain Management: Operative or Medical Procedures and Trauma. Clinical Practice Guideline (AHCPR 92-0032). Washington, DC, US Government Printing Office, 1992.

Agency for Health Care Policy and Research. Public Health Service. Department of Health and Human Services. Management of Cancer Pain: Adults (AHCPR 94-0592). Washington, DC, US Government Printing Office, 1994.

American Pain Society. Principles of Analgesic Use in the Treatment of Acute Pain and Chronic Cancer Pain. A Concise Guide to Medical Practice, 3rd ed. Skokie, IL, American Pain Society, 1992.

Greenwald P, Kramer BS, and Weed DL. Cancer Prevention and Control. New York, Marcel Dekker, 1995.

Groenwald SL et al (eds). Cancer Nursing: Principles and Practice, 3rd ed. Boston, Jones and Bartlett, 1993.

Klastasky J, Schimpff SC, and Senn H-J. Handbook of Supportive Care in Cancer. New York, Marcel Dekker, 1995

McKenna RJ and Murphy GP. Cancer Surgery. Philadelphia, JB Lippincott, 1994.

Niederhuber JE (ed). Current Therapy in Oncology. St Louis, BC Decker, Mosby Year Book, 1993.

Clark JC and McGee RF (eds). Oncology Nursing Society Core Curriculum for Oncology Nursing. Philadelphia, WB Saunders, 1992.

Journals

Asterisks indicate nursing research articles.

General

Bearhs OH. Staging of cancer. CA 1991 March/April; 41(2):121–125.

Blaese RM et al. Gene therapy: Sci-fi no longer. Patient Care 1993 June; 27(11):24–27, 30, 35, 38–39.

Ellison Derby S. Ageism in cancer care of the elderly. Oncol Nurs Forum 1991 July; 18(5):921–926.

Garden FH and Grabois M. Cancer rehabilitation. Phys Med Rehabil 1994 Jun; 8(2):229–440.

Holmes S. The oral complications of specific anti-cancer therapy. Int J Nurs Stud 1991; 28(4):343–360.

Irvine DM et al. A critical appraisal of the research literature investigating fatigue in the individual with cancer. Cancer Nurs 1991 Aug; 14(4):188–199.

Kusler DL and Rambur BA. Treatment for radiation-induced xerostomia: An innovative remedy. Cancer Nurs 1992 June; 15(3):191–195.

Montbriand MJ. An overview of alternate therapies chosen by patients with cancer. Oncol Nurs Forum 1994 Sep/Oct; 21(9): 1547–1554.

*Pickard-Holley S. Fatigue in cancer patients: A descriptive study. Cancer Nurs 1991 Feb; 14(1):13–19.

Skalla KA and Lacasse C. Patient education for fatigue. Oncol Nurs Forum 1991 Nov/Dec; 19(10):1537–1541.

Winningham ML. How exercise mitigates fatigue: Implications for people receiving cancer therapy. The Biotherapy of Cancer–V: Proceedings of a Symposium at the 16th Annual Oncology Nursing Society Congress 1992 May: 16–21.

Zaloznik AJ. Unproven (unorthodox) cancer treatments. Cancer Practice 1994 Jan/Feb; 2(1):19–24.

Cancer Process/Epidemiology

Applebaum JW. The role of the immune system in the pathogenesis of cancer. Semin Oncol Nurs 1992 Feb; 8(1):51–62.

Boring CC, et al. Cancer statistics 1994. CA 1994 Jan/Feb; 44(1):7–26.

Jenkins J. Biology of cancer: Current issues and future prospects. Semin Oncol Nurs 1992 Feb; 8(1):63–69.

Steile G et al. Clinical highlights from the national cancer data base:1993. CA 1993 March/April; 43(2):71–82.

Cancer Detection and Prevention

*Baulch Y et al. The relationship of visual acuity, tactile sensitivity and mobility of the upper extremity to proficient breast self exam in women 65 and older. Oncol Nurs Forum 1992 Oct; 19(9):1367–1372.

*Coleman EA et al. Efficacy of breast self-examination teaching methods among older women. Oncol Nurs Forum 1991 April; 18(3):561–566.

Frank-Stromborg M and Rohan K. Nursing's involvement in the primary and secondary prevention of cancer: Nationally and internationally. Cancer Nurs 1992 April; 15(2):79–108.

Levin B and Murphy G. Revision of American Cancer Society recommendations for early detection of colorectal cancer. CA 1992 Sept/Oct; 42(5):296–299.

Mettlin C and Dodd GD. The American Cancer Society guidelines for the cancer-related checkup: An update. CA 1991 Sept/Oct; 41(5):279–282.

*Underwood SM. African-American men: Perceptual determinants of early cancer detection and cancer risk reduction. Cancer Nurs 1991 Dec; 14(6):281–288.

Chemotherapy/Radiation Therapy

Boyle DM and Engelking C. Vesicant extravasation: Myths and realities. Oncol Nurs Forum 1995 Jan/Feb; 22(1):57–67.

Camp-Sorrell D. Controlling adverse effects of chemotherapy. Nursing 1991 April; 2(4):34–40.

Krakoff IH. Cancer chemotherapeutic and biologic agents. CA 1991 Sept/Oct; 41(5):264–278.

*Nail LM. Coping with intracavitary radiation treatment for gynecologic cancer. Cancer Practice 1993 Sep/Oct; 1(3):218–224.

Rieger PT and Haeuber D. A new approach to managing chemotherapy-related anemia: Nursing implications of epoetin alpha. Oncol Nurs Forum 1995 Jan/Feb; 22(1):71–81.

Biologic Response Modifiers

Brophy LR and Sharp EJ. Physical symptoms of combination biotherapy: A quality of life issue. Oncol Nurs Forum 1991 Supplement Jan/Feb; 18(1).

Bockheim CM and Jassak PF. The expanding world of colony-stimulating factors. Cancer Practice 1993 Sep/Oct; 1(3):205–216.

Gould Tseuat J and Lacasse CL. Understanding the special needs of patients receiving biotherapy: A conceptual model. The Biotherapy of Cancer–V, Proceedings of a Symposium; 16th Annual Oncology Nursing Society Congress 1992 August: 5–9.

Hogan CM. Coping with biotherapy: Physiological and psychosocial concerns. Oncol Nurs Forum 1991 Jan/Feb supplement; 18(1):19–23.

Moldewer NP and Figlin RA. Tumor necrosis factor: Current clinical status and implications for nursing management. Semin Oncol Nurs 1988 May; 4(2):120–125.

Oncologic Emergencies

Baker GL and Barnes HJ. Superior vena cava syndrome: Etiology, diagnosis and treatment. Am J Crit Care 1992 Jan; 1(1):54–64.

Byrne TN. Spinal cord compression from epidural metastasis. N Engl J Med 1992; 327(9):614–619.

Hilderlay LJ. Spinal cord compression: The nurse's role in early detection and rehabilitation. Proceedings of the 6th National Conference on Cancer Nursing: Challenges in Treatment and Management American Cancer Society 1992:81–86.

Jorgensen Huston C. Emergency! Disseminated Intravascular coagulation. Am J Nurs 1994 Aug; 94(8):51.

Kaplan M. Hypercalcemia of malignancy: A review of advances in pathophysiology. Onc Nurs Forum 1994 July; 21(6):1039–1046.

Kurtz A. Disseminated intravascular coagulation with leukemia patients. Cancer Nurs 1993 Dec; 16(6):456–463.

Lang-Kummer J. Hypercalcemia: Prevention of an emergency. Proceedings of the 6th National Conference on Cancer Nursing: Challenges in Treatment and Management American Cancer Society 1992:65–80.

Moroney Labovich T. Selected complications in the patient with cancer: Spinal cord compression, malignant bowel obstruction, malignant ascites and gastrointestinal bleeding. Semin Oncol Nurs 1994 Aug; 10(3):189–197.

Olopade OI and Ultmann JE. Malignant effusions. CA 1991 May/June; 41(3):166–179.

Peterson R. A nursing intervention for early detection of spinal cord compression in patients with cancer. Cancer Nurs 1993 March: 16(2):113–116.

Shuey KM Heart, lung and endocrine complications of solid tumors. Semin Oncol Nurs 1994 Aug; 10(3):177–188.

Stucky LA. Acute tumor lysis syndrome: Assessment and nursing implications. Oncol Nurs Forum 1993 Jan/Feb; 20(1): 49–59.

Truett L. The septic syndrome: An oncologic treatment challenge. Cancer Nurs 1991 August; 14(4):175–180.

Pain

Degner L and Barkwell D. Nonanalgesic approaches to pain control. Cancer Nurs 1991 April; 14(2):105–111.

*Diekmann JM and Wassem RA. A survey of nursing students' knowledge of cancer pain control. Cancer Nurs 1991 Dec; 14(6):314–320.

*Ferrell BR et al. Clinical decision making and pain. Cancer Nurs 1991 Dec; 14(6):289–297.

*Ferrell BR et al. Searching for the meaning of pain. Cancer patients', caregivers' and nurses' perspectives. Cancer Practice 1991 Sep/Oct; 1(3):185–194.

Ferrell B and Dean G. The meaning of cancer pain. Semin Oncol Nurs 1995 Feb; 11(1):17–22.

Greene PE. America responds to cancer pain: A survey of state pain initiatives. Cancer Practice 1993 May/June; 1(1):65–71.

Haviley C et al. Pharmacological management of cancer pain: A guide for the health care professional. Cancer Nurs 1992 Oct; 15(5):331–346.

Levy MH. Pain management in advanced cancer. Semin Oncol 1985 Dec; 12(4):394–410.

McCaffery M and Ferrell B. How to use the new AHCPR cancer pain guidelines. Am J Nurs 1994 July; 94(7):42–46.

Paice JA. Unraveling the mystery of pain. Oncol Nurs Forum 1991 July; 18(5):843–848.

*Sheidler VR et al. Analgesic decision-making skills of nurses. Oncol Nurs Forum 1992 Nov/Dec; 19(10):1531–1534.

Spross JA, McGuire DB, and Schmitt RM. Oncology Nursing Society position paper on cancer pain (part I). Oncol Nurs Forum 1990 July/August; 17(4):595–614.

Spross JA, McGuire DB, and Schmitt RM. Oncology Nursing Society position paper on cancer pain (part II). Oncol Nurs Forum 1990 Sept/Oct; 17(5):751–760.

Spross JA, McGuire DB, and Schmitt RM. Oncology Nursing Society position paper on cancer pain (part III). Oncol Nurs Forum 1990 Nov/Dec; 17(6):943–955.

Psychosocial/Home Care Concerns

Carpenter JS and Brockopp DY. Evaluation of self-esteem of women with cancer receiving chemotherapy. Oncol Nurs Forum 1994 May/June; 21(4):751–757.

Chekryn Reimer J, Davies B, and Martens N. Palliative care. Cancer Nurs 1991 Dec; 14(6):321–327.

Cooley ME. Bereavement care: A role for nurses. Cancer Nurs 1992 April; 15(2):125–129.

*Degner LF, Gow CM, and Thompson LA. Critical nursing behaviors in care for the dying. Cancer Nurs 1991 Oct; 14(5):246–253.

Hannigan Maloney C and Preston F. An overview of home care needs for patients with cancer. Oncol Nurs Forum 1992 Jan/Feb; 19(1):75–80.

Hull MM. Hospice nurses: Caring support for caregiving families. Cancer Nurs 1991 April; 14(2):63–70.

*Hull MM. Coping strategies of family caregivers in hospice homecare. Oncol Nurs Forum 1992 Sept; 19(8):1179–1187.

*Hunt Raleigh ED. Sources of hope in chronic illness. Oncol Nurs Forum 1992 April; 19(3):443–448.

*Krause K. Contracting cancer and coping with it: Patients' experiences. Cancer Nurs 1991 Oct; 14(5):240–245.

Mahon SM. Managing the psychosocial consequences of cancer recurrence: Implications for nurses. Oncol Nurs Forum 1991 April; 18(3):577–583.

Reimer JC, Davies B, and Martens N. Palliative care: The nurse's role in helping families through the transition of "fading away." Cancer Nurs 1991 Dec; 14(6):321–327.

Valente SM, Saunders JM, and Cohen MZ. Evaluating depression among patients with cancer. Cancer Practice 1994 Jan/Feb; 2(1):19–24.

Nutrition

Muscari Lin E. Nutrition support: Making the difficult decisions. Cancer Nurs 1991 Oct; 14(5):261–269.

Robuck JT and Fleetwood JB. Nutritional support of the patient with cancer. AACN Focus on Critical Care 1992 April; 19(2): 129–130, 132–134, 136–138.

Infection

Baird S (ed). New perspectives on the management for myelosuppression. Proceedings of a Symposium 1990 May. Oncol Nurs Forum 1991 Supplement to March; 18(2):1–24.

Brown KK. CE credit: Septic shock: Stopping the deadly cascade. Am J Nurs 1994 Sep; 94(9):20–26.

Buchsel PC. Managing infections in the neutropenic oncology patient: Challenges in treatment and management. Proceedings of the 6th National Conference on Cancer Nursing. American Cancer Society 1992:7–24.

DiJulio J. Hematopoiesis: An overview. Oncol Nurs Forum 1991 Supplement to March; 18(2):3–6.

Gawlikowski J. White cells at war. Am J Nurs 1992 March; 92(3): 45–51.

Rostad ME. Current strategies for managing myelosuppression in patients with cancer. Oncol Nurs Forum 1991 Supplement to March; 18(2):7–15.

Vascular Access Devices

Lucas AB. A critical review of venous access devices: The nursing perpectives. Current Issues in Cancer Nursing Practice 1992; 1(7):1–10.

Rountree D. The PIC catheter: A different approach. Am J Nurs 1991 August; 91(8):22–28.

Gene Therapy

Carroll-Johnson RM (ed). The genetic revolution: Promise and predicament for oncology nurses. Oncol Nurs Forum 1995 Mar (Suppl); 22(2):1–36.

PATIENT/FAMILY RESOURCES

Books

Altman B and Sarg M. The Cancer Dictionary. New York, Facts on File Inc., 1992.

Burning N. Coping with Chemotherapy. New York, Ballantine Books, 1993.

Fintel WA and McDermott GR. A Medical and Spiritual Guide to Living With Cancer. Dallas, Word Publishing, 1993.

Hirshaut Y and Pressman PI. Breast Cancer: The Complete Guide. New York, Bantam Books, 1992.

Johnson J and Klein L. I Can Cope: Staying Healthy With Cancer. Minneapolis, The Wellness Series, 1988.

Seigel B. Love, Medicine and Miracles. New York, Harper and Row, 1986.

Simonton OC, Matthews-Simonton S, and Creighton JL. Getting Well Again. New York, Bantam Books, 1981.

Organizations

American Cancer Society
1599 Clifton Rd NE, Atlanta, GA, (800) ACS-2345

American Foundation for Urologic Disease
1120 North Charles St, Suite 401, Baltimore, MD, 21201

Concern for Dying
250 West 57th Street, New York, NY 10107, (212) 246-6962

Hospice Foundation Institute
5 Essex Square, Suite 3-B, PO Box 713, Essex, CT 06426, (800) 331-1620

Leukemia Society of America
733 Third Avenue, New York, NY 10017, (212) 573-8484

Make Today Count
101 1/2 S Union St, Alexandria, VA 22314-3323, (703) 548-9714

National Alliance of Breast Cancer Associations
1180 Avenue of the Americas, 2nd Floor, New York, NY 10036, (212) 221-3300.

National Cancer Information Clearing House
Room 10A18 Building 31 NCI/NIH, Bethesda, MD 20205, (301) 496-4070

National Coalition for Cancer Survivorship
1010 Wayne Ave. Silver Spring, MD. 20910, (301) 585-2616

United Ostomy Association Inc
36 Executive Park Suite 120, Irvine CA 92714, (714) 660-8624

Support Groups: Check your local area.

17

Chronic Illness

CHAPTER OUTLINE

The Phenomenon of Chronic Illness
Definition of Chronic Illness
Causes of Chronic Illness

The Implications of Chronicity

The Problems of Managing Chronic Illness

Implications for Nursing

The Chronic Illness Trajectory Framework
Overview
Phases of Chronic Illness
Steps of the Trajectory Nursing Model

Patient Education and Home Care Considerations

Critical Thinking Exercises

LEARNING OBJECTIVES

On completion of this chapter, the learner will be able to:

1. Define chronic illness
2. Identify factors related to the increasing incidence of chronic illness
3. Describe characteristics of chronic illnesses and implications for people with chronic illness and their family
4. Describe the phases of chronic illness using the trajectory framework
5. Use the nursing process and the trajectory framework in the care of the patient with a chronic illness

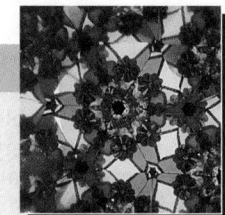

The Phenomenon of Chronic Illness

Chronic health problems affect persons across the life span. They occur in the very young as well as the middle-aged and very old persons. Many chronic illnesses and conditions are more common in one age group than others. However, chronic illnesses increase in frequency with age and many elderly persons develop multiple chronic illnesses. Chronic illness occurs across genders, socioeconomic levels, and ethnic, cultural, and racial groups. However, chronic health problems are more common in individuals from low socioeconomic groups because of less access to health care, poor nutrition, and often unhealthy lifestyles.

Chronic illnesses can have little if any impact on activity or lifestyle (as in very mild skin condition or chronic sinusitis) or can lead to dependence on advanced technology for survival (as in advanced amyotrophic lateral sclerosis [ALS] or end-stage renal disease). People with chronic health care problems may function independently and lead a full life with only minor disruption; others may require frequent and close monitoring or permanent placement in a long-term care facility.

Whereas each chronic condition has its own distinct set of characteristics and management problems, many chronic illnesses share similar characteristics. For example, many chronic conditions are associated with symptoms such as pain and fatigue. Severe or advanced chronic illnesses are likely to cause some degree of disability, which in turn limits the person's participation in activities. Many chronic conditions require management regimens to keep them under control. Unlike the term "acute," which implies a curable and relatively short disease course, "chronic" describes a long and often incurable course. It is this characteristic of *duration* that often makes managing chronic conditions so problematic for those who must live with them.

Psychological and emotional reactions of individuals to acute and chronic illnesses and change in health status have been described in detail in Chapter 10. Briefly, an individual who develops a chronic illness may react with shock and disbelief, depression, anger, resentment, or a number of other emotions. How individuals react and cope with chronic illness is usually similar to their reactions to other events in their lives. Responses and reactions depend, in part, on individuals' understanding of the chronic illness and their perceptions of its potential impact on their lives, their families, and their lifestyle.

Reactions to chronic illness are likely to occur at its initial onset, but also as symptoms reappear or worsen. Symptoms associated with chronic illnesses are often both unpredictable and perceived as crisis events by patients and their families as they deal with the uncertainty of chronic illness and the changes brought about in their lives. This chapter describes some of the problems of living with and managing chronic conditions and offers a framework to guide nursing assessment and intervention when providing care to persons with chronic health problems.

Definition of Chronic Illness

Chronic illness is defined as a medical condition or health problem with associated symptoms or disabilities that require long-term management. Part of that management includes learning to live with symptoms and disability, while coming to terms with any identity changes that illness brings. Another part consists of carrying out the lifestyle changes and regimens that are designed to keep signs and symptoms under control and to prevent complications. Although some persons take on what might be called a "sick role" identity, most people with chronic illness do not consider themselves sick or ill and try to live as normal a life as is possible (Robinson et al., 1993). It is only when complications or severe symptoms interfere with daily life activities that many chronically ill persons think of themselves as being "sick" (Forsyth, Delaney, & Gresham, 1984).

Causes of Chronic Illness

Chronic illness can be found in every age group, socioeconomic level, and culture. It has been reported that as many as 34.2 million people have activity limitations due to chronic conditions (Disability Abstracts, 1991). Table 17-1 presents a list of the chronic conditions most often cited by the general population as causing limitations in activity. Table 17-2 shows how such conditions are distributed by age group. As is apparent in Table 17-2, the incidence and type of condition vary by age, with those in the older age categories having the greatest numbers of conditions. This information is useful in planning health promotion and education programs and for allocating resources and services.

Many possible explanations exist as to why chronic illness has become a major health problem in developed countries, including the following reasons: (1) advances in modern medicine that have led to decreased mortality rates from infectious diseases such as smallpox and diphtheria, and from other serious conditions; (2) improved nutrition and stricter rules governing safety in the work place that have enabled people to live longer; and (3) lifestyles associ-

TABLE 17-1 Prevalence Of Major Reported Chronic Conditions, 1991

Condition	Prevalence (in 1000s)
Chronic sinusitis	32,167
Arthritis	31,148
Deformity or orthopedic impairment	28,725
Hypertension	27,800
Hay fever without asthma	24,248
Hearing impairment	22,680
Heart disease	20,536
Chronic bronchitis	12,549
Asthma	11,735
Migraine headaches	9,539
Visual impairment	7,988
Diabetes	7,223

(National Center for Health Statistics. Vital and Health Statistics. Hyattsville, MD, U.S. Department of Health and Human Services, 1992.)

TABLE 17-2 Prevalence of Top-Ranking Reported Chronic Conditions by Age, 1991

Selected Chronic Condition	Rate / 1000 By Age				
	Under 18 Yrs	18–44 Yrs	45–64 Yrs	65–74 Yrs	75 Yrs+
Hay fever without asthma	64.6	120.6	107.1		
Asthma	62.5				
Chronic sinusitis	59.6	151	171.1	156.4	113.7
Chronic bronchitis	53.1				
Acne	26.5				
Chronic disease of tonsils	24				
Deformity/orthopedic, back		89.9	99.3		
Migraine headache		55.5			
Hearing impairment		49.7	141.3	266.2	403.6
Arthritis		47.3	240.8	425.6	575.2
High blood pressure (hypertension)			244	376.6	365.5
Cataracts				127.6	242.3
Ischemic heart disease				127.2	155.3
Diabetes				103.8	
Visual impairment					113.3

(National Center for Health Statistics. Vital and Health Statistics. Hyattsville, MD, U.S. Department of Health and Human Services, 1992.)

ated with a modern society that have increased the incidence of chronic illness.

Advances in health care technology and pharmacology have extended life spans, without necessarily curing the underlying causes of chronic disease. Improved methods of screening and diagnosis enable early detection of disease while conditions are still treatable; thus, longevity is increased. Although an infectious disease, AIDS has become chronic in nature owing to the development and use of new medications for the treatment of opportunistic infections. Aggressive management of myocardial infarctions (heart attacks) and cardiac dysrhythmias has enabled people to survive medical crises and go on to lead productive and fulfilling lives.

Although technology may save lives, it can also result in chronic problems that are almost as debilitating as the ones it was designed to treat. For example, technology has greatly increased the survival rates of severely premature infants at the same time that it has made them vulnerable to complications, such as ventilator dependence and blindness. Certain medications can relieve symptoms of mental illness, but they often cause side effects, such as tardive dyskinesia. Medications used to prevent rejection of transplanted organs can place users at a higher than normal risk for the development of cancers.

The habits of modern society also have contributed to the increase in the incidence of chronic illness. Diets high in saturated fat and cholesterol, sedentary lifestyles, substance abuse, smoking, and high levels of stress, all have been related to the development of chronic conditions in genetically susceptible persons. Although greater emphasis has been placed on healthy lifestyles in recent years, it will be some time before any noticeable decrease in cases of chronic illness occurs.

The Implications of Chronicity

Chronic illness touches many people in many ways, either directly or indirectly. In a country where so much importance is placed on achievement and good health, it is important to understand the implications of chronic illness for individuals, families, and society. Only in this way can nurses, other health care providers, and society begin to address these problems. The implications include:

1. *Managing chronic illness involves more than managing medical problems.* Important *psychological* and *social* considerations also must be addressed. Living permanently or for long periods of time with symptoms and disability may lead to identity adjustments, role changes, and the need to cope with an altered body image or lifestyle. Adaptation to illness and disability is a continuous process. Each major change or decrease in functional ability requires further physical, emotional, and social adaptation (Bury, 1991), both for the individual and for the family.
2. *Chronic conditions can pass through many different phases over the course of the disease* (Rolland, 1987). There can be stable and unstable periods, flare-ups, and remissions. Each phase brings its own set of physical, psychological, and social problems, and each requires different regimens and types of management (Corbin & Strauss, 1988).
3. *Keeping chronic conditions under control requires persistent adherence to therapeutic regimens.* Failing to adhere to a treatment plan or following the regimen in an inconsistent manner can increase the risks of developing complications and accelerating the disease process. Yet, it is important to realize that the realities of

daily living, as well as culture, values, and socioeconomic factors affect the degree to which a person will adhere to a treatment regimen. Managing a chronic illness takes time, requires knowledge and planning, and can be uncomfortable and inconvenient. It is not unusual for people to discontinue taking medications or to alter dosages because the side effects are more disturbing or disruptive than the symptoms of the illness itself, and people frequently cut back on regimens they consider overly time-consuming or too fatiguing (Strauss et al., 1984).

4. *One chronic disease can lead to other chronic conditions.* For example, diabetes may eventually lead to neurologic and circulatory changes that may result in vision, cardiac, sexual, and kidney problems.
5. *Chronic illness affects the whole family.* Not only do family members become involved in managing the chronic illness of a loved one, but family life can be dramatically altered by chronic illness, especially if it is severe. Role reversals, unfilled roles, loss of income, time spent managing illness, decreases in family activities and socialization, and the cost of treatment can create tension, stress, and fatigue within the family. The effect on the family can be profound, sometimes drawing members closer together, other times driving them apart (Foxhall, Ekberg & Griffith, 1985; Stuifbergen, 1987).
6. *People with chronic illness and their families must assume major responsibility for the day-to-day management of the illness.* Unlike with acute conditions, the *home* rather than the hospital becomes the primary center of care in chronic illness. Outside support services are available from hospitals, clinics, doctors' offices, nursing homes, nursing centers, and community agencies (visiting nurse services, social services, and disease-specific associations and societies). These services enable a person to manage chronic illness at home (Strauss & Corbin, 1988).
7. *The management of chronic conditions is a process of discovery.* People can be taught how to manage their conditions. However "teaching about" symptoms is not the same as "experiencing" them. Each person must discover how his or her own body reacts under varying conditions, such as what it is like to feel hypoglycemic, what activities are likely to bring on a symptom, and how it can be prevented and managed in the best ways.
8. *Managing chronic conditions requires handling complex, interrelated problems that are medical, social, and emotional in nature.* The collaborative efforts of many different health care professionals are required to provide the full range of services that are often needed.
9. *The management of chronic conditions is expensive.* Billions of health care dollars are spent every year on equipment, medications, and services related to chronic illness. These expenditures cause a drain on the individual, the family, and the national financial resources.
10. *Chronic conditions pose ethical dilemmas for the individual, health care professionals, and society.* There are no easy solutions to questions and issues, such as when to terminate care, how to provide access to care, how to establish cost controls, and how to evaluate quality of life (Jennings, Callahan, & Caplan, 1986).
11. *Living with chronic illness means living with uncertainty* (Mishel, 1990; Yarcheski, 1988). Although health care professionals can identify the anticipated course of an illness, they cannot determine with certainty what that exact course will be for each individual. That is, it is often unknown and unpredictable how fast and how far a condition will progress or if and when complications might occur despite adherence to regimens. Even when a patient has been labeled as being "in remission" or "disease free," there is always that lingering doubt and dread that the illness will recur (Smeltzer, 1992).

The Problems of Managing Chronic Illness

The problems associated with managing chronic illness emerge as a person attempts to live with his or her condition over time. Naturally, it is preferable to prevent chronic disease through promotion of healthy lifestyles. However, once chronic illness occurs, the overall management problem shifts to controlling the course of the illness while maintaining an acceptable quality of life. Although the problems of chronicity are felt most acutely by the individual and family, they are also to some degree the problems of both health care providers and society at large. The problems of managing a chronic condition include the following:

- Preventing the occurrence of chronic conditions
- Alleviating and managing symptoms
- Preventing and handling disabilities
- Preventing and managing crises and complications
- Attaining, maintaining, and regaining illness stability
- Validating individual self-worth and family functioning
- Adapting to repeated identity threats and progressive loss of function
- Normalizing individual and family life as much as possible
- Living with altered time, social isolation, and loneliness
- Identifying and obtaining resources and establishing networks of support
- Returning to a satisfactory life after an acute phase of a chronic illness
- Dying with dignity and comfort

Implications for Nursing

Most people requiring nursing care have problems associated with chronic conditions. Even those persons who are hospitalized with acute or crisis conditions, such as myocardial infarctions or strokes, have an underlying chronic illness that led to or preceded the acute crisis or event.

Working with the chronically ill presents its own set of challenges. People living with an illness often act or respond in ways that are quite different from the way health practitioners believe they should act. Perception of quality of life is often *the* force driving the individual's behavior, and what is considered quality of life is determined by each person. Although it may be difficult for nurses and other health care providers to stand by while patients make unwise decisions about their health, they must accept the fact that individuals have the right to make their own choices about lifestyle and health care. Patients should be able to make such decisions and choices without fear of ridicule or refusal of treatment.

Given the implications of "living with" chronic illness, nurses need frameworks of practice to enable them to understand the impact of chronic illness on an individual and the family. Superimposing an "acute care framework" on a chronic condition ignores the differences between acute and chronic illness and increases the risk that the nurse will miss many of the more subtle and nonmedical problems associated with chronic illness.

The Chronic Illness Trajectory Framework

Overview

The Chronic Illness Trajectory Framework is one of several approaches developed for working with the chronically ill and their families. In this framework, the term *trajectory* refers to the course of action taken by a chronically ill person, the family, and health professionals to manage the chronic illness. This framework also addresses the impact of chronic illness and its management on everyday life activities and the individual's sense of identity. Additionally, it takes into account the degree to which the individual's and the family's identities and their needs and preferences about daily life activities influence treatment decisions. Chronically ill individuals and their families are considered active participants in the management process and have the right to make their own decisions about their lifestyles and well-being. Although this is true in all areas of nursing and patient care, it is of particular importance in chronic illness because the patient and family have the primary roles and responsibilities in managing the chronic illness.

The Chronic Illness Trajectory Framework is an approach to caring for a person with chronic illness that includes the social and psychological impact of the chronic illness on the patient and family along with the medical aspects of illness and its management. In other words, these aspects are related and therefore are not separated or isolated from each other. The trajectory framework identifies the specific *phase of illness*, the management strategies that are specific to each illness phase, and the impact of the chronic illness and its management on the everyday activities of the patient and the family.

Phases of Chronic Illness

As chronic illness progresses, the impact on the patient and family change as well. The trajectory framework identifies several phases of the chronic illness course and the medical, biographic, and everyday living problems that occur in different phases of the illness. Nine phases are identified: pre-trajectory, trajectory onset, stable, unstable, acute, crisis, comeback, downward, and dying phases (Table 17-3).

TABLE 17-3 Phases in the Trajectory Model of Chronic Illness

Pre-trajectory	Genetic factors or life-style behaviors that place an individual or community at risk for the development of a chronic condition.
Trajectory onset	Appearance of noticeable symptoms; includes period of diagnostic workup and announcement of diagnosis. May be accompanied by biographical limbo as person begins to discover and cope with implications of diagnosis.
Stable	Illness course and symptoms are under control. Biography and everyday life activities are being managed within limitations of illness. Illness management centered on the home.
Unstable	Period of inability to keep symptoms under control or reactivation of illness. Biographical disruption and difficulty in carrying out everyday life activities. Adjustments being made in regimen with care usually taking place at home.
Acute	Severe and unrelieved symptoms or the development of illness complications necessitating hospitalization or bed rest to bring illness course under control. Biography and everyday life activities temporarily placed on hold or drastically cut back.
Crisis	Critical or life-threatening situation requiring emergency treatment or care. Biography and everyday life activities suspended until the crisis passes.
Comeback	A gradual return to an acceptable way of life within limits imposed by disability or illness. Involves physical healing, stretching limitations through rehabilitative procedures, psychosocial coming to terms, and biographical re-engagement with adjustments in everyday life activities.
Downward	Illness course characterized by rapid or gradual physical decline accompanied by increasing disability or difficulty in controlling symptoms. Requires biographical adjustment and alterations in everyday life activity with each major downward step.
Dying	Final days or weeks before death. Characterized by gradual or rapid shutting down of body processes, biographical disengagement and closure, and relinquishment of everyday life interests and activities.

The **pre-trajectory phase** describes the stage at which the person is at risk for a chronic illness because of genetic factors or behaviors that increase the person's susceptibility to chronic illness. The **trajectory phase** is characterized by the appearance of symptoms associated with chronic illness. This phase is often accompanied by uncertainty as symptoms are being evaluated and diagnostic tests are performed. The **stable phase** occurs when symptoms and the illness course are under control. The **unstable phase** is characterized by instability of the chronic illness, recurrence of symptoms, or progression of the illness. During this phase, the person's everyday activities may be disrupted by the illness and the strategies needed to manage it. The **acute phase** is characterized by severe and unrelieved symptoms or complications that necessitate hospitalization for their management. This phase may require major modification of the person's usual activities. The **crisis phase** is characterized by a critical or life-threatening situation that requires emergency treatment or care. The **comeback phase** is a return to an acceptable way of living within the limitations imposed by the chronic condition. The **downward phase** occurs when the illness course progresses and is accompanied by increasing disability or difficulty in managing symptoms. The **dying phase** is characterized by the gradual or rapid decrease in function and disengagement of the individual.

Identifying the phase enables the individual with chronic illness, the family, and health care providers to identify factors that influence the daily problems involved in living with the chronic illness and the care, support, and teaching that are needed at different phases. The nurse using the trajectory model in practice would provide *supportive assistance*; this means that the nurse would support the person's efforts to manage the chronic conditions to whatever extent possible. Although there are times when nurses must take over aspects of management for the patient (during crisis or acute periods), it is necessary to prepare or assist the patient and the family to assume ultimate responsibility for managing the chronic illness.

Providing supportive assistance is guided by the nursing process. The collaborative aspects of the nursing process are specific to each illness. For a more detailed discussion of the framework and its application to specific chronic conditions the reader is referred to the following sources: Corbin and Strauss (1991); Rawnsley (1992; mental illness), Walker (1992; diabetes), Smeltzer (1992; multiple sclerosis), Nokes (1992; HIV infection and AIDS), and Hawthorne (1992; cardiac disease). For a description of how the framework has been operationalized, refer to Robinson et al. (1993).

Steps of the Trajectory Nursing Model

The care provided in the steps of the trajectory framework is similar to that provided in the nursing process—assessment, diagnosis, planning, implementation, and evaluation.

Step 1: Identifying the Trajectory Phase. The first step involves assessing the patient and determining the specific phase (see Table 17-3) of trajectory management (this is also referred to as *locating* the patient along the trajectory). This assessment enables the nurse to identify the general management needed because each management phase has its own set of medical, social, and psychological problems. For example, the problems and subsequent care of a client in a crisis phase of an acute myocardial infarction are quite different from the downward phase of a patient with a chronic-progressive form of multiple sclerosis.

Step 2: Identifying Problems and Establishing Goals. The second step involves identifying the specific problems experienced by the patient related to the phase of the trajectory and establishing goals. These problems and goals are validated with the patient. For example, a patient may report that frequent angina or chest pain interferes with the ability to carry out activities of daily living. Related nursing diagnoses might include the following: activity intolerance or alteration in activities of daily living related to discomfort or pain (angina) secondary to cardiac disease. Prevention and management of symptoms may be identified as an overall goal by the patient and nurse. A more specific goal would be to reduce the episodes of angina associated with activity. An example of a goal for a patient with impaired self-care related to fatigue associated with multiple sclerosis (MS) is: identifying strategies to improve self-care abilities.

Step 3: Establishing Plan to Meet Goals. The third step consists of establishing a realistic and mutually agreed on plan for reaching the goals. Specific criteria to be used to assess progress in meeting the goal would also be identified. For example, a plan of care for the client with angina might include assisting the patient to identify which activities of daily living are likely to precipitate angina and developing strategies to prevent or minimize the occurrence of such episodes. Criteria might include statements that indicate progress toward the goal, such as:

- At the end of the first nurse–patient session, the patient will be able to state four activities of daily living that usually precipitate angina and describe how those situations can be avoided or altered to minimize angina.
- Two weeks after discharge from the hospital, the patient will report fewer episodes of angina and greater ability to engage in desired activities of daily living.
- One month after discharge, the patient will report the ability to anticipate which activities of daily living are likely to cause angina and will identify specific preventive actions.

The idea is to help the patient improve the quality of life through participating in activities while keeping the episodes of angina to a minimum.

Criteria for a patient unable to participate in self-care activities because of fatigue secondary to MS might include the following:

- The patient will identify those self-care activities of highest personal priority by the time the home care nurse has completed the first visit.
- Strategies to minimize nonessential activities will be identified by the patient at the beginning of the second visit by the nurse.
- By the third home care visit the patient will report increased participation in those self-care activities that are personally important.

Step 4: Identifying Factors that Facilitate or Hinder Attainment of Goals. This step involves determining factors that may interfere with achieving the goal.

For example, in the instance of the person with angina, are there stairs in the house that must be climbed several times a day? Are symptoms related to other activities, such as eating? Are there certain activities, such as sexual activities, that the patient or spouse fears? Does the person carry nitroglycerin tablets at all times? How does the person use and store the tablets? Identifying barriers as well as factors that enhance the goal is important because these are factors the nurse can manipulate during the intervention phase.

In the example of the person with multiple sclerosis, the nurse and patient together would identify those factors that prevent the patient from establishing a schedule of self-care activities or a schedule that allows for alternating periods of rest and activity. Additionally, the nurse would assist the person in identifying resources that would decrease the level of fatigue.

Step 5: Implementing Interventions. The fifth step is the intervention phase. Intervention can include providing direct care or serving as advocate for the patient, teaching, counseling, making referrals, or arranging for resources or services. For example, if it is determined in the previous step that one of the situations most likely to precipitate angina is showering and shaving after breakfast, the nurse might assist the patient to pace activities, either showering and shaving before eating breakfast, or doing it late in the evening before retiring, or showering at one time and shaving at another time. If climbing the stairs precipitates angina, the nurse could assist the patient to plan activities to minimize the need to climb the stairs, or suggest that the stairs be climbed slowly, with stops to rest every few steps.

If the patient with multiple sclerosis attempts to complete self-care activities when fatigue is at its highest level, the nurse might suggest ways to reschedule and plan activities more efficiently.

There are many different strategies that a patient might use to prevent or minimize episodes of angina or fatigue; he or she has to discover which work best on an individual basis. Whereas the physician can prescribe appropriate medication and give advice on when and how to use it, it is the nurse who can best help patients develop the life-managing strategies needed to implement their regimens and carry out activities of daily living within the limits of the chronic illness.

Step 6: Evaluating the Effectiveness of Interventions. The final step involves evaluating the effectiveness of interventions to determine if the management goals have been met using the previously established criteria. In chronic illness, success is often measured as progress toward change rather than actual change. If no progress is made, the criteria and goals may need to be revised to make them more realistic given the patient's motivation and lifestyle. However, there are times when change is not possible, and the nurse must accept this. The nurse must also accept that the patient shares responsibility for management outcomes.

Patient Education and Home Care Considerations

The importance of patient and family teaching in care of patients with chronic illness cannot be overemphasized. It is one of the most important aspects of nursing care and often makes the difference between the patient's success or failure to adapt to a chronic health problem and cope with it. The well-informed, educated patient is more likely to recognize changes in symptoms and the onset of complications and to seek early health care than is the patient who does not receive adequate education. The patient who is poorly informed about a chronic health problem or chronic illness and its management is unlikely to recognize subtle changes in symptoms or early complications and to seek early treatment for those complications. Such a patient is more likely to develop complications that require hospitalization than a patient who is well informed. The patient who is well educated about an illness is better able to make informed choices and decisions.

Despite the importance of teaching the patient and family to adapt to chronic illness and to maintain health, the nurse must recognize that patients recently diagnosed with a serious chronic illness need time to grasp the significance of the illness and its impact on their lives. Teaching should be planned carefully so that it provides information that is important to the patient's well-being at the time but does not become overwhelming.

The nurse who cares for patients with a chronic illness in the hospital, clinic setting, or home needs to assess their knowledge about the illness and its management. The nurse cannot assume that because the patient has had an illness for a number of years that the patient has all the knowledge needed or that learning needs have not changed over time. The nurse must also consider that patients who have managed their own care at home are often more knowledgeable about its management than many health care providers.

CRITICAL THINKING EXERCISES

1. A 24-year-old woman has just been diagnosed with a chronic illness that has an uncertain, unpredictable course. She is very upset about the diagnosis and is threatening to kill herself. How would you respond to her reaction to the diagnosis?
2. A 46-year-old man has developed complications from a chronic health problem that he has had but largely ignored for the last 20 years. Describe how you would determine what factors and psychologic reactions to consider in developing a teaching plan to assist the patient in dealing with the complications.
3. How would the learning needs for a patient with a newly diagnosed chronic illness differ from those of a patient with a chronic illness that has been stable for many years, and one who has experienced progressive deterioration in health status? Describe those factors that would be the focus of your assessment in these three patients to assess their needs for patient education.

Nevertheless, the nurse's contact with the patient in the hospital, clinic, or home is often an ideal time to reassess the person's learning needs and ability to manage the health care problem and to provide additional information about its management.

Chronic illness management is a collaborative process in which the nurse plays an important part through the provision of supportive assistance. Collaboration, however, does not end when a patient leaves the hospital; rather, it continues throughout the illness trajectory. Keeping an illness stable over time requires careful and continued monitoring of symptoms and attention to management regimens. Detecting problems early with either the chronic illness itself or the management regimen and devising appropriate interventions can make a significant difference in patient outcomes.

Most chronic illnesses are managed in the home. Therefore, care and teaching during hospitalization focus on what the patient needs to know to manage personal care at home. Resources and services that the patient will require at home are discussed with both the patient and the family and arrangements are made to obtain these resources and services without delay. When appropriate, home care services are contacted directly. The home care nurse will continue with the plan of care and assess how well the patient and family are adapting to the chronic illness and its treatment.

REFERENCES AND BIBLIOGRAPHY

Books

Corbin J and Strauss A. Unending Work and Care. San Francisco, Jossey-Bass, 1988.

Dorsett DS. The trajectory of cancer recovery. In Woog P (ed). The Chronic Illness Trajectory Framework. New York, Springer, 1992, 29–38.

Hawthorne MH. Using the trajectory framework: Reconceptualizing cardiac illness. In Woog P (ed). The Chronic Illness Trajectory Framework. New York, Springer, 1992.

Lupkin IM. Chronic Illness: Impact and Interventions. Boston, Jones & Bartlett, 1986.

Miller JF. Coping with Chronic Illness: Overcoming Powerlessness. Philadelphia, FA Davis, 1983.

National Center for Health Statistics. Current estimates from the national health interview survey, 1991. Series 10 No. 184. US Department of Health and Human Services, 1992.

Nokes KM. Applying the chronic illness trajectory model to HIV/AIDS. In Woog P (ed). The Chronic Illness Trajectory Framework. New York, Springer, 1992, 51–58 .

Rawnsley MM. Chronic mental illness: The timeless trajectory. In Woog P (ed). The Chronic Illness Trajectory Framework. New York, Springer, 1992, 59–67.

Rolland JS. Chronic illness and the family: An overview. In Wright L and Leahey M (eds). Families and Chronic Illness. Springhouse, PA, Springhouse, 1987, 33–54.

Smeltzer SC. Use of the trajectory model of nursing in multiple sclerosis. In Woog P (ed). The Chronic Illness Trajectory Framework New York, Springer, 1992, 73–88.

Strauss A and Glaser B. Chronic Illness and the Quality of Life. St Louis, Mosby, 1975.

Strauss A et al. Chronic Illness and the Quality of Life, 2nd ed. St Louis, Mosby, 1984.

Strauss A and Corbin J. Shaping a New Health Care System. San Francisco, Jossey-Bass, 1988.

Walker EA. Shaping the course of a marathon: Using the trajectory framework for diabetes mellitus. In Woog P (ed), The Chronic Illness Trajectory Framework. New York, Springer, 1992, 89–96.

Journals

Bury M. The sociology of chronic illness: A review of research and prospects. Sociology of Health & Illness 1991; 13(4): 451–468.

Corbin J and Strauss A. A nursing model for chronic illness management based upon the trajectory framework. Scholarly Inquiry for Nursing Practice 1991; 5(3):155–174.

Disability Statistics Program. Disability statistics abstracts. (Prepared for US Department of Education, National Institute on Disability and Rehabilitation Research.) San Francisco, School of Nursing, University of California, 1991.

Feldman J. Chronic disabling illness: A holistic view. J Chronic Dis 1974; 27;287–291.

Forsyth G, Delaney K, and Gresham L. Vying for a winning position: Management style of the chronically ill. Res Nurs Health 1984; 7:181–188.

Foxhall M, Ekberg J, and Griffith N. Adjustment patterns of chronically ill middle-aged persons and spouses. West J Nurs Res 1985; 7(4):425–444.

Gerson E and Strauss A. Time for living: Problems in chronic illness care. Social Policy 1975; 36:12–18.

Haas DL. Application of Orem's self-care deficit theory to the pediatric chronically ill population. Issues in Comprehensive Pediatr Nurs 1990; 13(4):253–264.

Jennings B, Callahan D and Caplan A. Ethical challenges of chronic illness. Hastings Center Report Special Supplement. The Hastings Center, February/March 1986.

Jillings C. Is chronic illness a relevant topic for the critical care nurse? Crit Care Nurse 1987; 7(3):14–17.

Mishel MH. Reconceptualization of the uncertainty in illness theory. Image: J Nurs Scholarship 1990; 22:256–262.

Parsons T. The social system. New York, Free Press of Glencoe, 1951.

Pollock SE. Adaptation to chronic illness: A program of research for testing nursing theory. Nurs Sci Q 1993; 6(2):86–92.

Rankin SH and Weeks DP. Life-span development: A review of theory and practice for families with chronically ill members. Schol Inq Nurs Prac 1989; 3(1):3–22.

Robinson CA. Managing life with a chronic condition: The story of normalization. Qualitative Health Research 1993; 3(1):6–28.

Robinson L et al. Operationalizing the Corbin & Strauss Trajectory Model for elderly clients with chronic illness. Schol In Nurs Prac 1993 Winter; 7(4):253–264.

Shaw MC and Halliday PH. The family, crisis and chronic illness: An evolutionary model. J Adv Nurs 1992; 17(5):537–543.

Stuifbergen AK. The impact of chronic illness on families. Family Community Health 1987; 9(4):43–51.

Wiener Cl and Dodd MJ. Coping amid uncertainty: An illness trajectory perspective. Schol Inq Nurs Prac 1993.

Yarcheski A. Uncertainty in illness and the future. West J Nurs Res 1988; 10(4):401–413.

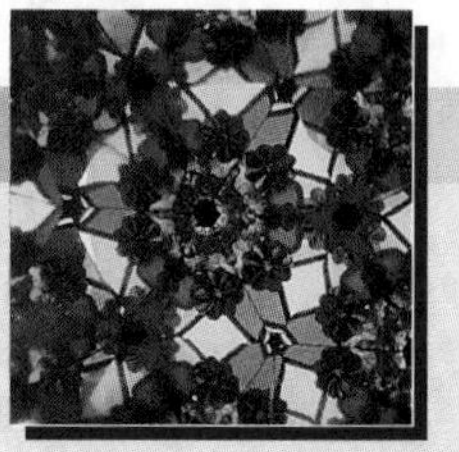

18

Principles and Practices of Rehabilitation

CHAPTER OUTLINE

LEARNING OBJECTIVES

On completion of this chapter, the learner will be able to:

1. Describe the current philosophy of rehabilitation
2. Discuss the interdisciplinary approach to rehabilitation
3. Identify the usual emotional reactions exhibited by patients with newly acquired disabilities
4. Use the nursing process as a framework for care of patients with self-care deficits, impaired physical mobility, impaired skin integrity, and altered patterns of elimination
5. Describe nursing strategies appropriate for promoting self-care through activities of daily living
6. Describe nursing strategies appropriate for promoting mobility and ambulation and the use of assistive devices
7. Describe risk factors and related nursing measures to prevent development of pressure ulcers
8. Incorporate bladder training and bowel training into the plan of care for patients with bladder and bowel problems.
9. Describe the significance of continuity of care from the health care facility to the home or extended care facility for patients who need rehabilitative assistance and services

Philosophy of Rehabilitation

Rehabilitation is a dynamic, health-oriented process that assists an ill or disabled individual to achieve the greatest possible level of physical, mental, spiritual, social, and economic functioning. The rehabilitation process helps the person to achieve an acceptable quality of life with dignity, self-respect, and independence. Rehabilitation programs are designed for individuals with physical, mental, and emotional disabilities. During rehabilitation, the individual is assisted to adjust to the disability by learning how to use resources and to focus on existing abilities. *Abilities, not disabilities, are emphasized.*

Rehabilitation is an integral part of nursing. Rehabilitation efforts should begin during the initial contact with the patient. Every major illness or injury carries with it the threat of disability. *The principles of rehabilitation are basic to the care of all patients.* The emphasis of rehabilitation is to restore the patient to independence or to the pre-illness or pre-injury level of function in as short a time as possible. If this is not possible, the aims of rehabilitation are maximal independence and quality of life acceptable to the patient. Realistic goals based on individual patient assessment are established with the patient to guide the rehabilitation program.

Rehabilitation services are required by more people than ever before because of advances in technology that save the lives of the seriously ill, injured, and disabled. Increasing numbers of patients who are recovering from serious illnesses or injuries are returning to their homes and communities with ongoing needs for rehabilitation. Every patient, regardless of age, socioeconomic status, or diagnosis, has a right to rehabilitation services.

The economic advantage of rehabilitation is readily apparent; instead of being unemployed, the person is rehabilitated into employment. Instead of being dependent on society, the person contributes to it.

Gerontologic Considerations

Dependency is of great concern to the older adult. Performing even simple activities may be very important to the frail elderly. Short-term rehabilitation goals of older adults must include maintaining independence. Older adults may have multiple pathologies, reduced physiologic reserve, impairments of mobility and balance, or mental status changes which must be considered when developing the rehabilitation plan. The older adult may require more time to learn self-care activities, exercises, transfer techniques, and independent mobility. In addition, very old adults require an extensive support system for successful rehabilitation.

Psychologic and Emotional Reactions to Disability

A person usually goes through a series of emotional reactions to a newly acquired disability. The reactions may progress from disorganization and confusion to denial of the disability, grief over the lost function or body part, depression, anger, and finally to acceptance of the disability. Not all individuals go through all the stages; however, most individuals exhibit grief, which is believed to be necessary to adapt to disability. The nurse should show a willingness to listen to the patient talk about the disability. Patients exhibiting grief should not be blithely encouraged to "cheer up."

Because the stages may occur in any order and some stages may not appear at all, the nurse must recognize when the patient is exhibiting ineffective coping and impaired adjustment to a disability. The goal of rehabilitation is to help the patient in revising the self image and to encourage the patient to direct energy into coping and physical functioning. The patient may require the assistance of a mental health professional to adjust to the disability.

Coping With Fatigue

Individuals with a disability frequently experience fatigue. Physical and emotional weariness may be caused by discomfort and pain associated with a chronic health problem, deconditioning associated with prolonged periods of bed rest and immobility, impaired motor function requiring excessive expenditure of energy to ambulate, and the frustrations of performing activities of daily living. Ineffective coping with the disability, unresolved grief, and depression can contribute to fatigue.

The patient can use coping strategies to deal with the psychologic impact of the disability and pain management techniques to control the associated discomforts. (Refer to Chapter 13 for discussion of pain management.) In addition, the nurse can teach the patient to manage fatigue through priority setting and energy conserving techniques.

The following may be useful in teaching patients how to reduce their energy output, thus conserving their strength to achieve a meaningful life style:

Take Control of Your Life
- Face the reality of your disability.
- Emphasize areas of strength.
- Remain outward looking.
- Seek inventive ways to tackle problems.
- Share concerns and frustrations.
- Maintain and improve general health.
- Plan for recreation.

Have Well-Defined Goals and Priorities
- Keep priorities in order; eliminate nonessential activities.
- Plan and pace your activities.

Organize Your Life
- Plan each day.
- Organize work.
- Perform tasks in steps.
- Distribute heavy work throughout the day or week.

Conserve Energy
- Rest before undertaking difficult tasks.
- Stop the activity before fatigue occurs.
- Continue with an exercise conditioning program to strengthen muscles.

Control Your Environment
- Try to be well organized.
- Keep possessions in the same place, so that they can be found with a minimum of effort.

- Store equipment (personal care, crafts, work) in a box or basket.
- Use energy conservation and work simplification techniques.
- Keep work within easy reach and in front of you.
- Use adaptive equipment, self-help aids, and labor-saving devices.
- Recruit assistance of others; delegate when necessary.
- Take safety precautions.

Sexuality Issues

Sexuality involves not only biologic sexual activity but also the person's concept of his masculinity or her femininity. Sexuality affects the way a person reacts to others and is perceived by them. It takes many forms: caring, reaching out, sharing, and emotional intimacy.

Sexual matters usually are considered to be very private and the patient may not want to talk about them. Sexuality problems faced by the disabled include limited access to information about sexuality, lack of opportunity to form friendships and loving relationships, impaired self-image, low self-esteem, and lack of social skills. Frequently, rehabilitation programs focus only on helping the patient to gain independence and forget that sexuality is part of the patient's identity. Recognizing and dealing with sexual issues will promote feelings of self-worth, which are essential to total rehabilitation. The nurse should give the patient permission to discuss sexuality issues and should show a willingness to listen and to help the patient deal with sexuality issues.

The disabled person may need further sex education, communication, and social and assertiveness skills to develop relationships in general. The specialized services of a sex counselor are available to help those with specific sexual needs or conflicts. Classes, books, movies, and support groups also may be useful.

The Rehabilitation Team

Rehabilitation is a creative, dynamic process that requires a team of professionals working together with the patient and the family. The team members represent a variety of disciplines, with each health professional making a unique contribution. Each health professional assesses the patient and identifies patient needs within the discipline's domain. Rehabilitative goals are set. Team members meet in group sessions at frequent intervals to collaborate, to evaluate progress, and to modify goals as needed to facilitate rehabilitation.

Patient. The patient is the key member of the rehabilitation team. The patient is the focus of the team effort and the one who determines the final outcomes of the process. The patient participates in goal setting, in learning to function using remaining abilities, and in adjusting to living with disabilities. The rehabilitation team promotes independence, self-respect, and an acceptable quality of life.

Family. The patient's family is incorporated into the team. The family is a dynamic system. Disability of one member affects other family members. Only by incorporating the family into the rehabilitation process can the family system adapt to the change in one of its members. The family provides ongoing support, participates in problem solving, and learns to provide necessary ongoing care.

Rehabilitation Nurse. The rehabilitation nurse develops a therapeutic and supportive relationship with the patient and the family. The nurse always emphasizes the patient's assets and strengths. During nurse–patient interactions, the nurse actively listens, encourages, and shares the patient's triumphs. The patient is praised for efforts to improve self-concept and self-care abilities.

Through application of the nursing process, the nurse develops a plan of care designed to facilitate rehabilitation, to restore and maintain optimum health, and to prevent complications. The nurse helps the patient to identify strengths and past successes and to develop new goals. Frequently, coping with the disability, self-care, mobility, skin care, and bowel and bladder management are areas for nursing intervention. The nurse assumes roles of caregiver, teacher, counselor, patient advocate, and consultant. Frequently the nurse is the case manager responsible for coordinating the total rehabilitative plan. The nurse collaborates with and coordinates the services provided by all members of the health care team including the home health nurse who is responsible for directing the patient's care after return to the home.

Other Team Members. The rehabilitation team also may include a physician, physiatrist, physical therapist, occupational therapist, speech-language pathologist, psychologist, social worker, vocational counselor, orthotist/prosthetist, rehabilitation engineer, and sex counselor.

Assessment for Rehabilitation

Comprehensive assessment is the basis for formulation of a rehabilitation program. Nursing assessment requires a holistic approach. Physical, mental, emotional, spiritual, social, and economic status must be assessed. The rehabilitation nurse focuses on coping patterns, functional ability, mobility, integrity of skin, and control of bowel and bladder function.

The nurse recognizes the patient as an individual and as a part of a family system. Because no two people react in the same way to a disability, the nurse must determine the patient's and family's perceptions and coping patterns.

Functional ability assessment focuses on self-care: feeding, bathing/hygiene, dressing/grooming, toileting, and mobility. Functional ability depends on good joint motion, muscle strength, and an intact neurologic system. Disabilities most likely to produce loss of function are those involving the musculoskeletal, neurologic, and cardiovascular systems. In addition, secondary problems related to the disability that affect functional ability, such as muscle atrophy and deconditioning, are assessed. Also, residual strengths unaffected by disease or disability are evaluated.

The nurse assesses the ability of an individual to function by observing the person perform the activity (eating, dressing) and noting the degree of independence, the time taken, and the amount of assistance required. The nurse notes the patient's mobility, coordination, and endurance.

There are numerous assessment tools and scales to evaluate the functional abilities of the patient. Generally these are used to assess the individual's ability to perform activities of daily living independently as well as to communicate. Rehabilitation centers use these tools to form an initial assessment of the patient's abilities and to monitor the patient's progress in independence.

The **PULSES** profile is used to assess *p*hysical condition (*e.g.*, health/illness status), *u*pper extremity functions (*e.g.*, eating, bathing), *l*ower extremity functions (*e.g.*, transfer, ambulation), *s*ensory function (*e.g.*, vision, hearing, speech), *e*xcretory function (*i.e.*, control of bowel/bladder), and *s*ituational factors (*e.g.*, social and financial support). Each of these areas is rated on a scale of 1 (independent) to 4 (greatest dependency).

The **Barthel Index** is used to measure the patient's level of independence in activities of daily living (feeding, bathing, dressing, grooming), continence, toileting, transfers, and ambulation (or wheelchair mobility). This scale does not address communicative or cognitive abilities.

The **Functional Independence Measure (FIM)** is used to assess the patient's level of independence. The six areas assessed are self-care, sphincter management, mobility, locomotion, communication and cognitive ability, and social cognition.

The **Patient Evaluation Conference System (PECS)** contains 15 categories. This comprehensive assessment scale includes such areas as medications, pain, nutrition, use of assistive devices, psychologic status, vocation, and recreation.

Other areas that require nursing assessment include potential for altered skin integrity, altered bowel and bladder control, and sexual dysfunction.

❑ NURSING PROCESS
Self-Care Deficit: Activities of Daily Living

Activities of daily living (ADLs) are those self-care activities that the patient must accomplish each day to meet personal needs and the demands of daily life. ADLs include personal hygiene/bathing, dressing/grooming, feeding, and toileting. Many patients are unable to perform these activities easily. An ADL program is started as soon as the rehabilitation process begins. The ability to perform ADLs is frequently the key to independence, return to the home, and reentry into the community.

Assessment

The nurse must observe and assess the patient's ability to perform ADLs to determine the level of independence in self-care and the need for nursing intervention. The activity of bathing requires obtaining bath water and utensils, undressing, washing, and drying the body after bathing. Dressing requires selecting, putting on and taking off clothing, fastening the clothing, and combing the hair. Self-feeding requires selecting foods, using utensils to bring food to the mouth, and chewing and swallowing the food. The activity of toileting includes the ability to get to the toilet, removing clothing to use the toilet, getting on and off the toilet, cleansing self, redressing self, and performing hand hygiene. Patients who can sit up and raise their hands to their head probably can begin to bathe and feed themselves. Balance and some muscle strength and coordination are required for dressing. Toileting requires transfer and dressing abilities.

In addition, the nurse needs to be aware of the patient's medical conditions and the effect that they have on the ability to perform activities of daily living. Assessment of the family's involvement in the patient's activities of daily living is also important. This information is valuable in goal setting and development of the plan of care to maximize self-care.

Diagnosis

Nursing Diagnoses

Based on the assessment data, major nursing diagnoses for the patient may include the following:

- Self-care deficit: bathing/hygiene, dressing/grooming, feeding, toileting related to disability (*e.g.*, paralysis, amputation, neuromuscular impairment)

Planning and Implementation

Goals. The major goals of the patient include bathing/hygiene independently or with assistance, using adaptive devices as appropriate; dressing/grooming independently or with assistance, using adaptive devices as appropriate; feeding independently or with assistance, using adaptive devices as appropriate; and toileting independently or with assistance, using adaptive devices as appropriate. In addition, the individual with a self-care deficit expresses satisfaction with the extent of independence in self-care activities.

Nursing Interventions

Self-Care: Bathing/Hygiene, Dressing/Grooming, Feeding, Toileting. To learn methods of self-care effectively, the patient must be motivated. An "I'd rather do it myself" attitude is encouraged. The nurse must also help the patient identify the safe limits of independent activity. Knowing when to ask for assistance is very important.

The nurse teaches, guides, and supports the patient learning how to perform self-care activities. Consistency in instructions and assistance given by the caregiver facilitates the learning process. Recording the patient's performance provides data for evaluating progress and may be used as a source of motivation and for morale building (Chart 18-1).

Self-care techniques need to be adapted to accommodate the individual patient differences and life style. Often a simple maneuver requires concentration and the exertion of considerable effort on the part of the individual with a disability. Common sense and a little ingenuity may promote increased independence. It is important to remember that there is usually more than one way to accomplish a self-care activity. For example, a person who cannot quite reach his or her head may be able to do so by leaning forward. Encouraging the patient to participate in a support group may help in discovering inventive solutions to self-care problems.

If the patient has difficulty in performing an activity of daily living, an adaptive/assistive device (self-help device) may be useful. A large variety of assistive devices are available commercially or can be fabricated by the nurse, the occupational therapist, the patient, or the family. The nurse

CHART 18-1
Guidelines for Teaching the Activities of Daily Living

1. Define the goal of the activity with the patient. Be realistic. Set short-term goals that can be accomplished in the near future.
2. Identify several approaches to accomplish the task. (Example: There are several ways to put on a given garment.)
3. Select the approach most likely to succeed.
4. Specify the approach on the patient's care plan and the patient's level of accomplishment on the progress notes.
5. Identify the motions necessary to accomplish the activity. (Example: To pick up glass, extend arm; place open hand next to glass; flex fingers around glass; move arm/hand holding glass vertically; flex arm toward body.)
6. Focus on gross functional movements initially and gradually include activities that use finer motions (*e.g.,* buttoning clothes, eating with a fork).
7. Encourage the patient to perform the activity up to maximal capacity within the limitations of the disability.
8. Monitor the patient's tolerance.
9. Minimize frustration and fatigue.
10. Support the patient by giving appropriate praise for effort put forth and for acts accomplished.
11. Assist the patient to perform and practice the activity in real-life situations.

should be alert to "gadgets" coming on the market that may be useful to the individual with a disability. The nurse must exercise professional judgment and caution in recommending these to vulnerable patients.

A wide selection of computerized assistive devices is available or can be designed to help individuals with severe disabilities to function more independently. The ABLEDATA* project offers a computerized listing of commercially available aids and equipment for individuals with disabilities.

If a person has a severe disability, independent self-care may be an unrealistic goal. The individual with the disability may require a personal attendant to perform activities of daily living. Because of the roles one assumes in life, family members may not be appropriate for providing bathing/hygiene, dressing/grooming, feeding, and toileting assistance. A personal caregiver may need to be hired. The individual with the disability is assisted in accepting self-care dependency. Independence in other areas such as social interaction would be emphasized to promote self-concept (*i.e.*, self-esteem, role performance, personal identity).

Evaluation

Expected Outcomes

1. Demonstrates independent self-care in bathing/hygiene or with assistance, using adaptive devices as appropriate
   a. Bathes self at maximal level of independence
   b. Uses adaptive devices effectively
   c. Reports satisfaction with level of independence in bathing/hygiene
2. Demonstrates independent self-care in dressing/grooming or with assistance, using adaptive devices as appropriate
   a. Dresses/grooms self at maximal level of independence
   b. Uses adaptive devices effectively
   c. Reports satisfaction with level of independence in dressing/grooming
   d. Demonstrates increased interest in appearance
3. Demonstrates independent self-care in feeding or with assistance, using adaptive devices as appropriate
   a. Feeds self at maximal level of independence
   b. Uses adaptive devices effectively
   c. Demonstrates increased interest in eating
   d. Maintains adequate nutritional intake
4. Demonstrates independent self-care in toileting or with assistance, using adaptive devices as appropriate
   a. Toilets self at maximal level of independence
   b. Uses adaptive devices effectively
   c. Indicates positive feeling regarding level of toileting independence
   d. Experiences adequate frequency of bowel and bladder elimination
   e. Does not experience incontinence, constipation, urinary tract infection, or other complications

*National Rehabilitation Information Center, 8455 Colesville Rd., Silver Spring, MD 20910-3319. Toll-free telephone number: 800-346-2742 (voice/TDD).

❑ NURSING PROCESS
Impaired Physical Mobility

Individuals who are ill or injured are frequently placed on bed rest or have their activities limited. Problems frequently associated with immobility include weakened muscles, joint contracture, and deformity. Each joint of the body has a normal range of motion. If the range is limited, the functions of the joint and of the muscles that move the joint are impaired and painful deformities may develop. Nurses must identify patients at risk for such complications.

Another problem frequently seen in rehabilitation nursing is an altered ambulatory/mobility pattern. The patient with a disability may be unable either temporarily or permanently to walk independently and unaided. The nurse assesses the mobility of the patient and designs care that promotes independent mobility within the prescribed therapeutic limits.

When a person is not able to exercise and move joints through the full range of motion, contractures may develop. A **contracture** is a shortening of the muscle and tendon that leads to deformity. Contractures limit joint mobility. When the contracted joint is moved, the patient experiences pain. In addition, it requires more energy to move when joints are contracted and deformed.

An **orthosis** is an external appliance that provides support, prevents or corrects deformities, and improves function. Orthoses include braces, splints, collars, corsets, or supports that are designed and fitted by an orthotist or prosthetist. Static orthoses (no moving parts) are used to stabilize joints and prevent contractures. Dynamic orthoses are flexible and are used to improve function by assisting weak muscles. The nurse recognizes the need for orthoses and works with the patient and orthotist to obtain maximum benefits from these devices.

Assessment

At times an individual's mobility is restricted because of pain, paralysis, loss of muscle strength, systemic disease, presence of an immobilizing device (*e.g.*, cast, brace), or prescribed limits to promote healing. Assessment of the patient's mobility includes positioning, ability to move, muscular strength, joint function, and the prescribed mobility limits. The nurse may need to collaborate with the physical therapist or other team members to assess mobility.

During position change, transfer, and ambulation activities, the nurse assesses the patient's abilities, the extent of disability, and residual capacity for physiologic adaptation. The nurse observes for orthostatic hypotension, pallor, diaphoresis, nausea, tachycardia, and fatigue.

If a patient is not able to ambulate independently, without assistance, the nurse assesses ability to balance, transfer, and use assistive devices (*e.g.*, crutches, walker). Crutch walking requires a high energy expenditure and produces considerable cardiovascular stress. Older persons with reduced exercise capacity, decreased arm strength, and problems with balance due to age and multiple diseases may be unable to use crutches. A walker is more stable and may be a better choice for the older patient. The nurse assesses the patient's ability to use various devices that promote mobility.

If a patient uses an orthosis, the nurse monitors the patient for effective use and potential problems associated with its use.

Diagnosis

Nursing Diagnoses

Based on the assessment data, major nursing diagnoses for the patient may include the following:

- Impaired physical mobility related to prescribed bed rest, neurologic or musculoskeletal disorder, immobilizing device, contracture, activity intolerance
- Activity intolerance

Planning and Implementation

Goals. The major goals of the patient may include absence of contracture and deformity, maintenance of muscle strength and joint mobility, independent mobility, and increased activity tolerance.

Nursing Interventions

Positioning. Deformities and contractures can often be prevented by proper positioning. Maintaining correct body alignment while in bed is essential regardless of the position selected. During each contact with the patient the nurse evaluates the patient's position. The nurse suggests and assists the patient to achieve proper positioning and alignment.

The most common positions that a patient assumes in bed are supine (dorsal), side-lying (lateral), and prone. The nurse helps the patient assume these positions and supports the body in correct alignment with pillows. Chart 18-2 summarizes these positions. At times, a splint (*e.g.*, wrist/hand splint) may be fabricated by the occupational therapist to support a joint and prevent deformity. The nurse must assure proper use of the splint and provide skin care.

Preventing External Rotation of the Hip. Patients who are in bed for any period of time may develop external rotation deformity of the hip. The ball-and-socket joint of the hip has a tendency to rotate outward when the patient lies on his or her back. A trochanter roll extending from the crest of the ilium to the midthigh will prevent this deformity. With correct placement, the trochanter roll serves as a mechanical wedge under the projection of the greater trochanter.

Preventing Footdrop. Footdrop is a deformity in which the foot is plantar flexed (the ankle bends in the direction of the sole of the foot). If the condition continues without correction, the patient will not be able to hold the foot in a normal position and will walk on his or her toes without touching the ground with the heel of the foot. The deformity is caused by contracture of both the gastrocnemius and the soleus muscles. Damage to the peroneal nerve may result in foot drop. It may also be produced by loss of flexibility of the Achilles tendon.

- Prolonged bed rest, lack of exercise, incorrect positioning in bed, and the weight of the bedding forcing the toes into plantar flexion are factors that contribute to footdrop.

To prevent this crippling deformity, a footboard or pillows are used to keep the feet at right angles to the legs when the patient is in a supine position. The feet are positioned so that both plantar surfaces are firmly against the footboard or pillows. High-top athletic shoes or positioning splints may be used to maintain the position.

The patient is encouraged to perform ankle exercises several times each hour. These exercises include dorsiflexion and plantar flexion of the feet, flexion and extension (curl and stretch) of the toes, and eversion and inversion of the feet at the ankles.

Maintaining Muscle Strength and Joint Mobility. Optimal functioning depends on the strength of the muscles and joint motion. Active participation in ADLs promotes maintenance of muscle strength and joint mobility. Range-of-motion exercises and specific therapeutic exercises may be included in the nursing plan of care.

Performing Range-of-Motion Exercises. Range of motion is movement of a joint through its full range in all appropriate planes (Chart 18-3). To maintain or increase the

CHART 18-2
Positioning a Patient in Bed

Supine (Dorsal) Position

1. The head is in line with the spine, both laterally and anteroposteriorly.
2. The trunk is positioned so that flexion of the hips is minimized.
3. The arms are flexed at the elbow with the hands resting against the lateral abdomen.
4. The legs are extended with a small, firm support under the popliteal area.
5. The heels are supported off the mattress with a small pillow or towel roll at the ankles.
6. The toes are pointed straight up, supported by an adjusted foot board used to prevent footdrop.
7. Trochanter rolls are placed under the greater trochanter in the hip joint areas to prevent external rotation of the hip.

Side-Lying (Lateral) Position

1. The head is in line with the spine, supported by a pillow.
2. The body is in alignment and is not twisted.
3. Shoulders and elbows are flexed and the upper arm is supported by a pillow.
4. The uppermost hip joint is slightly forward and the leg is supported in a position of slight abduction by a pillow.
5. The feet are placed and supported in neutral dorsiflexion.
6. The back may be supported by a pillow.

Prone (on Abdomen) Position

1. The head is turned laterally and is in alignment with the rest of the body.
2. The arms are abducted and externally rotated at the shoulder joint; the elbows are flexed.
3. A small flat support is placed under the pelvis, extending from the level of the umbilicus to the upper third of the thigh.
4. The lower extremities remain in a neutral position.
5. The toes are suspended over the edge of the mattress.

motion of a joint, range-of-motion exercises (Chart 18-4) are initiated as soon as the patient's condition permits. The exercises are planned for the individual to accommodate the wide variation in the degrees of motion that persons of varying body build and age groups can attain.

Range-of-motion exercises may be **active** (performed by the patient under supervision of the nurse), **assisted** (the nurse helps the patient if unable to do exercise independently), or **passive** (performed by the nurse). Unless prescribed otherwise, a joint should be moved through its range of motion three times, at least twice a day. The joint to be exercised is supported, the bones above the joint are stabilized, and the body part distal to the joint is moved through the range of motion of the joint. For example, when the elbow is taken through its range of motion, the humerus must be stabilized while the radius and ulna are moved through their range of motion at the elbow joint (Fig. 18-1).

The joint should not be moved beyond its free range of motion. Therefore, the joint is moved to the point of

Text continues on page 335.

CHART 18-3
Definition of Terms

Abduction movement away from the midline of the body

Adduction movement toward the midline of the body

Flexion bending of a joint so that the angle of the joint diminishes

Extension the return movement from flexion; the joint angle is increased

Rotation turning or movement of a part around its axis

- **Internal** turning inward, toward the center
- **External** turning outward, away from the center

Dorsiflexion movement that flexes or bends the hand back toward the body or foot toward the leg

Palmar flexion movement that flexes or bends the hand in the direction of the palm

Plantar flexion movement that flexes or bends the foot in the direction of the sole

Pronation rotation of the forearm so that the palm of the hand is down

Supination rotation of the forearm so that the palm of the hand is up

Opposition touching thumb to each finger tip on same hand

Inversion movement that turns the sole of the foot inward

Eversion movement that turns the sole of the foot outward

CHART 18-4
Range-of-Motion Exercises

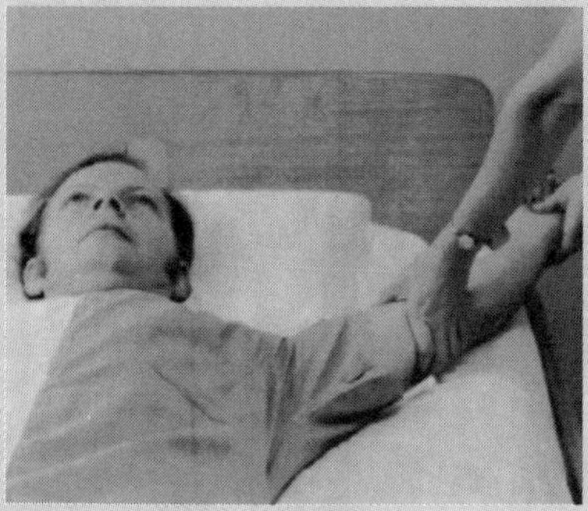

Abduction of shoulder. Move arm from side of body to above the head. Then return arm to side of body or neutral position (adduction).

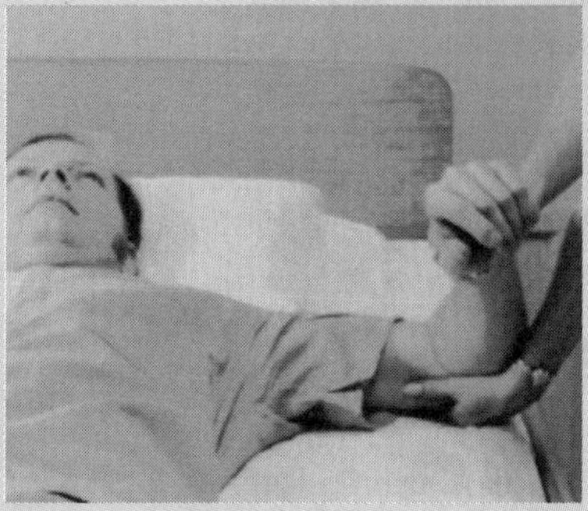

Internal rotation of shoulder. With arm at shoulder height, elbow bent at a 90-degree angle, and palm toward feet, turn upper arm until palm and forearm face backward.

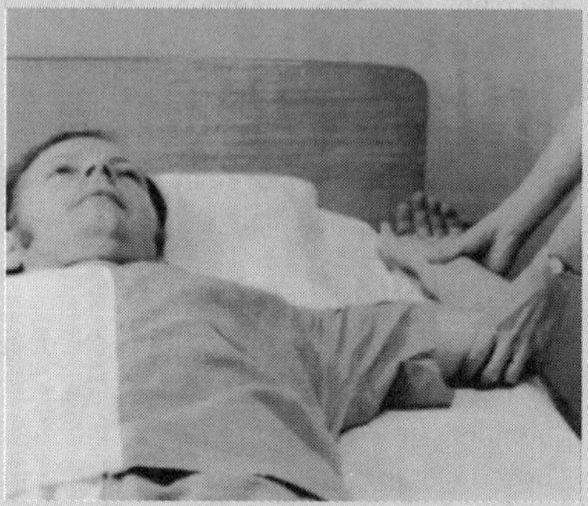

External rotation of shoulder. With arm at shoulder height, elbow bent at a 90-degree angle, and palm toward feet, turn upper arm until the palm and forearm face forward.

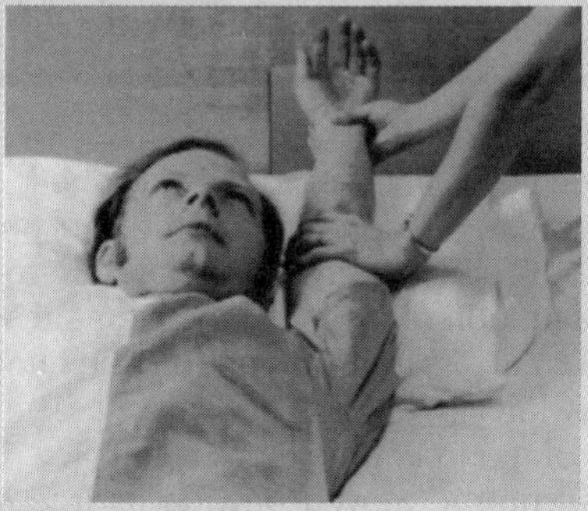

Forward flexion of shoulder. Move arm forward and upward until it is alongside of head.

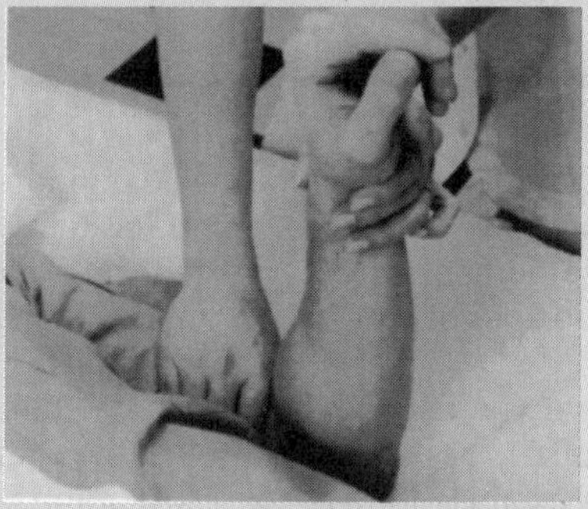

Pronation of forearm. With elbow at waist and bent at 90-degree angle, turn hand so that palm is facing down.

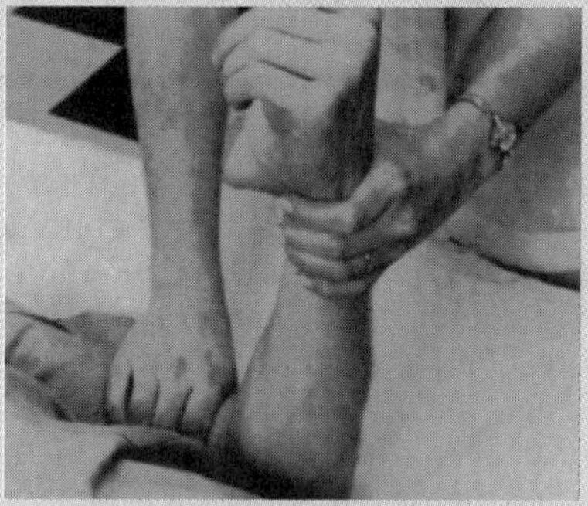

Supination of forearm. With elbow at waist and arm bent at 90-degree angle, turn hand so that palm is facing up.

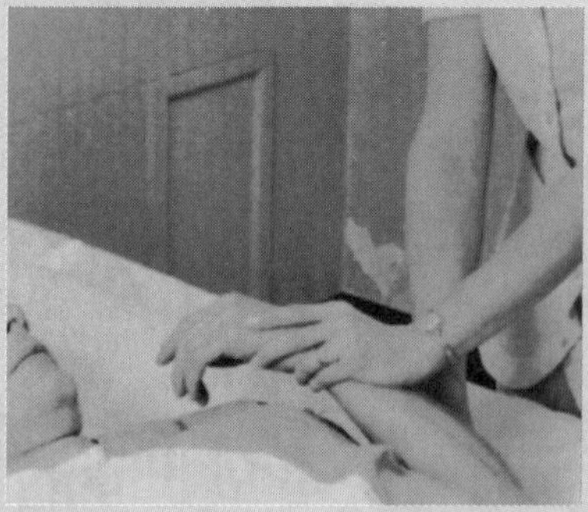

Flexion of elbow. Bend elbow, bringing forearm and hand toward shoulder. Then return forearm and hand to neutral position (arm straight).

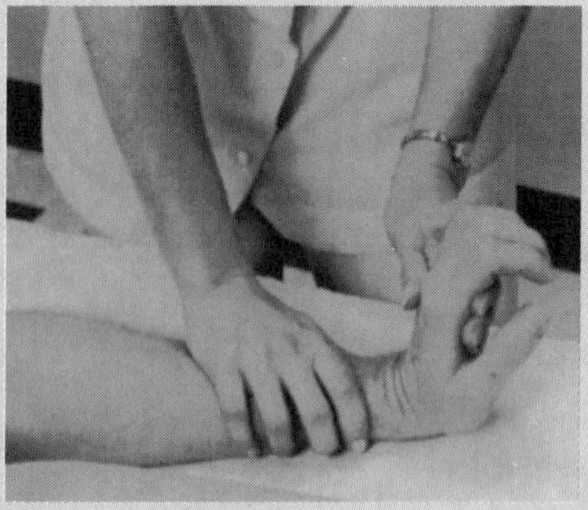

Wrist extension.

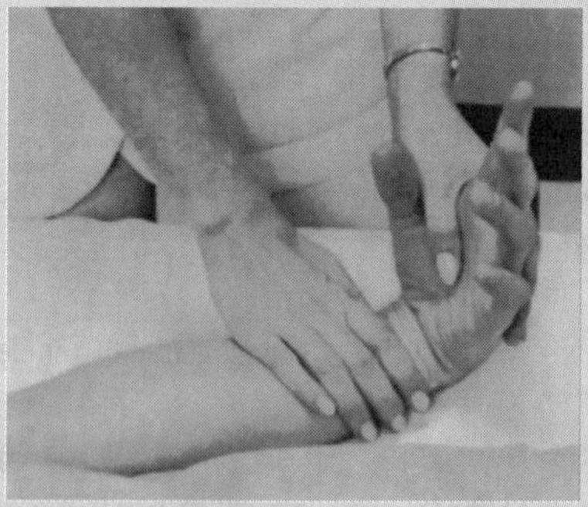

Flexion of wrist. Bend wrist so that palm is toward forearm. Straighten to a neutral position.

(continued)

CHART 18-4 *(continued)*

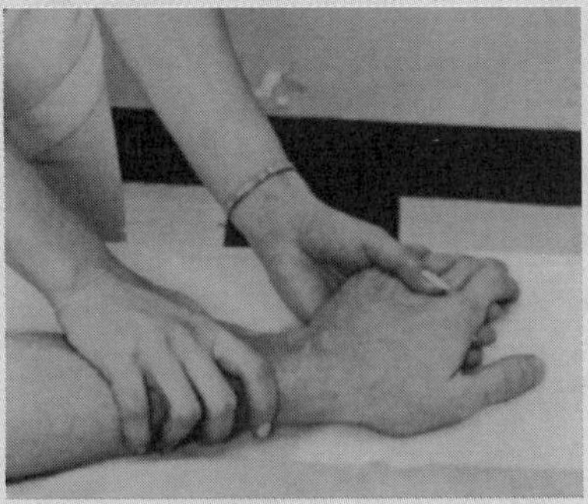

Ulnar deviation. Move hand sideways so that the side of hand on which little finger is located moves toward forearm.

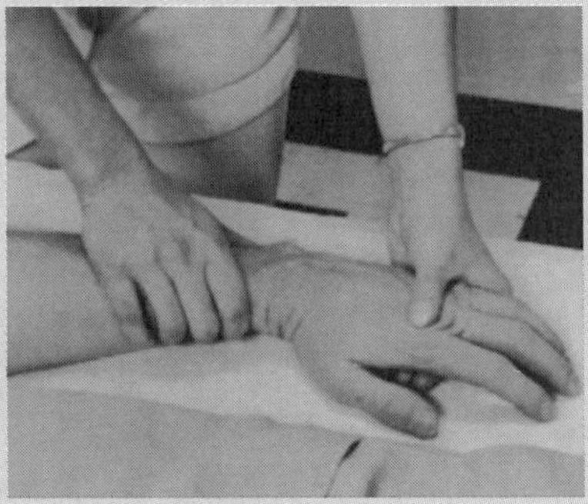

Radial deviation. Move hand sideways so that side of hand on which thumb is located moves toward forearm.

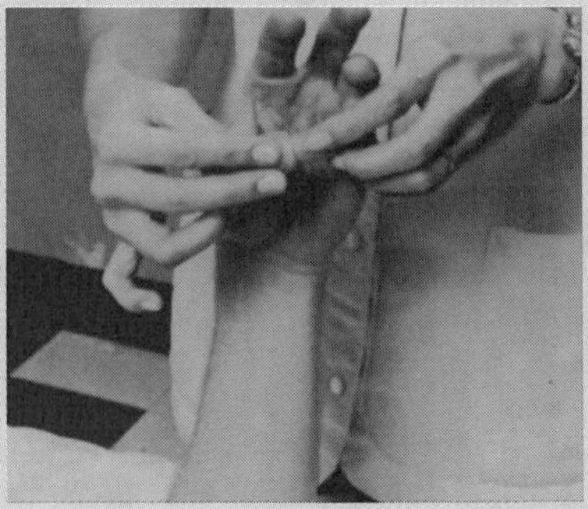

Thumb opposition. Move thumb out and around to touch little finger.

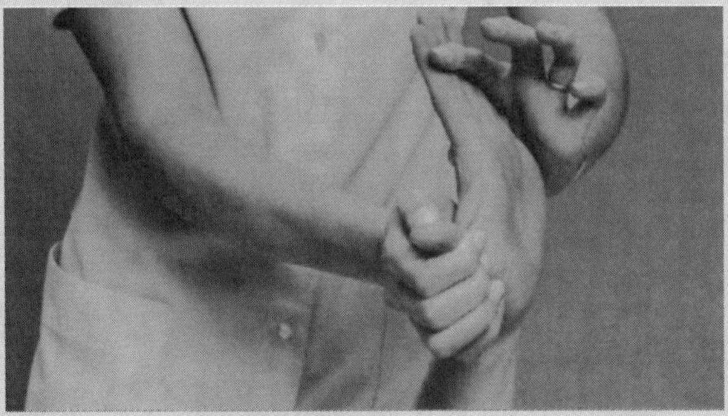

Extension of fingers.

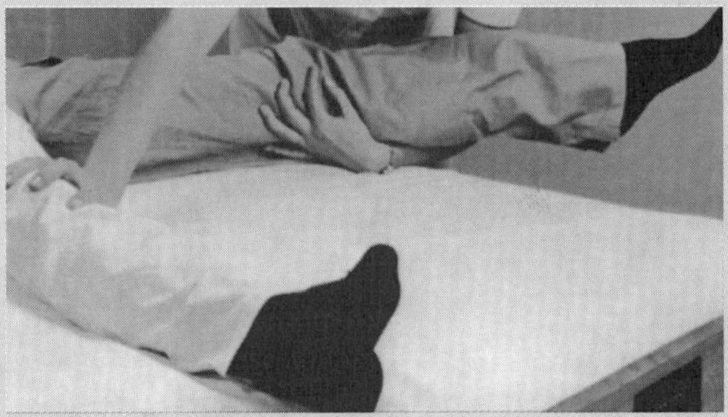

Abduction-adduction of hip. Move leg outward from the body as far as possible. Return leg from abducted position to neutral position and across the other leg as far as possible.

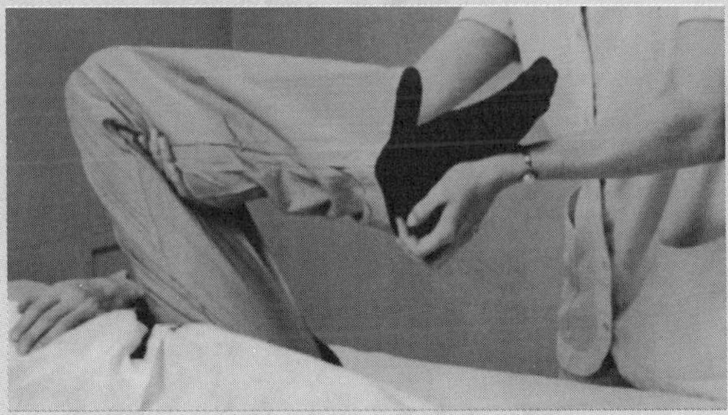

Flexion of hip and flexion of knee. Bend hip by moving the leg forward as far as possible. Return leg from the flexed position to the neutral position.

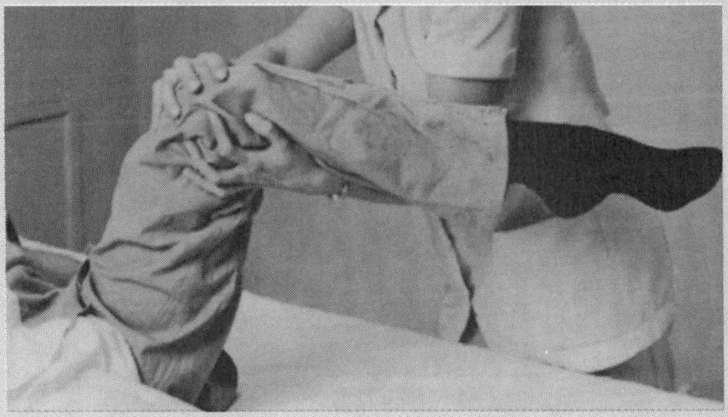

Internal-external rotation of hip. Turn leg in an inward motion so that toes point in. Turn leg in an outward motion so that toes point out.

(continued)

CHART 18-4 (continued)

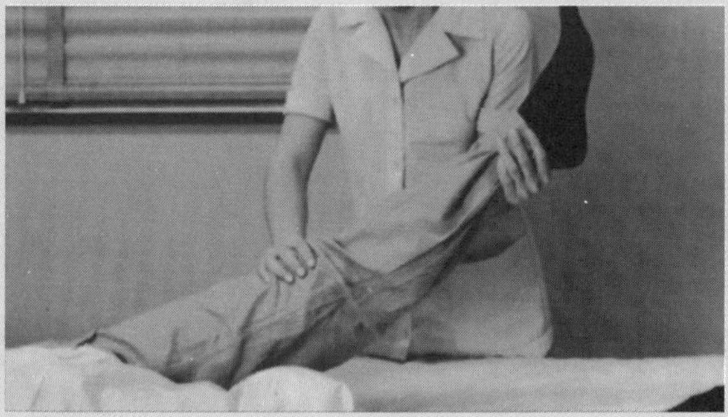

To stretch hamstring muscles, straighten leg and then raise the leg.

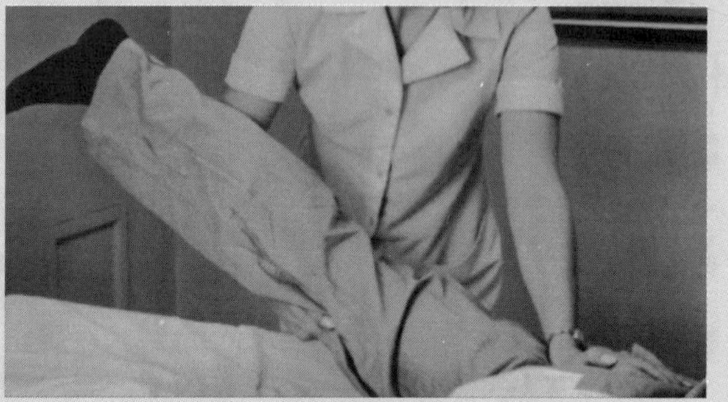

Hypertension of hip. Place the patient in a prone position, and move leg backward from the body as far as possible.

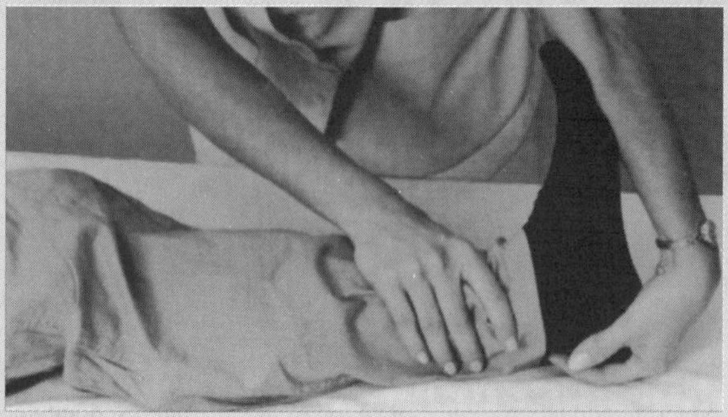

Dorsiflexion of foot. Move foot up and toward the leg. Then move the foot down and away from the leg (plantar flexion).

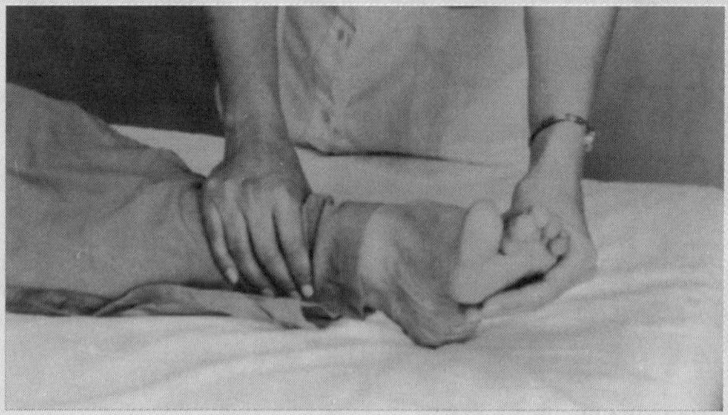

Inversion and eversion of foot. Move foot so that sole is facing outward (eversion). Then move foot so that sole is facing inward (inversion).

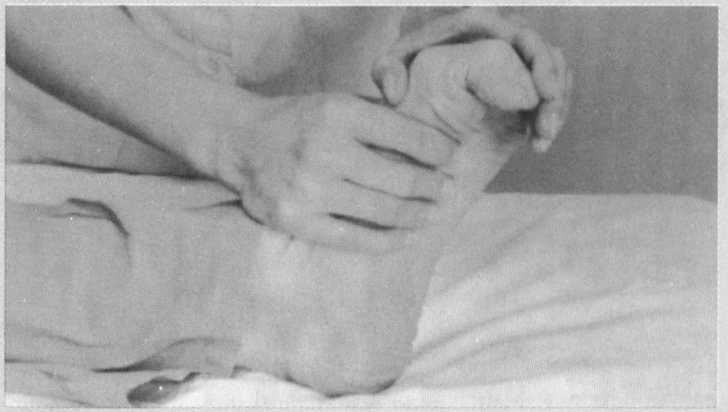

Flexion of toes. Bend the toes toward the ball of foot.

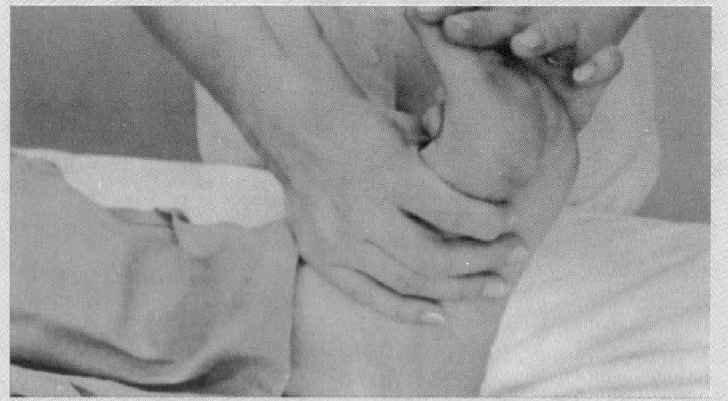

Extension of toes. Straighten toes and pull them toward the leg as far as possible.

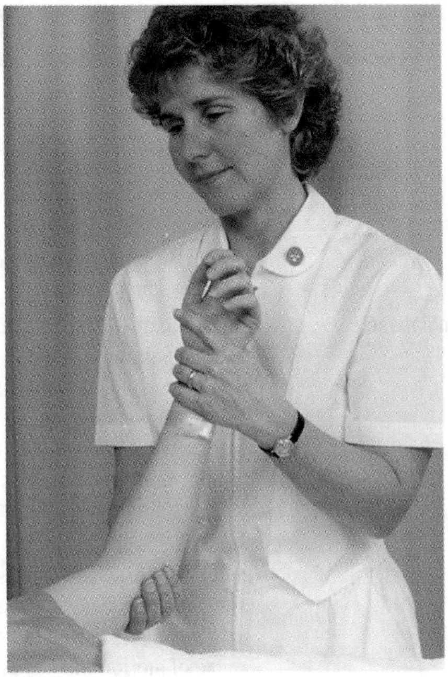

FIGURE 18-1. Supporting the elbow joint while moving through the range of motion.

resistance and stopped at the point of pain. If muscle spasms are present, move the joint slowly to the point of resistance, then apply gentle steady pressure until the muscle relaxes. Continue the motion to the joint's final point of resistance.

To perform assisted or passive range-of-motion exercises, the patient must be in a comfortable supine position with arms at the sides and knees extended. Good body posture is maintained during the exercises. The nurse also uses good body mechanics during the exercise session.

Performing Therapeutic Exercises. Therapeutic exercises are prescribed by the physician and performed with the assistance and guidance of a physical therapist or nurse.

The patient should have a clear understanding of the goal of the prescribed exercise. Written instructions about the frequency, duration, and number of repetitions, as well as simple line drawings of the exercise, help to assure adherence to the exercise program.

Exercise, when correctly performed, assists in (1) maintaining and building muscle strength, (2) maintaining joint function, (3) preventing deformity, (4) stimulating circulation, (5) developing endurance, and (6) promoting relaxation. Exercise is also valuable in helping restore motivation and well-being of the patient. There are five types of exercise: passive, active assistive, active, resistive, and isometric. The description, purpose, and action of each of these exercises are summarized in Table 18-1.

Promoting Independent Mobility. When the patient's condition stabilizes and the physical condition permits, the patient is assisted to sit up on the side of the bed and then to stand. The patient's tolerance of this activity is assessed.

Orthostatic (postural) hypotension may develop when the patient assumes a vertical position. Because of inadequate vasomotor reflexes, blood pools in the splanchnic (visceral) area and in the legs, resulting in inadequate cerebral circulation. If indicators of orthostatic hypotension (*i.e.*, drop in blood pressure, pallor, diaphoresis, nausea, tachycardia, dizziness) are present, the activity is stopped and the patient is assisted to a supine position in bed.

Some disabilities, such as spinal cord injury, brain damage, and conditions that require extended periods in the recumbent position, prevent patients from assuming an upright position at the bedside. A **tilt table,** a board that can be tilted in 5- to 10-degree increments from a horizontal to a vertical position, may be used. The tilt table promotes vasomotor adjustment to positional changes and helps the patient with standing balance and weight bearing activities to help prevent decalcification of bones associated with disuse syndrome.

The patient is transferred from the bed to the tilt table and position and secure the patient to prevent sliding or falling during standing. Elastic stockings are used to prevent venous stasis. At times, a compression leotard or snug-fitting abdominal binder and elastic compression bandaging of the legs are needed to prevent venous stasis and ensuing orthostatic hypotension. The nurse monitors the patient's blood pressure and pulse and observes for signs of orthostatic hypotension and cerebral insufficiency (*i.e.*, the patient reports feeling faint and weakness), which suggest intolerance of the upright position. If the patient does not tolerate the upright position, the nurse should return the patient to a horizontal position. When the patient is standing, the feet are protected with a pair of properly fitted shoes. Extended periods of standing are avoided because of venous pooling and pressure on the soles of the feet.

Assisting the Patient With Transfer. A **transfer** is the movement of the patient from one place to another (*e.g.*, bed to chair, chair to commode, wheelchair to tub). As soon as the patient is permitted out of bed, transfer activities are started. The nurse assesses the patient's ability to participate actively in the transfer.

While confined to bed, it is important that the patient maintain muscle strength and participate in "push-up" exercises to strengthen the arm and shoulder extensor muscles. The push-up exercise requires the patient to sit upright in bed; a book is placed under each of the patient's hands to provide a hard surface, and the patient is instructed to push down on the book raising the body. It is desirable that the patient be able to raise and move the body in different directions by means of these push-up exercises.

The nurse teaches the patient how to transfer. There are several methods of transferring from the bed to the wheelchair when the patient is unable to stand. The technique chosen should be appropriate for the patient, considering the abilities and disabilities. It is helpful for the nurse to demonstrate the technique. If the physical therapist is involved in teaching the patient to transfer, the nurse and the physical therapist must collaborate so that consistent instructions are given to the patient. During transfer, the nurse assists and coaches the patient. Figure 18-2 shows weight-bearing and non–weight-bearing transfer.

If the patient's muscles are not strong enough to overcome the resistance of body weight, a polished lightweight board (transfer board; sliding board) may be used to bridge the gap between the bed and the chair. The patient slides across on the board. This board may also be used to transfer

TABLE 18-1 Therapeutic Exercises

Exercise	Description	Purposes	Action
Passive	An exercise carried out by the therapist or the nurse without assistance from the patient	To retain as much joint range of motion as possible, to maintain circulation	Stabilize the proximal joint, and support the distal part. Move the joint smoothly, slowly, and gently through its full range of motion. Avoid producing pain.
Active assistance	An exercise carried out by the patient with the assistance of the therapist or the nurse	To encourage normal muscle function	Support the distal part, and encourage the patient to take the joint actively through its range of motion. Give no more assistance than is necessary to accomplish the action. Short periods of activity should be followed by adequate rest periods.
Active	An exercise accomplished by the patient without assistance; activities include turning from side to side and from back to abdomen and moving up and down in bed	To increase muscle strength	When possible, active exercise should be performed against gravity. The joint is moved through full range of motion without assistance. (Make sure that the patient does not substitute another joint movement for the one intended.)
Resistive	An active exercise carried out by the patient working against resistance produced by either manual or mechanical means	To provide resistance to increase muscle power	The patient moves the joint through its range of motion while the therapist resists slightly at first and then with progressively increasing resistance. Sandbags and weights can be used and are applied at the distal point of the involved joint. The movements should be performed smoothly.
Isometric or muscle setting	Alternately contracting and relaxing a muscle while keeping the part in a fixed position; this exercise is performed by the patient	To maintain strength when a joint is immobilized	Contract or tighten the muscle as much as possible without moving the joint, hold for several seconds, then let go and relax. Breathe deeply.

the patient from the chair to the toilet or bathtub bench. Safety is a primary concern during a transfer.

- Chairs and beds must be locked before the patient transfers.
- One end of the transfer board is placed under the patient's buttocks and the other end on the surface to which the transfer is being made (*e.g.*, the chair).
- The patient is instructed to push up with his or her hands to shift the buttocks and then to slide across the board to the other surface.

Frequently the nurse assists weak and incapacitated patients out of bed. The nurse supports and gently assists the patient during position changes, protecting the patient from injury. The nurse avoids pulling on the weak or paralyzed upper extremity, to prevent dislocation of the shoulder. The patient is assisted to move toward the stronger side. Chart 18-5 outlines techniques for assisting the patient out of bed.

In the home setting, getting in and out of bed and performing chair, toilet, and tub transfers are difficult for persons with weak musculature and loss of hip, knee, and ankle motion. A rope attached to the headboard of the bed helps the patient to pull toward the center of the bed, and the use of a rope attached to the footboard facilitates getting in and out of bed. The height of a chair can be raised with cushions on the seat or with hollowed-out blocks placed under the chair legs. Bars can be attached to the wall near the toilet and tub to provide leverage and stability.

Preparing for Ambulation. Regaining the ability to walk is a prime morale builder. To be prepared for ambulation—whether with brace, walker, cane, or crutches—the patient must strengthen the muscles required. Exercise is the foundation of preparation. The nurse instructs and supervises the patient in these exercises.

For ambulation, the quadriceps muscles and the gluteal muscles are strengthened. The quadriceps muscles stabilize the knee joint. To perform **quadricep setting exercises,** the patient contracts the quadriceps muscle by attempting to push the popliteal area against the mattress and at the same time raising the heel. The patient maintains

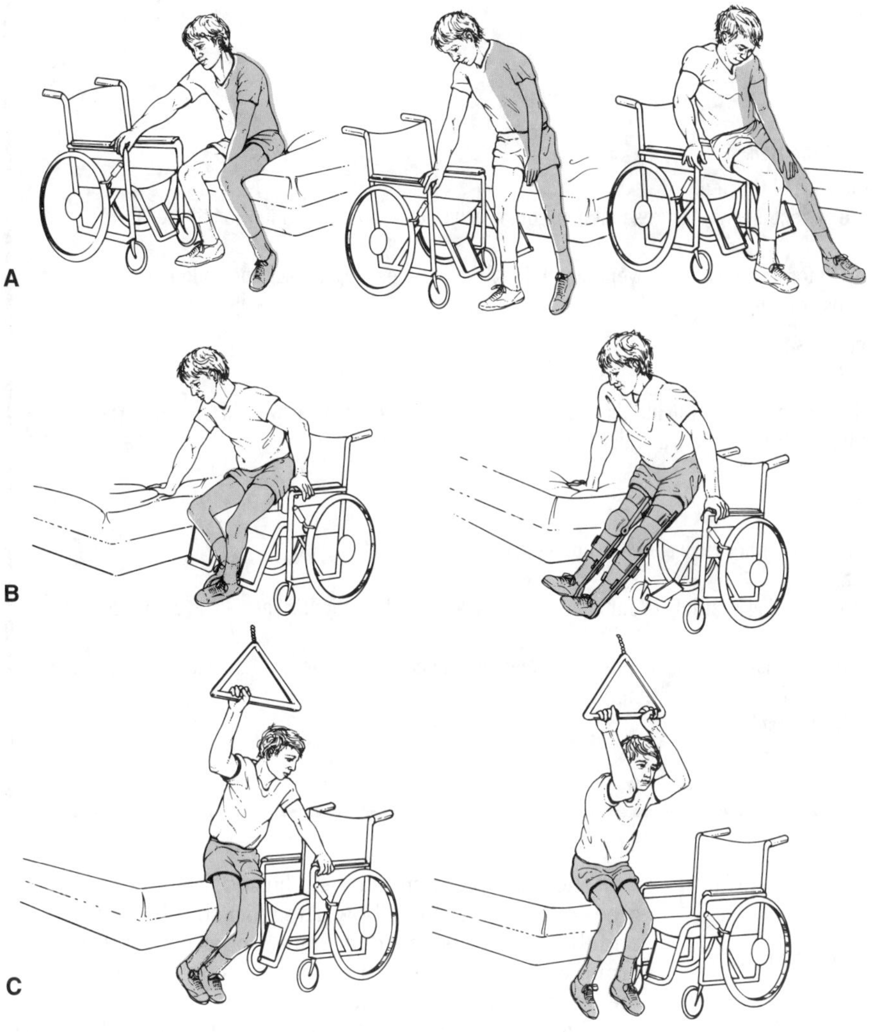

FIGURE 18-2. Methods of transferring the patient from the bed to a wheelchair. The wheelchair is in a locked position. *Shaded areas* indicate non–weight-bearing body parts. (**A**) Weight-bearing transfer from bed to chair. The patient stands up, pivots until his back is opposite the new seat, and sits down. (**B**) (*Left*) Non–weight-bearing transfer from chair to bed. (*Right*) With legs braced. (**C**) (*Left*) Non–weight-bearing transfer, combined method. (*Right*) Non–weight-bearing transfer, pull-up method.

the muscle contraction until a count of five and relaxes for a count of five. The exercise is repeated 10 to 15 times hourly. Exercising the quadriceps muscles prevents flexion contractures of the knee. In **gluteal setting,** the patient contracts or "pinches" the buttocks together until the count of five, relaxes for the count of five, and repeats 10 to 15 times hourly.

When ambulatory aids (*i.e.*, walker, cane, crutches) are used, the muscles of the upper extremities are exercised and strengthened. **Push-ups** are useful. While in a sitting position, the patient raises the body by pushing the hands against the chair seat or mattress. The patient should be encouraged to do push-ups while in a prone position also. **Pull-ups** on a trapeze, while lifting the body, are also effective conditioners. The patient is taught to raise the arms above the head and lower them in a slow, rhythmic manner while holding weights. Gradually the poundage of weight is increased. The hands are strengthened by squeezing a rubber ball.

The physical therapist designs exercises to help the patient develop sitting and standing balance, stability, and coordination needed for ambulation. After sitting and standing balance are achieved, the patient uses parallel bars. Under the supervision of the physical therapist, the patient practices shifting weight from side to side, lifting one leg while supporting weight on the other, and then walking between the parallel bars.

Using Ambulatory Aids. A patient who is ready to begin ambulation must be fitted with the appropriate ambulatory aid, instructed as to the prescribed weight-bearing limits (*e.g.*, non–weight-bearing, partial weight-bearing), and taught how to use the aid safely. The nurse continually assesses the patient for stability and protects the patient from falling. The patient should wear sturdy, well-fitting shoes and be advised of the dangers of wet and highly polished floors and throw rugs. The patient needs to learn how to ambulate on inclines, how to maneuver uneven surfaces, and how to manage stairs.

Crutches provide for support and balance and are a convenient method of getting from one place to another. Good balance and erect posture are essential for crutch walking. For safety, crutches should have large rubber suction tips and the patient should wear well-fitting shoes that have firm soles. Patients who are prescribed partial weight-bearing or non–weight-bearing ambulation may use crutches. The nurse or physical therapist determines if crutches are appropriate ambulatory aids for the patient.

Preparatory exercises are aimed at strengthening the shoulder girdle and upper extremity muscles, which bear the patient's weight when crutch walking.

CHART 18-5
Assisting the Patient Out of Bed

Technique for Moving the Patient to the Edge of the Bed

- Move head and shoulders of patient toward the edge of the bed.
- Move feet and legs to the edge of the bed. (The patient is now in a crescent position, which gives good range of motion to the lateral trunk muscles.)
- Place both arms well under the patient's hips. (Before the next maneuver, tighten [set] the muscles of your back and abdomen.)
- Straighten your back while moving the patient toward you.

Technique for Sitting Patient on the Edge of the Bed

- Place arm and hand under shoulders of the patient.
- Instruct the patient to push his or her elbow into the bed while you lift his or her shoulders with one arm and swing his or her legs over the edge of the bed with the other. (Gravity pulls the legs downward, which aids in raising the patient's trunk.)

Technique for Assisting Patient to Stand

- Place patient's feet well under him or her.
- Face the patient while firmly grasping each side of his or her rib cage with your hands.
- Push your knee against one knee of the patient.
- Rock the patient forward as he or she comes to a standing position. (Your knee is pushed against the patient's knee as he or she comes to the standing position.)
- Ensure that the patient's knees are "locked" (full extension) while he or she is standing. ("Locking" the knees of the patient is a safety measure for those who are weak or have been in bed for a period of time.)
- Give the patient *enough time* to balance himself or herself.
- Pivot the patient to position him or her to sit in the chair.

The following muscle groups are important for crutch walking (Fig. 18-3A):

- ❑ Shoulder depressors—to stabilize the upper extremity and prevent shoulder hiking
- ❑ Shoulder adductors—to hold the crutch top against the chest wall
- ❑ Arm flexors, extensors, and abductors (at the shoulder)—to move crutches forward, backward, and sideward
- ❑ Forearm extensors—to prevent flexion or buckling; important in raising the body for swinging gait
- ❑ Wrist extensors—to enable weight-bearing on hand pieces
- ❑ Finger and thumb flexors—to grasp the hand piece

Crutches must be adjusted to the patient. Adjustable crutches allow for optimal individual fit.

Measuring for Crutches. To determine the approximate crutch length, the patient may be measured standing or lying, or the patient's height may be used.

To measure a standing patient for crutches, the patient is positioned against the wall with the feet slightly apart and away from the wall. Five centimeters (2 in) are marked out to the side from the tip of the toe. Fifteen centimeters (6 in) are measured straight ahead from the first mark and this point is marked. Five centimeters (2 in) are measured below the axilla to the second mark for the approximate crutch length.

If the patient has to be measured while lying down, he or she is measured from the anterior fold of the axilla to the sole of the foot, and then 5 cm (2 in) are added. If the patient's height is used, 40 cm (16 in) are subtracted to obtain the approximate crutch length.

The hand piece should be adjusted to allow 20 to 30 degrees of flexion at the elbow. The wrist should be extended and the hand dorsiflexed. A foam rubber pad on the under arm piece may be used to relieve pressure of the crutch on the upper arm and thoracic cage.

Teaching the Patient to Ambulate With Crutches. Because crutch walking is not an inherent skill, it must be taught. All patient education is individualized to meet the patient's learning needs. The patient is instructed to wear sturdy, well-fitting shoes. The nurse or physical therapist explains and demonstrates to the patient how to manipulate the crutches before the patient attempts to do so. The patient learns standing balance by standing on the unaffected leg by a chair. To help the patient maintain balance, the nurse holds the patient near the waist or uses a transfer belt.

The patient is taught to support weight on the hand pieces. (For individuals unable to support weight through the wrist and hand because of arthritis or fracture, platform crutches that support the forearm and allow the weight to be borne through the elbow are available.) If weight is borne on the axilla, the pressure of the crutch can damage the brachial plexus nerves, producing "crutch paralysis."

Crutch Stance. For maximum stability, the patient learns to assume a tripod position. The crutches are placed approximately 20 cm to 25 cm (8 to 10 in) in front and to the side of the patient's toes (see Fig. 18-3B). This base of support is adjusted according to the height of the patient (*i.e.*, a tall person requires a broader base of support than a short person).

Crutch Gaits. Before walking, the patient learns how to shift weight and maintain balance. The selection of the crutch gait depends on the type and severity of the disability and on the patient's physical condition, arm and trunk

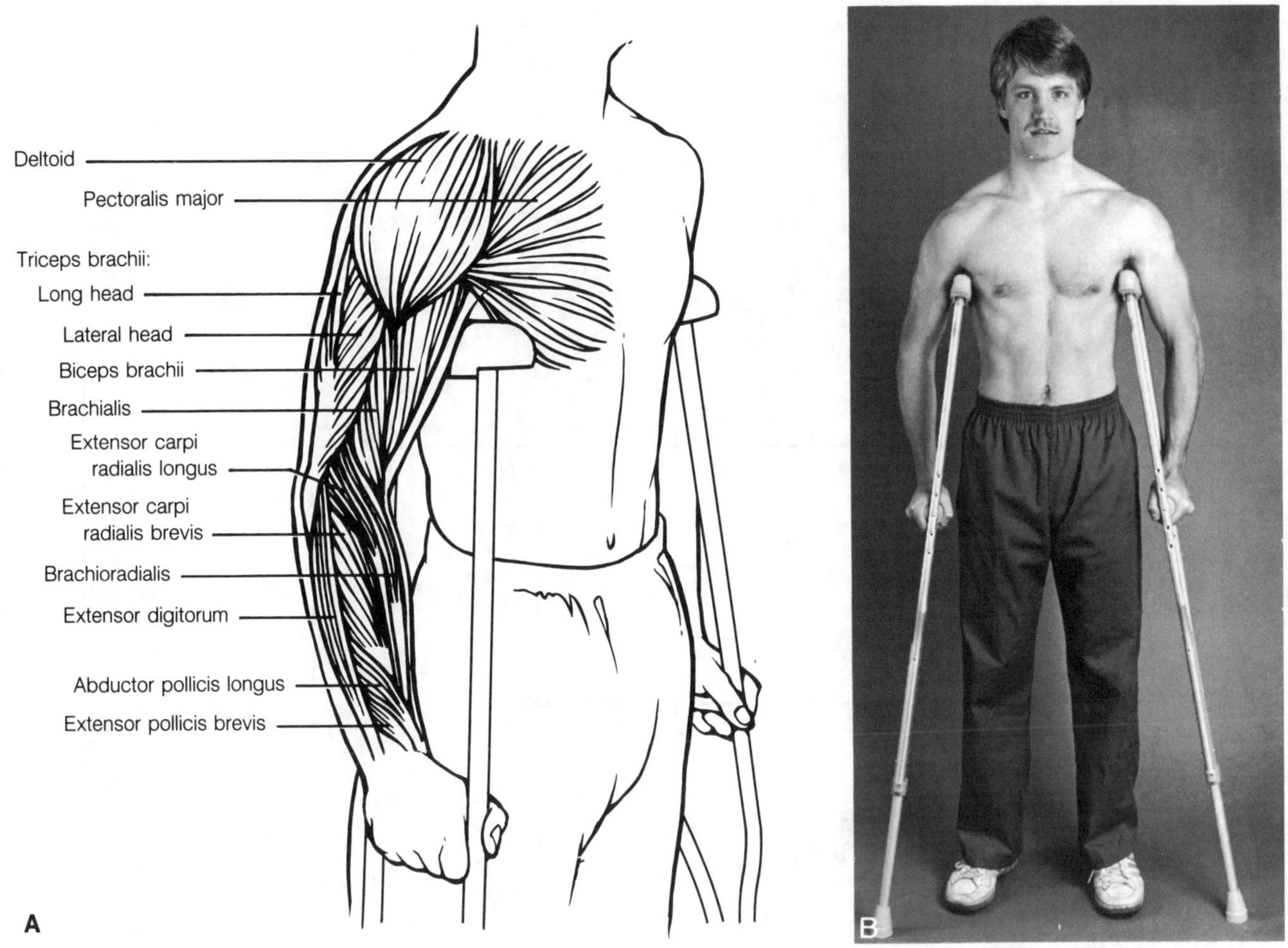

FIGURE 18-3. Crutch walking. (**A**) Muscle groups important for crutch walking. (**B**) The tripod position for the basic crutch stance.

strength, and body balance. The patient should be taught two gaits in order to change from one to another. Shifting crutch gaits relieves fatigue, as each gait requires the use of a different combination of muscles. (If a muscle is forced to contract steadily without relaxing, the circulation of the blood to that part is reduced.) A faster gait can be used for distances, whereas a slower one is used in crowded places.

All gaits begin in the tripod position. The more common gaits are the four-point, the three-point, the two-point, and the swinging-to and swinging-through gaits. The sequence of movements for each of these gaits is depicted in Chart 18-6.

The nurse continually assesses the patient's stability and protects the patient from falls. The nurse walks with the patient, holding the patient at the waist as needed for balance.

The nurse monitors the patient's tolerance of crutch walking. Prolonged periods of bed rest and inactivity affect the patient's strength and endurance. Sweating and shortness of breath are indications that crutch walking practice should be stopped and the patient permitted to rest.

Other Crutch-Maneuvering Techniques. Before a patient is considered independent in crutch walking, he or she needs to learn to sit in a chair, stand from sitting, and go up and down stairs. The following instructions are given to the patient:

1. To sit down:
   a. Grasp the crutches at the hand pieces for control.
   b. Bend forward slightly while assuming a sitting position.
   c. Place the affected leg forward to prevent weight-bearing and flexion.
2. To stand up:
   a. Move forward to the edge of the chair with the strong leg slightly under the seat.
   b. Place both crutches in the hand on the side of the affected extremity.
   c. Push down on the hand piece while raising the body to a standing position.
3. To go down stairs:
   a. Walk forward as far as possible on the step.
   b. Advance crutches to the lower step. The weaker leg is advanced first and then the stronger one. In this way, the stronger extremity shares with the arms the work of raising and lowering the body weight.
4. To go up stairs:
   a. Advance the stronger leg first up to the next step.
   b. Then advance the crutches and the weaker extremity. Note that the strong leg goes up first and comes down last. A memory device for the patients is "up with the good; down with the bad."

CHART 18-6
Crutch Gaits

Shaded areas are weight-bearing. ↑ indicates advance foot or crutch.

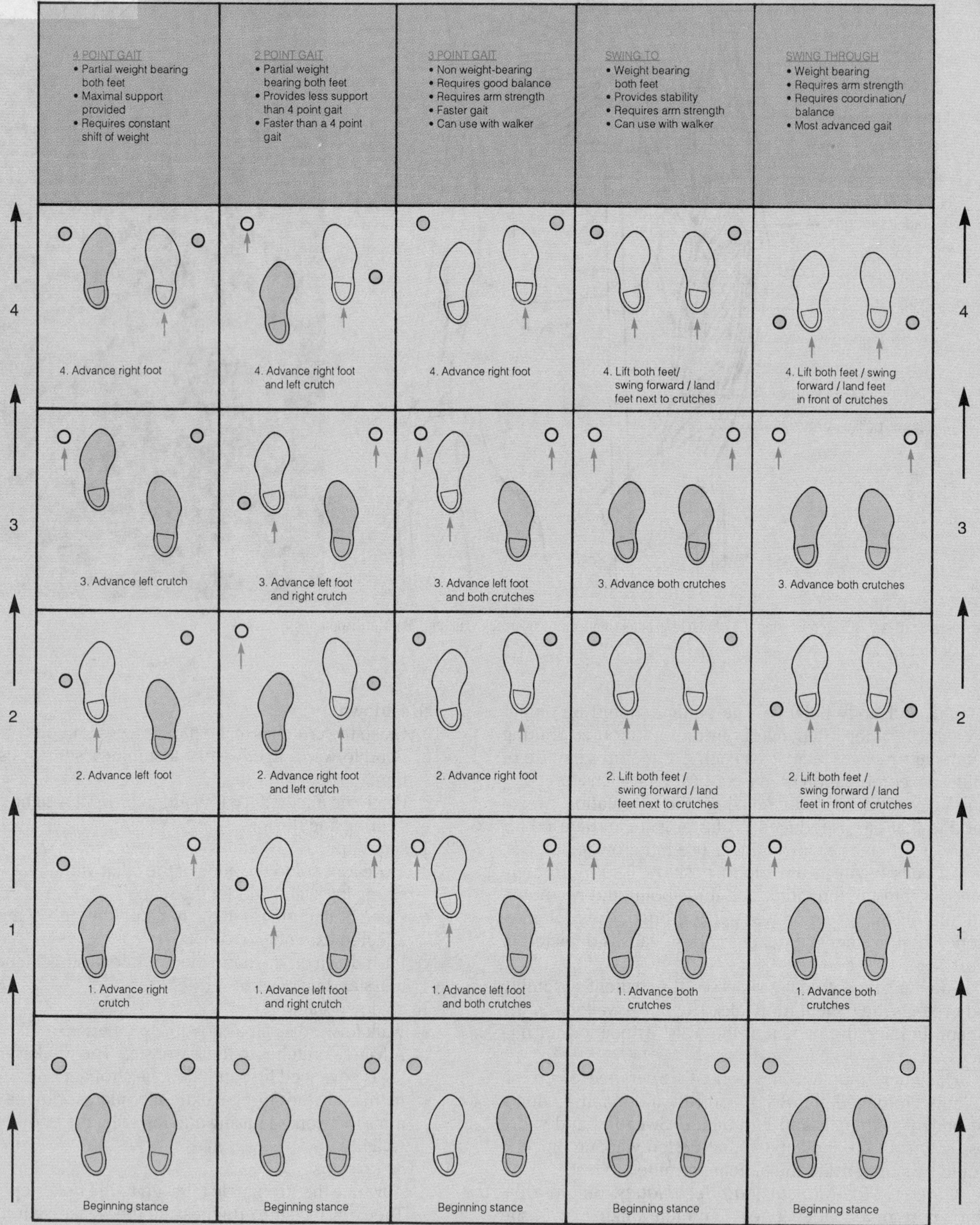

4 POINT GAIT
• Partial weight bearing both feet
• Maximal support provided
• Requires constant shift of weight
2 POINT GAIT
• Partial weight bearing both feet
• Provides less support than 4 point gait
• Faster than a 4 point gait
3 POINT GAIT
• Non weight-bearing
• Requires good balance
• Requires arm strength
• Faster gait
• Can use with walker
SWING TO
• Weight bearing both feet
• Provides stability
• Requires arm strength
• Can use with walker
SWING THROUGH
• Weight bearing
• Requires arm strength
• Requires coordination/ balance
• Most advanced gait
4
4. Advance right foot
4. Advance right foot and left crutch
4. Advance right foot
4. Lift both feet/ swing forward / land feet next to crutches
4. Lift both feet / swing forward / land feet in front of crutches
4
3
3. Advance left crutch
3. Advance left foot and right crutch
3. Advance left foot and both crutches
3. Advance both crutches
3. Advance both crutches
3
2
2. Advance left foot
2. Advance right foot and left crutch
2. Advance right foot
2. Lift both feet / swing forward / land feet next to crutches
2. Lift both feet / swing forward / land feet in front of crutches
2
1
1. Advance right crutch
1. Advance left foot and right crutch
1. Advance left foot and both crutches
1. Advance both crutches
1. Advance both crutches
1
Beginning stance
Beginning stance
Beginning stance
Beginning stance
Beginning stance

Walker. A walker provides more support and stability than a cane or crutches. A walker does not permit a natural reciprocal walking pattern. It is useful for patients who have poor balance or limited cardiovascular reserve, or who cannot use crutches. The height of the walker is adjusted to the patient. The patient's arms resting on the walker hand grips should exhibit 20 to 30 degrees of flexion at the elbows. The patient should wear sturdy, well-fitting shoes. The nurse continually assesses the patient's stability and protects the patient from falls. The nurse walks with the patient, holding at the waist as needed for balance

The patient is taught to ambulate with a walker as follows:

1. Hold the walker on the hand grips for stability.
2. Lift the walker, placing it in front of you while leaning your body slightly forward.
3. Walk into the walker, supporting your body weight on your hands when advancing your weaker leg, permitting partial weight-bearing or non–weight-bearing as prescribed.
4. Balance yourself on your feet.
5. Lift the walker and place it in front of you again. Continue this pattern of walking.

Cane. A cane is used to help the patient walk with greater balance and support and to relieve the pressure on weight-bearing joints by redistributing the weight. Quad canes (four-footed canes) provide more stability than straight canes.

The cane should be fitted with a gently flaring tip that has flexible and concentric rings; the tip with its concentric rings provides optimal stability, functions as a shock absorber, and enables the patient to walk with greater speed and less fatigue.

To fit the patient for a cane, the patient is instructed to flex the elbow at a 30-degree angle, hold the handle of the cane approximately level with the greater trochanter, and place the tip of the cane 15 cm (6 in) lateral to the base of the fifth toe. Adjustable canes make individualization easy.

The cane is held in the hand opposite to the affected extremity. In normal walking, the opposite leg and arm move together (reciprocal motion); such motion is to be carried through in walking with a cane.

The nurse continually assesses the patient's stability and protects the patient from falls. The nurse walks with the patient, holding at the waist as needed for balance. The patient is assessed for tolerance of walking and rest periods are provided as needed.

The patient is taught to ambulate with a cane as follows:

1. Cane–foot sequence:
   a. Hold the cane in the hand opposite the affected extremity to widen the base of support and to reduce the stress on the involved extremity. (If the patient for some reason is unable to use the cane in the opposite hand, the cane may be used on the same side.)
   b. Advance the cane at the same time the affected leg is moved forward.
   c. Keep the cane fairly close to the body to prevent leaning.
   d. Bear down on the cane when the unaffected extremity begins the swing phase.
2. To go up and down stairs using the cane:
   a. Step up on the unaffected extremity.
   b. Then place the cane and affected extremity up on the step.
   c. Reverse this procedure for descending steps ("up with the good, down with the bad").

Assisting the Patient Using an Orthosis/Prosthesis. Orthoses and prostheses are designed to facilitate mobilization and maximize the patient's quality of life. The nurse helps the patient develop an attitude of realistic hopefulness. If the patient has had an amputation, the nurse promotes tissue healing, uses compression dressings to promote residual limb shaping, and minimizes contracture formation. The nurse works with the patient and emphasizes the orthotist's/prosthetist's instructions related to skin care and care of the orthosis/prosthesis. Skin problems or pressure ulcers may develop if the device is applied too tightly or if it is adjusted improperly. The patient is taught to examine the orthosis periodically to see that it fits as designed, its shape is not distorted, and the padding distributes pressure evenly.

Learning to use a prosthesis successfully requires the efforts of the patient, physical therapist, nurse, and prosthetist. Efforts are directed at acceptance of the prosthesis and using it to maximize mobility and quality of life.

Evaluation

Expected Outcomes

1. Demonstrates improved physical mobility
   a. Maintains muscle strength and joint mobility
   b. Does not develop contractures
   c. Participates in exercise program
2. Transfers safely
   a. Demonstrates assisted transfers
   b. Performs independent transfers
3. Ambulates with maximum independence
   a. Uses ambulatory aid safely
   b. Adheres to weight-bearing prescription
   c. Requests assistance as needed
4. Demonstrates increased activity tolerance
   a. Does not experience orthostatic hypotension episodes
   b. Reports absence of fatigue associated with ambulatory efforts
   c. Gradually increases distance and speed of ambulation

❑ *NURSING PROCESS* *Impaired Skin Integrity*

Patients confined to bed for long periods, patients with motor or sensory dysfunction, and patients who experience muscular atrophy and reduction of padding between the overlying skin and the underlying bone are prone to pressure ulcers. Pressure ulcers are localized areas of infarcted soft tissue that occur when pressure applied to the skin over time is greater than normal capillary closure pressure, approximately 32 mm Hg. Critically ill patients have a lower capillary closure pressure and are at greater risk for pressure ulcers. The initial sign of pressure is erythema (redness of the skin) due to reactive hyperemia. Normally reactive hyperemia resolves in less than one hour. Unrelieved pressure results in tissue ischemia or anoxia. The cutaneous tissues become broken or destroyed, leading to progressive destruction and necrosis of underlying soft tissue. The resulting pressure ulcer is painful and slow to heal.

Contributing Factors

Factors that have been identified as contributing to the development of pressure ulcers include immobility, impaired sensory perception and/or cognition, decreased tissue perfusion, decreased nutritional status, friction and shear forces, increased moisture, and age-related skin changes.

Immobility. When a person is immobile and inactive, pressure is exerted on the skin and subcutaneous tissue by objects on which the person rests, such as a mattress, chair seat, or cast. The development of pressure ulcers is directly related to the duration of immobility. If pressure continues long enough, small vessel thrombosis and tissue necrosis occur, resulting in a pressure ulcer. Weight-bearing bony prominences are most susceptible to pressure ulcer development. These prominences are covered by skin and small amounts of subcutaneous tissue. Susceptible areas include the sacrum and coccygeal areas, ischial tuberosities (especially in persons who sit for prolonged periods), greater trochanter, heel, knee, malleolus, medial condyle of the tibia, the fibular head, scapula, and elbow (Fig. 18-4).

Impaired Sensory Perception and/or Cognition. Patients with sensory loss, impaired levels of consciousness, or paralysis may not be aware of the discomfort associated with prolonged pressure on the skin. Therefore, they will not change position themselves to relieve the pressure. This prolonged pressure impedes blood flow, reducing nourishment of the skin. A pressure ulcer may develop in a very short period.

Decreased Tissue Perfusion. Any condition that reduces the circulation and nourishment of the skin and subcutaneous tissue (altered peripheral tissue perfusion) increases the risk of pressure ulcer development. Persons with diabetes mellitus experience an alteration in microcirculation. Similarly, patients with edema have impaired circulation and poor nourishment of the skin tissue. Obese patients have large amounts of poorly vascularized adipose tissue, which is susceptible to breakdown.

Decreased Nutritional Status. Nutritional deficiencies, anemias, and metabolic disorders also contribute to pressure ulcer development. Anemia, regardless of its cause, decreases the blood's oxygen-carrying ability and predisposes to pressure ulcer formation. Patients who have low protein levels or who are in a negative nitrogen balance experience tissue wasting and inhibited tissue repair. Serum albumin is a sensitive indicator of protein deficiency. Albumin levels less than 3.0 g/ml are associated with hypoalbuminemic tissue edema and increased risk of pressure ulcers. Specific nutrients such as vitamin C and trace minerals are needed for tissue maintenance and repair.

Friction and Shear Forces. Mechanical forces contribute to the development of pressure ulcers. **Friction** is the resistance to movement that occurs when two surfaces are moved across each other. **Shearing force** is created by the interplay of gravitational forces (forces that push the body down) and friction. With shearing, tissue layers slide over one another, blood vessels stretch and twist, and the microcirculation of the skin and subcutaneous tissue is disrupted. Evidence of deep tissue damage may be slow to develop and may present through the development of a draining tract. The sacrum and heels are most susceptible to the effects of shear. Pressure ulcers from friction and shearing forces occur when the patient slides down in bed (Fig. 18-5) or when the patient is moved or positioned improperly (*e.g.*, dragging the patient up in bed). Spastic muscles and paralysis increase the patient's vulnerability to pressure ulcers related to friction and shearing forces.

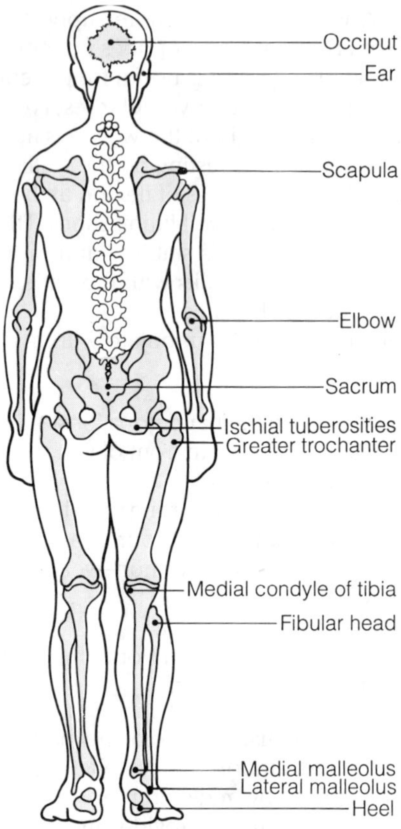

FIGURE 18-4. Areas susceptible to pressure ulcers.

Increased Moisture. Prolonged contact with moisture from perspiration, urine, feces, or drainage produces maceration (softening) of the skin. The skin reacts to the caustic substances in the excreta or drainage and becomes irritated. Moist, irritated skin is more vulnerable to pressure breakdown.

Once the skin is open, the area is invaded by microorganisms (*e.g.*, streptococci and staphylococci, *Pseudomonas aeruginosa, Escherichia coli*), and infection occurs. Foul-smelling infectious drainage is present. The lesion may enlarge and allow a continuous loss of serum, which may further deplete the body of essential protein needed for tissue repair and maintenance. The lesion may continue to enlarge and extend deep into the fascia, muscle, and bone, with multiple sinus tracts radiating from the pressure ulcer.

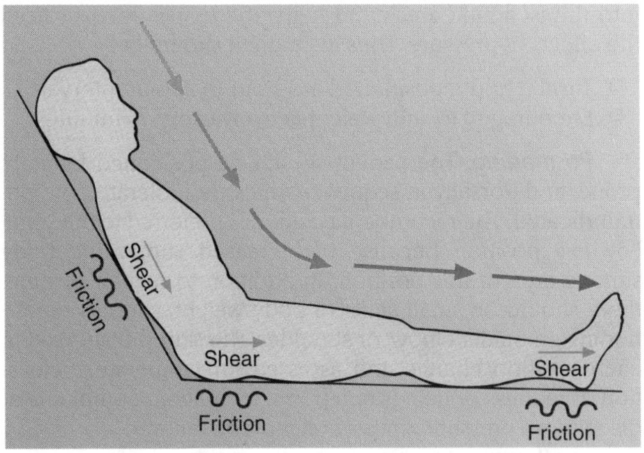

FIGURE 18-5. Mechanical forces contribute to pressure ulcer development. As the person slides down in bed, *friction* resists this movement. *Shearing* occurs when one layer of tissue slides over another, disrupting microcirculation of skin and subcutaneous tissue.

With extensive pressure ulcers, systemic infections may develop, frequently from gram-negative organisms.

Gerontologic Considerations. In the older adult, the skin has diminished epidermal thickness, dermal collagen, and tissue elasticity. The skin is drier as a result of diminished sebaceous and sweat gland activity. Cardiovascular changes result in decreased tissue perfusion. Muscles atrophy and bone structures become prominent. Diminished sensory perception and reduced ability to reposition oneself contribute to prolonged pressure on the skin. Therefore, the older adult is more susceptible to pressure ulcers, which cause pain and suffering and reduce quality of life (AHCPR, 1994).

An estimated 1.7 million patients develop pressure ulcers annually. Both prevention and treatment of pressure ulcers are costly in terms of health care dollars and quality of life for patients at risk. Since the cost in terms of pain and suffering for an individual with a pressure ulcer cannot be quantified, the old saying "an ounce of prevention is worth a pound of cure" is particularly applicable to pressure ulcers.

Assessment

In assessing the patient for potential risk for pressure ulcer development, the nurse assesses the patient's mobility, sensory perception and cognitive abilities, tissue perfusion, nutritional status, friction and shear forces, sources of moisture on the skin, and age (Chart 18-7). The nurse

- ❑ Assesses total skin condition at least twice a day
- ❑ Inspects each pressure site for erythema
- ❑ Assesses areas of erythema for blanching response
- ❑ Palpates the skin for increased warmth
- ❑ Inspects for dry skin, moist skin, breaks in skin
- ❑ Notes drainage and odor
- ❑ Evaluates level of mobility
- ❑ Notes restrictive devices (*e.g.*, restraints, splints)
- ❑ Evaluates circulatory status (*e.g.*, peripheral pulses, edema)
- ❑ Assesses neurologic status

CHART 18-7
Risk Factors for Development of Pressure Ulcers

Prolonged pressure on tissue
Immobility, compromised mobility
Loss of protective reflexes, sensory deficit/loss
Poor skin perfusion; edema
Malnutrition, hypoproteinemia, anemia, vitamin deficiency
Friction, shearing forces, trauma
Incontinence of urine or feces
Altered skin moisture: excessively dry, excessively moist
Advanced age, debilitation
Equipment: casts, traction, restraints, bedding, chairs

- ❑ Determines presence of incontinence
- ❑ Evaluates nutritional and hydration status
- ❑ Reviews the patient's record for hematocrit, hemoglobin, and blood chemistry (serum albumin values)
- ❑ Notes present health problems
- ❑ Reviews current medications

In order to facilitate systematic assessment and quantification of a patient's risk for pressure ulcer, scales such as the Braden or Norton scales may be used. The nurse needs to recognize that the reliability of these scales is not well established. They tend to overpredict those at risk and may promote unwarranted use of costly preventive equipment.

If a pressure area is noted, the nurse notes its size and location and may use a grading system to describe its severity (Chart 18-8). Generally, a **stage I pressure ulcer** is an area of nonblanchable erythema, tissue swelling, and congestion, with the patient complaining of discomfort. The skin temperature is elevated because of the increased vasodilation. The redness progresses to a dusky, cyanotic blue–gray appearance, which is the result of skin capillary occlusion and subcutaneous weakening.

A **stage II pressure ulcer** exhibits a break in the skin through the epidermis and/or the dermis. An abrasion, blister, or shallow crater may be seen. Necrosis occurs. There is venous sludging and thrombosis and edema with cellular extravasation and infiltration.

A **stage III pressure ulcer** extends into the subcutaneous tissues. Clinically, a deep crater with or without undermining of adjacent tissues is noted.

A **stage IV pressure ulcer** extends into the underlying structures, including the muscle and possibly the bone. The skin lesion may represent only the "tip of the iceberg," because a small surface ulcer may be present over a large undermining area.

The appearance of purulent drainage or foul odor suggests an infection. With an extensive pressure ulcer, deep pockets of infection are often present. Drying and crusting of exudate may be present. Infection of a pressure ulcer may advance to osteomyelitis, pyarthrosis (pus formation within a joint cavity), or generalized sepsis.

CHART 18-8
Assessment of Pressure Ulcer Stage

Stage I
- Area of erythema
- Erythema does not blanch with pressure
- Skin temperature elevated
- Tissue swollen and congested
- Patient complains of discomfort
- Erythema progresses to dusky, blue–gray

Stage II
- Skin breaks
- Abrasion, blister, or shallow crater
- Edema persists
- Ulcer drains
- Infection may develop

Stage III
- Ulcer extends into subcutaneous tissue
- Necrosis and drainage continue
- Infection develops

Stage IV
- Ulcer extends to underlying muscle and bone
- Deep pockets of infection develop
- Necrosis and drainage continue

Diagnosis

Nursing Diagnoses

Based on the assessment data, major nursing diagnoses for the patient may include the following:

- Impaired skin integrity related to any of the following factors: immobility, decreased sensory perception, decreased tissue perfusion, decreased nutritional status, friction and shear forces, increased moisture, or advanced age

Planning and Implementation

Goals. The major goals of the patient may include relief of pressure, improved mobility, improved sensory perception, improved tissue perfusion, improved nutritional status, minimized friction and shear forces, dry surfaces in contact with skin, and healing of pressure ulcer, if present.

Nursing Interventions

Relieving Pressure. The patient needs frequent changes of position to relieve and redistribute the pressure on the skin and to prevent prolonged reduced blood flow to the skin and subcutaneous tissues. This can be accomplished by teaching the patient to change position or by turning and repositioning the patient. Families of patients in the home should be taught how to position and turn patients to prevent pressure ulcers. Shifting weight allows the blood to flow into the ischemic areas and helps the tissues recover from the effects of pressure. Thus the patient should be:

- Turned and repositioned at 1-hour to 2-hour intervals
- Encouraged to shift weight actively every 15 minutes

Positioning. The patient should be positioned laterally, prone, and dorsally in sequence unless not tolerated or contraindicated. The recumbent position is preferred to the semi-Fowler's position because of increased supporting body surface area in this position. In addition to regular turning, there should be small shifts of body weight, such as repositioning an ankle, elbow, or shoulder. The skin is inspected at each position change and assessed for temperature elevation. If redness or heat is noted or if the patient complains of discomfort, pressure on the area must be relieved.

Another way to relieve pressure over bony prominences is the bridging technique, accomplished through the correct positioning of pillows. Just as a bridge is supported on pillars to allow traffic to move underneath, so can the body be supported by pillows to allow for space between bony prominences and the mattress. A pillow or commercial heel protector may be used to support the heels off the bed when the patient is supine. Placing pillows superior and inferior to the sacrum relieves sacral pressure. Supporting the patient in a 30 degree sidelying position avoids pressure on the trochanter.

Gerontologic Considerations. In the aging patient, frequent small shifts of body weight may be effective. Placing a small rolled towel or sheepskin under a shoulder or hip will allow a return of blood flow to the skin on which the patient is sitting or lying. The towel or sheepskin is moved around the patient's pressure points in a clockwise fashion.

Pressure-Relieving Devices. At times, special equipment and beds may be needed to help relieve the pressure on the skin. These are designed to provide support for specific body areas or for distributing pressure evenly and uniformly.

Patients sitting in wheelchairs for prolonged periods should have wheelchair cushions fitted and adjusted on an individualized basis, using pressure measurement techniques as a guide to selection and fitting. The aim is to redistribute pressure away from areas at risk for ulcers. However, no cushion is able to eliminate excessive pressure. The patient should be reminded to shift weight frequently and raise up for a few seconds every 15 minutes while sitting in a chair (Fig. 18-6).

Static support devices (*e.g.*, high density foam, air, or liquid mattress overlays) distribute pressure evenly by bringing more of the patient's body surface in contact with the supporting surface. The gel-type flotation pad and air fluidized beds reduce pressure. As the patient's body sinks into the fluid, additional surface becomes available for weight-bearing, thereby further decreasing body weight per unit area. (Pascal's law states that the weight of the body floating on a fluid system is evenly distributed over the entire supporting surface.) Thus, there is less pressure on the body parts.

Soft, moisture-absorbing padding is also useful because the softness and resilience of padding provides even distribution of pressure and the dissipation and absorption of moisture, along with freedom from wrinkles and friction. Bony prominences may be protected by gel pads, sheepskin padding, or soft foam rubber beneath the sacrum, the tro-

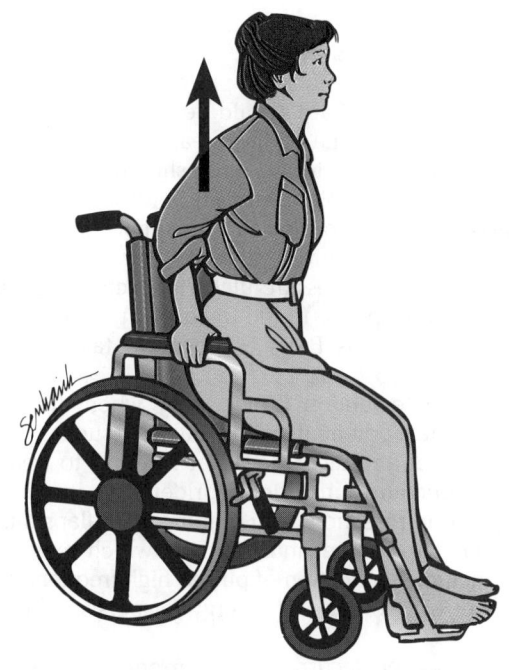

FIGURE 18-6. Wheelchair push-up to prevent ischial pressure ulcers. These push-ups should become an automatic routine (every 15 minutes) for the person with paraplegia. He should stay up, out of contact with the seat for several seconds. The wheels are kept in the locked position during the exercise.

chanters, heels, elbows, scapulae, and the back of the head when there is pressure on the sites.

Specialized beds have been designed to prevent pressure on the skin. Air-fluidized beds float the patient. Dynamic support surfaces, such as low-air-loss pockets, alternately inflate and deflate sections to change support pressure for very high-risk patients who are critically ill and debilitated, and cannot be repositioned to relieve pressure. Oscillating or kinetic beds change pressure by rocking movements of the bed. The constant movement redistributes the patient's weight and stimulates circulation. They are frequently used with patients who have experienced multiple trauma.

Improving Mobility. The patient is encouraged to remain active and is ambulated whenever possible. When sitting, the patient is reminded to change positions frequently to redistribute weight. Active and passive exercises increase muscular, skin, and vascular tone. Circulation is stimulated with activity, which relieves tissue ischemia, the forerunner of pressure ulcers.

For the patient at risk for pressure ulcers, turning schedules and exercise schedules are essential. Repositioning must occur around the clock.

Improving Sensory Perception. The nurse helps the patient recognize and compensate for altered sensory perception. Depending on the origin of the alteration (*e.g.*, decreased level of consciousness, spinal cord lesion), specific interventions are selected. Strategies to improve cognition and sensory perception may include stimulating the patient to increase awareness of self in the environment, encouraging the patient to participate in self-care, or supporting the patient's efforts toward active compensation for loss of sensation (*e.g.*, a paraplegic patient lifting himself or herself from the sitting position every 15 minutes). When decreased sensory perception exists, the patient/caregiver is taught to inspect potential pressure areas visually, using a mirror if needed, for evidence of pressure ulcer development.

Improving Tissue Perfusion. Exercise and repositioning improve tissue perfusion. Massage of erythematous areas is avoided, because damage to the capillaries and deep tissue may occur.

- ❑ Reddened areas are *not* massaged, as this may increase the damage to already traumatized skin.

If the patient has evidence of compromised peripheral circulation such as edema, positioning and elevation of the edematous body part to promote venous return and diminish congestion will improve tissue perfusion. In addition, the nurse or family must be alert to environmental factors (*e.g.*, wrinkles in sheets, pressure of tubes) that may contribute to pressure on the skin and diminished circulation; the source of pressure must be removed.

Improving Nutritional Status. The patient's nutritional status must be adequate and a positive nitrogen balance must be maintained. Pressure ulcers develop more quickly and are more resistant to treatment in patients suffering from nutritional disorders. A high-protein diet with protein supplements may be helpful. Iron preparations may be necessary to raise the hemoglobin level so that tissue oxygen levels will be maintained within acceptable limits. Ascorbic acid (vitamin C) is necessary for tissue healing.

Other nutrients associated with healthy skin include vitamin A, B vitamins, zinc, and sulfur. With balanced nutrition and hydration, the skin is able to maintain a healthy status and repair damaged tissues.

To assess nutritional status response to therapeutic strategies, the nurse monitors the patient's hemoglobin, albumin, and body weight weekly. Nutritional assessment is described in further detail in Chapter 7.

Reducing Friction and Shear Forces. Shearing forces occur when the patient is pulled, allowed to slump, or moves by digging heels or elbows into the mattress. Raising the head of the bed by even a few centimeters increases the shearing force over the sacral area. Therefore, the semireclining position is avoided for patients at risk. The patient can be protected from sliding down in bed by using a well-padded footboard and by placing extra protection on the heels. Proper positioning with adequate support is important when a patient is sitting in a chair. Polyester sheepskin pads are thought to reduce shearing and friction and may be used with at-risk patients.

- ❑ To avoid shearing forces when repositioning, the patient is lifted, not dragged across a surface.

Minimizing Moisture. Continuous moisture on the skin must be prevented by meticulous hygienic measures. Perspiration, urine, stool, and drainage must be removed from the skin promptly. The soiled skin should be promptly washed with mild soap and water and blotted dry with a soft towel. The skin may be lubricated with a bland lotion to keep it soft and pliable. Drying agents and powders are avoided. Topical barrier ointments (*e.g.*, Vaseline) may be helpful in protecting the skin of patients who are incontinent.

Absorbent pads which wick moisture away from the body should be used to absorb drainage. Patients who are incontinent need to be checked and their wet incontinence pads and linens changed promptly. All efforts must be made to keep the skin clean and dry.

Promoting Pressure Ulcer Healing. Regardless of the stage of the pressure ulcer, the pressure on the area must be eliminated. The ulcer will not heal until all pressure is removed. The patient must not lie or sit on the pressure ulcer, even for a few minutes. Individualized positioning and turning schedules must be written in the nursing care plan and followed meticulously.

In addition, inadequate nutritional status and fluid and electrolyte abnormalities must be corrected to promote healing. Wounds that drain body fluids and protein place the patient in a catabolic state and predispose to hypoproteinemia and serious secondary infections. Protein deficiency must be corrected to heal the pressure ulcer. Carbohydrates are necessary to "spare" the protein and to provide an energy source. Vitamin C and trace elements, especially zinc, are necessary for collagen formation and wound healing.

Stage I Pressure Ulcers. To permit healing of stage I pressure ulcers, the pressure is removed to permit increased tissue perfusion, improved nutritional and fluid and electrolyte status, reduction of friction and shearing forces, and avoidance of moisture to the skin.

❑ The reddened skin must not be massaged as increased tissue damage may result.

Stage II Pressure Ulcers. Stage II pressure ulcers have broken skin. In addition to measures listed for stage I pressure ulcers, a moist environment is desired to aid wound healing. A heat lamp is not used to dry the open wound. Migration of epidermal cells over the ulcer surface occurs more rapidly in a moist environment. The ulcer is gently cleansed with sterile saline solution. Use of antiseptic solutions which damage healthy tissues and delay wound healing is avoided. Semipermeable occlusive dressing, hydrocolloid wafers, or wet saline dressings are helpful in providing a moist environment for healing and in minimizing the loss of fluids and proteins from the body.

Stages III and IV Pressure Ulcers. Stage III and IV pressure ulcers have extensive damaged tissue. In addition to measures listed for stage I, these advanced draining, necrotic pressure ulcers must be cleaned (debrided) to create an area that will heal. Necrotic, devitalized tissue favors bacterial growth, delays granulation, and inhibits healing. Wound cleaning and dressing are uncomfortable; therefore, the nurse must prepare the patient, explain the procedure, and administer prescribed analgesia when needed.

Debridement may be accomplished by wet-to-damp dressing changes, mechanical flushing of necrotic and infective exudate, application of prescribed enzyme preparations that dissolve necrotic tissue, or surgical dissection. If an eschar covers the ulcer, it is removed surgically to ensure a clean, vitalized wound. Exudate may be absorbed by dressings or special hydrophilic powders, beads, or gels. Cultures of infected pressure ulcers are obtained to guide selection of antibiotic therapy.

After the pressure ulcer is clean, a topical treatment is prescribed. The goal of therapy is to promote granulation. New granulation tissue must be protected from reinfection, drying, and damage. Care should be taken to prevent pressure and further trauma to the area. Dressings, solutions, and ointments applied to the ulcer should not disrupt the healing process. Multiple agents and protocols are used to treat pressure ulcers. Consistency is an important key to success. In addition, objective evaluation of the pressure ulcer (*e.g.*, measuring the pressure ulcer, inspecting for granulation tissue) for response to the treatment protocol must be made every 4 to 6 days. Pressure ulcers can take a long time to heal.

Surgical intervention is necessary when the ulcer is extensive, when potential complications (such as fistula) exist, and when the ulcer does not respond to treatment. Surgical procedures include debridement, incision and drainage, bone resection, skin grafting, skin flaps, and myocutaneous flaps. Other interventions which may be prescribed include application of pulsed high-frequency, high–peak-power electromagnetic energy for persistent pressure ulcers.

Prevention of Recurrence. Recurrence of pressure ulcers should be anticipated; therefore, active, preventive intervention and frequent continuing assessment are essential. The patient's tolerance for sitting/lying on the healed pressure area is increased gradually; the time that pressure is allowed on the area is increased in 5- to 15-minute increments. The patient is taught to increase mobility and to follow a regimen of turning, weight shifting, and repositioning. The patient teaching plan includes instruction on strategies to reduce the risk for developing pressure ulcers and methods to detect, inspect, and minimize pressure areas. Early recognition and intervention are keys to long-term management of potential impaired skin integrity.

Evaluation

Expected Outcomes

1. Maintains intact skin
   a. Exhibits no areas of nonblanchable erythema at bony prominences
   b. Avoids massage of bony prominences
   c. Exhibits no breaks in skin
2. Avoids pressure on bony prominences
   a. Changes position every 1 to 2 hours
   b. Uses bridging techniques to remove pressure
   c. Uses special equipment as appropriate
   d. Raises self from seat/wheelchair every 15 minutes
3. Increases mobility
   a. Performs range of motion exercises
   b. Adheres to turning schedule
   c. Shifts weight frequently
4. Sensory and cognitive ability improved
   a. Demonstrates improved level of consciousness
   b. Inspects potential pressure ulcer areas
5. Demonstrates improved tissue perfusion
   a. Exercises to increase circulation
   b. Elevates body parts susceptible to edema
6. Attains/maintains adequate nutritional status
   a. Verbalizes the importance of protein and vitamin C in diet

b. Consumes balanced diet high in protein and vitamin C
c. Hemoglobin and albumin levels maintained at acceptable levels
7. Avoids friction and shearing forces
a. Avoids semi-reclining position
b. Uses sheepskin pad/heel protectors when appropriate
c. Lifts body instead of sliding across surfaces
8. Maintains clean, dry skin
a. Avoids prolonged contact with wet or soiled surfaces
b. Keeps skin clean and dry
c. Uses lotion to keep skin lubricated
9. Experiences healing of pressure ulcer
a. Avoids pressure on area
b. Improves nutritional status
c. Participates in therapeutic regimen
d. Demonstrates behaviors to prevent new pressure ulcers
e. States early indicators of pressure ulcer development

❑ NURSING PROCESS
Altered Elimination Patterns: Urinary/Bowel

Urinary and bowel incontinence are frequent problems in the disabled patient. Bladder and bowel control are important functions of the body and are influenced by social behavior and expectations. Incontinence curtails a person's independence, causing embarrassment, isolation, and often institutionalization of the elderly. It occurs in up to 15% of the community-based elderly population, whereas almost half of nursing home residents are either bowel or bladder incontinent or both.

In addition, constipation may be a problem for the person with a disability. Regularity is a goal. If a bowel routine is not established, the person may experience abdominal distention, small, frequent oozing of stool, or impaction.

Assessment

Urinary incontinence may be classified as urge, reflex, stress, functional, or total incontinence (AHCPR, 1992). **Urge incontinence** is involuntary elimination of urine associated with a strong perceived need to void. **Reflex (neurogenic) incontinence** is associated with a spinal cord lesion which interrupts cerebral control resulting in voiding. **Stress incontinence** is associated with weakened perineal muscles which permit leakage of urine when intra-abdominal pressure is increased (*e.g.*, with coughing or sneezing). **Functional incontinence** refers to individuals with intact excretory physiology who experience mobility impairment, environmental barriers, or cognitive problems. They are unable to reach and use the toilet before soiling themselves. **Total incontinence** occurs with individuals who are unable to control excreta due to physiologic or psychologic impairment; management of the excreta is the focus of nursing care. Urinary incontinence may result from multiple causes (*e.g.*, urinary tract infection, detrusor instability, bladder outlet obstruction/incompetence, neurologic impairment, bladder spasm/contracture, inability to reach the toilet in time).

The health history is used to explore excreta control status, symptoms associated with bladder and bowel function, physiologic risk factors for elimination problems, perception of micturition and defecation cues, and functional toileting abilities. Previous and current fluid intake and voiding patterns may be helpful in designing the nursing care plan. A record of times of voiding and amounts voided is kept for at least 48 hours. In addition, episodes of incontinence and associated activity (*e.g.*, coughing, sneezing, lifting), fluid intake time and amount, and medications are recorded. This record is analyzed and used to determine patterns and relationships of incontinence to other activities and factors.

The ability to get to the bathroom, manipulate clothing, and use the toilet are important functional factors that may be related to incontinence. Also, related cognitive functioning (perception of need to void, verbalization of need to void, and ability to learn to control urination) must be assessed. In addition, the nurse reviews the results of the diagnostic studies (*e.g.*, urinalysis, urodynamic tests, postvoiding residual volumes).

Bowel incontinence and constipation may result from multiple causes (*e.g.*, diminished/absent sphincter control, cognitive/perceptual impairment, neurogenic factors, diet, immobility). The origin of the bowel problem must be determined.

The nurse assesses the patient's normal bowel patterns, nutritional patterns, use of laxatives, gastrointestinal problems (*e.g.*, colitis), bowel sounds, anal reflex and tone, and functional abilities. The character and frequency of bowel movements are recorded and analyzed.

Gerontologic Considerations. Decreased bladder capacity, decreased muscle tone, increased residual volumes, and delayed perception of elimination cues are among the changes that occur with aging and affect elimination patterns in the older adult. In addition, various medications can alter elimination patterns by affecting the volume of urine produced (*e.g.*, diuretics), altering sensitivity to bladder cues (*e.g.*, sedatives), and causing urinary retention (*e.g.*, adrenergic agents, anticholinergics). Functional immobility and activity intolerance may limit the older adult's ability to reach and use the toilet before incontinence occurs.

Diagnosis

Nursing Diagnoses

Based on the assessment data, major nursing diagnoses for the patient may include the following:

- ❑ Altered pattern of elimination related to urinary incontinence, urinary retention, bowel incontinence, or constipation*

*Specific NANDA nursing diagnoses that may be appropriate for the individual with elimination problems are Constipation; Incontinence, bowel; Incontinence, functional; Incontinence, reflex; Incontinence, stress; Incontinence, total; Incontinence, urge; Self-care deficit, toileting; Altered patterns of urinary elimination; Urinary retention.

Planning and Implementation

Goals. The major goals of the patient may include control of urinary incontinence or urinary retention, control of bowel incontinence, and regular elimination patterns.

Nursing Interventions

Promoting Urinary Continence. Once the nature of the urinary incontinence has been identified, a nursing plan of care is developed based on analysis of the assessment data. Various approaches to promotion of urinary continence have been designed. Most approaches attempt to condition the body to successfully control urination or to minimize the occurrence of unscheduled urination. Selection of the approach depends on the cause of the patient's incontinence. For the program to be successful, the patient's participation and desire to avoid incontinence episodes are crucial. An optimistic attitude with positive feedback for even slight gains is essential for success. Accurate recording of intake and output and response to selected strategies is essential for evaluation.

To help maintain skin integrity, the skin is washed and dried thoroughly after each incontinence episode. Protective moisture barrier ointment may be needed for individuals with constant urinary leakage.

At no time should the fluid intake be restricted just to decrease frequency of urination. Sufficient fluid intake (2000 to 3000 ml/day according to patient needs) must be assured. To optimize the likelihood of voiding as scheduled, measured amounts of fluids may be administered approximately 30 minutes before voiding attempts. In addition, most of the fluids should be consumed before evening to minimize the need to void frequently during the night.

Approaches for Promoting Urinary Continence. The goal of **bladder training** is to restore the bladder to normal function. It can be used with cognitively intact individuals experiencing urge incontinence. A voiding/toileting schedule is formulated based on analysis of the assessment data. The schedule specifies times for the patient to try to empty the bladder using a toilet or commode. Privacy should be provided during voiding efforts. The interval between voidings in the early phase of the bladder training period is short (1½–2 hours). The patient is encouraged not to void until the specified voiding time. Voiding success and episodes of incontinence are recorded. As the patient's bladder capacity and control increase, the interval is lengthened. Usually there is a temporal relationship between drinking, eating, exercising, and voiding. The alert patient can participate in recording intake, activity, and voiding and can plan the schedule to achieve maximum continence.

Barrier-free access to the toilet and modification of clothing help the patient with functional incontinence to achieve self-care in toileting and continence.

Habit training is used to try to keep the patient dry by strictly adhering to a toileting schedule. It may be successful with stress, urge, or functional incontinence. With a confused elderly person, the caregiver takes the person to the toilet according to the schedule before involuntary voiding occurs. Simple cueing and consistency promote success. Periods of continence and successful voidings are praised and rewarded.

Biofeedback is a system through which the patient learns consciously to contract excretory sphincters and control voiding cues. Cognitively intact patients who have stress or urge incontinence may gain bladder control through biofeedback.

Pelvic floor exercises (Kegel exercises) strengthen the pubococcygeus muscle. The patient is instructed to tighten pelvic floor muscles for 4 seconds 10 times, 4 to 6 times a day. Stopping and starting the stream during urination is recommended to increase control. Daily practice is essential. These exercises are helpful for cognitively intact women who experience stress incontinence.

Cutaneous stimulation to stimulate bladder contraction and voiding may control reflex incontinence. Suprapubic tapping or stroking the inner thigh may initiate planned voiding by stimulating the voiding reflex arc.

Clean intermittent catheterization is an appropriate approach for managing urinary retention and incontinence associated with distended bladder urinary overflow incontinence. Aseptic intermittent catheterization technique is required in health care institutions due to the potential for bladder infection from resistant organisms.

Indwelling catheters are avoided if at all possible. The incidence of urinary tract infection with indwelling catheters is high. However, short-term use may be needed during treatment of severe skin breakdown due to continued incontinence.

External catheters (condom catheters) to collect spontaneous voidings are useful for male patients with reflex or total incontinence. The appropriate design and size must be chosen for maximal success. The patient or caregiver must be taught how to apply the condom catheter and how to provide daily hygiene, including skin inspection.

Incontinence pads (diapers) are used only as a last resort. They manage rather than solve the incontinence problem. Also, they have a negative psychologic effect on the patient. Every effort should be made to reduce the incidence of incontinence episodes through other methods that have been described. Incontinence pads may be useful at times for patients with stress or total incontinence to protect clothing, but should be avoided whenever possible. When incontinence pads are used, they should wick moisture away from the body to minimize contact of moisture and excreta with the skin. Wet incontinence pads must be changed promptly, the skin cleansed, and a moisture barrier applied to protect the skin.

Promoting Bowel Continence. The goals of a bowel training program are to develop regular bowel habits and to prevent uninhibited bowel elimination. Regular complete emptying of the lower bowel results in bowel continence. A bowel training program takes advantage of the patient's natural reflexes. Regularity, timing, nutrition and fluids, exercise, and correct positioning promote predictable defecation.

The nurse records defecation time, character of stool, nutritional intake, cognitive abilities, and functional self-care toileting abilities for 5 to 7 days. Analysis of this record is helpful when designing a bowel program for the individual with fecal incontinence.

Consistency in implementing the plan is essential. A regular time for defecation is established. Attempts at evacuation should be within 15 minutes of the designated time daily. Natural gastrocolic and duodenocolic reflexes occur about 30 minutes after a meal. Therefore, after breakfast is one of the best times to plan for bowel evacuation. If the patient had a previously established habit pattern at a different time of day, it should be followed.

The anorectal reflex may be stimulated by rectal suppository (*e.g.*, glycerin) or mechanical stimulation (*e.g.*, digital stimulation with a lubricated gloved finger or anal dilator). The suppository should be inserted about 30 minutes before the scheduled bowel elimination time. The interval between insertion of suppository and defecation is noted for subsequent modification of the bowel program. Once the bowel routine is well established, stimulation with a suppository probably will not be necessary.

The patient should assume the normal squatting position (knees higher than the hips) for defecation if at all possible. Bedpans should be avoided if possible. The patient is instructed to bear down and to contract the abdominal muscles. If necessary, the patient can lean forward to increase intra-abdominal pressure and massage the abdomen right to left to facilitate movement of feces in the lower tract.

To promote regular bowel elimination, the diet should be high in fiber with adequate fluid (2000 to 2400 ml/day). Natural stimulants such as prunes, fruits, vegetables, and whole grains are preferred to laxatives.

Preventing Constipation. The record of bowel elimination, character of stool, food and fluid intake, level of activity, bowel sounds, medications, and other assessment data are reviewed to develop the plan of care. Multiple approaches may be used to prevent constipation.

The diet should be well balanced and include adequate intake of high fiber foods (vegetables, fruits, bran) to prevent hard stools and stimulate peristalsis. Fluid intake should be between 2 and 3 liters per day unless contraindicated. Prune juice or fig juice (120 ml) taken 30 minutes before a meal once daily is helpful to some when constipation is a problem.

Physical activity and exercise are encouraged, as is self-care in toileting. The patient is encouraged to respond to the natural urge to defecate. Privacy during toileting is provided.

Stool softeners, bulk-forming agents, mild stimulants, and suppositories may be prescribed to stimulate defecation and to prevent constipation.

Evaluation

Expected Outcomes

1. Demonstrates control over excreta
   a. Experiences no episodes of incontinence
   b. Avoids constipation
   c. Achieves independence in toileting
   d. Expresses satisfaction in level of excreta control
2. Achieves urinary continence
   a. Uses therapeutic approach appropriate to type of incontinence
   b. Maintains adequate fluid intake
   c. Washes and dries skin after episodes of incontinence
3. Achieves bowel continence
   a. Participates in bowel program
   b. Verbalizes need for regular time for bowel evacuation
   c. Modifies diet to promote continence
   d. Uses bowel stimulators as prescribed and needed
4. Experiences relief of constipation
   a. Uses high-fiber diet, fluids, and exercise to promote defecation
   b. Responds to urge to defecate

Continuing Rehabilitation in the Home and Community

An important goal of rehabilitation is to assist the person to return to the home environment after learning to manage the disability. A referral system maintains continuity of care when the patient is transferred to the home or to an extended care facility. The plan for discharge is formulated when the patient is first admitted to the hospital, and discharge plans are made with the patient's functional potential in mind.

The patient's support system (family, friends) is assessed. The attitudes of family and friends toward the patient, the disability, and the return home are important in successful transition to home.

Not all families are able to carry on the arduous programs of exercise and physical training that a patient may need. They may not have the resources or stability to care for a severely disabled family member. Even a stable family may be overwhelmed by the physical, emotional, economic, and energy strains of a disabling disease. The family may require counseling to allow them to discuss and explore their feelings and attitudes (rejection, aversion, avoidance) toward the disabled family member. Every effort is made for successful transition to home.

The family will need to know as much as possible about the patient's condition and care so that they will not fear the patient's return home. The nurse plans with the patient and family methods for coping with problems that may arise. A skills checklist individualized for the patient and family can be developed to make certain that the family is proficient in assisting the patient with certain tasks.

The community health or home care nurse visits the patient in the hospital, interviews the patient and family, reviews the ADL sheet, and gains first-hand knowledge of the activities the patient can perform. This helps ensure continuity of care and that the patient does not "lose ground" but instead maintains the independence gained while in the hospital. The family may need to purchase, borrow, or improvise needed equipment such as safety rails, raised toilet seat or commode, or tub bench. Ramps may have to be built or doorways widened to achieve full access.

Family members are taught how to use equipment and are given a copy of the equipment manufacturer's instruction booklet, the names of resource persons, and lists of supplies and where these may be obtained. A written summary of the care plan is included in family teaching.

A network of support services and communication systems may be required to enhance opportunities for independent living. The nurse uses collaborative, administrative skills to coordinate these activities and to pull together the network of care. The nurse also provides skilled care, initiates additional referrals when indicated, and serves as the patient's advocate and counselor when obstacles are encountered. The nurse continues to reinforce the teaching that has been done and helps the patient to set and achieve attainable goals. The degree to which the patient adapts to the home and community environment depends on the confidence and self-esteem developed during the rehabilitation process and on the acceptance, support, and reactions of the family, employer, and community members.

There is a growing trend toward independent living by severely disabled people, either alone or in groups that share resources. Preparation for independent living should include training in managing a household and working with personal care attendants, as well as in mobility. The goal is integration into the community—living and working in the community with accessible housing, employment, public buildings, transportation, and recreation.

State rehabilitation administration agencies provide services to assist disabled persons in obtaining the help they need to engage in gainful employment. These services include diagnostic, medical, and mental health services. There are counseling, training, placement, and follow-up services available to help the individual with a disability select and attain a job.

If the patient is transferred to an extended care facility, the transition is planned to promote continued progress. Independence gained continues to be supported, and progress is fostered. Adjustment to the extended care facility is facilitated through communication. The family is encouraged to visit, to be involved, and to take the patient home on weekends and holidays if possible.

Americans With Disabilities Act

For years persons with disabilities have been discriminated against in employment, public accommodations, and public and private services. In 1990, Congress passed the Americans with Disabilities Act (ADA) (PL 101-336). This civil rights legislation is designed to permit those with disabilities access to the community and to job opportunities. It stipulates that communities must provide public transportation which is accessible to persons with disabilities. Public facilities (*e.g.*, stores, restaurants, hotels) must be accessible and accommodate those with disabilities. Telecommunication providers must offer communication devices for the deaf. Employers must evaluate an applicant's ability to perform the job and not discriminate on the basis of a disability. Employers also must make "reasonable accommodations," such as equipment or access ramps, to facilitate employment of an individual with a disability.

Although the regulations took effect in July, 1992, compliance has been slow. "Reasonable accommodation" and "without undue hardship" provisions in the law permit businesses to continue with inaccessible conditions. However, all new construction and modifications of public facilities must address access by persons with disabilities. With increased awareness of the needs of persons with disabilities, there will be changes to facilitate access and accommodate them. A higher quality of life for those with disabilities is an objective of the ADA.

Persons with disabilities are no longer an invisible minority. They are active members of society. Modification of the physical environment permits access to public and private facilities and services. Many employment opportunities require minimal modification for a qualified applicant with a disability to be successful. Nurses can serve as advocates for compliance with ADA legislation to eliminate discriminatory practices.

CRITICAL THINKING EXERCISES

1. You are caring for a patient who is recovering from a stroke. You are discussing the patient's level of functioning with the physical rehabilitation team. Describe the kinds of self-care activities that would help determine the rehabilitation plan for the patient.
2. An elderly patient who has limited mobility and ambulation abilities is to be discharged to his home to be cared for by his family. The family members express particular concern about how to prevent pressure ulcers. Describe the instructions you would give them. How might your teaching strategies differ if the family converses primarily in their native tongue, which is not English?
3. You are caring for a young adult patient who was injured in a motor vehicle crash. He is to return home to continue rehabilitation as an outpatient. You accompany the home health care nurse who is conducting an assessment of the patient's home environment in anticipation of his discharge. Compare the types of safety factors that might be considered if the patient lives in a single-story house, a two-story house, a two-room apartment in a high-rise building, or on a farm.

BIBLIOGRAPHY

Books

Agency for Health Care Policy and Research, Public Health Service, U.S. Department of Health and Human Services. Panel for the Prediction and Prevention of Pressure Ulcers in Adults. Pressure Ulcers in Adults: Prediction and Prevention. Clinical Practice Guideline, Number 3. AHCPR Publication No.92-0047. Rockville, MD, May 1992.

Agency for Health Care Policy and Research. Public Health Service, U.S. Department of Health and Human Services. Urinary Incontinence Guideline Panel. Urinary Incontinence in Adults: Clinical Practice Guideline. AHCPR Pub. No.92-0038. Rockville, MD, March 1992.

Agency for Health Care Policy and Research, Public Health Service, U.S. Department of Health and Human Services. Treatment of Pressure Ulcers: Clinical Practice Guidelines, Number 15. AHCPR Publication No. 95-0652. Rockville, MD, Dec 1994.

American Nurses Association and Association of Rehabilitation Nurses. Standards of Rehabilitation Nursing Practice. Kansas City, MO, American Nurses Association, 1986.

Bryant R et al. Pressure ulcers. In Bryant R (ed). Acute and Chronic

Wounds: Nursing Management (pp. 105–152). St. Louis, Mosby Year Book, 1992.
Dittmar S. Rehabilitation Nursing: Process and Application. St. Louis, CV Mosby, 1989.
Fraley A. Nursing and the Disabled: Across the Life Span. Boston, Jones Bartlett, 1992.
Hartke R. Psychological Aspects of Geriatric Rehabilitation. Gaithersburg, MD, Aspen, 1991.
Jeter K et al. Nursing of Continence. Philadelphia, WB Saunders, 1990.
Letts R. Principles of Seating the Disabled. Boca Raton, FL, CRC Press, 1991.
Marinelli R and Dell Orto A. The Psychological and Social Impact of Disability, 3rd ed. New York, Springer, 1991.
May B. Home Health and Rehabilitation: Concepts of Care. Philadelphia, FA Davis, 1993.
Miller J. Coping with Chronic Illness: Overcoming Powerlessness, 2nd ed. Philadelphia, FA Davis, 1992.
National Institute on Disability and Rehabilitation Research, Office of Special Education and Rehabilitative Services. Directory of National Information Sources on Disabilities. Washington, DC, U.S. Department of Education, 1991.
Rehabilitation Nursing Foundation. The Special Practice of Rehabilitation Nursing: A Core Curriculum. Evanston, IL, Rehabilitation Nursing Foundation, 1994.
Rothstein J et al. The Rehabilitation Specialist's Handbook. Philadelphia, FA Davis, 1991.
Young R et al. Health, Illness, and Disability in Later Life: Practice Issues and Interventions. Chicago, Sage, 1991.

Journals

Asterisks indicate nursing research articles.

Rehabilitation

Atchinson D. Restorative nursing: A concept whose time has come. Nurs Homes 1992 Jan/Feb; 41(1):8–12.
Butler M. Geriatric rehabilitation nursing. Rehabil Nurs 1991 Nov/Dec; 16(6):318–321.
*Gibbon B and Thompson A. The role of the nurse in rehabilitation. Nurs Stand 1992 May 27–Jun 2; 6(36):32–35.
Kilbury R et al. The interaction of legislation, public attitudes, and access to opportunities for persons with disabilities. J Rehabil 1992 Oct–Dec; 58(4):34–39.
Meyer C. The changing face of rehabilitation nursing. Am J Nurs 1993 Feb; 93(2):76–82.
Meyer C. Rehab: "Primary nursing as it was meant to be." Am J Nurs 1992 Feb; 92(2):59–60, 62, 64.
Phipps M. Assessment of neurologic deficits in stroke: Acute-care and rehabilitation implications. Nurs Clin North Am 1991 Dec; 26(4):957–970.
Swanson B et al. The impact of psychosocial factors on adapting to physical disability: A review of research literature. Rehabil Nurs 1989 Mar/Apr; 14(2):64–68.
Vance J. Learning readiness in rehabilitation patients. Rehabil Nurs 1992 May/Jun; 17(3):148–149.
Watson P. The Americans with Disabilities Act: More rights for people with disabilities. Rehabil Nurs 1990 Nov/Dec; 15(6):325–328.
Youngblood N et al. The influence of the family's perception of disability on rehabilitation outcomes. Rehabil Nurs 1992 Nov/Dec; 17(6):323–326.

Assessment

Calvani D and Douris K. Functional assessment: A holistic approach to rehabilitation of the geriatric patient. Rehabil Nurs 1991 Nov/Dec; 16(6):330–336.
Granger C et al. Functional assessment scales: A study of persons after stroke. Arch Phys Med Rehabil 1993 Feb; 74(2):133–138.

Self-Care Deficit

*Doyle D et al. Negotiating self-care in rehabilitation nursing. Rehabil Nurs 1992 Nov/Dec; 17(6):319–322, 326.
Osborn C et al. Promoting mealtime independence. Geriatr Nurs 1992 Sep/Oct; 13(5):254–256.
Price E. Independence and the individual with severe disability. J Rehabil 1990 Oct–Dec; 56(4):15–18.
Rourke A. Self care: Chore or challenge. J Adv Nurs 1991 Feb; 16(2): 233–241.

Impaired Physical Mobility

*Glick O. Interventions related to activity and movement. Nurs Clin North Am 1992 Jun; 27(2):541–568.
*Johnson P et al. Applying nursing diagnosis and nursing process to activities of daily living and mobility. Geriatr Nurs 1992 Jan/Feb; 13(1):25–27.

Impaired Skin Integrity

Alterescu V and Alterescu K. Pressure ulcers: Assessment and treatment. Orthop Nurs 1992 Mar/Apr; 11(2):37–49.
*Aronovitch S. A retrospective study of the use of specialty beds in the medical and surgical intensive care units of a tertiary care facility. Decubitus 1992 Jan; 5(1):36–42.
*Bergstrum N and Braden B. A prospective study of pressure sore risk among institutionalized elderly. J Amer Geriatr Soc 1992 Aug; 40(8):747–758.
*Curry K and Casady L. The relationship between extended periods of immobility and decubitus ulcer formation in the acutely spinal cord injured individual. J Neurosci Nurs 1992 Apr; 24(4):185–189.
Dugan M. Pressure areas: Standard protocols improve care. Nurs Mgt 1992 Nov; 23(11):78–80.
*Ferrell B et al. A randomized trial of low-air-loss beds for treatment of pressure ulcers. JAMA 1993 Jan 27; 269(4):494–497.
Goodridge D. Pressure ulcer risk assessment tools: What's new for gerontological nurses. J Geront Nurs 1993 Feb; 19(2):23–27.
Inman K et al. Clinical utility and cost-effectiveness of an air suspension bed in the prevention of pressure ulcers. JAMA 1993 Mar 3; 269(9):1139–1143.
*Itoh M et al. Accelerated wound healing of pressure ulcers by pulsed high peak power electromagnetic energy (Diapulse). Decubitus 1991 Feb; 4(1):24–25, 29–30, 32+.
Kuhn B and Coulter S. Balancing the pressure ulcer cost and quality equation. Nurs Econ 1992 Sep/Oct; 10(5):353–359.
Maklebust J. Pressure ulcer update. RN 1991 Dec; 54(12):56–63.
Perez E. Pressure ulcers: Updated guidelines for treatment and prevention. Geriatrics 1993 Jan; 48(1):39–44.
*Sideranko S et al. Effects of position and mattress overlay on sacral and heel pressures in a clinical population. Res Nurs Heal 1992 Aug; 15(4):245–251.
*Sparks S. Nurse validation of pressure ulcer risk factors for a nursing diagnosis. Decubitus 1992 Jan; 5(1):26–35.

Altered Elimination

*Colling J et al. The effect of patterned urge-response toileting (PURT) on urinary incontinence among nursing home residents. J Am Geriatr Soc 1992 Feb; 40(2):135–141.
*Dowd T. Discovering older women's experience of urinary incontinence. Res Nurs Health 1991 Jun; 14(3):179–186.
Doyle M. Continence. Suffering in secret. Nurs Times 1993 Jan 27–Feb 2; 89(4):64–66.
Hebel J and Warren J. The use of urethral, condom, and suprapubic catheters in aged nursing home patients. J Am Geriatr Soc 1990 Jul; 38(7):777–778.
Kunin C et al. The association between the use of urinary catheters and morbidity and mortality among elderly patients in nursing homes. Am J Epidemiol 1992 Feb 1; 135(3):291–301.
McCormick K et al. Urinary incontinence in adults. Am J Nurs 1992 Oct; 92(10):75–76, 78–82, 84–86.

Newman DK et al. Restoring urinary continence. Am J Nurs 1991 Jan; 91(1):28–36.

O'Brien J et al. Urinary incontinence: Prevalence, need for treatment, and effectiveness of intervention by nurse. Br Med J 1991 Nov 23; 303(6813):1308–1312.

Rousseau P and Fuentevilla-Clifton A. Urinary incontinence in the aged. Part 1: Patient evaluation. Part 2: Management strategies. Geriatrics 1992 Jun; 47(6):22–26, 33–34; 37–40, 45, 48.

Schnelle J et al. Assessment and quality control of incontinence care in long-term nursing facilities. J Am Geriatr Soc 1991 Feb; 39(2):165–171.

*Venn M et al. The influence of timing and suppository use of efficiency and effectiveness of bowel training after stroke. Rehabil Nurs 1992 May/Jun; 17(3):116-121.

Weiss B. Nonpharmacologic treatment of urinary incontinence. Am Fam Physician 1991 Aug; 44(2):579–586.

Wyman J. Bladder training in ambulatory care management of urinary incontinence. Urol Nurs 1991 Sep; 11(3):11–17.

Nursing Research Profile for Unit 4

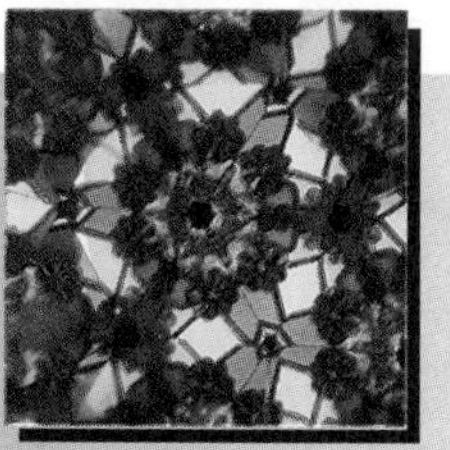

Concepts and Challenges in Patient Management

Overview

Nursing research highlighted in this section focuses on pain management and issues related to oncology and rehabilitation nursing.

Duggleby W and Lander J. Patient-controlled analgesia for older adults. Clin Nurs Research 1992 Feb; 1(1):107–113.

The purpose of this study was to compare analgesia management in patients using patient-controlled analgesia (PCA) and those with traditional nurse-controlled pain management among older adults undergoing hip arthoplasty. Sixty patients between the ages of 50 and 80 years were randomly assigned to either the PCA group or the traditional management group. The traditional management group patients were instructed about postoperative medication and how to ask for analgesia. The PCA patients were instructed in the use of the PCA pump. Both groups were instructed in how to use visual analogue scales (VAS), which were used to measure pain intensity, pain distress, satisfaction with pain relief, and sleep disturbance from pain. Patients in the PCA group were placed on the PCA pump upon their return to the nursing unit from the post-anesthesia unit. The pump was programmed to deliver a continuous infusion of morphine at the rate of 1 mg/hr, although the patient had the option to self-administer 1 mg every 15 minutes. Patients in the traditional management group received the standard analgesia regimen provided through the orthopedic service. Over 5 days, beginning on the day of surgery, the researchers assessed pain intensity and pain distress 14 times, satisfaction with pain relief 13 times, and sleep disturbance 4 times. Analgesic intake in mg/hr for the time intervals between pain assessments was reported.

The researchers found that patients in the PCA group received significantly more analgesia than did the patients in the traditional management group; however, they received a smaller percentage of the analgesia available to them. Patients in the PCA group received an average of 1.9 mg/hr of morphine over the first 48 hours; this was 33.8% of the medication available to them. Patients in the traditional management group received 0.9 mg/hr, which was 36.8% of the prescribed analgesia. During the first 24 hours when pain was most severe, PCA patients self-administered 41.3% of available analgesia, whereas nurses administered 25.3% of available analgesia to the traditional management group in the same time period. Although the researchers do not report mean VAS scores by treatment group, they do suggest that neither group received adequate pain control. They also note that elderly patients in the study had no more difficulty understanding the use of the PCA or VAS than did the middle-aged patients.

Nursing Implications. Findings of this study indicate that patients who self-administer postoperative analgesia receive more medication than those who receive nurse-administered medication. However, neither group in this study received enough medication to effectively control their pain. The findings also suggest that the elderly can safely use a PCA pump.

Belec R. Quality of life: Perceptions of long-term survivors of bone marrow transplantation. Oncol Nurs Forum 1992 Jan/Feb; 19(1):31–37.

Bone marrow transplantation (BMT) is a complex treatment option in cancer care that is demanding for patients in terms of length, morbidity, and mortality. Thus far, few nursing studies have examined the quality of life of those undergoing BMT. This study examined the perceived quality of life of 24 patients who received either an autologous or allogenic BMT at least 1 year prior to the study. The cancer version of the Quality of Life Index (QLI) was completed by each patient either at home or in the outpatient clinic setting.

Results of the study showed that approximately 92% of the participants' scores on the QLI fell in the upper half of the scale, indicating a perceived acceptable quality of life, and approximately 8% of scores fell in the lower half of the scale. The family subscale scores were also found to be in the upper half of the scoring range. The family subscale scores appeared to have the greatest positive impact on overall perceived quality of life of patients. Participants were generally most concerned regarding issues of health and employment. Despite the grueling therapy, only one participant reported that he would not make the same decision to receive BMT. Approximately 90% of the participants felt that the BMT experience gave greater meaning to their lives in terms of reassessing priorities and value.

Nursing Implications. As technology increases the treatment options in cancer care, nurses must not lose sight of the quality of life of patients undergoing these therapies. This study offers nurses some insight into understanding the BMT experience and its impact on quality of life, which will enable them to better anticipate needs and support patients through the experience. As indicated by the results of the study, nurses must also assess family functioning and assist with family coping since the influence of the family greatly affects the patient's quality of life.

Jansen C, et al. Family problems during cancer chemotherapy. Oncol Nurs Forum 1993 May; 20(4):689–694.

Cancer is a disease that affects the entire family, not only the patient. Few nursing research studies have examined the impact of cancer and its treatment on the family as a whole. To assess family needs, the investigators of this longitudinal study conducted three family interviews over a 6-month period, beginning at the initiation of chemotherapy. The sample comprised 226 participants: 100 adult patients with cancer and 126 family members. Participants completed the Problem Centered Family Coping Inventory (PCFCI), a semistructured interview tool, at 1½ weeks, 7½ weeks, and 6 months following chemotherapy.

The most frequently discussed issue (48%–52% of all interview times) was the patient's cancer-related health status. The side effects of chemotherapy, particularly fatigue, nausea/vomiting, pain, anorexia, and myelosuppression, were important family concerns. Other issues that affected the family unit included the patient's psychologic health, negative family affect, existential concerns, financial concerns, and employment. The total number of identifiable needs decreased from the time of the initial interview to the time of the 6-month interview, indicating that family needs change and evolve over the course of the disease and treatment.

Nursing Implications. As is evident from the results of this study, nurses must consider the family as a whole when assessing needs during the cancer experience. Family needs must be assessed over time to recognize changes in problem resolution or the development of new problems. Nurses can assist families by anticipating problems and by functioning proactively to reduce the negative impact of these issues and enhance family coping.

Bergstrom N and Braden B. A prospective study of pressure sore risk among institutionalized elderly. J Am Geriatr Soc 1992 Aug; 40(8):747–758.

The purpose of this prospective study was to determine if dietary intake, nutritional status, and other physiologic factors are risk factors for pressure ulcers in newly admitted nursing home residents. The subjects were 200 newly admitted skilled-level nursing home residents over 65 years of age who were identified as being at risk for pressure ulcers by a score on the Braden scale of less than 17, were free of existing pressure ulcers, and were expected to be in the nursing home for more than 10 days.

The subjects were assessed at weekly intervals for 12 weeks or until discharged. The Braden scale, which is used to score activity, mobility, sensory perception, friction and shear, skin moisture, and dietary intake, was completed for each subject weekly. Braden scale scores of less than 12 indicate high risk, scores of 13 to 15 indicate moderate risk, and scores of 16 to 17 indicate mild risk of pressure ulcer development. Complete blood counts and serum levels of iron, total protein, albumin, zinc, copper, and vitamin C were obtained weekly for 4 weeks and then biweekly. Anthropometric measurements (height/weight, triceps skinfold, midarm muscle circumference) were obtained weekly, as were blood pressure, body temperature, and dietary intake. Each subject's skin was assessed weekly and pressure ulcers, if present, were graded (Stage 1—non-blanchable erythema present greater than 24 hours after pressure relieved; Stage 2—superficial lesions such as blisters and abrasions; Stage 3—skin break with subcutaneous tissue exposed; Stage 4—lesion exposes muscle or bone). The research team informed the nursing staff of the presence of pressure ulcers so that nursing measures (*e.g.*, turning, protective devices, keeping skin dry and clean) could be implemented.

Seventy percent of the subjects developed pressure ulcers; 35% were stage 1; 38.5% were stage 2 or worse. The most prevalent sites included the coccyx and sacrum, heel, and ankle. Most (80%) of the pressure ulcers developed within 2 weeks of admission. Subjects who developed pressure ulcers had lower Braden scores the week prior to developing ulcers than those who did not. Subjects who developed pressure ulcers were older and had lower systolic and diastolic blood pressure and higher body temperatures than those who did not. Dietary intake of nutrients studied was lower among subjects who developed pressure ulcers. The mean protein intake was significantly lower among patients who developed stage 1 pressure ulcers ($p < .001$) and those who developed stage 2 or worse ulcers ($p < .01$) when these groups were compared with those who developed no ulcers. Serum albumin was the only nutritional marker that differed significantly between those who developed stage 1 pressure ulcers ($p = .001$) and stage 2 pressure ulcers ($p = .01$) when compared with those who did not.

Statistical analyses were conducted to identify predictors of pressure ulcer development. The best predictors were the Braden scale score, diastolic blood pressure, temperature, age, and dietary intake of protein or iron. Dietary intake of protein was a predictor of deep pressure ulcers, and dietary iron intake was a predictor of stage 1 and stage 2 or greater ulcers.

Nursing Implications. The results of this study support the value of weekly assessment of nursing home residents for risk of pressure ulcers during the first month following admission to the nursing home. The Braden scale, combined with information about the patient's temperature, blood pressure, age, and dietary protein intake during the week prior to the development of pressure ulcer, can be predictive of pressure ulcer development. Identifying those patients at highest risk enables aggressive implementation of strategies to prevent pressure ulcers.

UNIT 5

Perioperative Concepts and Management

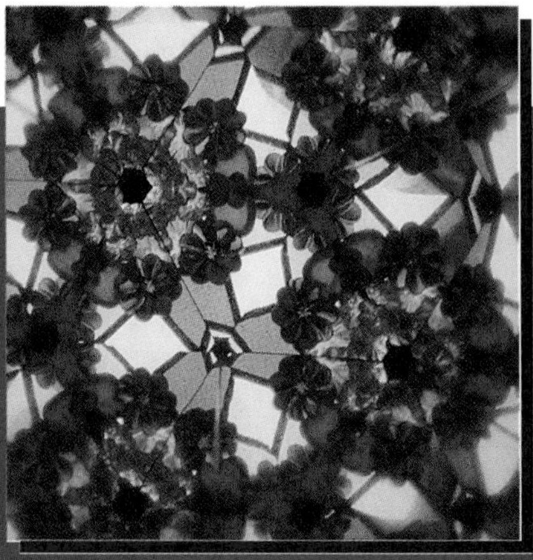

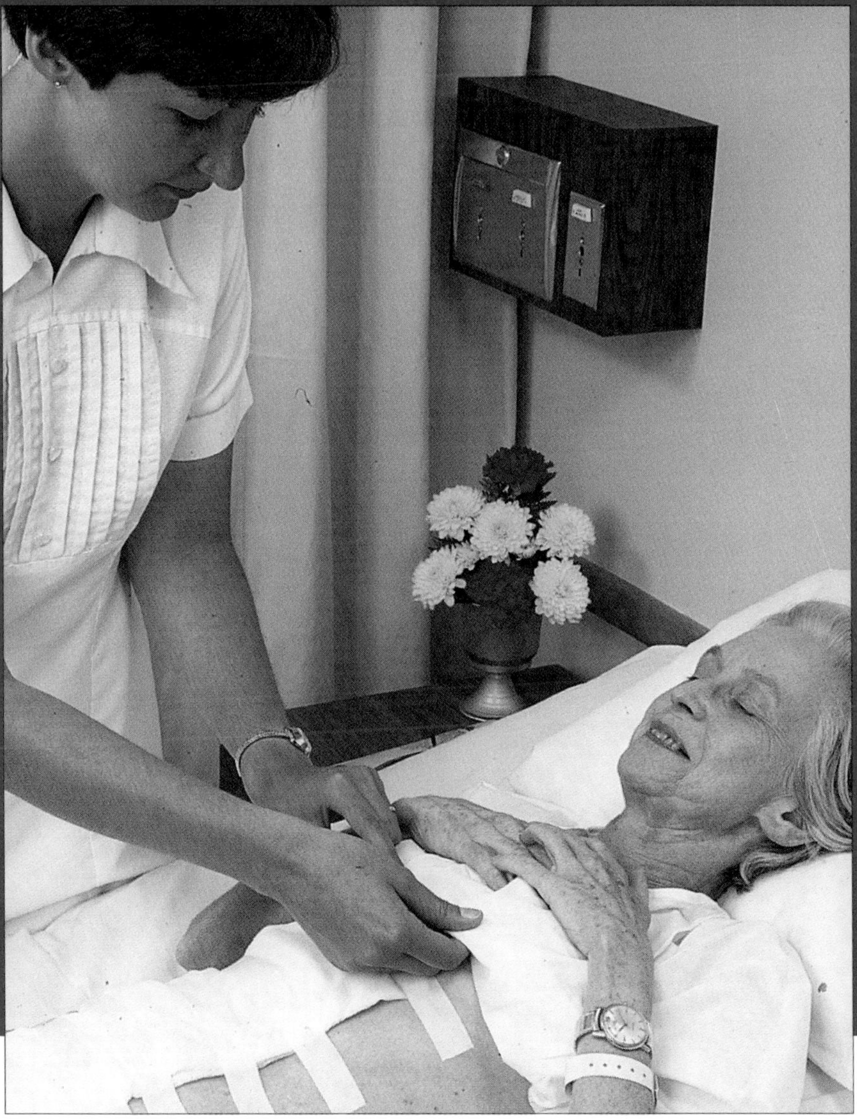

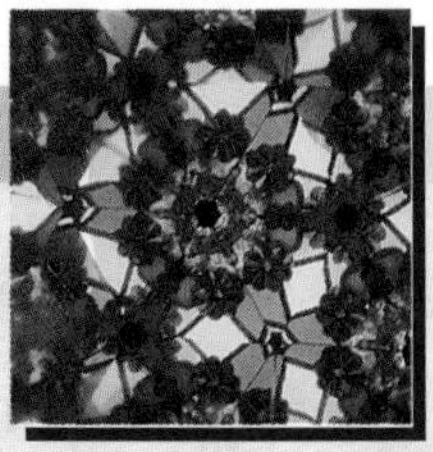

19

Preoperative Nursing Management

CHAPTER OUTLINE

LEARNING OBJECTIVES

On completion of this chapter, the learner will be able to:

1. Identify the causes of preoperative anxieties and nursing measures to ally anxiety
2. Use comprehensive preoperative assessment to identify surgical risk factors
3. Identify legal and ethical considerations related to the operative permit and informed consent
4. Describe preoperative nursing measures that decrease the risk for infection and other postoperative complications
5. Develop a preoperative teaching plan designed to promote the patient's recovery and to prevent postoperative complications
6. Describe the immediate preoperative preparation of the patient
7. Identify the nurse's responsibility in meeting the needs of the family of the preoperative/operative patient

Surgery, whether elective or emergency, is a stressful, complex event. Most surgical procedures are performed in a hospital operating room, although many simpler procedures that do not require hospitalization are carried out in surgical centers and ambulatory surgery units. The person with a health care problem that requires surgical intervention usually undergoes a surgical procedure that involves the administration of local, regional, or general anesthesia. The development of anesthetic agents has recently focused on short-acting and "faster recovery" drugs.

Recent technologic advances have led to more complex procedures, such as those requiring microsurgical techniques or the use of lasers; more sophisticated bypass equipment; and highly sensitive monitoring devices. Surgery has involved the transplantation of multiple human organs, the implantation of mechanical devices, and the reattachment of body parts.

Concurrent advances have also been made in the development of pharmaceutical preparations and nutritional supplements. Although these technologic advances have focused attention on the essential "high-tech" role of nursing personnel, the role of human touch is equally important.

At the same time that technologic advances have occurred, the delivery and payment for health care have changed, resulting in shorter hospital stays and cost-containment measures. As a result, many people scheduled for surgery undergo diagnostic and preoperative preparation before entering the hospital. They also leave the hospital sooner, increasing the need for patient teaching, discharge planning, preparation for self-care, and referral for home care and rehabilitation services. With the advent of cost-containment measures, same-day surgery, and early postoperative discharge, it is not unusual for a patient to be admitted to the hospital on the day of surgery, to receive general anesthesia and undergo a surgical procedure, and to be discharged home to the care of the family or friends the same day.

In the 1980s, seven out of every eight surgeries required at least one overnight stay in the hospital. Today, it is estimated that 60% of surgeries are performed on an outpatient basis. Ambulatory, or same-day, surgery requires the nurse to have a solid knowledge of all aspects of surgical patient care. No longer is preoperative and postoperative nursing knowledge sufficient; complete care must include an understanding of intraoperative activity.

This unit focuses on the application of the nursing process for the patient undergoing major surgery, same-day surgery, or surgery in a short-procedure unit. In each type of setting, the basic principles remain the same.

Perioperative Nursing

Perioperative nursing is the term used to describe the wide variety of nursing functions associated with the patient's surgical experience. The word "perioperative" is an encompassing term that incorporates the three phases of the surgical experience—preoperative, intraoperative, and postoperative. As shown in Chart 19-1, each of these phases begins and ends at a particular time in the sequence of events that constitute the surgical experience, and each includes a wide range of behaviors and nursing activities that the nurse performs using the nursing process and standards of practice.

The **preoperative phase** of the perioperative nursing role begins when the decision for surgical intervention is made and ends with the transfer of the patient to the operating room table. The scope of nursing activities during this time can include establishing a baseline assessment of the patient in the clinical setting or at home, carrying out a preoperative interview, and preparing the patient for the anesthetic to be given and the surgery. However, the nursing activities may be limited to performing a preoperative patient assessment in the holding area or surgical suite.

The **intraoperative phase** of perioperative nursing begins when the patient is admitted or transferred to the surgery department and ends when he or she is admitted to the recovery area. In this phase, the scope of nursing activity can include starting the IV infusion, administering IV medications, carrying out the full scope of physiologic monitoring throughout the surgical procedure, and providing for the patient's safety. In some instances, the nursing activities can be limited to holding the patient's hand during general anesthesia induction, acting in the role of scrub nurse, or assisting in positioning the patient on the operating room table using basic principles of body alignment.

The **postoperative phase** begins with the admission of the patient to the recovery area and ends with a follow-up evaluation in the clinical setting or at home. The scope of nursing covers a wide range of activities during this period. In the immediate postoperative phase, the focus includes assessing the effects of the anesthetic agents, monitoring vital functions, and preventing complications. Nursing activities then focus on promoting the patient's recovery and initiating the teaching, follow-up care, and referrals essential for successful recuperation and rehabilitation following discharge.

Each phase is reviewed in more detail in this unit. Where pertinent and possible, the nursing process of assessment, nursing diagnosis, planning, intervention, and evaluation is described.

Gerontologic Considerations

Surgery imposes physical and psychologic stress, but advances in assessment techniques, surgical procedures, anesthetic techniques, and monitoring capabilities allow older patients to tolerate elective surgery surprisingly well. The underlying principle that guides the preoperative assessment, surgery, and postoperative care is that the aged patient has less **physiologic reserve** (the ability of an organ to return to normal after a disturbance in its equilibrium) than the younger patient.

The special requirements for optimum results following surgery on an elderly patient include (1) skillful preoperative assessment and treatment, (2) careful anesthesia and surgery, and (3) meticulous and competent postoperative management. The hazards of surgery for the aged are proportional to the number and severity of coexisting health problems and the nature and duration of the operative procedure.

CHART 19-1

Examples of Nursing Activities in the Perioperative Role

Preoperative Phase

Preoperative Assessment
Clinic/Telephone
1. Initiates initial preoperative assessment
2. Plans teaching methods appropriate to patient's needs
3. Involves family in interview
4. Verifies completion of preoperative testing
5. Assesses patient's need for postoperative transportation and care

Surgical Unit
1. Completes preoperative assessment
2. Coordinates patient teaching with other nursing staff
3. Explains phases in perioperative period and expectations
4. Develops a plan of care

Operating Room
1. Assesses patient's level of consciousness
2. Reviews chart
3. Identifies patient
4. Verifies surgical site

Planning
1. Determines a plan of care
2. Coordinates appropriate services and resources

Psychologic Support
1. Tells patient what is happening
2. Determines psychologic status
3. Gives warning of noxious stimuli
4. Communicates patient's emotional status to other appropriate members of the health care team

Intraoperative Phase

Maintenance of Safety
1. Positions the patient
   a. Functional alignment
   b. Exposure of surgical site
   c. Maintenance of position throughout procedure
2. Applies grounding device to patient
3. Provides physical support
4. Ensures that the sponge, needle, and instrument counts are correct

Physiologic Monitoring
1. Calculates effects on patient of excessive fluid loss or gain
2. Distinguishes normal from abnormal cardiopulmonary data
3. Reports changes in patient's pulse, respirations, temperature, and blood pressure

Psychologic Support (Before Induction and if Patient is Conscious)
1. Provides emotional support to patient
2. Stands near or touches patient during procedures and induction
3. Continues to assess patient's emotional status
4. Communicates patient's emotional status to other appropriate members of the health care team

Nursing Management
1. Provides physical safety for the patient
2. Maintains aseptic, controlled environment
3. Effectively manages human resources

Postoperative Phase

Communication of Intraoperative Information
1. States patient's name
2. States type of surgery performed
3. Describes intraoperative factors (*i.e.*, insertion of drains or catheters, occurrence of unexpected events)
4. Describes physical limitations
5. Reports patient's preoperative level of consciousness
6. Communicates necessary equipment needs

Postoperative Assessment Recovery Area
1. Determines patient's immediate response to surgical intervention

Surgical Unit
1. Evaluates effectiveness of nursing care in the OR
2. Determines patient's level of satisfaction with care given during perioperative period
3. Evaluates products used on patient in the OR
4. Determines patient's psychologic status
5. Assists with discharge planning

Home/Clinic
1. Seeks patient's perception of surgery in terms of the effects of anesthetic agents, impact on body image, distortion, immobilization
2. Determines family's perception of surgery

(A model for perioperative nursing practice. AORN J Jan; 41:1. Reprinted with permission from AORN, Inc, 10170 E. Mississippi Avenue, Denver, CO 80231. All rights reserved.)

Surgical Indications and Classifications

Surgery may be performed for a variety of reasons. It may be **diagnostic**, such as when a biopsy is obtained or an exploratory laparotomy is performed; it may be **curative**, such as when a tumor mass is excised or an inflamed appendix is removed; it may be **reparative**, such as when multiple wounds must be repaired; it may be **reconstructive** or **cosmetic**, such as when a mammoplasty or a face lift is performed; or it may be **palliative**, such as when pain must be relieved or a problem corrected—for example, when a gastrostomy tube is inserted to compensate for the inability to swallow food.

Surgery may also be classified according to the degree of urgency involved, with use of the terms **emergency, urgent, required, elective,** and **optional.** These terms are defined in Table 19-1, along with examples of the types of surgery involved.

❑ NURSING PROCESS OVERVIEW

Assessment

Assessment of the surgical patient involves evaluating a wide range of physical and psychologic factors. Many

TABLE 19-1 Categories of Surgery Based on Urgency

Classification	Indications for Surgery	Examples
I. Emergency—Patient requires immediate attention; disorder may be life-threatening	Without delay	Severe bleeding Bladder or intestinal obstruction Fractured skull Gunshot/stab wounds Extensive burns
II. Urgent—Patient requires prompt attention	Within 24–30 h	Acute gallbladder infection Kidney or ureteral stones
III. Required—Patient needs to have surgery	Plan within a few weeks or months	Prostatic hyperplasia without bladder obstruction Thyroid disorders Cataracts
IV. Elective—Patient should be operated upon	Failure to have surgery not catastrophic	Repair of scars Simple hernia Vaginal repair
V. Optional—Decision rests with patient	Personal preference	Cosmetic surgery

parameters are considered in the overall assessment of the patient, and a variety of patient problems or nursing diagnoses can be anticipated or identified on the basis of the data. Detailed discussions of the psychosocial assessment and the physical examination of the surgical patient follow this section.

Nursing Diagnoses

Based on the assessment data, major preoperative nursing diagnoses of the surgical patient may include:

- Anxiety related to the surgical experience (anesthesia, pain) and the outcome of surgery
- Knowledge deficit regarding preoperative procedures and protocols and postoperative expectations

Planning and Implementation

Goals: The surgical patient's major goals may include relief of preoperative anxiety and increased knowledge of preoperative preparations and postoperative expectations.

Nursing Interventions

Reducing Preoperative Anxiety. Specific nursing interventions are discussed in detail under Psychosocial Nursing Assessment and Interventions.

Patient Education. Specific nursing interventions are discussed in detail in other sections of this chapter under Preoperative Patient Education. See also Preoperative Nursing Interventions and Immediate Preoperative Nursing Interventions.

Evaluation

Expected Outcomes

1. Anxiety is relieved
   a. Discusses concerns related to types of anesthesia and induction with anesthesiologist/anesthetist
   b. Verbalizes an understanding of the preanesthetic medication and general anesthesia
   c. Discusses last-minute concerns with nurse or physician
   d. Discusses financial concerns with social worker, when appropriate
   e. Requests visit with member of clergy when appropriate
   f. Relaxes quietly after being visited by health team members
2. Prepares for surgical intervention
   a. Participates in preoperative preparation
   b. Demonstrates and describes exercises he or she is expected to perform postoperatively
   c. Reviews information about postoperative care
   d. Accepts preanesthetic medication
   e. Remains in bed
   f. Relaxes during transportation to operating unit
   g. States rationale for use of side rails

Psychosocial Nursing Assessment and Interventions

Any surgical procedure is preceded by some type of emotional reaction by the patient, whether it is obvious or hidden, normal or abnormal. For example, preoperative anxiety may be an anticipatory response to an experience that the patient may view as a threat to his or her customary role in life, body integrity, or even life itself. It is known that a troubled mind directly influences the functioning of the body. Therefore, it is imperative to identify the anxieties that the patient is experiencing.

By taking a careful health history, the nurse elicits patient concerns that can have a direct bearing on the course of the surgical experience. Undoubtedly, a patient facing surgery is beset by fears, including fears of the unknown, of death, of anesthesia, of cancer. Concerns about loss of work time, the possible loss of job, the responsibility of family support, and the threat of permanent incapacity further contribute to the often enormous emotional strain created by the prospect of surgery. Less obvious concerns may occur because of previous experiences with the health care system and people the patient has known with the same condition. Consequently, the nurse must encourage verbalization, and must listen, be understanding, and provide information that helps to allay concerns.

The extent of the patient's reaction is based on many factors, including the discomforts and changes anticipated—whether physical, financial, psychologic, spiritual, or social—and the surgical outcome envisioned. Will the operation improve the condition? Will it result in disability? Is this just a temporary measure in a chronic condition?

An important part of the assessment is to determine the role of the patient's family or friends. The value and reliability of all available support systems are also determined. Other information, such as usual level of functioning and typical daily activities, may assist in the patient's care and rehabilitation plans.

Fear is expressed in different ways by different people. For example, fear may be expressed indirectly by the patient who repeatedly asks a lot of questions, even though answers were given previously. For another person, the reaction may be withdrawal—deliberately avoiding communication, perhaps by reading or watching television. Still others may talk incessantly about trivialities. When a patient expresses concern or worry about impending surgery, it is important to keep the lines of communication open. To respond to the patient's fears with unwarranted reassurance by saying, "Oh, there's nothing to be afraid of" immediately closes the door and causes the patient to lapse into less effective means of coping with his or her worries.

A preoperative patient may experience a number of fears. Fear of anesthesia, fear of pain or death, fear of the unknown, or fear of deformity or other threats to body image may cause unease and anxiety. The nurse can do much to dispel false conceptions and misinformation, and to provide reassurance when possible. In addition to the above fears, the patient often has other worries, such as financial problems, family responsibilities, and employment obligations, or fear of a poor prognosis or the probability of disability in the future. The nurse can explore these fears with the patient and arrange for the assistance of other health professionals if required. If the worry stems from fear of what the prognosis is likely to be, the physician is informed.

Spiritual beliefs play an important role in dealing with fears and anxiety. Regardless of religious affiliation of the patient, spiritual beliefs can be as therapeutic as medication. Every attempt must be made to help the patient obtain the spiritual help that he or she requests. Faith has great sustaining power; thus, the beliefs of each individual patient should be respected and supported. Some nurses avoid the subject of a clergy visit on the premise that the suggestion may alarm the patient. However, asking if the patient's minister, priest, or rabbi knows about the impending surgery is a caring, nonthreatening approach.

Respect for a patient's **cultural values** and beliefs facilitates rapport and trust. Some areas of assessment include the ethnic group that the patient relates to and the customs and beliefs toward illness and health care providers. For example, patients from some cultural groups are unaccustomed to expressing feelings openly. Nurses need to consider this pattern of self control when assessing pain. As a sign of respect, individuals from other cultural groups do not make direct eye contact with others. It is important for the nurse to know that this lack of eye contact is not avoidance or a lack of interest.

Perhaps the most valuable facility at the disposal of the nurse is the ability to *listen* to the patient, especially when obtaining the patient's history. By engaging in conversation and using the principles of communication and interviewing, the nurse can acquire invaluable information and insight. An unhurried, understanding, and caring nurse invites confidence on the part of the patient.

General Physical Assessment

Before treatment is initiated, a health history is obtained and a physical examination is performed during which vital signs are noted and a data base is established for future comparisons. Many diagnostic tests may be performed, such as blood analyses, x-ray studies, endoscopies, tissue biopsies, and stool and urine studies. In preparation for these tests, the nurse is in a position to help the patient understand the need for the diagnostic studies. There is also an opportunity during the physical examination to note significant physical findings, such as pressure ulcers, edema, or abnormal breath sounds that further describe the patient's overall condition.

These preliminary contacts with the health care team provide the patient with opportunities to ask questions and to become acquainted with those who might be providing care during and following surgery.

Nutritional Status and Chemical Substance Use

Nutritional needs are determined by measuring the patient's height and weight, triceps skin fold, upper arm circumference, serum protein levels, and nitrogen balance. Any nutrient deficiency should be corrected prior to surgery to provide enough protein for tissue repair.

Dehydration, hypovolemia, and electrolyte imbalances are common and should be carefully documented. The degree of severity is often difficult to determine. When a patient is being prepared for surgery, additional time may be needed to correct deficits to promote the best possible preoperative condition. Nutrients needed for wound healing are summarized in Table 19-2.

Obesity. Obesity greatly increases the risk and severity of complications associated with surgery. During surgery, fatty tissues are especially susceptible to infection. Additionally, obesity creates increased technical and mechanical problems. Therefore, dehiscence (wound separation) and wound infections are more common. The obese patient is often more difficult to care for because of the added weight; the patient breathes poorly when lying on his or her side

TABLE 19-2 Nutrients Important for Wound Healing and Recovery

Nutrient	Rationale for Increased Need	Possible Deficiency Outcome
Protein	To replace the lean body mass lost during the catabolic phase following surgery To restore blood volume and plasma proteins lost through exudates, bleeding from the wound, and possible hemorrhage To replace losses resulting from immobility (increased excretion) To meet the increased needs for tissue repair and resistance to infection	Significant weight loss Impaired/delayed wound healing Shock related to decreased blood volume Edema related to decreased serum albumin Diarrhea related to decreased albumin Anemia Increased risk of infection related to decreased antibodies, impaired tissue integrity Decreased lipoprotein synthesis → fatty infiltration of the liver → liver damage Increased mortality
Calories	To replace losses related to NPO, hypermetabolism during catabolic phase following surgery To spare protein To restore normal weight	Signs and symptoms of protein deficiency may develop when protein is used to meet energy requirements. Extensive weight loss
Water	To replace losses through vomiting, hemorrhage, exudates, fever, drainage, diuresis To maintain homeostasis	Signs, symptoms, and complications of dehydration such as poor skin turgor, dry mucous membranes, oliguria, anuria, weight loss, increased pulse rate, decreased central venous pressure (CVP)
Vitamin C	Important for tissue synthesis and wound healing through collagen formation	Impaired/delayed wound healing related to impaired collagen formation and increased capillary fragility and permeability
Thiamine, niacin, riboflavin	Requirements based on metabolic rate: increased metabolic rate→ increased requirements	Decreased enzymes available for energy metabolism
Folic acid, vitamin B_{12}	Needed for cell proliferation and therefore tissue synthesis Important for maturation of red blood cells Impaired folic acid synthesis related to some antibiotics; impaired vitamin B_{12} absorption related to some antibiotics	Decreased or arrested cell division Megaloblastic anemia
Vitamin A	Important for tissue synthesis and wound healing Enhances resistance to infection	Impaired/delayed wound healing related to decreased collagen synthesis Increased risk of infection
Vitamin K	Important for normal blood clotting Impaired intestinal synthesis related to antibiotics	Prolonged prothrombin time
Iron	To replace iron lost through blood loss	Signs, symptoms, and complications of iron deficiency anemia, such as fatigue, weakness, pallor, anorexia, dizziness, headaches, stomatitis, glossitis, cardiovascular and respiratory changes, possible cardiac failure
Zinc	Needed for protein synthesis and wound healing	Impaired/delayed wound healing

(Adapted from: Dudek SG. Nutrition Handbook for Nursing Practice, 2nd ed. Philadelphia, JB Lippincott, 1993, p. 395.)

and thus is subject to hypoventilation and postoperative pulmonary complications. In addition, abdominal distention, phlebitis, and cardiovascular, endocrine, hepatic, and biliary diseases occur more readily in obese patients. It has been estimated that for each 30 pounds of excess weight, about 25 additional miles of blood vessels are needed. The increased demands on the heart are obvious.

Drug or Alcohol Use. People who have an addiction to drugs or alcohol frequently deny or attempt to hide the habit. Often a variety of infections and trauma sites on the body can be noted. This situation calls for meticulous attention, patience, frank questions, and a nonjudgmental attitude on the part of the nurse who is assessing the patient.

The acutely intoxicated person is susceptible to injury. Therefore, surgery is postponed if possible. If emergency surgery is required, local or regional block anesthesia is used for minor surgery. Otherwise, to prevent vomiting and aspiration, the stomach must be intubated and aspirated before general anesthesia is administered.

The person with a history of chronic alcoholism often suffers from malnutrition and other systemic problems that increase the surgical risk. Additionally, alcohol withdrawal delirium (delirium tremens) may be anticipated on the second or third day after alcohol withdrawal, and it is associated with a significant mortality rate when it occurs postoperatively.

Respiratory Status

The goal for potential surgical patients is to have optimum respiratory function. All patients are urged to stop smoking 4 to 6 weeks before surgery; those undergoing upper abdominal and chest surgery are taught breathing exercises and how to use an incentive spirometer.

Because it is necessary to maintain adequate ventilation during all phases of surgical treatment, surgery is usually contraindicated when the patient has a respiratory infection.

Respiratory difficulties increase the possibility of atelectasis, bronchopneumonia, and respiratory failure when anesthetics are superimposed upon inadequate ventilation. Patients with pre-existing pulmonary problems are evaluated by means of pulmonary function studies and blood gas analysis to note the extent of respiratory insufficiency. Antibiotics may be prescribed for infections.

Cardiovascular Status

The goal in preparing any patient for surgery is to have a well-functioning cardiovascular system to meet the oxygen, fluid, and nutritional needs throughout the perioperative period.

Because cardiovascular disease increases risk, patients with these conditions demand greater than usual diligence during all phases of management and care. Depending on the severity of symptoms, surgery may be deferred until medical treatment can be instituted to improve the patient's condition. At times, surgical treatment can be modified to meet the cardiac tolerance of the patient. For example, in a patient with an obstruction of the descending colon and coronary artery disease, a temporary simple colostomy may be performed rather than a more extensive colon resection.

Of particular importance in the patient with cardiovascular disease is the need to avoid sudden changes of position, prolonged immobilization, hypotension or hypoxia, and overloading of the circulatory system with fluids or blood.

Hepatic and Renal Function

The goal is to have maximum functioning of the liver and urinary systems so that medications, anesthetic agents, and body wastes and toxins are adequately removed from the body.

The **liver** is important in the biotransformation of anesthetic compounds. Therefore, any disorder of the liver has an effect on how an anesthetic is metabolized. Because acute liver disease is associated with a high surgical mortality, preoperative improvement in liver function is desired. Careful assessment is made with various liver function tests (see Chapter 38).

The **kidneys** are involved in the excretion of anesthetic drugs and their metabolites.

Acid–base status and metabolism are also important considerations in anesthetic administration. Surgery is contraindicated when a patient has acute nephritis, acute renal insufficiency with oliguria or anuria, or other acute renal problems, unless the surgery is a lifesaving measure or is necessary to improve urinary function, as in an obstructive uropathy.

Endocrine Function

In uncontrolled **diabetes**, the chief life-threatening hazard is hypoglycemia, which may develop during anesthesia or from inadequate intake of carbohydrates postoperatively or excessive administration of insulin. Other hazards that threaten the patient but occur less rapidly are acidosis and glucosuria. In general, the surgical risk for the patient with controlled diabetes is not greater than that for the nondiabetic patient; however, frequent monitoring of blood glucose levels is important before, during, and after surgery (see Chapter 39).

Patients receiving **corticosteroids** are at risk for adrenal insufficiency; therefore, the use of steroid medications for any purpose during the preceding year must be reported to the anesthesiologist and surgeon. Additionally, the patient is monitored for signs of adrenal insufficiency.

Immunologic Function

An important function of preoperative assessment is to determine the existence of allergies, including previous allergic reactions. It is especially important to identify and document any sensitivities to certain medications and past adverse reactions to these agents. The patient is asked to identify any substances that precipitated previous allergic reactions, including medications, blood transfusions, and contrast agents, and to describe the signs and symptoms produced by these substances. A history of bronchial asthma is reported to the anesthesiologist.

Immunosuppression is common with corticosteroid therapy, renal transplantation, radiation therapy, chemotherapy, and disorders affecting the immune system (*e.g.*, AIDS, leukemia).

The mildest symptoms or slightest temperature elevation must be investigated. Because these patients are highly susceptible to infection, great care is taken to use meticulous asepsis.

Previous Medication Therapy

A medication history is obtained from each patient because of the possible effects of medications on the patient's perioperative course and the possibility of drug interaction effects. Any medication the patient is using or has used in the past is documented, including over-the-counter (OTC) preparations and the frequency with which they are taken. Potent medications have an effect on physiologic functions; interactions of such medications with anesthetic agents have caused serious problems, such as arterial hypotension and circulatory collapse or depression.

The potential effects of prior medication therapy are evaluated by the anesthesiologist, who considers the length of time the patient has used the medications, the patient, and the nature of the proposed surgery. Medications that cause particular concern include the following:

Adrenal corticosteroids—Corticosteroids are not to be discontinued abruptly before surgery. A person who has been taking steroids for some time may suffer cardiovascular collapse if the steroids are discontinued suddenly. Therefore, a bolus of steroid may be administered intravenously immediately before and after surgery.

Diuretics—Thiazide diuretics may cause excessive respiratory depression during anesthesia; this results from an associated electrolyte imbalance.

Phenothiazines—These medications may increase the hypotensive action of anesthetics.

Antidepressants—Monoamine oxidase (MAO) inhibitors increase the hypotensive effects of anesthetics.

Tranquilizers—Barbiturates, diazepam, and chlordiazepoxide may cause anxiety, tension, and even seizures if withdrawn suddenly.

Insulin: Interaction between anesthetics and insulin must be considered when a patient with diabetes is undergoing surgery.

Antibiotics—"Mycin" drugs such as neomycin, kanamycin, and, less frequently, streptomycin may present problems; when these medications are combined with a curariform muscle relaxant, nerve transmission is interrupted and apnea due to respiratory paralysis may result.

For the reasons cited, it is imperative that the patient's medication history be assessed by the nurse and anesthesiologist.

Gerontologic Considerations

An older person facing an operation may have a combination of chronic illnesses and health problems in addition to the specific one for which surgery is indicated. Elderly people frequently do not report symptoms, perhaps because they fear that a serious illness may be diagnosed or because they accept such symptoms as part of the aging process. A high level of awareness of subtle clues alerts the nurse to underlying problems.

In general, the elderly are considered poorer surgical risks than younger patients. Cardiac reserves are lower, renal and hepatic function are depressed, and gastrointestinal activity is likely to be reduced. Dehydration, constipation, and malnutrition may be evident.

Sensory limitations such as impaired vision or hearing and reduced sensitivity of touch are often the reasons for accidents, injuries, and burns. Therefore, the nurse must be alert to maintaining a safe environment. Arthritis is common in older persons and may affect mobility, making it difficult for the patient to turn from one side to the other without discomfort. Protective measures include adequate padding for tender areas, moving the patient slowly, protecting bony prominences from prolonged pressure, and providing gentle massage to promote adequate circulation.

The condition of the mouth is important to assess because of the frequent presence of dental caries, dentures, and partial plates. Such findings are particularly significant to the anesthesiologist.

Decreased perspiration leads to dry, itchy skin. Such fragile skin is easily abraded, so added precautions are taken in moving an elderly person. Decreased subcutaneous fat makes older people more susceptible to temperature changes. A lightweight cotton blanket is an appropriate cover when an elderly patient is moved to and from the operating room.

The elderly person has undoubtedly experienced many personal illnesses and possibly life-threatening illnesses of friends and family. Such experiences may result in fears about the future. Providing an opportunity to express these fears enables the patient to gain some peace of mind and a sense of being understood.

In summary, the overall goal in the preoperative period is to have as many positive health factors as possible. Every attempt is made to stabilize those conditions that otherwise hinder a smooth recovery. When negative factors such as those listed in Chart 19-2 dominate, the risks of surgery and postoperative complications increase.

Informed Consent

Voluntary and informed written consent from the patient is necessary before surgery can be done. Such written permission protects the patient against unsanctioned surgery and protects the surgeon against claims of an unauthorized op-

CHART 19-2
Risk Factors for Any Surgical Procedure

Systemic Factors
- Hypovolemia
- Dehydration or electrolyte imbalance
- Nutritional deficits
- Extremes of age
- Extremes of weight
- Infection and sepsis
- Toxic conditions
- Immunologic abnormalities

Pulmonary Disease
- Obstructive disease
- Restrictive disorder
- Respiratory infection

Renal or Urinary Tract Disease
- Decreased renal function
- Urinary tract infection
- Obstruction

Pregnancy
- Diminished maternal physiologic reserve

Cardiovascular Disease
- Coronary artery disease
- Cardiac failure
- Dysrhythmias
- Hypertension
- Prosthetic heart valve
- Thromboembolism
- Hemorrhagic diathesis
- Cerebrovascular disease

Endocrine Dysfunction
- Diabetes mellitus
- Adrenal disorders
- Thyroid malfunction

Hepatic Disease
- Cirrhosis
- Hepatitis

eration. In the best interests of all parties concerned, sound medicolegal principles are followed.

The nurse's responsibility is to ensure that an *informed* consent has been obtained voluntarily from the patient by the physician. Table 19-3 lists the criteria for a valid informed consent.

Before the patient signs the consent form, the surgeon should provide a clear and simple explanation of what the surgery will entail. The surgeon must also inform the patient of alternatives, possible risks, complications, disfigurement, disability, and removal of body parts, as well as what to expect in the early and late postoperative periods.

Informed consent is necessary when:

- The procedure is invasive, such as a surgical incision, a biopsy, a cystoscopy, or paracentesis
- Anesthesia is used
- A nonsurgical procedure is performed in which there is more than slight risk to the patient, such as an arteriogram
- A procedure is performed that involves radiation or cobalt therapy

The patient personally signs the consent if he or she is of legal age and is mentally capable. When the patient is a minor or is unconscious or incompetent, permission must be obtained from a responsible family member or legal

TABLE 19-3 Criteria for Valid Informed Consent

Component	Comments
Consent voluntarily given	Valid consent must be freely given, without coercion.
Incompetent subject	Legal definition: individuals who are *not* autonomous and cannot give or withhold consent (*e.g.,* individuals who are mentally retarded, mentally ill, or comatose)
Informed subject	Consent form should be in writing (although law does not require written documentation). It should contain the following: Explanation of procedure and its risks Description of benefits and alternatives An offer to answer questions about procedure Instructions that the patient may withdraw consent A statement informing the patient if the protocol differs from customary procedure
Subject able to comprehend	Information must be written and delivered in language understandable to the patient. Questions must be answered to facilitate comprehension if material is confusing.

(Adapted from Douglas S and Larson E. There's more to informed consent than information. Focus Crit Care 1986 Apr; 13[2]:44.)

guardian. An emancipated minor (married or independently earning own living) may sign the permit. State regulations and agency policy must be followed.

In an emergency, it may be necessary for the surgeon to operate as a lifesaving measure without the patient's informed consent. However, every effort must be made to contact the patient's family. In such a situation, contact can be made by telephone, telegram, fax, or other electronic means.

When the patient has doubts and has not had the opportunity to investigate alternative treatments, a second opinion may be requested. No patient should be forced to sign an operative permit. Refusing to undergo a surgical procedure is a person's legal right and privilege. However, such information must be documented and relayed to the surgeon so that other arrangements can be made; for instance, additional explanations may be provided to the patient and family, or the surgery may be rescheduled at a later time.

The consent process can be improved by providing audiovisual materials to supplement discussion, by ensuring that the wording of the consent form is understandable, and by using other strategies and resources as needed to help the patient understand.

- The signed consent form is placed in a prominent place on the patient's chart and accompanies the patient to the operating room.

Preoperative Patient Education

The value of preoperative instruction has long been recognized. Each patient is taught as an individual, with consideration for any unique anxieties, needs, and hopes. A program of instruction based on the individual's needs is planned and implemented at the proper time. If teaching sessions are held several days before surgery, the patient may not remember what was said. If instruction occurs too close to the time of surgery, the patient may not be able to concentrate or learn because of anxiety or the effect of the preanesthetic medication.

Ideally, instruction is spaced over a period of time to allow the patient to assimilate information and to ask questions as they arise. Frequently, teaching sessions are combined with various preparation procedures to allow for an easy flow of information. In reality, the nurse must make a judgment about how much the patient wants and needs to know. In some instances, too much detail raises the patient's anxiety level.

Teaching should go beyond descriptions of the various steps of a procedure and should include explanations of the sensations the patient will experience. For example, telling the patient only that preoperative medication will relax him or her before the operation is not as effective as also noting that the medication may result in a lightheaded and sleepy feeling. Knowing what to expect will help the patient anticipate these reactions and thus attain a higher degree of relaxation than might otherwise be expected.

The ideal timing for preoperative teaching is not realistic in the surgical center or same-day surgery setting. However, during the preadmission visit when diagnostic tests are being done, a nurse or resource person can answer questions and provide the opportunity for teaching the patient and building rapport. During this visit, the patient can meet and ask questions of the liaison nurse, view audiovisuals, receive written materials, and be given the telephone number to call as questions arise closer to the date of surgery.

Deep Breathing, Coughing, and Relaxation Exercises

One goal of preoperative nursing care is to teach the patient how to promote lung ventilation and blood oxygenation following general anesthesia. This is accomplished by demonstrating to the patient how to take a deep, slow breath (maximal sustained inspiration, MSI) and how to exhale slowly. The patient is placed in a sitting position to provide maximum lung expansion. After practicing deep breathing several times, the patient is instructed to breathe deeply, exhale through the mouth, take a short breath, and cough from deep in the lungs (see Figs. 19-1 and 19-2 in Chart 19-3). In addition to enhancing respiration, these exercises help the patient to relax.

If there is to be a thoracic or abdominal incision, the nurse demonstrates how the incision line can be splinted so that pressure is minimized and pain is controlled. The patient should put the palms of both hands together, interlacing the fingers snugly. Placing the hands across the incisional site acts as an effective splint when coughing. In addition, the patient is informed that medications will be administered to control pain.

The goal in promoting coughing is to mobilize secretions so they can be removed. When a deep breath is taken before coughing, the cough reflex is stimulated. If the patient does not cough effectively, hypostatic pneumonia and other lung complications may occur.

Turning and Active Body Movement

The goals of promoting deliberate body movement postoperatively are to improve circulation, to prevent venous stasis, and to contribute to optimal respiratory function.

The patient is shown how to turn from side to side and how to assume the lateral position. This position will be used postoperatively (even before the patient is conscious) and assumed every second hour.

Exercises of the extremities include extension and flexion of the knee and hip joints (similar to bicycle riding while lying on the side). The foot is rotated as though tracing the largest possible circle with the great toe (see Chart 19-3, Figs. 19-3 and 19-4). The elbow and shoulder are also put through range of motion. At first the patient will be assisted and reminded to perform these exercises, but later is encouraged to do them independently. Muscle tone is maintained so that ambulation will be easier.

The nurse is reminded to use proper body mechanics and to instruct the patient to do the same. When the patient is placed in any position, his or her body is maintained in proper alignment.

CHART 19-3
Preoperative Patient Instruction

A. Diaphragmatic Breathing

Diaphragmatic breathing refers to a flattening of the dome of the diaphragm during inspiration with resulting enlargement of the upper abdomen as air rushes in. During expiration, the abdominal muscles contract.

1. Practice in the same position you would assume in bed following surgery: a semi-Fowler's position, propped in bed with the back and shoulders well supported with pillows.
2. With the hands in a loose-fist position, allow the hands to rest lightly on the front of the lower ribs—fingernails against lower chest to feel the movement (Fig. 19-1).
3. Breathe out gently and fully as the ribs sink down and inward toward midline.
4. Then take a deep breath through your nose and mouth, letting the abdomen rise as the lungs fill with air.
5. Hold this breath for a count of five.
6. Exhale and let out *all* the air through the nose and mouth.
7. Repeat 15 times with a short rest after each group of five.
8. Practice this twice a day preoperatively.

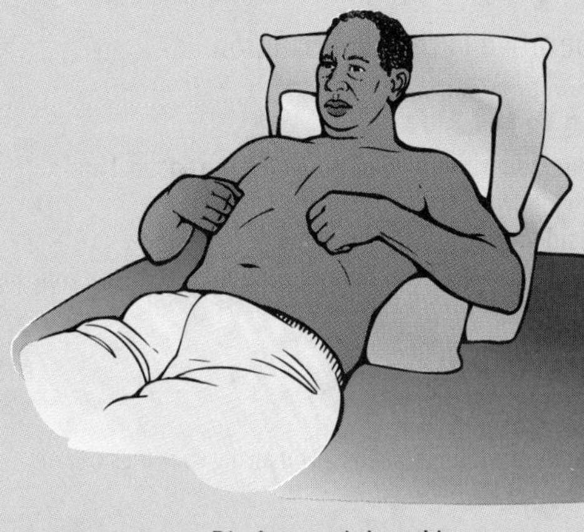

FIGURE 19-1. Diaphragmatic breathing.

B. Coughing

1. Lean forward slightly from a sitting position in bed, interlace the fingers together, and place the hands across the incisional site to act as a splint when coughing (Fig. 19-2).
2. Breathe with the diaphragm as described in *A*.
3. With the mouth slightly open, breathe in fully.
4. "Hack" out sharply for three short breaths.
5. Then, keeping the mouth open, take in a quick deep breath and immediately give a strong cough once or twice. This helps clear secretions from the chest. It may cause some discomfort but will not harm incision.

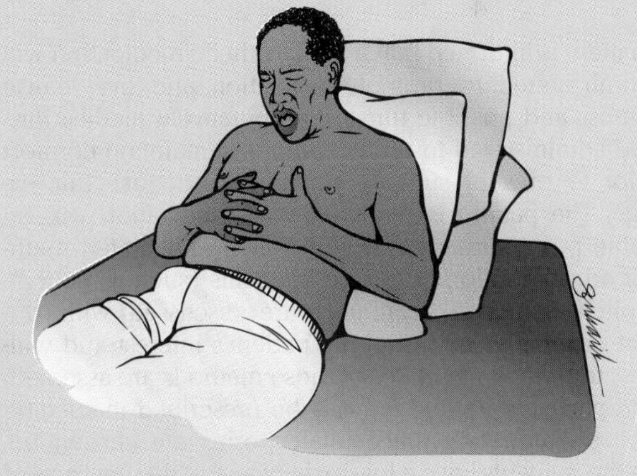

FIGURE 19-2. Splinting when coughing.

C. Leg Exercises

1. Lie in a semi-Fowler's position and perform the following simple exercises to improve circulation.
2. Bend the knee and raise the foot—hold it a few seconds, then extend the leg and lower it to the bed (Fig. 19-3).
3. Do this five times with one leg, then repeat with the other leg.
4. Then trace circles with the feet by bending them down, in toward each other, up, and then out (Fig. 19-4).
5. Repeat these movements five times.

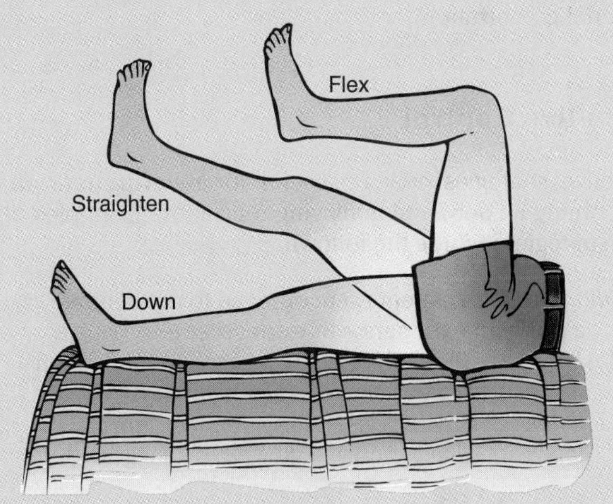

FIGURE 19-3. Leg exercises.

(continued)

CHART 19-3 *(continued)*
Preoperative Patient Instruction

D. Turning to the Side

1. Turn on your side with the uppermost leg flexed most and supported on a pillow.
2. Grasp the side rail as an aid to maneuver to the side.
3. Practice diaphragmatic breathing and coughing while on your side.

E. Getting Out of Bed

1. Turn on your side.
2. Push yourself up with one hand as you swing your legs out of bed.

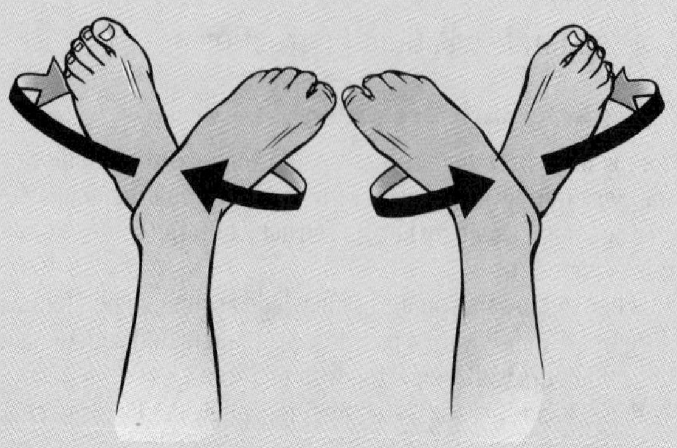

FIGURE 19-4. Foot exercise.

Pain Control and Medications

The patient is informed that a preanesthetic medication will be administered to promote relaxation and may cause sleepiness and possible thirst. Postoperatively, medications will be administered to reduce pain and maintain comfort but not to prevent suitable activity or adequate air exchange. The patient is reassured that medication will be available postoperatively for pain relief. Anticipated methods of administration of analgesic agents (such as patient-controlled analgesia, epidural) are discussed with the patient prior to surgery, and the patient's interest and willingness to participate in use of those methods are assessed.

Prophylactic antibiotics may be prescribed in specific instances. Frequently, the cephalosporins are chosen because these agents have a low toxicity and wide spectrum of action. However, use of short-term or single dose antimicrobial prophylaxis for clean surgical procedures must be carefully weighed as their use may increase rather than decrease bacterial colonization.

Cognitive Control

Cognitive strategies may be useful for relieving tension, overcoming anxiety, and achieving relaxation. Examples of such strategies include the following:

Imagery—The patient is encouraged to concentrate on a pleasant experience or restful scene.
Distraction—The patient is encouraged to think of an enjoyable story or recite a favorite poem.
Optimistic self-recitation—Recitation of optimistic thoughts ("I know all will go well") is suggested.

Other Information

The patient will benefit from knowing when family and friends will be able to visit following surgery and that a spiritual advisor will be available if so desired. Knowing ahead of time about the possible need for a ventilator or the presence of drainage tubes will help the patient accept these devices in the postoperative period.

Preoperative Nursing Interventions

Nutrition and Fluids

When surgery is scheduled for the morning, a light meal may be permitted on the preceding evening. In dehydrated patients, and especially in older ones, fluids by mouth often are encouraged before an operation. In addition, fluids may be prescribed intravenously, especially in patients who are unable to take fluids by mouth. If the surgery is scheduled to take place after noon and does not involve any part of the gastrointestinal tract, a soft breakfast may be prescribed. Most often, oral intake of food or water is withheld 8 to 10 hours before the operation. However, many ambulatory centers now allow clear fluids up to 3 to 4 hours before surgery.

The purpose of withholding food before surgery is to prevent aspiration. Aspiration occurs when food or fluid is regurgitated from the stomach and enters the pulmonary system. Such inhaled material acts as a foreign substance, is irritating, and causes an inflammatory reaction. At the same time, the inflammatory reaction interferes with adequate air exchange. Aspiration is a serious problem and carries a high mortality rate (60% to 70%) when it occurs. The elderly surgical patient is at even greater risk for aspiration.

Intestinal Preparation

A cleansing enema or laxative may be prescribed the evening before surgery and may be repeated if ineffective. This is to prevent defecation during anesthesia or to prevent accidental trauma to the intestine during abdominal surgery. Unless the condition of the patient presents some contraindication, the toilet or bedside commode, rather than the bedpan, is used for evacuation of the enema. Additionally, antibiotics may be prescribed to reduce intestinal flora.

Preoperative Skin Preparation

The goal of preoperative skin preparation is to decrease bacterial sources without injuring the skin. When there is time, such as in elective surgery, the patient may be instructed to use a soap containing a detergent–germicide to cleanse the skin area for several days before surgery to reduce the number of skin organisms; this preparation may be carried out at home.

Before surgery, the patient should take a warm, relaxing bath or shower, using povidone-iodine (Betadine) soap. Although it is preferable that this be done on the day of surgery, the time scheduled for surgery may require that the shower be taken the night before. The purpose of scheduling the cleansing shower as close as possible to the time of surgery is to reduce the risk of skin contamination of the surgical wound. A shampoo the day before the operation is advisable unless the condition of the patient prevents it.

It is preferred that the skin at and around the operative site *not* be shaved. During shaving, the skin may be injured by the razor and become a portal of entry for bacteria; this injured tissue may act as a substrate for bacterial growth. In addition, the longer the interval between the shave and the operation, the higher the rate of postoperative wound infection. Skin that is well cleansed but unshaven is less often implicated in wound infections than is shaved skin.

The protocols for skin preparation vary. Some surgeons prefer that hair be removed in and around the operative site. One approach involves the use of electric clippers to remove hair to within 1 to 2 mm of the skin to avoid abrading the skin. The clippers must be thoroughly cleaned after use. Another approach is the use of a depilatory cream (see below).

If agency protocol or the surgeon requires that the skin be shaved, the patient is told about the shaving procedure, placed in a comfortable position, and not exposed unnecessarily. Any adhesive or grease may be readily removed with a sponge moistened in benzene or ether, if the odor and cold temperature are not objectionable to the patient.

The skin may be shaved by a special prep team, by the nurse assigned to the patient, or by a member of the operating room team. Scissors can be used initially to remove the longer hair. An antimicrobial detergent can be used to produce a lather that makes hair easier to remove. The skin is held taut and shaved in the direction of hair growth. Long, continuous strokes are used. Scratches are avoided, and any potential sites of infection are reported. All actions and findings are documented.

Depilatory Cream. Chemical compounds (creams to remove hair) are safe for preparing the skin for surgery. If there is question about the possibility of an allergic reaction, a test patch should be tried first. As an economic measure, long hairs may be cut before the cream is applied to reduce the amount of cream used.

The cream is spread in a smooth layer of about 1.25 cm (½ inch) in depth over the entire operative site. A wooden tongue blade or a gloved hand can be used to apply the cream. After the cream has remained on the skin for 10 minutes (depending on directions), it is removed gently with the tongue blade or with multiple moistened gauze sponges. When all cream and hair have been removed, the skin is washed with soap and water and patted dry.

There are several advantages to using a depilatory cream for preoperative skin preparation. The end result is clean, smooth, and intact skin. Scrapes, abrasions, cuts, and inadequate hair removal are prevented. It is comfortable for the patient, and the patient may even apply the cream personally for selected operative procedures. Depilatory creams are more effective and safer for use on uncooperative or agitated patients. This method is no more expensive than other methods. A disadvantage is that a few patients have had some transient skin reactions if depilatory cream is used near the rectal and scrotal areas.

Immediate Preoperative Nursing Interventions

The patient is dressed in a hospital gown that is left untied and open in the back. If the patient has long hair, it may be braided; hairpins are removed, and the hair is completely covered with a disposable paper cap.

The mouth is inspected, and dentures or plates and chewing gum are removed. If left in the mouth, these items could easily fall to the back of the throat during induction of anesthesia and cause respiratory obstruction.

Jewelry is not worn to the operating room; even wedding rings should be removed. If a patient objects to the removal of a ring, a strip of narrow gauze can be looped through the ring and tied securely around the patient's wrist. All articles of value, including dentures and prosthetic devices, are labeled clearly with the patient's name and stored in a safe place according to agency policy.

All patients (except those with urologic disorders) should void immediately before going to the operating room to promote continence during low abdominal surgery and to make abdominal organs more accessible. Catheterization should not be resorted to, except in an emergency or when it is desirable to have an indwelling catheter in place to ensure an empty bladder. In this instance, such a catheter would be connected to a closed drainage system. The voided urine is measured, and the amount and the time of voiding are recorded on the preoperative record.

Preanesthetic Medication: Pharmacokinetics

Barbiturates/Tranquilizers. For sedation, barbiturates are commonly used—mainly pentobarbital (Nembutal) and secobarbital (Seconal Sodium)—as are hypnotics such as benzodiazepines (flurazepam, diazepam). However, the visit of the anesthesiologist and operating room nurse prior to surgery often has a more reassuring and calming effect than the barbiturates. Nonetheless, the night before surgery a hypnotic is usually prescribed to allay insomnia.

Opioids. Medications such as morphine and meperidine (Demerol) may be prescribed before an operation to reduce the amount of general anesthetic required. These medications can also be used to produce analgesia in patients who have pain prior to surgery. At the same time, it is important to realize that analgesic doses may depress respiration and the cough reflex and increase the risk of respiratory acidosis and aspiration pneumonitis. Full doses may cause hypotension, nausea, vomiting, constipation, and abdominal distention.

Anticholinergics. Anticholinergic medications may be prescribed to reduce respiratory tract secretions and to prevent or treat severe reflex slowing of the heart during anesthesia. They are administered also to counteract secretions that are anticipated with anesthetic induction and intubation. Atropine is frequently prescribed; however, it must be used with caution in patients with glaucoma, thyrotoxicosis, prostatic hyperplasia, or some forms of heart disease.

Because the belladonna alkaloids (atropine and scopolamine) have varying effects on pulse rate, as well as other shortcomings, glycopyrrolate (Robinul), a quaternary ammonium compound, is often used. It is an anticholinergic medication that is twice as potent an anti-sialagogue (reducing secretions) and acts three times as long.

Other Preanesthetic Medications. Other agents used as preanesthetic medication are droperidol, fentanyl, or a combination of these. They should not be used with sedatives because they may cause respiratory or circulatory depression and may potentiate depressants.

Prophylactic antibiotics are administered when bacterial contamination is expected, or for the patient with a clean wound in which a prosthetic device is being inserted.

Timing of Administration of Medications. Because preanesthetic medications should be given from 45 to 75 minutes before anesthesia is begun, it is most important that the nurse administer this medication precisely at the prescribed time; otherwise, its effect will have worn off, or it will not have begun to act when anesthesia is started.

After the preanesthetic medication is given, the patient is kept in bed with the side rails raised because the medication will cause lightheadedness or drowsiness. If atropine or glycopyrrolate (Robinul) is given, the patient is informed that it will make his or her mouth dry. During this time, the nurse observes the patient for any untoward reaction to the medications. The immediate surroundings are kept quiet to promote relaxation.

Very frequently, surgery is delayed or operating room schedules are changed, and it becomes impossible to request that a medication be given at a specific time. In these situations, the preoperative medication is prescribed "on call from operating room." The nurse can have the medication ready to give and administer it as soon as a call is received from the operating room staff. It usually takes 15 to 20 minutes to prepare the patient for the operating room. If the nurse gives the medication before attending to the other details of preoperative preparation, the patient will have at least partial benefit from the preoperative medication and will have a smoother anesthetic and operative course.

Preoperative Record

A preoperative checklist is shown in Figure 19-5. The completed chart accompanies the patient to the operating room. The informed consent form is also attached, as are all laboratory reports and nurses' records. Any unusual last-minute observations that may have a bearing on the anesthesia or surgery are placed at the front of the chart in a prominent place.

Transportation to the Presurgical Suite

The patient is transferred to the holding area or presurgical suite in a bed or on a stretcher about 30 to 60 minutes before the anesthetic is to be given. The stretcher should be as comfortable as possible, with a sufficient number of blankets to ensure against chilling in air-conditioned rooms. A small pillow at the head is usually provided. The top covers of the stretcher should be long enough to tuck in around the patient at both feet and shoulders. Ideally, the nurse who has cared for the patient up to this time accompanies him or her to the operating room.

The patient is taken to a waiting room in the surgical suite, and is greeted by name and made to feel in safe hands. The area must be quiet if the preoperative medication is to have maximal effect. Unpleasant sounds or conversation should be avoided as they might be misinterpreted by a sedated patient who overhears them.

- It is important that someone be with the preoperative patient at all times.

Even though the patient has had preoperative medication, appears to be dozing, and seems to be secure on

CRITICAL THINKING EXERCISES

1. A patient who has signed a consent form for surgery tells you that he is having second thoughts about having the surgery. Describe the actions you would take and the information you would document in the patient's medical record.
2. Prior to surgery, a patient tells you that he has been a chronic user of IV drugs and that his physician is unaware of this practice. What implications does this have for the safety and well-being of the patient, and what actions would you take?
3. A patient with a long history of asthma is scheduled for major surgery. How would you modify your preoperative care based on this history?
4. Two patients are admitted to the same-day surgery unit for diagnostic cardiac catheterization. One patient is 45 years old; the other is 75 years old. How would your assessments and preoperative preparation differ for these two patients?

1. Patient's name: ____________ Date: ________ Height: ______ Weight: ______
   Identification band present: ____________
2. Informed Consent signed: ________ Special permits signed: ____________
   (Ex: Sterilization)
3. History & Physical Examination report present: ________ Date: ____________
4. Laboratory records present: ____________
   CBC: ________ Hb: ________ Urinalysis: ________ Hct: ________

5. Item	Present	Removed
a. Natural teeth	______	______
Dentures: upper, lower, partial	______	______
Bridge, fixed; crown	______	______
b. Contact lenses	______	______
c. Other prostheses—type: ______	______	______
d. Jewelry:		
Wedding band (taped/tied)	______	______
Rings	______	______
Earrings: pierced, clip-on	______	______
Neck chains	______	______
e. Make-up	______	______
Nail polish	______	______
6. Clothing		
a. Clean patient gown	______	______
b. Cap	______	______
c. Sanitary pad, *etc.*	______	______

7. Family instructed where to wait? ____________
8. Valuables secured? ____________
9. Blood available? ________ Ordered? ________ Where? ____________
10. Preanesthetic medication given: ____________ Signature ____________ Time
11. Voided: ________ Amount: ________ Time: ________ Catheter: ________
    Mouth care given: ________
12. Vital signs: Temperature: ________ Pulse: ________ Resp: ________ Blood Press: ________
13. Special problems/precautions: (Allergies, deafness, *etc.*): ____________
14. Area of skin preparation: ____________
15. ____________ Date: ________ Time: ________
    Signature: Nurse releasing patient

FIGURE 19-5. Preoperative checklist.

the stretcher with a strap in place, someone should always be in attendance. Having someone with the patient provides reassurance as well as safety. Reassurance can be communicated verbally as well as nonverbally by facial expression, manner, the warm grasp of a hand, and seeing a familiar face—the nurse who helped prepare the patient prior to transfer to the surgical suite, or the anesthesiologist who visited the day before and discussed anesthetic management.

Helping the Family Cope

Most hospitals and surgicenters have a special surgical waiting room where the family can wait while the patient is undergoing surgery. This room may be equipped with comfortable chairs, television, telephones, and facilities for light refreshment. Volunteers may remain with the family, serve them coffee, and keep them informed of the patient's progress. After surgery, the surgeon may meet the family in the waiting room and discuss the outcome.

The family should never judge the seriousness of an operation by the length of time the patient is in the operating room. A patient may be in surgery much longer than the actual operating time for several reasons:

- It is customary to send for the patient some time in advance of the actual operating time.
- Anesthesiologists often make additional preparations that may take from 30 to 60 minutes.
- Occasionally the surgeon takes longer than expected with the preceding case, which delays the start of the next surgical procedure.
- After surgery, the patient is taken to the postanesthesia care unit (recovery room) to ensure satisfactory emergence from the anesthetic.

Those waiting to see the patient after surgery should be informed that the patient may have certain equipment or devices in place when returned to the room (*e.g.*, intravenous lines, indwelling urinary catheter, nasogastric tube, suction bottles, oxygen lines, monitoring equipment, and blood transfusion lines). When the patient returns to the room, the nurse provides accurate assurances regarding the frequent postoperative observations.

However, it is the responsibility of the surgeon, and not the prerogative or responsibility of the nurse, to relay the surgical findings and the prognosis, even when the findings are favorable.

BIBLIOGRAPHY

See Bibliography for unit following Chapter 21.

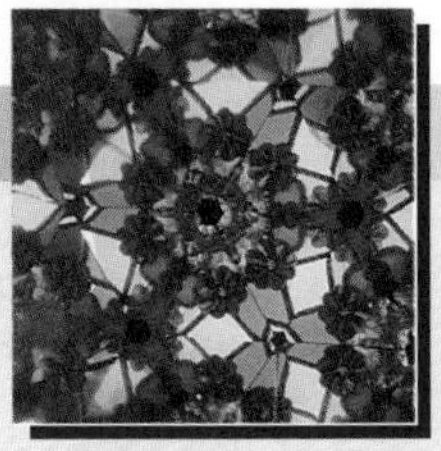

20 Intraoperative Nursing and Anesthesia

CHAPTER OUTLINE

LEARNING OBJECTIVES

On completion of this chapter, the learner will be able to:

1. Describe the interdisciplinary approach to the care of the patient during surgery
2. Describe the principles, protocols, and basic rules of surgical asepsis
3. Describe the role of the anesthesiologist in the preoperative and intraoperative care of the patient
4. Identify the risk factors related to surgery of elderly persons and nursing interventions to reduce risks to the elderly surgical patient
5. Compare the various types of anesthesia with regard to uses, advantages, disadvantages, and nursing responsibilities

Suzanne C. Smeltzer and Brenda G. Bare: Brunner and Suddarth's Textbook of Medical-Surgical Nursing, 8th Edition. © 1996 Lippincott-Raven Publishers.

Activity in the operating room centers on the patient who is undergoing a surgical procedure for the repair, correction, or relief of a physical problem. Attention focuses on the psychologic as well as physiologic reactions of the patient.

Throughout the surgical experience, the nurse functions as the patient's chief advocate. The caring and concern of the nurse extend from the time the patient is prepared for and instructed about the forthcoming surgical procedure, through the immediate preoperative period, into the operative phase and the recovery from anesthesia, and through convalescence. Because surgery is usually a stressful experience, the patient needs the security of knowing that someone is providing protection during the procedure and while he is anesthetized.

Studies have shown that a preoperative visit the day before (or the day of) surgery by the operating room nurse as well as the anesthesiologist or nurse anesthetist often is effective in helping the patient make a smooth transition from the hospital unit to the operating room. During the visit, time is provided for the patient to ask questions.

When a patient arrives in the operating room, essentially three different groups of personnel are preparing for his or her care: (1) the anesthesiologist or nurse anesthetist, who administers the anesthetic agent and places the patient in the proper position on the operating table; (2) the surgeon and assistants who scrub and perform the surgery; and (3) the intraoperative nurses who manage the operating room.

Intraoperative nurses are responsible for the safety and well-being of the patient, the coordination of the operating room personnel, and the performance of scrub nurse and circulating activities during the surgery. Another role of the nurse in the operating room is the **RN First Assistant** (RNFA). Although the practice of the RNFA depends on the scope of a state's Nurse Practice Act, the RNFA practices under the direct supervision of the surgeon. RNFA responsibilities may include handling tissue, providing exposure at the operative field, using instruments, suturing, and providing hemostasis.

To ensure optimal patient care during the surgical procedure, information about the patient must be shared by the anesthesiologist or nurse anesthetist, the nurse, and the surgeon. In addition, any pertinent developments that are related to patient care in the postanesthesia care unit (PACU) (*e.g.*, hemorrhage, unexpected findings, fluid and electrolyte problems, shock, or respiratory difficulties) must be noted, documented, and communicated to the staff of the PACU, formerly referred to as the postanesthesia recovery room (PARR).

Intraoperative Nursing Functions

Nursing functions in the operating room are frequently described in terms of circulating and scrub activities.

The **circulating nurse** manages the operating room and protects the safety and health needs of the patient by monitoring the activities of members of the surgical team and checking the conditions in the operating room. The main responsibilities include assuring cleanliness, proper temperature, humidity, and lighting; the safe functioning of equipment; and the availability of supplies and materials. The circulating nurse also monitors aseptic practices to avoid breaks in technique, while coordinating the movement of related personnel (medical, x-ray, and laboratory). The circulating nurse also monitors the patient throughout the operative procedure to ensure the person's safety and well being.

The activities of the **scrub nurse** include scrubbing for surgery; setting up the sterile tables; preparing sutures, ligatures, and special equipment; assisting the surgeon and the surgical assistants during the surgical procedure by anticipating the required instruments, sponges, drains, and other equipment; and keeping track of the time the patient is under anesthesia and the time the wound is open. As the surgical incision is closed, equipment and materials must be checked to ensure that all needles, sponges, and instruments are accounted for. Specimens must also be labeled and sent to the laboratory.

The entire process requires a thorough understanding of anatomy, tissue care, and the principles of asepsis; an awareness of the objectives of the surgery; the knowledge and ability to anticipate needs and to work as a skilled member of a team; and the capacity to handle any emergency situation in the operating room.

Principles of Health and Operating Room Attire

Good health is essential for any person in the operating room. Colds, sore throats, and skin infections are sources of pathogenic organisms and must be reported. In one instance, a series of wound infections in postoperative patients was traced to a mild throat infection in an operating room nurse (Barber & Brown, 1993). Therefore, the importance of promptly reporting even a slight ailment is apparent.

Clothing. Street clothes are never worn in the operating room. Only approved and clean operating room attire is permitted. Written policies describe the practice that all persons are required to follow. Dressing rooms are located near the operating suite and are reached from an outer corridor. Clothing is changed in the dressing room before entering and on leaving the operating suite. Operating suite attire is not worn out of the operating room.

Operating room attire includes close-fitting cotton dresses, pants suits, and jumpsuits. When pants are worn, the ankles should have close-fitting cuffs (drawstring or knitted) to prevent organisms shed from the perineum and legs from being released into the immediate surroundings. Shirts and waist drawstrings should be tucked inside the pants to prevent any accidental contact with sterile areas and again to contain skin sheddings. Garments that are wet or soiled should be changed. A fresh set of operating suite attire is put on each time the person enters the operating suite.

Mask. Masks are worn at all times in the operating room for the purpose of minimizing airborne contamination. Droplets containing microorganisms from the oropharynx and nasopharynx must be contained and filtered. Therefore, the mask must be tight-fitting and should cover the nose and mouth completely. At the same time, it should not interfere with breathing, speech, or vision, and it must be compact and comfortable. Forced expiration, such as that produced by laughing, sneezing, coughing, and unnecessary talking, should be avoided because it deposits additional organisms on the mask. Effective disposable masks that have a high filtration efficiency of greater than 95% are also available. Tests demonstrate their superiority over gauze masks. Masks are changed at a minimum between patients and are not to be worn outside the surgical department.

Because the mask loses much of its effectiveness when it becomes moistened, it is changed between surgical procedures and more often if necessary. Mask strings are tied snugly; top strings are tied at the back of the head, and bottom strings are tied at the back of the neck. The mask must be either on or off; it must not be allowed to hang around the neck. When the mask is removed, only the strings are handled to prevent contamination of the hands.

Headgear. Headgear should completely cover the hair (head and neckline, including beard) so that single strands of hair, bobby pins, clips, particles of dandruff, and dust do not fall on the sterile field. The styles of headgear available are all disposable, lint-free, and clothlike.

Shoes. Shoes should be comfortable and supportive; clogs, tennis shoes, sandals, and boots are not permitted because they are unsafe and difficult to clean. Shoes are covered with disposable or canvas shoe covers. Conductive covers establish an electrical ground for the wearer. The black strips provided with some conductive shoe covers should be placed inside the shoe in contact with the sole of the foot. Shoe covers are worn one time only and are removed upon leaving the restricted area.

Conductometers are usually located at the entrance to the operating room area.

Health Hazards. The presence of occupational hazards in the operating room is not a new concept, but the characteristics of these hazards are changing. Internal monitoring of the operating room includes the analysis of swipe samples for infectious and toxic agents. In addition, policies and procedures for laser and radiation safety in the operating room have been established.

Since 1987, the CDC (Centers for Disease Control) reported several cases of health care workers who contracted AIDS through occupational exposure. With the spread of HIV, operating room attire has changed drastically. Double gloving is routine, at least in trauma surgery where sharp bone fragments are present. Goggles are worn when the surgical wound is irrigated or bone drilling is performed. In addition to the routine scrub suit and double gloves, some surgeons wear rubber boots, a waterproof apron, and sleeve protectors. In bloody surgical cases, a wraparound face shield substitutes for goggles.

Principles of Perioperative Asepsis

Throughout all phases of the surgical experience, the main priority for all personnel is prevention of patient complications, which includes protecting the patient from infection. The possibility of infection is markedly reduced by strict adherence to the principles of asepsis during the patient's preoperative preparation, the course of the surgical procedure, and the healing of the surgical wound.

To provide the best possible conditions for surgery, the operating room is located in a section of the hospital that is free from such hazards as contaminating particles, dust, other pollutants, radiation, and noise. Electrical hazards, conductivity checks, emergency exit clearances, and storage of equipment and anesthetic gases are checked periodically by the state and the Joint Commission for the Accreditation of Healthcare Organizations (JCAHO).

In surgical practice, asepsis prevents the contamination of surgical wounds. Although postoperative wound infection may be caused by natural skin flora or a previously existing infection, operating room personnel have the responsibility of using aseptic principles to minimize this risk. The following discussion on protocols illustrates how principles of asepsis are carried out in practice.

Protocols

Preoperative. All surgical material—any instruments, needles, sutures, dressings, gloves, covers, and solutions that may come in contact with the surgical wound and exposed tissues—must be sterilized before they are used in surgery. In addition, the surgeon, surgical assistants, and nurses must prepare themselves by scrubbing their hands and arms with soap and water and donning long-sleeved, sterile gowns and gloves. Head and hair are covered with a cap, and a mask is worn over the nose and mouth to minimize the possibility of bacteria from the upper respiratory tract entering the wound.

The patient's skin, over an area considerably larger than that requiring exposure during the course of surgery, also requires meticulous cleansing followed by the application of an antiseptic agent. The remainder of the patient's body is covered with sterile drapes.

Intraoperative. During surgery, the personnel who have scrubbed and gowned touch only those objects that were sterilized. Nonscrubbed personnel refrain from touching or contaminating anything that is sterile.

Postoperative. Following surgery, the wound is protected from possible contamination by means of sterile dressings. Subsequently, the wound is cleansed with sterile saline and antiseptics are used when the wound is cleansed and the dressing changed. Particular care is taken to protect the unhealed wound from coming in contact with anything that is not sterile.

When infection has already developed in tissues, antimicrobials specific for the invading organism are prescribed and heat is applied or drainage established to assist the body in eliminating the organisms. It may be necessary to remove and destroy microorganisms that are already in the tissues by removing, or débriding, devitalized tissues. To prevent subsequent infection from external sources, rigid aseptic technique must be followed during the course of treatment.

Environmental Controls. In addition to the abovementioned protocols, the implementation of aseptic principles requires meticulous housekeeping in the operating room. Floors and horizontal surfaces are cleaned frequently with detergent soap and water or detergent germicide, and sterilizing equipment is inspected regularly to ensure optimal operation and performance.

Prepackaged sterilized linens, drapes, and solutions are used; instruments are cleaned and sterilized in a unit near the operating room. Individually wrapped sterile items are used when additional individual items are needed.

Many operating rooms are equipped with laminar air flow systems that filter out a high percentage of dust and bacteria. Originally designed for spacecraft, these systems use high efficiency particulate air (HEPA) filters to remove more than 99% of airborne particles measuring 0.3 μm or more. Laminar flow also exchanges air more effectively—about 200 times an hour—as compared with air conditioning, which exchanges air 12 times per hour.

Despite all these precautions, postoperative wound contamination may occasionally occur during surgery but become apparent days or weeks later in the form of an incisional infection or abscess. Constant surveillance and conscientious technique in carrying out aseptic practices must be stressed continually to reduce the risk for contamination and infection.

Basic Rules of Surgical Asepsis

General

- Sterile surfaces or articles may touch other sterile surfaces or articles and remain sterile; contact with unsterile objects at any point renders a sterile area contaminated.
- If there is any doubt about the sterility of an article or area, it is considered unsterile and contaminated.
- Whatever is sterile for one patient (an opened sterile tray or tables with sterile supplies) can be used for this patient only. Unused sterile supplies must be discarded or resterilized if they are to be used again.

Personnel

- Scrubbed personnel remain in the area of the surgical procedure; if a scrubbed person leaves the room, that person's sterile status is lost. To return to surgery, this person is required to go through the procedure of scrubbing, gowning, and gloving.
- Only a small part of a scrubbed person's body is considered sterile: from front waist to the shoulder area; forearms and gloves. Therefore, the gloved hands must be kept in front between the shoulders and waistline.
- In some operating rooms, a special wraparound gown is worn, which extends the sterile area.
- The circulating nurse and any unscrubbed personnel remain at a safe distance to avoid contamination of any sterile area.

Draping

- During draping of a table or patient, the sterile drape is held well above the surface to be covered and is positioned from front to back.
- Only the top of the patient or table that is draped is considered sterile; drapes hanging over the edge are not regarded as sterile.
- Sterile drapes are kept in position by the use of clips or adherent material; drapes are not moved during the surgical procedure.
- A tear or puncture of the drape permitting access to an unsterile surface underneath renders the area unsterile. Such a drape must be replaced.

Delivery of Sterile Supplies

- Packages are wrapped or sealed in such a way that they can be opened easily without risk of contaminating contents.
- Sterile supplies, including solutions, are delivered to a sterile field or handed to a "scrubbed" person in such a way that sterility of the object or fluid remains intact.
- Edges of wrappers covering sterile supplies or outer lips of bottles or flasks containing sterile solutions are not considered sterile.
- The unsterile arm of the circulating nurse must not extend over a sterile area. Sterile articles are to be dropped onto the sterile field, a reasonable distance from the edge of the sterile area.

Solutions

- Sterile solutions are poured from a point high enough to prevent accidental touching of the sterile receiving cup or basin, but not so high as to produce splashing. (When a sterile surface becomes wet, it is contaminated.)

The Patient Undergoing Anesthesia

The Patient and the Anesthesiologist

An **anesthesiologist** is a physician specifically trained in the art and the science of anesthesiology. After consulting with the surgeon, the anesthesiologist usually selects the anesthesia and deals with any technical problems relating to the administration of the anesthetic agent and supervision of the patient's condition during the surgical procedure.

An **anesthetist** is a qualified nurse, dentist, or physician who administers anesthetics. Most anesthetists are nurses who have graduated from an accredited nurse anesthesia program and have passed certification by the American Association of Nurse Anesthetists to become certified registered nurse anesthetists (CRNA).

The surgical patient is usually interested in and concerned about the anesthesia that will be administered. Hearsay of friends and relatives, written comments about anesthesia, and possible preconceived ideas can cause fear or anxiety. Therefore, it is helpful for the anesthesiologist/anesthetist to visit the patient before surgery to provide information, answer questions, and allay any fears that may exist in the patient's mind. Choice of anesthetic agent is discussed, and the patient has an opportunity to disclose previous reactions and information about any medication currently being taken that may affect the choice of an agent (see p. 378).

At this time, the anesthesiologist assesses the condition of the patient's cardiovascular system and lungs and inquires about any preexisting pulmonary infections and the extent to which the patient smokes. The patient's general physical condition must also be assessed because it may affect the management of anesthesia (Table 20-1).

On the day of surgery, the patient is transported to the operating room and transferred to the operating table, where the anesthesiologist or nurse anesthetist again assesses physical condition; blood pressure, pulse, and respiratory rate, in particular, are noted. Then the anesthetic is administered.

During the course of surgery, the anesthesiologist monitors the patient's blood pressure, pulse, and respirations as well as the electrocardiogram (ECG), tidal volume, blood gas levels, blood *p*H, alveolar gas concentrations, and body temperature.

Monitoring by electroencephalograph (EEG) may be required in some instances. Anesthetic levels in the body can also be determined; a mass spectrometer is able to provide instant readouts of the critical concentration levels on display terminals.

After surgery when the patient is recovering from the anesthetic, the mass spectrometer can reveal the concentration of gaseous anesthetic still remaining in the patient. The device also assesses the ability to breathe unassisted and indicates the need for mechanical assistance when the patient is breathing independently.

Gerontologic Considerations

By the year 2000, it is estimated that there will be 35 million people over the age of 65 in the United States. As the percentage of the elderly population grows, increasing numbers of older patients are undergoing surgical procedures.

Elderly patients face higher risks from anesthesia and surgery than do other adults. Statistically, perioperative risk increases with each decade over 60. However, with modifications tailored to the biologic changes that occur in the later decades of life (see Chapter 12) and the application of research findings for this population, the risks are lowered. The following examples illustrate some of these changes and interventions.

With aging, the heart and blood vessels have a decreased ability to respond to stress. Cardiac changes include reduced cardiac output and limited cardiac reserve. With intravenous infusions, an excessive amount or rapid rate of administration may cause pulmonary edema. A sudden or prolonged drop in blood pressure may lead to cerebral ischemia, thrombosis, embolism, infarction, and anoxemia. With a reduced vasculature, the elderly are prone to thermoregulatory problems and may require extra body covering to maintain body temperature. With diminished ciliary action and a less effective cough reflex, there is an increased risk of pneumonia. Reduced gas exchange adds to the risk of cerebral hypoxia.

In terms of surgery, an older person needs less anesthetic to produce anesthesia and takes longer to eliminate anesthetic agents. One reason for reduction of anesthesia dosage is that, as people age, the percentage of fatty tissue steadily increases (from 20% to 30% at age 20, to 35% to 45% at age 60 to 70); anesthetic agents that have an affinity for fatty tissue concentrate in body fat and the brain. Another reason is that the geriatric patient, particularly when malnourished, may have low plasma proteins. With decreased plasma proteins, more of the anesthetic agent remains free or unbound, resulting in a more potent action. In addition, there is a shrinkage of the body tissues that are made up predominantly of water and have a rich blood supply, such as skeletal muscle, liver, and kidney. Reduction in liver size decreases the rate at which the liver can inactivate many anesthetics. The decreased functioning of kidney cells reduces excretion of waste products and anesthetics.

Careful manipulation and positioning are required during surgery because of the normal bone loss in the elderly (25% in women; 12% in men).

The reduced ability of the elderly to adjust rapidly to physical and emotional stress influences surgical outcomes.

TABLE 20-1 Classification of Physical Status for Anesthesia Before Surgery

Classification	Description	Example
1. Good	No organic disease, no systemic disturbance	Uncomplicated hernias, fractures
2. Fair	Mild to moderate systemic disturbance	Mild cardiac (I and II) disease, mild diabetes
3. Poor	Severe systemic disturbance	Poorly controlled diabetes, pulmonary complications, moderate cardiac (III) disease
4. Serious	Systemic disease threatening life	Severe renal disease, severe cardiac disease (IV), decompensation
5. Moribund	Little chance of survival but submitting to operation in desperation	Massive pulmonary embolus, ruptured abdominal aneurysm with profound shock
E. Emergency	Any of the above when surgery is performed in an emergency situation	An uncomplicated hernia that is now strangulated and associated with nausea and vomiting; designation 1(E) If classification is 3 and an emergency, the designation is 3(E)

(American Society of Anesthesiology, Inc. Codes for the Collection and Tabulation of Data Relating to Anesthesia, Inhalation Therapy and Therapeutic Diagnostic Blocks.)

As expected, the mortality rate is higher with emergency surgery than it is with elective surgery. Consequently, continuous and careful monitoring and quick intervention when needed is essential for gerontologic surgical patients.

Anesthesia: An Overview

Anesthesia is a state of narcosis, analgesia, relaxation, and reflex loss. Inhalation anesthesia is the most common method of administration because it can be controlled. The intake and elimination of the anesthetic are in large measure affected by pulmonary ventilation. Greater depth (or plane) of anesthesia requires a stronger concentration of the agent.

Anesthetics are divided into two classes: (1) those that suspend sensation in the whole body (general anesthesia) or (2) those that suspend sensation in parts of the body (local, regional, epidural, or spinal anesthesia).

General Anesthesia

General anesthesia is most commonly achieved when the anesthetic is inhaled or administered intravenously.

Volatile liquid anesthetics produce anesthesia when their vapors are inhaled. Included in this group are halothane, enflurane, and isoflurane. All are administered with oxygen, and usually with nitrous oxide as well. Table 20-2 identifies the advantages, disadvantages, and implications of the different types of liquid anesthetics.

Gas anesthetics are administered by inhalation and are always combined with oxygen. This group of anesthetics includes nitrous oxide and cyclopropane. The advantages and disadvantages of these agents are spelled out in Table 20-3.

The substances, when inhaled, enter the blood through the pulmonary capillaries and, when in sufficient concentration, act on the cerebral centers to produce loss of consciousness and loss of sensation. When administration of the anesthetic is discontinued, the vapor or gas is eliminated by way of the lungs.

Physiologic and Physical Factors. General anesthetics produce anesthesia because they are delivered to the brain at high partial pressure. Relatively large amounts of anesthetic must be administered during induction and the early maintenance phases because the anesthetic is recirculated and deposited in body tissues. As these sites become saturated, smaller amounts of the anesthetic agent are required to maintain anesthesia because equilibrium or near equilibrium has been achieved between brain, blood, and other tissues.

Anything that diminishes peripheral blood flow, such as vasoconstriction or shock, may cause only small amounts of anesthetic to be required. Conversely, when peripheral blood flow is unusually high, as in the muscularly active or the apprehensive patient, induction is slower and larger quantities of anesthetic are required because the brain receives a smaller quantity of anesthetic.

Methods of Administration. Liquid anesthetics may be administered by mixing the vapors with oxygen or nitrous oxide–oxygen and then having the patient inhale the mixture. The vapor is administered to the patient via a tube and a mask.

The endotracheal technique for administering anesthetics consists of introducing a soft rubber or plastic en-

TABLE 20-2 Volatile Liquids as Agents of General Anesthesia

Agent	Administration	Advantages	Disadvantages	Implications
Halothane (Fluothane)	Inhalation; special vaporizer	Not explosive or flammable Induction rapid and smooth Useful in almost every type of surgery Low incidence of postoperative nausea and vomiting	Requires skillful administration to prevent overdosage May cause liver damage May produce hypotension Requires special vaporizer for administration	In addition to observation of pulse and respiration postoperatively, it is important that blood pressure be monitored frequently.
Methoxyflurane (Penthrane)	Inhalation; special vaporizer	Nonflammable Seldom causes postoperative nausea and vomiting Analgesic action continues several hours after surgery Excellent muscle relaxation	Requires skillful administration Renal damage may occur Unpleasant odor	Prolonged postoperative depressant action calls for careful observation by PACU/recovery room personnel.
Enflurane (Ethrane)	Inhalation	Rapid induction and recovery Potent analgesic Not explosive or flammable	Respiratory depression may develop rapidly along with EEG abnormalities Not compatible with epinephrine	Observe for possible respiratory depression. Administration with epinephrine may cause ventricular fibrillation.
Isoflurane (Forane)	Inhalation	Rapid induction and recovery Muscle relaxants are markedly potentiated	A profound respiratory depressant	Respirations must be monitored closely and supported when necessary.

TABLE 20-3 Gases as Agents of General Anesthesia

Agent	Administration	Advantages	Disadvantages	Implications
Nitrous oxide (N_2O)	Inhalation (semiclosed method)	Induction and recovery rapid Nonflammable Useful with oxygen for short procedures Useful with other agents for all types of surgery	Poor relaxant Weak anesthetic May produce hypoxia	Most useful in conjunction with other agents with longer action Observe precautions with "other agents"
Cyclopropane (C_3H_6)	Inhalation (closed method)	Good relaxant Useful for all types of surgery Rapid induction and emergence Wide margin of safety Pleasant	Explosive Powerful depressant; therefore must be administered skillfully Frequently produces disturbances in heart rhythm May cause bronchospasm and acidosis	Use precautions against explosions. Because cyclopropane may be followed by hypotension, it is important to observe blood pressure postoperatively.

dotracheal tube into the trachea by means of a flexible fiberoptic endoscope, either by exposing the larynx with a laryngoscope or by passing the tube "blindly." It may be inserted through either the nose or mouth (Fig. 20-1). When in place, the endotracheal tube seals the lungs off from the esophagus, so that if the patient vomits, none of the stomach contents enters the lungs.

Stages of General Anesthesia

Anesthesia consists of four stages, each of which presents a definite group of signs and symptoms. When narcotics and neuromuscular blockers (relaxants) are administered, several of the stages are absent.

Stage I: Beginning Anesthesia. As the patient breathes in the anesthetic mixture, warmth, dizziness, and a feeling of detachment may be experienced. The patient may have a ringing, roaring, or buzzing in the ears and, though still conscious, is aware of being unable to move the extremities easily. During this stage, noises are exaggerated; even low voices or minor sounds appear distressingly loud and unreal. For this reason, unnecessary noise or motion must be avoided when anesthesia is started.

Stage II: Excitement. The excitement stage—characterized variously by struggling, shouting, talking, singing, laughing, or even crying—frequently may be avoided if the anesthetic is administered smoothly and quickly. The pupils become dilated but contract if exposed to light; the pulse rate is rapid and respirations irregular.

Because of the uncontrolled movements of the patient during this stage, the anesthesiologist must always be attended by someone ready to help restrain the patient. A strap may be in place across the patient's thighs, and the hands are secured to an armboard. The patient should not be touched except for purposes of restraint, but restraints should not be applied over the operative site. Manipulation increases circulation to the operative site, thereby increasing the potential for bleeding.

Stage III: Surgical Anesthesia. Surgical anesthesia is reached by continued administration of the vapor or gas. The patient is unconscious, lying quietly on the table. The pupils are small but will contract further when exposed to light. Respirations are regular, the pulse rate and volume are normal and the skin is pink or slightly flushed. With proper administration of the anesthetic, this stage may be maintained for hours in one of several planes, ranging from light (1) to deep (4), depending on the depth of anesthesia needed.

Stage IV: Overdosage. This stage is reached when too much anesthesia has been administered. Respirations become shallow; the pulse is weak and thready; the pupils become widely dilated and no longer contract when exposed to light. Cyanosis develops and, unless prompt action is taken, death follows rapidly. If this stage should develop, the anesthetic is discontinued immediately, and respiratory and circulatory support are necessary to prevent death. Stimulants, although rarely used, may be administered if an overdosage of anesthetic has been administered. Narcotic antagonists can be used if overdosage is due to narcotics.

During smooth administration of an anesthetic there is, of course, no sharp division between the first three stages, and there is no Stage IV. The patient passes gradually from one stage to another, and it is only by close observation of the signs exhibited by the patient that an anesthesiologist can control the situation. The responses of the pupils, the blood pressure, and the respiratory and cardiac rates are probably the most reliable guides to the patient's condition.

Other Physiologic Changes

The administration of an anesthetic is attended by other physiologic activities. A few anesthetics may produce hyper-

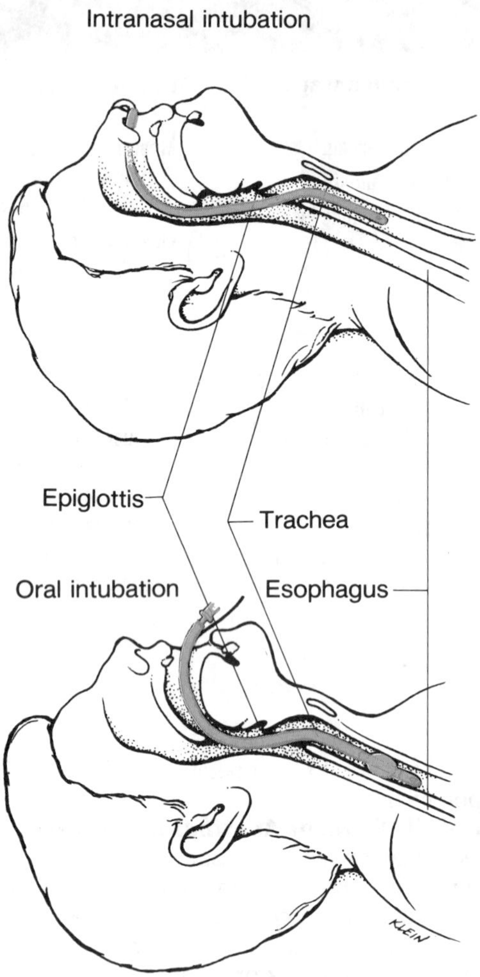

FIGURE 20-1. Endotracheal anesthesia. (**Top**) Nasal endotracheal catheter in proper position. (**Bottom**) Oral endotracheal intubation; tube in position with cuff inflated. For both methods, the head is tilted back to permit the airway to be open.

secretion of mucus and saliva. This may be minimized by the preoperative administration of atropine. Vomiting or regurgitation may occur, especially when the patient comes to the operating room with a full stomach. If gagging occurs, the patient is turned to the side, the head of the table is lowered, and a basin is provided to collect the vomitus. A suction apparatus is always available and is used to remove saliva and vomited gastric contents.

During anesthesia, the patient's temperature may fall, and therefore every precaution must be taken against chilling. Warm, cotton blankets should be available (see Hypothermia, p. 386). Glucose metabolism is reduced, and as a result, metabolic acidosis may develop.

In addition to the dangers of the anesthetic itself, the anesthesiologist must guard against asphyxia. This may be caused by foreign bodies in the mouth, spasm of the vocal cords, relaxation of the tongue, or aspiration of vomitus, saliva, or blood. These complications are avoided by using an endotracheal tube with an inflated cuff.

Intravenous Anesthesia

General anesthesia also can be produced by the intravenous injection of various substances, such as thiopental. A short-acting barbiturate, thiopental sodium (Pentothal) is the anesthetic most commonly used for this purpose. This substance leads to unconsciousness within 30 seconds. Other intravenous anesthetics are presented in Table 20-4.

Advantages. The onset of anesthesia is pleasant; there is none of the buzzing, roaring, or dizziness known to follow administration of an inhalation anesthetic. For this reason, induction of anesthesia with an intravenous agent is preferred by patients who have experienced various methods. The duration of action is brief, and the patient awakens with little nausea or vomiting. Thiopental is often administered with other anesthetic agents in prolonged procedures.

Intravenous anesthetic agents have the advantages of being nonexplosive, requiring little equipment, and being easy to administer. The low incidence of postoperative nausea and vomiting makes the method useful in eye surgery, because vomiting would increase intraocular pressure and endanger vision in the operated eye. Intravenous anesthesia is useful for short procedures but is used less often for the longer procedures of abdominal surgery. It is not indicated for children, who have small veins and require intubation because of their susceptibility to respiratory obstruction.

Disadvantages. Thiopental is a powerful respiratory depressant and its chief toxic effect results from this characteristic. It must be administered by skilled anesthesiologists and nurse anesthetists and only when some method of oxygen administration is available immediately should difficulty arise. Sneezing, coughing, and laryngospasm are sometimes noted with its use.

Adjunctive Agents: Neuromuscular Blockers

Neuromuscular blockers (muscle relaxants) are agents that block transmission of nerve impulses at the neuromuscular junction of skeletal muscles. Muscle relaxants are used to relax muscles in abdominal and thoracic surgery, relax eye muscles in certain kinds of eye surgery, facilitate endotracheal intubation, treat laryngospasm, and assist in mechanical ventilation.

Purified curare was the first widely used muscle relaxant; tubocurarine was isolated as the active principle. Succinylcholine was later introduced because it acts more rapidly than curare. Several other agents have since been introduced (Table 20-5). The ideal muscle relaxant has the following characteristics:

- Is nondepolarizing, with an onset time and duration of action similar to those of succinylcholine but without its problems of bradycardia and cardiac dysrhythmias
- Has a duration of action between those of succinylcholine and pancuronium
- Lacks cumulative and cardiovascular effects
- Is metabolizable and does not depend on the kidneys for its elimination

Regional Anesthesia

Regional anesthesia is a form of local anesthesia in which an anesthetic agent is injected around nerves so that the area supplied by these nerves is anesthetized. The effect depends on the type of nerve involved. Motor fibers are the

TABLE 20-4 Intravenous Anesthetic Agents

Agent	Administration	Advantages	Disadvantages	Implications
BARBITURATES				
Thiopental sodium (Pentothal)	Intravenous injection (or rectal)	Rapid induction Nonexplosive Requires little equipment Low incidence of postoperative nausea and vomiting	Powerful depressant of breathing Poor relaxant May produce coughing, sneezing, and laryngospasm Not useful for children because of small veins	Requires intelligent and close observation because of potency and rapidity of drug action.
OPIOIDS (NARCOTICS)				
Meperidine hydrochloride (Demerol)	Intravenously Subcutaneously Intramuscularly	Prompt onset Because of spasmolytic effect, it is drug of choice for surgery of bile duct, distal colon, and rectum; easily detoxified and excreted	May slow rate of respirations Adverse reactions: dizziness, nausea, and vomiting	In some patients, histamine may be released; treatment is diphenhydramine (Benadryl).
Morphine (high doses)	Intravenously	Not a myocardial depressant	Can depress arterial blood pressure by decreasing systemic vascular resistance Does not provide good amnesia Does not promote adequate muscular relaxation	Orthostatic hypotension may occur after morphine.
NEUROLEPTANALGESICS				
The term *neuroleptanalgesic* refers to the combination of a short-acting synthetic narcotic agent (fentanyl) and a butyrophenone (droperidol). Patient becomes very drowsy; responds to voice command, although analgesia is profound. Of significance, the combination produces peripheral vasodilation followed by a decrease in arterial blood pressure. If administered rapidly, it may cause skeletal muscular rigidity and possibly respiratory impairment.				
Fentanyl (Sublimaze; related chemically to meperidine)	Intravenously Transdermally	75–100 times more potent than morphine and about 25% of duration of morphine (IV) Little effect on cardiovascular system	In very high dosage, an alpha-adrenergic blocking effect Respiratory depression	Short duration of action is due to its more rapid redistribution and more active metabolism by liver than other narcotics.
Sufentanil	Injection	Onset, extremely rapid		Duration only about one third that of fentanyl.
DISSOCIATIVE AGENTS				
When under dissociative analgesia, the patient appears not to be asleep or anesthetized, but rather dissociated from the surroundings.				
Ketamine (Ketalar; Ketaject)	Intravenously Intramuscularly	Rapid induction and short action; often used to supplement nitrous oxide Useful when hypotension may be hazardous; can be administered as analgesic or anesthetic	May cause elevated blood pressure and depressed respirations Patient may experience hallucinations Vomiting and aspiration may occur	Avoid verbal, visual, or tactile stimulation because this may trigger psychic aberration. Droperidol or diazepam (see below) may eliminate such psychic phenomena. Observe for signs of respiratory depression. Keep resuscitation equipment nearby.

(continued)

TABLE 20-4 *(continued)*

Agent	Administration	Advantages	Disadvantages	Implications
TRANQUILIZERS				
Benzodiazepines Diazepam (Valium)	Intravenously Orally	Preoperative sedation Intraoperative tranquilization during regional anesthesia	Absorbed unpredictably when given intramuscularly	IV administration may produce thrombophlebitis (central vein therefore is preferred).
Chlordiazepoxide (Librium)	Intramuscularly	Production of hypnosis during anesthetic induction		
Droperidol (Inapsine)	Intravenously	Long duration of action	Weak antihistaminic action and alpha-adrenergic blocking action; inhibition of basic ganglionic dopaminergic pathways—may lead to extrapyramidal rigidity resembling parkinsonism	Major tranquilizer Keep IV fluids and vasopressors available for hypotension.

largest fibers and have the thickest myelin sheath. Sympathetic fibers are the smallest and have a minimal covering. Sensory fibers are intermediate. Thus, a local anesthetic blocks motor nerves least readily and sympathetic nerves most readily. An anesthetic cannot be regarded as having "worn off" until all three systems (motor, sensory, and autonomic) are no longer affected by the anesthetic.

The patient under spinal or local anesthesia is awake and aware of his or her surroundings. Careless conversation, unnecessary noise, and unpleasant odors must be avoided—these may be noticed by the patient in the operating room and may contribute to a negative view of the surgical experience by the patient. A quiet environment is therapeutic. Even the diagnosis must not be stated aloud if the patient is not to know it at this time.

Spinal Anesthesia

Spinal anesthesia is a type of extensive conduction nerve block that occurs by introducing a local anesthetic into the subarachnoid space at the lumbar level (usually between L4 and L5). It produces anesthesia of the lower extremities, perineum, and lower abdomen. For the lumbar puncture procedure, the patient lies on his or her side in a knee–chest position. Sterile technique is used as a spinal puncture is made and the medication is injected through the needle. As soon as the injection has been made, the patient is placed on his or her back. If a relatively high level of block is sought, the head and shoulders are lowered.

The spread of the anesthetic agent and the level of anesthesia depend on the amount of fluid injected, the speed with which it is injected, the positioning of the patient after the injection, and the specific gravity of the agent. If the specific gravity of the agent is greater than that of cerebrospinal fluid (CSF), the agent moves to the dependent position of the subarachnoid space; if the specific gravity is less than that of CSF, the anesthetic moves away from the dependent portion. These boundaries are controlled by the anesthesiologist. Generally, the agents used are procaine, tetracaine (Pontocaine), and lidocaine (Xylocaine) (Table 20-6).

In a few minutes, anesthesia and paralysis affect the toes and perineum and then gradually affect the legs and abdomen. If the anesthetic reaches the upper thoracic and cervical cord in high concentration, a temporary respiratory paralysis, partial or complete, may occur. Paralysis of the respiratory muscles is managed by maintaining artificial respiration until the effects of the anesthetic on the respiratory nerves have worn off.

Nausea, vomiting, and pain may occur during surgery when spinal anesthesia is used. As a rule, these reactions result from traction on various structures, particularly those within the abdominal cavity. Such reactions may be avoided by the simultaneous intravenous administration of a weak solution of thiopental and inhalation of nitrous oxide.

Headache may occur as a postoperative complication. Several factors are involved in the incidence of headache: the size of the spinal needle used, the leakage of fluid from the subarachnoid space through the puncture site, and the patient's hydration status. Measures that increase cerebrospinal pressure are helpful in relieving headache. These include keeping the patient lying flat, quiet, and well hydrated.

Nursing Assessment After Spinal Anesthesia. In addition to monitoring vital signs, the nurse observes these patients closely and records the time when motion and sensation of the legs and the toes return. When there is complete return of sensation in the toes, the patient may be considered to have recovered from the effects of the spinal anesthetic.

Serial (Continuous) Spinal Anesthesia. The tip of a plastic catheter may be left in the subarachnoid space during the surgical procedure so that more anesthetic may be

TABLE 20-5 Muscle Relaxants

Muscle Relaxant	Action	Advantages	Disadvantages	Uses and Comments
NONDEPOLARIZING NEUROMUSCULAR BLOCKING AGENTS				
Tubocurarine chloride (Tubarine)	Peaks at 30–60 min	50%–70% excreted unchanged in 3–6 hr	Histamine-like reaction Hypotension Increased airway resistance Skin erythema	Contraindicated with history of allergy, asthma
Gallamine (Flaxedil)	1/5 as potent as curare Lasts 25% shorter than curare Blocks vagal ganglia in heart	All excreted unchanged	Tachycardia	Used with cyclopropane or halothane
Pancuronium bromide (Pavulon)	Similar to curare but 5 times more potent Duration, 60–85 min	Safe; stable Good muscle relaxant Reversible by neostigmine and atropine		Excellent for situations requiring complete relaxation Avoid with myasthenia gravis or renal disease Avoid with patients sensitive to bromide
Vecuronium bromide (Norcuron)	Blocks depolarization	Facilitates endotracheal intubation; good muscle relaxant	Prolonged dose-related apnea	Related to Pavulon Well tolerated in patients with renal failure
DEPOLARIZING NEUROMUSCULAR BLOCKING AGENTS These mimic the action of acetylcholine at the neuromuscular junction. Acetylcholine is discharged almost immediately on release → repolarization of muscle takes place. When depolarizing neuromuscular blocking agents are used, skeletal muscle depolarizes.				
Succinylcholine (Anectine; Sucostrin)	Onset is rapid: 1 min Duration: 4–8 min	Ideal for endotracheal intubation, fracture reduction; treatment of laryngospasm	Contraindicated for patients with low pseudocholinesterase On second IV injection, bradycardia and various dysrhythmias May cause fasciculations of the muscles and pain	Used to treat larynogospasm, status asthmaticus, and toxic reactions to local anesthetic drugs
Decamethonium bromide (Syncurine)	Onset: 30–40 sec Duration: 15–20 min	Excreted unchanged by kidney	Some fasciculation of muscle: jaw masseter muscles; posterior calf muscles Difficult to reverse its action	Produces depolarization of end plate region

TABLE 20-6 Spinal Anesthetic Agents

Agent	Advantages of Spinal Anesthesia (Includes All Agents)	Disadvantages of Spinal Anesthesia (Includes All Agents)
Procaine (Novocaine) Tetracaine (Pontocaine) Lidocaine (Xylocaine)	Easily administered by a physician Inexpensive Minimum of equipment required Rapid onset Excellent muscular relaxation	Blood pressure may fall rapidly unless monitored carefully and treated with medications such as ephedrine. If the spinal anesthesia ascends to the chest, there may be respiratory distress. Occasionally postoperative complications occur, such as headache or, rarely, meningitis or paralysis.

injected as needed. This technique provides greater control of the dosage. However, there is greater potential for postanesthetic headache because of the large-gauge needle used.

Conduction Blocks

There are many types of conduction blocks depending on the various nerve groups that are injected.

Epidural Block. Epidural anesthesia is achieved by injecting a local anesthetic into the spinal canal in the space surrounding the dura mater. Epidural anesthesia blocks similar sensory, motor, and autonomic functions, but it is the injection site that differentiates it from spinal anesthesia. Epidural doses are much larger than those administered during spinal anesthesia because the epidural anesthetic does not make direct contact with the cord or nerve roots.

An advantage of epidural anesthesia is the absence of headache that occasionally results from subarachnoid injection. A disadvantage is the greater technical challenge of introducing the anesthetic into the epidural rather than the subarachnoid space. If accidental subarachnoid injection occurs during epidural anesthesia and the anesthetic travels toward the head, "high" spinal anesthesia can result. High spinal anesthesia can produce severe hypotension and respiratory depression and arrest. The treatment for these complications is airway support, intravenous fluids, and use of vasopressors.

Brachial Plexus Block. A brachial plexus block produces anesthesia of the arm.

Paravertebral Anesthesia. Paravertebral anesthesia produces anesthesia of the nerves supplying the chest, abdominal wall, and extremities.

Transsacral (Caudal) Block. A transsacral block produces anesthesia of the perineum and, occasionally, the lower abdomen.

Local Infiltration Anesthesia

Infiltration anesthesia is the injection of a solution containing the local anesthetic into the tissues at the planned incision site. Often, it is combined with a local regional block by injecting the nerves immediately supplying the area. The advantages of local anesthesia are as follows:

- It is simple, economical, and nonexplosive. The amount of equipment is minimal. Postoperative recovery is shortened.
- Undesirable effects of general anesthesia are avoided.
- It is ideal for short and superficial surgical procedures.

Local anesthesia is often administered in combination with epinephrine. Epinephrine causes constriction of blood vessels, which prevents rapid absorption of the anesthetic agent and thus prolongs its local action; rapid absorption into the bloodstream, which could cause seizures, is also prevented.

Different types of local anesthetic agents are listed in Table 20-7.

Contraindications. Local anesthesia is the anesthesia of choice in any surgical procedure in which it can be used. However, it is contraindicated for surgery on highly nervous, apprehensive patients, because surgery with local anesthesia may increase anxiety. A patient who begs to be put to sleep rarely does well under local anesthesia.

For some surgical procedures, local anesthesia is impractical because of the number of injections and the amount of anesthetic that would be required—as in breast reconstruction, for example.

Technique. Introduction of local infiltration requires the following:

- Solution of local anesthetic in various concentrations (0.5% to 2%)
- Sterile container
- Sterile syringes and needles
- Sterile sponges and drape

The skin is prepared as for any surgical procedure, and a small-gauge needle is used to inject a small amount of the anesthetic into the skin layers. This produces blanching or a wheal. Additional anesthetic is then injected in the skin until an area the length of the proposed incision is anesthetized. A larger, longer needle then is used to infiltrate deeper tissues with the anesthetic.

The action of the agent is almost immediate, so surgery may begin as soon as the injection is complete. Anesthesia lasts anywhere from 45 minutes to 3 hours, depending on the anesthetic and the use of epinephrine.

Patient Position on the Operating Table

The position in which the patient is placed on the operating table depends on the surgical procedure to be performed as well as on the physical condition of the patient (Fig. 20-2). Factors to consider include the following:

- The patient should be in as comfortable a position as possible, whether asleep or awake.
- The operative area must be adequately exposed.
- The vascular supply should not be obstructed by an awkward position or undue pressure on a part.
- There should be no interference with the patient's respiration as a result of pressure of the arms on the chest or constriction of the neck or chest caused by a gown.
- Nerves must be protected from undue pressure. Improper positioning of the arms, hands, legs, or feet may cause serious injury or paralysis. Shoulder braces must be well padded to prevent irreparable nerve injury, especially when the Trendelenburg position is necessary.
- Precautions for patient safety must be observed, particularly with thin, elderly, or obese patients.
- The patient needs *gentle* restraint before induction, in case of excitement.

Dorsal Recumbent Position. The usual position for surgery is flat on the back; one arm is at the side of the table, with the hand placed palm down; the other is carefully positioned on an armboard for intravenous infusion

TABLE 20-7 Local Anesthetic Agents

Agent	Administration and Action	Advantages	Disadvantages	Implications and Use
AMIDES				
Lidocaine (Xylocaine) and mepivacaine (Carbocaine)	Topical or injection	Rapid Longer duration of action (compared with procaine) Free from local irritative effect	Occasional idiosyncrasy	Useful topically for cystoscopy Injected for use in dental work and surgery Observe for untoward reactions—drowsiness, depressed respiration
Bupivacaine (Marcaine)	Infiltration Peripheral nerve block Epidural	Duration is 2–3 times longer than lidocaine or mepivacaine	Use cautiously in persons with known drug allergies or sensitivities.	A period of analgesia persists after return of sensation; therefore, need for strong analgesics is reduced
Etidocaine (Duranest)	Infiltration Block			Greater potency and longer action than lidocaine
ESTERS				
Procaine (Novocaine)	Subcutaneously, intramuscularly, intravenously, or spinal	Low toxicity Inexpensive	Some idiosyncrasies Skin rash Poor stability	Observe for reaction: hypotension, bradycardia, weak pulse Usually given with epinephrine, causing vasoconstriction, thereby slowing absorption and prolonging nerve-deadening effect
Tetracaine (Pontocaine)	Topical Infiltration Nerve block	Same as procaine	Same as procaine	More than 10 times as potent as procaine Usually administered with epinephrine

(see Fig. 20-2). This position is used for most abdominal surgery, except for surgery on the gallbladder and the pelvis. Positions for specific procedures are described below.

Trendelenburg Position. The Trendelenburg position usually is used for surgery on the lower abdomen and the pelvis to obtain good exposure by displacing the intestines into the upper abdomen. In this position, the head and body are lowered and the knees are flexed.

The patient is held in position by padded shoulder braces (see Fig. 20-2).

Lithotomy Position. In the lithotomy position, the patient is lying on the back with the legs and thighs flexed at right angles. The position is maintained by placing the feet in stirrups. Nearly all perineal, rectal, and vaginal surgical procedures require this posture (see Fig. 20-2).

For Kidney Surgery. The patient is placed on the nonoperative side in Sims's position with an air pillow 12.5 to 15 cm (5 or 6 in) thick under the loin, or on a table with a kidney or back lift (see Fig. 20-2).

For Chest and Abdominothoracic Surgery. The position varies with the surgery to be performed. The surgeon and the anesthesiologist place the patient on the operating table in the desired position.

Surgery on the Neck. Neck surgery—for example, surgery involving the thyroid—is performed with the patient on the back, the neck extended somewhat by a pillow beneath the shoulders, and the head and chest elevated to reduce venous pressure.

Surgery on the Skull and the Brain. Such procedures demand special positions and apparatus, usually adjusted by the surgeon.

Induced Hypotension

There are times during surgery when it is desirable to lower blood pressure in order to reduce bleeding at the operative site, because this allows the surgery to be carried out more quickly with less blood loss. In procedures such as brain surgery, radical neck dissection, and radical pelvic surgery, artificially induced hypotension has been used.

Deliberate hypotension is accomplished by inhalation or intravenous injection of medications that affect the sympathetic nervous system and peripheral smooth muscle. Halothane is the inhalation anesthetic agent commonly used. This anesthetic is supplemented with other measures to lower blood pressure, such as a head-up position, positive pressure applied to the airway, and administration of a ganglionic blocking agent such as pentolinium (Ansolysen) or sodium nitroprusside.

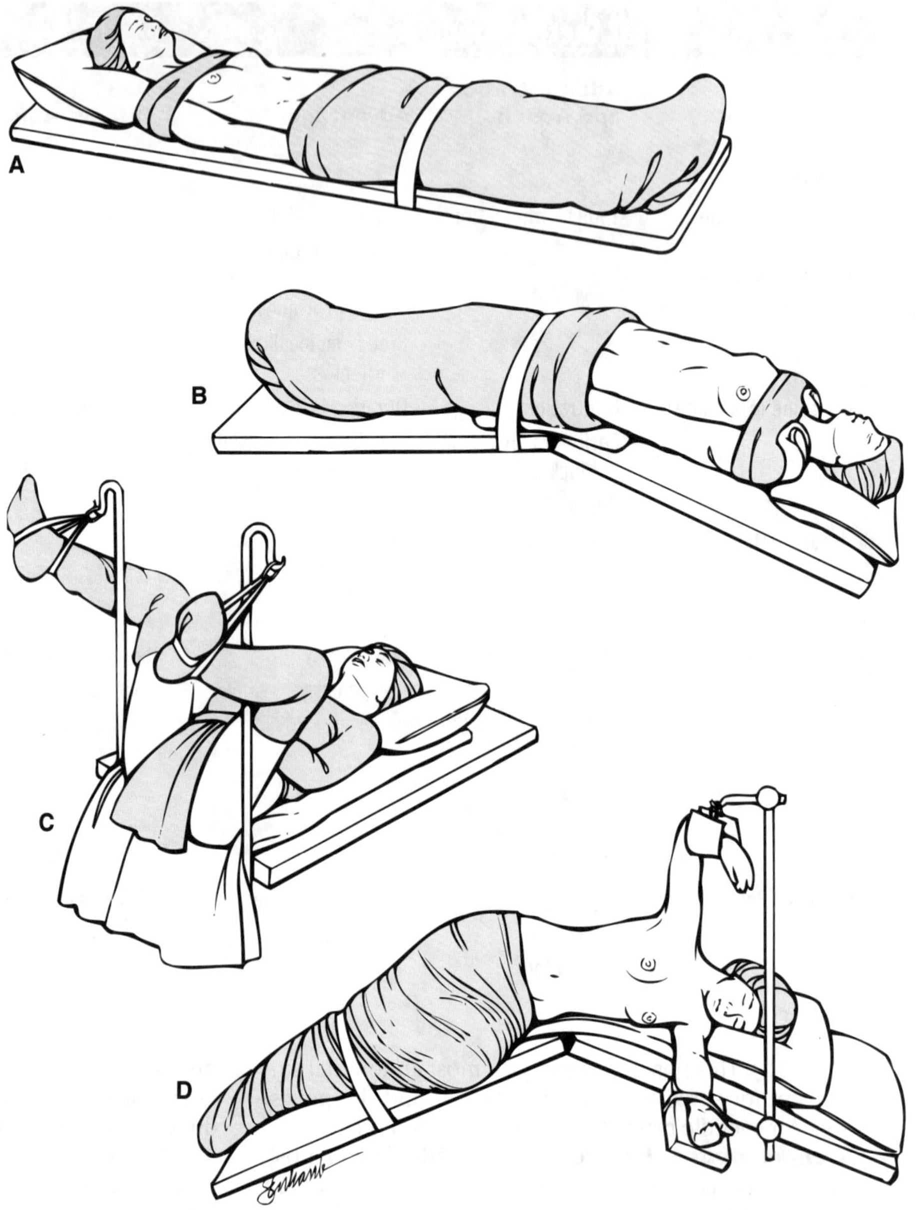

A Patient in position on the operating table as prepared for a laparotomy. Note the strap above the knees.

B Patient in Trendelenburg position on operating table. Note padded shoulder braces in place. Be sure that brace does not press on brachial plexus.

C Patient in lithotomy position. Note that the hips extend over the edge of the table.

D Patient on operating table for kidney operation, lying on his unaffected side. Table is broken to spread apart space between the lower ribs and the pelvis. The upper leg is extended; the lower leg is flexed at the knee and the hip joints; a pillow is placed between the legs. Note the sandbag, which helps to support the patient's chest.

FIGURE 20-2. Positions on the operating table. Captions call attention to safety and comfort features. All surgical patients wear caps to completely cover the hair.

Hypothermia

Hypothermia is the state of core body temperature below physiologic normal limits. **Normothermia** is 36.6° to 37.5°C (98.0° to 99.5°F). Inadvertent hypothermia may be experienced by the patient as a result of a low temperature in the operating room, infusion of cold fluids, inhalation of cold gases, open body wounds or cavities, decreased muscle activity, advanced age, or the pharmaceutical agents ¡used (vasodilators, phenothiazines, general anesthetics). Hypothermia may also be intentionally induced in selected surgical procedures to reduce the patient's metabolic rate.

Treatment. Prevention of hypothermia is a major objective; if hypothermia occurs, the goal of intervention is to minimize or reverse the physiologic process. With intentional hypothermia, the goal is safe return to normal body temperature.

Environmental temperature in the operating room should be set at 25° to 26.6°C (78° to 80°F). Intravenous and irrigating fluids are warmed to 37°C (98.6°F). Wet gowns and drapes are removed promptly and replaced with dry materials, because wet linens promote heat loss. Whatever methods are employed to rewarm the patient, warming must be accomplished gradually, not rapidly.

Conscientious monitoring of core temperature, urinary output, ECG, blood pressure, arterial blood gases, and serum electrolytes is required. Attention to hypothermia management extends into the postoperative period to prevent significant nitrogen loss and catabolism. Treatment includes oxygen administration, adequate hydration, and proper nutrition.

Gerontologic Considerations. Heat loss in older patients in the operating room can be prevented by covering the head of the patient with a heat-retaining cap during anesthesia. An ordinary disposable plastic shower cap can be effective and inexpensive.

Also, the operating room temperature should be maintained at 26.6°C (80°F). Antiseptic solutions used in the ini-

CHART 20-1
The Nursing Process in the Intraoperative Phase

Assessment

A. Use data from patient and the patient record to identify variables that can affect care and that serve as guidelines for developing an individualized plan of patient care.
  1. Identify patient.
  2. Validate necessary data with patient per department policy.
  3. Review patient record for:
    a. Correct informed surgical consent with patient's signature
    b. Completed records for health history and physical examination
    c. Results of diagnostic studies
    d. Completed health history and assessment
    e. Preoperative checklist
  4. Complete immediate preoperative nursing assessment.
    a. Physiologic status (*e.g.,* health-illness level, level of consciousness)
    b. Psychosocial status (*e.g.,* expressions of concern, anxiety level, verbal communication problems, coping mechanisms)
    c. Physical status (*e.g.,* operative site, skin condition and effectiveness of preparation, shave, or depilatory; immobile joints)

Planning

A. Interpret common variables and incorporate them into the plan of care.
  1. Age, size, sex, surgical procedure, type of anesthesia planned, surgeon, anesthesiologist, and team members
  2. Availability of necessary equipment specific to procedure and surgeon
  3. Need for nonroutine medications, blood components, instruments, etc.
  4. Readiness of room for patient; completeness of physical setup; completeness of instrument, suture, and dressing setups.

B. Identify aspects of the operating room environment that may negatively affect the patient.
  1. Physical
    a. Room temperature and humidity
    b. Electrical hazards
    c. Potential contaminants (dust, blood, and discharge on floor or surfaces; uncovered hair, faulty attire of personnel, jewelry worn by personnel, dirty footwear)
    d. Unnecessary traffic
  2. Psychosocial
    a. Noise
    b. Lack of recognition as a person
    c. Sense of abandonment—unchaperoned in waiting area
    d. Unnecessary conversation

Intervention

A. Provide nursing care based on priority of patient needs.
  1. Set up and maintain suction in working order.
  2. Set up invasive monitoring equipment.
  3. Assist with line insertion (arterial, Swan-Ganz, CVP, IV).
  4. Initiate appropriate physical comfort measures for patient.

Intervention

  5. Position patient correctly for anesthesia and surgical procedures; maintain functional body alignment.
  6. Follow steps in surgical procedure.
    a. Scrub/circulate competently.
    b. Respond to needs of patient by anticipating what supplies and equipment are required before they are requested.
    c. Assume role of RN First Assistant as required.
  7. Follow established procedures—for example:
    a. Care and use of blood and blood components
    b. Care and handling of specimens, tissue, and cultures
    c. Antiseptic skin preparation
    d. Donning gown—self; holding gown for surgeon
    e. Open and closed gloving
    f. Counts: sponge, instrument, needle, special
    g. Septic case technique
    h. Urinary catheter management
    i. Drainage/dressing management
  8. Communicate adverse situations to surgeon, anesthesiologist, or charge nurse, or act appropriately to control or reverse the situation.
  9. Use supplies judiciously for cost-effectiveness.
  10. Assist the surgeon and anesthesiologist in implementing their plans of care.

B. Act as the patient's advocate.
  1. Provide physical privacy.
  2. Maintain confidentiality.
  3. Provide physical safety and comfort.

C. Inform patient regarding intraoperative experience.
  1. Describe any sensory stimulation patient will experience.
  2. Use common, basic communication skills to reduce anxiety in the patient—for example:
    a. Touch
    b. Eye contact
    c. Assure the patient you will be present in the operating room
    d. Realistic verbal reassurance

D. Coordinate activities of others involved in patient care:
  1. X-ray, laboratory, PACU, intensive care unit, surgical nursing unit
  2. Technicians—cast, laboratory, etc.
  3. Pharmacist
  4. Ancillary operating room personnel and nonprofessional staff

E. Operate and troubleshoot all equipment commonly used in the operating room and assigned specialty service (including autoclaves).

F. Participate in patient care conferences.

G. Document all observations and appropriate actions on the required forms, including patient's record.

H. Communicate, orally and in writing, with the recovery room and outpatient surgical nursing staff (as pertinent) regarding the health status of the patient on transfer from the operating room.

(continued)

CHART 20-1 *(continued)*

The Nursing Process in the Intraoperative Phase

Evaluation

A. Evaluate the condition of the patient immediately prior to discharge from the operating room—for example:
   1. Respiratory condition: breathing easily (independently or assisted)
   2. Skin condition: color good; absence of abrasions, burns, bruises
   3. Functioning of invasive tubing: IV, drains, catheters, nasogastric—no kinks or obstruction, functioning normally, etc.
   4. Grounding pad site: good condition
   5. Dressings: adequate for drainage, fastened securely, not too tight, etc.

B. Participate in the identification of unsafe patient care practices and intervene appropriately.

C. Participate in evaluating the safety of the environment—for example, equipment, cleanliness.

D. Report and document any adverse behavior or problem.

E. Demonstrate understanding of principles of asepsis and technical nursing practices.

F. Recognize the legal accountability of perioperative nursing.

(Adapted from procedure and practices at Memorial Hospital Medical Center of Long Beach, California.)

tial preparation of the skin before the application of drapes should be comfortably warm, not cold.

Malignant Hyperthermia During General Anesthesia

Malignant hyperthermia is an inherited muscle disorder that is chemically induced by anesthetic agents.

Etiology and Pathophysiology. During anesthesia, potent agents such as inhalation anesthetics (halothane, enflurane) and muscle relaxants (succinylcholine) may trigger the symptoms of malignant hyperthermia. Such medications as sympathomimetics (epinephrine), theophylline, aminophylline, anticholinergics (atropine), and cardiac glycosides (digitalis) can also induce or intensify such a reaction. The process is also initiated by stress.

The pathophysiology is related to muscle cell activity. Muscle cells are composed of inner fluid (sarcoplasm) and an outer surrounding membrane. Calcium, an essential factor in the process of muscle contraction, is normally stored in sacs in the sarcoplasm. When nerve impulses stimulate the muscle, calcium is released, allowing contraction to occur. A pumping mechanism returns calcium to the sacs so that relaxation can take place. In malignant hyperthermia, this mechanism is disrupted. Calcium ions are not returned and they accumulate, causing clinical symptoms of hypermetabolism, which in turn increases muscle contraction (rigidity), hyperthermia, and damage to the central nervous system.

With the mortality rate exceeding 50%, identifying patients at risk is imperative. Persons susceptible to malignant hyperthermia include those with bulky, strong muscles, a history of muscle cramps or muscle weakness and unexplained temperature elevation, and an unexplained death of a family member during surgery that was accompanied by a febrile response.

Clinical Manifestations. The initial symptoms of malignant hyperthermia are related to cardiovascular and musculoskeletal activity. Tachycardia (heart rate above 150/min) is often the earliest sign. In addition to the tachycardia, sympathetic nervous stimulation leads to ventricular dysrhythmia, hypotension, decreased cardiac output, oliguria, and, later, cardiac arrest. With the abnormal transport of calcium, rigidity or tetany-like movements occur, often in the jaw. The rise in temperature is actually a late sign that develops rapidly, and it can increase 1° every 5 minutes.

Management. Early recognition of symptoms by the circulating nurse and the prompt discontinuation of anesthesia are imperative. It is also necessary to monitor all vital signs, arterial blood gases, electrolytes, and the ECG. Goals of treatment are to decrease metabolism, reverse metabolic and respiratory acidosis, correct dysrhythmias, decrease body temperature, provide oxygen and nutrition to tissues, and correct electrolyte imbalance.

CRITICAL THINKING EXERCISES

1. Your patient has been in the operating room three times longer than expected. Her family is becoming increasingly anxious about her. Upon checking with the Post Anesthesia Care Unit (PACU) staff, you find that she has been in the operating room the entire time because of unforeseen complications. Indicate how you would respond to the family and what information you would convey to them about the patient.
2. A patient in the operating room is about to receive general anesthesia. She states that she is very nervous and worried that she may say something while under anesthesia that will be embarrassing to her. Describe the type of explanation you would give to relieve her fears and concerns.

Although most instances occur about 10 to 20 minutes after induction of the anesthetic, malignant hyperthermia can also occur in the first 24-hour postoperative period. As soon as the diagnosis of malignant hyperthermia is made, anesthesia and surgery are halted and the patient is hyperventilated with 100% oxygen. Dantrolene sodium, a skeletal muscle relaxant, and sodium bicarbonate are administered immediately. Continued monitoring of all parameters is necessary to evaluate the patient's progress.

Although malignant hyperthermia occurs infrequently, enough is now known about the problem that, if it does occur, it can be recognized. It is imperative that the nurse identify patients at risk, recognize the problem, have the appropriate medication and equipment available, and know the protocol to follow. This information may be lifesaving if malignant hyperthermia occurs.

Intraoperative Nursing: The Nursing Process

The nursing process as applied to intraoperative nursing is summarized in Chart 20-1.

BIBLIOGRAPHY

See Bibliography for unit following Chapter 21.

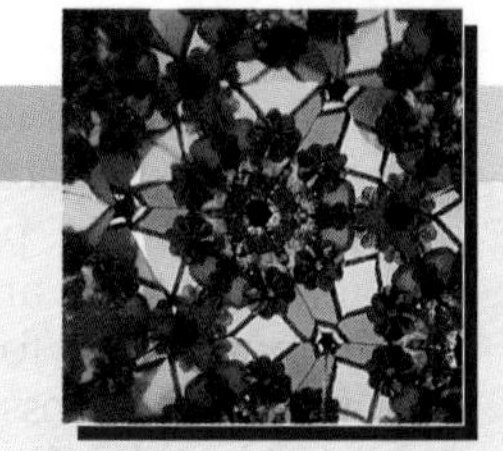

21 Postoperative Nursing Management

CHAPTER OUTLINE

Transferring the Patient to the Postanesthesia Care Unit

Postanesthesia Care Unit
Immediate Postoperative Assessment
Nursing Interventions
Postanesthesia Care Unit Criteria and Scoring Guide

Patient's Reception and Care on the Clinical Unit
NURSING PROCESS: Caring for the Postoperative Patient

Postoperative Complications
Shock
Hemorrhage
Deep Venous Thrombosis
Pulmonary Embolism
Respiratory Complications
Urinary Retention
Gastrointestinal Complications
Postoperative Psychosis
Gerontologic Considerations

Ambulatory Surgery
Types of Ambulatory Surgery Procedures
Patient Selection
Preoperative and Postoperative Care

Care of the Surgical Incision/Wound
Wound Classification
Physiology of Wound Healing
Dressings
Wound Complications

Critical Thinking Exercises

LEARNING OBJECTIVES

On completion of this chapter, the learner will be able to:

1. Describe the responsibilities of the postanesthesia care unit nurse in the prevention of immediate postoperative complications
2. Use the nursing process as a framework for care of postoperative patients
3. Identify common postoperative discomforts and their management
4. Describe the gerontologic considerations related to postoperative management of patients
5. Describe variables that affect wound healing
6. Demonstrate sterile dressing technique
7. Identify assessment parameters appropriate for the early detection of postoperative complications
8. Describe the advantages and process of ambulatory surgery

During the postoperative period, the nursing process is directed toward reestablishing the patient's physiologic equilibrium, alleviating pain, and preventing complications. Careful assessment and immediate intervention assist the patient in returning to optimal function quickly, safely, and as comfortably as possible.

Considerable effort is directed toward anticipating and preventing problems in the postoperative period. Prompt assessment prevents complications that prolong the hospital stay or endanger the patient. In this respect, the nursing care of the patient after surgery is equal in importance to the surgical procedure itself.

Transferring the Patient to the Postanesthesia Care Unit

The transfer from the operating room to the postanesthesia care unit (PACU), also referred to as the postanesthesia recovery room (PARR), involves special consideration of the patient's incision site, vascular changes, and exposure. The location of the surgical incision is considered every time the postoperative patient is moved. Many wounds are closed under considerable tension, and every effort is made to prevent further strain on the sutures. In addition, the patient is positioned so that he or she is not lying on and obstructing drains or drainage tubes.

Serious arterial hypotension may occur when a patient is moved from one position to another, such as from a lithotomy position to a horizontal position, from a lateral to a supine position, or from a prone to a supine position. Even moving the anesthetized patient to the stretcher can precipitate this problem. Thus, the patient must be moved *slowly* and *carefully*. As soon as the patient is placed on the stretcher or bed, the soiled gown is removed and replaced with a dry gown. The patient is covered with lightweight blankets and secured with straps above the knees and elbows. The straps serve the double purpose of anchoring the blankets and restraining the patient should he or she pass through a stage of excitement while recovering from the anesthetic. Side rails are raised to protect against falls.

Transferring the postoperative patient from the operating room to the postanesthesia care unit (PACU) is the responsibility of the anesthesiologist, with a member of the surgical team in attendance.

Additional assistance may be provided by a nurse assigned to this particular patient. The patient is transferred expediently with special attention paid to maintaining comfort and safety. Tubes and drainage equipment are handled carefully for optimal function.

Postanesthesia Care Unit

The PACU is usually located adjacent to the operating rooms. Patients who are still under anesthesia or recovering from it are placed in this unit for easy access to (1) nurses who are prepared in caring for the immediate postoperative patient, (2) anesthesiologists and surgeons, and (3) monitors and special equipment, medications, and replacement fluids. In this setting, the patient is given the specialized care available by those best qualified to provide it.

The room is kept quiet, clean, and free of unnecessary equipment. It should also be painted in soft, pleasing colors and have (1) indirect lighting; (2) a soundproof ceiling; (3) equipment that controls or eliminates noise (*e.g.*, plastic emesis basins, rubber bumpers on beds and tables); and (4) isolated quarters (glass encased) for disruptive patients. These features are of psychologic value to the patient to decrease anxiety.

Monitoring devices are available to provide accurate and instant appraisal of the patient's condition. Special equipment includes most types of breathing aids: oxygen, laryngoscopes, tracheotomy sets, bronchial instruments, catheters, mechanical ventilators, and suction equipment.

Other equipment is needed for meeting circulatory needs, such as blood pressure apparatus, parenteral equipment, plasma expanders, intravenous trays and cutdown trays, cardiac arrest equipment, defibrillator, venous catheters, and tourniquets. Surgical dressing materials, narcotics, and emergency medications are available, as well as catheterization sets and drainage equipment.

The recovery bed is one that provides easy access to the patient, is safe and easily movable, can readily be placed in shock position, and possesses features that facilitate care, such as intravenous poles, side rails, wheel brakes, and chart storage rack.

Room temperature should be 20° to 22.2°C (68° to 70°F), and the room should be well ventilated.

A patient remains in the PACU until fully recovered from the anesthetic agent, that is, until the patient has a stable blood pressure, adequate respiratory function, a minimum of 95% O_2 saturation, and a reasonable degree of consciousness. Criteria to determine the degree of recovery are provided in detail in Figure 21-1.

The nursing management objectives of the PACU are to provide care until the patient has recovered from the effects of anesthesia (*i.e.*, until return of motor and sensory functions), is oriented, has stable vital signs, and shows no evidence of hemorrhage. If a problem arises, the proximity to the surgeon, anesthesiologist, and operating room provides immediate access to expert assistance. The patient who progresses uneventfully is transferred from the PACU to the surgical nursing unit.

Immediate Postoperative Assessment

The PACU nurse who receives the patient reviews the following with the anesthesiologist/anesthetist:

1. Medical diagnosis and type of surgery performed
2. Patient's age and general condition, airway patency, vital signs
3. Anesthetic and other medications used (*e.g.*, narcotics, muscle relaxant, antibiotics)
4. Any problems that occurred in the operating room that might influence postoperative care (*e.g.*, extensive hemorrhage, shock, cardiac arrest)
5. Pathology encountered (if malignancy, whether the patient or family has been informed)

POSTANESTHESIA RECOVERY ROOM
Scoring

Patient: Final Score:

Room: Surgeon:

Date: R.R. Nurse:

Area of Assessment	Point Score	Upon Admission	After 1 hr	After 2 hr	After 3 hr
Respiration:					
• Ability to breathe deeply and cough	2				
• Limited respiratory effort (dyspnea or splinting)	1				
• No spontaneous effort	0				
Circulation: Systolic arterial pressure					
• >80% of preanesthetic level	2				
• 50% to 80% of preanesthetic level	1				
• <50% of preanesthetic level	0				
Consciousness Level:					
• Verbally responds to questions/ oriented to location	2				
• Aroused when called by name	1				
• Failure to respond to command	0				
Color:					
• Normal skin color and appearance	2				
• Altered skin color: pale, dusky, blotchy, jaundiced	1				
• Frank cyanosis	0				
Muscle Activity: Moves spontaneously or on command:					
• Ability to move all extremities	2				
• Ability to move 2 extremities	1				
• Unable to control any extremity	0				
Totals:					

Required for Discharge from Recovery Room: 7-8 points

Time of Release ____________ Signature of Nurse ____________

FIGURE 21-1. Postanesthesia recovery room chart.

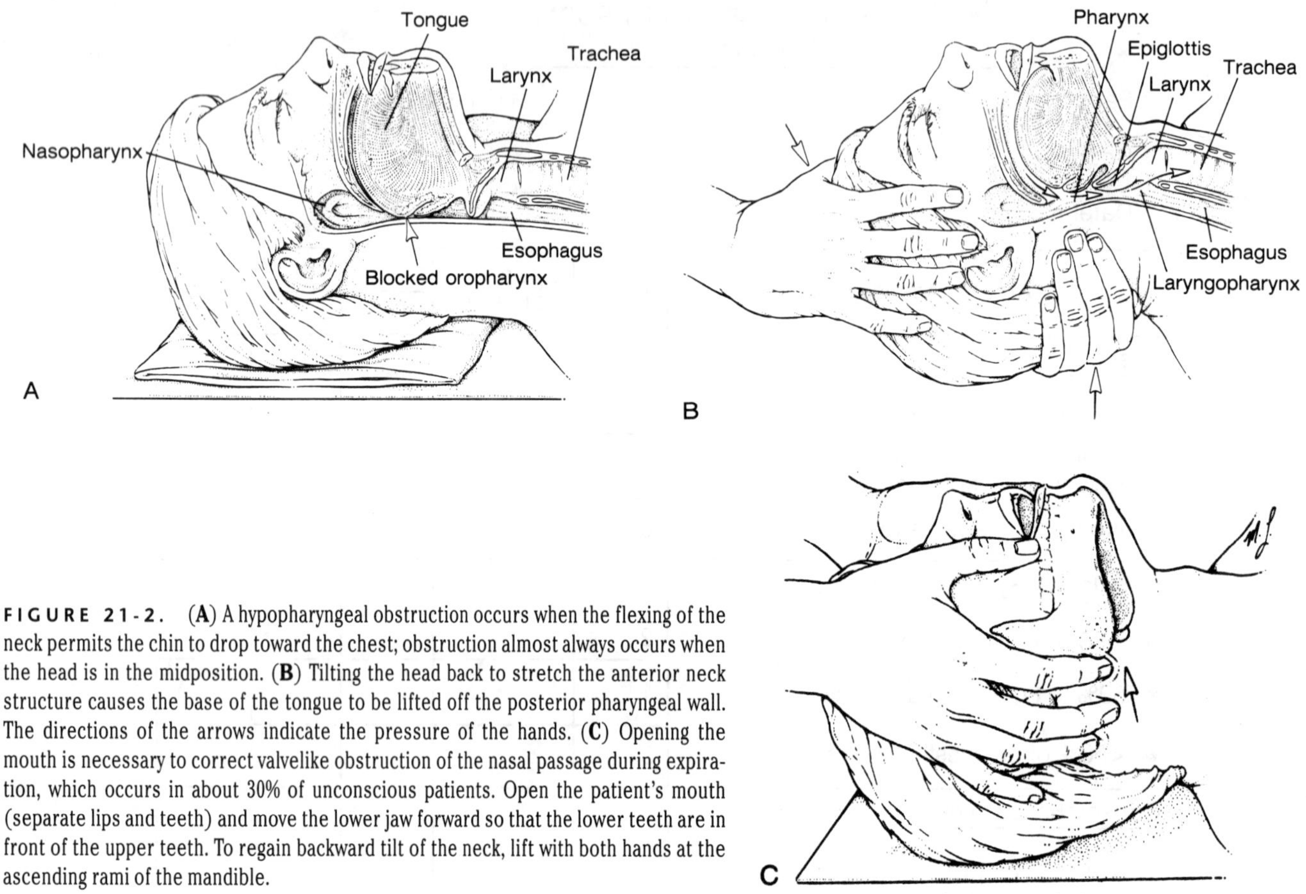

FIGURE 21-2. (**A**) A hypopharyngeal obstruction occurs when the flexing of the neck permits the chin to drop toward the chest; obstruction almost always occurs when the head is in the midposition. (**B**) Tilting the head back to stretch the anterior neck structure causes the base of the tongue to be lifted off the posterior pharyngeal wall. The directions of the arrows indicate the pressure of the hands. (**C**) Opening the mouth is necessary to correct valvelike obstruction of the nasal passage during expiration, which occurs in about 30% of unconscious patients. Open the patient's mouth (separate lips and teeth) and move the lower jaw forward so that the lower teeth are in front of the upper teeth. To regain backward tilt of the neck, lift with both hands at the ascending rami of the mandible.

6. Fluid administered, blood loss and replacement
7. Any tubing, drains, catheters, or other supportive aids
8. Specific information about which the surgeon or anesthesiologist wishes to be notified

This preliminary assessment of the patient includes evaluating oxygen saturation by pulse oximetry and monitoring pulse volume and regularity, depth and nature of respirations, skin color, level of consciousness, and the patient's ability to respond to commands. The operative site is checked for drainage or hemorrhage, and for any clamped tubing that needs to be unclamped and connected to a drainage receptacle.

It is also essential for the nurse to be aware of any pertinent information from the preoperative history that may be significant at this time (*e.g.*, patient is hard of hearing, has a history of seizures, has diabetes, is allergic to certain medications). This information may have been obtained in a preoperative visit with the patient.

Nursing Interventions

Vital signs are monitored and the patient's general physical status is assessed at least every 15 minutes. Patency of the airway and respiratory function are always evaluated first, followed by assessment of cardiovascular function (including vital signs), the condition of the surgical site, and function of the central nervous system.

- The primary objective is to maintain pulmonary ventilation and thus to prevent hypoxemia (reduced oxygen in blood) and hypercapnia (excess carbon dioxide in blood). These can occur if the airway is obstructed and ventilation is reduced (hypoventilation).

Shock can be avoided largely by the timely administration of intravenous fluids, blood, and medications that elevate blood pressure.

Respiratory Considerations. Respiratory difficulties are associated with specific types of anesthesia. Patients who received local anesthesia or nitrous oxide usually are awake within a few minutes of leaving the operating room. However, patients who have experienced prolonged anesthesia usually are unconscious, with all muscles relaxed. This relaxation extends to the muscles of the pharynx; therefore, when the patient lies on his or her back, the lower jaw and the tongue fall backward, and the air passages become obstructed (Fig. 21-2*A*). Signs of this difficulty include choking, noisy and irregular respirations, and, within minutes, a blue, dusky color (cyanosis) of the skin.

- The only sure way of knowing whether a patient is breathing or not is to place the palm of the hand over the patient's nose and mouth to feel the exhaled breath. Movements of the thorax and the diaphragm do not necessarily indicate that a patient is breathing.
- The treatment of hypopharyngeal obstruction involves tilting the head back and pushing forward on the angle

of the lower jaw, as if to push the lower teeth in front of the upper teeth (see Fig. 21-2*B,C*). This maneuver pulls the tongue forward and opens the air passages.

Often the anesthesiologist leaves a hard rubber or plastic airway in the patient's mouth (Fig. 21-3) to maintain a patent airway. Such a device should not be removed until signs, such as gagging, indicate that reflex action is returning.

The patient may be brought to the PACU with an endotracheal tube still in place and may require continued mechanical ventilation. The nurse then assists in initiating the use of the ventilator and in the weaning and extubation procedures.

Clearing Secretions From the Airway. Respiratory difficulty can result from excessive secretion of mucus. Turning the patient to one side allows the collected fluid to escape from the side of the mouth. If the patient's teeth are clenched, the mouth may be opened manually but cautiously with a padded tongue blade.

If vomiting occurs, the patient is turned to the side and the vomitus collected in the emesis basin. The face is wiped with gauze or paper wipes and the nature and amount of the vomitus are recorded.

Mucus or vomitus obstructing the pharynx or the trachea is suctioned with a pharyngeal suction tip or a nasal catheter introduced into the nasopharynx or the oropharynx.

Wall suction or suction machines are available for this purpose. The catheter can be passed into the nasopharynx or the oropharynx safely to a distance of 15 to 20 cm (6 to 8 in) if secretions are obtained at this level. Caution is necessary in suctioning the throat of a patient who has had a tonsillectomy, because the operative area may become irritated, causing bleeding and added discomfort. For infection control, a sterile disposable catheter is used each time the patient requires suctioning. For aesthetic reasons, the same catheter can be passed from mouth to nose but not from nose to mouth.

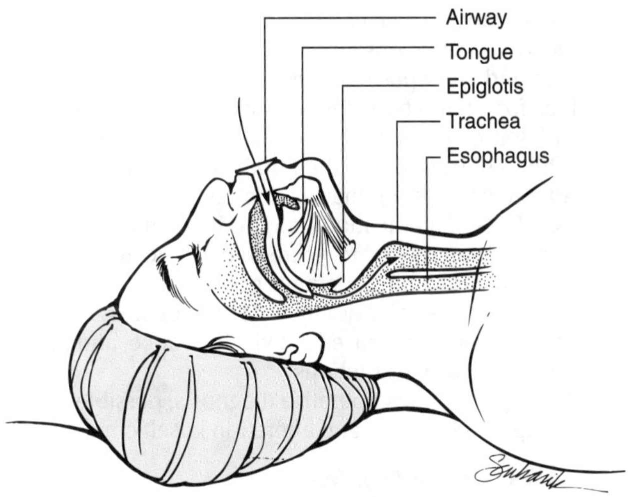

FIGURE 21-3. Diagrammatic view showing a method by which an airway prevents respiratory difficulty after anesthesia. The airway passes over the base of the tongue and permits passage of air into the pharynx in the region of the epiglottis. Patients are often brought from the operating room with an airway in place. This should remain in place until the patient recovers sufficiently to breathe normally. As the patient regains consciousness, the airway usually causes irritation; it should be removed.

Positioning. The bed is kept flat until the patient regains consciousness. Unless contraindicated, the unconscious patient is positioned on one side with a pillow at the back and with chin extended to minimize any danger of aspiration. Knees are flexed and a pillow positioned between the legs to reduce strain on abdominal sutures. If side-lying is contraindicated, only the patient's head is turned to the side.

Psychologic Support. The function of the PACU nurse is not limited to monitoring the patient's physiologic status. Providing psychologic support is also important. If one nurse has accompanied the patient through the immediate preoperative and operative experiences, that nurse can offer valuable information about the patient's mental status, such as any fears or concerns. If more than one nurse has provided care, then the PACU nurse can check the chart for any pertinent documentation that reflects the individual needs of the patient.

Postanesthesia Care Unit Criteria and Scoring Guide

Usually the following criteria are used to determine the patient's readiness for discharge from the PACU:

- Uncompromised pulmonary function
- Pulse oximetry readings of adequate O_2 saturation
- Stable vital signs, including blood pressure
- Orientation to place, events, time
- Urine output not less than 30 ml/hr
- Nausea and vomiting under control; pain minimal

Many hospitals use a scoring system to determine the patient's general condition and readiness to be transferred from the PACU. Throughout the recovery period, the patient's physical signs are observed and evaluated by means of a scoring system based on a set of objective criteria. This evaluation guide, a modification of the Apgar scoring system used for evaluating newborns, makes possible a more objective assessment of the patient's physical condition in the PACU (see Fig. 21-1).

The patient's score is taken at stated intervals, such as every 15 or 30 minutes, and totaled on the assessment record. Patients with a total score of less than 7 must remain in the recovery room until their condition improves or they are transferred to an intensive care area.

Patient's Reception and Care on the Clinical Unit

The patient's unit is readied by assembling the necessary equipment and supplies: intravenous pole, drainage receptacle holder, emesis basin, tissues, disposable pads (Chux), blankets, and postoperative charting sheets. When the call comes to the unit about the patient's transfer from the PACU, any additional items that might be needed are communicated.

The patient is transferred from the PACU to the clinical unit when the above criteria have been met and the PACU chart score confirms the patient's responsiveness. The recovery room nurse reports the baseline data of the patient's condition to the receiving nurse. The report includes medications prescribed and administered for pain, the type and amount of fluids received, whether the patient has voided, and information that the patient and family have received about the patient's condition. Usually the surgeon speaks to the family after surgery and relates the general condition of the patient and what to expect when the patient arrives on the unit. The receiving nurse also reviews the postoperative orders.

❑ NURSING PROCESS
Caring for the Postoperative Patient

Assessment

After the PACU report, the unit nurse performs an initial assessment and proceeds with any immediate nursing interventions. Usually the question "How are you feeling?" provides information about the patient's discomfort as well as the level of mental alertness. Often the physical transfer adds some temporary discomfort.

The nurse consults the patient's chart to determine when pain medication can be administered, and reminds the patient that the medication will be available when needed. An emesis basin is kept nearby, in case the patient is nauseated from the anesthetic agent.

Immediate assessment of the surgical patient on returning to the clinical unit consists of the following:

- *Respiratory:* Airway patency; depth, rate, and character of respirations; nature of breath sounds
- *Circulatory:* Vital signs including blood pressure; skin condition
- *Neurologic:* Level of responsiveness
- *Drainage:* Presence of drainage; need to connect tubes to a specific drainage system; presence and condition of dressings
- *Comfort:* Type of pain and location; nausea or vomiting; position change required
- *Psychologic:* Nature of patient's questions; need for rest and sleep; disturbance by noise, visitors; availability of call bell or call light
- *Safety:* Need for side rails; drainage tubes unobstructed; IV fluids properly infusing and IV sites properly splinted
- *Equipment:* Checked for proper functioning

Respiratory Assessment. On admission to the clinical unit, the patient is observed for patency of the airway. The quality of respirations is noted, such as depth, rate, and sound. Often, because of pain medications, respirations are slow. Shallow and rapid respirations may be due to pain, constricting dressings, gastric dilatation, or obesity. Noisy breathing may be due to obstruction by secretions or the tongue (see p. 394). The chest is auscultated and the findings are documented as a baseline for later comparisons. Crackles may indicate that secretions are present and need to be coughed up or removed by suctioning. The patient is instructed and assisted to turn, cough, and breathe deeply. Chest physical therapy may be prescribed if indicated.

Circulatory Assessment. The basic consideration in assessing cardiovascular function is monitoring the patient for signs of shock and hemorrhage. The patient's appearance, pulse, respirations, blood pressure, and temperature are used to determine cardiovascular function. Central venous pressure (CVP) and arterial blood gas values are monitored if the patient's condition requires such assessment.

Institutions have specific protocols for postoperative monitoring. Unless indicated more frequently, the pulse, blood pressure and respirations are recorded every 15 minutes for the first 2 hours, and every 30 minutes for the next 2 hours. Thereafter, they are measured less frequently if they remain stable. The temperature is monitored every 4 hours for the first 24 hours.

- A temperature above 37.7°C (100°F) or below 36.1°C (97°F), respirations over 30 or under 16 per minute, and a falling systolic blood pressure under 90 mm Hg are usually considered reportable at once. However, the patient's preoperative or baseline blood pressure is used to make informed postoperative comparisons.
- A previously stable blood pressure that shows a downward trend of 5 mm Hg at each 15-minute reading should also alert the nurse to a problem.

The general condition of the patient is assessed and recorded, including whether skin color is good or cyanotic, whether the skin is cold and clammy or warm and moist, or if there is excessive mucus in the throat and in the nose.

Diagnosis

Nursing Diagnoses

Based on the assessment data, major nursing diagnoses might include the following:

- Ineffective airway clearance related to depressant effects of medications and anesthetic agent
- Pain and other postoperative discomforts
- Risk for altered body temperature: hypothermia
- Risk for injury related to postanesthesia status
- Altered nutrition: Less than body requirements
- Altered urinary elimination related to decreased activity, effects of medications, and reduced intake of fluids
- Constipation related to decreased gastric and intestinal motility during intraoperative period
- Impaired physical mobility related to depressant effects of anesthesia, decreased activity tolerance, and prescribed activity restrictions
- Anxiety about postoperative diagnosis, possible changes in life-style, and alteration in self-concept

Collaborative Problems/ Potential Complications

Based on the assessment data, potential complications may include:

- Altered systemic tissue perfusion secondary to hypovolemia, peripheral blood pooling, and vasoconstriction
- Risk for fluid volume deficit
- Impaired skin integrity related to the surgical incision and drainage sites

- Risk for wound infection related to susceptibility to bacterial invasion

Planning and Implementation

Goals. The major goals of the patient may include optimal respiratory function, relief of pain and postoperative discomforts (nausea and vomiting, abdominal distention, hiccups), maintenance of normal body temperature, freedom from injury, maintenance of nutritional balance, return of normal urinary function, resumption of usual pattern of bowel elimination, restoration of mobility within limitations of postoperative and rehabilitative plan, reduction of anxiety and achievement of psychologic well-being, and absence of complications. These complications include, but are not limited to, impaired tissue perfusion, fluid imbalance, impaired skin integrity, and infection.

Nursing Interventions

Ensuring Optimal Respiratory Function. Measures to maintain a patent airway are carried out as described earlier in this chapter.

Promoting Lung Expansion. To encourage lung expansion and exchange of gas, a variety of measures may be followed. For example, having the patient yawn or take sustained maximal inspirations creates a negative intrathoracic pressure of –40 mm Hg and expands lung volume to total capacity.

At least every 2 hours, the patient is turned and encouraged to take deep breaths. Coughing is also encouraged to dislodge mucus plugs. Careful splinting of abdominal or thoracic incision sites helps the patient overcome the fear that the exertion of coughing might open the incision. Pain medications are administered to permit more effective coughing, and oxygen is administered as prescribed to prevent or relieve hypoxemia or hypoxia. Coughing is contraindicated in patients who have head injuries or who have undergone intracranial surgery (because of risk of increasing intracranial pressure), as well as in patients who have undergone eye surgery (because of increasing intraocular pressure) or plastic surgery (because of increasing tension on delicate tissues).

Incentive Spirometry. Incentive spirometry is a method by which the patient performs sustained maximal inspirations and at the same time sees the results of these efforts as registered on the spirometer. Such motivation encourages the patient to continue to take deep breaths to maximize voluntary lung expansion. The patient is taught how to use the device for maximum effectiveness.

An example of this type of equipment that demonstrates how well the patient is inhaling is shown in Figure 25-2. A goal is established toward which the patient strives. The patient first exhales, then places the lips around the mouthpiece and slowly inhales, trying to drive the piston on the device to a marked goal. Such a device offers several advantages: (1) the patient is encouraged to participate actively in the treatment; (2) it ensures that the maneuver is physiologically appropriate and is repeated; and (3) it is a cost-effective way of preventing complications.

Evaluation: Expected Outcomes. The patient maintains optimal respiratory function.

1. Performs deep-breathing exercises
2. Displays clear breath sounds
3. Uses incentive spirometer as prescribed
4. Exhibits normal body temperature
5. Maintains normal arterial blood gas values
6. Exhibits normal chest x-rays
7. Turns from one position to another as instructed
8. Coughs effectively to clear secretions
9. Exercises and ambulates as prescribed
10. Avoids persons with upper respiratory infections

Relieving Postoperative Discomforts

Relieving Pain. Many psychologic factors (motivational, affective, cognitive, and emotional) influence the patient's total pain experience. Research findings have led to a better understanding of how perception, learning, personality, ethnic and cultural factors, and environment can affect anxiety, depression, and pain. The degree and severity of postoperative pain depend on the physiologic and psychologic makeup of the person, the subsequent tolerance level for pain, the incision site, the nature of the surgical procedure, the extent of surgical trauma, and the type of anesthetic agent and how it was administered. The preoperative preparation received by the patient (including information about what to expect as well as reassurance and psychologic support) is a significant factor in decreasing anxiety, apprehension, and even the pain experienced in the postoperative period.

The reasons for effective pain control are compelling. There is a well known correlation between frequency of complications and localization of pain (Benedetti, 1990). Intense pain stimulates the stress response which adversely affects the cardiac and immune systems. When pain impulses are transmitted, muscle tension increases, as does local vasoconstriction. The ischemia in the affected area causes further stimulation of pain receptors. When these noxious impulses travel centrally, sympathetic activity is compounded, which increases myocardial demand and oxygen consumption. Research has shown that cardiovascular insufficiency occurs three times more frequently and the incidence of infection is five times greater in people with poor postoperative pain control (Benedetti, 1990). Hypothalamic stress response is also responsible for an increase in blood viscosity and platelet aggregation. This can lead to phlebothrombosis and pulmonary embolism.

Opioids. With regard to the need for opioids (narcotics), about one third of patients complain of severe pain, one third of moderate pain, and one third of little or no pain. These statistics do not mean that the patients in the last group have no pain; rather, they appear to activate psychodynamic mechanisms that impair the registering of pain ("gate closing" theory and impaired nociceptive transmission). See Chapter 13 for a more detailed discussion of the gate control theory and other factors that block the transmission of pain sensation.

Opioid analgesics are often prescribed for pain and immediate postoperative restlessness. Although the minimum time between prn doses is prescribed, the time of administration is frequently the function of nursing judgment. However, pain in the first 24 hours after surgery requires relief by opioids, and use of these medications should be encouraged. With the high profile of drug addiction in the last two decades, patients and nurses have underutilized the prn pain order. In reality, although prolonged opioid analgesic treatment for controlling chronic pain may precipitate addiction in a very small number of patients, this is not the case for short-term pain control.

PCA. In view of the negative impact of pain on recovery, nurses need to think "pain prevention" rather than sporadic pain control and encourage the use of patient-controlled analgesia (PCA). Because patients recuperate more quickly when adequate pain measures are utilized, the clinical practice guidelines for postoperative analgesia issued by the Agency for Health Care Policy and Research (AHCPR, 1992) stress prevention rather than pain control and advocate PCA. PCA permits patients to self-administer pain medication when needed. The amount of medication delivered via the intravenous or epidural route and the time span in which the opioid is released is controlled by the PCA device. Self-administration promotes patient participation in care, eliminates delayed administration of pain medications, and maintains a therapeutic level of opioid.

Most patients are candidates for PCA. The two requirements for PCA are (1) an understanding of the need to self dose and (2) the physical ability to self dose. Upon sensing pain, the patient activates the pump with a hand-held button. PCA enables the patient to move, turn, cough, and take deep breaths with less pain, thus reducing postoperative pulmonary problems.

Epidural Infusions and Interpleural Anesthesia. For thoracic and major abdominal surgery, certain opioids may be administered by epidural or intrathecal infusion. Epidural infusions produce a more profound analgesia. These infusions are useful in obstetric and orthopedic surgeries. Epidurals are used with caution in chest procedures because the effect of the analgesia may ascend along the spinal cord and affect respiration. Interpleural anesthesia employs the administration of local anesthetic via catheter between the parietal and visceral pleura. It provides sensory anesthesia without affecting motor function to the intercostal muscles. This anesthesia allows more effective coughing and deep breathing in conditions where pain in the thoracic region would interfere with these functions (*e.g.*, cholecystectomy, renal surgery, and rib fractures).

Interpleural anesthesia has fewer adverse effects than systemic or spinal opioids and less urinary retention, vomiting, and pruritus when compared with a thoracic epidural.

Other Pain Measures. Complete pain relief in the area of the surgical incision may not occur for a few weeks, depending on the site and nature of surgery (Table 21-1). However, changing the patient's position, using distraction, applying cool washcloths to the face, and rubbing the back with a soothing lotion may be useful in relieving general discomfort temporarily and rendering the medication more effective when it is administered.

- The legs should never be rubbed vigorously; vigorous rubbing may dislodge a thrombus and result in fatal embolism.

Relieving Restlessness. Postoperative restlessness may be a symptom of oxygen deficit or hemorrhage, which is also assessed by monitoring vital signs. However, the most common cause is probably general discomfort resulting from the patient lying in one position on the operating table, the surgeon's handling of tissues, and the body's reaction to recovery from the anesthetic. These discomforts may be relieved by administering the prescribed postoperative analgesics and changing the patient's position frequently.

TABLE 21-1 Approximate Incidence, Intensity, and Duration of Surgical Pain

Site	Moderate (%)	Severe (%)	Duration (days)
Upper abdominal	30	70	3
Thoracic	35	65	4
Lower abdominal	55	30	2
Back/lower extremities	30	70	3
Anorectal	40	50	3
Head and neck	45	15	1
Mastectomy	45	15	1

(Adapted from Benedetti C. The pathogenic effects of postoperative pain. In Lipton S, Tunks E, and Zoppi M [eds]. Advances in Pain Research and Therapy, Vol. 13. New York, Raven Press, 1990.)

At the same time, the nurse assesses other possible causes of discomfort, such as tight, drainage-soaked bandages. Reinforcing or changing the dressing completely makes the patient more comfortable. Urinary output is noted, and the bladder is palpated for distention; urinary retention can cause restlessness. If possible, the patient should be helped to assume as normal a position as possible for voiding. Various techniques are used to encourage voiding before catheterization is performed.

Relieving Nausea and Vomiting. Nausea is more common in women, people who are obese (fat cells act as reservoirs for the anesthesia), individuals prone to motion sickness, and patients who have undergone lengthy surgical procedures. With the advent of newer anesthetic agents and antiemetic medications, vomiting has become a less common postoperative phenomenon, although inadequate ventilation during anesthesia can increase the incidence of vomiting. Also, the vomiting that occurs as the patient emerges from anesthesia is frequently an attempt to relieve the stomach of the mucus and saliva swallowed during the anesthetic period.

After surgery, simple symptomatic therapy is usually all that is required. Many authorities believe that most antiemetic medications (usually derivatives of phenothiazine) produce more undesirable effects, such as hypotension and respiratory depression. If a medication is required, short-acting barbiturates are often prescribed. Droperidol (Inapsine) may be prescribed for intravenous or intramuscular use to produce sedation and reduce the incidence of nausea and vomiting. The medication may be administered preoperatively and during surgery; its effects carry over into the postoperative period.

- At the slightest indication of nausea, the patient is turned completely on one side to promote mouth drainage.
- The most important nursing intervention required when vomiting occurs is to prevent aspiration of vom-

itus, which can cause asphyxiation and death (see Chapter 25).

When vomiting is likely because of the nature of surgery, a nasogastric tube is inserted beforehand and remains in place throughout the surgery and the immediate postoperative period. In addition, a nasogastric tube may be inserted when a patient who has food in the stomach requires emergency surgery.

Other causes of postoperative vomiting include an accumulation of fluid in the stomach, inflation of the stomach, and the ingestion of food and fluid before peristalsis returns. Psychologic factors also may play a role; the patient who expects to vomit postoperatively frequently does. Thus, helpful preoperative instruction can reduce the probability of vomiting after surgery.

Some anesthesiologists administer preoperative oral antacids to counteract the **acid-aspiration syndrome**. Otherwise, if acid from the vomitus is aspirated into the lungs, it causes an asthma-like attack, with severe bronchial spasms and wheezing. Patients can subsequently develop pneumonitis and pulmonary edema and become extremely hypoxic.

Increasing medical attention is being paid to silent regurgitation of gastric contents because it occurs more frequently than was previously realized. The importance of *p*H in the etiology of acid aspiration is being studied, as is the value of preoperatively administering an H_2-receptor antagonist such as cimetidine or ranitidine.

Relieving Abdominal Distention. Postoperative distention of the abdomen results from the accumulation of gas in the intestinal tract. Manipulation of the abdominal organs during the surgical procedure may produce a loss of normal peristalsis for 24 to 48 hours, depending on the type and the extent of surgery. Even though nothing is given by mouth, swallowed air and gastrointestinal secretions enter the stomach and the intestines; if not propelled by peristaltic activity, they collect in the intestines, producing distention and causing the patient to complain of fullness or pain in the abdomen. Most often the gas collects in the colon. A rectal tube or catheter may be prescribed on occasion to provide relief.

After major abdominal surgery, distention may be avoided by having the patient turn frequently, exercise, and ambulate when permissible. When postoperative distention is anticipated, a nasogastric tube may be inserted prior to surgery. Swallowing air (often done by patients as part of an anxiety reaction) provides most of the gas that produces distention. The nasogastric tube may remain in place until full peristaltic activity (passage of flatus) has resumed. The nurse can determine when peristaltic bowel sounds return by listening to the abdomen with a stethoscope. The presence of bowel sounds is reported so that the proper diet progression can be prescribed.

Relieving Hiccups. A hiccup is produced by intermittent spasms of the diaphragm and is manifested by a coarse sound (an audible "hic"), a result of the vibration of the closed vocal cords as the air rushes suddenly into the lungs. The cause of the diaphragmatic spasm may be any irritation of the phrenic nerve from its center in the spinal cord to its terminal ramifications on the undersurface of the diaphragm. This irritation may be (1) direct—such as stimulation of the nerve itself by a distended stomach, peritonitis or subdiaphragmatic abscess, abdominal distention, pleurisy, or tumors in the chest pressing on the nerves; (2) indirect—such as from toxemia or uremia that stimulates the center; or (3) reflexive—such as irritation from a drainage tube, exposure to cold, drinking very hot or very cold fluids, or obstruction of the intestines.

Hiccups occur occasionally after abdominal surgery. Usually, these occurrences are mild, transitory attacks that cease spontaneously or with very simple treatment. When hiccups persist, they may produce considerable distress and serious effects, such as vomiting, exhaustion, and possibly wound dehiscence.

The multitude of remedies suggested for the relief of hiccups is proof that no one treatment is effective in every situation. The best remedy is to eliminate causes, such as fluids that are too hot or too cold. Probably the most efficient of the older and simpler remedies is to hold the breath while taking swallows of water. Prescription of phenothiazine medications has been helpful on occasion. Another method is finger pressure on closed eyelids for several minutes. Induced vomiting has helped in some instances.

Evaluation: Expected Outcomes. The patient experiences relief of pain and postoperative discomforts (restlessness, nausea and vomiting, abdominal distention, and hiccups).

1. Indicates that pain is decreased in intensity
2. Splints incision site when coughing to reduce pain
3. Participates in distraction strategies (*e.g.*, conversation, television)
4. Reports absence of nausea; no vomiting
5. Is free of abdominal distress and gas pains
6. Demonstrates the absence of hiccups

Maintaining Normal Body Temperature. Patients who have been anesthetized are susceptible to chills and drafts. A patient who has undergone prolonged exposure to cold in the operating room and received large amounts of intravenous infusions is monitored for potential hypothermia. Signs of hypothermia are reported to the physician. The room is maintained at a comfortable temperature and blankets are provided to prevent chilling. The patient is also monitored for cardiac dysrhythmias. The risks of hypothermia are greater in the elderly and in those patients who have been in the cool operating room environment for a prolonged period of time.

Evaluation: Expected Outcomes. The patient maintains normal body temperature.

1. Exhibits normal core body temperature
2. Is free of chills
3. Shows no signs of shivering
4. Experiences no cardiac dysrhythmias

Avoiding Injury. A patient emerging from anesthesia may display restless behavior. If at all possible, restraints should not be used. However, the patient must be protected from causing self injury or interfering with IV therapy, tubes, and monitoring equipment. To reduce the restlessness associated with pain, analgesics and sedatives are administered as prescribed. The possible causes of discomfort that can affect subconscious cognition include dressings that are too tight, pressure on a nerve due to improper positioning, irritating drainage, leakage of IV fluids, or a hot water bottle that is too hot. Through careful monitoring as the patient emerges from the anesthetic, the nurse can detect problems before they cause injury.

Evaluation: Expected Outcomes. The patient:

1. Avoids injury
2. Accepts side rails in raised position when required
3. Is free from injury related to faulty position, falling, other hazards
4. Attains normal sensorium

Maintaining Normal Nutritional Status. Following surgery, the sooner the patient can tolerate a usual diet, the more quickly normal gastrointestinal function will resume. Taking food by mouth stimulates digestive juices and promotes gastric function and intestinal peristalsis. Exercise in bed or early ambulation also assists the digestive process and prevents such problems as distention, "gas pains," and constipation.

The return to normal dietary intake should proceed at the pace set by the individual patient. Of course, the nature of surgery and the type of anesthesia directly affect the rate of return. Once the patient has completely recovered from the effects of anesthesia and is no longer nauseated, a normal diet is instituted.

Liquids are usually the first substances desired and tolerated by the patient after surgery. Water, fruit juices, and tea may be given in increasing amounts if vomiting does not occur and when peristalsis returns. The fluids administered should be cool, not ice cold or tepid. Because fluids supply relatively few calories, soft foods (gelatin, junket, custard, milk, and creamed soups) that supply additional calories and nutrients are added gradually after clear fluids have been tolerated. As soon as the patient tolerates soft foods well, solid food may be given.

- When surgery has been performed on the gastrointestinal tract, peristalsis takes longer to return.

Following gastrointestinal surgery, a nasogastric or gastrointestinal tube is usually in place for the first 24 to 48 hours. Such decompression tubes remove flatus and secretions. Attention is given to maintaining proper fluid and electrolyte balance. Parenteral fluids or total parenteral nutrition may be prescribed to provide nutrients, fluid, and electrolytes (see Chapter 35).

When nothing is given by mouth postoperatively, conscientious oral hygiene is required. A clean, refreshed mouth diminishes nausea and promotes the appetite when eating is resumed. Weighing the patient daily provides an indication of progress.

If the patient is unable to consume an adequate dietary intake, total parenteral nutrition or enteral feedings may be needed to assure that nutrients are available for healing to occur.

Evaluation: Expected Outcomes. The patient maintains nutritional balance.

1. Exhibits increased gastrointestinal motility and absence of paralytic ileus; bowel sounds normal
2. Resumes normal dietary patterns when appropriate
3. Gains weight to return to baseline

Promoting Normal Urinary Function. The time a patient may be permitted to go without voiding after surgery varies considerably with the type of surgical procedure performed.

- Generally, every effort is made to avoid the use of a catheter because of the risk of urinary tract infection.

All known methods to aid the patient in voiding should be tried (*e.g.*, letting water run, applying heat to the perineum). A bedpan should be warm; a cold bedpan causes discomfort and automatic tightening of muscles (including the urethral sphincter). When a patient complains of not being able to use the bedpan, it may be permissible to use a commode rather than resort to catheterization. Male patients are often permitted to sit up or stand beside the bed to use the urinal, but safeguards should be taken to prevent the patient from falling or fainting.

- All urine, whether voided or obtained by catheterization, is measured and the amount noted on the patient's record.
- Intake and output are recorded for all patients following urologic or complex operative procedures and for all elderly patients.
- A urine output of less than 30 ml for each of 2 consecutive hours is reported.

Evaluation: Expected Outcomes. Normal urinary function returns.

1. Voids adequately without use of a catheter
2. Demonstrates absence of frequent small amounts in voiding (indicative of retention)
3. Assumes responsibility for adequate intake of fluids

Promoting Bowel Elimination. Preoperative bowel preparation, immobility, possible intestinal manipulation during surgery, and reduced oral intake can all affect bowel function. Increased fluid intake and early ambulation can facilitate the return of bowel sounds and peristalsis. Abdominal auscultation with a stethoscope is used to detect the presence of bowel sounds; if bowel sounds are heard, the patient's diet is gradually increased.

Paralytic ileus is a complication that may occur after intestinal or abdominal surgery. It is characterized by the absence of bowel sounds (no peristalsis) and discomfort and distention of the abdomen (denoted by complaints of abdominal tightness and increased abdominal girth). The condition may even result in reverse peristalsis, which causes nausea and vomiting, and possibly the vomiting of fecal material. Insertion of a nasogastric tube is ordered and, depending on the patient's condition, intravenous fluids or total parenteral nutrition may be indicated.

Constipation. The causes of constipation after surgery may be minor or serious. Irritation and trauma to the bowel during surgery may inhibit intestinal movement for several days, but usually peristalsis returns after the third day, following the combined effect of early ambulation, an increase in diet, and perhaps a laxative, suppository, or enema (if prescribed). If constipation results from secondary conditions (*e.g.*, local inflammation, peritonitis, or abscess), treatment of the cause is indicated. Constipation has been described as difficult or infrequent passage of stools.

It is important to note that many people are constipated habitually and often give a history of daily laxative use for many years. Attempts should be made to correct their bowel habits as soon as is practical. However, in some instances, especially with elderly patients, these attempts may not be feasible. If fluids, roughage, and bulk laxatives are ineffective, enemas are used to evacuate the lower bowel. Laxatives may be prescribed by the physician.

Evaluation: Expected Outcomes. The patient resumes normal bowel function.

1. Exhibits normal and effective bowel sounds on auscultation
2. Is free of abdominal distress, gas pains, and constipation
3. Demonstrates usual bowel elimination pattern

Restoring Mobility. Hampered by dressings, splints, or drainage apparatus, the patient frequently is unable to change position. Lying constantly in the same position may lead to pressure ulcers or hypostatic pneumonia, to mention only two of the more serious resulting complications.

- The patient with limited mobility must be turned from side to side at least every 2 hours. The patient's position must be changed when discomfort occurs from lying in one position.

Positioning. Following surgery, the patient may be placed in a variety of positions (depending on the nature of the surgical procedure) to promote comfort and ease pain.

Supine Position. The patient lies on the back without elevation of the head. In most cases, this is the position in which the patient is placed immediately after surgery. Bed covers should not restrict the movement of the patient's toes and feet.

Lateral Position. The patient lies on either side with the upper arm forward. The bottom leg is slightly flexed, while the upper leg is flexed at the thigh and the knee. The patient's head is supported on a pillow, and a second pillow is placed longitudinally between the legs. This position is used when it is desirable to have the patient change positions frequently; to aid in the drainage of cavities, such as the chest and abdomen; and to prevent postoperative respiratory and circulatory complications.

Fowler's Position. Of all the positions prescribed for a patient, Fowler's position is perhaps the most common, as well as the most difficult to maintain. The difficulty in most instances lies in trying to make the patient fit the bed rather than having the bed conform to the needs of the patient.

The patient's trunk is raised to an angle of 60 to 70 degrees. This is a comfortable sitting position. Patients with abdominal drainage usually are put in Fowler's position as soon as they have recovered consciousness, but the head of the bed must be raised slowly to reduce the feeling of lightheadedness.

- It is not unusual for a patient to feel faint after the head of the bed is raised; for this reason, pulse rate and color must be assessed frequently. If the patient complains of any dizziness, the bed must be slowly lowered. If the dizziness ends, the head of the bed may be raised again in 1 to 2 hours.

The nurse must determine whether the patient is in correct position and comfortable. Often, very short people are most uncomfortable in the ordinary hospital bed and must be supported by pillows. It is advisable to place a support against the feet to prevent the patient from slipping down in bed and to make the patient feel more secure. Even with these measures, it will be necessary to move the patient up in bed frequently and to readjust the pillows.

Ambulation. Most surgical patients are encouraged to be out of bed as soon as indicated. This is determined by the stability of a patient's cardiovascular and neuromuscular systems, the usual level of physical activity, and the nature of the surgery performed. Following spinal anesthesia, minor surgery, and same-day surgery, the patient ambulates on the day of surgery.

- The advantage of early ambulation is that it reduces the incidence of postoperative complications such as atelectasis, hypostatic pneumonia, gastrointestinal discomfort, and circulatory problems.

Atelectasis and hypostatic pneumonia are relatively infrequent when the patient is ambulatory, because ambulation increases ventilation and reduces stasis of bronchial secretions in the lung. Ambulation also reduces the possibility of postoperative abdominal distention because it helps to increase the tone of the gastrointestinal tract and the abdominal wall and stimulates peristalsis.

Thrombophlebitis or phlebothrombosis occurs less frequently because early ambulation prevents stasis of blood by increasing the rate of circulation in the extremities. The rate of healing in abdominal wounds is more rapid when ambulation is started early; the occurrence of postoperative evisceration in a series of cases was actually less frequent when patients were allowed to be out of bed soon after surgery. Studies also indicate that pain is decreased when early ambulation is allowed. Comparative records show that the pulse rate and the temperature return to normal sooner when the patient attempts to regain normal preoperative activity as quickly as possible. Finally, the hospital stay is shorter and less costly, a further advantage to the patient and the hospital.

Early ambulation should not exceed the patient's tolerance. The condition of the patient must be the deciding factor, and a progression of steps is followed in mobilizing the patient:

- First, with nursing support and encouragement, and with safety as the main concern, the patient is helped to move gradually from the lying position to the sitting position until any evidence of dizziness has passed. This position can be achieved by raising the head of the bed.
- The patient may then be placed completely upright and turned so that both legs hang over the edge of the bed.
- After this preparation, the patient may be helped to stand beside the bed.

When accustomed to the upright position, the patient may start to walk. The nurse should be at the patient's side to give physical support and encouragement. Care must be taken not to tire the patient; the extent of the first few periods of ambulation varies with the type of surgical procedure and the patient's physical condition and age.

Bed Exercises. When early ambulation is not feasible, bed exercises may achieve some degree of desirable results. General exercises should begin as soon after surgery as possible—preferably within the first 24 hours—and are performed under supervision to ensure that they are done properly and in a safe manner. The purpose of these exercises is to promote circulation and prevent the development of contractures as well as to permit the patient the fullest return of physiologic functions. Such exercises include the following:

- Deep-breathing exercises for complete lung expansion
- Arm exercises through the full range of motion, with specific attention to abduction and external rotation of the shoulder
- Hand and finger exercises
- Foot exercises to prevent foot drop and toe deformities and to aid in maintaining good circulation
- Leg flexion and leg lifting exercises to prepare the patient for ambulation activities
- Abdominal and gluteal contraction exercises

Evaluation: Expected Outcomes. The patient resumes mobility within the limitations of the postoperative and rehabilitation plan.

1. Alternates periods of rest and activity
2. Progressively increases ambulation
3. Resumes normal activities within prescribed time frame
4. Performs activities related to self-care
5. Participates in a rehabilitation program (when appropriate)

Reducing Anxiety and Achieving Psychosocial Well-Being. Almost all postoperative patients need psychologic support during the immediate postoperative period. When the patient's condition permits, a close member of the family may visit for a few moments. Thus, the patient feels more secure and the family is reassured.

The questions posed by a patient in PACU often indicate concerns about the outcome of the surgery and thoughts about the future. Whatever the patient's concern, the nurse should be in a position to answer queries reassuringly without going into a discussion of details. While the immediate postoperative period is not the time for discussion of surgical findings or prognosis, these questions should not be dismissed lightly because they may offer clues to the patient's concerns.

As the patient moves through the early postoperative phases, measures are implemented to provide feelings of stability. This is accomplished by assuring the patient that a nurse is available to listen, to reinforce the explanations of the physician, and to correct any misconceptions. The patient is instructed in relaxation techniques and diversional activities. Significant others are included in instructional sessions to assist the patient at home. Projections are made about home care needs following discharge, and home-care visits may be arranged if needed.

Evaluation: Expected Outcomes. The patient attains/maintains psychosocial well-being.

- Participates in self-care activities
- Takes time for grooming
- Talks positively about future plans
- Asks questions about resuming sexual relations
- Expresses anticipation about seeing friends and family

Collaborative Interventions

Maintaining Adequate Tissue Perfusion. The patient is monitored for any signs and symptoms suggesting diminished tissue perfusion: a decreasing blood pressure; inadequate O_2 saturation; rapid or labored respirations; resting pulse greater than 100 beats per minute; restlessness; slow responses; cold, clammy, pale, or cyanotic skin; diminished or absent peripheral pulses; or urine output less than 30 ml/hr. Any one of these signs and symptoms is reported.

Measures are initiated to maintain adequate tissue perfusion. Depending on the cause of inadequate tissue perfusion, measures that may be initiated include fluid replacement, blood component therapy, medications to support or improve cardiac function (*e.g.*, coronary vasodilators, antidysrhythmics, inotropic agents), and administration of oxygen.

The patient's response to these measures is monitored and documented. In addition, the room temperature is kept comfortable and the patient is provided with sufficient clothing and blankets to prevent chilling, which causes vasoconstriction. The effects of fluid and blood component therapy are monitored.

Activities, such as leg exercises, are initiated to stimulate circulation and the patient is encouraged to turn and change position slowly and to avoid positions that compromise venous return. Venous return is compromised by a raised knee gatch or pillow under the knees, sitting for long periods, and dangling the legs with pressure at the back of the knees. Venous return is promoted by prescribed antiembolitic stockings and ambulation. The patient is assisted to get out of bed and walk; antiemboli stockings are applied before the patient gets out of bed and are removed only during daily bathing.

Maintaining Adequate Fluid Volume. A considerable loss of body fluids occurs with surgery as a result of increased perspiration, increased mucus secretion in the lungs, and loss of blood. To combat the loss of fluids, solutions are administered intravenously for the first few hours after surgery. Even though an adequate amount of fluid is taken by this method, often it does not relieve thirst.

Thirst is also a troublesome symptom after many general anesthetics, and even after local anesthesia. It stems largely from the dryness of the mouth and the pharynx caused by the inhibition of mucus secretion after the usual preoperative medication of atropine. Many patients who receive local anesthesia complain of thirst during the surgical procedure.

Because a sticky, dry mouth demands moisture, fluids may be given to most patients as soon as the postoperative nausea and vomiting have passed and bowel sounds are present. Sips of hot tea with lemon juice dissolve the mucus better than cold water does. As soon as the patient can take water by mouth in sufficient quantities, intravenous administration of fluids is discontinued.

The patient is observed for evidence of electrolyte imbalance: weakness, lassitude, nausea, vomiting, irritability, and possibly neuromuscular abnormalities. Monitoring of mental status, skin color, and temperature is continued, and the presence and quality of peripheral pulses are noted. Signs of decreasing tissue perfusion are reported. The elderly patient is especially at risk for fluid and electrolyte imbalances:

- *Signs of hypovolemia:* Decreased blood pressure, tachycardia, reduced urinary output, CVP less than 4 cm H_2O

- *Signs of hypervolemia:* Increased blood pressure, CVP greater than 15 cm H_2O, crackles in lung bases (wet), S_3 gallop

Intravenous administration of fluid and electrolyte solutions continues into the postoperative period to assure fluid and electrolyte balance. Electrolyte levels, vital signs, and urine output are monitored closely and abnormalities are reported so that appropriate treatment can be initiated.

Preventing Infection. Between 10% and 15% of surgical patients develop nosocomial (hospital-acquired) infections. Most of these are in one of four anatomic sites: surgical wound, urinary tract, bloodstream, or respiratory tract. The infections occur for several reasons:

- Intact skin and mucous membranes have been invaded by tubes and catheters, by the disease process, or by the surgical procedure.
- The effects of anesthesia and surgery reduce the resistance of the body to infection.
- The patient may be exposed to infectious agents during hospitalization.
- The organisms that are found in hospital-acquired infections are widespread and resistant to antibiotics (*e.g., Staphylococcus aureus,* methicillin-resistant *Staphylococcus aureus* [MRSA], *Escherichia coli, Pseudomonas, Klebsiella pneumoniae, Proteus* and *Clostridium difficile* [C-dif]).
- There are breaks in aseptic technique and may be inadequate hand-washing practices.

When postoperative infections occur, healing is delayed, convalescence is prolonged, functional recovery may be impaired, and death may occur. These complications impose serious burdens on the patient, the family, other patients (cross-contamination and consequent cross-infections), hospital staff (the increased patient care and hospitalization required), and society as a whole (increased hospitalization, insurance costs, and loss of work force).

Effective infection control is carried out postoperatively by encouraging the patient to cough and take deep breaths and by frequent turning. These measures prevent secretions from being retained and possibly causing atelectasis, lung congestion, and pneumonia. The use of sterile equipment (needles, cannulae, dressings), including equipment for respiratory care, prevents transmission of pathogenic organisms. Antibiotics may be prescribed prophylactically by the physician when infections are encountered, and antimicrobials may be prescribed for specific identified organisms in established infections.

The nurse plays a key role in infection control by practicing aseptic technique, by conscientiously monitoring and instructing others, and by administering antibiotics and antimicrobial medications as prescribed.

- Conscientious hand washing is essential for every person who comes in contact with patients and is performed before and after each patient contact.
- Prevention of skin breakdown and infection are of even greater importance in the patient with a compromised immune system (*i.e.,* AIDS, leukemia, cancer, malnutrition).

Dressings are inspected periodically to detect signs of hemorrhage or abnormal drainage. When incisions are on the anterior part of the body, the posterior area is inspected for bleeding, because gravity enables seepage to accumulate in an area quite removed from the incision. Dressings should be reinforced if necessary, and the time of dressing changes noted on the patient's chart. (Dressings and care of the incision are discussed in detail on p. 417.)

Judicious control of upper respiratory infections and skin lesions must be practiced. A common cause of infections is contamination related to intravenous infusions (see p. 243 for methods of control); therefore, recommendations for replacing intravenous lines and other invasive devices must be followed.

Decision Making Guidelines

Determining the significance of the signs and symptoms noted in assessing the patient requires judgment and critical thinking. When viewed in isolation, one sign may be of little importance, but in the broader context it may be significant in assessment of the patient.

There are a few general guidelines that may assist in guiding the nurse to make accurate judgments and determine when collaboration with the physician is warranted. Of course, any severe symptom is always important.

- Any apparently minor symptom that tends to recur repeatedly or to increase in severity should be regarded as significant—for example, hiccups may or may not be of importance, depending on their duration.
- A symptom may seem insignificant in itself but when associated with other definite changes may signal danger. For example, a repeated sigh, when accompanied by increasing restlessness, pallor, and a rising pulse rate, may be one of the clinical signs of dangerous hemorrhage.
- Any steadily progressive decline in the general condition of the patient, even with no outstanding symptoms evident, is of grave importance.
- The patient's complaints and statements should never be dismissed without investigation.

Documenting information accurately and concisely not only informs all medical and nursing personnel of the patient's condition but also satisfies medicolegal requirements.

If a physician is to be notified for any reason, all necessary information should be at hand before the physician is contacted by phone, including the patient's latest vital signs. It is also advisable to take the patient's chart, including nursing records, to the telephone to refer to them should questions arise.

Postoperative Complications

The danger inherent in surgery involves not only the risk of the surgical procedure but also the hazard of postoperative complications that may prolong convalescence or adversely affect the surgical outcome. The nurse plays an important part in the prevention of these complications and collaborates with the physician and other members of the health care team in their management, should they occur. Major postoperative complications include shock; hemorrhage; deep vein thrombosis; pulmonary embolism; respiratory complications, such as hypoxemia, atelectasis, and pneumonia, among others; urinary retention; intestinal obstruction; and possible postoperative psychosis. The signs and symptoms of these postoperative complications will be discussed, along with the most effective method of prevention and the usual medical and nursing management.

Shock

Shock is one of the most serious postoperative complications. Shock may be described as inadequate cellular oxygenation accompanied by the inability to excrete waste products of metabolism. Although there are many kinds of shock, the basic definition of shock in general centers on an inadequate blood flow to vital organs or the inability of the tissues of these organs to utilize oxygen and other nutrients (see Chapter 15 for a detailed discussion of shock).

The classic signs of shock are:

- Pallor
- Cool, moist skin
- Rapid breathing
- Cyanosis of the lips, gums, and tongue
- A rapid, weak, thready pulse
- Decreasing pulse pressure
- Usually, a low blood pressure and concentrated urine

Two classifications of shock that can occur in surgical patients are hypovolemic and neurogenic shock. **Hypovolemic shock** is caused by decreased fluid volume from blood or plasma loss; it is the most common type of shock in surgical patients. In the surgical patient, hypovolemic shock may be caused by frank hemorrhage, loss of blood and plasma from the circulation during the surgical procedure, or inadequate fluid replacement during and after surgery. Hypovolemic shock is characterized by a fall in venous pressure, a rise in peripheral resistance, and tachycardia.

Neurogenic shock is a less common cause of shock in the surgical patient; it may, however, occur as a result of decreased arterial resistance caused by spinal anesthesia. It is characterized by a fall in blood pressure due to pooling of blood in dilated capacitance vessels (those with the ability to change volume capacity). Heart activity increases in response and thus maintains a normal output (stroke volume); this helps to fill the dilated vascular system as it attempts to preserve perfusion pressure.

Prevention

The best treatment for shock is prophylaxis or prevention. This consists of assuring optimal physical status prior to surgery and anticipating any complication that may arise during or after surgery. Special equipment for the treatment of shock must be available. The proper type of anesthesia should be chosen by the anesthesiologist after careful consideration of the patient and the disorder. Blood and blood component therapy should be available if indicated. Blood loss should be measured as accurately as possible.

- If the amount of blood loss exceeds 500 ml (especially if the loss is rapid), replacement is usually indicated.

The individual patient and the particular circumstances must be considered in determining replacement therapy. An older, malnourished person is more likely to require this therapy than a younger patient whose health is generally good.

Surgical trauma should be kept at a minimum as the first step in avoiding shock. After surgery, the factors that may contribute to shock are avoided. For example, pain is controlled by making the patient as comfortable as possible and by using narcotics judiciously. Exposure is avoided, and lightweight, unheated bed linens are used to prevent vasodilation. In the PACU, the patient is monitored closely. In addition, a quiet room helps to reduce stress. The patient is moved gently and placed in a supine position to facilitate circulation. Vital signs are monitored continuously until the patient's recovery indicates that shock is unlikely.

Treatment

The patient is kept warm; however, overheating is avoided to prevent cutaneous vessels from dilating and depriving vital organs of blood. An infusion of lactated Ringer's solution is started. The patient is placed flat in bed with legs elevated. Respiratory and pulse rate, blood pressure, O_2 concentration, urinary output, level of consciousness, central venous pressure, pulmonary artery pressure, pulmonary capillary wedge pressure, and cardiac output provide information about the patient's respiratory and cardiovascular status.

The basic approach to the treatment of shock is to determine its cause and correct it if possible. Prevention strategies are described as follows.

Assure Respiratory Status. Blood gas determinations are made to assess pulmonary function, and oxygen is administered by intubation or nasal cannula if indicated.

Restore Blood/Fluid Volume. The type of fluid and blood replacement depends on the type and amount lost as well as the condition of the patient. Fluids are administered intravenously immediately when the nature of loss is determined. Fluid replacement is modified accordingly. Under normal conditions, 20% of the total blood volume is in the capillaries, 10% is in the arterial system, and the balance is in the veins and heart. In shock the capillary beds dilate, causing a considerable volume of blood to accumulate there.

Fluids administered may include crystalloids (*e.g.*, lactated Ringers's solution) and colloids (*e.g.*, blood component therapy, albumin, plasma, or plasma substitutes). Because large volumes of fluids may be administered intravenously, the patient must be monitored closely for desired effects as well as unanticipated, untoward effects. Several intravenous lines may be used for administering fluids, and arterial lines may be inserted for hemodynamic monitoring.

Drug Therapy. Cardiotonics are administered to correct dysrhythmias and improve cardiac efficiency. Diuretics are administered to reduce fluid retention and edema during and following neurosurgery.

Vasodilators are prescribed to reduce peripheral resistance, which in turn decreases the work of the heart and increases cardiac output and tissue perfusion. The medication frequently used is sodium nitroprusside (Nipride), which stimulates myocardial contractility and lowers peripheral resistance. An infusion pump is used to control the amount of sodium nitroprusside that is administered. Monitors are also available to measure the patient's blood pressure every 10 seconds and automatically adjust the drug dosage if there are any changes.

Some clinicians advocate the use of steroids, while others use combinations of pharmacotherapeutic agents. Some authorities believe that hypovolemic shock should not be treated with vasoactive medications, because they increase vascular resistance and decrease tissue perfusion, thus aggravating the effects of shock.

Nursing Interventions

The nurse assists in carrying out the prescribed treatments. When vasodilators are prescribed, the patient's blood pressure must be monitored constantly. The patient is kept flat while these medications are administered. If the systolic blood pressure continues to fall, the medication is stopped and fluids are increased.

The following nursing measures are indicated:

1. Psychologic support is provided, and the patient's energy expenditure is reduced. The patient's reactions to treatment are assessed, and rest is promoted. Support and reassurance are provided to relieve apprehension. Sedatives are administered cautiously so that circulation is not further depressed.
2. The patient is kept warm, because hypothermia decreases tissue oxygenation. Hypothermia also affects peripheral circulation.
3. The patient is turned every 2 hours, and deep breathing is encouraged to promote optimal cardiopulmonary function.
4. Complications are prevented by observing all parameters and monitoring the patient closely in the 24-hour period following onset of shock. The most common complications are peripheral and pulmonary edema due to fluid overload, resulting from administering fluids faster than the body can accommodate them.
5. All observations and interventions are documented.

See Chapter 15 for a detailed discussion of shock and its management.

Hemorrhage

Hemorrhage is classified as (1) **primary,** (2) **intermediary,** and (3) **secondary.** Primary hemorrhage occurs at the time of surgery. Intermediary hemorrhage occurs during the first few hours after surgery when the rise of blood pressure to its normal level dislodges insecure clots from untied vessels. Secondary hemorrhage may occur some time after surgery if a ligature slips because a blood vessel was insecurely tied or became infected or was eroded by a drainage tube.

A further classification frequently is made according to the kind of vessel that is bleeding. **Capillary hemorrhage** is characterized by a slow, general ooze; **venous hemorrhage** bubbles out quickly and is dark in color; **arterial hemorrhage** is bright and appears in spurts with each heartbeat.

Hemorrhage is also characterized by its visibility: when the hemorrhage is on the surface and can be seen, it is **evident;** when it cannot be seen, as in the peritoneal cavity, it is **concealed.**

Clinical Manifestations

The clinical signs presented by hemorrhage depend on the amount of blood lost and how quickly it is lost. The patient is apprehensive and restless, moves continually, and is thirsty; the skin is cold, moist, and pale. The pulse rate increases, the temperature falls, and respirations are rapid and deep, often of the gasping type spoken of as "air hunger." If the hemorrhage progresses untreated, cardiac output decreases, arterial and venous blood pressure and the hemoglobin of the blood fall rapidly, the lips and the conjunctivae become pallid, spots appear before the eyes, a ringing is heard in the ears, and the patient grows weaker but remains conscious until near death.

Management

Often the signs of hemorrhage after surgery are masked by the effects of the anesthetic or shock; therefore, the initial treatment of the patient is in a general way almost identical to that described for the patient with shock (see previous section).

The patient is placed in the shock position (lying flat on back with legs elevated at a 20° angle while knees are kept straight). Sedatives or analgesics are administered as prescribed. The wound should always be inspected for bleeding. If bleeding is evident, a sterile gauze pad and a snug bandage are applied and the site of the bleeding is elevated to the level of the heart, if possible.

- Giving a transfusion of blood or blood products and determining the cause of hemorrhage are the initial therapeutic measures.
- When intravenous fluids are given in cases of hemorrhage, it is important to remember that unless the hemorrhage has been well controlled, giving too large a quantity or administering the intravenous fluid too rapidly may raise the blood pressure enough to start the bleeding again.

Deep Venous Thrombosis (DVT)

Deep venous thrombosis (DVT) is a thrombosis of deep rather than superficial veins. Two serious complications of DVT are pulmonary embolism and postphlebitic syndrome (see p. 407).

Incidence

Postoperatively, those at greatest risk for DVT have been identified as follows:

- Orthopedic patients having hip surgery, knee reconstruction, and other lower extremity surgery
- Urologic patients having transurethral prostatectomy, and older patients having urologic surgery
- General surgical patients over age 40, those who are obese, those with a malignancy, those who have had

prior DVT or pulmonary embolism, or those undergoing extensive, complicated surgical procedures
- Gynecology (and obstetric) patients over age 40 with added risk factors (varicose veins, previous venous thrombosis, infection, malignancy, obesity)
- Neurosurgical patients, similar to other surgical high-risk groups (in patients with stroke, for example, the risk of DVT in the paralyzed leg is as high as 75%)

Pathophysiology

A mild to severe inflammation of the vein occurs in association with a clotting of blood. The complication may result from a number of causes, including injury to the vein caused by tight straps or leg-holders at the time of surgery, pressure from a blanket roll under the knees, hemoconcentration from loss of fluid or dehydration, or, more commonly, the slowing of the blood flow in the extremity due to a lowered metabolism and depression of the circulation after surgery. It is probable that several of these factors interact to produce thrombosis. The left leg is affected more frequently.

Clinical Manifestations

The first symptom of DVT may be a pain or a cramp in the calf as elicited by Homans' sign (Fig. 21-4). Pressure there causes pain, and a day or so later a painful swelling of the entire leg occurs, often accompanied by a slight fever and sometimes chills and perspiration. The swelling is a soft edema that pits easily on pressure.

A milder form of the same disease is termed **phlebothrombosis,** to indicate intravascular clotting without marked inflammation of the vein. The clotting occurs usually in the veins of the calf, often with few symptoms except slight soreness of the calf. The danger from this type of thrombosis is that the clot may be dislodged, producing an embolus. It is believed that most pulmonary emboli arise from this source. Figure 21-4 describes the methods for assessing the signs and symptoms of phlebothrombosis.

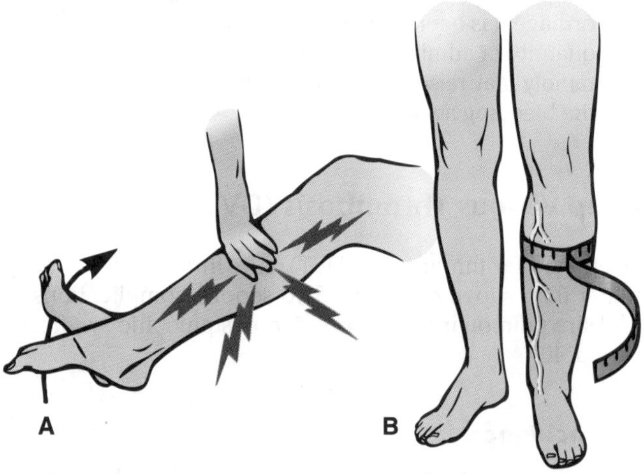

FIGURE 21-4. Assessment of signs and symptoms of phlebothrombosis. (**A**) With the knee flexed, the patient may complain of pain in the calf on dorsiflexion of foot (Homans' sign). This is a sign of early and subclinical thrombosis; it may or may not be present. Gentle compression reveals tenderness of the calf muscles (note arrow). (**B**) The affected leg may swell; veins are more prominent and may be palpated easily. (Suddarth DS. The Lippincott Manual of Nursing Practice, 5th ed. Philadelphia, JB Lippincott, 1991.)

Prevention

Efforts directed toward preventing the formation of a thrombus include such measures as leg exercises that can be taught before surgery (see Chapter 19, Figs. 19-3 and 19-4). A patient who recognizes the significance of these exercises in preventing circulatory complications often initiates the exercises without being prompted. To avoid thrombus formation, leg straps should not be fastened in the PACU. Stretchers that are equipped with side rails provide sufficient protection. Not only do the straps restrict patient motion, but they can constrict and impair circulation.

Low-dose heparin may be prescribed and administered subcutaneously until the patient is ambulatory. Low-dose warfarin is another possible anticoagulant. Dextran 40 and dextran 70 (low and high molecular weight, respectively) are plasma expanders that reduce the formation of microscopic clots triggered by hemoconcentration. Although comparable to anticoagulants in effectiveness, they are more expensive. External pneumatic compression and gradient elastic stockings can be used alone or in combination with low-dose heparin.

The adrenergic blocking agent dehydroergotamine has also been used with low-dose heparin; some claim that it is more efficacious, but the potential risks of vasoconstriction and its contraindications must be recognized. Aspirin alone has not been shown to be beneficial, but because aspirin increases the effect of anticoagulants, it should not be taken with them.

In addition to the nursing measures cited above, it is important to avoid the use of blanket rolls, pillow rolls, or any form of elevation that can constrict vessels under the knees. Even prolonged "dangling" (having the patient sit on the edge of the bed with legs hanging over the side) can be dangerous and is not recommended in susceptible individuals because pressure under the knees can impede circulation.

No one method is ideal, but prophylactic measures that are tailored to meet individual needs can be effective in markedly reducing what otherwise can be a serious, potentially lethal complication.

Treatment

Some surgeons consider ligation of the femoral veins to be an important therapeutic method. The rationale behind this method of therapy is to prevent pulmonary embolism by eliminating the cause (thrombi that could dislodge from the walls of the femoral veins and circulate in the blood).

Anticoagulant therapy has assumed a prominent place in the treatment of phlebitis and phlebothrombosis. Heparin (a thrombin inactivator), administered intravenously or subcutaneously, reduces the coagulability of the blood and is used most often when an immediate effect is desired. Repeated checks of the coagulation time or partial thromboplastin time of the blood are necessary to control its administration. Dicumarol or warfarin (Coumadin; a clotting factor inactivator) is used for the same purpose. It is given by mouth and does not become effective for about 24 hours. Dosage is controlled by daily estimations of the prothrombin time of the blood (see also p. 755).

High elastic (antiembolitic) stockings have been used as an active treatment of phlebitis and thrombosis. These toe-to-groin stockings prevent swelling and stagnation of venous blood in the legs and do much to relieve pain in the affected extremity. However, to be effective, elastic stockings must be used in combination with leg elevation and leg exercises. Early ambulation is helpful, but the nurse also needs to be aware that when a patient with a protruding abdomen walks a few steps and then sits with legs dependent, the pressure of the abdomen can obstruct venous flow.

Pulmonary Embolism

An **embolus** is a foreign body (blood clot, air, fat) that becomes dislodged from its original site and is carried along in the bloodstream.

When the embolus travels to the right side of the heart and completely occludes the pulmonary artery, the symptoms are sudden and startling. A patient experiencing an apparently normal convalescence suddenly cries out with sharp, stabbing pains in the chest and becomes breathless, diaphoretic, anxious, and cyanotic. The pupils dilate, the pulse becomes rapid and irregular; sudden death may occur.

Fortunately, pulmonary embolism usually causes partial, rather than complete, occlusion of the pulmonary vasculature, and the patient has signs of mild dyspnea (labored breathing), dysrhythmia, or seemingly innocent chest pain. Alertness on the part of the nurse is necessary to detect these small embolic episodes so that early treatment may be initiated and further embolization avoided.

- Early postoperative ambulation reduces the risk of pulmonary embolism.

See Chapter 24 for a full discussion of pulmonary embolus.

Respiratory Complications

Respiratory complications are among the most frequent and serious problems encountered by the surgical patient. Chart 21-1 lists the risk factors for pulmonary complications.

Prevention

Experience suggests that the incidence of these complications may be reduced by careful preoperative assessment and teaching and by taking precautions during and after surgery. It is well known that patients who have respiratory dysfunction before surgery are more likely to develop serious complications after surgery. Therefore, only emergency surgical procedures are performed when acute disease of the respiratory tract exists. Any cough, sneezing, inflamed conjunctivae, nasal discharge, and abnormal breath sounds are reported to the surgeon and anesthesiologist before the preoperative medications are administered.

CHART 21-1
Risk Factors for Postoperative Pulmonary Complications

Type of surgery—Greater incidence following all forms of abdominal surgery when compared with peripheral surgery
Location of incision—The closer the incision to the diaphragm, the higher the incidence of pulmonary complications
Preoperative respiratory problems
Age—Greater risk after age 40 than before age 40
Sepsis
Obesity—Weight greater than 110% of ideal body weight
Prolonged bed rest
Duration of surgical procedure—More than 3 hours
Aspiration
Dehydration
Malnutrition
Hypotension and shock
Immunosuppression

During and immediately after surgery, every effort is made to prevent chilling, which further lowers the patient's resistance. Suctioning of the nasopharynx in the recovery room removes secretions that would otherwise cause respiratory problems in the postoperative period. Occasionally, secretions form that cannot be coughed up by the patient and may be suctioned through an endotracheal tube or bronchoscope. In very debilitated patients in whom retained secretions are a complicating factor, a tracheostomy may be performed so that suctioning is accomplished directly through the trachea.

Types of Respiratory Complications

Respiratory complications that may arise include undetected hypoxemia, atelectasis, bronchitis, bronchopneumonia, lobar pneumonia, hypostatic pulmonary congestion, pleurisy, and superinfection.

Undetected Hypoxemia. The types of hypoxemia that can affect postoperative patients are subacute and episodic. Subacute hypoxemia is a constant low level of O_2 saturation, although the patient's breathing appears normal. Episodic hypoxemia happens suddenly and the patient may be at risk for cerebral dysfunction, myocardial ischemia, and cardiac arrest. These complications often occur the third to fourth postoperative night. Patients at risk for hypoxemia include those who have undergone major surgery (particularly abdominal), are obese, or have pre-existing pulmonary problems.

Hypoxemia can be detected by the accurate technique of pulse oximetry to determine O_2 saturation. Quantitative monitoring of O_2 saturation is mandated by the American Society of Anesthesiologists (ASA) in patients undergoing general anesthesia and in the PACU. The use of pulse oximetry is also expanding to general care units.

Atelectasis. When a mucus plug obstructs one of the bronchi entirely, the pulmonary tissue beyond the plug collapses and a massive atelectasis—an incomplete expansion of the lung—results. See the discussion of atelectasis in Chapter 24 for more information about treatment.

Bronchitis. Bronchitis may appear at any time after surgery but usually occurs within the first 5 or 6 days. The symptoms vary according to disease severity. Simple bronchitis is characterized by a productive cough but without marked temperature or pulse elevation.

A most effective method of treating bronchitis is the inhalation of cool mist or steam, which may be administered by vaporizers as prescribed. The vaporizer must be kept filled with water, and precautions are taken to prevent the patient from being burned.

Bronchopneumonia and Pneumonia. **Bronchopneumonia** is a frequent pulmonary complication. Along with a productive cough, there may be marked temperature elevation and an increase in the pulse and the respiratory rates.

Lobar pneumonia is a less frequent complication after surgery. Usually, it begins with a chill, followed by high temperature, pulse, and respiration. There may be little or no cough, but the respiratory distress, flushed cheeks, and obvious illness of the patient provide a combination of clinical signs that is distinctive. The disease runs its usual course but prolongs the surgical recovery.

In lobar pneumonia and bronchopneumonia, expectorant and antibiotic medications are prescribed and the patient is encouraged to take fluids. Breath sounds are assessed frequently to identify changes before further respiratory and cardiac dysfunction occurs.

Hypostatic Pulmonary Congestion. **Hypostatic pulmonary congestion** may develop in elderly or very weak patients. Its cause is a weakened heart and vascular system that permit stagnation of secretions at the base of both lungs. It occurs most frequently in elderly patients who are not mobilized effectively. The symptoms are often vague—perhaps a slight elevation of temperature, pulse, and respiratory rate and a cough. However, physical examination reveals dullness and crackles at the base of the lungs. If the condition progresses, the outcome may be fatal.

Many times the pulmonary complication of hypostatic pulmonary congestion becomes more serious than the original surgical condition. In this case, the prime objective of therapeutic management is to treat the hypostatic pneumonia.

Pleurisy. **Pleurisy** can occur after surgery. Its chief symptom is an acute, knifelike pain in the chest on the affected side that becomes excruciating when the patient takes a deep breath. Additionally, breath sounds are diminished or absent on the affected side. There is usually a slight fever and rise in pulse, and respirations are shallow and more rapid than normal.

For pleurisy, analgesics may be prescribed, or the physician may perform a procaine intercostal block to provide symptomatic relief. A search is made to detect any possible underlying disease (pneumonia, infarction).

Pleurisy with effusion may occur secondary to a primary pleurisy. In these patients, aspiration of the pleural space is frequently necessary.

Superinfections. **Superinfections** can occur when antimicrobial agents alter the bacterial flora of the respiratory tract. Susceptible bacteria are killed, and resistant bacteria multiply. These infections must be treated aggressively.

Nursing Management

Awareness of the many possible respiratory complications enables the nurse to initiate the preventive measures cited in the previous discussion (p. 397). Timely recognition of signs and symptoms allows the nurse to collaborate with the physician and other members of the health care team to combat specific respiratory problems. The patient requires close observation and careful management in the first postoperative week of recovery. If the patient has been discharged, patient teaching should alert the patient and family to possible early signs of respiratory problems.

The early signs of elevations in temperature, pulse, and respiratory rate are significant. The patient may seem to be restless and apprehensive and show signs of chest pain, dyspnea, and cough. These signs and symptoms are important and should be reported and documented so that appropriate interventions can be initiated.

Measures to Promote the Full Aeration of the Lungs. Strategies to prevent respiratory complications include measures to promote full aeration of the lungs. The nurse instructs the patient to take at least five deep inhalations every hour. The use of an incentive spirometer is prescribed to expand the lungs fully (see p. 397 for fuller discussion). Turning the patient from side to side can trigger coughing and the expectoration of a mucus plug and thereby increase aeration of the lungs.

Early ambulation is one of the best preventive measures for pulmonary complications; having the patient ambulate increases metabolism and pulmonary aeration and, in general, improves all body functions. When the patient's condition permits, the patient is encouraged to be out of bed on the first or second day after surgery, and frequently on the day of surgery. This practice is especially valuable in preventing pulmonary complications in older patients.

Urinary Retention

Although urinary retention may follow any surgical procedure, it occurs most frequently after surgery on the rectum, the anus, and the vagina, and after herniorrhaphies and surgery on the lower abdomen. The cause is thought to be a spasm of the bladder sphincter.

Management and Nursing Interventions

Quite often patients are unable to void while lying in bed, but when allowed to sit or stand up they do so without difficulty. When standing or sitting is not contraindicated, male patients are allowed to stand by the side of the bed and use a urinal. Female patients are allowed to sit on a bedpan on the edge of the bed with their feet on a chair or a stool. However, when sitting or standing is not possible, other means of encouraging urination must be tried. Some people cannot void with another person in the room. These patients should be left alone for a time after being provided with a warm bedpan or urinal.

Frequently the sound of running water relaxes the spasm of the bladder sphincter. Using a bedpan and irrigating the perineum with warm water often initiate urination for female patients. If the retention of urine continues for some hours and the patient complains of considerable abdominal discomfort, the distended bladder can be palpated and even seen in outline on the lower abdomen.

Catheterization may become necessary when all conservative measures have failed. If the patient has voided just before surgery, this procedure may be delayed for 8 to 12 hours, depending on the patient's intravenous and oral fluid intake and the physician's orders. Efforts are made to avoid catheterization because of the possibility of infecting the bladder and producing cystitis. Furthermore, experience has shown that once a patient has been catheterized, subsequent catheterizations are often needed.

At times the surgeon may anticipate voiding difficulties following extensive surgery, and an indwelling catheter is inserted before the patient emerges from anesthesia. The surgeon is notified if the catheter drains less than 30 ml of urine per hour.

Retention overflow may become a problem. Many patients exhibit lower abdominal discomfort, with a palpable bladder, and yet void only small amounts of urine at frequent intervals. The nurse should not mistake this for normal functioning of the bladder. This voiding of 30 to 60 ml (1 to 2 oz) of urine at intervals of 15 to 30 minutes is, rather, a sign of an overdistended bladder, which allows the escape of small amounts of urine at intervals. The condition is called retention overflow.

Incontinence of retention overflow may be evidenced by a constant dribble of urine while the bladder remains overdistended. Because distention compromises the vascular supply of the bladder wall and increases risk of infection, catheterization is indicated. Catheterization usually relieves the patient by draining 600 to 900 ml (20 to 30 oz) of urine from the bladder.

Gastrointestinal Complications

Nutritional Considerations

Surgery of the gastrointestinal tract frequently disrupts the normal physiologic processes of digestion and absorption. Complications arising from this disruption may take several forms, depending on the location and extent of surgery. For example, oral surgery may present problems of chewing and swallowing, requiring that diet be modified to accommodate this difficulty. Other surgical procedures, such as gastrectomy, small bowel resection, ileostomy, and colostomy, have a more drastic effect on the gastrointestinal system and require more extensive dietary considerations. These procedures are discussed in Chapters 36 and 37.

Intestinal Obstruction

Intestinal obstruction is a complication that may follow abdominal surgery. It occurs most often after surgery on the lower abdomen and pelvis, and especially after surgery in which drainage has been necessary. The symptoms usually appear between the third and fifth days but may occur at any time, even years after surgery. The cause is some obstruction of the intestinal flow—frequently a loop of intestine that has become kinked from inflammatory adhesions or is involved with peritonitis or generalized irritation of the peritoneal surface.

Clinical Manifestations. Often fever and pulse elevation are absent, but discomfort is present. At first the pains are localized. The painful area should be noted by the nurse because the localization of the early pains corresponds to the loop of intestine that is just above the obstruction. The patient continues to have abdominal pains, with shorter and shorter intervals between waves of pain. When a stethoscope is placed on the abdomen, sounds may reveal extremely active intestinal movements, especially during an attack of pain. The intestinal contents, unable to move forward, distend the intestinal coils, are carried backward to the stomach, and are vomited. Thus, vomiting and increasing distention gradually become more prominent symptoms. Hiccups often precede vomiting in many patients. Defecation does not occur, and enemas return nearly clear, indicating that only a small amount of the intestinal contents has reached the large bowel. Unless the obstruction is relieved, the patient continues to vomit, distention becomes more pronounced, the pulse becomes rapid, and death can result.

Management. Sometimes the distention of the intestine above the obstruction can be relieved by the use of intermittent-suction drainage with a nasoenteral or simple nasogastric tube. Sometimes the inflammatory bowel reaction may subside with subsequent relief of the obstruction. However, at other times it is necessary to relieve the obstruction surgically. Intravenous infusions are usually prescribed as well. (See Chapter 37 on intestinal obstruction for a more complete discussion of the treatment and postoperative care.)

Postoperative Psychosis

Postoperative psychosis (mental abnormalities) may be physiologic or psychologic in origin. Cerebral anoxia, thromboembolism, and fluid and electrolyte imbalances are recognized physical factors in postoperative central nervous system impairment and stress. Emotional factors such as fear, pain, and disorientation can contribute to postoperative depression and anxiety.

Older patients, particularly those with cerebrovascular atherosclerosis, are most susceptible to psychologic disturbances. Usually these patients manage fairly well until they have been subjected to the anesthetic and surgery. Postoperatively they may become very disturbed and disoriented. Disfiguring surgery and surgery for cancer also predispose the patient to intense emotional problems. Dressings that obscure vision or confinement in a body cast can result in behavioral changes because of the reduced sensory input.

Preoperative and Postoperative Management

The patient should be thoroughly informed before surgery about what to expect after surgery. Opportunities need to be provided for the patient to express thoughts and fears; misinformation can be corrected and reassurance provided. High-risk patients as described above may require special attention and support. Judicious use of narcotics postoperatively can also reduce confusion and disorientation.

Orienting the patient to time, day, and place can reduce confusion over being in new or strange surroundings. Studies have indicated that thorough preoperative briefing of both patient and family can usually diffuse many of the potential postoperative psychologic stresses. In addition, a positive attitude conveyed by all personnel who come in contact with the patient fosters positive feelings in the patient.

For overt psychosis, the patient may require a consultation, major tranquilizers, and therapy with mental health professionals. Because postoperative psychosis does occur, it is helpful to inform the family that these episodes are temporary. A patient with illusions or hallucinations is reassured that these aberrations occur occasionally, but are temporary and will resolve.

The patient's room should be adequately lighted to reduce the incidence of visual hallucinations. It may be desirable to have a family member stay with the patient as much as possible, because the presence of a familiar person has a reassuring and quieting effect.

Restraint. In the postoperative care of patients with psychologic disturbances, it is prudent for the nurse to explain why the patient must remain in bed. Often, patients try to get out of bed to void or to get a drink of water rather than bother the nurse. This may lead to serious complications that a brief explanation can prevent. However, some patients, especially elderly patients and those who are disoriented, may be unable to understand the explanation. For such patients, the simplest form of restraint is the use of beds with side rails or side protection. This permits patients to move about in bed but deters them from getting out of bed easily and injuring themselves.

To protect both patient and nurse, it may become necessary to apply some form of restraint in cases of delirium. These restraints require a physician's order. The psychologic effect of being restrained can be severe; therefore, any form of restraint is applied *only as a last resort.* All other means of quieting the patient are tried first. If possible, the patient should be isolated from other patients. Any potentially harmful article in the immediate surroundings is removed.

When restraints are used, the patient should be in a natural, comfortable position and the restraint must not interfere with chest expansion or circulation. The appearance of cyanosis of the hand or foot indicates that the restraint is too tight. The restraint is padded carefully and placed so as to prevent chafing or pressure ulcers. The skin underneath the restraint is inspected frequently, bathed carefully, and massaged at least every 2 hours. Any patient requiring restraint should have constant and careful nursing attention. Consideration is given to respecting the patient as a person.

Delirium

Postoperative delirium occurs occasionally in several groups of patients. The most common types of delirium are toxic, traumatic, and alcohol withdrawal delirium (delirium tremens).

Toxic Delirium. Toxic delirium occurs in conjunction with the signs and symptoms of general toxemia. The patient with toxic delirium is very ill and usually presents with a high temperature and rapid pulse rate. The face is flushed, and the eyes are bright and roving. The patient moves constantly, often attempting to get out of bed. A marked degree of mental confusion is apparent. Toxic delirium is seen most often in patients with general peritonitis or other septic conditions.

In such patients, the intake of fluids is encouraged and the causative condition is treated with antimicrobial therapy. At times, however, the patient does not survive.

Traumatic Delirium. Traumatic delirium is a mental state resulting from sudden trauma of any sort. It often occurs in highly nervous people. The malady may take the form of wild, manic excitement, simple confusion with hallucinations and delusions, or depression. Sedative medications (chloral hydrate, paraldehyde, and morphine) are used in treatment. Usually traumatic delirium begins and ends suddenly.

Alcohol Withdrawal Delirium (Delirium Tremens). Individuals who have used alcohol habitually over a long period of time are poor surgical risks. Not only is their resistance lower than normal, but the effects of alcohol have most likely caused multiple organ damage. In addition, these patients react poorly to anesthesia.

After surgery, the alcoholic patient may do well for a few days, but the prolonged abstinence from alcohol causes restlessness, nervousness, and irritability. Facial expression may change entirely. Sleep is poor and often disturbed by unreal dreams. When approached by the doctor or the nurse, the patient appears to wake suddenly and appear confused until oriented to time and place. After these episodes, the patient appears to be fairly normal for a short time. Patients who use alcohol regularly should be observed for such symptoms; with intervention at this stage, the more severe delirium may be avoided.

Active alcohol withdrawal delirium may occur suddenly or gradually. After a period of restless, nervous semidelirium, the patient loses control of mental functions. Attempts at restraint may prompt the patient to fight and cause bodily injury to self or others.

Management. When possible, the treatment of patients with alcohol withdrawal delirium should begin 2 or 3 days before surgery with an increased fluid intake. These measures should be continued postoperatively, especially if any of the early signs of the condition develop.

Administration of sedatives or tranquilizers is often indicated. The chief cause of the symptoms in patients with chronic alcoholism has been shown to be a depletion of the carbohydrate stores of the body and an inadequate ingestion of vitamins. Therefore, glucose is prescribed intravenously and vitamins are administered in concentrated form by mouth and by injection and infusion.

Gerontologic Considerations

The elderly patient who has undergone surgery is transferred from the operating room table to the bed *slowly* and *gently*. The effects of this action on blood pressure are monitored, and observation is made of facial expression (if the patient is awake) and evidence of hypoxia. Special attention is given to keeping the patient warm, because body temperature in the elderly is labile. Position is changed frequently to stimulate respirations and circulation and to promote comfort, because lying in one position can be uncomfortable.

Immediate postoperative care for the elderly patient is the same as that for any surgical patient, but additional support is given if there is impaired function of the cardiovascular, pulmonary, or renal systems. With invasive monitoring, it is possible to detect cardiopulmonary deficits before obvious signs and symptoms are apparent. Because of monitoring and improved individualized preoperative preparation, many older adults tolerate surgery well and have an unremarkable and uneventful recovery.

Confusion is one of the most common experiences of an older postoperative patient. This is aggravated by social isolation, restraints, and sensory deprivation. Nighttime confusion can be reduced by frequent nursing attention and caution in the use of medications, especially narcotic analgesics and sedatives. However, it is important to keep in mind that confusion may be the initial or only early indicator of deterioration of the elderly patient's condition.

Pneumonia, the most frequent respiratory complication in the elderly, often can be prevented by early ambulation or mobilization. Keeping the patient active also prevents atelectasis, irritation of pressure areas, deep venous thrombosis (DVT), and undue weakness. Sitting positions that promote venous stasis in the lower extremities are to be avoided. *Ambulation means walking, not sitting in a chair.* Adequate assistance is required to prevent bumping into objects and falling.

Urinary incontinence can be prevented by providing easy access to the call bell and the commode and by prompting voiding. Early ambulation and familiarity with the room help the patient to become self-sufficient sooner.

Gastrointestinal dysfunction, such as postoperative distention, reduced peristalsis, and fecal impaction can be prevented by promoting adequate hydration and activity.

Discomfort is a common complaint. During the early postoperative days, the patient may complain of sore muscles. This is common and usually due to maintaining a constant position during surgery. Massaging aching muscles *gently* and providing support with pillows can ease the discomfort.

Fluid and electrolyte status is monitored to avoid the extremes of fluid overload and dehydration. The nurse compares previous documentation with current records to note changes in fluid balance, breath sounds, and weight. It may be necessary to recommend physical therapy and intensive rehabilitation for patients undergoing prolonged convalescence.

Encouragement is provided. The nurse gently challenges the older adult to recognize that participation in all activities can enhance recovery and prevent complications.

Ambulatory Surgery

Although ambulatory surgery (same-day surgery, outpatient surgery) became popular in the 1970s, its recent growth is the result of advances in surgical practice and anesthesia techniques, prospective reimbursement, and government changes in Medicare and Medicaid provisions. Ambulatory surgery permits the patient to return home on the day of the surgery and is less costly than hospitalization.

Advantages of Ambulatory Surgery

- It is cost-effective for the patient, hospital, insurance carriers, and government agencies.
- There is less psychologic stress for the patient.
- Hospital-acquired infections are prevented or reduced in incidence.
- Recovery time is more rapid.

Types of Ambulatory Surgery Procedures

Ambulatory procedures are usually of short duration, from 15 to 90 minutes, in which minimal bleeding and minor physiologic disturbances are anticipated, as in the following examples:

General surgery—hernia repair, vasectomy, excision of small tumors, and laparoscopic cholecystectomies
Gynecology—dilation and curettage (D & C), tubal ligation, pregnancy termination, cervical diagnostic laparoscopy, biopsy, and conization
Dermatology—excision of warts and condylomata
Ophthalmology—cataract extraction, minor surgeries, laser treatments
Ear, nose, and throat—myringotomy, adenoidectomy, nasal polypectomy, oral surgery
Cardiac surgery—cardioversion, insertion and replacement of pacemakers
Orthopedic surgery—carpal tunnel surgery, ganglionectomy, arthroscopy

Patient Selection

The patient undergoing ambulatory surgery should be in stable medical condition and free of infection. It may be more practical for the person with a mild systemic disease to have a surgical procedure in the short-term facility than to be exposed to the greater risk of hospitalization. Usually age is not a factor; however, it is desirable that the patient be psychologically willing to accept this mode of treatment.

Preoperative and Postoperative Care

The similarities of inpatient and outpatient perioperative nursing include perioperative standards, adherence to aseptic technique, and an emphasis on patient safety. The differences in outpatient perioperative nursing include telephone assessment and teaching environment, even greater need for expert discharge planning skills, and follow-up home care.

The preoperative phase includes preoperative testing, the assessment interview, and teaching and usually occurs within 7 days of surgery. The interview may be conducted when the patient comes to the hospital or surgical center for testing or it may consist of a preoperative assessment telephone call. Preoperative teaching content may be presented in a group meeting, on a videotape, during night classes, or in conjunction with the preoperative interview. The instructions are presented in simple terms; for the elderly, the instructions should be in large print. The patient is told when and where to report, what to bring (insurance card, list of medications and allergies), what to leave at home (jewelry, watch, medications, contact lenses), and what to wear (loose-fitting, comfortable clothes; flat shoes). The surgeon's office is often an underutilized site for initiating teaching before the perioperative telephone contact. The last preoperative phone call is designed to remind the patient not to drink after midnight of the day before surgery; brushing teeth is permitted but no fluids should be swallowed.

On the day of surgery, the nurse monitors the patient's vital signs and administers the preanesthetic medication. After voiding, the patient is accompanied to the anesthesia unit. Following surgery, the patient remains in the recovery unit until recovered sufficiently from the anesthetic to go home, accompanied safely by a responsible person.

Criteria for discharge include a stable circulatory status, absence of bleeding, no nausea or vomiting, and no excessive pain.

Postoperative instructions, the necessary prescriptions, and an information sheet are provided to the patient. Although recovery time varies and is dependent on the type and extent of surgery and the patient's overall physical condition, instructions usually include "taking it easy" for 24 to 48 hours. During this time, the patient is not to drive a vehicle, drink alcoholic beverages, or perform tasks that require energy or skill. Fluids may be consumed as desired, and smaller than normal amounts eaten at mealtime. The patient is cautioned not to make important decisions at this time because the medications, anesthesia, and surgery may affect thinking ability.

Patient Education and Home Care Considerations

Expert patient teaching and discharge planning are necessary when a patient undergoes same-day surgery to assure patient safety and recovery. The patient and caregiver (*i.e.*, family member or friend) are informed about expected outcomes and immediate postoperative changes anticipated in the patient's capacity for self-care.

Because of the possibility of unexpected outcomes, the patient's caregiver at home is provided with verbal and written instructions about what to observe the patient for and about the actions to take if expected or unexpected events or complications occur. The nurse's or surgeon's telephone number is provided and the patient and caregiver are encouraged to call if questions arise; follow-up phone calls initiated at scheduled intervals are often reassuring to the patient and caregiver. Written instructions are also provided to the patient and caregiver about wound care, activity and dietary recommendations, medication, and follow-up visits to the same-day surgery unit or the surgeon.

The Elderly Surgical Outpatient

Third-party reimbursement policies often force the elderly into ambulatory surgery. If the elderly patient lives alone and self-care deficits related to the surgical experience are expected, then strong family or friend support is necessary. In the careful assessment of the home environment, this support provides the basis for a realistic discharge plan.

Many elderly individuals have short-term memory loss and a chronic disease such as arthritis, hearing loss, hypertension, or a cardiac condition. These long-term conditions and the medications taken for them affect preoperative preparation, anesthesia, and surgical outcomes. Therefore, it is the collaborative effort of the patient and the operating room, PACU, and home health staffs that makes ambulatory surgery a successful experience.

Care of the Surgical Incision/Wound

A **wound** may be described as a disruption in the continuity of cells; it follows, then, that **wound healing** is the restoration of that continuity.

When wounds occur, a variety of effects may result: (1) immediate loss of all or part of organ functioning, (2) sympathetic stress response, (3) hemorrhage and blood clotting, (4) bacterial contamination, and (5) death of cells. Careful asepsis is the most important factor in keeping these effects to a minimum and promoting the successful care of wounds.

Wound Classification

Wounds may be classified in two different ways: according to the mechanism of injury and the degree of wound contamination at the time of surgery.

Mechanism of Injury. Wounds may be described as incised, contused, lacerated, or puncture.

- **Incised wounds** are made by a clean cut with a sharp instrument—for example, those made by the surgeon in every surgical procedure. Clean wounds (those made aseptically) are usually closed by sutures after all bleeding vessels have been ligated carefully.
- **Contused wounds** are made by blunt force and are characterized by considerable injury of the soft parts, hemorrhage, and swelling.
- **Lacerated wounds** are those with jagged, irregular edges, such as would be made by glass or barbed wire.
- **Puncture wounds** result in small openings in the skin—for example, those made by bullets or knife stabs.

Degree of Contamination. Wounds may be described as clean, clean-contaminated, contaminated, or dirty or infected.*

- **Clean wounds** are uninfected surgical wounds in which there is no inflammation and the respiratory, alimentary, genital, or uninfected urinary tracts are not entered. Clean wounds are usually sutured closed; if necessary, a closed drainage system (*e.g.*, Jackson-Pratt) is inserted. The relative probability of wound infection is 1% to 5%.
- **Clean-contaminated wounds** are surgical wounds in which the respiratory, alimentary, genital, or urinary tract is entered under controlled conditions; there is no unusual contamination. The relative probability of wound infection is 3% to 11%.
- **Contaminated wounds** include open, fresh, accidental wounds, and surgical procedures with major breaks

*Centers for Disease Control: Guidelines for Prevention of Surgical Wound Infection. Washington, DC, U.S. Department of Health and Human Services, 1985.

in aseptic technique or gross spillage from the gastrointestinal tract; included in this category are incisions in which there is acute, nonpurulent inflammation. The relative probability of wound infection is 10% to 17%.

- **Dirty** or **infected wounds** are those in which the organisms that caused postoperative infection were present in the operative field before surgery. These include old traumatic wounds with retained devitalized tissue and those that involve existing clinical infections or perforated viscera. The relative probability of wound infection is over 27%. (See Wound Sepsis, p. 418.)

Treatment. Prophylactic antibiotics are administered when bacterial contamination is expected, or when a prosthetic device is being inserted into a clean wound. Infected wounds are not closed until every effort has been made to remove all devitalized and infected tissue, a procedure called **débridement**. Often a small drain is inserted before the wound is sutured to prevent lymph and blood from collecting and retarding the healing process.

Physiology of Wound Healing

Various continuous and overlapping cellular processes contribute to the restoration of a wound: cell regeneration, cell proliferation, and collagen production. The response of tissue to injury goes through several phases: inflammatory, proliferative, and maturation (Table 21-2).

Inflammatory Phase. Vascular and cellular responses occur immediately when tissue is cut or injured. Vasoconstriction of vessels occurs and a fibrinoplatelet clot forms in an attempt to control bleeding. This reaction lasts from 5 to 10 minutes and is followed by vasodilation of the venules. Microcirculation loses its vasoconstriction ability because norepinephrine is destroyed by the intracellular enzymes. Also, histamine is released, which increases capillary permeability.

When the microcirculation is damaged, blood elements such as antibodies, plasma proteins, electrolytes, complement, and water permeate the vascular space for 2 to 3 days, causing edema, warmth, redness, and pain. Neutrophils are the first leukocytes to move into damaged tissue. Monocytes that transform to macrophages engulf the debris and transport it from the area. Antigen-antibodies also appear. Basal cells at the wound edges undergo mitosis, and the resulting daughter cells migrate.

With this activity, proteolytic enzymes are secreted and dissolve the base of blood clots. The gap between both sides of the wound is progressively filled, and the sides eventually meet in 24 to 48 hours. At this point, cell migration is enhanced by hyperplastic bone marrow activity.

Proliferative Phase. Fibroblasts multiply and form a lattice framework for migrating cells. Epithelial cells form buds at the edges of the wound; these buds develop into capillaries, the nutritional source for the new granulation tissue.

Collagen is the primary component of replaced connective tissue. Fibroblasts initiate the synthesis of collagen and mucopolysaccharides. In a 2- to 4-week period, amino acid chains form into fibers of increasing length and diameter; these fibers become a well-structured pattern of packed bundles. The synthesis of collagen causes capillaries to decrease in number. Thereafter, collagen synthesis decreases in an attempt to balance the amount of collagen that is destroyed. Such synthesis and lysis result in increased tensile strength.

After 2 weeks, the wound has only 3% to 5% of the original skin strength. By the end of a month, only 35% to 59% of wound strength has been reached. Never more than 70% to 80% of strength is regained. Many vitamins, particularly vitamin C, aid in the metabolic process involved in wound healing.

Maturation Phase. About 3 weeks after injury, fibroblasts begin to leave the wound. The scar appears large, until collagen fibrils reorganize into tighter positions. This, along with dehydration, reduces the scar but increases its strength. Such tissue maturation continues and reaches maximum strength in 10 or 12 weeks, but it never reaches the original strength of the prewound tissue.

Forms of Healing

In the surgical management of wound healing, wounds are described as healing by first, second, or third intention.

Healing by First Intention (Primary Union). Wounds made aseptically, with a minimum of tissue destruction, and properly closed, as with sutures, heal with little tissue reaction by first intention (Fig. 21-5). When wounds heal

TABLE 21-2 Phases of Wound Healing

Phase	Length of Time	Events
Imflammatory (also called lag or exudative phase)	1–4 days	Blood clot forms Wound becomes edematous Debris of damaged tissue and blood clot are phagocytized
Proliferative (also called fibroblastic or connective tissue phase)	5–20 days	Collagen produced Granulation tissue forms Wound tensile strength increases
Maturation (also called differentiation, resorptive, remodeling, or plateau phase)	21 days to months or even years	Fibroblasts leave wound Tensile strength increases Collagen fibers reorganize and tighten to reduce scar size

by first intention, granulation tissue is not visible and scar formation is minimal.

Healing by Second Intention (Granulation). In wounds in which pus formation (suppuration) has occurred or in which the edges have not been approximated, the process of repair is less simple and takes longer.

When an abscess is incised it collapses partly, but the dead and the dying cells forming its walls are still being released into the cavity. For this reason, drainage tubes or gauze packing is often inserted into the abscess pocket to allow drainage to escape easily. Gradually the necrotic material disintegrates and escapes, and the abscess cavity fills with a red, soft, sensitive tissue that bleeds very easily. This tissue is composed of minute, thin-walled capillaries and buds that later form connective tissue. These buds, called granulations, enlarge until they fill the area left by the destroyed tissue (see Fig. 21-5). The cells surrounding the capillaries change their round shape to become long, thin, and intertwined with each other to form a ***scar*** or **cicatrix.** Healing is complete when skin cells (epithelium) grow over these granulations. This method of repair is called **healing by granulation,** and it takes place whenever pus is formed or when loss of tissue has occurred for any reason.

Healing by Third Intention (Secondary Suture). If a deep wound either has not been sutured early or breaks down and then is resutured later, two apposing granulation surfaces are brought together. This results in a deeper and wider scar (see Fig. 21-5).

Nursing Management and Its Effect on Wound Healing

As a wound undergoes the phases of healing, many elements, such as adequate nutrition, cleanliness, rest, and position, determine how quickly the process occurs. These factors are influenced by nursing interventions. Specific nursing assessments and interventions that address these factors and help to promote wound healing are presented in Chart 21-2. Methods for reducing the incidence of wound infection are described in Chart 21-3.

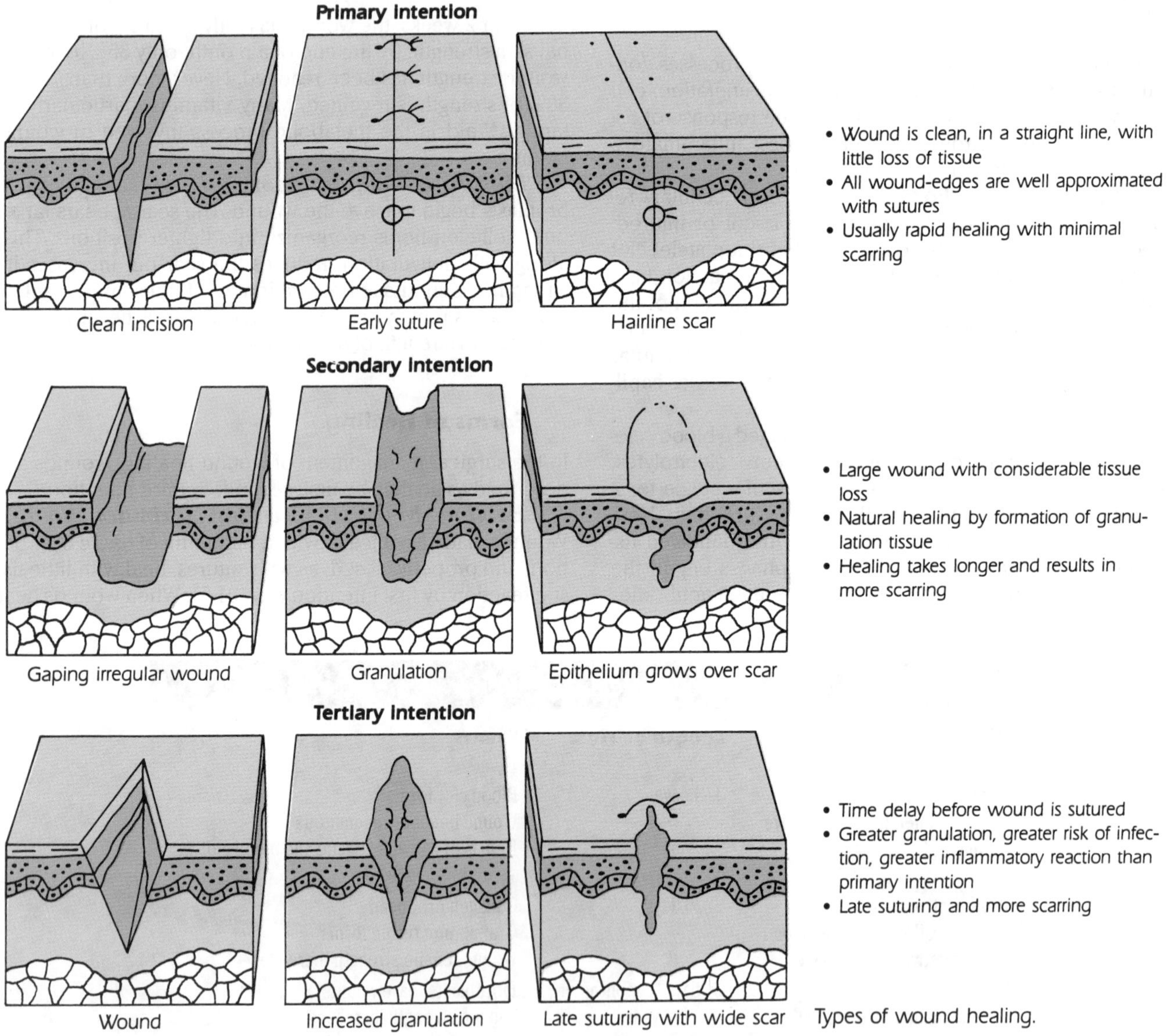

FIGURE 21-5. Types of wound healing: primary intention healing, secondary intention healing, and tertiary intention healing.

CHART 21-2
Factors Affecting Wound Healing

Factors	Rationale	Nursing Assessment/Interventions
Age of patient	The older the patient, the less resilient the tissues	Handle all tissues gently.
Handling of tissues	Rough handling causes injury and delayed healing	Handle tissues carefully and evenly.
Hemorrhage	Accumulation of blood creates dead spaces as well as dead cells that must be removed The area becomes a growth medium for infection	Monitor vital signs. Observe incision site for evidence of bleeding and infection.
Hypovolemia	Insufficient blood volume leads to vasoconstriction and reduced oxygen and nutrients available for wound healing	Monitor for volume deficit (circulatory impairment). Correct by fluid replacement as prescribed.
Local factors		
Edema	Reduces blood supply by exerting increased interstitial pressure on vessels	Elevate part; apply cool compresses.
Inadequate dressing technique		
Too small	Permits bacterial invasion and contamination	Follow guidelines for proper dressing technique.
Too tight	Reduces blood supply carrying nutrients and oxygen	
Nutritional deficits	Insulin secretion may be inhibited, causing blood glucose to rise	Monitor blood glucose levels. Administer vitamin A & C supplements as prescribed.
	Protein-calorie depletion may occur	Correct deficits: this may require parenteral nutritional therapy.
Foreign bodies	Foreign bodies retard healing	Keep wounds free of dressing threads, talcum, and powder from gloves.
Oxygen deficit		
Tissue oxygenation insufficient	Insufficient oxygen may be due to inadequate lung and cardiovascular function as well as localized vasoconstriction	Encourage deep breathing, turning, controlled coughing.
Drainage collection	Accumulated secretions hamper healing process	Monitor portable and other closed drainage systems for proper functioning. Institute measures to remove accumulated secretions.
Medications		
Steroids	May mask presence of infection by impairing normal inflammatory response	Be aware of action/effect of medications patient is receiving.
Anticoagulants	May cause hemorrhage	
Broad-spectrum/specific antibiotics	Effective if administered immediately before surgery for specific pathology or bacterial contamination If administered after wound is closed, ineffective because of intravascular coagulation	
Patient overactivity	Prevents approximation of wound edges Resting favors healing	Utilize measures to keep wound edges approximated: taping, bandaging, splints. Encourage rest.
Systemic disorders Hemorrhagic shock Acidosis Hypoxia Renal failure Hepatic disease Sepsis	These are depressants of cell function that directly affect wound healing	Be familiar with the nature of the specific disorder. Administer prescribed treatment. Cultures may be indicated to determine appropriate antibiotic.

(continued)

CHART 21-2 *(continued)*
Factors Affecting Wound Healing

Factors	Rationale	Nursing Assessment/Interventions
Immunosuppressed state	Patient is more vulnerable to bacterial/viral invasion; defense mechanisms are impaired	Provide maximum protection to prevent infection. Restrict visitors with colds; institute mandatory hand washing of all staff.
Wound stressors Vomiting Valsalva maneuver Heavy coughing Straining	Produce tension on wounds, particularly of the torso	Encourage frequent turning and ambulation, and administer antiemetic medications as prescribed. Assist patient in splinting of incision.

CHART 21-3
Effective Methods of Lowering Incidence of Wound Infection

GOALS: Reduce risks that inhibit wound healing. Lower incidence of wound infections.

Interventions	Rationale
Preoperative	
Short preoperative hospitalization	Reduces exposure of patient to nosocomial infections.
Treatment of coexistent infections	Infections, such as respiratory, can initiate pulmonary complications.
Avoid shaving of hair: if necessary, remove hair with clippers or depilatories rather than a razor	The fewer nicks and cuts in the skin, the less opportunity for infection.
If shaving is requested, it is performed immediately before the surgical procedure	The longer the time between shaving and the operation, the greater the incidence of infection.
Thorough cleansing of operative site—povidone-iodine (Betadine) shower the evening before and repeated preoperative cleansing with antiseptic detergents	Resident bacteria and skin contaminants are reduced to a minimum.
Prophylactic antibiotics with contaminated cases	
Intraoperative	
Thorough cleansing of operative site to remove superficial flora, soil, and debris	Reduces risk of contaminating the wound with patient's skin flora.
Flawless aseptic technique.	Any breaks in technique can initiate infection by introducing contaminants.
Powder or talcum washed off sterile gloves	Foreign particles in a wound, such as talcum or starch, will adversely affect the healing process.
Bleeding controlled with meticulous hemostasis	A clean wound heals without infection.
Drains eliminated in clean wounds	Drains are associated with higher wound infection rates.
Closure delayed in contaminated wounds	Permits healing from base of wound to exterior—otherwise, pocket of infection may develop.
Postoperative	
Meticulous aseptic technique during dressing changes	Help prevent microorganisms from entering the wound
Thoroughly cleanse the area around drainage tube	
Keep tubing away from incision	
Early discharge	Reduces exposure of patient to nosocomial infections

Dressings

The Purposes of an Effective Dressing

A dressing is applied to a wound for one or more of the following reasons: (1) to provide a proper environment for wound healing; (2) to absorb drainage; (3) to splint or immobilize the wound; (4) to protect the wound and new epithelial tissue from mechanical injury; (5) to protect the wound from bacterial contamination and from soiling by feces, vomitus, and urine; (6) to promote hemostasis, as in a pressure dressing; and (7) to provide mental and physical comfort for the patient.

In some instances dressings are eliminated during the immediate postoperative period. Examples of circumstances in which dressings are not necessary are facial lacerations, pedicle flaps, or skin grafts on a smooth surface.

When the initial dressing on a clean, dry incision is removed, often it is not replaced. Generally, initial dressings on clean, dry incisions are left in place until the wound edges are sealed and the wound is healing (usually 24 hours).

The advantages of not using any dressings include the following: (1) the conditions that promote growth of organisms (warmth, moisture, and darkness) are eliminated; (2) the wound can be readily observed; (3) bathing is easier; (4) reactions to tape are avoided; (5) patient comfort and activity are increased; (6) costs for dressings are reduced; and (7) psychologic impact of the surgical incision is reduced.

Surgical Dressings—Nursing Interventions

Although all initial postoperative dressings are changed by the surgeon, subsequent dressings in the immediate postoperative period are usually changed by the nurse. If necessary, the nurse can determine if the dressing needs to be reinforced before the first dressing change. Reinforcement keeps the outer dressing layer dry and clean, thus reducing contamination. The condition of surgical dressings and wounds is documented.

Preparation of the Patient. The patient is told that the dressing is to be changed and that changing the dressing is a simple procedure associated with little discomfort. The dressing change is scheduled for a suitable time. *Dressings should not be changed at mealtime.* If the patient is in an open unit, the curtains are drawn to ensure privacy; the patient should not be unduly exposed. The incision should not be referred to as a "scar," because for some patients the term has negative connotations. Assurance is given that the incision will shrink as it heals and the redness will fade.

Removal of Adhesive Dressings. Disposable gloves are worn. The adhesive is removed by pulling it parallel with the skin surface and in the direction of hair growth, rather than at right angles. Alcohol wipes or nonirritating solvents aid in removing adhesive painlessly and quickly. The old dressing is removed and then deposited in a plastic bag designated for biomedical waste disposal. In accordance with universal precautions, dressings are never touched by ungloved hands because of the danger of transmitting pathogenic organisms, including viruses such as HIV and hepatitis B. After instruments are used in the changing of dressings, they are placed in a bag or covered receptacle, not on surfaces where they might contaminate clean areas. Disposable instruments are discarded in the proper receptacle.

Simple Dressing. The tray for a routine dressing change includes gloves, cotton balls, a packet of antiseptic solution, dressings, and forceps. When the sterile tray has been properly opened, the nurse places additional dressings on the field, if needed, and moistens the cottonballs with the antiseptic. Forceps are used in cleansing the wound and surrounding skin with the moistened cottonballs. The new dressing is then applied.

- Soiled dressings must not be removed with ungloved hands.
- All wound dressings are applied with sterile gloves.
- If there is any doubt about the sterility of an instrument or a dressing, it is considered unsterile.

Completion of a Dressing. Dressings are held in place with tape that comes in many types and widths. If the patient is sensitive to adhesive material, hypoallergenic tape

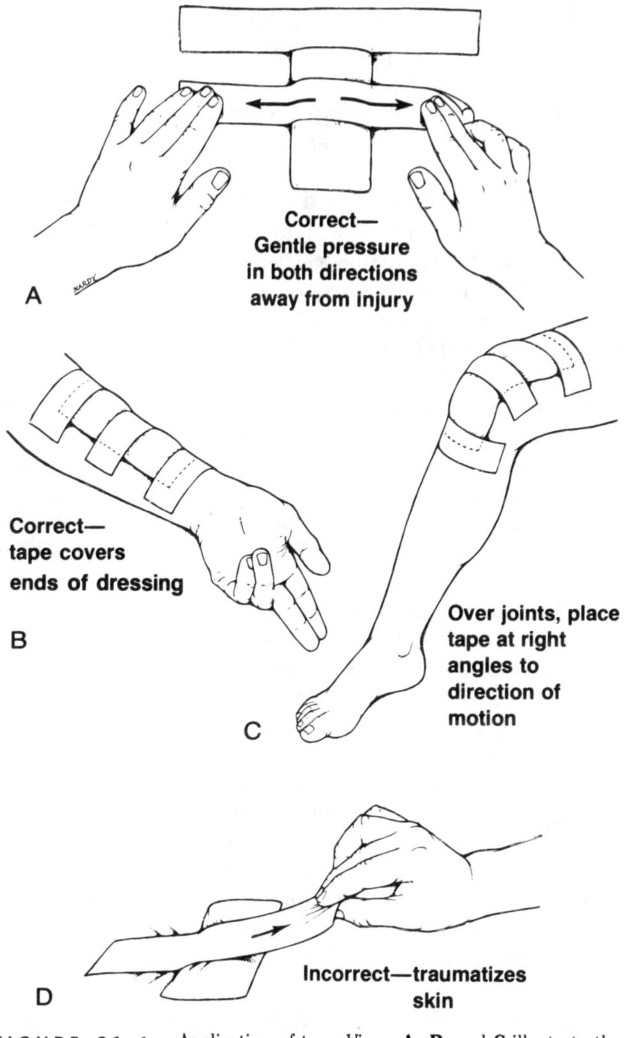

FIGURE 21-6. Application of tape. Views **A, B,** and **C** illustrate the correct method of application. The method shown in **D** is incorrect. (**A**) Pressure is applied evenly and directed away from the incision. (**D**) In the incorrect method, the tape is pulling against the skin and exerting pressure over the wound. (**B**) The proper way to cover the ends of a dressing for additional protection of the wound. (**C**) The correct way to position a dressing over a joint for maximum comfort and effectiveness.

is used. Many tapes are porous to permit ventilation and prevent maceration of the skin.

The correct way to apply tape is to place the tape at the center of the dressing and then press the tape down on both sides, applying tension evenly away from the midline (Fig. 21-6). The wrong method of applying tape—fixing one end of the tape to the skin and pulling it tight over the dressing—often wrinkles and pulls the skin in the process. The resulting continuous and forceful traction produces a shearing effect, causing the epidermal layer to slip sideways and become prematurely separated from the deeper dermal layers.

A commercial silicone aerosol is available that can be sprayed over the adhesive used to hold dressings in place; the silicone waterproofs the dressing so that the patient can bathe or swim, and it isolates the area from contamination. The spray is odorless, colorless, nonstaining, noninflammatory, heat stable, and hypoallergenic.

Elastic adhesive bandage (Elastoplast, Microfoam-3M) is preferable for holding dressings in place over mobile areas, such as the neck or the extremities, or where pressure is required.

When the dressing is completed, the soiled dressings are placed in a waterproof bag and deposited in a biomedical waste can for disposal.

Dressing of Draining Wounds. The risk of wound infection is reduced if there is adequate drainage. The wound needs to drain freely to release accumulated blood (clots), body fluids, pus, and necrotic material that otherwise would collect in the wound and provide a rich growth medium for microorganisms. If a wound is draining, the skin is not completely closed, so a pathway exists for microorganisms to enter and cause infection. Therefore, closed drainage is preferred to open drainage.

The drainage from an infected wound is frequently irritating to the surrounding skin. Often this situation can be avoided by using a protective ointment or dressing. Petrolatum gauze and zinc oxide ointment are effective preparations. If drainage is excessive, an enterostomal therapist (ET) or wound care nurse specialist may be consulted about strategies to contain the drainage and protect the skin.

Portable Wound Suction. The principle involved in portable wound suction is the use of gentle, constant suction to enhance drainage of serosanguineous fluid and to collapse the skin flaps against the underlying tissue. The **Hemovac** apparatus is a spring diaphragm evacuator for closed suction equipped with multiple small, perforated, inert polyethylene tubes. The tubes are inserted in the drainage areas in the operating room, and the wound is completely closed (Fig. 21-7). The **Surgivac** is a bellows-shaped evacuator for thicker drainage. These devices come in different sizes. The **Jackson-Pratt** is small and shaped like a grenade. Portable suction has several advantages: it is disposable, lightweight, inexpensive, silent, and space-saving.

Patient Education. While changing the dressing, the nurse has an opportunity to teach the patient how to care for the incision and change the dressings at home. The nurse observes for clues to the patient's readiness to learn, such as looking at the incision, expressing interest, or assisting in the dressing change. Information on self-care activities and possible signs of infection are summarized in Chart 21-4.

Wound Complications

Hematoma (Hemorrhage)

The dressings are inspected for hemorrhage at frequent intervals during the first 24 hours after surgery. Any undue amount of bleeding is reported. At times, concealed bleeding occurs in the wound, beneath the skin. This hemorrhage usually stops spontaneously but results in clot formation within the wound. If the clot is small, it will be absorbed and need not be treated. When the clot is large, the wound usually bulges somewhat, and healing will be delayed unless it is removed. After several sutures are removed by the physician, the clot is evacuated and the wound is packed lightly with gauze. Healing occurs usually by granulation, or a secondary closure may be performed.

Infection (Wound Sepsis)

Surgical wound infections are the second most frequent nosocomial infection in hospitals. Risk factors for wound infections are listed in Chart 21-5. The most important area of prevention lies in meticulous wound management and surgical technique. In addition, cleanliness and environmental disinfection are important.

Staphylococcus aureus accounts for many postoperative wound infections. Other infections may result from *Escherichia coli, Proteus vulgaris, Aerobacter aerogenes, Pseudomonas aeruginosa*, and other organisms (see Nosocomial Infections, Chapter 65).

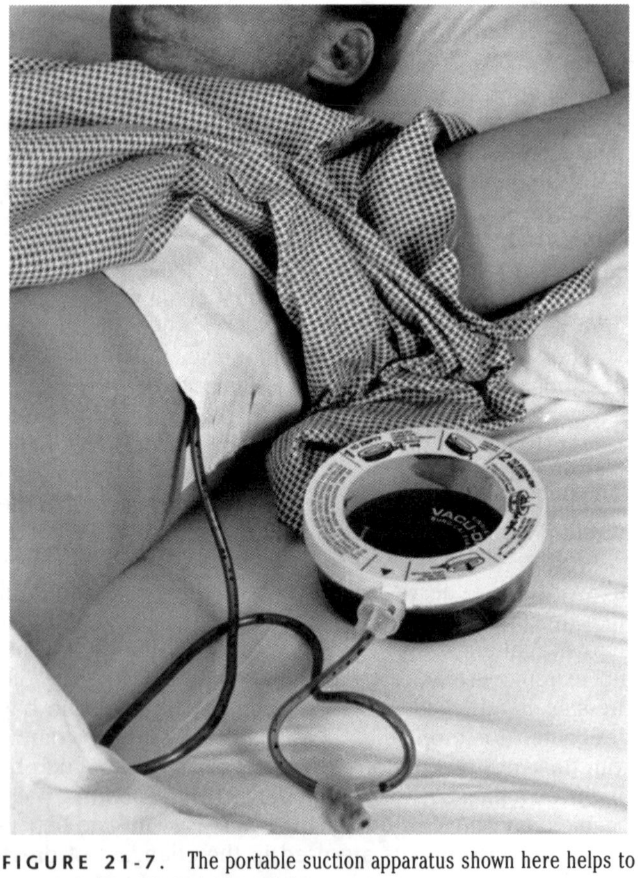

FIGURE 21-7. The portable suction apparatus shown here helps to remove drainage from the wound site.

CHART 21-4
Patient Education: Wound Care

Until Sutures Are Removed

1. Keep the wound dry and clean.
   a. If there is no dressing, ask your nurse or physician if you can bathe or shower.
   b. If a dressing or splint is in place, do not remove it unless it is wet or soiled.
   c. If wet or soiled, change dressing yourself if you have been taught to do so; otherwise, call your nurse or physician for guidance.
   d. If you have been taught, instruction might be as follows:
      (1) Cleanse area *gently* with 70% isopropyl alcohol once or twice daily.
      (2) Cover with a sterile Telfa pad or gauze square—sufficiently large to cover wound.
      (3) Apply hypoallergenic Dermacel or paper tape (adhesive is not recommended because it is difficult to remove without possible injury to incision site).
2. Report immediately if any of these signs of infection occur:
   a. Redness, marked swelling (beyond 2.5 cm [½ in] from incision site), tenderness, increased warmth around wound
   b. Red streaks in skin near wound
   c. Pus or discharge, foul odor
   d. Chills or fever (over 37.7°C [100°F])
3. If soreness or pain is causing discomfort, apply a dry cool pack (containing ice or cold water) or take prescribed acetaminophen tablets (2) every 4–6 hours. Avoid aspirin without direction or instruction because bleeding may be enhanced with its use.
4. Swelling following surgery is common. To help reduce swelling, elevate the affected part to the level of the heart.
   a. Hand or arm
      (1) Sleep—elevate arm on pillow at side.
      (2) Sitting—place arm on pillow on adjacent table.
      (3) Standing—rest affected hand on opposite shoulder; support elbow with unaffected hand.
   b. Leg or foot
      (1) Sitting—place a pillow on a facing chair; provide support underneath the knee.
      (2) Lying—place a pillow under affected leg.

After Sutures Are Removed

Although the wound appears to be healed when sutures are removed, it is still tender and will continue to heal and strengthen for several weeks.

1. Follow directives of physician or nurse as to extent of activity.
2. Keep suture line clean; do not rub vigorously; pat dry. Wound edges may look red and may be slightly raised. This is normal.
3. Massage around wound gently using a bland baby oil, petrolatum, or moisturizing cream (twice a day).
4. Report to the health care provider if after 8 weeks the site continues to be red, thick, painful to pressure. (This may be due to excessive collagen formation and should be checked.)

CHART 21-5
Risk Factors Contributing to Wound Sepsis

Local Factors

Wound contamination
Foreign body
Faulty suturing technique
Devitalized tissue
Hematoma
"Dead" space

General Factors

Debilitation
  Dehydration
  Malnutrition
  Anemia
Advanced age
Extreme obesity
Shock
Length of preoperative hospitalization
Duration of surgical procedure
Associated disorders (*e.g.,* diabetes mellitus; immunosuppression)

When the inflammatory process occurs, it usually causes symptoms in 36 to 48 hours. The patient's pulse rate and temperature increase, the WBC count rises, and the wound usually becomes swollen, warm, and tender with incisional pain. Local signs may be absent when the infection is deep.

When a diagnosis of wound infection in a postoperative wound is made, the surgeon usually removes one or more sutures and, under aseptic precautions, separates the wound edges with a pair of blunt scissors or a hemostat. Once the incision is opened, a drain is inserted.

Cellulitis is a bacterial infection that spreads into tissue planes. All the manifestations of inflammation are evident; streptococcus is frequently the responsible organism. Systemic antibiotics are usually effective. If an extremity is the site of the infection, elevation reduces dependent edema and the application of heat promotes local blood circulation. Rest decreases muscular contractions that could introduce the offending organisms into the circulatory system.

Abscess is a localized bacterial infection characterized by a collection of pus (bacteria, necrotic tissue, and WBCs). Usually a "point" develops that is tender. Because the area is under pressure, there is a tendency for the infection to seed bacteria that may invade adjacent tissues (cellulitis) or vascular spaces (bacteremia, sepsis). Treatment is surgical drainage or excision and the administration of antibiotics. Recurrence is prevented by allowing the treated wound to drain. Rest, elevation of the part, and heat are helpful.

Lymphangitis is a spread of infection from a cellulitis or abscess to the lymphatic system. This is treated by rest and antibiotics.

Dehiscence and Evisceration

The complications of dehiscence (disruption of surgical incision or wound) and evisceration (protrusion of wound contents) are especially serious when they involve abdominal incisions or wounds. These complications result from sutures giving way, from infection, and, more frequently, after marked distention or strenuous cough. They may also occur because of increasing age, poor nutritional status, and the presence of pulmonary or cardiovascular disease in patients who undergo abdominal surgery.

When the wound edges separate slowly, the intestines may protrude gradually, or not at all, and the earliest sign may be a gush of bloody (serosanguineous) peritoneal fluid from the wound. When the rupture of a wound occurs suddenly, coils of intestine may push out of the abdomen. Frequently, the patient may say that "something gave way." The evisceration causes pain and can be associated with vomiting.

- When disruption of a wound occurs, the surgeon is notified at once. The protruding coils of intestine are covered with sterile dressings moistened with sterile saline.

An abdominal binder, properly applied, is an excellent prophylactic measure against an evisceration of this kind, and often it is used along with the primary dressing, especially for surgery on patients with weak or pendulous abdominal walls, or when rupture of a wound has occurred.

CRITICAL THINKING EXERCISES

1. A patient with a poor nutritional status has undergone emergency surgery. How would you modify your assessment and nursing management in the postoperative period because of his poor nutritional status?
2. You are assigned to care for a patient who has undergone a nephrectomy. The patient experienced a thoracic spinal cord injury 20 years ago and has managed well since then. How will the presence of the spinal cord injury affect your postoperative care?
3. A patient who has undergone extensive orthopedic surgery is reporting excruciating pain and refuses to cough, deep breath, turn, or perform prescribed exercises until the pain has been relieved. When you check the patient's chart you find that medication cannot be given for two more hours. How would you deal with this situation?

Vitamin deficiency or lowered serum protein or chloride may require correction.

BIBLIOGRAPHY

Books

Agency for Health Care Policy and Research. Acute Pain Management: Operative or Medical Procedures and Trauma. Clinical Practice Guideline. Washington, DC, Public Health Service, U.S. Department of Health and Human Services, 1992.
American College of Surgeons. Care of the Surgical Patient. Vol 1, Critical Care. New York, Scientific American Inc, 1994.
American College of Surgeons. Care of the Surgical Patient. Vol 2, Elective Care. New York, Scientific American Inc, 1994.
American Society of Anesthesiology. ASA Standards for Post Anesthesia Care. Park Ridge, IL, American Society of Anesthesiology, 1992.
American Society of Post Anesthesia Nurses. Standards for Post Anesthesia Nursing Practice. Richmond, VA, American Society of Post Anesthesia Nurses, 1992.
Applegeet CJ. AORN Patient Classification Instrument for Perioperative Nursing. Denver, Association of Operating Room Nurses, 1993.
Benedetti C. The pathogenic effects of postoperative pain. In Lipton S, Tunks E, and Zoppi M (eds). Advances in Pain Research and Therapy, Vol. 13. New York, Raven Press, 1990:279–285.
Benedetti C et al (eds). Advances in Pain Research and Therapy. Vol 14. New York, Raven Press, 1990.
Burden N. Ambulatory Surgical Nursing. Philadelphia, WB Saunders, 1993.
Drain CB (ed). The Postanesthesia Care Unit: A Critical Care Approach to Postanesthesia Nursing. Philadelphia, WB Saunders, 1994.
Fairchild S. Perioperative Nursing: Principles and Practice. Boston, Jones and Bartlett, 1993.
Greenfield LJ (ed). Complications in Surgery and Trauma, 2nd ed. Philadelphia, JB Lippincott, 1990.
Kneedler JA and Dodge GH. Perioperative Patient Care: The Nursing Perspective, 3rd ed. Boston, Jones and Bartlett, 1994.
Litwack K. Postanesthesia Care Nursing. St. Louis, Mosby–Year Book, 1995.
McCredie JA. Basic Surgery, 2nd ed. New York, Macmillan, 1986.
McGoldrick KE. Ambulatory Anesthesiology: A Problem-Oriented Approach. Baltimore, Williams & Wilkins, 1995.
Merli G and Weitz H (eds). Medical Management of the Surgical Patient. Philadelphia, WB Saunders, 1992.
Miller R (ed). Anesthesia, 4th ed. New York, Churchill Livingstone, 1994.
Schwartz S et al. Principles of Surgery. New York, McGraw-Hill, 1994.
Summers S and Ebbert DW. Ambulatory Surgical Nursing: A Nursing Diagnosis Approach. Philadelphia, JB Lippincott, 1992.
Vender J and Spiess B (eds). Post Anesthesia Care. Philadelphia, WB Saunders, 1992.

Journals

Asterisks indicate nursing research articles.

General

Bailes BK. Disseminated intravascular coagulation: Principles, treatment, nursing management. AORN J 1992 Feb; 55(2):515, 517–520.
Bender BS and Bender JS. Surgical issues in the management of the HIV-infected patient. Surg Clin North Am 1993 Apr; 73(2): 373–388.

*Byra-Cook CJ, Dracup K, and Lazik AJ. Direct and indirect blood pressure in critical care patients. Nurs Res 1990 Sept/Oct; 39(5):285–288.

Carr P. "What am I going to do now?" Am J Nurs 1993 Nov; 93(11):24.

Davis AJ. Clinical nurses' ethical decision making in situations of informed consent. Adv Nurs Sci 1989 Apr; 11(3):63–69.

*Fawcett DL. Attitudes toward patients with AIDS: A comparison between urban and rural perioperative nurses. AORN J 1993 Feb; 57(2):489–492.

*Foreman MD, Theis SL and Anderson MA. Adverse events in the hospitalized elderly. Clin Nurs Res 1993 Aug; 2(3):360–370.

Kirkpatrick L et al. Surgical trends change nursing care: Operating room nurses share new procedures that will affect home health care. Home Healthcare Nurse 1991 Nov/Dec; 9(6):13–20.

*Llewellyn J et al. Analysis of falls in the acute surgical and cardiovascular surgical patient. Appl Nurs Res 1988 Nov; 1(3): 116–121.

Newhouse RP. Physician, nursing, facility implications of informed consent. AORN J 1993 Feb; 57(2):505–510.

*O'Connell M. Anxiety reduction in family members of patients in surgery and postanesthesia care: A pilot study. J Post Anesth Nurs 1989 Feb; 4(1):7–16.

Patterson P. New certification exams for first assistants. OR Manager 1992 Feb; 8(2):1, 9.

Revised AORN official statement on RN first assistants. AORN J 1993 Jan; 57(1):47–51.

*Richards ML. Perioperative nursing research. Part 6. Postoperative phase. AORN J 1989 Jul; 50(1):120–122.

Perioperative Nursing

*Bargagliotti LA. Perioperative nursing research: Issues in perioperative nursing. Part 8. AORN J 1989 Sept; 50(3):613–617.

Chana CH. Documenting the nursing process: A perioperative nursing care plan. AORN J 1992 May; 55(5):1231–1233, 1235.

Dellasega C and Burgunder C. Perioperative nursing care for the elderly surgical patient. Todays OR Nurse 1991 June; 13(6): 12–17, 30–31.

Drescher NI. An integrated care plan: Developing an innovative guideline for patient care. AORN J 1991 Dec; 54(6):1265–1270.

Falkenhagen K. Perioperative nursing in the new decade: What does the future hold? Dimensions in Oncology Nurs 1991 Spring; 5(1):4.

Groah L and Howery D. 25 predictions for perioperative nursing. Nursing 1992 Jan; 22(1):48–49.

Kam BW and Werner PW. Self-care theory: Application to perioperative nursing. AORN J 1990 May; 51(5):1365–1367, 1369–1370.

Kelly KB. Advances in perioperative nutritional support. Med Clin North Am 1993 Mar; 77(2):465–475.

Kjervik DK and Weisensee MG. Empowering older people is a perioperative nursing challenge. AORN J 1992 Apr; 55(4):1086–1089.

Leske JS. Practice-based perioperative research: Meeting the challenges. AORN J 1992 Feb; 55(2):501–507, 589–590.

Lunow K et al. Comprehensive perioperative care: Patient assessment, teaching, documentation. AORN J 1993 May; 57(3): 1167–1168, 1170–1171, 1173–1177.

Mathias JM. Trying new tools: Critical pathways, case management. OR Manager 1993 Jul; 9(7):1, 10–11.

*Noriega L et al. Perioperative nursing research. Part 7. AORN J 1989 Aug; 50(2):379–381.

O'Connell WD. The resuscitation OR: Priorities for the perioperative trauma nurse. Todays OR Nurse 1992 Dec; 14(12):9–12.

Palmer PN. Assessing ECG rhythms is part of perioperative nursing . . . electrocardiogram. AORN J 1990 Aug; 52(2):215–216.

*Parsons EC. Perioperative nurse caring behaviors: Perceptions of surgical patients. AORN J 1993 May; 57(5):1106–1107, 1110–1114.

Patterson P. Integrated model for perioperative nursing. OR Manage 1991 Oct; 7(10):23, 25.

Pobojewski BJ et al. Documenting nursing process in the perioperative setting: Continuity of care, patient evaluation. AORN J 1992 July; 56(1):98–104, 106–110, 112.

Recommended practices: Documentation of perioperative nursing care. AORN J 1991 Sept; 54(3):592, 594–596.

Reeder JM. Advancing perioperative nursing with Project 2000. AORN J 1991 Sept; 54(3):440, 442.

Smalley PJ. Laser nursing—a perioperative challenge. Can Oper Rm Nurs J 1992 Mar/Apr; 10(1):15–16, 18–19, 22.

Standards of perioperative nursing: Clinical practice/professional performance. AORN J 1992 Apr; 55(4):1047, 1051, 1053–1056.

Vidor KK. Perioperative nursing diagnosis: Potential for ineffective airway clearance. Todays OR Nurse 1991 May; 13(5):26–27.

Preoperative Nursing

*Biley C. Nurses' perception of stress in preoperative surgical patients. J Adv Nurs 1989 Jul; 14(7):575–581.

DeLong DL. Preoperative holding area: Personalizing patients' experiences. AORN J 1992 Feb; 55(2):563, 565–566.

*Gamotis PB et al. Inpatient vs outpatient satisfaction: A research study. AORN J 1988 June; 47(6):1424–1425.

Holloway G and Hall J. Planning for a more comfortable stay: Setting up a pre-admission visiting service. AORN J 1992 June; 55(6):1562–1568, 1570.

Leckrone L. Preparing your patient for surgery. Nursing 1991 Jul; 21(7):47–49.

*Rothrock JC. Perioperative nursing research: Preoperative psychoeducational interventions. Part 1. AORN J 1989 Feb; 49(2):597.

*Takahashi JJ et al. Preoperative assessment: A research study. AORN J 1989 Nov; 50(5):1024–1032.

Warner MA et al. Role of preoperative cessation of smoking and other factors in postoperative pulmonary complications: A blinded prospective study of coronary bypass patients. Mayo Clin Proc 1989 June; 64(6):609–616.

Intraoperative Nursing

*Bailes BK. Perioperative nursing research: Intraoperative phase. Part 4. AORN J 1989 May; 49(5):1397–1399.

Bateman F et al. One solution for pressure sores . . . pressure ulcer development in the operating room: Nursing implications. AORN J 1992 Nov; 56(5):832.

Fox V. Passing surgical instruments, sharps without injury . . . using hands-free techniques. AORN J 1992 Jan; 55(1):264–266.

Fox VJ. Preventing glove tears, sharp injuries. AORN J 1993 Mar; 57(3):703, 705–706.

Hoyman K and Gruber N. A case study of interdepartmental cooperation: Operating room–acquired pressure ulcers. J Nurs Care Qual 1992; Spec Rep:12–17.

Matthews K. Argon beam coagulation: New directions in surgery . . . the ABC is not a laser. AORN J 1992 Nov; 56(5):882, 885–886, 888–889.

Morris PB et al. Outpatient carbon dioxide laser mastectomy: Laser techniques, patient outcomes, cost containment. AORN J 1992 Apr; 55(4):984–990, 992.

Moss VA. Burnout: Symptoms, causes, prevention. AORN J Nov; 50(5):1071–1076.

Ratner LE and Smith GW. Intraoperative fluid management. Surg Clin North Am 1993 Apr; 73(2):229–242.

Scott SM, Mayhew PA and Harris EA. Pressure ulcer development in the operating room: Nursing implications. AORN J 1992 Aug; 56(2):242–245, 247, 249–250.

*Silo HM. Perioperative nursing research: Intraoperative recommended practices. Part 5. AORN J 1989 June; 49(6):1627–1636.

Sola JE and Bender JS. Use of the pulmonary artery catheter to reduce operative complications. Surg Clin North Am 1993 Apr; 73(2):253–264.

Stillman A. Laparoscopic cholecystectomy: An electrosurgical approach to biliary disease. AORN J 1993 Feb; 57(2):429–430, 432–436.

Vance A and Davidhizar R. The element of care in the operating room. Todays OR Nurse 1992 Nov; 14(11):24–27.

Weaver DW. Differential diagnosis and management of unexplained bleeding. Surg Clin North Am 1993 Apr; 73(2): 353–361.

Personnel and Communications

Bowen M and Davidhizar R. Anxiety in the operating room: The manager's dilemma. Today's OR Nurs 1990 June; 12(6):32–33.

*Kneedler JA et al. Perioperative nursing research. Part 2. Intraoperative chemical and physical hazards to personnel. AORN J 1989 Mar; 49(3):829–836.

*Kneedler JA et al. Perioperative nursing research. Part 3. Potential intraoperative biological hazard to personnel. AORN J 1989 Apr; 49(4):1066–1067.

Patterson P. OR managers face AIDS ethical dilemmas. Today's OR Nurs 1990 June; 12(6):31.

Scrubbing/Handwashing/Asepsis

Bruning LM. Disposables vs. reusables in OR practice: Weighing contributions to patient care. Part I. Nurs Manage 1992 Feb; 23(2):OR/Ambulatory Surg Ed: 80J-K, 80N, 80P.

Centers for Disease Control. Update: Universal precautions for prevention of human immunodeficiency virus, hepatitis B virus, and other blood-borne pathogens. MMWR 1988; 37(24): 377–390.

Fay MF and Dooher DT. Surgical gloves: Measuring cost and barrier effectiveness. AORN J 1992 June; 55(6):1500–1505, 1507, 1510–1516.

*Korniewicz DM et al. Integrity of vinyl and latex procedure gloves. Nurs Res 1989 May/June; 38(3):144–146.

Thompson S. Eliminating surgical masks...The surgical mask: another sacred cow. AORN J 1992 June; 55(6):1351–1352.

Young MA et al. Latex allergy: A guideline for perioperative nurses. AORN J 1992 Sept; 56(3):485, 488–493, 496–497.

Anesthesia and Surgery

Geniton DJ. A comparison of three anesthetic agents. AORN J 1992 June; 55(6):1562–1568, 1570.

Marco AP and Furman WR. Anesthetic problems: Venous air embolism, airway difficulties, and massive transfusion. Surg Clin North Am 1993 Apr; 73(2):213–228.

Rivellini D. Local and regional anesthesia: Nursing implications. Nurs Clin North Am 1993 Sept; 28(3):547–572.

Hypothermia and Malignant Hyperthermia

*Erickson RS, Yount ST. Comparison of tympanic and oral temperatures in surgical patients. Nurs Res 1991 Mar/Apr; 40(2):90–93.

Feroe DD and Augustine SD. Hypothermia in the PACU. Crit Care Nurs Clin North Am 1991 Mar; 3(1):135–144.

Frederick C, Rosemann D and Austin MJ. Malignant hyperthermia: Nursing diagnosis and care. J Post Anesth Nurs 1990 Feb; 5(1):29–32.

*Holtzclaw BJ. Effects of extremity wraps to control drug-induced shivering: A pilot study. Nurs Res 1990 Sept/Oct; 39(5): 280–284.

*Markin DA et al. Comparison between two types of body surface temperature devices: Efficiency, accuracy and cost. J Post Anesth Nurs 1990 Feb; 5(1):33–37.

Moody D. Hypothermic reaction during laser endometrial ablation: A follow-up study. Laser Nurs 1992 Winter; 6(4):134–136.

Newberry JE. Malignant hyperthermia in the postanesthesia care unit: A review of current etiology, diagnosis and treatment. J Post Anesth Nurs 1990 Feb; 5(1):25–28.

Norris MK. Action stat! Malignant hypothermia. Nurs 90 1990 June; 20(6):33.

Stoecker S. Malignant hyperthermia. AORN J 1992 Dec; 5(4): 13–16, 18–19.

Surkitt-Parr M. Hypothermia in surgical patients. Br J Nurs 1992 Oct 8–21; 1(11):543–545.

*White HE et al. Temperature in elderly surgical patients. Res Nurs Health 1987; 10:317–321.

Woody GS. Malignant hyperthermia. Crit Care Nurs Clin North Am 1991 Mar; 3(1):129–134.

Postoperative Nursing

Biga CD and Bethel SA. Hemodynamic monitoring in postanesthesia care units. Crit Care Nurs Clin North Am 1991 Mar; 3(1): 83–93.

Bines AS and Landron SL. Cardiovascular emergencies in the post anesthesia care unit. Nurs Clin North Am 1993 Sept; 28(3): 493–506.

Jones DH. Fluid therapy in the PACU. Crit Care Nurs Clin North Am 1991 Mar; 3(1):109–120.

Kane AM and Kurlowicz LH. Improving the postoperative care of acutely confused older adults. Medsurg Nurs 1994 Dec; 3(6): 453–458.

Lawler M. Preventing postop complications: Managing other complications. Nursing 1991 Nov; 21(11):33, 40–46.

Levin DF. Assessing and improving quality in the post anesthesia care unit. Nurs Clin North Am 1993 Sept; 28(3):581–596

Lipov EG. Emergency delirium in the PACU. Crit Care Nurs Clin North Am 1991 Mar; 3(1):145–149.

Litwack K. Bleeding and coagulation in the PACU. Crit Care Nurs Clin North Am 1991 Mar; 3(1):121–127.

Litwack K. Post-anesthesia assessment: What medical-surgical nurses need to know. Medsurg Nurs 1993 Aug; 2(4):294–300.

Litwack K, Saleh D and Schultz, P. Postoperative pulmonary complications. Crit Care Nurs Clin North Am 1991 Mar; 3(1):77–82.

McConnell EA. What's wrong with this patient? Nursing 1992 Apr; 22(4):110, 112, 114.

Odom JL. Airway emergencies in the post anesthesia care unit. Nurs Clin North Am 1993 Sept; 28(3):483–492.

Russell G B and Graybell J M. Hypoxemic episodes of patients in a postanesthesia care unit. Chest 1993 Sep; 104(3):899–903.

Saleh KL. The elderly patient in the post anesthesia care unit. Nurs Clin North Am 1993 Sept; 28(3):507-518.

Tremblay DR et al. Arrhythmias in the PACU: A review. Crit Care Nurs Clin North Am 1991 Mar; 3(1):95–108.

Van Sickel AD and Spadaccia K. Muscle relaxants and reversal agents. Crit Care Nurs Clin North Am 1991 Mar; 3(1):151–158.

Vissering TR. Narcotics and implications for the post anesthesia care unit. Nurs Clin North Am 1993 Sept; 28(3):573–580.

Walsh J. Postop effects of OR positioning. RN 1993 Feb; 56(2): 50–57.

Pain

Dean RJ Jr. Regional anesthetic techniques for postoperative analgesia. Crit Care Nurs Clin North Am 1991 Mar; 3(1):43–47.

Doody SB, Smith C, and Webb J. Nonpharmacologic interventions for pain management. Crit Care Nurs Clin North Am 1991 Mar; 3(1):69–75.

Eng JB and Sabanathan S. Postoperative wound pain. Br J Surg 1989 Jan; 76(10):101–102.

*Fortin JD, Schwartz-Barcott D and Rossi S. The postoperative pain experience. Clin Nurs Res 1992 Aug; 1(3):292–304.

Gilbert HC. Pain relief methods in the postanesthesia care unit. J Post Anesth Nurs 1990 Feb; 5(1):6–15.

*Hargraves A and Lander J. Use of transcutaneous electrical nerve stimulation for postoperative pain. Nurs Res 1989 May/June; 38(3):159–161.

Keeney SA. Nursing care of the postoperative patient receiving epidural analgesia. Medsurg Nurs 1993 June; 2(3):191–194.

Lubenow TR and Ivankovich AD. Patient-controlled analgesia for postoperative pain. Crit Care Nurs Clin North Am 1991 Mar; 3(1):35–41.

Lubenow TR and Ivankovich, AD. Postoperative epidural analgesia. Crit Care Nurs Clin North Am 1991 Mar; 3(1):25–32.

Polomano RC, Blumenthal NP and Riegler FX. Interpleural analgesia for the management of postoperative pain. Medsurg Nurs 1993 June; 2(3):185–190.

Rowland MA. Myths—and facts—about postop discomfort. Am J Nurse 1990 May; 90(5):60–64.

*Wilkie DJ. Use of the McGill Pain Questionnaire to measure pain: A meta-analysis. Nurs Res 1990 Jan/Feb; 39(1):36–41.

Wounds and Infection

Barber GR and Brown AE. Surveillance of surgical wound infections in cancer patients. Cancer Practice 1993 May/June; 1(1): 72–76.

Beck-Sague CM et al. Outbreak of surgical wound infections associated with total hip arthroplasty. Infect Control Hosp Epidemiol 1992 Sept; 13(9):526–534.

Boriskin MI. Primary care management of wounds: Cleaning, suturing, and infection control. Nurs Practitioner 1994 Nov; 19(11): 39, 40, 45–46, 49–51, 54, 57–58.

Boyce JM. Methicillin-resistant Staphylococcus aureus in hospitals and long-term care facilities: Microbiology, epidemiology, and preventive measures. Infect Control Hosp Epidemiol 1992 Dec; 13(12):725–737.

Crow S. Sterilization processes: Meeting the demands of today's health care technology. Nurs Clin North Am 1993 Sept; 28(3): 687–698.

Morita MM. Methicillin-resistant Staphylococcus aureus: Past, present, and future. Nurs Clin North Am 1993 Sept; 28(3):625–638.

Privitera G et al. Prospective study of Clostridium difficile intestinal colonization and disease following single dose antibiotic prophylaxis in surgery. Antimicrob Chemother 1991; 35:208–210.

Ambulatory Surgery and Same-Day Surgery

Bean M. Preparation for surgery in an ambulatory surgery unit. J Post Anesth Nurs 1990 Feb; 5(1):42–47.

Haines N. Same day surgery: Coordinating the education process. AORN J 1992 Feb: 55(2):573-576, 578–580.

Keithley J et al. The cost effectiveness of same-day admission surgery. Nurs Econ 1989; 7(2):90–93.

Masterson C. Increasing volume and decreasing costs in the ambulatory surgery unit. J Post Anesth Nurs 1990 Feb; 5(1):38–41.

Murphy EK. Liability exposure in ambulatory surgery settings. AORN J 1991 Dec; 54(6):1287–1289.

Parnass SM. Ambulatory surgical patient priorities. Nurs Clin North Am 1993 Sept; 28(3):531–546.

SDS units produce special risks for nursing liability. Same Day Surg 1992 Mar; 16(3):55–57.

Waldmeier-Veta. Open cholecystectomy: A same day surgery experience. Todays OR Nurse 1992 Sept; 14(9):19–23, 39–34.

Wiseman SJ. Patient advocacy: The essence of perioperative nursing in ambulatory surgery. AORN J 1990 Mar; 51(3):754, 756, 758–759.

Agencies

American Society of Anesthesiologists
500 North Michigan Avenue, Chicago, IL 60611

American Society of Postanesthesia Nurses
PO Box 11083, Richmond, VA 23230

Association of Operating Room Nurses, Inc.
10170 E. Mississippi Avenue, Denver, CO 80231

Malignant Hyperthermia Association of the United States (MHAUS)
163 Waverly Street, Arlington, MA 02174

Nursing Research Profile for Unit 5

Perioperative Nursing

Overview

Nursing research in perioperative nursing reviewed here addresses body temperature assessment and pain control.

Giuffre M, Heidenreich T, and Pruitt L. Rewarming cardiac surgery patients: Radiant heat versus forced warm air. Nurs Res 1994 May/Jun; 43(3):174–178.

During cardiac surgery, hypothermia is induced to protect vital organs from hypoxia. Before the cardiopulmonary bypass (CPB) machine is discontinued, core rewarming is initiated. Various methods of rewarming the patient have been used to minimize these negative consequences. The purpose of this study was to compare the postoperative rewarming times and incidence of shivering in postoperative cardiac patients treated with a forced air warmer or a non-infrared radiant heater. In addition, the preferences of nurses for these two rewarming methods were elicited.

The sample consisted of 38 cardiac surgery patients (29 men and 9 women) admitted to the surgical intensive care unit (SICU) with core temperatures of less than 96.8°F (36°C). The subjects ranged in age from 31 to 78 (M = 60.5 years) and were randomly assigned to either the warm air or radiant heat group. There were no significant differences in age, body surface area, length of cooling during CPB, duration of warming CPB, and baseline core temperatures at SICU admission of patients assigned to the two methods of rewarming. Six other patients (two men and four women) who met the criteria and had received only warmed blankets were used as a comparison group.

Radiant heat was provided by a large over-bed heater with a surface area suspended over the patient. The suspended surface of the heater was placed 28 inches away from the patient's exposed skin. Warm air was provided to the second group of patients by a commercial warming system consisting of a paper and plastic sheet placed over the patient and attached to a warm air blower. The paper and plastic sheet was placed over the patient's skin and covered with a blanket; this allowed warm air to flow onto and be maintained near the patient's skin.

Core temperature was measured by the thermistor (temperature sensitive component) of the pulmonary artery catheter. Skin temperature was measured by a non-contact infrared tympanic thermometer. Core and skin temperatures were taken within minutes (up to 15) of admission to the SICU, and temperature and shivering were assessed at 15-minute intervals until the patient's core temperature had reached and remained at 96.8°F for 30 minutes.

The mean time for rewarming was 100.3 minutes for the warm air group, 99.3 minutes for the radiant heat group, and 188.2 minutes for the warmed blanket group. There were no differences in mean time to rewarm to core temperature in the warm air and radiant heat groups; the only significant difference in the core rewarming times was detected when the blanket group was compared with the combined experimental groups ($p < .003$). The difference in mean skin temperature between the warm air and radiant heat groups was statistically significant at all measurements. The skin temperature of the warm air group was initially lower than the radiant heat group but exceeded the radiant heat group skin temperature within 15 minutes and remained higher throughout subsequent readings.

Afterdrop occurred in all subjects between the time that warming CPB was discontinued in the operating room until arrival in the SICU. Core temperatures continued to drop in 12 patients after rewarming was initiated. Five patients in the warm air group had further drops in core temperature (M = .12°C) in the first 30 minutes of rewarming therapy; seven patients in the radiant heat group had further afterdrop (M = .27°C) in the first 45 minutes of rewarming.

Shivering is not expected with cardiac surgery patients because high dosages of opiates are given intraoperatively. However, one subject in the warm air group and five subjects in the radiant heat group experienced shivering. Four patients developed shivering after reaching a core temperature of 36°C (96.8°F), and one subject from each group developed shivering before reaching 36°C.

SICU nurses caring for patients in this study had positive reactions to both methods of rewarming. Of the 12 nurses asked their preference for the methods on the last day of the study, all indicated a preference for the forced warm air method of rewarming.

Nursing Implications. This study found that the methods of forced warm air and radiant heat rewarmed patients at almost equal rates. However, after rewarming was initiated, the patients in the warm air group had consistently warmer skin and less afterdrop than the radiant heat group. Additionally, the afterdrop was of shorter duration than that of the radiant heat group. This correlates with the belief that afterdrop is inversely related to the effectiveness of total body warming and supports the assumption that the most effective peripheral warming will most effectively warm the core. No conclusion can be stated about the ineffectiveness of warmed blankets because these few subjects had intraoperative factors different from the experimental groups and were not randomly assigned to this method of rewarming.

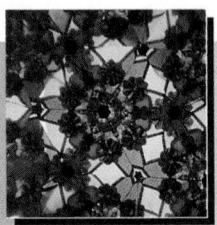

Erickson RS and Yount ST. Comparison of tympanic and oral temperatures in surgical patients. Nurs Res 1991 Mar/Apr; 40(2):90–93.

In the operating room (OR), a patient's core body temperature can drop during skin preparation, draping, and exposure of the surgical site. Two current methods of easily measuring core temperature are the tympanic thermometer and the oral thermometer. The tympanic measurement estimates core temperature, whereas the oral sublingual measurement is a more peripheral reflection of core temperature. This study compared infrared tympanic and thermistor oral temperatures at four times during the perioperative experience to assess their equivalence and stability.

The convenience sample (n = 60) consisted of 11 men and 49 women undergoing major nonvascular abdominal surgery under general anesthesia; they ranged in age from 25 to 80 years (M = 51.6, SD = 14.6 years). Tympanic and oral temperatures were measured (1) within thirty minutes before OR transport; (2) upon entry into the OR; (3) at entry in the postanesthesia care unit (PACU); and (4) before exit from PACU. Tympanic temperatures were also measured after surgical site preparation in the OR.

Oral temperature was measured with a predictive thermometer with the probe tip placed in the patient's posterior sublingual pocket. Tympanic temperature was measured with an infrared thermometer with the probe tip placed in the opening of the ear canal.

Findings indicated a similar pattern of change in temperature obtained with tympanic and oral thermometers and that the subjects' temperatures changed significantly over time at both sites. Temperatures obtained at the two sites had a moderately high correlation at each of the four measurement times ($r = .77$ to $.85$, $p < .0001$). Temperature did not change significantly during transport but had a significant fall of approximately 2°F in the OR during surgery and during preparation of the surgical site ($p = .01$) and a significant rise of about 1°F in PACU ($p = .01$). In 99% of the measurements, tympanic temperature readings were higher than oral readings, and the difference ranged from 1.1° to 1.5°F.

Nursing Implications. The findings suggest that both the infrared tympanic and the predictive thermistor oral thermometer are stable and provide generally similar readings in afebrile postoperative patients. However, consistency in site of measurement in an individual is important to provide a comparison of temperature over time. Suggestions for further research include comparison studies over a longer period of time, in different age groups, and in abnormal conditions such as fever and hypothermia.

Puntillo D and Weiss SJ. Pain: Its mediators and associated morbidity in critically ill cardiovascular surgical patients. Nurs Res 1994 Jan/Feb; 43(1):31–36.

This study examined the effects of age, sex, personality adjustment, and analgesic administration on the pain experience of cardiac surgery (CS) and abdominal vascular surgery (AVS) patients in their initial postoperative period. The majority (81%) of the convenience sample of 74 cardiovascular patients (44 males and 16 females) underwent cardiac bypass surgery. The remaining 14 subjects (13 males and 1 female) had abdominal vascular surgery. Eighty-four percent had a preoperative physical status rating of severe systemic disease, defined as a functional limitation that may be a constant threat to life.. There was no significant difference in age between men and women (M = 64 years), who ranged in age from 33 to 83 years.

Pain intensity was measured by a 10-cm horizontal numerical rating scale (NRS); sensory and affective components of pain were measured by the McGill pain questionnaire short form (MPQ-SF). Analgesic use was calculated by summing all dosages of intravenous and oral analgesic use during study participation. Personality adjustment was measured by the California Q-Set. A family member or a close friend who knew the patient well categorized the 100 items of the Q-Set according to how well the items described the subject's personality characteristics. The presence or absence of postoperative complications (infection, reintubation, atelectasis, pneumonia, pleural effusion, and psychologic disturbances) was used as an indicator of morbidity. Subjects participated in the study for 3 consecutive days during their postoperative stay in the critical care unit; 97% of subjects were entered in the study by their second postoperative day. Pain data were collected once each day but not within 2 hours of the last opiate administration.

Study findings revealed that pain intensity varied little over the 3 days but that the patients with AVS had more pain on all 3 postoperative days when compared with CS patients. Statistical analyses (hierarchial regression analyses) were used to determine how much the variables (age, gender, amount of analgesics, degree of personality adjustment, type of surgery) contributed to pain intensity, sensation, and affect. Three separate regression models were tested, one for each of the three pain dimensions (intensity, sensation, and affect). Analyses revealed that the amount of analgesics received over the 3 days was the only significant predictor of pain intensity and pain magnitude (or affect). The amount of analgesics received, along with gender and type of surgery (AVS vs. CS), explained significant portions of the variance of pain sensation.

Subjects were divided into two groups on each pain dimension by their pain scores to analyze the relationship of pain and postoperative complications. The magnitude of pain related to only one postoperative complication on one pain dimension: patients with higher pain intensity scores had significantly more atelectasis than those with lower pain intensity ($p < .05$).

Nursing Implications. Although these subjects did not have significantly less pain during the 3 days of participation, the amount of analgesics administered was small and decreased on each subsequent day. Analgesics received were not effective since the greater amount of pain medication received, the greater the magnitude of pain. A limiting factor in this study was that pain was assessed only once each day. Although research with a larger and more representative sample is required, this study does support the need to rethink the conservative use of analgesics and the use of nonpharmacologic methods to reduce pain. The relationship between pain intensity and atelectasis is an important finding and indicates the need for more effective postoperative analgesia to reduce the incidence of this important postoperative complication.

UNIT 6

Oxygen–Carbon Dioxide Exchange and Respiratory Function

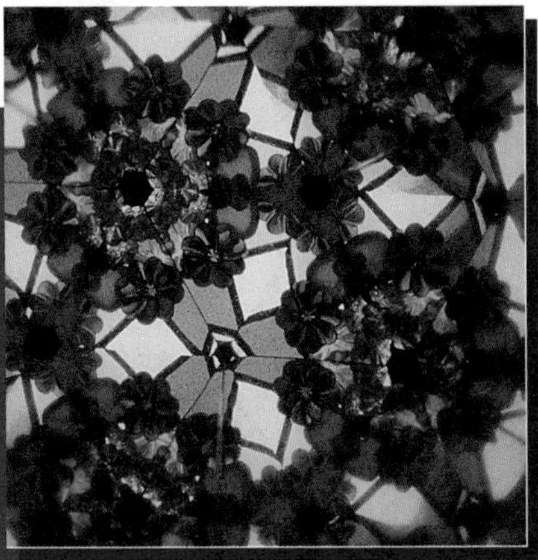

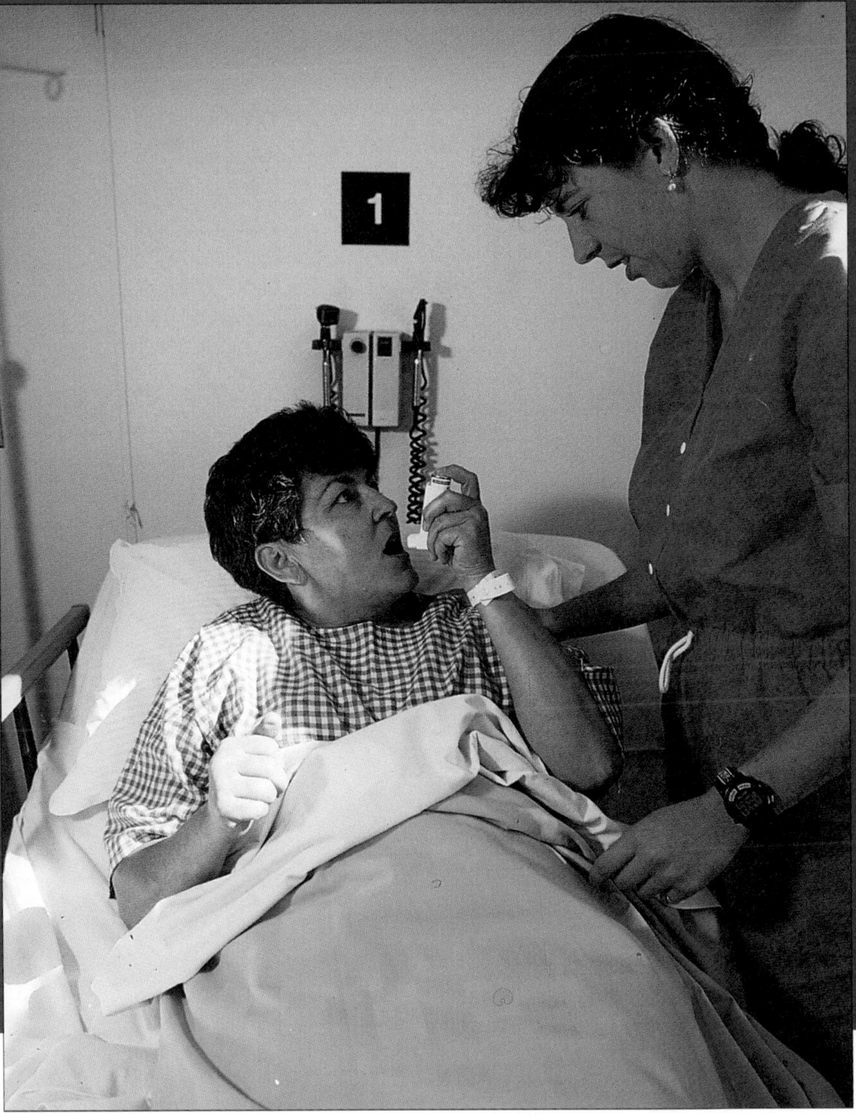

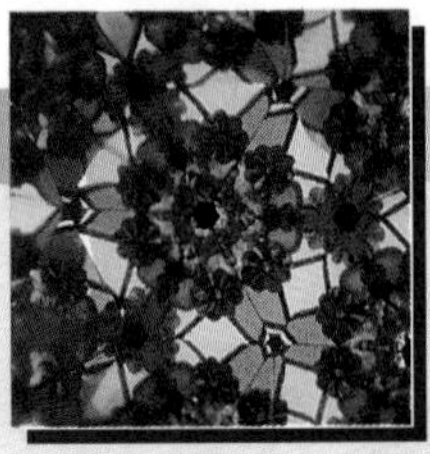

22

Assessment of Respiratory Function

CHAPTER OUTLINE

LEARNING OBJECTIVES

On completion of this chapter, the learner will be able to:

1. Describe structures of the upper airway and their functions
2. Describe ventilation, perfusion, diffusion, shunting, and the relationship of pulmonary circulation to these processes
3. Discriminate between normal and abnormal breath sounds
4. Use assessment parameters appropriate for determining the characteristics and severity of the major symptoms of respiratory dysfunction
5. Identify the nursing implications of the various procedures used for diagnostic assessment of respiratory function

Anatomy of the Upper Respiratory Airway

Nose

The nose is composed of an external and an internal portion. The external portion protrudes from the face and is supported by the nasal bones and cartilage. The anterior nares (nostrils) are the outside openings of the nasal cavities.

The internal portion of the nose is a hollow cavity separated into the right and left nasal cavities by a narrow vertical divider, the septum. Each nasal cavity is divided into three passageways by the projection of the turbinates (also called conchae) from the lateral walls. The nasal cavities are lined with highly vascular ciliated mucous membranes called the nasal mucosa. Mucus secreted continuously by goblet cells covers the surface of the nasal mucosa and is moved back to the nasopharynx by the action of the cilia.

The nose serves as a passageway for air to pass to and from the lungs. It filters impurities and it humidifies and warms the air as it is inhaled into the lungs. It is responsible for olfaction (smell) because the olfactory receptors are located in the nasal mucosa. This function diminishes with age.

Paranasal Sinuses

The paranasal sinuses include four pairs of bony cavities that are lined with nasal mucosa and ciliated pseudostratified columnar epithelium. These air spaces are connected by a series of ducts that drain into the nasal cavity. The sinuses are named by their location, namely, frontal, ethmoidal, sphenoidal, and maxillary (Fig. 22-1).

A prominent function of the sinuses is to serve as a resonating chamber in speech. The sinuses are a common site of infection.

Turbinate Bones (Conchae)

The turbinate bones, or conchae (the name suggested by their shell-like appearance), are adapted by shape and position to increase the mucous membrane surface of the nasal passages and to slightly obstruct the current of air flowing through them (Fig. 22-2).

The current of air entering the nostrils is deflected upward to the roof of the nose and follows a circuitous route before it reaches the nasopharynx. On its way, it comes into contact with a large surface of moist, warm mucous membrane that catches practically all of the dust and organisms in the inhaled air. This air is moistened and warmed to body temperature and brought into contact with sensitive nerves. Some of these nerves detect odors, and others provoke sneezing to expel irritating dust.

Pharynx, Tonsils, and Adenoids

The pharynx, or throat, is a tubelike structure that connects the nasal and oral cavities to the larynx. It is divided into three regions: nasal, oral, and laryngeal.

The nasopharynx is located posterior to the nose and is above the soft palate. The oropharynx houses the faucial, or palatine, tonsils. The laryngopharynx extends from the hyoid bone to the cricoid cartilage. The entrance of the larynx is formed by the epiglottis.

The adenoids, or pharyngeal tonsils, are located in the roof of the nasopharynx. The throat is encircled by the tonsils, the adenoids, and other lymphoid tissue. These structures are important links in the chain of lymph nodes guarding the body from invasion by organisms entering the nose and the throat. The function of the pharynx is to provide a passageway for the respiratory and digestive tracts.

Larynx

The larynx, or voice organ, is a cartilaginous epithelium-lined structure that connects the pharynx and the trachea.

The major function of the larynx is to permit vocalization. It also protects the lower airway from foreign substances and facilitates coughing. It is frequently referred to as the voice box and consists of the following:

- *Epiglottis*—a valve flap of cartilage that covers the opening to the larynx during swallowing
- *Glottis*—the opening between the vocal cords in the larynx

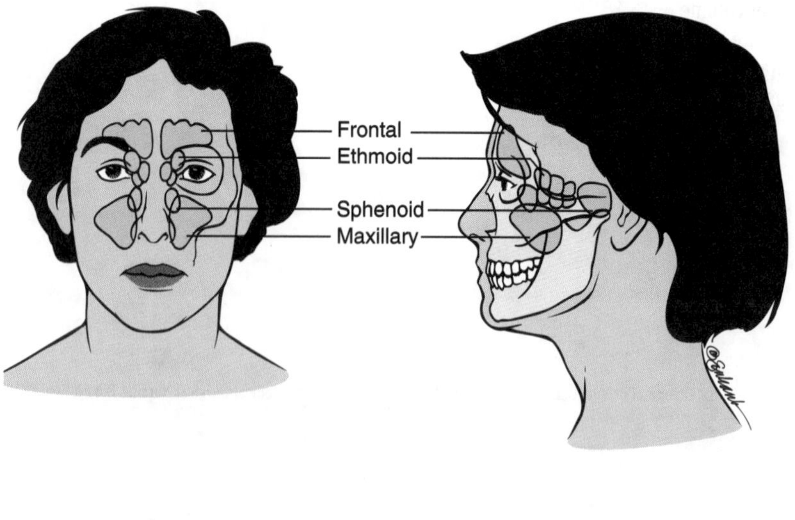

FIGURE 22-1. The paranasal sinuses.

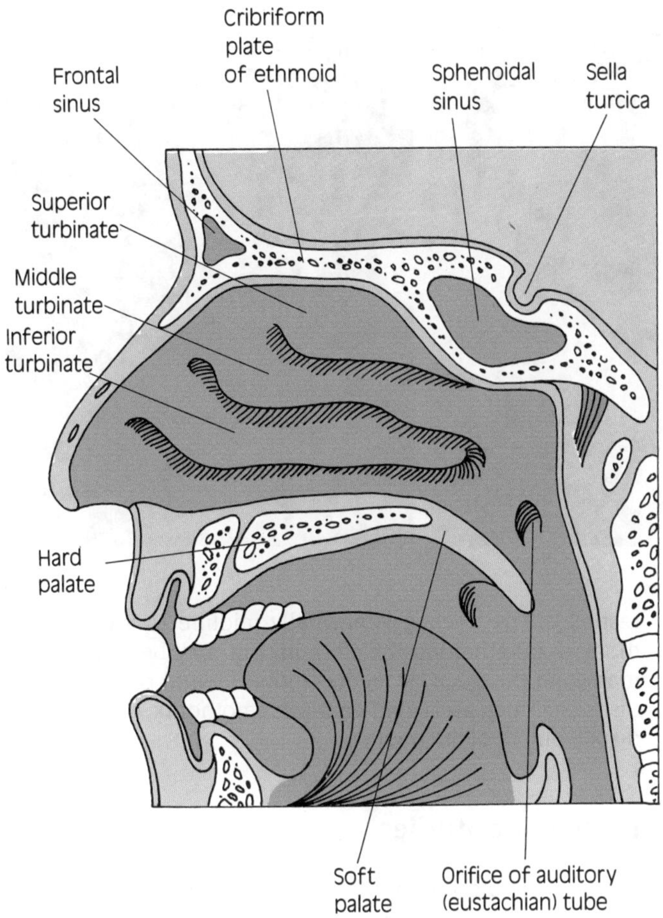

FIGURE 22-2. Cross section of the nasal cavity.

- *Thyroid cartilage*—the largest cartilage in the trachea, part of it forms the Adam's apple
- *Cricoid cartilage*—the only complete cartilaginous ring in the larynx (located below the thyroid cartilage)
- *Arytenoid cartilages*—used in vocal cord movement with the thyroid cartilage
- *Vocal cords*—ligaments controlled by muscular movements that produce vocal sounds; they are mounted in the lumen of the larynx

Assessment of the Upper Respiratory Airway

Nose and Sinuses

The nose and sinuses are examined by inspection and palpation. For a routine examination, only a simple light source, such as a penlight, is necessary. A more thorough examination requires the use of a nasal speculum.

The external nose is inspected for lesions, asymmetry, or inflammation. The patient is then instructed to tilt the head backward while the examiner gently pushes the tip of the nose upward to examine the internal structures of the nose. The mucosa is inspected for color, swelling, exudate, or bleeding. The nasal mucosa is normally more red than the oral mucosa but may appear swollen and hyperemic in the presence of the common cold. Allergic rhinitis, however, is suggested when the mucosa appears pale and swollen.

The septum is inspected for deviation, perforation, or bleeding. A slight degree of septal deviation is present in most people. Actual displacement of the cartilage into either the right or left side of the nose may produce nasal obstruction, but such deviation is usually asymptomatic.

With the patient's head tilted back, the examiner attempts to visualize the inferior and middle turbinates. In chronic rhinitis, nasal polyps may develop between the inferior and middle turbinates and are distinguished by their gray appearance. Unlike the turbinates, they are gelatinous and freely movable.

The frontal and maxillary sinuses are palpated for tenderness (Fig. 22-3). Using the thumbs, the examiner applies gentle pressure in an upward fashion at the supraorbital ridges (frontal sinuses) and in the cheek area adjacent to the nose (maxillary sinuses). Tenderness in either area suggests inflammation. The frontal and maxillary sinuses can be inspected by transillumination (passing a strong light through a bony structure such as the sinuses to inspect the cavity; Fig. 22-4).

Pharynx

A tongue blade, which often is used to depress the tongue so that the pharynx can be seen more clearly, is not always

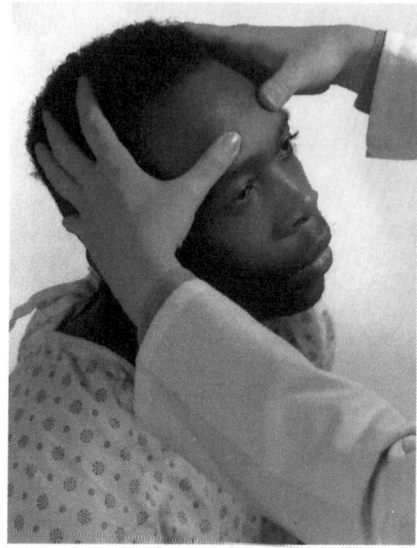

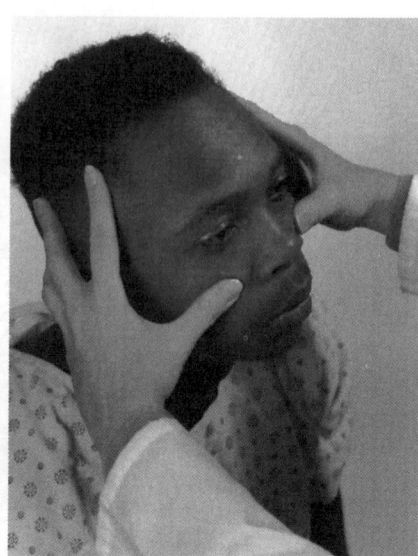

FIGURE 22-3. Technique for palpating the frontal sinuses (**left**) and the maxillary sinuses (**right**). (From Fuller J and Schaller-Ayers J. Health Assessment: A Nursing Approach, 2nd ed. Philadelphia, JB Lippincott, 1994.)

necessary. The patient is instructed to open the mouth wide and take a deep breath. Often this will flatten the posterior tongue and briefly expose a full view of the anterior and posterior pillars, tonsils, uvula, and posterior pharynx (Fig. 22-5). These structures are inspected for color, symmetry, and evidence of exudate, ulceration, or enlargement. If a 431tongue blade is used to visualize the pharynx, it is pressed firmly beyond the midpoint of the tongue. Proper placement avoids a gagging response.

Trachea

The position and mobility of the trachea are usually noted by direct palpation. This is performed by placing the thumb and index finger of one hand on either side of the trachea just above the sternal notch. The trachea is highly sensitive, and palpating too firmly may incite a coughing or gagging response. The trachea is normally midline as it enters the thoracic inlet behind the sternum but may be deviated by masses in the neck or mediastinum. Pleural or pulmonary disorders, such as a significant pneumothorax, may result in displacement of the trachea.

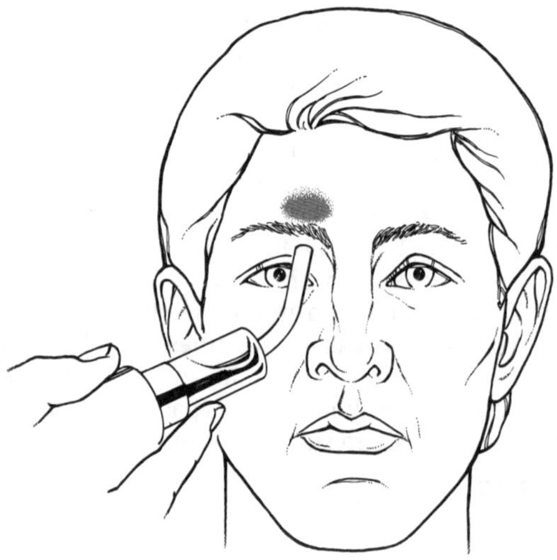

FIGURE 22-4. Method for transilluminating the frontal sinus. Light source is pressed against the supraorbital rim. A glow should appear above the eye. (From Fuller J and Schaller-Ayers J. Health Assessment: A Nursing Approach, 2nd ed. Philadelphia, JB Lippincott, 1994.)

Diagnostic Studies

Cultures and biopsies are the procedures used most often in the diagnosis of the upper airways. However, more extensive diagnostic testing may be indicated.

Cultures. Throat cultures may be performed to identify organisms responsible for pharyngitis. Additionally, throat culture may assist in identifying organisms responsible for infection of the lower respiratory tract. Nasal swabs may also be performed for the same purpose.

Biopsy. Biopsy, the excision of a small amount of tissue, may be performed to permit examination of cells from the pharynx, larynx, and nasal passages. Local, topical, or general anesthesia may be administered, depending on the site and the procedure.

Imaging Studies. Imaging studies, including soft tissue x-rays, computed tomography (CT) scans, contrast studies, and magnetic resonance imaging (MRI), may be performed as part of the diagnostic work-up to determine the extent of infection in sinusitis or of tumor growth in the case of cancer.

Physiologic Overview of Respiration

The cells of the body derive the energy they need from the oxidation of carbohydrates, fats, and proteins. As with any type of combustion, this process requires oxygen. Certain vital tissues, such as those of the brain and the heart, cannot survive for long without a continuing supply of oxygen. As a result of oxidation in the body tissues, carbon dioxide is produced and must be removed from the cells to prevent build-up of acid waste products.

Oxygen Transport. Oxygen is supplied to and carbon dioxide is removed from cells by way of the circulating

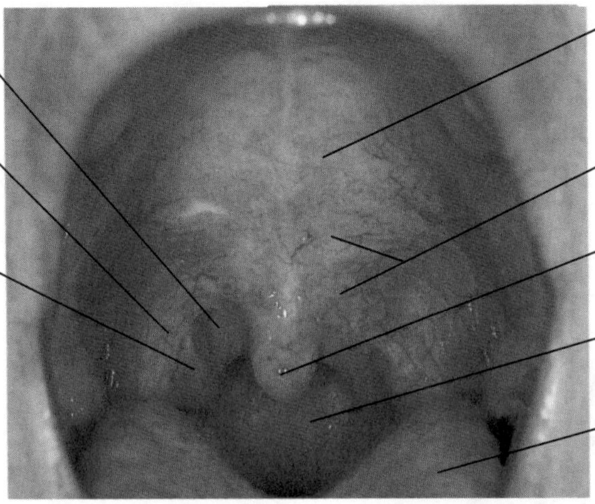

FIGURE 22-5. View of the pharynx showing the pillars, tonsils, uvula, hard and soft palates, posterior pharynx, and tongue. (From Bates B. A Guide to Physical Assessment and History Taking, 6th ed. Philadelphia, JB Lippincott, 1995.)

blood. Cells are in close contact with capillaries, whose thin walls permit easy passage or exchange of oxygen and carbon dioxide. Oxygen diffuses from the capillary, through the capillary wall to the interstitial fluid, and then through the membrane of tissue cells, where it can be used by mitochondria for cellular respiration. The movement of carbon dioxide also occurs by diffusion and proceeds in the opposite direction, from cell to blood.

Gas Exchange. After these tissue capillary exchanges, blood enters the systemic veins (where it is called *venous blood*) and travels to the pulmonary circulation. The oxygen concentration in blood within the capillaries of the lungs is lower than it is in the lungs' air sacs, which are called **alveoli**. As a result of this concentration gradient, oxygen diffuses from the alveoli to the blood. Carbon dioxide, which has a concentration in the blood higher than that in the alveoli, diffuses from the blood into the alveoli. Movement of air in and out of the airways (called **ventilation**) continually replenishes the oxygen and removes the carbon dioxide from the airways in the lung. This whole process of gas exchange between the atmospheric air and the blood and between the blood and cells of the body is called **respiration**.

Anatomy of the Lung

The lungs are elastic structures enclosed in the thoracic cage, which is an airtight chamber with distensible walls (Fig. 22-6). Ventilation requires movement of the walls of the thoracic cage and of its floor, the diaphragm. The effect of these movements is alternately to increase and decrease the capacity of the chest. When the capacity of the chest is increased, air enters through the trachea (*inspiration*), because of the lowered pressure within, and inflates the lungs. When the chest wall and diaphragm return to their previous positions (*expiration*), the elastic lungs recoil and force the air out through the bronchi and trachea. The inspiratory phase of respiration normally requires energy; the expiratory phase is normally passive. Inspiration occupies the first third of the respiratory cycle, expiration the latter two thirds.

Pleura. The outer surfaces of the lungs are surrounded by a smooth, slippery membrane, the pleura, which also extends to cover the interior wall of the thorax and the superior surface of the diaphragm (see Fig. 22-6). *Parietal pleura* lines the thorax, and *visceral pleura* covers the lungs. Between the two pleural surfaces is a space, called the *pleural space*, which contains a small amount of fluid that lubricates the surfaces and allows them to slide freely during ventilation.

Mediastinum. The mediastinum is the wall that divides the thoracic cavity into two halves. It is composed of two layers of pleura. All of the thoracic structures except the lungs are located between the two layers of pleura.

Lobes. Each lung is divided into lobes. The left lung consists of upper and lower lobes, whereas the right lung has upper, middle, and lower lobes (Fig. 22-7). Each lobe is further subdivided into two to five segments separated by fissures, which are extensions of the pleura.

Bronchi and Bronchioles. There are several divisions of the bronchi within each lobe of the lung. First are the lobar bronchi (three in the right lung and two in the left lung). Lobar bronchi divide into segmental bronchi (10 on the right and 8 on the left), which are the structures identified when choosing the most effective postural drainage position for a given patient. Segmental bronchi then divide into subsegmental bronchi. These bronchi are surrounded by connective tissue that contains arteries, lymphatics, and nerves.

The subsegmental bronchi then branch into *bronchioles*, which have no cartilage in their walls. Their patency depends entirely on the elastic recoil of the surrounding smooth muscle and on the alveolar pressure. The bronchioles contain submucosal glands, which produce mucus that forms an uninterrupted covering for the inside lining of the airway. The bronchi and bronchioles are lined also with cells that have surfaces covered with short "hairs" called *cilia*. These cilia create a constant whipping motion that serves to propel mucus and foreign substances away from the lung toward the larynx.

The bronchioles then branch into *terminal bronchioles*, which do not have mucous glands or cilia. Terminal bronchioles then become *respiratory bronchioles*, which are considered to be the transition passageways between the conducting airways and the gas exchange airways. Up to this point, the conducting airways contain about 150 ml of air in the tracheobronchial tree that does not participate in gas exchange. This is known as *physiologic dead space*. The respiratory bronchioles then lead into alveolar ducts and alveolar sacs and then alveoli. Oxygen and carbon dioxide exchange takes place in the alveoli.

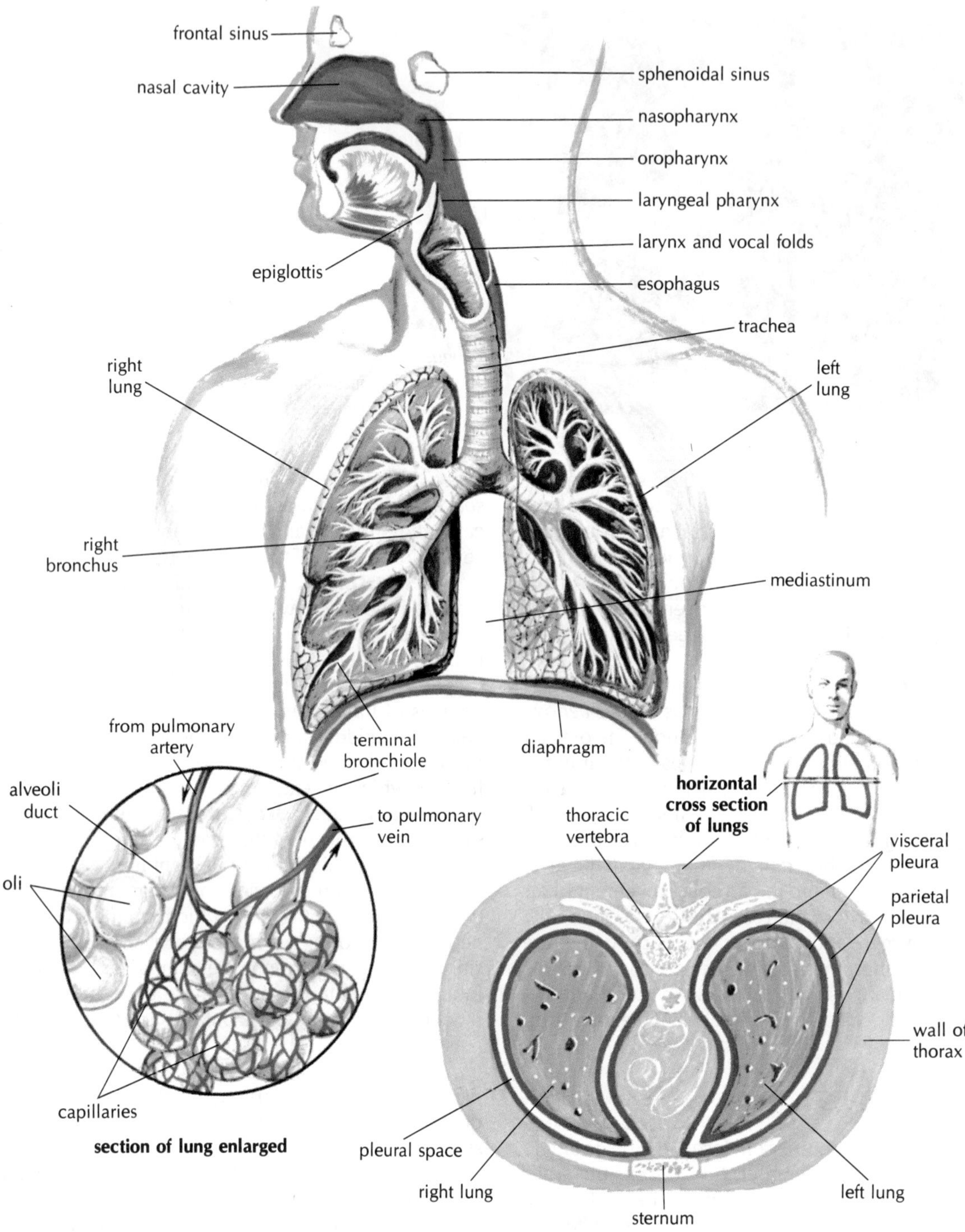

FIGURE 22-6. The respiratory system, showing upper respiratory structures and the structures of the thorax; *insets* show the alveoli and a horizontal cross-section of the lungs.

Alveoli. The lung is made up of about 300 million alveoli, which are arranged in clusters of 15 to 20. So numerous are these alveoli that if their surfaces were united to form one sheet, it would cover an area 70 square meters (the size of a tennis court).

There are three types of alveolar cells. Type I alveolar cells are epithelial cells that form the alveolar walls. Type II alveolar cells, metabolically active cells, secrete *surfactant*, a phospholipid that lines the inner surface and prevents alveolar collapse. Type III alveoli cell macrophages are large phagocytic cells that ingest foreign matter (*e.g.*, mucus, bacteria) and act as an important defense mechanism.

Mechanics of Ventilation

During inspiration, air flows from the environment into the trachea, bronchi, bronchioles, and alveoli. During expiration, alveolar gas travels the same route in reverse.

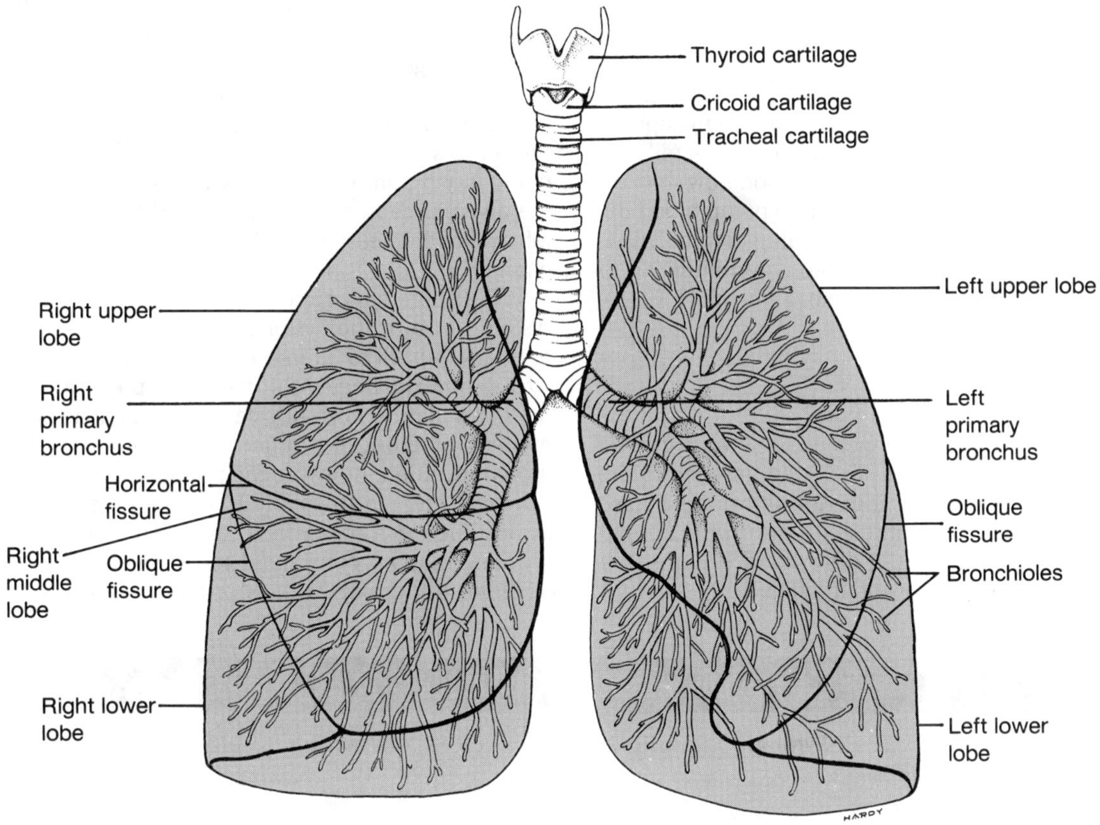

FIGURE 22-7. Anterior view of the trachea, bronchial tree, and lobes of the lungs.

The physical factors that govern air flow in and out of the lungs are collectively referred to as the mechanics of ventilation and include air pressure variances, resistance to air flow, and lung compliance.

Air Pressure Variances. Air flows from a region of higher pressure to a region of lower pressure. During inspiration, movement of the diaphragm and other muscles of respiration enlarges the thoracic cavity and thereby lowers the pressure inside the thorax to a level below that of atmospheric pressure. Therefore, air is drawn through the trachea and bronchi into the alveoli.

During normal expiration, the diaphragm relaxes, and the lungs recoil, resulting in a decrease in the size of the thoracic cavity. The alveolar pressure then exceeds atmospheric pressure, and air flows from the lungs into the atmosphere.

Airway Resistance. Resistance is determined chiefly by the radius or size of the airway through which the air is flowing. Any process that changes bronchial diameter or width therefore affects airway resistance and alters the rate of air flow for a given pressure gradient during respiration. Common factors that may alter bronchial diameter include contraction of bronchial smooth muscle, as in asthma; thickening of bronchial mucosa, as in chronic bronchitis; or obstruction of the airway due to mucus, a tumor, or a foreign body. Loss of lung elasticity, such as is seen in emphysema, also may alter bronchial diameter as the lung connective tissue encircles the airways and helps keep them open during both inspiration and expiration. With increased resistance, greater than normal respiratory effort is required by the patient to achieve normal levels of ventilation.

Compliance. The pressure gradient between the thoracic cavity and the atmosphere causes air to flow in and out of the lungs. When pressure changes are applied in the normal lung, there is a proportional change in the lung volume. A measure of the elasticity, expandibility, and distensibility of the lungs and thoracic structures is called *compliance*. Factors that determine lung compliance are the surface tension of the alveoli (normally low with the presence of surfactant) and the connective tissue, (*i.e.*, collagen and elastin) of the lungs.

Compliance is determined by examining the volume-pressure relationship in the lungs and the thorax. In normal compliance, (1.0 L/cm H_2O), the lungs and thorax easily stretch and distend when pressure is applied. High or increased compliance occurs when the lungs have lost their elasticity and the thorax is overdistended, (*i.e.*, emphysema). When the lungs and thorax are "stiff," there is low or decreased compliance. Conditions associated with this include pneumothorax, hemothorax, pleural effusion, pulmonary edema, atelectasis, pulmonary fibrosis, and adult respiratory distress syndrome (ARDS). Measurement of compliance is one method used for assessing the progression and improvement in ARDS. Lungs with decreased compliance require greater than normal energy expenditure to achieve normal levels of ventilation. Compliance is usually measured under static conditions.

Lung function, which reflects the mechanisms of ventilation, is viewed in terms of lung volumes and lung capacities. *Lung volumes* are divided into tidal volume, inspiratory reserve volume, expiratory reserve volume, and residual volume. *Lung capacity* is evaluated in terms of vital capacity, inspiratory capacity, functional residual capacity, and total lung capacity. The definition and effect of each of these terms are described in Table 22-1.

In the upright position, ventilation is greatest in the lower regions of the lungs and decreases toward the apices. This regional inequality is caused by gravity. The capillaries at the bases of the lungs receive greater blood flow than do the apices owing to the pressure needed to pump blood upward. In addition to this regional inequality of ventilation, there is uneven ventilation among alveoli, permitting air to be distributed more evenly among them.

Diffusion and Perfusion

Diffusion is the process by which oxygen and carbon dioxide are exchanged at the air–blood interface. The alveolar–capillary membrane is ideal for diffusion because of its large surface area and thin membrane. In the normal healthy adult, oxygen and carbon dioxide travel across the alveolar–capillary membrane without difficulty.

Pulmonary perfusion is the actual blood flow through the pulmonary circulation. The blood is pumped into the lungs by the right ventricle through the pulmonary artery. The pulmonary artery divides into the right and left branches to supply both lungs. These two branches divide further to supply all parts of each lung. Normally about 2% of the blood pumped by the right ventricle does not perfuse the alveolar capillaries. This *shunted blood* drains into the left side of the heart without participating in alveolar gas exchange.

The pulmonary circulation is considered a low pressure system because the systolic blood pressure in the pulmonary artery is 20 to 30 mm Hg and the diastolic pressure is 5 to 15 mm Hg. Because of these low pressures, the pulmonary vasculature normally can vary its capacity to accommodate the blood flow it receives. When a person is in an upright position, however, the pulmonary artery pressure is not great enough to supply blood to the apex of the lung against the force of gravity. Thus, when a person is upright, the lung may be considered to be divided into three sections: an upper part with poor blood supply, a lower part

TABLE 22-1 Lung Volumes and Lung Capacities

Term Used	Symbol	Description	Remarks
Lung Volumes			
Tidal volume	V_T or TV	The volume of air inhaled and exhaled with each breath	The tidal volume may not vary, even with severe disease.
Inspiratory reserve volume	IRV	The maximum volume of air that can be inhaled after a normal inhalation	
Expiratory reserve volume	ERV	The maximum volume of air that can be exhaled forcibly after a normal exhalation	Expiratory reserve volume is decreased with restrictive disorders, such as obesity, ascites, pregnancy.
Residual volume	RV	The volume of air remaining in the lungs after a maximum exhalation	Residual volume may be increased with obstructive diseases.
Lung Capacities			
Vital capacity	VC	The maximum volume of air exhaled from the point of maximum inspiration	A decrease in vital capacity may be found in neuromuscular disease, generalized fatigue, atelectasis, pulmonary edema, and COPD.
Inspiratory capacity	IC	The maximum volume of air inhaled after normal expiration	A decrease in inspiratory capacity may indicate restrictive disease.
Functional residual capacity	FRC	The volume of air remaining in lungs after a normal expiration	Functional residual capacity may be increased with obstructive disease (COPD) and decreased in ARDS.
Total lung capacity	TLC	The volume of air in the lungs after a maximum inspiration and equal to the sum of all four volumes (V_T, IRV, ERV, RV)	Total lung capacity may be decreased with restrictive disease (atelectasis, pneumonia) and increased in obstructive disease (COPD)

with maximal blood supply, and the section in between the two with an intermediate supply of blood. When a person lying down turns to one side, more blood passes to the dependent lung.

Perfusion is also influenced by alveolar pressure. The pulmonary capillaries are sandwiched between adjacent alveoli. If the alveolar pressure is sufficiently high, the capillaries will be squeezed. Depending on the pressure, some capillaries completely collapse, whereas others will narrow.

Pulmonary artery pressure, gravity, and alveolar pressure determine the patterns of perfusion. In lung disease these factors vary and the perfusion of the lung may become very abnormal.

Ventilation and Perfusion Balance and Imbalance

Ventilation is the flow of gas in and out of the lungs, and perfusion is the filling of the pulmonary capillaries with blood. Adequate gas exchange is dependent on an adequate ventilation–perfusion ratio. In different areas of the lung, the ratio may vary.

Alterations in perfusion may occur with a change in the pulmonary artery pressure, alveolar pressure, and gravity. Alteration in ventilation may occur with blockage of the airways, local changes in compliance of the lung, and gravity.

A **ventilation–perfusion (V–Q) imbalance** occurs when there is either inadequate ventilation or inadequate perfusion, or both. There are four possible ventilation–perfusion states in the lung: normal ventilation–perfusion ratio, low ventilation–perfusion ratio (shunt), high ventilation–perfusion ratio (dead space), and low ventilation–perfusion (silent unit) (Fig. 22-8).

It is important to understand the four possible ventilation–perfusion matches.

- *Normal: ventilation matches perfusion*. In the healthy lung, a given amount of blood passes an alveolus and is matched with an equal amount of gas. The ratio is 1:1 (ventilation matches perfusion).
- *Low ventilation–perfusion ratio: shunt-producing disorders*. When perfusion exceeds ventilation, a shunt exists. Blood bypasses the alveoli without gas exchange occurring. This is seen with obstruction of the distal airways, such as with pneumonia, atelectasis, tumor, or a mucus plug.
- *High ventilation–perfusion ratio: dead space–producing disorder*. When ventilation exceeds perfusion, dead space occurs. The alveoli have inadequate blood supply to allow gas exchange to occur. This is seen with a variety of disorders, including pulmonary emboli, pulmonary infarction, and cardiogenic shock.
- *Silent unit: absence of ventilation and perfusion*. When there is limited ventilation and perfusion, a silent unit occurs. This is seen with pneumothorax and severe adult respiratory distress syndrome (ARDS).

Ventilation and perfusion imbalance causes shunting of blood, resulting in **hypoxia**. It appears to be the main cause of hypoxia after thoracic or abdominal surgery and most types of respiratory failure. Severe hypoxia results when the amount of blood shunted exceeds 20%. Oxygen can

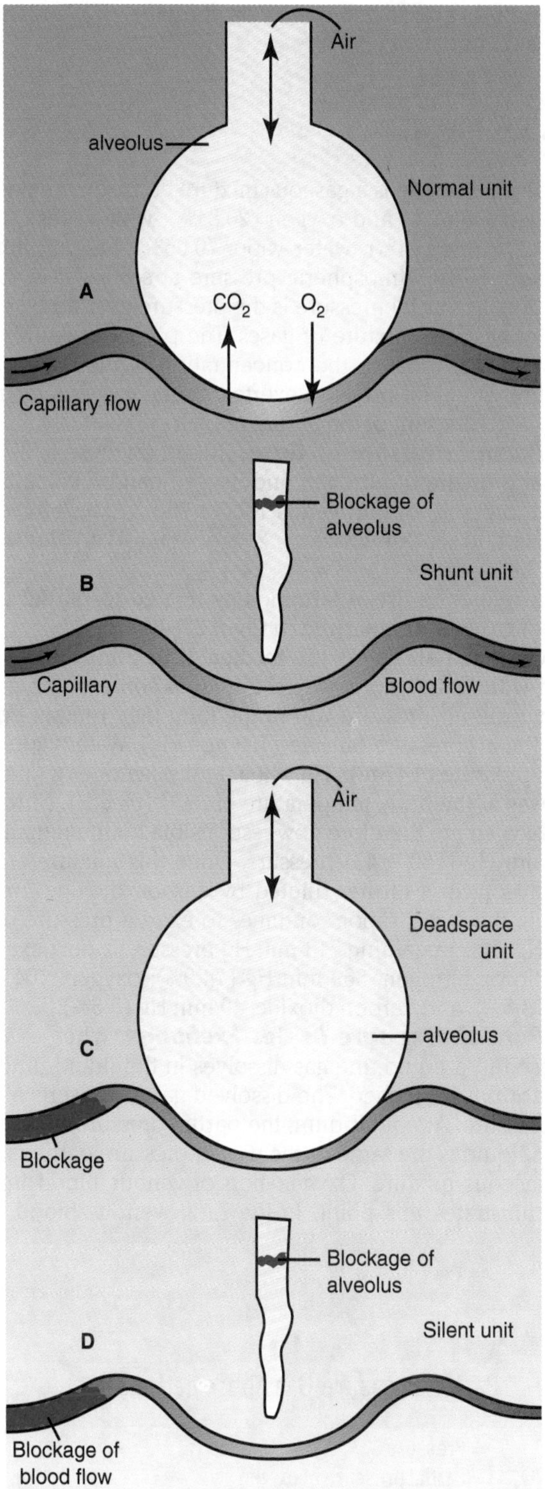

FIGURE 22-8. A schematic representation of various respiratory units showing ventilation–perfusion situations in (**A**) a normal unit with normal ventilation, normal perfusion; (**B**) a shunt unit with no ventilation, normal perfusion; (**C**) a dead space unit with normal ventilation, no perfusion, and (**D**) a silent unit with no ventilation and no perfusion.

eliminate hypoxia, depending on the type of ventilation–perfusion imbalance.

Gas Exchange

The air we breathe is a gaseous mixture consisting mainly of nitrogen (78.62%) and oxygen (20.84%), with traces of carbon dioxide (0.04%), water vapor (0.05%), helium, argon, and so on. The atmospheric pressure at sea level is about 760 mm Hg. Partial pressure is the pressure exerted by each type of gas in a mixture of gases. The partial pressure of a gas is proportional to the concentration of that gas in the mixture. The total pressure exerted by the gaseous mixture is equal to the sum of the partial pressures.

Partial Pressure of Gases. Based on these facts, the partial pressure of nitrogen and oxygen can be calculated. Partial pressure of nitrogen is 79% of 760 (.79 × 760) = 600 mm Hg and that of oxygen is 21% of 760 (.21 × 760) = 160 mm Hg.

A reference list of terminology related to partial pressure of gases is summarized in Chart 22–1.

Once the air enters the trachea, it becomes fully saturated with water vapor, which displaces some of the gases so that the air pressure within the lung may remain equal with the air pressure outside (760 mm Hg). Water vapor exerts a pressure of 47 mm Hg when it fully saturates a mixture of gases at the body temperature of 37°C (98.6°F). Nitrogen and oxygen are therefore now responsible for the remaining 713 mm Hg (760 – 47) pressure. Once this mixture enters the alveoli, it is further diluted by carbon dioxide. In the alveoli, the water vapor continues to exert a pressure of 47 mm Hg. The remaining 713 mm Hg pressure is now exerted as follows: nitrogen, 569 mm Hg (74.9%); oxygen, 104 mm Hg (13.6%), and carbon dioxide, 40 mm Hg (5.3%).

Partial Presssure in Gas Exchange. When a gas is exposed to a liquid, the gas dissolves in the liquid until an equilibrium is reached. The dissolved gas also exerts a partial pressure. At equilibrium, the partial pressure of the gas in the liquid is the same as the partial pressure of the gas in the gaseous mixture. Oxygenation of venous blood in the lung illustrates this point. In the lung, venous blood and alveolar oxygen are separated by a very thin alveolar membrane. Oxygen diffuses across this membrane to dissolve in the blood until the partial pressure of oxygen in the blood is the same as that in the alveoli (104 mm Hg). Because carbon dioxide is a by-product of oxidation in the cells, however, venous blood contains carbon dioxide at a higher partial pressure than that in the alveolar gas. In the lung, carbon dioxide diffuses out of venous blood into the alveolar gas. At equilibrium, the partial pressure of carbon dioxide in the blood and in alveolar gas is the same (40 mm Hg).

The entire sequence of changes in partial pressure readings (in milligrams) may be summarized as below. A graphic representation of the changes in partial pressure is shown in Figure 22-9.

	Atmospheric Air	Tracheal Air	Alveolar Air
PH_2O	3.7	47.0	47.0
PN_2	597.0	563.4	569.0
PO_2	159.0	149.3	104.0
PCO_2	0.3	0.3	40.0
Total	760.0	760.0	760.0

CHART 22-1

Partial Pressure Gas Abbreviations

P = Pressure
PO_2 = Partial pressure of oxygen
PCO_2 = Partial pressure of carbon dioxide
PAO_2 = Partial pressure of alveolar oxygen
$PACO_2$ = Partial pressure of alveolar carbon dioxide
PaO_2 = Partial pressure of arterial oxygen
$PaCO_2$ = Partial pressure of arterial carbon dioxide
PVO_2 = Partial pressure of venous oxygen
$PVCO_2$ = Partial pressure of venous carbon dioxide
P_{50} = Partial pressure of oxygen when the hemoglobin is 50% saturated

Oxygen Transport

Oxygen and carbon dioxide are carried simultaneously by virtue of their abilities to dissolve in blood or to combine with some of the elements of blood. Oxygen is carried in the blood in two forms: (1) as physically dissolved oxygen in the plasma and (2) in combination with the hemoglobin of the red blood cells. Each 100 ml of normal arterial blood carries 0.3 ml of oxygen *physically dissolved* in the plasma and 20 ml of oxygen in combination with hemoglobin. Large amounts of oxygen can be transported in the blood because it combines easily with hemoglobin to form oxyhemoglobin:

$$O_2 + Hb \leftrightarrows HbO_2$$

The volume of oxygen physically dissolved in the plasma varies directly with the partial pressure of oxygen in the arteries (PaO_2). The higher the PaO_2, the greater the amount of oxygen dissolved. For example, at a PaO_2 of 10 mm Hg, 0.03 ml of oxygen is dissolved in 100 ml of plasma. At 20 mm Hg, twice this amount is dissolved in plasma, and at 100 mm Hg, ten times this amount is dissolved. Therefore, the amount of dissolved oxygen is directly proportional to the partial pressure, regardless of how high the oxygen pressure rises.

The amount of oxygen that combines with hemoglobin also depends on PaO_2, but only up to a PaO_2 of about 150 mm Hg. When the PaO_2 is 150 mm Hg, hemoglobin is 100% saturated and will not combine with any additional oxygen. When hemoglobin is 100% saturated, 1 g of hemoglobin will combine with 1.34 ml of oxygen. Therefore, in a person with 14 g/dl of hemoglobin, each 100 ml of blood will contain about 19 ml of oxygen associated with hemoglobin. If the PaO_2 is less than 150 mm Hg, the percentage of hemoglobin saturated with oxygen is lower. For example, at a PaO_2 of 100

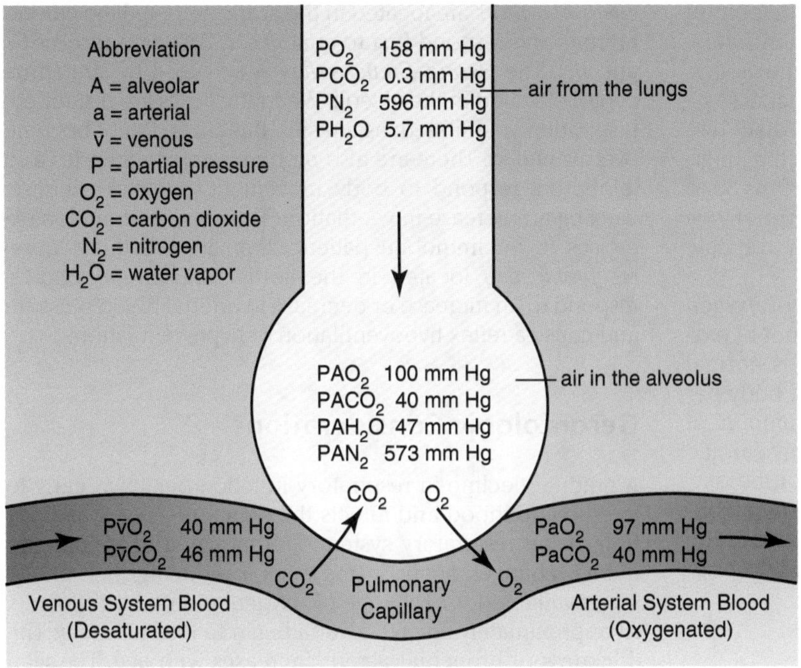

FIGURE 22-9. Changes in the partial pressure of gases during respiration, demonstrating the exchange of oxygen and carbon dioxide with the changes that occur in their partial pressures as blood from the venous system flows through the lungs.

mm Hg (normal value) saturation is 97%, and at a PaO_2 of 40 mm Hg, the saturation is 70%.

Oxyhemoglobin Dissociation Curve

The oxyhemoglobin dissociation curve (Fig. 22-10) shows the relationship between the partial pressure of oxygen (PaO_2) and the percentage of saturation of oxygen (SaO_2). The oxyhemoglobin dissociation curve in Figure 22-10 is marked to show three levels of sufficiency: (1) normal levels—PaO_2 above 70 mm Hg; (2) relatively safe levels—PaO_2 45 to 70 mm Hg; and (3) dangerous levels—PaO_2 below 40 mm Hg. The percentage of saturation can be affected by the following factors: CO_2, *p*H, temperature, and 2,3 diphosphoglycerate.

A rise in these factors shifts the curve to the right, so that more oxygen is then released to the tissues at the same PaO_2. A reduction in these factors causes the curve to shift to the left, making the bond between oxygen and hemoglobin stronger, so that less oxygen is given up to the tissues at the same PaO_2. In Figure 22-10, the normal (middle) curve shows that 75% saturation occurs at a PaO_2 of 40 mm Hg. If the curve shifts to the right, the same saturation (75%) occurs at the higher PaO_2 of 57 mm Hg. If the curve shifts to the left, 75% saturation occurs at a PaO_2 of 25 mm Hg.

The unusual shape of the oxyhemoglobin dissociation curve is a distinct advantage to the patient for two reasons:

1. If the arterial PO_2 decreases from 100 to 80 mm Hg as a result of lung disease or heart disease, the hemoglobin of the arterial blood remains almost maximally saturated (94%) and the tissues will not suffer from anoxia.
2. When the arterial blood passes into tissue capillaries and is exposed to the tissue tension of oxygen (about 40 mm Hg), hemoglobin gives up large quantities of oxygen for use by the tissues.

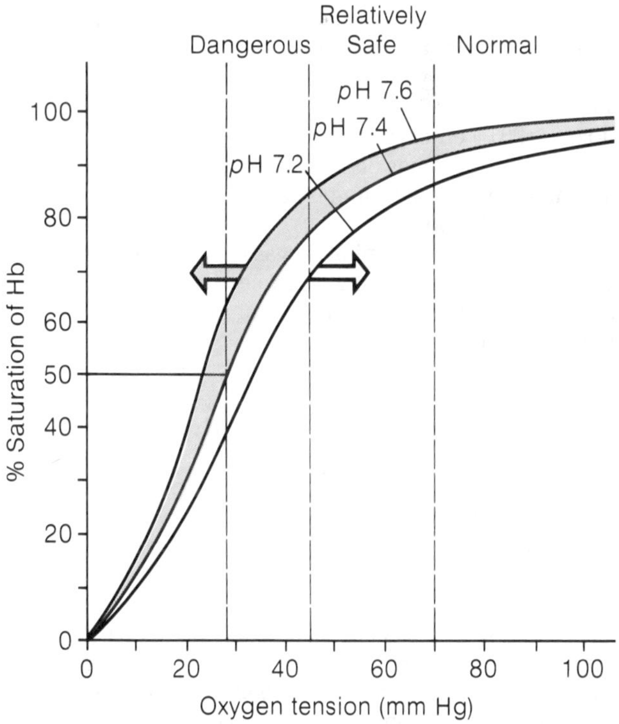

FIGURE 22-10. Oxygen–hemoglobin dissociation curve. The oxygen can attach to the hemoglobin more easily (higher oxygen saturation per Po_2) but has trouble coming off the hemoglobin at the tissues, resulting in less tissue oxygenation. Decreased oxygen affinity (shift to the right) means that it is more difficult for the oxygen to attach to the hemoglobin (there is lower oxygen saturation per Po_2), but it can come off at the tissues more easily. The P_{50} is normally 27 mm Hg. A shift to the right gives a higher P_{50}; a shift to the left gives a lower P_{50}.

Clinical Significance. With a normal hemoglobin of 15 g/100 ml and a PaO_2 level of 40 mm Hg (oxygen saturation 75%), there is adequate oxygen available for the tissues, but there is no reserve. When a serious incident occurs (*e.g.*, bronchospasm, aspiration, hypotension, or cardiac dysrhythmias) that reduces the intake of oxygen from the lungs, tissue hypoxia will result. The normal value of PaO_2 is 80 to 100 mm Hg (95% to 98% saturation). With this level of oxygenation, there is a 15% margin of excess oxygen available to the tissues.

An important consideration in the transport of oxygen is the cardiac output, which determines the amount of oxygen delivered to the body. If the cardiac output is normal (5 L/min), the amount of oxygen delivered to the body per minute will be normal. If cardiac output falls, the amount of oxygen delivered to the tissues also falls. This is why cardiac output measurements are so important. Not all of the oxygen delivered to the body is used. In fact, only 250 ml of oxygen is used per minute. The rest of the oxygen returns to the right side of the heart, and the PO_2 of venous blood drops to about 40 mm Hg.

Carbon Dioxide Transport

Simultaneously with the diffusion of oxygen from the blood into the tissues, carbon dioxide diffuses in the opposite direction (*i.e.*, from tissue cells to blood) and is transported to the lung for excretion. The amount of carbon dioxide in transit is one of the major determinants of the acid–base balance of the body. Normally, only 6% of the venous carbon dioxide is removed and enough remains in the arterial side to exert a pressure of 40 mm Hg. Most of the carbon dioxide (90%) enters the red blood cells, and the small portion (5%) that remains dissolved in the plasma (PCO_2) is the critical factor that determines carbon dioxide movement in or out of the blood.

In summarizing respiratory gas transport, it is important to emphasize that the many processes described do not take place in intermittent stages but occur rapidly, simultaneously, and continuously.

Neurologic Control of Ventilation

The rhythmicity of breathing is controlled by respiratory centers located in the brain. The inspiratory and expiratory centers located in the medulla oblongata and pons control the rate and depth of ventilation to meet the body's metabolic demands.

The *apneustic center* in the lower pons stimulates the inspiratory medullary center to promote deep, prolonged inspirations. The *pneumotaxic center*, located in the upper pons, is thought to control the pattern of respirations.

There are several groups of receptor sites that assist in the brain's control of respiratory function. The *central chemoreceptors* are located in the medulla and respond to chemical changes in the cerebrospinal fluid, which are in turn due to chemical changes in the blood. These receptors respond to an increase or decrease in the *p*H and convey a message to the lungs to change the depth and then the rate of ventilation to correct the imbalance. The *peripheral chemoreceptors* are located in the aortic arch and the carotid arteries and respond first to changes in PaO_2, then to $PaCO_2$ and *p*H. The *Hering–Breuer reflex* is activated by stretch receptors located in the alveoli. When the lungs are distended, inspiration is inhibited; as a result, the lungs do not become overdistended. There are also *proprioceptors* in muscles and joints that respond to body movements such as exercise, causing an increase in ventilation. Thus, range of motion exercises in an immobile patient stimulate breathing. *Baroreceptors*, also located in the aortic and carotid bodies, respond to an increase or decrease in arterial blood pressure and cause a reflex hypoventilation or hyperventilation.

Gerontologic Considerations

A gradual decline in respiratory function begins in early to middle adulthood and affects the structure as well as function of the respiratory system. During aging (40 years and older), changes occur in the alveoli reducing the surface area available for exchange of oxygen and carbon dioxide. At approximately age 50, alveoli begin to lose elasticity. The thickness of bronchial glands increases with age. The vital capacity of the lungs reaches a maximum at 20 to 25 years of age and decreases thereafter throughout life. A decrease in vital capacity occurs with loss of chest wall mobility, thus restricting tidal flow of air. The amount of respiratory dead space increases with age. These changes result in decreased diffusion capacity for oxygen with age, producing lower oxygen in the arterial circulation. Despite these changes, in the absence of chronic pulmonary disease, elderly persons are able to carry out activities of daily living, but they may have decreased tolerance for prolonged activity or excessive exertion and may require rest after prolonged or vigorous activity.

Assessment of Patients With Pulmonary Disorders

History

The health history focuses on the physical and functional problems experienced by the patient and the effect of these problems on the patient's life and life-style. The reason for the patient's seeking health care often is related to one of the following: dyspnea, pain, the accumulation of mucus, wheezing, hemoptysis, edema of the ankles and feet, cough, and general fatigue and weakness.

In addition to identifying the chief reason why the patient is seeking health care, it is important to determine when the health problem or symptom started, how long it lasted, if it was relieved at any time, and how relief was obtained. Information about precipitating factors, duration, severity, and associated factors or symptoms is collected.

In a respiratory history, factors that may contribute to the patient's lung condition are assessed:

- Smoking (the single most important factor that contributes to lung disease)
- Previous personal or family history of lung disease
- Occupational history

- Allergens and environmental pollutants
- Recreational exposure

Psychosocial factors that may affect the patient's life are evaluated and include anxiety, role changes, family relationships, financial problems, and employment or unemployment. Questions to consider in this assessment include: What are the patient's coping mechanisms? Is the patient exhibiting anxiety, anger, hostility, dependency, withdrawal, isolation, avoidance, noncompliance, acceptance, or denial? Finally, what are the support systems the patient uses to deal with the illness? Are supportive family members, friends, or community resources available?

Examination of the Thorax

If a patient has a known or suspected pulmonary condition, respiratory function must be assessed. Assessment of the thorax and lungs uses the skills of inspection, palpation, percussion, and auscultation. When these techniques are properly performed and the results logically interpreted, much can be learned that will help the nurse develop a plan of care. When recording or communicating findings, it is customary to refer to known anatomic landmarks as points of reference.

Thoracic Landmarks

With respect to the thorax, location is defined both horizontally and vertically. **Horizontal reference** is made in terms of the rib or the intercostal space under the examiner's fingers (Fig. 22-11). On the anterior surface, identifying the specific rib is facilitated by locating the angle (angle of Louis) at which the manubrium joins the body of the sternum in the midline. The second rib joins the sternum at this prominent landmark. Other ribs may be identified by counting down from the second rib. The intercostal spaces are referred to in terms of the rib immediately above the intercostal space.

Location of ribs on the posterior surface of the thorax (see Fig. 22-11) is more difficult. The first step is to identify

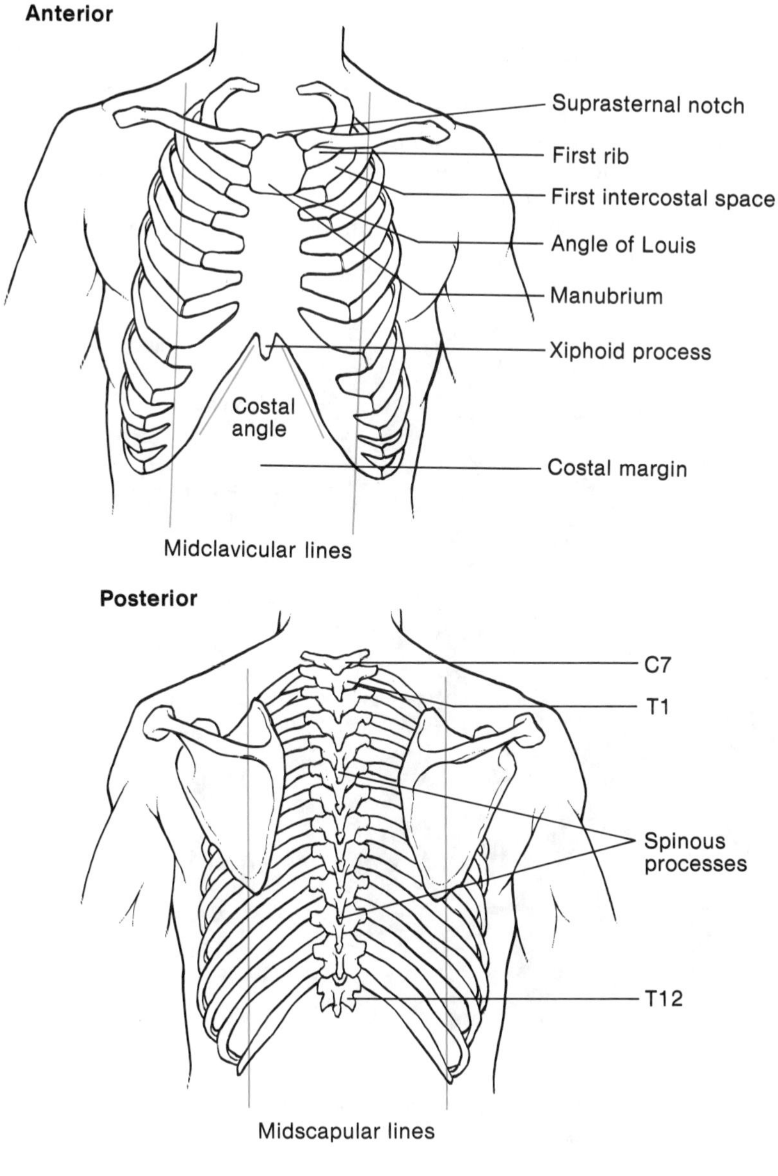

FIGURE 22-11. Landmarks of the anterior and posterior thorax are used in describing assessment findings.

the spinous process. This is accomplished by finding the most prominent of the spinous processes, the seventh cervical vertebra (*vertebra prominens*). When the neck is slightly flexed, the seventh cervical spinous process stands out. Other vertebrae are then identified by counting down.

Several imaginary lines are used as **vertical references** or landmarks to identify the location of thoracic findings (Fig. 22-12). The *midsternal line* is drawn down through the center of the sternum. The *midclavicular line* is an imaginary line drawn from the middle of the clavicle (Fig. 22-12*A*). The point of maximal impulse of the heart most generally lies along this line on the left thorax.

When the arm is abducted from the body at 90 degrees, imaginary vertical lines may be drawn from the anterior axillary fold, from the middle of the axilla, and from the posterior axillary fold. These lines are called, respectively, the *anterior axillary line,* the *midaxillary line,* and the *posterior axillary line* (Fig. 22-12*B*).

A line drawn vertically through the superior and inferior poles of the scapula is called the *scapular line*, and a line drawn down the center of the vertebral column is called the *vertebral line*. Using these landmarks, the examiner can easily be understood when referring to an area of dullness extending from the vertebral to the scapular line between the seventh and tenth ribs on the right.

The **lobes of the lung** may be located on the surface of the chest wall in the following manner (Fig. 22-13): The line between the upper and lower lobes on the left begins at the fourth thoracic spinous process posteriorly, proceeds around to cross the fifth rib in the midaxillary line, and meets the sixth rib at the sternum. This line on the right divides the right middle lobe from the right lower lobe. The line dividing the right upper lobe from the middle lobe is an incomplete one that begins at the fifth rib in the midaxillary line, where it intersects the line between the upper and lower lobes and traverses horizontally to the sternum. Thus, the upper lobes are dominant on the anterior surface of the thorax and the lower lobes are dominant on the posterior surface. There is no presentation of the middle lobe on the posterior surface of the chest.

Inspection of the Thorax

Inspection of the thorax provides information about musculoskeletal structure, nutrition, and the status of the respiratory system. The skin over the thorax is observed for color and turgor and for evidence of loss of subcutaneous tissue. Asymmetry, if present, is noted.

Chest Configuration

Normally, the anteroposterior diameter in proportion to the lateral diameter is 1:2. There are, however, four main deformities of the chest associated with respiratory disease: barrel chest, funnel chest (pectus excavatum), pigeon chest (pectus carinatum), and kyphoscoliosis.

Barrel Chest. Barrel chest occurs as a result of overinflation of the lungs. There is an increase in the anteroposterior diameter of the thorax. In a patient with emphysema, the ribs are more widely spaced and the intercostal spaces tend to bulge on expiration. The appearance of the patient with advanced emphysema is thus quite characteristic and often allows the observer to detect its presence easily, even from a distance.

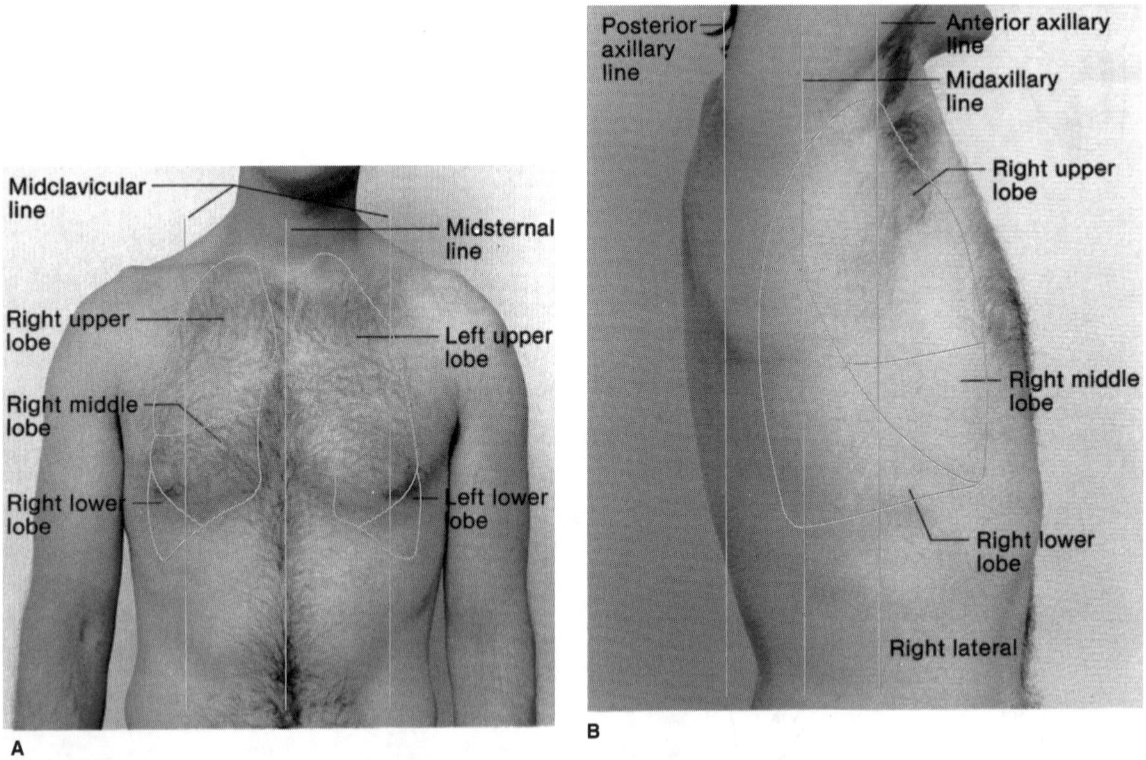

FIGURE 22-12. Imaginary reference lines for examination of the thorax. (From Fuller J and Schaller-Ayers J. Health Assessment: A Nursing Approach, 2nd ed. Philadelphia, JB Lippincott, 1994.)

Funnel Chest (Pectus Excavatum). Funnel chest occurs when there is a depression in the lower portion of the sternum. This may compress the heart and great vessels, resulting in murmurs. This condition may occur with rickets, Marfan's syndrome, or as an occupational hazard (as in cobbler's chest.)

Pigeon Chest (Pectus Carinatum). A pigeon chest occurs as a result of displacement of the sternum. There is an increase in the anteroposterior diameter. This may occur with rickets, Marfan's syndrome, or severe kyphoscoliosis.

Kyphoscoliosis. A kyphoscoliosis appears with an elevation of the scapula, with a corresponding S-shaped curved spine. This deformity limits the lung within the thorax; it may occur with osteoporosis and other skeletal disorders that affect the thorax.

Breathing Patterns

Observing the rate and depth of respiration is also important. In the adult, the normal respiratory rate is 12 to 18 breaths per minute; it is regular in depth and rhythm. An increase in the rate of respiration is called **tachypnea**; an increase in depth is called **hyperpnea**. An increase in both rate and depth that results in a lowered arterial PCO_2 is referred to as **hyperventilation**. With rapid breathing, inspiration and expiration are nearly equal. Hyperventilation that is marked by an increase in rate and depth, associated with severe acidosis of diabetic or renal origin, is called **Kussmaul** respiration. **Cheyne–Stokes** respiration is characterized by alternating episodes of apnea (cessation of breathing) and periods of deep breathing. It most frequently is associated with heart failure and damage to the respiratory center (drug-induced, tumor, trauma). A graphic representation of the rate and depth of different kinds of respiration is presented in Figure 22-14.

In thin persons, it is quite normal to note a slight retraction of the intercostal spaces during quiet breathing. Bulging during expiration implies obstruction of expiratory air flow, as in emphysema. Marked retraction on inspiration, particularly if asymmetric, implies blockage of a branch of the respiratory tree. Asymmetric bulging of the intercostal spaces, on one side or the other, is created by an increase in pressure within the hemithorax. This may be a result of air trapped under pressure within the pleural cavity where it does not normally appear (pneumothorax) or the pressure of fluid within the pleural space (pleural effusion).

Certain patterns of respiration are characteristic of specific disease states. Observing and documenting respiratory rhythms and their deviation from normal are important nursing functions.

Palpation of the Thorax

After inspection, the thorax is palpated for tenderness, masses, lesions, respiratory excursion, and vocal fremitus. If the patient has reported an area of pain, or if lesions are

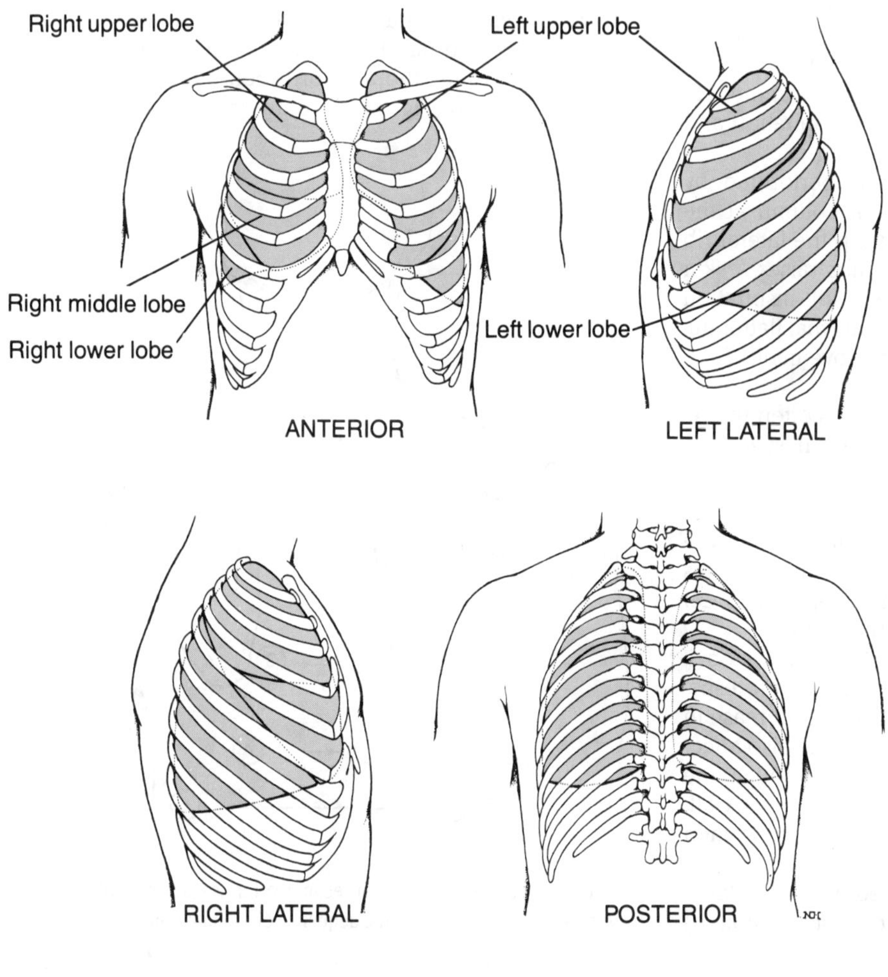

FIGURE 22-13. Topographic relationship of the ribs to the lobes of the lung.

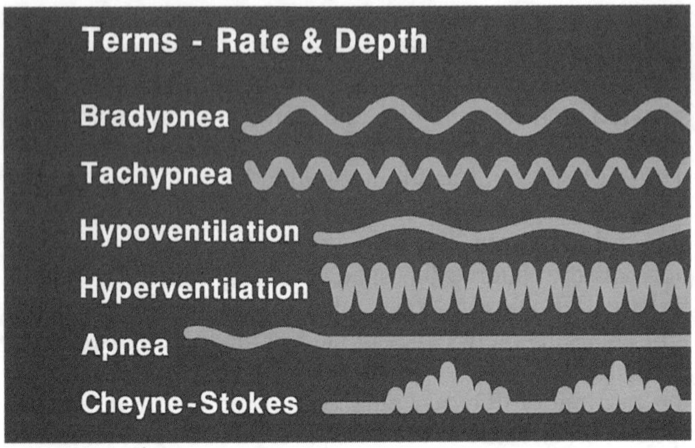

FIGURE 22-14. Different rates and depths of respiration.

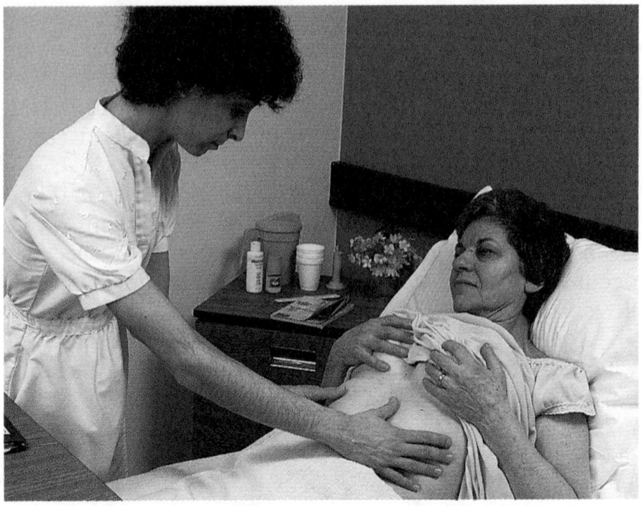

FIGURE 22-15. Method for assessing respiratory excursion. Hands are placed along the rib cage with thumbs extending along the costal margin below the xiphoid process.

apparent, direct palpation is performed with the fingertips (for skin lesions and subcutaneous masses) or with the ball of the hand (for deeper masses or generalized flank or rib discomfort).

Respiratory Excursion

Respiratory excursion is an estimation of thoracic expansion and may disclose significant information about thoracic movement during breathing. Differences in expansion are more readily detectable on the anterior thorax, where a fuller range of motion occurs during respiration. The examiner's thumbs are placed along each costal margin, below the xiphoid process, while the hands rest along the lateral rib cage (Fig. 22-15). Sliding the thumbs medially about 2.5 cm (1 in) raises a small skin fold between the thumbs. The patient is instructed to inhale deeply while the examiner observes the movement of the thumbs during inspiration and expiration. This movement is normally symmetric.

Procedure. A posterior assessment is performed by placing the thumbs adjacent to the spinal column at the level of the tenth rib. The hands lightly grasp the lateral rib cage. Again, a medial motion of the thumbs raises a skin fold, and the patient is instructed to take a full inspiration and expiration. The examiner observes for normal flattening of the skin fold and feels the symmetric movement of the thorax.

Findings. Respiratory lag or impairment is often the result of pleurisy, fractured ribs, or trauma to the chest wall.

Tactile Fremitus

Sound generated by the larynx travels distally along the bronchial tree to set the chest wall in resonant motion. This is especially true of consonant sounds. The capacity to *feel* sound on the chest well is called **tactile fremitus**.

There is a wide variation in normal fremitus. It is obviously influenced by the thickness of the chest wall, especially if that thickness is muscular, although the increase in subcutaneous tissue associated with obesity may also affect fremitus. Lower-pitched sounds travel better through the normal lung and produce greater vibration of the chest wall. Thus, fremitus is more pronounced in men than in women because of the deeper male voice.

Normally, fremitus is most pronounced where the large bronchi are closest to the chest wall and least palpable as the examiner progresses from the major bronchi to the distant lung fields. Therefore, it is most palpable in the upper thorax anteriorly and posteriorly.

Procedure. To elicit tactile fremitus, the examiner instructs the patient to repeat the words *ninety-nine* or *one, two, three*, or "eee, eee, eee" with each movement of the examiner's hands. The vibrations are detected by placing the palmar surfaces of the fingers and hands, or the ulnar aspect of the extended hands, on the thorax. To facilitate comparison, only one hand is used as the examiner moves in sequence down the thorax. Corresponding areas of the thorax are compared (Fig. 22-16). Bony areas are not tested.

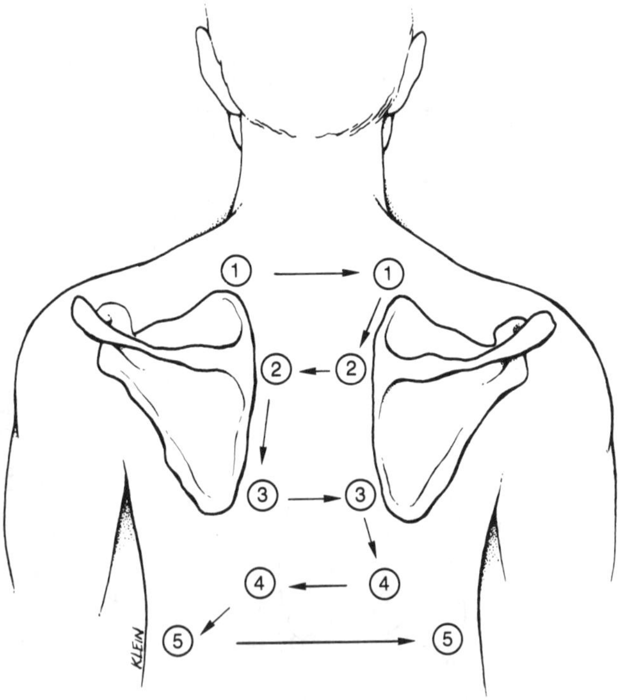

FIGURE 22-16. Palpation technique for assessing tactile fremitus. *Numbers* and *arrows* indicate the sequence of examination.

Findings. An understanding of the physics of sound transmission through the lung aids in interpreting the findings. Air does not conduct sound well; solid substance (tissue) does, provided that it has elasticity and is not conglomerated into a nonresonant mass. Thus, an increase in solid tissue per unit volume of lung will enhance fremitus. An increase in air per unit volume of lung will impede sound. Patients with emphysema, which results in the rupture of alveoli and trapping of air, exhibit almost no tactile fremitus. A patient with consolidation of a lobe of the lung due to pneumonia will have increased tactile fremitus over that lobe. Air in the pleural space will not conduct sound.

Percussion of the Thorax

Percussion sets the chest wall and underlying structures in motion, producing audible and tactile vibrations. The examiner uses percussion to determine whether or not underlying tissues are filled with air, fluid, or solid material. One also uses percussion to estimate the size and location of certain structures within the thorax (*e.g.*, diaphragm, heart, liver).

Procedure. Percussion usually begins with the *posterior thorax*. Ideally, the patient is in a sitting position with head flexed forward and arms crossed on the lap. This position separates the scapulae widely and exposes more lung area for assessment. The procedure is as follows: Percuss across each shoulder top, locating the 5-cm width of resonance overlying the lung apices (Fig. 22-17). Proceed down the posterior thorax, percussing symmetric areas at 5 to 6 cm (2 to 2.5 in) intervals. The middle finger is positioned parallel to the ribs in the intercostal space; the finger is placed firmly against the chest wall before striking it with the middle finger of the opposite hand. Percussion over the scapulae or rib surfaces yields a dull sound and only confuses findings.

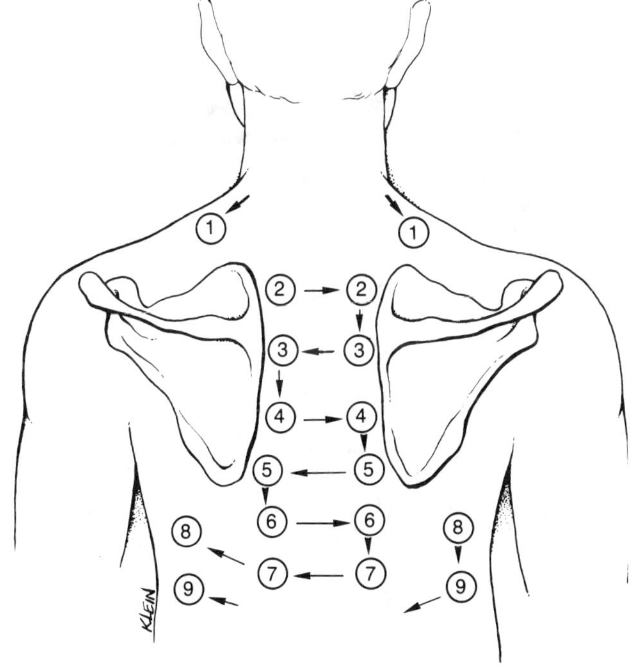

FIGURE 22-17. Percussion of the posterior thorax. With the patient in a sitting position, symmetric areas of the lungs are percussed at 5-cm intervals. This progression starts at the apex of each lung and concludes with percussion of each lateral chest wall.

Percussion over the anterior chest is performed with the patient in an upright position with shoulders arched backward and arms at the side. The examiner begins in the supraclavicular area and proceeds downward, from intercostal space to intercostal space. In the female patient, it may be necessary to displace the breasts for an adequate examination. Dullness noted to the left of the sternum between the third and fifth intercostal spaces is the heart and is a normal finding. Similarly, there is a normal span of liver dullness in the right thorax from the fifth intercostal space to the right costal margin at the midclavicular line.

The anterior and lateral thorax is examined with the patient in a supine position. If the patient is unable to sit up, percussion of the posterior thorax is performed with the patient positioned on the side.

Findings. *Dullness* over the lung occurs when air-filled lung tissue is replaced by fluid or solid tissue. Examples include lobar pneumonia, in which consolidation results from accumulation of fluid, blood, fibrous tissue, cells, or tumor in the pleural space. Pneumothorax produces a tympanic or drumlike sound, whereas emphysema is perceived as hyperresonance. Table 22-2 reviews percussion sounds and their characteristics.

Diaphragmatic Excursion

The normal resonance of the lung stops at the diaphragm. The position of the diaphragm is different during inspiration than during expiration.

Procedure. For assessment of its position and motion, the patient is instructed to take a deep breath and hold it while the maximal descent of the diaphragm is percussed. This is performed along the midscapular lines bilaterally. The point at which the percussion note changes from resonance to dullness is noted. If desired, this point can be marked with a pen. The patient is then instructed to exhale fully and hold it while the examiner again percusses downward to the dullness of the diaphragm. This location is marked. The distance between the two markings indicates the range of motion of the diaphragm.

Findings. Maximal excursion of the diaphragm may amount to as much as 8 to 10 cm (3 to 4 in) in healthy, tall, young men. For most persons, it is usually 5 to 7 cm (2 to 2.75 in). Normally, the diaphragm is 2 cm (0.75 in) or so higher on the right than on the left because of the position of the heart and the liver above and below the left and right segments of the diaphragm, respectively. Decreased diaphragmatic excursion may be apparent in patients with pleural effusion and emphysema. An increase in intra-abdominal pressure, such as occurs in pregnancy or ascites, may account for a diaphragm that is positioned high in the thorax.

Auscultation of the Thorax

Auscultation is useful in assessing the flow of air through the bronchial tree and in evaluating the presence of fluid or solid obstruction in the lung structures. To determine the condition of the lungs, the examiner auscultates for normal breath sounds, adventitious sounds, and voice sounds.

TABLE 22-2 Percussion Sounds and Their Characteristics

	Relative Intensity	Relative Pitch	Relative Duration	Example Location	Pathologic Examples
Flatness	Soft	High	Short	Thigh	Large pleural effusion
Dullness	Medium	Medium	Medium	Liver	Lobar pneumonia
Resonance	Loud	Low	Long	Normal lung	Simple chronic bronchitis
Hyperresonance	Very loud	Lower	Longer	None normally	Emphysema, pneumothorax
Tympany	Loud	High*	*	Gastric air bubble or puffed-out cheek	Large pneumothorax

*Distinguished mainly by its musical timbre
(Bates B. A Guide to Physical Examination and History Taking, 6th ed. Philadelphia, JB Lippincott, 1995.)

Procedure. A thorough examination includes auscultation of the anterior, posterior, and lateral thorax and is performed as follows: The diaphragm of the stethoscope is placed firmly against the chest wall as the patient breathes slowly and deeply through the mouth. Corresponding areas of the chest are auscultated in a systematic fashion from the apices to the bases and along midaxillary lines. The sequence of auscultation and the positioning of the patient are similar to those used for percussion. It often is necessary to listen to two full inspirations and expirations at each anatomic location to assure valid interpretation of the sound heard. Repeated deep breaths may result in symptoms of hyperventilation (*e.g.*, light-headedness) and can be avoided by having the patient rest and breathe normally once or twice during the examination.

Breath Sounds

Normal breath sounds are distinguished by their location over a specific area of the lung and are identified as vesicular, bronchial (tubular), and bronchovesicular breath sounds (Table 22-3).

Vesicular sounds are audible as quiet, low-pitched sounds that have a long inspiratory phase and a short expiratory phase. They are heard normally throughout the entire lung field, except over the upper sternum and between the scapulae. **Bronchial sounds** are usually louder and higher pitched than vesicular sounds. In comparison, the expiratory phase is longer than the inspiratory phase. Bronchial sounds are heard over the trachea. **Bronchovesicular sounds** are heard over the main bronchus area; specifically, they can be heard between the scapulae and on

TABLE 22-3 Characteristics of Breath Sounds

	Duration of Sounds	Intensity of Expiratory Sound	Pitch of Expiratory Sound	Locations Where Heard Normally
Vesicular*	Inspiratory sounds last longer than expiratory ones	Soft	Relatively low	Over most of both lungs
Broncho-vesicular	Inspiratory and expiratory sounds are about equal.	Intermediate	Intermediate	Often in the 1st and 2nd interspaces anteriorly and between the scapulae
Bronchial	Expiratory sounds last longer than inspiratory ones.	Loud	Relatively high	Over the manubrium, if heard at all
Tracheal	Inspiratory and expiratory sounds are about equal.	Very loud	Relatively high	Over the trachea in the neck

*The thickness of the bars indicates intensity; the steeper their incline, the higher the pitch.
(Bates B. A Guide to Physical Examination and History Taking, 6th ed. Philadelphia, JB Lippincott, 1995.)

either side of the sternum. Bronchovesicular breath sounds are medium in pitch; the inspiratory and expiratory phases are equal.

Findings. Bronchial and bronchovesicular sounds that are audible elsewhere in the lungs signify pathology, usually indicating consolidated areas in the lung (*e.g.*, pneumonia, heart failure), and necessitate further evaluation.

The quality and intensity of breath sounds are determined during auscultation. When air flow is decreased by bronchial obstruction (atelectasis) or when fluid (pleural effusion) or tissue (obesity) separates the air passages from the stethoscope, breath sounds are diminished or absent. For example, the breath sounds of the patient with emphysema are faint and often completely inaudible.

When heard, the expiratory phase is prolonged and may exhibit a high-pitched whistling tone called *wheezing*. This same sound is also heard in asthma and in any process associated with marked bronchoconstriction.

Adventitious Sounds

The presence of an abnormal condition that affects the bronchial tree and alveoli may produce adventitious (additional) sounds. Adventitious sounds are divided into two categories: discrete, noncontinuous sounds (**crackles**) and continuous musical sounds (**wheezes**). The duration of the sound is the important distinction to make in identifying the sound as noncontinuous or continuous. Pleural friction rubs are specific examples of crackles (Table 22-4).

Crackles (formerly referred to as *rales*) are discrete, noncontinuous sounds that result from delayed reopening of deflated airways. *Fine crackles*, usually audible at the end of inspiration and originating from the alveoli, typically are heard in patients with interstitial pneumonia or fibrosis. Their sound can be re-created by rubbing several strands of hair together next to one's ear. *Coarse crackles* have a harsh, moist sound. They are produced in the large bronchi and are audible in early to mid-inspiration. Crackles may or may not be cleared by coughing. Crackles reflect underlying inflammation or congestion and are often present in such conditions as pneumonia, bronchitis, congestive heart failure, bronchiectasis, and pulmonary fibrosis.

Wheezes (sibilant rhonchi) are continuous musical sounds that are longer in duration than crackles. They may be audible during inspiration, expiration, or both. These sounds result from air passing through narrowed or partially obstructed passages. Obstruction is often due to the presence of secretions or edema, and wheezes may clear with coughing. Wheezes originate in the smaller bronchi and

TABLE 22-4 Abnormal (Adventitious) Breath Sounds

Crackles

Crackles (formerly called rales) are soft, high-pitched, discontinuous popping sounds that occur during inspiration. The sounds are timed in relation to inspiration.

Crackles occur secondary to fluid in the airways or alveoli, or to opening of collapsed alveoli. Crackles in late inspiration are associated with restrictive pulmonary disease. Crackles in early inspiration are associated with obstructive pulmonary disease. *Fine crackles* in early inspiration are caused by small airway closure. *Coarse crackles* in early inspiration are associated with bronchitis or pneumonia.

Wheezes

Sonorous wheezes (formerly called rhonchi) are deep, low-pitched, rumbling sounds that are heard primarily during expiration and caused by air moving through narrowed tracheobronchial passages. Narrowing may be caused by secretions or tumor.

Sibilant wheezes (formerly called wheezes) are continuous, musical, high-pitched, whistle-like sounds that are heard during inspiration and expiration. They are caused by narrowed bronchioles and are associated with bronchospasm, asthma, and buildup of secretions.

Pleural Friction Rub

A *pleural friction rub* is a harsh crackling sound like two pieces of leather being rubbed together, and may be heard during inspiration alone or during both inspiration and expiration. This sound may disappear when the breath is held.

Pleural friction rubs are secondary to inflammation and loss of lubricating pleural fluid.

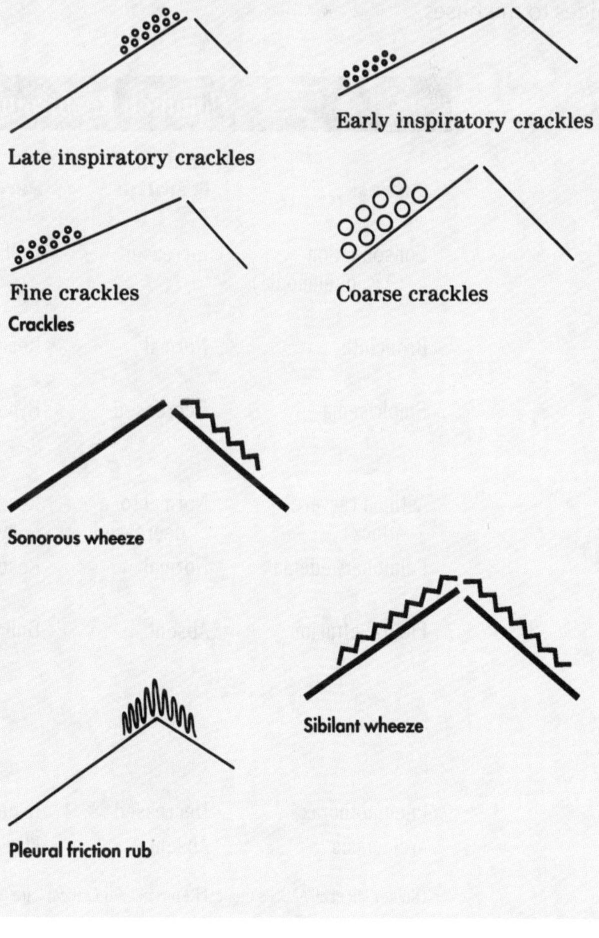

(Fuller J and Schaller–Ayers J. Health Assessment: A Nursing Approach, 2nd ed. Philadelphia, JB Lippincott, 1995.)

bronchioles; they are high pitched and whistling. *Rhonchi* originate in the larger bronchi or trachea and are lower pitched and sonorous. They are heard in patients with increased secretions. Wheezes are commonly heard in patients with asthma, chronic bronchitis, and bronchiectasis.

Friction rubs result from inflammation of the pleural surfaces that induces a crackling, grating sound that is usually heard in both inspiration and expiration. The sound is called a friction rub. It sounds quite close to the ear and is enhanced by applying pressure to the chest wall with the head of the stethoscope. The sound is imitated by rubbing the thumb and index finger together near the ear. The grating sound of a friction rub is not altered by coughing. If audible only during inspiration, it may be difficult to distinguish from crackles, which may be multiple and so frequent that a continuous sound is perceived. A friction rub is best heard over the lower lateral anterior surface of the thorax.

Voice Sounds

The sound heard through the stethoscope as the patient speaks is known as **vocal resonance**. The vibrations produced in the larynx are transmitted to the chest wall as they pass through the bronchi and alveolar tissue. During the process the sounds are diminished in intensity and altered so that syllables are not distinguishable. Voice sounds are usually assessed by having the patient repeat the phrase "ninety-nine" or "eee" while the examiner listens with the stethoscope in corresponding areas of the chest from the apices to the bases.

Bronchophony describes vocal resonance that is more intense and clearer than normal. **Egophony** describes voice sounds that are distorted. It is best appreciated by having the patient repeat the letter *e*. The distortion produced by consolidation transforms the sound into a clearly heard "a" rather than "e."

Findings. Bronchophony and egophony have precisely the same significance as bronchial breathing with an increase in tactile fremitus. When an abnormality is detected, it should be evident in more than one assessment method. A change in tactile fremitus is more subtle and can be missed, but bronchial breathing and bronchophony can be noted loudly and clearly.

Whispered pectoriloquy is a very subtle finding, heard only in the presence of rather dense consolidation of the lungs. Transmission of high-frequency components of sound is so enhanced by the consolidated tissue that even whispered words are heard, a circumstance not noted in normal physiology. The significance is the same as that of bronchophony.

The physical findings for the most common respiratory diseases are summarized in Table 22-5.

Assessment of Respiratory Signs and Symptoms

The major signs and symptoms of respiratory disease are dyspnea, cough, sputum production, chest pain, wheezing, clubbing of the fingers, hemoptysis, and cyanosis. These

TABLE 22-5 Common Respiratory Problems of Critically Ill Patients

Disease	Tactile Fremitus	Percussion	Auscultation
Consolidation (*e.g.*, pneumonia)	Increased	Dull	Bronchial breath sounds, crackles, bronchophony, egophony, whispered pectoriloquy
Bronchitis	Normal	Resonant	Normal to decreased breath sounds, wheezes
Emphysema	Decreased	Hyperresonant	Decreased intensity of breath sounds, usually with prolonged expiration
Asthma (severe attack)	Normal to decreased	Resonant to hyperresonant	Wheezes
Pulmonary edema	Normal	Resonant	Crackles at lung bases, possibly wheezes
Pleural effusion	Absent	Dull to flat	Decreased to absent breath sounds, bronchial breath sounds and bronchophony, egophony, and whispering pectoriloquy above the effusion over the area of compressed lung
Pneumothorax	Decreased	Hyperresonant	Absent breath sounds
Atelectasis	Absent	Flat	Decreased to absent breath sounds

(Kinney MR et al. AACN's Clinical Reference for Critical Care Nursing, 3rd ed. St. Louis, CV Mosby, 1993.)

clinical manifestations are related to the duration and severity of the disease.

Dyspnea

Dyspnea (difficult or labored breathing, shortness of breath) is a symptom common to many pulmonary and cardiac disorders, particularly when there is increased lung rigidity and airway resistance. The right ventricle of the heart will be affected ultimately by lung disease because it must pump blood through the lungs.

Significance. *Shortness of breath* or *dyspnea* may be a significant clinical sign. It may be the result of a cardiac or respiratory disease. In general, the acute diseases of the lungs produce a more severe grade of dyspnea than do the chronic diseases. *Sudden dyspnea* in a healthy person may indicate pneumothorax (air in the pleural cavity). In an ill patient or after surgery, sudden dyspnea may denote pulmonary embolism. *Orthopnea* (inability to breathe easily except in an upright position) may be found in patients with heart disease and, occasionally, in patients with chronic obstructive pulmonary disease (COPD). Dyspnea with an expiratory wheeze is seen in COPD (asthma, bronchitis, emphysema). *Noisy breathing* may result from a narrowing of the airway or localized obstruction of a major bronchus by a tumor or foreign body. The presence of both inspiratory and expiratory *wheezing* usually signifies asthma, if the patient is not in congestive heart failure.

The circumstance that produces the patient's dyspnea must be determined. Therefore, it is important to ask the patient:

- How much exertion triggers shortness of breath?
- Is there an associated cough?
- Is dyspnea related to other symptoms?
- Was the onset of shortness of breath sudden or gradual?
- At what time of day or night does the dyspnea occur?
- Is the shortness of breath worse when the patient is flat in bed?
- Does the shortness of breath occur at rest? With exercise? Running? Climbing stairs?
- Is the shortness of breath worse while walking? If so, when walking how far?

Relief Measures. The management of dyspnea is aimed at correcting its cause. Relief of the symptom sometimes is achieved by placing the patient at rest with the head elevated and, in severe cases, by administering oxygen.

Cough

Cough results from irritation of the mucous membranes anywhere in the respiratory tract. The stimulus producing a cough may arise from an infectious process or from an airborne irritant, such as smoke, smog, dust, or a gas. The cough is the patient's chief protection against the accumulation of secretions in the bronchi and bronchioles.

Significance. The presence of cough may indicate serious pulmonary disease. Of equal importance is the *type of cough*. A dry, irritative cough is characteristic of upper respiratory tract infection of viral origin. Laryngotracheitis causes an irritative, high-pitched cough. Tracheal lesions produce a brassy cough. A severe or *changing* cough may indicate bronchogenic carcinoma. Pleuritic chest pain accompanying coughing may indicate pleural or chest wall (musculoskeletal) involvement.

The *character of the cough* is evaluated. Is it dry? Hacking? Brassy? Wheezing? Loose? Severe? The *time of coughing* is noted. Coughing at night may herald the onset of left-sided heart failure or bronchial asthma. A cough in the morning with sputum production is indicative of bronchitis. A cough that worsens when the patient is supine may indicate a postnasal drip (sinusitis). Coughing after food intake may indicate aspirated material in the tracheobronchial tree. A cough of recent onset is usually from an acute infectious process.

Sputum Production

A patient who coughs long enough almost invariably produces sputum. Violent coughing causes bronchial spasm, obstruction, and further irritation of the bronchi and may result in syncope (fainting). A severe, repeated, or uncontrolled cough that is nonproductive is exhausting and potentially harmful. Sputum production is the reaction of the lungs to any constantly recurring irritant. It also may be associated with a nasal discharge.

Significance. A profuse amount of purulent sputum (thick and yellow or green) or a change in color of the sputum probably indicates a bacterial infection. Rusty sputum indicates the presence of bacterial pneumonia, if the patient has not received antibiotics. A thin, mucoid sputum frequently results from viral bronchitis. A gradual increase of sputum over time may indicate the presence of chronic bronchitis or bronchiectasis. Pink-tinged mucoid sputum is suggestive of a lung tumor, whereas profuse, frothy, pink material, often welling up into the throat, may indicate pulmonary edema. Malodorous sputum and bad breath point to the presence of lung abscess, bronchiectasis, or an infection caused by fusospirochetal or other anaerobic organisms.

Relief Measures. If the sputum is too thick to raise, it is necessary to decrease its viscosity by increasing its water content through adequate hydration (drinking water) and inhalation of aerosolized solutions, which may be delivered by any type of nebulizer. Methods of assisting the patient to cough productively are discussed on p. 367.

Smoking is definitely contraindicated because it interferes with ciliary action, increases bronchial secretions, causes inflammation and hyperplasia of the mucous membranes, and reduces production of surfactant. Thus, bronchial drainage is impaired. If smoking is stopped, sputum volume decreases and resistance to bronchial infections improves.

The patient's appetite may be decreased because of the odor of the sputum and the taste it leaves in the mouth. Adequate oral hygiene, proper environment, and wise selection of food will stimulate appetite. After the patient's mouth is carefully cleansed and rinsed, sputum cups and emesis basins should be removed before the next meal arrives.

Serving citrus juices at the beginning of the meal will make the mouth feel better and help the patient be more receptive to the rest of the meal.

Chest Pain

Chest pain or discomfort may be associated with pulmonary or cardiac disease. Chest pain associated with pulmonary conditions may be sharp, stabbing, and intermittent or it may be dull, aching, and persistent. The pain usually is felt on the side where the pathologic process is located, but it may be referred elsewhere, for example, to the neck, the back, or the abdomen.

Significance. Chest pain is experienced by many patients with pneumonia, pulmonary embolism with lung infarction, and pleurisy, and is a late symptom of bronchogenic carcinoma. In carcinoma the pain may be dull and persistent because the cancer has invaded the chest wall, mediastinum, or spine.

Lung disease does not always produce thoracic pain because the lungs and the visceral pleura lack sensory nerves and are insensitive to pain stimuli. But the parietal pleura has a rich supply of sensory nerves that are stimulated by inflammation and stretching of the membrane. **Pleuritic pain** due to irritation of the parietal pleura is sharp and seems to "catch" on inspiration; it is often described by patients as "like the stabbing of a knife." Patients are more comfortable when they lie on the affected side, a posture that tends to "splint" the chest wall, restrict the expansions and contractions of the lung, and reduce the friction between the injured or diseased pleurae on that side. Pain associated with cough may be lessened by manual splinting of the rib cage.

The **quality, intensity, and radiation** of pain are assessed and precipitating factors are identified and explored. Whether there is a relationship between pain and the patient's posture should be determined. Also, the inspiratory and expiratory phases of respiration and their effect on pain are evaluated.

Relief Measures. Analgesic medications are effective in relieving chest pain, but care must be taken not to depress the respiratory center or a productive cough. A regional anesthetic block is done at times to relieve extreme pain. A local anesthetic agent is injected along the intercostal nerves that supply the painful area.

Wheezing

Wheezing is often the major finding in a patient with bronchoconstriction or airway narrowing. It is heard with or without a stethoscope, depending on its location. Wheezing is a high-pitched, musical sound heard mainly on expiration (see p. 447 for assessment).

Clubbing of the Fingers

Clubbing of the fingers as a sign of lung disease is found in patients with chronic hypoxic conditions, chronic lung infections, and malignancies of the lung. This finding may be initially manifested as sponginess of the nailbed and loss of the nailbed angle (Fig. 22-18).

Hemoptysis

Hemoptysis (expectoration of blood from the respiratory tract) is a symptom of both pulmonary and cardiac disorders. It varies from blood-stained sputum to a large, sudden hemorrhage and always merits investigation.

The **most common causes** are (1) pulmonary infection, (2) carcinoma of the lung, (3) abnormalities of the heart or blood vessels, (4) pulmonary artery or vein abnormalities, and (5) pulmonary emboli and infarction. The onset of hemoptysis is usually sudden and may be intermittent or continuous.

Diagnostic evaluation includes several studies to determine the cause: inspection of the blood, chest angiography, chest x-ray, and bronchoscopy. A careful history and physical examination are necessary to establish a diagnosis of the underlying disease, irrespective of whether or not the bleeding produced involved a very small amount of blood in the sputum or a massive hemorrhage. The amount of blood produced is not always indicative of the seriousness of the cause.

Sources. First, it is important to determine the source of the bleeding: the gums, nasopharynx, lungs, or stomach. The nurse may be the only witness to the episode. The following points should be considered in making and recording observations.

- *Bloody sputum from the nose or the nasopharynx* is usually preceded by considerable sniffing, with blood possibly appearing in the nose.
- *Blood from the lung* is usually bright red, frothy, and mixed with sputum. Initial symptoms include a tickling sensation in the throat, a salty taste, a burning or bub-

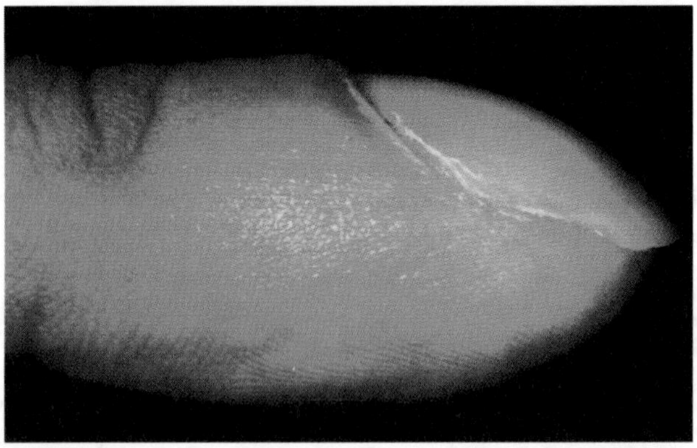

FIGURE 22-18. Clubbing of the fingers. In clubbing, the distal phalanx of each finger is rounded and bulbous. The nail plate is more convex, and the angle between the plate and the proximal nail fold increases to 180 degrees or more. The proximal nail fold, when palpated, feels spongy or floating. Causes are many, including chronic hypoxia and lung cancer. (From Bates B. A Guide to Physical Examination and History Taking, 6th ed. Philadelphia, JB Lippincott, 1995.)

bling sensation in the chest, and perhaps chest pain, in which case the patient tends to splint the bleeding side. The term **hemoptysis** is reserved for the coughing up of blood arising from a pulmonary hemorrhage. This blood has an alkaline *p*H (greater than 7.0).

- *If the hemorrhage is in the stomach,* the blood is vomited (**hematemesis**) rather than coughed up. Blood that has been in contact with gastric juice is sometimes so dark that it is referred to as "coffee ground" material. This blood has an acid *p*H (less than 7.0).

Cyanosis

Cyanosis, a bluish coloring of the skin, is a very late indicator of *hypoxia*. Cyanosis appears when there is 5 g/dl of unoxygenated hemoglobin. A patient whose hemoglobin is 15 g/dl will not demonstrate cyanosis until 5 g/dl of that hemoglobin becomes unoxygenated, reducing the effective circulating hemoglobin to two thirds of the normal level. The oxygenation of the blood determines cyanosis. As an illustration of this concept, the anemic patient rarely manifests cyanosis, and the polycythemic patient appears cyanotic even if adequately oxygenated. Therefore the presence of cyanosis is *not* a reliable sign of hypoxia.

Assessment of cyanosis is affected by room lighting, the patient's skin color, and distance of the blood vessels from the surface of the skin. In the presence of a pulmonary condition, central cyanosis is assessed by observing the color of the tongue and lips. This indicates a decrease in oxygen tension in the blood. Peripheral cyanosis results from decreased blood flow to a certain area of the body, as in vasoconstriction of the nail beds or ear lobes from exposure to cold, and does not necessarily indicate a central systemic problem.

Assessment of Breathing Ability

Tests of the patient's breathing ability are easily assessed at the bedside by measuring the respiratory rate, tidal volume, minute ventilation, vital capacity, inspiratory force, and compliance. These tests are particularly important for patients at risk for developing pulmonary complications, including those who have undergone chest or abdominal surgery, have experienced prolonged anesthesia, have preexisting pulmonary disease, or are elderly.

Patients whose chest expansion is limited by external restrictions such as obesity or abdominal distention and who are unable to breathe deeply because of postoperative pain or sedation will inhale and exhale a low volume of air (referred to as *low tidal volumes*. Ventilation at low tidal volumes without sigh inflations can produce alveolar collapse or atelectasis. The amount of air remaining in the lungs after a normal expiration (functional residual capacity) falls, the ability of the lungs to expand (compliance) is reduced, and the patient must breathe faster to maintain the same degree of tissue oxygenation. These events can be exaggerated in patients who have preexisting pulmonary diseases and in elderly patients whose airways are less compliant because the small airways may collapse during expiration.

Respiratory Rate

The normal adult who is resting comfortably breathes at 12 to 18 breaths per minute. Except for occasional sighs, the breathing is regular.

- *Bradypnea*, or slow breathing, is associated with increased intracranial pressure, brain injury, and drug overdose.
- *Tachypnea*, or rapid breathing, is commonly seen in patients with pneumonia, pulmonary edema, metabolic acidosis, septicemia, severe pain, and rib fracture.

Tidal Volume

The volume of each breath is referred to as the **tidal volume.** An instrument commonly used at the bedside to measure volumes is the Wright spirometer.

If the patient is breathing through an endotracheal tube or tracheostomy, the spirometer is directly attached to it and the exhaled volume is obtained from the reading on the gauge. In other patients, the spirometer is attached to a face mask, which is positioned to cover the nose and mouth so that it is airtight, and the exhaled volume is measured as before. Hand-held electronic spirometers that provide digital readouts of lung volumes are also available.

The tidal volume may vary from breath to breath. To make the measurement reliable, the volumes of several breaths are measured, and the range of tidal volumes together with the average tidal volume are noted. The normal tidal volume is approximately 8 to 10 ml per kilogram of body weight.

Minute Ventilation

Tidal volume and respiratory rates alone are unreliable indicators of adequate ventilation because both can vary widely from breath to breath. Together, however, the tidal volume and respiratory rate are important because they determine the minute ventilation, which is useful in the detection of respiratory failure. **Minute ventilation** ($\dot{V}_E$) is the volume of air expired per minute. It is equal to the product of the tidal volume (V_T) and respiratory rate or frequency (f) according to the following equation:

$$\dot{V}_E = V_T \times f$$

In practice, the minute ventilation is not calculated but is measured directly using a spirometer. Minute ventilation may be decreased by a variety of conditions that produce the following effects:

- Limit neurologic impulses transmitted from the brain to the respiratory muscles, such as spinal cord trauma, cerebrovascular accidents, tumors, myasthenia gravis, Guillain-Barré syndrome, polio, and drug overdose
- Depress the respiratory centers in the medulla, as with anesthesia and drug overdose
- Limit thoracic movement (kyphoscoliosis); limit lung movement (pleural effusion, pneumothorax); or

reduce functional lung tissue (chronic pulmonary diseases, severe pulmonary edema)

When the minute ventilation falls, alveolar ventilation in the lungs also must decrease, and the $PaCO_2$ increases.

- One should not rely on visual inspection of the rate and depth of a patient's respiratory excursions to determine the adequacy of ventilation. Respiratory excursions may appear normal or exaggerated, but the patient may actually be moving only enough air to ventilate the dead space.

Vital Capacity

Vital capacity is measured by having the patient take in a maximal breath and exhale fully through a spirometer. The normal value depends on age, sex, body build, and weight.

- Most patients can generate a vital capacity twice the volume they normally breathe in and out (tidal volume). If the vital capacity is less than 10 ml per kilogram of body weight, the patient will be unable to sustain spontaneous ventilation and respiratory assistance will be required.

When the vital capacity is exhaled at a maximal flow rate, the forced vital capacity (FVC) is measured. Most patients can exhale at least 75% of their vital capacity in 1 second (forced expiratory volume in 1 second, or FEV_1) and almost all of it in 3 seconds (FEV_3). A reduction in the FEV_1 suggests abnormal pulmonary air flow. If a patient's FEV_1 and FVC are proportionately reduced, maximal lung expansion is restricted in some way. If the reduction in FEV_1 greatly exceeds the reduction in FVC, the patient may have some degree of airway obstruction.

Inspiratory Force

Inspiratory force evaluates the effort a patient is making during inspiration. It does not require patient cooperation and hence is useful in the unconscious patient. The equipment needed for this measurement includes (1) a manometer that measures negative pressure and (2) adapters that are connected to an anesthesia mask or a cuffed endotracheal tube. The manometer is attached and the airway is completely occluded.

This process is continued for 10 to 20 seconds while the inspiratory efforts of the patient are registered on the manometer. The normal inspiratory pressure is –100 cm H_2O. If the negative pressure registered after 15 seconds of occluding the airway is less than –25 cm H_2O, mechanical ventilation is usually required, because the patient lacks sufficient muscle strength for deep breathing or effective coughing.

Diagnostic Assessment of Respiratory Function

A wide range of diagnostic studies, described on the following pages, may be performed in patients with respiratory conditions. Some of these procedures require a few seconds or minutes to complete; others are invasive procedures that require extensive patient preparation and use of local anesthetics.

Pulmonary Function Tests

Pulmonary function tests are performed to assess respiratory function and to detect and determine the extent of the abnormality. Such tests include measurements of lung volumes, ventilatory function, and the mechanics of breathing, diffusion, and gas exchange.

Pulmonary function tests are useful in following the course of a patient with established respiratory disease and assessing response to therapy. They are useful as screening tests in potentially hazardous industries, such as coal mining and those that involve exposure to asbestos and other noxious fumes, dusts, or gases. Preoperatively, they are useful for patients scheduled for thoracic and upper abdominal surgery, patients with a history of smoking and cough, obese patients, older patients, and patients with pulmonary disease.

Pulmonary function tests generally are performed by a technician. They require a spirometer that has a volume collecting device attached to a recorder that demonstrates volume and time simultaneously. Pulmonary function testing is becoming more automated (computerized); some systems measure multiple parameters. Smaller hospitals, by using a data transmitter, can send test information to a larger medical facility's computer for analysis.

A number of tests are carried out because no single measurement provides a complete picture of pulmonary function. Usually, test results are interpreted on the basis of degree of deviation from normal, taking into consideration the patient's height, weight, age, and gender.

Because there is a wide range of normal values, pulmonary function tests may not detect early localized changes. The patient with respiratory symptoms (dyspnea, wheezing, cough, sputum production) usually undergoes a complete diagnostic evaluation, even though the results of pulmonary function tests are "normal."

The most frequently used pulmonary function tests are described in Tables 22-1 and 22-6.

Arterial Blood Gas Studies

Measurements of blood *p*H and of arterial oxygen and carbon dioxide tensions are obtained when managing patients with respiratory problems and in adjusting oxygen therapy as needed. The arterial oxygen tension (PaO_2) indicates the degree of oxygenation of the blood, and the arterial carbon dioxide tension ($PaCO_2$) indicates adequacy of alveolar ventilation. Arterial blood gas studies aid in assessing the degree to which the lungs are able to provide adequate oxygen and remove carbon dioxide and the degree to which the kidneys are able to reabsorb or excrete bicarbonate ions to maintain normal body *p*H. Serial blood gas analysis also is a sensitive indicator of whether the lung has been damaged after chest trauma. Arterial blood gases are obtained

TABLE 22-6 Pulmonary Function Tests

Term Used	Symbol	Description	Remarks
Forced vital capacity	FVC	Vital capacity performed with a maximally forced expiratory effort	Forced vital capacity is often reduced in COPD because of air trapping.
Forced expiratory volume (qualified by subscript indicating the time intervals in seconds)	FEVt, usually FEV_1	Volume of air exhaled in the specified time during the performance of forced vital capacity	A valuable clue to the severity of the expiratory airway obstruction.
Ratio of timed forced expiratory volume to forced vital capacity	FEVt/FVC%, usually FEV_1/FVC%	FEVt expressed as a percentage of the forced vital capacity	Another way of expressing the presence or absence of airway obstruction.
Forced expiratory flow	$FEF_{200-1200}$	Mean forced expiratory flow between 200 and 1200 ml of the FVC	Formerly called maximum expiratory flow rate (MEFR). An indicator of large airway obstruction.
Forced midexpiratory flow	$FEF_{25\%-75\%}$	Mean forced expiratory flow during the middle half of the FVC	Formerly called maximum and midexpiratory flow rate. Slowed in small airway obstruction.
Forced end expiratory flow	$FEF_{75\%-85\%}$	Mean forced expiratory flow during the terminal portion of the FVC	Slowed in obstruction of smallest airways.
Maximal voluntary ventilation	MVV	Volume of air expired in a specified period (12 seconds) during repetitive maximal effort	Formerly called maximum breathing capacity. An important factor in exercise tolerance.

through an arterial puncture at the radial, brachial, or femoral artery or through an indwelling arterial catheter.

Pulse Oximetry

Pulse oximetry is a noninvasive method of continuously monitoring the oxygen saturation of hemoglobin (SaO_2). Although pulse oximetry does not replace arterial blood gases, it is an effective tool to monitor the patient for subtle or sudden changes in oxygen saturation. It is used in a variety of settings, including critical care units, general nursing units, and in diagnostic and treatment areas when there is a need to monitor the patient's oxygen saturation during procedures.

A disposable probe or sensor is attached to the finger tip (Fig. 22-19), forehead, earlobe, or bridge of the nose. A sensor detects changes in oxygen saturation levels by monitoring light signals generated by the oximeter and reflected by blood pulsing through the tissue at the probe. Normal SaO_2 values are 95% to 100%. Values below 85% indicate that the tissues are not receiving enough oxygen and the patient needs further evaluation. SaO_2 values obtained by pulse oximetry are unreliable in cardiac arrest, shock, use of vasoconstrictor medications, IV administration of dyes (*i.e.*, methylene blue) that tint the blood, severe anemia, and high carbon monoxide levels. Hemoglobin levels, arterial blood gases, and other laboratory tests are needed to validate the results of pulse oximetry in these situations.

Radiographic Examination of the Chest

Chest X-ray Studies. Normal pulmonary tissue is radiolucent; therefore, densities produced by fluid, tumors, foreign bodies and other pathologic conditions can be detected by means of x-ray examination. A chest x-ray film may reveal an extensive pathologic process in the lungs in the absence of symptoms. The routine chest x-ray consists of two views—the posteroanterior projection and the lateral projection. Chest x-rays are usually taken after full inspiration (deep breath because the lungs are

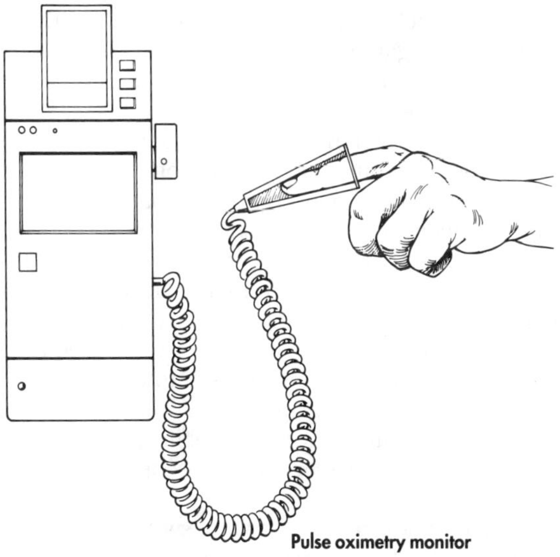

FIGURE 22-19. Pulse oximetry is an effective tool for measuring subtle changes in oxygen saturation (SaO_2). The finger, earlobe, or bridge of the nose can be used. A sensor detects changes in oxygen saturation levels in the blood pulsing through the tissue where the probe is attached. (From Fuller J and Schaller-Ayers J. Health Assessment: A Nursing Approach, 2nd ed. Philadelphia, JB Lippincott, 1994.)

best visualized when they are well aerated. Also, the diaphragm is at its lowest level and the largest expanse of lung is visible. Taken on expiration, x-ray films may accentuate an otherwise unnoticed pneumothorax or obstruction of a major artery.

Tomography (Planigraphy). Tomography provides images of sections of the lungs at different planes within the thorax. It is valuable in studying patients with pulmonary tuberculosis (TB), compressed lung tissue, and lung abscess. Tomography can show cavities, nodular infiltrates, and bronchiectasis associated with pulmonary tuberculosis, solid lesions seen in bronchogenic carcinoma, calcification, and bronchial occlusion.

Computed Tomography. Computed tomography (CT) is an imaging method in which the lungs are scanned in successive layers by a narrow-beam x-ray. The images produced provide a cross-sectional view of the chest. A regular chest x-ray film shows major contrast between body densities, such as bones, soft tissues, and air. CT scan, however, can distinguish fine tissue density. It may be used to define pulmonary nodules and small tumors adjacent to pleural surfaces that are not visible on routine chest x-ray films, and to demonstrate mediastinal abnormalities and hilar adenopathy, which are difficult to visualize with other techniques.

Contrast material is most useful when evaluating the mediastinum and its contents. A computer printout may be obtained of the absorption values of the tissues in the plane that is being scanned.

Positron Emission Tomography. Positron emission tomography (PET) uses high-energy physics and sophisticated computer techniques to study the way cells function in a living person. The patient inhales or is injected with a short-lived radioactive version of an element that occurs naturally in the body (oxygen, nitrogen, carbon, fluorine). The radioisotope emits subatomic particles called *positrons* (positively charged electrons). When a positron encounters an electron, which it does just after emission, both are destroyed and two gamma rays are released. These bursts of energy are recorded by the PET scanner, and its computer determines where in the body the radioactive material is located. PET is particularly useful for quantitative measurements of regional pulmonary perfusion and for studying ventilation–perfusion relationships. It is used in few centers because the technology is so costly.

Fluoroscopy. Fluoroscopy is used to assist with invasive procedures, such as a chest needle biopsy or transbronchial biopsy, in identifying lesions. It also may be used to study the movement of the chest wall, mediastinum, heart, and diaphragm. It may be used to detect diaphragm paralysis and locate lung masses. CT has replaced fluoroscopy for some indications. It is still used, however, in conjunction with fiberoptic bronchoscopy as a guide for biopsy.

Barium Swallow. A barium swallow outlines the esophagus and shows displacement of the esophagus and encroachment on its lumen by the heart, lungs, or mediastinal structures.

Bronchography. Bronchography is rarely used today since the advent of fiberoptic bronchoscopy and CT scans.

Angiographic Studies of the Pulmonary Vessels

Angiographic studies include pulmonary angiography, angiocardiography, aortography, bronchial arteriography, superior vena cava angiography, and azygography. Pulmonary angiography is most commonly used to investigate thromboembolic disease of the lungs, such as pulmonary emboli and congenital abnormalities of the pulmonary vascular tree.

Pulmonary angiography is the rapid injection of a radiopaque medium into the vasculature of the lungs for radiographic study of pulmonary vessels. It can be performed by injecting the radiopaque substance into a vein in one or both arms (simultaneously) or into the femoral vein, with a needle or catheter, or the medium can be injected into a catheter that has been placed into the main pulmonary artery or its branches or into the great veins proximal to the pulmonary artery.

Endoscopic Procedures

Bronchoscopy

Bronchoscopy is the direct inspection and examination of the larynx, trachea, and bronchi through either a flexible fiberoptic bronchoscope or a rigid bronchoscope. The fiberoptic scope is used more frequently in current practice.

The purposes of **diagnostic bronchoscopy** are (1) to examine tissues or collect secretions; (2) to determine the location and extent of the pathologic process and to obtain a tissue sample for diagnosis (by biting forceps, curettage, or brush biopsy); (3) determine whether or not a tumor can be resected surgically; and (4) to diagnose bleeding sites (source of hemoptysis).

Therapeutic bronchoscopy is used to (1) remove foreign bodies from the tracheobronchial tree, (2) remove secretions obstructing the tracheobronchial tree when the patient is unable to clear them, (3) provide postoperative treatment in atelectasis, and (4) destroy and excise lesions.

Procedure. The **fiberoptic bronchoscope** is a thin, flexible bronchoscope that can be directed into the segmental bronchi (Fig. 22-20). Because of its smaller size, flexibility, and excellent optical system, it allows increased visualization of the peripheral airways and is ideal for diagnosing pulmonary lesions. Cytologic examinations can be performed without surgical intervention.

Fiberoptic bronchoscopy is better tolerated by patients than rigid bronchoscopy, allows biopsy of previously inaccessible tumors, is safe to use in the very ill patient, and can be performed at the bedside or through endotracheal or tracheostomy tubes of patients on ventilators. Fiberoptic bronchoscopy allows direct intubation of the right upper lobe, which is impossible with the rigid bronchoscope.

The **rigid bronchoscope** is a hollow metallic tube with a light at its end; it is used mainly for removing foreign bodies, suctioning thick secretions, investigating the source of massive hemoptysis, or performing endobronchial surgical procedures.

Possible complications of bronchoscopy include reaction to the local anesthetic, infection, aspiration, broncho-

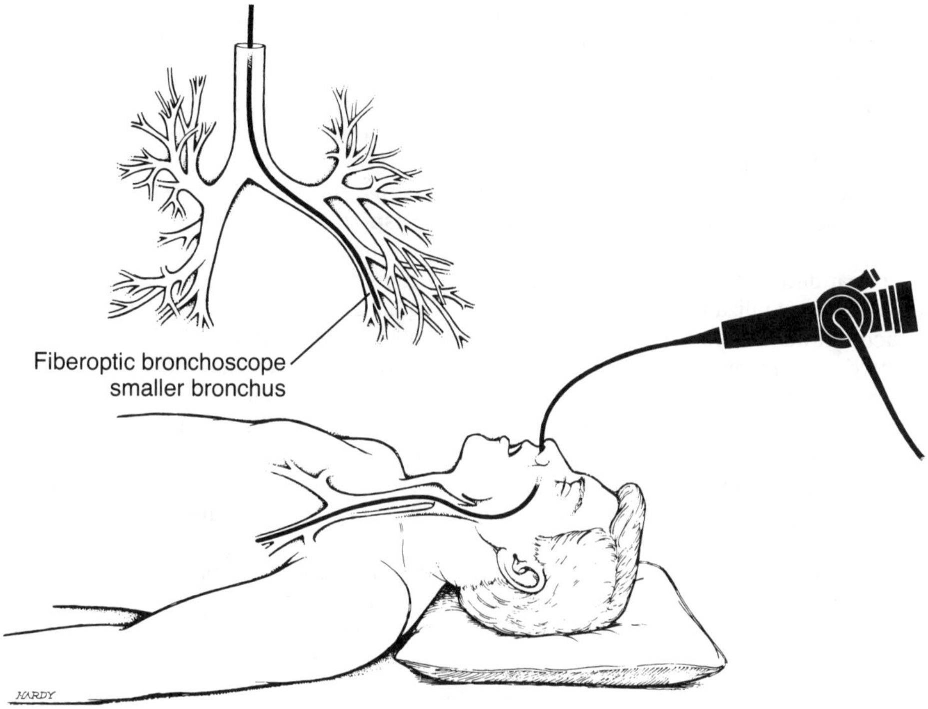

FIGURE 22-20. Fiberoptic bronchoscopy.

spasm, hypoxemia, pneumothorax, bleeding, and performation.

Nursing Interventions. An informed consent is obtained before the procedure. Food and fluids are withheld for 6 hours before the test to reduce the risk of aspiration when reflexes are blocked. The procedure is explained to the patient to reduce fear and correct misapprehensions. Preoperative medications (usually atropine and a sedative or opioid) are administered as prescribed to inhibit vagal stimulation (thereby guarding against bradycardia, dysrhythmias, hypotension), suppress the cough reflex, sedate the patient, and relieve anxiety.

- *Caution:* Sedation given to patients with respiratory insufficiency may precipitate respiratory arrest.

Contact lenses, dentures, and other prostheses are removed. The examination is usually performed under local anesthesia, but general anesthesia may be given.

A topical anesthetic such as lidocaine (Xylocaine) may be sprayed on the pharynx or dropped on the epiglottis and vocal cords and into the trachea to suppress the cough reflex and minimize discomfort. Sedatives or opioids are administered as prescribed, intravenously, for additional sedation.

After the procedure, the patient is given nothing by mouth until the cough reflex returns because the preoperative sedation and local anesthesia impair the protective laryngeal reflex and swallowing for several hours. Once the patient demonstrates a cough reflex, ice chips and eventually fluids may be given. The nurse assesses for confusion and lethargy in the elderly, which may be due to large doses of lidocaine given during the procedure. Respiratory status is monitored. The patient is observed for evidence of cyanosis, hypotension, tachycardia, dysrhythmias, hemoptysis, and dyspnea; any abnormality is reported promptly.

Thoracoscopy

Thoracoscopy is a diagnostic procedure in which the pleural cavity is examined with an endoscope (Fig. 22-21). Small incisions are made into the pleural cavity in an intercostal space; the location of the incision depends on clinical and diagnostic findings. After any fluid present in the

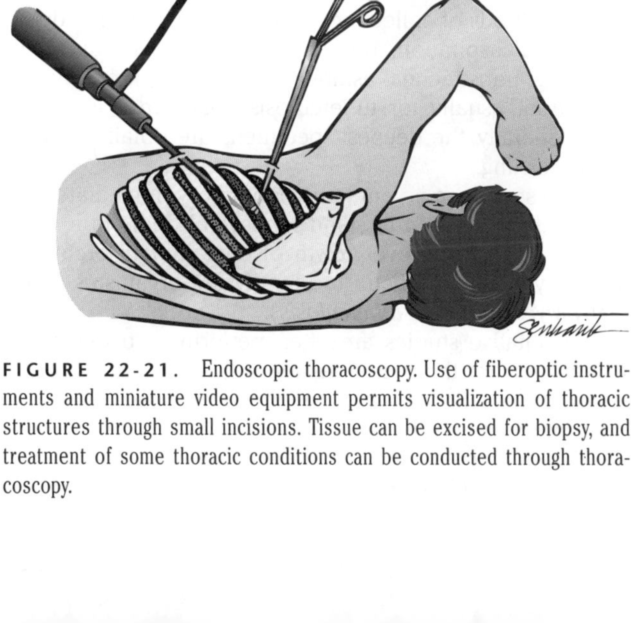

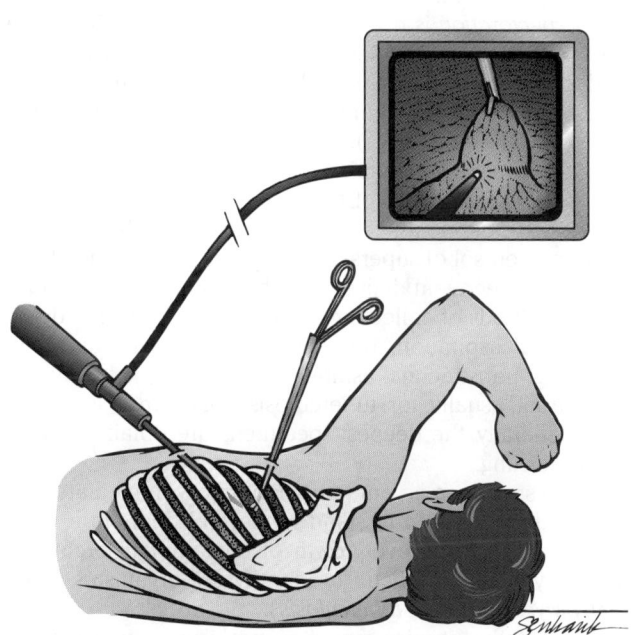

FIGURE 22-21. Endoscopic thoracoscopy. Use of fiberoptic instruments and miniature video equipment permits visualization of thoracic structures through small incisions. Tissue can be excised for biopsy, and treatment of some thoracic conditions can be conducted through thoracoscopy.

pleural cavity is aspirated, the fiberoptic mediastinoscope is inserted into the pleural cavity and its surface is inspected through the instrument. After the procedure, a chest tube may be inserted and the pleural cavity is drained by water-seal drainage.

Thoracoscopy is primarily indicated in the diagnostic evaluation of pleural effusions, pleural disease, and tumor staging. Biopsies of the lesions can be performed under visualization for diagnosis.

Thoracoscopic procedures have expanded with the availability of video monitoring, which permits visualization of the lung. It has, in some cases, replaced thoracotomy as the standard for diagnosis of diffuse lung disorders, pulmonary infiltrates, and lung biopsy. It also has been used with carbon dioxide laser in the removal of pulmonary blebs and bullae, and in the treatment of spontaneous pneumothorax. The Nd:YAG laser has been used in the excision of peripheral pulmonary nodules. Although it does not replace the need for thoracotomy in the treatment of some lung cancers, its use continues to expand because it is less invasive.

Sputum Studies

Sputum is obtained for study to identify pathogenic organisms and to determine whether or not malignant cells are present. It also may be used to assess for hypersensitivity states (in which there is an increase of eosinophils). Periodic sputum examinations may be necessary for patients receiving antibiotics, corticosteroids, and immunosuppressive medications for prolonged periods, as these agents give rise to opportunistic infections. In general, sputum cultures are used in diagnosis, for drug sensitivity testing, and as a guide in treatment.

Expectoration is the usual method for collecting a sputum specimen. The patient is instructed to clear the nose and throat and rinse the mouth to decrease contamination of the sputum. After taking a few deep breaths, the patient coughs (rather than spits), using the diaphragm, and expectorates into a sterile container.

If the sputum cannot be raised spontaneously, the patient often can be induced to cough deeply by breathing an irritating aerosol of supersaturated saline, propylene glycol, or some other agent delivered with an ultrasonic nebulizer. Other methods of collecting sputum specimens include endotracheal aspiration, bronchoscopic removal, bronchial brushing, transtracheal aspiration (see below), and gastric aspiration, usually for tuberculosis organisms (see Chap. 24). Generally, the deepest specimens are obtained in the early morning.

The specimen is sent to the laboratory immediately; allowing the specimen to stand for several hours in a warm room results in the overgrowth of contaminant organisms and may make it difficult to identify the organisms (especially *Mycobacterium tuberculosis*).

Qualitative studies are often performed to determine whether or not the secretions are saliva, mucus, or pus. A yellow-green color of the material expectorated usually implies infection (*i.e.*, pneumonia).

For quantitative studies, the patient is given a special container in which to expectorate. This is weighed at the end of 24 hours, and the amount and the character of the contents are described and recorded. Such a specimen is treated as biohazardous material and disposed of appropriately. To prevent odors, all sputum containers are covered. Malodorous mouth wipes are discarded and removed promptly, and good room ventilation is ensured. Frequent oral hygiene is a nursing priority for the patient.

Transtracheal aspiration of sputum is accomplished by puncturing the trachea through the cricothyroid membrane and by introducing a fine catheter through the neele into the trachea (Fig. 22-22). The needle is withdrawn, leaving the catheter in place. Sterile saline (2 to 5 ml) is injected into the catheter to loosen secretions and induce coughing. Then material is aspirated back through the catheter into a syringe. The contents of the syringe are expressed into a sterile culture tube. The catheter is withdrawn and pressure is applied over the puncture site for 5 to 10 minutes to minimize bleeding and prevent subcutaneous emphysema.

This technique is also used to promote coughing and sputum production in thoracotomy patients and in those patients with an absent cough reflex. In this instance, the catheter is left in place for periodic instillation of saline to induce coughing.

Transtracheal aspiration bypasses the orophrynx and thus avoids specimen contamination by mouth flora, particularly anaerobes. It is of special value to the immunocompromised patient with pneumonia who does not produce sputum.

The patient is observed for several hours after the procedure. Possible complications include intratracheal bleeding, hypoxemia, cardiac dysrhythmias, pneumomediastinum, subcutaneous emphysema, and infection.

Thoracentesis

A thin layer of pleural fluid normally remains in the pleural space. A sample of this fluid can be obtained by thoracentesis or by tube thoracotomy. Thoracentesis is the aspiration of pleural fluid for diagnosic or therapeutic purposes. The patient is positioned as shown in Figure 22-23.

A needle biopsy of the pleura may be performed at the same time. Guidelines for assisting the patient undergoing a thoracentesis are presented in Guideline 22-1. Studies of pleural fluid include Gram stain culture and sensitivity, acid-fast staining and culture, differential cell count, cytology, *p*H, specific gravity, total protein, and lactic dehydrogenase.

Pleural Biopsy

Pleural biopsy is accomplished by needle biopsy of the pleura or by pleuroscopy, which is a visual exploration through a fiberoptic bronchoscope inserted into the pleural space. Pleural biopsy is performed when there is pleural exudate of undetermined origin and when there is need to culture or stain the tissue to identify tuberculosis or fungi.

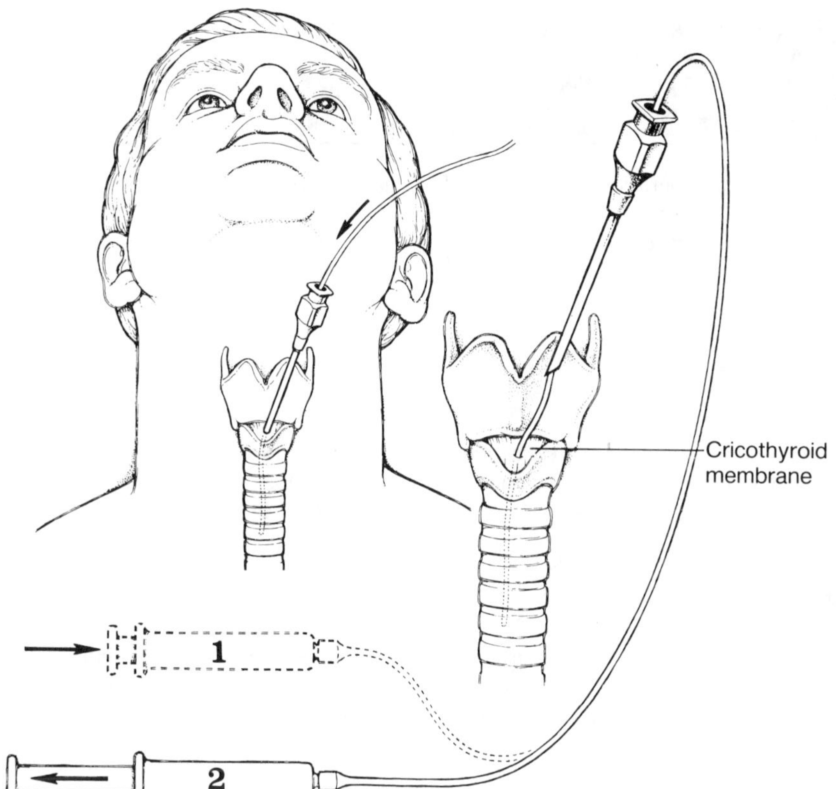

FIGURE 22-22. Transtracheal aspiration. After the catheter is positioned in the trachea, the needle is withdrawn, leaving the catheter in place. Sterile saline (2 to 5 ml) is injected into the catheter as indicated in (1) to loosen secretions and induce coughing. Then, as indicated at (2), the material is aspirated back through the catheter into the syringe.

Radioisotope Diagnostic Procedures (Lung Scan)

There are three types of lung scans: perfusion scan, ventilation scan, and inhalation scan. They are used to detect normal lung functioning, pulmonary vascular supply, and gas exchange.

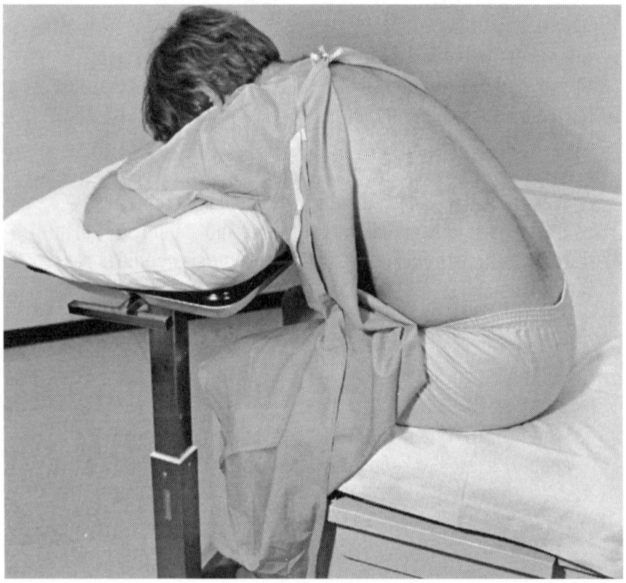

FIGURE 22-23. Position for a thoracentesis.

A **perfusion lung scan** is performed by injecting a radioactive agent (technetium) into a peripheral vein and then obtaining a scan of the chest and body to detect radiation. The isotope particles pass through the right side of the heart and are distributed into the lungs in amounts proportional to the regional blood flow, making it possible to trace and measure the blood perfusion through the lung. This procedure is used clinically to measure the integrity of the pulmonary vessels relative to blood flow and to evaluate blood flow abnormalities as seen in pulmonary emboli. The nurse informs the patient that the imaging time is 20 to 40 minutes, during which the patient will lie under the camera with a mask fitted over the nose and mouth for the duration of the test.

A **ventilation scan** is performed after the perfusion scan. The patient takes a deep breath of a mixture of oxygen and radioactive gas (xenon, krypton), which diffuses throughout the lungs. A scan is performed to detect ventilation abnormalities, especially in patients who have regional differences in ventilation. It may be helpful in the diagnosis of bronchitis, asthma, inflammatory fibrosis, pneumonia, emphysema, and lung cancer.

An **inhalation scan** is performed by administering droplets of radioactive material by a positive-pressure ventilator. This scan is helpful, particularly in visualizing the trachea and major airways.

The **gallium scan** is a radioisotope lung scan used to detect inflammatory conditions, abscesses, adhesions, and the presence, location, and size of tumors. It is used to stage bronchogenic cancer and record tumor regression after chemotherapy or radiation.

GUIDELINE 22–1
Assisting the Patient Having a Thoracentesis

A thoracentesis (aspiration of fluid or air from the pleural space) is performed on patients with various clinical problems. It may be a diagnostic or therapeutic procedure for

1. Removal of fluid and air from the pleural cavity
2. Diagnostic aspiration of pleural fluid
3. Pleural biopsy
4. Instillation of medication into the pleural space

The responsibilities of the nurse in relation to the patient having a thoracentesis and the rationale for participation are summarized below:

Nursing Activities	Amplification/Rationale
1. Ascertain in advance whether chest x-ray films have been prescribed and completed and the consent form has been signed.	1. Posteroanterior and lateral chest x-ray films are used to localize fluid and air in the pleural cavity and to aid in determining the puncture site. Ultrasound scanning is performed when fluid is loculated (isolated in a pocket of pleural fluid) to help select the best site for needle aspiration.
2. Assess the patient for allergy to the local anesthetic agent to be used. Give sedation if prescribed.	
3. Inform the patient about the procedure: a. The nature of the procedure b. The importance of remaining immobile c. Pressure sensations to be experienced d. That no discomfort is anticipated after the procedure	3. An explanation helps to orient the patient to the procedure, assists the patient to mobilize resources, and provides an opportunity to ask questions and verbalize anxiety.
4. Make the patient comfortable with adequate supports (see Fig. 22-23). If possible, place the patient upright and in one of the following positions: a. Sitting on the edge of the bed with the feet supported and arms and head on a padded over-the-bed table b. Straddling a chair with arms and head resting on the back of the chair c. Lying on the unaffected side with the bed elevated 30 to 45 degrees if unable to assume a sitting position	4. The upright position facilitates the removal of fluid that usually localizes at the base of the chest. A position of comfort helps the patient to relax.
5. Support and reassure the patient during the procedure. a. Prepare the patient for cold sensation of skin germicide solution and of pressure sensation from infiltration of local anesthetic agent. b. Encourage the patient to refrain from coughing.	5. Sudden and unexpected movement by the patient can cause trauma to the visceral pleura and lung.
6. Expose the entire chest. The site for aspiration is determined from chest x-ray films and by percussion. If fluid is in the pleural cavity, the thoracentesis site is determined by the chest x-ray films, ultrasound scanning, and physical findings, with attention to site of maximal dullness on percussion.	6. If air is in the pleural cavity, the thoracentesis site is usually in the second or third intercostal space in the midclavicular line because air rises in the thorax.
7. The procedure is performed under aseptic conditions. After the skin is cleansed, a local anesthetic is injected slowly with a small-caliber needle into the intercostal space by the physician.	7. An intradermal wheal is raised slowly; rapid injection causes pain. The parietal pleura is very sensitive and should be well infiltrated with anesthetic before the thoracentesis needle is passed through it.
8. The physician advances the thoracentesis needle with the syringe attached. When the pleural space is reached, suction may be applied with the syringe.	
a. A 20-ml syringe with a three-way adapter (stopcock) is attached to the needle (one end of the adapter is attached to the needle and the other to the tubing leading to a receptable that receives the fluid being aspirated).	a. When a large quantity of fluid is withdrawn, a three-way adapter serves to keep air from entering the pleural cavity.

(continued)

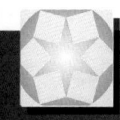

GUIDELINE 22–1 *(continued)*
Assisting the Patient Having a Thoracentesis

Nursing Activities	Amplification/Rationale
b. If a considerable quantity of fluid is removed, the needle is held in place on the chest wall with a small hemostat.	b. The hemostat steadies the needle on the chest wall. Sudden pleuritic chest pain or shoulder pain may indicate that the visceral or diaphragmatic pleura is being irritated by the needle point.
9. After the needle is withdrawn, pressure is applied over the puncture site and a small, sterile dressing is fixed in place.	
10. The patient is placed on bed rest. A chest x-ray is obtained after thoracentesis.	10. A chest x-ray verifies that there is no pneumothorax.
11. Record the total amount of fluid withdrawn and the nature of the fluid, its color, and its viscosity. If requested, prepare samples of fluid for laboratory evaluation. A specimen container with formalin may be needed if a pleural biopsy is to be obtained.	11. The fluid may be clear, serous, bloody, purulent, etc.
12. Evaluate the patient at intervals for increasing respiratory rate; asymmetry in respiratory movement; faintness; vertigo; tightness in chest; uncontrollable cough; blood-tinged, frothy mucus; a rapid pulse, and signs of hypoxemia.	12. Pneumothorax, tension pneumothorax, subcutaneous emphysema, or pyrogenic infection may result from a thoracentesis. Pulmonary edema or cardiac distress can be produced by a sudden shift in mediastinal contents when large amounts of fluid are aspirated.

Lung Biopsy Procedures

When the chest x-ray film is inconclusive or shows pulmonary density (indicating an infiltrate or lesion), it is desirable to examine lung tissue to establish the nature of the lesion. There are several nonsurgical lung biopsy techniques that are used because they yield accurate information with low morbidity: (1) transcatheter bronchial brushing, (2) percutaneous (through the skin) needle biopsy, or (3) transbronchial lung biopsy.

In **transcatheter bronchial brushing**, a fiberoptic bronchoscope is introduced into the bronchus under fluoroscopy. A small brush is attached to the end of a flexible wire, which is inserted through the bronchoscope. Under direct visualization, the area under suspicion is brushed back and forth, causing cells to slough off and adhere to the brush. The bronchoscopic catheter may be irrigated with saline to secure material for additional studies. The brush is removed from the bronchoscope and a microscopic slide is made. Sometimes the brush is cut off and sent to the laboratory for pathologic tests.

This procedure is useful for cytologic evaluations of lung lesions and for the identification of pathogenic organisms (*Nocardia, Aspergillus, Pneumocystis carinii*, and other pathogens). It is especially useful in the immunologically compromised patient.

A consent form is signed before this procedure; the nurse provides explanations and clarifies questions that the patient may have. After the procedure, the patient may have a mild sore throat and transient hemoptysis. Fluids and food are withheld for several hours after the procedure. Possible complications include anesthetic reactions, laryngospasm, hemoptysis, and, rarely, pneumothorax.

Another method of bronchial brushing involves the introduction of the catheter through the transcricothyroid membrane by needle puncture. After this procedure, the patient is instructed to hold a finger or thumb over the puncture site while coughing to prevent air from leaking into the surrounding tissues.

Percutaneous needle biopsy may be accomplished with a cutting needle or by aspiration with a spinal-type needle that provides a tissue specimen for histologic study. A **transbronchial lung biopsy** uses cutting forceps introduced by fiberoptic bronchoscope. A biopsy is indicated when a lung lesion is suspected and routine sputum samples and bronchoscopic washings are negative.

Analgesia may be administered before the procedure. The skin over the biopsy site is cleansed and anesthetized and a small incision is made. The biopsy needle is inserted through the incision into the pleura with the patient holding the breath in midexpiration. With flouroscopic monitoring, the surgeon guides the needle into the periphery of the lesion and obtains a tissue sample from the mass. Possible complications include pneumothorax, pulmonary hemorrhage, and empyema.

Lymph Node Biopsy

The scalene lymph nodes are enmeshed in the deep cervical pad of fat overlying the scalenus anterior muscle. They drain the lungs and mediastinum and may show histologic changes due to intrathoracic disease. When these nodes are palpable on physical examination, a **scalene node** biopsy may be performed. A biopsy of these nodes may be performed to detect lymph node spread of pulmonary disease

CRITICAL THINKING EXERCISES

1. Following a thoracentesis for diagnostic purposes, your patient reports shortness of breath and appears anxious. Based on your knowledge of the risks associated with thoracentesis, explain how you would focus your assessment because of those risks.
2. Your patient is scheduled for pulmonary function tests (PFTs) prior to heart surgery. You know that a patient who understands the purposes of the tests and what to expect during the procedures will be able to cooperate more while the tests are being conducted. Describe how you would teach this patient, and present the details of the explanations you would give.

and to establish a diagnosis or prognosis in such diseases as Hodgkin's disease, sarcoidosis, fungal disease, tuberculosis, and carcinoma.

Mediastinoscopy is the endoscopic examination of the mediastinum for exploration and biopsy of mediastinal lymph nodes that drain the lungs; this examination does not require a thoracotomy. Biopsy is usually performed through a suprasternal incision. Mediastinoscopy is carried out to detect mediastinal involvement of pulmonary malignancy and to obtain tissue for diagnostic studies of other conditions (*e.g.*, sarcoidosis).

An **anterior mediastinotomy** is thought to provide better exposure and diagnostic possibilities than a mediastinoscopy. An incision is made in the area of the second or third costal cartilage. The mediastinum is explored, and biopsies are performed on any lymph nodes found. Chest tube drainage is required after the procedure. This diagnostic modality is particularly valuable to determine whether a pulmonary lesion is resectable.

BIBLIOGRAPHY

Books

Bates B. A Guide to Physical Examination and History-Taking, 6th ed. Philadelphia, JB Lippincott, 1995.

Baum GL and Wolinsky E (eds). Textbook of Pulmonary Diseases, 5th ed. Boston, Little, Brown, 1993.

Brown WT. Atlas of Video-Assisted Thoracic Surgery. Philadelphia, WB Saunders, 1994.

Burton GG, Hodgkin JE, Ward JJ, (eds). Respiratory Care: A Guide to Clinical Practice, 2nd ed. Philadelphia, JB Lippincott, 1991.

Comroe JH et al. The Lung, Clinical Physiology and Pulmonary Function Tests, 2nd ed. Chicago, Year Book, 1977.

Fishman AP. Pulmonary Diseases and Disorders, 2nd ed, Vol 1. New York, McGraw-Hill, 1988.

Kinney MR et al. AACN's Clinical Reference for Critical Care Nursing, 3rd ed. New York, McGraw-Hill, 1993.

Murray JF and Nadel JA. Textbook of Respiratory Medicine, Vol. 1, 2nd ed. Philadelphia, WB Saunders, 1994.

Shapiro BA et al. Clinical Application of Blood Gases, 4th ed. Chicago, Mosby–Year Book, 1988.

Weinberger SE. Principles of Pulmonary Medicine, 2nd ed. Philadelphia, WB Saunders, 1988.

Wilkins RL, Hodgkin JE, and Lopez B. Lung Sounds: A Practical Guide. St Louis, CV Mosby, 1988.

Journals

Cherniack RM. Evaluation of respiratory function in health and disease. Disease-A-Month 1992 July; 505–576.

Crapo RO. Pulmonary function testing. N Engl J Med 1994 Jul 7; 331(1):25–30.

Grap MJ, Glass C, and Constantino S. Accurate assessment of ventilation and oxygenation. Medsurg Nurs 1994 Dec; 3(6): 435–442.

Keene A. Cardiovascular and respiratory assessment in the office setting. Plastic Surg Nurs 1994 Spring; 13(4):181–184.

Lewis RJ. Video-assisted thoracic surgery. Chest Surg Clin North Am 1993 May; 3(2):179–356.

McElvein RB. Procedures in the evaluation of chest disease. Clin Chest Med 1992 March; 13(1):1–9.

Qureshi N, Momin ZA, and Brandstetter RD. Thoracentesis in practice. Heart Lung 1994 Oct; 23(5):376–383.

Stiesmeyer JK. A four-step approach to pulmonary assessment. Am J Nurs 1993 Aug; 98(8):22–28.

Wood DE. Thorascopic surgery. Respiratory Care 1993 April; 38(4): 388–397.

INFORMATION/RESOURCES

Government Agencies

National Heart, Lung and Blood Institute
National Institutes of Health
900 Rockville Pike, Bldg 31,
Bethesda, MD 20892, (301) 496-5166

Voluntary Agencies

American Lung Association
1740 Broadway
New York, NY 10019, (212) 315-8700

American Thoracic Society
1740 Broadway
New York, NY 10019, (212) 315-8700

Respiratory Nursing Society
5700 Old Orchard Road, 1st Floor
Skokie, IL 60077-1057, (708) 966-8673

Voluntary American Association for Respiratory Care
1720 Regal Row
Dallas, TX 75235, (214) 630-3540

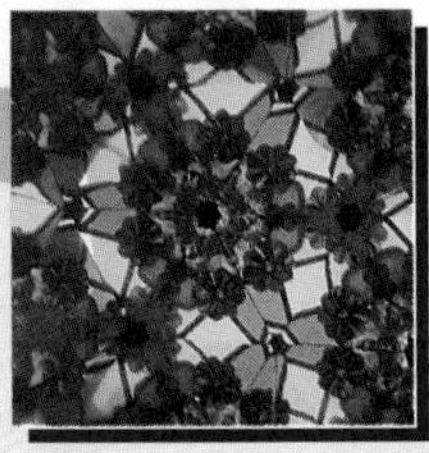

23

Management of Patients With Conditions of the Upper Respiratory Tract

CHAPTER OUTLINE

Upper Airway Infections
Common Cold
Herpes Simplex Infection
Sinusitis
Rhinitis
Acute Pharyngitis
Chronic Pharyngitis
Tonsillitis and Adenoiditis
Peritonsillar Abscess
Laryngitis
NURSING PROCESS: The Patient With Upper Airway Infection

Obstruction and Trauma of the Upper Respiratory Airway
Epistaxis (Nosebleed)
Nasal Obstruction
Fractures of the Nose
Laryngeal Obstruction

Cancer of the Larynx
Clinical Manifestations
Diagnostic Evaluation
Medical Management
NURSING PROCESS: The Patient Undergoing Laryngectomy

Critical Thinking Exercises

LEARNING OBJECTIVES

On completion of this chapter, the learner will be able to:

1. Describe nursing management of patients with upper respiratory airway disorders
2. Compare the upper respiratory tract infections with regard to cause, incidence, clinical manifestations, management, and the significance of preventive health care
3. Use the nursing process as a framework for care of patients with upper airway infection
4. Describe nursing management of the patient with epistaxis
5. Use the nursing process as a framework for care of patients undergoing laryngectomy

Upper Airway Infections

Upper airway infections are common conditions that affect most people on occasion. Some of these conditions are acute, with symptoms that last several days; others are chronic, with symptoms that last a long time or occur repeatedly. Seldom do patients with these conditions require hospitalization; however, nurses working in ambulatory centers or long-term care facilities may encounter patients who have these infections. Thus, it is important to recognize the signs and symptoms and to provide appropriate nursing care.

Common Cold

The phrase *common cold* usually is used when referring to symptoms of an upper respiratory tract infection, characterized by nasal congestion, sore throat, and cough. Colds are highly contagious because patients shed virus for about 2 days before the symptoms appear and during the first part of the symptomatic phase. Colds prevail among 15% of the work population at any time during the winter and account for almost half of all work absences and one fourth of the total time lost from work.

Three waves of colds appear yearly in the United States: in September, just after the opening of school; in late January; and toward the end of April. Immunity after recovery is variable and depends on many factors, including a person's natural host resistance and the specific virus causing the cold.

Clinical Manifestations. The signs and symptoms of a cold are nasal congestion, sore throat, sneezing, malaise, fever, chills, and often headache and muscle aches. As the cold progresses, cough usually appears. Most specifically, the term *cold* refers to an afebrile, infectious, acute inflammation of the mucous membranes of the nasal cavity. More broadly, the term refers to an acute upper respiratory tract infection, whereas terms such as *rhinitis, pharyngitis, laryngitis,* and *chest cold* distinguish the sites of the major symptoms.

The symptoms last 5 days to 2 weeks. If there is significant fever or more severe systemic respiratory symptoms, it is no longer a common cold but one of the other acute upper respiratory tract infections. More than 200 different viruses, classified into five major groupings, are known to produce the signs and symptoms of the common cold: picornaviruses, coronaviruses, myxoviruses, para viruses, and adenoviruses. Rhinovirus, "the classic head cold," and a member of the picornavirus group, accounts for 30% to 40% of all colds. Allergic conditions can also affect the nose and mimic the symptoms of a cold.

Medical Management. There is no specific treatment for the common cold. Management of the common cold consists of symptomatic therapy. Some measures may include providing adequate fluid intake, rest, prevention of chilling, aqueous nasal decongestants, vitamin C, and expectorants as needed. Warm salt water gargles soothe the sore throat, and aspirin or acetaminophen relieves the general constitutional symptoms. Antibiotics do not affect the virus or reduce the incidence of bacterial complications; however, they may be used prophylactically for high-risk respiratory patients.

Nursing Intervention: Patient Education. It is important to teach the patient how to break the chain of infection. Handwashing remains the most effective measure to prevent transmission of organisms. Using disposable tissues and discarding them hygienically, covering the mouth when coughing, and avoiding crowds are important measures to prevent the spread of an upper respiratory airway infection.

Herpes Simplex Infection

The herpes simplex virus (HSV-1) most commonly produces the familiar *herpes labialis* (cold sore, fever blister, or canker). Small vesicles, single or clustered, may erupt on the lips, inside the mouth, including the tongue, soft and hard palate, gums, buccal mucosa, and the pharynx. These soon rupture, forming sore, shallow ulcers (Fig. 23-1).

Herpes virus infections appear often in association with other febrile infections, such as streptococcal pneumonia, meningococcal meningitis, and malaria. The virus remains latent in cells of the lips or nose and is activated by febrile illnesses.

Medical Management. The herpes virus may subside spontaneously in 10 to 14 days. If it does not, acyclovir, an antiviral agent, may be administered orally or topically to decrease the severity of symptoms and the duration or length of the flare-up. Analgesics, such as acetaminophen (Tylenol) with codeine or aspirin with codeine, are helpful in relieving pain and discomfort. Topical anesthetics, such as lidocaine (Xylocaine), Orabase, or dyclonine (Dyclone) give a measure of relief for oral pain. Applications of drying lotions or liquids may help to dry the lesions.

Sinusitis

The sinuses are involved in a high proportion of upper respiratory tract infections. If their openings into the nasal passages are clear, the infections resolve promptly. However, if their drainage is obstructed by a deviated septum or by hypertrophied turbinates, spurs, or polyps, sinusitis may per-

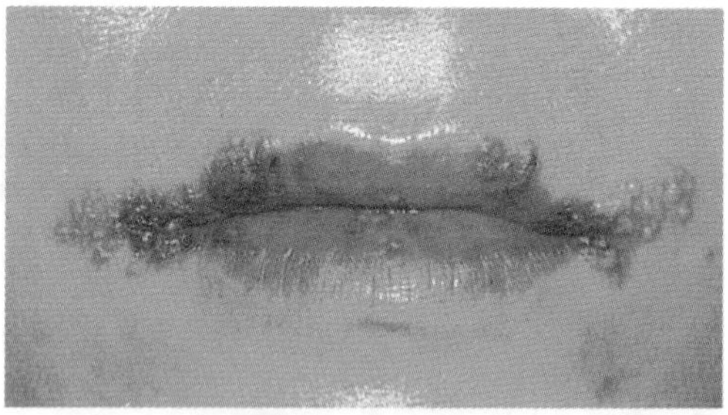

FIGURE 23-1. Herpes simplex (cold sore, fever blister). The herpes simplex virus (HSV) produces recurrent and painful vesicular eruptions of the lips and surrounding skin. A small cluster of vesicles first develops. As these break, yellow-brown crusts form, and healing ensues within 10 to 14 days. Both of these stages are visible. (From Bates B. A Guide to Physical Examination and History Taking, 6th ed. Philadelphia, JB Lippincott, 1995.)

sist as a smoldering secondary infection or progress to an acute suppurative process.

Acute Sinusitis

The symptoms of acute sinusitis include pressure, pain over the sinus area, and purulent nasal secretions.

Acute sinusitis frequently develops as a result of an upper respiratory tract infection, particularly, a viral infection or an exacerbation of allergic rhinitis. Nasal congestion, caused by inflammation, edema, and transudation of fluid, leads to obstruction of the sinus cavities. This provides an excellent medium for bacterial growth. Bacterial organisms account for greater than 60% of the cases of acute sinusitis, namely, *Streptococcus pneumoniae*, *Haemophilus influenzae*, and *Staphylococcus aureus*. Dental infections also have been associated with acute sinusitis.

A careful history and diagnostic assessment, including sinus x-ray studies, are performed to rule out other local or systemic disorders, such as tumor, fistula, and allergy. Complications of sinusitis, although uncommon, include severe orbital cellulitis, subperiosteal abscess, cavernous sinus thrombosis, meningitis, and brain abscess.

Medical Management. The goals of treatment of acute sinusitis are to control the infection, shrink the nasal mucosa, and relieve pain. The antibiotics of choice are amoxicillin and ampicillin. Alternatives for patients allergic to penicillin include trimethoprim/sulfamethoxazole (double strength) (Bactrim DS, Septra DS). Oral and topical decongestants may be administered. Heated mist and saline irrigation also may be effective for opening blocked passages, thereby allowing drainage of purulent discharge. The common oral decongestants are Drixoral and Dimetapp. Commonly used topical decongestants are Afrin and Otrivin. Topical decongestants should be administered with the patient's head back to promote maximal drainage. If the patient continues to have symptoms after 7 to 10 days, the sinuses may need to be irrigated.

Nursing Interventions/Patient Education. Patient teaching is an important aspect of nursing care for the patient with acute sinusitis. The nurse can instruct the patient on methods to promote drainage such as inhaling steam (steam bath, hot shower, facial sauna), increasing fluid intake, and applying local heat (hot wet packs). The patient is also instructed about the side effects of nasal sprays, such as rebound congestion which can occur with their overuse.

The nurse teaches the patient the early signs of a sinus infection and recommends preventive measures such as following healthy practices and avoiding contact with people who have upper respiratory infections (Chart 23-1).

Acute sinusitis, if left untreated, might lead to severe and, occasionally, life-threatening complications, such as meningitis, brain abscess, and osteomyelitis. The presence of fever, severe headache, and nuchal rigidity are signs of potential complications. If fever persists in spite of antibiotic therapy, the patient should seek additional care.

CHART 23-1

Patient Education: Prevention of Sinus Infections

1. Avoid allergens if allergies are suspected.
2. Maintain general health so that the body's natural resistance is not lowered.
   a. Eat a proper diet.
   b. Exercise.
   c. Get plenty of rest.
3. Avoid people with respiratory tract infections.
4. Seek medical attention if upper respiratory symptoms persist longer than 7 to 10 days.
5. Notify primary care provider if pain in sinus areas persists or if nasal discharge is present and is discolored and foul smelling.

Chronic Sinusitis

Clinical Manifestations. Chronic sinusitis usually is caused by chronic nasal obstruction due to discharge and edema of the nasal mucous membrane. The patient experiences cough, because of the constant dripping of the thick discharge backward into the nasopharynx, and chronic headaches in the periorbital area and facial pain, which are generally most pronounced on awakening in the morning. Fatigue is also common, as is nasal stuffiness.

Medical Management. The medical management of chronic sinusitis is the same as for acute sinusitis. Surgery may be indicated in chronic sinusitis to correct structural deformities that obstruct the ostia (openings) of the sinus. Surgery may include excising and cauterizing polyps, correcting a deviated septum, and incising and draining the sinuses.

Some patients with severe chronic sinusitis obtain relief only by moving to a dry climate.

Nursing Interventions/Patient Education. As with sinusitis, the patient will benefit from measures to drain the sinuses, such as increasing the humidity (steam bath, hot shower, facial sauna), increasing fluid intake, and applying local heat (hot wet packs).

The early signs of a sinus infection are described and preventive measures recommended.

Rhinitis

Rhinitis is an inflammation of the mucous membranes of the nose and may be classified as either nonallergic or allergic rhinitis. Non-allergic rhinitis is most commonly caused by upper respiratory infections, including viral rhinitis (common cold) and nasal and bacterial rhinitis. It also occurs as a result of foreign bodies entering the nose; structural deformities, neoplasms, and masses; chronic use of nasal decongestants; use of oral contraceptives, cocaine, and antihypertensives. Rhinitis may be a manifestation of an allergy (see Chapter 51), in which case it is referred to as *allergic rhinitis*. It is estimated that between 10% and 20% of the population of the United States have allergic rhinitis. Rhinitis may be an acute or chronic condition. Figure 23-2 provides a graphic respresentation of the pathologic processes involved in rhinitis and sinusitis.

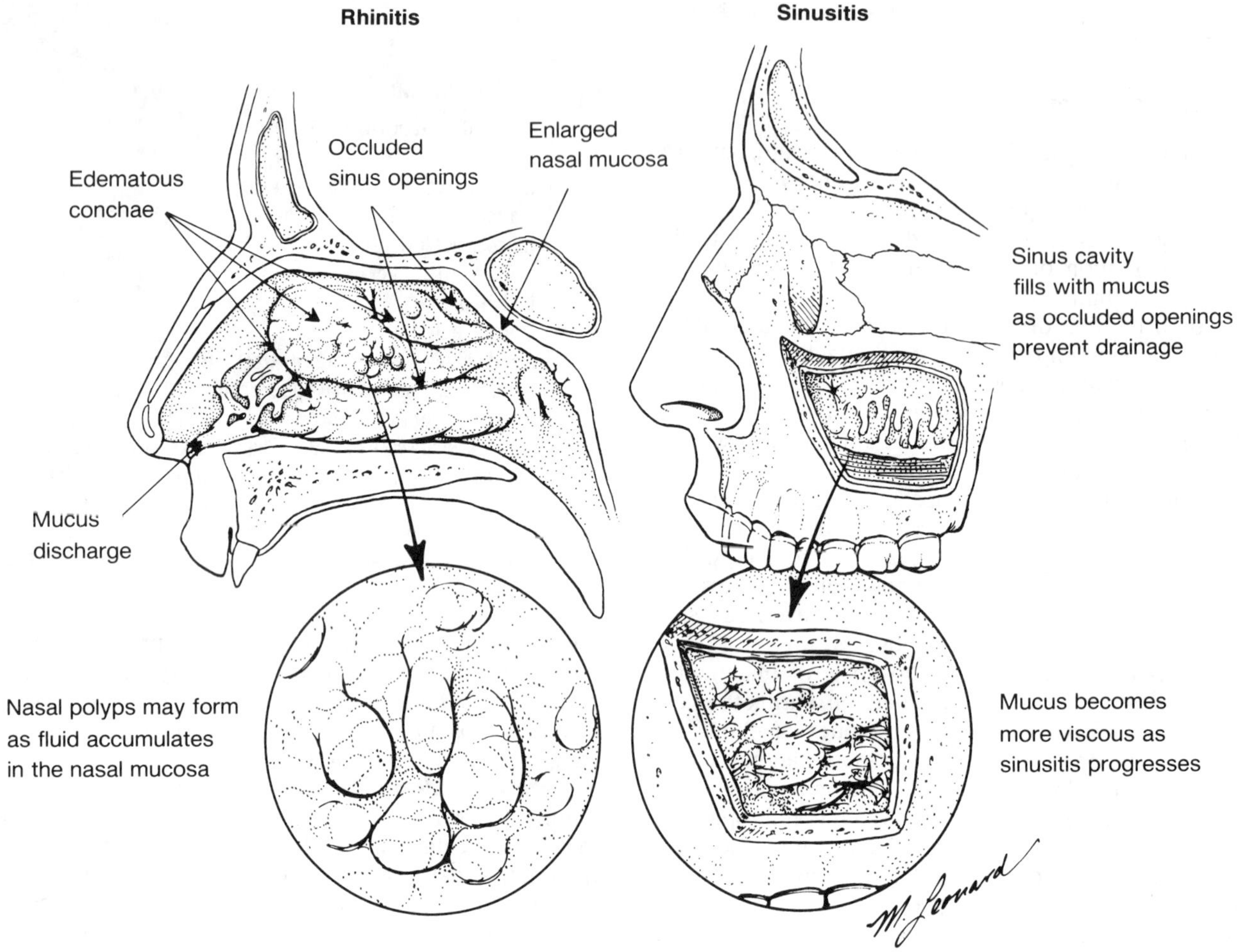

FIGURE 23-2. Pathophysiologic processes in rhinitis and sinusitis.

Clinical Manifestations. The signs and symptoms of rhinitis are nasal congestion, nasal discharge (purulent with bacterial rhinitis), nasal itchiness, and sneezing. Headache may occur, particularly if sinusitis is also present.

Medical Management. The management of rhinitis is dependent on the cause, which may be identified by taking a complete history and asking the patient about possible exposure to allergens in the home, environment, or work place. If symptoms suggest an allergic rhinitis, tests may be conducted to identify possible allergens. Medication therapy may include antihistamines, decongestants, topical corticosteroids, and cromolyn sodium. The prescribed medications are usually used in some combination, depending on the patient's symptoms.

Nursing Interventions/Patient Education. The patient with allergic rhinitis is instructed to avoid allergens and irritants, such as dusts, fumes, odors, powders, sprays, and tobacco smoke. Saline nasal sprays may be helpful in soothing mucous membranes, softening crusted secretions, and removing irritants. The patient is instructed in the proper use and technique for administration of medications, particularly nasal sprays or aerosols. To achieve maximal relief, the patient is instructed to blow the nose before applying any medication into the nasal cavity.

Acute Pharyngitis

Acute pharyngitis is a febrile inflammation of the throat that is caused by a viral organism 70% of the time. Group A streptococcus is the most common bacterial organism associated with acute pharyngitis, which is then referred to as "strep throat" (Fig. 23-3).

Clinical Manifestations. The signs and symptoms of acute pharyngitis include a fiery red pharyngeal membrane and tonsils; lymphoid follicles that are swollen and flecked with exudate; and enlarged and tender cervical lymph nodes. Fever, malaise, and sore throat also may be present. Hoarseness, cough, and rhinitis are not uncommon.

Uncomplicated viral infections usually subside promptly, within 3 to 10 days after the onset. However, pharyngitis caused by more virulent bacteria such as *Group A streptococcus* is a more severe illness during the acute stage, and far more important because of the incidence of dangerous complications. These complications include sinusitis, otitis media, peritonsillar abscess, mastoiditis, cervical adenitis, rheumatic fever, and nephritis. A throat culture is the chief means of determining the causative organism after which appropriate therapy is prescribed. Nasal swabbings and

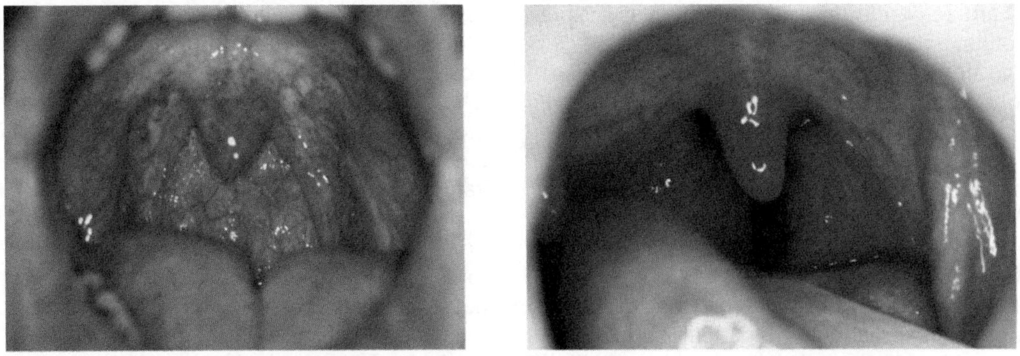

A B

FIGURE 23-3. Pharyngitis. These two photos show reddened throats without exudate. In **A,** redness and vascularity of the pillars and uvula are mild to moderate. In **B,** redness is diffuse and intense. Each patient would probably complain of a sore throat. Possible causes include several kinds of viruses and bacteria. (From Bates B. A Guide to Physical Examination and History Taking, 6th ed. Philadelphia, JB Lippincott, 1995.)

blood cultures may also be necessary to identify the organism.

Medical Management. If a bacterial cause is suggested or demonstrated, treatment may include the administration of antimicrobial agents. For group A streptococci, penicillin is the medication of choice. For those patients who are allergic to penicillin or have organisms that are resistant to erythromycin (one fifth of group A streptococci and most *S. aureus* organisms are resistant to penicillin and erythromycin), cephalosporins are used. Antibiotics are administered for at least 10 days to eradicate group A streptococci from the oropharynx.

A liquid or soft diet is provided during the acute stage of the disease, depending on the patient's appetite and the degree of discomfort that occurs with swallowing. Occasionally, the throat is so sore that liquids cannot be taken in adequate amounts by mouth. In severe situations, fluids are administered intravenously. Otherwise, the patient is encouraged to drink as much fluid as possible, with 2 to 3 L being the minimum per day.

Nursing Interventions/Patient Education. The patient is instructed to stay in bed during the febrile stage of illness and to rest frequently once up and about. Any tissues should be disposed of properly to prevent the spread of infection. The skin is examined once or twice daily for possible rash because acute pharyngitis may precede some other communicable diseases.

Warm saline gargles or irrigations are used, depending on the severity of the lesion and the degree of pain. The benefits of this treatment depend on the degree of heat that is applied. The nurse instructs the patient concerning the temperature of the solution. The temperature should be sufficiently high to be effective and should be as hot as the patient can tolerate, usually between 105°F and 110°F (40.6°C to 43.3°C). Irrigating the throat properly is an effective means of reducing spasm in the pharyngeal muscles and relieving soreness of the throat. Unless the purpose of the procedure and its technique are understood clearly by the patient and family, the results may be less than satisfactory.

Severe sore throats can also be relieved by an ice collar and analgesic medications, as prescribed; for example, aspirin or acetaminophen (Tylenol) can be taken at 3- to 6-hour intervals and, if required, Tylenol with codeine three or four times daily. Antitussive medication, in the form of codeine, dextromethorphan (Robitussin DM), or hydrocodone bitartrate (Hycodan), may be required to control a persistent and painful cough that often accompanies acute pharyngitis.

Mouth care may add greatly to the patient's comfort and may prevent the development of fissures of the lips and inflammation about the mouth when bacterial infection is present.

Resumption of activity is permitted gradually. A full course of antibiotic therapy is indicated in patients with hemolytic Streptococcus infection in view of the possible development of complications such as nephritis and rheumatic fever, which may have their onset 2 or 3 weeks after the pharyngitis has subsided. The patient or the family is advised about the importance of taking a full course of therapy and is informed about the symptoms to watch for that may indicate possible complications.

Chronic Pharyngitis

Chronic pharyngitis is common in adults who work or live in dusty surroundings, use the voice to excess, suffer from chronic cough, and habitually use alcohol and tobacco.

Three types of chronic pharyngitis are recognized: (1) hypertrophic, characterized by general thickening and congestion of the pharyngeal mucous membrane; (2) atrophic, probably a late stage of the first type (the membrane is thin, whitish, glistening, and, at times, wrinkled); and (3) chronic granular ("clergyman's sore throat"), with numerous swollen lymph follicles on the pharyngeal wall.

Clinical Manifestations. Patients with chronic pharyngitis complain of a constant sense of irritation or fullness in the throat; of mucus, which collects in the throat and can be expelled by coughing; and of difficulty in swallowing.

Medical Management. The treatment of chronic pharyngitis is based on relieving symptoms, avoiding exposure to irritants, and correcting any upper respiratory, pulmonary, or cardiac condition that might be responsible for a chronic cough.

Nasal congestion may be relieved by nasal sprays or medications containing ephedrine sulfate (Afrin) or phenylephrine hydrochloride (Neo-Synephrine). If there is a history of allergy, one of the antihistamine decongestant medications, such as Drixoral or Dimetapp, is taken orally every 4 to 6 hours. Malaise is controlled effectively by aspirin or acetaminophen. Contact with others should be avoided, at least until the fever has subsided completely.

Nursing Interventions/Patient Education. To prevent the infection from spreading, the patient is instructed to avoid contact with others until the fever has subsided and to avoid the use of alcohol, tobacco, secondhand smoke, and exposure to cold. Environmental/occupational pollutants should be avoided or exposure to them minimized by using disposable masks. The patient is encouraged to drink plenty of fluids. Gargling with warm saline solutions may relieve throat discomfort. Lozenges will keep the throat moistened.

Tonsillitis and Adenoiditis

The tonsils are composed of lymphatic tissue and are situated on each side of the oropharynx. They frequently serve as the site of acute infection. Group A streptococcus is the most common organism associated with tonsillitis and adenoiditis. Chronic tonsillitis is less common and may be mistaken for other disorders such as allergy, asthma, and sinusitis.

The adenoids consist of an abnormally large lymphoid tissue mass near the center of the posterior wall of the nasopharynx. Infection of the adenoids frequently accompanies acute tonsillitis.

Clinical Manifestations. The symptoms of tonsillitis include sore throat, fever, snoring, and difficulty in swallowing. Enlarged adenoids may cause mouth-breathing, earache, draining ears, frequent head colds, bronchitis, foul-smelling breath, voice impairment, and noisy respiration. Unusually enlarged adenoids may cause nasal obstruction. Infection can extend to the middle ears by way of the auditory (eustachian) tubes and may result in acute otitis media, which can lead to spontaneous rupture of the eardrums and further extension of the infection into the mastoid cells, causing acute mastoiditis. The infection also may reside in the middle ear as a chronic, low-grade, smoldering process that eventually may cause permanent deafness.

Diagnostic Evaluation. A thorough physical examination is performed, and a careful history is obtained to rule out related or systemic conditions. The tonsillar site is cultured to determine the presence of bacterial infection. In adenoiditis, if recurrent episodes of suppurative otitis media results in a hearing loss, the patient should be given a comprehensive audiometric examination (see Chapter 57).

Tonsillectomy and Adenoidectomy

Tonsillectomy is usually performed if medical treatment is unsuccessful and there is severe hypertrophy or peritonsillar abscess that occludes the pharynx, making swallowing difficult and endangering the airway. Enlargement of the tonsils is rarely an indication for their removal; most children normally have large tonsils, which decrease in size with age. Despite the continuing debate over the effectiveness of many tonsillectomies, the operation is still a common surgical procedure performed in the United States.

Tonsillectomy or adenoidectomy is performed only if the patient has had any of the following problems: repeated bouts of tonsillitis; hypertrophy of the tonsils and adenoids that could cause obstruction; repeated attacks of purulent otitis media; suspected hearing loss due to serous otitis media that has occurred in association with enlarged tonsils and adenoids; and some other conditions, such as an exacerbation of asthma or rheumatic fever. Appropriate antibiotic therapy is initiated for patients undergoing tonsillectomy or adenoidectomy. The most common antibiotic therapy is oral penicillin, which is taken for 10 days. Amoxicillin and erythromycin are alternatives.

Postoperative Nursing Interventions. Continuous nursing observation is required in the immediate postoperative and recovery period because of the significant risk of hemorrhage. In the immediate postoperative period, the most comfortable position is prone with the head turned to the side to allow for drainage from the mouth and pharynx. The oral airway is not removed until the patient demonstrates that the swallowing reflex has returned. An ice collar is applied to the neck, and a basin and tissues are provided for the expectoration of blood and mucus.

Bleeding may be bright red if the patient expectorates blood at once. Often, however, the blood is swallowed and immediately becomes brown because of the action of the acidic gastric juice.

Hemorrhage is a potential complication after a tonsillectomy and adenoidectomy. If the patient vomits large amounts of altered blood or bright red blood at frequent intervals, or if the pulse rate and temperature rise and the patient is restless, the surgeon is notified immediately. The nurse should have the following items ready to examine the surgical site for bleeding: a light, a mirror, gauze, curved hemostats, and a waste basin.

Occasionally, it may be necessary to suture or ligate the bleeding vessel. In such cases, the patient is taken to the operating room and given general anesthesia. After ligation, continuous nursing observation and postoperative care are required, as in the initial postoperative period.

If there is no bleeding, water and ice chips are given to the patient as soon as desired. The patient is instructed to refrain from too much talking and coughing because this can produce throat pain.

Nursing Interventions/Patient Education. Tonsillectomy or adenoidectomy, generally, do not require hospitalization and are performed as outpatient surgery with a short length of stay. Because the patient will be sent home soon after surgery, it is critical that the patient and family understand the signs and symptoms of hemorrhage. Hemorrhage usually occurs in the first 12 to 24 hours. The patient is instructed to report any bleeding to the physician.

Alkaline mouthwashes and warm saline solutions are useful in coping with the thick mucus that may be present after a tonsillectomy. A liquid or semi-liquid diet is given for several days. Sherbet and gelatin are acceptable foods. Spicy, hot, cold, acidic, or rough foods are avoided. Milk and mild products (ice cream) may be restricted because they tend to increase the amount of mucus produced.

Peritonsillar Abscess

Peritonsillar abscess develops above the tonsil in the tissues of the anterior pillar and soft palate. As a rule, it occurs several days after an acute tonsillar infection and usually is caused by a group A streptococcus.

Clinical Manifestations. The usual symptoms of an infection are present, together with such local symptoms as difficulty in swallowing anything other than liquids (dysphagia), thickening of the voice, drooling, and local pain. An examination shows marked swelling of the soft palate, often to the extent of half occluding the opening from the mouth into the pharynx.

Medical Management. Antibiotics (usually penicillin) are extremely effective in the control of the infection in peritonsillar abscess. If antibiotics are prescribed early in the course of the disease, the abscess may resolve without needing to be incised. If antibiotics are not prescribed until later, the abscess must be drained, but improvement in the inflammatory reaction is rapid.

The abscess is evacuated as soon as possible. The mucous membrane over the swelling is first sprayed with a topical anesthetic and then injected with a local anesthetic. Single or repeated needle aspirations are performed to decompress the abscess. The abscess may also be incised and drained. These procedures are performed best with the patient in the sitting position to make it easier to expectorate the pus and blood that accumulate in the pharynx. Almost immediate relief is experienced.

Some laryngologists advocate removing the tonsils for an acute peritonsillar abscess to prevent abscess from recurring and to eliminate unsuspected asymptomatic pockets of infection.

Nursing Interventions/Patient Education. Considerable relief may be obtained by topical anesthetics and throat irrigations or the frequent use of mouthwashes or gargles, using saline or alkaline solutions at a temperature of 105°F to 110°F (40.6°C to 43.3°C). The patient is instsructed to gargle at intervals of 1 or 2 hours for 24 to 36 hours. Liquids that are cool or at room temperature are usually well tolerated.

Laryngitis

Inflammation of the larynx often occurs as a result of voice abuse, exposure to dust, chemicals, smoke, and other pollutants, or as part of an upper respiratory tract infection. It also may be caused by isolated infection involving only the vocal cords.

The cause of this inflammation is almost always a virus. Bacterial invasion may be secondary. Laryngitis usually is associated with acute rhinitis or nasopharyngitis. The onset of infection may be associated with exposure to sudden temperature changes, dietary deficiencies, malnutrition, and lack of immunity. Laryngitis is common in the winter and is easily transmitted.

Clinical Manifestations. The signs and symptoms of acute laryngitis include hoarseness or complete loss of voice (aphonia) and severe cough. Chronic laryngitis is marked by persistent hoarseness. Laryngitis may be a complication of chronic sinusitis and chronic bronchitis.

Medical Management. Management of acute laryngitis includes resting the voice, avoiding smoking, resting in bed, and inhaling cool steam or an aerosol. If the laryngitis is part of a more extensive respiratory infection due to a bacterial organism or if it is severe, appropriate antibacterial therapy is instituted. The majority of patients recover with conservative treatment; however, laryngitis tends to be more severe in elderly patients and may be complicated by pneumonia.

For chronic laryngitis, the treatment includes resting the voice, eliminating any primary respiratory tract infection that may be present, and restricting smoking. The use of topical corticosteroids, such as beclomethasone dipropionate (Vanceril) inhalation, may also be used. These preparations have no systemic or long-lasting effects and may reduce local inflammatory reactions.

Nursing Interventions/Patient Education. The patient is instructed to rest the voice and to maintain a well-humidified environment. If laryngeal secretions are present during acute episodes, expectorants are suggested along with a daily fluid intake of 3 L to thin secretions.

❑ *NURSING PROCESS*
The Patient With Upper Airway Infection

Assessment

A complete history of the patient's problem reveals possible signs and symptoms of headache, sore throat, pain around the eyes and on either side of the nose, difficulty in swallowing, cough, hoarseness, fever, stuffiness, and generalized discomfort and fatigue. Determining when the symptoms began, what precipitated them, what if anything relieves them, and what aggravates them is part of the assessment, as well as identifying any history of allergy or the existence of a concomitant illness.

Inspection may reveal swelling, lesions, or asymmetry of the nose as well as bleeding or discharge. The nasal mucosa is inspected for as abnormal findings such as a reddened color, swelling, or exudate, and nasal polyps, which may develop in chronic rhinitis.

The frontal and maxillary sinuses are palpated for tenderness, which suggests inflammation. The throat is observed by having the patient open the mouth wide and take a deep breath. The tonsils and pharynx are inspected for the abnormal findings of reddened color, asymmetry, or evidence of drainage, ulceration, or enlargement.

The trachea is palpated for midline position in the neck, and any masses or deformities are identified. The neck lymph nodes also are palpated for associated enlargement and tenderness.

Diagnosis

Nursing Diagnoses

Based on all the assessment data, the patient's major nursing diagnoses may include the following:

- Ineffective airway clearance related to excessive secretions secondary to an inflammatory process
- Pain related to upper airway irritation secondary to an infection
- Impaired verbal communication related to upper airway irritation secondary to an infection or swelling
- Fluid volume deficit related to increased fluid loss secondary to diaphoresis associated with a fever
- Knowledge deficit regarding prevention of upper respiratory infections, treatment regimen, surgical procedure, or postoperative care

Collaborative Problems/ Potential Complications

Based on assessment data, potential complications may include:

- Sepsis
- Peritonsillar abscess
- Otitis media
- Sinusitis

Planning and Implementation

Goals. The major goals for the patient may include maintenance of a patent airway, relief of pain, maintenance of effective means of communication, absence of fluid volume deficit, and knowledge of how to prevent upper airway infections, and absence of complications.

Nursing Interventions

Clearing the Airways. An accumulation of secretions can block the airway in many patients with an upper airway infection. Changes in the respiratory pattern result, and the work of breathing required to get beyond the blockage is increased. There are several measures that can be used to loosen thick secretions or to keep the secretions moist so that they can be easily expectorated. Increasing fluid intake helps thin the mucus. Humidifying the environment with room vaporizers or inhaling steam also loosens secretions and reduces inflammation of the mucous membranes. The patient is instructed about the best position to assume to enhance drainage from the sinuses, which will depend on the location of the infection or inflammation. For example, drainage for sinusitis or rhinitis is achieved in the upright position. In some conditions, topical or systemic medications, when prescribed, help to relieve nasal or throat congestion.

Promoting Comfort Measures. Upper respiratory tract infections usually produce localized discomfort. In sinusitis, pain may occur in the area of the sinuses or may produce a general headache. In pharyngitis, laryngitis, or tonsillitis, a sore throat occurs. The nurse encourages the patient to take analgesics, such as acetaminophen (Tylenol) with codeine, as prescribed, which will help relieve this discomfort. Other helpful measures include topical anesthetics for symptomatic relief for herpes simplex blisters and sore throats; hot packs to relieve the congestion of sinusitis and promote drainage; and warm water gargles or irrigations to relieve the pain of a sore throat. Encouraging the patient to rest will help relieve the generalized discomfort or fever that accompanies many upper airway conditions (especially rhinitis, pharyngitis, and laryngitis). The nurse instructs the patient in general oral and nasal hygiene techniques to help relieve localized discomfort and to prevent the spread of infection. For postoperative care following a tonsillectomy and adenoidectomy, an ice collar can be applied to reduce swelling and decrease bleeding.

Promoting Communication. Upper airway infections may result in hoarseness or loss of speech. The patient is instructed not to try to speak, to refrain from speaking as much as possible, and to communicate instead in writing if appropriate. Additional strain on the vocal cords may further delay return of full voice.

Encouraging Fluid Intake. In upper airway infections, the work of breathing and the respiratory rate increase as inflammation and secretions develop. This, in turn, may increase insensible fluid loss. An associated fever increases the metabolic rate, which results in diaphoresis and increased fluid loss.

Sore throat, malaise, and fever may interfere with a patient's willingness to eat. The patient is encouraged to drink 2 to 3 L of fluid per day during the acute stage of airway infection, unless contraindicated, to thin secretions and promote drainage. Liquids (hot or cold) may be soothing, depending on the illness.

Patient Teaching. Patient teaching is important in preventing infection and its spread to others and in minimizing complications. Prevention of most upper airway infections is difficult because of the many potential causes. The responsible pathogen usually cannot be identified, and vaccines are unavailable except in rare instances. Allergies, pathologic conditions of the septum and the turbinates, emotional problems, and various systemic illnesses may be predisposing factors in isolated cases. Handwashing is still critical in preventing the spread of infection.

The nurse instructs the patient about the importance of good health measures. A nutritious diet, appropriate exercise, and adequate rest and sleep are important to support the body's defenses and reduce susceptibility to respiratory infections. Instructions on how to prevent cross-infection to other family members is also important. Handwashing remains the most important way to prevent the spread of infection. Proper disposal of tissues and covering the mouth when coughing are stressed. The major points to stress in a teaching program to prevent upper respiratory infection are highlighted in Chart 23-2.

Monitoring and Managing Potential Complications. If the patient seeks additional care because the symptoms become more severe the nurse will check vital signs and observe for a spike in temperature, as well as an increased pulse rate to detect impeding sepsis, otitis media, or sinusitis. Difficulty swallowing and a severe sore throat would be cardinal signs of peritonsillar abscess. The patient

CHART 23-2
Patient Education: Prevention of Upper Respiratory Infections

1. Practice good health measures.
   a. Eat a nutritious diet
   b. Exercise appropriately.
   c. Get adequate rest and sleep.
   d. Avoid smoking and excessive intake of alcohol.
2. Wash hands often.
3. Increase humidity in house air, especially during cold weather.
4. Avoid irritants (dust, chemical, tobacco smoke) when possible.
5. Avoid unnecessary chilling of the skin; chilling lowers resistance.
6. Get influenza vaccination if so advised, especially if you are elderly or have a chronic illness.
7. Avoid crowds during the flu season.
8. Practice adequate dental hygiene.

is instructed to measure morning and evening temperature until recovery is complete.

If antibiotics have been prescribed, the patient is instructed in their proper administration; additionally, the patient is reminded to complete the whole course of antibiotics even if symptoms resolve soon after therapy is initiated. The patient is also instructed about the signs and symptoms of complications and the need to contact the primary health care provider if early indicators of complications develop.

Evaluation

Expected Outcomes

1. Maintains a patent airway by managing secretions
   a. Reports decreased congestion
   b. Assumes best position to facilitate drainage of secretions for the condition
2. Reports feeling more comfortable
   a. Follows comfort measures—analgesics, hot packs, gargles, rest
   b. Demonstrates adequate oral hygiene
3. Demonstrates ability to communicate needs, wants, level of comfort
4. Maintains an adequate fluid intake
5. Identifies strategies to prevent upper airway infections and allergic reactions
6. Demonstrates an adequate level of knowledge and performs self-care adequately.
7. Becomes free of signs and symptoms of infection
   a. Exhibits normal vital signs (temperature, pulse and respiratory rate)
   b. Absence of purulent drainage
   c. Free of pain in ears, sinuses, and throat

Obstruction and Trauma of the Upper Respiratory Airway

Epistaxis (Nosebleed)

A hemorrhage from the nose, referred to as **epistaxis**, is caused by the rupture of tiny, distended vessels in the mucous membrane of any area of the nose. Rarely does epistaxis originate in the densely vascular tissue over the turbinates. Most commonly, the site is the anterior septum, where three major blood vessels enter the nasal cavity: (1) the anterior ethmoidal artery on the forward part of the roof (Kesselbach's plexus), (2) the sphenopalatine artery in the posterosuperior region, and (3) the internal maxillary branches (the plexus of veins located at the back of the lateral wall under the inferior turbinate).

There are a variety of causes associated with epistaxis, including trauma, infection, drugs, cardiovascular diseases, blood dyscrasias, nasal tumors, low humidity, a foreign body in the nose, and a deviated nasal septum. Additionally, vigorous nose-blowing and nose-picking have been associated with epistaxis.

Medical Management. The management of epistaxis depends on the location of the bleeding site. A nasal speculum or headlight may be used to determine the site of bleeding in the nasal cavity. The majority of nosebleeds originate from the anterior portion of the nose. Initial treatment may include applying direct pressure. The patient sits upright with the head tilted forward to prevent swallowing and aspiration of blood and is directed to pinch the soft outer portion of the nose against the midline septum for 5 or 10 minutes continuously. If this measure is unsuccessful, additional treatment is indicated. In anterior nosebleeds, the area may be treated with a silver nitrate applicator and Gelfoam, or by electrocautery. Topical vasoconstrictors, such as adrenaline (1:1000), cocaine (0.5%), and phenylephrine may be prescribed.

If bleeding is occurring from the posterior regions, cotton pledgets soaked in a vasoconstricting solution may be inserted into the nose to reduce the blood flow and improve the examiner's view of the bleeding site. Alternatively, a cotton tampon may be used to try to stop the bleeding. Suction can remove excess blood and clots from the field of inspection. The search for the bleeding site should shift from the anteroinferior quadrant to the anterosuperior, then to the posterosuperior, and finally to the posteroinferior area. The field is kept clear by using suction and by shifting the cotton tampons. Only about 60% of the total nasal cavity can actually be seen, however.

When the origin of the bleeding cannot be identified, the nose may be packed with gauze impregnated with petrolatum; a topical anesthetic spray and decongestant may be used prior to inserting the gauze packing or a balloon-inflated catheter may be used (Fig. 23-4). The packing may remain in place for 48 hours or up to 5 or 6 days if necessary to control bleeding.

Nursing Interventions/Patient Education. The nurse monitors the vital signs and assists in the control of bleeding. Tissues and an emesis basin are provided to allow the patient to expectorate any excess blood.

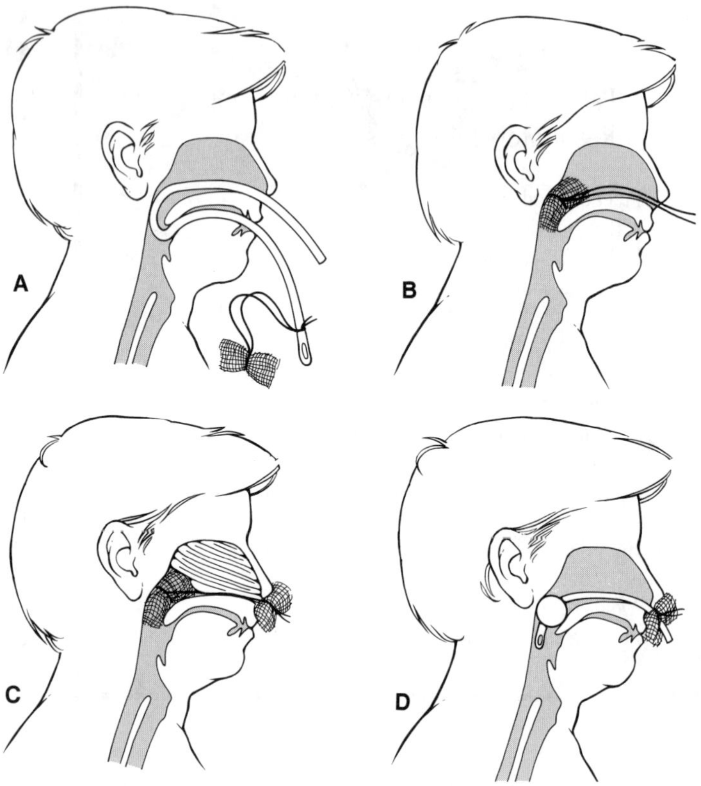

FIGURE 23-4. Packing to control bleeding from the posterior nose. (**A**) Catheter is inserted and packing is attached. (**B**) Packing is drawn into position as the catheter is removed. (**C**) Strip is tied over a bolster to hold the packing in place with anterior pack installed "accordian pleat" style. (**D**) Alternative method, using a balloon catheter instead of gauze packing.

It is not uncommon for patients to be anxious in response to a nosebleed. Blood loss on clothing and handkerchiefs can be frightening and the nasal examination and treatment are uncomfortable. Assuring the patient in a calm, efficient manner that bleeding can be controlled can help reduce anxiety.

Discharge teaching includes reviewing ways to prevent epistaxis: avoiding forceful nose blowing, straining, high altitudes, and nasal trauma (including nose-picking). Adequate humidification may prevent drying of the nasal passages. The patient is instructed how to apply direct pressure to the nose with the thumb and the index finger for 15 minutes in the case of a recurrent nosebleed. If recurrent bleeding cannot be stopped, the patient is instructed to seek additional medical attention.

Nasal Obstruction

The passage of air through the nostrils is frequently obstructed by a deviation of the nasal septum, hypertrophy of the turbinate bones, or the pressure of polyps, which are grapelike swellings that arise from the mucous membrane of the sinuses, especially the ethmoids. This obstruction also may lead to a condition of chronic infection of the nose and result in frequent episodes of nasopharyngitis. Frequently, the infection extends to the sinuses of the nose (mucus-lined cavities filled with air that drain normally into the nose). When sinusitis develops and the drainage from these cavities is obstructed by deformity or swelling within the nose, pain is experienced in the region of the affected sinus.

Medical Management. The treatment of nasal obstruction requires the removal of the obstruction, followed by measures to overcome whatever chronic infection exists. In many patients an underlying allergy requires treatment. At times surgery is necessary to drain the nasal sinuses. The specific procedure performed depends on the type of nasal obstruction found. Usually, surgery is performed under local anesthesia.

If a deviation of the septum is the cause of the obstruction, the surgeon makes an incision into the mucous membrane and, after raising it from the bone, removes the deviated bone and cartilage with bone forceps. The mucosa then is allowed to fall back in place and is held there by tight packing. Generally, the packing is soaked in liquid petrolatum so that it can be removed easily in 24 to 36 hours. This operation is called a *submucous resection* or septoplasty.

Nasal polyps are removed by clipping them at their base with a wire snare. Hypertrophied turbinates may be treated by applying astringent to shrink them close to the side of the nose.

Nursing Interventions. Most of these procedures are conducted on an out-patient basis. The head of the bed is elevated to promote drainage and to help alleviate discomfort from edema. Frequent oral hygiene is encouraged to overcome dryness caused by breathing through the mouth.

Fractures of the Nose

The location of the nose makes it susceptible to injury by a wide variety of causes. In fact, the nose sustains fractures more frequently than any other bone in the body. Fractures of the nose usually result from direct trauma. As a rule, no serious consequences result, but the deformity that may follow often gives rise to obstruction of the nasal air passages and to facial disfigurement.

Clinical Manifestations. The signs and symptoms of a nasal fracture are bleeding from the nose externally and internally into the pharynx, swelling of the soft tissues adjacent to the nose, and deformity.

Assessment. The nose is examined internally to rule out the possibility that the injury may be complicated by a fracture of the nasal septum and the presence of a submucosal septal hematoma. If a hematoma develops and is not drained, it eventually may become an abscess that destroys the septal cartilage. A saddle deformity of the nose results.

Immediately after the injury there is usually considerable bleeding from the nose externally and internally into the pharynx. There is marked swelling of the soft tissues adjacent to the nose and, frequently, a definite deformity. Because of this swelling and bleeding, an accurate diagnosis can be made only after the swelling has subsided.

Clear fluid draining from either nostril suggests a fracture of the cribriform plate with leakage of cerebrospinal fluid. Because cerebrospinal fluid contains glucose, it can readily be differentiated from nasal mucus by means of a dipstick (Dextrostix). Usually, careful inspection or palpation will disclose any deviations of the bone or disruptions of the nasal cartilages. An x-ray film may help to determine displacement of the fractured bones and help rule out extension of the fracture into the skull.

Medical Management. As a rule, bleeding is controlled with the use of cold compresses. The nose is assessed for symmetry either before swelling has occurred or after it has subsided. The patient will be referred to a specialist, usually 3 to 5 days after the injury, to evaluate the need to realign the bones. Nasal fractures are surgically reduced 7 to 10 days after the injury.

Nursing Interventions/Patient Education. The nurse instructs the patient to apply ice packs to the nose for 20 minutes four times each day to decrease swelling. The patient who experiences bleeding from the nose (epistaxis) because of injury or for unexplained reasons is usually frightened and anxious. The presence of packing to stop the bleeding may be uncomfortable and unpleasant; obstruction of the nasal passages by the packing forces the patient to breathe through the mouth; this in turn causes the oral mucous membranes to become dry. Mouth rinses will help to moisten the mucous membranes and to reduce the smell and taste of dried blood in the oropharynx and nasopharynx.

Laryngeal Obstruction

Edema of the larynx is a serious, often fatal, condition. The larynx is a stiff box that will not stretch. It contains a narrow space between the vocal cords (glottis), through which air must pass. Swelling of the laryngeal mucous membranes, therefore, may close off the opening tightly, leading to suffocation. Edema of the glottis occurs rarely in patients with acute laryngitis, occasionally in patients with urticaria, and more frequently in severe inflammations of the throat (*e.g.*, erysipelas and scarlet fever). It is an occasional cause of death in severe anaphylaxis (angioneurotic edema).

When caused by an allergic reaction, treatment includes administering subcutaneous epinephrine or an adrenal corticosteroid and applying an ice pack to the neck (see Chapter 51).

Foreign bodies frequently are aspirated into the pharynx, the larynx, or the trachea and cause a twofold problem. First they obstruct the air passages and cause difficulty in breathing, which may lead to asphyxia; later they may be drawn farther down, entering the bronchi or a bronchial branch and causing symptoms of irritation, such as a croupy cough, expectoration of blood or mucus, or labored breathing. The physical signs and x-ray findings confirm the diagnosis.

In emergencies, when the signs of asphyxia are evident, immediate treatment is necessary. Frequently, if the foreign body has lodged in the pharynx and can be visualized, it can be dislodged by the finger. If the obstruction is in the larynx or the trachea, the subdiaphragmatic abdominal thrust (Heimlich) maneuver is tried (Guideline 23-1 and Fig. 23-5). If all efforts are unsuccessful, an immediate tracheotomy is necessary.

Cancer of the Larynx

Cancer of the larynx is potentially curable if detected early. It represents 1% of all cancers and occurs about eight times more frequently in men than in women and most commonly in persons 50 to 70 years of age.

Each year in the United States, approximately 11,600 new cases are discovered and 4,090 persons with cancer of the larynx will die (American Cancer Society, 1995). Some carcinogens that have been associated with the development of laryngeal cancer include: tobacco (smoke, smokeless) and alcohol and their combined effects; exposure to asbestos; mustard gas; wood; leather and metals. Other contributing factors include: straining the voice, chronic laryngitis, nutritional deficiencies (riboflavin), and family predisposition.

A malignant growth may occur in three different areas of the larynx: the glottic area (vocal cords), supraglottic area (area above the glottis, including epiglottis and false cords), and subglottis (area below the glottis). Two thirds of the laryngeal cancers are in the glottic area. Supraglottic cancers account for approximately one third of the cases, and subglottic tumors account for less than 1%.

Clinical Manifestations

Hoarseness is noted early in the patient with cancer in the glottic area because the tumor impedes the action of the vocal cords during speech. The voice may sound harsh and lower in pitch. Affected voice sounds are not early signs of subglottic or supraglottic cancer; however, the patient may complain of pain and burning in the throat when drinking hot liquids and citrus juices. A lump may be felt in the neck. Later symptoms include difficulties in swallowing (dysphagia) or breathing (dyspnea), hoarseness, and foul breath. Enlarged cervical lymph nodes, weight loss, a general debilitated state, and pain radiating to the ear may occur with metastasis.

GUIDELINE 23–1
Performing the Abdominal Thrust Maneuver (Heimlich Maneuver)

1. Stand behind the person who is choking (Fig. 23-5).
2. Place both arms around the person's waist.
3. Make a fist with one hand with the thumb outside the fist.
4. Place thumb side of fist against the person's abdomen above the navel and below the ribs.
5. Grasp fist with other hand.
6. Quickly and forcefully exert pressure against the person's diaphragm, pressing upward with quick, firm thrusts.
7. Apply thrusts 6 to 10 times until the obstruction is cleared.
8. Pressure will compress the lungs and expel the aspirated object.

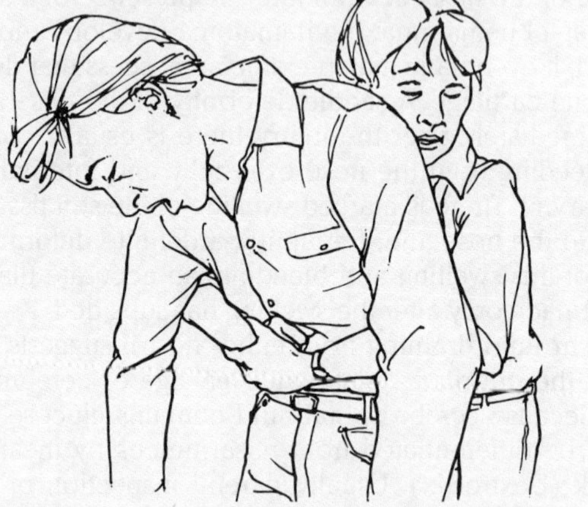

FIGURE 23-5. Abdominal thrust (Heimlich maneuver) administered to a conscious (standing) victim who has a foreign body obstructing the airway. (From Emergency Cardiac Care Committee and Subcommittees: AHA Guidelines for Cardiopulmonary Resuscitation and Emergency Cardiac Care. JAMA 268: 2193, 1992. Copyright 1992, American Medical Association.)

Diagnostic Evaluation

An initial assessment includes a complete history, and examination of the head and neck. An indirect laryngoscopy is performed to visually evaluate the extent of the tumor. Diagnostic tests, including soft tissue x-ray studies, tomograms, xerograms, contrast studies, and magnetic resonance imaging (MRI), are performed as part of the diagnostic work-up to determine the extent of the tumor growth. Direct laryngoscopic examination under general anesthesia, however, is the primary method for evaluating the larynx. All areas of the larynx can be inspected and biopsies performed. The growth may involve any of the three areas and may vary in appearance.

Most tumors are squamous cell. They are classified by the extent of the primary tumor (T), which includes size and invasion into other sites; location and extent of nodal involvement (N), and degree of metastasis (M). The classification of the tumor determines the suggested treatment modalities. Because many of these lesions are submucosal, biopsy may require that an incision be made with microlaryngeal techniques or laser to transect the mucosa and reach the tumor.

Mobility of the vocal cords is assessed; if normal movement is limited, the growth may affect muscle, other tissue, and even the airway. The lymph nodes of the neck and the thyroid gland are palpated to determine spread of the malignancy.

Medical Management

Treatment varies with the extent of the malignancy. Treatment options include radiation therapy and surgery. A complete dental examination is completed to rule out any oral disease. Any dental problems are resolved, if possible, prior to surgery.

If surgery is to be performed, a multidisciplinary team evaluates the needs of the patient and family to develop a successful plan of care.

Radiation Therapy

Excellent results have been achieved with radiation therapy in patients in whom only one cord is affected and is normally mobile (*i.e.*, moves with phonation). In addition, these patients retain a near normal voice. A few may develop chondritis (inflammation of the cartilage) or stenosis; a small number may later require laryngectomy. Radiation therapy may also be used preoperatively to reduce the tumor size.

Surgery: Laryngectomy

Partial Laryngectomy (Laryngofissure–Thyrotomy). A partial laryngectomy (laryngofissure–thyrotomy) is recommended in the early stages of cancer in the glottic area when only one vocal cord is involved. It has a very high cure rate. In this operation, one vocal cord is removed and all other structures remain intact. The patient's voice may be hoarse. The airway will remain intact and the patient should have no difficulty swallowing.

Supraglottic (Horizontal) Laryngectomy. A supraglottic laryngectomy is used in the management of supraglottic tumors. The hyoid bone, glottis, and false cords are removed. The vocal cords, cricoid cartilage, and trachea remain intact. During surgery, a radical neck dissection is performed on the involved side. A tracheostomy tube (see p. 554) is left in the trachea until the glottic airway is established. It is usually removed after a few days and the stoma is allowed to close. Nutrition is provided through a nasogastric tube until there is healing and no danger of aspiration. Postoperatively, the patient may experience some difficulty in swallowing for the first 2 weeks. The chief advantage of this operation is that it preserves the voice. The major problem is the risk that the cancer will recur. Therefore, patients are selected carefully.

Hemivertical Laryngectomy. A hemivertical laryngectomy is performed when the tumor extends beyond the vocal cord, but is less than 1 cm and is limited to the subglottic area. In this procedure, the thyroid cartilage of the larynx is split in the midline of the neck and the portion of the vocal cord (one true cord and one false cord) with tumor growth is removed. The arytenoid cartilage and one half of the thyroid are removed. The patient will have a tracheostomy tube and nasogastric tube in place following surgery. The patient is at risk for aspiration postoperatively. Some change may occur in the voice quality (hoarseness) and projection. The airway and swallowing remain intact, however.

Total Laryngectomy. A total laryngectomy is performed when cancer extends beyond the vocal cords. Additionally, the hyoid bone, epiglottis, cricoid cartilage, and two or three rings of the trachea are removed. The tongue, pharyngeal walls, and trachea are preserved. Many surgeons recommend that a neck dissection be performed on the same side as the lesion even if no lymph nodes are palpable. The rationale for this approach is that metastases to the cervical lymph nodes occur frequently. The problem is more complex when a lesion involves midline structures or both vocal cords. With or without neck dissection, a total laryngectomy requires a permanent tracheal stoma. This prevents aspiration of food and fluid into the lower respiratory tract, because the larynx that provides the protective sphincter is no longer present. The patient will have no voice but will have normal swallowing. A total laryngectomy changes the manner in which airflow is used for breathing and speaking as depicted in Figure 23-6.

❑ NURSING PROCESS
The Patient Undergoing Laryngectomy

Assessment

The nurse assesses the patient for the following symptoms: hoarseness, sore throat, dyspnea, dysphagia, or pain and burning in the throat. The patient's neck is palpated for swelling.

If treatment includes surgery, it is important for the nurse to know the nature of the surgery to plan appropriate care. If the patient is expected to have no voice, a preoperative evaluation by the speech therapist is indicated. The patient's ability to hear, see, read, and write is assessed. Visual impairment and functional illiteracy may create additional problems with communication and require creative approaches to assure that the patient is able to communicate any needs.

In addition, the nurse determines the psychological preparedness of the patient. The idea of cancer is terrifying to most people. Fear is compounded by the possibility of permanently losing one's voice and, in some cases, of having some degree of disfigurement. The nurse evaluates the patient's and family's coping methods to develop an

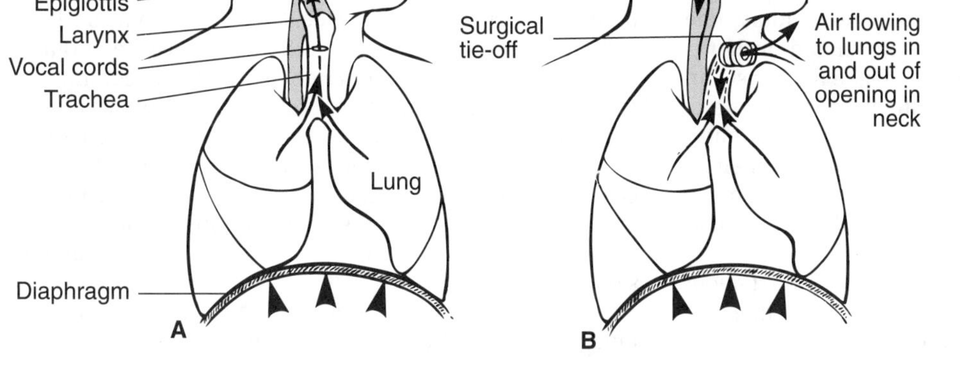

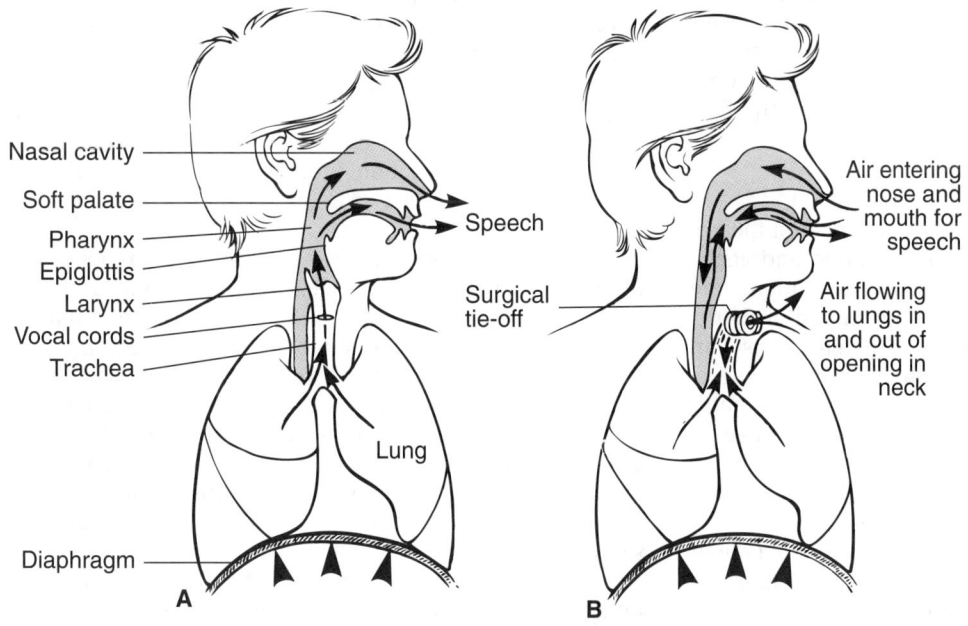

FIGURE 23-6. Laryngectomy requires a change in airflow for breathing and speaking. (**A**) Normal airflow. (**B**) Airflow after total laryngectomy.

effective approach to supporting them both preoperatively and postoperatively.

Diagnosis

Nursing Diagnoses

Based on all the assessment data, the patient's major nursing diagnoses may include the following:

- Knowledge deficit about the surgical procedure and postoperative course
- Anxiety related to the diagnosis of cancer and impending surgery
- Ineffective airway clearance related to surgical alterations in the airway
- Impaired verbal communication related to removal of larynx and to edema
- Altered nutrition: less than body requirements, related to swallowing difficulties
- Disturbance in body image, self-concept, and self-esteem related to major neck surgery
- Self-care deficit related to postoperative care
- Potential for noncompliance to rehabilitative program and home maintenance management

Collaborative Problems/ Potential Complications

Based on assessment data, potential complications that may develop include:

- Respiratory distress (hypoxia, airway obstruction, tracheal edema)
- Hemorrhage
- Infection

Planning and Implementation

Goals. The major goals for the patient may include attainment of an adequate level of knowledge, reduction in anxiety, maintenance of a patent airway (patient is able to handle own secretions), improvement in communication by use of alternative methods, attainment of optimal levels of nutrition and hydration, improvement in body image and self-esteem, adherence to rehabilitative program, home maintenance management, and prevention of complications.

Preoperative Nursing Interventions

Patient Education. The diagnosis of cancer of the larynx is associated with preconceived notions and fears. Many persons categorize it with other cancers and assume the worst. Others assume that loss of speech and disfigurement are inevitable with this condition. Once the physician explains the diagnosis to the patient, the nurse clarifies any misconceptions by identifying where the larynx is, what it does, what the particular procedure will be, and what effect surgery will have on the patient's speech. Educational materials (written and audiovisual) are given to the patient and family for review and reinforcement.

If a complete laryngectomy is to done, the patient should know that the natural voice will be lost, but that special training will provide a means for carrying on a fairly normal conversation. However, the ability to sing, laugh, or whistle will be lost. Until this training is initiated, the patient needs to know communication is possible by using the call light and by writing. The nurse answers questions about the nature of the surgery and reinforces the physician's explanation that the patient will lose the ability to vocalize, but that a rehabilitation program is available. The multidisciplinary team conducts an initial assessment of the patient and family. The team might include the nurse, physician, respiratory therapist, speech therapist, clinical nurse specialist, social worker, clinical dietitian, and home health care nurse.

Equipment and treatments that will be part of the postoperative care are reviewed. Additionally, coughing and deep breathing exercises are taught to the patient with opportunity provided for return demonstration. The patient's role in the postoperative and rehabilitative periods is explained.

Reducing Anxiety and Depression. Because surgery of the larynx is performed most commonly for a tumor that is malignant, the patient will have many questions: Will the surgeon be able to remove all of the tumor? Is it cancer? Will I die? Will I choke? Will I suffocate? Will I ever speak again? What will I look like? Therefore, the psychological preparation of the patient is as important as the physical preparation.

Any patient undergoing surgery may have many fears. (See Chapter 19 for further discussion.) The patient is given the opportunity to verbalize feelings and share perceptions. Any misconceptions the patient might have about the condition are addressed. Questions are answered as concisely and completely as possible. During the preoperative or postoperative period, a visit from someone who has had a laryngectomy is often helpful in conveying to the patient that there are people available and willing to help and that successful rehabilitation is possible.

Postoperative Nursing Interventions

Maintaining a Patent Airway. A patent airway is promoted by positioning the patient in the semi-Fowler's or Fowler's position after recovery from anesthesia. The patient is observed for restlessness, labored breathing, apprehension, and increased pulse rate, because these suggest respiratory or circulatory problems. Medications that depress respirations are avoided. As with other surgical patients, the laryngectomy patient is encouraged to turn, cough, and take deep breaths; suctioning may be necessary. Early ambulation is also encouraged to prevent atelectasis and pneumonia.

If a total laryngectomy was performed, a laryngectomy tube will most likely be in place. (In some instances a laryngectomy tube is not used; in others it is used temporarily; and in many it is used permanently.) The laryngectomy tube (which is shorter than a tracheostomy tube but has a larger diameter) is the only airway the patient has. The care of this tube is the same as for a tracheostomy tube (see Chapter 25, Guideline 25-4). The stoma is cleansed daily with saline solution or other prescribed solution; antibiotic ointment (of a nonoil base) may be prescribed and is applied around the stoma and suture line.

Wound drains may be in place to assist in removal of fluid and air from the surgical site. Suction may also be used but with caution to avoid trauma to the surgical site and incision. Drainage is observed, measured, and recorded; when drainage is less than 50 to 60 ml/day, the physician usually removes the drains.

The laryngectomy tube may be removed when the stoma is well healed, usually within 3 to 6 weeks after surgery. Until that time, the patient needs to be taught how to clean and change the laryngectomy tube (see p. 476) and how to clear the airway of secretions.

Promoting Communication and Speech Rehabilitation. The loss of speech or impaired speech is discussed preoperatively with the patient and family. The speech therapist conducts a preoperative evaluation. During this initial visit, the patient and family are educated about alternative forms of communication, and the postoperative rehabilitative plan. The inability to speak can be very frustrating. Postoperatively, the system of communication established preoperatively with the nurse, physician, and family is implemented.

Because a "magic slate" often is used for communication, it is helpful to document which hand the patient uses for writing so that the opposite arm can be used for intravenous infusions. Any notes used for communication should be destroyed to ensure the patient's privacy. If the patient is not able to write, a picture/word/phrase board or hand signals can be used.

An alternative to the call bell, such as a hand bell, may be required. This system is reviewed preoperatively with the patient. It can be very time-consuming to have to write everything or communicate through gestures. The patient may become impatient and angry when not understood. The nurse must be patient and understanding of such feelings. Other staff members should be alerted that the patient will be unable to use the intercom system.

The return of communication is generally the ultimate goal in the rehabilitation of the postlaryngectomy patient. Several methods of communication exist, such as writing, lip-speaking, and communication/word boards. The most commonly used and preferred methods at present include esophageal speech, the electrolarynx, and tracheoesophageal puncture. These techniques can be used once medical clearance is obtained from the physician.

Esophageal speech requires that the patient be able to compress air into the esophagus and expel it, setting off a vibration of the pharyngeal esophageal segment. This can be taught once the patient begins oral feedings or 1 week postoperatively. The patient first develops the ability to belch and is reminded to do so an hour after eating. This technique is practiced repeatedly. Later this conscious action is transformed into simple explosions of air from the esophagus for speech purposes. Thereafter, the speech–language pathologist works with the patient in an attempt to make speech intelligible and as close to normal as possible.

If esophageal speech is not successful, or until the technique is mastered, an *electric larynx* may be used for communication. This apparatus projects sound into the oral cavity. When words are formed by the mouth (articulated), the sound from the electric larynx becomes words that can be heard. The voice that is produced is obviously not a normal voice, but the patient is able to communicate with relative ease.

Another form of communication that will help the patient be better understood is called *tracheoesophageal puncture* (TEP) (Fig. 23-7). In this method the voice is restored by diverting air, which travels from the lungs through a puncture in the posterior wall of the trachea, into the esophagus, and out of the mouth. Once the puncture is surgically created and has healed, a voice prosthesis (Blom–Singer) is fitted over the puncture site. To prevent airway obstruction, the prosthesis is removed and cleaned when mucus builds up. A speech-language therapist teaches the patient how to produce sounds, but the speech is produced just as before by moving the tongue and lips to form the sound into words.

Promoting Adequate Nutrition. Postoperatively, the patient may not be permitted to eat or drink for 10 to 14 days. Alternative sources of nutrition and hydration include intravenous fluids, enteral feedings through a nasogastric tube, and total parenteral nutrition.

Once the patient is ready to start oral feedings, the nurse explains to the patient that thick fluids, such as Ensure and gelatin, will be used first because they are easy to swallow. The patient is instructed to avoid sweet foods, which increase salivation and suppress the appetite. Solid foods are introduced as tolerated. In addition, the patient is instructed to rinse the mouth with warm water or mouthwash and to brush the teeth frequently.

Promoting Self-Esteem. Disfiguring surgery and an altered communication pattern are a threat to a patient's self-concept, self-esteem, and body image. The reaction of family members is a major concern for the patient.

A positive approach is important when caring for the patient. Promoting self-care activities is part of this approach. The nurse reviews with the patient and family the tubes, dressings, and drains that are in place postoperatively. The patient is encouraged to express any negative feelings about the changes brought about by surgery. The patient often experiences anger, depression, and isolation.

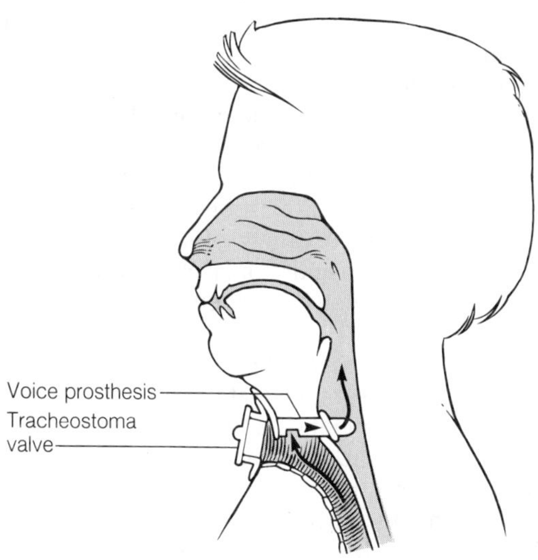

FIGURE 23-7. Schematic representation of tracheopharyngeal puncture speech (TEP). Air travels from the lung through a puncture in the posterior wall of the trachea into the esophagus and out the mouth. A voice prosthesis is fitted over the puncture site.

The nurse needs to be a good listener and a support to the family. Referral to a support group, such as The International Association of Laryngectomees and I Can Cope, may help the patient and family deal with the changes in their lives.

Monitoring and Managing Potential Complications. The immediate postoperative complications post-laryngectomy include *respiratory distress and hypoxia, bleeding,* and *infection.*

Respiratory Complications. The nurse monitors the patient for signs and symptoms of respiratory distress and hypoxia, particularly restlessness, irritation, agitation, confusion, tachypnea, use of accessory muscles, and decreased oxygen saturation. Any change in the patient's respiratory status requires immediate intervention. Obstruction needs to be ruled out immediately by suctioning and having the patient cough and breathe deeply. Hypoxia and airway obstruction, if not immediately treated, can be life-threatening. The physician is contacted immediately if nursing measures do not improve the patient's respiratory status.

Bleeding. Bleeding at the surgical site from the drains or with tracheal suctioning may be symptoms of hemorrhage. The surgeon should be notified of any active bleeding immediately. Bleeding may occur at a variety of sites, including the surgical site, drains, or trachea. Rupture of the carotid artery is especially dangerous. Should this occur, the nurse should apply direct pressure over the artery, summon assistance, and provide psychological support to the patient until the vessel can be ligated. Vital signs are monitored for changes, particularly, an increase in pulse and a decrease in blood pressure, or rapid deep respirations. Cold, clammy, pale skin may be signs of active bleeding.

Infection. The nurse observes for early signs and symptoms of postoperative infection. Early signs include an increase in temperature and pulse, change in the type of wound drainage, or increased areas of redness or tenderness at the surgical site. The nurse reports any significant change to the surgeon. Any increase in temperature, pulse, purulent drainage, odor, increase in wound drainage, and areas of redness or tenderness around the surgical site may indicate the presence of infection.

Patient Education and Home Care Considerations. The nurse has an important role in the rehabilitation of the laryngectomy patient. The patient will experience many emotions, physical changes, and changes in lifestyle. Discharge instruction begins as soon as the patient is able. The patient will learn a variety of self-care behaviors, including: tracheostomy and stoma care, wound care, and oral hygiene. The following patient education areas are addressed.

Tracheostomy and Stomal Care. The nurse conveys optimism, offering assurance that the patient will be able to carry on most preoperative activities. The patient needs specific information about what to expect from the tracheostomy. The patient frequently will cough up rather large amounts of mucus through this opening. Because air passes directly into the trachea without being warmed and moistened by the upper respiratory mucosa, the tracheobronchial tree compensates by secreting excessive amounts of mucus. Therefore, the patient will have frequent coughing episodes and may be somewhat troubled by the brassy sounding, mucus-producing cough. The patient should be assured that these problems will diminish in time as the tracheobronchial mucosa adapts to the altered physiology.

When the patient coughs, the orifice should be wiped clean and cleared of mucus. In addition, the skin around the stoma should be washed twice daily. If crusting occurs, the skin around the stoma is lubricated with a non–oil-based ointment (prescribed by the physician) and the crusts removed with sterile tweezers. It may be necessary that a bib be worn in front of the tracheostomy to keep the mucus from soiling the clothing. The bib may be a simple gauze dressing taped over the neck or one made of other porous fabric.

One of the most important factors in decreasing cough and mucus production as well as crusting around the stoma is adequate humidification of the environment. Mechanical humidifiers and aerosol generators (nebulizers) are excellent sources of humidification and are absolutely essential for the patient's comfort. Some system of humidification should be set up in the home before the patient is discharged from the hospital. An air-conditioned atmosphere may be distressing to the newly laryngectomized patient, because the air may be too cool or too dry and thus too irritating.

Changes in Taste and Smell. The patient can expect to have a diminished sense of taste and smell for a period of time after surgery. Because breathing occurs directly into the trachea, air is not passing through the nose to the olfactory end organs. Because taste and smell are so closely connected, taste sensations are altered. In time, however, the patient usually accommodates to this problem and olfactory sensation adapts.

Hygienic Measures. Special precautions need to be taken in a shower to prevent water from entering the stoma. Wearing a loose-fitting plastic bib or simply holding one's hand over the opening is effective. Swimming is not recommended, however, because the patient with a laryngectomy can drown without getting the face wet. Barbers and beauticians need to be cautioned so that hair sprays, loose hair, and powder do not get near the stoma because these substances can block or irritate the trachea and possibly cause infection. These self-care points are summarized in Chart 23-3.

Recreation Measures. Recreation and exercise are important. Golf, bowling, card and computer games, spectator activities, and walking can be enjoyed safely. Moderation to prevent fatigue is important because, when tired, the patient has more difficulty speaking, which can be discouraging.

Home Care and Safety Measures. Referral to a home health nurse for postoperative follow-up after discharge will assist in the transition and rehabilitative period. The nurse making the home visits will evaluate the patient's general status and ability to care effectively for the stoma and tracheostomy. Any additional teaching needs will be addressed at this time and key points about possible complications and problems repeated and reinforced. If the patient has a long history of smoking, referral to a smoking cessation program is suggested.

The nurse also encourages the person who has had a laryngectomy to have regular physical examinations and to seek advice concerning any problems relating to recovery and rehabilitation. Additional safety points include carrying proper identification, such as a card, to alert first-aid personnel to the special requirements of resuscitation should this need arise. On the back of the card can be included the name of a responsible person to notify in the event of emergency. For home emergency situations, prerecorded emergency messages for police, fire department, or other emergency services can be kept by the phone to be used quickly.

Evaluation

Expected Outcomes

1. Acquires an adequate level of knowledge
   a. Verbalizes an understanding of the surgical procedure and performs self-care adequately
2. Demonstrates less anxiety and depression
   a. Expresses a sense of hope
   b. Meets with someone from the Lost Chord or New Voice club
3. Maintains a clear airway and handles own secretions
   a. Demonstrates practical and correct technique involved in cleaning and changing the laryngectomy tube
4. Acquires effective communication techniques
   a. Uses assistive devices for communications: magic slate; call bell, picture board, sign language, lip reading, computer aids
   b. Practices the directives of the speech-language pathologist
5. Maintains balanced nutrition and adequate fluid intake
6. Exhibits improved body image, self-esteem, and self-concept
   a. Expresses feelings and concerns
   b. Participates in self-care and decision making
   c. Accepts information about support group
7. Adheres to rehabilitation and home care program
   a. Practices recommended speech therapy
   b. Demonstrates proper methods for caring for stoma and laryngectomy tube (if present)
   c. Verbalizes understanding of symptoms that require medical attention
   d. States safety measures to take in emergencies
8. Exhibits no complications
   a. Vital signs (blood pressure, temperature, pulse and respiratory rate) normal
   b. No redness, tenderness, or purulent drainage at surgical site
   c. Demonstrates a patent airway and appropriate respirations
   d. No bleeding from surgical site and minimal bleeding from drains

CHART 23-3
Patient Education: The Patient With a Laryngectomy

1. Expect frequent coughing at first because of the mucus present in the tracheobronchial tree.
2. After coughing, wipe the tracheal orifice and clear out the mucus.
3. Wash the skin around the stoma twice daily.
4. If crusting occurs around the stoma, lubricate with ointment as prescribed and remove crusts with sterile tweezers.
5. Consider wearing some kind of protection in front of the tracheostomy to keep the mucus from soiling the clothing.
6. Maintain adequate humidification with a humidifier or nebulizer.
7. Avoid air conditioning at first to prevent the cold air from irritating the airway.
8. When showering, cover the stoma to keep water from entering the airway passage.
9. Do not allow hair spray, powder, or loose hair to enter the stoma to avoid irritation and possible infection.
10. Wear or carry special identification to alert others in case of emergencies.
11. Have regular check-ups and report any problems immediately.

CRITICAL THINKING EXERCISES

1. You are caring for a patient who is scheduled for a complete laryngectomy for cancer of the larynx. In anticipating the altered speech that will result from this surgery, describe the information you would share with the patient about methods of communicating in the early postoperative period as well as in the long term.
2. In discussing methods to be used by the patient in the immediate postoperative period following a laryngectomy, you realize that the patient and his family do not fully understand the alterations in breathing and speech that will result from this surgery. How would you expand the discussion to explain these changes to the patient and his family?
3. A 21-year-old has experienced a continuous nosebleed since being hit in the face with a baseball more than an hour ago and comes to see you for first aid. Describe the actions you would take initially, and compare them to the actions you would take if your initial measures were ineffective in halting the bleeding.
4. Two patients have come to the clinic with upper respiratory infections. Both have a fever and sore throat. One is a 25-year-old mother with two small children; the other is a 68-year-old woman with a heart condition. How might the treatment plans and the patient teaching considerations for each of these patients differ?

REFERENCES AND SELECTED READINGS

Books

American Cancer Society. Cancer Facts and Figures—1994. Atlanta, American Cancer Society, 1994.

Baird SB. A Cancer Source Book for Nurses, 6th ed. Atlanta, American Cancer Society, 1991.

Carrieri-Kohlman V and Janson-Bjerklie S. Dyspnea. In Carrieri-Kohlman V, Lindsey AM, and West CM. Pathophysiological Phenomena in Nursing: Human Responses to Illness. Philadelphia, WB Saunders, 1993.

Eisele DW. Complications in Head and Neck Surgery. St. Louis, CV Mosby, 1993.

Fishman AP. Pulmonary Diseases and Disorders, 2nd ed, Vol 1. New York, McGraw-Hill, 1988.

Groenwald S. Cancer Nursing: Principles and Practice, 3rd ed. Boston, Jones and Barlett Publishers, 1993.

Jacobs C (ed). Carcinomas of the Head and Neck: Evaluation and Management. Boston, Kluwer Academic Publisher, 1990.

Meyers EM. Head and Neck Oncology. Diagnosis, Treatment, and Rehabilitation. Boston, Little, Brown and Company, 1991.

Murray JF and Nadel JA. The Textbook of Respiratory Medicine, 2nd ed, Vols 1 & 2. Philadelphia, WB Saunders, 1994.

Neiderman MS (ed). Respiratory Infections in the Elderly. New York, Raven Press, 1991.

Otto SE (ed). Oncology Nursing, 2nd ed. St Louis, Mosby–Year Book, 1993.

Rosen P (ed). Emergency Medicine Concepts and Clinical Practice, 3rd ed, Volume I & III. Chicago, Mosby–Year Book, 1992.

Swartz WM and Banis JC. Head and Microsurgery. Baltimore, Williams & Wilkins, 1992.

Journals

Ackerstaff AH et al. Improvements in the assessment of pulmonary function in laryngectomized patients. Laryngoscopy 1993 December; 103(12):1391–1394.

Baker CA. Factors associated with rehabilitation in head and neck cancer. Cancer Nurs 1992 June; 15(6):395–400.

Bernstein JA. Allergic rhinitis. Postgrad Med 1993 May; 93(6): 124–131.

Druce HM. Diagnosis of sinusitis in adults: History, physical examination, nasal cytology, echo, and rhinoscope. J Allergy Clin Immunol 1992 Sept; 90(3):436–441.

Elizondo E and Sanchez PD. Streptococcal pharyngitis: An update. Physician Assistant 1992 January; 16(1):79–85.

English GM. Sinusitis: Strategies to cope with acute infection. Consultant 1993 April; 33(4):118–130.

Esposito B et al. Facial trauma. AORN J 1992 June; 55(6):1467–1479.

Gantz NM. An update of sinusitis. Patient Care 1992 April 30; 26(8):141–163.

Hengerer AS, Hunt M, and Turner LM. Epistaxis. Patient Care 1992 November 15; 26(18):84–99.

Hilding DA. Literature review: The common cold. Ear, Nose and Throat 1994 Sep; 639–643.

Holley HP and Fowler SL. Update on herpes simplex infections. Hospital Medicine 1993 May; 29(5):28–45.

Kronenberger MB. Dysphagia. Dysphagia 1994 Fall; 9(4):236–244.

Kuo E et al. Tracheostomal stenosis after total laryngectomy: An analysis of pre-disposing clinical factors. Laryngoscope 1994 January; 104(1):59–63.

Langius A, Bjorvell H, and Lind MG. Oral- and pharyngeal-cancer patient's perceived symptoms of health cancer nursing. Cancer Nurs 1993 March; 16(3):214–221.

Lockhart JS, Troff JL, and Artim LS. Total laryngectomy and radical neck dissection. AORN J 1992 Feb; 55(2):458–479.

Mellette S and Parker GG. Future directions in cancer rehabilitation. Semin Oncol Nurs 1992 August; 8(3):219–223.

Moses BL, Eisele DW, and Jones BJ. Radiologic assessment of the early post-operative total laryngectomy patient. Laryngoscope 1993 October; 103(10):1157–1160.

Schwartz R. The diagnosis and management of sinusitis. Nurse Practitioner 1994 Dec; 19(12):58–63.

Schwartz RH, Seid AB, and Stool SE. Tonsillectomy today: Who needs it? Patient Care 1992 Jan; 26(1):173–194.

Shumrick KA et al. Extended access/internal approaches for the management of facial trauma. Otolaryngol Head Neck Surg 1992 October; 118(10):1105–1111.

Vukmir RB. Adult and pediatric pharyngitis: A review. J Emerg Med 1992 Sept/Oct; 10(5):607–616.

INFORMATION/RESOURCES

Agencies

American Cancer Society
1599 Clifton Road, NE
Atlanta, GA 30329-4251
(404) 320-3333
(800) ACS-2345

American Lung Association
1740 Broadway
New York, NY 10019–4374
(212) 315-8700

International Association of Laryngectomees
c/o American Cancer Society (above)

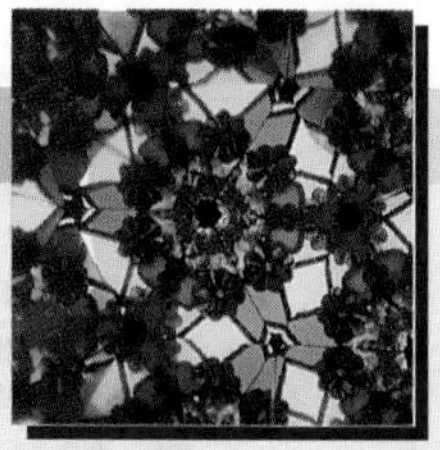

24

Management of Patients With Conditions of the Chest and Lower Respiratory Tract

CHAPTER OUTLINE

Atelectasis

Respiratory Infections
Acute Tracheobronchitis
Pneumonia
NURSING PROCESS: The Patient With Pneumonia
Pulmonary Tuberculosis
NURSING PROCESS: The Patient With Tuberculosis

Lung Abscess

Pleural Conditions
Pleurisy
Pleural Effusion
Empyema

Chronic Obstructive Pulmonary Disease
NURSING PROCESS: The Patient With COPD
Chronic Bronchitis
Bronchiectasis
Pulmonary Emphysema
Asthma
Status Asthmaticus

Acute Respiratory Failure

Adult Respiratory Distress Syndrome

Pulmonary Hypertension

Pulmonary Heart Disease (Cor Pulmonale)

Pulmonary Embolism

Breathing Disorders During Sleep

Sarcoidosis

Occupational Lung Diseases
Pneumoconioses

Chest Tumors
Lung Cancer (Bronchogenic Carcinoma)
Tumors of the Mediastinum

Chest Trauma
Rib Fractures
Flail Chest
Hemothorax and Pneumothorax
Tension Pneumothorax
Penetrating Wounds of the Chest
Pulmonary Contusion
Cardiac Tamponade
Subcutaneous Emphysema

Aspiration

Critical Thinking Exercises

LEARNING OBJECTIVES

On completion of this chapter, the learner will be able to:

1. Identify patients at risk for atelectasis and nursing interventions related to its prevention and management
2. Compare the various pulmonary infections with regard to causes, clinical manifestations, nursing management, complications, and prevention
3. Use the nursing process as a framework for care of the patient with pneumonia
4. Use the nursing process as a framework for care of the patient with pulmonary tuberculosis
5. Relate pleurisy, pleural effusion, and empyema to pulmonary infection
6. Discuss smoking and air pollution as causes of pulmonary disease
7. Compare and contrast chronic bronchitis, bronchiectasis, pulmonary emphysema, and asthma as chronic obstructive pulmonary diseases, and describe their relationship to pulmonary heart disease
8. Use the nursing process as a framework for care of the patient with chronic obstructive pulmonary disease (COPD)
9. Develop a teaching plan for patients with COPD
10. Describe risk factors and measures appropriate for prevention and management of pulmonary embolism
11. Describe preventive measures appropriate for controlling and eliminating the problem of occupational lung disease
12. Discuss the modes of therapy and related nursing management for patients with lung cancer
13. Describe the complications of chest trauma and their clinical manifestations and nursing management
14. Describe nursing measures to prevent aspiration
15. Relate the therapeutic management techniques of adult respiratory distress syndrome to the underlying pathophysiology of the syndrome

Atelectasis

Atelectasis refers to the collapse of an alveolus, a lobule, or larger lung unit. It may be caused by obstruction of a bronchus. The blockage impedes the passage of air to and from the alveoli that normally receive air through the bronchus. The trapped alveolar air becomes absorbed into the bloodstream but outside air cannot replace the absorbed air because of the obstruction. As a result, the isolated portion of the lung becomes airless and shrinks in size, causing the remainder of the lung to overexpand.

Atelectasis may follow bronchial obstruction by a foreign body or a plug of thick exudate. Also, the risk for atelectasis is increased by the supine position; splinting of the chest due to pain; respiratory depression from opioids, sedatives, and muscle relaxants; and abdominal distention. Atelectasis resulting from bronchial obstruction by secretions is the usual cause of the "massive collapse" occasionally observed postoperatively and in debilitated, bedridden patients. In these patients, there is likely to be long, continued respiratory depression, together with inadequate respiratory excursion and retention of bronchial secretions.

Atelectasis also may result from pressure on the lung tissue, which restricts normal lung expansion on inspiration. Such pressure may be produced by a variety of causes: fluid accumulating within the thorax (pleural effusion), air in the pleural space (pneumothorax), a very enlarged heart, a pericardium distended with fluid (pericardial effusion), tumor growth within the thorax, or an elevated diaphragm that is displaced upward as the result of abdominal pressure. Atelectasis caused by pressure is often encountered in patients with pleural effusion due to cardiac failure or pleural infection. Atelectasis is often one of the first signs of a tumor of the bronchi.

Assessment. If lung collapse occurs suddenly, and if sufficient lung tissue is involved, marked dyspnea, cyanosis, prostration, and pleural pain may be anticipated. Tachycardia and fever are common. The patient characteristically sits upright in bed, is anxious, and has difficulty breathing. The chest wall on the affected side moves little, if at all, whereas the excursion appears excessive on the opposite side.

Management. The goal is to improve ventilation and remove secretions. If atelectasis has resulted from a pleural effusion or pressure pneumothorax, the fluid or air may be removed by needle aspiration. If bronchial obstruction is the cause, the obstruction must be removed to permit air to enter that portion of the lung again. If respiratory care measures fail to remove the obstruction, a bronchoscopy is performed. Endotracheal intubation and mechanical ventilation may be necessary. Prompt treatment reduces the risk of pneumonia and lung abscess.

Prevention. Nursing measures to prevent bronchial obstruction include aspirating secretions, encouraging the patient to cough, and using an aerosol nebulizer, followed by postural drainage and chest percussion. The patient should be turned frequently to stimulate coughing. If possible, the patient is ambulated to aid in mobilizing and clearing secretions.

All stuporous, debilitated, and sedated patients are turned frequently in bed. Coughing and deep breathing (at least every 2 hours) assist in preventing and treating atelectasis. The use of incentive spirometry or voluntary deep breathing enhances inspiration and decreases the potential for airway closure. Nasopharyngeal and nasotracheal suction is also helpful in stimulating patients to cough, thereby removing tenacious secretions. (See Chart 24-1 for a summary of measures to prevent atelectasis.)

Respiratory Infections

Acute Tracheobronchitis

Acute tracheobronchitis is an acute inflammation of the mucous membranes of the trachea and the bronchial tree that often follows infections of the upper respiratory tract. A patient with a viral infection has a lessened resistance and can readily develop a secondary bacterial infection. Thus, the adequate treatment of upper respiratory tract infections is one of the major factors in the prevention of acute bronchitis. Aside from infection, inhalation of physical and chemical irritants, gases, and other air contaminants can also cause acute bronchial irritations.

Clinical Manifestations. The signs and symptoms of acute tracheobronchitis result from the mucopurulent sputum that is secreted by the inflamed mucosa of the bronchi. Initially, the patient has a dry, irritating cough and expectorates a scanty amount of mucoid sputum. The patient complains of sternal soreness from coughing and has fever, headache, and general malaise. As the infection progresses, inspiration may become noisy (inspiratory stridor) and more profuse purulent sputum may be present.

A culture of the sputum is essential to identify the specific causative organism. Although *Streptococcus pneumoniae* and *Haemophilus influenzae* often cause this infection, tracheobronchitis is the most common clinical syndrome that results from infection from *Mycoplasma pneumoniae*.

Medical Management. The treatment is largely symptomatic. The patient is advised to rest in bed. Cool vapor therapy or steam inhalations are beneficial in relieving

CHART 24-1
Prevention of Atelectasis

1. Encourage appropriate deep breathing and coughing to prevent secretions from collecting and to expel exudate.
2. Change patient's position frequently, especially from supine to upright position, to promote ventilation and prevent secretions from accumulating.
3. Promote proper expansion of chest during breathing to aerate lungs fully.
4. Administer opioids and sedatives judiciously to prevent respiratory depression.
5. Institute suctioning to remove tracheobronchial secretions.
6. Carry out postural drainage and chest percussion.
7. Encourage early ambulation.
8. Teach appropriate technique for incentive spirometry.

the laryngeal and tracheal irritation. Increasing the vapor pressure (moisture content) in the air will reduce irritation. Moist heat to the chest will relieve the soreness and pain.

Antihistamines may be excessively drying, making secretions more difficult to expectorate. Expectorants, such as Robitussin, may be prescribed, although their efficacy is subject to debate. Fluid intake is increased to thin the viscous and tenacious secretions. Antibiotic treatment is indicated when the sputum becomes purulent. If the copious, purulent secretions cannot be cleared by coughing, the patient may be in danger of complete obstruction. Nasotracheal intubation may be required.

Nursing Interventions. A primary nursing function is to encourage bronchial hygiene, such as coughing frequently to remove secretions. The elderly patient can easily develop bronchopneumonia from acute tracheobronchitis if adequate care is not implemented. The patient should be encouraged and assisted to sit up frequently to cough effectively and to prevent retention of mucopurulent sputum. The nurse cautions the patient against overexertion, which can induce a relapse or extension of the infection. To avoid recurrence, the patient is advised to allow adequate time for convalescence after the acute infection subsides.

Pneumonia

Pneumonia is an inflammatory process of the lung parenchyma that is commonly caused by infectious agents. Pneumonia is the most common cause of death from infectious diseases in the United States. It ranks fourth for men and fifth for women as a cause for hospitalization. It is also treated extensively on an outpatient basis.

Pneumonia is classified according to its causative agent and is categorized as bacterial and atypical pneumonia (Table 24-1). Pneumonia also may be caused by radiation therapy, ingestion of chemicals, and aspiration. Radiation pneumonia may follow radiation therapy for breast or lung cancer, usually 6 weeks or more after completion of treatment. Chemical pneumonitis or pneumonia may occur after ingestion of kerosene or inhalation of irritating gases. Aspiration pneumonia is discussed on p. 539.

If a substantial portion of one or more lobes is involved, the disease is referred to as **lobar pneumonia**. The term **bronchopneumonia** is used to describe pneumonia that is distributed in a patchy fashion, having originated in one or more localized areas within the bronchi and extending to the adjacent surrounding lung parenchyma. Bronchopneumonia is more common than lobar pneumonia (Fig. 24-1).

In general, patients with bacterial pneumonia usually have acute or chronic underlying disease that impairs host defenses. More often, pneumonia arises from normally present flora in a patient whose resistance has been altered, or it results from aspiration of flora present in the mouth. Although most atypical pneumonias, such as those caused by viral infections, occur in previously healthy persons, when bacterial pneumonia occurs in a healthy person there is usually a history of preceding viral illness.

Increasing numbers of patients who have compromised defenses against infections are susceptible to pneumonia. Included are people on corticosteroids or other immunosuppressive agents, those on broad-spectrum antimicrobials, those with AIDS, and those requiring the use of advanced life-support technology. These patients have suppressed immune systems and often acquire pneumonia from organisms of low virulence. In addition, increasing numbers of patients with impaired defenses develop hospital-acquired pneumonia from gram-negative bacilli *(Klebsiella, Pseudomonas, Escherichia coli,* Enterobacteriaceae, *Proteus, Serratia).* Gram-positive cocci, anaerobes, mycobacteria, nocardial species of bacteria, and viral, chlamydial, fungal, and parasitic agents can cause pneumonia. Commonly encountered pneumonias and their clinical features, treatment, and complications are presented in Table 24-1.

Prevention and Risk Factors

Being knowledgeable about the factors and circumstances that commonly predispose a person to pneumonia will aid in identifying those patients at high risk for pneumonia. Providing anticipatory and preventive care is an important nursing measure (Chart 24-2, p. 486).

- Any condition that produces mucus or bronchial obstruction and interferes with normal drainage of the lung (*e.g.*, cancer, chronic obstructive pulmonary disease [COPD]) increases the patient's susceptibility to pneumonia. *Preventive measure:* Promote coughing and expectoration of secretions.
- Immunosuppressed patients and those with a low neutrophil count (neutropenic) are at risk. *Preventive measure:* Initiate special precautions against infection.
- People who smoke are at risk because cigarette smoke disrupts both mucociliary and macrophage activity. *Preventive measure:* Encourage people to stop smoking.
- Any patient who is permitted to lie passively in bed for prolonged periods, relatively immobile and breathing shallowly, is at high risk for bronchopneumonia. *Preventive measure:* Change positions frequently.
- Any person who has a depressed cough reflex (due to medications, a debilitated state, or weak respiratory muscles), has aspirated foreign material into the lungs during a period of unconsciousness (head injury, anesthesia), or has an abnormal swallowing mechanism is very likely to develop bronchopneumonia. *Preventive measures:* Tracheobronchial suctioning, frequent position changes, judicious administration of medications that increase risk for aspiration, and chest physical therapy.
- Any hospitalized patient on a nothing-by-mouth (NPO) regimen or who is receiving antibiotics has increased pharyngeal colonization of organisms and is at risk. In very ill persons, the oropharynx is likely to be colonized by gram-negative bacteria. *Preventive measure:* Promote frequent oral hygiene.
- People who are intoxicated frequently are particularly susceptible to pneumonia, because alcohol suppresses the body's reflexes, white cell mobilization, and tracheobronchial ciliary motion. *Preventive measure:* Encourage people to reduce alcohol intake.
- Any person who receives a sedative or opioid may experience respiratory depression, which predisposes to

(text continues on page 484)

TABLE 24-1 Commonly Encountered Pneumonias

Type	Organism Responsible	Epidemiology
Bacterial Pneumonias		
Streptococcal pneumonia	*Streptococcus pneumoniae*	Highest occurrence in winter months. Incidence greatest in the elderly and in patients with COPD, CHF, alcoholism, splenectomy.
Staphylococcal pneumonia	*Staphylococcus aureus*	Incidence greatest in immunocompromised patients, IV drug users, and as a complication of epidemic influenza. Commonly nosocomial in origin. Accounts for 2% to 10% of community-acquired and 10% to 15% of hospital-acquired pneumonias. Mortality rate: 25% to 60%.
Klebsiella pneumonia	*Klebsiella pneumoniae* (Friedlander's bacillus-encapsulated gram-negative aerobic bacillus)	Incidence greatest in the elderly, alcoholics; patients with chronic disease, such as diabetes, CHF, COPD; patients in chronic care facilities and nursing homes. Accounts for 2% to 5% of community-acquired and 10% to 30% of hospital-acquired pneumonias. Mortality rate: 40% to 50%.
Pseudomonas pneumonia	*Pseudomonas aeruginosa*	Incidence greatest in those with pre-existing lung disease, cancer (particularly leukemia); those with homograft transplants, burns; debilitated persons; and patients receiving antimicrobial therapy and treatments such as tracheostomy, suctioning. It is almost always of nosocomial origin. Accounts for 5% to 15% of hospital-acquired pneumonias. Mortality rate: 40% to 60%.
Haemophilus influenza	*Haemophilus influenzae*	Incidence greatest in alcoholics, the elderly, patients in chronic care facilities and nursing homes, patients with diabetes or COPD and children less than 5 years old. Accounts for 5% to 20% of community-acquired pneumonias. Mortality rate: 33%.
Atypical Pneumonias		
Legionnaires' disease	*Legionella pneumophila*	Highest occurrence in summer and fall. May cause disease sporadically or as part of an epidemic. Incidence greatest in middle-aged and older men, smokers, and patients with chronic diseases, receiving immunosuppressive therapy, or those in close proximity to excavation site. Accounts for 15% of community-acquired pneumonia. Mortality rate: 15% to 50%.

Clinical Features	Treatment	Comments
Herpes simplex lesion often present on face. Usually involves one or more lobes. Bacteremia is common. Right lower lobe infiltrate common on chest x-ray, with occasional bronchopneumonia pattern.	Penicillin G IV Penicillin V PO Alternate antibiotic therapy, such as cefuroxime or a third generation cephalosporins (cefotaxime, ceftizoxime, ceftriaxone); erythromycin, clindamycin, other penicillins,trimethoprim-sulfamethoxazole (Bactrim).	Complications include: shock, pleural effusion, superinfections, pericarditis, and otitis media.
Severe hypoxemia, cyanosis, necrotizing infection. Bacteremia is common.	Nafcillin, methicillin, oxacillin, vancomycin for methicillin-resistant organisms, or for penicillin-allergic patients.	Complications include: pleural effusion/pneumothorax, lung abscess, empyema, meningitis, endocarditis. Frequently requires hospitalization. Treatment must be vigorous and prolonged because of disease's tendency to destroy the lungs.
Tissue necrosis occurs rapidly in lungs (mimics TB) with cavity formation in some patients.	Gentamicin, tobramycin, third-generation cephalosporins (cefotaxime, ceftizoxime, ceftriaxone).	Complications include: multiple lung abscesses with cyst formation, empyema, pericarditis, pleural effusion. May be fulminating, progressing to fatal outcome.
Diffuse consolidation on chest x-ray.	Piperacillin; ticarcillin combined with gentamicin or ortobramycin.	Complications include lung cavitation. Has capacity to invade blood vessels, causing hemorrhage and lung infarction. Usually requires hospitalization.
Frequently insidious onset associated with upper respiratory tract infection 2 to 6 weeks before onset of illness. Fever, chills, productive cough. Usually involves one or more lobes. Bacteremia is common. Infiltrate, occasional bronchopneumonia pattern in right lower lobe on chest x-ray.	Ampicillin, amoxicillin, Augmentin, cefaclor or cefuroxime. Trimethoprim-sulfamethoxazole for penicillin-allergic patients.	Complications include: lung abscess, pleural effusion.
Flulike symptoms. High fevers with a pulse-temperature deficit (relative bradycardia), mental confusion, headache, pleuritic pain, myalgias, dyspnea, productive cough, hemoptysis. Patchy infiltrates, consolidation, possible pleural effusion on chest x-ray.	Erythromycin; rifampin	Complications include hypotension, shock, and acute renal failure.

(continued)

TABLE 24-1 *(continued)*

Type	Organism Responsible	Epidemiology
Atypical Pneumonias *(continued)*		
Mycoplasma pneumonia	*Mycoplasma pneumoniae*	Highest occurrence in fall and early winter. Responsible for epidemics of respiratory illness that occur every 4 years. Most common type of atypical pneumonia. Accounts for 20% of community-acquired pneumonias. More common in children and young adults. Mortality rate: less than 0.1%.
Viral pneumonia	Influenza viruses types A, B, C	Incidence greatest in winter months. Epidemics occur every 2 to 3 years. Most common organism in adults. Other organisms in children (*e.g.,* cytomegalovirus [CMV] and respiratory syncytial virus [RSV]). Accounts for 17% of community-acquired pneumonias.
Pneumocystis carinii pneumonia (PCP)	*Pneumocystis carinii*	Incidence greatest in patients with AIDS and patients receiving immunosuppressive therapy for cancer, organ transplants, and other disorders. Frequently seen with CMV infection. Mortality rate 60% to 80%.
Fungal pneumonia	*Aspergillus fumigatus*	Incidence greatest in immunocompromised and neutropenic patients. Mortality rate: 15% to 20%.
Chlamydial pneumonia (TWAR pneumonia)	*Cipittaci*	Incidence reported mainly in college students and military recruits. May be a common cause of community-acquired pneumonia. Mortality rate: 1% to 5%.
Tuberculosis	*Mycobacterium tuberculosis*	Incidence increased in indigent, immigrant and prison populations, AIDS patients, and the homeless. Mortality rate 0.0006%.

the pooling of bronchial secretions and subsequent development of pneumonia. *Preventive measures:* Observe the respiratory rate and depth before giving the medication. If respiratory depression is apparent, withhold the medication and report the problem.

- Patients who are unconscious or have poor cough and gag reflexes are at risk for pneumonia from accumulated secretions or aspiration. *Preventive measure:* Carry out frequent suctioning of secretions.
- Elderly people are especially vulnerable to pneumonia because of depression of cough and glottic reflexes. Postoperative pneumonia should be anticipated in the elderly. *Preventive measures:* Frequent mobilization, effective coughing, and breathing exercises.
- Anyone receiving treatment with respiratory therapy equipment can develop pneumonia if the equipment has not been properly cleaned. *Preventive measure:* Asssure that respiratory equipment is cleaned properly.

Pneumonia has been known to be more prevalent with certain underlying disorders such as congestive heart failure, diabetes, alcoholism, COPD, and AIDS. Certain diseases also have been associated with specific pathogens. For example, staphylococcal pneumonia has been noted after epidemics of influenza, and patients with COPD are at increased risk for developing pneumonia caused by pneumococci or *Haemophilus influenzae*.

Cystic fibrosis is associated with respiratory infection with *Pseudomonas* and *Staphylococcus*. *Pneumocystis carinii* pneumonia (PCP) has been associated with AIDS. Pneumonias occurring in hospitalized patients often involve organisms not usually found in community-acquired pneu-

Clinical Features	Treatment	Comments
Onset is usually insidious. Patients not usually as ill as in other pneumonias. Sore throat, nasal congestion, ear pain, headache, low grade fever, pleuritic pain, myalgias, diarrhea, erythema rash, pharyngitis. Patchy infiltrate, small pleural effusion on chest x-ray.	Erythromycin; tetracycline derivatives (Doxycycline)	Complications include aseptic meningitis, meningoencephalitis, cerebral ataxia, Guillain-Barré syndrome, transverse myelitis, pericarditis, myocarditis.
In majority of patients, influenza begins as an acute upper respiratory infection; others have bronchitis, pleurisy, etc., and still others develop gastrointestinal symptoms.	Amantadine; Rimantadine Treated symptomatically. Does not respond to treatment with presently available antimicrobials.	Complications include a superimposed bacterial infection, bronchopneumonia.
Pulmonary infiltrates on chest x-ray.	Trimethoprim-sulfamethoxazole, Dapsone, pentamidine	Complications include respiratory failure.
Cough, hemoptysis, infiltrates, fungus ball on chest x-ray.	Flucytosine with amphotericin B in non-neutropenic patients. Ketoconazole Lobectomy of fungus ball	
Hoarseness, fever, pharyngitis, rhinitis, nonproductive cough, myalgias, arthralgia. Single infiltrate on chest x-ray; pleural effusion possible	Doxycycline, erythromycin, clarithromycin, azithromycin	Complications include reinfection and ARDS.
Weight loss, fever, night sweats, cough, sputum production, hemoptysis, nonspecific infiltrate (lower lobe), hilar node enlargement, pleural effusion on chest x-ray.	Rifampin, streptomycin, ethambutol, INH (Isoniazid), pyrazinamide	Complications include reinfection and ARDS.

monias, including enteric gram-negative bacilli and *Staphylococcus aureus.*

Preventive Measures. To reduce or prevent serious complications of pneumonia in high-risk groups, vaccination against pneumococcal and influenza viral infections has been recommended for persons over 50 years of age, nursing home residents, debilitated patients, those with cardiovascular disease, patients who have had a splenectomy, and those with sickle cell disease or alcoholism. The vaccine provides specific prevention against pneumonia that is caused by major organisms. Vaccines should be avoided in the first trimester of pregnancy.

Bacterial and Atypical Pneumonia

Bacterial Pneumonia. Pneumonia caused by *Streptococcus pneumoniae* is the most common bacterial pneumonia and is most prevalent during the winter and spring when upper respiratory tract infections are most frequent. It may occur as a lobar or bronchopneumonic form in patients of any age and may follow a recent respiratory illness.

S. pneumoniae is a gram-positive, capsulated, nonmotile coccus that resides naturally in the upper respiratory tract. It commonly is referred to as the *pneumococcus.*

Pathophysiology. Bacterial pneumonia affects both ventilation and diffusion. An inflammatory reaction initiated by pneumococci occurs in the alveoli and produces an exudate, which interferes with movement and diffusion of oxygen and carbon dioxide. White blood cells, mostly neutrophils, also migrate into the alveoli and fill the normally air-containing spaces. Areas of the lung are not adequately ventilated because of secretions, mucosal edema, and bronchospasm, causing partial occlusion of the

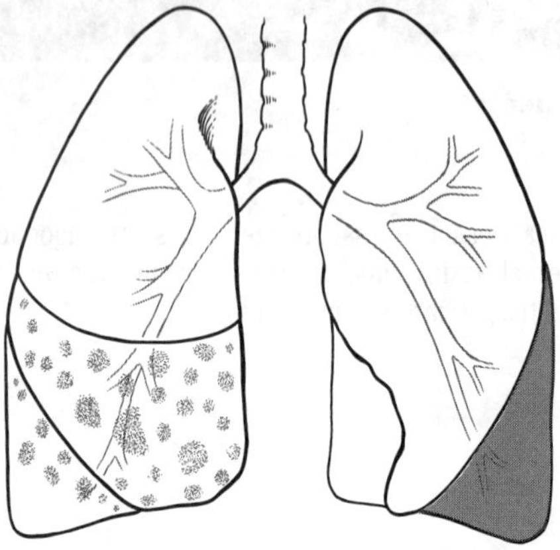

FIGURE 24-1. Distribution of lung involvement in lobar and bronchial pneumonia. In bronchopneumonia, patchy areas of consolidation occur. In lobar pneumonia, an entire lobe is consolidated. (From Porth C. Pathophysiology: Concepts of Altered Health States, 4th ed. Philadelphia, JB Lippincott, 1994.)

bronchi or alveoli with a resulting decrease in alveolar oxygen tension. Venous blood entering the lungs passes through the underventilated area and exits to the left side of the heart without being oxygenated. In essence, the blood is shunted from the right to the left side of the heart. This mixing of oxygenated and unoxygenated blood eventually results in arterial hypoxemia.

Atypical Pneumonia Syndromes. Pneumonias associated with mycoplasmas, fungus, chlamydia, Q fever, Legionnaires' disease, *Pneumocystis carinii*, and viruses are included in the atypical pneumonia syndromes (see Table 24-1).

Mycoplasma pneumoniae is the most common cause of primary atypical pneumonia. Mycoplasmas are small organisms surrounded by a triple-layered membrane without a cell wall. The organisms grow on a special culture medium but differ from viruses. Mycoplasma pneumonia occurs most frequently in older children and young adults.

Pneumonia probably is spread by infected respiratory droplets, through person-to-person contact. Patients can be tested for mycoplasma antibodies.

The inflammatory infiltrate is primarily interstitial rather than alveolar. It spreads throughout the entire respiratory tract, including the bronchioles. Generally, it has the characteristics of a bronchopneumonia. Earache and bullous myringitis are common. Atypical pneumonia may create some of the same problems in both ventilation and diffusion as described in bacterial pneumonia.

Clinical Manifestations

Bacterial (or pneumococcal) pneumonia typically starts with a sudden onset of shaking chills, rapidly rising fever (39.5° to 40.5°C [101° to 105°F]), and stabbing chest pain that is aggravated by breathing and coughing. The patient is severely ill with marked tachypnea (25 to 45 breaths/min) accompanied by respiratory grunting, nasal flaring, and the use of accessory muscles of respiration.

Atypical pneumonia varies in symptoms depending on the organism. Many patients have had an upper respiratory tract infection (nasal congestion, sore throat), and the onset of symptoms of pneumonia is gradual. The predominant symptoms are headache, low grade fever, pleuritic pain, myalgia, rash, and pharyngitis. After a few days, mucoid or mucopurulent sputum is expectorated.

The pulse is rapid and bounding. It usually increases about 10 beats/min for every degree of Celsius temperature elevation. A relative bradycardia for the amount of fever may suggest viral infection, *Mycoplasma* infection, or infection with *Legionella* species.

In many cases of pneumonia, the cheeks are flushed, the eyes bright, and the lips and nail beds cyanotic. The patient prefers to be propped up in bed leaning forward, trying to achieve adequate gas exchange without trying to cough or breathe deeply. The patient perspires profusely. The sputum is purulent and not a reliable indicator of the etiologic agent. Rusty, blood-tinged sputum is often produced in pneumococcal, staphylococcal, *Klebsiella,* and streptococcal pneumonia. *Klebsiella* pneumonia frequently also has viscous sputum; *H. influenzae* sputum is often green.

Other signs occur in patients with other conditions, such as cancer, or in those who are undergoing treatment with immunosuppressants, which lower the resistance to infection and to organisms previously not considered serious pathogens. Such patients present with fever, crackles, and physical findings that indicate solid areas (consolidation) in the lobes of the lung, including increased tactile fremitus, percussion dullness, bronchovesicular or bronchial breath sounds, egophony (auscultated bleating sounds), and whispered pectoriloquy (whispered sounds are auscultated through the chest wall). These changes occur because sound is transmitted better through solid or dense tissue

CHART 24-2
Prevention of Pneumonia

- Encourage frequent coughing and expectoration of secretions.
- Teach deep breathing exercises.
- Take special precautions to prevent infections.
- Change patient's position frequently.
- Institute tracheobronchial suctioning for patients at risk who are unable to cough up secretions.
- Carry out chest physical therapy to loosen secretions and improve expectoration of secretions.
- Promote frequent oral hygiene for patients who are on NPO regimens or antibiotics to minimize colonization of organisms.
- Administer sedatives and opioids judiciously to avoid suppressing respirations.
- Be especially alert to risk for pneumonia in the elderly, postoperative patients, those with a depressed immune system, those with compromised respiratory function, and those who are unconscious.
- Assure that respiratory equipment is properly cleaned.
- Encourage people to stop smoking and reduce alcohol intake.

(consolidation) than through normal tissue; they are described in Chapter 22.

In elderly patients or those with COPD, the symptoms may develop insidiously. Purulent sputum may be the only sign of pneumonia in these patients. It is difficult to detect subtle changes in their conditions because they already have seriously compromised pulmonary function.

Diagnostic Evaluation

The diagnosis of pneumonia is made by history (particularly of recent respiratory tract infection), physical examination, chest x-ray, blood culture (bloodstream invasion, called *bacteremia*, occurs frequently), and sputum examination.

- To obtain an adequate sample of sputum, the patient rinses the mouth with water to minimize contamination by normal oral flora. Then the patient is told to breathe deeply several times and then to cough deeply and expectorate the raised sputum into a sterile container.

Sputum also may be obtained by transtracheal aspiration (p. 456) or fiberoptic bronchoscopy (p. 454) in patients who cannot expectorate sputum or those who are unconscious, have abnormal immune mechanisms, or have developed pneumonia after taking antibiotics or while hospitalized.

Medical Management

Consolidation or dense areas in the lungs are seen on chest x-ray involving patchy areas or an entire lobe (lobar pneumonia). On physical examination, the findings vary depending on the severity of the pneumonia. The findings may include bronchovesicular or bronchial breath sounds, crackles, increased fremitus, positive egophony, and dullness on percussion.

The treatment of pneumonia includes administration of the appropriate antibiotic as determined by the results of the Gram stain. Penicillin G is clearly the antibiotic of choice for infection with *S. pneumoniae*. Other effective medications include erythromycin, clindamycin, the second and third generation cephalosporins, other penicillins, and trimethoprim-sulfamethoxazole (Bactrim). Treatment for other types of pneumonia is outlined in Table 24-1.

Mycoplasma pneumonia responds to erythromycin, tetracycline, and tetracycline derivatives (doxycycline). Other atypical pneumonias are viral in origin, and most do not respond to antimicrobials. *Pneumocystis carinii* responds best to pentamidine and trimethoprim-sulfamethoxazole (Bactrim, TMP-SMZ). Warm, moist inhalations are helpful in relieving bronchial irritation. The nursing care and treatment (with the exception of antimicrobial therapy) are the same as those given to the patient who has bacterial pneumonia.

The patient is placed on bed rest until infection shows signs of clearing. If hospitalized, the patient is observed carefully and continually until the clinical condition improves.

If hypoxemia develops, the patient is given oxygen. Arterial blood gas analysis is performed to determine the need for oxygen and to evaluate the effectiveness of the oxygen therapy. A high concentration of oxygen is contraindicated in patients with COPD because it may worsen alveolar ventilation by removing the patient's only remaining ventilatory drive and lead to respiratory decompensation. Respiratory support measures such as endotracheal intubation, high inspiratory oxygen concentrations, mechanical ventilation, and positive end expiratory pressure (PEEP) may be required for some patients. These treatment modalities are discussed in Chapter 25.

An example of a critical path for a patient with pneumonia is shown on pp. 488–489.

Gerontologic Considerations

Pneumonia in the elderly patient may occur spontaneously or as a complication of a chronic disease process. Pulmonary infections in the elderly frequently are difficult to treat and are associated with a higher mortality than such infections in younger patients. The onset of pneumonia may be signaled by general deterioration, weakness, abdominal symptoms, anorexia, confusion, tachycardia, and tachypnea. The diagnosis of pneumonia may be missed because the classic symptoms of cough, chest pain, sputum production, and fever often are absent in the elderly patient

The presence of some signs may be misleading. Abnormal breath sounds, for example, may be due to microatelectasis that occurs with aging. Because chronic congestive heart failure (CHF) is often seen in the elderly, chest x-rays may be obtained to assist in differentiating CHF from pneumonia as the cause of clinical signs and symptoms.

Supportive treatment includes increased fluid intake (with caution and frequent assessment in view of the risk of fluid overload in the elderly), oxygen therapy; and assistance with deep breathing, coughing, sputum production, and position changes, all of which are particularly important in nursing care of the elderly patient with pneumonia.

To reduce or prevent serious complications of pneumonia in the elderly, vaccination against pneumococcal and influenza viral infections has been recommended for persons over 50 years of age, nursing home residents, debilitated patients, and those with cardiovascular disease. The vaccine provides prevention against pneumonia that is caused by specific organisms.

The pneumococcal vaccine is recommended for high-risk groups, as well as for patients who have had a splenectomy and those with sickle cell disease or alcoholism.

❑ NURSING PROCESS
The Patient With Pneumonia

Assessment

Most patients with pneumonia are not hospitalized. However, because many hospitalized patients can develop pneumonia, a careful assessment by the nurse is critical to detect this problem. The presence of a fever in *any* hospitalized patient should alert the nurse to the possibility of bacterial pneumonia. A respiratory assessment will further identify

(*text continues on page 490*)

CRITICAL PATHWAY
Pneumonia Critical Path

(PLEASE NOTE: IN THIS EXAMPLE OF A CRITICAL PATH FOR PNEUMONIA, HOURS 24–72 HAVE BEEN CUT FROM PHASE II)

This critical path applies to all patients admitted with Community-Acquired or Institutional Pneumonia EXCEPT:

Patients with HIV, neutropenia, severe hypotension, steroid dependency > 20 mg/day, those requiring mechanical ventilation, or patients on immunosuppressive or chemotherapy.

Addressograph

	DATE:				DATE:							
	ER 1–4 Hours (Phase I)	**D**	**E**	**N**	**4–24 Hours (Phase II)**	**D**	**E**	**N**	**Day of Discharge (Phase III)**	**D**	**E**	**N**
Assessments Consults	Triage assessement*, HPI/per ER nursing standards*, notify attending physician Notify admitting resident				Assessment by resident and admission orders written within 4 hours of arrival on unit Resident to reassess diagnosis Nursing admission assessment w/focused respiratory assessment*				Review of systems assessment* Focused respiratory assessment*			
Labs and Diagnostics	AP&LAT CXR Time____, sputum CX & gram stain sent* Y__N__, pulse OX on room air result*____, ABG if pulse OX < 92% on R/A, blood CX x2*, CBC with diff*, SMA-7*, EKG female > 55/male> 45 or clinically indicated	— —	— —	— —	Sputum CX/gram stain if not obtained in ER or inadequate*	— —	— —	— —				
Interventions	VS per ER routine* Establish IV access*				VS q4 hours × 24 hours then q shift (unless ordered more frequently)*, I/O × 24 hours only (unless reordered)*				Vital signs*			

IV	IV fluids	IV fluids/heplock	D/C heplock*
Medication	*See Chart 24-3. Administer first dose of antibiotics after blood CXS obtained and sputum CX attempted time* ____, O_2 therapy	See Chart 24-3. Maintain O_2 for pOX < 92% per oxygen therapy protocol, tylenol/antipyretic PRN, review and document current medications	See Chart 24-3. Document need for pneumovax and administer if indicated but not contraindicated, tylenol/antipyretic PRN, oxygen therapy protocol per respiratory therapy pOX result* __
Diet/GI		As tolerated	
Activity	Bedrest/BRP	Bedrest/BRP, OOB to chair by 24 hours*, ambulate by 48 hours	Increase activity as tolerated*, patient and/or significant other able to accomplish ADL's* Y__ N__ Or appropriate support agency in place?* Y__ N__
Teaching	Instruct patient/significant other in disease process and treatment*	Smoking cessation encouraged*, instruct patient/significant other in disease process and treatment*	Instruct regarding completion of antibiotic prescription*, provide and review discharge instructions* Y__ N__
D/C, Planning & Follow-up		Assessment for SS consult* Elderly Y__ N__ Lives alone Y__ N__ Patient request Y__ N__ Social service consult called* X2270 Y__ N__	Has follow up appointment been made* Y__ N__ Arrange home oxygen therapy if pOX < 89% on room air Y__ N__
Key Patient Indicators	Clinically stable*: Pulse OX > 92% (w or w/o O_2) Y__ N__ Heart rate 60–135 Y__ N__ Respiratory rate 12–35 Y__ N__ SBP > 90 Y__ N__	Clinically stable*: Pulse OX > 92% (w or w/o O_2) Y__ N__ Heart rate 60–135 Y__ N__ Respiratory rate 12–35 Y__ N__ SBP > 90 Y__ N__	Afebrile* Y__ N__ Respiratory rate < 30* Y__ N__

*Indicates nursing activity. Signature sheet (last page) *must be signed.*
Initial in box or enter result as called for/or enter N/A if not applicable for the patient or the time frame.
This pathway was developed as a guideline. It is not intended to be used as a substitute for clinical judgment. Acceptable medical practice generally does include a variety of responses to a particular problem.
ABG = arterial blood gas; AP&LAT CXR = anterior/posterior chest x-ray; BRP = bathroom privileges; CBC with diff = complete blood count with differential; CX = culture; D/C = discontinue; EKG = electrocardiogram; GNR = gram-negative rods; HPI = history of present illness; I/O = intake and output; IV = intravenous; MRSA = methicillin-resistant *S. aureus*; OOB = out of bed; PCN = penicillin; pulse OX or pOX = pO_2 by pulse oximetry; SBP = systolic blood pressure; SMA-7 = electrolyte screen; SS = social service; TMP/SMX = trimethoprim/sulfamethoxazole; VS = vital signs.

CHART 24-3

Suggestions for Antibiotic Selection in the Patient with Pneumonia (see Critical Pathway)

Phase I (Hours 1–4)—Emergency Department

Community Acquired

Is the patient allergic to PCN?

- No → Ceftriaxone 1gm q24°
- Yes → TMP/SMX 2amps (320mg/1600mg) IV q12°

Institutional

Is the patient allergic to PCN?

- No → Ticarcillin/clavulanate 3.1gm q6°
- Yes → Ciprofloxacin 400mg IV q12° and Clindamycin 600mg IV q8°

Early Phase II (Hours 4–8)—Initial Housestaff Evaluation

Options based on clinical impression and/or Gram stain results

1. Consider broadening coverage or substituting erythromycin if Mycoplasma or Legionella is suspected.
2. Consider adding tobramycin if GNR is suspected.
3. Consider adding vancomycin if MRSA is suspected.
4. Consider adding anaerobic coverage to either ceftriaxone or TMP/SMX if clinically indicated.
5. Continue antibiotics as initiated in ED.

Phase III—Discharge

Options for oral antibiotics when no culture result is available

(Selection of oral antibiotic should be based on culture result when available.)

If parenteral antibiotic was:	Oral antibiotic choice is:
Ceftriaxone	Cefaclor or amoxicillin/clavulanate
TMP/SMX	TMP/SMX
Ceftriaxone and erythromycin	Cefaclor and erythromycin or clarithromycin alone
Ticarcillin/clavulanate	Amoxicillin/clavulanate
Ciprofloxacin and erythromycin	Ciprofloxacin and erythromycin

the clinical manifestations of pneumonia: pain; tachypnea; use of accessory muscles for breathing; rapid, bounding pulse or relative bradycardia; coughing; and purulent sputum. The severity, location, and cause of the chest pain must be identified as well as what relieves it. Any changes in temperature and pulse, amount, odor, and color of secretions, frequency and severity of the cough, and degree of tachypnea or shortness of breath also are monitored. Consolidation in the lungs is assessed by evaluating breath sounds (bronchial breathing, bronchovesicular rhonchi, or crackles), fremitus, egophony, whispered pectoriloquy, and the results of percussion (dullness in the affected area of the chest). (See Chapter 22 for a full discussion of these findings.)

The elderly patient is assessed for unusual behavior, alterations in mental status, prostration, and congestive heart failure. A restless, excited delirium may be exhibited, especially in patients with alcoholism.

Diagnosis

Nursing Diagnoses

Based on the assessment data, the patient's major nursing diagnoses may include:

- Ineffective airway clearance related to copious tracheobronchial secretions
- Activity intolerance related to altered respiratory function
- Risk for fluid volume deficit related to fever and dyspnea
- Knowledge deficit about the treatment regimen and preventive health measures

Collaborative Problems/ Potential Complications

Based on the assessment data, potential complications that may develop include:

- Hypotension and shock
- Respiratory failure
- Atelectasis
- Pleural effusion
- Delirium
- Superinfection

Planning and Implementation

Goals. The major goals for the patient may include improving airway patency, obtaining enough rest to conserve energy, maintaining proper fluid volume, understanding the treatment protocol and preventive measures, and absence of complications.

Nursing Interventions

Improving Airway Patency. *Removing secretions* is important because retained secretions interfere with gas exchange and may slow recovery. A high level of fluid intake (2 to 3 L/day) is encouraged, as adequate hydration thins and loosens pulmonary secretions and also replaces fluid losses resulting from fever, diaphoresis, dehydration, and a rapid respiratory rate. The air is humidified to loosen secretions and improve ventilation. A high-humidity face mask (using either compressed air or oxygen) delivers warm, humidified air to the tracheobronchial tree and liquefies secretions. The patient is encouraged to cough in the manner described for the postoperative patient (p. 367).

Chest physiotherapy is extremely important in loosening and mobilizing secretions. The patient is placed in the proper position to drain the involved lung, and then the chest is vibrated and percussed. After the lung has drained for 10 to 20 minutes (depending on tolerance), the patient is encouraged to breathe deeply and cough. If the patient is too weak to cough effectively, the mucus may need to be removed by nasotracheal suctioning or bronchoscopic aspiration as indicated.

Oxygen is administered as prescribed. The effectiveness of the oxygen concentration is monitored by assessing for the clinical manifestations of hypoxia and by arterial blood gas analysis.

Promoting Rest and Conserving Energy. The patient who is debilitated is encouraged to rest and remain in bed to avoid overexertion and possible exacerbation of symptoms. A comfortable position to promote rest and breathing (*e.g.*, semi-Fowler's) is assumed and is changed frequently. Outpatients are instructed not to overexert themselves and to engage in moderate activity only.

If sedatives or tranquilizers are prescribed, the patient's mental status (sensorium) is evaluated before the medications are administered. Restlessness, confusion, and aggression may be due to cerebral hypoxemia, in which case sedatives are contraindicated.

Promoting Fluid Intake. The respiratory rate of a patient with pneumonia increases because of dyspnea and fever. An increased rate leads to an increase in insensible fluid loss during exhalation. The patient can quickly become dehydrated. Therefore, fluids are encouraged (at least 2 L/day). Frequently, patients who are having difficulty breathing lose their appetite and will take only fluids. Fluids, then, are beneficial for volume replacement. Nutrients may also be administered by the IV route.

Patient Education and Home Care Considerations. After the fever subsides, the patient may gradually increase activities. Fatigue and weakness may be prolonged after pneumonia. Breathing exercises to clear the lungs and promote full lung expansion are encouraged. The patient is instructed to return to the clinic or physician's office for a follow-up chest x-ray and complete examination. A severely debilitated patient may require home care visits by the nurse to monitor status, prevent further complications, and provide ongoing patient teaching.

The nurse encourages the patient to stop tobacco smoking because it destroys tracheobronchial ciliary action, which is the first line of defense of the lungs. Smoking also irritates the mucous cells of the bronchi and inhibits the function of alveolar macrophage (scavenger) cells. The patient is instructed to avoid fatigue, sudden changes in temperature, and excessive alcohol intake, which lower resistance to pneumonia. The nurse reviews with the patient the principles of adequate nutrition and rest, because one episode of pneumonia may make the patient susceptible to recurring respiratory tract infections. The patient is encouraged to obtain influenza vaccine at the prescribed times, because influenza increases susceptibility to secondary bacterial pneumonia, especially that caused by *Staphylococcus*, *H. influenzae*, and *S. pneumoniae*. The patient is also encouraged to seek medical advice about receiving vaccine (Pneumovax) against *S. pneumoniae*. The care plan for the patient with bacterial pneumonia is found in Nursing Care Plan 24-1.

Monitoring and Managing Potential Complications

Persistent Symptoms. Lethal complications may develop during the first few days of antibiotic treatment. The patient is observed for response to antibiotic therapy and is monitored for persistent or recurrent fever. Inadequate lung drainage or insufficient blood supply to the involved lung may reduce the concentration of antibiotic agent reaching the invading organism.

Persistent or recurrent fever may be due to drug allergy (assess for rash); drug resistance or slow response of the susceptible organism; superinfection (a subsequent infection with another bacteria, which occurs during antibiotic therapy); pleural effusion; or pneumonia caused by unusual organisms (such as *Pneumocystis carinii* or *Aspergillus fumigatus*. Failure of the pneumonia to resolve, or persistence of symptoms in spite of improving on chest x-ray, raises the suspicion of underlying respiratory carcinoma.

Shock and Respiratory Failure. Patients usually respond to treatment within 24 to 48 hours after antibiotic therapy is initiated. Complications of pneumonia include *hypotension and shock* and *respiratory failure* (especially in gram-negative bacterial disease in the elderly).

These complications are encountered chiefly in patients who have received no specific treatment, received inadequate or delayed treatment or antimicrobial therapy to which the infecting organism is resistant, or in those with a preexisting disease that complicates the pneumonia.

If the patient is seriously ill, aggressive therapy may include hemodynamic and ventilatory support to combat peripheral collapse and maintain arterial blood pressure. A vasopressor agent may be administered intravenously by continuous infusion and at a rate that is readjusted in accordance with the pressure response. Corticosteroids may be administered parenterally to combat shock and toxicity in patients with pneumonia who are extremely ill and in apparent danger of succumbing to the infection. Patients may require endotracheal intubation and mechanical ventilation. Congestive heart failure, cardiac dysrhythmias, pericarditis, and myocarditis also are complications of pneumonia that may lead to shock.

Atelectasis and Pleural Effusion. *Atelectasis* (from obstruction of a bronchus by accumulated secretions) may occur at any stage of acute pneumonia. Pleural effusion, in

(text continues on page 495)

NURSING CARE PLAN 24–1
Care of the Patient With Bacterial Pneumonia

NURSING DIAGNOSIS: Ineffective airway clearance related to tracheobronchial secretions

GOAL: Improvement of airway patency

Nursing Interventions	Rationale	Expected Outcomes
1. Assist the patient to cough productively: a. Splint the patient's chest during coughing. b. Administer codeine as prescribed. c. Humidify air to loosen secretions and improve ventilation. Encourage increased fluid intake.	1. Depression of the cough reflex may produce retention of pulmonary secretions and lead to atelectasis. Elderly patients have a diminished cough reflex and may require vigorous measures (suctioning, bronchoscopy) for removal of secretions. Adequate hydration thins mucus and serves as an effective expectorant.	• Demonstrates effective coughing techniques. • States importance of drinking plenty of fluids. • Airway is clear of secretions. • Uses appropriate methods to reduce pleuritic pain. • Reports minimal pleuritic pain and uses methods to reduce it. • Verbalizes importance of taking antibiotics at prescribed intervals and reports side effects. • Arterial oxygen tension is 60 mm Hg or greater. • Temperature is normal. • Pulse and respiration are within normal limits. • Is normotensive. • Breath sounds are normal.
2. Perform postural drainage, percussion, and vibration to mobilize secretions.	2. Postural drainage uses gravity to remove secretions from the lung.	
3. Use measures to reduce pleuritic pain: a. Apply heat and cold as directed. b. Assist with intercostal nerve block with procaine when indicated. c. Use prescribed analgesics *with caution* to prevent depression of cough reflex and central nervous system respiratory drive. d. Treat dry cough and laryngospasm with aerosol therapy.	3. Pain and cough result from pleuritic invasion by pneumococci. The discomfort of pleuritic pain can interfere with the mechanics of ventilation and effective airway clearance.	
4. Administer prescribed antibiotic at correct time intervals. a. Penicillin is usually the drug of choice. Erythromycin or clindamycin can be prescribed if patient is allergic to penicillin. b. Observe patient for nausea, vomiting, diarrhea, anal pruritus, rash, and soft tissue reactions.	4. Treatment is based on results of sputum culture and sensitivity, and on the drainage of purulent secretions. Pneumococci are highly susceptible to the action of penicillin.	
5. Give oxygen as prescribed for dyspnea, circulatory disturbance, hypoxemia, or delirium. Monitor arterial blood gases and oxygen saturation through pulse oximetry to determine oxygen need and evaluate oxygen effectiveness.	5. Restlessness, confusion, and combative behavior may be due to cerebral hypoxia.	
6. Monitor the patient's response to therapy. a. Monitor temperature, pulse, respiration, and blood pressure every 4 hours and more frequently if indicated. Observe for continuing and recurring fever from drug allergy, drug resistance, or slow response to therapy, inadequate/inappropriate antimicrobial therapy, superinfection, or failure of pneumonia to resolve. b. Auscultate chest for crackles, signs of consolidation, or pleural effusion.	6. Lethal complications may develop during the early period of antimicrobial treatment. The temperature curve provides an index of the patient's response to therapy. Hypotension occurring early in the course of the illness may indicate hypoxia or bacteremia. Antipyretics are administered with caution, as they produce a decrease in temperature and thus interfere with evaluation of the temperature curve.	

(continued)

NURSING CARE PLAN 24–1 *(continued)*
Care of the Patient With Bacterial Pneumonia

NURSING DIAGNOSIS: Activity intolerance related to altered respiratory function

GOAL: Rest to conserve energy

Nursing Interventions	Rationale	Expected Outcomes
1. Encourage patient to rest as much as possible	1. Rest decreases oxygen demand.	• Remains at rest as needed. • Assumes best position for adequate breathing. • Oriented and alert.
2. Assist patient to assume a comfortable position and to change position frequently.	2. A comfortable position promotes rest. Semi-Fowler's position is desirable if patient is dyspneic. Changing positions frequently prevents pooling of secretions in the lungs.	
3. Evaluate sensorium before sedatives or tranquilizers are administered.	3. Restlessness, confusion, and aggression may indicate cerebral hypoxemia. If this is present, sedatives are inappropriate.	

NURSING DIAGNOSIS: High risk for fluid volume deficit related to fever and dyspnea

GOAL: Achieves adequate fluid balance

Nursing Interventions	Rationale	Expected Outcomes
1. Give patient 2 to 3 liters of fluid per day (unless patient has a fluid restriction).	1. Fever and tachypnea cause an increase in insensible water loss. Patient may become dehydrated. A poor appetite during bacterial pneumonia increases the need for increased fluid intake.	• Verbalizes the importance of drinking 2 to 3 liters of fluid per day. • Is adequately hydrated.
2. Monitor intake and output, skin, and vital signs.	2. Assists in assessment of fluid balance.	

NURSING DIAGNOSIS: Knowledge deficit about the treatment protocol and methods of prevention

GOAL: Acquisition of knowledge about the treatment protocol and preventive aspects

Nursing Interventions	Rationale	Expected Outcomes
1. Teach the patient about preventive measures: a. Avoid smoking b. Maintain natural resistance (adequate rest and nutrition and proper exercise). c. Obtain influenza vaccine and pneumococcal vaccine at prescribed times. d. Avoid fatigue, chilling, and excessive alcohol intake, which lower resistance to pneumonia. e. Report any signs and symptoms of a respiratory tract infection to primary care provider. f. Have follow-up examinations after discharge from the hospital.	1. Cigarette smoking destroys tracheobronchial ciliary action, stimulates mucosal cells, causes increased mucus production, and inhibits alveolar scavenger cells (macrophages). Susceptibility to recurring respiratory infections increases after initial exposure. Upper respiratory tract infections may lead to bacterial invasion of the respiratory tract. Pneumonia frequently coexists with other pathologic pulmonary conditions, namely, cancer of the lung.	• Identifies factors that contribute to development of pneumonia. • Stops smoking. • Makes an appointment for a follow-up chest x-ray and influenza and pneumococcal vaccinations. • Alternates rest periods with increasing activity.

(continued)

NURSING CARE PLAN 24-1 *(continued)*
Care of the Patient With Bacterial Pneumonia

Nursing Interventions	Rationale	Expected Outcomes
COLLABORATIVE PROBLEMS: Potential complications of pneumonia include superinfection; atelectasis; pleural effusion; hypotension/shock; and respiratory failure.		
Superinfection		
1. Asses vital signs. 2. Monitor WBC values. 3. Administer antibiotic therapy, as ordered, and instruct the patient concerning the importance of following the prescribed regimen.	1. A change in vital signs, including an elevated temperature, tachypnea, and tachycardia may be seen with superinfection. 2. An elevation in WBC while on antibiotics may indicate super infection. 3. Maintenance of therapeutic blood level of antibiotics is critical to treatment of an underlying infectious process.	• Afebrile. • Normal temperature and pulse. • Normal WBC. • Afebrile. • Follows antibiotic regimen, as prescribed.
Atelectasis		
1. Monitor respiratory status, including rate and pattern of respirations, breath sounds and signs/symptoms of respiratory distress. 2. Instruct and encourage diaphragmatic breathing and effective coughing techniques. 3. Uses incentive spirometry, as prescribed	1. A change in respiratory status, including tachypnea, dyspnea, and diminished or absent breath sounds, may indicate change in respiratory status. 2. These techniques improve ventilation by opening airways, thereby improving gas exchange. 3. Incentive spirometry promotes maximal lung expansion.	• Normal respiratory rate and pattern. • Normal breath sounds. • Demonstrates diaphragmatic breathing and coughing. • Uses incentive spirometry as prescribed.
Pleural Effusion		
1. Monitor respiratory status, including rate and pattern of respirations, breath sounds, signs/symptoms of respiratory distress, and percussion. 2. Monitor and assist with diagnostic tests. 3. Explain thoracentesis procedure to patient.	1. Dyspnea, coughing, decreased or absent breath sounds, egophony and dullness on the affected side may indicate a pleural effusion. 2. The presence of a pleural effusion is confirmed on chest x-ray and thoracentesis. 3. Knowledge of the procedure will assist patient in coping and alleviate anxiety about the unknown.	• Normal respiratory rate and pattern. • Diagnostic work-up is performed. • Knowledgeable about thoracentesis procedure.
Hypotension/Shock		
1. Assess vital signs. 2. Notify the physician immediately of any significant change in vital signs. 3. Administer IV therapy and medications, as prescribed.	1. A change in vital signs, including fever, tachycardia, tachypnea, and a decreased blood pressure may be the signs of impending septic shock. 2. Impending septic shock is a medical emergency requiring immediate intervention. 3. IV fluids (crystalloids) are given to maintain blood pressure. Cardiotonic agents may be given to improve cardiac efficiency.	• Normal vital signs. • Absence of shock. • IV and drug therapy administered as prescribed.

(continued)

NURSING CARE PLAN 24–1 (*continued*)
Care of the Patient With Bacterial Pneumonia

Nursing Interventions	Rationale	Expected Outcomes
Respiratory Failure		
1. Monitor respiratory status, including rate and pattern of respirations, breath sounds, and signs/symptoms of respiratory distress.	1. Recognition of a change in respiratory function will prevent further complications, such as respiratory failure, severe hypoxia, and hypercapnia.	• Normal respiratory rate and pattern. • Absence of indicators of hypoxia and hypercapnia. • Maintains normal ABGs. • Evidence of normal ABGs.
2. Monitor arterial blood gases.	2. Recognition of changes in oxygenation and acid–base balance will assist in correcting and preventing complications.	
3. Administer supplemental oxygen, including mechanical ventilation, as prescribed.	3. Respiratory failure is a medical emergency. Hypoxia is a hallmark sign. Administration of oxygen therapy and effective mechanical ventilation are critical to survival.	

which fluid collects in the pleural space (p. 502), is fairly common and may signal the beginning of empyema (purulent fluid within the pleural space). A diagnostic thoracentesis is usually necessary to confirm a *pleural effusion*. After the pleural effusion is visualized on chest x-ray, a chest tube may be inserted to treat pleural infection by establishing proper drainage of the empyema.

Delirium. Delirium is another possible complication and is considered a medical emergency when it occurs. It may be caused by hypoxia, meningitis, or alcohol withdrawal syndrome. The patient with delirium is given oxygen, adequate hydration, and mild sedation as prescribed and is observed constantly.

Superinfection. Superinfection may occur with the administration of very large doses of antibiotics, such as penicillin, or with the use of combinations of antibiotics. If the patient improves and the fever diminishes after initial antibiotic therapy, but subsequently there is a rise in temperature with increasing cough and evidence that the pneumonia has spread, a superinfection is likely. Antibiotics are changed appropriately or discontinued entirely in some cases.

Evaluation

Expected Outcomes

1. Demonstrates improved airway patency as evidenced by adequate blood gases, normal temperature, normal breath sounds, and effective coughing
2. Rests and conserves energy by remaining in bed while symptomatic.
3. Maintains an adequate fluid intake as evidenced by drinking appropriate amounts of fluid and having normal skin turgor
4. Complies with treatment protocol and prevention strategies
5. Is free of complications
   a. Normal vital signs and arterial blood gases
   b. Productive cough
   c. Exhibits no signs or symptoms of shock, respiratory failure, or pleural effusion
   d. Oriented and aware of surroundings

Pulmonary Tuberculosis

Tuberculosis (TB) is an infectious disease, which primarily affects the lung parenchyma. It may also be transmitted to other parts of the body, including the meninges, kidneys, bones, and lymph nodes. The primary infectious agent, *Mycobacterium tuberculosis*, is an acid fast aerobic rod that grows slowly and is sensitive to heat and ultraviolet (UV) light. *M. bovis* and *M. avium* have, on rare occasions, been associated with the development of a tuberculosis infection.

Tuberculosis is a worldwide public health problem. The mortality and morbidity rates continue to rise. TB is closely associated with poverty, malnutrition, overcrowding, substandard housing, and inadequate health care. In 1952, antituberculosis drugs were introduced and the rate of reported cases of TB in the United States declined an average of 6% each year between 1953 and 1985. It was thought that by the early part of the 21st century TB in the United States might be eliminated. However, since 1985 the trend has been reversed and the number of cases has increased. This change has been attributed to several factors, including increased immigration, the HIV epidemic, multidrug-resistant strains of TB, and inadequate funding of the United States public health system.

Transmission and Risk Factors

Tuberculosis is spread from person to person by airborne transmission. An infected person, through talking, coughing, sneezing, laughing, or singing, releases large (greater than 100 μ) and small (1 to 5 μ) droplets. The large droplets settle, while the small droplets remain suspended in the air and are inhaled by the susceptible person. Persons who are at greatest risk for acquiring tuberculosis are:

- Those in close contact with someone who has active TB
- Immunocompromised persons (including the elderly, patients with cancer, those on corticosteroid therapy, or those infected with HIV)
- IV drug users and alcoholics
- Any person without adequate health care (the homeless; impoverished; ethnic and racial minorities, particularly, children under 15 years of age and young adults between 15 and 44 years of age)
- Any person with pre-existing medical conditions (*e.g.*, diabetes, chronic renal failure, silicosis, malnourishment, gastrectomy or jejunoileal bypass)
- Immigrants from countries with a high incidence of TB (southeast Asia, Africa, Latin America, Caribbean)
- Any person who is institutionalized (*e.g.*, long-term care facilities, psychiatric institutions, prisons)
- Persons living in overcrowded substandard housing
- Healthcare workers

The risk for acquiring tuberculosis also depends on the density of the organisms in the air.

Pathophysiology

A susceptible person inhales mycobacterium bacilli and becomes infected. The bacteria are transmitted through the airways to the alveoli, where they are deposited and begin to multiply. The bacilli are also transported via the lymph system and bloodstream to other parts of the body (kidneys, bones, cerebral cortex), and other areas of the lungs (upper lobes).

The body's immune system responds by initiating an inflammatory reaction. Phagocytes (neutrophils and macrophages) engulf many of the bacteria; tuberculosis-specific lymphocytes lyse (destroy) the bacilli and normal tissue. This tissue reaction results in accumulation of exudate in the alveoli, causing bronchopneumonia. The initial infection usually occurs 2 to 10 weeks after exposure.

New tissue masses, called *granulomas*, which are clumps of live and dead bacilli, are surrounded by macrophages forming a protective wall. Granulomas are transformed to a fibrous tissue mass. The central portion of the fibrous mass is called *Ghon tubercle*. The material (bacteria and macrophages) become necrotic, forming a cheesy mass. It may become calcified, forming a collagenous scar. The bacteria become dormant, with no further progression of active disease.

After initial exposure and infection, the person may develop active disease because of a compromised or inadequate immune system response. Active disease may also occur with reinfection and activation of dormant bacteria. In this case, the Ghon tubercle ulcerates, releasing the cheesy material into the bronchi. The bacteria then become airborne, resulting in further spread of the disease. The ulcerated tubercle heals, forming scar tissue. The infected lung becomes more inflamed, resulting in further development of bronchopneumonia, tubercle formation, and so forth.

Unless the process can be arrested, it spreads slowly downward to the hilum of the lungs and later extends to adjacent lobes. The process may be prolonged and characterized by long remissions when the disease is arrested, only to be followed by periods of renewed activity. Only approximately 10% of persons who are initially infected develop active disease.

Clinical Manifestations

Pulmonary tuberculosis is insidious. Most patients present with low grade fever, fatigue, anorexia, weight loss, night sweats, chest pain, and a persistent cough. The cough initially may be nonproductive, but may progress to mucopurulent sputum with hemoptysis.

Tuberculosis may have atypical manifestations in the elderly, such as unusual behavior and an altered mental status, fever, anorexia, and weight loss. The TB bacilli may survive more than 50 years in a dormant state.

Diagnostic Evaluation

The diagnosis of tuberculosis is made by a complete history, physical examination, chest x-ray, acid-fast bacillus (AFB) smear, sputum culture, and tuberculin skin test. The chest x-ray usually will reveal lesions in the upper lobes. An early morning sputum for an AFB culture is obtained; the AFB smear will indicate whether mycobacterium is present, indicating the diagnosis of tuberculosis.

Tuberculin Skin Test. The Mantoux Test is a skin test that is used to determine if a person has been infected with the TB bacilli. Tubercle bacillus extract (tuberculin) is injected into the intradermal layer of the inner aspect of the forearm, approximately 4 inches below the elbow (Fig. 24-2). Intermediate strength (5 Tu) of purified protein derivative (PPD) is used. Using a tuberculin syringe, a ½-inch 26- or 27- gauge needle is inserted beneath the skin with the bevel of the needle up. Then 0.1 ml of PPD is injected, creating an elevation in the skin, a wheal. The site, antigen name, strength, lot number, and date and time of the test are recorded. The test is read 48 to 72 hours after injection. The tuberculin skin test is a delayed localized reaction, which indicates that the person is sensitive to tuberculin.

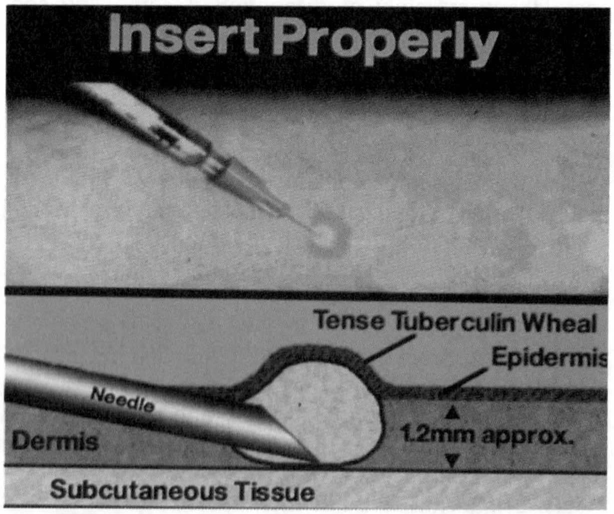

FIGURE 24-2. The Mantoux test for tuberculosis. Correct technique for inserting the needle.

A reaction occurs when both induration and erythema are noted. After the area is inspected for induration (hardening), it is lightly palpated across the injection site, from the area of normal skin to the margins of the induration. The diameter of the induration (*not erythema*) is measured in millimeters at its widest part (Fig. 24-3). Erythema, or redness without induration, is not considered to be significant. The size of the induration is documented.

Interpretation of Results. The size of the induration determines whether there has been a significant or nonsignificant reaction (versus positive or negative). A reaction of 0 to 4 mm is not considered significant; a reaction of 5 mm or greater *may* be significant (see Fig. 24-3). An induration of 10 mm or greater *is* usually considered significant. A significant reaction indicates that a patient has been exposed to *M. tuberculosis* recently or in the past or vaccinated with Bacilli Calmette-Guerin (BCG) vaccine. The BCG vaccine is given to produce a greater resistance to developing TB. It is effective in anywhere from 0% to 76% of those who receive it. It is used in Europe and Latin America, but is not routinely used in the United States.

A *significant* (positive) reaction does not necessarily mean that active disease is present in the body. Most (more than 90%) people who are tuberculin-significant reactors do *not* develop clinical tuberculosis. (However, all significant reactors are candidates for active tuberculosis.) In general, the more intense the reaction, the greater the likelihood of an active infection.

A *nonsignificant* (negative) skin test does not exclude tuberculous infection or disease as patients who are immunosuppressed are unable to mount an immune response adequate (anergy) to produce a positive skin test. Many elderly patients may have no reaction or delayed reactivity for up to a week. This is known as a recall phenomenon. A second skin test is repeated in 1 to 2 weeks.

Other Skin Tests. Multiple-puncture skin tests are used for surveying and screening large groups and are not intended to establish positive diagnosis, because there is no way to standardize the amount of tuberculin introduced. The test is conducted by introducing tuberculin into the skin either by puncturing the skin with a device with points coated with dried tuberculin or by puncturing the skin after a thin coat of liquid tuberculin has been spread on it. The test is read 48 to 72 hours after administration. If the reaction is in the form of papules, the diameter of the largest single papule or the largest diameter of coalescent induration is measured. If a blister is present, the person is sensitive to the tuberculin and is termed a *reactor*. However, not all reactors are infected with tuberculosis. All reactors should be retested with the Mantoux test and should have a chest x-ray obtained.

Medical Management

Pulmonary tuberculosis is treated primarily with chemotherapeutic agents (antituberculosis agents) for a period of 6 to 12 months. Five first-line medications are used: isoniazid (INH), rifampin (RIF), streptomycin (SM), ethambutol (EMB), and pyrazinamide (PZA) (Table 24-2). Capreomycin, kanamycin, ethionamide, para-aminosalicylate sodium, amikacin, and cyclizine are second-line medications.

Resistance of *M. tuberculosis* to medications continues to be a growing issue worldwide. Although TB drug resistance has been identified since the 1950s, the incidence of multidrug resistance has created a new challenge. Several types of drug resistance must be considered when planning effective therapy:

- *Primary drug resistance* is resistance to one of the first-line antituberculosis agents in a person who has not had previous treatment.
- *Secondary or acquired drug resistance* is resistance to one or more antituberculosis agents in a patient undergoing therapy.
- *Multidrug resistance* is resistance to two agents, namely, INH and RIF.

The recommended treatment for newly diagnosed cases of pulmonary tuberculosis is a multiple medication regimen, including INH, RIF, and PZA for 4 months, with INH and RIF continuing for an additional 2 months (total of 6 months). Currently, each agent is contained in a separate pill. A new three-in-one anti-tuberculosis pill of INH, RIF and PZA has been developed, which will have tremendous

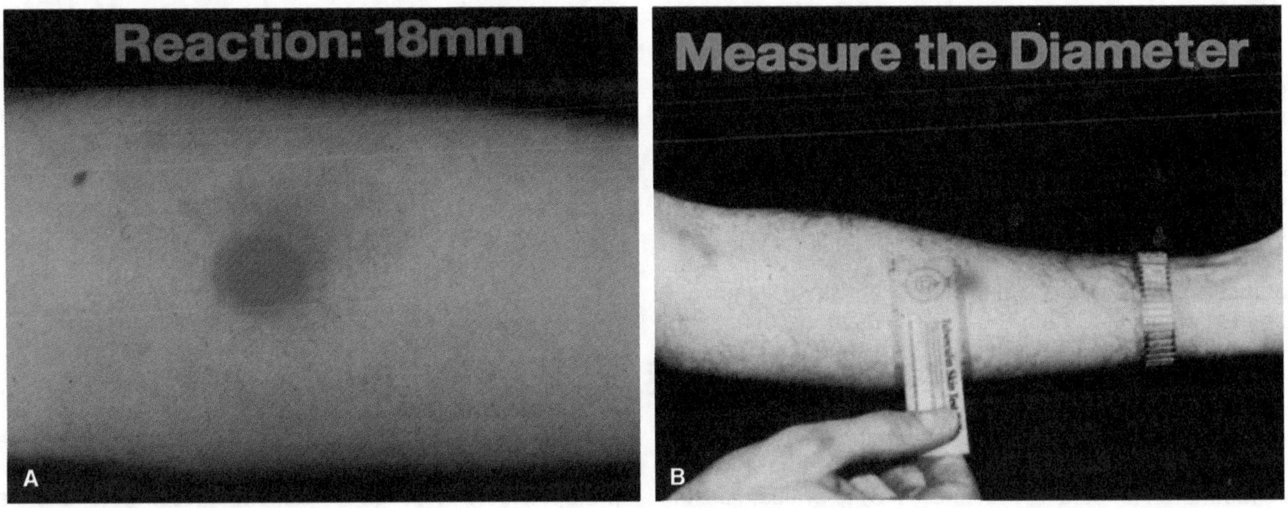

FIGURE 24-3. Reaction to Mantoux test. (**A**) Appearance of the reaction. (**B**) The area of the reaction is measured to determine the extent of the reaction.

TABLE 24-2 First-Line Antituberculosis Drugs

Commonly Used Agents	Adult Daily Dosage*	Most Common Side Effects	Drug Interactions†	Remarks*
Isoniazid (INH)	300 mg*	Peripheral neuritis, hepatitis, hypersensitivity	Phenytoin–synergistic Antabuse Alcohol	Bactericidal Pyridoxine as prophylaxis for neuritis. Monitor SGOT (AST) and SGPT (ALT).
Rifampin (RIF)	600 mg*	Hepatitis, febrile reaction, purpura (rare), nausea, vomiting	Rifampin increases metabolism of oral contraceptives, quinidine, corticosteroids, coumarin drugs and methadone, digoxin, oral hypoglycemics; PAS may interfere with absorption of rifampin.	Bactericidal. Orange urine and other body secretions. Discoloring of contact lenses. Monitor SGOT (AST) and SGPT (ALT).
Streptomycin (SM)	15 mg/kg* (1 gm maximum)*	8th cranial nerve damage (may lead to deafness), nephrotoxicity	Neuromuscular blocking agents—may be potentiated to cause prolonged paralysis.	Bactericidal in alkaline *p*H. Use with caution in elderly or in those with renal disease. Monitor vestibular function, audiograms, BUN/creatinine.
Pyrazinamide (PZA)	25 mg/kg* (2.5 g maximum)*	Hyperuricemia, hepatotoxicity, skin rash, arthralgias, GI distress		Bactericidal. Monitor uric acid, SGOT (AST) and SGPT (ALT).
Ethambutol (EMB)	15 mg/kg* (2.5 g maximum)*	Optic neuritis (may lead to blindness; very rare at 15 mg/kg), skin rash		Bacteriostatic. Use with caution with renal disease or when eye testing is not feasible. Monitor visual acuity, color discrimination.‡

*Check product labeling for detailed information on dose, contraindications, drug interaction, adverse reactions, and monitoring.
†Reference should be made to current literature, particularly on rifampin, because it indicates hepatic microenzymes and therefore interacts with many drugs.
‡Initial examination should be performed at start of treatment.
(Modified from Lordi GM and Reichman L. Treatment of tuberculosis. American Family Physician 1991; 44(1):220.

implications in terms of possible improved adherence to the drug regimen. Initially, ethambutol and streptomycin may be included in the initial therapy until drug resistance studies are available. The medication regimen, however, may continue for 12 months. A person is considered noninfectious after 2 to 3 weeks of continuous medication therapy.

Isoniazid (INH) may be used as a preventive measure for those persons who are known to be at risk for significant disease, for example, household family members of patients with active disease. This prophylactic treatment regimen involves taking daily doses of INH for 6 to 12 months. To minimize side effects, pyridoxine (vitamin B_6) may be administered. Liver enzymes, blood urea nitrogen (BUN), and creatinine are monitored monthly. Sputum culture results are monitored for acid-fast bacillus (AFB) to evaluate the effectiveness of treatment and the patient's compliance with therapy.

Chart 24-4 summarizes the recommendations of the Centers for Disease Control (CDC) to prevent transmission of TB in health care settings.

❑ NURSING PROCESS
The Patient With Tuberculosis

Assessment

A complete history and physical examination are performed. Clinical manifestations of fever, anorexia, weight loss, night sweats, fatigue, cough, and sputum production prompt a more thorough assessment of respiratory function.

CHART 24-4
Preventing the Transmission of Tuberculosis in Health-Care Settings

1. Early identification and treatment of persons with active tuberculosis (TB)
   a. Maintain a high index of suspicion for TB to identify cases rapidly.
   b. Promptly initiate effective multidrug anti-TB therapy based on clinical and drug-resistance surveillance data.
2. Prevention of spread of infectious droplet nuclei by source control methods and by reduction of microbial contamination of indoor air
   a. Initiate acid-fast bacilli (AFB) isolation precautions immediately for all patients who are suspected or confirmed to have active TB and who may be infectious. AFB isolation precautions include use of a private room with negative pressure in relation to surrounding areas and a minimum of six air exchanges per hour. Air from the room should be exhausted directly to the outside. Use of ultraviolet lamps and/or high-efficiency particulate air filters to supplement ventilation may be considered.
   b. Persons entering the AFB isolation room should use disposable particulate respirators that fit snugly around the face.
   c. Continue AFB isolation precautions until there is clinical evidence of reduced infectiousness (i.e., cough has substantially decreased, and the number of organisms on sequential sputum smears is decreasing). If drug resistance is suspected or confirmed, continue AFB precautions until the sputum smear is negative for AFB.
   d. Use special precautions during cough-inducing procedures.
3. Surveillance for TB transmission
   a. Maintain surveillance for TB infection among health-care workers (HCWs) by routine, periodic tuberculin skin testing. Recommend appropriate preventive therapy for HCWs when indicated.
   b. Maintain surveillance for TB cases among patients and HCWs.
   c. Promptly initiate contact investigation procedures among HCWs, patients, and visitors exposed to an untreated, or ineffectively treated, infectious TB patient for whom appropriate AFB procedures are not in place. Recommend appropriate therapy or preventive therapy for contacts with disease or TB infection without current disease. Therapeutic regimens should be chosen based on the clinical history and local drug-resistance surveillance data.

(Centers for Disease Control and Prevention. MMWR 1991; 40:586.)

Any change in temperature or respiratory rate, amount and color of secretions, frequency and severity of cough, and chest pain are assessed. The lungs are assessed for consolidation by evaluating breath sounds (diminished, bronchial, or bronchovesicular sounds, crackles), fremitus, egophony, and results of percussion (dullness). The patient may also have enlarged, painful lymph nodes. The patient's emotional readiness to learn, as well as perceptions and understanding of tuberculosis and its treatment are also assessed. The results of the physical and laboratory evaluations are also reviewed.

Diagnosis

Nursing Diagnoses

Based on the assessment data, the nursing diagnoses may include:

- Ineffective airway clearance related to copious tracheobronchial secretions
- Nonadherence to treatment regimen
- Activity intolerance related to fatigue, altered nutritional status, and fever
- Knowledge deficit about treatment regimen and preventive health measures

Collaborative Problems/ Potential Complications

Based on the assessment data, the potential complications may include:

- Malnutrition
- Side effects of medication therapy: hepatitis, neurologic changes (deafness or neuritis), skin rash, GI upset
- Multidrug resistance
- Spread of TB infection (miliary TB)

Planning and Implementation

Goals. The major goals for the patient include maintenance of a patent airway, knowledge about the disease and treatment regimen, adherence to the medication regimen, increased activity tolerance, and absence of complications.

Nursing Interventions

Promoting Airway Clearance. Copious secretions can block the airways in many patients with tuberculosis and interfere with adequate gas exchange. Increasing fluid intake provides systemic hydration and serves as an effective expectorant. The patient is instructed about the best position to assume to facilitate drainage. A high humidity face mask or a humidifier at home may assist in liquefying secretions.

Advocating Adherence to Treatment Regimen. The multiple drug regimen that a patient must follow can be quite complex. Understanding the medications, schedule, and side effects is important. The patient must understand that tuberculosis is a communicable disease and that taking medications is the most effective means of preventing transmission. The major reason treatment fails is that patients do not take their medications regularly and for the time prescribed. The patient is carefully instructed about important hygienic measures, including mouth care, covering of the mouth and nose when coughing and sneezing, proper disposal of tissues, and handwashing.

Promoting Activity and Adequate Nutrition. Patients with TB are often debilitated due to a prolonged chronic illness and impaired nutritional status. A progressive activity schedule is planned, which focuses on increasing activity tolerance and muscle strength.

Anorexia, weight loss, and malnutrition are common in patients with TB. The patient's willingness to eat may be altered by fatigue from excessive coughing, sputum production, chest pain, or a generalized debilitated state. A nutritional plan that allows for small frequent meals may be required. Liquid nutritional supplements, such as Ensure and Isocal, may assist in meeting the basic caloric requirements.

Patient Education and Home Care Considerations. The nurse has an important role in the care of the patient with TB and the family, including assessing the patient's ability to continue therapy at home. The nurse assesses the patient for adverse drug reactions and participates in surveying the patient's home and work environment to identify other persons who may have been in contact with the patient during the infectious stage. Follow-up screening for contacts may need to be arranged.

The nurse instructs the patient and family about infection control procedures, such as proper disposal of tissues, covering the mouth during coughing, and handwashing. In some cases when the ability of the patient to comply with the medication regimen is in question, referring the patient to an outpatient clinic for daily administration of medications may be required.

Monitoring and Managing Potential Complications

Inadequate Nutritional Intake and Malnutrition. This may be a consequence of the patient's life-style, lack of knowledge about adequate nutrition and its role in health maintenance, lack of resources, fatigue, or lack of appetite because of coughing and mucus production. To counter the effects of these factors, the nurse works in collaboration with the dietician, physician, social worker, and patient to identify strategies to ensure an adequate nutritional intake and to ensure availability of nutritious food. Identifying facilities (*e.g.*, shelters, soup kitchens) that provide meals in the patient's neighborhood may increase the likelihood that the patient with limited resources will have access to a more nutritious intake. Use of dietary supplements (*e.g.*, Ensure, Isocal) may be suggested as a strategy for increasing dietary intake.

Side Effects of Medication Therapy. These are assessed because they are often a reason the patient fails to adhere to the prescribed medication plan. Efforts are made to reduce the side effects in an effort to increase the patient's willingness to take the medications as prescribed.

Patients are instructed to take their medication either on an empty stomach or at least 1 hour before meals because food interferes with drug absorption. The result frequently is gastrointestinal upset. Patients on INH should avoid foods containing tyramine and histamine (tuna, aged cheese, red wine, soy sauce, yeast extracts), which may result in headache, flushing, hypotension, lightheadedness, palpitations, and diaphoresis.

The patient is monitored for other side effects of medications prescribed for TB; these include hepatitis, neurologic changes (deafness, neuritis), and skin rash. Liver enzymes, BUN, and serum creatinine are monitored to detect changes in liver and kidney function due to these medications. Sputum culture results are monitored for acid-fast bacillus (AFB) to evaluate effectiveness of the treatment regimen and compliance with therapy.

Rifampin can increase the metabolism of medications, making them less effective, particularly, beta blockers, oral anticoagulants, digoxin, quinidine, corticosteriods, coumadin, oral hypoglycemic agents, oral contraceptives, theophylline, and verapamil. Patients are informed that rifampin may discolor contact lenses; therefore, use of eye glasses is suggested during treatment.

Multidrug Resistance. The nurse carefully monitors vital signs and observes for spikes in temperature. Any change in the patient's respiratory status is reported to the physician. The patient is instructed about the risk of drug resistance if the medication regimen is not continuously followed.

The length of treatment frequently causes patients to stop taking their medicine. Failure to comply with the prescribed regimen has resulted in *multidrug resistance*. In some cities, such as New York City, multidrug resistance has caused extensive spread of the disease. Patients are instructed about the importance of taking medications as prescribed and reporting changes in symptoms.

Spread of Tuberculosis Infection. Spread of tuberculosis injection to nonpulmonary sites of the body is known as **miliary TB**. It is the result of invasion of the bloodstream by the tubercle bacillus (Ghon tubercle). Usually it results from late reactivation of a dormant infection in the lung or elsewhere and is spread through the blood to other organs. The origin of the bacilli that enter the bloodstream is either some chronic focus that has ulcerated into a blood vessel or multitudes of miliary tubercles lining the inner surface of the thoracic duct. The organisms migrate from these foci into the bloodstream, are carried throughout the body, and disseminate throughout all tissues, with tiny miliary tubercles developing in the lungs, spleen, liver, kidneys, meninges, and other organs.

The clinical course of miliary tuberculosis may vary from an acute, rapidly progressive infection with high fever to an indolent process with low-grade fever, anemia, and debilitation. At first, there may be no localizing signs except for an enlarged spleen and a reduced number of leukocytes. Within a few weeks, however, the chest x-ray reveals small densities scattered diffusely throughout both lung fields; these are the miliary tubercles, which gradually increase in size.

The possibility of TB in nonpulmonary sites in the body requires that the patient be carefully monitored for this very serious form of the infection. The nurse carefully monitors vital signs and observes for spikes in temperature as well as changes in renal and cognitive function. Few physical signs may be elicited on physical examination of the chest, but at this stage, the patient has a severe cough, dyspnea, and cyanosis. Treatment of miliary TB is the same as that of pulmonary TB.

Evaluation

Expected Outcomes

1. Maintains a patent airway by managing secretions with humidification, fluid intake, coughing, and postural drainage
2. Demonstrates an adequate level of knowledge

   a. Lists medications by name and the correct schedule for taking them
   b. Names expected side effects of medications
3. Adheres to treatment regimen by taking medications as prescribed and reporting for follow-up screening
4. Participates in preventive measures
   a. Disposes of used tissues properly
   b. Encourages persons who are close contacts to report for testing
5. Maintains activity schedule
6. Takes steps to minimize side effects
   a. Takes supplemental vitamins (vitamin B_6), as prescribed, to minimize peripheral neuropathy
   b. Avoids use of alcohol
   c. Avoids foods containing tyramine and histamine
   d. Has regular physical examinations and blood tests to evaluate liver and kidney function, neuropathy, and visual acuity
7. Exhibits no complications
   a. Maintains adequate weight or gains weight if indicated
   b. Exhibits normal results of tests of liver and kidney function

Lung Abscess

Pathogenesis

A lung abscess is a localized necrotic lesion of the lung parenchyma containing purulent material; the lesion collapses and forms a cavity.

Most lung abscesses occur because material has been aspirated from the nose or mouth. Abscesses also may occur secondary to mechanical or functional obstruction of the bronchi, including tumor, foreign body, or bronchial stenosis. Or they may result from necrotizing pneumonias, tuberculosis, pulmonary embolism, or chest trauma.

Patients who have impaired cough reflexes and are unable to close the glottis, or those who have swallowing difficulties, are at risk for aspirating foreign material and developing a lung abscess. Other at-risk patients include those with an altered state of consciousness from anesthesia, central nervous system disorders (seizure, stroke), drug addiction, alcoholism, or esophageal disease, as well as patients fed by nasogastric tube. Patients with compromised immune function are at great risk. Patients with pneumonia can also develop abscesses.

The site of the lung abscess is related to gravitational pull determined by the patient's position. For patients in a recumbant positon, the posterior segment of the upper right lobe is the most common site. The apical segments of both lower lobes are the next most frequent areas in which lung abscess occurs.

In the initial stages, the cavity in the lung may or may not extend directly into a bronchus. Eventually the abscess becomes surrounded, or *encapsulated,* by a wall of fibrous tissue, except at one or two points where the necrotic process extends until it reaches the lumen of some bronchus or the pleural space and thus establishes a communication with the respiratory tract, the pleural cavity, or both. If the bronchus is involved, the purulent contents are expectorated continuously in the form of sputum, whereas if the pleura is involved, empyema (collection of pus in the pleural cavity) results; if both types of communication or connection are present, the problem becomes a *bronchopleural fistula.*

The aerobic organism most frequently associated with lung abscesses is *Staphylococcus aureus*. Anaerobic organisms, however, are much more prevalent. They vary depending on the underlying predisposing factors.

Clinical Manifestations

The clinical presentations of a lung abscess may vary from a mild productive cough to acute illness. Patients may be acutely or chronically ill. Most patients have a fever and a productive cough of moderate to copious amounts of foul-smelling sputum that is often bloody. Pleurisy, or dull chest pain, dyspnea, weakness, anorexia, and weight loss are common.

Diagnostic Evaluation

Physical examination of the chest may reveal dullness on percussion and decreased or absent breath sounds with an intermittent pleural friction rub on auscultation. Crackles may be present. Confirmation of the diagnosis is made by chest x-ray, sputum culture, and in some cases, fiberoptic bronchoscopy. The chest x-ray will reveal an infiltrate with an air–fluid level. It most commonly occurs on the right side in the lower lobe.

Medical Management

The findings of the history, physical examination, chest x-ray, and sputum culture will indicate the type of organism and treatment required.

Intravenous antimicrobial therapy depends on the results of sputum culture and sensitivity and is administered for an extended period. The treatment of choice depends on the isolated organism.

Clindamycin is the medication of choice, followed by penicillin with metronidazole. Ceftazidime plus aminoglycoside or cefoperazone is used when the organism is *Pseudomonas aeruginosa*. *S. aureus* is treated with oxacillin, nafcillin, or a first generation cephalosporin (cefuroxime). Large intravenous doses are generally required, because the antibiotic must penetrate the necrotic tissue and the fluid in the abscess. This is followed by long-term therapy with an oral agent.

Adequate drainage of the lung abscess often is achieved through postural drainage and chest physiotherapy. The use of bronchoscopy to drain an abscess is controversial. It can be useful to rule out a foreign body or a tumor or to locate the site of the draining bronchus.

A *diet* high in protein and calories is necessary because chronic infection is associated with a catabolic state, necessitating increased intake of calories and protein to facilitate healing.

Oral antibiotics replace intravenous therapy, after the patient shows signs of improvement, in 3 to 4 days, as demonstrated by normal temperature, lowering of white blood cell count, and improvement in the chest x-ray results (resolution of surrounding infiltrate, reduction in the size of the cavity, and absence of fluid). If treatment is stopped too soon, a relapse may occur. The duration of antibiotic therapy may be from 6 to 16 weeks.

Surgical intervention is rare. However, pulmonary resection (lobectomy) is performed when there is massive hemoptysis, a malignancy, or no response to medical management.

Prevention

The following measures will reduce the risk of lung abscess:

- Patients who must have teeth extracted while their gums and teeth are infected may be given appropriate antibiotic therapy before any dental procedures.
- The patient is instructed to maintain adequate dental and oral hygiene, because anaerobic bacteria play a role in the pathogenesis of lung abscess.
- Appropriate antimicrobial therapy is prescribed for patients with pneumonia.

Nursing Interventions

The antibiotic and intravenous therapy are administered as prescribed and the patient is monitored for any adverse effects. Chest physiotherapy is initiated as prescribed to facilitate drainage of the abscess. The patient is taught deep breathing and coughing exercises to help expand the lungs. To ensure proper nutritional intake, a diet high in protein and calories is encouraged. Emotional support is provided because the abscess may take a long time to resolve.

Patient Education and Home Care Considerations. If surgery has been performed, the patient may return home before the wound closes entirely. It will be necessary to teach the patient or a caregiver how to change the dressings to prevent skin excoriation and an offensive odor. Deep breathing and coughing exercises are to be performed every 2 hours during the day. Postural drainage and percussion techniques are taught to a caregiver so that expectoration of lung secretions can be facilitated.

In some patients whose condition requires home care, a nurse may visit the home to provide the necessary therapy and to assess the patient's condition. Patient teaching is reinformed during these visits. Nutrition counseling is also provided for attaining and maintaining an optimal state of nutrition. To prevent a relapse, the importance of completing the antibiotic regimen and of following the suggestions for rest and appropriate activity levels is emphasized to the patient and family.

If intravenous antibiotic therapy is to continue at home, an intravenous therapy nurse may be arranged to administer the medication. On occasion, the patient may visit a nearby clinic for this treatment.

Pleural Conditions

Pleurisy

Pleurisy (pleuritis) refers to inflammation of both layers of the pleura: the parietal pleura, which covers the surface of the chest wall, the mediastinum, and the upper surfaces of the diaphragm; and the visceral pleura, which covers the entire surface of both lungs. When these inflamed membranes rub together during respiration (particularly inspiration), the result is severe, sharp, "knifelike" pain. The pain may become minimal or absent when the breath is held, or it may be localized or radiate to the shoulder or abdomen. Later, as pleural fluid develops, the pain lessens. In the early period, when little fluid has accumulated, the pleural friction rub can be heard with the stethoscope, only to disappear later as fluid accumulates and separates the inflamed pleural surfaces.

Pleurisy may develop with pneumonia or upper respiratory tract infection, tuberculosis, collagen disease, after trauma to the chest, pulmonary infarction or pulmonary embolism, in primary and metastatic cancer and after thoracotomy.

Diagnostic tests may include chest x-rays, sputum examinations, thoracentesis to obtain a specimen of pleural fluid for examination, and a pleural biopsy.

Medical Management. The objectives of treatment are to discover the underlying condition causing the pleurisy, and to relieve the pain. As the underlying disease (pneumonia, infection) is treated, the pleuritic inflammation usually resolves. At the same time it is necessary to monitor for signs and symptoms of pleural effusion, such as shortness of breath, pain, and decreased excursion of the chest wall.

Prescribed analgesics and topical applications of heat or cold will provide symptomatic relief. Indomethacin, a nonsteroidal anti-inflammatory drug, may provide pain relief while allowing the patient to cough effectively. If the pain is severe, a procaine intercostal block may be required.

Nursing Interventions. Because this patient has considerable pain on inspiration, the nurse can offer suggestions to enhance comfort, such as turning frequently on the affected side to splint the chest wall; this will lessen the stretching of the pleura. The nurse also can teach the patient to use the hands to splint the rib cage while coughing. Because pain on breathing may produce anxiety, the patient requires emotional support and understanding.

Pleural Effusion

Pleural effusion, a collection of fluid in the pleural space, which is located between the visceral and parietal surfaces, is rarely a primary disease process but is usually secondary to other diseases. Normally, the pleural space contains a small amount of fluid (5 to 15 ml) acting as a lubricant that allows the pleural surfaces to move without friction.

In certain disorders, fluid may accumulate in the pleural space to a point where it becomes clinically evident, and it is almost always of pathologic significance. The effusion can be composed of a relatively clear fluid, which may be a transudate or an exudate, or it can be bloody or purulent. A *transudate* (filtrates of plasma that move across intact capillary walls) occurs when factors influencing the formation and reabsorption of pleural fluid are altered, usually by imbalances in hydrostatic or oncotic pressures. A transudate indicates that a condition such as ascites or a systemic disease such as congestive heart failure or renal failure underlies the fluid accumulation. An *exudate* (extravasation of fluid into tissues or a cavity) usually results from inflammation by bacterial products or tumors involving the pleural surfaces.

Pleural effusion may be a complication of congestive heart failure, tuberculosis, pneumonia, pulmonary infections (particularly, viral), nephrotic syndrome, connective tissue disease, and neoplastic tumors. Bronchogenic carcinoma is the most common malignancy associated with a pleural effusion. Pleural effusion may also be seen in cirrhosis, pulmonary embolism, and parasitic infection.

Clinical Manifestations. Usually the clinical manifestations are those caused by the underlying disease. Pneumonia will cause fever, chills, and pleuritic chest pain, whereas a malignant effusion may result in dyspnea and coughing. The size of the effusion will determine the severity of symptoms. A large pleural effusion will cause shortness of breath. The areas that contain fluid or reveal minimal or no breath sounds produce a dull, flat sound when percussed. Egophony will be present above the effusion (see Chapter 22). Tracheal deviation away from the affected side may occur when significant accumulation of pleural fluid occurs. When a small-to-moderate pleural effusion is present, dyspnea may not be present.

The presence of fluid is confirmed by chest x-ray, ultrasound, physical examination, and thoracentesis. Pleural fluid is analyzed by bacterial cultures, Gram stain, acid-fast bacillus stain (for tuberculosis), red and white blood cell counts, chemistry studies (glucose, amylase, lactic dehydrogenase [LDH], protein), cytology analysis for malignant cells, and *p*H. A pleural biopsy may also be performed.

Medical Management. The objectives of treatment are to discover the underlying cause, to prevent reaccumulation of fluid, and to relieve discomfort and dyspnea. Specific treatment is directed to the underlying cause (*e.g.*, congestive heart failure, pneumonia, cirrhosis).

Thoracentesis is performed to remove fluid, to obtain a specimen for analysis, and to relieve dyspnea. If the underlying cause is a malignancy, however, the effusion may recur within a few days or weeks. Repeated thoracenteses result in pain, depletion of protein and electrolytes, and sometimes pneumothorax. In this event the patient may be treated with chest tube drainage connected to a water-seal drainage system or suction to evacuate the pleural space and reexpand the lung.

Chemically irritating agents, such as tetracycline, are instilled in the pleural space to obliterate the pleural space and prevent further accumulation of fluid. After the agent is instilled, the chest tube is clamped and the patient is assisted to assume various positions to ensure uniform distribution of the agent and to maximize its contact with the pleural surfaces. The tube is unclamped as prescribed, and chest drainage is usually continued several days longer to prevent reaccumulation of fluid and to promote the formation of adhesions between the visceral and parietal pleurae.

Other modalities of treatment for malignant pleural effusions include radiation of the chest wall, surgical pleurectomy, and diuretic therapy. If the pleural fluid is an exudate, more extensive diagnostic procedures are performed to determine the cause. Treatment for the primary cause is then instituted.

Nursing Interventions. The nurse's role in the care of the patient with a pleural effusion includes implementing the medical regimen. The nurse prepares and positions the patient for thoracentesis and offers support throughout the procedure. Because the pleura is involved, there will be considerable pain; therefore, the patient is assisted to assume positions that are the least painful, and pain medication is administered as prescribed and as needed.

If a chest tube drainage and water-seal system is used, the nurse is responsible for monitoring the system's function and recording the amount of drainage at prescribed intervals. Nursing care related to the underlying cause of the pleural effusion will be specific to that condition.

Empyema

Empyema is a collection of purulent liquid (pus) in the pleural cavity. At first, the pleural fluid is thin, with a low leukocyte count, but frequently it progresses to a fibropurulent stage and, finally, to a stage where it encloses the lung within a thick exudative membrane. It may occur if a lung abscess extends through to the pleural cavity. Although empyema is an unusual complication of a pulmonary infection, it may occur if treatment is delayed.

Clinical Manifestations. The patient has fever, night sweats, pleural pain, dyspnea, anorexia, and weight loss. Chest auscultation shows the absence of breath sounds and there is flatness on chest percussion, as well as decreased fremitus (vocal vibration detected on palpation). If the patient has received antimicrobial therapy, the clinical manifestations may be altered. The diagnosis is established on the basis of the results of chest x-rays and thoracentesis.

Medical Management The objectives of treatment are to drain the pleural cavity and to achieve full expansion of the lung. The fluid is drained and appropriate antibiotics are prescribed based on the causative organism. Large doses of the antibiotic are usually prescribed. Streptokinase may also be instilled into the space around the empyema to prevent further accumulation of fluid.

Drainage of the pleural fluid depends on the stage of the disease and is accomplished by the following:

- Needle aspiration (thoracentesis) with a thin percutaneous catheter, if the fluid is not too thick
- Closed-chest drainage using a large-diameter intercostal tube attached to water-seal drainage (see Chapter 25)
- Open drainage by means of rib resection to remove the thickened pleura, pus, and debris and to resect the underlying diseased pulmonary tissue

If the inflammation has been long-standing, an exudate can form over the lung and interfere with its normal expansion. This will have to be removed surgically (decortication). The drainage tube is left in place until the pus-filled space is obliterated completely. The complete obliteration of the pleural space is monitored by chest x-rays, and the patient should be informed that treatment may take a long time.

Nursing Interventions. Resolution of empyema is a prolonged process. The nurse helps the patient cope with the condition and instructs in breathing exercises (pursed lip and diaphragmatic breathing), which help to restore normal respiratory function. The nurse also provides care specific to the method of drainage of the pleural fluid, such as needle aspiration, closed chest drainage, or rib resection and drainage. (See nursing management following a thoracotomy, Chapter 25.)

Chronic Obstructive Pulmonary Disease (COPD)

COPD is a broad classification of disorders, including chronic bronchitis, bronchiectasis, emphysema, and asthma. It is an irreversible condition associated with dyspnea on exertion and reduced airflow in or out of the lungs. COPD is the fifth most common cause of death in the United States. It affects over 25% of the adult population.

The airway obstruction that causes a reduction in airflow varies according to the disease. In chronic bronchitis and bronchiolitis, excessive accumulation of mucus and secretions blocks the airway. In emphysema, the obstruction to oxygen and carbon dioxide exchange results from destruction of the walls of the alveoli caused by an overextension of the airspaces in the lung. In asthma, the bronchial airways narrow and restrict the amount of air flowing into the lungs. Certain treatment protocols are used in all these disorders, although the underlying pathophysiology of each disorder requires specific approaches.

COPD is considered to be a disease related to an interaction of genetics and the environment. Cigarette smoking, air pollution, and occupational exposure (to coal, cotton, grain) are important risk factors that contribute to its development. The process may occur over a 20- to 30-year span. COPD has also been found in persons who lack an enzyme inhibitor that normally prevents destruction of lung tissue by certain enzymes. COPD appears to begin fairly early in life and is a slowly progressive disorder that is present many years before the onset of clinical symptoms of impaired pulmonary function.

COPD often becomes symptomatic during the middle adult years, but its incidence increases with age. Although certain aspects of lung function, such as vital capacity and forced expiratory volume, decrease with age, COPD accentuates many of the physiologic changes associated with aging and results in airway obstruction (in bronchitis) and excessive loss of elastic lung recoil (in emphysema). Therefore, there are additional changes in ventilation–perfusion ratios in elderly patients with COPD. (For a discussion of ventilation–perfusion imbalances, see p. 437.)

❑ NURSING PROCESS
The Patient With COPD

Assessment

Assessment involves obtaining information about current symptoms as well as previous disease manifestations. The following is a list of questions that can be used as a guide to obtain a clear history of the disease process:

- ❑ How long has the patient had respiratory difficulty?
- ❑ Does exertion increase the dyspnea? What type of exertion?
- ❑ What are the patient's limits to exercise tolerance?
- ❑ At what times during the day does the patient complain most of fatigue and shortness of breath?
- ❑ Have eating and sleeping habits been affected?
- ❑ What does the patient know about the disease and his or her condition?

Additional data are obtained through observation and examination; questions to consider in obtaining further data include:

- ❑ What are the pulse and the respiratory rates?
- ❑ Are the respirations even and without effort?
- ❑ Does the patient contract the abdominal muscles during inspiration?
- ❑ Does the patient use accessory muscles when breathing?
- ❑ Does the patient take a long time to exhale (prolonged expiration)?
- ❑ Is cyanosis evident?
- ❑ Are the patient's neck veins engorged?
- ❑ Does the patient have peripheral edema?
- ❑ Is the patient coughing?
- ❑ What are the color, amount, and consistency of the sputum?
- ❑ What is the status of the patient's sensorium?
- ❑ Is there increasing stupor? Apprehension?

Diagnosis

Nursing Diagnoses

Based on all the assessment data, the patient's major nursing diagnoses may include the following:

- ❑ Impaired gas exchange related to ventilation–perfusion inequality
- ❑ Ineffective airway clearance related to bronchoconstriction, increased mucus production, ineffective cough, and bronchopulmonary infection
- ❑ Ineffective breathing pattern related to shortness of breath, mucus, bronchoconstriction, and airway irritants
- ❑ Self-care deficit related to fatigue secondary to increased work of breathing and insufficient ventilation and oxygenation
- ❑ Activity intolerance due to fatigue, hypoxemia, and ineffective breathing patterns
- ❑ Ineffective individual coping related to less socialization, anxiety, depression, lower activity level, and the inability to work
- ❑ Knowledge deficit of self-care procedures to be performed at home

Collaborative Problems/ Potential Complications

Based on the assessment data, potential complications that may develop include:

- ❑ Respiratory insufficiency/failure
- ❑ Atelectasis
- ❑ Pneumonia
- ❑ Pneumothorax
- ❑ Pulmonary hypertension

Planning and Implementation

Goals. The major goals for the patient may include improvement in gas exchange, achievement of airway clearance, improvement in breathing pattern, independence in self-care activities, improvement in activity tolerance, improvement in coping ability, adherence to therapeutic program and home care, and absence of complications.

Nursing Interventions

Improving Gas Exchange. Bronchospasm, which is present in many pulmonary diseases, reduces the caliber of the small bronchi, resulting in stasis of secretions and infection. Bronchospasm is detected when wheezing is heard on auscultation with a stethoscope. Increased mucus production along with decreased mucociliary action contributes to further reduction in the caliber of the bronchi and results in decreased air flow and decreased gas exchange, which is aggravated by the loss of lung elasticity.

These changes in the airway require that the patient be monitored for dyspnea and hypoxia. If bronchodilators or corticosteroids are prescribed, the nurse must properly administer the medications and be alert for potential side effects. The relief of bronchospasm is confirmed by measuring improvement in expiratory flow rates (how long it takes to exhale and the amount of air exhaled) and assessing whether the patient experiences less dyspnea.

Aerosol therapy helps loosen secretions so that they can be removed. Inhaled bronchodilators often are added to the nebulizer to provide direct bronchodilator action on the airways, thereby improving gas exchange. Inhalation or aerosol treatments should be given before meals to improve lung ventilation and thus reduce the fatigue that accompanies eating. After inhalation of nebulized bronchodilators, the patient is advised to inhale moisture to liquefy secretions further. Then expulsive coughing or postural drainage will aid in expectoration of secretions. The patient is assisted to do this in a manner that is not exhausting.

Oxygen is prescribed when hypoxemia is present. The nurse must monitor the effectiveness of the oxygen therapy and ensure that the patient is compliant in using the oxygen delivery device. The patient is instructed about the proper use of oxygen and about the dangers of increasing the oxygen flow rate without explicit directions from the physician

- ❑ Because hypoxia is the stimulus for respirations in the patient with long-standing COPD and CO_2 retention, increasing the oxygen flow rate may raise the oxygen level in the patient's blood and remove the stimulus for breathing.

Additionally, the patient is advised that smoking with or near oxygen is extremely dangerous. Oxygen may be required at home and can be supplied to the home by compressed gas, liquid, or concentrator systems. Portable oxygen systems are available that allow the patient to work and travel. Patient education includes reassuring the patient that oxygen is not "addicting" and explaining the precautions involved in using oxygen (no smoking) and the necessity of having regular measurements of arterial blood gases.

Continuous oxygen therapy has been demonstrated to prolong life for those with arterial oxygen pressure (PaO_2) of 55 mm Hg or less on room air because of the ability to maintain a constant oxygen saturation. Intermittent oxygen use has little value in the patient with COPD, except during an intensive exercise program or during the night while the patient is sleeping.

Removing Bronchial Secretions. A major goal in the treatment of COPD is to diminish the quantity and viscosity of sputum to improve pulmonary ventilation and gas exchange. All pulmonary irritants must be eliminated, particularly cigarette smoking, which is the most persistent source of pulmonary irritation. A *high fluid intake* (6 to 8 glasses) daily is encouraged to liquefy secretions. An added reason for encouraging fluid intake is the tendency for the patient to breathe through the mouth, which accelerates water loss. Inhaling nebulized water also is helpful because it humidifies the bronchial tree, adding water to the sputum and decreasing its viscosity, so that it can be coughed up more easily.

Postural drainage with percussion and vibration uses gravity to help raise secretions so that they can be expectorated or suctioned easily. Therapies that dilate the bronchioles, such as aerosol therapy, aerosolized bronchodilators, or an intermittent positive-pressure breathing (IPPB) treatment, should be administered before postural drainage because secretions will drain more readily after the tracheobronchial tree is dilated. The patient is instructed in effective breathing and coughing to help raise the secretions. Postural drainage usually is carried out when the patient wakes up, to remove secretions that have accumulated overnight, and before retiring, to promote sleep. The frequency of these measures throughout the day will be dictated by the patient's needs.

Preventing Bronchopulmonary Infections. Bronchopulmonary infections must be controlled to diminish inflammatory edema and to permit recovery of normal ciliary action. Minor respiratory infections that are of no consequence to the person with normal lungs can be life-threatening in the person with COPD. The cough associated with bronchial infection introduces a vicious cycle with further trauma and damage to the lungs, progression of symptoms, increased bronchospasm, and further increase in susceptibility to bronchial infection. Infection compromises lung function and is a common cause of respiratory failure in individuals with COPD.

In COPD, infection may be accompanied by subtle changes. The patient is instructed to report immediately if the sputum becomes discolored, because purulent expectoration or a change in the character, color, or amount of the sputum is a sign of infection. Any worsening of symptoms (increased tightness of the chest, increase in dyspnea, and fatigue) is also suggestive of infection and must be reported. Viral infections are hazardous to these patients because they are so often followed by infections caused by organisms, such as *S. pneumoniae*, and *H. influenzae*.

Patients with COPD are prone to respiratory infections and should be immunized against influenza and *S. pneumoniae*. During the spring when the pollen count is high or in areas with significant air pollution, these persons should avoid the outdoors because it may increase bronchospasm. Outdoor periods of high temperatures with high humidity should also be avoided.

Breathing Exercises and Respiratory Training

Breathing Exercises. Most people with COPD breathe shallowly from the upper chest in a rapid and inefficient manner. This type of upper chest breathing can be changed to *diaphragmatic breathing* with practice. Training in diaphragmatic breathing reduces the respiratory rate, increases alveolar ventilation, and sometimes helps expel as much air as possible during expiration (see Chapter 25 for technique).

Pursed-lip breathing slows expiration, prevents collapse of lung units, and helps the patient to control the rate and depth of respiration and to relax, which enables the patient to gain control of dyspnea and feelings of panic.

Pacing Activity. A patient with COPD has a decrease in exercise tolerance at definite periods of the day. This is especially true on arising in the morning, because bronchial secretions and edema collect in the lungs during the night while the person is lying down. The patient often will be unable to bathe or dress. Activities requiring the arms to be supported above the level of the thorax may produce fatigue or respiratory distress. These activities may be tolerated better after the patient has been up and moving around for an hour or more. Because of these limitations, the patient must participate in planning self-care activities with the nurse and in determining the best time for bathing and dressing. A hot beverage on arising, along with diaphragmatic breathing, will help to expectorate secretions and will shorten the period of disability experienced on arising.

Another period of increased disability occurs immediately after meals, particularly the evening meal. Fatigue from the day's activities coupled with abdominal distention limits the patient's exercise tolerance. The patient's chief complaint at this time is fatigue or dyspnea.

Inspiratory Muscle Training. Once the patient has learned diaphragmatic breathing, a program of inspiratory muscle training may be prescribed to help strengthen the muscles used in breathing. This program requires that the patient breathe against a resistance for 10 to 15 minutes every day. The resistance is gradually increased and the muscles become better conditioned. Conditioning of the respiratory muscles takes a long time, and the patient is instructed to continue practicing at home.

Performing Self-Care Activities. As gas exchange, airway clearance, and the breathing pattern improve, the patient is encouraged to assume self-care activities.The patient is taught to try to coordinate diaphragmatic breathing with activities such as walking, bathing, bending, or climbing stairs. The patient should begin to bathe, dress, and take short walks, resting as needed to avoid fatigue and excessive dyspnea. Fluids should be readily available, and the patient should begin to drink without having to be reminded. If postural drainage will be done at home, the patient is instructed and supervised by the nurse before discharge.

Promoting Physical Conditioning. Physical conditioning techniques include breathing exercises and general physical conditioning exercises intended to conserve and increase pulmonary ventilation. There is a close relationship between physical fitness and respiratory fitness. Graded exercises and physical conditioning programs employing treadmills, stationary bicycles, and measured level walks have been shown to improve symptoms and to increase work capacity and exercise tolerance. A physical activity that can be done on a regular sustained basis is helpful. A lightweight portable oxygen system is available for the ambulatory patient who requires oxygen therapy during physical activity to decrease hypoxia. This type of rehabilitation improves the quality of life.

Promoting Coping Measures. Any factor that interferes with normal breathing quite naturally induces anxiety, depression, and changes in behavior. Many patients find the slightest exertion exhausting. Constant shortness of breath and fatigue may make the patient irritable and apprehensive to the point of panic. Restricted activity (and reversal of family roles due to loss of employment), the frustration of having to work to breathe, and the realization that the disease is prolonged and unrelenting, may cause the patient to react with anger, depression, and demanding behavior. Sexual function may be compromised, which also diminishes self-esteem.

It is important that the nurse and other health care personnel encourage the patient to remain as active as possible without becoming fatigued. Emphasis should be on controlling symptoms and increasing self-esteem and a sense of mastery and well-being. Supportive medical and nursing care, ongoing patient teaching, exercise conditioning, and possibly group therapy sessions help somewhat to relieve an almost overwhelming burden.

The patient may also be directed to support groups conducted by the American Lung Association, to pulmonary rehabilitation programs, to smoking cessation programs (if still smoking), and to senior citizens' groups for social interaction. These groups will help improve the patient's knowledge and ability to cope with COPD, and will promote a sense of self-worth.

Patient Education and Home Care Considerations

Setting Realistic Goals. The patient with COPD can improve the quality of life by learning about the disease process. One of the major teaching factors is explaining the importance of setting and accepting realistic short-term and long-range goals. If the patient is severely disabled, the objectives of treatment are to preserve current pulmonary function and relieve symptoms as much as possible. If the disease is mild, the objectives are to increase exercise tolerance and prevent further loss of pulmonary function. The goals and expectations of treatment must be shared and planned with the patient. The patient and those providing care need patience to achieve these goals.

Avoiding Temperature Extremes. The patient is instructed to avoid extremes of heat and cold. Heat increases the body temperature, thereby raising the oxygen requirements of the body; cold tends to promote bronchospasm. Bronchospasm may be initiated also by air pollutants such as fumes, smoke, dust, and even talcum, lint, and aerosol sprays. High altitudes aggravate the hypoxia.

Smoking. Protection of the lung is basic for the preservation of lung function. Patients with COPD should be informed unequivocally that, for them, smoking is dangerous. Smoking depresses the activity of scavenger cells and affects the ciliary cleansing mechanism of the respiratory tract, the function of which is to keep the breathing passages free of inhaled irritants, bacteria, and other foreign matter. This is one of the major defense mechanisms of the body. When this cleansing mechanism is damaged by smoking, air flow is obstructed and air becomes trapped behind the obstructed airway. The alveoli greatly distend and the lung capacity is diminished. Smoking also irritates the goblet cells and mucous glands, causing an increased accumulation of mucus. The mucus accumulation produces more irritation, infection, and damage to the lung.

Frequently the patient is unaware of the magnitude of these changes until extra physical effort produces respiratory distress. At this point the damage may be irreversible. Therefore, patients with COPD should definitely refrain from smoking. There is a wide variety of smoking control strategies, including prevention, cessation, and behavior modification.

Lifestyle Changes. It is recommended that patients with COPD adopt a lifestyle of moderate activity, ideally in a climate with minimal shifts in temperature and humidity. Stressful situations that might trigger a coughing episode or emotional disturbance should be avoided. Compliance with a complex medication regimen to manage COPD can be difficult. In particular, patients who are receiving medication via aerosol delivery with a metered-dose inhaler (MDI) may particularly be challenged. One of every three patients incorrectly uses the MDI (DeBlaquiere et al, 1989). Review and return demonstration by the patient prior to discharge, during follow-up visits to the physician or nurse practitioner's office, and during visits to the patient or home care is critical.

Patients may be directed to community resources such as pulmonary rehabilitation programs, smoking cessation programs, and other programs to help improve their ability to cope with their chronic condition and their therapeutic regimen and to give them a sense of worth, hope, and well-being.

Monitoring and Managing Potential Complications. Because COPD is a broad classification of respiratory diseases, the potential complications may vary, depending on the underlying disorder. Respiratory insufficiency and failure are major life-threatening complications of COPD. Other complications of COPD (*i.e.*, pneumonia, atelectasis, pneumothorax) increase the risk for respiratory failure to the patient.

The acuity of the onset and the severity of *respiratory failure* depend on the patient's baseline pulmonary function, arterial blood gas values, and the severity of other complications of COPD. Respiratory insufficiency and failure may be chronic in nature (with long-standing emphysema) or acute (with severe asthma attack, pneumonia in the patient with long-standing COPD). Acute respiratory insufficiency and failure may necessitate ventilatory support until other acute complications, such as infection, can be treated and successfully resolved. Management of the patient requiring ventilatory support is discussed in Chapter 25.

Other complications of COPD include atelectasis and pneumonia, pneumothorax, mediastinal or subcutaneous emphysema, and pulmonary hypertension (cor pulmonale).

Chronic hypoxia due to complications may lead to symptoms and personality changes. The patient is assessed for the need for oxygen. Oxygen is used cautiously. The patient is monitored and taught the signs and symptoms of respiratory infection. See the following pages for further discussion of management of these complications: atelectasis, page 480; pneumonia, page 481; pneumothorax, page 536; pulmonary hypertension, page 523.

Breathing exercises, along with postural drainage and aerosol therapy, are prescribed to aid in removing retained secretions. IPPB is not advocated for acute asthma attacks because it can result in further bronchospasm. If the patient's condition worsens to the point of acute respiratory failure, intubation and mechanical ventilation will be necessary.

Evaluation

Expected Outcomes

1. Demonstrates improved gas exchange by using bronchodilators and oxygen therapy as prescribed
   a. Shows no signs of restlessness, confusion, or agitation
   b. Has stable arterial blood gas values (but not necessarily normal values due to chronic changes in the gas exchange ability of the lungs)
2. Achieves airway clearance
   a. Stops smoking
   b. Avoids noxious substances and extremes of temperature
   c. Increases fluid intake to 6 to 8 glasses of fluid a day
   d. Performs postural drainage correctly
   e. Knows signs of early infection and is aware of need to report them if they occur
3. Improves breathing pattern
   a. Practices and uses pursed-lip and diaphragmatic breathing
   b. Shows signs of decreased respiratory effort
4. Performs self-care activities within tolerance range
   a. Paces self to avoid fatigue and dyspnea
   b. Uses controlled breathing while performing activities
5. Achieves activity tolerance, and exercises and performs activities with less shortness of breath
6. Acquires effective coping mechanisms and participates in a pulmonary rehabilitation program
7. Adheres to therapeutic program
   a. Follows prescribed medication regimen
   b. Stops smoking
   c. Maintains acceptable activity level
8. Is free of complications
   a. Exhibits no evidence of respiratory failure or insufficiency
   b. Maintains appropriate arterial blood gases
   c. Shows no signs of infection

Chronic Bronchitis

Chronic bronchitis is defined as the presence of a productive cough that lasts 3 months a year for 2 consecutive years. The accumulated secretions in the bronchioles interfere with effective breathing. Cigarette smoking or exposure to pollution are major causes of chronic bronchitis. Patients with chronic bronchitis are more susceptible to recurring infections of the lower respiratory tract. A wide range of viral, bacterial, and mycoplasmal infections can produce acute episodes of bronchitis. Exacerbations of chronic bronchitis are most likely to occur during the winter. Inhaling cold air produces bronchospasm in those who are susceptible.

Pathophysiology

Smoke irritates the airways, resulting in hypersecretion of mucus and inflammation. Because of this constant irritation, the mucus-secreting glands and goblet cells increase in number, cilia function is reduced, and more mucus is produced. As a result, the bronchioles become narrow and clogged. Alveoli adjacent to the bronchioles may become damaged and fibrosed, resulting in altered function of the alveolar macrophages, which play an important role in destroying foreign particles, including bacteria. The patient then becomes more susceptible to respiratory infection. Further bronchial narrowing follows as a result of the fibrotic changes that occur in the airways. In time, irreversible lung changes may occur, possibly resulting in emphysema and bronchiectasis.

Clinical Manifestations

A chronic, productive cough in the winter months is the earliest sign of chronic bronchitis. The cough may be exacerbated by cold weather, dampness, and pulmonary irritants. The patient usually has a history of cigarette smoking and frequent respiratory infections.

Diagnostic Evaluation

A complete history, including family, environmental exposure to irritating substances, and occupational history is taken, including smoking habits (number of packs per day). In addition, arterial blood gases, x-ray, and pulmonary function studies are performed, as well as hemoglobin and hematocrit studies.

The pulmonary function studies reveal a decrease in vital capacity (VC), and forced expiratory volume (FEV; the amount of air exhaled), and an increased residual volume (RV; the air remaining in the lungs after maximal exhalation), with a normal to slightly increased total lung capacity (TLC). The hematocrit and hemoglobin may be slightly increased. The blood gas analysis may reveal hypoxia with hypercapnia. The chest x-ray may reveal an enlarged heart with a normal or flattened diaphragm. Consolidation in the lung fields may also be noted.

Medical Management

The main objectives of treatment are to keep the bronchioles open and functioning, to facilitate removal of bronchial secretions to prevent infection, and to prevent disability. Changes in the sputum pattern (nature, color, amount, thickness) and in the cough pattern are important signs to note. Recurrent bacterial infections are treated with antibiotic therapy based on culture and sensitivity studies.

To help in removing bronchial secretions, bronchodilators are prescribed to relieve bronchospasm and reduce airway obstruction; thus, more oxygen is distributed throughout the lungs, and alveolar ventilation is improved. Postural drainage and chest percussion after treatments are usually helpful, especially if bronchiectasis is present. Fluid (given orally or parenterally if bronchospasm is severe) is an important part of therapy, because proper hydration helps to loosen secretions so they can be removed by coughing. Corticosteroid therapy may be used when the patient fails to respond to more conservative measures. The patient must stop smoking because it causes bronchoconstriction, paralyzes the cilia, which are important in removing irritating particles, and inactivates surfactant, which plays an important role in enabling the lungs to expand. Smokers are also more susceptible to bronchial infection.

Prevention

Because of the disabling nature of chronic bronchitis, every effort is directed toward preventing its occurrence. One essential measure is to avoid respiratory irritants (particularly tobacco smoke). People who are prone to respiratory tract infections should be immunized against common viral agents with vaccines for influenza and for *S. pneumoniae.* All patients with acute upper respiratory tract infections should receive proper treatment, including antimicrobial therapy based on cultures and sensitivity studies at the first sign of purulent sputum.

For nursing management and patient education, see Nursing Process: The Patient With COPD, pp. 504-507.

Bronchiectasis

Bronchiectasis is a chronic dilation of the bronchi and bronchioles that may be caused by a variety of conditions, including pulmonary infections and obstruction of the bronchus; aspiration of foreign bodies, vomitus, or material from the upper respiratory tract; and pressure from tumors, dilated blood vessels, and enlarged lymph nodes. A person may be predisposed to bronchiectasis as a result of respiratory infection in early childhood, measles, influenza, tuberculosis, and immunodeficiency disorders. After surgery, bronchiectasis may develop when the patient is unable to cough effectively, with the result that mucus obstructs the bronchi and leads to atelectasis.

Pathophysiology

The infection damages the bronchial wall, causing a loss of its supporting structure and producing thick sputum that ultimately may obstruct the bronchi. The walls become permanently distended by severe coughing. The infection extends to the peribronchial tissues, so that in the case of saccular bronchiectasis, each dilated tube virtually amounts to a lung abscess, the exudate of which drains freely through the bronchus. Bronchiectasis is usually localized, affecting a lung lobe or segment. The lower lobes are most frequently involved.

The retention of secretions and subsequent obstruction ultimately cause the alveoli distal to the obstruction to collapse (atelectasis). Inflammatory scarring or fibrosis replaces functioning lung tissue. In time the patient develops respiratory insufficiency with reduced vital capacity, decreased ventilation, and an increased ratio of residual volume to total lung capacity. There is impaired mixing of inspired gas (ventilation–perfusion imbalance) and hypoxemia.

Clinical Manifestations

Characteristic symptoms of bronchiectasis include chronic cough and the production of purulent sputum in copious amounts. A sputum specimen will characteristically "layer out" into three layers on standing: a frothy top layer, a middle clear layer, and a dense particulate bottom layer. A high percentage of patients with this disease experience hemoptysis. Clubbing of the fingers is also very common because of respiratory insufficiency. The patient is likely to have repeated episodes of pulmonary infection.

Bronchiectasis is not readily diagnosed because the symptoms can be mistaken for those of simple chronic bronchitis. A definite sign is offered by the prolonged history of productive cough, with sputum consistently negative for tubercle bacilli. The diagnosis is established on the basis of bronchography and bronchoscopy (p. 454), and CT scan, which demonstrates either the presence or absence of bronchial dilatation.

Medical Management

The objectives of treatment are to prevent and control infection and to promote bronchial drainage to clear the affected portion of the lung or lungs of excessive secretions.

Infection is controlled with *antimicrobial therapy* based on results of sensitivity studies on organisms cultured from sputum. Patients may be put on a year-round regimen of antibiotics, with different types of antibiotics at alternated intervals. Some clinicians prescribe antibiotics throughout the winter or when acute upper respiratory tract infections occur. Patients should be vaccinated against influenza and pneumococcal pneumonia.

Postural drainage of the bronchial tubes underlies all treatment plans because draining the bronchiectatic areas by gravity reduces the amount of secretions and the degree of infection. (Sometimes mucopurulent sputum must be removed by bronchoscopy.) The affected chest area may be percussed or "cupped" to assist in raising secretions. Postural drainage is initially carried out for short periods and then increased steadily.

Bronchodilators may be given to persons who also have obstructive airway disease. Patients with bronchiectasis almost always have associated bronchitis. Sympathomimetics, particularly β-adrenergics, may be used for bronchodilation and to increase the mucociliary transport of secretions.

To promote sputum expectoration, the water content of the sputum is increased by *aerosolized nebulizer* treatments and by an increase in oral fluid intake. A face tent is ideal for providing extra humidification for aerosols. The patient should not smoke, as this impairs bronchial drainage by paralyzing ciliary action, increasing bronchial secretions, and causing inflammation of the mucous membranes, resulting in hyperplasia of the mucous glands.

Surgical intervention, although used infrequently, may be indicated for the patient who continues to expectorate fairly large amounts of sputum and experiences repeated bouts of pneumonia and hemoptysis in spite of the patient's adherence to the treatment regimen. However, the disease must involve only one or two areas of the lung that can be removed without producing respiratory insufficiency. The goal of surgical treatment is to conserve normal pulmonary tissue and avoid infectious complications.

All diseased tissue is removed, provided that the postoperative lung function will be adequate. It may be necessary to remove a segment of a lobe (segmental resection), a lobe (lobectomy), or an entire lung (pneumonectomy). *Segmental resection* is the removal of an anatomic subdivision of a pulmonary lobe. The chief advantage is that only diseased tissue is removed and healthy lung tissue is conserved. Bronchography aids in delineating the segment.

The surgery is preceded by a period of careful preoperative preparation. The objective is to obtain a dry (as dry as possible) tracheobronchial tree to prevent complications (atelectasis, pneumonia, bronchopleural fistula, and empyema). This is accomplished by means of postural drainage or, depending on the location of the abscess, by direct suction through a bronchoscope. A course of antibacterial therapy may be prescribed.

After the surgery, the care is the same as for any patient undergoing chest surgery, as discussed in Chapter 25. For nursing management and patient education, see Nursing Process: The Patient With COPD.

Pulmonary Emphysema

Pulmonary emphysema is defined as an abnormal distention of the air spaces beyond the terminal bronchioles with destruction of the walls of the alveoli. It is the end stage of a process that has progressed slowly for many years. In fact, by the time the patient develops symptoms, pulmonary function often is irreversibly impaired. Along with chronic obstructive bronchitis, it is a major cause of disability.

Smoking is the major cause of emphysema. In a small percentage of patients, however, there is a familial predisposition to emphysema associated with a plasma protein abnormality, a deficiency of α_1-antitrypsin, which is an enzyme inhibitor. Without it, certain enzymes will destroy lung tissue. The genetically susceptible person is sensitive to environmental factors (smoking, air pollution, infectious agents, allergens) and, in time, develops chronic obstructive symptoms. It is imperative that the carriers of this genetic defect be identified to permit modification of the environmental factors to delay or prevent overt symptoms of disease. Genetic counseling should also be offered.

Pathophysiology

In emphysema, several factors cause airway obstruction, namely: inflammation and swelling of bronchi; excessive mucus production; loss of elastic recoil of the airways; and collapse of bronchioles and redistribution of air to the functional alveoli.

As the walls of the alveoli are destroyed (a process accelerated by recurrent infections), the alveolar surface area that comes in direct contact with the pulmonary capillaries continually decreases, causing an increase in dead space (lung area where no gas exchange can occur) and resulting in impaired oxygen diffusion. Impaired oxygen diffusion results in hypoxemia. In the later stages of the disease, the elimination of carbon dioxide is impaired, resulting in increased carbon dioxide tension in arterial blood (called *hypercapnia*) and causing respiratory acidosis.

As the alveolar walls continue to break down, the pulmonary capillary bed is reduced. The pulmonary blood flow is increased and the right ventricle is forced to maintain a higher blood pressure in the pulmonary artery. Thus, *right-sided heart failure (cor pulmonale)* is one of the complications of emphysema. The presence of congestion, leg edema (dependent edema), distended neck veins, or pain in the region of the liver suggests the development of cardiac failure.

Secretions are increased and retained because the person is unable to generate a forceful cough to expel them. Chronic and acute infections thus persist in the emphysematous lungs, adding to the problem.

The person with emphysema has a chronic obstruction (marked increase in airway resistance) to the inflow and outflow of air from the lungs. The lungs are in a state of chronic hyperexpansion. To move air into and out of the lungs, negative pressure is required during inspiration and an adequate level of positive pressure must be attained and maintained during expiration. The resting position is one of inflation. Instead of being an involuntary passive act, expiration becomes active and requires muscular effort. The patient becomes increasingly short of breath, the chest becomes rigid, and the ribs are fixed at their joints. The "barrel chest" of many of these patients is due to loss of lung elasticity in the presence of the continued tendency of the chest wall to expand (Fig. 24-4).

In some instances, the barrel chest is due to kyphosis in which the upper spine becomes abnormally rounded or convex in shape. Some patients bend forward to breathe, using the accessory muscles of respiration. Retraction of the supraclavicular fossae occurs on inspiration causing the shoulders to heave upward (Fig. 24-5). In advanced disease, the abdominal muscles also contract on inspiration. There is a progressive reduction of the vital capacity. Normal exhalation becomes increasingly difficult and finally impossible. The total vital capacity (VC) may be normal, but the ratio of forced expiratory volume in 1-second to the vital capacity (FEV_1:VC) is low. This occurs because the elasticity of the alveoli is greatly diminished. The effort required by the patient to move air from the damaged alveoli and narrowed airway increases the work of breathing. The ability to adapt to changing oxygenation needs is greatly compromised.

Classification

There are two main types of emphysema, which are classified on the basis of the changes taking place in the lung: (1) panlobular (panacinar) and (2) centrilobular (centroacinar). Figure 24-6 contrasts the two types of emphysema.

In the **panlobular (panacinar) type**, there is destruction of the respiratory bronchiole, alveolar duct, and alveoli. All air spaces within the lobule are more or less enlarged, with little inflammatory disease. The patient with this type of emphysema typically has a hyperinflated chest and marked dyspnea on exertion, and weight loss. The term "pink puffer" is sometimes used in describing this patient, because the patient remains "pink," or well oxygenated, until the disease becomes terminal.

In the **centrilobular (centroacinar) form**, the pathologic changes take place mainly in the center of the secondary lobule, and the peripheral portions of the acinus are preserved. Frequently, there is a derangement of ventilation–perfusion ratios, producing chronic hypoxia, hypercapnia (increased CO_2 in the arterial blood), polycythemia, and episodes of right-sided heart failure. This leads to cyanosis, peripheral edema, and respiratory failure. The patient is referred to as a "blue bloater." In addition to the management outlined below, the blue bloater usually receives diuretic therapy for edema. Both types of emphysema very often occur in the same patient.

Clinical Manifestations

Dyspnea is the main symptom in emphysema and has an insidious onset. The patient usually has a history of cigarette smoking and a long history of chronic cough, wheezing, and increasing shortness of breath and rapid breathing (tachypnea). The symptoms are exacerbated with a respiratory infection.

On inspection, the patient usually has a "barrel chest" due to air being trapped, muscle wasting, and pursed lip breathing. Chest breathing, ineffective abnormal breathing, and use of accessory muscles (sternocleidomastoid) are common. In advanced stages dyspnea occurs on exertion with even simple activities of daily living, such as eating and bathing.

When the chest is examined, hyperresonance and decreased fremitus are found throughout the lung fields. Auscultation reveals diminished breath sounds with crackles, rhonchi, and prolonged expiration. Anorexia, weight loss, and weakness are common complaints. Low oxygen levels (hypoxemia) and high carbon dioxide levels (hypercapnia) are present in advanced stages of the disease.

In time, even the slightest exertion, such as bending over to tie one's shoelaces, produces dyspnea and fatigue (exertional dyspnea). The emphysematous lung does not contract on expiration and the bronchioles are not effectively emptied of their secretions.

The patient is prone to inflammatory reactions and infections due to the pooling of these secretions. After these infections occur, the patient experiences prolonged wheezing on expiration. Anorexia, weight loss, and weakness are common. The neck veins may be distended during expiration. Physical examination reveals diminished breath sounds with rhonchi and prolonged expiration, hyperresonance with percussion, and a decrease in tactile fremitus.

Diagnostic Evaluation

The patient's symptoms and the clinical findings on physical examination provide the initial clues to the patient's problem. Other diagnostic tests include chest x-rays, pulmonary function studies (particularly spirometry), arterial blood gases (to assess ventilatory function and pulmonary gas exchange), and complete blood count (CBC).

The pulmonary function studies usually reveal increased total lung capacity (TLC) and residual volume

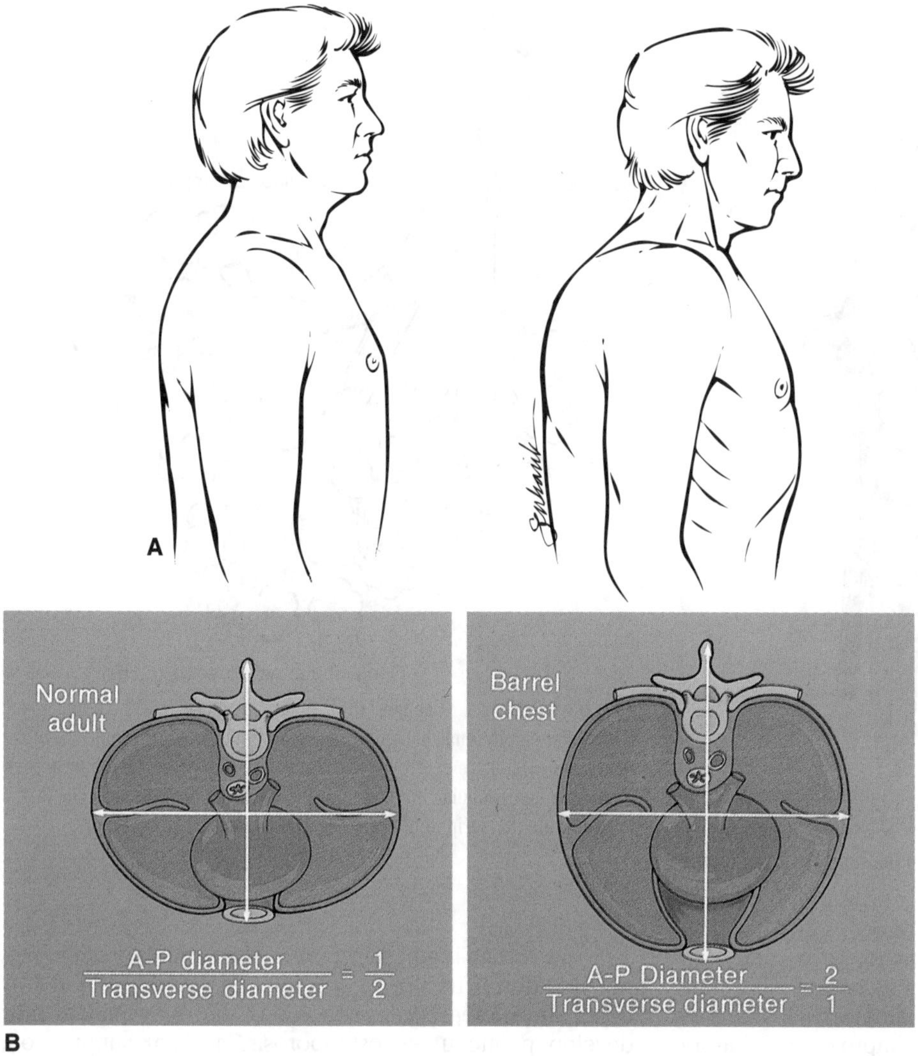

FIGURE 24-4. Changes in the chest wall resulting from COPD. (**A**) The chest assumes a "barrel" shape (barrel chest, *right*) characteristic of emphysema. (**B**) Cross sections of normal (*left*) versus barrel chest (*right*).

(RV). There is a decrease in the vital capacity (VC) and forced expiratory volume (FEV). These findings underscore the difficulty the patient has in pushing air out of the lungs. The hemoglobin and hematocrit may be normal in the early stages of the disease. The chest x-ray reveals hyperinflation, a flattened diaphragm, widened intercostal margin, and a normal heart. With advanced disease, the arterial blood gases may reveal mild hypoxia with hypercapnia.

Medical Management

The major objectives of treatment are to improve the quality of life, to slow the progression of the disease process, and to treat the obstructed airways to relieve hypoxia. The therapeutic approach includes:

- Treatment measures designed to improve ventilation and decrease the work of breathing
- Prevention and prompt treatment of infection
- Physical therapy techniques to conserve and increase pulmonary ventilation
- Maintenance of proper environmental conditions to facilitate breathing
- Psychologic support
- Ongoing patient education and rehabilitation

Bronchodilators. Bronchodilators are prescribed to dilate the airways because they combat both bronchial mucosal edema and muscular spasm and help both in reducing airway obstruction and in improving gas exchange.

These medications include the β-adrenergic agonists (metaproterenol, isoproterenol) and the methylxanthines (theophylline, aminophylline), which produce bronchial dilation by different mechanisms. Bronchodilators may be administered orally, subcutaneously, intravenously, rectally, or by inhalation. Inhaled medications may be delivered by pressurized aerosols, hand-bulb nebulizers, pump-driven nebulizers, metered-dose inhalers, or IPPB.

Bronchodilators may produce unwanted side effects, which include tachycardia, cardiac dysrhythmias, and central nervous system excitation. The methylxanthines may also produce gastrointestinal disturbances such as nausea and vomiting. Because side effects are common, the dosage is carefully adjusted in accordance with the patient's tolerance and clinical response.

Aerosol Therapy. Aerosolization (the process of dispensing particles in a fine mist) of saline bronchodilators and mucolytics frequently is used to aid in bronchodilation. The particle size in the aerosol mist must be small enough to allow the medication to be deposited deep within the tracheobronchial tree.

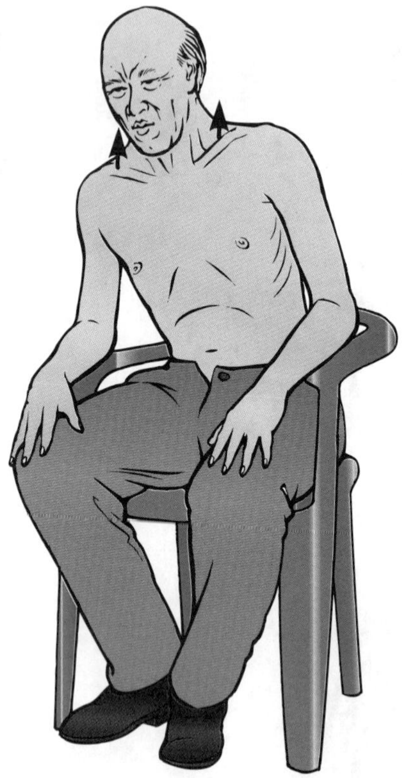

FIGURE 24-5. Typical posture of person with emphysema. The person tends to lean forward and uses accessory muscles of respiration to breathe, forcing the shoulder girdle upward and the supraclavicular fossae to retract on inspiration.

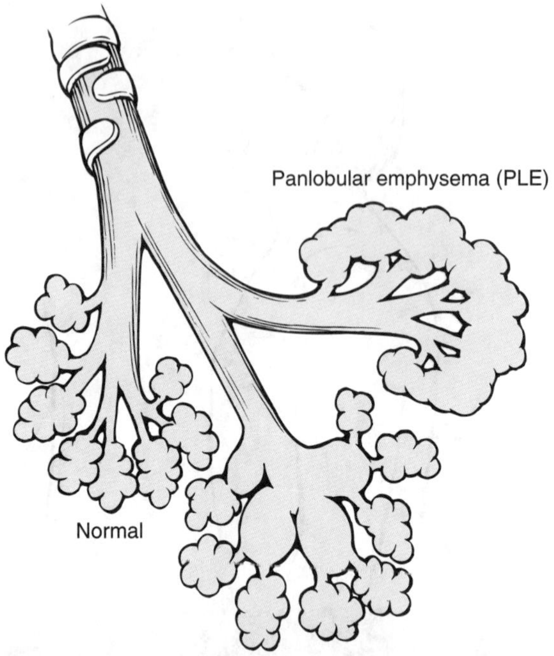

FIGURE 24-6. Changes in alveolar structure in centrilobular and panlobular emphysema. In panlobular emphysema, the bronchioles, alveolar ducts, and alveoli are destroyed and the air spaces within the lobule are enlarged. In centrilobular emphysema, the pathologic changes occur in the lobule, while the peripheral portions of the acinus are preserved.

Nebulized aerosols relieve bronchospasm, decrease mucosal edema, and liquefy bronchial secretions. This facilitates the process of clearing the bronchioles, helps to control the inflammatory process, and improves ventilatory function. Hand-bulb nebulizers and metered-dose aerosol devices give the patient quick relief. Electrically powered nebulizers and air-powered nebulizers are useful if the patient has more marked ventilatory impairment. The improvement of the oxygen saturation of the arterial blood and the reduction of its carbon dioxide content assist in relieving the patient's hypoxia and give considerable relief from constant respiratory fatigue.

Nebulizer treatments with oxygen must be given with extreme caution in patients who have chronically elevated carbon dioxide tensions and are breathing on hypoxic stimuli. There is a trend away from the use of IPPB, especially in the home.

Treatment of Infection. Patients with emphysema are susceptible to lung infections and must be treated at the earliest signs of infection. *S. pneumoniae*, *H. influenzae*, and *Branhamella catarrhalis* are the most common organisms involved. Antimicrobial therapy with tetracyclines, ampicillin, amoxicillin, or trimethoprim-sulfamethoxazole (Bactrim) is usually prescribed. An antimicrobial regimen is used at the first sign of respiratory infection, as evidenced by purulent sputum, increased cough, and fever.

Corticosteroids. Corticosteroids remain controversial in the treatment of emphysema. They are used after other measures to dilate the bronchioles and remove secretions have failed. Prednisone is usually prescribed.

The dosage is adjusted to keep the patient on the lowest possible dose. The side effects include gastrointestinal (GI) upset and increased appetite. Long term, the patient may develop peptic ulcer, osteoporosis, adrenal suppression, steroid myopathy, and cataract formation. See Chapter 40 for further description of the effects of corticosteroids.

Oxygenation. Oxygen therapy may increase survival in patients with severe emphysema. Severe hypoxemia is treated with low concentrations of oxygen to raise the PaO_2 to between 65 and 80 mm Hg. In severe emphysema, oxygen is administered at least 16 hours per day, with 24 hours preferable. This modality may alleviate the patient's symptoms and improve the quality of life. Some patients require long-term home use of oxygen The general nursing care of the patient with COPD is discussed in Nursing Care Plan 24-2 and in the Nursing Process section (pp. 504–507).

Asthma

Asthma is an intermittent, reversible, obstructive airway disease in which the trachea and bronchi respond in a hyperactive way to certain stimuli. It is manifested by a narrowing of the airways, resulting in dyspnea, cough, and wheezing. The degree of airway narrowing may change either spontaneously or because of therapy. Asthma differs from other obstructive lung diseases in that it is a reversible process. Acute exacerbations may occur, which last from minutes to hours, interspersed with symptom-free periods. When

(text continues on page 518)

NURSING CARE PLAN 24–2
Care of the Patient With Chronic Obstructive Pulmonary Disease

Nursing Interventions	Rationale	Expected Outcomes
NURSING DIAGNOSIS: Impaired gas exchange related to ventilation-perfusion inequality		
GOAL: Improvement in gas exchange		
1. Administer bronchodilators as prescribed: a. Can be given orally, intravenously, rectally, or by inhalation b. Administer oral or intravenous bronchodilators at alternate times to nebulizer, metered dose inhaler, or IPPB treatment to prolong the effectiveness of the medication. c. Observe for side effects: tachycardia, dysrhythmias, central nervous system excitation, nausea, and vomiting.	1. Bronchodilators dilate the airways and help to combat bronchial mucosa edema and muscular spasm. Because side effects are common, the drug dosage is carefully adjusted for each patient, in accordance with his tolerance and clinical response.	• Verbalizes need for bronchodilators and for taking them on prescribed schedule. • Evidences minimal side effects; heart rate near normal, absence of dysrhythmias, normal mentation. • Reports a decrease in dyspnea. • Shows an improved expiratory flow rate • Uses and cleans respiratory therapy equipment as applicable. • Demonstrates diaphragmatic breathing and coughing. • Uses oxygen equipment appropriately when indicated.
2. Evaluate effectiveness of nebulizer, metered dose inhaler, or IPPB treatments. a. Assess for decreased shortness of breath, decreased wheezing or crackles, secretions loosened, decreased anxiety. b. Ensure that treatment is given before meals to avoid nausea and to reduce fatigue that accompanies eating.	2. Combining medication with aerosolized bronchodilators is typically used to control bronchoconstriction. Improper administration of the treatment will render it ineffective. Aerosolization facilitates bronchial clearance, helps control the imflammatory process, and improves ventilatory function.	• Evidences normal arterial blood gases.
3. Instruct and encourage patient in diaphragmatic breathing and effective coughing.	3. These techniques improve ventilation by opening airways and clearing the airways of sputum. Gas exchange is improved.	
4. Administer oxygen by the method prescribed. a. Explain importance to patient. b. Evaluate effectiveness; observe for signs of hypoxia. Notify physician if restlessness, anxiety, somnolence, cyanosis, or tachycardia is present. c. Analyze arterial blood gases and compare with baseline values. When arterial puncture is performed and a blood sample is obtained, hold puncture site for 5 minutes to prevent arterial bleeding. d. Initiate pulse oximetry to monitor oxygen saturation. e. Explain that no smoking is permitted by patient or visitors while oxygen is in use.	4. Oxygen will correct the hypoxemia. Careful observation of the liter flow or the percentage administered and its effect on the patient is needed. If the patient has chronic CO_2 retention, then hypoxia is the stimulus to breathe. Excessive oxygen could suppress the hypoxic drive and death would occur. These patients generally need low-flow oxygen rates of 1 to 2 L/min. Periodic arterial blood gases and pulse oximetry help to evaluate adequacy of oxygenation.	

(*continued*)

NURSING CARE PLAN 24–2 *(continued)*
Care of the Patient With Chronic Obstructive Pulmonary Disease

NURSING DIAGNOSIS: Ineffective airway clearance related to bronchoconstriction, increased mucus production, ineffective cough, and bronchopulmonary infection

GOAL: Achievement of airway clearance

Nursing Interventions	Rationale	Expected Outcomes
1. Give patient 6 to 8 glasses of fluids/day unless cor pulmonale is present.	1. Systemic hydration keeps secretions moist and easier to raise. Fluids must be given with caution if right-sided heart failure is present.	• Verbalizes need to drink 6 to 8 glasses of fluids/day • Demonstrates diaphragmatic breathing and coughing. • Performs postural drainage correctly. • Coughs less. • Does not smoke. • Verbalizes that pollens, fumes, gases, dusts, and extremes of temperature and humidity are irritants to be avoided. • Identifies signs of early infection. • Is free of infection (no fever, no change in sputum, lessening of dyspnea). • Verbalizes need to notify physician at the earliest sign of infection. • Verbalizes need to stay away from crowds or people with colds in flu season. • Plans to discuss flu and pneumonia vaccines with physician to help prevent infection
2. Teach and encourage the use of diaphragmatic breathing and coughing techniques.	2. These techniques will help to improve ventilation and to produce secretions without causing breathlessness and fatigue.	
3. Assist in administering nebulizer, metered dose inhaler, or IPPB treatments.	3. These treatments add water to the bronchial tree and to the sputum, decreasing its viscosity, so that evacuation of secretions is facilitated.	
4. Perform postural drainage with percussion and vibration in the morning and at night as prescribed.	4. Uses gravity to help raise secretions so they can be more easily coughed up or suctioned.	
5. Instruct patient to avoid bronchial irritants such as cigarette smoke, aerosols, extremes of temperature, and fumes.	5. Bronchial irritants cause bronchoconstriction and increased mucus production, which then interferes with airway clearance.	
6. Teach early signs of infection that are to be reported to the physician immediately: a. Increased sputum b. Change in color of sputum c. Increased thickness of sputum d. Increased shortness of breath, tightness in chest, or fatigue e. Increased coughing	6. Minor respiratory infections that are of no consequence to the person with normal lungs can produce fatal disturbances in the lungs of the person with emphysema. Early recognition is crucial.	
7. Administer antibiotics as prescribed.	7. Antibiotics may be prescribed to prevent or treat infection.	
8. Encourage patient to be immunized against influenza and *Streptococcus pneumoniae.*	8. People with respiratory conditions are prone to respiratory infections and are encouraged to be immunized.	

NURSING DIAGNOSIS: Ineffective breathing pattern related to shortness of breath, mucus, bronchoconstriction, and airway irritants

GOAL: Improvement in breathing pattern

Nursing Interventions	Rationale	Expected Outcomes
1. Teach patient diaphragmatic and pursed lip breathing.	1. Helps patient prolong expiration time. With these techniques, patient will breathe more efficiently and effectively.	• Practices pursed lip and diaphragmatic breathing and uses them when short of breath and with activity. • Shows signs of decreased respiratory effort and paces activities. • Uses inspiratory muscle trainer, as prescribed, for 10 minutes every day.
2. Encourage alternating activity with rest periods. Let patient make some decisions (bath, shaving) about his care based on his tolerance level.	2. Pacing activities will permit patient to perform activities without excessive distress.	
3. Encourage use of an inspiratory muscle trainer if prescribed.	3. Strengthens and conditions the respiratory muscles.	

(continued)

NURSING CARE PLAN 24–2 *(continued)*
Care of the Patient With Chronic Obstructive Pulmonary Disease

Nursing Interventions	Rationale	Expected Outcomes
NURSING DIAGNOSIS: Self-care deficits related to fatigue secondary to increased work of breathing and insufficient ventilation and oxygenation		
GOAL: Independence in self-care activities		
1. Teach patient to coordinate diaphragmatic breathing with activity (*e.g.,* walking, bending). 2. Encourage patient to begin to bathe self, dress self, walk, and drink fluids. Discuss energy conservation measures. 3. Teach postural drainage if appropriate.	1. This will allow the patient to be more active and to avoid excessive fatigue or dyspnea during activity. 2. As condition resolves, patient will be able to do more but needs to be encouraged to avoid increasing dependence. 3. Encourages patient to become involved in own care. Builds self-esteem and prepares patient to manage at home.	• Uses controlled breathing while bathing, bending, and walking. • Paces activities of daily living to alternate with rest periods to reduce fatigue and dyspnea. • Describes energy conservation strategies. • Performs same self-care activities as before. • Performs postural drainage correctly.
NURSING DIAGNOSIS: Activity intolerance due to fatigue, hypoxemia, and ineffective breathing patterns		
GOAL: Improvement in activity tolerance		
1. Support patient in establishing a regular regimen of exercise using treadmill and exercycle, walking or other appropriate exercises, such as mall walking. a. Assess the patient's current level of functioning and develop exercise plan based on baseline functional status. b. Suggest consultation with a physical therapist to determine an exercise program specific to the patient's capability. Have portable oxygen unit available in case oxygen is needed during exercise.	1. Muscles that are deconditioned consume more oxygen and place an additional burden on the lungs. Through regular, graded exercise, these muscle groups become more conditioned, and the patient can do more without getting as short of breath. Graded exercise breaks this cycle of debilitation.	• Performs activities with less shortness of breath. • Verbalizes need to exercise daily and demonstrates an exercise plan to be carried out at home. • Walks and gradually increases walking time and distance to improve physical condition.
NURSING DIAGNOSIS: Ineffective individual coping related to less socialization, anxiety, depression, lower activity level, and the inability to work		
GOAL: Attainment of an optimal level of coping		
1. Adopt a hopeful and encouraging attitude toward patient. 2. Encourage activity to level of symptom tolerance. 3. Teach relaxation technique or provide a relaxation tape for patient. 4. Enroll patient in pulmonary rehabilitation program where available.	1. A sense of hope will give the patient something to work toward, rather than a defeated, hopeless attitude. 2. Activity reduces tension and decreases degree of dyspnea as patient becomes conditioned. 3. Relaxation reduces stress and anxiety and helps patient to cope with disability. 4. Pulmonary rehabilitation programs have been shown to promote a subjective improvement in a patient's status and self-esteem as well as increased exercise tolerance and decreased hospitalizations.	• Expresses interest in the future. • Participates in the discharge plan. • Discusses activities or methods that can be performed to ease shortness of breath. • Uses relaxation techniques appropriately. • Expresses interest in a pulmonary rehabilitation program.

(continued)

NURSING CARE PLAN 24–2 *(continued)*
Care of the Patient With Chronic Obstructive Pulmonary Disease

Nursing Interventions	Rationale	Expected Outcomes
5. Suggest vocational counseling to explore alternative avenues of employment (if applicable).	5. Work modification may need to be made and appropriate resources used to achieve this goal.	• Explores resources available for work modification.
NURSING DIAGNOSIS: Knowledge deficit about self-care procedures to be performed at home.		
GOAL: Compliance with therapeutic program and home care		
1. Help patient understand short- and long-term goals. a. Teach the patient about his disease and care.	1. Patient needs to see that there is a method and plan for care in which they play a major role. Needs to know what to expect. Teaching about the condition is one of the most important aspects of care; it will prepare the patient to live and cope with the condition and improve quality of life.	• Understands the disease and what affects it. • Verbalizes the need to preserve existing lung function by adhering to the prescribed program.
2. Discuss the need to stop smoking. Provide information about resource groups. (*e.g.*, Smoke Enders, American Cancer Society).	2. Tobacco smoking causes definite damage to the lung and diminishes the lungs' protective mechanisms. Air flow is obstructed and lung capacity is reduced.	• Stops smoking or enrolls in a smoking cessation program.
COLLABORATIVE PROBLEMS: Potential complications of COPD include atelectasis; pneumothorax; respiratory failure; pulmonary hypertension; and status asthmaticus.		
Atelectasis		
1. Monitor respiratory status, including rate and pattern of respirations, breath sounds, and signs/symptoms of respiratory distress. 2. Instruct and encourage diaphragmatic breathing and effective coughing techniques. 3. Promote use of incentive spirometry, as prescribed.	1. A change in respiratory status, including tachypnea, dyspnea, and diminished, or absent breath sounds, may indicate atelectasis. 2. These techniques improve ventilation by opening airways, thereby, improving gas exchange. 3. Incentive spirometry promotes maximal lung expansion.	• Normal respiratory rate and pattern. • Normal breath sounds. • Demonstrates diaphragmatic breathing and coughing. • Uses incentive spirometry, as prescribed.
Pneumothorax		
1. Monitor respiratory status, including rate and pattern of respirations, breath sounds, and signs/symptoms of respiratory distress. 2. Assess pulse. 3. Assess for chest pain and precipitating factors. 4. Palpate for tracheal deviation.	1. Dyspnea, tachypnea, tachycardia, acute pleuritic chest pain, tracheal deviation, and absence of breath sounds on the affected side may indicate a pneumothorax. 2. Tachycardia is associated with a pneumothorax. 3. Pain may accompany pneumothorax. 4. Early detection and prompt intervention of a pneumothorax will prevent other serious complications.	• Normal respiratory rate and pattern. • Normal pulse. • Absence of pain. • Trachea is midline.

(continued)

NURSING CARE PLAN 24–2 *(continued)*
Care of the Patient With Chronic Obstructive Pulmonary Disease

Nursing Interventions	Rationale	Expected Outcomes
5. Monitor arterial blood gases. 6. Administer supplemental oxygen therapy, as indicated. 7. Administer analgesics, as indicated, for chest pain. 8. Use pleural drainage system, as prescribed	5. Recognition of a change in respiratory function will prevent serious complications. 6. Oxygen will correct hypoxemia. 7. Pain interferes with chest movement, resulting in a decrease in lung expansion. 8. Removal of air and fluid from the pleural space will reexpand the lung.	• Maintains normal ABGs. • Exhibits no hypoxia and hypercapnia. • Maintains normal ABGs. • Absence of pain. • Adequate chest movement. • Lung is reexpanded. • Breath sounds are heard on the affected side.
Respiratory Failure		
1. Monitor respiratory status, including rate and pattern of respirations, breath sounds, and signs/symptoms of respiratory distress. 2. Monitor arterial blood gases. 3. Administer supplemental oxygen, including mechanical ventilation, as prescribed.	1. Recognition of a change in respiratory function will prevent further complications, such as respiratory failure, severe hypoxia, and hypercapnia. 2. Recognition of changes in oxygenation and acid–base balance will assist in correcting and preventing complications. 3. Respiratory failure is a medical emergency. Hypoxia is a hallmark sign. Administration of oxygen therapy and mechanical ventilation is critical to survival.	• Normal respiratory rate and pattern. • Recognizes hypoxia and hypercapnia. • Maintains normal ABGs. • Maintains normal ABGs.
Pulmonary Hypertension		
1. Monitor respiratory status, including rate and pattern of respirations, breath sounds, and signs/symptoms of respiratory distress. 2. Assess for signs and symptoms of right-sided heart failure, including peripheral edema, ascites, distended neck veins, rales, and a heart murmur. 3. Administer oxygen therapy, as prescribed.	1. Dyspnea is the main symptom of pulmonary hypertension. 2. Right-sided heart failure is a common clinical manifestation of pulmonary hypertension due to right ventricular hypertrophy. 3. Continuous oxygen therapy is a major component of management of pulmonary hypertension by preventing hypoxia and increased workload on heart.	• Normal respiratory rate and pattern. • Exhibits no signs and symptoms of right-sided failure. • Maintains normal ABGs.
Status Asthmaticus		
1. Monitor respiratory status, including rate and pattern of respirations, breath sounds, and signs/symptoms of respiratory distress. 2. Monitor arterial blood gases. 3. Administer supplemental oxygen therapy, as ordered. 4. Administer drug therapy (beta agonists and methylxanthenes), as prescribed.	1. Dyspnea, tachypnea, cyanosis, labored, wheezy breathing, sibilant rhonchi, or absent breath sounds are signs of respiratory distress due to status asthmaticus. 2. Hypoxia and hypercapnia are signs of bronchospasm. 3. Oxygen will correct hypoxia. 4. Beta agonists and methylxanthenes are used initially to dilate bronchial smooth muscle.	• Normal respiratory rate and pattern. • Normal breath sounds. • Maintains normal arterial blood gases. • Improvement in respiratory function.

asthma and bronchitis occur together, the obstruction is compounded and is called *chronic asthmatic bronchitis*.

Asthma can begin at any age; about half of the cases develop in childhood and another third before age 40. Approximately 17% of all Americans have had asthma at some time in their lives. Although asthma can be fatal, more often it is disruptive, affecting school attendance, occupational choices, physical activity, and many other aspects of life.

Types of Asthma

Asthma is often characterized as allergic, idiopathic, nonallergic, or mixed.

Allergic asthma is caused by a known allergen or allergens (*e.g.*, dust pollens, animals, dander, food, and mold). Most of the allergens are airborne and seasonal. Patients with allergic asthma usually have a family history of allergies and a past medical history of eczema or allergic rhinitis. Exposure to the allergen triggers an asthmatic attack. Children with allergic asthma often outgrow the condition by adolescence.

Idiopathic or nonallergic asthma is not related to a specific allergen. Factors, such as a common cold, respiratory tract infections, exercise, emotions, and environmental pollutants may trigger an attack. Some pharmacologic agents, such as aspirin and other nonsteroidal anti-inflammatory agents, hair dye, beta-adrenergic antagonists, and sulfite agents (food preservatives), also may be factors. The attacks of idiopathic or nonallergic asthma become more severe and frequent with time and can progress to chronic bronchitis and emphysema. Some patients will develop mixed asthma.

Mixed asthma is the most common form of asthma. It has characteristics of both the allergic and the idiopathic or nonallergic forms.

Pathophysiology

Asthma is a reversible diffuse airway obstruction. The obstruction is caused by one or more of the following: (1) contraction of muscles surrounding the bronchi, which narrows the airway; (2) swelling of membranes that line the bronchi; and (3) filling of the bronchi with thick mucus. In addition, the bronchial muscles and mucous glands enlarge; thick, tenacious sputum is produced and the alveoli hyperinflate, with air becoming trapped in the lung tissue. The exact mechanism for these changes is not known, but most of what is known involves the immunologic system and the autonomic nervous system.

Some persons with asthma develop exaggerated immune responses to their environments. The antibodies that are produced (IgE) then attach to mast cells in the lung. Reexposure to the antigen results in the antigen binding to the antibody, causing the release of mast cell products (called mediators) such as histamine, bradykinin, and prostaglandins and of the slow-reacting substance of anaphylaxis (SRS-A). The release of these mediators in the lung tissue affects the smooth muscle and glands of the airway, causing bronchospasm, mucous membrane swelling, and excessive mucus production.

The autonomic nervous system innervates the lung. Bronchial muscle tone is regulated by vagal nerve impulses through the parasympathetic system. In idiopathic or nonallergic asthma, when the nerve endings in the airway are stimulated by such factors as infection, exercise, cold, smoking, emotions, and pollutants, an increased amount of acetylcholine is released. This can directly cause bronchoconstriction as well as stimulate the production of the chemical mediators discussed above. Persons with asthma may have a low tolerance for parasympathetic responses.

In addition, α- and β-adrenergic receptors of the sympathetic nervous system are located in the bronchi. When the α-adrenergic receptors are stimulated, bronchoconstriction occurs; bronchodilation occurs when the β-adrenergic receptors are stimulated. The balance between α- and β-receptors is controlled primarily by cyclic adenosine monophosphate (cAMP). Alpha-receptor stimulation results in a decrease in cAMP, which leads to an increase of chemical mediators released by the mast cells and bronchoconstriction. Beta-receptor stimulation results in increased levels of cAMP, which inhibits release of chemical mediators and causes bronchodilation. A proposed theory is that β-adrenergic blockade occurs in persons with asthma. Consequently, asthmatics are prone to an increased release of chemical mediators and constriction of smooth muscle.

Clinical Manifestations

The three common symptoms of asthma are cough, dyspnea, and wheezing. In some instances, cough may be the only symptom. Asthma attacks frequently occur at night. The causes are not completely understood, but may be related to circadian variations, which influence airway receptor thresholds.

An asthmatic attack usually starts suddenly with coughing and a tight sensation in the chest, followed by slow, laborious, wheezy breathing. Expiration is always much more strenuous and prolonged than inspiration, which forces the patient to sit upright and use every accessory muscle of respiration. Obstructed air flow causes dyspnea. The cough at first is tight and dry but soon becomes more forceful. Sputum, consisting of thin mucus containing small, round, gelatinous masses is coughed up with much difficulty. Later signs include cyanosis secondary to severe hypoxia, and symptoms of carbon dioxide retention, including sweating, tachycardia, and a widened pulse pressure.

The asthma attack may last from 30 minutes to several hours and may subside spontaneously. Although asthma attacks are rarely fatal, occasionally a more severe continuous reaction, called "status asthmaticus" occurs. This condition is life threatening (see p. 520).

Related Reactions. Other possible allergic reactions that may accompany asthma include eczema, rashes, and temporary edema. Asthmatic attacks may occur periodically after exposure to a specific allergen, some medications, physical exertion, and emotional excitement.

Diagnostic Evaluation

No single test can confirm a diagnosis of asthma. A complete history, including a family, environmental, and occupational history, may disclose factors or substances that precipitate asthma attacks. A positive skin test that produces a wheal and flare reaction identifies specific allergens.

A positive family history frequently is associated with allergic asthma. Environmental factors, including seasonal changes, high pollen counts, and mold also are associated with allergic asthma. Climate changes, particularly cold air and air pollution are primarily associated with nonallergic asthma. A variety of occupation-related chemicals and compounds have been associated with the development of asthma, including metal salts, wood and vegetable dust, medications (*e.g.*, aspirin, antibiotics, piperazine and cimetidine), industrial chemicals and plastics, biologic enzymes, (*e.g.*, laundry detergents), animal and insect dusts, sera, and secretions.

During acute episodes, a chest x-ray may show hyperinflation and a flattened diaphragm. Sputum and blood studies may disclose eosinophilia (elevated levels of eosinophils). There is an elevation in serum levels of immunoglobulin E (IgE) in allergic asthma.

Sputum may be clear and foamy (allergic) or thick and white (nonallergic) and stringy (nonallergic).

Arterial blood gases reveal hypoxia during acute attacks. Initially, hypocapnia and respiratory alkalosis and low carbon dioxide partial pressure (PCO_2) are present. As the condition worsens and the patient becomes more fatigued, the PCO_2 may rise. A normal PCO_2 may be a signal of impending respiratory failure. Because PCO_2 is 20 times more diffusible than oxygen, it is rare for PCO_2 to be normal or elevated in a person who is breathing very rapidly.

Pulmonary function is usually normal between attacks. During an acute attack, there is an increase in the total lung capacity (TLC) and functional residual volume (FRV) secondary to air trapping. The FEV and forced vital capacity (FVC) are markedly decreased.

Medication Therapy

There are five categories of medications used in the treatment of asthma: beta agonists, methylxanthines, anticholinergics, corticosteroids, and mast cell inhibitors.

Beta Agonists. The beta agonists (β-adrenergic agents) are the initial medications used in the treatment of asthma because they dilate bronchial smooth muscles. Adrenergic agents also increase ciliary movements, decrease the chemical mediators of anaphylaxis and can potentiate the bronchodilating effects of corticosteroids. The most commonly used adrenergic agents include epinephrine, albuterol, metaproterenol, isoproterenol, isoetharine, and terbutaline. They usually are administered parenterally or by inhalation. The inhalation route is the route of choice because it affects the bronchioles directly and has fewer side effects.

Methylxanthines. Methylxanthines, such as aminophylline and theophylline, are used because of their bronchodilating effects. They relax bronchial smooth muscle, increase movement of mucus in the airways, and increase the contraction of the diaphragm. Aminophylline (the IV form of theophylline) is administered intravenously. Theophylline is given orally. Methylxanthines are not used in acute attacks because they are slower in onset than beta agonists. There are several factors that may alter the metabolism of methylxanthines, particularly theophylline, including tobacco smoking, heart failure, chronic liver disease, oral contraceptives, erythromycin, and cimetidine. Care should be taken when administering these medications intravenously. If they are given too rapidly, tachycardia or cardiac dysrhythmias may result.

Anticholinergics. Anticholinergics, such as atropine, have not historically been used in the routine treatment of asthma because of their systemic side effects, such as dryness of the mouth, blurred vision, urinary hesitancy, palpitations, and flushing. However, quaternary ammonium derivatives, such as atropine methylnitrate, and ipratropium bromide (Atrovent), have demonstrated excellent bronchodilator effects with minimal systemic side effects. These agents are given by inhalation. Anticholinergics may be particularly beneficial to asthmatics who are not candidates for beta agonists and methylxanthines because of underlying cardiac disease.

Corticosteroids. Corticosteroids are important in the treatment of asthma. These medications may be administered intravenously (hydrocortisone), orally (prednisone, prednisolone), or by inhalation (beclomethasone, dexamethasone). The mechanism of action is not certain; however, they are thought to reduce inflammation and bronchoconstriction. Corticosteroids (*not* by inhalation) may be administered for an acute asthmatic attack that does not respond to bronchodilator therapy. Corticosteroids have proved effective in the treatment of asthma and COPD. Prolonged use of corticosteroids can result in the development of serious side effects, including peptic ulcers, osteoporosis, adrenal suppression, steroid myopathy, and cataracts.

Inhaled corticosteroids may be effective in the treatment of patients with steroid-dependent asthma. A major advantage of this method of administration is the reduced effects of the corticosteroids on other body systems. Throat irritation, coughing, dry mouth, hoarseness, and fungal infection of the mouth and pharynx may occur. The patient is instructed to rinse the mouth and gargle immediately after using inhaled corticosteroids to decrease the incidence of fungal infection. The patient is instructed to report the incidence of redness or the presence of white patches in the mouth. Switching from systemic to inhaled corticosteroids puts the patient at risk for adrenal insufficiency. Therefore, the process must be accomplished gradually and under close supervision.

See Chapter 40 for detailed discussion of the effects of corticosteroids.

Mast Cell Inhibitors. Cromolyn sodium, a mast cell inhibitor, is an integral part of the treatment of asthma. It is administered by inhalation. It prevents the release of chemical mediators of anaphylaxis, thereby resulting in bronchodilation and a decrease in airway inflammation. Cromolyn sodium is most beneficial between attacks or while the asthma is in remission. It may result in the reduction of use of other medications and overall improvement in symptoms.

Prevention

Patients with recurrent asthma should undergo tests to identify the substances that precipitate the attacks. Possible causes could be pillows, mattresses, certain types of cloth, pets, horses, detergents, soaps, certain foods, molds, and pollens. If the attacks are seasonal, then pollens can be strongly suspected. Attempts should be made to avoid the causative agents whenever possible.

The *complications of asthma* may include status asthmaticus, rib fracture, pneumonia, and atelectasis. Airway obstruction, particularly during acute asthmatic episodes, often results in hypoxemia, requiring the administration of oxygen and the monitoring of arterial blood gases. Fluids are administered because persons with asthma are frequently dehydrated from diaphoresis and insensible fluid loss with hyperventilation. Management of status asthmaticus is further described below.

Status Asthmaticus

Status asthmaticus is severe and persistent asthma that does not respond to conventional therapy. The attacks can last longer than 24 hours. Infection, anxiety, overuse of tranquilizers, nebulizer abuse, dehydration, increased adrenergic block, and nonspecific irritants may contribute to these episodes. An acute episode may be precipitated by hypersensitivity to aspirin.

Pathophysiology. The basic characteristics of asthma (constriction of the bronchiolar smooth muscle, swelling of bronchial mucosa, and thickened secretions) decrease the diameter of the bronchi and are apparent in status asthmaticus. A ventilation–perfusion abnormality results in hypoxemia and respiratory alkalosis initially, followed by respiratory acidosis.

There is a reduced PaO_2 and an initial respiratory alkalosis with a decreased $PaCO_2$ and an increased *p*H. As the severity of status asthmaticus increases, the $PaCO_2$ increases and the *p*H falls, reflecting respiratory acidosis.

Clinical Manifestations. The clinical manifestations are the same as those seen in severe asthma—labored breathing, prolonged exhalation, engorged neck veins, and wheezing. However, the extent of wheezing does not indicate the severity of the attack. As the obstruction becomes greater, the wheezing may disappear, which is frequently a sign of impending respiratory failure.

Diagnostic Evaluation. Pulmonary function studies are the most accurate means of assessing acute airway obstruction. Arterial blood gases are obtained if the patient is unable to perform pulmonary function maneuvers because of severe obstruction or fatigue, or if the patient does not respond to treatment. Respiratory alkalosis (low CO_2) is the most common finding in asthmatic patients. A rising PCO_2 (to normal levels or levels indicating respiratory acidosis) frequently is a danger signal of impending respiratory failure.

Medical Management. In the emergency room setting, the patient is treated initially with beta agonists (*e.g.*, metaproterenol, terbutaline, and albuterol) and corticosteroids. The patient may also require supplemental oxygen and intravenous fluids for hydration.

Oxygen therapy is initiated to treat dyspnea, cyanosis, and hypoxemia. Low-flow humidified oxygen by either Venturi mask or nasal catheter is administered. The flow is based on arterial blood gas values. The PaO_2 is maintained between 65 and 85 mm Hg. Sedatives are contraindicated. If there is no response to repeated treatments, hospitalization is required.

Low pulmonary function results and deteriorating blood gases (respiratory acidosis), which may indicate that the patient is tiring and will require mechanical ventilation, are other criteria calling for hospitalization. Although most patients do not need mechanical ventilation, it is used when the patient is in respiratory failure or in those who tire and who are too fatigued by the attempt to breathe or whose condition does not respond to initial treatment.

Nursing Interventions. Signs of dehydration are identified by checking skin turgor. Fluid intake is essential to combat dehydration, to loosen secretions, and to facilitate expectoration. Intravenous fluids are administered as prescribed, up to 3 to 4 L/day, unless contraindicated.

Constant monitoring of the patient by the nurse is important for the first 12 to 24 hours, or until status asthmaticus is halted. The patient's energy needs to be conserved and the room should be quiet and free of respiratory irritants, including flowers, tobacco smoke, perfumes, or odors of cleaning agents. A nonallergenic pillow should be used.

Patient Teaching. Patient education is an important part of care if recurrences and rehospitalizations are to be kept to a minimum. Patients are instructed to report immediately troublesome signs and symptoms, such as awakening during the night with an acute attack, not gaining complete relief from the inhaler, or developing a respiratory infection. Bronchodilators may be required on an around-the-clock basis. Certain medications (*i.e.*, theophylline and corticosteroids) may be added or dosage increased when asthmatic attacks occur. Adequate hydration must be maintained at home to keep secretions from thickening. The patient needs to recognize that infection is to be avoided because it can trigger an attack.

Certain self-care activities are promoted to abort severe attacks and provide a measure of independence. If theophylline in a long-acting oral preparation is prescribed, careful instructions are given on the hazards of overuse. A β_2-selective adrenergic, such as metaproterenol or albuterol, may also be prescribed to be self-administered with a hand-held metered-dose inhaler. Should these bronchodilators fail, a corticosteroid (short, high dose), usually prednisone, is prescribed. Instructions on the use of these medications are also provided and the patient is advised to seek follow-up care as necessary.

Acute Respiratory Failure

Respiratory failure exists whenever the exchange of oxygen for carbon dioxide in the lungs cannot keep up with the rate of oxygen consumption and carbon dioxide production in the cells of the body. This results in a fall in arterial oxygen tension to less than 50 mm Hg (hypoxemia) and a rise in arterial carbon dioxide tension to greater than 45 mm Hg (hypercapnia).

One must distinguish between acute respiratory failure and acute exacerbation of chronic respiratory failure. *Acute respiratory failure* is the respiratory failure appearing in the patient whose lung was structurally and functionally normal before the onset of the present illness. *Chronic respiratory failure* is the respiratory failure seen in patients with chronic lung diseases such as chronic bronchitis, emphysema, and black lung disease (coal miner's disease). These patients develop a tolerance to the gradually worsening hypoxia and hypercapnia. After acute respiratory failure, the lung usually returns to its original state. In chronic respiratory failure the structural damage is irreversible. The principles of management of these two conditions are different; the following discussion will be confined to acute respiratory failure.

Causes

Acute respiratory failure can be caused by numerous circumstances, some of which result in inadequate ventilation. In some instances the lung itself remains structurally normal in the early stages. One of the most important causes of inadequate ventilation is *upper airway obstruction*. Its cause, diagnosis, and management are discussed on pp. 469–471.

Central nervous system depression also will result in inadequate ventilation. The respiratory center, which controls breathing, lies in the lower part of the brain stem (pons and medulla). Drug overdose, anesthesia, opioids, head injury, stroke, brain tumors, encephalitis, meningitis, hypoxia, and hypercapnia are all capable of depressing the respiratory center. In these patients, respiration becomes slow and shallow. Respiratory arrest may occur in severe cases.

Primary neurologic disorders can also affect respiratory function. The impulses arising in the respiratory center travel through nerves that extend from the brain stem down the spinal cord to receptors in the muscles of respiration. Any disease of the nerves, spinal cord, muscles, or neuromuscular junction involved in respiration will seriously affect ventilation. Guillain-Barré syndrome, myasthenia gravis, damage to the cervical segment of the spinal cord, large acute lesions in the brain stem in multiple sclerosis, and poliomyelitis are examples of such diseases.

In the *postoperative period,* especially after major thoracic or upper abdominal surgery, respiratory failure due to inadequate ventilation may occur. The reasons for respiratory failure during this period are numerous. The effects of anesthetic agents, analgesics, and sedatives (*e.g.*, pentobarbital) are long-lasting. They depress respiration by their own effects or by enhancing the effects of opioid analgesics. Pain in the thoracic and abdominal area interferes with deep breathing and coughing. Muscle relaxants frequently are used during anesthesia. Some patients may have difficulty in metabolizing or excreting these medications, so that their effects last longer than usual, causing muscle weakness in the postoperative period. Use of small intravenous doses of morphine is recommended in the postanesthesia room, because they are short acting and easily titrated. A mismatch of ventilation to perfusion also accounts for respiratory failure after major abdominal and thoracic surgery.

Pleural effusion, hemothorax, and *pneumothorax* are conditions that interfere with ventilation by preventing expansion of the lung. They usually are produced by an underlying lung disease, pleural disease, or trauma and injury and may cause respiratory failure.

Trauma caused by motor vehicle crashes is a very common cause of acute respiratory failure. Crashes resulting in head injury, unconsciousness, and bleeding from the nose and mouth may lead to upper airway obstruction and respiratory depression. Hemothorax, pneumothorax, and rib fractures may occur and may be responsible for inadequate ventilation. Flail chest also may occur and may lead to respiratory failure. The treatment is to repair the underlying pathology.

Acute diseases of the lung may lead to acute respiratory failure. Of these diseases, pneumonia is perhaps the most common. It usually is caused by viral or bacterial activity. Chemical pneumonitis or pneumonia is produced by the inhalation of irritant fumes or the aspiration of acidic gastric material. Bronchial asthma, atelectasis, pulmonary embolism, and pulmonary edema are some other conditions that can cause acute respiratory failure.

Adult Respiratory Distress Syndrome

Adult respiratory distress syndrome (ARDS), also known as noncardiogenic pulmonary edema, is a clinical syndrome characterized by a progressive decrease in arterial oxygen content occurring after a serious illness or injury. ARDS usually requires mechanical ventilation with a higher than normal airway pressure. There is a wide range of factors associated with the development of ARDS (Chart 24-5), including direct injury to the lungs (such as smoke inhalation) or indirect insult to the body (such as shock).

Pathophysiology. ARDS occurs as a result of injury to the alveolar capillary membrane resulting in leakage of fluid into the alveolar interstitial spaces and alteration in the capillary bed. Figure 24-7 represents a flow chart showing the sequence of pathophysiologic events that lead to ARDS. There is a marked ventilation–perfusion (V/Q) imbalance due to an impaired gas exchange and extensive shunting of blood in the lungs. ARDS causes a decrease in surfactant production, which leads to alveolar collapse. The lung compliance becomes markedly decreased (stiff lungs). The result is a characteristic decrease in functional residual capacity, severe hypoxia, and hypocapnia.

ARDS has been associated with a mortality rate of as high as 50% to 60%. The survival rate is somewhat improved when the cause can be determined, and early and aggres-

CHART 24-5
Etiologic Factors Related to ARDS

- Aspiration (gastric secretions, drowning, hydrocarbons)
- Drug ingestion and overdose
- Hematologic disorders (disseminated intravascular coagulopathy, massive transfusions, cardiopulmonary bypass)
- Prolonged inhalation of high concentrations of oxygen, smoke, or corrosive substances
- Localized infection (bacterial, fungal, viral pneumonia)
- Metabolic disorders (pancreatitis, uremia)
- Shock (any cause)
- Trauma (pulmonary contusion, multiple fractures, head injury)
- Major surgery
- Fat or air embolism
- Systemic sepsis

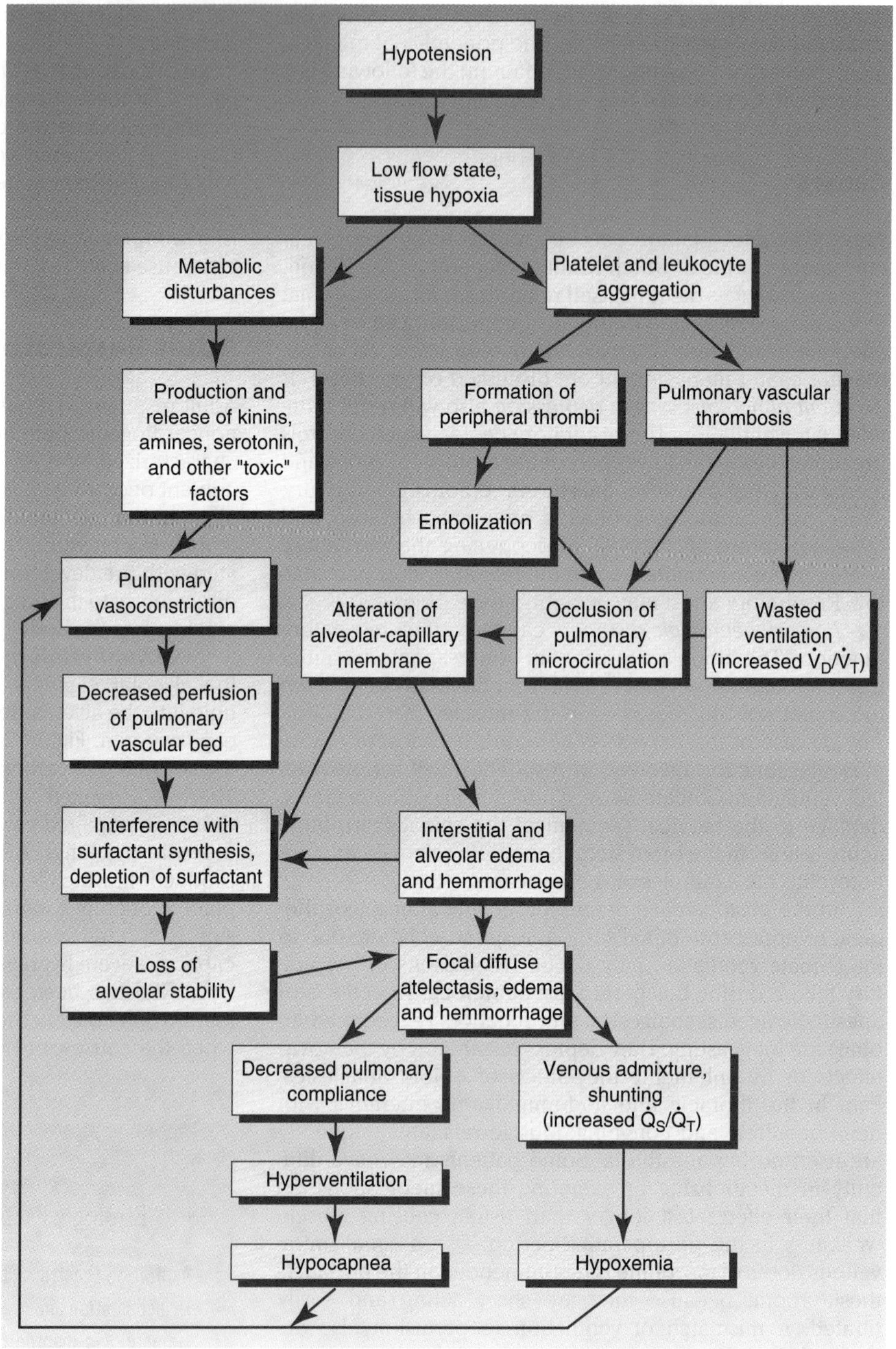

FIGURE 24-7. Pathogenesis and pathophysiology of adult respiratory distress syndrome. (From Burton G et al. Respiratory Care: A Guide to Clinical Practice. Philadelphia, JB Lippincott, 1991.)

sive treatment is implemented, especially the use of positive end-expiratory pressure (PEEP).

Diagnostic Criteria. A diagnosis of ARDS may be made based on the following criteria: (1) acute respiratory failure, (2) bilateral "fluffy" pulmonary infiltrates on chest x-ray, and (3) hypoxemia (PaO_2 below 50 to 60 mm Hg) despite FIO_2 of 50% to 60% (fraction of inspired oxygen).

Medical Management. The management of ARDS includes the following: (1) identifying and treating the cause, (2) assuring adequate ventilation, (3) providing circulatory support, (4) ensuring an adequate fluid volume, and (5) providing nutritional support.

Identifying and treating the cause and preventing infection are critical. *Ventilation* needs are equally as critical. Initially, the patient requires only supplemental oxygen. As the disease progresses, intubation and mechanical ventilation are instituted. The concentration of oxygen and ventilator settings are determined by the patient's status. This is monitored by arterial blood gases. Positive end-expiratory pressure (PEEP) or continuous positive air pressure (CPAP) is a critical part of the treatment of ARDS. PEEP and CPAP increase functional residual capacity (FRC) and reverse alveolar collapse by keeping the alveoli open, resulting in improved arterial oxygenation and a reduction in the V/Q imbalance. By using PEEP, a lower FIO_2 is required. The goal is an FIO_2 of greater or equal to 50%. Most problems of oxygenation are caused by collapsed alveoli. PEEP and CPAP are discussed in Chapter 25.

Systemic hypotension may occur in ARDS owing to hypovolemia secondary to leakage of fluid into the interstitial spaces. Hypovolemia must be carefully treated without causing further overload. Intravenous crystalloid solutions are administered with careful monitoring of pulmonary status. Inotropic or vasopressor agents may be required. Pulmonary artery pressure catheters are used to monitor the patient's fluid status.

The use of corticosteroids in the treatment of ARDS is controversial. Many, in fact, believe that their use may contribute to a deterioration in pulmonary function and the development of superinfections.

Adequate nutritional support is vital in the treatment of ARDS. Patients with ARDS require 35 to 45 kcal/kg a day to meet normal requirements. Enteral feeding is the first consideration; however, total parenteral nutrition also may be required.

Nursing Interventions. *General Measures.* The patient with acute respiratory failure and ARDS is critically ill and requires close monitoring because the condition could quickly change to a life-threatening situation. Most of the respiratory modalities discussed in Chapter 25 will be used in this situation (oxygen administration, mini-nebulizer therapy, chest physiotherapy, endotracheal intubation or tracheostomy, suctioning, tracheostomy care, and ventilator management). Frequent assessment of the patient's status is necessary to evaluate the effectiveness of treatment.

In addition to implementing the medical plan of care, the nurse considers other needs of the patient. If the patient is not being mechanically ventilated, the patient is placed in semi-Fowler's or high-Fowler's position to allow maximal excursion of the thorax. The patient is supported in whatever position feels most comfortable, using pillows, blankets, or an overbed table. If fluids are not restricted, fluid intake is encouraged to correct fluid loss that occurs during rapid breathing and to loosen secretions. The patient will be extremely anxious because of the hypoxemia and dyspnea. The nurse should offer reassurance about the ability and concern of the health care team, explain all procedures, and deliver care in a calm, patient manner. It is important to reduce the patient's anxiety because anxiety prevents rest and increases oxygen expenditure. Rest is essential to reduce oxygen consumption, thereby reducing oxygen needs.

Ventilator Considerations. If the patient is on PEEP, several unique considerations must be addressed. PEEP is an unnatural pattern of breathing and will feel strange to the patient. The patient may be anxious and fight the ventilator. Sedation may be required.

If the PEEP level cannot be maintained, neuromuscular blocking agents, such as vecuronium and atracuronium, may be administered to paralyze the respiratory muscles so the patient does not resist the ventilator and PEEP. In this situation, the patient loses motor function but retains sensation. The patient will be paralyzed and unable to breathe, talk, or blink. The patient will appear unconscious, but will be awake and able to hear. The patient is reassured that the paralysis is a result of the medication and is temporary.

The nurse must be sure the patient does not become disconnected from the ventilator, because the patient will be apneic. Consequently, the nurse ensures that the patient is closely monitored at all times. Expiratory volume alarms are essential. When the patient is removed from the ventilator for suctioning or measurements, it is done quickly to minimize the time without ventilation.

The patient also may experience discomfort or pain but will be unable to communicate these sensations. Analgesia is usually administered concurrently with neuromuscular blocking agents. The nurse must anticipate the patient's needs regarding pain and comfort. The nurse checks the patient's position to ensure it is comfortable, and talks *to* and not *about* the patient while in the patient's presence. Complete eye care is important because of the patient's inability to blink and the risk of corneal abrasions.

Pulmonary Hypertension

Pulmonary hypertension is a condition that is not clinically evident until late in its disease progression. Pulmonary hypertension exists when the systolic pulmonary artery pressure exceeds 30 mm Hg and the mean pulmonary artery pressure is above 15 mm Hg. These pressures, however, cannot be measured indirectly as can systemic blood pressure, but must be measured during right-sided heart catheterization. In the absence of these measurements, clinical recognition becomes the only indicator for the presence of pulmonary hypertension.

There are two forms of pulmonary hypertension: primary (or idiopathic) and secondary. **Primary pulmonary hypertension** is an uncommon disease in which the diagnosis is made by excluding all other possible causes. The exact cause is unknown. The clinical presentation of pulmonary hypertension exists with no evidence of pulmonary and cardiac disease or pulmonary embolism. It occurs most often in women between 20 and 40 years of age and is usually fatal within 5 years of diagnosis.

Secondary pulmonary hypertension is more common and results from existing cardiac or pulmonary disease. Its prognosis depends on the severity of the underlying disorder and the changes in the pulmonary vascular bed. The most common cause of pulmonary hypertension is pulmonary artery constriction due to hypoxia from COPD (Chart 24-6).

Pathophysiology. Normally, the pulmonary vascular bed can handle the blood volume delivered by the right ventricle. It has a low resistance to blood flow and compensates for increased blood volume by dilation of the vessels in the pulmonary circulation. If the pulmonary vascular bed is destroyed or obstructed, however, as in pulmonary hypertension, the ability to handle whatever flow or volume of blood it receives is lost and the increased blood flow then increases the pulmonary artery pressures. As the pulmonary arterial pressure increases, the pulmonary vascular resistance also increases. Both pulmonary artery constriction (as occurs in hypoxia or hypercapnia) and a reduction of the pulmonary vascular bed (which occurs with pulmonary emboli) result in an increase in pulmonary vascular resistance and pressure. This increased work load affects right

CHART 24-6

Causes of Pulmonary Hypertension

Primary or Idiopathic

Altered immune mechanisms
Silent pulmonary emboli
Raynaud's phenomenon
Oral contraceptives
Sickle cell disease
Collagen diseases

Secondary

Pulmonary Vasoconstriction Due to Hypoxia

Chronic obstructive pulmonary disease
Kyphoscoliosis
Obesity
Smoke inhalation
High altitude
Neuromuscular disorders
Diffuse interstitial pneumonia

Reduction of the Pulmonary Vascular Bed (Must Impair 50% to 75% of the Vascular Bed)

Pulmonary emboli
Vasculitis
Widespread interstitial lung disease (sarcoidosis, systemic sclerosis)
Tumor emboli

Primary Cardiac Disease

Congenital (patent ductus arteriosus, atrial septal defect, ventricular septal defect)
Acquired (rheumatic valvular disease, mitral stenosis, myxoma, left ventricular failure)

ventricular function. The myocardium ultimately is unable to meet the increasing demands imposed on it, leading to right ventricular hypertrophy (enlargement and dilatation) and failure (cor pulmonale).

Clinical Manifestations. Dyspnea is the main symptom of pulmonary hypertension, occurring at first with exertion and eventually at rest. Substernal chest pain is also common, affecting 25% to 50% of patients. Other signs and symptoms include weakness, fatigability, syncope, and signs of right-sided heart failure (peripheral edema, ascites, distended neck veins, liver engorgement, crackles, heart murmur). Electrocardiographic changes reveal right ventricular hypertrophy, right axis deviation, tall peaked P waves in inferior leads, and decreased PaO_2 (hypoxemia).

Diagnostic Evaluation. A complete diagnostic evaluation includes a history, physical examination, chest x-rays, ECG, cardiac catheterization, perfusion lung scan, pulmonary function studies, and a lung biopsy. Cardiac catheterization of the right side of the heart will reveal elevated pulmonary arterial pressures. Pulmonary angiography will detect defects in pulmonary vasculature, such as pulmonary emboli. Pulmonary function studies will show an increased residual volume and total lung capacity and a decreased forced expiratory volume (FEV_1) in obstructive pulmonary diseases and a decreased vital capacity and total lung capacity in restrictive lung diseases. A lung biopsy will confirm the diagnosis of pulmonary hypertension.

Medical Management. The goal of treatment is to manage the underlying cardiac or pulmonary condition. Because **hypoxia** is the most common cause of pulmonary vasoconstriction leading to increased pulmonary vascular resistance and pulmonary hypertension, continuous oxygen therapy is the major component of management. In acute conditions, appropriate oxygen therapy (see Chapter 25) will reverse the vasoconstriction and reduce the pulmonary hypertension in a relatively short time. In more chronic, progressive conditions, continuous oxygen therapy may be necessary to slow the progression of the disease.

In the presence of cor pulmonale, treatment should include fluid restriction, cardiac glycosides such as digitalis to improve cardiac function, rest, and diuretics to decrease fluid accumulation.

In *primary pulmonary hypertension,* vasodilators have been administered with variable success. Anticoagulants, such as coumadin, have been given to patients because of chronic pulmonary emboli. Heart–lung transplantation has been successful in a number of patients with primary hypertension who have not been responsive to other therapies.

Nursing Interventions. The major nursing goals are to identify those patients who are at high risk of developing pulmonary hypertension (*i.e.*, those with COPD, pulmonary emboli, congenital heart disease, and mitral valve disease); to be alert for signs and symptoms; to administer oxygen therapy appropriately; and to instruct patients and their families about the safe use of oxygen in the home.

Pulmonary Heart Disease (Cor Pulmonale)

Cor pulmonale is a condition in which the right ventricle of the heart enlarges (with or without right-sided heart failure) as a result of diseases that affect the structure or function of the lung or its vasculature. Any disease affecting the lungs and accompanied by hypoxemia may result in cor pulmonale. The most frequent cause is COPD in which changes in the airway and retained secretions reduce alveolar ventilation. Other causes are conditions that restrict or compromise ventilatory function, leading to hypoxia or acidosis (deformities of the thoracic cage, massive obesity) or conditions that reduce the pulmonary vascular bed (primary idiopathic pulmonary arterial hypertension, pulmonary embolus). Certain disorders of the nervous system, respiratory muscles, chest wall, and pulmonary arterial tree may also be responsible for cor pulmonale.

Pathophysiology. Pulmonary disease can produce physiologic changes that will in time affect the heart and cause the right ventricle to enlarge and eventually fail. Any condition that deprives the lungs of oxygen can cause hypoxemia (decreased arterial oxygen tension) and hypercapnia (increased carbon dioxide in the blood), resulting in ventilatory insufficiency. Hypoxia and hypercapnia cause pulmonary arterial vasoconstriction and possibly reduction of the pulmonary vascular bed, as in emphysema or pulmonary emboli. The result is increased resistance in the pulmonary circulatory system, with a subsequent rise in pulmonary blood pressure (pulmonary hypertension). Pulmonary arterial mean pressures of 45 mm Hg or more may occur in cor pulmonale. Right ventricular hypertrophy may result and be followed by right ventricular failure.

In short, cor pulmonale results from pulmonary hypertension that causes the right side of the heart to enlarge because of the increased work required to pump blood against high resistance through the pulmonary vascular system.

Clinical Manifestations. The symptoms of cor pulmonale are usually related to the underlying lung disease, such as COPD. Shortness of breath and cough are key signs in COPD. As the right ventricle fails, the patient develops edema of the feet and legs, distended neck veins, an enlarged, palpable liver, pleural effusion, ascites, and a heart murmur. Headache, confusion, and somnolence may occur as a result of increased levels of carbon dioxide.

Medical Management. The objectives of treatment are to improve the patient's ventilation and to treat both the underlying lung disease and the manifestations of heart disease. In COPD administration of oxygen may be necessary to improve gas exchange and reduce pulmonary arterial pressure and pulmonary vascular resistance. Improved oxygen transport will relieve the pulmonary hypertension that is causing the cor pulmonale. Administering oxygen is therefore a major part of treatment.

Better survival rates and greater reduction in pulmonary vascular resistance have been reported with continuous, around-the-clock oxygen therapy for patients with severe hypoxia. Substantial improvement may require 4 to 6 weeks of oxygen therapy, usually at home. Periodic assessment of arterial blood gases is necessary to determine adequacy of alveolar ventilation and to monitor the effectiveness of oxygen therapy.

Ventilation is further improved with bronchial hygiene to remove accumulated secretions, the administration of bronchodilators, and chest physical therapy. Further measures depend on the patient's condition. If the patient is in respiratory failure, endotracheal intubation and mechanical ventilation may be necessary. If the patient is in heart failure, hypoxemia and hypercapnia must be relieved to improve cardiac function and output. Bed rest, sodium restriction, and diuretic therapy are also instituted judiciously to reduce peripheral edema (to lower pulmonary arterial pressure through a decrease in total blood volume) and the circulatory load on the right side of the heart. Digitalis may be given if the patient also has left ventricular failure, a supraventricular dysrhythmia, or right ventricular failure that does not respond to other therapy to relieve pulmonary hypertension. Digitalis is administered with extreme caution, because pulmonary heart disease appears to enhance susceptibility to digitalis toxicity.

Electrocardiographic (ECG) monitoring may be indicated because of the high incidence of dysrhythmias in patients with cor pulmonale. Respiratory infection must be treated, as it commonly precipitates pulmonary heart disease. The patient's prognosis depends on whether the hypertensive process is reversible. (The management of the patient with respiratory failure is discussed on pp. 520–521.)

Patient Education and Home Care Considerations. Because management of pulmonary heart disease is related to treating the underlying cause, it is often a long-term process. Consequently, most of the care and monitoring is performed in the home. The patient with COPD is advised to avoid those things that irritate the airways. If continuous oxygen is administered, the patient and the family are instructed in its use. A home health care nurse may visit the home to evaluate the patient's status and understanding of the procedures involved. Most importantly, the patient is urged to stop smoking. Nutrition counseling is necessary if the patient is on a sodium-restricted diet or is taking diuretics. The family is counseled that restlessness, depression, irritability, or atypical behavior may be encountered with hypoxemia or hypercapnia and should decrease as the arterial blood gas values improve.

Pulmonary Embolism

Pulmonary embolism refers to the obstruction of one or more pulmonary arteries by a thrombus (or thrombi) that originates somewhere in the venous system or in the right side of the heart. It is estimated that over half a million people develop pulmonary emboli yearly, resulting in over 50,000 deaths each year. Pulmonary embolism is a common disorder and often is associated with trauma, surgery (orthopedic, pelvic, gynecologic), pregnancy, congestive heart failure, advanced age (over 60), and prolonged immobility. It may occur in an apparently healthy person. Persons who are at risk for developing a pulmonary embolus are identified in Chart 24-7.

Although most thrombi originate in the deep veins of the legs, other sites include the pelvic veins and the right atrium of the heart. A venous thrombosis can result from a slowing of blood flow (stasis), secondary to damage to the blood vessel wall (particularly the endothelial lining) and changes in the blood coagulation mechanism.

Pathophysiology. When a thrombus completely or partially obstructs a pulmonary artery, the alveolar dead space enlarges because the area, although continuing to be ventilated, receives little or no blood flow. In addition, a number of substances are released from the clot and cause the blood vessels and bronchioles to constrict. This reaction compounds the ventilation–perfusion imbalance, causing some blood to be shunted (no gas exchange occurs) and resulting in decreased O_2 and increased CO_2 levels.

The hemodynamic consequences are increased pulmonary vascular resistance due to the reduced size of the pulmonary vascular bed, resulting in an increase in pulmonary arterial pressure and, in turn, an increase in right

CHART 24-7
Pulmonary Embolism: Risk Factors

The following events and conditions predispose to thrombophlebitis and pulmonary embolism.

Venous Stasis (slowing of blood flow in veins)
Prolonged immobilization (especially postoperative)
Prolonged periods of sitting/traveling
Varicose veins
Spinal cord injury

Hypercoagulability (due to release of tissue thromboplastin after injury/surgery)
Injury
Tumor (pancreatic, GI, GU, breast, lung)
Increased platelet count (polycythemia, splenectomy)

Venous Endothelial Disease
Thrombophlebitis
Vascular disease
Foreign bodies (IV/central venous catheters)

Certain Disease States (combination of stasis, coagulation alterations, and venous injury)
Heart disease (especially congestive heart failure)
Trauma (especially fracture of hip, pelvis, vertebra, lower extremities)
Postoperative state/postpartum period
Diabetes mellitus
Chronic obstructive pulmonary disease

Other Predisposing Conditions
Advanced age
Obesity
Pregnancy
Oral contraceptive use
History of previous thrombophlebitis, pulmonary embolism
Constrictive clothing

ventricular work to maintain pulmonary blood flow. When the work requirements of the right ventricle exceed its capacity, right ventricular failure occurs, leading to a decrease in cardiac output followed by a decrease in systemic blood pressure and the development of shock.

Clinical Manifestations. The symptoms of pulmonary embolism depend on the size of the thrombus and the area of the pulmonary artery occluded by the thrombus. The symptoms may be nonspecific. Chest pain is the most common symptom and is usually sudden in onset and pleuritic in nature. It occasionally can be substernal and may mimic angina pectoris or a myocardial infarction. Dyspnea is the second most common symptom, followed by tachypnea (very rapid respiratory rate). Other symptoms include fever, tachycardia, apprehension, cough, diaphoresis, hemoptysis, and syncope.

A massive embolism occluding the bifurcation of the pulmonary artery can produce pronounced dyspnea, sudden substernal pain, rapid and weak pulse, shock, syncope, and sudden death.

Multiple small emboli can lodge in the terminal pulmonary arterioles, producing multiple small infarctions of the lungs. The clinical picture may simulate that of bronchopneumonia or heart failure. In atypical instances, the disease causes few signs and symptoms, whereas in other instances, it mimics various cardiopulmonary disorders.

Diagnostic Evaluation. Because the symptoms of pulmonary embolism can vary, a diagnostic work-up is performed to rule out other diseases. Deep vein thrombosis is closely associated with the development of pulmonary embolism.

The diagnostic work-up includes a chest x-ray, ECG, peripheral vascular studies, impedance plethysmography, arterial blood gases, ventilation–perfusion scan, and pulmonary angiography.

The chest x-ray results are usually normal but may show pneumoconstriction, infiltrates, atelectasis, elevation of the diaphragm on the affected side, or great dilation of the pulmonary artery and a pleural effusion. The ECG usually shows sinus tachycardia, atrial flutter or fibrillation and possible right axis deviation, right bundle branch block, or right ventricular strain. Radiofibrinogen leg scanning and impedance plethysmography are performed to determine the presence of deep vein thrombosis. Test results confirm or exclude the diagnosis of pulmonary embolism. Arterial blood gases may show hypoxemia and hypocapnia. A perfusion lung scan may indicate areas of diminished or absent blood flow. A ventilation scan may show whether there is also a perfusion abnormality present. If there is a ventilation–perfusion (V/Q) mismatch, the probability of a pulmonary embolism is high. If lung scanning is not definitive, pulmonary angiography will confirm the diagnosis of pulmonary emboli.

Prevention. The most effective approach in preventing pulmonary embolism is to prevent deep vein thrombosis. Active leg exercises to avoid venous stasis, early ambulation, and use of elastic stockings are general preventive measures (Chart 24-8). Two additional strategies are recommended:

- Anticoagulant therapy
- Intermittent pneumatic leg compression devices

Patients who are over 40 years of age and whose hemostasis is adequate and who are undergoing major elective abdominal or thoracic surgery frequently are given low

CHART 24-8
Prevention of Pulmonary Embolism

- Encourage active and passive leg exercises to prevent venous stasis in patients on bed rest or in postoperative period.
  Move legs in pumping action so leg muscles can help increase venous blood flow.
- Advise against habits that increase venous stasis:
  Crossing legs.
  Sitting or lying down for prolonged periods.
  Wearing constricting clothing.
  Dangling legs and feet over edge of bed.
- Avoid leaving IV catheters in veins for prolonged periods, if possible.
- Apply elastic stockings or intermittent pneumatic leg compression devices (if prescribed), to compress superficial veins and increase blood flow.
- Elevate legs above level of heart.

doses of heparin preoperatively to reduce the risk of postoperative deep vein thrombus and pulmonary embolism. It is recommended that heparin be administered subcutaneously 2 hours before surgery and continued every 8 to 12 hours until the patient is discharged. Low-dose heparin is thought to enhance the activity of antithrombin III, a major plasma inhibitor of clotting factor X. (This regimen is not recommended for patients who are experiencing an active thrombotic process or those undergoing major orthopedic surgery, open prostatectomy, or surgery on the eye or brain.) Coumadin also may be used prophylactically preoperatively to prevent the development of thromboembolism.

Intermittent pneumatic leg compression devices are very useful in preventing thromboembolism. The device inflates a bag that mechanically compresses the leg from the calf to the thigh, thereby improving venous return. It may be applied preoperatively and continued until the patient is ambulatory. The device is particularly useful for patients who are not candidates for anticoagulant therapy.

Emergency Interventions. Massive pulmonary embolism is a true life-threatening, medical emergency; the patient's condition tends to deteriorate rapidly. The immediate objective of treatment is to stabilize the cardiorespiratory system. The majority of patients who die of massive pulmonary embolism do so in the *first 2 hours* after the embolic event. Emergency management consists of the following:

- Nasal oxygen is administered immediately to relieve hypoxemia, respiratory distress, and cyanosis.
- An intravenous infusion is started to establish a route for drugs or fluids that will be needed.
- Pulmonary angiography, hemodynamic measurements, arterial blood gas determinations, and perfusion lung scans are performed. A sudden rise in pulmonary resistance increases the work of the right ventricle, which can cause acute right-sided heart failure with cardiogenic shock.
- If the patient has suffered massive embolism and is hypotensive, an indwelling urinary catheter is inserted to monitor urinary output.
- Hypotension is treated by a slow infusion of dobutamine (has a dilating effect on pulmonary vessels and bronchi) or dopamine.
- The ECG is monitored continuously for right ventricular failure, which may occur suddenly.
- Digitalis glycosides, intravenous diuretics, and antidysrhythmic agents are administered when appropriate.
- Blood is drawn for serum electrolytes, blood urea nitrogen, complete blood count, and hematocrit.
- If clinical assessment and arterial blood gases indicate the need, the patient is placed on a volume-controlled ventilator.
- Small doses of intravenous morphine are given to relieve the patient's anxiety, to alleviate chest discomfort, to improve tolerance of the endotracheal tube, and to ease adaptation to the mechanical ventilator.

Medical Management. The goal of the treatment is to dissolve (lyse) the existing emboli and prevent new ones from forming. The treatment of pulmonary embolism may include a variety of modalities:

- Anticoagulation therapy
- Thrombolytic therapy
- General measures to improve respiratory and vascular status
- Surgical intervention

Anticoagulation Therapy. Anticoagulant therapy (heparin, warfarin sodium) has traditionally been the primary method for managing acute deep vein thrombosis and pulmonary embolism.

Heparin is used to prevent recurrence of emboli but has no effect on emboli that are already present. It is administered as an IV bolus of 5,000 units followed by continuous infusion of 1,000 units per hour. The goal is to keep the partial thromboplastin time (PTT) 1.5 to 2 times normal. Heparin is administered for 5 to 7 days. *Coumadin* administration is started within 24 hours following the start of heparin therapy and continued for 3 months. The prothrombin time (PT) is maintained at 1.5 times normal. Anticoagulation therapy is contraindicated in patients who are at risk for bleeding (*e.g.*, GI, postoperative, or postpartum bleeding).

Thrombolytic Therapy. Thrombolytic therapy (urokinase, streptokinase) also may be used in treating pulmonary embolism, particularly in patients who are severely compromised.

Thrombolytic therapy resolves the thrombi or emboli more quickly and restores more normal hemodynamic functioning of the pulmonary circulation, thereby reducing pulmonary hypertension and improving perfusion, oxygenation, and cardiac output. Bleeding, however, is a significant side effect. Consequently, thrombolytic agents are advocated only for patients with thrombi affecting the popliteal vein or deep veins of the thigh and pelvis, and for patients with massive pulmonary emboli affecting a significant area of blood flow to the lung.

Before thrombolytic therapy is started, PT, PTT, hematocrit values, and platelet counts are obtained. During therapy all but absolutely essential invasive procedures are avoided, with the exception of careful venipuncture with a 22- or 23-gauge needle to obtain blood samples to monitor the effects of the therapy. If necessary, fresh whole blood, packed red cells, cryoprecipitate, or frozen plasma is given to replace blood loss and reverse the bleeding tendency.

After the thrombolytic infusion is completed (which varies in duration according to the agent used and the condition being treated), the patient is placed on anticoagulants.

General Measures. Other measures are initiated to improve the patient's respiratory and vascular status. Oxygen therapy is administered to correct the hypoxia and to relieve the pulmonary vascular vasoconstriction and reduce the pulmonary hypertension. Venous stasis is reduced by using elastic stockings or intermittent pneumatic leg compression devices. These measures compress the superficial veins and increase the velocity of blood in the deep veins by redirecting the blood through the deep veins. Venous stasis is thereby reduced. Elevating the leg (above the level of the heart) also increases venous flow. Some authorities believe elastic stockings are unnecessary if the patient's legs are elevated.

Surgical Intervention. A **pulmonary embolectomy** may be indicated in the following conditions: (1) if the patient has persistent hypotension, shock, and respiratory distress; (2) if pulmonary artery pressure is greatly elevated; and (3) if angiograms show obstruction of a large part of the pulmonary vasculature. Pulmonary embolectomy requires a thoracotomy with cardiopulmonary bypass technique.

Interrupting the inferior vena cava is another surgical technique used when pulmonary emboli recur or when the patient is intolerant of anticoagulant therapy. This approach prevents dislodged thrombi from being swept into the lungs while allowing adequate blood flow. The procedure can be performed by totally ligating the vena cava or applying Teflon clips to the vena cava to divide the lumen of the vena cava into small channels without occluding caval blood flow.

The use of transvenous devices that occlude or filter the blood through the inferior vena cava is a fairly safe procedure to prevent recurrent pulmonary embolism. One such technique involves inserting a filter (Greenfield filter) into the internal jugular vein or common femoral vein (Fig. 24-8). This filter is advanced through the superior vena cava into the inferior vena cava, where it is brought into an open position. The perforated umbrella permits the passage of blood but prevents the passage of large thrombi.

Transvenous catheter embolectomy is a technique in which a vacuum-cupped catheter is introduced transvenously into the affected pulmonary artery. Suction is applied to the end of the embolus, and the embolus is aspirated into the cup. The surgeon maintains suction to hold the embolus within the cup, and the entire catheter is withdrawn through the right side of the heart and out the femoral venotomy. An inferior caval filter often is inserted at the same time to protect against a recurrence.

Postoperative Nursing Care. Following surgery, the patient's pulmonary arterial pressure and urinary output are measured. The insertion site of the arterial catheter is assessed for hematoma formation and infection. An adequate blood pressure must be maintained to ensure perfusion of vital organs. To prevent peripheral venous stasis and edema of the lower extremities, the foot of the bed is elevated. Isometric exercises, elastic stockings, and walking are encouraged when the patient is permitted out of bed. Sitting is discouraged because hip flexion causes compression of the large veins in the legs.

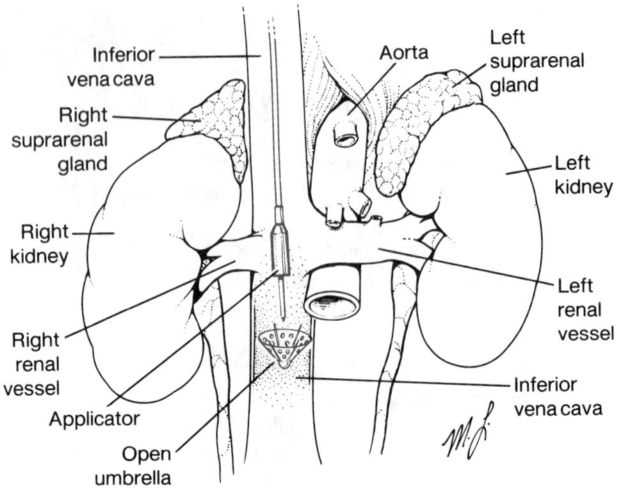

FIGURE 24-8. An umbrella filter is in place in the inferior vena cava to prevent pulmonary embolism. The filter (compressed within an applicator catheter) is inserted through an incision in the right internal jugular vein. The applicator is withdrawn when the filter fixes itself to the wall of the inferior vena cava after ejection from the applicator.

Nursing Assessment. Patients who are at risk for developing pulmonary embolism are examined for a positive Homans' sign, which may or may not indicate impending thrombosis of the leg veins (see Chapter 31). To test Homans' sign, the patient assumes a supine position. The leg is lifted and the foot is dorsiflexed (see Fig. 21-4). The patient is asked to report if calf pain occurs during this maneuver. The occurrence of pain is a positive Homans' sign, which may indicate deep venous thrombosis.

A key role of the nurse is to minimize the risk of pulmonary embolism in all patients and to identify those who are at high risk (see Charts 24-6 and 24-7). The nurse must have a high degree of suspicion for pulmonary embolism in any patient, but particularly those with conditions predisposing to a slowing of venous return. Such conditions include trauma to the pelvis (especially surgical trauma) and to the lower extremities (especially hip fractures), obesity, previous thromboembolic episodes, varicose veins, pregnancy, congestive heart failure, myocardial infarction, use of oral contraceptives, and malignant disease. Also, postoperative patients and the elderly often have a slower venous return.

Nursing Interventions. When caring for a patient who has had a pulmonary embolism, the nurse must be alert for the potential complication of cardiogenic shock or right ventricular failure subsequent to the effect of the pulmonary embolus on the cardiovascular system. Nursing activities for management of shock are found in Chapter 15.

Prevention. Preventing thrombus formation is a major nursing responsibility. Ambulation and active and passive leg exercises are encouraged to prevent venous stasis in patients on bed rest. The patient is instructed to move the legs in a "pumping" exercise so that the leg muscles can help increase venous flow. The patient also is advised not to sit or lie for prolonged periods, to cross the legs or wear constricting clothing. Legs should not be "dangled" nor feet placed in a dependent position while the patient sits on the edge of the bed. Instead, the patient's feet should rest on the floor or on a chair. Intravenous catheters (for parenteral therapy or measurements of central venous pressure) should not be left in place for prolonged periods.

Monitoring Thrombolytic Therapy. The nurse is responsible for monitoring thrombolytic and anticoagulant therapy. Thrombolytic therapy (streptokinase, urokinase) causes lysis of deep vein thrombi and pulmonary emboli, which helps resolve the clot. During thrombolytic infusion, the patient remains on bed rest, vital signs are assessed every 2 hours, and invasive procedures are limited. Tests to determine prothrombin time or partial thromboplastin time are performed 3 to 4 hours after the thrombolytic infusion is started to confirm that the fibrinolytic systems have been activated. Because of the prolonged clotting time, only essential arterial blood gas studies are performed. Pressure is applied by hand to the puncture site for at least 30 minutes. The infusion is immediately discontinued if uncontrolled bleeding occurs. (See Chapter 31 for nursing management for the patient receiving anticoagulant or thrombolytic therapy.)

Pain Management. Chest pain, if present, is usually pleuritic rather than cardiac in origin. The patient should be in semi-Fowler's position to make it easier to breathe and to distribute air throughout the lungs. Opioid (narcotic) analgesics are administered as prescribed for severe pain.

Oxygen Therapy. Careful attention is given to the proper use of oxygen. It is important to ensure that the patient understands the need for continuous oxygen therapy. The nurse assesses the patient frequently for signs of hypoxia to evaluate the effectiveness of the oxygen therapy. Nebulizer therapy, incentive spirometry, or postural drainage is administered if there is an accumulation of secretions complicating the pulmonary embolism.

Coping With Anxiety. The patient, once stabilized, is encouraged to talk about any fears or concerns growing out of this frightening episode. The patient's questions are answered concisely and accurately, the therapy is explained, and the early recognition of untoward effects is described.

Patient Education and Home Care Considerations. Prior to hospital discharge and at follow-up visits to the clinic or during home visits, the patient is instructed about how to prevent recurrence and what signs and symptoms should be reported immediately. Patient instructions, as presented in Chart 24-9, are intended to help prevent recurrences and side effects of treatment.

CHART 24-9
Patient Education: Preventing Recurrent Episodes of Pulmonary Embolism

- When taking anticoagulants, look for bruising and bleeding; try to avoid bumping into objects that can cause bruising (avoid sharps to prevent cuts, shave with electric shaver).
- Use a toothbrush with soft bristles.
- Do not take aspirin or antihistamine drugs while receiving warfarin sodium (Coumadin). Always check with your physician before taking any medication, including over-the-counter medications.
- Continue to wear elastic stockings as long as directed.
- Avoid laxatives, because they affect vitamin K absorption.
- Avoid sitting with your legs crossed or sitting for prolonged periods.
- When traveling, change your position regularly, walk occasionally, and do active exercises of the legs and ankles while sitting. Drink plenty of liquids while traveling to avoid hemoconcentration due to fluid deficit.
- Report dark, tarry stools to your primary health care provider immediately.
- Wear an identification bracelet (or carry a card) stating that anticoagulants are being taken.

Breathing Disorders During Sleep

A variety of respiratory disorders are associated with sleep, the most common being sleep apnea syndrome. **Sleep apnea syndrome** is defined as cessation of air flow (apnea) during sleep. Sleep apnea is classified into three types: (1) *obstructive*—lack of air flow due to pharyngeal occlusion; (2) *central*—simultaneous cessation of both air flow and respiratory movements; and (3) *mixed*—a combination of central and obstructive apnea within one apneic episode.

Clinical Manifestations. Sleep apnea usually occurs in men, especially those who are older and overweight. The patient snores loudly, stops breathing up to 10 seconds or more, and then awakens abruptly with a loud snort as blood oxygen level drops. Ten apneic episodes per hour to several hundred per night can occur. The effect can seriously tax the heart and lungs. Other symptoms include excessive daytime sleepiness, morning headache, sore throat, intellectual deterioration, personality changes, behavioral disorders, enuresis, impotence, obesity, and complaints by the partner that the patient snores loudly or is unusually restless during sleep (Chart 24-10).

Medical Management. Patients seek medical treatment because their partners express concern or they experience excessive sleeplessness at inappropriate times or settings, for example, while driving a car. A variety of treatments are used in the management of sleep apnea. In mild cases of obstructive sleep apnea, the patient is advised to avoid alcohol and medications that depress the upper airway and to lose weight. In more severe cases of obstructive sleep apnea, in which hypoxia with severe CO_2 retention (hypercapnia) is present, the treatment includes continuous positive airway pressure (CPAP) or bi-level positive airway pressure (BIPAP) with supplemental oxygen via nasal cannula. Medroxyprogesterone acetate has been used to stimulate respirations. Surgical procedures to correct the obstruction may be performed. As a last resort, a tracheostomy is performed to bypass the obstruction if the potential for

CHART 24-10
Clinical Features of Obstructive Sleep Apnea Syndrome

Excessive daytime sleepiness
Frequent nocturnal awakening
Insomnia
Loud snoring
Morning headaches
Intellectual deterioration
Personality changes, irritability
Impotence
Systemic hypertension
Dysrhythmias
Pulmonary hypertension, cor pulmonale
Polycythemia

life-threatening dysrhythmia exists. The tracheostomy is unplugged only during the patient's sleep.

The treatment of central sleep apnea includes using respiratory stimulants. Low-flow nasal oxygen taken at night can help relieve hypoxemia in some patients. Using a pacemaker to stimulate the phrenic nerves may be indicated in some patients.

Sarcoidosis

Sarcoidosis is a granulomatous disease that affects many body systems. Although the cause is unknown, patients with sarcoidosis have a number of immunologic abnormalities. It may involve almost any organ or tissue, but most commonly involves the lungs, lymph nodes, liver, spleen, skin, eyes and fingers, and parotid glands. Sarcoidosis is fairly common worldwide and usually occurs between the second and fourth decades.

The clinical picture includes dyspnea, cough, hemoptysis, and congestion. Generalized symptoms include anorexia, fatigue, and weight loss. The chest x-ray may show hilar adenopathy and disseminated miliary and nodular lesions in the lungs. Other signs include uveitis, joint pain, fever, and granulomatous lesions of the skin, liver, spleen, kidney, and central nervous system. The granulomas may disappear or gradually convert to fibrous tissue. With multiple organ system involvement, the patient experiences fatigue, fever, anorexia, weight loss, and joint pain.

The diagnosis is confirmed by biopsy of the skin and lymph nodes, which shows noncaseating granulomas. Pulmonary function tests are abnormal if there is restriction of lung function (reduction in total lung capacity). Arterial blood gases may be normal or may show reduced oxygen levels (hypoxemia) and increased carbon dioxide levels (hypercapnia).

The condition may resolve itself naturally. Corticosteroid therapy may benefit some patients because of its anti-inflammatory effect, which relieves symptoms and improves organ function. It is useful for patients with ocular and myocardial involvement, extensive pulmonary disease that compromises pulmonary function, and hypercalcemia. Isoniazid may be given to patients with positive tuberculin tests.

Occupational Lung Diseases

Diseases of the lungs occur in numerous occupations as a result of exposure to organic and inorganic (mineral) dusts and noxious gases (fumes and aerosols). The effects of inhaling these materials depends on the composition of the substance, its concentration, its ability to initiate an immune response, its irritating properties, the duration of exposure, and the individual's response or susceptibility to the irritant. Smoking may compound the problem and may increase the risk of lung cancers in people exposed to asbestos.

Pneumoconioses

Pneumoconiosis refers to a nonneoplastic alteration of the lung resulting from exposure to inorganic dust (*e.g.*, "dusty lung"). The most common pneumoconioses are silicosis, asbestosis, and coal worker's pneumoconiosis.

Silicosis. Silicosis is a chronic pulmonary disease caused by inhalation of silica dust (silicon dioxide particles). Exposure to silica and silicates occurs in almost all mining, quarrying, and tunneling operations. Stonecutting, the manufacture of abrasives and pottery, and foundry work are other occupations with exposure hazards.

Pathophysiology. When the silica particles, which have fibrogenic properties, are inhaled, nodular lesions are produced throughout the lungs. With the passage of time and further exposure, the nodules enlarge and coalesce. Dense masses form in the upper portion of the lungs, resulting in loss of pulmonary volume. Restrictive lung disease (inability of the lungs to expand fully) and obstructive lung disease from secondary emphysema result. Cavities can form as a result of superimposed tuberculosis. Exposure of 10 to 20 years is usually required before the disease develops and shortness of breath is manifested. Fibrotic destruction of pulmonary tissue can lead to emphysema, pulmonary hypertension, and cor pulmonale.

Clinical Manifestations. The patient may experience symptoms indicative of hypoxemia, severe airflow obstruction, and right-sided heart failure. Edema may occur because of the cardiac failure.

Medical Management. There is no specific treatment for silicosis. Therapy is directed at managing complications and preventing infection. Testing is performed to rule out tuberculosis. If tuberculosis is present, it is aggressively treated. Additional therapy might include oxygen, diuretics, β-antagonists, and bronchodilator therapy (theophylline and ipratropium bromide).

Asbestosis. Asbestosis is a disease characterized by diffuse pulmonary fibrosis due to the inhalation of asbestos dust. Laws have restricted the use of asbestos but many industries in the past used it so that exposure occurs in numerous occupations, including asbestos mining and manufacturing, demolition work, and roofing. Materials such as shingles, cement, vinyl asbestos tile, fireproof paint and clothing, brake linings, and filters all contained asbestos at one time.

Pathophysiology. The asbestos fibers, when inhaled, enter the alveoli, which eventually are obliterated by fibrous tissue that surrounds the asbestos particles. Fibrous changes also affect the pleura, which thickens and develops plaque. The result of these physiologic changes is a restrictive lung disease, with a decrease in lung volume, diminished exchange of oxygen and carbon dioxide, and hypoxemia.

Clinical Manifestations. The patient experiences dyspnea, which becomes progressively worse, mild to moderate chest pain, anorexia, and weight loss. Cor pulmonale and respiratory failure occur as the disease progresses. A fairly high proportion of workers who have been exposed to asbestos dust die of lung cancer, especially those who smoke. Cancer also can occur in other tissues.

Medical Management. There is no effective treatment for asbestosis. Management is directed at controlling infection and treating the lung disease. When oxygen–carbon dioxide exchange becomes severely impaired, continuous oxygen therapy may help improve exercise tolerance. Exposure to asbestos should be avoided and workers should be instructed to stop smoking.

Coal Worker's Pneumoconiosis. Coal worker's pneumoconiosis ("black lung disease") includes a variety of respiratory diseases found in coal workers who have inhaled coal dust over the years. Coal miners are exposed to dusts that are mixtures of coal, kaolin, mica, and silica.

Pathophysiology. When coal dust is deposited in the alveoli and respiratory bronchioles, macrophages engulf the particles (by phagocytosis) and transport them to the terminal bronchioles where they are removed by mucociliary action. In time, the clearance mechanisms are unable to handle the excessive dust load and the macrophages aggregate in the respiratory bronchioles and alveoli. Fibroblasts appear and a network of reticulin is laid down surrounding the dust-laden macrophages. The bronchioles and the alveoli become clogged with coal dust, dying macrophages, and fibroblasts, which leads to the formation of the coal macule, the primary lesion of the disorder. (Macules appear as blackish dots on the lungs.) As the macules enlarge, the weakening bronchioles dilate with subsequent development of a localized emphysema.

Patients with complicated coal worker's pneumoconiosis have massive lung lesions of dense fibrotic tissue containing black material. These masses eventually destroy blood vessels and the bronchi of the affected lobe.

Clinical Manifestations. The first signs are a chronic cough and sputum production, similar to the signs encountered in chronic bronchitis. As the disease progresses, the patient develops dyspnea and coughs up large amounts of sputum with varying amounts of black fluid (melanoptysis), particularly if the individual is a smoker. Eventually cor pulmonale and respiratory failure result. The treatment is symptomatic. (See also treatment of emphysema, pp. 509–512.)

Prevention

The occupational health nurse should act as an employee advocate, making every effort to promote measures to reduce the exposure of workers to industrial products. Laws require that the work environment be ventilated properly to remove any noxious agent. Dust control can prevent many of the pneumoconioses and includes ventilation, spraying an area with water to control release of dust, and effective and frequent floor cleaning. Air samples need to be monitored. Toxic substances should be enclosed and placed in restricted areas. Workers must wear or use protective devices (face masks, hoods, industrial respirators) to provide a safe air supply when a toxic element is present. Employees who are at risk should be carefully screened and followed. There is a risk of developing serious smoking-related illness (cancer) in industries in which there are unsafe levels of certain gases, dusts, fumes, fluids, and other toxic substances. Ongoing educational programs should teach workers to take responsibility for their own health and to stop smoking and get an influenza vaccination.

The "Right to Know" law stipulates that employees must be informed about all hazardous and toxic substances in the workplace. Specifically, they must be educated about any hazardous or toxic substances they work with, what effects these substances can have on their health, and the protective measures they can take to protect themselves. The responsibility for implementating these controls inevitably falls on the federal or state governments, as exemplified by the Coal Mine Health and Safety Act, the Occupational Safety and Health Act (OSHA), and the Federal Mine Safety and Health Amendment Act. The workplace is currently monitored by the Mining Safety and Health Administration (MSHA) of the Department of Labor, the National Coal Workers' Health Surveillance Program of the National Institute for Occupational Safety and Health (NIOSH), as well as state and local agencies.

Chest Tumors

Tumors of the lung may be benign or malignant. A malignant chest tumor can be *primary,* arising within the lung or the mediastinum, or it can be a *metastasis* from a primary tumor site elsewhere in the body. Metastatic lung tumors occur frequently because the bloodstream transports free cancer cells from primary cancers elsewhere in the body to the lungs. The tumors grow in and between the alveoli and the bronchi, pushing them apart as they grow. This process may occur over a long period, causing few or no symptoms.

Many tumors of the chest arise from the bronchial epithelium. Bronchial adenomas are slow-growing, usually benign tumors, but they are very vascular and, therefore, produce symptoms of bleeding and bronchial obstruction. Bronchogenic carcinoma is a malignant tumor arising from the bronchus. Such a tumor is epidermoid, usually located in the larger bronchi, or it may be an adenocarcinoma, arising farther out in the lung. There are also several intermediate or undifferentiated types of lung cancer, identifiable by cell type.

Lung Cancer (Bronchogenic Carcinoma)

Lung cancer is the number one cancer killer among men in the United States. However, it is increasing at a greater rate in women than it is in men and now exceeds breast cancer as the most common cause of cancer death in women. In approximately 70% of lung cancer patients the disease has spread to regional lymphatics and other sites by the time of diagnosis. As a result, the survival rate for lung cancer patients is low. Evidence indicates that carcinoma tends to arise at sites of previous scarring (tuberculosis, fibrosis) in the lung. Most cases of lung cancer could be prevented if cigarette smoking were eliminated.

Classification and Staging

Four major cell types of lung cancer (which differ significantly) have been identified: epidermoid (squamous cell) carcinoma, small cell (oat cell) carcinoma, adenocarcinoma, and large cell (undifferentiated) carcinoma. Many tumors contain more than one cell type. The different cell types act differently and differ in prognosis. Prognosis appears more favorable for epidermoid cancers and adenocarcinomas; undifferentiated small cell (oat cell) tumors have a poor prognosis.

In addition to cell type, lung cancers are also staged; the stage of the tumor refers to the size of the tumor, whether the lymph nodes are involved, and if the cancer has spread. Staging is determined by tissue biopsy, lymph node biopsy, and mediastinoscopy. Staging helps determine whether the tumor should be removed.

Risk Factors

A variety of factors have been associated with the development of lung cancer: tobacco smoke, second-hand smoke, air pollution, radon, and inadequate intake of vitamin A.

Tobacco Smoke. Tobacco use is responsible for more than one of every 6 deaths in the United States due to pulmonary and cardiovascular diseases; it is the most important single preventable cause of death and disease in this country (Healthy People 2000, 1990). Lung cancer is ten times more common in cigarette smokers than nonsmokers. Risk is determined by the pack-year history (number of packs of cigarettes used each day times the number of years smoked). In addition, the younger a person starts smoking, the greater the risk of developing lung cancer. Other factors that are considered include the type of cigarettes smoked (tar content, filter vs. nonfilter).

Second-Hand Smoke. Passive smoking has been identified as a possible cause of lung cancer in nonsmokers. In other words, persons who are involuntarily exposed to tobacco smoke in a closed environment (car, building) are at risk for developing lung cancer. Public opinion has led to numerous campaigns to restrict smoking in public places such as restaurants, offices, and airplanes.

Air Pollution. A variety of carcinogens have been identified in the atmosphere, including sulphur, motor vehicle emissions, and pollutants from refinery and manufacturing plants. Evidence suggests that the incidence of lung cancer is greater in urban areas as a result of build-up of pollutants and motor vehicle emissions.

Occupational Exposure. Chronic exposure to industrial carcinogens, such as arsenic, asbestos, mustard gas, chromates, coke oven fumes, nickel, oil, and radiation has been associated with the development of lung cancer. Laws have been passed to control exposure to such elements in the workplace.

Radon. Radon is a colorless, odorless gas found in soil and rocks. For many years, it has been associated with uranium mines but is now known to seep into homes through ground rock. Today, high levels of radon (greater than 4 picocuries/L) have been associated with the development of lung cancer. Home owners are advised to have radon levels checked in their houses and to arrange for special venting if the levels are high.

Vitamin A. Research suggests that there is a relationship between low dietary intake of vitamin A and the development of lung cancer. It is postulated that vitamin A is associated with the regulation of cell differentiation.

Other factors that have been associated with lung cancer include genetic predisposition and other underlying respiratory diseases, such as COPD and tuberculosis. A combination of risk factors, particularly cigarette smoking, greatly increases the risk of developing lung cancer.

Clinical Manifestations

Tumors of the bronchopulmonary system may affect the lining of the respiratory tract, lung parenchyma, pleura, or chest wall. The disease develops slowly (usually over several decades) and often is asymptomatic until late in its course. The signs and symptoms depend on the location and size of the tumor, the degree of obstruction, and the existence of metastases to regional or distant sites.

The most frequent symptom of lung cancer is cough, probably from irritation caused by the tumor mass. People frequently ignore this symptom and attribute it to smoking. The cough starts as a hacking cough, without producing any sputum, but progresses to a point where it produces a thick, purulent sputum in response to secondary infection.

- A cough that changes in character should arouse suspicion of lung cancer.

Wheezing can be noted (occurs when a bronchus becomes partially obstructed by the tumor) in about 20% of patients with lung cancer. Blood-tinged sputum is frequently coughed up, particularly in the morning. The sputum becomes streaked with blood as it passes over the ulcerated tumor surface. In some patients, a recurring fever occurs as an early symptom in response to a persisting infection in an area of pneumonitis distal to the tumor. In fact, cancer of the lung should be suspected in persons with repeated unresolved upper respiratory tract infections. Pain is a late manifestation and is often found to be related to bone metastasis.

If the tumor spreads to adjacent structures and regional lymph nodes, the patient may present with chest pain and tightness, hoarseness (involving the recurrent laryngeal nerve), dysphagia, head and neck edema, and symptoms of pleural or pericardial effusion. The most common sites of metastases are lymph nodes, bone, brain, contralateral lung, and adrenal glands. General symptoms of weakness, anorexia, weight loss, and anemia appear late.

Diagnostic Evaluation

If pulmonary symptoms occur in a heavy smoker, cancer of the lung is suspected. Chest x-ray is performed to search for pulmonary density, a solitary peripheral nodule (coin lesion), atelectasis, and infection. Cytologic examination of fresh sputum obtained by cough or saline washings from a bronchus that is suspected of being a cancer site is performed to search for malignant cells. Fiberoptic bronchoscopy provides a detailed study of the bronchial segments and aids in identifying the source of malignant cells and the probable extent of anticipated surgery. Fluorescent bronchofibroscopy is also used to detect small, early bronchogenic cancers. Hematoporphyrin is injected, absorbed by malignant cells, and appears as a red fluorescent glow when examined under ultraviolet light.

Lung scans are part of the diagnostic work-up and a bone scan or bone marrow study is performed to detect bone metastasis. Liver scanning may also be used to determine if the cancer has spread to the liver. Any central nervous system metastases are detected by brain scanning, CT scan, magnetic resonance imaging (MRI), and other neurologic diagnostic procedures. Mediastinoscopy may be used to determine if the tumor has spread to the hilar lymph nodes of the right lung, and a mediastinotomy gives access to the hilar lymphatics of the left lung.

Before surgery is performed, the patient is evaluated to determine whether the tumor is resectable and whether the physiologic impairment resulting from such surgery can be tolerated. Pulmonary function tests combined with split-function perfusion scans are performed to determine if the patient will have adequate pulmonary reserve after the procedure. The patient's ability to move air (vital capacity, FEV_1) is important because the ability to generate an effective cough is imperative in the postoperative period.

Gerontologic Considerations

Cancer of the lung is not unusual in the elderly; however, the presence of coronary artery disease or pulmonary insufficiency may contraindicate surgical intervention. If the patient's cardiovascular status and pulmonary function are satisfactory, surgery is generally well tolerated.

Medical Management

The objective of management is to provide a cure, if possible. The treatment depends on the cell type, the stage of the disease, and the physiologic status (particularly cardiac and pulmonary status) of the patient. In general, treatment may involve surgery, radiation therapy, chemotherapy, and immunotherapy, used separately or in combination.

Surgery. Surgical resection is the preferred method for patients with localized tumors with no evidence of metastatic spread and whose cardiopulmonary function is adequate. Three types of lung resection may be performed: *lobectomy* (a single lobe of lung is removed), *sleeve lobectomy* (cancerous lobe is removed and segment of main bronchus is resected), and *pneumonectomy* (removal of entire lung).

It is rare for a surgical resection to result in a complete cure. (Usually, surgery for small cell cancer of the lung is not advisable because this type of cancer grows rapidly and metastasizes early and extensively.) Unfortunately, in a large number of patients with bronchogenic cancer the lesion is inoperable at the time of diagnosis. The usual operation for small, apparently curable tumor of the lung is lobectomy (removal of a lobe of the lung). An entire lung may be removed (pneumonectomy) in combination with other surgical procedures, such as resection of involved mediastinal lymph nodes.

Before surgery, the cardiopulmonary reserve of the patient must be determined. (See pp. 566–576 for the preoperative and postoperative management of the patient undergoing chest surgery.)

Radiation Therapy. Radiation therapy may cure a small percentage of patients. It is useful in controlling neoplasms that cannot be resected but are responsive to radiation. The small cell and epidermoid tumors are usually radiation sensitive. Radiation may also be used to reduce the size of a tumor to make an inoperable tumor operable or radiation may be used as palliative treatment to relieve pressure of the tumor on vital structures. It can control symptoms of spinal cord metastasis and superior vena cava compression. Also, prophylactic brain irradiation is used on certain patients to treat microscopic metastases to the brain. Radiation may help relieve cough, chest pain, dyspnea, hemoptysis, and bone and liver pain. Relief of symptoms may last from a few weeks to many months and is important in improving the quality of the remaining period of life.

Radiation therapy usually is toxic to normal tissue within the radiation field. Complications of radiation therapy include esophagitis, pneumonitis, and radiation lung fibrosis, which may impair ventilatory and diffusion capacity and significantly reduce pulmonary reserve. Radiation also can affect the heart.

The patient's nutritional status and psychological outlook are monitored through the treatment, along with signs of anemia and infection. (See Chapter 16 for management of the patient receiving radiation therapy.)

Chemotherapy. Chemotherapy is used to alter tumor growth patterns, to treat patients with distant metastases or small-cell cancer of the lung, and to supplement surgery or radiation therapy. Combinations of two or more medications may be more beneficial than single-dose regimens. A large number of medications act against lung cancer. A variety of chemotherapeutic agents, including alkylating agents (ifosfamide), platinum analogues (cisplatin and carboplatin), mitomycin C, vinca alkaloids (vinblastine and vindesine) and etoposide (V-16) are used. The choice of agent depends on the growth of the tumor cell and the specific phase of the cell cycle that the drug affects. These agents are toxic and have a narrow margin of safety.

Chemotherapy may provide some relief, especially of pain, but it does not cure and rarely prolongs life. It is valuable in reducing pressure symptoms of lung cancer and in treating brain, spinal cord, and pericardial metastasis. (See Chapter 16 for chemotherapy for the patient with cancer.)

Potential Complications

A variety of complications may occur in the management of lung cancer. Surgical resection may result in respiratory failure, particularly when the cardiopulmonary system is compromised prior to surgery. Radiation therapy may result in diminished cardiopulmonary function. Pulmonary fibrosis, pericarditis, myelitis, and cor pulmonale are some of the known complications. Chemotherapy, particularly in combination with radiation therapy, can cause pneumonitis. Pulmonary toxicity and leukemia are potential side effects of chemotherapy.

The nurse instructs the patient and family about the potential side effects of the specific treatment plan and strategies to manage them. Symptom management will assist the patient to cope with the therapeutic measures.

Nursing Interventions

Nursing care of the patient with lung cancer is similar to that of other patients with cancer (see Chap. 16). Special attention is focused on the respiratory manifestations of the disease. Airway management is needed to maintain airway patency through the removal of secretions or exudate. As the tumor enlarges, it may compress a bronchus or involve a large area of lung tissue, resulting in an impaired breathing pattern and poor gas exchange. Deep breathing and coughing, aerosol therapy, oxygen therapy, and mechanical ventilation may be necessary when there is respiratory impairment.

The psychologic aspects of care for the patient with lung cancer are extremely important. The patient will have to cope with many issues during the course of the disease (see Chapter 16).

Tumors of the Mediastinum

Tumors of the mediastinum include neurogenic tumors, tumors of the thymus, and mesodermal and endocrine tumors. Of these tumors, tumors of the thymus have the highest percentage of malignancy.

Cysts of the mediastinum are usually small and benign. Dermoid cysts occasionally develop and may ulcerate into the air passages.

Clinical Manifestations. Nearly all the symptoms of mediastinal tumors are due to the pressure of the mass against important intrathoracic organs and include chest pain; bulging of the chest wall; orthopnea (an early sign due to pressure against the trachea, a main bronchus, the recurrent laryngeal nerve, or the lung); cardiac palpitation, angina, and various other circulatory disturbances; cyanosis; superior vena caval syndromes (*i.e.*, swelling of the face, the neck, and the upper extremities) and the marked distention of the veins of the neck and the chest wall (evidence of the obstruction of large veins of the mediastinum by extravascular compression or intravascular invasion); and dysphagia from pressure against the esophagus.

Diagnostic Evaluation. Chest x-rays are a major means of diagnosing mediastinal tumors and cysts. Lateral and oblique x-rays can localize the tumor. CT scans are used to detect hidden thymomas as well as to define a mass lesion. The biopsy of an enlarged lymph node removed from above the clavicle or one removed during mediastinoscopy may provide the diagnosis. Blood studies are of value in excluding other causes of lymph node enlargement, such as leukemia, and sputum examinations aid in ruling out tuberculosis.

Management. Many mediastinal tumors are benign and operable. The location of the tumor in the mediastinum will dictate the type of incision. Most incisions are median sternotomies. The care is the same as for any patient who is undergoing thoracic surgery (see pp. 566–576). The major complications, although infrequent, include hemorrhage, injury to the phrenic or recurrent laryngeal nerve, and infection. If the tumor is malignant and has infiltrated surrounding tissue, radiation therapy and chemotherapy are the therapeutic modalities used when complete surgical removal is not feasible.

Chest Trauma

Chest trauma accounts for approximately 25% of all trauma-related deaths in the United States and is closely associated with another 50% of trauma-related deaths involving multiple system injuries. Chest trauma is classified as either blunt or penetrating. Although blunt chest trauma is more common, it is often difficult to identify the extent of the damage because the symptoms may be generalized and vague. Patients may not seek immediate medical attention, which may further complicate the problem. Automobile crashes, falls, and bicycle handlebars are the most common mechanisms for blunt chest trauma. The most common mechanisms for penetrating chest trauma include gunshot wounds and stabbing.

Injuries to the chest are often life threatening and result in one or more of the following pathologic mechanisms:

- *Hypoxemia* due to disruption in the airway, injury to the lung parenchyma, rib cage, and respiratory musculature, collapsed lung, and pneumothorax
- *Hypovolemia* due to massive fluid loss from the great vessels, cardiac rupture, or hemothorax
- *Cardiac failure* due to cardiac tamponade, cardiac contusion, or increased intrathoracic pressure

These mechanisms frequently result in impaired ventilation and perfusion leading to acute respiratory failure, hypovolemic shock, and death.

Immediate Assessment and Management

Time is critical in treating chest trauma. The immediate factors to determine include: the time the injury occurred; the mechanism of injury; if the patient is responsive, the specific injuries; the estimated blood loss; whether drugs or alcohol have been used; and the prehospital treatment. A physical examination includes inspection of the airway, thorax, neck veins, breathing, vital signs, and skin color for signs of shock. The thorax is palpated for tenderness, crepitus, and the position of the trachea. Breath sounds and heart sounds are auscultated.

An initial diagnostic work-up includes a chest x-ray, CBC, clotting studies, type and cross-match, urinalysis, electrolytes and osmolality, oxygen saturation, arterial blood gases, and an ECG. A CT scan may also be obtained.

The patient is completely undressed to avoid missing additional injuries that can further complicate care. Many injuries involving the chest have associated head and abdominal injuries that require attention. Ongoing assessment is essential to monitor the patient's response to treatment and to detect early signs of a deteriorating condition.

The goals of treatment are to evaluate the patient's condition and initiate aggressive resuscitation. An airway is immediately established with oxygen support and, in some cases, ventilatory support. Reestablishing fluid volume, restoring the pleural seal in the chest, and draining intrapleural fluid and blood are essential.

The potential for massive blood loss and exsanguination with blunt and penetrating chest injuries is high because of injury to the great blood vessels. Many patients die at the scene or are in shock by the time help arrives. Agitation and irrational and combative behavior are signs of decreased oxygen delivery to the cerebral cortex. To restore and maintain cardiopulmonary function, an adequate airway is created and ventilation is initiated. This includes stabilizing and reestablishing chest wall integrity, plugging any hole in the chest (open pneumothorax), and draining or removing any air or fluid from the thorax to relieve pneumothorax/hemothorax and cardiac tamponade. Hypovolemia and low cardiac output are corrected. Many of these treatment efforts, along with the control of hemorrhage, are usually carried out simultaneously at the scene of the injury or in the emergency department.

Principles of management are essentially those pertaining to care of the postoperative thoracic patient (see pp. 569–576).

Rib Fractures

Rib fractures are the most common type of chest trauma, occurring in over 60% of patients admitted with blunt chest injury. Most rib fractures are benign and are treated conservatively. Fractures of the first three ribs are rare but can result in a high mortality rate because they are associated with laceration of the subclavian artery or vein. The fifth through ninth ribs are the most common sites of fractures. Fractures of the lower ribs are associated with injury to the spleen and liver, which may be lacerated by fragmented sections of the rib.

If conscious, the patient will experience severe pain, tenderness, and muscle spasm over the area of the fracture, which is aggravated by coughing, deep breathing, and motion. The area around the fracture may be bruised. A crackling, grating sound in the thorax (subcutaneous crepitus) may be detected. To reduce the pain, the patient will splint the chest by breathing in a shallow manner and will avoid sighs, deep breaths, coughing, and movement. This reluctance to move or breathe deeply results in diminished ventilation, collapse of unaerated alveoli (atelectasis), pneumonitis, and hypoxemia. Respiratory insufficiency and failure can be the outcomes of such a cycle. The diagnostic work-up may include a chest x-ray, rib series, ECG, and arterial blood gases.

Medical Management. The goals of treatment are to control pain and to detect and treat the injury. Sedation is used to relieve pain and to allow deep breathing and coughing. Care must be taken to avoid oversedation and suppression of the respiratory drive. Alternative strategies to relieve pain include intercostal nerve block and ice over the fracture site; a chest binder may decrease pain on movement. Usually the pain abates in 5 to 7 days and discomfort can be controlled with epidural analgesia, patient-controlled analgesia, or non-opioid analgesia. Most rib fractures heal in 3 to 6 weeks. The patient is monitored closely for signs and symptoms of associated injuries.

Flail Chest

Flail chest occurs when two or more adjacent ribs are fractured at two or more sites, resulting in a free-floating rib segment. As a result the chest wall loses stability, with subsequent respiratory impairment and usually severe respiratory distress.

During inspiration, as the chest expands, the detached part of the rib segment (flail segment) will move in a paradoxical manner in that it is pulled inward during inspiration, reducing the amount of air that can be drawn into the lungs. On expiration, because the intrathoracic pressure will exceed atmospheric pressure, the flail segment will bulge outward, impairing the patient's ability to exhale. The mediastinum then shifts back to the affected side (Fig. 24-9). This paradoxical action results in increased dead space that cannot participate in ventilation, retained airway secretions, increased lung resistance, decreased compliance, and a reduction in alveolar ventilation. Lung contusion and atelectasis frequently accompany flail chest. As a result, the oxygen content of the blood decreases and carbon dioxide content increases, producing respiratory acidosis. Often, hypotension, inadequate tissue perfusion, and metabolic acidosis follow as cardiac output is decreased by the paradoxical motion of the mediastinum.

Medical Management. Management includes providing ventilatory support, clearing secretions from the lungs, and controlling pain. The specific management depends on the degree of respiratory dysfunction. If only a small segment of the chest is involved, the objectives are to clear the airway (coughing, deep breathing, gentle suctioning) to aid in the expansion of the lung, and to relieve pain by intercostal nerve blocks, high thoracic epidural blocks, or careful use of intravenous narcotics.

For *mild to moderate flail chest injuries*, the underlying pulmonary contusion is treated by restricting fluid intake and prescribing diuretics, corticosteroids, and albumin, while relieving chest pain. Pulmonary physiotherapy is carried out and the patient is closely monitored.

When a *severe flail chest injury* is encountered, endotracheal intubation and mechanical ventilation with a volume-cycled ventilator and sometimes PEEP are used to splint the chest wall (internal pneumatic stabilization) and to correct abnormalities in gas exchange. This helps to treat the underlying pulmonary contusion, serves to stabilize the thoracic cage to allow the fractures to heal, and improves alveolar ventilation and intrathoracic volume by decreasing the work of breathing. This treatment modality requires long-term endotracheal intubation and ventilator support.

Regardless of the type of treatment, the patient will be carefully monitored by serial chest x-rays, arterial blood gases, pulse oximetry, and pulmonary function studies. Pain management is key to successful treatment. Patient-controlled analgesia, intercostal nerve blocks, epidural analgesia and intrapleural administration of narcotics may be used to control thoracic pain.

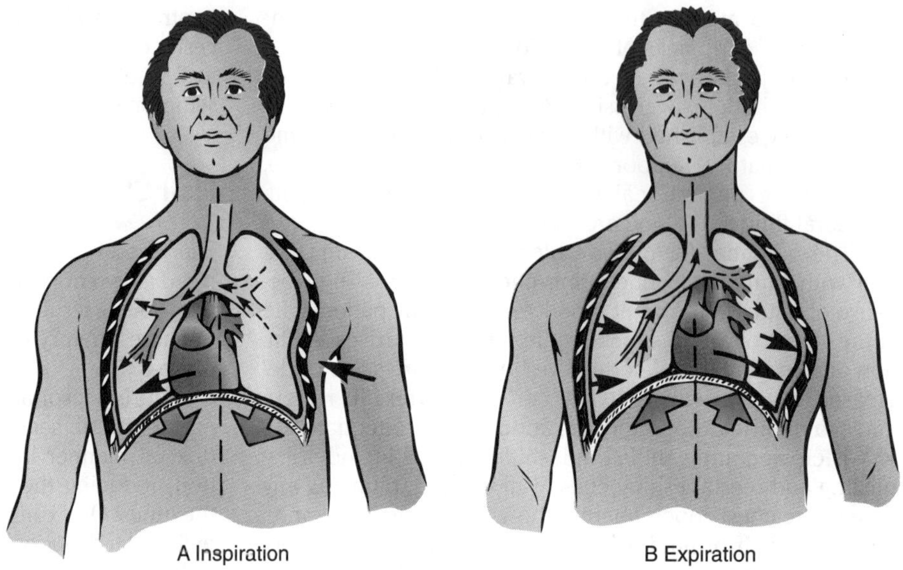

FIGURE 24-9. Flail chest is caused by a free-floating segment of rib cage resulting from multiple rib fractures. (**A**) Paradoxical movement on inspiration occurs when the flail rib segment is sucked inward and the mediastinal structures shift to the unaffected side. The amount of air drawn into the affected lung is reduced. (**B**) On expiration, the flail segment bulges outward and the mediastinal structures shift back to the affected side.

Hemothorax and Pneumothorax

In severe chest injuries, blood frequently collects in the chest cavity (*hemothorax*) because of torn intercostal vessels, lacerations of the lungs, or the escape of air from the injured lung into the pleural cavity (*pneumothorax*). Often, both blood and air are found in the chest cavity (*hemopneumothorax*). Chest injury may interfere with normal lung function.

The seriousness of the problem depends on the amount and rate of thoracic bleeding. The pleural cavity can be decompressed by needle aspiration (thoracentesis) or chest tube drainage of the blood or air. The lung is then able to reexpand and again perform its function in respiration.

The chest wall will be opened surgically (*thoracotomy*) when more than 1500 ml of blood is aspirated initially by thoracentesis, when 500 ml of drainage is collected for more than an hour, or 200 ml per hour for 5 to 6 hours. An emergency thoracotomy also may be performed in the emergency department if there is suggested cardiovascular injury secondary to chest or penetrating trauma.

Medical Management. The goal of treatment is to evacuate the air or blood from the pleural space. For a hemothorax, a large-diameter chest tube (up to 40F) is inserted usually in the fourth through sixth intercostal space between the anterior and posterior line. For a pneumothorax, a small chest tube (28F) is inserted near the second intercostal space. This space is used because it is the thinnest part of the chest wall, minimizes the danger of contacting the thoracic nerve, and will leave a less visible scar. Once the chest tubes are inserted, prompt and effective decompression of the pleural cavity (drainage of blood or air) usually occurs. If there is an excessive amount of blood in the chest tube in a relatively short period, an autotransfusion may be needed. This technique involves taking the patient's own blood that has been drained from the chest, filtering it, and then transfusing it back into the patient's vascular system.

Tension Pneumothorax

A tension pneumothorax occurs when air is drawn into the pleural space from a lacerated lung or through a small hole in the chest wall. In either case, the air that enters the chest cavity with each inspiration is trapped there; it cannot be expelled through the air passage or the small hole in the chest wall.

Thus, tension (pressure) is built up within the pleural space, which causes the lung to collapse and the heart, the great vessels, and trachea shift toward the unaffected side of the chest. Both respiration and circulatory function are impaired because with increased intrathoracic pressure, venous return to the heart is compromised, causing decreased cardiac output and impairment of peripheral circulation. In extreme cases, the pulse may be undetectable, known as *pulseless electrical activity* (PEA). The clinical picture is one of air hunger, agitation, hypotension, tachycardia, profuse diaphoresis, and cyanosis. A comparison of open and tension pneumothorax is shown in Figure 24-10.

- Relief of tension pneumothorax is considered an emergency measure.

Medical Management. If a tension pneumothorax is suspected, the patient should immediately be given a high concentration of oxygen to treat the hypoxia. In an emergency situation, a tension pneumothorax can be converted quickly to a simple pneumothorax by inserting a large-bore needle at the second intercostal space midclavicular line on the affected side. This will relieve the pressure and vent the intrathoracic air to the outside. A chest tube is then inserted and connected to suction to remove the remaining air and fluid and reexpand the lung.

If the lung expands and leakage from the lung stops, further drainage may be unnecessary. If the lung continues to leak, as evidenced by the reaccumulation of an inexhaustible volume of air during the thoracentesis, the air must be removed by a chest tube with water-seal drainage.

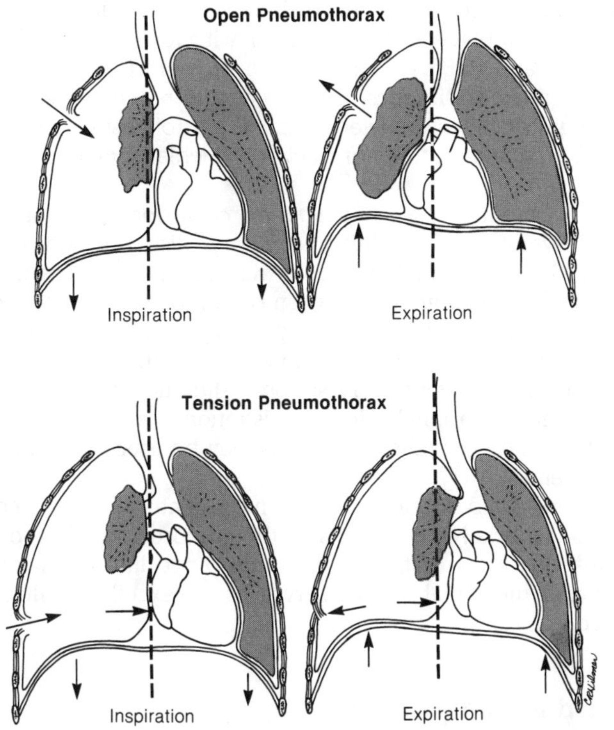

FIGURE 24-10. Open pneumothorax (**top**) and tension pneumothorax (**bottom**). In *open pneumothorax,* air enters the chest during inspiration and exits during expiration. A slight shift of the affected lung may occur because of a decrease in pressure as air moves out of the chest. In *tension pneumothorax,* air enters but cannot leave the chest. As the pressure increases, the heart and great vessels are compressed and the mediastinal structures are shifted toward the opposite side of the chest. The trachea is pushed from its normal midline position toward the opposite side of the chest, and the unaffected lung is compressed. (From Porth C. Pathophysiology: Concepts of Altered Health States, 4th ed. Philadelphia, JB Lippincott, 1994.)

Penetrating Wounds of the Chest

Open Pneumothorax

Open pneumothorax occurs when an opening in the chest wall is large enough to allow air to pass freely in and out of the thoracic cavity with each attempted respiration. Because the rush of air through the hole in the chest wall produces a sucking sound, such injuries are termed *sucking wounds* of the chest. In such patients, not only does the lung collapse, but the structures of the mediastinum (heart and great vessels) shift toward the uninjured side with each inspiration and in the opposite direction with expiration. This is termed *mediastinal flutter,* and it produces serious circulatory problems.

Medical Management. Open pneumothorax calls for emergency interventions.

- Stopping the flow of air through the opening in the chest wall is a life-saving measure.

In such an emergency, anything may be used that is large enough to fill the chest wound—a towel, a handkerchief, or the heel of the hand. If conscious, the patient is instructed to inhale and strain against a closed glottis. This action assists in reexpanding the lung and ejecting the air from the thorax. In the hospital, the opening is plugged by sealing it with gauze impregnated with petroleum. A pressure dressing is applied and secured with a circumferential strap. Usually, a chest tube connected to water-seal drainage is inserted to permit air and fluid to drain. Antibiotics usually are prescribed to combat infection from contamination.

Gunshot and Stab Wounds

Gunshot wounds (GSW) and stab wounds are the most common types of penetrating chest trauma. They are classified according to their velocity.

Stab wounds are generally considered low velocity because the weapon destroys a small area around the wound. Most stab wounds are caused by knives and switchblades. They are frequently associated with alcohol or substance abuse. The appearance of the external wound may be very deceptive, because pneumothorax, hemothorax, and cardiac tamponade along with severe and continuing hemorrhage can occur from any small wound, even one caused by a small-diameter instrument such as an ice pick.

Gunshot wounds to the chest may be classified as low, medium, or high velocity. The factors that determine the velocity and resulting extent of damage include the distance from which the gun was fired, the caliber of the gun, and construction and size of the bullet. A GSW can produce a variety of pathophysiologic changes. A bullet can cause damage at the site of penetration and along its pathway, and may ricochet off bony structures, which may damage the chest organs and great vessels. If the diaphragm is involved in either a GSW or stab wound, injury to the chest cavity must be considered.

Medical Management. The objective of immediate management is to restore and maintain cardiopulmonary function. After an adequate airway is ensured and ventilation is established, the patient is examined for shock and intrathoracic and intra-abdominal injuries. The patient is undressed completely so that additional injuries will not be missed. There is a high risk for associated intra-abdominal injuries with stab wounds below the level of the fifth anterior intercostal space. Death can result from exsanguinating hemorrhage or intra-abdominal sepsis.

After the status of the peripheral pulses is assessed, a large-bore intravenous line is inserted. A diagnostic work-up includes a chemistry profile, arterial blood gases, pulse oximetry, and an electrocardiogram. Blood typing and cross-matching are done in case blood transfusion is required. An indwelling catheter is inserted to monitor urinary output and to collect a urine sample for laboratory study. A nasogastric tube is inserted to prevent aspiration, minimize leakage of abdominal contents, and decompress the gastrointestinal tract.

Shock is treated simultaneously with colloid solutions, crystalloids, or blood, as indicated by the condition of the patient. Chest x-rays are obtained, and other diagnostic procedures are carried out (esophagogram, flat plate of the abdomen, arteriogram) as dictated by the needs of the patient.

A chest tube is inserted into the pleural space in most patients with penetrating wounds of the chest to achieve rapid and continuing reexpansion of the lungs. The chest tube will frequently result in a complete evacuation of hemothorax and will decrease the incidence of clotted hemothorax. The chest tube will also allow early recognition of continuing intrathoracic bleeding, which will make surgical exploration necessary.

If the patient has a penetrating wound of the heart and great vessels, the esophagus, and the tracheobronchial tree, surgical intervention is required.

Pulmonary Contusion

Pulmonary contusion is damage to the lung tissues resulting in hemorrhage and localized edema. It is associated with chest trauma when there is rapid compression and decompression to the chest wall, (*i.e.*, blunt trauma). It may not be evident initially on examination.

Pathophysiology. The primary pathologic defect is an abnormal accumulation of fluid in the interstitial and intra-alveolar spaces. It is thought that injury to the lung parenchyma and its capillary network results in a leak of serum protein and plasma. The leaking serum protein exerts an osmotic pressure that enhances loss of fluid from the capillaries. Blood, edema, and cellular debris (from cellular response to injury) enter the lung and accumulate in the bronchioles and alveolar surface, where they interfere with gas exchange. An increase in pulmonary vascular resistance and pulmonary artery pressure occurs. The patient experiences systemic hypoxia and carbon dioxide retention. Occasionally, a contused lung occurs on the other side of the point of body impact. This is called a *contrecoup contusion*.

Clinical Manifestations. Pulmonary contusion may be mild, moderate, or severe. The clinical manifestations vary from tachypnea, tachycardia, pleuritic chest pain, hypoxemia, and blood-tinged secretions to more severe tachypnea, tachycardia, crackles, frank bleeding, severe hypoxemia, and respiratory acidosis. Changes in sensorium, including increased agitation or combative irrational behavior, may be signs of hypoxia. The efficiency of gas exchange is determined by arterial blood gas measurements. The chest x-ray may show pulmonary infiltration. The initial chest x-ray may show no changes and, in fact, changes may not appear for one or two days after the initial insult.

Medical Management. The goal of treatment includes maintaining the airway, providing adequate oxygenation, and controlling pain. In *mild pulmonary contusion*, ultrasonic mist nebulization is used to keep the secretions fluid. Postural drainage, physiotherapy, and sterile endotracheal suctioning are used to remove the secretions. Pain is managed by intercostal nerve blocks or by opioids. Usually, antimicrobial therapy is administered because a damaged lung is susceptible to infection. Oxygen is usually given by mask or cannula for 24 to 36 hours. Fluids are restricted because the injury is thought to be due to abnormal collection of fluid in the interstices of the lung.

If *moderate pulmonary contusion* is encountered, in addition to the above symptoms, the patient will have a large amount of mucus, serum, and frank blood in the tracheobronchial tree. The patient coughs constantly but is unable to clear the secretions. This patient usually requires intubation and is placed on a ventilator with low-concentration oxygen and PEEP to maintain the pressure and keep the lungs inflated. Diuretics may be given to reduce edema. A nasogastric tube is inserted to relieve gastrointestinal distention. Frequent cultures of tracheobronchial secretions are obtained.

A patient with *severe pulmonary contusion* has the signs and symptoms of adult respiratory distress syndrome (ARDS), which include rapid respirations, tachycardia, cyanosis, agitation, combativeness, and continuous and productive coughing of mucoid, frothy, and bloody secretions. This patient is treated aggressively with endotracheal intubation and ventilatory support, diuretics, fluid restriction, and the prophylactic administration of antimicrobials. Colloids and crystalloid solutions may be used to treat hypovolemia.

The *complications* of pulmonary contusion are infections, especially pneumonia in the contused segment, because the extravasation of fluid and blood into the alveolar and interstitial spaces serves as an excellent culture medium.

Cardiac Tamponade

Cardiac tamponade is the compression of the heart as a result of fluid within the pericardial sac. It usually is caused by blunt or penetrating trauma to the chest. (A penetrating wound of the heart is associated with a high mortality.) Cardiac tamponade also may follow diagnostic cardiac catheterization, angiographic procedures, and pacemaker insertion, which can produce perforations of the heart and great vessels. Pericardial effusion also may develop from metastases to the pericardium from malignant tumors of the breast and lung and may occur with lymphomas and leukemias, renal failure, tuberculosis, and high-dose radiation to the chest.

Pathophysiology. If the fluid formation is slow, the pericardium will distend without producing noticeable clinical symptoms until enough fluid accumulates to raise the intrapericardial pressure. A rapidly developing effusion interferes with ventricular filling and causes impairment of circulation with reduced cardiac output and insufficient venous return to the heart. Circulatory collapse can result.

Clinical Manifestations. The clinical manifestations depend on the speed with which the fluid accumulates. Important signs include a falling blood pressure, rising venous pressure (distended neck veins), and distant (muffled) heart sounds from impaired diastolic filling of the heart. Pulsus paradoxus (systolic blood pressure drops and fluctuates with respiration) may occur early in the development of cardiac tamponade. The patient may be anxious, confused, and restless and may have dyspnea, tachypnea, and precordial pain. The central venous pressure is usually elevated; however, it may be low or normal if a large amount of blood has been lost as a result of associated injuries.

Medical Management. The treatment of cardiac tamponade is thoracotomy for penetrating cardiac injuries where cardiorrhaphy (suturing the heart muscle) is performed to stop hemorrhage, relieve tamponade, and repair associated lacerations and lesions. (See the care of the patient undergoing heart surgery [Chapter 30] and of the patient undergoing chest surgery [Chapter 25]). Pericardiocentesis (needle aspiration of fluid from the pericardium [Chapter 28]) may be performed to "buy time" before the patient is taken to surgery. This decompression of the pericardial sac permits the heart to resume effective action.

Subcutaneous Emphysema

When the lung or the air passages are injured, air may enter the tissue planes and pass for some distance under the skin (*e.g.*, neck, chest). The tissues give a crackling sensation when palpated, and the subcutaneous air produces an alarming appearance as face, neck, body, and scrotum become misshapen by subcutaneous air. Fortunately, subcutaneous emphysema is of itself not a serious complication. The subcutaneous air is spontaneously absorbed if the underlying air leak is treated or stops spontaneously.

Giving the patient inhalations of high concentrations of oxygen will promote the reabsorption of subcutaneous air by washing nitrogen from the blood and improving its diffusion from the subcutaneous tissues back into the circulation. In severe cases in which there is widespread subcutaneous emphysema, a tracheostomy is indicated to ensure patency of the airway.

Aspiration

Aspiration (inhalation) of stomach contents into the lungs is a serious complication that may cause death. It can occur when the protective airway reflexes are lost, such as is seen in patients who are unconscious from drugs, alcohol, stroke, or cardiac arrest, or in instances when a nonfunctioning nasogastric tube allows the gastric contents to drain around the tube and cause silent aspiration.

If untreated, massive inhalation of gastric contents will result, in a period of several hours, in the clinical syndrome of tachycardia, dyspnea, cyanosis, and hypertension, followed by hypotension and finally death. The primary factors responsible for morbidity and mortality after aspiration of gastric contents are the volume and character of the aspirated gastric contents. A full stomach contains solid particles of food. If these are aspirated, the problem then becomes one of mechanical blockage of the airways and secondary infection.

During periods of fasting, the stomach contains acidic gastric juice, which, if aspirated, may prove destructive to the alveoli and capillaries. The presence of fecal contamination (more likely seen in intestinal obstruction) will increase the likelihood of mortality because the endotoxins produced by intestinal organisms may be absorbed systemically, or the thick proteinaceous material found in the intestinal contents may obstruct the airway, leading to atelectasis and secondary bacterial invasion.

Chemical pneumonitis may develop from aspiration and result in the destruction of alveolar-capillary endothelial cells, with a consequent outpouring of protein-rich fluids into the interstitial and intra-alveolar spaces. This results in loss of surfactant, which in turn causes the airway to close. Finally, the impaired exchange of oxygen and carbon dioxide causes respiratory failure. Characteristics of aspiration include the following:

- Massive aspiration is usually fatal.
- Small, localized aspiration from regurgitation can cause pneumonia and respiratory distress.
- Silent regurgitation often occurs unobserved and may be more common than suspected.

Prevention

When Reflexes Are Lacking. Aspiration is likely to occur if the patient cannot adequately coordinate protective glottic, laryngeal, and cough reflexes. This hazard is increased if the patient has a distended abdomen, is in a supine position, has the upper extremities immobilized by intravenous infusions or hand restraints, receives local anesthetics to the oropharyngeal or laryngeal area for diagnostic procedures, or has been sedated.

When vomiting, a person can normally protect the airway by sitting up or turning on the side and coordinating breathing, coughing, gag, and glottic reflexes. If these reflexes are active, an oral airway should not be inserted. If an airway is in place, it should be pulled out the moment the patient gags on it so as not to stimulate the pharyngeal gag reflex and promote vomiting and aspiration. Suctioning of oral secretions with a catheter should be performed with minimal pharyngeal stimulation.

During Tube Feeding. The patient who is receiving tube feedings is positioned upright during the continuous feeding or at timed intervals. The patient receiving continuous infusion is given small volumes under low pressure in an upright position, which will help to prevent aspiration. Patients receiving tube feedings at timed intervals are maintained in an upright position during the feeding and for 30 minutes afterward to allow the stomach to partially empty. Tube feedings must be given only when it is certain that the feeding tube is positioned correctly in the stomach. Many patients today receive enteral feeding directly into the duodenum through a small-bore flexible feeding tube or surgically implanted tube. Feedings are given slowly and regulated by a feeding pump. Correct placement is confirmed by chest x-ray.

Assessing for Delayed Emptying Time of Stomach. A full stomach may cause aspiration because of increased intragastric or extragastric pressure. The following clinical situations cause delayed emptying time of the stomach and may contribute to aspiration: intestinal obstruction; increased gastric secretions during anxiety, stress, or pain; or abdominal distention because of ileus, ascites, peritonitis, use of opioids and sedatives, severe illness, or vaginal delivery.

When a feeding tube is present, contents are aspirated, usually every 4 hours, to determine the amount of the last feeding left in the stomach. If more than 50 ml is aspirated, there may be a problem with delayed emptying and the next feeding should be delayed or the continuous feeding stopped for a period of time.

After Prolonged Endotracheal Intubation. Prolonged endotracheal intubation or tracheostomy can depress the laryngeal and glottic reflexes because of disuse.

CRITICAL THINKING EXERCISES

1. Your patient has a diagnosis of chronic obstructive pulmonary disease (COPD) and is experiencing shortness of breath. Oxygen is prescribed at 2 L/min. His family keeps asking that the oxygen flow be increased to make it easier for him to breathe. What explanation would you give to the patient and family about the need to keep the oxygen at the prescribed rate? Indicate the actions you would take to assist the patient's breathing.
2. During a home visit, your patient explains that he is unable to do anything except sit in a chair because he gets short of breath during exertion. Describe the strategies you would plan with the patient to minimize his shortness of breath during activities and to improve the quality of his life.
3. Your patient, a 45-year-old worker at a boarding home, has been started on treatment for active tuberculosis at home with specific instructions about her medication. She states that she is unable to take time off from work, where she has some contact with the children of the boarding home residents. What are the public health issues that are of concern to you, and what instructions would you provide to the patient and to the boarding home residents?

Even when the patient is intubated, aspiration may well occur even with the presence of a nasogastric tube. This aspiration may result in a nosocomial pneumonia. Blue dye may be added to the tube feeding to assess for aspiration by monitoring the pulmonary secretions. Patients with prolonged tracheostomies are encouraged to phonate and exercise their laryngeal muscles. The pharynx is suctioned before the cuff is deflated to prevent aspiration of regurgitated material. It is important to remember that improperly administered IPPB treatments by mask can distend the stomach and promote aspiration.

BIBLIOGRAPHY

Books

Baum GL and Wolinsky E. Textbook of Pulmonary Diseases, 5th ed, Vols 1 & 2. Boston, Little, Brown, 1994.

Clochesy JM et al. Critical Care Nursing. Philadelphia, WB Saunders, 1993.

Groenwald SL. Cancer Nursing Principles and Practice, 3rd ed. Boston, Jones and Barlett Publishers, 1993.

Holloway NM. Nursing the Critically Ill Adult, 4th ed. New York, Addison Wesley Publishing, 1993.

Isselbacher K. Harrison's Principles of Internal Medicine, 13th ed. New York, McGraw–Hill, 1994.

Karetzky M, Cunha BA, and Brendstetter RD. The Pneumonias. New York, Springer-Verlag, 1993.

Kinney MR et al. AACN's Clinical Reference for Critical Care Nursing, 3rd ed. New York, McGraw-Hill, 1993.

Thelan LA et al. Critical Care Nursing: Diagnosis and Management. St Louis, Mosby, 1994.

U.S. Department of Health and Human Services. Healthy People 2000. National Health Promotion and Disease Prevention Objectives. U.S. Government Printing Office, Washington, DC, 1990.

Weinberger SE. Principles of Pulmonary Medicine. Philadelphia, WB Saunders, 1992.

Wilson RF. Critical Care Manual: Applied Physiology and Principles of Therapy. Philadelphia, FA Davis, 1992.

Journals

Asterisks indicate nursing research articles.

Pulmonary Infections

Brown RB. Community-acquired pneumonia: Diagnosis and therapy of older adults. Geriatrics 1993 February; 48(2):43–50.

Collins CM. Reducing occupational transmission of tuberculosis to health care workers. Medsurg Nurs 1993 May; 2(5) 389–395.

Couser JI and Glassroth J. Tuberculosis: An epidemic in older adults. Clin Chest Med 1993 March; 14(3):491–499.

Elpern EH and Girzadas AM. Tuberculosis update: New challenges of an old disease. Medsurg Nurs 1993 March; 2(3):176–183.

Gleeson K. Life-threatening pneumonia. Clin Chest Med 1994 Sep; 15(3):581–602.

Granton JT and Grossman RF. Community-acquired pneumonia in the elderly patient. Clin Chest Med 1993 March; 14(3):537–553.

Hecht A, et al. Diagnosis and treatment of pneumonia in the nursing home. Nurse Prac 1995 May; 20(5):24, 27, 28, 35–39.

Idell S. When pleural effusion defies diagnosis. Emerg Med 1993 June; 30:15–23.

Ismeurt RL and Leng CO. Tuberculosis: A new threat from an old nemesis. Home Healthcare Nurse 1993 April; 11(4):16–23.

Jacobs RF. Multiple-drug-resistant tuberculosis. Clin Infect Dis 1994 Jul; 19(1):1–8.

Johnson DH and Cunha BA. Atypical pneumonias. Postgrad Med 1993 May 15; (93):769–782.

Kent JH. The epidemiology of multidrug-resistant tuberculosis in the United States. Med Clin North Am 1993 June; 77(6):1391–1405.

Lordi GM and Reichman L. Treatment of tuberculosis. Am Fam Physician 1991; 44(1):220–224.

Long CO, Holmes NJ, and Ismeurt RL. The tuberculin skin test. Home Healthcare Nurse 1993 March; 11(3):13–18.

Malseed RT and Wilson BA. Isoniazid and Rifampin therapy for tuberculosis: What patients need to know. Medsurg Nurs 1993 March; 2(3):236–238.

Nadell EA. Environmental control of tuberculosis. Med Clin North Am 1993 June; 77(6):1315–1333.

Ruben FL. Viral pneumonias. Postgrad Med 1993 May 15; 1993 93(7):57–64.

Sahn SA. Pleural effusion in lung cancer. Clin Chest Med 1993 March; 14(3):189–197.

Schlick W. The problems of treating atypical pneumonia. J Antimicrob Chemother 1993; 31(Suppl C):111–120.

Sumortojo E. When tuberculosis treatment fails: A social behavioral account of patient adherence. Am Rev Respir Dis 1993; 147: 1311–1320.

Tsivitis MC. Resurgent tuberculosis. Cancer Practice 1993 March; 1(3):233-239.

Walsh K. Guidelines for the prevention and control of tuberculosis in the elderly. Nurse Pract 1994 Nov; 19(11):79–84.

Wisinger D. Bacterial pneumonia. Postgrad Med 1993 May 15; 93(7):43–52.

Chronic Obstructive Pulmonary Disease

Bone RC. Bronchial asthma: Diagnostic and treatment issues. Hosp Pract 1993 Sept; 30:45–52.

Borkgren MW and Gronkiewicz CA. Update your asthma care from hospital to home. Am J Nurs 1995 Jan; 95(1):26–34, 35.

*Breslin EH, Adams E, Lutz A, and Roy C. Standardization of a device-to-device to measure unsupported arm exercise endurance in chronic obstructive pulmonary disease. Nurs Res 1992 Sept/Oct; 41(5):292–295.

*Brundage DJ, Swearingen P, and Woody JW. Self-care instruction for patients with COPD. Rehabilitation Nursing 1993 Sept/Oct; 18(5):321–325.

DeBlaquiere P, Christensen DB, Carter WB, and Martin TR. Use and misuse of metered dose inhalers by patients with chronic lung diseases. Am Rev Resp Dis 1989; 140:110–116.

Fanta CH. Emergency management of acute asthma. Respir Care 1992 July; 37(6):551.

Janson-Bjerklie S. The nurse's role in asthma management. Perspec Respir Nurs 1993 Mar; 4(1):4–6.

*Kim MJ et al. Inspiratory muscle training in patients with chronic obstructive pulmonary disease. Nurs Res 1993 Nov/Dec; 42(6):356–362.

McFadden ER. Dosages of corticosteroids in asthma. Am Rev Respir Disease 1993 Oct; 148:1306–1310.

Miracle VA. Treating asthma in adults. Perspec Respir Nurs 1994 Nov; 5(4):1, 3–5.

Murphy S. Asthma etiology and management: Primary to tertiary prevention. Preventive Med 1994 Sep 23; 23(5):688–692.

Murphy TF and Sethi S. Preventing or treating COPD flare-ups. Emerg Med 1993 March; 65–68.

*Narsavage GL and Weaver TE. Physiologic status, coping, and hardiness as predictors of outcomes in chronic obstructive pulmonary disease. Nurs Res 1994 Mar/Apr; 43(2):90–94.

Perry AG. Discharge teaching for patients with COPD. Perspect Respir Nurs 1993 April; 4(2):1–4.

Prentice D and Ahrens T. Pulmonary complications of trauma. Crit Care Nurs Q 1994 Aug; 17(2):24–33.

Skorodin MS. Pharmacotherapy for asthma and chronic obstructive pulmonary disease: Current thinking, practices and controversies. Arch Intern Med 1993 April; 12;153(7):814–828.

*Weaver TI and Narsvage GL. Physiological and psychological variables related to functional status in chronic obstructive pulmonary disease. Nurs Res 1992 Sept/Oct; 41(5):286–291.

Lung Cancer

Beckett WS. Epidemiology and etiology of lung cancer. Clin Chest Med 1993 March; 14(1):1–15.

Johnson BE. Management of small cell lung cancer. Clin Chest Med 1993 March; 14(1):173–187.

Monntain CF. Lung cancer staging classification. Clin Chest Med 1993 March; 14(1):43–51.

Murren JR and Buzaid AC. Chemotherapy and radiation for the treatment of non-small cell lung cancer: A critical review. Clin Chest Med 1993 March; 14(1):161–187.

Shepard K. The relationship among nursing diagnoses in discharge planning for patients with lung cancer. Nurs Diag 1993 April; 4(4):148–154.

Stewart GS. Trends in radiation therapy for the treatment of lung cancer. Nurs Clin North Am 1992 Sept; 27(3):643–651.

White CS and Templeton PA. Radiologic manifestations. Clin Chest Med 1993 March; 14(1):55–67.

Yesner R. Lung cancer: Pathogenesis and pathology. Clin Chest Med 1993 March; 14(1):17–30.

Trauma

Harn PD and Hartsock. Blunt thoracic injuries. Crit Care Nurs Clin North Am 1993 Dec; 5(4):673–686.

Hurst JM. Thoracic trauma. Respir Care 1992 July; 37(7):708–717.

Jackimczyk K. Blunt chest trauma. Emerg Med Clin North Am 1993 Nov; 11(1):81–96.

Jordan RC. Penetrating chest trauma. Emerg Med Clin North Am 1993; 11(1):97–106.

Kshettry VR and Bolman RM III. Chest trauma: Assessment, diagnosis and management. Clin Chest Med 1994 Mar; 15(1):137–146.

Schrader KA. Penetrating chest trauma. Crit Care Nurs Clin North Am 1993; 5(4):687–696.

Stanik-Hutt JA. Strategies for pain management in traumatic thoracic injuries. Crit Care Nurs Clin North Am 1993 Dec; 5(4):713–722.

Acute Respiratory Failure and ARDS

Jones MA. A.R.D.S. revisited. New ways to fight an old enemy. Nursing 1994 Dec; 24(12):34–43.

Kearney ML. Adult respiratory distress syndrome following thoracic trauma. Crit Care Nurs Clin North Am 1993; 5(4):723–734.

Kollef MH and Schuster DP. The acute respiratory distress syndrome. N Engl J Med 1995 Jan 5; 332(1):27–37.

Occupational Lung Diseases

Coultas DB and Samet JM. Occupational lung cancer. Clin Chest Med 1992 June; 13(2):341–354.

Gaensler EA. Asbestos. Clin Chest Med 1992 June; 13(2):231–242.

Graham WG. Silicosis. Clin Chest Med 1992 June; 13(2):253–268.

Lapp NL and Porter JE. Coal workers' pneumoconiosis. Clin Chest Med 1992 June; 13(2):243–252.

Sherman CB. The health consequences of cigarette smoking. Pulmon Dis Med Clin North Am 1992 March; 76(2):355–375.

Miscellaneous

Andrews L. Medical management of pulmonary emboli. Medsurg Nurs 1994 Feb; 3(1):31–35.

Bradley TD and Phillipson EA. Central sleep apnea. Clin Chest Med 1992 Sept; 13(3):493–505.

Davis LA and O'Rourke NC. Pulmonary embolism: Early recognition and managment in the postanesthesia care unit. J Post Anesth Nurs 1993 Oct; 8(5):338–343.

Fox JM. Malignant pleural effusion. Medsurg Nurs 1994 Oct; 3(5):353–360.

*Gift AG and Pugh LC. Dyspnea and fatigue. Nurs Clin North Am 1993 June; 28(2):373–384.

Handler JA and Feied CF. Acute pulmonary embolism. Aggressive therapy with anticoagulents and antithrombolytics. Postgrad Med 1995 Jan; 97(1):61–62, 65–68, 71–72.

Humble A. Smoking: A disease prevention issue. Medsurg Nurs 1994 Aug; 3(4):286–289, 292.

Keep NB. Identifying pulmonary embolism. Am J Nurs 1995 Apr; 95(4):52.

Kryger MH. Management of obstructive sleep apnea. Clin Chest Med 1992 Sept; 13(3):481–492.

*McCabe SM and Smeltzer SC. Comparison of tidal volumes obtained by one-handed and two-handed ventilation techniques. Am J Crit Care 1993 Nov; 2(6):467–473.

Repasky TM. Tension pneumothorax. Am J Nurs 1994 Sept; 94(9):47.

Wiegard L and Zwillich CW. Obstructivre sleep apnea. Disease-a-Month 1994 Apr; 40(4):197–252.

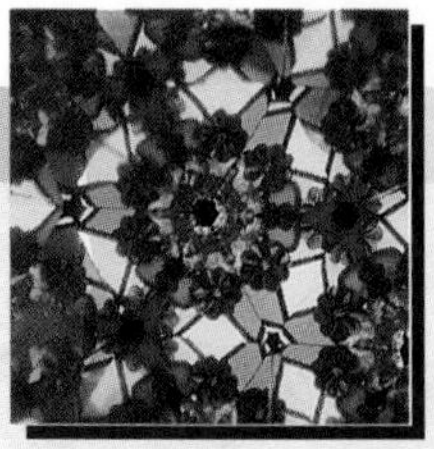

25 Respiratory Care Modalities

CHAPTER OUTLINE

Specific Modes of Management of Respiratory Conditions
- Oxygen Therapy
- Intermittent Positive-Pressure Breathing
- Mini-nebulizer Therapy
- Incentive Spirometry (Sustained Maximal Inspiration)
- Chest Physiotherapy
- Breathing Retraining

The Patient Requiring Airway Management
- Emergency Management of Upper Airway Obstruction
- Endotracheal Intubation
- Tracheostomy

The Patient Requiring Mechanical Ventilation
- Indications for Mechanical Ventilation
- Classification of Ventilators
- Features and Settings of Volume Ventilators
  - NURSING PROCESS: Care of the Mechanically Ventilated Patient
- Problems With Mechanical Ventilation
- Weaning the Patient From the Ventilator
- Mechanical Ventilation in the Home

The Patient Undergoing Thoracic Surgery
- Diagnostic Evaluation
- Operative Procedures
- Preoperative Management
- Postoperative Management
  - NURSING PROCESS: The Patient Undergoing Thoracic Surgery

Critical Thinking Exercises

LEARNING OBJECTIVES

On completion of this chapter, the learner will be able to:

1. Describe the nursing management for patients receiving oxygen therapy, intermittent positive-pressure breathing, mini-nebulizer therapy, incentive spirometry, chest physiotherapy, and breathing retraining
2. Describe the nursing care for a patient with an endotracheal tube and for a patient with a tracheostomy
3. Demonstrate the procedure of tracheal suctioning
4. Use the nursing process as a framework for care of patients who are mechanically ventilated
5. Describe the significance of preoperative nursing assessment and patient teaching for the patient who is to have thoracic surgery
6. Explain the principles of chest drainage and the nursing responsibilities related to the care of the patient with water-seal drainage
7. Describe the patient education and home care considerations for patients who have had thoracic surgery

Specific Modes of Management of Respiratory Conditions

Numerous treatment modalities are used when caring for patients with different types of respiratory conditions. The choice of modality is based on the oxygenation disorder and whether there is a problem with gas ventilation, diffusion, or both. Therapies range from simple and noninvasive modalities (oxygen and nebulizer therapy, chest physiotherapy, breathing retraining) to complex and highly invasive treatments (intubation, mechanical ventilation, surgery). Assessment and management of the respiratory patient is best accomplished when the approach is multidisciplinary and collaborative.

Oxygen Therapy

Oxygen therapy is the administration of oxygen at a concentration greater than that found in the environmental atmosphere. At sea level, the concentration of oxygen in room air is 21%. The goal of oxygen therapy is to provide adequate transport of oxygen in the blood while decreasing the work of breathing and reducing stress on the myocardium.

Oxygen transport to the tissues depends on factors such as cardiac output, arterial oxygen content, adequate concentration of hemoglobin, and metabolic requirements. All of these factors must be kept in mind when oxygen therapy is considered. (Respiratory physiology and oxygen transport are discussed in Chapter 22.)

Assessment

A change in the patient's respiratory rate or pattern may be one of the earliest indicators of the need for oxygen therapy; it may result from hypoxemia or hypoxia.

Hypoxemia (a decrease in the arterial oxygen tension in the *blood*) is manifested by changes in mental status (progressing through impaired judgment, agitation, disorientation, confusion, lethargy, and coma), dyspnea, increase in blood pressure, changes in heart rate, dysrhythmias, central cyanosis (late sign), diaphoresis, and cool extremities. Hypoxemia usually leads to **hypoxia**, which is a decrease in oxygen supply to the *tissues*. Hypoxia, if severe enough, can be life-threatening.

The signs and symptoms of the need for oxygen may depend on how suddenly this need develops. With rapidly developing hypoxia, changes occur in the central nervous system because the higher neurologic centers are more sensitive to oxygen deprivation. The clinical picture may resemble that of alcohol intoxication, with the patient exhibiting incoordination and impaired judgment. Long-standing hypoxia (as seen in chronic obstructive pulmonary disease [COPD] and chronic congestive heart failure) may produce fatigue, drowsiness, apathy, inattentiveness, and delayed reaction time. The need for oxygen is assessed by arterial blood gas analysis (p. 452) as well as by clinical evaluation.

Types and Treatment of Hypoxia

Hypoxia can occur from either severe pulmonary disease (inadequate oxygen supply) or from extrapulmonary disease (inadequate oxygen delivery) affecting gas exchange at the cellular level. The four general types of hypoxia are (1) hypoxemic hypoxia, (2) circulatory hypoxia, (3) anemic hypoxia, and (4) histotoxic hypoxia.

Hypoxemic hypoxia is a decreased oxygen level in the blood resulting in decreased oxygen diffusion into the tissues. It may be caused by hypoventilation, high altitudes, ventilation–perfusion mismatch (as in pulmonary embolism), shunts in which the alveoli are collapsed and cannot provide oxygen to the blood, (commonly caused by atelectasis), and pulmonary diffusion defects; it is corrected by increasing alveolar ventilation or providing supplemental oxygen.

Circulatory hypoxia is hypoxia resulting from inadequate capillary circulation. It may be caused by decreased cardiac output, local vascular obstruction, low-flow states such as shock, or cardiac arrest. Although tissue partial pressure of oxygen (PO_2) is reduced, arterial oxygen (PaO_2) remains normal. Circulatory hypoxia is corrected by identifying and treating the underlying cause.

Anemic hypoxia is a result of decreased effective hemoglobin concentration, which causes a decrease in the oxygen-carrying capacity of the blood. It is rarely accompanied by hypoxemia. Carbon monoxide poisoning, because it reduces the oxygen-carrying capacity of hemoglobin, produces similar effects but is not strictly anemic hypoxia because hemoglobin levels may be normal.

Histotoxic hypoxia occurs when a toxic substance, such as cyanide, interferes with the ability of tissues to use available oxygen.

Cautions in Oxygen Therapy

As with other medications, oxygen is administered with care, and its effects on each patient are carefully assessed. Oxygen is a medication and except in emergency situations is administered only when prescribed by a physician.

In general, patients with respiratory conditions are given oxygen therapy only to raise the arterial oxygen pressure (PaO_2) back to the patient's normal baseline, which may vary from 60 to 95 mm Hg. In terms of the oxyhemoglobin dissociation curve (see p. 439), the blood at these levels is 80% to 98% (also written as 0.80 to 0.98) saturated; higher inspired oxygen flow (FIO_2) values add no further significant amounts of oxygen to the red blood cells or plasma. Instead of helping, increased amounts of oxygen possibly may suppress ventilation in certain types of pulmonary patients.

Excessive oxygen may produce toxic effects on the lungs and central nervous system or may depress ventilation. For example, in patients with chronic obstructive pulmonary disease (COPD), the stimulus for respiration is a decrease in blood oxygen rather than an elevation in carbon dioxide levels. Thus, administration of a high concentration of oxygen will remove the respiratory drive that has been created largely by the patient's chronic low oxygen tension. The resulting decrease in alveolar ventilation can cause a progressive increase in arterial carbon dioxide pressure ($PaCO_2$), ultimately leading to death from carbon dioxide narcosis and acidosis (see p. 234).

Subtle indications of inadequate oxygenation must be observed for when oxygen is administered by any method. Therefore, the patient is assessed frequently for:

confusion, restlessness progressing to lethargy, diaphoresis, pallor, tachycardia, tachypnea, and hypertension.

Other precautions to be taken when administering oxygen involve the careful handling of the equipment. Because oxygen supports combustion, there is always a danger of fire when it is used. "No smoking" signs must be posted when oxygen is in use. Oxygen therapy equipment is also a potential source of bacterial cross-infection and thus the tubing is changed frequently, depending on infection control policy and the type of oxygen delivery equipment.

Oxygen Toxicity. Oxygen is a medication and can cause serious side effects, such as oxygen-induced hypoventilation (prevented by giving low-flow oxygen rates of 1 to 2 L/min) and atelectasis. Perhaps the most serious and insidious hazard is oxygen toxicity, which may occur when too high a concentration of oxygen (greater than 50%) is administered for an extended period (longer than 48 hours).

The pathophysiology of oxygen toxicity is not fully understood, but is related to destruction and decrease of surfactant, the formation of a hyaline membrane lining the lung, and the development of pulmonary edema that is not cardiac in origin.

Signs and symptoms of oxygen toxicity include substernal distress, paresthesias, dyspnea, restlessness, fatigue, malaise, progressive respiratory difficulty, and an alveolar pattern on chest x-ray.

Prevention of oxygen toxicity is achieved by using oxygen only as prescribed. If high concentrations of oxygen are necessary, the duration of administration is kept to a minimum and reduced as soon as possible. Often, positive end expiratory pressure (PEEP) or continuous positive airway pressure (CPAP) is used in conjunction with oxygen therapy to reverse or prevent microatelectasis, and thus allow a lower percentage of oxygen to be used. The level of PEEP that allows the best oxygenation without hemodynamic compromise is known as "best PEEP."

Methods of Oxygen Administration

Oxygen is dispensed from a cylinder or from a piped-in system. A reduction gauge is necessary to reduce the pressure to a working level, and a flowmeter regulates the flow of oxygen in liters per minute. When oxygen is used at high-flow rates, it should be moistened by passing it through a humidification system to prevent the mucous membranes of the respiratory tract from becoming dry.

Many different oxygen devices are used; all will deliver oxygen if used as prescribed and if the devices are used and maintained correctly (Table 25-1). The amount of oxygen delivered is expressed as a percentage concentration (as in 70%). The appropriate form of oxygen therapy is best determined by arterial blood gas levels, which indicate the patient's oxygenation status.

The **nasal cannula** is used when the patient requires a low-to-medium concentration of oxygen for which precise accuracy is not essential. This method is relatively simple and allows the patient to move about in bed, talk, cough, and eat without interrupting oxygen flow. Flow rates

TABLE 25-1 Oxygen Administration Devices

Device	Suggested Flow Rate (L/min)	O_2 Percentage Setting	Advantages	Disadvantages
Cannula	1–2 3–5 6	23–30 30–40 42	Lightweight, comfortable, inexpensive, continuous use with meals and activity	Nasal mucosal drying, variable FiO_2
Catheter	1–6	23–42	Inexpensive	Variable FiO_2, requires frequent change (q8h), gastric distention can occur
Mask, simple	6–8	40–60	Simple to use, inexpensive	Poor fitting, variable FiO_2, must remove to eat
Mask, partial rebreather	8–11	50–75	Moderate O_2 concentration	Warm, poor fitting, must remove to eat
Mask, non-rebreather	12	80–100	High O_2 concentration	Poor fitting
Mask, Venturi	4–6 6–8	24, 26, 28 30, 35, 40	Provides low levels of supplemental O_2 Precise FiO_2, additional humidity available	Must remove to eat
Mask, aerosol	8–10	30–100	Good humidity, accurate FiO_2	Uncomfortable for some
Tracheostomy collar	8–10	30–100	Good humidity, comfortable, fairly accurate FiO_2	
T-piece, Briggs	8–10	30–100	Same as tracheostomy collar	Heavy with tubing
Face tent	8–10	30–100	Good humidity, fairly accurate FiO_2	Bulky and cumbersome

in excess of 6 to 8 L/min may lead to the patient swallowing air and cause irritation and drying of the nasal and pharyngeal mucosa.

The **oropharyngeal catheter** is rarely used but may be prescribed for short-term therapy to administer low-to-moderate concentrations of oxygen. This method can lead to irritation of the nasal mucosa.

When oxygen is administered nasally (cannula or catheter), the percentage of oxygen reaching the lungs varies with the depth and rate of respirations, particularly if the nasal mucosa is swollen or the patient is a mouth breather.

Oxygen masks come in several forms, each used for different purposes (Fig. 25-1). *Simple masks* are used for low-to-moderate concentrations of oxygen, whereas *partial rebreathing or nonrebreathing masks* are used for moderate to high concentrations of oxygen. Although widely used, these masks cannot be used for controlled oxygen concentrations and must be adjusted for proper fit. They should not press too tightly against the skin, as this may cause a sense of claustrophobia; adjustable elastic bands are provided to ensure comfort and security. Bags on partial rebreathing and nonrebreathing masks must remain inflated during both inspiration and expiration. This is accomplished by adjusting the flow so the bag does not collapse on inspiration.

The *Venturi mask* is the most reliable and accurate method for delivering precise concentrations of oxygen through noninvasive means. The mask is constructed in a way that allows a constant flow of room air blended with a fixed flow of oxygen. It is used primarily for patients with COPD because it can provide low levels of supplemental oxygen, thus avoiding the risk of suppressing the hypoxic drive.

The Venturi mask employs the principle of air entrainment (trapping the air like a vacuum), which provides a high air flow with controlled oxygen enrichment. Excess gas leaves the mask through the perforated cuff, carrying with it the exhaled carbon dioxide. This method allows a constant oxygen concentration to be inhaled regardless of the depth or rate of respiration.

The mask should fit snugly enough to prevent oxygen from flowing into the eyes, and the patient's skin is checked for irritation. The mask must be removed so that the patient can eat, drink, and take medications.

Other oxygen devices include *aerosol masks, tracheostomy collars,* and *face tents*, which are used with aerosol devices (nebulizers) that can be adjusted for oxygen concentrations in ranges from 27% to 100% (0.27 to 1.00). If the gas mixture flow falls below patient demand, room air will be pulled in, diluting the concentration. The aerosol mist must be available constantly for the patient during the entire inspiratory phase.

Oxygen concentrators are another means of providing varying amounts of oxygen, especially in the home setting. These devices are relatively portable, easy to operate, and cost effective. However, they also require more maintenance than tank or liquid systems, and probably cannot deliver flows in excess of 4 liters, which provides an FIO_2 of approximately 36%.

Patient Education and Home Care Considerations

At times oxygen must be administered to the patient at home. The patient or family should be instructed in the methods for administering oxygen and should be informed that oxygen is available in gas, liquid, and concentrated forms. The gas and liquid forms come in portable devices so that the patient can leave home while receiving oxygen therapy. Humidity must be provided while oxygen is used (except with portable devices) to counteract the dry, irritating effects of compressed oxygen on the airway.

Home visits by a home health nurse may be arranged based on the patient's status and needs. The nurse evaluates the patient's situation and reinforces the teaching points on how to use the oxygen safely and effectively.

To maintain a consistent quality of care and to maximize the patient's financial reimbursement for home oxy-

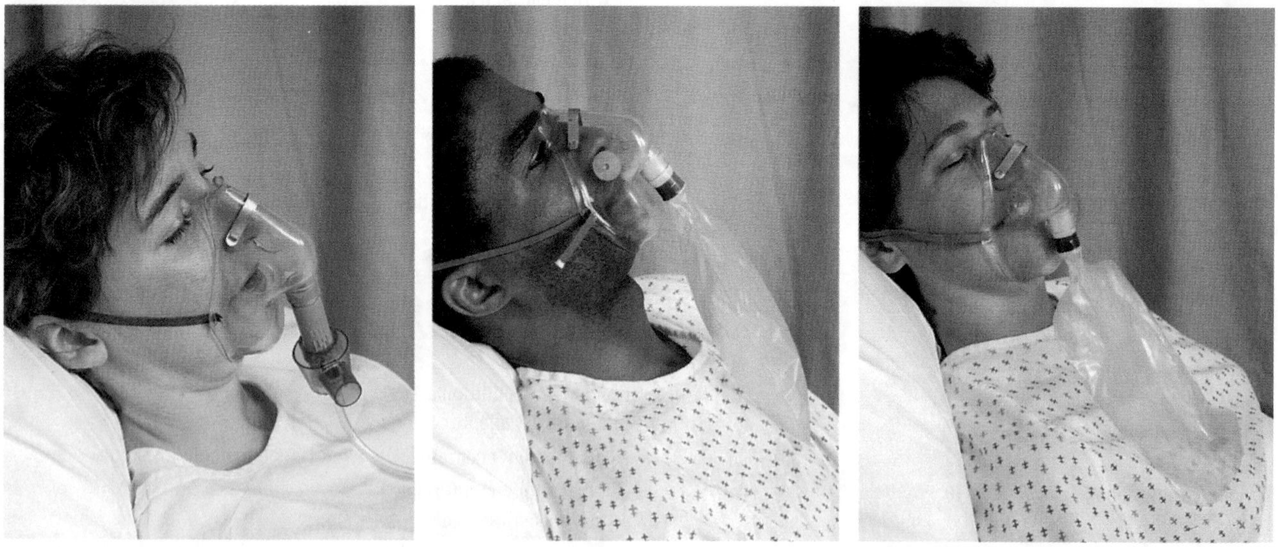

Venturi mask
Nonrebreather mask
Partial rebreather mask

FIGURE 25-1. Types of oxygen masks used to deliver varying concentrations of oxygen. (Photos © Ken Kaspar.)

gen therapy, the nurse ensures that the physician's order includes the disorder, the prescribed oxygen flow, and conditions for use (*e.g.*, continuous use, nighttime use only).

Intermittent Positive-Pressure Breathing

Intermittent positive-pressure breathing (IPPB) is the breathing of air or oxygen (or a combination of both) at a pressure higher than atmospheric pressure to produce air flow into the lungs during inhalation. IPPB is applied by a mechanical device that inflates the lungs through positive pressure, dispersing a prescribed medication. When the patient inhales, the negative inspiratory force triggers the machine to deliver a positive-pressure breath; after a preset pressure is reached on the machine, the machine cycles off and there is passive exhalation. The IPPB machine may be powered by electricity or gas and may be connected with a mouthpiece, mask, or tracheostomy adapter.

Indications. General indications include: difficulty in raising respiratory secretions, reduced vital capacity (VC) with ineffective deep breathing and coughing, or unsuccessful trials of simpler and cheaper methods for loosening secretions, delivering aerosol or expanding the lungs.

Complications. IPPB therapy is used less frequently than previously because of its inherent hazards, which may include pneumothorax, mucosal drying, increased intracranial pressure, hemoptysis, gastric distention, vomiting with possible aspiration, psychological dependency (especially with long-term use, as in COPD), hyperventilation, excessive oxygen administration, and cardiovascular problems.

Mini-nebulizer Therapy

The mini-nebulizer is a hand-held apparatus that disperses a moisturizing agent or medication, such as a bronchodilator or mucolytic agent, into microscopic particles and delivers it to the lungs as the patient inhales. The mini-nebulizer is usually air-driven by means of a compressor through connecting tubing. In some instances, the nebulizer is oxygen-driven rather than air-driven. To be effective, a visible mist must be available for the patient to inhale.

Indications. The indications for use of a mini-nebulizer are similar to the indications for IPPB except that the patient must be able to generate a deep breath without the aid of the positive-pressure machine. Diaphragmatic breathing is helpful as a technique to prepare for the proper use of the mini-nebulizer. Mini-nebulizers frequently are used for patients with COPD to dispense inhaled medications and commonly are used at home on a long-term basis.

Nursing Interventions/Patient Education. The patient is instructed to breathe through the mouth, taking slow, deep breaths and then to hold the breath for a few seconds at the end of inspiration to increase intrapleural pressure and reopen collapsed alveoli, thereby increasing functional residual capacity (see Chap. 22). The patient is encouraged to cough and to evaluate how well the therapy is working. The equipment must be cleaned and stored properly when used at home.

Incentive Spirometry (Sustained Maximal Inspiration)

The incentive spirometer gives visual feedback to guide the patient to inhale slowly and deeply to maximize lung inflation. The patient assumes a sitting or semi-Fowler's position to enhance diaphragmatic excursion. However, this treatment may be performed with the patient in any position.

Incentive spirometers may be one of two types: volume or flow. In the *volume type*, the tidal volume of the spirometer is set according to the manufacturer's instructions. The purpose of the device is to assure that the volume of air inhaled is increased gradually as the patient takes deeper and deeper breaths. The patient takes a deep breath through the mouthpiece, pauses at peak inflation, then relaxes and exhales. Taking several normal breaths before attempting another with the incentive spirometer helps avoid fatigue. The volume is periodically increased as tolerated.

A *flow spirometer* has the same purpose as a volume spirometer but the volume is not preset. The spirometer contains a number of movable balls that are pushed up by the force of the breath and held suspended in the air while the patient inhales. The amount of air inhaled and the flow of the air are estimated by how long and how high the balls are suspended (Fig. 25-2).

Indications. Incentive spirometry is used postoperatively, especially after thoracic and abdominal surgery to promote the expansion of the alveoli and to prevent or treat atelectasis. As a preventive measure, incentive spirometry may be more effective than IPPB because it maximizes the amount of air inhaled while maintaining relatively low airway pressures.

Nursing Interventions. Nursing management of the patient using incentive spirometry includes placing the patient in the proper position, teaching the technique for using the incentive spirometer, setting realistic goals for the patient, and recording the results of the therapy (Chart 25-1).

Chest Physiotherapy

Chest physiotherapy includes postural drainage, chest percussion and vibration, breathing exercises/breathing retraining, and effective coughing. The goals of chest physiotherapy are to remove bronchial secretions, improve ventilation, and increase the efficiency of the respiratory muscles.

Postural Drainage (Segmented Bronchial Drainage)

Postural drainage uses specific positions that allow the force of gravity to assist in the removal of bronchial secretions. The secretions drain from the affected bronchioles into the bronchi and trachea and are removed by coughing or suctioning. It is used to prevent or relieve bronchial obstruction caused by accumulation of secretions.

Because the patient usually sits in an upright position, secretions are likely to accumulate in the lower parts of the lungs. When postural drainage is used, the patient is placed

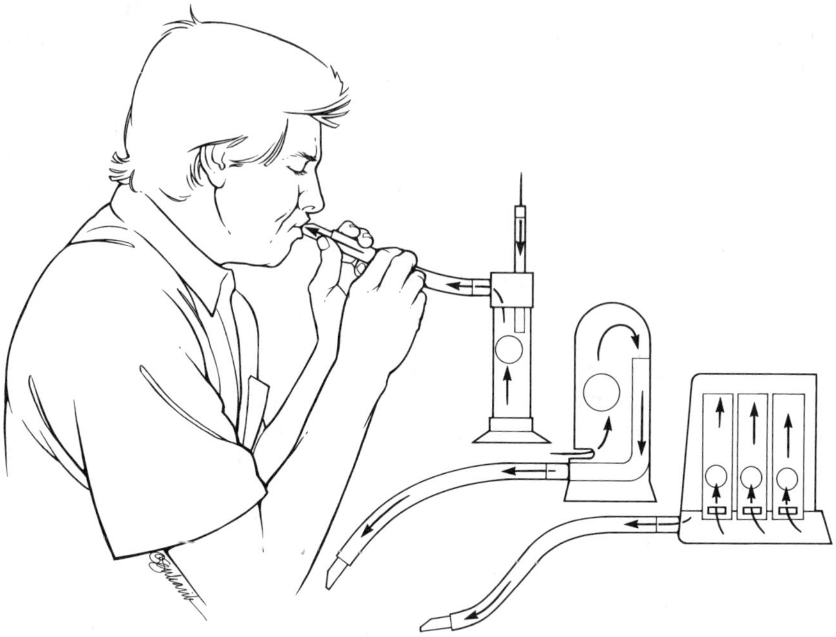

FIGURE 25-2. Flow incentive spirometer. Patients are instructed to inhale to elevate the balls and to keep them floating for as long as possible. The volume inhaled is estimated and variable.

sequentially in different positions (Fig. 25-3), so that the force of gravity helps to drain secretions from the smaller bronchial airways to the main bronchi and trachea. The secretions then are removed by coughing. Having the patient inhale prescribed bronchodilators and mucolytic agents before postural drainage assists in draining the bronchial tree.

Postural drainage exercises can be directed at any of the segments of the lungs. The lower and middle lobe bronchi empty more effectively when the head is down; the upper lobe bronchi empty more effectively when the head is up. Frequently, the patient is placed in five positions, one for drainage of each lobe: head down, prone, right and left lateral, and sitting upright.

Nursing Interventions. The nurse should be aware of the patient's diagnosis as well as the lung lobes or segments involved, the cardiac status, and any structural deformities of the chest wall and spine. Auscultating the chest before and after the procedure helps to identify the areas needing drainage and the effectiveness of treatment, thereby providing immediate feedback on the effectiveness of treatment.

Postural drainage is usually performed two to four times daily, before meals (to prevent nausea, vomiting, and aspiration) and at bedtime. If prescribed, bronchodilators, water, or saline may be nebulized and inhaled before postural drainage to dilate the bronchioles, reduce bronchospasm, decrease the thickness of mucus and sputum, and combat edema of the bronchial walls.

The patient is made as comfortable as possible in each position, and an emesis basin, sputum cup, and paper tissues are provided. The patient is instructed to remain in each position for 10 to 15 minutes and to breathe in slowly through the nose and then breathe out slowly through pursed lips to help keep the airways open so that secretions can be drained while the various positions are assumed. When the position cannot be tolerated, the patient is helped to assume a modified position.

Coughing Technique. When changing position, the patient is instructed to cough and remove secretions as follows:

1. Assume a sitting position and bend slightly forward because the upright position permits a stronger cough.

CHART 25-1
Patient Education: Using Incentive Spirometry

- Explain the reason for the therapy.
- Assess the patient's level of pain and administer pain medication if prescribed.
- Position the patient in semi-Fowler's position or in an upright position (although any position is acceptable).
- Teach the patient to use diaphragmatic breathing.
- Instruct the patient to hold his or her breath at the end of inspiration (for 3 seconds), and then to exhale slowly.
- Encourage approximately 10 breaths per hour with the spirometer during waking hours.
- Set a reasonable volume and repetitive goal (to provide encouragement and give the patient a sense of accomplishment).
- Encourage coughing during and after each session.
- Help the patient splint the incision while coughing postoperatively.
- Place the spirometer within the patient's reach.
- For the postoperative patient, begin the therapy immediately. (If the patient begins to hypoventilate, atelectasis can start to occur within an hour.)
- Record how effectively the patient performs the therapy and the number of breaths achieved with the spirometer every 2 hours.

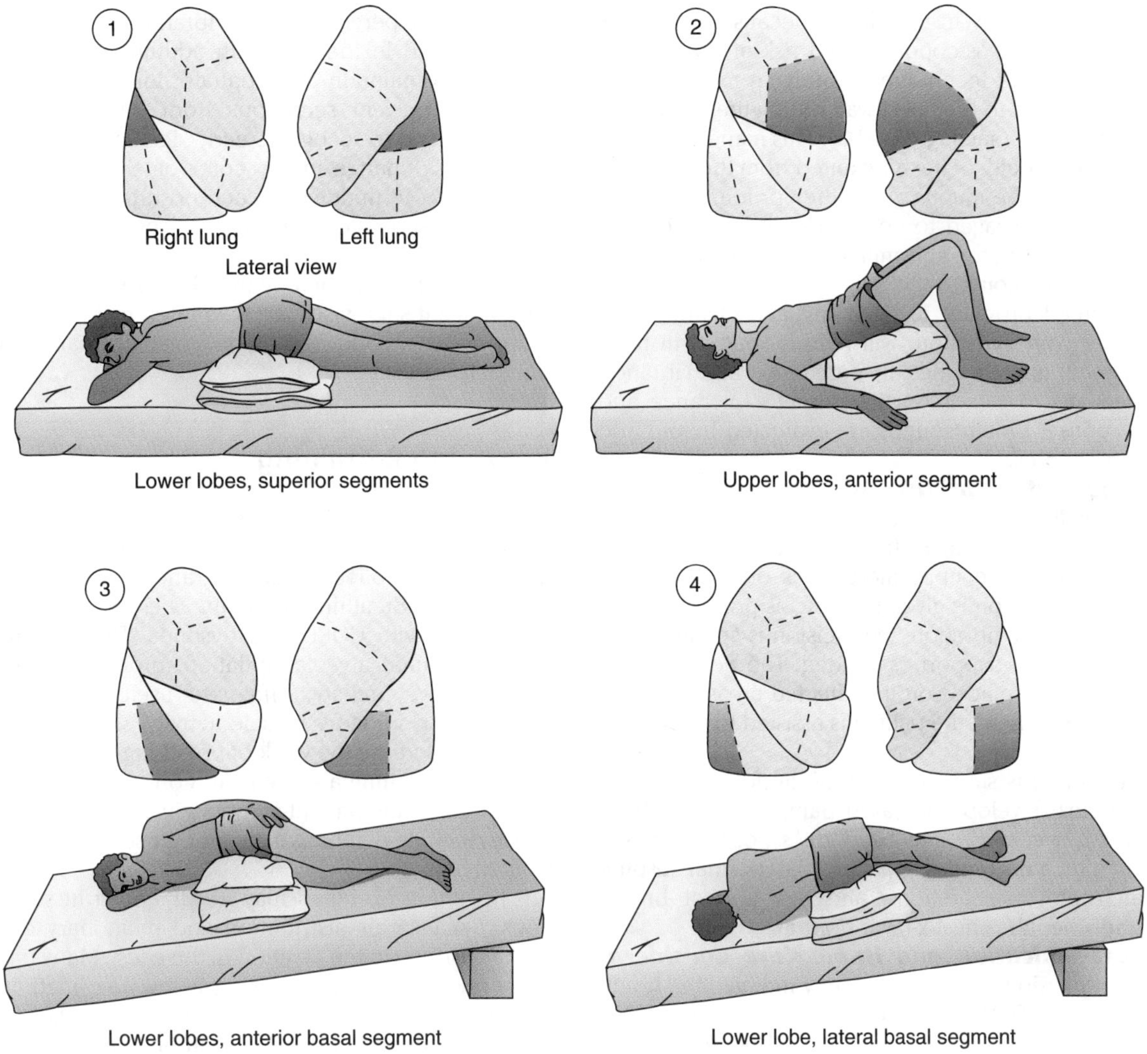

FIGURE 25-3. Postural drainage positions and the areas of lung drained by each position.

2. Keep the knees and hips flexed to promote relaxation and lessen the strain on the abdominal muscles while coughing.
3. Inhale slowly through the nose and exhale through pursed lips several times.
4. Cough twice during each exhalation while contracting (pulling in) the abdomen sharply with each cough.
5. Splint the incision, using pillow support, if necessary.

The secretions may need to be suctioned mechanically if the patient is unable to cough. It also may be necessary to use chest percussion and vibration to loosen bronchial secretions and mucus plugs that adhere to the bronchioles and bronchi and to propel sputum in the direction of gravity drainage.

After the procedure, the amount, color, viscosity, and character of the ejected sputum are noted; the patient's color and pulse are evaluated the first few times the procedure is performed. It may be necessary to administer oxygen during postural drainage.

If the sputum is foul smelling, postural drainage is carried out in a room away from other patients and deodorizers are used. After the procedure the patient may find it refreshing to brush the teeth and use a mouthwash before resting in bed.

Chest Percussion and Vibration

Thick secretions that are difficult to cough up may be loosened by tapping (percussing) and vibrating the chest. Percussion and vibration help to dislodge mucus adhering to the bronchioles and bronchi.

Percussion is carried out by cupping the hands and lightly striking the chest wall in a rhythmic fashion over the lung segment to be drained. The wrists are alternately flexed and extended so that the chest is cupped or clapped in a painless manner (Fig. 25-4*A*). A soft cloth or towel may be placed over the segment of the chest that is being cupped to prevent skin irritation and redness from direct contact. Percussion, alternating with vibration, is performed for 3 to 5 minutes for each position. The patient uses diaphragmatic breathing during this procedure to promote relaxtion (see Breathing Retraining) As a precaution, percussion over chest drainage tubes, the sternum, spine, liver, kidneys, spleen, or breasts (in women) is avoided. Percussion is performed cautiously in the elderly because of their increased incidence of osteoporosis and risk of rib fracture.

Vibration is the technique of applying manual compression and tremor to the chest wall during the exhalation phase of respiration (see Fig. 25-4*B,C*). This maneuver helps to increase the velocity of the air expired from the small airways, thus freeing the mucus. After three or four vibrations the patient is encouraged to cough, using the abdominal muscles. (Contracting the abdominal muscles increases the effectiveness of the cough.)

A scheduled program of coughing and clearing sputum, together with hydration, will reduce sputum in most patients. The number of times the percussion and vibration cycle is repeated depends on the patient's tolerance and clinical response. Breath sounds are evaluated before and after the procedures.

Nursing Interventions. When performing chest physiotherapy, it is important to make sure the patient is comfortable, is not wearing restrictive clothing, and has not just eaten a meal. The uppermost areas of the lung are treated first. Medication is given for pain, as prescribed, before percussion and vibration; the incision is splinted; and pillows are used for support as needed. The positions are varied, but focus is placed on the affected areas. On completion of the treatment, the patient is assisted to a comfortable position.

The treatment is stopped if any of the following untoward symptoms develop: increased pain, increased shortness of breath, weakness, light-headedness, or hemoptysis. Therapy is indicated until the patient has normal respirations, can mobilize secretions, and has normal breath sounds, and when the chest x-ray is normal.

Patient Education and Home Care Considerations. Chest physiotherapy is frequently indicated at home for patients with COPD, bronchiectasis, and cystic fibrosis. The techniques are the same as described above, but gravity drainage is achieved by placing the hips over a box, a stack of magazines, or pillows (unless a hospital bed is available). The patient and family are instructed in the positions and techniques of percussion and vibration, so that therapy can be continued in the home. In addition, the patient is instructed to maintain an adequate fluid intake and air humidity to prevent secretions from becoming thick and tenacious and to recognize early signs of infection such as fever and a change in the color or character of sputum. Resting 5 to 10 minutes in each postural drainage position prior to chest physiotherapy maximizes the amount of secretions obtained.

Chest physical therapy may be carried out by a home care nurse if such visits are warranted by the patient's condition. Further patient and family teaching can be provided during these visits.

Breathing Retraining

Breathing retraining consists of exercises and breathing practices designed and carried out to achieve a more efficient and controlled ventilation, and to decrease the work of breathing. Breathing retraining is especially indicated in the patient with COPD and dyspnea. These exercises enhance maximal alveolar inflation; promote muscle relaxation; relieve anxiety; eliminate useless, uncoordinated patterns of respiratory muscle activity; slow the respiratory rate; and decrease the work of breathing. Slow, relaxed, and rhythmic breathing also helps to control the anxiety that is present when the patient is dyspneic. Specific breathing exercises include diaphragmatic and pursed lip breathing (described below).

Breathing exercises may be practiced in several positions, because air distribution and pulmonary circulation vary according to the position of the chest. Many patients require additional oxygen, using a low-flow method, while performing breathing exercises. Emphysema-like changes in the lung occur as part of the natural aging process of the lung; therefore, breathing exercises are appropriate for all elderly hospitalized patients and those on restricted bed rest at home even in the absence of primary lung disease.

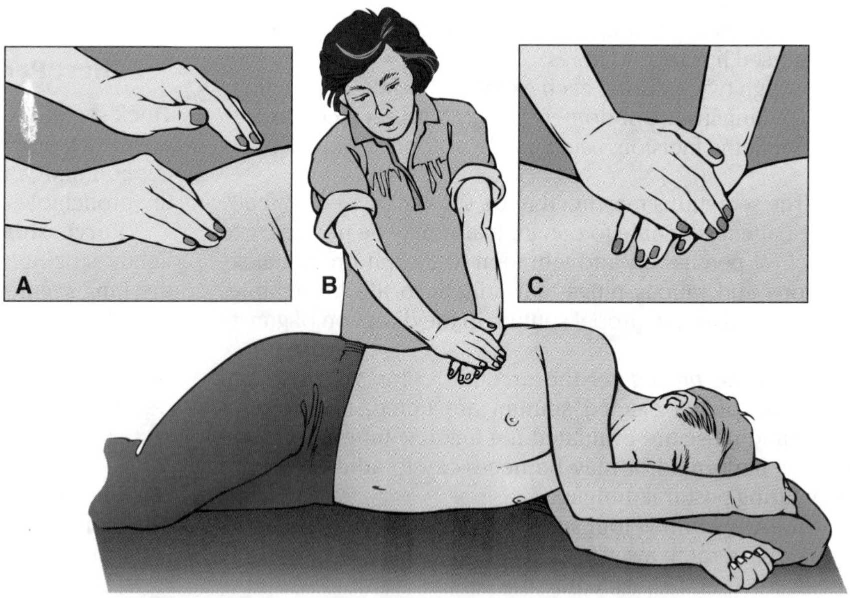

FIGURE 25-4. Percussion and vibration. (**A**) Proper hand positioning for percussion. (**B**) Proper technique for vibration. Note that the wrists and elbows are kept stiff and the vibrating motion is produced by the shoulder muscles. (**C**) Proper hand position for vibration.

Patient Teaching

The patient is instructed to breathe slowly and rhythmically in a relaxed manner and to exhale completely and empty the lungs. The patient is instructed to always inhale through the nose because this filters, humidifies, and warms the air. If short of breath, the patient should concentrate on breathing slowly and rhythmically. To avoid initiating a cycle of increasing shortness of breath and panic, it is often helpful to instruct the patient to concentrate on prolonging the length of exhalation, rather than merely slowing down the rate of breathing. Minimizing the amount of dust or particles in the air and providing adequate humidification may also make it easier for the patient to breathe.

Diaphragmatic Breathing. The goal of diaphragmatic breathing is to use and strengthen the diaphragm during breathing. Diaphragmatic breathing can become automatic with sufficient practice and concentration. The patient is instructed as described in Chart 25-2.

Pursed Lip Breathing. Pursed lip breathing, which improves oxygen transport, helps to induce a slow, deep breathing pattern and assists the patient to control breathing, even during periods of physical stress. This type of breathing helps prevent airway collapse secondary to loss of lung elasticity in emphysema. The goal of pursed lip breathing is to train the muscles of expiration to prolong exhalation and increase airway pressure during expiration, thus lessening the amount of airway trapping and resistance. Patient instructions are provided in Chart 25-2.

CHART 25-2

Patient Education: Breathing Exercises

General Instructions

- Breathe slowly and rhythmically to exhale completely and empty the lungs completely.
- Inhale through the nose to filter, humidify, and warm the air before it enters the lungs.
- If you feel out of breath, breathe more slowly by prolonging the exhalation time.
- Keep the air moist with a humidifier.

Diaphragmatic Breathing

Goal: To use and strengthen the diaphragm during breathing.

- Place one hand on the abdomen (just below the ribs) and the other hand on the middle of the chest to increase the awareness of the diaphragm and its function in breathing.
- Breathe in slowly and deeply through the nose, letting the abdomen protrude as far as possible.
- Breathe out through pursed lips while tightening (contracting) the abdominal muscles.
- Press firmly inward and upward on the abdomen while breathing out.
- Repeat for 1 minute; follow with a rest period of 2 minutes.
- Work up to 5 minutes, several times a day (before meals and at bedtime).

Pursed Lip Breathing

Goal: To prolong exhalation and increase airway pressure during expiration, thus reducing the amount of trapped air and the amount of airway resistance

- Inhale through the nose while counting to 3—the amount of time needed to say "Smell a rose."
- Exhale slowly and evenly against pursed lips while tightening the abdominal muscles. (Pursing the lips increases intratracheal pressure; exhaling through the mouth offers less resistance to expired air.)
- Count to 7 while prolonging expiration through pursed lips—the length of time to say "Blow out the candle."
- *While sitting in a chair:*
  - Fold arms over the abdomen.
  - Inhale through the nose while counting to 3.
  - Bend forward and exhale slowly through pursed lips while counting to 7.
- *While walking:*
  - Inhale while walking two steps.
  - Exhale through pursed lips while walking four or five steps.

The Patient Requiring Airway Management

Adequate ventilation is dependent on free movement of air through the upper and lower airways. In many conditions the airway becomes narrowed or blocked as a result of disease process, bronchoconstriction (narrowing of airway by contraction of muscle fibers), a foreign body, or secretions. Maintaining a patent (open) airway is achieved through meticulous airway management, whether in an emergency situation such as airway obstruction, or in long-term management, as in caring for a patient with an endotracheal or a tracheostomy tube.

Emergency Management of Upper Airway Obstruction

Upper airway obstruction has a variety of causes. Acute upper airway obstruction may be caused by food particles, vomitus, blood clots, or any other particle that enters and obstructs the larynx or trachea. It also may occur from enlargement of tissue in the wall of the airway, as in epiglottitis, laryngeal edema, laryngeal carcinoma, or peritonsillar abscess, or from thick secretions. Pressure on the walls of the airway, as occurs in retrosternal goiter, enlarged mediastinal lymph nodes, hematoma around the upper airway, and thoracic aneurysm also may result in upper airway obstruction.

The patient with an altered level of consciousness of any cause is at risk of having the upper airway obstructed owing to loss of the protective reflexes (cough and swallowing) and the tone of the pharyngeal muscles, causing the tongue to fall back and block the airway.

The nurse makes the following observations to assess for signs and symptoms of upper airway obstruction:

Inspection. Is the patient conscious? Is there any inspiratory effort? Does the chest rise symmetrically? Is there use

GUIDELINE 25–1
Clearing An Upper Airway Obstruction

- Hyperextend the patient's neck by placing one hand on the forehead and placing the fingers of the other hand underneath the jaw and lifting upward and forward. This action will pull the tongue away from the back of the pharynx (Fig. 25-5A).
- Assess the patient by observing the chest and listening and feeling for the movement of air.
- Use a cross-finger technique to open the mouth and observe for obvious obstructions such as secretions, blood clots, or food particles.
- If no passage of air is possible, apply five quick sharp abdominal thrusts just below the xyphoid process to expel the obstruction (Heimlich maneuver). Repeat this procedure until the obstruction is expelled (Fig. 25-5B).
- When the obstruction is relieved and the patient is able to breathe spontaneously, but cannot cough or swallow and does not have a gag reflex, insert an oral or nasopharyngeal airway.

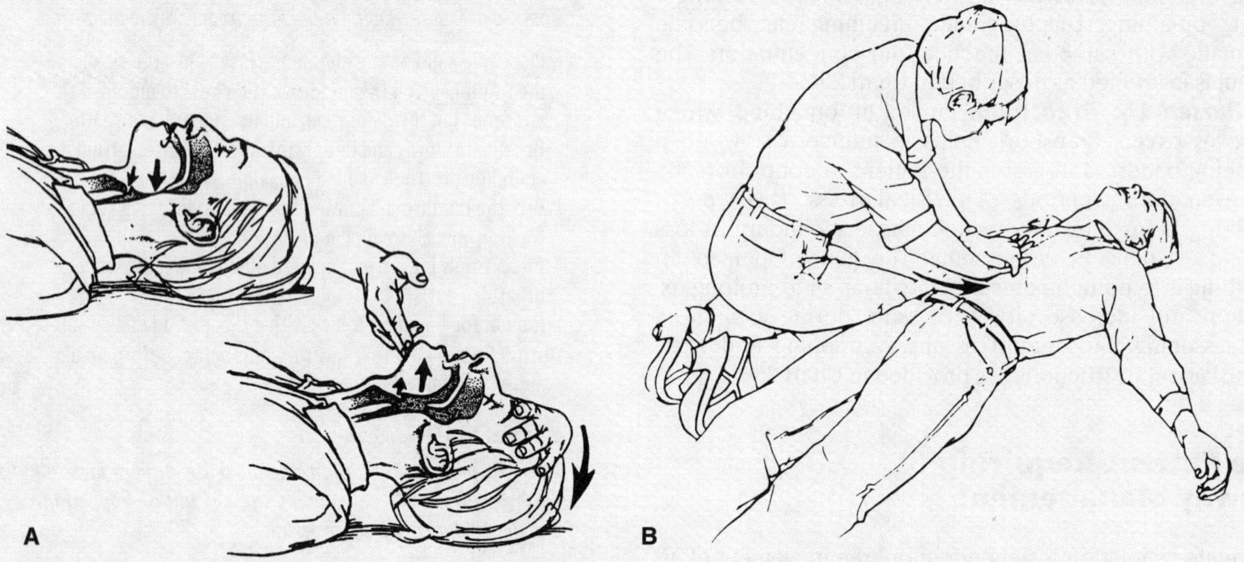

FIGURE 25-5. (A) Opening the airway. (*Top*) Airway obstruction produced by tongue and epiglottis; (*bottom*) relief by head tilt–chin lift maneuver. (B) Heimlich maneuver administered to unconscious victim with airway obstruction caused by foreign body. (From Emergency Cardiac Care Committee and Subcommittees: AHA Guidelines for Cardiopulmonary Resuscitation and Emergency Cardiac Care. JAMA 268: 2193. Copyright 1992, American Medical Association.)

Bag and Mask Resuscitation

- Use a resuscitator bag and mask if assisted ventilation is required.
- Apply the mask to the patient's face and create a seal by pressing the left thumb on the bridge of the nose and the index finger on the chin. Use the rest of the fingers on the left hand and pull on the chin and the angle of the mandible to maintain the head in extension (Fig. 25-6).
- Use the right hand to inflate the lungs by squeezing the bag to its full volume.

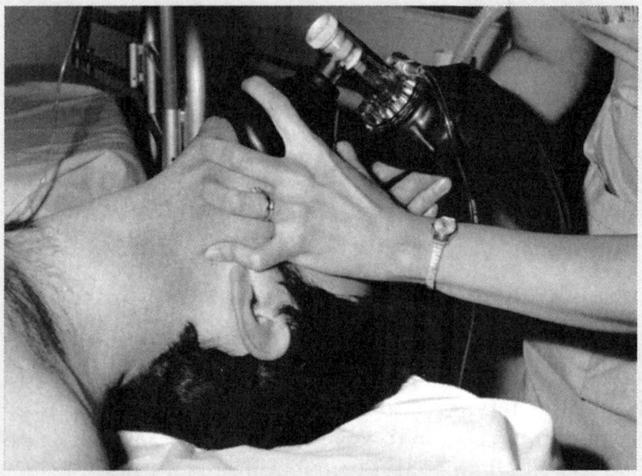

FIGURE 25-6. Bag and mask ventilation. The head is extended and the mask is sealed to the face by pressing the left thumb to the bridge of the nose and the index finger on the chin. The remaining three fingers pull the chin and mandible upward to maintain the head in extension. The right hand then squeezes the bag, while the chest is observed for symmetric expansion.

or retraction of accessory muscles? What is the skin color? Are there any obvious signs of deformity or obstruction (trauma, food, teeth, vomitus)? Is the trachea midline?

Palpation. Do both sides of the chest rise equally with inspiration? Are there any specific areas of tenderness, fracture, or subcutaneous emphysema (crepitus)?

Auscultation. Is there any audible air movement, stridor (inspiratory sound), or wheezing (expiratory sound)? Are breath sounds present bilaterally in all lobes?

As soon as an upper airway obstruction is identified, emergency measures are taken (Guideline 25-1).

Endotracheal Intubation

Endotracheal intubation involves passing an **endotracheal tube** through the mouth or nose into the trachea. Intubation provides a patent airway when the patient is having respiratory distress that cannot be treated by simpler methods. It is the method of choice in emergency care. Endotracheal intubation is a means of providing an airway for patients who cannot maintain an adequate airway on their own (comatose patients, those with upper airway obstruction), for mechanical ventilation, and for suctioning secretions from the pulmonary tree.

An endotracheal tube usually is passed with the aid of a laryngoscope by medical, nursing, or respiratory therapy personnel who are specifically trained in this technique. Once the tube is inserted, a cuff around the tube is inflated to prevent air from leaking around the outer part of the tube and to minimize the possibility of subsequent aspiration and prevent movement of the tube.

Suctioning of the tracheobronchial secretions is performed through the tube. Warmed, humidified oxygen should always be introduced through the tube, whether the patient is breathing spontaneously or is on ventilatory support. Endotracheal intubation may be used for up to 3 weeks, at which time a tracheostomy must be considered to decrease irritation of and trauma to the tracheal lining, to reduce the incidence of vocal cord paralysis (secondary to laryngeal nerve damage), and to reduce mechanical dead space.

Disadvantages exist with endotracheal or tracheostomy tubes as with many treatment modalities. For one thing, the tube causes discomfort. In addition, the cough reflex is depressed because closure of the glottis is hindered. Secretions tend to become thicker because the warming and humidifying effect of the upper respiratory tract has been bypassed. The swallowing reflexes, composed of the glottic, pharyngeal, and laryngeal reflexes, are depressed because of prolonged disuse and the mechanical trauma of the endotracheal or tracheostomy tube, which puts the patient at increased risk for aspiration. Ulceration and stricture of the larynx or trachea may develop.

Of great concern to the patient is the inability to talk and to communicate needs.

For nursing management of the patient with endotracheal intubation, see Guideline 25-2.

GUIDELINE 25–2
Nursing Management of the Patient With an Endotracheal Tube

Immediately After Intubation

1. Check symmetry of chest expansion
   a. Auscultate breath sounds of anterior and lateral chest bilaterally.
   b. Obtain order for chest x-ray to verify proper tube placement.
2. Ensure high humidity.
   A visible mist should be seen from the T-piece
3. Administer oxygen concentration as prescribed by physician.
4. Secure the tube to the patient's face with tape and mark the proximal end for position maintenance.
   a. Cut proximal end of tube if it is longer than 7.5 cm (3 in) to prevent kinking.
   b. An oral airway or mouth bite may be inserted to prevent the patient from biting and obstructing the tube.
5. Use sterile suction technique and airway care to prevent iatrogenic contamination and infection.
6. Continue to reposition patient every 2 hours and as needed to prevent atelectasis and to optimize lung expansion.
7. Provide oral hygiene and suction the oropharynx whenever necessary.

Extubation (Removal of Endotracheal Tube)

1. Explain procedure.
2. Have self-inflating bag and mask ready in case ventilatory assistance is required immediately after extubation.
3. Suction the tracheobronchial tree and oropharynx, remove tape, then deflate the cuff.
4. Give oxygen for a few breaths, then insert new, sterile suction catheter inside tube.
5. Have the patient inhale, and at peak inspiration remove the tube, suctioning the airway through the tube as it is pulled out.

Note: In some hospitals this procedure can be performed by respiratory therapists; in others, nurses perform it. Check hospital policy.

Care of Patient Following Removal of the Endotracheal Tube

1. Give heated humidity and oxygen by way of face mask.
2. Monitor respiratory rate and quality of chest excursions. Note stridor, color change, and change in mental altertness or behavior.
3. Keep NPO or give only ice chips for next few hours.
4. Provide mouth care.
5. Instruct patient in coughing and deep-breathing exercises.

Tracheostomy

A **tracheotomy** is a procedure in which an opening is made into the trachea. When an indwelling tube is inserted into the trachea, the term **tracheostomy** is used. A tracheostomy may be either temporary or permanent.

A tracheostomy is performed to bypass an upper airway obstruction, to remove tracheobronchial secretions, to permit the long-term use of mechanical ventilation, to prevent aspiration of oral or gastric secretions in the unconscious or paralyzed patient (by closing off the trachea from the esophagus), and to replace an endotracheal tube. There are many disease processes and emergency conditions that make a tracheostomy necessary.

Procedure. The procedure is usually performed in the operating room or in an intensive care unit, where the patient's ventilation can be well controlled and optimal aseptic technique can be maintained. An opening is made in the second and third tracheal rings. After the trachea is exposed, a cuffed tracheostomy tube of an appropriate size is inserted (Fig. 25-7*A*). The cuff is an inflatable attachment to the tracheostomy that is designed to occlude the space between the trachea walls and the tube to permit effective mechanical ventilation.

The tracheostomy tube is held in place by tapes fastened around the patient's neck. Usually, a square of sterile gauze is placed between the tube and the skin to absorb drainage and prevent infection (see Fig. 25-7*B*).

Complications. Complications may occur early or late in the course of tracheostomy tube management. They may even occur years after the tube has been removed. *Early complications* immediately after the tracheostomy is performed include bleeding, pneumothorax, air embolism, aspiration, subcutaneous or mediastinal emphysema, recurrent laryngeal nerve damage, or posterior tracheal wall penetration. *Long-term complications* include airway obstruction due to accumulation of secretions or protrusion of the cuff over the opening of the tube, infection, rupture of the innominate artery, dysphagia, tracheoesophageal fistula, tracheal dilation, or tracheal ischemia and necrosis. Tracheal stenosis may develop after the tube is removed.

Postoperative Nursing Interventions. The patient requires continuous monitoring and assessment. The newly made opening must be kept patent by proper suctioning of secretions as described in Guideline 25-3. After the vital signs are stable, the patient is placed in a semi-Fowler's position to facilitate ventilation, promote drainage, minimize edema, and prevent strain on the suture lines. Analgesic and sedative drugs are administered with caution because it is undesirable to depress the cough reflex.

A major objective of nursing care is to alleviate the apprehension of the patient and provide an effective means of communication. Reassurance will help allay the fear of asphyxiation if the patient is unable to call for help.

Paper and pencil or a "magic slate" and the patient call light are kept within reach to ensure a means of communication.

Tracheostomy Care

Tracheal Suctioning (Tracheostomy or Endotracheal Tube). When a tracheostomy or an endotracheal tube is present, it is usually necessary to suction the patient's secretions because the effectiveness of the cough mechanism is decreased. Tracheal suctioning is performed when adventitious breath sounds are detected or whenever secretions are obviously present. Unnecessary suctioning can initiate bronchospasm and cause mechanical trauma to the tracheal mucosa.

All equipment that comes into direct contact with the patient's lower airway must be sterile to prevent overwhelming pulmonary and systemic infections. The procedure for suctioning a tracheostomy is presented in Guideline 25-3.

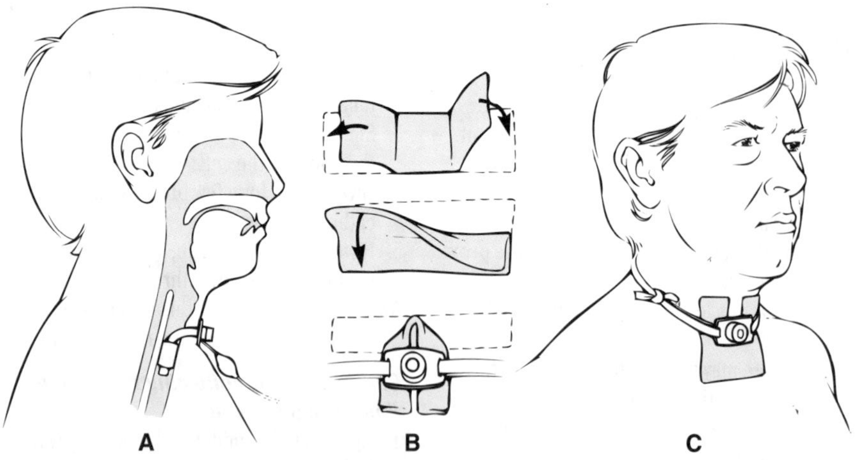

FIGURE 25-7. Tracheostomy tube dressing and tape changes. (**A**) The cuff of the tracheostomy tube fits smoothly within the tracheal wall. Pressure should be great enough to seal (above 20 cm H_2O) but not so great (below 25 cm H_2O) as to impair circulation. (**B**) How to fold a 4 × 4 gauze square so that it need not be cut (cut or frayed threads could be aspirated), yet will provide a comfortable neck pad. (**C**) A precut gauze tracheostomy dressing. Dressings are changed as often as necessary. Note how the neck twill tapes are fastened to the openings in the neck plate of the tracheostomy tube. Twill tapes should be tied to the side of the neck rather than in the back, eliminating the discomfort of lying on the knot.

GUIDELINE 25-3
Suctioning a Tracheostomy

Equipment

- Suction catheters
- Gloves
- Goggles for eye protection
- 5- to 10-ml syringe
- Sterile normal saline poured in a cup for irrigation
- The patient's own self-inflating bag (hand resuscitator) with supplemental oxygen (the bag is changed daily to reduce the chance of infection)
- Suction machine

Procedure

- Explain the procedure to the patient before beginning and offer reassurance during suctioning, as the patient may be apprehensive about choking and about an inability to communicate.
- Begin by washing hands thoroughly.
- Turn on suction source (pressure should not exceed 120 mm Hg).
- Open suction catheter kit.
- Fill basin with sterile normal saline.
- Ventilate the patient with manual resuscitation bag and high flow oxygen.
- Put sterile glove on dominant hand.
- Pick up suction catheter in gloved hand and connect to suction.
- Hyperinflate or hyperoxygenate the patient's lungs for several deep breaths with a self-inflating bag.
- Insert catheter at least as far as the end of the tube without applying suction, just far enough to stimulate the cough reflex.
- Apply suction while withdrawing the catheter, rotating it gently 360 degrees (no longer than 10 to 15 seconds, because the patient can become hypoxic and develop dysrhythmias, which can lead to cardiac arrest).
- Reoxygenate and inflate the patient's lungs for several breaths.
- Instill 3 to 5 ml normal saline into the airway only if cough reflex is depressed.
- Repeat previous four steps until the airway is clear.
- Rinse catheter in basin with sterile normal saline between suction attempts if necessary.
- Suction oropharyngeal cavity after completing tracheal suctioning.
- Rinse suction tubing.
- Discard catheter, gloves, and basin.

Cuff Management. As a general rule, the cuff on an endotracheal or tracheostomy tube should be inflated. The pressure within the cuff should be the lowest possible that allows delivery of adequate tidal volumes and prevents pulmonary aspiration. Usually the pressure is maintained below 25 cm H_2O to prevent injury and above 20 cm H_2O to prevent aspiration. Cuff pressure must be monitored at least every 8 hours by attaching a hand-held pressure gauge to the pilot balloon of the tube or through the use of minimal leak volume or minimal occlusion volume techniques. With long-term intubation, higher pressures may be needed to maintain an adequate seal.

Tracheostomy Care. The care of the patient with a tracheostomy tube is summarized in Guideline 25-4.

The Patient Requiring Mechanical Ventilation

A mechanical ventilator is a positive- or negative-pressure breathing device that can maintain ventilation and oxygen delivery for a prolonged period.

Caring for a patient on mechanical ventilation has become an integral part of nursing care in critical care units, on general medical-surgical units, in extended care facilities, and even in the home. Nurses, physicians, and respiratory therapists must understand each patient's specific pulmonary needs and work together to set realistic goals. Essential ingredients for positive patient outcomes include understanding the principles of mechanical ventilation and the care needs of the patient, as well as open communication among members of the health care team about the goals of therapy, weaning plans, and the patient's tolerance of changes in ventilator settings. (See the Ethical Question display.)

Indications for Mechanical Ventilation

If a patient is experiencing a continuous decrease in oxygenation (PaO_2), an increase in arterial carbon dioxide levels ($PaCO_2$), and a persistent acidosis (a decreased *p*H), then mechanical ventilation may be necessary. Conditions such as postoperative thoracic or abdominal surgery, drug overdose, neuromuscular diseases, inhalation injury, COPD, multiple trauma, shock, multisystem failure, and coma all may lead to respiratory failure and the need for mechanical ventilation. The criteria for mechanical ventilation (Chart 25-3) serve as guidelines for making the decision to place a patient on a ventilator. A patient with apnea that is not readily reversible is also a candidate for mechanical ventilation.

Classification of Ventilators

There are several types of mechanical ventilators. Ventilators are classified according to the manner in which they support ventilation. The two general categories are negative-pressure and positive-pressure ventilators.

By far the most common category in use today is the positive-pressure ventilator. Positive-pressure ventilators are

GUIDELINE 25-4
Care of the Patient With a Tracheostomy

Tracheostomy Care	***Rationale***
Tracheostomy Cuff	
1. Cuffed tube (air injected into cuff) is required during prolonged mechanical ventilation.	The purpose of a cuffed tube is to prevent air from leaking during positive-pressure ventilation and to prevent tracheal aspiration of gastric contents. An adequate seal is indicated by the disappearance of any air leakage from the mouth or tracheostomy or disappearance of the harsh, gurgling sound of air coming from the throat.
2. Low-pressure cuff	Low-pressure cuffs exert minimal pressure on the tracheal mucosa and thus reduce the danger of tracheal ulceration and stricture.
Tracheostomy Tube and Skin Care	
1. Inspect tracheostomy dressing for moisture or drainage.	The tracheostomy dressing is changed as needed to keep the skin clean and dry. Do not allow moist or soiled dressings to remain on the skin.
2. Wash hands.	Handwashing reduces bacteria on hands.
3. Explain procedure to patient.	A patient with a tracheostomy is apprehensive and requires ongoing assurance and support.
4. Wearing clean gloves, remove soiled dressing and discard.	Observing body substance isolation with contaminated dressings reduces cross-contamination.
5. Prepare sterile supplies, including hydrogen peroxide, normal saline or sterile water, cotton-tipped applicators, dressing.	Having necessary supplies and equipment readily available allows the procedure to be completed efficiently.
6. Put on sterile gloves.	Minimizes transmission of surface flora to sterile respiratory tract.
7. Cleanse wound and plate of tracheostomy tube with sterile applicators moistened with hydrogen peroxide. Rinse with sterile saline.	Hydrogen peroxide is effective in loosening crusted secretions. Rinsing prevents skin residue.
8. Use bacteriostatic ointment on the edge of the tracheostomy wound if prescribed.	Provides topical bacteriostatic protection.
9. If old tapes are soiled, place clean twill tapes in position to secure tracheostomy tube. Insert one end of tape through the side opening of the outer cannula. Wrap it around the patient's neck and thread it through the opposite opening of the outer cannula. Bring both ends around so that they meet on one side of the neck. Secure with a knot. Tighten until only two fingers can be comfortably inserted under tape.	This will provide a double thickness of tape around the neck. Tracheostomy tube can be dislodged by movement or forceful cough if left unsecured. It is difficult to reinsert the tracheostomy tube, and respiratory distress may occur if the tracheostomy tube is dislodged.
10. Remove old tapes and discard.	
11. Use sterile tracheostomy dressing, and fit securely under the twill tapes and flange of tracheostomy tube so that the incision is covered (see Fig. 25-7).	Dressings that will shred are not used around a tracheostomy because of the danger that pieces of material, lint, or thread may get into the tube, and eventually into the trachea, causing obstruction or abscess formation. Special dressings that do not have a tendency to shred are used.

also classified by the method of ending the inspiratory phase (pressure-cycled, time-cycled, and volume-cycled).

Negative-Pressure Ventilators

Negative-pressure ventilators exert a negative pressure on the external chest. Decreasing the intrathoracic pressure during inspiration allows air to flow into the lung, filling its volume. Physiologically, this type of assisted ventilation is similar to spontaneous ventilation. It is used mainly in chronic respiratory failure associated with neuromuscular conditions such as poliomyelitis, muscular dystrophy, amyotrophic lateral sclerosis, and myasthenia gravis. Its use is not appropriate for the unstable or complex patient or the patient whose condition requires frequent ventilatory changes.

Negative-pressure ventilators are simple to use and do not require intubation of the patient's airway. They are used most often for the patient with borderline pulmonary function due to neuromuscular disease. Consequently, they are especially adaptable for home use. There are several types of negative-pressure ventilators: iron lung, body wrap, and chest cuirass.

Drinker Respirator Tank (Iron Lung). The iron lung is a negative-pressure chamber used for ventilation. It

ETHICAL QUESTION:

Can Patients Refuse Mechanical Ventilation?

Situation

Mechanical ventilation is a life-support treatment that can be used in a variety of clinical settings for acute and chronic conditions. Does a patient have the right to refuse a life-support treatment that is keeping him or her alive, even when the prognosis with continued treatment is favorable? If the withdrawal of the ventilator results in the death of the patient, is the health care provider who removed the ventilator guilty of killing the patient?

Dilemma

The patient's right to refuse treatment conflicts with the health care provider's obligation to help the patient (autonomy versus beneficence).

Discussion

- What arguments would you pose *in favor of* withdrawing the ventilator at the patient's request?
- What arguments would you pose *against* withdrawing mechanical ventilation at the patient's request?

was used extensively during polio epidemics in the past and currently is used by polio survivors and other neuromuscularly impaired patients.

Body Wrap (Pneumowrap) and Chest Cuirass (Tortoise Shell). Both of these portable devices require a rigid cage or shell to create a negative-pressure chamber around the thorax and abdomen. Because of problems with proper fit and system leaks, these types of ventilators are used only with carefully selected patients.

Positive-Pressure Ventilators

Positive-pressure ventilators inflate the lungs by exerting positive pressure on the airway, similar to a bellows mechanism, and thus force the alveoli to expand during inspiration. Expiration occurs passively.

Endotracheal intubation or tracheostomy is necessary. These ventilators are widely used in the hospital setting and are increasingly used in the home for patients with primary lung disease. There are three types of positive-pressure ventilators: pressure-cycled, timed-cycled, and volume-cycled.

Pressure-Cycled Ventilators. The pressure-cycled ventilator is a positive-pressure ventilator that ends inspiration when a preset pressure has been reached. In other words, the ventilator cycles on, delivers a flow of air until a certain predetermined pressure is reached, and then cycles off. The major limitation with this type of ventilator is that the volume of air or oxygen can vary as the patient's airway resistance or compliance changes. The result is an inconsistency in the amount of tidal volume delivered and a possible compromise of ventilation. Consequently, in adults, pressure-cycled ventilators are intended only for short-term use in the recovery room. The most common type is the IPPB machine.

Time-Cycled Ventilators. Time-cycled ventilators terminate or control inspiration after a preset time. The volume of air the patient receives is regulated by the length of inspiration and the flow rate of the air. Most ventilators have a rate control that determines the respiratory rate, but pure time-cycling is rarely used for adults. These ventilators are used in newborns and infants.

Volume-Cycled Ventilators. Volume-cycled ventilators are by far the most commonly used positive-pressure ventilators in use today (Figs. 25-8 and 25-9). With this type of ventilator, the volume of air to be delivered with each inspiration is preset. Once this preset volume is delivered to the patient, the ventilator cycles off and exhalation occurs passively. From breath to breath, the volume of air delivered by the ventilator is relatively constant, assuring consistent, adequate breaths despite varying airway pressures.

CHART 25-3
Indications for Mechanical Ventilation

$PaO_2 < 50$ mm Hg with $FiO_2 > 0.60$
$PaO_2 > 50$ mm Hg with $pH < 7.25$
Vital capacity < 2 times tidal volume
Negative inspiratory force < 25 cm H_2O
Respiratory rate > 35/min

Features and Settings of Volume Ventilators

Numerous features are used in the management of the patient on a mechanical ventilator. The most crucial features and settings of a volume ventilator relative to nursing care are presented in Chart 25-4.

Adjustment of the Ventilator. The ventilator is adjusted so that the patient is comfortable and "in sync" with the machine. Minimal alteration of the normal cardiovascular and pulmonary dynamics is desired. If the volume ventilator is adjusted appropriately, the patient's arterial blood gas levels will be satisfactory and there will be little or no cardiovascular compromise. Guidelines to determine how to achieve adequate mechanical ventilation for each patient are described in Guideline 25-5.

❑ *NURSING PROCESS*
Care of the Mechanically Ventilated Patient

Assessment

The nurse has a vital role in assessing the patient's status and the functioning of the ventilator. In assessing the patient, the nurse evaluates the following:

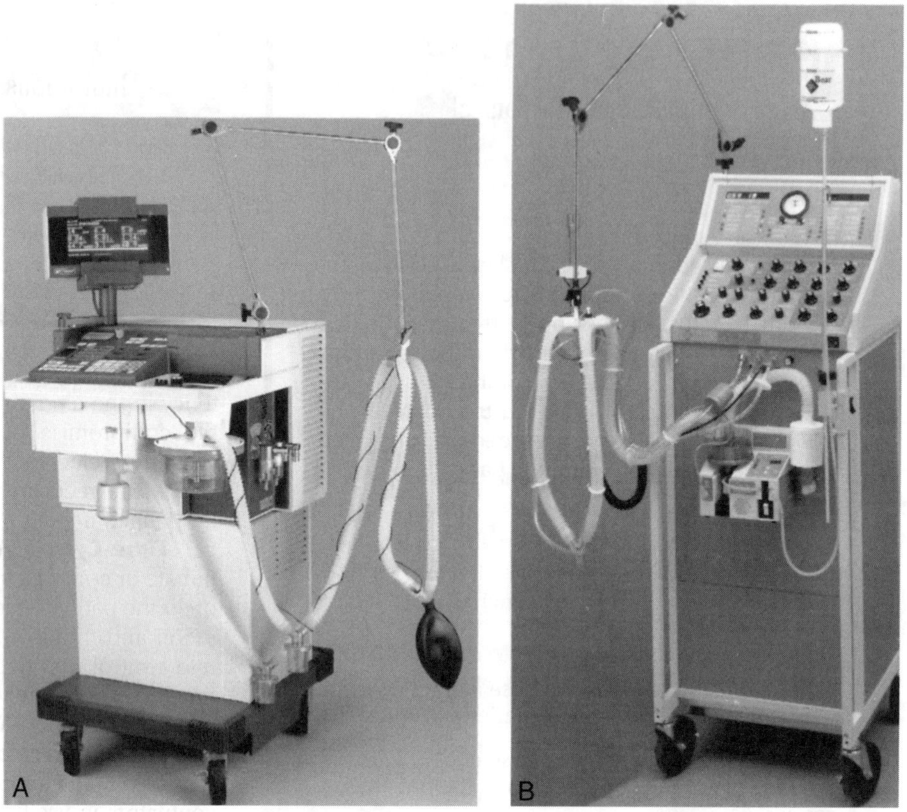

FIGURE 25-8. Two commonly used brands of volume-controlled ventilators: (**A**) Puritan-Bennett 7200A; (**B**) Bear 3 Adult. (**A** courtesy of Puritan Bennett Corp; **B** courtesy of Bear Medical Systems, Inc.)

- ❑ Vital signs
- ❑ Evidence of hypoxia (restlessness, anxiety, tachycardia, increased respiratory rate, cyanosis)
- ❑ Respiratory rate and pattern
- ❑ Breath sounds
- ❑ Neurologic status
- ❑ Tidal volume, minute ventilation, forced vital capacity
- ❑ Suctioning needs
- ❑ Patient's spontaneous ventilatory effort
- ❑ Nutritional status
- ❑ Psychologic status

Assessment of Cardiac Function. Alterations in cardiac output may occur as a result of positive-pressure ventilation. The positive intrathoracic pressure during inspiration compresses the heart and great vessels, thereby reducing venous return and cardiac output. This is usually corrected during exhalation when the positive pressure is off. Excessive positive pressure may cause a spontaneous *pneumothorax* due to trauma to the alveoli. This may quickly develop into a tension pneumothorax, further compromising venous return, cardiac output, and blood pressure.

To evaluate cardiac function, the nurse first looks for signs and symptoms of hypoxemia and hypoxia (restlessness, apprehension, confusion, tachycardia, tachypnea, labored breathing, pallor progressing to cyanosis, diaphoresis, transient hypertension, and decreased urine output). If a pulmonary artery catheter is in place, cardiac output, cardiac index, and other hemodynamic values can be determined.

Assessment of Equipment. The ventilator also needs to be assessed to make sure that it is functioning properly and that the settings are appropriate. Even though the nurse is not primarily responsible for adjusting the settings on the ventilator or measuring ventilator parameters (usually the responsibility of the respiratory therapist), the nurse is responsible for the patient and therefore needs to evaluate how the ventilator affects the patient's overall status. In monitoring the ventilator, the nurse should note the following:

- ❑ Type of ventilator (volume-cycled, pressure-cycled, negative-pressure)
- ❑ Controlling mode (control, assist/control, intermittent mandatory ventilation)
- ❑ Tidal volume and rate settings
- ❑ FIO_2 (fraction of inspired oxygen) setting
- ❑ Inspiratory pressure reached and pressure limit

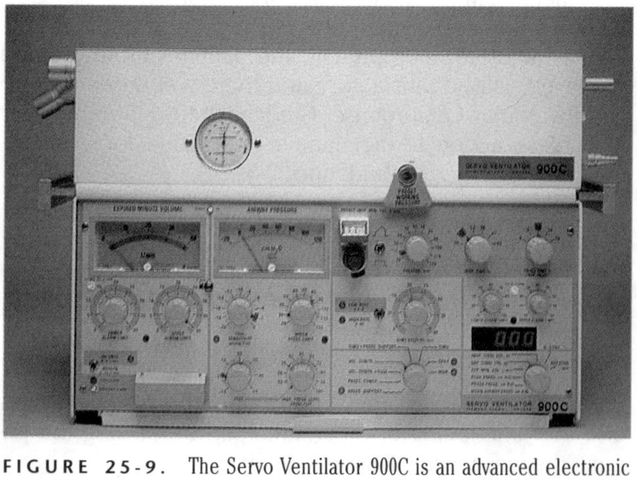

FIGURE 25-9. The Servo Ventilator 900C is an advanced electronic ventilator. (Courtesy Siemens Medical Systems, Inc.)

CHART 25-4
Features and Settings of a Volume Ventilator

A volume-controlled ventilator (MA1, Bear, Servo) will deliver set tidal volume with varying pressures.

Fraction of Inspired Oxygen (F_{IO_2})

The concentration of oxygen delivered is dependent on patient need, as determined by the physician and evaluated by arterial blood gas levels.

Tidal Volume (V_T)

10–15 ml/kg body weight

Respiratory Rate

12–16/min

Sensitivity Setting

- The patient should not have to generate more than –2 cm H_2O inspiratory force to trigger the ventilator.

Type of Ventilation

Controlled. The machine completely controls the patient's ventilation according to set tidal volumes and respiratory rate. Because of problems with synchrony, it is rarely used.

Assist/Control. The patient triggers the machine. If the patient fails to breathe, the machine will deliver a controlled breath at a minimum rate and preset volume.

Intermittent Mandatory Ventilation (IMV). Machine allows patient to breathe spontaneously while providing preset F_{IO_2} and number of ventilator breaths to ensure adequate ventilation without fatigue.

Inspiration to Exhalation Ratio (I:E Ratio)

- Should be 1:3, 1:2, or more (1 second of inspiration to 3 seconds of exhalation, etc.), in keeping with normal respiratory pattern

Minute Volume (V_E)

Tidal volume × respiratory rate/min
Normal = 6–8 L/min

Airway Pressure

Normal = 15–20 cm H_2O, but varies.
Low airway pressure is seen with air leak.
High airway pressure is seen in
- Increased secretions
- Airway obstruction
- Bronchospasms
- Pulmonary edema
- Pneumothorax
- Flail chest
- Patient exhaling when ventilator cycling

Sigh

- The lungs are hyperinflated periodically to open collapsed alveoli.
- Sigh volume is 1.5 times tidal volume 1–3 times/hr.
- Used only with assist-control mode.

Humidity and Temperature

- Heated humidity is provided for all patients with endotracheal tube or tracheostomy to avoid thick secretions
- Daily clinical evaluation of the viscosity of the patient's secretions provides a guideline for the effectiveness of humidification and nebulization.

Positive End-Expiratory Pressure (PEEP)

- A positive pressure of 5 cm, 10 cm, or 15 cm H_2O is maintained at the end of exhalation instead of a normal 0 cm H_2O pressure.
- Increases functional residual capacity (opens collapsed alveoli) and improves oxygenation with lower F_{IO_2}.

- ❑ Sigh settings (usually 1.5 times the tidal volume and range from 1 to 3/hr) if applicable
- ❑ Presence of water in the tubing, disconnection, or kinking of the tubing
- ❑ Humidification (humidifier filled with water)
- ❑ Alarms (functioning properly)
- ❑ PEEP (positive end-expiratory pressure) or pressure support level, if applicable

Note: If a malfunction of the ventilator system occurs, and if the problem cannot be identified and corrected immediately, the nurse must be prepared to ventilate the

GUIDELINE 25–5
Setting Initial Ventilator Setting

1. Set the machine to deliver tidal volume required (10 to 15 ml/kg).
2. Adjust the machine to deliver the lowest concentration of oxygen to maintain normal PaO_2 (80–100 mm Hg). This setting may be set high and gradually reduced based on arterial blood gas results.
3. Record peak inspiratory pressure.
4. Set mode (assist-control or intermittent mandatory ventilation) and rate according to physician order. (Modes of mechanical ventilation are described in Figure 25-10.)
5. If the ventilator is set on assist-control mode, adjust sensitivity so that the patient can trigger the ventilator with a minimal effort (usually 2 mm Hg negative inspiratory force).
6. Record minute volume and measure carbon dioxide partial pressure (PCO_2), *p*H, and PO_2 after 20 minutes of continuous mechanical ventilation.
7. Adjust setting (FIO_2 and rate) according to results of arterial blood gases to provide normal values or those set by the physician.
8. If patient suddenly becomes confused or agitated or begins "bucking" the ventilator for some unexplained reason, assess for hypoxemia and manually ventilate on 100% oxygen with a resuscitation bag.

patient with a manual resuscitation bag until the problem is resolved.

Diagnosis

Nursing Diagnoses

Based on the assessment data, the patient's major nursing diagnoses may include:

- Impaired gas exchange related to underlying illness, or ventilator setting adjustment during stabilization or weaning. (*Note:* The nursing diagnosis of impaired gas exchange is, by its complex nature, multidisciplinary and collaborative.)
- Ineffective airway clearance related to increased mucus production associated with continuous positive-pressure mechanical ventilation
- Risk for trauma and infection related to endotracheal intubation or tracheostomy
- Impaired physical mobility related to ventilator dependency
- Impaired verbal communication related to presence of endotracheal tube and attachment to ventilator
- Ineffective individual coping and powerlessness related to ventilator dependency

Collaborative Problems/ Potential Complications

- Fighting the ventilator
- Ventilator problems–increase in peak airway pressure; decrease in pressure; loss of volume
- Cardiovascular compromise
- Barotrauma and pneumothorax
- Pulmonary infection

Planning and Implementation

Goals. The major goals for the patient may include the following: optimal gas exchange; reduction of mucus accumulation; absence of trauma or infection; attainment of optimal mobility; adjustment to nonverbal methods of communication; acquisition of successful coping measures; and absence of complications.

Nursing Interventions

Nursing care of the mechanically ventilated patient requires unique technical and interpersonal skills. Nursing interventions are similar whether the patient is in an intensive care unit, a medical-surgical unit, or an extended care facility. The frequency of administering the care and the stability of the patient are the factors that vary from unit to unit.

Enhancing Gas Exchange. The entire purpose of mechanical ventilation is to optimize gas exchange by maintaining alveolar ventilation and oxygen delivery. The alteration in gas exchange may be due to the underlying illness or to mechanical factors related to the adjustment of the machine to the patient. The health care team, including the nurse, physician, and respiratory therapist, continually assesses the patient for adequate gas exchange, signs and symptoms of hypoxia, and response to treatment. It is imperative that the team members share goals and information freely. All other goals directly or indirectly relate to this primary goal.

Nursing interventions for the mechanically ventilated patient are not uniquely different from other pulmonary patients, yet the need for astute nursing observation and the establishment of a therapeutic nurse–patient relationship is of paramount importance. The constellation of interventions used by the nurse is determined by the underlying disease process and the patient's response. For example, poor gas exchange can be related to a wide variety of factors: altered level of consciousness, atelectasis, fluid overload, incisional pain, or primary disease processes such as pneumonia.

As a result, nursing interventions to promote optimal gas exchange include judicious administration of pain medications to *relieve pain* but not to significantly decrease the respiratory drive, and frequent *repositioning* to diminish the pulmonary effects of immobility.

The nurse also monitors for adequate *fluid balance* by assessing for the presence of peripheral edema, calculating daily intake and output, and monitoring daily weights. The nurse administers *medications* to control the primary disease and monitors for their potential side effects. *Sterile suctioning* of the lower airway combined with *chest physiother-*

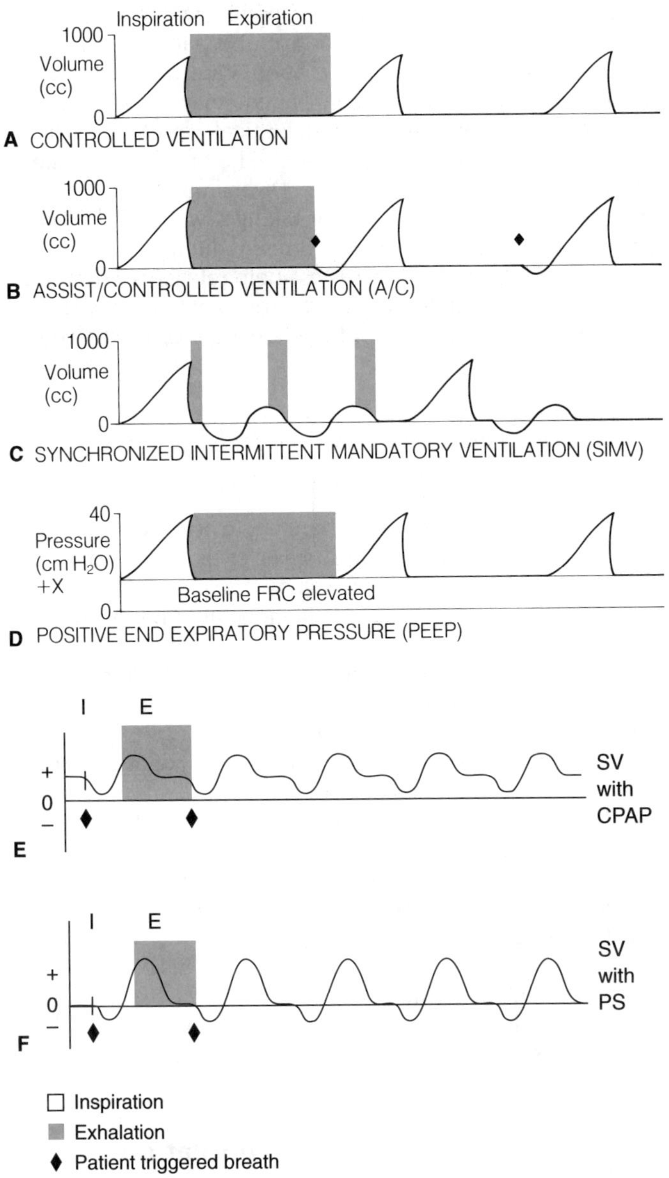

(**A**) Flow in the controlled ventilation mode. A preset volume of gas is delivered to the patient under positive pressure while spontaneous patient respiratory effort is "locked out."

(**B**) Gas flow in the assist/control ventilation mode. In this mode, a preset volume of gas is delivered to the patient at a preset rate, but the patient may trigger a ventilator breath with negative inspiratory effort.

(**C**) Gas flow in the synchronized intermittent mandatory ventilation (IMV) mode. A preset minimum number of breaths are synchronously delivered to the patient, but the patient may also take spontaneous breaths of varying volumes. Note how inspiratory and expiratory pressures differ between spontaneous and ventilator breaths.

(**D**) Airway pressure with varying levels of positive end-expiratory pressure (PEEP). Note that at end expiration, the airway is not allowed to return to zero.

(**E**) Spontaneous ventilation with continuous positive airway pressure (CPAP). This ventilatory adjunct is used only with spontaneous ventilation; the patient breathes spontaneously through the ventilator at an elevated baseline pressure throughout the breathing cycle.

(**F**) Spontaneous ventilation with pressure support (PS). The patient breathes spontaneously with pressure assistance to each spontaneous inspiration.

FIGURE 25-10. Modes of mechanical ventilation with air flow waveforms.

apy (percussion, vibration) are other strategies to clear the airway of excessive secretions. Because of well-documented damage to the intima of the tracheobronchial tree, suctioning should be performed when clinically indicated rather than on a routine schedule.

Two general nursing interventions that are of particular importance to the mechanically ventilated patient are *pulmonary auscultation* and interpretation of *arterial blood gases*. The nurse is often the first to notice changes in physical assessment findings or significant trends in blood gases that signal the development of a significant problem (pneumothorax, tube displacement, pulmonary embolus).

Airway Management. Continuous positive-pressure ventilation increases the production of secretions regardless of the patient's underlying condition. The nurse must identify the presence of secretions by lung auscultation at least every 2 to 4 hours. Measures to clear the airway of secretions include suctioning, chest physiotherapy, frequent position changes, and increased mobility as soon as possible.

The sigh mechanism on the ventilator may be adjusted to deliver at least 1 to 3 sighs per hour at 1.5 times the tidal volume if the patient is on assist-control. Because of the risk of hyperventilation and trauma to pulmonary tissue from excess ventilator pressure (barotrauma, pneumothorax), this feature is not being used as frequently in recent years. If the patient is on an intermittent mandatory ventilation (IMV) mode, the mandatory ventilations act as sighs because they are of greater volume than the patient's spontaneous breaths.

Periodic sighing prevents atelectasis and the further retention of secretions. Humidification by way of the ventilator is maintained to help liquefy secretions so they are more easily raised. Bronchodilators, either intravenous or inhaled, are administered as prescribed to dilate the bronchioles so that secretions are more easily mobilized.

Preventing Trauma and Infection. Airway management must involve maintaining the endotracheal or tracheostomy tube. The ventilator tubing is positioned so there is minimal pulling or distortion of the tube in the trachea; this reduces trauma to the trachea. Cuff pressure must be monitored every 8 hours to maintain the pressure under 25 cm H_2O. The presence of a cuff leak is evaluated at the same time.

Tracheostomy care is performed at least every 8 hours and more frequently if indicated because of the increased risk of infection. Oral hygiene is administered frequently because the oral cavity is a primary source of contamination of the lungs in the intubated and compromised patient. The presence of a nasogastric tube and the use of antacids in the mechanically ventilated patient also have been shown to predispose the patient to nosocomial pneumonia from subclinical aspiration. The patient also should be positioned with the head elevated above the stomach as much as possible to decrease the potential for aspiration of gastric contents.

Promoting Optimal Level of Mobility. The patient's mobility is limited because of being connected to the ventilator. A patient whose condition has become stable should be assisted out of bed and to a chair as soon as possible. Mobility and muscle activity are beneficial because they stimulate respirations and improve morale. If the patient is not able to get out of bed, then active or passive range of motion exercises are performed every 8 hours to prevent muscle atrophy, contractures, and venous stasis.

Promoting Optimal Communication. Alternative methods of communication must be developed for the patient on a ventilator. The nurse assesses the patient's communication abilities:

- ❏ Is the patient conscious and able to communicate? Can the patient nod or shake his or her head?)
- ❏ Is the patient's mouth unobstructed by the tube for mouthing words?
- ❏ Is the patient's hand strong and available for writing? (If right-handed, the intravenous line is placed in the left arm if possible.)

Once the patient's limitations are known, the nurse offers several appropriate communication approaches: lip reading (use single key words); pad and pencil or "magic slate"; communication board; gesturing; electric larynx. Use of a "talking" or fenestrated trach can be suggested to the physician to allow the patient to talk while on the ventilator.

Additionally, the patient's eye glasses and hearing aid and a translator are made available, if indicated, to enhance the patient's ability to communicate with others.

The patient must be assisted to find the most suitable communication method. Some methods may be frustrating to both the patient and the nurse, and they need to be identified and minimized. A speech-language therapist can assist in determining the most appropriate method for the patient.

Promoting Coping Ability. Dependence on a ventilator is frightening to both the patient and the family and will disrupt even the most stable families. Encouraging them to verbalize their feelings about the ventilator, the patient's condition, and the environment in general is beneficial. Explaining procedures every time they are performed helps to reduce anxiety and familiarize the patient with hospital routines. To restore a sense of control, the patient is encouraged to participate in decisions about care, schedules, and treatment when possible. The patient may become withdrawn or depressed during mechanical ventilation, especially if it is prolonged. Consequently, he or she is informed about progress when appropriate. Diversions such as watching television, playing music, or taking a walk (if appropriate and possible) are provided. Stress-reduction techniques (a back rub, relaxation measures) help release tension and enable the patient to deal with any anxieties and fears about both the condition and the dependence on the ventilator.

Evaluation

Expected Outcomes

1. Exhibits adequate gas exchange as evidenced by breath sounds, arterial blood gas levels, pulmonary artery pressures, and vital signs
2. Demonstrates adequate ventilation with minimal mucus accumulation
3. Is free of injury or infection as evidenced by temperature and white blood count
4. Is mobile within limits of ability
   a. Gets out of bed to chair, bears weight, or ambulates as soon as possible
   b. Performs range-of-motion exercises every 6 to 8 hours
5. Communicates effectively through written messages, gestures, or other communication devices
6. Copes effectively
   a. Verbalizes fears and concerns about his condition and the equipment
   b. Participates in decision making when possible
   c. Uses stress-reduction techniques when necessary

Problems With Mechanical Ventilation

Because of the seriousness of the patient's condition and the highly complex and technical nature of mechanical ventilation, a number of problems or complications can occur. Such situations basically fall into two categories: ventilator problems or actual patient problems. In either case, the patient must be supported while the problem is being identified and corrected. Ventilator problems include cardiovascular compromise, pneumothorax, and pulmonary infection. These problems, their probable causes, and solutions are listed in Table 25-2.

"Bucking" the Ventilator. The patient is in synchrony with the ventilator when thoracic expansion coincides with the inspiratory phase of the machine and exhalation occurs passively. The patient "fights" or "bucks" the ventilator when out of phase with the machine. This is manifested when the patient attempts to breathe out during the ventilator's mechanical inspiratory phase or when there is jerky and increased abdominal muscle effort. The following factors contribute to this problem: anxiety, hypoxia, increased secretions, hypercarbia, inadequate minute volume, and pulmonary edema. These problems must be corrected before resorting to use of paralyzing agents to re-

TABLE 25-2 Causes and Solutions of Ventilator Problems

Problem	Cause	Solution
Ventilator		
Increase in peak airway pressure	Coughing or plugged airway tube	Suction airway for secretions, empty condensation fluid from circuit.
	Patient "bucking" ventilator	Adjust sensitivity.
	Decreasing lung compliance	Manually ventilate patient. Assess for hypoxia or bronchospasm. Check blood gases. Sedate only if necessary
	Tubing kinked	Check tubing; reposition patient; insert oral airway if necessary.
	Pneumothorax	Manually ventilate patient; notify physician.
	Atelectasis or bronchospasm	Clear secretions.
Decrease in pressure or loss of volume	Increase in compliance	None.
	Leak in ventilator or tubing; cuff on tube/humidifier not tight	Check entire ventilator circuit for patency. Correct leak.
Patient		
Cardiovascular compromise	Decrease in venous return due to application of positive pressure to lungs	Assess for adequate volume status by measuring heart rate, blood pressure, central venous pressure, pulmonary capillary wedge pressure, and urine output. Notify physician if values are abnormal.
Barotrauma/pneumothorax	Application of positive pressure to lungs; high mean airway pressures lead to alveolar rupture.	Notify physician. Prepare patient for chest tube insertion. Avoid high pressure settings for patients with COPD, ARDS, or history of pneumothorax.
Pulmonary infection	Bypass of normal defense mechanisms; frequent breaks in ventilator circuit; decreased mobility; impaired cough reflex.	Meticulous aseptic technique. Frequent mouth care. Optimize nutritional status.

duce bucking, or else the underlying problem is masked and the patient's condition will continue to deteriorate.

Muscle relaxants, tranquilizers, analgesics, and paralyzing agents are given at times to a patient on mechanical ventilation. Their purpose is ultimately to increase the patient–machine synchrony by decreasing the patient's anxiety, hyperventilation, or excessive muscle activity. The selection and dose of the appropriate drug are determined carefully and are based on the individual patient's requirements and the cause of the patient's restlessness. Paralyzing agents (atracurium, vecuronium, and pancuronium) are always used as a last resort.

Weaning the Patient From the Ventilator

Weaning the patient from dependence on the ventilator takes place in three stages. The patient is gradually weaned from the (1) ventilator, (2) tube, and (3) oxygen. Weaning from mechanical ventilation is performed at the earliest possible time consistent with patient safety. It is essential that the decision be made from a physiologic rather than from a mechanical viewpoint. A thorough understanding of the patient's clinical status is required in making this decision.

Weaning is started when the patient is recovering from the acute stage of medical and surgical problems and when the cause of respiratory failure is sufficiently reversed.

Criteria for Weaning. The objective measurements of the patient's ventilatory capacities include the following:

1. An ability to generate a minimal vital capacity of 10 to 15 ml/kg of body weight or a vital capacity twice as large as the predicted normal resting tidal volume. The minimal required volume is usually in the range of 1000 ml in a normal adult.

2. A spontaneous inspiratory force of at least –20 cm H_2O pressure
3. A PaO_2 of greater than 60% with an FiO_2 of less than 40%
4. Vital signs that are stable

When the decision has been made that the patient has adequate ventilatory capacity, baseline measurements are noted: (1) vital capacity, (2) inspiratory force, (3) respiratory rate, (4) resting tidal volume, (5) minute ventilation (frequency times total volume, or $f \times V_T$), (6) arterial blood gases, and (7) FiO_2. It is important to follow the trend of these values as the weaning progresses, rather than to rely on isolated measurements.

Patient Preparation. To maximize the success of weaning, the nurse must also consider the patient as a whole. Factors that impair the delivery of oxygen and elimination of carbon dioxide, as well as those that increase oxygen demand (sepsis, seizures, thyroid imbalances) or negatively affect the patient's overall strength (nutrition, neuromuscular disease), must be considered. Adequate psychological preparation is necessary before and during the weaning process. Patients need to know what is expected of them during the procedure. They are frightened by having responsibility for their own breathing again and need the reassurance that they are improving and are well enough to handle spontaneous breathing. The nurse explains what will happen during weaning and what role the patient will play in the procedure. The nurse emphasizes to the patient that someone will be with or near at all times and allows time to answer any questions simply and concisely. Proper preparation of the patient can reduce the weaning time.

Methods of Weaning

Considerable effort has been devoted to finding the "best" method of weaning from mechanical ventilation. Actually, there is no "best" way. Success depends on the combination of adequate patient preparation, available equipment, and a interdisciplinary approach to solving patient problems. The two most common weaning methods in use today are described below.

Traditional Method. The traditional method involves switching from the assist-control or IMV mode to one or more T-piece trials. This method of weaning is usually used when there is short-term ventilatory assistance (less than 2 days) *and* when the patient is awake, alert, breathing without difficulty, has good gag and cough reflexes, and is hemodynamically stable. The patient breathes spontaneously with the aid of humidified oxygen. During the weaning process, the patient is maintained on the same or higher oxygen concentration than when on the ventilator.

While on the T-piece, the patient is observed for signs and symptoms of hypoxemia or increasing fatigue as manifested by the following: (1) tachycardia, premature ventricular contractions (PVCs), ischemic ECG changes or any other sign of increasing cardiac irritability; (2) restlessness; (3) a respiratory rate greater than 35/min; (4) use of accessory muscles, and (5) paradoxical chest movement. Fatigue or exhaustion is initially manifested by an increased respiratory rate associated with a gradual reduction in tidal volume. Later there is a slowing of the respiratory rate.

If the patient appears to be tolerating the T-tube trial, a second set of arterial blood gases is drawn 20 minutes after the patient has been on spontaneous ventilation at a constant FIO_2. (It takes 15 to 20 minutes for alveolar arterial equilibration to take place.)

Signs of exhaustion and hypoxemia correlated with a deterioration of the above measurements indicate the need for ventilatory support. The patient is placed back on the ventilator each time signs of fatigue or deterioration develop.

If clinically stable, the patient usually can be extubated within 2 or 3 hours of weaning and allowed spontaneous ventilation by means of a mask with humidified oxygen. Patients who have had prolonged ventilatory assistance usually require more gradual weaning, which may take days or even weeks. They are weaned primarily during the day and placed back on the ventilator at night to rest.

Intermittent Mandatory Ventilation (IMV) Method. Some patients are difficult to wean from mechanical ventilation. An IMV device incorporated into the ventilator allows the patient to breathe spontaneously as desired but also delivers a mandatory ventilation at regular intervals. IMV is indicated if the patient satisfies all the criteria for weaning but cannot sustain adequate spontaneous ventilation for long periods.

Before the IMV method is initiated, the same weaning criteria are assessed and met as with the traditional method. The patient is assessed for symptoms of hypoxemia and cardiovascular compromise.

After initiation of IMV, serial determinations of the following are made and recorded: (1) respiratory rate, (2) minute volume ($\dot{V}_E$), (3) V_T of patient and machine, (4) FiO_2, and (5) arterial blood gas values.

If no deterioration is apparent in these parameters, and if the patient maintains adequate tidal volumes, the rate of the ventilator is progressively decreased and the patient is allowed to rely more on spontaneous respiration until weaning is complete.

Successful weaning from the ventilator is supplemented by intensive pulmonary care. The following are continued: (1) oxygen therapy; (2) arterial blood gas evaluation; (3) pulse oximetry; (4) bronchodilator therapy; (5) chest physiotherapy; (6) adequate nutrition, hydration, and humidification; and (7) incentive spirometry. These patients still have borderline pulmonary function and need vigorous supportive therapy before their respiratory status returns to a level that supports activities of daily living.

Pulse oximetry has become a commonly used assessment technology because it is noninvasive, easily applied and tolerated, allows any changes or trends in oxygen saturation data to be quickly identified, and may decrease the need for more frequent ABG analyses. The pulse oximeter sensor contains two light sources (red and infrared), and a photodetector that is placed across a pulsating arteriolar bed such as the finger, toe, earlobe, or the bridge of the nose. Selected wavelengths of light are absorbed by hemoglobin and are transmitted through tissue to the sensor, which transforms the signal into a digital display of percent saturation of hemoglobin (SaO_2 normal: 97% to 99%) and pulse rate. To maximize the accuracy of the pulse oximeter data, the nurse ensures that the sensor is not placed on an extremity that has poor arterial flow or venous outflow, and that it is shielded from large amounts of ambient light. There should also be correlation between the pulse sensed by the pulse oximeter and that obtained by the nurse and the cardiac monitor.

Weaning From the Tube. The tracheostomy or endotracheal tube can be removed if the following criteria are present: (1) spontaneous ventilation is adequate; (2) the pharyngeal and laryngeal gag reflexes are active; (3) the patient is maintaining an adequate airway and can swallow, move the jaw, or clench the teeth; and (4) voluntary cough is effective in bringing up secretions. If these are ineffective, the tube is needed so that tracheobronchial secretions can be suctioned.

Before the patient is weaned from the tracheostomy tube a trial period of mouth- or nose-breathing is conducted. This is accomplished by (1) changing to a smaller size tube to increase the resistance to air flow and plugging the tracheostomy (deflate the cuff) at the same time; (2) switching to a cuffless tracheostomy tube; (3) changing to a fenestrated tube (one with an opening or window in the bend of the tube), which permits air to flow around and through the tube to the upper airway and permits talking; (4) changing to a tracheostomy button; or (5) removing the tracheostomy tube completely.

Weaning From Oxygen. The patient has been weaned from the ventilator, cuff, and tube. Respiratory function has been checked, and oxygen has been given according to the result of the blood gas determinations. The FIO_2 then is gradually reduced until the PO_2 is in the 70 to 100 mm Hg range while the patient is breathing room air. If the PO_2 is less than 70 mm Hg on room air, supplementary oxygen is recommended. The Health Care Financing Administration (HCFA) requires that the patient's PaO_2 on room air be below 55 mm Hg for the patient to be eligible for financial reimbursement for in-home oxygen.

Success in weaning the long-term ventilator-dependent patient requires early, aggressive yet judicious *nutritional support*. Respiratory musculature (diaphragm and especially intercostals) quickly become weak or atrophied after just a few days of mechanical ventilation, especially if nutrition is not supported. High carbohydrate loads increase carbon dioxide production and thus may increase the work of breathing in patients with borderline pulmonary function. Consultation with a dietitian or nutrition support team soon after admission to plan the best form of nutritional replacement may decrease the duration of mechanical ventilation and prevent other complications, especially sepsis.

Research is underway in a number of areas related to the mechanically ventilated patient and strategies for weaning. Areas of particular interest are effectiveness of respiratory muscle training, nutritional support, modes and pressures of mechanical ventilation, suctioning frequency, and patient–nurse interactions.

Mechanical Ventilation in the Home

Under certain physiologic, psychological, or economic conditions, it is possible that the patient may not be completely weaned from the ventilator, from the tube, or from oxygen before leaving the hospital. Patients are at times being discharged to extended-care facilities or to their homes on mechanical ventilators, with tracheostomy tubes, or on oxygen therapy. Patients on home ventilator care usually have neuromuscular conditions or COPD.

Mechanical ventilation in the home (or an extended-care facility) is increasing in frequency because of a number of influences:

1. Early diagnosis and treatment of pulmonary disorders has resulted in increased patient longevity.
2. Increasing numbers of health care professionals are becoming more proficient in providing rehabilitative and maintenance ventilator care in the home.
3. Prospective payment systems demand reductions in costs placed on the health care industry.
4. Concerned family members are willing to provide necessary support and care.
5. Technological advances have made ventilators simple, portable, versatile, compact, and safe for use by the homebound patient and caregivers.
6. In certain diseases such as kyphoscoliosis or COPD, patients may not require 24-hour mechanical ventilation, but only support through the night to maintain oxygenation and rest the respiratory muscles during sleep. Home ventilator therapy prevents the patient from having to remain hospitalized.

Caring for the patient with mechanical ventilator support at home can be accomplished quite successfully. Multiple factors must be considered for this endeavor to work. The family must be emotionally, educationally, and physically able to assume the role of primary caregiver. A home care team consisting of nurse, physician, respiratory therapist, social service or home care agency, and equipment supplier needs to be available. The home itself is evaluated to determine if it is adequate for the safe operation of all electrical equipment. A summary of the basic assessment criteria needed for successful home care is presented in Chart 25-5.

Once the decision is made to initiate mechanical ventilation at home, the patient and family are prepared for home care. Home health teaching includes information about the ventilator, suctioning, tracheostomy care, signs of pulmonary infection, cuff inflation and deflation, and assessment of vital signs. Family instruction begins in the hospital and continues in the home. Nursing responsibilities include evaluating the patient's and the family's understanding of the information presented.

Once the patient is at home, a community or home health nurse is involved in monitoring and evaluating how well the patient and family are adapting to providing care in the home environment. The adequacy of ventilation and oxygenation is assessed, as is airway patency. The nurse needs to address any unique adaptation problems the patient may have and to listen to the patient's and the family's anxieties and frustrations, offering appropriate support and encouragement where possible. The nurse helps identify and contact appropriate community resources that may assist in home management of the patient with mechanical ventilation.

The technical aspects of the ventilator are managed by vendor follow-up. A respiratory therapist usually is assigned to the patient and makes frequent home visits to evaluate

CHART 25-5
Summary of Assessment Criteria for Successful Home Ventilator Care

1. The family members and professional staff are competent, dependable, and willing to spend the time required for proper training.
2. The patient is willing to go home.
3. The family understands the diagnosis and prognosis.
4. There is evidence of chronic underlying pulmonary abnormalities.
5. The patient's clinical pulmonary status is stable.
6. The family has sufficient financial/support resources.
7. A psychological consultation with the patient and family is made before the patient is discharged.
8. The home environment is conducive to accepting the patient.
9. The electrical facilities are adequate to operate all equipment safely.
10. The patient environment is controlled, preventing drafts in cold weather and ensuring proper ventilation in warm weather.
11. Equipment cleaning and storage space is available.

(Adapted from O'Ryan JA and Burns DG. Pulmonary Rehabilitation: From Hospital to Home. Chicago, Year Book Medical Publishers, 1984)

CHART 25-6
Patient Education: Ventilator Care in the Home

Patient Care

- Monitor vital signs as directed.
- Observe physical signs such as color, secretions, breathing pattern, and state of consciousness.
- Perform physical care such as suctioning, postural drainage, and ambulation.
- Observe the tidal volume and pressure manometer regularly. Intervene when they are abnormal (*i.e.,* suction if airway pressure increases).
- Provide a communication method for the patient (*e.g.,* pad and pencil, electric larynx, talking trach)

Ventilator Care

- Check the ventilator settings twice each day and whenever the patient is removed from the ventilator.
- Adjust the volume and pressure alarms if needed.
- Fill humidifier as needed and check its level three times a day.
- Empty water in tubing as needed.

Ventilator Maintenance

- Use a clean humidifier when circuitry is changed.
- Keep exterior clean and free of any objects.
- Change external circuitry once a week or more.
- Report malfunction or strange noises immediately.

the patient and perform a maintenance check of the ventilator.

Transportation services are identified to determine the procedure for providing patient transportation in an emergency. These arrangements need to be made before an emergency arises because of the uniqueness of the situation.

The family is taught cardiopulmonary resuscitation, including mouth-to-tracheostomy tube (instead of mouth-to-mouth) breathing. Handling a power failure is also explained. This involves the conversion of most ventilators from an electrical power source to a battery power source. Conversion is automatic in most types of home ventilators and lasts approximately 1 hour. The family also is instructed in the use of a manual self-inflation bag should it be necessary.

Ultimately the patient and family responsibilities at home include those spelled out in Chart 25-6.

Providing the opportunity for ventilator-dependent patients and their families to return home to live in familiar surroundings can be a rich, rewarding experience for all. The technical ability now exists to accomplish this objective. The ultimate goal for the patient on home ventilator therapy is to enhance the quality of life, not simply to support or prolong it.

The Patient Undergoing Thoracic Surgery

Assessment and management are particularly important in the patient undergoing thoracic surgery. Thoracic surgical procedures are performed for a wide variety of reasons. Frequently these patients also have obstructive pulmonary disease with compromised breathing. Preoperative preparation and careful postoperative management are crucial for successful patient outcomes because these patients may have a very narrow range of what allows them to be functional and what causes distress.

Fortunately, the lungs have a large functional reserve. More advanced techniques of anesthesia, respiratory therapy, surgical techniques, and intensive postoperative care have made possible more extensive, and sometimes, less invasive thoracic surgery.

The objectives of preoperative care are to ascertain the patient's functional reserve to determine if the patient can survive the surgery and to ensure the optimal condition of the patient for surgery.

Diagnostic Evaluation

A number of tests are performed to determine the preoperative status of the patient and to assess physical assets and limitations. The assessment starts with the history and physical examination–the foundation of preoperative evaluation. The general appearance of the patient, including behavior and mental status, will indicate whether a significant surgical risk is involved.

The decision to perform any pulmonary resection is based on the patient's cardiovascular status and pulmonary reserve. Pulmonary function studies (especially lung volume and vital capacity) are performed to determine whether the contemplated resection will leave sufficient functioning lung tissue. Arterial blood gas values are assessed to provide a more complete picture of the functional capacity of the lung. Exercise tolerance tests have predictive value. Such tests are especially important to determine whether the patient who is a candidate for pneumonectomy can tolerate removal of one of the lungs.

Preoperative studies are performed to provide a baseline for comparison during the postoperative period and to reveal any unsuspected abnormalities. These studies include chest x-ray, electrocardiography (for arteriosclerotic heart disease, conduction defects), nutritional assessment, determination of blood urea nitrogen and serum creatinine (renal function), glucose tolerance or blood glucose (diabetes), assessment of serum electrolytes and protein levels, blood volume determinations, and complete blood cell count.

Operative Procedures

Pneumonectomy. The removal of an entire lung (pneumonectomy) is performed chiefly for cancer when the lesion cannot be removed by a lesser procedure. It also may be performed for lung abscesses, bronchiectasis, or extensive unilateral tuberculosis. The removal of the right lung is more dangerous than the removal of the left, because the right lung has a larger vascular bed and its removal imposes a greater physiologic burden.

A posterolateral or anterolateral thoracotomy incision is made, sometimes with resection of a rib. The pulmonary artery and the pulmonary veins are ligated and severed.

The main bronchus is divided and the lung removed. The bronchial stump is stapled, and usually no drains are used because the accumulation of fluid in the empty hemithorax is the desired end result because the volume of accumulated fluid prevents mediastinal shift (Fig. 25-11*B*).

Lobectomy. When the pathology is limited to one area of a lung, a lobectomy (removal of a lobe of a lung) is performed (Fig. 25-11*A*). This operation, which is more common than pneumonectomy, may be carried out for bronchogenic carcinoma, giant emphysematous blebs or bullae, benign tumors, metastatic malignant tumors, bronchiectasis, and fungus infections.

A thoracotomy incision is used, its exact location depending on the lobe to be resected. When the pleura is entered, the involved lung collapses and the lobar vessels and the bronchus are ligated and divided. After the lobe is removed, the remaining lobes of the lung are reexpanded. Usually, two chest catheters are inserted for drainage.

The upper tube is for the removal of air; the lower one is for drainage of fluid. Sometimes, only one catheter is needed. The chest tube is connected to a chest drainage apparatus for several days.

Segmentectomy (Segmental Resection). Some lesions are located in only one segment of the lung. Bronchopulmonary segments are subdivisions of the lung that function as individual units. They are held together by delicate connective tissue. Disease processes may be limited to a single segment. Care is used to preserve as much healthy and functional lung tissue as possible, especially in patients who already have limited cardiopulmonary reserve. Single segments can be removed from any lobe, except the right middle lobe, which has only two small segments, invariably is removed entirely. On the left side, corresponding to a middle lobe, is a "lingular" segment of the upper lobe. This can be removed as a single segment or by *lingulectomy*. This segment frequently is involved in bronchiectasis.

Wedge Resection. A wedge resection of a small, well-circumscribed lesion may be performed without regard for the location of the intersegmental planes. The pleural cavity usually is drained because of the possibility of an air or blood leak. This procedure is performed for diagnostic lung biopsy and for the excision of small peripheral nodules.

Bronchoplastic or Sleeve Resection. Bronchoplastic resection is a procedure in which only one lobar bronchus together with a part of the right or left bronchus is excised. The distal bronchus is reanastomosed to the proximal bronchus or trachea.

Video Thoracoscopy. A video thoracoscopy (see p. 455) is an endoscopic procedure that allows the surgeon, without an open incision, to look into the thorax, obtain specimens of tissue for biopsy, treat recurrent spontaneous pneumothorax, and diagnose either pleural effusions or

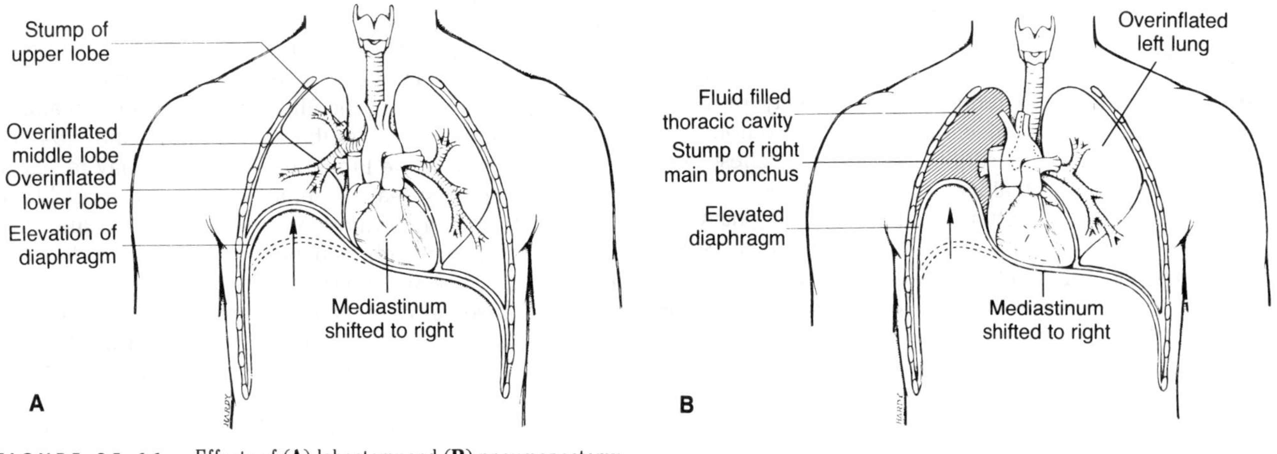

FIGURE 25-11. Effects of (**A**) lobectomy and (**B**) pneumonectomy.

pleural masses. The advantages of the video thoracoscopy may include rapid diagnosis and treatment of some conditions, possibly less intense postoperative care, and a shortened hospital stay.

Preoperative Management

Assessment

Chest auscultation provides an estimate of the intensity of breath sounds in the different regions of the lungs (see Chapter 22). When the chest is auscultated, it is important to note whether breath sounds are normal, indicating a free flow of air in and out of the lungs. (In the patient with emphysema, the breath sounds may be markedly decreased or even absent on auscultation.) Crackles and wheezes are noted; hyperresonance and decreased diaphragmatic motion are assessed. Unilateral diminished breath sounds and rhonchi can be the result of occlusion of the bronchi by mucus plugs. Evidence of retained secretions is evaluated during auscultation by asking the patient to cough. Any signs of rhonchi or wheezing are noted. The patient history and assessment include the following:

- What signs and symptoms are present—cough, sputum expectorated (amount), hemoptysis, chest pain, dyspnea?
- What is the smoking history? How long has the patient been smoking? How much is being smoked currently? Packs/day/years?
- What is the patient's cardiopulmonary tolerance while resting, eating, bathing, walking?
- What is the patient's breathing pattern? How much exertion is required to produce dyspnea?
- Does the patient need to sleep in an upright position?
- What is the physiologic status of the patient—for example, general appearance, mental alertness, behavior, nutritional status?
- What other medical conditions exist—allergies, cardiac disorders, or diabetes?
- What are the patient's personal preferences and dislikes?

Preoperative Nursing Interventions

Improving Airway Clearance

The underlying lung condition often is associated with increased respiratory secretions. Preoperatively, the airway is cleared of secretions to reduce the possibility of postoperative atelectasis or infection. This is accomplished through humidification, postural drainage, and chest percussion after bronchodilators are administered, if prescribed. The volume of sputum is estimated in patients who expectorate large amounts of secretions. Such measurements are carried out to determine if and when the amount decreases. Antibiotics are administered as prescribed for infection, which may be causing the excessive secretions.

Patient Education

The patient is informed of what to expect in the postoperative period, that is, the possible presence of a chest tube or tubes and drainage receptacles, the usual postoperative administration of oxygen to facilitate breathing, and the possible use of a ventilator. The importance of frequent turning to promote drainage of lung secretions is explained. Instruction in the use of incentive spirometry begins preoperatively to familiarize the patient with its correct use. Diaphragmatic and pursed lip breathing are taught and should be practiced at this time.

Because a coughing schedule will be necessary in the postoperative period to promote clearance or removal of secretions, the patient should be instructed in the technique of coughing and warned that the coughing routine may prove to be uncomfortable. The patient is taught to splint the incision with the hands, a pillow, or a folded towel.

Coughing Technique. The patient is taught coughing technique as follows:

1. Sit upright with knees flexed and body bent slightly forward.
2. Splint the incisional area with firm hand pressure or support it with a pillow or rolled blanket while coughing. (The nurse can initially demonstrate this by using the patient's hands).
3. Take three deep breaths followed by a deep inspiration (inhaling slowly and evenly through the nose).
4. Contract (pull in) the abdominal muscles and cough twice forcefully, with mouth open and tongue out.
5. If unable to sit, lie on one side with hips and knees flexed.

Forced Exhalation Technique (Huffing Technique). "Huffing" is the expulsion of air through an open glottis and may be helpful for the patient with diminished expiratory flow rates or for the patient in severe pain who refuses to cough. This type of forceful exhalation stimulates pulmonary expansion and assists in alveolar inflation. Instructions to the patient include:

1. Take a deep diaphragmatic breath and exhale forcefully against your hand. Exhale forcefully in a quick, distinct pant, or "huff."
2. Practice doing small huffs and progress to one strong huff during exhalation.

Relieving Anxiety

Increasingly, patients are admitted only 1 or 2 days before or even on the day of surgery, which does not provide much time for the nurse to talk with the patient. To use the time effectively before surgery, the nurse listens to the patient to evaluate feelings about the illness and proposed treatment. The nurse also determines the patient's motivation to return to normal or baseline function. The patient may reveal significant reactions: fear of hemorrhage because of bloody sputum, fear of discomfort of a chronic cough and chest pain, fear of ventilator dependence, or fear of death because of dyspnea and tumor.

The nurse helps the patient to overcome many of these fears and to cope with the stress of surgery. This is accomplished by correcting any false impressions, by supporting the patient's decision to undergo surgery, by reassuring the patient that the incision will "hold," and by dealing honestly with questions about pain and discomfort and their treatment. The management and control of pain begin before surgery when the patient is informed that many postoperative problems can be overcome by following certain routines related to deep breathing, coughing, turning, and moving. If patient-controlled analgesia (PCA) or epidural analgesia is to be used postoperatively, the patient is also instructed in this treatment modality.

Postoperative Management

Mechanical Ventilation

Depending on the nature of the surgery, the patient's underlying condition, the intraoperative course and the depth of anesthesia, the patient may require mechanical ventilation postoperatively. The physician is responsible for determining the ventilator settings and modes, as well as determining the overall method and pace of weaning. However, the physician, nurse, and respiratory therapist work together closely to assess the patient's tolerance and weaning progress. It is essential that each discipline have an understanding of the scope and function of each team member in relation to patient weaning to conserve patient strength, use resources efficiently, and maximize successful outcomes.

Chest Drainage

A crucial intervention for improving gas exchange and breathing in the postoperative period is the proper management of chest drainage. After thoracic surgery, chest tubes and a closed drainage system are used to reexpand the involved lung and to remove excess air, fluid, and blood.

Basic Principles. The normal breathing mechanism operates on the principle of negative pressure; that is, the pressure in the chest cavity is lower than the pressure of the atmosphere, causing air to move into the lungs during inspiration. Whenever the chest is opened, for any reason, there is a loss of negative pressure, which can result in the collapse of the lung. The collection of air, fluid, or other substances in the chest can compromise cardiopulmonary function and even cause the lung to collapse. Pathologic substances that collect in the pleural space include fibrin, or clotted blood; liquids (serous fluids, blood, pus, chyle); and gases (air from the lung, tracheobronchial tree, or esophagus).

Surgical incision of the chest wall almost always causes some degree of pneumothorax. Air and fluid collect in the intrapleural space, restricting lung expansion and reducing gas exchange. It is necessary to keep the pleural space evacuated postoperatively and to maintain negative pressure within this potential space. Therefore, during or immediately after thoracic surgery, chest catheters are positioned strategically in the pleural space, sutured to the skin, and connected to a drainage apparatus to remove the residual air and drainage fluid from the pleural or mediastinal space. This results in the reexpansion of remaining lung tissue.

Commercial Systems. A chest drainage system must be capable of removing whatever collects in the pleural space so that a normal pleural space and normal cardiopulmonary function may be restored and maintained. A commercially available system (*e.g.*, Pleur-Evac, Argyle, Atrium) is the most common method currently in use to provide water-seal drainage (Fig. 25-12); these systems use the same principles as a three-bottle water-seal system. The chest tube or catheter is attached to the drainage system, using a one-way valve. Water in the second chamber acts as a seal and allows air and fluid to drain from the chest into the first chamber, but air cannot reenter the chest tube. Drainage accumulates in the first chamber and air exits through and from the second chamber. The water level fluctuates as the patient breathes; it moves up when the patient inhales and it moves down when the patient exhales. Suction may be added to the second chamber to create a negative pressure to promote drainage of fluid and removal of air. The addition of suction creates constant bubbling in the third chamber; if constant bubbling occurs in the absence of suction, there may be leakage of air from the lung or a leak in the system. Care of the patient with water-seal chest drainage is discussed in Guideline 25-6.

Single-Bottle Water-Seal System. The end of the drainage tube from the patient's chest is submerged in water, which permits drainage of air and fluid from the pleural space but does not allow air to move back into the chest. Functionally, drainage depends on gravity and on the

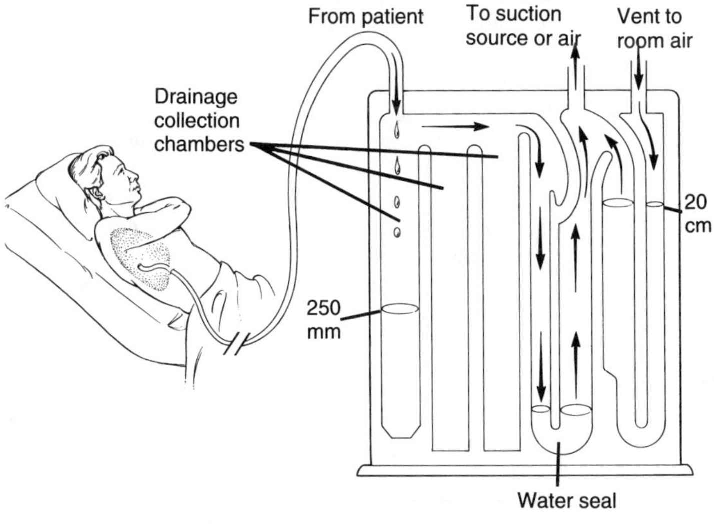

FIGURE 25-12. A disposable chest drainage system.

GUIDELINE 25–6
Guidelines to the Nurse's Role in the Management of the Patient With Water-Seal Chest Drainage*

An intrapleural drainage tube is used after most intrathoracic procedures. One or more chest catheters are held in the pleural space by suture to the chest wall and are attached to a drainage system. The purposes are

1. To remove liquids and gas from the pleural space or thoracic cavity and the mediastinal space
2. To bring about reexpansion of the lung and restore normal cardiorespiratory function after surgery, trauma, or medical conditions by establishing negative pressure in the pleural cavity

Procedure

Nursing Action	Rationale/Amplification
1. Fill the water-seal chamber with sterile water to the level equaling 2 cm H_2O.	Water-seal drainage provides for the escape of air and fluid into a drainage bottle. The water acts as a seal and keeps the air from being drawn back into the pleural space.
2. If suction is used, fill the suction control chamber with sterile water to the 20-cm level or as prescribed.	The water level will determine the degree of suction applied.
3. Attach the drainage catheter from the pleural space (the patient) to the tubing coming from the collection chamber of the water seal system. Tape securely.	In disposable units, the system is a closed system, with the only connection being the one to the patient's catheter.
4. If suction is used, connect the suction control chamber tubing to the suction unit. Turn on suction unit and increase pressure until slow but steady bubbling appears in the suction control chamber.	The degree of suction is determined by the amount of water in the suction control chamber and is *not* dependent on the rate of bubbling or the pressure gauge setting on the suction unit.
5. Mark the original fluid level with tape on the outside of the drainage unit. Mark hourly/daily increments (date and time) at the drainage level.	This marking will show the amount of fluid loss and how fast fluid is collecting in the drainage bottle. It serves as a basis for blood replacement, if the fluid is blood. Grossly bloody drainage will appear in the bottle in the immediate postoperative period; it gradually becomes serous and if excessive may require reoperation or autotransfusion. Drainage usually declines progressively in the first 24 hours.
6. Ensure that the tubing is not looping or interfering with the movements of the patient.	Kinking, looping, or pressure on the drainage tubing can produce back-pressure, and may thus possibly force drainage back into the pleural space or impede drainage from the pleural space.
7. Encourage the patient to assume a position of comfort. Encourage good body alignment. When the patient is in the lateral position, make sure that the tubing is not compressed by the weight of the patient's body. Encourage the patient to change position frequently.	The patient's position should be changed frequently to promote drainage, and the body should be kept in good alignment to prevent postural deformities and contractures. Proper positioning helps breathing and promotes better air exchange. Pain medication may be needed to enhance comfort and deep breathing.
8. Put the arm and shoulder of the affected side through range of motion exercises several times daily. Some pain medication may be necessary.	Exercise helps to prevent ankylosis of the shoulder and assists in lessening postoperative pain and discomfort.
9. Gently "milk" the tubing in the direction of the drainage chamber as needed.	"Milking" the tubing prevents it from becoming plugged with clots and fibrin. Constant attention to maintaining the patency of the tube facilitates prompt expansion of the lung and minimizes complications.
10. Make sure there is fluctuation ("tidaling") of the fluid level in the water-seal chamber.	Fluctuation of the water level in the tube shows that there is effective communication between the pleural cavity and the drainage bottle, provides a valuable indication of the patency of the drainage system, and is a gauge of intrapleural pressure.
11. Fluctuations of fluid in the tubing will stop when a. The lung has reexpanded. b. The tubing is obstructed by blood clots or fibrin, or kinking. c. A dependent loop develops. d. Suction motor or wall suction is not working properly.	

(continued)

GUIDELINE 25-6 *(continued)*
Guidelines to the Nurse's Role in the Management of the Patient With Water-Seal Chest Drainage*

12. Observe for leaks of air in the drainage system as indicated by constant bubbling in the water-seal chamber. a. Assess chest tube system for correctable external leaks. b. Notify physician immediately of excessive bubbling in the water-seal chamber not due to external leaks.	Leaking and trapping of air in the pleural space can result in tension pneumothorax.
13. Observe and immediately report rapid, shallow breathing; cyanosis; pressure in the chest; subcutaneous emphysema; symptoms of hemorrhage; significant changes in vital signs.	Many clinical conditions may cause these signs and symptoms, including tension pneumothorax, mediastinal shift, hemorrhage, severe incisional pain, pulmonary embolus, and cardiac tamponade. Surgical intervention may be necessary.
14. Encourage the patient to breathe deeply and cough at frequent intervals. Provide adequate pain medication. Request order for PCA pump if appropriate. Instruct in use of incentive spirometry.	Deep breathing and coughing help to raise the intrapleural pressure, which allows emptying of any accumulation in the pleural space and removes secretions from the tracheobronchial tree, so that the lung expands and atelectasis is prevented.
15. If the patient has to be transported to another area, place the drainage system below the chest level, if he is lying on a stretcher. If the tube becomes disconnected, cut off the contaminated tips of the chest tube and tubing, insert a sterile connector in the chest tube and tubing, and reattach to the drainage system. Do *not* clamp chest tube during transport.	The drainage apparatus must be kept at a level lower than the patient's chest to prevent backflow of fluid into the pleural space.
16. When assisting the surgeon in removing the tube: a. Instruct the patient to perform a gentle Valsalva maneuver or to breathe quietly. b. The chest tube is clamped and quickly removed. c. Simultaneously, a small bandage is applied and made airtight with petrolatum gauze covered by a 4 × 4-inch gauze pad and thoroughly covered and sealed with adhesive tape.	The chest tube is removed as directed when the lung is reexpanded (usually 24 hours to several days) depending on the cause of the pneumothorax. During removal of the tube the chief priorities are prevention of entrance of air into the pleural cavity as the tube is withdrawn and prevention of infection.

**There are commercial disposable chest drainage devices available that use the water-seal principle, and these guidelines refer to their use.*

mechanics of respiration. As the fluid level in the bottle increases, it becomes progressively more difficult for air and fluid to exit the chest. Therefore, suction may be added.

Two-Bottle System. The two-bottle system consists of the same water-seal chamber plus a fluid collection bottle. Drainage is similar to that of a single unit, except that when pleural fluid accumulates, the underwater seal system is not affected by the volume of drainage.

Effective drainage depends on gravity or on the amount of suction added to the system. When vacuum (suction) is added to the system from a vacuum source, such as wall suction, the connection is made at the vent stem of the underwater-seal bottle. The amount of suction applied to the system is regulated by the wall gauge.

Three-Bottle System. The three-bottle system is similar in all respects to the two-bottle system, except for the addition of a third bottle to control the amount of suction applied. The amount of suction is determined by the depth to which the tip of the venting glass tube is submerged. (For example, submersion to 10 cm below the surface of the water will equal 10 cm of water suction applied to the patient.)

In the three-bottle system (as in the other two), drainage depends on gravity or the amount of suction applied. The amount of suction in this system is controlled by the manometer bottle. The mechanical suction motor or wall suction creates and maintains a negative pressure throughout the entire closed drainage system.

The third bottle regulates the amount of vacuum in the system. This depends on the depth to which the tube is submerged—the usual depth is 20 cm (7.6 in).

When the vacuum in the system becomes greater than the depth to which the tube is submerged, outside air is sucked into the system. This results in constant bubbling in the manometer (or pressure-regulator) bottle, which indicates that the system is functioning properly.

- *Note:* When the wall vacuum is turned off, the drainage system must be open to the atmosphere so that intrapleural air can escape from the system. This can be done by detaching the tubing from the suction port to provide a vent.

The commercially available systems are safer because they are self-contained, unbreakable, and disposable, and have no connections (except to the chest catheter) that may become loose. Nursing care is easier to provide, and the convenience of the systems encourages easier and earlier ambulation for the patient.

❑ NURSING PROCESS
The Patient Undergoing Thoracic Surgery

Postoperative Assessment

The character and depth of respirations and the patient's color serve as important criteria in evaluating whether the lungs are being adequately expanded. The heart rate and rhythm are monitored by auscultation and electrocardiography, because major dysrhythmic episodes are common after thoracic and cardiac surgery. Dysrhythmias can occur at any time, but frequently are seen between the second and sixth postoperative days. The rate of occurrence of dysrhythmias increases with patients over 50 years of age and with those undergoing pneumonectomy or esophageal surgery.

An arterial line is maintained to facilitate frequent monitoring of blood gases, serum electrolytes, hemoglobin and hematocrit values, and arterial pressure. Central venous pressure is monitored to detect early signs of fluid volume disturbances.

Diagnosis

Nursing Diagnoses

Based on the assessment data, the patient's major postoperative nursing diagnoses may include:

- Impaired gas exchange related to lung impairment and surgery
- Ineffective airway clearance related to lung impairment, anesthesia, and pain
- Pain related to incision, drainage tubes, and the surgical procedure
- Impaired physical mobility of the upper extremities related to thoracic surgery
- Fluid volume imbalance related to the surgical procedure
- Altered nutritional status related to dyspnea and anorexia
- Knowledge deficit about care procedures at home

Collaborative Problems/ Potential Complications

- Respiratory distress
- Dysrhythmias
- Atelectasis, pneumothorax, and bronchopleural fistula
- Blood loss; hemorrhage
- Pulmonary edema

Planning and Implementation

Goals. The major goals for the patient may include improvement of gas exchange and breathing, improvement of airway clearance, relief of pain and discomfort, increased arm and shoulder mobility, maintenance of adequate fluid volume and nutritional status, understanding of self-care procedures and absence of complications.

Nursing Interventions

Improving Gas Exchange and Breathing. Gas exchange is determined by evaluating oxygenation and ventilation. In the immediate postoperative period, this is achieved by measuring *vital signs* (blood pressure, pulse, and respirations) at least every 15 minutes for the first 1 to 2 hours, then less frequently as the patient's condition stabilizes.

Arterial blood gases (ABGs) are drawn early in the postoperative period to establish a baseline to assess adequacy of oxygenation and ventilation and the possible retention of CO_2 The frequency of postoperative ABGs depends on whether the patient is mechanically ventilated or exhibits signs of respiratory distress, as ABG results help determine appropriate therapy. It is also common practice for patients to have an arterial line in place to obtain blood for ABGs and to monitor blood pressure closely. Hemodynamic monitoring may be used to assess the patient's hemodynamic stability.

Breathing techniques, such as diaphragmatic and pursed lip breathing, taught preoperatively should be practiced every 2 hours to expand alveoli and prevent atelectasis. Another technique to improve ventilation is sustained maximal inspiratory (SMI) therapy or incentive spirometry (p. 547). The SMI technique optimizes lung inflation, improves the cough mechanism, and provides for early assessment of acute pulmonary changes.

Positioning also improves breathing. When the patient is oriented and blood pressure is stabilized, the head of the bed is elevated 30 to 40 degrees during the immediate postoperative period. This facilitates ventilation, promotes chest drainage from the lower chest tube, and helps residual air to rise in the upper portion of the pleural space, where it can be removed through the upper chest tube.

The surgeon is consulted about individual *patient positioning*. The patient with unilateral lung pathology may not be able to turn well onto the operated side because of pain, thus limiting ventilation of the operated side. However, positioning the patient with the "good lung" (unoperated) down allows a better match of ventilation and perfusion, and therefore may actually improve oxygenation. The patient's position is changed from horizontal to semi-upright, because remaining in one position tends to promote the retention of secretions in the dependent portion of the lungs. After a pneumonectomy, the operated side should be dependent so that fluid in the pleural space remains below the level of the bronchial stump, and the unoperative side can fully expand.

The procedure for turning a patient is as follows:

1. Instruct the patient to bend the knees and use the feet to push.
2. Have the patient shift hips and shoulders to the opposite side of the bed while pushing with the feet.
3. Bring the patient's arm over the chest, pointing it in the direction toward which the patient is being turned and have the patient grasp the side rail with the hand.
4. Turn patient in "log roll" fashion to prevent twisting at the waist and possible pulling of the incision, which could be painful.

Improving Airway Clearance. Retained secretions are a threat to the thoracotomy patient postoperatively. Trauma to the tracheobronchial tree during surgery, diminished lung ventilation, and diminished cough reflex all result in the accumulation of excessive secretions. If the secretions are retained, airway obstruction will occur, which causes air in the alveoli distal to the obstruction to become absorbed and the affected portion of the lung to collapse. Atelectasis, pneumonia, and respiratory failure may result.

There are a few techniques that are used to maintain a patent airway. First, secretions are suctioned from the tracheobronchial tree before the endotracheal tube is removed (this begins in the recovery room). Secretions continue to be removed by suctioning until the patient can cough up secretions effectively. *Nasotracheal suctioning*, although a difficult skill to master, may be useful to stimulate a deep cough and aspirate secretions that the patient is unable to cough up. It should be used only after other methods to raise secretions have been unsuccessful, however (Guideline 25-7).

Coughing technique is another measure that is used in maintaining a patent airway. The patient is encouraged to cough effectively, as ineffective coughing results in exhaustion and retention of secretions. To be effective, the cough must be low pitched, deep, and controlled. Because it is difficult to cough in a supine position, the patient is helped to a sitting position on the edge of the bed, with the feet resting on a chair. Coughing is carried out at least every hour (as described on p. 568) during the first 24 hours and when necessary thereafter. If audible crackles are present, it may be necessary to use chest percussion with the cough routine until the lungs are clear. Aerosol therapy is helpful in humidifying and mobilizing secretions so that they can be readily cleared by coughing. To lessen incisional pain during coughing, the nurse supports the incision firmly over the operated side and against the opposite chest (Fig. 25-13).

After helping the patient to cough, the nurse should listen to both lungs, anteriorly and posteriorly, to determine whether there are any changes in breath sounds, as diminished sounds may indicate collapsed or hypoventilated alveoli.

Chest physiotherapy is the final technique for maintaining a patent airway. If a patient is identified as being at high risk for developing postoperative pulmonary complications, then chest physiotherapy is started immediately (perhaps even preoperatively). The techniques of postural drainage, vibration, and percussion help to loosen and mobilize the secretions so that they can be coughed up or suctioned.

Relieving Pain and Discomfort. Pain after a thoracotomy may be severe, depending on the type of incision and the patient's reaction to and ability to cope with pain. Deep inspiration is very painful after thoracotomy. Pain can lead to postoperative complications if it reduces the patient's ability to breathe deeply and cough, and if it further limits chest excursions so that effective ventilation is decreased.

Immediately after the surgical procedure and before the incision is closed, the surgeon may perform a nerve block with a long-acting local anesthetic, which can reduce postoperative pain. Small, intravenous or epidural doses of a narcotic are administered as prescribed and are titrated to relieve pain while allowing the patient to cooperate in deep breathing, coughing, and mobilization efforts. It is important to avoid depressing the respiratory system with excessive analgesia, however, as the patient should not be so somnolent as to be unable to cough.

Because of the need to maximize patient comfort without depressing the respiratory drive, use of *patient-controlled analgesia* (PCA) is increasing. Patient-controlled analgesia through an intravenous pump or epidural catheter allows the patient to control the frequency and total dose of opioid analgesia. Preset limits on the PCA pump avoid overdosage. With proper instruction, these methods are well tolerated and allow earlier mobilization and cooperation with the treatment regimen. (See Chapter 13 for a more extensive discussion of PCA and pain management.)

- *Note:* The restlessness of hypoxia should not be confused with restlessness due to pain. Dyspnea, restlessness, increasing respiratory rate, increasing blood

GUIDELINE 25-7
Nasotracheal Suctioning

Sterile Technique to Be Used

1. Explain procedure to the patient.
2. Medicate patient for pain if necessary.
3. Place the patient in a sitting or semi-Fowler's position. Make sure the patient's head is not flexed forward. Remove excess pillows if necessary.
4. Oxygenate the patient several minutes before initiating the suctioning procedure. Have oxygen source ready nearby during procedure.
5. Put on sterile gloves.
6. Lubricate catheter with water-soluble gel.
7. Gently pass catheter through the patient's nose to the pharynx. Check the position of the tip of the catheter by asking the patient to open the mouth and inspecting it; the tip of the catheter should be in the lower pharynx.
8. Instruct the patient to take a deep breath or stick out the tongue. This action opens the epiglottis and promotes downward movement of the catheter.
9. Advance the catheter into the trachea only during inspiration. Listen for cough or for passage of air through the catheter.
10. Attach the catheter to suction apparatus. Apply intermittent suction while slowly withdrawing the catheter. Do not let suction exceed 120 mm Hg.
11. Do not suction for longer than 10 to 15 seconds, as dysrhythmias, bradycardia, or cardiac arrest may occur in patients with borderline oxygenation.
12. If additional suctioning is needed, withdraw the catheter to the back of the pharynx. Reassure patient and oxygenate for several minutes before resuming suctioning.

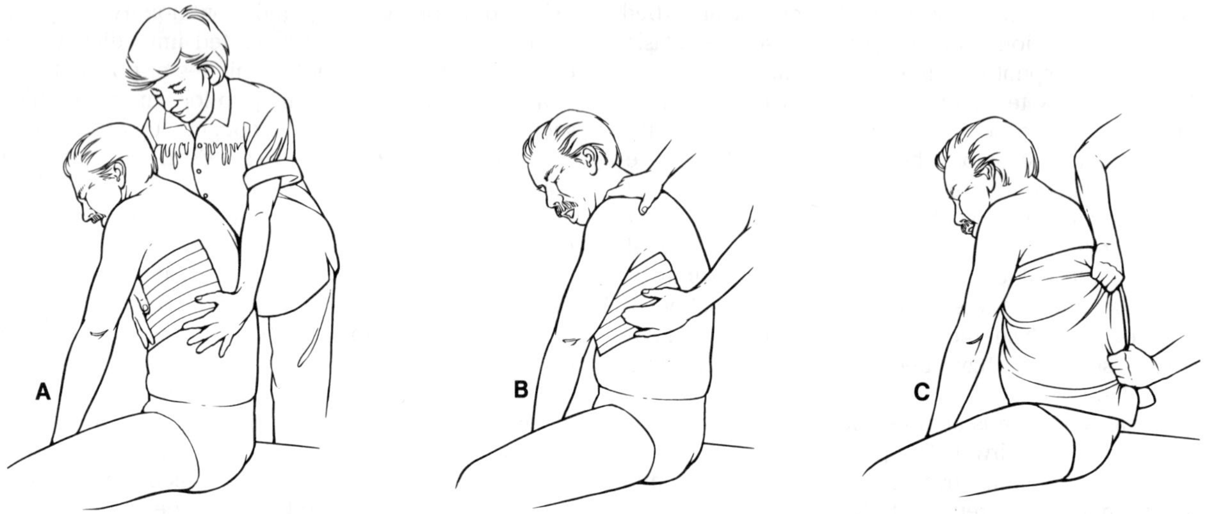

(**A**) The nurse's hands should support the chest incision anteriorly and posteriorly. The patient is instructed to take several deep breaths, inhale, and then cough forcibly.

(**B**) With one hand, the nurse exerts downward pressure on the shoulder of the affected side while firmly supporting beneath the wound with the other hand. The patient is instructed to take several deep breaths, inhale, and then cough forcibly.

(**C**) The nurse can wrap a towel or sheet around the patient's chest and hold the ends together, pulling slightly as the patient coughs, releasing as he takes deep breaths.

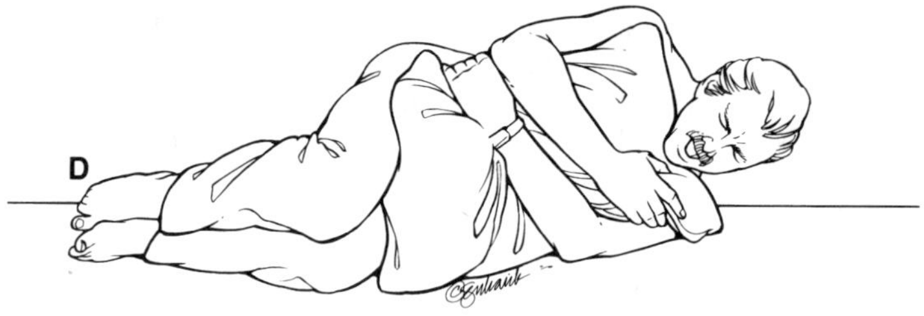

(**D**) The patient can be taught to hold a pillow firmly against his incision while coughing. This can be done while lying down or sitting in an upright position.

FIGURE 25-13. Techniques for support of incision while patient with thoracic surgery coughs.

pressure, and tachycardia are warning signs of impending respiratory insufficiency.

Promoting Mobility and Shoulder Exercises. When the patient is ready for activity, the patient is encouraged and assisted to get out of bed. Often this occurs on the evening of the day of surgery. Although this may be painful initially, the earlier the patient moves, the sooner the pain will subside. In addition to getting out of bed, the patient begins arm and shoulder exercises (Fig. 25-14) to restore movement and prevent painful stiffening of the affected arm and shoulder.

Maintaining Fluid Volume and Nutrition

IV Therapy. During the surgical procedure or immediately after, the patient may receive a blood transfusion, followed by a continuous intravenous infusion. The rate of administration must be titrated (as prescribed) based on the nurse's assessment of patient tolerance, especially when there is evidence of limited cardiopulmonary reserve and when the pulmonary vascular bed has been greatly reduced, as in pneumonectomy. Additional assessment includes monitoring of intake and output, vital signs, and jugular vein distention.

Diet. It is not unusual for patients undergoing thoracotomy to have poor nutritional status preoperatively, because of dyspnea, sputum production, and poor appetite. It is especially important therefore that the patient's nutrition be supported as soon as feasible postoperatively. A liquid diet is provided as soon as there is evidence of bowel sounds. The patient is progressed to a full diet as soon as possible. Small, frequent, well-balanced meals are better tolerated and crucial to the recovery and maintenance of lung function.

Patient Education and Home Care Considerations. Because large shoulder girdle muscles are transected during a thoracotomy, the arm and shoulder must be mobilized by full range of motion of the shoulder. This is accomplished by teaching the exercises necessary to improve function and encouraging the patient to continue them on discharge. The patient is taught to extend the arm (stretch and reach) and then reach behind the head, and to do these exercises five times daily (Fig. 25-14). This accelerates recovery of muscle function affected by incision, pain, and "splinting," and reduces long-term pain and discomfort and particularly the development of adhesions. All joints should be stretched and flexed. The patient is encouraged to as-

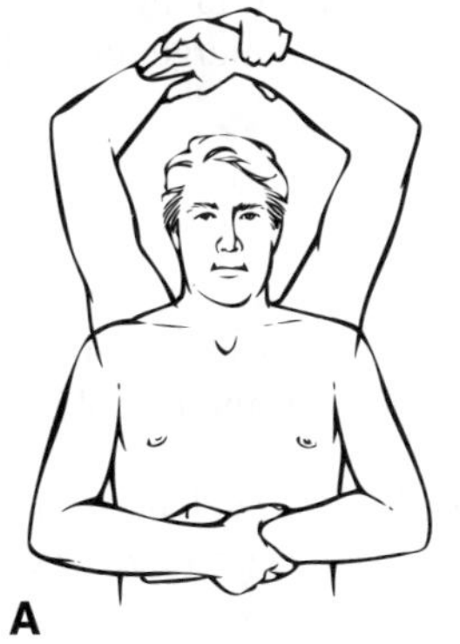

Hold hand of the affected side with the other hand, palms facing in. Raise the arms forward, upward, and then overhead, while taking a deep breath. Exhale while lowering the arms. Repeat five times.

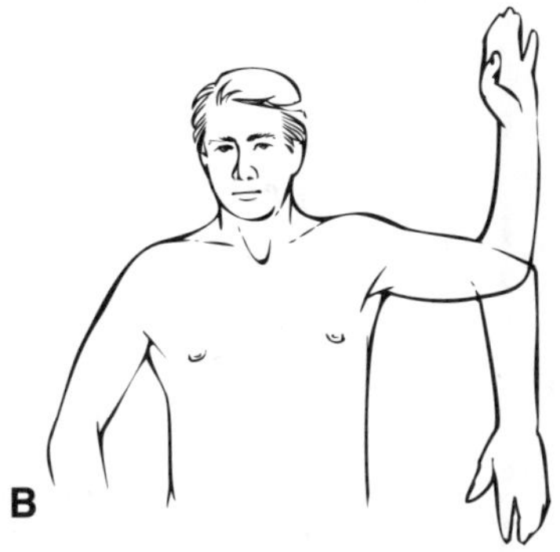

Raise arm sideward, upward, and downward in a waving motion.

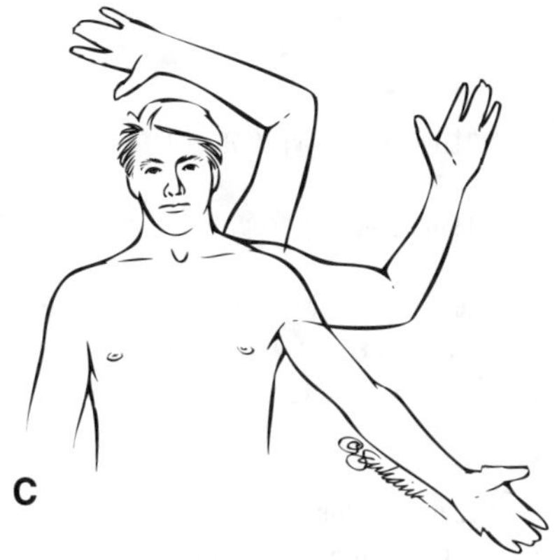

Place arm at side. Raise arm sideward, upward, and over the head. Repeat five times. These exercises can also be done while lying in bed.

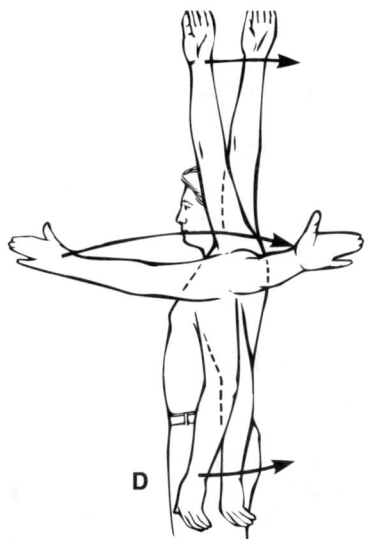

Extend the arm up and back, out to the side and back, down at the side and back.

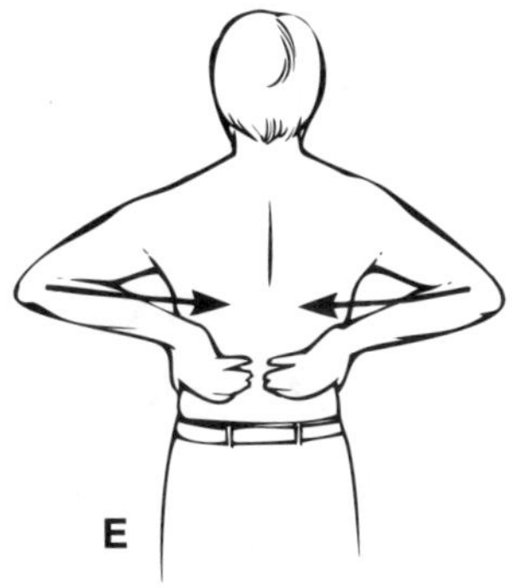

Place hands in small of back. Push elbows as far back as possible.

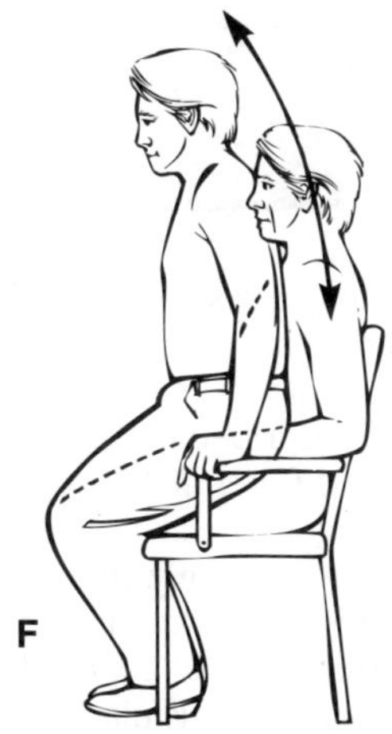

Sit erect in an armchair: place the hands on the arms of the chair directly opposite either side of the body. Press down on hands, consciously pulling the abdomen in and stretching up from the waist. Inhale while raising the body until the elbows are extended completely. Hold this position a moment, and begin exhaling while lowering the body slowly to the original position.

FIGURE 25-14. Arm and shoulder exercises are performed after thoracic surgery to restore movement, prevent painful stiffening of the shoulder, and improve muscle power.

CHART 25-7
Patient Education Following a Thoracotomy

1. Relieve intercostal pain that may occur by using local heat and oral analgesia.
2. Alternate walking and other activities with frequent rest periods. Be aware that weakness and fatigue are common for the first 3 weeks.
3. Practice breathing exercises several times daily for the first few weeks at home.
4. Avoid lifting more than 20 pounds until complete healing has taken place; the chest muscles and incision may be weaker than normal for 3 to 6 months after surgery.
5. Walk at a moderate pace, gradually extending walking time and distance. Be persistent.
6. Immediately stop any activity that causes undue fatigue, increased shortness of breath, or chest pain.
7. Avoid bronchial irritants (smoke, fumes, air pollution, aerosol sprays).
8. Prevent colds or lung infections.
9. Obtain an annual influenza vaccine. Also discuss vaccination against pneumonia with the physician.
10. Report for follow-up care by the surgeon or clinic as necessary.
11. Stop smoking.

sume a functional erect position to restore normal posture (preferably in front of a full-length mirror).

In addition to the arm and shoulder exercises, the patient is instructed in the points described in Chart 25-7.

Monitoring and Managing Potential Complications. Complications after thoracic surgery are always a possibility and must be identified and managed early. In addition, the patient is monitored at regular intervals for signs of respiratory distress or developing respiratory failure, dysrhythmias, the development of a bronchopleural fistula, hemorrhage and shock, atelectasis, and pulmonary infection.

Respiratory distress is treated by identifying and eliminating its cause while providing supplemental oxygen; if the patient progresses to respiratory failure, intubation and mechanical ventilation will be necessary, eventually requiring weaning (see section on weaning, pp. 563–565).

Dysrhythmias are often related to the effects of hypoxia or the surgical procedure, and are treated with anti-dysrhythmic medication and supportive therapy.

Pulmonary infections or effusion postoperatively, often preceded by *atelectasis,* may occur a few days into the postoperative course.

Bronchopleural fistula (BPF) is a serious although rare complication preventing the return of negative intrathoracic pressure and lung reexpansion. Depending on its severity, BPF is treated with closed chest drainage, mechanical ventilation, and possibly talc pleurodesis.

Hemorrhage and shock are managed by treating the underlying cause, whether by reoperation, or by administration of blood products or fluids.

Pulmonary edema due to overinfusion of intravenous fluids is a significant danger. The early symptoms are dyspnea, crackles, bubbling sounds in the chest, tachycardia, and pink, frothy sputum. This constitutes an emergency and is reported immediately.

Evaluation

Expected Outcomes

1. Demonstrates improved gas exchange as reflected in arterial blood gases, breathing exercises, and use of incentive spirometry
2. Improves airway clearance as evidenced by deep, controlled coughing and clear breath sounds or decreased presence of adventitious sounds
3. Experiences decreased pain and discomfort by splinting incision during coughing and increasing activity level
4. Improved mobility of shoulder and arm; demonstrates arm and shoulder exercises to relieve stiffening
5. Maintains adequate fluid intake and maintains nutrition for healing
6. Exhibits less anxiety by using appropriate coping skills and demonstrates a basic understanding of technology used in care
7. Adheres to therapeutic program and home care
8. Is free of complications as evidenced by normal vital signs and temperature, improved ABGs, clear lung sounds, and adequate respiratory function

For a detailed plan of nursing care for the patient who has had a thoracotomy, see Nursing Care Plan 25-1.

(*text continues on page 580*)

CRITICAL THINKING EXERCISES

1. Your patient will be discharged from the hospital with continuous oxygen. How would you develop a teaching plan with the patient to ensure correct and safe use of oxygen in the home? How might the plan change if the patient is very weak and debilitated?
2. You are the first person to see a patient who is brought to the emergency room with a stab wound to the chest. The patient is experiencing increasing difficulty breathing and is very anxious. His chest moves asymmetrically when he breathes. How would you describe the extent of the inury, and what would your initial action be? Describe the general treatment you would anticipate for this patient.
3. A patient with a cervical spinal cord injury has been on a mechanical ventilator for 3 days without experiencing any problems. However, he is becoming agitated and an alarm on the ventilator keeps sounding. What actions would you take to troubleshoot the ventilator? What actions would you take if you are unable to locate and correct the problem quickly?

NURSING CARE PLAN 25–1
Care of the Patient Following Thoracotomy

NURSING DIAGNOSIS: Impaired gas exchange related to lung impairment and surgery

GOAL: Improvement of gas exchange and breathing

Nursing Interventions	Rationale	Expected Outcomes
1. Monitor pulmonary status as directed and as needed: a. Auscultate breath sounds. b. Check rate, depth, and pattern of respirations. c. Assess blood gases for signs of hypoxemia or CO_2 retention. d. Evaluate patient's color for cyanosis.	1. Changes in pulmonary status indicate improvement or onset of complications.	• Lungs are clear on auscultation. • Respiratory rate is within normal range with no episodes of dyspnea. • Vital signs are stable. • Dysrhythmias are not present or are under control. • Demonstrates deep, controlled, effective breathing to allow maximal lung expansion. • Uses incentive spirometer every 2 hours while awake. • Demonstrates deep, effective coughing technique. • Lungs are expanded to capacity (evidenced by chest x-ray).
2. Monitor and record blood pressure, apical pulse, and temperature every 2–4 hours, central venous pressure (if indicated) every 2 hours.	2. Aid in evaluating effect of surgery on cardiac status.	
3. Monitor continuous electrocardiogram for pattern and dysrhythmias.	3. Dysrhythmias, (especially atrial fibrillation and atrial flutter) are more frequently seen after thoracic surgery. A patient with total pneumonectomy is especially prone to cardiac irregularity.	
4. Elevate head of bed 30–40 degrees when patient is oriented and hemodynamic status is stable.	4. Maximum lung excursion is achieved when patient is as close to upright as possible.	
5. Encourage deep breathing exercises (see section on Breathing Retraining) and effective use of incentive spirometer (sustained maximal inspiration).	5. Helps to achieve maximal lung inflation and to open closed airways.	
6. Encourage and promote an effective cough routine to be performed every 1–2 hours during first 24 hours.	6. Coughing is necessary to remove retained secretions.	
7. Assess and monitor the water-seal drainage system:* a. Assess for leaks and patency as needed. b. Monitor amount and character of drainage and document every 2 hours. Notify physician if drainage is 150 ml/hr or greater. c. See Guideline 25-6 for summary of nurse's role in management of water-seal drainage.	7. System is used to eliminate any residual air or fluid after thoracotomy.	

NURSING DIAGNOSIS: Ineffective airway clearance related to lung impairment, anesthesia, and pain

GOAL: Improvement of airway clearance and achievement of a patent airway

Nursing Interventions	Rationale	Expected Outcomes
1. Maintain an open airway.	1. Provides for adequate ventilation and gas exchange.	• Airway is patent. • Coughs effectively. • Splints incision while coughing.

*A patient with a pneumonectomy usually does not have water-seal chest drainage, because it is desirable that the pleural space fill with an effusion, which eventually obliterates this space. Some surgeons do use a modified water-seal system.

(*continued*)

NURSING CARE PLAN 25–1 *(continued)*
Care of the Patient Following Thoracotomy

Nursing Interventions	Rationale	Expected Outcomes
2. Perform endotracheal suctioning until patient is able to raise secretions effectively.	2. Endotracheal secretions are present in excessive amounts in post-thoracotomy patients due to trauma to the tracheobronchial tree during surgery, diminished lung ventilation, and cough reflex.	• Sputum is clear or colorless. • Lungs are clear on auscultation.
3. Assess and medicate for pain. Encourage deep breathing and coughing exercises. Assist in splinting the incision during coughing.	3. Helps to achieve maximal lung inflation and to open closed airways. Coughing is painful; incision needs to be supported.	
4. Monitor amount, viscosity, color, and odor of sputum. Notify physician if sputum is excessive or contains bright red blood.	4. Changes in sputum suggest presence of infection or change in pulmonary status. Colorless sputum is not unusual; opacification or coloring of sputum may indicate dehydration or infection.	
5. Administer humidification and mini-nebulizer therapy as prescribed.	5. Secretions must be moistened and thinned if they are to be raised from the chest with the least amount of effort.	
6. Perform postural drainage, percussion, and vibration as prescribed. Do not percuss or vibrate directly over operative site.	6. Chest physiotherapy uses gravity to help remove secretions from the lung.	
7. Auscultate both sides of chest to determine changes in breath sounds.	7. Indications for tracheal suctioning are determined by chest auscultation.	

NURSING DIAGNOSIS: Pain related to incision and surgical procedure

GOAL: Relief of pain and discomfort

Nursing Interventions	Rationale	Expected Outcomes
1. Evaluate location, character, quality and severity of pain. Administer pain medication as prescribed and as needed. Observe for respiratory effect of narcotic analgesic. Is patient too somnolent to cough? Are respirations depressed?	1. Pain limits chest excursions and thereby decreases ventilation.	• Asks for pain medication, but verbalizes that he expects some discomfort while deep breathing and coughing. • Verbalizes that he is comfortable and not in acute distress. • No signs of incisional infection evident.
2. Maintain care postoperatively in positioning the thoracotomy patient: a. Place patient in semi-Fowler's position. b. Patients with limited respiratory reserve may not be able to turn on unoperated side. c. Assist or turn patient every 2 hours.	2. If patient is comfortable and free of pain, he will be less likely to splint his chest while breathing. A semi-Fowler's position permits residual air to rise to upper portion of pleural space and be removed via the upper chest catheter.	
3. Assess incision area every 8 hours for redness, heat, induration, swelling, separation, and drainage.	3. These signs indicate possible infection.	
4. Request order for PCA pump if appropriate for patient.	4. Allowing patient control over frequency and dose improves comfort and compliance with treatment regimen.	

(continued)

NURSING CARE PLAN 25–1 *(continued)*
Care of the Patient Following Thoracotomy

NURSING DIAGNOSIS: Anxiety related to outcomes of surgery, pain, technology

GOAL: Reduction of anxiety to a manageable level.

Nursing Interventions	Rationale	Expected Outcomes
1. Explain all procedures in simple terms.	1. Explaining what can be expected in understandable terms decreases anxiety and increases cooperation.	• States that anxiety is at a manageable level. • Participates with health care team in treatment regimen. • Uses appropriate coping skills (verbalization, pain relief, use of support systems such as family, clergy). • Demonstrates basic understanding of technology used in care.
2. Assess for pain and medicate, especially before potentially painful procedures.	2. Premedication before painful procedures or activities improves comfort and minimizes undue anxiety.	
3. Silence all *unnecessary* alarms on technology (monitors, ventilators).	3. Unnecessary alarms increase the risk of sensory overload and may increase anxiety.	
4. Encourage and support patient while increasing activity level.	4. Positive reinforcement and encouragement improve patient motivation and independence.	
5. Mobilize resources (family, clergy, social worker) to help patient cope with outcomes of surgery (diagnosis, change in functional abilities).	5. A multidisciplinary approach promotes the patient's strengths and coping mechanisms.	

NURSING DIAGNOSIS: Impaired physical mobility of the upper extremities related to thoracic surgery

GOAL: Increased mobility of the affected shoulder and arm

Nursing Interventions	Rationale	Expected Outcomes
1. Assist patient with normal range of motion and function of shoulder and trunk. a. Teach breathing exercises to mobilize thorax. b. Encourage skeletal exercises to promote abduction and mobilization of shoulder (see Fig. 25-14). c. Assist out of bed to chair as soon as pulmonary and circulatory systems are stable (usually by evening of surgery).	1. Necessary to regain normal mobility of arm and shoulder and to speed recovery and minimize discomfort.	• Demonstrates arm and shoulder exercises and verbalizes intent to perform them on discharge.
2. Encourage progressive activities according to development of fatigue.	2. Increases the patient's use of affected shoulder and arm.	

NURSING DIAGNOSIS: Fluid volume imbalance related to the surgical procedure

GOAL: Maintenance of adequate fluid volume

Nursing Interventions	Rationale	Expected Outcomes
1. Monitor and record hourly intake and output. Urine output should be at least 30 ml or urine hourly after surgery.	1. Fluid management may be altered before, during, and after surgery, and patient's response to and need for fluid management must be assessed.	• Patient is adequately hydrated, as evidenced by: Urine output greater than 30 ml/hr Vital signs stable, heart rate and CVP approaching normal. No excessive peripheral edema
2. Administer blood component therapy and parenteral fluids or diuretics as prescribed to restore and maintain fluid volume.	2. Pulmonary edema due to transfusion or fluid overload is an ever-present threat; after pneumonectomy, the pulmonary vascular system has been greatly reduced.	

(continued)

NURSING CARE PLAN 25–1 *(continued)*
Care of the Patient Following Thoracotomy

Nursing Interventions	Rationale	Expected Outcomes
NURSING DIAGNOSIS: Knowledge deficit of care procedures at home		
GOAL: Increased ability to carry out care procedures at home		
1. Encourage patient to practice arm and shoulder exercises five times daily at home.	1. Exercise accelerates recovery of muscle function and reduces long-term pain and discomfort.	• Demonstrates arm and shoulder exercises.
2. Instruct patient to practice assuming a functionally erect position in front of a full-length mirror.	2. Practice will help restore normal posture.	• Verbalizes need to try to assume an erect posture.
3. Instruct patient in following aspects of home care:	3.	• Verbalizes the importance of relieving discomfort, alternating walking and rest, practicing breathing exercises, avoiding heavy lifting, avoiding undue fatigue, avoiding bronchial irritants, preventing colds or lung infections, getting flu vaccine, keeping follow-up visits, and stopping smoking.
a. Relieve intercostal pain by local heat or oral analgesia.	a. Some soreness may persist for several weeks.	
b. Alternate activities with frequent rest periods.	b. Weakness and fatigability are common for the first 3 weeks.	
c. Practice the breathing exercises at home.	c. Effective breathing is necessary to prevent splinting of affected side, which may lead to atelectasis.	
d. Avoid heavy lifting until complete healing has occurred.	d. Chest muscles and incision may be weaker than normal for 3–6 months.	
e. Avoid undue fatigue, increased shortness of breath, or chest pain.	e. Undue stress may prolong the healing process.	
f. Avoid bronchial irritants.	f. The lung's resistance is lowered and more susceptible to irritants.	
g. Prevent colds or lung infection.	g. The lung is more susceptible to infection during the recovery phase.	
h. Get annual influenza vaccine.	h. Vaccination helps prevent flu.	
i. Keep follow-up appointment with physician.	i. This allows timely follow-up assessment.	
j. Stop smoking.	j. Smoking will slow healing process by decreasing oxygen delivery to tissues and make lung susceptible to infection and other complications.	

BIBLIOGRAPHY

Books

Ahrens T, Rutherford K. Essentials of Oxygenation: Implications for Clinical Practice. Boston. Jones and Bartlett, 1993.

Alspach JG. Core Curriculum for Critical Care Nursing, 4th ed. Philadelphia, WB Saunders, 1991.

Boggs RL and Woolridge-King M. AACN Procedure Manual for Critical Care, 3rd ed. Philadelphia, WB Saunders, 1993.

Carpenito LJ. Nursing Diagnosis: Application to Clinical Practice, 6th ed. Philadelphia, JB Lippincott, 1995.

Clochesy JM, Breu C, Cardin S, Rudy EB, Whittaker AA. Critical Care Nursing. Philadelphia, WB Saunders, 1993.

Kersten LD. Comprehensive Respiratory Nursing: A Decision-Making Approach. Philadelphia, WB Saunders, 1989.

May DF. Rehabilitation and Continuity of Care in Pulmonary Disease. St Louis, MosbyYear Book, 1991.

Pierson DJ, Kacmarek RM. Foundations of Respiratory Care. New York, Churchill Livingstone, 1992.

Roberts SL. Behavioral Concepts and the Critically Ill Patient, 2nd ed. Norwalk, CT, Appleton-Century-Crofts, 1986.

Schneider CC and Slatten R. Thoracic surgery. In Vazquez M et al (eds): Critical Care Nursing, 2nd ed. Philadelphia, WB Saunders, 1992, pp. 233–239.

Sexton DL. Nursing Care of the Respiratory Patient. Norwalk, CT, Appleton and Lange, 1990.

Shapiro B, Kacmarek RM, Cane RD, Hauptmen D. Clinical Application of Respiratory Care, 4th ed. Chicago, Year Book Medical, 1991.

Journals

Asterisks indicate nursing research articles.

Airway Management

*Ackerman MH. The effect of saline lavage prior to suctioning. Am J Crit Care 1993; 2(4):326–330.

*Czarnik RE, Stone KS, Everhart CC, Preusser BA. Differential effects of continuous versus intermittent suction on tracheal tissue. Heart Lung 1991 Mar; 20(2):144–151.

DePew CL and Noll ML. Inline closed-system suctioning: A research analysis. Dimens Crit Care Nursing 1994 Mar-Apr; 13(2):73–83.

*Gunderson LP, Stone KS, and Hamlin RL. Endotracheal suctioning-induced heart rate alterations. Nurs Res 1991 May/Jun; 40(3):139–143.

*Harshbarger SA, Hoffman LA, Zullo TG, Pinsky MR. Effects of a closed tracheal suction system on ventilatory and cardiovascular parameters. Am J Crit Care 1992 Nov; 1(3):57–61.

Ledwidge MK, Corley M, Grap MJ, Glass C. Manual resuscitation bag oxygen delivery. Heart Lung 1991 May; 20(3):300.

*Lookinland S and Appel PL. Hemodynamic and oxygen transport changes following endotracheal suctioning in trauma patients. Nurs Res 1991 May/Jun; 40(3):133–138.

Macaluso S and Roman M. Managing post-intubation injuries. Medsurg Nurs 1994 Jun; 3(3):192–199, 202.

*McCabe SM and Smeltzer SC. Comparison of tidal volumes obtained by one-handed and two-handed ventilation techniques. Am J Crit Care 1993 Nov; 2(6):467–473.

*McIntosh D, Baun MM, and Rogge J. Effects of lung hyperventilation and presence of positive end-expiratory pressure on arterial and tissue oxygenation during endotracheal suctioning. Am J Crit Care 1993; 2(4):317–325.

*Noll ML and Byers JF. Comparison of SVO_2, SpO_2, and clinical parameters with arterial blood gases during ventilatory weaning after cardiac surger. Am J Crit Care 1994 Sep; 3(5):353–355.

*O'Donohue WJ. Effects of oxygen therapy on increasing arterial oxygen tension in hypoxemic patients with stable chronic obstructive pulmonary disease while breathing ambient air. Chest 1991; 100:968–972.

Pfister S. Management of a transtracheal oxygen catheter in a mechanically ventilated patient. Crit Care Nurse 1993 Aug; 13(4): 52–58.

Redick EL. Closed-system, in-line endotracheal suctioning. Crit Care Nurse 1993 Aug; 13(4):47–51.

*Rudy EB et al. Endotracheal suctioning in adults with head injury. Heart Lung 1991 Nov; 20(6):667–674.

Somerson SJ, Sicilia MR. Emergency oxygen administration and airway management. Crit Care Nurse 1992 Apr; 12(4):23–29.

*Stone KS et al. The effect of lung hyperinflation and endotracheal suctioning on cardiopulmonary hemodynamics. Nurs Res 1991 Mar/Apr; 40(2):76–85.

*Stone KS, Bell SD, and Preusser BA. The effect of repeated endotracheal suctioning on arterial blood pressure. Appl Nurs Res 1991 Nov; 4(4):152–158.

Williams ML. An algorithm for selecting a communication technique with intubated patients. Dimen Crit Care Nurs 1992 Jul-Aug; 11(4):222–229.

Mechanical Ventilation

*Abalos A, Leibowitz AB, Distefano D et al. Myocardial ischemia during the weaning period. Am J Crit Care 1992 Nov; 1(3): 32–36.

Briones TL. Pressure support ventilation: New ventilatory technique. Crit Care Nurse 1992 Apr; 12(4):51–58.

Bouley GH, Froman R, Shah H. The experience of dyspnea during weaning. Heart Lung 1992 Sept-Oct; 21(5):471–476.

Burns SM, Fahey SA, Barton DM, Slack D. Weaning from mechanical ventilation: A method for assessment and planning. AACN Clin Iss Crit Care 1991 Aug; 2(3):372–388.

Campbell ML, Carlson RW. Terminal weaning from mechanical ventilation: Ethical and practical considerations for patient management. Am J Crit Care 1992 Nov; 1(3):52–56.

Carroll KC and Magruder CC. The role of analgesics and sedatives in the management of pain and agitation during weaning from mechanical ventilation. Crit Care Nurs Q 1993 Feb; 15(4):68–77.

Dettenmeier PA and Jackson NC. Chronic hypoventilation syndrome: Treatment with non-invasive mechanical ventilation. AACN Clin Iss Crit Care 1991 Aug; 2(3):415–431.

Freichels TA. Cardiopulmonary effects of artificial ventilatory support. Dimen Crit Care Nurs 1993 Jul-Aug; 12(4):170–181.

Geisman LK and Ahrens T. Auto-PEEP: An impediment to weaning in the chronically ventilated patient. AACN Clin Iss Crit Care 1991 Aug; 2(3):391–397.

*Goodnough Hanneman SK. Multidimensional predictors of success or failure with early weaning from mechanical ventilation after cardiac surgery. Nurs Res 1994 Jan–Feb; 43(1):4–10.

Grossbach I. Pressure support ventilation. Crit Care Nurse 1992 Mar; 12(3):50–52.

Juarez P. Mechanical ventilation for the patient with severe ARDS: PC-IRV. Crit Care Nurse 1992 Apr; 12(4):34–39.

Knebel AR. When weaning from mechanical ventilation fails. Am J Crit Care 1992 Nov; 1(3):19–29.

Plummer AL and Gracey DR. Consensus conference on artificial airways in patients receiving mechanical ventilation. Chest 1989; 96:178–179.

Richless CI. Current trends in mechanical ventilation. Crit Care Nurse 1991 Mar; 11(3):41–50.

Rotello LC, Warren J, Jastremski MS, and Milewski A. A nurse-directed protocol using pulse oximetry to wean mechanically ventilated patients from toxic oxygen concentrations. Chest 1992 Dec; 102(6):1833–1835.

Shekleton ME. Respiratory muscle conditioning and the work of breathing: A critical balance in the weaning patient. AACN Clin Iss Crit Care 1991 Aug; 2(3):405–414.

Smith CE, Mayer LS, Parkhurst C et al. Adaptation in families with a member requiring mechanical ventilation at home. Heart Lung 1991 Jul; 20(4):349–356.

*Smith CE et al. Caregiver learning needs and reactions to managing home mechanical ventilation. Heart Lung 1994 Mar–Apr; 23(2):157–163.

St John RE and Eisenberg P. Nutrition and the use of metabolic assessment in the ventilator-dependent patient. AACN Clin Iss Crit Care Nurs 1991 Aug; 2(3):453–461.

Weilitz PB. Weaning a patient from mechanical ventilation. Crit Care Nurse 1993 Aug; 13(4):33–41.

Thoracic Surgery

*Carlson MM et al. Managing pain during mediastinal chest tube removal. Heart Lung 1994 Nov–Dec; 23(6):500–505.

Carroll P. Nursing the thoracotomy patient. RN 1992 Jun; 55(6): 34–38, 41–42.

Dajczman E, Gordon A, Kreisman H, and Wolkove N. Long-term postthoracotomy pain. Chest 1991 Feb; 99(2):270–274.

Langston WG. Surgical resection of lung cancer. Nurs Clin North Am 1992 Sep; 27(3):665–679.

Litwack K. Practical points in the care of the thoracic surgery patient. J Post Anesth Nurs 1990 Aug; 5(4):276–278.

Morey LB and Dungan JM. Chylothorax: A complication of thoracic trauma or surgery. Dimen Crit Care Nurs 1992 Jul-Aug; 11(4): 184–190.

Nicholson C, Coleman CA, and Mack M. Are you ready for video thoracoscopy? Am J Nurs 1993 Mar; 93(3):54–57.

Olsen GN, Bolton JWR, Weiman DS, and Hornung CA. Stair climbing as an exercise test to predict the postoperative complications of lung resection: two years' experience. Chest 1991 Mar; 99(3):587–590.

Tampinco-Golos I. Endoscopic thoracotomy: A new approach to thoracic surgery . . . thoracoscopy. AORN J 1992 May; 55(5): 1167, 1169–1172, 1174–1177.

Yeaw EMJ. Good lung down? Am J Nurs 1992 Mar; 92(3):26–29.

INFORMATION/RESOURCES

Governmental Agencies

National Heart, Lung and Blood Institute
National Institutes of Health
900 Rockville Pike, Bldg 31,
Bethesda, MD 20892, (301) 496-5166

Voluntary Agencies

American Association for Respiratory Care
1720 Regal Row
Dallas, TX 75235, (214) 630-3540

American Lung Association
1740 Broadway
New York, NY 10019, (212) 315-8700

American Thoracic Society
1740 Broadway
New York, NY 10019, (212) 315-8700

Respiratory Nursing Society
5700 Old Orchard Rd, 1st Floor
Skokie, IL 60077

Nursing Research Profile for Unit 6

Respiratory Nursing

Overview

Nursing research reviewed here addresses chronic obstructive pulmonary disease, manual resuscitation, and suctioning.

Breslin EH, et al. Standardization of a device to measure unsupported arm exercise endurance in chronic obstructive pulmonary disease. Nursing Research 1992; 41(5):292–295.

Persons with chronic obstructive pulmonary disease (COPD) often limit their participation in activities that require exertion or exercise because of dyspnea. Although all forms of exercise increase ventilatory demand, unsupported arm exercise (UAE) also leads to competitive recruitment of respiratory muscles to maintain increases in ventilation required by the exercise and to support arm weight during such exercise. Because of their inability to meet exercise-induced demands for ventilation with unsupported use of the arms (activities such as bathing and putting groceries on cabinet shelves), persons with COPD often avoid such activities to avoid increased dyspnea and fatigue.

Previous methods of evaluating exercise tolerance in patients with COPD have addressed lower leg exercise and supported rather than unsupported arm exercise. This study compared respiratory responses in COPD patients with UAE with a newly developed, electromechanical device. The device is designed to measure UAE endurance and permits control of the rate and rhythm of arm motion. Additionally, it allows measurement of UAE endurance with the arm in various positions.

The purpose of the study was to develop endurance limits and respiratory physiologic and sensory standards for UAE in COPD patients. During UAE, subjects lifted their fully extended arms at and above shoulder level at slow and moderate rates (21 and 42 times, respectively). Patients with moderately severe and severe COPD ($n = 21$) participated in the study. The following variables were measured after slow and moderate exercise: tidal volume (VT), respiratory rate (RR), respiratory muscle duty cycle (Ti/Titot), minute ventilation (Ve), oxygen uptake (VO_2), carbon dioxide production (VCO_2), inspiratory flow (VT/Ti), and heart rate (HR). Patients' sensations of dyspnea, arm fatigue, and respiratory effort were assessed before and after UAE using a horizontal, 100-mm visual analog scale.

The results of this study demonstrated a significant increase in VO_2, VCO_2, VT/Ti, Ve, RR, and HR at both slow and moderate UAE. There was an increase in VT with moderate exercise only; no change in Ti/Titot was observed. In addition, HR tended to increase in moderate UAE compared with slow UAE. Patients reported a significant increase in dyspnea, respiratory effort, and arm fatigue with both moderate and slow exercise.

Nursing Implications. The findings of this study increase understanding of the relationship between UAE, dyspnea, and activity tolerance in COPD. This study emphasizes the importance of standard measures of exercise tolerance in COPD that will provide clearer methods to define disability and help patients maintain activities of daily living. Subsequent studies with the device may lead to identification and testing of strategies to increase COPD patients' UAE tolerance and participation in activities of daily living requiring use of the arms.

Weaver TE and Narsavage GL. Physiological and psychological variables related to functional status in chronic obstructive pulmonary disease. Nursing Research 1992 Sep/Oct; 41(5):286–291.

Although a significant number (45%) of patients with COPD have restricted activities, physiologic variables alone do not fully account for these limitations. This study examined the relationship of psychologic and physiologic variables to functional status. Psychologic variables included causal attributions, mood, and self-esteem; physiologic variables included pulmonary function and exercise capacity.

A descriptive correlational design with a convenience sample of 104 subjects was used. All subjects had some form of COPD. Psychologic measures included mood (Multiple Affect Adjective Check List), self-esteem (Self-Esteem Scale), and causal attribution (Attributions Interview Schedule). Physiologic measures studied included pulmonary function utilizing spirometry (FEV_1) and exercise capacity (12-minute walking test). Functional status was measured using the Pulmonary Functional Status Scale, which measures daily behaviors such as self-care, grocery shopping, meal preparation, and dyspnea.

A two-way analysis of variance was used to examine functional status and causal attribution. A significant relationship ($p = .03$) was identified between functional status between those who did and those who did not ask "Why me?" Other physiologic variables and two psychologic variables (mood and self-esteem) were significantly correlated ($p < .01$) with functional status. When multiple regression was performed to identify the combination of variables that best predicted functional status, exercise capacity and depression were found to be the best predictors ($p < .0001$).

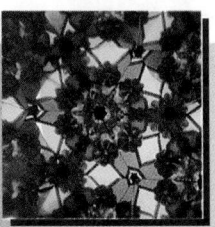

Nursing Implications. This results of this study illustrate how psychologic factors can affect the functional status of patients with COPD and clearly demonstrate the importance of assessing the psychologic as well as physical status of patients in order to effect the most positive health outcomes. COPD patients should routinely be assessed for a depressed mood, and interventions should be directed at alleviating the depression.

Kim MJ, et al. Inspiratory muscle training in patients with chronic obstructive pulmonary disease. Nursing Research 1993; 42(6):356–362.

Inspiratory muscle weakness has been described as a factor that limits the ability of COPD patients to meet the demands of exercise and predisposes them to fatigue. This weakness contributes to dyspnea and breathlessness. Pulmonary rehabilitation programs often employ inspiratory muscle training (IMT) to improve the strength and endurance of the muscles; however, previous studies have produced conflicting results regarding IMT.

The investigators of this study theorized that increasing muscle strength and endurance would delay respiratory muscle fatigue and dyspnea. This study used a double-blind design of 67 patients with COPD with training over a 6-month period. The sample included men (n = 51) and women (n = 16) who were assigned to either an experimental (n = 41) or control group (n = 26). Maximal inspiratory pressure (PI_{max}), respiratory muscle endurance time (RMET), bronchitis-emphysema symptom checklist, and the Sickness Impact Profile were used to assess outcomes of the training.

All patients were trained for 30 minutes on IMT daily for 6 months using a threshold inspiratory muscle training device. The threshold load was increased each month for the treatment group at a significantly greater rate than the control or sham training group; the changes in the threshold load were based on each patient's maximal inspiratory pressure. Measurements were taken prior to beginning the training and at the end of 3 and 6 months of IMT. Data obtained from interviews were analyzed to describe patients' perceptions of the effects of the training.

A wide range of responses was noted in both the experimental and control groups. Both groups demonstrated improvement in performance of PI_{max}, respiratory muscle endurance, 12-minute distance walk, and dyspnea. The researchers thought that improvements were related to better coordination of inspiratory muscles and desensitization to dyspnea. Compared with the control group, the treatment group did not demonstrate significant effects in results. Some possible explanations for the lack of differences between groups are the long-term training effects of sham training, multiple upper respiratory infections in both groups, inadequate training for the experimental group, and measurement problems with respiratory muscle endurance time (RMET). Final results indicated that patients may derive similar benefits from light loads of IMT as from moderate loads, but further research is needed to confirm these benefits and test higher loads.

Nursing Implications. Nurses need to recognize that disease processes are complex, and further research is needed to document the beneifts of different training modalities and to test theoretical concepts. COPD includes changes in physiologic measures and the perceptions of dyspnea. The interaction of physiologic and psychologic variables must be considered in the care of the patient.

McCabe S and Smeltzer SC. Comparison of tidal volumes obtained by one-handed and two-handed ventilation techniques. Am J Crit Care 1993; 2(6):467–473.

Objectives of this study were to compare tidal volumes delivered by one- and two-handed compressions of a manual resuscitation bag and to assess the effects of subject characteristics on those tidal volumes. The issue of one- versus two-handed ventilation is significant since varying tidal volumes may contribute either to hypoinflation (atelectasis, microatelectasis, retention of CO_2 and secretions) or hyperinflation (barotrauma, pneumothorax).

The sample comprised 108 health care workers randomly assigned to one of two procedures: one- followed by two-handed compressions or two- followed by one-handed compressions. The investigators also studied variables that could affect tidal volumes: subjects' hand size, grip strength, and experience with manual ventilation.

The subjects compressed a manual resuscitation bag to generate tidal volumes through a lung ventilator performance analyzer. This device, composed of rubber bellows and pressure gauges, could be adjusted to simulate total compliance and airway resistance. Generated volumes were measured with a Wright spirometer. Subjects' grip strength was measured while standing using a Jamar Dynameter; hand size was obtained by estimating the area of the hand using palm width and length from the middle fingertip to the distal skin crease at the wrist.

Paired *t* tests and one-way analysis of variance (ANOVA) were used to compare volumes obtained with one- and two-handed compressions and to determine if volumes differed by the variables of gender, category of health care provider, basic or advanced cardiac life support training, or manual ventilation experience. Stepwise regression analysis was used to determine which variables contributed more to volumes achieved.

Results showed a statistically significant difference ($p < .0001$) between volumes obtained by one- and two-handed compressions, with greater volume achieved with the two-handed procedure. Grip strength was more strongly correlated with one- and two-handed volumes than were any other variables, and a stronger correlation was found with one-handed than with two-handed tidal volumes.

Nursing Implications. Findings suggest that the two-handed technique is necessary to deliver minimal required tidal volumes; this can be accomplished either with two caregivers (one to ventilate, one to suction) or with the ventilator's sigh mechanism if two caregivers are not available. The investigators also suggest a training program to focus on effective delivery, with feedback on corrrect and incorrect technique to increase the reliability of the procedure.

UNIT 7

Cardiovascular, Circulatory, and Hematologic Function

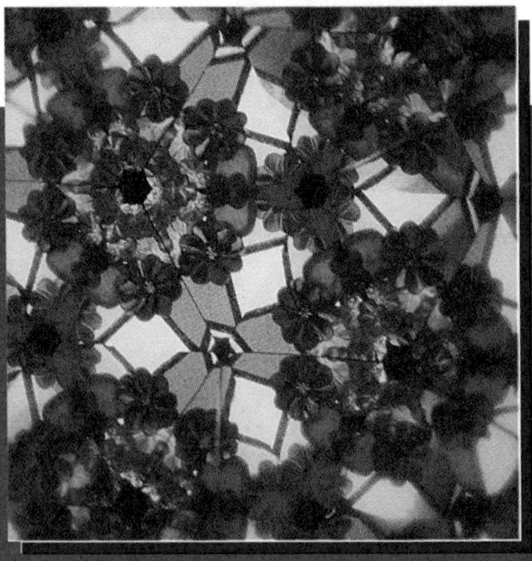

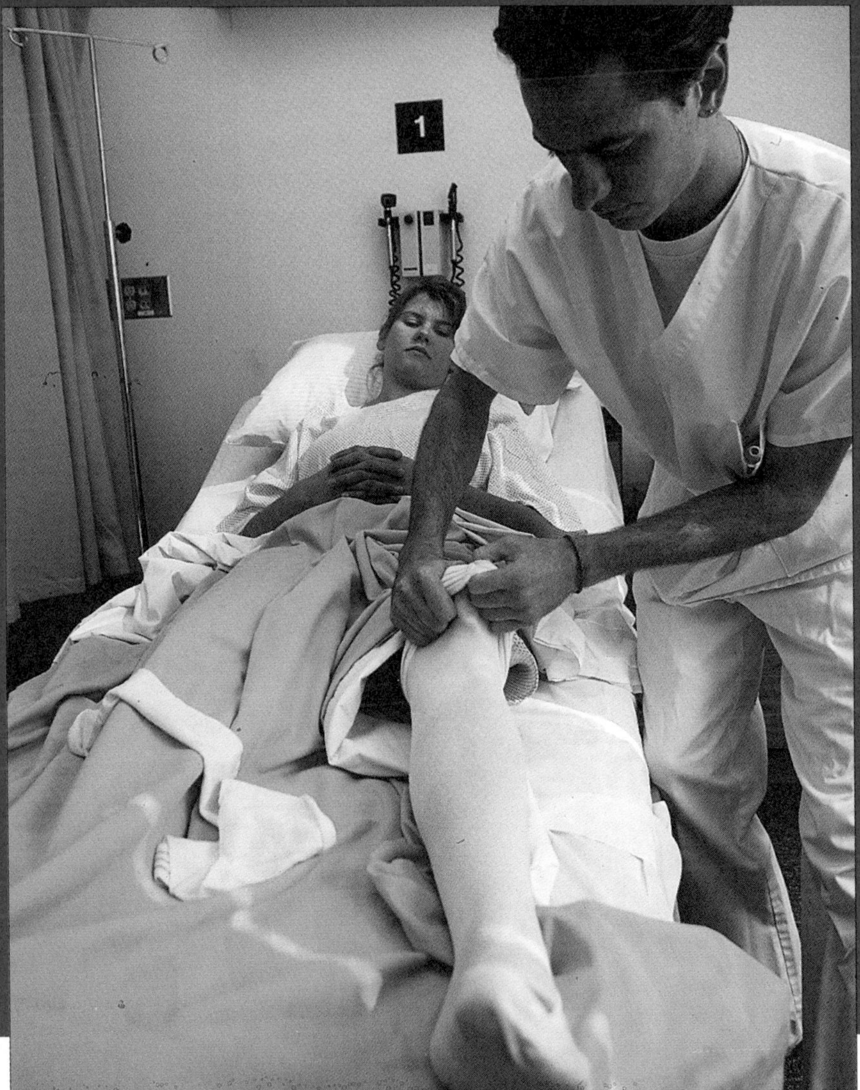

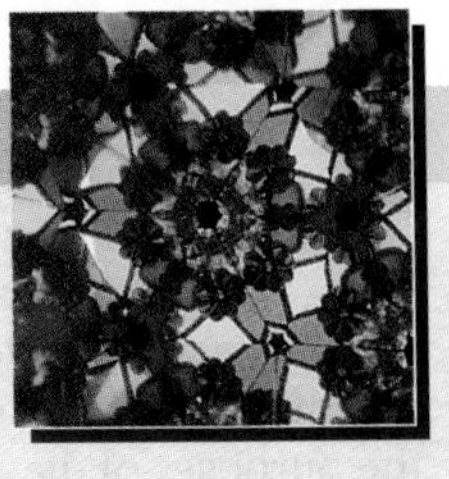

26

Assessment of Cardiovascular Function

CHAPTER OUTLINE

Overview of Cardiac Structure and Function
- Cardiac Anatomy
- Conduction System of the Heart
- Cardiac Physiology
- Gerontologic Considerations

Health History
- Risk Factors in Coronary Artery Disease

Physical Assessment
- General Appearance
- Examination of Blood Pressure
- Examination of the Pulse
- Hands
- Head and Neck
- Heart
- Other Assessment Parameters
- Gerontologic Considerations

Diagnostic Tests and Procedures
- Laboratory Tests
- Chest X-ray and Fluoroscopy
- Electrocardiography
- Exercise Tolerance Testing
- Cardiac Catheterization
- Echocardiography
- Radionuclide Imaging
- Electrophysiologic Testing
- Hemodynamic Monitoring

Critical Thinking Exercises

LEARNING OBJECTIVES

On completion of this chapter, the learner will be able to:

1. Explain cardiac physiology in relation to cardiac anatomy and the normal conduction system of the heart
2. Incorporate assessment of cardiac risk factors into the health history and physical assessment of the cardiac patient
3. Use assessment parameters appropriate for determining the status of cardiovascular function
4. Identify the clinical significance and related nursing implications of the various tests and procedures used for diagnostic assessment of cardiac function
5. Compare central venous pressure monitoring, pulmonary artery pressure monitoring, and systemic intra-arterial monitoring with regard to clinical usefulness and significance, nursing responsibilities, and possible complications

Nursing assessment of a patient with heart disease includes taking a history, performing a physical examination, and monitoring test results of cardiac functioning. Sound knowledge of cardiac anatomy, physiology, and pathophysiology is necessary for developing assessment skills, defining nursing diagnoses, planning nursing care, and understanding the purposes of diagnostic tests.

Overview of Cardiac Structure and Function

The heart is a hollow, muscular organ located in the center of the thorax, where it occupies the space between the lungs and rests on the diaphragm. It weighs approximately 300 g (10.6 oz), although heart weight and size are influenced by age, gender, body weight, extent of physical exercise and conditioning, and heart disease. The function of the heart is to pump blood to the tissues, supplying them with oxygen and other nutrients while removing carbon dioxide and other waste products of metabolism. There are actually two pumps within the heart, located on the right side and left side. The output of the right heart is distributed entirely to the lungs by the pulmonary artery, and the output of the left heart is distributed to the remainder of the body by the aorta. These two pumps eject blood simultaneously at approximately the same rate of output.

The pumping action of the heart is accomplished by the rhythmic contraction and relaxation of its muscular wall. During contraction of the muscle (**systole**), the chambers of the heart become smaller as the blood is ejected. During relaxation of the muscles of the heart wall (**diastole**), the heart chambers fill with blood in preparation for the subsequent ejection. A normal adult heart beats approximately 60 to 80 times per minute, ejects approximately 70 ml of blood from either ventricle per beat, and has a total output of approximately 5 L/min.

Cardiac Anatomy

The area in the middle of the chest between the two lungs is called the **mediastinum**. The bulk of the mediastinal space is occupied by the heart, which is encased in a thin, fibrous sac called the **pericardium**.

The pericardium protects the surface of the heart but is not essential for the heart to function properly. The space between the surface of the heart and the pericardial lining is filled with a very small amount of fluid, which lubricates the surface and reduces friction during contraction of the cardiac muscle.

Heart Chambers. The right and left sides of the heart are each composed of two chambers, an **atrium** (pl. atria) and a **ventricle**. The common wall between the right and left chambers is called the septum. The ventricles are the chambers that eject blood into the arteries. The functions of the atria are to receive incoming blood from the veins and to act as temporary storage reservoirs from which the blood will subsequently empty into the ventricles. The relationship of the four chambers of the heart is shown in Figure 26-1.

The varying thicknesses of the atrial and ventricular walls relate to the workload required by each chamber. The atrial walls are thinner than those of the ventricles because of the lower pressure produced by the atria holding the blood and then channeling it to the ventricles. Because the left ventricle has the greater workload of the two bottom chambers, it is about 2-½ times as thick as the right ventricle. The left ventricle ejects blood against the high systemic pressure, whereas the right ventricle ejects against the low pressure of the pulmonary vasculature.

Because the heart lies in a rotated position within the chest cavity, the right ventricle lies anteriorly (just beneath the sternum) and the left ventricle is situated posteriorly. The left ventricle is responsible for the apex beat or the point of maximum impulse (PMI), which is normally palpable in the left midclavicular line of the chest wall at the 5th intercostal space.

Cardiac Valves. Cardiac valves permit blood to flow in only one direction through the heart. Valves, which are composed of thin leaflets of fibrous tissue, open and close passively in response to pressure changes and blood movement. There are two types of valves: atrioventricular and semilunar.

Atrioventricular Valves. The valves that separate the atria from the ventricles are termed atrioventricular valves. The **tricuspid valve**, so named because it its composed of three cusps, or leaflets, separates the right atrium from the right ventricle. The **mitral** or **bicuspid valve** (two cusps) lies between the left atrium and left ventricle (see Fig. 26-1).

Normally, when the ventricles contract, ventricular pressure tends to push the atrioventricular valve leaflets upward into the atrial cavity. If enough pressure were to be exerted on the valves, blood would be ejected backward from the ventricles to the atria. Papillary muscles and chordae tendineae are responsible for keeping the blood flowing in one direction through the atrioventricular valves. **Papillary muscles** are muscle bundles that are located on the sides of the ventricular walls. **Chordae tendineae** are fibrous bands extending from the papillary muscles to the edges of the valve leaflets, acting to tether the free edges of the valves to the ventricular wall. Contraction of the papillary muscles causes the chordae tendineae to become taut. This keeps the valve leaflets closed during systole, preventing backflow of blood. Papillary muscles and chordae tendineae are attached only to the mitral and tricuspid valves and are notably absent from the semilunar valves.

Semilunar Valves. Semilunar valves are situated between each ventricle and its corresponding artery. The valve between the right ventricle and the pulmonary artery is called the **pulmonic valve**; the valve between the left ventricle and the aorta is called the **aortic valve**. Both of the semilunar valves are normally composed of three cusps, which function properly without papillary muscles and chordae tendineae. There are no valves between the large veins and the atria.

Coronary Arteries. The coronary arteries are the vessels that supply blood to the heart muscle, which has large metabolic requirements for oxygen and nutrients (Fig. 26-2). The heart uses approximately 70% to 80% of the oxygen delivered through the coronary arteries; in contrast, other or-

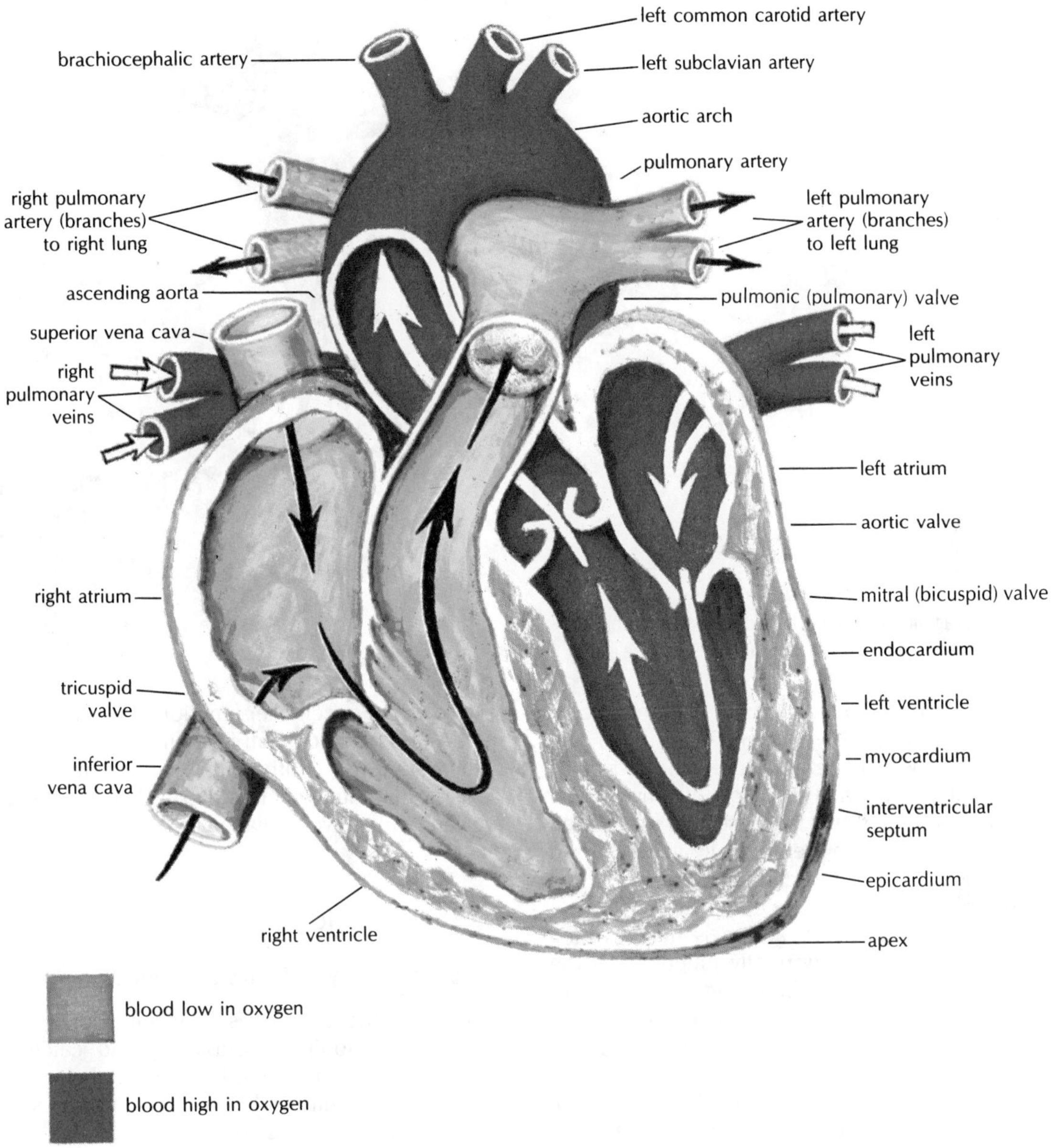

FIGURE 26-1. Structure of the heart and course of blood flow through the heart chambers, as indicated by *arrows.*

gans use, on the average, only one quarter of the oxygen delivered to them. The coronary arteries arise from the aorta near its origin at the left ventricle. The wall of the left side of the heart is supplied in large part through the **left main coronary artery**, which divides into several large branches that run down (**left anterior descending artery**) and across (**circumflex artery**) the left side of the myocardium. The right heart wall is supplied similarly from a separate **right coronary artery**. Unlike other arteries, the coronary arteries are perfused during diastole.

Cardiac Muscle. The specialized muscle tissue composing the wall of the heart is called cardiac muscle. Microscopically, cardiac muscle resembles striated (skeletal) muscle, which is under conscious control. Functionally, however, heart muscle resembles smooth muscle because it is involuntary.

The cardiac muscle fibers are arranged in an interconnected manner (called a syncytium) so that they can contract and relax in a coordinated manner. The sequential pattern of contraction and relaxation of individual muscle fibers ensures the rhythmic behavior of the heart muscle as a whole and enables it to function as a pump. The heart muscle itself is called the **myocardium**. The inner lining of the myocardium, which is in contact with the blood, is called the **endocardium**, and the outer layer of cells is called the **epicardium**.

Conduction System of the Heart

Cardiac muscle cells have an inherent rhythmic action (rhythmicity), which is illustrated by the fact that a segment

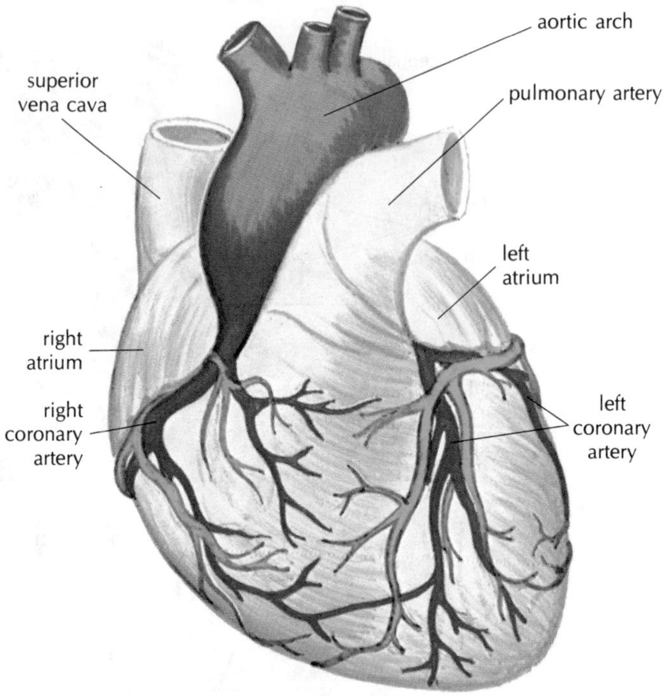

FIGURE 26-2. Diagram of the coronary arteries arising from the aorta and encircling the heart. Some of the coronary veins also are shown.

of myocardium removed from the rest of the heart will continue to contract rhythmically if maintained under the proper conditions. However, the atria and ventricles must contract sequentially to provide the most effective blood flow. Orderly contraction occurs because the specialized cells of the conduction system methodically generate and conduct electrical impulses to myocardial cells.

The **sinoatrial (SA) node**, located at the junction of the superior vena cava and the right atrium, is the beginning of the conduction system and normally functions as the pacemaker for the entire myocardium (Fig. 26-3). The SA node initiates approximately 60 to 100 impulses per minute in a resting normal heart, but can change its rate in response to the needs of the body.

The electrical signal initiated by the SA node is conducted along the myocardial cells of the atrium to the **atrioventricular (AV) node**. The AV node (located in the right atrial wall near the tricuspid valve) is another group of specialized muscle cells similar to the SA node, but with an intrinsic rate of about 40 to 60 impulses per minute. The AV node coordinates the incoming electrical impulses from the atria and, after a slight delay, relays an impulse to the ventricles. This impulse is conducted through a bundle of specialized muscle fibers (**the bundle of His**) that travel in the septum separating the left and right ventricles. The His bundle divides into right and left bundle branches, which terminate in fibers called **Purkinje fibers**. The right bundle fans out into the right ventricular muscle. The left bundle divides again into the left anterior and left posterior bundle branches, which fan out into the left ventricular muscle. Further spread of the impulse by depolarization through the rest of the myocardium takes place by conduction through the muscle fibers themselves.

The heart rate is determined by the myocardial cells with the fastest intrinsic rate. Normally, the SA node is fastest. If the SA node malfunctions, the AV node generally takes over the pacemaker function of the heart. Should both the SA and AV nodes fail in their pacemaker function, the myocardium will continue to beat at a rate of less than 40 beats per minute, which is the intrinsic pacemaker rate of the ventricular myocardial cells.

Cardiac Physiology

Electrophysiologic Overview

Cardiac electrical activity is the result of ions (charged particles such as sodium, potassium, and calcium) moving across the cell membrane. The electrical changes recorded within a single cell result in what is known as the **cardiac action potential** (Fig. 26-4).

In the resting state, cardiac muscle cells are **polarized**, which means an electrical difference exists between the negatively charged inside and the positively charged outside of the cell membrane. The cardiac cycle begins when an electrical impulse is released, beginning the phase of **depolarization**. The permeability of the cell membrane changes and ions move across it (see Fig. 26-4). With movement of ions into the cell, the inside of the cell becomes positive. Contraction of the muscle follows depolarization. A cardiac muscle cell is normally depolarized when a neighboring cell is depolarized (although it also can be depolarized by external electrical stimulation). Sufficient depolarization of a single specialized conduction system cell will therefore result in depolarization and contraction of the entire myocardium. **Repolarization** occurs as the cell returns to its baseline state (becomes more negative), and corresponds to relaxation of myocardial muscle.

After the rapid influx of sodium into the cell during depolarization, the permeability of the cell membrane to calcium is changed, allowing for uptake of calcium into the

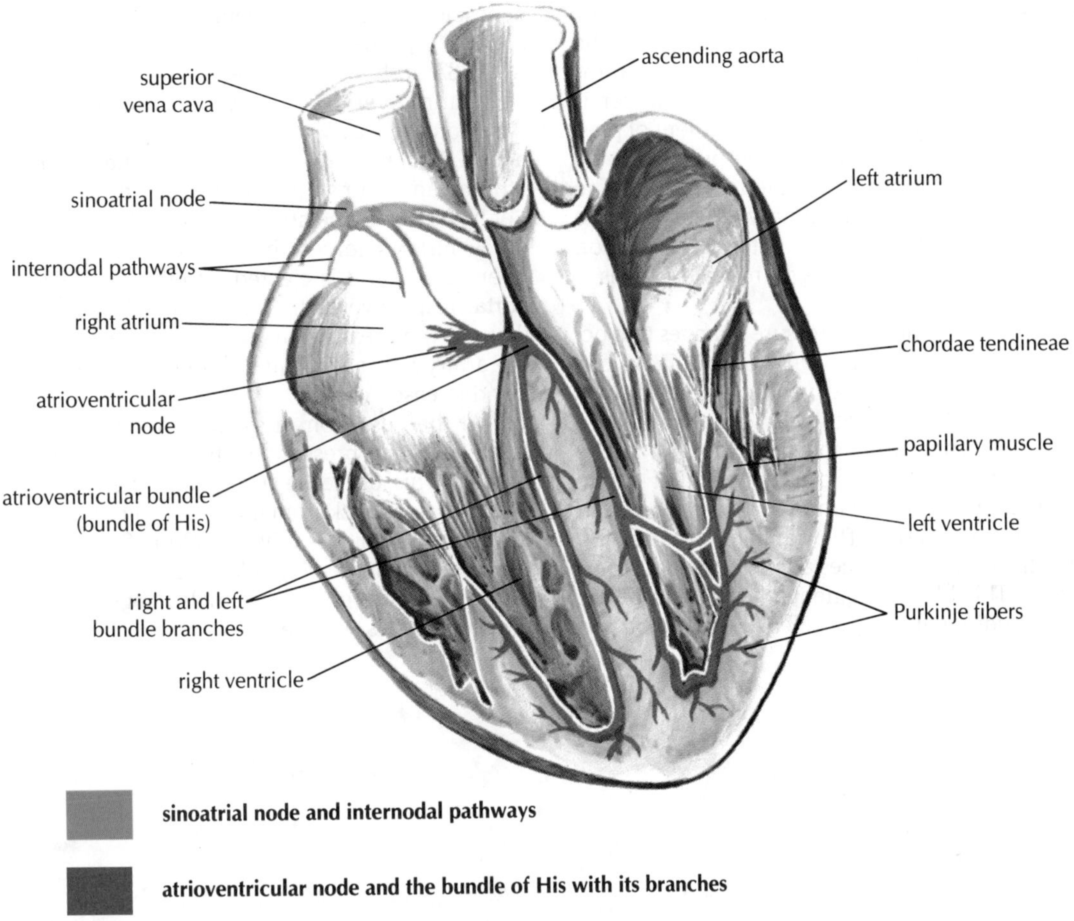

FIGURE 26-3. Conduction system. Diagram shows relationships of the sinoatrial node, the atrioventricular node, the common atrioventricular bundle, and its branches.

cell. The influx of calcium, occurring during the plateau phase of repolarization, is much slower than that of sodium and continues for a longer period. This interaction between changes in membrane voltage and muscle contraction is called electromechanical coupling.

Cardiac muscle, unlike skeletal or smooth muscle, has a prolonged refractory period during which it cannot be restimulated to contract. This protects the heart from sustained contraction (tetany), which would result in sudden cardiac death.

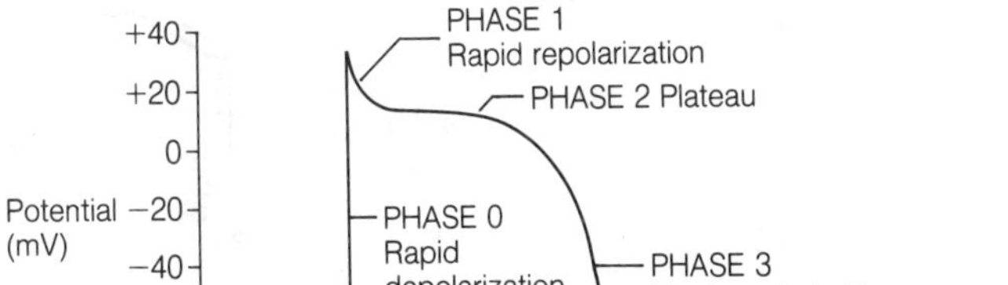

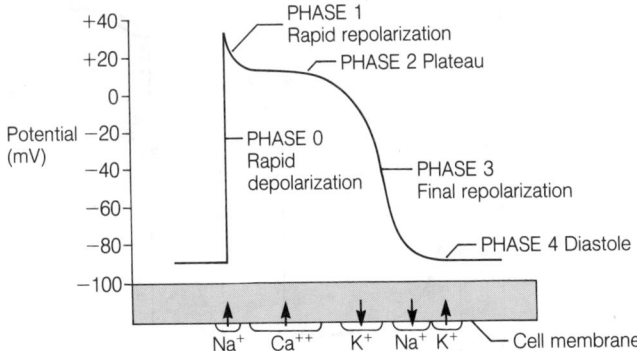

FIGURE 26-4. Cardiac action potential. The arrows below the diagram indicate the approximate time and direction of movement of each ion influencing membrane potential. The phase of Ca^{++} moving out of the cell is not well defined but is thought to occur during phase 4.

Normal electromechanical coupling and contraction of the heart are dependent on the composition of the interstitial fluid surrounding the heart muscle cells. The composition of this fluid is in turn influenced by the composition of the blood. A change in blood calcium concentration therefore may alter contraction of the heart muscle fibers. A change in blood potassium concentration is also important, because potassium affects the normal electrical voltage of the cell.

Cardiac Hemodynamics

An important principle that determines the direction of blood flow is that fluid flows from a region of higher pressure to a region of lower pressure. The pressures that are responsible for blood flow in the normal circulation are generated by contraction of the ventricular muscle. When the muscle contracts, blood is forced from the ventricle into the aorta during the period when left ventricular pressure exceeds aortic pressure. When these two pressures become equal, the aortic valve closes and output from the left ventricle ceases. The blood that has entered the aorta increases the pressure in that vessel. This provides a pressure gradient to force blood progressively through the arteries and capillaries and into the veins. The blood returns to the right atrium because pressure in this chamber is lower than pressure in the veins. Similarly, a gradient of pressure is responsible for blood flow from the pulmonary artery through the lung and back to the left atrium. The pressure gradients within the pulmonary circulation are considerably lower than those in the systemic circulation because the resistance to flow in the pulmonary vessels is lower.

Cardiac Cycle. Consider the pressure changes that occur in the chambers of the heart during the cardiac cycle, beginning with diastole when the ventricles are relaxed (Fig. 26-5). During **diastole** the atrioventricular valves are open, and blood returning from the veins flows into the atrium and then into the ventricle. Toward the end of this diastolic period, the atrial muscle contracts in response to a signal initiated by the SA node. The contraction raises the pressure inside the atrium and forces an increment of blood into the ventricle. This blood augments the volume of the ventricles by an additional 15% to 25%. At this point, the ventricles themselves begin to contract (systole) in response to propagation of the electrical impulse that began in the SA node some milliseconds previously.

During **systole**, the pressure inside the ventricle rapidly rises, forcing the AV valves to close. The consequence of this action is that no further filling of the ventricle from the atrium can occur, and blood ejected from the ventricle cannot flow back to the atrium. The rapid rise of pressure inside the ventricles forces the pulmonic and aortic valves to open, and blood is ejected into the pulmonary artery and aorta, respectively. The exit of blood is at first rapid, and then, as the pressures in each ventricle and its corresponding artery approach equalization, the flow of blood gradually decreases.

At the cessation of systole, the ventricular muscle relaxes and the pressure within the chamber rapidly decreases. This decrease in pressure creates a tendency for blood to flow back from the artery into the ventricle, which forces the semilunar valves to close. Simultaneously, as the pressure within the ventricle drops to below atrial pressure, the AV valves open, the ventricles begin to fill, and the entire sequence is repeated.

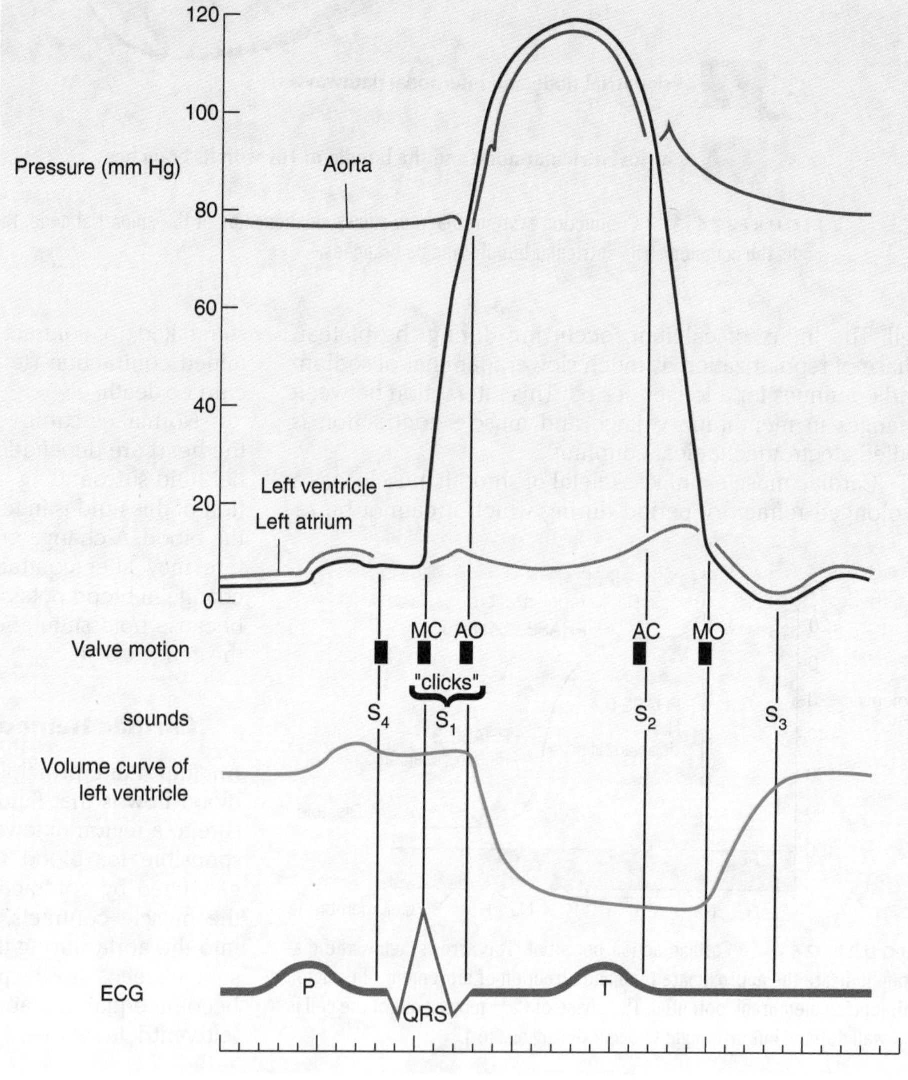

FIGURE 26-5. Events in the cardiac cycle. Three pressure curves are displayed: aortic, left ventricular, and left atrial. Electrocardiographic events precede the mechanical events (see Analysis of ECG in Chapter 27). Valve closure and opening are indicated, as is the relationship of the cardiac sounds to these events (see Auscultation of the Heart in this chapter).

It is important to note that the mechanical events related to filling and ejection by the heart are closely coupled to the corresponding electrical events that cause cardiac contraction and relaxation. When interpreting Figure 26-5, it is necessary to realize that the electrical events (ECG) precede the mechanical events (pressures). (See Analysis of the ECG, Chapter 27.)

The events just described lead to the repetitive rise and fall of pressures inside the ventricles. The maximum pressure reached is called systolic pressure and the minimum pressure diastolic pressure.

Cardiac Output

Cardiac output is the amount of blood pumped by the ventricles during a given period. The cardiac output of a typical adult is normally about 5 L/min but varies greatly, depending on the metabolic needs of the body. Cardiac output (CO) equals the stroke volume (SV) times the heart rate (HR).

$$CO = SV \times HR$$

Stroke volume is the amount of blood ejected per heartbeat. Cardiac output can be affected, therefore, by changes in either stroke volume or heart rate. The resting heart rate of an average adult is approximately 60 to 80 beats/min and the average stroke volume is about 70 ml/beat.

Control of Heart Rate. Because the function of the heart is to supply blood to all tissues of the body, its output must vary as the metabolic needs of the tissues themselves change. For example, during exercise the total cardiac output may increase fourfold, to 20 L/min. This increase is normally accomplished by approximately doubling both the heart rate and the stroke volume. Changes in heart rate are accomplished by reflex controls mediated by the autonomic nervous system, including its sympathetic and parasympathetic divisions. The parasympathetic impulses, which travel to the heart through the vagus nerve, can slow the cardiac rate, whereas sympathetic impulses increase it. These effects on heart rate result from action on the SA node to either decrease or increase its rate of intrinsic depolarization. The balance between these two reflex control systems normally determines the heart rate. The heart rate is stimulated also by an increased level of circulating catecholamines (secreted by the adrenal gland) and by the presence of excess thyroid hormone, which produces a catecholamine-like effect.

Control of Stroke Volume. Stroke volume is primarily determined by three factors: (1) intrinsic contractility of the cardiac muscle, (2) the degree of stretch of the cardiac muscle before its contraction (preload), and (3) the pressure against which the heart muscle has to eject blood during contraction (afterload).

Intrinsic contractility is a term used to denote the force that can be generated by the contracting myocardium under any given condition. It is increased by circulating catecholamines, sympathetic neuronal activity, and certain medications (such as digitalis). It is depressed by hypoxemia and acidosis. Increased contractility results in increased stroke volume.

The second factor influencing stroke volume is **preload**, which is the distending force that stretches the ventricular muscle before its excitation and contraction. Ventricular preload is determined by the volume of blood within the ventricle at the end of diastole. The larger the preload, the greater will be the stroke volume, until a point is reached when the muscle is so stretched it can no longer contract. The relationship between increased stroke volume and increased ventricular end-diastolic volume for a given intrinsic contractility is called **Starling's law** of the heart, which is based on the fact that the greater the initial length or stretch of the cardiac muscle, the greater the degree of shortening that will occur. This results from increased interaction between thick and thin filaments of the sarcomeres (similar to the interaction discussed more fully in the chapter on skeletal muscle physiology).

The third determinant of stroke volume is **afterload**, the pressure against which the ventricles must eject blood. The resistance to the left ventricle ejection is called **systemic vascular resistance** (SVR). The resistance by the pulmonary pressure to the right ventricle ejection is called pulmonary vascular resistance (PVR). Increased afterload leads to decreased stroke volume.

The heart can achieve a greatly increased stroke volume, as during exercise, by increasing preload (through increased venous return), by increasing contractility (through sympathetic nervous system discharge), and by decreasing afterload (through peripheral vasodilation with decreased aortic pressure).

The percentage of the end-diastolic volume that is ejected with each stroke is called the **ejection fraction**. With each stroke, 55% to 75% of the end-diastolic volume is ejected by the normal heart. The ejection fraction can be used as an index of myocardial contractility; it is decreased if contractility is depressed.

Gerontologic Considerations

Atherosclerosis or hardening of the coronary arteries and the resultant effects on the heart have long been associated with the aging process. Recent investigations, however, show little evidence that age alone is the precipitating factor. Current evidence indicates that the cardiac changes once attributed to aging can be minimized by modifying lifestyle and personal habits, that is, by following a low-sodium, low-fat diet, not smoking, and exercising regularly.

Studies have shown that the normal aging heart is able to provide an adequate cardiac output under ordinary circumstances, but may have limited functional ability to respond to situations that cause physical or emotional stress. In an elderly person who is less active, the left ventricle may become smaller in response to the decreased workload demand. Aging also results in decreased elasticity and widening of the aorta, thickening and rigidity of the cardiac valves, and increased connective tissue in the SA and AV nodes and bundle branches.

These changes lead to decreased myocardial contractility, increased left ventricular ejection time, and delayed conduction. Thus, stressful physical and emotional conditions, especially those that occur suddenly, may have adverse effects on the aged person. The heart is unable to respond to such conditions with an adequate increase in rate, and more time is required for the heart rate to return to basal levels after even a minimal increase. In some patients, heart failure may be precipitated.

Health History

Nursing assessment of cardiac patients who are acutely ill requires a different initial health history than that for cardiac patients with stable or chronic problems. A patient experiencing an acute myocardial infarction (commonly called a heart attack by the lay public) requires immediate, and possibly life-saving, medical and nursing interventions—for example, relief of chest discomfort or prevention of dysrhythmias. For this patient, a few well-chosen questions about chest discomfort, associated symptoms (such as shortness of breath or palpitations), medication allergies, and smoking history are asked at the same time one is assessing heart rate, rhythm, and blood pressure and inserting an intravenous line. When the patient's condition is more stable, a more extensive history is obtained.

When caring for an acutely ill cardiac patient, the nurse must first focus on assessing the heart and cardiac output. Patients with atherosclerotic coronary artery disease commonly experience the following symptoms:

- Chest discomfort (angina pectoris or myocardial infarction)
- Shortness of breath, fatigue, and reduced urine output (left ventricular failure with decreased cardiac output)
- Palpitations and dizziness (dysrhythmias due to ischemia [inadequate blood supply], aneurysm, stress, or electrolyte imbalance)
- Edema and weight gain (right ventricular failure)
- Postural hypotension with dizziness and lightheadedness upon standing (intravascular volume depletion from diuretic therapy)

Patients with valvular disease may have symptoms of heart failure, dysrhythmias, and chest discomfort.

When a patient is experiencing chest discomfort, questions should focus on differentiating a serious, life-threatening condition such as myocardial infarction from conditions that are less serious or that would be treated in a different manner. Not all chest discomfort is related to myocardial ischemia (inadequate blood flow to the heart). Table 26-1 summarizes the characteristics and patterns of the more common cardiac and noncardiac causes of chest pain. There are some important points to remember, however, when evaluating chest discomfort:

- There is little correlation between the severity of the chest discomfort and the gravity of its cause. Some patients, such as the elderly or those with diabetes, may not experience pain with angina or myocardial infarction. Fatigue may be the predominant symptom.
- There is poor correlation between the location of chest discomfort and its source.
- The patient may have more than one clinical problem occurring simultaneously.
- In a patient with a history of atherosclerotic coronary artery disease, it is assumed that the chest discomfort is secondary to ischemia until proven otherwise.

To facilitate the gathering of subjective information for a cardiovascular health history, the patient is questioned as indicated below. It is important to individualize the questions for each patient, however, and to pursue areas where further clarification is necessary.

Breathing
- Are you ever short of breath?
- When do you become short of breath?
- How do you make your breathing better?
- What makes it worse?
- How long has shortness of breath been a problem?
- What essential activities are you no longer able to do because of your breathing?
- Are you on any medication to improve your breathing?
- Does any medication you are taking affect your breathing?
- What time of day do you prefer to take your medication?

Circulation
- Describe the discomfort that you have in your chest.*
- Does the pain spread to your arms, neck, jaw, or back?
- Is there anything that seems to cause the pain?
- How long does the pain usually last?
- What relieves the discomfort?
- Have you gained or lost any weight recently?
- Have you noticed any swelling of your hands, feet, or legs (or sacrum, if bedridden)?
- Do you ever feel dizzy or lightheaded? Under what circumstances does this occur?
- Have you noticed any changes in your energy level? Fatigue level?
- Do you ever feel as if your heart is racing, skipping beats, or pounding?
- Have you had problems with your blood pressure?
- Do you have headaches? What seems to cause them?
- Have you noticed that your hands or feet get unusually cold? When does this seem to happen?

Urination
- Is the amount of your urine output normal for you?
- Do you ever get up at night to use the bathroom? How many times? When did you notice the change?
- Do you take a diuretic? When do you take it?

Mentation
- Do you think as fast as you used to? As clearly?
- Do you laugh or cry more easily than before?
- When did you notice the change?
- Are you taking any medication that might affect your thinking?

When the patient's condition permits, other functional areas are also assessed.

Information obtained in the health history is needed to plan individualized care while the patient is hospitalized, to aid in discharge planning, and to provide education appropriate for helping the patient to meet whatever needs exist

*Because patients do not always admit to having chest "pain," word equivalents of pain are used when eliciting the quality of discomfort. Common descriptions used by patients include strangling, constriction, tightness, aching, squeezing, pressing, heaviness, expanding sensation, choking in throat, indigestion, and burning.

TABLE 26-1 Assessment of Chest Pain

	Character, Location, and Radiation	Duration	Precipitating Events	Relieving Measures
ANGINA PECTORIS 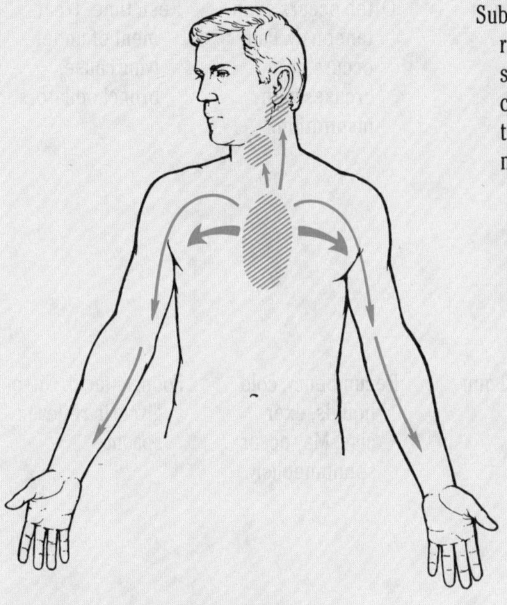	Substernal or retrosternal pain spreading across chest. May radiate to inside of arm, neck, or jaws.	5–15 min	Usually related to exertion, emotion, eating, cold.	Rest, nitroglycerin, oxygen
MYOCARDIAL INFARCTION 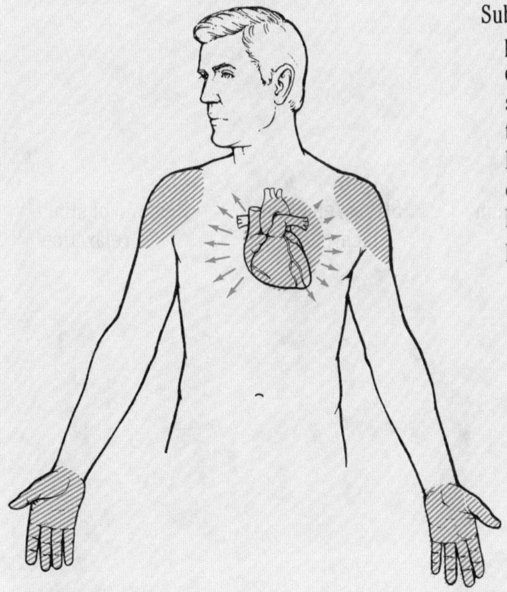	Substernal pain or pain over precordium. May spread widely throughout chest. Painful disability of shoulders and hands may be present.	>15 min	Occurs spontaneously but may be sequela to unstable angina.	Morphine sulfate, successful reperfusion of blocked coronary artery
PERICARDITIS 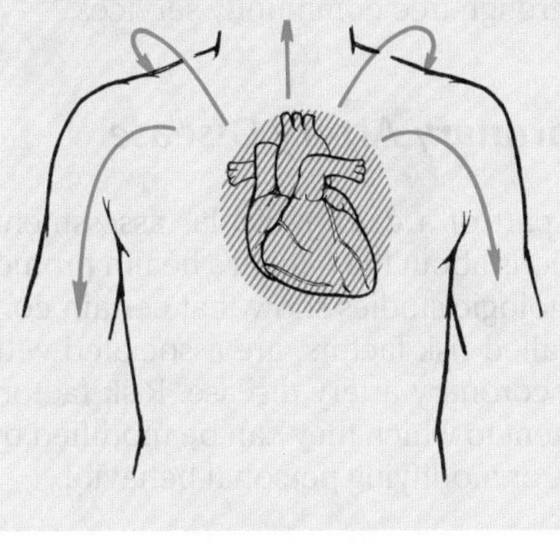	Sharp, severe substernal pain or pain to the left of sternum. May be felt in epigastrium and may be referred to neck, arms, and back.	Intermittent	Sudden onset. Pain increases with inspiration, swallowing, coughing, and rotation of trunk.	Sitting upright, analgesia, anti-inflammatory medications

(continued)

TABLE 26-1 *(continued)*

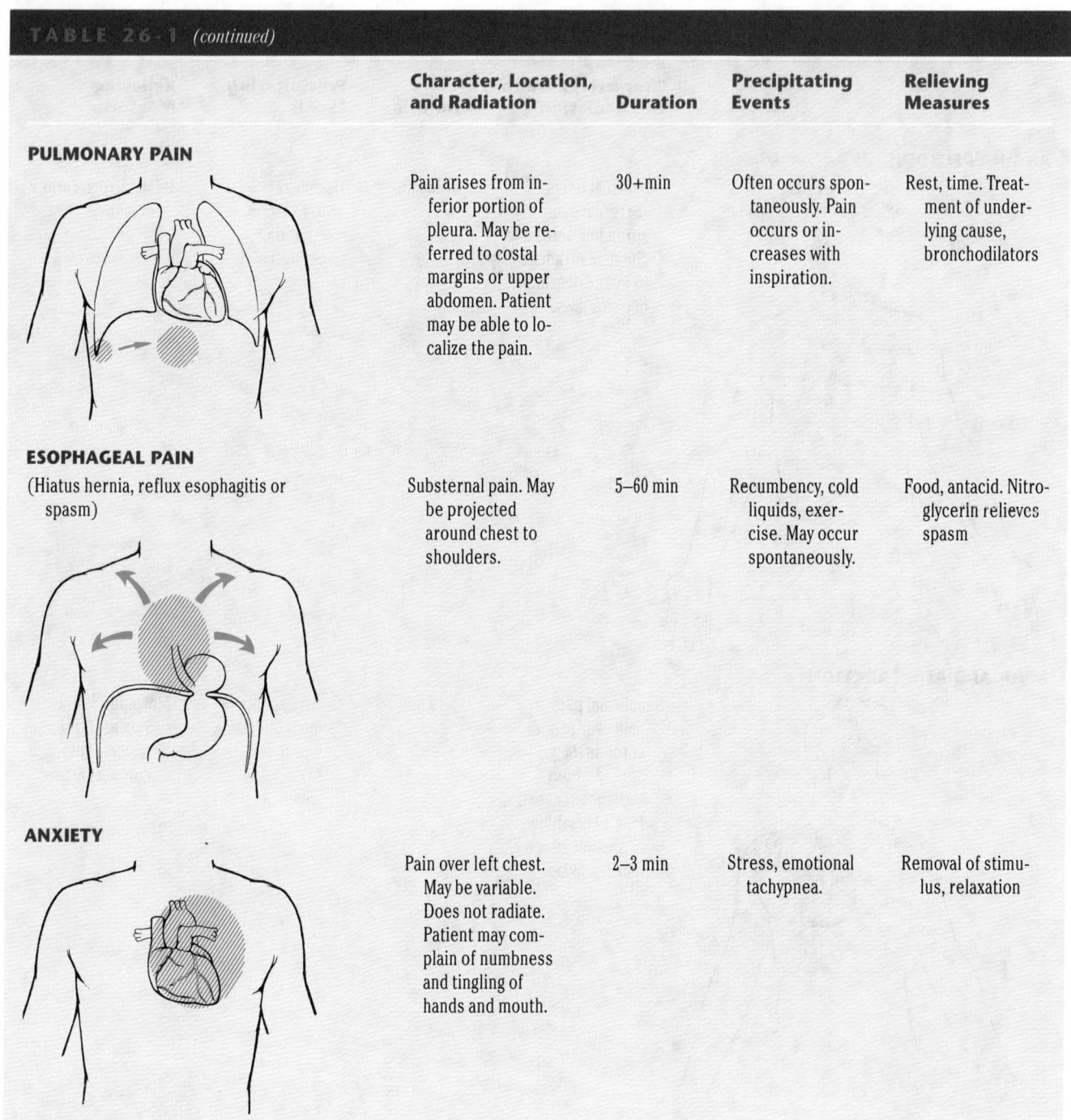

	Character, Location, and Radiation	Duration	Precipitating Events	Relieving Measures
PULMONARY PAIN 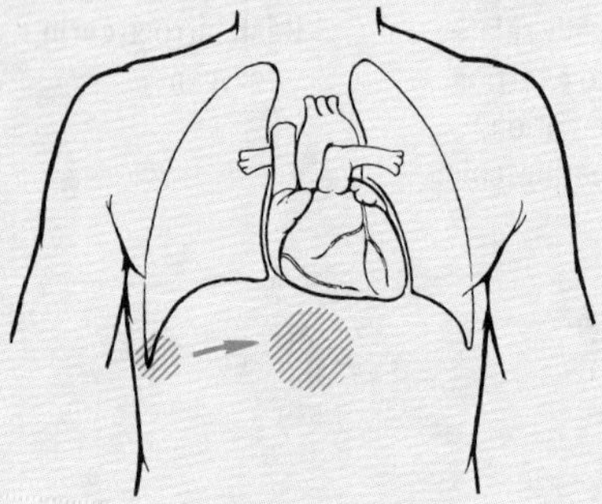	Pain arises from inferior portion of pleura. May be referred to costal margins or upper abdomen. Patient may be able to localize the pain.	30+min	Often occurs spontaneously. Pain occurs or increases with inspiration.	Rest, time. Treatment of underlying cause, bronchodilators
ESOPHAGEAL PAIN (Hiatus hernia, reflux esophagitis or spasm) 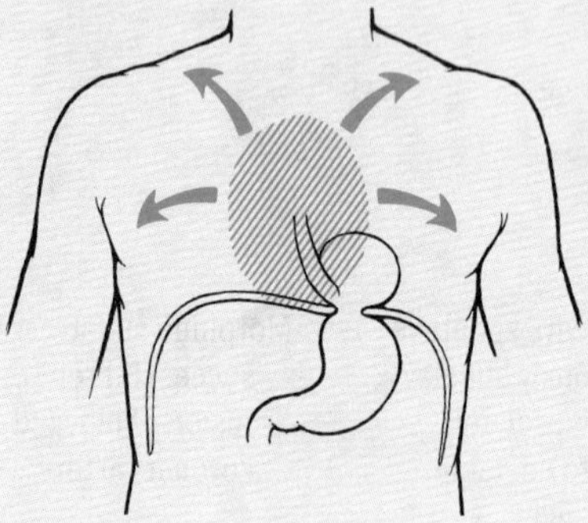	Substernal pain. May be projected around chest to shoulders.	5–60 min	Recumbency, cold liquids, exercise. May occur spontaneously.	Food, antacid. Nitroglycerin relieves spasm
ANXIETY 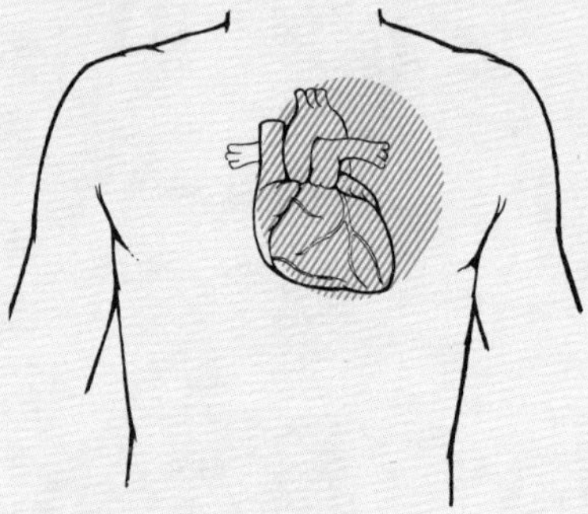	Pain over left chest. May be variable. Does not radiate. Patient may complain of numbness and tingling of hands and mouth.	2–3 min	Stress, emotional tachypnea.	Removal of stimulus, relaxation

upon return to the home setting. Knowing how the patient perceives the effects of the disease process on activities of daily living will help to identify specific aims for cardiac rehabilitation or strategies for modifying certain activities.

Because dietary modification (reducing intake of sodium, saturated fat, or calories) probably will be prescribed, the history should include the following: food preferences (including cultural or ethnic), eating habits (canned or commercially prepared foods versus fresh foods, and restaurant cooking versus home cooking), who shops for groceries, and who prepares the meals. Knowledge of the patient's financial status assists the nurse in planning an affordable therapeutic regimen—one that includes, for example, economical options for healthy eating, exercise, and obtaining education through free community services.

Risk Factors in Coronary Artery Disease

The health history, as part of a cardiovascular assessment, needs to include questions about the patient's health promotion practices. Epidemiologic studies show that certain conditions or behaviors, called risk factors, are associated with a greater incidence of coronary artery disease. Risk factors are classified by the extent to which they can be modified by changing one's lifestyle or modifying personal behavior.

Nonmodifiable risk factors include the following:

- Positive family history for heart problems
- Increasing age
- Gender (men at greater risk than premenopausal women)
- Race (higher incidence in African-Americans than in Caucasians)

Modifiable risk factors include the following:

- Elevated blood cholesterol
- Elevated blood pressure
- Cigarette smoking
- Elevated blood glucose (diabetes mellitus)
- Obesity
- Physical inactivity
- Stress
- Use of oral contraceptives

Assessment of these risk factors is an important and necessary part of cardiovascular assessment. Detailed discussion of these risk factors is presented in Chapter 28.

Primary Prevention

Effective patient teaching requires that the nurse have an adequate knowledge base supported by data from current research studies about risk factors. After effectively educating the patient about risk factors, the nurse assists the patient in setting realistic goals for modifying the risk factors. Although there is not complete agreement among health professionals about the effectiveness of modifying risk factors in patients with known coronary artery disease, it is generally accepted that making healthy changes (*e.g.*, reducing dietary fat intake and exercising regularly) promotes overall good health.

Physical Assessment

Assessing for physical findings is performed to confirm data obtained in the health history. Baseline information is obtained on admission. For the acutely ill cardiac patient, physical examination is performed with routine vital signs (every 4 hours, or more frequently if indicated). Because nurses in acute care settings spend 24 hours a day with the patient, they are in the best position to identify any changes that may occur. Changes must be detected early, before serious complications develop. These changes are reported to the physician and noted in detail in the patient's chart.

In addition to assessing the patient's appearance, a cardiac physical assessment should include an evaluation of the following:

- Effectiveness of the heart as a pump
- Filling volumes and pressures
- Cardiac output
- Compensatory mechanisms

Factors that indicate that the heart is not contracting sufficiently or functioning effectively as a pump include: reduced pulse pressure, cardiac enlargement, and the presence of murmurs and gallop rhythms (abnormal heart sounds).

The amount of blood filling the atria and ventricles and the resulting pressures (called filling volumes and pressures) are estimated by the degree of jugular vein distention (JVD) and the presence or absence of congestion in the lungs, peripheral edema, and postural changes in blood pressure that occur when the person sits up or stands.

Cardiac output is reflected by heart rate, pulse pressure, peripheral vascular resistance, urine output, and central nervous system manifestations.

Examples of compensatory mechanisms that help maintain cardiac output are increased filling volumes and elevated heart rate. Note that findings on physical examination are correlated with data obtained from diagnostic procedures, such as invasive hemodynamic monitoring, which will be discussed later in this chapter.

The order of examination proceeds logically from head to toe, and with practice can be performed in about 10 minutes: (1) general appearance, (2) blood pressure, (3) pulse, (4) hands, (5) head and neck, (6) heart, (7) lungs, (8) abdomen, and (9) feet and legs.

General Appearance

The patient's level of distress is observed. Level of consciousness is noted and described. It is particularly important to evaluate the ability of the patient to think logically as a way of determining if an adequate supply of oxygen is reaching the brain (cerebral perfusion). Family members who are most familiar with the patient can be helpful in alerting the examiner to subtle behavioral changes. The patient's anxiety level is noted, along with any effects these emotional factors may have on cardiovascular status. The nurse attempts to put the anxious patient at ease throughout the examination.

Examination of Blood Pressure

Blood pressure is the pressure exerted on the walls of the arteries. It is affected by factors such as cardiac output, distention of the arteries, and the volume, velocity, and thickness (viscosity) of the blood. Blood pressure occurs as a cyclic phenomenon. The peak pressure occurs when the ventricles are contracting and is called systolic pressure. Diastolic pressure is the lowest pressure, which occurs when the ventricles are resting. Blood pressure usually is expressed as the ratio of the systolic pressure over the diastolic pressure, with normal adult values ranging from 100/60 to 140/90. The average normal blood pressure usually cited is 120/80.

Pulse Pressure. The difference between the systolic and the diastolic pressures is called the **pulse pressure**. Normally, this amounts to approximately 40 mm Hg. An increase in blood pressure is called **hypertension**; a decrease is called **hypotension**. When only the systolic pressure is elevated (systolic hypertension), a widening of the pulse pressure results. This happens in atherosclerosis (hardening of the arteries) and in thyrotoxicosis. Elevation of the diastolic pressure is always associated with elevation of the systolic pressure. An increase in the diastolic pressure to 95 mm Hg gives rise to concern, particularly in younger patients; an increase in excess of 95 mm Hg in the diastolic pressure constitutes true hypertension and requires investigation and control.

Blood Pressure Measurement. Blood pressure can be measured directly or indirectly. In the direct method an arterial catheter is inserted into an artery, as discussed later in this chapter. The indirect measurement is performed with a sphygmomanometer and a stethoscope. The sphygmomanometer consists of an inflatable cuff and a pressure gauge that communicates with the hollow portion of the cuff. The device is calibrated in such a manner that the pressure read on the manometer is comparable to the pressure in millimeters of mercury that is being transmitted to the brachial artery. The cuff is wrapped snugly and smoothly around the upper arm and is inflated by a bulb. Pressure on the cuff is increased until the radial or brachial pulse disappears. The disappearance of the pulse signifies that systolic blood pressure has been exceeded and the brachial artery is occluded. The cuff is then inflated 20 to 30 mm Hg above the point at which radial pulsation disappears. The cuff is slowly deflated, and the reading is made either by auscultation or palpation. Auscultation enables a more accurate measurement of systolic and diastolic pressure.

To **auscultate the blood pressure**, the bell or diaphragm* of the stethoscope is placed over the brachial artery, just below the crease of the elbow (antecubital space), which is the point at which the brachial artery emerges from the two heads of the biceps muscle. The cuff is deflated by 2 to 3 mm Hg per second, while one listens for the onset of tapping sounds, which indicate the systolic blood pressure. These sounds, known as **Korotkoff sounds**, coincide with the heart beat, and will continue to emanate from the brachial artery until the pressure in the cuff has been reduced below diastolic pressure. At that point, the sound ceases. In actual practice, the sound more often becomes muffled (changes character) as diastolic pressure is reached and then disappears at approximately 10 mm Hg below normal diastolic pressure.

The disappearance of the sounds is closer to the true diastolic pressure. If there is greater than 10 mm Hg between the muffled sound and when it disappears, the blood pressure is recorded as a **tripartite pressure**, *e.g.*, 120/80/60, which implies that the sound became muffled at 80 mm Hg and disappeared at 60 mm Hg.

Sometimes, a temporary disappearance of sound occurs when auscultating the blood pressure. This is called an **auscultatory gap**. For example, Korotkoff sounds may be heard at 170 mm Hg, disappear at 150, return at 130, and disappear at 90. This patient has a 20-point auscultatory gap. It is common in patients with high blood pressure or severe aortic stenosis (narrowing of the valve opening between the left ventricle and the aorta, reducing the flow of blood into the aorta).

Palpation of blood pressure is similar to the procedure described above. When the cuff is deflated, the radial or brachial pulse is palpated. The reading at which the pulse returns is the systolic pressure. Palpation is used when the blood pressure is difficult to hear. However, with palpation the diastolic pressure cannot be accurately determined.

*The bell is better than the diaphragm in hearing the low-frequency Korotkoff sounds. In practice, however, the diaphragm is effective for blood pressure reading and is often used as well.

Cuff Size. Accurate recording of the blood pressure depends on using a cuff that is the appropriate size for the patient. If the cuff is too large for the arm, as with a child, the pressure reading will be substantially below the true pressure. If the cuff is too small, as with using a standard adult cuff on obese persons, the pressure reading will be higher than the true pressure. The patient may appear to be hypertensive when the actual pressure is normal. Special cuffs are manufactured for various arm circumferences.

Bilateral Readings. Initially, blood pressure is measured in both the right and the left arms. If a difference is found, the readings are reported to the physician and recorded. Subsequent measurements are taken on the arm with the higher pressure. If there is great difficulty in measuring the blood pressure in either arm, blood pressure also can be obtained in the lower extremities using an extrawide cuff.

Summary Points. Several important details must be observed to ensure the accurate assessment of blood pressure:

- Cuff size must be appropriate for the patient.
- Cuff is firmly wrapped around the arm, and cuff bladder is centered over the brachial artery.
- Patient's arm should be at heart level.
- Initial recordings are made on both arms, and subsequent measurements are taken on the arm with the higher pressure. Normally, in the absence of disease of the vasculature, there is no more than a difference of 5 mm Hg between arm pressures.
- Position of the patient and site of blood pressure measurement (*e.g.*, RA for right arm) are recorded.
- Palpation of the systolic pressure before auscultation helps to note an auscultatory gap more readily.
- The patient is asked not to talk during blood pressure measurements. Researchers have found a significant increase in blood pressure and heart rate when subjects are talking.

Pulse Pressure. Pulse pressure (difference between systolic and diastolic pressures) reflects stroke volume, ejection velocity, and systemic vascular resistance. Pulse pressure may serve as a noninvasive indicator of the patient's ability to maintain cardiac output. If the pulse pressure in the cardiac patient falls below 30 mm Hg, further assessment of the patient's cardiovascular status may be indicated.

Postural Blood Pressure Changes

Postural (orthostatic) hypotension occurs when the blood pressure drops significantly after an upright posture is assumed; it usually is accompanied by dizziness, lightheadedness, or syncope. Although there are many causes of postural hypotension, the three most commonly seen in the cardiac patient are a reduced amount of fluid or blood in the circulatory system (intravascular volume depletion); inadequate vasoconstrictor mechanisms; and insufficient autonomic effect on vascular constriction. Postural changes in blood pressure, along with appropriate history, can help the clinician differentiate between these causes. The following steps are important when assessing postural blood pressure changes:

- Position the patient supine and as flat as symptoms permit for 10 minutes before taking the initial blood pressure and heart rate measurements.
- Always check supine measurements before checking upright measurements.
- Always record both heart rate and blood pressure and indicate the corresponding position (*e.g.*, lying = o+; sitting = ⚲; standing = ♀)
- Do not remove the blood pressure cuff between position changes, but do check to see that it is still correctly placed.
- Assess postural blood pressure changes with the patient sitting on the edge of the bed with feet dangling and, if necessary, with the patient standing at the side of the bed.
- Wait 1 to 3 minutes after each postural change before recording blood pressure and heart rate.
- Be alert for any signs or symptoms of patient distress and, if necessary, return the patient to bed before test completion.
- Record any signs or symptoms that accompany the postural change.

Normal postural responses that occur when a person stands up or goes from a lying to a sitting position include (1) a heart rate of 15 to 20 beats above the resting rate (to offset reduced stroke volume and maintain cardiac output), (2) a drop in systolic pressure of up to 15 mm Hg, and (3) a slight drop to an increase of 5 to 10 mm Hg in diastolic pressure.

A decrease in the amount of blood or fluid in the circulatory system should be suspected after diuretic therapy or bleeding when a postural change results in an increased heart rate and either a decrease in systolic pressure by 15 mm Hg or a drop in the diastolic pressure by 10 mm Hg. Vital signs alone will not help differentiate between a decrease in intravascular volume or inadequate constriction of the blood vessels as a cause of postural hypotension. With intravascular volume depletion, the reflexes that maintain cardiac output (increased heart rate and peripheral vasoconstriction) will function correctly; the heart rate will increase and the peripheral vessels will constrict. But because of lost volume, the blood pressure falls. With inadequate vasoconstrictor mechanisms, the heart rate again responds appropriately but, because of diminished peripheral vasoconstriction, the blood pressure drops. The following is an example of a postural blood pressure recording showing either intravascular volume depletion or inadequate vasoconstrictor mechanisms:

	Blood Pressure	Heart Rate
Lying down o+	120/70	70
Sitting ⚲	100/55	90
Standing ♀	98/52	94

In autonomic insufficiency, the heart rate is unable to increase to compensate for the gravitational effects of an upright posture. Peripheral vasoconstriction may be absent or diminished. The presence of autonomic insufficiency does not rule out a concurrent decrease in intravascular volume. The following is an example of autonomic insufficiency as demonstrated by postural blood pressures changes:

	Blood Pressure	Heart Rate
Lying down o+	150/90	60
Sitting ⚲	100/60	60

Examination of the Pulse

In examining the pulse, the factors to be evaluated are rate, rhythm, quality, configuration of the pulse wave, and quality of the vessel itself.

Pulse Rate. The normal pulse rate varies from a low of 50 in healthy, athletic, young adults to rates well in excess of 100 after exercise or during times of excitement. Anxiety frequently elevates the pulse rate during the physical examination. If the rate is higher than expected, it is appropriate to reassess it near the end of the physical examination, at a time when the examiner has established better rapport with the patient.

Pulse Rhythm. The rhythm of the pulse is as important to assess as the pulse rate. Minor variations in the regularity of the pulse are normal. The pulse rate, particularly in young people, increases during inspiration and slows during expiration. This is called sinus dysrhythmia.

For the initial cardiac examination or if the pulse rhythm is irregular, the heart rate should be counted by auscultating the apical pulse for a full minute while simultaneously palpating the radial pulse.

Any discrepancy between contractions heard and pulses felt is noted. Disturbances of rhythm (dysrhythmias) often result in a **pulse deficit**, a difference between the apical rate (heart rate heard at the apex of the heart) and the peripheral rate. Pulse deficits commonly occur with atrial fibrillation, atrial flutter, premature ventricular contractions, and varying degrees of heart block. See Chapter 27 for a detailed discussion of these dysrhythmias.

An understanding of the complexity of dysrhythmias that may be encountered during the examination requires a sophisticated knowledge of cardiac electrophysiology, knowledge usually possessed by the nurse who specializes in cardiovascular nursing.

Pulse Quality. The quality, or amplitude, of the pulse can be described as normal, diminished, or absent. Some authorities suggest a numerical classification based on a 0 to 4 scale:

0—absence of pulsation
+1—marked impairment of pulsation
+2—moderate impairment of pulsation
+3—slight impairment of pulsation
+4—normal pulsation

Numerical classification is quite subjective; thus, when writing down the pulse quality, it is helpful to specify the scale range (*e.g.*, left radial +3/+4).

Pulse Configuration. The configuration, or contour, of the pulse frequently conveys important information. In stenosis of the aortic valve, in which the valve opening is narrowed, reducing the amount of blood ejected into the aorta, the pulse pressure is narrow and the pulse feels feeble. With aortic insufficiency, in which the aortic valve does not close completely, allowing blood to flow back or leak from the aorta into the left ventricle, the rise of the pulse wave is abrupt and its fall is precipitous—a "collapsing" pulse. The true configuration of the pulse is best appreciated by palpating over the carotid artery rather than the distal radial artery, because the dramatic characteristics of the pulse wave may be distorted when the pulse is transmitted to smaller vessels.

Vessel Quality. The condition of the vessel wall also influences the pulse and is of concern, especially in older patients. Once rate and rhythm have been determined, the quality of the vessel is assessed by palpating along the radial artery and comparing it with normal vessels. Does it appear to be thickened? Is it tortuous?

To assess peripheral circulation, locate and evaluate all arterial pulses. Arterial pulses are palpated at points where the arteries are near the skin surface and are easily compressible against bones or firm musculature. Pulses are detected over the temporal, carotid, brachial, radial, femoral, popliteal, dorsalis pedis, and posterior tibial arteries. A reliable assessment of the pulses of the lower extremities depends on accurately identifying the location of the artery and carefully palpating the area (see Fig. 31-2). Light palpation is essential. Firm finger pressure can easily obliterate the dorsalis pedis and posterior tibial pulses and confuse the examiner. In approximately 10% of the population, the dorsalis pedis pulses are not palpable. In such circumstances, both are usually absent together, and the posterior tibial arteries alone provide adequate blood supply to the feet.

Hands

In the cardiac patient, the following are the most important findings to note when examining the upper extremities:

- **Peripheral cyanosis**, in which the skin has a bluish tinge, implies decreased flow rate of blood in the periphery, allowing more time for the hemoglobin molecule to become desaturated. This may occur normally with the peripheral vasoconstriction associated with a cold environment, or pathologically in conditions that reduce blood flow, for example, cardiogenic shock.
- **Pallor** can denote anemia or an increased systemic vascular resistance.
- **Capillary refill time** provides the basis for estimating the rate of peripheral blood flow. To test capillary refill, briefly compress the tip of the finger and then release quickly. Normally, reperfusion occurs almost instantaneously as evidenced by a return of color to the finger. More sluggish reperfusion indicates a slower peripheral flow rate, as may occur in heart failure.
- **Hand temperature and moistness** are controlled by the autonomic nervous system. Normally hands are warm and dry. Under stress, they may be cool and moist. In cardiogenic shock, hands become cold and clammy due to stimulation of the sympathetic nervous system and resulting vasoconstriction.
- **Edema** stretches the skin and makes it less pliable.
- **Reduced skin turgor** occurs with dehydration and aging.
- **Clubbing of the fingers and toes** implies chronic hemoglobin desaturation, as in congenital heart disease.

Head and Neck

Examining the head as part of a cardiovascular assessment primarily involves assessing the lips and earlobes for peripheral cyanosis or blueness. Peripheral cyanosis is a result of reduced blood flow to the periphery. More oxygen is extracted from the hemoglobin, resulting in a bluish color.

An estimate of right heart function can be made by observing the pulsations of the jugular veins of the neck. This provides a means of estimating central venous pressure, which reflects right atrial or right ventricular end-diastolic pressure (the pressure immediately preceding the contraction of the right ventricle).

Jugular vein distention is caused by increased filling volume and pressure on the right side of the heart. Jugular vein pressure is measured as follows:

- Begin with the patient supine, with the head of the examination table or bed elevated 15 to 30 degrees.
- See that the patient's head is turned slightly away from the side of the neck that is being examined.
- Identify the external jugular vein.
- Locate the pulsations of the internal jugular vein. (Distinguish these pulsations from those of the adjacent carotid artery.)
- Identify the highest point at which the internal jugular vein pulsations can be seen.
- Using a centimeter ruler, measure the vertical distance between this point and the sternal angle (Fig. 26-6).
- Record the distance in centimeters and indicate the angle at which the patient was lying (*e.g.*, "The internal jugular vein pulse is 5 cm above the sternal angle, with the head elevated to 30 degrees").
- Measurements greater than 3 to 4 cm above the sternal angle are considered elevated.

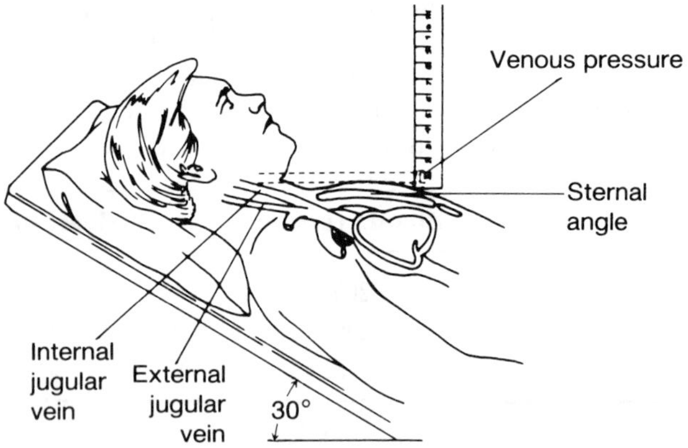

FIGURE 26-6. An assessment of jugular venous pressure. The highest point at which jugular vein pulsations can be seen is noted. The vertical distance between this point and the sternal angle is measured and recorded as centimeters above or below the sternal angle.

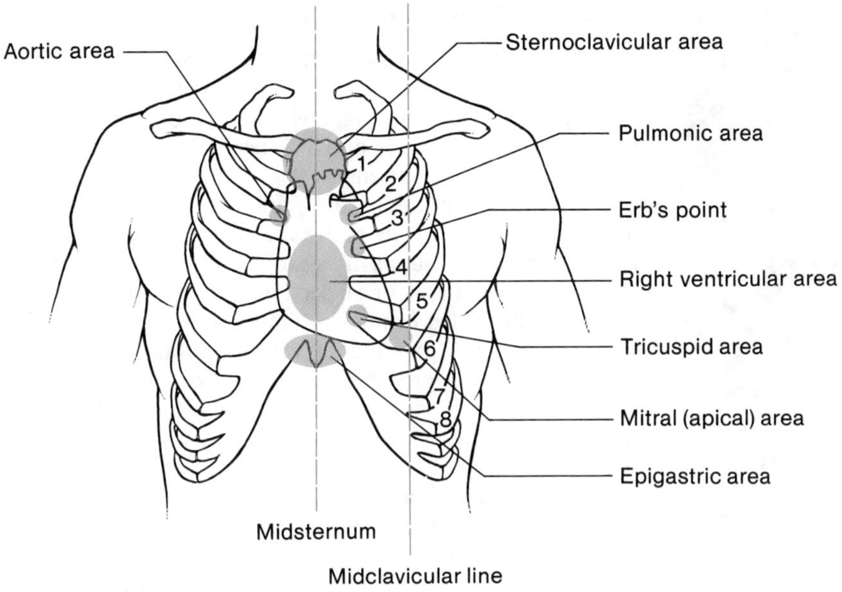

FIGURE 26-7. Areas of the precordium to be assessed when evaluating heart function.

When the internal jugular veins are difficult to see, the pulsations of the external jugular veins can be noted. These are more superficial and visible just above the clavicles adjacent to the sternocleidomastoid muscles. They are frequently distended while the patient lies supine on the examining table or bed. As the patient's head is elevated, the distention of the veins will disappear. The veins are not normally apparent if the head of the bed or examining table is elevated more than 30 degrees.

Obvious distention of the veins with the patient's head elevated 45 to 90 degrees indicates an abnormal increase in the volume of the venous system. This is associated with right-sided cardiac failure or, less commonly, with obstruction of blood flow in the superior vena cava, and although a rare event, acute massive pulmonary embolism.

Heart

The heart is examined indirectly by inspection, palpation, percussion, and auscultation of the chest wall. A systematic approach is the cornerstone of a thorough assessment. Examination of the chest wall is performed in the following six areas (Fig. 26-7).

1. Aortic area—second intercostal space* to the right of the sternum
2. Pulmonary area—second intercostal space to the left of the sternum
3. Erb's point—third intercostal space to the left of the sternum
4. Right ventricular or tricuspid area—fourth and fifth intercostal spaces to the left of the sternum
5. Left ventricular or apical area—fifth intercostal space to the left of the sternum
6. Epigastric area—below the xiphoid process

For the majority of the examination, the patient is supine, with his or her head slightly elevated. The right-handed examiner is positioned at the right side of the patient and the left-handed examiner is at the left side.

Inspection and Palpation

In a systematic fashion, each area of the precordium is inspected and then palpated. Oblique lighting is used to assist the examiner in identifying subtle pulsation. There is a normal impulse that is distinct and well localized directly over the apex of the heart; it may be observed in young persons and in older persons who are thin. This is called the **apical impulse** or **point of maximal impulse (PMI)** and is normally located in the left fifth intercostal space in the mid-clavicular line. The PMI is auscultated in this area (Fig. 26-8).

The apical impulse can often be palpated. It normally is felt as a light pulsation, 1 to 2 cm in diameter. It is felt at the onset of the first heart sound and lasts only half of systole. (See next section for discussion of heart sounds.) The palm of the hand is used initially to locate the apical impulse, and the finger pads are used to describe its size and quality. If the apical impulse is broad and forceful, it is often referred to as a **left ventricular heave** or lift. It is so named because it appears to "lift" the hand from the chest wall during palpation.

- Abnormal PMI. If the PMI is below the 5th intercostal space or lateral to the midclavicular line, the cause is left ventricular enlargement from left ventricular failure. Normally, the PMI is palpable in only one intercostal space. Palpation of the PMI in two or more adjacent intercostal spaces is indicative of left ventricular enlargement. If the PMI can be palpated in two distinctly separate areas and the pulsation movements

*Note: An accurate method of determining the correct intercostal space is first to locate the angle of Louis (see Fig. 26-7). This is done by locating the bony ridge near the top of the sternum at the junction of the body and the manubrium. From the angle of Louis, the second intercostal space is located by sliding one finger to the left or the right of the sternum. Subsequent intercostal spaces are located from this reference point by palpating down the rib cage.

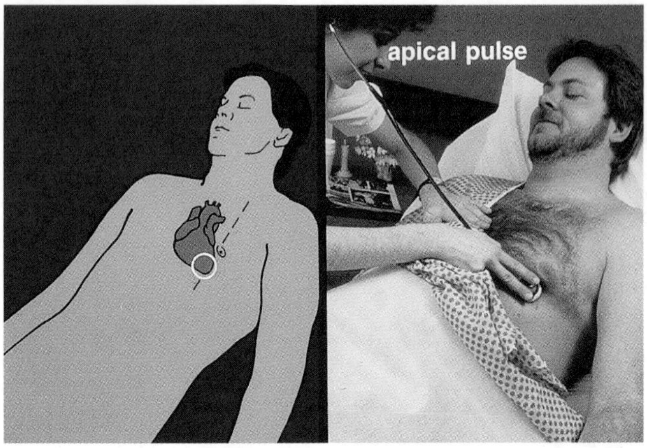

FIGURE 26-8. The apical impulse or point of maximal impulse (PMI) can be auscultated in the left intercostal space in the mid-clavicular line.

are paradoxical (not simultaneous), a ventricular aneurysm should be suspected.

Murmurs, when they are exceptionally loud, also may be palpated and are felt by the palm of the hand as a "purring" sensation. This phenomenon is called a **thrill** and is always indicative of significant pathology within the heart. Thrills also may be palpated over vessels when there is significant, substantial obstruction to blood flow, and will occur over the carotid arteries in the presence of narrowing (or stenosis) of the aortic valve.

Percussion

Normally, only the left border of the heart is detected by percussion. It extends from the sternum to the midclavicular line in the third to fifth intercostal space. The right border lies under the right margin of the sternum and is not detectable. Enlargement of the heart to either the left or right usually can be noted. In many persons who have very thick chests, are obese, or have emphysema, the heart may lie sufficiently far beneath the thoracic surface so that not even its left border can be noted unless the heart is enlarged.

Unless the examiner detects a displaced apical impulse and suspects cardiac enlargement, percussion is omitted.

Auscultation

All areas identified in Figure 26-7, except the epigastric area, are auscultated. These include the aortic area, the pulmonary area, Erb's point, the tricuspid area, and the apical area. The action of the four valves are uniquely reflected at specific locations on the chest wall. These locations do not correspond to the anatomic location of the valve within the chest. Rather, they reflect the patterns by which heart sounds radiate toward the chest wall. Sound in vessels through which blood is flowing is always reflected downstream. For example, actions of the mitral valve are usually heard best in the fifth intercostal space at the midclavicular line. This is called the mitral valve area.

The examiner seeks to identify normal and abnormal heart sounds, which is a sophisticated and challenging process.

Heart Sounds: General Description

The normal heart sounds, S_1 and S_2, are produced primarily by the heart valves closing. The time between S_1 and S_2 corresponds to systole (Fig. 26-9). This is normally shorter than the time between S_2 and S_1 (diastole). As the heart rate increases, diastole shortens.

In normal physiology, the periods of systole and diastole are silent. Pathology of the ventricle, however, can give rise to transient sounds in systole and diastole that are called gallops, snaps, or clicks. Significant pathologic narrowing of the valve orifices at times when they should be open or residual gapping of valves at times when they should be closed give rise to prolonged sounds that are called murmurs. A more detailed description of the various heart sounds follows below, and precedes a summary of the procedure for heart auscultation.

First Heart Sound. The first heart sound (S_1) is created by the simultaneous closure of the mitral and tricuspid valves, although vibration of the myocardial wall also may contribute to this sound. Although heard over the entire precordium, it is heard best at the apex of the heart (mitral area). It is increased in intensity when the valve leaflets are made rigid by calcium in rheumatic heart disease and in any circumstance in which ventricular contraction intervenes at a time when the valve is caught wide open. The latter circumstance will occur, for example, when a premature ventricular contraction interrupts the normal cardiac cycle. The first heart sound varies in intensity from beat to beat when atrial contraction is not synchronous with ventricular contraction. This is because the valve may be fully or partially closed on one beat and quite widely patent or open on the subsequent one as a function of irregular atrial activity. The first heart sound is easily identifiable and serves as the point of reference for the remainder of the cardiac cycle (see Fig. 26-5).

Second Heart Sound. The second heart sound (S_2) is produced by the closing of the aortic and pulmonic valves. Although these two valves close almost simultaneously, the pulmonic valve usually lags slightly behind. Therefore, under certain circumstances, the two components of the second sound may be heard separately (split S_2). The splitting is more likely to be accentuated on inspiration and to disappear on expiration. (More blood is ejected from the right ventricle during inspiration; less blood is ejected during expiration.)

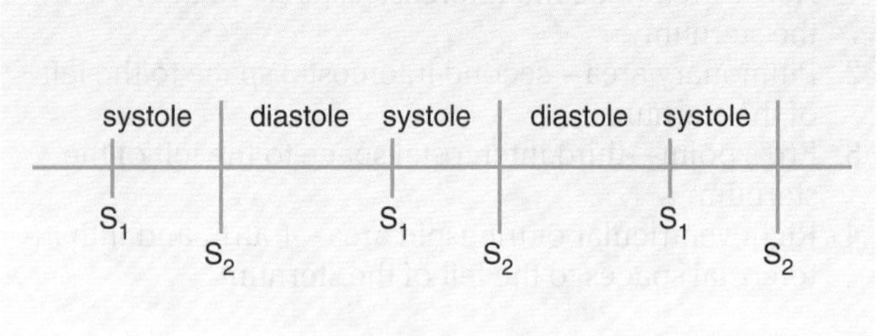

FIGURE 26-9. The normal heart sounds. The first heart sound (S_1) is produced by the simultaneous closing of the mitral and tricuspid valves and is best heard at the apex of the heart (mitral area). The second heart sound (S_2) is produced by the closing of the aortic and pulmonic valves and is heard loudest at the base of the heart. The time between S_1 and S_2 corresponds to systole. The time between S_2 and S_1 is diastole.

S_2 is heard loudest at the base of the heart. The aortic component of the second sound is heard clearly in both the aortic and pulmonic areas, and is heard less clearly at the apex. The pulmonic component of the second sound, if present, may be heard only over the pulmonic area. Thus, one may hear a "single" second heart sound in the aortic area and a split second heart sound in the pulmonic area.

Gallop Sounds. If the blood filling the ventricle is impeded during diastole, as occurs in certain disease states, then a temporary vibration may occur in diastole, similar to, although usually softer than, the first and second heart sounds. Heart sounds then come in triplets and have the acoustical effect of a galloping horse; they are therefore called gallops. This may occur early in diastole, during the rapid-filling phase of the cardiac cycle, or later at the time of atrial contraction.

A gallop sound occurring during rapid ventricular filling is called a third heart sound (S_3) and represents a normal finding in children and young adults (Fig. 26-10). Such a sound is heard in patients who have myocardial disease or in those who are in congestive heart failure and whose ventricles fail to eject all of their blood during systole. An S_3 gallop is heard best with the patient lying on the left side.

Gallop sounds heard during atrial contraction are called fourth heart sounds (S_4) (Fig. 26-11). An S_4 is often heard when the ventricle is enlarged or hypertrophied and therefore resistant to filling. Such a circumstance may be associated with coronary artery disease, hypertension, or stenosis of the aortic valve. On rare occasions all four heart sounds are heard within a single cardiac cycle, giving rise to what is called a quadruple rhythm.

Gallop sounds are very low-frequency sounds and may only be heard with the bell of the stethoscope placed very lightly against the chest. They are heard best at the apex, although occasionally, when emanating from the right ventricle, they may be heard to the left of the sternum.

Snaps and Clicks. Stenosis of the mitral valve resulting from rheumatic heart disease gives rise to an unusual sound very early in diastole that is high-pitched and best heard along the left sternal border. The sound is caused by high pressure in the left atrium with abrupt displacement of a rigid mitral valve. The sound is called an **opening snap**. It occurs too long after the second sound to be mistaken for a split second sound and too early in diastole to be mistaken for a gallop. It almost always is associated with the murmur of mitral stenosis and is specific for this disorder.

In a similar manner, stenosis of the aortic valve gives rise to a short, high-pitched sound immediately after the first heart sound that is called an **ejection click**. This is due to very high pressure within the ventricle, displacing a rigid and calcified aortic valve.

Murmurs. Murmurs are created by the turbulent flow of blood. The causes of the turbulence may be a critically narrowed valve; a malfunctioning valve, which allows regurgitant blood flow; a congenital defect of the ventricular wall or a defect between the aorta and the pulmonary artery; or an increased flow of blood through a normal structure (*e.g.*, with fever, pregnancy, hyperthyroidism).

Murmurs are characterized and consequently described by several characteristics, including timing in the cardiac cycle, location on the chest wall, intensity, pitch, quality, and pattern of radiation.

Timing. The timing of the murmur in the cardiac cycle is vital. First, the examiner determines whether the murmur is occurring in systole or in diastole. Does it begin simultaneously with the first heart sound, or is there some delay between the sound and the beginning of a systolic murmur? Does the murmur continue to (or through) the second heart sound, or is there again delay between the end of the murmur and the occurrence of the second heart sound? Are diastolic murmurs continuous, or do they disappear in mid- or late diastole?

Location. The location of the murmur or where it is detected on the chest wall is critical. Depending on the type of valvular disorder, a murmur can be heard only at the apex or more widely over the chest wall, or along the left sternal border between the third and fourth interspaces.

Intensity. The intensity of murmurs is conventionally graded from I through VI. It is sometimes difficult to hear a grade I murmur. A grade II cardiac murmur should be easily perceived. Murmurs of grades IV or louder are usually associated with thrills that may be palpated on the surface of the chest wall. A grade VI murmur often can be heard with the stethoscope off the chest. A murmur may vary in intensity from its beginning to its conclusion. This is very characteristic of certain valvular disorders.

Pitch. The next important quality of a murmur is its pitch, which may be a low, rumbling sound, often heard only with the bell placed lightly on the chest wall, or a very high-pitched murmur, occasionally "whistling" in character, heard best with the diaphragm. Other murmurs contain the full spectrum of sound frequency and make the murmur appear to be very harsh in quality.

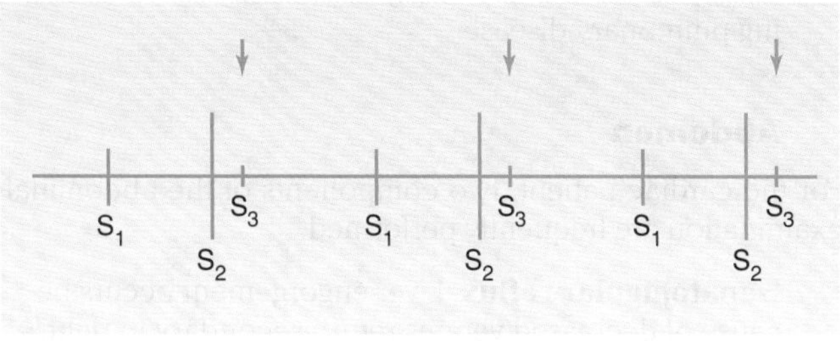

FIGURE 26-10. An S_3 gallop is heard immediately following the S_2 and occurs when the blood filling the ventricle is impeded during diastole, resulting in temporary vibrations. The heart sounds come in triplets and resemble the sound of a galloping horse. Myocardial disease and congestive heart failure are associated with this sound.

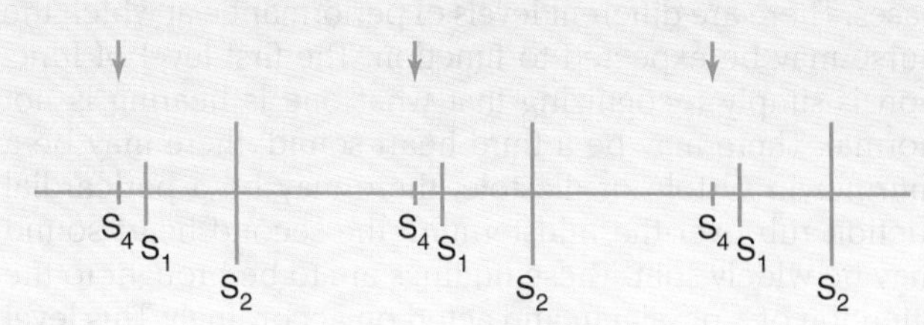

FIGURE 26-11. An S_4 gallop is heard immediately preceding the S_1. The S_4 sound occurs during atrial contraction and is often heard when the ventricle is enlarged or hypertrophied. Associated conditions include coronary artery disease, hypertension, and stenosis of the aortic valve.

Radiation of Sound. The last feature of concern is radiation of the murmur. A murmur can radiate into the axilla, the carotid arteries in the neck, the left shoulder, or the back.

Friction Rub. In pericarditis, a harsh grating sound that can be heard in both systole and diastole is called a friction rub. It is caused by the abrasion of the pericardial surfaces during the cardiac cycle. This may be confused with a murmur; care should be taken to identify the sound when appropriate and to distinguish it from murmurs that may be heard in both systole and diastole. A pericardial friction rub can be heard best using the diaphragm of the stethoscope, with the patient sitting up and leaning forward.

Summary of the Procedure for Auscultation

For auscultation, the patient remains supine and the examining room is as quiet as possible. A stethoscope with a diaphragm and a bell is necessary for accurate auscultation of the heart.

Using the diaphragm, the examiner starts at the apical area and progresses upward along the left sternal border to the pulmonic and aortic areas. If desired, the examiner may choose to begin the examination at the aortic and pulmonic areas and progress downward to the apex of the heart. Initially, S_1 is identified and evaluated with respect to its intensity and splitting. Next, S_2 is identified and its intensity noted. After concentrating on S_1 and S_2, the examiner listens for extra sounds in systole and then in diastole.

Sometimes it is useful to ask oneself the following questions: Do I hear snapping or clicking sounds? Do I hear any high-pitched blowing sounds? Is this sound in systole, or diastole, or both? The examiner again proceeds to move the stethoscope to all of the designated areas of the precordium, listening carefully for these sounds. Finally, the patient is turned on the left side and the stethoscope is placed on the apical area, where an S_3 and a mitral murmur are more readily detected.

If an abnormality is heard, the entire chest surface is reexamined to determine the exact location of the sound and its radiation. It is important to reassure the patient who may be concerned about the prolonged examination. Once the characteristics of each phase of the cycle have been determined, the relationship of one to another and the synthesis of events within the cardiac cycle may be summarized.

Interpretation of Cardiac Sounds

Interpreting cardiac sounds requires detailed knowledge of cardiac physiology and the pathophysiology of cardiac diseases. There are different levels of performance at which the nurse may be expected to function. The first level of function is simply recognizing that what one is hearing is not normal. There may be a third heart sound; there may be a murmur in systole or diastole; there may be a pericardial friction rub over the midsternum; the second heart sound may be widely split. These findings are to be brought to the attention of a physician and acted on accordingly. This level of function is useful in screening. It is the kind of activity involved in performing physical examinations in schools on normal children or in performing routine physical examinations or screening examinations.

The second level of function involves recognizing patterns. The nurse correctly observes the findings and is capable of recognizing the constellation of sounds and the diagnostic significance of common ones. The advanced-practice nurse is skilled in this level of function.

At its most sophisticated level, cardiac diagnosis can be interpretive. Highly skilled nurses can differentiate among dysrhythmias and respond accordingly. They can determine the significance of the appearance and disappearance of gallops during treatment of patients who have had myocardial infarctions or who are in heart failure. This is the role that the coronary care nurse and the cardiovascular clinical nurse specialist assume. They function with a team of other health professionals for whom the fine details of cardiovascular diagnosis have become highly tuned skills.

Other Assessment Parameters

Lungs

The details of respiratory assessment are described in Chapter 22. Findings frequently exhibited by cardiac patients include the following:

- **Tachypnea**. Rapid, shallow breathing may be noted in patients who have heart failure or pain, or who are extremely anxious.
- **Cheyne-Stokes respirations**. Patients in severe left ventricular failure may exhibit Cheyne-Stokes breathing, which is a pattern of rapid respirations alternating with apnea. It is important to note the duration of the apnea.
- **Hemoptysis**. Pink, frothy sputum is indicative of acute pulmonary edema.
- **Cough**. A dry, hacking cough from irritation of small airways is common in patients with pulmonary congestion from heart failure.
- **Crackles**. Heart failure or atelectasis associated with bedrest, splinting from ischemic pain, or the effects of pain medication and sedatives often results in the development of crackles. Typically, crackles are first noted at the bases (because of gravity's effect on fluid accumulation and decreased ventilation of basilar tissue) but may progress to all portions of the lung fields.
- **Wheezes**. Compression of the small airways by interstitial pulmonary edema may cause wheezing. Beta-blocking agents, such as propranolol, may precipitate airway narrowing, especially in patients with underlying pulmonary disease.

Abdomen

For the cardiac patient, two components of the abdominal examination are frequently performed.

- **Hepatojugular reflux**. Liver engorgement occurs because of decreased venous return secondary to right ventricular failure. The liver will be enlarged, firm, nontender, and smooth. Hepatojugular reflux may be demonstrated by pressing firmly over the liver for 30 to 60 seconds and noting a 1-cm rise in jugular vein pressure. This rise indicates an inability of the right side of the heart to accommodate increased volume.

- **Bladder distention**. Urine output is an important indicator of cardiac function; therefore, decreased urine output is a significant finding that must be investigated to determine if the decrease is a result of decreased production of urine (which occurs when renal perfusion is decreased) or if it is due to the inability of the patient to void. The suprapubic area is palpated for an oval-shaped mass and is percussed for dullness indicative of a full bladder.

Feet and Legs

Many patients with heart disease have associated peripheral vascular disease, or peripheral edema secondary to right ventricular failure. Therefore, in all cardiac patients it is important to assess peripheral arterial circulation and venous return. In addition, thrombophlebitis is a complication associated with bedrest and requires careful monitoring. Refer to Chapter 31 for a complete description of these techniques.

Gerontologic Considerations

When a cardiovascular physical examination is performed on an elderly client, a few considerations are noteworthy. Peripheral pulses in an elderly patient can be palpated more readily because of increased hardness of the arteries and a loss of adjacent connective tissue. Palpating the precordium in the elderly is affected by the changes in the shape of the chest. For example, a cardiac impulse may not be palpable in a patient with chronic obstructive pulmonary disease because these patients usually have an increased anterior–posterior diameter of the chest. Kyphoscoliosis, which is a spinal deformity that occurs frequently in elderly patients, may dislocate the cardiac apex downward so that the diagnostic significance of palpating the PMI is obscured.

Systolic blood pressure increases with age, but diastolic blood pressure usually plateaus after 50 years. Conventionally, medication therapy for high blood pressure begins when consistent systolic readings of 160 mm Hg or diastolic readings of 95 mm Hg are observed. For the elderly patient, however, many factors are considered before initiating treatment. Orthostatic hypotension may be present, reflecting a decreasing sensitivity of postural reflexes; this is considered when medication therapy is prescribed.

An S_4 is heard in about 90% of elderly patients, which is thought to be due to decreased compliance of the left ventricle. The S_2 is usually split. Murmurs are present in 60% or more of elderly patients. The most common murmur is a soft systolic ejection murmur due to sclerotic changes of the aortic leaflets.

Diagnostic Tests and Procedures

Diagnostic tests and procedures are used to confirm data obtained by history and examination. Some tests are easy to interpret, but others must be interpreted by expert clinicians. All tests should be explained to the patient. Some necessitate special preparation before they are done and special monitoring by the nurse after the procedure.

Laboratory Tests

Laboratory tests may be requested for the following reasons:

1. To assist in the diagnosis of acute myocardial infarction (angina pectoris, which is chest pain due to an insufficient supply of blood to the heart, cannot be confirmed by either blood or urine studies)
2. To measure abnormalities in blood chemistries that could affect the prognosis of a cardiac patient
3. To assess the degree of the inflammatory process
4. To screen for risk factors associated with the presence of atherosclerotic coronary artery disease
5. To determine baseline values before therapeutic intervention
6. To assess serum levels of medications
7. To assess the effects of medications (*e.g.*, the effects of diuretics on serum potassium levels)
8. To screen generally for any abnormalities. Because many different methods of measurement are used, normal values may differ from one laboratory to the next.

Cardiac Enzymes

Plasma cardiac enzyme analysis is part of a diagnostic profile, including history, symptoms, and electrocardiogram, to diagnose acute myocardial infarction. Enzymes are released from cells when the cells are injured and their membranes rupture. Most enzymes are nonspecific in relation to the particular organ that has been damaged. Certain isoenzymes, however, come only from myocardial cells and are released when the cells are damaged by sustained hypoxia, resulting in infarction. The isoenzymes leak into the interstitial spaces of the myocardium and are carried into the general circulation by the lymph system and the coronary circulation, resulting in elevated blood levels.

Because different enzymes are released into the blood at varying periods after myocardial infarction, it is crucial to evaluate the enzyme level in relation to the time of the onset of chest discomfort or other symptoms. Creatine kinase (CK) and its isoenzyme (CK-MB) are the most specific enzymes analyzed in the diagnosis of acute myocardial infarction, and they are the first enzymes to rise. Lactic dehydrogenase (LDH) and its isoenzymes also are analyzed for patients who have delayed seeking medical attention, because blood levels rise and peak in 2 to 3 days, much later than CK (see Table 28-1 for the time course of cardiac enzymes.)

Blood Chemistries

Lipid Profile. Total cholesterol, triglycerides, and lipoproteins are measured to evaluate a person's risk of developing atherosclerotic disease, especially if there is a positive family history of heart disease, or to diagnose a specific lipoprotein abnormality. Total serum cholesterol that is elevated above 200 mg/ml is one predictor of increased risk of coronary heart disease (CAD). Lipoproteins, which transport cholesterol in the blood, can be analyzed through electrophoresis. High-density lipoprotein (HDL), which takes cholesterol from the peripheral cells and brings it to the liver, has a protective influence. Conversely, low-density lipoproteins (LDL) transport cholesterol to the peripheral cells. Decreased levels of high-density lipoprotein and elevated levels of low-density lipoprotein increase the risk of atherosclerotic coronary artery disease. Although the total cholesterol value remains relatively constant over 24 hours, the measurement of a total lipid profile should be performed after a 12-hour fast. Prolonged stress may increase the total cholesterol.

Serum Electrolytes. Serum electrolytes can affect the prognosis of a patient with acute myocardial infarction or any cardiac condition. **Serum sodium** reflects relative fluid balance. Generally, hyponatremia indicates fluid excess and hypernatremia indicates fluid deficit. **Calcium** is necessary for blood coagulability and neuromuscular activity. Hypocalcemia and hypercalcemia can cause ECG changes and dysrhythmias.

Serum potassium is affected by renal function and may be decreased by diuretic agents that often are used to treat congestive heart failure. A decrease in potassium causes cardiac irritability and predisposes the patient receiving a digitalis preparation to digitalis toxicity and to the development of dysrhythmias. Elevated serum potassium has a myocardial depressant effect and a ventricular irritability effect. Hypokalemia and hyperkalemia each can lead to ventricular fibrillation or cardiac standstill.

Blood Urea Nitrogen. Blood urea nitrogen (BUN) is an end product of protein metabolism and is excreted by the kidneys. In the cardiac patient, elevated BUN could reflect reduced renal perfusion (due to decreased cardiac output) or intravascular fluid volume deficit (due to diuretic therapy).

Glucose. Serum glucose is important to monitor because many cardiac patients also have diabetes mellitus. Serum glucose may be mildly elevated in stressful situations when mobilization of endogenous epinephrine results in conversion of liver glycogen to glucose.

Chest X-ray and Fluoroscopy

A chest x-ray usually is obtained to determine the size, contour, and position of the heart. It reveals cardiac and pericardial calcifications and demonstrates physiologic alterations in the pulmonary circulation. It does not aid in the diagnosis of acute myocardial infarction, but can confirm the presence of some complications (*e.g.*, congestive heart failure). Correct placement of cardiac catheters, such as pacemakers and pulmonary artery catheters, is also confirmed by chest x-ray.

Fluoroscopy provides visual observation of the heart on a luminescent x-ray screen. It shows cardiac and vascular pulsations and is useful in assessing unusual cardiac contours. Fluoroscopy is a useful tool for the placement and positioning of intravenous pacing electrodes and for guiding the catheter insertion in cardiac catheterization.

Electrocardiography

The electrocardiogram (ECG) is a visual representation of the electrical activity of the heart as reflected from various angles to the skin surface.

The ECG is recorded as a tracing on a strip of paper or appears on the screen of an oscilloscope. To facilitate the interpretation of the ECG, data about the patient's age, sex, blood pressure, height, weight, symptoms, and medications (especially digitalis and antidysrhythmic agents) should be noted on the ECG requisition. Electrocardiography is particularly useful in the evaluation of conditions that interfere with normal heart functions, such as disturbances of rate or rhythm, disorders of conduction, enlargement of heart chambers, presence of a myocardial infarction, and electrolyte imbalances. The details of electrocardiography are covered in Chapter 27.

Ambulatory Electrocardiographic Monitoring

Continuous Monitoring. To have a patient's ECG continuously available for assessment, one of the 12 leads can be monitored on an oscilloscope. Two leads commonly used for continuous monitoring are lead II and a modification of V1 (MCL1) (Fig. 26-12). Lead II is selected when it is desirable to have accurate visualization of P waves which represent depolarization of the atria. MCL1 is selected when it is desirable to determine which ventricle is the site of origin of ectopic or abnormal beats. The patient's rhythm is transmitted to the cardiac monitor either by direct contact of the electrode wires to the monitor or by telemetry. With telemetry, the ECG signals are transmitted as radiowaves from a battery-operated transmitter worn by the patient. Patients can walk around the unit while being monitored. Continuous ECG monitoring is part of the standard treatment regimen in critical care units, and is also frequently used on step-down and general nursing units to detect dysrhythmias.

A few guidelines for electrode placement will ensure good conduction and a clear picture of the patient's rhythm on the monitor:

- Clean the skin surface with alcohol and gauze before applying the electrodes. If the patient has much hair where the electrodes need to be placed, shave the area.
- Apply a little benzoin to the skin if the patient is diaphoretic and the electrodes are not adhering well.
- Change the electrodes every 24 to 48 hours and examine the skin for irritation. Apply the electrodes to different locations each time they are changed.
- If the patient is sensitive to the electrodes, use hypoallergenic electrodes.

Portable Tape Recorders. One lead of the ECG can be monitored by a small tape recorder (Holter recorder) and recorded on a continuous (1 to 24 hours) magnetic tape recording. The patient can then be monitored day or night to detect dysrhythmias or evidence of myocardial ischemia during activities of daily living. The tape recorder weighs approximately 2 pounds and can be carried over the shoulder. The patient keeps a diary of activity, noting the

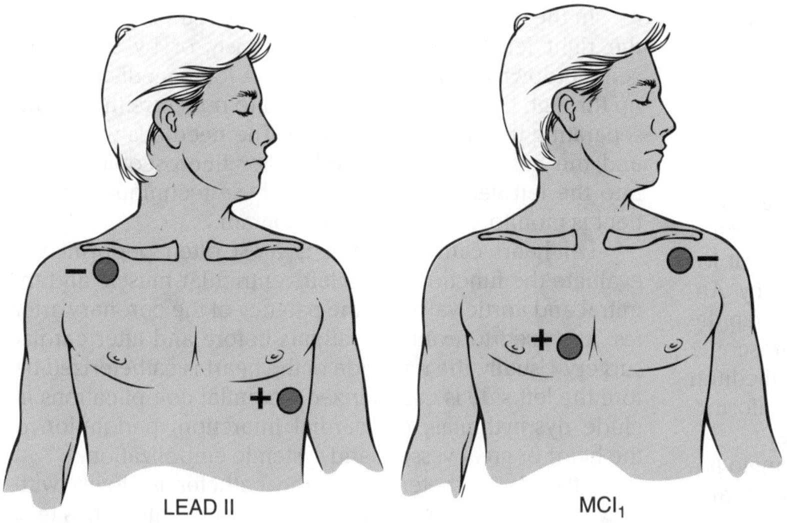

FIGURE 26-12. Two leads commonly used for continuous monitoring. Lead II—the negative electrode is placed on the right upper chest; the positive electrode is placed on the left lower chest. MCL_1—the negative electrode is placed on the left upper chest; the positive electrode is placed in the V_1 position. If a three-electrode system is used, the third electrode, which is the ground electrode, can be placed anywhere on the chest.

time of any symptoms, experiences, or unusual activities performed. The tape recording is then examined (using a specialized instrument called a scanner), analyzed, and interpreted. Evidence obtained in this way is helpful in diagnosing dysrhythmias and myocardial ischemia and in evaluating therapy such as antidysrhythmic and antianginal medications or pacemaker function.

Signal-Averaging ECG. For some patients considered at high risk for sudden cardiac death, a signal-averaged ECG is performed. This high resolution ECG assists in identifying risk for life-threatening dysrhythmias and helps to determine the need for further invasive diagnostic procedures. Signal averaging works by averaging about 150 to 300 QRS waveforms. (QRS waveforms represent depolarization of the ventricle.) The resulting averaged QRS complex is analyzed for certain characteristics that are likely to lead to lethal ventricular dysrhythmias. The recording is performed at the bedside and requires about 15 minutes.

Trans-telephonic Monitoring. Another method of evaluating the ECG of a patient at home is by trans-telephonic monitoring. The patient attaches a specific lead system for transmitting the signals and places a telephone mouthpiece over the transmitter box; the ECG is recorded and evaluated at another location. This method is often used for diagnosing dysrhythmias and in follow-up evaluation of permanent pacemakers.

Exercise Tolerance Testing

Exercise tolerance testing (ETT) is a noninvasive means of assessing certain aspects of cardiac function. By evaluating cardiac action during physical stress, the heart's response to an increased demand for oxygen can be determined. The test is used for the following purposes: (1) to assist in diagnosing the cause of chest pain, (2) to screen for ischemic heart disease, (3) to determine the functional capacity of the heart after an MI or after heart surgery, (4) to assess the effectiveness of antianginal or antidysrhythmia medication therapy, (5) to identify dysrhythmias that occur during physical exercise, and (6) to aid in the development of a physical fitness program.

Exercise tolerance testing may be performed by having the patient walk on a treadmill, pedal a stationary bicycle, or climb a set of stairs. The patient is exercised by increasing walking speed and the incline of the treadmill or by increasing the load against which the bicycle is pedaled. ECG electrodes are applied to the patient, and tracings are made before, during, and after exercise testing. Blood pressure, skin temperature, physical appearance, and the occurrence or worsening of chest pain are monitored closely during and after the test.

The test is continued until a predetermined target is achieved, based on the patient's pretest assessment and on the laboratory's protocols. The test is stopped early if the patient experiences chest pain, extreme fatigue, a drop in blood pressure or pulse rate, malignant ECG changes, or other complications.

The patient is instructed to avoid smoking, eating, and drinking for 4 hours before the test and to wear comfortable shoes suitable for walking. Women are advised to wear a bra that provides adequate support. The patient is instructed to rest after the test for a period and to avoid stimulants, eating, or extreme temperature changes (*e.g.*, hot or cold showers, going out into the cold). Blood pressure and ECG are monitored for 10 to 15 minutes after completion of the test, or until they return to baseline.

Cardiac Catheterization

Cardiac catheterization is an invasive diagnostic procedure in which one or more catheters are introduced into the heart and selected blood vessels to measure pressures in the various heart chambers and to determine oxygen saturation of the blood. By far the most common use of cardiac catheterization is to assess the patency of the patient's coronary arteries and to determine the appropriate treatment, *e.g.*, percutaneous transluminal coronary angioplasty (PTCA) or coronary bypass surgery if atherosclerosis is present (see Chapter 28). During cardiac catheterization the patient's electrocardiogram is monitored by means of an oscilloscope. Because the introduction of the catheter into the heart can induce potentially fatal dysrhythmias, resuscitation equipment must be readily available when the procedure is being performed.

Angiography

Cardiac catheterization is usually performed with angiography, a technique of injecting contrast media into the vascular system to outline the heart and blood vessels. When a particular heart chamber or blood vessel is singled out for study, the procedure becomes selective angiography. Angiography makes use of cineangiograms, a series of rapidly changing films or movies on an intensified fluoroscopic screen that records the passage of the contrast medium through the vascular site(s). The recording of the information allows for comparison of information over time.

Four of the more common sites for selective angiography are the aorta, the coronary arteries, and the right and left sides of the heart.

Aortography. An aortogram is a form of angiography that outlines the lumen of the aorta and the major arteries arising from it. In thoracic aortography, contrast media are used to study the aortic arch and its major branches. The translumbar or retrograde brachial or femoral approach may be used.

Coronary Arteriography. In coronary arteriography a radiopaque catheter is introduced into the right or left brachial or femoral artery and is passed into the ascending aorta and manipulated into the appropriate coronary artery under fluoroscopic control. Coronary arteriography is used to evaluate the degree of atherosclerosis and to determine the mode of treatment. It is also used to study suspected congenital anomalies of the coronary arteries.

Right-Heart Catheterization. Right-heart catheterization involves passing a radiopaque catheter from an antecubital or femoral vein into the right atrium, right ventricle, and pulmonary vasculature. This is performed under direct visualization with a fluoroscope. Pressures within the right atrium are measured and recorded, and blood samples are obtained for measurement of the hematocrit and oxygen saturation. The catheter is then passed through the tricuspid valve, and similar tests are performed on the blood in the right ventricle. Finally, the catheter is introduced into the pulmonary artery (through the pulmonic valve) and as far as possible beyond that point, where capillary samples are obtained and capillary pressures (also known as wedge pressures) are recorded. The catheter is then withdrawn.

- Right-heart catheterization is considered a relatively safe procedure. Potential complications, however, include cardiac dysrhythmias, venous spasm, infection of the insertion site, cardiac perforation, and, rarely, cardiac arrest.

Left-Heart Catheterization. Left-heart catheterization usually is performed by retrograde catheterization of the left ventricle or by transseptal catheterization of the left atrium. In the retrograde technique, the catheter is inserted under direct vision into the right brachial artery (arteriotomy) and advanced under fluoroscopic control into the ascending aorta and into the left ventricle; or the catheter may be introduced percutaneously by puncture of the femoral artery.

In the transseptal approach, the catheter is passed from the right femoral vein (percutaneously or by saphenous vein cutdown) into the right atrium. A long needle is passed up through the catheter and is used to puncture the septum separating the right and left atria. The needle is withdrawn and the catheter is advanced under fluoroscopic control into the left ventricle. In both of these techniques the patient is monitored by electrocardiogram.

Left-heart catheterization is most often performed to evaluate the function of the left ventricular muscle and the mitral and aortic valves or the patency of the coronary arteries. It is used to evaluate patients before and after cardiac surgery. Usually, the right side of the heart is catheterized before the left side is catheterized. Potential complications include dysrhythmias, myocardial infarction, perforation of the heart or great vessels, and systemic embolization.

After the catheterization, the catheter is slowly withdrawn. With the brachial approach, the cutdown site is closed and the area bandaged. With the femoral puncture method, manual pressure is applied until the bleeding is stopped.

Nursing Interventions

Precatheterization nursing responsibilities include the following:

- Instruct the patient to fast, usually for 8 to 12 hours, before the procedure.
- Prepare the patient for the expected duration of the procedure; indicate that it will involve lying on a hard table for about 2 hours.
- Prepare the patient to experience certain sensations during the catheterization. Knowing what to expect can help the patient cope with the experience.

An occasional pounding sensation (palpitation) may be felt in the chest because of extrasystoles that almost always occur, particularly when the catheter tip touches the myocardium. The patient may be asked to cough and breathe deeply, especially after the dye injection. Coughing may help to disrupt a dysrhythmia and help to clear the dye from the arteries. Breathing deeply and holding the breath helps to lower the diaphragm for better visualization of heart structures. The injection of contrast media into either side of the heart may produce a flushed feeling throughout the body and a feeling of voiding, which leaves in a minute or less.

- Encourage the patient to express fears and anxieties. Provide teaching and reassurance to reduce apprehension.
- Prepare the patient for the postcatheterization procedures.

Postcatheterization nursing interventions include the following:

- Observe the puncture (or cutdown) sites for bleeding or hematoma formation, and assess the peripheral pulses in the affected extremity (dorsalis pedis and posterior tibial pulses in the lower extremity, radial pulse in the upper extremity) every 15 minutes for 1 to 2 hours, and then every 1 to 2 hours until stable.

- Evaluate temperature and color of the affected extremity and any patient complaints of pain, numbness, or tingling sensations in the affected extremity to determine signs of arterial insufficiency. Report changes promptly.
- Observe for dysrhythmias by observing the cardiac monitor or by assessing the apical and peripheral pulses for changes in rate and rhythm. A vasovagal reaction, consisting of bradycardia, hypotension, and nausea, can be precipitated by pain or a distended bladder, usually when a femoral site has been used. Prompt intervention is critical, which includes raising the feet and legs above the head, and administering intravenous fluids and sometimes intravenous atropine.
- If the procedure was performed percutaneously through the femoral artery, the patient will need to remain supine with the affected leg straight and the head elevated no more than 30 degrees for several hours. Manual pressure is applied until the bleeding stops. The patient is turned from side to side as needed for comfort. Analgesic medication is administered as prescribed for discomfort at the site.
- Report any complaint of chest discomfort immediately.
- Encourage fluids to increase urinary output and flush out the dye.
- Instruct the patient to ask for help in getting out of bed the first time after prolonged bedrest. Orthostatic hypotension may occur.

Echocardiography

Echocardiography is a noninvasive ultrasound test used to examine the size, shape, and motion of cardiac structures. It involves the transmission of high-frequency sound waves into the heart through the chest wall and the recording of the return signals. The ultrasound is generated by a hand-held transducer applied to the front of the chest. The transducer picks up the echoes, converts them to electrical impulses, and transmits them to the echocardiography machine for display on an oscilloscope and for recording on a videotape. An ECG is recorded simultaneously to time events within the cardiac cycle.

M-mode (motion), the unidimensional mode that was first introduced, provides information about the cardiac structures and their motion. Two-dimensional or cross-sectional echocardiography (Fig. 26-13), an enhancement of the technique, creates a sophisticated, spatially correct image of the heart. Doppler and color flow imaging echocardiography, the most recently developed, allow visualization of the direction and velocity of the blood flow through the heart. All modes continue to be used.

Echocardiography is a safe, noninvasive test that provides information similar in many respects to the data obtained with angiocardiography. It is especially useful in the diagnosis and differentiation of heart murmurs. An echocardiogram can show whether the heart is dilated, the walls or septum are thickened, or pericardial effusion is present. It has also been used to study the motion of prosthetic heart valves.

Transesophageal Echocardiography (TEE). One significant limitation of traditional echocardiography has been the poor quality of images produced. Ultrasound loses its clarity as it passes through tissue, lung, and bone. A more recent echocardiographic technique involves threading a small transducer through the mouth and into the esophagus. This technique, called transesophageal echocardiography (TEE) provides clearer images because ultrasound waves are passing through less tissue.

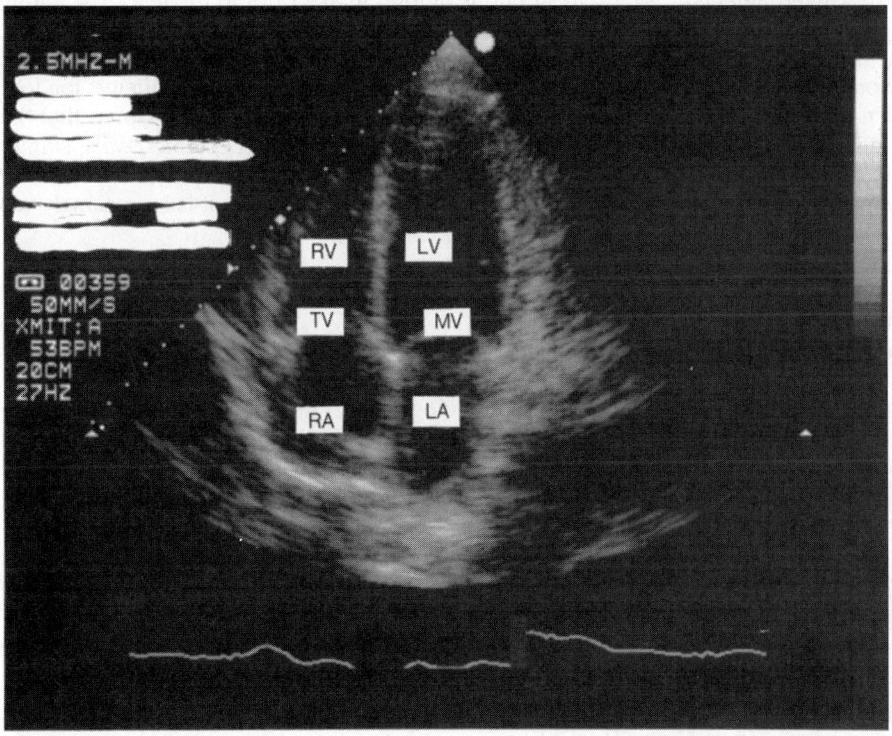

FIGURE 26-13. Two-dimensional echocardiographic view of the four chambers in a normal patient. (RV = right ventricle; LV = left ventricle; TV = tricuspid valve; MV = mitral valve; RA = right atrium; LA = left atrium.)

The patient is assured that the test is safe and painless. Position changes are necessary during the procedure, and the patient is asked to breathe slowly and periodically to hold respirations. In TEE a fasting state is recommended for a period before the study. Patients are also administered local anesthesia and a sedative if needed.

Radionuclide Imaging

Radionuclide studies are useful for detecting myocardial infarction and decreased myocardial blood flow, and for evaluating left ventricular function. The radioisotopes are injected intravenously, and scans are performed using a gamma scintillation camera.

Myocardial Perfusion Imaging. Thallium-201 can be used to improve the accuracy of diagnosing impaired myocardial perfusion. Thallium, which concentrates in normal myocardial tissue but not in ischemic or necrotic tissues, is extremely sensitive in detecting an acute MI, especially within the first 6 hours. However, since it is difficult to distinguish between myocardial ischemia and myocardial scar it is infrequently used for this purpose.

Often, thallium is used in conjunction with an exercise tolerance test to evaluate blood flow through vessels that are too small to visualize with coronary arteriography and to compare changes in myocardial perfusion immediately after exercise and at rest. One or two minutes before the end of the exercise test, a dose of thallium-201 is injected into the intravenous line to allow for distribution to the heart before the exercise is completed. Images are taken immediately and repeated in 2 to 4 hours. Areas that do not show uptake of thallium are noted as "defects" and indicate lack of perfusion. "Defects" that disappear in the follow-up images indicate ischemia with exercise. Persistent "defects" indicate areas of infarction and are noted as "fixed defects."

An alternative for patients who cannot tolerate exercise is the infusion of various pharmacologic agents to simulate the effects of exercise and resulting myocardial perfusion. Persantine (dipyridamole) is a selective coronary vasodilator which increases blood flow in the regions of the heart with normal coronary arteries. Those areas of the heart fed by stenosed arteries will not have increased blood flow. More recently, adenosine, a potent coronary vasodilator with a shorter half-life, has been used in selected patients to promote coronary dilation.

Although the most common thallium imaging is a one-dimensional view, a newer method with single photon emission tomography (SPECT) provides three-dimensional images. With SPECT, the camera moves around the patient in a 180- to 360-degree arc, to more precisely identify the areas of decreased myocardial perfusion.

The patient is assured that the thallium studies involve safe and acceptable radiation exposure, similar to other diagnostic x-rays.

Evaluation of Ventricular Function and Wall Motion. Equilibrium radionuclide angiocardiography (ERNA), also known as multiple-gated acquisition (MUGA) scanning, is a common noninvasive technique that uses a conventional scintillation camera interfaced with a computer to record images of the heart during several hundred heart beats. The computer processes the data and allows for sequential viewing of the functioning heart. The sequential images are analyzed to evaluate left ventricular function, wall motion, and ejection fraction. The ejection fraction (EF) is the percentage of the end-diastolic volume that is ejected with each stroke. Normal right ventricular EF (RVEF) is >42%; normal left ventricular EF (LVEF) is >50%. MUGA scanning can also be used to assess the differences in left ventricular function during rest and exercise.

The patient is assured that there is no known radiation danger and is instructed to remain motionless during the scan.

Positron Emission Tomography. Positron emission tomography (PET) is a noninvasive scan used in the past primarily to study neurologic dysfunction. More recently and with increasing frequency, PET is also used to diagnose cardiac dysfunction. For cardiac patients, including those who are asymptomatic, PET provides more specific information about myocardial perfusion and viability than do TEE or thallium scans. It is helpful in planning the course of treatment, *e.g.*, in determining if coronary artery bypass graft (CABG) surgery or angioplasty would be beneficial. It is also used to evaluate the patency of native and previously grafted vessels and collateral circulation.

In the patient undergoing a PET scan, radioisotopes are administered by injection; one compound is used to determine blood flow in the myocardium and another shows the metabolic function. The PET camera provides detailed three-dimensional images of the distributed compounds. Viability of the myocardium is determined by comparing the extent of glucose metabolism in the myocardium to the degree of blood flow. For example, ischemic but viable tissue would show decreased blood flow and elevated metabolism. For this patient, revascularization through surgery or angioplasty would likely improve heart function.

Restrictions of food intake prior to the test vary among institutions, but since PET evaluates glucose metabolism, the patient's blood sugar should be in the normal range. The patient should refrain from tobacco and caffeine for four hours before the procedure. The patient is assured that the radiation exposure is at safe and acceptable levels, similar to thallium studies. Although PET equipment is currently too costly for every institution to have, it is increasingly valued and available.

Electrophysiologic Testing

The electrophysiology study (EPS) is a noninvasive diagnostic serial procedure performed under laboratory conditions to record cardiac electrical activity during sinus rhythm and dysrhythmia. This test is most commonly performed to identify the point of origin (irritable foci) of unexplained dysrhythmias, palpitations, and syncope. It can also be used for patients who have survived cardiac arrest. EPS is used to evaluate the need for placement of a pacemaker or implantable cardioverter defibrillator (ICD). This test is also used in localizing and (when necessary) destroying arrythmogenic foci.

A catheter is introduced into the femoral or right subclavian vein to record the normal activation of heart activity and the activity of the heart during dysrhythmia. Fluoroscopy is used to guide a pacing electrode into the heart to stimulate the myocardium. The aim is to produce the patient's particular dysrhythmia and subsequently test antidysrhythmic medication therapy to determine if (and which) medication will control the dysrhythmia.

Local anesthesia is used and the patient's diet may need to be restricted prior to the procedure depending on the time of the study. Lethal dysrhythmias may be induced; therefore, the procedure is performed in a controlled environment with resuscitative equipment (*e.g.*, defibrillator) readily available. Possible complications include hematoma, pneumothorax (air in the pleural cavity), deep vein thrombosis (DVT), cerebral vascular accident (stroke), or sudden death.

Hemodynamic Monitoring

Hemodynamic monitoring involves the use of invasive catheters placed in the vascular system of patients to monitor closely heart function, blood volume, and circulation. Patients requiring hemodynamic monitoring are usually critically ill and in an intensive care unit, although some stable patients on an intermediate care unit may have a central venous pressure catheter or an arterial catheter. The patient may have any number of underlying medical conditions, but the failure of the heart as a pump or a major circulation disturbance necessitates the invasive monitoring.

The specific monitoring catheters discussed below are central venous pressure (CVP), pulmonary artery pressure, and systemic arterial pressure catheters.

Central Venous Pressure Monitoring

CVP is the pressure within the right atrium and in the great veins within the thorax. It represents the filling pressure of the right ventricle and indicates the ability of the right side of the heart to manage a fluid load. It serves as a guide to fluid replacement in seriously ill patients and is a measure of effective circulating blood volume. Although CVP is one of several measurements obtained through a pulmonary artery catheter as described below, occasionally a catheter will be inserted in a patient on a general unit to measure CVP only.

CVP is a dynamic or changing measurement. The change in CVP correlated with the patient's clinical status is a more useful indication of adequacy of venous blood volume and alterations of cardiovascular function than is a single measurement of CVP. CVP reflects right ventricular function. Most right ventricular failure is secondary to left ventricular failure. Therefore, an elevated CVP can be a late sign of left ventricular failure. A decreased CVP indicates that the patient is hypovolemic, and this is verified when a rapid intravenous infusion causes the CVP to rise. A rising CVP may be due to either hypervolemia or poor cardiac contractility.

The CVP site is prepared by shaving if necessary and cleansing with an antiseptic solution. A local anesthetic may be used. The catheter is threaded through the external jugular, antecubital, or femoral vein into the vena cava just above or within the right atrium. Once the CVP catheter is inserted, antiseptic ointment and a dry, sterile dressing are applied. The dressing, intravenous fluid, manometer, and tubing are changed according to hospital policy and protocol. The usual intervals for changing the various components are as follows: intravenous solution—every 24 hours; the line set-up—every 24 to 48 hours; the catheter insertion site dressing—every 24 to 72 hours.

CVP is measured by the height of a column of water in a manometer. When measuring CVP, it is crucial to assure that the zero mark on the manometer is placed at a standard reference point, called the phlebostatic axis (Fig. 26-14). When this position is located, an ink mark is made on the chest to indicate the location. If the phlebostatic axis is used, CVP can be measured correctly with the patient supine at any backrest position up to 45 degrees. Normal CVP is 4 to 10 cm H_2O. The most common complications of CVP monitoring are infection and air embolism.

Pulmonary Artery Pressure Monitoring

The pulmonary artery (PA) catheter is an important assessment tool that is useful to measure or calculate several right- and left-sided intracardiac pressures effectively. Patients with pulmonary artery catheters are monitored only in critical care units and not on general medical-surgical nursing units.

Many models of PA catheters are currently used, varying in the number of lumina and the types of measurement capability. All types involve a balloon-tipped, flow-directed catheter inserted into a large vein (usually the subclavian or jugular veins) that leads into the superior vena cava and right atrium. The balloon is inflated, and the catheter is carried rapidly by the flow of blood through the tricuspid valve, into the right ventricle, through the pulmonic valve, and into a branch of the pulmonary artery. When the catheter reaches a small pulmonary artery, the balloon is deflated and the catheter is secured with sutures.

With the PA catheter correctly positioned, several parameters can be measured, including CVP or right atrial pressure, PA systolic and diastolic pressures, mean PA pressure, and pulmonary capillary wedge pressure. If certain thermodilution catheters are used, the cardiac output, systemic vascular resistance, pulmonary vascular resistance, and oxygen saturation can be measured or calculated. It is beyond the scope of this chapter to describe all the hemodynamic parameters in detail. The reader is referred to the bibliography for more detailed information about this aspect of critical care nursing. Some parameters are discussed below.

Pulmonary artery systolic and diastolic pressures are obtained with a transducer and blood pressure monitor. Normal pulmonary artery pressure is 25/9 mm Hg, with a mean pressure of 15 mm Hg. When the balloon is inflated, the catheter is "wedged" in the pulmonary artery. Pressures transmitted to the catheter reflect left ventricular end-

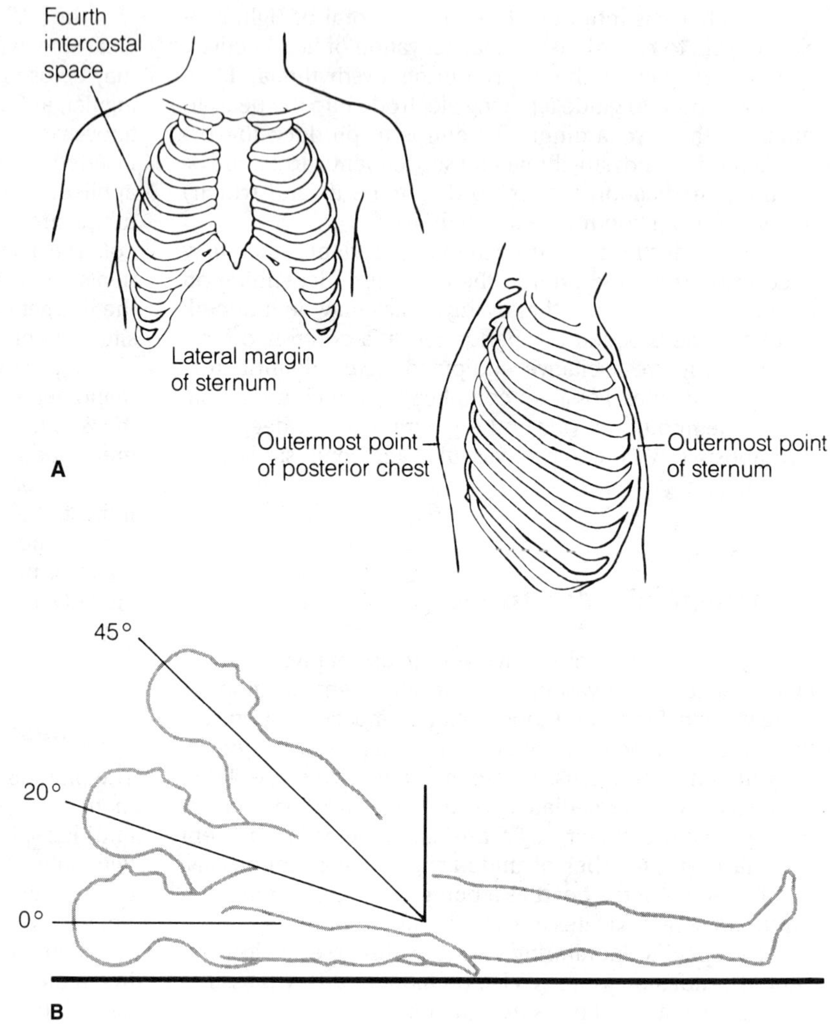

FIGURE 26-14. The phlebostatic axis and the phlebostatic level. (**A**) The phlebostatic axis is the crossing of two reference lines: (1) a line from the fourth intercostal space at the point where it joins the sternum, drawn out to the side of the body beneath the axilla; (2) a line midpoint between the anterior and posterior surfaces of the chest. (**B**) The phlebostatic level is a horizontal line through the phlebostatic axis. The transducer or the zero mark on the manometer must be level with this axis for accurate measurements. As the patient moves from the flat to erect positions, he moves his chest and therefore the reference level; the phlebostatic level stays horizontal through the same reference point. (After Shinn J et al: Heart Lung 8[2]:324.)

diastolic pressure. At end-diastole, when the mitral valve is open, pulmonary artery wedge pressure is the same as the pressure in the left atrium and the left ventricle, unless the patient has mitral valve disease or pulmonary hypertension. Pulmonary artery wedge pressure is a mean pressure and is normally 4.5 to 13 mm Hg.

Catheter site care is essentially the same as that for a CVP catheter. The catheter flush solution is heparinized normal saline, delivered in small amounts using a pressure bag and flush device. See Chapter 28 for more specific guidelines for caring for a patient with a pulmonary artery catheter. As in measuring CVP, it is essential to place the transducer at the phlebostatic axis to ensure accurate readings. Measurement of cardiac output can also be obtained by using a pulmonary artery catheter.

Complications of pulmonary artery monitoring include infection, pulmonary artery rupture, pulmonary thromboembolism, pulmonary infarction, catheter kinking, dysrhythmias, and air embolism.

Systemic Arterial Pressure Monitoring

Intra-arterial monitoring is used to obtain direct and continuous blood pressures in critically ill patients with severe high blood pressure or hypotension. Arterial catheters are also useful when obtaining arterial blood gases and serial blood samples. Intra-arterial monitoring is generally restricted to critical care units.

Once an arterial site is selected (radial, brachial, femoral, or dorsalis pedis), collateral circulation to the area must be confirmed before the catheter is placed. If no collateral circulation existed, and the cannulated artery became occluded, ischemia and infarction of the area distal to the cannulated site could occur. Collateral circulation can be checked by either the Allen test to evaluate the radial and ulnar arteries, or by using an ultrasonic Doppler test for any of the arteries. With the Allen test, the radial and ulnar arteries are simultaneously compressed, and the patient is asked to make a fist, causing the hand to blanch. After the patient opens the fist, the pressure on the ulnar artery is released while maintaining pressure on the radial artery. The hand will turn pink if the ulnar artery is patent.

Site preparation and care are the same as for CVP catheters. The catheter flush solution is the same as for pulmonary artery catheters. A transducer is attached, and pressures are obtained in millimeters of mercury. Complications include local obstruction with distal ischemia, external hemorrhage, massive ecchymosis, dissection, air embolism, blood loss, pain, arteriospasm, and infection.

CRITICAL THINKING EXERCISES

1. You are caring for a patient in the home setting who has a history of cardiac disease. How does the assessment of this patient differ from the assessment of the acutely ill cardiac patient in the acute care setting?
2. The son of a patient who has cardiac disease expresses concern over his own risks for developing cardiac problems. Based on your knowledge of cardiac risk factors, what explanation would you give him?
3. A middle-aged cardiac patient indicates that he believes that his disease process is a result of aging. Describe the teaching plan you would develop for this patient.

REFERENCES AND SELECTED READINGS

Books

Bates B. A Guide to Physical Examination, 6th ed. Philadelphia, JB Lippincott, 1995.

Fuller J and Schaller-Ayers J. Health Assessment, 2nd ed. A Nursing Approach. Philadelphia, JB Lippincott, 1994.

Guzzetta C and Dossey B. Cardiovascular Nursing. Holistic Practice. St. Louis, Mosby-Year Book, 1992.

Hurst JW et al. The Heart, 7th ed. New York, McGraw–Hill, 1990.

Stein E and Delman AJ. Rapid Interpretation of Heart Sounds and Murmurs, 3rd ed. Philadelphia, Lea & Febiger, 1990.

Wingate S. Cardiac Nursing: A Clinical Management and Patient Care Resource. Gaithersburg, MD, Aspen Publishers, 1991.

Woods S et al. Cardiac Nursing, 3rd ed. Philadelphia, JB Lippincott, 1995.

Zorb SL. Cardiovascular Diagnostic Testing: A Nursing Guide. Gaithersburg, MD, Aspen Publishers, 1991.

Journals

Anardi DM. Assessment of right heart function. J Cardiovasc Nurs 1991 Oct; 6(1):12–33.

Apple S and Thurkauf GE. Preparing for and understanding transesophageal echocardiography. Crit Care Nurse 1992 Aug; 12(6):29–34.

Beattie S and Meinhardt SL. Transesophagael echocardiography: Advanced technology for the cardiac patient. Crit Care Nurse 1992 Dec; 12(8):42–46.

Berry VA. Wolff-Parkinson-White syndrome and the use of radiofrequency catheter ablation. Heart Lung 1993 Jan/Feb; 22(1): 15–25.

Bubien RS et al. What you need to know about radiofrequency ablation. Am J Nurs 1993 July; 93(7):30–36.

Cheney AM and Maquindang ML. Patient teaching for X-ray and other diagnostics. RN 1993 April; 56(4):54–56.

Dault LH et al. Helping your patient through cardiac catheterization. Nursing 1992 Feb; 22(2):52–55.

Gillman PH. Continuous measurement of cardiac output: A milestone in hemodynamic monitoring. Focus on Critical Care 1992 Apr; 19(2):155–158.

Hill MN and Grim CM. How to take a precise blood pressure. Am J Nurs 1991 Feb; 91(2):38–42.

Hochrein MA and Sohl L. Heart smart: A guide to cardiac tests. Am J Nurs 1992 Dec; 92(12):22–25.

Kuecherer HF et al. Role of transesophageal echocardiography in diagnosis and management of cardiovascular disease. Cardiol Clin 1990 May; 8(2):377–387.

Moser D et al. Signal-averaged electrocardiography: Diagnostic uses and clinical implications. Crit Care Nurs Q 1991 Aug; 14(2):30–40.

Moser DK et al. Noninvasive identification of patients at risk for ventricular tachycardia with the signal-averaged electrocardiogram. AACN Clin Issues Crit Care Nurs 1990 May; 1(1):79–86.

Peterson M. Patient anxiety before cardiac catheterization: An intervention study. Heart Lung 1991 Nov; 20(6):643–647.

Proulx et al. Detection of right ventricular myocardial infarction. Crit Care Nurs 1992 June; 12(5):50–59.

Rossi L and Leary E. Evaluating the patient with coronary artery disease. Nurs Clin North Am 1992 Mar; 27(1):171–186.

Schactman M and Greene JS. Signal-averaged electrocardiography: A new technique for determining which patients may be at risk for sudden cardiac death. Focus on Critical Care 1991 June; 18(3):202–210.

Schultz SJ et al. Preparing your patient for cardiac PET scan. Nursing 1991 Sept; 21(9):63–64.

Sullivan-Witterschein K et al. Using transesophageal echocardiography to assess the heart. Nursing 1992 Aug; 22(8):63–64.

Weikart CJ. New eye into the heart. RN 1993 Oct; 56(10):36–40.

Zaret BL and Wackers FJ. Nuclear cardiology. Part I. N Engl J Med 1993 Sept 9; 329(11):775–783.

Zaret BL and Wackers FJ. Nuclear cardiology. Part II. N Engl J Med 1993 Sept 16; 329(12):855–863.

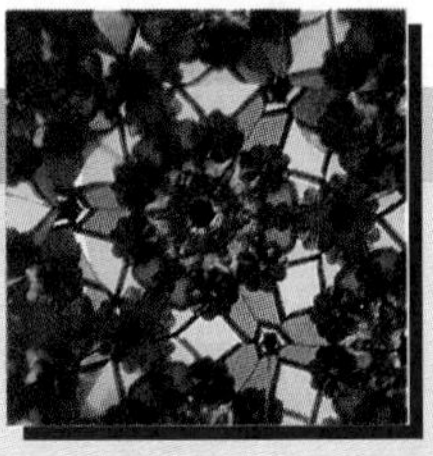

27

Management of Patients With Dysrhythmias and Conduction Problems

CHAPTER OUTLINE

LEARNING OBJECTIVES

On completion of this chapter, the learner will be able to:

1. Correlate the components of the ECG with physiologic events of the heart
2. Determine the following information from an ECG strip: rate, presence or absence of P waves, PR interval, QRS interval, presence or absence of dysrhythmia, origin of dysrhythmia
3. Define the different types of dysrhythmias including cause, characteristic ECG waveforms, and management
4. Use the nursing process as a framework for care of patients with dysrhythmias
5. Define the different types of heart blocks including cause, characteristic ECG waveforms, and management
6. Describe the key points to follow when using a defibrillator
7. Compare the different types of pacemakers, their uses, nursing implications, and possible complications
8. Use the nursing process as a framework for care of patients with pacemakers

Dysrhythmias

A dysrhythmia is a disorder of the heartbeat that includes a disturbance of rate or rhythm, or both. Dysrhythmias are derangements of the heart's conduction system and not of heart structure. They are identified by analyzing electrocardiogram (ECG) waveforms. Dysrhythmias are named according to the site of origin of the impulse and the mechanism of conduction involved. For example, a dysrhythmia that originates in the sinus node (SA node) and is slow in rate is called sinus bradycardia. There are four possible sites of origin of dysrhythmias, as indicated in Chart 27-1: the sinus node, the atria, the AV node or junction, and the ventricles. The possible altered conduction mechanisms that can occur include bradycardia, tachycardia, flutter, fibrillation, premature beats, and heart blocks.

Properties of Cardiac Muscle

The cardiac muscle possesses the physiologic properties of excitability, automaticity, conductivity, and contractility.

- **Excitability** is the ability of a myocardial cell to respond to a stimulus.
- **Automaticity** allows a cell to reach a threshold potential and generate an impulse without being stimulated by another source.
- **Conductivity** refers to the ability of the muscle to transmit an impulse from cell to cell.
- **Contractility** allows the muscle to shorten when stimulated.

When all of these properties are intact, the heart muscle is stimulated by impulses originating in the sinus node; hence, *the sinus node is referred to as the heart's pacemaker.*

If disequilibrium occurs in one of the heart's basic properties, a dysrhythmia may result. The disequilibrium can be caused by normal activity such as exercise or by a pathologic condition such as a myocardial infarction. In myocardial infarction, because reduced oxygenation to the myocardium can increase excitability, the myocardium has an increased response to stimuli. This is an example of one of the most common causes of a dysrhythmia.

Normal Conduction Pathway. Once an impulse originates in the sinus node, a normal electrical pathway is followed. The impulse travels from the sinus node through the atria to the AV node or junction, which also includes the bundle of His (see Fig. 26-3). The impulse is delayed in time at the AV node to allow the ventricles to fill with blood. From the AV node the impulse travels very quickly through the bundle branches, terminating in the Purkinje fibers of the ventricular walls to initiate systole. The cycle then begins again. It is important to remember that an electrical stimulus is followed by a mechanical event of the heart. A fuller explanation of the physiologic functioning of the heart can be found in Chapter 26.

Autonomic Nervous System. The heart is under the control of the autonomic nervous system, which consists of sympathetic and parasympathetic fibers. The **sympathetic** system is also referred to as **adrenergic,** a word derived from the root word adrenal. Thus, stimulation of the sympathetic system accelerates heart rate, raises blood pressure, and enhances the force of myocardial contraction. **Parasympathetic** stimulation, conversely, slows the heart rate, lowers blood pressure, and reduces the force of contraction.

Manipulation of the autonomic nervous system forms the foundation for much of the medication therapy in dysrhythmia control (*e.g.*, b-adrenergic blockers).

CHART 27-1
Identification of Dysrhythmias

Sites of Origin	Mechanisms of Conduction
Sinus node	Bradycardia
Atria	Tachycardia
AV node or junction	Flutter
Ventricles	Fibrillation
	Premature beats
	Heart blocks

ECG Interpretation

The electrical activity of the heart can be viewed by means of an electrocardiogram (ECG). Each phase of the cardiac cycle is reflected by specific waveforms that are captured and recorded on a strip of ECG paper. The tracings may also be viewed on the screen of an oscilloscope. The electrical activity is picked up by a set of leads or electrodes placed at specific points on the body.

Procedure for Obtaining an Electrocardiogram

The standard ECG consists of 12 leads. Information regarding the electrical activity of the heart is obtained by placing electrodes on the skin surface at standardized anatomic positions (Fig. 27-1). The various electrode positions that may be monitored are referred to as leads. For example, lead 1 measures the electrical activity between the left arm and the right arm. For a complete 12-lead ECG, the heart is viewed from each of 12 different anatomic positions.

To ensure good contact between skin and electrode, the limb electrodes are placed on a flat skin surface just above the wrists and ankles. The electrodes may be connected to the ECG machine in several ways, usually via a clip attached to the adhesive-tabbed electrode.

With the four extremity electrodes in place, the first six leads can be recorded: lead I, II, and III, and AVR, AVL, and AVF. The six precordial or V leads are attached similarly. Most ECG machines record all 12 leads simultaneously with all electrodes attached.

When an ECG is taken, additional leads may be recorded to obtain more complete information. Electrocardiographic changes consistent with ischemia or infarction

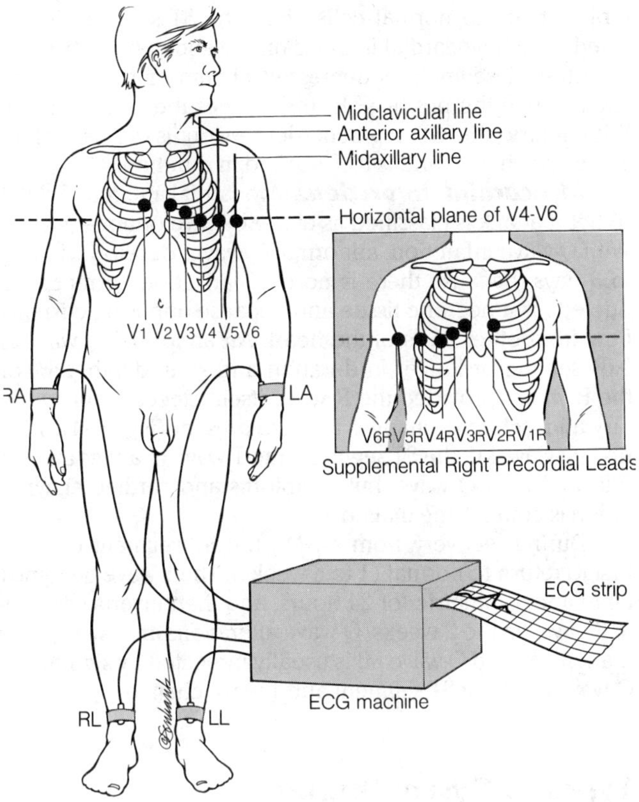

FIGURE 27-1. ECG electrode placement. The standard left precordial leads are V_1: 4th intercostal space, R sternal border; V_2: 4th intercostal space, L sternal border; V_3: diagonally between V_2 and V_4; V_4: 5th intercostal space, L midclavicular line, V_5: same line as V_4, anterior axillary line; V_6: same line as V_4 and V_5, midaxillary line. The right precordial leads, placed across the right side of the chest, are the mirror opposite of the left leads.

appear in specific leads which reflect the damaged area of the myocardium. Left precordial leads are standard. In patients with suspected right-sided heart damage, however, right-sided precordial leads may be required to better evaluate the right ventricle (see Fig. 27-1).

ECG Analysis

When analyzed accurately, the ECG offers important information about the electrical activity of the myocardium. ECG waveforms are printed on graph paper. Time or rate is measured on the horizontal axis of the graph, and amplitude or voltage is measured on the vertical axis. The ECG waveform represents the function of the heart's conduction system, which normally initiates and conducts the electrical activity.

Waves, Complexes, and Intervals

The ECG is composed of several waveforms, including the P wave, the QRS complex, the T wave, the ST segment, the PR interval, and possibly a U wave (Fig. 27-2).

The **P wave** represents atrial muscle depolarization. It is normally 2.5 mm high or less and 0.11 second or less in duration.

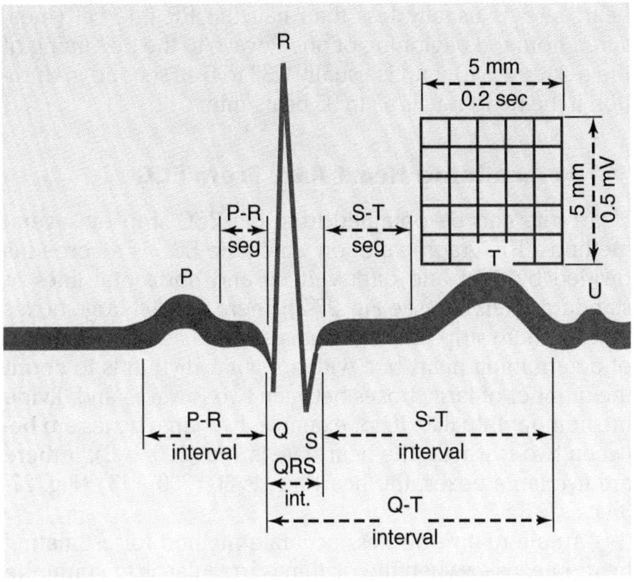

FIGURE 27-2. Commonly measured complex components. The PR interval is measured from the beginning of the P wave to the beginning of the QRS; the QRS is measured from the beginning of the Q wave to the end of the S wave; the QT interval is measured from the beginning of the Q wave to the end of the T wave.

The first negative deflection after the P wave is the *Q wave*, which is normally less than 0.03 second in duration and less than 25% of the R wave amplitude; the first positive deflection after the P wave is the *R wave*; and the *S wave* is the first negative deflection after the R wave.

The **QRS complex** (beginning of Q wave, or R wave if there is no Q wave, to end of S wave) represents ventricular muscle depolarization. The QRS complex is normally 0.04 to 0.10 second in duration. When a wave is less than 5 mm vertically, small letters (q, r, s) are used; when a wave is larger than 5 mm vertically, capital letters (Q, R, S) are used. Not all QRS complexes have all three waveforms.

The **T wave** represents ventricular muscle repolarization. It follows the QRS complex and is usually of the same deflection as the QRS complex.

The **U wave** is thought to represent repolarization of the Purkinje fibers but it sometimes is seen in patients with hypokalemia (low potassium levels). If present, the U wave follows the T wave and is approximately the same size as the P wave. It may be mistaken for an extra P wave.

The **ST segment,** which represents early ventricular repolarization, lasts from the end of the S wave to the beginning of the T wave. It is normally isoelectric (no variation in electric potential). It is analyzed for signs of reduced oxygen supply to the heart (ischemia).

The **PR interval** is measured from the beginning of the P wave to the beginning of the Q or R wave and represents the time required for atrial depolarization and the delay of the impulse in the AV node before ventricular depolarization. In adults, the PR interval normally ranges from 0.12 to 0.20 second in duration.

The **QT interval,** which represents the total time for ventricular depolarization and repolarization, is measured from the beginning of the Q wave, or R wave if no Q wave is present, to the end of the T wave. The QT interval varies with heart rate, is usually less than half the RR interval (measured from the beginning of one R wave to the beginning of the next R wave), and is usually 0.32 to 0.40 second in duration if the heart rate is 65 to 95 beats/min.

Determining Heart Rate From ECG

Heart rate can be obtained from the ECG strip by several methods. The graph paper on which the ECG is recorded is divided by light and dark vertical and horizontal lines at standard intervals (see Fig. 27-2). There are 300 large boxes in a 1-minute strip. Therefore, an easy and accurate method of determining heart rate with a regular rhythm is to count the number of large boxes between two R waves and divide the number into 300. If, for example, two large boxes are between two R waves, the heart rate is 150 (300 ÷ 2); if there are five large boxes, the heart rate is 60 (300 ÷ 5) (Fig. 27-3*A*).

An alternative but less accurate method for estimating heart rate, used when the rhythm is irregular, is to count the number of R-R intervals in 6 seconds and multiply that number by 10. The ECG paper is usually marked at 3-second intervals (15 large boxes, horizontally) by a vertical line at the top of the paper (see Fig. 27-3*B*). The RR intervals are counted rather than QRS complexes, because a computed heart rate based on the latter might be inaccurately high.

Abnormal Findings

Myocardial Ischemia and Injury. Myocardial ischemia, in which the heart is deprived of adequate oxygen, causes the T wave to be larger and inverted because of altered late repolarization. Possibly, the ischemic region remains depolarized, whereas adjacent areas have returned to the resting state. The change is seen in the leads closest to the involved surface of the heart. Ischemia also causes ST segment changes. If there is epicardial myocardial injury, the injured cells depolarize normally but repolarize more rapidly than do normal cells; thus, the ST segment is elevated. If the myocardial injury is on the endocardial surface, then the ST segment is depressed (1 mm or more) in the leads where the positive electrode faces the area of injury. With injury, the ST segment depression is horizontal or slopes downward and is 0.08 second in duration.

Myocardial Infarction. Myocardial infarction (MI) or heart attack is classified as either Q-wave or non–Q-wave. With Q-wave infarction, abnormal Q waves develop within 1 to 3 days, because there is no depolarization current conducted from necrotic tissue and because opposing currents flow from other parts of the heart. An abnormal Q wave is 0.04 second or longer in duration and is, in depth, 25% of the R wave (provided the R wave itself exceeds 5 mm). Injury and ischemic changes are also present (Fig. 27-4). With non–Q-wave MI, the ST segment and T wave changes are not followed by a Q wave, but symptoms and cardiac enzyme analysis confirm the diagnosis.

During recovery from an MI, the ST segment often is first to return to normal (1 to 6 weeks). The T wave becomes large and symmetric for 24 hours, and then inverts within 1 to 3 days for 1 to 2 weeks. Q wave alterations are usually permanent. An old Q-wave MI is usually indicated by significant Q waves without ST segment and T wave changes.

Types of Dysrhythmias

Sinus Node Dysrhythmias

Sinus Bradycardia

Sinus bradycardia may be due to vagal stimulation, digitalis toxicity, increased intracranial pressure, or myocardial infarction (MI). It also is seen in highly trained athletes, in persons in severe pain, in persons on medication (propranolol, reserpine, methyldopa), in hypoendocrine states (myxedema, Addison's disease, panhypopituitarism), in anorexia

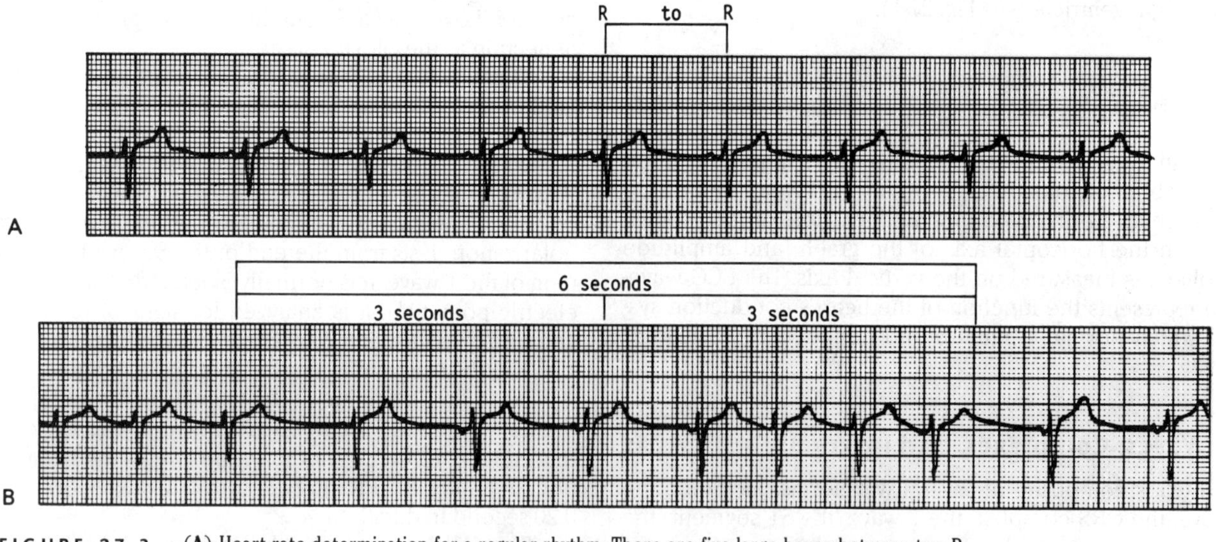

FIGURE 27-3. (**A**) Heart rate determination for a regular rhythm. There are five large boxes between two R waves. 300 divided by this number equals 60. The heart rate is approximately 60. (**B**) Heart rate determination if the rhythm is irregular. There are approximately seven RR intervals in 6 seconds. Seven times 10 equals 70. The heart rate is 70. (Woods et al. Cardiac Nursing, 3rd ed. Philadelphia, JB Lippincott, 1995, p 294.)

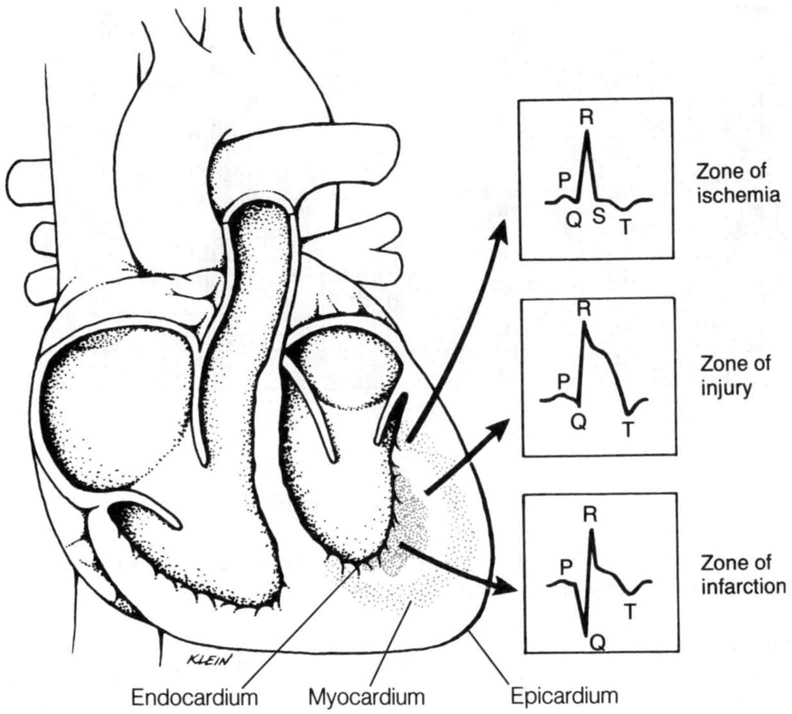

FIGURE 27-4. Effects of ischemia, injury, and infarction on ECG recording. Ischemia causes inversion of T wave because of altered repolarization. Cardiac muscle injury causes elevation of the ST segment. With Q-wave infarction, Q or QS waves develop because of the absence of depolarization current from the necrotic tissue and opposing currents from other parts of the heart.

nervosa, in hypothermia, and after surgical damage to the SA node.

The following are characteristics of this dysrhythmia (Fig. 27-5):

Rate: 40 to 60 beats per minute
P waves: Precede each QRS complex; PR interval normal
QRS complex: Usually normal
Conduction: Usually normal
Rhythm: Regular

All characteristics of sinus bradycardia are the same as those of normal sinus rhythm, except for the rate. If the slow heart rate is causing significant hemodynamic changes resulting in syncope (fainting), angina, or ectopic dysrhythmias, then treatment is directed toward increasing the heart rate. If the decrease in heart rate is due to vagal stimulation (stimulation of the vagus nerve) such as bearing down during defecation or vomiting, attempts are made to prevent further vagal stimulation. If the patient has digitalis toxicity, digitalis is withheld. The medication of choice in treating sinus bradycardia is atropine. Atropine blocks vagal stimulation, thus allowing a normal rate to occur.

Sinus Tachycardia

Sinus tachycardia (fast heart beat) may be caused by fever, acute blood loss, anemia, shock, exercise, congestive heart failure (CHF), pain, hypermetabolic states, anxiety, or sympathomimetic or parasympatholytic medications. The ECG pattern is as follows (Fig. 27-6):

Rate: 100 to 180 beats per minute
P waves: Precede each QRS complex; may be buried in the preceding T wave; PR interval normal
QRS complex: Usually has a normal duration

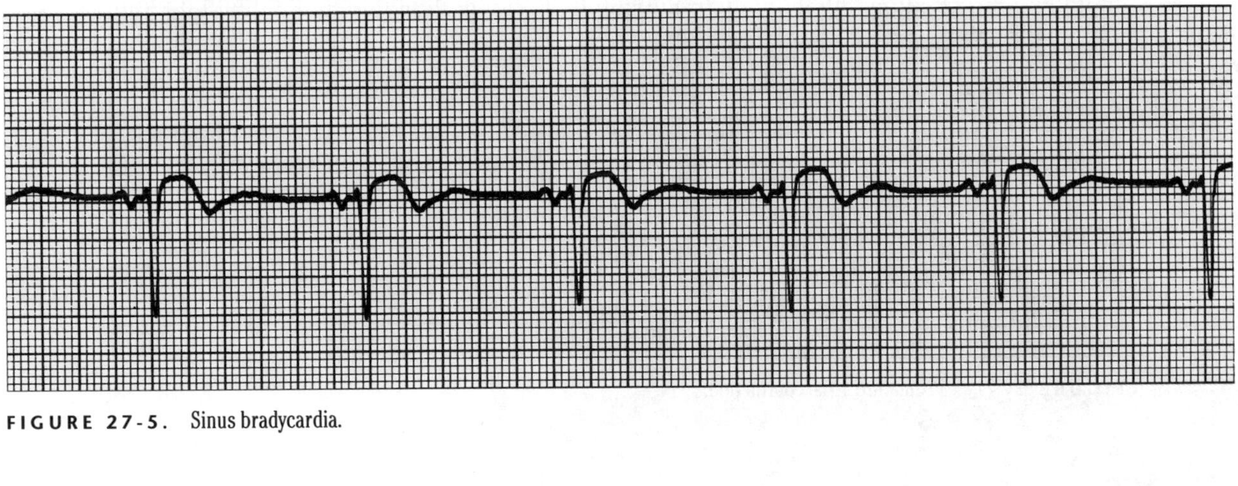

FIGURE 27-5. Sinus bradycardia.

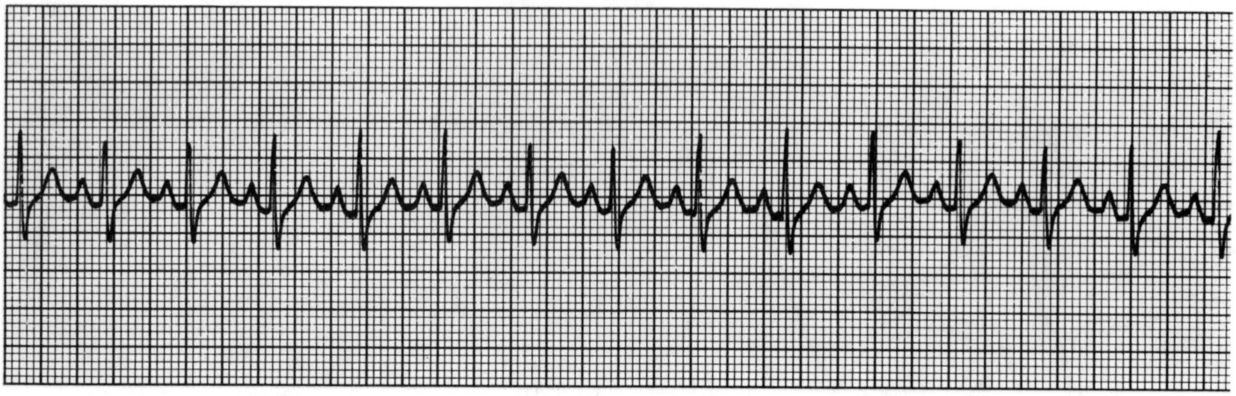

FIGURE 27-6. Sinus tachycardia.

Conduction: Usually normal
Rhythm: Regular

All aspects of sinus tachycardia are the same as those of normal sinus rhythm, except for the rate.

Carotid sinus pressure, applied to one side of the neck at a time, may be effective in slowing the rate temporarily, and thereby help to rule out other dysrhythmias. As heart rate increases, diastolic filling time decreases, resulting in reduced cardiac output and subsequent symptoms of syncope and low blood pressure. If the rapid rate persists and the heart is unable to compensate for the decreased ventricular filling, the patient may develop acute pulmonary edema.

Treatment of sinus tachycardia is usually directed at abolishing its cause. Propranolol (Inderal) may be used to reduce the heart rate quickly. Propranolol blocks the effect of adrenergic fibers, thus slowing the rate.

Atrial Dysrhythmias

Premature Atrial Contractions

Premature atrial contractions (PACs) may be due to irritability of the atrial muscle caused by caffeine, alcohol, nicotine, stretched atrial myocardium as in congestive heart failure (CHF), stress or anxiety, hypokalemia (low potassium levels), atrial ischemia, injury, infarction, or hypermetabolic states.

Premature atrial contractions have the following characteristics (Fig. 27-7):

Rate: 60 to 100 beats per minute
P waves: Usually have a configuration different from that of the P waves that originate in the SA node. Another site in the atria has become irritable (increased automaticity) and fires before the normal firing time of the SA node. PR interval may vary from the PR intervals of impulses originating in the SA node.
QRS complex: May be normal, aberrant, or absent. If the ventricles have completed their repolarization phase, they can respond to this early stimulus from the atria.
Conduction: Usually normal
Rhythm: Regular, except when the PACs occur. The P wave will occur early in the cycle and usually will not have a complete compensatory pause. (Time between the preceding complex and the following complex is less than the time for two RR intervals.)

Premature atrial contractions are frequently seen in normal hearts. The patient may say that the heart "skipped a beat." A pulse deficit (a difference between apical and radial pulse rate) may exist. If PACs are infrequent, no treatment is necessary. If they are frequent (more than 6 per

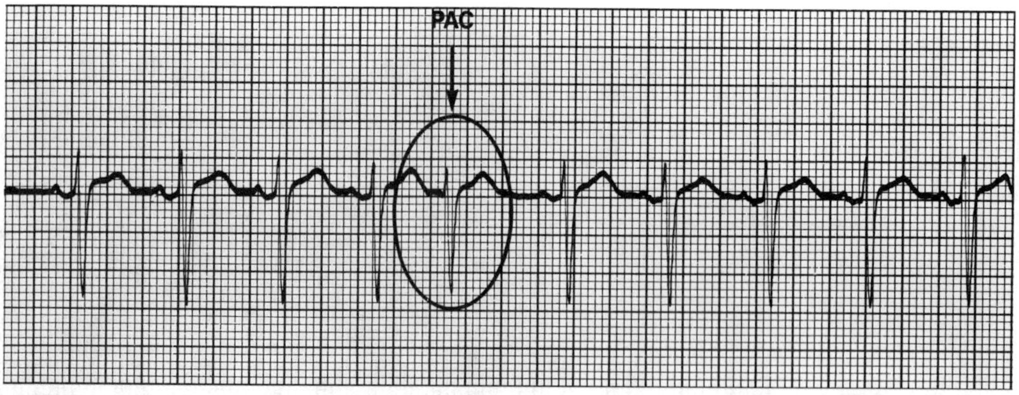

FIGURE 27-7. Premature atrial contraction.

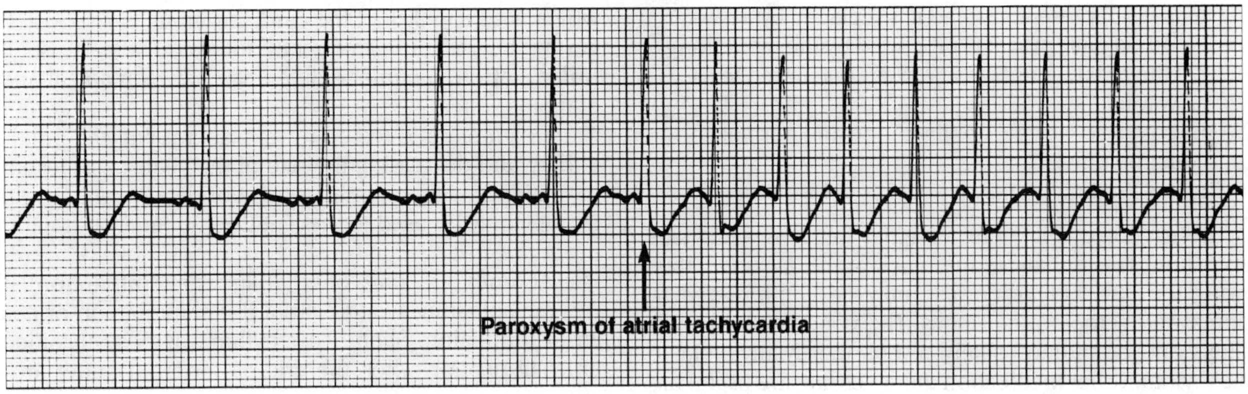

FIGURE 27-8. Paroxysmal atrial tachycardia.

minute) or occur during atrial repolarization, this may herald more serious dysrhythmias such as atrial fibrillation. Again, treatment is directed toward the cause.

Paroxysmal Atrial Tachycardia

Paroxysmal atrial tachycardia (PAT) is atrial tachycardia characterized by abrupt onset and abrupt cessation. It may be triggered by emotions, tobacco, caffeine, fatigue, sympathomimetic medications, or alcohol. Paroxysmal atrial tachycardia is not usually associated with organic heart disease. The rapid rate may produce angina due to decreased coronary artery filling. Cardiac output is reduced and heart failure may occur.

Paroxysmal atrial tachycardia is characterized by the following (Fig. 27-8):

Rate: 150 to 250 beats per minute
P waves: Ectopic and distorted as compared with normal P wave; may be found in the preceding T wave; PR interval shortened (less than 0.12 second)
QRS complex: Usually normal, but may be distorted if aberrant conduction is present
Conduction: Usually normal
Rhythm: Regular

The patient may not be aware of PAT. Treatment is directed toward eliminating the cause and decreasing the heart rate. Morphine may slow the rate without further treatment. Carotid sinus pressure, applied to one side at a time, slows the rate or stops the attack and is usually more effective after digitalis or vasopressors, which depress heart rate. The use of vasopressors has a reflex effect on the carotid sinus by elevating the blood pressure and thus slowing the heart rate. Short-acting digitalis preparations may be used. Propranolol may be tried if digitalis is unsuccessful. Quinidine may be effective, or the calcium channel blocker verapamil (Calan) can be used. Cardioversion may be necessary if the patient does not tolerate the fast heart rate.

Atrial Flutter

Atrial flutter occurs when a focal point in the atrium captures the heart rhythm and discharges impulses at a rate of between 250 and 400 times per minute. An important characteristic of this dysrhythmia is the occurrence of a therapeutic block at the AV node, which prevents some impulse transmission. Conduction of the impulse through the heart is otherwise normal, so the QRS complex is unaffected. This is an important feature of this dysrhythmia, because the 1:1 conduction of atrial impulses firing at 250 to 400 times per minute would result in ventricular fibrillation, a life-threatening dysrhythmia.

Atrial flutter is characterized by the following (Fig. 27-9):

Rate: Atrial rate between 250 and 400 beats per minute
Rhythm: Regular or irregular, depending on kind of block (*e.g.*, 2:1, 3:1, or a combination)

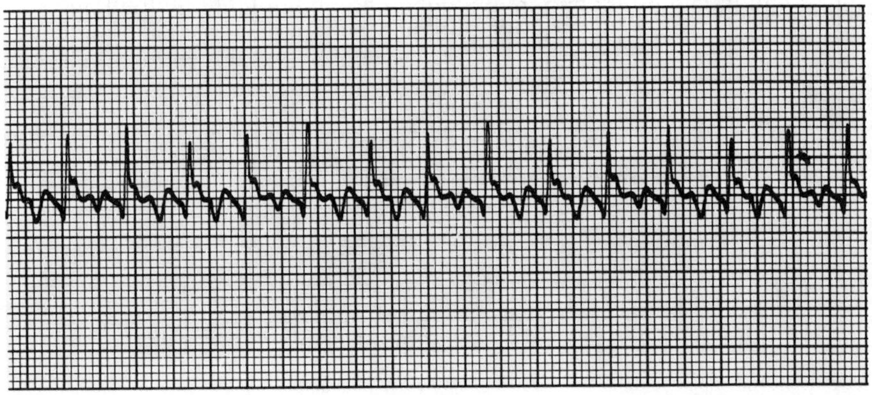

FIGURE 27-9. Atrial flutter.

P wave: Not present; instead it is replaced by a sawtoothed pattern that is produced by the rapid firing of the atrial focus. These waves are referred to as *F* waves.

QRS complex: Normal configuration and normal conduction time

T wave: Present but may be obscured by flutter waves

The accepted treatment for atrial flutter is a digitalis preparation. This enhances the block at the AV node, thus slowing the rate. Quinidine also may be administered to suppress the ectopic atrial focus. The concomitant use of digitalis and quinidine usually reverts the dysrhythmia to sinus rhythm. Other medication therapies that are useful are calcium channel blockers and beta-adrenergic blockers.

If medication therapy is unsuccessful, atrial flutter often will respond to electrical cardioversion.

Atrial Fibrillation

Atrial fibrillation (disorganized and uncoordinated twitching of atrial musculature) is usually associated with atherosclerotic heart disease, valvular heart disease, congestive heart failure, thyrotoxicosis, cor pulmonale, or congenital heart disease.

Atrial fibrillation (Fig. 27-10) is characterized by the following:

Rate: An atrial rate of 350 to 600 beats per minute; ventricular response usually 120 to 200 beats per minute.

P waves: No discernible P waves; irregular undulation, termed fibrillatory or *f* waves, is seen; PR interval cannot be measured.

QRS complex: Usually normal.

Conduction: Usually normal through the ventricles. Characterized by an irregular ventricular response, because the AV node does not respond to the rapid atrial rate. Impulses that are transmitted cause the ventricles to respond irregularly.

Rhythm: Irregular and usually rapid, unless controlled. Irregularity of rhythm is due to variable conduction within the AV node.

A rapid ventricular response reduces the time for ventricular filling and hence the stroke volume. The atrial kick, which is 25% to 30% of the cardiac output, is also lost. Congestive heart failure frequently follows. There is usually a **pulse deficit,** a numeric difference between apical and radial pulse rates.

Treatment is directed toward decreasing the atrial irritability and decreasing the rate of the ventricular response. In patients with chronic atrial fibrillation, anticoagulant therapy may be used to prevent thromboemboli from forming in the atria.

At times a mixture of atrial flutter and atrial fibrillation is seen, sometimes called atrial flutter-fibrillation or coarse atrial fibrillation. Such a dysrhythmia is best classified as atrial fibrillation when the criteria for atrial flutter are not met.

Medications of choice to treat atrial fibrillation are similar to those used in the treatment of PAT. A digitalis preparation is used to slow the heart rate, and an antidysrhythmic such as quinidine is used to suppress the dysrhythmia.

Ventricular Dysrhythmias

Premature Ventricular Contractions

Premature ventricular contractions (PVCs) are the result of increased automaticity of the ventricular muscle cells. PVCs can be due to digitalis toxicity, hypoxia, hypokalemia, fever, acidosis, exercise, or increased circulating catecholamines.

Infrequent PVCs are not serious in themselves. Usually, the patient feels a palpitating sensation but has no other complaints. The concern, however, lies in the fact that these premature contractions may lead to more serious ventricular dysrhythmias.

In the patient with acute myocardial infarction (MI), PVCs are considered serious precursors of ventricular tachycardia and ventricular fibrillation when they (1) occur in increasing number, more than 6 per minute; (2) are multifocal or originate from several areas in the heart; (3) occur in pairs or triplets; and (4) occur in the vulnerable phase of conduction. The T wave represents the period when the heart is most likely to respond to any stray beat and be excited in a dysrhythmic manner. This phase of T-wave conduction is said to be the vulnerable phase.

Premature ventricular contractions (Fig. 27-11) have the following characteristics:

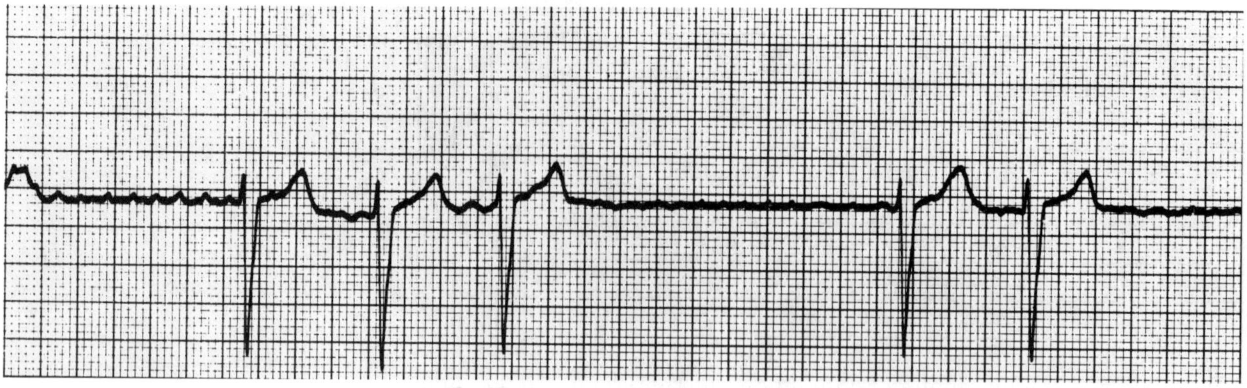

FIGURE 27-10. Atrial fibrillation.

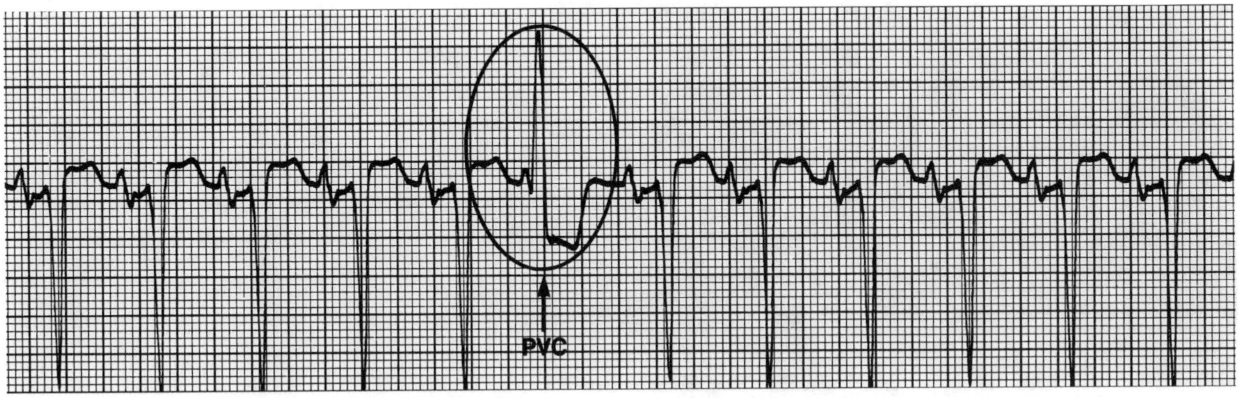

FIGURE 27-11. Premature ventricular contraction.

Rate: 60 to 100 beats per minute.
P waves: Will not be present because impulses originate in the ventricles.
QRS complex: Usually wide and bizarre. Usually longer than 0.10 second in duration. May have the same focus in the ventricle, or may have a wide variety of configurations if occurring from multiple foci in the ventricles.
Conduction: Occasionally retrograde through the junctional tissue and atria.
Rhythm: Irregular when the premature beat occurs.

To decrease the myocardial irritability, the cause must be determined and, if possible, corrected. An antidysrhythmic medication may be used for immediate and possibly long-term therapy. The medication most commonly used in acute care is lidocaine; for long-term therapy procainamide (Pronestyl) or quinidine may be effective.

Ventricular Bigeminy

Ventricular bigeminy is frequently associated with digitalis toxicity, coronary artery disease, acute MI, and CHF. The term **bigeminy** refers to a condition in which every other beat is premature.

Ventricular bigeminy (Fig. 27-12) has the following characteristics:

Rate: May occur at any heart rate, but rate is usually less than 90 beats per minute.
P waves: The same as described for PVCs; may be hidden within the QRS complex.
QRS complex: Every other beat is a PVC with a wide, bizarre QRS complex and a complete compensatory pause.
Conduction: The sinus beats are conducted from the sinus node in a normal fashion, but alternating PVCs start in the ventricles and may have retrograde conduction through the junctional tissue and atria.
Rhythm: Irregular.

If the ectopic beats occur every third beat, this is termed **trigeminy;** every fourth beat, **quadrigeminy.**

The treatment for ventricular bigeminy is the same as for PVCs. Because the underlying cause of ventricular bigeminy is frequently digitalis toxicity, this possible cause should be ruled out or treated if present. Ventricular bigeminy caused by digitalis toxicity is treated with phenytoin (Dilantin).

Ventricular Tachycardia

This dysrhythmia is caused by increased myocardial irritability, as are PVCs. It is usually associated with coronary artery disease and may precede ventricular fibrillation. Ventricular tachycardia is extremely dangerous and should be considered an emergency. The patient is generally aware of this rapid rhythm and is quite anxious. Accelerated

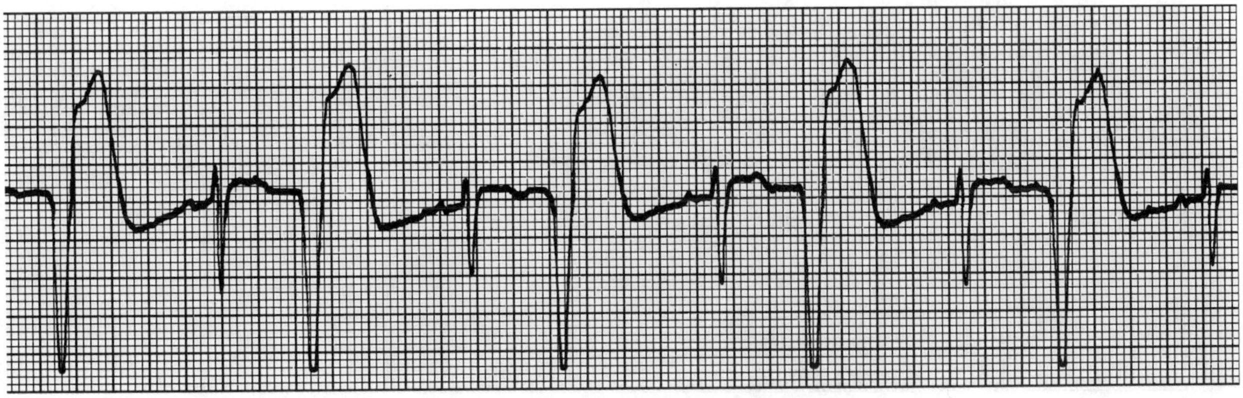

FIGURE 27-12. Ventricular bigeminy.

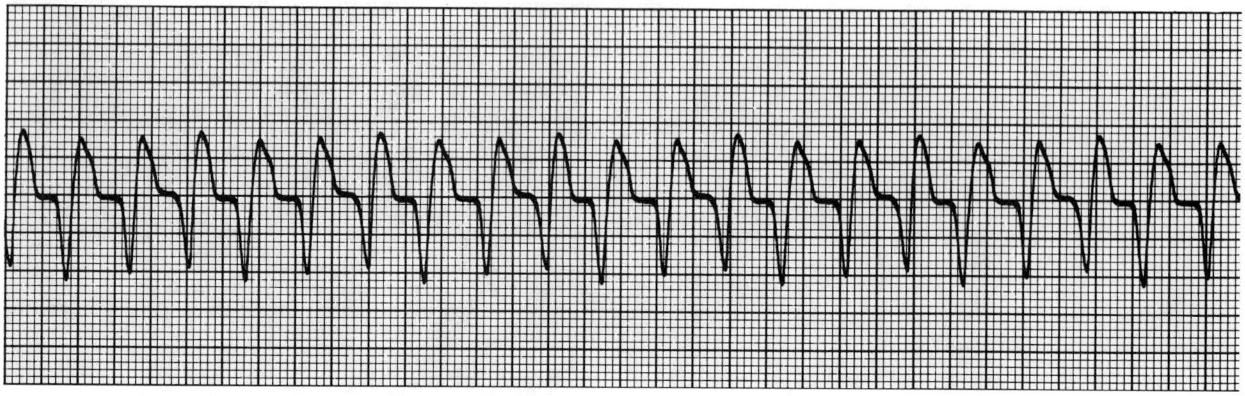

FIGURE 27-13. Ventricular tachycardia.

ventricular rhythm and ventricular tachycardia have the following characteristics (Fig. 27-13):

Rate: 150 to 200 beats per minute.
P waves: Usually buried in the QRS complex; if seen, they do not necessarily fall in the normal pattern with the QRS. The ventricular contractions are dissociated from the atrial contractions.
QRS complex: Have the same configurations as those of a PVC—wide and bizarre, with T waves in the opposite direction. A ventricular beat may fuse with a normal QRS, resulting in a fusion beat.
Conduction: Originates in the ventricle, with possible retrograde conduction to the junctional tissue and atria.
Rhythm: Usually regular, but irregular ventricular tachycardia is also seen.

The patient's tolerance or lack of tolerance for this rapid rhythm will dictate the therapy to be given. The cause of the myocardial irritability must be determined and corrected promptly, if possible. Antidysrhythmic medications may be used. Cardioversion (discussed on p. 628) may be indicated if the reduction in cardiac output is marked.

Ventricular Fibrillation

Ventricular fibrillation is rapid, ineffective quivering of the ventricles. With this dysrhythmia there is no audible heartbeat, no palpable pulse, and no respiration. This pattern is so grossly irregular it can hardly be mistaken for another type of dysrhythmia. Because there is no coordinated cardiac activity, cardiac arrest and death are imminent if ventricular fibrillation is not corrected immediately.

Ventricular fibrillation (Fig. 27-14) has the following characteristics:

Rate: Rapid, uncoordinated, ineffective.
P waves: Not seen.
QRS complex: Rapid, irregular undulation without specific pattern (multifocal). The ventricles have only a quivering motion.
Conduction: Foci are located in the ventricles, but so many foci are firing at one time that there is no organized conduction; no ventricular contractions occur.
Rhythm: Extremely irregular and uncoordinated, without specific pattern.

Immediate treatment is defibrillation (see page 628).

Conduction Abnormalities

First-Degree AV Block

First-degree AV block is usually associated with organic heart disease or may be due to the effect of digitalis. It is

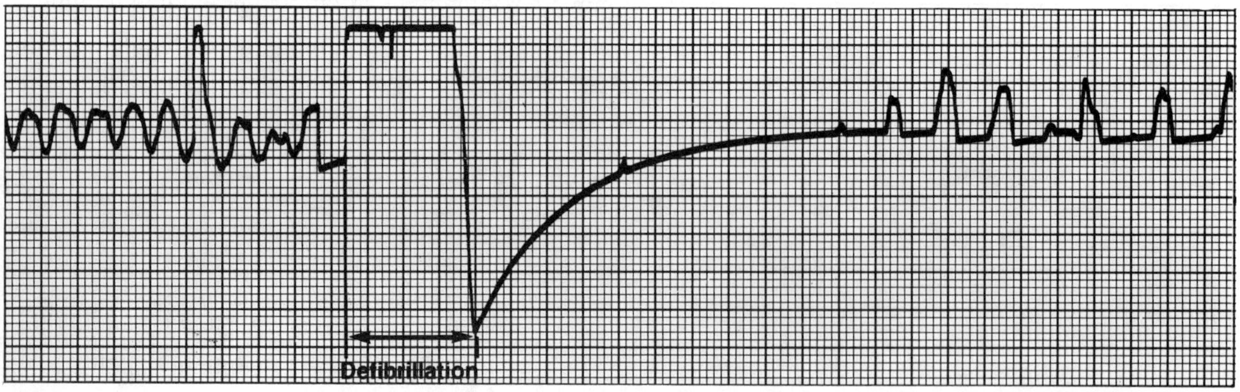

FIGURE 27-14. Ventricular fibrillation with defibrillation.

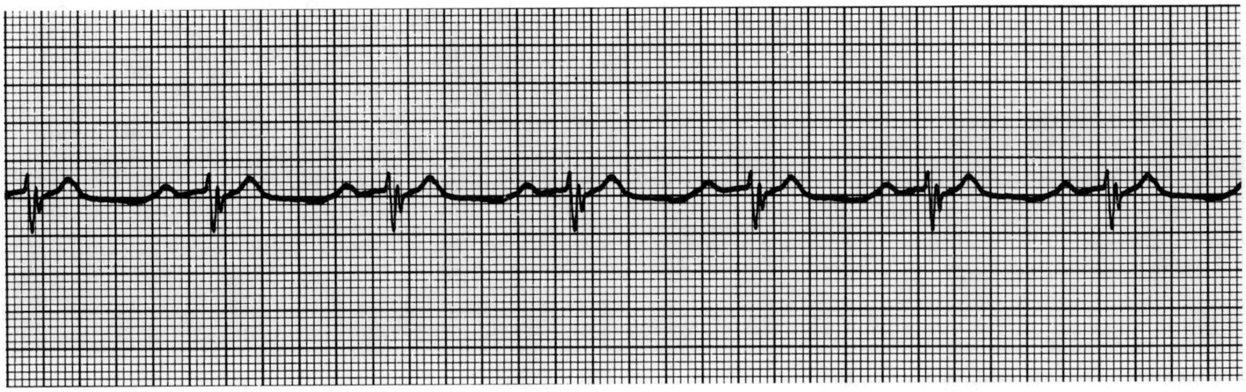

FIGURE 27-15. First-degree heart block.

seen frequently in patients with myocardial infarctions of the inferior wall of the heart.

First-degree heart block has the following characteristics (Fig. 27-15):

Rate: Variable, usually 60 to 100 beats per minute.
P waves: Precede each QRS complex. The PR interval is greater than 0.20 second in duration.
QRS complex: Follows each P wave; usually normal.
Conduction: Delayed conduction, usually anywhere between the junctional tissue and the Purkinje network, produces a prolonged PR interval. Ventricular conduction is usually normal.
Rhythm: Usually regular.

This dysrhythmia is important because it may lead to more serious forms of heart block. It is often a warning signal. Therefore, the patient should be monitored closely for any advancing block.

Second-Degree AV Block

Second-degree AV block is also caused by organic heart disease, myocardial infarction (MI), or digitalis intoxication. This type of block results in a reduced heart rate and usually a reduced cardiac output (cardiac output = stroke volume × heart rate).

Second-degree AV block has the following characteristics (Fig. 27-16):

Rate: 30 to 55 beats per minute. The atrial rate may be two, three, or four times faster than the ventricular rate.
P waves: There are two, three, or four P waves for each QRS complex. The PR interval of the conducted beat is usually normal in duration.
QRS complex: Usually normal.
Conduction: One or more of the impulses are not conducted through the ventricles.
Rhythm: Usually slow and regular. When an irregularity is present, it is due to the fact that the block is varying from 2:1 to 3:1 or to some other combination.

Treatment is directed toward increasing the heart rate to maintain a normal cardiac output. Digitalis toxicity should be ruled out and any medication that depresses myocardial activity should be withheld.

Third-Degree AV Block

Third-degree AV block (complete heart block) is also associated with organic heart disease, digitalis toxicity, and MI. The heart rate may be markedly decreased, resulting in a decrease in perfusion to vital organs, such as the brain, heart, kidneys, lungs, and skin.

Complete block—third-degree AV block—has the following characteristics (Fig. 27-17):

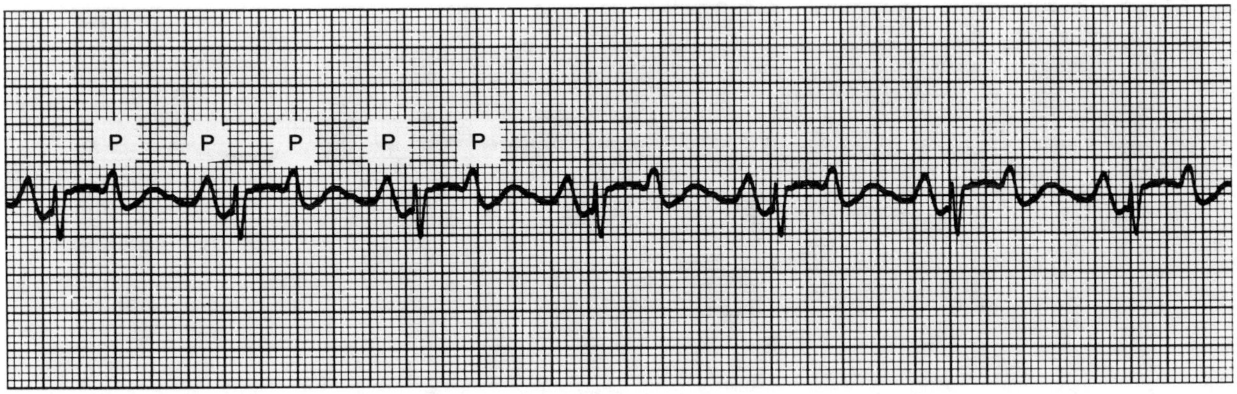

FIGURE 27-16. Second-degree heart block.

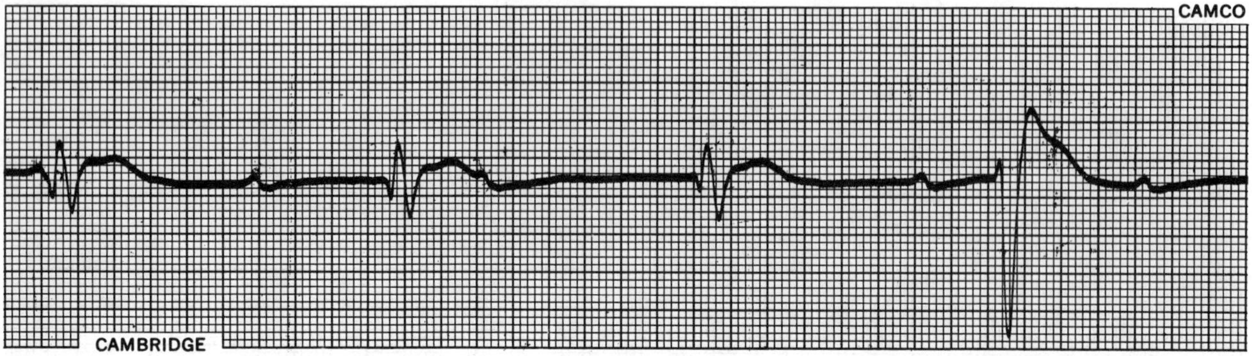

FIGURE 27-17. Third-degree heart block.

Origin: Impulses originate in the SA node, but are not conducted to the Purkinje fibers. They are completely blocked. An escape rhythm from either the junctional or the ventricular area therefore takes over as the pacemaker.

Rate: Atrial rate, 60 to 100 beats per minute; ventricular rate, 40 to 60 beats per minute if the escape rhythm originated in the junction, 20 to 40 beats per minute if the escape rhythm originated in the ventricle.

P waves: The P waves originating from the SA node are seen regularly throughout the rhythm, but they have no association with the QRS complexes.

QRS complex: If the escape rhythm originated in the junction, the QRS complexes have a normal supraventricular configuration, but have no association with the P waves. QRS complexes occur regularly. If the escape rhythm originated in the ventricle, the QRS complex is longer than 0.10 second in duration, and is usually broad and slurred. These QRS complexes have the same configuration as the QRS complexes of a PVC.

Conduction: The SA node is firing, and P waves can be seen. They are all blocked and not conducted to the ventricles. Escape rhythms originating in the junction are usually conducted normally through the ventricles. Escape rhythms from the ventricles are ectopic with aberrant configuration.

Rhythm: Usually slow but regular.

Treatment is directed toward increasing perfusion to vital organs. The use of a temporary pacemaker is the recommended treatment. A permanent pacemaker may be necessary if the block is persistent.

Ventricular Asystole

In ventricular asystole there are no QRS complexes. There is no heartbeat, no palpable pulse, and no respiration. Without immediate treatment, ventricular asystole is fatal.

Ventricular asystole (Fig. 27-18) has the following characteristics:

Rate: None.

P waves: May be visible, but they do not conduct through the AV node and ventricles.

QRS complex: None.

Conduction: Possibly, through the atria only.

Rhythm: None.

Cardiopulmonary resuscitation (CPR) is necessary to keep the patient alive. To decrease any vagal stimuli, atropine is administered intravenously. Epinephrine (intracardiac) should be administered and repeated at 5-minute intervals. Sodium bicarbonate may be administered intravenously. Insertion of a transthoracic, transvenous, or external pacemaker may be necessary.

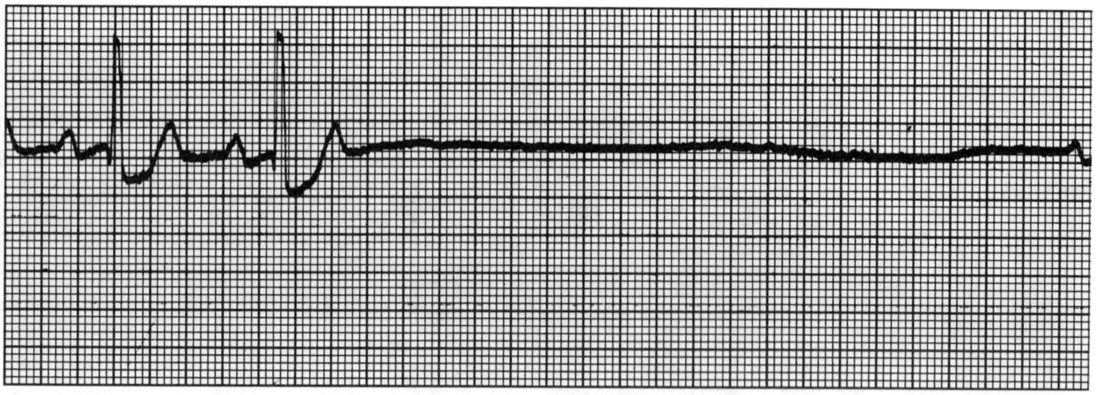

FIGURE 27-18. Ventricular asystole.

❑ NURSING PROCESS
The Patient With a Dysrhythmia

Assessment

The patient with a cardiac dysrhythmia is assessed through patient history and physical and psychosocial assessments. A major focus of assessment is the dysrhythmia and the effect it is having on cardiac output (heart rate × stroke volume). When cardiac output is reduced, the amount of oxygen reaching the tissues and vital organs is diminished. This diminished oxygenation produces the signs associated with dysrhythmias. A patient history is conducted to determine the past or present existence of syncope (fainting), lightheadedness, dizziness, fatigue, chest discomfort, and palpitations. Any one or all of these signs can be present when cardiac output is decreased.

Physical assessment is conducted to confirm the data obtained from the patient history and to observe for signs of diminished cardiac output. Attention is directed toward the skin, which can be pale and cool. Signs of fluid retention, such as neck vein distention and crackles and wheezes in the lungs are observed. The pulse is assessed apically and peripherally for rate and rhythm. The presence or absence of a pulse deficit is noted. The heart is auscultated for extra sounds, especially S_3 and S_4, which reflect reduced compliance of the myocardium seen in reduced cardiac output. Blood pressure is measured and pulse pressure is determined. A declining pulse pressure indicates reduced cardiac output.

An isolated assessment may not disclose significant changes in cardiac output; therefore, the nurse compares multiple observations over time to recognize subtle changes.

Diagnosis

Nursing Diagnoses

Based on assessment data, major nursing diagnoses of the patient may include:

- ❑ Anxiety related to fear of the unknown
- ❑ Knowledge deficit about the dysrhythmia and its treatment

Collaborative Problems/ Potential Complications

Based on the assessment data, potential complications that may develop include:

- ❑ Congestive heart failure

Planning and Implementation

Goals. The major goals of the patient may include minimization of anxiety, attainment of knowledge about the dysrhythmia and its treatment, and absence of potential complications.

Nursing Interventions

Minimizing Anxiety. The relationship between a dysrhythmia and cardiac output is explained so that the patient understands the rationale for the medical regimen. In particular, the relationship between myocardial oxygen demands and the subsequent effect on cardiac output is stressed.

During episodes of dysrhythmia, the nurse maintains a calm and reassuring attitude; this demeanor fosters a trusting relationship with the patient and assists in reducing anxiety. Small successes are shared with the patient to promote a sense of confidence in living with a dysrhythmia. For example, if a patient is experiencing episodes of dysrhythmia and a medication is administered that begins to lessen the number of ectopic beats, the nurse shares that information with the patient. The nursing goal is to maximize the patient's control and to make the unknown less threatening.

Patient Teaching. The patient will benefit from learning about the dysrhythmia and the necessary treatment. The information presented should be stated in terms that are understandable and offered in a manner that is not frightening. The importance of maintaining therapeutic serum levels of antidysrhythmic medications is explained instead of a statement such as, "Always take your medications at a regular time each day."

Providing the patient with a plan of action for emergency needs is an effective means of increasing patient knowledge. Advising the patient to predetermine which hospital to be taken to in the event of an emergency is strongly suggested.

Monitoring and Managing Potential Complications. Cardiac output is best protected by controlling episodes of the dysrhythmia. Administration of medications is managed carefully so that a constant serum blood level of the medication is maintained at all times. In the hospitalized patient with a threatening dysrhythmia, frequent rhythm strips are analyzed to track the dysrhythmia and prevent it from deteriorating into a more life-threatening dysrhythmia (*e.g.*, PVCs are aggressively managed before they become ventricular tachycardia). Rest is promoted for the patient so that myocardial oxygen needs are reduced. Blood pressure, rate and depth of respirations, and pulse rate and rhythm are evaluated regularly.

Evaluation

Expected Outcomes

1. Anxiety is minimized
   a. Expresses a positive attitude about living with the dysrhythmia
   b. Expresses confidence in knowing what to do in case of an emergency
2. Conveys knowledge of the dysrhythmia and its treatment
   a. Explains the dysrhythmia and its effect on cardiac output
   b. Articulates rationale for medication regimen and explains need for therapeutic serum level of the medication
   c. States actions to take in the event of an emergency
3. Shows no signs of complications
   a. Demonstrates minimal number of episodes of dysrhythmias

b. Demonstrates blood pressure, pulse, and respirations within normal parameters without wide variations

Adjunctive Management of Dysrhythmias

Dysrhythmias are most commonly treated with medication therapy, as previously described. In situations in which medications alone are not adequate, certain adjunctive mechanical therapies are available. The most common are elective cardioversion, defibrillation, and pacemakers. Surgical treatment, although less common, is also available.

Cardioversion

Cardioversion involves applying an electrical current to terminate dysrhythmias that have QRS complexes. It is usually an elective procedure. The patient is alert, and informed consent is obtained. Digoxin is usually withheld for 48 hours before cardioversion to prevent postcardioversion dysrhythmias. The patient is usually given conscious sedation intravenously before cardioversion to promote anesthesia, and is rarely intubated after being anesthetized. The amount of voltage used varies from 25 to 400 watt-seconds. The synchronizer is turned on.

The defibrillator is synchronized with a cardiac monitor so that an electrical impulse is discharged during ventricular depolarization (the QRS complex). If not synchronized, the defibrillator could discharge during the vulnerable period (T wave), resulting in ventricular tachycardia or fibrillation. There is no discernible QRS in ventricular fibrillation; the synchronizer is programmed to sense QRSs. If the synchronizer is left on, the machine will not fire as it waits to respond to a QRS.

If ventricular fibrillation occurs after cardioversion, the defibrillator must be recharged immediately, the synchronizer turned off, and defibrillation repeated. After use, the defibrillator must be turned off to prevent accidental discharge of the paddles. Oxygen flow should be stopped during cardioversion, if possible, to avoid the hazard of fire.

Indications of a successful response are conversion to sinus rhythm, strong peripheral pulses, and adequate blood pressure. Airway patency should be maintained, and the patient's state of consciousness assessed. Vital signs should be monitored and recorded until the patient is stabilized. ECG monitoring is required during and after cardioversion.

Defibrillation

Defibrillation is asynchronous cardioversion that is used in an emergency situation. It is usually confined to the treatment of ventricular fibrillation when there is no organized cardiac rhythm. Defibrillation completely depolarizes all the myocardial cells at once, allowing the sinus node to recapture its role as the pacemaker. The electrical voltage required to defibrillate the heart is much greater than that usually required for cardioversions. The following are some key points to remember when assisting with defibrillation or cardioversion:

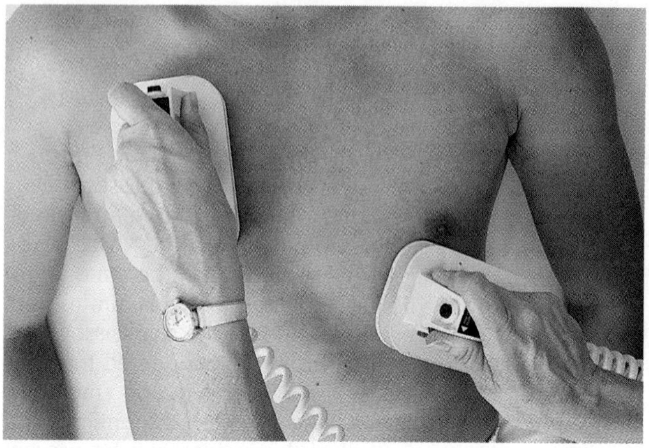

FIGURE 27-19. One method of paddle placement in cardioversion.

- Use a conducting agent between the skin and the paddles, such as saline pads or electrode paste.
- Position the paddles so as to create an effective arc (Fig. 27-19).
- Exert 20 to 25 pounds of pressure on each paddle to ensure good skin contact.
- Practice safety by being certain no one is touching the bed or the patient when the paddles are discharged.
- In the case of ventricular fibrillation, cardiopulmonary resuscitation (CPR) is initiated and continued until mechanical defibrillation is available and successful.

If defibrillation has been unsuccessful, cardiopulmonary resuscitation is resumed immediately. Epinephrine may be used if the pattern of ventricular fibrillation is fine; that is, no undulating waveform is discernible (Fig. 27-20*A*). Epinephrine may make the fibrillation coarser and thus easier to convert with defibrillation (see Fig. 27-20*B*). Sodium bicarbonate is prescribed to reverse the acidosis caused by lack of respiratory exchange. Epinephrine and sodium bicarbonate are incompatible when mixed together and must be administered separately. Blood pressure is supported using vasopressors. At no time during the resuscitation should the external cardiac massage and the assisted ventilation be stopped for longer than 5 seconds.

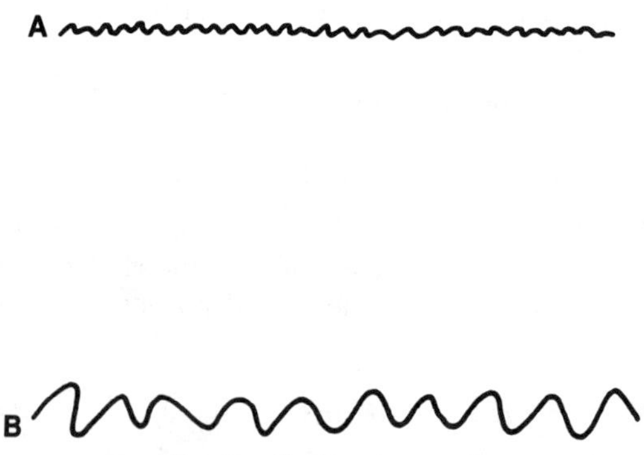

FIGURE 27-20. Very fine fibrillatory waves of ventricular fibrillation (**A**) can sometimes be coarsened into a more distinct fibrillatory pattern (**B**) by administration of epinephrine.

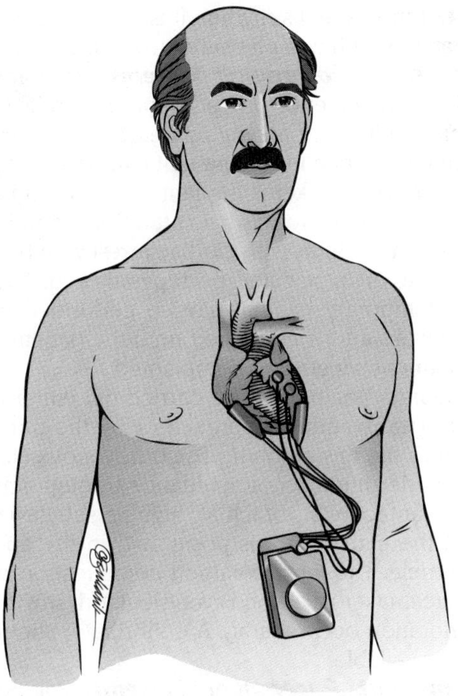

FIGURE 27-21. The implantable cardioverter-defibrillator mechanical system consists of a generator, two rate-sensing electrodes, and two epicardial patches.

Implantable Cardioverter Defibrillator

The implantable cardioverter defibrillator (ICD) is a device that detects and terminates life-threatening episodes of ventricular tachycardia or ventricular fibrillation in patients deemed at high risk. Patients at high risk are those who have survived sudden cardiac death syndrome, who have sustained ventricular tachycardia, or who have syncope secondary to ventricular tachycardia. Many of these patients are unresponsive to medications or surgical ablation of irritable myocardial tissue. This is the population of patients most suitable for ICD.

The mechanical system consists of a pulse generator, two rate-sensing leads, and two leads through which electrical shock can be delivered directly to the myocardium (Fig. 27-21). The device is implanted by thoracotomy under surgical conditions. The rate-sensing leads are designed to respond to two criteria: a rate change and an altered length of isoelectric line segments. When a dysrhythmia occurs, the rate sensors take 5 to 10 seconds to sense the dysrhythmia and another 5 to 7 seconds to charge the capacitors to deliver electrical shock to revert the rhythm. The device may deliver up to six shocks if necessary.

The use of the ICD does not eliminate the need for antidysrhythmic medication therapy. Medications are administered in conjunction with this technology.

The primary **complications** associated with the ICD are pulmonary in origin. The two most common complications are pulmonary dysfunctions, secondary to the thoracotomy required for insertion of the ICD, and surgical infections. There are lesser complications associated with the technical aspects of the equipment such as premature battery depletion or fractured leads. In spite of the possible complications, consensus among clinicians is that the benefit of this therapy to the patient exceeds the risks.

The **nursing interventions** for the patient with an ICD occur throughout three different phases: preoperative, postoperative, and predischarge. The first or preoperative phase may require management of acute episodes of life-threatening dysrhythmias in addition to providing the patient and family with explanations regarding the implantation of the ICD. The postoperative phase involves astute observation of the patient and his or her responses to the new technology. The predischarge phase involves more teaching and is vitally important to the patient's ability to live independently (Chart 27-2).

Pacemaker Therapy

A pacemaker is an electronic device that provides repetitive electrical stimuli to the heart muscle for the control of heart rate. It initiates and maintains the heart rate when the natural pacemakers of the heart are unable to do so. Pacemakers are generally used when a patient has a conduction disturbance or the forerunner of a conduction disturbance

CHART 27-2

Patient Education: The Patient With an Implantable Cardioverter Defibrillator

1. Avoid infection at the operative site.
   a. Observe incision site daily for redness, swelling, and heat.
   b. Avoid restrictive clothing that may produce friction over the wound site.
2. Avoid magnetic fields such as metal detectors at security check points, MRIs, and microwaves.
   a. Magnetic fields can deactivate the ICD, negating any effect on a dysrhythmia.
3. Maintain a log to record shocks; record events that precipitate the sensation of shock. This provides important data for the physician to use in readjusting the medical regimen.
4. Avoid danger to self and others.
   a. Discuss safety of activities (*e.g.,* driving) with physician.
   b. Adhere to appointments that are scheduled to test electronic performance of ICD.
   c. Call 911 for emergency assistance if you feel dizzy. Wear Medic-Alert identification that includes physician information.
5. Avoid frightening family or friends with unexpected shocks. Inform those closest to you that in the event they are touching you when a shock is delivered they may also feel the shock. It is especially important to warn sexual partners that this may occur.

that causes failure of cardiac output. Pacemakers can be permanent or temporary. Permanent pacemakers are used most commonly for irreversible complete heart block; temporary pacemakers are used as adjunctive therapy to support patients such as those who have had heart block after myocardial infarction or open-heart surgery. In some cases a pacemaker can also be used to control tachydysrhythmias that otherwise do not respond to medication therapy.

Pacemaker Design

Pacemakers consist of two component parts: (1) the electronic pulse generator, which contains the circuitry and batteries that generate the electrical stimulus; and (2) the pacemaker electrodes (also called leads or wires), which transmit the pacemaker impulses to the heart. The stimuli from the pacemaker travel through a flexible catheter electrode that is threaded through a vein into the right ventricle or introduced by direct penetration of the chest wall. The pulse generator is usually implanted in a subcutaneous pocket in the pectoral or axillary region; sometimes an abdominal site is selected.

Pacemaker generators are insulated to protect against body moisture and warmth. The pulse generator (or pacemaker) contains its own supply of power, which is provided by battery cells. The main power sources in current use are mercury-zinc batteries (lasting 3 to 4 years), lithium cell units (lasting up to 10 years), and a nuclear-powered pacemaker (^{238}plutonium source) that lasts 20 years to a lifetime. There are also pacemakers that can be recharged externally. Because pacemakers rely on batteries, battery exhaustion (with the exception of nuclear-powered and rechargeable batteries) is inevitable. Therefore, the generator that contains the batteries must be replaced periodically.

Types of Pacemakers

The most commonly used pacemaker is the **demand** (synchronous; noncompetitive) pacemaker, which is set for a specific rate and stimulates the heart when normal ventricular repolarization does not occur (Fig. 27-22). It functions only when the natural heart rate goes below a certain level. The **fixed rate** pacemaker (asynchronous; competitive) stimulates the ventricle at a preset constant rate that is independent of the patient's rhythm. It is used infrequently, usually in patients with complete and unvarying heart block.

Temporary Pacemaker Systems. Temporary pacing is usually an emergency procedure and permits the observation of the effects of pacing on heart function so that the optimum pacing rate for the patient can be selected before a permanent pacemaker is implanted. It is used in patients who have suffered myocardial infarction complicated by heart block, in patients with cardiac arrest with bradycardia and asystole, or in selected postoperative cardiac surgery patients. Temporary pacing may be performed for hours, days, or weeks and is continued until the patient improves or a permanent pacemaker is implanted.

Temporary pacing may be carried out either by an endocardial (transvenous) approach or by the transthoracic approach to the myocardium. The transvenous electrode is inserted under fluoroscopic guidance through any peripheral vein (antecubital, brachial, jugular, subclavian, femoral), and the catheter tip is positioned in the apex of the right ventricle. The most common complication occurring during pacemaker insertion is ventricular dysrhythmia. Cardiac perforation occurs rarely. A defibrillator should be immediately available.

Permanent Pacemaker Systems. For permanent pacing, the endocardial lead is passed transvenously into the right ventricle, and the pulse generator is implanted within the body underneath the skin below the right or left pectoral region or below the clavicle (Fig. 27-23). This is termed an endocardial or transvenous implant. This procedure is usually performed under local anesthesia. Another method of permanent pacing is implanting the pulse generator in the abdominal wall. The electrode is passed transthoracically to the myocardium, where it is sutured in place. For this method, termed an **epicardial** or **myocardial implant,** a thoracotomy is required to provide access to the heart.

Atrioventricular Pacemakers (Physiologic Pacing). Pacemaker technology, through the development of AV pacemakers, has fostered the growth of safe and effective pacemaker therapy for many complex cardiac problems. AV pacemakers are considered highly desirable because they can be programmed to mimic the patient's own intrinsic cardiac function; hence they are referred to as **physiologic pacemakers.**

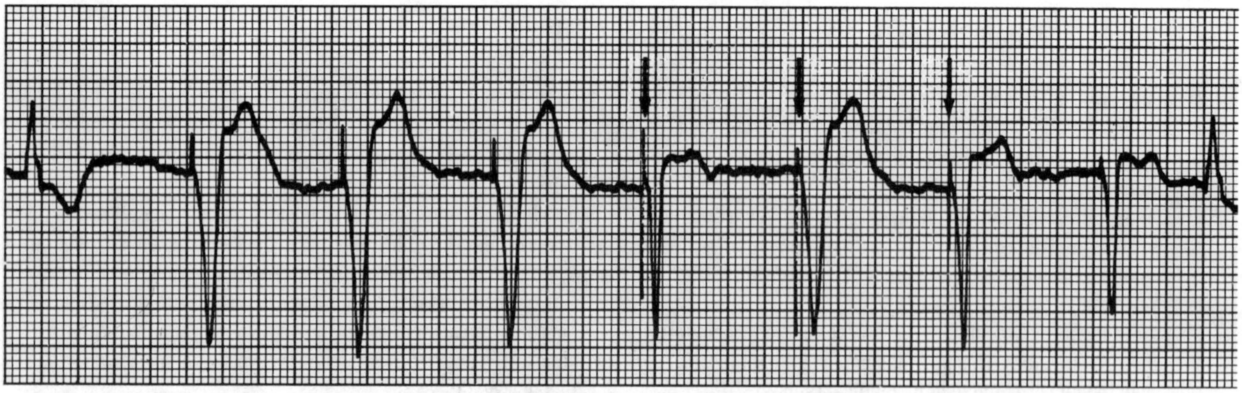

FIGURE 27-22. Synchronized pacemaker rhythm. *Arrows* indicate presence of sensed pacing spike.

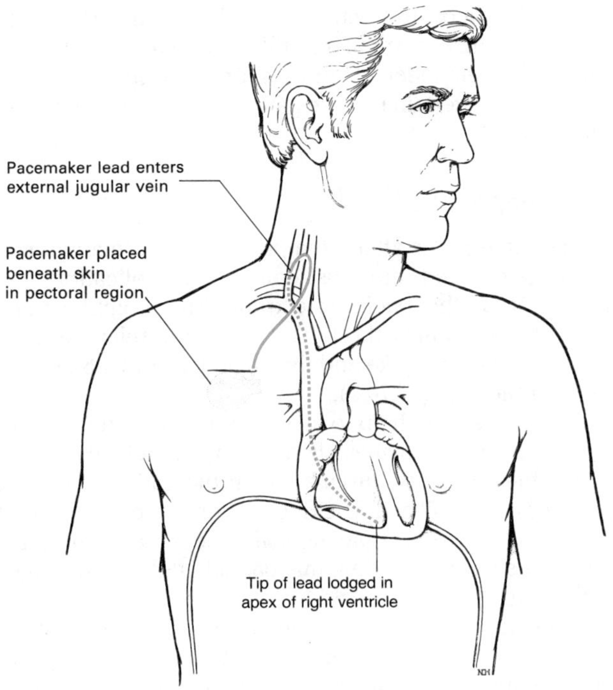

FIGURE 27-23. Implanted transvenous pacing electrode and pacemaker generator.

Because of the sophistication of pacemakers, a universal code has been adopted to provide a means of safe communication about their function. The coding is referred to as the **ICHD code** because it is sanctioned by the Inter-Society Commission for Heart Disease. The complete code consists of five letters, but only three are used in common practice.

The **first letter** of the code always describes the chamber being paced, that is, the chamber containing the pacing electrode. The possible letter characters for this code are A (atrium), V (ventricle), or D (dual, meaning both A and V).

The **second letter** describes the chamber being sensed by the pacemaker generator. Information sensed is dispatched to the generator for interpretation and action by the generator. The possible letter characters here are once again A (atrium), V (ventricle), and D (dual).

The **third letter** of the code always describes the type of response exhibited by the pacemaker. There are five characters used to describe this response, but of the five only two are in common use: I (inhibitory) and T (triggered). Inhibitory response means that the response of the pacemaker is controlled by the activity of the patient's own heart; that is, the pacemaker will not function when the patient's heart beats. In contrast, triggered response means that the pacemaker will trigger a response based on intrinsic heart activity.

An example of an ICHD-coded pacemaker is DVI:

D—Both the atrium and the ventricle have a pacing electrode in place.
V—The pacemaker is sensing the activity of the ventricle only.
I—The pacemaker's stimulating effect is being inhibited by the activity of the patient's ventricle.

Activity Response Pacemaker. A pacemaker that will alter cardiac rate in response to changes in activity is being investigated. The preliminary designs depend on parameters such as physical activity, acid–base changes, and oxygen saturation, instead of depending on sinus node function. This pacemaker will be capable of improving cardiac output during exercise.

Complications

Complications associated with pacemakers relate to (1) their presence within the body, and (2) improper functioning. The following complications may arise from the presence of the pacemaker:

- Local infection (sepsis or hematoma formation) may occur at the site of venous cutdown or subcutaneous pacemaker placement.
- Dysrhythmias—ventricular ectopic activity may follow irritation of the ventricular wall by the electrode.
- Perforation of the myocardium or right ventricle by the catheter may occur.
- Abrupt loss of pacing may be caused by high ventricular threshold.

Pacemaker malfunction can arise from failure in one or more components of the pacing system. The majority of pulse generator failures are from depletion of the power supply (*i.e.*, battery failure). The patient should be informed that the battery cells are sealed in the pulse generator. When it is time for a battery change, a new incision is made at the site of the old incision. The old pulse generator is removed, and the new unit is connected to the existing leads and reimplanted in the already existing pocket. This is usually performed under local anesthesia. Other complications include fracture (breakage) or dislocation of the electrodes and electronic failure.

Malfunction of the pacemaker can also occur with exposure to electromagnetic fields. Electromagnetic fields are produced by technologic equipment such as microwave ovens, magnetic resonance imaging (MRI) equipment, and the hand-held metal detectors found at security checkpoints such as those at airports and government buildings. The patient is cautioned to avoid situations that involve electromagnetic field exposure. The patient is advised to wear identification that will alert emergency health care personnel to the presence of the pacemaker.

Complications are manifested by abrupt changes in heart rate and rhythm. The degree to which these symptoms become apparent will depend on the patient's level of dependency on the pacemaker. The diagnosis of these complications is made by ECG analysis. Manipulating the electrodes or replacing the pacemaker generator may be necessary.

Pacemaker Surveillance

Pacemaker clinics have been established to monitor patients and to test pulse generators for warnings of impending pacemaker system failure. Testing of pacemaker pulse amplitude and duration and analysis of pulse contour require amplification equipment. With special equipment, lead fracture and insulation disruption can be detected. A 12-lead ECG is performed during each patient visit to the clinic.

Another method of follow-up is trans-telephone transmission of the generator's pulse rate. Special equipment is used to transmit the sound tone of the patient's pacemaker over the telephone to a receiving system at a pacemaker clinic. The sounds are converted into an electronic signal and permanently recorded on an ECG strip. The pacemaker rate and other data concerning pacemaker function are obtained and evaluated by a cardiologist. This simplifies the diagnosis of a failing generator, provides reassurance, and improves the management of the person who is physically remote from pacemaker testing facilities.

❑ NURSING PROCESS
The Patient With a Pacemaker

Assessment

After a temporary or a permanent pacemaker is inserted, the patient's heart rate and rhythm are monitored by electrocardiogram. The preset pacemaker rate is noted; the patient's heart rate may vary as much as five beats above or below the preset pacemaker rate. The appearance or increasing frequency of dysrhythmia is observed and reported to the physician.

The incision site where the pulse generator is implanted (or the entry site for the pacing electrode if the pacemaker is temporary) is observed for bleeding, hematoma formation, or infection. Infection is a major threat to the patient who has received a new pacemaker. The insertion site is observed primarily for swelling, unusual tenderness, and increased heat. The patient may complain of continuous throbbing or pain. Any unusual drainage is reported to the physician.

All electrical equipment used in the vicinity of the patient is grounded. Improperly grounded equipment can generate leakage currents capable of producing ventricular fibrillation.

The nurse observes for potential sources of electrical hazards. No metal parts of the output terminal or pacemaker wires should be exposed. All such bare metal must be carefully covered with nonconductive material to prevent accidental ventricular fibrillation from stray currents. A biomedical engineer, electrician, or other qualified person should make certain that the patient is in an electrically safe environment.

Complications

In the initial hours after a temporary or a permanent pacemaker is inserted, the most common complication is dislodgment of the pacing electrode. This complication is noted by examining the ECG pattern; the relationship between the pacing spike and the patient's P or QRS becomes asynchronous (Fig. 27-24).

The nurse can help to avoid this complication by minimizing patient activities. If a temporary electrode is in place, the extremity through which the catheter has been passed is immobilized. The ECG is monitored very carefully for the presence of a pacing spike. Because of the importance of such monitoring, this patient is ideally in a monitored unit.

The following data should be noted on the patient's record: the model of pacemaker, date and time of its insertion, location of the pulse generator, stimulation threshold, and pacer rate. This information is important for solving any unusual dysrhythmia problem.

Diagnosis

Nursing Diagnoses

Based on assessment data, major nursing diagnoses of the patient may include the following:

- Risk for infection related to catheter or generator insertion
- Knowledge deficit regarding self-care program

Collaborative Problems/ Potential Complications

Based on the assessment data, potential complications that may develop include:

- Pacemaker malfunction resulting in decreased cardiac output

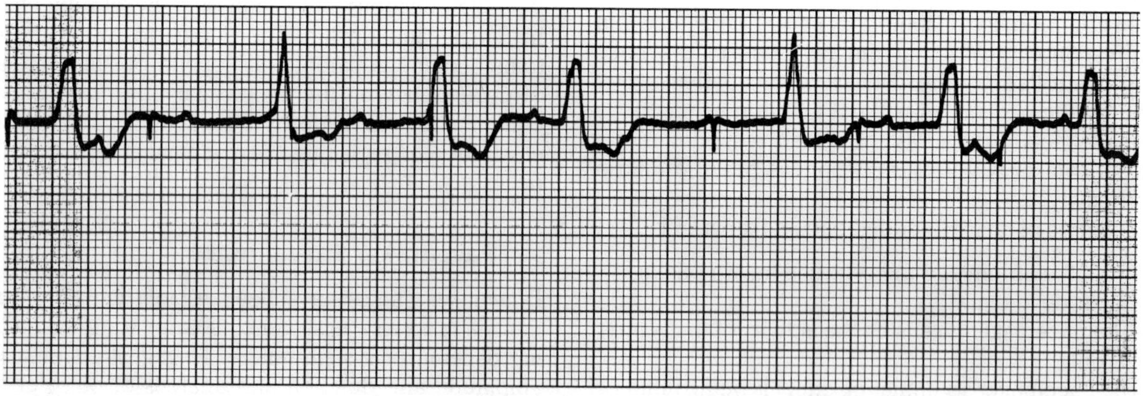

FIGURE 27-24. Loss of capture of pacemaker. Pacer discharge spike, but no mechanical activity follows.

Planning and Implementation

Goals. The major goals of the patient may include (1) absence of infection, (2) adherence to a self-care program, and (3) maintenance of pacemaker function.

Nursing Interventions

Preventing Infection. The wound site is inspected regularly for redness, edema, pain, or any unusual bleeding. The physician performs the initial dressing change and the nurse inspects and changes the dressing each day thereafter. Changes in the wound are reported to the physician.

Patient Education and Home Care Considerations. Because of need for a pacemaker, most patients are very compliant with the home health-care program. The patient follows a prescribed program of assessing and recording pulse rate. See Chart 27-3 for additional details of patient education and maintenance of pacemaker function.

Evaluation

Expected Outcomes

1. Free of infection
   a. Temperature normal
   b. WBCs within normal range (5,000 to 10,000/mm^3)
   c. Exhibits no redness or swelling of pacemaker insertion site
2. Adheres to a self-care program
   a. Responds appropriately when queried about the signs and symptoms of infection
   b. Knows when to seek medical attention (as demonstrated in responses to signs and symptoms)
3. Maintains pacemaker function
   a. Measures and records pulse rate at regular intervals
   b. Experiences no abrupt changes in pulse rate or rhythm
   c. See Chart 27-3 for additional outcomes related to maintaining pacemaker function

Electrophysiologic Studies

Electrophysiologic studies (EPSs) allow the clinician to induce troubling dysrhythmias in a controlled environment for the purpose of determining appropriate treatment. Catheters containing electrodes in the distal portion are placed within the heart. Stimulation of these electrode-containing catheters induces dysrhythmias. Once a dysrhythmia is induced, different medications are administered to determine which is the most effective in suppressing the dysrhythmia. The long-term benefit of EPS remains to be determined.

Patients who are to receive EPS are usually very anxious about the procedure and about its outcome. Prior to the procedure they should receive instructions about the procedure, what to expect, and what will be expected of them (*e.g.*, lying very still during the procedure). During the procedure they can benefit from a calm, reassuring approach.

Cardiac Conduction Surgery

Atrial and ventricular tachycardias that do not respond to medications and are not suitable for anti-tachycardia pacing may be treated by methods other than medications and pacemakers. Such methods include endocardial isolation, endocardial resection, cryoablation, electrical ablation, and radiofrequency ablation. An implantable cardioverter defibrillator (ICD) may be used in conjunction with these surgical interventions.

Endocardial isolation involves making an incision into the endocardium separating the area where the dys-

CHART 27-3
Patient Education: The Patient With a Pacemaker

1. Report to physician/pacemaker clinic periodically as prescribed, so that the rate of the pacemaker and its function can be monitored. This is especially important during the first month after implantation.
   a. Adhere to weekly monitoring schedule during the first month after implantation.
   b. Check pulse daily. Report *immediately* any sudden slowing or increasing of the pulse rate. This may indicate pacemaker malfunction.
   c. Resume weekly monitoring when battery depletion is anticipated. (The time for reimplantation depends on the type of battery in use.)
2. Wear loose-fitting clothing around the area of the pacemaker.
   a. State the reason for the slight bulge over the pacemaker implant.
   b. Notify physician if the area becomes reddened or painful.
   c. Avoid trauma to the area of the pacemaker generator.
3. Study the manufacturer's instructions and become familiar with the pacemaker.
4. Recognize that physical activity does not usually have to be curtailed, with the exception of contact sports.
5. Carry an identification card/bracelet indicating physician's name, type and model number of pacemaker, manufacturer's name, pacemaker rate, and hospital where pacemaker was inserted.
6. Avoid close exposure to microwave ovens, MRI, and other sources of magnetic fields.
7. Show identification card and request scanning by a hand scanner when going through security gates, *e.g.*, at airports, government buildings.
8. Remember that hospitalization is necessary periodically for battery changes/pacemaker unit replacement.

CRITICAL THINKING EXERCISES

1. You are working in a clinic when a patient enters complaining of dizziness and fatigue. She tells you that she has been diagnosed as having an atrial dysrhythmia. How would you focus your assessment of this patient, and what key assessment factors would you highlight in reporting to the primary care provider?
3. You are caring for a patient who is being prepared for cardioversion. He indicates that he is very anxious about the procedure because it is the same as the "defibrillation" that his brother had when he died. In offering an explanation to the patient, how would you describe the differences in the two treatments?

rhythmia originates from the surrounding endocardium. The edges of the incision are then sutured back together. The incision and its resulting scar tissue prevent the dysrhythmia from affecting the whole heart.

In **endocardial resection,** the origin of the dysrhythmia is identified and that area of the endocardium is peeled away. No reconstruction or repair is necessary.

Cryoablation involves placing a special probe, cooled to a temperature of –60°C (–76°F), on the endocardium at the site of the dysrhythmia's origin for 2 minutes. The frozen area becomes a small scar and the origin of the dysrhythmia is eliminated.

In **electrical ablation** a catheter is placed at or near the origin of the dysrhythmia, and one to four shocks of 100 to 300 joules are administered through the catheter directly to the endocardium and surrounding tissue. The cardiac tissue is burned and scars, thus eliminating the source of the dysrhythmia.

Radiofrequency ablation involves placing a special catheter at or near the origin of the dysrhythmia. High-frequency sound waves are passed through the catheter, destroying the dysrhythmic tissue. The tissue damage is more specific to the dysrhythmic tissue with less trauma to the surrounding cardiac tissue than occurs with cryoablation or electrical ablation.

REFERENCES AND SELECTED READINGS

Books and Pamphlets

American Heart Association. Textbook of Advanced Cardiac Life Support. Dallas, 1990.
Braunwald E. Heart Disease: A Textbook of Cardiovascular Medicine. Philadelphia, WB Saunders, 1992.
Chou T. Electrocardiography in Clinical Practice. Philadelphia, WB Saunders, 1991
Conover MB. Understanding Electrocardiography. St. Louis, CV Mosby, 1992.
Hurst JW (ed). The Heart. New York, McGraw-Hill, 1990.
Kinny M et al. AACN's Clinical Reference Manual. New York, McGraw-Hill, 1993.
Kinny M et al. Comprehensive Cardiac Care. St. Louis, CV Mosby, 1991.
Marriott HJL. Practical Electrocardiography. Baltimore, Williams and Wilkins, 1988.
Woods SL et al. Cardiac Nursing, 3rd ed. Philadelphia, JB Lippincott, 1995.

Journals

Asterisks indicate nursing research articles.

Allard KS. Current trends in defibrillation. Medsurg Nurs Q 1992 Summer; 1(1):26–43.
Berry S and Schleicher C. Adjusting the beat. Am J Nurs 1992 June; 92(6):55–60.
Brannon PH and Johnson R. The internal cardioverter defibrillator: Patient–family teaching. Focus on Critical Care 1992 Feb; 19(1):41–46.
Burke L et al. Living with recurrent ventricular dysrhythmias. Focus on Critical Care 1992 Feb; 19(1):60–66.
Collins M. When your patient has an implantable cardioverter-defibrillator. Am J Nurs 1994 Mar; 94(3):34–38.
Currier DS and Packa D. The patient with an implantable cardiac defibrillator: A case study. Focus on Critical Care 1992 April; 19(2):150–154.
DeAngelis R and Lessig ML. Hyperkalemia. Crit Care Nurs 1992 Mar; 12(3):55–59.
DeAngelis R and Lessig ML. Hypokalemia. Crit Care Nurs 1991 July; 11(7):71–75.
Dreifus LS et al. Guidelines for implantation of cardiac pacemakers and antiarrhythmia devices. Circulation 1991 July; 84(1): 455–467.
Fabiszewski R and Volosin KJ. Refusal of cardioverter defibrillator generator replacement: The nurse's role. Focus on Critical Care 1992 April; 19(2):97–100.
Friday BA. Magnesium metabolism: A case report and literature review. Crit Care Nurs 1991 May; 11(5):62–71.
Horowitz LN. The automatic implantable cardioverter defibrillator: Review of clinical results 1980–1990. Pace—Pacing and Clinical Electrophysiology 1992 April; 15(4 part 3):604–609.
Kleinschmidt KM and Stafford MJ. Dual-chamber cardiac pacemakers. J Cardiovasc Nurs 1991 April; 5(3):9–20.
Kuhrik N et al. Defibrillation over the phone. Am J Nurs 1992 Nov; 92(11):28–31.
Mason P and McPherson C. Implantable cardioverter defibrillator: A review. Heart Lung 1992 Mar; 21(2):141–147.
Nursing responsibilities during CPR. Medsurg Nurs Q 1992 Summer; 1(1):1–25.
Porterfield M and Porterfield JG. Digitalis toxicity: A common occurrence. Crit Care Nurs 1993 Dec; 13(6):40–43.
Saver CL. Decoding the ACLS algorithms. Am J Nurs 1994 Jan; 94(1):27–36.
Scrima D. Managing dobutamine infusions. Medsurg Nurs 1993 Dec; 2(6):459–465.
Smith DF and Bumann R. Assessing and treating decreased cardiac output. Medsurg Nurs 1993 Oct; 2(5):351–357.
Sommers MS. Potential for injury: Trauma after cardiopulmonary resuscitation. Heart Lung 1991 May; 20(3):287–293.
Sommers MS. Preventing complications of CPR. Medsurg Nurs Q 1992 Summer; 1(1):45–54.
Stahl L. How to manage common arrhythmias in medical patients. Am J Nurs 1995 Mar; 95(3):36–41.
Teplitz L. Cardiac pacing. J Cardiovasc Nurs 1991 April; 5(3):1–8.

INFORMATION/RESOURCES

Government Agencies

National Heart, Lung, and Blood Institute
National Institutes of Health
Building 31, Room 5A52
Bethesda, MD 20892

Independent Agencies

American Heart Association
7320 Greenville Ave.
Dallas, TX 75231

Coronary Club
9500 Euclid Ave.
Cleveland, OH 44106

Heartlife
PO Box 54305
Atlanta, GA 30308

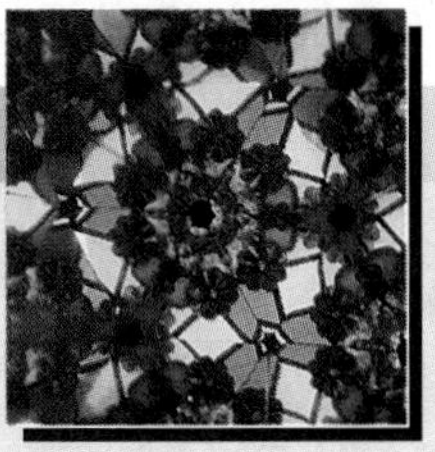

28

Management of Patients With Cardiac Disorders and Related Complications

CHAPTER OUTLINE

Coronary Artery Disease
Coronary Atherosclerosis
Angina Pectoris
- NURSING PROCESS: The Patient With Angina Pectoris

Myocardial Infarction
- NURSING PROCESS: The Patient With Myocardial Infarction

Complications
Acute Pulmonary Edema
Cardiac Failure: Congestive Heart Failure
- NURSING PROCESS: The Patient With Cardiac Failure

Cardiogenic Shock
Thromboembolic Episodes
Pericardial Effusion and Cardiac Tamponade
Myocardial Rupture
Cardiac Arrest
Cardiopulmonary Resuscitation
Critical Thinking Exercises

LEARNING OBJECTIVES

On completion of this chapter, the learner will be able to:

1. Describe the relationship between coronary atherosclerosis, angina pectoris, and myocardial infarction
2. Develop teaching plans for patients with angina pectoris and myocardial infarction
3. Use the nursing process as a framework for care of patients with angina pectoris
4. Use the nursing process as a framework for care of patients with myocardial infarction
5. Describe the management of patients with acute pulmonary edema
6. Use the nursing process as a framework for care of patients with cardiac failure
7. Demonstrate the techniques of cardiopulmonary resuscitation

Heart disease is a major cause of morbidity and mortality in America. Although some forms of heart disease, such as valvular disorders, have been significantly reduced as a result of sophisticated technology and treatment, others, such as coronary heart disease (CHD) or coronary artery disease (CAD), continue as a major threat to health and well-being.

In the past, the major focus of concern about heart disease concentrated on white, middle-aged males. More recently, studies have shown that other segments of the population are also affected by cardiac problems at an alarming rate. Women, in particular, and especially women after menopause, have been shown to have similar rates of mortality from coronary heart disease as men. Increasing attention has been focused on whether hormone replacement therapy (HRT) for women during and after menopause provides a means of reducing the incidence of coronary heart disease.

Because coronary heart disease is so prevalent in America, nurses need to become familiar with the various types of cardiac problems and the methods for assessing and possibly preventing these disorders.

Coronary Artery Disease

Coronary Atherosclerosis

The most common heart disease in the United States is coronary atherosclerosis. This pathologic condition of the coronary arteries is characterized by an abnormal accumulation of lipid or fatty substances and fibrous tissue in the vessel wall that leads to changes in arterial structure and function and reduction of blood flow to the myocardium. Atherosclerotic heart disease is probably caused by alterations in lipid metabolism, blood coagulation, and the biophysical and biochemical properties of the arterial walls.

Although there is disagreement among authorities about how atherosclerosis begins, there is agreement that atherosclerosis is a progressive disease and that it can be curtailed and in some cases reversed.

Pathophysiology

Atherosclerosis begins when waxy cholesterol becomes deposited on the intima of the major arteries. These deposits, called **atheromas** or **plaques** interfere with the absorption of nutrients by the endothelial cells that compose the vessel lining and obstruct blood flow by protruding into the lumen of the vessel (Fig. 28-1). The vascular endothelium in the involved areas becomes necrotic and then scarred, further compromising the lumen and impeding the flow of blood. At sites where the lumen is narrowed and the wall rough, there is a great tendency for clots to form, which explains why intravascular coagulation, followed by thromboembolic disease, is among the most important complications of atherosclerosis.

Several theories about how atherosclerotic lesions begin have been proposed, but none has been conclusively proven. Among suspected mechanisms are the formation of thrombi on the surface of the plaque; consolidation of the thrombus from the effects of fibrin; hemorrhage into a plaque; and continuing accumulation of lipid. If the fibrous cap of the plaque ruptures, the lipid debris is swept into the bloodstream and obstructs the arteries and capillaries distal to the ruptured plaque.

The anatomic structure of the coronary arteries makes them particularly susceptible to the mechanisms of atherosclerosis. As can be seen in Figure 28-2, they twist and turn as they supply the heart, thereby creating sites susceptible to atheroma development.

Clinical Manifestations

Coronary atherosclerosis produces symptoms and complications as a result of the narrowing of the arterial lumen and obstruction of blood flow to the myocardium. This impediment to blood flow is progressive, and the inadequate blood supply (**ischemia**) that results deprives the muscle cells of the blood components they need for their survival.

Varying degrees of cell damage are produced by ischemia. The major manifestation of ischemia of the myocardium is chest pain. **Angina pectoris** refers to recurrent chest pain that is not accompanied by irreversible damage to myocardial cells. More severe ischemia with cell damage is termed **myocardial infarction.** Irreversibly damaged myocardium undergoes degeneration and is replaced by scar tissue. If the damage to the myocardium is extensive, the heart may eventually fail, that is, it may be unable to support the body's needs for blood by providing an adequate cardiac output.

Other clinical manifestations of coronary artery disease may be ECG changes, ventricular aneurysms, dysrhythmias, and sudden death.

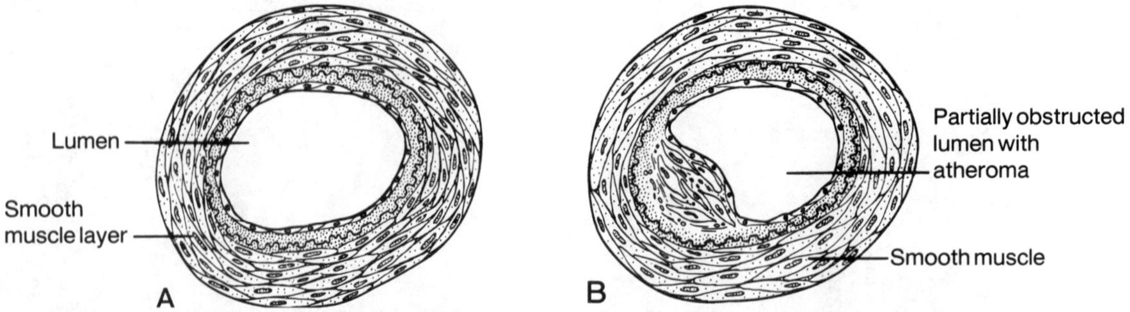

FIGURE 28-1. Cross-section of a normal and an atherosclerotic artery. (**A**) Cross-section of normal artery showing patent lumen. (**B**) Cross-section of artery showing atheroma and diminished patency of artery lumen.

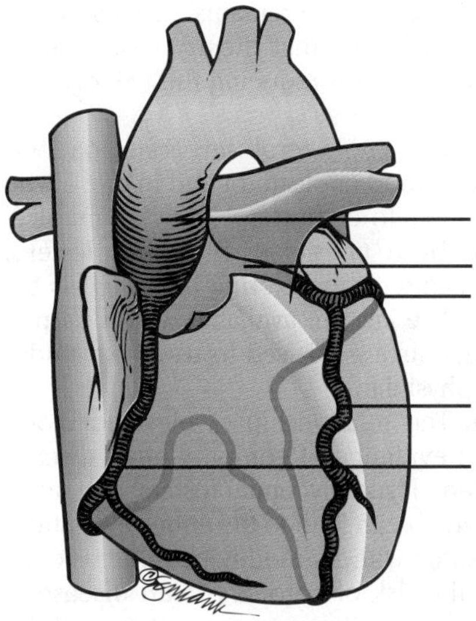

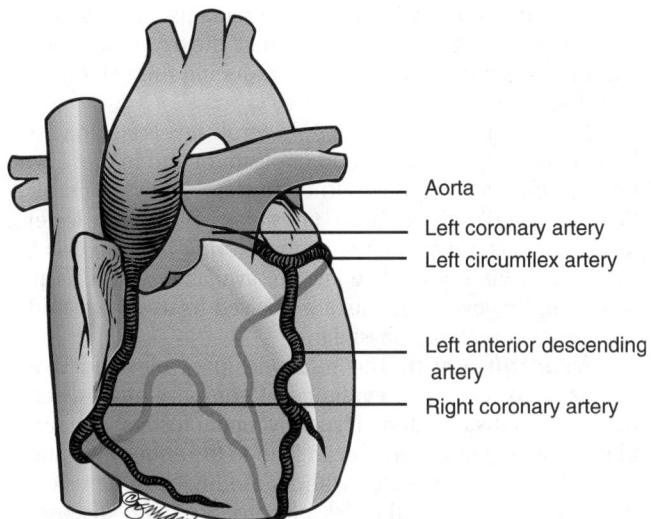

FIGURE 28-2. Angles of the coronary arteries. The many angles and curves of the coronary arteries contribute to the vessels' susceptibility to the development of atheromatous plaques. Arteries shown in color are behind the heart.

CHART 28-1
Risk Factors for Coronary Heart Disease

Nonmodifiable Risk Factors

- Positive family history
- Increasing age
- Gender—Occurs three times more often in men than in women
- Race—Higher incidence in African-Americans than in Caucasians

Modifiable Risk Factors

- High blood cholesterol
- Elevated blood pressure
- Cigarette smoking
- Elevated blood glucose (diabetes mellitus)
- Obesity
- Physical inactivity
- Stress
- Use of oral contraceptives
- Personality traits such as highly competitive, aggressive, or ambitious
- Geography—Higher incidence in industrialized regions

Risk Factors

Epidemiologic studies show that there are conditions that may precede or accompany the onset of coronary heart disease. These conditions are called risk factors because the presence of one or more is believed to increase one's risk of developing coronary heart disease.

A risk factor may be modifiable or nonmodifiable. A **modifiable risk factor** is one over which an individual may exercise control by changing a lifestyle or personal habit; a **nonmodifiable risk factor** is a consequence of genetics over which an individual has no control (Chart 28-1).

A risk factor may operate independently or in tandem with other risk factors. The more risk factors a person has, the greater is the likelihood of developing coronary artery disease. Persons at risk are advised to seek regular medical examinations and, where possible, to engage in a deliberate effort to reduce the number and extent of risks.

Prevention

A major goal in identifying and reducing risk factors is to prevent coronary heart disease. Prevention may be primary or secondary. Primary prevention involves measures taken before the development of symptoms of a disease process; secondary prevention involves those measures that may be taken to reduce the progress of or prevent the recurrence of a disease process.

Five modifiable risk factors—cigarette smoking, elevated blood pressure, high blood cholesterol, hyperglycemia, and certain behavior patterns—have received a great deal of attention in health promotion programs. Cigarette smoking and hypertension have been cited as *major* causes of coronary artery disease (CAD) and its consequent complications.

Cigarette Smoking. Cigarette smoking contributes to the development and severity of coronary artery disease in three ways.

First, the inhalation of smoke increases the blood carbon monoxide (CO) level. Hemoglobin, the oxygen-carrying component of blood, combines more readily with CO than with O_2. Thus, the oxygen being supplied to the heart is severely limited, which makes the heart work harder to produce the same amount of energy.

Second, nicotinic acid in tobacco products triggers the release of catecholamines, which cause arterial constriction. Blood flow and subsequent oxygenation are compromised.

Third, cigarette smoking increases platelet adhesion, leading to a higher probability of thrombus formation.

A person with increased risk for coronary heart disease is encouraged to stop smoking. The individual who successfully stops smoking reduces the risk of coronary heart disease by 50% within the first year. The risk continues to decline as long as the individual refrains from smoking. Exposure to passive smoke is discouraged since it may aggravate any existing cardiopulmonary disease.

Elevated Blood Pressure. Elevated blood pressure is the most insidious of all risk factors because it is asymptomatic until hypertension is well advanced. An elevated blood pressure creates a very high pressure gradient against which the left ventricle must pump. The continued high pressure forces the myocardial oxygen demands to exceed the supply. This initiates the vicious cycle of pain associated with coronary artery disease.

Early detection of high blood pressure and compliance with a therapeutic regimen can prevent the serious consequences associated with untreated elevated blood pressure. Blood pressure is discussed in detail in Chapter 31.

High Blood Cholesterol. The association of high blood cholesterol with coronary heart disease is well established and accepted. While the metabolism of fats is highly complex and difficult to understand, several key components are important in understanding the development of coronary heart disease (CHD).

Fats, which are insoluble in water, are encased in water-soluble lipoproteins to allow them to be transported within a circulatory system that is water-based. Three elements of fat metabolism—total cholesterol, low density lipoprotein (LDL), and high density lipoprotein (HDL)—are cited as primary factors affecting the development of CHD. Controlling the serum levels of total cholesterol and LDL and HDL within a therapeutic range is the goal of dietary management of CHD.

LDL exerts a harmful effect on the arterial wall and accelerates the process of atherosclerosis. In contrast, HDL assists the utilization of total cholesterol by transporting LDL to the liver where it is biodegraded and then excreted. The desired goal is to have low LDL values (<130 mg/dl) and high HDL values (>50 mg/dl) and a total cholesterol level of <200 mg/dl. These normal values are recommended in the absence of coronary heart disease and other significant risk factors.

Control and Prevention. Serum levels of cholesterol can usually be controlled by diet and exercise. Reducing the amount of fat eaten daily will reduce the fat available for metabolism and conversion to cholesterol.

Dietary control has been made easier because food manufacturers are required to provide comprehensive nutritional data on product labels. The label information that would be of interest to a person attempting to control cholesterol might be: (1) serving size expressed in household measure, (2) total calories from fat per serving, and (3) percent of daily value (DV) for fat. There are many resources available to assist persons who are attempting to control their cholesterol levels. Registered dieticians, self-help groups, and literature from the American Heart Association are a few examples of these resources.

Dietary soluble fiber may also help lower cholesterol. Soluble fibers such as pectin (found in fresh fruit) enhance the excretion of metabolized cholesterol. The effect of fiber to reduce serum cholesterol consistently continues to be investigated.

Exercise is known to raise HDL, which in turn helps to metabolize and reduce levels of LDL.

Medications may also be used in some instances to control cholesterol. For patients in whom diet alone cannot normalize serum cholesterol, there are several medications that have a synergistic effect when taken with the prescribed diet. These agents are shown to be biochemically effective by helping reduce elevated lipoprotein concentration and eliminating manifestations of abnormally high lipoprotein levels, such as xanthomas (yellow papules in the skin caused by lipid deposits).

The medications used are usually grouped into two types: those that decrease lipoprotein synthesis, such as nicotinic acid and clofibrate, and those that increase lipoprotein breakdown (catabolism), such as cholestyramine, sitosterol, and D-thyroxine.

Harmful side effects can occur from the use of these medications. Medication therapy is, therefore, reserved for the high-risk patient and is not regarded as a viable substitute for dietary modification. The usefulness of medications in reversing coronary heart disease remains under scrutiny. It is, however, broadly accepted that dietary modification can have a significant impact on reducing the risk of coronary heart disease.

Monitoring of blood cholesterol levels in patients known to have elevated blood cholesterol and in those who need to monitor responses to cholesterol-lowering medications is usually done by a physician. Blood cholesterol home test kits are available for monitoring blood levels between physician visits. The kits are available without a prescription; however, patients are advised to use them under the management of a physician.

Hyperglycemia. The relationship of elevated blood glucose and increased evidence of coronary heart disease has been substantiated. Hyperglycemia fosters increased platelet aggregation, which can lead to thrombus formation. Controlling hyperglycemia without modifying other risk factors does not reduce the risk of coronary heart disease. If other risk factors such as obesity are present, they must be brought under control.

Behavior Patterns. It is believed that stress and certain behaviors contribute to the pathogenesis of coronary heart disease. Psychobiologic and epidemiologic studies describe behaviors that characterize people who are prone to coronary heart disease: competitive striving for achievement, exaggerated sense of time urgency, aggressiveness, and hostility. A person who manifests these behaviors is classified as type A coronary prone. It appears that, in addition to reducing other risk factors (smoking, dietary fats), such a person should take steps to alter lifestyle and long-term habits.

The type A behavior pattern is widely accepted as a risk factor for coronary heart disease. Contemporary research indicates that it may not be as significant as was once thought, but there is not yet conclusive evidence of its precise role.

Gerontologic Considerations

Atherosclerotic coronary heart disease is not a function of aging. Aging does, however, produce changes in the integrity of the lining of the walls of arteries (arteriosclerosis), thus impeding blood flow and tissue nutrition. These changes are often sufficient to diminish oxygenation and increase myocardial oxygen consumption (MVO_2). The result can be debilitating angina pectoris and eventually congestive heart failure.

Angina Pectoris

Pathophysiology

Angina pectoris is a clinical syndrome characterized by episodes or paroxysms of pain or a feeling of pressure in the anterior chest. The cause is considered to be insufficient coronary blood flow, resulting in inadequate oxygen supply to the myocardium; in other words, myocardial oxygen demands exceed the supply of oxygen.

Angina is usually caused by atherosclerotic heart disease and almost invariably is associated with a significant obstruction of a major coronary artery. The characteristics of the various types of angina are listed in Chart 28-2.

A number of factors can produce anginal pain:

1. Physical exertion can precipitate an attack by increasing myocardial oxygen demands.
2. Exposure to cold can cause vasoconstriction and an elevated blood pressure, with increased oxygen demand.
3. Eating a heavy meal increases the blood flow to the mesenteric area for digestion, thus reducing the available blood supply to the heart. (In a severely compromised heart, the shunting of blood for digestion can be sufficient to induce anginal pain.)
4. Stress or any emotion-provoking situation causing the release of adrenaline and increased blood pressure may accelerate the heart rate, thus increasing myocardial workload.

Identifying angina requires a careful history; effective treatment begins with patient teaching.

Clinical Manifestations

Ischemia of the heart muscle produces **pain,** varying in severity from pressure in the upper chest to agonizing pain that is accompanied by severe apprehension and a feeling of impending death. The pain is usually felt deep in the chest behind the upper or middle third of the sternum (retrosternal). Although the pain frequently is localized, it may radiate to the neck, jaw, shoulders, and inner aspects of the upper extremities.

The patient often experiences a tightness, a choking or strangling sensation that has a viselike, insistent quality. A feeling of weakness or numbness in the arms, wrists, and hands may accompany the pain. Along with the physical pain, the patient may have a sense of impending death. An important characteristic of anginal pain is that it subsides when the precipitating cause is removed.

Gerontologic Considerations

The elderly person who experiences angina may not exhibit the typical pain profile because of changes in neuroreceptors. Pain is often manifested in the elderly as weakness or fainting. When exposed to cold temperatures, elderly persons may experience anginal symptoms more quickly than younger persons because they have less subcutaneous fat to provide insulation. They should be encouraged to dress with extra clothing and advised to recognize feelings of weakness as an indication that they should rest or take prescribed medications.

CHART 28-2

Types of Angina

Unstable Angina (Preinfarction Angina; Crescendo Angina)

Progressive increase in frequency, intensity, and duration of anginal attacks

Chronic Stable Angina

Predictable, consistent, occurs on exertion and is relieved by rest.

Nocturnal Angina

Pain occurs at night, usually during sleep; may be relieved by sitting upright.

Commonly due to left ventricular failure

Angina Decubitus

Angina while lying down

Intractable or Refractory Angina

Severe incapacitating angina

Prinzmetal's Angina (Variant: Resting)

Spontaneous type of anginal pain accompanied by ST-segment elevation in ECG

Thought to be due to coronary artery spasm

Associated with high risk of infarction

Silent Ischemia

Objective evidence of ischemia (such as stress test), but patient is asymptomatic

Diagnostic Evaluation

The diagnosis of angina is often made by evaluating the clinical manifestations of pain and the patient's history. In certain types of angina, electrocardiogram (ECG) changes are helpful in making a differential diagnosis of the angina. The patient's response to exertion or stress also may be tested by means of electrocardiographic monitoring while the patient exercises on a bicycle or treadmill.

Management

The objectives of medical management of angina are to decrease the oxygen demands of the myocardium and to increase the oxygen supply. Medically these objectives are met through pharmacologic therapy and control of risk factors. Surgically the objectives are met by revascularization of the blood supply to the myocardium through coronary artery bypass surgery or percutaneous transluminal coronary angioplasty (PTCA) (discussed below). Frequently a combination of medical and surgical therapies is employed.

As will be discussed later, several other approaches are currently being used to revascularize the myocardium. Three major techniques that offer relief for the patient with coronary artery disease include the application of intracoronary stents to enhance blood flow, the use of lasers to vaporize plaques, and the use of percutaneous coronary endarterectomy to extract obstructions. Studies that compare the outcomes of one or all of the above with the well-established bypass surgery and PTCA are being conducted. The advances of science continue to relieve symptoms and retard the disease process for patients experiencing angina.

Pharmacologic Therapy

Nitroglycerin. The nitrates remain the mainstay for treating angina pectoris. Nitroglycerin is administered to reduce myocardial oxygen consumption, which decreases ischemia and relieves anginal pain.

Nitroglycerin is a vasoactive agent that acts to dilate both the veins and the arteries and thus has an effect on the peripheral circulation. Dilation of the veins causes venous pooling of blood throughout the body. As a result, less blood is returned to the heart and there is a reduction in filling pressure (preload). Nitrates also relax the systemic arteriolar bed and thus cause a fall in blood pressure (decreased afterload). These effects decrease myocardial oxygen requirements, bringing about a more favorable balance between supply and demand.

Nitroglycerin is generally placed under the tongue (sublingually) or in the cheek (buccal pouch) and alleviates the pain of ischemia within 3 minutes.

- The patient is instructed to keep the tongue still and to avoid swallowing saliva until the nitroglycerin tablet is dissolved. If the pain is severe, the tablet can be crushed between the teeth to hasten sublingual absorption.
- As a precaution, the patient should carry the medication at all times. Nitroglycerin is very unstable and is kept in a securely capped dark glass bottle. Nitroglycerin is not stored in metal or plastic pillboxes.
- Nitroglycerin is volatile and is inactivated by heat, moisture, air, light, and time. If the nitroglycerin is fresh, the patient will feel a burning sensation under the tongue and often a feeling of fullness or throbbing in the head. The nitroglycerin supply should be renewed every 6 months.
- Instead of using a fixed dosage, the patient regulates usage, taking the smallest dose that relieves pain. The medication should be taken in anticipation of any activity that may produce pain. Because nitroglycerin will increase the patient's tolerance for exercise and stress when taken prophylactically (*e.g.*, before exercise, stair-climbing, and sexual intercourse), it is best that it be taken *before* the pain develops.
- The patient should note how long it takes for the nitroglycerin to relieve the discomfort. If the pain is not relieved by nitroglycerin, an impending myocardial infarction may be suspected.
- If pain persists after taking three (3) sublingual tablets at 5 minute intervals, the patient is advised to be taken to the nearest emergency care facility.

Side effects of nitroglycerin include flushing, throbbing headache, hypotension, and tachycardia. The use of long-acting nitrate preparations is controversial. Isosorbide dinitrate (Isordil) appears to be effective for up to 2 hours if taken sublingually, but has an uncertain effect if taken orally.

Topical Nitroglycerin Ointment. Nitroglycerin is also available in a lanolin-petrolatum base. In this form it is applied to the skin to protect against anginal pain and promote relief. It is especially useful when patients experience nocturnal angina or are involved in periods of extended activity (*e.g.*, golfing) because it has a prolonged effect of up to 24 hours. The dose is usually increased until headache or an excessive effect on blood pressure or heart rate occurs, and then the dose is reduced to the largest dose that does not produce these side effects. Instructions for applying the ointment accompany the various products. The user should be reminded to rotate the site of application to avoid skin irritation.

Beta-adrenergic Blockers. If the patient continues to have chest pain despite treatment with nitroglycerin and modification of lifestyle, a beta-adrenergic blocking agent is recommended. Propranolol hydrochloride (Inderal) remains the medication of choice. This medication appears to reduce myocardial oxygen consumption by blocking the sympathetic impulses to the heart. The result is a reduction in heart rate, blood pressure, and myocardial contractility that establishes a more favorable balance between myocardial oxygen needs and the amount of oxygen available. This helps to control chest pain and allows the patient to work or exercise. Propranolol may be administered with sublingual or oral isosorbide dinitrate to prevent anginal pain.

Propranolol is cleared by the liver at varying rates, depending on the individual patient. It is usually taken at 6-hour intervals. Side effects include musculoskeletal weakness, hypotension, bradycardia, and mental depression.

When propranolol is started, blood pressure and heart rate should be monitored (while the patient is in an upright position) 2 hours after the medication has been administered. This may need to be done at home by a family member or by a health care provider. If the blood pressure drops significantly, a vasopressor may be needed. If severe bradycardia occurs, atropine is the antidote of choice. It is also important to remember that propranolol can precipitate congestive heart failure and asthma.

- The patient is cautioned not to stop taking propranolol abruptly, because there is evidence that angina may worsen and myocardial infarction may develop if this medication is abruptly discontinued.

Calcium Ion Antagonists/Channel Blockers. The calcium channel blockers, or antagonists, possess properties that have profound effects on myocardial oxygen demand and supply, hence their value in the treatment of angina. Physiologically, the calcium ion performs at the cellular level to influence contraction of all types of muscle tissue and plays a role in the electrical stimulation of the heart.

Calcium ion antagonists/blockers increase myocardial oxygen supply by dilating the smooth muscle wall of the coronary arterioles, and decrease myocardial oxygen demands by reducing systemic arterial pressure and thus the workload of the left ventricle. The three calcium ion antagonists/blockers most commonly used are nifedipine (Procardia), verapamil (Isoptin, Calan) and diltiazem (Cardizem). The vasodilating effects of these agents, particularly on coronary circulation, have made them valuable in angina that results from coronary vasospasm (**Prinzmetal's angina**).

Calcium blockers should be used with great caution in individuals with heart failure because they block the calcium that supports contractility. Hypotension may occur after intravenous (IV) administration. Other side effects that may occur are constipation, gastric distress, dizziness, or headache associated with dizziness.

Calcium ion antagonists/blockers are usually administered every 6 to 12 hours. Therapeutic doses vary from one person to another.

Control of Risk Factors

Several other measures may be necessary to decrease the oxygen demands of the myocardium. It is important that the patient stop smoking, because smoking produces tachycardia and raises the blood pressure, thus increasing the work of the heart. Obese persons are advised to lose weight to reduce cardiac work. Other risk factors are identified in Chart 28-1.

❑ NURSING PROCESS
The Patient With Angina Pectoris

Assessment

The nurse gathers information about all facets of the patient's activities, especially those that have been found to precede and precipitate attacks of anginal pain. Appropriate questions may include:

- ❑ When do attacks tend to occur? Following a meal? After engaging in certain activities? After physical activities in general? After visits from members of the family or others?
- ❑ How does the patient describe the pain?
- ❑ Is the onset of pain gradual or sudden?
- ❑ How long does it last—seconds? minutes? hours?
- ❑ Is the pain steady and persistent in quality?
- ❑ Is the discomfort accompanied by other symptoms, such as excessive perspiration, lightheadedness, nausea, palpitation, shortness of breath?
- ❑ How many minutes after taking nitroglycerin does the pain last?
- ❑ What is the mode of pain relief?

The answers to these questions form a basis for designing a logical program of prevention.

When sensing that an attack is imminent, a patient should cease all movement to reduce to a minimum the oxygen requirements of the ischemic myocardium. This is done with the hope that oxygen needs can be met by the limited blood oxygen supply available at the moment and the impending attack can thus be averted.

Diagnosis

Nursing Diagnoses

Based on the assessment data, major nursing diagnoses for the patient may include the following:

- ❑ Pain related to myocardial ischemia
- ❑ Anxiety related to fear of death
- ❑ Knowledge deficit about the underlying nature of disease and methods for avoiding complications
- ❑ Potential noncompliance to therapeutic regimen related to nonacceptance of necessary life style changes

Collaborative Problems/ Potential Complications

Potential complications of angina include myocardial infarction and its complications as discussed in the next section.

Planning and Implementation

Goals. The major goals of the patient include prevention of pain, reduction of anxiety, awareness of the underlying nature of the disorder and understanding of the prescribed care, adherence to the self-care program, and absence of complications.

Nursing Interventions

Preventing Pain. The patient must understand the symptom complex and the need to avoid activities known to cause anginal pain, such as sudden exertion, exposure to cold, and emotional excitement. Learning to change, modify, or adapt to these stresses is essential.

For patients whose attacks occur predominantly in the morning, a change in the schedule of daily activities is indicated. As a first step, the patient should plan to rise earlier each morning to wash and dress in a more leisurely fashion. Ideally, this unhurried pace should be maintained throughout the entire day, so that scheduled tasks and commitments are handled without haste or a sense of pressure.

Any patient with angina pectoris should be instructed to initiate all movements with deliberation, avoid exposure to cold, avoid tobacco, eat regularly but lightly, and maintain weight within prescribed limits. Use of over-the-counter medications should be discouraged, especially diet pills, nasal decongestants, or other medications containing agents that will increase heart rate and blood pressure.

Reducing Anxiety. This patient often has a strong fear of death. For the hospitalized patient, nursing care is planned so that time away from the bedside is kept to a minimum, because this fear of death often is alleviated by the physical presence of another person. For the ambulatory patient at home, essential information about the illness and explanation of why it is important to follow prescribed directives are pr ovided.

Patient Education and Home Care Considerations. The teaching program for the patient with angina is designed to explain the basic nature of the illness and to furnish the facts needed to reorganize living habits in a way that will achieve the following goals: (1) reduce the frequency and severity of anginal attacks; (2) delay the progress of the underlying disease, if possible; and (3) provide protection from other complications. The factors outlined in Chart 28-3 are important in educating the patient with angina pectoris.

The self-care program is prepared in collaboration with the patient and family or friends. Activities should be planned to minimize the occurrence of angina episodes. The patient should understand that any pain unrelieved by the usual methods should be treated at the closest emergency center.

CHART 28-3
Patient Education for the Person With Angina

Goal: To improve the quality of life and promote health

Expected Outcomes

I. Patient reduces probability of an episode of anginal pain
 A. Uses moderation in all activities of life
  1. Participates in a regular daily program of activities that do not produce chest discomfort, shortness of breath, and undue fatigue
  2. Avoids exercises requiring sudden bursts of activity; avoids all isometric exercise
  3. Alternates activity with periods of rest. Some fatigue is normal and temporary
 B. Uses appropriate resources for support during emotionally stressful times, *e.g.*, counselor, nurse, clergy, physician
 C. Avoids overeating
  1. Eats smaller portions; may be necessary to eat frequently in smaller amounts to satisfy hunger
  2. Avoids excessive caffeine intake (coffee, cola drinks), which can increase the heart rate and produce angina
  3. Refrains from engaging in physical exercise for 2 h after meals
 D. Does not use diet pills, nasal decongestants, or any over-the-counter medication that can increase the heart rate
 E. Stops smoking, as smoking increases the heart rate, blood pressure, and blood carbon monoxide levels
 F. Avoids extremes of cold
  1. Wears scarf over nose/mouth during very cold weather to warm the air
  2. Walks more slowly in cold weather
  3. Dresses warmly in winter, including head, neck, and hand coverings

II. Patient manages an attack of anginal pain
 A. Carries nitroglycerin at all times
  1. Keeps nitroglycerin in a tightly capped, dark-colored glass bottle
  2. Discards the cotton filler/packing to allow prompt access to the pills
  3. Avoids opening the bottle unnecessarily
  4. Discards unused tablets after 5 months; obtains a fresh prescription
  5. States that when tablets are fresh, they cause a burning sensation when placed under the tongue
 B. Places nitroglycerin under the tongue at first sign of chest discomfort
  1. Does not swallow saliva until the tablet has dissolved
  2. Stops all activity and rests until all pain subsides
  3. States the significance of using the upright position to potentiate the effects of nitroglycerin
  4. Usually, another nitroglycerin tablet may be taken in 3 to 5 minutes for two times. If the discomfort is unrelieved by the usual number of nitroglycerin tablets, or if it recurs after a short interval, is taken to the nearest emergency facility
 C. Takes nitroglycerin prophylactically to avoid pain that may occur with certain activities (stair-climbing, sexual intercourse)
 D. Is alert for the side effects of nitroglycerin: headache, flushing, dizziness

Evaluation

Expected Outcomes

1. Is relieved of pain (see Chart 28-3 for specific outcomes related to patient education)
2. Demonstrates less anxiety
   a. Understands the illness and purpose of treatment
   b. Adheres to medical regimen
   c. Knows to seek medical assistance if pain persists or changes in quality
   d. Avoids being alone during painful episodes
3. Understands ways to avoid complications and demonstrates freedom from complications
   a. Describes the process of angina
   b. Explains reasons for measures to prevent complications
   c. Exhibits normal ECG and level of cardiac enzymes
   d. Is free of signs and symptoms of acute myocardial infarction
4. Adheres to self-care program
   a. Demonstrates an understanding of pharmacologic therapy
   b. Daily habits reflect modification of lifestyle (Chart 28-3)

Surgical Measures for Angina

Angina pectoris may persist for many years in a stable form with brief attacks. It is a serious disease, however, in the unstable stage. The episodes of chest pain become more frequent and intense, occurring without apparent provocation. When symptoms cannot be controlled despite an adequate trial of pharmacologic therapy, invasive measures such as percutaneous transluminal coronary angioplasty (PTCA) or revascularization are considered to correct the basic problem by either improving circulation or bringing a new blood supply to the ischemic myocardium.

Percutaneous Transluminal Coronary Angioplasty (PTCA)

Percutaneous transluminal coronary angioplasty attempts to improve blood flow within a coronary artery by cracking the plaque or atheroma that has built up and is interfering with circulation of blood to the heart. A balloon-tipped catheter is passed into the affected coronary artery and placed within the atherosclerotic area. The balloon is inflated and deflated rapidly to crack the plaque.

Candidates for PTCA are patients who have lesions that occlude at least 70% of the internal lumen of a major coronary artery, placing a large area of the myocardium at risk for ischemia. These patients are those whose conditions do not respond to medical treatments, and who meet the criteria for coronary artery bypass surgery. PTCA is attempted when the cardiologist believes that the procedure can improve blood flow to the myocardium.

PTCAs are seldom attempted in the following patients: (1) those with occlusions of the left main coronary artery that do not demonstrate collateral flow to the left anterior descending and circumflex arteries; (2) those with stenoses at the origin of the right coronary artery with the aorta; (3) those whose coronary arteries demo˘strate an aneurysm proximal or distal to the stenosis; (4) those who have a saphenous vein graft that was done more than 5 years ago or a graft that has become diseased; or (5) those with questionable left ventricular function.

The **procedure** for PTCA is usually carried out in the cardiac catheterization laboratory. Patient care for PTCA is very similar to that for a cardiac catheterization. The patient's coronary arteries are examined by angiography, as they were during the diagnostic cardiac catheterization. The lesions are verified for location, extent, and calcification before a guidewire is passed into the artery beyond the lesion. A guide catheter is passed over the guidewire to the lesion. A balloon-tipped dilation catheter is then passed over the guidewire (through the guide catheter) and positioned over the lesion. When the balloon-tipped dilation catheter is properly positioned, pressurized contrast solution fills the balloon for an average of 30 to 60 seconds, cracking and possibly compressing the atherosclerotic lesion (Fig. 28-3). The coronary artery's media and adventitia are also stretched.

Several inflations may be required to achieve the desired effect—usually defined as an increase in the artery's lumen of 20% or more. Other measures used to gauge the success of a PTCA are a residual stenosis of less than 50% or less than 20 mm Hg difference in blood pressure from one side of the lesion to the other and no clinically obvious arterial trauma.

Postprocedure Care. Many patients are admitted to the hospital the day of their PTCA. Those who experience no complications go home the next day. During the PCTA procedure, patients receive large amounts of heparin. The patient often returns to the unit with the large peripheral vascular access cannula in place. The patient is monitored closely for signs of bleeding. The cannulas are removed once the patient's clotting studies return to within 1.5 to 2 times the laboratory's normal values. Most patients receive intravenous heparin and nitroglycerine for a period after the procedure to prevent clot formation and arterial spasm. The patients are usually able to be weaned from the intravenous medications, resume self-care, and ambulate unassisted within 24 hours of the procedure.

Complications. Possible complications during the PTCA procedure or the recovery period include dissection of the artery, abrupt closure of the artery, and spasm of the coronary artery. These may require emergency surgical treatment. For this reason, all PTCA candidates also must be candidates for coronary artery bypass. A cardiac surgery operating room and surgical team are always on standby during a PTCA.

Alternative Procedures

Three alternative procedures to emergency cardiac surgery are being examined. The first is redilation via another PTCA. The second is redilation with an intravascular stent over the balloon. When the balloon is deflated the stent remains in

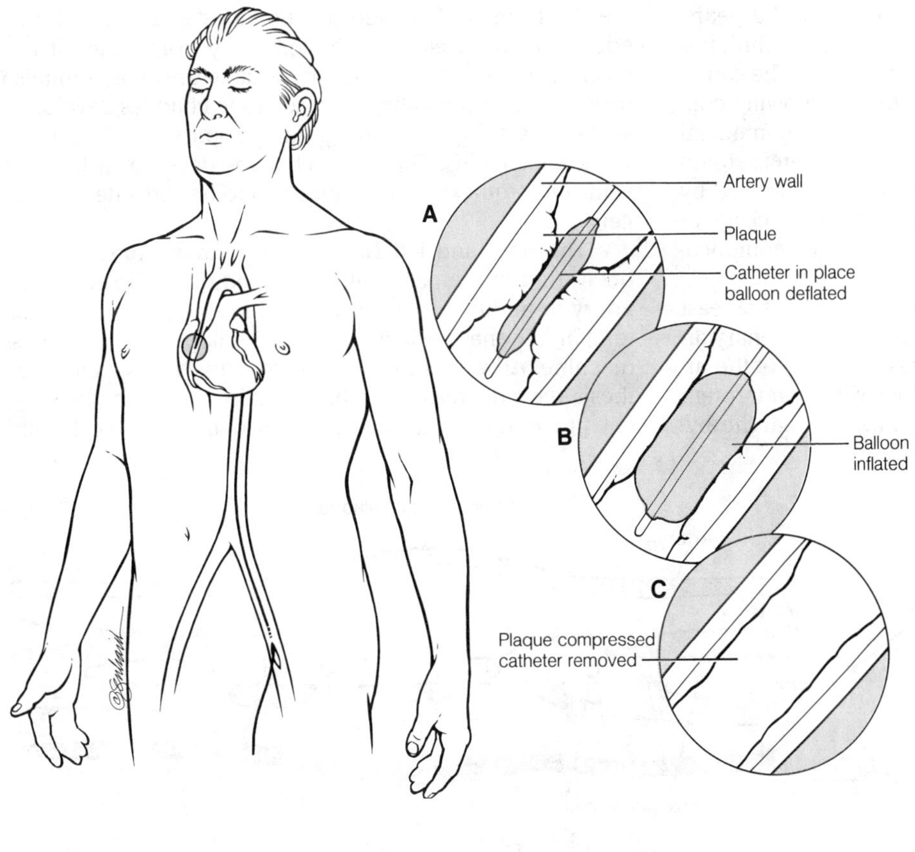

FIGURE 28-3. Percutaneous transluminal coronary angioplasty. (**A**) A balloon-tipped catheter is passed into the affected coronary artery and placed within the atherosclerotic lesion. (**B**) The balloon is then rapidly inflated and deflated with controlled pressure. (**C**) After the plaque is cracked, the catheter is removed, allowing improved blood flow through the vessel.

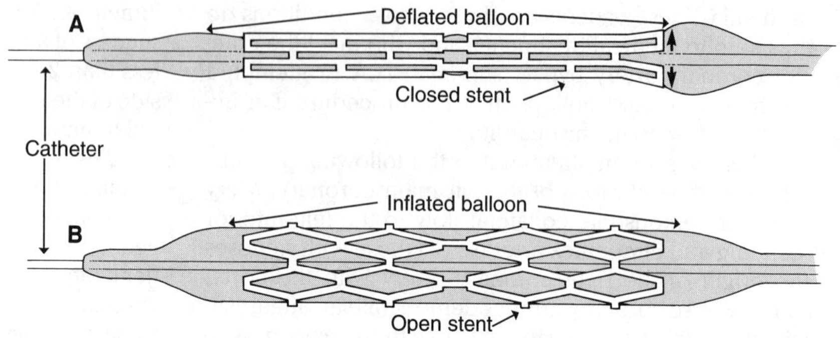

FIGURE 28-4. Schematic drawing of an intracoronary artery stent: (**A**) stent closed, before balloon inflation; (**B**) stent open, balloon inflated; stent will remain expanded after balloon is deflated and removed.

the artery, holding the artery open (Fig. 28-4). Eventually endothelium covers the stent and it is incorporated into the vessel wall. The third alternative is the use of a laser. There are numerous types of lasers being used experimentally today. The theory is that the laser is able to "weld" the artery open or "melt" the plaque by the heat it generates.

A shunt catheter may also be used to avoid the risks of emergency surgery. It is sometimes possible to pass a shunt catheter through a reoccluded coronary artery. This special catheter has numerous holes along its distal end. The catheter is placed in the occluded artery. The holes proximal to the lesion permit arterial blood to flow into the catheter while those distal to the lesion permit the arterial blood to flow out of the catheter (Fig. 28-5). The shunt catheter maintains a flow of blood distal to the occlusion while the patient is prepared for heart surgery. The shunt catheter is removed during the coronary artery bypass graft surgery.

Coronary Artery Revascularization

Coronary artery disease has been treated by some form of myocardial revascularization for approximately 30 years. Current coronary artery bypass graft (CABG) techniques have been performed for approximately 25 years. The candidates for CABG are usually patients with the following conditions: (1) angina that cannot be controlled by medical therapies, (2) unstable angina, (3) a positive exercise tolerance test and lesions or blockage that cannot be treated by PTCA, (4) a left main coronary artery lesion or blockage of more than 60%, and (5) individuals who have complications from or unsuccessful PTCAs.

The coronary arteries to be bypassed must have at least a 70% occlusive lesion (60% if it is the left main coronary artery) to be considered for CABG. If less than 70% of the artery is occluded then enough blood flow will occur through the artery to prevent adequate blood flow through the bypass. Thus, the CABG would clot, effectively negating the surgery performed.

Coronary artery bypass grafting is performed under general anesthesia. A median sternotomy incision is made and the patient is placed on cardiopulmonary bypass. A blood vessel from another part of the body (*e.g.*, saphenous vein, left internal mammary artery) is grafted distal to the coronary artery lesion—"bypassing" the obstruction (Fig. 28-6). Cardiopulmonary bypass is discontinued and the incision is closed. The patient then is admitted to a critical care unit.

Artery Selection. The most recent advances in the surgical procedure have been in the variety of blood vessels used to bypass the coronary artery lesion. The most common vessel has been the greater saphenous vein, followed by the lesser saphenous vein. Cephalic and basilic veins also have been used. The vein is removed from the leg (or arm) and grafted to the ascending aorta and to the coronary artery distal to the lesion. The saphenous veins are used in emergency CABG procedures because they can be obtained by one surgical team while another team performs the chest surgery. One side effect of using a large vein is that edema often develops in the extremity from which it was taken. The degree of edema is variable and may diminish over time. Symptomatic atherosclerotic changes develop in saphenous veins used for grafting approximately 5 to 10 years after CABG. The same changes develop in the arm veins more quickly, approximately 3 to 6 years after the surgery.

The right and left **internal mammary arteries** had been used in the past, but the procedure of dissecting the artery from the chest wall required keeping the patient too long under anesthesia and on the cardiopulmonary bypass machine. Advances in cardiopulmonary bypass and anesthesia have decreased the time required to begin the surgical procedures and have decreased the risks of lengthy

FIGURE 28-5. Schematic drawing of a shunt catheter. The catheter traverses the atherosclerotic plaque. Arterial blood pressure pushes blood through the proximal side holes of the catheter and out the distal side holes of the catheter.

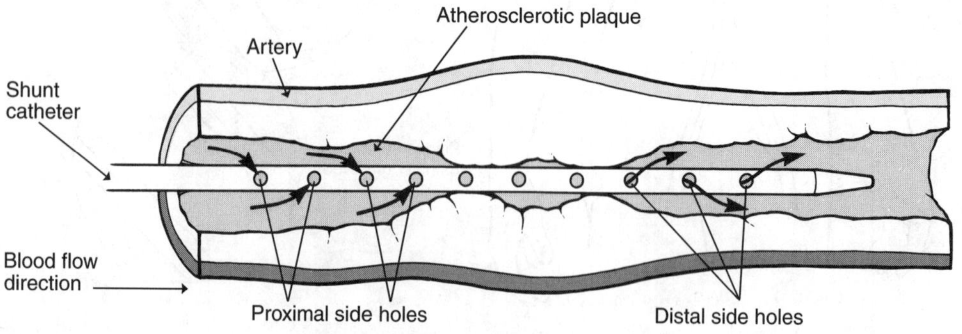

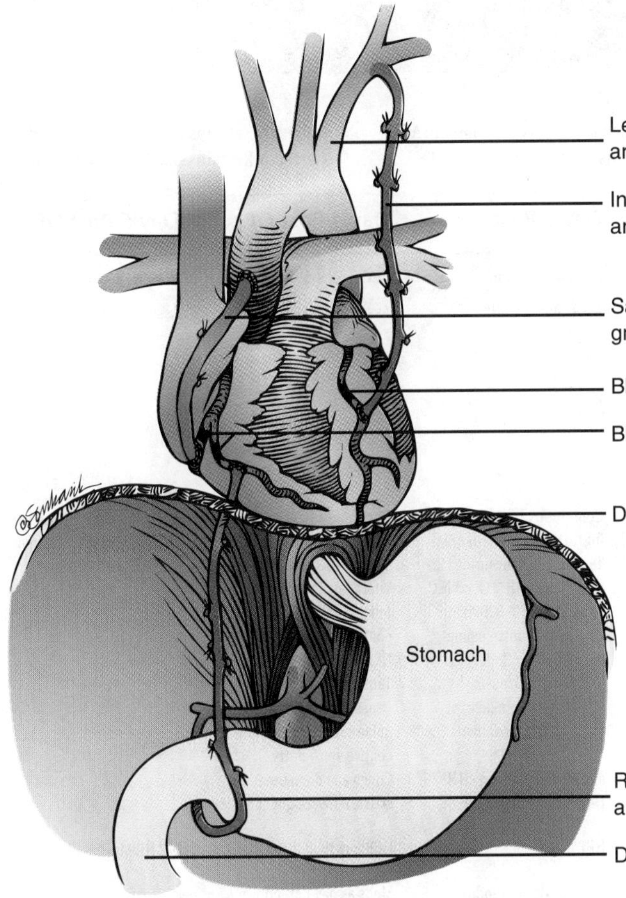

FIGURE 28-6. Schematic drawing of three coronary artery bypass grafts. One or more procedures may be performed. (**A**) Saphenous vein, the most frequently utilized bypass. (**B**) Left internal mammary artery, gaining in popularity because of its functional longevity. (**C**) Right gastroepiploic artery, rarely utilized because it has a more extensive blood supply to its wall and because of the risk of gastrointestinal tract contamination of the abdominal and/or mediastinal wound.

surgical times, thus renewing interest in using arteries for CABGs. Because research had shown that arterial grafts did not develop atherosclerotic changes as quickly and maintained patency longer than vein grafts, use of the right and left internal mammary arteries has regained popularity. The proximal end of the mammary artery is left intact. The distal end of the artery is dissected away from the chest wall. This distal end of the artery is then grafted to the coronary artery distal to the lesion.

The internal mammary arteries are not always long enough nor do they always have a sufficient diameter to be used for CABG. One side effect of the use of the internal mammary artery is ulnar nerve sensory damage, which can be temporary or permanent.

The **gastroepiploic artery** (located on the greater curvature of the stomach; see Fig. 28-6) also has been used for CABG. It has a much more extensive blood supply to its wall than the internal mammaries have, so it does not respond as well when used as a graft. Another disadvantage of using the gastroepiploic artery is that the chest incision must be extended to the abdomen, thus exposing the patient to the additional risks of an abdominal incision and infection from contamination of the gastrointestinal tract at the surgical site.

Postoperative Care. Initially the patient's care is focused on achieving or maintaining hemodynamic stability and recovery from general anesthesia. Within 48 hours the typical patient is transferred to a telemetry or surgical unit. The patient's care is focused on wound care, progressive activity, and diet. In addition, education about medications and risk factor modification is emphasized. Discharge from the hospital is usually 5 to 10 days after CABG. Patients can expect fewer symptoms from their coronary artery disease and should enjoy an increase in quality of life. However, CABG has not been shown to increase patients' lifespans.

Complications. Coronary artery bypass graft surgery may result in complications such as myocardial infarction, dysrhythmias, and hemorrhage. The patient's underlying coronary heart disease remains; therefore, the patient may develop angina, exercise intolerance, or other symptoms experienced before CABG. Medications required preoperatively may need to be continued. The lifestyle modifications recommended before surgery remain important, not just for the original pathology, but for the continued viability of the newly implanted grafts.

An example of a critical pathway for the postoperative management of the patient who has undergone a CABG procedure and has been transferred to the stepdown unit can be found on page 648. This critical pathway outlines the key points to be addressed in a 5-day postoperative period. The pathway also includes (not shown in this example) activities for preadmission, presurgery, and the first 24 hours in the postoperative period spent in the recovery room and SICU unit.

Myocardial Infarction

Pathophysiology

Myocardial infarction refers to the process by which myocardial tissue is destroyed in regions of the heart that are deprived of an adequate blood supply because of a reduced

CRITICAL PATHWAY
Coronary Artery Bypass Graft

The Graduate Hospital Nursing Services Department
1800 Lombard Street
Philadelphia, PA 19146

Outcome Criteria D/C to Home:

- ☐ Demonstrates Level of Endurance Necessary to Complete ADL's
- ☐ Ambulates Functional Rate and Distance
- ☐ Correctly Restates Home Walking Program
- ☐ Correctly Restates Discharge Instructions

	Day 1 Post OP Stepdown	Day 2 Post OP	Day 3 Post OP	Day 4 Post OP	Day 5 Post OP
Assessments	Review of systems Assessment Q4H*	Review of systems Assessment Q4H*	Review of systems Assessment Q4H*	Review of systems Assessment Q4H*	Review of systems Assessment*
Consults		Nutrition consult			
Labs and Diagnostics		K^+	K^+	Hg/Hct K^+, BUN/CREAT CXR PA & LAT	
Interventions	Continuous ECG monitoring*, Vital signs Q4H* ⊕, O_2 via N.C. to keep SaO_2 > 92%* ⊕ , Continuous pulse oximetry*, D/C chest tubes per guidelines if indicated ⊕, I&O* ⊕, Teds*, Safety measures*, Dressing/wound care*, Ankle exercises Q1H*, Incentive spirometry Q1H*, Cough and deep breathing Q1H*, Daily weight at 6AM*	Continuous ECG monitoring*, Vital signs Q4H* ⊕, O_2 via N.C. to keep SaO_2 > 92%* ⊕, Continuous pulse oximetry*, D/C chest tubes per guidelines if indicated, ⊕, I&O* ⊕, Teds*, Safety measures*, Dressing/wound care*, Ankle exercises Q1H*, Incentive spirometry Q1H*, Cough and deep breathing Q1H*, Daily weight at 6AM*	Continuous ECG monitoring*, D/C pacer wires* ⊕, Tamponade precautions*, Vital signs Q4H*, O_2 via N.C. to keep SaO_2 > 92%* ⊕, Continuous pulse oximetry*, I&O* ⊕, Teds*, Safety measures*, Dressing/wound care*, Ankle exercises Q1H*, Incentive spirometry Q1H*, Cough and deep breathing Q1H*, Daily weight at 6AM*	Continuous ECG monitoring*, D/C pacer wires* ⊕, Tamponade precautions*, Vital signs Q4H*, O_2 via N.C. to keep SaO_2 > 92%* ⊕, D/C continuous pulse oximetry if RA SAT > 92% ⊕, I&O* ⊕, Teds*, Safety measures*, Dressing/ wound care*, Ankle exercise Q1H*, Incentive spirometry Q1H*, Cough and deep breathing Q1H*, Daily weight at 6AM*	D/C continuous ECG monitoring* ⊕, Assess if outcome criteria have been met* Teds*, Dressing/wound care*, D/C sternal staples
IV's	HEP lock*	HEP lock*	HEP lock*	HEP lock*	D/C HEP lock*
Medication	P.O. SVT prophylaxis, diuretics/K^+ replacement if indicated, ABX until C.T. DC'D, Iron, ASA, Stool softeners, Analgesics, Non cardiac meds	Meds as day 1 stepdown	Meds as day 1 stepdown MOM @ HS*	Meds as day 1 stepdown Laxative supp if needed*	
Diet/GI	Clear liquid/cardiac diet	Cardiac diet	Cardiac diet	Cardiac diet	Cardiac diet
Activity	OOB to chair* Cardiac rehab: Level I progress as indicated	OOB to chair qid* Cardiac rehab progress as indicated	OOB qid* Cardiac rehab progress as indicated	OOB qid* Cardiac rehab progress as indicated	
Teaching	Family and patient education-orient patient to new unit, Discuss diet/activity, Meds/wound care*, Reinforce previous teaching*	Risk modification and energy conservation instruction (card-rehab) Reinforce all previous teaching*	Patient and family teaching by cardiac rehab; reinforce previous teaching*	Patient and family teaching by cardiac rehab; reinforce previous teaching*, Dietary instruction with patient and family	
D/C Planning & Follow-Up			Assess D/C needs Arrange transportation	Written D/C activity instructions per cardiac rehab D/C instructions for meds, F/U appt, Wound care. All Rx on chart	Review all D/C instructions* D/C_______Time
KEY: *NSG Activities ⊕ to be ordered by PHYSICIAN *V = Variance* *N = No Var.*	V V V N N N	V V V N N N	V V V N N N	V V V N N N	V V V N N N
NSG Care Performed:	☐ ☐ ☐	☐ ☐ ☐	☐ ☐ ☐	☐ ☐ ☐	☐ ☐ ☐
SIGNATURES: →	1. ________	1. ________	1. ________	1. ________	1. ________
→	2. ________	2. ________	2. ________	2. ________	2. ________
→	3. ________	3. ________	3. ________	3. ________	3. ________

LEGEND: ABG = arterial blood gas; ASA = salicylic acid; C.T. = chest tube; CBC = complete blood count; CXR = chest x-ray; D/C = discharge or discontinue; ECG = electrocardiogram; GLU = glucose; F/U = follow-up; Hg/Hct = hemoglobin and hematocrit; I&O = intake and output; IVF's = intravenous fluids; K^+ = potassium; MN = midnight; NA^+ = sodium; NGT = nasogastric tube; OOB = out of bed; PAT = preadmission testing; PLT = platelets; PT = prothrombin time; PTT = partial thromboplastin time; SICU = surgical intensive care unit; SMA-7 = electrolyte screen; SVT = superventricular tachycardia; T&C = type and crossmatch; U/A = urinalysis.

coronary blood flow. The cause of the reduced blood flow is either a critical narrowing of a coronary artery due to atherosclerosis or a complete occlusion of an artery due to embolus or thrombus. Decreased coronary blood flow may also result from shock and hemorrhage. In each case, there is a profound imbalance between myocardial oxygen supply and demand.

"Coronary occlusion," "heart attack," and "myocardial infarction" are all used synonymously, but the preferred term is **myocardial infarction** (MI). In the United States, well over a million of these attacks occur annually.

An MI is further described by the location of the injury to the myocardial wall: anterior, inferior (posterior), or lateral wall. Whereas the left ventricle is the usual site of injury, right ventricular infarctions occur. Differential diagnosis is made through an ECG. Regardless of the location, the goal of medical therapy is to prevent or minimize myocardial tissue necrosis.

The pathophysiology of coronary heart disease and the risk factors involved have already been discussed in the opening pages of this chapter.

Clinical Manifestations

Studies indicate that the patient with myocardial infarction is usually male, over 40, and has atherosclerosis of the coronary vessels, often with arterial hypertension. Attacks also occur in women and in younger men in their early 30s or even 20s. Women who take oral contraceptives and also smoke are at very high risk. Overall, however, the rate of myocardial infarction is greater in men than in women at all ages.

Chest pain that occurs suddenly and continues unabated, usually over the lower sternal region and the upper abdomen, is the primary presenting symptom. The pain may increase steadily in severity until it becomes almost unbearable. It is a heavy, viselike pain, which may radiate to the shoulders and down the arms, usually the left arm. Unlike the pain of true angina, it begins spontaneously (not after effort or emotional upset) persists for hours or days, and is relieved neither by rest nor by nitroglycerin. In some cases the pain may radiate to the jaw and neck. The pain is often accompanied by shortness of breath, pallor, diaphoresis, dizziness or lightheadedness, and nausea and vomiting.

The patient with diabetes mellitus may not experience severe pain with myocardial infarction. The neuropathy that accompanies diabetes can interfere with neuroreceptors, thus dulling the pain experience.

Although the typical patient is male and over 40, the female patient presenting with these signs and symptoms is taken seriously, especially if she is a smoker and also takes oral contraceptives. The incidence of MI also increases markedly in postmenopausal women.

Gerontologic Considerations

The elderly patient may not experience the typical viselike pain associated with myocardial infarction because of the diminished responses of neurotransmitters that occur in the aging process. Often the pain is atypical, such as jaw pain, or fainting may be experienced.

The arteriosclerosis that accompanies aging may compromise tissue perfusion because the stiffness of the arteries leads to increased peripheral vascular resistance. Because elderly patients may have a well-established collateral circulation of the myocardium, they often are spared the lethal complications associated with myocardial infarction.

Diagnostic Evaluation

Diagnosis of myocardial infarction is generally based on history of the present illness, electrocardiogram, and serial serum enzymes. Prognosis depends on the severity of coronary artery obstruction and hence the extent of myocardial damage. Physical examination is always conducted but alone is insufficient to confirm the diagnosis.

Patient History. The taking of a patient history occurs in two steps: (1) the history of the present illness, and (2) the history of previous illnesses and family health history, particularly related to the incidence of heart disease in the family. Previous history often can provide valuable information about the patient's risk factors for coronary heart disease. The history of the present illness (*e.g.*, the onset and description of pain) is in many cases conclusive for the diagnosis of myocardial infarction.

The patient's history provides subjective data. The careful practitioner will also obtain objective data in terms of ECG interpretation and serial enzyme studies.

Electrocardiogram. The ECG provides information about the electrophysiology of the heart. Through the use of readings over a period of time, the physician is able to monitor the evolution and resolution of an MI. The location and relative size of the infarction also may be determined by ECG. The details describing the ECG waveforms associated with an MI are covered in Chapter 27.

Although there are newer technologies that offer equivalent diagnostic data, the ECG remains the first diagnostic instrument of choice because it can be used at the bedside and is noninvasive.

Echocardiogram. The echocardiogram is used to further evaluate cardiac function, specifically ventricular function. The ejection fraction can be determined by echocardiogram (see Chapter 26).

Serum Enzymes and Isoenzymes. Serial enzyme studies include creatine kinase and lactic dehydrogenase.

Creatine Kinase and Its Isoenzymes. Creatine kinase (CK, with its isoenzyme CK-MB) is regarded as the most sensitive and reliable indicator of all cardiac enzymes in diagnosing myocardial infarction. There are three CK isoenzymes: CK-MM (skeletal muscle), CK-MB (heart muscle), and CK-BB (brain tissue). CK-MB is the cardiac-specific isoenzyme; that is, CK-MB is found only in cardiac cells and therefore rises only when there has been damage to these cells. CK-MB is the most specific index for the diagnosis of acute myocardial infarction. It is always increased in acute MI (AMI).

Lactic Dehydrogenase and Its Isoenzymes. Lactic dehydrogenase (LDH) is not as reliable an indicator of acute myocardial damage as CK. However, because it peaks later and is elevated longer than other cardiac enzymes, LDH is useful for diagnosing an MI in patients who may have sustained an acute MI but have delayed admission to the hospital.

TABLE 28-1 Time Course of Cardiac Enzymes Following Acute Myocardial Infarction

Enzyme	Onset	Peak	Return to Normal
CK	3–6 hr	12–24 hr	3–5 days
CK-MB	2–4 hr	12–20 hr	48–72 hr
LDH	24 hr	48–72 hr	7–10 days
LDH_1	4 hr	48 hr	10 days
LDH_2	4 hr	48 hr	10 days

CK, creatine kinase; CK-MB, creatine kinase-MB isoenzyme; LDH, lactic dehydrogenase.

There are five LDH isoenzymes, but only two (LDH_1 and LDH_2) are important in the diagnosis of an acute MI. Both LDH_1 and LDH_2 predominate in the heart, kidney, and brain, but normally the percentage of LDH_2 compared with LDH_1 is greater. When the percentage of LDH_1 exceeds that of LDH_2, the pattern is said to have "flipped," indicating an acute MI.

Table 28-1 shows the time courses of cardiac enzymes.

Medical Management

The goal of medical management is to minimize myocardial damage and thus reduce the probability of complications. Minimizing myocardial damage is accomplished by quickly bringing into balance myocardial oxygen demand and supply. Medication therapy, oxygen administration, and bedrest are initiated simultaneously to help preserve the myocardium. Medications and oxygen are used to increase oxygen supply; bedrest is used to reduce oxygen demand. The resolution of pain is the primary clinical indicator that demand and supply are in equilibrium.

Pharmacotherapy

Three classes of medications are used to increase oxygen supply: vasodilators (specifically nitrates), anticoagulants, and thrombolytics. Analgesics are helpful in relieving the pain but are not known to enhance coronary blood flow directly.

Vasodilators. The vasodilator of choice to treat myocardial pain is intravenous **nitroglycerine** (NTG). The dose of NTG required to abolish chest pain varies from one patient to another. Because doses vary, the prescribed amount of NTG is defined as the amount required to relieve pain while maintaining a systolic blood pressure within parameters therapeutic for the individual patient. Doses are calculated based on body weight and are designated as micrograms per kilogram of weight.

Nitroglycerine dilates both arteries and veins causing blood to pool or collect in the periphery, thereby reducing the amount of blood returning to the heart (preload) and reducing the workload of the heart. Because NTG also acts on the arteries, a fall in blood pressure is an anticipated outcome, thus reducing systemic blood pressure (afterload). The therapeutic effect of the nitrates also explains the primary side effect, which is clinical hypotension.

Anticoagulants. Heparin is the anticoagulant of choice to assist in preserving myocardial integrity. Heparin prolongs the clotting time of the blood, thus *reducing the probability of thrombus formation* and the subsequent diminished blood flow.

Thrombolytics. The purpose of thrombolytics is to *dissolve* any thrombus that may have formed in a coronary artery, minimizing the occlusion and hence the size of the infarction. To be effective these agents must be administered early after the onset of chest pain.

Three thrombolytic agents have proven to be valuable in dissolving thrombi (thrombolysis): streptokinase, tissue-type plasminogen activator (t-PA), and anistreplase.

Streptokinase. Streptokinase acts systemically on the body's clotting mechanism. Although this medication has demonstrated effectiveness in dissolving clots (clot lysis) the potential for systemic hemorrhage presents a significant risk. Streptokinase also entails a risk of allergic reactions and has proven to be maximally effective only when injected directly into the coronary arteries. Intracoronary administration requires a cardiac catheterization facility, a highly skilled physician, and a cardiothoracic surgery stand-by team.

Tissue-Type Plasminogen Activator. Tissue-type plasminogen activator, in contrast to streptokinase, has a specific action in dissolving the clot so the risk of systemic bleeding is reduced. The enzyme t-PA is a naturally occurring enzyme, so allergic reactions are minimized. Finally, studies thus far indicate that intracoronary and intravenous administration of t-PA are equally effective.

Anistreplase. Anistreplase, a clot-specific thrombolytic agent, parallels streptokinase and t-PA in clinical effectiveness. Anistreplase is growing in acceptance because of its ease of administration and low cost.

These medications are only effective if administered within 6 hours of the onset of chest pain, before transmural tissue necrosis occurs; thus the number of patients that this treatment benefits is limited. Coronary artery bypass surgery remains the viable alternative for revascularization of the myocardium in those persons for whom clot lysis is ineffective or contraindicated.

Oxygen Administration. Oxygen therapy is initiated at the onset of chest pain. Oxygen inhaled directly increases its saturation in the blood. The therapeutic effectiveness of oxygen is determined by observing the rate and rhythm of respiratory exchange. The patient is able to breath more easily. Oxygen saturation in the blood is concomitantly measured by pulse oximetry.

Analgesics. The need for analgesia is limited to those patients in whom nitrates and anticoagulants are ineffective in relieving pain. The analgesic of choice remains **morphine sulfate** administered in intravenous incremental doses of 1 to 2 mg. The cardiovascular response to morphine is monitored carefully, specifically the blood pressure, which can be lowered. However, because morphine reduces preload and afterload and relaxes bronchioles to enhance oxygenation, there are also therapeutic benefits other than pain relief to be derived from its administration.

An example of a critical pathway for an acute myocardial infarction (AMI) can be found on pages 652–653. The activities spelled out in this pathway cover an 8-day span, four of which are spent in the critical care unit and four of which are spent on a step down unit.

NURSING PROCESS
The Patient With Myocardial Infarction

Assessment

One of the most important aspects of care of the patient with an MI is the nursing assessment. This serves to establish a baseline of information on the present status of the patient, so that any deviations may be noted immediately. The nursing assessment is systematic and is aimed at identifying the needs of the cardiac patient and determining the priority of these needs.

Systematic assessment of the patient includes a careful history, particularly as it relates to the description of symptoms: chest pain, difficulty breathing (dyspnea), palpitations, faintness (syncope), or sweating (diaphoresis). Each symptom must be evaluated with regard to time, duration, and the factors that precipitate the symptom and relieve it.

In addition, a precise and complete physical assessment is critical to detect complications. Any change in patient status is reported immediately. A systematic method is used in carrying out the assessment and should include the following parameters.

Level of Consciousness. The patient's orientation to time, place, and person is monitored closely. Often changes in sensorium or mental status are produced by medication therapies or impending cardiogenic shock. An altered sensorium can mean that the heart is not pumping enough blood to oxygenate the brain. Because the patient may be receiving medications which alter blood coagulation function, observing for signs of cerebral bleeding is an important responsibility for the nurse. Two changes to watch for are slurred speech and deepening of snoring sounds in the sleeping patient. The patient who is receiving coagulation-altering medications should be aroused at frequent intervals to assess mentation.

Motor function and level of consciousness can be tested concomitantly by testing the ability to respond to simple commands. For example, the response of the patient to "squeeze my hands" allows the nurse to assess mentation as well as the grip strength in each hand.

Chest Pain. The presence or absence of chest pain is the single most important clinical finding of the patient with an acute MI. With each episode of chest pain a 12-lead ECG recording is obtained. The patient may be asked to rate the severity of pain on a numerical scale of 0 to 10, with 0 being the absence of pain and 10 being the most severe pain.

Heart Rate and Rhythm. Heart rate and rhythm are monitored continuously at the bedside and by a remote cardiac monitor. Rate is observed for any *unexplained* increase or decrease; rhythm is observed for deviation from sinus rhythm. The onset of dysrhythmia can indicate that not enough oxygen is being supplied to the myocardium. If dysrhythmia occurs in the absence of chest pain, other clinical parameters, aside from adequate oxygenation, are explored, such as the most recent serum potassium level. In some cases antidysrhythmia medication therapy may be necessary.

Heart Sounds. Heart sounds are auscultated with a good quality stethoscope. The bell portion of the chest piece is used to pick up low-pitched sounds. The diaphragm is used to auscultate high-pitched sounds. The bell of the stethoscope is applied to the skin lightly; the diaphragm is applied firmly.

The first heart sound (S_1), heard best over the apex of the heart and indicating the beginning of systole, should be identified first. The second sound (S_2), heard best at the base and indicating the beginning of diastole, is identified next (Fig. 28-7).

Abnormal sounds are noted. These include the third heart sound (S_3), known as ventricular gallop, and the fourth heart sound (S_4), known as an atrial or presystolic gallop. S_1 and S_2 together sound like the syllables "lub-dub." S_1 ("lub") is louder at the apex, and S_2 ("dub") is louder at the base. The S_3 sound follows closely after S_2 in a cadence similar to that of the word *Ken-tuck-y* (S_1-S_2-S_3). The S_4 sound precedes the S_1 in the cadence of the word *Ten-nes-see* (S_4-S_1-S_2).

Frequently after an MI, an S_3 sound will develop. The sound of the S_3 is produced when the blood in the ventricles hits against the noncompliant walls of a damaged myocardium. An S_3 can be an early sign of impending left ventricular failure. Early detection of an S_3 followed by aggressive medical management can prevent life-threatening pulmonary edema.

A **heart murmur** or a pericardial **friction rub** can be easily heard as extra sounds. These sounds are more complex to diagnose but can be heard readily and are reported promptly. The onset of a murmur not previously present can indicate a change in myocardial muscle function; a friction rub can indicate pericarditis.

Blood Pressure. The blood pressure is measured to determine response to pain and to therapeutic measures, especially to vasodilator therapy, which is known to lower blood pressure. Careful attention is given to pulse pressure measurements. Pulse pressure is the numeric difference between the systolic and diastolic pressures. A narrowing pulse pressure often is seen after an MI. Stroke volume (the amount of blood ejected with each ventricular contraction) may be inferred from the pulse pressure. A narrowing pulse pressure can indicate a decreasing stroke volume.

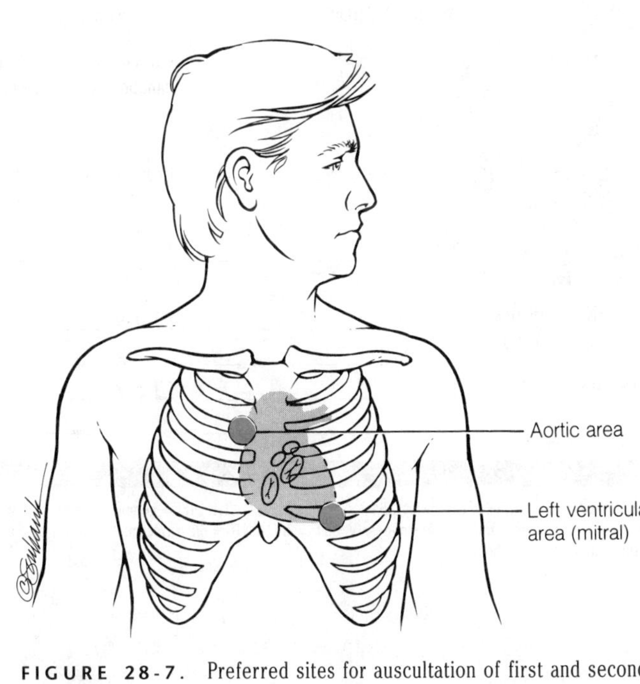

FIGURE 28-7. Preferred sites for auscultation of first and second heart sounds.

CRITICAL PATHWAY
AMI Uncomplicated With Intervention—Cardiac Care Unit

The Graduate Hospital Nursing Services Department
1800 Lombard Street
Philadelphia, PA 19146

Addressograph

	Day 1–CCU, Date: __	Day 2, Date: __	Day 3, Date: __	Day 4, Date: __
Assessments	History & Physical Nursing admission assessment* ROSA q shift & prn*	24 hr summary, PE ROSA q shift & prn*	24 hr summary, PE ROSA q shift & prn*	24 hr summary, PE ROSA q shift & prn*
Consults	Social work if indicated		Cardiac Rehab	Dietary
Labs, Diagnostics & Procedures	Total CK/iso's q 8h till peak, PTT (& with hep. changes), UA, EKG Echo (day 1 or 2)	Total CK/iso's if not baseline, PTT (if on heparin & with changes), Chem 7, CBC EKG Echo (day 1 or 2)	Total CK/iso's if not baseline, PTT (if on heparin & with changes) Schedule Stress test (ST)	Total CK/iso's if not baseline, PTT (if on heparin & with changes) Stress Test (Resting)
Interventions	Continuous EKG monitoring*, Noninvasive B/P monitoring*, Continuous pulse oximetry*, Rhythm strip q shift & prn*, VS per routine*, I & O per routine*, Chest pain protocol*, Guaiac stools*, Lytic therapy care per standard*, IV site care*, Immobility complication prevention*	Continuous EKG monitoring*, Noninvasive B/P monitoring*, Assess O_2 & D/C oximetry, Rhythm strip q shift & prn*, VS per routine*, I & O per routine*, Chest pain protocol*, Guaiac stools*, IV site care*, Immobility complication prevention*	Continuous EKG monitoring*, Noninvasive B/P monitoring*, Rhythm strip q shift & prn*, VS per routine*, I & O per routine*, Chest pain protocol*, Guaiac stools*, IV site care*, Immobility complication prevention*	Continuous EKG monitoring*, Rhythm strip q shift & prn*, VS per routine*, Chest pain protocol*, Guaiac stools*, IV site care*, Immobility complication prevention*
Medications & IV's	As indicated: Heparin drip, NTG, ASA, Beta blocker, Analgesics, Stool softener, Antiemetic, Sedative/Sleeper, Oxygen	As indicated: Heparin drip, NTG, ASA, Beta blocker, Analgesics, Stool softener, Antiemetic, Sedative/Sleeper, D/C Oxygen if indicated	As indicated: Heparin drip, NTG, ASA, Beta blocker, Analgesics, Stool softener, Antiemetic, Sedative/Sleeper	As indicated: Heparin drip, NTG, ASA, Beta blocker, Analgesics, Stool softener, Sedative/Sleeper
Diet	Low salt/low fat diet, house or ADA	Continue ordered diet	Continue ordered diet NPO post MN for ST	Continue ordered diet NPO post MN for ST
Activity	Bed rest with commode* Assist with ADLs*	Out of bed to chair* Assist with ADLs*	Ambulate with assist* Assist with ADLs*	Ambulate with assist* Assist with ADLs*
Teaching		Cardiac teaching: critical path, CCU handbook, pain scale per protocol*	Cardiac teaching* Differentiate CCU and Telemetry ST instructions*	Cardiac teaching* ST instructions*
D/C, Planning & Follow-up		Begin discharge teaching*	Discharge teaching* Request 4 South bed for day 4	Discharge teaching* Transfer to 4 South
Nursing Care Performed KEY: *NSG Activities V = Variance N = No Var.	☐ 1. V ____ N ____ ☐ 2. V ____ N ____ ☐ 3. V ____ N ____	☐ 1. V ____ N ____ ☐ 2. V ____ N ____ ☐ 3. V ____ N ____	☐ 1. V ____ N ____ ☐ 2. V ____ N ____ ☐ 3. V ____ N ____	☐ 1. V ____ N ____ ☐ 2. V ____ N ____ ☐ 3. V ____ N ____

LEGEND: ADL = activities of daily living; ASA = salicylic acid; CBC WITH DIFF = complete blood count with differential; CCU = cardiac care unit; ECHO = echocardiogram; EKG = electrocardiogram; H & H = hemoglobin and hematocrit; ISO = isoenzymes; IV = intravenous; NTG = nitroglycerin; PT = prothrombin time; PTT = partial thromboplastin time; ROSA = review of systems assessment; SAT = saturation; U/O = urine output; W/O = without.

CRITICAL PATHWAY
AMI Uncomplicated With Intervention—

Outcome Criteria for Discharge

1. Hemodynamically stable
2. Absence of chest pain, failure, ischemia or significant dysrhythmia
3. Able to carry-out ADL's
4. Able to demonstrate knowledge of discharge instructions/teaching

Day 5, Date: __	Day 6, Date: __	Day 7, Date: __	Day 8, Date: __
24 hr summary, PE ROSA q shift & prn*	24 hr summary, PE ROSA q shift & prn*	24 hr summary, PE ROSA q shift & prn*	24 hr summary, PE ROSA q shift & prn*
Total CK/iso's if not baseline, PTT (if on heparin & with changes) Stress Test (Exercise) Schedule Cardiac Cath if indicated—follow cath algorithm	Total CK/iso's if not baseline, PTT (if on heparin & with changes) Diagnostic Cardiac Cath Schedule PTCA/Interv. if indicated—follow PTCA. Intervention algorithm	Total CK/iso's if not baseline, PTT (if on heparin & with changes) PTCA / Interventional Tx	PTT, H/H, CK, BUN, Creatinine
Continuous EKG monitoring*, If (−) ST: D/C EKG monitoring, If (+) ST: Continue EKG monitor, Rhythm strip q shift & prn*, VS per routine*, Chest pain protocol*, Guaiac stools*, IV site care*, If (+) ST: Continue IV access*, If (−) ST: D/C IV access*, Immobility complication prevention*	Continuous EKG monitoring*, Rhythm strip q shift & prn*, VS per routine*, Chest pain protocol*, Guaiac stools*, IV site care*, Immobility complication prevention*	Continuous EKG monitoring*, Rhythm strip q shift & prn*, VS per routine*, Chest pain protocol*, Guaiac stools*, IV site care*, Immobility complication prevention*	Continuous EKG monitoring*, Rhythm strip q shift & prn*, VS per routine*, Chest pain protocol*, Guaiac stools*, IV site care*, Immobility complication prevention*
As indicated: Heparin drip, NTG, ASA, Beta Blocker, Analgesics, Stool softener, Sedative/Sleeper	As indicated: Heparin drip, NTG, ASA, Beta Blocker, Analgesics, Stool softener, Sedative/Sleeper	As indicated: Heparin drip, NTG, ASA, Beta Blocker, Analgesics, Stool softener, Sedative/Sleeper	As indicated: Heparin drip, NTG, ASA, Beta Blocker, Analgesics, Stool softener, Sedative/Sleeper, D/C IV access
Continue order diet Resume diet post ST	Continue ordered diet	Continue ordered diet	Continue ordered diet
Ambulate independently* Assist with ADLs*	Ambulate independently Assist with ADL*	Activity per cath standard Assist with ADL*	Activity per Intervention standard Assist with ADL*
Cardiac teaching* If (−) ST: Discharge meds & instructions*	Cardiac teaching per protocol* If (−) ST: Discharge meds & instructions*	If no PTCA: Discharge meds* Discharge instructions*	Discharge meds* Discharge instructions*
Discharge teaching*	Discharge teaching* If (−) ST: Discharge	If (−) Cath: discharge	
☐ 1. V ______ N ______ ☐ 2. V ______ N ______ ☐ 3. V ______ N ______	☐ 1. V ______ N ______ ☐ 2. V ______ N ______ ☐ 3. V ______ N ______	☐ 1. V ______ N ______ ☐ 2. V ______ N ______ ☐ 3. V ______ N ______	☐ 1. V ______ N ______ ☐ 2. V ______ N ______ ☐ 3. V ______ N ______

Peripheral Pulses. Peripheral pulses are evaluated for rate and volume. A difference between the peripheral pulse rate and the apical heart rate can confirm the presence of a dysrhythmia such as atrial fibrillation (see Chapter 27). Most often, peripheral pulses are evaluated to determine appropriate blood flow to an extremity. The patient with an acute MI is prone to thrombus formation in the peripheral arteries. A weakening peripheral pulse may be an indication that an obstruction to blood flow is occurring.

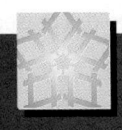

Intravenous sites are examined frequently for patency and signs of inflammation. Many medications are administered intravenously to avoid altering serum enzyme levels, which could occur if medications were injected intramuscularly. It is essential that at least one and possibly two intravenous lines be in place in any patient experiencing chest pain to assure that access is available for administering emergency medications.

Skin Color and Temperature. The skin is evaluated to see that it has a healthy pink color and is warm and dry, indicating good peripheral circulation. Because skin tones vary among individuals, the best places to observe color are nail beds, oral mucosa, and ear lobes. These sites may appear blue to purple in patients who are having difficulty maintaining oxygen demands. Patients who have cool, moist skin or are sweating (diaphoresis) may be responding to medication therapy or may be progressing to cardiovascular collapse as in cardiogenic shock (see Chapter 15).

Lungs. Any increase or decrease in rate of respiration is observed, along with any signs of labored breathing. Respiratory effort should be regular and without any impedance to air flow.

Shortness of breath, with or without exertion, and **cough** are key clinical signs to observe. A dry, hacking cough is often a sign of cardiac failure. The chest is auscultated for wheezes and crackles. **Wheezes** are produced when air crosses constricted passageways; **crackles** are produced when air moves through water and, in the presence of an acute MI, usually indicates heart failure.

Gastrointestinal Function. Nausea and vomiting can occur in AMI. The amount of any emesis is documented, and the emesis is tested for the presence of blood. Restricting intake to only fluids reduces myocardial work by minimizing blood flow required for digesting solid foods. If an invasive procedure becomes necessary, the possibility of aspirating stomach contents into the lungs is lessened if the patient has only been consuming liquids.

The abdomen is palpated for tenderness in all four quadrants. Each quadrant is auscultated for bowel sounds. The presence or absence of flatus is noted. The mesenteric artery is susceptible to ventricular thrombi secondary to AMI; loss of bowel motility is a cardinal sign of this problem. Any stool produced is tested for blood, especially for patients who are receiving coagulation-altering agents.

Fluid Volume Status. Measuring urinary output is important, especially in relation to intake. In most cases an equal or negative fluid balance is desirable for the patient with an AMI to avoid fluid overload and the possibility of cardiac failure. The patient is observed for edema. In the patient who is on bedrest, the sacrum and other dependent body parts should be observed for edema that results from circulatory stasis. The nurse must be particularly alert to reduced urine output (oliguria); an early sign of cardiogenic shock is hypotension accompanied by oliguria.

Diagnosis

Nursing Diagnoses

Based on the clinical manifestations, nursing history, and the diagnostic assessment data, the patient's major nursing diagnoses may include the following:

- Chest pain related to reduced coronary blood flow
- Potential ineffective breathing patterns related to fluid overload
- Potential altered tissue perfusion related to decreased cardiac output
- Anxiety related to fear of death
- Potential noncompliance with self-care program related to denial of diagnosis of MI

Collaborative Problems/ Potential Complications

Based on the assessment data, potential complications that may develop include:

- Dysrhythmias
- Acute pulmonary edema
- Congestive heart failure
- Thromboembolism

Planning and Implementation

Goals. The major goals of the patient include relief of chest pain, absence of respiratory difficulties, maintenance or attainment of adequate tissue perfusion, reduction of anxiety, adherence to the self-care program, and absence of complications.

Nursing Interventions

Relieving Chest Pain. Relieving chest pain is the top priority for the patient with an acute MI, and medication therapy is required to accomplish this goal. Thus, the management of chest pain is truly a collaborative effort between the physician and the nurse. However, because the chest pain is part of the patient's acute disease process and not a complication of the MI, management of the patient's chest pain is presented in this discussion of nursing interventions; collaboration between the nurse and the physician is critical in assessing the patient's response to medication therapy and in altering the medications accordingly.

The accepted method for relieving chest pain associated with MI is the intravenous administration of **vasodilator** and **anticoagulant medication** therapy. Nitroglycerine and heparin are the medications of choice, respectively. Thrombolytic therapy (*e.g.*, streptokinase, anistreplase) is highly desirable for those individuals who gain access to healthcare facilities immediately and who qualify clinically, that is, there is no major contraindication to the medication.

These therapies are important because, in addition to relieving pain, they aid in minimizing or avoiding permanent injury to the myocardium. Although analgesics, especially morphine, can be and are used, they do not directly preserve heart muscle as do vasodilators and anticoagulants.

Oxygen should be administered along with medication therapy to assure maximum relief of pain. Inhaling oxygen even in low doses raises the circulating level of oxygen and reduces pain associated with low levels of circulating oxygen. The route of administration, usually by nasal cannula, and the rate of flow of oxygen are documented. A flow rate of 2 to 4 liters per minute is usually adequate to maintain oxygen saturation levels of 96% to 100%, if no other disease process is present.

Vital signs are assessed frequently as long as the patient is experiencing pain.

Physical rest, in bed with the backrest elevated or in a cardiac chair, will assist in decreasing chest discomfort and dyspnea. The head-up position is beneficial for the following reasons: (1) tidal volume is improved because there is reduced pressure from abdominal contents on the diaphragm, and thus gas exchange is improved; (2) drainage of the upper lobes of the lungs is improved; and (3) venous return to the heart is reduced (preload), which reduces the work of the heart.

Improving Respiratory Function. Regular and careful assessment of respiratory function can help the nurse detect early signs of complications associated with the lungs. Scrupulous attention to fluid volume status will prevent overloading the heart and hence the lungs. Encouraging the patient to breathe deeply and change position frequently will prevent pooling of fluid in the lung bases.

Promoting Adequate Tissue Perfusion. Keeping the patient on bed or chair rest is particularly helpful in reducing myocardial oxygen consumption (MVO_2). Checking skin temperature and peripheral pulses frequently is important to assure adequate tissue perfusion. Oxygen may be administered to enrich the supply of circulating oxygen.

Reducing Anxiety. Developing a trusting and caring relationship with the patient is critical in reducing anxiety. Frequent private opportunities are provided for the patient to share concerns and fears. An atmosphere of acceptance helps the patient to know that these feelings are both realistic and normal.

Patient Education and Home Care Considerations. The most effective way to increase the probability that the patient will comply with a self-care regimen after discharge is to provide adequate education about the disease process. Working with patients in developing plans designed to meet their specific needs further enhances potential for compliance. The home health care program for the patient with acute myocardial infarction is presented in Chart 28-4.

Monitoring and Managing Potential Complications. Complications that can occur after acute myocardial infarction are due to the damage that occurs to the myocardium and to the conduction system as a result of the reduced coronary blood flow. Because these complications can be lethal, early identification of the cardinal signs and symptoms that signal their onset is critical.

The patient is monitored closely for changes in cardiac rate and rhythm, heart sounds, blood pressure, chest pain, respiratory status, urinary output, skin color and temperature, changes in sensorium, and changes in laboratory values. Any changes in the patient's condition are promptly reported to the physician and emergency measures are instituted when necessary. A detailed description of the complications that can result from acute myocardial infarction is presented on pages 656–676.

Evaluation

Expected Outcomes

1. Patient experiences relief of pain
2. Shows no signs of respiratory difficulties
3. Maintains adequate tissue perfusion

CHART 28-4
Home Health Care Program for the Patient With a Myocardial Infarction

A patient who has had an MI learns to regulate activity according to personal responses to each situation.

Goal: To extend and improve the quality of life

Expected Outcomes

I. Patient modifies activities during convalescence so that complete recovery is achieved.
   A. Myocardial healing starts early but is not complete for varying periods, usually 6 to 8 weeks.
   B. A myocardial infarction usually requires some modification of life style; adaptation to a heart attack is an ongoing process.
      1. Avoids any activity that produces chest pain, dyspnea, or undue fatigue
      2. Avoids extremes of heat and cold and walking against the wind
      3. Loses weight, if indicated
      4. Stops smoking
      5. Alternates activity with rest periods. Some fatigue is normal and expected during convalescence.
      6. Uses personal strengths to compensate for limitations
      7. Develops regular eating patterns
         a. Avoids large meals and hurrying while eating
         b. Restricts caffeine-containing beverages, because caffeine can affect heart rate, rhythm, and blood pressure
         c. Complies with prescribed diet, modifying calories, fat, and sodium as prescribed
      8. Makes every effort to adhere to medical regimen, especially in taking medications
      9. Pursues activities that afford release of tension

II. Patient undertakes an *orderly* program of increasing activity and exercise for long-term rehabilitation.
   A. Engages in a regimen of physical conditioning with a gradual increase in activity levels
      1. Walks daily, increasing distance and time as prescribed
      2. Monitors pulse during physical activity until the maximum level of activity is attained
      3. Avoids activities that tense the muscles: isometric exercise, weight-lifting, any activity that requires sudden bursts of energy
      4. Avoids physical exercise immediately after a meal
      5. Shortens work hours when first returning to work
   B. Participates in a *daily* program of exercise that develops into a program of regular exercise for a lifetime

III. Manages occurrences of symptoms
      1. Reports to nearest emergency facility if chest pressure or pain is not relieved in 15 min by nitroglycerin
      2. Contacts the physician when the following occur:
         a. Shortness of breath
         b. Fainting
         c. Slow or rapid heartbeat
         d. Swelling of feet and ankles

4. Expresses less anxiety
5. Complies with self-care program
6. Experiences absence of complications

Care of the patient with an uncomplicated MI is summarized in Nursing Care Plan 28-1.

Cardiac Rehabilitation

Once the patient who has experienced an acute MI becomes free of symptoms, an active rehabilitation program is initiated.

The goals of rehabilitation for the patient with an MI are to extend and improve the person's quality of life. The immediate objectives are to return the patient as rapidly as possible to a normal or near-normal lifestyle. These objectives are accomplished by encouraging physical activity and physical conditioning, educating both patient and family, and initiating psychosocial and vocational counseling when necessary.

Phases of Cardiac Rehabilitation. Cardiac rehabilitation actually occurs in four phases.

Phase 1 begins as soon as the acute episode of illness occurs, usually while the patient is still in the coronary care unit.

Phase 2 occurs during the remainder of the hospitalization. During these first two phases, the nurse can assist the patient toward realizing the goal of independence, even while on strict bedrest. This is achieved by directing the patient's thinking toward the time when he or she will be active again. The goal here is not to change the patient's lifestyle completely, but to encourage necessary modifications. It is best to avoid focusing on what the patient cannot do. Instead, encourage short-term and long-range goals based on individual needs. It is important to explain the nature of the disease, answer questions honestly, and reassure the patient that most persons resume their usual activities following an MI. These positive approaches help to keep the patient from becoming a cardiac invalid.

Phase 3 begins with the patient's discharge to home and continues throughout the convalescent period. The goal of phase 3 is to continue to restore the patient to activity levels that allow the return to work or the resumption of those activities performed before the illness occurred. This phase is usually accomplished by enrolling the patient in a formal rehabilitation program that provides supervised incremental increases in activities and exercise. These outpatient cardiac rehabilitation programs are designed to accommodate the work and activity schedules of patients. Many of these programs offer appointments early in the morning, late in the afternoon, and in the evening so that patients who have returned to work can schedule their appointments around their day's activities.

Phase 4 focuses on long-term conditioning and on maintaining cardiovascular stability. The patient is usually very self-directed during this phase and does not require a supervised program. The goals of each phase build on the accomplishments of the previous phase.

Physical Conditioning. Throughout all phases of rehabilitation the goals of activity and exercise tolerance are achieved through physical conditioning, aimed at improving cardiac efficiency. Cardiac efficiency is achieved when work and activities of daily living can be performed at reduced heart rates and lower blood pressure, thereby reducing the heart's oxygen requirements and reducing cardiac workload.

Physical conditioning occurs in phase 1 with range of motion exercises for the arms. Phase 2 includes chair sitting, walking, and some stair climbing. Phase 3 may include walking more vigorously. Finally, phase 4 may include jogging.

Physical conditioning is only conducted under the care of a physician. The patient is observed during activities for chest pain, dyspnea, weakness, fatigue, and an excessive increase in heart rate over the baseline rate. Should any of these signs or symptoms occur, the patient is cautioned to cease activity immediately and seek appropriate medical attention.

Complications

Acute Pulmonary Edema

Pathophysiology

Pulmonary edema is the abnormal accumulation of fluid in the lungs, either in the interstitial spaces or in the alveoli. Pulmonary edema represents the ultimate stage of pulmonary congestion, in which fluid has leaked through the capillary walls and is permeating the airways, giving rise to dyspnea of dramatic severity. Pulmonary congestion occurs when the pulmonary vascular bed has received more blood from the right ventricle than the left can accommodate and remove. The slightest imbalance between inflow on the right side and outflow on the left side of the heart may have drastic consequences.

Noncardiac pulmonary edema has a wide variety of causes: toxic inhalants, medication overdose, and neurogenic etiologies. Clinical management is directed toward reducing pulmonary blood flow and pulmonary arterial pressure.

The most common cause of pulmonary edema is cardiac disease—atherosclerotic, hypertensive, valvular, myopathic. Most patients with pulmonary edema have chronic heart disease of a type that imposes a strain on the left ventricle, such as arterial hypertension or aortic valve disease. The edema is particularly likely to arise from the damage to the heart muscle caused by acute MI. The development of pulmonary edema signifies that cardiac function has become grossly inadequate. There is an elevated left ventricular end-diastolic pressure and a rise in pulmonary venous pressure. This produces an increase in hydrostatic pressure, which results in seepage of fluid. Impaired lymphatic drainage contributes to the accumulation of fluid in the lung tissues.

The pulmonary capillaries, engorged with an excess of blood that the left ventricle is incapable of pumping, no longer are able to contain their contents. Fluid, first serous and later bloody, escapes into the adjacent alveoli through the communicating bronchioles and bronchi. It then mixes with air and, churned by respiratory agitation, is expelled from the mouth and nose. Because of the fluid buildup, the lungs become stiff and cannot expand, and air cannot enter. The result is severe hypoxia.

(text continues on page 660)

NURSING CARE PLAN 28–1
Care of the Patient With an Uncomplicated Myocardial Infarction

NURSING DIAGNOSIS: Chest pain related to reduced coronary blood flow

GOAL: Relief of chest pain

Nursing Interventions	Rationale	Expected Outcomes
1. Initially assess, document, and report to the physician the following:	1. These data assist in determining the cause and effect of the chest discomfort and provide a baseline with which post-therapy symptoms can be compared.	• Reports beginning relief of chest discomfort at once. • Appears comfortable and pain free: Is restful Respiratory rate, cardiac rate, and blood pressure return to prediscomfort level Skin warm and dry • Adequate cardiac output as evidenced by: Heart rate and rhythm Blood pressure Mentation Urine output Serum BUN and creatinine Skin color, temperature, and moisture
a. The patient's description of chest discomfort, including location, radiation, duration of pain, and factors that affect it	a. There are many conditions associated with chest discomfort. There are characteristic clinical findings of ischemic pain.	
b. The effect of chest discomfort on cardiovascular hemodynamic perfusion—to the heart, to the brain, to the kidneys, and to the skin	b. Myocardial infarction decreases myocardial contractility and ventricular compliance, and may produce dysrhythmias. Cardiac output is reduced, resulting in reduced blood pressure and decreased organ perfusion. The heart rate may increase as a compensatory mechanism to maintain cardiac output.	
2. Obtain a 12-lead ECG recording during pain, as prescribed, to determine extension of infarction.	2. An ECG during pain may be useful in the diagnosis of an extension of myocardial infarction versus an anginal episode.	
3. Administer oxygen as prescribed.	3. Oxygen therapy may increase the oxygen supply to the myocardium if actual oxygen saturation is less than normal.	
4. Administer medication therapy as prescribed and evaluate the patient's response continuously.	4. Medication therapy is the first line of defense in preserving myocardial tissue. The side effects of these medications can be hazardous and the patient's status must be assessed.	
5. Ensure physical rest: use of the bedside commode with assistance; backrest elevated to promote comfort; full liquid diet as tolerated; arms supported during upper extremity activity; use of stool softener to prevent straining at stool. Provide a restful environment, and allay fears and anxiety by being supportive, calm, and competent. Visitor privileges are individualized, based on patient response.	5. Physical rest reduces myocardial oxygen consumption. Fear and anxiety precipitate the stress response; this results in increased levels of endogenous catecholamines, which increase myocardial oxygen consumption. Also, with increased epinephrine the pain threshold is decreased and pain increases the myocardial oxygen consumption.	
6. Promote the patient's physical comfort by providing individualized basic nursing care.	6. Physical comfort promotes the patient's sense of well-being and reduces anxiety.	

NURSING DIAGNOSIS: Potential ineffective breathing pattern related to fluid overload

GOAL: Absence of respiratory difficulties

Nursing Interventions	Rationale	Expected Outcomes
1. Initially and every 4 h, and with chest discomfort, assess, document, and report to the physician abnormal heart sounds	1. These data are useful in diagnosing left ventricular failure. Diastolic filling sounds (S_3–S_4 gallop) result from	• Denies shortness of breath, dyspnea on exertion, orthopnea, or paroxysmal nocturnal dyspnea.

(continued)

NURSING CARE PLAN 28–1 *(continued)*
Care of the Patient With an Uncomplicated Myocardial Infarction

Nursing Interventions	Rationale	Expected Outcomes
(particularly S_3 and S_4 gallops and the holosystolic murmur of left ventricular papillary muscle dysfunction), abnormal breath sounds (particularly crackles), and patient intolerance to specific activities.	decreased left ventricular compliance associated with myocardial infarction. Papillary muscle dysfunction (from infarction of the papillary muscle) can result in mitral regurgitation and a reduction in stroke volume, leading to left ventricular failure. The presence of crackles (usually at the lung bases) may indicate pulmonary congestion from increased left heart pressures. The association of symptoms and activity can be used as a guide for activity prescription and a basis for patient teaching.	• Respiratory rate remains less than 20 breaths/min with physical activity and 16 breaths/min with rest. • Skin color is normal. • PaO_2 and $PaCO_2$ are within normal range. • Heart rate is less than 100 beats/min and greater than 60 beats/min with blood pressure within patient's normal limits. • Chest film normal. • Patient reports relief of chest discomfort. • Appears comfortable: Appears rested Respiratory rate, cardiac rate, and blood pressure return to prediscomfort level. Skin warm and dry
2. Promote the patient's physical comfort by providing individualized nursing care. Ensure physical rest.	2. Physical comfort promotes the patient's sense of well-being and reduces anxiety.	
3. Teach patient: a. To adhere to the diet prescribed (for example, explain low-sodium, low-calorie diet)	3. a. Low-sodium diet may reduce extracellular volume, thus reducing preload and afterload, and thus myocardial oxygen consumption. In the obese patient, weight reduction may decrease cardiac work and improve tidal volume.	
b. To adhere to activity prescription	b. The activity prescription is determined individually to maintain the heart rate and blood pressure within safe limits.	

NURSING DIAGNOSIS: Potential inadequate tissue perfusion related to decreased cardiac output

GOAL: Maintenance/attainment of adequate tissue perfusion

Nursing Interventions	Rationale	Expected Outcomes
1. Initially and every 4 h, and with chest discomfort, assess, document and report to the physician the following: a. Hypotension b. Tachycardia and other dysrhythmia c. Fatigability d. Mentation changes (use family input) e. Reduced urine output (less than 250 ml per 8 h) f. Cool, moist, cyanotic extremities	1. These data are useful in determining a low cardiac output state. An ECG with pain may be useful in the diagnosis of an extension of myocardial ischemia, injury, and infarction, and of variant angina.	• Blood pressure remains within the patient's normal range. • Ideally, normal sinus rhythm without dysrhythmia is maintained, or patient's baseline rhythm is maintained between 60 and 100 beats/min without further dysrhythmia. • No complaints of fatigue with prescribed activity • Remains fully alert and oriented and without personality change. • Appears comfortable a. Appears rested b. Respiratory rate, cardiac rate, and blood pressure return to prediscomfort level

(continued)

NURSING CARE PLAN 28–1 *(continued)*
Care of the Patient With an Uncomplicated Myocardial Infarction

Nursing Interventions	Rationale	Expected Outcomes
2. Promote the patient's physical comfort and rest by providing individualized nursing care.	2. Physical comfort promotes the patient's sense of well-being and reduces anxiety. Rest reduces myocardial oxygen consumption.	c. Skin warm and dry • Urine output is greater than 40 ml/h. • Extremities remain warm and dry with normal color.

NURSING DIAGNOSIS: Anxiety related to fear of death

GOAL: Reduction of anxiety

Nursing Interventions	Rationale	Expected Outcomes
1. Assess, document, and report to the physician the patient's and family's level of anxiety and coping mechanisms.	1. These data provide information about the psychological well-being and a baseline so that post-therapy symptoms can be compared. Causes of anxiety are variable and individual, and may include acute illness, hospitalization, pain, disruption of activities of daily living at home and at work, changes in role and self-image due to chronic illness, and lack of financial support. Because anxious family members can transmit anxiety to the patient, the nurse must also reduce the family's fear and anxiety.	• Reports less anxiety. • Patient and family discuss their anxieties and fears about death. • Patient and family appear less anxious. • Appears restful, respiratory rate less than 16/min, heart rate less than 100/min without ectopic beats, blood pressure within patient's normal limits, skin warm and dry. • Participates actively in a progressive rehabilitation program. • Practices stress-reduction techniques
2. Assess the need for spiritual counseling and refer as appropriate.	2. If a patient finds support in a religion, religious counseling may assist in reducing anxiety and fear.	
3. Allow patient (and family) to express anxiety and fear: a. By showing a genuine interest and concern b. By facilitating communication (listening, reflecting, guiding) c. By answering questions	3. Unresolved anxiety (the stress response) increases myocardial oxygen consumption.	
4. Use of flexible visiting hours allows the presence of a supportive family to assist in reducing the patient's level of anxiety.	4. The presence of supportive family members may reduce both patient's and family's anxiety.	
5. Encourage active participation in a cardiac rehabilitation program.	5. Prescribed cardiac rehabilitation may help to eliminate fear of death, may reduce anxiety, and may enhance feelings of well-being.	
6. Teach stress reduction techniques.	6. Stress reduction may help to reduce myocardial oxygen consumption and may enhance feelings of well-being.	

NURSING DIAGNOSIS: Potential noncompliance with self-care program related to denial of diagnosis of myocardial infarction

GOAL: Complies with the home health-care program

(See Chart 28-4.)

Death from pulmonary edema is by no means inevitable. If appropriate measures are taken promptly, attacks can be aborted and patients can survive this complication to benefit from measures directed against its recurrence. Fortunately, pulmonary edema usually does not develop precipitously but is preceded by the premonitory symptoms of pulmonary congestion.

Clinical Manifestations

The typical attack of pulmonary edema occurs after the patient has been lying down for a few hours. Recumbency increases the venous return to the heart and favors the resorption of edema from the legs. The circulating blood becomes diluted, and its volume expands. The venous pressure rises and the right atrium fills with increasing rapidity. There is a corresponding increase in the right ventricular output, which eventually surpasses the output from the left ventricle. The pulmonary vessels become engorged with blood and proceed to leak. Meanwhile, the patient has become increasingly restless and anxious.

There is a sudden onset of breathlessness and a sense of suffocation. The patient's hands become cold and moist, the nail beds become cyanotic, and the skin color turns gray. In addition, the pulse is weak and rapid and the neck veins are distended. There is incessant coughing, which produces increasing quantities of mucoid sputum. As the pulmonary edema progresses, anxiety develops into near panic and the patient becomes confused, then stuporous. Breathing is noisy and moist, and the patient, nearly suffocated by the blood-tinged, frothy fluid now pouring into the bronchi and trachea, is literally drowning in secretions. The situation demands immediate action.

Diagnostic Evaluation

The diagnosis is made by evaluating the clinical manifestations resulting from pulmonary congestion. A pulmonary artery catheter may be inserted to facilitate the monitoring of hemodynamic data essential to diagnosis and treatment. (See discussion of hemodynamic monitoring on page 665.)

Management

The goals of medical management for the patient with acute pulmonary edema are to reduce total circulating volume and to improve respiratory exchange. These goals are accomplished through a combination of oxygen and medication therapies and nursing support.

Oxygenation. Oxygen is administered in concentrations adequate to relieve hypoxia and dyspnea. If signs of hypoxia persist, oxygen may be delivered by intermittent or continuous positive pressure. If respiratory failure occurs despite optimal management, endotracheal intubation and mechanical ventilation are required. The use of positive end expiratory pressure (PEEP) is effective in reducing venous return, lowering pulmonary capillary pressure, and improving oxygenation. Oxygenation is monitored with pulse oximetry and by measurement of arterial blood gases.

Pharmacotherapy: Morphine. Morphine is administered intravenously in small doses to reduce anxiety and dyspnea and to decrease peripheral resistance so that blood can be redistributed from the pulmonary circulation to other parts of the body. This action decreases pressure in the pulmonary capillaries and decreases seepage of fluid into the lung tissue. The decrease in rate of respirations resulting from morphine is also beneficial.

- Morphine is not usually administered if pulmonary edema is caused by cerebral vascular accident or if chronic pulmonary disease or cardiogenic shock is present.
- The patient is observed for excessive respiratory depression; morphine antagonist (naloxone hydrochloride [Narcan]) is kept available.

Diuretics. Furosemide (Lasix) is administered intravenously to produce a rapid diuretic effect. Furosemide also causes vasodilation and the pooling of blood in peripheral blood vessels, which in turn reduces the amount of blood returned to the heart, even before the diuretic effect. Some physicians may prefer to use bumetanide (Bumex) and diuril in place of furosemide. (Table 28-2 lists commonly used diuretics with related nursing implications.) Dyspnea is rapidly relieved and pulmonary congestion is decreased. Because a large volume of urine will be formed within minutes after a potent diuretic is administered, an indwelling catheter may be indicated.

- Falling blood pressure, increasing heart rate, and decreasing urinary output indicate that the circulatory system is not tolerating diuresis and that measures must be taken to reverse the hypovolemia that has occurred.
- Patients with prostatic hyperplasia must be observed for signs of urinary retention.

Digitalis. To improve the contractile force of the heart, thus increasing the output of the left ventricle, the patient may be prescribed a rapid-acting digitalis preparation. The improved cardiac contractility will increase cardiac output, enhance diuresis, and reduce diastolic pressure. Thus pulmonary capillary pressure and the transudation or seepage of fluid into the alveoli will be reduced.

- Digitalis must be administered with extreme caution to patients with acute myocardial infarction, because these patients are sensitive to digitalis and may develop toxic dysrhythmias.
- The serum potassium level is measured at intervals because diuresis may have produced hypokalemia. The effect of digitalis in the presence of hypokalemia is enhanced, so digitalis toxicity may occur.
- If the patient has been on digitalis, the medication is usually withheld until the possibility of digitalis toxicity is ruled out.

An overview of digitalis and cardiac glycoside preparations along with nursing considerations and actions is presented in Chart 28-5.

Aminophylline. When the patient is wheezing and bronchospasm appears to play a significant role, aminophylline may be administered to relax bronchospasm.

- Aminophylline is administered by continuous intravenous drip in dosages based on body weight.

TABLE 28-2 Commonly Used Diuretics

Definition: Diuretics are agents that increase the rate of urine flow.

Action: Dependent on functionally active kidneys; most diuretics decrease the reabsorption of electrolytes (principally sodium) by the kidneys, promoting water loss as a secondary action. In the treatment of hypertension, the natriuretic (sodium excretion) effect is probably the action of importance. In edema states, the salt and water actions are both important.

Special Precaution: Some diuretics may produce electrolyte depletion, including potassium loss, which causes weakness and induces cardiac dysrhythmias. Vigorous diuresis can produce hypovolemia.

Dosage Determination: (1) Patient's daily weight; (2) clinical signs and symptoms; (3) state of renal function

Diuretic	Action	Nursing Implications
THIAZIDES AND RELATED DRUGS		
Chlorothiazide (Diuril) Hydrochlorothiazide (HydroDIURIL, Esidrix, Oretic) Methyclothiazide (Enduron) Polythiazide (Renese) Chlorthalidone (Hygroton) Quinethazone (Hydromox)	Increases renal excretion of sodium (natriuresis), potassium, chloride, bicarbonate (alkaline urine), with accompanying "osmotic" water loss Used principally in states of edema and hypertension Most widely used for prolonged administration	Monitor for electrolyte depletion: hyponatremia, hypokalemia, hypochloremic alkalosis Observe for signs and symptoms of electrolyte imbalance, dizziness, lightheadedness. Adverse reactions may occur, manifested by gastrointestinal, central nervous system, hematologic, and cardiovascular signs and symptoms. Supplementary potassium is usually prescribed with these diuretics.
POTASSIUM-SPARING DIURETICS		
Spironolactone (Aldactone)	Inhibits action of aldosterone in distal tubule and reduces reabsorption of sodium and chloride Produces gradual diuretic effect Used in treatment of cirrhosis and edema when other diuretics are toxic or ineffective	Monitor for electrolyte depletion. Usually used in combination with thiazide diuretic Observe for side effects—skin rash, gynecomastia.
Triamterene (Dyrenium)	Inhibits reabsorption of sodium ions in exchange for potassium and hydrogen ions in distal tubule	Usually used as an adjunct to thiazide therapy May cause elevation in blood uric acid Observe for nausea, vomiting, diarrhea, weakness, headache, and skin rash.
POTENT DIURETICS		
Furosemide (Lasix) Bumetanide (Bumex)	Usually reserved for patients who do not respond to thiazide diuretics Blocks the reabsorption of sodium and water in proximal renal tubule and interferes with reabsorption of sodium in ascending limb of loop of Henle and in the most proximal portion of the distal tubule Associated with sodium, potassium, chloride, and hydrogen ion loss (acid urine) Has an almost immediate action (within 5 min) when given IV	Monitor for electrolyte depletion: may produce *profound diuresis* with hyponatremia, hypokalemia, hypochloremic alkalosis, and circulatory collapse. Potent and rapid acting Especially useful in acute pulmonary edema Observe for nausea, vomiting, diarrhea, skin rash, pruritus, blurring of vision, postural hypotension, vertigo, hearing loss. Furosemide is chemically related to sulfonamides; consider cross-allergies. Administer early in the day to avoid nocturia and consequent loss of sleep. Some patients may benefit from taking diuretics at bedtime to avoid paroxysmal nocturnal dyspnea.

Positioning. Proper positioning can help reduce venous return to the heart.

- The patient is positioned upright, with legs and feet down, preferably with legs dangling over the side of the bed. This has the immediate effect of decreasing venous return, lowering the output of the right ventricle, and decreasing lung congestion (*e.g.*, reducing preload).
- If unable to sit with lower extremities dependent, the patient may be placed in an upright position in bed.

Rotating Tourniquets and Phlebotomy. The use of **rotating tourniquets** to mechanically reduce the

CHART 28-5
Digitalis and Cardiac Glycoside Preparations

Actions of Digitalis

Increases force of myocardial contractions

- Increases cardiac output by enhancing force of contraction of ventricle
- Slows heart rate
- Decreases heart size
- Decreases venous pressure
- Promotes diuresis
- Slows the ventricular rate in the setting of supraventricular dysrhythmias

Clinical Uses

- Congestive heart failure
- Atrial fibrillation; atrial flutter
- Supraventricular tachydysrhythmias
- Before cardiac surgery

Preparations

The choice of drug depends on the speed of onset desired, duration of action required, and individual patient response. The recommended dosage varies considerably.

Oral	Parenteral
Digitalis	Ouabain
Digoxin (Lanoxin)	Digoxin (Lanoxin)

Nursing Considerations and Actions

Special Precautions: The incidence of digitalis toxicity is high. Toxic effects do not always appear in a predictable manner.

- Monitor for toxic effects: dysrhythmias (most important toxic effect), anorexia, nausea, vomiting, bradycardia, headache, malaise.
- Assess clinical response of patient by relief of symptoms (dyspnea, orthopnea, crackles, hepatomegaly, peripheral edema).
- Elderly patients may tolerate digitalis therapy poorly; assess for bradycardia, impaired renal function.
- Monitor serum potassium levels in patients receiving digitalis, especially those receiving both digitalis and diuretics. There is a predisposition to dysrhythmias if a potassium imbalance is not detected and corrected.
- Assess for symptoms of electrolyte depletion in patients taking digitalis: lassitude, apathy, mental confusion, anorexia, decreasing urinary output, azotemia.
- The following factors may increase sensitivity to digitalis: myocardial infarction, myocarditis, potassium depletion, kidney or hepatic disease, diuretic therapy, diarrhea, loss of appetite, advancing age, hypoxia and hypercapnia in pulmonary disease, acidosis, alkalosis.
- Check apical rate before each dose. A rate of 60 or above with no dysrhythmias is desirable. Check with the physician regarding specific guidelines for each individual patient.

volume of blood returning to the heart (preload) was once a first-line treatment for acute pulmonary edema. Tourniquets were applied to three of four extremities securely enough to impede venous return to the heart but not so tightly that they interfered with arterial flow to each extremity. To avoid the hazard of impaired oxygenation to an extremity, the tourniquets were rotated every 15 minutes in a clockwise pattern. The tourniquets were confining and disturbing to patients already struggling to breathe. In addition, the stagnation of blood in the extremities fostered the development of serious thromboembolic sequelae.

In recent years, the development of newer, more efficient pharmacologic agents in tandem with the ability to monitor fluid volume status via a multilumen pulmonary artery catheter (see discussion of hemodynamic monitoring, p. 665) has replaced the use of rotating tourniquets in most settings.

Therapeutic phlebotomy, the removal of a specified volume of blood for therapeutic reasons, was once used in severe cases of pulmonary edema. Although phlebotomy is a therapeutic technique for some hematologic conditions (*e.g.*, polycythemia vera), it is no longer an accepted standard of treatment for pulmonary edema.

Psychologic Support. Extreme fear and anxiety are cardinal features of pulmonary edema. These emotions, which are self-perpetuating, make the condition more severe. Reassuring the patient and providing skillful anticipatory nursing care are integral parts of the therapy. Because this patient experiences a sense of impending doom, it is essential that the nurse remain with the patient as much as possible. Nursing care should be organized to maximize the nurse's presence at the bedside. The patient is frequently given simple, concise information about what is being done to treat the condition and how he or she is responding to the treatment.

Prevention

Like most complications, pulmonary edema is easier to prevent than to treat. To recognize it in its early stages, when the presenting signs and symptoms are solely those of pulmonary congestion, the nurse auscultates the lung fields of hospitalized patients with cardiac disease each day or more frequently if indicated by the patient's condition. A dry, hacking cough and the presence of a third heart sound (S_3) are often the earliest indicators of pulmonary congestion. The S_3 is best heard at the apex with the patient lying in the left lateral decubitus position.

In an early stage, the condition may be corrected by relatively simple measures. These include (1) placing the patient in an upright position with the feet and legs dependent, (2) eliminating overexertion and emotional stress to reduce the left ventricular load, and (3) administering morphine to reduce anxiety, dyspnea, and preload.

The long-range approach to the prevention of pulmonary edema must be directed at its precursor, pulmonary congestion. Measures to prevent congestive heart failure and the various facets of patient teaching are discussed in the next section.

In addition to these measures, the patient is advised to sleep with the head of the bed elevated on 25-cm (10-inch) blocks. It is especially important to use extreme caution when administering infusions and transfusions to cardiac patients and elderly persons.

- To prevent circulatory overload, which could precipitate acute pulmonary edema, intravenous fluids are administered slowly, with the patient positioned upright in bed and under close nursing surveillance.
- Intravenous infusion control devices are used to restrict the rate and volume of fluid that can be delivered.

Surgical treatment may be necessary to eliminate or to minimize valvular defects that limit the flow of blood into or out of the left ventricle, because such defects impair the cardiac output and predispose the patient to the development of pulmonary congestion and edema.

Cardiac Failure: Congestive Heart Failure

Cardiac failure, often referred to as congestive heart failure, is the inability of the heart to pump sufficient blood to meet the needs of the tissues for oxygen and nutrients. The term **congestive heart failure** is most commonly used when referring to left-sided and right-sided failure.

Pathophysiology

The underlying mechanism of cardiac failure involves impairment of the contractile properties of the heart, which leads to a lower-than-normal cardiac output. The concept of cardiac output is best explained by the equation $CO = HR \times SV$, where cardiac output (CO) is a function of heart rate (HR) × stroke volume (SV).

Heart rate is a function of the autonomic nervous system. When cardiac output falls, the sympathetic nervous system accelerates the heart rate to maintain adequate cardiac output. When this compensatory mechanism fails to maintain adequate tissue perfusion, the properties of stroke volume must adjust to maintain cardiac output.

However, in cardiac failure in which the primary problem is damaged and inhibited myocardial muscle fibers, stroke volume is impaired and normal cardiac output cannot be maintained.

Stroke volume, the amount of blood pumped with each contraction, is dependent on three factors: preload, contractility, and afterload.

- **Preload** is synonymous with Starling's Law of the Heart, which states that the amount of blood filling the heart is directly proportional to pressure created by the length of the stretch of the myocardial fibers.
- **Contractility** refers to an alteration in the force of contraction that occurs at the cellular level and is related to changes in myocardial fiber length and calcium levels.
- **Afterload** refers to the amount of pressure the ventricle must create to pump blood across the pressure gradient created by arteriole resistance.

In cardiac failure, any one or more of these three factors may be altered such that cardiac output is impaired. The relative ease of determining hemodynamic measurements through invasive monitoring procedures has made it easier to diagnose congestive heart failure and to implement effective pharmacologic therapy.

Etiology

Cardiac Muscle Disorders. Cardiac failure most commonly occurs with disorders of cardiac muscle that result in decreased contractile properties of the heart. Common underlying conditions that lead to disordered muscle function include coronary atherosclerosis, arterial hypertension, and inflammatory or degenerative muscle disease.

Coronary atherosclerosis leads to myocardial dysfunction by interfering with the normal supply of blood to cardiac muscle. Hypoxia and acidosis (due to accumulation of lactic acid) result. Myocardial infarction (death of myocardial cells) frequently precedes the development of overt cardiac failure.

Systemic or pulmonary hypertension (increased afterload) increases the work requirement of the heart, and this in turn leads to hypertrophy of myocardial muscle fibers. This effect (myocardial hypertrophy) can be considered a compensatory mechanism because it increases the contractility of the heart. For reasons that are not clear, however, the hypertrophied cardiac muscle does not function normally, and cardiac failure may eventually result.

Inflammatory and **degenerative diseases of the myocardium** associated with cardiac failure lead to direct damage to myocardial fibers, with a resultant decrease in contractility.

Other Heart Disease. Cardiac failure may occur as a result of heart disease that only secondarily affects the myocardium. The mechanisms involved include impediment to flow of blood through the heart (*e.g.*, stenosis of a semilunar valve), inability of the heart to fill with blood (*e.g.*, pericardial tamponade, constrictive pericarditis, or stenosis of AV valves), or abnormal emptying of the heart (*e.g.*, insufficiency of AV valves). Sudden increase in afterload due to elevated systemic blood pressure ("malignant" hypertension) may result in cardiac failure in the absence of myocardial hypertrophy.

Systemic Factors. A number of systemic factors can contribute to the development and severity of cardiac failure. Increased metabolic rate (*e.g.*, fever, thyrotoxicosis), hypoxia, and anemia require an increased cardiac output to satisfy systemic oxygen demand. Hypoxia or anemia also may decrease the supply of oxygen to the myocardium. Acidosis (respiratory or metabolic) and electrolyte abnormalities may decrease myocardial contractility. Cardiac dysrhythmias, which may be present independently or secondary to cardiac failure, decrease the overall efficiency of myocardial function.

Clinical Manifestations

The dominant feature in cardiac failure is increased intravascular volume. Congestion of tissues results from increased arterial and venous pressures due to decreased cardiac output in the failing heart. Increased pulmonary venous pressure can cause fluid to pass from the pulmonary capillaries to the alveoli resulting in pulmonary edema, manifested by cough and shortness of breath. Increased systemic venous pressure can result in generalized peripheral edema and weight gain.

The diminished cardiac output from cardiac failure has widespread manifestations because not enough blood reaches the tissues and organs (low perfusion) to provide the necessary oxygen. Some commonly encountered effects related to low perfusion are dizziness, confusion, fatigue, exercise or heat intolerance, cool extremities, and reduced urine output (oliguria). Renal perfusion pressure falls, which results in the release of renin from the kidney, which in turn leads to aldosterone secretion, sodium and fluid retention, and increased intravascular volume.

Left- and Right-Sided Cardiac Failure

The left and right ventricles can fail separately. Left ventricular failure most often precedes right ventricular failure. Pure left ventricular failure is synonymous with acute pulmonary edema. Because the outputs of the ventricles are coupled or synchronized, failure of either ventricle may lead to decreased tissue perfusion. The congestive manifestations, however, may differ according to whether left or right ventricular failure exists.

Left-Sided Cardiac Failure

Pulmonary congestion predominates when the left ventricle fails, because the left ventricle is unable to pump adequately the blood coming to it from the lungs. The increased pressure in the pulmonary circulation causes fluid to be forced into the pulmonary tissues. The clinical manifestations that ensue include dyspnea, cough, fatigability, rapid heart beat (tachycardia) with an S_3 heart sound, and anxiety and restlessness.

Dyspnea results from the accumulation of fluid in the alveoli, which impairs gas exchange. Dyspnea may occur even at rest or may be precipitated by minimal to moderate exertion. **Orthopnea,** difficulty in breathing when lying flat, may be present. The patient who experiences orthopnea will not lie flat, but instead will use pillows to be propped up in bed or will sit in a chair, even to sleep.

Some patients experience orthopnea only at night, a condition known as **paroxysmal nocturnal dyspnea** (PND). This occurs when the patient, who has been sitting for a long period with the feet and legs in a dependent position, goes to bed. After several hours the fluid that accumulated in the dependent extremities begins to be reabsorbed, and the impaired left ventricle is unable to empty the increased volume adequately. As a result, the pressure in the pulmonary circulation increases and causes further shifting of fluid into the alveoli.

The **cough** associated with left ventricular failure may be dry and nonproductive, but is most often moist. Large quantities of frothy sputum, which is sometimes blood-tinged, may be produced.

Fatigability results from the low cardiac output that deprives tissues of normal circulation and oxygen and decreases the removal of catabolic waste products. It is also a result of the increased energy expended for breathing and the insomnia that results from respiratory distress and coughing.

Restlessness and anxiety result from the impaired oxygenation of tissues, the stress associated with respiratory difficulty, and the knowledge that the heart is not functioning properly. As anxiety increases, so does dyspnea, which in turn further enhances the anxiety, creating a vicious cycle.

Right-Sided Cardiac Failure

When the right ventricle fails, congestion of the viscera and the peripheral tissues predominates. This occurs because the right side of the heart is unable to empty its blood volume adequately and thus cannot accommodate all of the blood that normally returns to it from the venous circulation.

The clinical manifestations that ensue include edema of the lower extremities (dependent edema), which is usually pitting edema, weight gain, hepatomegaly (enlargement of liver), distended neck veins, ascites (accumulation of fluid in the peritoneal cavity), anorexia and nausea, nocturia, and weakness.

Edema begins in the feet and ankles (dependent edema) and can gradually progress up the legs and thighs

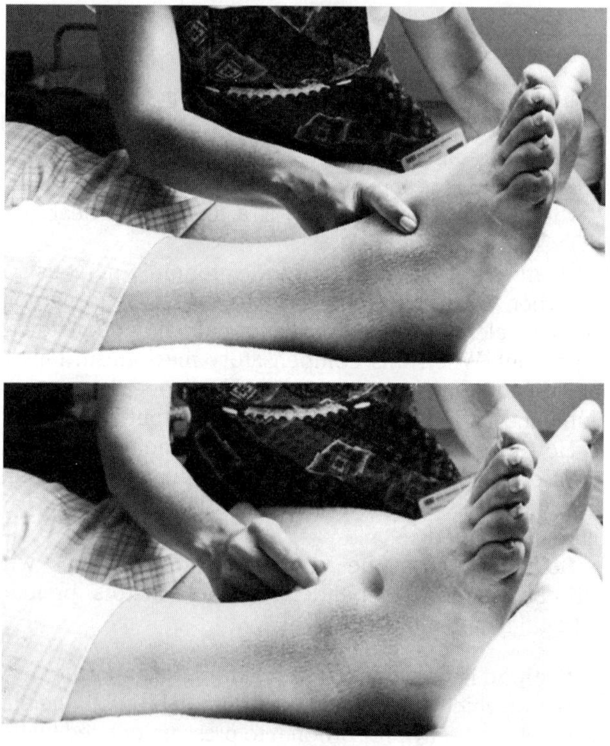

FIGURE 28-8. Example of pitting edema. An area near the ankle is pressed. When the pressure is released, an indentation of the edematous tissue remains.

and eventually into the external genitalia and lower trunk. Sacral edema is not uncommon for patients who are on bedrest, as the sacral area is dependent. **Pitting edema,** edema in which pits remain after even slight compression with the fingertips (Fig. 28-8) is obvious only after retention of at least 4.5 kg (10 lb) of fluid.

Hepatomegaly and tenderness in the right upper abdominal quadrant results from venous engorgement of the liver. As this process progresses, pressure within the portal vessels can become great enough to cause fluid to be forced into the abdominal cavity, a condition known as **ascites.** This collection of fluid in the abdominal cavity can cause pressure on the diaphragm and respiratory distress.

Anorexia (loss of appetite) and **nausea** result from the venous engorgement and venous stasis within the abdominal organs.

Nocturia, or the need to urinate at night, occurs because renal perfusion is promoted by periods of recumbency. Diuresis results and is most common at night because cardiac output is improved with physical rest.

Weakness that accompanies right-sided failure is due to the reduced cardiac output, impaired circulation, and inadequate removal of catabolic waste products from the tissues.

Diagnosis

Hemodynamic Monitoring

The diagnosis of cardiac failure is made by evaluating the clinical manifestations of pulmonary and systemic congestion. An important method for evaluating stroke volume is the use of the pulmonary artery catheter (Fig. 28-9). This catheter may be inserted at the bedside. The catheter contains several lumena, which allows for the measurement of more than one hemodynamic parameter via a single catheter. The catheter is inserted into the superior vena cava and threaded into the right atrium. A balloon at the end of the catheter is then inflated, allowing the catheter to follow the blood flow through the tricuspid valve, the right ventricle, the pulmonic valve, into the main pulmonary artery, and then into the right or left pulmonary artery, ultimately wedging into a small branch of the pulmonary artery.

Waveform and pressure readings are noted during insertion to identify where the catheter is located within the heart. The balloon is deflated once the catheter is in the pulmonary artery. It is then properly secured. The methods for inserting the pulmonary artery catheter, obtaining pressure readings, and providing follow-up care are described in Guideline 28-1.

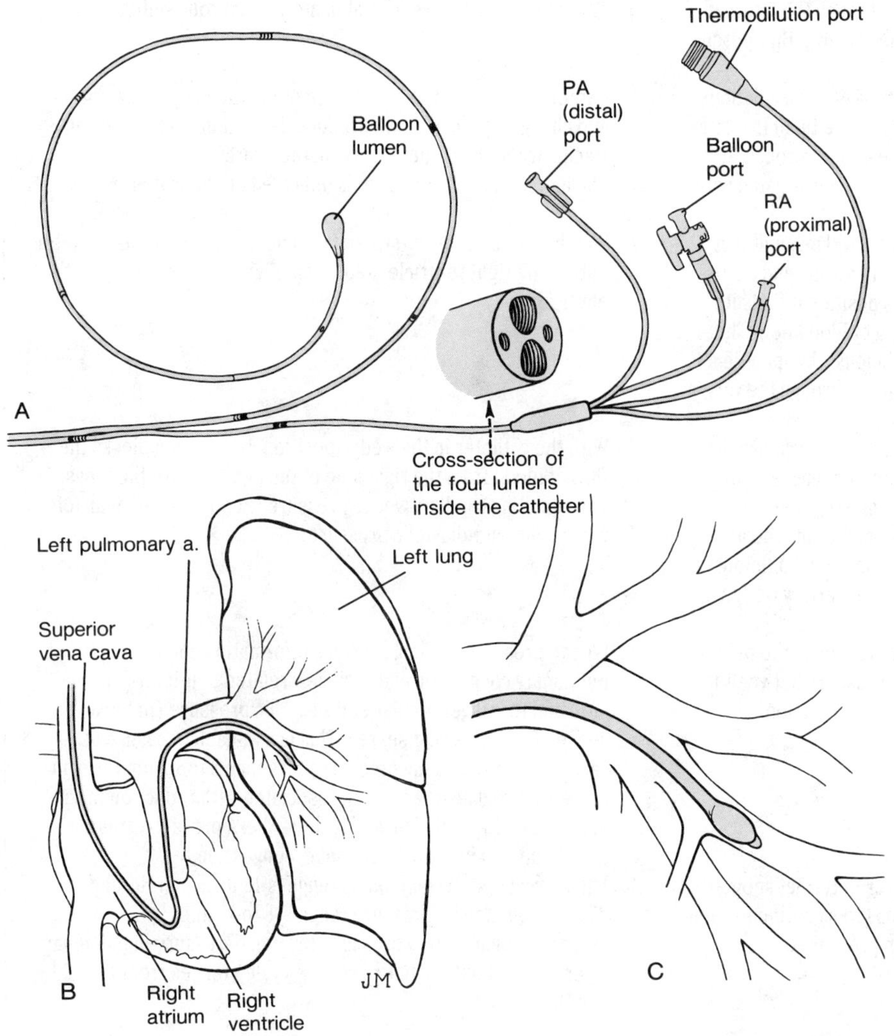

FIGURE 28-9. (**A**) The multilumen pulmonary artery catheter. (**B**) Location of the catheter within the heart. The catheter enters the right atrium via the superior vena cava. The balloon is then inflated, allowing the catheter to follow the blood flow through the tricuspid valve, through the right ventricle, through the pulmonic valve, and into the main pulmonary artery. Waveform and pressure readings are noted during insertion to identify location of the catheter within the heart. The balloon is deflated once the catheter is in the pulmonary artery and properly secured. (**C**) Pulmonary artery wedge pressure (PAWP). The catheter floats into a distal branch of the pulmonary artery when the balloon is inflated, and becomes "wedged." The wedged catheter occludes blood flow from behind, and the tip of the lumen records pressures in front of the catheter. The balloon is then deflated, allowing the catheter to float back into the main pulmonary artery. (Suddarth DS. The Lippincott Manual of Nursing Practice, 5th ed. Philadelphia, JB Lippincott, 1991.)

GUIDELINE 28–1
Hemodynamic Monitoring: Multilumen Pulmonary Artery Catheter

Nursing Action	Rationale/Amplification
Preparatory Phase	
1. Explain procedure to patient and family/significant other.	1. Explain that it is normal to feel the catheter moving through the vein.
2. Check vital signs and apply ECG electrodes.	2. An initial assessment offers a baseline for comparison.
3. Place patient in a position of comfort; this is the baseline position.	3. Document the angle of elevation if patient cannot lie flat, as subsequent pressure readings are taken from this baseline position to ensure consistency.
4. Set up equipment according to manufacturer's directives:	4.
a. The pulmonary artery catheter requires a transducer, recording, amplifying, and flush systems.	a. Monitoring systems may vary greatly. The complexity of equipment requires an understanding of the equipment in use.
b. The pressure equipment is calibrated and flushed according to manufacturer's directives.	b. Flushing of the catheter system ensures patency and eliminates air bubbles.
c. The balloon is inflated with air or sterile water or saline to test for leakage (bubbles).	c. Testing is indicated to ensure that the balloon is intact.
5. Prepare the skin over insertion site.	5. Decreases risk of infection at insertion site.
Performance Phase (by the Physician)	
1. The pulmonary artery catheter is inserted through the internal jugular, subclavian, or any easily accessible vein by either percutaneous puncture or venotomy.	1. The internal jugular vein establishes a short route into the central venous system.
2. The catheter is advanced to the superior vena cava. Oscillations of the pressure waveforms will indicate when the tip of the catheter is within the heart. The patient may be asked to cough.	2. Catheter placement is determined by characteristic waveforms and changes. Coughing will produce deflections in the pressure tracing when the catheter tip is in the heart.
3. When the catheter is in the superior vena cava, it is inflated with air and advanced gently.	3. The amount of air to be used is indicated on the catheter.
4. The inflated balloon at the tip of the catheter will be guided by the flowing stream of blood through the right atrium and tricuspid valve into the right ventricle. From this position it finds its way into the main pulmonary artery, carried by blood flow. The catheter tip pressures are recorded continuously by specific pressure waveforms as the catheter advances through the various chambers of the heart.	4. Watch ECG monitor for signs of ventricular irritability as catheter enters the right ventricle. Report any signs of dysrhythmia to the physician.
5. The flowing blood will continue to direct the catheter more distally into the pulmonary tree. When the catheter reaches a pulmonary vessel that is approximately the same size or slightly smaller in diameter than the inflated balloon, it cannot be advanced any further. This is the wedge position, called pulmonary capillary wedge pressure (PCWP) or pulmonary artery wedge pressure (PAWP).	5. With the catheter in the wedge position, the balloon blocks the flow of blood from the right side of the heart toward the lungs. The resulting capillary wedge pressure is equal to the mean left ventricular end-diastolic pressure.
6. The pressure is recorded with the balloon wedged in the pulmonary vascular bed. A mean capillary wedge pressure between 14 and 18 mm Hg indicates optimal left ventricular function.	6. Wedge pressure reading provides information about the level of pulmonary congestion and is closely related to left atrial pressure and to left ventricular end-diastolic pressure (in the absence of mitral valve disease). This is a valuable measure of cardiac function. Filling pressures less than 8 to 10 mm Hg in an acutely injured heart are often associated with reduction in cardiac output, hypotension, and tachycardia. A pressure greater than 18 mm Hg indicates pulmonary congestion.
7. The balloon is deflated, causing the catheter to retract spontaneously into a larger pulmonary artery. This gives continuous pulmonary artery systolic, diastolic, and mean pressures.	7. The normal systolic pulmonary range is 15 to 25 mm Hg, and the diastolic pulmonary pressure range is 8 to 12 mm Hg. The normal mean pulmonary artery pressure (average pressure in pulmonary artery throughout the entire cardiac cycle) ranges from 10 to 20 mm Hg.

(continued)

GUIDELINE 28–1 *(continued)*
Hemodynamic Monitoring: Multilumen Pulmonary Artery Catheter

Nursing Action	Rationale/Amplification
Performance Phase (by the Physician)	
8. The catheter is sutured in place.	8. An antibiotic ointment may be placed around the site and covered with a sterile dressing.
9. The patency of the catheter is maintained with low-flow continuous irrigation.	9. A chest x-ray to confirm catheter position and as a baseline for future reference is obtained after catheter insertion.
To Obtain a Wedge Pressure Reading	
1. Close off the microdrip.	1. The transducer converts the pressure wave into an electronic wave that is displayed on a screen.
2. Inflate the balloon slowly until the contour of the pulmonary arterial pressure changes to that of pulmonary wedge pressure. As soon as a wedge pattern is observed, no more air is introduced. Do not introduce more air into balloon than specified.	2. *Caution: Do not allow catheter to remain in the wedge position when patient is unattended or when not directly making the measurement. Segmental lung infarction may occur if the catheter balloon is left inflated for long periods.*
3. Deflate the balloon as soon as the pressure reading is obtained.	
To Obtain a Central Venous Pressure Reading	
1. Turn the stopcock so that the CVP port is connected to the transducer.	1. Confirm the waveform to be that of the right atrium.
2. The pressure recorded is the central venous pressure.	2. Flush the tubing to ensure patency and return the stopcock to the continuous drip position.
Follow-Up Phase	
1. Inspect the insertion site daily. Observe for signs of infection, swelling, and bleeding.	1. A foreign body (catheter) in the vascular system increases the risk of sepsis.
2. Record data and time of dressing change and IV tubing change.	
3. If a peripheral vessel access site is used, assess the extremity for color, temperature, capillary filling, and sensation.	3. Ischemia (with possible loss of digits) may occur from inadequate arterial flow.
4. Evaluate pulse.	
5. Assess for complications: pulmonary embolism, dysrhythmias, heart block, damage to tricuspid valve, intracardiac knotting of catheter, thrombophlebitis, infection, balloon rupture, rupture of pulmonary artery.	
For Removal of the Catheter	
1. Be sure that the balloon is not inflated.	
2. The catheter is removed without excessive force of traction; pressure dressing is applied over the site.	2. This site should be checked periodically for bleeding.

Pressure measurements of preload, afterload, and cardiac output can be obtained through ports located at various intervals along the catheter. One port lies at the level of the right atrium. Because **preload** is the amount of venous return to the heart and is therefore equal to the central venous pressure measurement, measuring the pressure at the proximal port yields an accurate preload and hence **central venous pressure** (CVP) measurement.

The tip of the catheter rests in the pulmonary artery where left ventricular pressure measurements are made. The balloon is inflated and flows into a small pulmonary artery, occluding or wedging the artery. Pulmonary artery wedge pressures (PAWP) are then obtained. A pressure measurement is made that is the left ventricular end-diastolic pressure.

Cardiac output is measured with a thermodilution lumen connected to a computer.

Measurements of the various pressures are made at intervals prescribed by the physician, and medication therapy is adjusted based on the readings.

Nursing Management. Nursing management of the patient who has a hemodynamic catheter is highly specialized and is best managed in an intensive care environment (see Guideline 28-1).

Management

The basic objectives in the treatment of patients with cardiac failure are the following:

1. To promote rest to reduce the workload on the heart
2. To increase the force and efficiency of myocardial contraction through the action of pharmacologic agents
3. To eliminate the excessive accumulation of body water by means of diuretic therapy, diet, and rest

Pharmacologic Therapy

Cardiac glycosides, diuretics, and vasodilators form the basis of the pharmacologic treatment of cardiac failure. Chart 28-5 summarizes the major cardiac glycosides, along with their actions and the nursing surveillance required when these medications are administered.

Digitalis. Digitalis increases the force of myocardial contraction and slows the heart rate. Several effects are produced: an increase in cardiac output; a decrease in venous pressure and blood volume; and an increase in diuresis, which removes fluid and relieves edema. The effect of a given dose of digitalis depends on the state of the myocardium, electrolyte and fluid balance, and renal and hepatic function.

A loading dose of digitalis may be administered to induce the full therapeutic effect of the medication. This is usually administered in the treatment of more severe forms of cardiac failure. Otherwise, the digitalis is started without a loading dose. A maintenance dose is administered and continued daily.

In either case, the patient is observed closely and administered a daily dose just adequate to replace the amount of medication that is metabolized or excreted, to maintain the digitalis effect without producing toxicity. The optimal dosage is the amount that relieves the patient's signs and symptoms of cardiac failure or slows the ventricular response therapeutically *without causing toxicity.*

The patient is observed closely for relief of signs and symptoms: lessening dyspnea and orthopnea, decrease in crackles, and relief of peripheral edema.

Digitalis Toxicity. Anorexia, nausea, and vomiting are early effects of **digitalis toxicity**. There may be alterations in the heart rhythm, bradycardia, premature ventricular contractions, ventricular bigeminy (coupling of normal and premature beat), and paroxysmal atrial tachycardia.

- The apical heart rate is assessed before digitalis is administered. If there is excessive slowing of the heart rate or change in rhythm, the medication is withheld and the physician is notified. Frequently the physician withholds the digitalis preparation if the rate is 60 or less.
- If prescribed, the serum digitalis level is checked before the medication is administered.

Other symptoms of digitalis toxicity include blurred, yellow, or green vision; weakness; drowsiness; and mental depression.

Diuretic Therapy. Diuretics are prescribed to promote the excretion of sodium and water through the kidneys. These medications may not be necessary if the patient responds to restricted activity, digitalis, and a low-sodium diet.

- When diuretics are prescribed they should be administered early in the morning so that the resultant diuresis does not interfere with the patient's nighttime rest.
- An intake and output record is kept, because the patient may lose a large volume of fluid after a single dose of a diuretic.
- As a basis for evaluating the effectiveness of therapy, a patient receiving diuretic medications is weighed daily at the same time. In addition, skin turgor and mucous membranes are examined for evidence of edema or dehydration. The pulse rate is also monitored.

The dosage schedule is determined by the patient's daily weight, physical findings, and symptoms. Table 28-2 summarizes the diuretics in common use. Furosemide (Lasix) is a particularly useful diuretic in the treatment of heart failure because it dilates the venules, thereby increasing venous capacity, which in turn reduces preload (venous return to the heart).

Prolonged diuretic therapy may produce **hyponatremia** (deficiency of sodium in the blood), which results in apprehension, weakness, fatigue, malaise, muscle cramps and twitching, and rapid, thready pulse.

Profuse and repeated diuresis can also lead to **hypokalemia** (potassium depletion). Signs are weak pulse, faint heart sounds, hypotension, muscle flabbiness, diminished tendon reflexes, and generalized weakness. Hypokalemia poses new problems for the cardiac patient, because among the complications of hypokalemia are marked weakening of cardiac contractions and the precipitation of digitalis toxicity in persons receiving digitalis, both of which increase the likelihood of dangerous dysrhythmias.

- Periodic assessment of the electrolytes will alert health team members to hypokalemia and hyponatremia.
- To lessen the risk of hypokalemia and its attendant complications, patients receiving diuretic medications may be given a potassium supplement (potassium chloride). Bananas, orange juice, dried prunes, raisins, apricots, dates, figs, peaches, and spinach are good dietary sources of potassium.

Other problems associated with diuretic administration are hyperuricemia (excessive uric acid in the blood), volume depletion from excessive urination, and hyperglycemia.

The elderly male patient requires ongoing nursing surveillance because the incidence of urethral obstruction due to an enlarged prostate gland is high in this age group. Signs of bladder distention should be observed for regularly by palpating over the bladder.

Vasodilator Therapy. Of particular significance in the management of cardiac failure are the vasoactive medications.

Vasodilator medications have been used to reduce impedance (resistance) to left ventricular ejection of blood. The medications promote ventricular emptying and increase venous capacity, so left ventricular filling pressure is reduced and a dramatic decrease in pulmonary congestion may be achieved rapidly.

Sodium nitroprusside may be administered intravenously by means of carefully monitored infusions. The dosage is titrated to keep the arterial systolic pressure at the prescribed level, and the patient is monitored by measuring pulmonary artery pressures and cardiac output. Another commonly used vasodilator medication is nitroglycerin.

Dietary Support

The rationale for dietary support is to provide a diet that will cause the heart the least possible work effort and muscular strain and maintain good nutritional status, taking into consideration the patient's likes, dislikes, and cultural food patterns.

Sodium Restriction. Restriction of sodium is indicated for the prevention, control, or elimination of edema, as in hypertension or cardiac failure. The sources of sodium should be specified in describing the regimen, rather than "low-salt" or "salt-free," and the quantity should be indicated in milligrams. Very often mistakes are made because of inconsistencies in the translation of salt to sodium. It is important to realize that salt is not 100% sodium. There are 393 mg, or approximately 400 mg, of sodium in 1 g (1000 mg) of salt.

Although the major source of sodium in the average American diet is salt, many types of natural foods contain varying amounts of sodium. Therefore, even if no salt is added in cooking and if salty foods are avoided, the daily diet may still contain approximately 1000 to 2000 mg of sodium.

Other sources of sodium can be found in some processed foods. Added food substances—such as sodium alginate, which improves food texture; sodium benzoate, which acts as a preservative; and disodium phosphate, which improves cooking quality in certain foods—increase the sodium intake when included in the daily diet. Therefore, patients on low-sodium diets should be advised not to buy processed foods and to check labels carefully for such words as "salt" or "sodium," especially on canned foods. For diets that call for less than 1000 mg of sodium, low-sodium milk and bread and salt-free butter should be considered.

Patients on sodium-restricted diets also should be cautioned against using nonprescription medications, such as antacids, cough syrups, laxatives, sedatives, or salt substitutes, because these products contain sodium or excessive amounts of potassium. Over-the-counter medications should not be used without first consulting the physician.

When diets are very restricted in both fat and sodium content, the patient may find the food unpalatable and may refuse to eat. A variety of flavorings such as lemon juice and herb seasonings may be used to improve the taste of the food and encourage the person to accept the diet. Every effort should be made to take into account the individual's food preferences.

❑ NURSING PROCESS
The Patient With Cardiac Failure

Assessment

The focus of the nursing assessment for the patient with cardiac failure is directed toward observing for signs and symptoms of pulmonary and systemic fluid overload. All untoward signs are recorded and reported.

Respiratory. The lungs are auscultated at frequent intervals to determine the presence or absence of crackles and wheezes. Crackles are produced by the movement of air through fluid, and therefore indicate that pulmonary congestion is developing. The rate and depth of respirations are also noted.

Cardiac. The heart is auscultated for the presence of an S_3 or S_4 heart sound. The presence of these signs may mean that the pump is beginning to fail and that there is increased blood volume remaining in the ventricle with each beat. The rate and rhythm are also noted. Rapid rates indicate that the ventricle has had less time to fill, indicating that some stagnation of blood is occurring in the atria and eventually in the pulmonary bed.

Sensorium/Level of Consciousness. As the volume of blood and fluid within the blood vessels increases, the circulating blood becomes dilute and its oxygen transport capacity is compromised. The brain tolerates inadequate oxygenation poorly, and the patient becomes confused.

Periphery. The dependent parts of the patient's body are assessed for edema. If the patient is sitting upright, the feet and lower legs are examined; if the patient is supine in bed, the sacrum and back are assessed for edema. Fingers and hands may also become edematous. In extreme cases of cardiac failure the patient may develop periorbital edema, in which the eyelids may be swollen shut.

The liver is examined for hepatojugular reflux (HJR). The patient is asked to breathe normally while manual pressure is applied over the liver for 30 to 60 seconds. If neck vein distention increases more than 1 cm, the test is positive for increased venous pressure.

Jugular Vein Distention. JVD is also assessed. This is performed by elevating the patient to a 45-degree angle. The distance between the angle of Louis and the level of jugular vein distension is estimated. (The **angle of Louis** is the junction between the body of the sternum and the manubrium.) A distance greater than 3 cm is said to be abnormal. Remember that this is an estimate and not an exact measurement.

Urinary Output. The patient may become oliguric (diminished urine output between 100 and 400 ml/24 hr) or anuric (urine output of less than 100 ml/24 hr). It is important to measure output frequently to develop a baseline against which to measure the effectiveness of diuretic therapy. Intake and output records are rigorously maintained and the patient is weighed daily, at the same time and on the same scales.

Diagnosis

Nursing Diagnoses

Based on the assessment data, major nursing diagnoses for the patient may include the following:

- ❑ Activity intolerance related to fatigue and dyspnea secondary to decreased cardiac output
- ❑ Anxiety related to breathlessness and restlessness secondary to inadequate oxygenation
- ❑ Altered peripheral tissue perfusion related to venous stasis
- ❑ Potential knowledge deficit of self-care program related to nonacceptance of necessary lifestyle changes

Collaborative Problems/ Potential Complications

Based on the assessment data, potential complications that may develop include:

- ❑ Cardiogenic shock

- ❑ Thromboembolic episodes
- ❑ Pericardial effusion and pericardial tamponade

These complications are discussed on pages 672–674.

Planning and Implementation

Goals. The major goals of the patient may include promotion of rest, relief of anxiety, attainment of normal tissue perfusion, knowledge of self-care program, and absence of complications.

Nursing Interventions

Promoting Rest. It is essential that the patient have both physical and emotional rest. Rest reduces the work of the heart, increases cardiac reserve, and reduces blood pressure. Periods of recumbency also promote diuresis by improving renal perfusion. Rest also decreases the work of the respiratory muscles and the utilization of oxygen. The heart rate is slowed, which prolongs the diastolic period of recovery and thus improves the efficiency of heart contraction.

Positioning. The head of the bed may be elevated on 20- to 30-cm (8- to 10-in) blocks or the patient may be placed in a comfortable armchair. In this position the venous return to the heart (preload) and the lungs is reduced, pulmonary congestion is alleviated, and impingement of the liver on the diaphragm is minimized. The lower arms should be supported with pillows to eliminate the fatigue caused by the constant pull of their weight on the shoulder muscles.

The patient who can breathe only in the upright position (orthopnea) may sit on the side of the bed with feet supported on a chair, the head and arms resting on an over-the-bed table, and lumbosacral spine supported by a pillow (Fig. 28-10). If pulmonary congestion is present, positioning the patient in an armchair is advantageous because this position favors the shift of fluid away from the lungs. Edema, which usually occurs in dependent parts of the body, shifts from the extremities to the sacral areas when the patient is confined to bed.

Relieving Anxiety. Because patients in cardiac failure have difficulty maintaining adequate oxygenation, they are likely to be restless and anxious and feel overwhelmed by breathlessness. These symptoms tend to become exaggerated at night.

Raising the head of the bed and keeping a night light on are often helpful. The presence of a member of the family provides necessary reassurance to some persons. Oxygen may be administered during the acute stage to diminish the work of breathing and to increase the comfort of the patient. Small doses of morphine may be prescribed for extreme dyspnea, and hypnotics may be administered as prescribed for sleep.

- ❑ In a patient with hepatic congestion, the liver is unable to detoxify medications within a normal time frame. Therefore, medications must be administered with caution.
- ❑ Cerebral hypoxia with superimposed nitrogen retention is also a problem in cardiac failure and may cause the patient to react unfavorably to sedative and hypnotic medications as evidenced by signs of confusion and increased anxiety.

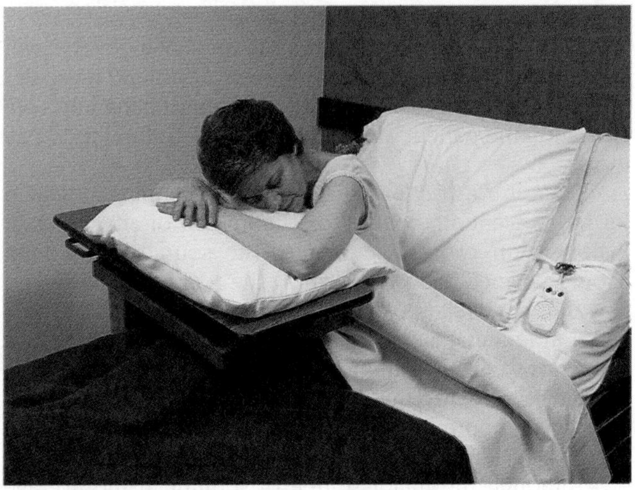

FIGURE 28-10. A patient with congestive heart failure can assume the position shown to relieve breathing difficulties and to reduce the amount of blood returning to the heart, which alleviates pulmonary congestion.

- ❑ Use of restraints is avoided; restraints are likely to be resisted, and resistance inevitably increases the cardiac load.

The patient who insists on getting out of bed at night can be seated comfortably in an armchair. As cerebral and systemic circulation improves, the quality of sleep will improve.

Avoiding Stress. A highly anxious patient is not able to rest properly. Emotional stress produces vasoconstriction, elevates arterial pressure, and speeds the heart. Promoting physical comfort and avoiding situations that tend to promote anxiety and agitation may help the patient to relax. Rest is continued for a few days to a few weeks until the cardiac failure is controlled.

Promoting Normal Tissue Perfusion. The decreased tissue perfusion that occurs in cardiac failure results from inadequate levels of circulating oxygen and stagnation of blood in the peripheral tissues. Moderate daily exercise will enhance the blood flow to peripheral tissues. Adequate oxygenation and appropriate diuresis will serve also to provide good tissue perfusion. Effective diuresis reduces dilution of the blood, thus providing more oxygen-carrying capacity to the vascular system. Adequate rest is essential to promote adequate tissue perfusion.

- ❑ There are dangers inherent in bedrest, such as pressure ulcers (especially in edematous patients), phlebothrombosis, and pulmonary embolism. Changes of position, deep breathing, elastic stockings, and leg exercises all help to improve muscle tone and at the same time aid venous return to the heart.

Patient Education and Home Care Considerations. After cardiac failure is under control, the patient is encouraged gradually to resume as much as possible the lifestyle and activities engaged in prior to illness. Activities of daily living should be planned to minimize breathlessness and fatigue. Some modifications in daily habits, work, and interpersonal relationships usually have to be made. Any activity that produces symptoms must be curtailed or other adaptations made. The patient should be helped to identify emotional stresses and to explore ways to resolve them.

All too frequently patients keep returning to the clinic and hospital for recurring episodes of cardiac failure. Not only does this create psychologic, sociologic, and financial problems, but the physiologic burden on the patient can be serious. Ultimately body organs may be damaged. Repeated attacks can lead to pulmonary fibrosis, liver cirrhosis, enlargement of the spleen and kidneys, and even brain damage due to insufficient oxygen during acute episodes.

Providing patient education and involving the patient in implementing the therapeutic regimen will promote cooperation and compliance. Many recurrences of cardiac failure occur because the patient does not follow the therapeutic recommendations, such as failing to follow the medication therapy properly, straying from dietary restrictions, failing to obtain adequate medical follow-up, engaging in excessive physical activity, and failing to recognize recurring symptoms. A summary of patient education teaching points for the patient with cardiac failure is presented in Chart 28-6.

The patient should be assisted to understand that cardiac failure can be controlled. Arranging for regular medical follow-up, maintaining correct weight, restricting sodium intake, preventing infection, avoiding noxious agents such as coffee and tobacco, and avoiding unregulated or excessive exercise all aid in preventing the onset of cardiac failure. In patients with valvular heart disease, surgery to correct the defect at the appropriate time may spare the heart and prevent failure.

Evaluation

Expected Outcomes

1. Experiences reduced fatigue and dyspnea
   a. Obtains adequate physical and emotional rest
   b. Assumes positions that reduce fatigue and dyspnea
   c. Adheres to medication regimen
2. Experiences less anxiety
   a. Avoids situations that produce stress
   b. Sleeps comfortably at night
   c. Reports decreased stress and anxiety

CHART 28-6
Patient Education: Cardiac Failure

A patient with heart disease can learn to regulate activity according to individual response.

Goal: To deter progression of disease and the development of cardiac failure

The patient learns to do the following to achieve these goals:

I. Live within the limits of the cardiac reserve.
   A. Obtain adequate rest.
      1. Have a regular daily rest period.
      2. Shorten working hours if possible.
      3. Avoid emotional upsets.
   B. Accept the fact that taking digitalis and restricting sodium intake may be a permanent way of life.
      1. Take digitalis daily, exactly as prescribed.
         a. Avoid substituting another brand of digitalis for the one prescribed.
         b. Check own pulse rate daily.
         c. Have a check-off system to ensure that medicine(s) has been taken.
      2. Take diuretic as prescribed.
         a. Weigh at the same time daily to detect any tendency toward fluid accumulation.
         b. Report weight gain of more than 0.9 to 1.4 kg (2–3 pounds) in a few days.
         c. Know the signs and symptoms of potassium depletion; if taking oral potassium, keep a check-off system along with diuretic medication.
      3. Take vasodilator as prescribed.
         a. Learn to take own blood pressure at prescribed intervals.
         b. Know signs and symptoms of orthostatic hypotension and how to prevent it.
   C. Restrict sodium as directed.
      1. Consult the written diet plan and the list of permitted and restricted foods.
      2. Examine labels to ascertain sodium content (antacids, laxatives, cough, remedies, and the like).
      3. Avoid using salt.
      4. Avoid excesses in eating and drinking.
   D. Review activity program.
      1. Increase walking and other activities gradually, provided that they do not cause fatigue and dyspnea.
      2. In general, continue at whatever activity level can be maintained without the appearance of symptoms.
      3. Avoid extremes of heat and cold, which increase the work of the heart. Air conditioning may be essential in a hot, humid environment.
      4. Keep regular appointments with physician or clinic.

II. Be alert for symptoms that may indicate recurring failure.
   A. Recall the symptoms experienced when illness began. Reappearance of previous symptoms may indicate a recurrence.
   B. Report immediately to the physician or clinic any of the following:
      1. Gain in weight
      2. Loss of appetite
      3. Shortness of breath with activity
      4. Swelling of ankles, feet, or abdomen
      5. Persistent cough
      6. Frequent urination at night

3. Attains normal tissue perfusion
   a. Obtains adequate rest
   b. Performs activities that promote venous return: moderate daily exercise; active range of motion of extremities if immobile or in bed for long periods; wearing support stockings
   c. Skin warm and dry with normal color
   d. Exhibits no peripheral edema
4. Adheres to self-care regimen (see Chart 28-6)

Cardiogenic Shock

Cardiogenic shock, the end stage of left ventricular dysfunction or congestive heart failure, occurs when the left ventricle is extensively damaged. The heart muscle loses its contractile power, resulting in a marked reduction in cardiac output with inadequate tissue perfusion to the vital organs (heart, brain, kidneys). The degree of shock is proportional to the level of left ventricular dysfunction. Although cardiogenic shock is seen most commonly as a complication of MI, it also can occur with cardiac tamponade, pulmonary embolism, cardiomyopathy, and dysrhythmias.

Pathophysiology

The signs and symptoms of cardiogenic shock reflect the circular nature of the pathophysiology of cardiac failure. The damage to the myocardium results in a decrease in cardiac output, which in turn reduces arterial blood pressure in the vital organs. Flow to the coronary arteries is reduced, resulting in a decrease in the oxygen supply to the myocardium, which in turn increases ischemia and further reduces the heart's ability to pump. Thus, a vicious circle is set in motion.

- The classic signs of cardiogenic shock are low blood pressure, rapid and weak pulse, cerebral hypoxia manifested by confusion and agitation, decreased urinary output, and cold, clammy skin.

Dysrhythmias are common and result from a decrease in oxygen to the myocardium. As in cardiac failure, the use of a pulmonary artery catheter to measure left ventricular pressure and cardiac output is important in assessing the severity of the problem and evaluating management. Continuing elevation of left ventricular end-diastolic pressure (LVEDP) accompanied by a fall in arterial blood pressure indicates that the heart is failing to function as an effective pump.

Management

General Measures. There are many approaches to the treatment of cardiogenic shock. Any major dysrhythmias are corrected because they may have caused or contributed to the shock. If hypovolemia or low intravascular volume is suggested or detected through pressure readings, the patient is given IV infusions to expand the amount of fluid in the circulatory system. If hypoxia is present, oxygen is administered, often under positive pressure when regular flow is insufficient to meet tissue demands.

Pharmacotherapy. Medication therapy is selected and guided according to cardiac output and mean arterial blood pressure. One group of medications used is the catecholamines, which raise blood pressure and increase cardiac output. However, they tend to increase the workload of the heart by increasing oxygen demand.

Vasoactive agents such as sodium nitroprusside and nitroglycerin are effective medications that lower blood pressure and thus cardiac work. They cause the arteries and veins to dilate, thereby shunting much of the intravascular volume to the periphery and causing a reduction in preload and afterload. These vasoactive agents are usually administered with dopamine, a vasopressor that assists in maintaining an adequate blood pressure.

Intra-aortic Balloon Pump. Other therapeutic modalities employed in treating cardiogenic shock involve the use of circulatory assist devices. The most frequently used mechanical support system is the **intra-aortic balloon pump** (IABP). The IABP uses internal counterpulsation to augment the pumping action of the heart through the regular inflation and deflation of a balloon located in the descending thoracic aorta (Fig. 28-11). The device is connected to a control box that synchronizes its activities with the electrocardiogram. Hemodynamic monitoring is

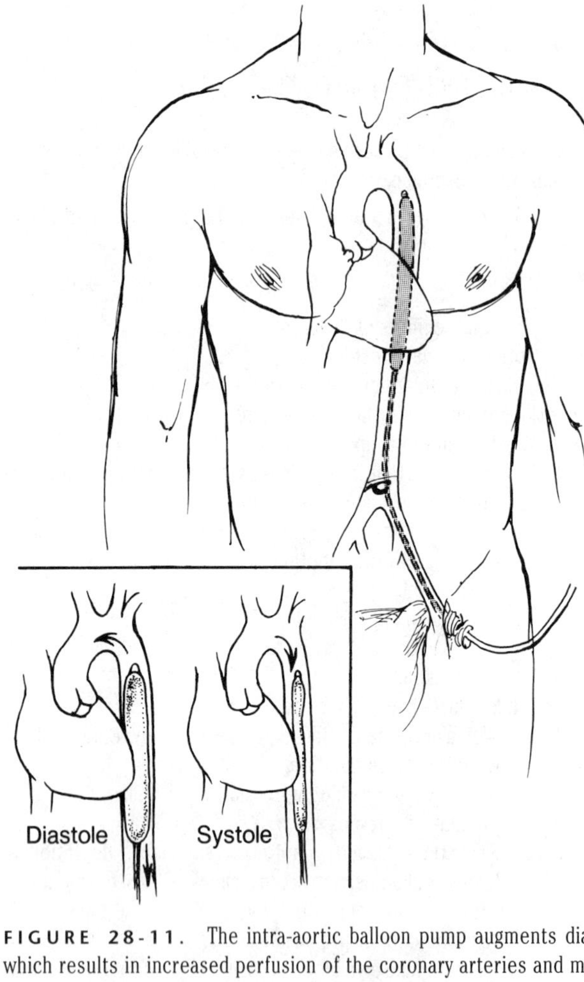

FIGURE 28-11. The intra-aortic balloon pump augments diastole, which results in increased perfusion of the coronary arteries and myocardium and a decrease in the left ventricular workload.

ETHICAL QUESTION:

When is it appropriate to consider withholding or withdrawing life support?

Situation

Life-support devices include intra-aortic balloon pumps, ventilators, vasoactive infusions, CPR, and antibiotics. Patients who receive these treatments include the acutely, chronically, and terminally ill. When dependent on life support, a patient may be unable to make decisions about his or her own care, and the patient's family may be too confused and upset to make choices for the patient. At what point is it appropriate to raise the delicate issue of withholding or withdrawing life support?

Dilemma

The patient's right to choose or refuse treatment conflicts with the obligation to do what is best for the patient (autonomy versus beneficence). The patient's right to choose or refuse treatment conflicts with the obligation not to harm the patient with threatening or inappropriate questions at the wrong time (autonomy versus non-maleficence).

Discussion

- What arguments would you offer to support the view that discussions about the limitations of life-supporting treatment should be held when patients are admitted to the hospital?
- What arguments would you offer to support the view that discussions about the limitations of life-supporting treatment should be done only when certain circumstances arise?

also essential to determine the patient's circulatory status during the use of the IABP.

The balloon inflates during ventricular diastole and deflates during systole at a rate equal to the heart rate. The IABP augments diastole, which results in increased perfusion of the coronary arteries and myocardium. IABP deflates during systole, which decrease left ventricular workload.

Nursing Implications

The patient with cardiogenic shock requires constant nursing care and observation. Carefully assessing the patient, measuring hemodynamic parameters, and recording fluid intake and urinary output are essential. The patient must be closely monitored for dysrhythmias, which must be corrected immediately.

Because of the technology required for effective medical management in such cases, the patient is always treated in a critical care environment. Critical care nurses with highly developed skills are responsible for the nursing management. Every nurse, however, needs to understand the concepts of treatment modalities. (For further details about shock, see Chapter 15.)

Thromboembolic Episodes

The decreased mobility of the patient with cardiac disease and the impaired circulation that accompany these disorders contribute to the development of intracardiac and intravascular thrombosis. As the patient increases activities after a period of immobility, a thrombus may become detached (the detached thrombus is called an **embolus**) and may be carried to the brain, kidneys, intestines, or lungs.

The most common embolic episode is that of a **pulmonary embolism.** The symptoms of pulmonary embolism include chest pain, cyanosis, shortness of breath, rapid respirations, and hemoptysis (bloody sputum). The pulmonary embolus may block the circulation to a part of the lung, producing an area of pulmonary infarction. The pain experienced is usually pleuritic—that is, it increases with respiration and may disappear when the patient holds his or her breath. Cardiac pain is continuous, however, and usually does not vary with respirations. The treatment of pulmonary embolism is discussed in Chapter 24.

Systemic embolism may occur from the left ventricle. The resulting vascular occlusion may present as stroke or renal infarction; it can also compromise the blood supply to an extremity.

The nurse must be aware of such possible complications and prepared to identify and report signs and symptoms.

Pericardial Effusion and Cardiac Tamponade

Pathophysiology

Pericardial effusion refers to the escape of fluid into the pericardial sac. This occurrence may accompany pericarditis, advanced congestive heart failure, or cardiac surgery.

Normally, the pericardial sac contains less than 50 ml of fluid. Pericardial fluid may accumulate slowly without causing noticeable symptoms. A *rapidly* developing effusion, however, can stretch the pericardium to its maximum size and can cause decreased cardiac output and decreased venous return to the heart. The result is **cardiac tamponade** (compression of the heart). The assessment findings in cardiac tamponade are depicted in Figure 28-12.

Clinical Manifestations

The patient may complain of a feeling of fullness within the chest or have substantial or ill-defined pain. The feeling of pressure in the chest is due to the stretching of the pericardial sac. Other signs include shortness of breath and a drop and fluctuation in blood pressure. Blood pressure is lowest on inspiration (**pulsus paradoxus**), at which point the pulse may not be perceptible. The venous pressure tends to rise, as evidenced by engorged neck veins.

The cardinal signs are falling arterial blood pressure, narrowing pulse pressure, rising venous pressure, and distant heart sounds.

- Pericardial tamponade is a life-threatening situation, demanding immediate intervention.

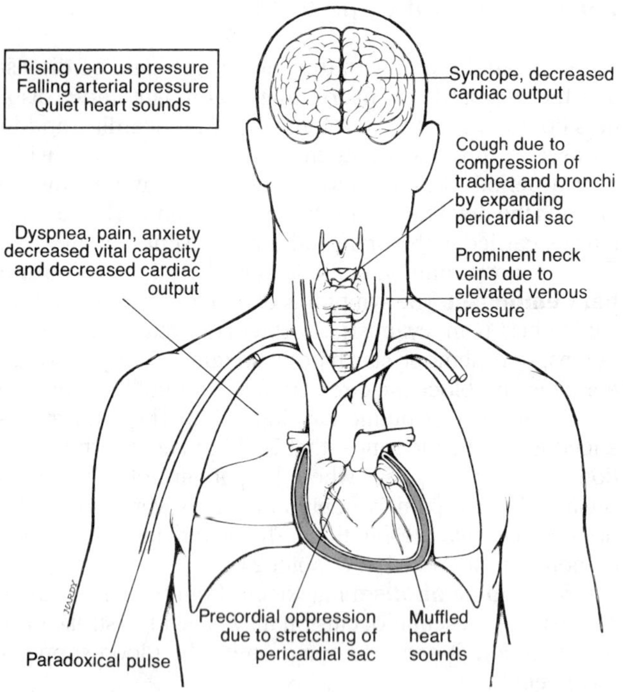

FIGURE 28-12. Assessment for cardiac tamponade due to pericardial effusion.

Diagnostic Evaluation

Pericardial effusion is detected by percussing the chest and noting an extension of flatness across the anterior aspect of the chest. If the clinical manifestations are not immediately life-threatening, the physician may prescribe an echocardiogram to confirm the diagnosis. The clinical signs and symptoms and chest x-ray are usually sufficient to diagnose pericardial effusion.

Management: Pericardial Aspiration (Pericardiocentesis)

If cardiac function becomes seriously impaired, a pericardial aspiration (puncture of the pericardial sac) is performed to remove fluid from the pericardial sac. The major goal is to prevent cardiac tamponade, which restricts normal heart action.

During the procedure the patient is monitored by ECG and hemodynamic pressure measurements. Emergency resuscitative equipment should be readily available. The head of the bed is elevated to a 45- to 60-degree angle, placing the heart in close proximity to the chest wall so that the needle can be inserted into the pericardial sac more easily. If a peripheral intravenous device is not already in place, one is inserted and a slow intravenous infusion is started in case it becomes necessary to administer emergency medications or blood products.

The pericardial aspiration needle is attached to a 50-ml syringe by a three-way stopcock. The V lead (precordial lead wire) of the ECG may be attached to the hub of the aspirating needle with alligator clips, because the ECG will help determine whether or not the needle has contacted the myocardium. Contact is evidenced by an elevation of the ST segment or stimulation of premature ventricular contractions.

Several possible sites are used for pericardial aspiration. The needle may be inserted in the angle between the left costal margin and the xiphoid, near the cardiac apex; at the fifth or sixth interspace at the left sternal margin; or on the right sternal margin of the fourth intercostal space. The needle is advanced slowly until fluid is obtained.

A fall in central venous pressure associated with a rise in blood pressure indicates that the cardiac tamponade has been relieved. The patient almost always feels immediate relief. If there is a substantial amount of pericardial fluid, a small catheter may be left in place to drain recurrent bleeding or effusion.

During the procedure, it is important to check the drainage for any bloody fluid. Pericardial blood does not clot readily, whereas blood obtained from inadvertent puncture of one of the heart chambers does clot.

Pericardial fluid is sent to the laboratory for examination for tumor cells, bacterial culture, chemical and serologic analysis, and differential cell count.

After pericardiocentesis, the patient's blood pressure, venous pressure, and heart sounds are monitored to detect any possible recurrence of cardiac tamponade. If it recurs, repeated aspiration is necessary. Cardiac tamponade may require treatment by open pericardial drainage. The patient is ideally in an intensive care unit.

Pericardiotomy

Recurrent pericardial effusions, usually associated with neoplastic diseases, may be treated by a pericardiotomy (pericardial window). General anesthesia is used, but cardiopulmonary bypass is seldom necessary. A portion of the pericardium is excised to permit the pericardial fluid to drain through the lymphatic system into the abdominal cavity. More rarely, catheters may be placed between the pericardium and abdominal cavity to drain the pericardial fluid. The nursing care is the same as that described for other cardiac surgery. (See Chapter 30.)

Myocardial Rupture

Myocardial rupture is a rare event. However, it can occur when a myocardial infarction, infectious process, pericardial disease, or other myocardial dysfunction weakens the cardiac muscle substantially. In most cases the result is immediate death.

Death is caused by cardiac tamponade (the heart is bleeding into its pericardial sac). Pericardiocentesis and repair of the myocardium can be life-saving measures.

Cardiac Arrest

Cardiac arrest occurs when the heart suddenly stops beating, resulting in the cessation of effective circulation. All heart action may stop, or asynchronized muscular twitchings (ventricular fibrillation) may occur.

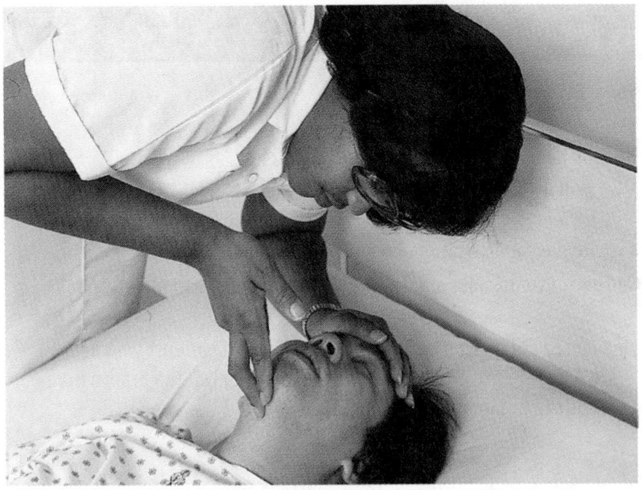

FIGURE 28-13. The chin lift or jaw-thrust maneuver is carried out in cardiopulmonary resuscitation to open the airway.

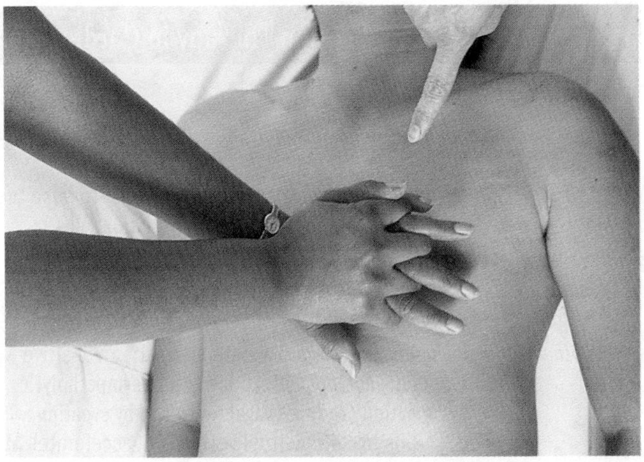

FIGURE 28-15. Positioning of the hands for cardiac compression in CPR. The heel of one hand is placed on the lower half of the sternum. The other hand is placed on top of the first hand.

There is an immediate loss of consciousness and an absence of pulses and audible heart sounds. The pupils of the eyes begin dilating within 45 seconds. Seizures may or may not occur.

There is an interval of approximately 4 minutes between the cessation of circulation and the development of irreversible brain damage. The interval varies with the age of the patient. During this period, the diagnosis of cardiac arrest must be made and the circulation must be restored.

- *The most reliable sign of arrest is the absence of a carotid pulsation.* Valuable time should not be wasted taking the blood pressure or listening for the heartbeat.

Cardiopulmonary Resuscitation

The ABCs of basic CPR consist of the following sequence: Airway, Breathing, and Circulation. The resuscitation process consists of (1) maintaining an open airway, (2) providing artificial ventilation by means of rescue breathing, and (3) providing artificial circulation by external cardiac compression.

Airway and Ventilation. The first step in CPR is to secure an airway. Remove any material from the mouth or throat and lift the jaw forward (Fig. 28-13). An oropharyngeal airway is inserted if available. Ventilate the patient with 12 breaths per minute using the bag and mask technique (Fig. 28-14).

Cardiac Compression. The next step after ventilation is external cardiac compression. This must be performed with the patient on a firm surface. Place the heel of one hand on the lower half of the sternum, 3.8 cm (1½ in) from the tip of the xiphoid, and toward the patient's head. Place the other hand on top of the first one (Fig. 28-15). Do not allow the fingers to touch the chest wall. Using the body weight while keeping the elbows straight, apply quick, forceful compressions to the lower sternum, 3.8 cm to 5 cm (1½ to 2 in) toward the spine (Fig. 28-16). Regular compression and release are made 60 times per minute.

Two-Person Technique. When two persons are available, the first person performs the cardiac compressions

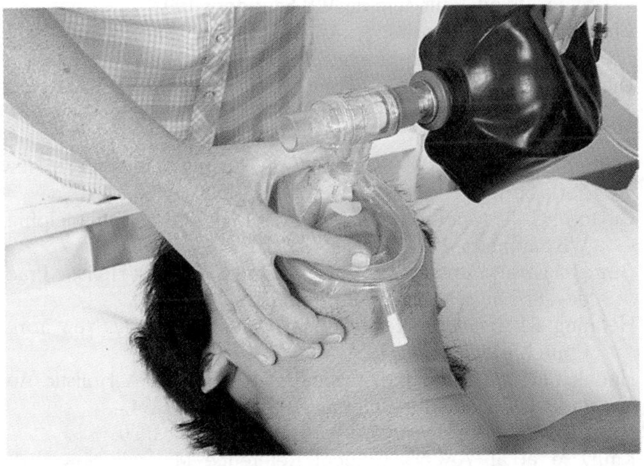

FIGURE 28-14. Bag-and-mask technique for ventilating patients needing cardiopulmonary resuscitation.

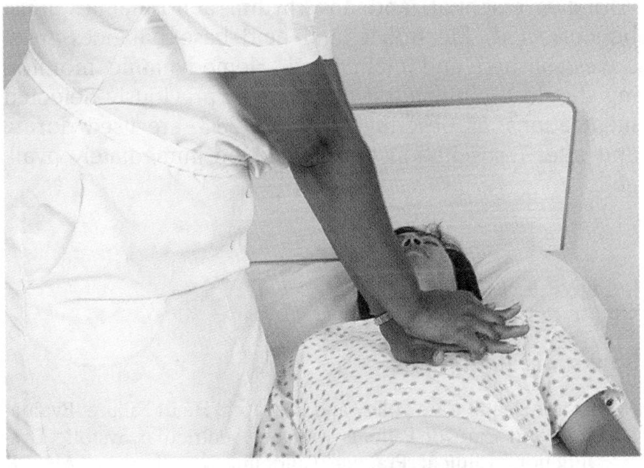

FIGURE 28-16. Elbows are kept straight and body weight is used to apply quick, forceful compressions to the lower sternum.

TABLE 28-3 Medication Therapy in Cardiopulmonary Resuscitation

Drug	Objective	Side Effects and Comments
Oxygen	To correct hypoxemia	No lung damage when used for less than 24 hr
Lidocaine	To suppress ventricular dysrhythmias. To raise the threshold for ventricular fibrillation (VF)	Myocardial and circulatory depression. CNS changes: drowsiness, disorientation, decreased hearing ability, paresthesias, muscle twitching, and agitation. Focal and grand mal seizures.
Procainamide hydrochloride	To suppress ventricular dysrhythmias when lidocaine is ineffective	Can cause ventricular asystole or fibrillation when administered IV.
Atropine	To accelerate cardiac rate by creating a positive chronotropic effect due to parasympatholytic action (reduces vagal tone) and by creating a positive dromotropic effect that accelerates AV conduction.	This increased heart rate may be deleterious in patients with acute MI. Atropine should be used with acute MI only if the bradycardia results in hemodynamic changes.
Epinephrine	To increase perfusion pressure during cardiac compressions To improve the myocardial contractile state To stimulate spontaneous contractions (*e.g.,* in asystole) To increase the vigor of VF	Epinephrine should not be added directly to a bicarbonate infusion, because catecholamines may be inactivated by alkaline solution.
Sodium bicarbonate ($NaHCO_3$)	To correct metabolic and respiratory acidosis	Because CO_2 production is increased, adequate ventilation is required. Excessive $NaHCO_3$ leads to metabolic alkalosis with displacement of oxyhemoglobin dissociation curve and consequent impairment of oxygen release to tissues. Hyperosmolality may also develop. Catecholamines and calcium salts should not be added to bicarbonate infusions because inactivation results. Because bicarbonate has a high *p*H, avoid mixing any drugs with it.

and the second ventilates the patient after five compressions. If only one person is available, the rate is two ventilations to every 15 cardiac compressions.

The decision to terminate resuscitation is based on medical considerations and will take into account the cerebral and cardiac status of the patient.

Follow-Up Monitoring. Once the patient is successfully resuscitated following cardiac arrest, the nurse should carefully monitor the situation because the patient is at great risk for another cardiac arrest. Continuous ECG monitoring is essential, and any rhythm abnormalities must be corrected. Electrolyte and acid–base balances must be established and maintained. Hemodynamic monitoring should be initiated if not done so previously. Selected medications, as described in Table 28-3, are used during and after resuscitation and should be immediately available.

REFERENCES AND SELECTED READINGS

Books and Pamphlets

Agency for Health Care Policy and Research. Heart Failure: Evaluation and Care of Patients with Left-Ventricular Systolic Dysfunction. Clinical Practice Guideline, Number 11, AHCPR Publication No. 94-0612. Public Health Service, U.S. Department of Health and Human Services, Rockville, MD, June 1994.

Agency for Health Care Policy and Research. Unstable Angina: Diagnosis and Management. Clinical Practice Guideline, Number 10, AHCPR Publication No. 94-0602. Public Health Service, U.S. Department of Health and Human Services, Rockville, MD, March 1994.

American Heart Association. Textbook of Advanced Cardiac Life Support. Dallas, AHA, 1990.

American Heart Association. Heart Facts. Dallas, AHA, 1991.

Bates B. A Guide to Physical Examination and History Taking. Philadelphia, JB Lippincott, 1995.

Braunwald E. Heart Disease: A Textbook of Cardiovascular Medicine, 4th ed. Philadelphia, WB Saunders, 1992.

Chatterjee K et al. Cardiology: An Illustrated Text Reference, vol. 1. Philadelphia, JB Lippincott, 1991.

Diethrich EB and Cohan C. Women and Heart Disease: What You Can Do to Stop the No. 1 Killer of American Women. New York, Times Books, 1994.

Fulmer TT and Walker MK. Critical Care Nursing of the Elderly. New York, Springer Publishing Company, 1992.

Guyton AC. Textbook of Medical Physiology, 8th ed. Philadelphia, WB Saunders, 1991.

Guzzetta CE and Dossey BM. Cardiovascular Nursing: Holistic Practice. St. Louis, Mosby-Year Book, 1992.

Henning RJ and Grenik A. Critical Care Cardiology. New York, Churchill-Livingston, 1991.

Hudak CM and Gallo BM. Critical Care Nursing: A Holistic Approach, 6th ed. Philadelphia, JB Lippincott, 1994.

Hurst JW (ed). The Heart. New York, McGraw-Hill, 1990.

Kinny M et al. AACN's Clinical Reference Manual. New York, McGraw-Hill, 1993.

Kinny M et al. Comprehensive Cardiac Care, 7th ed. St. Louis, CV Mosby, 1991.

CRITICAL THINKING EXERCISES

1. You are caring for a patient who was admitted to the hospital 6 hours earlier with angina pectoris. He complains of chest pain and states that he has received no relief from three nitroglycerin tablets. How would you determine what actions to take? How would your actions differ if this is a patient in a walk-in clinic?
2. A patient who had a myocardial infarction 2 days ago begins to complain of shortness of breath and coughing. Describe the assessment data you would gather in preparing to report this development.
3. Prior to administering a patient's daily maintenance dose of digitalis, you assess his heart rate and rhythm. His apical pulse rate is 122 beats/minute and the rhythm is irregular. Explain the rationale behind the actions you will take.
4. The wife of a patient who is preparing for discharge following a myocardial infarction approaches you and expresses concern about what to do if her husband suffers another heart attack. How might you instruct her in preparation for such an event? How would your instruction vary if the wife is in her 40s versus her late 60s or lives in a rural community versus a suburban development?

Seidel HM et al. Mosby's Guide to Physical Examination. St. Louis, Mosby-Year Book, 1991.
Woods SL et al. Cardiac Nursing. Philadelphia, JB Lippincott, 1995.

Journals

Asterisks indicate nursing research articles.

Altman LK. New recommendations on clot-busting drugs for heart victims. The New York Times, Feb 8 1994.
*Anderson KO and Masur FT. Psychologic preparation for cardiac catheterization. Heart Lung 1989 Mar; 18(2):154–163.
Aragon D and Martin M. What you should know about thrombolytic therapy for acute MI. Am J Nurs 1993 Sept; 93(9):24–31.
Bavin T and Self MA. Weaning from intra-aortic balloon pump support. Am J Nurs 1991 Oct; 91(10):54–59.
*Beach EK et al. The spouse: A factor in recovery after acute myocardial infarction. Am J Crit Care 1992 Jan; 21(1);30–38.
*Beattie S and Geden E. Reducing pain and discomfort following percutaneous transluminal coronary angioplasty. DCCN 1990 May–Jun; 9(3):150–155.
Bevans M and McLimore E. Intracoronary stents: A new approach to coronary dilation. J Cardiovasc Nurs 1992 Oct; 7(1):34–49.
Bubien RS et al. What you need to know about radiofrequency ablation. Am J Nurs 1993 July; 93(7):30–36.
Chyun D et al. Silent myocardial ischemia. Focus Crit Care 1991 Aug; 18(4):295–302.
Collings S. Coronary atherectomy takes a new direction. Am J Nurs 1991 Oct; 91(8):16.
Cupples SA. Effects of timing and reenforcement of preoperative education on knowledge and recovery of patients having coronary artery bypass graft surgery. Heart Lung 1991 Nov; 20(6):654–660.
Dailey EK. Clinical management of patients receiving thrombolytic therapy. Heart Lung 1991 Sept; 20(5):559–565.
DeAngelis R and Lessig ML. Hyperkalemia. Crit Care Nurs 1992 Mar; 12(3):55–59.
DeAngelis R and Lessig ML. Hypokalemia. Crit Care Nurs 1991 July; 11(7):71–75.
Dougherty KG et al. Laser ablation of coronary arteries: Preliminary findings. AORN Journal 1991 Aug; 54(2):244–261.
*Duryee R. The efficacy of inpatient education after myocardial infarction. Heart Lung 1992 May; 21(3):217–224.
Forman R and Aronow W. Pharmacologic therapy for acute MI in the elderly. Pharm Thera 1993 Nov; 18(11):1080–1090.
Friday BA. Magnesium metabolism: A case report and literature review. Crit Care Nurs 1991 May; 11(5):62–71.
*Funk M and Pooley-Richards RL. Predicting hospital mortality in patients with acute myocardial infarction. Am J Crit Care 1994 May; 3(3):168–176.
Gaw B. Motivation to change life-style following PTCA. DCCN 1992 Mar–Apr; 11(2):68–74.
Gawlinski A and Jensen G. The complications of cardiovascular aging. Am J Nurs 1991 Nov; 91(11):26–30.
Green E. Solving the puzzle of chest pain. Am J Nurs 1992 Jan; 92(1):32–37.
Hadley SA and Saarmann L. Lipid physiology and nutritional considerations in coronary heart disease. Crit Care Nurs 1991 Nov/Dec; 11(10):28–37.
Hanisch PJ. Identification and treatment of acute myocardial infarction by electrocardiographic site classification. Focus on Critical Care 1991 Dec; 18(6):480–488.
Hanson MJS. Modifiable risk factors for coronary heart disease in women. Am J Crit Care 1994 May; 3(3):177–186.
Heart disease: Women at risk. Consumer Reports 1993 May; 300–304.
Kater KM et al. Corralling atrial fibrillation with 'maze' surgery. Am J Nurs 1992 July; 92(7):34—38.
Kerner-Slemons S et al. Bypass-supported angioplasty: What your patient needs to know at discharge. Crit Care Nurs 1992 Feb; 12(2):55–57.
*King KB et al. Coronary artery bypass graft surgery in older women and men. Am J Crit Care 1992 Sept; 1(2):28–35.
Kronick-Mest C. Postpericardiotomy syndrome: Etiology, manifestations, and interventions. Heart Lung 1989 Mar; 18(2):92–98.
Levin R. Caring for the cardiac spouse. Am J Nurs 1993 Nov; 93(11): 51–53.
Lewandowski DM. Congestive heart failure. Am J Nurs 1995 May; 95(3):36.
McCauley K. Cognitive strategies for emotional distress after myocardial infarction. Medsurg Nurs Q 1992 Fall; 1(2):56–59.
McKenna M. Management of the patient undergoing myocardial revascularization: Percutaneous transluminal coronary angioplasty. Nurs Clin North Am 1992 Mar; 27(1):231–242.
McMillan JY and Little CD. Right ventricular infarction. Focus on Critical Care 1991 April; 18(2):158–163.
Messerli FH and McLoughlin M. Calcium channel antagonists: What do they offer? Pharm Thera 1993 Nov; 18(11):1051–1063.
Meyer C. New drugs in the cardiovascular arena. Am J Nurs 1993 June; 93(6):55–60.
*Miracle VA and Hovekamp G. Needs of families of patients undergoing invasive cardiac procedures. Am J Crit Care 1994 Mar; 3(2):155–157.
*Mooney J et al. Are coronary angioplasty and coronary bypass patients different in medical status and psychosocial perception at 2 year follow-up? Heart Lung 1992 May; 21(3):289.

New cholesterol guidelines released. Heart Memo. NIH Pub 1993 Fall.
Norton M et al. Right ventricular infarction vs. left ventricular infarction: Review of pathophysiology, medical treatment and nursing care. Medsurg Nurs 1993 June; 2(3):203–209.
*Nyamathi A et al. Coping and adjustment of spouses of critically ill patients with cardiac disease. Heart Lung 1992 Mar; 21(2): 160–166.
Palarski V and Washburn S. Overcoming LVD in cardiac rehab. AJN 1992 Sept; 92(9):52–57.
Porterfield M and Porterfield JG. Digitalis toxicity: A common occurrence. Crit Care Nurs 1993 Dec; 13(6):40–43.
Proulx R et al. Detection of right ventricular myocardial infarction in patients with inferior wall myocardial infarction. Crit Care Nurs 1992 June; 12(6):50–59.
Rappaport E. Overview: Rationale of thrombolysis in treating acute myocardial infarction. Heart Lung 1991 Sept; 20(5):538–541.
*Robertson D and Keller C. Relationships among health beliefs, self-efficacy and exercise adherence in patients with coronary artery disease. Heart Lung 1992 Jan; 21(1):56–63.
Saver CL. Decoding the ACLS algorithms. Am J Nurs 1994 Jan; 94(1):27–36.
Scrima D. Managing dobutamine infusions. Medsurg Nurs 1993 Dec; 2(6):459–465.
Shinn JA. Management of a patient undergoing myocardial revascularization: Coronary artery bypass graft surgery. Nurs Clin North Am 1992 Mar; 27(1):243–256.
Smith A and Fitzpatrick E. Penetrating cardiac trauma: Surgical and nursing management. J Cardiovasc Nurs 1993 Jan; 7(2): 52–70.
Smith DF and Bumann R. Assessing and treating decreased cardiac output. Medsurg Nurs 1993 Oct; 2(5):351–357.
Sommers MS. Potential for injury: Trauma after cardiopulmonary resuscitation. Heart Lung 1991 May; 20(3):287–293.
Sommers MS. Preventing complications of CPR. Medsurg Nurs Q 1992 Summer; 1(1):45–54.
Strimike CL. Caring for a patient with an intracoronary stent. Am J Nurs 1995 Jan; 95(1):40–46.
Summary of the second report of the national cholesterol education program (NCEP) expert panel on detection, evaluation and treatment of high blood cholesterol in adults (adult treatment panel II). JAMA 1993 June; 269(23):3015–3023.
Teplitz L. Surgical treatment of ventricular arrhythmias: Historical and current perspectives. Crit Care Nurs Q 1991 Aug; 14(2): 41–59.
Tess MM. Acute confusional states in critically ill patients: A review. J Neuroscience Nurs 1991 Dec; 23(6):398–402.
Trotter DJ and Kochar MS. Hypertension and high cholesterol: A dangerous synergy. Am J Nurs 1992 Nov; 92(11):40–43.
Veseth-Rogers J. A practical approach to teaching the automatic cardioverter-defibrillator patient. J Cardiovasc Nurs 1990 Feb; 4(2):7–19.
Wingate S. Women and coronary heart disease: Implications for the critical care setting. Focus on Critical Care 1991 June; 18(3): 212–218.
Wirebaugh SR. Long-term compliance with lipid-lowering therapy. Pharm Thera 1993 June; 18(6):559–571.
Women and heart disease. Helix 1993 Spring:31–33.

INFORMATION/RESOURCES

Government Agencies

National Heart, Lung, and Blood Institute
National Institutes of Health
Building 31, Room 5A52
Bethesda, MD 20892

Independent Agencies

American Heart Association
7320 Greenville Ave.
Dallas, TX 75231

Coronary Club
9500 Euclid Ave.
Cleveland, OH 44106

Heartlife
PO Box 54305
Atlanta, GA 30308

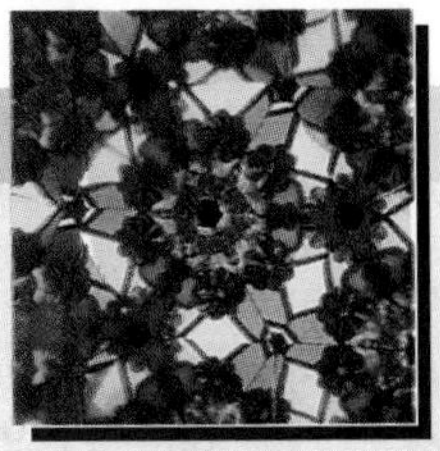

29

Management of Patients With Structural, Infectious, or Inflammatory Cardiac Disorders

CHAPTER OUTLINE

Acquired Valvular Disorders of the Heart
Types of Valvular Problems
Valve Repair and Replacement
Septal Repair
Cardiomyopathies
NURSING PROCESS: The Patient With a Cardiomyopathy
Infectious Diseases of the Heart
Rheumatic Endocarditis
Infective Endocarditis
Myocarditis
Pericarditis
NURSING PROCESS: The Patient With Pericarditis
Critical Thinking Exercises

LEARNING OBJECTIVES

On completion of this chapter, the learner will be able to:

1. Define the various types of valvular disorders of the heart and describe the pathophysiology, clinical manifestations and management of each one
2. Describe the types of valve repair and replacement procedures that are done to correct valvular problems and the type of care needed by patients who undergo these corrective procedures
3. Distinguish between congestive, hypertrophic, and restrictive cardiomyopathies and describe the patient problems that accompany these disorders and the corresponding care needed
4. Compare the infectious diseases of the heart, identifying their causes, pathologic changes, clinical manifestations, management, and prevention
5. Describe the significance of prophylactic antibiotic therapy for patients with rheumatic endocarditis, infective endocarditis, myocarditis, mitral prolapse, and mitral stenosis
6. Describe the collaborative management of patients with pericarditis

Acquired Valvular Disorders of the Heart

The valves of the heart control the flow of blood through the heart and into the pulmonary artery and aorta by opening and closing at appropriate times as the heart contracts and relaxes through the cardiac cycle.

The atrioventricular valves separate the atria from the ventricles and include the **tricuspid valve**, which separates the right atrium from the right ventricle, and the **mitral or bicuspid valve**, which separates the left atrium from the left ventricle.

The semilumar valves are located between the ventricles and their corresponding arteries. The **pulmonic valve** lies between the right ventricle and the pulmonary artery, whereas the **aortic valve** lies between the left ventricle and the aorta. Figure 29-1 shows the shapes of these various valves in the closed position.

When any of the heart valves do not open or close properly, blood flow is affected. When valves to not open completely (usually because of stenosis), the result is reduced blood flow through the valve. When valves do not close completely, blood leaks back through the valve in a process termed *regurgitation* or *insufficiency*.

Disorders of the mitral valve fall into the following categories: mitral valve prolapse, mitral stenosis, and mitral insufficiency or regurgitation. Disorders of the aortic valve are categorized as aortic stenosis and aortic insufficiency or regurgitation. These different valvular disorders lead to a variety of symptoms, depending on their severity, and may require surgical repair or replacement to correct the problem.

Types of Valvular Problems

Mitral Valve Prolapse Syndrome

Pathophysiology. The mitral valve prolapse syndrome is a dysfunction of the mitral valve leaflets that may prevent the mitral valve from closing completely and result in valvular regurgitation in which blood from the left ventricle seeps back into the left atrium. This syndrome may produce no symptoms or it may progress rapidly and result in sudden death. In recent years the syndrome has been diagnosed more frequently, ostensibly as a result of improved diagnostic methods.

Clinical Manifestations. Many individuals have the syndrome but no symptoms. Often the symptoms are first identified during a physical examination of the heart, which discloses an extra heart sound referred to as a **mitral click.** The presence of a click is an early sign that the valve tissue is bulging into the left atrium and that blood flow is being disrupted. The mitral click may deteriorate into a murmur over time as the valve leaflets become progressively dysfunctional. Concomitant with the progression of the murmur may be signs and symptoms of heart failure as mitral regurgitation (back flow of blood) ensues. Mitral valve prolapse occurs more frequently in women than in men.

Management. Medical management is directed at controlling the associated symptoms. Some persons experience worrisome dysrhythmias and require antidysrhythmic agents. Others experience mild heart failure and require therapy (see Chap. 28 for a discussion of heart failure). In advanced stages, mitral valve replacement may be necessary.

It is important to educate patients with this syndrome about the need for prophylactic antibiotic therapy before undergoing invasive procedures (*e.g.*, dental work, genitourinary or gastrointestinal procedures, intravenous [IV] therapy) that may introduce infectious agents systemically. If in doubt about risk factors and the need for antibiotics, patients are advised to consult their physician.

Mitral Stenosis

Pathophysiology. Mitral stenosis is the progressive thickening and contracting of the mitral valve cusps, which causes narrowing of the orifice and progressive obstruction to blood flow.

Normally, the mitral valve opening is as wide as three fingers. In cases of marked stenosis, the opening narrows to the width of a lead pencil. The left ventricle is not affected, but the left atrium has great difficulty in emptying blood through the narrow orifice into the ventricle. Therefore, it dilates and hypertrophies. Because no valve protects the pulmonary veins from a backward flow from this atrium, pulmonary circulation becomes markedly congested. As a result the right ventricle must maintain an abnormally high pulmonary arterial pressure and is thus subjected to excessive strain. Eventually it fails.

Clinical Manifestations. Patients with mitral stenosis are likely to show progressive fatigue as a result of low cardiac output, may expectorate blood (hemoptysis), and experience breathing difficulty (dyspnea) on exertion owing to pulmonary venous hypertension, cough, and repeated respiratory infections.

FIGURE 29-1. The valves of the heart (aortic or semilunar, tricuspid, and mitral) shown in closed position.

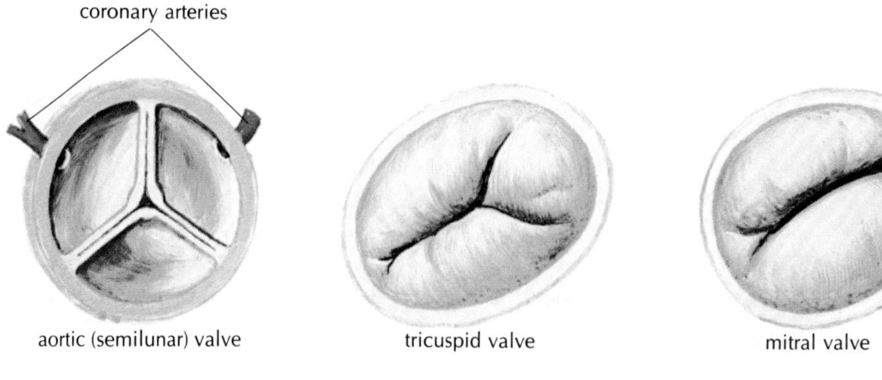

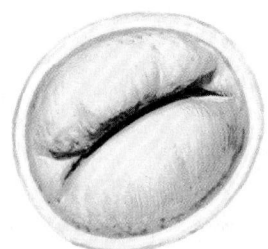

The pulse is weak and often irregular because of atrial fibrillation caused by the atrium's dilation and hypertrophy. As a result of these changes, the atrium becomes electrically unstable, resulting in a permanent atrial dysrhythmia. Diagnostic aids for the cardiologist are electrocardiography, echocardiography, and cardiac catheterization with angiography to verify the severity of the mitral stenosis.

Management. Antibiotic therapy is instituted to prevent recurrence of infections. Congestive heart failure is treated with cardiotonics and diuretics. Surgical intervention consists of a commissurotomy to open or "rupture" the fused commissures of the mitral valve or replacement of the mitral valve with a prosthetic valve. In some cases where surgery is contraindicated and medical therapy is not producing the desired results, percutaneous transluminal valvuloplasty may offer some relief of symptoms.

Mitral Insufficiency (Regurgitation)

Pathophysiology. Mitral insufficiency results when the margins of the mitral valve are unable to close during systole. The chordae tendinae may become shortened, preventing complete closure of the leaflets, resulting in mitral regurgitation or back flow of blood from the left ventricle into the left atrium.

Shortening or tearing of one or both of the mitral valve leaflets prevents the perfect closure of the mitral orifice while the powerful left ventricle is forcing the blood into the aorta. At each beat the left ventricle forces some of the blood back into the left atrium. Because this blood is added to the blood that is beginning to flow into this chamber from the lungs, the left atrium must dilate and hypertrophy. This backward flow of blood from the ventricle diminishes the volume of blood flowing from the lungs. As a result, the lungs become congested, which adds an extra strain on the right ventricle. Therefore, the result of even a slight mitral leak always involves both lungs and the right ventricle.

Clinical Manifestations. Palpitation of the heart, shortness of breath on exertion, and cough due to chronic passive pulmonary congestion are common symptoms. The pulse may be regular and of good volume, but frequently it becomes irregular as a result of either extrasystoles or atrial fibrillation, which may persist indefinitely.

Management. Management is the same as that for congestive heart failure. Surgical intervention consists of mitral valve replacement.

Aortic Valve Stenosis

Pathophysiology. Aortic valve stenosis is the narrowing of the orifice between the left ventricle and the aorta. In adults the stenosis may be congenital, or it may be a result of rheumatic endocarditis or cusp calcification of unknown cause. There is progressive narrowing of the valve orifice over a period of several years to several decades.

The leaflets of the aortic valve fuse and partially close the opening between the heart and the aorta. The left ventricle overcomes this obstruction to circulation by contracting more slowly but with greater energy than normal, forcibly squeezing the blood through the very small orifice. The heart's compensatory mechanisms begin to fail and clinical signs develop.

The obstruction to the aortic outflow tract places a pressure load on the left ventricle, which results in a thickening of the muscle wall. The heart muscle increases in size (hypertrophy) in response to all degrees of obstruction; cardiac failure occurs when obstruction is severe.

Clinical Manifestations. In moderate to severe cases of aortic stenosis, the patient first experiences exertional dyspnea, which is a manifestation of left ventricular decompensation with pulmonary congestion. Other signs are dizziness and fainting because of reduced volume of blood going to the brain. Angina pectoris is a frequent symptom that results from the increased oxygen demands imposed by the increased work of the left ventricle and by myocardial hypertrophy. Blood pressure can be low but is usually normal; often there is a low pulse pressure (30 mm Hg or less) because of diminished blood flow.

On physical examination, a loud, rough systolic murmur may be heard over the aortic area. The sound to listen for is a systolic crescendo–decrescendo murmur, which may radiate into the carotid arteries and to the apex of the left ventricle. The murmur is low-pitched, rough, rasping, and vibrating. If one rests a hand over the base of the heart, a vibration is felt that is the most intense of all cardiac thrills and resembles the purring of a cat. The purring is related to the turbulence caused by the blood flow across a narrowed valve orifice. The evidence of left ventricular hypertrophy may be seen on a 12-lead electrocardiogram (ECG) and echocardiogram.

Left-heart catheterization is necessary to measure accurately the severity of this valvular abnormality. Pressure tracings are taken from the left ventricle and the base of the aorta. The systolic pressure in the left ventricle is considerably higher than that in the aorta during systole.

Management. Definitive treatment for aortic stenosis is surgical replacement of the aortic valve. A significant risk of sudden death exists for those patients who are treated medically without surgical repair. The uncorrected condition can lead to irreversible heart failure that is nonresponsive to medical therapies.

Aortic Insufficiency (Regurgitation)

Pathophysiology. Aortic insufficiency is caused by inflammatory lesions that deform the flaps of the aortic valve, preventing them from completely sealing the aortic orifice during diastole and thus allowing a backflow of blood from the aorta into the left ventricle. This valvular defect may result from endocarditis, congenital abnormalities, or diseases such as syphilis and a dissecting aneurysm that cause dilation or tearing of the ascending aorta.

Because of the leak in the aortic valve during diastole, some of the blood in the aorta, which is always under high pressure, flows into the left ventricle, which must handle both the blood normally delivered by the left atrium into the ventricle through the mitral orifice and that returning from the aorta. The left ventricle dilates to accommodate this increased volume, hypertrophies to expel it, and does so with more than normal force, thus raising systolic blood pressure. The cardiovascular system attempts to compensate through reflex vasodilation; the peripheral arterioles become relaxed, so peripheral resistance is reduced and diastolic pressure greatly lowered.

Clinical Manifestations. Aortic insufficiency develops insidiously, and the earliest manifestation is the patient's awareness of the increased force of the heartbeat. There may be marked arterial pulsations that are visible or palpable over the precordium. Arterial pulsation in the neck also will be marked. This is a result of the increased force and volume of the blood ejected from the hypertrophied left ventricle. Exertional dyspnea and easy fatigability follow. Signs and symptoms of left ventricular failure include breathing difficulties, especially at night (orthopnea, paroxysmal nocturnal dyspnea) and they occur with moderate to severe regurgitation.

The pulse pressure (the difference between systolic and diastolic pressures) is considerably widened in these patients. One of the characteristic signs of the disease is the manner in which the pulse strikes the palpating finger with quick, sharp strokes and then suddenly collapses (**water-hammer pulse**). The nature of the pulse wave is quite unmistakable, because it rises rapidly to a peak and collapses quickly.

Diagnosis is made through ECG, echocardiogram, and cardiac catheterization.

Management. Aortic valve replacement is the treatment of choice, but the optimal time for valve replacement remains controversial. Surgery is recommended for any patient with left ventricular hypertrophy regardless of the presence or absence of other symptoms. If the patient has symptoms of congestive heart failure, medical management is required until surgery can be performed. (Management of the patient undergoing cardiac surgery is discussed in Chap. 30.)

Valve Repair and Replacement

Valvuloplasty

The repair, rather than replacement, of a cardiac valve is referred to as **valvuloplasty.** The type of valvuloplasty depends on the cause and type of valve dysfunction. Repair may be to the commissures between the leaflets (commissurotomy), to the annulus of the valve (annuloplasty), or to the leaflets and the chordae (chordoplasty).

Most valvuloplasty procedures require general anesthesia and most also require cardiopulmonary bypass. Some procedures, however, can be performed in the cardiac catheterization laboratory; these procedures do not always require general anesthesia or cardiopulmonary bypass. A newly developed percutaneous, partial cardiopulmonary bypass technique is now used in some cardiac catheterization laboratories.

The patient is managed in a critical care unit for the first 24 to 72 hours postoperatively. Care focuses on hemodynamic stabilization and recovery from anesthesia. Most patients are then transferred to a telemetry or surgical unit for continued postsurgical care and teaching. Patients are discharged from the hospital in 2 to 10 days. In general, valves that have undergone valvuloplasty function longer than replacement valves and the patients do not require continuous anticoagulation. An example of a critical or clinical pathway for a patient who has undergone a valve procedure is presented on p. 684.

Commissurotomy. The most common valvuloplasty procedure is the commissurotomy. Each valve has leaflets; the site where the leaflets meet each other is the commissure. The leaflets may adhere to one another and close the commissure—**stenosis.** Less commonly the leaflets fuse in such a way that there is not only a stenosis, but the leaflets are also prevented from closing completely, resulting in a backward flow of blood—**regurgitation.** A commissurotomy is the procedure performed to separate the fused leaflets.

Closed commissurotomies do not require cardiopulmonary bypass. The patient is placed under general anesthesia, a midsternal incision is made, a small hole is cut into the heart, and the surgeon's finger or a dilator is used to break open the commissure. The valve is not directly visualized. This type of commissurotomy has been performed for mitral, aortic, tricuspid, and pulmonary valve disease.

Balloon valvuloplasty (Fig. 29-2) is another procedure that has been beneficial for mitral valve stenosis in younger patients, as well as aortic valve stenosis in elderly patients and individuals with complex medical conditions that place them at high risk for the complications of more extensive surgical procedures. Most commonly used for mitral and aortic valve stenosis, balloon valvuloplasty also has been used for tricuspid and pulmonic valve stenosis. The procedure is performed in the cardiac catheterization laboratory and may be performed with local anesthesia. Patients remain in the hospital 24 to 48 hours after the procedure.

The **mitral procedure** involves passing one or two catheters into the right atrium, through the atrial septum

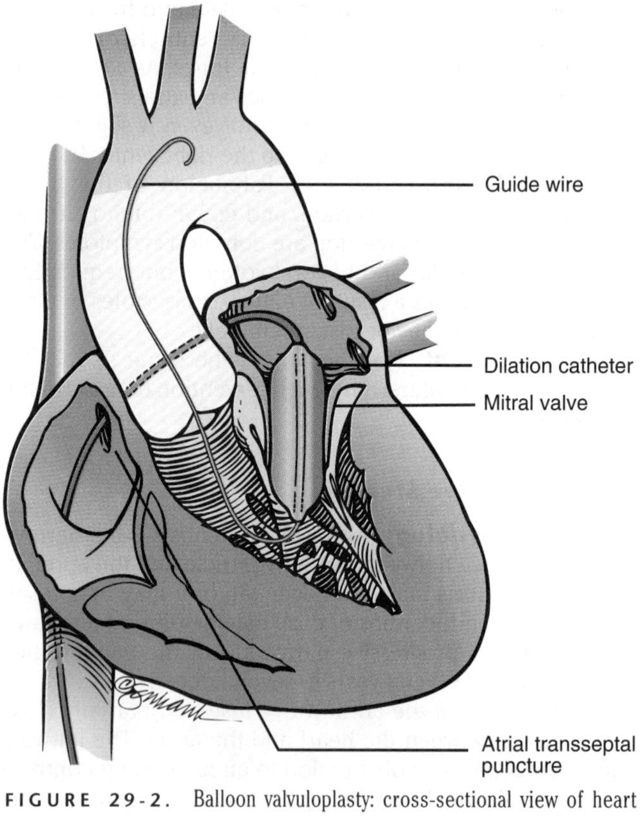

FIGURE 29-2. Balloon valvuloplasty: cross-sectional view of heart illustrating guide wire and dilatation catheter placed through an atrial transseptal puncture and across the mitral valve. The guide wire is extended out from the aortic valve into the aorta for catheter support.

into the left atrium, across the mitral valve into the left ventricle, and out into the aorta. A guidewire is placed through each catheter and the original catheter is removed. A large balloon catheter is then placed over the guidewire and positioned with the balloon across the mitral valve. The balloon is then inflated with a dilute liquid angiographic solution. When two balloons are used, they are inflated simultaneously. The advantage of two balloons is that they are each smaller than the one large balloon often used, making smaller atrial septal defects. Also, as the balloons are inflated they usually do not completely occlude the mitral valve, thus permitting some forward flow of blood during the inflation period. All patients will experience some degree of mitral regurgitation after the procedure.

Other possible complications include bleeding from the catheter insertion sites, emboli resulting in complications such as strokes, and, rarely, left-to-right atrial shunts through an atrial septal defect caused by the procedure.

The **aortic procedure** also may be performed by passing the balloon or balloons through the atrial septum, but it is performed more commonly by introducing a catheter through the aorta, across the aortic valve, and into the left ventricle. Either the one-balloon or the two-balloon technique can be used for aortic stenosis. Unfortunately the procedure is not as effective as with the mitral valve, and the rate of restenosis is nearly 50% in the first 12 to 15 months after the procedure.

Possible complications include aortic regurgitation, emboli, ventricular perforation, rupture of the aortic valve annulus, ventricular dysrhythmias, mitral valve damage, and bleeding from the catheter insertion sites.

Open commissurotomies are performed with direct visualization of the valve. The patient is under general anesthesia and a median sternotomy or left thoracic incision is made. The patient is placed on cardiopulmonary bypass, and an incision is made into the heart. A finger, scalpel, balloon, or dilator may be used to open the commissures. The added advantage of direct visualization of the valve is that thrombus may be noted and removed, calcifications seen, and if the valve has chordae or papillary muscles they also may be surgically repaired (see chordoplasty section of this chapter, page 684).

The patient is admitted to a critical care unit after surgery. The care focuses on the patient's recovery from anesthesia and on maintaining hemodynamic stability. The patient is usually transferred to a telemetry or surgical unit in 24 to 48 hours. Wound care and patient teaching regarding diet, activity, medications, and self-care continue until discharge from the hospital about 7 to 10 days after surgery.

Annuloplasty. An **annuloplasty** is the repair of the valve annulus (the junction of the valve leaflets and the muscular heart wall). General anesthesia and cardiopulmonary bypass are required for all annuloplasties. The procedure narrows the diameter of the valve's orifice and is useful for the treatment of regurgitation.

There are two different annuloplasty techniques. One technique is to use an annuloplasty ring (Fig. 29-3). The leaflets of the valve are sutured to a ring, creating an annulus of the desired size. When the ring is in place, the tension created by the moving blood and the contracting heart is borne by the ring rather than by the valve or a suture line. Thus, progressive regurgitation is prevented by the repair. The other technique involves tacking the valve leaflets to the atrium with sutures or taking "tucks" to tighten the annulus. The valve's leaflets and the suture lines are subjected to the direct forces of the blood and heart muscle movement, so the repair may degenerate more quickly than with the annuloplasty ring technique.

Leaflet Repair. Cardiac valve leaflets may be damaged by being stretched out of shape, being shortened, or developing holes. The repair for elongated, ballooning, or other excess tissue leaflets is to remove the extra tissue. The

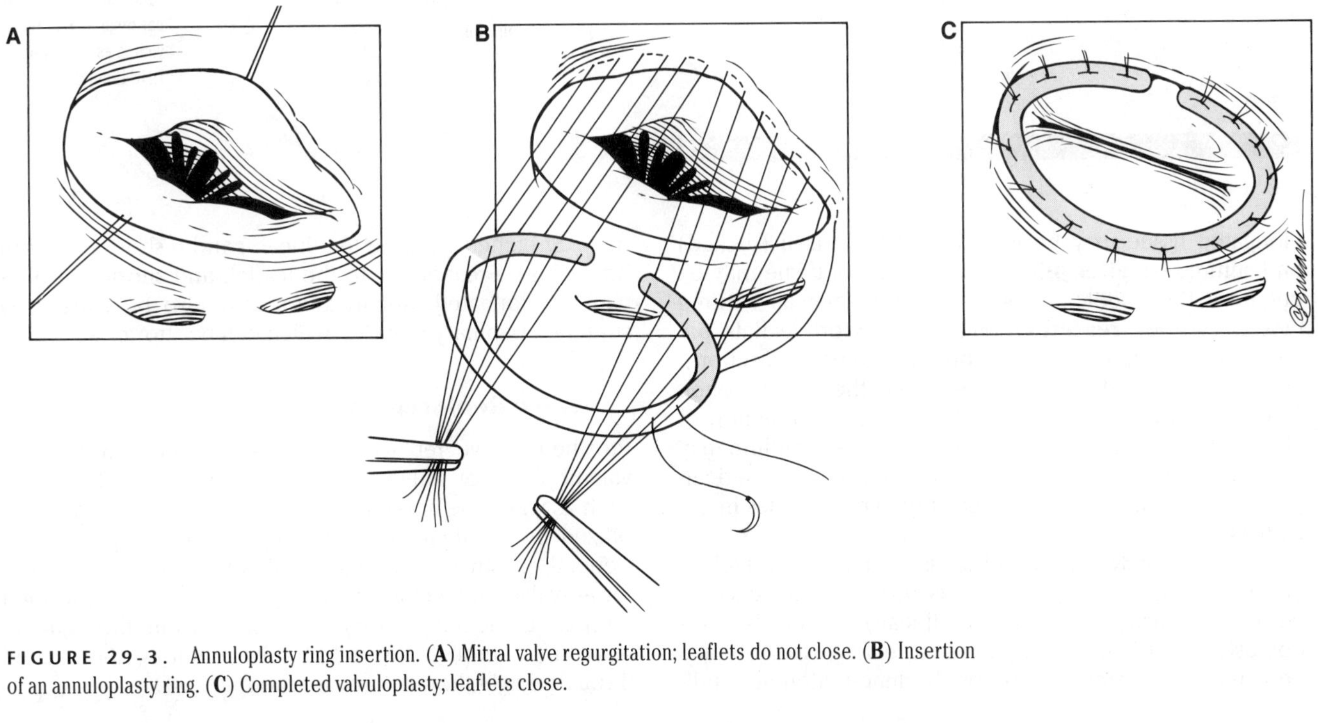

FIGURE 29-3. Annuloplasty ring insertion. (**A**) Mitral valve regurgitation; leaflets do not close. (**B**) Insertion of an annuloplasty ring. (**C**) Completed valvuloplasty; leaflets close.

CRITICAL PATHWAY
Cardiac Valve Procedure

Hahnemann University Hospital
Broad and Vine Streets
Philadelphia, PA

Discharge date: ______
Smoker: Y N Redo: Y N
Diabetic: Y N MI: Y N

LVEF > 50: Y N COPD: Y N
LVEF 36–49: Y N Emer: Y N
LVEF < 35: Y N PULM HTN: Y N

Day	1	2	3
POD #	OR	1	2
Locations	8CTICU	8CTICU	17ICTU
Tests	EKG, CBC, H + H q6⁰ × 24⁰, K^+ q4 × 24⁰, PT, PTT, Platelets, ABG with each vent change, SMA-7, Enzymes q8⁰ × 3, CxR, MVB, Glucose q6⁰	EKG, CBC, SMA-7, ABG, H + H, CXR, PT, PTT, platelets	EKG, CBC, CXR, SMA-7, SaO_2, PT/PTT
Procedures/ Treatments	VS q 15 min × 4 till stable then q1⁰, Hemodynamic Monitoring q1⁰, CO/CI q 1⁰ till stable then q 2⁰, milk CT q 15 min × 4 then q1⁰, ETT suction PRN, NGT irrigation q2⁰, Vent changes, Urine output q1⁰, wean FIO_2, T piece, Extubate, A&V wires to pacer settings.	T-piece, Extubate, Nebs q4⁰, Face mask, CPT QID, dsg. Change d/c Cordis, A-line & foley; Incentive spirometry, TED stockings, Insert Heplock	Nasal Cannula, d/c dsgs, d/c CT's, CPT + Nebs q4⁰, IS, Daily weight
Medications	IV antibiotics, IV medications/infusions, KCL replacement, Sedation, Volume Replacement, Tagamet	IV antibiotics until last dose, Start P.O. meds, pain meds, wean IV meds	PO meds, IV antibiotics, 5 mg coumadin
Activity	Bedrest, Turn patient PRN Dangle side of bed (if extubated)	OOB-Chair × 1 Consult Cardiac Rehab	OOB-Chair TID Start Cardiac Rehab.
Dietary	NPO	Clear liquids	Cardiac Prudent
Outcomes	Patient will: 1. View pre-op video 2. Receive patient pathway	Patient will be extubated	Patient will: 1. Do IS, C&DB q1⁰ 2. Begin to ambulate
Dschrg/ Planning Teaching	Orient patient and family to CT-ICU and explain all procedures.	Cough & deep breathing Incentive spirometer, incision splinting	Reinforce pulmonary toilet and fluid modification. Social Services visit & assessment/ HHC if needed

elongated tissue may be folded over onto itself (tucked) and sutured—**leaflet plication.** A wedge of tissue may be cut from the middle of the leaflet and the gap sutured closed—**leaflet resection** (Fig. 29-4). Short leaflets are most often repaired by chordoplasty (see next section). Once the short chordae are released, the leaflets often "unfurl" and are able to resume their normal function of closing the valve during systole. A piece of pericardium may also be sutured to the leaflet. Most commonly the pericardial patch is used when it is necessary to repair holes in the leaflets.

Chordoplasty. Chordoplasty is the repair of the chordae tendineae. The mitral valve is involved with chordoplasty (as it has the chordae tendineae); seldom is chordoplasty required for the tricuspid valve. Regurgitation may be caused by stretched, torn, or shortened chordae tendineae. Stretched chordae tendineae can be shortened; torn ones can be reattached to the leaflet; and shortened ones can be elongated. Regurgitation may also be caused by stretched papillary muscles, which can be shortened.

Valve Replacement

Prosthetic valve replacement began in the 1960s. When valvuloplasty or valve repair is not a viable alternative, such as when the annulus or leaflets of the valve are immobilized by calcifications, valve replacement is performed. General anesthesia and cardiopulmonary bypass are used for all valve replacements. Most procedures are performed through a median sternotomy (an incision through the sternum), although the mitral valve often is approached through a right thoracotomy incision.

CRITICAL PATHWAY
Cardiac Valve Procedure

DRG: 105 Cardiac Valve Procedure w/o Cath
MLOS: 6
Clinical Path Los: 7

Surgeon: ________
Date of Surgery: ____
Addressograph

4	5	6	7
3	4	5	6
17ICTU	**17ICTU**	**17ICTU**	**17ICTU Discharge**
SMA-7, SaO_2, CBC, PT/PTT, CXR	PT/PTT M-W-F: SMA-7, CBC	PT/PTT	PT/PTT
Nebs-if still needed (reevaluate) O_2prn, wound care, IS, Daily weight	Nebs-re-evaluate q4⁰, O_2 prn, wound care, IS Daily weight DC wires (PT</=18)	O_2 prn, wound care, IS. Daily weight ECHO	Wound care Daily weight IS
PO meds 5mg coumadin	PO meds 5mg coumadin	PO meds coumadin	PO meds coumadin
Cardiac Rehab OOB-TID	Ambulate TID Cardiac Rehab	Ambulate QID	Ambulate PRN
Cardiac Prudent	Dietary teaching class Pt & significant other prior to d/c	Teaching	Teaching
Patient will ambulate with assistance in hallway	Patient will: 1. Perform ADLs with minimal assistance; 2. Ambulate with supervision	Patient will progress to fitness center/stair climbing	Patient will: 1. ID critical S&S to report to MD 2. State date/time of f/u visit
Coumadin teaching, Medications, advise pt. & significant others of dietary + rehab classes, wound care, video library, Social Service visit and assessment/HHC if needed.	Advise of possible day of d/c, instruct pt's family to bring in clothes for d/c., d/c teaching re: wound care, meds, and activity	Reinforce previous teaching	Reinforce previous teaching PT level f/u with cardiologist/pcp & HHC

Once the valve is visualized, the leaflets and other valve structures such as chordae and papillary muscles are removed. (There is some evidence to suggest that the posterior mitral valve leaflet, its chordae, and papillary muscles should be left in place to maintain the shape and function of the left ventricle.) Sutures are placed around the annulus and then into the valve prosthesis. The replacement valve is slid down the suture into position and tied into place (Fig. 29-5). The incision is closed and the surgeon evaluates the function of the heart and the quality of the prosthetic repair. The patient is weaned from cardiopulmonary bypass and surgery is completed. Complications unique to valve replacement are related to the sudden changes in intracardiac blood pressures; before surgery the heart gradually adjusted to the pathology, but the surgery abruptly "corrects" the way blood flows through the heart.

Types of Valve Prostheses. Four types of valve prostheses may be used—mechanical valves, xenografts, homografts, and autographs. (Figure 29-6 shows mechanical and xenograft valves.)

The **mechanical valves** are of the ball and cage or disc design. Mechanical valves are thought to be more durable than the other types of prosthetic valves and often are used for younger patients. Thromboemboli are significant complications associated with mechanical valves, so long-term anticoagulation with warfarin is required.

Xenografts are tissue valves (bioprostheses, heterografts); most are from pigs (porcine) but valves from cows (bovine) may also be used. Their viability is 7 to 10 years. They do not generate thrombi thus eliminating the need for long-term anticoagulation. They are used for women of child-bearing age because the potential complications of long-

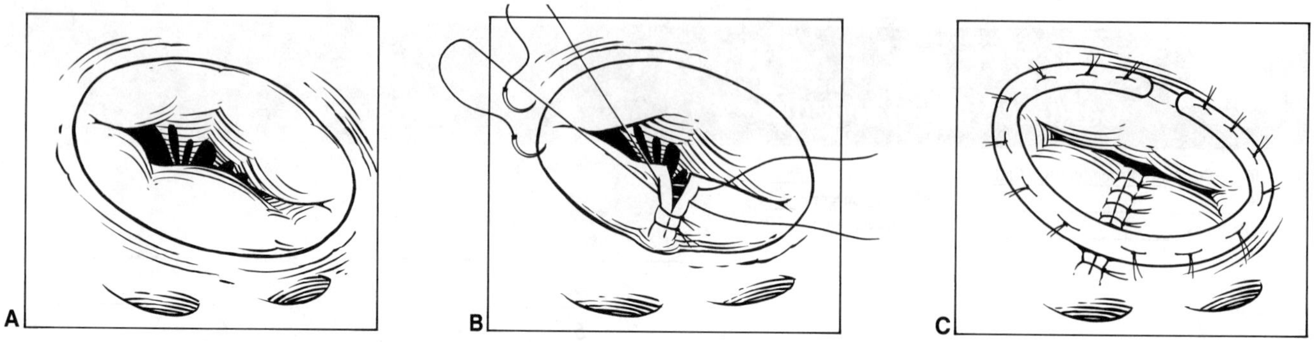

FIGURE 29-4. Valve leaflet resection and repair with a ring annuloplasty. (**A**) Mitral valve regurgitation; the section indicated by dashed lines will be excised. (**B**) Approximation of edges and suturing. (**C**) Completed valvuloplasty, leaflet repair, and annuloplasty ring.

term anticoagulation associated with menses and placental transfer to a fetus and those associated with delivery of a child do not exist. Xenografts also are used for patients over 70 years of age, individuals with a history of peptic ulcer disease, and others who cannot tolerate long-term anticoagulation. Xenografts are used for all tricuspid valve replacements.

Homografts (human valves) are obtained from cadaver tissue donations. The aortic valve and a portion of the aorta or the pulmonic valve and a portion of the pulmonary artery are harvested and stored cryogenically. Homografts are not always available and are very expensive. Homografts last for 10 to 15 years, somewhat longer than xenografts. The homografts are not thrombogenic and are resistant to subacute bacterial endocarditis. Homografts are used for aortic and pulmonic valve replacement.

Autografts (autologous valves) are obtained by excising the patient's own pulmonic valve and a portion of the pulmonary artery for use as the aortic valve. Anticoagulation is not necessary as the valve is the patient's own tissue and not thrombogenic. The autograft is an alternative for children, women of childbearing age, young adults, individuals with a history of peptic ulcer disease, and those who cannot tolerate anticoagulation. Aortic valve autografts have remained viable for more than 20 years.

Most aortic valve autograft surgeries are double valve replacement procedures, as a homograft also is performed for pulmonic valve replacement. If pulmonary vascular pressures are normal, some surgeons elect not to replace the pulmonic valve. The patient is able to recover without a valve between the right ventricle and the pulmonary artery.

FIGURE 29-5. Illustration of a valve replacement. (**A**) The native valve excised and prosthetic valve being sutured. (**B**) Once all sutures are placed through the ring, the prosthetic valve is slid down the sutures and into the natural orifice. The sutures are then tied off and trimmed.

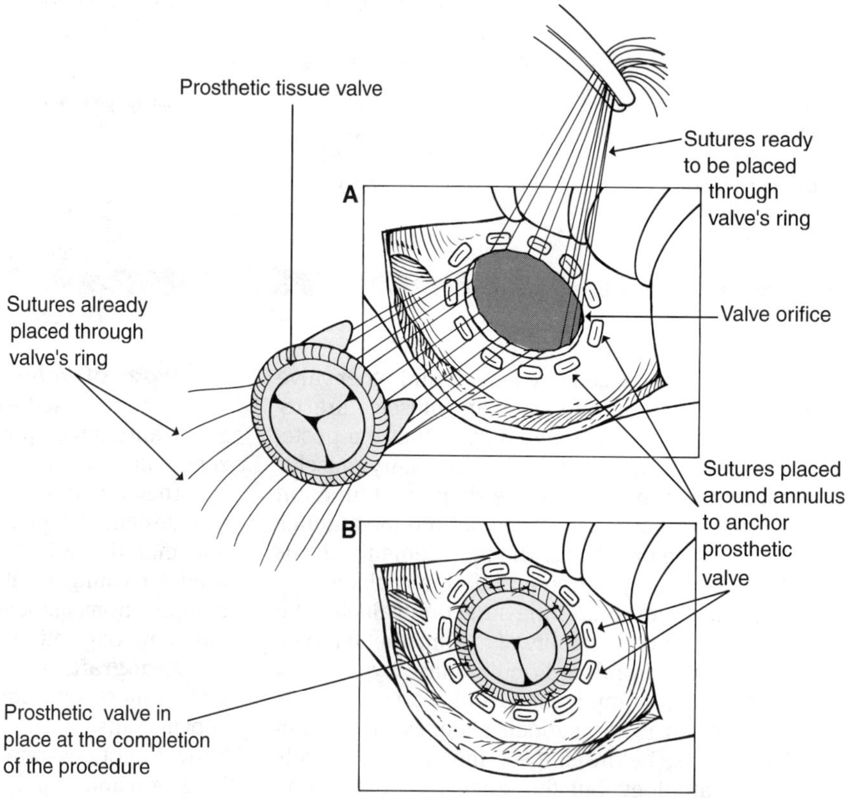

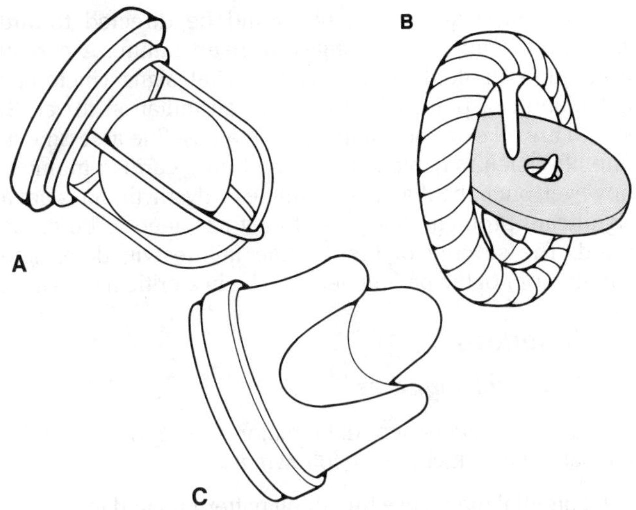

FIGURE 29-6. Common mechanical and biologic valve replacements. (**A**) Caged ball valve (Starr-Edwards/mechanical). (**B**) Tilting-disc valve (Medtronic-Hall/mechanical). (**C**) Porcine heterograft valve (Carpenter-Edwards/biologic).

Complications. The sudden change in hemodynamics, as well as the procedure, puts the patient at risk for many postoperative complications. These include bleeding, thromboembolism, infection, congestive heart failure, hypertension, dysrhythmias, hemolysis, and mechanical obstruction.

Nursing Considerations. Patients who have had valve replacements are admitted to the critical care unit; their care is directed toward recovery from anesthesia and promotion of hemodynamic stability.

The patient is usually transferred to a telemetry or surgical unit within 24 to 72 hours after valve replacement. The nursing care continues as for most postsurgical patients, including wound care and patient education regarding diet, activity, medication, and self-care. In addition to education about long-term anticoagulant therapy, patients with a mechanical valve prosthesis require education regarding antibiotic prophylaxis for bacterial endocarditis before all dental and surgical interventions.

Septal Repair

The atrial or ventricular septum may have an abnormal opening between the right and left sides of the heart: **a septal defect.** Although most septal defects are congenital and are repaired during infancy and childhood, adults may not have undergone early repair or may develop septal defects as a result of myocardial infarctions or diagnostic and treatment procedures.

Repair of septal defects requires general anesthesia and cardiopulmonary bypass. The heart is opened and a pericardial or synthetic (usually Dacron) patch is used to close the opening. Atrial septal defect repairs have low morbidity and mortality. When the mitral or tricuspid valve is involved, however, the procedure is more complicated. Generally, ventricular septal repairs are uncomplicated, but the proximity of the defect to the intraventricular conduction system and the valves may make this repair more complex.

Cardiomyopathies

Pathophysiology

Myopathy is a disease of muscle. The cardiomyopathies are a group of diseases that affect the structure and function of the myocardium.

The cardiomyopathies are categorized by pathologic, physiologic, and clinical signs. They are defined as (1) dilated cardiomyopathy, or sometimes congestive cardiomyopathy; (2) hypertrophic cardiomyopathy; and (3) restrictive cardiomyopathy. Regardless of the category and the cause, these diseases lead to severe heart failure and often death.

Dilated or congestive cardiomyopathy is the most commonly occurring form of the cardiomyopathies. It is distinguished by a dilated and enlarged ventricular cavity along with decreasing muscle wall thickness, left atrial enlargement, and blood stasis in the ventricle. Microscopic examination of the muscle tissue shows a diminishing of the contractile elements of the muscle fibers. Excessive chronic alcohol intake is often implicated in this type of cardiomyopathy.

Hypertrophic cardiomyopathy occurs less frequently. In hypertrophic cardiomyopathies, the heart muscle actually increases in mass weight, especially along the septum. The septal size increase may obstruct the flow of blood from the atria to the ventricles; hence, this category is divided further into obstructive and nonobstructive types.

Restrictive cardiomyopathy is the last and least frequently occurring category. This form is characterized by an impairment of ventricular stretch and hence volume. Restrictive cardiomyopathy can be associated with amyloidosis (in which amyloid, a protein substance, is deposited within the cells) and other such infiltrative diseases.

Regardless of the distinguishing features, the pathophysiology of cardiomyopathy is a series of progressive events that culminates in impaired pumping of the left ventricle. As the stroke volume becomes less and less, the sympathetic nervous system is stimulated, resulting in increased systemic vascular resistance. As in the pathophysiology of heart failure from any cause, the left ventricle enlarges to accommodate the demands and eventually fails. Failure of the right ventricle usually accompanies this process (Fig. 29-7).

Clinical Manifestations

The cardiomyopathies may occur at any age and affect both men and women. Most persons with cardiomyopathy present initially with signs and symptoms of heart failure. Dyspnea on exertion, paroxysmal nocturnal dyspnea (PND), cough, and easy fatigability are early symptoms. A physical examination usually reveals systemic venous congestion, jugular vein distention, pitting edema of dependent body parts, an enlarged liver, and tachycardia.

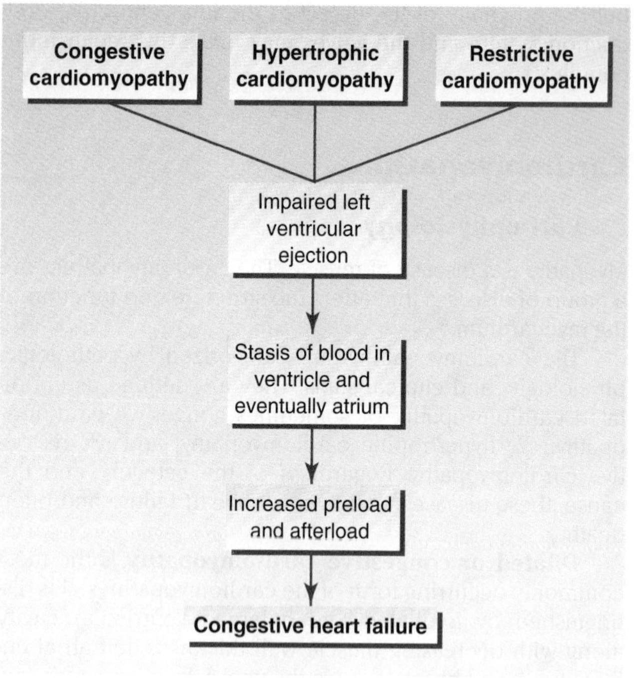

FIGURE 29-7. Cardiomyopathy and the development of congestive heart failure.

Diagnostic Evaluation

Diagnosis of cardiomyopathy is usually made from findings disclosed by patient history and by ruling out other causes of the failure, such as myocardial infarction. The ECG will demonstrate changes consistent with left ventricular hypertrophy. The echocardiogram is probably one of the most helpful diagnostic tools in that the functioning of the left ventricle can be observed easily. Cardiac catheterization is sometimes used to rule out coronary artery disease as a causative factor.

Management

Medical management is directed toward correcting the heart failure. When heart failure has progressed to a point where medical treatment is not effective, heart transplantation is the patient's only hope for survival. In some cases ventricular assist devices are necessary to support the failing heart until a suitable donor becomes available (see Chapter 30).

❑ NURSING PROCESS
The Patient With Cardiomyopathy

Assessment

Nursing assessment for the patient with cardiomyopathy begins with a detailed history of the presenting signs and symptoms. Because of the chronic nature of this problem, a careful psychosocial history is also important. The patient's family support system should be identified very early and involved in the management of the patient.

The physical assessment should be directed toward signs and symptoms of congestive heart failure. A careful evaluation of fluid volume status, vital signs (including calculation of pulse pressure), and auscultation for an S_3 sound are all extremely important in a baseline assessment. The physician may place the patient on a cardiac monitor; however, once the diagnosis is made or dysrhythmia is not a significant problem, the patient may not need to be monitored. The severity of the cardiac failure will determine whether or not the patient needs to be in a critical care unit.

Diagnosis

Nursing Diagnoses

Based on the assessment data, major nursing diagnoses for the patient may include the following:

- ❑ Potential ineffective breathing pattern related to myocardial failure
- ❑ Activity intolerance related to excessive fluid volume
- ❑ Anxiety related to the disease process
- ❑ Potential noncompliance with the self-care program

Collaborative Problems/ Potential Complications

Based on the assessment data, potential complications that may develop include:

- ❑ Cardiac failure

Planning and Implementation

Goals. The major goals of the patient include absence of respiratory difficulties, increased activity tolerance, reduction of anxiety, compliance with the self-care program, and absence of complications.

Nursing Interventions

Relieving Respiratory Difficulties. Because many of the patient's signs and symptoms are corrected by pharmacologic agents, attention to the timeliness of administering prescribed medications is vitally important. Careful documentation of the patient's response is critical. Supporting respiratory exchange with oxygen by way of nasal prongs is also indicated.

The patient may be most comfortable if allowed to rest at the bedside in a chair. This position is helpful in pooling venous blood in the periphery and reducing preload. Helping the patient to keep warm and to change position frequently stimulates circulation and reduces the possibility of skin breakdown. Maintaining an environment free of dust, lint, flowers, and perfumes will also support easier respiratory exchange.

Increasing Activity Tolerance. Planning nursing care so that the patient participates frequently in activities of short duration is important. Allowing the patient to accomplish a goal, no matter how small, also enhances a sense of well-being. For example, working with the patient to determine what part of the bath can be completed without aid, and then providing a period of rest before completing the bath, helps the patient conserve energy that is in short supply. Activities that deplete the patient's energy are avoided.

Reducing Anxiety. The patient is provided with appropriate information about the signs and symptoms of the cardiomyopathy and encouraged to accomplish certain self-care activities. An atmosphere in which the patient feels free to verbalize any fears is provided, as is offering assurance that these concerns are legitimate. If the patient is facing death or awaiting transplant surgery, time must be provided to discuss these issues. Spiritual, psychological, and emotional support may be indicated for the patient and significant others.

Patient Education and Home Care Considerations. It is particularly important for the patient with cardiomyopathy to learn what self-care activities are necessary and how to perform them at home. An optimal health status is very desirable should the patient be a candidate for a heart transplant. Satisfactory improvement can be obtained by meticulous attention to a medication program, which usually consists of several different medications to maintain a state free of cardiac failure.

The nurse can be integral to the process as patients review lifestyle and work to incorporate the above therapeutic activities with minimal intrusion. Helping patients to accept their disease status makes it easier for them to follow the self-care program at home.

Establishing trust is vital to the relationship with these chronically ill and debilitated patients. Providing realistic hope helps reduce their anxiety while awaiting a donor heart when transplant is an acceptable treatment modality.

When a patient can no longer be helped by any therapeutic technique, allowing the patient and significant others the freedom to begin the grieving process is vitally important.

Evaluation

Expected Outcomes

1. Demonstrates improved respiratory function
   a. Respiratory rate is within normal limits
   b. Blood gases are normal
   c. Reports decreased dyspnea and increased comfort
   d. Uses oxygen therapy as prescribed
2. Increases activity tolerance
   a. Carries out activities of daily living (*e.g.*, brushes teeth, feeds self)
   b. Transfers self from chair to bed
   c. Reports increased tolerance to activity
3. Experiences reduction of anxiety
   a. Discusses prognosis freely
   b. Verbalizes fears and concerns
   c. Participates in support groups if appropriate
4. Complies with the program of self-care
   a. Takes medications according to prescribed schedule
   b. Modifies lifestyle to accommodate activity limitations
   c. Identifies signs and symptoms to be reported to the health care professional

Cardiomyopathy Surgery

Hypertrophic cardiomyopathies (cardiac disorders that involve an enlarged area of the heart muscle) may impair outflow of blood from the left ventricle to the aorta. When the patient becomes symptomatic despite medical therapy and when a difference in pressure of 50 mm Hg or more exists between the left ventricle and the aorta, surgery is considered. The most common procedure is a **myectomy** (sometimes referred to as a myotomy–myectomy), in which some of the heart tissue is excised. Septal tissue approximately 1 cm wide and deep is cut from the enlarged septum below the aortic valve. The length of septum removed depends on the degree of obstruction caused by the hypertrophied muscle.

Instead of a septal myectomy, the left ventricle's outflow tract to the aortic valve may be opened by removing the mitral valve, chordae, and papillary muscles. The mitral valve then is replaced with a low-profile disc valve. The space taken up by the mitral valve is substantially reduced and blood is able to move around the enlarged septum to the aortic valve in the area that the mitral valve previously occupied.

The primary complication of both procedures is dysrhythmia; in addition, the patient is at risk for the surgical complications.

Infectious Diseases of the Heart

Rheumatic Endocarditis

Pathophysiology

The development of rheumatic endocarditis is directly attributed to rheumatic fever, a systemic disease caused by a group A streptococcal infection. Rheumatic fever affects all bony joints, producing a polyarthritis. The heart is also a target organ and is where the most serious damage occurs.

The heart damage and the joint lesions are not infectious in origin, in the sense that these tissues are not invaded and directly damaged by destructive organisms; rather, they represent a sensitivity phenomenon or reaction occurring in response to **hemolytic streptococcus.** Blood leukocytes accumulate in the affected tissues and form nodules, which eventually are replaced by scars. The myocardium is certain to be involved in this inflammatory process; that is, **rheumatic myocarditis** develops, which temporarily weakens the contractile power of the heart. The pericardium likewise is affected; that is, **rheumatic pericarditis** also occurs during the acute illness. These myocardial and pericardial complications usually are without serious sequelae. **Rheumatic endocarditis,** on the other hand, results in permanent and often crippling side effects.

Rheumatic endocarditis anatomically manifests itself first by tiny translucent vegetations or growths, which resemble beads about the size of the head of a pin, arranged in a row along the free margins of the valve flaps. These tiny beads look harmless enough and may disappear without injuring the valve leaflets, but more often they have serious effects. They are the starting point of a process that gradually thickens the leaflets, rendering them shorter and thicker than normal, which prevents them from closing completely. The result is leakage, a condition called **valvular regurgitation.** The most common site of valvular regurgitation is the mitral valve.

In other patients, the inflamed margins of the valve leaflets become adherent, resulting in **valvular stenosis,** a narrowed or "stenotic" valvular orifice. A small percentage of patients with rheumatic fever become critically ill with intractable heart failure, serious dysrhythmias, and rheumatic pneumonia. These patients are treated in an intensive care unit.

Most patients recover quickly and usually completely. However, although the patient is free of symptoms, certain permanent residual effects remain that often lead to progressive valvular deformities. The extent of cardiac damage, or even its existence, may not have been apparent in clinical examinations during the acute phase of the disease. Eventually, however, the heart murmurs that are characteristic of valvular stenosis, regurgitation, or both, become audible on auscultation and, in some patients, even detectable as "thrills" on palpation. The myocardium usually can compensate for these valvular defects very well for a time. As long as the myocardium can compensate, the patient remains in apparent good health. Sooner or later, however, the myocardium fails to compensate. Decompensation, when it occurs, is signaled by the manifestations of congestive heart failure, as described in Chapter 28.

Clinical Manifestations

The cardiac symptoms that appear are dependent on which side of the heart is involved. The mitral valve is most often affected, producing the symptoms of **left-sided heart failure:** shortness of breath with crackles and wheezes in the lungs. See Chapter 28 for a discussion of left-sided versus right-sided failure. The severity of the symptoms depends on the size and location of the lesion.

The systemic symptoms that are present will be proportionate to the virulence of the invading organism. When a new murmur is detected in an individual with a systemic infection, infectious endocarditis should be suspected.

Management

The objectives of medical management are to aggressively eradicate the causative organism and prevent additional complications, such as a thromboembolic event. Long-term antibiotic therapy is the treatment of choice. Penicillin administered parenterally remains the medication of choice.

The patient with rheumatic endocarditis, whose valve function is faulty but whose disease is quiescent, does not require therapy as long as the heart pumps effectively. Nevertheless, the danger exists for recurrent attacks of acute rheumatic fever; bacterial endocarditis; embolism from vegetations or mural thrombi in the heart; and eventual cardiac failure. (The relationship between valvular disease and congestive failure and the treatment of heart failure are presented in Chapter 28.)

Prevention

Rheumatic endocarditis is prevented through early and adequate treatment of streptococcal infections in all persons.

A first-line approach in preventing initial attacks of rheumatic endocarditis is to recognize streptococcal infections, treat them adequately, and control epidemics in the community. Every nurse should be familiar with the signs and symptoms of streptococcal pharyngitis: high fever (38.9° to 40°C, or 101 to 104°F), chills, sore throat, redness of throat with exudate; enlarged lymph nodes, abdominal pain, and acute nasal infection. (Chart 29-1 presents a summary overview of these symptoms.)

- A throat culture is the only method by which an accurate diagnosis can be made.

Susceptible patients may require long-term oral antibiotic therapy or, more commonly, be required to take prophylactic antibiotics before procedures that can potentiate invasion by a microorganism. Penicillin taken before dental checkups is an excellent example. The patient also must be reminded of less common procedures such as cystoscopy that may also require prophylactic antibiotics.

Infective Endocarditis

Pathophysiology

Infective endocarditis (bacterial endocarditis) is an infection of the valves and endothelial surface of the heart caused by direct invasion by bacteria or other organisms and leading to deformity of the valve leaflets. Causative microorganisms include bacteria (streptococci, enterococci, pneumococci, staphylococci) fungi, rickettsiae, and *Streptococcus viridans.*

Infective endocarditis usually develops in patients who have a history of valvular heart disease. At great risk are patients with rheumatic heart disease or mitral valve prolapse and individuals who have had prosthetic valve surgery.

Infective endocarditis is more common in older persons, probably because of decreased immunologic responses to infection, metabolic alterations arising from

CHART 29-1
Prevention of Rheumatic Fever

Rheumatic fever is a preventable disease. Eradicating rheumatic fever, would eliminate *rheumatic heart disease.* Penicillin therapy in patients with streptococcal infections can prevent almost all primary attacks of rheumatic fever. A throat culture is the only method by which an accurate diagnosis can be determined.

The signs and symptoms of streptococcal pharyngitis are the following:

- Fever (38.9° to 40°C, or 101° to 104°F)
- Chills
- Sore throat (sudden in onset)
- Diffuse redness of throat with exudate on oropharynx (may not appear until after the first day)
- Enlarged and tender lymph nodes
- Abdominal pain (more common in children)
- Acute sinusitis and acute otitis media (may be due to streptococcus)

changes in the aging body, and increased invasive diagnostic procedures, especially in genitourinary disease. There is a high incidence of staphylococcal endocarditis among intravenous drug users, the disease occurring for the most part on otherwise normal valves.

Hospital-acquired endocarditis occurs most often in patients with debilitating disease, those with indwelling catheters, and those on prolonged intravenous or antibiotic therapy. Patients on immunosuppressive medications or steroids may develop fungal endocarditis.

Clinical Manifestations

The onset of infective endocarditis usually is insidious. The signs and symptoms develop from the toxic effect of the infection, from destruction of the heart valves, and from embolization of fragments of vegetative growths on the heart.

The **general manifestations,** which may be mistaken for influenza, include vague complaints of malaise, anorexia, weight loss, cough, and back and joint pain. Fever is intermittent and may be absent in patients who are receiving antibiotics or corticosteroids or in those who are elderly or have congestive heart failure or renal failure. Splinter hemorrhages (hemorrhagic lines and streaks) may be noted under the fingernails and toenails, and petechiae may appear in the conjunctiva and mucous membranes. Hemorrhages with pale centers (Roth's spots) that may be seen in the fundi of the eyes are caused by emboli in the nerve fiber layer of the eye.

The **cardiac manifestations** include heart murmurs, which may be absent initially. Progressive changes in murmurs over time may be encountered and indicate valvular damage due to vegetations or to perforation of the valve or the chordae tendineae. Enlargement of the heart or evidence of congestive heart failure is also seen.

The **central nervous system manifestations** include headache, temporary or transient cerebral ischemia, and strokes, which may be caused by emboli involving the cerebral arteries.

Embolization may be a presenting symptom, occurring at any time and involving other organ systems. The embolic phenomena may be manifested in the lung (recurrent pneumonia; pulmonary abscesses), kidney (hematuria; renal failure), spleen (left upper quadrant pain), heart (myocardial infarction), brain (stroke), or peripheral vessels.

Management

The objective of treatment is to totally eradicate the invading organism through adequate doses of an appropriate antimicrobial agent. The causative organism can be isolated through serial blood cultures. It is treated with a bactericidal agent or other appropriate medication that is known to be effective against the causative agent. The antibiotic is usually administered parenterally in a continuous intravenous infusion for a period of 4 to 6 weeks. Usually this therapy is delivered in a home setting and is monitored by the home care nurse. Bactericidal serum levels of the selected antibiotic are monitored by titrating it against the causative organism. If the serum does not demonstrate bactericidal activity, increased dosages of the antibiotic are given or a different antibiotic is tried. There are numerous antimicrobial regimens currently in use, but penicillin is usually the medication of choice. Blood cultures are taken periodically to monitor the course of therapy.

In fungal endocarditis, an antifungal agent, such as amphotericin B, is the usual treatment. The patient's temperature is monitored at regular intervals because the course of fever is one indication of the effectiveness of treatment. However, febrile reactions also may occur as a result of medication therapy. After adequate antimicrobial therapy is initiated, bacteria usually disappear. The patient should begin to feel better, regain an appetite and feel less tired. During this time, patients require a great deal of psychosocial support because, although they feel well, they may find themselves confined to the hospital or home with restrictive IV therapy.

After the patient has recovered from the infectious process, the valves may need to be replaced if they have been seriously damaged and cause severe symptoms.

Complications. Even if the patient responds to the antimicrobial therapy, endocarditis can be very destructive to the heart and other organs. Congestive heart failure and cerebral vascular complications such as strokes may occur before, during, or after therapy. Valve stenosis or regurgitation, myocardial damage, and mycotic (fungal) aneurysms are some potential heart complications. Many other organ complications can result from septic or nonseptic emboli, immunologic responses, or hemodynamic deterioration.

Surgery. Surgical valve replacement greatly improves the prognosis for patients with severely damaged heart valves. Usually, valve excision and replacement are required for (1) patients who develop congestive heart failure as a result of aortic or mitral valve involvement despite adequate medical treatment; (2) patients who have more than one serious systemic embolic episode; and (3) persons with uncontrolled infection, recurrent infection, or fungal endocarditis. Many patients who have prosthetic valve endocarditis (infected prostheses) require valve replacement.

Prevention

Infective endocarditis occurs most often in persons with structural abnormalities of the heart and great vessels, especially valvular heart disease. Any procedure that is associated with transient bacteremia may cause bacteria to lodge on damaged or abnormal valves. Persons at risk are those with prosthetic cardiac valves; previous bacterial endocarditis, even in the absence of heart disease; most congenital malformations; rheumatic and other acquired valvular dysfunction, even after valvular surgery; hypertrophic cardiomyopathy; and mitral valve prolapse with valvular regurgitation.

Antibiotic prophylaxis is recommended for persons at risk who undergo the following procedures:*

- Dental procedures known to induce gingival or mucosal bleeding, including professional cleaning
- Tonsillectomy or adenoidectomy

*A Statement for Health Professionals by the Committee on Rheumatic Fever, Endocarditis, and Kawasaki Disease of the Council on Cardiovascular Disease in the Young of the American Heart Association. JAMA 1990 Dec 12; 264(22):2919–2922.

- Surgical operations that involve intestinal or respiratory mucosa
- Bronchoscopy with a rigid bronchoscope
- Sclerotherapy for esophageal varices
- Esophageal dilation
- Gallbladder surgery
- Cystoscopy
- Urethral dilation
- Urethral catheterization if urinary tract infection is present
- Urinary tract surgery if urinary tract infection is present
- Prostatic surgery
- Incision and drainage of infected tissue
- Vaginal hysterectomy
- Vaginal delivery in the presence of infection

Myocarditis

Pathophysiology

Acute myocarditis is an inflammatory process involving the myocardium. The heart is a muscle; hence, its efficiency depends on the health of the individual muscle fibers. When the muscle fibers are healthy, the heart can function well in spite of severe valvular injuries; when the muscle fibers are damaged, life is threatened.

Myocarditis usually results from an infectious process, particularly of viral, bacterial, mycotic, parasitic, protozoal, or spirochetal origin, or it may be produced by hypersensitivity states such as rheumatic fever. Therefore, myocarditis may be seen in patients with acute systemic infections, those receiving immunosuppressive therapy, or those with infective endocarditis.

Myocarditis can cause heart dilatation, thrombi on the heart wall (mural thrombi), infiltration of circulating blood cells around the coronary vessels and between the muscle fibers, and degeneration of the muscle fibers themselves.

Clinical Manifestations

The symptoms of acute myocarditis depend on the type of infection, the degree of myocardial damage, and the capacity of the myocardium to recover. Symptoms may be mild or absent. The patient may complain of fatigue and dyspnea, palpitations, and occasional discomfort in the chest and upper abdomen. Clinical examination may show cardiac enlargement, faint heart sounds, gallop rhythm, and a systolic murmur. A pericardial friction rub may be heard if the patient has associated pericarditis. Pulsus alternans (a pulse in which there is a regular alternation of weak and strong beats) may be present. Fever and tachycardia are frequently seen and symptoms of congestive heart failure may develop. Diagnosis can be confirmed by endomyocardial biopsy.

Management

The patient is given specific treatment for the underlying cause, if it is known (*e.g.*, penicillin for hemolytic streptococci), and is placed on bed rest to decrease cardiac work. Bed rest also helps to decrease residual myocardial damage and the complications of myocarditis. The treatment is essentially the same as that used for congestive heart failure (see Chapter 28).

Cardiac function and temperature are evaluated to determine whether the disease is subsiding and whether congestive heart failure has occurred. If a dysrhythmia occurs, the patient should be cared for in a unit with continuous cardiac monitoring so that personnel and equipment are readily available if a life-threatening dysrhythmia occurs.

When there is evidence of congestive heart failure, medication is administered to slow the heart rate and augment myocardial contractility.

- Patients with myocarditis are sensitive to digitalis. Therefore, the patient must be closely monitored for digitalis toxicity (evidenced by dysrhythmia, anorexia, nausea, vomiting, bradycardia, headache, malaise).

Elastic stockings and passive and active exercises should be used, because embolization from venous thrombosis and mural thrombi can occur.

Prevention

Prevention of infectious diseases by means of appropriate immunizations and early treatment appears to be important in decreasing the incidence of myocarditis. After an episode of myocarditis, there is usually some residual heart enlargement. Physical activity is increased slowly, and the patient is instructed to report any symptoms that occur with increasing activity, such as a rapidly beating heart. Competitive sports and alcohol must be avoided.

Pericarditis

Pathophysiology

Pericarditis refers to an inflammation of the pericardium, the membranous sac enveloping the heart. It may be a primary illness, or it may develop in the course of a variety of medical and surgical diseases. The following are some of the causes underlying or associated with pericarditis:

1. Idiopathic or nonspecific causes
2. Infection
   a. Bacterial (*e.g.*, streptococcus, staphylococcus, meningococcus, gonococcus)
   b. Viral (*e.g.*, coxsackie, influenza)
   c. Mycotic (fungal) (*e.g.*, rickettsia, parasite)
3. Disorders of connective tissue—systemic lupus erythematosus, rheumatic fever, rheumatoid arthritis, polyarteritis
4. Hypersensitivity states—immune reactions, drug reactions, serum sickness
5. Diseases of adjacent structures—myocardial infarction, dissecting aneurysm, pleural and pulmonary disease (pneumonia)
6. Neoplastic disease
   a. Secondary to metastasis from lung cancer, breast cancer
   b. Leukemia
   c. Primary (mesothelioma)

7. Radiation therapy
8. Trauma—chest injury, cardiac surgery, during cardiac catheterization, pacemaker implantation
9. Renal failure and uremia
10. Tuberculosis

Clinical Manifestations

The characteristic symptom of pericarditis is **pain** and the characteristic sign is a **friction rub.** Pain is almost always present in acute pericarditis and is most common over the precordium. The pain may be felt beneath the clavicle and in the neck and left scapular region. Pericardial pain is aggravated by breathing, turning in bed, and twisting the body; it is relieved by sitting up. In fact, the patient prefers to adopt a forward-leaning or a sitting posture. Dyspnea may occur as the result of pericardial compression of the heart's movements, which leads to a decreased cardiac output. The patient may appear extremely ill. Pericarditis *per se* often gives rise to no signs other than fever and the production of a friction rub.

Diagnostic Evaluation

Diagnosis is most often made on the basis of signs and symptoms. The ECG and echocardiogram assist in confirming the diagnosis.

Management

The objectives of management are to (1) determine the cause, (2) administer therapy for the specific cause (when known), and (3) be alert for **cardiac tamponade** (compression of the heart from fluid in the pericardial sac; see Chapter 28). The patient is placed on bed rest when cardiac output is impaired, until the fever, chest pain, and friction rub have disappeared.

Analgesics may be prescribed for pain relief during the acute phase. Salicylates relieve pain and hasten reabsorption of fluid in the patient with rheumatic pericarditis. Corticosteroids may be prescribed to control symptoms, hasten resolution of the inflammatory process in the pericardium, and prevent recurring pericardial effusion.

- Be alert to the possibility of cardiac tamponade. Use nursing assessment skills to anticipate and identify the triad of symptoms—falling arterial pressure, rising venous pressure, and distant heart sounds.

Patients with infections of the pericardium are treated with the antimicrobial agent of choice once the organism causing the infection is identified. Pericarditis associated with rheumatic fever may respond to penicillin. Pericarditis resulting from tuberculosis is treated with isoniazid, ethambutol hydrochloride, rifampin, and streptomycin, in various combinations. Amphotericin B is used in fungal pericarditis, and corticosteroids are used in disseminated lupus erythematosus.

As the patient's condition improves, activity may be increased gradually. If pain, fever, or friction rub reappear, however, bed rest must be resumed.

❑ NURSING PROCESS
The Patient With Pericarditis

Assessment

Pain is the primary symptom of the patient with pericarditis. The pain of pericarditis is assessed by observing and evaluating the patient in various positions in bed.

While observing the patient, the examiner tries to discover whether or not the pain is influenced by respiratory movements, with or without the actual passage of air; by flexion, extension, or rotation of the spine, including the neck; by movements of the shoulders and arms; by coughing; or by swallowing. Recognizing those events that precipitate or intensify pain may be very helpful in establishing a diagnosis and differentiating the pain of pericarditis from the pain of myocardial infarction.

A pericardial friction rub occurs when the pericardial surfaces lose their lubricating fluid because of inflammation. The rub is audible on auscultation and is synchronous with the heartbeat. A pericardial friction rub is diagnostic of pericarditis and should be searched for diligently.

- ❑ The diaphragm of the stethoscope is placed tightly against the thorax; the left sternal edge in the fourth intercostal space, the site where the pericardium comes into contact with the left chest wall, is auscultated. A pericardial friction rub has a scratching or leathery sound. The rub is louder at the end of expiration and may be heard best with the patient in a sitting position.

If there is difficulty in distinguishing a pericardial friction rub from a pleural friction rub, patients are asked to hold their breath. A pericardial friction rub will continue.

The patient's temperature is monitored frequently. Pericarditis will cause an abrupt onset of fever in a patient who has been afebrile.

Diagnosis

Nursing Diagnoses

Based on the assessment data, major nursing diagnoses of the patient may include the following:

- ❑ Pain related to inflammation of the pericardium

Collaborative Problems/ Potential Complications

Based on the assessment data, potential complications that may develop include:

- ❑ Pericardial effusion
- ❑ Cardiac tamponade

Planning and Implementation

Goals. The patient's major goals may include relief of pain and absence of potential complications.

Nursing Interventions

Relief of Pain. Relief of pain is achieved by having the patient remain on bed rest or chair rest, whichever is more comfortable. Because sitting upright and leaning forward is the posture that tends to relieve pain, chair rest may be more comfortable. As the chest pain and friction rub abate, activities of daily living may be resumed gradually.

If the patient is receiving medications for the pericarditis, such as analgesics, antibiotics, or corticosteroids, the patient's responses are monitored and recorded.

If chest pain and friction rub recur, bed rest is resumed.

Monitor and Manage Potential Complications

Pericardial Effusion. If the patient does not respond to medical management, fluid may develop or accumulate between the pericardial linings or in the sac. This condition is called pericardial effusion (see Chapter 28). Fluid in the pericardial sac can cause constriction of the myocardium and interrupt its ability to pump. Thus, the cardiac output will decline with each contraction. Failure to identify the onset of this problem can lead to **cardiac tamponade** and the possibility of sudden death.

Early signs and symptoms of this event for which to observe are those that indicate a falling arterial pressure. Usually the systolic pressure falls while the diastolic pressure remains stable; hence the pulse pressure narrows. Heart sounds may progress from being distant to being imperceptible. Neck vein distention and other signs of rising central venous pressure are observed. These signs and symptoms occur because, as the fluid-filled pericardial sac compresses the myocardium, blood continues to return to the heart from the periphery but cannot be pumped back into the circulation.

The physician must be notified immediately. The nurse should prepare for a pericardiocentesis (see Chapter 28). The nurse stays with the patient and continues to assess and record signs and symptoms until the physician arrives to prescribe more definitive therapy.

Evaluation

Expected Outcomes

1. Patient is free of pain
   a. Performs activities of daily living comfortably
   b. Temperature returns to patient's normal range
   c. Pericardial friction rub is absent
2. Experiences absence of complications
   a. Blood pressure remains in patient's normal range
   b. Heart sounds are strong and can be auscultated
   c. Neck veins are not distended

Chronic Constrictive Pericarditis

Chronic constrictive pericarditis is a condition in which chronic inflammatory thickening of the pericardium compresses the heart and prevents it from expanding to normal size. The ventricles are unable to fill completely and therefore less blood is pumped into the circulatory system.

Often the adherent pericardium becomes calcified. The heart action is greatly restricted by this tough, unyielding enclosure, and edema, ascites, and hepatic enlargement result. The fixation of the heart to the pericardium may produce a retraction of the chest wall with every beat.

Chronic restrictive pericarditis is caused by long-standing pyogenic infections, postviral infections, tuberculosis, or blood in the pericardial cavity (hemopericardium).

CRITICAL THINKING EXERCISES

1. One of your neighbors has just had a mitral valve replacement and indicates that he does not understand why he has been instructed to take antibiotics before undergoing any dental work. How would you explain the rationale for these instructions?
2. Discharge plans are being made for a middle-aged male patient with cardiomyopathy. His wife indicates that she is prepared to care for him at home and that she expects he will be unable to participate extensively in his care. Based on your knowledge about developmental tasks of the middle years, how would you explain the husband's emotional and physical needs to the wife and the ways she can address these needs, as well as her own?
3. You are caring for a patient with pericarditis. His systolic blood pressure begins to fall and heart sounds cannot be heard. Describe the actions you would take and why.

The signs and symptoms are predominantly those of congestive heart failure (see Chapter 28), but dyspnea on exertion is the most prominent symptom. Chronic atrial fibrillation is commonly present.

Surgical removal of the tough encasing pericardium (pericardiectomy) is the only treatment of any benefit. The objective of the surgery is to release both ventricles from the constrictive and restrictive inflammation.

BIBLIOGRAPHY

Books and Pamphlets

American Heart Association. Heart Facts. Dallas, AHA, 1991.

Bates B. A Guide to Physical Examination and History Taking. Philadelphia, JB Lippincott, 1995.

Braunwald E. Heart Disease: A Textbook of Cardiovascular Medicine, 4th ed. Philadelphia, WB Saunders, 1992.

Chatterjee K, et al. Cardiology: An Illustrated Text Reference, Vol I. Philadelphia, JB Lippincott, 1991.

Fulmer TT and Walker MK. Critical Care Nursing of the Elderly. New York, Springer Publishing Company, 1992.

Guyton AC. Textbook of Medical Physiology, 8th ed. Philadelphia, WB Saunders, 1991.

Henning RJ and Grenik A. Critical Care Cardiology. New York, Churchill Livingstone, 1991.

Hudak CM and Gallo BM. Critical Care Nursing A Holistic Approach, 6th ed. Philadelphia, JB Lippincott, 1994.

Hurst JW (ed). The Heart. New York, McGraw-Hill, 1990.

Kinny M et al. AACN's Clinical Reference Manual. New York, McGraw-Hill, 1993.

Kinny M et al. Comprehensive Cardiac Care, 7th ed. St Louis, CV Mosby, 1991.

Seidel HM et al. Mosby's Guide to Physical Examination. St Louis, Mosby-Year Book, 1991.

Woods SL et al. Cardiac Nursing, 3rd ed. Philadelphia, JB Lippincott, 1995.

Journals

Constancia PE. The Ross procedure: Aortic valve replacement using autologous pulmonary valve. Crit Care Clin 1991 Dec; 3(4):717–721.

Ohler L et al. Aortic valvuloplasty: Medical and critical care nursing perspectives. Focus Crit Care 1989 Aug; 16(4):275–287.

Rafalowski M. Cardiac valve replacement: The homograft. Focus Crit Care 1990 Apr; 17(2):111–114.

Usznski HJ et al. Hypertrophic cardiomyopathy: Medical, surgical, and nursing management. J Cardiovasc Nurs 1993 Jan; 7(2): 13–22.

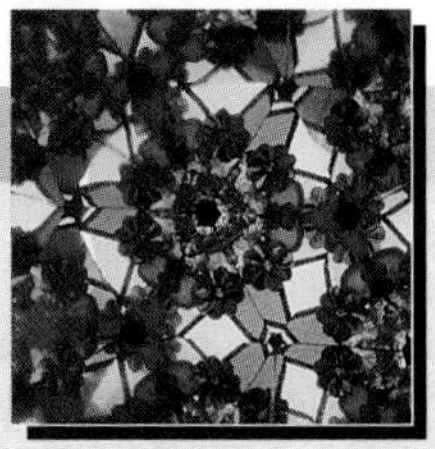

30 Management of the Cardiac Surgery Patient

CHAPTER OUTLINE

LEARNING OBJECTIVES

On completion of this chapter, the learner will be able to:

1. Discuss the various types of cardiac surgery and the nursing care involved
2. Describe the essential elements of nursing assessment, patient teaching, and psychologic support during preoperative preparation of the patient for cardiac surgery
3. Use the nursing process as a framework for the care of patients before cardiac surgery
4. Describe the critical nature of the components of postoperative management of the patient who has had cardiac surgery
5. Identify the possible complications of cardiac surgery, the measures to prevent these complications and assessment parameters appropriate for their identification
6. Use the nursing process as a framework for the care of patients after cardiac surgery

Today, the patient with heart disease and related complications can be assisted to achieve a quality of life far greater than anticipated even as recently as a decade ago. Through sophisticated diagnostic procedures that allow for earlier and more accurate diagnosis, treatment can begin well before significant debilitation takes place. New treatment technologies and pharmacotherapeutics are being developed rapidly and with increasing safety. Many of these therapies have been discussed in the preceding chapters.

Perhaps no therapeutic intervention has contributed as much as cardiac surgery to the improved quality of life for the patient with heart disease.

The first successful cardiac surgery, closure of a right ventricular stab wound, was performed in 1895 by the Italian surgeon de Vecchi. In the United States the first such successful surgery, also a repair of a stab wound, was performed in 1902. Valvular surgery followed in 1923 and 1925, closure of a patent ductus in 1937 and 1938, and resection of a coarctation of the aorta in 1944. The current era of coronary artery bypass grafting began in 1954.

The most revolutionary development in the advancement of cardiac surgery has been the technique for cardiopulmonary bypass. It was first used successfully in humans in 1951. Currently more than 250,000 procedures a year are performed, using cardiopulmonary bypass. Most (over 200,000) occur in North America. The majority of procedures are coronary artery bypass grafts (CABG) and valve repair or replacement.

The advances in diagnostics, medical management, surgical and anesthesia techniques, and cardiopulmonary bypass, as well as the care provided in critical care units and rehabilitation programs have assisted in making surgery a viable treatment option for patients with cardiac disease.

Cardiopulmonary Bypass

Many cardiac surgical procedures are possible because of cardiopulmonary bypass (extracorporeal circulation). The procedure provides a mechanical means of circulating and oxygenating blood for the body while "bypassing" the heart and lungs. The heart–lung machine allows for a bloodless surgical field while maintaining perfusion to the other body organs and tissues.

Cardiopulmonary bypass is accomplished by placing a cannula in the right atrium, vena cava, or femoral vein to withdraw blood from the body. The cannula is connected to tubing filled with an isotonic crystalloid solution (usually 5% dextrose in lactated Ringer's solution). Venous blood removed from the body by this cannula is filtered, oxygenated, cooled or warmed, and then returned to the body. The cannula used to return the oxygenated blood is usually inserted in the ascending aorta, but may be inserted in the femoral artery (Fig. 30-1).

Although cardiopulmonary bypass is a common technique in heart surgery, it is very complex. The patient requires anticoagulation with heparin to prevent thrombus formation and possible embolization that could occur when blood contacts the foreign surfaces of the cardiopulmonary bypass circuit and is pumped into the body

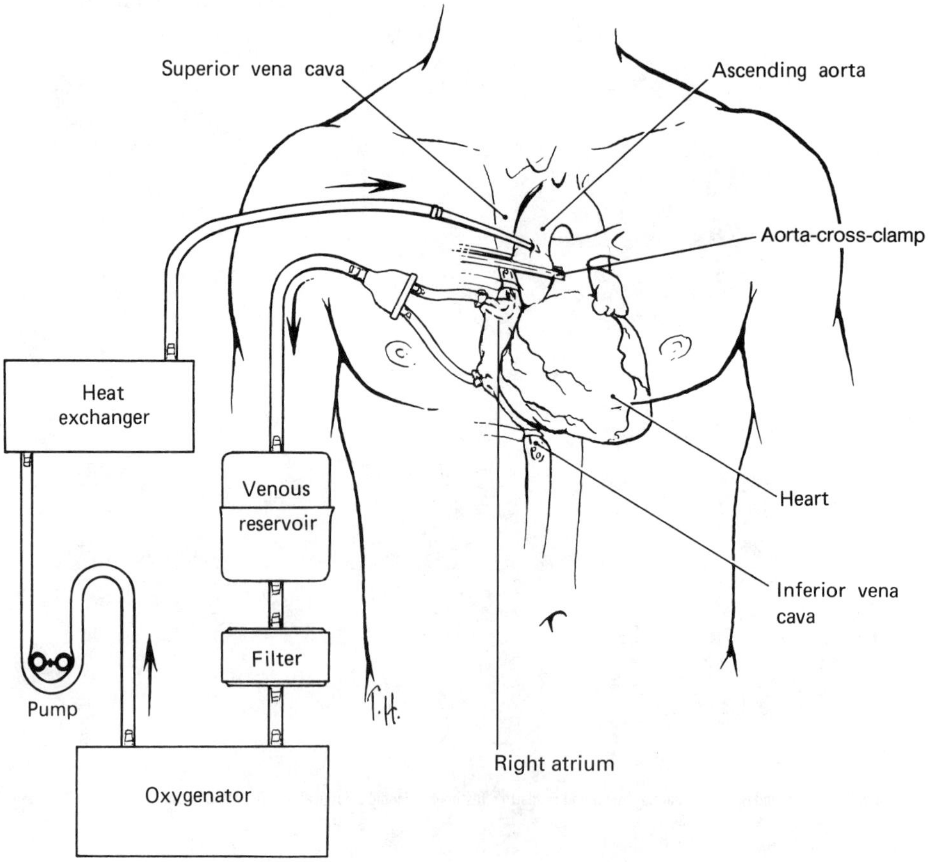

FIGURE 30-1. Schematic drawing of the cardiopulmonary bypass system. In this approach, cannulae are placed through the right atrium into the superior and inferior vena cava to divert blood from the body into the bypass system. The pump system creates a vacuum, pulling blood into the venous reservoir; the blood is cleared of air bubbles, clots, and particulates by the filter. The blood then passes through the oxygenator, releasing carbon dioxide and obtaining oxygen. The blood is pulled to the pump, then pushed out to the heat exchanger, where its temperature is regulated, and then returned to the body via the ascending aorta.

by a mechanical pump (not the normal blood vessels and heart). After the patient is removed from the bypass machine, protamine sulfate is used to reverse the effects of heparin.

During the procedure, hypothermia is maintained, usually 28°C to 32°C (82.4°F to 89.6°F). The blood is cooled during cardiopulmonary bypass and returned to the body. The cooled blood slows the body's basal metabolic rate, thereby decreasing its demand for oxygen. Cooled blood usually would have a higher viscosity, but the crystalloid solution used to prime the bypass tubing dilutes the blood. When the surgical procedure is completed, the blood is rewarmed as it passes through the cardiopulmonary bypass circuit.

Urine output, blood pressures, arterial blood gases, electrolytes, coagulation studies, and the electrocardiogram (ECG)all are used to monitor the patient's status during cardiopulmonary bypass.

There are still many things to learn about cardiopulmonary bypass. Numerous types of bypass circuits and pumping mechanisms are used today. Attempts are being made to increase the time a patient can safely spend on the heart–lung machine. Researchers continue to refine cardiopulmonary bypass to avoid or minimize the following problems: hemolysis, increased capillary membrane permeability, fluid and electrolyte shifts, tissue hypoxia or anoxia, thrombus or emboli formation, cardiac and vascular dissection, elevations of catecholamines and antidiuretic hormone (ADH), and the systemic inflammatory responses that complicate the procedure.

Types of Cardiac Surgery

Cardiac surgery is used to treat a variety of cardiac problems. The most common procedures include percutaneous transluminal coronary angioplasty (p. 644), coronary artery revoscularization (p. 646), and repair and replacement of defective cardiac valves (p. 682). These procedures have been discussed with the disorders with which they are associated—angina and valvular problems.

Surgical procedures discussed in this chapter include transplantation, cardiac tumor excision, and trauma repair.

Transplantation

The first human-to-human heart transplant was performed in 1967. Since then transplant procedures, equipment, and medications have continued to improve. In 1983, cyclosporine became available for general use. Cyclosporine is an immunosuppressant that greatly decreases the body's ability to reject foreign proteins such as transplanted organs. Unfortunately cyclosporine also decreases the body's ability to resist infections, so a fine balance must be achieved between suppressing rejection and avoiding infection. Since the advent of cyclosporine in 1983, heart transplantation has become a therapeutic option for patients with end-stage heart disease.

Cardiomyopathy, ischemic heart disease, congenital heart disease, valvular disease, and rejection of previously transplanted hearts are the most common indications for transplantation. Candidates usually have severe symptoms uncontrolled by medical therapy, no other surgical options, and a prognosis of less than 12 months to live. A patient is screened by a multidisciplinary team before becoming a candidate for heart transplant. The patient's age, pulmonary status, other chronic health conditions, infections, history of other transplants, compliance, and current health status are considered in evaluating the patient for transplantation.

When a donor heart becomes available, a computer generates a list of potential recipients on the basis of ABO blood group compatibility, sizes of donor and candidate, and the distance between the donor and potential recipient (distance is a variable because the transplanted heart's function is dependent on its being implanted within 4 hours of being harvested from the donor).

An **orthotopic transplant** is the most common surgical procedure for cardiac transplantation (Fig. 30-2). A portion of the recipient's atria (with the vena cava and pulmonary veins) is left in place; the remainder of the candidate's heart is removed from the mediastinum. The donor heart, which usually has been preserved in ice, is prepared for implant by cutting away a small section of the atria that corresponds with the sections of the recipient's heart that were left in place. The donor heart is implanted by suturing the donor atria to the residual atrial tissue of the recipient's native heart. The pulmonary artery and aorta are then anastomosed or connected.

The **heterotopic technique** is less commonly performed (Fig. 30-3). The donor heart is placed to the right and slightly anterior to the recipient's heart; the recipient's heart is not removed. Initially it was thought that the original heart might provide some protection for the patient in the event that the transplanted heart was rejected. Although the protective effect has not necessarily been proved, other reasons for retaining the original heart have been identified: a small donor heart, a prolonged ischemic time for the donor

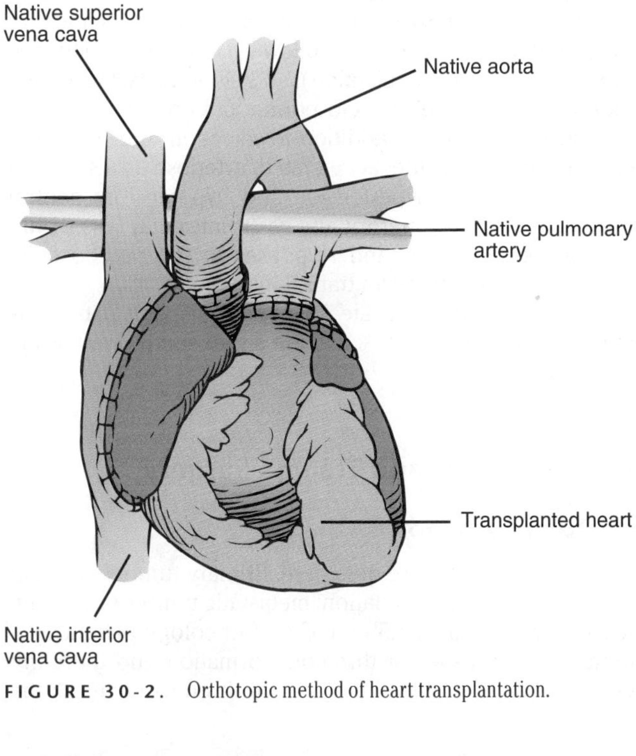

FIGURE 30-2. Orthotopic method of heart transplantation.

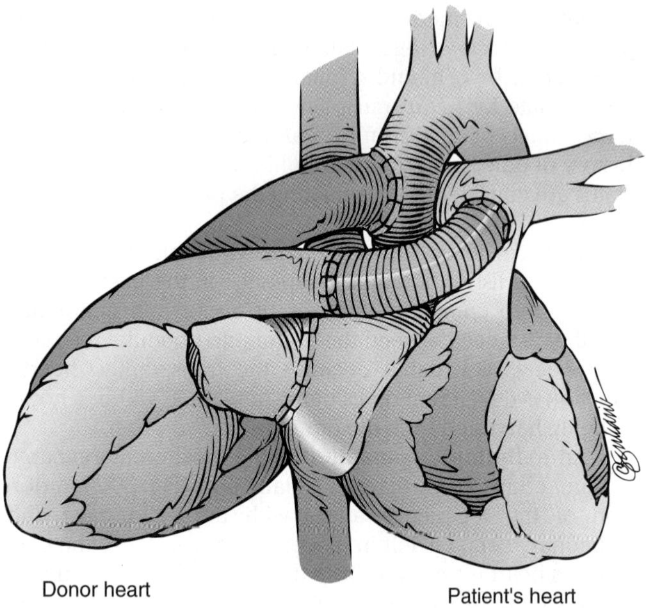

FIGURE 30-3. Heterotopic method of heart transplantation.

heart, or a donor heart that may have been otherwise compromised but must be used in an emergency.

The transplanted heart does not have nerve connections with the recipient's body (denervated heart); thus the sympathetic and vagus nerves do not affect the transplanted heart. The resting rate of the transplanted heart is approximately 70 to 90 beats per minute, but will increase gradually if catecholamines are in the circulation. Patients must **gradually** increase and decrease their exercise (extended warm-up and cool-down periods), as 20 to 30 minutes may be required to achieve the desired heart rate. Atropine will not increase the heart rate of these patients.

Postoperative Course. Heart transplant patients are constantly balancing the risk of rejection with the risk of infection. They must comply with a complex regimen of diet, medications, activity, follow-up laboratory studies, biopsies (to diagnose rejection), and clinic visits. Most commonly, patients receive cyclosporine and corticosteroids to minimize rejection. In addition to rejection and infection, complications include accelerated arteriosclerosis of the coronary arteries; hypertension and hypotension; central nervous system, respiratory, and gastrointestinal (GI) disturbances; renal failure; and responses to the psychosocial stresses imposed by organ transplantation.

The 1-year survival rate for heart transplant patients is approximately 80% to 90% and the 5-year survival rate is approximately 60% to 70%.

Cardiac Tumor and Trauma Surgery

Tumor Excision

Tumors of the heart are quite rare. Primary tumors occur in less than 1% of the population; metastatic tumors have been reported to occur in 1.5% to 35% of oncology patients. Tumors may be a site for thrombus formation and therefore create a risk of embolism. Dysrhythmias may occur as the myocardium or conduction system is affected. Most cardiac tumors are benign.

Surgical excision is performed only to prevent obstruction of a chamber or valve. Cardiopulmonary bypass is used, except for epicardial tumors, which can be excised without entering the heart and without stopping the heart from beating. The tumor location may necessitate valve replacement, myocardial patching, or pacemaker implantation. The nursing care is the same as that described for other cardiac surgery.

Trauma Repair

Patients who require surgical treatment for cardiac trauma have survived blunt force, gunshot, or stab injuries. The repairs are typically to the valves or septum in blunt force injuries, and to the ventricular and atrial walls in penetrating injuries. The wound is debrided and closed surgically when possible, but valve repair and replacement or patch grafts of the septum and atrial or ventricular walls may be required. The surgery is often an emergency procedure, so the risk of complications from the injury and surgery is high.

Mechanical Assist Devices and Total Artificial Hearts

The use of cardiopulmonary bypass for cardiovascular surgery and the possibility of performing heart transplantation for end-stage cardiac disease have increased the need for cardiac assist devices. Patients who cannot be weaned from cardiopulmonary bypass or patients who are in cardiogenic shock may benefit from a period of mechanical heart assistance. The most commonly used device is the **intra-aortic balloon pump** (IABP). The IABP decreases the work of the heart during contraction, but does not perform the actual work of the heart.

More complex devices that actually perform some or all of the pumping function for the heart also are being used. These more sophisticated **ventricular assist devices** (Fig. 30-4) can circulate as much, if not more, blood per minute as the patient's heart. Each ventricular assist device is used to support one ventricle. Today's most commonly used device is the **centrifugal pump.** Many pneumatically driven devices are being used, and the clinical results are very encouraging. Some ventricular assist devices can be combined with an oxygenator–extracorporeal membrane oxygenation (ECMO). The oxygenator–ventricular assist device combination is used for patients whose heart cannot pump adequate blood through their lungs or their body.

Total artificial hearts are designed to replace both ventricles. The patient's heart must be removed to implant the total artificial heart. All of these devices are experimental. The Jarvik-7 had some short-term success, but the long-term results have been disappointing. Most total artificial heart researchers are hoping to develop a device that can be permanently implanted and that will eliminate the need for donated human heart transplantation for the treatment of end-stage cardiac disease.

Ventricular assist devices and total artificial hearts currently are being used as temporary treatments while the pa-

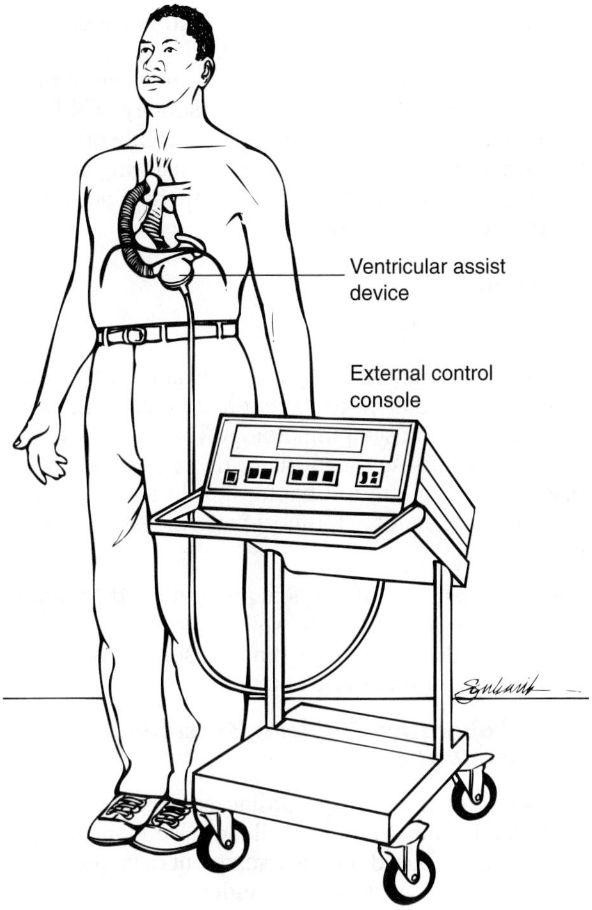

FIGURE 30-4. Left ventricular assist device.

tient's own heart recovers or until a donor heart becomes available for transplant. Bleeding disorders, hemorrhage, thrombus, emboli, hemolysis, infection, and mechanical failure are some of the complications of ventricular assist devices and total artificial hearts. The nursing care for these patients focuses not only on assessing and minimizing these complications, but also involves emotional support and education about the mechanical assist device.

Perioperative Nursing Management

The cardiac surgery patient has many of the same needs and requires the same perioperative care as other surgical patients (see Chapters 19 to 21). In addition, the patient and family are experiencing a major life crisis. The association of the heart with life and death intensifies their emotional and psychological needs. Patients frequently are admitted the same day as the procedure. For these patients it is crucial that their needs be carefully prioritized. Then, in the time allowed, the nurse focuses on those needs that have the highest priority.

Preoperatively, physical and psychologic assessment establishes the baseline for future reference. The patient's understanding of the surgical procedure, informed consent, and compliance with treatment protocols are evaluated. Assisting the patient to cope, understand the procedure, and maintain dignity during a safe operative period are nursing responsibilities. Postoperatively, close observation and specialized care begin in the critical care unit. Nurses continue to assist the patient and family through the recovery process on the step-down unit and through the rehabilitation phases until the patient and family are able to manage the care.

Preoperative Nursing Management

The preoperative phase of cardiac surgery usually begins before hospitalization. Other disease conditions (diabetes, high blood pressure, chronic obstructive pulmonary disease, and respiratory, endocrine, gastrointestinal, genitourinary, integumentary, and hematologic disorders) are treated and stabilized. Cardiac function is optimized; heart failure, dysrhythmias, and fluid and electrolyte imbalances are minimized. Sources of infection (dental, periodontal, integumentary, and gastrointestinal) are investigated and treated.

Patients may be instructed to alter their medication regimen before surgery, such as tapering steroids and digoxin, as well as decreasing or discontinuing anticoagulants. Medications for control of blood pressure, angina, diabetes, and dysrhythmia often are maintained until surgery. Maintaining activity patterns, a balanced diet, good sleep habits, and cessation of smoking are essential for minimizing the risks of surgery. Medications to reduce anxiety may be prescribed before surgery to prevent the sympathetic responses of increased heart rate and blood pressure that may increase the patient's cardiac symptoms.

❑ *NURSING PROCESS*
The Patient Awaiting Cardiac Surgery

Assessment

Patients with nonacute heart disease may be admitted to the hospital the day before or the day of their surgery. Most of the preoperative evaluation is completed before the patient enters the hospital. Many surgeons' offices or hospitals will have mailed an information packet to the patient's home.

A history and physical examination are performed by nursing and medical personnel. A chest x-ray, electrocardiogram, laboratory analyses, typing and cross-matching of blood, and autologous blood donation may also be done. The health assessment focuses on obtaining baseline physiologic, psychologic, and social information. The patient and family's learning needs are identified and addressed as necessary. Of particular importance is the patient's usual functional level, coping mechanisms, and support systems. The family support system and coping mechanisms are also assessed. These are important because the support of the family or significant others will affect the patient's postoperative course and rehabilitation. Discharge plans will be influenced by the lifestyle demands of the home situation and the physical environment of the home.

Health Assessment. The preoperative history and health assessment should be thorough and well documented because they provide a basis for postoperative comparison. A systematic assessment of all systems is performed, with emphasis on cardiovascular functioning.

Functional status of the cardiovascular system is determined by reviewing the patient's symptomatology, including past and present experiences with chest pain, hypertension, palpitations, cyanosis, breathing difficulty (dyspnea), leg pain that occurs with walking, orthopnea, paroxysmal nocturnal dyspnea, peripheral edema, and intermittent claudication. Because alterations in cardiac output can affect renal, respiratory, gastrointestinal, integumentary, hematologic, and neurologic functioning, these systems also are assessed thoroughly. History of major illnesses, previous surgeries, medication therapies, and use of drugs, alcohol, and tobacco are also explored.

A complete physical examination is performed, with special emphasis on the following parameters:

- General appearance and behavior
- Vital signs
- Nutritional and fluid status, weight, and height
- Inspection and palpation of the heart, noting the point of maximal impulse (PMI), abnormal pulsations, thrills
- Auscultation of the heart, noting pulse rate, rhythm, and quality, S_3, S_4, snaps, clicks, murmurs, friction rub
- Jugular venous pressure
- Peripheral pulses
- Peripheral edema

Psychosocial Assessment. The psychosocial assessment and the assessment of teaching—learning needs of the patient and family are as important as the physical examination. Anticipation of cardiac surgery is a source of great stress to the patient and family. They will be anxious and fearful and often have many unanswered questions. Their anxiety usually increases with the patient's admission to the hospital and the immediacy of surgery. An assessment of the level of anxiety is important. If it is low, this may indicate denial. If it is extremely high, it may interfere with the use of effective coping mechanisms and with preoperative teaching. Questions are asked to obtain the following information about both the patient and the family:

- The meaning of the surgery to the patient and family
- Coping mechanisms that are being used
- Measures used in the past to deal with stress
- Anticipated changes in lifestyle
- Support systems in effect
- Fears regarding the present and the future
- Knowledge and understanding of the surgical procedure, postoperative course, and long-term rehabilitation

Adequate time should be allowed for the patient and family to express their fears. The fears most often expressed are fear of the unknown, fear of pain, fear of body image change, and fear of dying.

During the assessment, the nurse determines how much the patient and family know about the impending surgery and the expected postoperative events. They are encouraged to ask questions and to indicate how much information they wish to have. Some patients prefer not to have detailed information, whereas others want to know as much as possible. Patients should be approached as unique individuals with their own specific learning needs, learning styles, and levels of understanding.

Patients requiring emergency heart surgery may have both cardiac catheterization and surgery within several hours of admission. The nurse will have little opportunity to assess and meet their emotional and learning needs before surgery. As a result, they will need extra help postoperatively to adjust to the situation.

Diagnosis

Nursing Diagnoses

The nursing diagnoses for patients awaiting cardiac surgery will vary from patient to patient according to their cardiac disease and their symptomatology. The majority of patients will have a nursing diagnosis of decreased cardiac output (see Cardiac Failure in Chapter 28). In addition, preoperative nursing diagnoses for most patients will include the following:

- Fear related to the surgical procedure, its uncertain outcome, and the threat to well-being
- Knowledge deficit regarding the surgical procedure and the postoperative course

Collaborative Problems/Potential Complications

The stress of impending cardiac surgery may precipitate complications that require collaborative management with the physician. Based on the assessment data, potential complications that may develop include:

- Angina (or anginal equivalent)
- Severe anxiety requiring an anxiolytic (anxiety-reducing) medication
- Cardiac arrest

Planning and Implementation

Goals. The major goals of the patient may include reduction of fear, learning about the surgical procedure and postoperative course, and absence of complications.

Nursing Interventions

During the preoperative phase of cardiac surgery, the nurse develops a plan of care that includes emotional support and teaching for the patient and family. Establishing rapport, answering questions, listening to fears and concerns, clarifying misconceptions, and providing information about what to expect are all interventions the nurse uses to prepare the patient and family emotionally for the surgery and for the postoperative events.

Reducing Fear. The patient and family are allowed adequate time and repeated opportunities to express their fears. If there is fear of the unknown, other surgical experiences that the patient has had can be compared with the impending surgery. It is often helpful to describe to the patient the sensations that are expected (Anderson & Masur, 1989). If the patient has already had a cardiac catheterization, the similarities and differences between that procedure and the surgery may be compared. Also, the patient is encouraged to talk about any concerns related to previous experiences.

Discussion of the patient's fears about pain is initiated. A comparison between the pain experienced with cardiac surgery and other pain experiences is made. The preoperative sedation, the anesthetic, and the postoperative pain medications are described. The patient is reassured that the fear of pain is normal. It is explained that some pain will be experienced, but that the patient will be closely observed and that the use of medication, positioning, and relaxation will make the pain more tolerable.

Patients who have a fear of scarring from surgery are encouraged to discuss this concern; misconceptions are corrected. It may be helpful to indicate that the health care team members will keep the patient informed about the healing process.

The patient and family are encouraged to talk about their fear of dying. They should be reassured that this fear is normal. For those who only hint about this concern despite efforts to encourage them to talk about their fear, coaching is helpful (*e.g.*, "Are you worrying about not making it through surgery? Most people who have heart surgery at least think about the possibility of dying."). Once the fear is expressed, the patient and family can be helped to explore their feelings.

By alleviating undue anxiety and fear, preparing the patient emotionally for surgery lessens the chance of preoperative problems, promotes smooth anesthesia induction, and enhances the patient's involvement postoperatively in care and recovery. In addition, preparing the family for the events to come helps them to cope, be supportive to the patient, and participate in the postoperative and rehabilitative care.

Patient Education and Home Care Considerations. Patient and family teaching is based on assessed learning needs. Teaching usually includes information about hospitalization, about the surgery (the preoperative and postoperative care, the length of the surgery, pain and discomfort that can be expected, the visiting hours, and procedures in the critical care unit), and information about the recovery phase (length of hospitalization, when normal activities, such as housework, shopping, and work, can be resumed). Any changes made in medical therapy and preoperative preparations need to be explained and reinforced.

The patient is informed that physical preparation usually involves several showers or scrubs with an antiseptic solution. A sedative will be given the night before surgery and the morning of surgery. Most cardiac surgical teams use prophylactic antibiotic therapy, and the antibiotics are started preoperatively.

If the preoperative hospitalization period is very short, teaching the patient and family together may be most effective. The patient's anxiety often increases with the admission process and the impending surgery. Unless the nurse has met the patient before the day of hospitalization, the time may be too short to establish a relationship that contributes to patient learning. Teaching the patient and family together capitalizes on their established support relationship. Teaching in this phase should be directed primarily by the patient's and family's questions. Too much detail may only increase anxiety.

The patient may be offered a tour of the intensive care unit, the postanesthesia recovery room, or both. (In some hospitals, the patient will initially go to the postanesthesia care unit.) The patient recovering from anesthesia is reassured by having already seen the surroundings and having met someone from the unit. The patient and family are informed about the equipment, tubes, and lines that will be present postoperatively and their purposes. They should know to expect monitors, several intravenous lines, chest tubes, and a urinary catheter. Explaining the purpose and the approximate time that these devices will be in place helps to reassure the patient. Most patients will remain intubated and on mechanical ventilation for 4 to 48 hours postoperatively. They need to be aware that this prevents them from talking, and they should be reassured that the staff will be able to assist them with other means of communication.

The patient's questions about postoperative care and procedures should be answered. Deep breathing and coughing, use of the incentive spirometer, and foot exercises are explained and practiced by the patient preoperatively. The family's questions at this time will focus primarily on the length of the surgery, who will discuss the results of the procedure with them and when this may occur, where to wait during the surgery, the visiting privileges in the intensive care unit, and how they can support the patient preoperatively and in the intensive care unit.

Monitoring and Managing Potential Complications. The patient who develops angina usually responds to normal angina therapy, most commonly nitroglycerine placed under the tongue. Some patients require oxygen and intravenous nitroglycerine drips (see Chapter 28).

For patients who experience excessive anxiety and fear and for whom emotional support and education do not seem adequate to allay those feelings, medication therapy may be a helpful adjunct. Antianxiety or anxiolytic agents most commonly used for preoperative cardiac surgery are diazepam and lorazepam.

Should cardiac arrest occur in the preoperative period, advanced cardiac life support is provided.

Evaluation

Expected Outcomes

1. Demonstrates reduced fear
   a. Identifies fears
   b. Discusses fears with family
   c. Uses past experiences as a focus for comparison
   d. Expresses positive attitude about outcome of surgery
   e. Expresses confidence in measures to be used to relieve pain
2. Acquires knowledge about the surgical procedure and postoperative course
   a. Identifies the purposes of the preoperative preparation procedure
   b. Tours the intensive care unit, if desired.
   c. Identifies limitations expected after surgery
   d. Discusses expected immediate postoperative environment, *e.g.*, tubes, machines, nursing surveillance
   e. Demonstrates expected activities after surgery (*e.g.*, deep breathing, coughing, foot exercises)

Intraoperative Nursing Management

Most of the cardiac surgical procedures are performed through a median sternotomy incision. The patient is prepared for continuous monitoring: electrodes, indwelling catheters, and probes are placed before the procedure to facilitate assessment of the patient's status and the need for changes in therapy. Intravenous lines will be inserted as needed to administer fluids, medications, and blood products. In addition, the patient will be intubated and placed on mechanical ventilation.

Before the chest incision is closed, chest tubes are positioned to evacuate air and drainage from the mediastinum and the thorax. Epicardial pacemaker electrodes are implanted on the surface of the right atrium and the right ventricle. These epicardial electrodes can be used postoperatively to pace the heart or to monitor it for dysrhythmias via the atrial leads.

In addition to assisting with the surgical procedures, the surgical nurses are responsible for the comfort and safety of the patient. Some areas of intervention include positioning, skin care, wound care, and emotional support of the patient and family.

Possible intraoperative complications include dysrhythmias, hemorrhage, myocardial infarction, cerebral vascular accident, embolization, and organ failure secondary to shock, embolus, or adverse drug reactions. Astute intraoperative patient assessment is critical in preventing these complications as well as detecting symptoms and initiating prompt therapy.

Postoperative Nursing Management

The immediate postoperative period for the patient who has undergone cardiac surgery presents many challenges to the health care team. All efforts are made to facilitate the transition from the operating room to the intensive care unit or postanesthesia suite with minimal risk. Specific information about the operation and important factors about postoperative management are communicated by the surgical team and anesthesia personnel to the critical care nurse, who then assumes responsibility for the patient's care. Figure 30-5 presents a graphic overview of the many aspects of postoperative care of the cardiac surgical patient.

❑ NURSING PROCESS
The Patient Who Has Had Cardiac Surgery

Assessment

When the patient is admitted to the critical care unit, and at least every 4 to 12 hours thereafter, a complete assessment of all systems is performed to determine the postoperative status of the patient as compared with the preoperative baseline and to note anticipated changes since surgery. The following parameters are assessed;

- *Neurologic status*—level of responsiveness, pupil size and reaction to light, reflexes, movement of extremities, and hand grip strength
- *Cardiac status*—heart rate and rhythm, heart sounds, arterial blood pressure, central venous pressure (CVP), pulmonary artery pressure, pulmonary artery wedge pressure (PAWP), left atrial pressure (LAP), waveforms from the invasive blood pressure lines, cardiac output or index, systemic and pulmonary vascular resistance, pulmonary artery oxygen saturation ($S\bar{v}O_2$) if available, chest tube drainage, and pacemaker status and function
- *Respiratory status*—chest movement, breath sounds, ventilator settings (rate, tidal volume, oxygen concentration, mode [*e.g.*, SIMV], positive end-expiratory pressure [PEEP]), respiratory rate, ventilatory pressure, arterial oxygen saturation (SaO_2), end-tidal CO_2, chest tube drainage, arterial blood gases
- *Peripheral vascular status*—peripheral pulses; color of skin, nail beds, mucosa, lips and earlobes; skin temperature; edema; condition of dressings and invasive lines
- *Renal function*—urinary output, urine specific gravity and osmolarity
- *Fluid and electrolyte status*—intake; output from all drainage tubes; all cardiac output parameters, and the following indications of electrolyte imbalance:
  Hypokalemia: digitalis toxicity, dysrhythmias (U wave, AV block, flat or inverted T waves)
  Hyperkalemia: mental confusion, restlessness, nausea, weakness, paresthesias of extremities, dysrhythmias (tall, peaked T waves; increased amplitude, widening QRS complex; prolonged QT interval)
  Hyponatremia: weakness, fatigue, confusion, convulsions, coma
  Hypocalcemia: paresthesias, carpal pedal spasm, muscle cramps, tetany
  Hypercalcemia: digitalis toxicity, asystole
- *Pain*—nature, type, location, duration (incisional pain must be differentiated from anginal pain); apprehension; response to analgesics
- Note: Some patients who have had CABG with an internal mammary artery experience ulnar nerve paresthesia on the same side of the body as the graft. The paresthesia may be temporary or permanent. Also, patients who have had CABG with the gastroepiploic artery may experience an ileus for a longer period postoperatively and will have abdominal pain at the site of the incision as well as chest pain.

Assessment also includes observing all equipment and tubes to determine if they are functioning properly: endotracheal tube, ventilator, end-tidal CO_2 monitor, SaO_2 monitor, pulmonary artery catheter, $S\bar{v}O_2$ monitor, arterial and intravenous lines, intravenous infusion devices and tubings, cardiac monitor, pacemaker, chest tubes, and urinary drainage system.

As the patient regains consciousness and progresses through the postoperative period, the nurse expands the assessment to include parameters indicative of psychological and emotional status. The patient may exhibit behavior that reflects denial or depression or may experience postcardiotomy psychosis. Characteristic signs of psychosis include (1) transient perceptual illusions, (2) visual and auditory hallucinations, and (3) disorientation and paranoid delusions.

The needs of the family also should be assessed. The nurse ascertains how they are coping with the situation;

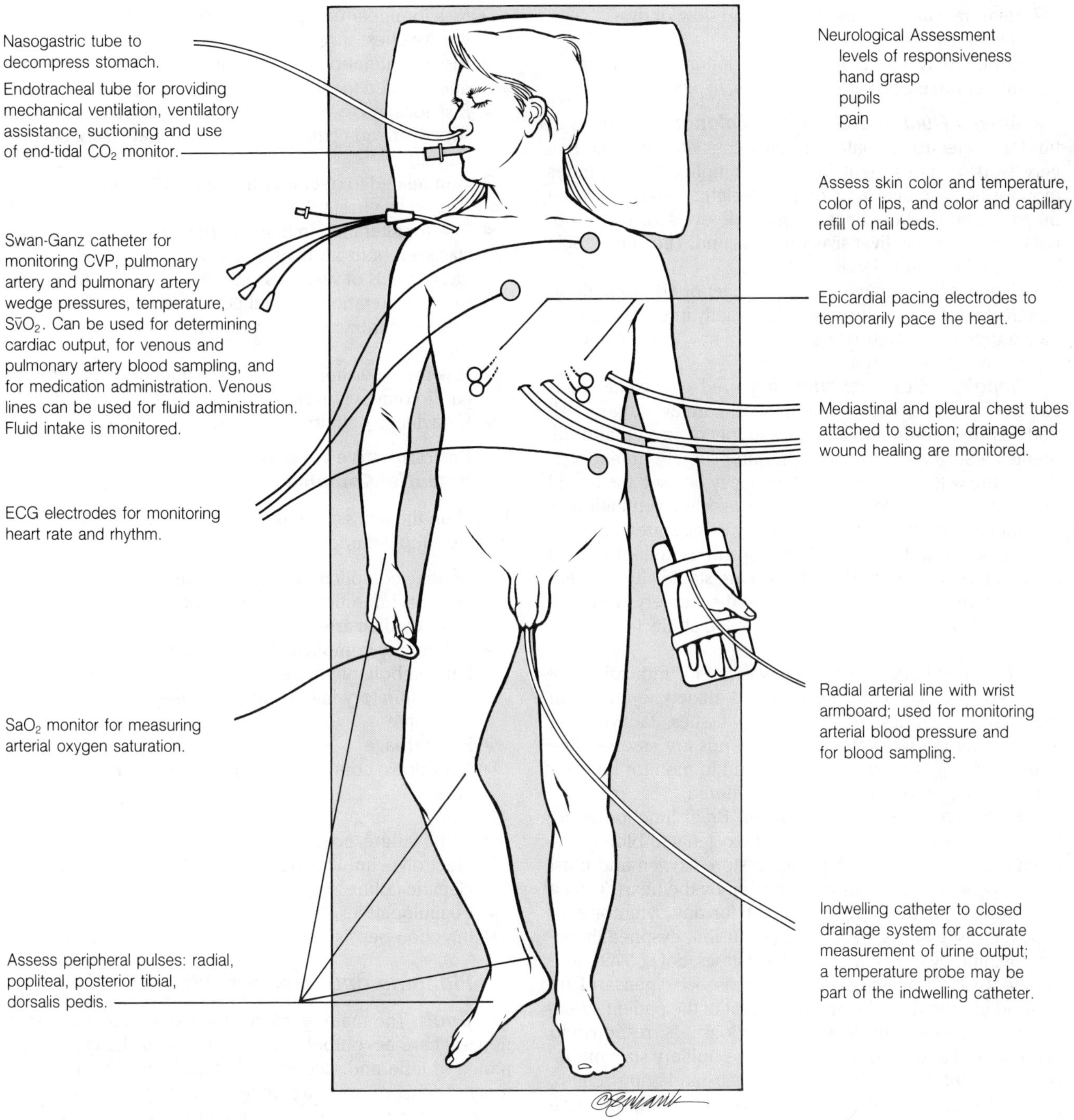
Nasogastric tube to
decompress stomach.
Endotracheal tube for providing
mechanical ventilation, ventilatory
assistance, suctioning and use
of end-tidal CO_2 monitor.
Swan-Ganz catheter for
monitoring CVP, pulmonary
artery and pulmonary artery
wedge pressures, temperature,
$S\bar{v}O_2$. Can be used for determining
cardiac output, for venous and
pulmonary artery blood sampling, and
for medication administration. Venous
lines can be used for fluid administration.
Fluid intake is monitored.
ECG electrodes for monitoring
heart rate and rhythm.
SaO_2 monitor for measuring
arterial oxygen saturation.
Assess peripheral pulses: radial,
popliteal, posterior tibial,
dorsalis pedis.
Neurological Assessment
levels of responsiveness
hand grasp
pupils
pain
Assess skin color and temperature,
color of lips, and color and capillary
refill of nail beds.
Epicardial pacing electrodes to
temporarily pace the heart.
Mediastinal and pleural chest tubes
attached to suction; drainage and
wound healing are monitored.
Radial arterial line with wrist
armboard; used for monitoring
arterial blood pressure and
for blood sampling.
Indwelling catheter to closed
drainage system for accurate
measurement of urine output;
a temperature probe may be
part of the indwelling catheter.

FIGURE 30-5. Postoperative care of the cardiac surgical patient.

what their psychological, emotional, and spiritual needs are; and whether or not they are receiving adequate information about the patient's condition.

Assessing for Complications

The patient is continuously assessed for indications of impending complications. The nurse and the physician function collaboratively to recognize early signs and symptoms of complications and to institute measures to reverse their progression.

Decreased Cardiac Output. A decrease in cardiac output is always a threat to the patient who has had cardiac surgery. It can be due to a variety of causes:

- Preload alterations—too little or too much blood volume returning to the heart because of hypovolemia, persistent bleeding, cardiac tamponade, or fluid overload
- Afterload alterations—arterioles and capillaries that are too constricted or too dilated because of alterations in body temperature or hypertension

- Heart rate alterations—too fast, too slow, or dysrhythmias
- Contractility alterations—cardiac failure, myocardial infarction, electrolyte imbalances, hypoxia

Altered Fluid and Electrolyte Balance. Alterations in fluid and electrolyte balance may occur after cardiac surgery. Nursing assessment for these complications includes monitoring of intake and output, weight, PAWP, left atrial pressure and CVP readings, hematocrit levels, distention of neck veins, edema, liver size, breath sounds (*i.e.*, fine crackles, wheezing), and electrolyte levels.

Changes in serum electrolytes are reported promptly so that treatment can be instituted. Especially important are either dangerously high or dangerously low levels of potassium, sodium, and calcium.

Impaired Gas Exchange. Impaired gas exchange is another possible complication after cardiac surgery. All body tissues require an adequate supply of oxygen and nutrients for survival. To achieve this after surgery, an endotracheal tube with ventilator assistance may be used for 4 to 48 or more hours postoperatively. The assisted ventilation is continued until the patient's blood gas measurements are acceptable and the patient demonstrates the ability to breathe independently. Patients who are stable after surgery may be extubated as early as 4 hours after surgery, which reduces their anxiety regarding their limited ability to communicate.

The patient is continuously assessed for indications of impaired gas exchange: restlessness, anxiety, cyanosis of mucous membranes and peripheral tissues, tachycardia, and fighting the ventilator. Breath sounds are assessed frequently to detect fluid in the lungs and to monitor lung expansion. Arterial blood gases are monitored.

Impaired Cerebral Circulation. Brain function is dependent on a continuous supply of oxygenated blood. The brain does not have the capacity to store oxygen and must rely on adequate continuous perfusion by the heart. Thus it is important to observe the patient for any symptoms of hypoxia: restlessness, headache, confusion, dyspnea, hypotension, and cyanosis. Arterial blood gases, SaO_2, $S\bar{v}O_2$, and end-tidal CO_2 are assessed for decreased oxygen and increased carbon dioxide. An assessment of the patient's neurologic status includes level of consciousness, response to verbal commands and painful stimuli, pupillary size and reaction to light, movement of extremities, hand grip strength, presence of pedal and popliteal pulses, as well as temperature and color of extremities. Any indication of a changing status is documented and any abnormal findings are reported to the surgeon immediately because they may signal the beginning of a complication in the postoperative period. Hypoperfusion or microemboli may produce central nervous system damage after cardiac surgery.

Diagnosis

Nursing Diagnoses

Based on the assessment data and the type of surgical procedure performed, major nursing diagnoses of the patient may include the following:

- Decreased cardiac output related to blood loss and compromised myocardial function
- Risk for impaired gas exchange related to trauma of extensive chest surgery
- Risk for alteration in fluid volume and electrolyte balance related to alteration in circulating blood volume
- Risk for sensory–perceptual alterations related to sensory overload (critical care environment, surgical experience)
- Pain related to operative trauma and pleural irritation caused by chest tubes
- Risk for alteration in tissue perfusion related to venous stasis, embolization, underlying atherosclerotic disease, effects of vasopressors, or coagulation problems
- Risk for alteration in renal perfusion related to decreased cardiac output, hemolysis, or vasopressor drug therapy
- Risk for hyperthermia related to infection or postpericardiotomy syndrome
- Knowledge deficit about self-care activities

Collaborative Problems/ Potential Complications

Based on the assessment data, potential complications that may develop include:

- Cardiac complications: congestive heart failure, myocardial infarction, stunned myocardium, dysrhythmias, cardiac arrest
- Pulmonary complications: pulmonary edema, pulmonary emboli, pleural effusions, pneumo- or hemothorax, respiratory failure, adult respiratory distress syndrome
- Hemorrhage
- Neurologic complications: cebrovascular accident, air emboli
- Pain
- Renal failure, acute or chronic
- Electrolyte imbalances
- Hepatic failure
- Coagulopathies
- Infection, sepsis

Planning and Implementation

Goals. The major goals for the patient include restoration of cardiac output, adequate gas exchange, maintenance of fluid and electrolyte balance, reduction of symptoms of sensory overload, relief of pain, promotion of rest, maintenance of adequate tissue perfusion, maintenance of adequate renal perfusion, maintenance of normal body temperature, learning self-care activities, and absence of complications.

Nursing Interventions

Restoring Cardiac Output. Nursing management of the patient involves continuously observing the patient's cardiac status and immediately notifying the surgeon of any changes that indicate decreased cardiac output. The nurse and the surgeon then work collaboratively to correct the problem.

In evaluating the patient's cardiac status, the nurse primarily determines the effectiveness of cardiac output through clinical observations and routine measurements: serial readings of blood pressure, heart rate, central venous pressure, arterial pressure, and left atrial or pulmonary artery pressure.

Renal function is related to cardiac function, as blood pressure and heart rate drive glomerular filtration; therefore, urinary output is measured and recorded. If urine output falls below 30 ml/hr, this may indicate a decrease in cardiac output. Urine specific gravity also is assessed (normal: 1.010 to 1.025), as is urine osmolality. Inadequate fluid volume may be manifested by low urinary output and a high specific gravity, whereas overhydration is exhibited by high urinary output with low specific gravity.

The growth and function of body cells depend on adequate cardiac output to provide a continuous supply of oxygenated blood to meet the changing demands of the organs and body systems. Because the buccal mucosa, nail beds, lips, and earlobes are sites with rich capillary beds, they should be observed for cyanosis or duskiness as possible signs of reduced heart action. Moist or dry skin may indicate either vasodilation or vasconstriction, respectively. Venous distention of the neck veins or of the dorsal surface of the hand raised to heart level may signal a changing demand or diminishing capacity of the heart. If cardiac output has fallen, the skin becomes cool, moist, and cyanotic or mottled.

Dysrhythmias, which may arise when poor perfusion of the heart exists, also serve as important indicators of cardiac function. The most common dysrhythmias encountered during the postoperative period are bradycardias, tachycardias, and ectopic beats. Continuous observation of the cardiac monitor for various dysrhythmias is an essential part of patient care and management.

Any indications of decreased cardiac output are reported promptly to the physician. These assessment data and results of diagnostic tests are used by the physician to determine the cause of the problem. Once a diagnosis has been made, the physician and the nurse work collaboratively to restore cardiac output and prevent further complications. When indicated, the physician prescribes blood components, fluids, digitalis, diuretics, vasodilators, or vasopressors. When further surgery is necessary, the patient and family are prepared for the procedure.

Promoting Adequate Gas Exchange. To assure adequate gas exchange, the nurse assesses and maintains the patency of the endotracheal tube. The patient is suctioned when wheezes or coarse crackles (rhonchi) are present. Suctioning may be performed with an in-line suction catheter; the nurse and respiratory therapist determine if the ventilator's fractional inspired oxygen (FiO_2) should be increased for three or more breaths before the patient is suctioned. Alternately, 100% oxygen is delivered to the patient by a manual resuscitation bag (Ambu) before and after suctioning to prevent hypoxia that can result from the suctioning procedure. Arterial blood gas determinations are compared with baseline data and changes are reported to the physician promptly.

Because a patent airway is essential for O_2 and CO_2 exchange, the endotracheal tube must be secured to prevent it from slipping into the right mainstem bronchus and occluding the airway. Frequent change of position also provides for optimal pulmonary ventilation and perfusion by allowing the lungs to expand more fully. When the patient's condition stabilizes, body position is changed every 1 to 2 hours and the nurse listens to breath sounds to detect the presence of crackles, wheezes, and fluid in the lungs. Deep breathing and coughing also are encouraged to open the alveolar sacs and provide for increased perfusion. The patient should be taught and assisted to splint the surgical chest incision before and during coughing to minimize the discomfort.

The patient may be ready for extubation when gagging or "fighting or bucking" the ventilator is observed. Before being extubated, the patient should have a cough–gag reflex and stable vital signs; be able to lift the head off the bed or give firm hand grasps; have adequate vital capacity, negative inspiratory force, and minute volume for body size; and have acceptable arterial blood gases while breathing warmed humidified oxygen without the assistance of the ventilator. Extubation has been performed within these parameters without any adverse effects on the patient's condition or prognosis. During this time the nurse assists with the weaning process and, eventually, the removal of the endotracheal tube.

Maintaining Fluid and Electrolyte Balance. To promote fluid and electrolyte balance, the nurse carefully assesses intake and output. Flow sheets are used to determine positive or negative fluid balance. All fluid intake is recorded, including intravenous fluids, flush solutions used in arterial and venous catheters and the nasogastric tube, and oral fluids. In addition, all output is recorded, including urine, nasogastric drainage, and chest drainage.

Hemodynamic parameters (blood pressure, pulmonary wedge and left atrial pressures, and CVP) are correlated with intake, output, and weight to determine the adequacy of hydration and cardiac output. Serum electrolytes are monitored and the patient is observed for signs of potassium, sodium, or calcium imbalances (hypokalemia, hyperkalemia, hyponatremia, and hypocalcemia).

Any indications of dehydration, fluid overload, or electrolyte imbalance are reported promptly, and the physician and nurse work collaboratively to restore fluid and electrolyte balance. The patient's response to fluid and electrolyte replacements or restrictions is monitored closely.

Reducing Symptoms of Sensory Overload. Sensory overload is a common effect associated with the surgical experience and environmental factors in the critical care unit. **Postcardiotomy psychosis** may occur after cardiac surgery. The term refers to a group of abnormal behaviors that occur in varying intensity and duration in a large number of patients. In the early years of cardiac surgery this phenomenon occurred more frequently than it does today. At that time it was attributed to inadequate cerebral perfusion during surgery, microemboli, and the length of time that the patient remained on the cardiopulmonary bypass machine. Advances in surgical techniques have significantly decreased these factors. Today, when it occurs, it is thought to be caused by anxiety, sleep deprivation, increased sensory input, and disorientation to night and day when the patient loses track of time. An important finding is that patients who do not or cannot express anxiety before surgery are more prone to develop psychosis in the postoperative period. Psychosis may appear after a brief lucid interval.

The nurse monitors the patient for signs of denial and provides an opportunity for emotional expression during the preoperative period. Careful explanations of all procedures and of the need for cooperation help to keep the patient oriented throughout the postoperative course. Continuity of care is desirable; a familiar face and a nursing staff with a consistent approach promote the delivery of quality nursing care. The use of a well-designed and individualized nursing care plan will provide guidelines to assist the nursing team coordinate their efforts for the emotional well-being of the patient.

Relieving Pain. Deep pain may not be reflected in the immediate area of injury but in a broader, more diffuse area. Patients who have had cardiac surgery experience pain caused by the interruption of intercostal nerves along the incision route and irritation of the pleura by the chest catheters. (Also, patients with internal mammary artery CABG may report ulnar nerve paresthesias on the same side of their body as the graft.)

It is essential to observe and listen to the patient for verbal and nonverbal clues about pain. The nurse accurately records the nature, type, location, and duration of the pain. (Incisional pain must be differentiated from anginal pain.) The patient is encouraged to accept medication as often as it is prescribed to reduce the amount of pain. The patient should then be able to participate in deep breathing and coughing exercises and to progressively increase self-care.

Pain produces tension, which may stimulate the central nervous system to release adrenaline, which results in constriction of the arterioles. This can cause increased afterload and decreased cardiac output. Morphine sulfate alleviates anxiety and pain and induces sleep, which reduces metabolic rate and oxygen demands. After the administration of opioids (narcotics), any observations indicating relief of apprehension and pain are documented in the patient's record. The patient is observed for any respiratory depressant effects of the analgesic. If respiratory depression occurs, an opioid antagonist (*e.g.*, naloxone [Narcan]) is used to counteract the effect.

Promoting Rest. Basic comfort measures used in conjunction with prescribed analgesics will potentiate the effects of the analgesics and promote rest. The patient is assisted in changing positions every 1 to 2 hours and is positioned in such a way that strain on the incisional line and chest tubes is avoided. Physical support of the incision during coughing and deep breathing helps to minimize pain. Nursing activities are scheduled as much as possible to provide undisturbed periods of rest. As the condition stabilizes and the patient is disturbed less frequently for monitoring and therapeutic procedures, rest periods can become extended.

Maintaining Adequate Tissue Perfusion. Peripheral pulses (pedal, tibial, popliteal, femoral, radial, brachial) are routinely palpated to assess for arterial obstruction. If a pulse is absent in any extremity, the cause may be prior catheterization of that extremity. The newly identified absence of any pulse is immediately reported to the physician.

After surgery, measures are taken to prevent venous stasis that can cause thrombus formation and subsequent embolization: (1) applying elastic stockings or elastic bandage wrap, (2) discouraging crossing of legs, (3) avoiding use of the knee gatch on the bed, (4) omitting pillows in the popliteal space, and (5) instituting passive exercises followed by active exercises to promote circulation and prevent loss of muscle tone.

Thrombus formation and resulting embolization also can result from injury to the intima of the blood vessels, dislodging of a clot from a damaged valve, loosening of mural thrombi, and coagulation problems. Air embolism may occur as a result of cardiopulmonary bypass. The usual embolic sites are the lungs, coronary arteries, mesentery, extremities, kidneys, spleen, and brain.

Symptoms of embolization, which vary according to site, should be observed for (1) midabdominal or midback pain; (2) pain, cessation of pulses, blanching, numbness, or coldness in an extremity; (3) chest pain and respiratory distress with pulmonary embolus or myocardial infarction; and (4) one-sided weakness and pupillary changes, such as occur in cerebral vascular accident. All such symptoms are promptly reported.

Maintaining Adequate Renal Perfusion. Inadequate renal perfusion can occur as a complication of open-heart surgery. One possible cause is low cardiac output. In addition, trauma to blood cells during cardiopulmonary bypass can cause hemolysis of red blood cells. This leads to a build-up of toxic substances because the glomeruli are occluded by the debris of the damaged red cells. Use of vasopressor agents to increase blood pressure can also lead to reduction of the blood flow to the kidneys.

Nursing management includes accurate measurement of urine output. An output of less than 20 ml/hr can indicate hypovolemia. Specific gravity tests should be carried out to determine the kidneys' ability to concentrate urine in the renal tubules. Rapid-acting diuretics or inotropic medications (digitalis, isoproterenol) may be prescribed to increase cardiac output and renal blood flow. The nurse should be aware of the blood urea nitrogen (BUN) and serum creatinine levels as well as urine and serum electrolyte levels. Abnormalities in these studies are reported promptly because it may be necessary to restrict fluids and limit the use of medications that are normally excreted by the kidneys.

If efforts to maintain renal perfusion are not effective, the patient may require peritoneal dialysis or hemodialysis (see Chapter 42).

Maintaining Normal Body Temperature. Patients are usually hypothermic when admitted to the critical care unit from the cardiac surgical procedure. The patient must be gradually warmed to a normal temperature. This is accomplished partially by the patient's own basal metabolic processes and often with the assistance of warmed ventilator air, warm blankets, or heat lamps. While the patient is hypothermic, the clotting process is less efficient, the heart is prone to dysrhythmias, and oxygen does not readily transfer from the hemoglobin to the tissues. Because anesthesia suppresses the basal metabolism, oxygen supply usually meets the cellular demand.

After cardiac surgery the patient is at risk for developing elevated body temperature caused by infection or postpericardiotomy syndrome. The resultant increase in metabolic rate increases tissue oxygen demands and thus increases cardiac workload. Measures are taken to prevent this sequence of events or to halt it as soon as it is recognized.

Sites of infection include the lungs, urinary tract, incisions, and intravascular catheters. Meticulous care is used to prevent contamination at the sites of catheter and tube insertions. Sterile technique is used when changing dressings and when providing endotracheal tube and catheter care. Clearance of pulmonary secretions is accomplished by frequent repositioning of the patient, chest physical therapy, and suctioning. A closed system is used to maintain all intravenous and arterial lines.

Postpericardiotomy syndrome occurs in approximately 10% to 40% of patients who undergo cardiac surgery. Its precise cause is unknown. A common factor appears to be trauma, with residual blood in the pericardial sac after surgery. The syndrome is characterized by fever, pericardial pain, pleural pain, dyspnea, pleural effusion and pericardial friction, and arthralgia. There may be a combination of these signs and symptoms. Leukocytosis is present, along with elevation of the sedimentation rate. These symptoms frequently appear after the patient is discharged from the hospital.

The syndrome must be differentiated from other postoperative complications (incisional pain, myocardial infarction, pulmonary embolus, bacterial endocarditis, pneumonia, or atelectasis). The treatment is dependent on the severity of the symptoms. Bed rest and anti-inflammatory agents, such as salicylates and corticosteroids, lead to a dramatic improvement in symptoms.

Evaluation

Expected Outcomes

See Nursing Care Plan 30-1 for specific outcomes.

1. Achieves adequate cardiac output
2. Maintains adequate gas exchange
3. Maintains fluid and electrolyte balance
4. Experiences decreased symptoms of sensory overload; is reoriented to person, place, and time
5. Experiences relief of pain
6. Maintains adequate tissue perfusion
7. Achieves adequate rest
8. Maintains adequate renal perfusion
9. Maintains normal body temperature
10. Performs self-care activities

A typical postoperative nursing care plan for the cardiac surgery patient is presented in Nursing Care Plan 30-1.

Potential Complications of Cardiac Surgery

Cardiac Complications

Cardiac complications following heart surgery may be diagnosed and treated according to the four components of cardiac output: preload, afterload, heart rate, and contractility. Each of these elements will be considered separately. However, the patient may require interventions for more than one component at a time. Collaboration between the nurses, physicians, pharmacists, and respiratory therapists is necessary to achieve the desired patient outcomes.

Preload Alterations. **Hypovolemia** is the most common cause of decreased cardiac output after cardiac surgery. The surgical procedure may have involved blood loss, although some of it will have been replaced to provide the patient with sufficient hemoglobin to carry oxygen to the tissues. As the hypothermic patient's body temperature rises, the blood vessels dilate and more volume is needed to fill the vessels. The capillary beds are more permeable as a result of cardiopulmonary bypass, and intravenous fluid is lost to the interstitial spaces. Arterial hypotension with low pulmonary artery wedge pressure (PAWP) and low central venous pressures (CVP) often are seen with an increased heart rate. The physician usually prescribes fluid replacement with a colloid (albumin or protein) or starch (hetastarch), but packed red blood cells or a crystalloid solution (normal saline, lactated Ringer's solution) may be prescribed.

Persistent bleeding can cause hypovolemia. The cardiopulmonary bypass procedure may cause platelets to function abnormally, therefore blood may not clot normally. Also, the clotting mechanisms do not work well when a patient is hypothermic. The patient has experienced a surgical procedure that causes trauma to tissues and blood vessels that continue to ooze bloody drainage. In addition, the patient usually has received anticoagulants.

Accurate measurement of wound and drainage tube bleeding is essential. Bloody drainage should not exceed 200 ml/hr for the first 4 to 6 hours. The drainage should decrease and stop within a few days, while progressing from sanguineous to serosanguineous and serous drainage. Bleeding may be treated with protamine sulfate to neutralize the heparin. Vitamin K and blood products may be used to replace deficiencies of the hematologic system. If the bleeding persists, the patient will be returned to the operating room for exploratory surgery; any bleeding sites are then controlled.

Cardiac tamponade also may decrease preload to the heart by preventing the available blood from getting into the heart. Fluid accumulates in the pericardial sac, which compresses the heart from the outside, preventing blood from filling the ventricles. Arterial hypotension, tachycardia, muffled heart sounds, and decreasing urine output are seen with an equalizing of the PAWP, CVP, and pulmonary artery diastolic (PAD) pressures. The arterial and pulmonary artery pressure waveforms also may demonstrate a pulsus paradoxus (a decrease of more than 10 mm Hg during inspiration). The chest tube drainage is usually decreased, suggesting that the drainage is trapped or clotted in the mediastinum.

Efforts are made to assure that there are no kinks or obstructions in the tubing. The nurse may try to reestablish patency of the drainage system by milking the tubing (care must be taken not to strip the tubing, creating massive negative pressure within the chest, which may cause harm to the surgical repair or stimulate a dysrhythmia). A chest x-ray may show a widening mediastinum. Emergency medical management is required, which may include a pericardiocentesis (see Chapter 28).

Fluid overload is a less common problem for postcardiac surgery patients. High PAWP, CVP, and PAD pressures as well as crackles indicate fluid overload. Diuretics are usually prescribed and the rate of intravenous fluid administration is slowed. The patient may be placed on a fluid restriction. Alternative treatments are continuous arterial–venous hemofiltration, dialysis, and phlebotomy.

Afterload Alterations. Afterload is the force that the ventricle must overcome to move blood forward. Vascular

(text continues on page 716)

NURSING CARE PLAN 30–1
Postoperative Nursing Care of the Cardiac Surgery Patient

NURSING DIAGNOSIS: Decreased cardiac output related to blood loss and compromised myocardial function.

GOAL: Restoration of cardiac output to maintain/attain desired lifestyle.

Nursing Interventions	Rationale	Expected Outcomes
1. Monitor cardiovascular status. Serial readings of blood pressures (arterial, left atrial, pulmonary artery, pulmonary artery wedge pressure [PAWP], central venous pressure [CVP]), cardiac output/index, systemic and pulmonary vascular resistance, and cardiac rhythm and rate are obtained, recorded and correlated with the patient's condition.	1. Effectiveness of cardiac output is determined by hemodynamic monitoring.	The following parameters are within the patient's normal ranges: • Arterial pressure • Left atrial pressure • PAWP • Pulmonary artery pressures • CVP • Heart sounds • Pulmonary and systemic vascular resistance • Cardiac output and cardiac index • Peripheral pulses • Cardiac rate and rhythm • Cardiac enzymes • Urine output • Skin and mucosal color • Skin temperature
a. Assess arterial pressure every 15 minutes until stable, and as directed thereafter.	a. Blood pressure is one of the most important physiologic parameters to follow; vasoconstriction after cardiopulmonary bypass may make auscultatory blood pressure unobtainable.	
b. Auscultate for heart sounds and rhythm.	b. Auscultation provides evidence of cardiac tamponade (muffled distant heart sounds), pericarditis (precordial rub), dysrhythmias.	
c. Assess all peripheral pulses (pedal, tibial, popliteal, femoral, radial, brachial, carotid).	c. Presence or absence and quality of pulses provide data about cardiac output as well as obstructive lesions.	
d. Measure left atrial pressure, pulmonary artery diastolic (PAD) pressure, PAWP to determine left ventricular end-diastolic volume and to assess cardiac output (see Guideline 28-1).	d. Rising pressures may indicate congestive heart failure or pulmonary edema.	
e. Monitor PAWP, PAD, left atrial pressure, and CVP to assess blood volume, vascular tone, and pumping effectiveness of the heart. *Remember: Trends are more important than isolated readings;* mechanical ventilator may elevate CVP.	e. High PAWP, PAD, left atrial pressure, or CVP may result from hypervolemia, heart failure, cardiac tamponade; if blood pressure drop is due to low blood volume, PAWP, PAD, left atrial pressure, and CVP will show corresponding drop.	
f. Monitor ECG pattern for cardiac dysrhythmias (see Chap. 27 for discussion of dysrhythmias).	f. Dysrhythmias may occur with coronary ischemia, hypoxia, alterations in serum potassium, edema, bleeding, acid–base or electrolyte disturbances, digitalis toxicity, cardiac failure. ST segment changes may indicate myocardial ischemia or coronary artery spasm. Pacemaker capture and antidysrhythmic medication effects are used to maintain a heart rate and rhythm to support stable blood pressures.	
g. Assess cardiac enzymes daily (if ordered).	g. Elevations may indicate myocardial infarction.	

(continued)

NURSING CARE PLAN 30–1 *(continued)*
Postoperative Nursing Care of the Cardiac Surgery Patient

Nursing Interventions	Rationale	Expected Outcomes
h. Measure urine output every ½ to 1 hour at first, then with vital signs.	h. Urine output less than 30 ml/hr indicates decreased cardiac output and decreased renal perfusion.	
i. Observe buccal mucosa, nail beds, lips, ear lobes, and extremities.	i. Duskiness and cyanosis may indicate decreased cardiac output.	
j. Assess skin; note temperature and color.	j. Cool moist skin indicates vasoconstriction and decreased cardiac output.	
2. Observe for persistent bleeding: steady, continuous drainage of blood; hypotension; low CVP; tachycardia. Prepare to administer blood products, IV solutions.	2. Bleeding can result from cardiac incision, tissue fragility, trauma to tissues, clotting defects.	• Less than 300 ml/hr of drainage through chest tubes during first 4 to 6 hours • Vital signs stable
3. Observe for cardiac tamponade: hypotension; rising PAWP, PAD, left atrial pressure, or CVP; muffled heart sounds; weak, thready pulse; jugular vein distention; decreasing urinary output. Check for diminished amount of blood in chest drainage collection system. Prepare for pericardiocentesis (see Chap. 28). Assess for pulsus paradoxus.	3. Cardiac tamponade results from bleeding into the pericardial sac or accumulation of fluid in the sac, which compresses the heart and prevents adequate filling of the ventricles. Decrease in chest drainage may indicate fluid is accumulating in the pericardial sac.	• Vital signs stable • Chest tube drainage expected amount • CVP and left atrial pressures within normal limits • Urinary output within normal limits
4. Observe for cardiac failure: hypotension, rising PAWP, PAD, CVP, and left atrial pressure, tachycardia, restlessness, agitation, cyanosis, venous distention, dyspnea, ascites. Prepare to administer diuretics and digitalis.	4. Cardiac failure results from decreased pumping action of the heart; can cause deficient blood perfusion to vital organs.	• Vital signs stable • CVP and left atrial pressures within normal limits • Skin color normal • Respirations unlabored, clear breath sounds
5. Observe for myocardial infarction: ST segment elevations, T wave changes, decreased cardiac output in presence of normal circulating volume and filling pressures. Obtain serial ECGs and isoenzymes. Differentiate myocardial pain from incisional pain.	5. Symptoms may be masked by the patient's level of consciousness and pain medication.	• Vital signs stable • Pain limited to incision • ECG and isoenzymes negative for ischemic changes

NURSING DIAGNOSIS: Risk for impaired gas exchange related to trauma of extensive chest surgery

GOAL: Adequate gas exchange

Nursing Interventions	Rationale	Expected Outcomes
Assess respiratory status and provide for adequate ventilation and tissue oxygenation.		
1. Maintain assist-controlled, or intermittent (synchronous if possible) ventilation.	1. Ventilatory support is used the first 4 to 48 hours to decrease work of the heart, to maintain effective ventilation, and to provide an airway in the event of cardiac arrest.	• Airway patent • ABGs within normal range • Endotracheal tube correctly placed, as evidenced by x-ray • Breath sounds clear
2. Monitor arterial blood gases, tidal volumes, peak inspiratory pressures, and extubation parameters.	2. ABGs and tidal volume indicate effectiveness of ventilator and changes that need to be made to improve gas exchange.	• Ventilator synchronous with respirations. • Breath sounds clear after suctioning. • Nail beds and mucous membranes pink.
3. Auscultate chest for breath sounds.	3. Crackles indicate pulmonary congestion; decreased or absent breath sounds indicate pneumothorax.	• Mental acuity consistent with amount of sedatives and analgesics received

(continued)

Postoperative Nursing Care of the Cardiac Surgery Patient

Nursing Interventions	Rationale	Expected Outcomes
4. Sedate patient adequately, as prescribed, and monitor respiratory rate and depth if ventilations are not "controlled."	4. Sedation helps the patient to tolerate the endotracheal tube and to cope with ventilatory sensations; sedatives can depress respiratory rate and depth.	• Oriented to person; able to respond yes and no appropriately
5. Provide chest physiotherapy as prescribed.	5. Aids in preventing retention of secretions and atelectasis	
6. Promote deep breathing, coughing, and turning. Encourage use of incentive spirometer and compliance with breathing treatments. Teach incisional splinting with a "cough pillow" to decrease discomfort during deep breathing and coughing.	6. Aids in keeping airway patent, preventing atelectasis, and facilitating lung expansion.	
7. Suction tracheobronchial secretions as needed, using strict aseptic technique.	7. Retention of secretions leads to hypoxia and possible cardiac arrest; retained secretions promote infection.	
8. See Chapter 23 for weaning process and endotracheal tube removal.		

NURSING DIAGNOSIS: Risk for alteration in fluid volume and electrolyte balance related to alternations in blood volume

GOAL: Fluid and electrolyte balance

Nursing Interventions	Rationale	Expected Outcomes
1. Maintain fluid and electrolyte balance.	1. Adequate circulating blood volume is necessary for optimum cellular activity; metabolic acidosis and electrolyte imbalance can occur after use of cardiopulmonary bypass.	• Fluid intake and output balanced • Hemodynamic assessment parameters negative for fluid overload and dehydration • Exhibits normal blood pressure with position changes • Absence of dysrhythmia
a. Keep intake and output flow sheets; record urine volume every ½ to 2 hours while in critical care unit; then every 4 hours.	a. Provides a method to determine positive or negative fluid balance and fluid requirements	
b. Assess the following parameters: pulmonary artery pressures, left atrial pressures, blood pressure, CVP, pulmonary artery wedge pressure, weight, electrolyte levels, hematocrit, jugular venous pressure, tissue turgor, liver size, breath sounds, urinary output, and nasogastric tube drainage.	b. Provides information about state of hydration	
c. Measure postoperative chest drainage (should not exceed 300 ml/hr for first 4 to 6 hours); cessation of drainage may indicate kinked or blocked chest tube. Assure patency and integrity of the drainage system. Maintain autotransfusion system if in use.	c. Excessive blood loss from chest cavity can cause hypovolemia.	
2. Be alert to changes in serum electrolyte levels.	2. A specific concentration of electrolytes is necessary in both extracellular and intracellular body fluids to sustain life.	• Blood *p*H 7.35 to 7.45 • Serum potassium 3.5 to 5.0 mEq/L (3.5–5.0 mmol/L)

(continued)

NURSING CARE PLAN 30–1 *(continued)*
Postoperative Nursing Care of the Cardiac Surgery Patient

Nursing Interventions	Rationale	Expected Outcomes
a. Hypokalemia (low potassium) *Effects:* dysrhythmias, digitalis toxicity, metabolic acidosis, weakened myocardium, cardiac arrest Observe for specific ECG changes. Administer IV potassium replacement as directed.	a. *Causes:* inadequate intake, diuretics, vomiting, excessive nasogastric drainage, stress from surgery	• Serum sodium 135 to 145 mEq/L (135–145 mmol/L) • Serum calcium 8.8 to 10.3 mg/100 ml (2.20–2.58 mmol/L)
b. Hyperkalemia (high potassium) *Effects:* mental confusion, restlessness, nausea, weakness, paresthesias of extremities Be prepared to administer an ion-exchange resin (sodium polystyrene sulfonate [Kayexalate]), IV sodium bicarbonate or IV insulin and glucose.	b. *Causes:* Increased intake, hemolysis from cardiopulmonary bypass/mechanical assist devices, acidosis, renal insufficiency, tissue necrosis, adrenal cortical insufficiency. The resin binds potassium and promotes intestinal excretion of it. IV sodium bicarbonate drives potassium into the cells from extracellular fluid. Insulin assists the cells with glucose absorption. The glucose provides the energy to activate the sodium/potassium pumps, which pull potassium into the cell while pumping sodium out.	
c. Hyponatremia (low sodium) *Effects:* weakness, fatigue, confusion, convulsions, coma Administer sodium or diuretics as directed.	c. *Causes:* reduction of total body sodium, or increased water intake causing dilution of sodium	
d. Hypocalcemia (low calcium) *Effects:* numbness and tingling in fingertips, toes, ears, nose; carpopedal spasm; muscle cramps; tetany Administer replacement therapy as directed.	d. *Causes:* alkalosis, multiple blood transfusions of citrated blood products	
e. Hypercalcemia (high calcium) *Effects:* dysrhythmias, digitalis toxicity, asystole Institute treatment as directed.	e. *Cause:* prolonged immobility	

NURSING DIAGNOSIS: Risk for sensory-perceptual alterations related to sensory overload

GOAL: Reduction of symptoms of sensory overload; prevention of postcardiotomy syndrome

Nursing Interventions	Rationale	Expected Outcomes
1. Use measures to prevent postcardiotomy syndrome: a. Explain all procedures and the need for patient cooperation. b. Plan nursing care to provide for periods of uninterrupted sleep with day–night pattern. c. Decrease sleep-preventing environmental stimuli as much as possible.	1. Postcardiotomy syndrome may result from anxiety, sleep deprivation, increased sensory input, disorientation to night and day. Normally, sleep cycles are at least 50 minutes long. The first cycle may be as long as 90 to 120 minutes and then shorten during successive cycles. Sleep deprivation results when the sleep cycles are interrupted or there are not enough of them.	• Patient cooperates with procedures. • Sleeps for long, uninterrupted intervals • Oriented to person, place, time • Experiences no perceptual distortions, hallucinations, disorientation, delusions

(continued)

NURSING CARE PLAN 30–1 *(continued)*
Postoperative Nursing Care of the Cardiac Surgery Patient

Nursing Interventions	Rationale	Expected Outcomes
d. Promote continuity of care from nurse to nurse. e. Orient to time and place frequently. Encourage family to visit at regular times. f. Assess for medications that may contribute to delirium g. Teach relaxation techniques and diversions. h. Encourage self-care as much as tolerated to enhance self-control. Assess support systems and coping mechanisms 2. Observe for symptoms: perceptual distortions, hallucinations, disorientation, paranoid delusions.		

NURSING DIAGNOSIS: Pain related to operative trauma and pleural irritation caused by chest tubes

GOAL: Relief of pain

Nursing Interventions	Rationale	Expected Outcomes
1. Record nature, type, location, and duration of pain.	1. Pain and anxiety increase pulse rate, oxygen consumption, and cardiac workload.	• States pain is decreasing in severity • Reports absence of pain • Restlessness decreased • Vital signs stable • Participates in deep breathing and coughing exercises • Verbalizes fewer complaints of pain each day • Positions self; participates in care activities • Gradually increases activity
2. Assist patient to differentiate between surgical pain and anginal pain.	2. Anginal pain requires immediate treatment.	
3. Encourage routine pain medication dosing for the first 24 to 72 hours and observe for side effects of lethargy, hypotension, tachycardia, respiratory depression.	3. Analgesia promotes rest, decreases oxygen consumption caused by pain, and aids patient in performing deep breathing and coughing exercises.	

NURSING DIAGNOSIS: Risk for alteration in renal perfusion related to decreased cardiac output, hemolysis, or vasopressor drug therapy

GOAL: Maintenance of adequate renal perfusion

Nursing Interventions	Rationale	Expected Outcomes
1. Assess renal function:	1. Renal injury can be caused by deficient perfusion, hemolysis, low cardiac output, and use of vasopressor agents to increase blood pressure.	• Urine output consistent with fluid intake; greater than 20 ml/hr • Urine specific gravity 1.015 to 1.025 • BUN, creatinine, electrolytes within normal limits
a. Measure urine output every ½ to 1 hour.	a. Less than 20 ml/hr indicates decreased renal function.	
b. Measure urine specific gravity	b. Indicates kidneys' ability to concentrate urine in renal tubules.	
c. Monitor and report lab results: BUN, serum creatinine, urine and serum electrolytes.	c. Indicate kidneys' ability to excrete waste products	
2. Prepare to administer rapid-acting diuretics or inotropic drugs (dopamine, dobutamine).	2. Promote renal function and increase cardiac output and renal blood flow	
3. Prepare patient for peritoneal dialysis or hemodialysis if indicated.		

(continued)

NURSING CARE PLAN 30–1 *(continued)*
Postoperative Nursing Care of the Cardiac Surgery Patient

Nursing Interventions	Rationale	Expected Outcomes
NURSING DIAGNOSIS: Risk for hyperthermia related to infection or postpericardiotomy syndrome		
GOAL: Maintenance of normal body temperature		
1. Assess temperature every hour.	1. Fever can indicate infectious process or postpericardiotomy syndrome.	• Normal body temperature • Incisions are free of infection and are healing • Absence of symptoms of postpericardiotomy syndrome
2. Use sterile technique when changing dressings, suctioning endotracheal tube; maintain closed system for all intravenous and arterial lines and for indwelling catheter.	2. Decreases chance of infection	
3. Observe for symptoms of postpericardiotomy syndrome: fever, malaise, pericardial effusion, pericardial friction rub, arthralgia.	3. Occurs in 10% to 40% of patients after cardiac surgery	
4. Administer anti-inflammatory agents as directed.	4. Relieve symptoms of inflammation (*e.g.*, warmth or feverish sensation, swelling, fullness, stiffness or aching sensation, and fatigue).	
NURSING DIAGNOSIS: Knowledge deficit about self-care activities		
GOAL: Ability to perform self-care activities		
1. Develop teaching plan for patient and family. Provide specific instructions for the following: • Diet • Activity progression • Exercise • Deep breathing, coughing, lung expansion exercises • Temperature monitoring • Medication regimen • Pulse taking • CPR, if appropriate for the family to learn • Entry to the emergency medical system • Need for Medic-Alert identification	1. Each patient will have unique learning needs.	• Patient and family members explain and comply with all aspects of therapeutic regimen • Patient and family members identify lifestyle changes necessitated by therapeutic regimen • Has copy of discharge instructions • Makes follow-up phone calls weekly • Keeps follow-up appointments with surgeon
2. Provide verbal and written instructions; provide several teaching sessions for reinforcement and answering questions.	2. Repetition promotes learning by allowing for clarification of misinformation. After cardiac surgery, patients have short-term memory difficulty; written information is helpful because it can be used as a resource even after discharge. The less familiar or greater the amount of the content the patient and family need to learn, the more time it will take to learn.	
3. Involve family in all teaching sessions	3. Family member responsible for home care is usually anxious and requires adequate time for learning.	

(continued)

NURSING CARE PLAN 30-1 *(continued)*
Postoperative Nursing Care of the Cardiac Surgery Patient

Nursing Interventions	Rationale	Expected Outcomes
4. Provide information regarding follow-up phone call to surgeon or cardiologist and assigned liaison nurse; follow-up visit with surgeon in 4 to 6 weeks. 5. Make appropriate referrals: home care agency, community support groups, Mended Hearts Club.	4. Arrangements for phone contacts with health-care personnel help to allay anxieties.	

resistance may be calculated to assess afterload and the effects of any vasoactive treatments. The patient's body temperature is the most common cause of alterations in afterload after cardiac surgery. With **hypothermia,** the blood vessels are constricted, increasing afterload. The treatment is to rewarm the patient gradually, although vasodilators may be required if the resistance is too great to wait for rewarming. Conversely, a fever or other hyperthermic condition dilates blood vessels, decreasing afterload. The treatment is to restore normothermia, but the patient may require vasopressor or volume support during a fever or if the vasodilatation is severe.

Hypertension is another cause of increased afterload. Some patients will have a history of this condition and the nurse can anticipate treatment postoperatively. Other patients experience transient hypertension. Vasodilators (nitroglycerine, nitroprusside) may be used to treat hypertension. If hypertension was present before surgery, the patient is returned to the preoperative management regimen as soon as possible.

Heart Rate Alterations. **Tachydysrhythmias** should first be assessed to establish that they are not the result of preload or afterload alterations. If a tachydysrhythmia is the primary symptom, the heart rhythm is assessed and medications (*e.g.*, digoxin, quinidine, verapamil, esmolol, propranolol, lidocaine, procainamide, bretylium) are prescribed. Carotid massage may be performed by a physician to assist with diagnosing or treating the dysrhythmia. Cardioversion and defibrillation are alternatives for symptomatic tachydysrhythmias.

Bradycardias also may cause symptoms. Many postoperative patients will have temporary pacer wires that can be attached to a pulse generator (pacemaker) to stimulate the heart to beat at a faster rate. Less commonly, atropine, epinephrine, or isoproterenol may be used to increase the heart rate.

Dysrhythmias may or may not affect cardiac output. Those that do affect cardiac output are treated with medications, pacemakers, carotid massage, cardioversion, or defibrillation. The primary goal of treatment is to return the heart to a normal sinus rhythm. Some patients are unable to attain a normal sinus rhythm, so an alternate goal may be to establish a stable rhythm that produces a cardiac output sufficient for the patient.

Contractility Alterations. **Cardiac failure** results when the heart fails as a pump and the chambers cannot adequately empty (see Chapter 28). The nurse observes for and reports falling mean arterial pressure; rising PAWP, PAD, and CVP; increasing tachycardia; restlessness and agitation; peripheral cyanosis; venous distention; labored respirations; and edema. Medical management includes diuretics and digitalization.

Myocardial infarction may occur intraoperatively or postoperatively. A portion of the cardiac muscle dies, therefore contractility decreases. Until the infarcted area becomes edematous, the ventricular wall moves paradoxically during contractions, further decreasing cardiac output. Symptoms may be masked by the postoperative surgical discomfort or the anesthesia–analgesia regimen. Careful assessment of pain must be made to determine the type of pain the patient is experiencing. A myocardial infarction should be suspected if the mean blood pressure is low with normal preload. The systemic vascular resistance (afterload) and heart rate may be elevated to compensate for poor contractility. Serial ECGs and cardiac enzymes assist in making the diagnosis. Analgesics are prescribed in small amounts while the patient's blood pressure and respiratory rate are monitored (because vasodilatation secondary to analgesics or decreasing pain may occur and compound the hypotension). Activity progression depends on the patient's tolerance.

Hypoxia and electrolyte imbalances, such as hypokalemia (see the following section), decrease contractility of the cardiac muscle. Tachycardia and hypotension may be seen. The patient's ventricular stroke work index may be calculated to assist with assessment of contractility.

Pulmonary Complications

Pulmonary complications are often detected during assessment of breath sounds, oxygen saturation levels, and end-tidal CO_2 levels, as well as by monitoring peak pressure and exhaled tidal volumes on the ventilator. Arterial blood gas results and mixed venous saturations also are monitored when available. Extended periods of mechanical ventilation are often required while the complications are treated and until they are resolved.

Hemorrhage

Hemorrhage usually requires surgical intervention. Blood products are often administered, in addition to autotransfusion if it is available. PEEP may be used to increase pressure on the mediastinum.

Neurologic Complications

Neurologically, most patients begin to recover from anesthesia within 1 to 6 hours. Patients who are unable to follow simple commands within 6 hours or who demonstrate different capabilities between the right side and left sides of their bodies should be evaluated for possible stroke (CVA) or air embolization. Patient who are elderly or have renal or hepatic failure may take longer to recover.

Pain

The management of pain has been the subject of AHCPR guidelines (discussed in Chapter 13). All patients have the right to effective pain management. A collaborative effort of pharmacologic and nonpharmacologic interventions must be provided.

Renal Failure and Electrolyte Imbalances

Renal failure may be responsive to diuretics or may require hemodialysis. Renal failure is usually acute and resolves within 3 months, but may become chronic and require ongoing hemodialysis. Acute tubular necrosis (ATN) is often the result of hypoperfusion of the kidneys but may result from the kidneys attempting to clear medication or from exacerbation of a pre-existing condition. Fluid, electrolyte, and urine output are monitored continuously. Major electrolyte imbalances (hypokalemia, hyperkalemia, hypernatremia, hyponatremia, hypocalcemia, or hypercalcemia) must be detected and treated immediately.

Hypokalemia. ***Hypokalemia*** (low potassium) may be caused by inadequate intake, diuretics, vomiting, diarrhea, excessive nasogastric drainage, and stress due to surgery (increased aldosterone secretion produces decreased potassium ion [K^+] and increased sodium ion [Na^+] retention). The patient must be observed carefully when serum potassium rises or falls outside the normal level (normal K^+ = 3.5 to 5.0 mEq/L [3.5 to 5.0 mmol/L]). Some cardiac surgeons believe that it is important to maintain the K^+ level at 4.0 mEq/L (4.0 mmol/L) or higher to avoid dysrhythmias in the postoperative period. The following effects of low K^+ may be noted: digitalis toxicity, dysrhythmias, metabolic alkalosis, a weakened myocardium, and cardiac arrest. One possible specific ECG change is the presence of a **U wave** (a positive deflection following the T wave) that is more than 1 mm high. Additional signs are AV block, flat or inverted T waves, and low voltage. When necessary, the physician prescribes intravenous potassium replacement.

Hyperkalemia. ***Hyperkalemia*** (high potassium) may be caused by increased intake, red cell hemolysis caused by cardiopulmonary bypass or mechanical assist devices, acidosis, renal insufficiency, tissue necrosis, and adrenal cortical insufficiency. The following effects of high K^+ may be exhibited: mental confusion, restlessness, nausea, weakness, and paresthesias of the extremities. ECG changes specific for hyperkalemia are tall, peaked T waves, increased amplitude, a widening of the QRS complex, and a prolonged QT interval.

The physician may prescribe an ion exchange resin, sodium polystyrene sulfonate (Kayexalate), which binds the potassium in the GI tract and results in decreased serum potassium. Alternative treatments are intravenous (IV) sodium bicarbonate or IV insulin and glucose to temporarily drive the potassium back into the cells from the extracellular fluid. Hemodialysis or peritoneal dialysis may be used.

Hypernatremia and Hyponatremia. Both **hypernatremia** (high sodium) and **hyponatremia** (low sodium) may occur after cardiac surgery; however, hyponatremia is more common. Hyponatremia may result from a reduction of total body sodium or from an increase in water intake, which causes a dilution of body sodium. The patient must be observed for sodium values that vary from the normal ranges (*i.e.*, normal Na^+ = 135 to 145 mEq/L [135 to 145 mmol/L]). The nurse observes for symptoms of hyponatremia: weakness, fatigue, confusion, convulsions, and coma. When there is a true loss of sodium from the body, the physician prescribes sodium replacement. Diuretics are prescribed when reduction in sodium is due to increased water intake.

Hypocalcemia. ***Hypocalcemia*** (low calcium) can be caused by alkalosis, which reduces the amount of Ca^{++} in the extracellular fluid. Another cause may be transfusions of large amounts of citrated blood products—packed red blood cells or whole blood. (Most blood banks now use very little citrate to store blood as compared with the amounts used before 1985.) Citrate binds with calcium, reducing the amount of circulating ionized calcium.

The calcium level is monitored to determine if it is within normal limits (normal Ca^{++} = 8.8 to 10.3 mg/100 ml [2.20 to 2.58 mmol/L]). The nurse assesses the patient for symptoms of reduced calcium: numbness and tingling in the fingertips, toes, ears, and nose; carpopedal spasm; and muscle cramps and tetany. Any symptoms of hypocalcemia are reported promptly so that the physician can institute calcium replacement immediately.

Hypercalcemia. ***Hypercalcemia*** (high calcium) can cause dysrhythmias that imitate those caused by digitalis toxicity. Calcium is known to potentiate, or enhance, the action of digitalis. Therefore, the nurse assesses the patient for signs of digitalis toxicity and reports these immediately so that the physician can institute treatment to prevent asystole and death.

Other Complications

Hepatic failure, although rare, is most common in patients with cirrhosis, hepatitis, or prolonged right-sided heart failure. Medications metabolized by the liver must be minimized. Coagulopathies may develop and require treatment. Bilirubin, albumin, and amylase levels are monitored and nutritional support must be provided. If hepatic failure cannot be reversed, the patient will die.

Coagulopathies may be the result of hypothermia, blood component depletion, anticoagulation, or liver dysfunction. Each patient must be carefully evaluated to determine the cause. Appropriate therapy is then provided.

Infection is a risk for any patient undergoing surgery. Cardiopulmonary bypass and anesthesia alter the patient's immune system. Many invasive devices are used to monitor and support the patient's recovery and may serve as a source of infection. The following parameters must be monitored to detect signs of possible infection: body temperature, white blood cell counts and differential counts, suture and puncture sites, cardiac output and systemic vascular resistance, urine (clarity, color, and odor), sputum (color, odor, amount), as well as nasogastric secretions. Antibiotic therapy may be expanded or modified to meet the situation. Invasive devices must be discontinued as soon as they are no longer required. Institutional protocols for maintaining and replacing invasive lines and devices must be followed to minimize the patient's risk for infection.

Patient Education and Home Care Considerations

Depending on the type of surgery and postoperative progress, the patient may be discharged from the hospital as early as 5 days after surgery. Although the patient may be anxious to return home, usually both patient and family have apprehensions about this transition. The family often expresses the fear that they are not capable of caring for the patient at home. They often are concerned that complications will occur that they are unprepared to handle.

The nurse helps the patient and family to set realistic, achievable goals. A teaching plan that meets the patient's individual needs is developed with the patient and family. This is done several days before discharge to allow ample time for periodic review of the plan and answering of questions. Specific instructions are provided about diet; activity progression and exercise; coughing, deep breathing, and lung expansion exercises; weight and temperature monitoring; the medication regimen; and follow-up visits with the surgeon as well as the cardiologist or internist.

Some patients may have difficulty learning and retaining information after cardiac surgery. Studies have documented that many patients experience difficulties in cognitive function after cardiac surgery that do not occur after other types of major surgery (Kronick-Mest, 1989; Mravinac, 1991; Tess, 1991). The patient may experience recent memory loss, short attention span, difficulty with simple math, poor handwriting, and visual disturbances. Patients who experience these difficulties often become frustrated when they try to resume normal activities and learn how to care for themselves at home. The patient and family are reassured that the difficulty is temporary and will subside, usually in 6 to 8 weeks.

In the meantime, instructions are given to the patient at a much slower pace than normal, and a family member assumes responsibility for making sure that the prescribed regimen is followed.

If necessary, arrangements are made for a home care nurse to provide care such as dressing changes, monitoring of vital signs, diet counseling, and support for the patient and family.

Patient education postoperatively does not end at the time of discharge. The patient is encouraged to maintain telephone contact with the surgeon, cardiologist, and nurse. This provides the patient and family with reassurance that questions can be answered and problems can be resolved when they arise. Many hospitals provide family support sessions that help family members to cope with their own stress related to the patient's home health care management. The patient is expected to have a follow-up visit with the surgeon 4 to 6 weeks after discharge.

Many patients and families benefit from supportive programs such as the postcardiac surgery rehabilitation programs offered by many medical centers. These programs provide exercise monitoring, instructions about diet and stress reduction; information about resuming exercise, work, driving, and sexual activity; and support groups for patients and families. The American Heart Association sponsors the Mended Hearts Club, which provides information as well as an opportunity for families to share experiences.

CRITICAL THINKING EXERCISES

1. You are caring for an elderly patient who is 5 days post open heart surgery and is progressing well. After ambulating in the corridor with his daughter he returns to his room and bumps his nose, which begins to bleed profusely. His daughter is visibly upset. Explain what your first action will be and why. If your initial actions are not successful in decreasing the bleeding, how would you proceed? How would you explain the episode to the daughter to provide her with an understanding of the bleeding?
2. You are caring for a patient who is scheduled to have coronary artery bypass graft surgery. He appears quite anxious and states that he is afraid of the pain after surgery. His wife tends to minimize the significance of his concerns about pain. How would you respond to this patient and his wife? How might your response differ if the wife shares her husband's concerns?
3. A patient is recovering from heart transplantation and indicates that he feels he has a "new lease on life" and is "looking forward to a normal life." What further information about the patient will be helpful in identifying his teaching and discharge planning needs? Another patient who has undergone the same operation seems depressed and apprehensive. How would you explain the different reactions, and how would your teaching strategies for these two patients differ?

REFERENCES AND SELECTED READINGS

Books

Braunwald E. Heart Disease: A Textbook of Cardiovascular Medicine, 4th ed. Philadelphia, WB Saunders, 1992

Guzzetta CE and Dossey BM. Cardiovascular Nursing: Holistic Practice. St Louis, Mosby-Year Book, 1992.
Hurst JW. The Heart, Arteries and Veins, 7th ed. New York, McGraw Hill, 1990.
Sigardson-Poor KM and Haggerty LM. Nursing Care of the Transplant Recipient. Philadelphia, WB Saunders, 1990.

Journals

Asterisks indicate nursing research articles.

*Anderson KO and Masur FT. Psychologic preparation for cardiac catheterization. Heart Lung 1989 Mar; 18(2):154–163.
Bell PE and Diffee GT. Cardiopulmonary bypass: Principles, nursing implications. AORN J 1991 Jun; 53(6):1480–1496.
Cifani L and Vargo R. Teaching strategies for the transplant recipient: A review and future directions. Focus Crit Care 1990 Dec; 17(6):476–479.
Holmquist T and Gamberg PL. Heart and heart-lung transplantation. Todays OR Nurse 1992 Feb; 14(2):12–17.
Jurf JB and Nirschl AL. Acute postoperative pain management: A comprehensive review and update. Crit Care Nurs Q 1993 May; 16(1):8–25.
Kern LS. The elderly heart surgery patient. Crit Care Nurs 1991 Dec; 3(4):749–756.
Komeda M et al. Operative risks and long-term results of operation for left ventricular aneurysm. Ann Thorac Surg 1992 Jan; 53(1):22–28.
Kronick-Mest C. Postpericardiotomy syndrome: Etiology, manifestations, and interventions. Heart Lung 1989 Mar; 18(2):92–98.
*Lange SS et al. Issues in transplantation: Infection control practices in cardiac transplant recipients. Heart Lung 1992 Mar; 21(2):101–105.
Manaois LA. Aortic aneurysm. In Vazquez M et al. Critical Care Nursing, 2nd ed. Philadelphia, WB Saunders, 1992:254–259.
McRae ME. Care plan for the patient undergoing intracardiac myxoma excision. Crit Care Nurs 1990 Oct; 10(9):58–63.
Mravinac CM. Neurologic dysfunctions following cardiac surgery. Crit Care Nurs Clin 1991 Dec; 3(4):691–698.
Muirhead J. Heart and heart-lung transplantation. Crit Care Nurs Clin 1992 Mar; 4(1):97–109.
*Ruiz BA et al. Predictors of general activity 8 weeks after cardiac surgery. Appl Nurs Res 1992 May; 5(2):59–65.
Ruzevich S. Heart assist devices: State of the art. Crit Care Clin 1991 Dec; 3(4):723–732.
Smith A and Fitzpatrick E. Penetrating cardiac trauma: Surgical and nursing management. J Cardiovasc Nurs 1993 Jan; 7(2):52–70.
Sweeney MS et al. Cardiac surgical emergencies. Crit Care Clin 1989 Jul; 5(3):659–678.
Tess MM. Acute confusional states in critically ill patients: A review. J Neurosci Nurs 1991 Dec; 23(6):398–402.
Ulicny KS and Hiratzka LF. Nutrition and the cardiac surgical patient. Chest 1992 Mar; 101(3):836–842.
Vaska PL. Fluid and electrolyte imbalances after cardiac surgery. AACN Clinical Issues in Critical Care Nursing 1992 Aug; 3(3): 664–671.

INFORMATION/RESOURCES

Agencies

American Heart Association
7320 Greenville Ave, Dallas, TX 75231

International Society for Heart Transplantation, Thoracic and Cardiovascular Surgery
Newark Beth Israel Hospital
201 Lyons Ave, Newark, NJ 07112

Mended Hearts
7320 Greenville Ave, Dallas, TX 75231

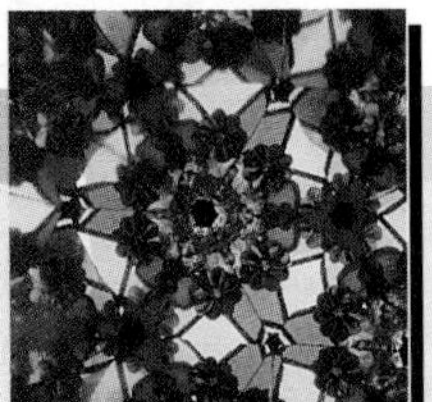

31

Assessment and Management of Patients With Vascular Disorders and Problems of Peripheral Circulation

CHAPTER OUTLINE

Physiologic Overview
Anatomy of the Vascular System
Circulatory Needs of Tissues
Blood Flow
Capillary Filtration and Reabsorption
Hemodynamic Resistance
Peripheral Vascular Regulating Mechanisms

Pathophysiology of the Vascular System
NURSING PROCESS: The Patient With Circulatory Insufficiency of the Extremities

Diseases of the Arteries
Arteriosclerosis and Atherosclerosis
Peripheral Arterial Occlusive Disease
Thromboangiitis Obliterans (Buerger's Disease)
Aortic Diseases
Arterial Embolism and Arterial Thrombosis
Raynaud's Disease

Hypertension
Definition, Incidence, and Etiology
Pathophysiology of Essential Hypertension
NURSING PROCESS: The Patient With Hypertension
Hypertensive Emergencies

Vein Disorders
Venous Thrombosis, Thrombophlebitis, Phlebothrombosis, and Deep Vein Thrombosis
Anticoagulant Therapy for Thromboembolism
Chronic Venous Insufficiency
Leg Ulcers
NURSING PROCESS: The Patient With Leg Ulcers
Varicose Veins

The Lymphatic System
Diagnostic Evaluation
Lymphangitis and Lymphadenitis
Lymphedema and Elephantiasis

Critical Thinking Exercises

LEARNING OBJECTIVES

On completion of this chapter, the learner will be able to:

1. Identify anatomic and physiologic factors that affect peripheral blood flow and tissue oxygenation
2. Use appropriate parameters for assessment of peripheral circulation
3. Use the nursing process as a framework of care for patients with circulatory insufficiency of the extremities
4. Compare the various diseases of the arteries, their causes, pathologic and physiologic changes, clinical manifestations, management, and prevention
5. Describe the "stepped care" approach to medication therapy for hypertension and the goals of health teaching for patients with hypertension
6. Use the nursing process as a framework of care for patients with hypertension
7. Describe the prevention and management of venous thrombosis
8. Compare the preventive management of venous insufficiency, leg ulcers, and varicose veins
9. Use the nursing process as a framework of care for patients with leg ulcers
10. Describe the relationship between lymphangitis and lymphedema

Physiologic Overview

Adequate perfusion results in oxygenation and nutrition of body tissues and is dependent in part on a properly functioning cardiovascular system. Adequate blood flow depends on the efficient pumping action of the heart, patent and responsive blood vessels, and an adequate circulating blood volume. Nervous system activity, blood viscosity, and the metabolic needs of tissues influence the rate of blood flow and hence the adequacy of blood flow.

The **vascular system** consists of two interdependent systems: the right heart pumps blood through the lungs to the pulmonary circulation, and the left heart pumps blood to all other body tissues through the systemic circulation. The blood vessels in both systems provide channels for transporting the blood from the heart to the tissues and back to the heart. Contractions of the ventricles supply the driving force for moving blood through the vascular systems. **Arteries** distribute oxygenated blood from the left side of the heart to the tissues, whereas the **veins** carry deoxygenated blood from the tissues to the right side of the heart. **Capillary vessels,** located within the tissues, connect the arterial and venous systems and constitute the site of exchange of nutrients and metabolic wastes between the circulatory system and the tissues. **Arterioles** and **venules** immediately adjacent to the capillaries, together with the capillaries, comprise the **microcirculation.** A schematic representation of the circulation system is shown in Figure 31-1.

The **lymphatic system** complements the function of the circulatory system. Lymphatic vessels transport **lymph** (a fluid similar to plasma) and tissue fluids (containing smaller proteins, cells, and cellular debris) from the interstitial space to systemic veins.

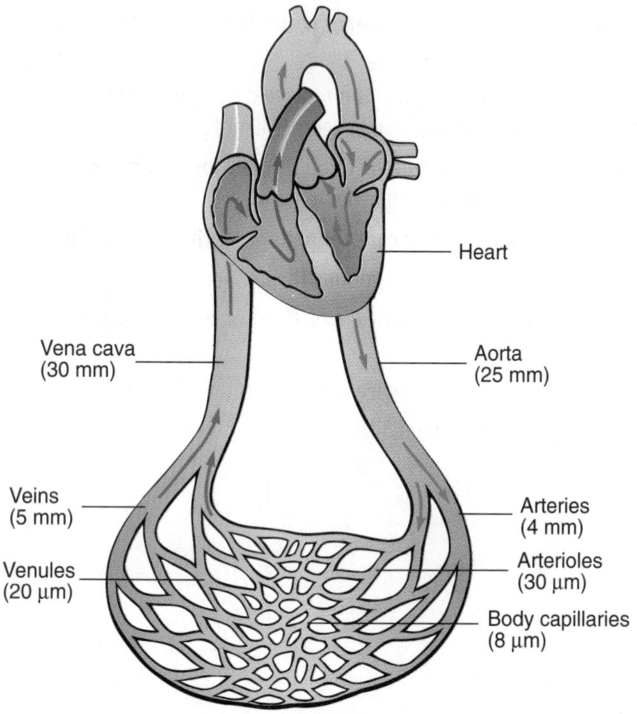

FIGURE 31-1. Schematic drawing of systemic circulation. Oxygen-rich blood leaves the heart, goes through the aorta into the systemic arterial circulation until it reaches the capillaries, where the exchange of nutrients takes place. The deoxygenated blood returns to the heart by way of the venous system. Comparison of vessel size is demonstrated.

Anatomy of the Vascular System

Arteries and Arterioles. Arteries are thick-walled structures that carry blood from the heart to the tissues. The aorta, which has a diameter of approximately 25 mm (1 inch), gives rise to numerous branches, which in turn divide into smaller vessels, arteries, and arterioles, that measure 4 mm (0.16 inch) in diameter by the time they reach the tissues. Within the tissues, the vessels divide further, diminishing to approximately 30 µm in diameter; these vessels are called *arterioles*.

The walls of the arteries and arterioles are composed of three layers: an inner endothelial cell layer called the *intima;* a middle layer of smooth elastic tissue called the *media;* and an outer layer of connective tissue called the *adventitia.* The intima, a very thin layer, provides a smooth surface for contact with the flowing blood.

The media makes up the major portion of the vessel wall in the aorta and other large arteries of the body. This layer is composed chiefly of elastic and connective tissue fibers that give the vessels considerable strength and allow them to constrict and dilate to accommodate the blood ejected from the heart (stroke volume) and maintain an even, steady flow of blood. The adventitia is a layer of connective tissue that anchors the vessel to its surroundings. There is much less elastic tissue in the smaller arteries and arterioles and the media in these vessels is composed primarily of smooth muscle.

Smooth muscle controls vessel diameter by contracting and relaxing. Chemical, hormonal, and nervous system factors influence the activity of smooth muscle. Because arterioles can alter their diameter, thereby offering resistance to blood flow, they are often referred to as *resistance vessels.* Arterioles regulate the volume and pressure in the arterial system and rate of blood flow to the capillaries.

Because of the large amount of muscle, the walls of the arteries are relatively thick, accounting for approximately 25% of the total diameter of the artery. The walls of the arterioles account for approximately 67% of the total diameter of arterioles.

The intima and the inner third of the smooth muscle layer are in such close contact with the blood that the blood vessel receives its nourishment from direct diffusion. The adventitia and the outer media layers have a limited vascular system for nourishment and require their own blood supply to meet their metabolic needs.

Capillaries. Capillary walls lack smooth muscle and adventitia and are composed of a single layer of endothelial cells. This thin-walled structure permits rapid and efficient transport of nutrients to the cells and removal of metabolic wastes. The diameter of capillaries ranges from 5 to 10 µm, requiring red blood cells to alter their shape to pass through these vessels. Changes in a capillary's diameter are passive and are influenced by contractile changes in the blood vessels that carry blood to and from a capillary. The capillary's diameter also changes in response to chemical stimuli. In some tissues, a cuff of smooth muscle, called the *precapil-*

lary sphincter, is located at the arteriolar end of the capillary and is responsible, along with the arteriole, for controlling capillary blood flow.

Some capillary beds, such as in the fingertips, contain **arteriovenous anastomoses,** through which blood passes directly from the arterial to the venous system. These vessels are believed to regulate heat exchange between the body and the external environment.

The distribution of capillaries throughout the tissues varies with the type of tissue. For example, skeletal tissue, which is metabolically active, has a more dense capillary network than does less active tissue such as cartilage.

Veins and Venules. Capillaries join together to form larger vessels called *venules*, which in turn join to form the veins. The venous system is therefore structurally analogous to the arterial system; venules correspond to arterioles, veins to arteries, and the vena cavae to the aorta. Analogous types of vessels in the arterial and venous systems have approximately the same diameters (see Fig. 31-1).

The walls of the veins, in contrast to those of the arteries, are thinner and considerably less muscular. The wall of the average vein amounts to only 10% of the vein diameter, in contrast to 25% in the artery. The walls of a vein, like those of arteries, are composed of three layers; however, these layers are not as well defined.

The thin, less muscular structure of the vein wall allows these vessels to distend more than arteries. Greater distensibility and compliance permit the large volumes of blood to be "stored" in the veins under low pressure. For this reason, veins are referred to as *capacitance vessels.* Approximately 75% of total blood volume is contained in the veins. The sympathetic nervous system, which innervates the vein musculature, can stimulate the veins to constrict (venoconstriction), thereby reducing venous volume and increasing the volume of blood in the general circulation.

Some veins, unlike arteries, are equipped with valves. In general, veins that transport blood against the force of gravity, as in the lower extremities, have one-way valves that interrupt the column of blood to prevent blood from seeping backward as it is propelled toward the heart. Valves are composed of endothelial leaflets, the competency of which depends on the integrity of the vein wall.

Lymphatic Vessels. The lymphatic vessels are a complex system of thin-walled vessels similar to the blood capillaries. This network serves to collect lymph fluid from tissues and organs and to transport the fluid to the venous circulation. The lymphatic vessels converge into two main trunks, the thoracic duct and the right lymphatic duct. These ducts empty into the junction of the subclavian and the internal jugular veins. The right lymphatic duct conveys lymph primarily from the right side of the head, neck, thorax, and upper arms. The thoracic duct conveys lymph from the remainder of the body. Peripheral lymphatic vessels join larger lymph vessels and pass through regional lymph nodes before entering the venous circulation. The lymph nodes play an important role in the filtration of foreign particles.

The lymphatic vessels are permeable to large molecules and provide the only means whereby interstitial proteins can return to the venous system. With muscular contraction, lymph vessels become distorted to create spaces between the endothelial cells, which allow protein and particles to enter. Muscular contraction of the lymphatic walls and surrounding tissues aids in propelling the lymph toward venous drainage points.

Circulatory Needs of Tissues

The amount of blood flow needed by body tissues constantly changes. The percentage of blood flow received by individual organs or tissues is determined by the rate of tissue metabolism, the availability of oxygen, and the function of the tissues (Table 31-1). When metabolic requirements increase, blood vessels dilate to increase the flow of oxygen

TABLE 31-1 Typical Values for Blood Flow and Oxygen Consumption for Various Human Organs

		Blood Flow During Rest		Oxygen Usage During Rest	
Organ	Organ Weight (kg)	Organ Blood Flow (ml/min)	% Total Cardiac Output	Organ O_2 Usage (ml/min)	% Total O_2 Usage
Brain	1.4	750	14	45	18
Heart	0.3	250	5	25	10
Liver	1.5	1,300	23	75	30
GI tract	2.5	1,000			
Kidneys	0.3	1,200	22	15	6
Muscle	35.0	1,000	18	50	20
Skin	2.0	200	4	5	2
Remainder (*e.g.,* skeleton, bone marrow, fat, connective tissue)	27.0	800	14	35	14
TOTAL	70	6,500	100	250	100

(Folkow B and Neil E. Circulation. New York, Oxford University Press.)

and nutrients to the tissues. When metabolic needs decrease, vessels constrict and blood flow to the tissues decreases. Metabolic demands of tissues increase with physical activity or exercise, local heat application, fever, and infection. Reduced metabolic requirements of tissues accompany rest or decreased physical activity, local cold application, and cooling of the body. If the blood vessels fail to dilate in response to the need for increased blood flow, tissue **ischemia** (deficient blood supply) results. The mechanism by which blood vessels dilate and constrict to adjust for metabolic changes assumes that a normal arterial pressure is maintained.

As blood passes through tissue capillaries, oxygen is removed and carbon dioxide is added. The amount of oxygen extracted by each tissue is different. For example, the myocardium tends to extract about 50% of the oxygen from arterial blood in one passage through its capillary bed, whereas the kidneys extract only about 7% of the oxygen from the blood that passes through them. The average amount of oxygen removed collectively by all of the body tissues is about 25%. This means that the blood in the vena cavae contains about 25% less oxygen than aortic blood. This is known as the *systemic arteriovenous oxygen difference.* It increases when the amount of oxygen delivered to the tissues is decreased relative to their metabolic needs. See Table 31-1 for more detailed information about blood flow and oxygen extraction as blood passes through capillary beds in various tissues.

Blood Flow

Blood flow through the cardiovascular system always proceeds in the same direction: left heart to aorta, arteries, arterioles, capillaries, venules, veins, vena cavae, and finally to the right heart. This unidirectional flow is caused by a pressure difference that exists between the arterial and venous systems. Because arterial pressure (approximately 100 mm Hg) is greater than venous pressure (approximately 4 mm Hg), and fluid always flows from an area of high pressure to an area of low pressure, blood flows from the arterial to the venous system.

The pressure difference (ΔP) between the two ends of the vessel provides the impetus for the forward propulsion of blood. Impediments to blood flow offer the opposing force, which is known as *resistance* (R). Thus, the rate of blood flow is determined by dividing the pressure difference by the resistance:

$$\text{Flow} = \Delta P/R$$

From this equation it is clear that when resistance increases, a greater driving pressure is required to maintain the same degree of flow. Physiologically, an increase in driving pressure is accomplished by an increase in the force of contraction of the heart. If arterial resistance is chronically elevated, the myocardium hypertrophies to sustain the greater contractile force.

In the majority of long smooth blood vessels, flow is laminar or streamlined, with blood in the center of the vessel moving slightly faster than the blood near the vessel walls. Laminar flow is silent. Laminar flow becomes turbulent when the rate of blood flow increases, when blood viscosity increases, when the diameter of the vessel becomes greater than normal, or when segments of the vessel become narrowed or constricted. Turbulent blood flow creates sounds, called *bruits,* that can be heard superficially with a stethoscope.

Blood Pressure. See Chapter 26 for physiology and measurement of blood pressure.

Capillary Filtration and Reabsorption

Fluid exchange across the capillary wall is continuous. This fluid, which has the same composition as plasma without the proteins, forms the interstitial fluid. The equilibrium between hydrostatic and osmotic forces of the blood and interstitium, as well as capillary permeability, govern the amount and direction of fluid movement across the capillary. **Hydrostatic force** is a driving pressure that is generated by the blood pressure. **Osmotic pressure** is the pulling force that is created by plasma proteins. Normally, the hydrostatic pressure at the arterial end of the capillary is relatively high compared with that at the venous end. This high pressure at the arterial end of the capillaries tends to drive fluid out of the capillary and into the tissue space. Osmotic pressure tends to pull fluid back into the capillary from the tissue space, but this osmotic force cannot overcome the high hydrostatic pressure at the arterial end of the capillary. At the venous end of the capillary, however, the osmotic force predominates over the low hydrostatic pressure and there is a net reabsorption of fluid from the tissue space back into the capillary.

Virtually all of the fluid that is filtered at the arterial end of the capillary bed is reabsorbed at the venous end, except for a very small amount. This excess filtered fluid enters the lymphatic circulation. These processes of filtration, reabsorption, and lymph formation aid in maintaining tissue fluid volume and removing tissue waste and debris. Capillary permeability, under normal conditions, remains constant.

Under certain abnormal conditions, the fluid filtered out of the capillaries may greatly exceed the amounts reabsorbed and carried away by the lymphatic vessels. This imbalance can result from damage to capillary walls and subsequent increased permeability, obstruction of lymphatic drainage, elevation of venous pressure, or decrease in plasma protein osmotic force. The accumulation of fluid that results from these processes is known as *edema.*

Hemodynamic Resistance

The most important factor in the vascular system that determines resistance is the vessel radius. Small changes in vessel radius lead to large changes in resistance. The predominant sites of change in the caliber or width of blood vessels, and therefore in resistance, are the arterioles and the precapillary sphincter.

Peripheral vascular resistance is the opposition to blood flow provided by the blood vessels. Poiseuille's law provides the method by which resistance can be calculated.

$$R = 8\eta\, L/\pi r^4$$

where R = resistance, r = radius of the vessel, L = length of the vessel, η = viscosity of the blood, and $8/\pi$ = a constant.

This equation shows that the resistance is proportional to the viscosity or thickness of the blood and the length of the vessel, but inversely proportional to the fourth power of the vessel radius.

Blood viscosity and vessel length, under normal conditions, do not change significantly. Therefore, these factors do not usually play an important role in blood flow. A large increase in hematocrit, however, may increase blood viscosity and reduce capillary blood flow.

Peripheral Vascular Regulating Mechanisms

Because the metabolic needs of body tissues, even at rest, are continuously changing, an integrated and coordinated system of regulation is necessary so that blood flow to individual areas is maintained in proportion to the needs of that area. As might be expected, this regulatory mechanism is complex and consists of central nervous system influences, circulating hormones and chemicals, and independent activity of the arterial wall itself.

Sympathetic (adrenergic) nervous system activity, mediated by the hypothalamus, is the most important factor in regulating the caliber, and thus the blood flow, of peripheral blood vessels. All vessels are innervated by the sympathetic nervous system except the capillary and precapillary sphincters. Stimulation of the sympathetic nerves causes vasoconstriction. The neurotransmitter responsible for sympathetic vasoconstriction is **norepinephrine.** Sympathetic activation occurs in response to a number of physiologic and psychological stressors. Removal of sympathetic activity by medications or sympathectomy results in vasodilation.

Other hormonal substances also affect peripheral vascular resistance. **Epinephrine**, released from the adrenal medulla, acts like norepinephrine in constricting peripheral blood vessels in most tissue beds. In low concentrations, however, epinephrine causes vasodilation in skeletal muscles, the heart, and the brain. **Angiotensin,** a potent substance formed from the interaction of renin (synthesized in the kidney) and a circulating serum protein, stimulates arterial constriction. Although the blood concentration of angiotensin is usually small, its profound vasoconstrictor effects become important in certain pathophysiologic states, such as congestive heart failure and hypovolemia.

Alterations in local blood flow are influenced by a number of circulating substances that have vasoactive properties. Potent vasodilator substances include histamine, bradykinin, prostaglandin, and certain muscle metabolites. A reduction in available oxygen and nutrients and changes in local *p*H also affect local blood flow. **Serotonin**, a substance liberated from platelets that aggregate at the site of vessel wall damage, constricts arterioles. The application of heat to parts of the body surface causes local vasodilation, whereas the application of cold causes vasoconstriction.

Pathophysiology of the Vascular System

Reduced blood flow through peripheral blood vessels characterizes all peripheral vascular diseases. The physiologic effects of altered blood flow depend on the extent to which tissue demands exceed the supply of oxygen and nutrients available. If tissue needs are high, even modestly reduced blood flow may be inadequate to maintain tissue integrity, and tissues then become **ischemic** (deficient in blood supply) and malnourished and ultimately die if adequate blood flow is not restored.

Heart Failure. Inadequate peripheral blood flow occurs whenever the heart's pumping action becomes inefficient. Left-sided heart failure causes an accumulation of blood in the lungs and a reduction in forward flow or cardiac output, which results in inadequate arterial blood flow to the tissues. Right-sided heart failure causes systemic venous congestion and a reduction in forward flow (see Chapter 28).

Alterations in Blood and Lymphatic Vessels. Blood vessels that are intact, patent, and responsive are necessary to deliver adequate amounts of oxygen to tissues and to remove metabolic wastes. Arteries can become obstructed by atherosclerotic plaque, a thrombus, or an embolus. Arteries can become damaged or obstructed as a result of chemical or mechanical trauma, infections or inflammatory processes, vasospastic disorders, and congenital malformations. A sudden arterial occlusion causes profound and frequently irreversible tissue ischemia and tissue death. When arterial occlusions develop gradually, there is less risk for sudden tissue death because collateral circulation has an opportunity to develop.

Venous blood flow can be reduced by a thrombus obstructing the vein, by incompetent venous valves, or by a reduction in the effectiveness of the pumping action of surrounding muscles. A decrease in venous blood flow results in an increase in venous pressure, a subsequent rise in capillary hydrostatic pressure, a net filtration of fluid out of the capillaries into the interstitial space, and subsequent edema. Edematous tissues cannot receive adequate nutrition from the blood and consequently are more susceptible to breakdown or injury and to infection.

Obstruction of lymphatic vessels also results in edema. Lymphatic vessels can become obstructed by tumor or by damage resulting from mechanical trauma or inflammatory processes.

Gerontologic Considerations. The aging process produces changes in the walls of the blood vessels that affect the transportation of oxygen and nutrients to the tissues. The intima thickens as a result of cellular proliferation and fibrosis. Elastin fibers of the media become calcified, thin, and fragmented, and collagen accumulates in both the intima and the media. These changes cause stiffening of the vessels, which results in increased peripheral resistance, impairment of blood flow, and increased left ventricular workload.

❑ NURSING PROCESS
The Patient With Circulatory Insufficiency of the Extremities

Assessment

Although many types of peripheral vascular diseases exist, most result in ischemia (deficiency of blood supply to a body part) and produce some of the same symptoms: pain,

TABLE 31-2 Differentiating Characteristics and Treatment of Arterial and Venous Insufficiency

	Arterial	Venous
Pain	Intermittent claudication to sharp, unrelenting, constant	Aching, cramping
Pulses	Diminished or absent	Present
Skin characteristics	Dependent rubor—elevational pallor of foot, thickened nails, dry, shiny skin, cool to cold temperature	Pigmentation in gaitor area (area of medial and lateral malleolus), skin thickened and tough, may be reddish blue in color, associated dermatitis frequent
Ulcer characteristics		
Location	Tip of toes, toe webs, heel or other pressure areas if confined to bed	Medial malleolus; infrequently lateral malleolus or anterior tibial area
Pain	Very painful	Minimal pain if superficial
Depth of Ulcer	Deep, often involving joint space	Superficial
Shape	Perfectly circular	Irregular in shape
Ulcer Base	Pale to black and dry gangrene	Granulation tissue—beefy red to yellow fibrinous in chronic long term ulcer
Edema	Minimal unless extremity kept in dependent position constantly to relieve pain	Moderate to severe
Ulcer treatment	Reconstructive surgery, interventional radiology procedure; maintain ulcer or digital gangrene by decreasing bacteria and keeping wound dry: 1. Wash daily with soap and water 2. Betadine swab to area 3. 2 × 2s between toes After surgery: 1. Debride demarcated necrotic or gangrene areas 2. Promote moist wound healing with: damp-to-dry dressings, calcium alginate dressing, hydrocolloid	Provide cleanliness 1. Wash with gentle soap and water Provide compression: 1. Ace wrap 2. Coban 3. Dome paste Often combinations of 1. Dome paste and Coban 2. Hydrocolloidal dressing with Coban

skin changes, diminished pulse, and possible edema. The type and severity of symptoms experienced depends in part, on the type, stage, and extent of the disease process as well as the speed with which the disorder develops. The distinguishing features of arterial and venous insufficiency are presented in Table 31-2.

Pain. A severe cramp-type pain in the extremities after activity or exercise is experienced by patients with peripheral arterial insufficiency. This pain, referred to as *intermittent claudication,* is due to the inability of the arterial system to provide adequate blood flow to the tissues in the face of increased demands for nutrients during exercise. As the tissues are forced to complete the energy cycle without the nutrients, muscle metabolites and lactic acid are produced. Pain is experienced as the metabolites aggravate the nerve endings of the surrounding tissue. Usually 75% of the vessel must be obstructed before intermittent claudication is experienced. When the patient rests, and thereby decreases the metabolic needs of the muscles, the pain subsides. The progression of the vascular disease can be monitored by documenting the amount of exercise or the distance a patient can walk before pain is produced. Persistent pain in the forefoot when the patient is resting indicates a severe degree of arterial insufficiency and a critical state of ischemia. This **rest pain** is often worse at night and may interfere with sleep. This pain frequently requires that the extremity be lowered to a dependent position.

The site of arterial disease can be deduced from the location of claudication. Calf pain may accompany reduced blood flow through the superficial femoral or popliteal artery, whereas pain in the hip or buttock may result from reduced blood flow in the abdominal aorta, common iliac, or hypogastric arteries.

Changes in Skin Appearance and Temperature. Adequate blood flow warms the extremities and gives them a rosy coloring. Inadequate blood flow results in cool and pale extremities. Further reduction of blood flow to these tissues, such as would occur when the extremity is elevated, results in an even whiter or more blanched appearance. A reddish blue discoloration of the extremities (**rubor**) may be observed within 20 seconds to 2 minutes after the extremity is dependent and is indicative of severe peripheral arterial damage in which vessels that are unable to constrict remain dilated. Even with rubor present, the extremity begins to pale with elevation. **Cyanosis,** a bluish coloring of the skin, is manifested when the amount of oxygenated hemoglobin contained in the blood is reduced.

Additional adverse changes seen in the extremities as a result of chronically reduced nutrient supply include loss of hair, brittle nails, dry or scaling skin, atrophy, and ulcerations. **Edema** may be apparent either bilaterally or unilaterally and is related to the affected extremity being in a chronically dependent position owing to severe rest pain. Gangrenous changes appear after prolonged severe ischemia and represent tissue necrosis. In the geriatric population gangrene may be the first sign of disease. Circulation is decreased, but is not apparent to the patient until trauma occurs. At this point, gangrene develops when minimal arterial flow is impaired further by edema formation resulting from the traumatic event.

Pulses. Determining the presence or absence, as well as the quality, of peripheral pulses is important in assessing the status of peripheral arterial circulation (Fig. 31-2). Absence of a pulse indicates that the site of obstruction is proximal to that location. Occlusive arterial disease impairs blood flow and can reduce or obliterate palpable pulsations in the extremities. When pulses cannot be reliably palpated, it may be helpful to use a Doppler ultrasound device to detect peripheral flow (Fig. 31-3).

Gerontologic Considerations. In the elderly person, the symptoms of peripheral vascular disease may be more pronounced than in the younger person because of the duration of the condition and the presence of coexisting chronic disease. Intermittent claudication may occur after walking only a few short blocks or after walking up a slight incline. Any prolonged pressure on the foot can cause pressure areas that become ulcerated, infected, and gangrenous. Chronic venous insufficiency can also lead to ulceration. The outcome of either arterial or venous insufficiency in the elderly person is reduced mobility and activity, and loss of independence.

Risk Factors for Peripheral Vascular Disease. Primary prevention may significantly decreased the incidence of peripheral vascular disease. When nurses provide health information, they make a significant impact on the prevention of peripheral vascular disorders. Risk factors for peripheral vascular disease are often poorly understood and are thought to occur only with advancing age. However, as indi-

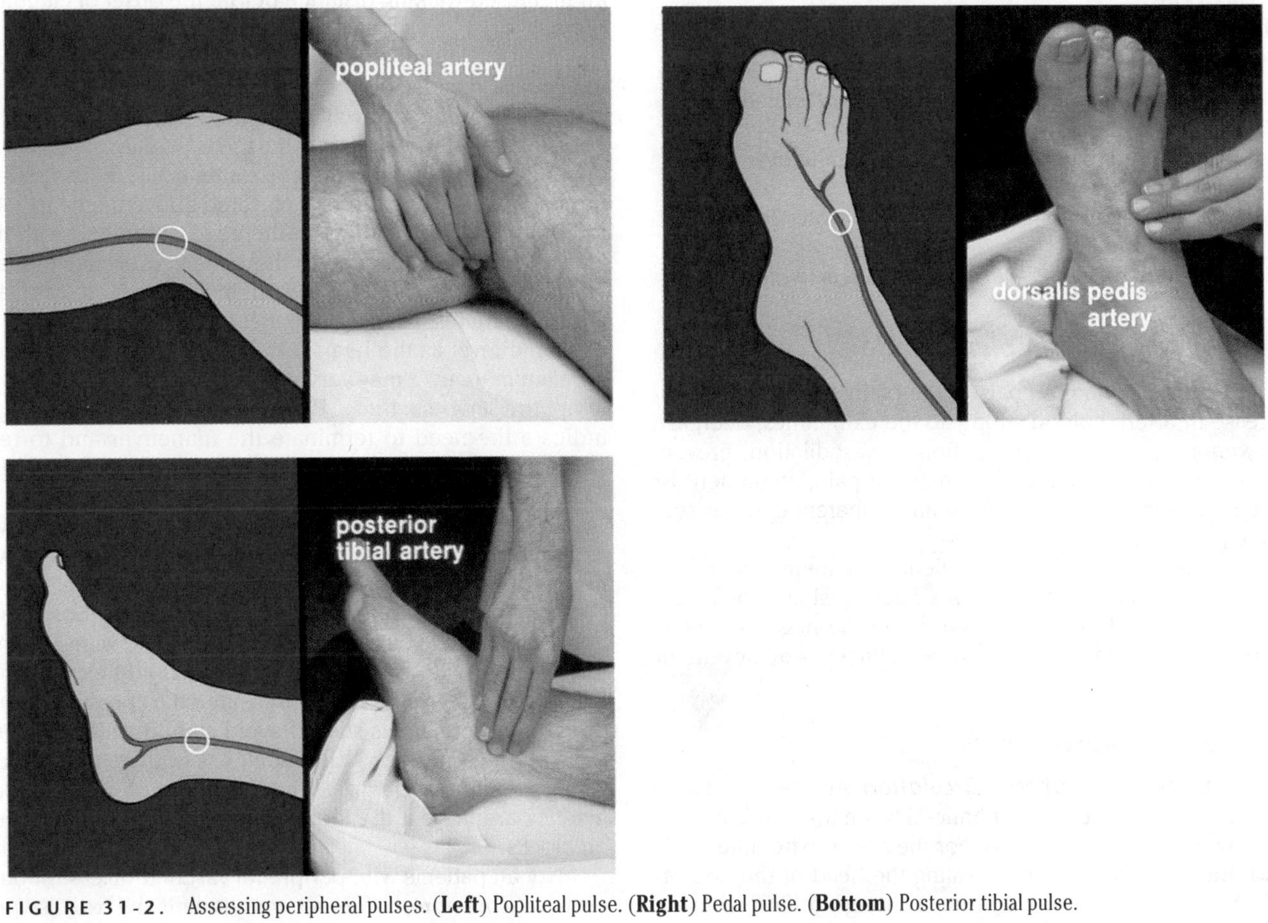

FIGURE 31-2. Assessing peripheral pulses. (**Left**) Popliteal pulse. (**Right**) Pedal pulse. (**Bottom**) Posterior tibial pulse.

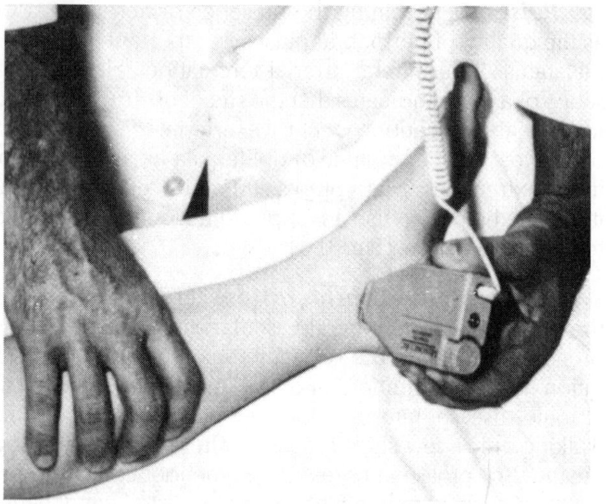

FIGURE 31-3. Doppler ultrasound transducer being used to detect posterior tibialis blood flow. (Suddarth DS. The Lippincott Manual of Nursing Practice, 5th ed. Philadelphia, JB Lippincott, 1991.)

CHART 31-1
Risk Factors for Peripheral Vascular Disease

Controllable Risk Factors

Tobacco use
Hypertension
Obesity
Sedentary lifestyle
Stress
Diabetes mellitus

Noncontrollable Risk Factors

Age
Gender
Familial predisposition

cated in Chart 31-1, risk factors apply to adults in general. Some of these risk factors are noncontrollable. Others, however, such as tobacco use, hypertension, obesity, a sedentary lifestyle, and stress are controllable.

Diagnosis

Nursing Diagnoses

Based on assessment data, major nursing diagnoses for the patient may include the following:

- Alteration in peripheral tissue perfusion related to compromised circulation
- Pain related to impaired ability of peripheral vessels to supply tissues with oxygen
- Risk for impairment of skin integrity related to compromised circulation
- Knowledge deficit regarding self-care activities

Planning and Implementation

Goals. The major goals of the patient may include increase in arterial blood supply to the extremities, decrease in venous congestion, promotion of vasodilation, prevention of vascular compression, relief of pain, attainment or maintenance of tissue integrity, and adherence to the self-care program.

Measures used by the patient and members of the health care team to accomplish a single goal must be evaluated in terms of both the positive and the negative effects these measures may have on the simultaneous achievement of other goals.

Nursing Interventions

Improving Peripheral Circulation. Arterial blood supply to a body part can be enhanced when the part is placed below the level of the heart. For the lower extremities, this can be accomplished by elevating the head of the bed on 15-cm (6-in) blocks or assuming a sitting position with the feet resting on the floor. Walking or other moderate or graded isometric exercises may be prescribed to promote blood flow and thus to encourage the development of collateral circulation. Pain can serve as a guide in determining the amount of exercise appropriate for an individual. The onset of pain indicates that the tissues are not receiving adequate oxygen, signaling the patient to rest before continuing activity. However, a regular exercise program can result in an increased walking distance before the onset of claudication.

Active postural exercises, such as the **Buerger-Allen exercises**, may be prescribed for the patient with arterial insufficiency of the lower extremities. These exercises involve placing the extremities in three positions: elevation, dependency, and then at the horizontal position. The patient lies flat in bed with both legs elevated above the heart for 2 to 3 minutes. Then, sitting on the edge of the bed with the legs relaxed and dependent, the patient exercises the feet and toes (upward and downward, inward and outward) for about 3 minutes. Finally, the patient lies flat with the legs at the same level as the heart for about 5 minutes. The times for each maneuver may vary, although the patient should attempt the series six times. Pain and dramatic color changes indicate the need to terminate the maneuver and to rest. This routine may be repeated (Fig. 31-4) four times per day or as tolerated.

In patients with venous insufficiency, placing the lower extremities in a dependent position will only worsen the venous pooling associated with this condition. The pull of gravity impedes venous return to the heart and promotes venous stasis (the accumulation of blood in the veins). Therefore, persons with venous insufficiency should elevate their legs above the level of the heart as much as possible. When upright, these patients should avoid standing still or sitting for prolonged periods. Walking aids venous return by activating the "muscle pump." When patients with venous insufficiency are in bed, the foot of the bed should be elevated on blocks.

Not all patients with peripheral vascular disease should exercise. Therefore, before recommending any exercise pro-

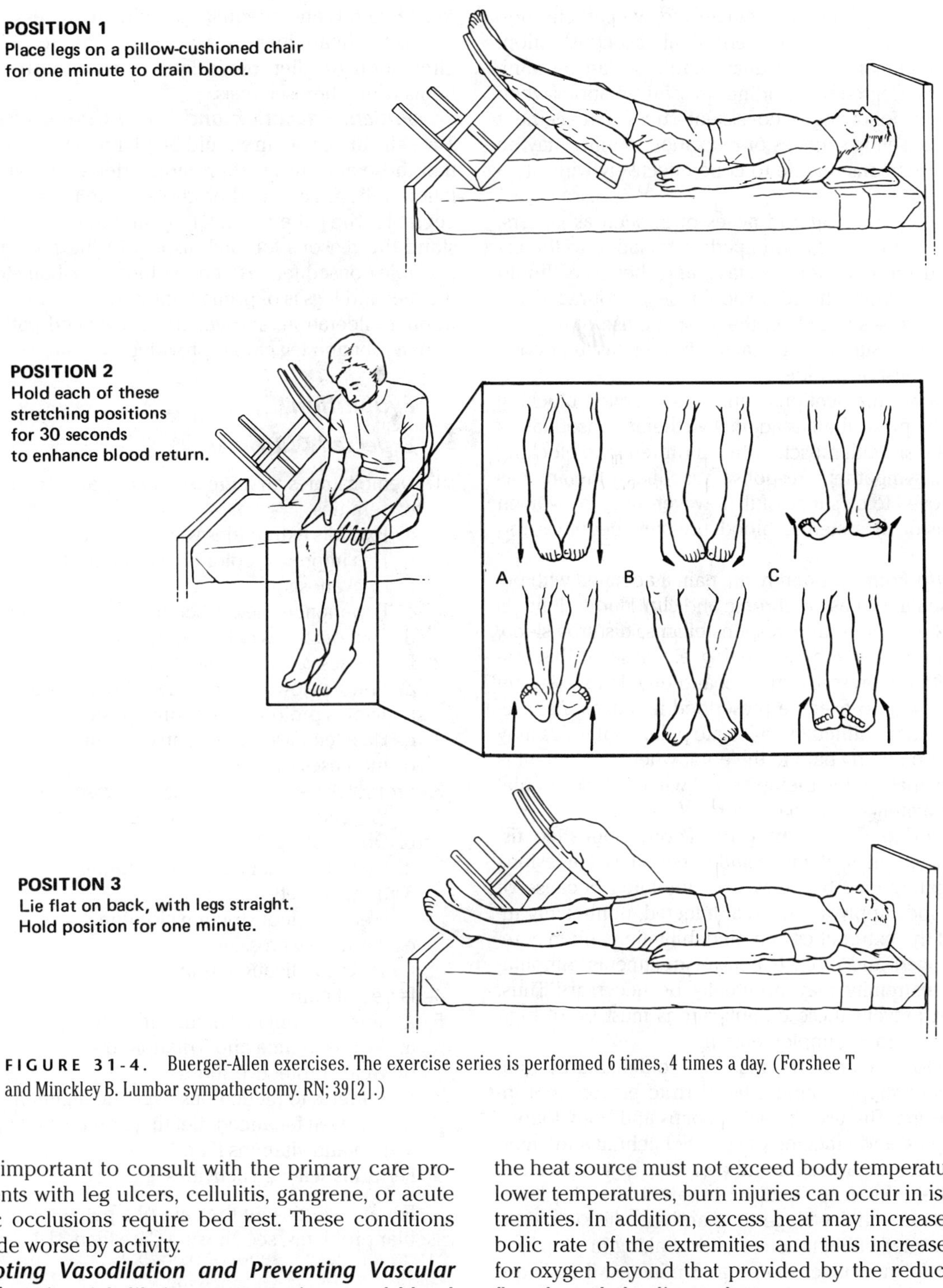

FIGURE 31-4. Buerger-Allen exercises. The exercise series is performed 6 times, 4 times a day. (Forshee T and Minckley B. Lumbar sympathectomy. RN; 39[2].)

gram, it is important to consult with the primary care provider. Patients with leg ulcers, cellulitis, gangrene, or acute thrombotic occlusions require bed rest. These conditions can be made worse by activity.

Promoting Vasodilation and Preventing Vascular Compression. Arterial dilation promotes increased blood flow to the extremities and is therefore a desirable goal in people who have peripheral arterial disease. However, in instances where the arteries are severely sclerosed, inelastic, or damaged, dilation is not possible. For this reason, measures to promote vasodilation, such as medications or surgery, may be only minimally effective.

Warmth promotes arterial flow; exposure to cold temperatures causes vasoconstriction. Adequate clothing and warm temperatures protect the patient from chilling. If chilling occurs, a warm bath or drink is helpful. When heat is applied directly to ischemic extremities, the temperature of the heat source must not exceed body temperature. Even at lower temperatures, burn injuries can occur in ischemic extremities. In addition, excess heat may increase the metabolic rate of the extremities and thus increase the need for oxygen beyond that provided by the reduced arterial flow through the diseased artery.

- ❑ Patients are instructed to test the temperature of bath water and to avoid using hot water bottles and heating pads on the extremities. Applying a heating pad to the abdomen can cause reflex vasodilation in the extremities and is safer than direct application of heat to affected extremities.

Nicotine causes vasospasm and can thereby dramatically reduce circulation to the extremities. Patients with arterial insufficiency who smoke must be fully informed of the effects of nicotine on circulation and encouraged to stop smoking. Emotional upsets stimulate the sympathetic nervous system, which results in peripheral vasoconstriction. Although emotional stress is unavoidable, it can be minimized to some degree by avoiding stressful situations when possible or by following a consistent stress management program. Counseling services or relaxation training may be indicated for persons unable to cope effectively with situational stressors.

Constricting clothing and accessories such as garters, belts, girdles, and shoe laces impede circulation to the extremities and promote venous stasis and therefore should be avoided. Crossing the legs should be discouraged because it compresses vessels in the legs. The use of the bed knee gatch to elevate the legs causes further vascular compression and must be avoided.

Vasodilator medications and adrenergic blocking agents may be prescribed as adjunctive therapy. Vasodilators relax vascular smooth muscle, whereas adrenergic blocking agents block sympathetic response. Vasodilator therapy has not been proved to be successful, however, and may worsen tissue perfusion if systemic blood pressure becomes too low.

Relieving Pain. Frequently, the pain associated with peripheral vascular disease is chronic and continuous. It limits activities, affects work and responsibilities, disturbs sleep, and alters one's sense of well-being. Because of this, patients are often depressed, irritable, and unable to exert the energy necessary to execute prescribed therapies. As a result it can be more difficult to alleviate pain. Analgesics may be helpful in reducing pain to the point where the patient is able to participate in the therapies that will increase circulation and ultimately relieve pain more effectively.

Maintaining Tissue Integrity. Poorly nourished tissues are susceptible to damage and infection. When lesions develop, healing may be delayed or inhibited because of the poor blood supply to the area. Infected, nonhealing ulcerations of the extremities can be debilitating and may require prolonged and often expensive treatments. Amputation of the extremity may eventually be necessary. Thus, measures to prevent these complications must be of high priority and vigorously implemented.

Trauma to the extremities must be avoided. Sturdy, well-fitting shoes or slippers should be worn to prevent foot injury and blisters. The use of neutral soaps and body lotions prevents drying and cracking of skin. Scratching and vigorous rubbing can abrade skin and create a site for bacterial invasion; therefore feet should be patted dry. Stockings should be clean and dry. Fingernails and toenails should be carefully trimmed straight across after soaking in soap and warm water for no longer than 3 to 5 minutes. If nails are thick and brittle and cannot be trimmed safely, a podiatrist should be consulted. Corns and callouses need to be removed by a health care professional. Special shoe inserts may be needed to prevent calluses from recurring. All signs of blisters, ingrown toenails, infection, or other problems should be reported to health care professionals for treatment and follow-up. Persons with diminished vision may require assistance in periodically examining the lower extremities for trauma.

Good nutrition promotes healing and prevents tissue breakdown and is thus included in the overall preventive program for persons with peripheral vascular disease. Vitamins B and C and adequate protein are necessary. (Obesity strains the heart, increases venous congestion, and reduces circulation.) A diet low in lipids may be indicated for patients with atherosclerosis.

Patient Education and Home Care Considerations. The self-care program should be planned with the patient so that those activities that promote arterial and venous circulation, relieve pain, and promote tissue integrity will be acceptable. The patient and family should be helped to understand the reasons for each aspect of the program and the possible consequences of nonadherence. Long-term care of the feet and legs is of prime importance in the prevention of trauma, ulceration, and gangrene. Detailed patient instruction in foot and leg care is provided in Chart 31-2.

Evaluation

Expected Outcomes

1. Demonstrates an increase in arterial blood supply to extremities
   a. Exhibits extremities warm to touch
   b. Has improved color of extremities (is free of rubor or cyanosis)
   c. Experiences decreased muscle pain with exercise
   d. Demonstrates palpable peripheral pulses
2. Decreases venous congestion
   a. Elevates lower extremities as prescribed
   b. Avoids prolonged standing or sitting
   c. Has decreased edema in extremities
   d. Increases walking time
3. Promotes vasodilation; prevents vascular compression
   a. Protects extremities from exposure to cold
   b. Does not smoke
   c. Uses stress management program to minimize emotional upset
   d. Wears nonconstricting clothing
   e. Avoids leg crossing
   f. Takes medication as prescribed
4. Is free of pain
5. Attains or maintains tissue integrity
   a. Avoids trauma and irritation to skin
   b. Wears protective shoes
   c. Adheres to meticulous hygienic regimen
   d. Eats well-balanced diet that contains adequate protein and vitamins B and C
6. Performs self-care activities

For an overview of the care of a patient with peripheral vascular problems, see Nursing Care Plan 31-1.

Diseases of the Arteries

Arteriosclerosis and Artherosclerosis

Arteriosclerosis is the most common disease of the arteries; it literally means "hardening of the arteries." It is a diffuse process whereby the muscle fibers and the endothelial lining of the walls of small arteries and arterioles become thickened. **Atherosclerosis** involves a different process, affecting the intima of the large and medium-sized arteries. These changes consist of the accumulation of lipids, cal-

CHART 31-2

Patient Education: Care of the Feet and Legs for the Person with a Peripheral Vascular Problem

Cleanliness

1. Wash feet daily especially between toes
2. Use mild soap and lukewarm water
3. Rinse thoroughly
4. Dry feet thoroughly, especially between the toes; pat dry rather than rub

Warmth

1. Wear clean, loose, soft cotton socks because they are comfortable and will absorb moisture
2. Do not use a heating pad
3. Wear extra socks in cold weather in extra large shoes
4. Avoid sunburn

Safety

1. Inspect feet daily with a mirror for redness, dryness, cuts, blisters, etc.
2. Always wear soft shoes or slippers when out of bed
3. Trim nails straight across after showering
4. Consult podiatrist to trim nails if vision is decreased; also for care of corns, blisters, or ingrown nails
5. Clear pathways in house to prevent injury

Comfort Measures

1. Wear shoes with extra depth toebox and made of leather. Synthetic shoes do not allow air to circulate
2. If feet become dry and scaly, use cream with lanolin. Never put cream between the toes.
3. If feet perspire, especially between the toes, use powder daily and/or lamb's wool between the toes to promote drying

Prevent Constriction of Blood Vessels

1. Avoid circular compression around feet or knees, such as knee-high stockings, pantyhose, or garters
2. Do not cross legs at knees
3. Use lamb's wool between toes if they overlap or rub each other
4. Quit smoking (nicotine causes vasoconstriction and vasospasm)

Exercise

1. Participate in a regular walking exercise program which will stimulate circulation

Seeking Medical Attention

1. Contact health care provider at the onset of skin breakdown such as abrasions, blisters, athlete's foot, or pain
2. Do not use any medication on feet or legs unless prescribed by a health care provider

cium, blood components, carbohydrates, and fibrous tissue on the intimal layer of the artery. These accumulations are referred to as *atheromas* or *plaques*. Although the pathologic processes of arteriosclerosis and atherosclerosis differ, rarely does one occur without the other, and thus the terms are often used interchangeably. Because atherosclerosis is a generalized disease of the arteries, when it is present in the extremities it is usually present elsewhere in the body.

Pathophysiology and Etiology

The most common direct results of atherosclerosis in arteries include narrowing (stenosis) of the lumen, obstruction by thrombosis, aneurysm (abnormal dilation of a blood vessel), ulceration, and rupture. Its indirect results are malnutrition and the subsequent fibrosis of the organs that the sclerotic arteries supply with blood. All actively functioning tissue cells require an abundant supply of nutrients and oxygen and are sensitive to any reduction in the supply of these nutrients. If such reductions are severe and permanent, these cells undergo ischemic necrosis (death of cells due to deficient blood flow) and are replaced by fibrous tissue, which requires much less nutrition.

Atherosclerosis primarily affects the main arteries throughout the entire arterial tree in varying degrees, usually in a patchy manner. Branch arteries are affected usually only at their bifurcations.

Many theories attempt to explain why and how atherosclerosis develops. The primary lesion, the atheroma, is a lipid plaque with a fibrous covering that slowly occludes the lumen of the vessel. No single theory has fully explained the pathogenesis; however, parts of several theories have been combined into the reaction-to-injury theory. According to this theory, vascular endothelial cell injury results from prolonged hemodynamic forces, such as shearing stresses and turbulent flow, radiation, chemicals, or chronic hyperlipidemia present in the arterial system. Injury to the endothelium increases the aggregation of platelets and monocytes at the site of the injury. Smooth muscle cells migrate and proliferate, allowing a matrix of collagen and elastic fibers to form. It may be that there is no single cause or mechanism for the development of atherosclerosis; rather, multiple processes may be involved.

Morphologically, atherosclerotic lesions are of two types: fatty streaks and fibrous plaque. **Fatty streaks** are yellow and smooth, protrude slightly into the lumen of the artery, and are composed of lipids and elongated smooth muscle cells. These lesions have been found in the arteries of persons of all age groups, including infants. It is not clear whether fatty streaks predispose to the formation of fibrous plaques or if they are reversible. They do not usually cause clinical symptoms.

The **fibrous plaque** characteristic of atherosclerosis is composed of smooth muscle cells, collagen fibers, plasma

NURSING CARE PLAN 31–1
Care of the Patient With Peripheral Vascular Problems

Nursing Interventions	Rationale	Expected Outcomes
NURSING DIAGNOSIS: Alteration in peripheral tissue perfusion related to compromised circulation		
GOAL: Increased arterial blood supply to extremities		
1. Lower the extremities below the level of the heart. 2. Encourage moderate amount of walking or graded extremity exercises. 3. Encourage active postural exercise (Bueger-Allen exercises).	1. Dependency of lower extremities enhances arterial blood supply 2. Muscular exercise promotes blood flow and the development of collateral circulation. 3. With postural exercises, gravity alternately fills and empties the blood vessels.	• Extremities are warm to touch • Color of extremities improved • Experiences decreased muscle pain with exercise • Performs Bueger-Allen exercise series 6 times, 4 times per day as tolerated
GOAL: Decrease in venous congestion		
1. Elevate extremities above heart level. 2. Discourage standing still or sitting for prolonged periods. 3. Encourage walking.	1. Elevation of extremities counteracts gravitational pull, promotes venous return, and prevents venous stasis. 2. Prolonged standing still or sitting promotes venous stasis. 3. Walking promotes venous return by activating the "muscle pump."	• Elevates lower extremities as prescribed • Decreased edema of extremities • Avoids prolonged standing still or sitting • Gradually increases walking time daily
GOAL: Promotion of vasodilation and prevention of vascular compression		
1. Maintain warm temperature and avoid chilling. 2. Discourage smoking. 3. Counsel in ways to avoid emotional upsets; stress management. 4. Encourage avoidance of constrictive clothing and accessories (*e.g.,* constricting seat belts) 5. Encourage avoidance of leg crossing 6. Administer vasodilator drugs and adrenergic blocking agents as prescribed, with appropriate nursing considerations	1. Warmth promotes arterial flow by preventing the vasoconstriction effects of chilling 2. Nicotine causes vasospasm, which impedes peripheral circulation 3. Emotional stress causes peripheral vasoconstriction by stimulating the sympathetic nervous system 4. Constrictive clothing and accessories impede circulation and promote venous stasis 5. Leg crossing causes compression of vessels with subsequent impediment of circulation, resulting in venous stasis 6. Vasodilators relax smooth muscle, adrenergic blocking agents block the response to sympathetic nerve impulses or circulating catecholamines	• Protects extremities from exposure to cold • Does not smoke • Uses stress management program to minimize emotional upset • Avoids constricting clothing and accessories • Avoids leg crossing • Takes medication as prescribed
NURSING DIAGNOSIS: Pain related to impaired ability of peripheral vessels to supply tissues with oxygen		
GOAL: Relief of pain		
1. Promote increased circulation.	1. Enhancement of peripheral circulation increases the oxygen supplied to the muscle and decreases the accumulation of metabolites that cause muscle spasms	• Uses measures to increase arterial blood supply to extremities

(*continued*)

NURSING CARE PLAN 31–1 *(continued)*
Care of the Patient With Peripheral Vascular Problems

Nursing Interventions	Rationale	Expected Outcomes
2. Administer analgesics as prescribed, with appropriate nursing considerations.	2. Analgesics help to reduce pain and allow the patient to participate in activities and exercises that promote circulation	• Uses analgesics as prescribed
NURSING DIAGNOSIS: Risk for impaired skin integrity related to compromised circulation		
GOAL: Attainment/maintenance of tissue integrity		
1. Instruct in ways to avoid trauma to extremities.	1. Poorly nourished tissues are susceptible to trauma and bacterial invasion; healing of wounds is delayed or inhibited due to poor tissue perfusion	• Inspects skin daily for evidence of injury or ulceration • Avoids trauma and irritation to skin • Wears protective shoes • Adheres to meticulous hygienic regimen • Eats well-balanced diet that contains adequate protein and vitamins B and C
2. Encourage wearing protective shoes and padding for pressure areas.	2. Protective shoes and padding prevent foot injuries and blisters	
3. Encourage meticulous hygiene; bathing with neutral soaps, applying lotions, carefully trimming nails.	3. Neutral soaps and lotions prevent drying and cracking of skin	
4. Caution to avoid scratching or vigorous rubbing.	4. Scratching and rubbing can cause skin abrasions and bacterial invasion	
5. Promote good nutrition; adequate intake of vitamins B and C and protein; control of obesity.	5. Good nutrition promotes healing and prevents tissue breakdown	
NURSING DIAGNOSIS: Knowledge deficit regarding self-care activities		
GOAL: Adherence to the self-care program		
1. Include family/significant others in teaching program.	1. Adherence to the self-care program is enhanced when the patient receives support from family and from appropriate self-help groups and agencies.	• Practices frequent position changes as prescribed • Practices postural exercises as prescribed • Takes medications as prescribed • Avoids vasoconstrictors • Uses measures to prevent trauma • Uses stress management program • Accepts condition as chronic but amenable to therapies that will decrease symptomatology
2. Provide written instructions about foot care, leg care, and exercise program.	2. Written instructions serve as reminder and reinforcement of information.	
3. Assist to secure properly fitting clothing, shoes, stockings.		
4. Refer to self-help groups as indicated, *e.g.*, smoking cessation clinics, stress management, weight management, and exercise program.		

components, and lipids. It is white to whitish-yellow and protrudes in varying degrees into the arterial lumen, at times completely obstructing it. These plaques are found predominantly in the abdominal aorta, coronary, popliteal, and internal carotid arteries. This plaque is believed to be an irreversible lesion (Fig. 31-5).

Gradual narrowing of the arterial lumen as the disease process progresses stimulates the development of collateral circulation (Fig. 31-6).

This vascular "bypass" allows continued perfusion to the tissues beyond the arterial obstruction, but it is often inadequate to meet imposed metabolic demands, and ischemia results. The collateral vessels may or may not provide adequate perfusion to distal tissues.

Risk Factors

Many factors are associated with the development of atherosclerosis. Although it is not completely clear whether modification of these risk factors prevents the development of cardiovascular disease, evidence indicates that it may slow the disease process. Some risk factors, such as age or gender, cannot be modified. It is believed, however, that genetic factors can be modified indirectly by altering other risk fac-

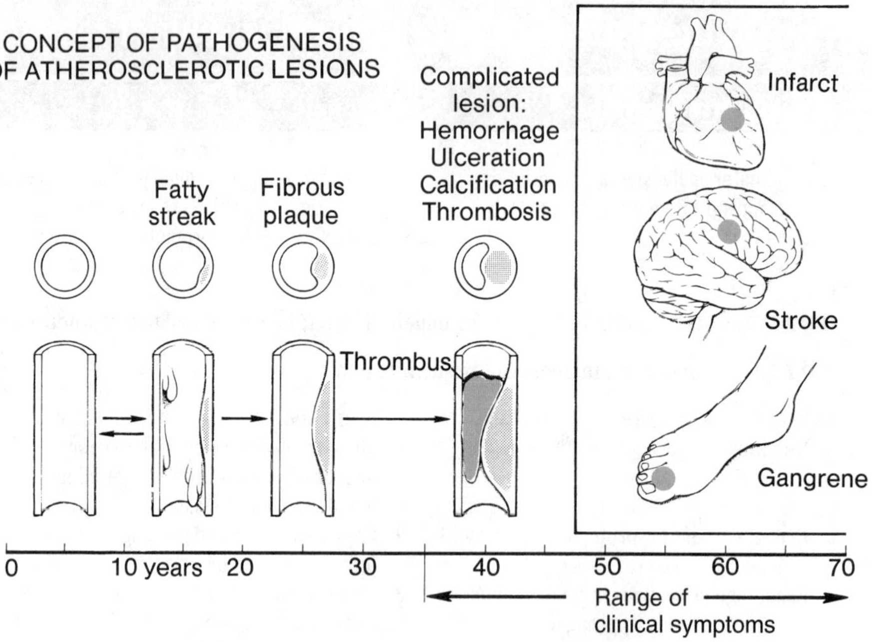

FIGURE 31-5. Schematic concept of the progression of atherosclerosis. Fatty streaks constitute one of the earliest lesions of atherosclerosis. Many fatty streaks regress, whereas others progress to fibrous plaques and eventually to atheromata. These may then bccomc complicated by hemorrhage, ulceration, calcification, or thrombosis and may produce myocardial infarction. (Adapted from Hurst JW and Logue RB. The Heart. New York, McGraw-Hill.)

tors. These controllable risk factors include dietary factors, high blood pressure, diabetes, and smoking.

A diet high in fat has been strongly implicated in causing atherosclerosis. Approximately 39% of the calories Americans ingest are derived from fats. A complete explanation of the relationship between high cholesterol and cardiovascular disease can be found in Chapter 28. The American

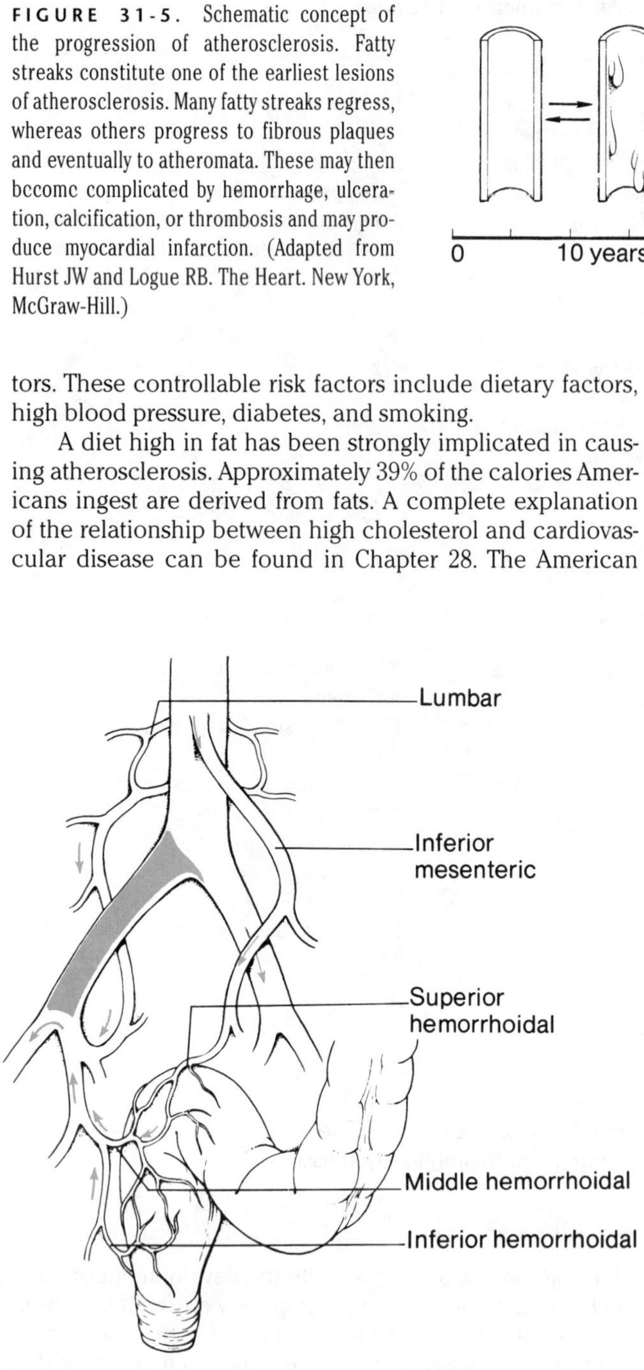

FIGURE 31-6. Development of collateral channels in response to occlusion of the right common iliac artery and the terminal aortic bifurcation.

Heart Association recommends that, to reduce the risk of cardiovascular disease, persons should reduce the total amount of fat ingested in the diet, substitute unsaturated fats for saturated fats, and decrease the intake of cholesterol to no more than 300 mg per day.

Certain medications are now being used to reduce blood lipid levels in conjunction with dietary modification and exercise. Several medication classifications are used: bile acid sequestrants (cholestyramine or colestipol), nicotinic acid, statins (lovastatin, pravastin, and simvastatin), fibric acids (gemfibrozil), probucol, and estrogen replacement therapy. Close supervision of patients on long-term therapy with these medications is required.

Hypertension, which accelerates the rate at which atherosclerotic lesions form in high-pressure vessels, can lead to stroke. The use of antihypertensive medication reduces the incidence of stroke. **Diabetes** also speeds up the atherosclerotic process by thickening the basement membranes of both the large and small vessels.

Smoking is one of the strongest risk factors in the development of atherosclerotic lesions. Nicotine decreases blood flow to the extremities and increases heart rate and blood pressure by stimulating the sympathetic nervous system. In addition, it increases the chances of clot formation by increasing the aggregation of platelets. By combining more readily with the hemoglobin, carbon monoxide deprives the tissues of oxygen. The number of cigarettes smoked is directly related to the extent of the disease. Cessation of smoking reduces the risks. Many other factors such as **obesity, stress,** and **lack of exercise** have been identified as contributing to the disease process.

Although no single risk factor has been identified as the primary contributor to the development of atherosclerotic cardiovascular disease, it is clear that the greater the number of risk factors, the greater the likelihood of developing the disease. Therefore, the elimination of all controllable risk factors is strongly emphasized.

Clinical Manifestations

The clinical signs and symptoms resulting from the atherosclerotic process depend on the organ or tissue affected. Coronary atherosclerosis (heart disease), angina, and acute myocardial infarction are discussed in Chapter 28. Cerebrovascular disease, including transient cerebral ischemic attacks and stroke, is discussed in Chapter 60. Atherosclerosis of the aorta, including aneurysm, and atherosclerotic lesions of the extremities are discussed later in this chapter.

Management

The traditional management of atherosclerosis depends on modification of risk factors, medication, surgical graft procedures (connecting two vessels with good blood flow to each other), and the nursing measures previously discussed. The surgical graft procedure to be performed is determined from the angiogram that identifies the level of obstruction.

Vascular surgical procedures are divided into two groups: inflow procedures that provide blood supply from the aorta into the femoral artery, and outflow procedures that provide blood supply to vessels below the femoral artery.

If the obstruction is at the level of the aorta or iliac artery, new inflow of blood is required. The surgical procedure of choice is the aorta-bi-iliac graft. If possible, the distal anastomosis is made to the iliac artery and therefore the entire surgical procedure can be performed within the abdomen. If, however, the iliacs are aneurysmal or occluded, the distal anastomosis must be to the femoral arteries (aorta-bifemoral). If inflow is needed and the patient's physical condition does not warrant abdominal surgery, which causes wide variations in blood pressure and is a lengthy procedure, an inflow procedure can be from the axillary artery to the femoral artery.

Either axillary artery may be used for inflow. This is important because many of these patients have occluded vessels due to other conditions such as chronic renal failure requiring hemodialysis. For example, if the right axillary artery is used it can be connected by a graft placed to the left femoral artery (if this femoral artery is adequate) to supply blood to the left leg. Thus the patient would receive a right axillary femoral and a femoral-to-femoral graft going right to left. If both sides require blood, an axillary bifemoral graft is necessary.

If the atherosclerotic occlusion is below the inguinal ligament in the superficial femoral artery, the surgical procedure of choice is the femoral-to-popliteal graft. If the distal anastomosis is above the knee, prosthetic material may be used for the graft. If however, the distal anastomosis is below the knee, the saphenous vein is required to ensure patency.

Lower leg or ankle vessels with occlusions may also require grafts. Occasionally the entire popliteal artery is occluded and only collateral circulation is identified. The graft would be from the femoral to either the posterior tibial, anterior tibial, or peroneal artery. These grafts require native vein to ensure patency. Native vein is autologous vein, usually the short or long saphenous vein, or a combination of veins to meet the required length. How long the graft remains patent is determined by several facts including size of graft, graft location, and development of intimal hyperplasia at anastomosis sites.

Several x-ray techniques have been shown to be important adjunctive therapies to surgical procedures. Laser angioplasty is a technique whereby amplified light waves are transmitted by fiberoptic catheters. The laser beam heats the tip of a percutaneous catheter and vaporizes the atherosclerotic plaque. The rotational arthrectomy device removes lesions by abrading plaque that has completely occluded the artery. The advantage to laser, angioplasty, and arthrectomy is the decreased length of hospital stay required for the treatment.

Peripheral Arterial Occlusive Disease

Arterial insufficiency of the extremities is usually found in individuals over 50 years of age, most often in men. The legs are most frequently affected. The age of onset and severity are influenced by the type and number of atherosclerotic risk factors. In peripheral vascular disease, obstructive lesions are predominantly confined to segments of the arterial system extending from the aorta, below the renal arteries, to the popliteal artery (Fig. 31-7). However, distal occlusive disease is frequently seen in patients with diabetes mellitus and in the geriatric population.

Clinical Manifestations

The hallmark of peripheral arterial insufficiency is **intermittent claudication.** This pain is insidious and may be described as aching, cramping, fatigue, or weakness. **Rest pain** is persistent, aching, or boring, and is usually present in the distal portions of the extremities. Elevating the extremity or placing it in a horizontal position will increase the pain, whereas placing the extremity in a dependent position reduces the pain. Some patients sleep with the affected leg hanging over the side of the bed in an attempt to relieve the pain.

A sensation of coldness or numbness in the extremities may accompany intermittent claudication and is a result of the reduced arterial flow. When the extremity is examined it may feel cool and look pale when elevated or ruddy and cyanotic when placed in a dependent position. Skin and nail changes, ulcerations, gangrene, and muscle atrophy may be evident. Bruits may be auscultated with a stethoscope (a **bruit** is the sound produced by turbulent flow of blood through an irregular, stenotic vessel or through a dilated segment of the vessel—an aneurysm). Peripheral pulses may be diminished or absent.

Examining the peripheral pulses is an important part of assessing for arterial occlusive disease. Unequal pulses between extremities or the absence of a normally palpable pulse is a reliable sign of occlusion. The femoral pulse in the groin and the posterior tibial pulse beside the medial malleolus are most easily found. The popliteal pulse is sometimes difficult to palpate behind the knee in an obese patient; the location of the pedal artery on the dorsum of the foot varies and is normally absent in about 7% of the population.

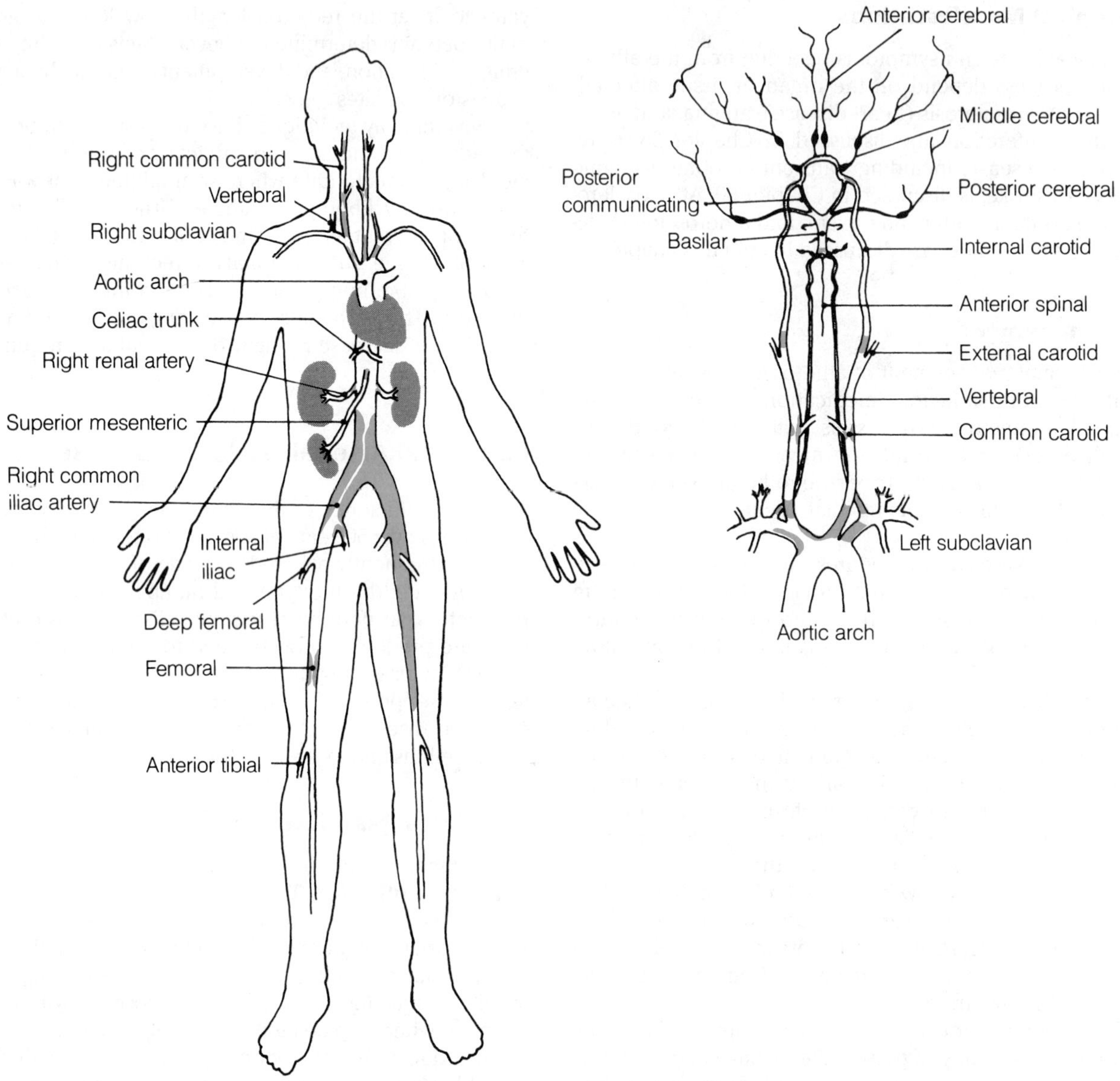

FIGURE 31-7. Common sites of atherosclerotic obstruction in major arterial systems of the body. (Figure at *left* redrawn from Crawford ES and DeBakey ME. Surgical treatment of occlusive cerebrovascular disease. Mod Treat 2:36. Figure at *right* from Beeson PB and McDermott W. Textbook of Medicine. Philadelphia, WB Saunders.)

Assessment

The presence, location, and extent of arterial occlusive disease are determined by a careful history of the patient's symptoms and by physical examination. The color and temperature of the extremity are noted and the pulses palpated. The nails may be thickened and opaque, and the skin shiny, atrophic, and dry with sparse hair growth. A comparative assessment is made of the two extremities.

Diagnostic Evaluation and Management

Doppler ultrasonic flow studies help determine the qualitative and quantitative aspects of the problem. The Doppler is an electronic stethoscope that can reflect the sound of blood flow even when pulses are not palpable. In addition, the Doppler can be coupled with a standard pneumatic cuff to provide lower extremity blood pressure measurements. When leg blood pressures are compared with arm pressures in a patient with arterial occlusive disease of the lower extremities, the pressure in the legs will be lower than that in the arms.

Oscillometry is used to measure variations in pulse volumes at different levels of the extremity. Two measurement indices may be taken: the ankle–arm index (AAI) or the ankle–brachial index (ABI). A Doppler and blood pressure cuff are used to obtain the systolic pressure in the arms. A blood pressure cuff is then placed around the ankle and Doppler signals are obtained in both the posterior tibialis and dorsalis pedis arteries. The highest ankle pressure obtained is divided by the arm pressure.

For example, if the right arm pressure is 160 mm Hg and the right dorsalis pedis pressure is 90 mm Hg, while the right posterior tibialis pressure is 120 mm Hg, the ABI is 120 divided by 160 or 0.75. Normal ABI is 0.95 to 1.0. The ABI provides a quick reference to the severity of the disease. Patients with an ABI below 0.75 to 0.40 frequently experience claudication. If the ABI is below 0.40, the limb is considered to be ischemic.

Calcified vessels are incompressible and yield false high readings of ankle brachial indices. The pulse volume wave recording, which normally appears in the shape of an arterial wave form, will change shape with the presence of occlusion. The pulse volume wave recordings are more accurate than the ankle brachial index if calcified vessels are present.

Angiography may be used to confirm the diagnosis of occlusive arterial disease if surgery is considered. The procedure involves injecting a contrast medium directly into the vascular system to visualize the vessels as the radiopaque material flows through them. The location of vascular obstructions or aneurysms and the presence of collateral circulation can be demonstrated. Usually patients experience a temporary sensation of warmth as the contrast medium is injected. Local irritation at the injection site may occur. Infrequently, a patient may have an allergic reaction to the iodine contained in the contrast material. This reaction may appear immediately after the injection or may be delayed. Manifestations may include dyspnea, nausea and vomiting, sweating, tachycardia, and numbness of the extremities. Any such reaction is reported at once; treatment may include the administration of epinephrine (adrenalin), antihistamines, or steroids. In addition, there are risks of vessel injury, bleeding, and possibly stroke.

Digital subtraction angiography (DSA) is a visualization of arterial vessels using radiographic and computer technology. Usually, angiography requires hospital admission from the day before the test until 24 hours after the test, and there are risks of severe complications after the procedure. With DSA, no hospitalization is necessary and the risks are fewer because the arterial system is not entered. An image-intensifier video system displays the vessels on a TV monitor. The computer eliminates those images not required so that the final image of the desired area is intensified.

If an isolated lesion or lesions are identified during the angiogram, **percutaneous transluminal angioplasty (PTA)** may be performed. Under local anesthesia, a balloon catheter is maneuvered across the area of stenosis or occlusion. The balloon is inflated and cracks the lesion, compressing it back up against the vessel wall. Angioplasty can be performed for many different levels of lesions but is most successful in stenosis of the iliac arteries. Complications from PTA include hematoma formation, embolus, arterial dissection, and bleeding.

If an occluded vessel or graft can be cannulated with a guide wire during the arteriogram, **thrombolytic therapy** may be instituted. In some cases of total occlusion, thrombolytic therapy is useful to dissolve a clot and to identify an underlying stenosis that can be treated with PTA. Combined use of these two therapies is referred to as *thrombolysoangioplasty*. Because surgery and general anesthesia are not required for PTA, the morbidity and mortality are less than for surgical corrective procedures, as are the length and cost of hospitalization. If restenosis occurs, subsequent PTAs can be performed, or if that is not feasible, operation may be required.

In some cases of arterial insufficiency an **exercise test** may be helpful to determine the amount of activity possible before the onset of intermittent claudication. A **lumbar sympathetic block** is a test used to evaluate peripheral circulation. An injection of a local anesthetic is made into the lumbar epidural space to block the sympathetic nerves that go to the legs. Because the sympathetic nerves control the tension in the muscles of the blood vessels, a block of these nerves should produce vasodilation and increased temperature in the legs. Because atherosclerotic vessels are incapable of vasodilation, there is either no increase in the temperature in the legs or only a slight increase. This test is often used to determine if **sympathectomy** (interruption of afferent pathways in the sympathetic division of the autonomic nervous system) would be of benefit to the patient with impaired circulation of the legs. Sympathectomy eliminates vasospasm and improves peripheral blood flow. Sympathectomy may be used if there are no other surgical options available and in cases of reflex sympathetic dystrophy. Reflex sympathetic dystrophy is a form of causalgic (intense burning) pain. This pain may be caused by ischemic damage to peripheral nerves following delayed revascularization, or it may follow inadvertant injury during surgery.

The general care measures for patients with peripheral arterial disorders were described earlier in this chapter and are summarized in Chart 31-2. Generally, patients feel better on some type of exercise program. If this program is combined with weight reduction and the cessation of smoking, patients often can improve their activity tolerance. Patients should not be promised that their symptoms will be relieved if they stop smoking. If claudication persists, they may lose their motivation not to smoke.

In most patients, when intermittent claudication has become severe and disabling or when the limb is at risk for amputation owing to tissue loss, vascular **grafting** or **endarterectomy** is the treatment of choice. A graft is created by connecting two vessels with good flow to each other. For example, a portion of the femoral artery is connected to the posterior tibial artery. Material used for arterial bypass grafts may be synthetic (*e.g.*, Dacron) or may be from autogenous veins (*e.g.*, saphenous vein). Specific types of grafts are discussed earlier in this chapter. When an endarterectomy is performed, an incision is made into the artery and the atheromatous obstruction is "removed." The artery is then sutured closed to restore vascular integrity.

Postoperative Nursing Management. The primary objective in postoperative management of patients who have undergone vascular procedures is to maintain adequate circulation through the arterial repair. Pulses of the affected extremities are checked and recorded frequently and compared with those of the other extremity. Disappearance of a pulse may indicate thrombotic occlusion of the graft, so the surgeon is immediately notified. The color and temperature of the extremity are also monitored and any changes reported. An adequate circulating blood volume should be established and maintained. Continuous monitoring of urine output, central venous pressure, mental status, and pulse rate and volume permits the early recognition and treatment of fluid imbalances. Leg crossing and prolonged extremity dependency are avoided to prevent thrombosis. Leg elevation reduces edema.

Thromboangiitis Obliterans (Buerger's Disease)

Buerger's disease is characterized by recurring inflammation of the intermediate and small arteries and veins of the lower and (in rare cases) upper extremities, and results in thrombus formation and occlusion of the vessels. It is differentiated from other vessel diseases by its microscopic appearance. In contrast to atherosclerosis, Buerger's disease is believed to be an autoimmune disease that results in occlusion of distal vessels. Although this condition is different from atherosclerosis, in older patients with Buerger's disease atherosclerosis of the larger vessels may occur after involvement of the smaller vessels.

Etiology and Clinical Manifestations

The cause of Buerger's disease is unknown, but it is believed to be due to autoimmune vasculitis. It occurs most often in men between the ages of 20 and 35, and it has been reported in all races in many areas of the world. There is considerable evidence that heavy smoking is either a causative or aggravating factor. Generally, the lower extremities are affected, but arteries in the upper extremities or viscera can also be involved. Superficial thrombophlebitis may be present. Arteriography confirms arterial occlusive disease.

Pain is the outstanding symptom of Buerger's disease. The patient complains of cramps in the feet (especially the arches) or legs after exercise (intermittent claudication), which are relieved by rest; often there is considerable burning pain that is aggravated by emotional disturbances, smoking, or chilling. Rest pain, a sensation of burning or sensitivity to cold, may be early symptoms. Rest pain is present all the time. The characteristic of the pain does not change between activity and rest. Various types of paresthesia may develop, and pulses may be diminished or absent.

As the disease progresses, definite redness or cyanosis of the part appears when the extremity is in a dependent position. Color changes may affect only one extremity or only certain digits. This may progress to ulceration. Ulceration with gangrene eventually occurs.

Management and Nursing Interventions

The treatment of Buerger's disease is essentially the same as that for atherosclerotic peripheral vascular disease. The main objectives are to improve circulation to the extremities, prevent the progression of the disease, and protect the extremities from trauma and infection. Smoking is highly detrimental, and patients are advised to stop completely. Smoking cessation programs are helpful for many patients. Symptoms are often relieved by cessation of smoking.

Vasodilators are rarely prescribed because these medications cause dilation of only healthy vessels; therefore, vasodilators may even divert blood away from the partially occluded vessels, which makes the situation worse. Regional sympathetic block or ganglionectomy may be useful in some instances to produce vasodilation and thereby increase blood flow.

Prognosis

If gangrene of a toe develops as a result of arterial occlusive disease in the leg, it is unlikely that toe amputation or even transmetatarsal amputation will be sufficient. Usually a below-knee amputation, or occasionally an above-knee amputation, is necessary. The indications for amputation are worsening gangrene, especially if moist; severe rest pain; or fulminating sepsis. If any of these is present amputation becomes necessary.

Aortic Diseases

The aorta, which is the main trunk of the arterial system, is divided into the ascending aorta (5 cm [2 inches] contained in the pericardium), the aortic arch (extending upward, backward, and downward), and the descending aorta. The aorta is designated as thoracic above the diaphragm and abdominal below the diaphragm.

Aortitis

Aortitis is inflammation of the aorta, particularly of the aortic arch. Two types are known to occur: Takayasu's disease and syphilitic aortitis. Takayasu's disease, or occlusive thromboaortopathy, is uncommon; syphilitic aortitis is rarely seen today.

Takayasu's Disease. Takayasu's disease is a chronic inflammatory disease of the aortic arch and its branches seen primarily in young or middle-aged women. It results in ischemic symptoms affecting the upper extremities, brain, and eyes. In the early stages, it may respond to corticosteroids.

Syphilitic Aortitis. Syphilitic aortitis usually begins before the age of 50. It affects the aortic root and ascending aorta. In most cases, the inflammatory process produces moderate dilation of the aorta, but it can produce more serious complications such as aortic insufficiency, aneurysm, or occlusion of the coronary ostia. Symptoms experienced by patients include angina or substernal heaviness due to coronary involvement; shortness of breath and congestive heart failure may be present if aortic insufficiency is present.

Aortic Aneurysms

Classification of Aneurysms

An aneurysm is a localized sac or dilation involving an artery formed at a weak point in the vessel wall (Fig. 31-8); it may be classified by either the shape or the form of the defect. The most common forms of aneurysms are those that are saccular or fusiform. A saccular aneurysm projects from one side of the vessel only. If an entire arterial segment becomes dilated, a *fusiform aneurysm* develops. Very small aneurysms due to a localized infection are called *mycotic aneurysms*. The most common cause of aneurysm is atherosclerosis. Other causes include trauma to the wall of the ar-

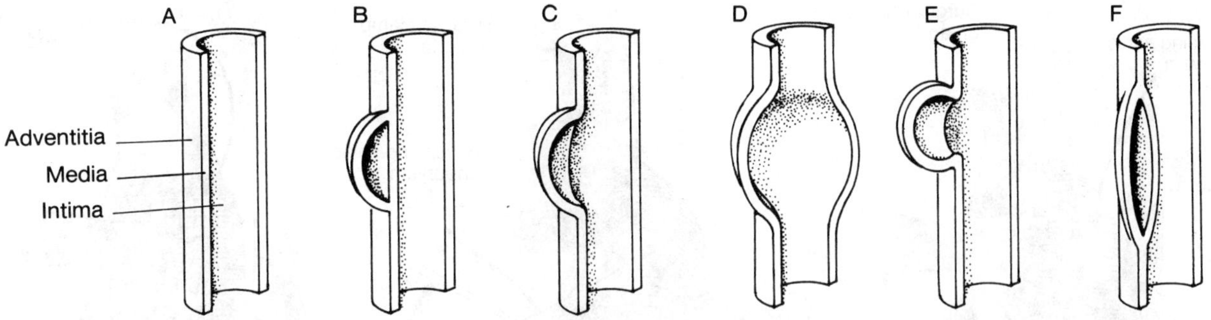

FIGURE 31-8. Characteristics of arterial aneurysm. (**A**) Normal artery. (**B**) False aneurysm—actually a pulsating hematoma. The clot and connective tissue are outside the arterial wall. (**C**) True aneurysm. One, two, or all three layers may be involved. (**D**) Fusiform aneurysm—symmetrical, spindle-shaped expansion of entire circumference of involved vessel. (**E**) Saccular aneurysm—a bulbous protrusion of one side of the arterial wall. (**F**) Dissecting aneurysm—this usually is a hematoma that splits the layers of the arterial wall.

tery, infection (pyogenic or syphilitic), and congenital defects of the artery wall. Aneurysms are serious because they can rupture, leading to hemorrhage and death.

Aneurysm of the Thoracic Aorta

Approximately 85% of all cases of thoracic aortic aneurysm are caused by atherosclerosis. They occur most frequently in men between the ages of 40 and 70 years. The thoracic area is the most common site for the development of a dissecting aneurysm. About one third of patients with thoracic aneurysms die from rupture of the aneurysm.

Clinical Manifestations. Symptoms are variable and depend on how rapidly the aneurysm dilates and how the pulsating mass affects surrounding intrathoracic structures. Some patients are asymptomatic. In most cases *pain* is the most prominent symptom. The pain is usually constant and boring in character and may occur only when the person is lying in a supine position. Other conspicuous symptoms are *dyspnea,* the result of pressure of the sac against the trachea, a main bronchus, or the lung itself; *cough,* frequently paroxysmal and with a brassy quality; *hoarseness,* stridor, weakness or complete loss of the voice (aphonia), resulting from pressure against the left recurrent laryngeal nerve; and *dysphagia* (difficulty in swallowing) due to impingement on the esophagus.

When large veins in the chest are compressed by the aneurysm, the superficial veins on the chest, neck, or the arms become dilated and edematous areas on the chest wall and cyanosis are often evident. Pressure against the cervical sympathetic chain can result in unequal pupils in the eyes. Diagnosis of a thoracic aortic aneurysm is principally by chest x-ray, sonography, and computed tomography (CT) scan.

Management. In most cases, an aneurysm is treated by surgical repair. General measures such as controlling blood pressure and correcting risk factors may be useful. It is very important to control blood pressure in patients with dissecting aneurysms. Systolic pressure is maintained at about 100 to 120 mm Hg with antihypertensive drugs (*e.g.,* labetalol, nitroprusside). Pulsatile flow is reduced by medications that reduce cardiac contractility (*e.g.,* propranolol). The goal of surgery is to remove the aneurysm and restore vascular continuity with a vascular graft (Fig. 31-9). Intensive monitoring is usually required after this type of surgery, and the patient is cared for in the critical care unit.

Abdominal Aortic Aneurysm

The most common cause of abdominal aortic aneurysm is atherosclerosis. The condition is more common among Caucasians, affects men four times more often than women, and is most prevalent after the age of 60. Most of these aneurysms occur below the renal arteries. Untreated, the eventual outcome may be rupture and death.

Pathophysiology. All aneurysms involve a damaged media layer of the vessel. This may be caused by congenital weakness, trauma, or disease process. Once an aneurysm develops, it tends to increase in size. Risk factors include genetic predisposition, smoking, and hypertension. More than half of these patients exhibit hypertension.

Clinical Manifestations and Diagnosis. About two fifths of patients with abdominal aortic aneurysms have symptoms; the remainder are asymptomatic. Some patients complain that they can feel their "heart beating" in their abdomen when lying down, or they may claim to feel the presence of an abdominal mass or abdominal throbbing. If the abdominal aortic aneurysm is associated with thrombus, a major vessel may be occluded or smaller distal occlusions may result from emboli. An occlusion of a digital vessel causes "blue toe syndrome."

The most important diagnostic indication of an abdominal aortic aneurysm is the presence of a pulsatile mass in the middle and upper abdomen. About 80% of these aneurysms can be palpated. A systolic bruit may be heard over the mass. An abdominal x-ray study may confirm the existence of an aneurysm, if the aneurysm is calcified. Ultrasonography or CT scan is useful for determining the size of the aneurysm. When the aneurysm is small, serial ultrasonography is conducted at 6-month intervals until the aneurysm reaches a size where operation to prevent rupture is of more benefit than the possible complications of a surgical procedure. Some aneurysms remain stable over many years of observation.

Management. An expanding or enlarging abdominal aneurysm is likely to rupture. Therefore, surgery is the treatment of choice for abdominal aneurysms larger than 5 cm (2 in) in diameter or those that are enlarging. The aneurysm

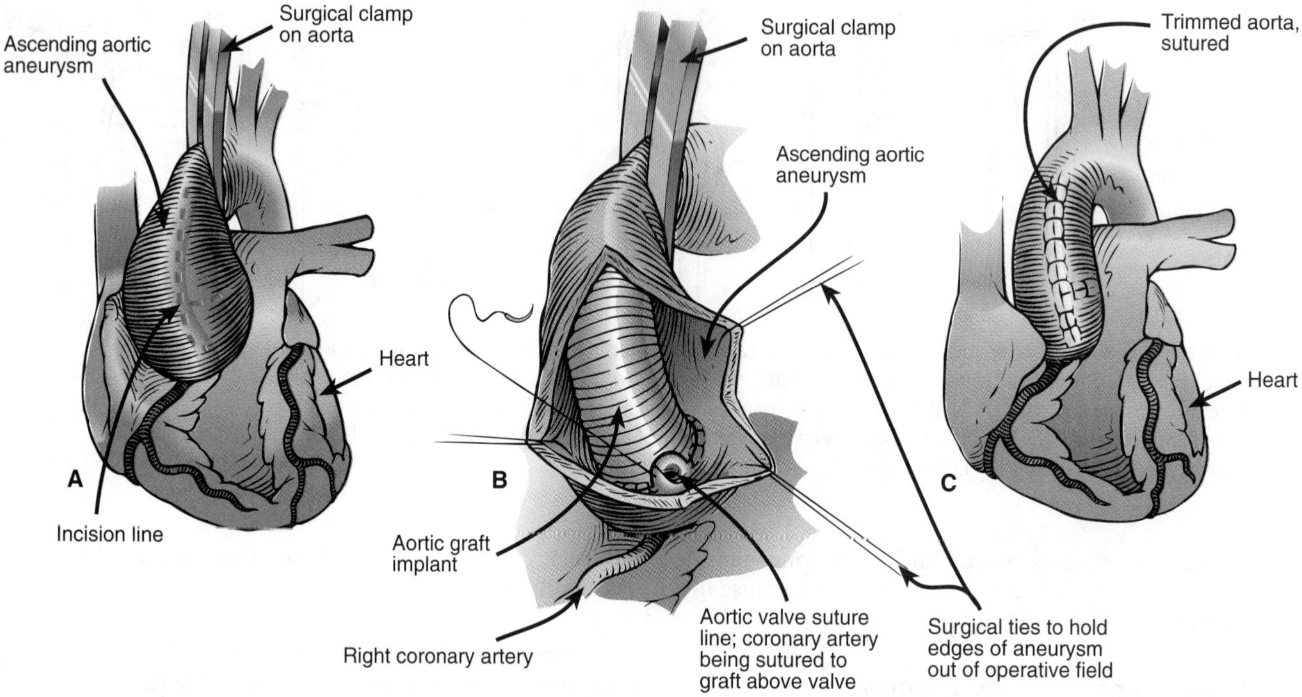

FIGURE 31-9. Repair of an ascending aortic aneurysm and aortic valve replacement: (**A**) incision into aortic aneurysm; (**B**) aortic valve replacement with aortic graft implant to repair ascending aortic aneurysm; (**C**) aortic aneurysm trimmed and closed over graft.

is resected and a bypass (synthetic) graft is inserted (Fig. 31-10). Elective aneurysm repair, a major surgical procedure, has a reported mortality rate of 1% to 4%. The prognosis for a patient with a ruptured aneurysm is poor, and surgery is performed immediately.

Preoperatively, nursing assessment should be guided by the fact that the aneurysm might rupture and by the recognition that the patient may have cardiovascular, cerebral, pulmonary, and renal impairment secondary to atherosclerosis. Therefore, the functional capacity of all organ systems should be established. Medical therapies designed to stabilize physiologic function should be promptly implemented. Postoperative care requires intense monitoring of pulmonary, cardiovascular, renal, and neurologic status. Possible complications of surgery include arterial occlusion, hemorrhage, infection, ischemic colon, renal failure, and impotence.

Signs of impending rupture include severe back pain or abdominal pain, which may be persistent or intermittent and is often localized in the middle or lower abdomen to the left of the midline. Low back pain may also be present owing to pressure of the aneurysm on the lumbar nerves. This is a serious symptom, usually indicating that the aneurysm is expanding rapidly and is about to rupture. Indications of a rupturing abdominal aortic aneurysm include a constant intense back pain, falling blood pressure, and decreasing hematocrit. A retroperitoneal rupture of an aneurysm may result in hematomas in the scrotum, perineum, flank, or penis. Signs of heart failure or a loud bruit may suggest a rupture into the vena cava. Rupture into the peritoneal cavity is rapidly fatal. The overall surgical mortality rate with ruptured aneurysm is 50% to 75%.

Dissecting Aneurysm of the Aorta

Pathophysiology. Occasionally, in an aorta diseased by arteriosclerosis, a tear develops in the intima or the media degenerates, resulting in a dissection. Dissecting aneurysms are often associated with poorly controlled hypertension; they are three times more common in men than in women and occur in the 50- to 70-year-old age group. A dissecting aneurysm is caused by rupture in the intimal layer resulting in blood dissecting in the layers of media. A rupture may occur through adventitia or into the lumen through the intima, thereby allowing blood to re-enter the main channel, resulting in chronic dissection, or the dissection can result in occlusion of branches of the aorta. Death is usually caused by external rupture of the hematoma.

Clinical Manifestations and Assessment. As the dissection progresses, the arteries branching from the involved area of the aorta become sheared and occluded. The tear occurs most commonly in the region of the aortic arch, with the highest mortality associated with ascending aortic dissection. The dissection of the aorta may progress backward in the direction of the heart, obstructing the opening to the coronary arteries or producing hemopericardium (effusion of blood into the pericardial sac) or aortic insufficiency, or it may extend in the opposite direction, causing occlusion of the arteries supplying the gastrointestinal tract, the kidneys, the spinal cord, and even the legs.

The onset of symptoms is usually sudden. Severe and persistent pain, described as "tearing" or "ripping," may be reported in the anterior chest or back and extends to shoulders, epigastric area, or abdomen. Cardiovascular, neurologic, and gastrointestinal symptoms are responsible for other clinical manifestations, depending on the loca-

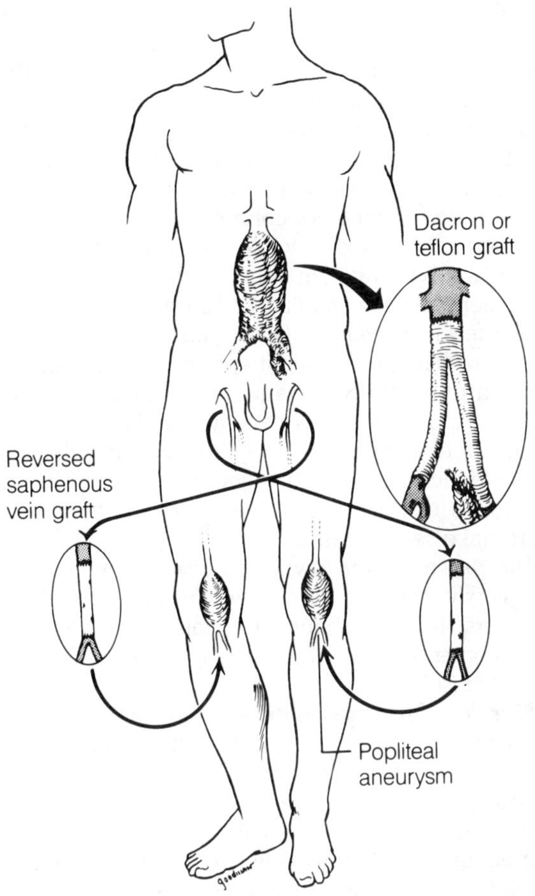

FIGURE 31-10. Surgical treatment of a large abdominal aneurysm involving the iliac arteries plus bilateral symptomatic popliteal aneurysms. Following resection, the abdominal aneurysm is replaced with a Goretex graft; the popliteal aneurysms are replaced by saphenous vein grafts, which appear to function much better at the flexion crease than the synthetic graft. (Hardy JD et al. Aneurysms of the popliteal artery. Surg Gynecol Obstet Mar; 140:402. By permission of Surgery, Gynecology & Obstetrics.)

tion and extensiveness of the dissection. The patient may manifest pallor, sweating, and tachycardia. Blood pressure may be elevated or markedly different from one arm to the other if dissection involves the orifice of the subclavian artery on one side. Because of the variable clinical picture associated with this condition, early diagnosis is often difficult.

Angiogram, CT scan, ultrasound, and magnetic resonance imaging (MRI) aid in the diagnosis. Medical or surgical treatment of a dissecting aneurysm depends on the type of aneurysm present and follows the general principles outlined for treatment of thoracic aortic aneurysms.

Other Aneurysms

Aneurysms may also arise in the peripheral vessels, most often as a result of atherosclerosis. These may involve such vessels as the renal artery, the subclavian artery, or (most frequently) the popliteal artery in the area of the knee. Such aneurysms may be bilateral.

The aneurysm produces a pulsating mass and a disturbance of peripheral circulation distal to it. Pain and swelling develop because of pressure on adjacent nerves and veins. Surgical repair of such aneurysms is performed with replacement grafts.

Gerontologic Considerations

Most abdominal aneurysms occur in patients between the ages of 60 and 90 years. Aneurysm rupture is likely if there is coexisting hypertension or if the aneurysm is larger than 6 cm. The likelihood of rupture increases with size. There is a 30% chance of rupture per year when the aneurysm reaches 6 cm. At this point the chances of rupture are greater than the chance of mortality during the surgical procedure in most cases. At present aneurysms that are 4 cm are repaired in patients who are good candidates for surgery. If the patient is considered at moderate risk for complications related to surgery or anesthesia, the aneurysm is not repaired until it reaches 5 cm. If the patient is a poor surgical risk, the aneurysm is not repaired until it reaches 6 cm. Some aneurysms remain the same size for many years.

Arterial Embolism and Arterial Thrombosis

Pathophysiology. Acute vascular occlusion may be due to an embolus or to acute thrombosis. An embolus is usually diagnosed on the basis of the sudden or acute nature of the onset of symptoms and an apparent source for the embolus. Arterial emboli arise most commonly from thrombi that develop in the chambers of the heart as a result of atrial fibrillation, myocardial infarction, infective endocarditis, or chronic congestive heart failure. These thrombi become detached and are carried from the left side of the heart into the arterial system, where they obstruct an artery that is smaller in size than the embolus. Emboli may also develop in advanced aortic atherosclerosis because the atheromatous plaques ulcerate or become rough. The symptoms of arterial emboli depend primarily on the size of the embolus, the organ involved, and the state of the collateral vessels. The immediate effect is cessation of distal blood flow. The clot can progress above and below the obstruction. Secondary vasospasm can contribute to the ischemia. The embolus can fragment or break apart, resulting in occlusion of distal vessels.

Emboli tend to lodge at arterial bifurcations and areas narrowed by atherosclerosis. Cerebral, mesenteric, renal, and coronary arteries are often involved in addition to the large arteries of the extremities.

Acute thrombosis frequently occurs in patients with pre-existing ischemic symptoms. **Arterial thrombosis** can also acutely occlude an artery. A thrombosis is a slowly developing clot that usually occurs where the arterial wall has become damaged, generally as a result of atherosclerosis. Thrombi may also develop in an arterial aneurysm. The manifestations of an acute thrombotic arterial occlusion are similar to those described for embolic occlusion. However, treatment is more difficult with a thrombus because the arterial occlusion has occurred in a degenerated vessel and requires more extensive reconstructive surgery to restore flow than is required with an embolic event.

Clinical Manifestations. The symptoms of acute arterial embolism in extremities with poor collateral flow are acute, severe pain and a gradual loss of sensory and motor function. The five Ps associated with acute arterial embolism are pain, pallor, pulselessness, paresthesia, and paralysis. Eventually superficial veins may collapse because of decreased blood flow to the extremity. The part of the limb below the occlusion is markedly colder and paler than the part above the occlusion because of ischemia.

Management. Management of arterial thrombois depends on its cause. Acute embolic occlusion usually requires surgery because time is of the essence. Because onset of the event is acute, collateral circulation has not developed and the patient quickly moves through the list of five Ps to paralysis, which is the most advanced stage. With the limb at risk, emergency embolectomy is the surgical procedure of choice. This involves incising the vessel and removing the clot. Before surgery, the patient remains on bed rest with the extremity level or slightly (15 degrees) dependent. The affected part is kept at room temperature and protected from trauma.

When collateral circulation is present, treatment may include intravenous anticoagulation with heparin, which will prevent the clot from spreading and thus reduce muscle necrosis. Thrombolytic agents, such as streptokinase, urokinase, and tissue-type plasminogen activator (t-PA), help to dissolve the embolus. Although these agents differ in their pharmacokinetics, they are administered in a similar manner. A catheter is advanced under x-ray visualization to the clot and the thrombolytic agent is then infused. Thrombolytic therapy should not be used when there are known contraindications to therapy or when the extremity could not tolerate several additional hours of ischemia that would be required for the agent to cause lysis of the clot. Contraindications to thrombolytic therapy include active internal bleeding, stroke, recent major surgery, uncontrolled hypertension, and pregnancy.

Postoperative Nursing Management. During the postoperative period, the nurse collaborates with the surgeon about the appropriate level of activity warranted, which is based on the patient's condition. Generally every effort is made to encourage the patient to move the leg to stimulate circulation and prevent stasis. Anticoagulants may be continued after surgery to prevent thrombosis of the affected artery and to diminish the development of subsequent thrombi at the initiating site. The nurse assesses the surgical incision frequently for evidence of hemorrhage, which can occur when anticoagulants are administered.

Raynaud's Disease

Raynaud's disease is a form of intermittent arteriolar vasoconstriction that results in coldness, pain, and pallor of the fingertips, toes, or tip of the nose. The cause is unknown, although many patients with the disease seem to have immunologic disorders. Recent studies indicate that the symptoms may be the result of a defect in basal heat production that eventually decreases the ability of cutaneous vessels to dilate. Episodes may be triggered by emotional factors or by unusual sensitivity to cold. The disease is most common in women between the ages of 16 and 40 years and is seen much more frequently in cold climates and during the winter months. The classic clinical picture reveals pallor brought on by sudden vasoconstriction. The skin then become bluish (cyanotic) as small amounts of blood enter the capillaries. Vasodilation then produces a red color. Thus the characteristic sequence of color change of Raynaud's phenomenon is described as white, blue, and red. Numbness, tingling, and burning pain occur as the color changes. The involvement tends to be bilateral and symmetric.

The term *Raynaud's phenomenon* is currently used to refer to localized, intermittent episodes of vasoconstriction of small arteries of the feet and hands that cause color and temperature changes. It is generally unilateral and affects only one or two digits. It is always associated with an underlying systemic disease. It may occur with scleroderma, systemic lupus erythematosus, rheumatoid arthritis, obstructive arterial disease, or trauma.

The prognosis for Raynaud's disease varies; some patients slowly improve, some become progressively worse, and others show no change. Ulceration and gangrene are rare; however, chronic disease may cause atrophy of the skin and muscles.

Nursing Management. Avoiding the particular stimuli that provoke vasoconstriction is the prime objective in controlling Raynaud's disease. Efforts should be made to avoid situations that may be upsetting. Concern about serious complications such as gangrene and amputation is common and certainly upsetting. The patient should be reassured that serious sequelae are not usual with Raynaud's disease. Smoking should be avoided.

Exposure to cold must be minimized. In areas where the fall and winter months are cold, the patient should remain indoors as much as possible and wear protective clothing when outdoors. Fabrics specially designed for cold climates (*e.g.*, Thinsulate) are recommended. Sharp objects should be handled carefully to avoid injuring the fingers. The physician may prescribe vasodilators, calcium channel blockers, and sympatholytic agents, such as procardia, nifedipine, or other rauwolfia derivatives, although their effectiveness varies. The patient is cautioned about postural hypotension that can result from these medications and can be affected by alcohol, exercise, and hot weather.

Interrupting the sympathetic nerves by removing the sympathetic ganglia or dividing their branches (**sympathectomy**) may offer some improvement in patients with Raynaud's disease.

Hypertension

Definition, Incidence, and Etiology

Hypertension can be defined arbitrarily as persistent levels of blood pressure in which the systolic pressure is above 140 mm Hg and the diastolic pressure is above 90 mm Hg. In the elderly population, hypertension is defined as systolic pressure above 160 mm Hg and diastolic pressure above 90 mm Hg. Hypertension is a major cause of heart failure, stroke, and kidney failure. It is called the "silent killer" because people with hypertension are often symptom free. The National Heart, Lung, and Blood Institute has estimated that half of the people with hypertension are unaware of the condition. Once it develops, a patient's blood pressure should be monitored at regular intervals because hypertension is a lifetime condition.

About 20% of the adult population develops hypertension; more than 90% of these have *essential* (primary) hypertension, which has no identifiable medical cause. The remainder develop elevations in blood pressure with specific cause (secondary hypertension), such as narrowing of the renal arteries or disease of the parenchyma of the kidneys, certain medications, organ dysfunctions, tumors, and pregnancy.

Hypertension carries the risk of premature morbidity and mortality, which increases as the systolic and diastolic pressures rise. The Fifth Report of the Joint National Committee on Detection, Evaluation, and Treatment of High Blood Pressure (1993) issued new guidelines regarding the detection, evaluation, and treatment of hypertension. The Committee also presented a classification of blood pressure for persons aged 18 years and older that is helpful in establishing follow-up criteria when it is used with the knowledge that a diagnosis is based on the average of two or more readings on two or more occasions (Table 31-3). The American College of Physicians has developed an algorithm illustrating a strategy for measuring blood pressure in nonphysician ambulatory settings as a means of diagnosing hypertension (Fig. 31-11). The Joint National Committee also developed recommendations for follow-up monitoring of individuals whose initial blood pressures readings were elevated (Table 31-4).

Essential hypertension usually begins as a labile (intermittent) process in individuals in their late 30s to early 50s and gradually becomes "fixed." On occasion it appears abruptly and severely and takes an accelerated or "malignant" course that causes the patient's condition to deteriorate rapidly.

Emotional disturbances, obesity, excessive alcohol intake, and overstimulation with coffee, tobacco, and stimulatory drugs play a role, but the disease is strongly familial. It affects more women than men; however, men, especially African-American men, are less able to tolerate the disease. In the United States, the incidence of hypertension increases with the aging process and the incidence for African-Americans far exceeds that of whites.

Prolonged elevation of blood pressure eventually damages blood vessels throughout the body, most notably in the eyes, heart, kidneys, and brain. Therefore, the usual consequences of prolonged, uncontrolled hypertension are failing vision, coronary occlusion, renal failure, and strokes. In addition, the heart becomes enlarged as it is forced to increase its workload in pumping against the sustained high pressure. This hypertrophy is noted on electrocardiogram and chest x-ray.

Increased peripheral resistance controlled at the arteriolar level is the basic cause for elevated blood pressure. The causes of increased resistance are poorly understood. Medication therapy is aimed at decreasing peripheral resistance

TABLE 31-3 Classification of Blood Pressure for Adults Aged 18 Years and Older*

Category	Systolic, mm Hg	Diastolic, mm Hg
Normal†	<130	<85
High normal	130–139	85–89
Hypertension‡		
Stage 1 (mild)	140–159	90–99
Stage 2 (moderate)	160–179	100–109
Stage 3 (severe)	180–209	110–119
Stage 4 (very severe)	≥210	≥120

*Not taking antihypertensive drugs and not acutely ill. When systolic and diastolic pressures fall into different categories, the higher category should be selected to classify the individual's blood pressure status. For instance, 160/92 mm Hg should be classified as stage 2, and 180/120 mm Hg should be classified as stage 4. Isolated systolic hypertension is defined as a systolic blood pressure of 140 mm Hg or more and a diastolic blood pressure of less than 90 mm Hg and staged appropriately (e.g., 170/85 mm Hg is defined as stage 2 isolated systolic hypertension).

In addition to classifying stages of hypertension on the basis of average blood pressure levels, the clinician should specify presence or absence of target-organ disease and additional risk factors. For example, a patient with diabetes and a blood pressure of 142/94 mm Hg, plus left ventricular hypertrophy should be classified as having "stage 1 hypertension with target-organ disease (left ventricular hypertrophy) and with another major risk factor (diabetes)." This specificity is important for risk classification and management.

†Optimal blood pressure with respect to cardiovascular risk is less than 120 mm Hg systolic and less than 80 mm Hg diastolic. However, unusually low readings should be evaluated for clinical significance.

‡Based on the average of two or more readings taken at each of two or more visits after an initial screening.

(The Fifth Report of the Joint National Committee on Detection, Evaluation, and Treatment of High Blood Pressure. Arch Intern Med 1993 Jan 25; 153:161.)

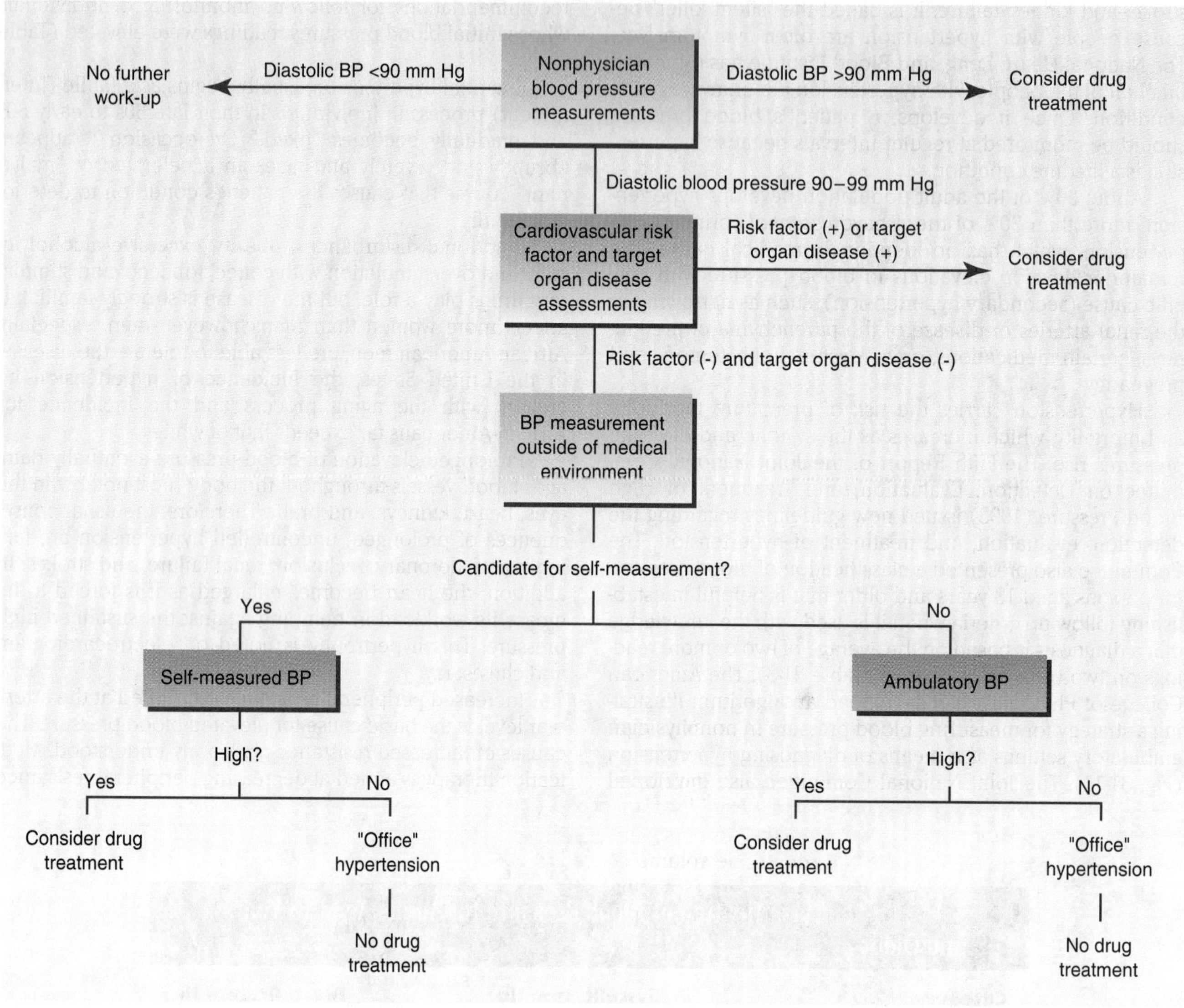

FIGURE 31-11. Algorithm from the American College of Physicians illustrating a strategy for integrating nonphysician self-measured, ambulatory blood pressure measurements in the diagnosis of hypertension.

to lower the blood pressure and reduce the stresses on the vascular system.

Pathophysiology of Essential Hypertension

The mechanism that controls the constriction and relaxation of blood vessels rests in the vasomotor center, situated in the medulla of the brain. Emanating from this vasomotor center are the sympathetic nervous system tracks, which go down the spinal cord and emerge from the spinal column at the sympathetic ganglia in the thorax and abdomen. Stimulation of the vasomotor center sets in motion impulses that travel down through the sympathetic nervous system to the sympathetic ganglia. At this point, the preganglionic neurons release acetylcholine, which stimulates the postganglionic nerve fibers in the blood vessels, where the release of norepinephrine results in constriction of the vessels. Numerous influences such as anxiety and fear may affect the response of the blood vessel to these vasoconstrictor stimuli. People with hypertension are very sensitive to norepinephrine, although it is not known exactly why.

At the same time that the sympathetic nervous system is stimulating the blood vessels in response to emotional stimuli, the adrenal gland is stimulated, resulting in additional vasoconstrictive activity. The adrenal medulla secretes epinephrine, which causes vasoconstriction. The adrenal cortex secretes cortisol and other steroids, which may enhance the vasoconstrictor response of the blood vessels. Vasoconstriction results in reduced blood flow to the kidney, causing the release of renin. Renin leads to the formation of angiotensin I, which converts to angiotensin II, a potent vasoconstrictor, which in turn stimulates secretion of aldosterone by the adrenal cortex. This hormone causes sodium and water to be retained by the kidney tubules, leading to an increase in intravascular volume. All these factors tend to perpetuate the hypertensive state.

TABLE 31-4 Recommendations for Follow-up Based on Initial Set of Blood Pressure Measurements for Adults

Initial Screening Blood Pressure, mm Hg*		
Systolic	**Diastolic**	**Follow-up Recommended†**
<130	<85	Recheck in 2 y
130–139	85–89	Recheck in 1 y‡
140–159	90–99	Confirm within 2 mo
160–179	100–109	Evaluate or refer to source of care within 1 mo
180–209	110–119	Evaluate or refer to source of care within 1 wk
≥210	≥120	Evaluate or refer to source of care immediately

*If the systolic and diastolic categories are different, follow recommendation for the shorter-time follow-up (e.g., 160/85 mm Hg should be evaluated or referred to source of care within 1 month).

†The scheduling of follow-up should be modified by reliable information about past blood pressure measurements, other cardiovascular risk factors, or target-organ disease.

‡Consider providing advice about life-style modifications.

(The Fifth Report of the Joint National Committee on Detection, Evaluation, and Treatment of High Blood Pressure. Arch Intern Med 1993 Jan 25; 153:162.)

Gerontologic Considerations. Structural and functional changes in the peripheral vascular system are responsible for the changes in blood pressure that occur with age. These changes include atherosclerosis, the loss of connective tissue elasticity, and a decrease in the relaxation of vascular smooth muscle, which in turn reduce the ability of the vessels to distend and recoil. Consequently, the aorta and large arteries are less able to accommodate the volume of blood pumped out by the heart (stroke volume), resulting in a decrease in cardiac output and an increase in peripheral resistance.

Clinical Manifestations

Physical examination may reveal no abnormalities other than high blood pressure, but changes may be noted in the retina, such as hemorrhages, exudates (fluid accumulation), narrowed arterioles, and, in severe cases, papilledema (edema of the optic disc).

Persons with hypertension can be asymptomatic and remain so for many years. Symptoms, when they do appear, usually indicate vascular damage, with specific manifestations related to the organ systems served by the involved vessels. Coronary artery disease with angina is the most common sequela in hypertensive individuals. Left ventricular hypertrophy occurs in response to the increased workload placed on the ventricle as it is forced to contract against higher systemic pressures. When the heart can no longer sustain the increased workload, left heart failure ensues. Pathologic changes in the kidneys may be manifested as nocturia (increased urination at night) and azotemia (increased blood urea nitrogen [BUN] and creatinine). Cerebral vascular involvement may produce a stroke or transient ischemic attack manifested by temporary paralysis on one side (hemiplegia), or alterations in vision. Cerebral infarctions account for 80% of the strokes and transient ischemic attacks in hypertensive persons.

Diagnostic Evaluation

A thorough history and physical examination are necessary. The retinas are examined, and laboratory studies are performed to assess possible damage to organs, such as the kidney or heart, that may be affected by the increased blood pressure. Left ventricular hypertrophy can be assessed by electrocardiography; protein in the urine can be detected by urinalysis. Inability to concentrate the urine and an increase in the blood urea nitrogen may also be present. Special studies, such as renogram, intravenous pyelogram, renal arteriogram, split renal function studies, and the determination of renin levels, may also be performed to identify patients with renovascular disease. The presence of additional risk factors is assessed and evaluated.

Management

The objective of any treatment program selected for individual patients is to prevent associated morbidity and mortality by achieving and maintaining an arterial blood pressure below 140/90 mm Hg whenever possible. The effectiveness of any program is determined by the degree of hypertension, complications, cost of care, and perceived quality of life associated with the therapy.

Some studies have indicated that nonpharmacologic approaches, including weight reduction; restriction of alcohol, sodium, and tobacco; exercise; and relaxation are definitive interventions that should be used in all antihypertensive therapy. When an individual with mild hypertension is at high risk (men, smokers) or when diastolic blood pressure is persistently elevated over 85 to 89 mm Hg and the systolic is 130 to 139 mm Hg, medication therapy should be initiated.

The *treatment algorithm* issued by the Joint National Committee on Detection, Evaluation and Treatment of High Blood Pressure allows the practitioner to select the drug class that has the greatest effectiveness, fewest side effects, and best chance of acceptance by the patient (Fig. 31-12). Two classes of medications are available as first-line therapy: diuretics and beta-blockers. When the patient with mild hypertension has had it controlled for a year, the therapy can be reduced. To promote adherence to the recommended therapeutic regimen, complicated medication therapy schedules should be avoided. Table 31-5 describes the various pharmacologic agents used in the treatment of hypertension.

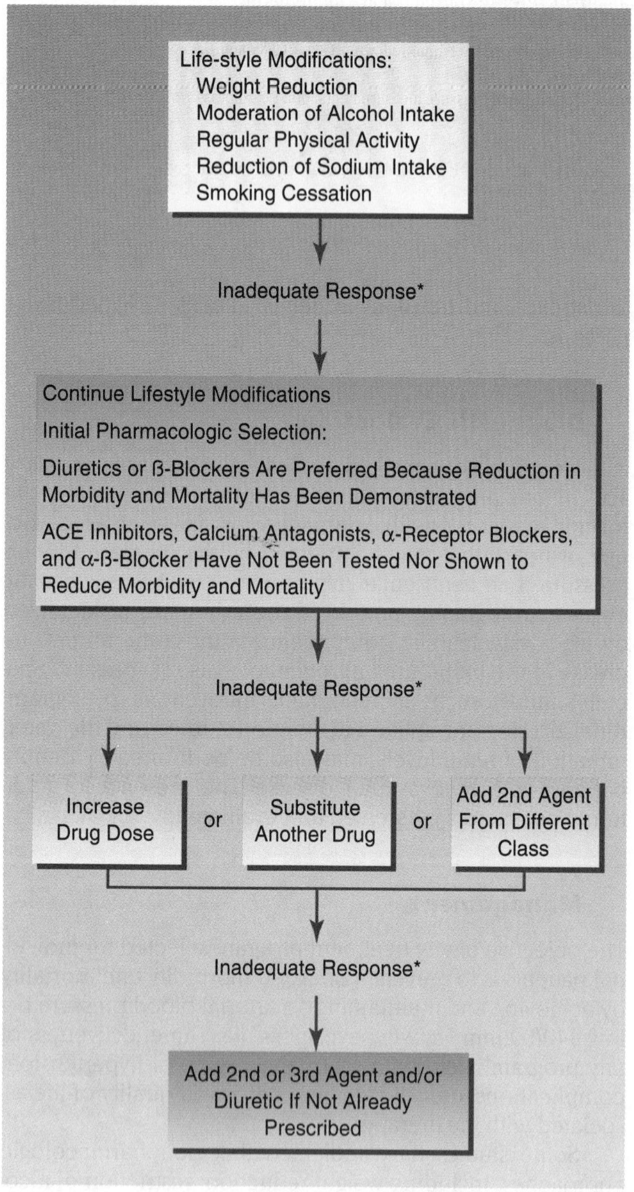

FIGURE 31-12. Treatment algorithm for hypertension. *Asterisk* indicates that response means the patient achieved goal blood pressure or is making considerable progress toward this goal. ACE, angiotensin-converting enzyme. (From Fifth Report of the Joint National Committee on Detection, Evaluation, and Treatment of High Blood Pressure. Arch Intern Med 1993 Jan; 153:163.)

❑ NURSING PROCESS
The Patient With Hypertension

Assessment

Assessing the patient when hypertension is initially detected involves carefully monitoring the blood pressure at frequent intervals and then at routine, scheduled intervals. The 1993 report of the Joint National Committee on Detection, Evaluation, and Treatment of High Blood Pressure developed guidelines it issued at an earlier date concerning conditions required before blood pressure measurements are taken, equipment specifications, and techniques for measuring blood pressure to obtain a reliable value that reflects the patient's normal blood pressure (Table 31-6). When the patient is placed on an antihypertensive medication regimen, blood pressure readings are imperative to determine if the medication has been effective and to reveal if any changes in blood pressure require a change in medication.

A complete history should be obtained to assess for symptoms that indicate if other body systems have been affected by the hypertension. These would include signs such as nosebleeds, anginal pain, shortness of breath, alterations in vision, vertigo, headaches, or nocturia. The physical examination must also pay specific attention to the rate, rhythm, and character of the apical and peripheral pulses to detect effects of the hypertension on the heart and the peripheral vessels. A thorough assessment can yield valuable information about the extent to which the hypertension has affected the body as well as any psychological factors related to the problem.

Diagnosis

Nursing Diagnoses

Based on the assessment data, nursing diagnoses for the patient may include the following:

- ❑ Knowledge deficit regarding the relationship between the treatment regimen and control of the disease process
- ❑ Potential noncompliance to the self-care program related to side effects of prescribed therapy

Collaborative Problems/ Potential Complications

Based on the assessment data, potential complications that may develop include:

- ❑ Retinal hemorrhage
- ❑ Congestive heart failure
- ❑ Renal insufficiency
- ❑ Cerebrovascular accident (CVA) or stroke

Planning and Implementation

Goals. The major goals for the patient include understanding the disease process and its treatment, compli-

(text continues on page 752)

TABLE 31-5 Medication Therapy for Hypertension

Purpose: To maintain blood pressure within normal ranges by the simplest and safest means possible with the fewest side effects for each individual patient

Medication	Major Action	Advantages	Contraindications	Effects and Nursing Considerations
Diuretics and Related Drugs				
Thiazide Diuretics				
Chlorthalidone (Hygroton) Quinethazone (Hydromox) Chlorothiazide (Diuril) Hydrochlorothiazide (Esidrix; HydroDIURIL)	Decrease of blood volume, renal blood flow, and cardiac output Depletion of extracellular fluid Negative sodium balance (from natriuresis), mild hypokalemia Directly affect vascular smooth muscle	Effective orally Effective during long-term administration Mild side effects Enhance other antihypertensive drugs Counter sodium retention effect of other antihypertensive medications	Gout Known sensitivity to sulfonamide-derived medications Severely impaired kidney function	Dry mouth, thirst, weakness, drowsiness, lethargy, muscle aches, muscular fatigue, tachycardia, GI disturbance. Postural hypotension may be potentiated by alcohol, barbiturates, or narcotics. Because thiazides cause sodium loss, patient is instructed to watch for postural hypotension in hot weather. (Eating salted pretzels in hot weather may avert this.) Administer supplementary potassium. **Gerontologic Considerations:** Risk of postural hypotension is significant because of volume depletion; measure blood pressure in three positions; caution patient to rise slowly.
Loop Diuretics				
Furosemide (Lasix)	Volume depletion Block reabsorption of sodium and water in kidney Antagonize action of aldosterone	Action rapid Potent To be used only when thiazides fail	Same as for thiazides	Volume depletion is rapid–profound diuresis can occur. Electrolyte depletion–replacement is required. Thirst, nausea, vomiting, skin rash, postural hypotension. Sweet taste noted; oral and gastric burning. **Gerontologic Considerations:** Same as thiazides.
Potassium-Sparing Diuretics				
Spironolactone (Aldactone)	Competitive inhibitors of aldosterone	Spironolactone is effective in treating hypertension accompanying primary aldosteronism.	Renal disease Azotemia Severe hepatic disease	Drowsiness, lethargy, headache—decrease the dosage.

(continued)

TABLE 31-5 *(continued)*

Medication	Major Action	Advantages	Contraindications	Effects and Nursing Considerations
Diuretics & Related Drugs *(continued)*				
Triamterene (Dyrenium)	Act on distal tubule independently of aldosterone	Both spironolactone and triamterene cause retention of potassium.		Diarrhea and other GI symptoms—administer medication after meals. Skin eruptions, urticaria. Mental confusion, ataxia—dosage may need to be reduced. Gynecomastia (not for triamterene).
Adrenergic Inhibitors				
Reserpine (alkaloid of *Rauwolfia serpentina*)	Impairs synthesis and reuptake of norepinephrine	Slows pulse, which counteracts tachycardia of hydralazine	History of depression Psychosis Obesity Chronic sinusitis Peptic ulcer	May cause severe depression; report manifestations, as this may require that drug be omitted. Nasal stuffiness, which may require nasal vasoconstrictor. Increases appetite—therefore, weight control may be difficult. Recurrence of peptic ulcer. Administer with meals or milk. **Gerontologic Considerations:** Depression and postural hypotension common in elderly.
Methyldopa (Aldomet)	Dopa-decarboxylase inhibitor; displaces norepinephrine from storage sites	Effective in patients not controlled with thiazide-reserpine (with or without hydralazine) Useful in patients with renal failure Does not decrease cardiac output or renal blood flow Does not induce oliguria	Liver disease	Drowsiness, dizziness. Dry mouth; nasal stuffiness (troublesome at first but then tends to disappear). Hemolytic anemia (a hypersensitization reaction)—positive Coombs' test. **Gerontologic Considerations:** May produce mental and behavioral changes in the elderly.
Propranolol (Inderal)	Blocks the sympathetic nervous system (β-adrenergic receptors), especially the sympathetics to the heart, producing a slower heart rate and lowered blood pressure	Reduces pulse rate in patients with tachycardia and blood pressure elevation and is useful as an adjunct with medications that act at the neuroeffector site of the blood vessel	Bronchial asthma Allergic rhinitis Right ventricular failure due to pulmonary hypertension Congestive heart failure	Mental depression manifested by insomnia, lassitude, weakness, and fatigue. Lightheadedness and occasional nausea, vomiting, and epigastric distress.

(continued)

TABLE 31-5 *(continued)*

Medication	Major Action	Advantages	Contraindications	Effects and Nursing Considerations
Adrenergic Inhibitors *(continued)*				
				Blood dyscrasias such as agranulocytosis and thrombocytopenic purpura do occur, but are uncommon. **Gerontologic Considerations:** Risk of toxicity is increased for elderly with decreased renal and liver function. Take blood pressure in three positions and observe for hypotension.
Prazosin hydrochloride (Minipress)	Peripheral vasodilator acting directly on the blood vessel; similar to hydralazine	Acts directly on the blood vessel and is an effective agent in patients with adverse reactions to hydralazine	Angina pectoris and coronary artery disease. Induces tachycardia if not preceded by administration of propranolol and a diuretic	Occasional vomiting and diarrhea, urinary frequency, and cardiovascular collapse, especially if given in addition to hydralazine without lowering the dose of the latter. Patients occasionally experience drowsiness, lack of energy, and weakness.
Clonidine hydrochloride (Catapres)	Exact mode of action not understood, but acts through the central nervous system, apparently through centrally mediated α-adrenergic stimulation in the brain, producing blood pressure reduction	Little or no orthostatic effect. Moderately potent, and sometimes is effective when other drugs fail to lower blood pressure	Severe coronary artery disease, pregnancy, children	Most common side effects are dry mouth, drowsiness, sedation, and occasional headaches and fatigue. Anorexia, malaise, and vomiting with mild disturbance of liver function have been reported. Skin rash, dreams and nightmares, insomnia, and anxiety have been reported but are not common.
Metoprolol (Lopressor)	Blocks access of norepinephrine to β_1-adrenergic receptors, especially in myocardium; decreases blood pressure by decreasing cardiac output and peripheral resistance	Rapid absorption	Cardiac failure Sinus bradycardia A-V conduction defects Diabetes mellitus	May cause bradycardia, congestive heart failure, intensification of heart block—take apical pulse before administration. May cause severe depression; report manifestations, as this may require that medication be omitted.

(continued)

TABLE 31-5 *(continued)*

Medication	Major Action	Advantages	Contraindications	Effects and Nursing Considerations
Adrenergic Inhibitors *(continued)*				
				Instruct patient to take radial pulse before each dose and report slow or irregular pulse to physician.
Nadolol (Corgard)	Blocks β-adrenergic receptors within the heart; reduces cardiac rate and output and decreases myocardial automaticity; exact mode of action for decreasing standing and supine blood pressures unknown	Can be used alone to treat hypertension, or in combination with a diuretic Long half-life; once daily administration	Cardiac failure Sinus bradycardia Bronchial asthma COPD	May cause bradycardia; instruct patient to take pulse before each dose and report slow pulse to physician. May cause dizziness, sedation, behavioral changes, depression; caution patient to avoid driving and other dangerous activities until response is known.
Guanethidine (Ismelin)	Prevents release of sympathetic transmitter, norepinephrine. Is a depressant of adrenergic activity Depletes tissue stores of norepinephrine Causes venous pooling, decreased venous return, and decreased cardiac output Decreases pulse rate, cardiac output, and renal blood flow	Potency	Pheochromocytoma, because greatly enhances pressor effect of catecholamines	Severe postural hypotension accentuated by alcohol, exercise, hot weather Warn against standing suddenly or standing for a long time. Diarrhea and nausea, nocturia. Failure of ejaculation; counsel about possible sexual dysfunction. Fatigue and giddiness; blackout.
Labetalol hydrochloride (Normodyne, Trandate) Phentolamine camsylate (Arfonad) Phentolamine mesylate (Regitine)	By blocking adrenergic receptors causes peripheral dilation and decreases peripheral vascular resistance	Fast acting No decrease in renal blood flow	Asthma Cardiogenic shock Severe tachycardia, heart block	Orthostatic hypotension, tachycardia.
Vasodilators				
Hydralazine hydrochloride (Apresoline)	Decreases peripheral resistance but concurrently elevates cardiac output Acts directly on smooth muscle of blood vessels	Used as a third medication of choice when patient does not respond to thiazide-reserpine, thiazide-methyldopa, or thiazide-guanethidine	Angina or coronary disease Congestive heart failure Hypersensitivity	Headache, tachycardia, flushing, and dyspnea may occur—can be prevented by pretreating with reserpine. Peripheral edema may require diuretics. May produce lupus erythematosus-like syndrome.

(continued)

TABLE 31-5 *(continued)*

Medication	Major Action	Advantages	Contraindications	Effects and Nursing Considerations
Vasodilators *(continued)*				
Minoxidil	Direct vasodilating action on arteriolar vessels, causing decreased peripheral vascular resistance; reduces systolic and diastolic pressures	Hypotensive effect more pronounced than hydralazine No effect on vasomotor reflexes; thus does not cause postural hypotension	Pheochromocytoma	Tachycardia, angina pectoris, ECG changes, edema; take blood pressure and apical pulse before administration; monitor I&O and daily weights.
Sodium nitroprusside (Nipride, Nitropress) Nitroglycerin Diazoxide (Hyperstat)	Peripheral vasodilation by relaxation of smooth muscle	Fast acting	Sepsis	Dizziness, headache, nausea, edema, tachycardia, palpitations.
Angiotensin-Converting Enzyme Inhibitor				
Captopril (Capoten)	Inhibits conversion of angiotensin I to angiotensin II Lowers total peripheral resistance	Fewer cardiovascular side effects Can be used with thiazide diuretic and digitalis Hypotension can be reversed by fluid replacement	Renal impairment	**Gerontologic Considerations:** Requires reduced dosages and loop diuretics with renal dysfunction.
Calcium Antagonist				
Diltiazem Hydrochloride (Cardizem)	Inhibits calcium ion influx Reduces cardiac afterload	Inhibits coronary artery spasm not controlled by β-blockers or nitrates	Sick sinus syndrome; second or third degree AV block; hypotension; congestive heart failure	Do not discontinue suddenly. Observe for hypotension. Report irregular heartbeat, dizziness, edema. Instruct on regular dental care because of potential gingivitis.
Nifedipine (Procardia: Adalat)	Inhibits calcium ion influx across membranes Vasodilating effects on coronary and peripheral arteriole Decreases cardiac work and energy consumption, increases delivery of oxygen to myocardium	Rapid action Effective by oral or sublingual route No tendency to slow SA nodal activity or prolong AV node conduction	None	Administer on empty stomach. Use with caution in diabetic patients. Small frequent meals if complains of nausea. Muscle cramps, joint stiffness, sexual difficulties may disappear when dose decreased. Report irregular heartbeat, constipation, shortness of breath, edema. May cause dizziness.
Verapamil (Calan, Isoptin)	Inhibits calcium ion influx Slows velocity of conduction of cardiac impulse	Effective antidysrhythmic Rapid IV onset Blocks SA and AV node channels	Sinus or AV node disease; severe heart failure Severe hypotension	Administer on empty stomach or before meal. Do not discontinue suddenly.

(continued)

TABLE 31-5 *(continued)*

Medication	Major Action	Advantages	Contraindications	Effects and Nursing Considerations
Calcium Antagonist *(continued)*				
				Depression may disappear when medication discontinued. For headaches: reduce noise, monitor electrolytes. Decrease dose for liver or renal failure. **Gerontologic Considerations:** Requires reduced dose.

ance with the self-care program, and absence of complications.

Nursing Interventions

Patient Education for Self-Care. The objective of treatment for hypertension is to lower the blood pressure to as close to normal levels as possible without introducing adverse effects. Adherence to therapy must be promoted in a cost-effective manner.

The treatment regimen consists of antihypertensive medications, dietary restrictions of sodium and fat, weight control, lifestyle changes, exercise program, and follow-up health care at regular intervals. Because the therapeutic regimen becomes the responsibility of the patient (if the person is able) or a significant other, counseling and education on an ongoing basis are imperative. Many patients benefit from attending hypertension clinics and attending support group meetings in which they can share their concerns with other patients and find the needed support for making the lifestyle changes that are part of therapy. The family is involved in the educational and counseling programs to enable them to support the patient's efforts to control hypertension.

Regular follow-up care is imperative so that the disease process can be assessed in terms of control or progression and treated accordingly. A history and physical examination should be completed at each clinic visit. The history should include all data that pertain to any potential problem, but specifically problems with medications such as dizziness or lightheadedness when standing.

Compliance With the Self-Care Program. Noncompliance with the therapeutic program is a significant problem in people with hypertension. It is estimated that 50% discontinue their medication therapy within 1 year of its initiation. Adequate blood pressure control is maintained by only 20%. However, when patients actively participate in the program, including self-monitoring of blood pressure and diet, compliance has been shown to increase because immediate feedback is obtained along with a greater sense of control.

Considerable effort is required by patients with hypertension to adhere to lifestyle, diet, and activity restrictions and to take regularly prescribed medications. The effort needed may seem unreasonable to some, particularly when they experience no symptoms without medications but experience side effects with the medications. Continued supervision, education, and encouragement are often needed

TABLE 31-6 Conditions, Equipment, and Techniques for Measuring Blood Pressure

Conditions Before Measurement

No smoking or caffeine for 30 minutes.

Five minutes of quiet rest.

Patient seated with bare arm positioned at heart level and supported.

Equipment

For clinician's use: mercury sphygmomanometer, recently calibrated aneroid manometer, or validated electronic device.

For patient's use (at home): automatic and semiautomatic devices using acoustic or oscillometric methods and digital display of readings.

Several sizes of cuffs with appropriate cuff chosen so that rubber bladder encircles at least two thirds of arm (for children, bladder should encircle circumference of arm).

Techniques

Assessment based on average of at least two readings (if two readings differ by more than 5 mm Hg, additional readings are taken and used to calculate the average).

Conditions After Measurement

Inform patient of numeric BP value and need for periodic reassessment based on established follow-up criteria (wallet-sized cards designed for these purposes serve as useful reminders).

(Update on High Blood Pressure: Highlights from 1988 National Report. Nurs Prac 1988 Dec; 13[12]: 10.)

to enable those with hypertension to arrive at an acceptable plan for them to live with their hypertension and adhere to the treatment regimen. Compromises may have to be made on some aspects of the therapy to achieve success in higher-priority goals.

A thorough understanding of the disease process as well as how medication and health habits can control hypertension are important. The concept of controlling hypertension rather than curing it is important to explain. The temporary nature of medication side effects should be emphasized. Consultation with a dietitian may be useful in exploring the various ways to modify salt and fat intake. Providing lists of low-salt foods and beverages and identifying inexpensive salt substitutes can be helpful. The patient should be advised to avoid beverages that contain caffeine and alcohol and informed that alcohol may have synergistic effects with the medications. Tobacco should also be avoided because nicotine causes vasoconstriction. Support groups for controlling weight, smoking, and stress may be beneficial for some patients. Others benefit from support of family and friends.

Written information about the expected effects and side effects of medications is very useful in maintaining a safe self-administration program. When side effects do occur, patients need to know when and whom to contact. In addition, patients should be advised of the possibility of both rebound hypertension that may occur if antihypertensive medication is suddenly stopped and sexual dysfunction related to the medications.

The patient may be taught to measure blood pressure at home. Some authorities believe that this involves patients in their own care and emphasizes the fact that failing to take the medication can lead to a rise in blood pressure. However, it is difficult to convince many patients that blood pressure tends to vary and does not stay fixed at one measurement.

Gerontologic Considerations. Compliance with the therapeutic program is even more difficult for elderly people than for the general population. Medication therapy can be a significant problem because it must be taken daily, may need to be taken several times a day, and is expensive for someone on a fixed income. Treatment with a single agent (monotherapy) may be appropriate in the elderly population and may simplify the medication regimen and make it less expensive. Special care must be taken to make sure that the patient understands the medication regimen and is able to read the instructions, and that provisions are made for having prescriptions refilled as needed. The elderly patient's family should always be included in the teaching program so that they can understand the patient's needs, support adherence to the therapeutic program, and know when to seek guidance from health professionals.

The patient and family should be especially cautioned that the antihypertensive medication therapy may cause problems of hypotension, which should be reported immediately. Because elderly people have impaired cardiovascular reflexes, they are often more sensitive than younger people to the volume depletion caused by diuretic therapy and by the sympathetic inhibition effect of adrenergic antagonists. In an attempt to prevent the postural hypotension that may ensue, the patient should be very careful to change positions slowly and to use supportive devices (*e.g.* handrails, walker), if necessary to prevent falls that could result from dizziness and syncope.

Monitoring and Managing Potential Complications. Symptoms that the disease is progressing and involving other body systems must be detected early so that the treatment regimen can be changed accordingly. When the patient returns to the outpatient setting for follow-up care, all body systems must be assessed to detect any evidence that vascular damage may be occurring to vital organs. Examining the eyes is particularly important because blood vessel damage in the retina is indicative of similar damage elsewhere in the vascular system. The patient is questioned about blurred vision, spots in front of the eyes, and diminished visual acuity. The heart, nervous system, and kidneys must also be carefully assessed and examined. Any significant findings are promptly reported to determine if additional diagnostic studies are required. Based on the findings, medications may be changed in an attempt to control the hypertension.

Evaluation

Expected Outcomes

1. Maintains adequate tissue perfusion
   a. Maintains blood pressure within acceptable range with medication, diet therapy, and lifestyle changes
   b. Demonstrates no evidence of symptoms of angina, palpitations, vision changes
   c. Has stable BUN and serum creatinine levels
   d. Peripheral pulses present
2. Complies with the self-care program
   a. Takes medication as prescribed and reports any side effects
   b. Adheres to the dietary regimen as prescribed: sodium, cholesterol, and calorie reduction
   c. Exercises regularly and as appropriate
   d. Takes own blood pressure routinely
   e. Abstains from tobacco, caffeine, and alcohol
   f. Keeps follow-up clinic or physician appointments
3. Is free of complications.
   a. Reports no changes in vision
   b. Eye grounds reveal no retinal hemorrhage
   c. Pulse rate and rhythm and respiratory rate are within normal range
   d. Reports no dyspnea or edema
   e. Maintains urine output consistent with intake
   f. Renal function studies within normal range
   g. Demonstrates no motor, speech, or sensory deficits
   h. Reports no headaches, dizziness, weakness, or changes in gait

Hypertensive Emergencies

A hypertensive emergency exists when an elevated blood pressure must be lowered within 1 hour. These acute, life-threatening elevations in blood pressure require prompt treatment in an intensive care setting because of the serious damage that may occur to other organs in the body.

Hypertensive emergencies occur in patients whose hypertension has been poorly controlled or in those who have abruptly discontinued their medications. The presence of acute left ventricular failure or cerebral dysfunction indicates the need for immediate reduction in blood pressure.

The medications of choice in hypertensive emergencies are those that have immediate effect. Intravenous nitroprusside and labetalol hydrochloride have an immediate vasodilating action that is short-lived, and are thus widely used as the initial treatment in crisis. The effects of most antihypertensive agents are increased by diuretics. Extremely close hemodynamic monitoring of the patient's blood pressure and cardiovascular status is required during treatment with these medications. A precipitous drop in blood pressure can occur and requires immediate action to restore blood pressure to an acceptable level.

Vein Disorders

Venous Thrombosis, Thrombophlebitis, Phlebothrombosis, and Deep Vein Thrombosis

Although the above terms do not necessarily represent an identical pathology, for clinical purposes they are often used interchangeably.

Pathophysiology and Etiology

Although the exact cause of **venous thrombosis** remains unclear, three factors are believed to play a significant role in its development: stasis of blood, vessel wall injury, and altered blood coagulation. The presence of at least two factors appears to be necessary for thrombosis to occur.

Venous stasis occurs when blood flow is retarded, such as occurs with heart failure or shock; when veins are dilated, as a result of medication therapy; and when skeletal muscle contraction is reduced, as with immobility, extremity paralysis, or anesthesia. Bed rest has been shown to reduce blood flow in the legs by at least 50%.

Damage to the intimal lining of blood vessels creates a site for clot formation. Direct trauma to the vessels, such as occurs following a fracture or dislocation, diseases of the veins, and chemical irritation of the vein from intravenous medications or solutions, all can damage veins.

Increased coagulability of blood occurs most commonly in patients who have been abruptly withdrawn from anticoagulant medications. Oral contraceptives and a number of blood dyscrasias also can lead to hypercoagulability.

Thrombophlebitis is inflammation of the walls of the veins and is frequently accompanied by the formation of a clot. When a clot develops initially in the veins as a result of stasis or hypercoagulability, but without inflammation, the process is referred to as **phlebothrombosis**. Venous thrombosis can occur in any vein but occurs most frequently in the veins of the lower extremities. Both the superficial and deep veins of the legs may be affected. Of the superficial veins, the saphenous vein is most frequently affected. Of the deep leg veins, the iliofemoral, popliteal, and small calf veins are most often involved.

Venous thrombi are composed of an aggregate of platelets attached to the vein wall, along with a tail-like appendage containing fibrin, white blood cells, and many red blood cells. The "tail" can grow larger or propagate in the direction of blood flow as successive layers of the clot occur. This propagating venous thrombosis is dangerous because parts of the clot can become detached and produce an embolic occlusion of the pulmonary blood vessels. Fragmentation of the thrombus can occur spontaneously as the clot dissolves naturally, or it can occur in association with an elevation in venous pressure, such as occurs when a person stands suddenly or engages in muscular activity after prolonged inactivity. Other complications of venous thrombosis are described in Figure 31-13.

All surgical patients are at risk for **deep vein thrombosis** (DVT). Many studies have been performed over the years to document the incidence of DVT and the usefulness of prophylactic measures in preventing its occurrence. The rate of DVT in surgical patients without any therapy is 27%, with subcutaneous heparin 9.7%, with elastic stockings 11.1%, with an intermittent pneumatic compression device 17.7%, with heparin and stockings combined 6.3%, and with stockings and intermittent compression device 4.5%.

Clinical Manifestations

As many as 50% of all patients with venous thrombosis of the lower extremities have no symptoms. In others, symptoms are variable and not usually specific for thrombophlebitis. Despite this variability, however, the presence of clinical signs should always be investigated.

Deep Veins. Obstruction of the deep veins of the legs produces edema and swelling of the extremity because

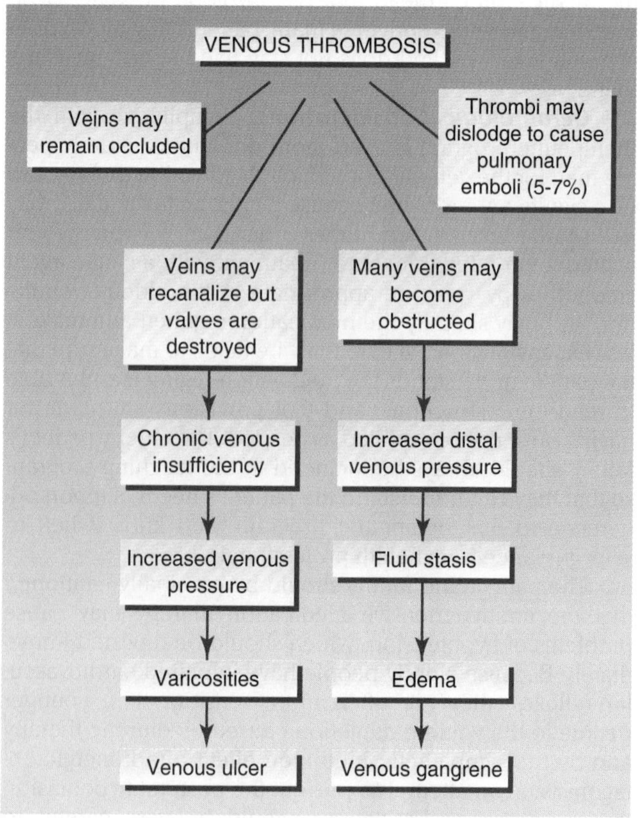

FIGURE 31-13. Complications of venous thrombosis.

the outflow of venous blood is inhibited. The amount of swelling can be determined by measuring the circumference of the leg at various levels with a tape measure. One leg is compared with the other at the same level to determine size differences. If both legs are swollen, a difference in size may be difficult to detect. The affected leg may feel warmer than the unaffected leg, and the superficial veins may appear to be more prominent. Tenderness, which usually occurs later, is produced by inflammation of the vein wall and can be detected by gently palpating the leg. *Homans' sign* (pain in the calf after the foot is sharply dorsiflexed) is not specific for deep venous thrombosis because it can be elicited in any painful condition of the calf. In some cases, signs of a pulmonary embolus are the first indication of a deep venous thrombosis.

Superficial Veins. Thrombosis of superficial veins produces pain or tenderness, redness, and warmth in the involved area. The risk of the superficial venous thrombi becoming dislodged or fragmenting into emboli is very low because most of them dissolve spontaneously. Thus, this condition can be treated at home with bed rest, elevation of the leg, analgesics, and possibly anti-inflammatory medication. A comparison of superficial and deep thrombophlebitis is presented in Table 31-7.

Assessment

Careful assessment is invaluable in detecting early signs of venous disorders of the lower extremities. Patients with a history of varicose veins, hypercoagulation, neoplastic disease, cardiovascular disease, or recent major surgery or injury are at high risk. Also, the obese, the elderly, and women taking oral contraceptives are at risk. Chart 31-3 lists the risk factors for developing deep vein thrombosis.

The following parameters are included in the nursing assessment:

- Question the patient about the presence of leg pain, heaviness, any functional impairment, or edema.
- Inspect the legs from the groin to the feet, noting any difference between the two and measuring and recording calf circumference. (One early indication of edema is engorgement around the ankle.)
- Note any increase in temperature in the affected leg. (To determine temperature differences most effectively, cool hands in cold water, dry, and place simultaneously on both of the patient's ankles and then on the calves.)
- To identify areas of tenderness and any thromboses (as evidenced by cordlike venous segments), palpate the medial aspect of the leg carefully using three or four fingers, advancing the hands back and forth from the ankle to the knee and then to the groin.

Diagnostic Evaluation

Many techniques, both noninvasive and invasive, are available to aid in verifying, defining, and localizing the presence of venous thrombosis.

TABLE 31-7 Comparison of Superficial and Deep Thrombophlebitis

Superficial	Deep
Clinical Manifestations	
Local swelling; bumpy and knotty	"Heaviness" on standing
Red, tender, local induration	Cramping leg pain
Saphenous vein (medial side of leg) feels like a cord	Swelling: Calf vein thrombus—none Femoral vein thrombus—mild to moderate Ileofemoral vein thrombus—severe
	Positive Homans' sign
Diagnostic Evaluation	
Venography—to rule out deep vein thrombosis	Blood flow studies to show inflow, filling, and emptying
Duplex venous scanning	Venography—to determine presence of phlebitis, recanalization, occlusion
	Duplex Venous Scanning
Management	
Bed rest	Bed rest
Warm, moist compresses	Warm, moist compresses
Legs elevated; then elastic support after acute stage	Foot of bed elevated to 15 cm (6 in)
	Surgery, possibly, to prevent embolic development
Heparin, intermittent or continuous	Thrombolytic therapy
Acetaminophen for pain	Venous valvuloplasty
Antibiotics if necessary	
If deep veins are patent, superficial phlebitic veins may be removed	

CHART 31-3
Risk Factors For Deep Vein Thrombosis and Pulmonary Embolism

Endothelial Damage

Leg trauma
Surgery
Pacing wires
Central venous catheters
Local vein damage

Venous Stasis

Bed rest or immobilization
Obesity
History of varicosities
Spinal cord injury
Over 65 years of age

Coagulopathy

Malignancy
Pregnancy
Oral contraceptives
Polycythemia, leukocytosis, thrombocytosis

Noninvasive Techniques. The noninvasive techniques of Doppler ultrasonography, impedance plethysmography, and duplex imaging rely on the thrombus to create abnormalities of venous flow.

Doppler ultrasonography involves placing a Doppler probe over veins that are obstructed. The Doppler flow reading will be diminished in comparison to the opposite leg or it will be absent. This method is relatively inexpensive, portable, simple, rapid, and noninvasive. Duplex venous imaging is used to obtain anatomic information as well as to assess physiologic parameters.

Impedance plethysmography is used to measure changes in blood volume in the veins. A blood pressure cuff is applied to the patient's thigh and inflated sufficiently to impede venous flow (about 50 to 60 mm Hg) but not enough to impede arterial flow. Calf electrodes are used to measure electrical resistance that results from changes in the blood volume in the vein. In the presence of deep vein thrombosis, the increase in venous volume that normally results from blood trapped below the level of the cuff will be less than expected. False-positive results can stem from factors that cause vasoconstriction, increased venous pressure, decreased cardiac output, or external compression of the vein. False-negative readings can result from the existence of an old thrombus that has led to the development of adequate collateral circulation or from superficial phlebitis.

The use of Doppler ultrasonography, duplex venous scanning, and impedance plethysmography can significantly increase the accuracy of diagnosis. Duplex venous scanning is the procedure of choice because it shows both the vessel and the clot and is noninvasive.

Invasive Techniques. Invasive techniques rely on the injection of contrast media into the venous system, which then binds with structural elements of the thrombus. I^{251}-labeled fibrinogen and contrast phlebography are examples of these tests.

I^{251}-labeled fibrinogen scanning is a more recently developed diagnostic procedure that provides a sensitive method for early detection of venous thrombosis. The test relies on the fact that radioactive fibrinogen, when injected intravenously, concentrates in the forming clot. The level of radioactivity can then be serially measured by an external counter and the progression of the clot can be monitored. However, this test will not reveal thrombi that have already formed nor thrombi in the groin or pelvic areas. A further drawback is the costliness of the test.

Contrast phlebography (venography) involves the injection of radiographic contrast media into the venous system through a dorsal foot vein. When a thrombus exists, an x-ray will show an unfilled segment of vein in an otherwise completely filled vein with its connecting collaterals. Injection of the contrast agent can cause a brief but painful inflammation of the vein. This test is generally accepted as the hallmark for diagnosing venous thrombosis.

Preventive Measures

Venous thrombosis, thrombophlebitis, and deep vein thrombosis can often be prevented, especially if patients who are considered at high risk are identified and preventive measures are instituted without delay.

Elastic Stockings. One preventive approach is to use elastic stockings, which are usually prescribed for patients with venous insufficiency. These stockings exert a sustained, evenly distributed pressure over the entire surface of the calves, and thus reduce the caliber of the superficial veins in the legs, resulting in increased flow in the deeper veins. It is important to note that any type of stocking, including the elastic type, can inadvertently become tourniquets if applied incorrectly (*i.e.*, rolled tightly at the top). In such instances, the stockings will produce stasis instead of preventing it. Elastic stockings are removed at night and reapplied before the legs are lowered from the bed to the floor in the morning.

When the stockings are off, the skin is inspected for signs of irritation and the calves are examined for possible tenderness. Any skin changes or signs of tenderness are reported. Stockings are contraindicated in patients with severe pitting edema because they can produce severe pitting at the knee.

Intermittent pneumatic compression (IPC) devices can be used with the elastic stocking for the prevention of deep vein thrombosis. The IPC device consists of an electric controller that is attached by air hoses to plastic leg sleeves. The leg sleeves are divided into compartments, which sequentially fill to apply pressure to the ankle, calf, and thigh at 35 to 55 mm Hg pressure. The advantage of IPC is its ability to increase blood velocity beyond that produced by the elastic stockings. Nursing measures include ensuring that prescribed pressures are not exceeded and assessing for patient comfort.

A further method to prevent venous thrombosis in surgical patients is administration of subcutaneous heparin.

Gerontologic Considerations. Because of decreased strength and manual dexterity, elderly patients may be unable to apply elastic stockings properly. If such is the case, a family member should be taught how to assist the patient to apply the stockings so that they do not cause undue pressure on any part of the feet or legs.

Body Position and Exercise. When the patient is on bed rest, the feet and lower legs should be elevated periodically above the level of the heart. This position allows the superficial and tibial veins to empty rapidly and to remain collapsed. Active and passive leg exercises, particularly those involving calf muscles, should be performed preoperatively and postoperatively to increase venous flow. Early ambulation is most effective in preventing venous stasis. Deep-breathing exercises are beneficial because they produce increased negative pressure in the thorax, which assists in emptying the large veins.

Management

The objectives of medical treatment of thrombophlebitis are to prevent the thrombus from growing and fragmenting, with the inherent risk of pulmonary embolism, and to prevent recurrent thromboemboli.

Therapeutic anticoagulation can accomplish both of these goals. Heparin, which is administered for 10 to 12 days by intermittent intravenous infusion or by continuous infusion, prevents the extension of a clot and the development of new clots. Medication dosage is regulated by monitoring the partial thromboplastin time (PTT). (A more detailed discussion of anticoagulation therapy is presented below.)

Four to 7 days before intravenous heparin therapy is scheduled to be completed, an oral anticoagulant is started. The patient receives the oral anticoagulant for 3 months or longer for long-term prevention.

Unlike heparin, thrombolytic (fibrinolytic) therapy causes the clot to decompose and dissolve in 50% of patients. Thrombolytic therapy is given within the first 3 days after acute occlusion, with either streptokinase, urokinase, or tissue-type plasminogen activator (t-PA). The advantages of lytic therapy are that it preserves the venous valves and reduces the incidence of postphlebotic syndrome (see p. 760) and chronic venous insufficiency. However, thrombolytic therapy results in approximately a threefold greater incidence of bleeding than does heparin.

The patient's PTT, prothrombin time, hemoglobin, hematocrit, platelet count, and fibrinogen level are monitored frequently. Close nursing observation is required to detect bleeding. If bleeding occurs and cannot be stopped, the thrombolytic agent is discontinued.

Surgical Management. Surgery for deep vein thrombosis is necessary when (1) anticoagulant or thrombolytic therapy is contraindicated; (2) the danger of pulmonary embolism is extreme; and (3) the venous drainage is so severely compromised that permanent damage to the extremity will probably result. A thrombectomy (removal of the thrombosis) is the treatment of choice when surgery is necessary. A vena cava filter may be placed at the time of the thrombectomy, which will trap large emboli and prevent pulmonary emboli (for further details see Chapter 25).

Nursing Management. Bed rest, elevation of the affected extremity, elastic stockings, and analgesics for pain are adjuncts to therapy. Usually, bed rest is required for 5 to 7 days after a deep venous thrombosis occurs. This is approximately the length of time necessary for the thrombus to adhere to the vein wall, thus preventing embolization. When the patient begins to ambulate, elastic stockings are used. Walking is better than standing or sitting for long periods. Bed exercises, such as dorsiflexion of the foot against a foot board, are also recommended.

Warm, moist packs to the affected extremity reduce discomfort associated with deep venous thrombosis. Mild analgesics for pain control, as prescribed, provide additional relief.

Anticoagulant Therapy for Thromboembolism

Anticoagulant therapy is the administration of a medication to delay the clotting time of blood, prevent the formation of a thrombus in postoperative patients, and forestall the extension of a thrombus once it has formed. Anticoagulants cannot dissolve a thrombus that has already formed.

Measures for preventing or reducing blood clotting within the vascular system are indicated in the following patients: those with thrombophlebitis; those believed to have recurrent embolus formation; those with persistent leg edema secondary to heart failure; and the elderly person with a hip fracture who is likely to be immobilized for a considerable time. The usual treatment consists of the single or combined administration of heparin or coumarin derivatives, which reduce the normal activity of the clotting mechanism (Table 31-8).

Administration. *Continuous IV infusion* by pump is the preferred method of administration to prevent inadvertent infusion of large volumes of heparin which could cause hemorrhagic complications. Dosage is calculated on the basis of weight, and any possible bleeding tendencies are detected by a pretreatment clotting profile. If renal insufficiency exists, lower doses of heparin are required. Periodic coagulation tests and hematocrit evaluations are obtained. Heparin is in the effective range when the PTT is one and a half times the control.

Intermittent intravenous injection is another means of administering heparin; a dilute aqueous solution of heparin is given every 4 hours. Administration may be facilitated by using a "heparin lock"—a small, butterfly-type scalp vein needle with an injection site at the end of the tubing (see Chapter 14).

Oral anticoagulants, such as Coumadin, are monitored by the prothrombin time. Because the effect of Coumadin is delayed for 3 to 5 days, it is usually administered in conjunction with heparin until desired anticoagulation has been achieved (*i.e.*, when the prothrombin time [PT] is achieved at one and a half to two times the normal).

Precautions and Nursing Assessment. The principal complication of anticoagulant therapy is spontaneous bleeding anywhere in the body. Bleeding from the kidneys will be manifested by microscopic hematuria and is often the first sign of anticoagulant overdose. Bruises, nosebleeds, and bleeding gums are also early signs of bleeding. To reverse the effects of heparin promptly, intravenous injections of protamine sulfate may be prescribed. Reversing the effects of coumarin derivatives is more difficult, but effective

TABLE 31-8 Comparison of Heparin and Coumarin Derivatives

Heparin Sodium	Coumarin Derivatives
Physiologic Action	
Interferes with clotting reaction at many points but primarily acts as an antagonist to thrombin and prevents conversion of fibrinogen to fibrin	Blocks the formation of prothrombin from vitamin K, a conversion that normally occurs in the liver
Therapeautic Action	
Advantages	
Used for short-term therapy primarily (may also be used for long-term therapy) Action is prompt and predictable. It can be used outside the body as well as inside: it may be used in certain dialysis procedures and in place of sodium citrate in donor blood.	Used for long-term therapy Is given orally and provides efficient absorption from gastrointestinal tract Uniform strength of medication because of synthetic production Less expensive than heparin sodium Control better than with heparin sodium Sodium warfarin more completely absorbed than bishydroxycoumarin
Disadvantages	
Must be given parenterally, intravenously, or subcutaneously. A few patients have developed allergic reactions; transient hair loss and osteoporosis have been reported (after several months of therapy).	Prolonged lag period (2–3 days) before the appearance of its effect Unpredictable duration of anticoagulant action (at times persisting up to 3 weeks)
Administration	
Test clotting and partial thromboplastin time (PTT) first. PTTs are obtained every 4 to 6 hours, at which time repeat doses of heparin are given. The object is to attain a PTT 1½ to 2½ times the normal control. *Subcutaneous route*-least recommended because of erratic absorption, possible puncture of vessels, and discomfort The average therapeutic dose is 20,000 to 30,000 units daily either by *continuous infusion* with an infusion pump or in divided doses by *intermittent IV injection* every 4 to 6 hours. *Prolonged therapy:* May be given deep subcutaneously in mid abdomen. Use a fine, short, sharp needle (No. 25-27 gauge, 1.27 cm—1.60 cm [0.5–0.62 inches]). Grasp roll of fat gently, and in dartlike fashion insert needle at right angle to the skin surface. After injection, do not rub site but firmly press site with an alcohol sponge. Use a new site on lower abdomen for each injection. *Note:* Intramuscular administration of heparin is avoided because of likelihood of local hematomas and tissue irritation.	Test prothrombin time first (see below). Warfarin: The average initial dose is 15 to 25 mg. A second dose, somewhat smaller (10 mg), is prescribed on the following day. Subsequent doses are adjusted on the basis of daily prothrombin levels. Average dose is usually 5 mg/day Therapeutic level of hypoprothrombinemia may be reached in 3 to 5 days
Action for Adverse Effects	
Discontinue heparin. Protamine sulfate (acts as a base to neutralize acidic heparin) Blood transfusion when hemorrhage occurs	Administer vitamin K preparations: *For mild bleeding control:* Phytonadione tablets (oral use) (Mephyton) (vitamin K_1) *For moderate to severe control:* Phytonadione solution (Aqua-MEPHYTON) IV or IM. Transfusion may be required

Prothrombin time is measured in seconds or percent of normal.
Normal: 12.5 seconds or 100%.
Desired Therapeutic Range: 25 to 30 seconds when the control is 12 seconds (approximately 1½–2½ times the control in seconds). When the prothrombin time is measured in percentage of normal, the desired therapeutic range is thought to be 20% to 30%.

measures that may be prescribed include vitamin K and possibly transfusion of fresh whole blood or plasma.

A further possible complication of heparin therapy is that of heparin-induced *thrombocytopenia* (decrease in platelets), which generally occurs 7 to 10 days after the treatment has been started. The thrombocytopenia is thought to be the result of an immunologic mechanism that causes aggregation of platelets. This serious complication results in thromboembolic manifestations, and the prognosis is extremely guarded. Prevention of thrombocytopenia is dependent on regular monitoring of platelet counts. If thrombocytopenia does occur, platelet aggregation studies are conducted, the heparin will be discontinued, and protamine sulfate will be administered to reverse the heparin effects.

Because oral anticoagulants interact with many other medications, close monitoring of the patient's medication schedule is necessary. Medications that potentiate oral anticoagulants include salicylates, anabolic steroids, chloral hydrate, glucagon, chloramphenicol, neomycin, quinidine, and phenylbutazone (Butazolidin). Medications that decrease the anticoagulant effect include phenytoin, barbiturates, diuretics, and estrogen. It is advisable to identify medication interactions for patients taking specific oral anticoagulants.

Contraindications to anticoagulant therapy are summarized in Chart 31-4.

Patient Education About Oral Anticoagulants. The patient should be informed about the medication, its purpose, and the need to take the correct amount at the specific times prescribed. The patient should also be aware that blood tests are scheduled periodically to determine whether a change in medication dosage is required. If the patient is unable or unwilling to cooperate with the therapeutic regimen, continuation of the medication therapy should be questioned. A person who refuses to discontinue the use of alcohol should not be on anticoagulants because chronic alcohol use decreases the effectiveness of oral anticoagulants. In addition, if hepatic impairment has occurred, the patient has the potential for bleeding tendencies that can be exacerbated with anticoagulants. Specific teaching directives should include the points listed in Chart 31-5.

CHART 31-4

Contraindications to Anticoagulant Therapy

Lack of patient cooperation
Bleeding from the following systems:
- Gastrointestinal
- Genitourinary
- Respiratory

Hemorrhagic blood dyscrasias
Aneurysms
Severe trauma
Alcoholism
Recent or impending surgery of:
- Eye
- Spinal cord
- Brain

Severe hepatic or renal disease
Recent cerebrovascular hemorrhage
Infections
Open ulcerative wounds
Occupations that involve a significant hazard of injury

Chronic Venous Insufficiency

Pathophysiology and Clinical Manifestations

Venous insufficiency is a disease state resulting from the obstruction of the venous valves in the legs or a reflux of

CHART 31-5

Patient Teaching: The Patient on Anticoagulation Therapy

1. Take the anticoagulant tablet at the same time each day, usually between 8:00 and 9:00 AM
2. Wear or carry identification indicating the anticoagulant being taken.
3. Keep all appointments for blood tests.
4. Because other medications affect the way the anticoagulant normally acts, do not take any of the following medications without the physician's consent: vitamins, cold medicines, antibiotics, aspirin, mineral oil, and anti-inflammatory agents. The physician should be contacted before taking any over-the-counter drugs.
5. Avoid alcohol because it may alter the body's response to an anticoagulant.
6. Avoid food fads, crash diets, or marked changes in eating habits.
7. Do not take Coumadin unless so directed by the physician.
8. Do not stop taking Coumadin (when prescribed) unless so directed by the physician or nurse.
9. When seeking treatment from another physician, a dentist, or a podiatrist, indicate that an anticoagulant is being taken.
10. Contact personal physician before dental extraction or elective surgery.
11. If any of the following signs appear, report them immediately to the physician:
    a. Faintness, dizziness, or increased weakness
    b. Severe headaches or abdominal pain
    c. Red or brown color of urine
    d. Any bleeding, such as cuts that do not stop bleeding
    e. Bruises that increase in size, nosebleeds, or unusual bleeding from any part of the body
    f. Red or black bowel movements
    g. Skin rash
12. Avoid injury that can cause bleeding.
13. Women should notify their physicians if they suspect that they are pregnant.

blood back through the valves. Both superficial and deep leg veins can be involved. The resulting venous hypertension can occur whenever there has been a prolonged increase in venous pressure, such as occurs with deep venous thrombosis.

Because the walls of veins are thinner and more elastic than walls of arteries, they distend readily when venous pressure is consistently elevated. In this state, leaflets of the venous valves are stretched and prevented from closing completely, thereby allowing a backflow or reflux of blood in the veins. Venography confirms the presence of obstruction and identifies the level of valvular incompetence.

When the valves in the deep veins in the legs become incompetent after a thrombus has formed, **postphlebotic syndrome** may develop. This disorder is characterized by chronic venous stasis, resulting in edema, altered pigmentation, pain, stasis dermatitis, and stasis ulceration. Superficial veins may be dilated. The disorder is long-standing, difficult to treat, and often disabling.

Stasis ulcers develop as a result of the rupture of small skin veins and subsequent ulcerations. When these vessels rupture, red blood cells escape into surrounding tissues and then degenerate, leaving a brownish discoloration of the tissues. The pigmentation and ulcerations usually occur in the lower part of the extremity in the area of the medial malleolus of the ankle. The skin becomes dry, cracks, and itches; subcutaneous tissues fibrose and atrophy. The risk of injury and infection of the extremities is increased.

Venous ulceration is the most serious complication of chronic venous insufficiency and can be associated with other conditions affecting the circulation of the lower extremities. The potential complications and the principles of care are the same.

Management and Patient Education

Management of the patient with venous insufficiency is directed at reducing venous stasis and preventing ulcerations. Measures that increase venous blood flow are antigravity activities, such as elevating the leg, and compression of superficial veins with elastic stockings.

Elevating the legs decreases edema, promotes venous return, and provides symptomatic relief. The legs should be elevated frequently throughout the day (at least 30 minutes every 2 hours). At night, the patient should sleep with the foot of the bed elevated about 15 cm (6 inches). Prolonged sitting or standing still is detrimental, but walking should be encouraged. When sitting, the patient should avoid placing pressure on the popliteal spaces, such as occurs when crossing the legs or sitting with the legs dangling over the side of the bed. Constricting garments such as girdles or garters should be avoided.

Elastic compression of the legs reduces pooling of venous blood and enhances venous return to the heart. Thus, elastic stockings are recommended for people with venous insufficiency. The fit of the stocking is important. It should provide for a greater pressure at the foot and ankle, gradually declining to a lesser pressure at the knee or groin. If the top of the stocking is too tight or becomes twisted, a tourniquet effect is created, which worsens venous pooling. Stockings should be applied after the legs have been elevated for a period of time when the amount of blood in the leg veins is at its lowest.

Extremities with venous insufficiency are carefully protected from trauma. The skin is kept clean, dry, and soft. Signs of ulceration are immediately reported to the health care provider for treatment and follow-up.

Leg Ulcers

Definition and Etiology

A *leg ulcer* is an excavation of the skin surface that is produced when inflammed necrotic tissue sloughs off. Approximately 75% of all leg ulcers are due to chronic venous insufficiency. Lesions due to arterial insufficiency account for approximately 20% and the remaining 5% are due to burns, sickle cell anemia, and other factors.

Pathophysiology

Inadequate exchange of oxygen and other nutrients in the tissue is the metabolic abnormality underlying the development of leg ulcers. When the cellular metabolism cannot maintain energy balance, cell death (necrosis) results. Alterations in blood vessels at the arterial, capillary, and venous levels may affect cellular processes and lead to the formation of ulcers.

Clinical Manifestations

The clinical appearance and associated characteristics of leg ulcers are determined by the cause of the ulcer. It is important to note that most ulcers, especially in a geriatric patient, have more than one cause. The symptoms vary depending on whether the problem is arterial or venous in origin (see Table 30-2). The severity of the symptoms depends on the extent and duration of the vascular insufficiency. The ulcer itself appears as an open inflamed sore. Drainage may be present or the area may be covered by eschar (dark, hard crust).

Chronic arterial disease is often characterized by pain. If the onset of arterial occlusion is acute, ischemic pain is unrelenting and rarely relieved even with narcotics. Chronic arterial disease is characterized by intermittent claudication, which is pain caused by activity that is relieved after a few minutes of rest.

Typically, arterial ulcers are small, circular, deep ulcerations on the tips of toes or in the web spaces between toes. Ulcers often occur on the medial side of the hallux or lateral fifth toe and may be due to a combination of ischemia and pressure.

Chronic venous insufficiency is characterized by pain described as aching or heaviness. Edema of the foot and ankle is often present. Ulcerations are either in the area of the medial or lateral malleolus (gaitor area). These ulcers are typically large, superficial, and highly exudative. Venous hypertension causes extravasation of blood, which will cause pigment discoloration in the gaitor area.

Patients with neuropathy frequently have ulcerations on the side of the foot over the metatarsal heads. These ulcers are painless and are described in further detail in Chapter 39.

Diagnostic Evaluation

Because ulcers result from many causes, it is important that the reason for the ulcer be identified so that appropriate therapy can be prescribed. The history of the condition is important in determining the presence of venous or arterial insufficiency. The pulses of the lower extremities (femoral, popliteal, posterior tibial, and pedal) are carefully assessed. More conclusive diagnostic aids are Doppler ultrasound studies, arteriography, and venography. Cultures of the ulcer drainage may be necessary to determine whether infection is the primary cause of the ulcer.

Management

Patients with ulcers are effectively managed by advanced practice nurses in collaboration with physicians. All ulcers have the potential to become infected.

Antibiotic Therapy. Antibiotic therapy is prescribed when infection is present; the specific antibiotic is determined by culture and sensitivity tests. Oral antibiotics are usually prescribed because topical antibiotics have not proved to be effective for leg ulcers.

Debridement. To promote healing, the wound is kept clean of drainage and necrotic tissue. The usual method is to flush the area with normal saline; if this is unsuccessful, debridement may be necessary. **Debridement** is the removal of nonviable tissue from wounds. Removing the dead tissue is important particularly in the presence of infection. Debridement can be accomplished by several different methods:

- *Sharp surgical debridement* is the fastest method and can be accomplished by the trained advanced practice nurse in collaboration with the physician.
- *Nonselective debridement* can be accomplished by applying isotonic saline dressings of fine mesh gauze to the ulcer. When the dressing dries, it is removed along with the debris adhering to the gauze.
- *Enzymatic debridement* and the application of enzyme ointments may be prescribed to treat the ulcer. The ointment is applied to the lesion but not to normal surrounding skin. The lesion and ointment are then covered with a saline-soaked sponge that has been thoroughly wrung out. A gauze dressing and a loose bandage are then applied. The moist saline dressings are continued (without enzyme ointments) when pink granulating tissue develops.
- *Debriding agents* can be used. Dextranomer (Debrisan) beads are small, highly porous, spherical beads (0.1 to 0.3 mm in diameter) that can absorb wound secretions. Bacteria and the products of tissue necrosis and protein degradation are absorbed into the bead layer. When the beads are completely saturated they take on a grayish yellow color, at which point their cleansing action stops. They are then removed and a fresh layer is applied.
- *Calcium alginate dressings* can also be used for debridement and absorption of exudate. These dressings are changed daily or when the exudate seeps through the cover dressing. The dressing can also be used on areas that are bleeding because the material helps stop the bleeding. As the dry fibers absorb exudate, they become a gel that is painlessly removed from the ulcer bed.

A variety of topical agents and soaps can be used in conjunction with washing and debridement therapies to promote healing of leg ulcers. The goals of treatment are to remove devitalized tissue and to keep the ulcer clean and moist while healing takes place. The treatment should not destroy developing tissue. For topical treatments to be successful, adequate nutritional therapy must be maintained in these patients.

Wound Dressing. Once circulatory status has been assessed and determined to be adequate for healing (ABI above 0.5), surgical dressings can be used to promote a moist environment. The simplest method is to use a wound contact material (*e.g.*, Tegapore) next to the wound bed and cover it with gauze. Tegapore maintains a moist environment, can be left in place for several days, and does not disrupt the capillary bed when removed for evaluation. Hydrocolloids (Duoderm CGF, Restore, Comfeel, Tegasorb) are also good choices to promote granulation tissue and re-epithelization. They also provide a barrier for protection because they adhere to the wound bed and surrounding tissue. However, a deep wound or an infected wound should never be covered with a hydrocolloid. The hydrocolloid dressing promotes an anaerobic environment and may increase the incidence of anaerobic infection.

Hyperbaric oxygen therapy may be considered in addition to topical therapy. The increase in the level of oxygen tension to 30 mm Hg increases fibroblast and collagen proliferation.

Gangrene of the Toe. Arterial insufficiency may result in gangrene of the toe (digital gangrene), which is usually caused by trauma. The toe is stubbed and then "turns black." Frequently patients with this problem are elderly people who do not have adequate circulation to provide revascularization. Debridement is contraindicated in these instances. Although the toe is gangrenous it is dry, which is preferable to debriding the toe and causing an open wound that does not have adequate circulation and therefore will not heal. If the toe were to be amputated, the lack of adequate circulation would prevent healing and might make further amputation necessary—either a below-knee amputation or even an above-knee amputation. A higher-level amputation in the elderly could result in a loss of independence and possible institutional care. Therefore, gangrene of the toe in an elderly person with poor circulation is usually left undisturbed.

❑ NURSING PROCESS
The Patient With Leg Ulcers

Assessment

A careful nursing history and assessment of symptoms are important. The extent and type of pain are carefully assessed, as are the appearance and temperature of the skin of both legs. The quality of all peripheral pulses is assessed, and comparisons are made of the pulses in both legs. The legs are checked for edema. If the extremity is edematous, the degree of edema is determined. Any limitation of mobility and activity that results from the vascular insufficiency is identified. In addition, the patient's nutritional status is assessed and a history of the following conditions is obtained: diabetes, collagen disease, or varicose veins.

Diagnosis

Nursing Diagnoses

Based on the assessment data, major nursing diagnoses for the patient may include the following:

- Impairment of skin integrity related to vascular insufficiency
- Impaired physical mobility related to the activity restrictions of the therapeutic regimen and the presence of pain
- Altered nutrition, less than body requirements, related to increased need for nutrients that promote wound healing

Collaborative Problems/ Potential Complications

Based on the assessment data, potential complications that may develop include:

- Infection
- Gangrene

Planning and Implementation

Goals. The major goals of the patient may include restoration of skin integrity, improvement of physical mobility, attainment of adequate nutrition, and absence of complications.

The nursing challenge in caring for these patients is great, whether the patient is in the hospital, in a long-term care facility, or at home. The physical problem is often a long-term one that causes a substantial drain on the patient's physical, emotional, and economic resources.

Nursing Interventions

Restoring Skin Integrity. To promote wound healing, measures are used to keep the area clean. Cleansing requires very gentle handling, a mild soap, and lukewarm water. Positioning of the legs depends on whether the cause of the ulcer is of arterial or venous origin. If there is arterial insufficiency, the patient should be referred to be evaluated for vascular reconstruction. If there is venous insufficiency, dependent edema can be avoided by elevating the lower extremities. A decrease in edema will promote the exchange of cellular nutrients and waste products in the area of the ulcer; thus healing is promoted.

Avoiding trauma to the lower extremities is imperative in promoting skin integrity. Protective boots may be used (*i.e.*, the Rooke Vascular boot, which is soft and provides warmth and protection). If the patient is on bed rest it is important to relieve pressure on the heels, which can lead to ulcerations. When the patient is in bed, a bed cradle can be used to relieve pressure from bed linens and to prevent anything from touching the legs. When the patient is ambulatory, all obstacles are moved from the path so that the patient's legs will not be bumped. Heating pads, hot water bottles, or hot baths are avoided. Heat increases the oxygen demands and thus the blood flow demands of the tissue, which in this case are already compromised. The patient with diabetes mellitus suffers from neuropathy with decreased sensation; thus, heating pads may produce injury before the patient is aware of being burned.

Improving Physical Mobility. Generally, physical activity is initially restricted to promote healing. When infection has resolved and healing has begun, ambulation will be resumed gradually and progressively. Activity promotes arterial flow and venous return and is encouraged after the acute phase of the ulcer process.

Until full activity can be resumed, the patient is encouraged to move about when in bed, to turn from side to side frequently, and to exercise the upper extremities to maintain muscle tone and strength. Meanwhile, diversional activities that interest the patient are encouraged. Consultation with an occupational therapist may be helpful if a prolonged period of limited mobility and activity is anticipated.

If pain limits the patient's activity, analgesics are often prescribed by the physician. The pain of peripheral vascular disease is often chronic in nature. Analgesics may be taken prior to scheduled activity periods to help the patient participate more comfortably.

Attaining Adequate Nutrition. Nutritional deficiencies are determined from the patient's report of usual dietary intake. Alterations in the diet are made to remedy these deficiencies. In addition, a diet that is high in protein, vitamin C, and iron is encouraged in an attempt to promote the healing process.

Many patients with peripheral vascular disease are elderly. Their caloric intake may need to be adjusted because of their decreased metabolic rate and level of activity. Particular consideration should also be given to their iron intake because many elderly people are anemic. Once a diet plan has been developed that meets the individual's nutritional needs for promotion of the healing process, diet instruction is provided to the patient and family. The diet plan is designed to be compatible with the patient's and family's lifestyle and preferences.

Evaluation

Expected Outcomes

1. Skin integrity is restored
   a. Absence of inflammation
   b. Absence of drainage; negative wound culture
   c. Avoids trauma to the legs
   d. Elevates legs to promote circulation
2. Increases physical mobility
   a. Progresses gradually to optimal level of activity
   b. Reports that pain does not impede activity
3. Attains adequate nutrition
   a. Selects foods high in protein, vitamins, iron
   b. Discusses with family member dietary modifications that need to be made at home
   c. Plans, with family, a diet that is nutritionally sound

Varicose Veins

Incidence

Varicose veins (varicosities) are abnormally dilated, tortuous, superficial veins caused by incompetent venous valves (Fig. 31-14). Most commonly, this condition occurs in the lower extremities, the saphenous veins, or the lower trunk; however, it can occur elsewhere in the body (*e.g.*, esophageal varices; see Chapter 37).

It is estimated that varicose veins of the lower extremities affect one of five persons in the world. The condition is most common in women and in persons whose occupations require prolonged standing, such as salespeople, barbers, beauticians, elevator operators, nurses, and dentists. A hereditary weakness of the vein wall may contribute to the development of varicosities, and it is not uncommon to see this condition occur in several members of the same family.

Pathophysiology and Manifestations

Varicose veins may be considered *primary* (without involvement of deep veins) or *secondary* (resulting from obstruction of deep veins). A reflux of venous blood in the veins results in venous stasis. If only the superficial veins are affected, the person may have no symptoms but may be troubled by the cosmetic appearance of the dilated veins. Symptoms, if present, may take the form of dull aches, muscle cramps, and increased muscle fatigue in the lower legs. Ankle edema and a feeling of heaviness of the legs may occur. Nocturnal cramps are common.

When deep venous obstruction results in varicose veins, patients may demonstrate the signs and symptoms of chronic venous insufficiency: edema, pain, pigmentation, and ulcerations. Susceptibility to injury and infection is increased.

Diagnostic Evaluation

The **Brodie-Trendelenburg test** is a common diagnostic test for varicose veins. This test demonstrates the backward flow of blood through the incompetent valves of the superficial veins and of the branches that communicate with the deep veins of the leg. With the patient lying down, the affected leg is elevated to empty the veins. A soft, rubber tourniquet is then applied around the upper thigh to occlude the veins, and the patient is asked to stand. If the valves of the communicating veins are incompetent, blood flows into the superficial veins from the deep veins. If, on release of the tourniquet, blood flows rapidly from above into the superficial veins, the implication is that the valves of the superficial veins are also incompetent. This test is used to determine the type of treatment to be recommended for the varicose veins.

Perthes' test is a diagnostic procedure that easily indicates whether the deeper venous system and communicating veins are competent. A tourniquet is applied just below the knee and the patient is asked to walk. If the varicose veins disappear, the deep system and communicating vessels are competent. If the vessels do not empty but become even more distended on walking, incompetency or obstruction is inferred.

Additional diagnostic tests for the presence of varicose veins are the Doppler flow meter, venography, and plethysmography. The *Doppler flowmeter* can detect the retrograde flow of blood in superficial veins with incompetent valves after the leg is compressed. *Venography* involves injecting radiographic contrast media into the leg veins so that the vein anatomy can be visualized by x-ray studies during various leg movements. *Plethysmography* measures changes in venous blood volume.

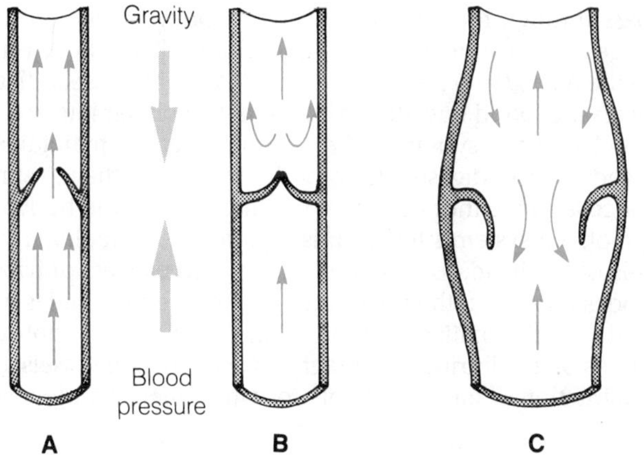

FIGURE 31-14. Competent valves showing blood flow patterns when the valve is open (**A**) and closed (**B**), allowing blood to flow against gravity. (**C**) With faulty, or incompetent, valves, the blood is unable to move toward the heart.

Prevention and Health Promotion

Activities that cause venous stasis should be avoided, such as wearing tight garters or a constricting panty girdle, crossing the legs at the thighs, and sitting or standing for long periods. Changing position frequently, elevating the legs when they are tired, and getting up to walk for several minutes of every hour promote circulation. The patient should be encouraged to walk 1 or 2 miles a day if there are no contraindications. Walking up the stairs rather than using the elevator or escalator is helpful in promoting circulation. Swimming is also good exercise for the legs.

Elastic stockings are useful, especially knee-high stockings. Patients are more likely to use knee-high stockings than thigh-high stockings. The overweight patient should be encouraged to enter or develop a weight-reduction plan.

Management

Surgery for varicose veins requires that the deep veins be patent and functional. The patient is placed under general anesthesia, and the saphenous vein is ligated and divided. The vein is ligated high in the groin where the saphenous vein meets the femoral vein. An incision is then made in the ankle, and a metal or plastic wire is passed the full length of the vein, "stripping" as it passes (Fig. 31-15). Pressure and elevation keep bleeding at a minimum during surgery.

Postoperative Nursing Management. Surgery can be performed in an outpatient setting, or patients can be admitted to the hospital on the day of surgery and discharged

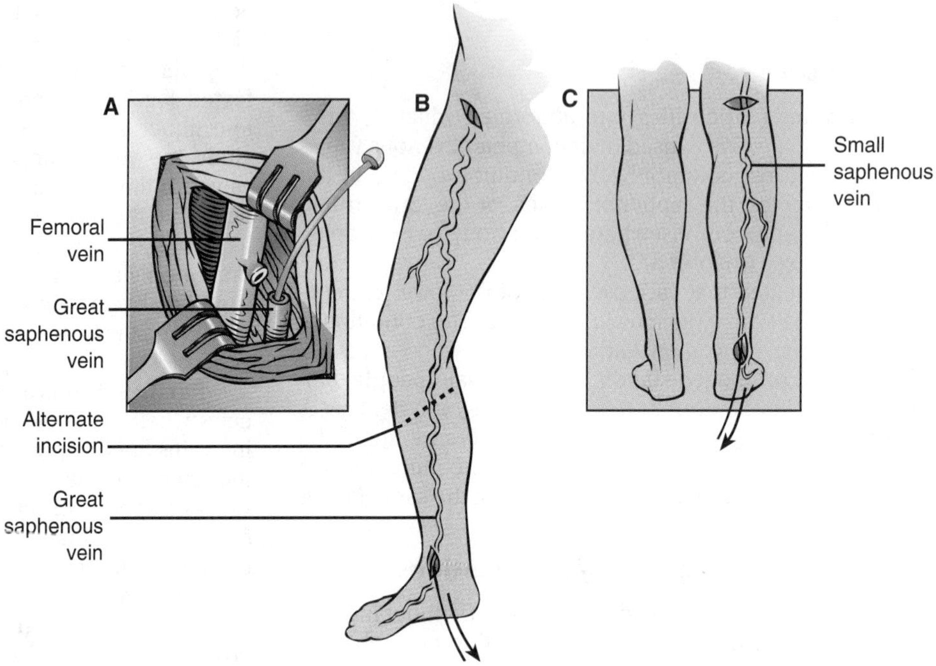

FIGURE 31-15. Ligation and stripping of the great and the small saphenous veins. (**A**) The tributaries of the saphenous vein have been ligated, and the saphenous vein has been ligated at the saphenofemoral junction. (**B**) Vein stripper has been inserted from the ankle superiorly to the groin. The vein is stripped from above downward. A number of alternate incisions may be needed to remove separate varicose masses. (**C**) The small saphenous vein is stripped from its junction with the popliteal vein to a point posterior to the lateral malleolus. (Rhoads et al. Surgery. Philadelphia, JB Lippincott.)

the following day. Bed rest is maintained for 24 hours, after which the patient begins walking every 2 hours for 5 to 10 minutes. Elastic compression of the leg is maintained continuously for about 1 week after vein stripping. Exercise and movement of the legs and elevation of the foot of the bed are necessary. Standing still and sitting are contraindicated.

Analgesics may help patients move affected extremities more easily. The dressings are inspected for bleeding, particularly at the groin where the risk of bleeding is greatest. Sensations of "pins and needles" or hypersensitivity to touch in the involved extremity may indicate a temporary or permanent nerve injury resulting from surgery. The saphenous vein and nerve are in close proximity in the leg.

Patients will require long-term elastic support of the leg after discharge, and plans are made to obtain adequate supplies of elastic stockings or bandages as appropriate. Exercises of the legs also will be necessary; the development of an individualized plan will require consultation with the patient and the health care team.

Sclerotherapy. In sclerotherapy, an irritating chemical, such as 0.5% sodium tetradecyl sulfate (Sotradecol), is injected into the vein, which irritates the venous endothelium and produces localized phlebitis and fibrosis, thereby obliterating the vein lumen. This treatment may be performed alone for small varicosities or may follow vein ligation or stripping. Sclerosing is palliative rather than curative. After the sclerosing agent is injected, elastic compression bandages are applied to the leg. These are worn for approximately 5 days. Compression stockings are then worn for an additional 5 weeks. Walking is important to maintain blood flow in the leg and should be emphasized.

If the patient experiences a burning sensation in the injected leg for 1 or 2 days, a mild sedative and walking usually provide relief. The bandage should be removed for the first time by the health care provider. Because bathing may be a problem during this time, a plastic bag may be placed over the bandaged leg and secured above the bandage to allow the patient to shower.

Sclerotherapy lost its popularity because of the possible complications of thrombosis, necrosis at the injection site, vasospasm, hemolysis, and allergic reactions associated with stronger solutions. However, lower concentrations of sclerosing solutions are available and have helped sclerotherapy, with or without surgery, regain some of its popularity.

The Lymphatic System

The lymphatic system consists of a set of vessels that spread throughout most of the body. These vessels start as lymph capillaries that drain unabsorbed plasma from tissue spaces. They unite to form the lymph vessels, which in turn pass through the lymph nodes and finally empty into the large thoracic duct that joins the jugular vein on the left side of the neck. *Lymph* is the fluid found in lymph vessels. *Tissue fluids* are found outside of vessels in the cellular interspace. The lymphatic system of the abdominal cavity maintains a steady flow of digested fatty food (chyle) from the intestinal mucosa to the thoracic duct. In other parts of the body the lymphatic system's function is regional; the lymphatic vessels of the head, for example, empty into clusters of lymph nodes located in the neck, and those of the extremities into nodes in the axillae and the groin. The flow of lymph depends on the intrinsic contractions of the lymph vessels, the contraction of muscles, respiratory movements, and gravity.

Diagnostic Evaluation

The lymphatic system can be viewed by x-ray following the injection of contrast media directly into lymphatic vessels in the hands and feet. This technique, *lymphangiography*, affords a means of detecting lymph node involvement by metastatic carcinoma, lymphoma, or infection in sites that are otherwise inaccessible to the examiner except by the direct surgical approach.

This procedure localizes a lymphatic vessel in each foot (or hand) when Evans blue contrast media is injected intradermally between the first and second digits. A blue lymphatic segment is identified, isolated, cannulated with a 25- to 30-gauge needle, and infused very slowly with a contrast agent containing iodine and oil. A series of x-rays is taken at the conclusion of the injection, 24 hours later, and periodically thereafter, as indicated. The identified lymphomatous lymph nodes retain the contrast agent for up to 1 year after the injection and any change in their size that may occur in response to radiation or chemotherapy can be measured and used as a criterion in determining therapeutic effect.

Lymphoscintigraphy is a reliable alternative to lymphangiography. A radioactive labeled colloid is injected subcutaneously in the second interdigital space. The extremity is then exercised to facilitate the uptake of the media by the lymph system. Serial images then are obtained at preset intervals. No adverse reactions have been reported.

Lymphangitis and Lymphadenitis

Lymphangitis is an acute inflammation of the lymphatic channels. It arises most commonly from a focus of infection in an extremity. Usually, the infectious organism is the hemolytic streptococcus. The characteristic red streaks that extend up the arm or the leg from an infected wound outline the course of the lymphatic vessels as they drain.

The lymph nodes located along the course of the lymphatic channels also become enlarged, red, and tender (*acute lymphadenitis*), and can become necrotic and form an abscess (*suppurative lymphadenitis*). The nodes involved most often are those in the groin, the axilla, or the cervical region.

Because these infections are nearly always caused by organisms that are sensitive to antibiotics, it is unusual to see abscess formation. Recurrent episodes of lymphangitis are often associated with progressive lymphedema.

After acute attacks, an elastic stocking or sleeve should be worn on the affected extremity for several months to prevent long-term edema.

Lymphedema and Elephantiasis

Lymphedemas are classified as primary (congenital malformations), or secondary (acquired obstruction). A swelling of tissues in the extremities occurs owing to an increased quantity of lymph that results from an obstruction of lymphatic vessels. It is especially marked when the extremity is in a dependent position. Initially the edema is soft, pitting, and relieved by treatment. As the condition progresses, the edema becomes firm, nonpitting, and unresponsive to treatment. The most common type is congenital lymphedema (lymphedema praecox), which is caused by hypoplasia of the lymphatic system of the lower extremity. This disorder is usually seen in women and first appears between the ages of 15 and 25 years.

The obstruction may be in both the lymph nodes and the lymphatic vessels. At times it is seen in the arm, after a radical mastectomy for carcinoma, and in the leg in association with varicose veins or chronic phlebitis. In the latter case, the lymphatic obstruction usually is due to a chronic lymphangitis. Lymphatic obstruction caused by a parasite (*Filaria*) is seen frequently in the tropics. When chronic swelling is present, there may be frequent bouts of acute infection characterized by high fever and chills and increased residual edema after the inflammation has resolved. These lead to chronic fibrosis, thickening of the subcutaneous tissues, and hypertrophy of the skin. This condition, in which chronic swelling of the extremity recedes only slightly with elevation, is referred to as *elephantiasis*.

Management

The goal of therapy is to reduce and control the edema and prevent infection. Strict bed rest with the leg elevated may aid in mobilizing the fluids. Active and passive exercises assist in moving lymphatic fluid into the bloodstream. External compression devices milk the fluid proximally from the foot to the hip. When the patient is ambulatory, custom-fitted elastic stockings are worn.

In the initial therapy, furosemide (Lasix) is taken intermittently to prevent fluid overload that can result from the mobilization of extracellular fluid. Diuretics have also been used palliatively for lymphedema in conjunction with elevating the leg and wearing compression stockings. However, the use of diuretics is controversial.

If lymphangitis or cellulitis is present, antibiotic therapy is initiated. The patient is taught to inspect the skin for evidence of infection.

Surgical treatment of lymphedema is performed if the edema is severe and uncontrolled by medical therapy, if mobility is severely compromised, or if there is persistent infection. One surgical approach involves the excision of the affected subcutaneous tissue and fascia, with skin grafting to cover the defect. Another procedure involves the surgical relocation of superficial lymphatic vessels into the deep lymphatic system by means of a buried dermal flap to provide a conduit for lymphatic drainage.

Postoperatively, the management of skin grafts and flaps is the same as when these therapies are used for other conditions. Prophylactic antibiotics may be prescribed for 5 to 7 days. Constant elevation of the affected extremity and observations for complications are essential. Complications may include flap necrosis, hematoma or abscess under the flap, and cellulitis.

BIBLIOGRAPHY

Bates B. A Guide to Physical Examination. Philadelphia, JB Lippincott, 1995.

Bell WR et al. Coagulation, coagulation disorders, and antithrombotic therapy. In Peripheral Vascular Diseases. St Louis, CV Mosby, 1991.

Berne R and Levy M. Physiology. St Louis, Mosby-Year Book, 1993.

Dossey BM et al. Essentials of Critical Care Nursing: Body, Mind, Spirit. Philadelphia, JB Lippincott, 1990.

Fahey VA. Vascular Nursing. Philadelphia, WB Saunders, 1994.

CRITICAL THINKING EXERCISES

1. You are assigned to a medical clinic where a large number of elderly patients receive care. Two patients, both of whom have peripheral vascular disease, are overheard comparing their symptoms and their medical management. When they realize that many of their symptoms are similar but their medical management is distinctly different, they question you about this. What further information will be helpful in determining an accurate explanation to give to these two patients?
2. You are assigned to a hypertension clinic. During a physical assessment of a middle-aged African-American male patient, he questions why he must have a complete physical examination every time he comes to the clinic. Describe the underlying rationale for the explanation you would give this patient.
3. You are caring for an elderly patient with hypertension who appears to be having difficulty taking the prescribed medication at home. How would you direct your assessment to identify those factors that might be interfering with this patient's ability to follow the medication regimen?

Guyton A. Textbook of Medical Physiology. Philadelphia, WB Saunders, 1991.

Hazzard WR et al. Principles of Geriatric Medicine and Gerontology, 2nd ed. New York, McGraw-Hill, 1994.

Jarrett F and Hirsch SA. Vascular Surgery of the Lower Extremity. St Louis, CV Mosby, 1985.

Lambert WC and Doty OB. Peripheral Vascular Surgery. Chicago, Year Book Medical, 1987.

Loscalzo J et. al. Vascular Medicine: A Textbook of Hypertension and Vascular Disease. St Louis, Mosby-Year Book, 1992.

Page IH. Hypertensive Mechanisms. Orlando, Grune & Stratton, 1987.

Rakel RE (ed). Conn's Current Therapy. Philadelphia, WB Saunders, 1988.

Robbins S et al. Pathologic Basis of Disease. Philadelphia, WB Saunders, 1989.

Strandness DE (ed). Vascular Diseases: Current Research and Clinical Applications. Orlando, Grune & Stratton, 1987.

Veith FJ et al. Vascular Surgery. St Louis, McGraw-Hill, 1994.

Journals

Anticoagulant and Thrombolytic Therapy

Eason JD et al. Hypercoagulable states in arterial thromboembolism. Surg Gynecol Obstet 1992 Mar; 174(3):211–215.

Harrington L et al. Heparin-induced thrombocytopenia and thrombosis syndrome: A case study. Heart Lung 1990 Jan; 19(1): 93–101.

Troyer-Caudle J. Reperfusion Injury. Journal of Vascular Nursing 1993 Sept; 11(3):76–79.

Arterial Conditions

Butler L et al. Acute arterial occlusion of the lower extremity. Journal of Vascular Nursing 1991; 11(1):19–22.

Capasso VC et al. The management of patients undergoing arterial reconstructive surgery. Medsurg Nursing 1993 Feb; 2(1):11–20.

Ciaccia JM. Benefits of a structured peripheral arterial vascular rehabilitation program. Journal of Vascular Nursing 1991; 11(1):1–4.

Coffman JD. Pathogenesis and treatment of Raynaud's phenomenon. Cardiovasc Drugs Ther 1990; 4:45–51.

Criqui MH et al. Mortality over a period of 10 years in patients with peripheral arterial disease. N Engl J Med 1992 Feb; 326: 381–386.

Crosby FE et al. Well-being and concerns of patients with peripheral arterial occlusive disease. Journal of Vascular Nursing 1991; 11(1):5–11.

Davis E. The diagnostic puzzle and management challenge of Raynaud's syndrome. Nurse Pract 1993 Mar; 18(3):18, 21, 22, 25.

DeMaioribus CA et al. A reevaluation of intraarterial thrombolytic therapy for acute lower extremity ischemia. Journal of Vascular Surgery 1993 May; 17(5):888–895.

Feinberg RL et al. The ischemic window: A method for the objective quantitation of the training effect in exercise therapy for intermittent claudication. Journal of Vascular Surgery 1992 Aug; 16(2):244–250.

Fellows E. Abdominal aortic aneurysm: Warning flags to watch for. Am J Nurs 1995 May; 95(5):26–32.

Fujitani R. Revision of the failing vein graft: Outcome of secondary operations. Seminars in Vascular Surgery 1993 Jun; 6(2): 118–129.

Hill SL. Discharge planning for the vascular patient: Where does home care fit in. Journal of Vascular Nursing 1991 Sept; 9(3):6–7.

Katz S et al. The use of epidural anesthesia and analgesia in aortic surgery. Am Surg 1992; 5(8):470–473.

Kwolek CJ et al. Peripheral vascular bypass in juvenile-onset diabetes mellitus: Are aggressive revascularization attempts justified? Journal of Vascular Surgery 1992 Feb; 15(2):394–400.

Miller L et al. Vasospastic disorders: Etiology, recognition, and treatment. Vascular Disorders 1993 Feb; 9(1):171–187.

Mills JL et al. The characteristics and anatomic distribution of lesions that cause reversed vein graft failure: A five-year prospective study. Journal of Vascular Surgery 1993 Feb; 17(1): 195–206.

Nishikimi N et al. Microcirculatory characteristics in patients with Buerger's disease. Journal of Vascular Diseases 1992 April; 43(4):312–319.

Orchard TJ et al. Assessment of peripheral vascular disease in diabetes. Circulation 1993 Aug; 88(2):819–828.

Provan JL. Peripheral vascular disease: What's urgent and what's not. Med Clin North Am 1993 Nov; 16(10):772–774, 776, 778.

Sandler RL. Abdominal aortic aneurysm. Am J Nurs 1995 Jan; 95(1): 38–39.

Whitaker L et al. Raynaud's syndrome: Diagnosis and treatment. Journal of Vascular Nursing 1994 Mar; 14(1):12–18.

Assessment and Diagnosis

Foldes MS. The role of duplex and color Doppler imaging in the operating room. Journal of Vascular Surgery 1993 Dec; 11(4): 108–110.

O'Flynn I. Three methods of taking the brachial systolic pressure to measure the ankle/brachial index: Which one is best? Journal of Vascular Surgery 1993 Sept; 11(3):71–75.

Wyffels PL. Increased limb salvage with intraoperative and postoperative ankle level urokinase infusion in acute lower extremity ischemia. Journal of Vascular Surgery 1992 May; 15(5): 771–779.

Sabatino KA et al. Research: Conception to completion. Journal of Vascular Surgery 1993 Dec; 11(4):111–115.

Hypertension

Johannsen JM. Update: Guidelines for treating hypertension. Am J Nurs 1993 Mar; 93(3):42–54.

Medical Research Council, Working Party. Medical Research Council trial of treatment of hypertension in older adults: Principal results. BMJ 1992 Feb; 304:405–412.

Moser M. Hypertension in the elderly. Physiology & Therapeutics 1992 Nov; 1727–1736.

Nash CA and Jensen PL. When your surgical patient has hypertension. Am J Nurs 1994 Dec; 94(12):38–44.

Systolic Hypertension of the Elderly Program, Cooperative Research Group. Prevention of stroke by antihypertensive drug treatment in older persons with isolated systolic hypertension: Final results. JAMA 1991 Jun; 265:3255–3264.

Thomas SA et al. Nursing blood pressure research, 1980–1990: A bio-psycho-social perspective. Image: Journal of Nursing Scholarship 1993; 25(2):157–164.

Trottier DJ et al. Hypertension and high cholesterol: A dangerous synergy. Am J Nurs 1992 Nov; 92(11):40–43.

Van Buskirk MC et al. Monitoring blood pressure. Am J Nurs 1993 Jun; 93(6):44–47.

Leg Ulcers

Bright LD et al. Is it arterial or venous? Am J Nurs 1992 Sept; 92(9):34–43.

Helt J. Foot care and footwear to prevent amputation. Journal of Vascular Nursing 1991 Dec; 11(4):3–8.

Redford JB et al. Foot orthoses: For your patients? Patient Care 1993 Jul; 87–106.

Troyer-Caudle J. The wound clinic connection. Ostomy/Wound Management 1992 Oct; 38(8):10–15.

Troyer-Caudle J. Debridement: Removal of non-viable tissue. Ostomy/Wound Management 1993 Jul/Aug; 39(6):24–32.

Trujillo EB. Effects of nutritional status on wound healing. Journal of Vascular Nursing 1993 Mar; 11(1):12–19.

Venous Conditions

Bright LD and Georgi S. How to protect your patient from DVT. Am J Nurs 1994 Dec; 94(12):28–32.

Interchange Forum: Developments in prophylactic therapy for venous thromboembolic disease. Pharmacy and Therapeutics 1994 Feb; 19:(2).

Lang W et al. Results of long-term venacavography study after placement of a Greenfield vena caval filter. J Cardiovasc Sur 1992 Sept–Oct; 33:573–578.

Lovell MB et al. The management of chronic venous disease. Journal of Vascular Nursing 1993 June; 11(2):43–47.

Notowitz LB. Normal venous anatomy and physiology of the lower extremity. Journal of Vascular Nursing 1993 Jun; 11(2):39–42.

Nunnelee JD et al. Interruption of the inferior vena cava for venous thromboembolic disease. Journal of Vascular Surgery 1993 Sept; 11(3):80–82.

Agency for Health Care Policy and Research (AHCPR) Guidelines

Acute Pain Management: Operative and Medical Procedures and Trauma. Clinical Practice Guidelines. AHCPR Publication No. 92-0032. Rockville, MD: Agency for Health Care Policy and Research, Public Health Service, U.S. Department of Health and Human Services, 1992.

INFORMATION/RESOURCES

Agencies

Joint National Committee on Detection, Evaluation and Treatment of High Blood Pressure
National Heart, Lung and Blood Institute, Building 31, Room 4A05, Bethesda, MD 20892

National Heart, Lung and Blood Institute
Education Programs Information Center, 4733 Bethesda Ave, Suite 530, Bethesda MD 20814

Agency for Health Care Policy and Research,
Public Health Service,
US Department of Health and Human Services
Center for Research Dissemination and Liaison
AHCPR Publication Clearinghouse
P.O. Box 8547
Silver Spring, MD 20907

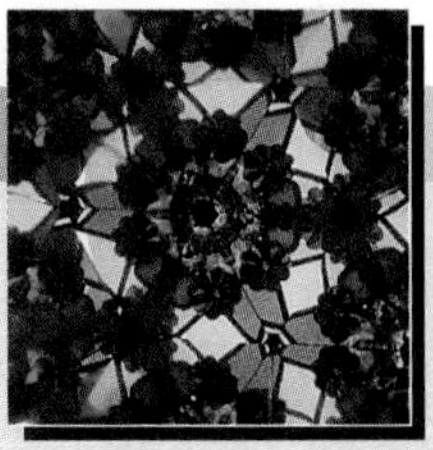

32

Assessment and Management of Patients With Hematologic Disorders

CHAPTER OUTLINE

Physiologic Overview
Bone Marrow
Erythrocytes
Leukocytes
Platelets
Blood Coagulation
Blood Plasma
Pathophysiology of the Hematologic System

Blood Study Procedures
Methods of Obtaining Blood
Bone Marrow Aspiration

Anemia
Pathophysiology
Gerontologic Considerations
Clinical Manifestations
Diagnostic Evaluation
Medical Management
Complications
NURSING PROCESS: The Patient With Anemia
Classification of Anemias
Hypoproliferative Anemias
Hemolytic Anemias
Inherited Hemolytic Anemias
NURSING PROCESS: The Patient With Sickle Cell Anemia
Acquired Hemolytic Anemias

Polycythemia
Polycythemia Vera
Secondary Polycythemia

Leukopenia and Agranulocytosis

Hematopoietic Malignancies
Leukemia
NURSING PROCESS: The Patient With Leukemia

Malignant Lymphomas
Hodgkin's Disease
Non-Hodgkin's Lymphomas

Multiple Myeloma

Bleeding Disorders
Pathophysiology
Vascular Disorders
Platelet Defects
Clotting Factor Defects
NURSING PROCESS: The Patient With Hemophilia

Therapeutic Measures in Blood Disorders
Splenectomy
Blood and Blood Component Therapy
Transfusion Techniques
Bone Marrow Transplantation

Critical Thinking Exercises

LEARNING OBJECTIVES

On completion of this chapter, the learner will be able to:

1. Compare the hypoproliferative anemias to the hemolytic anemias
2. Use the nursing process as a framework for care of patients with anemia
3. Use the nursing process as a framework for care of patients with sickle cell anemia
4. Compare the leukemias, their incidence, physiologic alterations, clinical manifestations, management, and prognosis
5. Use the nursing process as a framework for care of patients with leukemia
6. Describe the stages of Hodgkin's disease in relation to extent of disease process, clinical manifestations, and therapeutic management
7. Differentiate between bleeding disorders that are vascular disorders, those that are platelet defects, and those that are clotting factor defects
8. Use the nursing process as a framework for care of patients with hemophilia
9. Describe the therapeutic usefulness of whole blood and each of its components
10. Develop a plan of care for the patient receiving blood or blood component therapy

Physiologic Overview

The hematologic system consists of the blood and the sites where blood is produced, including the bone marrow and lymph nodes. The blood is a specialized organ that differs from other organs in that it exists in a fluid state.

The fluid consists of cellular components suspended in blood plasma (Fig. 32-1). The blood cells are divided into **erythrocytes** (red blood cells, normally 5 million per mm^3 of blood) and **leukocytes** (white blood cells, normally 5,000 to 10,000 per mm^3 of blood). There are approximately 500 to 1000 erythrocytes for each leukocyte. The leukocytes exist in several forms: eosinophils, basophils, monocytes, neutrophils, and lymphocytes. Also suspended in the plasma are small, nonnucleated cell fragments called **platelets** (normally 150,000 to 450,000 platelets per mm^3 of blood). These cellular components of blood normally make up 40% to 45% of the blood volume. The fraction of the blood occupied by erythrocytes is called the **hematocrit.** Blood appears as a thick, opaque, red fluid. Its color is imparted by the **hemoglobin** contained within the red blood cells. (See Chart 32-1 for a glossary of terms used in this chapter.)

The volume of blood in humans is approximately 7% to 10% of the normal body weight and amounts to about 5 liters. The blood circulates through the vascular system and serves as a link between body organs, carrying oxygen absorbed from the lungs and nutrients absorbed from the gastrointestinal tract to the body cells for cellular metabolism.

The blood also carries waste products produced by cellular metabolism to the lungs, skin, liver, and kidneys where they are transformed and eliminated from the body. The blood also carries hormones and antibodies to their sites of action or utilization.

To perform its functions, blood must remain in its normally fluid state. Because it is fluid, the danger always exists that trauma can lead to loss of blood from the vascular system. To prevent this danger, the blood has an intricate clotting mechanism that is activated when necessary to seal leaks in the blood vessels.

Excessive clotting is equally dangerous because it potentially obstructs blood flow to vital tissues. To prevent this complication, the body has a fibrinolytic mechanism that eventually dissolves the clots formed within blood vessels.

Bone Marrow

The bone marrow occupies the interior of spongy bones and the central cavity of the long bones of the skeleton. The marrow accounts for 4% to 5% of the total body weight and therefore is one of the larger organs of the body. The marrow can be either red or yellow. **Red marrow** is the site of active blood cell production and constitutes the major hematopoietic (blood-producing) organ. **Yellow marrow,** however, is composed mainly of fat and is not active in the production of blood elements. During childhood, the major portion of the marrow is red. As a person ages, a large portion of the marrow in the long bones is converted into yellow marrow, but it retains the potential for reverting to hematopoietic tissue if necessary. Red marrow in the adult

FIGURE 32-1. Types of blood cells.

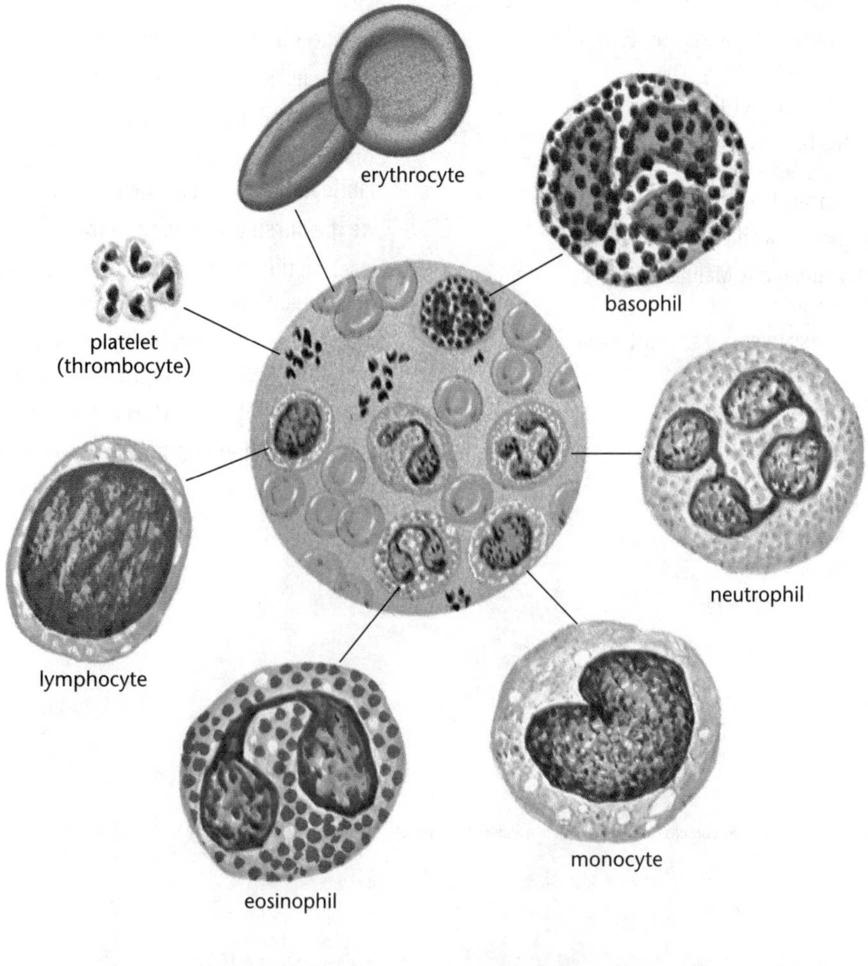

CHART 32-1
Glossary

Agranulocytosis acute disease in which the white blood cell count decreases to extremely low levels and neutropenia is pronounced

Aplasia failure of an organ or tissue to develop normally

Band cell immature granulocyte

Basophil a granular leukocyte

Ecchymosis a blue-black macula that results from seepage of blood into skin or mucous membrane

Eosinophil a granular leukocyte

Erythrocyte red blood cell

Erythropoiesis the formation of red blood cells

Erythropoietin hormone that regulates red blood cell production

Glossitis inflammation of the tongue

Granulocyte granular leukocyte: polymorphonuclear leukocyte (neutrophil, basophil, or eosinophil)

Granulocytopenia abnormal reduction of granulocytes in the blood

Hematocrit fraction of the blood occupied by erythrocytes

Hematopoiesis production and development of blood cells

Hematopoietic blood-producing

Hemoglobin iron-containing pigment of red blood cells

Hemolysis destruction of red blood cells with liberation of hemoglobin into the surrounding fluid

Histiocyte cell of loose connective tissue that shows phagocytic activity

Hyperplasia excessive proliferation of normal cells in normal tissue

Hypochromia blood possessing less than normal color and hemoglobin content

Leukocyte white blood cell

Leukopenia abnormal decrease of white blood cells

Lymphocyte a mononuclear leukocyte

Lysis disintegration or dissolution of cells

Macrocyte a large red blood cell

Macrophage cells of the reticuloendothelial system that have the ability to phagocytose particulate matter

Megaloblast abnormally large red blood cells

Microcyte a small red blood cell

Monocyte a mononuclear leukocyte

Mononuclear leukocyte agranulocyte (lymphocyte, monocyte)

Neutrophil a granular leukocyte

Normochromic normal color of cells

Normocytic normal size of cells

Oxyhemoglobin hemoglobin combined with oxygen

Pancytopenia reduction in all cellular elements of the blood

Petechiae pinpoint red or purple hemorrhagic spots on the skin

Phagocytosis the process of ingestion and digestion of bacteria and particles

Plasma liquid part of the blood

Platelet thrombocyte; cell fragment found in the blood that plays an important role in coagulation, hemostasis, and thrombus formation

Reticulocyte immature red blood cell

Reticuloendothelial system cells scattered throughout the body that have the ability to phagocytose particulate matter (bacteria, colloidal particles)

Serum the fluid portion of the blood that remains after coagulation

Spherocyte erythrocyte that assumes a spheroid shape

Thrombocyte platelet

Thrombocytopenia abnormal decrease in number of platelets

is confined chiefly to the ribs, vertebral column, and other flat bones.

The marrow is highly vascularized and consists of connective tissue containing free cells. The most primitive of this population of free cells are the **stem cells,** which are precursors of two different cell lines. The myeloid line includes erythrocytes, several types of leukocytes, and platelets. The lymphoid line differentiates into lymphocytes.

Erythrocytes

The normal red blood cell is a biconcave disc, its configuration resembling that of a soft ball compressed between two fingers (see Fig. 32-1). It has a diameter of about 8 μm but is a very flexible cell, so flexible that it is capable of passing easily through capillaries that may be as small as 4 μm in diameter. The volume of a red blood cell is about 90 μm^3. The red blood cell membrane is so thin that gases such as oxygen and carbon dioxide can easily diffuse across it. Mature red blood cells consist primarily of hemoglobin, which makes up 95% of the cell mass. These cells have no nuclei and have many fewer metabolic enzymes than do most other cells. The presence of a large amount of hemoglobin enables the cell to perform its principal function, the transport of oxygen between the lungs and tissues.

The oxygen-carrying pigment **hemoglobin** is a protein with a molecular weight of 64,000. The molecule is made up of four subunits, each containing a heme portion attached to a globin chain. Iron is present in the heme component of the molecule. An important property of the heme portion is its ability to bind to oxygen loosely and reversibly. When hemoglobin is combined with oxygen, it is called **oxyhemoglobin.** Oxyhemoglobin has a brighter red color than hemoglobin that does not contain oxygen (reduced hemoglobin), so arterial blood is brighter red than venous blood. Whole blood normally contains about 15 g of hemoglobin per 100 ml of blood, or 30 μm of hemoglobin per million erythrocytes.

Production of Erythrocytes (Erythropoiesis). Erythroblasts arise from the primitive stem cells in bone marrow. The **erythroblast** is a nucleated cell that in the process of maturing within the bone marrow accumulates hemoglobin and gradually loses its nucleus. At this stage, the cell is known as a **reticulocyte.** Further maturation into an erythrocyte entails the loss of dark staining material and a slight shrinkage in size. The mature erythrocyte is then released into the circulation. Under conditions of rapid erythropoiesis, reticulocytes and other immature cells may be released prematurely into the circulation.

Differentiation of the primitive multipotential stem cell of the marrow into an erythroblast is stimulated by **erythropoietin,** a substance produced primarily by the kidney. Under conditions of prolonged hypoxia, as in the case of persons living at high altitudes or after severe hemorrhage, erythropoietin levels are increased and red blood cell production is stimulated.

For normal erythrocyte production, the bone marrow requires iron, vitamin B_{12}, folic acid, pyridoxine (vitamin B_6), and other factors. A deficiency of these factors during erythropoiesis results in decreased red blood cell production and anemia.

Iron Stores and Metabolism. Total body iron content in the average adult is approximately 3 g, most of which is present in hemoglobin or one of its breakdown products. Normally, about 0.5 to 1 mg of iron is absorbed per day from the intestinal tract to replace losses of iron in the feces. Additional amounts of iron, up to 2 mg per day, must be absorbed by the adult female to replace blood lost during menstruation. Iron deficiency in the adult (decreased total body iron content) generally indicates that blood has been lost from the body—for example, by hemorrhage or excessive menstruation.

The concentration of iron in blood is normally about 80 to 180 μg/dl (SI:14–32 μmol/L) for men and 60 to 160 μg/dl (SI:11–29 μmol/L) for women. With iron deficiency, bone marrow iron stores are rapidly depleted, hemoglobin synthesis is depressed, and the red blood cells produced by the marrow are small and low in hemoglobin.

Vitamin B_{12} and Folic Acid Metabolism. Vitamin B_{12} and folic acid are required for DNA synthesis in many tissues, but deficiencies of either of these vitamins have the greatest effect on erythropoiesis. Vitamin B_{12} or folic acid deficiency is characterized by the production of abnormally large red blood cells called **megaloblasts.** Because these cells are abnormal, many are sequestered in the bone marrow and their rate of release is decreased. This condition results in **megaloblastic anemia.**

Both vitamin B_{12} and folic acid are derived from the diet. Vitamin B_{12} combines with intrinsic factor produced in the stomach. The vitamin B_{12} intrinsic factor complex is absorbed in the distal ileum. Folic acid is absorbed in the proximal small intestine.

Red Blood Cell Destruction. The average life span of a circulating red blood cell is 120 days. Aged red blood cells are removed from the blood by the reticuloendothelial system, particularly in the liver and the spleen. The reticuloendothelial cells produce a pigment called bilirubin from the hemoglobin that is released from the destroyed red blood cells. Bilirubin is a waste product that is excreted in the bile. The iron, freed from the hemoglobin during bilirubin formation, is carried in plasma bound to the protein called transferrin to the bone marrow, where it is reclaimed for production of new hemoglobin.

Function of Erythrocytes. The major function of the red blood cells is to transport oxygen from the lungs to the tissues. Erythrocytes are uniquely capable of performing this function because of their high concentration of hemoglobin. If hemoglobin were not present, the oxygen-carrying capacity of blood would be decreased by 99% and would not be sufficient to meet the metabolic needs of the body. An important property of hemoglobin is that is binds oxygen loosely and reversibly. As a result, oxygen readily binds to hemoglobin in the lungs, is carried as oxyhemoglobin in arterial blood, and readily dissociates from hemoglobin in the tissues. In venous blood, hemoglobin combines with hydrogen ions produced by cellular metabolism and thus buffers excess acid.

Leukocytes

Leukocytes are divided into two general categories, granulocytes and mononuclear cells (agranulocytes). In normal blood, the total leukocyte count is 5,000 to 10,000 cells per mm^3. Of these, approximately 60% are granulocytes and 40% are mononuclear cells. Leukocytes can be readily differentiated from erythrocytes by the presence of a nucleus, their larger size, and different staining properties.

Granulocytes. Granulocytes are defined by the presence of granules in their cytoplasm. The diameter of a granulocyte is generally two to three times that of an erythrocyte. Granulocytes are divided into three subgroups, which are characterized by their staining properties as seen on microscopic examination (see Fig. 32-1). *Eosinophils* have bright red granules in their cytoplasm, whereas the granules in *basophils* stain deep blue. The third, and by far the most numerous, cell in this series is the *neutrophil,* with granules that show a dull violet hue.

The nucleus of the mature granulocyte generally has multiple lobes (usually two to four) connected by thin filaments of nuclear material. Because of their nuclear characteristics, these cells are called *polymorphonuclear (PMN) leukocytes.* The immature granulocyte has a single-lobed ovoid nucleus and is called a band cell. Ordinarily, band cells account for only a small percentage of circulating granulocytes, although their percentage can increase greatly under conditions in which the rate of production of PMN leukocytes is increased.

The number of circulating granulocytes found in the healthy person is relatively constant, but in the presence of infection large numbers of these cells are rapidly released into the circulation. Granulocyte production from the stem cell pool is thought to be controlled in a manner similar to the regulation of erythrocyte production by erythropoietin.

Mononuclear Leukocytes (Agranulocytes). Mononuclear leukocytes (lymphocytes and monocytes) are white blood cells with a single-lobed nucleus and a granule-free cytoplasm. In normal adult blood, lymphocytes account for approximately 30% and monocytes approximately 5% of the total leukocytes. Mature *lymphocytes* are small cells with scanty cytoplasm. They are produced primarily in the lymph nodes and in the lymphoid tissue of the intestine, spleen, and thymus gland from precursor cells that originated as marrow stem cells. *Monocytes* are the largest of the blood leukocytes. They are produced by the bone marrow and give rise to tissue histiocytes, including Kupffer cells of the liver, peritoneal macrophages, alveolar macrophages, and other components of the reticuloendothelial system.

Function of the Leukocytes. The function of the leukocytes is to protect the body from invasion by bacteria and other foreign entities. The major function of neutrophilic PMNs is to ingest foreign material (phagocytosis) (Fig. 32-2). Neutrophils arrive at the site within an hour of the onset of an inflammatory reaction and initiate phagocytosis, but are relatively short-lived. The influx of monocytes is later, but these cells continue their phagocytic activities for long periods.

The function of lymphocytes is primarily to produce substances that aid in the attack of foreign material. One group of lymphocytes (*T lymphocytes*) kills foreign cells directly or releases a variety of lymphokines, substances that enhance the activity of phagocytic cells. The other group of lymphocytes (*B lymphocytes*) produces antibodies, protein molecules that destroy foreign material by several mechanisms.

Eosinophils and basophils function as reservoirs of potent biologic materials such as histamine, serotonin, and heparin. Release of these compounds alters the blood supply to tissues, such as occurs during inflammation, and helps to mobilize body defense mechanisms. The increase in the number of eosinophils in allergic states indicates that these cells are involved in the hypersensitivity reaction.

Platelets

Platelets are small particles, 2 to 4 μm in diameter, that are present in the circulating blood plasma. Because they disintegrate quickly and easily, their number varies normally between 150,000 and 450,000 per mm^3 of blood, depending on the numbers that are produced, how they are used, and how quickly they are destroyed. They are formed from the fragmentation of giant cells of the bone marrow, called *megakaryocytes*. Platelet production is regulated by *thrombopoietin*.

Platelets play an essential role in the control of bleeding. When vascular injury occurs, platelets collect at the site. Substances released from platelet granules and other blood cells cause the platelets to adhere to each other and form a patch or plug, which temporarily stops bleeding. Additional substances released from platelets activate coagulation factors in the blood plasma.

Blood Coagulation

Blood coagulation is the process whereby the components of the liquid blood are transformed into a semisolid material called a blood clot. The blood clot is composed mainly of blood cells entrapped in a meshwork of fibrin. Fibrin is formed from proteins in the plasma as the result of a complex series of reactions.

Many factors are involved in the reaction cascade that forms fibrin. The *clotting factors* are listed in Table 32-1, and the extrinsic and intrinsic pathways for fibrin generation are shown diagrammatically in Figure 32-3.

When tissue is injured, the *extrinsic pathway* is activated by the release from the tissue of a substance called thromboplastin. As the result of a series of reactions, prothrombin is converted to thrombin, which in turn catalyzes the conversion of fibrinogen to fibrin. Calcium (factor IV) is a necessary cofactor for many of these reactions. Clotting by the *intrinsic pathway* is activated when the collagen lining blood vessels is exposed. Clotting factors are then activated sequentially until, as with the extrinsic pathway, fibrin is ultimately formed. Although longer, this sequence is probably most often responsible for clotting *in vivo*.

The intrinsic pathway is also responsible for initiating the clotting of blood that comes into contact with glass or

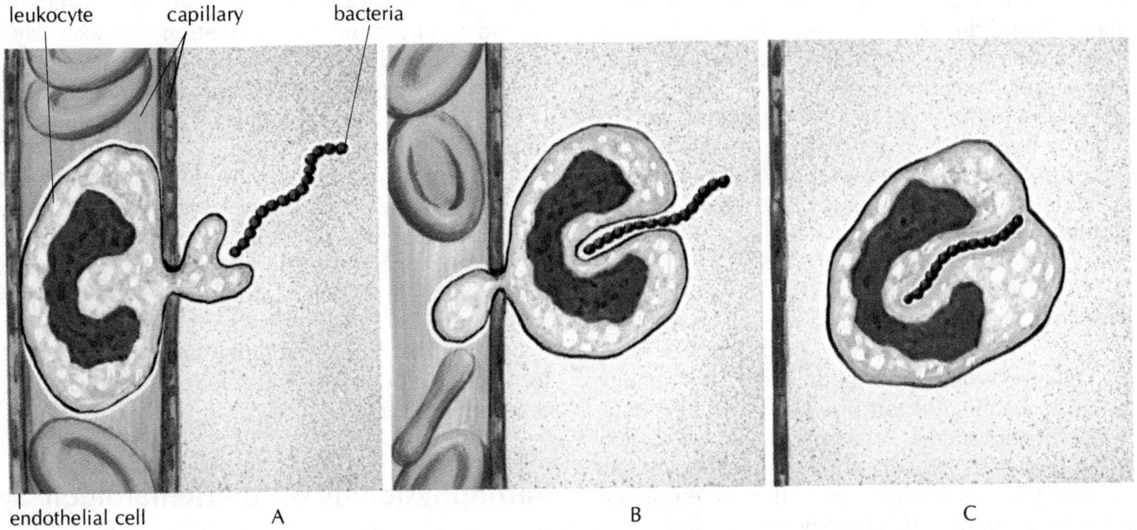

FIGURE 32-2. The process of phagocytosis for fighting infection. (**A**) The white cell exits from a capillary and (**B,C**) engulfs the bacteria in the process of destroying it.

TABLE 32-1 Clotting Factors

Official Number	Synonym	Contemporary Version	
I	Fibrinogen	I	(Fibrinogen)
II	Prothrombin	II	(Prothrombin)
III	Tissue thromboplastin	III	(Tissue factor)
IV	Calcium	IV	(Calcium)
V	Labile	V	(Labile factor)
		VI	PF_3 (platelet coagulant activities)
		VI	PF_4
VII	Stable factor	VII	(Stable factor)
VIII	Antihemophilic factor	VIII	AHF (antihemophilic factor)
		VIII	vWF (von Willebrand factor)
		VIII	RAg (related antigen)
IX	Christmas factor	IX	(Christmas factor)
X	Stuart-Prower factor	X	(Stuart-Prower factor)
XI	Plasma thromboplastin (antecedent)	XI	(Plasma thromboplastin antecedent)
XII	Hageman factor	XII	HF (Hageman factor)
		XII	PK (Prekallikrein Fletcher)
		XII	HMWK (High-molecular-weight kininogen)
XIII	Fibrin-stabilizing factor	XIII	Fibrin-stabilizing factor

The Roman numerals and synonyms designating each clotting factor accepted by the International Committee on Blood Clotting Factors are located in the left-hand columns. Note the absence of factor VI. The version in the right-hand column incorporates more recently recognized clotting factors but is not officially recognized.
(Green D. General considerations of coagulation proteins. Ann Clin Lab Sci 8[2]: 95–105.)

other foreign surfaces, as when blood is withdrawn from the body into a test tube. It is for this reason that anticoagulants often must be used in test tubes when drawing a specimen of blood for diagnostic tests. The anticoagulants usually used are either citrate, which binds the plasma calcium, or heparin, which prevents the conversion of prothrombin to thrombin. Citrate cannot be used as an anticoagulant *in vivo* because binding of plasma calcium would cause hypocalcemia and death. Heparin can be used clinically as an anticoagulant. Coumarins also are used clinically for their anticoagulant action of interfering with the production of several of the plasma-coagulating factors.

Clots that form in the body are eventually dissolved by the action of the fibrinolytic system, which consists of plasmin and other proteolytic enzymes. Through the action of this system, clots are dissolved as tissue is repaired, and the vascular system is returned to its normal baseline state.

Blood Plasma

After cellular elements are removed from blood, the remaining liquid portion is called **blood plasma.** It contains ions, proteins, and other substances. If plasma is allowed to clot, the remaining fluid is called **serum.** Serum has essentially the same composition as plasma, except that its fibrinogen and several of the clotting factors have been removed.

Plasma Proteins. Plasma proteins consist primarily of albumin and globulins. The globulins in turn consist of alpha, beta, and gamma fractions derived by a laboratory test called serum protein electrophoresis. Each of these groups is made up of distinct proteins.

The **gamma globulins,** which consist mainly of antibodies, are called immunoglobulins. These proteins are produced by the lymphocytes and plasma cells. Important proteins in the alpha and beta fractions are the transport globulins and the clotting factors that are made in the liver. The transport globulins carry various substances in the bound form around the circulation. For example, thyroid-binding globulin carries thyroxin, and transferrin carries iron. The clotting factors, including fibrinogen, remain in an inactive form in the blood plasma until activated by the clotting cascade.

Albumin is particularly important for the maintenance of fluid volume within the vascular system. Capillary walls are impermeable to albumin, so its presence in the plasma creates an osmotic force that keeps fluid within the vascular space. Albumin, which is produced by the liver, has the capacity to bind to a number of substances that are often present in plasma. In this way, it functions as a transport protein for metals, fatty acids, bilirubin, and medications, among other substances.

Pathophysiology of the Hematologic System

Anemias. A frequent disorder of the hematologic system is a decrease in the number of circulating red blood

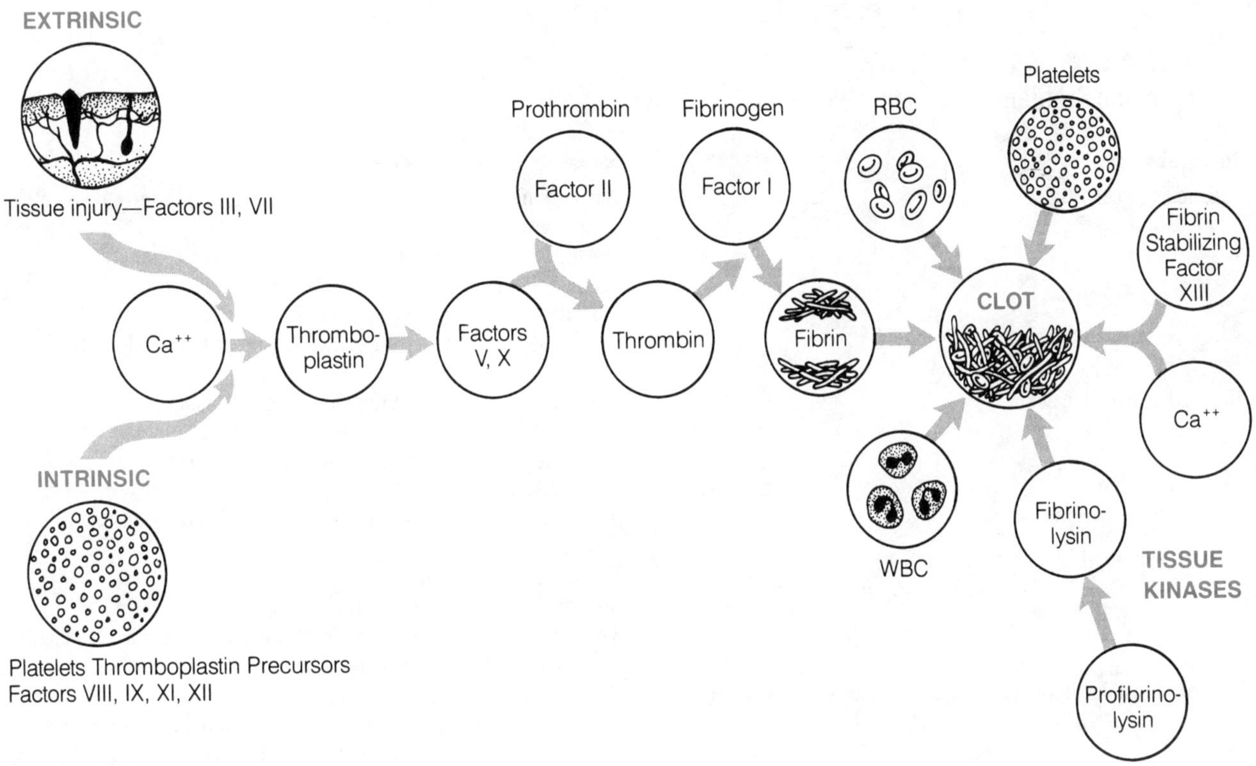

FIGURE 32-3. The blood-clotting mechanism. The schematic drawing represents the factors essential to change blood into a solid gel. The entire chain reaction in which fibrinogen (a plasma protein) is converted to fibrin (the clot) takes place at the site of vessel damage. (Adapted from Feller I and Archambeault C. Nursing the Burn Patient. Ann Arbor, The Institute for Burn Medicine.)

cells. This condition, called *anemia*, can result from either underproduction of red blood cells by the bone marrow or increased destruction of circulating red blood cells. Underproduction of red blood cells can be due to a deficiency in cofactors for erythropoiesis, including folic acid, vitamin B_{12}, and iron. Red blood cell production may also be reduced if bone marrow is suppressed (by tumor or medications) or is inadequately stimulated because of lack of erythropoietin, as occurs in chronic renal disease. Increased destruction of red blood cells may occur because of an overactive reticuloendothelial system (*e.g.*, hypersplenism) or because the bone marrow produces abnormal red blood cells (*e.g.*, sickle cell anemia). Because the red blood cell and its hemoglobin are important for the delivery of oxygen to tissues, anemias may result in tissue hypoxia.

Bleeding Disorders. Bleeding disorders can be attributed to deficiency in either platelets or clotting factors in the circulating blood. Platelet function in the blood plasma can be reduced as the result of bone marrow insufficiency, increased splenic destruction, or abnormal circulating platelets. Deficiencies of clotting factors are usually due to underproduction of these factors by the liver. Hemophilia is a hereditary disorder that results from deficiency of clotting factors VIII and IX.

Manifestations of Blood Disorders. Problems commonly seen in patients with blood disorders include fatigue and weakness; hemorrhagic tendencies; ulcerative lesions of the tongue, gums, or mucous membranes; dyspnea; bone and joint pains; fever; pruritus; and anxiety. The nursing interventions for these problems are presented in Chart 32-2.

Blood Study Procedures

Methods of Obtaining Blood

Venipuncture. Most routine hematologic studies are performed on venous blood, which is usually obtained from an antecubital vein. Occasionally, in very obese persons or those whose veins have been thrombosed by chemotherapy, it may be necessary to use one of the veins on the dorsum of the hand. (See Chapter 14 for procedure.)

Blood is immediately placed in the collection tube appropriate for the particular test required. The tubes are color coded to specify what, if any, additive they contain. For some tests the blood is allowed to coagulate; for others it is kept fluid by the presence of an anticoagulant in the collection tube.

Finger Puncture. The finger puncture method is used frequently for blood smears and counts. This method uses capillary blood, but for practical purposes the results are identical to those obtained with venous blood. Lancets of various shapes are available. These make a puncture of 1 to 2 mm. Best results are obtained if the patient's hand is warm and if the pulp of the index or middle finger is punctured. The skin should be cleaned with alcohol first and then carefully wiped dry with a lint-free sponge. If any alcohol remains, it will alter red cell morphology. The drops of blood

CHART 32-2
Common Problems of Patients With Blood Disorders

Problem	Nursing Interventions
Fatigue and weakness	Plan nursing care to conserve the patient's strength and emotional energy. Provide frequent rest periods. Encourage ambulation and other activities as tolerated. Avoid disturbing activities, noise, and stress. Encourage optimal nutrition—high-protein and high-calorie foods and drinks.
Hemorrhagic tendencies	Keep the patient at rest during the bleeding episodes. Apply gentle pressure to the bleeding sites. Apply cold compresses to the bleeding sites when indicated. Do not disturb clots. Use small-gauge needles when administering medications by injection. Support the patient during transfusion therapy. Observe for symptoms of internal bleeding. Have a tracheostomy set available for the patient who is bleeding from the mouth or the throat.
Ulcerative lesions of the tongue, gums, or mucous membranes	Avoid irritating foods and beverages. Provide frequent oral hygiene with mild, cool mouthwash solutions. Use applicators or soft-bristled toothbrush. Keep the lips lubricated. Provide mouth care both before and after meals. Encourage regular visits to the dentist.
Dyspnea	Elevate the head of the bed. Use pillows to support the patient in the orthopneic position. Administer oxygen when indicated. Prevent unnecessary exertion. Avoid gas-forming foods.
Bone and joint pains	Relieve pressure of bedding by using a cradle. Administer either hot or cold compresses as prescribed. Administer analgesic as prescribed on a regular basis. Provide for joint immobilization when prescribed.
Fever	Provide cool baths. Administer antipyretic (acetaminophen) medications as prescribed. Encourage fluid intake unless contraindicated. Maintain a cool environmental temperature.
Pruritus or skin eruptions	Keep the patient's fingernails short. Use soap sparingly. Apply emollient lotions in skin care.
Anxiety of the patient and family	Explain the nature, the discomforts, and the limitations of activity associated with the diagnostic procedures and treatments. Encourage the patient and family to express their anxieties. Provide an atmosphere of acceptance and understanding. Promote the patient's relaxation and comfort. Consider the patient's individual preferences. Promote independence and self-care within the patient's limitations. Encourage the family to participate in the patient's care (as desired). Create a comfortable atmosphere for family visits with the patient.

obtained by this method can be gently touched to glass slides or cover slips, for peripheral smears. Capillary blood can also be drawn into calibrated red cell and white cell pipettes and into microhematocrit tubes.

The most common hematologic tests are described in Chart 32-3.

Bone Marrow Aspiration

Bone marrow is usually aspirated from the sternum or iliac crest in adults. Most patients need no more preparation than a careful explanation of the procedure, but for some very anxious patients, meperidine (Demerol) or an antianxiety

CHART 32-3
Common Hematologic Laboratory Tests

Test	Definition
Complete blood count (CBC)	Includes enumeration of number of white cells, red cells, and platelets per cubic millimeter of venous blood, as well as a differential count, percentage of each type of nucleated cell in the blood (*e.g.*, percentage of polymorphonuclears, percentage of lymphocytes).
Reticulocyte count	Percentage of young (1–2 days old), nonnucleated erythrocytes in peripheral blood; they are recognized in special stains of blood smears as cells with lacy inclusions, which consist of RNA.
Hemoglobin electrophoresis	A drop of blood placed on a solid medium (paper, starch block, gel, or cellulose acetate) is exposed to a current of electricity while being bathed by a buffer solution. The different hemoglobins (*e.g.*, A, A-2, F, S) travel at varying speeds, depending on their charge. At the end of the procedure, the paper or gel is stained, and the hemoglobins in each sample can be identified.
Sickling test	A drop of blood is mixed with a drop of a reducing agent (sodium metabisulfite). This substance deprives the red cells of oxygen and induces sickling if S hemoglobin is present. Sickling of red cells is observed under the microscope in 30 minutes if the blood was obtained from a person with either sickle trait or sickle cell anemia. Normal blood does not undergo any change.
Leukocyte alkaline phosphatase (LAP)	LAP is an enzyme present in high concentrations in granules of neutrophils. A special stain of peripheral blood smears is used to estimate the amount of LAP present per cell. The normal value is 20 to 130. Untreated chronic myelogenous leukemia patients have values of less than 20, and the test is useful to help diagnose CML. High values are seen in infection and steroid-induced leukocytosis.
Coombs' test	Determines the presence of immune globulin (hence, antibodies) on the surface of erythrocytes (direct Coombs' test) or in the plasma (indirect Coombs' test).
Bleeding time	A screening test for disorders of platelet function. It is the time taken for bleeding to cease after a standardized skin wound is produced, usually on the forearm. A prolonged time suggests an inherited or acquired platelet defect (*e.g.*, von Willebrand's disease or aspirin ingestion).
Platelet aggregation	A measure of the time and completeness of the formation of platelet aggregates in a sample of plasma, after the addition of an agent such as epinephrine or ADP.
Prothrombin time	Measures the coagulant activity of the "extrinsic" system, including fibrinogen, prothrombin, and factors V, VII, and X. It is used to monitor therapy of coumarin derivatives, as well as to screen for liver disease.
Partial thromboplastin time	A screening test for deficiencies of all plasma coagulation factors except VII and XIII. It is usually considered abnormally prolonged if levels of factors are less than 30% of normal. It is often used to monitor heparin therapy.

medication may be useful. It is always important for the physician or nurse to describe and explain the procedure and the sensations that will be experienced during the procedure.

First, the skin area is cleansed as for any minor surgery. Then a small area is anesthetized with lidocaine (Xylocaine) through the skin and subcutaneous tissue to the periosteum of the bone. The bone marrow needle is introduced with a stylet in place. When the needle is felt to go through the outer cortex of bone and enter the marrow cavity, the stylet is removed, a syringe is attached, and a small volume (0.5 ml) of blood and marrow is aspirated. The actual aspiration always causes brief pain, and the patient should be warned of this. Taking deep breaths or using relaxation techniques often helps.

If a bone marrow biopsy is necessary, it is best performed after the aspiration and with a special needle.

Several types of needles are available, the procedure varying according to the type of needle used. Because these needles are large, the skin is punctured first with a surgical blade (no. 9 or 11) to make a 3- or 4-mm incision. Only the iliac bone is used for this procedure, because the sternum is too thin.

The major hazard of these procedures is a slight risk of hemorrhage. This risk is increased if the patient's platelet count is low; therefore a platelet count is obtained before the procedure. After bone marrow aspiration, pressure is applied to the site for several minutes. After a biopsy, pressure is applied to the posterior iliac crest for 60 minutes by the combination of a pressure dressing and having the patient lie recumbent in bed. Most patients have no discomfort after a bone marrow aspiration, but the site of a biopsy may ache for a day or two.

Anemia

Anemia is a term that indicates a low red cell count and a below-normal hemoglobin or hematocrit level. It is not a disease but rather reflects a disease state or altered body function. Physiologically, anemia exists when there is an insufficient amount of hemoglobin to deliver oxygen to the tissues.

There are many different kinds of anemias. Some are due to inadequate production of red blood cells, and others are due to premature or excessive destruction of red blood cells. Other etiologic factors include blood loss, deficits in nutrients, hereditary factors, and chronic diseases. Iron deficiency anemia is the most common anemia in the world.

Pathophysiology

The appearance of anemia reflects either marrow failure or excessive red cell loss, or both. Marrow failure (*i.e.*, reduced erythropoiesis) may occur as a result of nutritional deficiency, toxic exposure, tumor invasion, or, as in many instances, from causes unknown. Red cells may be lost through hemorrhage or hemolysis (destruction). In the latter case, the problem may be due to a red cell defect that is incompatible with normal red cell survival or to some factor extrinsic to the red cell that promotes red cell destruction.

Red cell lysis (dissolution) occurs mainly within the phagocytic cells of the reticuloendothelial system, notably in the liver and spleen. As a byproduct of this process, bilirubin, formed within the phagocyte, enters the bloodstream. Any increase in the destruction of red blood cells (hemolysis) is promptly reflected by an increase in plasma bilirubin. (This concentration normally is 1 mg/dl or less; levels above 1.5 mg/dl produce visible jaundice of the sclerae.)

If, as happens in certain specific hemolytic disorders, red cells are destroyed within the circulating bloodstream, hemoglobin appears in the plasma (hemoglobinemia). If the plasma concentration exceeds the capacity of the plasma haptoglobin (a binding protein for free hemoglobin) to bind it all (*i.e.*, if the amount is more than about 100 mg/dl), hemoglobin diffuses through the renal glomeruli and into the urine (hemoglobinuria). Thus the presence or absence of hemoglobinemia and hemoglobinuria provides information about the location of abnormal blood destruction in a patient with hemolysis and can be a clue to the nature of the hemolytic process.

A conclusion as to whether the anemia in a particular patient is caused by destruction of red blood cells or inadequate production of red blood cells usually can be reached on the basis of (1) the reticulocyte count in the circulating blood; (2) the degree to which young red cells proliferate in the bone marrow and the manner in which they mature, as observed on biopsy; and (3) the presence or absence of hyperbilirubinemia and hemoglobinemia.

Erythropoiesis (red cell production) can be quantified by measuring the rate at which injected radioactive iron is incorporated into circulating erythrocytes. The life span of the patient's red cells (therefore, the rate of hemolysis) can be measured by tagging a portion of these with radioactive chromium, reinjecting them, and following their disappearance from the circulating blood over the course of days or weeks. Methods by which one particular type of marrow failure can be distinguished from another type, and one hemolytic disease from another, are discussed later in this chapter.

Gerontologic Considerations

Anemia is common in older persons and is the most common hematologic condition that affects the elderly, but studies indicate that the aging process does not cause changes in hematopoiesis. The cause is usually unexplained. Anemia is generally considered to be part of a pathologic process that results in blood loss rather than a result of aging. Because the elderly person may be unable to respond adequately to the anemia with increased cardiac output or pulmonary ventilation, anemia can have serious effects on cardiopulmonary function if not properly treated. Thus, it is important to identify the cause of the anemia rather than to consider it an inevitable consequence of aging.

Clinical Manifestations

Aside from the severity of the anemia, several factors affect the severity and presence of symptoms: (1) the speed with which the anemia has developed, (2) its duration (*i.e.*, its chronicity), (3) the metabolic requirements of the particular patient, (4) the presence of other disorders or disabilities, and (5) special complications or concomitant features of the condition that produced the anemia.

The more rapidly an anemia develops, the more severe its symptoms. An otherwise normal person can tolerate as much as a 50% *gradual* reduction in hemoglobin, red count, or hematocrit without pronounced symptoms or significant incapacity, whereas the *rapid* loss of as little as 30% may precipitate profound vascular collapse in the same individual. A person who has been anemic for a very long time, with hemoglobin levels between 9 and 11 mg/dl, experiences few or no symptoms other than slight tachycardia on exertion. Exertional dyspnea is likely to occur below, but not above, 7.5 g/dl; weakness, only below 6 g/dl; dyspnea at rest, below 3 g/dl; and cardiac failure, only at the extremely low level of 2 to 2.5 g/dl.

Patients who customarily are very active are more likely to experience symptoms, and symptoms that are more pronounced, than a more sedentary person. A patient with hypothyroidism with decreased oxygen needs may be completely asymptomatic, without tachycardia or increased cardiac output, at a hemoglobin level of 10 g/dl.

Finally, many anemic disorders are complicated by various other abnormalities that do not result from the anemia but are inherently associated with these particular diseases. These abnormalities may give rise to symptoms that completely overshadow those of the anemia, as is exemplified by the painful crises of sickle cell anemia (see p. 784).

Diagnostic Evaluation

A variety of hematologic studies are performed to determine the type and cause of the anemia. These include hemoglobin and hematocrit levels, red blood cell indices, white blood cell studies, serum iron level, measurement of total iron-binding capacity, folate level, vitamin B_{12} level, platelet count, bleeding time, prothrombin time, and partial thromboplastin time. Bone marrow aspiration and biopsy may be performed. In addition, diagnostic studies are carried out to determine the presence of acute or chronic illness and the source of any chronic blood loss.

Medical Management

Management of anemia is directed toward reversing the cause and replacing blood that has been lost. The management of the various types of anemia will be covered in the discussions of each type presented in the following pages.

Complications

General complications of anemia include congestive heart failure, paresthesias, and confusion. At any given level of anemia, patients with underlying heart disease are far more likely to experience angina or symptoms of congestive failure than someone without heart disease.

Complications associated with specific types of anemia are included with their separate descriptions.

❑ NURSING PROCESS
The Patient With Anemia

Assessment

The health history and physical examination will provide data about the patient's problems and concerns. Weakness, fatigue, and general malaise are common, as are pallor of the skin and mucous membranes. Jaundice may be present in patients with pernicious anemia or hemolytic anemia. Dryness of the skin and hair are often seen in iron-deficiency anemia.

Cardiac status is carefully assessed. When the hemoglobin is low, the heart will attempt to compensate by pumping faster and harder in an effort to deliver more blood to hypoxic tissue. This increased cardiac workload results in such symptoms as tachycardia, palpitations, dyspnea, dizziness, orthopnea, and exertional dyspnea. Congestive heart failure will eventually develop, as evidenced by an enlarged heart (cardiomegaly) and liver (hepatomegaly), and peripheral edema.

Neurologic examination is also important because of the effect of pernicious anemia on the central and peripheral nervous systems. The patient is assessed for peripheral numbness and paresthesias, ataxia, poor coordination, and confusion. Assessment of gastrointestinal function may disclose complaints of nausea, vomiting, diarrhea, anorexia, and glossitis (inflammation of the tongue).

The health history includes information about any medications the patient may be taking that could depress bone marrow activity or interfere with folate metabolism. Accurate history of alcohol intake, including amount and duration of drinking, is obtained. The patient is also questioned about any loss of blood, as evidenced by blood in the stools, or, for women, excessive menstrual flow. Family history is important because certain anemias are inherited. Athletic endeavors are significant because exercise can decrease erythropoiesis and red cell survival in a small percentage of athletes. A nutritional assessment may indicate deficiencies in essential nutrients such as iron, vitamin B_{12}, and folic acid. Children of homeless families are at high risk for anemias because of malnutrition.

Diagnosis

Nursing Diagnoses

Based on the assessment data, major nursing diagnoses for the patient may include the following:

- ❑ Activity intolerance related to weakness, fatigue, and general malaise
- ❑ Altered nutrition, less than body requirements, related to inadequate intake of essential nutrients

Collaborative Problems/ Potential Complications

Based on the assessment data, potential complications that may develop include:

- ❑ Congestive heart failure
- ❑ Paresthesias
- ❑ Confusion

Planning and Implementation

Goals. The major goals of the patient may include tolerance of normal activity, attainment or maintenance of adequate nutrition, and absence of complications.

Nursing Interventions

Promoting Rest and Activity. The patient is encouraged to conserve strength and physical and emotional energy. Frequent rest periods are encouraged, and family support is elicited to promote a restful environment. A regular schedule of rest and sleep is imperative for restoring strength and activity tolerance. Ambulation and activities of daily living are encouraged as tolerated. As the anemia is treated and blood values return to normal, the patient is encouraged to resume normal activities gradually. Activities that are found to cause undue fatigue are postponed until endurance increases. Conditioning exercises may be used to increase endurance. Safety precautions are used to prevent falls resulting from poor coordination, paresthesias, and weakness.

Maintaining Adequate Nutrition. Inadequate intake of essential nutrients, such as iron and folic acid, can cause some anemias. The symptoms associated with anemias, such as fatigue and anorexia, can in turn also interfere with nutrition. A well-balanced diet high in protein and high-calorie foods, fruits, and vegetables is encouraged. Alcohol interferes with the utilization of essential nutrients; therefore the patient is advised to avoid alcoholic beverages or to limit their intake. Spicy foods that can cause gastric irritation and foods that are gas producing are avoided. Dietary teaching sessions are planned for the patient and the family because the diet plan should be acceptable to both the patient and family. Dietary supplements (*e.g.*, vitamins, iron, folate) may be prescribed.

Monitoring and Managing Complications. With longstanding reduction of oxyhemoglobin, the heart may be less able to supply blood to hypoxic tissue. The heart will begin to enlarge, cardiac output will decrease, and congestive heart failure will ensue. Nursing measures are directed toward decreasing activities and stimuli that cause an increase in heart rate and increased cardiac output. The patient is encouraged to identify those situations that precipitate palpitations and dyspnea and to avoid them until the anemia is resolved. If dyspnea is a problem, measures such as elevation of the head of the bed and the use of pillows for support are used. Unnecessary exertion is avoided. Oxygen may need to be administered. Vital signs are monitored frequently and the patient is observed for indications of fluid retention (*e.g.*, peripheral edema, decreased urinary output, and neck vein distention).

The patient is monitored for signs of *paresthesia* (*e.g.*, unexplained bruises or burns on lower extremities), poor coordination, ataxia, and *confusion*. Safety measures are implemented to prevent injury.

Evaluation

Expected Outcomes

1. Tolerates normal activity
   a. Follows a progressive plan of rest, activities, and exercises
   b. Paces activities according to energy level
2. Attains/maintains adequate nutrition
   a. Eats foods high in protein, calories, and vitamins
   b. Avoids foods that cause gastric irritation
   c. Develops a meal plan that promotes optimal nutrition
3. Experiences absence of complications
   a. Avoids activities that cause tachycardia, palpitations, dizziness, and dyspnea
   b. Uses rest and comfort measures to alleviate dyspnea
   c. Has normal vital signs
   d. Experiences no signs of fluid retention (*e.g.*, peripheral edema, decreased urinary output, neck vein distention)
   e. Is oriented to name, time, place, and situation
   f. Remains free of injury

Classification of Anemias

Anemia may be classified in several ways. The physiologic approach is to determine whether the deficiency in red cells is due to a defect in production of red cells (hypoproliferative anemia) or to destruction of the red cells (hemolytic anemia).

In the hypoproliferative anemias, red cells usually survive normally, but the marrow is unable to produce adequate numbers of cells; thus, the reticulocyte count is depressed. This situation may be a result of marrow damage by medications or chemicals (*e.g.*, chloramphenicol, benzene) or may be due to lack of erythropoietin (as in renal disease), iron, vitamin B_{12}, or folic acid.

When hemolysis (dissolution of red blood cells with liberation of hemoglobin into surrounding plasma) is the major cause of anemia, the abnormality is usually within the red cell itself (as in sickle cell anemia or G-6-PD [glucose-6-phosphate dehydrogenase] deficiency), in the plasma (as in immune hemolytic anemias), or in the circulation (as in heart valve hemolysis). With hemolytic anemias, the reticulocyte count and indirect bilirubin level are elevated, often enough to cause clinical jaundice.

Hypoproliferative Anemias

Aplastic Anemia

Pathophysiology. Aplastic anemia is caused by a decrease in precursor cells in the bone marrow and replacement of the marrow with fat. It can be congenital or acquired. It may be idiopathic (*i.e.*, without apparent cause), and this accounts for the majority of cases. Certain infections and pregnancy can trigger it; or it may be caused by medications, chemicals, or radiation damage. Agents that regularly produce marrow aplasia include benzene and benzene derivatives (*e.g.*, airplane glue); antitumor agents such as nitrogen mustard; the antimetabolites, including methotrexate and 6-mercaptopurine; and certain toxic materials, such as inorganic arsenic.

Other agents occasionally responsible for aplasia or hypoplasia include certain antimicrobials, anticonvulsants, antithyroid medications, oral hypoglycemic agents, antihistamines, analgesics, sedatives, phenothiazines, insecticides, and heavy metals. The most common offenders are the antimicrobials, chloramphenicol and the organic arsenicals, the anticonvulsants mephenytoin (Mesantoin) and trimethadione (Tridione), the anti-inflammatory analgesic agent phenylbutazone, sulfonamides, and gold compounds.

In many situations, aplastic anemia occurs when a medication or chemical is ingested in toxic amounts. However, in a small number of persons, it develops after a medication has been taken in the recommended dosage. These latter cases may be considered a type of idiosyncratic medication reaction in persons who are highly susceptible for unknown reasons. Provided that their exposure is ended early (*i.e.*, on the first appearance of reticulocytopenia, anemia, granulocytopenia, or thrombocytopenia), a prompt and complete recovery may be anticipated. Young adolescent males who have hepatitis are at risk for a severe form of aplastic anemia that carries a high mortality rate, 90% at one year with a median survival rate of six months; bone marrow transplant is the preferred treatment.

Whatever the offending agent, if exposure continues after signs of hypoplasia have appeared, bone marrow depression almost certainly progresses to the point of complete and irreversible failure—hence the importance of frequent complete blood counts for every patient receiving a medication or exposed regularly to any chemical that has been implicated in aplastic anemia.

Diagnostic Evaluation. Because of the reduced number of cells in the bone marrow, attempts at bone marrow aspiration frequently yield only a few drops of blood. A biopsy is usually necessary to demonstrate a severe decrease in normal marrow elements and replacement by fat. The abnormality is probably in the stem cell, the precursor for granulocytes, erythrocytes, and platelets. As a result, pancytopenia (deficiency in all of the cellular elements of the blood) occurs.

Clinical Manifestations. The onset of aplastic anemia characteristically is a gradual one, marked by weakness, pallor, breathlessness on exertion, and other manifestations of anemia. Abnormal bleeding due to thrombocytopenia is a presenting symptom in about a third of the patients. When granulocytes are also involved, the patient is likely to present with fever, acute pharyngitis, or some other form of sepsis, and bleeding. Physical signs, except for pallor and skin hemorrhages, are unremarkable. The blood count reveals deficiencies in the various types of blood cells (pancytopenia). Red cells are normocytic and normochromic, that is, of normal size and color. Frequently, patients have no characteristic physical findings; adenopathy (enlargement of glands) and hepatosplenomegaly (liver and spleen enlargement) may be absent.

Management. As might be expected from a condition that affects all hematopoietic cells, aplastic anemia carries a very poor prognosis. Two methods of treatment are currently employed: (1) bone marrow transplantation and (2) administration of immunosuppressive therapy with antithymocyte globulin (ATG).

Bone marrow transplantation is performed to provide the patient with a supply of functioning hematopoietic tissue. Successful transplantation requires the ability to match donor and recipient cells and to prevent complications during recovery. With the use of the immunosuppressant cyclosporine, incidence of graft rejection is less than 10%.

Immunosuppressive therapy with ATG is prescribed to interrupt the immunologic functions that prolong the aplasia and thus allow the patient's bone marrow to recover. ATG is administered through a central venous catheter daily for 7 to 10 days. Patients who respond to the therapy usually do so within weeks to 3 months, but response may be as late as 6 months after treatment. Patients who have severe aplastic anemia and are treated early in the course of their disease have the best chance of responding to ATG.

Several studies have demonstrated that when ATG is combined with high-dose methylprednisolone, 3-year and 5-year survival rates range between 50% and 80%. Facon and colleagues (1991) reported that when androgens are added to ATG (with or without high-dose corticosteroids) 3-year survival rates are 77%. Not all researchers have met with such success in this treatment for severe aplastic anemia.

Supportive therapy plays a major role in the management of aplastic anemia. Any offending agent is discontinued. The patient is supported with transfusions of red cells and platelets as necessary to manage symptoms. Eventually, such patients may develop antibodies to minor red cell antigens and to platelet antigens, so that transfusions no longer raise the counts sufficiently. Death is usually caused by hemorrhage or infection, although antibiotics, especially those active against gram-negative bacilli, have been a major advance for these patients. Patients with pronounced leukopenia (abnormal decrease of white blood cells) are protected from contact with people who have infections. Antibiotics should not be used prophylactically in patients with abnormally low levels of neutrophils (neutropenia) because antibiotics can promote the emergence of resistant bacteria and fungi.

Preventive Management. Prevention of medication-induced aplastic anemia is extremely important. Because it is not possible to predict which patients will react adversely to a particular agent, potentially toxic medications should be used only when alternative therapies are not available. Blood cell counts must be carefully monitored in patients receiving potentially marrow-toxic medications, such as chloramphenicol. Persons taking toxic medications on a long-term basis should understand the need for periodic blood studies and know what symptoms to report.

Nursing Interventions. Patients with aplastic anemia are vulnerable to problems related to leukocyte, erythrocyte, and platelet deficiencies. They should be assessed carefully for signs of infection, tissue hypoxia, and bleeding. Any wound, abrasion, or ulcer of mucous membrane or skin is a potential site of infection and should be guarded against. Oral hygiene also is very important. Depending on the degree of weakness and fatigue, care should be planned to preserve the patient's energy. When platelet counts are low (thrombocytopenia), minor trauma, including subcutaneous and intramuscular (IM) injections, must be avoided. Regular bowel movements without straining or enemas are important, because hemorrhoids can develop and become infected or bleed.

Anemias in Renal Disease

The degree of anemia seen in patients with end-stage renal disease varies greatly, but in general, patients with a blood urea nitrogen (BUN) greater than 100 mg/dl are anemic. The symptoms of anemia are often the most disturbing of the patient's symptoms. The hematocrit usually falls to between 20% and 30%, although in rare cases it may fall below 15%. The red cells appear normal on peripheral smear.

This anemia is due to both a mild shortening of red cell survival and a deficiency of erythropoietin. Some erythropoietin is evidently produced outside the kidney, because some erythropoiesis does continue, even in patients whose kidneys have been removed.

- Patients undergoing long-term hemodialysis lose blood into the dialyzer (artificial kidney) and may thus become iron deficient. Folic acid deficiency develops because this vitamin passes into the dialysate.
- Dialysis patients should be treated with iron and folic acid.
- The availability of recombinant erythropoietin (Epoetin alfa) has dramatically altered the management of anemia in end-stage renal disease. With this therapy, in

combination with oral iron supplements, hematocrit levels can often be maintained at between 33% and 38%. This treatment has been successfully carried out with selected dialysis patients. Many patients report decreased fatigue, increased energy levels, increased feelings of well-being, improved exercise tolerance, and better tolerance of dialysis treatments. Hypertension is the most serious side effect and may require antihypertensive therapy. This therapy has decreased the need for transfusion and its risks.

Anemias in Chronic Diseases

Many chronic inflammatory diseases are associated with anemia of a normochromic, normocytic type (red cells are normal in color and size). These disorders include rheumatoid arthritis, lung abscesses, osteomyelitis, tuberculosis, and many malignancies.

The anemia is usually mild and nonprogressive. It develops gradually over a period of 6 to 8 weeks and then stabilizes at hematocrit levels that are seldom below 25%. The hemoglobin rarely falls below 9 g/dl, and the bone marrow has normal cellularity with increased stores of iron. Erythropoietin levels are low, perhaps because of decreased production, and there is a block in the utilization of iron by erythroid cells. A moderate shortening of red cell survival also occurs.

Most of these patients are asymptomatic and do not require treatment for the anemia. With successful treatment of the underlying disorder, the bone marrow iron is used to make red cells, and the hemoglobin rises.

HIV-positive patients who receive zidovudine (Retrovir) are at risk for anemia from bone marrow suppression. Epoetin alfa, a recombinant form of human erythropoietin, has been effective in treating this anemia when patients' endogenous erythropoietin levels are low. Adequate serum iron stores are necessary for this medication to be effective in raising hematocrit levels.

Iron-Deficiency Anemia

Iron-deficiency anemia is a condition in which the total body iron content is decreased below a normal level. (Iron is needed for the synthesis of hemoglobin.) It is the most common type of anemia in all age groups.

Etiology. The common cause of iron deficiency in men and postmenopausal women is bleeding (*e.g.*, from ulcers, gastritis, or gastrointestinal tumors) or malabsorption, especially after gastric resection. Iron cannot be adequately absorbed when a patient ingests a diet very high in fiber. The most common cause of iron deficiency anemia in premenopausal women is menorrhagia (excessive menstrual bleeding). Patients with chronic alcoholism often have inadequate iron intake and lose iron through blood loss from the GI tract, precipitating anemia.

Clinical and Laboratory Manifestations. Persons who are iron deficient have reduced counts of blood hemoglobin and red blood cells. The hemoglobin is reduced more than the red cell count, and for this reason the red cells tend to be small and relatively devoid of pigment, that is, they are hypochromic. *Hypochromia* is the hallmark of iron deficiency.

The cause of iron deficiency is the failure of the patient to ingest or absorb sufficient dietary iron to compensate for the iron requirements associated with body growth or for the loss of iron that attends bleeding, whether the bleeding is physiologic (*e.g.*, menstrual) or pathologic.

Patients with iron deficiency present primarily with the symptoms of anemia. If the deficiency is severe, they may also have a smooth, sore tongue and pica (a craving to eat unusual substances, such as clay, laundry starch, or ice). These symptoms subside after therapy.

The laboratory studies show a hemoglobin level that is proportionately lower than the hematocrit and red count, because of the small, poorly hemoglobinized red cells (microcytosis and hypochromia). The serum iron concentration is low, the total iron-binding capacity is high, and the serum ferritin (a measure of the iron stores) is low. The white count is usually normal, and the platelet count is variable.

Management. Except in the case of pregnancy, it is always important to search for a cause of iron deficiency. Anemia may be a sign of a curable gastrointestinal malignancy or of uterine fibroids or cancer. Stool specimens should be tested for occult blood.

Several oral iron preparations are available for treatment: ferrous sulfate, ferrous gluconate, and ferrous fumarate. The least expensive and most effective preparation is ferrous sulfate. Tablets with enteric coating may be poorly absorbed and should be avoided. Generally, the iron is continued for a year after the source of bleeding has been controlled. This allows for replenishing of the iron stores.

Nursing Interventions. *Preventive education* is important because iron-deficiency anemia is so common in menstruating and pregnant women. Food sources high in iron include organ meats (liver from cow, chicken, or calf), other meats, beans (black, pinto, and garbanzo), leafy vegetables, raisins, and molasses. Taking iron-rich foods with a source of vitamin C enhances absorption. Antacids should not be taken with iron because the phosphates may form complexes with iron.

The selection of a well-balanced diet is encouraged. Nutritional counseling is provided for those whose normal diet is less than adequate. Patients who have a history of eating fad diets are counseled that such diets often contain inadequate amounts of absorbable iron.

In some cases, IM or IV administration of iron dextran may be prescribed, that is, when oral iron is not absorbed or is poorly tolerated or when iron is needed in large amounts. The IV route is preferred. The IM injection causes some local pain and can stain the skin. Iron dextran should be injected deeply into each buttock using the Z-track technique. Prior to parenteral administration of a full dose, a small test dose should be administered to avoid the risk of anaphylaxis, which is greater with IM injections than with IV injections.

Patients with iron-deficiency anemia are encouraged to continue their iron therapy as long as it is prescribed, even though they may no longer be fatigued. If the iron supplement causes gastric distress, the patient is advised to take it with meals until the symptoms subside, and then to resume the between-meal schedule for maximum absorption.

The patient is informed that iron salts often change the stool to a dark green or black color. Liquid forms of iron stain teeth; thus, patients are instructed to take this medication through a straw, to rinse their mouth with water, and to practice good oral hygiene. Because ferrous sulfate is likely to be deposited on the teeth and gums, the patient is advised to use frequent oral hygiene measures.

Megaloblastic Anemias

The anemias caused by deficiencies of the vitamins B_{12} and folic acid show identical bone marrow and peripheral blood changes, because both vitamins are essential for normal DNA synthesis. In each case, hyperplasia (abnormal increase in the number of normal cells) of the marrow occurs, and the precursor erythroid and myeloid cells are large and bizarre; some are multinucleated. Many of these cells die within the marrow, however, so the mature cells which leave the marrow are decreased in number. Thus, a pancytopenia (deficiency of all cellular elements of the blood) develops. In an advanced situation, the hemoglobin may be as low as 4 to 5 g/dl, the white blood count 2000 to 3000 per mm^3, and the platelet count less than 50,000 per mm^3. The red cells are large and the PMNs are hypersegmented.

Vitamin B_{12} Deficiency

A deficiency of vitamin B_{12} can occur in several ways. Inadequate dietary intake is very rare but can develop in vegetarians who consume no meat. Faulty absorption from the gastrointestinal tract is more common.

An absence of intrinsic factor normally secreted by cells of the stomach is called *pernicious anemia*. This is primarily a disorder of elderly persons and has a familial tendency. The abnormality is in the gastric mucosa: the stomach wall becomes atrophic and fails to secrete intrinsic factor. This substance ordinarily binds with the dietary vitamin B_{12} and travels with it to the ileum, where the vitamin is absorbed. Without intrinsic factor, no orally administered B_{12} can be absorbed by the body. Even if adequate B_{12} and intrinsic factor are present, a deficiency can occur if disease involving the ileum or pancreas impairs absorption. Gastrectomy can also cause vitamin B_{12} deficiency.

Clinical Manifestations. After the body stores of vitamin B_{12} are depleted, patients begin to show signs of the anemia. They gradually become weak, listless, and pale. The hematologic effects of deficiency are accompanied by effects on other organ systems, particularly the gastrointestinal tract and nervous system. Patients with pernicious anemia develop a smooth, sore, red tongue and mild diarrhea. They may become confused, but more often have paresthesias in the extremities and difficulty maintaining their balance because of damage to the spinal cord; they also lose position sense. These symptoms are progressive, although the course may be marked by spontaneous partial remissions and exacerbations. Without treatment, patients die after several years, usually from congestive heart failure secondary to anemia.

Diagnostic Evaluation. One means of determining the cause of vitamin B_{12} deficiency is the *Schilling test.* After fasting for 12 hours, the patient is administered a small dose of radioactive B_{12} in water to drink, followed by a large, nonradioactive IM dose. When the oral vitamin is absorbed, it will be excreted in the urine; the IM dose helps to flush it into the urine. A 24-hour urine specimen is collected and measured for radioactivity. If very little has been excreted, the test is repeated several days later (the "second stage"), with a capsule of oral intrinsic factor added to the oral B_{12}. If the patient has pernicious anemia, this time much more radioactivity will be found in the 24-hour urine specimen. If the problem is due to an ileal or pancreatic defect, administration of digestive enzymes will increase absorption and subsequently increase urine radioactivity.

Management. Vitamin B_{12} deficiency is treated by B_{12} replacement. Vegetarians can prevent or treat deficiency with oral supplementation through vitamins or fortified soy milk. When, as is much more common, the deficiency is due to defective absorption or absence of intrinsic factor, replacement is by IM injections of vitamin B_{12}.

At first, B_{12} is administered daily, but eventually most patients are managed with 100 μg IM monthly. This can produce dramatic recovery in desperately ill patients. The reticulocyte count rises within a week, and in several weeks the blood counts are all normal. The tongue improves in several days. The neurologic manifestations require more time for recovery; if there is severe neuropathy, paralysis, or incontinence, the patient may never recover fully.

- To prevent recurrence of the anemia, vitamin B_{12} therapy must be continued for the life of the patient who has had pernicious anemia or noncorrectable malabsorption.

Nursing Interventions. These patients may need support during the diagnostic tests and nursing care for several aspects of their disease: anemia, congestive heart failure, and neuropathy. When they are incontinent or paralyzed, care must be taken to prevent pressure ulcers and contracture deformities. The Schilling test is useful only if the urine collections are complete; therefore, the nurse's assistance is essential. Patients must be taught about the chronicity of their disorder and the necessity for monthly injections even when they are asymptomatic. The gastric atrophy associated with pernicious anemia increases the risk of gastric carcinoma, so these patients need to understand that ongoing medical follow-up is important.

Folic Acid Deficiency

Folic acid is another vitamin that is necessary for normal red blood cell production. It is stored as different compounds, referred to as folates. The folate stores in the body are much smaller than those of vitamin B_{12}, so it is much more common to see dietary folate deficiency. This deficiency occurs in patients who rarely eat uncooked vegetables or fruits (*i.e.*, primarily elderly people living alone, the poor, or persons with alcoholism). Alcohol increases folic acid requirements, and at the same time persons suffering from alcoholism usually have a diet that is deficient in the vitamin. Folic acid requirements are also increased in persons with chronic hemolytic anemias and women who are pregnant.

- Patients on prolonged intravenous feeding or total parenteral nutrition may become folate deficient after several months, unless the vitamin is administered intramuscularly. Some patients with diseases of the small bowel may not absorb folic acid normally.

Clinical Manifestations. All of these patients have the characteristic findings of megaloblastic anemia along with a sore tongue. Symptoms of folic acid and vitamin B_{12} deficiencies are quite similar, and the two anemias may coexist. However, the neurologic manifestations of vitamin B_{12} deficiency do not occur with folic acid deficiency, and persist if B_{12} is not replaced. Therefore, careful distinction between the two anemias must be made. Serum levels of both vitamins can be measured.

Management. Treatment includes a nutritious diet and administration of 1 mg of folic acid a day. Folic acid is administered intramuscularly only in patients with malabsorption. With the exception of the vitamins administered during pregnancy, most proprietary vitamin preparations do not contain folic acid, so it must be administered as a separate tablet. When the hemoglobin returns to normal, the folic acid replacement can be stopped. However, persons who have alcoholism should continue receiving folic acid as long as they continue alcohol consumption.

Hemolytic Anemias

In hemolytic anemias, the erythrocytes have a shortened life span. The bone marrow is usually able to compensate partially by producing new red cells at three or more times the normal rate. Consequently, all of these anemias share certain laboratory features: (1) the reticulocyte count is elevated, (2) the fraction of indirect bilirubin is increased, and (3) the haptoglobin (a binding protein for free hemoglobin) is often low. The bone marrow is hypercellular with a proliferation of erythrocytes.

The only truly diagnostic test for hemolysis is the *red cell survival study*. This is usually necessary only for difficult diagnostic problems. About 20 to 30 ml of the patient's blood is removed, incubated with radioactive chromium-51, and then reinjected. The chromium-51 labels the red cells exclusively. After these cells have mixed with the circulating blood, small samples are taken at intervals over the next days and weeks, and the radioactivity is measured. A normal chromium-51 survival time is 28 to 35 days. Red cells of patients with severe hemolysis (such as sickle cell anemia) have survival times of 10 days or less.

Inherited Hemolytic Anemias

Hereditary Spherocytosis

Hereditary spherocytosis is a hemolytic anemia characterized by small, sphere-shaped red cells and splenomegaly (enlarged spleen). This is an uncommon disorder inherited in a dominant fashion. The disorder is usually diagnosed in childhood, but may be missed until adulthood because there are few symptoms. Surgical removal of the spleen is the treatment.

Sickle Cell Anemia

Sickle cell anemia is a severe hemolytic anemia resulting from a defective hemoglobin molecule and associated with attacks of pain. This disabling disease is found predominantly in those of African heritage; it affects 1 in 375 African-American infants. It also occurs in people of Mediterranean, Caribbean, and South and Central American heritage and those of Arab and East Indian ancestry.

Pathophysiology. The defect is a single amino acid substitution in the β chain of hemoglobin. Because normal hemoglobin A contains two α and two β chains, there are two genes for synthesis of each chain.

Sickle Cell Trait. Persons with *sickle cell trait* have inherited only one abnormal gene, so their red cells can synthesize both normal β chains and β^s chains; thus, they have A and S hemoglobin. They have no anemia and look and feel well. Between 8% and 12% of African-Americans have sickle cell trait.

If two people with sickle trait marry, some of their children may inherit two abnormal genes and will then have only β^s chains and only S hemoglobin; these children have sickle cell anemia.

Clinical Manifestations. The sickle hemoglobin has the unfortunate property of acquiring a crystal-like formation when exposed to low oxygen tension. The oxygen in venous blood is low enough to cause this change; consequently, the cell containing S hemoglobin becomes deformed, rigid, and sickle-shaped when in the venous circulation (Fig. 32-4). These long, rigid cells can become lodged in small vessels and, when they pile up against each other, blood flow to a region or an organ may be slowed. When ischemia or infarction results, the patient may experience pain, swelling, and fever. Such a chain of events is presumed to explain the painful crises of this disease, but what triggers the chain or how to prevent it is not understood.

Symptoms are secondary to *hemolysis* and *thrombosis*. The sickled red blood cells have a short life span of 15 to 25 days; normal is 120 days. Patients are always anemic, with hemoglobin values in the 7 to 10 g/dl range. Jaundice is characteristic and is usually obvious in the sclerae. The bone marrow expands in childhood in a compensatory effort, sometimes leading to enlargement of the bones of the face and skull. The chronic anemia is associated with tachycardia, cardiac murmurs, and often an enlarged heart (car-

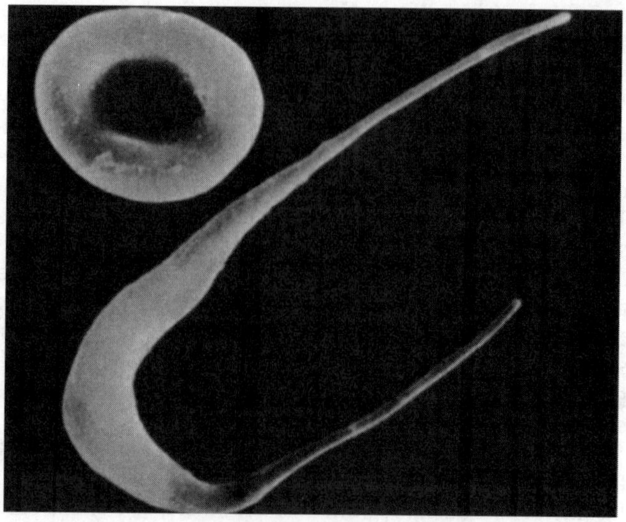

FIGURE 32-4. Photograph of a sickled cell and a normal red blood cell taken under the auspices of the Comprehensive Sickle Cell Center, University of Miami. (Photo by Dr. Bruce R. Cameron.)

diomegaly). Dysrhythmias and heart failure may occur in adults.

All the tissues and organs are constantly vulnerable to microcirculatory interruptions by the sickling process, and therefore are susceptible to hypoxic damage or true ischemic necrosis. There is marked viscosity of the blood.

Diagnostic Evaluation. The diagnosis can be made by hemoglobin electrophoresis or by isoelectric focusing and high performance liquid chromatography techniques. A definitive diagnosis for infants cannot be made until further laboratory tests are conducted on a second sample of the infant's blood and correlated with the clinical history. Only electrophoresis can distinguish between sickle cell trait or sickle cell anemia. The patient with sickle cell trait has normal hemoglobin and hematocrit levels as well as a normal blood smear. In contrast, the patient with sickle cell anemia has a low hematocrit and sickled cells on smear.

The AHCPR Sickle Cell Disease Clinical Practice Guidelines (1993) recommend screening all newborns, because some affected infants will be missed if only specific groups are targeted.

Prognosis of Sickle Cell Anemia. Patients with sickle cell anemia are usually diagnosed in childhood, because they are anemic in infancy and begin to have sickle cell crises at 1 or 2 years of age. Many die in the first years of life, but antibiotics and increased knowledge about this disease coupled with patient education have probably improved the outlook in the last 20 to 25 years. Although the average life expectancy is 40 years, some patients live into the sixth decade. All siblings of a patient with sickle cell anemia should be tested for the disease.

Management. Treatment for this hemoglobin abnormality is still evolving. Many trials of medications that have antisickling properties are being conducted. Although sample sizes are small, some promising results have been shown with hydroxyurea. This medication increases fetal hemoglobin (Hb F) production in patients with sickle cell disease. The percent of irreversible sickled cells is decreased and the number of pain crises is lessened. The medication also reduces hemolysis and prolongs red cell survival. This medication is still considered experimental and has risks such as carcinogenesis and teratogenesis that are poorly understood.

Cetiedil citrate, a red blood cell membrane modifier, has also shown effective antisickling effects. Pentoxifylline, a medication that reduces blood viscosity and peripheral vascular resistance, shows some promise for decreasing the length of sickle cell crisis. Vanillin, a food additive, has antisickling properties and is being evaluated as adjunctive therapy for sickle cell anemia.

Counseling about childbearing should be offered to all persons of childbearing age who have sickle cell anemia or sickle cell trait. Education may be more effective if carried out by members of the community who are from the same ethnic group as the high risk populations. Crises cannot always be prevented. However, when infants with sickle cell disease are immunized against *Haemophilus influenza* at the age of 2 months and prescribed prophylactic treatment with penicillin, the morbidity and mortality rates are decreased.

Because infection seems to predispose to crises, all infections should be promptly treated or prevented when possible. Because dehydration and hypoxia promote sickling, patients are instructed to avoid high altitudes, anesthesia, or fluid loss. Because of a renal defect, these patients easily become dehydrated. Folic acid therapy is administered daily, because the marrow has an increased requirement.

Sickle Cell Crisis. When sickle cell crisis occurs, the mainstays of therapy are hydration and analgesia. Increased fluid intake helps to dilute the blood and reverse the agglutination of sickled cells within the small blood vessels. Patients and families can learn to handle minor crises at home, but if there is no relief after several hours, hospital admission may be necessary.

The patients with sickle cell crisis often have fever and leukocytosis, so infection, appendicitis, or cholecystitis must be ruled out. Intravenous fluids (3 to 5 L/day for adults) are essential. Small gauge catheters lessen trauma to veins; after many crises, the veins become sclerosed. Opioid analgesics are often necessary because of the severity of pain and should be prescribed in adequate doses. Patient-controlled analgesia (PCA) with morphine sulfate may be the best choice. However, narcotics should never be used for long-term pain relief because of the risk of dependency. Non-steroidal anti-inflammatory agents can relieve mild pain. Referral to a pain clinic is appropriate for the patient with chronic pain.

Transfusions are reserved for particular situations: (1) aplastic crisis, when the patient's hemoglobin falls rapidly; (2) severe painful crisis not responsive to any other therapy after several days; (3) as a preoperative measure to dilute the amount of sickled blood; and (4) sometimes during the latter half of pregnancy in an attempt to prevent crises.

Complications. Complications of sickle cell anemia include infection, hypoxia and ischemia, thrombic episodes, stroke, renal failure, and priapism (abnormal, painful, continued erection of the penis).

Patients with sickle cell anemia are unusually susceptible to infection, particularly pneumonias and osteomyelitis. They may develop aplastic crises with infections and may have gallstones (due to increased hemolysis that leads to bilirubin stones) and leg ulcers. The ulcers may be chronic and painful and require skin grafting. Infection has been one of the most common causes of death.

Thrombotic episodes may result in pulmonary infarction or in the sudden appearance of a stroke with paralysis on one side. These episodes are completely unpredictable; they can occur monthly or very rarely and may last for hours, days, or weeks. Events that seem to precipitate crises include dehydration, fatigue, intake of alcohol, emotional stress, and acidosis. Certain effects of infarction are permanent, such as hemiplegia, aseptic necrosis of the head of the femur, and renal concentrating defects. Renal failure is a major cause of death in adults with this disease.

❑ NURSING PROCESS
The Patient With Sickle Cell Anemia

Assessment

Because the sickling process can interrupt circulation in any tissues and organs, with resultant hypoxia and ischemia, a careful assessment of all body systems is necessary. Particular emphasis is placed on assessing for pain, swelling, and fever. All joint areas are carefully examined for pain and swelling, as is the abdomen. A careful neurologic examination is important to elicit symptoms of cerebral hypoxia. The patient is also questioned about symptoms indicative of gallstones, such as food intolerances, epigastric distress, and pain in the right upper abdominal quadrant.

Because patients with sickle cell anemia are so susceptible to infections, they are assessed for the presence of any infectious process. Particular attention is given to examination of the chest and long bones and femoral head, as pneumonia and osteomyelitis are especially common. Leg ulcers, which may be infected and are slow to heal, are sometimes present. Chronic anemia, another common problem associated with sickle cell anemia, is also considered during the physical examination.

Patients in crisis are questioned about factors that could have precipitated the crisis. They are asked to recall whether they have recently had symptoms of infection or dehydration or have been experiencing situations that promote fatigue or emotional stress. History of alcohol intake is also assessed. In addition, patients are asked to recall factors that seemed to precipitate previous crises and measures that they use to prevent crises. This information will provide guidelines for identifying and meeting their learning needs.

Diagnosis

Nursing Diagnoses

Based on the assessment data, major nursing diagnoses for the patient may include the following:

- Pain related to agglutination of sickled cells within blood vessels
- Knowledge deficit regarding prevention of crisis
- Self-esteem disturbance related to altered body image
- Powerlessness related to illness-induced helplessness

Collaborative Problems/ Potential Complications

Based on the assessment data, potential complications may include:

- Sickle cell crisis
- Infection
- Hypoxia and ischemia
- Priapism

Planning and Implementation

Goals. The major goals are relief of pain, avoidance of situations that can precipitate crisis, enhanced feelings of self-esteem and power, and absence of complications.

Nursing Interventions

A care plan detailing the interventions for the patient with sickle cell disease is presented in Nursing Care Plan 32-1.

Monitoring and Managing Potential Complications. During sickle cell crisis, the patient is allowed to rest undisturbed as much as possible. Swollen extremities should not be exercised and pain should be relieved. The patient's subjective description of pain, using a rating scale, must guide the use of analgesics. Relaxation techniques, breathing exercises, transcutaneous nerve stimulation, and whirlpool baths are helpful for some patients.

The nurse can help the patient and family adjust to this chronic disease and understand the importance of hydration and prevention of infection. Compliance with prophylactic penicillin for infants requires constant reinforcement by the nurse. Patients and parents are taught to seek prompt medical care for signs of infection and other complications. When leg ulcers are present, they require careful dressing and protection from trauma and wound contamination. If they fail to heal, skin grafting may be necessary. Scrupulous aseptic technique is warranted to prevent nosocomial infections.

Male patients may develop sudden, painful episodes of priapism (persistent penile erection). The patient is taught to empty his bladder at the onset of the attack, exercise, and take a warm bath. If an episode persists more than 3 hours, medical attention is recommended. Repeated episodes may lead to extensive vascular thrombosis resulting in impotence.

Promoting Coping Skills. This illness, with its acute exacerbations that often result in chronic health problems, frequently leaves the patient feeling powerless and with a sense of decreased self-esteem. The patient's ability to use normal coping resources of physical strength, psychologic stamina, and positive self-esteem is dramatically diminished. Nursing care that focuses on the patient's strengths rather than deficits can enhance effective coping skills. Providing the patient with opportunities to make decisions about daily care increases feelings of control.

Other Hemoglobinopathies

C Hemoglobin. C hemoglobin is less common among African-Americans than S hemoglobin. Patients with the C trait are asymptomatic, and homozygous C disease is a mild hemolytic anemia with splenomegaly (enlarged spleen) but no serious complications.

Thalassemia. Thalassemia is a group of hereditary disorders associated with defective hemoglobin-chain synthesis. These anemias occur worldwide, but the highest prevalence is found in persons of Mediterranean, African, and Southeast Asian ancestry. The incidence is increasing in the United States with immigration of persons from Southeast Asia. Thalassemias are characterized by abnormal decrease in hemoglobin content of erythrocytes (hypochromia), smaller than normal erythrocytes (microcytosis), destruction of blood elements (hemolysis), and variable degrees of anemia.

The thalassemias are classified into two major groups according to the affected globin chain of hemoglobin: α-thalassemias and β-thalassemias, which are associated with decreased or absent α-chain synthesis and β-chain synthesis, respectively. The α-thalassemias occur mainly in people from Southeast Asia and Africa, and the β-thalassemias are most prevalent in Mediterranean populations. The α-thalassemias are milder than the β-forms and are often without symptoms. Patients with severe β-thalassemia will die within the first few years of life if untreated; if treated with regular transfusion therapy, they may survive into their 20s and 30s. Patient education during reproductive years

(text continues on page 791)

NURSING CARE PLAN 32–1
Care of the Patient With Sickle Cell Disease

NURSING DIAGNOSIS: Pain related to agglutination of sickled cells within small blood vessels

GOAL: Relief of pain

Nursing Interventions	Rationale	Expected Outcomes
1. Assess severity and location of pain. Common sites of pain are joints and extremities, chest, abdomen.	1. Tissues and organs are susceptible to microcirculatory thrombosis with resulting hypoxic damage; hypoxia causes pain.	• Verbalizes that pain is relieved after administration of analgesics • Moves body parts slowly and carefully to minimize pain • Increases fluid intake • Gradually experiences longer pain-free periods • Expresses interest in diversional activities
2. Administer analgesics as prescribed. Consider use of patient-controlled analgesia (PCA).	2. Opioid analgesics are necessary to relieve severe pain; avoid use of opioids for chronic pain because of the possibility of dependency. PCA provides patient with more control over pain relief.	
3. Encourage oral intake of fluids and administer IV fluids as prescribed; monitor intake and output.	3. Fluids promote hemodilution and reverse agglutination of sickled cells within small blood vessels.	
4. Carefully position and support painful areas; encourage use of relaxation techniques and breathing exercises; apply moist heat to painful areas; discourage crossing legs when sitting.	4. Joint pain can be minimized during a crisis by careful movement and with the use of moist heat; relaxation techniques and breathing exercises may serve as a distraction. Vessel occlusion by sickle cells decreases circulation.	

NURSING DIAGNOSIS: Knowledge deficit regarding prevention of sickle cell crisis

GOAL: Avoidance of situations that can precipitate sickle cell crisis

Nursing Interventions	Rationale	Expected Outcomes
1. Discuss factors that commonly precipitate crisis: a. Infection b. Dehydration c. Trauma d. Strenuous physical exertion e. Pregnancy f. Exposure to cold g. Hypoxia (*e.g.,* high altitudes) h. Emotional stress	1. Avoidance of situations that precipitate crisis can often increase the intervals between crisis attacks.	• Patient identifies factors that can precipitate crisis • Identifies acceptable life-style changes necessary to prevent crisis • Elicits support of family in making changes in life style • Maintains adequate fluid intake • Avoids alcohol and caffeine • Identifies sources of infection that can be avoided • Identifies the need to seek prompt medical attention when infection occurs • Seeks prenatal counseling if appropriate
2. Discuss the chronic nature of the disease with patient and family; stress the importance of adequate hydration and avoidance of infection.	2. Understanding of the chronicity of the disorder and the ability to minimize crises promotes adherence to the therapeutic regimen.	

NURSING DIAGNOSIS: Self-esteem disturbance related to altered body image

GOAL: Verbalization of increased feelings of worth

Nursing Interventions	Rationale	Expected Outcomes
1. Spend time with patient to convey acceptance.	1. The feeling of acceptance by others increases self-esteem.	• Identifies strengths • Identifies characteristics liked about self • Develops goals that increase sense of control and are age appropriate • Verbalizes positive self-perception • Demonstrates effective problem-solving skills
2. Assist in identifying strengths.	2. Low self-esteem impedes recognition of strengths.	
3. Encourage problem-solving in areas patient has identified he or she would like to change.	3. Problem solving is hampered by low self-esteem.	

(*continued*)

NURSING CARE PLAN 32–1 *(continued)*
Care of the Patient With Sickle Cell Disease

Nursing Interventions	Rationale	Expected Outcomes
4. Provide recognition for accomplishments.	4. Self-esteem is increased by positive reinforcement.	• Contacts member of support group prior to discharge from hospital
5. Avoid assuming the role of caregiver in situations patients can perform independently.	5. Increased independence enhances self-esteem.	
6. Assess for signs of depression a. Changes in sleep patterns b. Decreased appetite, weight loss c. Sad mood d. Lack of interest in normal activities	6. Patients with sickle cell disease have an increased incidence of clinical depression.	
7. Assess for developmental delays, especially in adolescents.	7. Increased dependence on parents and health care providers can delay successful completion of developmental tasks.	
8. Encourage participation in support group for patients with sickle cell disease.	8. Acceptance and a feeling of adequacy can evolve when patients feel safe in a support group, thus increasing self-esteem.	

NURSING DIAGNOSIS: Powerlessness related to illness-induced helplessness

GOAL: Effective problem solving to increase control of chronic illness

Nursing Interventions	Rationale	Expected Outcomes
1. Assess knowledge of disease and provide information to add to knowledge base.	1. Knowledge is empowering.	• Verbalizes accurate knowledge of disease • Develops goals that increase sense of control • Appropriate choices are made independently • Practices assertive communication techniques • Participates in decision making about own care • Demonstrates effective problem-solving skills • Verbalizes feelings about aspects of disease that cannot be changed
2. Include patient in setting realistic goals of care. a. Give patient the responsibility for establishing own schedule for ADLs. b. Provide patient with choices. c. Encourage participation in activities that patient can successfully achieve.	2. Active participation in health care contributes to positive adaptation to chronic illness; feelings of control increase when patients have more choices; success increases self-esteem.	
3. Provide positive feedback for achievements.	3. Increases self-esteem and encourages attempts at other activities.	
4. Teach assertiveness skills to improve effectiveness of communication with others.	4. Improved ability to communicate needs increases sense of control.	
5. Involve in opportunities to increase the awareness of health care providers about the disease (e.g., at health fairs, speaking to medical and nursing students).	5. Active participation in health care contributes to positive adaptation to chronic illness.	
6. Encourage verbalization of feelings about potential drug dependence to control painful crises.	6. Painful crises require treatment with opioid analgesics, but long-term use increases risk of dependence. Use of opioid analgesics often becomes a source of conflict between health care providers and patients.	
7. Encourage verbalization of concerns of death.	7. SCD has life-threatening complications that most patients are aware of; verbalizing these concerns can decrease anxiety.	

(continued)

NURSING CARE PLAN 32-1 *(continued)*
Care of the Patient With Sickle Cell Disease

Nursing Interventions	Rationale	Expected Outcomes
COLLABORATIVE PROBLEMS: Infection, hypoxia and ischemia, renal failure, priapism		
GOAL: Prevention of infection		
1. Assess for signs and symptoms of infection. Common sites of infection are lungs long bones; head of the femur, leg ulcers.	1. The physiologic stress that results from infection often precipitates crises; resolution of infection at its onset can prevent or limit the duration of a crisis episode.	• Temperature normal • Breath sounds clear • WBCs within normal range (5,000–10,000/mm^3) • Absence of pain of long bones • Cultures of wound drainage negative • Immunizations are received as appropriate
2. Encourage early ambulation and pulmonary hygiene.	2. Activity mobilizes pulmonary secretions; stagnant secretions are a prime medium for bacterial growth.	
3. Use aseptic technique when changing wound dressings.	3. Aseptic technique deters introduction of microorganisms into wound areas.	
4. Promote adequate nutrition and fluid intake.	4. Optimal nutrition and fluid balance promote tissue integrity.	
5 Inquire about date of most recent immunization against *Haemophilus influenza*.	5. Immunizations increase protection against infection.	
GOAL: Absence of hypoxia and ischemia		
1. Assess respiratory status.	1. Infection and infarction can result in acute chest syndrome.	• Lungs clear to auscultation, no chest pain or dyspnea; no evidence of acute chest syndrome • No evidence of deteriorating neurologic signs • No evidence of acute splenic sequestration crisis • Joints are free of pain • Skin integrity is maintained • Patient adheres to bedrest • Fluid intake is adequate • No complications occur from blood transfusions • Environmental temperature is comfortable for patient • Avoids cold and caffeinated beverages
2. Administer oxygen, if prescribed.	2. Oxygen decreases sickling. When blood oxygen levels increase, most sickle cells resume normal shape.	
3. Assess neurologic status to elicit symptoms of cerebral hypoxia.	3. Sickling causes inflammatory changes in the walls of vessels and vascular occlusions, which can cause cerebrovascular accident.	
4. Assess abdomen for distention and pain.	4. Acute splenic sequestration crisis occurs when sickle cells block the flow of blood from the spleen. This causes severe pain and is accompanied by tachycardia and tachypnea.	
5. Assess all joints for swelling and pain.	5. Sickling causes inflammatory changes in the walls of vessels and vascular occlusions, which can cause cerebrovascular accident.	
6. Assess lower extremities for stasis ulcers.	6. Poor venous return increases risk of ulcers.	
7. Promote bedrest during crisis.	7. Decreases oxygen demand.	
8. Encourage oral intake of fluids and administer IV fluids as prescribed; monitor intake and output.	8. Adequate fluid intake helps dilute the blood and reverse agglutination of sickled cells within small blood vessels.	
9. Administer packed red blood cells, if prescribed. Monitor: a. Signs of fluid overload b. Hematocrit c. Signs of transfusion reaction	9. Packed red blood cells increase oxygen with minimal effect on fluid volume. Increased hemoglobin concentration may become greater than desired when cells that were trapped in the spleen are released. Hematocrit should not exceed 45%.	

(continued)

NURSING CARE PLAN 32–1 *(continued)*
Care of the Patient With Sickle Cell Disease

Nursing Interventions	Rationale	Expected Outcomes
10. Keep room warm. 11. Encourage intake of warm, caffeine-free beverages.	10. Prevents peripheral vasoconstriction. 11. Cold and caffeine constrict blood vessels.	
GOAL: Absence of renal failure		
1. Assess renal function: a. Monitor BUN, serum creatinine b. Assess for flank pain c. Assess color of urine	1. Glomerular filtration is decreased due to renal ischemia. These tests measure the retention of metabolic wastes, an indicator of renal function. Hemolysis causes pain in the kidneys. Hematuria occurs with acute papillary necrosis. Dark yellow urine occurs as increased RBC destruction causes bilirubin levels to increase.	• Intake and output are balanced • Electrolytes are within safe limits • Weight is within acceptable range • Renal function test results return to normal range
2. Manage fluid balance; monitor intake and output.	2. When the kidneys are in failure, fluid intake is based on the patient's weight, blood pressure, and fluid losses. Dialysis may be initiated to prevent complications from uremia.	
3. Assess for presence of edema.	3. Assessment provides baseline and continuing data for monitoring changes in fluid and electrolyte balance.	
4. Weigh daily.	4. Most accurate method to assess hydration.	
5. Monitor serum electrolytes, especially potassium.	5. Hyperkalemia (K> 6.0 mEq/L) is life threatening due to dysrhythmia and possible cardiac arrest.	
6. Limit dietary proteins to 1 g/kg during oliguric phase.	6. Protein breakdown is minimized and the buildup of toxic end products is prevented.	
7. Provide high-carbohydrate diet.	7. Spares protein and meets caloric requirements.	
GOAL: Absence of priapism		
1. Teach patient to report persistent penile erections. 2. Notify physician of persistent penile erection.	1. Sickle cells can obstruct the blood vessels in the penis causing extreme pain. 2. Impotence can occur from repeated episodes of vascular thrombosis. A surgically created shunt may be necessary to relieve the obstruction.	• Penis resumes flaccid state • Impotence is avoided • Verbalizes that pain is relieved after administration of analgesics • Returns to prepriapism pattern of urinary elimination
3. Administer analgesics as prescribed.	3. Opioid analgesics are necessary to relieve pain of engorgement, which can last up to 24 hours.	
4. Teach patient to empty bladder at onset of priapism.	4. Engorgement of corpora cavernosa can cause temporary inability to initiate voiding.	
5. Administer oxygen, if prescribed.	5. Oxygen decreases sickling. When blood oxygen levels increase, most sickle cells resume normal shape.	

(continued)

NURSING CARE PLAN 32–1 *(continued)*
Care of the Patient With Sickle Cell Disease

Nursing Interventions	Rationale	Expected Outcomes
6. Provide emotional support and privacy.	6. Initially, this is an embarrassing experience for the patient; then pain and fear become the dominant emotions.	
7. Suggest a warm bath.	7. Warm water is relaxing and causes vasodilation, which can decrease pain.	

should include preconception counseling about the risk of congenital thalassemia major.

Thalassemia Minor. The majority of patients with thalassemia minor are asymptomatic but are carriers of thalassemia major. Pregnancy causes significant anemia that requires transfusion therapy.

Thalassemia Major. Thalassemia major (Cooley's anemia) is characterized by severe anemia, marked hemolysis, and ineffective production of erythrocytes (erythropoiesis). With early regular transfusion therapy, growth and development through childhood is facilitated. Organ dysfunction due to iron overload occurs. Regular chelation therapy with subcutaneous desferrioxamine has reduced the complications of iron overload and prolonged the life of these patients. The overall survival of patients receiving iron chelation continuously from the first few years of life is unknown, however.

Glucose-6-Phosphate Dehydrogenase Deficiency

The abnormality in this disorder is in G-6-PD, an enzyme within the red cell that is essential for membrane stability. A few patients have inherited an enzyme so defective that they have a chronic hemolytic anemia, but the most common type of defect results in hemolysis only when the red cells are stressed by certain situations, such as fever or the presence of certain medications. The disorder came to the attention of researchers during World War II, when some soldiers developed hemolysis while taking primaquine, an antimalarial agent.

Medications that have hemolytic effects for people with G-6-PD deficiency are antimalarial agents, sulfonamides, nitrofurantoin, the common coal tar analgesics (including aspirin), the thiazide diuretics, the oral hypoglycemic agents, chloramphenicol, para-aminosalicylic acid (PAS), and vitamin K.

African-Americans and persons of Greek or Italian origin are those primarily affected by this disorder. The type of deficiency found in the Mediterranean population is more severe than that in the African-American population, resulting in greater hemolysis and sometimes in life-threatening anemias.

All types of G-6-PD deficiency are inherited as X-linked defects; thus, many more men are at risk than women. In the United States, about 15% of African-American males are affected.

Clinical Manifestations. The patients are asymptomatic and have normal hemoglobin levels and reticulocyte counts most of the time. Several days after exposure to an offending medication, they may develop pallor, jaundice, and hemoglobinuria (hemoglobin in the urine), and the reticulocyte count will rise. Special strains of the peripheral blood may then show Heinz bodies (degraded hemoglobin). Hemolysis continues for a week and then spontaneously the counts begin to improve because the new young red cells are resistant to lysis. In the Mediterranean type, this recovery does not occur.

Diagnostic Evaluation and Management. The diagnosis is made by a screening test or a quantitative assay of G-6-PD. The treatment is to stop the medication. Transfusion is necessary only in the Mediterranean variety. The patient should be educated about the disease and given a list of medications to avoid. These include sulfonamides, hypoglycemic agents, antimalarials, nitrofurantoin, phenacetin, aspirin (in high doses), and para-aminosalicylic acid.

Acquired Hemolytic Anemias

There are a variety of acquired hemolytic anemias, including paroxysmal nocturnal hemoglobinuria, immune hemolytic anemia, microangiopathic hemolytic anemia, heart valve hemolysis, and spur cell anemia, as well as those associated with infections and hypersplenism. Table 32-2 identifies the causes, manifestations, and treatment of these anemias.

Immune Hemolytic Anemia

When antibodies combine with red cells they can be either isoantibodies, reacting with foreign cells (as in transfusion reactions or erythroblastosis fetalis), or autoantibodies, which react with the person's own cells. The immune hemolysis that results may be very severe. Antibodies coat the red cells, producing a positive Coombs' test. These cells are then removed by the spleen and the rest of the reticuloendothelial system. Many cells are destroyed, and others return to the circulation as spherocytes with reduced membrane and a shortened survival rate.

In idiopathic autoimmune hemolytic states, the reason the immune system is induced to produce the antibodies is not known. The disease usually begins suddenly, often in persons over 40 years of age. In some cases, the hemolysis

TABLE 32-2 Acquired Hemolytic Anemias

Name	Cause	Manifestations and Treatment
Paroxysmal nocturnal hemoglobinuria	Unknown—sometimes occurs with aplastic anemia	Dark urine (hemoglobinuria), especially in morning Sometimes pancytopenia Multiple venous thrombosis No treatment known
Immune hemolytic anemia	Antibodies produced, sometimes secondary to medications (methyldopa [Aldomet], penicillin)	Jaundice, spherocytes Responds to corticosteroids
Microangiopathic hemolytic anemia	RBC damaged during flow through abnormal small blood vessels, as in malignant hypertension	Fragmented RBC seen on smears Treat primary disease
Cardiac valve hemolysis	RBC damaged by regurgitant flow through incompetent valve prosthesis	Fragmented RBC Treatment: replace valve
Spur cell anemia	Severe liver disease, hypertension Increased lipid in RBC membrane	Spur-shaped RBC No treatment
Infections	Malaria, *Clostridium welchii,* especially after septic abortion	Hemoglobinuria possible Treat the infection
Hypersplenism	Large spleen from any cause: cirrhosis, lymphomas	Sometimes pancytopenia Treatment: splenectomy

is associated with systemic disease (especially systemic lupus erythematosus, chronic lymphatic leukemia, or lymphoma). Other people, with identical clinical features, can be shown to be producing antibodies to a medication (especially penicillin, cephalosporins, or quinidine). The antibodies or the medication–antibody complexes then attach to red cells, resulting in destruction of the cells (hemolysis). Patients taking large doses of methyldopa may develop antibodies to their own red cells; only a few of these patients have a significant hemolytic anemia.

Clinical Manifestations. Clinical manifestations can vary. A positive Coombs' test may be the only manifestation in mild cases. More often, signs of anemia are present. These include fatigue, dyspnea, palpitations, and jaundice. Occasionally, the anemia is so severe that the patient has an overwhelming hemolysis and is in shock.

Management. Any possibly offending medication should be discontinued. The treatment consists of high doses of corticosteroids until hemolysis decreases. When the hemoglobin has returned toward normal, usually after several weeks, the steroid dose can be lowered or, in some cases, tapered and discontinued. In severe cases, blood transfusions may be required. Because the antibody may react with all possible donor cells, careful blood typing is necessary and the transfusion should be administered slowly and cautiously.

Splenectomy (removal of the spleen) removes a major site of red cell destruction; therefore, it may be performed if corticosteroids do not produce a remission. If neither corticosteroid therapy nor splenectomy is successful, immunosuppressive agents may be administered.

Polycythemia

Polycythemia refers to an increased concentration of red cells. It is a term used when the red cell count is greater than 6 million/mm^3 or the hemoglobin exceeds 18 g/dl.

Polycythemia Vera

Polycythemia vera, or *primary polycythemia,* is a proliferative disorder in which all the marrow cells seem to have escaped from the normal control mechanisms. The bone marrow has a large number of cells, and the red cell, white cell, and platelet counts in the peripheral blood are often elevated. Patients typically have a ruddy complexion and hepatosplenomegaly (enlarged liver and spleen). The symptoms are due to the increased blood volume (headache, dizziness, fatigue, and blurred vision) or to increased blood viscosity (angina, claudication, thrombophlebitis). Bleeding is also a complication, possibly because of the engorged capillaries. Another common and unexplained problem is pruritus.

Management

The objective of management is to reduce the high blood viscosity. Phlebotomy (removing blood from a vein) is an important part of therapy and can be performed repeatedly to keep the hemoglobin within normal range. Radioactive phosphorus or chemotherapeutic agents can be used to suppress marrow function but may increase the risk of leukemia. When the patient has an elevated uric acid level, allopurinol is used to prevent gouty attacks. Antihistamines may be administered to control itching.

Secondary Polycythemia

Secondary polycythemia is caused by excessive production of erythropoietin. This may occur in response to a reduced amount of oxygen, which acts as a hypoxic stimulus, as in chronic obstructive pulmonary disease or cyanotic heart disease, or in certain hemoglobinopathies in which the hemoglobin has an abnormally high affinity for oxygen (*e.g.*, hemoglobin Chesapeake).

Management of secondary polycythemia involves treating the primary problem. If the cause cannot be corrected, phlebotomy (withdrawal of blood) may be necessary to reduce the blood volume and the viscosity of the blood.

Leukopenia and Agranulocytosis

Leukopenia is a condition in which the white cells are fewer in number than normal. **Agranulocytosis** is a potentially fatal condition in which there is almost complete absence of polymorphonuclear leukocytes (PMNs). A leukocyte count of fewer than $5000/mm^3$ or a granulocyte count of fewer than $2000/mm^3$ is abnormal and may be a signal of a generalized bone marrow disorder, such as megaloblastic anemia, aplasia, metastatic tumor, myelofibrosis, or acute leukemia. Viral infections and overwhelming bacterial sepsis also can cause leukopenia. Most commonly, the cause is medication toxicity; phenothiazines are implicated frequently, as is Clozapine, an atypical neuroleptic. Antithyroid agents, sulfonamides, phenylbutazone, and chloramphenicol are also contributing agents.

The patient has no symptoms unless infection develops, which usually occurs when the granulocytes are fewer than $1000/mm^3$. Fever and severe sore throat with ulcerations are common complaints. Bacteremia may develop.

Any possibly offending medications are withdrawn. If the granulocyte count is very low, the patient is protected from any obvious sources of infection. Cultures of all orifices (*e.g.*, nose, mouth) and the blood are essential, and when fever occurs it is treated with broad-spectrum antibiotics until the specific organism is known. Good oral hygiene is important.

Hot saline irrigations of the throat are used to keep the throat clear of necrotic exudate. Comfort is provided by supplying an ice collar and analgesic, antipyretic, and sedative medications that may be indicated. The goal of treatment, apart from eradicating the infection, is to eliminate, if possible, the cause of the bone marrow depression. Bone marrow function returns spontaneously (except in the case of neoplastic diseases) within 2 or 3 weeks, if death from infection can be prevented.

Hematopoietic Malignancies

Blood-forming tissues are characterized by rapid continuous turnover of cells. Normally, production of specialized blood cells from their stem cell precursors is carefully regulated according to the body's needs. If the mechanisms that control the production of these cells are disrupted, the cells will proliferate to a dangerous degree (neoplastic proliferation). A wide variety of hematopoietic malignancies can develop and they are often classified according to the cells involved. Leukemia, literally "white blood," is a neoplastic proliferation of one particular cell (granulocytes, monocytes, lymphocytes, or megakaryocytes). The defect is believed to originate in the hematopoietic stem cell. The lymphomas are neoplasms of lymphoid tissue. Hodgkin's disease accounts for 40% of all lymphomas and is believed to result from defective T lymphocytes. Many other lymphomas are derived from B lymphocytes. Both Waldenström's macroglobulinemia and multiple myeloma are neoplasms affecting plasma cells produced by B lymphocytes.

Leukemia

The common feature of the leukemias is an unregulated proliferation or accumulation of white cells in the bone marrow, replacing normal marrow elements. There is also proliferation in the liver, spleen, and lymph nodes, and invasion of nonhematologic organs, such as the meninges, gastrointestinal tract, kidney, and skin.

The leukemias are often classified according to the cell line involved, as either lymphocytic or myelocytic, and according to the maturity of the malignant cells, as either acute (immature cells) or chronic (differentiated cells). The cause is unknown, but there is some evidence that genetic influence and viral pathogenesis may be involved. Bone marrow damage due to radiation exposure or chemicals (benzene) can cause leukemia.

Acute Myelogenous Leukemia

Acute myelogenous leukemia (AML) affects the hematopoietic stem cell that differentiates into all myeloid cells: monocytes, granulocytes (basophils, neutrophils, eosinophils), erythrocytes, and platelets. All age groups are affected; incidence rises with age. It is the most common nonlymphocytic leukemia.

Clinical Manifestations. Most of the signs and symptoms evolve from insufficient production of normal blood cells. Vulnerability to infection results from granulocytopenia, a deficiency of granulocytes; weakness and fatigue occur due to anemia; and bleeding tendencies arise as a result of thrombocytopenia, a deficiency in the number of platelets. The proliferation of leukemic cells within organs leads to a variety of additional symptoms: pain from an enlarged liver or spleen; lymph gland problems; headache or vomiting secondary to meningeal leukemia (most common in lymphocytic leukemia); and bone pain from expansion of marrow.

The disorder develops without warning, with symptoms occurring over a period of 1 to 6 months. Blood counts will show a decrease in both erythrocytes and platelets. Although the total leukocyte count can be low, normal, or high, the percentage of normal cells is usually vastly decreased. A bone marrow specimen is diagnostic, disclosing an excess of immature blast cells. The presence of Auer rods in the cytoplasm indicates acute myelogenous leukemia (AML).

Management. Chemotherapy is the major form of therapy and in some instances results in remissions lasting a year or longer. Agents commonly used include daunorubicin hydrochloride (Cerubidine), cytarabine (Cytosar-U), and mercaptopurine (Purinethol). Supportive care consists of administering blood products and promptly treating infections. When a tissue match with a close relative can be obtained, a bone marrow transplantation is performed to provide normal bone marrow, following destruction of leukemic marrow by chemotherapy.

Prognosis. Patients who receive treatment survive an average of only 1 year, with death usually a result of infection or hemorrhage. Schiller (1992) reports that in patients under 40 years old, the 5-year survival rate is about 35% when the patient is treated with high dose cytarabine-anthracycline consolidation chemotherapy, without maintenance therapy. Untreated patients survive only about 2 to 5 months. Research trials with new combinations of chemotherapeutic agents are being conducted at oncology treatment centers throughout the world.

Chronic Myelogenous Leukemia

Chronic myelogenous leukemia (CML) is also believed to be a malignancy of myeloid stem cells. However, more normal cells are present than in the acute form, and therefore the disease is milder. A genetic abnormality termed the Philadelphia chromosome is found in 90% to 95% of patients with CML. CML is uncommon in people under 20, but the incidence rises with age.

Manifestations. The clinical picture of CML is similar to that of AML, but signs and symptoms are less severe. Many patients are without symptoms for years. An increase in leukocytes is always present, sometimes at extraordinary levels. The spleen is frequently enlarged.

Management and Prognosis. Therapies of choice for chronic myelogenous leukemia are busulfan (Myleran), hydroxyurea, and chlorambucil (Leukeran) alone or with corticosteroids. Survival has been significantly improved with bone marrow transplantation for patients younger than 50 years of age who have a suitable HLA donor. Alpha-interferon is an alternative choice of treatment, but is expensive, has unpleasant side effects, and has not provided evidence of prolonged survival. Fludarabine (Fludara) has been effective for patients whose disease has not responded to existing treatments or continues to progress after treatment. For most patients, acute myelogenous leukemia develops and is usually resistant to all therapy. Overall, patients live for 3 to 4 years. Death usually results from infection or hemorrhage.

Acute Lymphocytic Leukemia

Acute lymphocytic leukemia (ALL) is believed to be a malignant proliferation of lymphoblasts. It is most common in young children, with males affected more than females, and with a peak incidence at 4 years of age. After age 15, ALL is uncommon.

Manifestations. Immature lymphocytes proliferate in the marrow and peripheral tissue and crowd the development of normal cells. As a result, normal hematopoiesis is inhibited, resulting in reduced numbers of leukocytes, red blood cells, and platelets. Erythrocyte and platelet counts are low, and leukocyte counts may be either low or high but always include immature cells. Manifestations of leukemic cell infiltration into other organs are more common with ALL than with other forms of leukemia and include pain from an enlarged liver or spleen, headache, vomiting because of meningeal involvement, and bone pain.

Management and Prognosis. Therapy for ALL has improved to the extent that approximately 60% of children survive at least 5 years. The major form of treatment is chemotherapy with combinations of vincristine, prednisone, daunorubicin, and asparaginase used for initial therapy and combinations of mercaptopurine, methotrexate, vincristine, and prednisone for maintenance. Irradiation of the craniospinal region and intrathecal injection of chemotherapeutic agents help prevent central nervous system recurrence.

Chronic Lymphocytic Leukemia

Chronic lymphocytic leukemia (CLL) tends to be a mild disorder that primarily affects persons between 50 and 70 years of age. Western countries report this as the most common leukemia.

Clinical Manifestations. Many patients are asymptomatic and are diagnosed during physical examination or treatment for another disease. Possible manifestations are those of anemia, infection, or enlargement of lymph nodes and abdominal organs. The erythrocyte and platelet counts may be normal or decreased. A decreased lymphocyte count (lymphocytopenia) is always present.

Medical Management and Prognosis. If mild, CLL may require no treatment. When symptoms are severe, chemotherapy with corticosteroids and chlorambucil (Leukeran) is often used. A significant number of patients who do not respond to these medications have achieved remission by treatment with fludarabine monophosphate, 2-chlorodeoxyadenosine (2-CDA), or pentostatin. The major side effect of these medications is bone marrow suppression, manifested in such infections as *Pneumocystis carinii*, listeria, mycobacteria, herpes viruses and cytomegalovirus. Intravenous treatment with immunoglobulin is effective in preventing these problems in selected patients. The average survival for patients with CLL is 7 years.

Complications. Complications of leukemia include bleeding and infection, which is the major cause of death. Renal stone formation, anemia, and gastrointestinal problems are other complications.

The risk of bleeding correlates with the level of platelet deficiency (thrombocytopenia). The low platelet count can result in bruising (ecchymoses) and petechiae (pinpoint red or purple hemorrhagic spots on the skin). Patients may also develop major hemorrhages when their platelet counts drop below 20,000 per mm^3 of blood. For undetermined reasons, fever or infection also increases the likelihood of bleeding.

Because of the lack of mature and normal granulocytes, these patients are always threatened by infection. The likelihood of infection increases with the degree of neutropenia, so granulocyte counts under 100/ml of blood make the development of systemic infection highly probable. Immune dysfunction compounds the risk of infection.

The massive cell destruction resulting from chemotherapy increases uric acid levels and makes patients vulnerable to renal stone formation and renal colic. Therefore, patients require a high fluid intake to prevent crystallization of uric acid and subsequent stone formation.

Gastrointestinal problems may result from the infiltration of abnormal leukocytes into the abdominal organs as well as from the toxicity of the chemotherapeutic agents. Anorexia, nausea, vomiting, diarrhea, and mucosal lesions in the mouth are common.

❑ NURSING PROCESS
The Patient With Leukemia

Assessment

Although the clinical picture will vary with the type of leukemia involved, the health history may reveal a range of signs and symptoms reported by the patient and noted during the physical examination. Included in the clinical manifestations may be weakness and fatigue, bleeding tendencies, petechiae and ecchymoses, pain, headache, vomiting, fever, and infection. Blood studies may show alterations of the white blood cells, anemia, and a low platelet count (thrombocytopenia). Specific manifestations are identified under the discussion of each of the types of leukemia.

Diagnosis

Nursing Diagnoses

Based on the assessment data, nursing diagnoses for the patient may include:

- ❑ Pain related to leukocytic infiltration of systemic tissues
- ❑ Altered nutrition: less than body requirements, related to gastrointestinal proliferative changes and toxic effects of chemotherapeutic agents
- ❑ Fatigue and activity intolerance related to anemia
- ❑ Grieving related to anticipatory loss and altered role functioning
- ❑ Impaired skin integrity: alopecia related to toxic effects of chemotherapy
- ❑ Disturbance in body image related to change in appearance, in function and roles

Collaborative Problems/ Potential Complications

Based on the assessment data, potential complications that may develop include:

- ❑ Infection
- ❑ Bleeding

Planning and Implementation

Goals. The major goals of the patient may include attainment or maintenance of comfort, attainment or maintenance of adequate nutrition, tolerance of activity, ability to cope with the diagnosis and prognosis, promotion of positive body image, and absence of complications.

Nursing Interventions

Refer to the nursing care plan Care of The Patient With Cancer (Chapter 16) for interventions, rationale, and evaluation.

Monitoring and Managing Potential Complications. It is essential to monitor the patient for the following signs and symptoms of infection: temperature elevation, flushed appearance, chills, tachycardia, appearance of white patches in the mouth; redness, swelling, heat, or pain of eyes, ears, throat, skin, joints, abdomen, rectal, and perineal areas; cough; changes in character or color of sputum or stool; and skin rash.

The usual manifestations of infection are altered in patients with leukemia. Corticosteroid therapy may blunt the normal febrile and inflammatory responses to infection.

Preventing bleeding should be approached in the same manner as for patients with aplastic anemia. Any increase in petechiae and any blood in the stools or urine (melena, hematuria) or nosebleeds should be reported. Injections must be avoided and safety precautions taken to avoid trauma. Acetaminophen, rather than aspirin, should be used for analgesia. Hormonal therapy may be prescribed to prevent menses. Hemorrhage is treated by bed rest and transfusions of red blood cells and platelets.

Administering analgesics helps manage pain that results from infiltration and enlargement of abdominal organs, lymph nodes, bones, and joints.

Patient Education and Home Care Considerations. It is important that patients and their families have a clear understanding of the disease and prognosis. The nurse acts as an advocate to assure that this information is provided. For patients who no longer respond to therapy, it is important to respect the patient's choices about treatment, including measures to prolong life. Advance directives and living wills provide patients with some measure of control during the terminal phase of illness.

Many patients choose to be cared for at home. Families often need support when considering this option. Coordination of home care services can help to alleviate anxiety about managing the patient's care in the home.

It is often helpful to begin teaching family members about home care while the patient is still in the hospital. Gradual involvement in basic care and comfort measures increases the caregivers' confidence. In addition, family members often need to be encouraged to take care of themselves, allowing time for adequate rest and accepting emotional support. Hospice staff can assist in providing respite for family members as well as care for the patient. Patients and families need assistance to cope with changes in their roles and responsibilities. Anticipatory grieving is an essential task during this time.

There may come a time when the family can no longer care for the patient in the home setting. Hospital-based hospice programs provide palliative care.

Malignant Lymphomas

The lymphomas are neoplasms of the cells of lymphoid origin. They are often classified according to the degree of cell differentiation and the origin of the predominant malignant cell. These tumors usually start in lymph nodes, but can involve lymphoid tissue in the spleen, the gastrointestinal tract (for example, the wall of the stomach), the liver, or the bone marrow. They often spread to all of these areas and to extralymphatic tissues (lungs, kidneys, skin) by the time of death. The cause of these tumors is unknown.

Hodgkin's Disease

Hodgkin's disease, like other lymphomas, is a malignant disease of unknown origin that originates in the lymphatic system and involves predominantly the lymph nodes. It is somewhat more common in men than women and has two peaks of incidence: one in the early 20s and the other after age 50. Because many manifestations are similar to those occurring with infection, diagnostic studies are performed to rule out an infectious origin for the disease.

The malignant cell of Hodgkin's disease is the "Reed-Sternberg cell," a gigantic atypical tumor cell, morphologically unique and of uncertain lineage. It is the pathologic hallmark and essential diagnostic criterion for Hodgkin's disease.

Hodgkin's disease is customarily classified into subgroups based on pathologic criteria that reflect the grade of malignancy and suggest the prognosis. When lymphocytes predominate, for example, with few Reed-Sternberg cells and minimal involvement of the nodes, the prognosis is much more favorable than when the lymphocyte count is low and the lymph nodes are virtually replaced by tumor cells of the most primitive type. The majority of patients (those with conditions currently designated "nodular sclerosis" and "mixed cellularity") are in an intermediate position with respect to the number and destructiveness of tumor cells, the degree to which they respond to therapy, and the overall prognosis.

Clinical Manifestations

Hodgkin's disease usually begins as a painless enlargement of the lymph nodes on one side of the neck, which becomes increasingly conspicuous. The individual nodes are rubbery and painless. Soon the lymph nodes of other regions, usually the other side of the neck, also enlarge in the same manner. The mediastinal and retroperitoneal lymph nodes may also enlarge, causing severe pressure symptoms: pressure against the trachea results in breathing difficulties; pressure against the esophagus causes swallowing problems; pressure on the nerves causes laryngeal paralysis and brachial, lumbar, or sacral neuralgias; pressure on the veins results in edema of one or both extremities and effusions into the pleura or peritoneum; and pressure on the bile duct causes obstructive jaundice. Later the spleen may become palpable, and the liver may enlarge. In some patients the first nodes to enlarge are those under one of the arms or in one groin. Occasionally, the disease starts in mediastinal or peritoneal nodes and may remain limited to them. In still other cases the enlargement of the spleen is the only conspicuous lesion.

Eventually a progressive anemia develops. The leukocyte count is often high, with an abnormally high polymorphonuclear (PMN) count and an elevated eosinophil count. About half of the patients have a slight fever, with the temperature seldom rising above 38.3°C (101°F). Patients with mediastinal and abdominal involvement, however, develop a significant intermittent fever. The temperature goes as high as 40.0°C (104°F) for periods of 3 to 14 days, returning to normal within a few weeks.

If the disease is not treated, it progresses in its course; the patient loses weight and becomes cachectic (physically wasted), infections develop, anemia becomes marked, anasarca (severe generalized edema) appears, the blood pressure falls, and death is likely in 1 to 3 years without treatment.

Diagnostic Evaluation

The diagnosis of Hodgkin's disease depends on identifying the characteristic presence of the Reed-Sternberg cell in an excised lymph node. Once the diagnosis is confirmed, it is necessary to assess the total extent of tumor involvement and to identify every tumor lesion inside and outside the lymphatic system. This is a difficult, expensive, and uncertain undertaking but an extremely important one because these are the factors on which treatment is based.

Laboratory tests include a complete blood count, platelet count, sedimentation rate, and liver and renal function studies. A bone marrow biopsy and liver and spleen scans are performed to determine if these organs are involved. Chest x-ray and bone scans of the pelvis, vertebrae, and long bones are performed to identify any involvement in these areas.

Management

Current concepts of treatment stem from the following observations and premises:

1. Hodgkin's disease spreads from its original location (usually a single node) by way of the lymphatic channels to contiguous lymph nodes, which in turn become the sites of tumor growth; it rarely skips lymph nodes en route to more distant sites of metastasis.
2. Hodgkin's disease rarely spreads beyond the lymphatic system to involve other organs and tissues until late in the disease.
3. Hodgkin's disease can be completely and permanently eradicated 95% of the time from any site that has received a radiation dose of 3500 to 4500 rad within the space of about 4 weeks. Megavoltage radiation techniques permit the delivery of such a dose to one or more entire lymph node chains.
4. Areas of the body in which the lymph node chains are located can tolerate doses of this magnitude without serious damage (as can the area of the spleen and the oronasopharynx, both of which may be involved in Hodgkin's disease), provided that vital structures such as the lungs, liver, gastrointestinal tract, kidneys, and bone marrow are protected by lead shields.

Treatment is primarily determined by the stage of the disease, instead of the histologic type. Hodgkin's disease is potentially curable by radiotherapy, provided it has not extended beyond the lymph node chains, spleen, and oronasopharynx. Patients whose disease has not spread should have the benefit of "curative" radiotherapy in which doses large enough to destroy the tumors are delivered not only to obvious tumor nodes but to all adjacent nodes and lymph node chains as well. Any sign of spread beyond the treatable areas automatically disqualifies the Hodgkin's patient from such a program, in which case a combination of chemotherapy and palliative radiotherapy is indicated.

Staging of Hodgkin's Disease

For the sake of simplicity, and to determine treatment, the extent of Hodgkin's disease is classified, or "staged" as follows:

Stage I: Disease is limited to a single node and contiguous structures, or a single organ or site outside the lymphatic system.
Stage II: Disease involves more than a single node or group of contiguous nodes, but is confined to one side of the diaphragm only.
Stage III: Disease is present both above and below the diaphragm and may involve only the spleen, one site outside the lymphatic system, or both.
Stage IV: Disease has disseminated diffusely to one or more extralymphatic sites with or without associated lymph node involvement.

Stages are further subdivided by the presence or absence of one or more of the following symptoms: fever, night sweats, and unexplained weight loss. Patients without these symptoms are designated A and patients with them are designated B. The size or bulk of tumor masses is also determined, as they may require separate therapy. Chemotherapy is often added for stage IIB and for stage IIIA. For stages IIIB and IV, combination chemotherapy is used, and radiation is generally reserved for the palliative treatment of local lesions that are especially destructive or painful. Currently patients diagnosed at stage IA or IIA have a 5-year survival rate of 90% and can essentially be considered cured. Survival rates decrease progressively with more advanced stages.

Nursing Interventions

Radiation therapy often requires many weeks of daily trips to the hospital. The dose to the tumor and adjacent lymph node areas is generally 4500 rad (45 grays).

Patients often develop esophagitis, anorexia, loss of taste, dry mouth, nausea and vomiting, diarrhea, skin reactions, and lethargy secondary to radiation therapy. Much ingenuity is needed to help patients cope with these unpleasant side effects. They should be encouraged to make a concerted effort to eat. Bland, soft foods that they normally like are usually most palatable and are tolerated best when served at mild temperatures. Anesthetic throat lozenges may be helpful in relieving the mouth and throat discomfort that often interferes with eating. Decreased saliva increases the risk of dental caries and requires proper dental hygiene. The antiemetic that is prescribed should be administered during the peak times of nausea.

Skin reactions that give the appearance of sunburn or tan are common. Patients are alerted that these reactions are expected and that rubbing the area and applying heat, cold, or lotions must be avoided. If the reaction is severe, they should notify the physician or nurse.

The lethargy that accompanies radiation may cause patients to become discouraged about their progress. They should be informed that they will feel tired and that they must increase periods of rest and sleep to maintain a reasonable energy level. The family is encouraged to help patients in their attempts to rest. Diversional activities that require minimal energy expenditure may help to prevent boredom.

A commonly used chemotherapeutic regimen is a combination of nitrogen mustard, vincristine (Oncovin), prednisone, and procarbazine (MOPP). Survival rates for patients with advanced Hodgkin's disease have been improved by the combination of medications. Canellos (1992) demonstrated that ABVD therapy (adriamycin [doxorubicin], bleomycin, vinblastine and dacarbazine) for 6 to 8 months was as effective as 12 months of MOPP alternating with ABDV; and both were superior to MOPP alone. Other agents that have also shown favorable responses, in combination with standard medications, are erythropoietin and etoposide.

As with any patient receiving chemotherapy (see Chapter 16), support is necessary to help these patients tolerate the toxic effects, which include bone marrow depression, gastrointestinal disturbances, and hair loss (alopecia). Many patients experience anticipatory nausea and vomiting. Recognizing this side effect and treating it promptly can offset its impact. It often helps if patients are informed that the therapy will end at a specific time. This, along with the knowledge that there is a high likelihood of cure, often serves as an incentive for them to continue with the therapy. Helping patients to prepare for the alopecia by encouraging them to purchase a wig that is acceptable to them before the problem occurs often averts some of the distress commonly associated with the loss of hair.

Patients with Hodgkin's disease are extremely vulnerable to infection, both as a result of radiation and chemotherapy and as a consequence of defective immune responses caused by the tumor. They are urged to report fever or any other signs of infection (skin redness, tenderness, lesions, cough) immediately so that treatment can be instituted. They are also informed of the importance of avoiding contact with persons with infections. Use of contraception during treatment is necessary because chemotherapy would have a cytotoxic effect on the fetus if pregnancy occurred.

Follow-up appointments with the physician are important to determine the effectiveness of the treatment and to detect complications. A high incidence of acute leukemia can occur several years after treatment with radiation and chemotherapy. For this reason, the patient is encouraged to keep all follow-up appointments.

Non-Hodgkin's Lymphomas

Non-Hodgkin's lymphomas are a heterogeneous group of disorders that can be defined as malignancies of the lymphoid tissue other than Hodgkin's disease. The cause is unknown; viral etiology has been suggested. There is an association with immunosuppressed states (*e.g.*, AIDS and immunosuppressive therapy for organ transplantion). It is common in persons with AIDS; as persons with AIDS live longer, the risk for lymphoma increases.

Manifestations are similar to those of Hodgkin's disease, but these disorders are more likely to have spread throughout the lymphatic system and beyond by the time the disorder is first diagnosed. If the disease is localized, radiation is the treatment of choice. If there is generalized involvement, combination chemotherapy is used. Administration of a lower dosage for HIV-positive patients is recommended to avoid severe, potentially lethal infections. As with Hodgkin's disease, infection is a major problem. Central nervous system involvement is also common.

Gerontologic Considerations. Non-Hodgkin's lymphoma is more common in the older adult. Older people with the disease also seem to have an increased incidence of herpes zoster. The elderly may be more sensitive to the effects of radiation and require careful assessment for signs of complications.

Multiple Myeloma

Multiple myeloma is a malignant disease of plasma cells that infiltrate bone, lymph nodes, liver, spleen, and kidneys. It is not classified as a lymphoma. The malignant cell is the plasma cell, the neoplastic proliferation taking place mainly in the bone marrow.

Patients generally complain of back pain and have a normochromic, normocytic anemia (the red blood cells have a normal color and size). They may have reduced counts of leukocytes and platelets because the bone marrow is infiltrated by malignant plasma cells. The diagnosis of myeloma can be made by aspiration or biopsy of the bone marrow. X-rays showing destructive lesions of many bones may suggest myeloma but are not diagnostic for this disease. The malignant plasma cells produce large quantities of abnormal globulins, which appear on the serum electrophoresis as a paraprotein "spike." Fragments of these globulins are excreted in urine as Bence Jones proteins.

Patients may be incapacitated by constant bone pain. The lesions destroy the bone and are often associated with hypercalcemia. Bone fractures are common, especially in the vertebrae or ribs. Median survival is between 2 to 5 years, with death usually resulting from infection or renal failure.

Management. Melphalan (Alkeran), cyclophosphamide, and corticosteroids are the agents used to decrease the tumor mass and relieve bone pain. They can prolong life from 1 year to 2 or 3 years. Radiation is very useful in relieving bone pain and reducing the size of plasma cell tumors that occur outside the skeletal system. Hydration is essential to prevent renal damage resulting from the Bence Jones protein precipitating in the renal tubules and from excessive calcium and uric acid in the blood. Thus, it is important to assess these patients for signs and symptoms of renal insufficiency. Allopurinol is used to prevent uric acid crystallization. When patients have severe pain they need opioid analgesics and local radiation, and sometimes back braces to relieve pressure. Pathologic fractures are also possible. It is important to keep the patient as active as possible, because bed rest only increases the likelihood of excess calcium levels in the blood (hypercalcemia). Bacterial infections, especially pneumonia, are common in these patients because antibody production is impaired. Patients with multiple myeloma should not be put on fasting regimens for diagnostic tests because dehydrating procedures can precipitate acute renal failure.

Gerontologic Considerations. The incidence of multiple myeloma increases with age, rarely occurring before age 40. Because of the increasing older population, more patients are seeking treatment for this disease. Back pain should be closely investigated in elderly patients, as it often is a presenting complaint.

Bleeding Disorders

Pathophysiology

The body normally protects against excessive and lethal blood loss through numerous complex and interrelated mechanisms. As indicated in Figure 32-3, the mechanisms that halt bleeding (hemostasis) include three phases. In the first phase, the *vascular phase,* the injured vessels immediately constrict. This vessel spasm is sufficient to stop capillary bleeding. In the second phase, or *platelet phase,* the platelets aggregate at the bleeding site. These tiny cells are rapidly attracted to the damaged endothelium and form loose plugs. More platelets gather and eventually fuse and contract, forming stable plugs. The platelet plug effectively stops bleeding from small vessels such as venules, and provides temporary protection in larger injuries.

Complete and permanent sealing of vascular wounds is accomplished through the clotting of the blood, which results in the production of an adherent, gel-like mass that effectively controls most types of hemorrhage. This third phase, or *coagulation phase,* is initiated through either the intrinsic or the extrinsic pathway. A chain reaction occurs in which blood proteins are sequentially activated until factor Xa is formed. At this point, factor Xa interacts with factor V, calcium, and a platelet substance to convert prothrombin to thrombin. Thrombin is a very active enzyme that has several functions: one is to encourage further platelet aggregation; another is to convert fibrinogen to fibrin.

Strands of fibrin begin to form in the vicinity of the platelet plug, reinforcing the plug and producing a larger clot. The fibrin clot is then further stabilized by the formation of bonds between the molecules, catalyzed by another plasma protein, factor XIII. As a result, the damaged vessel is sealed and blood flow in the area is slowed. Tissue repair of the vessel endothelium can then proceed. Eventually, much of the fibrin clot will be lysed or dissolved by another plasma protein system—the plasmin system, which produces fibrinolysis.

Abnormalities that predispose a person to hemorrhagic diseases can affect vessels, platelets, and any of the plasma coagulation factors, fibrin, or plasmin. Some patients can have defects at several sites simultaneously. Bleeding may be a manifestation of a primary coagulation defect (as in hemophilia), may occur secondary to another disease (as in cirrhosis, renal failure, or leukemia), or may be due to medications (overdose of warfarin sodium).

Clinical Manifestations

The symptoms and signs of bleeding disorders vary, depending on the type of defect. A careful history can often give clues to the diagnosis.

Abnormalities of the vascular system give rise to local bleeding, usually into the skin. Because platelets are primarily responsible for stopping bleeding from small vessels, patients with low platelet counts will develop *petechiae*, often in clusters, seen on the skin and mucous membranes. Trauma results in excessive *bruising* but not large, uncontrolled hematomas. After cuts or skin puncture, bleeding can be stopped promptly when local pressure is applied and does not recur when the pressure is released.

In contrast, in hemophilia and abnormalities of other coagulation factors, the platelets function normally so that there are no petechial or superficial hemorrhages. Instead, deep bleeding occurs after minor trauma, such as intramuscular hematomas and hemorrhage into joint spaces. External bleeding recurs several hours after pressure is removed. For example, severe bleeding will start several hours after a tooth extraction.

Patients who have bleeding disorders or who have the potential for developing such disorders as a result of disease processes or therapeutic agents are observed carefully and frequently for bleeding. All drainage and excreta such as feces, urine, emesis, and gastric drainage are observed for occult as well as obvious blood. The skin is observed for petechiae and ecchymoses or bruises, and the nose and gums are assessed for bleeding. Abdominal, flank, or joint pain is promptly reported because it may be indicative of internal bleeding. In addition, the patient is closely observed for evidence of hypovolemia (low blood volume) manifested by hypotension, tachycardia, pallor, cool clammy skin, altered responsiveness, and oliguria (reduced urine output).

Vascular Disorders

Spontaneous rupture of small vessels that are defective or injured results in blood leaking into the skin and mucous membranes. The smallest hemorrhages, pinhead in size, are called petechiae. Larger lesions are termed ecchymoses or bruises. Platelet count and coagulation tests are usually normal.

Vascular dysfunction can be caused by a variety of mechanisms. Alterations in the connective tissue framework that supports blood vessels may explain the bleeding associated with vitamin C deficiency and adrenocortical hormone excess. Vascular injury can result from systemic diseases such as diabetes mellitus or the action of bacterial toxins. Vascular injury may also be influenced by immunologic factors, or may occur as a consequence of medication reactions, bacterial infections, allergic disorders, or collagen-vascular diseases. In general, bleeding from vascular disorders is mild.

Platelet Defects

The sudden onset of petechiae or excessive bruising or bleeding from the nose or gums should stimulate a search for a platelet defect. Deficiencies in the number of platelets (thrombocytopenias) are most common in platelet disorders; in some rare disorders of platelet function, the platelet count is normal but the clinical picture is identical to that seen in thrombocytopenia. The platelet function disorders can be diagnosed by special tests for platelet factor 3 and platelet adhesiveness and aggregation.

An important functional platelet disorder is that induced by aspirin; even small amounts of aspirin prevent normal platelet aggregation, and the bleeding time is prolonged for several days after aspirin ingestion. Although this defect does not cause bleeding in most normal people, patients with another coagulation disorder (such as thrombocytopenia or hemophilia) can experience life-threatening hemorrhage after taking aspirin; in addition, patients undergoing extensive surgery may experience bleeding postoperatively.

Thrombocytopenia

Thrombocytopenia is the most common cause of abnormal bleeding. It can result either from decreased production of platelets by the bone marrow or from increased destruction of platelets. Some of the causes are listed in Table 32-3. A platelet deficiency that is secondary to an underlying disease can usually be diagnosed from examining the patient or the patient's bone marrow. When platelet destruction is the cause of thrombocytopenia, the marrow shows increased megakaryocytes (the stem cells from which the platelets come) and normal platelet production. Bleeding and petechiae usually do not occur with platelet counts above 50,000/mm^3, although excessive bleeding can follow surgery.

When the platelet count drops below 20,000/mm^3, petechiae appear, along with nose bleeds, excessive menstrual bleeding, and hemorrhage after surgery or dental extractions. When the platelet count is less than 5000/mm^3, spontaneous fatal central nervous system hemorrhage or gastrointestinal hemorrhage can occur.

Management. The management for secondary thrombocytopenia is usually to treat the underlying disease. If platelet production is impaired, platelet transfusions may raise platelet counts and stop bleeding or prevent intracranial hemorrhage. If excessive platelet destruction occurs, transfused platelets will also be destroyed and will not raise the count.

Idiopathic Thrombocytopenic Purpura

Idiopathic thrombocytopenic purpura (ITP) is a disease that affects people of all ages but is more common among children and young women. Although the precise cause remains unknown, viral infections sometimes precede the disease in children. Antibodies that attack the platelets are produced, so the life span of the platelets is markedly shortened. Occasionally, the antibodies can be demonstrated *in vitro*, but usually the diagnosis is made from the decreased platelet count and survival time and increased bleeding time. Other overt causes of thrombocytopenia must be excluded.

Symptoms may begin suddenly, with petechiae, mucosal bleeding, and heavy menses in women. The platelet

TABLE 32-3 Thrombocytopenias

Cause	Medical Management
Failure of Production	
Leukemia	Treat the leukemia.
Tumor invasion of marrow	
Aplastic anemia	Bone marrow transplant, androgens, antithymocyte globulin
Megaloblastic anemia	Vitamin B_{12} or folic acid
Toxins	Discontinue toxin.
Medications: heparin, chloramphenicol, cytotoxic drugs	Discontinue drug.
Infection, especially septicemia, viral infections, tuberculosis	Treat infection.
Alcohol	Discontinue alcohol.
Increased Destruction	
Due to antibodies	
Idiopathic thrombocytopenia purpura	Corticosteroids, splenectomy
Lupus erythematosus	Corticosteroids, immunosuppressive drugs
Malignant lymphoma	Corticosteroids
Medications: quinine, quinidine, digoxin, phenytoin, aspirin, sulfonamides, alcohol, gold	Discontinue drug.
Due to entrapment in large spleen	Splenectomy
Due to infections	Treat infection.
Bacteremia	
Postviral infections	
Increased Utilization	
Disseminated intravascular coagulopathy	Heparin

count is generally below 20,000/mm^3. Individuals with chronic ITP who do not respond to treatment are at increased risk for serious intracranial bleeding.

Management. Corticosteroids are the treatment of choice for ITP; the bleeding ceases in 1 to 2 days, and platelet counts rise in a week or so. About three fourths of patients respond to corticosteroids, but many have a relapse when the medication is withdrawn. Intravenous immunoglobulin is administered to patients who do not respond to corticosteroids. Removing the spleen (splenectomy) is an alternate treatment that produces a lasting remission in 75% of patients, although transient recurrences of thrombocytopenia may occur months or years later. The rare patients who do not respond to splenectomy may be treated with the immunosuppressive agents azathioprine or cyclophosphamide. Patients are instructed to avoid all medications that interfere with platelet function.

Clotting Factor Defects

Hemophilia

Two hereditary bleeding disorders are clinically indistinguishable but can be separated by laboratory tests: hemophilia A and hemophilia B. *Hemophilia A* is due to a deficiency of factor VIII clotting activity, whereas *hemophilia B* stems from a deficiency of factor IX. Factor VIII deficiency is about five times more common. Both types of hemophilia are inherited as X-linked traits, so almost all affected persons are males; their mothers and some of their sisters are carriers but are asymptomatic.

Clinical Manifestations. The disease, which may be very severe, is manifested by large, spreading bruises and bleeding into muscles, joints, and soft tissues after even minimal trauma. Patients often note pain in a joint before they are aware of swelling and limitation of motion. Recurrent joint hemorrhages can result in damage so severe that chronic pain or ankylosis (fixation) of the joint occurs. Many of the patients are crippled by the joint damage before they become adults. Spontaneous hematuria and gastrointestinal bleeding can occur. The disease is recognized in early childhood, usually in the toddler age group.

Before factor VIII concentrates became available, many patients died of the complications of hemophilia before they could reach adulthood. Some patients with hemophilia have a milder deficiency, having between 5% and 25% of the normal level of factor VIII or IX. These patients do not experience painful and disabling muscle and joint hemorrhages, but bleed only after dental extractions or surgery. Nevertheless, such hemorrhages can prove fatal if the cause is not recognized quickly.

Management. In the past, the only treatment for hemophilia was fresh frozen plasma, which had to be administered in such large quantities that the patients experienced an overload of fluid volume. Now factor VIII and IX concentrates are available to all blood banks. Patients are given concentrates when they are actively bleeding or as a preventive measure before dental extractions or surgery. The patient and family are taught how to administer the concentrate at home, at the first sign of bleeding.

A few patients eventually develop antibodies to the concentrates, so their factor levels cannot be increased. Treatment of this problem is extremely difficult and often unsuccessful. Aminocaproic acid is an inhibitor of fibrinolytic enzymes. This agent can slow the dissolution of blood clots that do form, and it is sometimes used after oral surgery in patients with hemophilia.

In terms of general care, patients with hemophilia should never be administered aspirin or IM injections. Dental hygiene is very important as a preventive measure, because dental extractions are so hazardous. Splints and other orthopedic devices may be very useful in patients who have suffered joint or muscle hemorrhages.

Complications. Complications of hemophilia include bleeding episodes with decreased tissue perfusion, ankylosis of joints from hemorrhage, and spontaneous hematuria and gastrointestinal bleeding. In recent years it has been found that patients with hemophilia are at high risk for developing AIDS as a result of the transfusions of blood and blood components that they previously received. All donated blood is now tested for the presence of antibodies to the AIDS virus. Commercial factor concentrates are heat-treated to reduce the possible transmission of blood-borne infectious diseases.

❑ NURSING PROCESS
The Patient With Hemophilia

Assessment

Patients with hemophilia are carefully assessed for evidence of internal bleeding (abdominal, chest, or flank pain; blood in the urine, bowel, or emesis), muscle hematomas, and hemorrhage into joint spaces. Vital signs and hemodynamic pressure readings are monitored for indications of hypovolemia. All extremities and the torso are carefully examined for hematomas. All joints are assessed for swelling, limitation of mobility, and pain. Range of motion of the joints is performed slowly and carefully to avoid further damage. At the first indication of pain, joint motion is stopped. Patients are questioned about any limitations of activities and movement experienced in the past and any need they have had for assistive devices such as splints, a cane, or crutches.

If the patient has had recent surgery, the surgical site is frequently and carefully assessed for bleeding. Frequent monitoring of vital signs may be necessary until it is certain that excessive postoperative bleeding is not present.

All patients with hemophilia are questioned about how they and their family cope with their condition, measures that they use to prevent bleeding episodes, and any limitations that the condition imposes on their life style and daily activities. The patient who has been hospitalized frequently for bleeding episodes due to traumatic injury is carefully questioned about the factors that have led to these episodes. Such data are particularly helpful in determining the extent to which the patient has accepted the condition and the need for providing patient and family education regarding measures to prevent unnecessary trauma.

Diagnosis

Nursing Diagnoses

Based on the assessment data, major nursing diagnoses for the patient may include the following:

- ❑ Pain related to joint hemorrhage and subsequent ankylosis
- ❑ Altered health maintenance related to ongoing need for preventive health practices
- ❑ Ineffective coping related to the chronicity of the condition and its effects on life-style

Collaborative Problems/ Potential Complications

Based on the assessment data, potential complications may include:

- ❑ Bleeding

Planning and Implementation

Goals. The major goals of the patient may include relief or minimization of pain, compliance with measures to prevent bleeding, coping with chronicity and altered life style, and absence of complications.

Nursing Interventions

Relieving Pain. Generally, analgesics are required to alleviate the pain associated with large muscle hematomas and joint hemorrhage. Oral non-opioid analgesics are prescribed when possible, because pain may be of long duration, and dependency on narcotics becomes a problem with chronic pain. It is often helpful to administer the analgesic before activities that are known to precipitate pain. This not only helps the patient to accomplish the activity, but also tends to decrease the amount of analgesic that the patient requires.

All efforts possible are taken to prevent or minimize pain due to activity. The patient is encouraged to move slowly and to prevent undue stress on involved joints. Many patients report that warm baths promote relaxation, improve mobility, and lessen pain. Heat is avoided during bleeding episodes, however, because it potentiates further bleeding.

Because joint pain restricts mobility, patients with excessive pain during activity may benefit from assistive devices. Splints, canes, or crutches are helpful in some cases in shifting body weight off joints that are particularly painful. Splints must be properly applied and crutches must be properly fitted to prevent undue pressure on body surfaces that could cause tissue trauma and bleeding.

Monitoring and Managing Complications. The patient is assessed frequently for signs and symptoms of decreased tissue perfusion as evidenced by hypoxia to vital organs: restlessness; anxiety; confusion; pallor; cool, clammy skin; chest pain; and decreased urinary output. Hypotension and tachycardia will occur as a result of volume depletion. The blood pressure, pulse, respiration, central venous pressure, and pulmonary artery pressure are monitored, as are the hemoglobin and hematocrit, coagulation and bleeding times, and platelet counts.

The patient is observed frequently for bleeding from the skin, mucous membranes, and wounds and for internal bleeding. During bleeding episodes, the patient is kept at rest and gentle pressure is applied to any external bleeding sites. Cold compresses are applied to bleeding sites when indicated.

Parenteral medications are administered with small-gauge needles to decrease trauma and the risk of bleeding. All possible efforts are made to protect the patient from trauma. The environment is kept free of obstacles that could cause falls, and the patient is turned and moved with care. Side rails are padded when necessary. Blood and blood components are administered as prescribed, and precautions are taken to avoid complications (see p. 808).

Patient Education and Home Care Considerations

Measures to Prevent Bleeding. The patient and family are informed of the risk of bleeding and the necessary safety precautions to be taken. They are encouraged to alter the home environment as necessary to prevent physical trauma. Obstacles that could cause falls are removed. An electric razor is used for shaving and a soft toothbrush is used for oral hygiene. Forceful nose blowing and coughing and straining at stool are avoided. A stool softener is used if necessary. Aspirin and aspirin-containing medications are to be avoided.

Physical activity is encouraged, but with proper safety measures. Noncontact sports such as swimming, hiking, and golf are acceptable activities, whereas contact sports are always to be avoided. Strength training of the legs can be effective in rehabilitation following acute hemarthrosis.

The necessity for regular checkups and laboratory studies is explained. With knowledge of the reasons for continued medical evaluation, the patient will be more likely to keep appointments.

Coping With Chronicity and Altered Life Style. Patients with hemophilia often require assistance in coping with the condition because it is chronic, places restrictions on their lives, and is an inherited disorder that can be passed to future generations. From childhood, patients are helped to accept themselves and the disease and to identify the positive aspects of their lives. They are encouraged to be self-sufficient and to maintain independence by preventing unnecessary trauma that can cause acute bleeding episodes and temporarily interfere with normal activities. As they work through feelings about the condition and progress to accepting it, they will assume more and more responsibility for maintaining optimal health. Because of an increase in the percent of persons with hemophilia who are HIV positive, patients and families need to learn how to deal effectively with their anger about the fatal illness of AIDS. The increased mortality rate of persons with hemophilia who develop AIDS has changed the role of the nurse. Nurses need to recognize the effects of this stress professionally and personally and explore sources of support for themselves as well as for these patients and their families.

Ideally, all patients with hemophilia will cooperate with health care providers, keep regular medical and dental appointments, and strive toward a healthy, productive life. Many patients benefit from the services of hemophilia care centers and support groups. These provide coordinated, ongoing care and the opportunity to interact with others who are faced with the same situation.

Evaluation

Expected Outcomes

1. Experiences relief or minimization of pain
   a. Reports decrease in pain after taking analgesic
   b. Exhibits increased ability to tolerate joint motion
   c. Uses assistive devices (when necessary) to decrease pain
2. Uses measures to prevent bleeding
   a. Avoids physical trauma
   b. Alters home environment to increase safety
   c. Keeps appointments with health care professional
   d. Keeps appointments for laboratory studies
   e. Avoids contact sports
   f. Avoids aspirin and aspirin-containing medications
   g. Wears Medic-Alert bracelet
3. Copes with chronicity and altered life style
   a. Identifies the positive aspects of present life
   b. Involves family members in decisions about the future and changes to be made in life style
   c. Strives toward independence
   d. Makes specific plans for continuation of health care
4. Experiences absence of complications
   a. Vital signs and hemodynamic pressure readings remain normal
   b. Laboratory studies remain within normal ranges
   c. Experiences no active bleeding

Von Willebrand's Disease

Von Willebrand's disease is a common bleeding disorder, usually inherited as a dominant trait and affecting males and females equally. It is due to a mild deficiency of factor VIII (15% to 50% of normal) associated with an impairment of platelet function. The laboratory tests show normal platelet count, prolonged bleeding time, and slightly prolonged partial thromboplastin time. Patients commonly have nosebleeds, excessively heavy menses, bleeding from cuts, and postoperative bleeding. They do not suffer from massive soft tissue or joint hemorrhages. Both the factor deficiency and the platelet impairment can be corrected either by the administration of cryoprecipitate, which contains factor VIII, fibrinogen, and factor XIII, or desmopressin (DDAVP), a synthetic vasopressin analogue that is used in hemorrhagic disorders related to platelet dysfunction.

Hypoprothrombinemia

Prothrombin, as previously noted, is essential for clotting. This protein is produced in the liver by a vitamin K–dependent chemical process. Vitamin K comes from food sources as well as from synthesis by bacteria that reside in the intestine. Normal prothrombin activity in the blood depends on adequate absorption of vitamin K from the gastrointestinal tract and adequate liver function. Therefore, prothrombin deficiency may arise from factors that affect vitamin K absorption, such as diarrhea; a lack of bile in the gastrointestinal tract (necessary for absorption of fat-soluble vitamin K) due to biliary tract obstruction; surgical removal of or mucosal damage to a large part of the small intestine; prolonged antibiotic therapy; or liver disease.

The principal manifestation of prothrombin deficiency is prolonged hemorrhage from blood vessels that are damaged by trauma or disease. This explains the characteristic occurrence of ecchymoses, blood in the urine (hematuria), gastrointestinal bleeding, and postoperative hemorrhages.

Coumarin Toxicity. The coumarins are agents that often are employed to induce a partial depression of prothrombin activity, because they interfere with the action of vitamin K in the liver. Therapy is usually calculated to prolong the prothrombin time by 1.5 to 2 times normal. In this range, thrombosis is inhibited and thrombophlebitis is prevented. However if the medications are taken in excessive dosages, whether intentionally or by mistake, or if certain other agents that interfere with metabolism are administered simultaneously, the complete picture of prothrombin deficiency, with a severe hemorrhagic disorder, may result. Agents that enhance coumarin-induced anticoagulation include phenylbutazone, indomethacin, phenytoin, and salicylates. Other agents, such as barbiturates, decrease coumarin effects.

Management. Hypoprothrombinemia, if due to vitamin K deficiency, responds to treatment with oral or parenteral administration of vitamin K. When corrective measures are urgently required, however, particularly in patients with liver disease or coumarin toxicity, fresh frozen plasma will promptly correct the deficit.

Liver Disease. The liver produces all the plasma protein coagulation factors except factor VIII. Therefore, in severe hepatic disease of any sort, deficiencies in these factors may occur. The prothrombin time and partial thromboplastin time will both be prolonged. If the spleen is enlarged as well (as in cirrhosis), the platelet count also may be depressed. Patients with liver diseases frequently bruise easily and may have life-threatening hemorrhage from peptic ulcers or esophageal varices. Treatment includes administering fresh frozen plasma, cryoprecipitate, and platelets. Vitamin K does not improve the disorder.

Gerontologic Considerations. The older patient is likely to be taking several medications because of chronic illness. If the patient is also taking a coumarin agent, the possibility of a medication interaction increases. Changes in schedules or dosages can be confusing to the elderly. Clear instructions should be written for the patient to refer to later. Special emphasis is placed on helping the patient to avoid taking medications that can have harmful interactions.

Disseminated Intravascular Coagulopathy (DIC)

Occasionally, widespread clotting in small vessels of the body occurs, causing clotting factors and platelets to be used up. Thus, paradoxically, the patient develops a bleeding disorder characterized by low fibrinogen, prolonged prothrombin time and partial thromboplastin time, reduced platelet count, and elevated fibrin split products.

Such patients may bleed from mucous membranes, venipuncture sites, and the gastrointestinal and urinary tracts. The bleeding can range from minimal occult internal bleeding to profuse hemorrhage from all orifices. Patients may also develop organ dysfunction, such as renal failure and pulmonary and multifocal CNS infarctions due to micro- and macrothromboses.

Many serious illnesses may predispose to DIC, including septicemia, premature separation of the placenta in pregnancy, metastatic malignancies (see presentation of DIC in Chapter 16), hemolytic transfusion reactions, massive tissue trauma, and shock. DIC should be suspected in any patient with a predisposing cause who develops purpura, a bleeding tendency, signs of tissue hypoxemia and hypovolemia, and signs of renal damage. It can also occur during surgery.

There is a 68% mortality rate in confirmed cases. Nurses who recognize patients at risk for DIC and the early clinical manifestations of this syndrome may ensure earlier medical intervention, which improves the prognosis.

Goals of management include controlling hemorrhage and clotting and restoring acid–base balance and hemostasis. Serious hemorrhage requires replacement therapy: packed red cells, platelet concentrates, and volume expanders without clotting proteins (*e.g.*, albumin), plasma protein fraction, and hydroxyethyl starch. If blood products with clotting factors are used, administering heparin prior to the transfusion to reduce intravascular clotting is recommended. The best treatment is to correct the underlying disease, but in the meantime intravenous heparin may be administered to retard the coagulation process and permit clotting tests to return to normal and hemorrhagic manifestations to decrease.

Therapeutic Measures in Blood Disorders

Splenectomy

The surgical removal of the spleen (splenectomy) is sometimes necessary after trauma to the abdomen. Because the spleen is very vascular, severe hemorrhage can result if the spleen ruptures. Under such circumstances, splenectomy becomes an emergency procedure.

Splenectomy is also often performed as a treatment for a number of hematologic disorders. An enlarged spleen may be the site of excessive destruction of blood cells; when this destruction is life-threatening, surgery may be lifesaving. This is the case in autoimmune hemolytic anemia or idiopathic thrombocytopenia purpura when these disorders do not respond to corticosteroids. Some patients with severe anemia due to inherited red cell defects, such as thalassemia, may benefit from splenectomy. In some patients with rheumatoid arthritis the spleen may enlarge, resulting in destruction of granulocytes and granulocytopenia; removal of the spleen may improve the blood count and reduce the tendency toward infection.

When the spleen is large, the surgery can be difficult, but generally there is a very low mortality following splenectomy. Complications may result from postoperative atelectasis, pneumonia, abdominal distention, and abscess formation. Although young children are at the highest risk following splenectomy, all age groups are vulnerable to overwhelming lethal infections and should receive pneumococcal vaccine before undergoing a surgical procedure if possible. Patients are instructed to seek prompt medical attention when even relatively minor symptoms of infection occur. Patients with high platelet counts often are found to have even higher counts after splenectomy—greater than a million—which can predispose the patient to serious thrombotic or hemorrhagic problems.

Blood and Blood Component Therapy

Blood Donation

Because blood and blood components are used so frequently, nearly all hospitals have blood banks, and most large hospitals also have facilities for blood donation. Nurses employed in these departments screen prospective donors, perform the phlebotomies, and assure the health and safety of the donors.

Donor Interviewing

To protect both the donor and the recipients, all prospective donors are examined and interviewed before they are allowed to donate their blood. The questioning must be tactful but complete, and an experienced interviewer will learn how to ask each question in several ways to obtain the most complete answers. Donors should be in good health and should be free of any of the following disqualifying factors:

- A history of viral hepatitis, recently or at any time in the past, or a history of close contact with a hepatitis or dialysis patient within 6 months
- A history of receiving a blood transfusion or injection of any fraction of blood other than serum albumin or immune globulin within 6 months
- A history of untreated syphilis or malaria, because these diseases can be transmitted by transfusion even years later. A person who has been free of symptoms and off therapy for 3 years after malaria may be a donor.
- A history or evidence of drug abuse in which substances were self-injected, because many intravenous drug users are hepatitis carriers and because the risk of AIDS is high in this group.
- A history of possible exposure to the AIDS virus. A test for the presence of antibodies to AIDS virus in donated blood is now available. The population at risk includes those persons who engage in anal sex practices, persons with multiple sexual partners, intravenous drug users, sexual partners of individuals at risk for AIDS, and persons with hemophilia.
- A skin infection, because of the possibility of contaminating the phlebotomy needle
- A history of recent asthma, urticaria, or allergy to medications, because hypersensitivity can be passively transferred to the recipient
- Pregnancy within 6 months, because of the nutritional demands of pregnancy on the mother
- A history of tooth extraction or oral surgery within 72 hours, because such procedures are frequently associated with transient bacteremia
- A history of recent tattoo, because of the risk of hepatitis
- A history of exposure to infectious disease within the past 3 weeks, because of the risk of transmission to the recipient
- Recent immunizations, because of the risk of transmitting live organisms (2-week waiting period for live, attenuated organisms; 1 month for rubella; 1 year for rabies)
- Presence of cancer, because of the uncertainty about transmission
- A history of whole blood donation within the past 56 days

Blood donors who pass this screening procedure are then examined with regard to blood pressure, pulse, oral temperature, weight, and hemoglobin level. Persons under 17 and over 65 years of age are usually disqualified.

ETHICAL QUESTION:

Should a Jehovah's Witness Patient Receive Life-saving Blood Transfusions against His Wishes?

Situation

Blood transfusions are performed in the event of serious, often life-threatening health crises. They have the potential to save life in an otherwise hopeless situation. Jehovah's Witnesses are a sect of Christians who consent to aggressive medical treatment in case of illness or trauma, yet consistently refuse any blood or blood products because of their unique interpretation of the Bible. Should a Jehovah's Witness patient suffering from acute blood loss be allowed to die because of a religious belief if a relatively simple and accessible treatment (blood transfusion) could be performed that would most likely save his life?

Dilemma

The patient's right to refuse treatment conflicts with the professional obligation to help the patient (autonomy versus beneficence).

Discussion

- What arguments would you offer in support of the view that Jehovah's Witnesses *should* receive life-saving transfusions against their will?
- What arguments would you offer to support the view that Jehovah's Witnesses *should not* receive blood transfusions if they refuse them?

At times friends and family of a patient will donate blood for that person. These blood donations are termed directed donations. However, there is no evidence to support the belief that these donations are safer than those provided by other donors. Directed donors may not be as willing to identify themselves as having a history of any of the factors that disqualify a person from donating blood.

All donors are expected to meet the following minimal requirements:

1. The body weight should exceed 50 kg (110 pounds) for a standard 450-ml donation. Donors weighing less than 50 kg (110 pounds) donate proportionately less blood.
2. The oral temperature should not exceed 37.5°C (99.6°F).
3. The pulse rate should be regular and between 50 and 100 beats per minute.
4. The systolic arterial pressure should be between 90 and 180 mm Hg, and the diastolic pressure between 50 and 100 mm Hg.
5. The hemoglobin level in the case of a woman should be at least 12.5 g/dl, and in the case of a man, 13.5 g/dl.

Phlebotomy

Phlebotomy consists of venipuncture and the withdrawal of blood. Universal precautions are used. Donors are placed in a semirecumbent position. The skin over the antecubital fossa is carefully cleansed with an iodine preparation. A tourniquet is applied, and venipuncture is performed. Withdrawal of 450 ml of blood takes less than 15 minutes. After the needle is removed, donors are asked to hold the involved arm straight up, and firm pressure is applied with sterile gauze for 2 or 3 minutes or until bleeding stops. A firm bandage is then applied. Donors are asked to remain recumbent until they feel able to sit up, usually within 1 or 2 minutes. If weakness or faintness is experienced, they should rest for a longer period. After resting, they are given food and fluids in a reception area and asked to remain another 15 minutes.

Donors should be instructed to leave the dressing on and avoid heavy lifting for several hours, to avoid smoking for 1 hour and alcoholic beverages for 3 hours, to increase fluid intake for 2 days, and to be sure to eat well-balanced meals for 2 weeks.

The labels on the blood bag and tubes are checked carefully before and after donation to avoid any error that could prove fatal to a recipient.

Complications of Blood Donation

Excessive bleeding at the site of venipuncture in a blood donor is sometimes due to a bleeding disorder in the donor, but more often results from a technical error: laceration of the vein, excessive tourniquet pressure, or failure to apply enough pressure after the needle is withdrawn.

Fainting is relatively common following blood donation and may be related to emotional factors, a vasovagal reaction, or prolonged fasting before donation. Because of the loss of blood volume, hypotension and syncope may occur when the donor assumes an erect position.

- A donor who appears pale or complains of faintness should immediately lie down or sit with head lowered below the knees. The nurse should observe the donor for another 30 minutes.

Anginal chest pain may be precipitated in patients with unsuspected coronary artery disease. *Seizures* may occur in patients with epilepsy. Both angina and seizures require further medical evaluation.

Autologous Transfusions

A patient's blood may be collected for future transfusion (autologous transfusion) in one of three ways: preoperative donation, intraoperative blood salvage, and acute normovolemic hemodilution.

Preoperative donations are best collected 4 to 6 weeks prior to surgery. Iron supplements are prescribed during this period. Individual blood components can also be collected. Phlebotomies are not performed within 72 hours of surgery.

Intraoperative blood salvage provides replacement for patients unable to donate preoperatively and for patients undergoing vascular surgery, repair of traumatic injuries, and organ transplants. Salvaged blood cannot be stored because bacteria cannot be completely removed from the blood.

The collection of *normovolemic hemodilution transfusions* are initiated prior to or following induction of anesthesia. One or two units of blood are removed through a venous or arterial line and simultaneously replaced with a colloid or crystalloid solution. The blood is then reinfused after surgery. The advantage of this method is that the patient loses fewer red blood cells during surgery.

The primary *advantage* of these autologous transfusions is the prevention of viral infections from another person's blood. Other advantages include safe transfusion for patients with a history of transfusion reactions, stockpiling of rare blood type, prevention of alloimmunization and avoidance of complications in patients with alloantibodies, and maintenance of a supply of blood in isolated communities.

Contraindications to autologous transfusion are acute infection, severely debilitating chronic disease, hemoglobin less than 11 g/L, hematocrit less than 33%, a history of active epilepsy, cardiac dysrhythmias, and acute cardiovascular or cerebrovascular disease.

Blood and Blood Components

A unit of blood that has been drawn from a donor consists of approximately 450 ml of whole blood and 60 to 70 ml of preservative–anticoagulant, which serves as an anticoagulant and also provides the red cells with a sugar for metabolism. This blood can be maintained at 1°C to 6°C in the blood bank for 21 to 35 days, depending on the type of preservative–anticoagulant used; after that time it is discarded if unused, because too many of the red cells are unable to survive *in vivo*. Whole blood stored more than 24 hours does not contain functional platelets or practical amounts of coagulation factors V and VIII.

Blood Testing. Samples of the unit of blood are always taken immediately after donation so that the blood can be typed and tested. Each donation is tested for antibodies to human immunodeficiency virus (HIV), hepatitis B

TABLE 32-4 Summary of Blood Components

Component	Major Indications	Action	Not Indicated for—	Special Precautions	Hazards	Rate of Infusion
Whole Blood	Symptomatic anemia with large volume deficit	Restoration of oxygen-carrying capacity, restoration of blood volume	Condition responsive to specific component	Must be ABO-identical Labile coagulation factors deteriorate within 24 hours after collection	Infectious diseases; septic/toxic, allergic, febrile reactions; circulatory overload	For massive loss, fast as patient can tolerate
Red Blood Cells	Symptomatic anemia	Restoration of oxygen-carrying capacity	Pharmacologically treatable anemia Coagulation deficiency	Must be ABO-compatible	Infectious diseases; septic/toxic, allergic, febrile reactions	As patient can tolerate but less than 4 hours
Red Blood Cells, Leukocytes Removed	Symptomatic anemia, febrile reactions from leukocyte antibodies	Restoration of oxygen-carrying capacity	Pharmacologically treatable anemia Coagulation deficiency	Must be ABO-compatible	Infectious diseases; septic/toxic, allergic reaction (unless plasma also removed, *e.g.*, by washing)	As patient can tolerate but less than 4 hours
Red Blood Cells, Adenine-Saline Added	Symptomatic anemia with volume deficit	Restoration of oxygen-carrying capacity	Pharmacologically treatable anemia Coagulation deficiency	Must be ABO-compatible	Infectious diseases; septic/toxic, allergic, febrile reactions; circulatory overload	As patient can tolerate but less than 4 hours
Fresh Frozen Plasma	Deficit of labile and stable plasma coagulation factors and TTP	Source of labile and nonlabile plasma factors	Condition responsive to volume replacement	Should be ABO-compatible	Infectious diseases, allergic reactions, circulatory overload	Less than 4 hours
Liquid Plasma and Plasma	Deficit of stable coagulation factors	Source of nonlabile factors	Deficit of labile coagulation factors or volume replacement	Should be ABO-compatible	Infectious diseases, allergic reactions	Less than 4 hours
Cryoprecipitated AHF	Hemophilia A von Willebrand's Disease Hypofibrinogenemia Factor XIII deficiency	Provides Factor VIII, fibrinogen, vWF, Factor XIII	Conditions not deficient in contained factors	Frequent repeat doses may be necessary	Infectious diseases, allergic reactions	Less than 4 hours
Platelets: Platelets, Pheresis	Bleeding from thrombocytopenia or platelet function abnormality	Improves hemostasis	Plasma coagulation deficits and some conditions with rapid platelet destruction (*e.g.*, ITP)	Should not use some microaggregate filters (check manufacturer's instructions)	Infectious diseases; septic/toxic, allergic, febrile reactions	Less than 4 hours
Granulocytes	Neutropenia with infection	Provides granulocytes	Infection responsive to antibiotics	Must be ABO-compatible, do not use depth-type microaggregate filters	Infectious diseases, allergic reactions, febrile reactions	One pheresis unit over 2–4 hour period—closely observe for reactions

(American Association of Blood Banks. Circular of information for the use of human blood and blood components. ARC 1751 Aug. 1992.)

surface antigen (HBsAG), hepatitis B core antigen (anti-HBc), hepatitis C virus (anti-HCV), and human T-cell lymphotropic virus, type I (anti-HTLV-I) and anti-HIV 2. Alanine aminotransferase (ALT [SGPT]) should be within normal limits as a prevention against viral hepatitis. The blood is also tested for the presence of syphilis. Negative reactions are required for the blood to be used and each unit of blood is labeled certifying these results.

Blood Components. Whole blood is a complex tissue with both cellular and many noncellular plasma components. Whole blood is necessary only in certain clinical situations; many times, component therapy can replace the particular deficiency without subjecting the patient to unnecessary risks, such as circulatory overload. In addition, the use for components is more economical because the needs of more than one patient can be met from a single blood donation. Many blood banks are able to separate whole blood into these fractions, and all of the components are available from the American Red Cross. Table 32-4 describes the major indications, actions, special precautions, hazards, and rate of infusion for the most commonly prescribed blood components.

Hemophilia. Two additional components are used to treat hemophilia. Factor VIII concentrate (antihemophilic factor) is a lyophilized (freeze-dried) concentrate of pooled fractionated human plasma. It is used in the treatment of hemophilia A. Factor IX concentrate (prothrombin complex) is similarly prepared and contains factors II, VII, IX, and X. It is used primarily for the treatment of patients with factor IX deficiency (hemophilia B or Christmas disease). It is also useful for the treatment of patients with congenital factor VII and X deficiencies. Both components are heat treated to reduce the risk of transmitting infectious diseases.

Albumin. Plasma albumin is a large protein molecule that usually stays within vessels and is a major contributor to plasma oncotic pressure. This material is used to expand the blood volume of patients in hypovolemic shock and to elevate the level of circulating albumin in patients with hypoalbuminemia. These preparations, in contrast to all other fractions of human blood, cellular or soluble, are subjected to heating at 60°C (140°F) for 10 hours to free them of viral contaminants.

Transfusion Techniques

Administration of blood and blood components demands knowledge of correct administration techniques and knowledge of possible complications. The method for administering a transfusion is presented in Guideline 32-1.

GUIDELINE 32–1
Transfusion of Blood or Blood Products

Preprocedure

1. Verify that patient has signed a written consent form.
2. Check that patient's blood has been typed and cross matched.
3. Confirm that the transfusion has been prescribed.
4. Explain the procedure to the patient.
5. Obtain the blood or blood components.
   a. Double check the labels with another nurse to make sure that the ABO group and RH type agree with the compatibility record.
   b. Check the blood for gas bubbles and any unusual color or cloudiness.
      Gas bubbles may indicate bacterial growth.
      Abnormal color or cloudiness may be a sign of hemolysis.
   c. Check to see that the number and type on the donor blood label and on the recipient chart are correct.
6. Check the patient's identification by asking the patient's name and checking the identification wristband.
7. Double check the patient's chart for blood type and number.
8. Take patient's temperature, pulse, respiration, and blood pressure to establish a baseline for comparing vital signs at a later time.

Procedure

1. Wear gloves in accordance with Universal Precautions that stipulate that gloves be worn during all procedures involving possible contact with blood or other body fluids.
2. Record vital signs before beginning the transfusion.
3. Never add medications to blood or blood products.
4. Make sure blood is administered within 30 minutes of removing it from the refrigerator.
5. If blood must be warmed, heat it by an in-line blood warmer with a monitoring system.
   Blood is never warmed in water or a microwave oven.
6. Use a 19-gauge or larger needle for placement in a large vein.
7. Use special tubing that contains a blood filter to screen out fibrin clots and other particulate matter.
8. Do not vent the blood container.
9. For first 15 minutes, run the transfusion slowly—no faster than 5 ml/minute.
10. Observe the patient carefully for adverse effects.
11. If no adverse effects occur during the first 15 minutes, increase the flow rate unless the patient is at high risk for circulatory overload.
12. Observe the patient frequently throughout the transfusion.
    a. Monitor closely for 15–30 minutes to detect signs of reaction or circulatory overload.
    b. Monitor vital signs at regular intervals.
13. Note that administration time does not exceed 4 hours because of the increased risk for bacterial proliferation.
14. Be alert for signs of adverse reactions:
    a. Circulatory overload
    b. Sepsis
    c. Febrile reaction
    d. Allergic reaction
    e. Acute hemolytic reaction

Home Care Considerations

Blood transfusions are being administered at home by nurses employed by some home health care agencies. Patients with sickle cell anemia, chronic anemia, AIDS, and cancer are the most appropriate candidates for a home blood transfusion. Verification and administration of the blood product follow a procedure similar to that in a hospital setting.

Complications and Nursing Management

Every patient who receives a blood transfusion may develop complications from the transfusion therapy. When explaining the reasons for the transfusion to the patient, the nurse should include the risks and benefits and what to expect during and after the transfusion. Patients must be informed that the supply of blood is not completely risk-free but that it has been tested carefully. Nursing management is directed toward preventing complications and promptly initiating measures to control any complications that occur. Transfusion complications include the following:

Circulatory overload
Sepsis
Febrile, non-hemolytic reaction
Allergic reaction
Acute hemolytic reaction
Delayed hemolytic reaction
Diseases transmitted by the transfusion

Circulatory Overload. In patients with normal blood volume (as in chronic anemia) or increased blood volume (as in renal failure or heart failure), the addition of whole blood or packed cells can precipitate pulmonary edema. Packed red cells are safer to use; if the rate of administration is sufficiently slow, circulatory overload may be prevented.

- The *signs of circulatory overload* include dyspnea, orthopnea, tachycardia, or sudden anxiety. If the transfusion is continued, severe dyspnea and coughing of pink, frothy sputum can occur. Neck vein distention, crackles at the base of the lungs, and a rise in central venous pressure will occur.
- The patient is placed in an upright position with the feet in a dependent position, the blood is discontinued, and the physician is notified. The intravenous line is kept patent with a very slow infusion of normal saline to retain access to the vein in case intravenous medications are necessary. Phlebotomy or diuretics, oxygen, morphine, and aminophylline may be necessary if improvement does not occur rapidly.

Sepsis. Patients may develop a fever during transfusion because of the presence of contaminated blood products. Because of the widespread use of disposable transfusion equipment, bacterial pyrogens are rarely a cause.

Preventive measures include administering blood within a 4-hour period before warm room temperatures promote bacterial growth, and inspecting blood or components for gas bubbles, clotting, or abnormal color. Infrequently, blood can be grossly contaminated with large numbers of microorganisms that survive in the 4°C (39.2°F) storage. If such blood is infused, the patient develops fever and shaking chills within 30 minutes, and shock soon follows. Even when the cause of this reaction is recognized early (by Gram stain of the donor blood), mortality is high.

As soon as the reaction is recognized, the transfusion is discontinued and the intravenous line is kept open with normal saline. The physician and blood bank are notified and the blood container is returned to the blood bank. The patient's temperature is monitored 30 minutes after the chill and as indicated thereafter. Antipyretics are administered as prescribed. Aspirin is not administered to patients with thrombocytopenia. Septicemia is treated with intravenous fluids, corticosteroids, and vasopressors.

Febrile, Non-hemolytic Reaction. This is the most common type of reaction to a transfusion. It is caused by sensitivity to donor WBCs, platelets, or plasma proteins. It is often seen in previously transfused patients or women who have borne children. The patient's temperature rises during the administration of blood or shortly afterward and may be associated with chills and malaise. This type of reaction has a good prognosis; the treatment is an antipyretic medication. Subsequent transfusions should use blood with reduced amounts of leukocytes.

Allergic Reaction. Some patients may develop urticaria (hives) or generalized itching or, rarely, wheezing or anaphylaxis. The cause of these reactions is thought to be sensitivity to a plasma protein in the transfused blood, or passive transfer of antibodies from the donor that react with some antigen to which the recipient is exposed. The reactions are usually mild and respond to antihistamines. If a skin rash and itching (urticaria) are the only symptoms, the transfusion can sometimes be continued at a slower rate. If the reaction is severe, parenteral epinephrine is used.

Future reactions may be prevented by giving the patient antihistamines prior to the transfusion. Subsequent transfusions consist of leukocyte-reduced (leukocyte-poor) blood products. There are several methods to produce this product: red blood cell washing, administration of blood products through specially designed filters, and laboratory techniques that filter the blood prior to administration.

Acute Hemolytic Reaction. The most dangerous type of transfusion reaction occurs when the donor blood is incompatible with that of the recipient. Antibodies in the recipient's plasma rapidly combine with antigens on donor erythrocytes, and the cells are hemolyzed (destroyed) either in the circulation or in the reticuloendothelial system. The most rapid hemolysis occurs in ABO incompatibility (*e.g.*, if the donor is group A and the recipient is group O, and therefore has anti-A and anti-B antibodies). Rh incompatibility is often less severe. This reaction can occur after transfusion of as little as 10 ml of blood.

- *Symptoms* consist of chills, low back pain, headache, nausea, or chest tightness, followed by fever, hypotension, and vascular collapse, and may result in death. Severe reactions usually start within 15 minutes after the transfusion is begun. Hemoglobinuria (red urine) appears at the next voiding.
- The reaction must be recognized promptly and the transfusion discontinued immediately. The most common causes of this reaction are the result of administration errors in labeling and patient identification.

Treatment is directed toward correcting the hypotension and preventing the renal damage that can follow hemoglobinuria.

The patient is supported with intravenous colloid and administered mannitol as an osmotic diuretic to maintain adequate urine flow, glomerular filtration, and renal blood flow. An indwelling urinary catheter often is necessary to measure output accurately. If, after 24 hours, urine flow cannot be maintained, mannitol is contraindicated because it can be assumed that acute tubular necrosis has occurred. The subsequent management will be that for the renal disorder and will include fluid restriction and possibly dialysis until spontaneous recovery of normal function occurs.

Delayed Hemolytic Reaction. Delayed hemolytic reactions usually occur at about 2 to 14 days and are recognized by fever, mild jaundice, a gradual fall in hemoglobin level, and a direct anti–human globulin test. Rarely is there hemoglobinuria, and generally these reactions are not dangerous. Recognition is important, however, because subsequent transfusions may cause an acute hemolytic reaction. Patients should be alerted to the possibility of this reaction and instructed to report it immediately.

Diseases Transmitted by Blood Transfusion. The following diseases are transmittable by blood transfusion even with donor screening and blood testing prior to infusion:

Hepatitis. Hepatitis is an important risk of transfusion therapy, both for whole blood and for most components. Blood and blood products obtained from paid donors carry a higher risk than those from volunteer donors. Pooled blood products also constitute a significantly higher risk. Tests are used to detect hepatitis B virus, as well as hepatitis C. Hepatitis is further discussed in Chapter 38.

Malaria. Malaria may be transmitted in blood donated by asymptomatic persons who have been exposed to the disease. Recipients develop high fever and headache several weeks after the transfusion.

Acquired Immunodeficiency Syndrome (AIDS). The human retroviruses (HIV and HTLV) have been associated with transfusion of blood products. For this reason persons who engage in high risk behaviors (*i.e.*, sex with multiple partners, anal sex, intravenous drug use, sex with persons at risk for AIDS), and persons with signs and symptoms suggestive of the disease should not donate blood. All donated blood is now tested for the presence of antibodies to the AIDS virus.

Graft-Versus-Host Disease. Blood transfusion is a type of tissue transplant. Engraftment of donor lymphocytes in immunocompromised recipients could result in graft-versus-host disease when transfused lymphocytes attack the lymphocytes or body tissues of the recipient. It occurs 2 to 30 days following the transfusion. High fever, skin rash that is diffuse, nausea, vomiting, and diarrhea are symptoms of this disease. Irradiating blood products inactivates donor lymphocytes, lessening the chance of this complication. There are no known risks of radiation to the person receiving or administering this type of blood product.

Cytomegalovirus (CMV). CMV can be transmitted to premature newborns who have a CMV antibody-negative mother and in other immunocompromised recipients of cellular blood products. Leukocyte-reduced blood transfusions have been effective in reducing the transmission of this virus.

Gerontologic Considerations. The elderly patient who is receiving blood products is assessed for signs of circulatory overload. Rapid infusions of large volumes can result in congestive heart failure. Nursing care should include careful assessment of cardiac and pulmonary function and monitoring of fluid intake and output.

Nursing Interventions in Transfusion Reactions

If it is suspected that a transfusion reaction is occurring because of any of the conditions mentioned previously, the nurse should stop the transfusion and notify the physician immediately. The following steps are taken so that a diagnosis may be made regarding the type and severity of the reaction:

- The transfusion set is disconnected, but the intravenous line is kept patent with a normal saline solution (0.9%) in case intravenous medication should be needed rapidly.
- The blood container and tubing are saved, not discarded. They are sent to the blood bank for repeat typing and culture. The identifying tags and numbers are verified.
- The symptoms are treated as prescribed by the physician and vital signs are monitored.
- The patient's blood is drawn for plasma hemoglobin, culture, and retyping.
- A urine sample is collected as soon as possible and sent to the laboratory for a hemoglobin determination. Subsequent voidings of urine should be observed.
- The blood bank is notified that a suspected transfusion reaction has occurred.
- The reaction is documented according to the institution's policy.

Pharmacologic Alternatives to Blood Transfusions

Erythropoietin (Epoetin Alfa) has been an effective alternative treatment for patients with chronic anemia secondary to chronic renal disease. The major effect of this medication is to stimulate erythropoiesis. It has also been used for patients who are anemic from chemotherapy or AZT therapy, or who have diseases with bone marrow suppression or sickle cell disease. The medication can be administered intravenously or subcutaneously. More sustained plasma levels are achieved by the subcutaneous route.

DDAVP is a synthetic form of L-arginine vasopressin, an antidiuretic that occurs naturally in the body. It is effective in treating hemorrhagic disorders related to platelet dysfunction or thrombocytopenia. The primary uses of this medication are to manage bleeding episodes in patients with hemophilia A and von Willebrand's disease. Other uses include bleeding in patients with acute or chronic renal failure, and bleeding due to aspirin ingestion, cirrhosis of the liver, and cardiac and orthopedic surgeries.

Routes of administration for DDAVP are intravenous, subcutaneous, and intranasal. There are few serious side effects. Facial flushing, nausea, mild headache, abdominal cramps, and vulval pain have been reported.

Research continues to seek a red cell substitute that is practical and safe.

Bone Marrow Transplantation

Bone marrow transplantation (BMT) is a therapeutic possibility for some patients with hematologic disorders, specifically severe aplastic anemia, some forms of leukemia, and thalassemia. Success of the treatment depends on tissue compatibility and the patient's tolerance of immunosuppression if the donor cells are not autologous. Patients require intensive nursing care that is directed toward prevention of infection and assessment for early signs and symptoms of complications. See Chapter 16 for a detailed presentation of care of the patient who has received bone marrow transplantation.

CRITICAL THINKING EXERCISES

1. An elderly patient who is anemic indicates that she believes that the anemia is due to her age, and she questions why she must have so many tests performed. What explanation would you give this patient about the importance of the diagnostic tests?
2. You are caring for a young adult patient who has had repeated hospitalizations for sickle cell crisis. What factors should be assessed to determine the patient's teaching needs?
3. You are caring for a patient who is being treated for leukemia. The family members are very concerned about the patient's risk for infection when she returns home from the hospital. What instructions should they be given about decreasing the risks for infection?
4. You are caring for a patient who is to receive a transfusion of packed red blood cells. The patient expresses anxiety about receiving the blood and indicates that the physician has not explained to her the risks, benefits, and alternatives of the transfusion. What actions would you take?

BIBLIOGRAPHY

Books

Agency for Health Care Policy and Research (AHCPR) Guidelines. Sickle Cell Disease: Screening, Diagnosis, Management, and Counseling in Newborns and Infants. Clinical practice guideline, Number 6. AHCPR Publication No. 93-0562. Rockville, MD, Agency for Health Care Policy and Research, Public Health Service, U.S. Department of Health and Human Services, April 1993.

Baird SB et al. Cancer Nursing: A Comprehensive Textbook. Philadelphia, WB Saunders, 1991.

Brain MC and Carbone PP. Current Therapy in Hematology Oncology 4. St. Louis, Mosby-Year Book, 1991.

Burke MB et al. Cancer Chemotherapy: A Nursing Process Approach. Boston, Jones and Bartlett, 1991.

Mankad VN and Moore RB (ed). Sickle Cell Disease: Pathophysiology, Diagnosis and Management. Westport, CT, Praeger, 1992.

Whedon MB. Bone Marrow Transplantation: Principles, Practice and Nursing Insights. Boston, Jones and Bartlett, 1991.

Journals

Asterisks indicate nursing research articles.

General

Canellos GP et al. Chemotherapy of advanced Hodgkin's disease with MOPP and ABVD or MOPP alternating with ABVD. N Engl J Med 1992 Nov 19; 327(21):1478–1484.

Hutman S. New approaches to the diagnosis and treatment of AIDS-related lymphoma. AIDS Patient Care 1992 Oct; 6(5):214–219.

Keating MJ et al. New drugs in the treatment of chronic lymphocytic leukemia. Leukemia 1992 Nov; 6 suppl(4):140–141.

Meyer C. The new drugs. The class of 1991. Am J Nurs 1991 Dec; 91(12):40–43.

Ready N and Freeman NJ. Treatment choices in chronic myelogenous leukemia. Hospital Practice 1992 Sep 30; 27(9A):95–98.

Schiller G et al. Long-term outcome of high-dose cytarabine-based consolidation chemotherapy for adults with acute myelogenous leukemia. Blood 1992 Dec 15; 80(12):2977–2982.

Timmerman PR. Intravenous immunoglobulin in oncology nursing practice. Onc Nurs Forum 1993 Jan/Feb; 20(1):69–74.

*White KS. Patient awareness of health precautions after splenectomy. Am J Infect Control 1991 Feb; 19(1):36–41.

York S and Jones D. Monitoring a home epogen program. American Nephrology Nurses Association Journal 1992 Apr; 19(2):164.

Anemia

Adams PC and Zauderer B. Sickle cell anemia: Clinical update. Medsurg Nurs Q 1993 Spring; 1(4):2–20.

Anand A. Future directions in sickle cell disease. West J Med 1993 May; 158(5):536–537.

*Armstrong FA et al. Impact of children's sickle cell history on nurse and physician ratings of pain and medicine decisions. J Pediatr Psychol 1992 May; 17(5):651–664.

Auerhahn C. Recognition and management of alcohol-related nutritional deficiencies. Nurse Practitioner 1992 Dec; 17(12): 40–49.

Bacigalupo A et al. Treatment of aplastic anaemia (AA) with antilymphocyte globulin (ALG) and methylprednisolone (MPred) with or without androgens; a randomized trial from the EBMT SAA working party. British Journal of Haematology 1993 Jan; 83(1):145–151.

Bolivar E. Hemophilia and AIDS: Dealing with nurse burnout. Caring Magazine 1991 July; 10(7):50–54.

Bushnell FKL. A guide to primary care of iron-deficiency anemia. Nurse Practitioner 1992 Nov; 17(11):68–74.

Butler DJ and Beltran LR. Functions of an adult sickle cell group: Education, task orientation, and support. Health and Social Work 1993 Feb; 18(1):49–55.

Cerrato PL. Your patient's anemic—but the problem isn't iron. RN 1991 Jul; 54(7):61–64.

Charache S. Experimental therapy of sickle cell disease. Use of hydroxyurea. American Journal of Pediatric Hematology-Oncology 1994 Feb; 16(1):62–66.

Charache S. Pharmacological modification of hemoglobin F expression in sickle cell anemia: An update on hydroxyurea studies. Experimentia 1993 Feb 15; 49(2):126–132.

Crump M et al. Treatment of adults with severe aplastic anemia: Primary therapy with antithymocyte globulin [ATG] and rescue of ATG failures with bone marrow transplantation. Am J Med 1992 June; 92(6):596–602.

Doheny MO et al. Caring for the orthopaedic patient with sickle cell disease. Orthopaedic Nursing 1992 Jan/Feb; 11(1):41–48.

Esposito NW. Thalassemias: Simple screening for hereditary anemias. Nurse Practitioner 1992 Feb; 17(2):52–57.

Facon et al. Treatment of severe aplastic anemia with antilymphocyte globulin and androgens: A report on 38 patients. Annals of Hematology 1991 Aug; 63(2):89–93.

Goldberg MA et al. Treatment of sickle cell anemia with hydroxyurea and erythropoietin. N Engl J Med 1990 Aug 9; 328(6): 366–372.

Kojima S et al. Treatment of aplastic anemia with antithymocyte globulin, Lymphoser Berna. Japanese Journal of Clinical Hematology 1993 Jul; 34(7):815–820.

London F. Nursing diagnoses and caring for patients with sickle cell disease. Advancing Clinical Care 1990 Sep–Oct; 5(5):12–16.

Meyer C. Erythropoietin fights anemia, for some. Am J Nurs 1993 Jan; 93(1):12.

Pollin S and DeLuca E. How to use the new weapon against anemia. RN 1992 Jan; 55(1):36–38.

Rivers R and Williamson N. Sickle cell anemia: Complex disease, nursing challenge. RN June 1990; 53(6):24–29.

Blood Transfusion Therapy

American Association of Blood Banks et al. Circular of information for the use of human blood and blood components. ARC 1751 August 1992.

Autologous transfusion for elective surgery. Emergency Medicine 1992 Oct; 1524(14):73,77.

Baranowski L. Current trends in blood component therapy: The evolution of a safer, more effective product. Journal of Intravenous Nursing 1992 May/June; 15(3):136–151.

Educator suggests guidelines for home blood transfusions. Hospital Home Health 1991 Feb; 8(2):17–19.

Transfusion nursing: Trends and practices for the '90s. Choosing blood components and equipment. Am J Nurs 1991 June; 91(6):42–55.

Disseminated Intravascular Coagulopathy

Bailes BK. Disseminated intravascular coagulation: Principle, treatment, nursing management. Association of Operating Room Nursing Journal 1992 Feb; 55(2):517–529.

Epstein C and Bakanauskas A. Clinical management of DIC: Early nursing interventions. Critical Care Nurse 1991 Nov/Dec; 11(10):43, 45–53.

Huston CJ. Disseminated intravascular coagulation. Am J Nurs 1994; 94(8):51.

AGENCIES

American Cancer Society
1599 Clifton Rd NE
Atlanta, GA 30329

American Red Cross
1730 E Street NW,
Washington, DC 20006

Leukemia Society of America
733 Third Avenue,
New York, NY 10017

National Association for Sickle Cell Disease, Inc.
4221 Wilshire Boulevard, Suite 360,
Los Angeles, CA 90010-3503

National Hemophilia Foundation
104 East 40th Street, Room 306,
New York, NY 10016

Nursing Research Profile for Unit 7

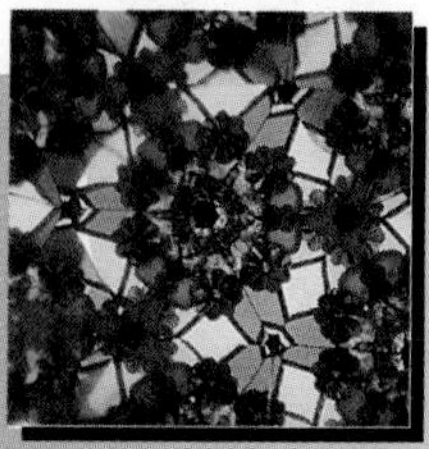

Overview

Nursing research here focuses on the physiologic responses, educational needs, and coping abilities of patients who have medical and surgical problems related to cardiovascular dysfunctions.

Duryee R. The efficacy of inpatient education after myocardial infarction. Heart Lung 1992 May; 21(3):217–224.

Educating the patient who has experienced a myocardial infarction (MI) has long been a challenge for the professional nurse. Nurses have prepared volumes of teaching materials to enlighten the patient who has experienced an MI.

The purpose of this study was to review the research literature on in-patient education after MI published between 1975 and 1989. The review of 21 studies sought to determine what information is most important to patients; whether in-patient teaching increases patient knowledge; the effect, if any, of anxiety upon learning; whether life-style changes are affected by education; and which instructional methods were most effective.

The information needs determined as being most important to the patient were those that are described as management versus explanatory. For example, patients were more interested in what to do about chest pain than in knowing about the cause of the pain. The primary concern for patients across all studies was that of risk factor management. Other areas of concern to patients were medications, activities, and control of symptoms. One study identified a disparity between what the nurse ranked as most important and what the patient ranked as most important.

Twelve of the 21 studies reviewed assessed the effect of in-patient education on patient knowledge after MI. In general the studies reveal that in-patient education can positively affect learning, especially with regard to activity. The studies reviewed documented some behavioral changes following discharge, especially related to activity and smoking. Dietary habits were least altered.

Nurses have held that anxiety precludes the patient's ability to learn during the acute hospital phase. One study reviewed supported an inverse relationship between anxiety and learning; that is, when anxiety is high, learning is low. This study has not been replicated.

Multiple teaching methods were used across the 21 studies reviewed: individual and group sessions led by nurse rehabilitators, slide-sound presentations, videotape presentations, programmed instructions, and individual sessions with a nurse. The studies demonstrated that audiovisual methods are as effective as presentations by an educator.

Nursing Implications. Further studies are required to validate the reported effect of anxiety on learning. In addition, information directed toward what the patient needs to do at home, rather than topics such as anatomy and physiology, is of most benefit to the patient. The support of dietitians in developing creative ways to encourage dietary modifications is essential. The utilization of audiotapes can be as effective as one-to-one counseling and may be more efficient for nursing staff, particularly in light of short hospital stays.

Robertson D and Keller C. Relationships among health beliefs, self-efficacy, and exercise adherence in patients with coronary artery disease. Heart Lung 1992 Jan; 21(1):56–63.

Many nursing care hours are dedicated to educating patients with coronary artery disease about their disease process and requisite life-style changes in order to maximize life expectancy. New therapies may abort life-threatening events; however, control of the progression of coronary artery disease is ultimately dependent upon the patient's cooperation in modifying risk factors. Too often health care recommendations go unheeded.

The purpose of this study was to develop a model that would explain relationships among several variables that determined adherence to an exercise regimen. The variables were chosen from the Health Belief Model (HBM) and the self-efficacy theory. Self-efficacy, perceived severity, barriers, benefits, and cues to action as they applied to exercise adherence were the variables selected for study.

A convenience sample of 51 men and women was selected. These subjects had undergone either a PTCA or CABG in the previous 4 to 8 months. The subjects responded to five different instruments. The scales were designed to measure a person's perception of (1) benefits of a recommended health behavior, (2) identified barriers to a health behavior, (3) the seriousness of the illness, (4) confidence in performing the activity, and (5) whether they performed the activity and how often.

Study findings revealed a significant positive correlation ($r = 0.229$, $p = 0.016$) between activity and perceived benefits and between activity and perceived self-efficacy. There was a significant negative relationship ($r = -0.390$, $p = 0.005$) between activity and perceived barriers. In addition, subjects who had had CABG were found to walk for longer periods of time than subjects who had had PTCA ($p = 0.014$). Perceived barriers, self-efficacy, and type of surgery explained 31% of the variance in exercise adherence, with perceived barriers providing the greatest degree of variance.

Nursing Implications. The study results confirm the difficulty in gaining compliance with health behavior modification after a diagnosis of coronary artery disease is made.

The need to assess each patient as an individual and to evaluate the patient's perception of benefits, barriers, severity of illness, and self-efficacy is important. Such assessment data can be used to identify patients who may have unrealistic expectations about the nature of their disease and who are likely to be noncompliant with their discharge exercise program. The nurse can encourage the patient by assessing his strengths and limitations and using these to plan a more realistic health care regimen with which he can choose to comply.

Beach EK et al. The spouse: A factor in recovery after acute myocardial infarction. Heart Lung 1992 Jan; 21(1):30–38.

Many studies have reported the increased potential of recovery for patients with strong family support systems. This study examines spouses of patients who have had an acute MI to determine the role of the spouse in the patient's recovery from acute MI. In particular, the social support of the spouse, family stress, marital satisfaction, and sexual comfort were researched.

The investigators used a longitudinal, descriptive methodology. Seventeen spouses (14 women and 3 men) participated in the study. The Social Support Inventory was used to measure social support; Family Inventory of Life Events Scale was used to measure family stress; Spanier's Dyadic Adjustment Scale was used to measure marital satisfaction; and comfort with sexual activity was measured with a Likert-type scale developed by the investigators. Recovery of the patient was defined by the score on the Myocardial Infarction Recovery Index. Data were collected four times: before discharge, at home visit 3 weeks following discharge and 3 months following acute MI, and at 6 months following acute MI (via telephone interview).

Findings of the study revealed a weak but statistically significant positive relationship between the spouse's family stress ($r = 0.42$, $p = 0.09$) and marital satisfaction ($r = 0.42$, $p = 0.10$) and the patient's recovery. In addition, the spouse's comfort with sexual activity was found to be significantly ($p = 0.10$) positively correlated with the patient's recovery from acute MI. The researchers concluded that the patient's recovery process after acute MI is influenced by the spouse's ability to cope with situational stressors.

Nursing Implications. Because the study did not address whether strategies that help spouses to deal with their stresses during the patient's recovery from acute MI improve recovery, the findings cannot be used to guide specific clinical treatment. However, the findings do provide data that indicate spouses should be assessed to determine if referral for support and follow-up are indicated. Further studies are needed to identify the most beneficial responses by spouses during the recovery period following acute MI.

Miracle VA and Hovekamp G. Needs of families of patients undergoing invasive cardiac procedures. Am J Crit Care 1994 Mar; 3(2):155–157.

This study was directed toward examining the specific needs of families waiting for patients undergoing percutaneous transluminal coronary angioplasty (PTCA) or cardiac catheterization. A descriptive design using convenience sampling and a survey approach was used by the investigator. Two hundred family members of patients having invasive cardiac procedures were asked to participate at the time that the patient was being prepared to leave the recovery room. These family members were given a 25-item questionnaire rated on a 4-point Likert scale; they were asked to return the survey within 2 weeks. Ninety-five subjects (48%) returned the survey. The majority (61%) were spouses of patients having cardiac catheterization and had no prior experience with this procedure.

The results demonstrated findings similar to those of studies of the needs of families of patients in ICUs during longer waiting periods of time. The need that was rated highest was information—about the procedure, the patient's condition, results of the procedure, prognosis, and possible complications. Subjects also indicated a need to feel that the staff were concerned about them. Comfort measures such as a private, comfortable waiting place and availability of beverages were rated lowest.

Nursing Implications. It is helpful to family members to receive explanations about the patient's condition and the procedure. A visit with the patient before and after the procedure is comforting to the family. If the nurse is not free to provide information to the family during or immediately after a procedure, this can be delegated to a responsible individual such as a clergy member or a patient representative. Further study is required to confirm the findings of the study.

Gaw B. Motivation to change life-style following PTCA. DCCN 1992 Mar; 11(2):68–74.

The purpose of this study was to determine if patients who have had successful PTCAs consider themselves cured of coronary artery disease. Fourteen PTCA patients were interviewed to gather qualitative data regarding their perceptions of cardiac disease, pre-procedure concerns, post-procedure concerns, and family concerns. There were seven men and seven women in the sample. Four of the patients had had a previous PTCA, eight a coronary angiogram, and two were having their first experience with PTCA. There were three interviews, one prior to the procedure and two after (one in the hospital, the other after discharge).

Seven of the 14 patients were able to identify their risk factors for coronary artery disease. Two patients did not identify that they had heart disease. Patients with a history of myocardial infarction had a higher level of knowledge regarding heart disease than did the other patients. During the post-procedure hospital interview, five patients reported intentions to modify their life-style. However, all five indicated that upon returning home and feeling better, they no longer felt it necessary to modify their life-styles. The researchers concluded that patients who have had successful PTCAs do consider themselves cured of coronary artery disease.

Nursing Implications. Pre-PTCA education should include an assessment of the patient's understanding of the diagnosis of coronary artery disease. Education regarding risk factor and life-style modification should be provided to all patients diagnosed with coronary artery disease and reinforced prior to and after PTCA. Each patient's motivations for PTCA and life-style changes should be identified. The recommendations for life-style changes should be discussed with the physician and family members. Cardiac rehabilitation should be encouraged for all patients diagnosed with coronary artery disease.

Hixon M. Perceived quality of life before and after percutaneous balloon valvuloplasty. Heart Lung 1992 May; 21(3):290.

Balloon valvuloplasty is used as a treatment modality for patients with stenotic valvular heart disease. The purpose of this study was to describe patients' perceived quality of life (QOL) before and after valvuloplasty. A non-randomized sample of 15 patients participated in this descriptive study. Their perceptions of quality of life were measured by use of the Quality of Life Index–Cardiac III on two occasions: before the procedure and 4 weeks after the procedure.

A significant ($p < 0.05$) improvement was found in the mean QOL scores after valvuloplasty. Significant ($p < 0.05$) improvements were also found in the QOL areas of health and functioning. Improvement in the psychological/spiritual area fo QOL was also found, although this improvement did not reach significance.

Nursing Implications. The findings of this study can provide nurses with knowledge about life-style changes that require patient teaching, intervention, and supportive measures that could improve patient outcomes.

Cupples SA. Effects of timing and reinforcement of preoperative education on knowledge and recovery of patients having coronary artery bypass graft surgery. Heart Lung 1991 Nov; 20(6):654–660.

Patient education is an essential nursing role. This study attempted to identify if the timing of preoperative teaching for coronary artery bypass surgery patients resulted in differences in knowledge, postoperative anxiety and mood, and recovery. A convenience sample ($n = 40$) of two groups was studied. The experimental group of 20 patients attended 45- to 60-minute class at the surgeon's office 5 to 14 days before admission. Both the control and experimental groups received the routine preoperative education after admission to the hospital. The patients completed a knowledge assessment questionnaire and anxiety scale after their initial education session. Anxiety was reevaluated after surgery. Assessments of mood and physiologic recovery were completed on the fourth postoperative day.

Analysis of the data revealed that the experimental group had significantly higher knowledge scores preoperatively, more positive mood states, and more favorable physiologic recovery. The anxiety levels were not significantly different between the groups postoperatively, and subjects of both groups were found to have elevated anxiety levels as late as the fourth postoperative day.

Nursing Implications. Preoperative teaching for coronary artery bypass surgery patients should be provided before the patient's admission to the hospital, with review of the information after admission. In addition, evaluation of the patient's anxiety level is important postoperatively, followed by appropriate interventions. Further studies are needed on larger samples and with length of hospitalization as an outcome measure.

King KB et al. Coronary artery bypass graft surgery in older women and men. Am J Crit Care 1992 March; 1(2):28–35.

This retrospective study of first-time CABG patients compared 465 women with the same number of age-matched men. The sample was further divided into individuals younger than 70 years of age and 70 years or older. The purpose of the study was to compare the women and men with regard to demographics, presence of pre-existing co-morbidities, risk factors documented at the time of admission, perioperative and postoperative complications, mortality, and length of stay. Data were obtained from hospital records.

The elderly (70 years of age or older) women and men had a higher incidence of congestive heart failure, renal disease, and hypertension preoperatively than did the younger subjects. The older patients also had longer lengths of ICU and hospital stays. The older patients had a lower incidence of smoking history. Older women had more hypertension and less diabetes preoperatively, fewer bypass grafts and shorter ischemic times, and more congestive heart failure postoperatively than the younger women. The incidence of postoperative congestive heart failure in the elderly women was also greater than in the elderly male subjects. More older men demonstrated diabetes. There was no difference in mortality between older and younger women. When compared with younger men, older men had increased mortality as well as postoperative ventricular dysrhythmias, pulmonary complications, strokes, and confusion.

Nursing Implications. Patients 70 years of age or older were found to require approximately 1 more ICU day and 2 more hospital days to recover from coronary artery bypass surgery than were younger patients. These data can be utilized for patient and family education and are important for case management, critical pathway development, and bed utilization decisions. Assessments should include particular attention to heart rate and rhythm as well as urine output and weights for patients 70 years of age or older recovering from CABG surgery.

UNIT 8

Digestive and Gastrointestinal Function

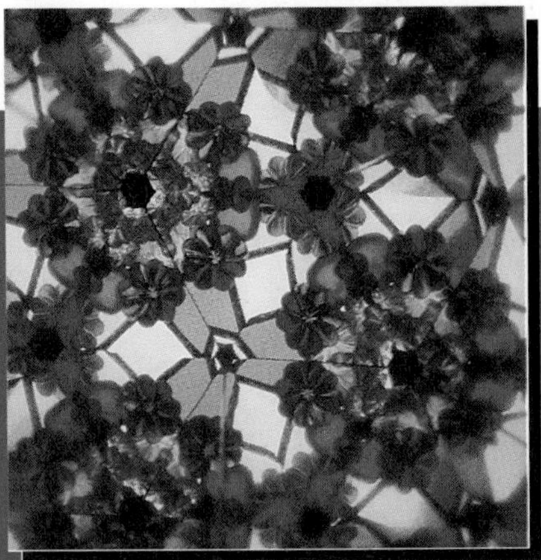

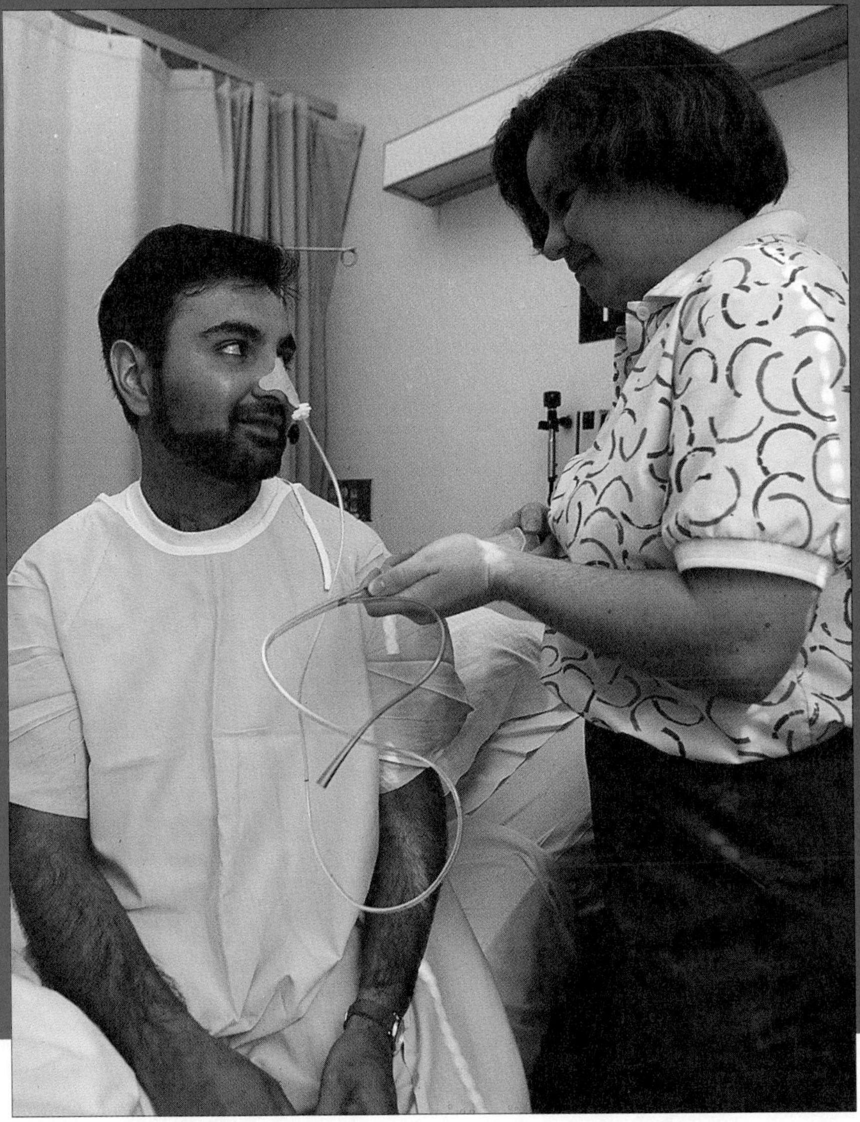

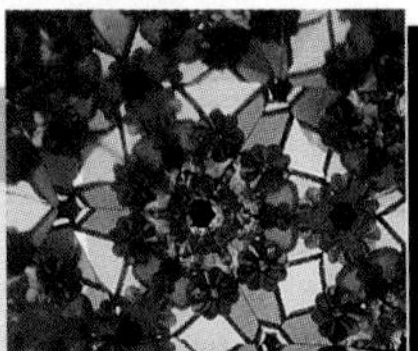

33

Assessment of Digestive and Gastrointestinal Function

CHAPTER OUTLINE

LEARNING OBJECTIVES

On completion of this chapter, the learner will be able to:

1. Describe the mechanical and chemical processes involved in digesting and absorbing foods and eliminating waste products
2. Use assessment parameters appropriate for determining the status of gastrointestinal function
3. Describe the patient preparation, teaching, and follow-up care appropriate for patients having diagnostic testing of the gastrointestinal tract.

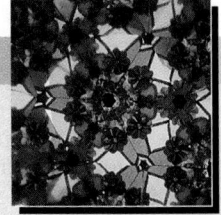

Anatomy and Physiology

The gastrointestinal (GI) tract (Fig. 33-1) is a pathway (23 to 26 feet in total length) that extends from the mouth through the esophagus, stomach, and intestines to the anus. The **esophagus** is located in the mediastinum in the thoracic cavity, anterior to the spine and posterior to the trachea and heart. This collapsible tube, which is about 25 cm (10 in) in length, becomes distended when food passes through it.

The remaining portion of the gastrointestinal tract is located within the peritoneal cavity. The **stomach** is situated in the upper portion of the abdomen to the left of the midline, just under the left diaphragm. It is a distensible pouch with a capacity of approximately 1500 ml. The inlet to the stomach is called the *esophagogastric junction*. It is surrounded by a ring of smooth muscle, called the *lower esophageal sphincter* (or cardiac sphincter), which, on contraction, closes off the stomach from the esophagus. The stomach can be divided into four anatomic regions: the cardia (entrance), fundus, body, and pylorus (outlet). Circular smooth muscle in the wall of the pylorus forms the **pyloric sphincter** and controls the opening between the stomach and small intestine.

The **small intestine** is the longest segment of the GI tract, accounting for about two thirds of the total length of the tract. It folds back and forth on itself allowing for approximately 7000 cm of surface area for secretion and absorption. The small intestine is divided into three anatomic parts: an upper part, called the *duodenum*; the middle part, called the *jejunum*; and the lower part, called the *ileum*. The common bile duct, which allows for the passage of both bile and pancreatic secretions, empties into the duodenum at the ampulla of Vater.

The junction between the small and large intestine is located in the right lower portion of the abdomen. It is called the **cecum**. At that junction is the **ileocecal valve**, which functions to control the passage of intestinal contents into the large intestine and to prevent reflux of bacteria into the small intestine. It is in this area that the **vermiform appendix** is located. The **large intestine** consists of an *ascending* segment on the right side of the abdomen, a *transverse* segment that extends from right to left in the upper abdomen, and a *descending* segment on the left side of the abdomen. The terminal portion of the large intestine consists of two parts: the **sigmoid colon** and the **rectum**. The rectum is continuous with the **anus**. The anal outlet is regulated by a network of striated muscle that forms both the **internal** and the **external anal sphincters** .

Blood Supply and Innervation of the Gastrointestinal Tract

The gastrointestinal tract receives its blood supply from many arteries that originate along the entire length of the thoracic and abdominal aorta. Of particular importance are the **gastric artery** and the **superior** and **inferior mesenteric arteries**. Oxygen and nutrients are supplied to the stomach by the gastric artery. These essential components are supplied to the intestine by the mesenteric arteries (Fig. 33-2). Blood is drained from these organs by veins that merge with others in the abdomen to form a large vessel called the **portal vein**. Nutrient-rich blood is then carried to the liver. The blood flow to the entire GI tract is about 20% of the total cardiac output; it increases significantly after eating.

The gastrointestinal tract is innervated by both the sympathetic and parasympathetic portions of the **autonomic nervous system**. In general, sympathetic nerves exert an inhibitory effect on the GI tract. Gastric secretion and motility are decreased. The sphincters and blood vessels constrict under the influence of sympathetic stimulation. Parasympathetic nerve stimulation causes peristalsis to occur and increases secretory activities. The sphincters relax under the influence of parasympathetic stimulation. The only portions of the tract under voluntary control are the upper esophagus and the external anal sphincter.

The Digestive Process

To perform their functions, all cells of the body require nutrients. These nutrients must be derived from the intake of food that contains protein, fat, carbohydrates, vitamins, and minerals, as well as cellulose fibers and other vegetable matter of no nutritional value.

The primary digestive functions of the gastrointestinal tract are specifically related to providing these body needs:

- To break down food particles into the molecular form for digestion
- To absorb into the bloodstream the small molecules produced by digestion
- To eliminate undigested and unabsorbed foodstuffs and other waste products from the body

As the food is propelled through the gastrointestinal tract, it comes into contact with a wide variety of secretions that aid in digesting, absorbing, or eliminating it from the gastrointestinal tract.

Oral Digestion

The process of digestion begins with the act of chewing, in which food is broken down into small particles that can be swallowed and mixed with digestive enzymes. Eating, or even the sight, smell, or taste of food can cause reflex salivation. Saliva is the first secretion that comes in contact with food. It is secreted in the mouth by the salivary glands at the rate of about 1.5 L daily. Saliva contains the enzyme **ptyalin**, or salivary amylase, which begins the digestion of starches (Table 33-1). Saliva also contains mucus that helps to lubricate the food as it is chewed, thereby facilitating swallowing.

Swallowing

Swallowing begins as a voluntary act that is regulated by a swallowing center in the medulla oblongata of the central nervous system. As the food is swallowed, the epiglottis moves to cover the tracheal opening and thus prevents aspiration of food into the lungs. Swallowing, which results in propelling the bolus of food into the upper esophagus, thus ends as a reflex action. The smooth muscle in the wall of the esophagus contracts in a rhythmic sequence from the upper

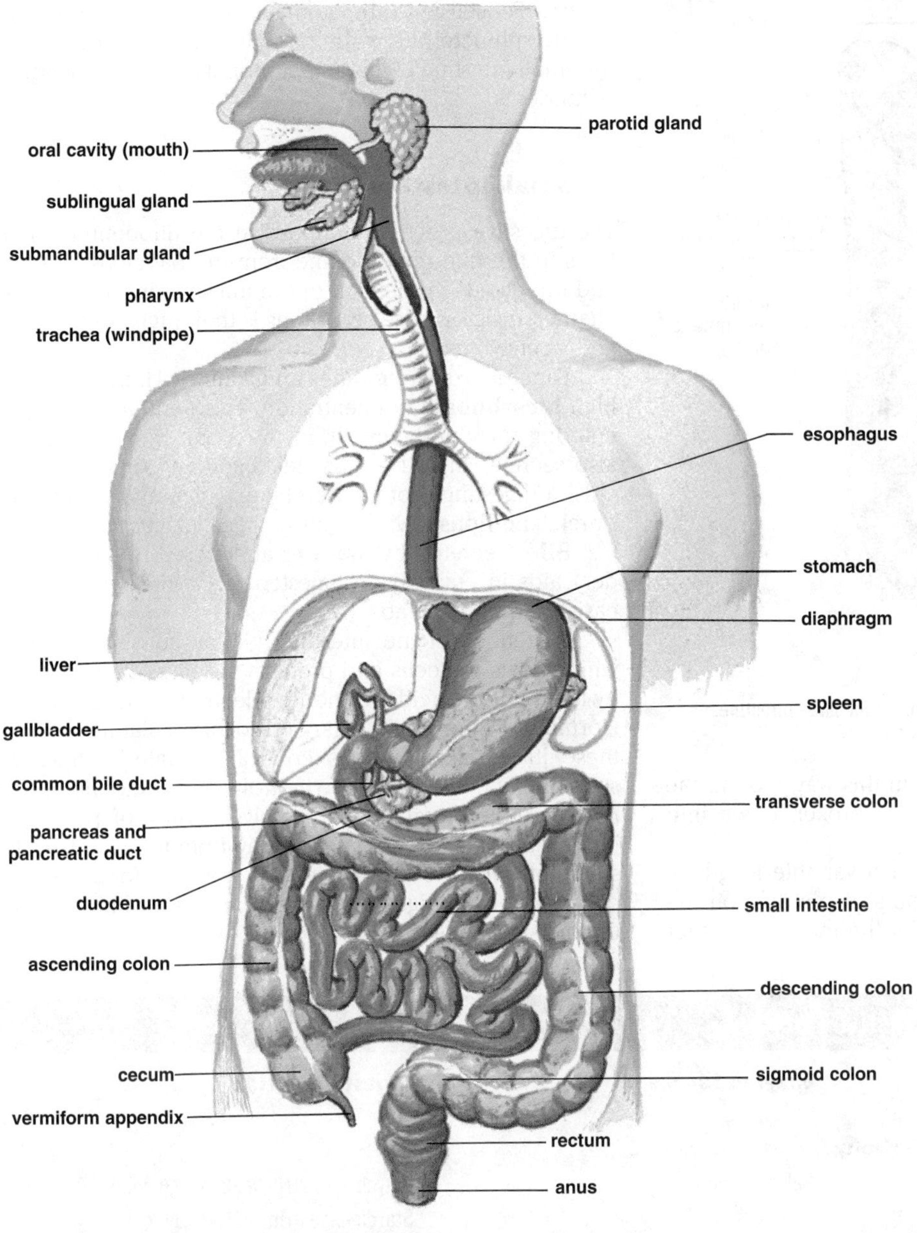

FIGURE 33-1. Organs of the digestive system and associated structures.

esophagus toward the stomach to propel the bolus of food along the tract. During this process of esophageal peristalsis, the lower esophageal sphincter relaxes and permits the bolus of food to enter the stomach. Subsequently, the lower esophageal sphincter closes tightly to prevent reflux of stomach contents into the esophagus.

- When there is reflux of the acidic contents of the stomach into the esophagus, an uncomfortable sensation occurs beneath the sternum. This sensation is commonly called *heartburn*.

Gastric Action

The stomach secretes a highly acidic fluid in response to the presence or anticipated ingestion of food. This fluid, which may have a *p*H as low as 1, derives its acidity from the **hydrochloric acid** secreted by the glands of the stomach. The function of this gastric secretion is twofold: (1) to break down food into more absorbable components and (2) to aid in the destruction of most ingested bacteria. The stomach can produce about 2.4 L/day of these gastric secretions.

Gastric secretions also contain the enzyme **pepsin**, which is important for initiating protein digestion. **Intrinsic factor** is also secreted by the gastric mucosa. This compound combines with dietary vitamin B_{12}, so that the vitamin can be absorbed in the ileum.

- In the absence of intrinsic factor, vitamin B_{12} cannot be absorbed and pernicious anemia results (see Chapter 32).

Hormones, neuroregulators, and local regulators found in the gastric secretions control the rate of gastric secretions and influence gastric motility (Table 33-2).

Peristaltic contractions in the stomach propel its contents toward the pylorus. Because large food particles cannot pass through the pyloric sphincter, they are churned

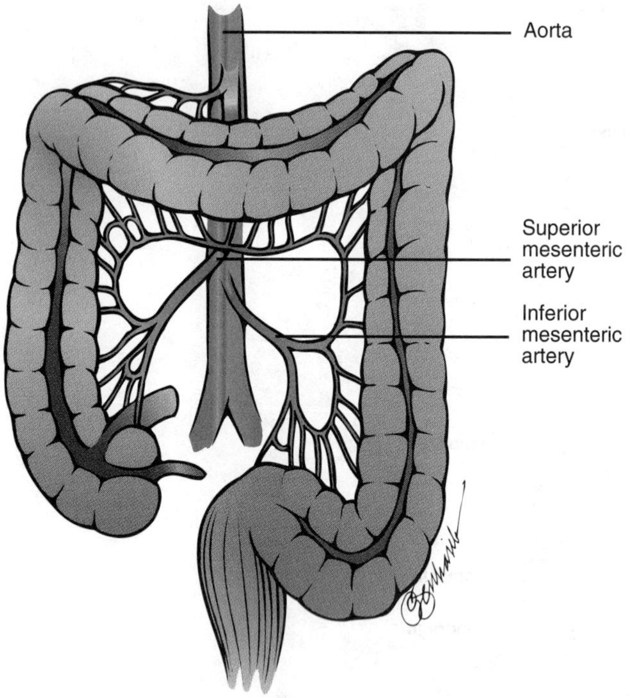

FIGURE 33-2. Anatomy and blood supply of the large intestine.

back into the body of the stomach. In this way, food in the stomach is mechanically agitated and broken down into smaller particles.

Food remains in the stomach for a variable length of time, from a half hour to several hours, depending on the size of food particles, composition of the meal, and other factors. Peristalsis in the stomach and contractions of the pyloric sphincter allow the partially digested food to enter the small intestine at a rate that permits efficient absorption of nutrients.

Small Intestine Action

The digestive process continues in the duodenum. Secretions in the duodenum come from the pancreas, the liver, and the glands in the wall of the intestine itself. The major characteristic of these secretions is their high content of digestive enzymes.

Pancreatic secretion has an alkaline *p*H, because of its high **bicarbonate** concentration. This neutralizes the acid entering the duodenum from the stomach. The pancreas also secretes digestive enzymes, including **trypsin**, which aids in digesting protein; **amylase**, which aids in digesting starch; and **lipase**, which aids in digesting fats.

Bile (secreted by the liver and stored in the gallbladder) aids in emulsifying ingested fats, which makes them easier to digest and absorb.

Secretions of the intestinal glands consist of mucus, which coats the cells and protects the mucosa from attack by hydrochloric acid, hormones, electrolytes, and enzymes. Hormones, neuroregulators, and local regulators found in these intestinal secretions control the rate of intestinal secretion and also influence gastrointestinal motility. Intestinal secretions total approximately 1 L/day of pancreatic juice, 0.5 L/day of bile, and 3 L/day from the glands of the small intestine. Refer to Tables 33-1 and 33-2 for summaries of the actions of digestive enzymes and gastrointestinal regulatory substances.

TABLE 33-1 The Major Digestive Enzymes

Enzyme	Enzyme Source	Digestive Action
Action of Enzymes that Digest Carbohydrates		
Ptyalin (salivary amylase)	Salivary glands	Starch→dextrin, maltose, glucose
Amylase	Pancreas	Starch→dextrin, maltose, glucose Dextrin→maltose, glucose
Maltase	Intestinal mucosa	Maltose→glucose
Sucrase	Intestinal mucosa	Sucrose→glucose, fructose
Lactase	Intestinal mucosa	Lactose→glucose, galactose
Action of Enzymes that Digest Protein		
Pepsin	Gastric mucosa	Protein→polypeptides
Trypsin	Pancreas	Proteins and Polypeptides→polypeptides, dipeptides, amino acids
Aminopeptidase	Intestinal mucosa	Polypeptides→dipeptides, amino acids
Dipeptidase	Intestinal mucosa	Dipeptides→amino acids
Action of Enzymes that Digest Fat (Triglyceride)		
Pharyngeal lipase	Pharynx mucosa	Triglycerides→fatty acids, diglycerides, monoglycerides
Steapsin	Gastric mucosa	Triglycerides→fatty acids, diglycerides, monoglycerides
Pancreatic lipase	Pancreas	Triglycerides→fatty acids, diglycerides, monoglycerides

TABLE 33-2 The Major Gastrointestinal Regulatory Substances

Substance	Stimulus for Production	Target Tissue	Effect on Secretions	Effect on Motility
Neuroregulators				
Acetylcholine	Sight, smell, chewing food, stomach distention	Gastric glands, other secretory glands, gastrointestinal muscle	Increased gastric acid	Generally increased; decreased sphincter tone
Norepinephrine	Stress, other various stimuli	Secretory glands, gastrointestinal muscle	Generally inhibitory	Generally decreased; increased sphincter tone
Hormonal Regulators				
Gastrin	Stomach distention with food	Gastric glands	Increased secretion of gastric juice, which is rich in HCl	Increased motility of stomach, decreased time required for gastric emptying Relaxation of ileocecal sphincter Excitation of colon Constriction of gastroesophageal sphincter
Cholecystokinin	Fat in duodenum	Gallbladder	Release of bile into duodenum	
		Pancreas	Increased production of enzyme-rich pancreatic secretions	
		Stomach	Inhibits gastric secretion somewhat	Inhibits stomach contractions
Secretin	*p*H of chyme in duodenum below 4–5	Stomach	Inhibits gastric secretion somewhat	
		Pancreas	Increased production of bicarbonate-rich pancreatic juice	
Local Regulator				
Histamine	Unclear; substances in food	Gastric glands	Increased gastric acid production	

There are two types of contractions that occur regularly in the small intestine. **Segmentation contractions** produce mixing waves that move the intestinal contents back and forth in a churning motion. **Intestinal peristalsis** propels the contents of the small intestine toward the colon.

Food, initially ingested in the form of fats, protein, and carbohydrates, is broken down into its constituent nutrients by the process of digestion. Carbohydrates are broken down into disaccharides (*e.g.*, sucrose, maltose, and galactose) and monosaccharides (*e.g.*, glucose and fructose).

- Glucose is the major carbohydrate that the tissue cells use as fuel.

Proteins are broken down into amino acids and peptides. Ingested fats are emulsified into monoglycerides and fatty acids. These smaller molecules are then ready to be absorbed. Vitamins and minerals are not digested, but rather absorbed essentially unchanged. Absorption takes place in the jejunum and is accomplished by both active transport and diffusion.

Colonic Action

Within 4 hours after eating, residual waste material passes into the terminal ileum and slowly passes into the proximal portion of the colon through the ileocecal valve.

This valve, which is normally closed, helps prevent colonic contents from refluxing back into the small intestine. With each peristaltic wave of the small intestine, the valve opens briefly and permits some of the contents to pass into the colon.

The bacterial population is a major component of the contents of the large intestine. Bacteria assist in completing the breakdown of waste material and bile salts. Two types of colonic secretions are added to the residual material—mucus and an electrolyte solution. The electrolyte solution is chiefly a bicarbonate solution that acts to neutralize the end products formed by the colonic bacterial action. The mucus protects the colonic mucosa from the interluminal contents and also provides adherence for the fecal mass.

Weak peristaltic activity moves the colonic contents slowly along the tract. This slow transport allows efficient reabsorption of water and electrolytes. Intermittent strong peristaltic waves propel the contents for considerable distances. This generally occurs after another meal is eaten, when intestine-stimulating hormones are released. The waste materials from a meal eventually reach and distend the rectum, usually in about 12 hours. As much as one fourth of the waste materials from a meal may still be in the rectum 3 days after the meal was ingested.

Defecation, Feces, and Flatus

Distention of the rectum reflexively initiates contractions of its musculature and relaxes the internal anal sphincter, which is ordinarily closed. The internal sphincter is controlled by the autonomic nervous system; the external sphincter is under the conscious control of the cerebral cortex. During defecation, the external anal sphincter voluntarily relaxes, to allow colonic contents to be expelled. Normally, the external anal sphincter is maintained in a state of tonic contraction. Thus, defecation is seen to be a spinal reflex that can be voluntarily inhibited by keeping the external anal sphincter closed. Contracting the abdominal muscles (straining) facilitates emptying of the colon.

The average frequency of defecation in humans is once daily, but the frequency varies among individuals.

- Changes in bowel habits may signify colonic disease. An increase in frequency of defecation is called *diarrhea*, whereas decreased frequency is called *constipation*.
- The aged population is prone to changes in frequency of defecation. See Chapter 37 for a detailed discussion of constipation in the elderly.

Feces consist of undigested foodstuffs, inorganic materials, water, and bacteria. Fecal matter is about 75% fluid and 25% solid material. The composition is relatively unaffected by alterations in diet, because a large portion of the fecal mass is of nondietary origin, derived from the secretions of the GI tract. The brown color of the feces is due to breakdown of bile by the intestinal bacteria.

Chemicals formed by intestinal bacteria (especially **indole** and **skatole**) are responsible in large part for the fecal odor. Gases formed contain methane, hydrogen sulfide, and ammonia, among others. The GI tract normally contains approximately 150 ml of these gases. These gases are either absorbed into the portal circulation and detoxified by the liver or expelled from the rectum (flatus).

- Patients with liver disease frequently are treated with antibiotics to reduce the number of colonic bacteria and thereby inhibit the production of toxic gases.

Nursing Assessment

Health History

The nurse begins by taking a complete history, focusing on symptoms common to gastrointestinal dysfunction. Symptoms on which the assessment focuses include pain, indigestion, intestinal gas, nausea and vomiting, hematemesis, and changes in bowel habits and stool characteristics.

Pain. Pain can be a major symptom of gastrointestinal disease. The character, duration, pattern, frequency, and time of the pain vary greatly, depending on the underlying cause, which also affects the location and distribution of referred pain (Fig. 33-3). Other factors, such as meals, rest, defecation, and vascular disorders, may directly affect this pain.

Indigestion. Indigestion can result from disturbed nervous control of the stomach or from a disorder in the GI tract or elsewhere in the body. Fatty foods tend to cause the most discomfort because they remain in the stomach

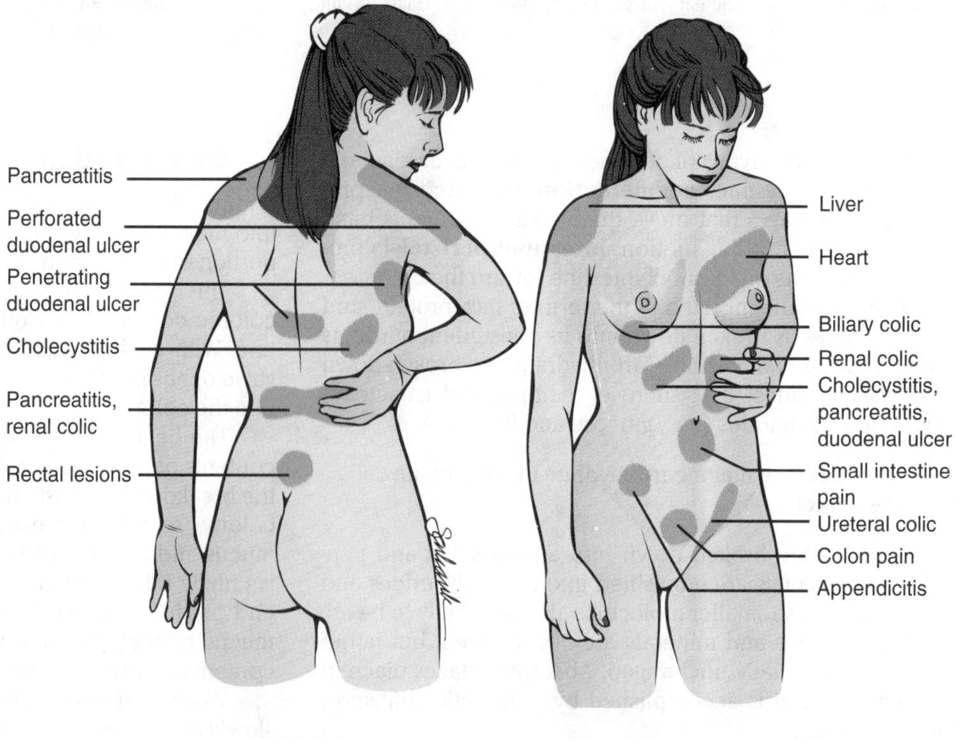

FIGURE 33-3. Common sites of referred abdominal pain.

longer than proteins or carbohydrates. Coarse vegetables and highly seasoned foods can also cause considerable distress.

Upper abdominal discomfort or distress associated with eating is the most common complaint of patients with gastrointestinal dysfunction. The basis for this abdominal distress may be the patient's own gastric peristaltic movements. Bowel movements may or may not relieve the pain.

Intestinal Gas (Belching and Flatulence). The accumulation of gas in the gastrointestinal tract may result in **belching**, the expulsion of gas from the stomach through the mouth, or **flatulence**, the expulsion of gas from the rectum. It is through belching that swallowed air is quickly expelled when it reaches the stomach. Usually, gases in the small intestine pass into the colon and are released as flatus. Patients often complain of bloating, distention, or being "full of gas."

Nausea and Vomiting. The involuntary act of vomiting is another major symptom of gastrointestinal disease. Vomiting is usually preceded by nausea, which can be triggered by odors, activity, or food intake. The emesis, or vomitus, may vary in color and content. It may contain undigested food particles or blood (hematemesis). When this happens soon after hemorrhage, the vomitus is bright red. If blood has been retained in the stomach, it takes on a coffee-ground appearance due to the action of the digestive enzymes.

Change in Bowel Habits and Stool Characteristics. *Diarrhea* is defined as an abnormal increase in the liquid of the stool and in daily stool weight (volume). Diarrhea commonly occurs when the contents move so rapidly through the intestine and colon that there is inadequate time for the gastrointestinal secretions to be absorbed. Fluid content of the diarrheal stool is thus increased. Diarrhea is sometimes associated with abdominal pain or cramping and nausea or vomiting.

Constipation is the retention of or a delay in expulsion of fecal content from the rectum. Excess water is absorbed from the fecal matter, producing stools that are hard, dry, and of smaller volume than normal. A person who strains at stool more than 25% of the time or passes two or fewer stools per week is said to be constipated. Constipation may be associated with anal discomfort and rectal bleeding.

The chacteristics of the stool may vary greatly; they may be brown, contain bright red blood, be black and tarry, or pale yellow and greasy (see Chapter 37 for an in-depth discussion of diarrhea and constipation). Refer to the discussion of stool chacteristics in the stool examination section later in this chapter.

Physical Examination

Physical findings are then assessed to confirm the subjective data obtained from the patient. The abdomen is inspected, auscultated, palpated, and percussed (Fig. 33-4). The patient is placed in the supine position. Contour and symmetry of the abdomen are noted with the identification

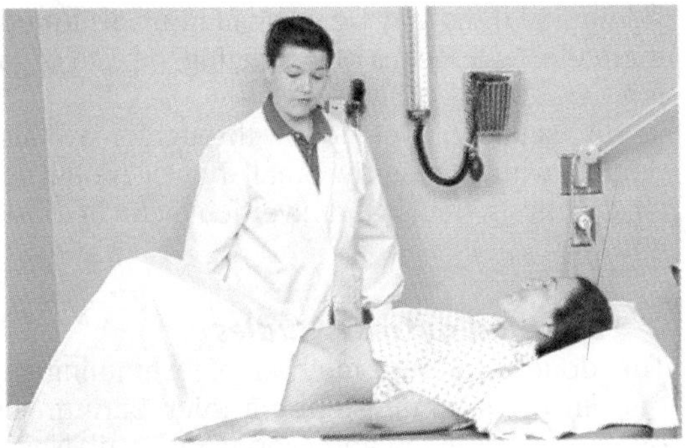

Inspecting the abdomen

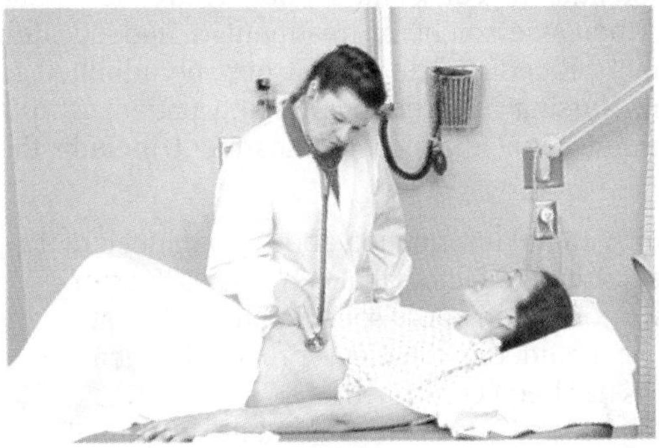

Auscultating the abdomen

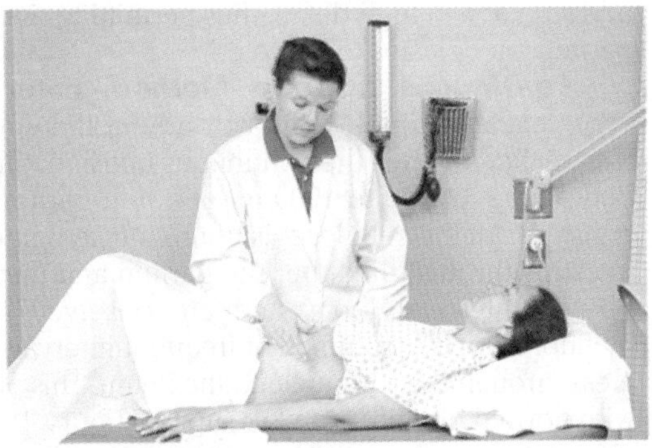

Palpating the abdomen

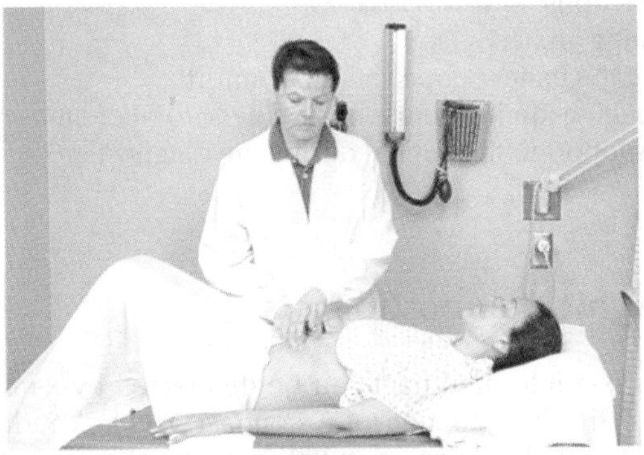

Percussing the abdomen

FIGURE 33-4. Examination of the abdomen includes inspection, palpation, auscultation, and percussion. (From Fuller J and Schaller-Ayers J. Health Assessment: A Nursing Approach, 2nd ed. Philadelphia, JB Lippincott, 1994.)

of localized bulging, distention, or peristaltic waves. Auscultation is performed prior to percussion and palpation (which can increase intestinal motility and thereby change bowel sounds). The character, location, and frequency of bowel sounds are noted. Tympany or dullness is noted during percussion. Palpation is used to identify abdominal masses or areas of tenderness. Any abnormal finding should be noted in relationship to the surface landmarks (xiphoid process, costal margins, anterior iliac spine, and symphysis pubis) or the four quadrants commonly used to describe the abdomen (RUQ—right upper quadrant, RLQ—right lower quadrant, LUQ—left upper quadrant, and LLQ—left lower quadrant).

Diagnostic Evaluation and Related Nursing Interventions

Diagnostic assessment of the gastrointestinal tract includes the use of x-ray and ultrasound studies and the passage of various gastric and intestinal tubes. The majority of these tests and procedures are now performed on an outpatient basis in special units designed for this purpose (*e.g.*, endoscopy or gastrointestinal lab). In general, the nurse supports and educates patients undergoing diagnostic evaluation, whether it be on an inpatient or outpatient basis. Patients requiring such tests are frequently anxious, elderly, or debilitated. The preparation for many of these studies includes fasting and the use of laxatives or enemas, measures that are poorly tolerated by weak patients and which have the potential to cause fluid and electrolyte imbalances. If further assessment or treatment is needed after any outpatient procedure, the patient may be admitted to the hospital. Nursing interventions for the patient who is having gastrointestinal diagnostic assessment include the following:

- Providing general information about a balanced diet and the nutritional factors that can cause GI disturbances. Information about specific nutrients that should be included in the diet is provided after a diagnosis has been confirmed.
- Providing needed information about the test and the activities required of the patient; providing instructions about postprocedure care, as well as dietary and activity restrictions.
- Alleviating anxiety
- Helping the patient cope with discomfort
- Encouraging family members, or others, to offer emotional support to the patient during the diagnostic testing

Radiographic Diagnostic Tests

The entire gastrointestinal tract can be delineated by x-ray studies, after the introduction of a contrast agent. A radiopaque liquid (such as barium sulfate) is one of the most commonly used media. This tasteless, odorless, nongranular, and completely insoluble (hence, not absorbable) powder is ingested in the form of a thick or thin aqueous suspension for the purpose of studying the upper gastrointestinal tract (**upper GI series**); when it is instilled rectally to visualize the colon, it is called a **barium enema**.

Upper Gastrointestinal Tract Studies

The upper GI series enables the examiner to detect or exclude any anatomic or functional derangement of the upper gastrointestinal organs or sphincters. It also aids in the diagnosis of ulcers, varices, tumors, regional enteritis, and malabsorption syndromes.

Patient Preparation. To prepare for this procedure, the patient may be asked to maintain a low-residue diet for several days prior to the test. The patient should receive nothing by mouth after midnight before the test. A laxative may be prescribed to clean out the intestinal tract. Because smoking can stimulate gastric motility, the patient is discouraged from smoking the morning before the examination. All medications are withheld.

Procedure. For purposes of examining the upper GI tract, the patient is required to swallow barium under direct fluoroscopic examination. As the barium descends into the stomach, the position, patency, and caliber of the esophagus are visualized, enabling the examiner to detect or exclude any anatomic or functional derangement of that organ.

Fluoroscopic examination next extends to the stomach, as its lumen fills with barium. The motility and the thickness of the gastric wall and the mucosal pattern are observed. The patency of the pyloric valve and the anatomy of the duodenum are also observed.

During this procedure, many x-ray films are obtained. Additional films may be taken at intervals for up to 24 hours thereafter as a means of estimating the rate of gastric emptying.

A small bowel follow-through may also be conducted with this study. Small bowel motility is observed. Obstructions, ileitis, and diverticula can be observed if present.

Double-Contrast Studies

The double-contrast method of examining the upper GI tract involves administering a thick barium suspension to outline the stomach and esophageal wall. Next, tablets that release carbon dioxide in the presence of water are given. This technique has the advantage of showing the esophagus and stomach in finer detail, thus permitting signs of early superficial neoplasms to be noted.

Continuous Infusion Method. **Enteroclysis** is a very detailed, double-contrast study of the entire small intestine that involves the continuous infusion, through a duodenal tube, of 500 to 1000 ml of a thin barium sulfate suspension. Methylcellulose is then infused into the small intestine through the tube. The barium and methylcellulose fill the intestinal loops and are observed continuously by fluoroscope and filmed at frequent intervals as they progress through the jejunum and the ileum. This process (even with normal motility) can take up to 6 hours. The procedure aids in diagnosing patients with partial small bowel obstructions or diverticula.

Postprocedure Care. Follow-up care is needed after any of the above procedures to ensure that the ingested barium has been completely eliminated. Stools must be monitored until they return to their normal color (the barium will look like clay). A laxative or enema may be needed.

Lower Gastrointestinal Tract Studies

The purpose of a barium enema is to detect the presence of polyps, tumors, and other lesions of the large intestine and to demonstrate any abnormal anatomy or malfunction of the bowel.

Patient Preparation. Preparing the patient includes performing those measures necessary to produce an empty and clean lower bowel. Usually, this includes a low-residue diet 1 to 2 days before the test; a clear liquid diet and a laxative the evening before, with the patient taking nothing by mouth after midnight; and cleansing enemas until returns are clear the following morning.

- Barium enemas should be scheduled before any upper GI studies.
- If the patient has active inflammatory disease of the colon, enemas are contraindicated. Active gastrointestinal bleeding may prohibit the use of laxatives and enemas. Barium enema is contraindicated in patients with signs of perforation or obstruction. Instead, a water-soluble contrast study may be performed in these situations.

Procedure. In the radiology department, the radiopaque substance is instilled rectally; it is viewed under fluoroscopy and then films are obtained. If the patient has been prepared adequately and the colon evacuated completely, the contour of the entire colon, including cecum and appendix (if patent), is clearly visible and the motility of each portion readily observed. The procedure generally takes about 15 to 30 minutes.

Double-Contrast Study. A double-contrast or air-contrast barium enema may be conducted. A thicker barium solution is instilled, followed by the instillation of air. The patient may feel some cramping or discomfort with this process. This test provides a contrast between the air-filled lumen and the barium-coated mucosa. Smaller lesions can be more easily detected with this technique.

Postprocedure Care. An enema or laxative is administered after these tests to facilitate barium removal. As with any barium study, the patient must be monitored for complete elimination of the barium.

Water-Soluble Contrast Study. When it is suspected that the patient has active inflammatory disease, fistulas, or perforation of the colon, a water-soluble iodinated contrast medium (*i.e.*, Gastrografin) can be used. This procedure is the same as for a barium enema. The patient, however, must be assessed for iodine or contrast media sensitivity prior to the procedure. The contrast is readily eliminated after the procedure, so there is no need for postprocedure laxatives. A few patients may complain of some diarrhea until the contrast media is totally eliminated.

Gastric Analysis, Gastric Acid Stimulation Test, and *p*H Monitoring

Gastric Analysis. Analysis of the gastric juice offers a means of estimating the secretory activity of the gastric mucosa and of determining the presence, or the degree, of gastric retention in patients thought to have pyloric or duodenal obstruction.

A small nasogastric tube, with a catheter tip marked at various points from the distal end, is inserted through the nose of the fasting patient. When the tube is at a point slightly less than 50 cm (21 in) distant, the tube should be within the stomach lying along the greater curvature. Once in place, the tube is secured to the patient's cheek and the patient is placed in a semireclining position. The entire stomach contents are aspirated by gentle suction into a syringe. Gastric samples are collected every 15 minutes for the next hour.

Gastric Acid Stimulation Test. Histamine or pentagastrin is given subcutaneously to stimulate gastric secretions. The patient is informed that this injection may produce a flushed feeling. Blood pressure and pulse are monitored frequently to detect hypotension.

Gastric specimens are collected after the injection—every 15 minutes for 1 hour. Specimens are labeled to indicate the time before and after histamine injections. The volume and *p*H of the specimen are analyzed. In certain instances, cytologic study by the Papanicolaou technique may be used to determine the presence or absence of malignant cells. Enzyme analysis of the gastric juice may be indicated.

One of the most important items of information to be gained from gastric analysis is the ability of the mucosa to secrete hydrochloric acid.

- Patients with pernicious anemia secrete no acid under basal conditions or after stimulation.
- Patients with severe chronic atrophic gastritis secrete little or no acid. Some patients with gastric cancer secrete little or no acid.
- Patients with peptic ulcer invariably secrete some acid; patients with duodenal ulcers usually secrete an excess amount.

Ambulatory pH Monitoring. Newer 24-hour ambulatory *p*H monitoring methods have been developed to assist in detecting esophageal reflux of the acidic gastric contents. Patients are maintained NPO (given nothing by mouth) for 6 hours, with all H_2 blockers held for 36 hours. A probe that measures *p*H is placed through the nose and into position about 5 inches above the lower esophageal sphincter. It is connected to an external recording device and is worn for 24 hours while the patient continues normal daily activities. The end result is a computer analysis and graphic display of results.

Endoscopic Procedures

Upper Gastrointestinal Fiberoscopy/ Esophagogastroduodenoscopy(EGD)

Fiberoscopy of the upper GI tract allows for direct visualization of the esophageal, gastric, and duodenal mucosa through a lighted endoscope (gastroscope) (Fig. 33-5). This procedure is especially valuable when esophageal, gastric, or duodenal abnormalities; and inflammatory, neoplastic, or infectious processes are suspected. Esophageal and gas-

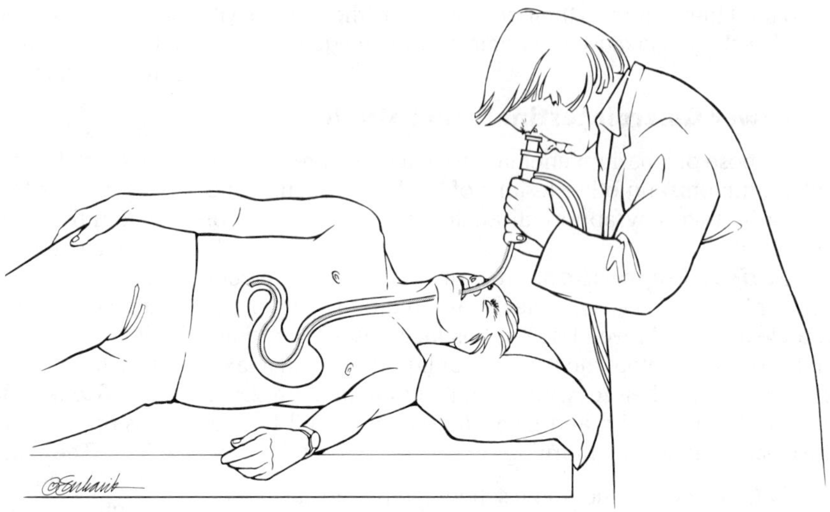

FIGURE 33-5. Patient undergoing gastroscopy.

tric motility can be evaluated. Secretions and tissue specimens can be collected for further analysis. Still or video photography taken through the scopes allows for documentation of findings.

Fiberscopes are flexible scopes equipped with fiberoptic lenses. Precautions must be taken to protect the scope, because the fiberoptic bundles may be broken if the scope is bent at an acute angle. Mouth guards are essential to prevent the patient from biting the scope. The gastroenterologist views the procedure through a viewing lens.

There are electronic video endoscopes available that attach directly to a video processor, which converts electronic signals into pictures that are visible on a television screen. This allows for larger and continuous viewing capabilities, as well as the simultaneous recording of the procedure.

Side-viewing flexible scopes are used to visualize the common bile, and pancreatic and hepatic ducts through the ampulla of Vater in the duodenum. This procedure is helpful in evaluating jaundice, pancreatitis, tumors of the pancreas, common duct stones, and biliary tract disease. This procedure is called endoscopic retrograde cholangiopancreatography (ERCP).

Upper gastrointestinal fiberoscopy also can be a therapeutic procedure when combined with other procedures. Therapeutic endoscopy can be used to remove common bile duct stones, dilate strictures, and treat gastric bleeding and esophageal varices. Laser-compatible scopes provide laser therapy for upper GI neoplasms.

Patient Preparation. The patient is instructed to fast for 6 to 12 hours before the examination. Patient preparation includes spraying or gargling with a local anesthetic, along with administering diazepam (Valium) intravenously just before the scope is introduced. Atropine may be administered to reduce secretions. Glucagon may be given to relax smooth muscle. The patient is positioned on the left side to facilitate saliva drainage and to provide easy access for the endoscope.

Procedure. The gastroscope is lubricated with a water-soluble lubricant and then passed smoothly and slowly along the back of the mouth and down into the esophagus. The gastroenterologist views the gastric wall as well as the sphincters. The endoscope is then advanced into the duodenum for further examination. Biopsy forceps to obtain tissue specimens or cytology brushes to obtain cells for microscopic study can be passed through the scope. The procedure generally takes about 30 minutes.

During the EGD it is important to monitor and maintain the patient's oral airway. Supplemental oxygen may be used if needed. Emergency equipment must be readily available.

Postprocedure Care. After a gastroscopy the patient is instructed not to eat or drink until the gag reflex returns (in 1 to 2 hr) to prevent aspiration of food or fluids into the lungs. Postgastroscopy assessment by the nurse includes observing for signs of perforation, such as pain, bleeding, unusual difficulty swallowing, and an elevated temperature. Minor throat discomfort can be relieved with lozenges, saline gargle, and oral analgesic medications after the gag reflex has returned. Patients who were sedated for the procedure are maintained on bed rest until fully alert.

Anoscopy, Proctoscopy, and Sigmoidoscopy

Procedures for the study of the lower portion of the colon make use of instruments that use small beams of light that allow the lumen of the lower bowel to be viewed directly. These can be rigid scopes or flexible fiberoptic scopes. The anoscope is a rigid scope used to examine the anal canal. Proctoscopes and sigmoidoscopes are rigid scopes used to inspect the rectum and the sigmoid colon, respectively, for evidence of ulceration, tumors, polyps, or other pathologic processes. It is an important part of the cancer screening process (Table 33-3).

The flexible fiberoptic sigmoidoscope (Fig. 33-6) permits the colon to be examined up to 40 to 50 cm (16 to 20 in) from the anus. This is more than the 25 cm (10 in) that can be seen with the rigid sigmoidoscope. The flexible scope has many of the same adaptabilities and capabilities as the scopes used for the upper GI study. Still or video images can be used to document findings.

Patient Preparation. These examinations require only limited bowel preparation. A warm tap water enema or Fleet's enema is given until returns are clear. Dietary restrictions are not usually necessary. Sedation is not usually required.

TABLE 33-3 Guidelines for Diagnostic GI Testing for Cancer Screening and Early Detection

Diagnostic Test	Guidelines
Digital rectal examination	Should be performed annually after age 40
Stool for occult blood	Should be performed annually after age 50
Proctosigmoidoscopy	Should be performed annually at ages 50 and 51, then every 3–5 years if initial two studies are normal and patient is asymptomatic
Colonoscopy	Should be performed if any of the above tests are positive or a polyp is found

Rigid Scope Procedures. The patient assumes the knee–chest position at the edge of the bed or the examining table. With the back inclined at about a 45-degree angle, the patient is in proper position for the introduction of an anoscope, proctoscope, or sigmoidoscope.

During a proctosigmoidoscopic examination, the patient is kept informed about the progress of the examination. The patient is informed that the pressure exerted by the instrument will create the urge to have a bowel movement.

Flexible Scope Procedures. The patient is placed in a comfortable position on the left side with the right leg bent and placed anteriorly. Biopsies and polypectomies also can be performed during this procedure. The same nursing implications apply as for the rigid scope procedures.

As part of the endoscopic examination, one or more small pieces of tissue may be removed for histologic study, a procedure referred to as a **biopsy**. This is performed with small biting forceps introduced through the instrument. Rectal and sigmoidal polyps, if present, may be removed with a wire snare, which is used to grasp the pedicle, or stalk. An electrocoagulating current is then used to sever the polyp and prevent bleeding.

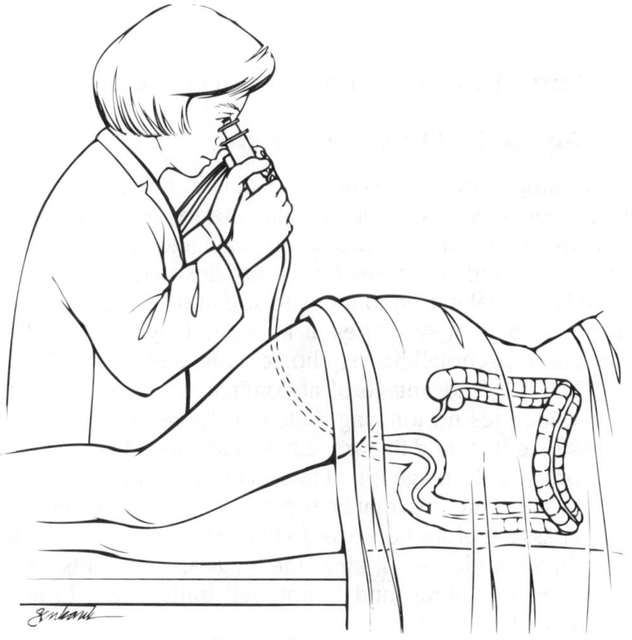

FIGURE 33-6. Flexible fiberoptic sigmoidoscopy. The instrument is advanced past the proximal sigmoid and then deflected into the descending colon.

- It is extremely important that all tissue that is excised by the endoscopist be placed immediately in moist gauze or in an appropriate receptacle, labeled correctly, and delivered without delay to the pathology laboratory for examination.

Postprocedure Care. After this procedure the patient is monitored for rectal bleeding and signs of intestinal perforation (*i.e.*, fever, rectal drainage, abdominal distention, and pain). On completion of this examination, the patient can resume regular activities and dietary practices.

Fiberoptic Colonoscopy

Direct visual inspection of the colon to the cecum is possible by means of a flexible fiberoptic colonoscope (Fig. 33-7). This procedure is commonly used as a diagnostic aid and screening device for patients at high risk for cancer (see Table 33-3). Tissue biopsies can be obtained as needed. During this procedure, polyps can be evaluated and inflammatory disease or other bowel disease can be diagnosed. These scopes have the same adaptabilities and capabilities as those used for the EGD; however, they are larger in diameter and longer in length. Still and video recordings can be used to observe and document the procedure and findings.

Therapeutically, the procedure can be used to remove polyps with a special snare and cautery through the colonoscope. Many colon cancers begin with adenomatous polyps of the colon; therefore, one goal of colonoscopic polypectomy is early detection and prevention of colorectal cancer. All visible polyps are removed. This procedure also can be used to treat areas of bleeding or stricture. Laser-compatible scopes provide laser therapy for colonic neoplasms. Bowel decompression can also be completed during the procedure.

Patient Preparation. The success of the procedure depends on how well the colon is prepared. For best results, the intestinal tract is prepared by limiting the patient's intake to liquids (for 1 to 3 days prior to the examination). Cleansing of the colon can be accomplished in various ways. The physician may order a laxative for 2 nights prior to the examination and a Fleet's or saline enema until the return runs clear the morning of the test.

Currently, polyethylene glycol electrolyte lavage solutions (GoLYTELY, Colyte) are being used as effective intestinal lavages for cleansing the bowel. The patient is placed on a clear liquid diet starting at noon the day before the procedure. The lavage solutions are then ingested orally at intervals over the next 3 to 4 hours. If necessary, this solution can be given through a feeding tube. Cleansing of the bowel is

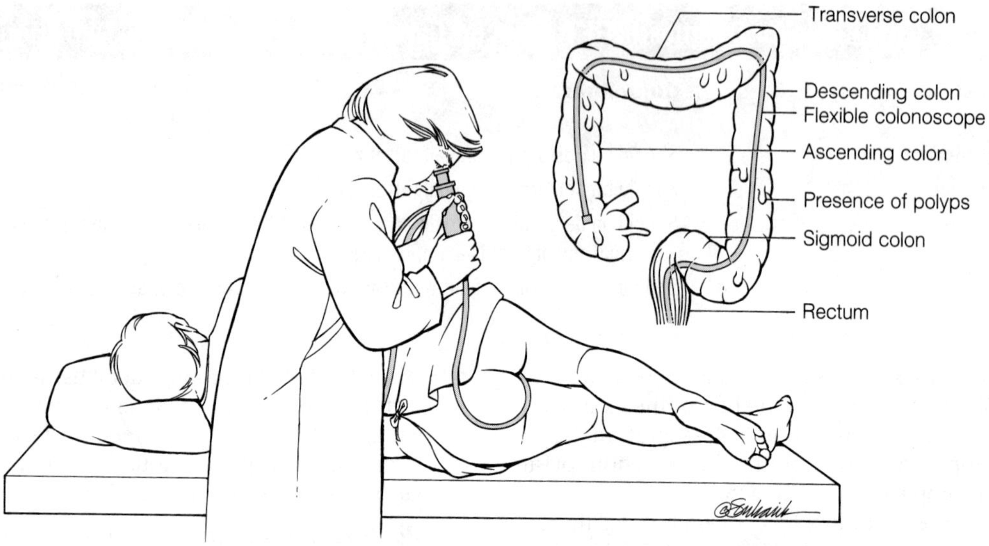

FIGURE 33-7. Colonoscopy. Flexible scope passes through rectum and sigmoid colon into the descending, transverse, and ascending colon.

fast (rectal effluent is clear in about 4 hours) and tolerated fairly well by most patients. Some side effects of the electrolyte solutions are nausea, fluid and electrolyte imbalance, and hypothermia (patients are often told to drink the preparation as cold as possible to make it more palatable). The side effects are especially problematic for elderly patients.

- The patient is instructed not to take routine medications when the lavage solution is ingested, as the medications will not be digested and thus are rendered ineffective.
- The use of lavage solutions is contraindicated in patients with intestinal obstructions and inflammatory bowel disease.

Before the examination, a narcotic analgesic, usually meperidine (Demerol), may be administered. During the examination, diazepam (Valium) may be useful in relieving anxiety. Glucagon may be used to relax colonic musculature.

Procedure. Colonoscopy is performed with the patient lying on the left side with the legs drawn up toward the chest. The procedure generally takes about 1 hour. Discomfort may result from instilling air to expand the colon or from inserting and moving the scope. Biopsy forceps or a cytology brush may be passed through the scope to obtain specimens for histology and cytology examinations. Potential complications of colonoscopy include cardiac dysrhythmias and respiratory depression resulting from medications administered, vasovagal reactions, and circulatory overload or hypotension resulting from overhydration or underhydration during bowel preparation. Therefore, it is important to continuously monitor the patient's cardiac and respiratory function. Supplemental oxygen may be used as necessary.

Postprocedure Care. Patients who were sedated for the procedure will be maintained on bed rest until fully alert. The patient must be observed for signs and symptoms of bowel perforation (*e.g.*, rectal bleeding, abdominal pain or distention, fever, or focal peritoneal signs).

Small Bowel Enteroscopy

A small-caliber transnasal endoscope allows direct observation of the small intestine wall. The endoscope used for this procedure is very long and flexible and has a balloon at its tip. When inflated, the balloon tip advances the scope by peristalsis through the small intestine. This procedure may take 10 or more hours to complete. The patient may be kept in the recovery area or sent home.

Once the scope has entered the distal ileum, it is slowly retracted while the endoscopist examines the intestinal wall. This lengthy procedure is usually conducted on a limited basis for those patients having continued bleeding even after extensive diagnostic testing has identified no other problem area.

Radiographic and Nonradiographic Imaging

Abdominal Ultrasonography

Ultrasonography is a noninvasive diagnostic technique in which sound waves are passed into internal body structures and are deflected back, producing an image of the abdominal organs and structures on the oscilloscope. This procedure is generally used to indicate size and configuration of these abdominal structures. It is particularly useful in the detection of cholelithiasis, cholecystitis, and appendicitis.

The chief advantage of abdominal ultrasonography is that it requires no ionizing radiation. There are no noticeable side effects and the procedure is relatively inexpensive.

One disadvantage is that this technique cannot be used to examine structures that lie behind bony tissue, which prevents passage of sound waves to deeper structures. Gas and fluid in the abdomen or air in the lungs also presents problems because ultrasound is not well transmitted through gas, air, or fluid.

- If barium studies are to be performed, they must be scheduled after this test; otherwise, the barium will interfere with the transmission of sound waves used for this procedure.

Endoscopic ultrasonography is a specialized enteroscopic procedure that aids in the diagnosis of GI disorders by providing direct imaging of a target area. It also helps to stage various gastrointestinal cancers preoperatively. A high-frequency ultrasonic beam is added to the tip of the fiberoptic scope so that a transintestinal study can be completed. Intestinal gas, bone, and thick layers of adipose tissue—all of which hamper conventional ultrasonography—are not problematic when this technique is used.

Computed Tomography

Computed tomography (CT) is a diagnostic method that provides cross-sectional images to allow the abdominal organs and structures to be more directly observed. Multiple x-rays are taken from many different angles, computerized, reconstructed, then viewed on a computer monitor. Indications for abdominal CT scanning are diseases of the liver, spleen, kidney, pancreas, and pelvic organs.

Because adequacy of detail in the test depends on the presence of fat, this diagnostic tool is not useful for very thin, cachectic patients. This procedure is completely painless. Radiation doses, however, are considerable. Because a scanning time of 5 seconds is required, motion artifacts produced by heartbeat and respiration cannot be avoided and pictures that are less than clear result.

- If barium studies are to be performed, they must be scheduled after CT scanning so as not to interfere with imaging.

Magnetic Resonance Imaging

Magnetic resonance imaging (MRI) for gastroenterology is currently used to supplement, not replace, ultrasonography and CT scanning. The development of oral contrast agents is, however, increasing the application of this technique for diagnosis of gastrointestinal diseases.

For this procedure, the patient lies in a machine that constructs an image based on the magnetic field created between the machine and the structures it is studying. The entire procedure takes 30 to 90 minutes. The patient has nothing by mouth for 6 hours prior to the test. The patient must be warned in advance that the close-fitting scanners used in most MRI facilities may induce feelings of claustrophobia and that the machine will make odd, possibly frightening sounds during the procedure. The physiologic artifacts of heartbeat, respiration, and peristalsis can cause a less than clear picture. Newer ultrafast MRI techniques may help to eliminate these physiologic motion artifacts.

- MRI is *contraindicated* for patients with permanent pacemakers, artificial heart valves and defibrillators, implanted insulin pumps, and transcutaneous electrical nerve stimulation (TENS) devices because the magnetic field could cause malfunction.
- MRI is also *contraindicated* for patients with internal metal devices (*e.g.*, aneurysm clips).

Radionuclide Imaging

Radionuclide testing is presently used to assess gastric emptying, colonic transit, and localization of inflammation and tumors in the gastrointestinal tract.

Gastric Emptying. The liquid and solid components of a meal are tagged with radionuclide markers. After ingesting the meal, the patient is positioned under a scintiscanner, which measures the rate of passage of the radioactivity out of the stomach. This is useful in diagnosing disorders of gastric motility.

Colonic Transit Studies. This procedure is used to evaluate colonic motility in instances of chronic constipation and obstructive defecation syndromes. It is usually an outpatient study. The patient is given a capsule containing 20 radionuclide markers. Following a regular diet and normal daily activities for 3 to 5 days, the patient returns and an abdominal x-ray is taken. The amount of time it takes for the radioactive material to move through the colon indicates colonic motility.

Tagged Red Blood Cells and Leukocytes. Red blood cells or leukocytes are tagged by radionuclide injection. They are then tracked to areas of inflammation, abscess, or neoplasm.

Manometry and Electrophysiologic Studies

Manometry. Tests of manometry are diagnostic tools used to evaluate the function of portions of the GI tract as well as their response to therapeutic interventions. Pressure transducers are used to measure motility and intraluminal pressures. These pressures can be recorded manually or on a physiograph or a computer.

Esophageal manometry is used to detect motility disorders of the esophagus as well as the lower esophageal sphincter. Patients must be NPO for 8 to 12 hours before the test. Medications that could have a direct affect on the motility are held for 24 to 48 hours (*i.e.*, calcium channel blockers, anticholinergics, and sedatives). The patient is awake during the procedure.

Gastroduodenal and small intestine manometry is used to evaluate delayed gastric emptying and gastric and intestinal motility disorders. This is often an ambulatory outpatient procedure lasting 24 to 72 hours.

Anorectal manometry is used to measure the resting tone of the internal anal sphincter and the contractibility of the external anal sphincter. It is helpful in evaluating patients with chronic constipation or fecal incontinence.

Electrogastrography (EGG). These newer studies assist in detecting and measuring the electrical signals that are initiated by the distal two thirds of the stomach, which can be useful in detecting motor/neurologic dysfunction in the stomach.

Stool Tests

The basic examination of the stool includes an inspection of the specimen for its amount, consistency, and color, and a screening test for occult blood. The nurse can perform these tests at the bedside. Special tests, including tests for fecal urobilinogen, fat, nitrogen, parasites, pathogens, food residues, and other substances, require that the specimen be sent to the laboratory.

Stool samples are usually collected on a random basis unless a quantitative study such as fecal fat or urobilinogen is performed. Random specimens need to be sent directly to the laboratory for analysis. The quantitative 24- to 72-hour collections must be kept refrigerated until taken to the laboratory.

Some stool collections require that a special diet be followed prior to the collection or that certain medications be withheld. It is important to follow test guidelines closely for accurate results.

Stool Color

The color of stools can vary from light to dark brown. Various foods and medications affect stool color as follows: meat protein produces a dark brown coloration; spinach, a green hue; carrots and beets, red; cocoa, dark red or brown; senna, a yellowish hue; bismuth, iron, licorice, and charcoal, black; and barium, a milky white appearance.

- If shed in sufficient quantities into the upper GI tract, blood produces a tarry black color (melena).
- Blood entering the lower portion of the GI tract or passing rapidly through it will appear bright or dark red.
- Lower rectal or anal bleeding is suspected if there is streaking of blood on the surface of the stool or if blood is noted on toilet tissue.

Stool Consistency and Appearance

In various disorders the stool assumes a typical appearance:

- In **steatorrhea**, the stools are generally bulky, greasy, foamy, and foul in odor; stool color is gray, with a silvery sheen.
- With **biliary obstruction**, the stool becomes "acholic" and is light gray or clay colored because of the absence of urobilin.
- In **chronic ulcerative colitis**, mucus threads or pus may be visible on gross inspection of the stool.
- **Constipation**, **obstipation** (extreme constipation), or **fecal impaction** may result in the passage of small, dry, rocky-hard masses called scybala. This type of stool may traumatize the rectal mucosa sufficiently to cause bleeding, in which case the fecal masses are streaked with blood.

Test for Occult Blood. This test is probably one of the most frequently performed stool tests. It is most useful in cancer screening programs and early cancer detection (see Table 33-3). The test can be performed at the bedside, in the laboratory, or at home. Tests for occult blood detect heme–the iron-containing portion of the hemoglobin molecule that is altered during transit through the intestines.

Probably the most widely used occult blood test is the Hemetest. It is inexpensive, noninvasive, and carries no risk to the patient. It should not, however, be performed when there is hemorrhoidal bleeding. The stool specimen is smeared on a dry, guiac-impregnated paper slide. The slide is mailed to the physician in an envelope provided for that purpose, and the stool specimen is examined. Serial 3-day testing is recommended.

The test, however, is not perfect. There are factors that interfere with the sensitivity and specificity of the test. False-positive results may occur if the patient has eaten rare meats, poultry, turnips, melons, salmon, sardines, or horseradish within 48 hours before or during the test. Medications such as iron, iodides, indomethacin, colchicine, salicylates, corticosteroids, and vitamin C may also cause false-positive results. Careful assessment of diet and the medication regimen is necessary to eliminate the chance of false-positive results.

New alternative occult blood tests are presently becoming available for public use. Hemetest II SENSA and HemoQuant are two examples of the tests that are being developed to provide more specific and more sensitive readings.

Newer Techniques

Newer and more sophisticated testing specific to the GI tract is becoming available. The following are only a few that will be seen in greater frequency in the next few years.

Laparoscopy (Peritoneoscopy). The use of laparoscopic techniques for the diagnosis of gastrointestinal disease has been expanded. The procedure is performed by using a special fiberoptic laparoscope that allows direct visualization of the organs and structures within the abdomen. It also allows for the biopsy of these structures and organs as necessary. This procedure is used to evaluate peritoneal disease, chronic abdominal pain, abdominal masses, and gallbladder and liver disease. The procedure is also being used in a therapeutic manner surgically to excise certain structures and masses.

Hydrogen Breath Test. This breath test was developed to evaluate carbohydrate absorption. It can also be used to aid in the diagnosis of bacterial overgrowth in the intestine, and short bowel syndrome. This test is specific to the amount of hydrogen expelled in the breath after it is produced in the colon (on contact of galactose with fermenting bacteria) and absorbed into the blood.

Rectal Sensory Function Test. This test is used to evaluate rectal sensory function and neuropathy. A catheter and balloon are passed into the rectum. The balloon is inflated until the patient feels distention. The tone and pressure of the rectum and anal sphincter are measured. The results are especially helpful in the evaluation of patients with chronic constipation, diarrhea, or incontinence.

Defecography. This is another test used to measure anorectal function. Very thick barium paste is instilled into the rectum. Fluoroscopy is performed and the function of the rectum and anal sphincter is visualized while the patient attempts to expel the barium.

Pathophysiologic and Psychologic Considerations

Abnormalities of the GI tract are numerous and exemplify every type of major pathology that can affect other organ

CRITICAL THINKING EXERCISES

1. You are caring for a patient who is to have a barium enema. The patient received a clear liquid diet and a laxative the evening before the test. On the morning of the test, she indicates that the laxative had caused her to have diarrhea during the night, and she refuses to have a cleansing enema. Based on your knowledge of intestinal physiology, how would you explain to this patient what has happened and why? Describe what the goals would be in this situation and the interventions that could be implemented to achieve them.
2. You accompany your patient to an endoscopy suite where the patient is to have a colonoscopy. You notice that emergency equipment is readily available. After the procedure is completed, the nurse, who assisted with the procedure and must now assist with another procedure, asks you to monitor the patient's vital signs. You agree to carry out this function because you have a thorough understanding of the complications that can occur. Describe the changes in vital signs that you might detect as an indication that complications are developing and the reasons these changes may occur.

systems: bleeding, perforation, obstruction, inflammation, and cancer. Congenital, inflammatory, infectious, traumatic, and neoplastic lesions have been encountered in every portion, and at every site, along the length of the gastrointestinal tract. The GI tract, as with all other organ systems, is subject to circulatory disturbances, faulty nervous system control, and aging.

Apart from the many organic diseases to which the GI tract is susceptible, there are many extrinsic factors that can interfere with its normal function and produce symptoms. Stress and anxiety, for example, often find their chief expression in indigestion, anorexia, or motor disturbances of the intestines, sometimes producing constipation or diarrhea.

In addition to the state of mental health, physical factors such as fatigue and an unbalanced or abruptly changed dietary intake can markedly affect the GI tract. In both assessing and instructing the patient, the nurse should realize that a combination of mental and physical factors affect the status of the gastrointestinal tract.

BIBLIOGRAPHY

Books

Beck M and Evans N (eds). Gastroenterology Nursing: A Core Curriculum. St Louis, Mosby-Year Book, 1993.

Eisenburg RL. Gastrointestinal Radiology. Philadelphia, JB Lippincott, 1990.

Gitnick C (ed). Current Gastroenterology. Vol 12. St. Louis, Mosby-Year Book, 1992.

Jarvis C. Physical Examination in Health Assessment. Philadelphia, WB Saunders, 1992.

Johnson L (ed). Gastrointestinal Physiology, 4th ed. St Louis, Mosby-Year Book, 1991.

Sodeman WA, Saladin VA, Boyd WP. Geriatric Gastroenterology. Philadelphia, WB Saunders, 1989.

Yamada T. Atlas of Gastroenterology. Philadelphia, JB Lippincott, 1992.

Journals

Archker E. Screening patients for colorectal cancer. Pract Gastroenterol 1989 Jan/Feb; 25(1):37, 41–42.

Clarke B. Making sense of bowel prep for diagnostic procedures. Nursing Times 1989 Feb 1–7; 85(5):46–47.

Holmgren C. Abdominal Assessment. RN 1992 March; 55(3):28–34.

Massoni M. Nurses' GI Handbook. Nursing 1990 Nov; 20(11):65–80.

McConnell E. Auscultating bowel sounds. Nursing 1990 May; 20(5):106.

O'Toole M. Advanced assessment of the abdomen and GI problems. Nurs Clin North Am 1990 Dec; 25(4):771–776.

Roberts A. The digestive system, Part 1. Nursing Times 1991 March 13; 87(11):45–48.

Roberts A. The digestive system, Part 2. Nursing Times 1991 April 10; 87(15):65–68.

Roberts A. The digestive system, Part 3. Nursing Times 1991 May 8; 87(19):61–64.

Roberts A. The digestive system, Part 4. Nursing Times 1991 June 12; 87(24):61–64.

Sweeney JP. Assessing the patient undergoing GI endoscopy. Gastroenterol Nurs 1992 April; 14(5):266–269.

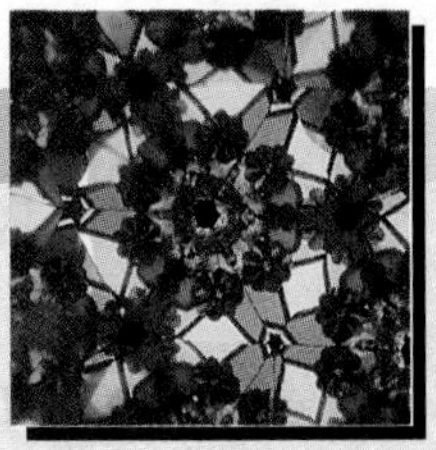

34

Management of Patients With Ingestive Problems and Upper Gastrointestinal Disorders

CHAPTER OUTLINE

Conditions of the Oral Cavity
Abnormalities of the Lips, Gums, and Mouth
Abnormalities of the Teeth
Jaw Repositioning and Reconstruction
Abnormalities of the Salivary Glands

Cancer of the Oral Cavity
NURSING PROCESS: Patients With Conditions of the Oral Cavity

Neck Dissection
NURSING PROCESS: The Patient Undergoing a Neck Dissection

Conditions of the Esophagus
Motility Disorders
Gastroesophageal Reflux
Hiatal Hernia
Diverticulum
Rings and Webs
Perforation
Foreign Bodies
Chemical Burns
Esophageal Varices
Benign Tumors
Cancer of the Esophagus
NURSING PROCESS: Patients With Conditions of the Esophagus

Critical Thinking Exercises

LEARNING OBJECTIVES

On completion of this chapter, the learner will be able to:

1. Use the nursing process as a framework for care of patients with conditions of the oral cavity
2. Describe the relationship of dental hygiene and dental problems to nutrition
3. Describe the nursing management of patients with abnormalities of the lips, gums, teeth, mouth, and salivary glands
4. Use the nursing process as a framework for care of patients with cancer of the oral cavity
5. Identify the physical and psychosocial long-term needs of patients with oral cancer
6. Use the nursing process as a framework for care of patients undergoing neck dissection
7. Use the nursing process as a framework for care of patients with conditions of the esophagus
8. Describe the various conditions of the esophagus, their clinical manifestations, management, and rehabilitation

Because the process of ingestion normally begins in the mouth, adequate nutrition is related to good dental health and the general condition of the mouth. Any discomfort or adverse condition in the oral cavity can affect a person's nutritional status. Changes in the oral cavity may influence the type and amount of food ingested as well as the degree to which food particles are properly mixed with salivary enzymes. Esophageal problems related to the act of swallowing can also adversely affect food and fluid intake, thereby jeopardizing general health and well-being.

Given the close interrelationship between adequate nutritional intake and all of the structures of the upper gastrointestinal tract (lips, mouth, teeth, pharynx, esophagus), preventive health teaching should emphasize helping people to prevent disorders associated with any of these structures.

Conditions of the Oral Cavity

Abnormalities of the Lips, Gums, and Mouth

Many diseases are manifested as alterations in the oral cavity, which includes areas of the lips, mouth, or gums. Table 34-1 reviews abnormalities that may occur in these areas, as well as possible causes and nursing interventions.

Abnormalities of the Teeth

Dental Plaque and Caries

Tooth decay is an erosive process that results from the action of bacteria on fermentable carbohydrates in the mouth, which in turn produces acids that dissolve tooth enamel. The extent of damage to the teeth depends on several factors, the most significant of which are (1) the presence of dental plaque; (2) the strength of the acids and the ability of the saliva to neutralize them; (3) the length of time the acids are in contact with the teeth; and (4) susceptibility of the teeth to decay. Dental plaque is a gluey, gelatin-like substance that adheres to the teeth. The initial action that causes damage to a tooth occurs under dental plaque.

Dental decay begins with a small hole, usually in a fissure (a break in the tooth's enamel) or in an area that is hard to clean. Left unchecked, the affected area penetrates the enamel into the dentin. Because the dentin is not as hard as the enamel, decay progresses somewhat more rapidly and in time reaches the pulp. When the blood, lymph vessels, and nerves are exposed, they become infected, and an abscess may form, either within the tooth or at the tip of the root. Soreness and pain usually accompany the abscess. As the infection increases, the patient's face may become swollen, and there may be pulsating pain. The dentist can determine by x-ray the extent of damage and the type of treatment needed. If treatment is not successful, it may be necessary to extract the tooth.

Preventive Management. Measures used to prevent and control dental caries include practicing effective mouth care, reducing the intake of sugars (refined carbohydrates), applying fluoride to the teeth or drinking fluoridated water, and using pit and fissure sealants.

Mouth Care. Healthy teeth must be conscientiously and effectively cleaned on a daily basis. Brushing is particularly effective in mechanically breaking up the bacterial plaque that collects around teeth. See Chart 34-1 for a more detailed list of instructions for practicing preventive oral hygiene.

The normal movement of the muscles of mastication and the normal flow of saliva also aid greatly in keeping the teeth clean. Because many ill patients do not eat normally, they produce less saliva, which in turn reduces the natural cleaning process of the teeth. The nurse must therefore assume the responsibility for brushing the patient's teeth. In any case, merely wiping the patient's mouth and teeth with a swab is ineffective. The most effective method is mechanical cleansing (brushing). If it is not possible to brush, it is better to wipe the teeth with a washcloth than to have the patient swish an antiseptic mouthwash several times before emitting it into the emesis basin. A soft bristle toothbrush is more effective than a sponge or foam stick. Lemon glycerin swabs, popular several years ago, are avoided because they are very drying to the patient's oral mucosa. Instead, the lips may be coated with a water-soluble gel to prevent drying.

Diet. Dental caries may be prevented by decreasing the amount of sugar in the diet. Patients who snack should be encouraged to choose less cariogenic alternatives such as fruits, vegetables, nuts, and possibly cheeses.

Fluoridation. Fluoridation of public water supplies may decrease the amount of dental caries by 60%. Some areas of the country have natural fluoridation; other communities have mandated the addition of fluoride to public water supplies. Fluoridation may be attained by having a dentist apply a concentrated gel or solution to the teeth; adding fluoride to home water supplies; using fluoridated toothpaste; or ingesting sodium fluoride tablets, drops, or lozenges.

Pit and Fissure Sealants. The occlusal surfaces of the teeth have pits and fissures, areas that are prone to caries. Some dentists apply a special coating to fill and seal these areas from potential exposure to cariogenic processes. These sealants may last up to 7 years.

Management. Treatment for dental caries includes fillings, extraction, dental implants, and dentures.

Dentoalveolar Abscess or Periapical Abscess

Periapical abscess, more commonly referred to as an *abscessed tooth*, involves the collection of pus in the apical dental periosteum (fibrous membrane supporting the tooth structure) and the tissue surrounding the apex of the tooth (where it is suspended in the jaw bone). It may appear in two forms: acute and chronic. *Acute periapical abscess* is usually secondary to a suppurative pulpitis (a pus-producing inflammation of the dental pulp) that arises from an infection extending from dental caries. The infection of the dental pulp extends through the apical foramen of the tooth to form an abscess around the apex. The abscess produces a dull, gnawing, continuous pain, often with a surrounding cellulitis and edema of the adjacent facial structures, and mobility of the involved tooth. The gum opposite the apex of the tooth is usually swollen on the cheek side. Swelling and cellulitis of the facial structures may make it difficult to open the mouth. In well-developed abscesses there may be a systemic reaction, fever, and malaise.

TABLE 34-1 Abnormalities of the Lip, Mouth, and Gums

Condition	Signs and Symptoms	Possible Causes	Nursing Management
Abnormalities of the Lip			
Actinic cheilitis	Irritation of lips associated with scaling, crusty, fissure. White overgrowth of horny layer of epidermis (hyperkeratosis).	Cumulative effect of exposure to sun. More frequently occurring in fair-skinned persons and in those whose occupations involve sun exposure, such as farmers. May lead to squamous cell cancer.	Teach patient importance of protecting lips from the sun by using protective ointment such as sun block. Instruct patient to have a periodic check-up by physician.
Herpes simplex 1—cold sore or fever blister	Symptoms may be delayed up to 20 days after exposure. Singular or clustered painful vesicles that may rupture.	Herpes simplex virus—an opportunistic infection. Frequently seen in immunosuppressed patients. May recur with menstruation, fever, or sun exposure.	Acyclovir ointment or systemic administration as prescribed. Administer analgesics as prescribed. Instruct patient to avoid irritating foods.
Chancre	Reddened circumscribed lesion that ulcerates and becomes crusted.	Primary lesion of syphilis. Very contagious.	Comfort measures: cold soaks to lip, mouth care. Administer antibiotics as prescribed. Instruct patient regarding contagion.
Contact dermatitis	Red area or rash. Itching.	Allergic reaction to lipstick, cosmetic ointments, or even toothpaste.	Instruct patient to avoid possible causes. Administer corticosteroids as prescribed.
Abnormalities of the Mouth			
Leukoplakia	White patches; may be hyperkeratotic. Usually in buccal mucosa. Usually painless.	Fewer than 2% are malignant.	Instruct patient to consult a physician if it persists longer than 2 weeks.
Hairy leukoplakia	White patches with rough hairlike projections. Typically found on lateral border of the tongue.	Possibly viral. Smoking and use of tobacco. Often seen in persons who are HIV positive.	Instruct patient to consult a physician if it persists longer than 2 weeks.
Lichen planus	White papules at the intersection of a network of interlacing lesions. Usually ulcerated and painful.	Recurrences are common. May lead to a malignant process.	Administer viscous lidocaine for pain. Instruct the patient to hold this in the mouth for 2–3 minutes. Apply tiramicinolone (Kenalog) or Orabase after meals or at bedtime to assist with healing. Administer corticosteroids systemically or intralesionally as prescribed. Instruct the patient of need for follow-up if condition is chronic.
Candidiasis—moniliasis/thrush	Cheesy white plaque that looks like milk curds. When rubbed off, it leaves erythematous and often bleeding base.	*Candida ablicans* fungus. Predisposing factors include diabetes, antibiotic therapy, and immunosuppression.	Antifungal medications such as nystatin (Mycostatin), clotrimazole, or ketoconazole may be prescribed. These may be taken in pill form or as a suspension. When used as a suspension, instruct the patient to swish vigorously for at least 1 minute and then swallow.

(continued)

TABLE 34-1 *(continued)*

Condition	Signs and Symptoms	Possible Causes	Nursing Management
Abnormalities of the Mouth *(continued)*			
Aphthous stomatitis—canker sore	Shallow ulcer with a white or gray center and red border. Seen on the inner side of the lip and cheek or on the tongue. It begins with a burning or tingling sensation and slight swelling. Painful. Usually lasts 7-10 days and heals without a scar.	It is associated with emotional or mental stress, fatigue, hormonal factors, minor trauma (such as biting), allergies, acidic foods, and juices. Associated with HIV infection. May recur.	Instruct the patient in comfort measures, such as saline rinses, and a soft or bland diet. Antibiotics or corticosteroids may be prescribed.
Leukoplakia buccalis—smoker's patch	This has two stages. Stage I has one or two thick pearly patches on the mucous membrane of the tongue or mouth. Over time the tongue and mouth become covered with a creamy thick white mucous membrane, which may slough, leaving a beefy red base.	Chronic irritation by carious, infected, poorly repaired teeth; tobacco; highly spiced foods; and occasionally due to syphilis.	Correction of the underlying cause will lead to disappearance.
Krythoplakia	Red patch on the oral mucous membrane.	Nonspecific inflammation. More frequently seen in the elderly.	
Kaposi's sarcoma	Appears first on the oral mucosa as a red, purple, or blue lesion. May be a singular lesion or multiple lesions. May be flat or raised.	HIV infection.	Instruct patient regarding side effects of planned treatment.
Abnormalities of the Gum			
Gingivitis	Painful, inflamed, swollen gums. Usually the gums bleed in response to light contact.	Poor oral hygiene: food debris, bacterial plaque, and calculus (tartar) accumulate. The gums may also swell in response to normal processes such as puberty and pregnancy.	Teach patient proper oral hygiene (see Chart 34-1).
Necrotizing gingivitis (Trench mouth)	Gray-white pseudomembranous ulcerations affecting the edges of the gums, mucosa of the mouth, tonsils, and pharynx. Foul breath. Painful, bleeding gums. Swallowing and talking are painful.	Poor oral hygiene. Bacterial infection, inadequate rest, overwork, emotional stress, and poor nutrition may contribute to development	Teach patient proper oral hygiene (see Chart 34-1). Irrigate with 2% to 3% hydrogen peroxide or normal saline.
Herpetic gingivostomatitis	Burning sensation with the appearance of small vesicles 24–48 hours later. Vesicles may rupture, forming sore, shallow ulcers covered with a gray membrane.	Herpes simplex virus. This occurs most frequently in persons who are immunosuppressed. May occur in other infectious processes such as streptococcal pneumonia, meningococcal meningitis, and malaria.	Apply topical anesthetics as prescribed. May need parenteral opioids if pain is severe. Saline or 2% to 3% hydrogen peroxide irrigations. Antiviral agents such as acyclovir may be prescribed.
Periodontitis	Little discomfort at onset. May have bleeding, infection, gum recession, and loosening of teeth. Later in the disease the teeth may fall out.	May result from untreated gingivitis. Poor or inadequate dental hygiene and inadequate diet contribute to development.	Instruct patient in proper oral hygiene (see Chart 34-1). Instruct patient to consult a dentist.

CHART 34-1
Preventive Oral Hygiene

1. Brush teeth using a soft toothbrush at least 2 times daily. Hold toothbrush at a 45-degree angle between brush and the gums and teeth. Gums and tongue surface should be brushed.
2. Floss at least once daily.
3. Use an antiplaque mouth rinse.
4. Visit a dentist at least every 6 months, or when you have a chipped tooth, oral sore that persists longer than 2 weeks, or a toothache.
5. Avoid alcohol and tobacco products, including smokeless tobacco.
6. Maintain adequate nutrition and avoid sweets.
7. Replace toothbrush at first signs of wear.

Chronic dentoalveolar abscess is a slowly progressive infectious process. It differs from the acute form in that the process may progress to a fully formed abscess without the patient's knowing it. The infection eventually leads to a "blind dental abscess" that is really a periapical granuloma. It may enlarge to as much as 1 cm in diameter. It is often discovered on x-ray and is treated by extraction or root canal therapy, often with apicectomy (excision of the apex of the tooth root).

Management. In the early stages of an infection, a dental surgeon may drill an opening into the pulp chamber to relieve tension and pain and to provide drainage. Usually, the infection has progressed to a periapical abscess. Drainage is provided by an incision through the gingivae down to the jaw bone. Pus (purulent material) escapes under pressure. This procedure is usually performed in the dental office. Occasionally, the patient is admitted to the hospital for same-day surgery. After the inflammatory reaction has subsided, the tooth may have to be extracted or appropriate root canal therapy performed.

Nursing Interventions. The nurse assesses the patient for bleeding after treatment and instructs the patient to use a warm saline or water mouth rinse to keep the area clean. The patient is also instructed in the use of antibiotics and analgesics and to advance from a liquid diet to a soft diet as tolerated.

Malocclusion

Malocclusion is a misalignment of the teeth of the upper and lower dental arcs when the jaws are closed. Fifty percent of the population has some form of malocclusion. Correction of malocclusion requires several factors: an orthodontist who has special training, a patient who is motivated and cooperative and has adequate time. Most treatments begin when the patient has shed the last primary tooth and the last permanent successor has erupted, usually around 12 or 13 years of age; but, treatment may occur in adulthood.

Preventive orthodontics may be started at age 5 if malocclusion is diagnosed early. Studies have shown the reduced need for teeth straightening in adolescence if preventive orthodontics is started with the primary teeth.

Management. To realign the teeth, the orthodontist gradually forces the teeth into a new location by using wires or plastic bands (braces). Although these devices may negatively affect the patient's appearance, this psychological burden must be overcome if good results are to be achieved in the future. In the final phase of treatment, a retaining device is worn for several hours each day to support the tissues as they adjust to the new alignment of the teeth.

Nursing Interventions. It is essential that the patient practice meticulous oral hygiene. The nurse encourages the patient to persist in this most important part of the treatment. An adolescent undergoing orthodontal correction admitted to the hospital for some other problem may have to be reminded to continue wearing the retainer if it does not interfere with the problem requiring hospitalization.

Jaw Repositioning and Reconstruction

The jaw may have to be repositioned or reconstructed for a variety of reasons. Simple fractures of the mandible without displacement, resulting from a blow on the chin, and planned surgical intervention, as in the correction of long or short jaw syndrome, may require treatment by these means. Jaw reconstruction may be necessary in the aftermath of trauma from a severe accident or cancer, both of which can cause loss of tissue and bone.

Mandibular fractures are usually closed fractures. In the past, immobilizing the lower jaw by wiring it to the upper jaw (internal maxillary fixation [IMF]) was the method used for treatment of mandibular fractures. This procedure is associated with several negative outcomes. Because the jaws remain wired for approximately 6 weeks, patients who have had this procedure experience difficulty in maintaining adequate nutrition. They also have difficulties with oral hygiene, masticatory muscle atrophy, and temporomandibular joint dysfunction. They are also at high risk for aspiration– especially in the immediate postoperative period.

Rigid plate fixation (placement of metal plates and screws into the bone to approximate and stabilize the bone) is the current treatment of choice in many cases of mandibular fracture and in some mandibular reconstructive surgery.

Nursing Interventions. Immediately after surgery, patients with IMF are placed on their side, with the head slightly elevated. The nasogastric suction tube inserted during surgery is connected to low-pressure suction to remove stomach contents and reduce the danger of aspiration. Wire cutters are kept at the patient's bedside. If the patient vomits, the nurse must cut the wires to prevent aspiration. Surgery and rewiring will be repeated later. Antiemetic drugs are administered to prevent vomiting.

Secretions of the nasopharyngeal area are cleared with a small catheter inserted through the nasal orifice. Mouth care and suctioning of oral secretions are performed with care.

The diet must necessarily be liquid, but sufficient caloric and fluid intake can be given easily to these patients. They can be fed through a straw without much difficulty, and soft foods are given by spoon. Water is given after each liquid feeding, followed by a mouthwash.

The patient with rigid fixation should not chew food in the first 1 to 4 postoperative weeks.

Patient Education and Home Care Considerations. The patient needs very specific guidelines for mouth care and feeding. It may be necessary to remind the patient to see a physician for scheduled visits to make sure the fixation appliance is functioning properly. Any irritated areas are to be reported. For patients discharged after IMF, a wire cutter is readily available and the patient and a family member are instructed about how to cut the wires in an emergency.

Abnormalities of the Salivary Glands

The **salivary glands** consist of the *parotid glands*, one on each side of the face below the ear; the *submaxillary and sublingual glands*, both in the floor of the mouth; and the *buccal gland*, beneath the lips. About 1200 ml of saliva are produced daily. The glands' primary functions are lubrication, antibacterial protection, and digestion.

Parotitis

Parotitis (inflammation of the parotid gland) is the most common inflammatory condition of the salivary glands; however, infection can occur in the other salivary glands as well. The essential lesion of mumps (epidemic parotitis) is an inflammation of the salivary gland (usually the parotid) and is primarily a pediatric communicable disease caused by viral infection.

Elderly, acutely ill, and debilitated people with decreased salivary flow due to general dehydration or medications are at high risk for developing parotitis. The infecting organisms travel from the mouth through the salivary duct.

The offending organism usually is *Staphylococcus aureus* (except in mumps). The onset of this complication is sudden, with an exacerbation of both the fever and the symptoms of the primary condition. The gland swells and becomes tense and tender. Pain is felt in the ear, and the swollen glands interfere with swallowing. The swelling increases rapidly, and the overlying skin soon becomes red and shiny.

Nursing Interventions. Preventive mechanisms are essential. To prevent postoperative parotitis, patients are advised to have necessary dental work performed before surgery. In addition, optimal patient preparation includes maintaining an adequate nutritional and fluid intake along with good oral hygiene, and if possible discontinuing medications that may cause a decrease in salivation (*e.g.*, tranquilizers and diuretics). If parotitis occurs, antibiotic therapy is necessary. Analgesics may also be prescribed to control pain. If antibiotic therapy is not effective, incision and drainage (I & D) of the gland are necessary.

Sialadenitis

Sialadenitis (inflammation of the salivary glands) may be caused by dehydration, radiation therapy, stress, malnutrition, salivary gland calculi (stones), or improper oral hygiene and is associated with infection with *Staphylococcus aureus, Streptococcus viridans,* or pneumococcus. Symptoms include pain, swelling, and a purulent discharge.

Management. Antibiotics are used to relieve acute symptoms. Massage, hydration, and corticosteroids frequently cure the problem. Chronic sialoadenitis, with uncontrolled pain, is treated by surgically draining the gland or excising the gland and its duct.

Salivary Calculus (Sialolithiasis)

Salivary calculi occur in the submandibular gland. Salivary gland ultrasound or sialograms (x-ray films taken with a radiopaque substance injected into the duct) may be required to demonstrate obstruction of the duct by stenosis. Salivary stones are formed mainly from calcium phosphate. If located within the gland, they are irregular and vary in diameter from 3 to 30 mm. Stones in the duct are small and oval shaped.

Calculi within the salivary gland cause no symptoms unless infection arises; but a calculus that obstructs the gland's duct causes sudden, local, and often colicky pain, which is suddenly relieved by a gush of saliva. This characteristic complaint can be elicited in a health history. When this condition exists, the gland is swollen and quite tender, the stone itself often is palpable, and its shadow may be seen on x-ray films.

The calculus can be extracted fairly easily from the duct in the mouth; sometimes enlarging the ductal orifice permits the stone to pass spontaneously. Surgery may be necessary to remove the gland if there are repeated recurrences of symptoms and calculi in the gland itself.

Lithotripsy (or disintegration of the stone by shockwaves) may be used instead of surgical extraction. Lithotripsy requires no anesthesia, sedation, or analgesia. Side effects may include local hemorrhage and swelling.

Neoplasms

Although uncommon, neoplasms (tumors or growths) of almost any type may develop in the salivary gland. Tumors occur more frequently in the parotid gland. The incidence of salivary gland tumors is similar in men and women. Diagnosis is based on the history and physical examination and biopsy results.

Management. There is controversy regarding the best way to manage salivary gland tumors. The common procedure involves partially excising the gland, along with all of the tumor and a wide margin. Dissection is carefully performed to preserve the vulnerable seventh cranial nerve (facial nerve). For more involved tumors, it may not be possible to preserve the nerve when a parotidectomy is performed. If the tumor is malignant, radiation therapy may follow surgery. Chemotherapy is usually used for palliative purposes. Local recurrences are common; the recurrent growth usually is more aggressive than the original. It has also been observed that these patients have an increased incidence of second primary cancers.

Cancer of the Oral Cavity

Cancer of the oral cavity, which may occur in any part of the mouth or throat, is curable if discovered early. This type of cancer is associated with the use of alcohol and tobacco. Many feel that the combination of alcohol and tobacco has a synergistic carcinogenic effect. Age is also a risk factor, with 75% of oral cancers occurring in persons over age 60; but it is increasing in men under age 30 because of the use of smokeless tobacco–especially snuff.

Cancer of the oral cavity accounts for less that 2% of all cancer deaths in the United States. Men are afflicted more often than women; however, the incidence in women is increasing, possibly because they use tobacco and alcohol more frequently than they did in the past. The 5-year survival rate for cancer of the oral cavity and pharynx is 54% for Caucasians and 32% for African-Americans. Of the 8370 annual deaths from oral cancer (Wingo et al., 1995), the distribution by site is estimated as follows:

Lip 100
Tongue 1870
Mouth 2300
Pharynx 4100

Chronic irritation by a warm pipe stem or prolonged exposure to the sun and wind may predispose one to lip cancer. Predisposing factors for other oral cancers are exposure to tobacco, including smokeless tobacco, and alcohol.

Clinical Manifestations. Many oral cancers exhibit no symptoms in the early stages. The most frequent complaint of the patient is a painless sore or mass that will not heal. A typical lesion in oral cancer is a painless indurated (hardened) ulcer with raised edges. Any ulcer of the oral cavity that does not heal in 2 weeks should be examined through biopsy. As the cancer progresses, the patient may complain of tenderness; difficulty in chewing, swallowing, or speaking; coughing of blood-tinged sputum; or enlarged cervical lymph nodes.

Diagnostic Evaluation. Diagnostic evaluation consists of an oral examination as well as an assessment of cervical lymph nodes to evaluate for possible metastasis. Biopsies are performed on lesions suggestive of cancer. Suspicious lesions are those that have not healed in 2 weeks. Oral areas of high risk include the buccal mucosa and gingiva for persons who use snuff or smoke a cigar or pipe. For persons who smoke cigarettes and drink alcohol, high-risk areas include the floor of the mouth, ventrolateral tongue, and soft palate complex (which includes the soft palate, the anterior and posterior tonsillar area, uvula, and the area behind the molar and tongue junction).

Management. Management varies with the nature of the lesion, preference of the physician, and patient choice. Resectional surgery, radiation therapy, chemotherapy, or a combination of these therapies may be effective.

In cancer of the lip, small lesions are usually excised liberally; larger lesions involving greater than one third of the lip may be more appropriately treated by radiation therapy because of superior cosmetic results. The choice depends on the extent of the lesion, the skill of the surgeon or radiologist, and what is necessary to cure the patient while preserving the best appearance. For tumors larger than 4 cm there is a high recurrence rate.

Cancer of the tongue is usually treated aggressively, as the recurrence rate is high. For cancer of the lateral margin of the tongue, the two major treatments of choice are radiation therapy and surgery. It is often necessary to perform a hemiglossectomy (surgical removal of half of the tongue).

When cancer is present at the base of the tongue, surgical resection is more debilitating. Often radiation therapy may be the primary treatment. A combination of radioactive interstitial implants and external beam radiation may be employed. For larger lesions, external beam therapy alone is used.

Often cancer of the oral cavity has metastasized through the extensive lymphatic channel in the neck region (Fig. 34-1), thereby requiring a neck dissection (see p. 843) and possibly reconstructive surgery of the oral cavity. A commonly used intraoral reconstructive technique involves use of a radial forearm free flap (use of a thin layer of skin from the forearm along with the radial artery).

Nursing Interventions. The patient's nutritional status is assessed preoperatively. A dietary consult may be necessary. The patient may require enteral (through the in-

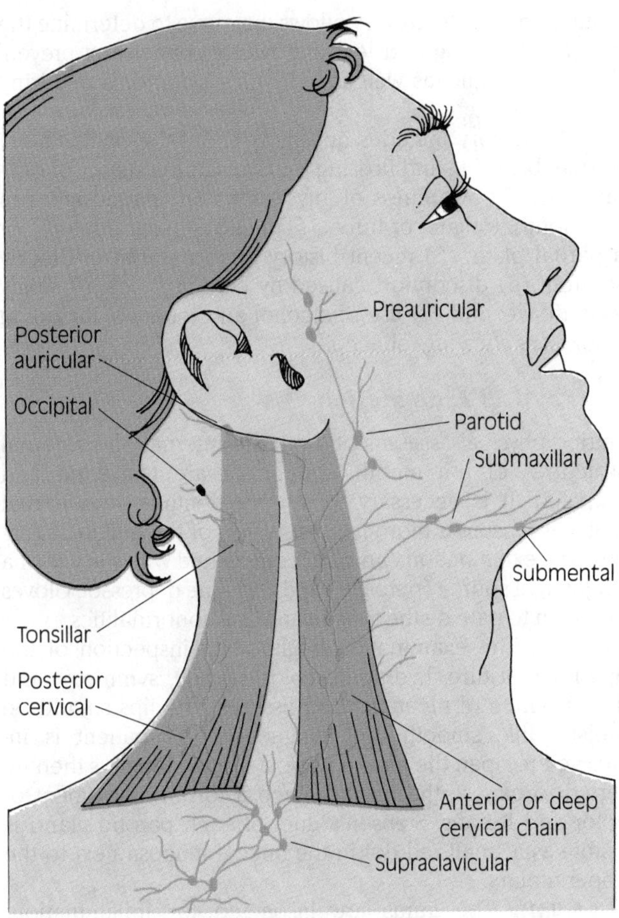

FIGURE 34-1. Lymphatic drainage of the head and neck.

testine) or parenteral (through any extra-alimentary route) feedings preoperatively and postoperatively to maintain adequate nutrition. If a radial graft is to be done, an Allen test on the donor arm must be performed to assure ulnar artery patency to provide blood flow to the hand after removal of the radial artery. (An Allen test is done by manually compressing the radial artery and asking the patient to make a fist. The patient's hand should turn pink indicating ulnar artery patency.)

Postoperatively the patient is assessed for maintenance of the airway. The patient may be unable to manage oral secretions and suctioning may be necessary. If grafting was done, suctioning must be performed with care to prevent damage to the graft. The graft is assessed postoperatively for viability. Although color should be assessed (white may indicate arterial occlusion and blue mottling may indicate venous congestion), it may be difficult to adequately assess the graft by looking into the mouth. A Doppler ultrasound may be used to locate the radial pulse at the graft site and to assess graft perfusion.

❑ NURSING PROCESS
Patients With Conditions of the Oral Cavity

Assessment

History

Obtaining a health history allows the nurse to determine the patient's teaching and learning needs concerning preventive oral hygiene, as well as to identify symptoms requiring medical evaluation.

The history includes questions about the patient's (1) normal brushing and flossing routine; (2) frequency of dental visits; (3) awareness of any lesions or irritated areas in the mouth, tongue, or throat; (4) need to wear dentures or a partial plate; (5) recent history of sore throat or bloody sputum; (6) discomfort caused by certain foods; (7) daily food intake; and (8) use of alcohol and tobacco, including smokeless chewing tobacco.

Physical Examination

During physical assessment, both the internal and external structures of the mouth and throat are inspected and palpated. It is necessary to remove dentures and partial plates to ensure a thorough inspection of the gums. In general, the examination can be accomplished with the use of a bright light source (penlight) and a tongue depressor. Gloves are worn to palpate the tongue and any abnormalities.

Lips. The examination begins with inspection of the lips for moisture, hydration, color, texture, symmetry, and the presence of ulcerations or fissures. The lips should be moist, pink, smooth and symmetric. The patient is instructed to open the mouth wide; a tongue blade is then inserted to expose the buccal mucosa for an assessment of color and lesions. Stensen's duct of each parotid gland is visible as a small red dot in the buccal mucosa next to the upper molars.

Gums. The gums are inspected for inflammation, bleeding, retraction, and discoloration. The odor of the breath is also noted. The hard palate is examined for color and shape.

Tongue. The dorsum (back) of the tongue is inspected for texture, color, and lesions. A thin, white coat and large, vallate papillae in a V formation on the distal portion of the dorsum of the tongue are normal findings. The patient is instructed to protrude his or her tongue and move it laterally. This provides the examiner with an opportunity to estimate the tongue's size as well as its symmetry and strength (assesses the integrity of the 12th cranial nerve [**hypoglossal**]).

Further inspection of the ventral surface of the tongue and the floor of the mouth is accomplished by asking the patient to touch the roof of the mouth with the tip of the tongue. Any lesions of the mucosa or any abnormalities involving the frenulum or superficial veins on the undersurface of the tongue are noted. This is a common area for oral cancer, which presents as a white or red plaque, an indurated ulcer, or a warty growth.

A tongue blade is used to depress the tongue for adequate visualization of the pharynx. It is pressed firmly beyond the midpoint of the tongue. Proper placement avoids a gagging response and minimizes the patient's aversion to future oral examinations. The patient is told to tip the head back, open the mouth wide, take a deep breath, and say "ah." Often this will flatten the posterior tongue and briefly expose a full view of the anterior and posterior pillars, the tonsils, uvula, and posterior pharynx (Fig. 34-2). These structures are inspected for color, symmetry, and evidence of exudate, ulceration, or enlargement. Normally, the uvula and soft palate rise symmetrically with a deep inspiration or "ah" and indicate an intact vagus nerve (10th cranial nerve).

A complete assessment of the oral cavity is essential, as many disorders such as cancer, diabetes, and immunosuppressive conditions from drug therapy or acquired immunodeficiency syndrome (AIDS) may be manifested by changes in the oral cavity. The neck is examined for enlarged lymph nodes (adenopathy).

Diagnosis

Nursing Diagnoses

Based on all the assessment data, major nursing diagnoses may include the following:

- ❑ Altered oral mucous membrane related to a pathologic condition, infection, or chemical or mechanical trauma (*e.g.*, drugs, ill-fitting dentures)
- ❑ Altered nutrition, less than body requirements, related to inability to ingest adequate nutrients secondary to oral or dental conditions.
- ❑ Body image disturbance related to a physical change in appearance resulting from a disease condition or its treatment
- ❑ Fear of pain and social isolation related to disease or change in physical appearance
- ❑ Pain related to oral lesion or treatment
- ❑ Impaired verbal communication related to treatment
- ❑ Risk for infection related to disease or treatment
- ❑ Knowledge deficit about disease process and treatment plan

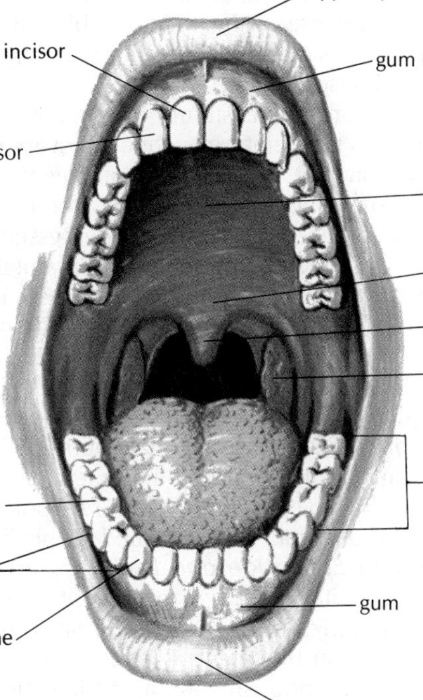

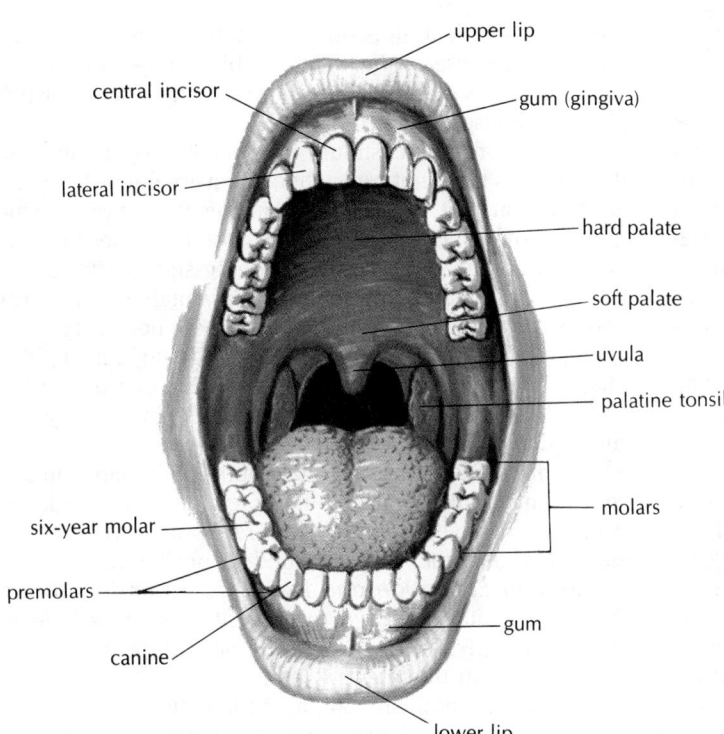

FIGURE 34-2. Structures of the mouth, including the tongue and palate.

Planning and Implementation

Goals. The major goals for the patient may include improvement in the condition of the oral mucous membrane, improvement in nutritional intake, attainment of a positive self-image, attainment of comfort, alternative communication methods, absence of infection, and understanding of the disease and its treatment.

Nursing Interventions

Promoting Mouth Care. Titler and colleagues (1991) stressed the need for the nurse to identify patients at risk for oral complications and to assist the patient with methods to decrease complications (see Nursing Research Profile for Unit 8.) The nurse instructs the patient in the importance and techniques of preventive mouth care (see Chart 34-1). The use of a soft tooth brush is preferable to the use of a foam sponge stick. If a patient cannot tolerate brushing or flossing, an irrigating solution of 1 teaspoon of baking soda to 8 ounces of warm water, half-strength hydrogen peroxide, or normal saline solution is recommended. The nurse reinforces the need to perform oral self-care, and actually provides such care to patients who are unable to do so themselves.

Any oral mucous membrane disorder is referred to the primary care provider for treatment. In the case of bacterial or fungal infections, the nurse administers the appropriate medication and instructs the patient in how to administer these same medications at home. The nurse monitors the patient's physical and psychological response to treatment.

Xerostomia. Dryness of the mouth (xerostomia) is a frequent sequela of oral cancer, particularly when the salivary glands have been exposed to radiation or major surgery. It is also noted in patients who are receiving psychopharmacologic agents, those with HIV infection, or those who are unable to close the mouth and therefore become mouth-breathers.

To minimize this problem, the patient is advised to avoid dry, bulky, and irritating foods and fluids, as well as alcohol and tobacco. The patient is also encouraged to increase intake of fluids, when it is not contraindicated, and to use a humidifier during sleep. The use of synthetic saliva, a moisturizing antibacterial gel such as Oral Balance, or a saliva production stimulant such as Salagen may be helpful. Kusler and Rambur (1992) report that coating the oral mucous membranes two to three times a day with 1/16 to 1/8 teaspoon of butter, margarine, or vegetable oil may help patients experiencing xerostomia secondary to radiation therapy, although there is no research to support this treatment.

Stomatitis or Mucositis. Stomatitis or mucositis (breakdown of the oral mucosa) is often a side effect of chemotherapy or radiation therapy. Prophylactic mouth care is started when the patient begins receiving treatment; however, mucositis may become so severe that a break in treatment is necessary. Some research studies suggest that using benzydamine hydrochloride rinse or topical prostaglandin E_2 may decrease mucositis (Calman & Langdon, 1991). If a patient receiving radiation therapy has poor dentition, extraction of the teeth is often recommended to prevent infection before treatment to the oral cavity is initiated. Many radiation therapy centers recommend the use of fluoride treatments for patients receiving radiation to the head and neck.

Assuring Adequate Food and Fluid Intake. The patient's weight, age, and level of activity are recorded to determine if nutritional intake is adequate. A daily calorie count may be necessary to determine the exact quantity of food and fluid ingested. The frequency and pattern of eating are recorded to determine if any psychosocial or physiologic factors are influencing ingestion.

The nurse recommends changes in the consistency of foods and the frequency of eating, based on the disease condition and the patient's preferences. Consultation with a dietitian can be helpful. The goal is to help the patient attain and maintain desirable body weight and level of energy, as well as to promote the healing of tissue. Research with patients receiving treatment for cancer of the head and neck has determined that (1) eating disabilities are common and (2) patients develop strategies to maintain adequate nutrition. (See Wilson et al., 1991, and Languis et al., 1993.)

Supporting a Positive Self-Image. A patient who has a disfiguring oral condition or has undergone disfiguring surgery may experience an alteration in self-image. The patient is encouraged to verbalize the perceived change in body appearance and realistically discuss actual changes or losses. The nurse offers support while the patient verbalizes fears and negative feelings (withdrawal, depression, anger). The nurse listens attentively and determines if the patient's needs are primarily psychosocial or cognitive-perceptual. This determination will help to individualize a plan of care. The patient's strengths, achievements, and positive attributes are reinforced.

The nurse should determine the patient's major anxieties concerning interpersonal relationships, for only then can the nurse recommend specific ways for the patient to interact with others. Referral to support groups, a psychiatric liaison nurse, social worker, or clergy may be useful in helping the patient to cope with anxieties and fears. Emphasizing that the patient's worth is not diminished by a physical change in a body part can be a helpful approach.

The patient's progress toward developing positive self-esteem is recorded. The nurse should be alert to signs of grieving and should record emotional changes. By providing an atmosphere of acceptance and support the nurse encourages the patient to express changes in feelings of self-esteem.

Minimizing Discomfort and Pain. Oral lesions may be painful. The nurse instructs the patient to minimize discomfort by avoiding foods that are spicy, hot, or hard (pretzels, nuts). The patient is also instructed about mouth care. It may be necessary to provide the patient with an analgesic such as viscous lidocaine (Xylocaine Viscous 2%) or opioids as prescribed. The nurse can reduce fear of pain by advising the patient regarding pain control methods.

Promoting Effective Communication. For the patient undergoing radical surgical procedures for oral cancer, the potential for loss of verbal communication is high. It is, therefore, vital that the patient's ability to communicate in writing be assessed preoperatively. A magic slate or pen and paper are provided postoperatively to those patients who can use them to communicate successfully. A communication board with commonly used words or pictures is obtained preoperatively and given to postoperative patients who are unable to write so that they may point to needed items. A speech therapist is also consulted postoperatively.

Promoting Infection Control. Leukopenia (a decrease in white blood cells) may result from radiation, chemotherapy, AIDS, and some medication used to treat AIDS. This reduces defense mechanisms, making the patient more susceptible to infections. Malnutrition, also common, may further decrease the patient's ability to resist infection. If the patient is diabetic, the risk of infection due to hyperglycemia is also a factor.

Laboratory results should be evaluated frequently, and the patient's temperature is checked every 6 to 8 hours for an elevation that may indicate an infection. Visitors who may transmit microorganisms are prohibited because the patient's immunologic system is depressed. Sensitive skin tissues are protected from trauma to maintain skin integrity and prevent infection. Aseptic technique is necessary when changing dressings. Desquamation (shedding of the epidermis) is a reaction to radiation therapy that causes dryness and itching and can lead to a break in skin integrity and subsequent infection.

As discussed above, adequate nutrition is helpful in preventing infection. Signs of wound infection such as redness, swelling, drainage, or tenderness are reported to the physician. Antibiotics may be prescribed prophylactically.

Patient Education and Home Care Considerations. The posthospital objectives of patient care are similar to those that apply during hospitalization. The patient who is recovering from treatment of a mouth condition needs to breathe, obtain nourishment, avoid infection, and be alert for adverse signs and symptoms. The patient, family members or the person responsible for home care, the nurse, and other health care professionals (such as a speech therapist, dietitian, and psychologist) need to work together to prepare an individualized plan of care.

If suctioning the mouth or tracheostomy tube is required, it is important to determine what equipment is needed and where it can be obtained. The patient and family are taught how to use the equipment. It may be necessary to humidify and aerate the room, as well as to control odors.

Methods of preparing foods that are nutritious, properly seasoned, and of the right temperature can be explained. It may be more convenient for some patients to use commercial baby food than to prepare liquid and soft diets in a blender. The patient who is unable to take foods orally may need to be instructed in the use of enteral or parenteral feedings.

For cancer patients, the use and care of prostheses must be understood. The importance of keeping the dressings clean is reviewed, as is the need to practice strict oral hygiene. The patient and the care provider at home need to know the signs of obstruction, hemorrhage, infection, depression, and withdrawal, as well as what to do about these problems.

Follow-up visits to the clinic or physician are important to determine progression or regression and to provide the patient and caregiver with instructions about any modifications in medication or general care.

Evaluation

Expected Outcomes

1. Shows evidence of intact oral mucous membranes
   a. Is free of pain and discomfort in the oral cavity
   b. Has no visible alteration in membrane integrity
   c. Identifies and avoids foods that are irritating (nuts, pretzels, spicy foods)

d. States measures necessary for preventive mouth care
e. Complies with medication regimen
f. Limits or avoids use of alcohol and tobacco (including smokeless tobacco)

2. Attains and maintains desirable body weight
3. Has a positive self-image
   a. Verbalizes anxieties
   b. Is able to accept change and modify self-concept accordingly
4. Attains an acceptable level of comfort
   a. Verbalizes that pain is absent or tolerable
   b. Avoids foods and liquids that cause discomfort
   c. Adheres to medication regimen
5. Experiences decreased fears related to pain, isolation, and the inability to cope
   a. Accepts that pain will be managed if not eliminated
   b. Freely expresses fears and concerns
6. Is free of infection
   a. Exhibits normal laboratory values
   b. Is afebrile
   c. Performs oral hygiene after every meal and at bedtime
7. Acquires information about disease process and course of treatment

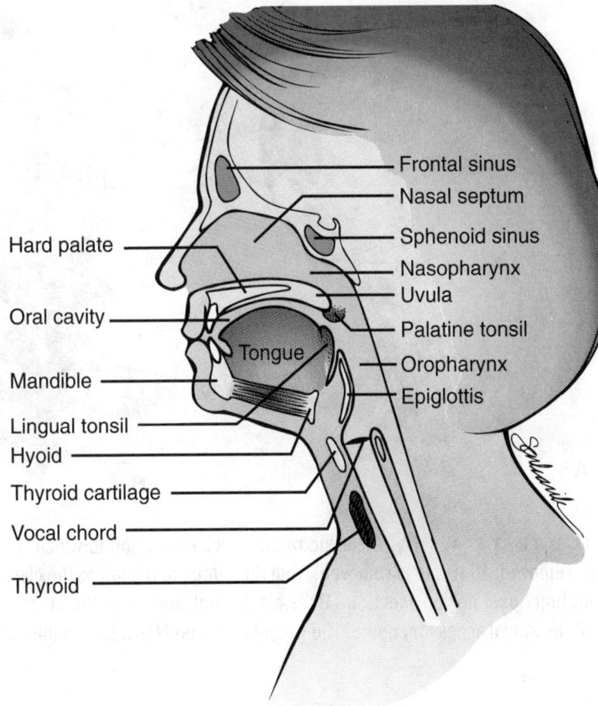

FIGURE 34-3. Anatomy of the head and neck.

Neck Dissection

Malignancies of the head and neck, include those of the oral cavity, oropharynx, hypopharynx, nasopharynx, nasal cavity, paranasal sinus, and larynx (Fig. 34-3). (Laryngeal cancer is discussed in Chapter 23.) These cancers account for less than 5% of all cancers. Depending on the location and stage, treatment may consist of radiation therapy, chemotherapy, surgery, or a combination of these modalities. Most observers agree that such patients do not die of recurrence at the site of the primary growth, but rather of metastasis to the cervical lymph nodes in the neck, which often takes place by way of the lymphatics before the primary lesion has been treated.

A radical neck dissection involves removal of all cervical lymph nodes from the mandible to the clavicle, removal of the sternocleidomastoid muscle, internal jugular vein, and the spinal accessory muscle. The associated morbidities include shoulder drop and poor cosmesis (visible neck depression). A surgical approach used more often is a modified radical neck dissection, which by definition preserves one or more of the nonlymphatic structures (Robbins et al, 1991). Many surgeons perform a modified radical neck dissection by preserving the internal jugular vein, the sternocleidomastoid muscle and the spinal accessory nerve. A selective neck dissection (in comparison to a radical dissection) preserves one or more of the lymph node groups (Fig. 34-4).

Reconstructive techniques may be performed with a variety of grafts. A cutaneous flap (skin and subcutaneous tissue), such as the deltopectoral flap may be used. A more frequently used graft for head and neck reconstruction is a myocutaneous flap (muscle and skin). This is usually done using the pectoralis major muscle. For large defects some surgeons use a microvascular free flap. This involves transfer of muscle, skin, or bone with an artery and vein to the area of reconstruction using microinstrumentation. Areas used for a free flap include the scapula, radial area of the forearm, or the fibula. The fibula provides a larger bone area if mandibular reconstruction is involved.

❑ NURSING PROCESS
The Patient Undergoing a Neck Dissection

Assessment

Preoperatively, the patient's physical and psychological preparation for major surgery is assessed. The patient is also assessed for knowledge related to the preoperative and postoperative procedures. Postoperatively, the patient is assessed for complications such as altered respiratory status, wound infection, and hemorrhage. As healing occurs, the patient's range of motion (ROM) of the neck is assessed.

Diagnosis

Nursing Diagnoses

Based on all the assessment data, major nursing diagnoses may include the following:

- ❑ Knowledge deficit about preoperative and postoperative procedures
- ❑ Ineffective airway clearance related to obstruction secondary to mucus, hemorrhage, or edema
- ❑ Risk for infection related to surgical intervention secondary to decreased nutritional status, or immunosuppression from chemotherapy or radiation therapy
- ❑ Impaired skin integrity secondary to surgery and graft
- ❑ Altered nutrition, less than body requirements, related to disease process or treatment
- ❑ Ineffective coping related to diagnosis or prognosis

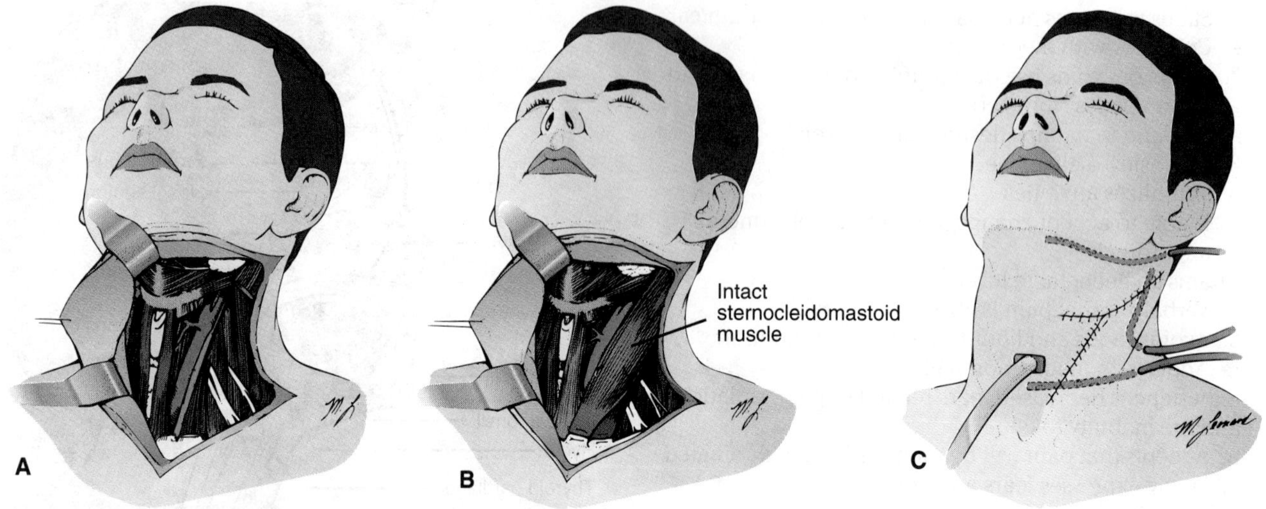

FIGURE 34-4. (A) A classic radical neck dissection in which the sternocleidomastoid and smaller muscles are removed. All tissue is removed, from the ramus of the jaw to the clavicle. The jugular vein has also been removed. The functional neck dissection (B) is similar but preserves the sternocleidomastoid muscle, internal jugular vein, and the spinal accessory nerve. The wound is closed (C), and portable suction drainage tubes are in place.

- Pain related to surgical incision and the presence of abnormal epithelial cells
- Impaired communication secondary to surgical treatment
- Impaired physical mobility secondary to nerve injury

Collaborative Problems/ Potential Complications

Potential postoperative complications that may develop include:

- Hemorrhage
- Nerve injury

Planning and Implementation

Goals. The major goals for the patient may include participation in the treatment plan, maintenance of respiratory status, absence of infection, graft viability, maintenance of adequate intake of food and fluids, effective coping strategies, attainment of comfort, effective communication, and absence of complications.

Nursing Interventions

Preoperative Patient Education

Before surgery, the patient should be informed about the impending surgery, what is to be done in the operating room (clarification of the surgeon's explanation), and what the postoperative period will be like. At the same time, the patient is encouraged to express concerns about the upcoming surgery. During this exchange, the nurse has an opportunity to assess the patient's coping abilities, answer questions, and develop a plan for offering assistance. A sense of mutual understanding and rapport will make the postoperative experience less traumatic for the patient. After the operation, the patient's expressions of concern, anxieties, and fears can guide the nurse in providing additional support.

General Postoperative Care

The general postoperative nursing intervention activities are similar to those described in Chapter 21. For the patient who has had extensive neck surgery, the specific postoperative nursing interventions include maintenance of a patent airway and continuous assessment of respiratory status; wound care and oral hygiene; nutritional needs; and observation for hemorrhage or nerve injury.

Maintaining the Airway. After the endotracheal tube or airway has been removed and the effects of the anesthesia have worn off, the patient may be placed in Fowler's position to facilitate breathing and promote comfort. This position also increases lymphatic and venous drainage, facilitates swallowing, and decreases venous pressure on the skin flaps.

Signs of respiratory distress, such as dyspnea, cyanosis, and changes in vital signs, are assessed because they may suggest edema, hemorrhage, or inadequate drainage. Temperature should not be taken orally.

In the immediate postoperative period, the nurse may be able to detect the presence of stridor (coarse, high-pitched sound on inspiration) by listening frequently over the trachea with a stethoscope. These findings should be reported immediately.

Pneumonia may occur in the postoperative phase if pulmonary secretions are not removed. Coughing and deep breathing are encouraged to aid in the removal of secretions. The patient should assume a sitting position, with the nurse supporting the neck so that the patient may be able to bring up excessive secretions. If this technique fails, the patient's respiratory tract may have to be suctioned. Care is exerted to protect the suture lines during suctioning. If a tracheostomy tube is in place, suctioning is performed through this tube using sterile technique. The patient may also be instructed on how to use the Yankauer suction (tonsil tip suction) to remove oral secretions.

Providing Wound Care. Drainage tubes are usually inserted during surgery to prevent collection of fluid subcutaneously. The drainage tubes are usually connected to portable suction. During the first 24 hours there may be 80 to 120 ml of serosanguineous secretions. If dressings are present, they may need to be reinforced from time to time. Dressings are observed for evidence of hemorrhage and constriction, which may affect respiration and graft perfusion. The graft is assessed for color and temperature, and presence of a pulse if applicable, to determine viability. The graft should be pale pink in color and warm to the touch. The wound is also assessed for signs and symptoms of infection. Any such signs are reported immediately. The patient may be placed on prophylactic antibiotics.

Maintaining Adequate Nutrition. Nutritional status is assessed preoperatively to decrease postoperative complications. Frequently, nutrition is less than optimal because of inadequate intake. Therefore, the patient often requires enteral or parenteral supplements preoperatively to attain a positive nitrogen balance. This may need to be continued postoperatively if the patient is unable to take enough calories by mouth.

The patient may attain a positive nitrogen balance by taking supplemental substances such as Ensure, Sustacal, or Carnation Instant Breakfast (as a few examples). These nutritional supports may be taken enterally either by mouth, by nasogastric feeding tube, or by gastrostomy feeding tube.

The patient who is able to chew may take food by mouth, although the level of the patient's chewing ability will determine if some diet modification (such as providing soft, pureed, or liquid foods) is necessary. Food preferences should also be discussed with the patient. Oral care before eating may enhance the patient's appetite. Oral care after eating is important to prevent infection.

Supporting Coping Measures. Preoperatively, the patient is given information about the planned surgery. The psychological postoperative nursing intervention is aimed at supporting the patient who has had a change in body image or who has major concerns regarding the prognosis. Such a patient may have difficulty communicating and be concerned about the ability to breathe and swallow normally. The nurse enlists the support of family or friends in encouraging and reassuring the patient that adjusting to the results of this surgery will take time.

The person who has had extensive neck surgery often is sensitive about his or her appearance, either when the operative area is covered by bulky dressings or when the incision line is visible. If the nurse accepts the patient's appearance and expresses a positive, optimistic attitude, the patient is more likely to be encouraged. The patient also needs an opportunity to express concerns regarding the success of the surgery and the prognosis. Most patients are able to maintain and gain weight.

Persons with cancer of the head and neck are frequently ones who used alcohol or tobacco before surgery; postoperatively, the patient is encouraged to abstain from these substances. Alternative methods of coping need to be explored and introduced slowly.

Relieving Pain. Pain and the patient's fear of pain are assessed and managed. Patients with head and neck cancer often report less pain than patients with other types of cancer; however, the nurse needs to be aware that each person's pain experience is individual. The nurse offers analgesics as prescribed and periodically assesses their effectiveness.

Promoting Effective Communication. If a laryngectomy was performed, the nurse explores other methods of communicating with the patient and obtains a consultation with a speech therapist.

Maintaining Physical Mobility. Excising muscles and nerves results in weakness at the shoulder that can cause "shoulder drop," a forward curvature of the shoulder.

Many problems can be avoided with a conscientious exercise program. These exercises are usually begun when drains are removed and the neck incision is sufficiently healed. The purpose of the exercises depicted in Figure 34-5 is to promote maximal shoulder function and neck motion after surgery.

Monitoring and Managing Potential Complications. **Hemorrhage** may occur from carotid artery rupture as a result of necrosis of the graft or damage to the artery itself from tumor or infection. The following measures are indicated to prevent or manage hemorrhage:

- Vital signs are assessed. Tachycardia, tachypnea, and hypotension may indicate impending hypovolemic shock subsequent to hemorrhage.
- The patient is instructed to avoid the Valsalva maneuver to prevent stress on the graft and carotid artery.
- Signs of impending rupture such as high epigastric pain or discomfort are reported.
- Dressings and wound drainage are observed for excessive bleeding.
- If hemorrhage occurs, assistance is summoned immediately.
- Hemorrhage requires the continuous application of pressure to the bleeding site or major associated vessel.
- The head of the patient's bed is elevated to maintain airway patency and prevent aspiration.
- A controlled, calm manner will allay the patient's anxiety.
- A physician is notified immediately because vascular or ligature tear requires surgical intervention.

Nerve injury can occur if the cervical plexus or spinal accessory nerves are severed during surgery. Because lower facial paralysis may occur as a result of injury to the facial nerve, this complication is observed for and reported. Likewise, if the superior laryngeal nerve is damaged, the patient may have difficulty swallowing liquids and food because of the partial lack of sensation of the glottis. Speech therapy may be indicated to assist with the problems related to nerve injury.

Patient Education and Home Care Considerations. The patient and family are instructed on how to administer enteral or parenteral nutrition if the patient is unable to take food by mouth. Home care by a visiting nurse may be necessary in the early period following discharge to assure that the feedings are being administered properly, to assess wound healing, and to detect any possible complications. Physical and speech therapy also may be continued at home.

The patient is given information regarding local support groups such as "I Can Cope" or "New Voice Club." The local chapter of the American Cancer Society may be contacted for information and equipment for the patient.

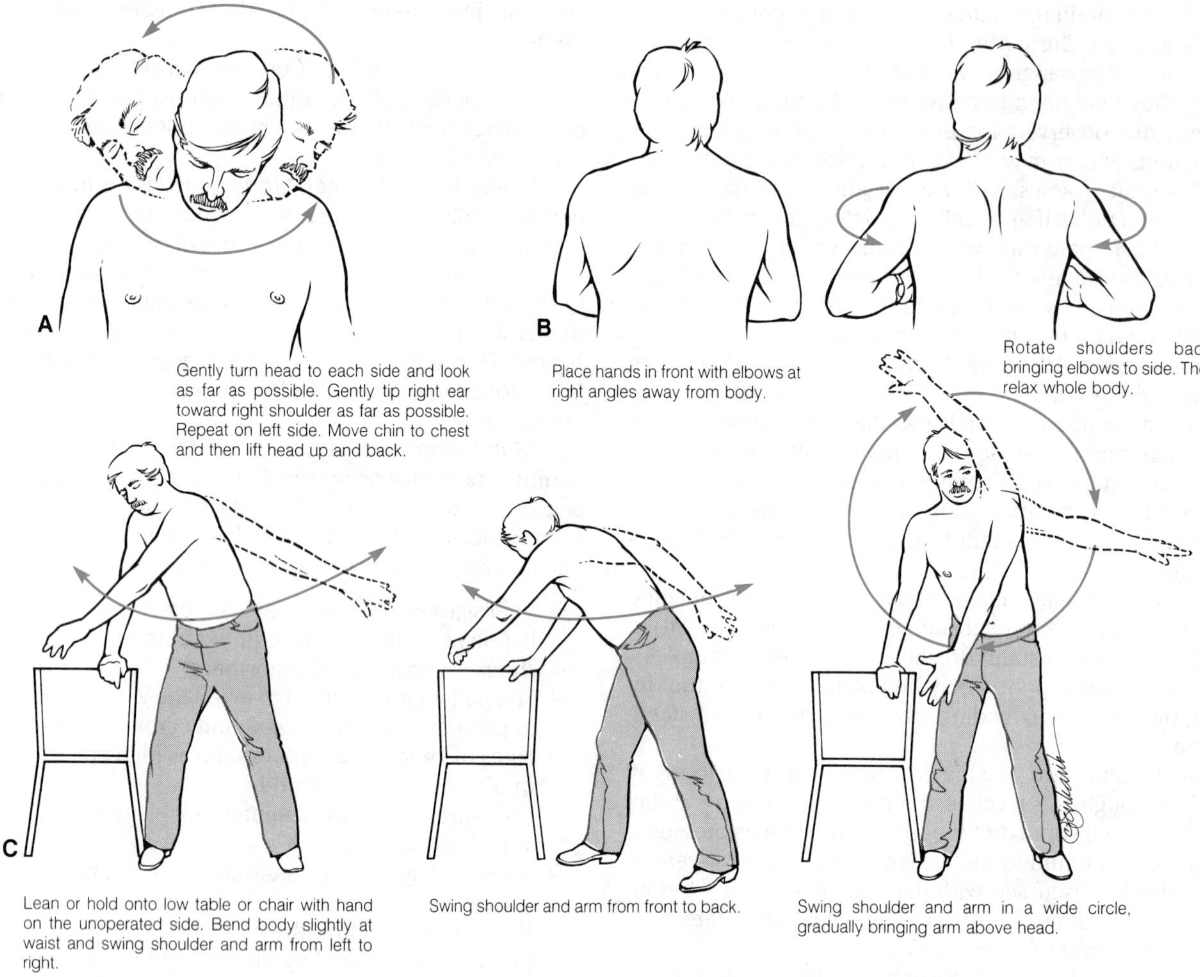

FIGURE 34-5. Three rehabilitation exercises after head and neck surgery. The objective is to regain maximum shoulder function and neck motion after neck surgery. (Exercise for Radical Neck Surgery Patients. Head and Neck Service, Department of Surgery, Memorial Hospital, New York, NY.)

Evaluation

Expected Outcomes

1. Acquires information about course of treatment
2. Demonstrates good respiratory exchange
   a. Lungs are clear to auscultation
   b. Breathes easily with no shortness of breath
   c. Demonstrates ability to use suction effectively
3. Is free of infection
   a. Maintains normal laboratory values
   b. Is afebrile
4. Graft is pink and warm to touch
5. Maintains adequate intake of foods and fluids
   a. Accepts altered route of feeding
   b. Is well hydrated
   c. Maintains or gains weight
6. Demonstrates ability to cope
   a. Verbally discusses emotional responses to the diagnosis
   b. Attends support groups
7. Verbalizes comfort
8. Attains maximal mobility
   a. Is compliant with physical therapy exercises
   b. Attains maximal range of motion

Nursing Care Plan 34-1 presents an overview of the care of a patient undergoing a neck dissection.

Conditions of the Esophagus

The esophagus is a mucus-lined, muscular tube that carries food from the mouth to the stomach. It begins at the base of the pharynx and ends about 4 cm below the diaphragm. Its ability to transport food and fluid is facilitated by two sphincters. The upper esophageal sphincter (UES), also called the hypopharyngeal sphincter, is located at the junction of the pharynx and the esophagus. The lower esophageal sphincter (LES), also called the gastroesophageal sphincter, is located at the junction of the esophagus and the stomach. An incompetent LES allows reflux (backward flow) of gastric contents.

Difficulty in swallowing (*dysphagia*) is the most common symptom of esophageal disease. This symptom may range from an uncomfortable feeling that a bolus of food is "caught" in the upper esophagus (before it eventually passes into the stomach) to acute pain on swallowing (*odynophagia*). Obstruction to the passage of food (solid and soft) and

(text continues on page 850)

NURSING CARE PLAN 34–1
Care of the Patient Who Has Undergone Neck Dissection

Nursing Interventions	Rationale	Expected Outcomes
NURSING DIAGNOSIS: Ineffective airway clearance related to obstruction secondary to edema, secretions, hemorrhage, or inadequate wound drainage.		
GOAL: Maintenance of normal respiratory function.		
1. Place the patient in high Fowler's position.	1. High Fowler's position facilitates expansion of the lungs because the diaphragm is pulled downward and the abdominal viscera are pulled away from the lungs. Breathing is promoted. This position also increases lymphatic and venous drainage, facilitates swallowing, and decreases venous pressure on the graft. Regurgitation and aspiration of stomach contents is prevented postoperatively.	• Achieves a normal respiratory rate. • Breathes comfortably. • Avoids use of accessory muscles of respiration. • Demonstrates full thoracic excursion.
2. Monitor vital signs according to postoperative routine.	2. Edema, hemorrhage, or inadequate drainage will alter heart rate and respirations. Tachypnea and restlessness may indicate respiratory distress.	• Maintains vital signs within normal range.
3. Auscultate breath sounds as needed. In the immediate postoperative period, place the stethoscope over the trachea to assess for the presence of stridor.	3. Abnormal breath sounds may indicate ineffective ventilation, decreased perfusion, and fluid accumulation. Stridor, a harsh, high-pitched sound primarily heard on inspiration, indicates airway obstruction.	• Shows evidence of normal breath sounds.
4. Encourage deep breathing and coughing. Place the patient in a sitting position and support the neck area with both hands.	4. Deep breathing before coughing promotes expansion of the airways and a more forceful cough. The coughing mechanism assists airway cilia with removal of secretions. Splinting the incision during coughing reduces strain and promotes the expulsion of secretions by allowing for deeper inspirations.	• Coughs effectively. • Maintains a patent airway.
5. Suction as needed using sterile technique and soft catheter.	5. Suctioning assists in removal of secretions that the patient may not be able to remove, thereby assisting with patent airway.	• Maintains a patent airway.
6. Provide humidified air or oxygen if patient has a tracheostomy.	6. Humidity helps keep secretions loose.	• Does not develop mucus plug.
NURSING DIAGNOSIS: Risk for infection.		
GOAL: Absence of infection.		
1. Instruct the patient in preoperative and postoperative oral hygiene using slightly alkaline solutions, such as 8 oz. of water mixed with 1 teaspoon of baking soda or normal saline solution every 4 hours.	1. Oral care decreases oral bacteria, therefore decreasing the risk of bacterial infection postoperatively. Hydrogen peroxide should not be used, as it may break down fresh granulation tissue.	• Performs oral hygiene preoperatively and postoperatively every 4 hours. • Mouth remains clean.

(*continued*)

NURSING CARE PLAN 34–1 *(continued)*
Care of the Patient Who Has Undergone Neck Dissection

Nursing Interventions	Rationale	Expected Outcomes
2. Monitor wound suction drainage.	2. Suction drainage negates the need for pressure dressings because the skin flaps are pulled down tightly. Drainage should approximate 80–120 ml of serosanguineous secretions for the first 24 hours; then the secretions should decrease daily. Continuous bloody drainage indicates small vessel oozing.	• Wound drains less than 200 ml of serosanguineous fluid the first postoperative day. • No hematoma at skin graft.
3. Note drainage quantity and odor.	3. Purulent, malodorous drainage indicates an infection. Drainage greater than 300 ml in the first 24 hours is considered abnormal.	• Serosanguineous drainage is within normal limits.
4. Assess condition of dressing and reinforce pressure dressings as needed.	4. If portable wound suction is not used, then pressure dressings may be applied to obliterate dead spaces and provide immobilization. These are reinforced (not changed) as needed. Assess for any possible constrictions that would affect respirations or decrease blood flow to graft.	• Dressing will remain intact with no constriction of airway or blood flow.
5. Use aseptic technique to cleanse skin around the drains; change the dressings as prescribed by physician (usually the second through fifth postoperative days).	5. Aseptic technique prevents wound contamination. Sterile saline effectively cleans the skin around the drains.	• Wound and surrounding skin remain clean and free of infection.
6. Monitor vital signs. Assess for symptoms of infection: chills, diaphoresis, altered level of consciousness.	6. An elevated temperature, tachypnea, and tachycardia may indicate an infection.	• Patient is afebrile with normal respirations and a normal heart rate. • Patient is alert and aware of surroundings.

NURSING DIAGNOSIS: Impaired skin integrity.

GOAL: Maintenance of intact skin and viability of graft.

1. Assess condition of graft for viability.	1. Cyanotic, cool, graft indicates possible necrosis. (Pale graft indicates arterial thrombosis; purple graft indicates venous congestion.)	• Graft will be pink in color and warm to touch. • Tissue will blanch to gentle touch. • Graft has pulse via Doppler ultrasound.

NURSING DIAGNOSIS: Altered nutrition, less than body requirements, related to anorexia and dysphagia.

GOAL: Attainment/maintenance of adequate nutrition.

1. Assess nutritional status preoperatively; consult with dietitian.	1. Poor nutrition preoperatively decreases wound healing and increases potential for infection.	• Does not experience weight loss greater than 10% of body weight. If patient does have weight loss of 10% to 20%, supplements are taken to maintain/increase weight and obtain positive nitrogen balance.

(continued)

NURSING CARE PLAN 34–1 *(continued)*
Care of the Patient Who Has Undergone Neck Dissection

Nursing Interventions	Rationale	Expected Outcomes
2. Administer tube feedings as prescribed. Keep head of bed elevated during feeding to prevent aspiration. Monitor for signs of tracheosophageal fistula (tube feeding formula in tracheal secretions).	2. A nasogastric tube may be in place for several days to administer enteral feedings.	• Tolerates tube feedings. • No signs of aspiration. • No signs of fistula.
3. Provide oral hygiene before and after meals.	3. Oral hygiene enhances the appetite.	• Expresses a desire for food.
4. Assist with oral intake: a. Offer easily chewed foods; mash or blenderize if necessary. b. Suggest that the head be tilted to the unaffected side when swallowing. c. Provide privacy if desired. d. Provide altered utensils as needed.	4. Soft-textured foods facilitate swallowing. Passage of food may be tolerated better when pressure occurs on the side opposite the surgery. Self-feeding difficulties may cause embarrassment and interfere with digestion.	• Swallows food easily. • Is comfortable eating alone or with others

NURSING DIAGNOSIS: Disturbance in self-concept and body image related to changes in appearance.

GOAL: Attainment of positive self-image.

Nursing Interventions	Rationale	Expected Outcomes
1. Assist the patient to communicate effectively. a. Provide materials for writing messages. b. Make certain that the call bell is readily accessible. c. Develop nonverbal ways to communicate (*e.g.,* finger-tapping, sign language, sign board, magic slate). d. Consult speech pathologist.	1. Temporary hoarseness is common after neck surgery. A tracheostomy may be performed and verbal communication may not be possible. Communication with head movement may be impossible because of incisional pain and need to maintain position of neck for graft. Speech pathologist may assist with others forms of communication such as esophageal speech or electro-larynx.	• Recognizes that hoarseness is temporary. • Develops alternative forms of communication.
2. Encourage verbalization of fears: a. Provide time to listen. b. Project a positive, optimistic attitude. c. Reinforce reality. d. Collaborate with family members to elicit their support and encouragement. e. Consult support groups such as New Voice Club through the American Cancer Society.	2. Listening conveys acceptance and encourages further verbalization. An optimistic approach conveys interest and hope. Honesty will promote a trusting relationship. This includes confirming cosmetic and functional limitations. Family members or significant others can provide valuable support to the patient.	• Willingly conveys fears and concerns. • Accepts prognosis with realistic limitations. • Accepts support as offered.
3. Observe for facial paralysis.	3. Injury to facial nerve will cause lower facial paralysis.	• Absence of facial paralysis.
4. Observe for excessive drooling.	4. Damage to the hypoglossal nerve will result in excessive drooling and decreased ability to swallow.	• Absence of drooling and dysphagia.
5. Check for normal shoulder position and function.	5. Damage to the spinal accessory nerve will result in drooping of the shoulder. Rehabilitation exercises are begun when the incision is healed.	• Maintains normal shoulder function.

even liquids may occur anywhere along the esophagus. Often the patient can indicate if the problem is located in the upper, middle, or lower third of the esophagus.

There are many pathologic conditions of the esophagus including motility disorders, gastroesophageal reflux, hiatal hernias, diverticula, rings and webs, perforation, foreign bodies, chemical burns, benign tumors, and carcinoma.

Motility Disorders

Achalasia

Achalasia is absent or ineffective peristalsis of the distal esophagus accompanied by failure of the esophageal sphincter to relax in response to swallowing. Narrowing of the esophagus just above the stomach results in a gradually increasing dilation of the esophagus in the upper chest. Achalasia may progress slowly. It occurs most often in persons aged 40 or older. It is thought that there may be a familial incidence of achalasia.

Clinical Manifestations. The primary symptom of achalasia is difficulty in swallowing both liquids and solids. The patient has a sensation of food "sticking" in the lower portion of the esophagus. As the condition progresses, food is commonly regurgitated, either spontaneously or on purpose to relieve the discomfort that is produced by the prolonged distention of the esophagus by food that will not pass into the stomach. The patient may also complain of chest pain and heartburn (*pyrosis*). Pain may or may not be associated with eating. There may be secondary pulmonary complications due to aspiration of gastric contents.

Diagnostic Evaluation. Diagnostic x-ray studies show esophageal dilation above the narrowing at the gastroesophageal junction. Barium swallow and endoscopy may be used for diagnosis; however, the diagnosis is confirmed by manometry, a process in which the esophageal pressure is measured by a radiologist or gastroenterologist.

Management. The patient should be instructed to eat slowly and drink fluids with meals. Calcium channel blockers and nitrates have been used to decrease esophageal pressure and improve swallowing. If these methods are unsuccessful, pneumatic (forceful) dilation or surgical separation of the muscle fibers may be recommended.

Achalasia may be treated conservatively by stretching the narrowed area of the esophagus by pneumatic dilation (Fig. 34-6). Pneumatic dilation has a good success rate. Perforation is a potential complication, but has a low incidence. The procedure can be painful; therefore, an analgesic or tranquilizer is administered before the treatment. The patient is monitored for perforation. Complaints of abdominal tenderness and fever may indicate that perforation has occurred (see later discussion on perforation).

Surgically, achalasia may be treated through an esophagomyotomy (Fig. 34-7). A thoracotomy may be performed to provide access and an incision is made through the muscularis of the lower esophagus. The esophageal muscle fibers are separated to relieve the lower esophageal stricture. Although patients with a history of achalasia have a slightly higher incidence of esophageal cancer, long-term follow-up with esophagoscopy has not proved beneficial.

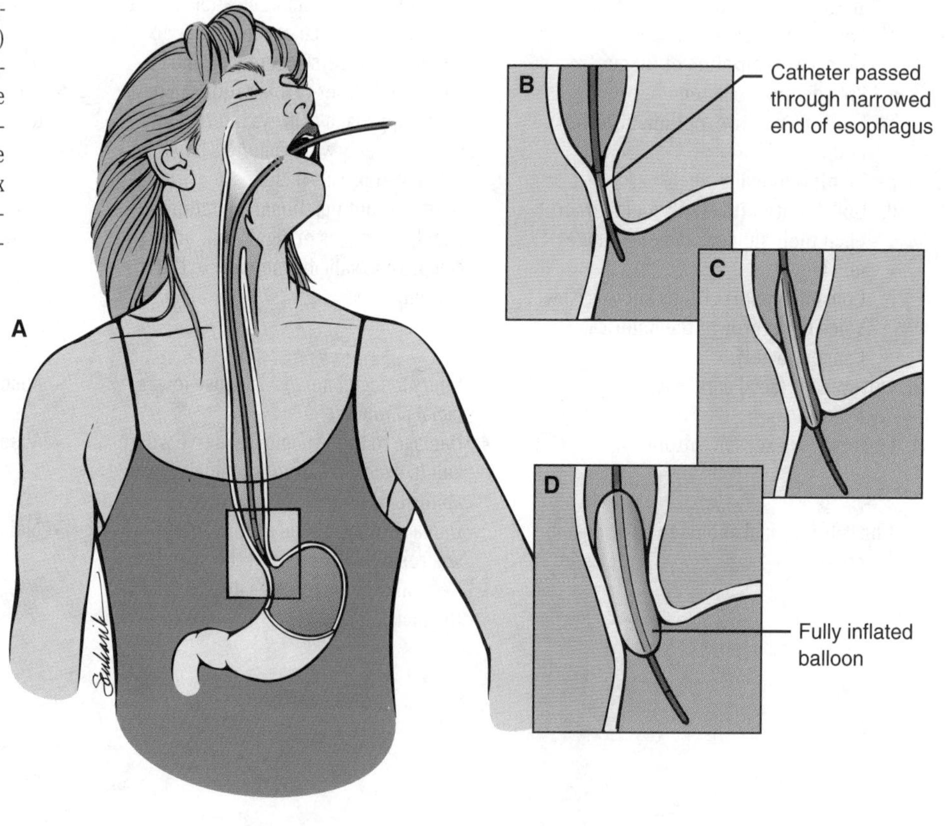

FIGURE 34-6. Treatment of achalasia by the conservative approach. (**A–C**) The dilator is passed, guided by a previously inserted guidewire. (**D**) When the balloon is in proper position, it is distended by pressure sufficient to dilate the narrowed area of the esophagus. (Rigiflex TTS Esophageal Balloon Dilatation Catheter courtesy of Microvasive/Boston Scientific Corporation.)

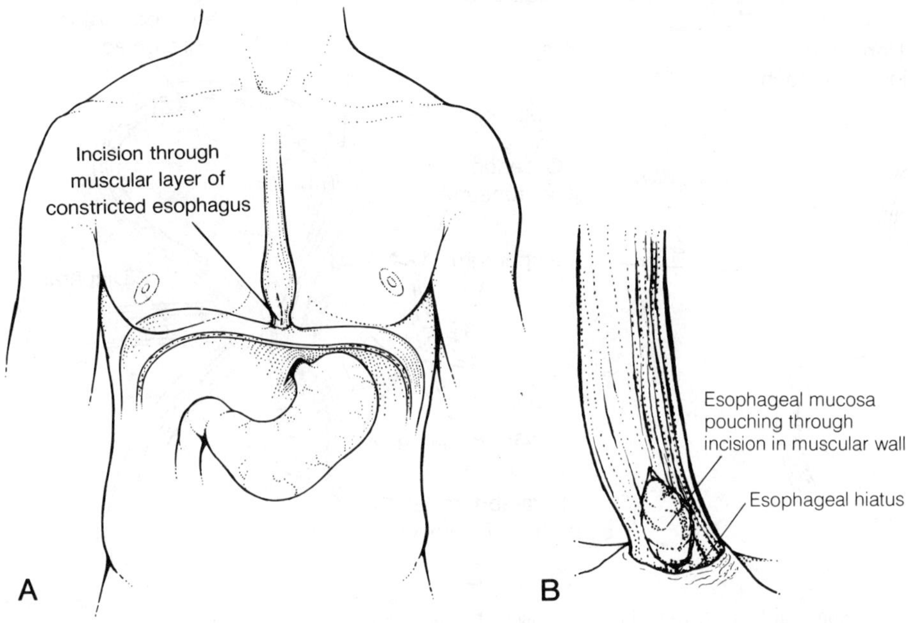

FIGURE 34-7. Treatment of achalasia: esophagomyomotomy. (**A**) The esophagus is approached via thoracotomy from the front, on the left side. An incision is made through the muscularis of the esophagus extending about 1 cm into the gastric area. (**B**) The incision is of sufficient size to allow a pouching of the esophageal mucosa. Separation of the muscular fibers relieves the narrowing at the lower end of the esophagus and permits the patient to swallow normally again.

Diffuse Spasm

Diffuse spasm is a motor disorder of the esophagus characterized by difficulty or pain on swallowing (dysphagia, odynphagia), and chest pain similar to that of coronary artery spasm. Esophageal manometry, which measures the motility of the esophagus and the pressure within the esophagus, indicates that simultaneous contractions of the esophagus occur irregularly.

Diagnostic Evaluation and Management. Diagnostic x-ray studies show separate areas of spasm. Conservative therapy includes administering sedatives and long-acting nitrates to relieve pain. Small, frequent feedings and a soft diet are usually recommended to decrease the esophageal pressure and irritation that lead to spasm. Dilation performed by bougienage (progressively sized mercury filled rubber dilators), pneumatic dilation, or esophagomyomotomy may be necessary if pain becomes intolerable.

Gastroesophageal Reflux

Some degree of gastroesophageal reflux (GER), or back flow of gastric or duodenal contents into the esophagus, is normal in both adults and children. Excessive reflux may occur owing to an incompetent lower esophageal sphincter, pyloric stenosis, or a motility disorder. The occurrence of reflux seems to increase with age.

Clinical Manifestations. Symptoms may include pyrosis (burning sensation in the esophagus), dyspepsia (indigestion), regurgitation, dysphagia, or odynophagia (difficulty swallowing; pain on swallowing), hypersalivation, or esophagitis. The symptoms may mimic those of a heart attack.

Diagnostic Evaluation and Management. Patient history aids in obtaining an accurate diagnosis. Diagnostic testing may include 12- to 36-hour esophageal *p*H monitoring to evaluate the degree of acid reflux; other tests may include endoscopy or barium swallow.

Management begins with patient teaching to avoid factors that decrease lower esophageal sphincter pressure or cause esophageal irritation. The patient is instructed to eat a low fat, high fiber diet; avoid caffeine, tobacco, and peppermint; avoid food or drink 2 hours before bedtime; avoid being overweight; and to elevate the head of the bed on 6- to 8-inch (15 to 20 cm) blocks. If gastroesophageal reflux persists, the patient may be placed on medications such as antacids, histamine receptor blockers, or gastric acid pump inhibitors (discussed in Chapter 36). In addition, the patient may receive prokinetic agents, which accelerate gastric emptying. These agents include bethanechol (Urecholine), domperidone (Moxilum), metachlopromide (Reglan), and cisapride (Propulsid).

If medical management is unsuccessful, surgical intervention may be necessary. Surgical management is achieved with a fundoplication (wrapping a portion of the gastric fundus around the sphincter area of the esophagus).

Hiatal Hernia

The esophagus enters the abdomen through an opening in the diaphragm, and empties at its lower end into the upper part of the stomach. Normally, the opening in the diaphragm encircles the esophagus tightly, and the stomach lies completely within the abdomen. In a condition known as **hiatus** (or **hiatal**) **hernia**, the opening in the diaphragm through which the esophagus passes becomes enlarged and part of the upper stomach tends to move up into the lower portion of the thorax. Hiatal hernia occurs more often in women than men. There are two types of hernias: *axial* and *paraesophageal.*

Axial. Axial, or sliding hiatal, hernias occur when the upper stomach and the gastroesophageal junction are dis-

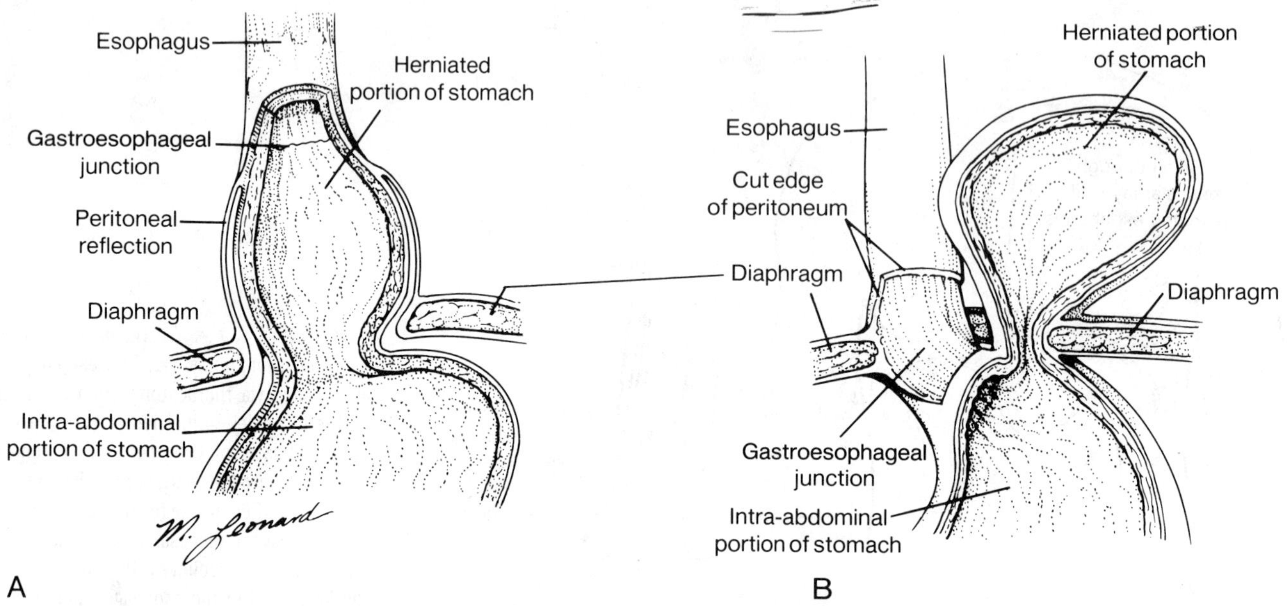

FIGURE 34-8. Sliding esophageal and paraesophageal hernias. (**A**) Sliding esophageal hernia. The upper stomach and cardioesophageal junction have moved upward and slide in and out of the thorax. (**B**) Paraesophageal hernia. All or part of the stomach pushes through the diaphragm next to the gastroesophageal junction.

placed upward and slide in and out of the thorax (Fig. 34-8*A*). About 90% of patients with esophageal hiatal hernias have sliding hernias.

Clinical Manifestations. The patient may experience heartburn, regurgitation, and dysphagia. At least 50% of patients are asymptomatic. Sliding hiatal hernia is often implicated in reflux.

Diagnosis and Management. Diagnosis is confirmed by x-ray studies and fluoroscopy. Management includes frequent, small feedings that can pass easily through the esophagus. The patient is advised not to recline for 1 hour after eating to prevent reflux or movement of the hernia and to elevate the head of the bed on 4- to 8-inch (10- to 20-cm) blocks to prevent the hernia from sliding upward. Surgery is indicated in about 15% of patients.

Paraesophageal Hernias. Paraesophageal hernias are less common than axial hernias. They occur when all or part of the stomach pushes through the diaphragm next to the gastroesophageal junction (see Fig. 34-8*B*). Fewer than 10% of patients experience paraesophageal herniation.

Clinical Manifestations. The patient usually experiences a sense of fullness after eating or may be asymptomatic. Reflux usually does not occur because the gastroesophageal sphincter is intact. The complications of hemorrhage, obstruction, and strangulation can occur.

Diagnostic Evaluation and Management. Diagnosis is confirmed by x-ray studies and fluoroscopy. Paraesophageal diverticula may require emergency surgery. Medical and surgical management are similar to that for gastroesophageal reflux.

Diverticulum

A **diverticulum** is an outpouching of mucosa and submucosa that protrudes through a weak portion of the musculature. Diverticula may occur in one of the three areas of the esophagus—(1) the pharyngoesophageal or upper part of the esophagus, (2) the midesophageal, or (3) the epiphrenic or lower part of the esophagus—or they may occur along the border of the esophagus intramurally.

Pharyngoesophageal Pulsion Diverticulum. The most common type of diverticulum, which is found three times more frequently in men than in women, is *pharyngoesophageal pulsion diverticulum* (Zenker's diverticulum). It occurs posteriorly through the cricopharyngeal muscle in the midline of the neck. It is usually seen in people over 60 years of age.

Clinical Manifestations. The patient first notices difficulty in swallowing and a fullness in the neck and may then complain of belching, regurgitation of undigested food, and gurgling noises after eating. The diverticulum, or pouch, becomes filled with food or liquid. When the patient assumes a recumbent position, undigested food is regurgitated and may also cause coughing, owing to irritation of the trachea. Halitosis and a sour taste in the mouth are also common, because of the decomposition of food retained in the diverticulum.

Diagnostic Evaluation and Management. A barium swallow may be obtained to determine the exact nature and location of a diverticulum. Esophagoscopy usually is contraindicated because of the danger of perforating the diverticulum, with resulting mediastinitis. The blind passing of a nasogastric tube should be avoided.

Because the condition is progressive, the only means of cure is surgical removal of the diverticulum. During surgery care is taken to avoid trauma to the common carotid artery and internal jugular veins. The sac is dissected free and amputated flush with the esophageal wall. In addition to a diverticulectomy, a myotomy of the cricopharyngeal muscle is often performed to relieve spasticity of the musculature, which otherwise seems to contribute to a continuation of the previous symptoms. Postoperatively, food and fluids are withheld until x-ray studies show no leakage at the surgical site. The diet is then begun with liquids and progresses as tolerated.

Midesophageal, Epiphrenic, and Intramural Diverticula. *Midesophageal diverticula* are uncommon. Symptoms are less acute, and usually the condition does not require surgery.

Epiphrenic diverticula are usually larger diverticula occurring in the lower esophagus just above the diaphragm. They are thought to be related to the improper functioning of the lower esophageal sphincter. One third of patients are asymptomatic, with the remaining two thirds complaining of dysphagia and chest pain.

Intramural diverticulosis is the occurrence of numerous small diverticula associated with a stricture in the upper esophagus.

Management. Surgery is indicated for epiphrenic and midesophageal diverticula only if the symptoms are troublesome and growing progressively worse. Treatment consists of a diverticulectomy and long myotomy. Intramural diverticula usually regress when the esophageal stricture is dilated.

Nursing Interventions. After surgery the patient receives nutrients through a nasogastric tube that usually is inserted at the time of operation. The feedings may include any liquid, but a careful record of the kind, amount, and character must be documented. After each feeding, the tube is flushed carefully with water. The surgical incision must be observed for evidence of leakage from the esophagus and a developing fistula.

Rings and Webs

Esophageal rings are thin concentric membranes consisting of mucosal tissue at the gastroesophageal junction. The patient with esophageal rings may complain of symptoms of dysphagia and food impaction. Esophageal webs consist of mucosa and submucosal tissue forming concentric shelves along the entire esophagus. The patient with esophageal webs usually complains of dysphagia.

Diagnosis and Management. The diagnosis is generally confirmed by a barium swallow. Esophageal webs may regress with iron treatment. Both esophageal rings and webs may require dilation, either with bougienage or a pneumatic balloon.

Perforation

The esophagus is not an uncommon site of injury. Perforation may result from stab or bullet wounds of the neck or chest, as well as from accidental puncture by a surgical instrument during examination or dilation. Spontaneous perforation of the esophagus has been known to occur during vomiting.

Clinical Manifestations. The patient experiences persistent pain followed by dysphagia. Infection, fever, leukocytosis, and severe hypotension may be noted. In some instances, signs of pneumothorax are observed.

Diagnostic Evaluation and Management. Diagnostic x-ray studies and fluoroscopy can localize the site of the injury. Because of the high risk of infection, broad-spectrum antibiotic therapy is initiated. A nasogastric tube is inserted to provide suction and to reduce the amount of gastric juice that can reflux into the esophagus and mediastinum. Nothing is given by mouth, but nutritional needs are met by total parenteral nutrition. Total parenteral nutrition is preferred to gastrostomy because the latter might cause reflux into the esophagus.

Surgery may be necessary to close the wound, and postoperative nutritional support then becomes a primary concern. Depending on the incisional site and nature of surgery, the postoperative nursing management is similar to that for patients who have had thoracic or abdominal surgery.

Foreign Bodies

Many swallowed foreign bodies pass through the gastrointestinal (GI) tract without the need for medical intervention. Some swallowed foreign bodies (dentures, fishbones, pins, small batteries, items containing mercury or lead) may injure the esophagus or obstruct its lumen and must be removed. Pain and dysphagia may be present and dyspnea may occur as a result of pressure on the trachea.

Diagnostic Evaluation and Management. X-ray findings are useful in identifying the foreign body. An endoscope with a covered hood or overtube may be used to remove objects from the esophagus.

If an impacted bolus of food is lodged in the esophagus, tartaric acid and sodium bicarbonate may be given to form a gas, thereby increasing the intraluminal pressure and possibly allowing the bolus to be dislodged. Glucagon also may be injected intramuscularly. This medication has a relaxing effect on the esophageal muscle. If these treatments are unsuccessful, an endoscopic procedure is performed to remove the impacting food.

Chemical Burns

Chemical burns of the esophagus may be caused by undissolved medications in the esophagus. This occurs more frequently in the elderly than it does among the general adult population. Chemical burns of the esophagus occur most often when a patient, either accidentally or intentionally, swallows a strong acid or base (such as lye). This patient is emotionally distraught as well as in acute physical pain. An acute chemical burn of the esophagus may be accompanied by severe burns of the lips, mouth, and pharynx, with pain on swallowing. There is sometimes difficulty in breathing due either to edema of the throat or to a collection of mucus in the pharynx.

Management. The patient, who may be profoundly toxic, febrile, and in shock, is treated immediately for shock, pain, and respiratory distress. Esophagoscopy and barium swallow are performed as soon as possible to determine the extent and severity of damage. The patient is kept NPO (given nothing by mouth) and intravenous fluids are administered. A nasogastric tube may be inserted by the physician. Emesis and gastric lavage are avoided.

The use of corticosteroid therapy to reduce inflammation and minimize subsequent scarring and stricture formation is of questionable value. The value of prophylactic use of antibiotics for this patient has also been questioned; however, these treatments continue to be prescribed.

After the acute phase has subsided, the patient may require further treatment to prevent or manage strictures of the esophagus. Dilation using bougies may be sufficient. Dilation treatment may need to be repeated periodically. For strictures that do not respond to dilation, surgical management is necessary. Reconstruction may be performed with an esophagectomy or colon interposition to replace the portion of esophagus removed.

Esophageal Varices

Varices of the lower esophagus are a complication of cirrhosis of the liver and portal hypertension (see Chapter 38).

Benign Tumors

Benign tumors may arise anywhere along the esophagus. The most common lesion is a leiomyoma (tumor of the smooth muscle), which can occlude the lumen of the esophagus. Most benign tumors are asymptomatic and are distinguished from cancerous lesions by a biopsy. Small lesions are excised during esophagoscopy; lesions that occur within the wall of the esophagus may require a thoracotomy.

Cancer of the Esophagus

In the United States, carcinoma of the esophagus occurs more than twice as often in men as in women. It is seen more frequently in African-Americans than in Caucasians and usually occurs in the fifth decade of life. Cancer of the esophagus has a much higher incidence in other parts of the world, including China and northern Iran.

Chronic irritation is considered to be a risk factor for esophageal cancer. In the United States, cancer of the esophagus has been associated with the ingestion of alcohol and the use of tobacco. In other parts of the world, esophageal cancer has been associated with the use of opium pipes, ingestion of excessively hot beverages, and nutritional deficiencies–especially lack of fruits and vegetables. It is thought that fruits and vegetables promote repair of irritated tissue.

Pathophysiology and Clinical Manifestations. Unfortunately, the patient may have an advanced ulcerated lesion of the esophagus before symptoms present. Malignancy, usually of the squamous cell epidermoid type, may spread beneath the esophageal mucosa, or it may spread directly into, through, and beyond the muscle layers into the lymphatics. In the latter stages, obstruction of the esophagus is noted, with possible perforation into the mediastinum and erosion into the great vessels.

When symptoms occur that are related to esophageal cancer, the disease is generally advanced. Symptoms include dysphagia, initially with solid foods and eventually with liquids; a feeling of a mass in the throat; painful swallowing; substernal pain or fullness; and, later, regurgitation of undigested food with foul breath and hiccoughs. The patient is first aware of intermittent and increasing difficulty in swallowing. At first only solid food causes distress, but as the growth progresses and the obstruction becomes more complete, even liquids cannot pass into the stomach. Regurgitation of food and saliva occurs, hemorrhage may take place, and progressive loss of weight and strength occurs owing to starvation. Later symptoms include substernal pain, hiccough, respiratory difficulty, and foul breath. The delay between the onset of early symptoms and the time when the patient seeks medical advice is often 12 to 18 months. Anyone with swallowing difficulties should be encouraged to consult a physician immediately.

Diagnostic Evaluation. Diagnosis is confirmed in 95% of the cases by esophagogastroduodenoscopy (EGD) with biopsy and brushings. Bronchoscopy usually is performed, especially in tumors of the middle and the upper third of the esophagus, to determine whether the trachea has been affected and to help in determining whether the lesion can be removed. Mediastinoscopy is used to determine if the cancer has spread to the nodes and other mediastinal structures. Cancer of the lower end of the esophagus may be due to adenocarcinoma of the stomach extending upward into the esophagus.

Management. If esophageal cancer is found at an early stage, treatment goals may be directed toward cure; however, it is often found in late stages, making palliation the only reasonable goal of therapy. Treatment may include surgery, radiation, chemotherapy, or a combination of these modalities and depends on the extent of the disease.

Standard surgical management includes a total resection of the esophagus (*esophagectomy*) with removal of the tumor plus a wide tumor-free margin of the esophagus and the lymph nodes in the area. The surgical approach may be through the thorax or the abdomen depending on the location of the tumor. When tumors occur in the cervical or upper thoracic area, esophageal continuity may be maintained by free jejunal graft transfer, in which the tumor is removed and the area replaced with a portion of the jejunum (Fig. 34-9). A segment of the colon may be used or the stomach can be elevated into the chest and the proximal section of the esophagus implanted into the stomach.

Tumors of the lower thoracic esophagus are more amenable to surgery than are tumors located higher in the esophagus, and GI tract integrity is maintained by implanting the lower esophagus into the stomach.

Surgical resection of the esophagus has a relatively high mortality rate because of infection, pulmonary complications, or leakage through the anastomosis. Postoperatively, the patient will have a nasogastric tube in place that should not be manipulated. The patient is kept NPO until x-ray studies confirm that the anastomosis is secure and not leaking.

The use of radiation therapy, either alone or in conjunction with surgery preoperatively or postoperatively, may be the treatment of choice. The use of chemotherapy combined with radiation or surgery is also being studied.

Palliative treatment may be necessary to keep the esophagus open, and to assist with nutrition and control saliva. Palliation may be accomplished with dilation of the

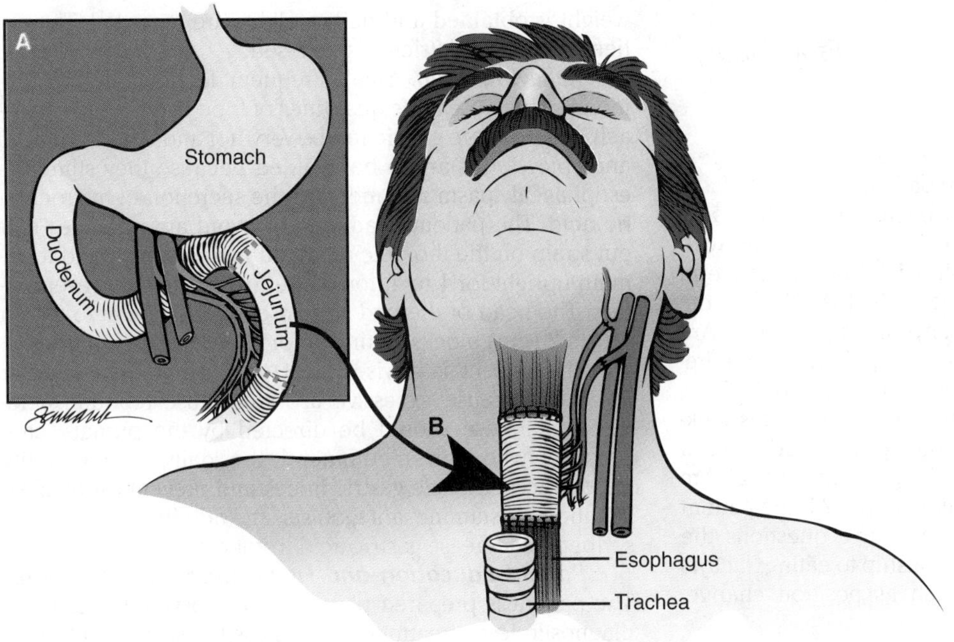

FIGURE 34-9. Esophageal reconstruction with free jejunal transfer. A portion of the jejunum is harvested and anastomosed between the esophagus and pharynx to replace the affected portion of the esophagus. Anastomosis of the vascular structures is also performed. A portion of the harvested jejunum may be externalized through the neck wound to evaluate graft viability. (Adapted from Foster J. Intensive care of the patient with cancer after reconstructive surgery. Focus on Critical Care 1992 April; 19(2): 126.)

esophagus, laser therapy, placement of an endoprosthesis (stent), radiation, and chemotherapy. Because the ideal method of treating esophageal cancer has not yet been found, each patient is treated using an individualized care plan.

Nursing Interventions. Intervention is directed toward improving the patient's nutritional and physical condition in preparation for surgery, radiation therapy, or chemotherapy. A program to promote weight gain based on a high-caloric and high-protein diet, in liquid or soft form, is provided if adequate foods can be taken by mouth. If not, total parenteral nutrition is initiated. Nutritional status is monitored throughout treatment.

The patient is informed about the nature of the postoperative equipment that will be used, including that required for closed chest drainage, nasogastric suction, parenteral fluid therapy, and gastric intubation. Immediate postoperative care is similar to that provided for patients undergoing thoracic surgery (see Chap. 25). After recovering from the effects of anesthesia, the patient is placed in a semi-Fowler's position, and later Fowler's position, to assist in preventing reflux of gastric secretions. The patient is then observed carefully for regurgitation and dyspnea. A common postoperative complication is aspiration pneumonia. Temperature is monitored to detect any elevation that may indicate seepage of fluid through the operative site into the mediastinum.

If grafting has been performed, the nurse checks for graft viability hourly for at least the first 12 hours. To make the graft visible the surgeon will usually bring a portion of the jejunum to the exterior neck by way of a small incision. A moist gauze covers the external portion of the graft. The gauze is removed briefly to assess the graft for color and to assess for the presence of a pulse by means of Doppler ultrasonography.

If an endoprosthesis has been placed or an anastomosis has been performed, a functioning continuum will exist between the throat and the stomach. Immediately postoperatively the nasogastric tube should be marked for position and the physician notified if displacement occurs. The nurse does not attempt to reinsert a displaced nasogastric tube, as damage to the anastomosis may occur. The nasogastric tube is removed 5 to 7 days after surgery and a barium swallow is performed to evaluate for any anastomotic leak before the patient is fed.

Once feeding begins, the nurse will encourage the patient to swallow small sips of water and, later, small amounts of pureed food. When the patient is able to increase food intake to a significant amount, parenteral fluids are discontinued. If an endoprosthesis is used, it may easily become obstructed if food is not chewed sufficiently. After each meal, the patient is to remain upright for at least 2 hours to allow the food to move through the GI tract. The nurse is challenged to encourage this patient to eat, because appetite is usually poor. Family involvement and home-cooked favorite foods may help the patient to eat. Antacids may help those who complain of gastric distress. When radiation is part of the therapy, the patient's appetite is further depressed and esophagitis may occur, causing the patient pain when food is eaten. Liquid supplements may be more easily tolerated.

Often, in either the preoperative or postoperative period, an obstructed or nearly obstructed esophagus causes difficulty with excess saliva, so that drooling becomes a problem. A wick-type of gauze may be placed at the corner of the mouth to direct secretions to a dressing or emesis basin. The possibility that the patient may aspirate saliva into the tracheobronchial tree, and thus increase the danger of pneumonia, is of great concern.

When the patient is ready to go home, the family is instructed in the following: how to promote nutrition, what observations to make, what measures to take if complications occur, how to keep the patient comfortable, and how to obtain needed physical and emotional support.

❑ NURSING PROCESS
Patients With Conditions of the Esophagus

Assessment

A complete health history may reveal a possible esophageal disorder. The nurse asks about the patient's appetite. Has it remained the same, increased, or decreased? Is there any discomfort with swallowing? If so, does it occur only with certain foods? Is it associated with pain? Does a change in position affect the discomfort? The patient is asked to describe the pain experience. Does anything aggravate it? Are there any other symptoms that occur regularly, such as regurgitation, nocturnal regurgitation, eructation (belching), heartburn, substernal pressure, a sensation that food is sticking in the throat, a feeling of becoming full after eating a small amount of food, nausea, vomiting, or weight loss? Are the symptoms aggravated by emotional upset? If the patient reports any of these complaints, the nurse questions the time of their occurrence; their relationship to eating; factors that relieve or aggravate them–such as position change, belching, antacids, or vomiting.

This history also includes questions about the existence of past or present causative factors, such as infections and chemical, mechanical, or physical irritants; the degree to which alcohol and tobacco are used; and the amount of daily food intake. The nurse determines if the patient appears emaciated and auscultates the patient's chest to determine if pulmonary complications exist.

Diagnosis

Nursing Diagnoses

Based on the assessment data, the nursing diagnoses may include the following:

- Altered nutrition, less than body requirements, related to difficulty swallowing
- Pain, related to difficulty swallowing, ingestion of an abrasive agent, a tumor, or frequent episodes of gastric reflux
- Knowledge deficit about the esophageal disorder, diagnostic studies, medical management, surgical intervention, and rehabilitation

Planning and Implementation

Goals. The major goals for the patient may include attainment of an adequate nutritional intake, relief of pain, and increased knowledge level.

Nursing Interventions

Encouraging Adequate Nutritional Intake. The patient is encouraged to eat slowly and to chew all food thoroughly so that it can pass easily into the stomach. Small, frequent feedings of nonirritating foods are recommended to promote digestion and to prevent tissue irritation. Sometimes liquid swallowed with food will help the food pass through the esophagus. Food should be prepared in an appealing manner to help stimulate the appetite. Irritants such as tobacco and alcohol should be avoided. A baseline weight is obtained and daily weights are recorded. The patient's intake of nutrients is assessed.

Relieving Pain. Small, frequent feedings are recommended because large quantities of food overload the stomach and promote gastric reflux. Very hot and cold beverages and spicy foods are to be avoided because they stimulate esophageal spasm and increase the secretion of hydrochloric acid. The patient is advised to avoid any activities that put strain on the thoracic area and increase pain and to remain upright for 1 to 4 hours after each meal to prevent reflux. The head of the bed should be placed on 4- to 8-inch (10- to 20-cm) blocks. Eating before bedtime is discouraged.

The patient is advised not to abuse over-the-counter antacids because excessive use can cause rebound acidity. Antacid use should be directed by the primary care provider who can recommend the daily, safe quantity needed to neutralize gastric juices and prevent esophageal irritation. Histamine antagonists are administered as prescribed to decrease gastric acid irritation.

Patient Education and Home Care Considerations. The patient is prepared physically and psychologically for diagnostic tests, treatments, and possible surgical intervention. The principal nursing interventions include reassuring the patient and discussing the procedures and their purposes. Some disorders of the esophagus evolve over time, whereas others are the result of trauma (*e.g.*, chemical burns or perforation). In instances of trauma, the emotional and physical preparation for treatment is more difficult because of the short time available and the circumstances of the injury. Treatment interventions must be evaluated continually; the patient is provided with sufficient information to participate in care and diagnostic efforts. If surgery is involved, immediate and long-term evaluation is similar to that of a patient undergoing thoracic surgery.

The goals of rehabilitation depend on whether surgery or more conservative measures, such as diet, positioning, or medications were instituted. If the condition is corrected, short-term evaluation may be sufficient. If an ongoing condition exists, the nurse must help the patient plan for needed physical and psychological adjustment and for follow-up care. Many elderly patients may experience ongoing conditions. These patients need support to plan meals realistically, to use medications as prescribed, and to participate in a full life. A multidisciplinary team, which includes a nutritionist, social worker, and family members, is helpful in these cases.

Chronic esophageal conditions require an individualized approach to home management. There may be a need to prepare food in a special way (blenderized foods; soft diets) and to eat more frequently (four to six small servings per day). The medication schedule is adjusted to the patient's daily activities as much as possible. Analgesics and antacids can be taken as needed every 3 to 4 hours.

Postoperative home health care focuses on nutritional support, management of pain, and respiratory function. Some patients are discharged from the hospital with enteral feeding by means of gastrostomy or jejunostomy tubes or total parenteral nutrition. The patient and family need specific instruction on the management of equipment and treatments. Home care visits by a nurse may be necessary to assure that the patient is doing well and that the family is able to provide the necessary care. (See Chapter 35 for more information on parenteral nutrition and management of the patient with a gastrostomy.)

Emergency conditions of the esophagus (perforation, chemical burns) usually occur in the home or away from medical help and require emergency medical care. The patient is treated for shock and respiratory distress and transported as quickly as possible to a medical facility.

Foreign bodies in the esophagus do not pose an immediate threat to life unless pressure is exerted on the trachea, resulting in dyspnea or interferring with respiration. Educating the public to prevent accidental swallowing of foreign bodies or corrosive agents is a major health issue. (See Chapter 66 for emergency resuscitation measures.)

Evaluation

Expected Outcomes

1. Achieves an adequate nutritional intake
   a. Eats small, frequent meals
   b. Drinks water with small servings of food
   c. Avoids irritants (alcohol, tobacco, very hot beverages)
   d. Maintains desired weight
2. Is free of pain or able to control pain within a tolerable level
   a. Avoids large meals and irritating foods
   b. Takes medications as prescribed
   c. Maintains an upright position after meals for 1 to 4 hours
   d. States that there is less eructation and chest pain
3. Increases knowledge level of esophageal condition, treatment, and prognosis
   a. States cause of condition
   b. Discusses rationale for medical or surgical management and diet or medication regimen
   c. Describes treatment program
   d. Practices preventive measures so accidental injuries are avoided

CRITICAL THINKING EXERCISES

1. You are interviewing a patient in the medical clinic who has been treated in the clinic previously for gastroesophageal reflux. He complains that his symptoms are worse but that he has been taking his medications as prescribed. He states that he has tried many different kinds of antacids but none of them are helping him. Describe how you would continue to assess this patient to obtain the additional information that is needed. Speculate as to the different causes that may underlie this patient's inability to obtain relief.
2. You are caring for two postoperative patients. One patient is being treated for cancer of the mouth, the other for cancer of the esophagus. How will the nutritional care of these two patients differ?

REFERENCES AND BIBLIOGRAPHY

Books

American Cancer Society. A Cancer Source Book for Nurses, 6th ed. Atlanta, The American Cancer Society, 1991.

Ahlgren J and McDonald J. Gastrointestinal Oncology. Philadelphia, JB Lippincott, 1992.

Baily BJ et al (eds). Head and Neck Surgery: Otolaryngology. Philadelphia, JB Lippincott, 1993.

Bates B. A Guide to Physical Examination and History Taking, 6th ed. Philadelphia, JB Lippincott, 1995.

Castell DO (ed). The Esophagus. Boston, Little, Brown & Co, 1993.

DeVita VT, Hellman S, and Rosenberg SA (eds). Cancer. Principles and Practice of Oncology, 4th ed. Philadelphia, JB Lippincott, 1993.

Groenwald S (ed). Cancer Nursing: Principles and Practices, 3rd ed. Boston, Jones & Bartlett, 1993.

Van Schaik T (ed). Gastroenterology Nursing. St Louis, Mosby-Year Book, 1993.

Wood NK and Goaz PW. Differential Diagnosis of Oral Lesions. St Louis, Mosby-Year Book, 1991.

Journals

Asterisks indicate nursing research articles.

Conditions and Cancer of the Oral Cavity

Calman FMB and Langdon J. Oral complications of cancer: Preventive treatment is vital and many specialties are required. BMJ 1991 Mar 2; 302(6775):485–486.

Esberger KK. Guide to gastrointestinal problems of elders. Geriatr Nurs 1991 Mar-Apr; 12(2):74–75.

Jansma J et al. Protocol for the prevention and treatment of oral sequelae resulting from head and neck radiation therapy. Cancer 1992 Oct 15; 70(8):2171–2180.

Just JK et al. Treating TM disorders: A survey on diagnosis, etiology and management. J Am Dent Assoc 1991 Sep; 122(10):55–60.

Kusler DL and Rambur BA. Treatment for radiation-induced xerostomia: An innovative remedy. Cancer Nurs 1992 Jun; 15(3): 191–195.

LaBlance GR et al. Rehabilitation of swallowing and communication following glossectomy. Rehabil Nurs 1991 Sep-Oct; 16(5): 266–270.

Ladd L. The dry mouth dilemma. Oncol Nurs Forum 1991; 18(4): 785–786.

*Langius A et al. Oral—and pharyngeal—cancer patients' perceived symptoms and health. Cancer Nurs 1993 Jun; 16(3): 214–221.

Limitone E. Reconstructive surgery for squamous cell carcinoma of the floor of the mouth: A case report. Dimens Oncol Nurs 1991 Spring; 5(1):33–35.

Pollard C. Practical approach to the GI evaluation in AIDS. Physician Assist 1992 May; 16(5):29–30, 33–34, 103–105.

Rogers RS. Common lesions of the oral mucosa. A guide to diseases of the lips, cheeks, tongue, and gingivae. Postgrad Med 1992 May; 91(6):141–148, 151–153.

Safro AJ. Dental care for the elderly. J Am Dent Assoc 1992 Aug; 123(8):18–22.

Stack BC Jr and Stack BC Sr. Temporomandibular joint disorder. Am Fam Physician 1992 Jul; 46(1):143–150.

Tami TA and Tarkington A. Rigid fixation in the management of maxillofacial trauma. Todays OR Nurse 1991 Mar; 13(3):8–14.

*Titler MG et al Classification of nursing interventions for care of the integument. Nurs Diagn 1991 Apr-Jun; 2(2):45–56.

Wingo PA et al. Cancer statistics, 1995. CA 1995 Jan/Feb, 45(1): 8–30.

Conditions and Treatment of the Head and Neck

Becker SP and Drucker C. Nonsquamous tumors of the head and neck in the geriatric population. Otolaryngol Clin North Am 1990 Dec; 23(6):1141–1157.

Cummings CW et al. Neck cancer: What's optimal therapy? Patient Care 1990 Feb 28; (4)44–48, 53–54, 57.

Droughton ML and Krech RL. Head and neck cancer resection and reconstruction: From past to present. Todays OR Nurse 1992 Sep; 14(9):25–34.

Foster J. Intensive care of the patient with cancer after reconstructive surgery. Focus Crit Care 1992 Apr; 19(2):122–127.

Koopman CF Jr. Otolaryngologic (head and neck) problems in the elderly. Med Clin North Am 1991 Nov; 75(6):1373–1388.

Lockhart JS et al. Total laryngectomy and radical neck dissection: A case study. AORN J 1992 Feb; 55(2):458–459, 462–464, 466.

*Wilson PR et al. Eating strategies used by persons with head and neck cancer during and after radiotherapy. Cancer Nurs 1991 Apr; 14(2):98–104.

Conditions and Treatment of the Esophagus

Daniel BT amd Shuey KM. Role of the nurse in managing the patient with esophageal cancer. Nursing Interventions in Oncology 1993; 5:14–22.

Esberger KK. Guide to gastrointestinal problems of elders. Geriatr Nurs 1991 Mar/Apr; 12(2):74–75.

Foster J. Intensive care of the patient with cancer after reconstructive surgery. Focus Crit Care 1992 Apr; 19(2):122–127.

Galindo M. Assessing three esophageal disorders. Nursing 1992 Jan; 22(1):32C–D.

Kauvar D and Brandt LJ. Treatment of common GI disorders in the elderly. Physician Assist 1992 Feb; 16(2):105–108, 111–112, 181.

Morton LS and Fomkes JJ. Gastroesophageal reflux disease: Diagnosis and medical therapy. Geriatrics 1993 Mar; 48(3):60–66.

Rex DK. Gastroesophageal reflux disease in adults: Pathophysiology, diagnosis, and management. J Fam Pract 1992 Dec; 35(6):673–681.

Wright K. Esophageal endoprosthesis therapy. Gastroenterol Nurs 1991 Dec; 14(3):127–131.

AGENCIES

American Association of Public Health Dentists
New York University Dental Center,
325 East 24th St,
New York, NY 10010

American Cancer Society
1599 Clifton Rd NE,
Atlanta, GA 30329

American Dental Association
211 E Chicago Ave,
Chicago, IL 60611

American Society of Geriatric Dentistry
1121 W Michigan St,
Indianapolis, IN 46202

National Institute of Dental Research
National Institutes of Health,
900 Rockville Pike,
Bethesda, MD 20892

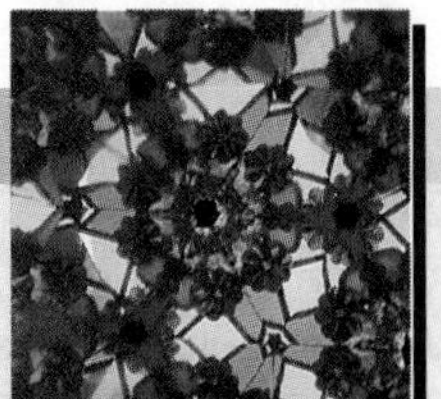

35 Gastrointestinal Intubation and Special Nutritional Management

CHAPTER OUTLINE

LEARNING OBJECTIVES

On completion of this chapter, the learner will be able to:

1. Describe the purposes of gastrointestinal intubation and the care of patients with these therapies
2. Use the nursing process as a framework for care of the patient receiving a tube feeding
3. Explain the preoperative and postoperative care of the patient with a gastrostomy
4. Use the nursing process as a framework for care of the patient with a gastrostomy
5. Identify the purposes and uses of total parenteral nutrition
6. Use the nursing process as a framework for care of the patient receiving total parenteral nutrition
7. Describe the nursing measures that are used to prevent complications of total parenteral nutrition

Nasogastric and nasoenteric tubes are commonly used for hospitalized patients, as well as for those in skilled nursing facilities and in the home setting. This chapter discusses several topics related to nasogastric and gastrointestinal intubation including managing patients with nasogastric and nasoenteric tubes, the various uses of these tubes, and the teaching points related to home health care; managing patients with gastrostomies; and the general indications for total parenteral nutrition (TPN) and the nursing care of patients receiving these support measures.

Gastrointestinal Intubation

Gastrointestinal intubation is the insertion of a short or a long flexible rubber or plastic tube into the stomach or intestine by way of the mouth or nose to (1) decompress the stomach and remove gas and fluid, (2) diagnose gastrointestinal motility, (3) administer medications and feedings, (4) treat an obstruction or bleeding site, or (5) obtain gastric contents for analysis. Any solution administered through a tube is either poured through a syringe or delivered by drip regulated by gravity or by an electric pump. Aspiration (suctioning) to remove gas and fluids is accomplished by using a syringe, an electric suction machine, or a built-in wall suction outlet.

A variety of tubes are used for decompression, aspiration, and irrigation (lavage) (Miller-Abbott, Cantor, Harris, Ewald, Levin, Moss, Salem sump), and to control bleeding from esophageal varices (Sengstaken-Blakemore); various other tubes are used to administer feedings and medications (Levin, Moss, Dobhoff, Keofeed, Flexiflo, Nutriflex, and Entriflex). The tubes are made of different material (rubber, polyurethane, silicone) and vary in length (90 cm to 3 m [36 inches to 10 feet]), size (6 to 18 Fr), purpose, and placement in the gastrointestinal tract (stomach, duodenum, jejunum).

Nasogastric Tubes

A nasogastric tube or short tube, is introduced through the nose or the mouth into the stomach. Commonly used short tubes include the Levin tube, gastric sump tube, Nutriflex tube, Moss tube, and the Sengstaken-Blakemore tube, which are described below.

Levin Tube. The Levin tube has a single lumen (No. 14 to 18 Fr) and is made of plastic or rubber with openings near its tip. The tube is used in adults to remove fluid and gas from the upper gastrointestinal (GI) tract, to obtain a specimen of gastric contents for laboratory studies, and to administer medications or feeding (gavage) directly into the gastrointestinal tract.

Circular markings at specific points on the tube serve as guides for insertion. A marking is made on the tube to indicate the midpoint (Fig. 35-1). The tube is advanced cautiously until this marking reaches the patient's nostril, indicating that the tube is in the stomach.

Placement may be checked further by aspirating gastric contents with a syringe and testing the *p*H of the aspirated material. (The *p*H will vary according to the source of origin.) An x-ray is the only sure way to verify the tube's location.

Gastric Sump Tube. The gastric sump tube (Salem, VENTROL) is a radiopaque, clear-plastic, double-lumen nasogastric tube. It is used to decompress the stomach and keep it empty. The inner, smaller tube vents the larger suction-drainage tube to the atmosphere by means of an opening at the distal end of the tube. It is passed into the stomach in the same way as the Levin tube. It can protect gastric suture lines because, when used properly, the sump tube never allows the force of suction at the drainage openings, or outlets, to exceed 25 mm Hg, the level of capillary fragility. This action is controlled by a small vent tube (blue pigtail). Continuous suction is set at a low pressure of 30 mm Hg with the vent outlet kept open. If available suction is intermittent, rather than continuous, it may be set at 80 to 120 mm Hg. Because of the cyclic setting, the suction will be reduced to about 25 mm Hg by the time it reaches the gastric mucosa.

To prevent reflux of gastric contents through the vent lumen (blue pigtail), the vent lumen is kept above the patient's midline; otherwise it will act as a siphon. Irrigation may be performed through either the main lumen or the vent lumen; if the vent lumen is used, irrigation is followed with injection of 20 ml of air, to clear the lumen.

Nutriflex Tube. The Nutriflex nasogastric feeding tube is 76 cm (30 in) long and has a mercury-weighted tip to facilitate insertion. It is coated with a hydromer lubricant that is activated when moistened.

Moss Tube. The Moss nasoesophageal gastric decompression tube is 90 cm (35 in) long and has a triple lumen (Fig. 35-2). It is anchored in the stomach by inflating the balloon. The decompression catheter provides for esophageal and gastric aspiration as well as lavage. The third lumen is an avenue for duodenal feedings.

Sengstaken-Blakemore (S-B) Tube. The S-B tube is used to treat bleeding esophageal varices (see Chapter 38 and Fig. 38-9). The S-B Tube has three lumina with two balloons. The balloons are checked for air leakage and proper inflation before the tube is inserted. One lumen is used to inflate the gastric balloon; the other is used to inflate the esophageal balloon. The desired pressure in each balloon is 25 to 30 mm Hg. The tube should be clamped to secure set pressures. Frequent pressure checks should be made to guard against undetected air leaks in the system. The third lumen is used for gastric lavage to monitor bleeding. A pair of scissors is taped near the bedside so that the tube may be cut to deflate the balloons if the patient develops respiratory distress. If this occurs, the physician is notified promptly because of the risk of rebleeding.

Nasoenteric Tubes

A nasoenteric tube, or long tube, is introduced through the nose and passed through the esophagus and stomach into the intestinal tract. It is used to aspirate intestinal contents to prevent gas and fluid from distending the coils of intestine. This process is called **decompression**. Three major nasoenteric tubes that are used for aspiration and decompression are the Miller-Abbott tube, the Harris tube, and the

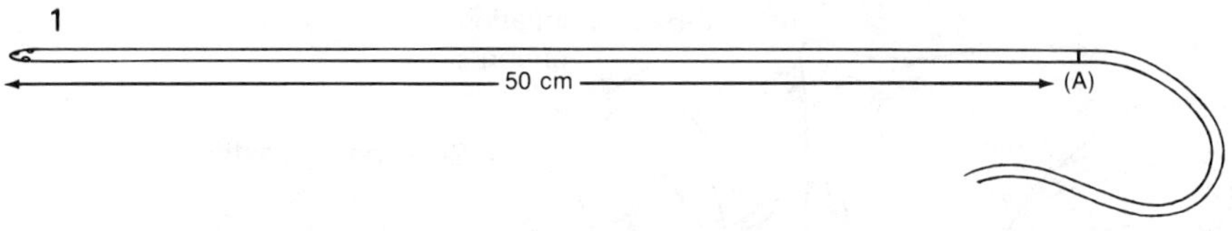

1. Mark the nasogastric tube at a point 50 cm. from the distal tip; call this point 'A'.

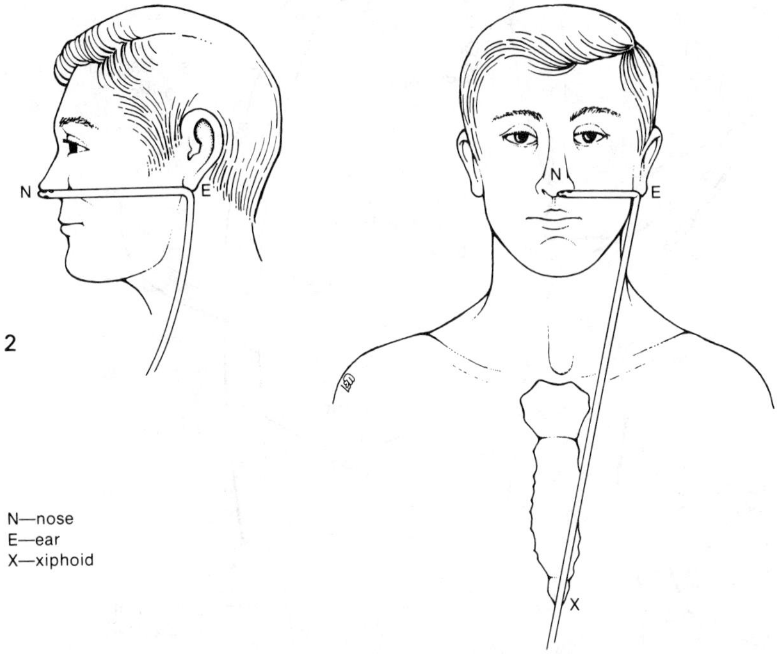

2. Have the patient sit in a neutral position with head facing forward. Place the distal tip of the tubing at the tip of the patient's nose (N); extend tube to the tragus (tip) of his ear (E), and then extend the tube straight down to the tip of his xiphoid (X). Mark this point 'B' on the tubing.

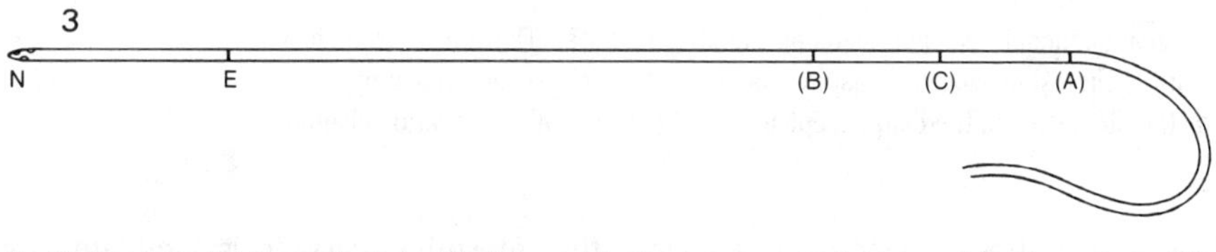

3. To locate point C on the tube, find the midpoint between points A and B. The nasogastric tube is passed to point C to ensure optimum placement in the stomach.

FIGURE 35-1. Nasogastric intubation using the Levin tube (short tube) or the Salem sump tube. (Based on research reported in Hanson RI. Predictive criteria for length of nasogastric tube insertion for tube feeding. J Parenteral Enteral Nutr 3[3]:160–163.)

Cantor tube. These tubes are used to relieve obstruction of the small intestine. They are also used prophylactically. They may be inserted the night before a gastrointestinal operation to prevent postoperative obstruction.

Because peristalsis is either absent or slowed for 24 to 48 hours after surgery as a result of the effects of anesthesia and of visceral manipulation, nasogastric or nasoenteric suction is used for the following reasons:

- To evacuate fluids and flatus, so that vomiting is prevented and tension is reduced along the incision line
- To reduce edema, which can cause obstruction
- To enhance blood supply to the suture line, thereby providing nutrition to the surgical site

Usually, the tubes are allowed to remain in place after surgery until peristalsis is resumed, as determined by the presence of bowel sounds and the passage of flatus.

Decompression Tubes

Miller-Abbott Tube. The Miller-Abbott tube is a double-lumen (No. 16 Fr), 3-m (10-ft) tube, one lumen of which is used to introduce mercury or air into the balloon at the end of the tube; the other lumen is used for aspiration. Before the tube is inserted, the balloon should be tested and its capacity measured; it is then deflated completely. The tube should be lubricated sparingly, and chilled well, before the tip is inserted through the patient's nose. Markings on the tube indicate the distance it has been passed. Prior to removal, the Miller-Abbott tube's balloon at the end of the lumina must be completely deflated.

Harris Tube. The Harris tube is a single-lumen (No. 14 Fr), mercury-weighted tube of about 1.8 m (6 ft). This tube has a metal tip that is lubricated and introduced through the nose. The mercury-weighted bag follows. The weight of

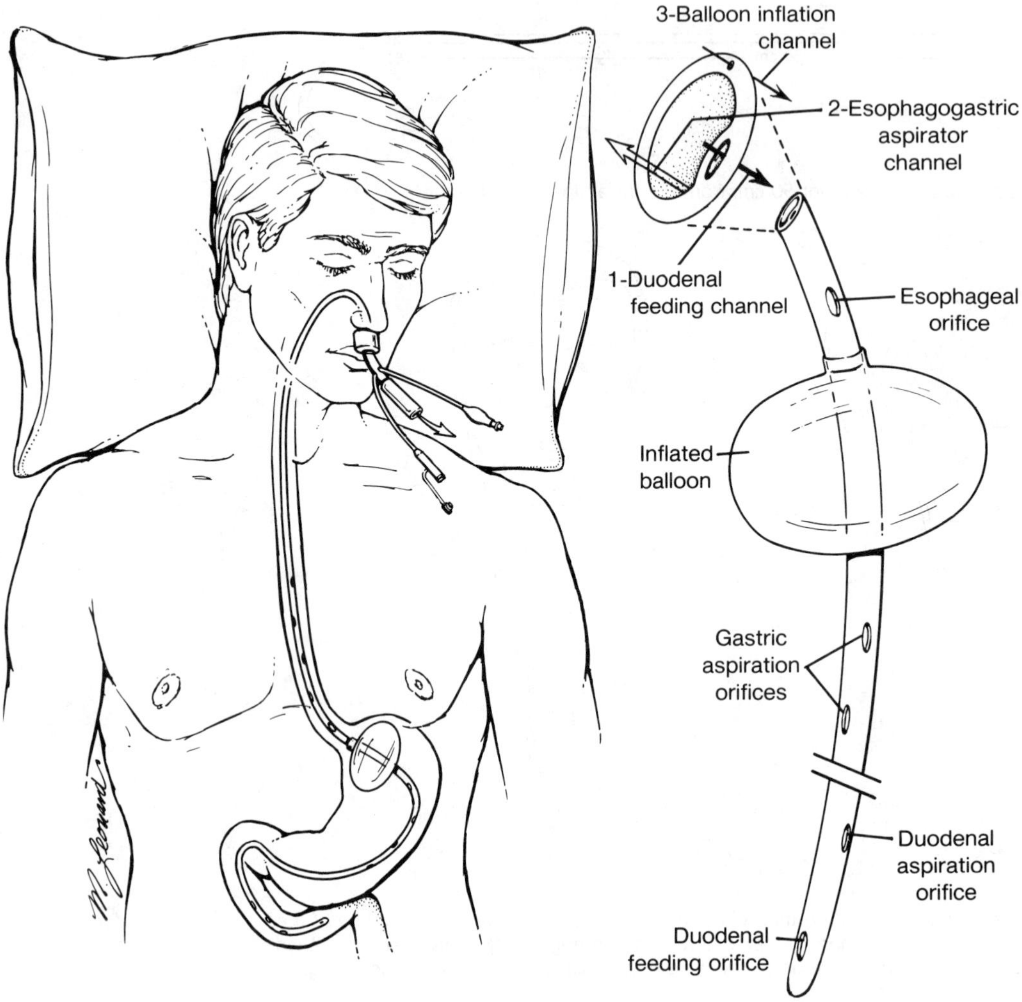

FIGURE 35-2. The Moss esophageal/duodenal decompression and feeding catheter. There are three channels: (1) the duodenal feeding channel; (2) the esophagogastric aspiration channel, which has additional openings into the proximal duodenum as well as the stomach and the distal esophagus; and (3) the balloon inflation channel.

the mercury carries the bag by gravity. This tube is used solely for suction and irrigation. Usually, a Y-tube is attached to the end of the Harris tube, so that the suction apparatus is attached to one side and an outlet with a clamp is available on the other side for irrigating purposes.

Cantor Tube. The Cantor tube is 3 m (10 ft) long with a No. 18 Fr lumen. Its distinguishing feature is that it is larger than the other long tubes and has 4 or 5 ml of mercury in the bag at the extreme end of the rubber tubing. Before the tube is inserted, the bag is wrapped around the tube. After the tube is lubricated, it is passed through the nose and advanced to the esophagus (Fig. 35-3). The patient is in a sitting position and is offered sips of water to facilitate passage of the tube. Fluoroscopy is helpful in verifying that the tube has passed into the duodenum.

Feeding Tubes

Several nasoenteric tubes that are commonly used for feeding include the Keofeed, Nyphus/Nelson, Moss, and Dubbhoff tubes (Fig. 35-4). It usually takes 24 hours for the Dobhoff and the Keofeed tubes to pass through the stomach and into the intestines. Passage is facilitated by having the patient lie on the right side. The Nyhus/Nelson nasoenteral tube uses a twin-balloon design to provide both gastric decompression and jejunal feeding. Both the Nyhus/Nelson and the Moss tubes are inserted in the operating room and are used frequently for postoperative enteral feeding to avoid negative nitrogen balance, to enhance wound healing, and to promote gastric motility and peristalsis, therefore reducing the length of postoperative hospital stay.

The polyurethane or silicone rubber feeding tubes have small diameters (6 to 12 Fr) and tungsten tips (rather than weighted mercury-filled bags); some have a water-activated lubricant that makes it easier to place the tube and insert and remove the stylet. The tubing may kink when a stylet is not used, particularly if the patient is uncooperative or unable to swallow. The stylet is used with caution in patients who are predisposed to esophageal punctures (elderly and frail with thin tissue). Essentially, such a tube is passed in the same way a nasogastric tube is passed, that is, with the patient in high Fowler's position. If this is not feasible, the patient is placed on the right side.

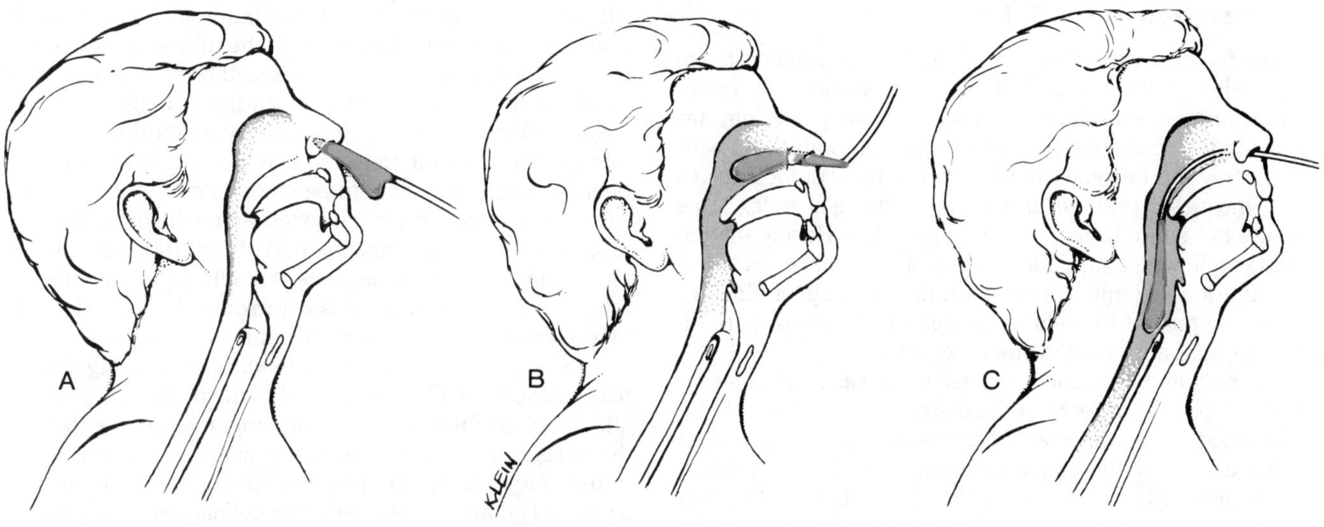

FIGURE 35-3. Passage of Cantor tube. (**A**) Tube with weighted mercury bag is introduced through the nose. Note the natural lift of the tubing. (**B**) After the mercury bag has entered the nostril, the catheter is tilted upward (head can also be tilted slightly upward) to facilitate gravity pull on the weighted bag. (**C**) The weight of the mercury pulls the bag downward.

Nursing Interventions for Nasogastric and Nasoenteric Intubation

Nursing interventions are organized into the following areas:

- Instructing the patient about the purposes of the tube and the procedures required for inserting and advancing it
- Identifying sensations to be expected during tube insertion
- Inserting the nasogastric tube and assisting with the insertion of the nasoenteric tube
- Confirming the placement of the nasogastric tube
- Advancing the nasoenteric tube
- Monitoring the patient
- Providing oral and nasal hygiene and care
- Monitoring potential complications
- Removing the tube

Providing Instruction

Before the patient is intubated, the nurse explains the purpose for using the tube. This information may make the patient more cooperative and tolerant of what is initially an unpleasant procedure. The general activities related to inserting the tube are then reviewed, including the fact that the patient may have to breathe through the mouth and a warning that the procedure may cause gagging until the tube has passed the patient's gag reflex.

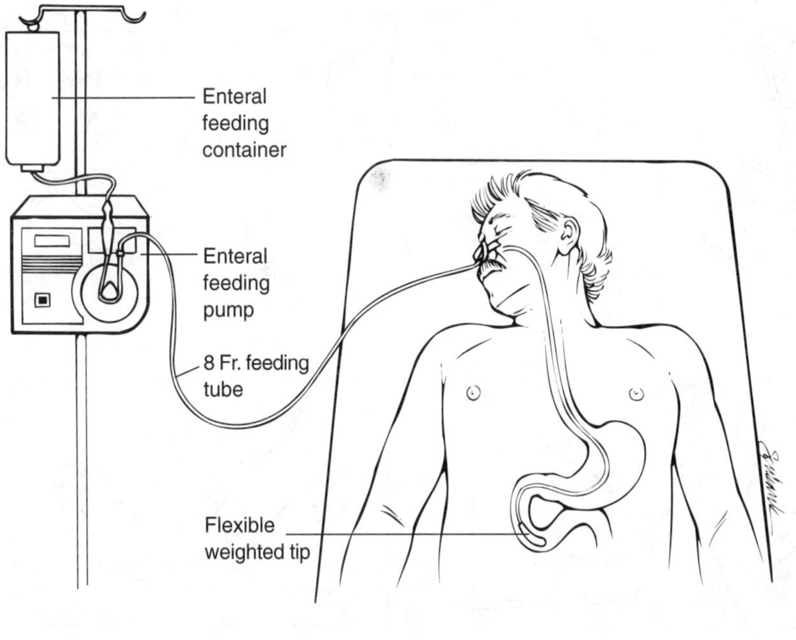

FIGURE 35-4. The enteral feeding tube (8 Fr) with a flexible weighted tip is readily passed into the stomach and through the pylorus into the duodenum or proximal jejunum. A pump is used for continuous tube feedings.

Insertion of the Tube

While the tube is being inserted, the patient usually sits upright with a towel spread bib-fashion over the chest. Tissue wipes are made available. Privacy and adequate light are provided. Occasionally, the physician will swab the nostril and spray the oropharynx with tetracaine (Pontocaine) to dull the nasal passage and suppress the gag reflex. This makes the entire procedure more tolerable. Having the patient gargle with a liquid anesthetic or hold ice chips in the mouth for a few minutes can have the same effect. Encouraging the patient to breathe through the mouth or pant often helps, as does swallowing water, if permitted.

A polyurethane tube may need to be warmed to make it more pliable. To make the tube easier to insert, it should be lubricated with a water-soluble substance (K-Y jelly) unless it has a dry coating called hydromer, which, when moistened, provides its own lubrication. The patient is placed in high Fowler's position. The nurse wears gloves during the procedure. The nostrils are inspected for any obstruction and the more patent nostril is selected for use. The tip of the patient's nose is raised and the tube is aligned to enter the oropharynx. When the tube reaches the nasopharynx, the patient is instructed to lower the head slightly and begin to swallow as the tube is advanced. The patient may also sip water through a straw to facilitate advancement of the tube. The oropharynx is inspected to ensure that the tube has not coiled in the pharynx or mouth.

Confirming Placement of the Nasogastric Tube

To ensure patient safety, it is important to confirm that the tube has been placed correctly. Initially, an x-ray may be taken for this purpose. However, each time liquids or medications are administered, the tube must be checked to assure that it is properly placed. The traditional recommendation has been to inject air through the tube and then to auscultate the epigastric area with a stethoscope to detect air insufflation. However, recent studies (Metheny, 1990a, 1990b) indicate that this auscultatory method is not accurate in differentiating between whether or not the tube has been inserted into the stomach or intestines or into the stomach or respiratory tract. Determining the *p*H of the tube aspirate is a more accurate method of confirming tube placement. The *p*H of gastric aspirate is acidic (approximately 3); the *p*H of intestinal aspirate is approximately 6.5; and the *p*H of respiratory aspirate is more alkaline (7 or greater).

Using gastric aspiration as a means of verifying that the nasogastric tube has been placed correctly may be problematic because of the characteristic properties and diameter of the tubes. A recent study suggests that aspiration may be performed more easily with polyurethane tubes and tubes with a size 10 Fr diameter. Metheny and colleagues (1993) recommend the following steps if problems occur with aspirating fluid from small-bore feeding tubes: (1) insufflate 20 ml air through the tube with a large syringe (30 to 60 ml); (2) pull back on the plunger; (3) if ineffective, insufflate another 20 ml of air and replace the large syringe with a smaller one (12 ml) and attempt to aspirate; (4) if still ineffective, repeat step 3; and finally (5) change the patient's position.

When the correct position of the tip in the stomach is confirmed, the nasogastric tube is secured to the nose or cheek (Fig. 35-5*A*). It is recommended that tincture of benzoin be applied to the skin where the nasogastric tube will be secured. The prepared area is covered with a strip of hypoallergenic tape or Op-site; the tube is then placed over the tape and secured with a second piece of tape. The nasoenteric tube can be secured by taping it to the cheek (use a slight U-shaped loop) or to the forehead (see Fig. 35-5*B*).

This technique secures the tube so that it does not dislodge when the patient moves. Nasoenteric tubes are *not*

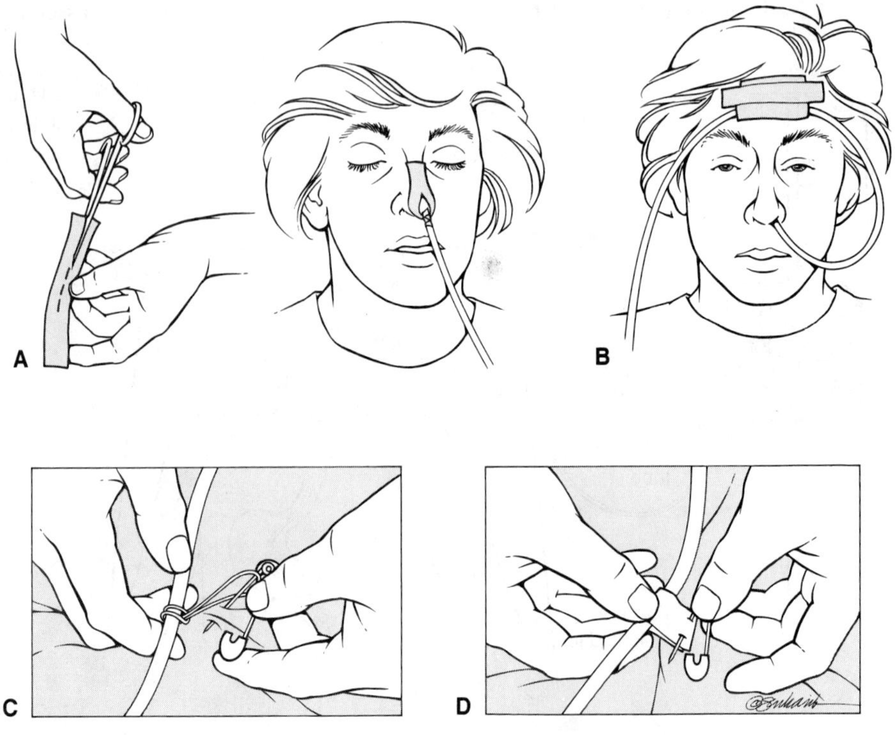

FIGURE 35-5. Securing nasogastric and nasoenteric tubes. (**A**) The nasogastric tube is secured to the nose with tape to prevent injury to the nasopharyngeal passages; the cheek may also be used. (**B**) Tape is placed on the forehead and the nasoenteric tube is taped to it, thereby allowing the Cantor tube to be advanced until desired placement is achieved. (**C, D**) Secure tubing to the patient's gown with either an elastic band or tape attached to a safety pin to prevent tension on the line during movement.

taped immediately, because it takes approximately 24 hours for these tubes to progress into the intestine.

Advancement of the Nasoenteric Tube

After the tube has passed through the pyloric sphincter, it may be advanced 5 to 7.5 cm (2 to 3 in) every hour. To enable gravity and peristalsis to assist in the passage of the tube, the patient is generally asked to lie in the following positions in the stated order: on right side for 2 hours, on the back for 2 hours, and then on the left side for 2 hours. Ambulation, if possible, also helps to advance the tube. If the tube is advanced too rapidly, it will curl and kink in the stomach. The tube is also irrigated with normal saline every 6 to 8 hours to prevent blockage.

Monitoring the Patient

If the nasogastric tube is used for decompression, it is attached to intermittent low suction. If it is used for enteral nutrition, the end of the tube is wrapped in gauze and clamped closed or plugged between feedings. Confirming tube placement is essential before any fluids or medications are instilled. Displacement of the tube may be caused by tension on the tube (when the patient moves around in the bed or room), coughing, tracheal or nasotracheal suctioning, and airway intubation.

An accurate record is kept of all fluid intake, feedings, and irrigation. Irrigation with normal saline is recommended to avoid electrolyte loss through gastric drainage. The amount, color, and type of all drainage are recorded every 8 hours.

When double- or triple-lumen tubes are used, each lumen is labeled according to its intended use: aspiration, feeding, or balloon inflation. To avoid tension on the tube, the portion of the tube from the nose to the drainage unit is fixed in position, either with a safety pin or with adhesive tape loops that are pinned to the patient's pajamas or gown. The tube must be looped loosely to prevent tension and dislodgment (see Fig. 35-5*C,D*).

Providing Oral and Nasal Hygiene and Care

Regular and conscientious oral and nasal hygiene is a vital part of patient care, as the tube may be in place for several days. Moistened cotton-tipped swabs can be used to clean the nose, followed by cleansing with water-soluble oil for lubrication. Frequent mouth care is comforting for the patient. The nasal tape is changed every other day and the nose is inspected for skin irritation. If the nasal and pharyngeal mucosa are excessively dry, steam or cool vapor inhalations may be beneficial. Throat lozenges, an ice collar, chewing gum (if permitted), and frequent movement also assist in relieving patient discomfort. These activities keep the mucous membranes moist and help prevent infection of the parotid glands.

Monitoring and Managing Potential Complications

Patients with nasogastric or nasoenteric intubation are susceptible to a variety of problems, including fluid volume deficit, pulmonary complications, and tube-related irritations. These potential complications require careful ongoing assessment, as follows:

Fluid Volume Deficit

1. Symptoms indicating a fluid volume deficit include
   a. Dryness of skin and mucous membranes
   b. Decreasing urinary output
   c. Lethargy and exhaustion
   d. Decrease in body temperature
2. Assessment of fluid volume deficit involves maintaining an accurate record of the following:
   a. Drainage—amount, color, and type, every 8 hours
   b. Amount of fluid instilled by irrigation of the nasogastric tube and the amount of water taken by mouth. An isotonic solution, such as normal saline, is used for irrigations to avoid electrolyte loss through gastric drainage
   c. Amount and character of vomitus, if any
   d. Fluid balance for 24 hours (intake versus output)
   e. Water administered with tube feedings
   f. Duration of any period in which the suction apparatus did not appear to function
   g. Effects produced by the treatment

Pulmonary Complications

1. Nasogastric intubation increases the incidence of postoperative pulmonary complications by interfering with coughing and clearing of the pharynx.
2. The nurse assesses the lung fields regularly, through auscultation, to determine the presence of congestion. In addition, the patient is encouraged to cough and to take deep breaths regularly. The nurse also carefully confirms the proper placement of the tube before instilling any fluids or medications.

Tube-Related Irritations

1. When providing oral hygiene, the nurse carefully inspects the mucous membranes for signs of irritation or excessive dryness. In addition, the nurse palpates the area around the parotid glands to detect any soreness or lumps and any skin or mucous membrane irritation or necrosis.
2. The nostrils, oral mucosa, esophagus, and trachea are susceptible to irritation and necrosis. Visible areas are inspected frequently and the adequacy of hydration is assessed. In addition, the patient is assessed for the presence of esophagitis and tracheitis. Symptoms include sore throat and hoarseness.

Removing the Tube

Prior to removing a tube, the nurse may intermittently clamp and unclamp the nasogastric tube for a trial period of 24 hours to assure that the patient does not experience nausea, vomiting, or distention. Gloves are used for removing the tube. Before it is removed, the tube is flushed with 10 ml of normal saline to ensure that it is free of debris and away from the gastric lining; then the balloon (if present) is deflated. The tube is withdrawn gently and slowly, for 15 to 20 cm (6 to 8 in), at intervals of 10 minutes, until the tip reaches the esophagus; the remainder is withdrawn rapidly from the nostril. If the tube does not come out easily, force should not be used and the problem is reported.

As the tube is withdrawn, it is concealed in a towel, because the sight of it may be unpleasant to the patient. After the tube is removed, oral hygiene is provided.

Nasogastric and Nasoenteric Tube Feedings

Tube feedings are given to meet nutritional requirements when oral intake is inadequate or not possible, as long as the GI tract is functioning normally. Tube feedings have several advantages: they are low in cost, safe, tolerated by the patient, and easy to use both in extended care facilities and in the home setting. Tube feedings are delivered to the stomach (nasogastric or gastrostomy) or to the distal duodenum or proximal jejunum (nasoenteric) when it is necessary to bypass the esophagus and stomach and when the patient is at risk for aspiration. The numerous conditions requiring enteral nutrition are summarized in Table 35-1.

Liquid formulas, taken either by mouth or through a tube, are designed to improve nutritional intake. Tube feedings have several advantages:

- Intraluminal delivery of nutrients preserves gastrointestinal integrity.
- Tube feedings preserve the normal sequence of intestinal and hepatic metabolism before nutrients are delivered to the arterial circulation.
- The intestinal mucosa and liver are important in fat metabolism and are the only sites of lipoprotein synthesis.
- Normal insulin-glucagon ratios are maintained when carbohydrates are administered through the intestines.

Osmosis and Osmolality

Highly concentrated solutions and certain foods can upset the normal fluid balance within the body. Fluid balance is maintained by the process of **osmosis,** which is accomplished within the body by moving water through membranes from a dilute solution of lower osmolality (ionic concentration) to a more concentrated one of higher osmolality until the solutions are of nearly equal osmolality. The osmolality of normal body fluids is approximately 300 mOsm/kg. The body attempts to keep the osmolality of the contents of the stomach and intestines at approximately this level.

Proteins are extremely large particles and therefore have little or no osmotic effect. Individual amino acids and carbohydrates are smaller particles and have greater osmotic effect. Fats are not water-soluble and do not form a solution in water; thus, they have no osmotic effect. Electrolytes such as sodium and potassium are comparatively small particles; they have a great effect on osmolality, and consequently on the patient's ability to tolerate a given solution.

Osmolality is an important consideration for patients who receive tube feedings through the duodenum or jejunum. When a concentrated solution of high osmolality is taken in large amounts, water will move to the stomach and intestines from fluid surrounding the organs and from the vascular compartment. The patient experiences a feeling of fullness, nausea, and diarrhea, which can bring about dehydration, resulting, in some cases, in hypotension and tachycardia. Collectively, these symptoms have been termed the **dumping syndrome**. This problem can generally be alleviated by starting with a more dilute solution and then increasing the concentration over several days.

Patients vary in the degree to which they can tolerate the effects of osmolality. Usually, debilitated patients are more sensitive to such disorders. Therefore, the nurse

TABLE 35-1 Conditions Requiring Enteral Nutrition

Condition or Need	Cause
Preoperative preparation with elemental diet	
Gastrointestinal problems with elemental diet	Fistulas, short bowel syndrome, Crohn's disease, ulcerative colitis, nonspecific maldigestion or malabsorption
Cancer therapy	Radiation, chemotherapy
Convalescent care	Surgery, injury, severe illness
Coma, semiconsciousness*	Stroke, head injury, neurologic disorders
Hypermetabolic conditions	Burns, trauma, multiple fractures, sepsis, AIDS, organ transplantation
Alcoholism, chronic depression, anorexia nervosa*	Chronic illness, psychiatric or neurologic disorder
Debilitation*	Disease or injury
Maxillofacial or cervical surgery	Disease or injury
Oropharyngeal or esophageal paralysis*	Disease or injury
Mental retardation*	

*Some of these patients will be at risk for regurgitating or vomiting and aspirating administered formula. Accordingly, each case must be considered individually.

(Jensen T. Home enteral nutrition. Dietetic Currents, Ross Timesaver Jul/Aug; 9:15–20.)

ETHICAL QUESTION

Is It Permissible to Withhold or Withdraw Nutrition and Hydration From Patients Who Cannot Eat or Drink?

Situation

It is generally agreed that patients (or their designated decision-makers) can refuse life-saving treatment. Nutrition and hydration, however, are perceived as food and drink because they can be provided often by low-tech means and because withdrawing or withholding them can result in the patient becoming dehydrated or even literally starving to death. Thus, some have argued that nutrition and hydration should always be provided to every patient, regardless of the patient's preference or condition.

Dilemma

The patient's desire to have nutrition or hydration withdrawn or withheld conflicts with the reluctance of others to harm the patient by withdrawing the food and water he needs for survival (autonomy versus nonmaleficence).

Discussion

- What arguments would you offer *against* the withholding and withdrawing of nutrition and hydration?
- What arguments would you offer in *favor* of withholding and withdrawing nutrition and hydration?

should be knowledgeable about the osmolality of formulas and should observe for and actively prevent such disorders.

Tube Feeding Formulas

The tube feeding formula chosen is influenced by the status of the gastrointestinal tract and the nutrient needs of the patient. Certain formula characteristics are evaluated when an enteral formula is considered: chemical composition of nutrient source (protein, carbohydrates, fat), caloric density, osmolality, residue, bacteriologic safety, vitamins, minerals, and cost.

Five major tube feeding types are available for use. Blenderized formulas can be made by the nurse or obtained in a ready-to-use form that is carefully prepared according to directions. Commercially prepared polymeric formulas are composed of protein, carbohydrates, and fats in a high molecular weight form (Ensure Plus, Sustacal). Chemically defined formulas contain predigested and easy-to-absorb nutrients (Isocal, Omolite). Modular products contain only one major nutrient such as protein or carbohydrate (Pomod). Disease-specific formulas are available for various conditions, such as severe chronic obstructive pulmonary disease (Pulmocare). Pulmocare is high in fat and low in carbohydrates. Its high density (1.5 calories/ml) is ideal for patients who require fluid restriction, and it is also designed to reduce carbon dioxide production. Fiber has also been added to formulas (Jevity, Enrich) in an attempt to decrease the occurrence of diarrhea.

Some feedings are given as supplements and others are provided to meet the patient's total nutritional needs. Nutritionists collaborate with physicians and nurses in determining the best formula for the individual patient.

Commercial formulas frequently present problems because the composition is "fixed." Some patients may not be able to tolerate certain ingredients, such as sodium, protein, or potassium. Modular products may be substituted and the critical constituents of sodium, potassium, and fat can be added. Attention is given to including all essential minerals and vitamins. Total intake of calories, nutrients, and fluids is assessed when there is a reduction in total intake or excessive dilution of feedings.

Tube Feeding Administration Methods

Many patients do not tolerate nasogastric and nasoenteric tubes feedings well. Often a medium- or fine-bore Silastic nasoenteric tube is tolerated better than a plastic or rubber tube. The finer-bore tube, however, requires a finely dispersed formula to prevent the tube from clogging. For long-term tube feeding therapy, a gastrostomy or jejunostomy is used (refer to page 871).

The tube feeding method chosen depends on the location of the tube, patient tolerance, convenience, and cost. Intermittent bolus feedings are administered into the stomach (usually by gastrostomy) in large amounts at designated intervals. The intermittent gravity drip is another method for administering tube feedings into the stomach and is commonly used when the patient is at home. The tube feeding is administered over 30 minutes at designated intervals. Both of these tube feeding methods are practical and inexpensive. However, the feedings delivered at variable rates may be poorly tolerated and time consuming.

The continuous infusion method is used when feedings are administered into the small intestine. This method is preferred when patients are at risk for aspiration or poor tolerance of tube feedings. The feedings are given continuously at a constant rate by means of a pump. Cyclic continuous infusions may be particularly suitable for patients at home. The infusion is given at a more rapid rate over a shorter period of time (usually 8 to 12 hours at night) so as not to interrupt the patient's lifestyle. The continuous tube feeding method decreases abdominal distention, gastric residuals, and the risk of aspiration. These methods are expensive (pumps) and permit the patient less flexibility.

A wide variety of containers, feeding tubes and catheters, delivery systems, and pumps (Kangaroo 2, IMED-430, Dobhoff, Keofeed II, Flexiflo II) are available for use in tube feedings.

Tube feeding solutions vary in terms of required preparation, consistency, and the number of calories and supplemental vitamins they contain. The type chosen depends on the size and location of the tube, the patient's nutrient needs, type of nutritional supplement, method of delivery, and convenience for the patient at home.

❑ NURSING PROCESS
The Patient Receiving a Tube Feeding

Assessment

A preliminary assessment of patients with suspected nutritional problems includes several considerations, as well as the family's need for information:

- What is the patient's nutritional status as judged by current physical appearance; dietary history, including a history of food intolerances especially milk or lactose intolerance; and recent weight loss or gain?
- Are there any existing chronic illnesses or factors that will increase metabolic demands on the body (*e.g.*, surgical stress, fever)?
- Is the patient's fluid and electrolyte balance in order?
- Is the patient's digestive tract functioning? Does it have good absorptive capacity?
- Are the kidneys and urinary system functioning normally?
- Are weight and fluid requirements (*i.e.*, 30 to 40 ml/kg body weight) being met?
- What medications and other therapies is the patient receiving that may affect digestive intake and function of the digestive system?
- Does the dietary prescription fulfill the patient's needs?

In addition, a more elaborate assessment is performed on those patients who may require extensive nutritional therapy. This is conducted by a team that includes the nurse, physician, and nutritionist. In addition to the history and physical examination (which includes anthropometric measurements), nutritional assessment consists of recording any weight change, determining serum albumin and transferrin levels and total lymphocyte count, testing of delayed hypersensitivity reaction, and evaluating muscle function. (See Chapter 7 for a detailed description of nutritional assessment.)

Diagnosis

Nursing Diagnoses

Based on all the assessment data, the major nursing diagnoses may include the following:

- Altered nutrition, less than body requirements, related to inadequate intake of nutrients
- Diarrhea related to the dumping syndrome or tube feeding intolerance
- Potential ineffective airway clearance related to aspiration of tube feeding
- Risk for fluid volume deficit related to hypertonic dehydration
- Potential ineffective individual coping related to the discomfort imposed by the presence of the nasogastric or nasoenteric tube
- Knowledge deficit about home tube feeding regimen

Collaborative Problems/ Potential Complications

Complications of nasogastric and nasoenteric tube feeding therapy are commonly classified as one of three types: gastrointestinal, mechanical, and metabolic (Table 35-2).

Planning and Implementation

Goals. The major goals of the patient may include attainment and maintenance of nutritional balance, maintenance of a normal bowel pattern, maintenance of a patent airway, maintenance of adequate hydration, improvement of individual coping, knowledge of and skill in self-care, and absence of complications.

Nursing Interventions

Maintaining Nutritional Balance. Temperature and volume of the feeding, flow rate, and adequate fluid intake are critically important when tube feedings are administered. The schedule determining the quantity and frequency of tube feedings is maintained. The nurse must carefully monitor the rate of drip and avoid administering fluids too rapidly. Electrical pumps commonly used to control the rate and pressure of the delivery of viscous fluids are relatively heavy and must be attached to an intravenous (IV) pole. Several pumps specifically designed for enteral tube feedings are lightweight and easy to handle and require minimal instructions for use. Some examples are the Kangaroo Easy-Cap II (Cheeseborough-Pond); the Flexiflo II Portable Enteral Nutrition Pump (Ross Laboratories), which can be carried by using a nylon adjustable strap and can operate for 8 hours on a rechargeable battery; the Enteroport (Diatek), designed for continuous home feedings and available with a portable shoulder strap; the IMED 430 Enteral Delivery System (IMED); and the Flo Gard 2000 peristaltic pump (Travenol Laboratories).

Residual gastric content is measured before each intermittent feeding and every 4 to 8 hours during continuous feedings. (This solution is readministered to the patient.) If the amount of aspirated gastric content is greater than 100 ml or more than 10% to 20% above the hourly continuous feeding rate, the feeding is delayed and the patient's condition is reassessed in 1 hour. If this occurs twice, the problem is reported.

To ensure patency and to decrease the chance of bacterial growth and crusting or occlusion of the tube, about 50 ml of water is administered in each of the following instances: (1) before and after each dose of medication and each tube feeding, (2) after checking for gastric residuals and gastric *p*H, and (3) every 4 to 6 hours with continuous feedings. Some studies (Wilson & Haynes-Johnson, 1987) have demonstrated that water is superior to other liquids in preventing tube occlusion. When different types of medications are administered, each type is given separately using a bolus method that is compatible with its preparation (Table 35-3). The tube is flushed with 5 ml of water after each dose. Medications are not to be mixed with each other or with the tube feeding formula.

When small-bore feeding tubes for continuous rates are irrigated, a 30-ml or larger syringe is used because pressure generated by smaller syringes can cause the tube to rupture. The bag and tubing are changed according to the agency's policy, usually every 24 to 48 hours; tube feeding solution is changed every 4 hours to reduce bacterial contamination.

Feedings are administered either by gravity (drip), bolus, or by continuous controlled pump that is either volumetric (ml/hr) or peristaltic (drops/hr). Gravity feedings are placed above the level of the stomach, and the speed of administration is determined by gravity. Bolus feedings are

TABLE 35-2 Complications of Enteral Therapy

Complications	Cause
Gastrointestinal	
Diarrhea (most frequent)	Hyperosmolar feedings Rapid infusion/bolus feedings Bacteria-contaminated feedings Lactase deficiency Medications/antibiotic therapy Decreased serum osmolality level Food allergies Cold formula
Nausea/vomiting	Change in rate Offensive smell Hyperosmolar formula Inadequate gastric emptying
Gas/bloating/cramping Dumping syndrome	Air in tube Bolus feedings/rapid rate Cold formula
Constipation	High milk content Lack of fiber Inadequate fluid intake
Mechanical	
Aspiration pneumonia (atelectasis)	Improper tube placement Vomiting and aspirated tube feeding Flat in bed Tube too large
Tube displacement	Excessive coughing/vomitus Tension on the tube/unsecured tube Tracheal suctioning Airway intubation
Tube obstruction Residue	Inadequate flushing/formula rate Inadequate crushing of medications and flushing after administration
Nasopharyngeal irritation	Tube position Large tubes
Metabolic	
Hyperglycemia	Glucose intolerance High carbohydrate feeding content
Dehydration and azotemia (excessive urea in the blood)	Hyperosmolar feedings with insufficient fluid intake
Tube feeding syndrome	Excessive urea from high-protein mixture and formulas lacking fat Dehydration

TABLE 35-3 Medication Administration Via Feeding Tube

Type	Preparation
Liquid	None
Simple compressed tablets	Crushed and dissolved in water
Buccal or sublingual tablets	Give as intended
Enteric-coated tablets	Cannot be crushed; change in form required
Time-released tablets	Some can be opened; cannot be crushed

given in large volumes, 300 to 400 ml every 4 to 6 hours. Continuous feeding is the preferred method; allowing the feeding to be given in small set amounts over long periods reduces the risk of aspiration, distention, nausea, vomiting, and diarrhea.

Feedings are lactose free, with an osmolality of only 300 mOsm/kg; a feeding may be given undiluted and provides 1 calorie/ml. Feeding rates of about 100 to 150 ml/hr (2400 to 3600 calories/d) are effective in inducing positive nitrogen balance and progressive weight gain, without producing abdominal cramps and diarrhea. If the feeding is intermittent, 200 to 350 ml are given in 10 to 15 minutes.

The tube-feeding regimen must be monitored continuously to determine its nutritional effectiveness. The following nursing measures are implemented:

- Assess tubing placement, patient's position, and flow rate.
- Observe patient's ability to tolerate the formula (assess for feeling of fullness, bloating, urticaria, nausea, vomiting, diarrhea, and constipation).
- Check clinical responses, as noted in laboratory findings: blood urea nitrogen, serum protein, hemoglobin, and hematocrit.
- Assess the patient's general condition by noting the appearance of the skin (turgor, dryness, color) and mucous membranes; urinary output; state of hydration; and weight gain or loss.
- Observe for signs of dehydration (dry mucous membranes, thirst, decreased urine output).
- Record the actual formula intake by the patient.
- Record incidents of vomiting and diarrhea or distention.
- Report a urine glucose concentration of +3 or +4, decreased urinary output, sudden weight gain, and periorbital or dependent edema.
- Replace tube formula every 4 hours with fresh formula.
- Change tube feeding container and tubing every 24 to 48 hours.
- Assess residual volumes before each feeding or, in the case of continuous feedings, every 4 hours.
- Monitor intake and output.
- Weigh patient two to three times a week.
- Consult dietician.

Maintaining Bowel Pattern. Patients receiving nasogastric or nasoenteric tube feedings frequently experience diarrhea (watery stools occurring three times in 24 hours). Pasty, unformed stool is expected with enteral therapy because many formulas have little or no residue. The dumping syndrome also leads to diarrhea. To confirm that the dumping syndrome is causing the diarrhea, other possible causes must be ruled out: zinc deficiency (adding 15 mg of zinc to the tube feeding every 24 hours is recommended to maintain a normal serum level of 50 to 150 μg/dl [7.65 to 22.95 μmol/L]); contaminated formula; malnutrition (a decrease in the intestinal absorptive area resulting from malnutrition can cause diarrhea); and medication therapy. Antibiotics such as clindamycin (Cleocin) and lincomycin (Lincocin), antidysrhythmic drugs (quinidine, propranolol [Inderal]), aminophylline (theophylline), and digitalis have been found to increase the frequency of the dumping syndrome in certain patients.

The dumping syndrome results from the rapid distention of the jejunum when hypertonic solutions are administered quickly (over 10 to 20 minutes). Foods high in carbohydrates and electrolytes draw extracellular fluid from the vascular system into the jejunum so that dilution and absorption can occur. The gastrointestinal symptoms (diarrhea, nausea) associated with the dumping syndrome can be managed in the following manner:

- Decreasing the instillation rate to provide time for carbohydrates and electrolytes to be diluted
- Administering the feedings at room temperature, because temperature extremes stimulate peristalsis
- Administering the feeding by continuous drip (if tolerated) rather than by bolus to prevent sudden distention of the intestine
- Advising the patient to remain in semi-Fowler's position for 30 minutes after the feeding (this position prolongs transit time by decreasing the influence of gravity)
- Instilling the minimal amount of water needed to flush the tubing before and after a feeding because fluid given with a feeding increases transit time

Managing the Airway. Airway obstruction occurs when stomach contents or enteral feedings are regurgitated and aspirated or when a nasogastric tube is improperly placed and feedings are instilled into the pharynx or the trachea. Nasoenteric tubes, especially those that provide for gastric and esophageal or duodenal decompression (Nyhus/Nelson, Moss), have helped decrease the frequency of regurgitation and aspiration.

To maintain a patent airway, the nurse must check tube placement before giving every feeding and always administer the feeding with the patient in the proper position to prevent regurgitation. To reduce the risk of reflux and pulmonary aspiration, the semi-Fowler's position is necessary for a nasogastric feeding; the patient's head should be elevated at least 30 degrees for a nasoenteric feeding. This position is maintained at least 30 minutes after completion of intermittent tube feedings; it is maintained at all times for patients receiving continuous tube feedings.

If aspiration is suspected, the feeding is stopped, the pharynx and trachea are suctioned, and the patient is placed on his or her right side with the head of the bed down. The physician is notified immediately.

Maintaining Adequate Hydration. The hydration of the patient is monitored carefully because the patient often cannot communicate the need for water. Water is given every 4 to 6 hours and after feedings to prevent hypertonic dehydration (at least 2 l/d). At the beginning of administration, the feeding is diluted to at least half-strength and not more than 50 to 100 ml is given at a time, or 40 to 60 ml/hr is given in continuous drip administration. This gradual administration helps the patient to develop tolerance, especially for hyperosmolar solutions. The following nursing measures are important:

- Observe for signs of dehydration (dry mucous membranes, thirst, decreased urine output).
- Administer water routinely and as needed.
- Monitor intake, output, and fluid balance (24-hour intake versus output).

Promoting Coping Ability. The psychosocial goal of nursing care is to support, encourage, and accept the patient, while conveying hope that daily progressive improvement is possible. If the patient is having difficulty adjusting to the treatment, the nurse intervenes by

- Praising the patient who adheres to the medical plan of care
- Encouraging self-care within the parameters of the patient's activity level (*e.g.*, recording daily weight and intake and output)
- Reinforcing an optimistic approach by identifying signs and symptoms that indicate progress (daily weight gain, electrolyte balance, absence of nausea and diarrhea)

Patient Education and Home Care Considerations. Some patients receive tube feedings in the home care setting. The need for long-term tube feeding may be a result of an obstruction of the upper GI tract, malabsorption syndrome, surgery of the GI tract or head or neck region, or decreased level of consciousness.

Young and White (1992) have determined that patients who are to be considered for tube feeding therapy at home must meet the following criteria: be medically stable, successfully complete a tube feeding trial (tolerate 70% of feeding), be capable of self-care or have a caregiver willing to assume the responsibility, and have access to and interest in education for self and caregiver.

Preparing the patient for home administration of enteral feedings begins while the patient is still hospitalized. The nurse teaches while administering the feedings so that the patient can observe the mechanics of the procedure, which reinforces them in the patient's mind prior to discharge. Before discharge, information is provided about the equipment, formula purchase and storage, and administration of the feedings (frequency, quantity, rate of instillation). Family members who will be active in the patient's home care are invited to participate in all teaching sessions. Available printed information about the delivery equipment and formula is reviewed. The patient is encouraged to learn to use the equipment with the supervision of the nurse.

A visiting nurse will monitor the progress (weight, vital signs, activity level, electrolyte values) of the homebound patient and assess for any complications (dumping syndrome, nausea or vomiting, weight loss, lethargy, confusion, excessive thirst). The patient is encouraged to keep a diary to record times and amounts of feedings and any symptoms that occur. The nurse reviews the diary with the patient during home visits.

Evaluation

Expected Outcomes

1. Attains or maintains nutritional balance
   a. Has positive nitrogen balance
   b. Diagnostic studies within normal limits (*i.e.*, blood urea nitrogen [BUN], hemoglobin, hematocrit, serum protein)
   c. Attains or maintains hydration of body tissue
   d. Attains or maintains desired body weight
2. Is free of episodes of diarrhea
   a. Has fewer than three watery stools a day
   b. Does not have a bowel movement after a bolus feeding
   c. States that there is no intestinal cramping
   d. Has normal bowel sounds
3. Maintains a patent airway
   a. Lungs are clear to auscultation
   b. Normal heart rate and respirations
4. Attains or maintains hydration of body tissue
   a. Has a balanced intake and output every 24 hours
   b. Does not have dry skin or mucous membranes
5. Copes effectively with tube feeding regimen
6. Demonstrates skill in managing tube feeding regimen
7. Is free of complications
   a. Has no gastrointestinal disturbances
   b. Tube remains intact and patent for duration of therapy
   c. Metabolic balance is maintained within normal limits.

Gastrostomy

A gastrostomy is a surgical procedure performed to create an opening into the stomach for the purpose of administering food and fluids. In some instances, a gastrostomy is used for prolonged nutrition, as in the elderly or debilitated patient. Gastrostomy is preferred to nasogastric feedings in the comatose patient because the gastroesophageal sphincter remains intact. Also, regurgitation is less likely to occur with a gastrostomy than with nasogastric feedings.

Different types of feeding gastrostomies may be used: the Stamm (temporary and permanent), Janeway (permanent), and percutaneous endoscopic gastrostomy (temporary). The Stamm and Janeway gastrostomies (Fig. 35-6) require either an upper abdominal midline incision or a left upper quadrant transverse incision. The *Stamm procedure* requires the use of concentric purse-string sutures to secure a tube to the anterior gastric wall. A stab wound exit is created in the left upper abdomen to provide for the gastrostomy. The *Janeway procedure* necessitates the creation of a tunnel (called a gastric tube) that is brought out through the abdomen to form a permanent stoma.

A *percutaneous endoscopic gastrostomy* (PEG) requires the services of two physicians. One inserts a cannula into the stomach through an abdominal incision, using local anesthesia and then threads a nonabsorbable suture through the cannula, while a second physician, looking

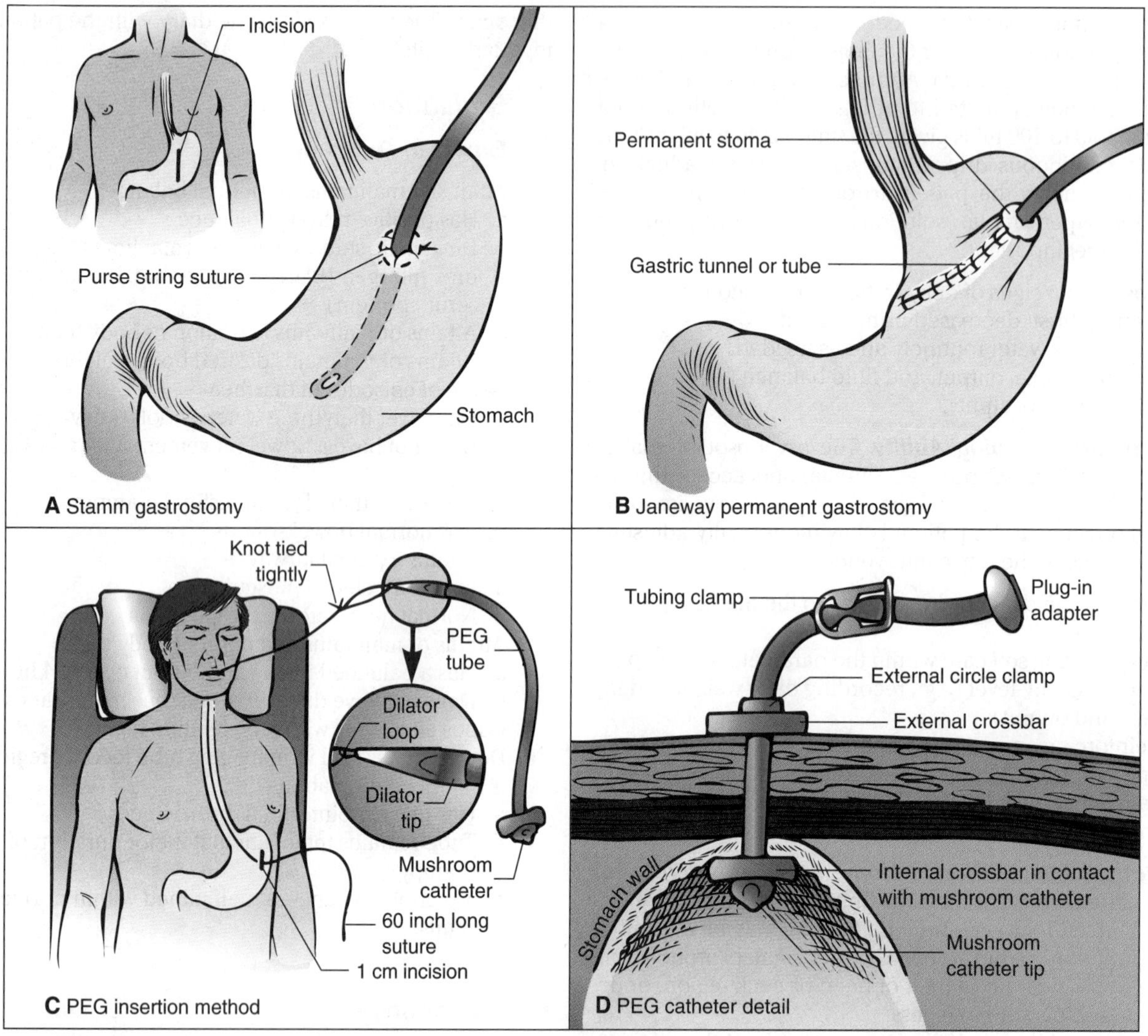

FIGURE 35-6. (**A**) Stamm gastrostomy, showing incision line and purse-string suture. (**B**) Janeway permanent gastrostomy. (**C**) Percutaneous endoscopic gastrostomy (PEG). (**D**) A detail of the abdomen and the PEG tube, showing catheter fixation.

through an endoscope that has been passed into the upper GI tract, uses the endoscopic snare to grasp the end of the suture and guide it up through the patient's mouth. The suture is knotted to the dilator tip at the end of the PEG tube. The endoscopist then advances the dilator tip through the patient's mouth while the other physician pulls the suture through the cannula site. The attached PEG tube is guided down the esophagus, into the stomach, and out through the abdominal incision. The mushroom catheter tip and internal crossbar secure the tube against the stomach wall. An external crossbar keeps the catheter in place. A tubing adaptor is in place between feedings and a clamp is used to close or open the tubing.

The PEG device can be removed and replaced once the tract is well established (10 to 14 days after insertion). Replacing the PEG device is indicated if it is used for long-term nutritional support, to replace a clotted tube, or to enhance patient comfort. The replacement device should be fitted securely to the stoma to prevent leakage of gastric acid; the stoma is gently cleaned and topical antibiotic ointment is applied around the insertion site. Skin-level replacement devices, such as the PEG button or the Gastro-port, are inserted flush with the skin. These devices have an anti-reflux valve and a cap to close completely between feedings. A major drawback to these devices is the need to obturate (insert a tube that is larger than the actual stoma). An alternative to this device is a MIC-KEY tube, a nonobturated skin-level silicone tube that is designed like a short indwelling catheter. The MIC-KEY is inserted into the stoma without force and a balloon is inflated to secure placement. There are also prepackaged gastrostomy tube kits available to insert and stabilize the tube. A Foley catheter may be used temporarily to maintain stoma patency until a proper replacement device can be obtained.

Patients with severe gastroesophageal reflux are at risk for aspiration pneumonia and therefore are not candidates for a gastrostomy. A jejunostomy is preferred, or jejunal feeding through a nasojejunal tube may be recommended.

❑ NURSING PROCESS
The Patient With a Gastrostomy

Assessment

Preoperative

The focus of the preoperative assessment is to determine the patient's ability both to understand and to deal with the impending surgical experience. The ability to adjust to a change in body image and to participate in self-care is evaluated, along with the patient's and the family's psychological status. Is the patient depressed, angry, withdrawn, or optimistic? Will the family be supportive?

The purpose of the operative procedure is explained so that the patient will have a better understanding of the expected postoperative course. The patient needs to know that the purpose of this surgery is to bypass the esophagus and that liquid feedings will be administered directly into the stomach by means of a rubber or plastic tube or a prosthesis. If the prosthesis is to be permanent, the patient should be made aware of this. Psychologically, this is often difficult for the patient to accept. When the procedure is being performed to relieve discomfort, prolonged vomiting, debilitation, and an inability to eat, the patient finds it more acceptable. Frequently, a gastrostomy is performed on an elderly or a comatose patient who cannot tolerate nasogastric feedings.

The nurse evaluates the patient's skin condition and determines whether a delay in wound healing may be anticipated because of a systemic disorder (*e.g.*, diabetes mellitus, cancer).

Postoperative

In the postoperative period the patient's fluid and nutritional needs are assessed to ensure proper food and fluid intake. The nurse observes the status of the tube and the wound for proper maintenance and any signs of infection. At the same time, the patient is evaluated for change in body image and an understanding of the methods for carrying out the feeding procedure. In this way interventions are determined that help the patient cope with the presence of the tube and learn self-care measures.

Diagnosis

Nursing Diagnoses

Based on all the assessment data, the major nursing diagnoses in the postoperative period may include the following:

- Altered nutrition, less than body requirements, related to enteral feeding problems
- Risk for infection related to presence of wound and tube
- Impairment of skin integrity at tube site
- Ineffective coping related to the inability to eat normally
- Disturbance in body image related to the presence of the tube
- Knowledge deficit about home care and the feeding procedure

Collaborative Problems/ Potential Complications

Based on the assessment data, potential complications that may develop include:

- Wound infection, cellulitis, and abdominal wall abscess
- Gastrointestinal bleeding
- Premature removal of the tube

Planning and Implementation

Goals. The major goals of the patient may include attainment of the desired level of nutrition, absence of infection, maintenance of skin integrity, improvement in coping methods, adjustment to changes in body image, knowledge of and skill in self-care, and absence of complications.

Nursing Interventions

Meeting Nutritional Needs. The first fluid nourishment is administered soon after surgery and usually consists of tap water and 10% glucose. At first only 30 to 60 ml (1 to 2 oz) is given at a time, but the amount is gradually increased. By the second day, from 180 to 240 ml (6 to 8 oz) may be given at one time, provided it is tolerated and no leakage of fluid occurs around the tube. Water and milk can be instilled after 24 hours for a permanent gastrostomy. High-calorie liquids are added gradually. In some settings, during the early postoperative period the nurse aspirates gastric secretions and reinstills them, after adding enough feeding to bring the volume to the desired total. By this method, gastric dilation is avoided.

Blenderized foods are gradually added to clear liquids until a full diet is reached. Powdered feedings that are easily liquified are commercially available. A food blender can be used to liquefy a normal diet, which then can be fed through the tube. The patient who receives blenderized tube feedings typically is not forced to give up usual dietary patterns, which may prove to be psychologically more acceptable. In addition, near-normal bowel function is promoted, as the fiber and residue are similar to that of a normal diet. Intake of milk is avoided in patients with lactase deficiency.

Providing Tube Care and Preventing Infection. The tube can be held in place by a thin strip of adhesive tape that is first twisted about the tube and then firmly attached to the abdomen. A catheter plug or rubber-tipped hemostat may close the outlet of the tube immediately after a feeding to prevent leakage. A small dressing can be applied over the tube outlet; the tube can be coiled and held in place by Montgomery straps or a firm abdominal binder. This protects the skin surrounding the incision from the seepage of gastric acid contents and the spillage of feedings (Fig. 35-7). Thereafter, the dressing is changed every 2 or 3 days and the patient is taught how to perform this self-care activity.

Providing Skin Care. The skin surrounding a gastrostomy requires special care, beacuse it may become irritated as a result of the enzymatic action of gastric juices that leak around the tube. If untreated, the skin becomes macerated, red, raw, and painful. Washing the area around the tube with soap and water daily and applying a bland ointment, such

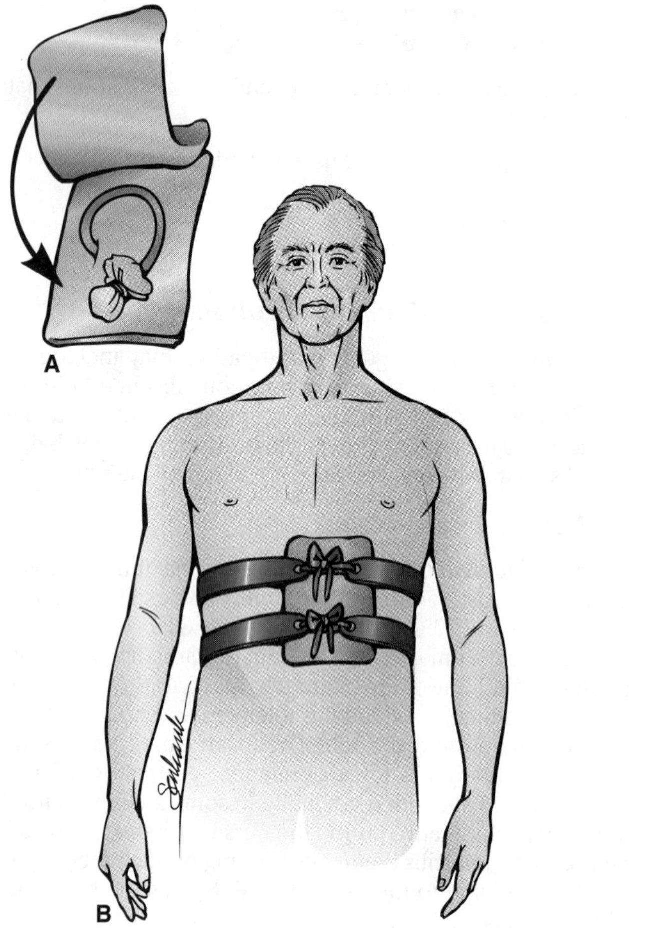

FIGURE 35-7. Tube care. (**A**) After a feeding, the opening of the tube is covered with a sterile gauze square held by a rubber band. (**B**) The tubing is coiled on a dressing, covered, and secured with Montgomery straps.

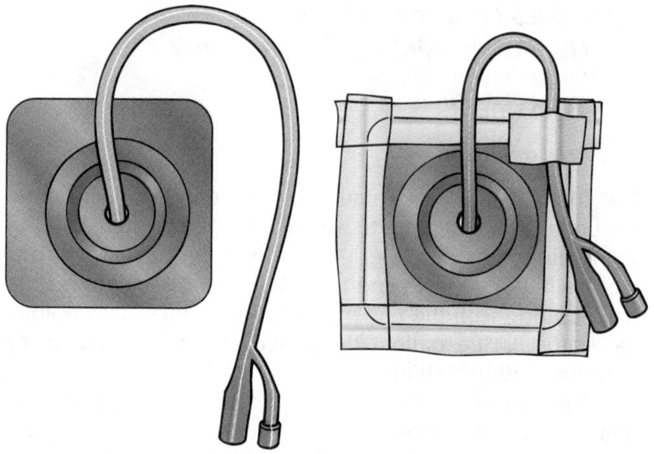

FIGURE 35-8. Securing a gastrostomy tube. (**Left**) An opening is cut in the stomahesive wafer the same shape as the exit site but one-eighth larger. The gastrostomy tube is then threaded through the hole and sealed. (**Right**) The wafer is framed with tape; the gastrostomy tube is then taped to the wafer to anchor and protect it.

as zinc oxide or petrolatum, are protective measures. A long-term gastrostomy may require application of a stomahesive wafer to maintain the integrity of the skin around the tube, protect it from gastric secretions, and stabilize the entry site (Fig. 35-8).

Skin status is evaluated daily for signs of breakdown, irritation, or excoriation (abrasion). The patient and family members should be encouraged to participate in this inspection and in hygiene activities. If skin problems do occur, the nurse will consult an enterostomal therapist.

Assisting With Body Image Adjustment. The patient with a gastrostomy has experienced a major assault to body image. Eating, which is a normal physiologic and social function, can no longer be taken for granted. The patient is also aware that gastrostomy as a therapeutic intervention is performed only in the presence of a major, chronic, or perhaps terminal illness.

Calm discussion of the purposes and routines of gastrostomy feeding can help keep a gastrostomy from becoming an overwhelming situation. Talking with a person who has had a gastrostomy can also help the patient to accept the expected changes. Adjusting to a change in body image takes time and requires family support and acceptance. Evaluating the existing family support system is necessary. One family member may emerge as the primary support person who will become the major communicator between the patient and health care personnel.

Monitoring and Managing Potential Complications. During the postoperative course the nurse monitors the patient for potential complications. The most frequent complications include wound infection and other wound problems including cellulitis at the wound site and abscesses in the abdominal wall. Because many patients who receive tube feedings are debilitated and have compromised nutritional status, any signs of infections are promptly reported to the physician so that appropriate antibiotic therapy can be instituted.

Gastrointestinal bleeding from the puncture site in the stomach may also occur. The patient's vital signs are monitored closely and all drainage from the operative site, vomitus, and stool are observed for evidence of bleeding. Any signs of bleeding are reported promptly.

Premature removal of the tube, whether it is done by the patient, by the caregiver, or inadvertently, is another complication (Rombeau & Caldwell, 1990). If the tube is removed prematurely, the skin is cleansed and a sterile dressing is applied; the physician is notified immediately.

Patient Education and Home Care Considerations. The nurse assesses the patient's level of knowledge, interest in learning about the tube feeding, and ability to understand and apply the information. Detailed instructions about how to prepare the formula and manage the tube feeding are provided. Standardized references for patients and caregivers are designed to outline the care instructions. To facilitate self-care, the patient is instructed in posthospital care and encouraged to establish as normal a routine as possible. These goals are achieved by teaching the patient about tube feedings and tube and skin care; also, the patient's understanding of the instructions is evaulated based on questioning and return-demonstrations. The patient (and the care-giver in the home setting) must be capable of and responsible for performing care; know the method and frequency with which self-care activities are administered; and have adequate supplies, including the physical, financial, and social resources to maintain care. In addition to individual teaching, the use of printed instruction is necessary as a reinforcement. Adequate supervision and support must be arranged. Home visits by the nurse may be arranged to evaluate the patient's status and to reinforce teaching points.

The demonstration begins by showing the patient how to check for residual gastric content before the feeding. The patient then learns how to determine the patency of the tube by administering water at room temperature before the feeding and afterwards to clear the tube of food particles, which could decompose if allowed to remain in the tube. All feedings are given at room temperature or near body temperature.

For a bolus feeding, the patient is shown how to introduce the liquid into the catheter by using a funnel or the barrel of a syringe. The receptacle is tilted to allow air to escape while the liquid is initially being instilled. As the syringe or barrel fills with liquid, the feeding is allowed to flow into the stomach by gravity by holding the barrel or syringe perpendicular to the abdomen (Fig. 35-9). The rate of flow is regulated by raising or lowering the receptacle to no higher than 45 cm (18 in) above the abdominal wall.

A bolus feeding of 300 to 500 ml usually is given for each meal and requires 10 to 15 minutes to complete. The amount is often determined by the patient's reaction. If the patient feels "full," it may be desirable to give smaller amounts more frequently.

- *Keeping the head of the bed elevated for at least a half hour after feeding facilitates digestion and decreases the risk of aspiration*. Any obstruction requires that the feeding be stopped and the physician notified.

The tube is marked at skin level to provide the patient a baseline for later comparison. The patient is advised to monitor the tube's length and notify the physician or home care nurse if the segment of the tube outside the body becomes shorter or longer. The tube is flushed with 30 ml of water after each bolus or medication administration, and otherwise flushed daily to keep it patent. Each day the irrigation set is cleaned with warm, soapy water and rinsed after each use.

Some patients smell, taste, and chew small amounts of food before taking their tube feedings. This procedure stimulates the flow of salivary and gastric secretions and may

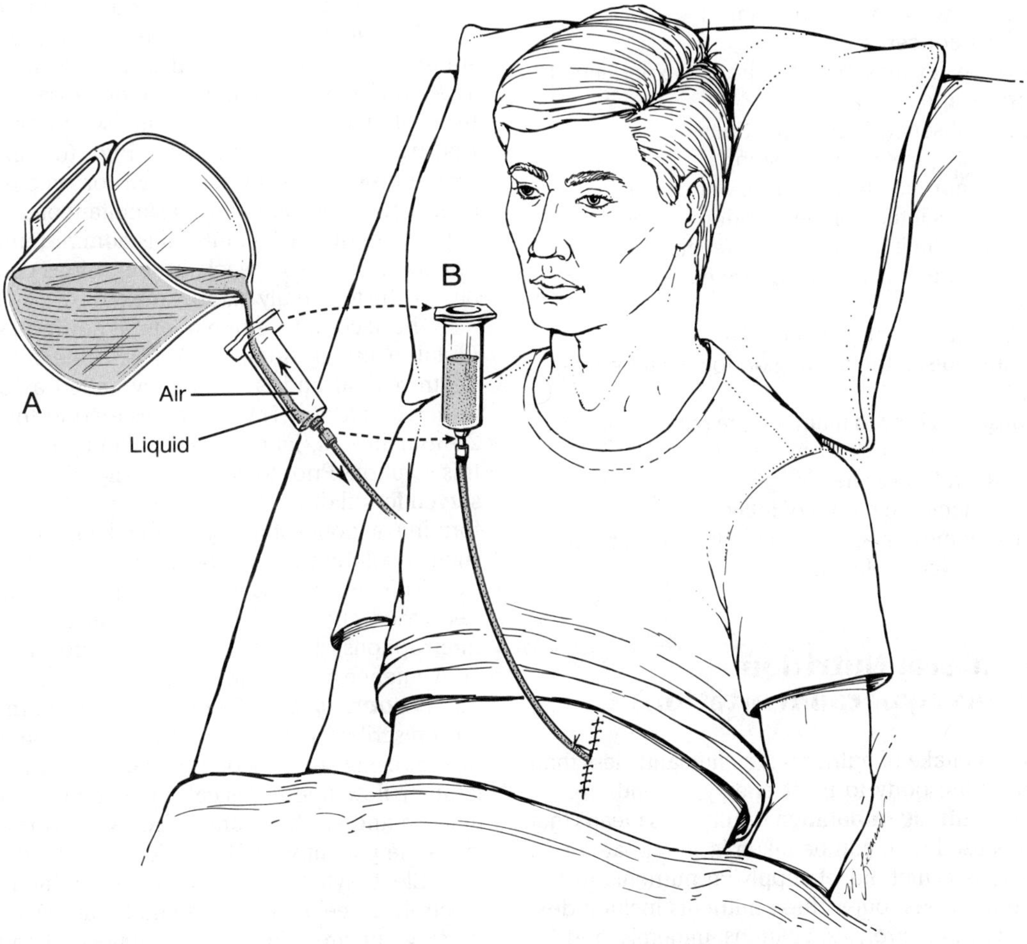

FIGURE 35-9. Gastrostomy feeding by gravity. (**A**) Feeding is instilled at an angle so that air does not enter the stomach. (**B**) Syringe is raised perpendicular to the stomach so that feeding can enter by gravity.

give some sensation of normal eating. The chewed food is then deposited by the patient into a funnel attached to the gastrostomy tube for administration into the stomach, rather than swallowed.

A tube feeding may also be given by intermittent or continuous pressure by a feeding pump. Instruction in the use of the particular pump is essential. Most enteral feeding systems have built-in alarms that signal when the bag is empty, when the battery is low, or if an occlusion is present.

Evaluation

Expected Outcomes

1. Achieves a balanced intake of nutrients
   a. Tolerates quantity and frequency of tube feedings
   b. Has 50 ml or less of residual gastric content before each feeding
   c. Has no diarrhea
   d. Maintains or gains weight
   e. Has normal electrolyte values
2. Is free from infection and skin breakdown
   a. Is afebrile
   b. Has no drainage from the wound
   c. Demonstrates intact skin surrounding the incision
   d. Inspects incision twice a day
3. Adjusts to change in body image
   a. Is able to discuss expected changes
   b. Verbalizes concerns
   c. Asks to speak with someone who has experienced this procedure
4. Experiences absence of complications
   a. Exhibits adequate wound healing
   b. Has no abnormal bleeding from puncture site
   c. Tube remains intact for the duration of therapy
5. Demonstrates skill in managing the feeding regimen
   a. Helps prepare the prescribed formula or blenderized food
   b. Handles equipment competently
   c. Helps administer the feeding or does so independently
   d. Demonstrates how to maintain the patency of the tube
   e. Cleans the tubing as needed
   f. Keeps an accurate record of intake
   g. Is able to remove and reinsert the tube as appropriate and needed for feedings

Total Parenteral Nutrition (Intravenous Hyperalimentation)

When a patient's intake of nutrients is significantly less than that required by the body to meet energy expenditures, a state of **negative nitrogen balance** results. This means that more protein is used than can be taken in. Total parenteral nutrition (TPN) is a method of supplying nutrients to the body by an intravenous route. These nutrients include dextrose, amino acids, electrolytes, vitamins, minerals, and fat emulsions. The goals of TPN are to attain improved nutritional status and weight gain and to enhance the healing process.

Traditional IV fluids do not provide sufficient calories or nitrogen to meet the body's daily requirements. In response, the body begins to convert protein to carbohydrates by the process of gluconeogenesis. TPN solutions, however, provide enough calories and nitrogen to meet the patient's daily nutritional needs. In general, TPN provides 30 to 35 kcal and 1.0 to 1.5 g/kg protein.

The average postoperative adult patient requires approximately 1500 calories a day to keep the body from using its own store of protein. The patient who has conditions such as fever, trauma, burns, major surgery, or hypermetabolic disease may require up to 10,000 additional calories daily. The amount of volume necessary to provide these calories would surpass fluid tolerance and lead to pulmonary edema or congestive heart failure. To provide the required calories in small volume, it is necessary to increase the concentration and to use a route of administration that will rapidly dilute incoming nutrients to the proper levels of body tolerance.

When *hypertonic glucose* is administered, it satisfies caloric requirements and allows amino acids to be released for protein synthesis, rather than being used for energy. Additional potassium is added to provide proper electrolyte balance and to transport glucose and amino acids across cell membranes. To prevent deficiencies and fulfill requirements for tissue synthesis, other elements, such as calcium, phosphorus, magnesium, and sodium chloride, are added.

TPN and TNA. Two types of nutritional intravenous solutions are currently used in clinical practice: TPN and TNA. TPN refers to amino acid-dextrose formulas. Two to three liters of solution are administered over a 24-hour period using a fine bacteria filter. Prior to administration, the TPN infusion must be inspected for precipitate. Fat emulsions (Intralipid) are infused simultaneously with TPN. Usually 500 ml of a 10% emulsion is administered over 6 hours, one to three times a week. Fat emulsions can provide up to 30% of the total daily calorie intake.

The second type of parenteral nutrition solution is TNA (Total Nutrient Admixture). TNA refers to amino acid-dextrose-lipid and is commonly called a "3-in-1" formulation. One liter of TNA is administered to the patient over a 24-hour period. Fine bacteria filters cannot be used with this solution. Prior to administering TNA, the solution is observed for oil droplets that have separated from the solution forming a noticeable layer (cracking of lipid emulsion); such a solution should be discarded. Advantages of TNA over TPN are cost savings in preparation and equipment, decreased chance of contamination with minimal IV line interruptions, less nursing time, and increased patient convenience and satisfaction.

Preparing the Solutions. The pharmacist prepares the prescribed nutritional intravenous solutions. These are mixed, using strict aseptic precautions, under a filtered-air laminar flow hood. Basically, the solution consists of 25% glucose and synthetic amino acids (FreAmine), which provides the patient with 1000 calories and 6 g of nitrogen per liter. Electrolytes are added as determined by the serum electrolyte needs of the patient. Solutions delivered to the nursing unit are refrigerated until needed and then allowed to warm to room temperature. Commercial preparations (Amigen, Aminosol, FreAmine, Hyprotigen C, and others) are available and can be modified to meet individual needs.

Clinical Indications

TPN is indicated for the following patients:

- Those whose intake is insufficient to maintain an anabolic state (*e.g.*, those with severe burns, malnutrition, short-bowel syndrome, AIDS, sepsis, cancer)
- Those who are unable to ingest food orally or by tube (*e.g.*, those with paralytic ileus, Crohn's disease with obstruction, postradiation enteritis, severe hyperemesis gravidarum in pregnancy)
- Those who refuse to ingest adequate nutrients (*e.g.*, patients with anorexia nervosa, postoperative elderly patients)
- Those who should not be fed orally or by tube (*e.g.*, patients with acute pancreatitis or high enterocutaneous fistula)
- Those who need sustained preoperative and postoperative nutritional support (*e.g.*, after bowel surgery)

Criteria that may be used to evaluate a patient's need for total parenteral nutrition include a 10% deficit in body weight; an inability to take oral food or fluids within 7 postoperative days; and hypercatabolic situations, such as major infection with fever.

Management

A nutritional support nurse, nutritionist, or physician determines the patient's need for TPN by evaluating certain criteria: the degree of weight loss, the nitrogen balance, the amount of muscle loss and the total lean body mass, as well as the patient's inability to tolerate ingestion of food through the GI tract. Ideally, the nutritional support nurse, pharmacist, nutritionist, and physician collaborate to determine the specific formula needed.

TPN solutions are initiated slowly and gradually advanced each day to the desired rate and as the patient's fluid and glucose tolerance permits. The patient's response to TPN therapy and lab values are monitored on an ongoing basis by the nutritional support team. Standing orders are initiated for weighing the patient, obtaining complete blood count, platelet count, prothrombin time, electrolytes (SMA-18), magnesium, and fingerstix glucose. In most hospitals, TPN solutions are prescribed by the physician on a daily parenteral nutrition order form. Formulation of the TPN solutions must be carefully calculated to meet the complete individualized needs of the patient.

Methods of Administration

Various methods and routes are used to administer TPN solution in clinical practice: peripheral, central, and atrial. The method depends on the patient's condition and the anticipated length of therapy.

Peripheral. TPN solution is used to supplement oral intake when complete bowel rest is not indicated and nasogastric or nasoenteric suction is not required; it is referred to as partial peripheral nutrition (PPN). PPN is administered by peripheral vein; this is possible because the solution used is less hypertonic than the solution used for TPN. Dextrose concentrations above 10% should not be administered through peripheral veins because they irritate the intima (innermost walls) of small veins. The usual length of therapy for PPN is less than 2 weeks.

Central. Because TPN solutions have five or six times the solute concentration of blood (and exert an osmotic pressure of about 2000 mOsm/l), they are injurious to the intima of peripheral veins. Therefore, to prevent phlebitis and other venous complications, these solutions are administered into the circulatory system through a catheter inserted into a high-flow large blood vessel (often the subclavian vein). Concentrated solutions are then very rapidly diluted to isotonic levels by the blood in this vessel.

Peripherally inserted central (PIC) catheters are used for moderate to long-term intravenous therapy in the hospital or home setting. PIC catheters are inserted by a certified skilled nurse at the bedside. The basilic or cephalic vein is accessed through the antecubital space and tubing is threaded to a designated location depending on the type of solution that is to be infused (superior vena cava for TPN).

Percutaneously placed central venous catheters are also used for moderate to long-term intravenous therapy. These catheters are inserted at the bedside by the physician. The subclavian vein and the internal jugular vein are the two most common vessels used. The subclavian vein is used more frequently than the jugular vein because the area provides a stable insertion site to which the catheter can be anchored, allows the patient freedom of movement, and provides easy access to the dressing site.

Single-, double-, and triple-lumen central venous catheters are available for subclavian lines. To ensure accessibility, it is recommended that a triple-lumen subclavian catheter be used because it offers three ports for various uses (Fig. 35-10). The distal lumen (16-gauge) is used to infuse blood or other viscous fluids and for drawing blood. The 18-gauge middle lumen is reserved for TPN infusion. The proximal port (18-gauge) is used for giving blood, administering medications, and for drawing blood.

If a single-lumen catheter is used, various restrictions apply. Medications cannot be administered through the main catheter because they would mix with the nutritional solution with which they might be incompatible (insulin is an exception). If medications must be given, they must be infused through a peripheral IV line, not by piggyback at the TPN line. Transfusions of blood products also cannot be given through the main line, as red cells may possibly coat the lumen of the catheter, thereby reducing the flow of the nutritional solution.

Atrial. Two devices that are used for long-term home IV therapy are external right atrial catheters and subcutaneous ports. External right atrial catheters can have single or double lumens; two types are the Hickman/Broviac catheter and the Groshong catheter. These catheters are inserted surgically. They are threaded under the skin (reduces risk of ascending infection) to the subclavian vein, and the distal end of the catheter is advanced into the superior vena cava 2 to 3 cm above the junction with the right atrium (see Chapter 16, Fig. 16-4).

The second type of device used for long-term home intravenous therapy is the subcutaneous port. Instead of exiting from the skin (as do the Hickman/Broviac and

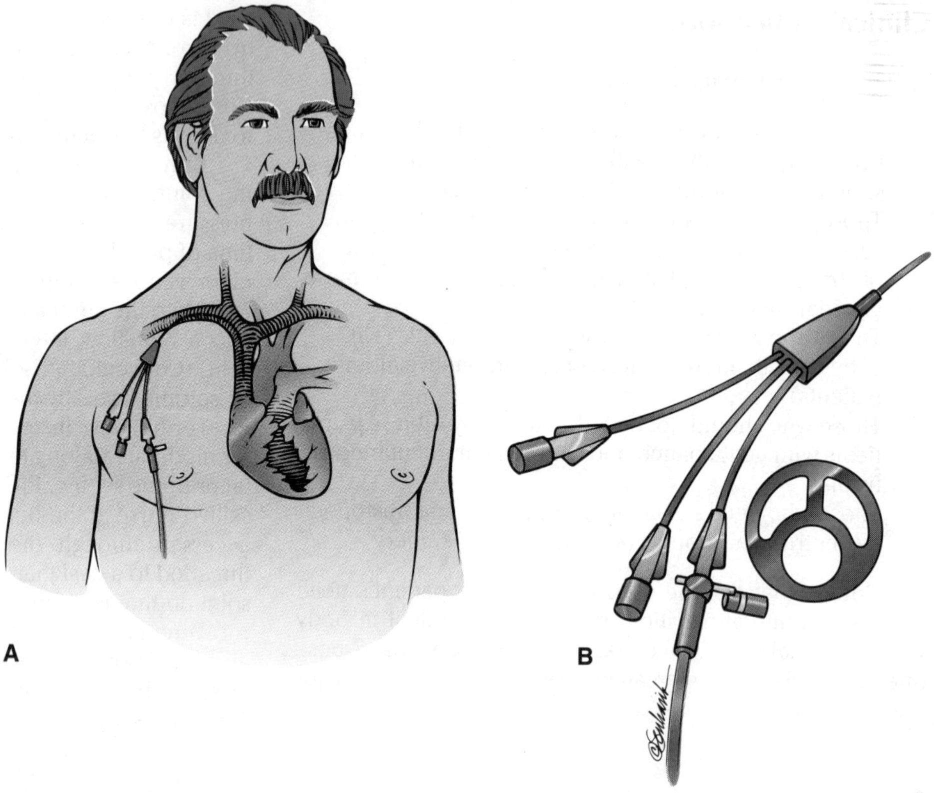

FIGURE 35-10. Subclavian triple lumen catheter used for total parenteral nutrition and other adjunct therapy. (**A**) The catheter is threaded through the subclavian vein and placed in the vena cava. (**B**) Each lumen is an avenue for solution administration; these are secured with Luer-Lok caps when not in use.

Groshong catheters), the end of the catheter is attached to a small chamber that is placed in a subcutaneous pocket either on the anterior chest wall or on the forearm. The subcutaneous port requires minimal care and allows the patient complete freedom of activity. They are more expensive than the external catheters and venous access requires passing a needle (Huber) through the skin into the chamber to initiate IV therapy (see Chapter 16, Fig. 16-5).

Central Venous Catheter Insertion/Subclavian

Patient Preparation. The procedure is explained so that the patient understands the importance of not touching the catheter insertion site and is aware of what to expect during the insertion procedure. To insert the catheter, the patient is placed supine, in head-low position (to produce dilation of neck and shoulder vessels, which makes entry easier and prevents air embolus). The area is shaved, if necessary, and the skin prepared with acetone or alcohol to remove surface oils. Final skin preparation includes scrubbing with tincture of iodine or povidone-iodine solution. To afford maximal accuracy in the placement of the tube, the patient is instructed (1) to turn the head away from the site of venipuncture and (2) to remain motionless while the catheter is inserted and the wound is dressed.

Insertion of the Central Venous Catheter. The preferred route is by way of the subclavian vein, which leads into the superior vena cava. An alternate route to the superior vena cava is through the internal jugular vein. Because an indwelling catheter is a constant source of potential infection, it is recommended that the site be changed every 4 weeks.

Sterile drapes are applied to the upper chest. The patient may be asked to wear a face mask to prevent the spread of microorganisms. Procaine or lidocaine is injected to anesthetize the skin and underlying tissues. The target area is the inferior border at the midpoint of the clavicle. A large-bore needle on a syringe is inserted and moved parallel to and beneath the clavicle until it enters the vein. The syringe is then detached and a radiopaque catheter is inserted through the needle into the vein.

When the catheter is positioned, the needle is withdrawn and the catheter is attached to the intravenous tubing. Until the syringe is detached from the needle and the catheter inserted, the patient may be asked to perform the Valsalva maneuver. (To do this, the patient is instructed to take a deep breath, hold it, and bear down with mouth closed. Compression of the abdomen may also accomplish the maneuver.) The Valsalva maneuver is performed to produce a positive phase in central venous pressure to lessen the possibility of air being drawn into the circulatory system (air embolism). The physician sutures the catheter to the skin to avoid accidental dislodgment.

The catheter insertion site is swabbed with a germicide solution, and antibiotic ointment is applied directly to the insertion site. A gauze or transparent dressing is applied using strict aseptic technique. An isotonic intravenous solution (*e.g.*, D_5W) is administered to keep the vein patent.

The position of the tip of the catheter is checked at this point with x-ray study to confirm its location in the superior vena cava and to rule out a pneumothorax resulting from accidental puncture of the pleura. Once the catheter position is confirmed, the prescribed TPN solution is started. The initial rate of infusion is usually set at 50 ml/hr and gradually increased to the maintenance rate or predetermined dose (100 to 125 ml/hr).

Each lumen of the catheter is secured with Luer-Lok caps and labeled according to location (proximal, middle, distal). To ensure patency, all lumina are flushed with a diluted heparin flush initially and twice a day when not in use, after each intermittent infusion, after blood drawing, and whenever an infusion is disconnected. Force is *never* used to flush the catheter. If resistance is met, the physician is notified; a clot may need to be dissolved with urokinase. If attempts to clear the lumen do not work, the lumen is labeled as "clotted off."

Discontinuing Total Parenteral Nutrition

TPN is discontinued gradually to allow the patient to adjust to decreased levels of glucose. After terminating the TPN solution, isotonic glucose is administered for several hours to protect against rebound hypoglycemia. Oral carbohydrates will shorten tapering time. Specific symptoms of rebound hypoglycemia include weakness, faintness, sweating, shakiness, feeling cold, confusion, and increased heart rate. Once all IV therapy is completed, the nurse may remove the subclavian catheter and apply an occlusive dressing to the exit site.

❑ NURSING PROCESS
The Patient Receiving Total Parenteral Nutrition

Assessment

The nurse assists in identifying a patient who may be a candidate for TPN. Indicators to observe for include any significant weight loss (10% or more of weight when healthy), a decrease in oral food intake for longer than 1 week, any significant sign of protein loss (serum albumin levels below 3.2 g/dl [32 g/L], muscle wasting, decreased tissue healing, or abnormal urea nitrogen excretion), and persistent vomiting and diarrhea. The nurse carefully monitors the patient's hydration, electrolyte balance, and calorie intake.

Diagnosis

Nursing Diagnoses

Based on all the assessment data, the major nursing diagnoses may include the following:

- Altered nutrition, less than body requirements, related to inadequate intake of nutrients
- Risk for infection related to contamination of the catheter site or infusion line
- Risk for fluid volume excess or deficit related to altered infusion rate
- Risk for activity intolerance related to fear that the catheter will become dislodged or occluded.
- Knowledge deficit about home TPN therapy

Collaborative Problems/ Potential Complications

Complications of TPN therapy are commonly classified into four groups:

- Mechanical or technical (catheters, pumps)
- Infectious
- Metabolic (glucose, fluid, electrolyte)
- Nutritional (deficiency or excess)

The most common complications include pneumothorax, air embolism, a clotted or displaced catheter, sepsis, hyperglycemia, rebound hypoglycemia, and fluid overload. These problems and the associated collaborative interventions are described in Table 35-4.

Planning and Implementation

Goals. The major goals for the patient may include attainment of an optimal level of nutrition, absence of infection, maintenance of adequate fluid volume, achievement of an optimal level of activity within individual limitations, knowledge of and skill in self-care, and absence of complications.

Nursing Interventions

Maintaining Optimal Nutrition. A continuous, uniform infusion of TPN solution over a 24-hour period is desired. In some cases, however (*e.g.*, home care patients), cyclic parenteral nutrition may be appropriate. With cyclic total parenteral nutrition there is a set time during a 24-hour period when TPN is infused and a set time when it is not. The time periods for infusion are sufficient to meet the patient's nutritional and pharmacologic needs. Ideally, cyclic TPN is infused over an 8- to 10-hour period during the night.

The patient is weighed two to three times a week at the same time of the day under the same conditions, for accurate comparison. Under the TPN regimen (without additional energy expenditure), a satisfactory weight gain is usually achieved. Accurate intake and output records and fluid balances are kept. A caloric count is kept of any oral nutrients. Trace elements (copper, zinc, chromium, manganese, and selenium) are included in TPN solutions and are individualized for each patient. The TPN solutions are evaluated and ordered daily by the physician on a parenteral nutrition order form according to laboratory values and patient tolerance.

Preventing Infection. Total parenteral nutrition solutions are ideal culture media for bacterial and fungal growth, and central venous catheters provide a port of entry. *Candida albicans* is the most common infectious organism. Other infectious organisms include *Staphylococcus aureus*, *S. epidermidis*, and *Klebsiella pneumoniae*. Therefore, meticulous technique is essential to reduce the risk of infection.

Dressings are changed aseptically, usually two to three times a week and as needed. The patient is placed in low Fowler's position for a dressing change. The nurse and patient may reduce the possibility of airborne contamination by wearing masks during dressing changes. Old dressings are removed carefully to prevent the catheter from becoming dislodged. The area is checked for leakage, kinked catheter, and skin reactions such as inflammation, redness, swelling, tenderness, or purulent drainage. The nurse puts on sterile gloves and cleanses the area with acetone or alcohol swabs, followed by tincture of iodine swabs. Cleaning begins from the center and moves outward. Alcohol may be used in the same manner to remove iodine. Antibiotic ointment is applied to the insertion site if prescribed, and the site is covered with a small dressing, slit to fit around the

TABLE 35-4 Complications of Total Parenteral Nutrition (TPN)

Complication	Cause	Nursing Actions and Collaborative Interventions
Pneumothorax	Improper catheter placement and inadvertent puncture of the pleura	Place in Fowler's position Offer reassurance Monitor vital signs Prepare for thoracentesis or chest tube insertion
Air embolism	Disconnected tubing	Tape all tubing connection sites securely Replace tubing immediately and notify physician
	Cap missing from port	Replace cap and notify physician
	Blocked segment of vascular system	Turn patient on left side and place in the head-low position. Notify physician
Clotted catheter line	Inadequate/infrequent heparin flushes	Administer heparin flush in unused lines twice a day
	Disruption of infusion	Monitor infusion rate hourly and inspect the integrity of the line On *rare* occasions, flush with urokinase as prescribed
Catheter displacement	Excessive movement, possibly with a nonsecured catheter	Stop the infusion and notify the physician
	Separation of tubing and contamination	Tape all tubing connection sites Avoid interrupting the main line or piggybacking other lines
Sepsis	Separation of dressings	Reinforce or change dressing quickly using aseptic technique
	Contaminated solution	Discard. Notify pharmacist
	Infection at insertion site of catheter	Notify physician. Monitor vital signs every 4 hours Change catheter site every 4 weeks
Hyperglycemia	Glucose intolerance	Monitor glucose levels (blood and urine) Monitor urine output Observe for stupor, confusion, lethargy. Notify physician; the addition of insulin to the TPN solution may be prescribed.
Fluid overload	Fluid infusing rapidly	Decrease infusion rate Monitor vital signs Notify physician Treat respiratory distress by sitting patient upright and administering oxygen as needed, if prescribed
Rebound hypoglycemia	Feedings stopped too abruptly	Monitor for symptoms (weakness, tremors, diaphoresis, headache, hunger, and apprehension); notify physician if necessary Gradually wean patient from TPN

catheter. A gauze pad or transparent dressing is centered over the area.

The advantages of using a transparent dressing over the gauze pad are that it allows for frequent examination of the catheter site, adheres well, and is more comfortable for the patient. When the IV tubing extension is changed, it is replaced quickly to prevent buildup of organisms along the lumen of the tubing. The union of the catheter and tubing is then covered and secured with adhesive tape to prevent separation and exposure to air. Main-line IV tubing and filters are changed every 24 hours, and all connections are taped securely to avoid breaks in the integrity of the system. The dressing and tubing are labeled with the date, time of dressing change, and the initials of the person carrying out the procedure.

If the patient has a draining wound, such as a tracheostomy, in the nearby area, additional precautions are taken to keep the wound dry by applying transparent plastic operating room adhesive drape over the dressings, to ensure waterproofing. Hypoallergenic adhesive tape can be used if the patient complains of itching from conventional tape. The dressing change is documented, and the condition of the area and the patient's reaction are reported.

Maintaining Adequate Fluid Volume Balance. An infusion pump is recommended for TPN to maintain an accurate prescribed rate. Rates are set at a designated rate of milliliters per hour. The rate is checked every half hour to 1 hour; an alarm signals a problem. The infusion rate cannot be increased or decreased to compensate for fluids that are infusing too quickly or too slowly. If the IV runs out, 10% dextrose and water is infused until the next TPN container is available from the pharmacy.

If the rate is too rapid, hyperosmolar diuresis occurs (excess sugar will be excreted), which if severe enough may cause intractable seizures, coma, and death. Symptoms of rapid hypertonic fluid intake include headache, nausea, fever, chills, and increasing lassitude.

If the flow rate is too slow, the patient does not get the maximal benefit of calories and nitrogen.

Intake and output are recorded every 8 hours so that fluid imbalance can be readily detected. The patient is weighed two to three times a week; in ideal situations, the patient will show neither weight loss nor significant weight gain. The nurse assesses for signs of dehydration (thirst, decreased skin turgor, lowered central venous pressure reading) and reports these findings to the physician immediately. It is essential to monitor blood glucose status because hyperglycemia can cause diuresis and excessive fluid loss.

Encouraging Activity. Activities and ambulation are encouraged when the patient is physically capable. With a plastic catheter in the subclavian vein, the patient is free to move the extremities and should be encouraged to maintain good muscle tone. The teaching and exercise program initiated in the occupational and physical therapy departments should be reinforced.

Patient Education and Home Care Considerations. Successful home TPN requires teaching the patient and family specialized skills by means of an intensive training program and follow-up supervision in the home. This is accomplished through a team effort. The financial costs of such programs, though high, are less than those incurred in a hospital. Initiation of a home program may be the only way the patient can be discharged from the hospital. Grant (1992) identifies ideal candidates for home TPN as those who have intestinal failure, have a reasonable life expectancy following transfer into the home, suffer from no other or a limited number of other medical illnesses (it is particularly important that the patient not be suffering from failure of major organ systems), and are highly motivated and fairly self-sufficient. In addition, ability to learn, availability of family interest and support, adequate finances, and the physical plan of the home are factors that must be assessed when the decision for home TPN is made. Institutions sponsoring home TPN programs have developed teaching brochures for every aspect of the treatment, including catheter and dressing care, use of an infusion pump, administration of fat emulsions, and instillation of heparin flushes.

The nurse should be aware that the average patient needs about 2 weeks of instruction and reinforcement. Additional time will be needed from a nutritional support nurse or pharmacist for patients who are going to mix their own solutions at home instead of using a premixed solution obtained from a pharmacy or commercial supplier.

Managing TPN. A home care teaching program prepares the patient to manage the appropriate form of TPN. The patient is taught how to store solutions, set up the infusion, flush the line with heparin, change the dressings, and troubleshoot for complications. The most frequent complication is infection. The nurse emphasizes handwashing and strict asepsis in handling equipment, changing the dressing, and preparing the solution.

Managing Mechanical Difficulties. Mechanical problems usually arise from technical complications found within the infusion pump or catheter site. The patient is taught how to troubleshoot for catheter problems (leakage, loose cap, tear in the tubing, blood clot) and is given a list of directions explaining what to do for each problem. Malfunctioning pumps usually can be replaced in 24 hours.

Recognizing Metabolic Complications. The patient is given a list of symptoms indicative of metabolic complications (neuropathies, mentation changes, diarrhea, nausea, skin changes, urine output) and directed to contact the home health care nurse or physician if any of these complications occurs. The patient is instructed to have weekly serum chemistry and hematology monitoring and to check the urine glucose level every day.

Psychosocial Support. The psychosocial aspects of home parenteral nutrition are as important as the physiologic and technical concerns. These patients must cope with the loss of eating and the changes in lifestyle brought on by sleep disturbances (frequent urination during infusions, usually two to three times during the night). Major psychosocial reactions include depression, anger, withdrawal, anxiety, and altered self-image. A successful home parenteral nutrition program depends on motivation, emotional stability, and technical competence. Support groups are also available in the community to help patients and families cope with the transition and to minimize disruption of the patient's lifestyle.

Evaluation

Expected Outcomes

1. Attains or maintains nutritional balance
2. Is infection free
   a. Is afebrile
   b. Has no purulent drainage from the catheter insertion site
   c. IV line integrity is maintained
3. Is hydrated as evidenced by good skin turgor
4. Achieves an optimal level of activity within self-limitations
5. Demonstrates skill in managing TPN regimen
6. Experiences absence of complications
   a. Catheter and equipment function properly
   b. Has no symptoms of sepsis or infection
   c. Metabolic balance is maintained within normal limits
   d. Nutritional status improves and stabilizes

REFERENCES AND SELECTED READINGS

Books

Fischer FE (ed). Total Parenteral Nutrition, 2nd ed. Boston, Little, Brown and Company, 1991.

Grant JP. Handbook of Total Parenteral Nutrition, 2nd ed. Philadelphia, WB Saunders, 1992.

CRITICAL THINKING EXERCISES

1. You are caring for a patient who has a nasogastric feeding tube. Before administering the medications, you must confirm that the tube is placed correctly. Based on research findings, how will you check to make sure that the tube is properly placed?
2. A patient who is receiving nasogastric tube feedings begins to have diarrhea. Explain what you think might be causing the diarrhea, and describe the assessment data that will be important in determining its possible causes and ways to control it.
3. When conducting a home visit of a patient who is receiving nightly 10-hour parenteral nutrition feedings, you find that the patient is experiencing chills, diarrhea, and a fever of 100°F. The patient's sister states that the previous evening's feeding solution looked "funny" and that she sped up the rate of the feeding so it would finish early. Analyze this situation and determine the actions you would take, explaining the reasoning behind your decision.

Rombeau JL and Caldwell MD. Clinical Nutrition Enteral and Tube Feeding, 2nd ed. Philadelphia, WB Saunders, 1990.

Schaik TV. Gastroenterology Nursing: A Core Curriculum. St Louis, Mosby-Year Book, 1993.

Spiro HM. Clinical Gastroenterology, 4th ed. New York, McGraw-Hill, 1993.

Zeman FJ. Clinical Nutrition and Dietetics, 2nd ed. New York, Macmillan, 1991.

Journals

Asterisks indicate nursing research articles.

Nasogastric and Nasoenteric Intubation and Feeding

Ackerman MH et al. Current trends in enteral feeding. Gastroenterology Nursing 1992 April; 14(5):233–236.

Bockus S. Trouble shooting your tube feedings. Am J Nurs 1991 May; 91(5):24–28.

Boyles RJ and Kruse JA. Nasogastric and nasoenteric intubation. Critical Care Clinics 1992 Oct; 8(4):865–878.

Camp D and Otten N. How to insert and remove nasogastric tubes quickly and easily. Nursing 1990 Sept; 20(9):59–64.

Davis AE et al. Preventing feeding-associated aspiration. Medsurg Nurs 1995 Apr; 4(2):141–145.

*Eisenberg P et al. Nasoenteral feeding-tube properties and the ability to withdraw fluid via syringe. Appl Nurs Res 1989 Nov; 2(4):168–172.

*Heather DJ. Effect of bulk-forming cathartic on diarrhea in tube-fed patients. Heart Lung 1991 July; 20(4):409–413.

Kohn CL and Keithley JK. Enteral nutrition. Potential complications and patient monitoring. Nurs Clin N Am 1989 June; 24(2):339-353.

Martyn-Nemeth P and Fitzgerald K. Tube feeding in the elderly. Journal of Gerontological Nursing 1992 Feb; 18(2):30–36.

Meehan M. Nursing dx: potential for aspiration. RN 1992 Jan; 55(1):30–34.

*Metheny N. Measures to test placement of nasogastric feeding tubes: A review. Nurs Res 1988 Nov/Dec; 37(6):324–329.

*Metheny N et al. How to aspirate fluid from small-bore feeding tubes. Am J Nurs 1993 May; 93(5):86–88.

*Metheny N et al. Detection of inadvertent respiratory placement of small-bore feeding tubes: A report of 10 cases. Heart Lung 1990a Nov; 19(6):631–638.

*Metheny N et al. Effectiveness of the auscultatory method in predicting feeding tube location. Nurs Res 1990b Sept/Oct; 39(5):262–267.

*Metheny N et al. Effect of feeding tube properties and three irrigants on clogging rates. Nurs Res 1988 May/June; 37(3):165–169.

*Metheny N et al. Aspiration pneumonia in patients fed through nasoenteral tubes. Heart Lung 1986 May; 15(3):256-261.

*Oie S et al. Microbial contamination of enteral feeding solution and its prevention. Am J Infect Control 1992 Aug; 20(4): 202–295.

*Sands JA. Incidence of pulmonary aspiration in intubated patients receiving enteral nutrition through wide and narrow bore nasogastric feeding tubes. Heart Lung 1991 Jan; 20(1): 75–80.

Surrant S. Troubleshooting a sump tube. AJN 1993 Jan; 93(1):42–47.

*Wilson DM. Ethical concerns in a long-term tube feeding study. IMAGE: Journal of Nursing Scholarship 1992 Fall; 24(3): 195–199.

*Wilson MF and Haynes-Johnson V. Cranberry juice or water? A comparison of feeding tube irrigant. Nutr Supp Serv 1987 Jul; 7(7):23–24.

Wurzbach ME. The dilemma of withholding or withdrawing nutrition. Image: Journal of Nursing Scholarship 1990 Winter; 22(4):226–230.

Young CK and White S. Preparing patients for tube feeding at home. Am J Nurs 1992 April; 92(4):46–53.

Gastrostomies

Barnie DC. Percutaneous endoscopic gastrostomy tubes: The nurse's role in a moral, ethical, and legal dilemmas. Gastroenterology Nursing 1990 Spring; 12(4):250–254.

Beck ML. Percutaneous endoscopic gastrostomy. Nursing 1989 April; 19(4):76–77.

Davis B. Effective and inexpensive management of a PEG tube. Ostomy/Wound Management 1989 Fall; 24:62–65.

McConnell EA. Administering a bolus gastrostomy feeding. Nursing 1990 Nov; 20(11):102.

Noble AC. Going home with a percutaneous endoscopic gastrostomy: A reference for patients and care givers. Gastroenterology Nursing 1992 Oct; 15(2):90–91.

Ricciardi E and Brown D. Managing PEG tubes. Am J Nurs 1994 Oct; 94(10):29–31.

Total Parenteral Nutrition

ASPEN Board of Directors. Guidelines for the use of parenteral and enteral nutrition in adult and pediatric patients. J Parenteral Enteral Nutr 1993 July–Aug:17(4)(Supplement).

*Capka MB. Nursing observations of central venous catheters. Journal of Intravenous Nursing 1991 July/Aug; 14(4):243–246.

Geels W and Bowens B. Nutrition that's "3 in 1." Nursing 1989 April; 19(4):78.

Holder C and Alexander J. A new and improved guide to IV therapy. Am J Nurs 1990 Feb; 90(2):43–47.

Lin EM. Nutrition support. Making the difficult decisions. Cancer Nursing 1991; 14(5):261-269.

Murray EW. Probing the safety of central venous catheters. Am J Nurs 1993 May; 93(5):72–76.

Rountree D. The PIC catheter: A different approach. Am J Nurs 1991 Aug; 91(8):22–28.
Worthington PH and Wagner BA. Total parenteral nutrition. Nurs Clin North Am 1989 June; 24(2):355–369.
Wroblewski B and Young LE. Topics in parenteral nutrition for the 1990s. Focus on Critical Care 1991 April; 19(4):278–285.

INFORMATION/RESOURCES

Agencies

Society of Gastroenterology Nurses & Associates, Inc.
1070 Sibley Towers,
Rochester, NY 14604

American Cancer Society
1599 Clifton Road NE,
Atlanta, GA, 30329

American Institute of Nutrition
9650 Rockville Pike,
Bethesda, MD 20014

American Society for Gastrointestinal Endoscopy
PO Box 1565, 13 Elm St,
Manchester, MA 01944

Nutrition Institute of America
200 W 86th St, Ste 17A,
New York, NY 10024

American Society of Parenteral and Enteral Nutrition
8630 Fenton Street, Suite 412,
Silver Spring, Maryland 20910-3805

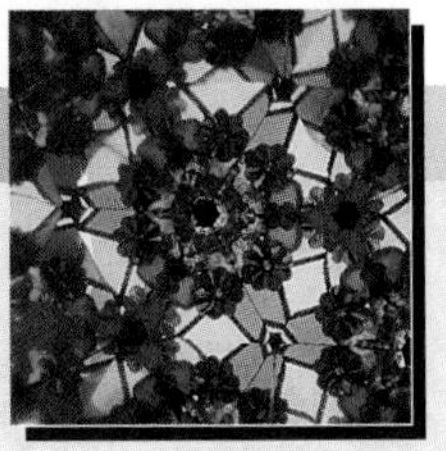

36

Management of Patients With Gastric and Duodenal Disorders

CHAPTER OUTLINE

Gastritis
Acute Gastritis
Chronic Gastritis
Management
NURSING PROCESS: The Patient With Gastritis
Peptic Ulcer
Etiology and Incidence
Pathophysiology
Clinical Manifestations
Diagnostic Evaluation
Management
Surgical Intervention
Managing Other Ulcer Conditions
NURSING PROCESS: The Patient With a Peptic Ulcer
Morbid Obesity
Surgical Management
Gastric Cancer
Clinical Manifestations
Diagnostic Evaluation
Management
NURSING PROCESS: The Patient With Gastric Cancer
Gastric Surgery
NURSING PROCESS: The Patient Undergoing Gastric Surgery
Critical Thinking Exercises

LEARNING OBJECTIVES

On completion of this chapter, the learner will be able to:

1. Compare the etiology, clinical manifestations, and management of acute gastritis, chronic gastritis, and peptic ulcer
2. Use the nursing process as a framework for care of patients with gastritis
3. Use the nursing process as a framework for care of patients with peptic ulcer
4. Describe the dietary, pharmacologic, and surgical treatment of peptic ulcer
5. Describe the nursing management of patients who undergo surgical procedures to treat obesity
6. Use the nursing process as a framework for care of patients with gastric cancer
7. Use the nursing process as a framework for care of patients undergoing gastric surgery
8. Identify the complications of gastric surgery and their prevention and management
9. Describe the home health care needs of the patient who has had gastric surgery

Gastritis

Acute Gastritis

Gastritis (inflammation of the stomach mucosa) is most often due to dietary indiscretion. The person eats too much or too rapidly or eats food that is too highly seasoned or contaminated with disease-causing microorganisms. Other causes of acute gastritis include alcohol, aspirin, bile reflux, or radiation therapy.

A more severe form of acute gastritis is caused by the ingestion of strong acids or alkalies, which may cause the mucosa to become gangrenous or to perforate. Scarring can occur, resulting in pyloric obstruction. Gastritis also may be the first sign of an acute systemic infection.

Pathophysiology and Clinical Manifestations. The gastric mucous membrane becomes edematous and hyperemic (congested with tissue, fluid, and blood) and undergoes superficial erosion; it secretes a scanty amount of gastric juice, containing very little acid but much mucus. Superficial ulceration may occur and can lead to hemorrhage. The patient may have abdominal discomfort, with headache, lassitude, nausea, and anorexia, often accompanied by vomiting and hiccuping. Some patients, however, are asymptomatic.

The gastric mucosa is capable of repairing itself after a bout of gastritis. Occasionally, hemorrhage may require surgical intervention. If the irritating food is not vomited but reaches the bowel, colic and diarrhea may result. As a rule, the patient recovers in about a day, although the appetite may be diminished for an additional 2 or 3 days.

Chronic Gastritis

Prolonged inflammation of the stomach may be caused by either benign or malignant ulcers of the stomach, or by the bacteria *Helicobacter pylori* (*H. pylori*).

Pathophysiology. Chronic gastritis may be classified as type A or type B. Type A (often referred to as *autoimmune gastritis*) results from parietal cell changes, leading to atrophy and cellular infiltration. It is associated with autoimmune diseases such as pernicious anemia and occurs in the fundus or body of the stomach. Type B (sometimes referred to as *H. pylori* gastritis) affects the antrum and pylorus (lower end of the stomach near the duodenum). It is associated with the *H. pylori* bacteria; dietary factors such as hot drinks or spices; use of drugs and alcohol; smoking; or reflux of intestinal contents into the stomach.

Clinical Manifestations. The patient with type A gastritis is essentially asymptomatic except for symptoms of vitamin B_{12} deficiency (see Chapter 32). In type B gastritis, the patient may complain of anorexia (poor appetite), heartburn after eating, belching, sour taste in the mouth, or nausea and vomiting.

Diagnostic Evaluation. Type A gastritis is associated with achlorhydria or hypochlorhydria (absence or low levels of hydrochloric acid), whereas type B gastritis is associated with hyperchlorhydria (high levels of hydrochloric acid). Diagnosis can be determined by endoscopy, upper gastrointestinal (GI) x-ray series, and histologic examination. Diagnostic measures for detecting *H. pylori* include serologic testing for antibodies for the *H. pylori* antigen and a breath test.

Management

Acute gastritis is managed by instructing the patient to refrain from alcohol and food until symptoms subside. When the patient is able to take nourishment by mouth, a nonirritating diet is recommended. If the symptoms persist, fluids may need to be administered parenterally. If bleeding is present, management is similar to the procedures used for upper gastrointestinal tract hemorrhage (see p. 895). If gastritis is due to ingestion of strong acids or alkalies, treatment consists of diluting and neutralizing the offending agent.

- To neutralize acids, common antacids (*e.g.*, aluminum hydroxide) are used; to neutralize an alkali, diluted lemon juice or diluted vinegar is used.
- If corrosion is extensive or severe, emetics and lavage are avoided because of the danger of perforation.

Therapy is supportive and may include nasogastric intubation, analgesics and sedatives, antacids, and intravenous fluids. Fiberoptic endoscopy may be necessary. Emergency surgery may be required to remove gangrenous or perforated tissue. Gastrojejunostomy or gastric resection may be necessary to treat pyloric obstruction.

Chronic gastritis is managed by modifying the patient's diet, promoting rest, reducing stress, and initiating pharmacotherapy. *H. pylori* may be treated with antibiotics (such as tetracycline or amoxicillin) and bismuth salts (Pepto-Bismol). Patients with type A gastritis usually have evidence of malabsorption of vitamin B_{12} caused by the presence of antibodies against intrinsic factor.

❑ NURSING PROCESS
The Patient With Gastritis

Assessment

During the history, the nurse asks about the patient's presenting signs and symptoms. Does the patient experience heartburn, indigestion, nausea, or vomiting? Do the symptoms occur at any specific time of the day, before or after meals, after ingesting spicy or irritating foods, or after the ingestion of certain drugs or alcohol? Are the symptoms related to anxiety, stress, allergies, eating or drinking too much, or eating too quickly? How are the symptoms relieved? Is there a history of previous gastric disease or surgery? A diet history plus a 72-hour diet recall is helpful. A thorough history is important in that it helps the nurse to identify whether known dietary excesses or other indiscretions are associated with the current symptoms, whether others in the patient's environment have similar symptoms, whether the patient is vomiting blood, and whether any known caustic element has been swallowed.

Signs to note during the physical examination include abdominal tenderness, dehydration (altered skin turgor, dry mucous membranes), and evidence of any systemic disorder that might be responsible for the symptoms of gastritis.

The length of time that the current symptoms last and any methods used by the patient to treat these symptoms, and their effects, are also identified.

Diagnosis

Nursing Diagnoses

Based on all the assessment data, the patient's major nursing diagnoses may include the following:

- Anxiety related to treatment
- Altered nutrition, less than body requirements, related to inadequate intake of nutrients
- Risk for fluid volume deficit related to insufficient fluid intake and excessive fluid loss subsequent to vomiting
- Knowledge deficit about dietary management and disease process
- Pain related to irritated stomach mucosa

Planning and Implementation

Goals. The major goals of the patient may be to reduce anxiety, avoid irritating foods and assure adequate intake of nutrients, maintain fluid balance, increase awareness of dietary management, and relieve pain.

Nursing Interventions

Reducing Anxiety. If the patient has ingested acids or alkalies, emergency measures may be needed. Supportive therapy is offered to the patient and family during treatment and after the ingested acid or alkali has been neutralized or diluted. The patient may need to be prepared for additional diagnostic studies (endoscopy) or surgery. Anxiety about the pain and treatment modalities is usually present as well as fear of permanent damage to the esophagus. The nurse uses a calm approach to assess the patient and answer all questions as completely as possible. All procedures and treatments are explained according to the patient's interest and level of understanding.

Promoting Nutrition. For acute gastritis, physical and emotional support is provided and the patient is helped to deal with the symptoms, which may include nausea, vomiting, heartburn, and fatigue. Foods and fluids are not permitted by mouth for hours or days until the acute symptoms subside. If intravenous therapy is necessary, it is monitored regularly, as are serum electrolyte values. When the symptoms subside, the patient is offered ice chips followed by clear liquids. Solid food is introduced as soon as possible to provide oral nutrition, decrease the need for intravenous therapy, and minimize irritation to the gastric mucosa. As food is introduced, any symptoms suggesting a repeat episode of gastritis are evaluated and reported.

The intake of caffeinated beverages is discouraged because caffeine is a central nervous system stimulant that increases gastric activity and pepsin secretion. The use of alcohol is also discouraged, as is cigarette smoking because nicotine reduces the secretion of pancreatic bicarbonate and thus inhibits the neutralization of gastric acid in the duodenum. Nicotine also increases parasympathetic stimulation, which increases muscular activity in the bowel and can lead to nausea and vomiting.

Promoting Fluid Balance. Daily fluid intake and output are monitored to detect early signs of dehydration (minimal urine output of 30 ml/hr, minimal intake of 1.5 L/d). If food and fluids are withheld, intravenous fluids (3 L/d) are usually prescribed. Fluid intake plus caloric value is measured (1 L 5% dextrose in water = 170 calories of carbohydrate). Electrolyte values (sodium, potassium, chloride) may be assessed every 24 hours to detect early indicators of imbalance.

The nurse must always be alert for any indicators of hemorrhagic gastritis: hematemesis (vomiting of blood), tachycardia, and hypotension. If these occur, the physician is alerted, vital signs are monitored as the patient's condition warrants, and the guidelines for managing upper GI tract bleeding are followed (see p. 895).

Relieving Pain. The patient is instructed to avoid foods and beverages that may be irritating to the gastric mucosa (see above). The nurse assesses the patient's level of pain and the extent of comfort attained from the use of medications and avoidance of irritating substances.

Patient Education and Home Care Considerations. The patient's knowledge about gastritis is evaluated so that a teaching plan can be individualized. A diet is prescribed that takes into account the patient's daily caloric needs, food preferences, and pattern of eating.

The patient is given a list of substances to avoid (*e.g.*, caffeine; nicotine; spicy, irritating, or highly seasoned foods; alcohol). Antibiotics, bismuth salts, medications to decrease gastric secretion, and medications to protect mucosal cells from gastric secretion are administered as prescribed. Patients with pernicious anemia are given instructions about the need for long-term vitamin B_{12} injections.

Evaluation

Expected Outcomes

1. Exhibits less anxiety
2. Avoids eating irritating foods or drinking caffeinated beverages or alcohol
3. Maintains fluid balance
   a. Tolerates intravenous therapy of at least 1.5 L daily
   b. Drinks 6 to 8 glasses of water daily
   c. Has a urinary output of about 1 L daily
   d. Displays adequate skin turgor
4. Adheres to medical regimen
   a. Selects nonirritating foods and beverages
   b. Takes medications as prescribed
5. Reports less pain

Peptic Ulcer

A peptic ulcer is an excavation (hollowed-out area) formed in the mucosal wall of the stomach, the pylorus, the duodenum, or the esophagus (Fig. 36-1). A peptic ulcer is frequently referred to as a *gastric, duodenal,* or *esophageal ulcer*, depending on its location. It is caused by the erosion of a circumscribed area of mucous membrane. This erosion may extend as deeply as the muscle layers or through the muscle to the peritoneum. Peptic ulcers are more likely to be in the duodenum than in the stomach. As a rule, they occur singularly, but they may occur in multiples. Chronic

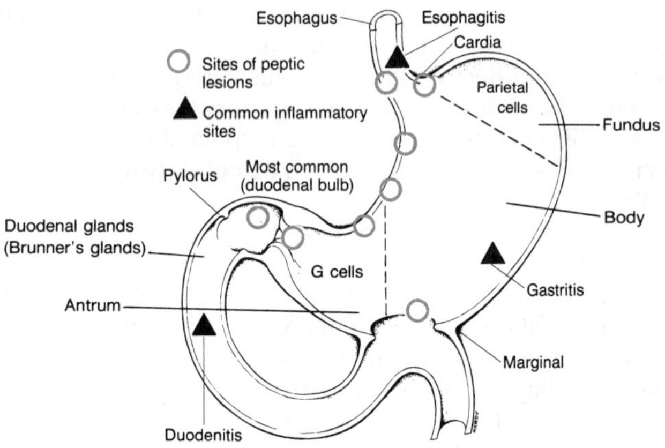

FIGURE 36-1. Peptic lesions may occur in the esophagus (esophagitis), stomach (gastritis), or duodenum (duodenitis). Note peptic ulcer sites and common inflammatory sites. Hydrochloric acid is formed by parietal cells in the fundus; gastrin is secreted by G cells in the antrum. The duodenal glands secrete an alkaline mucous solution.

gastric ulcers tend to occur in the lesser curvature of the stomach, near the pylorus. See Table 36-1 for a comparison of the features of gastric and duodenal ulcers.

Zollinger–Ellison syndrome is often considered a type of peptic ulceration. Stress ulcers, which are clinically different from peptic ulcers, are ulcerations in the mucosa that can occur in the gastroduodenal area. Both of these conditions will be addressed with peptic ulcers.

Etiology and Incidence

The etiology of peptic ulcers is poorly understood, although the gram negative bacteria *H. pylori* has been strongly implicated as a causative factor. It is known that peptic ulcers occur only in the areas of the GI tract that are exposed to hydrochloric acid and pepsin. The disease occurs with the greatest frequency in persons between the ages of 40 and 60 years but is relatively uncommon in women of childbearing age, although it has been observed in children and even in infants. Men are affected three times more often than women, but there is some evidence that the incidence in women is increasing. After menopause, the incidence of peptic ulcers in women is almost equal to that in men. Peptic ulcers in the body of the stomach can occur without excessive acid secretion.

It is estimated that 5% to 15% of the population in the United States have ulcers, but only about half of these are recognized. The incidence has declined by 50% over the past 20 years. Duodenal ulcers are 5 to 10 times more common than gastric ulcers.

Predisposition. Attempts are still made to delineate the "ulcer personality." Some claim that stress or anger, with no opportunity to express hostility, is a predisposing factor. Ulcers do seem to develop in persons who are emotionally tense, but whether this is a contributing factor to the condition is uncertain. Familial tendency also appears as a significant predisposing factor. A further hereditary link is noted in the finding that persons with blood type O are more susceptible than persons with blood type A, B, or AB.

TABLE 36-1 Comparison of Duodenal and Gastric Ulcer

Duodenal Ulcer	Gastric Ulcer
Incidence	**Incidence**
Age 30–60	Usually 50 and over
Male:female 3:1	Male:female 2:1
Occurs more frequently than gastric ulcers	
Signs and Symptoms/Clinical Findings	**Signs and Symptoms/Clinical Findings**
Hypersecretion of stomach acid	Normal to hyposecretion of stomach acid
May have weight gain	Weight loss may occur
Pain occurs 2–3 hours after a meal; often awakened between 1 and 2 am	Pain occurs ½ to 1 hour after a meal; rarely occurs at night; may be relieved by vomiting
Ingestion of food relieves pain	Ingestion of food does not help and sometimes increases pain
Vomiting is uncommon	Vomiting is common
Hemorrhage is less likely than with gastric ulcers; but, if present melena more common than hematemesis	Hemorrhage is more likely to occur than with duodenal ulcer, hematemesis more common than melena
More likely to perforate than gastric ulcers	
Malignancy Possibility	**Malignancy Possibility**
Rare	Occasionally
Risk Factors	**Risk Factors**
Blood group O, COPD, chronic renal failure, alcohol, smoking, cirrhosis, stress	Gastritis, alcohol, smoking, NSAID, stress

Other predisposing factors associated with peptic ulcer include chronic use of nonsteroidal anti-inflammatory drugs (NSAIDs), alcohol ingestion, and excessive smoking. Recent research suggests that gastric ulcers may be associated with bacterial infection with agents such as *H. pylori.* The presence of this bacteria increases with age. Rarely, ulcers are due to excessive amounts of the hormone gastrin, produced by tumors (gastrinomas—Zollinger-Ellison syndrome). Stress ulcers may also occur in patients exposed to stressful conditions.

Pathophysiology

Peptic ulcer occurs mainly in the gastroduodenal mucosa because this tissue is unable to withstand the digestive action of gastric acid (hydrochloric acid) and pepsin. The erosion is due to an increase in concentration or activity of acid-pepsin, or to a decrease in the normal resistance of the mucosa. A damaged mucosa is unable to secrete enough mucus to act as a barrier against hydrochloric acid.

Gastric Secretion. Gastric secretion occurs in three concurrent phases: (1) cephalic, (2) gastric, and (3) intestinal. Because these phases are interactive and not independent of one another, a disturbance in any one phase may be ulcerogenic.

Cephalic (Psychic) Phase. The first phase is initiated by stimuli such as the sight, smell, or taste of food acting on cerebral cortical receptors that, in turn, stimulate the vagal nerves. Essentially, an unappetizing meal has little effect on gastric secretion, whereas a tastier, more appealing meal evokes high secretion. This accounts for the traditional emphasis on serving a bland meal to the patient with a peptic ulcer. Today many gastroenterologists agree that the bland diet has no significant effect on gastric acidity or ulcer healing. However, excessive vagal activity during the night when the stomach is empty, is a significant irritant.

Gastric Phase. In the gastric phase, gastric acid is released as a result of chemical and mechanical stimulation of receptors in the wall of the stomach. The vagal reflex causes acid secretion in response to stomach distention by food.

Intestinal Phase. Food in the small intestine causes the release of a hormone (thought to be gastrin), which in turn stimulates the secretion of gastric acid.

Gastric Mucosal Barrier. In humans, gastric secretion is a mixture of mucopolysaccharides and mucoproteins secreted continuously by the mucosal glands. This mucus adsorbs pepsin and protects the mucosa against acid. Hydrochloric acid is secreted continuously, but secretions increase because of neurogenic and hormonal mechanisms that are initiated by gastric and intestinal stimuli. If hydrochloric acid were not buffered and neutralized, and if the outer layer of mucosa did not offer protection, hydrochloric acid, along with pepsin, would destroy the stomach. Hydrochloric acid comes into contact with only a small portion of the gastric mucosal surface; it diffuses into it very slowly. This impenetrability of the mucosa is called the **gastric mucosal barrier.** It is the stomach's chief defense against being digested by its own secretions. Other factors that influence mucosal resistance are blood supply, acid–base balance, integrity of the mucosal cells, and epithelial regeneration.

Therefore, a person is likely to develop a peptic ulcer from one of two causes: (1) hypersecretion of acid–pepsin and (2) a weakened gastric mucosal barrier. Anything that decreases the production of gastric mucus or damages gastric mucosa is ulcerogenic; salicylates and other nonsteroidal anti-inflammatory drugs, alcohol, and anti-inflammatory drugs fall into this category.

Zollinger–Ellison Syndrome (Gastrinoma). Zollinger–Ellison syndrome is suspected when a patient presents with several peptic ulcers or ulcers that are resistant to standard medical therapy. It is identified by the following findings: hypersecretion of gastric juice, duodenal ulcers, and gastrinomas (islet cell tumors) in the pancreas. Ninety percent of tumors are found in the "gastric triangle," which encompasses the cystic and common bile ducts, the second and third portions of the duodenum, and the neck and body of the pancreas. Approximately one third of gastrinomas are malignant.

Diarrhea and steatorrhea (unabsorbed fat in the stool) may be evident. These patients may have coexistent parathyroid adenomas or hyperplasia and may therefore exhibit signs of hypercalcemia. The patient's most frequent complaint is epigastric pain.

Stress Ulcer. Stress ulcer is the term given to acute mucosal ulceration of the duodenal or gastric area that occurs following physiologically stressful events. Stressful conditions such as burns, shock, severe sepsis, and multiple organ trauma can initiate the development of stress ulcers. Fiberoptic endoscopy within 24 hours of injury shows shallow erosions of the stomach wall; by 72 hours, multiple gastric erosions are observed. As the stressful condition continues, the ulcers spread. When the patient recovers, the lesions are reversed. This pattern is typical of stress ulceration.

Differences of opinion exist as to the actual cause of mucosal ulceration. Usually, it is preceded by shock; this leads to a decrease in gastric mucosal blood flow and to a reflux of duodenal contents into the stomach. In addition, large quantities of pepsin are released. The combination of ischemia, acid, and pepsin creates an ideal climate to produce ulceration. Stress ulcers should be distinguished from Cushing's ulcers and Curling's ulcers, two other types of gastric ulcers. Cushing's ulcers are common in patients with trauma to the brain. They may occur in the esophagus, stomach, or duodenum and are usually deeper and more penetrating than stress ulcers. Curling's ulcer is frequently observed about 72 hours after extensive burns.

Clinical Manifestations

Symptoms of an ulcer may last for a few days, weeks, or months and may even disappear only to reappear, often without an identifiable cause. Many persons have symptomless ulcers, and in 20% to 30%, perforation or hemorrhage may occur without any preceding manifestations.

Pain. As a rule, the patient with an ulcer complains of dull, gnawing pain or a burning sensation in the midepigastrium or in the back. It is believed that the pain occurs when the increased acid content of the stomach and duodenum erodes the lesion and stimulates the exposed nerve endings. Another theory suggests that contact of the lesion with acid stimulates a local reflex mechanism that initiates contraction of the adjacent smooth muscle.

Pain is usually relieved by eating, as food neutralizes the acid, or by taking alkali; however, once the stomach has emptied or the alkali wears off, the pain returns. Sharply localized tenderness can be elicited by applying gentle pressure to the epigastrium at or slightly to the right of the midline. Some relief is obtained by applying local pressure on the epigastrium.

Pyrosis (Heartburn). Some patients experience a burning sensation in the esophagus and stomach, which moves up to the mouth, occasionally with sour eructation. Eructation, or burping, is common when the patient's stomach is empty.

Vomiting. Although rare in uncomplicated duodenal ulcer, vomiting may be a symptom of peptic ulcer. It is due to obstruction of the gastric outlet caused by either muscular spasm of the pylorus or mechanical obstruction, which may be due to scarring or to acute swelling of the inflamed mucous membrane adjacent to the acute ulcer. Vomiting may or may not be preceded by nausea; usually it follows a bout of severe pain, which is relieved by ejection of the acid gastric contents.

Constipation and Bleeding. Constipation may occur in the patient with an ulcer, probably as a result of diet and medications. Patients may also present with gastrointestinal bleeding. A small portion of patients who bleed from an acute ulcer have had no previous digestive complaints, but they develop symptoms thereafter.

Diagnostic Evaluation

A physical examination may reveal pain, epigastric tenderness, or abdominal distention. Bowel sounds may be absent. A barium study of the upper GI tract may show an ulcer; however, endoscopy is the preferred diagnostic procedure.

Upper gastrointestinal endoscopy is used to identify inflammatory changes, ulcers, and lesions. Through endoscopy, the mucosa can be directly visualized and a biopsy obtained. Endoscopy has been found to detect some of those lesions not evident in x-ray studies because of the size or location of the lesion. Stools may be collected daily until the laboratory reports are negative for occult blood. Gastric secretory studies are of value in diagnosing achlorhydria (the absence of hydrochloric acid in gastric juices) and Zollinger–Ellison syndrome. Pain that is relieved by ingesting food or antacids and the absence of pain on arising are also highly suggestive of an ulcer.

The presence of *H. pylori* may be determined by biopsy and histology with culture, although this is a specialized laboratory test. There is also a breath test that detects *H. pylori*, as well as a serologic test for antibodies to the *H. pylori* antigen.

Management

From the beginning, once the diagnosis is established, the patient is informed that the problem can be kept under control, although remissions and recurrences may occur. The goal is to manage gastric acidity. Some methods used to control gastric acidity include lifestyle changes, medication, and surgical intervention.

Stress Reduction and Rest. Reducing environmental stress is a difficult task requiring physical and mental interventions on the patient's part and the aid and cooperation of family members and significant others. The patient may need help in identifying situations that are stressful or exhausting. A rushed lifestyle and an irregular schedule may aggravate symptoms and interfere with regular meals taken in relaxed settings and with regular administration of medications. In addition to suggestions for stress reduction, the patient also may benefit from suggestions to take regular rest periods during the day, at least during the acute phase of the disease. Biofeedback, hypnosis, or behavior modification may be helpful in some situations.

Smoking Cessation. Studies have shown that smoking decreases the secretion of bicarbonate from the pancreas into the duodenum. As a result, the acidity of the duodenum is higher when one smokes. Research indicates that continuing to smoke cigarettes may significantly inhibit ulcer repair. Therefore, the patient is strongly encouraged to stop smoking. Smoking cessation support groups are helpful for many patients.

Dietary Modification. Because there is little evidence to support the theory that bland diets are more beneficial than regular meals, patients have been encouraged to eat whatever agrees with them. There are, however, a few precautions to consider in the early stages of healing. The goal of the diet for patients with peptic ulcers is to avoid oversecretion of acid and hypermotility in the GI tract. These can be minimized by avoiding extremes of temperature and overstimulation by meat extracts, alcohol, and coffee (including decaffeinated coffee, which also stimulates acid secretion). In addition, an effort is made to neutralize acid by eating three regular meals a day. Small, frequent feedings are not necessary as long as an antacid or a histamine blocker is taken.

Diet compatibility becomes an individual matter. The patient eats foods that can be tolerated and avoids those that produce pain. Milk and cream are no longer considered central to therapy. In fact, diets rich in milk and cream are potentially harmful because they are potent acid stimulants.

Medications. Currently, the most frequently used medications in the treatment of ulcers include histamine receptor antagonists (H_2 receptor antagonists), which decrease the acid secretion in the stomach; proton pump inhibitors, which also decrease acid secretion; cytoprotective agents, which protect the mucosal cells from acid or NSAIDs; antacids; anticholinergics, which inhibit acid secretion; or a combination of antibiotics with bismuth salts, which suppress *H. pylori* bacteria. Table 36-2 provides a summary of some of the medications that may be used in the treatment of peptic ulcers.

The patient is counseled to adhere to the drug program to ensure complete healing of the ulcer. Because most patients become symptom free in a week, it becomes a nursing goal to stress the importance of following the prescribed regimen so that the healing process can continue uninterrupted and the return of chronic ulcer symptoms can be averted. Rest, sedatives, and tranquilizers may add to the

TABLE 36-2 Drug Therapy for Duodenal Ulcer Disease

Medication	Major Action	Effects and Nursing Considerations
Antacids*		
Magnesium-based (Milk of Magnesia) Aluminum-based (Amphojel, AlternaGEL, Alu-Caps, Basaljel) Magnesium-plus aluminum-based (Maalox, Maalox Plus, Gelusil, Mylanta, Riopan, Riopan Plus, Gaviscon, Di-gel) Calcium carbonate (Titralac, Titralac Plus, Tums, Rolaids)	Neutralizes acid secretions Provides some cytoprotective (cell protective) activity	Magnesium-based may cause diarrhea Aluminum-based may cause constipation Calcium carbonate may cause gastric hypersecretion and acid rebound Require frequent dosing as they are of short duration (some contain simethicone, an antiflatulent)
Histamine Receptor Antagonists (H_2 Receptor Antagonists)		
Cimetidine (Tagament)	Inhibits acid secretion by blocking the action of histamine on the histamine receptors of the parietal cells in the stomach	Least expensive of the H_2 receptor antagonists May cause confusion, agitation, or coma in the elderly or those with renal or hepatic insufficiency Long-term use may cause gynecomastia, impotence, and diarrhea
Ranitidine (Zantac)	Inhibits acid secretion by blocking the action of histamine on the histamine receptors of the parietal cells in the stomach	Prolonged half-life in patients with renal and hepatic insufficiency Causes fewer side effects than cimetidine Rarely causes constipation, diarrhea, dizziness, and depression
Famotidine (Pepcid)	Inhibits acid secretion by blocking the action of histamine on the histamine receptors of the parietal cells in the stomach	Best choice for critically ill patient as it is known to have less risk of interaction with other drugs than cimetidine (Unclear if other H_2 receptor antagonists are as safe as famitidine) Does not alter drug metabolism in the liver Prolonged half-life in patients with renal insufficiency Short-term relief for gastroesophageal reflux (GER) Dilute prior to IV injection On rare occasions causes constipation or diarrhea
Nizatidine (Axid)	Inhibits acid secretion by blocking the action of histamine on the histamine receptors of the parietal cells in the stomach	Used for duodenal ulcers Prolonged half-life in patients with renal insufficiency On rare occasions causes sweating, increased liver enzymes, nausea, urticaria
Antibiotics and Bismuth Salts		
Tetracycline (plus Flagyl and bismuth salts)	Exerts bacteriostatic effects to eradicate *H. pylori* bacteria in the gastric mucosa	May cause photosensitivity reaction Patient should use sunscreen Must be used with caution in patients with renal or hepatic impairment When taken with milk or dairy products effectiveness of drug may be reduced
Amoxicillin (plus Flagyl and bismuth salts)	A bactericidal antibiotic that assists with the eradication of *H. pylori* bacteria in the gastric mucosa	May cause diarrhea Do not use in patients allergic to penicillin
Metronidazole (Flagyl)	An amebocide that assists with the eradication of *H. pylori* bacteria in the gastric mucosa	Given with meals to decrease GI distress
Bismuth subsalicylate (Pepto-Bismol) (use with antibiotics)	Supresses *H. pylori* bacteria in the gastric mucosa and assists with healing of mucosal lesions	Given concurrently with antibiotics for cure of infection of *H. pylori* Should be taken on an empty stomach

(continued)

TABLE 36-2 *(continued)*

Medication	Major Action	Effects and Nursing Considerations
Proton (Gastric Acid) Pump Inhibitor		
Omeprazole (Prilosec)	Decreases gastric acid secretion by slowing the hydrogen–potassium adenosine triphosphatase (H^+, K^+–ATPase) pump on the surface of the parietal cells	Long-term use may cause gastric tumors and bacterial invasion
Cytoprotective Drugs		
Misoprostol (Cytotec)	A synthetic prostaglandin Protects the gastric mucosa from ulcerogenic agents Increases mucus production and bicarbonate levels	Used as a preventive method in patients using NSAID agents Should be taken with food May cause diarrhea and cramping (including uterine cramping)
Sucralfate (Carafate)	In the presence of gastric acid, sucralfate creates a viscous protective substance forming a protective layer at the site of the ulcer and prevents digestion by pepsin	May cause constipation or nausea Approved for duodenal ulcers, not gastric ulcers
Anticholinergics/Antimuscarin		
Pirenzepine	Inhibits the action of acetylcholine (which stimulates the gastric parietal cells to secrete acid) and thus reduces acid secretion	Fewer side effects than older, commonly used anticholinergics Investigational

*This listing of antacids is a sampling of available products.

patient's comfort and are used as needed. Maintenance dosages of H_2 receptor antagonists are usually recommended for 1 year.

Surgical Intervention

The introduction of H_2 receptor antagonists as a treatment for ulcers has greatly reduced the need for surgical interventions. However, surgery is usually recommended for patients with intractable ulcers (those who fail to heal after 12 to 16 weeks of medical treatment), life-threatening hemorrhage, perforation, or obstruction. Surgical procedures include vagotomy, vagotomy with pyloroplasty, or Billroth I or II (Fig. 36-2 and Table 36-3; see also Nursing Process: The Patient Undergoing Gastric Surgery, p. 901). Patients requiring ulcer surgery may have had a long illness, be discouraged, have interruptions in their work role, and experience pressures in their family life.

Nursing Interventions. Preoperative nursing care for the patient undergoing surgery for peptic ulcer disease includes the following:

- *Preparing the patient for diagnostic tests:* The patient undergoes laboratory analyses, x-ray series, and a general physical examination before surgery. The nurse prepares the patient for each of these diagnostic measures by explaining their nature and significance.
- *Attending to the patient's fluid and nutritional needs:* The nutritional and fluid needs of the patient are of major importance. In those patients with pyloric obstruction, there usually is prolonged vomiting, with resultant weight and fluid loss. Every effort is made to restore an adequate nutritional level and to maintain an optimal fluid and electrolyte balance.
- *Clearing and emptying the gastrointestinal tract:* Nasogastric suction often is required to empty the stomach, especially in patients with pyloric obstruction resulting from the ulcer. The tube is inserted before the operation and left in place for operative and postoperative use.

  It is important that the colon be empty when the patient goes to surgery; this is ensured by giving the patient an enema the day before surgery. If gastrointestinal x-rays with barium have been obtained shortly before the day of surgery, enemas are given to remove any traces of barium that may remain in the colon.
- *Limiting oral intake:* The patient's oral intake is usually limited to fluids during the 24-hour period before surgery.

Postoperative care is the same as that for gastric surgery, which is covered later in this chapter. (See Nursing Process: The Patient Undergoing Gastric Surgery and Nursing Care Plan 36-2: Care of the Patient Undergoing a Gastric Resection.)

Managing Other Ulcer Conditions

Zollinger–Ellison Syndrome. Hypersecretion of acid may be controlled with high doses of H_2 receptor antagonists as reviewed in Table 36-2. Patients may require twice the normal dose, and dosages usually need to be in-

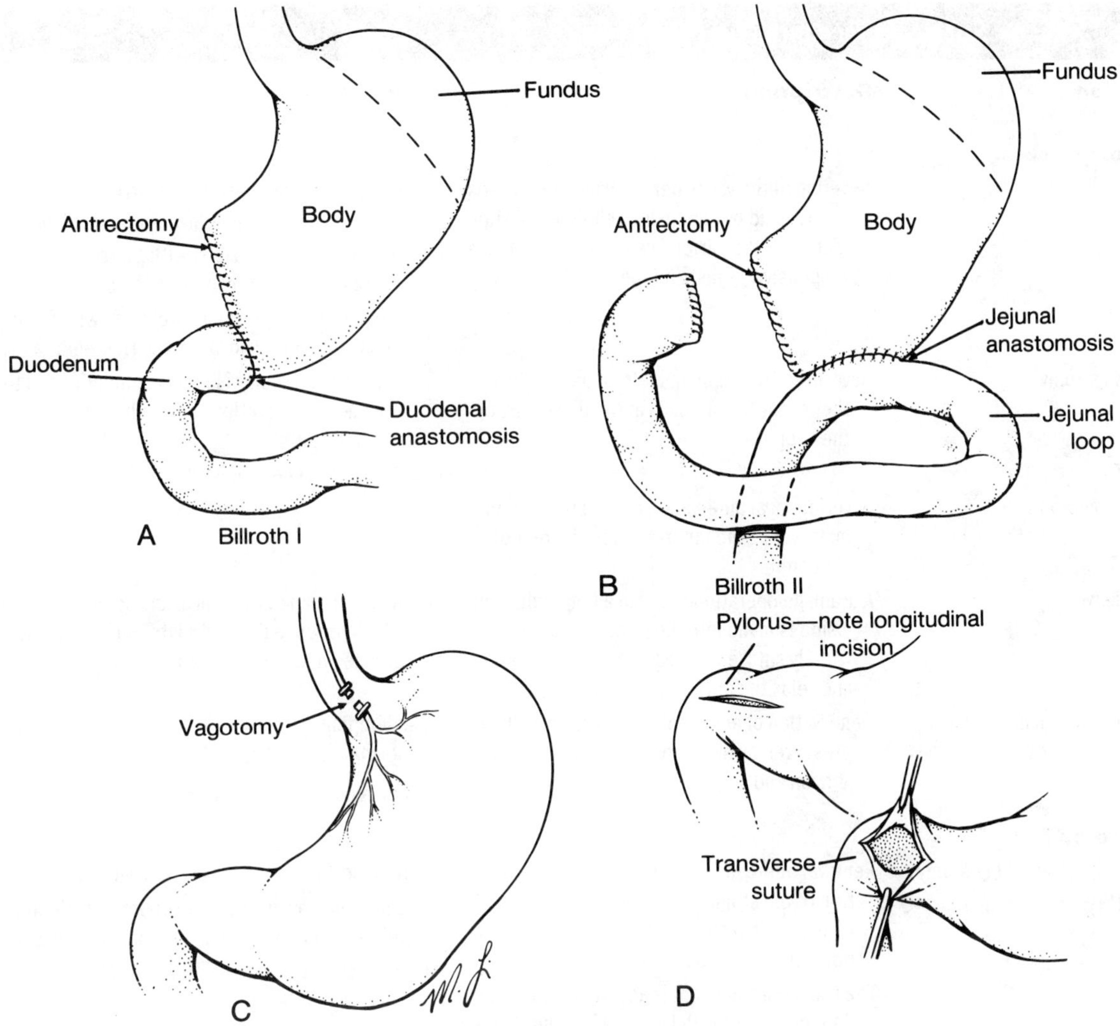

FIGURE 36-2. Surgical procedures for ulcer disease. (**A**) Antrectomy with anastomosis to the duodenum (gastroduodenostomy or Billroth I). (**B**) Antrectomy with anastomosis to the jejunum (gastrojejunostomy or Billroth II). (**C**) Severing of the vagus nerves (vagotomy). (**D**) Pyloroplasty—a longitudinal incision into the pylorus followed by a transverse suture to enlarge the opening.

creased with prolonged use. Patients may also be placed on the drug octreotide (Sandostatin), which has been found to suppress gastrin levels.

Surgical treatment may be helpful for patients not responding to medications. Total gastrectomy or parietal-cell vagotomy are the recommended surgical procedures (Table 36-3).

Stress Ulcers. Patients at risk for stress ulcers are treated prophylactically with intravenous H_2 receptor antagonists, cytoprotective agents, and perhaps antacids (see Table 36-2), as these patients are at high risk for upper GI tract hemorrhage. If the patient is acutely ill, antacids may be given through the nasogastric tube. Frequent gastric aspiration is performed to monitor *p*H. Antacid therapy also can inhibit the activity of pepsin.

Prognosis. There is the possibility that the ulcer will recur within 1 year. This incidence may be reduced with prophylactic use of H_2 receptor antagonists. The likelihood of recurrence is reduced if the person avoids smoking, tea, coffee and cola (including decaffeinated), alcohol, and ulcerogenic drugs (such as anti-inflammatory agents).

❑ NURSING PROCESS
The Patient With a Peptic Ulcer

Assessment

The history serves as an important base for diagnosis. The patient is asked to describe the pain and the methods used to relieve it (food, antacids). Peptic ulcer pain is usually described as "burning" or "gnawing" and occurs about 2 hours after a meal. It frequently awakens the patient between midnight and 3:00 AM. The patient usually states that the pain is relieved by taking antacids, eating foods, or by vomiting. The patient is asked if vomiting has occurred. If so, how much? Is emesis bright red or does it resemble coffee grounds? Has the patient noted any bloody stools? During the history the nurse asks the patient to list the usual food intake for a 72-hour period and to include all food habits (speed of eating, regularity of meals, preference for spicy foods, use of seasonings, use of caffeinated beverages). The patient's level of tension or nervousness is assessed. Does the patient smoke cigarettes? If yes, how many? How does

TABLE 36-3 Surgical Procedures for Peptic Ulcers

Operation	Description	Comments
Vagotomy		
	Severing of the vagus nerves, which decreases gastric acid by diminishing cholinergic stimulation to the parietal cells making them less responsive to gastrin (see Fig. 36-2)	May be performed to reduce gastric acid secretion A drainage type of procedure (see pyloroplasty) is usually performed to assist with gastric emptying (as there is total denervation to the stomach) Some patients experience problems with feeling of fullness, dumping syndrome, diarrhea, and gastritis
Truncal vagotomy	Severing of the right and left vagus nerves as they enter the stomach at the distal part of the esophagus	This type of vagotomy is most commonly used to decrease acid secretions and reduce gastric and intestinal motility Ulcer recurrence rate is 10% to 15%
Selective vagotomy	Severing vagal innervation to the stomach but maintaining the innervation to the rest of the abdomen	
Pyloroplasty	A drainage operation in which a longitudinal incision is made into the pylorus and transversely sutured closed to enlarge the outlet and relax the muscle (see Fig. 36-2)	Usually accompanies truncal and selective vagotomies, which produce delayed gastric emptying due to decreased innervation
Proximal (parietal cell) gastric vagotomy without pyloroplasty	Denervation of acid-secreting parietal cells but preserves vagal innervation to the gastric antrum and pyloris	No dumping syndrome Needs long-term follow-up Ulcer recurrence rate is 10% to 15%
Antrectomy		
Billroth I (gastroduodenostomy) Billroth II (gastrojejunostomy)	Removal of the lower portion of the antral portion of the stomach (which contains the cells that secrete gastrin) as well as a small portion of the duodenum and pylorus The remaining segment is anastomosed to the duodenum (Billroth I) or the jejunum (Billroth II) (see Fig. 36-2)	May be performed in conjunction with a truncal vagotomy The patient may experience problems with feeling of fullness, dumping syndrome, and diarrhea Ulcer recurrence rate is <1%
Subtotal gastrectomy with Billroth I or II anastomosis	Removal of distal third of stomach; anastomosis with duodenum or jejunum (removes gastrin-producing cells in the antrum and part of the parietal cells)	Dumping syndrome, anemia, malabsorption, and weight loss may occur Ulcer recurrence rate is 10% to 15%

the patient express anger, particularly within the context of work and family life? Is there occupational stress or are there problems within the family? Is there a family history of ulcer disease?

Vital signs are assessed for indicators of anemia (tachycardia, hypotension), and the stool is examined for occult blood. A physical examination is performed, and the abdomen is palpated for localized tenderness.

Diagnosis

Nursing Diagnoses

Based on all the assessment data, the patient's nursing diagnoses may include the following:

- Pain related to the effect of gastric acid secretion on damaged tissue
- Anxiety related to coping with an acute disease
- Knowledge deficit about prevention of symptoms and management of the condition

Collaborative Problems/ Potential Complications

Peptic ulcers may lead to the following complications.

- Hemorrhage—upper gastrointestinal
- Perforation
- Penetration
- Pyloric obstruction (gastric outlet obstruction)

Planning and Implementation

Goals. The major goals of the patient may include relief of pain, reduction of anxiety, acquisition of knowledge about management and prevention of ulcer recurrence, and absence of complications.

Nursing Interventions

Relieving Pain. Pain relief can be attained with prescribed medications. Aspirin and foods and beverages that contain caffeine (cola, tea, coffee, chocolate) are avoided. The patient is encouraged to take regularly spaced meals in a relaxed atmosphere. The patient is further encouraged to learn relaxation techniques to help manage stress and pain and to enhance smoking cessation efforts.

Reducing Anxiety. The nurse assesses what the patient knows and wants to know about the diagnosed disease, in addition to evaluating the level of anxiety. Patients with peptic ulcers are usually anxious, but their anxiety is not always obvious. Attempts at coping frequently aggravate the disease process. Information is provided at the patient's level of learning, and all questions are answered. The patient is encouraged to express fears openly. Diagnostic tests are explained, and medications are administered on schedule. These patients are frequently time oriented, and any schedule deviation or disruption can cause anxiety and increase gastric secretion. The patient is assured that nurses are always available to help with a problem. The nurse interacts with the patient in a relaxing manner and helps in identifying stressors and explaining effective coping techniques and relaxation methods, such as biofeedback, hypnosis, or behavior modification. The nurse encourages the patient's family to participate in care and to provide emotional support when appropriate.

Patient Education and Home Care Considerations. To deal successfully with ulcer disease, the patient must understand the situation and those factors that will help or aggravate the diagnosed condition. The following are areas that should be considered and perhaps modified, along with pertinent evaluative questions:

1. *Medication:* Does the patient know what medications are to be taken at home, including name, dosage, frequency, and possible side effects? Does the patient understand the importance of continuing to take medications even after signs and symptoms decrease? Does the patient know which drugs to avoid?
2. *Diet:* Does the patient know which particular foods tend to cause symptoms? Does the patient know that coffee, tea, colas, and alcohol have acid-producing potential? Does the patient understand the need to avoid overeating as well as the importance of taking regular meals in a relaxed setting?
3. *Smoking:* Does the patient know that smoking increases irritation to the ulcer and may interfere with ulcer healing? Has the nurse made the patient aware of programs to assist with smoking cessation?
4. *Rest and stress reduction:* Is the patient aware of sources of stress in family and work environments? Have this illness and other situations produced symptoms of stress or poor coping in the family or work setting? Can the patient take rest periods during the day? Can the patient plan for added periods of rest or relaxation after unavoidable periods of stress? Does the patient need extended psychological counseling?
5. *Awareness of complications:* Is the patient alert to signs and symptoms of complications that should be reported?
   a. *Hemorrhage:* cool skin, confusion, increased heart rate, labored breathing, blood in the stool
   b. *Penetration and perforation:* severe abdominal pain, rigid and tender abdomen, vomiting, elevated temperature, increased heart rate
   c. *Pyloric obstruction:* nausea, vomiting, distended abdomen, abdominal pain
6. *Post-treatment care:* Does the patient understand that follow-up supervision is necessary for about 1 year and that the ulcer could recur? Does the patient know to seek medical assistance if symptoms recur? The patient and family are informed that surgery is no guarantee that an ulcer is cured. Possible postoperative sequelae, such as intolerance to dairy products and sweet foods, are also discussed.

Monitoring for Hemorrhage—Upper Gastrointestinal. Gastritis and hemorrhage from peptic ulcer are the two most common causes of upper GI tract bleeding. (Upper GI bleeding may also occur with esophageal varices, as discussed in Chapter 38.) Hemorrhage is the most frequent complication of peptic ulcers and occurs in about 20% of patients with ulcers. The most frequent site is the distal portion of the duodenum. It may be manifested by **hematemesis** (vomiting of blood) or **melena** (tarry stools). The vomited blood can be bright red or have a "coffee ground" appearance (by way of an oxidizing process hemoglobin changes to methemoglobin, which is dark in color, in the stomach). Melena indicates upper gastrointestinal tract bleeding. When the hemorrhage is of large proportions (2000 to 3000 ml), most of the blood is vomited. The patient may lose large quantities of blood; therefore immediate correction of blood loss may be required to save the patient's life. When the hemorrhage is small, much or all of the blood may be passed in the stools, which will appear tarry black because of the digested hemoglobin. Management depends on the amount of blood lost and the rate of bleeding.

Assessment. The nurse assesses the patient for early symptoms of faintness or dizziness; nausea may precede or accompany bleeding. Dyspepsia may not be present. Vital signs are evaluated for tachycardia, hypotension, and tachypnea. The hemoglobin and hematocrit are monitored. The stool is tested for gross or occult blood, and 24-hour urinary output is recorded to detect anuria or oliguria (absence or reduction of urine production).

Management. Many times the bleeding from a peptic ulcer stops spontaneously; however, recurrence of bleeding is high. Because bleeding can be fatal, the cause and severity of the hemorrhage are quickly identified and the blood loss is treated to prevent hypovolemic shock. Management of upper GI tract bleeding consists of (1) quickly determining the amount of blood lost and the rate of bleeding, (2) rapidly replacing the blood that has been lost, (3) stopping the bleeding with water or saline lavage, (4) stabilizing the patient, and (5) diagnosing and treating the cause.

- ❑ Preparations are made for a peripheral intravenous line for infusion of saline or lactated Ringer's solution and blood. The nurse may need to assist with the placement of a pulmonary artery catheter for hemodynamic monitoring. Blood component therapy is initiated if there are signs of tachycardia, sweating, and coldness of the extremities.

- The hemoglobin and hematocrit are monitored to assist in evaluating bleeding.
- An indwelling urinary catheter is inserted to monitor urinary output.
- Nasogastric intubation may be used to distinguish fresh blood from "coffee ground" material, to aid in the removal of clots and acid, to prevent nausea and vomiting, and to provide a means of monitoring further bleeding. The *p*H of gastric secretions may be monitored hourly through the nasogastric tube, and antacids may be administered for a *p*H less than 4. The nasogastric tube may also be used to administer saline or water for lavage. The lavage solution is given at room temperature.
- Oxygen therapy may be required, especially for elderly patients.
- The patient is placed in the recumbent position to prevent hypovolemic shock; however, to prevent aspiration from vomiting, the patient may be placed on the left side.
- Vital signs are monitored as warranted by the patient's condition.
- Hypovolemic shock is treated as described in Chapter 15.

If bleeding cannot be managed by the measures just described, the following may be performed:

1. *Endoscopic therapy:* Control of bleeding may be accomplished by using several endoscopic therapies such as coagulation by laser, heat probes, or injection or sclerotherapy techniques (injection of drugs to control the bleeding, such as epinephrine or alcohol; or sclerosing [hardening] agents, such as Scleromate, Sotradecol, or Ethamolin). A combination of these therapies may be employed. There is much debate regarding how soon endoscopy should be performed. Some believe endoscopy should be performed in the first 24 hours after hemorrhage has been stabilized. Others believe endoscopy can be performed during acute bleeding, as long as the esophageal or gastric area can be visualized (visibility may be decreased owing to the presence of blood).
2. *Intra-arterial infusions:* Vasopressin is infused by pump, directly into a bleeding artery for 24 to 36 hours. A repeat arteriogram is needed to evaluate the efficacy of treatment.
3. *Selective embolization:* Emboli of autologous blood clots with or without Gelfoam (absorbable gelatin sponge) or a mixture of the patient's own blood or blood products are forced through a catheter to a point above the bleeding lesion. This procedure is performed by a radiologist.

Once the patient has been stabilized, if an endoscopy has not been performed during the acute phase, it can be used to determine the cause and precise site of bleeding. If the diagnosis is inconclusive, an upper gastrointestinal x-ray can provide more information.

Rebleeding may occur and warrants surgical intervention. The patient is carefully monitored so that indicators of bleeding can be quickly detected. These signs include tachycardia, tachypnea, hypotension, mental confusion, thirst, and oliguria.

Surgical Treatment. If bleeding recurs in 48 hours after medical therapy has begun, or if more than 6 to 10 units of blood are required in 24 hours to maintain blood volume, the patient is likely to be scheduled for surgery. Some physicians recommend surgical intervention if a patient with peptic ulcer hemorrhages three times.

Other determining factors for surgery are the patient's age (in those over 60, massive hemorrhaging is three times more likely to be fatal), a history of chronic duodenal ulcer, and a coincidental gastric ulcer.

The area of the ulcer is removed, or the bleeding vessels are ligated. In many patients a procedure is included that is aimed at controlling the underlying causes of the ulcer (*e.g.*, vagotomy and pyloroplasty, or gastrectomy).

Monitoring for Perforation. Perforation is the erosion of the ulcer through the gastric serosa into the peritoneal cavity without warning. Perforation is an abdominal catastrophe and an indication that surgery is required.

Signs and symptoms to note include the following:

- Sudden, severe upper abdominal pain (persisting and increasing in intensity)
- Pain, which may be referred to the shoulders, especially the right shoulder, because of irritation of the phrenic nerve in the diaphragm
- Vomiting and collapse (fainting)
- Extremely tender and rigid (boardlike) abdomen
- Shock

Immediate surgical intervention is indicated. Because chemical peritonitis develops within a few hours after perforation and is followed by a bacterial peritonitis, the perforation must be closed as quickly as possible. In a few patients, it may be deemed safe and advisable to perform surgery for the ulcer disease, in addition to suturing the perforation.

Postoperatively, the stomach contents are drained by means of a nasogastric tube. The nurse monitors fluid and electrolyte balance and assesses the patient for peritonitis or localized infection (increased temperature, abdominal pain, paralytic ileus, increased or absent bowel sounds, abdominal distention). Antibiotic therapy is given parenterally as prescribed.

Monitoring for Penetration or Obstruction. *Penetration* is erosion of the ulcer through the gastric serosa into adjacent structures such as the pancreas, biliary tract, or gastrohepatic omentum. The patient usually complains of back and epigastric pain that is not relieved by medications that were effective in the past. Like perforation, penetration usually requires surgical intervention.

Pyloric obstruction occurs when the area distal to the pyloric sphincter becomes scarred and stenosed from spasm or edema or from scar tissue that is formed when the ulcer alternately heals and breaks down. The patient has symptoms of nausea and vomiting, constipation, epigastric fullness, anorexia, and (later) weight loss.

In treating the patient with pyloric obstruction, the first consideration is to insert a nasogastric tube to decompress the stomach. At the same time, attempts are made to confirm that obstruction is the cause of discomfort. This may be done by checking the amount of fluid aspirated from the nasogastric tube. A residual of over 200 ml is strongly suggestive of obstruction. Usually an upper GI study or endoscopy is performed to confirm gastric outlet obstruction.

Decompressing the stomach and managing extracellular fluid volume and electrolyte balance may improve the patient's condition and avert the need for surgical intervention. If the obstruction is unrelieved by medical management, surgery (in the form of a vagotomy and antrectomy) may be required.

Evaluation

Expected Outcomes

1. Is free of pain between meals
2. Experiences less anxiety by avoiding stress
3. Complies with therapeutic regimen
   a. Avoids irritating foods and beverages
   b. Eats regularly scheduled meals
   c. Takes prescribed medications as scheduled
   d. Uses coping mechanisms to deal with stress
4. Experiences absence of complications

A summary of nursing care of the patient with a peptic ulcer is presented in Nursing Care Plan 36-1.

Morbid Obesity

Morbid obesity is a term applied to people who are more than 100 pounds over their ideal body weight. Patients with morbid obesity are at higher risk for health complications such as cardiovascular disease, arthritis, asthmatic bronchitis, and diabetes. Conservative management consists of placing the person on a very low calorie diet in conjunction with behavioral modification; however, diet therapy is usually unsuccessful. When these conservative measures have been tried and have failed, a surgical procedure may be performed. (Some physicians recommend acupuncture and hypnosis before recommending surgery.)

Surgical Management

Intragastric Balloon. The intragastric balloon is a soft polyurethane sac that is inserted into the stomach to reduce the space available for food. It has been found that this method of treatment is unsuccessful because the stomach expands over time. There is also the potential for rupture of the balloon leading to obstruction. Owing to the failure rate and risk of obstruction, this procedure is no longer available in the United States.

Intestinal Bypass. Intestinal bypass induces weight loss by means of malabsorption. This is sometimes performed with a biliopancreatic diversion, which entails a partial resection of the stomach (partial gastrectomy) and excision of the gallbladder (cholecystectomy) with transection of the jejunum. The proximal jejunum is anastomosed (surgically connected) to the distal ilium, and the distal jejunum is anastomosed to the remaining portion of the stomach. The proximal duodenum is anastomosed to the pancreas. A jejunoileal bypass (where the proximal jejunum is anastomosed to the terminal ileum) is a second surgical method of intestinal bypass. The jejunoileal bypass is no longer used in the United States because it has a high morbidity rate.

Long-term side effects of malabsorption surgery include the dumping syndrome, hepatic cirrhosis, renal stones, and hypoproteinemia (protein deficiency). The biliopancreatic diversion has fewer complications; however, a gastric reduction surgery is more commonly performed for the patient with morbid obesity.

Gastric Reduction. Gastric bypass and vertical banded gastroplasty are the current gastric reduction operations of choice. In gastric bypass surgery, the proximal segment of the stomach is transected to form a small pouch with a small gastroenterostomy stoma. The Roux-en-Y gastric bypass is the recommended procedure for long-term weight loss. In this procedure, a horizontal row of staples creates a stomach pouch with a 1-cm stoma that is anastomosed with a portion of distal jejunum, creating a gastroenterostomy. The transected proximal portion of the jejunum is anastomosed to the distal jejunum (Fig. 36-3*A*).

In vertical banded gastroplasty, a double row of staples is applied vertically along the lesser curvature of the stomach, beginning at the angle of His. A small stoma is created at the end of the staples by adding a circle of staples or a band of polypropylene mesh or silicone tubing (Fig. 36-3*B*).

Nursing Interventions. General postoperative nursing care is similar to that for a patient experiencing gastric resection (see Nursing Care Plan 36-2). Patients are usually discharged in 1 week with detailed dietary instruction. Patients are usually given six small feedings consisting of a total of 600 to 800 calories. Fluid intake is encouraged to prevent dehydration. Patients are instructed to report any excessive thirst or concentrated urine to their physician. Outpatient visits are scheduled monthly.

Psychosocial considerations are essential for these patients. All efforts are directed toward helping them modify their eating behaviors and cope with changes in body image. Noncompliance usually results in patients eating too much or too fast. If this happens, vomiting and painful esophageal distention may occur.

Postoperative complications may occur in the immediate postoperative period and include peritonitis, stomal obstruction, stomal ulcers, atelectasis and pneumonia, thromboembolism, and metabolic sequelae resulting from prolonged vomiting and diarrhea.

After weight loss, the patient may need surgical intervention for body contouring. This may include lipoplasty to remove fat deposits or a panniculectomy to remove excess abdominal skin folds.

Gastric Cancer

Cancer of the stomach continues to decrease in the United States. However, it is still a serious problem accounting for 14,700 deaths annually, mostly in people over the age of 40, and occasionally in younger people. Most stomach cancers occur in the lesser curvature or antrum of the stomach and are adenocarcinomas. The incidence of gastric cancer is much greater in Japan, which has led to mass screening for earlier diagnosis in that country. Diet appears to be a significant factor. A diet high in smoked foods and lacking in fruits

NURSING CARE PLAN 36–1
Care of the Patient with Peptic Ulcer Disease

Nursing Interventions	Rationale	Expected Outcomes
NURSING DIAGNOSIS: Knowledge deficit regarding the prevention of symptoms and management of the condition		
GOAL: Acquisition of knowledge about prevention and management		
1. Assess the patient's level of knowledge and "readiness to learn."	1. Attending to learning is dependent on the patient's physical condition, level of anxiety, and mental readiness.	• Expresses an interest in learning how to manage the disease.
2. Teach necessary information: a. Use words at the level of learner. b. Choose a time when the patient is rested and interested. c. Limit teaching sessions to 30 minutes or less.	2. Individualization of the teaching plan promotes learning.	• Participates in teaching sessions. • Asks questions.
3. Reassure the patient that the disease can be managed.	3. Reassurance can have a positive influence on behavior modification.	• States a desire to be responsible for self-care.
NURSING DIAGNOSIS: Pain related to irritated mucosa and muscle spasms		
GOAL: Relief of pain		
1. Administer medication therapy as prescribed: a. Histamine antagonists b. Antibiotics/bismuth salts c. Cytoprotective agents d. Proton pump inhititors e. Antacids f. Anticholinergics	1. Pharmacotherapy helps reduce pain as follows: a. Histamine antagonists interfere with the secretion of gastric acid. b. Antibiotics given in conjunction with bismuth salts eradicate *H. pylori.* c. Cytoprotective agents protect the mucosa of the stomach. d. Proton pump inhibitors decrease gastric acid. e. Antacids neutralize acidity of gastric secretions. f. Anticholinergics inhibit the release of gastric acid.	• Takes medications as prescribed. • Experiences less pain.
2. Recommend avoidance of ulcerogenic over-the-counter drugs.	2. Drugs that contain salicylates are irritating to the gastric mucosa.	• Substitutes acetaminophen (Tylenol) for aspirin. • Avoids over-the-counter drugs that contain acetylsalicylic acid (Contac, Alka-Seltzer).
3. Advise patient to avoid foods/beverages that are irritating to the stomach lining: caffiene and alcohol.	3. Foods/beverages that contain caffiene stimulate the secretion of hydrochloric acid.	• Complies with recommended restrictions • Identifies foods and beverages to be avoided.
4. Advise patient to space meals and snacks at regular intervals.	4. Regularly scheduled meals helps keep food particles in the stomach, which helps to neutralize the acidity of gastric secretions.	• Adheres to a schedule of regularly spaced meals and snacks.
5. Advise patient to stop smoking.	5. Smoking increases the possibility of recurrence of ulcer.	• Stops smoking • Participates in smoking cessation program if necessary.

(continued)

NURSING CARE PLAN 36–1 *(continued)*
Care of the Patient with Peptic Ulcer Disease

Nursing Interventions	Rationale	Expected Outcomes
NURSING DIAGNOSIS: Anxiety related to the nature of the disease and its long-term management		
GOAL: Reduction of anxiety		
1. Encourage the patient to express concerns and fears and ask questions as needed.	1. Open communication fosters a trusting relationship, which helps reduce anxiety and stress.	• Expresses fears and concerns.
2. Explain the reasons for adhering to a planned treatment schedule: a. Pharmacotherapy b. Diet restriction c. Modified activity levels d. Reduction or cessation of smoking	2. Knowledge reduces the anxiety found with "fear of the unknown." Knowledge can have a positive influence on behavior modification.	• Understands rationale for various treatments, and restrictions. • Modifies behavior appropriately.
3. Assist the patient to identify anxiety-producing situations.	3. Stressors need to be identified before they can be managaed.	• Identifies anxiety–producing situations.
4. Teach stress management strategies: *e.g.,* medication, distraction, and imagery.	4. Decreased anxiety decreases hydrochloric acid secretion.	• Uses stress management strategies appropriately
NURSING DIAGNOSIS: Altered nutrition, less than body requirements, related to pain associated with eating		
GOAL: Attainment of an optimal level of nutrition		
1. Recommend nonirritating foods and beverages.	1. Nonirritating foods reduce epigastric pain.	• Avoids irritating foods and beverages.
2. Suggest that meals be eaten at regularly scheduled times: avoid snacks before bedtime.	2. Regular meals help neutralize gastric secretions; snacks before bedtime increase acid secretion of the stomach.	• Eats meals and snacks at regularly scheduled intervals.
3. Encourage eating meals in a relaxed atmosphere.	3. A relaxed atmosphere is less anxiety producing. Decreasing anxiety helps decrease the secretion of hydrochloric acid.	• Chooses a relaxed atmosphere for meals.

and vegetables may increase the risk of gastric cancer. Other factors related to the incidence of gastric cancer include chronic inflammation of the stomach, pernicious anemia, achlorhydria (absence of hydrochloric acid), gastric ulcers, *H. pylori* bacteria, and heredity. The prognosis is poor, as most patients have metastases at the time of diagnosis.

Clinical Manifestations

The early symptoms of gastric cancer are often nondefinitive because most of these tumors begin on the lesser curvature, where they cause little disturbance of gastric functions. In the early stages of gastric cancer, symptoms may be absent. Some studies have shown that early symptoms, such as pain relieved with antacids, may resemble those of patients with benign ulcers. Symptoms of progressive disease may include indigestion, anorexia, dyspepsia, weight loss, abdominal pain, constipation, anemia, and nausea and vomiting.

Diagnostic Evaluation

Physical examination is usually not helpful, as most gastric tumors are not palpable. Ascites may be present if there is metastasis to the liver. Endoscopy for biopsy and cytologic washings is the usual diagnostic study. X-ray examination of the upper GI tract with barium may also be done. Because metastasis frequently occurs before warning signs present themselves, computed tomography (CT) scan, bone scan, and liver scan are valuable in determining the extent of the metastasis. Indigestion (dyspepsia) of more than 4 weeks' duration in any person over age 40 calls for complete x-ray examination of the GI tract.

Management

There is no successful treatment of gastric carcinoma except removal of the tumor. If the tumor can be removed while it is still localized to the stomach, the patient can be cured. If the tumor has spread beyond the area that can be

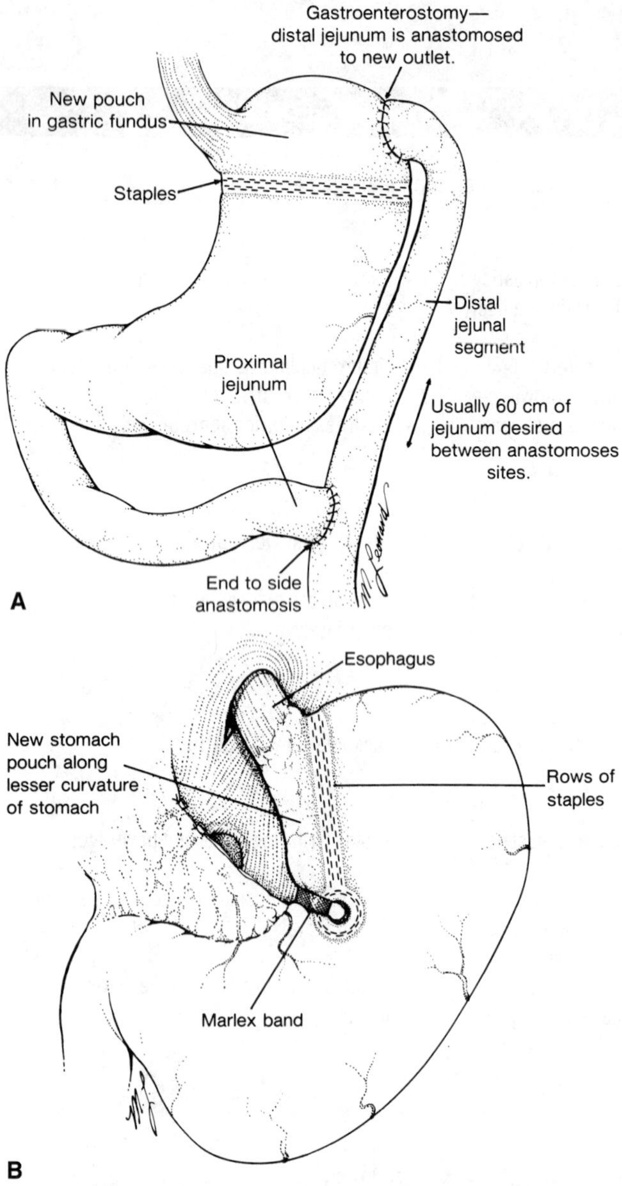

FIGURE 36-3. Surgical procedures for morbid obesity. (**A**) Gastric bypass with Roux-en-Y. A horizontal row of staples creates a pouch with a capacity of 50 ml or less. The proximal jejunum is transected and the distal end anastomosed to the new pouch. The proximal segment is anastomosed to the jejunum. (**B**) Vertical banded gastroplasty. A vertical row of staples along the lesser curvature of the stomach creates a new, smaller stomach pouch of 10–15 ml.

excised surgically, cure cannot be effected. In many of these patients, however, effective palliation, to prevent symptoms such as obstruction, may be obtained by resection of the tumor (see Nursing Process: The Patient Undergoing Gastric Surgery).

If a **radical subtotal gastrectomy** is performed, the stump of the stomach is anastomosed to the jejunum, as in the gastrectomy for ulcer. When **total gastrectomy** is performed, gastrointestinal continuity is restored by an anastomosis between the ends of the esophagus and jejunum. Palliative, rather than radical, surgery is performed if there is metastasis to other vital organs, such as the liver. Palliative surgery is performed to relieve symptoms of obstruction or dysphagia.

For patients in whom surgical treatment does not offer cure, treatment with chemotherapy may offer further control of the disease or palliation. Frequently used chemotherapeutic drugs include a combination of 5-fluorouracil (5FU), Adriamycin, and mitomycin-C. Radiation may be used for palliation in gastric cancer.

❑ NURSING PROCESS
The Patient With Gastric Cancer

Assessment

The nurse elicits a dietary history from the patient, focusing on issues such as high intake of smoked or cured foods and low intake of fruits and vegetables. Has the patient lost weight; if so, how much?

Does the patient smoke cigarettes? If so, how many a day and for how long? Does the patient notice any stomach discomfort during or after smoking? Does the patient drink alcohol? If so, how much?

The nurse asks the patient if there is a family history of cancer. If so, are immediate family members or close or distant relatives affected? What is the patient's marital status? Is there someone who can provide emotional support?

During the physical examination it may be possible to palpate a mass. The nurse should observe for the presence of ascites. Other organs are examined for tenderness or masses. Pain is usually a late symptom.

Diagnosis

Nursing Diagnoses

Based on all the assessment data, the patient's major nursing diagnoses may include the following:

- Anxiety related to the disease and anticipated treatment
- Altered nutrition, less than body requirements, related to anorexia
- Pain, related to the presence of abnormal epithelial cells
- Anticipatory grieving related to the diagnosis of cancer
- Knowledge deficit regarding self-care activities

Planning and Implementation

Goals. The major goals of the patient may include reduction of anxiety, attainment of optimal nutrition, relief of pain, and adjustment to the diagnosis and to anticipated lifestyle changes.

Nursing Interventions

Reducing Anxiety. A relaxed, nonthreatening atmosphere is provided so that the patient can express fears, concerns, and possibly anger with the diagnosis and prognosis. The nurse encourages the family in their efforts to support the patient, offering assurance and supporting positive coping measures. The nurse advises the patient about any procedures and treatments so that the patient knows what to expect; the nurse also may suggest that the patient who needs to discuss personal feelings do so with a support person (*e.g.* clergy) if desired.

Promoting Optimal Nutrition. Small, frequent feedings of nonirritating foods are encouraged to decrease gastric irritation. Food supplements should be high in calories as well as vitamins A and C and iron so that tissue repair is facilitated. If a total gastrectomy is to be performed, parenteral vitamin B_{12} will need to be administered indefinitely. The nurse monitors the rate and frequency of intravenous therapy. The nurse records intake, output, and daily weights to make sure the patient is maintaining or gaining weight. Signs of dehydration (thirst, dry mucous membranes, poor skin turgor, tachycardia) are assessed and results of daily laboratory studies are reviewed to note any metabolic abnormalities (sodium, potassium, glucose, blood urea nitrogen). Antiemetics are administered as prescribed.

Relieving Pain. Analgesics are administered as prescribed. A continuous infusion of an opioid may be necessary for severe pain. The frequency, intensity, and duration of the pain are assessed to determine the effectiveness of the analgesic being administered. The nurse works with the patient to manage pain (*e.g.*, position changes). Nonpharmacologic methods for pain relief such as imagery, distraction, relaxation tapes, backrubs, and massage are suggested, and periods of rest and relaxation are encouraged.

Providing Psychosocial Support. The nurse helps the patient express fears and concerns about the diagnosis, while allowing the freedom to grieve. The patient's questions are answered honestly, and the patient is encouraged to participate in treatment decisions. Some patients mourn the loss of a body part and perceive their surgery as a type of mutilation. Some express disbelief and need time and support to accept the diagnosis.

The nurse offers emotional support and involves family members and significant others whenever possible. This includes recognizing mood swings and defense mechanisms (denial, rationalization, displacement, regression) and reassuring the patient and family members that emotional responses are normal and expected. The services of clergy, psychiatric clinical nurse specialists, psychologists, social workers, and psychiatrists are made available, if needed. The nurse projects an empathic approach and spends time with the patient. Most patients will begin to participate in self-care activities when they have acknowledged their loss.

Patient Education and Home Care Considerations. The patient is advised that it may take 6 months before regular meals can be eaten after a partial gastric resection. Small, frequent feedings are given initially, or nutrients are administered through a tube; total parenteral nutrition may be necessary. With any enteral feeding, the possibility of the dumping syndrome exists, so it must be explained and ways to manage it reviewed.

The patient is informed that it may take 3 months before normal activities can be resumed. Daily periods of rest are necessary, and frequent visits to the physician after discharge will be required. Lifestyle will be affected by chemotherapy and radiation therapy, if prescribed, so the patient needs to know what to expect: length of treatments, expected reactions (nausea, vomiting, anorexia, fatigue), and need for transportation for treatments. Psychologic counseling may be necessary as well.

Nutritional counseling is started in the hospital and reinforced at home. Any enteral or parenteral feeding is supervised by a visiting nurse, who teaches the patient and family members how to use the equipment and formulas as well as how to detect complications. (See Chapter 35 to review management of tube feedings.) The patient learns to record daily intake, output, and weight and is instructed on how to cope with pain, nausea, vomiting, and bloating. The patient also is taught to recognize and report those complications that require medical attention, such as bleeding (overt or covert hematemesis, melena), obstruction, perforation, or any symptoms that become consistently worse.

The nurse teaches the patient how to care for the incision and how to examine the wound for signs of infection (malodorous drainage, pain, heat, inflammation, swelling). Any chemotherapy or radiation therapy regimen is explained. The patient and the family need to know what kind of care will be needed during and after treatments.

Evaluation

Expected Outcomes

1. Experiences less anxiety
   a. Expresses fears and concerns about surgery
   b. Seeks emotional support
2. Attains optimal nutrition
   a. Eats small, frequent meals high in calories, iron, and vitamins A and C
   b. Complies with enteral or parenteral nutrition as needed
3. Experiences less pain
4. Performs self-care activities and adjusts to lifestyle changes
   a. Resumes normal activities within 3 months
   b. Alternates periods of rest and activity
   c. Manages tube feedings

Gastric Surgery

Gastric surgery may be performed on patients with peptic ulcers who have life-threatening hemorrhage, obstruction, perforation, or penetration or do not respond to medication. It also may be indicated for patients with gastric cancer or trauma. Operative procedures may include a partial gastrectomy (removal of the stomach) or total gastrectomy with either end-to-end or end-to-side esophagojejunostomy anastomosis.

❑ *NURSING PROCESS*
The Patient Undergoing Gastric Surgery

Assessment

Preoperatively, the patient is assessed for knowledge of preoperative and postoperative surgical routines. The patient's and family's knowledge of the rationale for surgery is assessed. Also preoperatively, the nutritional status is assessed: Has the patient lost weight? How much? Over how much time? Does the patient have nausea and vomiting? Has the patient had hematemesis? The patient is assessed for presence of bowel sounds. Palpation of the abdomen is performed to determine if masses can be felt or if there is tenderness.

Postoperatively, the patient is assessed for complications secondary to the surgical intervention such as hemorrhage, infection, abdominal distention, or decreased nutritional status. (See Nursing Process: Caring for The Postoperative Patient in Chap. 21 and The Patient Undergoing Thoracic Surgery in Chap. 25 for the patient who has had a total gastrectomy, as the chest cavity may be entered).

Diagnosis

Nursing Diagnoses

Based on all the assessment data, the patient's major nursing diagnoses may include the following:

- Anxiety related to surgical intervention
- Knowledge deficit about surgical procedures and postoperative course
- Altered nutrition, less than body requirements related to poor nutrition preoperatively and altered gastrointestinal system postoperatively
- Pain related to surgical incision
- Knowledge deficit regarding home care

Collaborative Problems/ Potential Complications

The following are potential complications arising from gastric surgery:

- Hemorrhage
- Steatorrhea

Planning and Implementation

Goals. The major goals of the patient may include reduction of anxiety; knowledge and understanding about the surgical procedure and postoperative course; attainment of optimal nutrition; relief of pain; absence of hemorrhage, dumping syndrome, and steatorrhea; and ability to care for self at home. General postoperative care for the patient who received general anesthesia, as discussed in Chapter 21, should be followed.

Nursing Interventions

Reducing Anxiety. An important part of the preoperative nursing care involves allaying the patient's fears and anxieties about the impending surgery and its implications. The nurse encourages the patient to express feelings and answers all questions. If the patient is experiencing hemorrhage, perforation, or acute obstruction, adequate psychologic preparation may not be possible. In this event, the nurse caring for the patient postoperatively should anticipate the concerns, fears, and questions that are likely to surface. For all postoperative patients the nurse should be available for support and further explanations.

Increasing Knowledge. It is also necessary to explain the routine preoperative and postoperative activities to the patient such as preoperative medications, nasogastric intubation, intravenous fluids, abdominal dressings, and pulmonary care. These procedures need to be reinforced postoperatively—especially if the patient had emergency surgery.

Maintaining Adequate Nutrition. The patient should be evaluated preoperatively for nutritional status. Many patients with gastric cancer are malnourished and may require preoperative enteral or, more frequently, total parenteral nutrition (see Chapter 35). Postoperatively, parenteral nutrition may be continued to provide caloric needs as well as provide fluids lost in drainage and vomitus.

After the return of bowel sounds and removal of the nasogastric tube, fluids may be given, followed by food in small portions. Foods are gradually added until the patient is able to eat six small meals a day and drink 120 ml of fluid between meals. The key to increasing the dietary content is to offer food and fluids gradually as tolerated and to recognize that each person's tolerance is different.

Dysphagia. Dysphagia may be noticed in those patients who have had truncal vagotomy, which causes trauma to the lower esophagus. If regurgitation occurs in patients who have had gastric surgery, the patient may be eating too much or too fast. It also may indicate that edema along the suture line is preventing fluids and food from moving into the intestinal tract. If gastric retention does occur, it may be necessary to reinstate nasogastric suction; pressure must be low to avoid disruption of the suture line.

Bile Reflux. With the removal of the pylorus, which acts as a barrier to the reflux of duodenal contents, bile reflux gastritis and esophagitis may occur. This is manifested by burning epigastric pain and vomiting of bile material. Eating or vomiting does not relieve the situation. Binding agents such as cholestyramine (Questran), aluminum hydroxide gel, or metoclopramide hydrochloride (Reglan) have been used with some success.

Dumping Syndrome. The term dumping syndrome designates an unpleasant set of vasomotor and gastrointestinal symptoms that occur after meals in 10% to 50% of patients who have had gastrointestinal surgery or a form of vagotomy. There may be several causes for its occurrence. One cause is the mechanical result of surgery in which a small gastric remnant connects into the jejunum through a large opening. Foods that are high in carbohydrates and electrolytes have to be diluted in the jejunum before absorption can take place; yet the passage of food from the stomach remnant into the jejunum is too rapid. The ingestion of fluid at mealtime is another factor that causes the stomach contents to empty rapidly into the jejunum. The symptoms that occur are probably a result of rapid distention of the jejunal loop anastomosed to the stomach. The hypertonic intestinal contents draw extracellular fluid from the circulating blood volume into the jejunum to dilute the high concentration of electrolytes and sugars.

Early symptoms may include a sensation of fullness, weakness, faintness, dizziness, palpitations, diaphoresis, cramping pains, and diarrhea. Later, there is a rapid elevation of blood glucose, followed by a compensatory reaction of insulin secretion. This results in a reactive hypoglycemia, which also is unpleasant for the patient. Symptoms that occur 10 to 90 minutes after eating are vasomotor and are manifested by pallor, perspiration, palpitations, headache, and feelings of warmth, dizziness, and even drowsiness. Anorexia may also be due to the dumping syndrome.

NURSING CARE PLAN 36-2
Care of the Patient Undergoing Gastric Resection

Nursing Interventions	Rationale	Expected Outcomes
Preoperative		
NURSING DIAGNOSIS: Knowledge deficit regarding the surgical procedure and postoperative course		
GOAL: Attainment of information about the procedure and postoperative course		
1. Ascertain that the patient understands what type of surgery is planned.	1. Preoperative knowledge helps the patient understand the reasons for postoperative procedures.	• Discusses the surgery and what to expect postoperatively. • Practices deep breathing and coughing. • Describes the importance of early postoperative ambulation.
2. Advise the patient that a modified Fowler's position will be required after recovery from anesthesia.	2. Modified Fowler's position promotes comfort and drainage of the stomach.	
3. Advise the patient that requests will be made to breathe deeply and cough, postoperatively.	3. Coughing and deep breathing will prevent pulmonary complications.	
4. Advise the patient that a nasogastric tube will be placed postoperatively and fluids will be withheld until peristalsis returns.	4. The nasogastric tube provides for gastric drainage that may contain some blood for the first 12 hours.	
5. Inform the patient that parenteral fluids will be given. Oral fluids will be withheld until the nasogastric tube is removed and peristalisis returns.	5. Parenteral fluids meet fluid and nutritional needs and compensate for fluids lost in drainage and vomitus.	
6. Inform the patient that foods are advanced gradually, and that supplemental enteral or parenteral feedings may be necessary.	6. Small increments of fluid advancing to solid foods are initiated to determine the patient's tolerance.	
7. Inform the patient that there will be assisted ambulation on the first postoperative day.	7. Early ambulation prevents venous stasis and thrombophlebitis.	
8. Inform the patient that wound dressings may have drainage. Excessive drainage or bright red blood will be reported immediately.	8. Serosanguineous drainage is expected postoperatively, especially if tubes are left in the wound.	
Postoperative		
NURSING DIAGNOSIS: Pain related to the surgical incision		
GOAL: Relief of pain		
1. Administer analgesics as prescribed.	1. Pain control results from selective depression of the central nervous system.	• Patient requests pain medication as needed, or uses patient-controlled analgesia appropriately. • States that pain is relieved by analgesics
2. Promote frequent turning for comfort and for the prevention of pulmonary and vascular complications.	2. Inactivity encourages the pooling of pulmonary secretions and venous stasis.	• Cooperates with pulmonary routine.
3. Withhold oral fluids until prescribed.	3. Sealing of the suture line is enhanced if patient is NPO. Withholding fluid prevents unnecessary distention and pain.	• Remains NPO until physician allows intake of fluids.
4. Use gastric suction to remove liquids, blood, and gas from stomach.	4. Promotes healing of suture line. Prevents unnecessary distention and pain.	• Nasogastric tube remains patent. • Exhibits no evidence of abdominal distention.

(continued)

NURSING CARE PLAN 36–2 *(continued)*
Care of the Patient Undergoing Gastric Resection

NURSING DIAGNOSIS: Fluid volume deficit, related to shock or hemorrhage

GOAL: Experiences no fluid volume deficit, shock, or hemorrhage

Nursing Interventions	Rationale	Expected Outcomes
1. Monitor for signs of hemorrhage: a. Observe gastric aspirate for evidence of blood. b. Observe the suture line for bleeding. c. Evaluate blood pressure, pulse, and respiratory rate. d. Administer blood products as prescribed. e. If bleeding continues, prepare patient for surgical intervention.	1. Decreased circulating blood volume can lead to hypovolemic shock.	• Alerts nurse to any signs of bleeding. • Experiences no hemorrhage. • Vital signs within normal ranges.
2. Assess patient for signs of shock: a. Evaluate drainage from dressing and drainage receptacles. b. Evaluate blood pressure, pulse, and respiratory rate. c. Administer blood and fluids as prescribed. d. Instruct patient regarding symptoms to report.	2. Decreased circulating blood volume can lead to hypovolemic shock.	• Alerts nurse to any dizziness, increased heart rate, confusion, excessive fatigue or clammy skin. • Vital signs within normal ranges.

NURSING DIAGNOSIS: Altered nutrition, less than body requirements, related to the surgical procedure

GOAL: Attainment of optimal nutrition

Nursing Interventions	Rationale	Expected Outcomes
1. Administer intravenous fluids as prescribed.	1. Intravenous fluids help prevent shock and maintain fluid and electrolyte balance.	• Cooperates with intravenous therapy.
2. Administer oral fluids as prescribed when audible bowel sounds are present.	2. Positive bowel sounds indicate peristalsis is present.	• Bowel sounds audible • Gradually increases intake of fluids.
3. Increase fluids according to patient's tolerance.	3. Maintain fluid balance.	• Accepts fluids as tolerated.
4. Maintain supplementary iron and vitamin therapy as prescribed.	4. Iron and vitamin therapy is necessary to supplement postoperative diet to promote tissue repair and prevent anemia. (Removal of the stomach prevents the absorption of vitamin B_{12})	• Takes vitamin supplements as prescribed.
5. Discourage foods that may initiate development of dumping syndrome; encourage moderate amount of fat, low carbohydrates.	5. Decreased hypertonicity of intestinal contents prevents the osmotic pull of extracellular fluid into the intestinal area.	• Adheres to diet therapy. • Exhibits no symptoms of dumping syndrome.
6. Administer supplemental enteral or parenteral nutrition as prescribed.	6. Patient may require supplemental feedings if oral intake is inadequate.	• Attains adequate caloric intake.

NURSING DIAGNOSIS: Risk for infection related to surgical incision

GOAL: Free of infection

Nursing Interventions	Rationale	Expected Outcomes
1. Assess wound for signs and symptoms of infection such as redness, swelling, tenderness, purulent drainage; fever. Report signs and symptoms if present.	1. Wound should be clean; some serosanguinous drainage may occur the first 24 hours and then subside.	• Absence of signs and symptoms of infection.

(continued)

NURSING CARE PLAN 36–2 *(continued)*
Care of the Patient Undergoing Gastric Resection

Nursing Interventions	Rationale	Expected Outcomes
2. Assess abdomen for signs of peritonitis: tenderness, rigidity, distention.	2. Peritonitis may occur secondary to gastric surgery.	• Absence of symptoms of peritonitis.
3. Administer prophylactic antibiotics as prescribed.	3. Antibiotics are frequently administered to the patient following abdominal surgery to prevent infection.	• No reaction to antibiotics.
NURSING DIAGNOSIS: Potential noncompliance with the therapeutic regimen related to denial		
GOAL: Adherence to therapeutic regimen		
1. Help patient to modify any environmental stresses.	1. Stress increases the secretion of hydrochloric acid, which irritates a compromised/damaged gastric mucosa.	• Uses stress reduction methods (biofeedback, imagery, distraction).
2. Encourage patient to remain under health care supervision.	2. Periodic hematologic studies are necessary to monitor for anemia. A complete physical examination may yield data about possible metastasis.	• Sees physician every 6 to 12 months as scheduled.
3. Arrange for resources to help the patient cope: home health worker, clergy, psychologist, nurse practitioner.	3. Effective coping may require a support system.	• Aware of resources and seeks help when needed.

Related Dietary Deficiencies. Other dietary deficiencies the nurse should be aware of include (1) malabsorption of organic iron, which may require supplementation with oral or parenteral iron, and (2) low serum level of vitamin B_{12}, which may require supplementation by the intramuscular route. Total gastrectomy brings to a complete halt the production of "intrinsic factor," a gastric secretion that is required for the absorption of vitamin B_{12} from the GI tract. Therefore, unless this vitamin is supplied by parenteral injection following gastrectomy, the patient inevitably suffers from vitamin B_{12} deficiency, which leads in time to a condition identical to that of a patient with pernicious anemia. All manifestations of pernicious anemia, including macrocytic anemia and combined system disease, may be expected to develop within a period of 5 years or less, to progress in severity thereafter, and, in the absence of therapy, to prove fatal. This complication is avoided by the regular monthly intramuscular injection of 100 to 200 µg of vitamin B_{12}, a regimen that should be started without delay after gastrectomy. With regard to long-term management of these patients, weight loss is a common problem because the patient experiences early fullness that curbs the appetite.

In anticipation of the possibility of the patient's experiencing any of the above conditions affecting nutrition, nursing intervention is directed toward proper dietary instruction. The following teaching points are emphasized:

- The patient should be positioned in a semirecumbent position during mealtime. After the meal, the patient should lie down for 20 to 30 minutes to delay stomach emptying.
- Fluids are discouraged with meals but may be given up to 1 hour before or 1 hour after mealtime.
- Fat may be given to tolerance, but carbohydrate intake should be kept low (sucrose and glucose are avoided).
- Antispasmodics, as prescribed, also may aid in delaying the emptying of the stomach.
- Smaller but more frequent meals should be eaten.
- Meal composition should contain more dry than liquid items.
- Dietary supplements of vitamins and medium chain triglycerides, or injections of Vitamin B_{12} and iron may be prescribed.
- Instructions are given regarding enteral or parenteral supplementation.

Relieving Pain. The patient is given analgesics postoperatively as prescribed by the physician to maintain an acceptable level of comfort. Care must be taken to maintain the patient's ability to perform pulmonary care activities (deep breathing and coughing) adequately and to ambulate. The nurse assesses the effectiveness of analgesic intervention. Positioning the patient in a modified Fowler's position promotes comfort as well as allows for easy drainage of the stomach following a partial gastrectomy.

The function of the nasogastric tube is maintained to prevent distention and resultant pain. The amount of nasogastric drainage from the patient following a total gastrectomy is normally small.

Patient Education and Home Care Considerations. Patient teaching is based on assessment of the patient's physical and psychological readiness to return to the home and the community. (If the patient has gastric cancer, goals may be for maintenance and palliation.) The patient and family will benefit from a team approach to discharge care. The team members include the home care nurse, physician, nutritionist, and the social worker. Written instructions about meals, activities, medications, and follow-up care are often useful for the patient and family.

Monitoring and Managing Potential Complications. **Hemorrhage** is occasionally a complication after gastric surgery. The patient exhibits the usual signs (see Chapter 21) and may vomit considerable amounts of bright red blood. Nasogastric drainage should be assessed for the type and amount; some bloody drainage is expected for the first 12 hours, but excessive bleeding should be reported. The abdominal dressing should also be assessed for bleeding.

Because this situation is likely to be upsetting to the patient and family, the nurse should remain calm and reassure the patient. Emergency measures are performed, such as nasogastric lavage and administration of blood and blood products.

Steatorrhea may also occur in the patient with gastric surgery and is partially the result of rapid gastric emptying, which prevents adequate mixing with pancreatic and biliary secretions. In mild cases, steatorrhea can be controlled by reducing the intake of fat and administering an antimotility drug.

Evaluation

Expected Outcomes

1. Experiences less anxiety—expresses fears and concerns about surgery
2. Demonstrates knowledge regarding postoperative course by discussing the surgical procedure and postoperative course
3. Attains optimal nutrition
   a. Maintains a reasonable weight
   b. Does not experience excessive diarrhea
4. Attains optimal level of comfort
5. Is compliant with home care needs

For an overview of care of the patient undergoing gastric resection, refer to Nursing Care Plan 36-2.

CRITICAL THINKING EXERCISES

1. You are visiting a resident of a retirement community. She tells you that she has begun to have symptoms of a peptic ulcer just like she had many years ago and that she is treating the ulcer as she did before, with a bland diet and antacids. Based on your knowledge of current theories about peptic ulcers, how would you advise her? If she is skeptical of your explanations, how might you convince her?
2. You are caring for a patient who has had a gastrectomy to treat gastric cancer. The patient's wife indicates that she is eager for him to return home so that she can give him all of his favorite foods and help him to regain the weight that he has lost. Describe the conclusions you would draw from these statements, and explain how you would devise an instructional program that you feel would be helpful for this patient and his wife.

REFERENCES AND SELECTED READINGS

Books

Ahlgren J and McDonald J. Gastrointestinal Oncology. Philadelphia, JB Lippincott, 1992.
Ackar E et al (eds). Clinical Gastroenterology, 2nd ed. Philadelphia, Lea & Febiger, 1992.
American Cancer Society. A Cancer Source Book for Nurses, 6th ed. Atlanta, The American Cancer Society, 1991.
Baird SB et al (eds). Cancer Nursing. Philadelphia, WB Saunders, 1991.
Bates B. A Guide to Physical Examination and History Taking, 6th ed. Philadelphia, JB Lippincott, 1995.
DeVita VT et al (eds). Cancer: Principles and Practice of Oncology, 4th ed. Philadelphia, JB Lippincott, 1993.
Groenwald S (ed). Cancer Nursing: Principles and Practices, 3rd ed. Boston, Jones & Bartlett, 1993.
McEvoy GK (ed). AHFS Drug Information. Bethesda, MD, American Society of Hospital Pharmacists, 1993.
Polk HC et al (eds). Basic Surgery, 4th ed. St Louis, Quality Medical Publishing, 1993.
Van Schaik T (ed). Gastroenterology Nursing. St Louis, Mosby-Year Book, 1993.
Yamada T (ed). Atlas of Gastroenterology. Philadelphia, JB Lippincott, 1992.
Yamada T (ed). Textbook of Gastroenterology. Philadelphia, JB Lippincott, 1991.
Zuidema G (ed). Shackelford's Surgery of the Alimentary Tract, 3rd ed. WB Saunders, Philadelphia, 1991.

Journals

Asterisks indicate nursing research articles.

Peptic Ulcers and Gastritis

Berg CL and Wolfe MM. Zollinger-Ellison syndrome. Med Clin North Am 1991 Jul; 75(4):903–921.
Carey J. What Barry Marshall knew in his gut. Science and Technology 1992 Aug; 10:68–69.
Cook DJ et al. Endoscopic therapy for acute nonvariceal upper gastrointestinal hemorrhage: A meta-analysis. Gastroenterology 1992 Jan; 102(1):139–148.
Dye KR et al. Gastritis ulcers and *Helicobacter pylori*. Physician Assist 1991 May; 15(5):95–101.
Esberger KK. Guide to gastrointestinal problems of elders. Geriatr Nurs 1991 Mar–Apr; 12(2):74–75.
Feldman M et al. Treating ulcers and reflux: What's new? Patient Care 1992 Aug 15; 26(13):53–55, 59–64, 67–70.
Frucht H et al. Use of omeprazole in patients with Zollinger-Ellison syndrome. Dig Dis Sci 1992 Apr; 36(4):394–404.
Gervin AG et al. Upper GI bleeding: Treatment options. Patient Care 1991 Jan 30; 25(2):59–62, 68–70, 75–77.

Gilbert G et al. Peptic ulcer disease: How to treat it now. Postgrad Med 1991 Mar; 89(4):91–93, 96, 98.
Handerhan B. Managing patients with stress ulcers. Nursing 1991 Sept; 21(9):77–78, 81.
Holt L et al. Gastroduodenal injury from nonsteroidal anti-inflammatory drugs: Risk management issues. Gastroenterol Nurs 1991 Dec; 14(3):124–126.
Hopkins S. Undermining ulcers. Nursing Times 1992 April 15; 88(16):62–64.
Jaffe BM. Current issues in the management of Zollinger–Ellison syndrome. Surgery 1992 Mar; 111(3):241–243.
Johns J. When the patient has an ulcer . . . peptic ulcers. RN 1991 Nov; 54(11):44–51.
Kandel G. Management of nonvariceal upper GI hemorrhage. Hosp Pract (Off Ed) 1990 Jan 15; 25(1):167–171, 174, 177–184.
Kauvar D and Brandt LJ. Gastrointestinal disorders in the elderly. Pharmacy and Therapeutics 1992 Nov; 17:49–55, 60.
Kauvar D and Brandt LJ. Treatment of common GI disorders in the elderly. Physician Assist 1992 Feb; 16(2):105–108, 111–112, 181.
Keithley JR. Histamine H2-receptor antagonists. Nurs Clin North Am 1991 Jun; 26(2):361–373.
Loogman EA. Therapies for acid peptic disease. Gastroenterol Nurs 1991 Spring; 13(4):198–201.
Marotta RB and Floch MH. Diet and nutrition in ulcer disease. Med Clin North Am 1991 July; 75(4):967–979.
National Institutes of Health. NIH Consensus Statement. *Helicobacter pylori* in peptic ulcer disease. U.S. Dept. of Health and Human Services. 1994 Feb 7–9; 12(1).
Sachdeva AK et al. Surgical treatment of peptic ulcer disease. Med Clin North Am 1991 July; 75(4):999–1012.
Sweeney JP. Assessing the patient undergoing GI endoscopy. Gastroenterol Nurs 1992 Apr; 14(5):266–269.
Wardell TL. Assessing and managing a gastric ulcer. Nursing 1991 Mar; 21(3):34–42.
Williams SG and DiPalma JA. Medication induced digestive system injury in the elderly. Geriatr Nurs 1992 Jan–Feb; 13(1): 39–42.
Wilson V. Action STAT! Complications of thrombolytic therapy. Nursing 1991 Jan; 21(1):41.

Morbid Obesity

Black J and Mangan M. Body contouring and weight loss surgery for obesity. Nurs Clin North Am Sep 1991; 26(3):777–788.
Gastrointestinal surgery for severe obesity: National Institutes of Health Consensus Development Conference Statement. Am J Clin Nutr 1992 Feb; 55(Suppl 2):615S–619S.
Kral JG et al. Assessment of quality of life before and after surgery for severe obesity. Am J Clin Nutr 1992 Feb; 55(Suppl 2):611S–614S.
Kuzmak LI et al. Surgery for morbid obesity. AORN J 1990 May; 51(5):1307–1324.
MacLean LD et al. Results of the surgical treatment of obesity. Am J Surg 1993 Jan; 165(1):155–160.
O'Leary JP. Gastrointestinal malabsorptive procedures. Am J Clin Nutr 1992 Feb; 55(Suppl 2):567S–570S.
Sugerman HJ et al. Gastric bypass for treating severe obesity. Am J Clin Nutr 1992 Feb; 55(Suppl 2):560S–566S.

Gastric Cancer

Hoebler L and Irwin M. Gastrointestinal tract cancer: Current knowledge, medical treatment, and nursing management. Oncol Nurs Forum 1992 Oct; 19(9):1403–1413.
Kiyabu M et al. Effects of preoperative chemotherapy on gastric adenocarcinomas. Cancer 1992 Nov 1; 70(9):2239–2245.
Nakamura K et al. Pathology and prognosis of gastric carcinoma. Findings in 10,000 patients who underwent primary gastrectomy. Cancer 1992 Sep 1; 70(5):1030–1037.
Parsonnet J et al. Helicobacter pylori infection and the risk of gastric carcinoma. N Engl J Med 1991 Oct 17; 325(16):1127–1131.
Talley NJ et al. Gastric adenocarcinoma and *Helicobacter pylori* infection. J Natl Cancer Inst 1991 Dec 4; 83(23):1734–1739.
Wingo PA et al. Cancer statistics, 1995. CA 1995 Jan/Feb; 45(1):8–30.

INFORMATION/RESOURCES

Agencies

American Cancer Society
1599 Clifton Rd, NE,
Atlanta, GA 30329

American Digestive Disease Society
420 Lexington Ave,
New York, NY 10017

American Gastroenterological Association
6900 Grove Rd,
Thorofare, NJ 08086

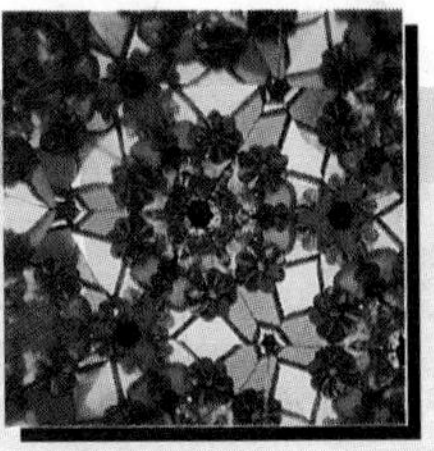

37 Management of Patients With Intestinal and Rectal Disorders

CHAPTER OUTLINE

LEARNING OBJECTIVES

On completion of this chapter, the learner will be able to:

1. Identify the health care teaching needs of patients with constipation and those with diarrhea
2. Use the nursing process as a framework for care of patients with constipation and patients with diarrhea
3. Compare the primary conditions of malabsorption with regard to their pathophysiology, clinical manifestations, and management
4. Use the nursing process as a framework for care of patients with diverticulitis
5. Compare regional enteritis and ulcerative colitis with regard to their pathophysiology, clinical manifestations, diagnostic evaluation, and medical, surgical, and nursing management
6. Use the nursing process as a framework for care of the patient with a chronic inflammatory bowel disease
7. Describe the responsibilities of the nurse in meeting the needs of the patient with a fecal diversion
8. Use the nursing process as a framework for care of the patient with cancer of the colon or rectum
9. Describe the various types of intestinal obstruction and their management
10. Use the nursing process as a framework for care of the patient with an anorectal condition

Suzanne C. Smeltzer and Brenda G. Bare: Brunner and Suddarth's Textbook of Medical-Surgical Nursing, 8th Edition. © 1996 Lippincott-Raven Publishers.

Gastrointestinal (GI) diseases constitute a major health problem, afflicting more than 34 million Americans. About 20 million of them have a chronic disorder and about 2 million are permanently disabled. The number of lives lost annually due to GI disease is 200,000. Gastrointestinal diseases are significant because the majority of the digestive process occurs on the intestinal surface and in the intestinal cell where absorption occurs. The types of diseases and disorders that affect the lower GI tract are many and varied.

In all age groups, a fast-paced life style, high levels of stress, irregular eating habits, insufficient intake of fiber and water, and lack of daily exercise contribute to these problems. Nurses can have an impact on these chronic problems by identifying behavior patterns that put patients at risk, by educating the public about prevention and management, and by helping those afflicted improve their condition and prevent complications.

Abnormalities of Fecal Elimination

Constipation

Constipation refers to an abnormal infrequency of defecation, and also to abnormal hardening of stools that makes their passage difficult and sometimes painful. This type of constipation is referred to as **colonic constipation.**

Most individuals have at least one bowel movement a day. The range of normal, however, extends from three movements per day to three or fewer per week. In persons who are constipated, defecation is irregular and is complicated by hardened stools. Some constipated persons occasionally produce liquid stools as a result of the irritation caused by hard, dry fecal masses in the colon. Such stools contain a good deal of mucus, secreted by glands in the colon in response to these irritating masses.

Constipation can be caused by certain medications (tranquilizers, anticholinergics, antihypertensives, opioids, antacids with aluminum); rectal/anal disorders (hemorrhoids, fissures); obstruction (cancer of the bowel); metabolic, neurologic, and neuromuscular conditions (diabetes mellitus, Parkinsonism, multiple sclerosis); endocrine conditions (hypothyroidism, pheochromocytoma); lead poisoning; and connective tissue disorders (scleroderma, lupus erythematosus). Constipation is a *major* problem for patients taking opioids for chronic pain. Diseases of the colon commonly associated with constipation are irritable bowel syndrome and diverticular disease.

Other causative factors include weakness, immobility, debility, fatigue, and inability to increase intra-abdominal pressure to facilitate the passage of stools, such as occurs with emphysema. Many people develop constipation because they do not take the time to defecate. In the United States constipation is also seen as a result of dietary habits (low consumption of fiber and inadequate fluid intake), lack of regular exercise, and a stress-filled life.

Perceived constipation can also be a problem. This is a subjective problem that occurs (Doughty & Jackson, 1993), when an individual's bowel elimination pattern is not consistent with what the person perceives as normal. Chronic laxative use is attributed to this problem and is a major health concern in the United States, especially among the elderly population.

- Constipation can also occur with acute processes such as appendicitis. Laxatives administered in this instance may produce perforation of the inflamed appendix. In general, a cathartic should not be administered while the patient has fever, nausea, or pain merely because the bowels fail to move. A cathartic should *never* be administered in the presence of inflammatory bowel disease.

Gerontologic Considerations. Elderly persons report problems with constipation five times more frequently than do younger persons. A number of factors contribute to this increased frequency. Persons who have loose-fitting dentures or have lost their teeth have difficulty chewing and frequently choose soft, processed foods that are low in fiber. Convenience foods, also low in fiber, are widely used by those who have lost interest in eating. Some older people reduce their fluid intake if they are not eating regular meals. Lack of exercise and prolonged bed rest also contribute to constipation by decreasing abdominal muscle tone and motility as well as intestinal and anal sphincter tone. Nerve impulses are dulled and there is decreased sensation to defecate. In addition, many older persons who overuse laxatives in an attempt to have a daily bowel movement become dependent upon them.

Pathophysiology. The pathophysiology of constipation is poorly understood. It is believed, however, to be related to interference with one of three major functions of the colon: (1) mucosal transport (mucosal secretions facilitate movement of colon contents), (2) myoelectric activity (mixing of the rectal mass and propulsive actions), or (3) the processes of defecation. The urge to defecate is normally stimulated by rectal distention, which initiates a series of four actions: stimulation of the inhibitory rectoanal reflex, relaxation of the internal sphincter muscle, relaxation of the external sphincter muscle and muscles in the pelvic region, and increased intra-abdominal pressure. Interference with any of these four processes can thus lead to constipation.

When the urge to defecate is ignored, the rectal mucous membrane and musculature become insensitive to the presence of fecal masses, and consequently a stronger stimulus is required to produce the necessary peristaltic rush for defecation. The initial effect of this fecal retention is to produce irritability of the colon, which at this stage frequently goes into spasm, especially after meals, giving rise to colicky midabdominal or low abdominal pains. After several years of this process, the colon loses muscular tone and becomes essentially unresponsive to normal stimuli. Constipation then becomes a problem. Atony of the bowel also occurs with aging, and this can be complicated when laxatives are overused.

Clinical Manifestations. Clinical manifestations include abdominal distention, borborygmus (intestinal rumbling), pain and pressure, decreased appetite, headache, fatigue, indigestion, a sensation of incomplete emptying, straining at stool, and the elimination of small-volume, hard, dry stool.

Diagnostic Evaluation. Diagnosis of constipation is based on a complete physical examination, a barium enema, a sigmoidoscopy, and stool testing for occult blood. These tests are completed to determine whether this symptom is due to spasm or narrowing of the bowel. Anorectal manometry (pressure studies) may be performed to determine malfunction of the muscle and sphincter. Defecography and bowel transit studies can also be completed (see Chapter 33 for discussion of these diagnostic studies). **Idiopathic constipation** is diagnosed only after all organic causes are eliminated.

Management. Treatment is aimed at the underlying cause of constipation. Management includes discontinuing abusive laxative use, recommending the inclusion of fiber in the diet with an increase in fluid intake, and prescribing an exercise routine to strengthen abdominal muscles. Biofeedback is a technique that can be used to help patients learn to relax the sphincter mechanism to expel stool. The daily addition to the diet of 6 to 12 teaspoonfuls of unprocessed bran is recommended, especially for the treatment of constipation in the elderly. Dietary counseling should encourage a high-residue diet to induce rapid movement through the colon and a large, soft stool.

If laxative use is necessary, one of the following may be prescribed: bulk-forming agents, saline and osmotic agents, lubricants, stimulants, or fecal softeners. The physiologic action and patient teaching related to these laxatives are described in Table 37-1. Enemas and rectal suppositories are generally not recommended for constipation and should be reserved for the treatment of impaction or for preparing the bowel for surgery or diagnostic procedures. If long-term laxative use is absolutely necessary, a

TABLE 37-1 Laxatives: Classification, Agent, Action, and Patient Education

Classification	Sample Agent	Action	Patient Education
Bulk-Forming	Psyllium hydrophilic muciloid (Metamucil)	Polysaccharides and cellulose derivatives mix with intestinal fluids, swell, and stimulate peristalsis.	Take with 8 ounces of water and follow with 8 ounces of water. Do not take dry. Report abdominal distention or unusual amount of flatulence.
Saline Agent	Magnesium hydroxide (Milk of Magnesia)	Nonabsorbable magnesium ions alter stool consistency by drawing water into the intestines by osmosis; peristalsis is stimulated. Action occurs within 2 hours.	The liquid preparation is more effective than the tablet form. Only short-term use is recommended because of toxicity (CNS or neuromuscular depression, electrolyte imbalance). Magnesium laxatives should not be taken by patients with renal insufficiency.
Lubricant	Mineral oil	Nonabsorbable hydrocarbons soften fecal matter by lubricating the intestinal mucosa. The passage of stool is facilitated. Action occurs within 6–8 hours.	Do not take with meals because mineral oils may impair the absorption of fat-soluble vitamins and delay gastric emptying. Swallow carefully because drops of oil that gain access to the pharynx may produce a lipid pneumonia.
Stimulant	Bisacodyl (Dulcolax)	Irritates the colon epithelium by stimulating sensory nerve endings and increasing mucosal secretions. Action occurs within 6–8 hours.	Catharsis may cause fluid and electrolyte imbalance, especially in the elderly. Tablets should be swallowed, not crushed or chewed. Avoid milk or antacids within 1 hour of taking the drug because the enteric coating may dissolve prematurely.
Fecal Softener	Dioctyl sodium sulfosuccinate (Colace)	Hydrates the stool by its surfactant action on the colonic epithelium (increases the wetting efficiency of intestinal water). Aqueous and fatty substances are mixed. The medication does not exert a laxative action.	Can be used safely by patients who should avoid straining (cardiac patients, patients with anorectal disorders).
Osmotic Agent	Polyethyleneglycol and electrolytes (Colyte)	Cleanses colon rapidly & induces diarrhea	This is a large volume product. It takes time to consume it safely. It may cause considerable nausea and bloating.

bulk-forming agent may be prescribed in combination with an osmotic laxative.

Specific medication therapy can be used to increase the intrinsic motor function of the intestine. New studies indicate that use of prokinetic agents such as Cisapride can increase stool frequency.

Complications. Complications of constipation include arterial hypertension, fecal impaction, hemorrhoids and fissures, and megacolon.

Increased arterial pressure can occur with defecation. Straining at stool, which results in the Valsalva maneuver (forcibly exhaling with the glottis closed), has a striking effect on the arterial blood pressure. During active straining, the flow of venous blood in the chest is temporarily impeded because of an increase in intrathoracic pressure. This pressure tends to collapse the large veins in the chest. The atria and the ventricles receive less blood, and consequently less is delivered by the systolic contractions of the left ventricle; the cardiac output is decreased, and there is a transient drop in arterial pressure. Almost immediately after this period of hypotension, a rise in arterial pressure occurs; the pressure is elevated momentarily to a point far exceeding the original level (the "rebound" phenomenon). In patients with arterial hypertension, this compensatory reaction may be exaggerated greatly, and the peaks of pressure attained may be dangerously high—sufficient to rupture a major artery in the brain or elsewhere.

Fecal impaction occurs when an accumulated mass of dry feces cannot be expelled. The mass may be palpable on digital examination, may produce pressure on the colon mucosa that results in ulcer formation, and may cause the frequent seepage of liquid stools.

Hemorrhoids and *anal fissures* can develop as a result of constipation. Anal fissures may result from the passage of the hard stool through the anus, tearing the lining of the anal canal. Hemorrhoids develop as a result of perianal vascular congestion caused by straining.

Megacolon is a dilated and atonic colon caused by a fecal mass that obstructs the passage of colon contents. Symptoms include constipation, liquid fecal incontinence, and abdominal distention. Megacolon can lead to perforation of the bowel.

❏ NURSING PROCESS
The Patient With Constipation

Assessment

When talking with patients about their bowel habits, it is important to keep in mind that some people may be embarrassed to discuss such a personal body function. Tact and respect are generally appreciated. Questions of a more personal matter may be asked later after rapport has been established.

A health history is taken to obtain information about the onset and duration of constipation, current and past elimination patterns, and the patient's expectation of normal bowel elimination. Life-style information should be assessed, including exercise and activity level, occupation, nutrition and fluid intake, and stress. Past medical and surgical history, current medication therapy, and laxative and enema use are important. The patient should be questioned about the presence of rectal pressure or fullness, abdominal pain, excess straining at defecation, flatulence, or watery diarrhea.

Objective assessment includes inspecting the stool for color, odor, consistency, size, shape, and components. The abdomen is auscultated for the presence and character of bowel sounds. Abdominal distention is noted. The perineal area is inspected for hemorrhoids, fissures, and skin irritation.

Diagnosis

Nursing Diagnoses

Based on all the assessment data, the patient's major nursing diagnoses may include the following:

- Colonic constipation or fecal impaction related to health habits or the effect of immobility on peristalsis
- Knowledge deficit about health maintenance practices to prevent constipation
- Anxiety related to concern about irregular elimination pattern

Collaborative Problems/ Potential Complications

Based on assessment data, potential complications that may develop include:

- Arterial hypertension
- Fecal impaction
- Anorectal disease (hemorrhoids, anal fissures)
- Megacolon

Planning and Implementation

Goals. The major goals of the patient may include restoration or maintenance of a regular pattern of normal bowel elimination, adequate intake of fluids and high-fiber foods, understanding of methods for avoiding constipation, relief of anxiety about bowel elimination patterns, and the absence of complications.

Nursing Interventions

Maintaining Elimination. Maintaining elimination is basic to the care of every patient. To facilitate elimination, the patient is assisted to assume the normal position for defecation. The semi-squatting position maximizes the use of the abdominal muscles and the force of gravity. Hospitalized patients who cannot use the bathroom experience less strain if assisted to a bedside commode, or if they are seated on a bedpan at the side of the bed with feet supported on a chair. If the patient cannot sit up, a small support should be placed under the lumbosacral curve to minimize strain and increase comfort while the bedpan is used. The frequency and consistency of the stool should be carefully monitored and documented. Setting up a routine schedule for bowel elimination (*e.g.*, after breakfast) may be helpful.

Patient Education and Home Care Considerations. Most of the patient's goals can be achieved through a thorough teaching program that presents information about the causes of constipation and the dietary practices and exercise activity that can promote healthy bowel habits. The patient who has limited activity, whether in the home setting or in an acute care or extended care facility, should be carefully assessed to determine if constipation is a problem. A teaching program that is designed specifically to meet the patient's needs can then be helpful in preventing constipation.

The role of the nurse is to initiate health teaching. The physiology of defecation should be explained carefully, with particular emphasis on the importance of promptly heeding the urge to defecate. The patient is instructed to have a regular time for defecation and to provide adequate time for defecation. The most preferable time is usually after breakfast. Thinking about the act of defecation (*i.e.*, "autosuggestion") may be an aid in initiating the reflex.

The patient must know what constitutes the prescribed diet. In general, a high-residue, high-fiber diet is prescribed. The patient should be aware that the addition of bran daily can markedly increase the number of spontaneous bowel movements and decrease the use of cathartics, stool softeners, and enemas. The patient must understand the need to gradually increase the amount of bran used. Increased fluid intake must also be emphasized (unless contraindicated).

The nurse encourages frequent ambulation and teaches abdominal muscle toning exercises to promote defecation. Abdominal toning exercises consist of contracting abdominal muscles (four times daily) and performing leg-to-chest lifts while sitting in a chair or lying in bed (10–20 times a day). A patient confined to bed is encouraged to perform range-of-motion exercises (6–10 times a day), turn frequently from side to side, and lie prone (if not contraindicated) for 30 minutes every 4 hours. These exercises increase abdominal muscle tone, which helps propel colon contents.

Reducing Anxiety. Patients who worry about having a *daily* bowel movement need reassurance. It is helpful to explain carefully that some healthy persons have a bowel movement three times daily while others do so only two or three times a week. Knowing that some of the food eaten may normally remain in the intestinal tract 48 hours after it is ingested will help the patient to understand and accept the fact that a daily bowel evacuation is not always necessary.

Explaining the preventive measures identified above often reduces the anxiety associated with constipation. A discussion about the concept of normal bowel elimination may also be beneficial.

Monitoring and Managing Potential Complications. The patient is monitored closely for evidence of arterial hypertension related to the Valsalva maneuver and for evidence of anorectal disease. Stool softeners can be administered to decrease the amount of straining necessary. If a fecal impaction is present, mineral oil and saline enemas may be prescribed. The stool may need to be extracted manually. Emergency colectomy may be required if signs and symptoms of megacolon or perforation are present.

Evaluation

Expected Outcomes

1. Establishes a regular pattern of bowel elimination
   a. Includes a time for defecation as part of daily routine
   b. Participates in a regular exercise program
   c. Avoids laxative abuse
   d. Drinks 2 to 3 liters of water daily
   e. Includes foods high in bulk in the diet (fresh fruits, bran, nuts, whole grain breads and cereals, cooked fruits and vegetables)
   f. Reports soft, formed stool every day or every 2 to 3 days
2. Demonstrates understanding of measures appropriate for preventing constipation
   a. Identifies measures that promote defecation
   b. Explains importance of ingesting fluids and foods high in bulk
   c. States the need to heed promptly the urge to defecate
   d. Performs abdominal muscle toning exercises
3. Experiences less anxiety about bowel function
   a. Identifies measures that can be used to prevent or relieve constipation
   b. Explores concerns and questions about normal bowel elimination
   c. Alters life style to promote normal bowel function
   d. Avoids use of laxatives unless prescribed
4. Experiences absence of complications
   a. No signs and symptoms of vascular damage from arterial hypertension related to Valsalva maneuver
   b. No fecal impaction
   c. No evidence of anal fissures or hemorrhoids
   d. No intestinal obstruction related to megacolon

Diarrhea

Diarrhea is a condition in which there is an unusual frequency of bowel movements (more than 3/day), as well as changes in the amount (more than 200 g/day) and consistency (liquid stool). It is usually associated with urgency, perianal discomfort, incontinence, or a combination of these factors. Any condition that causes a change in intestinal secretions, mucosal absorption, or motility can produce diarrhea.

Diarrhea can be acute or chronic in nature. It can be classified as high volume, low volume, secretory, osmotic, or mixed. *High volume* diarrhea exists when there is more than a liter of liquid stool per day. *Low volume* diarrhea exists when there is less than a liter of liquid stool produced per day.

Diarrhea can be caused by certain medications (thyroid hormone replacements, stool softeners and laxatives, antibiotics, chemotherapy, and antacids), tube feedings, metabolic and endocrine disorders (diabetes, Addison's, thyrotoxicosis), and viral/bacterial infectious processes (dysentery, Shigellosis, food poisoning). Other disease processes that are associated with diarrhea are nutritional and malabsorptive disorders (irritable bowel syndrome, ulcerative colitis, regional enteritis, and celiac disease), anal sphincter deficit, Zollinger–Ellison syndrome, paralytic ileus, and intestinal obstruction.

Pathophysiology. *Secretory diarrhea* is usually high volume diarrhea and is caused by an increased production and secretion of water and electrolytes by the intestinal mucosa into the intestinal lumen. *Osmotic diarrhea* occurs when water is pulled into the intestines by the osmotic pressure of nonabsorbed particles, slowing the reabsorption of water. *Mixed diarrhea* is caused by increased peristaltic action of the intestines (usually due to inflammatory bowel disease) and a combination of increased secretion or decreased absorption in the bowel. The physiology of diarrhea related to infection is discussed in Chapter 65.

Clinical Manifestations. The frequency of stool is increased along with the fluid content of the stool. The patient complains of abdominal cramps, distention, intestinal rumbling (borborygmus), anorexia, and thirst. Painful spasmodic contractions of the anus and ineffectual straining (tenesmus) may occur with each defecation.

The diarrhea may be explosive or gradual in nature and onset. Associated symptoms are those directly attributable to the diarrhea, namely, dehydration and weakness.

Watery stools are characteristic of small-bowel disease, whereas loose, semisolid stools are associated more often with disorders of the colon. Voluminous, greasy stools suggest intestinal malabsorption, and the presence of mucus and pus in the stools denotes inflammatory enteritis or colitis. Oil droplets on the toilet water are almost always diagnostic of pancreatic insufficiency. Nocturnal diarrhea may be a manifestation of diabetic neuropathy.

Diagnostic Evaluation. When the cause of the diarrhea is not evident the following diagnostic tests are performed: complete blood count (CBC), chemical profile, urinalysis, and a routine stool examination as well as a stool exam for infectious or parasitic organisms. Proctosigmoidoscopy and barium enema may also be necessary.

Management. Primary medical management is directed at controlling or curing the underlying disease. Certain medications (*e.g.*, prednisone) may reduce the severity of the diarrhea and the disease.

For mild diarrhea, oral fluids are immediately increased and an oral glucose and electrolyte solution may be prescribed to rehydrate the patient. For moderate diarrhea of a noninfectious source, nonspecific medications such as diphenoxylate (Lomotil) and loperamide (Imodium) are also prescribed to decrease motility. Antimicrobial agents are prescribed when an infectious agent has been identified or when the diarrhea is severe.

Intravenous fluid therapy may be necessary for rapid hydration, especially for the very young or the elderly.

Complications. Complications of diarrhea include the potential for cardiac dysrhythmias because of significant fluid and electrolyte loss (especially loss of potassium). Urinary output of less than 30 ml/hour for 2 to 3 consecutive hours as well as muscle weakness, paresthesia, hypotension, anorexia, and drowsiness with a potassium level below 3.0 mEq/L (SI: 3 mmol/L) must be reported. Decreased potassium levels cause cardiac dysrhythmias (atrial and ventricular tachycardia, ventricular fibrillation, and premature ventricular contractions) that can lead to death.

❑ NURSING PROCESS
The Patient With Diarrhea

Assessment

A health history is obtained to identify the onset and pattern of diarrhea as well as the patient's past elimination pattern. Current medication therapy, past medical and surgical history, daily dietary intake, and eating schedules are discussed. Reports of recent exposure to an acute illness or recent travel to another geographic area are important. The patient is also questioned about abdominal cramping and pain, the frequency and urgency of passing stools, the presence of watery or greasy stools, or mucus, pus, or blood in the stool.

Objective assessment includes weighing the patient, assessing for postural hypotension or tachycardia, and inspecting the stool for consistency, odor, and color. Abdominal auscultation reveals the presence and character of bowel sounds. Abdominal distention or tenderness is noted. The mucous membranes and skin are inspected to determine hydration status. The perianal skin is inspected for irritation.

Diagnosis

Nursing Diagnoses

Based on all the assessment data, the patient's major nursing diagnoses may include the following:

- ❑ Diarrhea related to infection, ingestion of irritating foods, or disorder of the bowel
- ❑ Risk for fluid volume deficit related to frequent passage of stools and insufficient fluid intake
- ❑ Anxiety related to frequent, uncontrolled elimination
- ❑ Risk for impaired skin integrity related to the passage of frequent, loose stools

Collaborative Problems/ Potential Complications

Based on the assessment data, a potential complication is:

- ❑ Cardiac dysrhythmia related to electrolyte depletion

Planning and Implementation

Goals. The major goals of the patient may include regaining normal bowel patterns, avoidance of fluid deficit, reduction of anxiety, maintenance of perianal skin integrity, and absence of complications.

Nursing Interventions

Measures to Control Diarrhea. During an episode of acute diarrhea, the patient is encouraged to rest in bed and take liquids and foods that are low in bulk until the acute period subsides. When food intake is tolerated, a bland diet of semisolids and solids is recommended. Caffeine and carbonated beverage intake is limited because these stimulate intestinal motility. Very hot and very cold foods should be avoided. Milk products, fat, whole grain products, fresh fruits, and vegetables may be restricted for several days. Antidiarrheal medications such as diphenoxylate (Lomotil) are administered as prescribed.

Maintaining Fluid Balance. Fluid balance is difficult to maintain during an acute episode of diarrhea because the feces are propelled through the intestines too quickly to allow for water absorption; output exceeds intake. When a patient experiences diarrhea the nurse assesses for dehydration (decreased skin turgor, tachycardia, weak pulse, decreased serum sodium, thirst) and keeps an accurate record of intake and output. Urine specific gravity can be monitored to assess hydration status. The patient is weighed daily. The nurse encourages oral fluid replacement in the form of water, juices, bouillon, and commercial preparations such as Gatorade. Parenteral fluids are administered as prescribed.

- Older persons can quickly become dehydrated and suffer from low potassium levels (hypokalemia) as a result of diarrhea. The older person taking digitalis must be aware of how quickly dehydration and hypokalemia can occur with diarrhea. This person is also instructed to recognize the signs of hypokalemia, because low levels of potassium intensify the action of digitalis, which can lead to digitalis toxicity.

Reducing Anxiety. An opportunity is provided for the patient to express fears and worry about being embarrassed by lack of control over bowel elimination. This fear of embarrassment is often a major concern.

The patient is assisted to identify irritating foods and stressors that precipitate an episode of diarrhea. Eliminating or reducing these factors helps control defecation. The patient is encouraged to be sensitive to body clues that warn of impending urgency (abdominal cramping, hyperactive bowel sounds). Special absorbent underwear, which will protect clothes if there is accidental fecal discharge, may be helpful.

An understanding, tolerant, and relaxed demeanor on the part of the nurse is essential. The patient's efforts to use coping mechanisms are supported and encouraged. Antianxiety medications are administered as prescribed.

Skin Care. The perianal area becomes excoriated because diarrheal stool contains digestive enzymes that can irritate the skin. The nurse instructs the patient to follow a perianal care routine such as the following: wipe or pat the area dry after defecation, cleanse with a mild soap and warm water, pat dry immediately with cotton balls, and apply skin sealants and moisture barriers as needed.

- The older person's skin is very sensitive because of decreased turgor and reduced subcutaneous fat layers.

Preventing Infection. All patients with diarrhea should be treated as potentially infectious until they are proven to be otherwise. Proper precautions, including Universal Precautions, must be taken to prevent the spread of the disease through contaminated hands, clothing, bed linens, and other objects.

Monitoring and Managing Potential Complications. Serum electrolyte levels are monitored daily. Vital signs, including apical pulse and changes in tendon reflexes and muscle strength, are monitored frequently. Electrolyte replacements are administered as prescribed. Evidence of dysrhythmias or a change in the level of consciousness is reported immediately.

Evaluation

Expected Outcomes

1. Reports normal bowel patterns
2. Maintains fluid balance
   a. Takes sufficient fluids orally
   b. Reports absence of fatigue and muscle weakness
   c. Exhibits moist mucous membranes and normal tissue turgor
   d. Has a balanced intake and output
   e. Has normal urine specific gravity
3. Experiences reduced level of anxiety
4. Maintains skin integrity
   a. Keeps skin clean after defecation
   b. Uses lotion or ointment as a skin barrier
5. Experiences absence of complications
   a. Electrolytes remain within a normal range
   b. Vital signs are stable
   c. No dysrhythmias or change in level of consciousness noted

Irritable Bowel Syndrome

Irritable bowel syndrome is one of the most common gastrointestinal problems. It affects 8% to 14% of the population and occurs more frequently in women than in men. While the cause is still unknown, there are various factors frequently associated with the syndrome. These include heredity, psychological stress or illness, diet high in rich and stimulating/irritating foods, alcohol consumption, and smoking.

Pathophysiology. Irritable bowel syndrome results from a functional disorder of intestinal motility. The change in motility may be related to the neurologic regulatory system, infection or irritation, or a vascular or metabolic disturbance. The peristaltic waves are affected at specific segments of the intestine and in the intensity with which they propel the fecal matter forward. There is no evidence of inflammation or tissue changes in the intestinal mucosa.

Clinical Manifestations. The primary symptom is an alteration in bowel patterns—constipation, diarrhea, or a combination of both. This is often accompanied by pain, bloating, and abdominal distention. These symptoms vary in intensity and duration. The abdominal pain is sometimes precipitated by eating and is frequently relieved by defecation.

Diagnostic Evaluation. Stool studies, contrast radiologic studies, and proctoscopy may be performed to rule out other colon diseases. Barium enema and colonoscopy may reveal spasm, distention, and/or mucus accumulation in the intestine (Fig. 37-1). Manometry and electromyography are used to study interluminal pressure changes generated by spasticity.

Management. The goals of treatment include relieving the abdominal pain, controlling the diarrhea and/or constipation, and reducing stress. A diet is prescribed to determine what types of food may be acting as irritants (*e.g.*, beans, caffeinated products, fried foods, alcohol, spicy foods). A well-balanced, high-fiber diet is also prescribed to help control the diarrhea and constipation.

Exercise is planned to assist in reducing anxiety and to increase intestinal motility. Patients often find it helpful to participate in a stress reduction/behavior modification program.

Hydrophylic colloids (bulk) and antidiarrheal agents are prescribed to control the diarrhea and fecal urgency. Antidepressants can assist in treating underlying anxiety and depression. Anticholinergics and calcium channel blockers are prescribed to decrease smooth muscle spasm, decreasing cramping and constipation.

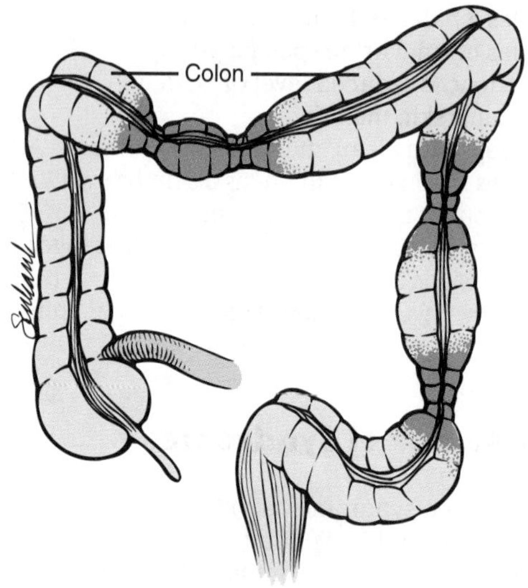

FIGURE 37-1. In irritable bowel syndrome the spastic contractions of the bowel can be seen in x-ray contrast studies.

Nursing Interventions. The nurse's role is to provide patient and family education. Emphasis is placed on teaching and reinforcing good dietary habits. The patient should be encouraged to eat at regular times and to chew food slowly and thoroughly. The patient should understand that although adequate fluid intake is necessary, fluid should not be taken with meals because this results in abdominal distention. Alcohol and cigarette consumption are discouraged.

Conditions of Malabsorption

Interruptions in the complex digestive process may occur anywhere in the digestive system and may cause malabsorption. Malabsorption is the inability of the digestive system to absorb one or more of the major nutrients—carbohydrates, fats, and proteins. Malabsorption occurs when the digestive process has been altered by:

- The inability of nutrients to be readily catabolized and transported (gastric resection, Zollinger–Ellison syndrome, pancreatic insufficiency)
- The decreased absorption of nutrients by the intestinal mucosa (jejunal diverticula, ileal dysfunction, loss of absorptive bowel mucosa through surgical resection)
- A combination of causes (parasitic diseases, Whipple's disease, celiac disease)

In addition to these causes, certain inflammatory bowel disorders, such as ulcerative colitis and regional enteritis (Crohn's disease), cause increased protein breakdown (catabolism) in the small intestine, resulting in a loss of protein into the lumen of the intestine (protein-losing enteropathy).

Pathophysiology. Three primary malabsorption diseases are (1) tropical sprue, (2) adult celiac disease (nontropical sprue, gluten-induced celiac disease), and (3) lactose intolerance. Tropical sprue and adult celiac disease are similar in clinical manifestations and pathologic changes, but differ in their geographic incidence and causes.

In **adult celiac disease,** protein malabsorption is frequently seen as an allergic reaction to gluten, which is found in wheat, rye, oats, and barley. Gluten causes the villi of the mucosa to atrophy, thus restricting their absorptive abilities and causing diarrhea to occur.

Lactose intolerance occurs when there is a deficiency of lactase, a digestive enzyme that breaks down milk sugar (the disaccharide lactose). The resulting high concentration of lactose in the intestines causes an osmotic retention of water, which results in abdominal cramping, nausea, and possibly diarrhea. Fermentation of the lactose in the bowel increases intestinal gas and causes distention.

Short bowel syndrome, a cause of malabsorption syndrome, is the result of massive small bowel resection (70%–80%). It results when the length of the functioning small bowel is insufficient to provide adequate absorption of nutrients and fluids.

Clinical Manifestations. The hallmarks of malabsorption syndrome, from whatever cause, are diarrhea or frequent loose, bulky, foul stools that have increased fat content and are often grayish in color. Associated weakness, weight loss, and lack of well-being are often present. The chief result of malabsorption is malnutrition, manifested by weight loss.

Patients with the malabsorption syndrome, if untreated, become weak and emaciated because of starvation and dehydration. Failure to absorb the fat-soluble vitamins A, D, and K causes these patients to develop a corresponding avitaminosis.

See Table 37-2 for the clinical and pathophysiologic aspects of malabsorption and maldigestion diseases.

Diagnostic Evaluation. Several diagnostic tests may be ordered. Lactulose tolerance tests, xylose absorption tests, and Schilling tests can be diagnostic of certain malabsorption diseases. Biopsy of the small intestine mucosa may be performed to diagnose tropical sprue or celiac sprue. Ultrasound and radiologic testing can reveal pancreatic or intestinal tumors that may be the cause. A complete blood count (CBC) is used to monitor for anemia. Fecal fat analysis will indicate a disorder in the digestion or absorption of fat.

Management. Intervention is aimed at avoiding dietary substances that aggravate malabsorption as well as supplementing nutrients that have been lost. Common supplements are water-soluble vitamins (B_{12}, folic acid); fat-soluble vitamins (A, D, K); and minerals (calcium, iron). Primary disease states may be managed surgically or nonsurgically. Antibiotics are used to treat those diseases involving bacterial overgrowth. Antidiarrheal agents may be used to decrease intestinal spasms. Parenteral fluids may be necessary to treat dehydration.

Nursing Interventions. The nurse provides patient and family education regarding dietary teaching and the use of nutritional supplements. Patients with diarrhea must be monitored for fluid and electrolyte imbalances. Ongoing assessment needs to be conducted to determine if the clinical manifestations related to the nutritional deficits have abated.

Acute Inflammatory Intestinal Disorders

Any part of the lower gastrointestinal tract is susceptible to acute inflammation caused by infection due to bacteria,

TABLE 37-2 Pathophysiologic and Clinical Aspects of Diseases of Malabsorption and Maldigestion

Diseases/Disorders	Physiologic Pathology	Clinical Features
Gastric resection with gastrojejunostomy	Decreased pancreatic stimulation because of duodenal bypass; poor mixing of food, bile, pancreatic enzymes; decreased intrinsic factor, bacterial stasis in afferent loop	Weight loss, moderate steatorrhea, anemia (combination of iron deficiency, vitamin B_{12} malabsorption, folate deficiency)
Pancreatic insufficiency (chronic pancreatitis, pancreatic carcinoma, pancreatic resection, cystic fibrosis)	Reduced intraluminal pancreatic enzyme activity, with maldigestion of lipids and proteins	History of abdominal pain followed by weight loss; marked steatorrhea, azotorrhea; also frequent glucose intolerance (70% in pancreatic insufficiency)
Ileal dysfunction (resection or disease)	Loss of ileal absorbing surface leads to reduced bile-salt pool size and reduced vitamin B_{12} absorption; bile in colon inhibits fluid absorption.	Diarrhea, weight loss with steatorrhea, especially when greater than 100 cm resection, decreased vitamin B_{12} absorption
Stasis syndromes (surgical strictures, blind loops, enteric fistulas, multiple jejunal diverticula, scleroderma)	Overgrowth of intraluminal intestinal bacteria, especially anaerobic organisms, to greater than 10^6/ml, results in deconjugation of bile salts, leading to decreased effective bile-salt pool size, also bacterial utilization of vitamin B_{12}.	Weight loss, steatorrhea; low vitamin B_{12} absorption; may have low D-xylose absorption
Zollinger-Ellison syndrome	Hyperacidity in duodenum inactivates pancreatic enzymes.	Ulcer diathesis, steatorrhea
Lactose intolerance	Deficiency of intestinal lactase results in high concentration of intraluminal lactose with osmotic diarrhea.	Varied degrees of diarrhea and cramps after ingestion of lactose-containing foods; positive lactose intolerance test, decreased intestinal lactase
Celiac disease (gluten enteropathy)	Toxic response to a gluten fraction by surface epithelium results in destruction of absorbing surface.	Weight loss, diarrhea, bloating, anemia (low iron, folate), osteomalacia, steatorrhea, azotorrhea, low D-xylose absorption; folate and iron malabsorption; diagnostic biopsy change
Tropical sprue	Unknown toxic factor results in mucosal inflammation, partial villous atrophy.	Weight loss, diarrhea, anemia (low folate, vitamin B_{12}); steatorrhea; low D-xylose absorption, low vitamin B_{12} absorption; typical but nonspecific biopsy change
Whipple's disease	Bacterial invasion of intestinal mucosa	Arthritis, hyperpigmentation, lymphadenopathy, serous effusions, fever, weight loss; steatorrhea, azotorrhea, diagnostic biopsy change
Certain parasitic diseases (giardiasis, strongyloidiasis, coccidiosis, capillariasis)	Damage to, or invasion of, surface mucosa	Diarrhea, weight loss; steatorrhea; organism may be seen on jejunal biopsy or recovered in stool
Immunoglobulinopathy	Decreased local gut defenses, lymphoid hyperplasia, lymphopenia	Frequent association with *Giardia:* hypogammaglobulinemia or isolated IgA deficiency; diagnostic or typical biopsy changes

(Halsted JA. The Laboratory in Clinical Medicine, Philadelphia, WB Saunders.)

virus, or fungus. Two such situations are appendicitis and diverticulitis. These two conditions can lead to peritonitis, an inflammatory process that can also result from abdominal surgery.

Appendicitis

The appendix is a small, finger-like appendage about 10 cm (4 in) long, attached to the cecum just below the ileocecal valve. The appendix fills with food and empties regularly into the cecum. Because it empties inefficiently, and its lumen is small, the appendix is prone to becoming obstructed and is particularly vulnerable to infection (appendicitis).

Appendicitis, the most common cause of acute inflammation in the right lower quadrant of the abdominal cavity, is the most common reason for emergency abdominal surgery. About 7% of the population will have appendicitis at some time in their lives; males are affected more than females, and teenagers more than adults. Although it can occur at any age, it occurs most frequently between the ages of 10 and 30 years.

Pathophysiology. The appendix becomes inflamed and edematous as a result of becoming either kinked or occluded, possibly by a fecalith (hardened mass of stool), tumor, or foreign body. The inflammatory process increases intraluminal pressure, initiating a progressively severe generalized or upper abdominal pain that, within a few hours, becomes localized in the right lower quadrant of the abdomen. Eventually, the inflamed appendix fills with pus.

Clinical Manifestations. Lower quadrant pain is present and is usually accompanied by a low-grade fever, nausea, and often vomiting. Loss of appetite is common. Local tenderness is noted at **McBurney's point** (Fig. 37-2) when pressure is applied. **Rebound tenderness** (production or intensification of pain when pressure is released) may be present. Just how much tenderness there will be, how much muscle spasm, and whether or not constipation or diarrhea occurs depend not so much on the severity of the appendiceal infection as on the location of the appendix. If the appendix curls around behind the cecum, pain and tenderness may be felt in the lumbar region; if its tip is in the pelvis, these signs may be elicited only on rectal examination. Pain on defecation suggests that the tip of the appendix is resting against the rectum; pain on urination suggests that the tip is near the bladder or impinges on the ureter. Some rigidity of the lower portion of the right rectus muscle may occur.

Rovsing's sign may be elicited by palpating the left lower quadrant (see Fig. 37-2), which, paradoxically, causes pain to be felt in the right lower quadrant. If the appendix has ruptured, the pain becomes more diffuse; abdominal distention develops as a result of paralytic ileus, and the patient's condition worsens.

- In the elderly patient, the signs and symptoms of appendicitis may vary greatly. They may be very vague, suggesting bowel obstruction or another process. The patient may experience no symptoms until the appendix ruptures. The incidence of perforated appendix is higher in the elderly population because many of these patients do not seek health care as quickly as younger patients.

Diagnostic Evaluation. Diagnosis is based on a complete physical examination and lab and x-ray tests. A CBC is performed and will demonstrate an elevated white blood count. The leukocyte count may be greater than 10,000/mm3 and the neutrophil count greater than 75%. Abdominal x-rays and ultrasound studies may reveal a right lower quadrant density or localized air-flow levels.

Management. Surgery is indicated if appendicitis is diagnosed. Antibiotics and IV fluids are administered until surgery is performed. Analgesics can be administered after the diagnosis is made.

An appendectomy (surgical removal of the appendix) is performed as soon as possible to decrease the risk of perforation. The appendectomy may be performed under a general or spinal anesthetic with a low abdominal incision or by laparoscopy, which is a recent, highly effective method.

Complications. The major complication of appendicitis is perforation of the appendix, which can lead to peritonitis or an abscess. The incidence of perforation is 10% to 32%. The incidence is higher in young children and the elderly. Perforation generally occurs 24 hours after the onset of pain. Symptoms include fever of 37.7°C (100°F) or greater, toxic appearance, and continued abdominal pain or tenderness.

Nursing Interventions. Nursing goals include relieving pain, preventing fluid volume deficit, reducing anxiety,

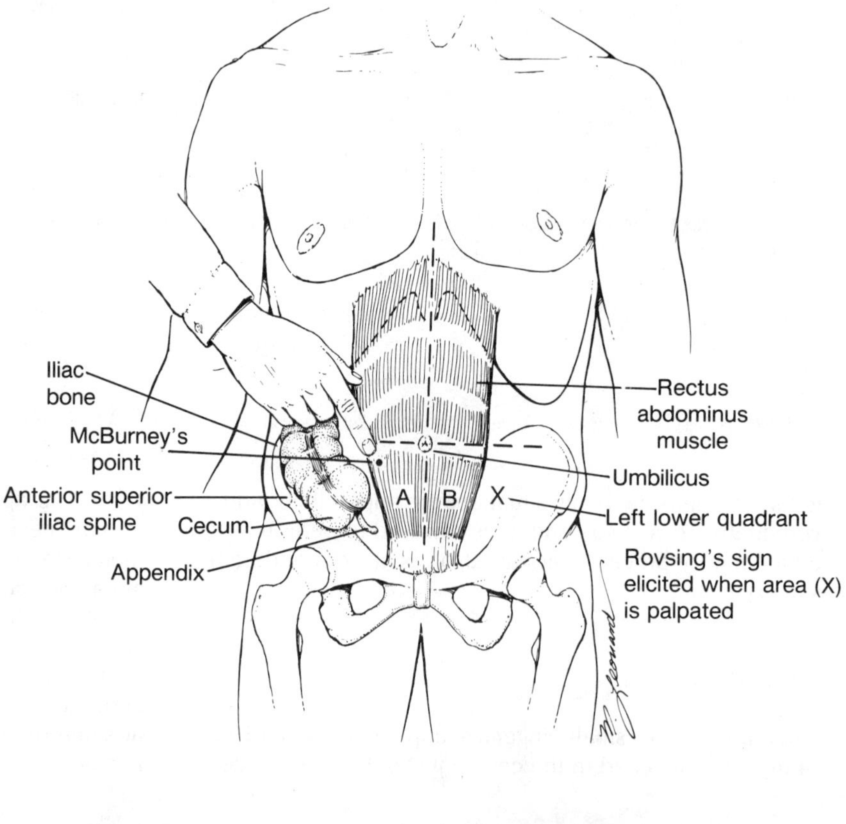

FIGURE 37-2. McBurney's point. When the appendix is inflamed, tenderness can be noted in the right lower quadrant at McBurney's point (*A*), which is between the umbilicus and the anterior superior iliac spine. Rovsing's sign occurs when pain is felt in the right lower quadrant after the left lower quadrant has been palpated (*B*).

eliminating infection due to the potential or actual disruption of the gastrointestinal tract, maintaining skin integrity, and attaining optimum nutrition.

Preoperatively, the nurse prepares the patient for surgery. An intravenous infusion is used to promote adequate renal function and replace existing fluid loss. Aspirin may be prescribed to reduce the elevated temperature. Antibiotic therapy may be administered to prevent infection. If there is evidence or likelihood of paralytic ileus, a nasogastric tube may be inserted. An enema is not administered, as it can lead to perforation.

Postoperatively, the patient is placed in semi-Fowler's position. This position reduces the tension on the incision and abdominal organs, helping to reduce pain. An opioid, usually morphine sulfate, is administered for the relief of pain. Oral fluids are usually administered when they can be tolerated. Any patient who was dehydrated before surgery is given fluids intravenously. Food may be given as desired on the day of surgery if tolerated.

If the appendectomy is uncomplicated, the patient may be discharged on the day of surgery provided the temperature is within normal limits and there is no undue discomfort in the operative area. Discharge teaching for the patient and family is imperative. The patient is instructed to make an appointment to have the surgeon remove the sutures between the fifth and seventh days. Incision care and activity guidelines are discussed. Normal activity can usually be resumed within 2 to 4 weeks.

If there is a possibility of peritonitis, a drain is left in place at the area of the incision. Patients at risk for this complication are kept in the hospital for several days and monitored carefully for signs of intestinal obstruction or secondary hemorrhage. Secondary abscesses may form in the pelvis, under the diaphragm, or in the liver causing an elevation of temperature and pulse rate, with an increase in the leukocyte count.

When the patient is ready for discharge, the patient and family must be taught to care for the wound and perform dressing changes and irrigations as prescribed. A home health nurse may be needed to assist with this care and to monitor the patient for complications and wound healing.

Other potential complications after treatment are identified in Chart 37-1.

Diverticulitis

A **diverticulum** is a saclike outpouching of the lining of the bowel that extends through a defect in the muscle layer. Diverticula may occur anywhere along the gastrointestinal tract.

Diverticulosis exists when multiple diverticula are present without inflammation or symptoms. **Diverticulitis** results when food and bacteria retained in a diverticulum produce infection and inflammation that can impede drainage and lead to perforation or abscess formation. Diverticulitis is most common in the sigmoid colon (95%). It has been estimated that approximately 20% of patients with diverticulosis experience diverticulitis at some point. Diverticulitis is most common in those over 60 years of age. Its incidence is approximately 60% in those over 80 years of age. A congenital predisposition is suspected when the disorder is present in those under 40 years of age. A low intake of dietary fiber is considered a major cause of the disease. Diverticulitis may occur in acute attacks or may persist as a long-continued, smoldering infection.

Pathophysiology. A diverticulum forms when the mucosa and submucosal layers of the colon herniate through

CHART 37-1
Potential Complications Following Appendectomy

Complication	Nursing Assessment and Interventions
Peritonitis	Observe for abdominal tenderness, fever, vomiting, abdominal rigidity, and tachycardia. Employ constant nasogastric suction. Correct dehydration as prescribed. Administer antibiotic agents as prescribed.
Pelvic or lumbar abscess	Evaluate for anorexia, chills, fever, and diaphoresis. Observe for diarrhea, which may indicate pelvic abscess. Prepare patient for rectal examination. Prepare patient for operative drainage procedure.
Subphrenic abscess (abscess under the diaphragm)	Assess patient for chills, fever, and diaphoresis. Prepare for x-ray examination. Prepare for surgical drainage of abscess.
Ileus (paralytic and mechanical)	Assess for bowel sounds. Employ nasogastric intubation and suction. Replace fluids and electrolytes by intravenous route as prescribed. Prepare for surgery, if diagnosis of mechanical ileus is established.

the muscular wall because of high intraluminal pressure, low volume in the colon (fiber-deficient contents), and decreased muscle strength in the colon wall (muscular hypertrophy from hardened fecal masses). A diverticulum can become obstructed and then inflamed if the obstruction continues. The inflammation tends to spread to the surrounding bowel wall, giving rise to irritability and spasticity of the colon. An abscess may develop, leading to peritonitis, and erosion of the blood vessels (arterial) may produce bleeding.

Clinical Manifestations. Constipation often precedes the development of diverticulosis by many years. Signs of acute diverticulosis are bowel irregularity and intervals of diarrhea, dull, crampy pain in the left lower quadrant of the abdomen, and a low-grade fever. Nausea and anorexia may be present. With repeated local inflammation of the diverticula, the large bowel may narrow with fibrotic stricture, leading to cramps, narrow stools, and increased constipation. Occult bleeding may occur, producing iron-deficiency anemia. In addition, weakness and fatigue are evident.

Gerontologic Considerations. The incidence of diverticular disease increases with age because of degeneration and structural changes in the circular muscle layers of the colon as well as cellular hypertrophy. The symptoms are less pronounced in the elderly than in other adults. The elderly may not experience abdominal pain until infection occurs. They may delay reporting symptoms because they fear surgery or are afraid that they may have cancer.

Blood in the stool may frequently be overlooked because of a failure to examine the stool or the inability to see changes because of diminished vision.

Diagnostic Evaluation. Diverticulosis may be diagnosed from x-ray studies such as barium enema that show narrowing of the colon and thickened muscle layers.

- Barium enema is contraindicated in diverticulitis because of the potential for perforation.

An abdominal x-ray may demonstrate free air under the diaphragm if a perforation has occurred from the diverticulitis. A computed tomography (CT) scan can reveal abscesses. A colonoscopy is performed to observe for the diverticula and also to rule out other possible diseases. Laboratory tests that will help in diagnosis are CBC (WBCs will be elevated) and sedimentation rate (which will be elevated).

Management. The bowel is rested by withholding oral intake, administering intravenous fluids, and instituting nasogastric suctioning if vomiting or distention is present. Broad-spectrum antibiotics are prescribed for 7 to 10 days. Meperidine (Demerol) is prescribed for pain relief. (Morphine is not used because it increases segmentation and intraluminal pressures.) Oral intake is increased as symptoms subside. A low-fiber diet may be necessary until signs of infection decrease.

Antispasmodics such as propantheline bromide (Pro-Banthine) and oxyphencyclimine (Daricon) may be prescribed. Normal stools can be achieved by using bulk preparations (Metamucil) or stool softeners (Colace), by instilling warm oil into the rectum, or by inserting an evacuant suppository (Dulcolax). Such a prophylactic plan will reduce the bacterial flora of the bowel, diminish the bulk of the stool, and soften the fecal mass, so that it moves more easily through the area of inflammatory obstruction.

Surgical Management. Although acute diverticulitis usually subsides with medical management, about 25% of the cases require surgical intervention for perforation, peritonitis, abscess formation, hemorrhage, and obstruction.

Two types of surgery are considered: (1) one-stage resection of the involved sigmoid section for recurrent attacks, and (2) multiple-staged procedures for complications, such as obstruction, perforation, and fistulas (Fig. 37-3).

In preparing the patient for surgery, it is important to avoid irritating the colon, which is already sensitive and susceptible to perforation. A mild saline laxative and carefully administered cleansing enemas may be sufficient.

The type of surgery performed varies according to the extent of complications found during surgery. When possible, the area of diverticulitis is resected and the remaining bowel is joined end to end (primary resection and end-to-end anastomosis). A two-stage resection may be performed, in which the diseased colon is resected (as in a one-stage procedure) but no anastomosis is performed. Both ends of the bowel are brought out onto the abdomen as stomas. This "double-barrel" colostomy is then reanastomosed in a later procedure. Fecal diversions are discussed later in this chapter.

Complications. Complications of diverticulitis include peritonitis, abscess formation, and bleeding. If an abscess develops, there is tenderness, a palpable mass, fever, and leukocytosis. An inflamed diverticulum that perforates

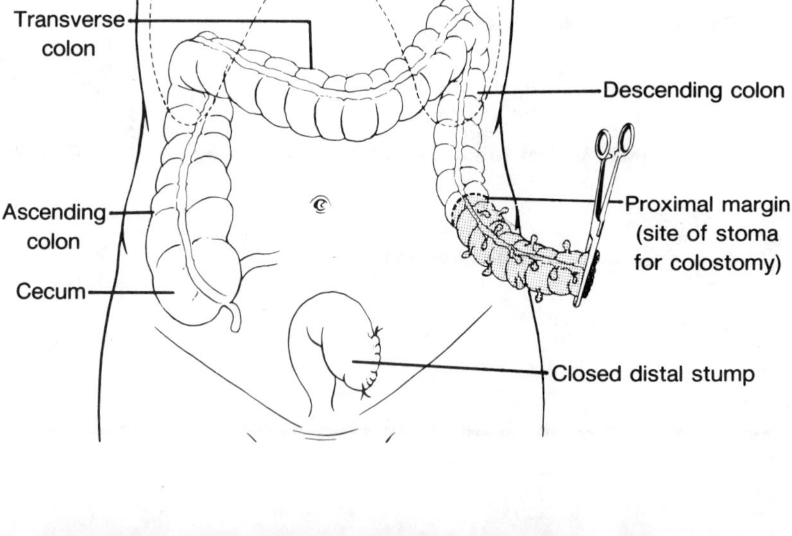

FIGURE 37-3. The Hartmann procedure for diverticulitis: primary resection for diverticulitis of the colon. The affected segment (*shaded*) has been divided at its distal end. If primary anastomosis is to be done, the proximal margin (*dotted line*) is transected, and the bowel is anastomosed end-to-end. If a two-stage procedure will be used, a colostomy is formed at the proximal margin, and the distal stump is oversewn (Hartmann procedure, as shown) or exteriorized as a mucous fistula. The second stage consists of colostomy takedown and anastomosis. (Way LW [ed]. Current Surgical Diagnosis and Treatment, 9th ed. Los Altos, CA, Lange Medical Publishers, 1991.)

results in abdominal pain that is localized over the involved segment, usually the sigmoid; local abscess or peritonitis follows. Abdominal pain, a rigid board-like abdomen, loss of bowel sounds, and signs and symptoms of shock occur with peritonitis. Noninflamed or slightly inflamed diverticula may erode areas adjacent to arterial branches, thus causing massive rectal bleeding.

❑ NURSING PROCESS
The Patient With Diverticulitis

Assessment

During the health history, the patient is queried about the onset and duration of pain as well as past and present elimination patterns. Dietary habits are reviewed to determine fiber intake. The patient should be questioned about straining at stool, presence of constipation with periods of diarrhea, tenesmus (spasms of the anal sphincter with pain and persistent urge to defecate), abdominal bloating, and distention.

Objective assessment includes auscultating for the presence and character of bowel sounds and palpating for lower left quadrant pain, tenderness, or firm mass. The stool is inspected for the presence of pus, mucus, and/or blood. Temperature, pulse, and blood pressure are monitored for abnormal variations.

Diagnosis

Nursing Diagnoses

Based on all the assessment data, the patient's major nursing diagnoses may include the following:

- ❑ Constipation related to narrowing of the colon secondary to thickened muscular segments and strictures
- ❑ Pain related to inflammation and infection
- ❑ Altered gastrointestinal tissue perfusion related to the infection process

Collaborative Problems/ Potential Complications

Based on assessment data, potential complications that may develop include:

- ❑ Peritonitis
- ❑ Abscess formation
- ❑ Bleeding

Planning and Implementation

Goals. The major goals of the patient may include attainment and maintenance of normal elimination, reduction in pain, improvement in gastrointestinal tissue perfusion, and absence of complications.

Nursing Interventions

Maintaining Normal Elimination Patterns. A fluid intake of 2 L/day (within limits of the patient's cardiac reserve) is recommended. Foods that are soft but have increased fiber are suggested to increase the bulk of the stool and to facilitate peristalsis, thereby promoting defecation. An individualized exercise program is encouraged to improve abdominal muscle tone. The patient's daily routine is reviewed to establish a schedule for meals and a set time for defecation. The patient is assisted in identifying habits that may have been used to suppress the urge to defecate. The daily intake of bulk laxatives such as Metamucil, which helps to propel feces through the colon, is encouraged. Stool softeners are administered as prescribed to decrease straining at stool, which in turn decreases intestinal pressure. Oil-retention enemas may be prescribed to soften the stool and decrease inflammation.

Pain Relief. Analgesics (*e.g.*, Demerol) are administered for pain. Antispasmodic agents are administered as prescribed to decrease intestinal spasm. The intensity, duration, and location of pain are recorded to determine if the inflammatory process becomes more severe or subsides.

Improving Gastrointestinal Tissue Perfusion. Vital signs and urine output are monitored for evidence of decreased tissue perfusion. IV fluids are administered to replace volume loss as needed.

Monitoring and Managing Potential Complications. The major nursing focus is to prevent complications by identifying persons at risk and managing their symptoms as needed. The nurse assesses for signs of perforation: an increase in abdominal pain and tenderness accompanied by abdominal rigidity; an elevated white blood cell count; an elevated sedimentation rate; increased temperature; tachycardia; and hypotension. Perforation constitutes a surgical emergency. Clinical manifestations of perforation and peritonitis and care of the patient with peritonitis are presented on pages 922 to 923.

Evaluation

Expected Outcomes

1. Attains a normal pattern of elimination
   a. Reports less abdominal cramping and pain
   b. Reports the passage of soft, formed stool, without pain
   c. Adds unprocessed bran to foods
   d. Drinks at least 10 glasses of fluid a day (if fluid intake is tolerated)
   e. Exercises daily
2. Experiences less pain
   a. Requests analgesics as needed
   b. Adheres to a low-fiber diet during acute episodes
3. Achieves normal gastrointestinal tissue perfusion
   a. Complies with food restrictions
   b. Urine output is adequate
   c. Blood pressure remains normal
4. Experiences absence of complications
   a. Is afebrile
   b. Has a soft, nontender abdomen with normal bowel sounds
   c. Stool is negative for occult blood

Peritonitis

Peritonitis is inflammation of the peritoneum—the serous membrane lining the abdominal cavity and covering the viscera. Usually, it is a result of bacterial infection; the organisms come from disease of the gastrointestinal tract or, in women, from the internal reproductive organs. Peritonitis can also result from external sources such as injury or trauma (*i.e.*, gunshot or stab wound) or by an inflammation that extends from an organ outside the peritoneal area, such as the kidney. The most common bacteria implicated are *E. coli, Klebsiella, Proteus,* and *Pseudomonas.* Inflammation and paralytic ileus are the direct effects of the infection. Other common causes of peritonitis are appendicitis, perforated ulcer, diverticulitis, and bowel perforation (Fig. 37-4). Peritonitis may also be associated with abdominal surgical procedures and peritoneal dialysis.

Pathophysiology. Peritonitis is caused by leakage of contents from abdominal organs into the abdominal cavity usually as a result of inflammation, infection, ischemia, trauma, or tumor perforation. Bacterial proliferation occurs. Edema of the tissues results, and in a short while exudation of fluid develops. Fluid in the peritoneal cavity becomes turbid with increasing amounts of protein, white cells, cellular debris, and blood. The immediate response of the intestinal tract is hypermotility, soon followed by paralytic ileus, with an accumulation of air and fluid in the bowel.

Clinical Manifestations. Symptoms depend on the location and extent of the inflammation. The early clinical manifestations of peritonitis frequently are the symptoms of the disorder causing the condition. At first a diffuse type of pain is felt. The pain tends to become constant, localized, and more intense near the site of the inflammation. It is usually aggravated by movement. The affected area of the abdomen becomes extremely tender, and the muscles become rigid. Rebound tenderness and paralytic ileus may be present. Usually, nausea and vomiting occur and peristalsis is diminished. The temperature and pulse rate increase, and there is almost always an elevation of the leukocyte count.

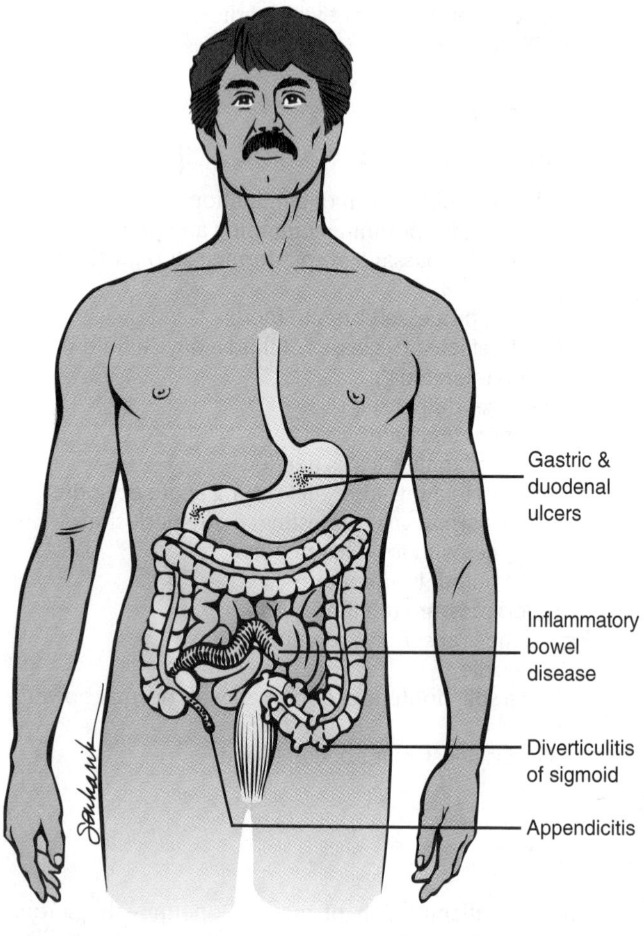

FIGURE 37-4. Common gastrointestinal causes of peritonitis.

Diagnostic Evaluation. The leukocytes will be elevated. The hemoglobin and hematocrit may be low if blood loss has occurred. Serum electrolytes may demonstrate altered levels of potassium, sodium, and chloride.

An abdominal x-ray is obtained and may show air and fluid levels as well as distended bowel loops. A CT scan of the abdomen may show abscess formation. Peritoneal aspiration and culture and sensitivity studies of the aspirated fluid may reveal infection and identify the causative organisms.

Management. Fluid, colloid, and electrolyte replacement is the major focus of medical management. Several liters of an isotonic solution are prescribed. Hypovolemia occurs because massive amounts of fluid and electrolytes move from the intestinal lumen into the peritoneal cavity and deplete the fluid in the vascular space.

Analgesics are prescribed for pain. Antiemetics can be administered as prescribed for nausea and vomiting. Intestinal intubation and suction assist in relieving abdominal distention and in promoting intestinal function. Fluid in the abdominal cavity can cause pressure that restricts expansion of the lungs and causes respiratory distress. Oxygen therapy by nasal cannula or mask will promote adequate oxygenation, but occasionally airway intubation and ventilatory assistance may be required.

Massive antibiotic therapy is usually initiated early in the treatment of peritonitis. Large doses of a broad-spectrum antibiotic are administered intravenously until the organism causing the infection is identified and the specific appropriate antibiotic therapy can be initiated.

Surgical objectives include removing the infected material and correcting the cause. Surgical treatment is directed toward excision (appendix), resection with or without anastomosis (intestine), repair (perforation), and drainage (abscess). With extensive sepsis, a fecal diversion may need to be created.

Complications. Frequently, the inflammation is not localized and the whole abdominal cavity becomes involved in a generalized sepsis. Sepsis is the major cause of death from peritonitis. Shock may result from septicemia or hypovolemia. The inflammatory process may cause intestinal obstruction, which is primarily due to the development of bowel adhesions.

The two most common postoperative complications are wound evisceration and abscess formation. Any suggestion from the patient that an area of the abdomen is tender, painful, or "feels as if something just gave way" must be reported. The sudden occurrence of serosanguineous wound drainage strongly suggests wound dehiscence (see Chapter 21).

Nursing Interventions. Ongoing assessment of pain, vital signs, gastrointestinal function, and fluid and electrolyte balance is important. A description of the nature of the pain, its location in the abdomen, and any shifts in location are reported. Administering analgesic medication and positioning the patient for comfort are helpful in decreasing pain. The patient should be placed on his or her side with knees flexed. This will decrease tension on the abdominal organs.

Accurate recording of all intake and output and central venous pressure assists in calculating fluid replacement. Intravenous fluids must be administered and monitored closely.

Signs that the peritonitis is subsiding include a decrease in temperature and pulse rate, softening of the abdomen, return of peristaltic sounds, passing of flatus, and bowel movements. Fluid and food intake will be gradually increased and parenteral fluids reduced. On the other hand, a worsened clinical condition may indicate a complication and the nurse will need to prepare the patient for emergency surgery.

Drains are frequently inserted during the surgical procedure, and postoperatively it is essential that the nurse observe and record the character of the drainage. Care must be taken when moving and turning the patient to prevent the drains from being dislodged accidentally.

Postoperatively, it is important for the nurse to prepare the patient and family for discharge. They must be taught to care for the incision and drains if the patient will be discharged with the drains still in place.

Chronic Inflammatory Bowel Disease

The term **inflammatory bowel disease** (IBD) is used to designate two chronic inflammatory gastrointestinal disorders: *regional enteritis* (Crohn's disease or granulomatous colitis) and *ulcerative colitis*.

The incidence of chronic inflammatory bowel disease in the United States is estimated to be between 4% and 10%, with 25,000 new cases occurring annually. The disease is seen more frequently in Caucasians and most frequently in the Jewish population. A familial history is found in 20% to 40% of patients.

The current belief is that regional enteritis and ulcerative colitis are separate entities with similar etiologies. Both are characterized by exacerbations and remissions. Neither disease has been associated with a specific chromosomal abnormality. Each disease may be triggered by environmental agents such as pesticides, food additives, tobacco, and radiation. An immunologic influence has been suggested because of studies that show abnormalities in humoral and cell-mediated immunity in people with these disorders. Lymphocytotoxic antibodies have been found in patients with inflammatory bowel disease, but more definitive research is needed to link immunologic and environmental factors. Recent research (Gitnick, 1992) implicates a mycobacterium as the causative agent for these diseases.

A psychologic factor has also been suggested. Many individuals with ulcerative colitis are found to be dependent or passive perfectionists, and anxious to please. Coping behaviors are often inappropriate and can include withdrawal, denial, and repression. Some people have a decreased level of tolerance for the pain and discomfort associated with intestinal cramping and diarrhea. Some clinicians suggest that the personality traits are the cause—not the result—of the disease symptoms, but more clinical research is needed to establish a causal relationship.

Regional Enteritis (Crohn's Disease)

Pathophysiology. Regional enteritis commonly occurs in adolescents or young adults, but can appear at any time of life. It is now seen frequently in the older population (50–80 years). Even though it can occur anywhere along the gastrointestinal tract, the most common areas in which it is found are the distal ileum and colon.

Regional enteritis is a subacute and chronic inflammation that extends through all layers of the bowel wall from the intestinal mucosa; it is therefore transmural. Formation of fistulas, fissures, and abscesses occurs as the inflammation extends into the peritoneum. The lesions (ulcers) are not in continuous contact with one another and are separated by normal tissue. Granulomas occur in half of the cases. In advanced cases the intestinal mucosa has a "cobblestone" appearance. As the disease advances, the bowel wall thickens and becomes fibrotic, and the intestinal lumen narrows.

Clinical Manifestations. With regional enteritis, the onset of symptoms is usually insidious, with prominent abdominal pain and diarrhea that are unrelieved by defecation. Diarrhea is present in 90% of patients. Scar tissue and formation of granulomas interfere with the ability of the intestine to transport products of the upper intestinal digestion through the constricted lumen, resulting in crampy abdominal pains. Because intestinal peristalsis is stimulated by eating food, the crampy pains occur after meals. To avoid these bouts of crampy pain, the patient tends to limit food intake, reducing the amounts and types of food to such a degree that normal nutritional requirements are not met. The result is weight loss, malnutrition, and secondary anemia. In addition, ulcers form in the membranous lining of the intestine and other inflammatory changes take place, resulting in a constant irritating discharge that is emptied into the colon from the weeping, swollen intestine, causing chronic diarrhea. Nutritional deficits may develop because absorption is disrupted. The end result is a person who is thin and emaciated from inadequate food intake and constant fluid loss. In some patients, the inflamed intestine may perforate and form intra-abdominal and anal abscesses. Fever and leukocytosis occur. Abscesses, fistulas, and fissures are common.

The clinical course and symptoms vary. In some patients periods of remission and exacerbation occur, while in others the disease follows a fulminating course.

Symptoms extend beyond the gastrointestinal tract and commonly include joint problems (arthritis), skin lesions (erythema nodosum), ocular disorders (conjunctivitis), and oral ulcers.

Diagnostic Evaluation. The most conclusive diagnostic aid for regional enteritis is a barium study of the upper gastrointestinal tract that shows the classic "string sign" on x-ray of the terminal ileum, indicating the constriction of a segment of intestine. A barium enema may also demonstrate ulceration and "cobblestone" appearance as well as the presence of fissures and fistulas. A CT scan may show bowel wall thickening and fistula tracts.

A proctosigmoidoscopic examination is usually performed initially to determine if the rectosigmoid area is inflamed. A stool examination is also performed and may be positive for occult blood and steatorrhea (excess fat in the feces).

A complete blood count (CBC) is performed to assess hematocrit and hemoglobin levels (which are usually decreased) as well as the WBC (which may be elevated). The sedimentation rate will usually be elevated. Albumin and protein levels may be decreased, indicating malnutrition.

Ulcerative Colitis

Pathophysiology. Ulcerative colitis is a recurrent ulcerative and inflammatory disease of the mucosal layer of the colon and rectum. It most commonly affects Caucasions, including people of Jewish heritage. The peak incidence is 30 to 50 years of age. It is a serious disease, accompanied by systemic complications and a high mortality rate. Eventually 10% to 15% of the patients develop carcinoma of the colon.

Ulcerative colitis affects the superficial mucosa of the colon and is characterized by multiple ulcerations, diffuse inflammations, and desquamation or shedding of the colonic epithelium. Bleeding occurs as a result of the ulcerations. The lesions are continuous, occurring one after the other. The disease process begins in the rectum and eventually may involve the entire colon. Eventually the bowel narrows, shortens, and thickens because of muscular hypertrophy and fat deposits.

Clinical Manifestations. The clinical course is usually one of exacerbations and remissions. The predominant symptoms of ulcerative colitis are diarrhea, abdominal pain, intermittent tenesmus, and rectal bleeding. The bleeding may be mild or severe. In addition, anorexia, weight loss, fever, vomiting, and dehydration may be evident, as well as cramping and the feeling of an urgent need to defecate. The patient may report passing 10 to 20 liquid stools daily. Hypocalcemia and anemia frequently develop. Rebound tenderness may occur in the right lower quadrant.

Other symptoms include skin lesions (erythema nodosum), eye lesions (uveitis), joint abnormalities (arthritis), and liver disease.

Diagnostic Evaluation. In the diagnosis of chronic ulcerative colitis, careful stool examination is performed to rule out dysentery caused by common intestinal organisms, especially *Entamoeba histolytica.* The stool is positive for blood. Laboratory tests will reveal a low hematocrit and hemoglobin, an elevated WBC, low albumin, and electrolyte imbalance. Sigmoidoscopy and barium enema are valuable in distinguishing this condition from other diseases of the colon with similar symptoms. A barium enema will show mucosal irregularities, shortening of the colon, and dilation of bowel loops. Endoscopy may demonstrate friable, inflamed mucosa with exudate and ulcerations.

- In acute ulcerative colitis, cathartics are contraindicated when the patient is being prepared for barium enema or endoscopy because they may exacerbate the condition, which may lead to megacolon (excessive dilation of the colon), perforation, and death.
- If the patient is required to have these diagnostic tests, a liquid diet for a few days before the x-ray and a gentle tap water enema on the day of examination may be prescribed. Colonoscopy is contraindicated in severe disease because of risk of perforation.

Medical Management of Chronic Inflammatory Bowel Disorders

Medical treatment for both regional enteritis and ulcerative colitis is aimed at reducing inflammation, suppressing inappropriate immune responses, and providing rest for a diseased bowel, so that healing may take place. (See Table 37-3 for a comparison of regional enteritis and ulcerative colitis.)

Diet and Fluid Intake. Oral fluids and a low-residue, high-protein, high-calorie diet with supplemental vitamin therapy and iron replacement are prescribed to meet nutritional needs. Fluid and electrolyte imbalance due to dehydration caused by diarrhea is corrected by intravenous therapy as necessary. Any foods that exacerbate diarrhea are avoided. Milk may contribute to diarrhea in those with lactose intolerance. In addition, cold foods are avoided, along with smoking, because both increase intestinal motility. Total parenteral nutrition may be indicated.

Medication Therapies. Sedative and antidiarrheal/antiperistaltic medications are used to reduce peristalsis to a minimum to rest the inflamed bowel. They are continued until the patient's stools approach normal frequency and consistency. Sulfonamides such as sulfasalazine (Azulfidine) or sulfisoxazole (Gantrisin) are often effective for mild or moderate inflammation. Antibiotics are used for secondary infections, particularly for purulent complications such as abscesses, perforation, and peritonitis. Azulfidine is helpful in preventing recurrences.

Parenteral adrenocorticotropic hormone (ACTH) and corticosteroids are effective in the treatment of acute inflammatory bowel disease. When corticosteroids are reduced or stopped, the symptoms of disease may return. If corticosteroids are continued, adverse sequelae such as hypertension, fluid retention, cataracts, hirsutism (abnormal hair growth), and adrenal suppression may develop.

New topical and oral aminosalicylates (*e.g.*, mesalamine [Asacol], olsalazine [Dipentum]) have been shown to be very effective in treatment. Immunosuppressive agents are also used; these agents help to prevent relapses and they allow the patient to receive lower doses of corticosteroids for shorter periods of time.

Psychotherapy is aimed at determining the factors that distress the patient, dealing with these factors, and attempting to resolve conflicts so that they no longer aggravate the patient's condition.

Complications. Complications of *regional enteritis* include intestinal obstruction or stricture formation, perianal disease, fluid and electrolyte imbalance, malnutrition from malabsorption, and fistula and abscess formation. A fistula is an abnormal communication between two body structures, either internal (between two structures) or external (between an internal structure and the outside surface of the body). The most common type of small bowel fistula that results from regional enteritis is the enterocutaneous fistula (between the small bowel and the skin). Abscesses

TABLE 37-3 Comparison of Regional Enteritis and Ulcerative Colitis

	Regional Enteritis	Ulcerative Colitis
Course	Prolonged, variable	Exacerbations, remissions
Pathology		
Early	Transmural thickening	Mucosal ulceration
Late	Deep, penetrating granulomas	Mucosal minute ulceration
Clinical Manifestations		
Location	Ileum, right colon (usually)	Rectum, left colon
Bleeding	Usually not, but may occur	Common—severe
Perianal involvement	Common	Rare—mild
Fistulas	Common	Rare
Rectal involvement	About 20%	Almost 100%
Diarrhea	Less severe	Severe
Diagnostic Study Findings		
X-ray	Regional, discontinuous lesions	Diffuse involvement
	Narrowing of colon	No narrowing of colon
	Thickening of bowel wall	No mucosal edema
	Mucosal edema	Stenosis rare
	Stenosis, fistulas	Shortening of colon
Sigmoidoscopy	May be unremarkable unless accompanied by perianal fistulas	Abnormal inflammed mucosa
Colonoscopy	Distinct ulcerations separated by relatively normal mucosa in right colon	Friable mucosa with pseudopolyps or ulcers in left colon
Therapeutic Management		
	Corticosteroids, sulfonamides (Sulfasalazine [Azulfidine])	Corticosteroids, sulfonamides; Azulfidine is useful in preventing recurrence
	Antibiotics	Bulk, hydrophylic agents
	Total parenteral nutrition	Antibiotics
	Partial or complete colectomy, with ileostomy or anastomosis	Proctocolectomy, with ileostomy
	Rectum can be preserved in some patients.	Rectum can be preserved in only a few patients "cured" by colectomy.
	Recurrence common	
Systemic Complications		
	Small bowel obstruction	Toxic megacolon
		Perforation
		Hemorrhage
		Malignant neoplasms
	Right-sided hydronephrosis	Pyelonephritis
	Nephrolithiasis	Same
	Cholelithiasis	Cholangiocarcinoma
	Arthritis	Same
	Retinitis, iritis	Same
	Erythema nodosum	Same

can be the result of an internal fistula tract into an area that results in fluid accumulation and infection.

Complications of *ulcerative colitis* include perforation and bleeding as a result of ulceration, vascular engorgement, and highly vascular granulation tissue.

For many patients surgery becomes necessary to relieve the effects of the disease and to avoid more serious complications. Usually an ileostomy is performed. The surgical procedures involved and the care of patients with this type of fecal diversion are discussed on pages 928 to 936.

NURSING PROCESS
The Patient With Chronic Inflammatory Bowel Disease

Assessment

A health history is taken to identify the onset, duration, and characteristics of abdominal pain; the presence of diarrhea or fecal urgency, straining at stool (tenesmus), nausea, anorexia, or weight loss; and family history of inflammatory bowel disease. Dietary patterns are discussed including the amounts of alcohol, caffeine, and nicotine used daily and weekly. Patterns of bowel elimination are assessed including character, frequency, and presence of blood, pus, fat, or mucus. Allergies are important to document, especially milk or lactose intolerance. The patient may indicate sleep pattern disturbances if diarrhea or pain occur at night.

Objective assessment includes auscultating the abdomen for bowel sounds and their characteristics; palpating the abdomen for distention, tenderness, or pain; and inspecting the skin for evidence of fistula tracts or symptoms of dehydration. The stool is inspected for blood and mucus.

With regional enteritis, pain is usually localized in the right lower quadrant where hyperactive bowel sounds can be heard because of borborygmus (gurgling bowel sounds caused by passage of gas through the intestine) and increased peristalsis. Abdominal tenderness is noted on palpation. The most prominent symptom is intermittent pain that occurs with diarrhea but does not decrease after defecation. Pain in the periumbilical region usually indicates involvement of the terminal ileum. With ulcerative colitis, the abdomen may be distended and rebound tenderness may be present. Rectal bleeding is a dominant sign.

Diagnosis

Nursing Diagnoses

Based on all the assessment data, the patient's major nursing diagnoses may include the following:

- Diarrhea related to the inflammatory process
- Abdominal pain, related to increased peristalsis and inflammation
- Fluid volume and electrolyte deficits related to anorexia, nausea, and diarrhea
- Altered nutrition, less than body requirements, related to dietary restrictions, nausea, and malabsorption
- Activity intolerance related to fatigue
- Anxiety related to impending surgery
- Ineffective individual coping related to repeated episodes of diarrhea
- Risk for impaired skin integrity related to malnutrition and diarrhea
- Knowledge deficit concerning the process and management of the disease

Collaborative Problems/ Potential Complications

Based on assessment data, potential complications that may develop include:

- Cardiac dysrhythmia related to electrolyte depletion
- GI bleeding with fluid volume loss
- Perforation of the bowel

Planning and Implementation

Goals. The major goals of the patient include attainment of normal bowel elimination, relief of abdominal pain and cramping, prevention of fluid volume deficit, maintenance of optimal nutrition and weight, avoidance of fatigue, reduction of anxiety, effective coping, prevention of skin breakdown, acquisition of knowledge and understanding of the disease process and therapeutic regimen, and absence of complications.

Nursing Interventions

Maintaining Normal Elimination Patterns. The nurse determines if there is a relationship between diarrhea and certain foods, activity, or emotional stress. Any precipitating factors are identified, as well as the frequency of bowel movements and the character, consistency, and amount of stool passed. Ready access to a bathroom or bedpan is provided, and the environment is kept clean and odor free. Antidiarrheal medications are administered as prescribed, and the frequency and consistency of stools are recorded after therapy is initiated. Bed rest is encouraged to decrease peristalsis.

Relieving Pain. The character of the pain is described as dull, burning, or cramplike. Its onset is relevant: Does it occur before or after meals, during the night, or before elimination? Is the pattern constant or intermittent? Is it relieved with medications?

Anticholinergic medications are administered as prescribed 30 minutes before a meal to decrease intestinal motility, and analgesics are administered as prescribed for pain. Pain can also be reduced by position changes, the local application of heat (as prescribed), diversional activities, and the prevention of fatigue.

Maintaining Fluid Intake. To detect fluid volume deficit, an accurate record of oral and intravenous fluids is kept as well as a record of output (urine, liquid stool, vomitus, wound or fistula drainage). Daily weights are monitored because they indicate rapid fluid gains or losses. The patient is assessed for signs of fluid volume deficit: dry skin and mucous membranes, decreased skin turgor, oliguria, exhaustion, decreased temperature, increased hematocrit, elevated urine specific gravity, and hypotension. Oral intake of fluids is encouraged, and intravenous flow rate is monitored. Measures to decrease diarrhea are initiated: dietary restrictions, stress reduction, and administration of antidiarrheal agents.

Nutritional Measures. Total parenteral nutrition (TPN) is used when the symptoms of inflammatory bowel disease are severe. With TPN, the nurse maintains an accurate record of fluid intake and output as well as the patient's daily weight. The patient should gain 0.5 kg daily during therapy. The urine is tested for glucose, acetone, and specific gravity daily when TPN is being used. Elemental feedings that are high in protein and low in fat and residue are instituted after TPN therapy because they are digested primarily in the jejunum, do not stimulate intestinal secretions, and allow the bowel to rest. Intolerance is noted if the patient exhibits nausea, vomiting, diarrhea, or abdominal distention.

If oral foods are tolerated, small, frequent, low-residue feedings are given to avoid overdistending the stomach and stimulating peristalsis. Activities are restricted to conserve energy, reduce peristalsis, and reduce calorie requirements.

Promoting Rest. Intermittent rest periods during the day are recommended and activities are scheduled and/or restricted to conserve energy and reduce the metabolic rate. Activity within the limit of the patient's capacity is encouraged. Bed rest is suggested for a patient who is febrile, has frequent diarrheal stools, or is bleeding. The patient on bed rest is encouraged to perform active and passive exercises to maintain muscle tone and prevent thromboembolic complications. Activity restrictions are modified as needed on a day-to-day basis.

Reducing Anxiety. Rapport can be established by being attentive and displaying a calm, confident manner. Time is provided for the patient to ask questions and express feelings. Careful listening and sensitivity to nonverbal indicators of anxiety (restlessness, tense facial expressions) are helpful. The patient may be emotionally labile because of the consequences of the disease, so information about impending surgery should be tailored to the patient's level of understanding and desire for detail. Some persons need to know everything to lessen their anxiety, whereas others want to know very little. Pictures and illustrations help to explain the surgical procedure and assist the patient to visualize what a stoma looks like.

Coping Measures. Because the patient may feel isolated, helpless, and out of control, understanding and emotional support are essential. The patient may respond to stress in a variety of ways that may alienate others, including anger, denial, and social self-isolation.

The nurse needs to recognize that the patient's behavior may be affected by innumerable factors unrelated to inherent emotional characteristics. Any patient who is suffering from the discomforts of frequent bowel movements and rectal soreness is anxious, discouraged, and depressed. Thus, it is important to develop a relationship with the patient that supports all attempts to deal with these stresses. It is important to communicate that the patient's feelings are understood: the patient is encouraged to talk and ventilate feelings, and to discuss any disturbing matters. Attention is directed to the patient rather than to the intestinal tract. Stress-reduction measures that may be used include relaxation techniques, breathing exercises, and biofeedback.

Professional counseling may be needed to help the patient and family deal with issues associated with chronic illness.

Preventing Skin Breakdown. The patient's skin should be examined frequently, especially the perianal skin. Perianal care, including use of a skin barrier, is provided after each bowel movement. Reddened or irritated areas over bony prominences must be given immediate attention. Pressure-relieving devices should be used to avoid possible skin breakdown. Consultation with a wound care specialist or enterostomal therapist is often helpful.

Patient Education and Home Care Considerations. The patient's understanding of the disease process and need for additional information about medical management (medications, diet) and surgical interventions are assessed.

Information about nutritional management is provided. A bland, low-residue, high-protein, high-calorie, and high-vitamin diet relieves symptoms and decreases diarrhea. The rationale for the use of corticosteroids, anti-inflammatory agents, antibacterial and antidiarrheal medications, and antispasmodics is provided. The importance of taking medications as prescribed and not abruptly discontinuing them (especially the corticosteroids) is emphasized as serious medical problems may result.

If surgery is required, the nurse explains the procedure and the preoperative and postoperative care. Ileostomy care is reviewed as necessary.

Patients who are being medically managed at home need to understand that their disease can be controlled and that they can lead a healthy life between exacerbations. Control implies management based on an understanding of inflammatory bowel disease and its treatment.

During a flare-up, patients are encouraged to rest as needed and modify activities according to energy levels. They are advised to limit tasks that impose strain on the lower abdominal muscles. Patients should sleep in a room close to the bathroom because of the frequent diarrhea (10 to 20 a day). Quick access to a toilet helps alleviate the worry of embarrassment if an accident occurs. Room deodorizers help control odors.

Patients in the home setting need information about their medications (name, dosage, side effects, frequency of administration) and need to take medications on schedule. Medication reminders are helpful (containers that separate pills according to day and time, daily checklists).

Dietary modifications can control but not cure the disease. A low-residue, high-protein, high-calorie diet is recommended, especially during an acute phase. Patients are encouraged to keep a record of those foods that irritate the bowel and to eliminate them from their diet. Fluid intake of at least 8 glasses of water per day is encouraged.

The prolonged nature of the disease often strains family life and financial resources. Family support is vital; however, some family members experience resentment, guilt, fatigue, and an inability to continue coping with the emotional demands of the illness as well as with the physical demands of caring for another.

Some persons will not socialize for fear of being embarrassed. Many prefer to eat alone. Because they have lost control over elimination they may fear losing control over other aspects of their life. They need time to ventilate their fears and frustrations.

Information that can be used for patient education can be obtained from the National Foundation for Ileitis and Colitis.

Monitoring and Managing Potential Complications. Serum electrolyte levels are monitored daily. Evidence of dysrhythmias or change in level of consciousness is reported immediately. Electrolyte replacements are administered as prescribed.

Rectal bleeding is monitored closely. Blood component therapy and volume expanders are administered as prescribed to prevent hypovolemia. The blood pressure is monitored for hypotension. Coagulation and hematocrit and hemoglobin profiles will be performed frequently. Vitamin K may be prescribed to increase clotting factors.

The patient must be monitored closely for indications of perforation (acute increase in abdominal pain, rigid abdomen, vomiting, or hypotension).

Evaluation

Expected Outcomes

1. Reports a decrease in the frequency of diarrheal stools
   a. Complies with dietary restrictions; maintains bed rest
   b. Takes medications as prescribed
2. Experiences less pain
3. Maintains fluid volume balance
   a. Drinks 1 to 2 liters of oral fluids daily
   b. Has a normal body temperature
   c. Displays adequate skin turgor and moist mucous membranes
4. Attains optimal nutrition—tolerates small, frequent feedings without diarrhea
5. Avoids episodes of fatigue
   a. Rests periodically during the day
   b. Adheres to activity restrictions
6. Experiences less anxiety
7. Copes successfully with diagnosis
   a. Ventilates feelings freely
   b. Uses appropriate stress-reduction behaviors
8. Maintains skin integrity
   a. Cleans perianal skin after defecation
   b. Uses lotion or ointment as skin barrier
9. Acquires an understanding of the disease process
   a. Modifies diet appropriately to decrease diarrhea
   b. Adheres to medication regimen
10. Experiences absence of complications
    a. Electrolytes are within normal range
    b. No dysrhythmias noted
    c. Fluid volume is maintained
    d. No evidence of perforation or rectal bleeding

Surgical Management of Chronic Inflammatory Bowel Disorders

When conservative measures fail to relieve the severe symptoms of inflammatory bowel disease, surgery may be recommended. A more recent technique that can be helpful is stricture plasty, in which the blocked or narrowed section of the bowel is widened, leaving the bowel intact.

If a lesion can be delineated in regional enteritis, or if a complication has occurred, it is resected and the remaining portions of the bowel are anastomosed. Surgical removal of up to 50% of the small bowel can usually be tolerated. The surgical procedures of choice are the following:

- Total colectomy (excision of the entire colon) with ileostomy
- Segmental colectomy (removal of a segment of the colon) with anastomosis (joining of the remaining portions of the colon)
- Subtotal colectomy (removal of nearly all of the colon) with ileorectal anastomosis (joining of the ileum and rectum)
- Total colectomy with continent ileostomy (formation of internal pouch)
- Total colectomy with ileoanal anastomosis (formation of a pouch with the anal sphincter intact)

The rate of recurrence after surgery is 20% to 40% in the first 5 years. Patients under 25 years of age have the highest recurrence rate.

Approximately 15% to 20% of the patients with ulcerative colitis require surgical intervention. Indications for surgery include lack of improvement and continued deterioration, profuse bleeding, perforation, stricture formation, and indications that carcinoma has developed. The procedure of choice is a total colectomy and ileostomy; any procedure more limited will prove to be of only temporary benefit in most patients. A proctocolectomy (complete excision of colon, rectum, and anus) is recommended when the rectum is severely involved.

Types of Fecal Diversions

An **ileostomy** is the surgical creation of an opening into the ileum or small intestines usually by means of an ileal stoma on the abdominal wall. It allows for drainage of fecal matter (effluent) from the ileum to the outside of the body. The drainage is very mushy and occurs at frequent intervals. The ileostomy may be temporary or permanent. A permanent ileostomy is created after a total colectomy.

Another procedure is the **continent ileal reservoir** (Kock's pouch). This procedure eliminates the need for an external fecal collection bag. Approximately 30 cm of the distal ileum is reconstructed to form a reservoir with a nipple valve that is created by pulling a portion of the terminal ileal loop back into the ileum (Fig. 37-5*A*). Gastrointestinal effluent (fecal matter) can accumulate in the pouch for several hours and then be removed by means of a catheter inserted through the nipple valve. The major problem with the Kock's pouch is malfunction of the nipple valve, which occurs in 20% to 40% of the patients.

An **ileoanal anastomosis** is another surgical procedure that eliminates the permanent ileostomy. It establishes an ileal reservoir and retains anal sphincter control of elimination. The procedure involves connecting a portion of the ileum to the anus (ileoanal anastomosis) in conjunction with removal of the colon and the rectal mucosa (a total abdominal colectomy and a mucosal proctectomy) (see Fig. 37-5*F*). A temporary diverting-loop ileostomy is constructed at the time of surgery and closed about 3 months later.

With ileoanal anastomosis, the diseased colon and rectum are removed, voluntary defecation is maintained, and anal continence is preserved. The ileal reservoir decreases the number of bowel movements by 50%, from approximately 14 to 20 per day to 7 to 10 per day. Nighttime elimination is gradually reduced to one bowel movement. Complications of ileoanal anastomosis include irritation of the perianal skin from leakage of fecal contents, stricture formation at the anastomosis site, and small bowel obstruction.

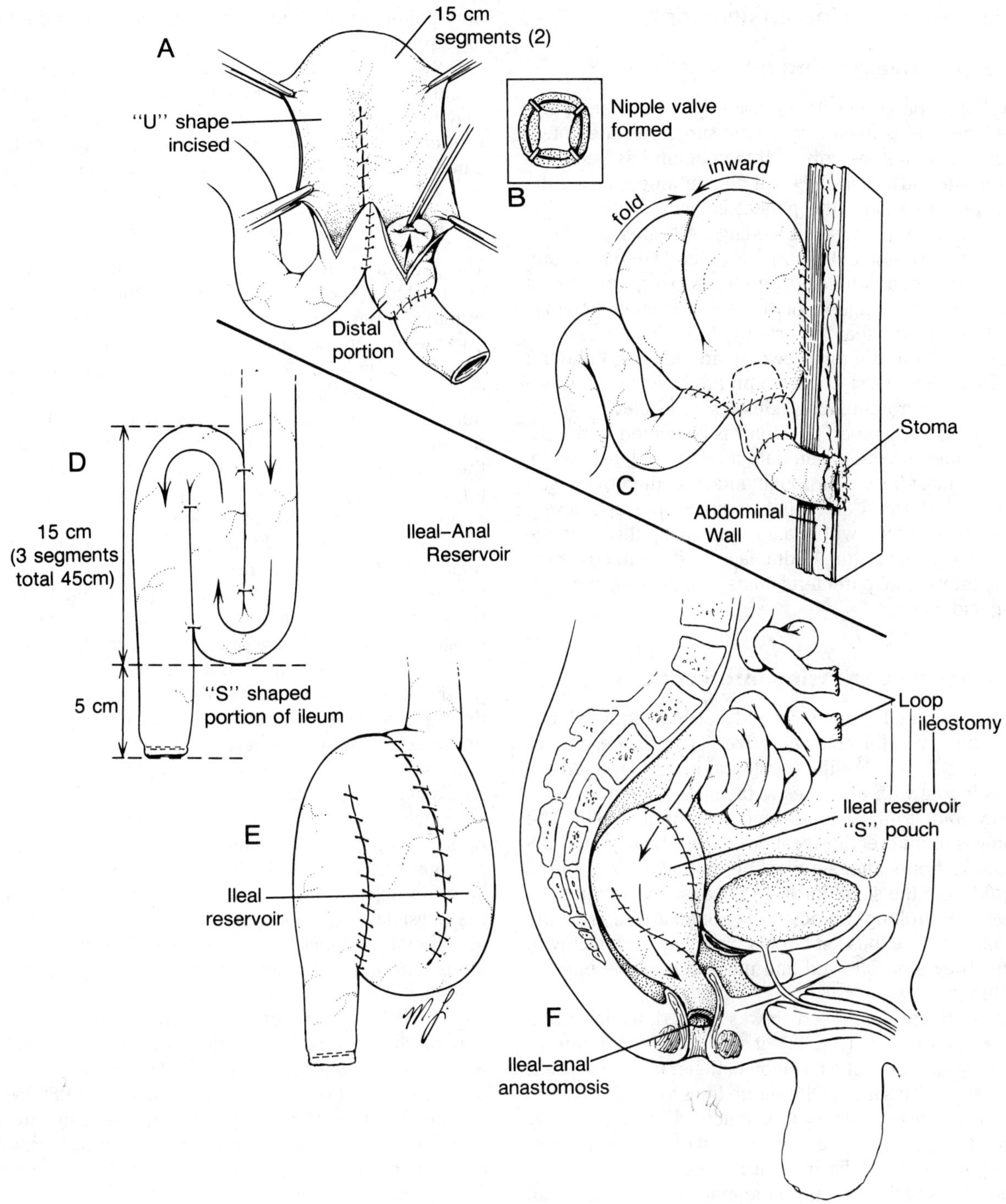

FIGURE 37-5. An ileal reservoir for the Kock pouch and for an ileoanal anastomosis. *For the Kock pouch:* (**A**) A 30-cm portion of the ileum is sutured together to form a U shape. It is then excised open and the distal portion is pulled back into the ileum (similar to intussusception). (**B**) A nipple value is formed by suturing the pulled-back portion of the intestine to itself. (**C**) The top of the ileum is folded onto itself and a stoma is formed from the distal portion. *For the ileoanal anastomosis:* (**D**) A 50-cm portion of the distal ileum is aligned in an S shape. (**E**) The bowel is opened along the antimesenteric surface, and then adjacent walls are anastomosed to create a reservoir. (**F**) A mucosal proctectomy precedes anastomosis of the ileal reservoir. A temporary loop ileostomy diverts effluent discharge for several months.

The Patient Requiring an Ileostomy

Preoperative Nursing Interventions

A period of preparation with intensive fluid, blood, and protein replacement is necessary before surgery is attempted. Antibiotics may be prescribed. If the patient has been taking corticosteroids, then they will be continued during the surgical phase. Usually, the patient is given a low-residue diet offered in frequent small feedings. All other preoperative measures are similar to those for general abdominal surgery. The abdomen is marked for the proper placement of the stoma by the surgeon or the enterostomal therapist. Care is taken to see that the ostomy stoma is conveniently placed—usually in the right lower quadrant (RLQ) about 2 inches below the waist crease in an area away from previous scars, bony prominences, skinfolds, or fistulae.

Information about an ileostomy is presented to the patient by means of written materials, models, and discussion. The patient must have a thorough understanding of the surgery to be performed and what to expect postoperatively. Preoperative teaching will relate to managing the drainage from the stoma, the nature of drainage, and the need for nasogastric intubation, parenteral fluids, and possibly perineal packing and care.

Postoperative Nursing Interventions

General abdominal surgery wound care is required. The stoma is observed for color and size. It should be pink to bright red and shiny. For the traditional ileostomy, a temporary plastic bag with an adhesive facing is placed over the ileostomy and firmly pressed onto surrounding skin. The ileostomy is monitored for fecal drainage, which should begin about 72 hours after surgery. The drainage is a continuous liquid from the small intestine because the stoma does not have a controlling sphincter. The contents drain into the plastic bag and are thus kept from coming into contact with the skin. They are collected and measured as the bag becomes full.

If a continent ileal reservoir was created, as described for the Kock's pouch (p. 928), it will require continuous drainage by an indwelling reservoir catheter for 2 to 3 weeks postoperatively. This allows the suture lines to heal.

Because these patients lose much fluid in the early postoperative period, an accurate record of fluid intake, urinary output, and fecal discharge is necessary to help gauge the fluid needs of the patient. There may be 1000 to 2000 ml of fluid lost each day. With this loss, sodium and potassium are depleted. Laboratory values must be monitored and electrolyte replacements administered as prescribed. Fluids are given intravenously to replace fluid losses for 4 to 5 days.

Nasogastric (NG) suction is also a part of immediate postoperative care, with the tube requiring frequent irrigation, as prescribed. The purpose of nasogastric suction is to prevent a buildup of gastric contents. After the NG tube is removed, sips of clear liquids are offered, and the diet is progressed gradually. Nausea and abdominal distention are observed as signs of an obstruction and are reported immediately.

As with other patients undergoing abdominal surgery, those with ileostomies are encouraged to engage in early ambulation. Prescribed pain medications are administered as required.

By the end of the first week, rectal packing is removed. Because this procedure may be uncomfortable, the patient may be administered an analgesic an hour before it is performed. After the packing is removed, the perineum is irrigated two to three times daily until full healing takes place.

Psychosocial Considerations

The patient understandably may think that everyone is aware of the ileostomy, and may view the stoma as a mutilation in comparison with other abdominal incisions that heal and are hidden. Because there is loss of a body part and a major change in anatomy, the ileostomy patient often goes through the various phases of grieving: shock, disbelief, denial, rejection, anger, and restitution. Nursing support through these phases is important, and understanding of the patient's emotional outlook in each instance should determine the approach taken. For example, teaching may be of no avail until the patient is ready to learn.

Concern over body image may lead to questions related to family relationships, sexual function, and for women the ability to become pregnant and to deliver a baby normally. Research shows that the sooner the patient masters the physical care of the ileostomy, the sooner he or she will psychologically accept it (Long, 1991).

Finally, such patients need to know that someone understands and cares about them. A calm, nonjudgmental attitude exhibited by the nurse will aid in gaining the patient's confidence. It is important to recognize the dependency needs of these patients.

Such patients may be particularly challenging to the nurse. Their prolonged illness can make them irritable, anxious, and depressed. The nurse can coordinate patient care through conferences attended by consultants such as the physician, psychologist, psychiatrist, social worker, enterostomal therapist, and dietitian. The team approach lends support in approaching the often complex care of this patient.

Conversely, a surgical procedure to create an ileostomy can produce dramatic positive changes in patients who have suffered from colitis for several years. Once the continuous discomfort of the disease has decreased and patients learn how to take care of the ileostomy, they often develop a more positive outlook. But until they progress to this phase, an empathic and tolerant approach by the nurse will play an important part in recovery.

The support of other ostomates is also of help. An agency that is dedicated to the rehabilitation of ostomates is the United Ostomy Association. This organization gives patients useful information about living with an ostomy through an educational program of literature, lectures, and exhibits. Local associations offer visiting services by qualified members who provide hope, as well as rehabilitation services, to new ostomy patients. Hospitals and other health care agencies may have an enterostomal therapy nurse on the staff who can serve as another valuable resource person for the ileostomy patient.

See Nursing Care Plan 37-1 for a summary overview of caring for the patient with a fecal diversion.

(text continues on page 934)

NURSING CARE PLAN 37–1
Care of the Patient With a Fecal Diversion

Nursing Interventions	Rationale	Expected Outcomes
Preoperative		
NURSING DIAGNOSIS: Knowledge deficit about the surgical procedure and preoperative preparation		
GOAL: Understands the surgical process and the necessary preoperative preparations		
1. Ascertain if the patient has had a previous surgical experience and ask for recollections of positive and negative impressions.	1. Fear of a repeated negative experience increases anxiety. Talking about the experience with a nurse helps clarify misconceptions and helps the patient ventilate any repressed emotions. Positive experiences are reinforced.	• Expresses anxieties and fears about the surgical process • Projects a positive attitude toward the surgical procedure • Repeats in own words information given by the surgeon • Identifies normal anatomy and physiology of gastrointestinal tract and how it will be altered. Can point to expected location of abdominal wound and stoma. Describes stoma appearance and size • Adheres to "bowel prep" regimen of antimicrobials or mechanical cleansing • Tolerates the presence of nasogastric/nasoenteric tube
2. Determine what information the surgeon gave the patient and family and whether it was understood. Clarify and elaborate as necessary. Determine whether the stoma is permanent or temporary. Be aware of the patient's prognosis if carcinoma exists.	2. Clarification prevents misunderstandings and alleviates anxiety. A positive affect may be more difficult to project if the ostomy is permanent or the prognosis poor.	
3. Use pictures or drawings to illustrate the location and appearance of the wounds (abdominal, perineal) and the stoma if the patient is interested and receptive.	3. Knowledge, for some, alleviates anxiety becuase fear of the unknown is decreased. Others choose not to know because it makes them more anxious.	
4. Explain that oral/parenteral antimicrobials will be administered to cleanse the bowel preoperatively. Mechanical cleansing may also be required.	4. Antimicrobials and mechanical cleansing will reduce intestinal bacterial flora.	
5. Assist the patient during nasogastric/nasoenteric intubation. Measure drainage from the tube.	5. Nasoenteral intubation is used for decompression and drainage of gastrointestinal contents before surgery.	
NURSING DIAGNOSIS: Body image disturbance		
GOAL: Attainment of a positive self-concept		
1. Encourage the patient to verbalize feelings about the stoma.	1. Free expression of feelings allows the patient the opportunity to verbalize and identify concerns. Expressed concerns can be therapeutically addressed by health care team members.	• Freely expresses concerns • Accepts support • Seeks help as needed • States is willing to talk with an ostomate
2. Offer to be present when the stoma is first viewed and touched.	2. Anxiety can be reduced if questions are immediately answered.	
3. Suggest that the spouse or significant other view the stoma.	3. Helps patient to overcome fears about partner's response.	
4. Offer counseling, if desired.	4. Provides opportunity for additional support.	
5. Arrange for a visit with an ostomate.	5. Ostomates can offer support and share mutual feelings.	

(*continued*)

NURSING CARE PLAN 37–1 *(continued)*
Care of the Patient With a Fecal Diversion

Nursing Interventions	Rationale	Expected Outcomes
Postoperative		
NURSING DIAGNOSIS: Anxiety related to the loss of bowel control		
GOAL: Reduction of anxiety		
1. Provide information about expected bowel function: a. Characteristics of effluent b. Frequency of discharge	1. Emotional adjustment is facilitated if adequate information is provided at the level of the learner.	• Expresses interest in learning about altered bowel function • Handles equipment correctly • Changes the pouch unassisted • Irrigates colostomy successfully • Progresses toward a regular schedule of elimination
2. Teach the patient how to prepare the pouch for an adequate fit.		
a. Choose the drainage pouch that will provide a secure fit around the stoma. Measure the stoma size with a measuring guide provided by the ostomy manufacturer and compare with the opening on the pouch. About 3-mm (1/8-in) clearance should be provided around the stoma.	a. The pouch opening should be larger than the stoma for an adequate fit. Available brands come in different sizes to fit the stoma. Adjustments are made as necessary.	
b. Remove any plastic covering that protects the pouch adhesive. *Note:* The pouch is applied by pressing the adhesive for 30 seconds to the skin or skin barrier.	b. The pouch is ready to apply directly to the skin or skin protector.	
3. Demonstrate how to change the pouch before leakage occurs. Be aware that the elderly person may have diminished vision and difficulty handling equipment.	3. Manipulation of the appliance is a learned motor skill that requires practice and positive encouragement.	
4. Demonstrate how to irrigate the colostomy (usually on the 4th–5th day.) Recommend that irrigating be done at a regular time, depending on the type of colostomy.		
NURSING DIAGNOSIS: Risk for impaired skin integrity related to irritation of the peristomal skin by the effluent		
GOAL: Attainment of skin integrity		
1. Provide information about signs/symptoms of irritated or inflamed skin. Use pictures if possible.	1. Peristomal skin should be slightly pink without abrasions and similar to that of the entire abdomen.	• Describes appearance of healthy skin • Correctly cleanses the skin • Successfully applies a skin barrier • Gently removes the drainage pouch without skin damage • Demonstrates intact skin around the colostomy stoma
2. Teach patient how to gently cleanse the peristomal skin.	2. Mild friction with warm water and a gentle soap cleanses the skin and minimizes irritation and possible abrasions. Patting the skin dry prevents tissue trauma.	
3. Demonstrate how to apply a skin barrier (powder, gel, paste, wafer).	3. Skin barriers protect the peristomal skin from enzymes and bacteria.	
4. Demonstrate how to remove the pouch.	4. Gently separate adhesive from the skin to avoid irritation. Never pull!	

(continued)

NURSING CARE PLAN 37–1 *(continued)*
Care of the Patient With a Fecal Diversion

NURSING DIAGNOSIS: Potential alteration in nutrition, less than body requirements, related to avoidance of foods that may cause gastrointestinal discomfort

GOAL: Achievement of an optimal nutritional intake

Nursing Interventions	Rationale	Expected Outcomes
1. Conduct a complete nutritional assessment to identify any foods that may increase peristalsis by irritating the bowel.	1. Patients react differently to certain foods because of individual sensitivity.	• Modifies diet to avoid offensive foods yet maintains a balanced nutritional intake • Avoids foods such as peanuts • Modifies intake of certain fruits
2. Advise the patient to avoid food products with a cellulose or hemicellulose base (nuts, seeds).	2. Cellulose food products are the nondigestable residue of plant foods. They hold water, provide bulk, and stimulate elimination.	
3. Recommend moderation in intake of certain irritating fruits such as prunes, grapes, and bananas.	3. These fruits tend to increase the quantity of effluent.	

NURSING DIAGNOSIS: Sexual dysfunction related to altered body image

GOAL: Attainment of satisfactory sexual performance

Nursing Interventions	Rationale	Expected Outcomes
1. Encourage the patient to verbalize fears. The sexual partner is welcomed to participate in the discussion.	1. Expressed needs help the therapist develop a plan of care.	• Expresses fears and concerns • Discusses alternative sexual positions • Accepts services of a professional counselor
2. Recommend alternative sexual positions.	2. Avoid patient embarrassment with the visual appearance of the stoma. Avoid peristomal skin irritation secondary to friction.	
3. Seek assistance from a sexual therapist or psychiatric clinical specialist.	3. Some patients need professional sexual counseling.	

NURSING DIAGNOSIS: Risk for fluid volume deficit related to anorexia and vomiting and increased loss of fluids and electrolytes from GI tract

GOAL: Attainment of fluid balance

Nursing Interventions	Rationale	Expected Outcomes
1. Estimate fluid intake and output:	1. Provides indication of fluid balance.	• Maintains fluid balance • Maintains normal serum and urinary values for sodium and potassium • Normal skin turgor • Surface of tongue is pink with a moist mucous membrane
a. Strict intake and output	a. An early indicator of fluid imbalance is a daily, significant difference between intake and output. The average person ingests (food, fluids) and loses (urine, feces, lungs) about 3 liters of fluid every 24 hours.	
b. Daily weights	b. A gain/loss of 1 liter of fluid is reflected in a body weight change of 2.2 pounds.	
2. Assess serum and urinary values of sodium and potassium.	2. Sodium is the major electrolyte regulating water balance. Vomiting results in decreased urinary and serum sodium levels. Urinary sodium values, in contrast to serum values, reflect early, sensitive changes in sodium balance.	

(continued)

NURSING CARE PLAN 37-1 *(continued)*
Care of the Patient With a Fecal Diversion

Nursing Interventions	Rationale	Expected Outcomes
	Sodium works in conjunction with potassium, which is also decreased with vomiting. A significant deficiency in potassium is associated with a decrease in intracellular potassium bicarbonate, which lead to acidosis and compensatory hyperventilation.	
3. Observe and record skin turgor and the appearance of the tongue.	3. Adequate hydration is reflected by the skin's ability to return to its normal shape after being grasped between the fingers. *Note:* In the older person, it is normal for the return to be delayed. Changes in the mucous membrane covering of the tongue are accurate and early indicators of hydration status.	

Rehabilitation After an Ileostomy

Stoma Care. There are certain rehabilitation problems unique to the ileostomy patient, one of which is irregularity of bowel evacuation. The patient with a traditional ileostomy cannot establish regular bowel habits because the contents of the ileum are fluid and are discharged continuously. Therefore, the patient must wear a pouch day and night. The pouch is regarded, then, as an intestinal prosthesis. By using this pouch, the patient can carry on normal activities without fear of leakage or odor. After the ileostomy has had a chance to heal, a permanent appliance is obtained and held in place on the skin with a special cement. The stomal size should be rechecked in 3 weeks, when the edema has subsided. The final size and type of appliance may be selected in 3 months, after the patient's weight has stabilized and the stoma shrinks to a stable shape.

The location and length of the stoma are significant in the management of the ileostomy by the patient. The surgeon positions the stoma as close to the midline as possible and at a location where even an obese patient with a protruding abdomen can care for it easily. Usually, the ileostomy stoma is about 2.5 cm (1 in) long, which makes it convenient for the attachment of an appliance.

Diet and Fluids. The ileostomy may be noisy at first because of slight obstruction of tissues caused by edema. Eventually it will become quieter. A low-residue diet is followed for the first six to eight weeks. Strained fruits and vegetables are given. These foods are important as sources of vitamins A and C. Later there are few dietary restrictions, except for avoiding foods that are high in fiber or hard-to-digest kernels, such as celery, popcorn, corn, poppy seeds, caraway seeds, and coconut. Foods are reintroduced one at a time. The patient's tolerance for these foods is assessed and he or she is taught to chew food thoroughly.

Fluids may be a problem during the summer, when perspiration adds to the fluid lost through the ileostomy. Fluids such as Gatorade are helpful in maintaining electrolyte balance. If the effluent (fecal discharge) is too watery, fibrous foods (such as whole grain cereals, fresh fruit skins, beans, corn, and nuts) are restricted. If the effluent is excessively dry, salt intake is increased. An increased intake of water or fluid will not increase the effluent because excess water is excreted in the urine.

Skin Care. Another possible problem is skin excoriation around the stoma. Periostomal skin integrity may be complicated by several factors, such as allergic reaction to the ostomy appliance, skin barrier or paste; chemical irritation from the effluent; mechanical injury from the removal of the appliance; and possible infection. If irritation and yeast growth are present, nystatin powder (Mycostatin) is dusted lightly on the peristomal skin.

Changing an Ileostomy Appliance. A regular schedule for changing the pouch before leakage occurs must be established for those with a traditional ileostomy. The patient can be taught to change the pouch in a manner similar to that described in Guideline 37-1.

The amount of time that a person can keep the appliance sealed to the body surface depends on the location of the stoma and on body structure. Usually, the normal wearing time is 5 to 7 days. The appliance is emptied every 4 to 6 hours, or at the same time the patient empties the bladder. An emptying spout at the bottom of the appliance is closed with a special clip made for this purpose.

Most pouches are disposable and odorproof. Foods such as spinach and parsley act as deodorizers in the intestinal tract; foods that cause odors include cabbage, onions, and fish. Bismuth subcarbonate tablets, which may be prescribed and taken by mouth three or four times a day, are effective in reducing odor. A stool thickener, such as diphenoxylate (Lomotil), may also be prescribed to be taken by mouth to assist in odor control.

Continent Ileostomy. For a continent ileostomy, the patient must be taught to drain the pouch as described in Guideline 37-2. A catheter is inserted into the reservoir to

GUIDELINE 37–1
Changing an Ileostomy Appliance

Changing an ileostomy appliance is necessary to prevent leakage (the bag is usually changed every 2 to 4 days), to allow for examination of the skin around the stoma, and to assist in controlling odor if this becomes a problem. The appliance should be changed at any time that the patient complains of burning or itching under the disc or pain in the area of the stoma; routine changes should be performed early in the morning before breakfast or 2 to 4 hours after a meal, when the bowel is least active.

Nursing Action	Rationale/Amplification
1. Promote patient comfort and involvement in the procedure. A. Have the patient assume a relaxed position. Provide privacy. B. Explain details of the procedure. C. Expose the ileostomy area; remove the ileostomy belt (if worn).	Providing a relaxed atmosphere and adequate explanations help the patient to become an active participant in the procedure.
2. Remove the appliance.	
A. Have the patient sit on the toilet or on a chair facing the toilet. A patient who prefers to stand should face the toilet.	These positions facilitate disposal or drainage.
B. The appliance (pouch) can be removed by gently pushing the skin away from the adhesive.	
3. Cleanse the skin.	
A. Wash the skin gently with a soft cloth moistened with tepid water and mild soap; the patient may prefer to bathe before putting on a clean appliance.	The patient may shower with or without the pouch. Micropore or waterproof tape applied to the sides of the faceplate will keep it secure during bathing.
B. Rinse and dry the skin thoroughly after cleansing.	Moisture or soap residue will interfere with appliance adhesion.
4. Apply appliance (when there is *no* skin irritation):	
A. An appropriate skin barrier is applied to the peristomal skin before the pouch is applied.	Many pouches have a built-in skin barrier.
B. Remove cover from adherent surface of disc of disposable plastic pouch and apply directly to the skin.	The skin should be thoroughly dried before applying the pouch.
C. Press firmly in place for 30 seconds to ensure adherence.	
5. Apply appliance (when there is skin irritation):	
A. Cleanse the skin thoroughly but gently; pat dry.	To remove debris.
B. Apply Kenalog spray; blot excess moisture with a cotton pledget and dust lightly with nystatin (Mycostatin) powder.	The corticosteroid preparation (Kenalog) helps to decrease inflammation. The antifungal agent (nystatin) treats those types of infections that are common around stomas. A prescription is required for both medications.
(1) An alternate effective measure is to apply a wafer of Stomahesive (Squibb), which is available in 10 × 10-cm (4 × 4-in) and 20 × 20-cm (8 × 8-in) pieces. The stomal opening should be cut the same size as the stoma; use a cutting guide (supplied with Stomahesive). The wafer is applied directly to the skin.	Stomahesive is a substance that facilitates healing of excoriated skin. It adheres well even to moist, irritated skin.
(2) A second alternative is to moisten a karaya gum washer and apply when it is tacky. If the skin is moist, karaya powder may be applied first and any excess dusted off gently.	Karaya also facilitates skin healing. Tackiness promotes adherence.
C. The pouch is then applied to the treated skin.	This will allow skin to heal while the appliance is in place.
6. Check the pouch bottom for closure; use the rubber band or clip provided.	Proper closure controls leakage.

drain the fluid. The length of time between drainage periods is gradually increased until the reservoir need only be drained every 4 to 6 hours and irrigated once a day. A pouch is not necessary; instead most patients wear a dressing over the opening.

When the fecal discharge is thick, water can be injected through the catheter to loosen and soften it. The consistency of the effluent is affected by food intake. At first drainage is only 60 to 80 ml, but as time goes on it will increase significantly. The internal Kock's pouch will stretch, eventually accommodating 500 to 1000 ml. The sensation of pressure in the pouch is the gauge to use to determine the frequency with which the pouch should be drained.

GUIDELINE 37–2
Draining a Continent Ileostomy (Kock's Pouch)

A **continent ileostomy** is the surgical creation of a pouch of small intestine that can serve as an internal receptacle for fecal discharge; a nipple valve is constructed at the outlet. Postoperatively, a catheter extends from the stoma and is attached to a closed drainage suction system. To assure patency of the catheter, usually every 3 hours 10 to 20 ml of normal saline are instilled gently into the pouch; return flow is not aspirated but is allowed to drain by gravity.

After approximately 2 weeks, when the healing process has progressed to the point at which the catheter is removed from the stoma, the patient is taught to drain the pouch. The equipment required includes a catheter, tissues, water-soluble lubricant, gauze squares, a syringe, irrigating solution in a bowl, and an emesis or receiving basin.

The following procedure is used to drain the pouch; the patient is assisted to participate in this procedure in order to learn to perform it unassisted.

Nursing Action	Rationale/Amplification
1. Lubricate the catheter and gently insert it about 5 cm (2 in), at which some resistance may be felt at the valve or "nipple."	When gentle pressure is used, the catheter usually will enter the pouch.
2. If there is much resistance, fill a syringe with 20 ml of air or water and inject it through the catheter, while still exerting some pressure on the catheter.	This will permit the catheter to enter the pouch.
3. Place the other end of the catheter in a drainage basin held below the level of the stoma. Later this process can be carried out at the toilet with drainage delivered into the toilet bowl.	Gravity facilitates drainage. Drainage may include flatus as well as effluent.
4. After drainage, the catheter is removed and the area around the stoma is gently washed with warm water. Pat dry and apply an absorbent pad over the stoma. Fasten the pad with hypoallergenic tape.	The entire procedure requires about 5 to 10 minutes; at first it is performed every 3 hours. The time between procedures is gradually lengthened to three times daily.

Patient Education and Home Care Considerations

The spouse and family should be familiar with the adjustment that will be necessary when the patient returns home. They need to know why it is necessary for the patient to occupy the bathroom for 10 minutes or more at certain times of the day, and why certain equipment is needed. Their understanding is necessary to reduce tension; a relaxed patient tends to have fewer problems. Visits from an enterostomal therapy nurse may be arranged to assure that the patient is progressing as expected and to provide additional guidance and teaching as needed.

The patient needs to be given the commercial name of the pouch to be used, in order to obtain a ready supply, and information about obtaining other supplies. The name of the local enterostomal therapy nurse and local self-help groups are often helpful. Any special restrictions on driving or working also need to be reviewed, if applicable. The patient should be taught about common postoperative complications as well as how to recognize and report them.

Complications of Ileostomy

Minor complications occur in about 40% of patients who have an ileostomy; less than 20% of the complications require surgical intervention.

Peristomal skin irritation, the most common complication of an ileostomy, is due to leakage of effluent. An ill-fitting pouch is frequently the cause. The pouch is adjusted by the nurse or an enterostomal therapist and skin barriers are applied.

Diarrhea, manifested by very irritating effluent that rapidly fills the pouch (every hour or sooner), can quickly lead to dehydration and electrolyte losses. Supplemental water, sodium, and potassium are administered to prevent hypovolemia and hypokalemia. Antidiarrheal agents are administered.

Stenosis is caused by circular scar tissue that forms at the stoma site. The scar tissue must be surgically released.

Urinary calculi occur in about 10% of ileostomy patients because of dehydration secondary to decreased fluid intake. Intense lower abdominal pain that radiates to the legs, hematuria, and signs of dehydration indicate that the urine should be strained. Fluid intake is encouraged. Sometimes small stones are passed during urination; otherwise, treatment is necessary to crush or remove the calculi.

Cholelithiasis (formation of gallstones) due to cholesterol occurs three times more frequently than in the general population because of changes in the absorption of bile acids that occur preoperatively. Spasm of the gallbladder causes severe upper right abdominal pain that can radiate to the back and right shoulder.

Ileitis is usually seen with a recurrence of inflammatory bowel disease.

Intestinal Obstruction

Intestinal obstruction exists when blockage prevents the normal flow of intestinal contents through the intestinal tract. This flow can be impeded by two types of processes:

1. *Mechanical*—an intraluminal obstruction or a mural obstruction from pressure on the intestinal walls occurs. Examples of conditions that can cause mechanical obstruction are intussusception, polypoid tumors and neoplasms, stenosis, strictures, adhesions, hernias, and abscesses.
2. *Functional*—the intestinal musculature is unable to propel the contents along the bowel. Examples are amyloidosis, muscular dystrophy, endocrine disorders such as diabetes mellitus, or neurologic disorders such as Parkinson's disease. It also can be temporary and the result of the handling of the bowel during surgery.

The obstruction can be partial or complete. Its severity depends on the region of bowel that is affected, the degree to which the lumen is occluded, and, especially, the degree to which the blood circulation in the bowel wall is disturbed.

Most bowel obstructions (85%) occur in the small intestine. Adhesions are the most common cause of small bowel obstruction (60% incidence), followed by hernias and neoplasms. Other causes include intussusception, volvulus (twisting of the bowel), and paralytic ileus. Table 37-4 and Figure 37-6 present a list of mechanical causes of obstruction and a graphic depiction of how they occur.

About 15% of intestinal obstructions occur in the large bowel, and most are found in the sigmoid. The most common causes are carcinoma, diverticulitis, inflammatory bowel disorders, and benign tumors.

Small Bowel Obstruction

Pathophysiology. An accumulation of intestinal contents, fluid, and gas develops above the intestinal obstruction. The distention and retention of fluid reduce the absorption of fluids and stimulate more gastric secretion. With increasing distention, pressure within the intestinal lumen increases, causing a decrease in venous and arteriolar capillary pressure. This, in turn, causes edema, congestion, necrosis, and eventual rupture or perforation of the intestinal wall with resultant peritonitis.

Reflux vomiting may occur from the abdominal distention. Vomiting results in a loss of hydrogen ions and potassium from the stomach, leading to a reduction of chlorides and potassium in the blood and to metabolic alkalosis. Then dehydration and acidosis develop because of loss of water and sodium. With acute fluid losses, hypovolemic shock may occur.

Clinical Manifestations. The initial symptom is usually crampy pain that is wavelike and colicky in character. The patient may pass blood and mucus, but no fecal matter and no flatus. Vomiting occurs. This pattern is often characteristic.

If the obstruction is complete, the peristaltic waves initially become extremely vigorous and will eventually assume a reverse direction, the intestinal contents being propelled toward the mouth instead of toward the rectum. If the obstruction is in the ileum, fecal vomiting takes place. First, the patient vomits the stomach contents, then the bile-stained contents of the duodenum and the jejunum, and finally, with each paroxysm of pain, the darker, fecal-like contents of the ileum.

The unmistakable signs of dehydration become evident: the patient experiences intense thirst, drowsiness, generalized malaise, and aching, and the tongue and mucous membranes become parched. The abdomen becomes

TABLE 37-4 Mechanical Causes of Intestinal Obstruction

Cause	Course of Events	Result
Adhesions	Loops of intestine become adherent to areas that heal slowly or scar after abdominal surgery.	3 or 4 days post-op this produces a kinking of an intestinal loop.
Intussusception	One part of the intestine slips into another part located below it (like a telescope shortening) (Fig. 37-6*A*).	Narrowing of the intestinal lumen
Volvulus	Bowel twists and turns upon itself (Fig. 37-6*B*).	Intestinal lumen becomes obstructed. Gas and fluid accumulate in the trapped bowel.
Hernia	Protrusion of intestine through a weakened area in the abdominal muscle or wall (Fig. 37-6*C*).	Intestinal flow may be completely obstructed. Blood flow to the area may be obstructed as well.
Tumor	A tumor that exists within the wall of the intestine extends into the intestinal lumen, or a tumor outside the intestine causes pressure on the wall of the intestine.	Intestinal lumen becomes partially obstructed; if the tumor is not removed complete obstruction results.

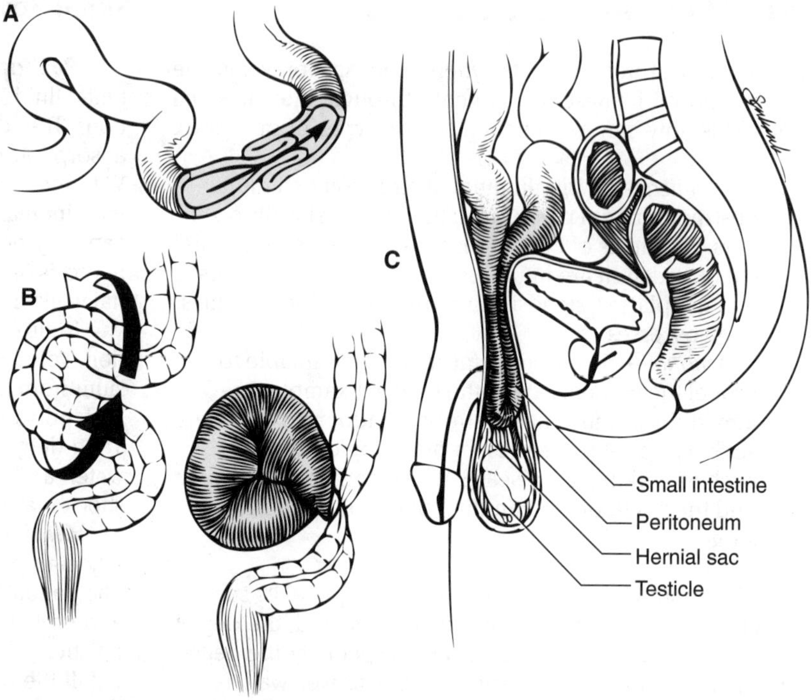

FIGURE 37-6. Three causes of intestinal obstruction. (**A**) Intussusception. Note invagination or shortening of colon by the movement of one segment of bowel into another. (**B**) Volvulus of the sigmoid colon. The twist is counterclockwise in most cases of sigmoid volvulus. Note the edematous bowel. (**C**) Hernia (inguinal). Note that the sac of the hernia is a continuation of the peritoneum of the abdomen and that the hernial contents are intestine, omentum, or other abdominal contents that pass through the hernial opening into the hernial sac.

distended. The lower the obstruction in the gastrointestinal tract, the more marked is the abdominal distention. If the obstruction continues uncorrected, shock occurs due to dehydration and loss of plasma volume.

Diagnostic Evaluation. Diagnosis is based on the symptoms described above as well as on x-ray studies. Abdominal x-rays will show abnormal quantities of gas and/or fluid in the bowel. Laboratory studies (*i.e.*, electrolyte studies and complete blood count) will reveal a picture of dehydration and loss of plasma volume, and possibly infection.

Management. Decompression of the bowel through a nasogastric or small bowel tube (see Chapter 35) is successful in the majority of cases. When the bowel is completely obstructed, the possibility of strangulation warrants surgical intervention. Prior to surgery, intravenous therapy is necessary to replace the depleted water, sodium, chloride, and potassium.

The surgical treatment of intestinal obstruction depends largely on the cause of the obstruction. In the most common causes of obstruction, such as hernia and adhesions, the surgical procedure involves repairing the hernia or dividing the adhesion to which the intestine is attached. In some instances, the portion of affected bowel may be removed and an anastomosis performed. The complexity of the surgical procedure for intestinal obstruction depends on the duration of the obstruction and the condition of the intestine found during surgery.

Large Bowel Obstruction

Pathophysiology. As in small bowel obstruction, large bowel obstruction results in an accumulation of intestinal contents, fluid, and gas proximal to the obstruction. Obstruction in the colon can lead to severe distention and perforation unless some gas and fluid can flow back through the ileal valve.

Large bowel obstruction, even if complete, is comparatively undramatic if the blood supply to the colon is not disturbed. If the blood supply is cut off, however, intestinal strangulation and necrosis (tissue death) occur; this condition is life threatening.

In the large intestine, dehydration occurs more slowly than in the small intestine because the colon is able to absorb its fluid contents and can distend to a size considerably beyond its normal full capacity.

Clinical Manifestations. Large bowel obstruction differs clinically from small bowel obstruction in that the symptoms develop and progress relatively slowly. In patients with obstruction in the sigmoid or the rectum, constipation may be the only symptom for days. Eventually, the abdomen becomes markedly distended, loops of large bowel become visibly outlined through the abdominal wall, and the patient suffers from crampy lower abdominal pain. Finally, fecal vomiting develops. Symptoms of shock may occur.

Diagnostic Evaluation. Diagnosis is based on symptomatology and on x-ray studies. Abdominal x-rays (flat and upright) will show a distended colon. Barium studies are contraindicated.

Medical and Surgical Management. If the obstruction is relatively high in the colon, a colonoscopy may be performed to untwist and decompress the bowel. A **cecostomy**, in which a surgical opening is made into the cecum, may be performed for those patients who are poor surgical risks and urgently need relief from the obstruction. The procedure provides an outlet for releasing gas and a small amount of drainage. A rectal tube may be used to decompress an area that is lower in the bowel.

The usual treatment, however, is **surgical resection** to remove the obstructing lesion. A temporary or permanent colostomy may be necessary (see p. 943). Sometimes an ileoanal anastomosis is performed if it is necessary to remove the entire large colon.

Nursing Interventions. The nurse's role is to monitor the patient for symptoms indicating that the intestinal obstruction is worsening, as well as to provide emotional support and comfort. IV fluids and electrolyte replacement are administered as ordered. If the patient's condition does not respond to medical treatment, the nurse must prepare the patient for surgery. This preparation includes preoperative teaching as the patient's condition indicates. Postoperatively, general abdominal wound care is given. Routine postoperative nursing care is required.

A critical pathway for a patient undergoing a colon resection without a colostomy is presented on pages 940 and 941. This pathway shows a 5-day postoperative plan.

Cancer of the Large Intestine: Colon and Rectum

Tumors of the small intestine are rare; conversely, tumors of the colon and rectum are relatively common. In fact, cancer of the colon and rectum is now the second most common type of internal cancer in the United States. It is a disease of Western cultures. It is estimated that 156,000 new cases of colorectal cancer are diagnosed in this country each year. Colon cancer affects more than twice as many people as does rectal cancer.

The incidence increases with age (most patients are over age 55) and is higher in persons with a family history of colon cancer, and in those with chronic inflammatory bowel disease or polyps. The distribution of cancer sites throughout the colon can be seen in Figure 37-7. Changes in the percentage distribution have occurred in recent years. The incidence of cancer in the sigmoid and rectal areas has decreased, whereas the incidence in the ascending and descending colon has increased.

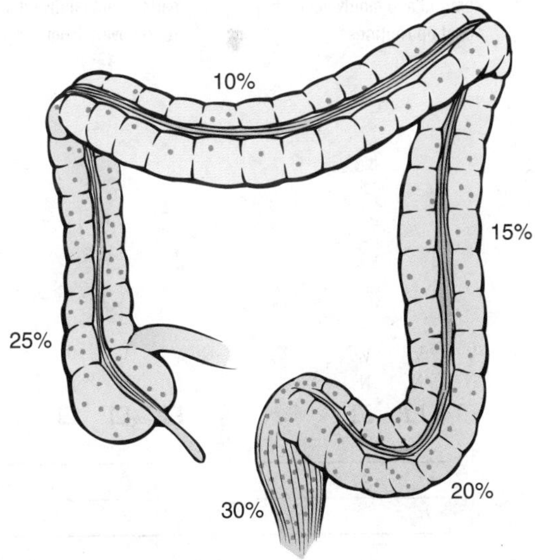

FIGURE 37-7. Percentage distribution of cancer sites in the colon and rectum.

Of the more than 156,000 people diagnosed each year, about half that number die annually—although almost three out of four patients could be saved by early diagnosis and prompt treatment. The low 5-year survival rate of 40% to 50% is due primarily to late diagnosis and metastasis. Most people are asymptomatic for long periods and seek health care only when they notice a change in bowel habits or rectal bleeding.

The exact cause of colon and rectal cancer is unknown, but risk factors have been identified, including a history or family history of colon cancer or polyps; a history of chronic inflammatory bowel disease; and a diet high in fat, protein, and beef and low in fiber (Chart 37-2).

Pathophysiology. Cancer of the colon and rectum is predominantly (95%) adenocarcinoma (arising from the epithelial lining of the intestine). It may start as a benign polyp but may become malignant and invade and destroy normal tissues and extend into surrounding structures. Cancer cells may break away from the primary tumor and spread to other parts of the body (most often to the liver).

Clinical Manifestations. The symptoms are greatly determined by the location of the cancer, the stage of the disease, and the function of the intestinal segment in which it is located. The most common presenting symptom is a change in bowel habits. The passage of blood in the stools is the second most common symptom. Symptoms may also include unexplained anemia, anorexia, weight loss, and fatigue.

The symptoms most commonly associated with right-sided lesions are dull abdominal pain and melena (black, tarry stools). The symptoms most commonly associated with left-sided lesions are those associated with obstruction (abdominal pain and cramping, narrowing stools, constipation, and distention), as well as bright red blood in the stool. Those symptoms associated with rectal lesions are tenesmus (ineffective, painful straining at stool), rectal pain, the feeling of incomplete evacuation after a bowel movement, alternating constipation and diarrhea, and bloody stool.

Gerontologic Considerations. The incidence of carcinoma of the colon and rectum increases with age. These cancers are considered the most common malignancies in old age except for prostatic cancer in men. Symptoms are

(text continues on page 942)

CHART 37-2
Risk Factors for Cancer of the Colon

- Age—over 40
- Blood in stool
- History of rectal polyps or colon polyps
- Presence of adenomatous polyps or villous adenomas
- Family history of colon cancer or familial polyposis
- History of chronic inflammatory bowel disease
- Diet—high in fat, protein, beef, and low in fiber

CRITICAL PATHWAY
Colon Resection W/O Colostomy

The Graduate Hospital Nursing Services Department
1800 Lombard Street
Philadelphia, PA 19146

	PAT Visit	Pre-Surgery Day -1•	Day 0 O.R. Day	Post OP Day 1
Assessments	History & physical with breast, rectal and pelvic exam Nursing assessment	Nursing admission assessment	Nursing admission assessment on TBA patients in holding area; post-op review of systems assessment*	Review of systems assessment*
Consults	Social service consult, physical therapy consult	Notify referring physician of impending admission		
Labs and Diagnostics	CBC with DIFF, ECG,CXR, PT/PTT, CEA, Bio chem profile, CT ABC w/wo contrast, CT pelvis, U/A, BaEnema & Flex Sigmoidoscopy/Colonoscopy; biopsy report	Type & screen for patients with Hg < 10	Type & screen for TBA patients in holding area with Hg <10	CBC
Interventions	Many or all of the above labs/diagnostics will have already been done. Check all results and fax to the surgeon's office.	Admit by 8AM, check for bowel prep orders Bowel Prep*, TEDS*, incentive spirometry, Ankle exercises*, IV access*, routine VS*	Shave & prep in O.R.; NG tube maintenance*, I/O*, vs per routine*, Foley care*, TEDS/Kendalls*, incentive spirometry*, ankle exercises*, IV site care*, HOB 30°*, safety measures*, wound care*, mouth care*	NG tube maintenance*, I/O*, vs per routine*, Foley care*, TEDS/ Kendalls*, incentive spirometry*, ankle exercises*, IV site care*, HOB 30°*, safety measures*, wound care*, mouth care*
IVs		IVF's	IVF's	IVF's
Medication	Prescribe Golytely/Nulytely 10A-2P, Neomycin @ 2P, 3P, & 10P Erythromycin @ 2P, 3P & 10P	Golytely/Nulytely 10A-2P, Erythromycin-2P, 3P & 10P, Neomycin-2P, 3P & 10P	Pre-op ABX in holding area, Post-op ABX, PCA (basal rate 0.5mg), S.Q heparin	PCA (basal rate 0.5mg) SQ heparin
Diet/GI	Clears presurgery day, NPO after midnight	Clears presurgery day, NPO after midnight	NPO/NG tube	NPO/NG tube
Activity			4 hours after surgery ambulate with abdominal binder*	Ambulate TID with abdominal binder*, may shower, physical therapy bid
Teaching	Instruct:* Golytely-1 gallon, 10a-2p preop day, Neomycin-@2P, 3P, 10P, Erythromycin @2P, 3P, 10P Instruct:* Incentive spirometry, ankle exercises for DVT prophylaxis, post op activity; clears pre surgery day; NPO after midnight	Instruct*/administer: Golytely-1 gallon 10a-2P preop day, Neomycin-2P, 3P, 10P, Erythromycin-2P, 3P, 10P Instruct*: Incentive spirometry, ankle exercises for DVT prophylaxis, post op activity, clears then NPO after midnight	Reinforce pre-op teaching*, patient and family education-post op routines*	Reinforce pre op teaching*, patient and family education-re: recovery from surgery*
D/C, Planning & Follow-up	Follow-up pre-op phone call 8A preop day			

Key: *NSG Activities

V = Variance	V V V	V V V	V V V	V V V
N = No Var.	N N N	N N N	N N N	N N N
	☐ ☐ ☐	☐ ☐ ☐	☐ ☐ ☐	☐ ☐ ☐
NSG Care Performed: →	1. ________	1. ________	1. ________	1. ________
SIGNATURES: →	2. ________	2. ________	2. ________	2. ________
→	3. ________	3. ________	3. ________	3. ________

ABX = antibiotics; CBC with DIFF = complete blood count with differential; CEA = carcinoembryonic antigen; CT = computerized tomography; CXR = chest x-ray; D/C = discontinue or discharge; IVF = intravenous fluids; NGT = nasogastric tube; PCA = patient-controlled analgesia; PT = prothrombin time; PTT = partial thromboplastin time; RR = respiratory rate; Rx = prescription;

CRITICAL PATHWAY
Colon Resection W/O Colostomy

Outcome Criteria for Discharge to Home
- □ Tolerating Diet/+ BM
- □ Afebrile
- □ Ambulates Functional Rate Independently
- □ Independent with ADL's
- □ Adequate Pain Control on Oral Analgesics

Post OP Day 2	Post OP Day 3	Post OP Day 4	Post OP Day 5
Review of systems assessment*	Review of systems assessment*	Review of systems assessment*	Review of systems assessment*
	Dietary consult		Oncology consult if indicated (Dukes B2 or C or high risk lesion) (or to be done as out patient)
EL-7 CXR if indicated	CBC EL-7	Pathology results on chart	CBC EL-7
D/C NG tube if possible* (per guidelines), I/O*, vs per routine*, D/C foley*, TEDS/ D/C Kendalls if ambulating*, Incentive spirometry*, ankle exercises*, IV site care*, HOB 30°*, safety measures*, wound care*, mouth care*	I/O*, vs per routine*, TEDS*, incentive spirometry*, ankle exercises*, IV site care*, safety measures*, wound care*	I/O*, vs per routine*, TEDS*, incentive spirometry*, ankle exercises*, IV site care*, safety measures*, wound care*	Consider staple removal; replace with steri strips, assess that patient has met D/C criteria*
IVF's	IV->heplock	Heplock	D/C heplock
PCA (.5mg basal rate)	D/C PCA, P.O. analgesia, resume routine home meds	P.O. Analgesia, Pre-op meds	P.O. analgesia Pre-op meds
D/C NG tube per guidelines: (clamp tube at 8am if no N/V and residual <200cc, D/C tube @12noon)* (Check with physician first)	Clears if +BM/Flatus, advance to post-op diet if tolerating clears (at least one tray of clears)*	House	House
Ambulate QID with abdominal binder*, may shower, physical therapy bid	Ambulate at least QID with abdominal binder*, may shower, physical therapy BID	Ambulate at least QID with abdominal binder*, may shower, physical therapy BID	
Reinforce pre-op teaching*, patient and family education PRN* Re: Family screening	Reinforce pre-op teaching*, patient and family education PRN*, Re: Family screening, begin D/C teaching*	Reinforce pre-op teaching*, patient and family education PRN*, D/C teaching re: reportable S/S, F/U and wound care*	Review all D/C instructions & Rx including:* Follow up appointments: with surgeon within 3 weeks, with oncologist within 1 month if indicated
Home care referral Social services visit		All Rx on chart, D/C order on chart, physician D/C instructions on chart, social service visit, home care visit	Discharge to home ______(time); follow up phone call, 48° after D/C
V V V N N N □ □ □ 1. ______ 2. ______ 3. ______	V V V N N N □ □ □ 1. ______ 2. ______ 3. ______	V V V N N N □ □ □ 1. ______ 2. ______ 3. ______	V V V N N N □ □ □ 1. ______ 2. ______ 3. ______

ECG = electrocardiogram; EL-7 = electrolyte screen; F/U = follow-up; Hg = hemoglobin; HOB = head of bed; HR = heart rate; I/O = intake and output; IV = intravenous; S/S = signs/symptoms; SBP = systolic blood pressure; SQ = subcutaneous; TBA = to be admitted; U/A = urinalysis; VS = vital signs; WNL = within normal limits.

often insidious. Fatigue is almost always present, due primarily to iron-deficiency anemia. The symptoms most commonly reported by the elderly are abdominal pain, obstruction, tenesmus, and rectal bleeding.

Colon cancer in the elderly has been closely associated with dietary carcinogens. Lack of fiber is a major causative factor because the passage of feces through the intestinal tract is prolonged, which in turn prolongs exposure to possible carcinogens. Excess fat is believed to alter bacterial flora and convert steroids into compounds that have carcinogenic properties.

Diagnostic Evaluation. Along with the abdominal and rectal examination, the most important diagnostic procedures for cancer of the colon are fecal occult blood testing, barium enema, proctosigmoidoscopy, and colonoscopy (these diagnostic procedures are described in Chapter 33). As many as 60% of colorectal cancer cases can be identified by sigmoidoscopy with biopsy or cytology smears.

Carcinoembryonic Antigen Studies. Carcinoembryonic antigen (CEA) studies may also be performed, although carcinoembryonic antigen may not be a highly reliable indicator in diagnosing colon cancer because not all lesions secrete CEA. Studies show that CEA levels are reliable in predicting prognosis. With complete excision of the tumor, the elevated levels of CEA should return to normal within 48 hours. Elevations of CEA at a later date suggest recurrence.

Medical Management. The patient with symptoms of intestinal obstruction is treated with IV fluids and nasogastric suction. If there has been significant bleeding, blood component therapy may be required.

Treatment depends on the stage of the disease and related complications. Endoscopy, ultrasonography, and laparoscopy have proven successful in staging colorectal cancer preoperatively. The most widely used staging method is Duke's classification:

- Class A—tumor limited to mucosa and submucosa
- Class B—penetration through bowel wall
- Class C—invasion into regional draining lymph system
- Class D—advanced and widespread regional metastasis

Medical treatment for colorectal cancer is most often in the form of supportive or adjuvant therapy. Adjuvant therapy is usually administered in addition to surgical treatment. Options include chemotherapy, radiation therapy, and/or immunotherapy.

The standard adjuvant therapy administered to patients with Class C colon cancer is the 5-FU/Levamesole regimen. Patients with Class B and C rectal cancer are given 5-FU and methyl CCNU and high doses of pelvic radiation.

Radiation therapy is now being used preoperatively, intraoperatively, and postoperatively to shrink the tumor, to achieve better results from the surgery, and to reduce the risk of recurrence. For inoperative or nonresectable tumors, radiation is used to give significant relief from the symptoms. Intracavity and implantable radiation devices are used.

Most recent data demonstrate delays in tumor recurrence and increases in survival time for those patients receiving some form of adjuvant therapy.

Complications. Tumor growth may cause partial or complete bowel obstruction. Growth and ulceration may

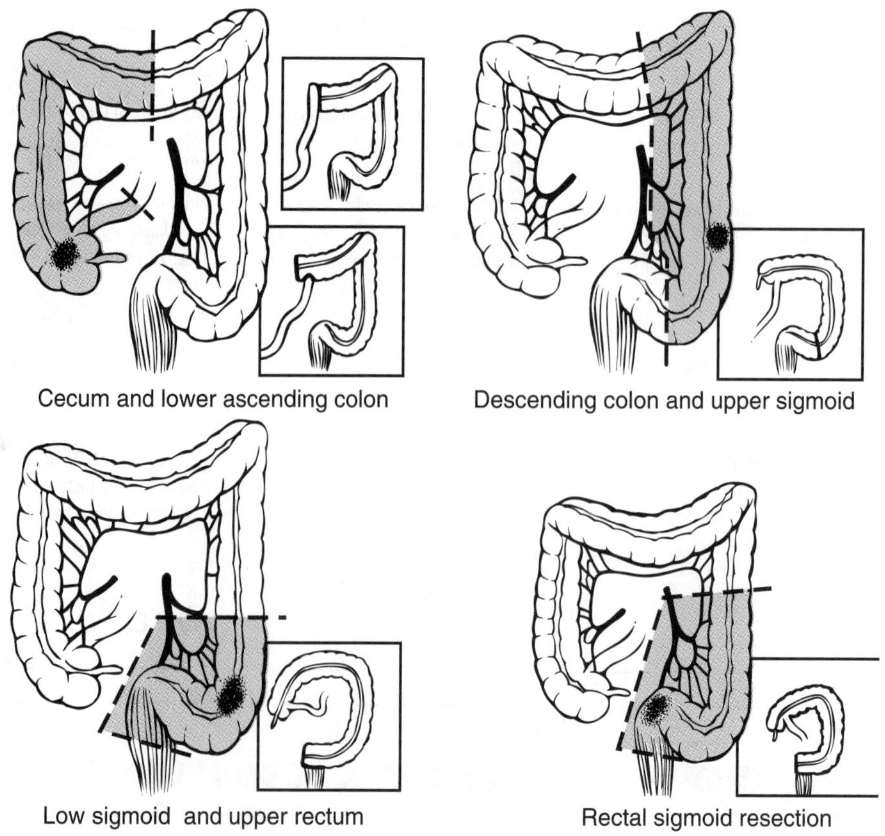

FIGURE 37-8. Examples of areas where cancer can occur, the area that is removed, and (in the very small diagrams) how the anastomosis is performed. (Adapted from American Cancer Society.)

also invade the blood vessels surrounding the colon causing hemorrhage. Perforation may occur, resulting in the formation of abscess. Peritonitis and/or sepsis may lead to shock.

Surgical Management. Surgery is the primary treatment for most colon and rectal cancers. Surgery may be curative or palliative. Cancers limited to one site are removable through the colonoscope. Laparoscopic colotomy with polypectomy is a more recently developed procedure that minimizes the extent of surgery needed in some cases. A laparoscope is used as a guide in making an incision into the colon; the tumor mass is then excised. The Nd:YAG laser has proved effective with some lesions as well. Bowel resection is indicated for most class A lesions and all class B and C lesions. Surgery is sometimes recommended for class D colon cancer. The goal of surgery in this instance is palliative. If the tumor has spread and involves surrounding vital structures, it is considered to be inoperable.

The type of surgery depends on the location and size of the tumor. The surgical procedures of choice are the following (Doughty & Jackson, 1993):

- Segmental resection with anastomosis (removal of the tumor and portions of the bowel on either side of the growth, as well as the blood vessels and lymphatic nodes) (Fig. 37-8)
- Abdominoperineal resection with permanent sigmoid colostomy (removal of the tumor and a portion of the sigmoid and all of the rectum and anal sphincter) (Fig. 37-9)
- Temporary colostomy followed by segmental resection and anastomosis and subsequent reanastomosis of the colostomy (allowing for initial bowel decompression and bowel preparation before resection)
- Permanent colostomy or ileostomy (for palliation of unresectable obstructing lesion)

Fecal Diversions for Cancer of the Colon and Rectum. Due to improved surgical techniques, **colostomies** are performed on less than one-third of patients with colorectal cancer. A colostomy is the surgical creation of an opening (stoma) into the colon. It can be created as a temporary or permanent diversion. It allows for the drainage or evacuation of colon contents to the outside of

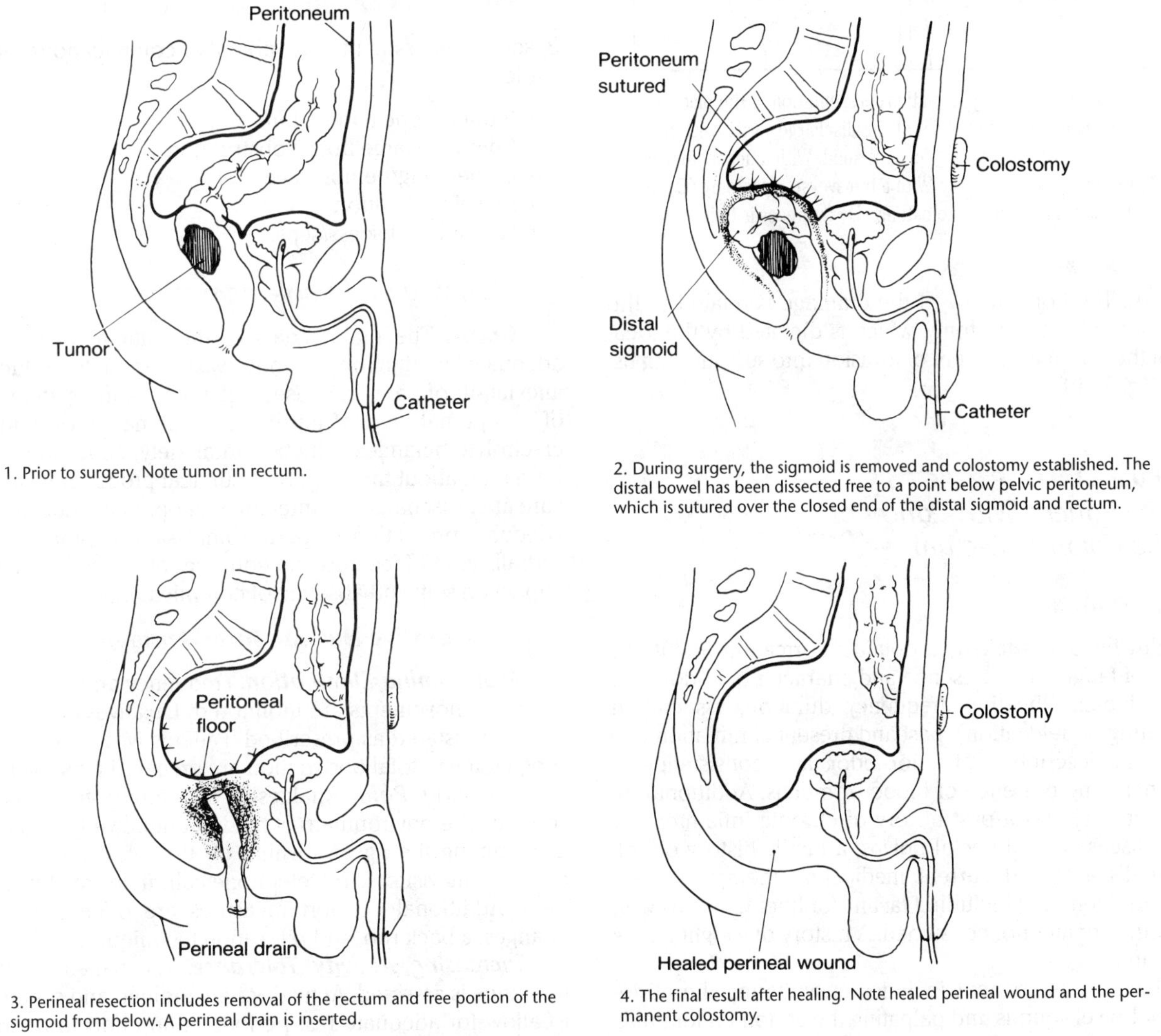

1. Prior to surgery. Note tumor in rectum.

2. During surgery, the sigmoid is removed and colostomy established. The distal bowel has been dissected free to a point below pelvic peritoneum, which is sutured over the closed end of the distal sigmoid and rectum.

3. Perineal resection includes removal of the rectum and free portion of the sigmoid from below. A perineal drain is inserted.

4. The final result after healing. Note healed perineal wound and the permanent colostomy.

FIGURE 37-9. Abdominoperineal resection for carcinoma of the rectum.

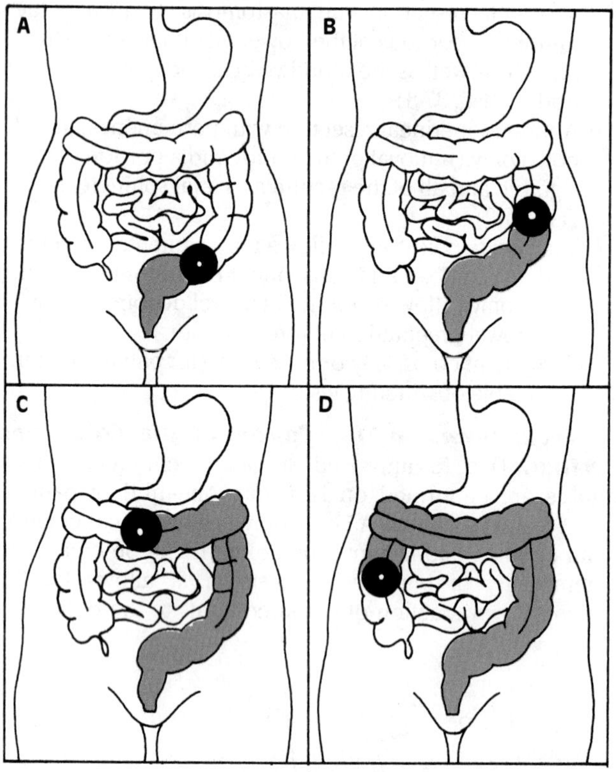

FIGURE 37-10. A diagrammatic representation of the placement of permanent colostomies. The nature of the discharge varies with the site. With a sigmoid colostomy (**A**) the feces is solid. With a descending colostomy (**B**) the feces is semimushy. With a transverse colostomy (**C**) the feces is mushy. With an ascending colostomy (**D**) the feces is fluid.

the body. The consistency of the drainage is related to the placement of the colostomy, which is dictated by the location of the tumor and extent of invasion into surrounding tissues (Fig. 37-10).

❑ NURSING PROCESS
The Patient With Cancer of the Colon or Rectum

Assessment

A health history is taken to obtain information about the feeling of fatigue; the presence and character of abdominal or rectal pain (location, frequency, duration, association with eating or defecation); past and present elimination patterns; and description of color, odor, and consistency of stool including presence of blood or mucus. Additional information includes a past history of chronic inflammatory bowel disease or colorectal polyps; a family history of colorectal disease; and current medication therapy. Dietary habits are identified including fat and/or fiber intake as well as amounts of alcohol consumed. A history of weight loss is important.

Objective assessment includes auscultating the abdomen for bowel sounds and palpating the abdomen for areas of tenderness, distention, and solid masses. Stool specimens are inspected for character and presence of blood.

Diagnosis

Nursing Diagnoses

Based on all the assessment data, the patient's major nursing diagnoses may include the following:

- ❑ Constipation related to obstructing lesion
- ❑ Pain related to tissue compression secondary to obstruction
- ❑ Fatigue related to anemia and anorexia
- ❑ Altered nutrition, less than body requirements, related to nausea and anorexia
- ❑ Risk for fluid volume deficit related to vomiting and dehydration
- ❑ Anxiety related to impending surgery and the diagnosis of cancer
- ❑ Knowledge deficit concerning the diagnosis, the surgical procedure, and self-care after discharge
- ❑ Impaired skin integrity related to the surgical incisions (abdominal and perianal), the formation of a stoma, and frequent fecal contamination of periostomal skin
- ❑ Body image disturbance related to colostomy

Collaborative Problems/ Potential Complications

Based on assessment data, potential complications may include:

- ❑ Intraperitoneal infection
- ❑ Complete large bowel obstruction
- ❑ GI bleeding/hemorrhage
- ❑ Bowel perforation
- ❑ Peritonitis/abscess/sepsis

Planning and Implementation

Goals. The major goals of the patient may include adequate elimination of body waste products; reduction/alleviation of pain; increased activity tolerance; attainment of an optimal level of nutrition; maintenance of fluid and electrolyte balance; reduction in anxiety; acquisition of information about the diagnosis, surgical procedure, and self-care after discharge; maintenance of optimal tissue healing; adequate protection of periostomal skin; exploration and verbalization of feelings and concerns about colostomy and impact on self; and absence of complications.

Preoperative Nursing Interventions

Maintaining Elimination. Frequency and consistency of bowel movements are monitored. Laxatives and enemas are administered as prescribed. Patients who show signs of progressing to total obstruction are prepared for surgery.

Relieving Pain. Analgesics are administered as prescribed. The environment is made conducive to relaxation by dimming the lights, turning off the television or radio, and limiting visitors and telephone calls if desired by the patient. Additional comfort measures are offered: position changes, a back rub, and relaxation techniques.

Increasing Activity Tolerance. The patient's activity tolerance is assessed. Activities are modified and scheduled to allow for adequate rest periods in an effort to decrease patient fatigue. Blood component therapy is administered as prescribed if the patient is severely anemic. When a blood transfusion is administered, normal safety guidelines and agency policy regarding safety are followed. Postoperatively, activity is progressed and tolerance is monitored.

Providing Nutritional Measures. If the patient's condition permits, a diet high in calories, protein, and carbohydrates and low in residue is given preoperatively for several days to provide adequate nutrition and minimize cramping by decreasing excessive peristalsis. A full-liquid diet may be prescribed 24 hours before surgery to decrease bulk. Total parenteral nutrition is required for some patients to replace depleted nutrients, vitamins, and minerals. Daily weights are recorded and the physician is notified if the patient continues to lose weight while receiving parenteral nutrition.

Maintaining Fluid and Electrolyte Balance. Intake and output, including vomitus, are measured and recorded, to provide an accurate record of fluid balance. The patient's intake of oral food and fluids is restricted to prevent vomiting. Antiemetics are administered as prescribed. Full or clear liquids may be tolerated, or the patient may be allowed nothing by mouth. A nasogastric tube will be inserted preoperatively to drain accumulated fluids and prevent abdominal distention. An indwelling urinary catheter may be inserted to allow for monitoring of hourly output. An output of less than 30 ml/hr is reported so that intravenous fluid therapy can be adjusted as necessary.

Intravenous administration of fluids and electrolytes is monitored. Serum electrolyte levels are monitored to detect hypokalemia and hyponatremia, which occur with gastrointestinal fluid loss. Vital signs are assessed to detect signs of hypovolemia: tachycardia, hypotension, and decreased pulse volume. Hydration status is assessed, and decreased skin turgor, dry mucous membranes, concentrated urine, and increased urine specific gravity are reported.

Reducing Anxiety. The patient's level of anxiety is assessed, as are coping mechanisms used to deal with stress. Supportive efforts include providing privacy if desired and instructing the patient in relaxation exercises. Time is set aside to listen to the patient who wishes to ventilate, cry, or ask questions. The nurse will arrange meetings with a member of the clergy if the patient so desires, with the physicians if the patient wishes to discuss the treatment or prognosis, and with an enterostomal therapist. An ostomate may be asked to visit if the patient expresses an interest in talking with one.

In order to promote patient comfort, the nurse projects a relaxed and empathetic attitude. Questions are answered honestly. All tests and procedures are explained in language the patient understands. Any information the physician has provided is clarified, if necessary. Sometimes anxiety is relieved if the patient knows what physical preparation is necessary preoperatively and what to expect postoperatively. Some patients appreciate seeing pictures or drawings, whereas others would prefer not to know details. The patient's needs and desires for information are assessed and used as a guide for teaching.

Preventing Infections. Antibiotics such as kanamycin sulfate (Kantrex), erythromycin (Erythrocin), and neomycin sulfate are administered as prescribed to reduce intestinal bacteria in preparation for bowel surgery. These are administered by mouth to reduce the bacterial content of the colon and to soften and decrease the bulk of the contents of the colon. In addition, the bowel can be cleansed by laxatives, enemas, or colonic irrigations. Antibiotics may be administered postoperatively to assist in preventing infection.

Preoperative Patient Education. The patient's present knowledge about the diagnosis, prognosis, surgical procedure, and expected level of functioning postoperatively is assessed. Information that is needed, how it should be presented, when the patient would be most receptive to it, and who should be present during the instruction are determined.

Information that the patient needs about the physical preparation for surgery, the expected appearance and care of the wound postoperatively, the technique of ostomy care, dietary restrictions, pain control, and medication management are included in the teaching plan (see Nursing Care Plan 37-1).

Postoperative Nursing Interventions

Wound Care. The abdominal wound is examined frequently during the first 24 hours to make sure that it is healing without complications (infection, dehiscence, hemorrhage, excessive edema). Dressings are changed as needed to prevent infection. The patient is assisted to splint the abdominal incision during coughing and deep breathing to lessen tension on the edges of the incision. Temperature, pulse, and respiratory rate are monitored for elevations that may indicate an infectious process.

The stoma is examined for swelling (slight edema due to surgical manipulation is normal), color (a healthy stoma is pink), discharge (a small amount of oozing is normal), and bleeding (an abnormal sign). The peristomal skin is cleansed gently and patted dry to prevent irritation. A protective skin barrier should be applied before attaching the drainage bag.

If the malignancy has been removed by the perineal route, the wound is observed carefully for signs of hemorrhage. This wound may contain a drain or packing that is removed gradually. There may be sloughing of bits of tissue for a week. This process is hastened by the mechanical irrigation of the wound or with sitz baths performed two or three times a day initially. The condition of the perineal wound and any bleeding, infection, or necrosis is documented.

Patient Education and Home Care Considerations. Discharge planning requires the combined efforts of the physician, nurse, enterostomal therapist, social worker, and dietitian. Patients being discharged from the hospital are given specific information, individualized to their needs, about ostomy care and complications for which to observe. Dietary instructions are essential to help patients identify and eliminate irritating foods that can cause diarrhea or constipation. Patients are taught about their prescribed medications (action, purpose, and possible side effects of each).

Treatments (irrigations, wound cleansing) and dressing changes are reviewed, and the family is encouraged to participate. Patients need very specific directions about when to call the physician. They need to know exactly which complications require prompt attention (bleeding, abdominal distention and rigidity, diarrhea, and the dumping syndrome). If radiation therapy is necessary, the possible side effects (anorexia, vomiting, diarrhea, and exhaustion) are reviewed.

Often home health care is required to provide essential care for debilitated patients or to carry out initial follow-up care of the wound. These visits provide an opportunity for additional patient teaching and observation of the patient's general condition.

Positive Body Image. The patient is encouraged to verbalize feelings and concerns as well as to discuss the surgery and the stoma (if one was created). Colostomy care must be learned and the patient must begin to plan for incorporating stoma care into daily life. A supportive environment and attitude on the nurse's part is crucial in promoting the patient's adaptation to the changes brought about by the surgery.

Monitoring and Managing Complications. The patient's condition is observed for symptoms of complications.

Frequent assessment of the abdomen, including decreasing or changing bowel sounds and increasing abdominal girth, is completed. The patient may need to be prepared for emergency surgery. Vital signs are monitored for increased pulse and respiration and decreased blood pressure, as well as rectal bleeding that would be indicative of hemorrhage. Hematocrit and hemoglobin are monitored. Blood component therapy is administered as prescribed. Any abrupt change in abdominal pain is reported because it may indicate perforation. Increase in WBCs and temperature and/or symptoms of shock are reported as they may indicate sepsis. Antibiotics are administered as ordered. See Chart 37-3 for possible postoperative complications.

Evaluation

Expected Outcomes

1. Maintains adequate bowel elimination
2. Experiences less pain
3. Activity tolerance increases
4. Achieves an optimal level of nutrition
   a. Eats a low-residue, high-protein, high-calorie diet
   b. Reports less abdominal cramping
5. Achieves fluid balance
   a. Restricts oral intake of foods and fluids when nauseated
   b. Urinates at least 1.5 L/24 hr
6. Experiences reduced anxiety
   a. Verbalizes concerns and fears freely
   b. Uses coping measures to deal with stress
7. Acquires information about the diagnosis, surgical procedure, and self-care after discharge
   a. Discusses the diagnosis, surgical procedure, and postoperative self-care
   b. Demonstrates technique of ostomy care
8. Maintains clean incision, stoma, and perineal wound
   a. Gradually increases participation in stoma and peristomal skin care
9. Verbalizes feelings and concerns about self
10. Experiences absence of complications
   a. Takes oral antibiotics as prescribed
   b. Cooperates with bowel cleansing protocol
   c. Is afebrile
   d. Bowel sounds are present
   e. Abdominal girth remains constant or decreases
   f. No evidence of perforation or bleeding noted

The Patient Requiring a Colostomy

Preoperative Nursing Interventions

Psychosocial Support. A patient diagnosed with cancer of the colon or rectum may require a permanent colostomy and may grieve about the diagnosis and the impending surgery. Patients undergoing surgery for a temporary colostomy may express fears and concerns similar to those of a person with a permanent stoma. All members of the health team, including the enterostomal therapy nurse, and the family should be available for assistance and support.

Speaking with a person who is successfully managing a colostomy is often helpful to the patient. The United Ostomy Association provides useful information about living with an ostomy, through literature, lectures, and exhibits. Visiting services by qualified members and rehabilitation services for new ostomy patients are provided.

Anticipated changes in body image and life style often are profoundly disturbing, and patients may need empathetic support in trying to adjust to them. Because the stoma is located on the abdomen, the patient may think that everyone will be aware of the ostomy. The nurse can help reduce this apprehension by presenting factual information about the surgical procedure and the creation and management of the ostomy. If the patient is receptive, diagrams, photographs, and appliances may be used to explain and clarify. Because the patient is experiencing emotional stress, the nurse may need to repeat some of the information. Time should be provided for the patient to ask questions. The nurse's acceptance and understanding of the patient's concerns and feelings convey a caring, competent attitude that promotes confidence and cooperation. Consultation with an enterostomal therapist during the preoperative period can be extremely helpful.

Preparation for Surgery. Usually, a high-calorie, low-residue diet is given for several days before surgery if time and the patient's condition permit. If an emergency does not exist, preoperative measures taken are similar to those for general abdominal surgery. Blood component therapy may be prescribed because anemia is common. Preoperative nasogastric intubation may be indicated and minimizes postoperative distention. An indwelling catheter is inserted to aid in keeping postoperative perineal dressings dry.

Postoperative Nursing Interventions

Postoperative nursing care for patients undergoing a colostomy is similar to nursing care for any abdominal surgery patient (see Chapter 21). In addition, the patient is monitored for signs of the complications discussed earlier in this section. These include leakage from an anastomotic site, prolapse of the stoma, perforation, stoma retraction, fecal impaction, and skin irritation, as well as pulmonary complications associated with abdominal surgery. The abdomen is monitored for signs of returning peristalsis and initial stool characteristics are assessed. Patients undergoing a colostomy are assisted out of bed on the first postoperative day and encouraged to begin participating in managing the colostomy. The return to normal diet is rapid. At least 2 L of fluid/day is suggested. Every effort is made to encourage the patient to live as he or she did before surgery.

CHART 37-3
Potential Complications After Intestinal Surgery

Complication	Nursing Assessment and Interventions
Paralytic ileus	Initiate or continue nasogastric intubation. Prepare patient for x-ray study. Ensure adequate fluid and electrolyte replacement. Administer prescribed antibiotics if patient has symptoms of peritonitis.
Mechanical obstruction	Evaluate patient for intermittent colicky pain, nausea, and vomiting.
Intraperitoneal infection and abdominal wound infection	Monitor for evidence of constant or generalized abdominal pain, rapid pulse, and elevation of temperature. Prepare for tube decompression of bowel. Administer fluids and electrolytes by IV route as prescribed. Administer antibiotics as prescribed
Intra-abdominal septic conditions	
Peritonitis	Evaluate patient for nausea, hiccups, chills, spiking fever, tachycardia. Administer antibiotics as prescribed. Prepare patient for drainage procedure. Institute intravenous fluid and electrolyte therapy as prescribed. Prepare patient for surgery if condition deteriorates.
Abscess formation	Administer antibiotics as prescribed. Apply warm compresses as prescribed. Prepare for surgical drainage.
Wound complications	
Infection	Monitor temperature; report temperature elevation. Observe for redness, tenderness, and pain around wound. Assist in establishing local drainage. Obtain specimen of drainage material for culture and sensitivity studies.
Wound disruption	Observe for sudden appearance of profuse serous drainage from wound. Cover wound area with sterile towels held in place with binder. Prepare patient immediately for surgery.
Anastomotic complications	
Dehiscence of anastomosis Fistulas	Prepare patient for surgery. Assist in bowel decompression. Administer parenteral fluids as prescribed to correct fluid and electrolyte defects.

Gerontologic Considerations. Elderly patients may have some degree of decreased vision and impaired hearing, as well as difficulty with skills that require fine motor coordination. Therefore, it may be helpful for the patient to handle the ostomy equipment preoperatively and simulate cleaning the peristomal skin and irrigating the stoma.

Accidents resulting from falls occur frequently among the elderly. Therefore, it is important to determine whether the patient can walk unassisted to the bathroom.

Skin care is a major concern for the elderly ostomate because of skin changes that occur with aging. The epithelial and subcutaneous fatty layers become thin and skin is easily irritated. To prevent breakdown, special attention is paid to skin cleansing and the proper fit of an appliance. Arteriosclerosis causes decreased blood flow to the wound and stoma site. As a result, transport of nutrients is delayed, and healing time may be prolonged.

Some patients experience delayed elimination after irrigation because of decreased peristalsis and mucus production. Most require 6 months before they feel comfortable with their ostomy care.

Managing the Colostomy

Colostomy function will begin 3 to 6 days postoperatively. The nurse manages the colostomy until the patient can take over its care. Skin care must be taught along with how to apply the drainage pouch and manage irrigation.

Skin Care. The effluent discharge will vary with the type of ostomy. With a transverse colostomy, the stool is soft and mushy and irritating to the skin. With a descending or sigmoid colostomy, the stool is fairly solid and slightly irritating to the skin. The patient is advised to protect the peristomal skin by frequently washing the area with a mild soap, applying a protective skin barrier around the stoma, and securely attaching the drainage pouch. Nystatin powder (Mycostatin) can be dusted lightly on the peristomal skin if irritation or yeast growth is present.

The skin is cleaned gently with a moist, soft cloth and a mild soap. Any excess skin barrier is removed. Soap acts as a mild abrasive agent to remove enzyme residue from fecal spillage. During the time the skin is being cleansed, a gauze dressing may cover the stoma or a vaginal tampon can be inserted gently to absorb excess drainage.

The patient may be permitted to bathe or shower before putting on the clean appliance. Micropore tape applied to the sides of the pouch will keep it secure during bathing. The skin is patted completely dry with a gauze pad; rubbing the area is avoided. A skin barrier (wafer, paste, or powder) is used around the stoma to protect the skin from fecal drainage.

Applying the Drainage Pouch. The stoma is measured to determine the correct size for the pouch. The pouch opening should be about 0.3 cm (⅛ inch) larger than the stoma. The skin is cleansed according to the above procedure. A peristomal skin barrier is applied. The backing from the adherent surface of the pouch is removed and the bag is pressed down over the stoma for 30 seconds (Fig. 37-11). Mild skin irritation may require dusting the skin with Karaya powder or stomahesive powder before attaching the pouch.

Managing the Drainage Pouch. Colostomy bags may be worn immediately after irrigation; then a change to a simple dressing may be effective. Patients can choose from a wide variety of pouches, depending on their individual needs. Most pouches are disposable and odor resistant. Commercially prepared deodorizers are available for use.

As a rule, colostomy bags are not necessary. As soon as the patient has learned a routine for evacuation, bags may be dispensed with and a closed ostomy pouch or a simple dressing of disposable tissue (often covered with plastic wrap) is used, held in place by an elastic belt or girdle. Except for gas and a slight amount of mucus, nothing will escape from the colostomy opening between irrigations; therefore, a colostomy bag is unnecessary. Colostomy plugs (which expand upon insertion to prevent passage of flatus and feces) are available.

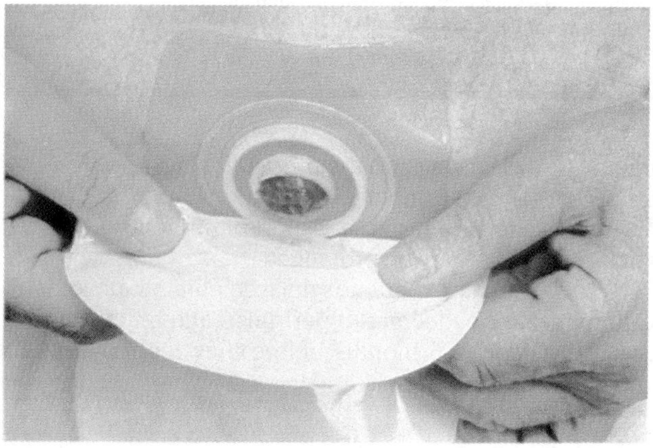

FIGURE 37-11. The colostomy appliance is pressed into place. (Courtesy of Convatec, A Squibb Company.)

Removing the Appliance. The drainage appliance is changed when it is one-third to one-fourth full so that the weight of its contents does not cause the pouch to separate from the adhesive disc and spill the contents. The patient assumes a comfortable sitting or standing position and *gently* pushes the skin down from the faceplate while pulling the pouch up and away from the stoma. Gentle pressure prevents the skin from being traumatized and any liquid fecal contents from spilling out.

Irrigating the Colostomy. A stoma on the abdomen does not have voluntary muscular control and may empty at irregular intervals. Regulating the passage of fecal material is achieved either by irrigating the colostomy or allowing the bowel to evacuate naturally without irrigations. The choice often depends on the individual and the nature of the colostomy.

The purpose of irrigating a colostomy is to empty the colon of gas, mucus, and feces so that the patient can go about social and business activities without fear of fecal drainage. By irrigating the stoma at a *regular* time, there is less gas and retention of irrigating fluids.

The time for irrigating the colostomy should be consistent with the schedule the person will follow after leaving the hospital. Refer to Guideline 37-3 for the irrigating procedure and Figure 37-12 for the equipment.

Patient Education and Home Care Considerations

Family members should be informed of the procedure involved in stoma care and the adjustments they will need to make in their daily lives once the patient comes home. They need to be encouraged to verbalize their concerns. They also need to understand the importance of making the necessary adjustments to enable the patient to deal with the change in body image and the need to take proper care of the colostomy.

Before the patient's discharge from the hospital, an individualized routine for stoma care and irrigation is reviewed with the patient and family. Supplemental literature is helpful, because those involved may have questions when the patient is back in the home setting. Someone in the family should assume responsibility for purchasing the equipment and supplies that will be needed at home.

Because the hospital stay is so limited, the patient may not be able to become proficient in stoma care techniques before discharge. Many patients benefit from referral to a home care agency or from the services of the local chapter of The American Cancer Society. The home care nurse will come to the home to provide further care and teaching and to assess how well the patient and family are adjusting to the colostomy.

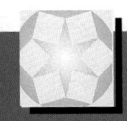

GUIDELINE 37-3
Irrigating a Colostomy

A colostomy is irrigated to empty the colon of feces, gas, or mucus, cleanse the lower intestinal tract, and establish a regular pattern of evacuation so that normal life activities may be pursued. A suitable time for the irrigation is selected, preferably after a meal, so that this time is compatible with the patient's posthospital pattern of activity. Irrigation should be performed at the same time each day.

Before the procedure the patient sits on a chair in front of the toilet or on the toilet itself. An irrigating reservoir with 500 to 1500 ml lukewarm tap water is hung 45 to 50 cm (18 to 20 in) above the stoma (shoulder height when the patient is seated). Dressings or pouch are removed. The following procedure is used; the patient is assisted to participate in the procedure in order to learn to perform it unassisted.

Nursing Action	Rationale/Amplification
1. Apply an irrigating sleeve or sheath to the stoma. Place the end in the commode (see Fig. 37-12).	This helps to control odor and splashing and allows feces and water to flow directly into the commode.
2. Allow some of the solution to flow through the tubing and catheter/cone.	Air bubbles in the setup are released so that air is not introduced into the colon, which would cause crampy pain.
3. Lubricate the catheter/cone and gently insert it into the stoma. Insert the catheter no more than 8 cm (3 in). Hold the shield/cone gently, but firmly, against the stoma to prevent backflow of water.	These steps are necessary to prevent intestinal perforation.
4. If the catheter does not advance easily, allow water to flow slowly while advancing catheter. *Never force the catheter!*	A slow rate of flow helps to relax the bowel and facilitates passage of the catheter.
5. Allow tepid fluid to enter the colon slowly. If cramping occurs, clamp off the tubing and allow the patient to rest before progressing. Water should flow in over a 5- to 10-minute period.	Painful cramps are usually caused by too rapid a flow or by too much solution. 300 cc of fluid may be all that is needed to stimulate evacuation. Volume may be increased with subsequent irrigations to 500, 1000, or 1500 ml as needed by the patient for effective results.
6. Hold the shield/cone in place 10 seconds after the water has been instilled; then gently remove it.	
7. Allow 10 to 15 minutes for most of the return; then dry the bottom of the sleeve/sheath and attach it to the top, or apply the appropriate clamp to the bottom of the sleeve.	Most of the water, feces, and flatus will be expelled in 10 to 15 minutes.
8. Leave the sleeve/sheath in place about 30–45 minutes while the patient gets up and moves around.	Ambulation stimulates peristalsis and completion of the irrigation return.
9. Cleanse the area with a mild soap and water; pat the area dry.	Cleanliness and dryness will provide the patient with hours of comfort.
10. Replace the colostomy dressing or pouch.	The patient should use a pouch until the colostomy is sufficiently controlled. A dressing may be all that is needed.

Nutritional Status

In general, the patient is reminded that good health practices, including consuming a healthy diet, will promote feelings of well-being and positive adjustment to the colostomy. The diet is individualized as long as it is well balanced and does not cause diarrhea or constipation.

A complete nutritional assessment is performed. Foods that cause excessive odor and gas are avoided. These include foods in the cabbage family, eggs, fish, beans, and cellulose products such as peanuts. It is important to determine if the elimination of specific foods is causing any nutritional deficiency. Nonirritating foods are substituted for those that are restricted so that deficiencies are corrected. The patient is advised to experiment with an irritating food several times before restricting it, because the reaction may be an initial sensitivity that will decrease with time.

Hydration status is assessed (skin turgor, mucous membranes, intake and output, weight) and signs of dehydration are reported. If the patient experiences diarrhea, the frequency of the diarrhea is noted, along with the occurrence of abdominal cramping, urgency, and hyperactive bowel sounds. The patient is assisted to identify any foods or fluids that may be causing diarrhea, such as fruits, high-fiber foods, soda, coffee, tea, or carbonated beverages. Paregoric, bismuth subgallate, bismuth subcarbonate, or diphenoxylate with atropine (Lomotil) will help control the diarrhea. For constipation, prune or apple juice or a mild laxative is effective.

Sexuality and Sexual Function

The patient is encouraged to discuss feelings about sexuality and sexual function. Some patients may initiate questions about sexual activity directly or give indirect clues about their fears. Some may view the surgery as mutilating and a threat to their sexuality; some fear impotence. Others

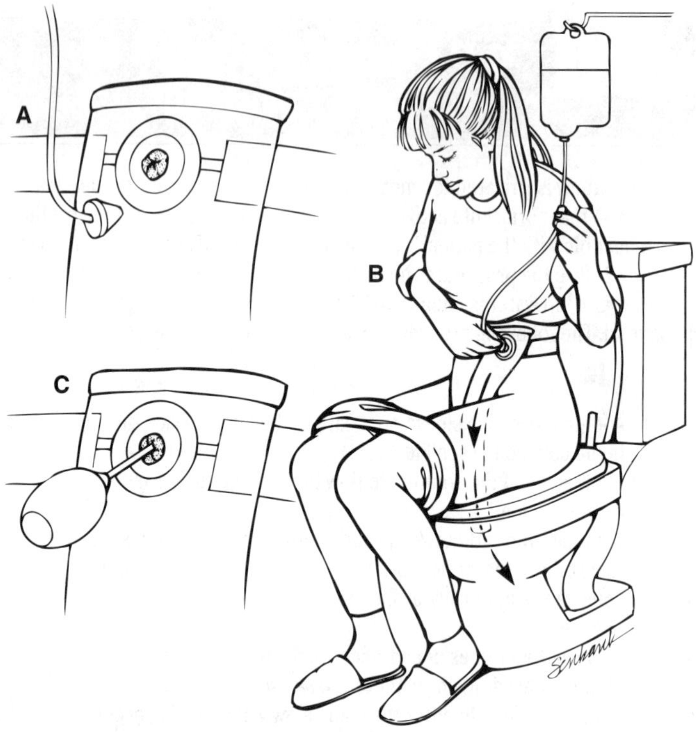

FIGURE 37-12. Colostomy irrigation. (**A**) Irrigating catheter has a cone attachment to prevent injury to stomal tissue. (**B**) Irrigating fluid is instilled with sleeve in place. Drainage contents empty into toilet. (**C**) The bulb syringe method can be used to stimulate fecal drainage. Note that a portion of the hard nozzle is removed and a catheter attached to minimize stomal irritation.

may express worry about odor or leakage from the pouch during sexual activity. Alternative sexual positions are recommended as well as alternative methods of stimulation to satisfy sexual drives. The nurse assesses the patient's needs and attempts to identify specific concerns. If the nurse is uncomfortable with this, or if the patient's concerns seem complex, it may be appropriate for the nurse to seek assistance from an enterostomal therapy nurse, sex counselor, or clinical nurse specialist.

Complications of Colostomy

The incidence of complications for patients with colostomies is about half that seen with ileostomies. Some common complications are **prolapse of the stoma** (usually due to obesity), **perforation** (due to improper stoma irrigation), **stoma retraction, fecal impaction,** and **skin irritation.** Leakage from an anastomotic site can occur if remaining bowel segments are diseased or weakened. Leakage from an intestinal anastomosis causes abdominal distention and rigidity, temperature elevation, and signs of shock. Surgical repair is necessary.

Pulmonary complications are always a concern with abdominal surgery. Patients over 50 years of age are considered to be at risk, especially if they are or have been receiving antibiotics or sedatives, or are being maintained on bed rest for a prolonged period. Two primary pulmonary complications are pneumonia and atelectasis. These complications can be prevented by frequent activity (turning the patient from side to side every 2 hours), deep breathing, coughing, and early ambulation.

See Chart 37-3 for a list of potential complications after intestinal surgery.

Polyps of the Colon and Rectum

A polyp is a mass of tissue that protrudes into the lumen of the bowel and can be found anywhere in the intestinal tract and rectum. Polyps can be classified as neoplastic (adenomas and carcinomas) or non-neoplastic (mucosal and hyperplastic). Adenomatous polyps (benign epithelial growths) are common in the western world. They occur more frequently in the large intestine than in the small intestine. Although the vast majority of them do not develop into invasive neoplasms, their presence must be identified and closely followed. Polyps occur in 10% to 60% of the population; they occur most frequently in the fifth decade of life.

Clinical manifestations depend on the size of the polyp and the amount of pressure it exerts on intestinal tissue. The most common symptom is rectal bleeding. Lower abdominal pain may also occur. If the polyp is large enough, symptoms of obstruction will be present.

The diagnosis is based on history and digital rectal exam, barium enema studies, sigmoidoscopy, or colonoscopy. Once a polyp is identified, it is removed through a colonoscope by the use of special equipment (*i.e.*, biopsy forceps and snares). Microscopic exam of the polyp then identifies the type of polyp and indicates if surgery is required. The principal reason for performing a colonic polypectomy is the possibility that malignancy is already present or may develop.

Diseases of the Anorectum

Patients with anorectal disorders seek medical care primarily because of pain and rectal bleeding. Other frequent complaints are protrusion of hemorrhoids, anal discharge, itching, swelling, anal tenderness, stenosis, and ulceration. Constipation results from delaying defecation because of pain.

Anorectal Abscess

Anorectal abscess is an infection in the pararectal spaces. Persons with regional enteritis and other immunodeficient states such as AIDS are particularly susceptible to these infections. Many of these abscesses will result in fistulas.

Clinical Manifestations. An abscess may occur in a variety of spaces in and around the rectum. Often it contains a quantity of foul-smelling pus and is painful. If the abscess is superficial, swelling, redness, and tenderness are observed. A deeper abscess may result in toxic symptoms and even lower abdominal pain, as well as fever. More than half of rectal abscesses will result in fistulas.

Management. Palliative therapy consists of sitz baths and analgesics. However, prompt surgical treatment to incise and drain the abscess is the treatment of choice. When deeper infection exists, with the possibility of a fistula, the fistulous tract must be removed. If possible, the fistula is removed when the abscess is incised and drained, or a second procedure to do so may be necessary. The wound may be packed with gauze and allowed to heal by granulation.

Anal Fistula

An anal fistula is a tiny, tubular, fibrous tract that extends into the anal canal from an opening located beside the anus (Fig. 37-13*A*). Fistulas usually result from an infection. They may also develop from trauma, fissures, or regional enteritis.

Clinical Manifestations. Pus or stool may leak constantly from the cutaneous opening. Other symptoms may be the passage of flatus or feces from the vagina or bladder depending on the fistula tract. Untreated fistulas may cause systemic infection with related symptoms.

Management. Surgery is always recommended because few fistulas heal spontaneously. A **fistulectomy** (excision of the fistulous tract) is the recommended surgical procedure. The lower bowel is evacuated thoroughly with several prescribed enemas.

During surgery, the sinus tract is identified by inserting a probe into it or by injecting the tract with methylene blue solution. The fistula is dissected out or laid open by an incision from its rectal opening to its outlet. The wound is packed with gauze.

Anal Fissure

An anal fissure is a longitudinal tear or ulceration in the lining of the anal canal (see Fig. 37-13*B*). Fissures are usually caused by the trauma of passing a large firm stool or from persistent tightening of the anal canal secondary to stress and anxiety (leading to constipation). Other causes include childbirth, trauma, and overuse of laxatives.

Clinical Manifestations and Management. Fissures are characterized by extremely painful defecation, burning, and bleeding. Most of these fissures will heal if treated by conservative measures, which include stool softeners and bulk agents, an increase in water intake, sitz baths, and emollient suppositories. A suppository combining an anesthetic with a corticosteroid helps relieve the discomfort. Anal dilation under anesthesia may be required.

If fissures do not respond to conservative treatment, surgery is indicated. Several types of procedures may be performed: in some cases, the anal sphincter is dilated and the fissure is excised; in others, a part of the external sphincter is divided. This produces a paralysis of the external sphincter, with consequent relief of spasm, and permits the ulcer to heal.

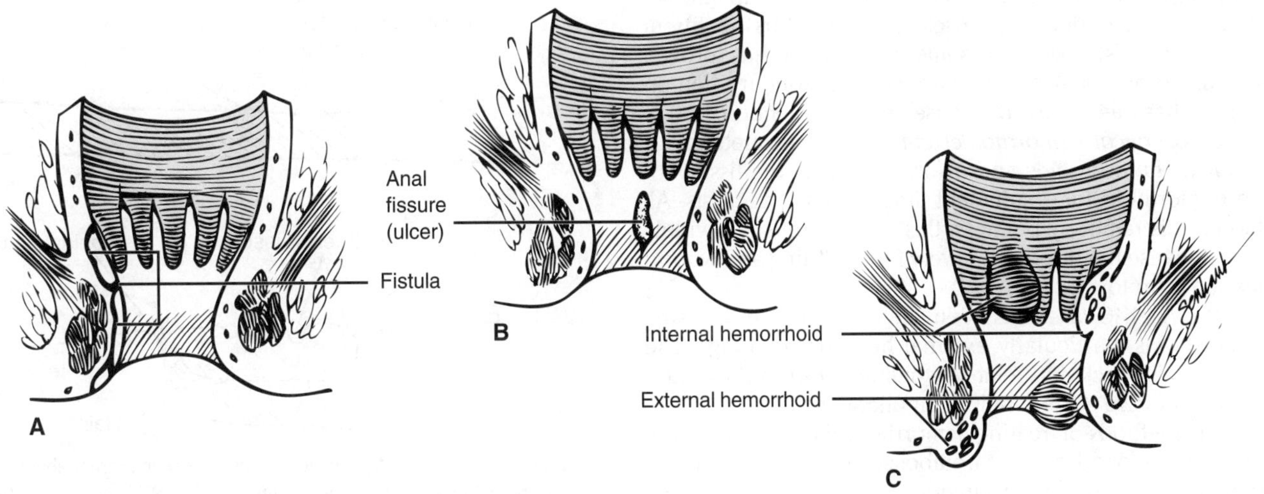

FIGURE 37-13. Various types of anal lesions. (**A**) Fistula. (**B**) Fissure. (**C**) External and internal hemorrhoids.

Hemorrhoids

Hemorrhoids are dilated portions of veins in the anal canal. They are very common. By the age of 50, 50% of people have hemorrhoids to some extent. Pregnancy is known to initiate or aggravate existing hemorrhoids. Hemorrhoids are classified into two types. Those occurring above the internal sphincter are called *internal hemorrhoids,* and those appearing outside the external sphincter are called *external hemorrhoids* (see Fig. 37-13C).

Clinical Manifestations. Hemorrhoids cause itching and pain, and are the most common cause of bright red bleeding that occurs with defecation. External hemorrhoids are associated with severe pain due to inflammation and edema caused by thrombosis. Thrombosis is the clotting of blood within the hemorrhoid. This may lead to ischemia of the area and eventual necrosis. Internal hemorrhoids are not usually painful until they bleed or prolapse when they become enlarged.

Management. Hemorrhoid symptoms and discomfort can be relieved by good personal hygiene and by avoiding excessive straining during defecation. A high-residue diet that contains fruit and bran may be all the treatment that is necessary; failing this, a laxative that absorbs water as it passes through the intestines may help. Sitz baths, ointments, and suppositories containing anesthetics, astringents (witch hazel), and bed rest are measures that allow the engorgement to subside.

There are several types of *nonoperative treatments* for hemorrhoids. Infrared photocoagulation, bipolar diathermy, and laser therapy are newer techniques that are used to affix the mucosa to the underlying muscle. Injecting sclerosing solutions is also effective for small, bleeding hemorrhoids. These procedures assist in preventing prolapse.

A conservative surgical treatment of internal hemorrhoids is the *rubber-band ligation* procedure. The hemorrhoid is visualized through the anoscope, and its proximal portion above the mucocutaneous lines is grasped with an instrument. A small rubber band is then slipped over the hemorrhoid. Tissue distal to the rubber band becomes necrotic after several days and sloughs off. Fibrosis occurs resulting in the lower anal mucosa being drawn up and adhering to the underlying muscle. Although this treatment has been satisfactory for some patients, it has proven painful for others and may cause some secondary hemorrhage. It has been known to cause perianal infection.

Cryosurgical hemorrhoidectomy is another method for removing hemorrhoids and involves freezing the tissues of the hemorrhoid for a sufficient time to cause necrosis. Although it is relatively painless, this procedure is not widely used because the discharge is very foul-smelling and wound healing is prolonged.

The *Nd:YAG laser* has been useful recently in excising hemorrhoids, particularly external hemorrhoidal tags. The treatment is quick and relatively painless. Hemorrhage and abscess are rare postoperative complications.

The methods of treating hemorrhoids just described are not effective for advanced thrombosed veins, which must be treated by more extensive surgery.

Hemorrhoidectomy, or surgical excision, can be performed to remove all of the redundant tissue involved in the process. During surgery the rectal sphincter is usually dilated digitally and the hemorrhoids are removed with a clamp and cautery or by being ligated and then excised. After the operative procedures are completed, a small tube may be inserted through the sphincter to permit the escape of flatus and blood; pieces of Gelfoam or Oxycel gauze may be placed over the anal wounds.

Pilonidal Sinus/Cyst

A pilonidal sinus or cyst is found in the intergluteal cleft on the posterior surface of the lower sacrum (Fig. 37-14). Current theories postulate that it results from the penetration of hairs into the epithelium and subcutaneous tissue. It may also be formed congenitally by an infolding of epithelial tissue beneath the skin, which may communicate with the skin surface through one or several small sinus openings. Hair frequently is seen protruding from these openings, and this gives the cyst its name—*pilonidal*—a nest of hair. The cysts rarely cause symptoms until adolescence or early adult life, when infection produces an irritating drainage or an abscess. This area is easily irritated by perspiration and friction.

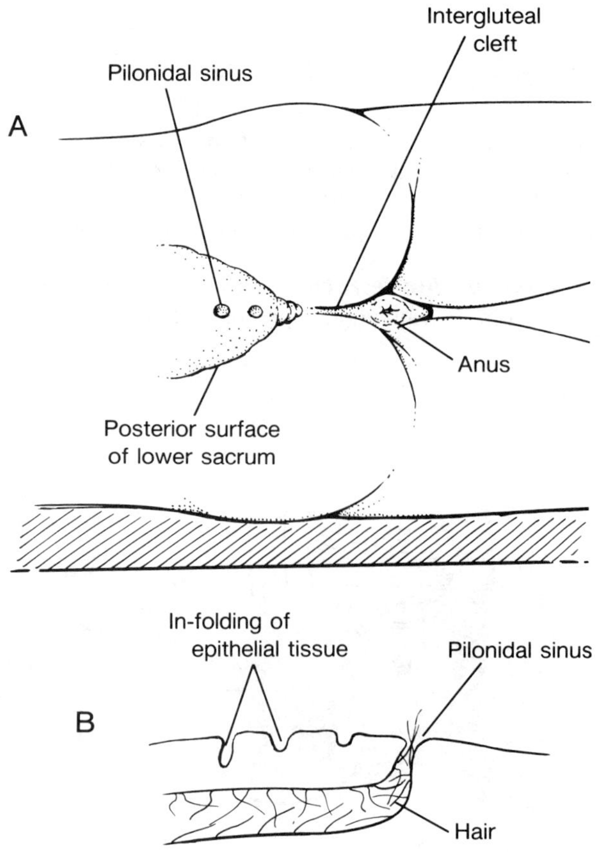

FIGURE 37-14. (**A**) Pilonidal sinus on lower sacrum about 5 cm (2 in) above the anus in the intergluteal cleft. (**B**) Note hair particles emerging from the sinus tract. Localized indentations of the skin (pits) can occur near the sinus openings.

Management. In the early stages of the inflammation, the infection may be controlled by antibiotic therapy. Once an abscess has formed, surgery is indicated. The abscess is incised and drained under local anesthetic. After the acute process resolves, further surgery is performed to excise the cyst and the secondary sinus tracts. The wound is allowed to heal by granulation. Gauze dressings are placed in the wound to keep its edges separated while healing occurs.

❑ NURSING PROCESS
The Patient With an Anorectal Condition

Assessment

A health history is taken to determine the presence and characteristics of any itching, burning, and pain. Does it occur during bowel movements? How long does it last? Is any abdominal pain associated with it? Does any bleeding occur from the rectum? How much? How frequently? What color is it? Is there any other discharge such as mucus or pus? Other questions relate to elimination patterns and laxative use; diet history, including fiber intake; the amount of exercise; activity levels; and occupation (especially if there is required prolonged sitting or standing).

Objective assessment includes inspecting the stool for blood or mucus, and the perianal area for hemorrhoids, fissures, irritation, or pus.

Diagnosis

Nursing Diagnoses

Based on all the assessment data, the patient's major nursing diagnoses may include the following:

- Constipation related to ignoring the urge to defecate because of pain during elimination
- Anxiety related to impending surgery and embarrassment
- Pain, related to irritation, pressure, and sensitivity in the rectal/anal area secondary to anorectal disease and sphincter spasms postoperatively
- Altered urinary elimination related to postoperative fear of pain
- Risk for ineffective management of the therapeutic regimen

Collaborative Problems/ Potential Complication

Based on assessment data, the following potential complication may develop:

- Hemorrhage

Planning and Implementation

Goals. The major goals of the patient may include attainment of adequate elimination patterns, reduction in anxiety, relief of pain, promotion of urinary elimination, compliance with the therapeutic regimen, and absence of complications.

Nursing Interventions

Relieving Constipation. The intake of at least 2 L of water daily is encouraged to provide adequate hydration. High-fiber foods are recommended to promote bulk in the stool and to make it easier to pass fecal matter through the rectum. Bulk laxatives such as Metamucil and stool softeners are administered as prescribed. The patient is advised to set aside a time for moving the bowels and to heed the urge to defecate as promptly as possible. It may be helpful to have the patient perform relaxation exercises before defecating to relax the abdominal perineal muscles that may be constricted or in spasm. Administering an analgesic before a bowel movement will be beneficial.

Reducing Anxiety. Patients facing rectal surgery may be upset and irritable because of discomfort, pain, and embarrassment. Specific psychosocial needs are identified and the plan of care is individualized. Privacy is provided by limiting visitors if the patient so desires. The patient's privacy is maintained when giving care. Soiled dressings are removed from the room promptly to prevent unpleasant odors. Room deodorizers may be needed if dressings are foul smelling.

Relieving Pain. During the first 24 hours after rectal surgery, painful spasms of the sphincter and perineal muscles may occur. Control of pain is a prime consideration. The patient is encouraged to assume a comfortable position. Flotation pads under the buttocks when sitting will help decrease the pain, as may ice and analgesic ointments. Warm compresses may promote circulation and soothe irritated tissues. Sitz baths, three or four times a day, will relieve soreness and pain by relaxing sphincter spasm. Twenty-four hours after surgery, topical anesthetic agents may be beneficial in relieving local irritation and soreness. Medications may include suppositories that contain anesthetics, astringents, antiseptics, tranquilizers, and antiemetics. Patients will be more compliant and less apprehensive if they are free of pain.

Wet dressings saturated with equal parts of cold water and witch hazel help relieve edema. When wet compresses are being used continuously, petrolatum should be applied around the anal area to prevent skin maceration. The patient is instructed to assume a prone position at intervals, because this position promotes dependent drainage of edematous fluid.

Promoting Urinary Elimination. Voiding may be a problem postoperatively, because of a reflex spasm of the sphincter at the outlet of the bladder and a certain amount of muscle-guarding from apprehension and pain. All methods to encourage voluntary voiding (increasing fluid intake, listening to running water, dripping water over the urinary meatus) should be tried before resorting to catheterization. After rectal surgery, urinary output should be monitored closely.

Monitoring and Managing Complications. The operative site must be examined frequently for rectal bleeding. The patient is assessed for systemic indicators of excessive bleeding (tachycardia, hypotension, restlessness, thirst). After hemorrhoidectomy, hemorrhage may occur from the veins that were cut. If a tube has been inserted through the sphincter after surgery, evidence of bleeding should be apparent on the dressings. If bleeding is obvious, direct pressure is applied to the area and the physician is notified. Moist heat is avoided as it will encourage vessel dilation and bleeding.

Patient Education and Home Care Considerations. The patient should keep the perianal area as clean as possible, by gently cleansing it with warm water and then drying it with absorbent cotton wipes. The patient is instructed to avoid rubbing the area with toilet tissue.

The patient is encouraged to respond quickly to the urge to defecate in order to prevent constipation. Diet is modified to increase fluids and fiber. The patient is informed about the prescribed diet, made aware of the significance of proper eating habits, instructed about laxatives that can be taken safely, and told why exercise is important. The patient is encouraged to ambulate as soon as possible. Moderate exercise is encouraged.

When it is time for discharge from the hospital, the patient should know how to take sitz baths and how to test the temperature of the water. Sitz baths may be given in a bathtub three or four times a day, or a plastic sitz bath unit can be used. Sitz baths should be taken after each bowel movement for 1 to 2 weeks after surgery.

Evaluation

Expected Outcomes

1. Attains a normal pattern of elimination
   a. Sets aside a time for defecation, usually after a meal or at bedtime
   b. Responds to the urge to defecate and takes the time to sit on the toilet and try to defecate
   c. Uses relaxation exercises as needed
   d. Increases fluid intake to 2 L/24 hr
   e. Adds high-fiber foods to diet
   f. Reports passage of soft, formed stools
   g. Reports decrease in abdominal discomfort
2. Experiences less anxiety
3. Experiences less pain
   a. Modifies body position and activities to minimize pain and discomfort
   b. Applies warmth/cold to rectal/anal area
   c. Takes sitz baths four times a day
4. Voids without difficulty
5. Adheres to the therapeutic regimen
   a. Keeps perianal area dry
   b. Eats bulk-forming foods
   c. Has soft, formed stools on a regular basis
6. Is free of any bleeding problems
   a. Has a clean incision
   b. Exhibits normal vital signs
   c. Shows no signs of hemorrhage

CRITICAL THINKING EXERCISES

1. You are visiting a resident in an extended-care facility. She complains that she has had pain throughout her abdomen for the past day. She has not had a bowel movement in 4 days, and she complains of loss of appetite. Physical examination reveals that her abdomen is distended and rigid and that bowel sounds are absent. Analyze these findings, indicate what you think the possible causes may be for these findings, and explain the actions you would take and why.
2. During a conversation with an elderly gentleman at a senior citizen's community center, he tells you that he cannot have a bowel movement without taking a laxative each day. He asks if this is acceptable, given that he also takes "blood pressure medicine, a heart pill and aspirin each day." Explain how you would advise this patient and the rationale behind your advice.
3. You are caring for a patient who has been treated medically for ulcerative colitis for 5 years. The patient is now 1 day post total colectomy and ileostomy. What are the similarities and differences between the care of this patient and that of a patient who has had a colon resection and colostomy? Explain how you would meet the emotional and health education needs of the patient with an ileostomy and the patient with a colostomy.

BIBLIOGRAPHY

Books

Allan RN et al. Inflammatory Bowel Diseases, 2nd ed. New York, Churchill Livingstone, 1990.

American Cancer Society. Cancer Facts and Figures. Atlanta, American Cancer Society, Inc., 1992.

Bryant R and Hampton B. Ostomies and Continent Diversions: Nursing Management. Baltimore, Mosby Year Book, 1992.

Corman ML. Colon and Rectal Surgery, 3rd ed. Philadelphia, JB Lippincott, 1993.

Doughty D and Jackson D. Gastrointestinal Disorders. St. Louis, Mosby, 1993.

Gitnick G (ed). Current Gastroenterology. Boston, Mosby Year Book, 1992.

Gitnick G. Inflammatory Bowel Disease—Diagnosis and Treatment. New York, Igaku-Shoin, 1991.

Gordon P and Nivatvongs S. Principles and Practices of Surgery for the Colon, Rectum, and Anus. St. Louis, Quality Medical Publishers, 1992.

NIH Consensus Statement—Adjuvant Therapy for Patients with Colon and Rectal Cancer. Califon, NJ, Gardiner-Caldwell Syner Med, 1990.

Phillips S et al. The Large Intestine: Physiology, Pathophysiology, and Disease. New York, Raven Press, 1991.

Shackelford RT and Zuidema GD. Surgery of the Alimentary Tract, 2nd ed. Philadelphia, WB Saunders, 1990.

Society of Gastroenterology Nurses and Associates. Gastroenterology Nursing, A Core Curriculum. Baltimore, Mosby Year Book, 1993.

Sodeman WA, Saladin TA, and Boyd WP. Geriatric Enterology. Philadelphia, WB Saunders, 1989.

Way LW. Current Surgical Diagnosis and Treatment. Los Altos, CA, Appleton and Lange, 1991.

Yamada T (ed). Atlas of Gastroenterology. Philadelphia, JB Lippincott, 1992.

Yamada T (ed). Textbook of Gastroenterology. Philadelphia, JB Lippincott, 1991.

Journals

Bayless TM et al. Malabsorption: Fine tuning the workup. Patient Care 1991 Nov 30; 25(19):17–53.

Beck M. Under the scope: A new surgical alternative. HELIX Winter 1992/1993:11–16.

Bryant G. When the bowel is blocked. RN 1992 Jan; 55(1):58–67.

Cooke DM. Inflammatory bowel disease: Primary health care management of ulcerative colitis and Crohn's disease. Nurse Pract 1991 Aug; 16(8):27–8, 30, 35–36.

Deeny P and McCrea H. Stoma care: The patient's perspective. J Adv Nurs 1991; 16(1):39–46.

Freidman L (ed). Gastrointestinal disorders in the elderly. Gastroenterol Clin North Am 1990; 19(2):15–22.

Frnka J. Ostomy appliances and equipment. Dimen Oncol Nur 1991 Fall; 5(3):20–5.

Handerhan B. Protecting your patient from ileus. Nurs 1991 Apr; 21(4):92–3, 95.

Hennessy K. Nutritional support and GI disease. Nurs Clin North Am 1989; 24(2):373–380.

Jansson JM. Dermatologic complications of ostomy care. Dimen Oncol Nur 1991 Fall; 5(3):10–13.

Leiback JR and Cerda JJ. Hemorrhoids: Modern treatment methods. Hosp Med 1991 Aug; 27(8):53–55, 59–60, 63.

Little MB et al. Measurement of pain in postoperative abdominal surgery patients. Applied Nurs Res 1992 Feb; 5(1):26–31.

Long L. Ileostomy care. Overcoming obstacles. Nursing 1991 Oct; 21(10):73–77.

McConnell EA. How to irrigate a colostomy. Nurs 1990 Sept; 20(9):78.

Meize-Grochowski R. When the diagnosis is Crohn's disease. RN 1991 Feb; 54(2):52–55.

O'Toole M. Advanced assessment of the abdomen and GI problems. Nurs Clin North Am 1990 Dec; 25(4):771–776.

Peppercorn M. Newer agents for the treatment of inflammatory bowel disease. Pharmacy & Therapeutics 1993; 18(6):583–595.

Rideout B. The patient with ileostomy: Nursing management and patient education. Nurs Clin North Am 1987; 22(2):253–262.

Roberts MI. Diarrhea: A symptom. Holistic Nurs Pract 1993 Jan; 7(2):73–80.

Roberts MK. Assessing and treating volvulus. Nurs 1992 Feb: 22(2):56–57.

Spollett G. Irritable bowel syndrome: Diagnosis and management. Nurs Pract 1989 Aug; 14(8):32–44.

Walker A and Whynes D. The cost of nursing care: A study of 65 colorectal patients. J Adv Nurs 1990 Nov; 15(11):1305–1309.

*Weinrich S et al. Knowledge of colorectal care among older persons. Cancer Nursing 1992 May; 15(5):322–330.

Witt ME. Current management of adults with colorectal cancer. Medsurg Nursing 1993 Apr; 2(2):105–111.

Zuro LM et al. Laparoscopic colostomy. Polypectomy. AORN J 1992 Dec; 56(6):1068, 1070–1073.

INFORMATION/RESOURCES

Agencies

American Cancer Society
1599 Clifton Rd. NE,
Atlanta, GA 30329

Crohn's and Colitis Foundation of America
44 Park Avenue So.,
New York, NY 10016-7374

International Association for Enterostomal Therapy
2081 Business Circle Dr., Suite 290,
Irvine, CA 92715

National Foundation for Ileitis and Colitis
444 Park Ave. South,
New York, NY 10016

United Ostomy Association
36 Executive Park, Irvine,
CA 92714

Nursing Research Profile for Unit 8

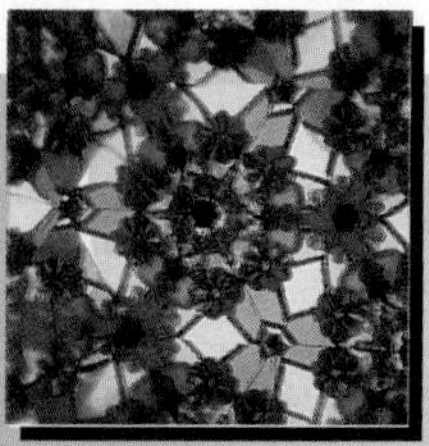

Digestive and Gastrointestinal Function

Overview

Nursing research reviewed here focuses on specific disease processes, health maintenance, and therapeutic modalities related to digestive and gastrointestinal function.

Metheny N et al. Detection of inadvertent respiratory placement of small-bore feeding tubes: A report of 10 cases. Heart Lung 1990 Nov; 19(6):631–638.

Small-bore enteral feeding tubes are often inserted by nurses at the bedside. These tubes may inadvertently enter the respiratory tract without clinically obvious signs. To assure proper placement, methods to confirm proper feeding tube position need to be determined.

The subjects of this small study were 10 patients with documented respiratory placement of small-bore feeding tubes. These tubes were inserted by unit personnel (nurses and physicians) of five intensive care units and two general medical units. The investigator either observed the procedures or interviewed the involved clinicians after the procedure, noting the types of placement testing methods used and their results. Placements were followed by x-rays to establish the actual location of the tubes. X-ray findings in all 10 of the subjects revealed inadvertent respiratory placement (*i.e.*, right or left main stem bronchus) of the feeding tubes.

The following methods were used by the clinicians to verify proper tube placement in the subjects: auscultatory method (nine subjects), changes in respiratory status (10 subjects), fluid aspiration from the tube (six subjects), *p*H testing of the aspirant (three subjects), and observing for bubbling when the end of the tube was held under water (one subject). In eight of the nine subjects for whom the auscultatory method was used, the clinicians reported hearing air insufflations; these sounds were identified as soft in one subject, muffled in two subjects, and loud in five subjects. Eight of the 10 subjects were reported to have no changes in respiratory status; the other two coughed during tube insertion but had no other reported signs of change in respiratory status. Fluid was aspirated from the tubes of all six subjects for whom aspiration was attempted; the aspirant from two of the tubes had *p*H values of 7 or greater and the aspirant from one of the tubes had a *p*H of 6.74.

Nursing Implications. Nurses confirm proper feeding tube placement using various bedside methods. In this study, these methods often gave false reassurance that the tubes were properly positioned. It is critical that all health care professionals be aware that x-ray is the only consistently reliable method of detecting inadvertent respiratory placement of feeding tubes and that these x-rays must be taken prior to any infusion of tube feeding.

Sands JA. Incidence of pulmonary aspiration in intubated patients receiving enteral nutrition through wide- and narrow-bore nasogastric feeding tubes. Heart Lung 1991 Jan; 20(1):75–80.

Nurses caring for patients receiving enteral nutrition must continually monitor for and use measures to prevent complications. A mechanical complication, pulmonary aspiration, has been found to be caused by various factors, including use of a feeding tube that is too large, improper patient position, improper feeding tube placement, or the patient vomiting and aspirating emesis. Attempts have been made by researchers to determine the safest type of tube to use to supply enteral nutrition. The purpose of this descriptive study was to compare the incidence of pulmonary aspiration in intubated patients receiving enteral nutrition through a narrow-bore nasogastric tube with that in patients with a wide-bore nasogastric tube.

A convenience sample of 25 patients in critical care units who had endotracheal tubes in place and who received tube feedings for a minimum of 3 days (15 wide-bore and 10 narrow-bore tubes) was studied. All subjects received the continuous method of tube feeding with a feeding pump. Each patient was followed by the investigator for a period of 3 days. The following clinical information significant to aspiration was collected: amount and rate of tube feeding infusion, residual volumes, tube displacement, and any occurrence of stained tracheal aspirant.

The findings of the study revealed that there was no significant difference ($p < 0.05$) in the incidence of pulmonary aspiration between the two groups (narrow-bore nasogastric tube group and wide-bore nasogastric tube group). Aspiration occurred in one subject. During the 3-day period of study for the 25 subjects, 72 chest x-rays and 1 abdominal x-ray were taken. The existence and placement of the nasogastric tube was reported on the x-ray results significantly more frequently ($p < 0.001$) in the group of subjects who had wide-bore nasogastric tubes in place than in the group with narrow-bore tubes.

The frequency of times that the nurses checked residual volumes and tube placement was significantly greater ($p < 0.05$) with patients with wide-bore tubes than with patients with narrow-bore tubes. Difficulty with checking residual volumes for patients with narrow-bore tubes was documented by the nurses.

Nursing Implications. Residual volumes and tube placement must be checked and recorded routinely while patients are receiving tube feedings. The study results raise questions about the use of narrow-bore feeding tubes for critically ill intubated patients.

Heather DJ. Effect of bulk-forming cathartic on diarrhea in tube-fed patients. Heart Lung 1991 July; 20(4):409–413.

Enteral feedings are administered to many patients in hospitals, extended-care facilities, and home settings. One of the most common gastrointestinal complications associated with enteral tube feedings is diarrhea. If diarrhea is not controlled properly, patients may experience problems with skin breakdown and pressure ulcer formation as well as fluid and electrolyte disturbances.

The purpose of this study was to determine whether giving a bulk-forming cathartic to patients receiving enteral nutrition via nasogastric or nasoduodenal tube would result in firmer stools.

An experimental design was used with a study sample of 49 patients who were randomly assigned to either a control or an experimental group. The subjects were unable to take nutrients by mouth either because of the presence of an endotracheal tube or because of debilitation.

During a 6-day period, all patients received tube feedings (Osmolite, Isocal, or Isocal HCN) via continuous infusion. The patients in the experimental group were given 5 ml of Hydrocil, a bulk-forming cathartic, three times a day. The patients in the control group received no bulk-forming-cathartic. Stool consistency and frequency were recorded for 6 consecutive days. A 7-point scale was used to determine consistency of stool, with 1 indicating watery stool and 7 indicating hard, formed stool. A significant difference ($p < 0.01$) in stool consistency (firmness) was found, with the experimental group that received Hydrocil having the firmer stool consistency. There was no significant difference between the groups with regard to stool frequency.

Nursing Implications. Patients with tube feedings may benefit from receiving bulk-forming cathartics to help control diarrhea and to help prevent skin breakdown that often results from diarrhea.

Wilson DM. Ethical concerns in a long-term tube feeding study. IMAGE: J Nurs Scholarship 1992 Fall; 24(3):195–199.

The researchers designed an exploratory study for the purpose of gathering data on recorded practices of long-term tube feeding. A chart review was conducted on the charts of 10 patients in a long-term care facility who had been tube fed for longer than 6 months; reviews were conducted by two investigators. The questions that were used to guide the chart review were as follows:

(1) Are nurses involved in decisions to initiate and continue tube feeding? (2) Are decisions made to continue tube feeding after its implementation, and are these decisions documented? (3) What are the patients' functional reasons for long-term tube feeding and medical diagnoses? (4) What are the types of feeding solutions, tubes, and methods used for long-term tube feeding? (5) What changes in mental and physical conditions of the patients have occurred since initiation of tube feeding?

The results of the study revealed that tube feeding practices were not standardized, patients did not appear to gain functionality (ability to perform ADLs) from tube feedings, and the tube feedings were capable of sustaining life for a long period of time. Secondary analysis raised five ethical concerns regarding decision making: (1) who should make the decision to tube feed? (2) how should tube feeding decisions be made? (3) what are valid reasons for initiating and continuing tube feedings? (4) is it permissible to withdraw tube feeding once it is initiated? and (5) is tube feeding an effective and appropriate life-supporting technology?

Nursing Implications. Nurses caring for patients in long-term care facilities should be involved in decision-making with regard to tube feedings for their patients. These nurses, who care for the patients on a day-to-day basis, have key information that can be helpful to physicians and family members as they make decisions about the benefits and burdens of treatment. In addition, nurses need to be aware of ethical issues regarding the use of tube feedings to sustain a patient's life. Many decisions need to be considered when tube feeding therapy is being considered.

Wilson PR, Herman J, and Chubon SJ. Eating strategies used by persons with head and neck cancer during and after radiotherapy. Cancer Nurs 1991 Apr; 14(2):98–104.

Persons with head and neck cancer frequently experience alterations in nutrition as a result of the disease and its treatment. The purpose of this descriptive study was to identify eating difficulties experienced by patients treated with radiation for head and neck cancer and to identify methods used by patients to overcome these difficulties. To obtain information the researchers interviewed 11 subjects within 6 months of completion of radiation therapy for head and neck cancer. The researcher-developed Eating During/After Treatment (EDT) interview form was used to guide the interviews; three open-ended questions were used to determine what the subject did to help himself to eat during and after treatment and what problems he encountered during treatment. In addition, demographic and nutritional status data were collected from the subjects' medical records.

The study revealed that most patients reported weight loss, sore mouth/throat, taste changes, loss of appetite, and difficulty swallowing. Strategies most commonly used by the patients to overcome these problems included eating only specific foods, having other people prepare their meals, using nutritional supplements, changing the texture of foods, and obtaining advice from others.

Nursing Implications. Patients with head and neck cancer are at risk for alteration in nutrition due to difficulties with eating. It is helpful for the nurse to determine the patient's perception of his eating difficulties and to identify eating strategies that he has found to be of help. Additional eating strategies can then be suggested and encouraged in an attempt to promote nutrition.

Weinrich P et al. Knowledge of colorectal cancer among older persons. Cancer Nursing 1992 May; 15(5):322–330.

Colorectal cancer is the second leading cause of death due to cancer in the United States. It has been found that survival rates could be greatly increased with screening, early detection, and appropriate management. The American Cancer Society has developed colorectal cancer screening guidelines to facilitate screening and early detection. The segment of the population that has been found by researchers to be the least likely to participate in colorectal screening is socioeconomically disadvantaged persons over 50 years of age.

The purpose of this study was to determine the level of knowledge about colorectal cancer among the socioeconomically disadvantaged population. The following question was posed: Is colorectal cancer knowledge a predictor for participation in fecal occult blood testing (FOBT)? The study sample consisted of 211 participants, the majority (77%) of whom were female, with an average age of 72 years; almost equal proportions were African Americans and Caucasians. The average educational level was eighth grade, and over 50% had incomes below the poverty level.

A quasi-experimental pretest-posttest design was utilized to measure the effect of knowledge on participation in FOBT. The Colorectal Cancer Knowledge Questionnaire was adapted for the study population and used as a pretest-posttest. The American Cancer Society's colorectal cancer slide-tape presentation was used as the educational program for all participants. Hemoccult II kits were given to all participants at no cost; these kits were collected from the participants 6 days after the educational program, and the posttest was administered at that time.

Results of the study revealed that Caucasian subjects had more knowledge about colorectal cancer than did African Americans, and persons with higher incomes had more knowledge than those with lower incomes. Six days after the colorectal cancer education program, the subjects' knowledge about colorectal cancer increased significantly ($p < 0.01$). This increased knowledge was a predictor of participation in FOBT ($p < 0.02$). Generalizations are limited only to persons similar to the socioeconomically disadvantaged study participants.

Nursing Implications. This study supported other research findings that show that many of the socioeconomically disadvantaged poor do not have knowledge about colorectal cancer and do not participate in screening processes. Nurses working in acute care settings and in community and home settings must be acutely aware of this knowledge deficit and include preventive education in interactions with this particular population of patients. Opportunities should also be sought to disseminate educational materials to churches, libraries, community centers, senior citizen communities, and other sites where older socioeconomically disadvantaged persons can be reached.

Tittle MB, Long MC, and McMillan SC. Measurement of pain in postoperative abdominal surgery patients. Appl Nurs Res 1992 Feb; 5(1):26–31.

Pain is one of the common symptoms experienced by patients during the postoperative period. The purpose of this study was to examine whether pain decreased between the first and the third postoperative days and to identify the words used by patients to describe the quality of their pain.

The study sample consisted of 100 patients who had undergone abdominal surgery. A visual analog scale (VAS) was used to document pain intensity. At the same time, the subjects were asked to answer questions from the Present Pain Intensity and the Pain Rating Index of the McGill Pain Questionnaire. These measures were used on the first and third postoperative days once it had been determined that subjects had received no analgesics within the past two hours.

Mean scores on the VAS decreased significantly ($p < 0.01$) over time from the first to the third postoperative day. However, for some subjects pain intensity increased: 19% experienced an increase in pain from the first to the third postoperative day. Of those patients who experienced a decrease in pain, pain was not completely absent on postoperative day three. It was also found that certain words were chosen most frequently to describe pain: *tender, sore, cramping, pulling,* and *tiring.*

Nursing Implications. This study confirms a common assumption of nurses that postoperative pain following abdominal surgery usually decreases as the patient recovers; however, this is very individualized, and patients may continue to have pain on the third postoperative day. Pain management interventions must be implemented on an individual basis. Nurses must listen to the words used by patients to describe pain and medicate patients according to their perceptions of pain, not according to the nurse's expectations of the pain that the patient should be experiencing. Also, nurses cannot assume that patients with similar surgical procedures will experience the same type and intensity of pain.

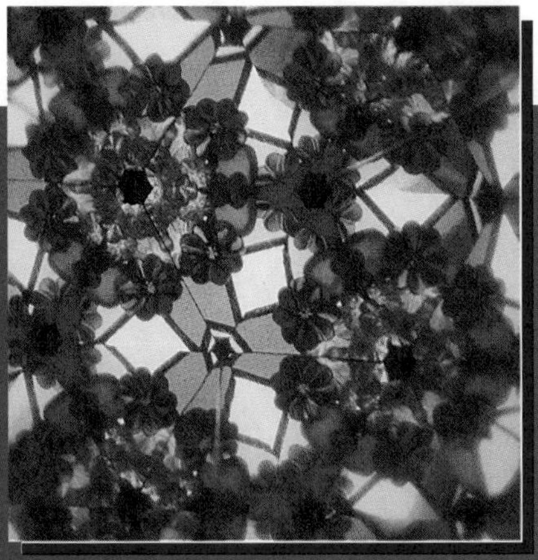

UNIT 9 Metabolic and Endocrine Function

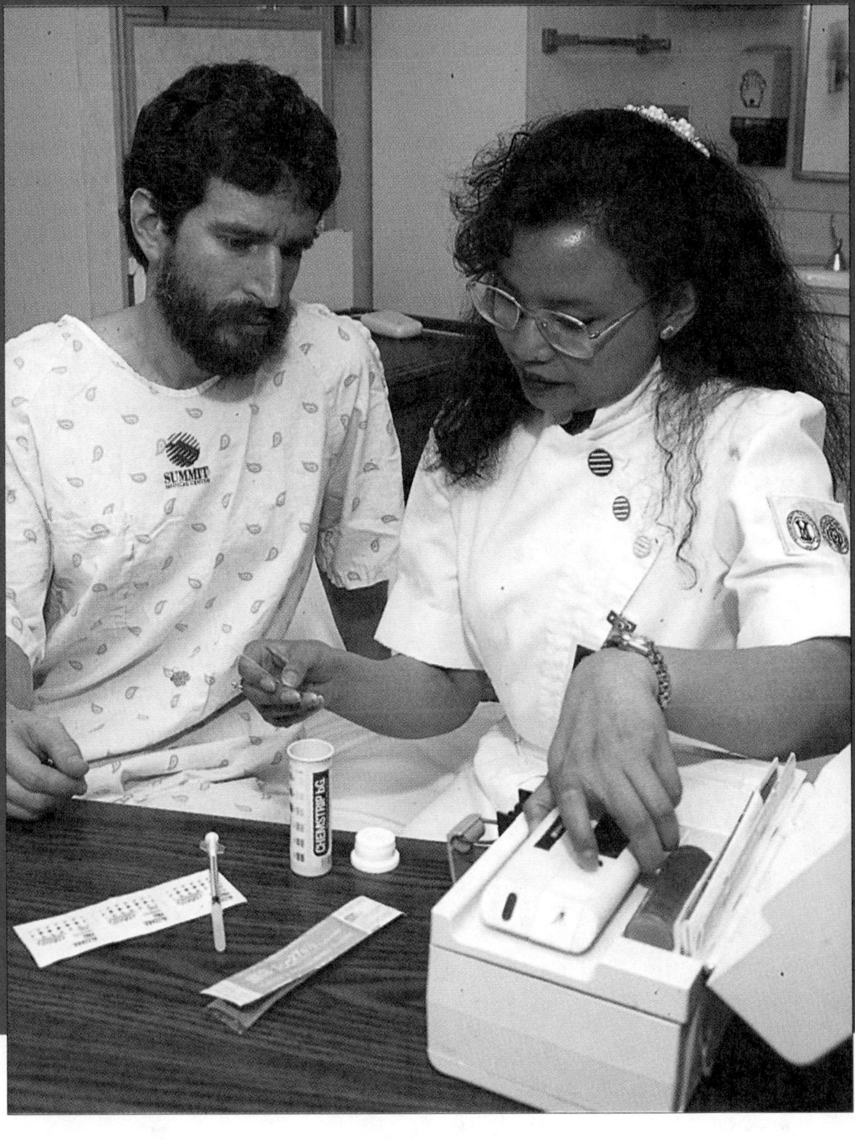

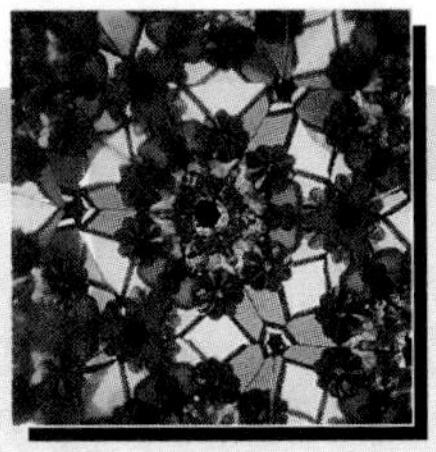

38

Assessment and Management of Patients With Hepatic and Biliary Disorders

CHAPTER OUTLINE

LEARNING OBJECTIVES

On completion of this chapter, the learner will be able to:

1. Identify the metabolic functions of the liver and the alterations in these functions that occur with liver disease
2. Explain liver function tests and clinical manifestations of liver dysfunction in relation to pathophysiologic alterations of the liver
3. Relate jaundice, portal hypertension, ascites, nutritional deficiencies, and hepatic coma to pathophysiologic alterations of the liver
4. Compare the various types of hepatitis and their causes, prevention, clinical manifestations, management, prognosis, and home health care needs
5. Use the nursing process as a framework for care of the patient with cirrhosis of the liver
6. Describe the medical and nursing management of patients with esophageal varices
7. Compare the nonsurgical and surgical management of patients with cancer of the liver
8. Describe the postoperative nursing care of the patient undergoing liver transplantation
9. Compare approaches to management of cholelithiasis
10. Use the nursing process as a framework for care of patients with cholelithiasis and those undergoing cholecystectomy

Physiologic Overview

The liver, the largest gland of the body, can be considered a chemical factory that manufactures, stores, alters, and excretes a large number of substances involved in metabolism. The location of the liver is essential in this function, because it receives nutrient-rich blood directly from the gastrointestinal tract and then either stores or transforms these nutrients into chemicals that are used elsewhere in the body for metabolic needs. The liver is especially important in the regulation of glucose and protein metabolism. The liver manufactures and secretes bile, which has a major role in the digestion and absorption of fats in the gastrointestinal tract. It removes waste products from the bloodstream and secretes them into the bile. The bile produced by the liver is stored temporarily in the gallbladder until it is needed for the process of digestion, at which time the gallbladder empties and bile enters the intestine. Figure 38-1 shows the liver and biliary system and their relation to the pancreas and spleen.

Anatomy

The liver is located behind the ribs in the upper right portion of the abdominal cavity. It weighs about 1500 g and is divided into four lobes. Each lobe is surrounded by a thin layer of connective tissue, which extends into the lobe itself and divides the liver mass into small units, called **lobules.** (see Fig. 38-1).

The circulation of the blood into and out of the liver is of major importance in its function. The blood that perfuses the liver comes from two sources. Approximately 75% of the blood supply comes from the portal vein, which drains the gastrointestinal tract and is rich in nutrients. The remainder of the blood supply enters by way of the hepatic artery and is rich in oxygen. Terminal branches of these two blood supplies join to form common capillary beds, which constitute the sinusoids of the liver (Fig. 38-2). Liver cells (hepatocytes) are thus bathed by a mixture of venous and arterial blood. The sinusoids empty into a venule that occupies the center of each liver lobule and is called the **central vein.** The central veins join to form the hepatic vein, which constitutes the venous drainage from the liver and empties into the inferior vena cava, close to the diaphragm. Thus, there are two sources of blood flowing into the liver and only one exit pathway.

In addition to hepatocytes, phagocytic cells belonging to the reticuloendothelial system are present in the liver. Other organs that contain reticuloendothelial cells are the spleen, bone marrow, lymph nodes, and lungs. In the liver, these cells are called **Kupffer cells.** Their main function is to engulf particulate matter (such as bacteria) that enters the liver through the portal blood.

The smallest bile ducts, called **canaliculi,** are located between the lobules of the liver. The canaliculi receive secretions from the hepatocytes and carry them to larger bile ducts, which eventually form the **hepatic duct.** The hepatic duct from the liver and the cystic duct from the gallbladder join to form the **common bile duct,** which empties into the small intestine. The flow of bile into the intestine is controlled by the sphincter of Oddi, located at the junction where the common bile duct enters the duodenum.

The **gallbladder,** a pear-shaped, hollow, saclike organ, 7.5 to 10 cm (3–4 in) long, lies in a shallow depression on the inferior surface of the liver, to which it is attached by loose connective tissue. The capacity of the gallbladder is 30

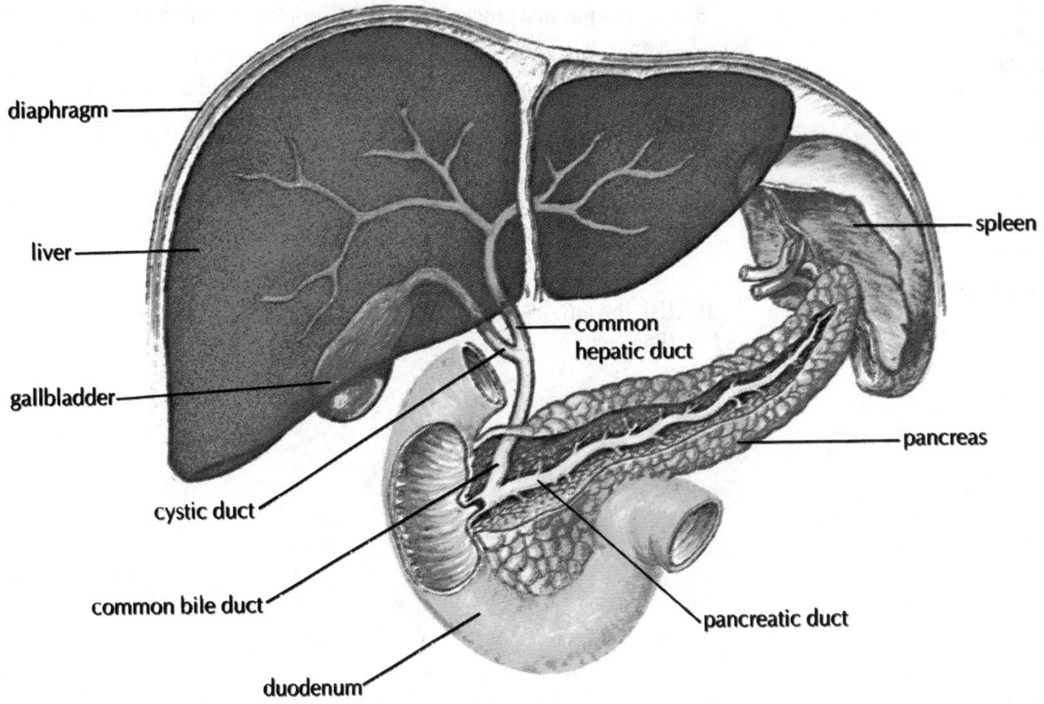

FIGURE 38-1. The liver and biliary system.

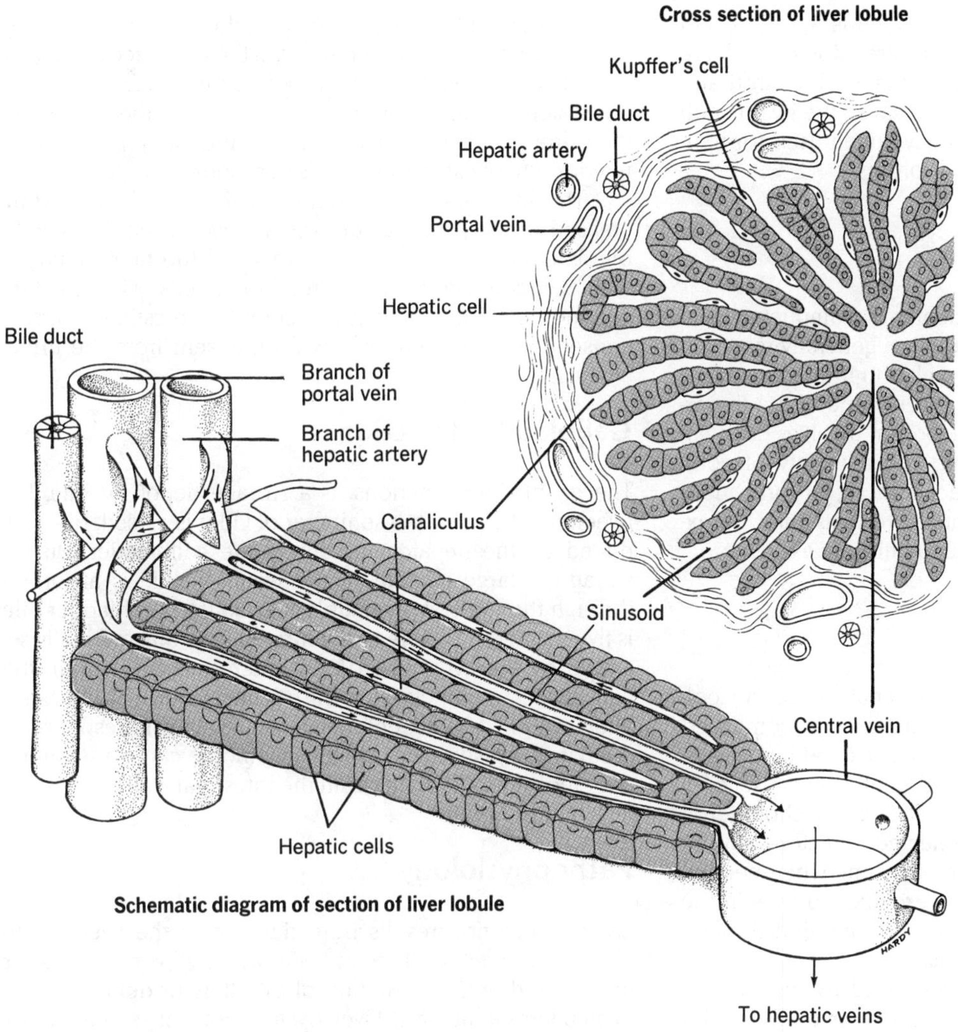

FIGURE 38-2. A section of liver lobule showing the location of hepatic veins, hepatic cells, liver sinusoids, and branches of the portal vein and hepatic artery.

to 50 ml of bile. Its wall is composed largely of smooth muscle. The gallbladder is connected to the common bile duct by the cystic duct (see Fig. 38-1).

Metabolic Functions of the Liver

Glucose Metabolism. The liver plays a major role in the metabolism of glucose and the regulation of blood glucose concentration. After a meal, glucose is taken up from the portal venous blood by the liver and converted into glycogen, which is stored in the hepatocytes. Subsequently, the glycogen is converted back to glucose and released as needed into the bloodstream to maintain normal levels of blood glucose. Additional glucose can be synthesized by the liver through a process called **gluconeogenesis.** For this process, the liver uses amino acids from protein breakdown or lactate produced by exercising muscles.

Ammonia Conversion. Use of amino acids for gluconeogenesis results in the formation of ammonia as a by-product. The liver converts this metabolically generated ammonia into urea. Ammonia produced by bacteria in the intestines is also removed from portal blood for urea synthesis. In this way, the liver converts ammonia, a potential toxin, into urea, a compound that can be excreted in the urine.

Protein Metabolism. The liver also plays an important role in protein metabolism. It synthesizes almost all of the plasma proteins (except τ-globulin), including albumin, α- and β-globulins, blood clotting factors, specific transport proteins, and most of the plasma lipoproteins. Vitamin K is required by the liver for synthesis of prothrombin and some of the other clotting factors. Amino acids serve as the building blocks for protein synthesis.

Fat Metabolism. The liver is also active in fat metabolism. Fatty acids can be broken down for the production of energy and production of ketone bodies (acetoacetic acid, β-hydroxybutyric acid, and acetone). **Ketone bodies** are small compounds that can enter the bloodstream and provide a source of energy for muscles and other tissues. Breakdown of fatty acids into ketone bodies occurs predominantly when the availability of glucose for metabolism is limited, as during starvation or in uncontrolled diabetes. Fatty acids and their metabolic products are also used for the synthesis of cholesterol, lecithin, lipoproteins, and other complex lipids. Under some conditions, lipids may accumulate in the hepatocytes and result in the abnormal condition called fatty liver.

Vitamin and Iron Storage. Vitamins A, B_{12}, D, and several of the B-complex vitamins are stored in large amounts in the liver. Certain substances, such as iron and copper, are also stored in the liver. Because the liver is rich in these substances, liver extracts have been used for therapy of a wide range of nutritional disorders.

Medication Metabolism

Many medications, such as barbiturates and amphetamines, are metabolized by the liver. Metabolism generally results in loss of activity of the medication, although in some cases activation of the medication may occur. One of the important pathways for medication metabolism involves conjugation (binding) of the medication with a variety of compounds, such as glucuronic or acetic acid, to form more soluble substances. The conjugated products may be excreted in the feces or urine, similar to bilirubin excretion.

Bile Formation

Bile is continuously formed by the hepatocytes and collected in the canaliculi and bile ducts. It is composed mainly of water and electrolytes, such as sodium, potassium, calcium, chloride, and bicarbonate, and also contains significant amounts of lecithin, fatty acids, cholesterol, bilirubin, and bile salts. Bile is collected and stored in the gallbladder and is emptied into the intestine when needed for digestion. The functions of bile are excretory, as in the excretion of bilirubin, and as an aid to digestion through the emulsification of fats by bile salts.

Bile Salts. Bile salts are synthesized by the hepatocytes from cholesterol. After conjugation or binding with amino acids (taurine and glycine), they are excreted into the bile. The bile salts, together with cholesterol and lecithin, are required for emulsification of fats in the intestine. This process is necessary for efficient digestion and absorption. Bile salts are then reabsorbed, primarily in the distal ileum, into portal blood for return to the liver and are again excreted into the bile. This pathway from hepatocytes to bile to intestine and back to the hepatocytes is called the **enterohepatic circulation.** Because of the enterohepatic circulation, only a small fraction of the bile salts that enter the intestine is excreted in the feces. This decreases the demand for active synthesis of bile salts by the liver cells.

Bilirubin Excretion

Bilirubin is a pigment derived from the breakdown of hemoglobin by cells of the reticuloendothelial system, including the Kupffer cells of the liver. Hepatocytes remove bilirubin from the blood and chemically modify it through conjugation to glucuronic acid, which makes the bilirubin more soluble in aqueous solutions. The conjugated bilirubin is secreted by the hepatocytes into the adjacent bile canaliculi and is eventually carried in the bile into the duodenum.

In the small intestine, bilirubin is converted into **urobilinogen,** which is in part excreted in the feces and in part absorbed through the intestinal mucosa into the portal blood. Much of this reabsorbed urobilinogen is removed by the hepatocytes and is secreted into the bile once again (enterohepatic circulation). Some of the urobilinogen enters the systemic circulation and is excreted by the kidneys in the urine. Elimination of bilirubin in the bile represents the major route of excretion for this compound.

The bilirubin concentration in the blood may be increased in the presence of liver disease, when the flow of bile is impeded (*i.e.*, with gallstones in the bile ducts), or with excessive destruction of red blood cells. With bile duct obstruction, bilirubin does not enter the intestine and, as a consequence, urobilinogen will be absent from the urine.

Gallbladder Function

The gallbladder functions as a storage depot for bile. Between meals, when the sphincter of Oddi is closed, bile produced by the hepatocytes enters the gallbladder. During storage, a large portion of the water in bile is absorbed through the walls of the gallbladder, so that gallbladder bile is five to ten times more concentrated than that originally secreted by the liver. When food enters the duodenum, the gallbladder contracts and the sphincter of Oddi relaxes, allowing the bile to enter the intestine. This response is mediated by secretion of the hormone cholecystokinin–pancreozymin (CCK-PZ) from the intestinal wall.

Pathophysiology

Liver dysfunction results from damage to the liver parenchymal cells, either directly, from primary liver diseases, or indirectly, due to obstruction of bile flow or derangements of hepatic circulation. Liver dysfunction may be acute or chronic; however, chronic dysfunction is far more common than acute.

Chronic liver disease, including cirrhosis, is the ninth most frequent cause of death in the United States. Approximately 46% of those deaths are associated with alcohol. The rates of chronic liver disease for men are two times higher than for women; it is more common among African-Americans than whites (CDC, 1993).

Causes. Disease processes that lead to hepatocellular dysfunction may be caused by infectious agents, such as bacteria and viruses, and by anoxia, metabolic disorders, toxins and medications, nutritional deficiencies, and states of hypersensitivity. The most common cause of parenchymal damage is malnutrition, especially in alcoholism.

The parenchymal cells respond to most noxious agents by replacing glycogen with lipids, producing fatty infiltration, with or without cell death or necrosis. This is commonly associated with inflammatory cell infiltration and growth of fibrous tissue. Cell regeneration can occur if the disease process is not too toxic to the cells. The end result of chronic parenchymal disease is the shrunken, fibrotic liver seen in cirrhosis.

Manifestations. Hepatocellular dysfunction is manifested by alteration of the metabolic and excretory functions of the liver. Serum bilirubin concentration rises, leading to **jaundice** (yellowing of the skin, mucous membranes, sclerae, and other tissues); this results from intrahepatic obstruction of bile channels. Abnormalities of carbohydrate, fat, and protein metabolism occur with liver dysfunction. Abnormal protein metabolism results in decreased serum albumin concentration and edema. Ammonia, a by-product of metabolism, is absorbed from the gastrointestinal tract but is not converted to urea by the damaged liver cells. An increased serum ammonia level may impair central nervous system function.

Hematologic Effects. The vascular architecture of the liver may be disturbed, causing increased portal vein blood pressure, which results in leakage of fluid into the peritoneal cavity (**ascites**) and **esophageal varices**. The lack of normal production of various blood-clotting factors can lead to bleeding from any site, but the patient with hepatic disease is particularly prone to gastrointestinal bleeding because of the changes in the liver's vasculature (development of collateral blood vessels) and increased pressure in the portal system (see discussion of portal hypertension on page 973).

Endocrine Imbalances. Many endocrine abnormalities also occur with liver dysfunction because the liver is unable to metabolize hormones normally, including androgens or sex hormones. Gynecomastia, amenorrhea, testicular atrophy, and other disturbances of sexual function and sex characteristics are thought to result from failure of the damaged liver to inactive estrogens normally.

Liver Failure. Acute liver damage may cause acute liver failure, may be completely reversible, or may progress to chronic liver disease. The end result of chronic liver damage is **cirrhosis,** characterized by replacement of parenchymal cells with fibrotic tissue. Liver failure occurs when the liver is unable to carry out its excretory functions, and metabolic functions of the liver are inadequate to meet the needs of the body. **Hepatic encephalopathy** or **coma** results when liver dysfunction is so severe that the liver is unable to remove ammonia, an end-product of protein metabolism from the bloodstream. Ammonia accumulates in the circulation and nervous system, producing severe, life-threatening signs and symptoms.

Gerontologic Considerations

The most common change in the liver in the elderly is a decrease in size and weight accompanied by a decrease in total hepatic blood flow. In general, however, these decreases are in proportion to the decreases in body size and weight seen in normal aging. Results of liver function tests do not normally change in the elderly; abnormal results in an elderly patient indicate abnormal liver function and are not the result of the aging process itself.

The immune system is altered in the aged, and a less responsive immune system may be responsible for the increased incidence and severity of hepatitis B in the elderly and the increased incidence of liver abscesses secondary to decreased phagocytosis by the Kupffer cells.

Metabolism of medications by the liver appears to be decreased in the elderly, but such changes are usually also accompanied by changes in intestinal absorption, renal excretion, and altered body distribution of some medications secondary to changes in fat deposition. These alterations necessitate careful administration and monitoring of all medications with reduction of dosage to prevent medication toxicity.

Diagnostic Evaluation of Hepatic Function

Examination of the Liver

The liver may be palpable in the right upper quadrant. A palpable liver presents as a firm, sharp ridge with a smooth surface (Fig. 38-3). The size of the liver is estimated by percussing the liver's upper and lower borders. When the liver is not palpable, but tenderness is suspected, tapping the lower right thorax briskly may elicit tenderness. The patient's response is then compared by performing a similar maneuver on the left lower thorax.

If the liver is palpable, the examiner notes and records its size and consistency, whether it is tender, and whether its outline is regular or irregular. If the liver is enlarged, the degree to which it descends below the right costal margin is recorded to provide some indication of its size. The examiner determines if the liver's edge is sharp and smooth or blunt and if the enlarged liver is nodular or smooth. The liver of a patient with cirrhosis is small and hard, while the liver of a patient with acute hepatitis is quite soft and the edge is easily moved by the hand.

Tenderness of the liver implies recent acute enlargement with consequent stretching of the liver capsule. The absence of tenderness may imply that the enlargement is of longstanding duration. The liver of a patient with viral hepatitis is tender, whereas that of a patient with alcoholic hepatitis is not. Enlargement of the liver is an abnormal finding requiring further evaluation.

Liver Function Tests

Over 70% of the parenchyma of the liver may be damaged before liver function tests become abnormal. Function is generally measured in terms of serum enzyme activity (*i.e.*, alkaline phosphatase, lactic dehydrogenase, serum

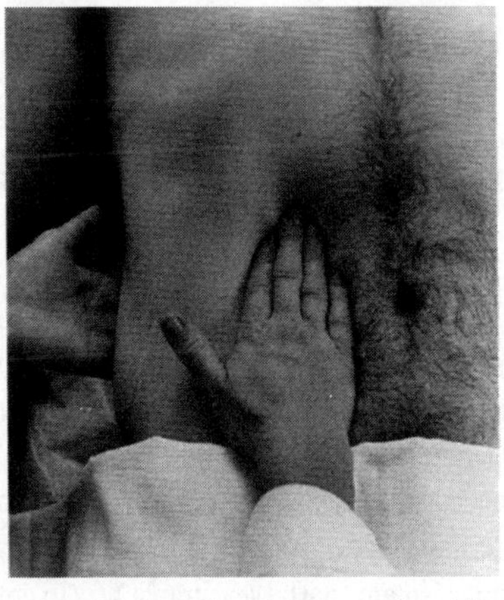

FIGURE 38-3. Technique for palpating the liver. The examiner places one hand under the right lower rib cage and presses downward with light pressure with the other hand.

TABLE 38-1 Liver Function Studies

Test	Normal	Clinical Functions
Pigment Studies		
Serum bilirubin, direct	0–0.3 mg/dl (0–5.1 μmol/L)	These studies measure the ability of liver to conjugate and excrete bilirubin. Results are abnormal in liver and biliary tract disease and are associated with jaundice clinically.
Serum bilirubin, total	0–0.9 mg/dl (1.7–20.5 μmol/L)	
Urine bilirubin	0 (0)	
Urine urobilinogen	0.05–2.5 mg/24 hr (0.09–4.23 μmol/24 hr)	
Fecal urobilinogen (infrequently used)	40–200 mg/24 hr (0.068–0.34 mmol/24 hr)	
Protein Studies		
Total serum protein	7.0–7.5 g/dl (70–75 g/L)	Proteins are manufactured by the liver. Their levels may be affected in a variety of liver impairments.
Serum albumin	3.5–5.5 g/dl (35–55 g/L)	Albumin: Cirrhosis; Chronic hepatitis; Edema, ascites
Serum globulin	1.5–3.0 g/dl (15–30 g/L)	Globulin: Cirrhosis; Liver disease; Chronic obstructive jaundice; Viral hepatitis
Serum protein electrophoresis	3.2–5.6 g/dl (32–56 g/L)	
Albumin		
α_1-Globulin	0.1–0.4 g/dl (1–4 g/L)	
α_2-Globulin	0.4–1.2 g/dl (4–12 g/L)	
β-Globulin	0.5–1.1 g/dl (5–11 g/L)	
γ-Globulin	0.5–1.6 g/dl (5–16 g/L)	
Albumin/globulin (A/G) ratio	A > G or 1.5:1–2.5:1	A/G ratio is reversed in chronic liver disease (decreased albumin and increased globulin).
Prothrombin Time		
Response of prothrombin time to vitamin K	100% return to normal	Prothrombin time may be prolonged in liver disease. It will not return to normal with vitamin K in severe liver cell damage.
Serum alkaline phosphatase	Varies with method: 2–5 Bodansky units 20–90 IU/L at 30° (20–90 U/L at 30°)	Serum alkaline phosphatase is manufactured in bones, liver, kidneys, and intestine and excreted through biliary tract. In absence of bone disease, it is a sensitive measure of biliary tract obstruction.
Serum Transferase or Transaminase Studies		
AST or SGOT	10–40 units (4.8–19 U/L)	The studies are based on release of enzymes from damaged liver cells. These enzymes are elevated in liver cell damage.
ALT or SGPT	5–35 units (2.4–17 U/L)	
LDH	165–400 units (80–192 U/L)	
Serum ammonia	20–120 μg/dl (11.1–67.0 μmol/L)	Liver converts ammonia to urea. Ammonia level rises in liver failure.
Cholesterol		
Ester	150–250 mg/dl (3.90–6.50 mmol/L) 60% of total (fraction of total cholesterol: 0.60)	Cholesterol levels are elevated in biliary obstruction and decreased in parenchymal liver disease.

Additional Studies	Clinical Functions
Radiologic Studies	
Barium study of esophagus	For varices, which indicate increased portal pressure
Abdominal x-ray	To determine gross liver size
Liver scan with radio-tagged iodinated rose bengal, gold, or technetium	To show size and shape of liver; to show replacement of liver tissue with scars, cysts, or tumor
Cholecystogram and cholangiogram	For gallbladder and bile duct visualization
Celiac axis arteriography	For liver and pancreas visualization
Splenoportogram (splenic portal venography)	To determine adequacy of portal blood flow

(continued)

TABLE 38-1 *(continued)*

Additional Studies	Clinical Functions
Laparoscopy	Direct visualization of anterior surface of liver, gallbladder, and mesentery through a trocar
Liver Biopsy	To determine anatomic changes in liver tissue
Measurement of Portal Pressure	Elevated in cirrhosis of the liver
Esophagoscopy/Endoscopy	To search for esophageal varices and abnormalities
Electroencephalogram	Abnormal in hepatic coma and impending hepatic coma
Ultrasonography	To show size of abdominal organs and presence of masses
Computed Tomography (CT Scan)	To detect hepatic neoplasms; diagnose cysts, abscesses, and hematomas; and distinguish between obstructive and nonobstructive jaundice
Angiography	Visualizes hepatic circulation and detects presence and nature of hepatic masses
Magnetic Resonance Imaging (MRI)	To detect hepatic neoplasms; diagnose cysts, abscesses, and hematomas
Endoscopic Retrograde Cholangiopancreatography (ERCP)	Visualizes biliary structures via endoscopy

aminotransferases [transaminases]), and serum concentrations of proteins, bilirubin, ammonia, clotting factors, and lipids. Several of these tests may be helpful for assessing patients with liver disease; however, the nature and extent of hepatic dysfunction cannot be determined by these tests alone as many other disorders can affect their results.

Serum aminotransferases (also called transaminases) are sensitive indicators of injury to the liver cells and are useful in detecting acute liver disease such as hepatitis. Alanine aminotransferase (ALT) (also called serum glutamic-pyruvic transaminase [SGPT]) and aspartate aminotransferase (AST) (also called serum glutamic-oxalocetic transaminase [SGOT]) are the most frequently used tests of liver damage. ALT (SGPT) levels increase primarily in liver disorders and may be used to monitor the course of hepatitis, cirrhosis, or the effects of treatments that may be toxic to the liver. AST (SGOT) is present in tissues that have high metabolic activity; thus it may be increased in damage or death of tissues of organs such as the heart, liver, skeletal muscle, and kidney. Although not specific to liver disease, AST (SGOT) may be increased in cirrhosis, hepatitis, and liver cancer.

Other Diagnostic Tests

Ultrasonography, computed tomography (CT) scanning, and **magnetic resonance imaging** (MRI) are used to identify normal structures and abnormalities of the liver and biliary tree. A radioisotope liver scan may be performed to assess liver size and hepatic blood flow and obstruction.

Laparoscopy (insertion of a fiberoptic endoscope through a small abdominal incision) is used to examine the liver and other pelvic structures. It is also used to perform guided liver biopsy, to determine the etiology of ascites, and to diagnose and stage tumors of the liver and other abdominal tumors.

A list of the commonly used liver function tests is shown in Table 38-1.

Liver Biopsy. Liver biopsy, the removal of a small amount of liver tissue usually through needle aspiration, permits examination of liver cells. The most common indication is to confirm suspected malignancy of the liver. Bleeding following liver biopsy is the major complication; therefore, coagulation studies are obtained and their values noted before liver biopsy is performed. Nursing responsibilities related to liver biopsy are summarized in Guideline 38-1. A graphic presentation is found in Figure 38-4.

Clinical Manifestations of Hepatic Dysfunction

The consequences of liver disease are numerous and varied. Their ultimate effects are incapacitating or life threatening; their presence is ominous, and their treatment is often difficult. Among the most frequent and important of consequences of liver disease are the following:

- Jaundice, resulting from increased bilirubin concentration in the blood.
- Portal hypertension and ascites, resulting from circulatory changes within the diseased liver and producing severe gastrointestinal hemorrhages and marked sodium and fluid retention.
- Nutritional deficiencies, which result from the inability of the damaged liver cells to metabolize certain vitamins, and which are responsible for impaired functioning of the central and peripheral nervous systems and for abnormal bleeding tendencies.
- Hepatic encephalopathy or coma, reflecting accumulation of ammonia in the serum due to impaired protein metabolism by the diseased liver.

Nursing care of the patient with impaired liver function is summarized in Nursing Care Plan 38-1.

(text continues on page 972)

GUIDELINE 38–1
Assisting with Liver Biopsy

Nursing Activities	Rationale
Preprocedure	
1. Ascertain that results of coagulation tests (prothrombin time, PTT, and platelet count) are available and that compatible donor blood is available.	Many patients with liver disease have clotting defects and are at risk for bleeding.
2. Check for signed consent.	
3. Measure and record the patient's pulse, respirations, and arterial pressure immediately before biopsy.	Prebiopsy values provide a basis on which to compare the patient's vital signs and evaluate status after the procedure.
4. Describe to the patient in advance: steps of the procedure; sensations expected; after-effects anticipated; restrictions of activity and monitoring procedures to follow.	Explanations serve to allay fears and ensure cooperation.
During Procedure	
5. Support the patient during the procedure.	The presence of a supportive nurse enhances comfort and promotes a sense of security.
6. Expose the right side of the patient's upper abdomen (right hypochondriac).	The skin at the site of penetration will be cleansed and infiltrted with local anesthetic.
7. Instruct the patient to inhale and exhale deeply several times, finally to exhale, and to hold breath at the end of expiration. The physician promptly introduces the biopsy needle by way of the transthoracic (intercostal) or transabdominal (subcostal) route, penetrates the liver, aspirates, and withdraws (Fig. 38-4). The entire procedure is completed within 5 to 10 seconds.	Holding the breath immobilizes the chest wall and the diaphragm; penetration of the diaphragm thereby is avoided, and the risk of lacerating the liver is minimized.
8. Instruct the patient to resume breathing.	

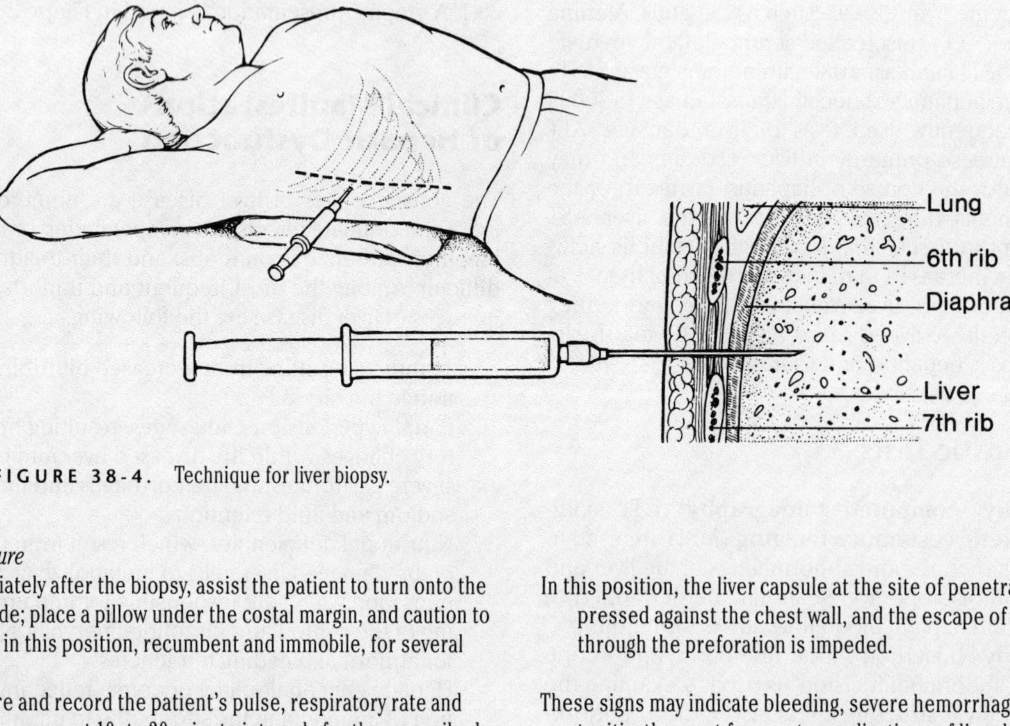

FIGURE 38-4. Technique for liver biopsy.

Nursing Activities	Rationale
Postprocedure	
9. Immediately after the biopsy, assist the patient to turn onto the right side; place a pillow under the costal margin, and caution to remain in this position, recumbent and immobile, for several hours.	In this position, the liver capsule at the site of penetration is compressed against the chest wall, and the escape of blood or bile through the preforation is impeded.
10. Measure and record the patient's pulse, respiratory rate and blood pressure at 10- to 20-minute intervals for the prescribed period, or until stable. Be alert to and report promptly any increase in pulse rate or any decrease in arterial pressure, any complaint of pain, or manifestations of apprehension.	These signs may indicate bleeding, severe hemorrhage, or bile peritonitis, the most frequent complications of liver biopsy.

NURSING CARE PLAN 38–1
Care of the Patient With Impaired Liver Function

NURSING DIAGNOSIS: Activity intolerance related to fatigue, lethargy, and malaise

GOAL: Increased activity tolerance

Nursing Interventions	Rationale	Expected Outcomes
1. Assess level of activity tolerance and degree of fatigue, lethargy, and malaise.	1. Provides baseline for further assessment and criteria for assessment of effectiveness of interventions.	• Exhibits increased interest in activities and events.
2. Assist with activities and hygiene when fatigued.	2. Promotes some exercise and hygiene within patient's level of tolerance.	• Participates in activities and gradually increases exercise within physical limits.
3. Encourage rest when fatigued or when abdominal pain or discomfort occurs.	3. Conserves energy and protects the liver.	• Reports increased strength and well-being.
4. Assist with selection and pacing of desired activities and exercise.	4. Stimulates patient's interest in selected activities.	• Reports absence of abdominal pain and discomfort.

NURSING DIAGNOSIS: Altered nutrition related to abdominal distention and discomfort and anorexia

GOAL: Improved nutritional status

Nursing Interventions	Rationale	Expected Outcomes
1. Assess dietary intake and nutritional status through diet history and diary, daily weight measurements, laboratory data, and anthropometric assessment.	1. Identifies deficits in nutritional intake and adequacy of nutritional state.	• Exhibits improved nutritional status by increased weight (without fluid retention), improved laboratory data and anthropometric measurements.
2. Provide diet high in carbohydrates with protein intake consistent with liver function.	2. Provides calories for energy, "sparing" protein for healing.	• States rationale for dietary modifications.
3. Assist patient in indentifying low sodium foods.	3. Reduces edema and ascites formation.	• Identifies foods high in carbohydrates and within protein requirements (high in cirrhosis and hepatitis, low in hepatic failure).
4. Elevate the head of the bed during patient's meals.	4. Reduces discomfort from abdominal distention and decreases sense of fullness produced by pressure of abdominal contents and ascites on the stomach.	• Reports improved appetite.
5. Provide oral hygiene before meals and pleasant environment for meals at meal time.	5. Promotes positive environment and increased appetite.	

NURSING DIAGNOSIS: Impaired skin integrity related to jaundice and edema

GOAL: Improved skin integrity

Nursing Interventions	Rationale	Expected Outcomes
1. Assess degree of discomfort related to pruritus and edema experienced by patient.	1. Assists in determining appropriate strategies.	• Exhibits intact skin without redness, excoriation, or breakdown.
2. Note and record degree of jaundice and extent of edema.	2. Provides baseline for detecting changes and evaluating effectiveness of interventions.	• Reports relief of pruritus.
3. Keep patient's fingernails short and smooth.	3. Prevents skin excoriation and infection from scratching.	• Exhibits no skin excoriation from scratching.
4. Provide frequent skin care; avoid use of soaps and alcohol-based lotions.	4. Removes waste products deposited in skin while preventing dryness of skin.	• Uses nondrying soaps and lotions. States rationale for use of nondrying soaps and lotions.
5. Massage bony prominences; turn frequently.	5. Promotes mobilization of edema.	• Turns self periodically. Exhibits reduced edema of dependent parts of the body.
6. Initiate use of alternating-pressure mattress.	6. Minimizes prolonged pressure on bony prominences susceptible to breakdown.	

(continued)

NURSING CARE PLAN 38–1 *(continued)*
Care of the Patient With Impaired Liver Function

NURSING DIAGNOSIS: High risk for injury related to altered clotting mechanisms and altered level of consciousness

GOAL: Reduced risk of injury

Nursing Interventions	Rationale	Expected Outcomes
1. Assess level of consciousness and cognitive level.	1. Assists in predicting patient's ability to protect self and comply with required self-protective actions; may detect deterioration of hepatic function.	• Is oriented to time, place, and person. • Exhibits no ecchymoses (bruises), cuts, or hematoma. • Exhibits no hallucinations, and demonstrtes no efforts to get up unassisted or to leave hospital. • Uses electric razor rather than sharp-edged razor
2. Provide safe environment (pad side rails, remove obstacles in room, prevent falls).	2. Minimizes falls and accidents and damage if falls occur.	
3. Provide frequent surveillance to orient patient and avoid use of restraints.	3. Protects patient from harm while stimulating and orienting patient; avoids use of restraints, which may disturb patient further.	
4. Replace sharp objects (razors) with safer items.	4. Avoids accidental cuts.	

NURSING DIAGNOSIS: Body image disturbance related to changes in appearance, sexual dysfunction, and role function

GOAL: Improvement of body image and self-esteem

Nursing Interventions	Rationale	Expected Outcomes
1. Assess changes in appearance and the meaning these changes have for patient and family.	1. Provides information for assessing impact of changes in appearance, sexual function, and role on the patient and family.	• Verbalizes concerns related to changes in appearance, life, and lifestyle. • Shares concerns with significant others. • Identifies past coping strategies that have been effective. • Uses past effective coping strategies to deal with changes in appearance, life, and lifestyle. • Maintains good grooming and hygiene. • Identifies short-term goals and strategies to achieve them. • Exercises an active role in decision making about self and care. • Identifies resources that are not harmful. • Verbalizes that some of previous lifestyle practices have been harmful. • Uses healthy expressions of frustration, anger, and so forth.
2. Encourage patient to verbalize reactions and feelings about these changes.	2. Enables patient to identify and express concerns; encourages patient and significant others to share these concerns.	
3. Assess patient's and family's previous coping strategies.	3. Permits encouragement of those coping strategies that are familiar to patient and have been effective in the past.	
4. Assist and encourage patient to maximize appearance and explore alternatives to previous sexual and role functions.	4. Encourages patient to continue safe roles and functions while encouraging exploration of alternatives.	
5. Assist patient in identifying short-term goals.	5. Accomplishing these goals serves as positive reinforcement and increases self-esteem.	
6. Encourage and assist patient in decision-making about care.	6. Promotes patient's control of life and improves sense of well-being and self-esteem.	
7. Identify with patient resources to provide additional support (counselor, clergy).	7. Assists patient in identifying resources and accepting assistance from others when indicated.	
8. Assist patient in identifying previous practices that may have been harmful to self (alcohol and drug abuse).	8. Recognition and acknowledgment of the harmful effects of these practices is necessary for identifying a more healthy lifestyle.	

(continued)

NURSING CARE PLAN 38–1 *(continued)*
Care of the Patient With Impaired Liver Function

COLLABORATIVE PROBLEM: Gastrointestinal bleeding and hemorrhage

GOAL: Prevention of gastrointestinal bleeding and hemorrhage; early detection of bleeding

Nursing Interventions	Rationale	Expected Outcomes
1. Assess patient for evidence of gastrointestinal bleeding or hemorrhage: a. Monitor vital signs (blood pressure, pulse, respiratory rate). b. Assess skin temperature, level of consciousness. c. Monitor gastrointestinal secretions and output (emesis, stool) for occult or obvious bleeding). d. Monitor hematocrit and hemoglobin levels.	1. Allows early detection of signs and symptoms of bleeding and hemorrhage.	• Experiences no episodes of bleeding and hemorrhage. • Vital signs are within acceptable range for patient. • No evidence of bleeding from gastrointestinal tract. • Hematocrit and hemoglobin levels within acceptable limits. • Patient turns and moves without straining and increasing intra-abdominal pressure. • No straining with bowel movements. • No further bleeding episodes if aggressive treatment of bleeding and hemorrhage was needed. • Patient and family state rationale for treatments. • Patient and family identify supports available to them.
2. Avoid activities that increase intra-abdominal pressure (straining, turning). a. Assist patient to turn. b. Keep all needed items within easy reach. c. Use measures to prevent constipation. d. Assure adequate fluid intake.	2. Minimizes increases in intra-abdominal pressure that could lead to rupture and bleeding of esophageal or gastric varices.	
3. Have equipment (Blakemore tube, medications, intravenous fluids) available if indicated.	3. Equipment, medications, and supplies will be readily available if patient experiences bleeding from ruptured esophageal or gastric varices.	
4. Assist with procedures and therapy needed to treat gastrointestinal bleeding and hemorrhage.	4. Gastrointestinal bleeding and hemorrhage require emergency measures by entire health care team.	
5. Monitor respiratory status and minimize risk of respiratory complications if esophageal tamponade is needed.	5. The patient is at high risk for respiratory complications, including asphyxiation if gastric balloon of Blakemore tube ruptures.	
6. Prepare patient physically and psychologically for other treatment modalities if needed.	6. The patient who experiences hemorrhage is very anxious and fearful; minimizing anxiety assists in control of hemorrhage.	
7. Monitor patient for recurrence of bleeding and hemorrhage.	7. Risk of rebleeding is high with all treatment modalities used to halt gastrointestinal bleeding.	
8. Keep family informed of patient's status.	8. Family members are likely to be anxious about the patient's status; providing information will reduce their anxiety level and promote more effective coping.	

COLLABORATIVE PROBLEM: Hepatic encephalopathy

GOAL: Prevention of hepatic encephalopathy

Nursing Interventions	Rationale	Expected Outcomes
1. Assess cognitive status at regular intervals: a. Assess patient's orientation to person, place, and time.	1. Data will provide baseline of patient's cognitive status and enable detection of changes.	• Remains awake, alert, and aware of surroundings. • Is oriented to time, place, and person.

(continued)

NURSING CARE PLAN 38–1 *(continued)*
Care of the Patient With Impaired Liver Function

Nursing Interventions	Rationale	Expected Outcomes
b. Monitor patient's level of activity, restlessness, and agitation. c. Obtain and record daily sample of patient's handwriting. d. Assess neurologic signs (deep tendon reflexes, ability to follow instructions).		• Exhibits no restlessness or agitation. • Record of handwriting demonstrates no deterioration in cognitive function. • States rationale for treatment used to prevent or treat hepatic encephalopathy. • Demonstrates stable serum ammonia level within acceptable limits. • Consumes adequate caloric intake and adheres to protein restriction. • Takes medications as prescribed. • Breath sounds are normal without adventitious sounds • Skin and tissue intact without evidence of pressure or breaks in integrity.
2. Monitor medications to prevent administration of those that may precipitate hepatic encephalopathy (sedatives, hypnotics, analgesics).	2. Medications are a common precipitating factor in development of hepatic encephalopathy in patients at risk.	
3. Monitor laboratory data, especially serum ammonia level.	3. Increases in serum ammonia level are associated with hepatic encephalopathy and coma.	
4. Notify physician of even subtle changes in patient's neurologic status and cognitive function.	4. Allows early initiation of treatment of hepatic encephalopathy and prevention of hepatic coma.	
5. Limit sources of protein from diet if indicated.	5. Reduces breakdown and conversion of protein to ammonia.	
6. Administer medications prescribed to reduce serum ammonia level (*e.g.,* lactulose, antibiotics, glucose)	6. Reduces serum ammonia level.	
7. Assess respiratory status and initiate measures to prevent complications.	7. The patient who develops hepatic coma is at risk for respiratory complications (*i.e.,* pneumonia, atelectasis, infection).	
8. Protect patient's skin and tissue from pressure and breakdown.	8. The patient in coma is at risk for skin breakdown and pressure ulcer formation.	

Jaundice

When the bilirubin concentration in the blood becomes abnormally increased, all the body tissues, including the sclerae and the skin, become yellow-tinged or greenish yellow. This condition is called **jaundice.** Jaundice becomes clinically evident when the serum bilirubin level exceeds 2 to 2.5 mg/dl (SI: 34–43 μmol/L). Increased serum bilirubin levels and jaundice may result from impairment of hepatic uptake, conjugation of bilirubin, or excretion of bilirubin into the biliary system.

There are several types of jaundice: (1) hemolytic, (2) hepatocellular, (3) obstructive, and (4) jaundice due to hereditary hyperbilirubinemia. Hepatocellular and obstructive jaundice are the two types commonly associated with liver disease.

Hemolytic Jaundice

Hemolytic jaundice is the result of an increased destruction of the red blood cells, the effect of which is to flood the plasma with bilirubin so rapidly that the liver, although functioning normally, cannot excrete the bilirubin as quickly as it is formed. This type of jaundice is encountered in patients with hemolytic transfusion reactions and other hemolytic disorders. The bilirubin in the blood of these patients is predominantly of the unconjugated, or "free," type. Fecal and urine urobilinogen are increased; conversely, the urine is free of bilirubin.

Patients with this type of jaundice, unless their hyperbilirubinemia is extreme, do not experience symptoms or complications as a result of the jaundice *per se.* Very prolonged jaundice, however, even if mild, predisposes to the formation of "pigment stones" in the gallbladder, and extremely severe jaundice (*i.e.,* in patients with levels of free bilirubin above 20–25 mg/dl) poses definite risk of possible brain stem damage.

Hepatocellular Jaundice

Hepatocellular jaundice is caused by the inability of damaged liver cells to clear normal amounts of bilirubin from the blood. The cellular damage may be from infection, such as in viral hepatitis (*e.g.,* hepatitis A, B, C, D, or E) or other viruses that affect the liver (*e.g.,* yellow fever virus, Epstein–Barr virus), from medication or chemical toxicity (*e.g.*, carbon tetrachloride, chloroform, phosphorus, arsenicals, certain medications), or from alcohol.

Cirrhosis of the liver is a form of hepatocellular disease that may produce jaundice. It is usually associated with excessive alcohol intake; however, it may also be a late result of liver cell necrosis caused by viral infection. In prolonged obstructive jaundice, cell damage eventually develops, so that both types appear together.

Clinical Manifestations. Patients with hepatocellular jaundice may be mildly or severely ill, with lack of appetite, nausea, malaise, fatigue, weakness, and possible weight loss. In some instances of hepatocellular disease, jaundice may not be obvious.

The serum bilirubin concentration and urine urobilinogen level may be elevated. In addition, AST (SGOT) and ALT (SGPT) levels may be increased, indicating cellular necrosis.

The patient may report headache, chills, and fever, if the cause is infectious. Depending on the cause and extent of the liver cell damage, hepatocellular jaundice may or may not be completely reversible.

Obstructive Jaundice

Obstructive jaundice of the extrahepatic type may be caused by occlusion of the bile duct by a gallstone, an inflammatory process, a tumor, or pressure from an enlarged organ. The obstruction may also involve the small bile ducts within the liver (*i.e.*, intrahepatic obstruction), caused, for example, by pressure on these channels from inflammatory swelling of the liver or by an inflammatory exudate within the ducts themselves.

Intrahepatic obstruction due to stasis and inspissation (thickening) of bile within the canaliculi may occur following the ingestion of certain medications, which are referred to as "cholestatic" agents. These include phenothiazines, antithyroid medications, sulfonylureas, tricyclic antidepressants, nitrofurantoin, androgens, and estrogens.

Clinical Manifestations. Whether the obstruction is intrahepatic or extrahepatic and whatever its cause may be, if bile cannot flow normally into the intestine but is backed up into the liver substance, it is reabsorbed into the blood and carried throughout the entire body, staining the skin, the mucous membranes, and the sclerae. It is excreted in the urine, which becomes deep orange and foamy. Because of the decreased amount of bile in the intestinal tract, the stools become light or clay-colored. The skin may itch intensely, requiring repeated soothing baths. Dyspepsia and an intolerance to fatty foods may develop because of impaired fat digestion in the absence of intestinal bile. The AST (SGOT) and ALT (SGPT) levels generally rise only moderately, but the bilirubin and alkaline phosphatase levels are elevated.

Hereditary Hyperbilirubinemia

Increased serum bilirubin levels (hyperbilirubinemia) due to several inherited disorders can also produce jaundice. **Gilbert's syndrome** is a familial disorder characterized by an increased unconjugated bilirubin level that causes jaundice. Although serum bilirubin levels are increased, liver histology and liver function test results are normal, and there is no hemolysis.

Other conditions that are probably caused by inborn errors of biliary metabolism include **Dubin–Johnson syndrome** (chronic idiopathic jaundice, with pigment in the liver) and **Rotor's syndrome** (chronic familial conjugated hyperbilirubinemia without pigment in the liver); "benign" cholestatic jaundice of pregnancy, with retention of conjugated bilirubin, probably secondary to unusual sensitivity to the hormones of pregnancy; and probably also benign recurrent intrahepatic cholestasis.

Portal Hypertension and Ascites

Obstruction to blood flow through the damaged liver results in increased blood pressure (**portal hypertension**) throughout the portal venous system. Although portal hypertension is commonly associated with hepatic cirrhosis, it can also occur with noncirrhotic liver disease.

Two major sequelae result from portal hypertension:

1. *The formation of esophageal, gastric, and hemorrhoidal varicosities (varices).* These varices develop because of the elevated pressures transmitted to all of the veins that drain into the portal system. These varicosities are prone to rupture and often are the source of massive hemorrhages from the upper gastrointestinal tract and the rectum (see p. 988). The likelihood of bleeding is increased by the blood clotting abnormalities often seen in patients with cirrhosis.
2. *The accumulation of fluid (ascites) in the abdominal cavity.* As ascites develops, intravascular volume tends to fall and renin is released by the kidneys. The renin causes increased secretion of the hormone aldosterone by the adrenal glands, which in turn causes the kidneys to retain sodium and water in an attempt to return intravascular volume to normal. As portal hypertension continues, fluid retention contributes to the formation of even more ascites as the albumin in the ascitic fluid creates an osmotic gradient and pulls more fluid into the peritoneal cavity (Fig. 38-5). (Although ascites is often a result of liver damage, it may also occur with other disorders including cancer, kidney disease, and heart failure.)

Assessment

The presence and extent of ascites are assessed by percussing the abdomen. When fluid has accumulated in the peritoneal cavity, the flanks will bulge when the patient assumes a supine position. The presence of fluid can be confirmed either by percussing for shifting dullness or by detecting a fluid wave (Fig. 38-6). A fluid wave is likely to be found only when there is a large amount of fluid present. Daily measurement and recording of abdominal girth and body weight are essential to assess the progression of ascites and its response to treatment. The roles of dietary modification, medication therapy, paracentesis, and shunting in controlling ascites are discussed below.

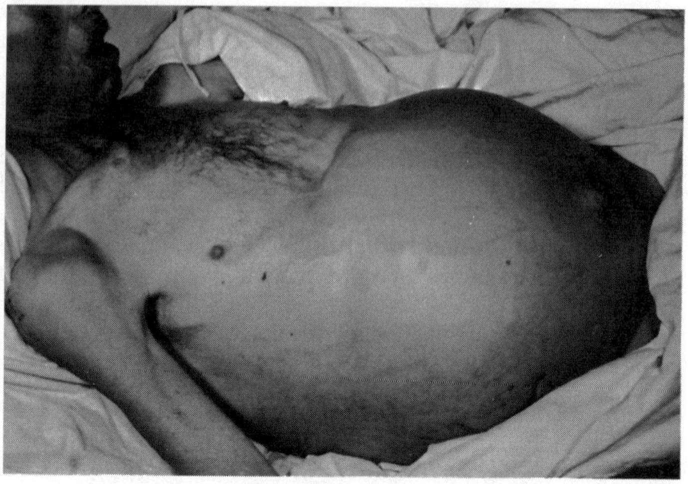

FIGURE 38-5. Example of ascites in patient with liver disease. (Schiff L and Schiff ER. Diseases of the Liver, 7th ed. Philadelphia, JB Lippincott, 1993.)

Management

Dietary Modification. The goal of treatment for the patient with ascites is a negative sodium balance to reduce fluid retention. Table salt, salty foods, salted butter and margarine, and all ordinary canned and frozen foods (those foods that are not specifically prepared for low-sodium/salt diets) should be avoided. The taste of unsalted foods can be improved by using salt substitutes, such as lemon juice, oregano, and thyme. Commercial salt substitutes need to be cleared with the physician as those containing ammonia could precipitate hepatic coma. Liberal use should be made of powdered, low-sodium milk and milk products. If fluid accumulation is not controlled on this regimen, the daily sodium allowance may be reduced further to 500 mg and diuretics administered.

Dietary control of ascites via strict sodium restriction is difficult to achieve at home. The likelihood of the patient following even a 2 g sodium diet is increased if the patient and the person preparing meals understand the rationale for the diet and receive periodic guidance about selecting and preparing appropriate foods.

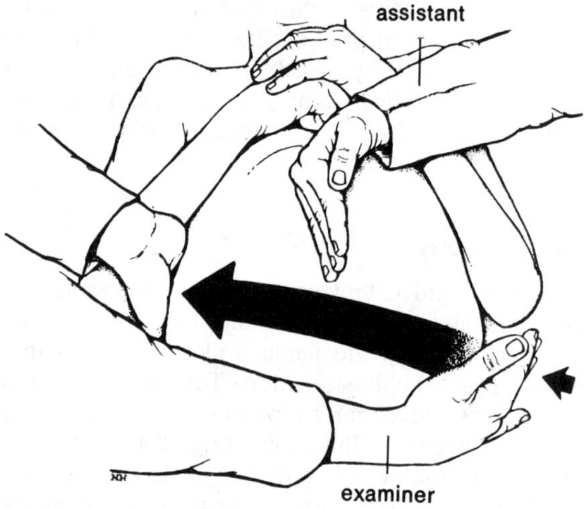

FIGURE 38-6. Assessing for abdominal fluid wave. The examiner places the hands along the side of the patient's flank, then strikes one flank sharply, detecting any fluid wave with the other hand. An assistant's hand is placed (ulnar side down) along the patient's midline to prevent the fluid wave from being transmitted through the tissues of the abdominal wall.

Diuretics. Use of diuretics along with sodium restriction is successful in 90% of patients with ascites. Spironolactone (Aldactone), an aldosterone-blocking agent, is often considered the first-line therapy in patients with ascites due to cirrhosis. When used with other diuretics, it helps prevent potassium loss. Oral diuretics such as furosemide (Lasix) may be added but should be used cautiously, because with long-term use they may also induce severe sodium depletion (hyponatremia). Ammonium chloride and acetazolamide (Diamox) are contraindicated because of the possibility of precipitating hepatic coma. Daily weight loss should not exceed 0.227 kg (less than ½ lb) daily. Fluid restriction is not attempted unless the serum sodium concentration is very low.

Complications. Possible complications of diuretic therapy include fluid and electrolyte disturbances and encephalopathy. Possible fluid and electrolyte problems include hypovolemia, hypokalemia, hyponatremia, and hypochloremic alkalosis. Encephalopathy may be precipitated by dehydration and hypovolemia. Additionally, when potassium stores are depleted, the amount of ammonia in the systemic circulation increases, which may cause impaired cerebral functioning and encephalopathy. If a patient with ascites from liver disease is hospitalized, nursing measures include assessment and documentation of intake and output, abdominal girth, and daily weight to assess fluid status. Serum ammonia and electrolyte levels are monitored to assess electrolyte balance, response to therapy, and risk of encephalopathy.

Skin Care. Skin integrity will be affected if skin care is not adequate. Pressure over bony prominences and edematous tissue must be relieved by frequently changing body position; use of an alternating-pressure mattress may assist in preventing skin breakdown. Elevation of the lower extremities and use of elastic stockings are warranted. Lower extremities may have to be elevated and support hose applied.

Salt-poor albumin may be prescribed intravenously to temporarily elevate the serum albumin level, which increases serum osmotic pressure. This helps reduce edema by causing the ascitic fluid to be drawn back into the bloodstream and ultimately eliminated by the kidneys.

Patient Education and Home Care Considerations. The patient treated for ascites is likely to be discharged home with some ascites still present. Follow-up by a home care nurse is helpful to assess the patient's adherence to the therapeutic regimen, to identify problems with preparing appropriate foods, and to assess the patient's weight, abdominal girth, skin, and cognitive and emotional status.

Prior to hospital discharge and during visits to the patient at home, the nurse assesses the patient's and family's understanding of the therapeutic regimen and its role in controlling ascites. The patient is instructed to monitor changes in weight, intake and output, and general sense of well-being. The instructions about signs and symptoms to report to the physician or nurse are reinforced to the patient and family.

Paracentesis

Paracentesis is the removal of fluid (ascites) from the peritoneal cavity through a small surgical incision or puncture made through the abdominal wall. Paracentesis was once considered a routine form of treatment for ascites but is now performed primarily for diagnostic examination of ascitic fluid, for treatment of massive ascites that is resistant to nutritional and diuretic therapy and causing severe problems to the patient, and as a prelude to diagnostic imaging studies, peritoneal dialysis, or surgery.

A sample of the ascitic fluid may be sent to the laboratory for analysis. Cell count, albumin and total protein levels, culture, and occasionally other tests are performed.

If paracentesis is performed to remove fluid, the aspiration is usually limited to the slow removal of 2 to 3 liters to relieve acute symptoms; however, it has been shown that removal of up to 4 to 6 liters of fluid may be done safely in some patients (Runyon, 1993). Ascitic fluid tends to form again, necessitating repeated removal.

Nursing Interventions. The nursing support of the patient undergoing a paracentesis is presented in Guideline 38-2.

Other Methods of Treatment

Intravenous infusion of ascitic fluid and insertion of a peritoneovenous shunt to redirect ascitic fluid from the peritoneal cavity into the systemic circulation was once a treatment modality for ascites, but these procedures have largely been abandoned because of the high complication rate and high incidence of shunt failure.

Nutritional Deficiencies

Another group of problems common to patients with severe chronic liver disease of all types results from inadequate intake of proper vitamins. Among the specific deficiency states that occur on this basis are (1) vitamin A deficiency; (2) beriberi, polyneuritis, and Wernicke–Korsakoff psychosis, all attributable to a deficiency of thiamine; (3) skin and mucous membrane lesions characteristic of riboflavin deficiency; (4) pyridoxine deficiency; (5) hypoprothrombinemia (see p. 802), characterized by spontaneous bleeding and ecchymoses, due to vitamin K deficiency; (6) the hemorrhagic lesions of scurvy (*i.e.,* vitamin C deficiency); and (7) the macrocytic anemia of folic acid deficiency.

- The threat of these avitaminoses provides the rationale for supplementing the diet of every patient with chronic liver disease (especially when alcoholism is involved) with ample quantities of vitamins A, B complex, C, K, and folic acid.

Hepatic Encephalopathy and Hepatic Coma

Hepatic encephalopathy, one of the dreaded complications of liver disease, occurs with profound liver failure and results from the accumulation of ammonia and other toxic metabolites in the blood. **Hepatic coma** represents the most advanced stage of hepatic encephalopathy. Ammonia accumulates because damaged liver cells fail to detoxify and convert to urea the ammonia that is constantly entering the bloodstream as a result of its absorption from the gastrointestinal tract and its liberation from kidney and muscle cells. The increased ammonia concentration in the blood causes brain dysfunction and damage, resulting in hepatic encephalopathy. **Portal-systemic encephalopathy** (PSE) is the most common type of hepatic encephalopathy and it occurs primarily in patients with cirrhosis with portal hypertension and portal-systemic shunting (page 998).

Assessment and Clinical Manifestations. The earliest symptoms of hepatic encephalopathy include minor mental changes and motor disturbances. The patient appears to be slightly confused, experiences alterations in mood, becomes unkempt in appearance, and experiences altered sleep patterns. The patient tends to sleep during the day and to experience restlessness and insomnia at night. As hepatic coma progresses, the patient may be difficult to awaken.

Asterixis (flapping tremor of the hands) may occur (Fig. 38-8). Simple tasks, such as handwriting, become difficult. A sample of handwriting, taken daily, may provide graphic evidence of progression or reversal of hepatic encephalopathy. In the early stages of hepatic encephalopathy, the patient's reflexes are hyperactive; with worsening of hepatic encephalopathy these reflexes disappear and the extremities may become flaccid.

The electroencephalogram (EEG) shows generalized slowing and an increase in amplitude of brain waves and the appearance of characteristic triphasic waves. Occasionally, **fetor hepaticus,** a characteristic breath odor like freshly mowed grass, acetone, or old wine, may be noticed. In a more advanced stage there are gross disturbances of consciousness and the patient is completely disoriented with respect to time and place. With further progression of the disorder, the patient lapses into frank coma and may have seizures. Approximately 35% of all patients with cirrhosis of the liver die in hepatic coma.

GUIDELINE 38-2
Assisting with a Paracentesis

Preprocedure

1. Prepare the patient by providing the necessary information and instructions about the procedure and by offering reassurance.
2. Gather appropriate sterile equipment and collection receptacles.
3. Place patient in upright position on edge of bed with feet supported on stool or place in chair.
4. Place sphygmomanometer cuff around patient's arm to monitor blood pressure during the procedure.

Procedure

1. The physician, using aseptic technique, inserts the trocar through a puncture wound in the midline below the umbilicus. The fluid drains from the abdomen through a drainage tube into a container (Fig. 38-7).
2. Help the patient maintain position throughout procedure.
3. Take and record blood pressure at frequent intervals from the beginning of the procedure.
4. Monitor the patient closely for signs of vascular collapse: pallor, increased pulse rate, or decreased blood pressure.

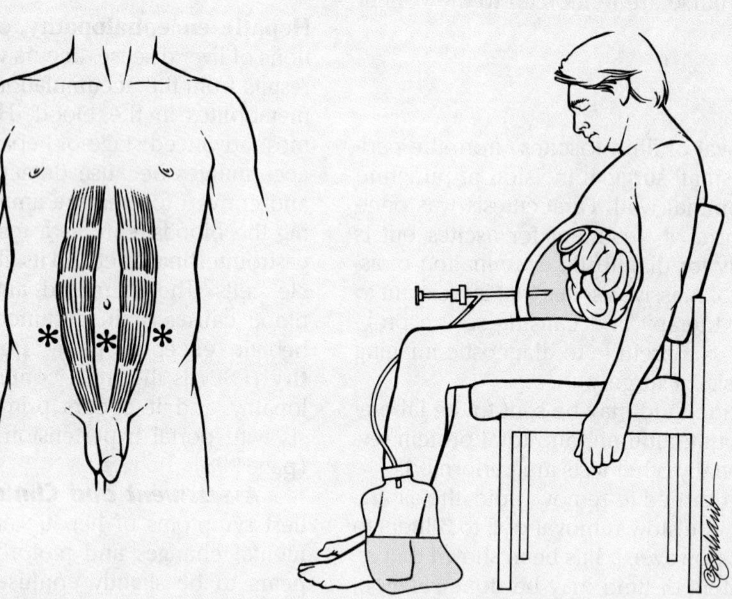

FIGURE 38-7. Paracentesis. Drawing on the *left* shows possible trocar insertion sites. Drawing on the *right* shows a patient with ascites undergoing paracentesis.

Postprocedure

1. Return patient to bed or to a comfortable sitting position.
2. Measure the fluid collected, describe, and record.
3. Label samples of fluid and send to laboratory.

Aggravating and Precipitating Factors. Circumstances that increase blood ammonia content tend to aggravate or precipitate hepatic encephalopathy. The largest source of blood ammonia is the enzymatic and bacterial digestion of dietary and blood proteins in the gastrointestinal tract. Ammonia from these sources is *increased* as a result of gastrointestinal (GI) bleeding (*i.e.*, bleeding esophageal varices or chronic GI bleeding), a high-protein diet, bacterial infections, and uremia. The ingestion of ammonium salts will also increase the blood ammonia level. In the presence of alkalosis or hypokalemia, increased amounts of ammonia are absorbed from the gastrointestinal tract and from the renal tubular fluid.

Conversely, serum ammonia is *decreased* by elimination of protein from the diet and by the administration of antibiotics, such as neomycin sulfate, that reduce the number of intestinal bacteria capable of converting urea to ammonia.

Other factors unrelated to increased blood ammonia that may induce hepatic encephalopathy in susceptible patients include excessive diuresis, dehydration, infections, surgery, fever, and some medications (sedatives, tranquilizers, analgesics, and diuretics that cause potassium loss). Table 38-2 presents the stages of hepatic encephalopathy, common signs and symptoms, and potential nursing diagnoses for each stage.

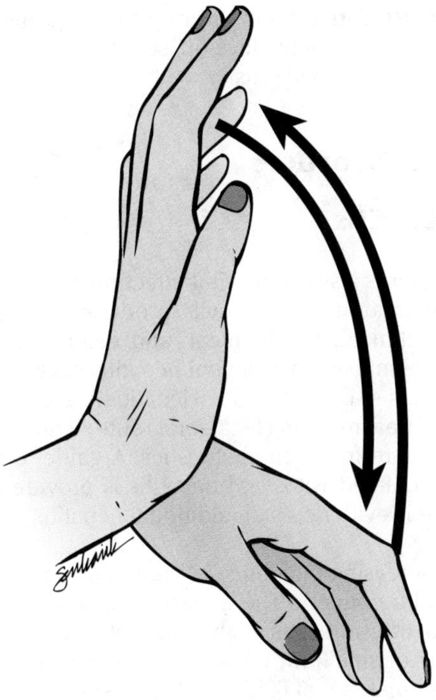

FIGURE 38-8. Asterixis or "liver flap" may occur in hepatic encephalopathy. The patient is asked to hold the arm out with the hand held upward (dorsiflexed). Within a few seconds, the hand falls forward involuntarily and then quickly returns to the dorsiflexed position.

Management

Principles of management of hepatic encephalopathy include the following:

- Therapy is directed toward treating or removing the offending cause.
- The patient with hepatic encephalopathy and impending coma is observed frequently to assess neurologic status. A daily record is kept of handwriting and performance in arithmetic to monitor mental status.
- Fluid intake and output and body weight are recorded each day.
- Vital signs are measured and recorded every 4 hours.
- Evidence suggesting pulmonary or other infection is assessed frequently and reported promptly if observed.
- Serum ammonia level is monitored daily.
- If signs of impending hepatic encephalopathy and coma occur, the patient's protein intake is reduced sharply or eliminated altogether, for a time.
- To reduce ammonia absorption from the gastrointestinal tract, an enema may be prescribed. (Dilute acetic acid solutions are preferable to soapsuds enemas as the alkaline environment created by soapsuds enemas favors passage of ammonia into the blood).
- In addition, nonabsorbable antibiotic agents such as neomycin, sulfasuxidine, or sulfathalidine are administered to suppress the activity of the bacterial flora of the intestinal tract.
- Electrolyte status is carefully monitored and corrected if abnormal.
- Medications that may precipitate hepatic encephalopathy (*i.e.*, sedatives, tranquilizers, analgesics) are discontinued.

Lactulose (Cephulac) is administered to reduce blood ammonia; it acts by several mechanisms that promote the excretion of ammonia in the stool: (1) ammonia is kept in the ionized state, resulting in a fall in colon *p*H, reversing the normal passage of ammonia from the colon to the blood; (2) evacuation of the bowel takes place, which decreases the ammonia absorbed from the colon; and (3) the fecal flora are changed to organisms that do not produce ammonia from urea.

Two or three soft stools per day are desirable; this indicates that lactulose is performing as intended. Watery diarrheal stools, however, indicate medication overdose.

TABLE 38-2 Stages of Hepatic Encephalopathy and Possible Nursing Diagnoses*

Stage	Clinical Symptoms	Clinical Signs and EEG Changes	Selected Potential Nursing Diagnoses
1	Normal level of consciousness with periods of lethargy and euphoria; reversal of day–night sleep patterns	Asterixis; impaired writing and ability to draw line figures. Normal EEG.	Activity intolerance Self-care deficit Sleep pattern disturbances
2	Increased drowsiness; disorientation; inappropriate behavior; mood swings; agitation	Asterixis; fetor hepaticus. Abnormal EEG with generalized slowing.	Impaired social interaction Altered role performance Risk for injury
3	Stuporous; difficult to arouse; sleeping most of time; marked confusion; incoherent speech	Asterixis; increased deep tendon reflexes; rigidity of extremities. EEG markedly abnormal.	Altered nutrition Impaired mobility Impaired communication
4	Comatose; may not respond to painful stimuli	Absence of asterixis; absence of deep tendon reflexes; flaccidity of extremities. EEG markedly abnormal.	Risk for aspiration Impaired gas exchange Impaired tissue integrity

*Nursing diagnoses are likely to progress so that most nursing diagnoses present at earlier stages will occur during later stages as well.

Possible side effects include intestinal bloating and cramps, which usually disappear in a week. To mask the sweet taste to which some patients object, lactulose can be diluted with fruit juice. The patient is closely monitored for hypokalemia and dehydration. Other laxatives are not prescribed during lactulose administration because their effects would disturb dosage regulation. Lactulose enemas have also been used effectively in acute hepatic encephalopathy for patients who are comatose or in whom oral administration is contraindicated or impossible.

Other aspects of management include intravenous administration of glucose to minimize protein breakdown, administration of vitamins to correct vitamin deficiencies, and correction of electrolytes (especially potassium). Oxygen is administered if oxygen desaturation occurs.

Home Care Considerations

If the patient has recovered from hepatic encephalopathy and is to be discharged home, the family must be instructed to observe the patient for subtle signs of recurrent encephalopathy. The importance of periodic follow-up is also emphasized. The home care nurse assesses the patient's physical and mental status and adherence to the prescribed therapeutic regimen.

Other Manifestations of Liver Dysfunction

Edema and Bleeding. Many patients with liver dysfunction develop generalized edema due to hypoalbuminemia that results from decreased hepatic production of serum albumin. The production of blood clotting factors by the liver is also reduced, leading to an increased incidence of bruising, nosebleeds, bleeding from wounds, and, as described above, gastrointestinal bleeding.

Vitamin Deficiency. Decreased production of several clotting factors may be due, in part, to deficient absorption of vitamin K from the gastrointestinal tract. This probably is caused by the inability of liver cells to use vitamin K to make prothrombin. Absorption of the other fat-soluble vitamins (vitamins A, D, and E) as well as dietary fats may also be impaired, because of decreased secretion of bile salts into the intestine.

Metabolic Abnormalities. Abnormalities of *glucose* metabolism also occur; the blood glucose level may be abnormally high shortly after a meal (a diabetic-type glucose tolerance test result), but hypoglycemia may occur during fasting because of decreased hepatic glycogen reserves and decreased gluconeogenesis.

- Because the ability to metabolize *medications* is decreased, medications must be used cautiously and usual medication dosages must be reduced for the patient with liver failure.

Decreased metabolism of *estrogens* by the damaged liver can lead to gynecomastia, testicular atrophy, loss of pubic hair in the male, and menstrual irregularities in the female, as well as spider angiomata and reddened palms ("liver palms").

Splenomegaly. Splenomegaly (enlarged spleen) with possible hypersplenism occurs commonly as a manifestation of portal hypertension.

Pruritus. Patients with liver dysfunction due to biliary obstruction commonly develop severe itching (pruritus) due to retention of bile salts.

Hepatic Disorders

Viral Hepatitis

Viral hepatitis is a systemic, viral infection in which necrosis and inflammation of liver cells produce a characteristic cluster of clinical, biochemical, and cellular changes. To date, five definitive types of viral hepatitis have been identified: hepatitis A, B, C, D, and E. Hepatitis A and E are similar in mode of transmission (fecal–oral route) while hepatitis B, C, and D share many characteristics. A guide to the terminology associated with viral hepatitis is provided in Chart 38-1. There is evidence that additional hepatitis viruses may exist.

The increasing incidence of viral hepatitis is a growing public health concern. The disease is important because it is easy to transmit, has high morbidity, and causes prolonged loss of time from school or employment.

It is estimated that 60% to 90% of cases of viral hepatitis go unreported. The occurrence of subclinical cases, failure to recognize mild cases, and misdiagnosis are thought to contribute to the underreporting. Although approximately 50% of adults in the United States have antibodies against hepatitis A virus, many are unable to recall an earlier episode or the occurrence of the symptoms of hepatitis.

Nursing Implications. The nurse is especially concerned with three major problem areas of viral hepatitis: (1) the care of the patient with hepatitis; (2) the fact that many people who have the disease are asymptomatic, which may present serious epidemiologic problems; and (3) the apparent health needs of the community that are required to eliminate the various forms of the disease. The last category includes the following considerations:

- Proper community and home sanitation
- Conscientious individual hygiene at all times (especially hand washing)
- Safe practices for preparing and dispensing food
- Effective health supervision in schools, dormitories, extended care facilities, barracks, and camps
- Continuous health education programs
- Reporting of every case of viral hepatitis to the local health department

For a comparison of the many aspects of the major forms of viral hepatitis, see Table 38-3.

Hepatitis A Virus

Hepatitis A, formerly designated **infectious hepatitis,** is caused by an RNA virus of the enterovirus family. The mode of transmission of this disease is the fecal–oral route, primarily through the ingestion of food or liquids infected by the virus. The virus has been found in the stool of infected patients before the onset of symptoms and during the first few days of illness. Typically, a young adult acquires the infection at school and brings it home, where haphazard sanitary habits spread it through the family. It is more

CHART 38-1
Glossary

Hepatitis A

HAV	Hepatitis A virus; etiologic agent of hepatitis A (formerly infectious hepatitis).
Anti-HAV	Antibody to hepatitis A virus; appears in serum soon after onset of symptoms; disappears after 3–12 months.
IgM anti-HAV	IgM antibody to HAV; indicates recent infection with HAV; positive up to 6 months after infection.

Hepatitis B

HBV	Hepatitis B virus; etiologic agent of hepatitis B (formerly serum hepatitis).
HB_sAg	Hepatitis B surface antigen (Australian antigen); indicates acute or chronic hepatitis B or carrier state; indicates infectious state.
Anti-HB_s	Antibody to hepatitis B surface antigen; indicates prior exposure and immunity to hepatitis; may indicate passive antibody from HBIG or immune response from hepatitis B vaccine.
HB_eAg	Hepatitis B e-antigen; present in serum early in course; indicates highly infectious stage of hepatitis B; persistence in serum indicates progression to chronic hepatitis.
Anti-HB_e	Antibody to hepatitis B e-antigen; suggests low titer of HBV.
HB_cAg	Hepatitis B core antigen; found in liver cells; not easily detected in serum.
Anti-HB_c	Antibody to hepatitis B core antigen; most sensitive indicator of hepatitis B; appears late in the acute phase of the disease; indicates infection of HBV at some time in the past.
IgM anti-HB_c	IgM antibody to HB_cAg; present for up to 6 months after HBV infection.

Hepatitis C

HCV	Hepatitis C virus (formerly non-A, non-B virus); may be more than one virus.

Hepatitis D

HDV	Hepatitis D virus (delta agent); etiologic agent to hepatitis D; HBV is required for replication.
HDAg	Hepatitis delta antigen; detectable in early acute HDV infection.
Anti-HDV	Antibody to HDV; indicates past or present infection with HDV.

Hepatitis E

HEV	Hepatitis E virus; etiologic agent of hepatitis E.

prevalent in underdeveloped countries or in instances of overcrowding and poor sanitation. An infected food handler can spread the disease, and people can contract it by consuming water or shellfish from sewage-contaminated waters. Outbreaks have occurred in day care centers and institutions for the developmentally delayed because of lapses in hygiene. It is rarely, if ever, transmitted by blood transfusions.

The incubation period is estimated to be from 1 to 7 weeks, with an average of 30 days. The course of the illness may be prolonged, lasting from 4 to 8 weeks. It generally lasts longer and is more severe in those over the age of 40.

The virus is present only briefly in the serum; by the time jaundice occurs, the patient is likely to be noninfectious.

Assessment and Clinical Manifestations. Many patients are anicteric (without jaundice) and symptomless. When symptoms appear, they are of a mild, flulike upper respiratory tract infection, with low-grade fever. Anorexia is an early symptom and is often severe. It is thought to result from release of a toxin by the damaged liver or by failure of the damaged liver cells to detoxify an abnormal product. Later, jaundice and dark urine may become apparent. Indigestion is present, in varying degrees, marked by vague epigastric distress, nausea, heartburn, and flatulence. The patient may also develop a strong aversion to the taste of cigarettes or the presence of cigarette smoke and other strong odors.

These symptoms tend to clear as soon as the jaundice reaches its peak—perhaps 10 days after its initial appearance. The liver and the spleen are often moderately enlarged for a few days after onset; otherwise, apart from jaundice, there are few physical signs to be elicited.

Although symptoms may be very mild in children, adults are more likely to be symptomatic, with the symptoms more severe and the course of the disease prolonged.

Management. Bed rest during the acute stage and a diet that is both acceptable and nutritious are part of the treatment and nursing care. During the period of anorexia, the patient should receive frequent small feedings, supplemented, if necessary, by intravenous infusions of glucose. Because this patient often has an aversion to food, gentle persistence and creativity may be required to stimulate the appetite. Optimal food and fluid levels are necessary to counteract weight loss and slow recovery. Even before the icteric phase, however, many patients recover their appetites and may not need reminders to maintain a good diet.

TABLE 38-3 Comparison of Types of Viral Hepatitis

	Hepatitis A	Hepatitis B	Hepatitis C	Hepatitis D	Hepatitis E
Previous names	Infectious hepatitis	Serum hepatitis	Non-A, non-B hepatitis		
Epidemiology					
Cause	hepatitis A virus (HAV)	hepatitis B virus (HBV)	hepatitis C virus (HCV)	hepatitis D virus (HDV)	hepatitis E virus (HEV)
Mode of transmission	Fecal–oral route; poor sanitation. Person-to-person contact. Water borne; foodborne.	Parenterally; or by intimate contact with carriers or those with acute disease; sexual and oral–oral contact. Perinatal transmission from mothers to infants. An important occupational hazard for health care personnel.	Transfusion of blood and blood products; exposure to contaminated blood through equipment or drug paraphenalia	Same as HBV. HBV surface antigen necessary for replication; pattern similar to that of hepatitis B.	Fecal–oral route; person-to-person contact may be possible although risk appears low.
Incubation (days)	15–49 days. Average: 30 days	28–160 days. Average: 70–80 days	15–160 days. Average: 50 days	21–140 days. Average: 35 days	15–65 days. Average: 42 days
Immunity	Homologous	Homologous	Second attack may indicate weak immunity or infection with another agent	Homologous	Unknown
Nature of Illness					
Signs and Symptoms	May occur with or without symptoms: flulike illness. *Preicteric phase:* Headache, malaise, fatigue, anorexia, fever. *Icteric phase:* Dark urine, jaundice of slcera and skin, tender liver.	May occur without symptoms. May develop arthralgias, rash	Similar to HBV; less severe and anicteric	Similar to HBV	Similar to HAV. Very severe in pregnant women
Outcome	Usually mild with recovery. Fatality rate: <1%. No carrier state or increased risk of chronic hepatitis, cirrhosis, or hepatic cancer.	May be severe. Fatality rate: 1%–10%. Carrier state possible. Increased risk of chronic hepatitis, cirrhosis, and hepatic cancer.	Frequent occurrence of chronic carrier state and chronic liver disease. Increased risk of hepatic cancer.	Similar to HBV but greater likelihood of carrier state, chronic active hepatitis, and cirrhosis.	Similar to HAV except very severe in pregnant women.

The patient's sense of well-being as well as laboratory test results are generally appropriate guides to bed rest and restriction of physical activity. Gradual but progressive ambulation seems to hasten recovery, provided the patient rests after activity and does not participate in activities to the point of fatigue.

Prognosis. Recovery from hepatitis type A is the rule; hepatitis A rarely progresses to acute liver necrosis or fulminant hepatitis, terminating in cirrhosis of the liver or death. Hepatitis A confers immunity against itself; however, the person may contract other forms of hepatitis. The mortality rate of hepatitis A is approximately 0.5%. No carrier state exists, and no chronic hepatitis is associated with hepatitis A.

Patient Teaching. The patient is usually managed at home unless symptoms are particularly severe. Therefore, the patient and family need to be assisted to cope with the temporary disability and fatigue that are common problems in hepatitis and to be aware of the indications to seek additional health care if the symptoms persist or worsen. Additionally, the patient and family need specific guidelines about diet, rest, follow-up blood work, and the importance of avoiding alcohol, as well as sanitation and hygiene measures, particularly hand washing, to prevent spread of the disease to other family members.

Specific teaching to patients and families about reducing the risk of contracting hepatitis A include:

- Good personal hygiene, stressing careful hand washing (after bowel movement and before eating)
- Environmental sanitation—safe food and water supply, as well as effective sewage disposal

Prevention

- *Hepatitis A vaccine:* In February 1995, the first vaccine against hepatitis A was approved by the Food and Drug Administration for use in the US. It is recommended that the two-dose vaccine be given to adults 18 years of age or older, with the second dose 6 to 12 months after the first. Protection against hepatitis A develops within several weeks after the first dose of the vaccine. Children and adolescents 2 to 18 years of age will receive three doses, with the second dose 1 month after the first and the third dose 6 to 12 months later. It is estimated that protection against hepatitis A may last for at least 20 years (Marwick, 1995).

  Hepatitis A vaccine is recommended for travelers to locations where sanitation and hygiene are unsatisfactory. Additionally, vaccination is recommended for those from other high-risk groups (homosexual men, intravenous drug users, staff of day care centers, and health care personnel). As with other vaccinations, precautions must be taken to ensure prevention, detection, and treatment of hypersensitivity reactions to the vaccine.
- *Administration of immune globulin:* Type A hepatitis can be prevented in those not previously vaccinated by the administration of globulin intramuscularly during the period of incubation, if this treatment is instituted within 2 weeks of exposure. This bolsters the person's own antibody production and provides 6 to 8 weeks of passive immunity. Immune globulin may suppress overt symptoms of the disease; the resulting subclinical case of hepatitis A would produce active immunity to subsequent episodes of the virus.

Although rare, systemic reactions to immune globulin may occur. (Caution is required when anyone who has previously had angioedema, hives, or other allergic reactions is treated with any human immune globulin. Epinephrine should be available for use in systemic or anaphylactic reactions.)

- *Preexposure prophylaxis* is recommended for those traveling to developing countries and settings with poor or uncertain sanitation conditions but who do not have sufficient time to acquire protection by administration of hepatitis A vaccine.
- Immune globulin is also recommended for household members and sexual contacts of persons with hepatitis A. (Susceptible people in the same household as the patient with hepatitis A are usually also infected by the time the diagnosis is made and should receive immune globulin.)

Hepatitis B Virus

Components. Hepatitis B virus (HBV) is a DNA virus that is composed of the following antigenic particles:

HBcAg—hepatitis B core antigen (antigenic material in an inner core)
HBsAg—hepatitis B surface antigen (antigenic material on surface of HBV)
HBeAg—an independent protein circulating in the blood
HBxAg—gene product of X gene of HBV/DNA

Each antigen elicits its specific antibody:

anti-HBc—antibody to core antigen or HBV; persists during the acute phase of illness; may indicate continuing hepatitis B virus in the liver
anti-HBs—antibody to surface determinants on HBV; detected during late convalescence; usually indicates recovery and development of immunity
anti-HBe—antibody to hepatitis B e antigen; usually signifies reduced infectivity
anti-HBxAg—antibody to the hepatitis B x antigen; may indicate ongoing replication of HBV

HBsAg appears in the circulation in 80% to 90% of infected patients 1 to 10 weeks after exposure to HBV and 2 to 8 weeks before the onset of symptoms or an increase in transferase (transaminase) levels. Those persons with HBsAg that persists for 6 or more months after acute infection are referred to as HBsAg carriers.

HBeAg is the next antigen of HBV to appear in the serum. It usually appears within a week of the appearance of HBsAg and before changes in aminotransferase levels, disappearing from the serum within 2 weeks. HBV DNA, detected by polymerase chain reaction (PCR) testing, appears in the serum at about the same time as HBeAg. HBcAg is not always detected in the serum in HBV infection.

About 15% of American adults are positive for anti-HBs, which indicates that they have had hepatitis B. Anti-HBs may be positive in as many as two thirds of IV drug users.

Disease Course and Risk Factors. Unlike hepatitis A, which is transmitted primarily by the fecal–oral route, hepatitis B is transmitted primarily through blood (percutaneous and permucosal routes). The virus has been found in blood, saliva, semen, and vaginal secretions and can be transmitted through mucous membranes and breaks in the skin.

Hepatitis B has a long incubation period. It replicates in the liver and remains in the serum for relatively long periods, allowing transmission of the virus. Therefore, those at risk of developing hepatitis B include surgeons, clinical laboratory workers, dentists, nurses, and respiratory therapists. Staff and patients in hemodialysis and oncology units and sexually active homosexual and bisexual males and IV drug users are also at increased risk.

Screening of blood donors for HBsAg has greatly reduced the occurrence of hepatitis B after blood transfusion.

Assessment and Clinical Manifestations. Clinically, the disease closely resembles hepatitis A. The incubation period, however, is much longer (between 1 and 6 months). The mortality is appreciable, ranging from 1% to 10%.

Signs and symptoms of hepatitis B may be insidious and variable. Fever and respiratory symptoms are rare; some patients have arthralgias and rashes. The patient may experience loss of appetite, dyspepsia, abdominal pain, generalized aching, malaise, and weakness. Jaundice may or may not be evident. If jaundice occurs, it is accompanied by light-colored stools and dark urine. The patient's liver may be tender and enlarged to 12 to 14 cm vertically. The spleen is enlarged and palpable in a small number of patients; the posterior cervical lymph nodes may also be enlarged.

Gerontologic Considerations. The elderly patient who contracts hepatitis B has a serious risk of severe liver cell necrosis or fulminant hepatic failure, particularly if other illnesses are present. The patient is seriously ill and the prognosis is poor.

Management. Clinical trials with **interferon** have shown that early treatment with daily injections of interferon induces remission of hepatitis B in over one third of patients and eliminates hepatitis B surface antigen (indicates carrier state) in 10% of patients. Although these results are very promising, interferon is ineffective in a sizable number of patients, must be administered by daily injection, and has significant side effects, including liver toxicity. Therefore, interferon should be used only under carefully controlled conditions.

Bed rest is usually recommended, regardless of other treatment, until the symptoms of hepatitis have subsided. Subsequently, the patient's activities are restricted until the hepatic enlargement and elevation of the levels of serum bilirubin and liver enzymes have disappeared.

Adequate nutrition should be maintained; proteins are restricted when the ability of the liver to metabolize protein by-products is impaired, as demonstrated by symptoms. *Therapeutic measures* to control the dyspeptic symptoms and general malaise include the use of antacids, belladonna, and antiemetics. However, all medications should be avoided if vomiting is a problem. If vomiting persists, the patient should be hospitalized and treated with fluid therapy. Because of the mode of transmission, the patient is evaluated for other blood-borne diseases.

Convalescence may be prolonged, with complete symptomatic recovery sometimes requiring 3 to 4 months or longer. During this stage, gradual restoration of physical activity is permitted and encouraged, after the jaundice has resolved.

Psychosocial considerations are identified by the nurse, particularly the effects of isolation and separation from family and friends during the acute and infective stages. Special planning is required to minimize alterations in sensory perception. The family is included in planning to decrease the fears and anxieties of the patient and family about the spread of the disease.

Prognosis. Mortality of hepatitis B has been reported to be as high as 10%. Another 10% of patients who have hepatitis B progress to a carrier state or develop chronic hepatitis. It remains the chief cause of cirrhosis and hepatocellular carcinoma worldwide.

Patient Education and Home Care Considerations. Because of the prolonged period of convalescence, the patient and family must be prepared for home care. Provision for adequate rest and nutrition must be ensured before the patient's discharge. Those family members and friends who have had intimate contact with the patient should be informed about the risks of contracting hepatitis B, and arrangements should be made for them to receive hepatitis B vaccine or hepatitis B immune globulin. Those at risk must be aware of early signs of hepatitis B and of ways to reduce risk to themselves.

Follow-up visits by a home health nurse are indicated to assess the patient's progress and answer family members' questions about transmission of the disease. A home visit also permits evaluation of the understanding of the patient and family about the importance of adequate rest and nutrition. Because of the risk of transmission through sexual intercourse, use of strategies to prevent exchange of body fluids is advised; these include abstinence or the use of condoms.

- Patients with all forms of hepatitis are cautioned to avoid use of alcohol.

Control and Prevention. The goals of prevention are (1) to interrupt the chain of transmission, (2) to protect those people at high risk with active immunization through the use of hepatitis B vaccine, and (3) to use passive immunization for unprotected people exposed to hepatitis B virus.

Preventing Transmission. Continued screening of potential blood donors for the presence of HBAg will further decrease the risk of transmission by blood transfusion. The use of disposable syringes, needles, and lancets and the introduction of needleless intravenous delivery systems reduce the risk of spreading this infection from one patient to another during the collection of blood samples or the administration of parenteral therapy. Good personal hygiene practices are fundamental to infection control. In the clinical laboratory, work areas should be disinfected daily. Gloves are worn when handling all blood and body fluids as well as HBAg-positive specimens or when there is potential exposure to blood (blood drawing) or to patients' secretions. Eating and smoking are prohibited in the laboratory and in other areas exposed to patients' secretions, blood, or blood products.

Active Immunization: Hepatitis B Vaccine. Active immunization is recommended for individuals at high risk for hepatitis B (*e.g.*, health care personnel, hemodialysis patients). A yeast-recombinant hepatitis B vaccine (Recombivax HB) is used to provide active immunity. Protection resulting from hepatitis B vaccine may last 5 to 7 years; annual testing of anti-HBs level is recommended to determine the need for booster doses.

A hepatitis B vaccine prepared from plasma of humans chronically infected with HBV is used only rarely and in patients who are immunodeficient or allergic to recombinant yeast-derived vaccines.

Both forms of the hepatitis B vaccine are administered in three doses, the second and third doses 1 and 6 months after the first dose. The third dose is very important in producing prolonged immunity. Hepatitis B vaccination should be administered to adults in the deltoid muscle, as administration in the gluteal region may result in suboptimal response.

Persons at high risk, including nurses and other health care personnel exposed to blood or blood products, should receive active immunization. (See Chart 38-2 for a list of other persons at risk for HBV who should receive hepatitis B vaccine.) Health care workers who have had frequent contact with blood are screened for anti-HBs to determine if immunity is already present from previous exposure. Studies have shown that the vaccine produces active immunity to HBV in 90% of healthy persons. It does not provide protection to those already exposed to HBV and provides no protection against hepatitis A or hepatitis C. Side effects of immunization are infrequent. Soreness and redness at the injection site are the most common postinjection complaints.

Passive Immunity: Hepatitis B Immune Globulin. Hepatitis B immune globulin (HBIG) provides passive immunity to hepatitis B and is indicated for persons exposed to HBV who have never had hepatitis B and have never received hepatitis B vaccine.

Specific indications for postexposure vaccine with HBIG include: (1) accidental exposure to HBAg-positive blood through percutaneous (needle-stick) or transmucosal (splashes in contact with mucous membrane) routes, (2) sexual contact with persons who are positive for HBAg, and (3) perinatal exposure.

HBIG, which provides passive immunity, is prepared from plasma selected for high titers of anti-HBs. Again, there has been no evidence that HIV infection can be transmitted by HBIG. Prompt immunization with HBIG, that is, within hours to a few days after exposure to hepatitis B, increases the likelihood of protection.

Both active and passive immunization are recommended for persons exposed to hepatitis B through sexual contact or through percutaneous or transmucosal routes. If HBIG and hepatitis B vaccine are administered at the same time, separate sites and separate syringes should be used.

CHART 38-2
Persons at Increased Risk for Hepatitis B

- Health care workers with frequent exposure to blood, blood products, or other body fluids
  - Hemodialysis staff
  - Oncology/chemotherapy nurses
  - All health care personnel at risk for needlesticks
  - Operating room staff
  - Respiratory therapists
  - Surgeons
  - Dentists
- Hemodialysis patients
- Sexually active homosexual and bisexual men
- Users of illicit intravenous drugs
- Household personnel or people in sexual contact with carriers of HBV
- Travelers to areas with poor or uncertain sanitary conditions
- Heterosexuals with multiple sexual partners
- Recipients of blood products (*i.e.,* clotting factor concentrate)

Hepatitis C

A significant proportion of cases of viral hepatitis are neither hepatitis A, hepatitis B, nor hepatitis D; as a result they are classified as hepatitis C (formerly referred to as non-A, non-B hepatitis or NANB hepatitis). Another agent, distinct from and unrelated to hepatitis C virus, is thought to be responsible for some cases of "non-A-non-B hepatitis" associated with blood transfusions. In the United States, over 90% of cases are a result of blood transfusion, and hepatitis C is the primary form of hepatitis associated with transfusions.

Individuals at special risk for hepatitis C include children receiving frequent transfusions or those who require large volumes of blood. Hepatitis is more likely to be transmitted from commercial or paid blood donors than from volunteer donors. Hepatitis C occurs not only in patients after blood transfusions and among IV drug users, but also in health care personnel associated with renal dialysis units.

The incubation period is variable and may range from 15 to 160 days. The clinical course of acute hepatitis C is similar to that of hepatitis B; symptoms are usually mild. A chronic carrier state occurs frequently, however, and there is an increased risk of chronic liver disease, including cirrhosis or liver cancer, after hepatitis C. Long-term, low-dose interferon therapy has been effective in preliminary trials in some patients with hepatitis C; however, beneficial responses have been temporary. The combination of interferon and ribavirin, a nucleoside analogue, is being tested to determine if a more prolonged benefit may occur (Fried & Hoofnagle, 1995).

Screening of blood transfusions for hepatitis C has reduced the number of cases of hepatitis associated with blood transfusions.

Hepatitis D

Hepatitis D (delta agent) occurs in some cases of hepatitis B. Because the virus requires hepatitis B surface antigen for its replication, only individuals with hepatitis B are at risk for hepatitis D. Anti-delta antibodies in the presence of HBAg on testing confirm the diagnosis. It is also common among IV drug users, hemodialysis patients, and recipients of multiple blood transfusions. Sexual contact with those with hepatitis B is considered to be an important mode of transmission of hepatitis B and D. The incubation period varies between 21 and 140 days.

The symptoms of hepatitis D are similar to those of hepatitis B except that patients are more likely to have fulminant hepatitis and to progress to chronic active hepatitis and cirrhosis. Treatment is similar to that of other forms of hepatitis, although interferon as a specific treatment for hepatitis D is under investigation.

Hepatitis E

Hepatitis E virus, the newest of the hepatitis viruses to be identified, is believed to be transmitted by the fecal–oral route. The incubation period of hepatitis E is variable and is estimated to range between 15 and 65 days. Its onset and symptoms are similar to those of other types of viral hepatitis.

Avoiding contact with the virus through good hygiene, including hand washing, is the major method of prevention of hepatitis E. The effectiveness of immune globulin in protecting against hepatitis E virus is uncertain.

Toxic Hepatitis and Drug-Induced Hepatitis

Certain chemicals have toxic effects on the liver and when taken by mouth or injected parenterally produce acute liver cell necrosis, or **toxic hepatitis.** The chemicals most commonly implicated in this disease are carbon tetrachloride, phosphorus, chloroform, and gold compounds. These substances are true hepatotoxins.

Many medications may induce hepatitis but are sensitizing rather than toxic. The result, **drug-induced hepatitis,** is similar to acute viral hepatitis; however, parenchymal destruction tends to be more extensive. Some examples of medications that can lead to hepatitis are isoniazid, halothane, acetaminophen, and certain antibiotics, antimetabolites, and anesthetic agents.

Toxic Hepatitis: Manifestations and Management. Toxic hepatitis resembles viral hepatitis in onset. Obtaining a history of exposure to hepatotoxic chemicals, medications, or other agents assists in early initiation of treatment and removal of the offending agent. Anorexia, nausea, and vomiting are the usual symptoms; jaundice and hepatomegaly are noted on physical assessment. Symptoms are more intense for the more severely toxic patient.

Recovery from acute toxic hepatitis is rapid if the hepatotoxin is identified early and removed or if exposure to the agent has been limited. Recovery, however, is unlikely if there is a prolonged period between exposure and onset of symptoms. There are no effective antidotes. The fever rises; the patient becomes very toxic and prostrated. Vomiting may be persistent, with the emesis containing blood. Clotting abnormalities may be severe, and hemorrhages may appear under the skin. The severe gastrointestinal symptoms may lead to vascular collapse. Delirium, coma, and convulsions develop, and within a few days the patient usually dies of fulminant hepatic failure (discussed below).

Short of liver transplantation, few treatment options are available. Therapy is directed toward restoring and maintaining fluid and electrolyte balance, blood replacement, and provision of comfort and supportive measures. A few patients recover from acute toxic hepatitis only to develop chronic liver disease. In the event that the liver heals, there may be scarring, followed by postnecrotic cirrhosis.

Drug-Induced Hepatitis: Manifestations and Management. Medication-induced hepatitis is responsible for up to 25% of cases of fulminant hepatic failure in the United States. Manifestations of sensitivity to a medication may occur on the first day of its use or not until several months later, depending on the medication. Usually, the onset is abrupt, with chills, fever, rash, pruritus, arthralgia, anorexia, and nausea. Later, there may be jaundice and dark urine and an enlarged and tender liver. When the offending medication is withdrawn, symptoms may gradually subside. Reactions may be severe, however, and even fatal, even though the medication is stopped. If fever, rash, or pruritus occurs from any medication, its use should be stopped immediately.

Although any medication can affect liver function, those most commonly associated with liver injury include but are not limited to anesthetic agents, medications used to treat rheumatic and musculoskeletal disease, antidepressants, psychotropic medications, anticonvulsants, and antituberculosis agents.

Halothane (Fluothane), a commonly used nonexplosive inhalation anesthetic, may cause serious, and sometimes fatal, liver damage; therefore, its use is contraindicated in (1) patients with known liver disease; (2) repeated instances, particularly in patients who have had a fever of unknown cause after the first administration of halothane; and (3) patients with evidence of prior sensitization. Such sensitization would have been evident during the second postoperative week, with such manifestations as fever, rash, eosinophilia, arthralgia, or jaundice.

Fulminant Hepatic Failure

Fulminant hepatic failure is characterized by the development of hepatic encephalopathy within weeks of the onset of disease in a patient without prior evidence of hepatic dysfunction. A new classification of acute liver failure based on the speed of development of encephalopathy in relation to the first appearance of jaundice has been proposed. In this classification system, there are three categories: hyperacute, acute, and subacute liver failure. In hyperacute liver failure, the duration of jaundice before the onset of encephalopathy is 0 to 7 days; in acute liver failure, it is 8 to 28 days; and in subacute liver failure, the duration is 28 to 72 days. The cause (viral vs. nonviral) and prognosis of the three categories of acute liver failure vary (Tibbs & Williams, 1995). All three types of fulminant liver failure are characterized by dramatic and rapid clinical deterioration caused by massive hepatocellular injury and necrosis. Mortality is extremely high (60% to 85%), despite intensive treatment.

Causes. Viral hepatitis is the most common cause of fulminant hepatic failure; other causes include toxic medications (*e.g.*, acetaminophen [Tylenol)] and chemicals (*e.g.*, carbon tetrachloride), metabolic disturbances (Wilson's disease), and structural changes (Budd–Chiari syndrome).

Clinical Manifestations. The presence of jaundice and profound anorexia may be the initial reason for the patient to seek health care. Fulminant hepatic failure is often accompanied by coagulation defects, renal failure and electrolyte disturbances, infection, hypoglycemia, encephalopathy, and cerebral edema.

Management. Treatment modalities have included blood or plasma exchanges, charcoal hemoperfusion, and corticosteroids. Despite these treatment modalities, however, mortality remains high. Consequently, liver transplantation has become the treatment of choice for persons with fulminant hepatic failure. Liver transplantation is discussed on p. 1003.

Hepatic Cirrhosis

There are three types of cirrhosis or scarring of the liver:

1. *Laennec's portal cirrhosis* (alcoholic, nutritional), in which the scar tissue characteristically surrounds the portal areas. This is most frequently due to chronic alcoholism and is the most common type of cirrhosis.
2. *Postnecrotic cirrhosis,* in which there are broad bands of scar tissue, as a late result of a previous acute viral hepatitis.
3. *Biliary cirrhosis,* in which scarring occurs in the liver around the bile ducts. This type usually is the result of chronic biliary obstruction and infection (cholangitis); its incidence is considerably lower than that of Laennec's and postnecrotic cirrhosis.

The portion of the liver chiefly involved in cirrhosis consists of the portal and the periportal spaces, where the bile canaliculi of each lobule communicate to form the liver bile ducts. These areas become the site of inflammation, and the bile ducts become occluded with inspissated (thickened) bile and pus. An attempt is made by the liver to form new bile channels; hence, there is an overgrowth of tissue made up largely of disconnected, newly formed bile ducts and surrounded by scar tissue.

Clinical manifestations of this disease include intermittent jaundice and fever. Initially the liver is enlarged, hard, and irregular; eventually it becomes atrophic. The treatment is the same as that for any form of chronic liver insufficiency.

Pathophysiology

Although several factors have been implicated in the etiology of cirrhosis, alcohol consumption is considered the major causative factor. Cirrhosis occurs with greatest frequency among alcoholics. Although nutritional deficiency with reduced protein intake contributes to liver destruction in cirrhosis, excessive alcohol intake is the major causative factor in fatty liver and its consequences. Cirrhosis, however, has also occurred in people who do not consume alcohol and in those who consume a normal diet and have a high alcohol intake.

Some people appear to be more susceptible than others to this disease, whether or not they are alcoholics or malnourished. Other factors may play a role, including exposure to certain chemicals (carbon tetrachloride, chlorinated naphthalene, arsenic, or phosphorus) or infectious schistosomiasis. Twice as many men as women are affected, and the majority of patients are between 40 and 60 years of age.

Laennec's cirrhosis is a disease characterized by episodes of necrosis involving the liver cells, sometimes occurring repeatedly throughout the course of the disease. The destroyed liver cells are gradually replaced by scar tissue; eventually the amount of scar tissue exceeds that of the functioning liver tissue. Islands of residual normal tissue and regenerating liver tissue may project from the constricted areas, giving the cirrhotic liver its characteristic hobnail appearance. The disease usually has a particularly insidious onset and a very protracted course, occasionally proceeding over a period of 30 or more years.

Clinical Manifestations

Liver Enlargement. Early in the course of cirrhosis, the liver tends to be large and its cells loaded with fat. The liver is firm and has a sharp edge noticeable on palpation. Abdominal pain may be present because of recent, rapid enlargement of the liver, producing tension on the fibrous covering of the liver (Glisson's capsule). Later in the course of the disease, the liver decreases in size as scar tissue contracts the liver tissue. The liver edge, if palpable, is nodular.

Portal Obstruction and Ascites. The late manifestations are due partly to chronic failure of liver function and partly to obstruction of the portal circulation. Practically all the blood from the digestive organs is collected in the portal veins and carried to the liver. Because a cirrhotic liver does not allow the blood free passage, it is backed up into the spleen and the gastrointestinal tract, with the result that these organs become the seat of chronic passive congestion; that is, they are stagnant with blood and thus cannot function properly. Such patients are likely to have chronic dyspepsia (indigestion) and constipation or diarrhea. There is gradual weight loss.

Fluid rich in protein may accumulate in the peritoneal cavity, producing ascites. This can be demonstrated through percussion for shifting dullness or a fluid wave (see Fig. 38-6). Splenomegaly may also be present. Spider telangiectases, or dilated superficial arterioles resembling bluish-red spiders, are frequently observed on inspection of the face and trunk.

Gastrointestinal Varices. The obstruction to blood flow through the liver resulting from the fibrotic changes also results in the formation of collateral blood vessels in the gastrointestinal system and shunting of blood from the portal vessels into blood vessels with lower pressures. As a result, the patient with cirrhosis will often have prominent, distended abdominal blood vessels, which are visible on abdominal inspection (caput medusae), and distended blood vessels throughout the gastrointestinal tract. The esophagus, stomach, and lower rectum are common sites of collateral blood vessels. These distended blood vessels form varices or hemorrhoids, depending on their location.

Because these vessels were not intended to carry the high pressure and volume of blood imposed by cirrhosis, they may rupture and bleed. Therefore, assessment must include observation for occult and frank bleeding from the gastrointestinal tract. Approximately 25% of patients develop small hematemesis; others have profuse hemorrhage from gastric and esophageal varices.

Edema. Other late symptoms of cirrhosis are attributable to chronic liver failure. The concentration of plasma albumin is reduced, predisposing to the formation of edema. Overproduction of aldosterone occurs, causing sodium and water retention and potassium excretion.

Vitamin Deficiency and Anemia. Because of inadequate formation, use, and storage of certain vitamins (notably vitamins A, C, and K), signs of their deficiency frequently are encountered, particularly hemorrhagic phenomena associated with vitamin K deficiency. Chronic gastritis and impaired gastrointestinal function, together with inadequate dietary intake and impaired liver function, account for the anemia often associated with this disease. The anemia and the patient's poor nutritional status and poor state of health result in severe fatigue, which interferes with the ability to carry out routine daily activities.

Mental Deterioration. Additional clinical manifestations include deterioration of mental function with impending hepatic encephalopathy and hepatic coma. Therefore, neurologic assessment is indicated and includes the patient's general behavior, cognitive abilities, orientation to time and place, and speech patterns.

Diagnostic Evaluation

The extent of liver disease and the type of treatment are determined after studying the laboratory findings. Because the functions of the liver are complex, there are many diagnostic tests that may provide information about liver function (see Table 38-1). The patient needs to know why these tests are being performed, why they are important, and how to cooperate.

In severe parenchymal liver dysfunction, the serum albumin level tends to decrease, and the serum globulin level rises. Enzyme tests indicate liver cell damage: serum alkaline phosphatase, AST (SGOT) and ALT (SGPT) levels increase, and the serum cholinesterase level may decrease. Bilirubin tests are performed to measure bile excretion or bile retention. Laparoscopy, in conjunction with biopsy, permits direct visualization of the liver.

Ultrasound scanning will measure the difference in density of parenchymal cells and scar tissue. Computed tomography (CT scan), MRI and radioisotopic liver scans give information about liver size and hepatic blood flow and obstruction.

Arterial blood gases may reveal a ventilation-perfusion imbalance and hypoxia in cirrhosis.

Management

The management of the patient with cirrhosis is usually based on the patient's presenting symptoms. For example, antacids are prescribed to decrease gastric distress and minimize the possibility of gastrointestinal bleeding. Vitamins and nutritional supplements promote healing of damaged liver cells and improve the patient's general nutritional status. Potassium-sparing diuretics (spironolactone) may be indicated to decrease ascites, if present, and minimize fluid and electrolyte changes common with other diuretic agents. Adequate intake of protein and calories is an essential part of treatment, along with the avoidance of further alcohol use. Although the fibrosis of the cirrhotic liver cannot be reversed, its progression may be halted or slowed by such measures.

Preliminary studies indicate that colchicine, an anti-inflammatory agent used to treat the symptoms of gout, may increase the length of survival in patients with mild to moderate cirrhosis.

❑ NURSING PROCESS
The Patient With Hepatic Cirrhosis

Assessment

Nursing assessment focuses on onset of symptoms and history of precipitating factors, particularly long-term alcohol abuse, as well as dietary intake and changes in the patient's physical and mental status. The patient's past and current patterns of alcohol use (duration and amount) are assessed and documented. It is also important to document any exposure to toxic agents encountered in the workplace or during recreational activities. Exposure to potentially hepatotoxic medications or general anesthetic agents is documented and reported.

Mental status is assessed through interview and other interaction with the patient; orientation to person, place, and time is noted. The patient's ability to carry on a job or household activities provides some information about physical and mental status. Additionally, the patient's relationships with family, friends, and coworkers may give some indication about incapacitation secondary to alcohol abuse and cirrhosis. Abdominal distention and bloating, gastrointestinal bleeding, bruising, and weight changes are noted.

Nutritional status, of major importance in cirrhosis, is assessed by daily weights, anthropometric measurements (see Chapter 7), and monitoring of plasma proteins, transferrin, and creatinine levels.

Diagnosis

Nursing Diagnoses

Based on all the assessment data, the patient's major nursing diagnoses may include the following:

- ❑ Activity intolerance related to fatigue, general debility, muscle wasting, and discomfort
- ❑ Altered nutrition related to chronic gastritis, decreased gastrointestinal motility, and anorexia
- ❑ Impaired skin integrity related to compromised immunologic status, edema, and poor nutrition
- ❑ Risk for injury related to altered clotting mechanisms and portal hypertension

Collaborative Problems/ Potential Complications

Based on assessment data, potential complications may include:

- ❑ Bleeding and hemorrhage
- ❑ Hepatic encephalopathy

Planning and Implementation

Goals. The goals of the patient may include independence in activities, improvement of nutritional status, improvement of skin integrity, decreased potential for injury, improvement of mental status, and absence of complications.

Nursing Interventions

Providing Rest. The patient with active liver disease requires rest and other supportive measures to permit the liver to reestablish its functional ability. If the patient is hospitalized, weight and fluid intake and output are measured and recorded daily. The patient's position in bed is adjusted for maximal respiratory efficiency, which is especially important if ascites is marked, as it interferes with adequate thoracic excursion. Oxygen therapy may be required in liver failure to oxygenate the damaged cells and prevent further cell destruction.

Rest reduces the demands on the liver and increases the liver's blood supply. Because the patient is susceptible to the hazards of immobility, efforts to prevent respiratory, circulatory, and vascular disturbances need to be initiated. These measures may help prevent such problems as pneumonia, thrombophlebitis, and pressure ulcers. When nutritional status improves and strength increases, the patient is encouraged to increase activity gradually. Activity and mild exercise, as well as rest, are planned.

Improving Nutritional Status. The patient with cirrhosis who has no ascites or edema and exhibits no signs of impending coma should receive a nutritious, high-protein diet supplemented by vitamins of the B complex and others as indicated (including vitamins A, C, and K and folic acid). Because proper nutrition is so important, every effort is made to encourage the patient to eat. This is as important as any medication. Often small, frequent meals are tolerated better than three large meals because of the abdominal pressure exerted by ascites.

Patient preferences are considered. Patients with prolonged or severe anorexia, or those who are vomiting or eating poorly for any reason, may receive nutrients by nasogastric tube or total parenteral nutrition (TPN).

Patients with fatty stools (steatorrhea) should receive water-soluble forms of fat-soluble vitamins—A, D, and E (Aquasol A, D, and E). Folic acid and iron are prescribed to prevent anemia. If the patient shows signs of impending or advancing coma, a low-protein diet is given temporarily. In the absence of hepatic encephalopathy, a moderate protein intake is provided with protein foods of high biologic value (*i.e.*, eggs, meat, dairy products).

A high-calorie intake should be maintained, and supplementary vitamins and minerals should be provided (*i.e.*, oral potassium, if the serum potassium is normal or low and if renal function is normal). As soon as the patient's condition permits, the protein intake should be restored to normal, or above. Diet therapy is determined on an individualized basis.

Providing Skin Care. Careful skin care is provided because of the presence of subcutaneous edema, the immobility of the patient, jaundice, and increased susceptibility to skin breakdown and infection. Frequent position changes are necessary to prevent pressure ulcers. Irritating soaps and use of adhesive tape are avoided to prevent trauma to the skin. Lotion may be soothing to irritated skin; measures are taken to minimize the patient's scratching of the skin.

Reducing Risk of Injury. The patient with cirrhosis is protected from falls and other injuries. The side rails are in place and padded with soft blankets to minimize risks if the patient becomes agitated or restless. The patient is oriented to time and place and all procedures are explained to minimize the patient's agitation. The patient is instructed to ask for assistance to get out of bed. Any injury is evaluated carefully because of the possibility of internal bleeding.

Because of risk of bleeding due to abnormal clotting, the patient is instructed and assisted to use an electric rather than safety razor. Bleeding of the gums is minimized by use of a soft bristled toothbrush. Pressure is applied to all venipuncture sites to minimize bleeding.

Monitoring and Managing Potential Complications

Preventing Bleeding. Bleeding and hemorrhage may occur because of decreased production of prothrombin and the decreased ability of the diseased liver to synthesize substances necessary for blood coagulation.

Precautionary measures include protecting the patient with padded side rails, applying pressure to any injection site, and avoiding injury from sharp objects. The nurse should observe for melena and assess stools for blood as signs of possible internal bleeding. Vital signs also are monitored regularly. Precautions are taken to minimize rupture of esophageal varices by avoiding further increases in portal pressure. Dietary modification and appropriate use of stool softeners may help prevent straining during defecation. The patient is monitored closely for gastrointestinal bleeding; equipment (Sengstaken–Blakemore tube), intravenous fluids, and medications needed to treat hemorrhage from esophageal varices are kept readily available (see pp. 996–999).

If hemorrhage occurs, the nurse assists the physician in initiating measures to halt the bleeding, administering fluid and blood component therapy and medications. The patient who experiences massive hemorrhage from bleeding esophageal or gastric varices may be transferred to the intensive care unit and may require emergency surgery or other treatment modalities (see pp. 998–999). The patient with cirrhosis who experiences hemorrhage and the patient's family require explanations about the event and necessary treatment.

Hepatic encephalopathy is a possible neurologic complication of cirrhosis that includes deteriorating mental status and dementia as well as physical signs such as abnormal voluntary and involuntary movements. Hepatic encephalopathy is mainly caused by accumulation of ammonia in the blood and its effect on cerebral metabolism. Many factors predispose the patient with cirrhosis to hepatic encephalopathy; therefore, the patient may require extensive diagnostic testing to identify hidden sources of bleeding and ammonia.

Treatment may include use of lactulose and nonabsorbable intestinal tract antibiotics to decrease ammonia levels, modification in medications to eliminate those that may precipitate or worsen hepatic encephalopathy, and bed rest to minimize energy expenditure.

Monitoring is an essential nursing function to identify early deterioration in mental status. The nurse monitors the patient's mental status closely and reports changes so that treatment of encephalopathy can be initiated promptly. Because electrolyte disturbances can contribute to encephalopathy, serum electrolyte levels are carefully monitored and corrected if abnormal. Oxygen is administered if oxygen desaturation occurs.

Patient Education and Home Care Considerations. During hospitalization, the patient is prepared for discharge by the nurse and other health care providers through dietary instruction. Of greatest importance is the exclusion of alcohol from the diet. The patient may need referral to

Alcoholics Anonymous, psychiatric care, or support from a trusted spiritual advisor.

Sodium restriction will continue for a considerable time, if not permanently. If this diet is to be followed correctly, the patient will require written instructions, teaching, reinforcement, and support from the staff as well as the family members.

The success of treatment depends on convincing the patient of the need to adhere completely to the therapeutic plan. This includes rest; probably a change in life-style; an adequate, well-balanced diet; and the elimination of alcohol. The patient and family are also instructed about the symptoms of impending encephalopathy and the possibility of bleeding tendencies and easy susceptibility to infection.

Recovery is neither rapid nor easy; there are frequent setbacks and apparent lack of improvement. Many patients find it difficult to refrain from using alcohol for comfort or escape. The understanding nurse can play a significant role in offering support and encouragement to this patient.

Referral of the patient to a home health nurse who visits the patient in the home after discharge may assist the patient in dealing with the transition from hospital to home, where use of alcohol may have been an important part of the patient's normal home and social life. The community health nurse or home care nurse assesses the patient's progress at home and the manner in which the patient and family cope with the elimination of alcohol and the dietary restrictions. Additionally, the nurse reinforces previous teaching and answers questions that may not have occurred to the patient or family until the patient is back home and trying to reestablish new patterns of eating, drinking, and life-style.

For an overall view of the nursing management of the patient with cirrhosis, refer to Nursing Care Plan 38-2.

Evaluation

Expected Outcomes

1. Demonstrates ability to participate in activities
   a. Plans activities and exercises to allow alternating periods of rest and activity
   b. Reports increased strength and well-being
   c. Displays increased weight gain without increased edema and ascites formation
   d. Participates in hygienic care
2. Increases nutritional intake
   a. Demonstrates intake of appropriate nutrients and avoidance of alcohol as reflected by diet log
   b. Gains weight without increased edema and ascites formation
   c. Reports decrease in gastrointestinal disturbances and anorexia
   d. Identifies foods and fluids that are nutritious and allowed on diet or restricted from diet
   e. Adheres to vitamin therapy regimen
   f. Describes the rationale for small, frequent meals
3. Demonstrates improved skin integrity
   a. Shows intact skin without evidence of breakdown, infection, or trauma
   b. Demonstrates normal turgor of skin of extremities and trunk, without edema
   c. Changes position frequently and inspects bony prominences daily
   d. Uses lotions to decrease pruritus
4. Experiences no injury
   a. Is free of ecchymotic areas or hematoma formation
   b. States rationale for side rails and asks for assistance to get out of bed
   c. Uses measures to prevent trauma (*i.e.*, uses soft toothbrush, blows nose gently, arranges furniture to prevent bumps and falls, avoids straining during defecation)
5. Is free of complications
   a. Reports absence of frank bleeding from gastrointestinal tract (*i.e.*, absence of melena and hematemesis)
   b. Is oriented to time, place, and person and demonstrates normal attention span
   c. Has serum ammonia level within normal limits
   d. Identifies early, reportable signs of impaired thought processes

Bleeding Esophageal Varices

Bleeding or hemorrhage from esophageal varices occurs in approximately one third of patients with cirrhosis and varices. The mortality rate resulting from the first bleeding episode is 45% to 50%; it is one of the major causes of death in patients with cirrhosis.

Pathophysiology and Clinical Manifestations

Esophageal varices are dilated, tortuous veins usually found in the submucosa of the lower esophagus; however, they may develop higher in the esophagus or extend into the stomach. Such a condition nearly always is caused by portal hypertension, which, in turn, is due to obstruction of the portal venous circulation within the cirrhotic liver (see p. 973).

Because of increased obstruction of the portal vein, venous blood from the intestinal tract and spleen seeks an outlet through collateral circulation (new pathways of return to the right atrium). The effect is increased pressure, particularly in the vessels in the submucosal layer of the lower esophagus and upper part of the stomach. These collateral vessels are not very elastic but rather are tortuous and fragile and bleed easily. Other less common causes of varices are abnormalities of the circulation in the splenic vein or superior vena cava and hepatic venothrombosis.

Bleeding esophageal varices are life threatening and can result in hemorrhagic shock, producing decreased cerebral, hepatic, and renal perfusion. In turn, there will be an increased nitrogen load from bleeding into the gastrointestinal tract and an increased serum ammonia level, which increase the risk of encephalopathy. Bleeding esophageal varices should be suspected in the presence of hematemesis and melena, especially in the patient who has abused alcohol. Usually, the dilated veins cause no symptoms unless the portal pressure increases sharply and the mucosa or supporting structures become thin. Then massive hemorrhage takes place.

(text continues on page 995)

NURSING CARE PLAN 38–2
Care of the Patient With Cirrhosis

Nursing Interventions	Rationale	Expected Outcomes
NURSING DIAGNOSIS: Activity intolerance related to fatigue and weight loss		
GOAL: Increased energy and increased participation in activities		
1. Offer high-protein, high-calorie diet.	1. Provides calories for energy and protein for healing.	• Reports increased strength and well-being.
2. Give supplementary vitamins (A, B-complex, C, and K).	2. Provides additional nutrients.	• Plans activities to allow ample periods of rest.
3. Encourage alternating periods of rest and exercise.	3. Conserves patient's energy while encouraging exercise within patient's tolerance.	• Increases activity and exercise as strength increases. • Gains weight without increased edema or ascites formation.
4. Encourage and assist with gradually increasing periods of exercise.	4. Improves general well-being and self-esteem.	• Demonstrates adequate intake of nutrients and excludes alcohol from diet.
NURSING DIAGNOSIS: Altered body temperature: hyperthermia related to inflammatory process of cirrhosis		
GOAL: Maintenance of normal body temperature		
1. Record temperature regularly.	1. Provides baseline to detect fever and to evaluate interventions.	• Reports normal temperature and absence of chills or sweating.
2. Encourage fluid intake.	2. Corrects fluid loss from perspiration and fever and increases patient's level of comfort.	• Demonstrates adequate intake of fluids.
3. Apply cool sponges or icebag for elevated temperature.	3. Promotes reduction of fever by conduction and evaporation and increases patient's comfort.	
4. Administer antibiotics as prescribed.	4. Promotes appropriate serum concentration of antibiotics to treat infection.	
5. Avoid exposure to infections.	5. Minimizes risk of further infection and further increases in body temperature and metabolic rate.	
6. Keep patient at rest while temperature is elevated.	6. Reduces metabolic rate.	
NURSING DIAGNOSIS: Impaired skin integrity related to edema formation		
GOAL: Improve skin integrity and protection of edematous tissue		
1. Restrict sodium as prescribed.	1. Minimizes edema formation.	• Exhibits normal turgor of skin of extremities and trunk.
2. Give careful attention and care to the skin.	2. Edematous skin and tissue has compromised nutrient supply and is very vulnerable to pressure and trauma.	• Exhibits absence of skin breakdown. • Exhibits normal tissue without evidence of redness, discoloration, or increased warmth over bony prominences.
3. Turn and change position of patient frequently.	3. Minimizes prolonged pressure and promotes mobilization of edema.	• Changes position frequently.
4. Weigh patient daily and record intake and output.	4. Permits best estimate of fluid status and monitoring of fluid retention and loss from tissues.	
5. Carry out passive range of motion exercises; elevate edematous extremities.	5. Promotes mobilization of edema.	
6. Provide small foam, rubber supports under heels, malleoli, and other bony prominences.	6. Protects bony prominences and minimizes trauma *if used correctly.*	

(*continued*)

NURSING CARE PLAN 38–2 *(continued)*
Care of the Patient With Cirrhosis

NURSING DIAGNOSIS: Impaired skin integrity related to jaundice and compromised immunologic status

GOAL: Improved skin integrity and minimization of skin irritation

Nursing Interventions	Rationale	Expected Outcomes
1. Note and record degree of jaundice of skin and sclerae.	1. Provides baseline for detecting changes and evaluating interventions.	• Exhibits intact skin without evidence of breakdown or infection.
2. Provide frequent skin care, bathing without soap, and massage with emollient lotions.	2. Prevents dryness of skin and minimizes pruritus.	• Reports absence of pruritus. • Demonstrates decreasing jaundice of skin and sclerae.
3. Keep patient's fingernails short.	3. Prevents skin excoriation from scratching.	• Uses emollients and avoids soaps in daily hygiene.

NURSING DIAGNOSIS: Altered nutrition, less than body requirements, related to anorexia and gastrointestinal disturbances

GOAL: Improved nutritional status

Nursing Interventions	Rationale	Expected Outcomes
1. Encourage patient to eat meals and supplementary feedings.	1. Encouragement is essential for the patient with anorexia and gastrointestinal discomfort.	• Demonstrates intake of sufficient high-protein, high-calorie meals. • Identifies foods and fluids that are nutritious and permitted on diet.
2. Offer frequent, small feedings.	2. Small meals are frequently easier for the anorexic patient to tolerate.	• Gains weight without increased edema or ascites formation.
3. Provide attractive meals and an aesthetically pleasing setting at meal time.	3. Promotes appetite and sense of well-being.	• Identifies the rationale for small, frequent meals.
4. Eliminate alcohol.	4. Eliminates "empty calories" and avoids the gastric irritation produced by alcohol.	• Reports increased appetite and well-being.
5. Provide oral hygiene before meals.	5. Reduces unpleasant taste and stimulates appetite.	• Excludes alcohol from diet. • Participates in oral hygiene measures before meals and to counteract nausea.
6. Apply an ice collar for nausea.	6. May reduce incidence of nausea.	
7. Administer medications prescribed for nausea, vomiting, diarrhea, or constipation.	7. Reduces gastrointestinal symptoms and discomforts that decrease the appetite and interest in food.	• Takes medications for gastrointestinal disorders as prescribed. • Reports normal gastrointestinal function with regular bowel function.
8. Encourage increased fluid intake and exercise if the patient reports constipation.	8. Promotes normal bowel pattern and reduces abdominal discomfort and distention.	• Identifies reportable symptoms of abnormal gastrointestinal function: melena, gross bleeding.
9. Observe for evidence of gastrointestinal bleeding.	9. Detects serious gastrointestinal complications.	

NURSING DIAGNOSIS: Risk for injury related to portal hypertension, altered clotting mechanisms, and impaired detoxification of drugs

GOAL: Decreased risk of injury

Nursing Interventions	Rationale	Expected Outcomes
1. Observe each stool for color, consistency, and amount.	1. Permits detection of bleeding in gastrointestinal tract.	• Exhibits absence of frank bleeding from gastrointestinal tract.
2. Be alert for symptoms of anxiety, epigastric fullness, weakness, and restlessness.	2. May indicate early signs of bleeding and shock.	• Exhibits absence of restlessness, epigastric fullness, and other indicators of hemorrhage and shock.
3. Test each stool and emesis for occult blood.	3. Detects early evidence of bleeding.	• Exhibits negative results of test for occult gastrointestinal bleeding.
4. Observe for hemorrhagic manifestations: ecchymosis, epistaxis, petechiae, and bleeding gums.	4. Indicates altered clotting mechanisms.	• Is free of ecchymotic areas or hematoma formation. • Exhibits normal vital signs.

(continued)

NURSING CARE PLAN 38–2 *(continued)*
Care of the Patient With Cirrhosis

Nursing Interventions	Rationale	Expected Outcomes
5. Record vital signs at frequent intervals.	5. Provides baseline and evidence of hypovolemia, shock.	• Maintains rest and remains quiet if active bleeding occurs.
6. Keep patient quiet and limit activity.	6. Minimizes risk of bleeding and straining.	• Identifies rationale for blood transfusions and measures to treat bleeding.
7. Assist physician in passage of tube for esophageal balloon tamponade.	7. Promote nontraumatic insertion of tube in anxious and combative patient for immediate treatment of bleeding.	• Uses measures to prevent trauma (*e.g.,* uses soft toothbrush, blows nose gently, avoids bumps and falls, avoids straining during defecation).
8. Observe during blood transfusions.	8. Permits detection of transfusion reactions (risk is increased with multiple blood transfusions needed for active bleeding from esophageal varices).	• Experiences no side effects of medications.
9. Measure and record nature, time, and amount of vomitus.	9. Assists in evaluating extent of bleeding and blood loss.	• Takes all medications as prescribed. • Identifies rationale for precautions with use of all medications.
10. Maintain patient in fasting state, if indicated.	10. Reduces risk of aspiration of gastric contents and minimizes risk of further trauma to esophagus and stomach by preventing vomiting.	
11. Administer vitamin K as prescribed.	11. Promotes clotting by providing fat-soluble vitamin necessary for clotting mechanism.	
12. Stay in constant attendance during episodes of bleeding.	12. Reassures anxious patient and permits monitoring and detection of further needs of the patient.	
13. Offer cold liquids by mouth when bleeding stops (if prescribed).	13. Minimizes risk of further bleeding by promoting vasoconstriction of esophageal and gastric blood vessels.	
14. Institute measures to prevent trauma:	14. Promotes safety of patient.	
a. Maintain safe environment.	a. Minimizes risk of trauma and bleeding by avoiding falls and cuts, etc.	
b. Encourage *gentle* blowing of nose.	b. Reduces risk of nosebleed (epistaxis) secondary to trauma and decreased clotting.	
c. Provide soft toothbrush and avoid use of toothpicks.	c. Prevents trauma to oral mucosa while promoting good oral hygiene.	
d. Encourage intake of foods with high content of vitamin C.	d. Promotes healing.	
e. Apply cold compresses where indicated.	e. Minimizes bleeding into tissues by promoting local vasoconstriction.	
f. Record location of bleeding sites.	f. Permits detection of new bleeding sites and monitoring of previous sites of bleeding.	
g. Use small-gauge needles for injections.	g. Minimizes oozing and blood loss from repeated injections.	
15. Administer medications carefully; monitor for side effects.	15. Reduces risk of side effects secondary to damaged liver's inability to detoxify (metabolize) drugs and medications normally.	

NURSING DIAGNOSIS: Pain and discomfort related to enlarged tender liver and ascites

GOAL: Increased level of comfort

1. Maintain bed rest when patient experiences abdominal discomfort.	1. Reduces metabolic demands and protects the liver.	• Maintains bed rest and decreases activity in presence of pain.

(continued)

NURSING CARE PLAN 38–2 *(continued)*
Care of the Patient With Cirrhosis

Nursing Interventions	Rationale	Expected Outcomes
2. Administer antispasmodics and sedatives as prescribed.	2. Reduces irritability of the gastrointestinal tract and decreases abdominal pain and discomfort.	• Takes antispasmodices and sedatives as indicated and as prescribed. • Reports decreased pain and abdominal discomfort.
3. Observe, record, and report presence and character of pain and discomfort.	3. Provides baseline to detect further deterioration of status and to evaluate interventions.	• Reports pain and discomfort if present. • Reduces sodium and fluid intake to prescribed levels if indicated to treat ascites.
4. Reduce sodium and fluid intake if prescribed.	4. Minimizes further formation of ascites.	• Obtains pain relief. • Exhibits decreased abdominal girth and appropriate weight changes.
NURSING DIAGNOSIS: Fluid volume excess related to ascites and edema formation		
GOAL: Restoration of normal fluid volume		
1. Restrict sodium and fluid intake if prescribed.	1. Minimizes formation of ascites and edema.	• Consumes diet low in sodium and within prescribed fluid restriction.
2. Administer diuretics, potassium, and protein supplements as prescribed.	2. Promotes excretion of fluid through the kidneys and maintenance of normal fluid and electrolyte balance.	• Takes diuretics, potassium, and protein supplements as indicated without experiencing side effects.
3. Record intake and output.	3. Assesses effectiveness of treatment and adequacy of fluid intake.	• Exhibits increased urine output. • Exhibits decreasing abdominal girth.
4. Measure and record abdominal girth daily.	4. Monitors changes in ascites formation and accumulation.	• Identifies rationale for sodium and fluid restriction.
5. Explain rationale for sodium and fluid restriction.	5. Promotes patient's understanding of restriction and cooperation with it.	
NURSING DIAGNOSIS: Altered thought processes related to deterioration of liver function and increased serum ammonia level		
GOAL: Improved mental status		
1. Restrict dietary protein as prescribed.	1. Reduces source of ammonia (protein foods).	• Demonstrates improved mental status: • Exhibits serum ammonia level within normal limits.
2. Give frequent, small feedings of carbohydrates.	2. Promotes adequate carbohydrate for energy requirements and "spares" protein from breakdown for energy.	• Is oriented to time, place, and person. • Reports normal sleep patterns. • Demonstrates an interest in events and activities in environment.
3. Protect from infection.	3. Minimizes risk of further increase in metabolic requirements.	• Demonstrates normal attention span.
4. Keep environment warm and draft-free.	4. Minimizes shivering, which would increase metabolic requirements.	• Follows and participates in conversations appropriately.
5. Pad the side-rails of the bed.	5. Provides protection for the patient in the event that hepatic coma and seizure activity occur.	• Reports urinary and fecal continence. • Experiences no seizures.
6. Limit visitors.	6. Minimizes patient's activity and metabolic requirements.	
7. Provide careful nursing surveillance to ensure patient's safety.	7. Provides close monitoring of new symptoms and minimizes trauma to the confused patient.	

(continued)

NURSING CARE PLAN 38–2 *(continued)*
Care of the Patient With Cirrhosis

Nursing Interventions	Rationale	Expected Outcomes
8. Avoid opioids and barbiturates.	8. Prevents masking of symptoms of hepatic coma and prevents drug overdose secondary to reduced ability of the damaged liver to metabolize narcotics and barbiturates.	
9. Arouse at intervals.	9. Provides stimulation to the patient and opportunity for observing the patient's level of consciousness.	

NURSING DIAGNOSIS: Ineffective breathing pattern related to ascites and restriction of thoracic excursion secondary to ascites, abdominal distention, and fluid in the thoracic cavity

GOAL: Improved respiratory status

Nursing Interventions	Rationale	Expected Outcomes
1. Elevate head of bed.	1. Reduces abdominal pressure on the diaphragm and permits fuller thoracic excursion and lung expansion.	• Experiences improved respiratory status: • Reports decreased shortness of breath.
2. Conserve patient's strength.	2. Reduces patient metabolic and oxygen requirements.	• Reports increased strength and sense of well-being.
3. Change position at intervals.	3. Promotes expansion and oxygenation of all areas of the lungs.	• Exhibits normal respiratory rate (12–18/min) with no adventitious sounds.
4. Assist patient during paracentesis or thoracentesis.	4. Paracentesis and thoracentesis (performed to remove fluid from the thoracic cavity) may be frightening to the patient. Helps obtain patient's cooperation with the procedure, minimizing discomfort and risks.	• Exhibits full thoracic excursion without shallow respirations. • Exhibits normal blood gases. • Experiences absence of confusion or cyanosis.
a. Support and maintain position during procedure.		
b. Record both the amount and the character of fluid aspirated.	b. Provides record of fluid removed and indication of severity of limitation of lung expansion by fluid.	
c. Observe for evidence of coughing, increasing dyspnea, or pulse rate.	c. Indicates irritation of the pleural space and evidence of ventilatory function compromised by pneumothorax or hemothorax (air or blood accumulating in pleural space).	

COLLABORATIVE PROBLEM: Bleeding and hemorrhage

GOAL: Prevention of bleeding and hemorrhage; early detection of bleeding

Nursing Interventions	Rationale	Expected Outcomes
1. Assess patient for evidence of bleeding or hemorrhage a. Monitor vital signs (blood pressure, pulse, respiratory rate). b. Assess skin temperature, level of consciousness. c. Monitor gastrointestinal secretions and output (emesis, stool) for occult or obvious bleeding).	1. Allows early detection of signs and symptoms of bleeding and hemorrhage.	• Experiences no episodes of bleeding and hemorrhage. • Vital signs are within acceptable range for patient. • No evidence of bleeding from gastrointestinal tract. • No evidence of bruising and hematoma formation in subcutaneous tissue. • Urine output within acceptable limits.

(continued)

NURSING CARE PLAN 38–2 *(continued)*
Care of the Patient With Cirrhosis

Nursing Interventions	Rationale	Expected Outcomes
d. Monitor hematocrit and hemoglobin levels. e. Monitor skin for bruising and hematoma formation. f. Monitor urine intake and output.		• Hematocrit and hemoglobin levels within acceptable limits. • Patient turns and moves without straining and increasing intra-abdominal pressure.
2. Protect patient from falls and injury. a. Raise side rails to prevent falls. b. Pad side rails. c. Keep light on in patient's room. d. Remove unnecessary furniture and equipment from room. e. Replace sharp objects with safe items.	2. Minimizes risk of bleeding secondary to abnormalities of clotting, portal hypertension, and esophageal and gastric varices.	• No further bleeding episodes if aggressive treatment of bleeding and hemorrhage was needed. • Patient and family state rationale for treatments. • Patient and family identify supports available to them.
3. Avoid activities that require patient to strain, lift, or turn. a. Assist patient to turn. b. Keep all needed items within easy reach. c. Use measures to prevent constipation.	3. Minimizes increases in intra-abdominal pressure that could lead to rupture and bleeding of esophageal or gastric varices.	
4. Have Blakemore tube and medications available if indicated.	4. Tube and medications will be readily available if patient experiences bleeding from ruptured esophageal or gastric varices.	
5. Assist physician with insertion and maintenance of Blakemore tube if indicated.	5. Bleeding requiring esophageal tamponade or other emergency treatment to stem hemorrhage requires rapid and efficient response by entire health care team.	
6. Monitor respiratory status and minimize risk of respiratory complications if esophageal tamponade is needed.	6. The patient is at high risk of aspiration because of bleeding and asphyxiation if gastric balloon ruptures.	
7. Prepare patient physically and psychologically for other treatment modalities if needed.	7. The patient who experiences hemorrhage is very anxious and fearful; minimizing anxiety assists in control of hemorrhage.	
8. Keep family informed of patient's status.	8. Family members are likely to be anxious about the patient's status; providing information will reduce their anxiety level and promote more effective coping.	

COLLABORATIVE PROBLEM: Hepatic encephalopathy

GOAL: Prevention of hepatic encephalopathy

Nursing Interventions	Rationale	Expected Outcomes
1. Assess cognitive status at regular intervals: a. Determine patient's orientation to person, place, and time. b. Assess patient's awareness of reason for health care and/or hospitalization.	1. Data will provide baseline of patient's cognitive status and enable detection of changes.	• Awake, alert, and aware of surroundings. • Oriented to time, place, and person. • Exhibits no restlessness or agitation. • Record of handwriting demonstrates no deterioration in cognitive function. • States rationale for treatment used to prevent or treat hepatic encephalopathy.

(continued)

NURSING CARE PLAN 38–2 *(continued)*
Care of the Patient With Cirrhosis

Nursing Interventions	Rationale	Expected Outcomes
c. Observe patient's level of activity, restlessness, and agitation. d. Obtain and record daily sample of patient's handwriting. e. Assess neurologic signs (deep tendon reflexes, ability to follow instructions).		• Demonstrates stable serum ammonia level within acceptable limits. • Consumes adequate caloric intake and adheres to protein restriction. • Takes medications as prescribed.
2. Monitor medications to prevent administration of those that may precipitate hepatic encephalopathy (sedatives, hypnotics, analgesics).	2. Medications are a common precipitating factor in development of hepatic encephalopathy in patients at risk.	
3. Monitor laboratory data, especially serum ammonia level.	3. Increases in serum ammonia level are associated with hepatic encephalopathy and coma.	
4. Notify physician of changes in neurologic status and cognitive function.	4. Allows early initiation of treatment of hepatic encephalopathy and hepatic coma.	
5. Limits sources of protein from diet if indicated.	5. Reduces breakdown and conversion of protein to ammonia.	
6. Administer medications prescribed to reduce serum ammonia level (*e.g.,* lactulose, antibiotics, glucose).	6. Reduces serum ammonia level.	

Factors that contribute to hemorrhage are muscular exertion from lifting heavy objects; straining at stool; sneezing, coughing, or vomiting; esophagitis; or irritation of vessels by poorly chewed foods or irritating fluids. Salicylates and any medication that erodes esophageal mucosa or interferes with cell replication also may contribute to bleeding.

Diagnostic Evaluation

The patient's history and physical examination will assist in identifying the cause of the bleeding. Endoscopy is used to identify the bleeding site, along with barium swallow, ultrasound, CT scan, and angiography.

Endoscopy. Immediate endoscopy is indicated to identify the cause and the site of bleeding; at least 30% of patients suspected of bleeding from esophageal varices bleed from other sources (gastritis, ulcers).

Nursing support before and during endoscopic examination can be effective in relieving anxiety during this often stressful experience. Careful monitoring can detect early signs of cardiac dysrhythmias, perforation, and hemorrhage.

After the examination, fluids are not given until the patient's gag reflex returns. Lozenges and gargles may be used to relieve throat discomfort if the patient's physical condition and mental status permit. If the patient is actively bleeding, oral intake will not be permitted and the patient will be prepared for further diagnostic and therapeutic procedures.

Neurologic Assessment. Neurologic assessment will assist in identifying possible hepatic encephalopathy resulting from the breakdown of blood in the gastrointestinal tract and a rising serum ammonia level. Manifestations range from drowsiness to encephalopathy and coma.

Portal Hypertension Measurements. Portal hypertension may be suspected if dilated abdominal veins and rectal hemorrhoids are detected. A palpable enlarged spleen (splenomegaly) and ascites may also be present.

Portal venous pressure (PVP) can be measured directly or indirectly. *Indirect measurement* of the hepatic vein pressure gradient (HVPG) is the most commonly used procedure; it requires insertion of a fluid-filled balloon catheter into the antecubital or femoral vein. The catheter is advanced under fluoroscopy to a hepatic vein. A "wedged" pressure (similar to pulmonary artery wedge pressure) is obtained by occluding the blood flow in the blood vessel; pressure in the unoccluded vessel is also measured. Although the HVPG values obtained may underestimate portal pressure, this measurement may be obtained several times to evaluate the results of therapy.

Direct measurement of portal vein pressure can be obtained by several methods. One method is used when the patient is undergoing laparotomy by introducing a needle into the spleen; a manometer reading above 20 ml saline is abnormal. Another direct measurement requires insertion of a catheter into the portal vein or one of its branches. Endoscopic measurement of pressure within varices is used only in conjunction with endoscopic sclerotherapy (see page 998).

Laboratory Tests. Laboratory tests that may be required include various liver function tests, such as serum aminotransferase (transaminase), bilirubin, alkaline phosphatase, and serum proteins. Blood flow and clearance studies also may be performed to assess cardiac output and hepatic blood flow.

Splenoportography involves serial or segmental x-ray films to detect extensive collateral circulation in esophageal vessels, which would be indicative of varices. Other tests are hepatoportography and celiac angiography. These are usually performed in the operating room or radiology department.

Nursing Management

Overall nursing assessment includes monitoring the patient's physical condition and evaluating emotional responses and cognitive status. Vital signs are monitored and recorded, and the patient's nutritional status is assessed.

Bleeding anywhere in the body is anxiety provoking, resulting in a crisis situation for the patient and family. If the patient is an alcoholic, delirium secondary to alcohol withdrawal can further complicate the situation. The nurse provides support and pertinent explanations regarding medical and nursing interventions. Monitoring the patient closely will help in detecting and managing complications.

Management

Bleeding from esophageal varices can quickly lead to hemorrhagic shock and should be considered an emergency. See Chapter 15 for discussion of care of the patient in shock.

The patient with bleeding varices is critically ill, requiring aggressive medical care and expert nursing care. The patient is often transferred to the intensive care unit for close monitoring and management.

Assessment requires that the extent of bleeding be evaluated and vital signs monitored continuously when hematemesis and melena are present. Signs of potential hypovolemia are noted, such as cold, clammy skin; tachycardia; a drop in blood pressure; decreased urine output; restlessness; and increased or shallow peripheral pulses. Blood volume is monitored by means of a central venous pressure or arterial catheter. Oxygen is administered to prevent hypoxia and to maintain adequate blood oxygenation.

Because patients with bleeding esophageal varices are subject to electrolyte imbalance, intravenous fluids and volume expanders are provided to restore fluid volume and replace electrolytes. Transfusion of blood components also may be required. An indwelling urinary catheter is usually inserted to permit monitoring of intake and output.

A variety of pharmacologic, endoscopic, and surgical approaches are used to treat bleeding esophageal varices; however, none of them is ideal and most are associated with considerable risk to the patient.

Nonsurgical Management

Nonsurgical treatment of bleeding esophageal varices is preferable because of the high mortality of emergency surgery for control of bleeding esophageal varices and because of the poor physical condition of the patient with severe liver dysfunction.

Pharmacologic Therapy. *Vasopressin* (Pitressin) may be the initial mode of therapy because of its constriction of the splanchnic arterial bed and resulting decrease in portal pressure. It may be administered intravenously or by intra-arterial infusion. Either method requires close monitoring by the nurse. The presence or absence of blood in the gastric aspirate and vital signs offer indices of the effectiveness of vasopressin. Electrolyte evaluation and monitoring of fluid intake and output are necessary, as hyponatremia may occur and vasopressin may have an antidiuretic effect.

Coronary artery disease in this patient is a contraindication to the use of vasopressin, because coronary vasoconstriction is a side effect that may precipitate myocardial infarction.

The combination of vasopressin and nitroglycerin (administered by intravenous, sublingual, or transdermal routes) has been effective in reducing or preventing the side effects (constriction of coronary vessels and angina) caused by vasopressin alone.

Somatostatin has been reported to be more effective than vasopressin in decreasing bleeding from esophageal varices without the vasoconstrictive effects of vasopressin. *Propranolol*, a β-blocking agent that decreases portal pressure, has been shown to prevent bleeding from esophageal varices in some patients; however, it is recommended that it be used only in combination with other treatment modalities such as sclerotherapy or balloon tamponade. Further studies of these and other medications are necessary to evaluate their use in treatment and prevention of bleeding episodes.

Balloon Tamponade. To control the hemorrhage in certain patients, pressure is exerted on the cardia (upper orifice of the stomach) and against the bleeding varices by a double-balloon tamponade (Sengstaken–Blakemore tube) (Fig. 38-9). The tube has four openings, each with a specific purpose: gastric aspiration, esophageal aspiration, inflation of the gastric balloon, and inflation of the esophageal balloon.

The balloon in the stomach is inflated, and the tube is pulled gently to exert a force against the cardia. Irrigation of the tubing is performed to detect bleeding; if returns are clear, the esophageal balloon is not inflated. If bleeding continues, the esophageal balloon is inflated. The desired pressure in both balloons is 25 to 30 mm Hg, as measured by the manometer. After the balloon is inflated, there is a possibility of injury or rupture of the esophagus. Constant nursing surveillance is necessary at this time. Traction may be placed on the tube. A chest x-ray is obtained to confirm the correct position of the tube and balloons.

A cathartic such as magnesium sulfate may be administered through the tube to eliminate blood in the gastrointestinal tract; otherwise, ammonia absorption could occur, which may lead to hepatic coma and death. Thereafter, neomycin is administered to reduce intestinal bacterial flora, which are a source of ammonia-forming enzymes.

Gastric suction is provided by connecting the proper catheter outlet to suction. The tubing is irrigated hourly, and drainage will indicate whether bleeding has been controlled. Iced saline lavage or irrigation may be used in the gastric balloon to constrict the gastric vessels. In such instances, the nurse anticipates possible chilling of the patient and provides comfort measures. The pressures on the tubes and traction are released periodically, as prescribed. Bal-

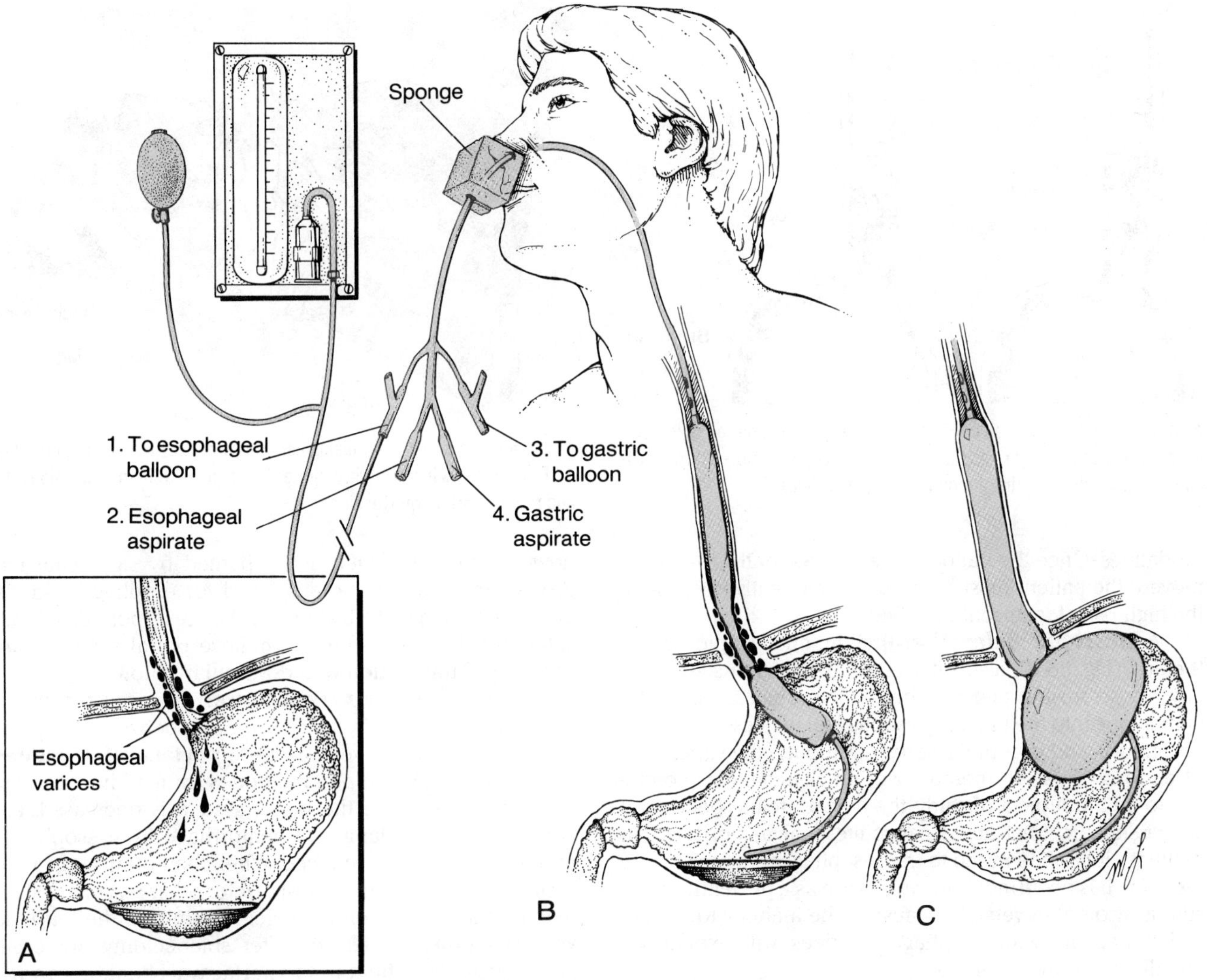

FIGURE 38-9. Esophageal balloon tamponade to treat esophageal varices. **(A)** Dilated, bleeding esophageal veins (varices) of the lower esophagus. **(B)** A four-lumen esophageal tamponade tube with balloons (uninflated) in place. **(C)** Compression of bleeding esophageal varices by inflated esophageal and gastric balloons. The gastric and esophageal outlets permit aspiration of secrettions.

loon tamponade is continued for several days and then cautiously released, followed by removal of the tube if no bleeding recurs.

Potential Complications. Although balloon tamponade has been fairly successful, it is important to note some inherent dangers. *Ulceration and necrosis* of the mucosa of the stomach or esophagus may occur if the tube is left in place or inflated too long or at too high a pressure. *Sudden rupture of the balloon* is disastrous—airway obstruction and aspiration of gastric contents into the lungs can occur. Using a new, tested tube may minimize this risk. *Asphyxiation* is another problem, caused by accidental pulling of the tube and inflated balloon into the oropharynx.

Aspiration of blood and secretions into the patient's lungs is frequently associated with the use of balloon tamponade, especially in the stuporous or comatose patient. Endotracheal intubation before insertion of the tube protects the airway and minimizes the risk of aspiration.

Nursing Measures. These potential complications necessitate intensive and expert care. A confused or restless patient with this tube in place and balloons inflated should not be left alone because of these risks.

The balloon may be deflated at intervals if prescribed to prevent erosion and necrosis of the mucosa of the stomach and esophagus and to determine if bleeding has ceased.

Nursing measures also include frequent mouth and nasal care. For secretions that accumulate in the mouth, tissues should be within easy reach of the patient. Oral suction may be necessary to remove oral secretions. The patient who has experienced esophageal hemorrhage is usually extremely anxious and frightened. Knowing that the nurse is nearby and will respond immediately can help alleviate some of this anxiety. The experience of having the tube inserted is uncomfortable and never pleasant. Explanations during the procedure and while the tube is in place may be reassuring to the patient.

Although use of balloon tamponade effectively stops the bleeding in most patients (90%), bleeding recurs in the majority of patients, necessitating other treatment

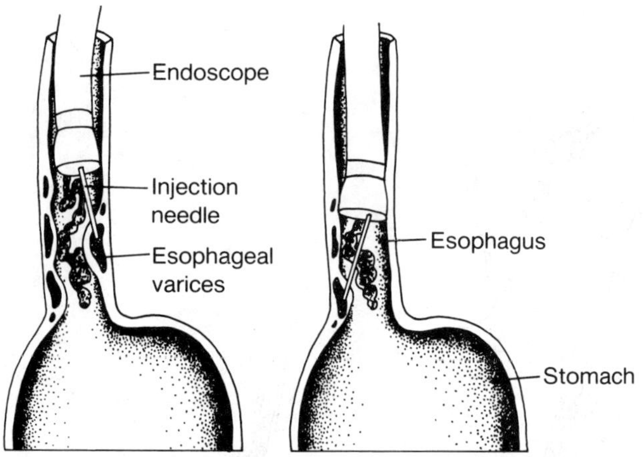

FIGURE 38-10. Injection sclerotherapy. Injection of sclerosing agent into esophageal varices through an endoscope promotes thrombosis and eventual sclerosis, thereby obliterating the varices.

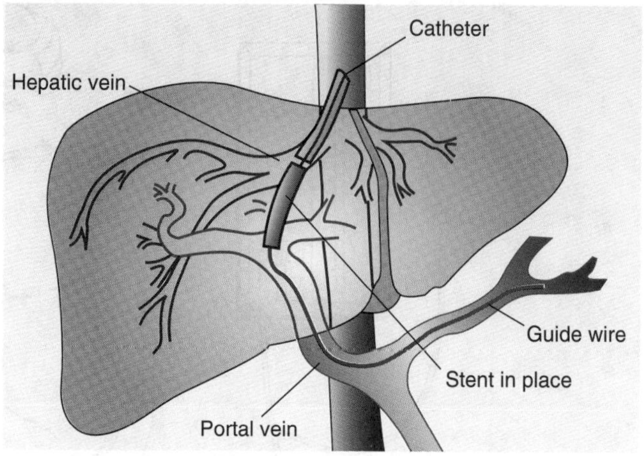

FIGURE 38-11. Transjugular intrahepatic portosystemic shunt (TIPS). A stent is inserted via catheter to the portal vein to divert blood flow and reduce portal hypertension.

modalities. Once the balloons are deflated or the tube is removed, the patient must be assessed frequently because of the high risk of recurrent bleeding.

Endoscopic Sclerotherapy. In endoscopic sclerotherapy (Fig. 38-10; also referred to as injection sclerotherapy), a sclerosing agent is injected through a fiberoptic endoscope into the bleeding esophageal varices to promote thrombosis and eventual sclerosis. Although the superiority of endoscopic sclerotherapy over other treatments continues to be the subject of study, the procedure has been used successfully to treat acute gastrointestinal hemorrhage. In addition, it has been used to treat esophageal varices before bleeding has occurred; however, its use as a preventive measure is also controversial because of the inability to predict which patients with esophageal varices will experience bleeding and which will not.

After treatment, the patient must be observed for bleeding, perforation of the esophagus, aspiration pneumonia, and esophageal stricture. Antacids may be administered after the procedure to counteract the effects of peptic reflux.

Repeated courses of sclerotherapy may be needed to obliterate all the varices. The patient and family need to be aware of the importance of these additional treatments and continued long-term follow-up, even though the patient may not be actively bleeding.

Transjugular Intrahepatic Portosystemic Shunting. Transjugular intrahepatic portosystemic shunting (TIPS) is a method of treatment for esophageal varices in which a cannula is threaded into the portal vein by the transjugular route. An expandable stent is inserted and serves as an intrahepatic shunt between the portal circulation and the hepatic vein (Fig. 38-11), thereby reducing portal hypertension. Because results of studies of the effectiveness of TIPS are inconclusive, this approach is generally reserved for situations in which other approaches are unavailable or unsuccessful.

Surgical Management

Several surgical procedures have been developed and used to treat esophageal varices and to minimize rebleeding; however, they are often accompanied by significant risk. Procedures that may be employed for esophageal varices are direct surgical ligation of varices, portacaval and splenorenal venous shunts to relieve portal pressure, and esophageal transection with devascularization.

Surgical Bypass Procedures. The most common procedure is to create an anastomosis between the portal vein and the inferior vena cava—a **portacaval anastomosis** (Fig. 38-12). When portal blood is shunted into the vena cava, the pressure in the portal system is decreased, and consequently the danger of hemorrhage from esophageal and gastric varices is reduced. When the portal vein cannot be used because of thrombosis, or for other reasons, a shunt may be made between the splenic vein and the left renal vein (**splenorenal shunt**) after splenectomy. Some surgeons prefer this shunt to the portacaval shunt, even when the portal vein can be used.

A **mesocaval** shunt is a third type of bypass procedure, in which the inferior vena cava is severed and the proximal end of the vena cava is anastomosed to the side of the superior mesenteric vein.

These procedures are extensive and are not always successful because of secondary clotting in the veins used for the shunt. Nevertheless, a shunt results in a lowering of pressure in the portal system. Because hemorrhages from the esophageal varices are often fatal, many of these relatively poor-risk patients must be subjected to these attempts to save their lives.

Devascularization and Transection. Devascularization and staple-gun transection procedures to separate the bleeding site from the high-pressure portal system have been used in emergency management of variceal bleeding. The lower end of the esophagus is reached through a small gastrostomy incision; a staple gun permits anastomosis of the transected ends of the esophagus. Rebleeding is a risk and outcomes of these procedures vary among patient populations.

Postoperative Nursing Interventions. Postoperative care is similar to that for any abdominal surgery, but the risk for complications is high, including hypovolemic or hemorrhagic shock, hepatic encephalopathy, electrolyte im-

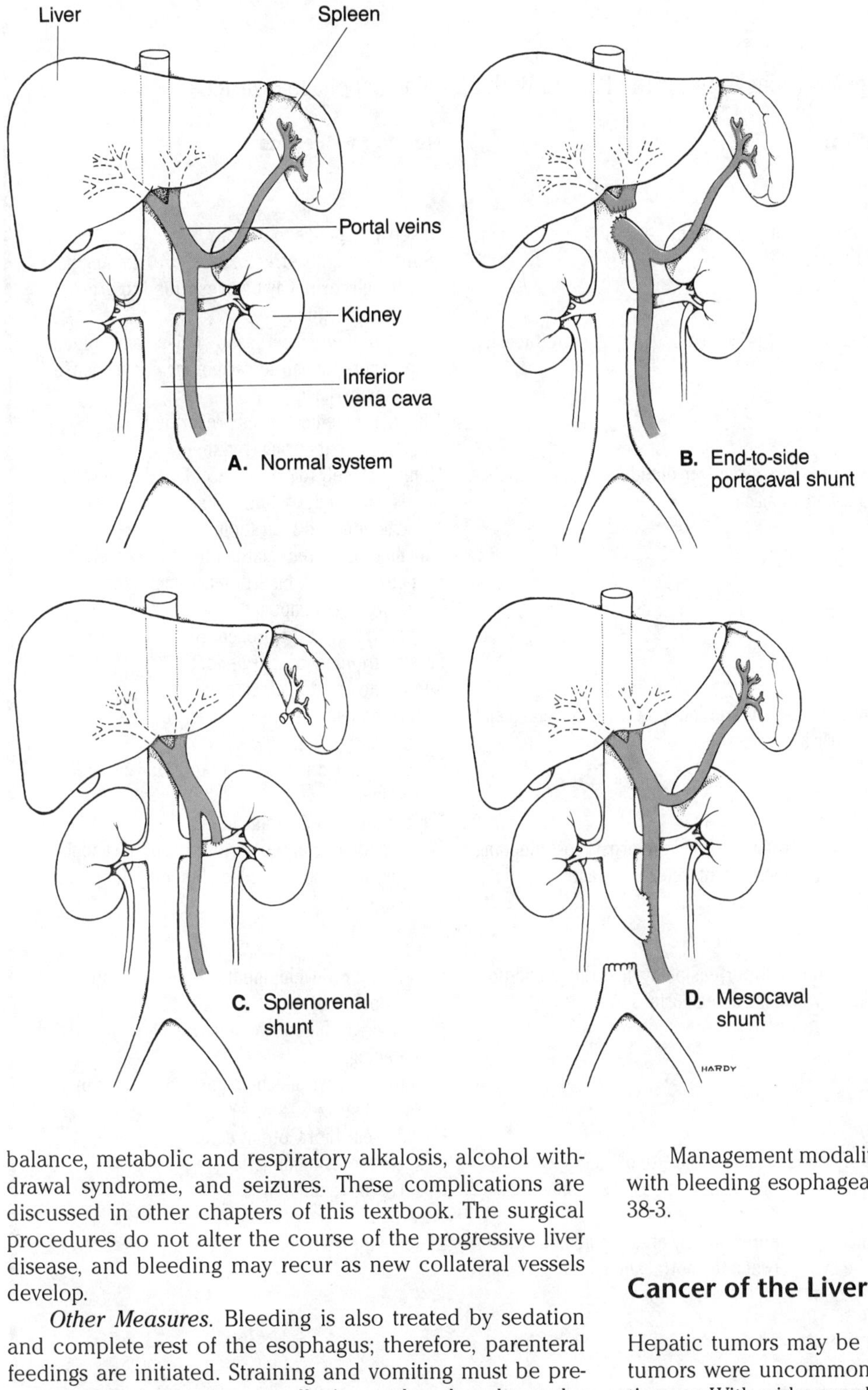

FIGURE 38-12. Portal systemic shunts. Normal portal system is shown in **A**; examples of portal shunts to reduce portal pressure are shown in **B** to **D**.

balance, metabolic and respiratory alkalosis, alcohol withdrawal syndrome, and seizures. These complications are discussed in other chapters of this textbook. The surgical procedures do not alter the course of the progressive liver disease, and bleeding may recur as new collateral vessels develop.

Other Measures. Bleeding is also treated by sedation and complete rest of the esophagus; therefore, parenteral feedings are initiated. Straining and vomiting must be prevented. Gastric suction usually is employed to keep the stomach as empty as possible. The patient often complains of severe thirst, which may be relieved by frequent oral hygiene and moist sponges to the lips. The nurse keeps close surveillance on the patient's blood pressure. Vitamin K therapy and multiple blood transfusions often are indicated because of blood loss. A quiet environment and calm reassurance will help to relieve the patient's anxiety and reduce agitation.

Management modalities and nursing care of the patient with bleeding esophageal varices are summarized in Chart 38-3.

Cancer of the Liver

Hepatic tumors may be malignant or benign. Benign liver tumors were uncommon until widespread oral contraceptive use. With widespread use of oral contraceptives, benign tumors of the liver occur most frequently in women in their reproductive years.

Primary Tumors. As for cancerous tumors, few cancers originate in the liver. Those that are primary liver tumors usually occur in patients with chronic liver disease, most frequently with cirrhosis. **Hepatocellular carcinoma** (HCC) is by far the most common type of primary liver cancer. HCC is usually nonresectable because of rapid

CHART 38-3
Management Modalities and Nursing Care for the Patient With Bleeding Esophageal Varices

Treatment Modality*	Action	Nursing Priorities
Nonsurgical Modalities		
Pharmacologic agents		
Vasopressin (Pitressin)	Reduces portal pressure by constricting splanchnic arteries	Observe response to therapy. Monitor for side-effects. (*Vasopressin:* angina. Nitroglycerin may be prescribed to prevent or treat angina.
Propranolol (Inderal)	Reduces portal pressure by β-adrenergic blocking action	*Propranolol:* decreased pulse and blood pressure, impaired cardiovascular response to hemorrhage.)
Somatostatin		Administer medication as prescribed. Support patient during treatment.
Balloon tamponade	Exerts pressure directly to bleeding sites in esophagus and stomach	Monitor closely to prevent accidental removal or displacement of tube, subsequent airway obstruction, and aspiration. Explain procedure to patient briefly to obtain cooperation with insertion and maintenance of esophageal-tamponade tube and reduce patient's fear of the procedure. Provide frequent oral hygiene. Report the onset of chest pain.
Iced saline lavage	Produces vasoconstriction of the esophageal and gastric blood vessels	Ensure patency of the nasogastric tube to prevent aspiration. Observe gastric aspirate for blood and cessation of bleeding. Protect the patient from chilling.
Injection sclerotherapy	Promotes thrombosis and sclerosis of bleeding sites by injection of sclerosing agent into the esophageal varices	Observe for aspiration, perforation of the esophagus, and recurrence of bleeding following treatment.
Surgical Modalities		
Portal-systemic shunts	Reduces portal hypertension by diverting blood flow away from obstructed portal system	Observe for development of portal systemic encephalopathy (altered mental status, neurologic dysfunction), hepatic failure, and rebleeding. Requires intensive, expert nursing care for prolonged period. Provide post-thoracotomy care.
Surgical ligation of varices	Ties off blood vessels at the site of bleeding	Observe for rebleeding.
Esophageal transection and devascularization	Separates bleeding site from portal system	Observe for rebleeding.
Transjugular intrahepatic portosystemic shunts (TIPS)	Reduces portal pressure by creating a shunt within the liver between the portal and systemic venous system	Observe for rebleeding.

*Several modalities may be used concurrently or in sequence.

growth and metastasis elsewhere. Other types of primary liver cancer include **cholangiocellular carcinoma** (CCC) and combined hepatocellular and cholangiocellular carcinoma. If found early, resection may be possible, but the likelihood of early detection is small.

Causes. Cirrhosis, hepatitis B and C, and exposure to certain chemical toxins (*e.g.*, vinyl chloride, arsenic) have been implicated in the etiology of HCC. Cigarette smoking has also been identified as a risk factor, especially when combined with alcohol use. Other substances that have been implicated include aflatoxins or carcinogens in herbal medicines, and nitrosamines.

Metastases. Metastases from other primary sites are found in the liver in about one half of all advanced cancer cases. Malignant tumors are likely to reach the liver eventually by way of the portal system or lymphatic channels, or by direct extension from an abdominal tumor. Moreover, the liver apparently is an ideal place for these malignant cells to thrive. Often the first evidence of cancer in an abdominal organ is the appearance of liver metastases, and, unless exploratory surgery or autopsy is performed, the primary tumor may never be identified.

Clinical Manifestations

The early manifestations of malignancy of the liver include signs and symptoms of impaired nutrition: recent loss of weight, loss of strength, anorexia, and anemia. Abdominal pain may be present and accompanied by rapid enlargement of the liver and an irregular surface upon palpation. Jaundice is present only if the larger bile ducts are occluded by the pressure of malignant nodules in the hilum of the liver. Ascites occurs if such nodules obstruct the portal veins or if tumor tissue is seeded in the peritoneal cavity.

Diagnostic Evaluation

The diagnosis of cancer of the liver is made on the basis of clinical signs and symptoms, history and physical examination, and results of laboratory and x-ray studies. Increased serum levels of bilirubin, alkaline phosphatase, aspartate aminotransferase (AST; glutamic oxalocetic transaminase [SGOT]), and lactic dehydrogenase (LDH) may occur. Leukocytosis (increased white blood cells), erythrocytosis (increased red blood cells), hypercalcemia, hypoglycemia, and hypocholesterolemia may also be seen on laboratory assessment. The serum level of alpha fetoprotein (AFP), which serves as a tumor marker, is abnormally elevated in 30% to 40% of patients with liver cancer. Carcinoembryonic antigen (CEA), which serves as a marker of advanced cancer of the digestive tract, may be elevated. CEA and AFP together are useful to distinguish between metastatic liver disease and primary liver cancer.

Many patients have metastases from the primary liver tumor to other sites by the time diagnosis is made; metastases occur primarily to the lung, but may also occur to regional lymph nodes, adrenals, bone, kidneys, heart, pancreas, and stomach.

X-rays, liver scans, CT scans, ultrasounds, MRI, and laparoscopy may be part of the diagnostic workup and may be performed to determine the extent of the cancer.

Nonsurgical Management

Although surgical resection of the liver tumor is possible in some patients, the underlying cirrhosis so prevalent in cancer of the liver increases the risks associated with surgery. Radiation therapy and chemotherapy have been used in the treatment of malignant disease of the liver with varying degrees of success. Although these therapies may prolong survival and improve the patient's quality of life by reducing pain and discomfort, the major effect remains palliative.

Radiation Therapy. Pain and discomfort have been effectively reduced in 70% to 90% of patients with radiation therapy; anorexia, weakness, and fever also have been reduced. Liver function tests may improve temporarily. Methods of delivering radiation include (1) intravenous injection of antibodies that are tagged with radioactive isotopes and specifically attack tumor-associated antigens and (2) percutaneous placement of a high-intensity source for interstitial radiation therapy. Their purpose is to deliver radiation directly to the tumor cells. External radiation therapy combined with chemotherapy has also been attempted, with no additional benefit demonstrated.

Chemotherapy. Chemotherapy has been used to improve the patient's quality of life and prolong survival; it also may be used as adjuvant therapy after surgical resection of hepatic tumors. Systemic chemotherapy and regional infusion chemotherapy are two methods used to administer antineoplastic agents to patients with primary and metastatic hepatic tumors.

An implantable pump has been used to deliver a high concentration of chemotherapy to the liver through the hepatic artery. This method provides a reliable, controlled, and continuous infusion of medication that can be carried out in the patient's home.

Patient Education and Home Care Considerations. The patient and family are instructed about the management strategies and their role in implementing them. They are instructed to assess and report complications and side effects of the chemotherapy that may be used. Therefore, they need to be well informed about its actions and desired and undesirable effects. They are instructed by the nurse about the importance of follow-up visits to permit frequent assessments of the response of the patient and the tumor to chemotherapy, the condition of the site of the pump insertion, and the occurrence of toxic effects. The patient is encouraged to resume routine activities as soon as possible, but warned to avoid activities that may damage the pump.

Because of the poor prognosis associated with liver cancer, the home care nurse serves a vital role in assisting the patient and family to cope with the symptoms that may occur and the prognosis. The home care nurse collaborates with the other members of the health care team, the patient, and family to identify and implement pain-management strategies and approaches to management of other problems that may occur: weakness, pruritus, inadequate dietary intake, jaundice, and symptoms associated with metastasis to other sites. The home care nurse also assists the patient and family in decision making about hospice care and assists with initiation of referrals.

Percutaneous Biliary Drainage. Percutaneous biliary or transhepatic drainage is used to bypass biliary ducts obstructed by liver, pancreatic, or bile duct tumors in patients with inoperable tumors or in those considered poor surgical risks. Under fluoroscopy, a catheter is inserted through the abdominal wall, past the obstruction into the duodenum. Such procedures are used to reestablish biliary drainage, relieve pressure and pain from buildup of bile behind the obstruction, and decrease pruritus and jaundice. As a result, the patient is made more comfortable and quality of life and survival are improved. For several days after its insertion, the catheter is opened to external drainage. The bile is observed closely for amount, color, and the presence of blood and debris.

Complications of percutaneous biliary drainage include sepsis, leakage of bile, hemorrhage, and reobstruction of the biliary system by debris in the catheter or from encroaching tumor. Therefore, the patient is observed for fever and chills, bile drainage around the catheter, changes in vital signs, and evidence of biliary obstruction, including increased pain or pressure, pruritus, and recurrence of jaundice.

Patient Education and Home Care Considerations. The patient being managed at home with a biliary drainage system in place and the family often fear that the catheter will be dislodged. They need reassurance and instruction to reduce their fear that the catheter will fall out easily. Additionally, the patient and family require instruction on catheter care. They are instructed in techniques to keep the catheter site clean and dry and to assess the catheter and its insertion site. Irrigation of the catheter with sterile normal saline or water may be prescribed to keep the catheter patent and free of debris. The patient and caregivers are taught proper technique to avoid introducing bacteria into the biliary system or catheter during irrigation. They are instructed not to aspirate or draw back on the syringe during irrigation to prevent entry of irritating duodenal contents into the biliary tree or catheter. The patient and caregivers are also instructed about the signs of complications and are encouraged to notify the nurse or physician if problems or questions occur.

Other Nonsurgical Treatment Modalities. **Hyperthermia** has been used as a treatment modality for hepatic metastases. Heat has been directed to tumors through several methods to cause necrosis of the tumors while sparing normal tissue. Freezing hepatic tumor cells by **cryosurgery** and use of **laser surgery** are in the early stages of development as treatment modalities. **Embolization** to interrupt the arterial blood flow to the tumor by inserting Gelfoam particles into the artery supplying the tumor has been effective in patients with small tumors. **Immunotherapy** is another treatment modality under investigation. In this therapy, lymphocytes with antitumor reactivity are administered to the patient with a hepatic tumor. Regression of the tumor, the desired outcome, has been demonstrated in patients with metastatic cancer in whom standard treatment has failed. These newer modes of therapy require further study before their benefits and side effects are known.

Surgical Management

Successful hepatic lobectomy for cancer can be performed when the primary hepatic tumor is localized or when, in the case of metastasis, the primary site can be completely excised and the metastasis is limited. Metastases to the liver, however, are rarely limited or solitary. Capitalizing on the regenerative capacity of the liver cells, some surgeons have successfully removed 90% of the liver. However, the presence of cirrhosis limits the ability of the liver to regenerate.

Preoperative Evaluation and Preparation. In preparation for surgery, the patient's nutritional, fluid, and general physical status is assessed and efforts are undertaken to assure as optimal a physical condition as possible. Support, explanation, and encouragement are provided to help the patient prepare psychologically for the surgery.

Meanwhile, extensive and exhausting diagnostic studies may be performed. It may be necessary to prepare the intestinal tract by way of cathartics, colonic irrigation, and intestinal antibiotics to minimize the possibility of ammonium accumulation and to anticipate the possibility of incision into the intestines at surgery. Specific studies may include liver scan, liver biopsy, cholangiography, selective hepatic angiography, percutaneous needle biopsy, peritoneoscopy, laparoscopy, ultrasound, CT scans, MRI, and blood tests, particularly determinations of serum alkaline phosphatase and AST (SGOT).

Staging of liver tumors aids in predicting the likelihood of surgical cure. The TNM staging system for liver tumors is summarized in Table 38-4.

Surgical Intervention. If it is necessary to restrict blood flow from the hepatic artery and portal vein beyond 15 minutes, it is likely that hypothermia will be used. Most surgeons prefer the anatomic (surgical) division of the lobes. Here the liver is divided into a right and a left lobe by a lobar fissure that is almost in line with the gallbladder bed and the inferior vena cava on the visceral surface. According to this division, the branching of hepatic vessels and the portal vein

TABLE 38-4 TNM Staging for Hepatoma

Stage I	T1	N0	M0
Stage II	T2	N0	M0
Stage III	T1	N1	M0
	T2	N1	M0
	T3	N0	M0
	T3	N1	M0
Stage IVA	T4	Any N	M0
Stage IVB	Any T	Any N	M1

T1 Solitary tumor 2 cm or less in greatest dimension without vascular invasion

T2 Solitary tumor 2 cm or less in greatest dimension with vascular invasion, *or*
Multiple tumors limited to one lobe none more than 2 cm in greatest dimension without vascular invasion, *or*
A solitary tumor more than 2 cm in greatest dimension without vascular invasion

T3 Solitary tumor more than 2 cm in greatest dimension with vascular invasion, *or*
Multiple tumors limited to one lobe, none more than 2 cm in greatest dimension, with vascular invasion, *or*
Multiple tumors limited to one lobe, any more than 2 cm in greatest dimension, with or without vascular invasion

T4 Multiple tumors in more than one lobe *or*
Tumor(s) involve(s) a major branch of portal or hepatic vein(s)

Lymph Node (N)

N0 No regional lymph node metastasis
N1 Regional lymph node metastasis

Distant Metastasis (M)

M0 No distant metastasis
M1 Distant metastasis

(From Beahrs OH et al [eds]. Manual for Staging of Cancer, 4th ed. Philadelphia, JB Lippincott, 1992.)

lend themselves to a more even segmentation. A right-liver lobectomy according to the surgical division is less extensive than it would be in the functional division.

For a right-liver lobectomy or an extended right lobectomy (including medial left lobe), a thoracoabdominal incision is used. An extensive abdominal incision is made for a left lobectomy.

Postoperative Nursing Interventions. There are potential problems related to cardiopulmonary involvement, vascular complications, and respiratory and liver dysfunction. Metabolic abnormalities require careful attention. A constant infusion of 10% glucose may be required in the first 48 hours to prevent a precipitous fall in blood sugar, resulting from decreased gluconeogenesis. Protein synthesis and lipid metabolism are also altered, necessitating infusions of albumin. Extensive blood loss may occur, and, as a result, the patient will receive infusions of blood and intravenous fluids.

The patient requires constant, close monitoring and care for the first 2 or 3 days, as described for abdominal and thoracic postsurgical nursing care (see Chapter 21). Early ambulation is encouraged. Liver regeneration is rapid; in one patient who had a 90% resection of the liver, a normal liver size was restored in 6 months.

Liver Transplantation to Treat Liver Tumors. Removal of the liver and its replacement by a healthy donor organ has been successful. Recurrence of the primary liver malignancy after transplantation, however, has been reported to be 80% to 85%. Therefore, it has been recommended that the patient be treated with systemic chemotherapy or radiation therapy along with liver transplantation.

Liver Transplantation

Liver transplantation involves total removal of the diseased liver and its replacement with a healthy liver. Removal of the patient's liver leaves a space for the new liver and permits anatomic reconstruction of the hepatic vasculature and biliary tract as close to normal as possible.

Liver transplantation is used to treat life-threatening, end-stage liver disease for which no other form of treatment is available. The success of liver transplantation depends on successful immunosuppression. Immunosuppressants currently in use include cyclosporine, corticosteroids, azathioprine, OKT3 (a monoclonal antibody), and FK506. Studies are underway to find the most effective combination of immunosuppressive agents.

Limitations. Despite the success of immunosuppression in reducing rejection of transplanted organs, liver transplantation is not a routine procedure and may be accompanied by complications related to the lengthy surgical procedure, immunosuppressive therapy, infection, and technical difficulties encountered in reconstruction of blood vessels and the biliary tract. Additionally, long-standing systemic problems resulting from the patient's primary liver disease may complicate the patient's preoperative and postoperative course. Previous surgery of the abdomen, including procedures to treat complications of advanced liver disease (*i.e.*, shunt procedures used to treat portal hypertension and esophageal varices), increase the complexity of the transplantation procedure.

Indications. The indications for liver transplantation are not as limited today as a result of the use of veno-venous bypass, advances in immunosuppressive therapy, and improvements in biliary tract reconstruction.

General indications for liver transplantation include irreversible advanced chronic liver disease, fulminant hepatic failure, metabolic liver diseases, and hepatic malignancies, where resection for cure requires complete removal of the liver. Examples of disorders that are indications for liver transplantation include hepatocellular liver disease (*e.g.*, viral hepatitis, medication- and alcohol-induced liver disease, and Wilson's disease) and cholestatic diseases (*i.e.*, primary biliary cirrhosis, sclerosis cholangitis, and biliary atresia).

The patient being considered for liver transplantation frequently has many systemic problems that influence preoperative and postoperative care. Because success of transplantation is more difficult when the patient has developed severe gastrointestinal bleeding and advanced hepatic coma, efforts are made to perform the procedure before this stage.

Liver transplantation is now recognized as an established therapeutic modality rather than as an experimental procedure to treat these disorders. As a result, centers where liver transplantation is performed are increasing. Patients requiring transplantation are often referred from distant hospitals to these sites. To prepare the potential patient and family for liver transplantation, nurses in all settings require an understanding of the process and the procedure of liver transplantation.

Psychosocial Considerations. The patient considering transplantation and the family have difficult decisions to make about treatment, use of financial resources, and relocating to another area to be closer to the medical center. Additionally, they have to deal with long-standing health problems and perhaps social and family problems associated with those behaviors that may be responsible for the patient's liver failure. Therefore, the time during which the patient and family are considering liver transplantation and awaiting the news that a liver is available is often very stressful.

The nurse must be aware of these issues and attuned to the emotional and psychologic status of the patient and family. Referral of the patient and family to a psychiatric liaison nurse, psychologist, psychiatrist, or clergy may be in order to help them deal with the stressors associated with chronic liver disease and liver transplantation.

Preoperative Nursing Interventions

Once irreversible, severe liver dysfunction has been diagnosed, the patient may be considered a potential candidate for transplantation. Extensive diagnostic evaluation will be carried out to determine if the patient is a suitable candidate for transplantation. The patient and family are given full explanations about the procedure and about the chances of success of transplantation and its risks, including the side effects of long-term immunosuppression. The need for close follow-up and lifelong compliance with the therapeutic regimen, including immunosuppression, is explained to the patient and family.

Once the patient is accepted as a suitable candidate for transplantation, the patient's name is placed on a waiting

ETHICAL QUESTION:

Should Patients with "Self-inflicted" Liver Disease Receive Liver Transplants?

Situation

Liver disease can develop as a result of drug and alcohol abuse. Should patients with so-called self-inflicted liver disease be considered for rare liver transplants? Should patients with idiopathic liver disease receive preference for organs over patients with self-inflicted disease?

Dilemma

The patient's desire for treatment of his disease conflicts with the obligation to distribute scarce resources in a fair manner (autonomy versus justice).

Discussion

- What arguments would you offer in support of the view that patients with self-inflicted liver disease *should* be considered for liver transplants?
- What arguments would you offer in support of the view that patients with self-inflicted liver disease *should not* be considered for liver transplants?

list at the transplant center; patient information is entered into the United Network Organ Sharing (UNOS) computer system so that candidates may be identified and matched when appropriate organs become available.

Because a liver becomes available for transplantation only with the death of another individual, usually healthy except for severe brain injury and brain death, the patient and family undergo a stressful waiting period. The nurse is often the major source of support for the patient and family during this period. The patient must be accessible at all times in case an appropriate liver becomes available. During this time, liver function may deteriorate further and the patient may experience other complications from the primary liver disease. Because of the current shortage of donor organs, patients sometimes die awaiting transplantation.

Malnutrition, massive ascites, and fluid and electrolyte disturbances are treated before surgery to increase the patient's chances of a successful outcome. If the patient's liver dysfunction has a very rapid onset, as in fulminant hepatic failure, there is little time or opportunity for the patient to consider and weigh options and their consequences; often this patient has developed coma, and the decision to proceed with transplantation is made by the patient's family.

The nurse coordinator is an integral member of the transplant team and plays an important role in preparing the patient for liver transplantation. The nurse serves as a patient and family advocate and assumes the important role of link between the patient and the other members of the transplant team. Additionally, the nurse serves as a resource to other nurses and health care team members involved in evaluating and caring for the patient undergoing this procedure.

Surgical Procedure

The donor liver is freed from other structures; the bile is flushed from the gallbladder to prevent damage to the walls of the biliary tract; and the liver is perfused with a preservative and cooled. Before the donor liver is placed in the recipient, it is flushed with cold lactated Ringer's solution to remove potassium and air bubbles.

Anastomoses of the blood vessels and bile duct between the donor and the recipient's liver are performed. Biliary reconstruction is performed with an end-to-end anastomosis of the donor and recipient common bile ducts; a stented T-tube is inserted to permit external drainage of bile. If an end-to-end anastomosis is not possible because of diseased or absent bile ducts, an end-to-side anastomosis will be made between the common bile duct of the graft and a loop (Roux-en-Y portion) of jejunum; in this case, bile drainage will be internal and a T-tube will not be inserted.

Liver transplantation is a long surgical procedure, partly because the patient with liver failure often has portal hypertension and subsequently many venous collateral vessels that must be ligated. Blood loss during the surgical procedure may be extensive. If the patient has adhesions from previous abdominal surgery, lysis of adhesions is often necessary. If a shunt procedure was performed previously, it must be surgically reversed to permit adequate portal venous blood supply to the new liver.

During the lengthy surgery, the family is often very anxious about the patient's well being. Updating the family about the progress of the surgery and the patient's status is often helpful during the procedure.

Postoperative Nursing Interventions

The patient is maintained in an environment as free from bacteria, viruses, and fungi as possible because immunosuppressive medications reduce the body's natural defenses.

Monitoring. In the immediate postoperative period, the patient is monitored continuously for cardiovascular, pulmonary, renal, neurologic, and metabolic function. Mean arterial and pulmonary artery pressures are monitored continuously. Cardiac output, central venous pressure, pulmonary capillary wedge pressure, arterial and mixed venous blood gases, urine output, heart rate, and blood pressure are used to evaluate the patient's hemodynamic status and intravascular fluid volume. Liver function tests, electrolyte levels, the coagulation profile, chest x-ray, cardiogram, and fluid output including urine, bile, and drainage from chest tubes and Jackson-Pratt tubes are monitored closely. Because the liver is responsible for storage of glycogen and synthesis of protein and clotting factors, monitoring and replacement of these substances in the immediate postoperative period are essential.

Mechanical Ventilation. Because of the likelihood of atelectasis and an altered ventilation–perfusion ratio due to insult to the diaphragm during the surgical procedure, prolonged anesthesia, immobility, postoperative pain, and the presence of chest tubes, the patient will have an endotracheal tube in place and require mechanical ventilation during the initial postoperative period. Suctioning is performed as required and sterile humidification is provided.

Postoperative Complications. The postoperative complication rate is high and is related primarily to technical complications or infection. Immediate postoperative complications may include bleeding, infection, rejection, and impaired biliary drainage. Disruption, infection, or obstruction of biliary anastomosis may occur.

Bleeding is common in the postoperative period and may result from coagulopathy, portal hypertension, and fibrinolysis caused by ischemic injury to the donor liver. Hypotension may occur in this phase secondary to blood loss. Administration of platelets, fresh frozen plasma, and other blood products may be necessary. Hypertension is more common; however, its cause is uncertain. This is treated if blood pressure elevation is significant or sustained.

Infection is the leading cause of death after liver transplantation. Pulmonary and fungal infections are common; susceptibility to infection is increased by immunosuppression needed to prevent rejection. Therefore, precautions must be taken to prevent nosocomial infections by strict asepsis when manipulating arterial, urinary, bile, and other drainage systems; obtaining specimens; and changing dressings.

Rejection is a key concern. A transplanted liver is perceived by the immune system as a foreign antigen. It triggers an immune response, leading to the activation of T lymphocytes that attack and destroy the transplanted liver. Immunosuppressive agents are used to prevent this response and rejection of the transplanted liver. These agents inhibit the activation of immunocompetent T lymphocytes to prevent the production of effector T cells.

Although the 1- and 5-year survival rates have increased dramatically since the advent of new immunosuppressive therapy, it is not without major side effects. A major side effect of cyclosporine, widely used in transplantation, is **nephrotoxicity;** this problem seems to be dose related, and renal dysfunction can be reversed if the dose of cyclosporine is appropriately decreased or if its use is not initiated immediately.

Corticosteroids, azathioprine, antilymphocytic globulin, OKT3, and FK506 are also part of the regimen of immunosuppression and may be used early in the postoperative course in place of cyclosporine until good urine output and creatinine clearance are established. Liver biopsy and ultrasound may be required to investigate suspected episodes of rejection.

Retransplantation is usually attempted if failure of the transplanted liver occurs. The success rate of retransplantation does not approach that of the initial transplantation, however.

Patient Teaching. Teaching the patient and family about long-term measures to promote health is an important function of the nurse. The patient and family must understand the reasons for the need to adhere continuously to the therapeutic regimen, with special emphasis on the methods of administration, rationale, and side effects of the prescribed immunosuppressive agents. The patient is given written as well as verbal instructions about how and when to take the medications and is instructed to take steps to be sure that an adequate supply of mediation is available so that there is no chance of running out of the medication or skipping a dose. Instructions are also provided about the signs and symptoms that are indications of problems requiring consultation with the transplant team. The patient with a T-tube in place will be instructed in care of the tube.

The importance of follow-up blood work and visits to the transplant team is emphasized. Cyclosporine trough levels will be obtained along with other blood tests that indicate the function of the liver and kidneys. During the first months, the patient is likely to require blood work two to three times a week. As the patient's condition stabilizes, blood work and visits to the transplant team will be scheduled less frequently. The importance of routine ophthalmology examinations is emphasized because of the increased incidence of cataracts and glaucoma with long-term steroid therapy. Regular oral hygiene and follow-up dental care, with administration of prophylactic antibiotics before dental treatments, are recommended because of the immunosuppression.

The patient is advised that while a successful transplantation will not return him or her to normal, it does increase the chances for survival and a more normal life than before transplantation, if rejection and infection can be prevented. Many patients have lived successful and productive lives after liver transplantation. Several women have had normal pregnancies and delivered normal infants after liver transplantation.

Liver Abscesses

Two categories of liver abscess have been identified: amebic and pyrogenic. **Amebic liver abscesses** are most commonly caused by *Entamoeba histolytica.* Most amebic liver abscesses occur in the developing countries of the tropics and subtropics because of poor sanitation and hygiene. **Pyrogenic liver abscesses** are much less common, but are more common in more developed countries than the amebic type.

Pathophysiology. Whenever an infection develops anywhere along the gastrointestinal tract, infecting organisms may reach the liver through the biliary system, portal venous system, or hepatic arterial or lymphatic systems. Most bacteria are promptly destroyed, but occasionally some gain a foothold. The bacterial toxins destroy the neighboring liver cells, and the resulting necrotic tissue serves as a protective wall for the organisms.

Meanwhile, leukocytes migrate into the infected area. The result is an abscess cavity full of a liquid containing living and dead leukocytes, liquefied liver cells, and bacteria. Pyogenic abscesses of this type may be either single or multiple and small. Examples of causes of pyrogenic liver abscess include cholangitis and abdominal trauma.

Clinical Manifestations. The clinical picture is one of sepsis with few or no localizing signs. Fever with chills and diaphoresis, malaise, anorexia, nausea, vomiting, and weight loss may occur. The patient may complain of dull abdominal pain and tenderness in the right upper quadrant of the abdomen. Hepatomegaly, jaundice, anemia, and pleural effusion may develop. Sepsis and shock may be severe and life threatening. In the past, mortality was 100% because of the vague clinical symptoms, inadequate diagnostic tools, and inadequate surgical drainage of the abscess. With the aid of ultrasound, CT scanning, and liver scans, early diagnosis and surgical drainage of the abscess have greatly reduced the mortality formerly associated with liver abscess.

Diagnostic Evaluation. Blood cultures are obtained, but may not identify the organism. Aspiration of the liver abscess guided by ultrasound or CT scan may be performed to assist in diagnosis and to obtain cultures of the organism. Percutaneous drainage of pyrogenic abscesses is carried out to evacuate the abscess material and promote healing. A catheter may be left in place for continuous drainage.

Management. Treatment includes intravenous antibiotic therapy; the specific antibiotic used in treatment depends on the organism identified. Continuous supportive care is indicated because of the serious condition of the patient.

Biliary Conditions

Several disorders affect the biliary system and interfere with normal drainage of bile into the duodenum. These disorders include carcinoma that obstructs the biliary tree and infection of the biliary system. Gallbladder disease with gallstones, however, is the most common disorder of the biliary system. Although not all occurrences of gallbladder infection (**cholecystitis**) are related to gallstones (**cholelithiasis**), more than 90% of patients with acute cholecystitis have gallstones. Most of the 15 million Americans with gallstones have no pain, however, and are unaware of the presence of stones. For a guide to the terminology associated with biliary disorders and procedures, see Chart 38-4.

CHART 38-4
Glossary: Biliary Disorders and Procedures

Cholecystitis inflammation of the gallbladder
Cholelithiasis the presence of calculi in the gallbladder
Cholecystectomy removal of the gallbladder
Cholecystostomy opening and drainage of the gallbladder
Choledochotomy opening into the common duct
Choledocholithiasis stones in the common duct
Choledocholithotomy incision of common bile duct for removal of stones
Choledochoduodenostomy anastomosis of common duct to duodenum
Choledochojejunostomy anastomosis of common duct to jejunum
Lithotripsy disintegration of gallstones by shock waves
Laparoscopic cholecystectomy removal of gallbladder through endoscopic procedure
Laser cholecystectomy removal of gallbladder using laser rather than scalpel and traditional surgical instruments

Cholecystitis

The gallbladder may be the site of an acute infection (cholecystitis) that causes acute pain, tenderness, and rigidity of the upper right abdomen, associated with nausea and vomiting and the usual signs of an acute inflammation. This condition is referred to as **acute cholecystitis.** If the gallbladder is found to be filled with pus, there is an **empyema** of the gallbladder.

Calculous cholecystitis occurs in more than 90% of patients with acute cholecystitis. In calculous cholecystitis, a gallbladder stone obstructs bile outflow. Bile remaining in the gallbladder initiates a chemical reaction; autolysis and edema occur; and the blood vessels in the gallbladder are compressed, compromising its vascular supply. Consequently, gangrene of the gallbladder with perforation may result. Bacteria play a minor role in acute cholecystitis; however, secondary infection with *E. coli* and other enteric organisms occurs in about 40% of patients.

Acalculous cholecystitis describes acute gallbladder inflammation in the absence of obstruction by gallstones. Acalculous cholecystitis occurs after major surgical procedures, severe trauma, or burns. Other factors associated with this type of cholecystitis include torsion cystic duct obstruction, primary bacterial infections of the gallbladder, and multiple blood transfusions. It is speculated that acalculous cholecystitis results from alterations in fluids and electrolytes and in regional blood flow in the visceral circulation. Its occurrence with major procedures or trauma makes its diagnosis difficult.

Cholelithiasis

Cholelithiasis (calculi, or gallstones) usually form in the gallbladder from the solid constituents of bile and vary greatly in size, shape, and composition (Fig. 38-13). Gallstones are uncommon in children and young adults but become increasingly prevalent after age 40. The incidence of cholelithiasis increases thereafter to such an extent that it has been estimated that by the age of 75, one of every three people will have gallstones.

Pathophysiology

There are two major types of gallstones: those composed predominantly of pigment and those composed primarily of cholesterol.

Pigment stones probably form when unconjugated pigments in the bile precipitate to form stones; these stones account for about one third of patients in the United States with gallstones. The risk of developing such stones is increased in patients with cirrhosis, hemolysis, and infections of the biliary tree. These stones cannot be dissolved and must be removed surgically.

Cholesterol stones account for most remaining cases of gallbladder disease in the United States. Cholesterol, a normal constituent of bile, is insoluble in water. Its solubility depends on bile acids and lecithin (phospholipids) in bile.

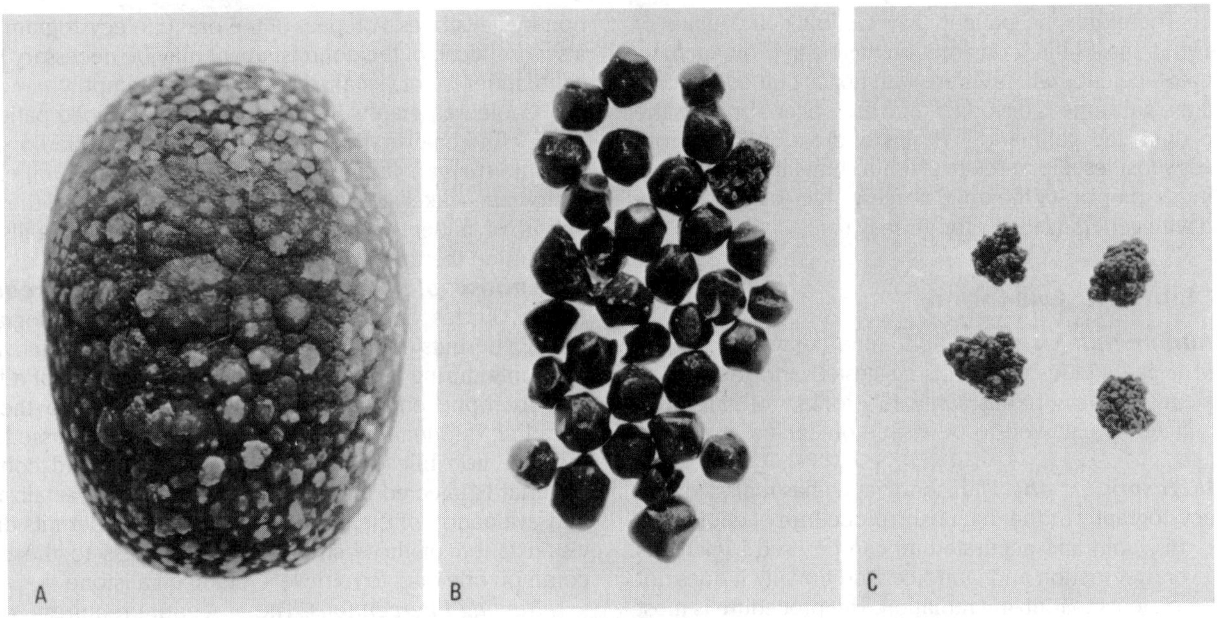

FIGURE 38-13. Common types of gallstones. **(A)** Solitary cholesterol gallstones made up of a coalescence of multiple small stones. **(B)** Faceted gallstones, the main constituent of which is cholesterol (about 70%). **(C)** Segment stones; typical "mulberry" caclium bilirubinate stones. (Schiff L. and Schiff E R.Diseases of the Liver, 7th ed. Philadelphia, JB Lippincott, 1993.)

In gallstone-prone patients, there is decreased bile acid synthesis and increased cholesterol synthesis in the liver, resulting in a bile supersaturated with cholesterol, which precipitates out of the bile to form stones. The cholesterol-saturated bile predisposes to the formation of gallstones and acts as an irritant, producing inflammatory changes in the gallbladder.

Four times more women than men develop cholesterol stones and gallbladder disease; they are usually over 40 years of age, multiparous, and obese. The incidence of stone formation is increased in users of oral contraceptives, estrogens, and clofibrate, which are known to increase biliary cholesterol saturation. The incidence of stone formation increases with age as a result of increased hepatic secretion of cholesterol and decreased bile acid synthesis. In addition, there is increased risk because of malabsorption of bile salts in patients with gastrointestinal disease or T-tube fistula or in those who have had ileal resection or bypass. There is also an increased incidence in persons with diabetes.

Clinical Manifestations

Gallstones may be silent, producing no pain and only mild gastrointestinal symptoms. Such stones may be detected incidentally during surgery or evaluation for nonrelated problems.

The patient with gallbladder disease due to gallstones may develop two types of symptoms: those due to disease of the gallbladder itself and those due to obstruction of the bile passages by a gallstone. The symptoms may be acute or chronic. Epigastric distress, such as fullness, abdominal distention, and vague pain in the right upper quadrant of the abdomen, may occur. This distress may follow a meal high in fried or fatty foods.

Pain and Biliary Colic. If a gallstone obstructs the cystic duct, the gallbladder becomes distended and eventually infected. The patient develops a fever and may have a palpable abdominal mass. The patient may experience biliary colic with excruciating upper right abdominal pain that radiates to the back or right shoulder, is usually associated with nausea and vomiting, and is noticeable several hours after a heavy meal. The patient moves about restlessly, unable to find a comfortable position. In some patients the pain is constant rather than colicky in nature.

Such a bout of biliary colic is caused by contraction of the gallbladder, which cannot release bile because of obstruction by the stone. When distended, the fundus of the gallbladder comes in contact with the abdominal wall in the region of the right ninth and tenth costal cartilages. This produces marked tenderness in the right upper quadrant on deep inspiration and prevents full inspiratory excursion.

The pain of acute cholecystitis may be so severe that analgesics such as meperidine are required. Morphine is thought to increase spasm of the sphincter of Oddi, and its use is therefore avoided.

Jaundice. Jaundice occurs in a small percentage of patients with gallbladder disease and usually occurs with obstruction of the common bile duct. Obstruction of the flow of bile into the duodenum results in the following characteristic symptoms: the bile, no longer carried to the duodenum, is absorbed by the blood, giving the skin and mucous membrane a yellow color. This is frequently accompanied by marked itching of the skin.

Changes in Urine and Stool Color. The excretion of the bile pigments by the kidneys gives the urine a very dark color. The feces, no longer colored with bile pigments, are grayish, like putty, and usually described as "clay-colored."

Vitamin Deficiency. Obstruction of bile flow also interferes with absorption of the fat-soluble vitamins A, D, E, and K. Therefore, the patient may exhibit deficiencies of these vitamins if biliary obstruction has been prolonged. Vitamin K deficiency will interfere with normal blood clotting.

If the gallstone is dislodged and no longer obstructs the cystic duct, the gallbladder drains and the inflammatory process subsides after a relatively short time. If the gallstone continues to obstruct the duct, abscess, necrosis, and perforation with generalized peritonitis may result.

Diagnostic Evaluation

Abdominal X-ray. An abdominal x-ray may be obtained if gallbladder disease is suggested and to exclude other causes of symptoms. Only 15% to 20% of gallstones are sufficiently calcified to be visible on such x-rays, however.

Ultrasonography. Ultrasonography has replaced oral cholecystography as the diagnostic procedure of choice because it is rapid and accurate and can be used in patients with liver dysfunction and jaundice. Additionally, it does not expose patients to ionizing radiation. The procedure is most accurate if the patient fasts overnight so that the gallbladder is distended. The use of ultrasound is based on reflected sound waves. Ultrasonography can detect calculi in the gallbladder or a dilated common bile duct. It is reported to detect gallstones with 95% accuracy.

Radionuclide Imaging or Cholescintography. Cholescintography is used successfully in the diagnosis of acute cholecystitis. In this procedure, a radioactive agent is administered intravenously. It is then taken up by the hepatocytes and rapidly excreted through the biliary system. The biliary tract is then scanned, and images of the gallbladder and biliary tree are obtained. This test is more expensive than ultrasonography, takes longer to perform, exposes the patient to radiation, and cannot detect gallstones. Its use may be limited to those cases in which ultrasonography is not conclusive.

Cholecystography. Although it has been replaced by ultrasonography as the test of choice, cholecystography is still used if ultrasound equipment is not available or if the ultrasound results are inconclusive. Oral cholangiography may be performed to detect gallstones and to assess the ability of the gallbladder to fill, concentrate its contents, contract, and empty. An iodide-containing contrast medium that is excreted by the liver and concentrated in the gallbladder is administered to the patient. The normal gallbladder fills with this radiopaque substance. If gallstones are present, they appear as shadows on the x-ray.

Medications administered as contrast agent include iopanoic acid (Telepaque), iodipamide meglumine (Cholografin), and sodium ipodate (Oragrafin). These preparations are administered in oral doses, 10 to 12 hours before x-ray study. The patient is permitted nothing by mouth after the contrast agent is administered to prevent contraction and emptying of the gallbladder.

The patient is asked about allergies to iodine or seafood. If no allergy is identified, the patient receives the oral form of the contrast agent the evening before the radiographs are obtained. An x-ray of the right upper abdomen is obtained. If the gallbladder is found to fill and empty normally and to contain no stones, it is concluded that no gallbladder disease is present. If gallbladder disease is present, the gallbladder may not be visualized because of obstruction by gallstones. A repeat of the oral cholecystogram with a second dose of the contrast agent may be necessary if the gallbladder is not visualized on the first attempt.

Cholecystography in the obviously jaundiced patient is not useful because the liver cannot excrete the radiopaque dye into the gallbladder in a jaundiced patient. Oral cholecystogram is likely to continue to be used as part of the evaluation of patients who have been treated with gallstone dissolution therapy or lithotripsy.

Endoscopic Retrograde Cholangiopancreatography. Endoscopic retrograde cholangiopancreatography (ERCP) permits direct visualization of structures once available only during laparotomy. It involves insertion of a flexible fiberoptic endoscope into the esophagus to the descending duodenum (Fig. 38-14). A cannula is passed into the common bile duct and pancreatic duct and contrast material is injected into the ducts, permitting visualization and evaluation of the biliary tree. ERCP also permits direct visualization of these structures and access to the distal common bile duct to retrieve a retained gallstone.

Nursing Interventions. The procedure requires a cooperative patient to permit insertion of the endoscope without damage to the gastrointestinal tract structures, including the biliary tree. Before the procedure, the patient is given an explanation of the procedure and his or her role in it. Sedation is administered immediately before the procedure. During ERCP, the nurse monitors intravenous fluids, administers medications, and positions the patient.

After the procedure, the nurse monitors the patient's condition, observing vital signs and monitoring for signs of perforation or infection. The nurse also monitors the patient for side effects of any medications received during the procedure and return of the patient's gag reflex after the use of local anesthetics.

Percutaneous Transhepatic Cholangiography. Percutaneous transhepatic cholangiography (PTC) involves the injection of dye directly into the biliary tree. Because of the relatively large concentration of dye that is introduced

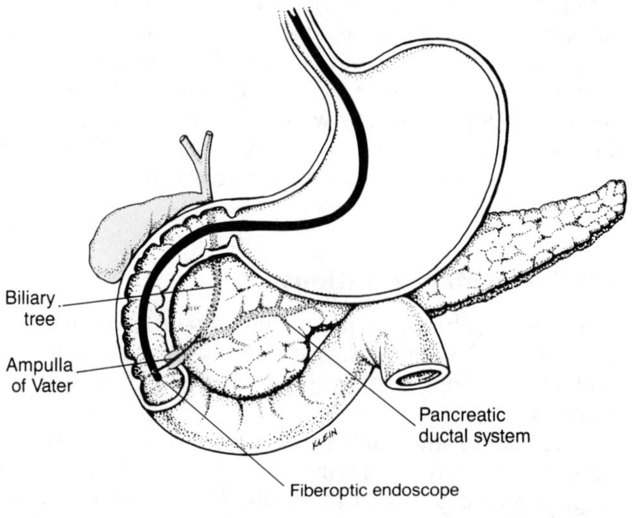

FIGURE 38-14. Endoscopic retrograde cholangiopancreatography (ERCP). A fiberoptic duodenoscope, with side-viewing apparatus, is inserted into the duodenum. The ampulla of Vater is catheterized and the biliary tree injected with contrast agent. The pancreatic ductal system is also assessed, if indicated. This procedure is of special value in visualizing neoplasms of the ampulla area and extracting a biopsy specimen.

into the biliary system, all components of the system, including the hepatic ducts within the liver, the entire length of the common bile duct, the cystic duct, and the gallbladder, are clearly outlined.

This procedure can be carried out even in the presence of liver dysfunction and jaundice. It is useful in distinguishing jaundice caused by liver disease (hepatocellular jaundice) from that due to biliary obstruction; for investigating the gastrointestinal symptoms of patients whose gallbladders have been removed; for locating stones within the bile ducts; and in diagnosing cancer involving the biliary system.

Procedure. The patient, who is fasting and well sedated, lies supine on the x-ray table. The injection site, which is usually in the midclavicular line immediately beneath the right costal margin, is disinfected and anesthetized with lidocaine (Xylocaine). A small incision is made at this point and a thin, flexible needle with stylet is inserted posteriorly at a 45-degree angle and parallel to the midline. When the needle has penetrated to a depth of approximately 10 cm (4 in), the stylet is removed and replaced by a plastic connector tube with a 50-ml syringe attached. Gentle suction is applied while the needle is slowly withdrawn, until bile appears in the syringe. As much bile as possible is withdrawn, a radiopaque dye is injected, and an x-ray film obtained.

Before the needle is removed, as much dye and bile as possible are aspirated to forestall subsequent leakage into the needle tract and eventually into the peritoneal cavity, to minimize the risk of bile peritonitis.

Nursing Interventions. Although the complication rate after this procedure is low, the patient must be observed closely for symptoms of bleeding, peritonitis, and septicemia. Pain and indicators of these complications should be reported immediately. Antibiotics should be administered as prescribed to minimize the risk of sepsis and septic shock.

Management of Cholecystitis

Surgical removal of the gallbladder through traditional surgical approaches was considered the standard approach to management for over 100 years. However, dramatic changes have occurred in surgical and nonsurgical management of gallbladder disease. Although nonsurgical approaches have the advantage of eliminating surgical risk, they are associated with persistent symptoms or recurrent stone formation. Most of the nonsurgical approaches, including lithotripsy and dissolution of gallstones, provide only temporary solutions to the problems associated with gallstones. With the widespread use of laparoscopic cholecystectomy, whereby the gallbladder is removed through a small incision through the umbilicus, surgical risks have decreased along with lengths of hospital stay and the long recovery period associated with the standard surgical cholecystectomy. However, other approaches discussed below may be indicated with specific patients.

Nonsurgical Management

The major objectives of medical therapy are to reduce the incidence of acute episodes of gallbladder pain and cholecystitis by supportive and dietary management, and, if possible, to remove the cause of cholecystitis by pharmacotherapy, endoscopic procedures, or surgical intervention.

Supportive and Dietary Management. Approximately 80% of the patients with acute gallbladder inflammation achieve a remission with rest, intravenous fluids, nasogastric suction, analgesia, and antibiotics. Unless the patient's condition deteriorates, surgical intervention is delayed until the patient's acute symptoms subside and complete evaluation can be carried out.

The diet immediately after an episode is usually limited to low-fat liquids. Powdered supplements high in protein and carbohydrate can be stirred into skim milk. The following may then be added as tolerated: cooked fruits, rice or tapioca, lean meats, mashed potatoes, non—gas-forming vegetables, bread, coffee, or tea. Eggs, cream, pork, fried foods, cheese and rich dressings, gas-forming vegetables, and alcohol are avoided. The patient may need to be reminded that fatty foods may bring on an episode.

Dietary management may be the major mode of therapy in those patients who have experienced only dietary intolerance to fatty foods and vague gastrointestinal symptoms.

Pharmacotherapy. Ursodeoxycholic acid (UDCA) and chenodeoxycholic acid (chenodiol or CDCA) have been used to dissolve small, radiolucent gallstones composed primarily of cholesterol. UDCA has fewer side effects than chenodiol and can be administered in smaller doses to achieve the same effect. The mechanism of action is the inhibition of liver synthesis and secretion of cholesterol, thereby desaturating bile. Existing stones can be decreased in size, small ones dissolved, and new stones prevented from forming. Six to 12 months of therapy are required in many patients to dissolve stones, and monitoring of the patient is required during this time. The effective dose of medication depends on body weight; this method of treatment is generally indicated for those patients who refuse surgery or for whom it is considered too risky.

Certain other medications, such as estrogens, oral contraceptives, clofibrate, and dietary cholesterol, may adversely affect the results of this method of treatment; therefore, the physician should be notified if the patient is taking any of these medications.

Recurrence of stones has been reported in 20% to 50% of patients after treatment is terminated; therefore, a low dose of this medication may be continued to prevent recurrence. Patients' adherence to this mode of therapy requires further study and follow-up.

If acute symptoms of cholecystitis continue or recur, pharmacotherapy is inappropriate as a substitute for more definitive treatment, and surgical intervention or lithotripsy is indicated.

Long-term follow-up and monitoring of the patient's liver enzymes are indicated. The patient is instructed to report adverse side effects of medications and the recurrence of symptoms of cholecystitis.

Nonsurgical Removal of Gallstones

Dissolving Gallstones. Several methods have been used to dissolve gallstones by infusion of a solvent (monooctanoin or methyl tertiary butyl ether [MTBE]) into the gallbladder. The solvent can be infused through the following routes: through a tube or catheter inserted percutaneously directly into the gallbladder, through a tube or drain inserted through a T-tube tract to dissolve stones not removed at the time of surgery, through an ERCP endoscope, or through a transnasal biliary catheter.

In this last procedure, the catheter is introduced through the mouth and inserted into the common bile duct. The upper end of the tube is then rerouted from the mouth to the nose and left in place. This enables the patient to eat and drink normally while passage of stones is monitored or chemical solvents are infused to dissolve the stones. This method of dissolution of stones is not widely used in patients with gallstone disease.

Nonsurgical Removal. Several nonsurgical methods are used to remove stones that were not removed at the time of cholecystectomy or have become lodged in the common bile duct (Fig. 38-15). A catheter and instrument with a basket attached are threaded through the T-tube tract or fistula formed at the time of T-tube insertion; the basket is used to retrieve and remove the stone lodged in the common bile duct.

A second procedure is use of the ERCP endoscope. After the endoscope is inserted, a cutting instrument is passed through the endoscope into the ampulla of Vater of the common bile duct. It may be used to cut the submucosal fibers, or papilla, of the sphincter of Oddi, enlarging the opening, which may allow the lodged stone to pass spontaneously into the duodenum. Another instrument with a small basket or balloon at its tip may be inserted through the endoscope to retrieve the stone (Fig. 38-15). Although complications after this procedure are rare, the patient must be observed closely for bleeding, perforation, and the development of pancreatitis.

The ERCP endoscope procedure is particularly useful in the diagnosis and treatment of patients presenting with symptoms after biliary tract surgery, for those patients with intact gallbladders, and for patients in whom surgery is particularly hazardous.

Extracorporeal Shock-Wave Lithotripsy. Extracorporeal shock-wave therapy (lithotripsy or ESWL) has been successfully used for nonsurgical fragmentation of gallstones. The word lithotripsy is derived from *lithos,* meaning stone, and *tripsis,* meaning rubbing or friction.

This noninvasive procedure uses repeated shock waves directed at the gallstone located in the gallbladder or common bile duct to fragment the stones. Shock waves are generated in a liquid medium by electric spark, piezoelectric, or electromagnetic discharges. The energy is transmitted to the body through a water bath or fluid-filled bag (Fig. 38-16). The converging shock waves are directed to the stones to be fragmented; because of differences in impedance among tissues, little shock-wave energy is absorbed before reaching the stone, and thus minimal tissue damage to surrounding tissue is expected if those tissues with large air contents or solid tissue (lung, GI tract, bone) are avoided.

After the stones are gradually broken up, the stone fragments pass from the gallbladder or common bile duct spontaneously, are removed by endoscopy, or are dissolved with oral bile acid or solvents. Because the procedure requires no incision and no hospitalization, patients are usually treated as outpatients; most return to their usual routines within 48 hours of treatment.

If the lithotriptor uses high total shock wave energy, a general, spinal, or epidural anesthetic is administered to the patient. If the lithotriptor uses low total shock wave energy, the treatment can be administered without anesthesia; how-

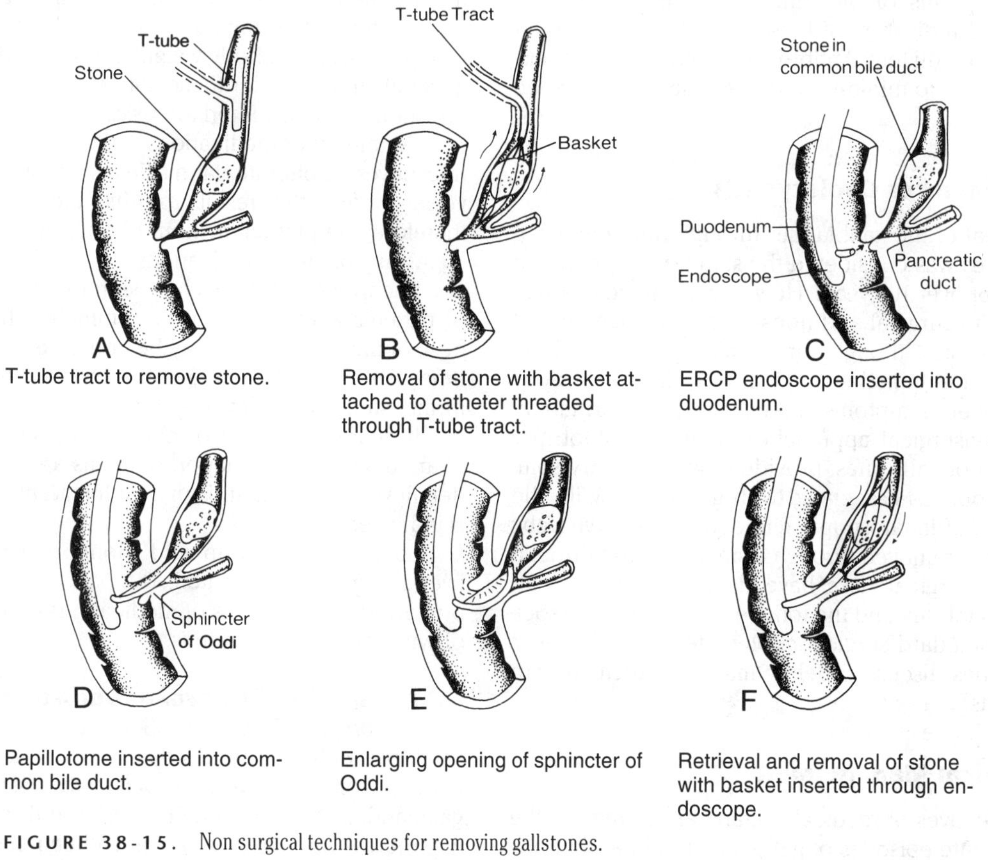

FIGURE 38-15. Non surgical techniques for removing gallstones.

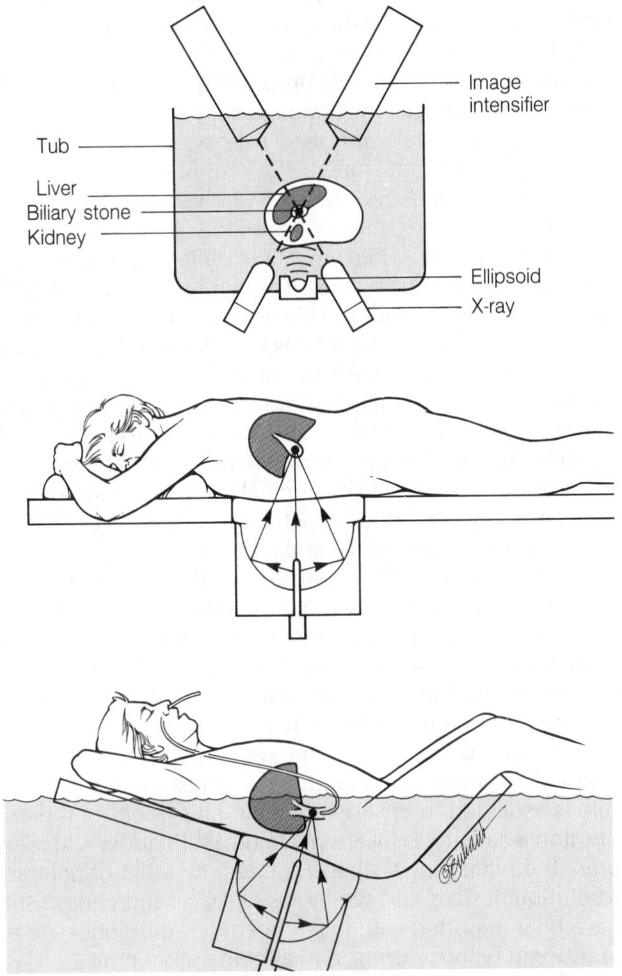

FIGURE 38-16. **(A)** Schematic illustration of extracorporeal shock wave therapy. The gallbladder stone is localized by imaging. Shock waves are generated in the ellipsoid reflector and transmitted through the water to the stone. **(B)** Positioning of the patient for treatment of stones located in the gallbladder. The fluid-filled bag is recessed in the table and transmits the shock wave from the generator to the patient's skin. **(C)** Positioning of the patient for treatment of stones located in the common bile duct. The patient is partially submerged in a water bath. A nasobiliary tube is used to introduce contrast material to permit visualization and localization of the stone and to decompress the biliary tree.

ever, more shocks must be used with this equipment before stones are fragmented.

Procedure. The patient with gallbladder stones is placed in a prone position over the shock wave generator (see Fig. 38-16). A fluid-filled cushion is placed between the patient and the lithotriptor. If treatment is for bile duct stones, the patient may be partially immersed in a water bath; a nasobiliary catheter or other biliary catheter is inserted to permit radiocontrast material to be introduced into the biliary tree and to decompress the bile duct during the treatment. Ultrasound is used to visualize the stones. The shock waves are timed with the electrocardiogram to reduce the risk of dysrhythmias.

Side Effects. Side effects of lithotripsy used to treat gallstones have included cutaneous petechiae (14%) and gross hematuria (3%), probably caused by microscopic injury to the right kidney from passage of shock waves through it. More serious side effects, such as pancreatitis or bile duct obstruction, are possible, but their incidence is small. The patient is monitored after the procedure for the occurrence of these symptoms.

Patient Education. Because the patient returns home soon after completion of the treatment, preparation for discharge and self-care is provided. Teaching includes information about the symptoms that should be reported. Use of ursodeoxycholic acid (UDCA) following the procedure increases the effectiveness of ESWL in reducing recurrence. If oral bile salts or UDCA is prescribed, the patient is instructed about the importance of compliance and follow-up.

Intracorporeal Lithotripsy. With intracorporeal lithotripsy, stones in the gallbladder or common bile duct may be fragmented by ultrasound, pulsed laser, or hydraulic lithotripsy applied through an endoscope directly to the stones. The stone fragments or debris are then removed by irrigation and aspiration. The procedure may be followed by removal of the gallbladder through an incision or by laparoscopy. If the gallbladder is not removed, a drain may be inserted for 7 days.

Surgical Management

Surgical treatment of gallbladder disease and gallstones is carried out to relieve long-continued symptoms, to remove the cause of biliary colic, and to treat acute cholecystitis. Surgery may be elective when the patient's symptoms have subsided or may be performed as an emergency procedure if the patient's condition necessitates it.

Preoperative Management. In addition to x-ray studies of the gallbladder, chest x-rays, electrocardiogram, and liver function tests (see Table 38-1) may be performed. Vitamin K may be administered if the patient's prothrombin level is low. Blood component therapy may be administered before surgery.

Nutritional requirements are considered; if the patient is not eating properly, it may be necessary to provide intravenous glucose with protein hydrolysate supplements to aid wound healing and help prevent liver damage.

Preparation for gallbladder surgery is similar to that for any upper abdominal laparotomy. Instruction and explanation are given before surgery with regard to turning and deep breathing. Because the abdominal incision is high, the patient is often reluctant to move and turn; pneumonia and atelectasis are possible postoperative complications that are often avoided by deep-breathing exercises and frequent turning. The patient should be informed that with some of these surgical procedures, drainage tubes are usually required and that a nasogastric tube and suction will also be required during the immediate postoperative period.

Surgical Intervention and Drainage Systems. Patients usually are placed on the operating table with the upper abdomen raised somewhat by an air pillow or sandbag to make the biliary area more accessible.

Cholecystectomy. Cholecystectomy is one of the most frequent surgical procedures, with over 600,000 performed each year in the United States. In this procedure, the gallbladder is removed after the cystic duct and artery are ligated. The procedure is performed in most cases of acute and chronic cholecystitis. A drain (Penrose) is placed in the gallbladder bed and brought out through a stab wound to drain blood, serosanguineous fluids, and bile into absorbent dressings.

Minicholecystectomy. Minicholecystectomy is a surgical procedure in which the gallbladder is removed through a 4-cm incision. If needed, the surgical incision is extended to remove large gallbladder stones. Drains may or may not be used with minicholecystectomy. Cost savings resulting from patients' shorter hospital stays have been identified as major reasons for pursuing this type of procedure. Debate exists about this procedure because it limits exposure to all the involved biliary strictures.

Laparoscopic Cholecystectomy. Laparoscopic (or endoscopic) cholecystectomy (LC) has dramatically changed the approach to management of cholecystitis. Approximately 600,000 patients require surgery each year for removal of the gallbladder and about 70% to 80% of them are candidates for laparoscopic cholecystectomy.

LC is performed through a small incision or puncture made through the abdominal wall in the umbilicus. In the LC procedure the abdominal cavity is insufflated with carbon dioxide (pneumoperitoneum) to assist in inserting the endoscope and to aid the surgeon in visualizing the abdominal structures. A fiberoptic endoscope is inserted through the small umbilical incision. Several additional punctures or small incisions are made in the abdominal wall to introduce other surgical instruments into the operative field. The surgeon is able to visualize the biliary system through the endoscope; a camera attached to the endoscope permits a view of the intra-abdominal field to be transmitted to a television monitor.

A traditional abdominal surgical procedure may be necessary if problems are encountered during the endoscopic procedure. The patient is informed that an open abdominal procedure may be necessary and general anesthesia is administered. The advantage of this procedure is that the patient does not experience the paralytic ileus that occurs with open abdominal surgery and has less postoperative abdominal pain. The patient is often discharged from the hospital on the day of surgery or within a day or two and is able to resume full activity and employment within a week of the surgery.

Although an open abdominal procedure has been necessary only occasionally, the need to resort to a full surgical procedure may result from an inability to identify and select patients at low risk for problems. With wider use of the procedure, there may be an increase in the number of patients who are found during the laparoscopy procedure to require an abdominal surgical approach.

Postoperative Patient Education. Because of the short hospital stay, written as well as verbal instructions must be provided for the patient and family. Information is provided about management of postoperative pain. The patient is also informed about signs and symptoms of intra-abdominal complications that should be reported, including loss of appetite, vomiting, pain, distention of the abdomen, and temperature elevation. Although patients do recover quickly from laparoscopic cholecystectomy, the patient will be drowsy afterwards and arrangements must be planned to ensure that the patient has assistance at home during the first 24–48 hours.

Choledochostomy. In choledochostomy, an incision is made into the common duct for removal of stones. After the stones have been evacuated, a tube usually is inserted into the duct for drainage of bile until edema subsides. This tube is connected to gravity drainage tubing. The gallbladder also contains stones and, as a rule, a cholecystectomy is performed at the same time.

Surgical Cholecystostomy. Cholecystostomy is performed when the patient's condition prevents more extensive surgery or when an acute inflammatory reaction obscures the biliary system. The gallbladder is surgically opened, the stones and the bile or the purulent drainage are removed, and a drainage tube is secured with a purse-string suture. The drainage tube is connected to a drainage system to prevent bile from leaking around the tube or escaping into the peritoneal cavity. After recovery from the acute episode, the patient may return for cholecystectomy.

Despite its lower risk, surgical cholecystostomy has a high mortality (reported as high as 20% to 30%) because of the patient's underlying disease process.

Percutaneous Cholecystostomy. Percutaneous cholecystostomy has been used in the treatment and diagnosis of acute cholecystitis in patients who are poor risks for any surgical procedure or for general anesthesia. These may include patients with sepsis or severe cardiac, renal, pulmonary, or liver failure. Under local anesthesia, a fine needle is inserted through the abdominal wall and liver edge into the gallbladder under the guidance of ultrasound or CT scan. Bile is aspirated to ensure adequate placement of the needle, and a catheter is inserted into the gallbladder to decompress the biliary tract. Almost immediate relief of pain and resolution of signs and symptoms of sepsis and cholecystitis have been reported with this procedure. Antibiotics are administered before, during, and after the procedure.

Gerontologic Considerations. Surgical intervention for disease of the biliary tract is the most common operative procedure performed in the elderly. Although the incidence of gallstones increases with age, the symptoms experienced by the elderly patient may not be the typical picture of fever, pain, chills, and jaundice. Biliary tract disease in the elderly may be accompanied or preceded by symptoms of septic shock: oliguria, hypotension, mental changes, tachycardia, and tachypnea.

Although surgery in the elderly presents risk because of preexisting associated diseases, the mortality from serious complications from biliary tract disease itself is also high. The risk of mortality and morbidity is increased in the elderly patient who undergoes emergency surgery for life-threatening disease of the biliary tract. Despite the presence of chronic illness in many elderly patients, elective cholecystectomy is usually well tolerated and can be carried out with low risk if expert assessment and care are provided before, during, and after the surgical procedure.

Because of recent changes in the health care system, there has been a decrease in the number of elective surgical procedures performed, including cholecystectomies. As a result, patients requiring the procedure are seen in the later stages of disease. Simultaneously, patients undergoing surgery are increasingly over 60 years of age and are presenting with complicated acute cholecystitis. The higher risk of complications and shorter hospital stays make it essential that older patients and their family members receive specific information about signs and symptoms of complications and measures to prevent them.

❑ NURSING PROCESS
The Patient Undergoing Surgery for Gallbladder Disease

Assessment

The patient who is to undergo surgical treatment of gallbladder disease is often admitted to the hospital or same-day-surgery unit on the morning of surgery. Preadmission testing has often been completed a week or more before admission. Therefore, little time is available to conduct an extensive history or physical assessment. As a result, the health history and examination should focus on those issues of most importance to the patient and to the health care team who will be managing the patient's care during and after surgery.

Assessment should focus on the patient's respiratory status. If a traditional surgical approach is planned, the high abdominal incision required during surgery may interfere with full respiratory excursion. A history of smoking or previous respiratory problems is noted. Shallow respirations, a persistent or ineffective cough, and the presence of adventitious breath sounds are noted. Nutritional status is evaluated through dietary history, general examination, and monitoring the previously obtained laboratory results.

Diagnosis

Nursing Diagnoses

Based on all the assessment data, the major nursing diagnoses for the patient undergoing surgery for gallbladder disease may include the following:

- Pain and discomfort related to surgical incision
- Impaired gas exchange related to the high abdominal surgical incision (if traditional surgical cholecystectomy is performed)
- Impaired skin integrity related to altered biliary drainage after surgical intervention (if a T-tube is inserted because of stones located in the common bile duct)
- Altered nutrition related to inadequate bile secretion
- Knowledge deficit about self-care activities after discharge

Collaborative Problems/ Potential Complications

Based on assessment data, potential complications may include:

- Bleeding
- Gastrointestinal symptoms

Planning and Implementation

Goals. The patient's goals include relief of pain, absence of respiratory complications, intact skin and normal biliary drainage, improved nutritional intake, understanding of self-care routines, and absence of complications.

Postoperative Nursing Interventions

As soon as the patient has recovered from anesthesia, he or she is placed in low Fowler's position. Fluids may be given intravenously, and nasogastric suction (nasogastric tube probably inserted immediately before surgery) may be instituted to relieve abdominal distention. Water and other fluids may be given in about 24 hours, and a soft diet started later, after bowel sounds return.

Relieving Pain. The location of the subcostal incision in gallbladder surgery is likely to cause the patient to avoid turning and moving and to splint the operative site by taking shallow breaths to prevent pain. Because full aeration of the lungs and gradually increased activity are necessary to prevent postoperative complications, analgesics should be administered as prescribed and the patient assisted to turn, cough, breathe deeply, and ambulate as indicated. Use of a pillow or binder over the incision may reduce pain during these maneuvers.

Improving Respiratory Status. Patients undergoing biliary tract surgery are especially prone to pulmonary complications, as are all patients with upper abdominal incisions. Thus, they should be reminded to take deep breaths every hour to expand the lungs fully and prevent atelectasis. Early ambulation prevents pulmonary complications as well as other complications, such as thrombophlebitis. Pulmonary complications are more likely to occur in the elderly and the obese patient.

Promoting Skin Care and Biliary Drainage. As previously mentioned, in patients who have undergone a cholecystostomy or choledochostomy, the drainage tubes must be connected immediately to a drainage receptacle. In addition, tubing should be fastened to the dressings or to the bottom sheet, with enough leeway for the patient to move without dislodging or kinking it. Because a drainage system remains attached when the patient is ambulating, the drainage bag may be placed in a bathrobe pocket or fastened so that it is below the waist or common duct level. If a Penrose drain is used, as it is for standard abdominal surgical cholecystectomy, the dressings are changed as required.

After these surgical procedures, the patient is observed for indications of infection, leakage of bile into the peritoneal cavity, and obstruction of bile drainage. If bile is not draining properly, an obstruction is probably causing bile to be forced back into the liver and bloodstream. Because jaundice may result, the nurse should be particularly observant of the color of the patient's sclerae. The nurse should also note and report right upper quadrant abdominal pain, nausea and vomiting, bile drainage around the T-tube, clay-colored stools, and a change in vital signs.

Bile may continue to drain from the drainage tract in considerable quantities for a time, necessitating frequent changes of the outer dressings and protection of the skin from irritation. Skin pastes of zinc oxide, aluminum, or petrolatum prevent the bile from literally digesting the skin.

To prevent total loss of bile, the physician may want the drainage tube or collecting receptacle elevated above the level of the abdomen, so that the bile drains externally only if pressure develops in the duct system. The bile collected is measured every 24 hours; the amount, color, and character of the drainage are documented. After several days of drainage, the tube may be clamped for an hour before and after each meal, with the purpose being to deliver bile to the duodenum to aid in digestion. Within 7 to 14 days, the drainage tube is removed. The patient who goes home with a drainage tube in place requires instruction and reassurance about its function and care of the tube (see page 1002).

In all patients with biliary drainage, the stools should be observed daily and their color noted. Specimens of both urine and stool may be sent to the laboratory for examination for bile pigments. In this way, it is possible to determine that the bile pigment is disappearing from the blood and is draining again into the duodenum. A careful record of fluid intake and output is maintained.

Improving Nutritional Status. The patient's diet may be low in fats and high in carbohydrates and proteins immediately after surgery. At the time of hospital discharge, there are usually no special dietary instructions, other than to maintain a nutritious diet and avoid excessive fats. Fat restriction usually is lifted in 4 to 6 weeks when biliary ducts dilate to accommodate the volume of bile once held by the gallbladder and when the ampulla of Vater again functions effectively. After this, when one eats fat, adequate bile will be released into the digestive tract to emulsify the fats and allow their digestion. Before surgery, fats may not be digested completely or adequately, and flatulence might occur. However, one purpose of gallbladder surgery is ultimately to allow for a normal diet.

Patient Education and Home Care Considerations. Because the patient may be discharged from the hospital while the drainage system is still in place, the patient and family will need instructions about its management. They must be instructed in proper care of the drainage tube and should know to report to the physician promptly changes in the amount or characteristics of drainage. Assistance in securing the appropriate dressings will reduce the patient's anxiety about going home with the drain or tube still in place.

The patient should be instructed about which medications are required (vitamins, anticholinergics, and antispasmodics) and their actions. The patient and family also should be aware of symptoms that are reportable to the physician—jaundice, dark urine, pale-colored stools, pruritus, or signs of inflammation and infection, such as pain or fever.

Some patients note "looseness of the bowels," consisting of one to three bowel movements a day—the result of a continual trickle of bile through the choledochoduodenal junction after cholecystectomy. Usually, such frequency diminishes over a period of a few weeks to several months. Follow-up visits are essential for this patient.

Monitoring and Managing Potential Complications. *Bleeding* may occur as a result of inadvertent puncture or nicking of a major blood vessel. Postoperatively, the patient's vital signs are monitored closely. Drainage (if T-tube is present) and the surgical incisions are inspected for bleeding. The patient is also assessed periodically for increased tenderness and rigidity of the abdomen. If these signs and symptoms occur, they are reported to the surgeon. The patient and family are instructed to report change in color of stools to the surgeon as this may indicate complications.

Gastrointestinal symptoms, although unexpected, may occur with manipulation of the intestines during surgery. Following laparoscopic cholecystectomy, the patient is assessed for loss of appetite, vomiting, pain, distention of the abdomen, and temperature elevation. These may indicate infection or disruption of the gastrointestinal tract and should be reported to the surgeon promptly. Because the patient is discharged soon after laparoscopic surgery, the patient and family must be instructed verbally and in writing about the importance of reporting these symptoms promptly.

Evaluation

Expected Outcomes

1. Reports decrease in pain
   a. Splints abdominal incision to decrease pain
   b. Avoids foods that cause pain
   c. Uses postoperative analgesia as prescribed
2. Demonstrates appropriate respiratory function
   a. Is able to achieve full respiratory excursion, with deep inspiration and expiration
   b. Coughs effectively, using pillow to splint abdominal incision
   c. Uses postoperative analgesia as prescribed
   d. Exercises as prescribed (*e.g.*, turns, ambulates)
3. Exhibits normal skin integrity around biliary drainage site
   a. Is free of fever, abdominal pain, change in vital signs, or bile around drainage tube
   b. Exhibits or reports gradual decrease in bile drainage and normal color in urine and stool
   c. Demonstrates proper management of catheter
   d. Identifies signs and symptoms of biliary obstruction to be noted and reported
   e. Has serum bilirubin level within normal range
4. Obtains relief of dietary intolerance
   a. Maintains adequate dietary intake and avoids foods that cause gastrointestinal symptoms
   b. Reports decreased incidence or absence of nausea, vomiting, diarrhea, flatulence, and abdominal discomfort
5. Is free of complications
   a. Has normal vital signs (blood pressure, pulse, respiratory rate and pattern, and temperature.
   b. Reports absence of bleeding from gastrointestinal tract or T-tube (if present) and no evidence of bleeding in stool
   c. Reports return of appetite and no evidence of vomiting, abdominal distention, and pain
   d. Lists symptoms that should be reported to surgeon promptly

BIBLIOGRAPHY

Books

Arias IM. The Liver: Biology and Pathobiology. New York, Raven Press, 1994.

Blumgart LH. Surgery of the Liver and Biliary Tract. New York, Churchill Livingstone, 1994.

CRITICAL THINKING EXERCISES

1. A 48-year-old patient who lives by herself is to be discharged from the hospital on the evening following her laparoscopic cholecystectomy. In preparing this patient for discharge, how would you formulate your instructions to ensure adequate recovery following the procedure? Describe how you would alert the patient to possible complications that would need to be reported to the health care provider. How would your instructions and discharge planning differ if the patient has family members caring for her?
2. A patient has been informed that he has hepatitis B. He explains that as a child he had hepatitis A. How would you explain the differences between these two types of hepatitis, and how would you caution the patient about preventing transmission to others? If this patient has a history of alcoholism, how might the treatment be modified and how might you modify your patient teaching plans?
3. A 58-year-old man with a long history of alcohol abuse is admitted to the hospital because he is vomiting blood. Describe the precautions and assessment and management strategies you would anticipate in the care of this patient and the reason for these strategies.

Fabry TL and Klion FM (eds). Guide to Liver Transplantation. New York, Igaku-Shoin, 1992.
International Symposium on Viral Hepatitis and Liver Disease. New York, Springer-Verlag, 1994.
Kaplowitz N. Liver and Biliary Diseases. Baltimore, Williams & Wilkins, 1992.
Rector WG. Complications of Chronic Liver Disease. St. Louis, Mosby Year Book, 1992.
Rustgi VK and Van Thiel DH. The Liver in Systemic Disease. New York, Raven Press, 1993.
Schiff L and Schiff ER. Diseases of the Liver, 7th ed. Philadelphia, JB Lippincott, 1993.
Summers S and Ebbert DW. Ambulatory Surgical Nursing: A Nursing Diagnosis Approach. Philadelphia, JB Lippincott, 1992.
Surawicz C and Owen R. Gastrointestinal and Hepatic Infections. Philadelphia, WB Saunders, 1995.

Journals

General Liver

el-Newihi and Nihas AA. Alcoholic hepatitis. Recent advances in pathogenesis and therapy. Postgrad Med 1994 Dec; 96(8): 61–64, 68–70.
Knechtle SJ et al. Portal hypertension: Surgical management in the 1990s. Surgery 1994 Oct; 116(4):687–693.
Mezey E. Treatment of alcoholic liver disease. Semin Liver Dis 1993 May; 13(2):210–216.
Moulds-Merritt C and Frazee RC. Therapeutic approach to hepatic abscesses. South Med J 1994 Sep; 87(9):884–888.
Muñoz SJ. Difficult management problems in fulminant hepatic failure. Semin Liver Dis 1993 Nov; 13(4):395–413.
Ochsner MG et al. Major hepatic trauma. Surg Clin North Am 1993 Apr; 73(2):337–352.
Pizzi CL and Mion LC. Alcoholism in the elderly: Implications for hospital nurses. Medsurg Nurs 1993 Dec; 2(6):453–458.
Riegler JL and Lake JR. Fulminant hepatic failure. Med Clin North Am 1993 Sep; 77(5):1057–1083.
Runyon BA. Refractory ascites. Semin Liver Dis 1993 Nov; 13(4): 343–351.
Schenker S and Halff GA. Nutritional therapy in alcoholic liver disease. Semin Liver Dis 1995 May; 13(2):196–209.
Tibbs C and Williams R. Viral causes and management of acute liver failure. J Hepatol 1995; 22(Suppl 1):68–73.
Young LM. Managing the patient with liver failure. MedSurg Nurs 1992 Aug; 2(4):275–281.

Cirrhosis

Butler RW. Managing the complications of cirrhosis. Am J Nurs 1994 Mar; 94(3):46–49.
Centers for Disease Control and Prevention. Deaths and hospitalizations from chronic liver disease and cirrhosis—United States, 1980–1989. MMWR 1993 Jan 8; 41(52 & 53):969–973.
Covington H. Nursing care of patients with alcoholic liver disease. Crit Care Nurse 1993 June; 13(3):47–57.
Hillaire S et al. Peritoneovenous shunting of intractable ascites in patients with cirrhosis: Improving results and predictive factors of failure. Surgery 1993 Apr; 113(4):373–379.
Kondrup J, Nielsen K, and Hamberg O. Nutritional therapy in patients with liver cirrhosis. Eur J Clin Nutr 1992 Apr; 46(4):239–246.

Liver Transplantation

Bismuth H et al. Surgical treatment of hepatocellular carcinoma in cirrhosis: Liver resection or transplantation? Transplant Proc 1993 Feb; 25(1):1066–1067.
Bonet H et al. Survival of patients transplanted with alcoholic hepatitis plus cirrhosis as compared with those with cirrhosis alone. Transplant Proc 1993 Feb; 25(1):1126–1127.
Gholson CF, McDonald J, and McMillan R. Liver transplantation. When is it indicated and what can be expected afterwards? Postgrad Med 1995 Feb; 97(2):101–104, 107–109, 113–114.
Laifer SA and Guido RS. Reproductive function and outcome of pregnancy after liver transplantation in women. Mayo Clin Proc 1995 Apr; 70(4):388–394.
Lake JR (ed). Advances in liver transplantation. Gastroenterol Clin North Am 1993 June; 22(2):213–473.
O'Connor TP, Lewis WD, and Jenkins RL. Biliary tract complications after liver transplantation. Arch Surg 1995 Mar; 130(3): 312–317.
Smith SL and Ciferni M. Liver transplantation for acute hepatic failure: A review of clinical experience and management. Am J Crit Care 1993 2(2):137–144.
Whiteman K et al. Liver transplantation. Am J Nurs 1990 June 90(6): 68–72.
Wood RP et al. Liver transplantation. The last ten years. Surg Clin North Am 1994 Oct; 74(5):1133–1154.

Esophageal Varices

Adams L and Soulen MC. TIPS: A new alternative for the variceal bleeder. Am J Crit Care 1993; 2(3):196–201.
Burns SM et al. Evaluation and revision of a vasopressin/nitroglycerin protocol for use in variceal bleeding. Am J Crit Care 1993; 2(3):202–207.
Burns SM and Martin M. VP/NTG therapy in the patient with variceal bleeding. Crit Care Nurse 1990; 10(9):42–49.

Doherty MM and Carver DK. New relief for esophageal varices. Am J Nurs 1993 Apr; 93(4):58–63.

Goff JS. Gastroesophageal varices: Pathogenesis and therapy of acute bleeding. Gastroenterol Clin North Am 1993 Dec; 22(4): 779–798.

Ink O et al. Does elective scherotherapy improve the efficacy of long-term propranolol for prevention of recurrent bleeding in patients with severe cirrhosis? A prospective multicenter, randomized trial. Hepatology 1992; 16(4):912–919.

Lopes GM and Grace ND. Gastroesophageal varices: Prevention of bleeding and rebleeding. Gastroenterol Clin North Am 1993 Dec; 22(4):801–818.

Marshall JB. Bleeding esophagogastric varices: Ways to treat active episodes and prevent recurrence. Postgrad Med 1991 May 1; 89(6):147–150, 155–158.

Rikkers LF and Gongliang J. Variceal hemorrhage: Surgical therapy. Gastroenterol Clin North Am 1993 Dec; 22(4):821–842.

Sanyal AJ et al. Bleeding gastroesophageal varices. Semin Liver Dis 1993 Nov; 13(4):328–342.

Hepatitis

Alter MJ. Epidemiology of hepatitis C in the West. Semin Liver Dis 1995 Feb; 15(1):5–14.

Davis GL. Hepatitis C virus antibody in patients with chronic autoimmune hepatitis: Pitfalls in diagnosis and implications for treatment [editorial]. Mayo Clin Proc 1991 June; 66(6):647–650.

Davis GL et al. Treatment of chronic hepatitis C with recombinant interferon alfa. A multicenter randomized, controlled trial. N Engl J Med 1989 Nov 30; 321(22):1501–1506.

De Medina M and Schiff ER. Hepatitis C: Diagnosis assays. Semin Liver Dis 1995 Feb; 15(1):33–40.

Di Biscegli AM et al. Recombinant interferon alfa therapy for chronic hepatitis C. A randomized, double-blind, placebo-controlled trial. N Engl J Med 1989 Nov 30; 321:1506–1510.

Fried MW and Hoofnagle JH. Therapy of hepatitis C. Semin Liver Dis 1995 15(1):82–91.

Gitlin N and Serio KM. Ischemic hepatitis: Widening horizons. Am J Gastroenterol 1992 July; 87(7):831–836.

Jackson MM and Rymer TE. Viral hepatitis. Anatomy of a diagnosis. Am J Nurs 1994 Jan; 94(1):43–48.

Koff RS. Seroepidemiology of hepatitis A in the United States. J Infec Dis 1995 Mar; 171 (Supp 1):S19–S23.

Liang TJ et al. Fulminant or subfulminant non-A, non-B viral hepatitis: The role of hepatitis C and E viruses. Gastroenterology 1993 Feb; 104(21):556–561.

Lisanti P and Talotta D. Hepatitis D: Yet another reason to get your HBV vaccine. Am J Nurs 1990 Apr; 90(4):29–30.

Marwick C. Hepatitis A vaccine set for 2-year-olds to adults. JAMA 1995 Mar 22/29; 273(12):906–907.

Morgan TR. Treatment of alcoholic hepatitis. Semin Liver Dis 1993 Nov; 13(4):384–393.

Roop JA. Implementation of a hepatitis B vaccine program: A how-to guide for home care providers. Home Healthcare Nurse 1993; 11(4):24–29.

Liver Cancer

Greene FL and Dorsay D. Laparoscopic evaluation of abdominal malignancy. Cancer Practice 1993 May/June; 1(1):29–34.

Keehn DM and Frank-Stromborg M. A worldwide perspective on the epidemiology and primary prevention of liver cancer. Cancer Nurs 1991 Aug 14(4):163–174.

La Vecchia C et al. Medical history and primary liver cancer. Cancer Res 1990 Oct 1; 50(19):6274–6277.

Schneider PD. Liver resection and laser hyperthermia. Surg Clin North Am 1992 June; 72(3):623–639.

Vauthey JN et al. Factors affecting long-term outcome after hepatic resection for hepatocellular carcinoma. Am J Surg 1995 Jan;169(1):28–34.

Gallbladder Disease

Bordelon BM, Hobday KA, and Junter JG. Laser vs electrosurgery in laparoscopic cholecystectomy: A prospective randomized trial. Arch Surg 1993 Feb; 128(2):233–236.

Frazee RC et al. What are the contraindications for laparoscopic cholecystectomy. Am J Surg 1992 Nov; 164(5):491–495.

Gallstones and Laparoscopic Cholecystectomy. NIH Consensus Statement 1992 Sep 14–16; 10(3):1–26.

Saunders-Kirkwood KD et al. Cholecystectomy: The impact of social change. Ann Surg 1992 Apr; 215(4):318–325.

Van Steenbergen W et al. Percutaneous transhepatic cholecystostomy for acute complicated calculous cholecystitis in elderly patients. J Am Geriatr Soc 1993 Feb; 41(2):157–162.

Vauthey JN et al. Indications and limitations of percutaneous cholecystostomy for acute cholecystitis. Surgery 1993 Jan; 176(1):49–54.

Wilson RG et al. Laparoscopic cholecystectomy as a safe and effective treatment for severe acute cholecystitis. Br Med J 1992 Aug 15; 305(6850):394–396.

Zuker KA, Bailey RW, and Flowers J. Laparoscopic management of acute and chronic cholecystitis. Surg Clin North Am 1992 Oct; 72(5):1045–1067.

INFORMATION/RESOURCES

Agencies

Alcoholics Anonymous World Service (AA)
PO Box 459, Grand Central Station, New York, NY 10163

American Liver Foundation
998 Pompton Ave., Cedar Grove, NJ 07009

National Council on Alcoholism, Inc.
12 W 21st St., New York, NY 10010

National Institute on Alcohol Abuse and Alcoholism
Rockville, MD 20857

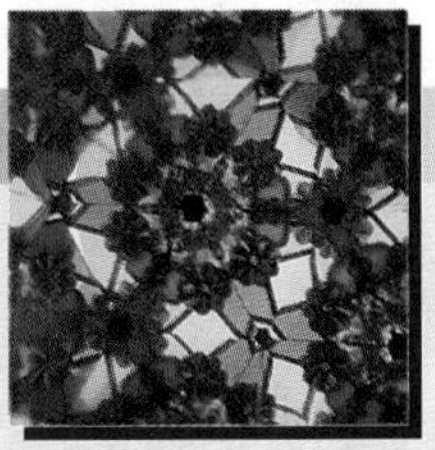

39

Assessment and Management of Patients With Diabetes Mellitus

CHAPTER OUTLINE

Definition

Types of Diabetes

Epidemiology

Overview of Physiology and Pathophysiology

Normal Physiology

Pathophysiology of Diabetes

Etiology

Type I Diabetes

Type II Diabetes

Diagnostic Evaluation

Management

The Diabetes Control and Complications Trial

Dietary Management

Exercise

Monitoring of Glucose and Ketones

Insulin Therapy

Oral Antidiabetic Agents

Patient Education and Home Care Considerations

Acute Complications of Diabetes

Hypoglycemia (Insulin Reactions)

Diabetic Ketoacidosis

Hyperglycemic Hyperosmolar Nonketotic Syndrome

NURSING PROCESS: The Patient With Newly Diagnosed Diabetes Mellitus

Long-Term Complications of Diabetes

Macrovascular Complications

Microvascular Complications

Foot and Leg Problems in Diabetes

Special Issues in Diabetes

The Patient With Diabetes Undergoing Surgery

Management of Hospitalized Diabetic Patients

Stress

Gerontologic Considerations

NURSING PROCESS: The Patient With Diabetes as a Secondary Diagnosis

Critical Thinking Exercises

LEARNING OBJECTIVES

On completion of this chapter, the learner will be able to:

1. Differentiate between type I and type II diabetes
2. Describe etiologic factors associated with diabetes
3. Relate the clinical manifestations of diabetes to the associated pathophysiologic alterations
4. Identify the diagnostic and clinical significance of blood glucose tests
5. Explain the dietary modifications used for management of persons with diabetes
6. Describe the relationship between diet, exercise, and medication (*i.e.,* insulin or oral hypoglycemic agents) for persons with diabetes
7. Develop a plan for teaching insulin self-administration
8. Identify the role of oral hypoglycemic agents in diabetic therapy
9. Differentiate between hypoglycemia and diabetic ketoacidosis, and hyperosmolar nonketotic syndrome
10. Describe management strategies for a person with diabetes to use during "sick days"
11. Describe the major macrovascular, microvascular, and neuropathic complications of diabetes and the self-care behaviors important in their prevention
12. Identify the teaching aids and community support groups that are available for persons with diabetes
13. Use the nursing process as a framework for care of the patient with diabetes

Definition

Diabetes mellitus is a group of heterogeneous disorders characterized by elevated levels of glucose in the blood, or hyperglycemia. Normally a certain amount of glucose circulates in the blood. This glucose is formed in the liver from ingested food. Insulin, a hormone produced by the pancreas, controls the level of glucose in the blood by regulating the production and storage of glucose.

In diabetes the body's ability to respond to insulin may decrease or the pancreas may stop producing insulin entirely. This leads to hyperglycemia, which may result in acute metabolic complications such as diabetic ketoacidosis and hyperglycemic hyperosmolar nonketotic (HHNK) syndrome. Long-term hyperglycemia may contribute to chronic microvascular complications (kidney and eye disease) and neuropathic complications (diseases of the nerves). Diabetes is also associated with an increased occurrence of macrovascular diseases, including myocardial infarction, strokes, and peripheral vascular disease.

Types of Diabetes

There are several different types of diabetes mellitus; they may differ in cause, clinical course, and treatment. The major classifications of diabetes are

- Type I: Insulin-dependent diabetes mellitus (IDDM)
- Type II: Non–insulin-dependent diabetes mellitus (NIDDM)
- Diabetes mellitus associated with other conditions or syndromes
- Gestational diabetes mellitus (GDM)

Approximately 5% to 10% of people with diabetes have type I, insulin-dependent diabetes. In this form of diabetes, the beta cells of the pancreas that normally produce insulin are destroyed by an autoimmune process. As a result, insulin injections are needed to control the blood glucose levels. Type I diabetes is characterized by a sudden onset, usually before the age of 30 years.

Approximately 90% to 95% of people with diabetes have type II, non–insulin-dependent diabetes. Type II diabetes results from a decreased sensitivity to insulin (called insulin resistance) or from a decreased amount of insulin production. Type II diabetes is first treated with diet and exercise. If elevated glucose levels persist, diet and exercise are supplemented with oral hypoglycemic agents. In some individuals with type II diabetes, oral agents do not control hyperglycemia, and insulin injections are required. In addition, some individuals who usually can control their type II diabetes with diet, exercise, and oral agents may require insulin injections during periods of acute physiologic stress (such as illness or surgery). Type II diabetes occurs most frequently in people who are older than 30 years of age and obese.

Diabetes complications may develop in any person with type I or type II diabetes—not only in patients who take insulin. Some persons with type II diabetes who are treated with oral medications may have the impression that they do not really have diabetes or that they simply have "borderline" diabetes. They may believe that, compared with diabetic patients who require insulin injections, their diabetes is not a "serious" problem. It is important for the nurse to emphasize to these individuals that they actually do have diabetes and not a borderline problem with sugar. ("Borderline" diabetes is classified as impaired glucose tolerance and refers to a condition in which blood glucose levels fall between normal and those levels considered diagnostic for diabetes [see p. 1022].)

Table 39-1 summarizes the major classifications of diabetes, current terminology, old labels, and major clinical characteristics. It is important to recognize that this classification system is dynamic in two ways. First, as research findings become available, it appears that there are many differences among individuals within each category. Second, with time, patients may move from one category to another. For example, a woman with gestational diabetes may, after delivery, move into the non–insulin-dependent (type II) category. These types also differ in their etiology, clinical course, and management.

Epidemiology

Diabetes mellitus is a chronic disease that affects approximately 12 million people. Seven million of the 12 million people with diabetes have been diagnosed; the remainder are undiagnosed. In the United States, approximately 650,000 new cases of diabetes are diagnosed yearly (*Healthy People 2000,* 1990).

Diabetes is especially prevalent in the elderly. Among people older than 65 years of age, 8.6% have type II diabetes. This figure includes 15% of the nursing home population. Hispanic, black, and some Native American populations have a higher rate of diabetes than the white population. Some Native American populations, such as the Pima, have adult diabetes rates of 20% to 50%.

In the United States diabetes is the leading cause of new blindness among 25- to 74-year-olds and also the leading cause of nontraumatic amputations. Thirty percent of patients beginning dialysis each year have diabetes. Diabetes is the third leading cause of death by disease, mostly because of the high rate of coronary artery disease among people with diabetes.

The economic cost of diabetes continues to rise because of increasing medical costs and an aging population. Costs directly related to diabetes are estimated to be *at least* $20 billion annually, including direct medical care expenses and indirect costs attributable to disability and premature death.

Hospitalization rates for people with diabetes are 2.4 times greater for adults and 5.3 times greater for children than for the general population. Half of all persons with diabetes who are older than 65 years are hospitalized each year. Severe and life-threatening complications often contribute to increased rates of hospitalization for patients with diabetes.

Overview of Physiology and Pathophysiology

Normal Physiology

Insulin is secreted by **beta** cells, which are one of four types of cells in the islets of Langerhans in the pancreas. Insulin is

TABLE 39-1 Classification of Diabetes Mellitus and Related Glucose Intolerances

Current Classification	Previous Classifications	Clinical Characteristics
Type I: Insulin-dependent diabetes mellitus (IDDM) (5%–10% of all diabetes)	Juvenile diabetes Juvenile-onset diabetes Ketosis-prone diabetes Brittle diabetes	Onset any age, but usually young (<30 yrs) Usually thin at diagnosis; with recent weight loss Etiology includes genetic, immunologic, or environmental factors (*e.g.*, virus) Often have islet cell antibodies Often have antibodies to insulin even before insulin treatment Little or no endogenous insulin Need insulin to preserve life Ketosis-prone when insulin absent Acute complication of hyperglycemia: diabetic ketoacidosis
Type II: Non–insulin-dependent diabetes (NIDDM) (90%–95% of all diabetes: obese—80% of type II; nonobese—20% of type II)	Adult-onset diabetes Maturity-onset diabetes Ketosis-resistant diabetes Stable diabetes	Onset any age, usually over 30 years Usually obese at diagnosis Etiology includes obesity, heredity, or environmental factors No islet cell antibodies Decrease in endogenous insulin or increased with insulin resistance Majority can control blood glucose through weight loss if obese Oral hypoglycemic agents may improve blood glucose levels if dietary modification and exercise are unsuccessful May need insulin on a short- or long-term basis to prevent hyperglycemia Ketosis rare, except in stress or infection Acute complication: hyperosmolar nonketotic syndrome
Diabetes mellitus associated with other conditions or syndromes	Secondary diabetes	Accompanied by conditions known or suspected to cause the disease: pancreatic diseases; hormonal abnormalities; drugs such as glucocorticoids and estrogen-containing preparations Depending on the ability of the pancreas to produce insulin, the patient may require treatment with oral agents or insulin.
Gestational diabetes	Gestational diabetes	Onset is during pregnancy, usually in the second or third trimester Due to hormones secreted by the placenta, which inhibit the action of insulin Above-normal risk of perinatal complications, especially macrosomia (abnormally large babies) Treat with diet and, if needed, insulin to strictly maintain normal blood glucose levels Occurs in about 2%–5% of all pregnancies Glucose intolerance transitory but may recur: · In subsequent pregnancies · 30%–40% will develop overt diabetes (usually type II) within 10 years (especially if obese) Risk factors include: obesity, age older than 30 years, family history of diabetes, previous large babies (over 9 lb) Screening tests (glucose challenge test) should be performed on ALL pregnant women between 24 and 28 weeks' gestation
Impaired glucose tolerance	Borderline diabetes Latent diabetes Chemical diabetes Subclinical diabetes Asymptomatic diabetes	Blood glucose levels between normal and that of diabetes 25% eventually develop diabetes Above-normal susceptibility to atherosclerotic disease Renal and retinal complications usually not significant May be obese or nonobese; obese should reduce weight Should be screened for diabetes periodically

(continued)

TABLE 39-1 *(continued)*

Current Classification	Previous Classifications	Clinical Characteristics
Previous abnormality of glucose tolerance (PrevAGT)	Latent diabetes Prediabetes	Current normal glucose metabolism Previous history of hyperglycemia (*e.g.*, during pregnancy or illness) Periodic blood glucose screening after age 40 if there is a family history of diabetes or if symptomatic Encourage ideal body weight because loss of 10–15 lbs may improve glycemic control
Potential abnormality of glucose tolerance (PotAGT)	Prediabetes	No history of glucose intolerance Increased risk of diabetes if: · Positive family history · Obesity · Mothers of babies over 9 pounds at birth · Members of certain Native American Indian tribes with high prevalence of diabetes (*e.g.*, Pima) Screening and weight advice as in PrevAGT

an anabolic, or storage, hormone. When a meal is eaten, insulin secretion increases and moves glucose from the blood into muscle, liver, and fat cells. In those cells, insulin has the following effects:

- Stimulates storage of glucose in the liver and muscle (in the form of glycogen)
- Enhances storage of dietary fat in adipose tissue
- Accelerates transport of amino acids (derived from dietary protein) into cells

Insulin also inhibits the breakdown of stored glucose, protein, and fat.

During "fasting" periods (between meals and overnight), the pancreas continuously releases a small amount of insulin along with another pancreatic hormone called glucagon (which is secreted by the **alpha** cells of the islets of Langerhans). The insulin and the glucagon together maintain a constant level of glucose in the blood by stimulating the release of glucose from the liver.

Initially, the liver produces glucose through the breakdown of glycogen (**glycogenolysis**). After 8 to 12 hours without food, the liver forms glucose from the breakdown of noncarbohydrate substances, including amino acids (**gluconeogenesis**).

Pathophysiology of Diabetes

Type I Diabetes. In type I diabetes there is inability to produce insulin because pancreatic beta cells have been destroyed by an autoimmune process. Fasting hyperglycemia occurs as a result of unchecked glucose production by the liver. In addition, glucose derived from food cannot be stored in the liver, but instead remains in the bloodstream and contributes to postprandial (after meal) hyperglycemia.

If the concentration of glucose in the blood is sufficiently high, the kidneys may not reabsorb all of the filtered glucose; the glucose then appears in the urine (**glucosuria**). When excess glucose is excreted in the urine, it is accompanied by excessive loss of fluids and electrolytes. This is called **osmotic diuresis**. As a result of the excess loss of fluid, the patient experiences increased urination (**polyuria**) and increased thirst (**polydipsia**).

Insulin deficiency also impairs the metabolism of proteins and fats, leading to weight loss. Patients may experience an increased appetite (**polyphagia**) because of the decreased storage of calories. Other symptoms include fatigue and weakness.

Because insulin normally controls glycogenolysis (breakdown of stored glucose) and gluconeogenesis (production of new glucose from amino acids and other substrates), in people with insulin deficiency, these processes occur unrestrained and contribute further to hyperglycemia. In addition, fat breakdown occurs, resulting in an increased production of ketone bodies, which are the byproducts of fat breakdown. **Ketone bodies** are acids that disturb the acid–base balance of the body when they accumulate in excess amounts. The resulting diabetic ketoacidosis (DKA) may cause signs and symptoms such as abdominal pain, nausea, vomiting, hyperventilation, fruity odor of the breath, and, if left untreated, altered level of consciousness, coma, and even death. Initiation of insulin treatment along with fluid and electrolytes as needed rapidly improves the metabolic abnormalities and resolves symptoms of hyperglycemia and DKA. Diet and exercise with frequent monitoring of blood glucose levels are also important components of therapy.

Type II Diabetes. In type II diabetes there are two main problems related to insulin: insulin resistance and impaired insulin secretion. **Insulin resistance** refers to a decreased sensitivity of the tissues to insulin. Normally, insulin binds to special receptors on cell surfaces. As a result of insulin binding to these receptors, a series of reactions involved in glucose metabolism occurs within the cell. The insulin resistance of type II diabetes is associated with a decrease in these intracellular reactions. The insulin thus becomes less effective at stimulating glucose uptake by the tissues.

To overcome insulin resistance and to prevent the buildup of glucose in the blood, there must be an increase in the amount of insulin secreted. In people with impaired glucose tolerance this occurs through excess secretion of insulin, and the glucose level is maintained at normal or slightly elevated. However, if the beta cells are unable to keep up with the increased demand for insulin, the glucose level rises, and type II diabetes develops.

Despite the impaired insulin secretion that is characteristic of type II diabetes, there is enough insulin present to prevent the breakdown of fat and the accompanying production of ketone bodies. Therefore, DKA does not occur in type II diabetes. Uncontrolled type II diabetes may, however, lead to another acute problem called hyperglycemic hyperosmolar nonketotic (HHNK) syndrome (see pp. 1049–1050).

Type II diabetes occurs most commonly in people older than 30 years of age who are obese. Because it is associated with a slow (over years), progressive glucose intolerance, the onset of type II diabetes may go undetected for many years. If symptoms are experienced, they are frequently mild and may include fatigue, irritability, polyuria, polydipsia, skin wounds that heal poorly, vaginal infections, or blurred vision (if glucose levels are very high).

For most patients (approximately 75%), type II diabetes is detected incidentally (*e.g.*, when routine laboratory tests are performed). One consequence of diabetes going undetected for many years is that long-term diabetes complications (*e.g.*, eye disease, peripheral neuropathy, peripheral vascular disease) may have developed before the actual diagnosis of diabetes is made.

Because insulin resistance is associated with obesity, the primary treatment of type II diabetes is weight loss. Exercise is also important in enhancing the effectiveness of insulin. Oral hypoglycemic agents may be added if diet and exercise are not successful in controlling blood glucose levels. If the use of maximum doses of oral agents fails to reduce glucose levels to satisfactory levels, insulin is used. Some patients require insulin on an ongoing basis, and a few may require insulin on a temporary basis during periods of acute physiologic stress, such as illness or surgery.

Diabetes and Pregnancy. Diabetes that occurs during pregnancy is a special concern. Women who have diabetes diagnosed before conception should be counseled about the management of diabetes during pregnancy. Poor control of diabetes (hyperglycemia) at conception has been associated with the occurrence of congenital malformations. For this reason women with diabetes should be in excellent diabetes control before conception and throughout pregnancy. It is recommended that women with diabetes begin a program of intensive therapy (testing blood glucose four times per day and taking three to four injections of insulin per day) with the goal of achieving a normal hemoglobin A_{1C} (described on p. 1029) 3 months before conception. Close monitoring and care by physicians who specialize in high-risk pregnancy are recommended.

Uncontrolled diabetes at the time of delivery has been associated with an increased incidence of fetal macrosomia (very large babies), difficult labor and delivery, cesarean section, and stillbirth. In addition, infants born to hyperglycemic mothers may become hypoglycemic at birth. This can occur because the infant's normal pancreas has been secreting insulin to compensate for the mother's hyperglycemia. These infants require close monitoring in the nursery, and their blood glucose levels should be measured frequently. If hypoglycemia occurs, feedings of glucose water are administered.

Gestational diabetes occurs in women who did not have diabetes before pregnancy. Hyperglycemia develops during pregnancy because of the secretion of placental hormones. All pregnant women should be screened for diabetes between the 24th and 27th weeks of gestation. Initial management includes dietary modification and blood glucose monitoring. If hyperglycemia persists, insulin is prescribed. Oral hypoglycemic agents should not be used during pregnancy. Goals for blood glucose during pregnancy are 70 to 100 mg/dl before meals and less than 165 mg/dl at 2 hours after meals.

After delivery of the infant, blood glucose levels in the woman with gestational diabetes return to normal. However, many women who have had gestational diabetes develop type II diabetes later on in life. Therefore, all women who have had gestational diabetes should be counseled to maintain their ideal body weight and to exercise regularly to attempt to avoid the onset of type II diabetes.

Etiology

Type I Diabetes

Type I diabetes is characterized by destruction of the pancreatic beta cells. It is thought that a combination of genetic, immunologic, and possibly environmental (*e.g.*, viral) factors contribute to beta cell destruction.

Genetic Factors. People do not inherit type I diabetes itself; rather, they inherit a genetic predisposition, or tendency, toward developing type I diabetes. This genetic tendency has been found in people with certain HLA (human leukocyte antigen) types. HLA refers to a cluster of genes responsible for transplantation antigens and other immune processes. Ninety-five percent of Caucasian patients with type I diabetes exhibit specific HLA types (DR3 or DR4). The risk of developing type I diabetes is increased three to five times in people who have one of these two HLA types. The risk is increased 10 to 20 times in people who have both DR3 and DR4 HLA types (as compared with the general population).

Immunologic Factors. In type I diabetes there is evidence of an autoimmune response. This is an abnormal response in which antibodies are directed against normal tissues of the body, responding to these tissues as if they are foreign. Autoantibodies against islet cells and against endogenous (internal) insulin have been detected in people at the time of diagnosis and even several years before the development of clinical signs of type I diabetes. Research is being conducted to evaluate the effect of immunosuppressive agents on progression of disease in persons with newly diagnosed type I diabetes or persons with prediabetes (those with detectable antibodies but no clinical symptoms of diabetes). Other research is examining the protective effect of small doses of insulin on beta cell function.

Environmental Factors. There are ongoing investigations into possible external factors that may initiate destruction of the beta cell. For example, it has been proposed that certain viruses or toxins may precipitate the autoimmune process that leads to beta cell destruction.

The interaction of genetic, immunologic, and environmental factors in the etiology of type I diabetes is the subject of continuing research. Although the events that lead to beta cell destruction are not fully understood, it is generally accepted that a genetic susceptibility is a common underlying factor in the development of type I diabetes.

Type II Diabetes

The exact mechanisms that lead to insulin resistance and impaired insulin secretion in type II diabetes are unknown. Genetic factors are thought to play a role in the development of insulin resistance. In addition, there are certain risk factors that are known to be associated with the development of type II diabetes. These include

- Age (insulin resistance tends to increase with age over 65)
- Obesity
- Family history
- Ethnic group (in the United States, there is a higher chance of type II diabetes developing in Hispanic and certain Native American populations, and, to a lesser degree, in the African-American population)

Diagnostic Evaluation

The presence of abnormally high blood glucose levels is the criterion on which the diagnosis of diabetes should be based. Fasting plasma glucose levels above 140 mg/dl (SI: 7.8 mmol/L) or random plasma glucose levels over 200 mg/dl (SI: 11.1 mmol/L) on more than one occasion is diagnostic of diabetes. If fasting glucose levels are normal or nearly normal, the diagnosis must be based on a glucose tolerance test.

Glucose Tolerance Test. Currently, the oral glucose tolerance test (OGTT) is more sensitive than the intravenous glucose tolerance test (IVGTT), which is used only in special circumstances (*e.g.*, for the patient who has had gastric surgery). The OGTT is carried out through administration of a simple carbohydrate solution.

The patient ingests high-carbohydrate (150 to 300 g) meals for 3 days preceding the test. After an overnight fast, a blood sample is drawn. Then a 75-g carbohydrate load, usually in the form of a carbonated sugar beverage (Glucola), is administered to the patient. The patient is instructed to sit quietly during the test and to avoid exercise, smoking, coffee, and any other oral intake except water.

The World Health Organization (WHO) recommends that blood samples be drawn 2 hours after glucose ingestion. Recommendations from the National Diabetes Data Group include also drawing blood samples at 30 and 60 minutes after glucose ingestion. See Chart 39-1 for specific WHO diagnostic criteria for diabetes mellitus.

Several factors affect the OGTT, including the method of analysis, source of the specimen (whole blood, plasma, or serum, capillary or venous blood), diet, activity level, amount of bed rest, presence of chronic disease, medication, and amount of the glucose load. In the elderly, diet, activity level, and medications present particular problems in interpreting the test results.

Dietary preparation for the test is very important because food intake may affect test results. It may be necessary to give written instructions to the patient to ensure the required intake of carbohydrate. If the diet is normal and the person's weight is stable, 150 g/day is usually sufficient.

CHART 39-1
World Health Organization Diagnostic Criteria for Diabetes Mellitus in Nonpregnant Adults

On at least two occasions:

1. *Random* plasma glucose > 200 mg/dl (11.1 mmol/L)

or

2. *Fasting* plasma glucose > 140 mg/dl (7.8 mmol/L)

or

3. *2-hour sample* during 75-g OGTT (Oral Glucose Tolerance Test) > 200 mg/dl (11.1 mmol/L)

(World Health Organization. Diabetes mellitus. Report of a WHO study group. Tech Report Series No. 727, 1985.)

Medications that affect glucose tolerance should be discontinued, if possible, for about 3 days before the test. Four commonly prescribed medications affect the OGTT: diuretics (usually thiazides), corticosteroids, synthetic estrogens, and phenytoin (Dilantin). Other interfering agents include high doses of nicotinic acid, alcohol, and the chronic ingestion of salicylates and monoamine oxidase (MAO) inhibitors (especially hydrazine derivatives).

Special circumstances that affect the OGTT are pregnancy, gastric surgery, and advanced age. There is a special modification of the diagnostic criteria for the pregnant patient. In patients who have had gastric surgery, the IVGTT is necessary because an oral glucose load passes quickly into the small intestine, leading to a rapid absorption of glucose and therefore to glucose levels that are abnormal.

Gerontologic Considerations. Elevated blood glucose levels appear to be age related and occur in both men and women throughout the world. Elevation of blood glucose appears in the fifth decade of life and increases in frequency with advancing age. When elderly people with overt diabetes are excluded from the statistics, approximately 10% to 30% of elderly people have age-related hyperglycemia.

The question then arises whether age-related hyperglycemia is part of the normal aging process and benign or pathologic and requiring therapeutic intervention. Several studies have suggested that the hyperglycemia is pathologic because it leads to macrovascular complications.

The cause of age-related changes in carbohydrate metabolism is still not resolved. Apparently, delayed absorption from the gastrointestinal tract is not a factor. Other possibilities include poor diet, physical inactivity, a decrease in the lean body mass in which ingested carbohydrate may be stored, altered insulin secretion, and insulin resistance.

Management

The main goal of the treatment of diabetes is to try to normalize insulin activity and blood glucose levels in an attempt to reduce the development of the vascular and neuropathic complications. The therapeutic goal within each type of diabetes is to achieve normal blood glucose levels (euglycemia) without hypoglycemia and without seriously disrupting the patient's usual activity patterns.

There are five components of management for diabetes:

Diet
Exercise
Monitoring
Medication (as needed)
Education

Treatment is variable throughout the course of the disease because of changes in lifestyle and physical and emotional status as well as advances in treatment methods resulting from research. Therefore, the management of diabetes involves constant assessment and modification of the treatment plan by health professionals as well as daily adjustments in therapy by the patient. Although the health care team directs the treatment, it is the patient who is faced with the daily charge of managing the intricacies of a complex therapeutic regimen. For this reason, patient and family education is seen as an essential component of diabetes treatment—equal in importance to other components of the treatment regimen.

The Diabetes Control and Complications Trial

The Diabetes Control and Complications Trial (DCCT) was a 10-year prospective clinical trial designed to determine the impact of intensive glucose control on the development and progression of complications such as retinopathy, nephropathy, and neuropathy. A cohort of 1,441 people with type I diabetes was randomly assigned to conventional treatment (1 to 2 insulin injections per day) or intensive treatment (3 to 4 insulin injections per day or insulin pump therapy). End-point data were collected for 9 years (1993).

The results of the DCCT demonstrated that the risk for developing retinopathy was reduced by 76%. In addition, the incidences of microalbuminuria and albuminuria, early signs of nephropathy, were reduced by 39% and 54%, respectively. Further, the incidence of neuropathy was decreased by 60% through control of serum glucose levels to normal or near-normal levels. On the basis of these results, it is now recommended that all patients with diabetes strive to achieve the most optimal glucose control to reduce their risks for complications.

The major adverse effect of intensive therapy was a threefold increase in incidence of severe hypoglycemia (severe enough to require assistance from another person), coma, or seizure. Because of these adverse effects, intensive therapy must be initiated with caution and must be accompanied by intensive education of the patient and family and by responsible behavior on the part of the patient. Careful screening of patients is a key step in initiating intensive therapy. There are other situations that preclude the initiation of very tight control of blood glucose (see discussion of insulin, pp. 1034–1035.)

Dietary Management

General Principles. Diet and weight control constitute the foundation of diabetes management. Nutritional management of the patient with diabetes is geared toward the following goals:

1. Provision of all the essential food constituents (*e.g.*, vitamins, minerals)
2. Achievement and maintenance of reasonable weight
3. Meeting energy needs
4. Prevention of wide daily fluctuations in blood glucose levels with blood glucose levels as close to normal as is safe and practical
5. Decrease of blood lipid levels, if elevated

For patients who require insulin to help control blood glucose levels, maintaining as much consistency as possible in the amount of calories and carbohydrates eaten at different meal times is important for control of blood glucose. In addition, consistency in the approximate time intervals between meals, with the addition of snacks, if necessary, helps in the prevention of hypoglycemic reactions and in overall blood glucose control.

For obese patients (especially those with type II diabetes), weight loss is the key to the treatment of diabetes. For obese patients in general, weight loss is the major preventive factor for the development of diabetes. Obesity is associated with an increased resistance to insulin and is one of the main etiologic factors associated with type II diabetes. Some obese type II diabetic patients who require insulin or oral agents for control of blood glucose may be able to significantly reduce or completely eliminate the need for medication through weight loss. Even as small a weight loss as 10% of total weight can significantly improve blood glucose levels. For obese diabetic patients who do not take insulin, consistency of meal content or timing is not as critical. Rather, the major focus is on decreasing the overall number of calories eaten. However, meals should not be skipped. Spacing food throughout the day places more manageable demands on the pancreas.

Long-term adherence to the meal plan is one of the most challenging aspects of diabetes management. For obese patients it may be more realistic to only moderately restrict calories. For those who have lost weight, maintaining the weight loss is often difficult. To assist these patients in incorporating new dietary habits into their lifestyles, participation in behavioral therapy, group support, and ongoing nutrition counseling is encouraged.

For all diabetic patients, the meal plan must take into consideration the patient's food preferences, lifestyle, usual eating times, and ethnic and cultural background. For patients using intensive insulin therapy regimens, there may be a greater flexibility in the timing and content of meals by making adjustments for changes in eating and exercise habits.

Meal Planning

Calorie Requirements. The first step in preparing a meal plan is to obtain a thorough diet history to identify the patient's eating habits and lifestyle. It is also necessary to assess the need for weight loss, gain, or maintenance. In most instances, the person with type II diabetes requires weight reduction. The most important objective in dietary management of diabetes is control of total calorie intake to attain or maintain a reasonable body weight and control of blood glucose levels. Success of this alone is often associated with reversal of hyperglycemia in type II diabetes. However, achieving this goal is not always easy. Calorie-controlled diets can be used by first calculating the individual's calorie requirements. Age, gender, height, and weight are used in the Harris-Benedict formula to determine basal energy expenditure (BEE), reflecting minimal energy needs. An activity factor is then factored into the BEE to provide the actual number of calories required for weight maintenance. To promote a 1- to 2-pound weight loss, 500 to 1000 calories are subtracted from the total. The calories are distributed into carbohydrates, proteins, and fats, and a meal plan can then be developed.

The 1986 Exchange Lists for Meal Planning are presented to the patient using the appropriate amount of calories with strict diet adherence as the goal. Unfortunately, calorie-controlled diets are often confusing and difficult to comply with as they require patients to measure precise portions and to eat specific foods and amounts at each meal and snack. In this instance, developing a meal plan based on the individuals usual eating habits and lifestyle is often a more realistic approach to glucose control and weight loss or weight maintenance. Both instances require the patient to work closely with a registered dietitian to assess current eating habits and to achieve realistic, individualized goals.

In a young patient with type I diabetes, priority should be given to providing a diet with enough calories to maintain normal growth and development. Some patients may be underweight at the onset of type I diabetes because of rapid weight loss from severe hyperglycemia. The goal with these patients initially may be to provide a higher-calorie diet to regain lost weight.

Calorie Distribution. A diabetic meal plan focuses on the percentage of calories to come from carbohydrates, proteins, and fats. There are two main types of carbohydrates—complex and simple. Starches such as bread, cereal, rice, and pasta are complex carbohydrates; fruit and sugars are examples of simple carbohydrates. In general, carbohydrate foods have the greatest effect on blood glucose levels because they are more quickly digested than other foods and are converted into glucose rapidly. Several decades ago it was recommended that diabetic diets contain more calories from protein and fat foods than from carbohydrates to reduce postmeal increases in blood glucose levels. However, more recently it has been found that complex carbohydrates are absorbed more gradually from the gastrointestinal tract and cause less of a rise in blood glucose level than initially thought. In addition, diets that contained fewer calories from carbohydrates contained increased calories from fats—a problem in trying to reduce the cardiovascular disease commonly associated with diabetes.

The caloric distribution currently recommended is higher in carbohydrates than in fat and protein. However, research into the appropriateness of a higher-carbohydrate diet in patients with decreased glucose tolerance is ongoing, and recommendations may be changed accordingly. Currently, the American Diabetes and American Dietetic Associations recommend that for all levels of caloric intake, 50% to 60% of calories be derived from carbohydrates, 20% to 30% from fat, and the remaining 12% to 20% from protein. These recommendations are also consistent with those of the American Heart Association and American Cancer Society.

Carbohydrates. The goal of the diabetic diet is to emphasize the intake of complex carbohydrates (especially those high in fiber), such as whole-grain breads, cereals, pastas, and beans. However, because certain nutritious foods such as milk and fruit contain simple sugars (lactose and fructose), encouraging complete avoidance of simple sugars is inappropriate. In addition, the use of moderate amounts of sucrose (table sugar) is gaining wider acceptance provided the patient can maintain adequate blood glucose levels, blood lipid levels (including all types of cholesterol and triglycerides), and weight control. For some patients, a more liberal use of simple carbohydrates can be a major factor in promoting adherence to a meal plan. However, they should be used in moderation and incorporated into meals rather than consumed separately.

Fat. The recommendations regarding fat content of the diabetic diet include both reduction in the total percentage of calories from fat sources to less than 30% of the total calories and limitation of the amount of saturated fats to 10% of total calories. In addition, limitation of total intake of dietary cholesterol to less than 300 mg/day is recommended. These recommendations may help in the reduction of risk factors, such as elevated serum cholesterol levels, which are associated with the development of coronary artery disease (CAD), the leading cause of death and disability among persons with diabetes.

Protein. The meal plan may include the use of some nonanimal sources of protein (*e.g.,* legumes, whole grains) to help in the reduction of saturated fat and cholesterol intake. In addition, recommendations for the amount of protein intake may be reduced in patients with early signs of developing renal disease.

Fiber. The use of fiber in diabetes has received increasing attention recently as researchers study the effects on diabetes of a high-carbohydrate, high-fiber diet. This type of diet plays a role in lowering total cholesterol and LDL (low-density lipoprotein) cholesterol in the blood. Increasing fiber in the diet may also improve blood glucose levels, leading to a decrease in the need for exogenous insulin.

There are two classifications of dietary fibers: soluble and insoluble. **Soluble fiber**—in foods such as legumes, oats, and some fruits—plays more of a role in lowering blood glucose and lipid levels than does insoluble fiber.

The mechanism of action of soluble fiber is thought to be related to the formation of a gel in the gastrointestinal tract. This gel slows the emptying of the stomach and the movement of food through the upper digestive tract. The potential glucose-lowering effect of fiber may be caused by the slower rate of glucose absorption from food that contains soluble fiber.

Insoluble fiber is found in whole-grain breads and cereals and in some vegetables. This type of fiber plays more of a role in increasing stool bulk and preventing constipation. Both insoluble and soluble fibers increase satiety, which is helpful for weight loss.

One risk involved in suddenly increasing fiber intake is that it may require adjusting the dosage of insulin or oral agents to prevent hypoglycemia. Other problems may include abdominal fullness, nausea, diarrhea, increased flatulence, and constipation if fluid intake is inadequate. If fiber is added to or increased in the meal plan, it should be done gradually and in consultation with a dietitian. The 1986 Exchange Lists for Meal Planning is an excellent guide for increasing fiber intake. Food choices high in fiber within the vegetable, fruit, and starch/bread exchanges are highlighted in the lists.

It appears that adding more fiber to the meal plan is beneficial. However, research is ongoing to determine how fiber works, which fibers are best, and the amount of fiber that is optimal for blood glucose and lipid control.

Alcohol. The ingestion of alcohol by diabetic patients need not be completely restricted. It is important, however, for patients and health care professionals to be aware of the potential adverse effects of alcohol specific to diabetes.

In general, the same precautions regarding the use of alcohol by the general public should be applied to patients with diabetes. Moderation in the amount of alcohol consumed is recommended. The main danger with the use of alcohol by a diabetic patient is hypoglycemia. This is especially true for patients who take insulin. Alcohol may decrease the normal physiologic reactions in the body that produce glucose (gluconeogenesis). Thus, if a diabetic patient takes alcohol on an empty stomach, there is an increased likelihood of hypoglycemia developing. In addition, excessive alcohol intake may impair a person's ability to recognize and appropriately treat hypoglycemia and to follow a prescribed meal plan to prevent hypoglycemia.

For the person with type II diabetes treated with oral agents, a potential side effect of alcohol consumption is a disulfiram (Antabuse) type of reaction. Depending on the amount of alcohol consumed, the person taking chlorpropamide (Diabinese) may experience facial flushing, warmth, headache, nausea, vomiting, sweating, or thirst within minutes of consuming alcohol. This reaction seems to be less common with other oral agents.

In addition to these immediate potential effects, alcohol consumption may also lead to excessive weight gain (because of the high caloric content of alcohol), hyperlipidemia, and (especially if mixed drinks and liqueurs are consumed) elevated glucose levels.

Patient teaching regarding alcohol intake must emphasize moderation in the amount of alcohol consumed; lower-calorie or less sweet drinks such as "light" beer or dry wine, and the intake of food along with alcohol, are advised. For type II diabetic patients especially, incorporating the calories from alcohol into the overall meal plan is important for weight control.

Food Classification Systems

To teach diet principles and to help patients in meal planning, several systems have been developed in which foods are organized into groups with common characteristics, such as number of calories, composition of foods (*i.e.*, amount of protein, fat, or carbohydrate in the food), or effect on blood glucose levels.

Exchange Lists. A common tool in use is the Exchange Lists for Meal Planning. There are six main exchange lists: bread/starch, vegetable, milk, meat, fruit, and fat. Foods included on one list (in the amounts specified) contain equal numbers of calories and are approximately equal in grams of protein, fat, and carbohydrate.

Patients are given meal plans (tailored to their individual needs and preferences) based on a recommended number of choices from each exchange list. Foods on one list may be interchanged with one another, allowing the patient to choose a variety while maintaining as much consistency as possible in the nutrient content of foods eaten. Table 39-2 presents three sample lunch menus that are interchangeable in terms of carbohydrate, protein, and fat content.

Information on combination foods such as pizza, chili, and chow mein is now available in the exchange list information from the American Dietetic Association. In addition, exchanges for a variety of foods, including convenience packaged foods, dessert foods, snack foods, and foods from "fast food" restaurants are available. Some food manufacturing companies publish exchange lists that describe their products. For more nutrition information, contact the American Diabetes Association, 1660 Duke St, Alexandria, VA 22314, 800-ADA-DISC.

The Food Guide Pyramid. The Food Guide Pyramid, another tool used to develop meal plans, has replaced the Basic Four Food Groups. It is commonly used for patients with type II diabetes who have a difficult time complying with a calorie-controlled diet. The food pyramid consists of six food groups: (1) bread, cereal, rice, and pasta; (2) fruit; (3) vegetable; (4) meat, poultry, fish, dry beans, eggs, and nuts; (5) milk, yogurt, cheese; and (6) fats, oils, and sweets (see Chapter 7). The pyramid shape was chosen to emphasize that the foods in the largest area or base of the pyramid (starches, fruit and vegetable groups) are lowest in calories and fat and highest in fiber. For those with diabetes, as well as for the general population, 50% to 60% of the daily caloric intake should be from these three groups. As one moves up the pyramid, foods higher in fat (particularly saturated fat) are illustrated;

TABLE 39-2 Sample Menus Based on the Exchange Lists

Exchanges	Sample Lunch #1	Sample Lunch #2	Sample Lunch #3
2 starch	2 slices bread	Hamburger bun	1 cup cooked pasta
3 meat	2 oz sliced turkey and 1 oz lowfat cheese	3 oz lean beef patty	3 oz boiled shrimp
1 vegetable	Lettuce, tomato, onion	Green salad	½ cup plum tomatoes
1 fat	1 tsp mayonnaise	1 tbsp salad dressing	1 tsp olive oil
1 fruit	1 medium apple	1 ¼ cup watermelon	1 ¼ cup fresh strawberries
"Free" items (optional)	Iced tea	Diet soda	Ice water with lemon
	Mustard, pickle, hot pepper	1 tbsp catsup, pickle, onions	Garlic, basil

these foods should account for a smaller percentage of the daily caloric intake. The very top of the pyramid illustrates fats, oils and sweets, foods that should be used sparingly by persons with diabetes to obtain weight and blood glucose control and to reduce the risk for cardiovascular disease.

The Food Guide Pyramid can be used to teach patients how to control the portions of foods and to emphasize which foods contain carbohydrate, protein, and fat. Menu planning should include meals with all three types of foods, emphasizing complex carbohydrates (starches) and limiting simple sugars and fat.

Glycemic Index. One of the main goals of diet therapy in diabetes is to avoid sharp, rapid increases in blood glucose levels after food is eaten. The term **glycemic index** is used to describe how much a given food raises the blood glucose level compared with an equivalent amount of glucose. Studies of the glycemic index of certain carbohydrates have raised questions regarding what we know about a food's effect on blood sugar levels. Although more research is necessary, the following guidelines can be followed when making dietary recommendations:

- Combining starch foods with protein- and fat-containing foods tends to slow their absorption and lower the glycemic response
- Eating foods that are raw and whole, in general, results in a lower glycemic response than eating chopped, pureed, or cooked foods
- When adding foods with simple sugars to the diet, a lower glycemic response may result if they are eaten with other more slowly absorbed foods

Patients can create their own glycemic index by monitoring their blood glucose level after ingesting a particular food. This can help patients improve blood glucose levels through individualized manipulation of the diet. Many patients who use frequent monitoring of blood glucose levels can use this information to adjust their insulin doses for variations in food intake.

Sweeteners and Food Labels. The use of sweeteners is acceptable for patients with diabetes, especially if it assists in overall dietary adherence. Moderation in the amount of sweetener used is encouraged to avoid potential adverse effects.

There are two main types of sweeteners: nutritive and non-nutritive. The **nutritive sweeteners** contain calories, and the **non-nutritive sweeteners** have few or no calories in the amounts normally used.

Nutritive Sweeteners

- Include fructose (fruit sugar), sorbitol, xylitol
- Are not calorie free
- Provide calories in amounts similar to those in sucrose (table sugar)
- Cause less elevation in blood sugar levels than sucrose
- Are often used in "sugar-free" foods
- May have a laxative effect (sorbitol)

Non-nutritive Sweeteners

- Have minimal or no calories
- Are used in food products and are also available for table use
- Produce minimal or no elevation in blood sugar levels
- Have been approved by the FDA as safe for people with diabetes
- Saccharin—no calories
- Aspartame (NutraSweet)—packaged with dextrose, 4 calories/packet, loses sweetness with heat
- Acesulfame-K (Sunnette)—packaged with dextrose, 1 calorie/packet

Food Labeling. Foods that are labeled "sugarless" or "sugar-free" may still provide calories equal to those of the equivalent non—sugar-free products if they are made with nutritive sweeteners. Thus, for weight loss, these products may not always be useful. In addition, patients must not consider them "free" foods to be eaten in unlimited quantity because they may cause elevations in blood glucose levels.

Foods that are labeled "dietetic" are not necessarily reduced-calorie foods. They may be lower in sodium or have other special dietary uses. Patients are advised that foods labeled "dietetic" may still contain significant amounts of sugar or fat.

Patients must also be taught to read labels of "health" foods—especially snacks—because they often contain sugar products such as honey, brown sugar, and corn syrup. In addition, these "health" snacks frequently contain saturated vegetable fats (such as coconut or palm oil), hydrogenated vegetable fats, or animal fats, which may be contraindicated in the patient with elevated blood lipids.

Health Teaching About Diet

The clinical dietitian uses various educational tools, teaching materials, and approaches to meal planning. Initial education will address the importance of consistency in eating habits, the relationship of food and insulin, and the provision of an individualized meal plan. Follow-up education will then focus on more in-depth management skills, such as restaurant eating, reading food labels, and adjusting the meal plan for exercise, illness, and special occasions. The nurse plays an important role in communicating pertinent information to the dietitian and reinforcing the patient's understanding.

For some patients, learning to use the exchange system may be too difficult. This may be related to limitations in what the patient is intellectually capable of understanding or it may be related to emotional issues, such as difficulty accepting the diagnosis of diabetes or feelings of deprivation and undue restriction in eating. It is important to simplify information as much as possible and to provide opportunities for practice and repetition of information. In addition, it should be emphasized that using the exchange system (or any food classification system) provides a new way of thinking about food rather than a completely new way of eating.

Exercise

Exercise is extremely important in the management of diabetes because of its effects on lowering blood glucose and reducing cardiovascular risk factors. Exercise lowers blood glucose by increasing the uptake of glucose by body muscles and by improving insulin utilization. It also improves circulation and muscle tone. Resistance training can increase lean muscle mass, thereby increasing the resting metabolic rate. These effects are useful in diabetes in relation to losing weight, easing stress, and maintaining a feeling of well-being. Exercise also alters blood lipids—increasing levels of high-density lipoproteins (HDL) and decreasing total cholesterol and triglyceride levels. This is especially important to the person with diabetes because of the increased risk of cardiovascular disease.

However, patients with blood glucose levels over 250 mg/dl (14 mmol/L) who have ketones in their urine should not begin exercising until the urine ketone test is negative and the blood glucose level is closer to normal. Exercising with elevated blood glucose levels causes increased secretions of glucagon, growth hormone, and catecholamines. The liver then releases more glucose, resulting in an increase in blood glucose.

Initially, the insulin-requiring patient should be taught to eat a 15-g carbohydrate snack (a fruit exchange) or a snack of complex carbohydrate with a protein before engaging in moderate exercise, to prevent unexpected hypoglycemia. The exact amount of food needed varies from person to person and should be determined by blood glucose monitoring. Some patients find that they do not require a pre-exercise snack if they exercise within 1 to 2 hours after a meal. Other patients may require extra food regardless of the timing of exercise. If extra food is required, it need not be deducted from the regular meal plan.

Another potential problem for patients who take insulin is hypoglycemia that occurs many hours *after* exercise. To avoid postexercise hypoglycemia, especially after strenuous exercise, the patient may need to eat a snack at the end of the exercise session. In addition, it may be necessary to have the patient reduce the dosage of insulin that peaks at the time of exercise.

Patients participating in extended periods of exercise should test blood glucose before, during, and after the exercise period, and they should eat carbohydrate snacks as needed to maintain blood glucose levels. Other participants or observers should be aware that the person exercising has diabetes, and they should know what assistance to give if severe hypoglycemia occurs.

In obese persons with type II diabetes, exercise in addition to dietary management both improves glucose metabolism and enhances loss of body fat. Exercise coupled with weight loss improves insulin sensitivity and may decrease the need for insulin or oral agents. Eventually, the patient's glucose tolerance may return to normal. The type II diabetic patient who is not taking insulin or an oral agent may not need extra food before exercise.

Persons with diabetes should be taught to exercise at the same time (preferably when blood glucose levels are at their peak) and in the same amount each day. Regular daily exercise, rather than sporadic exercise, should be encouraged. Exercise recommendations must be altered as necessary for patients with diabetic complications such as retinopathy, autonomic neuropathy, sensorimotor neuropathy, and cardiovascular disease; these disorders are discussed later in this chapter. Increased blood pressure associated with exercise may aggravate diabetic retinopathy and increase the risk of a hemorrhage into the vitreous or retina. In patients with ischemic heart disease, there is a risk of triggering angina or a myocardial infarction. Avoidance of trauma to the lower extremities is especially important in the patient with numbness related to neuropathy.

In general, a slow, gradual increase in the length of the exercise period is encouraged. For many patients, walking is a safe and beneficial form of exercise that requires no special equipment (except for proper shoes) and can be performed anywhere. Persons with diabetes should discuss an exercise program with their physician before undertaking it.

If the patient is older than 30 years of age and has two or more of the risk factors for heart disease, an exercise stress test is recommended. Risk factors for heart disease include hypertension, obesity, high cholesterol levels, abnormal resting electrocardiogram, sedentary lifestyle, smoking, and a family history of heart disease. General guidelines for exercise in diabetes are presented in Chart 39-2.

Gerontologic Considerations

Physical activity that is consistent and realistic is beneficial to the elderly person with diabetes. Advantages include a decrease in hyperglycemia, a general sense of well-being, and the utilization of ingested calories, resulting in weight reduction. Because there is an increased incidence of cardiovascular problems in the elderly, a pattern of gradual, consistent exercise should be planned that does not exceed the patient's physical capacity. Physical impairment from other chronic diseases must also be considered.

Monitoring of Glucose and Ketones

Self-Monitoring of Blood Glucose

With the use of frequent self-monitoring of blood glucose (SMBG) people with diabetes are now able to adjust the treatment regimen to obtain optimal blood glucose control. This allows for detection and prevention of hypoglycemia and hyperglycemia and plays a crucial role in normalizing blood glucose levels, which will possibly reduce long-term diabetic complications.

Various methods are available for SMBG. Most of them involve obtaining a drop of blood from the fingertip, apply-

CHART 39-2
General Guidelines for Exercise in Diabetes

- Use proper footwear and, if appropriate, other protective equipment.
- Avoid exercise in extreme heat or cold.
- Inspect feet daily after exercise.
- Avoid exercise during periods of poor metabolic control.

ing the blood to a special reagent strip, and allowing the blood to stay on the strip for a specific amount of time (usually between 45 and 60 seconds, as specified by the manufacturer). For some of the products, the blood is then wiped off the strip (using cotton or tissue per manufacturer specifications). The reagent pad of the strip changes color and can then be matched to a color chart on the product package (Fig. 39-1) or is inserted into a meter that gives a digital readout of the blood glucose value.

Several newer blood glucose monitors are available that have eliminated the step of blood removal from the strip. The strip is placed in the meter first, before blood is applied to it. Once the blood is placed on the strip, it remains there for the duration of the test. The meter automatically displays the blood glucose level after a short time (less than 1 minute). One of the newest products uses a glucose sensor cartridge (instead of strips) onto which the blood is placed. These new types of meters tend to give blood glucose results in a shorter period, and most of them have automatic timers that do not need to be activated by the user.

Meters have been developed that can be used by patients with visual impairments. They have audio components that assist the patient in performing the test and obtaining the result.

Advantages and Disadvantages of SMBG Systems. It is very important that the method used by patients be appropriately matched to their skill level. Factors affecting SMBG performance include visual acuity, fine motor coordination, intellectual capability, comfort with technology, willingness, and cost.

Visual methods are the least expensive and require less equipment. However, they require the ability to distinguish colors and to be exact in timing the procedures. Meters in general are more expensive (at least initially), but they eliminate the subjective aspect of trying to match colors visually.

Meters that require removal of blood from the reagent strip have more steps that must be performed in an exact sequence. However, they allow for double-checking the results through visual reading of the strips. The newer generation of meters that do not require removal of blood from the strip generally are simpler to use. However, most of them do not provide a backup method for visually assessing the meter results. Figure 39-2 illustrates a system available for glucose monitoring.

A potential hazard of all methods of SMBG is that the patient may obtain and report erroneous blood glucose values as a result of using incorrect techniques. Some common sources of error include

- Improper application of blood (*e.g.*, drop too small)
- Improper timing
- Improper blood removal (*e.g.*, wiping too hard or too lightly or not using recommended material for wiping)
- Improper cleaning and maintenance of meters (*e.g.*, allowing dust or blood to accumulate on the optic window)

The nurse plays an important role in providing initial education in SMBG techniques. Equally important is evaluating the techniques of patients who are "experienced" in self-monitoring. Patients should be discouraged from purchasing SMBG products from stores or catalogs that do not provide direct education. Every 6 to 12 months, patients should conduct a comparison of their meter with a simultaneous laboratory-measured blood glucose level in their physician's office. Additionally, the accuracy of the meter and strips should be assessed with control solutions specific to that meter whenever a new vial of strips is used or whenever the validity of the readings is in doubt.

Candidates for SMBG. Blood glucose monitoring is a useful procedure for all people with diabetes. It is a cornerstone of treatment for any intensive insulin therapy regimen (including two to four injections per day or insulin pumps) and for managing pregnancy complicated by diabetes. It is also highly recommended for patients with

- Unstable diabetes
- A tendency for severe ketosis or hypoglycemia
- Hypoglycemia without warning symptoms
- Abnormal renal glucose thresholds

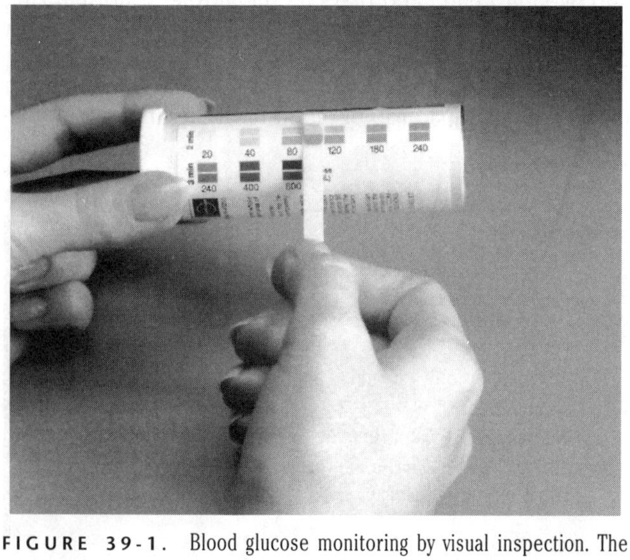

FIGURE 39-1. Blood glucose monitoring by visual inspection. The user visually compares the color on the reagent strip to a chart.

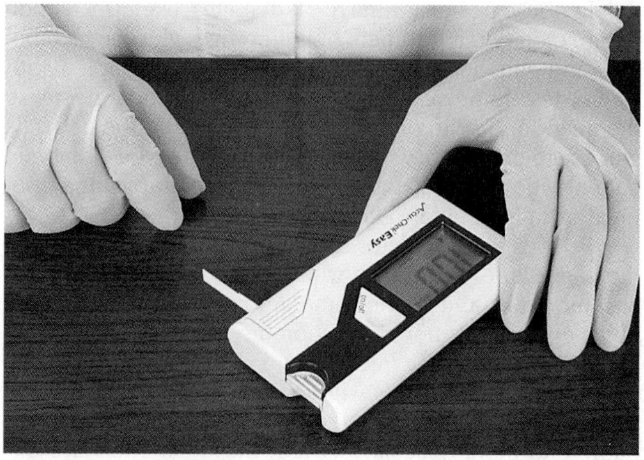

FIGURE 39-2. Example of a blood glucose monitor.

For patients not taking insulin, SMBG is helpful for monitoring the effectiveness of exercise, diet, and oral agents. It can also help to motivate patients to continue with treatment. For type II diabetic patients, SMBG should also be recommended during periods of suspected hyperglycemia (*e.g.*, illness) or hypoglycemia (*e.g.*, unusual increased activity levels).

Frequency of SMBG. For most patients who require insulin, testing two to four times per day is recommended (usually before meals and at bedtime). For patients who take insulin before each meal, testing at least three times per day is required for safely determining each insulin dose. Patients not on insulin may be instructed to assess blood glucose levels a minimum of two to three times per week.

For all patients, testing is recommended whenever hypoglycemia or hyperglycemia is suspected.

Interpretation of SMBG Results Patients should be instructed to keep a record or log book of blood glucose results so they can begin to see "patterns" emerge. The ideal testing schedule is 30 minutes before meals and at bedtime. Patients who take insulin at bedtime or who are on an insulin infusion pump must also test at 3:00 AM once a week to document that the blood glucose level is not decreasing overnight.

If a patient is unwilling or cannot afford to test frequently, then once or twice a day may be sufficient if the patient varies the time of day to test (*e.g.*, test before breakfast one day, before lunch the next day, etc.)

The tendency to discontinue SMBG may be seen in patients who were never instructed on how to use the results for altering their treatment regimen. Instructions vary according to the patient's understanding and the physician's philosophy of diabetes management. At the very least, patients should be given parameters for calling the physician. Patients using intensive insulin therapy regimens may be instructed in use of algorithms (rules or decision trees) for changing the insulin doses based on patterns of values greater or less than the target range.

Morning Hyperglycemia

An elevated blood glucose level on arising in the morning may be caused by an insufficient level of insulin, the dawn phenomenon, or the Somogyi effect. The **dawn phenomenon** is characterized by a relatively normal blood glucose level until approximately 3:00 AM, when blood glucose levels begin to rise. The phenomenon is thought to result from nocturnal surges in growth hormone secretion that create a greater need for insulin in the early morning hours in patients with type I diabetes. It must be distinguished from **insulin waning** (the progressive increase in blood glucose from bedtime to morning), or the **Somogyi effect** (nocturnal hypoglycemia followed by rebound hyperglycemia).

It is often difficult to tell from the patient's history which of these causes is responsible for morning hyperglycemia. To determine the cause, the patient must be awakened once or twice during the night to test blood glucose levels. Testing the blood glucose level at bedtime, at 3:00 AM, and on awakening provides information that can be used in making an insulin adjustment to avoid morning hyperglycemia caused by the dawn phenomenon. Table 39-3 summarizes the differences among insulin waning, the dawn phenomenon, and the Somogyi effect.

Glycosylated Hemoglobin

Glycosylated hemoglobin is a blood test that reflects average blood glucose levels over a period of approximately 2 to 3 months. When blood glucose levels are elevated, a glucose molecule attaches itself to hemoglobin in a red blood cell. The longer the glucose in the blood remains above normal, the more glucose binds to the red blood cell and the higher the glycosylated hemoglobin level. This complex (the hemoglobin attached to the glucose) is permanent and lasts for the life of the red blood cell, approximately 120 days. If near-normal blood glucose levels are maintained, with only occasional increases in blood

TABLE 39-3 Causes of Morning Hyperglycemia

Characteristic	Treatment
Insulin Waning	
Progressive rise in blood glucose from bedtime to morning	Increase evening (pre-dinner or bedtime) dose of intermediate- or long-acting insulin or institute a dose of insulin before the evening meal if one is not already in use.
Dawn Phenomenon	
Relatively normal blood glucose until about 3 AM, when the level begins to rise	Change time of injection of evening intermediate-acting insulin from dinner time to bedtime.
Somogyi Effect	
Normal or elevated blood glucose at bedtime, a decrease at 2–3 AM to hypoglycemic levels, and a subsequent increase caused by the production of counter-regulatory hormones	Decrease evening (pre-dinner or bedtime) dose of intermediate-acting insulin or increase bedtime snack.

glucose, the overall value will not be greatly elevated. However, if the blood glucose values are consistently high, then the test result will also be elevated. If patients report mostly normal results on records of self-glucose monitoring but the glycosylated hemoglobin is high, there may be errors in the methods used for glucose monitoring, errors in recording results, or frequent elevations in glucose levels at times during the day when the patient is not usually monitoring the blood.

There are various tests that measure the same thing but have different names, including hemoglobin A_{1C} and hemoglobin A_1. The normal values differ slightly from test to test and from laboratory to laboratory and normally range from 4% to 8%. Values within the normal range indicate consistently near-normal blood glucose levels, a goal made easier by patients' self-monitoring of blood glucose levels.

Urine Testing for Glucose

Before the availability of SMBG methods, urine glucose testing was the only method available for day-to-day monitoring of diabetes. Today its use is limited to those patients who cannot or will not perform blood glucose testing.

The general procedure involves applying urine to a reagent strip or tablet and matching colors on the strip with a color chart at the end of a specified period. The disadvantages of urine testing include

- Results do not reflect the blood glucose level at the time of the test
- It is impossible to detect hypoglycemia because a "negative" urine glucose result may occur when blood glucose ranges from 0 to 180 mg/dl (10 mmol/L) or higher
- Patients may have a false sense of being in "good" control when results are always negative
- Various medications (*e.g.*, aspirin, vitamin C, some antibiotics) may interfere with test results
- In the elderly and in patients with kidney disease, the renal threshold (*i.e.*, the level of blood glucose at which glucose starts to appear in the urine) is raised; thus, falsely negative readings may occur at dangerously elevated glucose levels

The advantages of urine glucose testing are that it is less expensive than SMBG and it is not invasive.

Urine Testing for Ketones

Ketones (or ketone bodies) in the urine signal that control of type I diabetes is deteriorating. When there is almost no effective insulin available, the body starts to break down stored fat for energy. Ketone bodies are by-products of this fat breakdown, and they accumulate in the blood and urine. The only method available for self-testing of ketone bodies by patients is urine testing.

The most commonly used method to detect ketonuria is to use a urine "dipstick" (Ketostix or Chemstrip uK), which measures one type of ketone body. The reagent pad on the strip turns a purplish color when ketones are present. (Note: one of the ketone bodies is called "acetone," and this term is frequently used interchangeably with the term "ketones.") There are also strips available that measure both glucose and ketones (Keto-Diastix or Chemstrip uGK). Large amounts of ketones may depress the color development of the glucose test area.

Urine ketone testing should be performed whenever patients with type I diabetes have glucosuria or unexplained elevated blood glucose levels (over 250 mg/dl or 14 mmol/L), and during illness and pregnancy.

Insulin Therapy

As stated earlier, insulin is secreted by the beta cells of the islets of Langerhans. It works to lower blood glucose after meals by facilitating the uptake and utilization of glucose by muscle, fat, and liver cells. During periods of fasting, insulin inhibits the breakdown of stored glucose, protein, and fat.

In type I diabetes, the body loses the ability to produce insulin. Thus, exogenous insulin must be administered indefinitely. In type II diabetes, insulin may be necessary on a long-term basis to control glucose levels if diet and oral agents have failed. In addition, some patients whose type II diabetes is usually controlled by diet alone or by diet and an oral agent may require insulin temporarily during illness, infection, pregnancy, surgery, or some other stressful event.

Frequently, insulin injections are taken two times per day (or even more often) to control postmeal and overnight

TABLE 39-4 Categories of Insulin

Time Course	Agent	Onset	Peak	Duration	Indications
Short-Acting	Regular ("R")	½–1 hr	2–3 hr	4–6 hr	Usually administered 20–30 minutes before a meal; may be taken alone or in combination with longer-acting insulin
Intermediate-Acting	NPH (neutral protamine Hagedorn) Lente ("L")	3–4 hr	4–12 hr	16–20 hr	Usually taken after food
Long-Acting	Ultralente ("UL")	6–8 hr	12–16 hr	20–30 hr	Used primarily to control fasting glucose level

Rapid Acting 3-5MIN Humulog short use immed. before meals inject + eat increases in blood glucose. Because the insulin dose required by the individual patient is determined by the level of glucose in the blood, accurate monitoring of blood glucose levels is essential. Self-monitoring of blood glucose levels has become the cornerstone of insulin therapy.

Insulin Preparations. A number of insulin preparations are available. They vary according to four main characteristics: time course of action, concentration, species (source), and manufacturer.

Time Course. Insulins may be grouped into three main categories based on the onset, peak, and duration of action (Table 39-4). (It is important to note that human insulin preparations have a shorter duration of action than insulin from animal sources.)

Short-Acting Insulins

- Regular insulin (marked "R" on the bottle)

The onset of regular human insulin action is ½ to 1 hour; peak, 2 to 3 hours; duration, 4 to 6 hours. Another name for regular insulin is crystalline zinc insulin (CZI).

Regular insulin is clear in appearance and is usually administered 20 to 30 minutes before a meal, either alone or in combination with a longer-acting insulin.

Intermediate-Acting Insulins

- NPH insulin (neutral protamine Hagedorn)
- Lente insulin ("L")

The onset of intermediate-acting human insulins is 3 to 4 hours; peak, 4 to 12 hours; duration, 16 to 20 hours.

Both insulins are similar in their time course of action and are white and milky in appearance. If NPH or Lente insulin is taken alone, it is not critical that it be taken a half-

(text continues of page 1034)

TABLE 39-5 Insulin Preparations Available in the United States

Manufacturer	Product	Species Source	Type
Rapid-Acting			
Lilly	Iletin I	Beef/pork	Regular
Lilly	Iletin II	Beef or pork	Regular
Lilly	Humulin Regular	Human	Regular
Novo Nordisk	Regular	Pork	Regular
Novo Nordisk	Purified Pork Regular	Pork	Regular
Novo Nordisk	Novolin R	Human	Regular
Novo Nordisk	Velosulin	Human	Regular
Intermediate-Acting			
Lilly	Iletin I NPH	Pork	NPH
Lilly	Iletin II NPH	Beef or pork	NPH
Lilly	Humulin NPH	Human	NPH
Novo Nordisk	NPH	Beef	NPH
Novo Nordisk	Purified Pork N	Pork	NPH
Novo Nordisk	Novolin N	Human	NPH
Lilly	Iletin I Lente	Beef/pork	Lente
Lilly	Iletin II Lente	Beef or pork	Lente
Lilly	Humulin L	Human	Lente
Novo Nordisk	Lente	Beef	Lente
Novo Nordisk	Purified Pork L	Pork	Lente
Novo Nordisk	Novolin L	Human	Lente
Long-Acting			
Lilly	Humulin U	Human	Ultralente
Novo Nordisk	Ultralente	Beef	Ultralente
Mixed			
Lilly	Humulin70/30, 50/50	Human	70% NPH/30% Reg; 50% NPH/50% Reg
Novo Nordisk	Novolin 70/30	Human	70% NPH/30% Reg

In the near future all insulins will be human, made from a recombinant DNA process in a laboratory.
Insulin analogues, very rapid-acting insulins, are currently in clinical trials; they will eliminate the need to wait 30 minutes after the injection to eat.

TABLE 39-6 Insulin Regimens

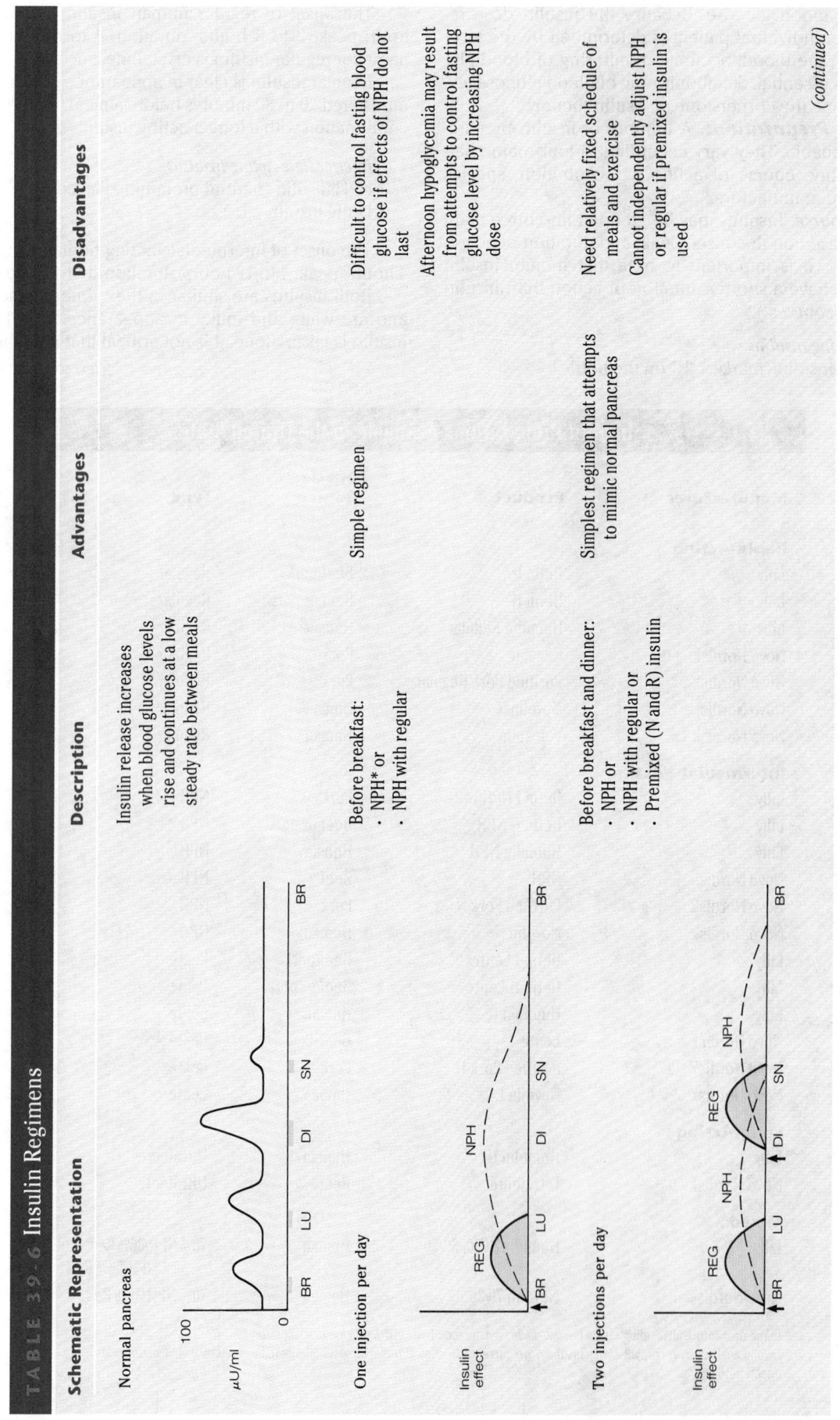

Schematic Representation	Description	Advantages	Disadvantages
Normal pancreas 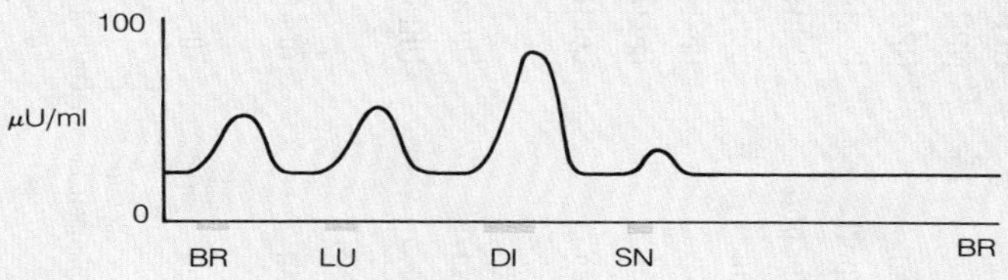	Insulin release increases when blood glucose levels rise and continues at a low steady rate between meals		
One injection per day 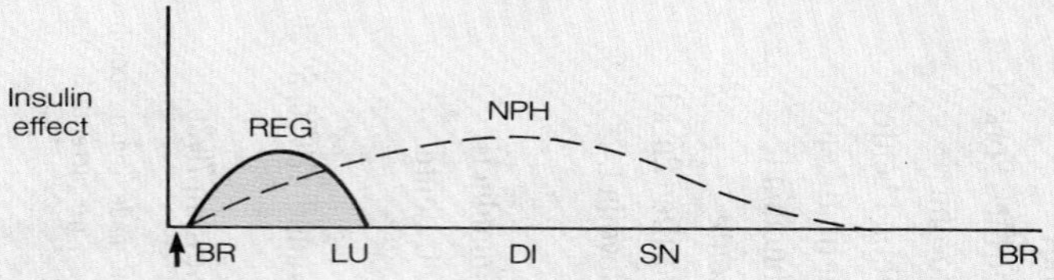	Before breakfast: · NPH* or · NPH with regular	Simple regimen	Difficult to control fasting blood glucose if effects of NPH do not last Afternoon hypoglycemia may result from attempts to control fasting glucose level by increasing NPH dose
Two injections per day 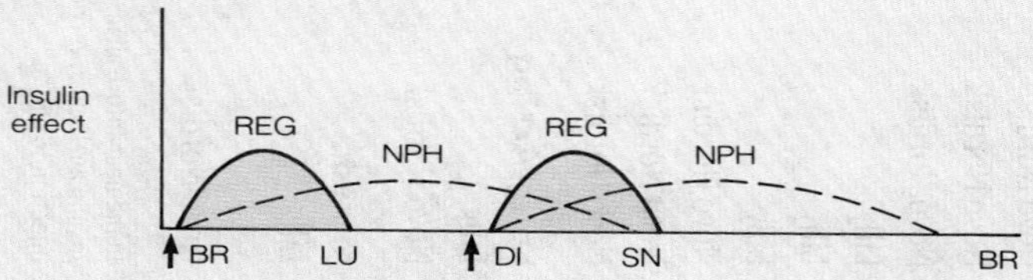	Before breakfast and dinner: · NPH or · NPH with regular or · Premixed (N and R) insulin	Simplest regimen that attempts to mimic normal pancreas	Need relatively fixed schedule of meals and exercise Cannot independently adjust NPH or regular if premixed insulin is used

(continued)

TABLE 39-6 *(continued)*

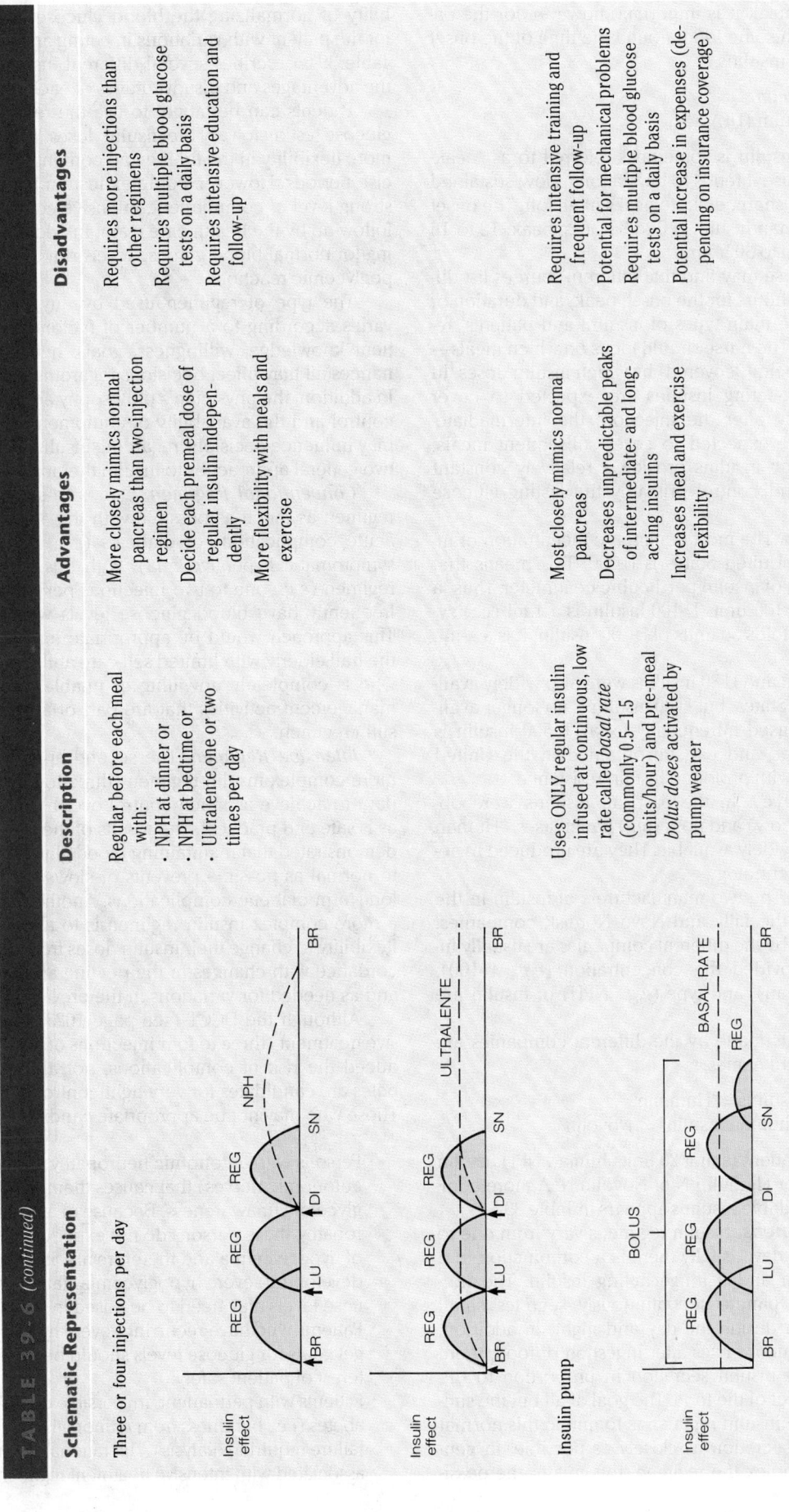

Schematic Representation	Description	Advantages	Disadvantages
Three or four injections per day 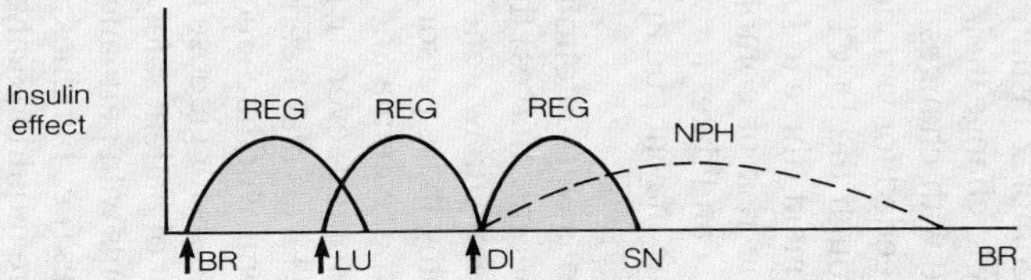 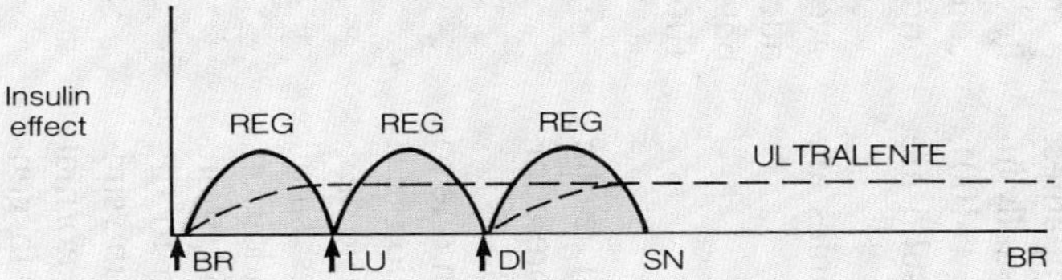	Regular before each meal with: · NPH at dinner or · NPH at bedtime or · Ultralente one or two times per day	More closely mimics normal pancreas than two-injection regimen Decide each premeal dose of regular insulin independently More flexibility with meals and exercise	Requires more injections than other regimens Requires multiple blood glucose tests on a daily basis Requires intensive education and follow-up
Insulin pump 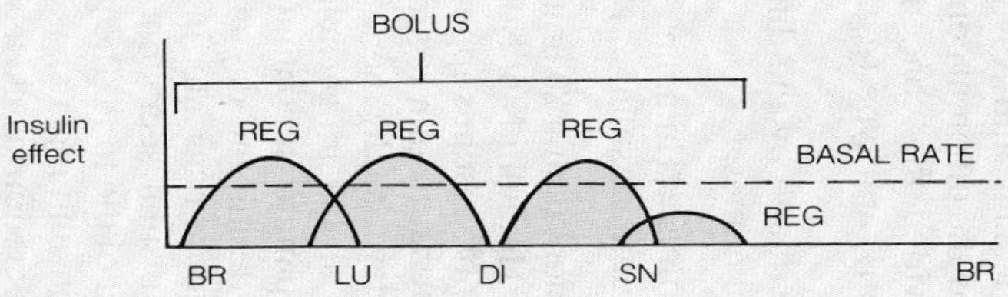	Uses ONLY regular insulin infused at continuous, low rate called *basal rate* (commonly 0.5–1.5 units/hour) and pre-meal *bolus doses* activated by pump wearer	Most closely mimics normal pancreas Decreases unpredictable peaks of intermediate- and long-acting insulins Increases meal and exercise flexibility	Requires intensive training and frequent follow-up Potential for mechanical problems Requires multiple blood glucose tests on a daily basis Potential increase in expenses (depending on insurance coverage)

*Where NPH appears, Lente insulin may also be used (however, the rate of absorption of regular insulin may be decreased when mixed with Lente preparations).
BR, breakfast; LU, lunch; DI, dinner; SN, snack; ↑ indicates insulin injection.

hour before the meal. It is important, however, for the patient to have eaten some food around the time of the onset and peak of these insulins.

Long-Acting Insulin

- Ultralente insulin (UL)

Long-acting insulin is sometimes referred to as "peakless" insulin because it tends to have a long, slow, sustained action rather than sharp, definite peaks in action. The onset of long-acting human insulin is 6 to 8 hours; peak, 12 to 16 hours; duration, 20 to 30 hours.

(Note: the nurse may find that different sources list differing numbers of hours for the onset, peak, and duration of action of the three main types of insulin, and patients' responses may vary. The nurse should focus on which meals—and snacks—are being "covered" by which insulin doses. In general, the short-acting insulins are expected to cover meals immediately after the injection; the intermediate-acting insulins are expected to cover subsequent meals; and the long-acting insulins provide a relatively constant level of insulin and control primarily the fasting glucose level.)

Concentration. The most common concentration of insulin used in the United States is U-100. This means that there are 100 units of insulin per 1 cubic centimeter. Thus, a syringe that holds 100 units U-100 insulin is a 1-ml (cc) syringe. If a syringe holds 50 units of U-100 insulin, it is a ½-ml, U-100 syringe.

Years ago, U-40 and U-80 insulins were also widely available in the United States, but U-80 insulin is no longer available, and U-40 is used infrequently today. U-500 insulin is available in Europe and can be obtained in the United States for patients with profound insulin resistance.

Species (Source). In the past, all insulins were obtained from beef (cow) and pork (pig) pancreases. "Human insulins" are now widely available. They are produced by recombinant DNA technology.

Manufacturer. The two manufacturers of insulin in the United States are the Lilly and Novo Nordisk companies. The insulins made by the different companies are usually interchangeable, provided the concentration (*e.g.,* U-100), species (*e.g.,* human), and type (*e.g.,* NPH) of insulin are the same.

Human insulins made by the different companies are given different brand names:

- Lilly human insulins = "Humulin"
- Novo Nordisk human insulins = "Novolin"

Therefore, a patient taking 20 units human NPH insulin may be using either Humulin N or Novolin N. A more complete list of the available insulins appears in Table 39-5.

Insulin Regimens. Insulin regimens vary from one to four injections per day. Usually there is a combination of a short-acting insulin and a longer-acting insulin. The normally functioning pancreas continuously secretes small amounts of insulin during the day and night. In addition, whenever blood glucose rises after ingestion of food, there is a rapid burst of insulin secretion in proportion to the glucose-raising effect of the food. The goal of all but the simplest, one-injection insulin regimen is to mimic this normal pattern of insulin secretion as closely as possible. In general, the more complex the regimen, the greater the possibility of normalizing the blood glucose levels—especially for the patient with variations in eating and activity patterns. Table 39-6 describes several different insulin regimens and the advantages and disadvantages of each one.

Patients can be taught to use the results of self–blood glucose testing to vary the insulin doses. This allows patients more flexibility in the timing and content of meals and exercise periods. However, complex insulin regimens require a strong level of commitment, intensive education, and close follow-up by the health care team. In addition, patients aiming for normal blood glucose levels run the risk of more hypoglycemic reactions.

The type of regimen used by any particular patient varies according to a number of factors. For example, patient knowledge, willingness, goals, health status, and finances all may affect decisions regarding insulin treatment. In addition, the physician's philosophy about blood glucose control and the availability of equipment and support staff may influence decisions regarding insulin therapy. There are two general approaches to insulin therapy.

Conventional Regimen. One is to simplify the insulin regimen as much as possible with the aim of avoiding the acute complications of diabetes (*i.e.,* hypoglycemia and symptomatic hyperglycemia). With this type of simplified regimen (*e.g.,* one to two injections per day), patients may frequently have blood glucose levels well above normal. This approach would be appropriate for the terminally ill, the frail elderly with limited self-care abilities, or any patient who is completely unwilling or unable to engage in self-management activities that are part of a more complex insulin regimen.

Intensive Regimen. The second approach is to use a more complex insulin regimen (three to four injections per day) to achieve as much control over blood glucose levels as is safe and practical. The results of the DCCT (1993) have demonstrated that maintaining blood glucose levels as close to normal as possible prevents or slows the progression of long-term diabetic complications. Another reason for using a more complex insulin regimen is to allow patients more flexibility to change their insulin doses from day to day in accordance with changes in their eating and activity patterns and as needed for variations in the prevailing glucose level.

Although the DCCT (see page 1023) found that intensive treatment (three to four injections of insulin per day) reduced the risk of complications, not all people with diabetes are candidates for very tight control of blood glucose. Those who may not be appropriate candidates include

- Persons with autonomic neuropathy (disease of the autonomic nerves) that causes them to have hypoglycemic unawareness. Because of autonomic neuropathy, these persons do not experience symptoms of hypoglycemia and therefore are at increased risk of developing severe hypoglycemia. Target goals for glucose levels may need to be raised in these persons.
- Patients who have recurring severe hypoglycemia. Target goals for glucose levels should be raised in the interest of patient safety.
- Patients with permanent, irreversible complications of diabetes (*i.e.,* blindness from retinopathy or chronic renal failure requiring dialysis). The rationale is that the risks associated with intensive treatment regimens may out-

weigh the benefits. An exception is the patient who has received a kidney transplant because of nephropathy and chronic renal failure; this patient should be on an intensive regimen to preserve function of the new kidney.

- Patients with cerebrovascular and cardiovascular complications. It is feared that an occurrence of severe hypoglycemia may trigger another cerebrovascular or cardiovascular event in patients with significant preexisting vascular changes.
- Patients who do not take full responsibility in their care. Failure to take responsibility for self-care increases the risk of severe hypoglycemia as a result of poor decision making.

It is very important for patients to be involved in the decision regarding which insulin regimen to use. Patients need to compare the potential benefits of different regimens with the potential costs (such as time involved, number of injections or fingersticks for glucose testing, amount of record keeping, etc.). There are no set guidelines as to which insulin regimen should be used for which patients. It must not be assumed that an elderly patient or a patient with visual impairment should automatically be given a simplified regimen. Likewise, it must not be assumed that all young people will want to be involved in a complex treatment regimen.

Nurses play an important role in educating patients about the availability of different approaches to insulin therapy. Nurses should refer patients to diabetes specialists or diabetes education centers for further training and education in the various insulin treatment regimens.

Patient Teaching—Insulin Injection

Insulin injections are administered into the subcutaneous tissue with the use of special insulin syringes. A variety of syringes and injection-aid devices are available. Charts 39-3 and 39-4 summarize important factors to include in teaching patients about insulin.

Equipment

Insulin. Short-acting insulins are clear in appearance, and longer-acting insulins are cloudy and white. The longer-acting insulins must be mixed (gently inverted or rolled in the hands) before use.

Some sources specify that insulin bottles in use be refrigerated, and others simply suggest that insulin be kept at room temperature. There is agreement that extremes of temperature are to be avoided; thus, insulin should not be allowed to freeze and should not be kept in direct sunlight or in a hot car. Before injection, it is recommended that insulin be at room temperature (which may require rolling it in the hands or removing it from a refrigerator for a time before the injection).

Insulin bottles should also be assessed for **flocculation,** which is a frosted, whitish coating inside the bottle of intermediate- or long-acting insulins. This occurs most commonly with human insulins that are not refrigerated. If a frosted, adherent coating is present, some of the insulin is bound and should not be used.

Syringes. Syringes must be matched with the insulin concentration (*e.g.,* U-100). Currently, three sizes of U-100 insulin syringes are available:

- 1-ml (cc) syringes—hold 100 units
- ½-ml syringes—hold 50 units
- 3/10-ml syringes—hold 30 units

Most insulin syringes have a 27- to 29-gauge needle that is approximately ½ inch in length. The smaller syringes are marked in 1-unit increments and may be easier to use for patients with visual deficits or patients taking very small doses of insulin. Some 1-ml syringes are marked in 2-unit increments. A small disposable insulin needle (29- to 30-gauge, 8 mm in length) is now available.

Preparing the Injection

Mixing Insulins. When short- and longer-acting insulins are to be given simultaneously, they are usually mixed together in the same syringe.

There is some question as to whether the two insulins are stable if the mixture is kept in the syringe for more than 5 to 15 minutes. This may depend on the ratio of the insulins as well as the time between mixing and injecting. Some research studies have suggested that when mixing regular insulin with the long-acting insulin, there is a binding reaction that slows the action of the regular insulin. This may also occur to a greater degree when mixing regular insulin with one of the Lente insulins. Patients are advised to consult their diabetes health care professionals for advice on this matter. The most important issue is that patients be consistent in how they prepare their insulin injections from day to day.

There are varying opinions regarding which type of insulin (short- or longer-acting) should be drawn up into the syringe first when they are going to be mixed. Most of the printed materials from pharmaceutical companies recommend drawing up the regular insulin first. The most important issues are that the patient be consistent in technique so as not to accidentally draw up the wrong dose or the wrong type of insulin, and that patients not inject one type of insulin into the bottle containing a different type of insulin.

For patients who have difficulty mixing insulins, two options are available: They may use a premixed insulin or they may have prefilled syringes prepared. Premixed insulins are available in several different ratios of NPH insulin to regular insulin. The ratio of 70/30 (70% NPH and 30% regular insulin in one bottle) is the most common and is available as Novolin 70/30 (Novo Nordisk) and Humulin 70/30 (Lilly). Other ratios available include 80/20, 60/40, and 50/50. The appropriate initial dosage of premixed insulin must be calculated so that the ratio of NPH to regular insulin most closely approximates the separate doses needed.

For patients who are able to inject insulin but who have difficulty drawing up a single or mixed dose, syringes can be prefilled with the help of home health nurses or family and friends. A 3-week supply of insulin syringes may be prepared and kept in the refrigerator. The prefilled syringes should be kept flat or with the needle in an upright position to avoid clogging of the needle.

Withdrawing Insulin. Most (if not all) of the printed materials available on insulin dose preparation instruct patients to inject air into the bottle of insulin equivalent to the number of units of insulin to be withdrawn. The rationale behind this is to prevent the formation of a vacuum inside the bottle, which would make it difficult to withdraw the proper amount of insulin.

CHART 39-3
Teaching Insulin Administration

Equipment

Insulin

1. Identifies information on label of insulin bottle
   - Type (*e.g.*, NPH, regular, 70/30)
   - Species (human, beef/pork)
   - Manufacturer (Lilly, Novo Nordisk)
   - Concentration (*e.g.*, U-100)
   - Expiration date
2. Checks appearance of insulin
   - Clear or milky white
   - Checks for flocculation (clumping, frosted appearance)
3. Identifies where to purchase and store insulin
   - Indicates approximately how long bottle will last (1000 units per bottle U-100 insulin)
   - Indicates how long opened bottles can be used

Syringes

1. Identifies concentration (U-100) marking on syringe
2. Identifies size of syringe (*e.g.*, 100-unit, 50-unit, 30-unit)
3. Describes appropriate disposal of used syringe

Preparation and Administration of Insulin Injection

1. Draws up correct amount and type of insulin
2. Properly mixes two insulins if necessary
3. Inserts needle, and injects insulin
4. Describes site rotation
   - Demonstrates injection with all anatomic areas to be used
   - Describes pattern for rotation, such as using abdomen only or using certain areas at the same time of day
   - Describes system for remembering site locations, such as horizontal pattern across the abdomen as if drawing a dotted line

Knowledge of Insulin Action

1. Lists prescription
   - Type and dosage of insulin
   - Timing of insulin injections
2. Describes approximate time course of insulin action
   - Identifies long- and short-acting insulins by name
   - States approximate time delay until onset of insulin action
   - Identifies need to delay food until 15–30 minutes after the injection (indicated when injecting regular insulin)
   - Knows that longer time delays are safe when blood glucose level is high and time delays may need to be shortened when blood glucose level is low

Incorporation of Insulin Injections Into Daily Schedule

1. Recites proper order of pre-meal diabetes activities
   - May use mnemonic devise such as the word "tie," which helps the patient remember the order of activities ("t" = test [blood glucose], "i" = insulin injection, "e" = eat)
   - Describes daily schedule, such as test, insulin, eat, before breakfast and dinner; test and eat, before lunch and bedtime
2. Describes information regarding hypoglycemia
   - Symptoms: shakiness, sweating, nervousness, hunger, weakness
   - Causes: too much insulin, too much exercise, not enough food
   - Treatment: 10–15 g simple carbohydrate, such as 2–3 glucose tablets, 1 tube glucose gel, ½–1 cup juice
   - After initial treatment, follow with snack including starch and protein, such as cheese and crackers, milk and crackers, half sandwich
3. Describes information regarding prevention of hypoglycemia
   - Avoid delays in meal timing
   - Eat a meal or snack approximately every 4–5 hours (while awake)
   - Do not skip meals
   - Increase food intake before exercise
   - Check blood glucose regularly
   - Change insulin doses only with medical supervision
   - Carry a form of fast-acting sugar at all times
   - Wear a medical ID bracelet
   - Teach family, friends, coworkers about signs and treatment of hypoglycemia
   - Have family, roommates, traveling companions learn to use injectable glucagon for severe hypoglycemic reactions
4. Regular follow-up for evaluation of diabetes control
   - Keeps written record of blood glucose, insulin doses, hypoglycemic reactions, variations in diet
   - Keeps all appointments with health professionals
   - Sees physician regularly (usually 2–4 times per year)
   - States how to contact physician in case of emergency
   - States when to call physician to report variations in blood glucose levels

Some nurses specializing in diabetes have found that some patients (who have been taking insulin for many years) have stopped injecting air before withdrawing the insulin. These patients found that the extra step was not necessary for accurately drawing up the insulin doses. Most patients find it easier to withdraw the insulin by eliminating the step and report no difficulty in preparing the proper insulin dose.

Elimination of this step (or alteration of this practice, *e.g.*, injecting a syringe full of air into the vial once per week) facilitates the teaching process for some patients learning to draw up insulin for the first time. Some patients become confused with the sequence of steps involved in injecting air into two separate bottles in two different amounts before drawing up a mixed dose. For many individuals, including the elderly, simplification of the procedure for

CHART 39-4
Self-Injection of Insulin

1. With one hand, stabilize the skin be spreading it or pinching up a large area.

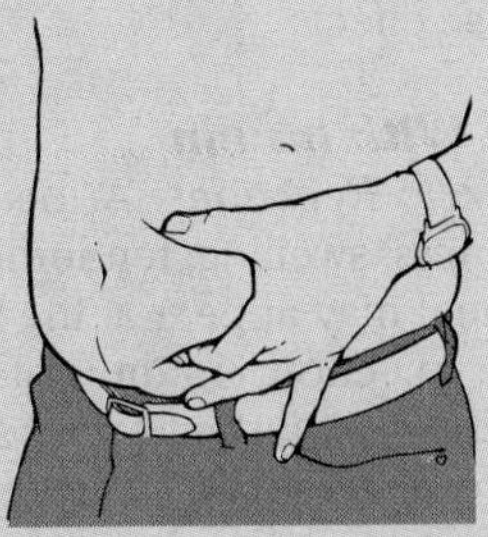

2. Pick up syringe with the other hand and hold it as you would a pencil. Insert needle straight into the skin.*

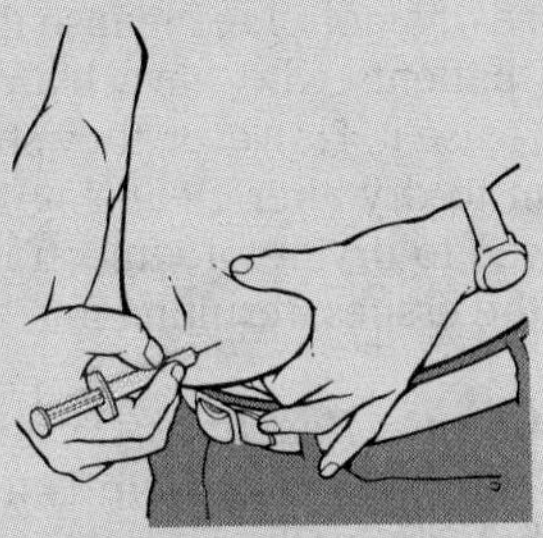

3. To inject the insulin, push the plunger all the way in.

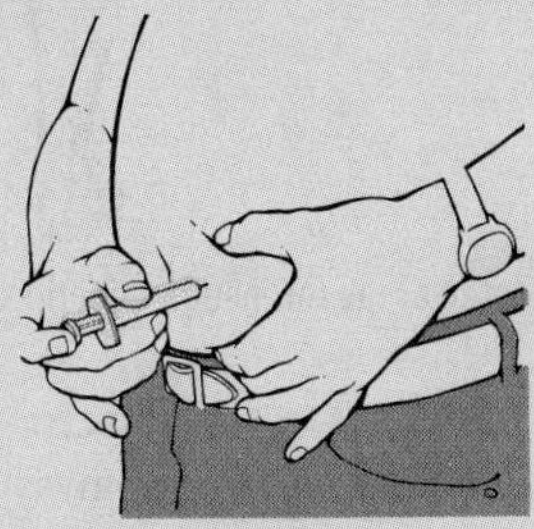

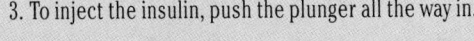

4. Pull needle straight out of skin. Press cotton ball over injection site for several seconds.

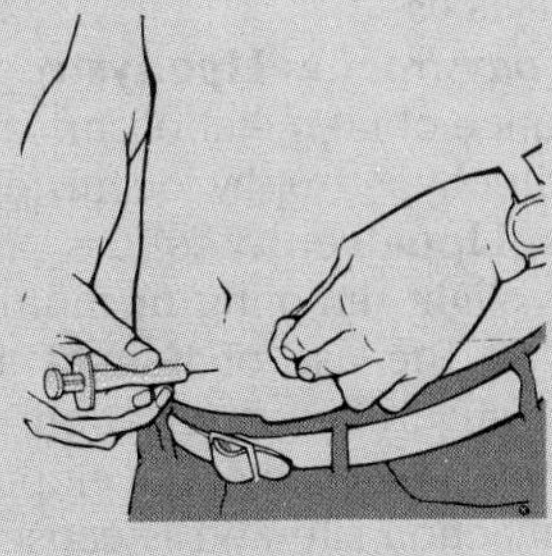

5. Use disposable syringe only once and discard into hard plastic container (with a tight-fitting top) such as an empty bleach or detergent container.†

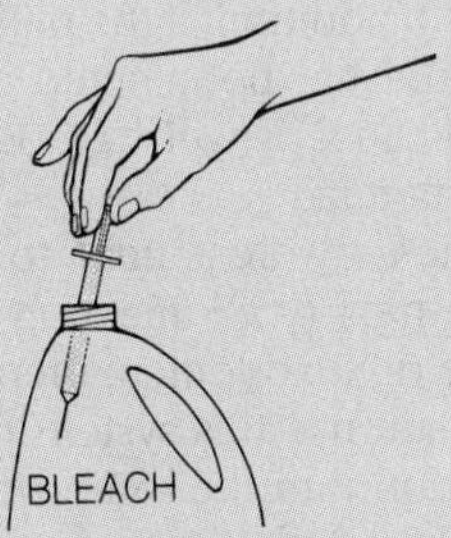

*Some patients may be taught to insert the needle at a 45-degree angle.
†Some studies suggest that it may be safe to reuse disposable syringes.

preparing insulin injections may have a major impact on maintaining independence in daily living.

As with other variations in insulin injection technique, the most important factor is that the patient maintain consistency in the procedure and that nurses be flexible when teaching new patients or assessing the skills of patients experienced with insulin injections.

Administering the Injection

Site Selection and Rotation. The four main areas for injection are the abdomen, arms (posterior surface), thighs (anterior surface), and hips (Fig. 39-3). Insulin is absorbed faster when injected into certain areas. Speed of absorption is greatest in the abdomen and decreases progressively in the arm, thigh, and hip.

Systematic rotation of injection sites within an anatomic area is recommended to prevent localized changes in fatty tissue (lipodystrophy). In addition, to promote consistency in insulin absorption, patients should be encouraged to use all available injection sites within one area rather than randomly rotating sites from area to area. For example, some patients almost exclusively use the abdominal area,

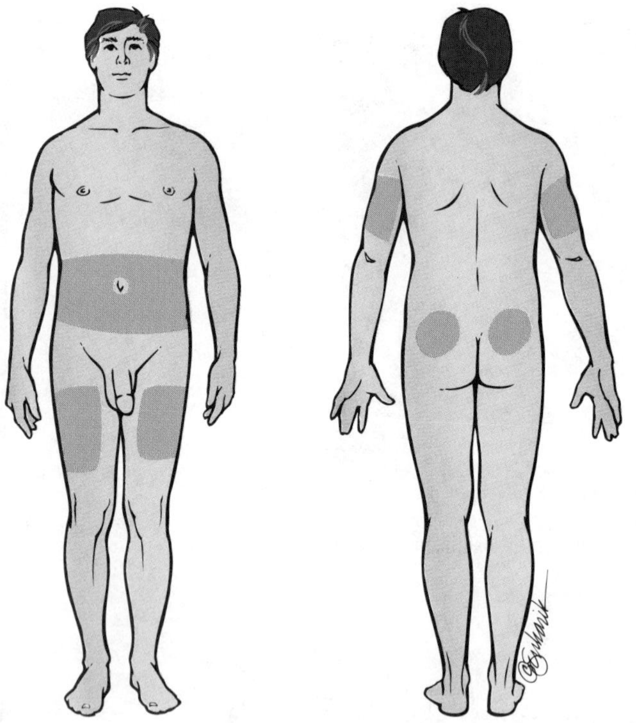

FIGURE 39-3. Suggested areas for insulin injection.

administering each injection ½ to 1 inch away from the previous injection. Another approach to rotation is to always use the same area at the same time of day. For example, patients may inject morning doses into the abdomen and evening doses into the arms or legs.

A few general principles apply to all rotation patterns. First, patients should try not to use the same site more than once in 2 to 3 weeks. In addition, if the patient is planning to exercise, insulin should not be injected into the limb that will be exercised, because it will be absorbed faster and may result in hypoglycemia.

In the past, patients were taught to rotate injections from one area to the next (*e.g.*, injecting once in the right arm, then once in the right abdomen, then once in the right thigh). Patients who still use this system must be taught to avoid repeated injection into the same site within an area. However, as previously stated, it is preferable for the patient to use the same anatomic area at the same time of day consistently; this reduces day-to-day variation in blood glucose levels because of different absorption rates.

Needle Insertion. There are varying approaches to insertion of the needle for insulin injections. These include spreading versus bunching the skin and using a 45-degree versus a 90-degree angle. The technique used for holding the skin and inserting the needle is based on the need to ensure that the insulin is injected into the subcutaneous tissue. Injection that is too deep (*e.g.*, intramuscular) or too shallow may affect the rate of absorption of the insulin.

The necessity of aspiration (inserting the needle and then pulling back on the plunger to assess for blood being drawn into the syringe) with self-injection of insulin has been questioned. For some patients, aspiration is a difficult and unsafe procedure. Patients with visual impairments or deficits in fine motor coordination may accidentally withdraw all or some of the needle while attempting to aspirate, and aspiration is virtually impossible for the patient limited to the use of one hand (*e.g.*, after a stroke). In addition, patients who use injection-aid devices into which the syringe is loaded are not able to visualize the syringe during the injection. Patients using insulin "pen" devices do not have the ability to pull back on the plunger at all. Many patients who have been using insulin for an extended period have eliminated this step from their insulin injection routine with no apparent adverse effects.

Problems With Insulin

Local Allergic Reactions. A local allergic reaction in the form of redness, swelling, tenderness, and induration or a 2- to 4-cm wheal may appear at the site of injection 1 to 2 hours after the injection is administered. These reactions usually occur during the beginning stages of therapy and disappear with continued use of insulin. These allergic reactions are becoming less frequent because of the increased purity of insulins. The physician may prescribe an antihistamine to be taken 1 hour before the injection if such a local reaction occurs.

Although use of alcohol to cleanse the skin is no longer recommended, patients who have learned this technique often continue to use it. However, they should be cautioned to allow the skin to dry after cleansing with alcohol. If the skin is not allowed to dry before injection, the alcohol may be carried into the tissues, resulting in a localized reddened area.

Systemic Allergic Reactions. Systemic allergic reactions to insulin are rare. First, there is an immediate local skin reaction that gradually spreads into generalized urticaria. The treatment is desensitization, with small doses of insulin administered in gradually increasing amounts. These rare reactions are occasionally associated with generalized edema or anaphylaxis.

Insulin Lipodystrophy. **Lipodystrophy** refers to a localized disturbance of fat metabolism, in the form of either lipoatrophy or lipohypertrophy, occurring at the site of insulin injections. **Lipoatrophy** is loss of subcutaneous fat and appears as slight dimpling or more serious pitting of subcutaneous fat. The use of human insulin has almost eliminated this disfiguring complication.

Lipohypertrophy is the development of fibrofatty masses at the injection site and is caused by the repeated use of an injection site. If insulin is injected into scarred areas, the absorption may be delayed. This is one reason why rotation of injection sites is so important. The patient should avoid injecting insulin into these areas until the hypertrophy disappears.

Insulin Resistance. Most patients at one time or another have some degree of insulin resistance. This may occur for various reasons, the most common being obesity, which can be overcome by weight loss.

Clinical insulin resistance has been defined as a daily insulin requirement of 200 units or more. In most diabetic patients taking insulin, immune antibodies develop and bind the insulin, thereby decreasing the insulin available for use. All animal insulins, as well as human insulins to a lesser degree, cause antibody production in humans.

Very few of these patients develop high levels of antibodies. Many of these patients give a history of insulin therapy interrupted for several months or more. Treatment consists of administering a purer insulin preparation, and occasionally prednisone may be needed to block the production of antibodies. This may be followed by a gradual reduction in insulin requirement. Therefore, patients need to monitor themselves for hypoglycemia.

Alternative Methods of Insulin Delivery

Injection Ports. These devices are subcutaneous access ports that are inserted into the subcutaneous tissue by the patient and remain in place for up to 3 days. The Button Infuser has a 27-gauge needle attached to a resealable injection port. A device called the Insuflon has a flexible Teflon catheter with an injection port attached. Similar to an IV catheter, there is an introducer needle that is removed once the catheter is in place. Patients tape the device in place and then give their insulin injections through the resealable port rather than puncturing their skin multiple times daily.

Insulin Pens. These devices use small (200-unit) prefilled insulin cartridges that are loaded into a penlike holder. A disposable needle is attached to the device for insulin injection. Insulin is delivered by dialing in a dose or pushing a button for every 1- or 2-unit increment administered. People using these devices still need to insert the needle for each injection; however, they do not need to carry insulin bottles or to draw up insulin before each injection. These devices are most useful for patients who need to inject only one type of insulin at a time (*e.g.*, premeal regular insulin three times a day and bedtime NPH insulin) or who can use the premixed insulins. These pens are convenient for those who administer insulin before dinner if eating out rather than at home.

Jet Injectors. As an alternative to needle injections, jet injection devices deliver insulin through the skin under pressure in an extremely fine stream. These devices are more expensive than other alternative devices mentioned above and require thorough training and supervision when first used. In addition, patients should be cautioned that absorption rates, peak insulin activity, and insulin levels may be different when changing to a jet injector. (Insulin administered by jet injector is usually absorbed faster.) Bruising has occurred in some patients with use of the jet injector.

Insulin Pumps. These are small, externally worn devices that closely mimic the functioning of the normal pancreas. Insulin pumps contain a 3-ml syringe that is attached to a long (42-inch), thin, narrow-lumen tube with a needle or Teflon catheter attached to the end (Figs. 39-4 and 39-5). The patient inserts the needle or Teflon catheter into the subcutaneous tissue (usually on the abdomen) and secures it with tape or a transparent dressing. The needle or Teflon catheter is changed at least every 3 days. The pump is then worn either on a belt or in a pocket. Some women keep the pump tucked into the front or side of the bra or wear it on a garter belt on the thigh.

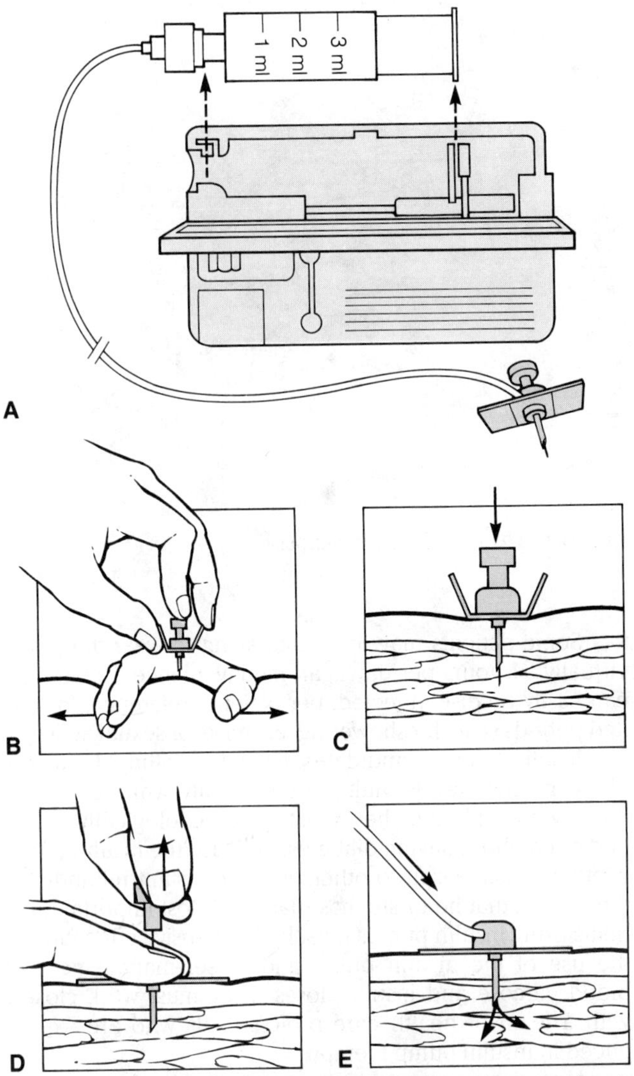

FIGURE 39-4. **(A)** Diagram of an insulin pump showing syringe in place inside pump and connection of pump via tubing to needle site. **(B–E)** Actual insertion site before, during, and after the needle and catheter have been inserted.

The pump uses only regular insulin, which is delivered in two different ways. First, there is a continuous "basal rate" of insulin that infuses typically at a rate of 0.5 to 2.0 units/hr. Then, before each meal, the patient activates the pump (through a series of button pushes) to deliver a "bolus" dose of insulin. The patient can decide on the amount of insulin bolus to infuse based on blood glucose levels and anticipated food intake and activity level.

There has been debate in the diabetes literature as to whether insulin pumps offer better control of blood glucose than other multiple-dose regimens (*e.g.*, three or four injections per day). One advantage of insulin pumps is that patients do not have to use intermediate- or long-acting insulins, which may have unpredictable peaks of action and may therefore cause unexpected swings in blood glucose. Some of the other advantages of insulin pumps include increased flexibility in lifestyle (in terms of timing and amount of meals, exercise, and travel) and, for some patients, improved blood glucose control.

A disadvantage of insulin pumps is that unexpected disruptions in the flow of insulin from the pump may occur if the tubing or needle becomes occluded, if the supply of insulin runs out, or if the battery is depleted. Another disadvantage is the potential for infection at needle insertion sites. Hypoglycemia may occur with insulin pump therapy; however, this is usually related to the lowered blood glucose levels many patients achieve rather than to a specific problem with the pump itself. The tight diabetic control associated with use of an insulin pump may increase the incidence of hypoglycemia awareness because of the gradual decline in serum glucose level from levels greater than 70 mg/dl (3.9 mmol/L) to those less than 60 mg/dl (3.3 mmol/L).

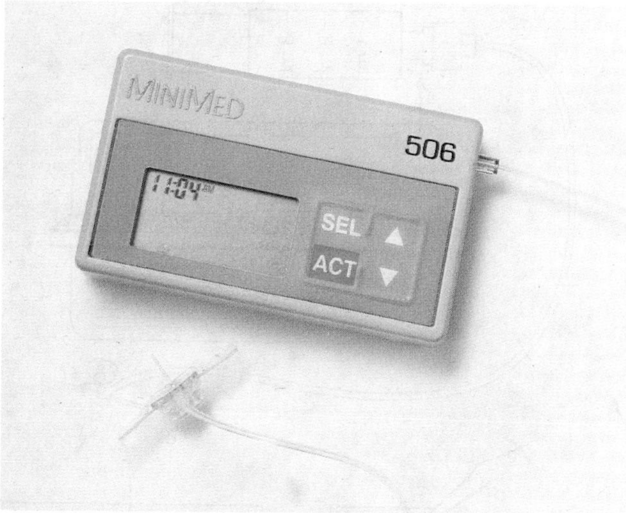

FIGURE 39-5. MiniMed insulin pump.

Some patients may find that having to wear the pump virtually 24 hours per day is an inconvenience. However, it can easily be disconnected, per patient preference, for limited periods (*e.g.*, for showering, exercise, or sexual activity).

Insulin pump candidates must be willing to assess blood glucose levels multiple times daily while on pump therapy. In addition, they must be psychologically stable and open about having diabetes, because the insulin pump is often a visible sign to others and a constant reminder to the patient that he or she has diabetes. Most important, patients using insulin pumps must have extensive education in the use of the insulin pump and in self-management of blood glucose and insulin doses. They must work closely with a team of health care professionals who are experienced in insulin pump therapy.

Many insurance policies cover the cost of pump therapy; if it is not covered, the extra expense of the pump and associated supplies may be a deterrent for some patients.

Research Into Alternative Insulin Delivery. Research into mechanical delivery of insulin has involved implantable insulin pumps that can be externally programmed according to blood glucose testing. Clinical trials with these devices are in progress. In addition, there is research into the development of implantable devices that both measure the blood glucose and deliver insulin as needed.

Research into nasal delivery of insulin has demonstrated this method of administration to be less effective and less consistent than hoped.

Transplantation. Transplantation of the whole pancreas or a segment of the pancreas is being performed on a limited population (mostly diabetic patients receiving kidney transplantations simultaneously). One main issue regarding pancreatic transplantation is weighing the risks of antirejection medications against the advantages of pancreas transplantation. Another approach under investigation is the implantation of insulin-producing pancreatic islet cells. This latter approach involves a less extensive surgical procedure and a potentially lower incidence of immunogenic problems. However, thus far independence from exogenous insulin has been limited to 2 years after transplantation of islet cells.

Oral Antidiabetic Agents

Oral antidiabetic agents may be effective for type II diabetic patients who cannot be treated by diet and exercise alone; however, they cannot be used during pregnancy. In the United States, oral antidiabetic agents include the sulfonylureas and biguanides (Table 39-7).

Sulfonylureas. The sulfonylureas exert their primary action by directly stimulating the pancreas to secrete insulin. Therefore, a functioning pancreas is necessary for these agents to be effective, and they cannot be used in patients with type I diabetes and who are prone to ketoacidosis. An additional important action of these agents, unrelated to a direct pancreatic effect, is to improve insulin action at the cellular level. They may also directly decrease glucose production by the liver.

The sulfonylureas can be divided into short-, intermediate-, and long-acting agents with varying duration of action.

TABLE 39-7 Oral Antidiabetic Agents Used in the United States

Generic Name (Trade Name)	Tablet Size (mg)	Usual Daily Dose Range (mg)	Maximum Dose (mg)	Duration of Action (hr)
Sulfonylurea Agents				
Acetohexamide (Dymelor)	250, 500	250–1500 (single or divided)	1500	12–24
Chlorpropamide (Diabinese)	100, 250	100–500 (single)	750	60
Glipizide (Glucotrol)	5, 10	5–25 (single or divided)	40	10–24
Glipizide (Glucotrol XL)	5, 10	5 mg single	10	24
Glyburide (Micronase, Diabeta)	1.25, 2.5, 5	2.5–10 (single or divided)	20	12–24
Tolazamide (Tolinase)	100, 250, 500	100–750 (single or divided)	1000	12–24
Tolbutamide (Orinase)	250, 500	500–2000 (divided)	3000	6–12
Biguanides				
Metformin (Glucophage)	500	1500 (divided)	2500	8

The most common side effects of these medications include gastrointestinal symptoms and dermatologic reactions. Hypoglycemia may occur when an excessive dose of a sulfonylurea is used or when meals are omitted or food intake is decreased. Because of the prolonged hypoglycemic effects of these agents (especially chlorpropamide), some patients need to be hospitalized for treatment of oral agent–induced hypoglycemia. Another side effect of chlorpropamide is a disulfiram (Antabuse)–type reaction when alcohol is ingested (see section on alcohol for more information).

Some medications may directly interact with sulfonylureas, potentiating their hypoglycemic effects (*e.g.*, sulfonamides, chloramphenicol, clofibrate, phenylbutazone, and bisohydroxycoumarin). In addition, certain medications may independently affect blood glucose levels, thereby indirectly interfering with these agents. Medications that may cause an elevation of glucose levels include potassium-losing diuretics, glucocorticoids, estrogen compounds, and diphenylhydantoin (Dilantin). Medications that may cause hypoglycemia include salicylates, propranolol, MAO (monoamine oxidase) inhibitors, and pentamidine.

Biguanides. Another category of oral antidiabetic agents is the biguanides. Metformin (Glucophage), a biguanide now approved for use in the U.S., produces its antidiabetic effects by facilitating insulin's action on peripheral receptor sites. Therefore, it can be used only in the presence of insulin. Biguanides have no effect on pancreatic beta cells. Lactic acidosis is a potential serious complication of biguanide therapy; the patient must be monitored closely when therapy is initiated or when dosage changes. Medications that may interact with biguanides include anticoagulants, corticosteroids, diuretics, and oral contraceptives. Metformin is contraindicated in patients with renal impairment; it should not be administered for 2 days before any diagnostic testing that may require use of a contrast agent. Both of these situations increase the risk for lactic acidosis.

It is important for patients to realize that oral agents are prescribed as an addition to (and not as a substitute for) other treatment modalities such as diet and exercise. Oral antidiabetic medications may need to be abandoned temporarily in favor of insulin if the patient develops hyperglycemia attributable to infection, trauma, or surgery.

If, as time goes on, a patient's blood glucose values that were once responsive to oral antidiabetic agents are no longer responsive to these agents, the patient is then treated with insulin. Approximately half of all patients who initially use oral antidiabetic agents eventually require insulin. This is referred to as a **secondary failure. Primary failure** occurs when the blood glucose level remains high a month after initial medication use.

Using a combination of oral agents with insulin has been proposed as a treatment for some patients with type II diabetes. However, the effectiveness of this approach has not yet been demonstrated.

Patient Education and Home Care Considerations

Diabetes mellitus is a chronic illness requiring a lifetime of special self-management behaviors. Because diet, physical activity, and physical and emotional stress can affect diabetic control, patients must learn to balance a multitude of factors. Not only must patients learn daily self-care skills for avoidance of acute decreases or increases in blood glucose, but they must also incorporate into their lifestyle many preventive behaviors for avoidance of long-term diabetic complications. An appreciation for the knowledge and skills that diabetic patients must acquire can help the nurse in providing effective patient education and counseling.

Approaches to Teaching. Changes in the health care delivery system as a whole have had a major impact on diabetes education and training. Patients with new-onset diabetes have much shorter hospital stays or may be managed completely on an outpatient basis. In recent years there has been a proliferation of outpatient diabetes education and training programs with increasing support of third-party reimbursement. Nonetheless, *for some patients, the only exposure to diabetes education is during hospitalization. This may be the only opportunity the patient has for learning skills of self-management and avoidance of diabetic complications.*

At many hospitals there are nurses who specialize in diabetes education and management. However, because of the large number of diabetic patients that are admitted to every unit of a hospital, the staff nurse plays a vital role in identifying diabetic patients, assessing self-care skills, providing basic education, reinforcing teaching provided by the specialist, and referring patients for follow-up after discharge.

Organizing Information. There are various schemes for organizing and prioritizing the vast amount of information that must be taught to diabetic patients. In addition, many hospitals and outpatient diabetes centers have devised written guidelines, care plans, and documentation forms (often based on guidelines from the American Diabetes Association) that may be used to document and evaluate diabetes teaching.

A general approach to organizing diabetes education is to divide information and skills into two main types: (1) basic, initial, or "survival" skills and information, and (2) in-depth ("advanced") or continuing education.

Survival Skills. This information must be taught to any patient with newly diagnosed type I diabetes or any type II diabetic patient starting on insulin for the first time. This basic survival information is literally that which the patient must know to "survive" (*i.e.*, avoid severe hypoglycemic or acute hyperglycemic complications) after discharge. Categories of survival information include:

1. Simple pathophysiology
   a. Basic definition of diabetes (having high blood glucose)
   b. Normal blood glucose ranges
   c. Effect of insulin and exercise (decrease glucose)
   d. Effect of food and stress, including illness and infections (increase glucose)
   e. Basic treatment approaches
2. Treatment modalities
   a. Insulin administration
   b. Basic diet information (*e.g.*, food groups and timing of meals)
   c. Monitoring of blood glucose, urine ketones
3. Recognition, treatment, and prevention of acute complications
   a. Hypoglycemia
   b. Hyperglycemia

4. Pragmatic information
   a. Where to buy and store insulin, syringes, glucose-monitoring supplies
   b. When and how to reach the physician

Newly diagnosed type II diabetic patients also need to learn some of this basic information. Most of the emphasis is initially placed on diet. For patients started on oral sulfonylureas, it is also very important to teach about hypoglycemia. If the diabetes has gone undetected for many years, the patient may already be experiencing some of the chronic diabetic complications. Thus, for some patients with newly diagnosed type II diabetes, the basic diabetes teaching must include information on preventive skills such as foot care and eye care (*i.e.*, planning yearly or more frequent examinations by the ophthalmologist and understanding that retinopathy is largely asymptomatic until the advanced stages). It is important for patients to realize that once they master the basic skills and information, further diabetes education must be pursued. Acquiring in-depth and advanced diabetes knowledge occurs throughout the patient's lifetime both informally (through experience and sharing of information with other people with diabetes) and formally (through programs of continuing education).

In-Depth/Continuing Education. This involves teaching more detailed information related to survival skills (such as learning to vary diet and insulin and preparing for travel) as well as learning preventive measures for the avoidance of long-term diabetic complications. These preventive measures include:

- Foot care
- Eye care
- General hygiene (*e.g.*, skin care, oral hygiene)
- Risk factor management (control of blood pressure and blood lipids, normalizing blood glucose levels)

More advanced continuing education may include the use of alternative methods for insulin delivery (*e.g.*, the insulin pump and learning algorithms or decision rules for evaluating and adjusting insulin doses). For example, patients can be taught to increase or decrease insulin doses based on a several-day pattern of blood glucose levels.

The amount of "advanced" diabetes education to be provided depends on patient interest and ability. However, learning preventive measures (especially foot care and eye care) is mandatory and vitally important for reducing the occurrence of amputations and blindness in the diabetic population.

Timing of Teaching. Before initiating diabetes education, it is important to assess the patient's (and family's) readiness to learn. When patients are first diagnosed with diabetes (or first told of their need for insulin), they go through various stages of the grieving process. These stages may include shock and denial, depression, negotiation, anger, and acceptance. The amount of time it takes for patients and family members to work through the grieving process varies from patient to patient. They may experience helplessness, guilt, altered body image, loss of self-esteem, and concern about the future. The nurse must assess the patient's coping strategies and reassure patients and families that feelings of depression and shock are normal.

Asking the patient and family about their major concerns or fears is an important way to learn about any misinformation that may be unnecessarily contributing to feelings of anxiety. Some common misconceptions regarding diabetes and its treatment are listed in Chart 39-5. Simple, direct information should be provided to dispel misconceptions. More in-depth information can be provided once survival skills are mastered.

After dispelling misconceptions or answering questions that concern the patient the most, the nurse must use a firm, but caring, approach to focus attention on concrete survival skills. Because of the immediacy of needing to learn multiple new skills, initiating teaching as soon as possible after diagnosis is crucial. For patients who are in the hospital, there is not usually the luxury of waiting until the patient feels ready to learn. Early discharge necessitates initiation of survival skill education as early as possible in the hospital stay. Early teaching allows the patient ample opportunity to practice skills with supervision by the nurse before discharge. Follow-up by home health nurses is often necessary for reinforcement of survival skills.

A goal of patient teaching is an educated consumer. The patient is informed about wide variations in prices of medications and supplies and about the importance of comparing prices.

Teaching Methods. Maintaining flexibility in teaching approaches is important. Teaching skills and information in a "logical" sequence is not always the most helpful for patients. For example, many patients are focused on their fear of the injection. Before they learn how to draw up, purchase, store, and mix insulins, they should be taught to insert the needle and inject insulin (or practice with saline). Furthermore, numerous demonstrations by the nurse or practice injections before the patient (or family) gives the first injection may actually increase the patient's anxiety and fear of self-injection.

For most patients, once they have actually performed the injection, they are more prepared to hear and to comprehend other information. (If the patient then wants to practice further using a pillow or an orange, that would be appropriate). Thus, having the patient self-inject first or having the patient perform a fingerstick for glucose monitoring first may enhance learning to draw up the insulin or to operate the glucose monitor.

Various tools can be used to aid in teaching. Many of the companies that manufacture products for diabetes self-care also provide booklets and videotapes to assist in patient teaching. It is important to use a variety of written handouts that are matched to the patient's ability (including different languages, low-literacy information, information with large print). Patients can be encouraged to continue learning about diabetes care by participating in activities sponsored by local hospitals and diabetes organizations. In addition, there are many magazines geared toward people with diabetes that provide information on all aspects of diabetes management.

Ample opportunity should be provided for the patient and family to repeatedly practice skills under supervision (including self-injection, self-testing, meal selection, verbalization of symptoms, and treatment of hypoglycemia). Once skills have been mastered, participation in ongoing support groups may assist patients in incorporating new habits and maintaining adherence to the treatment regimen.

Teaching the "Experienced" Diabetic Patient. The nurse should continue to assess skills of patients who have had diabetes for many years, because it has been esti-

CHART 39-5
Misconceptions Related to Diabetes and Its Treatment

Misconception	Nurse's Response
Diabetes is caused by eating too much sugar.	Once diabetes develops, eating too much sugar can cause the glucose level to rise. However, the reason that diabetes develops initially is that there is a decrease in the amount of insulin in the body or a decrease in the ability of insulin to control the blood glucose level. These problems are *not* caused by eating too much sugar. In type I diabetes, in which the pancreatic beta cells produce little or no insulin, various factors contribute to beta-cell damage, including genetics, a defect in the immune system, or an external factor (such as a virus). In type II diabetes, the body is resistant to the effect of insulin. The amount of insulin released by the beta cells is not enough to overcome this insulin resistance, and hyperglycemia results. Insulin resistance and decreased insulin release are *not* caused by eating too much sugar. Two factors that do contribute to the development of type II diabetes are obesity and a family history of diabetes.
Sugar is found only in dessert foods.	There are several different types of sugars (simple carbohydrates) that increase blood glucose levels. Dessert foods often contain sucrose, one type of sugar. Many other packaged foods (such as flavored yogurt, cereals, canned beans, sauces, salad dressing, "health food bars") also contain some form of sugar. Patients should be instructed to check labels for sources of sugar such as corn syrup, dextrose, brown sugar, honey. *Fruit and fruit juices also contain sugar.* Even if the juice is labeled "unsweetened" or "no sugar added," there is still natural fruit sugar in the product, which causes elevations in the glucose level.
The only diet change needed in the treatment of diabetes is to stop eating sugar.	First, it is important for the patient to realize that it is not feasible (nor is it advisable) to remove *all* sources of sugar from the diet. There are nutritional foods (such as fruit) that contain some form of sugar and that should be included in the meal plan. In addition, recent research has shown that increasing the amount of simple sugars (including table sugar) allowed in the diabetic meal plan may not adversely affect glucose levels. For patients requiring insulin, the meal plan includes limiting concentrated sweets as well as maintaining consistency in time intervals between meals. In addition, patients need to learn to adjust the insulin dose if there are variations in the amount of food eaten or in the carbohydrate content of meals. For patients receiving oral antidiabetic agents, it is important to avoid skipping meals and to limit intake of sugars. If the patient is obese, the meal plan emphasizes limiting total calories, which is best achieved by decreasing the fat content of meals.
Once insulin injections are started (for treatment of type II diabetes) they can never be discontinued.	During periods of acute stress (such as illness, infection, or surgery) or when receiving certain medications that cause elevations in blood glucose, some patients with type II diabetes require insulin. If the diabetes had previously been well controlled with diet alone or diet with oral antidiabetic agents, the patient should be able to resume previous methods for control of diabetes when the stress is resolved. In addition, insulin is sometimes used to control blood glucose levels in obese type II diabetic patients who have been unsuccessful at weight loss. If the patient is able to lose weight after insulin therapy is initiated, the insulin doses may be tapered and the patient may be able to switch to diet and exercise alone or with oral antidiabetic agents for control of blood glucose. (For patients with type I diabetes, insulin is needed on an ongoing basis. For thin patients with type II diabetes, once insulin has to be started, it is usually required permanently).
If increasing doses of insulin are needed to control the blood glucose, the diabetes must be getting "worse."	Explain to the patient that, unlike other medications that are given in standard doses, there is not a standard dose of insulin that is effective for all patients. Rather, the dose must be adjusted according to blood glucose test results. If the initial insulin dose prescribed for the patient does not adequately decrease the glucose level, the patient may assume that he or she has a "bad" case of diabetes or that the diabetes is getting worse. It is important to instruct patients that many different factors may affect the ability of insulin to lower the glucose, including obesity, puberty, pregnancy, illness, and certain medications.

(continued)

CHART 39-5 *(continued)*

Misconception	Nurse's Response
	In addition, to avoid hypoglycemia, physicians frequently initiate insulin therapy with smaller dosages than will eventually be needed. The doses are then increased in small increments until blood glucose levels are in the desired range.
Insulin causes blindness (or other diabetic complications).	When patients have a diabetic acquaintance in whom the initiation of insulin therapy happened to coincide with the onset of diabetic complications, the patient may view insulin as the cause of complications such as blindness or amputation. In these situations, the acquaintance probably had type II diabetes that was no longer controllable with diet and oral hypoglycemic agents. It must be explained to the patient that factors such as elevated blood glucose and elevated blood levels (and not insulin therapy) contribute to some of the diabetic complications. Furthermore, emphasize that insulin is a natural hormone that is present in every person's body, helps control blood glucose levels, and definitely does not cause long-term complications of diabetes.
Insulin must be injected directly into the vein.	When patients first learn that one area used for insulin injections in the arm, they may envision inserting the needle directly into a vein in the antecubital area, as in blood withdrawal. The patient must be reassured that insulin is injected into the fat tissue on the *back* of the arm (or on the abdomen, thigh, or hip) and that the needle is much shorter than that used for venipuncture.
There is extreme danger in injecting insulin if there are any air bubbles in the syringe.	Patients may have a fear of dying if air bubbles are injected with a syringe. (This may be related to the misconception that insulin is injected directly into the vein.) Reassure patients that the main danger in having air bubbles in the insulin syringe is that the amount of insulin being injected is less than the required dosage. It is often difficult to remove every small "champagne" bubble from the syringe. Thus, the patient should be reassured that injection of insulin when these bubbles are present will not cause any harm.
Urine and blood glucose testing are interchangeable (*i.e.,* they provide the same information).	Explain to the patient that directly testing the blood is the most accurate method of measuring the glucose level. The *urine* glucose test, which measures the amount of glucose that has "spilled" into the urine since the bladder was last emptied, is only an indirect way of determining the glucose level in the *blood.* The kidneys will not allow sugar to spill into the urine until the blood glucose reaches a level about 180 to 200 mg/dl (10–11.1 mmol/L). Therefore, the urine will test negative for glucose when the *blood* glucose is at any level between 0 and 200 mg/dl. Hypoglycemia cannot be detected with urine testing, nor can the blood glucose level be strictly controlled.
Blood glucose levels remain the same throughout the day.	Explain to patients that there is normally a variation in blood glucose levels—with the lowest levels before meals and the highest levels 1 to 2 hours after eating. The goal of the diabetes treatment plan is to minimize wide swings in glucose levels, not to eliminate the normal variations.

(Pearce MA, Rosenberg CS, and Davidson MB. Patient education. In Davidson MB [ed]. Diabetes Mellitus: Diagnosis and Treatment, 3rd ed. New York, Churchill Livingstone, 1991.)

mated that up to 50% of patients may make errors in self-care skills. Assessment of these patients must include **direct observation** of skills, not just asking patients to describe self-care behaviors. In addition, it is imperative that these patients be fully aware of preventive measures related to foot care, eye care, and risk factor management. If patients are experiencing long-term diabetic complications for the first time, they may go through the grieving process again. Some of these patients may experience a renewed interest in diabetes self-care in the hope of delaying further complications. Other patients may be overwhelmed by feelings of guilt and depression. The patient is encouraged to discuss feelings and fears related to complications; appropriate information regarding diabetic complications is provided by the nurse.

Promoting Adherence. Patients who are having difficulty adhering to the diabetes treatment plan must be approached with a sense of caring and understanding. The use of "scare" tactics (such as threats of blindness or amputation if the patient does not adhere to the treatment plan) or making the patient feel guilty is not productive and may interfere with establishing a trusting relationship with the patient. Using judgmental terminology, such as asking the patient if he or she has "cheated" on his or her diet, only promotes feelings of guilt and low self-esteem.

If problems exist with glucose control or with the development of preventable complications, it is important to distinguish between nonadherence, knowledge deficit, and a self-care deficit. It should not be assumed that problems with diabetes management are related to nonadherence. The patient may simply have forgotten or never learned certain information. The problem may be correctable simply through providing complete information and assuring patient comprehension of information.

If knowledge deficit is not the problem, certain physical or emotional factors may be impairing the patient's ability to perform self-care skills. For example, decreased visual acuity may impair the patient's ability to accurately administer insulin, measure blood glucose, or inspect skin and feet. In addition, decreased joint mobility (especially in the elderly) impairs the ability to inspect the bottom of the feet. Emotional factors such as denial of the diagnosis or depression may impair the patient's ability to carry out multiple daily self-care measures. In other circumstances, family, personal, or work problems and issues may seem urgent and may be perceived as higher priority by the patient. The patient facing competing demands for time and attention may benefit from assistance in establishing priorities.

It is also important to assess the patient for signs of infection or emotional stress that may lead to elevated blood glucose levels despite adherence to the treatment regimen.

The following approaches by the nurse are helpful for promoting adherence:

1. Deal with any underlying factors (*e.g.*, knowledge deficit, self-care deficit, illness) that may affect diabetic control
2. Simplify the treatment regimen if it is too difficult for the patient to follow
3. Adjust the treatment regimen to meet patient requests (*e.g.*, adjust diet or insulin schedule to allow for increased flexibility in meal content or timing)
4. Establish a specific plan or contract with the patient with simple, measurable goals
5. Provide positive reinforcement of self-care behaviors performed instead of focusing on behaviors that were neglected (*e.g.*, praise a patient for blood glucose testing that was performed instead of focusing on the number of "missed" tests)
6. Help the patient to identify personal motivating factors rather than focusing on wanting to please the doctor or nurse
7. Encourage pursuit of life goals and interests; discourage undue focus on diabetes

Encouraging Participation in Support Groups. Participation in support groups is encouraged for those who have had diabetes for many years as well as those who are newly diagnosed. Such participation may assist the patient and family in coping with changes in lifestyle that occur with the onset of diabetes and with its complications. In addition, those who participate in support groups often have an opportunity to share valuable information and experiences and to learn from others. Support groups provide opportunity for discussion of strategies to deal with diabetes and its management and to clarify and verify information with the nurse or other health care professionals. The support provided through participation in support groups may help patients and their families to become more knowledgeable about diabetes and its management and may promote adherence to the management plan.

Acute Complications of Diabetes

There are three major acute complications of diabetes related to short-term imbalances in blood glucose: hypoglycemia, DKA, and HHNK syndrome (also known as hyperglycemic hyperosmolar nonketotic coma—HHNKC).

Hypoglycemia (Insulin Reactions)

Hypoglycemia (abnormally low blood glucose level) occurs when the blood glucose falls below 50 to 60 mg/dl (2.7 to 3.3 mmol/L). It can be caused by too much insulin or oral hypoglycemic agents, too little food, or excessive physical activity. Hypoglycemia may occur at any time of the day or night. It often occurs before meals, especially if meals are delayed or snacks are omitted. For example, midmorning hypoglycemia may occur when the morning regular insulin is peaking, whereas hypoglycemia that occurs in the late afternoon coincides with the peak of the morning NPH or Lente insulin. Middle-of-the-night hypoglycemia may occur because of peaking evening NPH or Lente insulins, especially in patients who have not eaten a bedtime snack.

Symptoms. The symptoms of hypoglycemia may be grouped into two categories: adrenergic symptoms and central nervous system symptoms.

In **mild hypoglycemia,** as the blood glucose level falls, the sympathetic nervous system is stimulated. The surge of adrenalin causes symptoms such as sweating, tremor, tachycardia, palpitation, nervousness, and hunger.

In **moderate hypoglycemia,** the fall in blood glucose level deprives the brain cells of needed fuel for functioning. Signs of impaired function of the central nervous system may include inability to concentrate, headache, lightheadedness, confusion, memory lapses, numbness of the lips and tongue, slurred speech, incoordination, emotional changes, irrational behavior, double vision, and drowsiness. Any combination of these symptoms (in addition to adrenergic symptoms) may occur with moderate hypoglycemia.

In **severe hypoglycemia,** central nervous system function is so impaired that the patient needs the assistance of another person for treatment of hypoglycemia. Symptoms may include disoriented behavior, seizures, difficulty arousing from sleep, or loss of consciousness.

Hypoglycemic symptoms may occur suddenly and unexpectedly. The combination of symptoms varies considerably from person to person. To some degree, this may be related to the actual level to which the blood glucose drops or to the rate at which it is dropping. For example, patients who usually have blood glucose in the hyperglycemic range (*e.g.*, in the 200s or greater) may feel hypoglycemic (adrenergic) symptoms when their blood glucose quickly drops to 120 mg/dl (6.6 mmol/L) or less. Conversely, patients who frequently have glucose in the low range of normal may be asymptomatic when the blood glucose slowly falls under 50 mg/dl (2.7 mmol/L).

Another factor contributing to altered hypoglycemic symptoms is a decreased hormonal (adrenergic) response to hypoglycemia. This occurs in some patients who have had diabetes for many years. It may be related to one of the chronic diabetic complications—autonomic neuropathy (see section on hypoglycemic unawareness). As the blood glucose falls, the normal surge in adrenalin does not occur. The patient does not feel the usual adrenergic symptoms, such as sweating and shakiness. The hypoglycemia may not be detected until moderate or severe central nervous system impairment occurs. It is imperative that these patients perform self-monitoring of blood glucose on a frequent regular basis, especially before driving or engaging in other potentially dangerous activities.

Treatment. Immediate treatment must be given when hypoglycemia occurs. The usual recommendation is for 10 to 15 g of a fast-acting sugar orally:

2–4 commercially prepared glucose tablets
4–6 oz fruit juice or regular soda
6–10 Life Savers or other hard candies
2–3 tsp sugar or honey

(It is not necessary to add sugar to juice, even if it is labeled as "unsweetened" juice. The fruit sugar in juice contains enough simple carbohydrate to sufficiently raise the blood glucose level. Adding table sugar to juice may cause a sharp increase in the blood glucose, and the patient may experience hyperglycemia for hours after treatment.)

If the symptoms persist more than 10 to 15 minutes after initial treatment, the treatment is repeated. Once the symptoms resolve, a snack containing protein and starch (such as milk or cheese and crackers) is recommended unless the patient plans on eating a regular meal or snack within 30 to 60 minutes.

It is important for diabetic patients (especially those on insulin) to carry some form of simple sugar with them at all times. There are many different commercially prepared glucose tablets and gels that patients may find convenient to carry. If the patient experiences a hypoglycemic reaction and does not have any of the recommended emergency foods available, any available food (preferably a simple carbohydrate food) should be consumed.

Patients are encouraged to refrain from eating high-calorie, high-fat dessert foods (such as cookies, cakes, donuts, ice cream) to treat hypoglycemia. The high fat content of these foods may slow the absorption of the glucose, and the hypoglycemic symptoms may not be resolved as quickly as they are with the intake of simple carbohydrates. The patient may subsequently eat more of the foods when symptoms do not resolve rapidly. This in turn may cause very high levels of blood glucose for several hours after the reaction and may also contribute to weight gain.

Patients who feel unduly restricted by their meal plan may view hypoglycemic episodes as a time to "reward" themselves with desserts. It may be more prudent to teach these patients to incorporate occasional desserts into the meal plan. This may make it easier for them to limit their treatment of hypoglycemic episodes to simple (low-calorie) carbohydrates such as juice or glucose tablets.

Treatment of Severe Hypoglycemia. For patients who are unconscious, are unable to swallow, or refuse treatment, an injection of glucagon 1 mg can be administered either subcutaneously or intramuscularly. Glucagon is a hormone produced by the alpha cells of the pancreas that stimulates the liver to release glucose (through the breakdown of glycogen, the stored glucose). It is packaged as a powder in 1-mg vials and must be mixed with a diluent before being injected. After injection of glucagon, it may take up to 20 minutes for the patient to regain consciousness. A simple sugar followed by a snack should be given to the patient on awakening to prevent recurrence of hypoglycemia, because the duration of the action of 1 mg of glucagon is brief (its onset is 8 to 10 minutes and its action lasts 12 to 27 minutes) and to replenish liver stores of glucose. Some patients experience nausea after the administration of glucagon. The patient should be instructed to notify the physician after severe hypoglycemia has occurred.

Glucagon is sold by prescription only and should be part of the emergency supplies kept available by persons with diabetes who require insulin. Family members, neighbors, or co-workers should be instructed in the use of glucagon. This is especially true for patients who receive little or no warning of hypoglycemic episodes.

In the hospital or emergency room, patients who are unconscious or unable to swallow may be treated with 25 to 50 ml 50% dextrose in water ("D-50"), which is administered intravenously. The effect is usually seen within minutes. Patients may complain of a headache and of pain at the IV site. Assuring patency of the intravenous line used for injection of 50% dextrose is important; hypertonic solutions such as 50% dextrose are very irritating to the vein.

Patient Education and Home Care Considerations. Hypoglycemia is prevented by following a regular pattern for eating, administering insulin, and exercising. Between-meal and bedtime snacks may be needed to counteract the maximum insulin effect. In general, the patient should cover the time of peak activity of insulin by eating a snack and by taking additional food when engaging in an increased level of physical activity. Routine blood glucose tests are performed so that changing insulin requirements may be anticipated and adjusted.

Because unexpected hypoglycemia may occur, all patients treated with insulin should wear an identification bracelet or tag indicating that they have diabetes.

Patients and family members must be instructed on the various potential symptoms of hypoglycemia. Family members especially must be made aware that any subtle (but unusual) change in behavior may be an indication that hypoglycemia is occurring. They should be taught to encourage and even insist that the person with diabetes assess blood glucose levels if hypoglycemia is suspected. Some patients (when hypoglycemic) become very resistant to testing or eating and become angry at family members trying to treat the hypoglycemia. Family members must be taught to persevere and to understand that the hypoglycemia can cause irrational and unintentional behavior.

Some patients with autonomic neuropathy or those taking propranolol for the treatment of hypertension or cardiac dysrhythmias may not experience the typical symptoms of hypoglycemia. It is very important for these patients to perform blood glucose tests on a frequent and regular basis.

Type II diabetes patients who take oral hypoglycemic agents may also develop hypoglycemia (especially those taking chlorpropamide, which is a long-lasting oral hypoglycemic agent).

Gerontologic Considerations. In the elderly, hypoglycemia is a particular concern for many reasons:

Elderly people frequently live alone and may not recognize the symptoms of hypoglycemia
With decreasing renal function, it takes longer for oral hypoglycemic agents to be excreted by the kidneys
Skipping meals may occur because of decreased appetite or financial limitations on meal planning

Decreased visual acuity may lead to errors in insulin administration

Diabetic Ketoacidosis

Pathophysiology. Diabetic ketoacidosis (DKA) is caused by an absence or markedly inadequate amount of insulin. This results in disorders in the metabolism of carbohydrate, protein, and fat. The three main clinical features of DKA are

- Dehydration
- Electrolyte loss
- Acidosis

When insulin is lacking, the amount of glucose entering the cells is reduced. In addition, there is unrestrained production of glucose by the liver. Both of these factors lead to hyperglycemia. In an attempt to rid the body of the excess glucose, the kidneys excrete the glucose along with water and electrolytes (such as sodium and potassium). This osmotic diuresis, which is characterized by excessive urination (polyuria), leads to **dehydration** and marked **electrolyte loss.** Patients with severe DKA may lose an average of 6.5 liters of water and up to 400 to 500 mEq each of sodium, potassium, and chloride over a 24-hour period.

Another effect of insulin deficiency is the breakdown of fat (lipolysis) into free fatty acids and glycerol. The free fatty acids are converted into ketone bodies by the liver. In DKA there is an excess production of ketone bodies because of the lack of insulin that would normally prevent this from occurring. Ketone bodies are acids, and when they accumulate in the circulation they lead to metabolic **acidosis.**

Clinical Manifestations. The signs and symptoms of DKA are outlined in Figure 39-6. The hyperglycemia of DKA leads to polyuria and polydipsia (increased thirst). In addition, patients may experience blurred vision, weakness, and headache. Patients with marked intravascular volume depletion may have orthostatic hypotension (drop in systolic blood pressure of 20 mm Hg or more on standing). Volume depletion may also lead to frank hypotension with a weak, rapid pulse.

The ketosis and acidosis characteristic of DKA lead to gastrointestinal symptoms such as anorexia, nausea, vomiting, and abdominal pain. The abdominal pain and physical findings on examination can be so severe that it appears that there is an intraabdominal process occurring that will require surgery. Patients may have acetone breath (a fruity odor), which occurs with elevated levels of ketone bodies. In addition, hyperventilation (with very deep, but not labored, respirations) may occur. These **Kussmaul respirations** represent the body's attempt to decrease the acidosis, counteracting the effect of the ketone buildup.

Mental status changes in DKA vary widely from patient to patient. Patients may be alert, lethargic, or comatose, most likely depending on the plasma **osmolarity** (concentration of osmotically active particles).

Laboratory Values. Blood glucose levels may vary from 300 to 800 mg/dl (16.6 to 44.4 mmol/L). Some patients may have lower glucose values, and others may have values as high as 1000 mg/dl (55.5 mmol/L) or more (usually depending on the degree of dehydration).

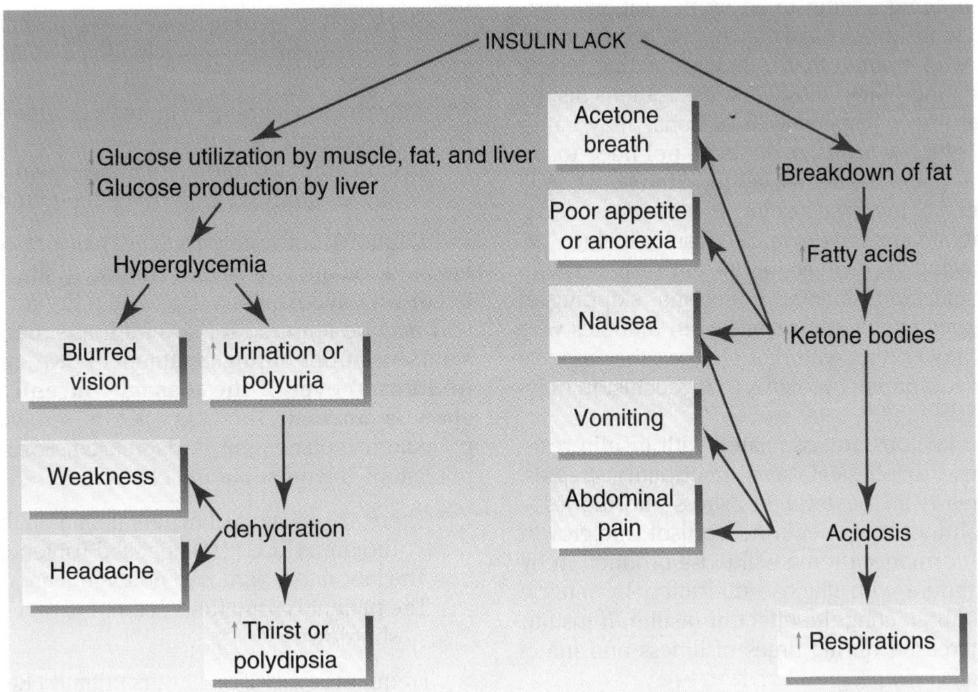

FIGURE 39-6. Abnormal metabolism that causes signs and symptoms of diabetic ketoacidosis: ↑, increased; ↓, decreased. (Pearce MA, Rosenberg CS, and Davidson MD. Patient education. In Davidson MB [ed]. Diabetes Mellitus: Diagnosis and Treatment, 3rd ed. New York, Churchill Livingstone, 1991.)

- It is important to realize that the severity of DKA is not necessarily related to the blood glucose level.
- Some patients may have severe acidosis with blood glucose levels in the high 100- to low 200-mg/dl (5.5 to 11.1 mmol/L) range, whereas others may have no evidence of DKA despite blood glucose levels of 400 to 500 mg/dl (22.2 to 27.7 mmol/L).

Evidence of ketoacidosis is reflected in low serum bicarbonate (0 to 15 mEq/L) and low *p*H (6.8 to 7.3) values. A low pCO_2 level (10 to 30 mm Hg) reflects respiratory compensation (Kussmaul respirations) for the metabolic acidosis. Accumulation of ketone bodies (which precipitates the acidosis) is reflected in blood and urine ketone measurements.

Sodium and potassium levels may be low, normal, or high, depending on the amount of water loss (dehydration). It is important to remember that despite the plasma concentration there has been a marked total body depletion of these (and other) electrolytes. Ultimately, these electrolytes will need to be replaced.

Elevated levels of creatinine, blood urea nitrogen (BUN), hemoglobin, and hematocrit may also be seen with dehydration. After rehydration, continued elevation in the serum creatinine and BUN levels will be present in the patient with underlying renal insufficiency.

Causes. Three main causes of DKA are

- A decreased or missed dose of insulin
- An illness or infection
- The initial manifestation of undiagnosed and untreated diabetes

A decrease in insulin may result from an insufficient dosage of insulin being prescribed or from an insufficient dosage of insulin being administered by the patient. Erroneous decreases in insulin dosage may be made by patients who are ill and who assume that if they are eating less or if they are vomiting, they must decrease their insulin doses. (Because illness [especially infections] may cause increased blood glucose levels, patients do not need to decrease doses to account for decreased food intake when ill and may even need to increase insulin.)

Other potential causes of decreased insulin include patient error in drawing up or injecting insulin (especially in patients with visual impairments); intentional skipping of insulin doses (especially in adolescents with diabetes who are having difficulty coping with diabetes or other aspects of their lives); or equipment problems (*e.g.*, occlusion of insulin pump tubing).

Illness and infections are associated with insulin resistance. In response to physical (and emotional) stresses, there is an increase in the level of "stress" hormones—glucagon, epinephrine, norepinephrine, cortisol, and growth hormone. These hormones promote glucose production by the liver and interfere with glucose utilization by muscle and fat tissue, counteracting the effect of insulin. If insulin levels are not increased during times of illness and infection, hyperglycemia may progress to DKA.

Treatment. Treatment of DKA is aimed at correction of the three main problems: dehydration, electrolyte loss, and acidosis.

Dehydration. Rehydration is important for maintaining tissue perfusion. In addition, fluid replacement enhances the excretion of excess glucose by the kidneys. Patients may need up to 6 to 10 liters intravenous fluid to replace fluid loss caused by polyuria, hyperventilation, diarrhea, and vomiting.

Initially, 0.9% normal saline is administered at a very high rate—usually 0.5 to 1 L/hr for 2 to 3 hours. Hypotonic normal saline (0.45%) may be used for patients with hypertension or hypernatremia or those at risk for congestive heart failure. After the first few hours, 0.45% normal saline is the fluid of choice for continued rehydration, provided the blood pressure is stable and the sodium level is not low. Moderate to high rates of infusion (200 to 500 ml/hr) may continue for several more hours.

Monitoring fluid volume status involves frequent measurement of vital signs (including monitoring for orthostatic changes in blood pressure and heart rate), lung assessment, and monitoring intake and output. Initial urine output will lag behind intravenous fluid intake as dehydration is corrected. Plasma expanders may be necessary for correction of severe hypotension that does not respond to intravenous fluid treatment. Monitoring for signs of fluid overload is especially important for the older patient or patients at risk for congestive heart failure.

Electrolyte Loss. The major electrolyte of concern during treatment of DKA is potassium. Although the initial plasma concentration of potassium may be low, normal, or even high, there is a major loss of potassium from body stores. Furthermore, the level of potassium drops during the course of treatment of DKA and therefore must be monitored frequently.

Some of the factors related to treatment of DKA that reduce the serum potassium concentration include

Rehydration leading to increased plasma volume and subsequent decreases in the concentration of serum potassium
Rehydration leading to increased urinary excretion of potassium
Insulin administration enhancing the movement of potassium from the extracellular fluid into the cells

Cautious but timely replacement of potassium is vital for the avoidance of severe cardiac dysrhythmias that may occur with hypokalemia. Up to 40 mEq/hr (added to IV fluids) may be required for several hours. Because the potassium level drops during treatment of DKA, **potassium must be infused even if the plasma concentration of potassium is normal.** Then, as DKA is resolving, the rate of potassium replacement is decreased. For safe infusion of potassium, the nurse should check that

There are no signs of hyperkalemia on the electrocardiogram (ECG) (tall, peaked [or tented] T waves)
The laboratory values of potassium are normal or low
The patient is urinating (*i.e.*, not experiencing renal shutdown)

Frequent (every 2 to 4 hours initially) ECG readings and laboratory measurements of potassium are necessary during the first 8 hours of treatment. Potassium replacement is withheld only if hyperkalemia is present or if the patient is not urinating. However, because the potassium level may drop quickly as a result of rehydration and insulin treatment, potassium replacement must be initiated as soon as potassium levels drop to normal.

Acidosis. The accumulation of ketone bodies (acids) is the result of fat breakdown. The acidosis that occurs in DKA is reversed with insulin. Insulin inhibits the fat breakdown, thereby stopping the buildup of acids.

Insulin is usually infused intravenously at a slow, continuous rate (*e.g.*, 5 units per hour). Hourly blood glucose values must be measured. Dextrose is added to IV fluids (*e.g.*, D_5NS or D_5.45NS) when blood glucose levels reach 250 to 300 mg/dl (13.8 to 16.6 mmol/L) to avoid too rapid a drop in the blood glucose level.

Various intravenous mixtures of regular insulin may be used. The nurse must convert hourly rates of insulin infusion (frequently ordered as "units per hour") to IV drip rates. For example, if 100 units regular insulin are mixed in 500 ml 0.9NS, then 1 unit insulin equals 5 ml. Thus, an initial insulin infusion rate of 5 units per hour would equal 25 ml/hr. It is best to infuse the insulin separately from the rehydration solutions to allow for frequent changes in rate and content of rehydration solutions.

- When mixing the insulin drip, it is important to flush the insulin solution through the entire IV infusion set and to discard the first 50 ml fluid. Insulin molecules adhere to the glass and plastic of IV infusion sets; thus, the initial fluid may contain a decreased concentration of insulin.
- It is imperative that the IV insulin be infused *continuously* until subcutaneous administration of insulin is resumed. Any interruption in insulin administration may result in the reaccumulation of ketone bodies and worsening acidosis. Even if blood glucose levels are dropping to normal, the insulin drip must not be turned off. Rather, the rate or concentration of the dextrose infusion should be increased.

It is important to remember that blood glucose levels are usually corrected before the acidosis is corrected. Thus, IV insulin may be continued for 12 to 24 hours, until the serum bicarbonate improves (to at least 15 to 18 mEq/L) and until the patient can eat.

In general, bicarbonate infusion for correction of severe acidosis is avoided during treatment of DKA because it precipitates further, sudden (and potentially fatal) decreases in serum potassium levels. Continuous insulin infusion is usually sufficient for reversing the acidosis of DKA.

Prevention and Education. For prevention of DKA related to illness, patients must be taught "sick day rules" for managing their diabetes when ill (Chart 39-6). The most important issue is to teach patients not to eliminate insulin doses when nausea and vomiting occur. Rather, they should take their usual insulin dose (or previously prescribed special "sick day" doses) and then attempt to consume frequent small portions of carbohydrates (including foods usually avoided, such as juices, regular sodas, and gelatin). Drinking fluids every hour—including broth—is important for avoidance of dehydration. Blood glucose and urine ketones must be assessed every 3 to 4 hours.

If the patient is unable to take fluids without vomiting, or if elevated glucose or ketone levels persist, the physician must be contacted. Patients are taught to plan ahead and to have available foods for use on sick days. In addition, a supply of urine test strips (for ketone testing) and blood glucose test strips should be available. Patients must know how to contact their physician 24 hours a day.

Diabetes self-management skills (including insulin administration and blood glucose testing) should be assessed to ensure that accidental error in insulin administration or blood glucose testing did not occur. Psychologic counseling is recommended for patients and family members if intentional alteration in insulin dosing was the cause of the DKA.

Hyperglycemic Hyperosmolar Nonketotic Syndrome

Pathophysiology and Clinical Manifestations. Hyperglycemic hyperosmolar nonketotic (HHNK) syn-

CHART 39-6

Guidelines to Follow During Periods of Illness ("Sick Day Rules")

- Take insulin or oral antidiabetic agents as usual.
- Test blood glucose and (for type I diabetic patients) test urine ketones every 3 to 4 hours.
- Report elevated glucose levels (greater than 300 mg/dl, 16.6 mmol/L, or as otherwise specified) or urine ketones to the physician.
- Insulin-requiring patients may need supplemental doses of regular insulin every 3 to 4 hours.
- If usual meal plan cannot be followed, substitute soft foods (*e.g.*, ½ cup regular gelatin, 1 cup cream soup, ½ cup custard, 3 squares graham crackers) six to eight times per day.
- If vomiting, diarrhea, or fever persists, take liquids (*e.g.*, ½ cup regular cola or orange juice, ½ cup broth, 1 cup Gatorade) every ½ to 1 hour to prevent dehydration and to provide calories.
- Report nausea, vomiting, and diarrhea to the physician because extreme fluid loss may be dangerous.
- For patients with type I diabetes, inability to retain oral fluids may warrant hospitalization to avoid diabetic ketoacidosis and possibly coma.

drome is a situation in which hyperosmolarity and hyperglycemia predominate, with alterations of the sensorium (sense of awareness). At the same time, ketosis is minimal or absent. The basic biochemical defect is lack of effective insulin. The patient's persistent hyperglycemia causes osmotic diuresis, resulting in losses of water and electrolytes. To maintain osmotic equilibrium, water shifts from the intracellular fluid space to the extracellular fluid space. With glucosuria and dehydration, hypernatremia and increased osmolarity occur.

One major difference between HHNK syndrome and DKA is that ketosis and acidosis do not occur in HHNK syndrome. Differences in the amount of insulin present in each condition are thought to be partially responsible for this. In DKA there is virtually no insulin present; thus, breakdown of stored glucose, protein, and fat occurs (the latter leading to production of ketone bodies and subsequent ketoacidosis). In HHNK syndrome, the level of insulin is not as low. Although there is not enough insulin to prevent hyperglycemia (and subsequent osmotic diuresis), the small amount of insulin present is enough to prevent fat breakdown. Patients with HHNK syndrome do not experience the gastrointestinal symptoms related to ketosis that cause the patient with DKA to seek medical attention. Often, patients developing HHNK syndrome tolerate polyuria and polydipsia for weeks, and only when neurologic changes occur or when an underlying illness worsens do they (or more often family or staff at an extended care facility) seek medical attention. Thus, the hyperglycemia and dehydration are more severe in HHNK syndrome secondary to delays in treatment.

The clinical picture of HHNK syndrome is one of hypotension, profound dehydration (dry mucous membranes, poor skin turgor), tachycardia, and variable neurologic signs (*e.g.*, alteration of sensorium, seizures, hemiparesis). This is a serious condition with a mortality rate ranging from 5% to 30%, usually related to an underlying illness.

Causes. This condition occurs most frequently in older people (50 to 70 years of age) who have had no previous history of diabetes or only mild type II diabetes. The acute development of the condition can be traced to some precipitating event, such as an acute illness (pneumonia, myocardial infarction, stroke), ingestion of medications known to provoke insulin insufficiency (thiazide diuretics, propranolol), or therapeutic procedures (peritoneal dialysis/hemodialysis, total parenteral nutrition). There is a history of days to weeks of polyuria, with inadequate fluid intake.

Management. The overall approach to the treatment of HHNK syndrome is similar to that of DKA: fluids, electrolytes, and insulin. Because of the increased age of the typical patient with HHNK syndrome, close monitoring of volume and electrolyte status may be needed for prevention of congestive heart failure and cardiac dysrhythmias. Fluid treatment is started with 0.9% or 0.45% normal saline, depending on the sodium level and severity of volume depletion. Central venous or arterial pressure monitoring may be necessary to guide fluid replacement. Potassium is added to replacement fluids when urinary output is adequate and is guided by continuous ECG monitoring and frequent laboratory determinations of potassium.

Extremely elevated blood glucose levels drop as the patient is rehydrated. Insulin plays a less crucial role in the treatment of HHNK syndrome because it is not needed for reversal of acidosis, as in DKA. Nonetheless, insulin is usually administered at a continuous low rate to treat hyperglycemia, and dextrose is added to replacement fluids (as in DKA) when the glucose level decreases to the 250- to 300-mg/dl range (13.8 to 16.6 mmol/L).

Other therapeutic modalities are determined by the underlying illness of the patient and the results of continuing clinical and laboratory evaluation. Treatment is continued until metabolic abnormalities are corrected and neurologic symptoms clear. It may take as many as 3 to 5 days for neurologic symptoms to resolve; thus, treatment of HHNK usually continues well beyond the time when metabolic abnormalities are resolved.

After recovery from HHNK syndrome, many patients can control diabetes with diet alone or with diet and oral hypoglycemic agents. Insulin may not be needed once the acute hyperglycemic complication is resolved.

❑ NURSING PROCESS
The Patient With Newly Diagnosed Diabetes Mellitus

Assessment

The history and physical assessment focus on the signs and symptoms of prolonged hyperglycemia and on physical, social, and emotional factors that may affect the patient's ability to learn and perform diabetes self-care activities.

The patient is interviewed and asked for a description of symptoms that preceded the diagnosis of diabetes, such as polyuria, polydipsia, polyphagia, skin dryness, blurred vision, weight loss, vaginal itching, and nonhealing ulcers. The blood glucose and, for patients with type I diabetes, urine ketone levels are measured.

Patients with type I diabetes are assessed for signs of DKA, including ketonuria, Kussmaul respirations, orthostatic hypotension, and lethargy. The patient is questioned about symptoms of DKA, such as nausea, vomiting, and abdominal pain. Laboratory values are monitored for signs of metabolic acidosis, such as decreased *p*H and decreased bicarbonate, and for signs of electrolyte imbalance.

Patients with type II diabetes are assessed for signs of HHNK syndrome, including hypotension, altered sensorium, seizures, and decreased skin turgor. Laboratory values are monitored for signs of hyperosmolarity and electrolyte imbalance.

(**Note:** If the patient exhibits signs and symptoms of DKA or HHNK syndrome, nursing care first focuses on treatment of these acute complications as outlined in previous sections. Once these complications are resolving, nursing care then focuses on long-term management of diabetes as discussed in this section.)

The patient is assessed for physical factors that may impair ability to learn or perform self-care skills, such as

- ❑ Visual deficits (the patient is asked to read numbers or words on the insulin syringe, menu, newspaper, or written teaching materials)

- Deficits in motor coordination (the patient is observed eating or performing other tasks or handling a syringe or finger-lancing device)
- Neurologic deficits (*e.g.*, due to stroke) (from history in chart; the patient is assessed for aphasia or decreased ability to follow simple commands)

The nurse evaluates the patient's social situation for factors that may influence the diabetes treatment and education plan, such as

- Decreased literacy (may be assessed while assessing for visual deficits by having patient read from teaching materials)
- Limited financial resources/lack of health insurance
- Presence or absence of family support
- Typical daily schedule (patient is asked about timing and number of usual daily meals, work and exercise schedule, plans for travel)

The patient's emotional status is assessed through observation of general demeanor (*e.g.*, withdrawn, anxious) and body language (*e.g.*, avoids eye contact). The patient is asked about major concerns and fears about diabetes (this allows for assessment of any misconceptions or misinformation regarding diabetes). Coping skills are assessed by asking how the patient has dealt with difficult situations in the past.

Diagnosis

Nursing Diagnoses

Based on the assessment data, the patient's major nursing diagnoses may include the following:

- Risk for fluid volume deficit related to polyuria and dehydration
- Altered nutrition related to imbalance of insulin, food, and physical activity
- Knowledge deficit about diabetes self-care skills/information
- Potential self-care deficit related to physical impairments or social factors
- Anxiety related to loss of control, fear of inability to manage diabetes, misinformation related to diabetes, fear of diabetes complications

Collaborative Problems/ Potential Complications

Based on assessment data, potential complications may include:

- Fluid overload, pulmonary edema, congestive heart failure
- Hypokalemia
- Hyperglycemia and ketoacidosis
- Hypoglycemia
- Cerebral edema

Planning and Implementation

Goals. The major goals of the patient may include attainment of fluid and electrolyte balance, optimal control of blood glucose, regaining weight lost, ability to perform basic (survival) diabetes skills and self-care activities, reduction in anxiety, and absence of complications.

Nursing Interventions

Maintaining Fluid and Electrolyte Balance. Intake and output are measured. Intravenous fluids and electrolytes are administered as ordered, and oral fluid intake is encouraged. Laboratory values of serum electrolytes (especially sodium and potassium) are monitored. The patient's vital signs are monitored to detect signs of dehydration: tachycardia, orthostatic hypotension.

Improving Nutritional Intake. The diet is planned with the control of glucose as the primary goal; however, it must also take into consideration the patient's lifestyle, cultural background, activity level, and food preferences. The patient is encouraged to eat full meals and snacks as prescribed per diabetic diet. Arrangements are made with the dietitian for extra snacks before increased physical activity. It is important for the nurse to ensure that insulin orders are altered as needed for delays in eating because of diagnostic and other procedures.

Reducing Anxiety. The nurse provides emotional support and sets aside time to sit with the patient who wishes to vent, cry, or ask questions about this new diagnosis. Any misconceptions the patient or family may have regarding diabetes are dispelled (see Chart 39-5). The patient and family are assisted to focus on learning self-care behaviors. The patient is encouraged to perform the skills that are feared most, and must be reassured that once a skill such as self-injection or puncturing a finger for glucose monitoring is performed for the first time, anxiety will be relieved. The patient is given positive reinforcement for the self-care behaviors attempted, even if the technique is not yet completely mastered.

Improving Self-Care. Patient teaching is the major strategy used to prepare the patient for self-care. Special equipment is used for instruction on diabetes survival skills, such as a magnifying glass for insulin preparation or an injection aid device for insulin injection. Low-literacy information is used as needed. The family is instructed to enable them to assist in diabetes management (*e.g.*, to prefill syringes, to monitor blood glucose). The diabetes specialist is consulted regarding various blood glucose monitors and other equipment for use with patients with physical impairments. Follow-up education is arranged with a home health nurse or an outpatient diabetes education center. The patient is assisted in identifying community resources for education and supplies as needed; consideration is given to financial limitations or physical limitations (such as centers for the visually impaired). Other members of the health care team are informed about variations in the timing of meals and the work schedule (*e.g.*, if patient works at night or in the evenings and sleeps during the day) so that the diabetes treatment regimen can be adjusted accordingly.

Patient Education and Home Care Considerations. The patient is taught survival skills, including simple pathophysiology; treatment modalities (insulin administration, monitoring of blood glucose and—for type I diabetes—urine ketones, diet); recognition, treatment, and prevention of acute complications (hypoglycemia and hyperglycemia); and pragmatic information (where to obtain supplies, when to call physician). If the patient has signs of long-term diabetes complications at the time of diagnosis of diabetes, teaching about appropriate preventive behaviors (*e.g.*, foot care or eye care) should be included at this time.

Monitoring and Managing Potential Complications

Fluid Overload. Fluid overload can occur because of the administration of large volume of fluid at a rapid rate that is often required to treat the patient with DKA or HHNK syndrome. This risk is increased in elderly patients and in those with preexisting cardiac disease. To avoid fluid overload and resulting congestive heart failure and pulmonary edema, the nurse monitors the patient closely during treatment by measuring vital signs at frequent intervals. Central venous pressure (CVP) monitoring and hemodynamic monitoring may be initiated to provide additional measures of the patient's fluid status. Physical examination focuses on assessment of cardiac rate and rhythm, breath sounds, venous distention, skin turgor, and urine output. The nurse monitors intravenous fluid intake and keeps careful records of intravenous and other fluid intake along with urine output measurements. The patient is monitored for orthostatic hypotension secondary to dehydration.

Hypokalemia. As previously described, hypokalemia is a potential complication during treatment of DKA as potassium is lost from body stores. Low potassium levels may result from rehydration, increased urinary excretion of potassium, and movement of potassium from the extracellular fluid into the cells with insulin administration. Prevention of hypokalemia includes cautious replacement of potassium; before its administration, however, it is important to ensure that the patient's kidneys are functioning. Because of the adverse effects of hypokalemia on cardiac function, monitoring of the cardiac rate, cardiac rhythm, ECG, and serum potassium levels is essential.

Hyperglycemia and Ketoacidosis. Although the hyperglycemia and ketoacidosis that may have led to the new diagnosis of diabetes may be resolved, the patient is at risk for their subsequent recurrence. Therefore, blood glucose levels and urine ketones are monitored, and medications (insulin, oral hypoglycemic agents) are administered as prescribed. The patient is monitored for signs and symptoms of impending hyperglycemia and ketoacidosis; if they occur, insulin and intravenous fluid are administered.

Hypoglycemia. Hypoglycemia may occur if the patient skips or delays meals or does not follow the prescribed diet or greatly increases the amount of exercise without modifying diet and insulin.

Additionally, the hospitalized patient or outpatient who fasts in preparation for diagnostic testing is at risk for hypoglycemia. Juice or glucose tablets are used for treatment of hypoglycemia. The patient is encouraged to eat full meals and snacks as prescribed per diabetic diet. If hypoglycemia is a recurrent problem, the patient's total therapeutic regimen should be reevaluated.

Because of risk of hypoglycemia, it is important for the nurse to review with the patient its signs and symptoms, possible causes, and measures to prevent and treat it. The importance of the patient having readily available information regarding diabetes is stressed by the nurse.

Cerebral Edema. Although the cause of cerebral edema is unknown, it is thought to be caused by correcting hyperglycemia too rapidly, resulting in fluid shifts. Cerebral edema can be prevented by gradual reduction in the blood glucose level. Use of an hourly flow sheet is initiated to enable close monitoring of the patient's blood glucose level, serum electrolyte levels, urine output, mental status, and neurologic signs. Precautions are taken to minimize activities that could increase intracranial pressure.

Evaluation

Expected Outcomes

1. Achieves fluid and electrolyte balance
   a. Demonstrates intake and output balance
   b. Exhibits electrolyte values that are within normal limits
   c. Vital signs remain stable with resolution of orthostatic hypotension and tachycardia
2. Achieves metabolic balance
   a. Avoids extremes of glucose levels (hypoglycemia or hyperglycemia)
   b. Demonstrates rapid resolution of hypoglycemic episodes
   c. Avoids further weight loss (if applicable) and begins to approach desired weight
3. Demonstrates/verbalizes diabetes survival skills, including:

Simple Pathophysiology

a. Defines diabetes as a condition in which high blood glucose is present
b. States normal blood glucose range
c. Identifies factors that cause the blood glucose level to fall (insulin, exercise)
d. Identifies factors that cause the blood glucose level to rise (food, illness, and infections)
e. Describes the major treatment modalities—diet, exercise, monitoring, medication, education

Treatment Modalities (Insulin, Diet, Monitoring, Education)

a. Demonstrates proper technique for drawing up and injecting insulin (including mixing two types of insulin if necessary)
b. Verbalizes insulin injection rotation plan
c. Verbalizes understanding of classification of food groups (depending on system used)
d. Verbalizes appropriate schedule for eating snacks and meals
e. Orders appropriate foods on menus and identifies foods that may be substituted for one another on the meal plan
f. Demonstrates proper technique for monitoring blood glucose, including using finger-lancing device; obtaining large, hanging drop of blood; applying blood properly to strip; removing blood from strip at appropriate interval (if necessary); obtaining value of blood glucose; and recording blood glucose value. If meter is used, patient is able to calibrate and clean meter, change batteries, and identify alarms and warnings on meter.
g. Demonstrates proper technique for disposing of needles used for blood glucose monitoring and insulin

injections (*e.g.*, discarding needles into hard plastic container such as empty bleach or detergent container)

h. Demonstrates proper technique for urine ketone testing (for patients with type I diabetes) and verbalizes appropriate times to assess for ketones—when ill or when glucose test results are repeatedly and unexplainably over 250 to 300 mg/dl (13.8 to 16.6 mmol/L)

i. Identifies community, outpatient resources for obtaining further diabetes education

Acute Complications (Hypoglycemia and Hyperglycemia)

a. Verbalizes symptoms of hypoglycemia (shakiness, sweating, headache, hunger, numbness or tingling of lips or fingers, weakness, fatigue, difficulty concentrating, change of mood) and dangers of untreated hypoglycemia (seizures and coma)

b. Identifies appropriate treatment of hypoglycemia, including 10 to 15 g simple carbohydrate (*e.g.*, 2 to 4 glucose tablets, 4 to 6 oz juice or soda, 2 to 3 tsp sugar, or 6 to 10 Life Savers) followed by a snack of protein and carbohydrate, such as cheese and crackers or milk, or by a regularly scheduled meal

c. Identifies potential causes of hypoglycemia—too much insulin, delayed or decreased food intake, increased physical activity

d. Verbalizes preventive behaviors, such as frequent monitoring of blood glucose when daily schedule is changed, taking snack before exercise. Verbalizes importance of wearing medical identification and carrying a source of simple carbohydrate **at all times.**

e. Verbalizes symptoms of prolonged hyperglycemia—increased thirst and urination

f. Verbalizes rules for sick-day management (see Chart 39-6)

Pragmatic Information

a. Verbalizes where to purchase and store insulin, syringes, and glucose-monitoring supplies

b. Identifies appropriate circumstances for calling the physician, including when ill, when glucose levels are repeatedly over a certain level (per physician guidelines), or when skin wounds fail to heal

c. Identifies name and phone number to reach physician or other member of health care team 24 hours per day

4. Absence of complications
   a. Exhibits normal cardiac rate and rhythm and normal breath sounds
   b. Jugular venous pressure and distention within normal limits
   c. Blood glucose and urine ketones within normal limits
   d. Exhibits no manifestations of hypo- or hyperglycemia
   e. Mental status improved without signs of cerebral edema
   f. States measures to prevent occurrence of complications

Long-Term Complications of Diabetes

There has been a steady decline in deaths of diabetic patients attributable to ketoacidosis and infection but an alarming rise in deaths of cardiovascular and renal complications. Long-term complications are becoming more common as more persons live longer with diabetes.

The long-term complications of diabetes can affect almost every organ system of the body. The general categories of chronic diabetic complications are

Macrovascular disease
Microvascular disease
Neuropathy

The specific causes and pathogenesis of each type of complication are still being investigated. It appears, however, that increased levels of blood glucose may play a role in neuropathic disease, microvascular complications, and risk factors contributing to macrovascular complications. Hypertension may also be a major contributing factor, especially in macrovascular and microvascular diseases.

Long-term complications are seen in both type I and type II diabetes, usually not occurring within the first 5 to 10 years of the diagnosis. Renal (microvascular) disease is more prevalent among type I diabetic patients, and cardiovascular (macrovascular) complications are more prevalent among older type II diabetic patients.

Macrovascular Complications

Atherosclerotic changes in the larger blood vessels commonly occur in diabetes. These atherosclerotic changes are similar to those seen in nondiabetic patients except that they tend to occur at an earlier age and with greater frequency in diabetic patients. Depending on the location of the atherosclerotic lesions, different types of macrovascular diseases may result.

Coronary Artery Disease. Atherosclerotic changes in the coronary arteries lead to an increased occurrence of myocardial infarctions in persons with diabetes (twice as frequent in diabetic men and three times as frequent in diabetic women). In diabetes there is an increased likelihood of complications resulting from myocardial infarction and increased likelihood of a second myocardial infarction occurring. Some studies suggest that coronary artery disease may account for 50% to 60% of all deaths in patients with diabetes.

One unique feature of coronary artery disease in patients with diabetes is that the typical ischemic symptoms may be absent. Thus, patients may not experience the early warning signs of decreased coronary blood flow and may have "silent" myocardial infarctions in which chest pain or other typical symptoms are not experienced. These "silent" myocardial infarctions may be discovered only as changes on the electrocardiogram. This lack of ischemic symptoms may be secondary to autonomic neuropathy.

Cerebrovascular Disease. Atherosclerotic changes in cerebral blood vessels or the formation of an embolus elsewhere in the vasculature that then lodges in a cerebral blood vessel can lead to the occurrence of transient ischemic attacks and strokes. Cerebrovascular disease in diabetic patients is similar to that of nondiabetic patients except that people with diabetes may have twice the risk of developing cerebrovascular disease, and studies suggest that there may be a greater likelihood of death due to cerebrovascular disease in diabetes. In addition, recovery from a stroke may be impaired in patients who have elevated blood glucose levels at the time of diagnosis and immediately after a cerebrovascular accident.

Symptoms of cerebrovascular disease may be quite similar to those of the acute diabetic complications (HHNK syndrome or hypoglycemia). These may include dizziness, decreased vision, slurred speech, and weakness. It is very important that patients reporting these types of symptoms be assessed for blood glucose levels (and treated as indicated for blood glucose abnormalities) before the initiation of extensive diagnostic testing for cerebrovascular disease.

Peripheral Vascular Disease. Atherosclerotic changes in the large blood vessels of the lower extremities are responsible for the increased incidence (two to three times higher than in nondiabetic persons) of occlusive peripheral arterial disease in diabetic patients. Signs and symptoms of peripheral vascular disease may include diminished peripheral pulses and intermittent claudication (pain in the buttock, thigh, or calf during walking). The severe form of arterial occlusive disease in the lower extremities is largely responsible for the increased incidence of gangrene and amputation in diabetic patients.

Neuropathy and impairments in wound healing also play a role in diabetic foot disease (see next sections).

Role of Diabetes in Macrovascular Diseases. Diabetes researchers continue to investigate the relationship between diabetes and macrovascular diseases. The atherosclerotic changes that occur in the blood vessels of diabetic patients are no different from those that occur in the nondiabetic population. Although diabetic patients are more likely to develop macrovascular diseases, there is no clear-cut explanation for why they are more prone to develop atherosclerotic changes than their nondiabetic counterparts. The main feature unique to diabetes is an elevated level of blood glucose. However, a direct link has not been found between hyperglycemia and atherosclerosis.

There are certain risk factors that are associated with accelerated atherosclerosis. These include elevated blood lipids, hypertension, cigarette smoking, obesity, lack of exercise, and family history. These risk factors appear to play equal roles in the development of macrovascular diseases in both the diabetic and nondiabetic population. Although certain risk factors may be more common among diabetic patients (*e.g.*, obesity, increased triglyceride levels, hypertension), there continues to be a higher rate of macrovascular diseases among diabetic patients as compared with nondiabetic patients possessing the same risk factors. Thus, diabetes itself is seen as an independent risk factor for the development of accelerated atherosclerosis.

Other potential factors that may play a role in diabetes-related atherosclerosis are the subject of debate among diabetes researchers. These include platelet and clotting-factor abnormalities, decreased flexibility of red blood cells, decreased oxygen release, changes in the arterial wall related to hyperglycemia, and possibly hyperinsulinemia.

Treatment and Prevention of Macrovascular Diseases. Prevention and treatment of the commonly accepted risk factors for atherosclerosis are recommended. Diet is important in the management of obesity, hypertension, and hyperlipidemia. In addition, the use of medications for control of hypertension and hyperlipidemia may be indicated. There is some evidence that increased triglyceride levels may improve with the control of blood glucose levels.

Regular exercise is important; however, there may be certain limitations that need to be considered. The presence of intermittent claudication may limit the patient's ability to exercise. These patients need to be given recommendations for slowly increasing the amount of exercise so as to increase blood flow to the lower extremities, thereby increasing exercise tolerance. In addition, pentoxifylline (Trental) may be prescribed for relief of pain from claudication. This medication improves blood flow to ischemic areas through its effect on red blood cell flexibility, platelet adhesiveness, and blood viscosity.

As discussed earlier (see Exercise, p. 1026), the presence of other diabetic complications (*e.g.*, neuropathy, retinopathy) may limit the types of exercises that can be performed. Exercise is timed to promote lowering of postmeal hyperglycemia while avoiding hypoglycemia at peak times of insulin action.

Risk factor management is an important aspect of diabetes treatment. For patients on insulin, attention is often focused exclusively on blood glucose levels and adjustment of insulin doses. However, it is important to teach patients that risk factor management is an equally important part of diabetic treatment and must not be forgotten, even by patients who successfully maintain strict blood glucose control.

When macrovascular complications do occur, treatment is the same as with nondiabetic patients. In addition, it is important to pay attention to blood glucose control. Physiologic stress that accompanies illnesses such as strokes and myocardial infarctions, as well as the stress of surgical procedures, may cause an increase in blood glucose levels. Appropriate adjustment of medications is important. For some type II diabetic patients there may be a need to switch from oral hypoglycemic medications to insulin.

The ability to perform diabetes self-care skills may be adversely affected in patients who have experienced a stroke and who have a deficit in upper extremity function. The use of special equipment for assistance in blood glucose monitoring and insulin administration may be indicated.

Microvascular Complications

Although macrovascular atherosclerotic changes are seen in both diabetic and nondiabetic patients, the microvascular changes are unique to diabetes. Diabetic microvascular disease (or microangiopathy) is characterized by capillary basement membrane thickening. The basement membrane surrounds the endothelial cells of the capillary. Researchers postulate that increased blood glucose levels react through a series of biochemical responses to thicken the basement membrane to several times its normal thickness.

Two places where impaired capillary function may have devastating effects are the microcirculation of the retina of the eye and the kidney. The resulting diabetic retinopathy is the leading cause of blindness in people between 20 and 74 years of age in the United States. Similarly, about one in every four individuals starting dialysis has diabetic nephropathy.

Diabetic Retinopathy

The eye pathology referred to as diabetic retinopathy is caused by changes in the small blood vessels in the retina of the eye (Fig. 39-7). The retina is the area of the eye that receives images and sends information about the images to the brain. It is richly supplied with blood vessels of all kinds—small arteries and veins, arterioles, venules, and capillaries.

There are three main stages of retinopathy: nonproliferative (background) retinopathy, preproliferative retinopathy, and proliferative retinopathy. Most diabetic patients develop some degree of background retinopathy within 5 to 15 years of the diagnosis of diabetes. A very small percentage of these patients go on to develop the more serious proliferative stage or the condition called **macular edema,** in which visual impairment is common.

The results of the DCCT (1993) demonstrated that maintenance of blood glucose to a normal or near-normal level through intensive insulin therapy decreased the risk for development of retinopathy by 76% when compared with conventional therapy in patients without preexisting retinopathy. The progression of retinopathy was decreased by 54% in patients with very mild to moderate nonproliferative retinopathy at the time of initiation of treatment.

Nonproliferative (Background) Retinopathy. As many as 90% of diabetic patients (with poorly controlled blood glucose) may develop clinical evidence of background retinopathy. Most of these patients will have no visual impairments and have little risk of developing blindness in the future. A complication of nonproliferative retinopathy, macular edema, occurs in approximately 10% of people with type I and type II diabetes and may lead to visual distortion and loss of central vision.

Preproliferative Retinopathy. This advanced form of background retinopathy is considered a precursor to the more serious proliferative retinopathy. Epidemiologic evidence suggests that 10% to 50% of patients with preproliferative retinopathy will develop proliferative retinopathy within a short time (maybe as little as 1 year). As with background retinopathy, if visual changes occur during the preproliferative stage, they are usually caused by macular edema.

Proliferative Retinopathy. The greatest threat to vision occurs in this advanced stage of retinopathy. The visual loss associated with proliferative retinopathy is caused by vitreous hemorrhage or retinal detachment. The vitreous is normally clear, allowing light to be transmitted to the retina. When there is a hemorrhage, the vitreous becomes clouded and cannot transmit light; the result is loss of vision. Another consequence of vitreous hemorrhaging is that resorption of the blood in the vitreous leads to the formation of fibrous scar tissue. This scar tissue may place traction on the retina, resulting in retinal detachment and subsequent visual loss.

Patients may have a fairly significant degree of proliferative retinopathy and may even have some hemorrhaging without major visual changes. It is important, however, if they report any symptoms indicative of hemorrhaging, such as "floaters" or "cobwebs" in the visual field, or if they report sudden visual changes, that they be referred immediately for an ophthalmologic evaluation and possible laser treatment.

Diagnostic Evaluation. Diagnosis is by direct visualization with an ophthalmoscope or with a technique known as fluorescein angiography. Fluorescein angiography can document the type and activity of the retinopathy. It is a technique in which a dye is injected into an arm vein. The dye is carried to various parts of the body through the blood, but especially through the vessels of the retina of the eye. This technique allows the ophthalmologist, using special instruments, to see the retinal vessels in bright detail and gives useful information that cannot be obtained with just an ophthalmoscope.

Side effects of this diagnostic procedure performed in an outpatient setting may include

- Nausea during the dye injection
- A yellowish, fluorescent discoloration of the skin and urine that may last 12 to 24 hours
- An occasional allergic reaction, usually hives or itching

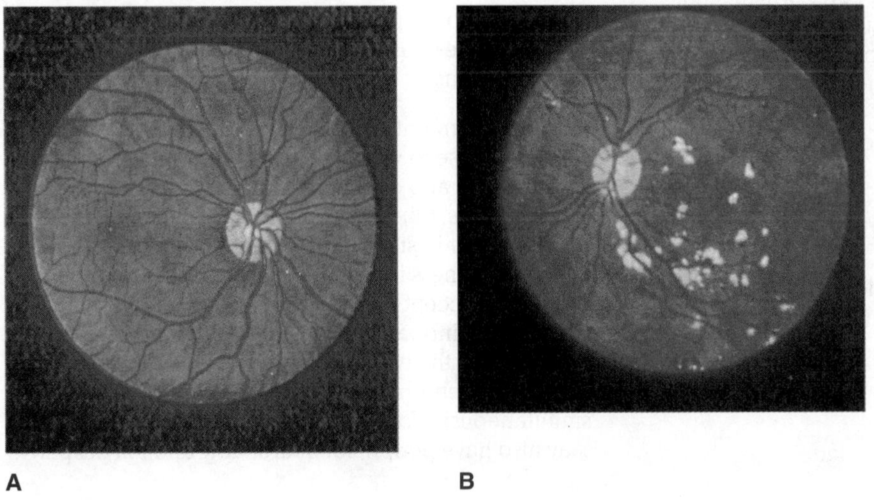

FIGURE 39-7. Diabetic retinopathy. **(A)** In the fundus photograph of a normal eye, the light circular area over which a number of blood vessels converge is the optic disc, where the optic nerve meets the back of the eye. **(B)** The fundus photograph of a patient with diabetic retinopathy shows characteristicf waxy-looking retinal lesions, microaneurysms of the vessels, and hemorrhages. (Fuller J and Schaller-Ayers J. Health Assessment: A Nursing Approach, 2nd ed. Philadelphia, JB Lippincott, 1994. Courtesy of American Optometric Association.)

However, it is generally a safe diagnostic procedure. Patient preparation includes explaining the following:

- The sequence of the steps of the procedure
- The fact that the procedure is painless
- The potential side effects
- The type of information the technique can provide
- That the flash of the camera may be slightly uncomfortable for a short time

Management

Photocoagulation ("Laser"). The main treatment of diabetic retinopathy is **argon-laser photocoagulation.** The laser treatment destroys leaking blood vessels and areas of neovascularization. For patients at increased risk for hemorrhaging, **panretinal photocoagulation** may significantly reduce the rate of progression to blindness. Panretinal photocoagulation involves the systematic application of multiple (more than 1000) laser burns throughout the retina (except in the macular region). This stops the widespread growth of new vessels and hemorrhaging of damaged vessels.

The role of "mild" panretinal photocoagulation (with one-third to one-half as many laser burns) in the early stages of proliferative retinopathy or in patients with preproliferative changes is being investigated.

For macular edema, "focal" photocoagulation is used to apply smaller laser burns to specific areas of microaneurysms in the macular region. Recent studies have shown that this may reduce the rate of visual loss from macular edema by 50%.

Photocoagulation treatments are usually performed on an outpatient basis, and most patients can return to their usual activities by the next day. For some patients, limitations may be placed on activities involving weight bearing or bearing down. For most patients, the treatment does not cause intense pain, although they may report varying degrees of discomfort. Usually an anesthetic eye drop is all that is needed during the treatment. A small percentage of patients may experience slight visual loss, loss of peripheral vision, or impairments in adaptation to the dark. For most patients, however, the risk of slight visual changes from the laser treatment itself is much less than the potential for loss of vision from progression of retinopathy.

Vitrectomy. When a major hemorrhage into the vitreous occurs, the vitreous fluid becomes mixed with blood and prevents light from passing through the eye, which can cause blindness. A vitrectomy is a surgical procedure in which vitreous humor filled with blood or fibrous tissue is removed with a special drill-like instrument and replaced with saline or another liquid.

A vitrectomy is performed on patients who already have a visual loss and in whom the vitreous hemorrhage has not cleared on its own after 6 months. The purpose is to restore useful vision; recovery to near-normal vision is not usually expected.

Other (Medical) Treatments. Studies continue into other ways to slow the progression of diabetic retinopathy. These include:

- Control of hypertension
- Control of blood glucose
- Cessation of smoking

Other Ophthalmologic Complications

Diabetic retinopathy is not the only complication of diabetes that can affect the vision. Cataracts, hypoglycemia and hyperglycemia, neuropathy, and glaucoma may also affect vision.

- **Cataracts:** Opacity of the lens of the eye; cataracts occur at an earlier age in patients with diabetes.
- **Lens changes:** The lens of the eye can swell when blood glucose levels are elevated. For some patients, visual changes related to lens swelling may be the first symptoms of diabetes. It may take up to 2 months of blood glucose control before hyperglycemic swelling subsides and vision stabilizes. Therefore, patients are advised not to change eyeglass prescriptions during the 2 months after discovery of hyperglycemia.
- **Hypoglycemia:** Temporary visual disturbances such as blurring and double vision may occur during episodes of hypoglycemia. These symptoms should subside after blood glucose levels return to normal.
- **Extraocular muscle palsy:** This may occur as a result of diabetic neuropathy. The involvement of various cranial nerves responsible for ocular movements may lead to double vision. This usually resolves spontaneously.
- **Glaucoma:** Glaucoma may occur with slightly higher frequency in the diabetic population.

Patient Education and Home Care Considerations. In all forms of therapy for retinopathy, something is destroyed in the process of saving vision. The facts must be presented to the patient and family as honestly as possible. The course of the retinopathy will be long and stressful. In counseling the patient, it is important to stress the following:

- The appearance of retinopathy can be expected after many years of diabetes, and its appearance does not necessarily mean that the diabetes is on a downhill course
- The odds for maintaining vision are in the patient's favor
- Frequent eye examinations are the best way to preserve vision, because they allow for the detection of any retinopathy

Some additional points to keep in mind when the patient with diabetes has some type of visual impairment include the following:

- Visual impairment can be a shock to anyone. A person's response to vision loss depends on personality, self-concept, and coping mechanisms.
- As in any loss, blindness and its acceptance by the patient occur in stages; some patients may learn to accept blindness in a rather short period, and others may never accept it.
- Although retinopathy occurs bilaterally, the severity may differ in the two eyes.
- Many of the chronic complications of diabetes occur simultaneously. For example, a blind diabetic patient may also have peripheral neuropathy and may experi-

ence impairment of manual dexterity and tactile sensation.

Medical management and nursing care of patients with visual disturbances are discussed in detail in Chapter 56.

Nephropathy

People with diabetes account for approximately 25% of patients with end-stage renal disease requiring dialysis or transplantation each year in the United States. Persons with diabetes have a 20% to 40% chance of developing renal disease.

People with type I diabetes frequently show initial signs of renal disease after 15 to 20 years, whereas patients with type II diabetes develop renal disease within 10 years of the diagnosis of diabetes. Many of these patients with type II diabetes may have had diabetes for many years before it was diagnosed and treated.

There is no reliable method to predict whether a person will develop renal disease. The DCCT (1993) results showed that intensive treatment of diabetes with a goal of achieving a hemoglobin A_{1C} as close to the nondiabetic range as possible reduced the occurrence of early signs of nephropathy, such as microalbuminuria, by 39%, and albuminuria by 54%.

Pathology. Evidence suggests that soon after the onset of diabetes, and especially if the blood glucose levels are elevated, the kidney's filtration mechanism is stressed, allowing blood proteins to leak into the urine. As a result, the pressure in the blood vessels of the kidney increases. It is thought that the elevated pressure serves as the stimulus for the development of nephropathy. Various medications and diets are being tested to prevent these complications.

Diagnostic Evaluation. One of the most important blood proteins that begins leaking into the urine is albumin. Small amounts may leak undetected for years. Early microalbuminuria may be discovered in a 24-hour urine sample. In patients with microalbuminuria, more than 85% eventually develop clinical nephropathy. However, if microalbuminuria is not present, fewer than 5% will develop nephropathy. Carefully designed low-protein diets appear to reverse early leakage of small amounts of protein from the kidney.

When a urine dipstick test reads consistently positive for significant amounts of albumin, the patient is tested for serum creatinine and blood urea nitrogen levels. At this point in the development of renal disease, diagnostic testing for cardiac or other systemic problems may also be required. Some of the tests involve injection of special dyes that are not easily cleared by the damaged kidney. Therefore, the value of the diagnostic test must be weighed against the potential risks.

Persons (both diabetic and nondiabetic) who are in the early stages of renal disease frequently develop hypertension. However, essential hypertension occurs in up to 50% of all individuals with diabetes (for unknown reasons); thus, it should not be assumed that someone with diabetes who has hypertension also has renal disease. Other diagnostic criteria must also be present.

Clinical Manifestations. Most of the signs and symptoms of renal dysfunction in the person with diabetes are similar to those seen in patients without diabetes. (See Chapter 43 for the management of patients with renal disorders.) Additionally, as renal failure progresses, the catabolism (breakdown) of both exogenous and endogenous insulin decreases, and frequent hypoglycemic episodes may result. Insulin needs change as a result of changes in the catabolism of insulin and also as a result of changes in diet related to the treatment of nephropathy. The stress of renal disease affects self-esteem, family relationships, marital relations, and virtually all aspects of daily life. As renal function decreases, the patient frequently experiences multiple-system failure (*e.g.*, declining visual acuity, impotence, foot ulcerations, congestive heart failure, and nocturnal diarrhea).

Prevention and Management. In addition to achieving and maintaining near-normal blood glucose levels, management for all patients with diabetes should include careful attention to the following:

- Control of hypertension (the use of angiotensin-converting enzyme [ACE] inhibitors, such as captopril, for control of hypertension may also decrease early proteinuria)
- Prevention or vigorous treatment of urinary tract infections
- Avoidance of nephrotoxic substances
- Adjustment of medications as renal function changes
- A diet low in sodium
- A diet low in protein

In renal failure, two types of treatment are available: dialysis (hemodialysis or peritoneal dialysis) and transplantation from a relative or a cadaver.

Hemodialysis for the patient with diabetes is similar to that for patients without the disease (see Chapter 42). Because hemodialysis creates additional stress on patients with cardiovascular disease, it may not be indicated in certain patients. In addition, it is extremely intrusive into a patient's life.

Both **continuous ambulatory peritoneal dialysis** (CAPD) and **intermittent peritoneal dialysis** are being used by an increasing number of patients with diabetes, mainly because of the independence they allow patients. In addition, insulin can be mixed into the dialysate, which may result in better blood glucose control and end the need for insulin injections. However, these patients may require more insulin because the dialysate contains glucose. A major risk of peritoneal dialysis is infection and peritonitis.

Renal disease is frequently accompanied by advancing retinopathy that may require laser treatments and surgery. Severe hypertension also worsens eye disease because of the additional stress it places on the blood vessels. Patients being treated by hemodialysis who require eye surgery may be changed to peritoneal dialysis and have their hypertension aggressively controlled for several weeks before surgery. The rationale for this change is that hemodialysis requires anticoagulants that can increase the risk of bleeding after the surgery, and peritoneal dialysis minimizes pressure changes in the eyes.

The success rate for kidney transplantation in patients with diabetes has improved. In medical centers performing large numbers of transplants, the chances are 75% to 80% that the transplanted kidney will continue to function in the patient with diabetes for at least 5 years. Like the original kidneys, transplanted kidneys in patients with diabetes can eventually be damaged if blood glucose levels are consistently high after the transplantation. Therefore, monitoring blood glucose levels frequently and adjusting insulin levels in diabetic patients with transplanted kidneys are essential for long-term success.

The mortality rate for diabetic patients undergoing dialysis is higher than that in nondiabetic patients undergoing dialysis and is closely related to the severity of cardiovascular problems.

The Neuropathies of Diabetes

Neuropathy in diabetes refers to a group of diseases that affect all types of nerves, including peripheral (sensorimotor), autonomic, and spinal nerves. The disorders appear to be clinically diverse and depend on the location of the affected nerve cells.

The prevalence increases with the age of the patient and the duration of the disease and may be as high as 50% in patients who have had diabetes for 25 years. Elevated blood glucose levels over a period of years have been implicated in the etiology of neuropathy.

The pathogenesis of neuropathy in diabetes may be attributable to either a vascular or a metabolic mechanism or both, but their relative contributions have not yet been determined. Capillary basement membrane thickening and capillary closure may be present. In addition, there may be demyelinization of the nerves, which is thought to be related to hyperglycemia. Nerve conduction is disrupted when there are aberrations of the myelin sheaths.

The two most common types of diabetic neuropathy are **sensorimotor polyneuropathy** and **autonomic neuropathy.** Cranial mononeuropathies, for example affecting the oculomotor nerve, also occur in diabetes, especially among the elderly. (See section on eye disorders in diabetes, p. 1056.)

Control of serum glucose levels to normal or near-normal levels was shown in the DCCT (1993) to decrease the incidence of neuropathy by 60%.

Clinical Manifestations of Sensorimotor Polyneuropathy. This type of neuropathy is also called **peripheral neuropathy.** It most commonly affects the distal portions of the nerves and especially the lower extremities. It affects both sides of the body in a symmetrical fashion and may progressively spread in a proximal direction.

Initial symptoms include paresthesias (prickling, tingling, or heightened sensation) and burning sensations (especially at night). As the neuropathy progresses, the feet become numb. In addition, a decrease in proprioception (awareness of posture and movement of the body and of position and weight of objects in relation to the body) and decreased sensation of light touch may lead to an unsteady gait. Decreased sensations of pain and temperature place patients with neuropathy at increased risk for injury and undetected foot infections.

On physical examination, a decrease in deep tendon reflexes and vibratory sensation is found. For some patients who have few or no symptoms of neuropathy, these physical findings may be the only indication that neuropathic changes are taking place. For patients with signs or symptoms of neuropathy, it is important to rule out other possible neuropathies, including alcohol-induced or vitamin-deficiency neuropathies.

Management of Sensorimotor Polyneuropathy. The results of the DCCT (1993) demonstrate that intensive insulin therapy and control of blood glucose levels delay the onset and slow the progression of neuropathy.

Pain, particularly of the lower extremities, is a disturbing symptom in some persons with neuropathy secondary to diabetes. For some patients, neuropathic pain spontaneously resolves within 6 months. For other patients, pain persists for many years. Various approaches to pain management can be tried. These include analgesics (preferably non-narcotic); tricyclic antidepressants, phenytoin or carbamazepine (anticonvulsants); mexiletine (an antidysrhythmic); or transcutaneous electrical nerve stimulation (TENS).

The use of aldose reductase inhibitors is currently under study to determine if they block the damaging effects of hyperglycemia. The topical medication capsaicin (Axscain) also has been shown in preliminary reports to decrease lower extremity neuropathic pain. Studies of the role of this topical medication in neuropathy continue.

Clinical Manifestations of Autonomic Neuropathy. Neuropathy of the autonomic nervous system results in a broad range of dysfunctions affecting almost every organ system of the body. Generally, treatment of specific problems is the same as it would be for similar problems in the nondiabetic population. Six main effects of autonomic neuropathy are described here.

Cardiovascular. Three manifestations of autonomic neuropathy are a fixed, slightly tachycardiac heart rate; orthostatic hypotension; and "silent," or painless, myocardial infarction.

Gastrointestinal. Delayed gastric emptying may occur with the typical symptoms of early satiety, bloating, nausea, and vomiting. In addition, there may be unexplained wide swings in blood glucose levels related to inconsistent absorption of the glucose from ingested foods. "Diabetic" constipation or diarrhea (especially nocturnal diarrhea) is also associated with gastrointestinal autonomic neuropathy.

Urinary. Urinary retention, a decreased sensation of bladder fullness, and other urinary symptoms of neurogenic bladder result from autonomic neuropathy. Patients with a neurogenic bladder are predisposed to developing urinary tract infections. This is especially true in patients with poorly controlled diabetes because hyperglycemia impairs resistance to infection.

Adrenal Gland ("Hypoglycemic Unawareness"). Autonomic neuropathy of the adrenal medulla is responsible for diminished or absent adrenergic symptoms of hypoglycemia. Patients may report that they no longer feel the typical shakiness, sweating, nervousness, and palpitations associated with hypoglycemia. Strict blood glucose control is recommended for these patients. Their inability to detect and appropriately treat these warning signs of hypoglycemia puts them at risk for developing dangerously low blood glucose levels.

Sudomotor Neuropathy. This neuropathic condition refers to a decrease or absence of sweating ("anhidrosis") of the extremities with a compensatory increase in upper body sweating. The dryness of the feet increases the risk for development of foot ulcers.

Sexual Dysfunction. Sexual dysfunction, especially impotence in men, is one of the most well-known and feared complications of diabetes. The effects of autonomic neuropathy on female sexual functioning are not well documented. Reduced vaginal lubrication has been mentioned as a possible neuropathic effect; however, research studies to support this and other potential female sexual dysfunctions are lacking.

Impotence, the difficulty or inability of the penis to become rigid and sustain an erection, occurs with greater frequency in diabetic men than in nondiabetic men of the same age. It is important for the nurse and patient to realize, however, that in diabetic men neuropathy is not the only cause of impotence. Medications such as antihypertensives, psychologic factors, and other medical conditions (*e.g.*, vascular insufficiency) that may affect nondiabetic men also play a role in impotence in diabetic men.

A thorough evaluation of possible factors affecting erectile dysfunction is extremely important. Treatment of potential underlying causes, such as changing antihypertensive medications or providing sexual or marital counseling, must take place before more extensive, invasive treatments such as surgical penile implants.

Many patients may be embarrassed to discuss sexual issues. A sensitive and straightforward approach to obtaining a sexual history is important. Some patients may be unaware that sexual dysfunction commonly occurs for medical reasons and may simply assume it is due to increasing age or stress. Conversely, psychogenic impotence may result from undue worry or misinformation about diabetes-related impotence. Providing correct information about various causes of impotence in diabetes is important.

The role of hyperglycemia and vascular disease in impotence is not clearly defined. Poorly controlled blood glucose, pain, and other symptoms related to diabetic complications may contribute to an overall feeling of malaise and weakness. These symptoms may contribute to decreased interest in sexual relations. In autonomic neuropathy, libido, the ability to ejaculate, and the sensation of orgasm are usually diminished.

In recent years, several nonsurgical options have been developed for impotence caused by diabetic autonomic neuropathy. There are external vacuum erection aid devices that manually draw blood into the penis. The erection is maintained through the use of a constrictor band, which is placed around the base of the penis. It is important for patients to realize that ejaculation may still occur even with the band in place and that contraception should be used if indicated.

Another nonsurgical treatment for impotence is self-injection of a vasodilating medication, such as papaverine. The patient injects the medication into the corpus cavernosum of the penis, causing an erection.

Surgical approaches include insertion of penile implants such as an inflatable penile prosthesis, which can be activated by the patient when erection is desired (see Chapter 47).

Some men with autonomic neuropathy have normal erectile function and are able to experience orgasm but do not ejaculate. Retrograde ejaculation occurs, in which seminal fluid is propelled backward through the posterior urethra and into the urinary bladder. Examination of the urine confirms the diagnosis because of the large number of active sperm present. Fertility counseling is necessary for couples attempting conception.

Foot and Leg Problems in Diabetes

Fifty percent to 75% of lower extremity amputations are performed on people with diabetes. As many as 50% of these amputations are thought to be preventable, provided patients are taught preventive foot care measures and practice preventive foot care on a daily basis.

Three diabetic complications contribute to the increased risk of foot infections. They are

Neuropathy: Sensory neuropathy leads to loss of pain and pressure sensation, and autonomic neuropathy leads to increased dryness and fissuring of the skin (secondary to decreased sweating).

Peripheral vascular disease: Poor circulation of the lower extremities contributes to poor wound healing and the development of gangrene.

Immunocompromise: Hyperglycemia impairs the ability of specialized leukocytes to destroy bacteria. Thus, in poorly controlled diabetes there is a lowered resistance to certain infections.

The typical sequence of events in the development of a diabetic foot ulcer begins with a soft-tissue injury of the foot, formation of a fissure between the toes or in an area of dry skin, or formation of a callus (Fig. 39-8). Injuries are not felt by the patient with an insensitive foot and may be thermal (*e.g.*, from using heating pads, walking barefoot on hot concrete, or testing bath water with the foot), chemical

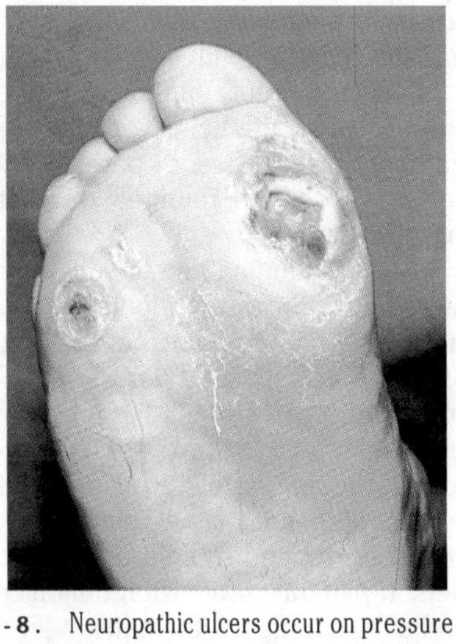

FIGURE 39-8. Neuropathic ulcers occur on pressure points in areas with diminished sensation in diabetic polyneuropathy. Pain is absent (and therefore the ulcer may go unnoticed). (Bates B. Guide to Physical Examination and History Taking, 6th ed. Philadelphia, JB Lippincott, 1995.)

(*e.g.*, burning the foot while using caustic agents on calluses, corns, or bunions), or traumatic (*e.g.*, injuring skin while cutting nails, walking with an undetected foreign object in the shoe, or wearing ill-fitting shoes and socks).

If the patient is not in the habit of thoroughly inspecting both feet on a daily basis, the injury or fissure may go unnoticed until a serious infection has developed. Drainage, swelling, redness (from cellulitis) of the leg, or gangrene may be the first sign of foot problems that the patient notices.

Treatment of foot ulcers involves bed rest, antibiotics, and debridement. In addition, controlling glucose levels that tend to increase when infections occur is important for promoting wound healing. In patients with peripheral vascular disease, foot ulcers may not heal because of the decreased ability of oxygen, nutrients, and antibiotics to reach the injured tissue. Amputation may be necessary to prevent further spread of infection.

Foot assessment and foot care instruction are most important when dealing with patients who are at high risk for developing foot infections. Some of the high-risk characteristics include:

- Duration of diabetes over 10 years
- Age older than 40 years
- History of smoking
- Decreased peripheral pulses
- Decreased sensation
- Anatomic deformities or pressure areas (such as bunions and calluses)
- History of previous foot ulcers or amputation

Foot Care. Preventive foot care includes properly bathing, drying, and lubricating feet; care must be taken not to allow moisture (water or lotion) to accumulate between the toes. Feet must be inspected on a daily basis for any redness, blisters, fissures, calluses, or ulcerations. For patients who have a visual impairment or have decreased joint mobility (especially the elderly), use of a mirror for inspection of the bottom of the feet or instruction of a family member in foot inspection may be necessary. The interior surfaces of shoes should be inspected for any rough spots or foreign objects. Visual and manual (with the hand) inspection on a daily basis is important. Feet should be examined on a regular basis by a podiatrist, physician, or nurse. Patients with pressure areas, such as calluses, or patients with thick toenails should see the podiatrist routinely for treatment of calluses and trimming of nails.

Patients should be taught to wear well-fitting, closed-toe shoes. Podiatrists can provide patients with inserts to remove pressure from pressure points on the foot. New shoes should be broken in slowly (*i.e.*, worn for 1 to 2 hours initially with gradual increases in the length of time worn) to avoid blister formation. High-risk behaviors should be avoided, such as walking barefoot, using heating pads on the feet, wearing open-toed shoes, and shaving calluses. Toenails should be trimmed straight across without rounding the corners. If patients have visual deficits or thickened toenails, a podiatrist should cut the nails.

Patients should be counseled on reducing risk factors, such as smoking and elevated blood lipids, that contribute to peripheral vascular disease. Blood glucose control is important for avoiding decreased resistance to infections and for avoiding diabetic neuropathy.

Special Issues in Diabetes

The Patient With Diabetes Undergoing Surgery

During periods of physiologic stress, such as surgery, blood glucose levels tend to rise as a result of an increase in the level of stress hormones (epinephrine, norepinephrine, glucagon, cortisol, and growth hormone). If hyperglycemia is not adequately controlled during surgery, the resulting osmotic diuresis may lead to excessive loss of fluids and electrolytes. Type I diabetic patients also risk developing ketoacidosis during periods of stress.

Hypoglycemia is also a concern in diabetic patients undergoing surgery. This is especially a concern during the preoperative period if surgery is delayed beyond the morning in a patient who received a morning injection of intermediate-acting insulin.

There are various approaches to the management of glucose control during the perioperative period. Frequent capillary glucose monitoring of the diabetic patient is vitally important throughout the preoperative and postoperative periods, regardless of the method used for glucose control.

For patients who usually take insulin, one-half to two-thirds of the usual morning dose (either intermediate-acting insulin alone or both short- and intermediate-acting insulins) may be administered subcutaneously in the morning before surgery. The remainder is then administered after surgery. Another approach with subcutaneous insulin is to divide the total number of units of insulin taken daily into four equal doses of regular insulin. This is then administered at 6-hour intervals.

The use of intravenous insulin and dextrose has become more widespread with the increased availability of meters for intraoperative glucose monitoring. The morning of surgery, all subcutaneous insulin doses are usually withheld (unless the blood glucose level is elevated, for example, above 200 mg/dl [11.1 mmol/L], in which case a small dose of subcutaneous regular insulin may be prescribed).

Blood glucose is controlled during surgery with the intravenous infusion of regular insulin, which is balanced by an infusion of dextrose. The insulin and dextrose infusion rates are adjusted according to frequent (hourly) capillary glucose determinations. Postoperatively, the insulin infusion may be continued until the patient is able to eat. If intravenous insulin is discontinued, subcutaneous regular insulin may be administered at set intervals (every 4 to 6 hours), or intermediate-acting insulin may be administered every 12 hours with supplemental regular insulin as necessary until the patient is eating and the usual pattern of insulin dosing is resumed.

The nurse taking care of a diabetic patient who is receiving intravenous insulin must carefully monitor the insulin infusion rate and blood glucose levels. Intravenous insulin has a much shorter duration of action than subcutaneous insulin. Thus, if the infusion is interrupted or discontinued, hyperglycemia will result within a few hours. The nurse must ensure that subcutaneous insulin is administered either immediately before or by 1 hour after the intravenous insulin infusion is discontinued.

Type II diabetic patients who do not usually take insulin may require insulin during the perioperative period to control blood glucose elevations. Patients who are taking chlorpropamide, a long-acting oral hypoglycemic agent, may be instructed to discontinue the oral agent 1 day before surgery. Some of these patients may resume their usual regimen of diet and oral agent during the recovery period. Other patients (who are probably not well controlled with diet and an oral hypoglycemic agent before surgery) will need to continue with insulin injections after discharge.

For type II diabetic patients who are undergoing minor surgery but who do not normally take insulin, glucose levels may remain stable provided no dextrose is infused during the surgery. Postoperatively, they may require small doses of regular insulin until the usual diet and oral agent are resumed.

During the postoperative period, diabetic patients must also be closely monitored for cardiovascular complications because of the increased prevalence of atherosclerosis in patients with diabetes, wound infections, and skin breakdown (especially in the patient with decreased pain sensation in the extremities caused by neuropathy). Maintaining adequate nutrition and blood glucose control promotes wound healing.

Management of Hospitalized Diabetic Patients

At any one time, 10% to 20% of general medical–surgical patients in the hospital have diabetes. This number may increase as the elderly make up a greater proportion of the population. Although some hospitals may have a specialized diabetic/metabolic unit, typically diabetic patients are admitted to all units of the hospital.

Often diabetes is not the primary medical diagnosis, yet problems with the control of diabetes frequently result from changes in the patient's normal routine or from illness or surgery. Some of the main issues pertinent to nursing care of the hospitalized diabetic patient are presented in the following section.

Self-Care Issues. All patients admitted to the hospital must relinquish control of most aspects of daily care to the hospital staff. For the diabetic patient who is actively involved in diabetes self-management (especially insulin dose adjustment), relinquishing control over meal timing, insulin timing, and insulin dosage may be particularly difficult. The patient may fear hypoglycemia and express much concern over possible delays in receiving attention from the nurse when hypoglycemic symptoms are experienced.

It is important for the nurse to acknowledge the patient's concerns and to involve the patient as much as possible in the plan of care. If the patient disagrees with certain aspects of the nursing or medical care related to diabetes, the nurse must communicate this to other members of the health care team and, where appropriate, make changes in the plan to meet patient needs.

Hyperglycemia During Hospitalization. Hyperglycemia may occur in the hospitalized patient as a result of the original illness that led to the need for hospitalization. In addition, a number of other factors may contribute to hyperglycemia, such as

- Changes in the usual treatment regimen (*e.g.*, increased food, decreased insulin, decreased activity)
- Medications (*e.g.*, glucocorticoids such as prednisone, which are used in the treatment of a variety of inflammatory disorders)
- Intravenous dextrose, which may be part of the maintenance fluids or may be used for intravenous administration of antibiotics and other medications
- Overly vigorous treatment of hypoglycemia
- Mismatched timing of meals and insulin (*e.g.*, postmeal hyperglycemia may occur if insulin is administered immediately before or even after meals)

Nursing action to correct some of these factors is important for the avoidance of unnecessary hyperglycemia. Assessment of the patient's usual home routine is important. The nurse should try to approximate as much as possible the home schedule of insulin, meals, and activities. Monitoring blood glucose levels and obtaining orders for extra doses of insulin (at times when insulin is usually taken by the patient) are important nursing functions.

- Insulin doses must not be withheld when blood glucose levels are normal.

Regular insulin is usually needed to avoid postmeal hyperglycemia (even in the patient with normal premeal glucose levels), and NPH insulin does not peak until many hours after the dose is given. Intravenous antibiotics should be mixed in normal saline (if possible) to avoid excess infusion of dextrose (especially in the patient who is eating). It is important to avoid overly vigorous treatment of hypoglycemia, which may lead to hyperglycemia. Treatment of hypoglycemia should be based on the established hospital protocol (usually 10 to 15 g carbohydrate in the form of juice, glucose tablets, or, if necessary, ½ to 1 ampule 50% dextrose administered intravenously). Adding extra sugar to the juice is unnecessary. If the initial treatment does not adequately increase the glucose level, the same treatment may be repeated.

Common Causes of Hypoglycemia. Hypoglycemia in a hospitalized patient is usually the result of too much insulin or delays in eating. Specific examples include

- Overuse of "sliding scale" regular insulin, particularly as a supplement to regularly scheduled, twice-daily short- and intermediate-acting insulins
- Lack of dosage change when dietary intake is changed (*e.g.*, in patient taking nothing by mouth)
- Overly vigorous treatment of hyperglycemia (*e.g.*, giving too frequent successive doses of regular insulin before the time of peak insulin activity is reached) so that there is an accumulated effect

Nurses must assess the pattern of glucose values and avoid giving doses of insulin that repeatedly lead to hypoglycemia. Successive doses of subcutaneous regular insulin should be administered no more frequently than every 3 to

4 hours. For patients receiving NPH or Lente insulin before breakfast and dinner, the nurse must use caution in administering supplemental doses of regular insulin at lunch and bedtime. Hypoglycemia may occur when two insulins peak at similar times (*e.g.*, morning NPH peaks with lunchtime regular insulin and may lead to late afternoon hypoglycemia, and dinnertime NPH peaks with bedtime regular insulin and may lead to nocturnal hypoglycemia). To avoid hypoglycemic reactions caused by delayed food intake, the nurse should arrange for a snack to be given to the patient if meals are going to be delayed because of procedures, physical therapy, or other activities.

Common Alterations in Diet. Dietary modifications common during hospitalization require special consideration when the patient has diabetes.

NPO (Nothing by Mouth). For the patient who must have nothing by mouth in preparation for a procedure, the nurse must ensure that the usual insulin dosage has been changed. These changes may include eliminating the regular insulin and giving a decreased amount (*e.g.*, half of the usual dose) of intermediate-acting NPH or Lente insulin. Another approach is to use frequent (every 3 to 4 hours) dosing of regular insulin only. Intravenous dextrose may be ordered to provide calories and to avoid the development of hypoglycemia.

It is important to remember that even when no food is taken, glucose levels may rise as a result of hepatic glucose production, especially in type I and lean type II diabetic patients. Furthermore, in type I diabetic patients, complete elimination of the insulin dose may lead to the development of diabetic ketoacidosis. Thus, administering insulin to the type I diabetic patient who is receiving nothing by mouth is an important nursing action.

For type II diabetic patients taking insulin, DKA does not develop when insulin doses are eliminated because the patient's own pancreas produces some insulin. Thus, skipping the insulin dose altogether when the patient has type II diabetes (and is receiving intravenous dextrose) may be safe.

For patients who receive nothing by mouth for extended periods, glucose testing and insulin administration should be performed at regular intervals, usually two to four times per day. Insulin regimens for the patient who is fasting for an extended period may include NPH insulin every 12 hours (with regular insulin added to the NPH depending on the results of glucose testing) or regular insulin only every 4 to 6 hours. These patients should receive dextrose infusions to provide some calories and limit ketosis.

Clear Liquid Diet. When the diet is advanced to include clear liquids, the diabetic patient will be receiving more simple carbohydrate foods, such as juice and gelatin desserts, than are usually included in the diabetic diet. It is important for hospitalized patients to maintain their nutritional status as much as possible to promote healing. Thus, the use of reduced-calorie substitutes such as diet soda or diet gelatin desserts would not be appropriate when the only source of calories is clear liquids. Simple carbohydrates, when eaten alone, cause a rapid rise in glucose levels; thus, it is important to try to match peak times of insulin with peaks in glucose. If a patient was receiving insulin at regular intervals while receiving nothing by mouth, the scheduled times for glucose tests and insulin injections must be changed to match meal times.

Enteral Tube Feedings. Solutions used for tube feedings in patients with nasogastric tubes or other feeding tubes contain more simple carbohydrates and less protein and fat than the typical diabetic diet. This results in increased levels of glucose. It is important that insulin doses be administered at regular intervals (*e.g.*, NPH every 12 hours or regular insulin every 4 to 6 hours) when tube feedings are administered at a continuous rate. If insulin is administered at routine (prebreakfast and predinner) times, hypoglycemia during the day may result from patients receiving more insulin without more calories, and hyperglycemia may occur during the night when feedings continue but insulin action wanes.

A common cause of hypoglycemia in patients receiving continuous tube feedings and insulin is inadvertent or purposeful discontinuation of the feeding. The nurse must discuss with the medical team any plans for temporarily discontinuing the tube feeding (*e.g.*, when the patient is away from the unit). Planning ahead may allow alterations to be made in the insulin dose, or it may allow for intravenous dextrose to be initiated. In addition, if problems with the tube feeding develop unexpectedly (*e.g.*, the patient pulls out the tube, the tube clogs, or the feeding is discontinued when residual gastric contents are found), the nurse must notify the physician, assess glucose levels more frequently, and administer intravenous dextrose if indicated.

Total Parenteral Nutrition (TPN). The diabetic patient receiving TPN may receive both intravenous insulin (added to the TPN container) and subcutaneous intermediate-acting or short-acting insulins. Similar to the patient receiving continuous nasogastric tube feedings, the blood glucose monitoring and insulin administration should be performed at regular intervals if the TPN infuses continuously. If the TPN is infused over a limited number of hours, subcutaneous insulin should be administered such that peak times of insulin action coincide with times of TPN infusion.

Hygiene. The nurse caring for a hospitalized diabetic patient must focus attention on oral hygiene and skin care. Because diabetic patients commonly develop periodontal disease, it is important for the nurse to assist patients with daily dental care. The patient should also be assisted in keeping skin clean and dry—especially in areas of contact between two skin surfaces (such as groin, axilla, and, in obese women, under the breasts), where chafing and fungal infections tend to occur.

For the bedridden diabetic patient, nursing care must emphasize the prevention of skin breakdown at pressure points. The heels are particularly susceptible to breakdown because of loss of sensation of pain and pressure associated with sensory neuropathy.

Feet should be cleaned, dried, lubricated (except in the area between the toes), and inspected frequently. If the patient is in the supine position, pressure on the heels can be alleviated by elevating the lower legs on a pillow with the heels hanging over the edge of the pillow. When the patient is seated in a chair, the feet should be positioned so that pressure is not placed on the heels. If the patient has a foot ulcer, it is important to perform preventive foot care of the unaffected foot as well as to carry out special care of the infected foot.

As always, every opportunity should be taken to teach the patient about diabetes self-management, including daily oral, skin, and foot care. Female diabetic patients should also be instructed about measures for the avoidance of vaginal infections, which occur more frequently when blood glucose levels are elevated. Patients often take their cues from the nurse and realize the importance of daily personal hygiene if this is emphasized during the course of their hospitalization.

Stress

As mentioned earlier, physiologic stress, such as infections and surgery, contribute to hyperglycemia and may precipitate DKA or HHNK syndrome. Emotional stress may have a negative impact on diabetic control as well. An increase in "stress" hormones leads to an increase in glucose levels, especially when the intake of food and insulin remains unchanged. In addition, during periods of emotional stress, the person with diabetes may alter the usual pattern of meals, exercise, and medication. This contributes to hyperglycemia or even hypoglycemia (*e.g.*, in the patient on insulin or oral hypoglycemic agents who stops eating in response to stress).

People who have diabetes must be made aware of the potential deterioration in diabetic control that can accompany emotional stress. They must be encouraged to try to adhere to the diabetes treatment plan as much as possible during times of stress. In addition, learning strategies for minimizing stress and coping with stress when it does occur are important aspects of diabetes education.

Gerontologic Considerations

People with diabetes are living longer; therefore, both type I and type II diabetes are seen more frequently in the elderly population. Regardless of the type or duration of diabetes, the goals of diabetes treatment may need to be altered when caring for the elderly. The focus is on quality-of-life issues, such as maintaining independent functioning and promoting general well-being. Although striving for strict blood glucose control may not be safe or appropriate, prolonged symptomatic hyperglycemia should be avoided.

Some elderly patients will not be able to manage a detailed diabetes treatment plan. However, it must not be assumed that all patients older than a certain age can adhere only to the simplest regimen. Although the goal may be simply to avoid hypoglycemia and symptomatic hyperglycemia, certain patients may prefer more complex regimens that allow more flexibility in meals and daily schedule. As with all people with diabetes, individualization of the treatment plan with frequent follow-up by the health care team is important.

Some of the barriers to learning and self-care that may be seen in the elderly include decreased vision, hearing loss, memory deficits, decreased mobility and fine motor coordination, increased tremors, depression and loneliness, decreased financial resources, and limitations related to other medical illnesses.

Assessing patients for these barriers as well as discussing any misconceptions or folk beliefs regarding the cause and treatment of diabetes is important in setting up a diabetes treatment plan and educational activities. Presenting brief, simplified instructions with ample opportunity for practice of skills is important. The use of special devices such as a magnifier for the insulin syringe, an insulin pen, or a mirror for foot inspection is helpful. If necessary, family members and other community resources are called on to assist with basic diabetes survival skills. If possible, it is preferable to teach patients or family members to test blood glucose at home, because urine glucose tests are usually less accurate in the elderly as a result of increased renal threshold and increased frequency of renal and urinary problems. Frequent evaluation of self-care skills (insulin administration, blood glucose monitoring, foot care, diet planning) is essential, especially in patients with deteriorating vision and memory.

Dietary adherence is difficult for some elderly patients because of decreased appetite, poor dentition, and decreased physical and financial ability to prepare meals. In addition, patients may be unwilling to change long-standing dietary habits. Altering the meal plan to incorporate these eating habits or other limitations may be necessary.

Careful monitoring for diabetes complications must not be neglected in the elderly. Hypoglycemia is especially dangerous because it may go undetected and result in falls. Dehydration is a concern in patients who have chronically elevated blood glucose levels. Assessment for long-term complications—especially eye and foot problems—is important. Avoiding blindness and amputation through early detection and treatment of retinopathy and foot ulcers may mean the difference between institutionalization and continued independent living for the elderly person with diabetes. Changes seen in the elderly person with diabetes are summarized in Chart 39-7.

❑ *NURSING PROCESS*
The Patient With Diabetes as a Secondary Diagnosis

People with diabetes frequently seek medical attention for problems not directly related to blood glucose control. However, during the course of treatment of the primary medical diagnosis, the blood glucose control may worsen. In addition, the only opportunity for some diabetic patients to update their knowledge in diabetes self-care and prevention of complications is during the time of hospitalization. Therefore, it is important for the nurse taking care of the diabetic patient to focus attention on diabetes, regardless of the primary problem. Furthermore, control of blood glucose levels is important because hyperglycemia impairs resistance to certain infections and may contribute to impaired wound healing.

Assessment

Assessment of the diabetic patient with a primary problem such as cardiac disease, renal disease, cerebrovascular disease, peripheral vascular disease, surgery, or any other type of illness is the same as that for a nondiabetic patient and is described in other chapters. In addition to nursing assessment for the primary problem, assessment of the diabetic patient must also focus on hypoglycemia and hyperglycemia, skin breakdown, and diabetes self-care skills, including

CHART 39-7

Factors in the Elderly That May Affect Diabetes

Sensory Changes
- Decreased vision
- Decreased smell
- Taste changes
- Decreased proprioception
- Diminished thirst

Gastrointestinal Changes
- Dental problems
- Appetite changes
- Delayed gastric emptying
- Decreased bowel motility

Activity/Exercise Pattern Changes
- More sedentary

Renal Function Changes
- Decreased function
- Decreased drug clearance

Affective/Cognitive Changes
- Medications/meals omitted or taken erratically

Socioeconomic Factors
- Fad diets
- Loneliness/living alone
- Lack of money

Chronic Diseases
- Hypertension
- Arthritis
- Neoplasms
- Acute/chronic infections

Potential Drug Interactions
- Use of another person's medications
- Consulting multiple physicians for different illnesses
- Alcohol

survival skills and measures for prevention of long-term complications.

The patient is assessed for hypoglycemia and hyperglycemia with frequent capillary glucose monitoring (usually ordered before meals and at bedtime) and with monitoring for signs and symptoms of hypoglycemia or prolonged hyperglycemia (including DKA or HHNK syndrome) as described in previous sections.

Careful assessment of the skin, especially at pressure points and on the lower extremities, is important. The skin is assessed for dryness, cracks, skin breakdown, and redness. The patient is asked about symptoms of neuropathy, such as tingling and pain or numbness of the feet. Deep tendon reflexes are assessed.

Assessment of diabetes self-care skills is performed as early as possible to determine if the patient requires further diabetes teaching. The nurse *observes* the patient preparing and injecting the insulin, monitoring blood glucose, and performing foot care. (Simply questioning the patient about these skills without actually observing performance of the skills is not sufficient.) Knowledge about diet can be assessed with the help of the dietitian through direct questioning and review of patient choices on the menu. The patient is questioned regarding signs, treatment, and prevention of hypoglycemia and hyperglycemia. The patient's knowledge of risk factors for macrovascular disease, including hypertension, increased lipids, and smoking, is assessed. The patient is questioned regarding the date of the last eye examination (including dilation of the pupils).

Diagnosis

Nursing Diagnoses

Based on the assessment data, the patient's major nursing diagnoses may include the following:

- Altered nutrition related to increase in stress hormones (caused by primary medical problem) and imbalances in insulin, food, and physical activity
- Risk for impaired skin integrity related to immobility and lack of sensation (caused by neuropathy)
- Potential knowledge deficit about diabetes self-care skills (caused by lack of basic diabetes education or lack of continuing in-depth diabetes education)

Collaborative Problems/ Potential Complications

Based on the assessment data, potential complications may include

- Inadequate control of glucose levels
- Development of short-term complications of diabetes because of inadequate control of glucose levels

Planning and Implementation

Goals. The major goals of the patient may include attainment of improved nutritional status, maintenance of skin integrity, ability to perform basic diabetes self-care skills as well as preventive care for the avoidance of long-term diabetes complications, and absence of complications.

Nursing Interventions

Improving Nutritional Status. The patient's diet is planned with the primary goal of glucose control; however, the dietary prescription must also consider the patient's primary health problem in addition to lifestyle, cultural background, activity level, and food preferences. If alterations are needed in the patient's diet because of the primary health problem (gastrointestinal problems, for example), alternative strategies to assure adequate nutritional intake must be implemented. The patient's nutritional intake is monitored carefully along with blood glucose, urine ketones, and daily weight. Blood glucose records are assessed for patterns of hypoglycemia and hyperglycemia at the same time of day, and findings are reported to the physician for alteration in insulin orders. In the patient with prolonged elevated blood glucose levels, laboratory values and the patient's physical condition are monitored for signs of DKA or HHNK syndrome.

Skin Care. The skin is assessed daily for dryness or breaks in skin. The feet are cleaned with warm water and soap. Excessive soaking of the feet is avoided. The feet are dried thoroughly, especially between the toes, and lotion is applied to the entire foot except between the toes. For bedridden patients (especially those with a history of neuropathy), the heels are elevated off the bed with a pillow placed under the lower legs and the heels resting over the edge of the pillow. Dermal ulcers are treated as indicated and prescribed. The nurse promotes optimal blood glucose control in patients with skin breakdown.

Patient Education and Home Care Considerations. Even if the patient has had diabetes for many years, it is important to carefully assess the patient's knowledge and adherence to the plan of care. It may be necessary to plan and implement a teaching plan that includes basic information about diabetes, its cause and symptoms, and long- and short-term complications and their treatment. The nurse requests that the patient give repeated return demonstrations of skills that were not performed correctly during the initial assessment. The patient is taught self-care activities for the prevention of long-term complications, including foot care, eye care, and risk factor management.

Monitoring and Managing Potential Complications. Inadequate control of glucose levels may adversely affect the patient's recovery from the immediate health problem. Blood glucose is monitored, and insulin is administered as prescribed. It is important for the nurse to ensure that insulin orders are altered as needed to compensate for changes in the patient's schedule or eating pattern. Treatment is given for hypoglycemia (with oral glucose) or hyperglycemia (with supplemental regular insulin not more often than every 3 to 4 hours). Blood glucose records are assessed for patterns of hypoglycemia and hyperglycemia at the same time of day, and findings are reported to the physician for modification in insulin orders. In the patient with prolonged elevated blood glucose levels, laboratory values and the patient's physical condition are monitored for signs of DKA or HHNK syndrome.

Development of short-term complications of diabetes secondary to inadequate control of glucose levels may be associated with other health care problems because of changes in activity level and diet and physiologic alterations related to the primary health problem itself. Therefore, it is essential that the patient be monitored for short-term complications (hyperglycemia, hypoglycemia) and that measures be implemented for their prevention and early treatment.

Evaluation

Expected Outcomes

1. Achieves optimal control of blood glucose
   a. Avoids extremes of hypoglycemia and hyperglycemia
   b. Hypoglycemic episodes are rapidly resolved
2. Maintains skin integrity
   a. Skin remains smooth without dryness and cracking
   b. Avoids ulcers caused by pressure and neuropathy
3. Demonstrates/verbalizes diabetes survival skills and preventive care

   Treatment Modalities
   a. Demonstrates proper technique for administering insulin and assessing blood glucose
   b. Demonstrates appropriate knowledge of diet through proper menu selections and identification of pattern used for selection of foods at home
   c. Verbalizes appropriate signs, treatment, and prevention of hypoglycemia and hyperglycemia

   Proper Foot Care
   a. Inspects feet (using mirror if necessary to see bottom of foot), including inspection for cracks between toes
   b. Washes feet with warm water and soap; dries feet thoroughly
   c. Applies lotion to entire foot except between toes
   d. Verbalizes behaviors that decrease the risk of foot ulcers, including
      (1) Wearing shoes at all times
      (2) Using hand or elbow, *not foot,* to test bath water
      (3) Avoiding use of heating pad on feet
      (4) Wearing cotton socks
      (5) Avoiding constrictive shoes
      (6) Wearing new shoes for brief periods
      (7) Avoiding home remedies for treatment of corns and calluses
      (8) Having feet examined at every appointment with the physician
      (9) Consulting a podiatrist for regular nail hygiene if necessary

   Measures and Information Regarding Prevention of Eye Disease
   a. Necessity of *yearly* or more frequent eye examinations by an ophthalmologist (starting at 5 years after diagnosis for type I diabetes or the year of diagnosis for type II diabetes)
   b. Relates that retinopathy usually does not cause change in vision until serious damage to the retina has occurred
   c. Relates that early laser treatment along with good control of blood glucose and blood pressure may prevent visual loss from retinopathy
   d. Identifies hypoglycemia and hyperglycemia as two causes of (temporary) blurred vision

   Measures for Controlling Macrovascular Risk Factors
   a. Smoking cessation
   b. Dietary limitation of fats and cholesterol
   c. Control of hypertension
   d. Exercise
4. Absence of complications
   a. Blood glucose and urine ketones within normal limits
   b. Experiences no signs or symptoms of hypoglycemia or hyperglycemia
   c. Identifies signs and symptoms of hypoglycemia or hyperglycemia
   d. Reports appearance of symptoms so that treatment can be initiated

CRITICAL THINKING EXERCISES

1. A diabetic diet has been prescribed for a newly diagnosed diabetic patient. Compare and contrast the modifications that would be made in the diet in the following situations: (1) the patient is a pregnant woman; (2) the patient is a devout Muslim; (3) the patient is a 55-year-old woman with osteoporosis.
2. A patient is brought to the emergency department by his coworkers because he has become drowsy and has developed slurred speech over the last hour. You learn that he has diabetes and takes insulin, but no other medical information is available. Describe how you would gather additional assessment data to help you distinguish between hypoglycemia and hyperglycemia. Before conducting an in-depth history or physical examination, the physician administers glucose to the patient. How would you explain the rationale for administering glucose before the definitive cause of the patient's symptoms is identified?
3. Your patient has been informed by her physician that intensive insulin therapy is going to be instituted. How would you explain to her the purpose of intensive insulin therapy and how it is carried out?
4. Your patient has been started on insulin therapy. He tells you that he would prefer to take oral medications, as a friend of his does. How would you explain to him the differences in the rationale for therapy with insulin and oral hypoglycemic agents?

BIBLIOGRAPHY

Books

Biermann J and Toohey B. The Diabetic's Book. Los Angeles, J Tarcher, 1990.

Biermann J and Toohey B. The Diabetic's Total Health Book. Los Angeles, J Tarcher, 1988.

Davidson M. Diabetes Mellitus: Diagnosis and Treatment, 3rd ed. New York, John Wiley & Sons, 1990.

Dunning T. Care of People With Diabetes: A Manual of Nursing Practice. Boston, Blackwell Scientific Publications, 1994.

Kahn CR and Weir GC (eds). Joslin's Diabetes Mellitus. Philadelphia, Lea & Febiger, 1994.

Kozak GP et al. Management of Diabetic Foot Problems. Philadelphia, Saunders, 1995.

Peterson C and Jovanovic L. The Diabetes Self-Care Method, 2nd ed. New York, Simon & Schuster, 1991.

Physician's Guide to Insulin-Dependent (Type I) Diabetes: Diagnosis and Treatment. Alexandria, VA, American Diabetes Association, 1994.

Physician's Guide to Non-Insulin-Dependent (Type II) Diabetes: Diagnosis and Treatment. Alexandria, VA, American Diabetes Association, 1994.

U.S. Department of Health and Human Services. Healthy People 2000: National Health Promotion and Disease Prevention Objectives. Washington, DC, U.S. Government Printing Office, 1990.

Journals

Asterisks indicate nursing research articles.

General

American Diabetes Association. Clinical practice recommendations. Diabetes Care 1995 Jan 18 Suppl 1:1–96.

Anderson R. The challenge of translating scientific knowledge into improved diabetes care in the 1990s. Diabetes Care 1991 May; 14(5):418–421.

Berry R, Mohn KR, Holzmeister LA. Monitoring diabetes therapy. Home Healthcare Nurse 1995 Jan–Feb; 13(1):39–42.

Betschart J. Children and adolescents with diabetes. Nurs Clin North Am 1993 Mar; 28(1):35–44.

*Boehm S et al. Behavioral analysis and behavioral strategies to improve self-management of type II diabetes. Clin Nurs Res 1993 Aug; 2(3):327–344.

*Brown SA, Hedges LV. Predicting metabolic control in diabetes: A pilot study using meta-analysis to estimate a linear model. Nurs Res 1994 Nov–Dec; 43(6):362–368.

Brown S, Thompson W. Therapeutic role of exercise in diabetes mellitus. Diabetes Educator; 1988 May/Jun; 14(3):202–206.

Deakins DA. Teaching elderly patients about diabetes. Am J Nurs 1994 Apr; 94(4):38–43.

Fain JA. National trends in diabetes: An epidemiologic perspective. Nurs Clin North Am 1993 Mar; 28(1):1–7.

Funnell MM, Merritt JH. The challenges of diabetes and older adults. Nurs Clin North Am 1993 Mar; 28(1):45–60.

*Goff J, Rogers BP. Selecting a bedside glucose monitor for outpatient clinics. Clin Nurs Res 1995 Feb; 4(1):105–113.

Haire-Joshu D, Funnell MM, Maschak-Carey BJ. Competencies for diabetes care for schools of nursing. Diabetes Spectrum 1993 Nov/Dec; 6(6):355–364.

Harris MD. Medicare and the nurse. Current research findings related to individuals with diabetes mellitus. Home Healthcare Nurse 1995 Jan–Feb; 13(1):79–81.

Hough DO. Diabetes mellitus in sports. Med Clin North Am 1994 Mar; 78(2):423–437.

*Joseph DH, Patterson B. Risk taking and the influence on metabolic control: A study of adult clients with diabetes. J Adv Nurs 1994 Jan; 19(1):77–84.

Krug L M, Haire-Joshu D, Heady SA. Exercise habits and exercise relapse in persons with non-insulin-dependent diabetes mellitus. Diabetes Educator 1994 May/Jun; 17(3):185–187.

*LeMone P. Assessing psychosexual concerns in adults with diabetes: Pilot project using Roy's modes of adaptation. Iss Mental Health Nurs 1995 Jan–Feb; 16(1):67–78.

LeMone P. Responses of the older adult to the effects and management of diabetes mellitus. Medsurg Nurs 1994 Apr; 3(2):122–127.

*LeMone P. Human sexuality in adults with insulin-dependent diabetes mellitus. Image: J Nurs Scholarship 1993 Summer; 25(2):101–105.

Martinez NC. Diabetes and minority populations: Focus on Mexican Americans. Nurs Clin North Am 1993 Mar; 28(1):87–95.

*Parker JG. The lived experience of Native Americans with diabetes within a transcultural nursing perspective. J Transcultural Nurs 1994 Summer; 6(1):5–11.

*Schwab T, Meyer J, Merrell R. Measuring attitudes and health beliefs among Mexican-Americans with diabetes. Diabetes Educator 1994 May/Jun; 20(3):221–227.

Walker EA. Quality assurance for blood glucose monitoring. Nurs Clin North Am 1993 Mar; 28(1):61–70.

Watts RJ. Sexual function of diabetic and nondiabetic African American women: A pilot study. J National Black Nurses Assoc 1994; 7(1):50–59.

Wells S. Postoperative recovery: How diabetes complicates care. J Cardiovasc Nurs 1993 Jul; 7(4):47–58.

*Zaldivar A, Smolowitz J. Perceptions of the importance placed on religion and folk medicine by non-Mexican-American Hispanic adults with diabetes. Diabetes Educator 1994 Jul/Aug; 20(4):303–306.

Management

Abrams R, Coustan D, Jovanovic-Peterson L. Gestational diabetes: Strategies for management. Diabetes Spectrum 1992; 5:17–51.

Anderson S. Seven care tips for managing patients with diabetes. Am J Nurs 1994 Sep; 94(9):36–38.

Collo MB, Johnson JL, Kabadi UM. Combination sulfonylurea and insulin therapy in non–insulin-dependent diabetes mellitus. Nurse Practitioner: Am J Primary Health Care 1993 Jul; 18(7):40, 43–44, 47–48.

Delahanty LM, Halford BN. The role of diet behaviors in improved glycemic control in intensively treated patients in the Diabetes Control and Complications Trial. Diabetes Care 1993 Nov; 16(11):1453–1459.

Galloway J. New directions in drug development: Mixtures, analogues, and modeling. Diabetes Care, 1993 Dec; 16(Suppl 3): 16–23.

Graham C. Exercise and aging: Implications for persons with diabetes. Diabetes Educator 1991 May/Jun; 17(3):189–195.

Hirsch IB, Farkas-Hirsch R. Intensive insulin therapy for the treatment of Type I diabetes. Diabetes Care 1992; 13(11):1265–1283.

Hirsch IB, Farkas-Hirsch R. Type I diabetes and insulin therapy. Nurs Clin North Am 1993 Mar; 28(1):9–23.

Hoyson PM. Diabetes 2000: Oral medications. RN 1995 May; 58(5):34–40.

Kestal F. Are you up to date on diabetes medications? Am J Nurs 1994 Jul; 94(7):48–52.

Kros S. Contraception in women with diabetes mellitus. Diabetes Spectrum 1993; 6(2):80–86.

Melkus GD. Type II non-insulin-dependent diabetes mellitus. Nurs Clin North Am 1993 Mar; 28(1):25–33.

Parker C. Responding quickly to hypoglycemia. Am J Nurs 1994 Jun; 94(6):46.

Spollett GR. Intensive insulin therapy in insulin dependent diabetes and combination therapy. Nurse Practitioner: Am J Primary Health Care 1993 Jul; 18(7):27–28, 33, 36–38.

Thom SL. Nutritional management of diabetes. Nurs Clin North Am 1993 Mar; 28(1):97–112.

Zinman B. Insulin regimens and strategies for IDDN. Diabetes Care 1993 Dec; 16(Suppl 3):24–28.

Patient and Family Education

Coonrod B, Betschart J, Harris M. Frequency and determinants of diabetes patient education among adults in the U.S. population. Diabetes Care 1994; 17(8):852–858.

Deakins DA. Teaching elderly patients about diabetes. Am J Nurs 1994 Apr; 94(4):38–42.

Funnell M et al. Empowerment: An idea whose time has come in diabetes education. Diabetes Educator 1991 Jan/Feb; 17(1): 37–41.

Hinnen D. Issues in diabetes education. Nurs Clin North Am 1993 Mar; 28(1):113–120.

*Leggett-Frazier N, Turner MS, Vincent PA. Measuring the diabetes knowledge of nurses in long-term care facilities. Diabetes Educator 1994 Jul/Aug; 20(4):307–310.

Mulhauser I, Berger M. Diabetes education and insulin therapy: When will they ever learn? J Intern Med 1993; 233:321–326.

Powers M. Facilitating nutritional changes in difficult patients. Diabetes Spectrum 1991; 4(4):186–192.

*Tu KS, McDaniel G, Templeton J. Diabetes self-care knowledge, behaviors, and metabolic control of older adults: The effect of a posteducational follow-up program. Diabetes Educator 1993 Jan/Feb; 19(1):25–29.

Complications

Bienkowski J. An overview of the progression of diabetic retinopathy with treatment recommendations. Nurse Practitioner: Am J Primary Health Care 1994 Jul; 19(7):50–58.

Clark AP. Complications and management of diabetes: A review of current research. Crit Care Nurs Clin North Am. 1994 Dec; 6(4):723–734.

DCCT Research Group. The effect of intensive treatment of diabetes on the development and progression of long-term complications in insulin-dependent diabetes mellitus. N Engl J Med 1993 Sep 30; 329(14):977–986.

DCCT Research Group. Epidemiology of severe hypoglycemia in the Diabetes Control and Complications Trial. Am J Med 1991 April; 90:450–459.

Fore WW. Non–insulin-dependent diabetes mellitus. The prevention of complications. Med Clin North Am 1995 Mar; 79(2): 287–298.

Haas LB. Chronic complications of diabetes mellitus. Nurs Clin North Am 1993 Mar; 28(1):71–85.

Haire-Joshu D. Smoking, cessation, and the diabetes health care team. Diabetes Educator 1991 Jan/Feb; 17(1):54–65.

Harley JR. Preventing diabetic foot disease. Nurse Practitioner: Am J Primary Health Care 1993 Oct; 18(10):37–38, 41–42, 44.

Jones TL. From diabetic ketoacidosis to hyperglycemic hyperosmolar nonketotic syndrome: The spectrum of uncontrolled hyperglycemia in diabetes mellitus. Crit Care Nurs Clin North Am 1994 Dec: 6(4):703–721.

Kitabchi AE, Wall BM. Diabetic ketoacidosis. Med Clin North Am 1995 Jan; 79(1):9–37.

Klein R. Hyperglycemia and microvascular disease in diabetes. Diabetes Care 1995 Feb; 18(2):258–268.

Lorber D. Nonketotic hypertonicity in diabetes mellitus. Med Clin North Am 1995 Jan; 79(1):39–52.

Machea Knight MK. Diabetic hypoglycemia: How to keep the threat at bay. Am J Nurs 1993 Apr; 93(4):26–30.

Murray R. Home before dark: One nurse's personal experience with diabetic neuropathy. Am J Nurs 1993 Nov; 93(11):36–42.

Nathan DM. Inferences and implications. Do results from the Diabetes Control and Complications Trial apply in NIDDM? Diabetes Care 1995 Feb; 18(2):251–257.

Rosenberg C. Wound healing in the patient with diabetes mellitus. Nurs Clin North Am 1990 Mar; 25(1):247–261.

Service FJ. Hypoglycemia. Med Clin North Am 1995 Jan; 79(1):1–8.

Smitherman KO, Peacock JE Jr. Infectious emergencies in patients with diabetes mellitus. Med Clin North Am 1995 Jan; 79(1): 53–77.

Pregnancy and Gestational Diabetes

Avery MD, Rossi MA. Gestational diabetes. J Nurse-Midwifery 1994 Mar–Apr; 39(2 Suppl):9S–19S, 3S–8S.

Barnes LP. Gestational diabetes: Teaching aspects of self care. MCN: Am J Maternal Child Nurs 1994 May–June; 19(3):175.

Jackson P, Bash DM. Management of the uncomplicated pregnant diabetic client in the ambulatory setting. Nurse Practitioner. Am J Primary Health Care 1994 Dec; 19(12):64, 66–73.

Janz NK et al. Diabetes and pregnancy. Factors associated with seeking pre-conception care. Diabetes Care 1995 Feb; 18(2): 157–165.

Niesen KM, Rajan MJ. Pregnancy complicated by diabetes mellitus, superimposed preeclampsia, and adult respiratory distress syndrome: A case study. Crit Care Nurs Clin North Am 1994 Dec; 6(4):841–854.

INFORMATION/RESOURCES

Agencies

American Association of Diabetes Educators
444 North Michigan Ave
Suite 1240,
Chicago, IL 60611
(312) 644-AADE

American Diabetes Association
1660 Duke St,
Alexandria, VA 22314
1-800-232-3472
See issues of Diabetes Care for Position Statements and Consensus Statements of the American Diabetes Association.

American Dietetic Association
216 West Jackson Boulevard,
Chicago, IL 60606
1-800-877-1600

American Foundation for the Blind
15 West 16th St,
New York, NY 10011
1-800-232-5463

Juvenile Diabetes Foundation
423 Park Ave S,
New York, NY 10016
(212) 889-7575, 1-800-JDF-CURE

Medic Alert Foundation International
2323 Colorado St,
Turlock CA 95381-1009
(209) 668-3333

National Library Services for the Blind and Physically Handicapped
1291 Taylor St, NW
Washington, DC 20542
(202) 287-5100

National Diabetes Information Clearing House
Box NDIC, 1801 Rockville Pike,
Bethesda, MD 20892
301-468-2162

Journals for Patients

Diabetes '90,
Subscription Department,
American Diabetes Association, 1660 Duke St,
Alexandria, VA 22314

Diabetes Forecast,
American Diabetes Association,
Membership Center,
PO Box 2055,
Harlan, IA 51593–0238

Diabetes in the News,
Ames Center for Diabetes Education,
Miles Inc,
PO Box 3105,
Elkhart, IN 46515

Diabetes Self-Management,
PO Box 51125,
Boulder, CO 80321-1125

Living Well With Diabetes,
Diabetes Center,
13911 Ridgedale Dr,
Suite 250,
Minnetonka, MN 55343

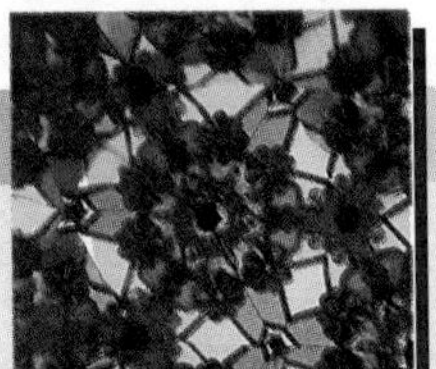

40

Assessment and Management of Patients With Endocrine Disorders

CHAPTER OUTLINE

LEARNING OBJECTIVES

On completion of this chapter, the learner will be able to:

1. Describe the functions and hormones secreted by each of the endocrine glands
2. Identify the diagnostic tests used to determine alterations in function of each of the endocrine glands
3. Compare hypothyroidism and hyperthyroidism: their causes, clinical manifestations, management, and nursing interventions
4. Develop a nursing care plan for the patient undergoing thyroidectomy
5. Compare hyperparathyroidism and hypoparathyroidism: their causes, clinical manifestations, management, and nursing interventions
6. Compare Addison's disease with Cushing's syndrome: their causes, clinical manifestations, management, and nursing interventions
7. Use the nursing process as a framework for care of patients with adrenal insufficiency
8. Use the nursing process as a framework for care of patients with Cushing's syndrome
9. Identify the teaching needs of patients requiring corticosteroid therapy
10. Differentiate between acute and chronic pancreatitis
11. Use the nursing process as a framework for care of patients with acute pancreatitis
12. Identify the limitations of surgical treatment of tumors of the pancreas

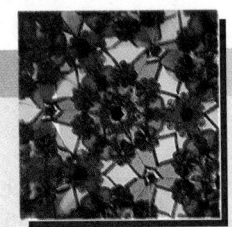

Physiologic Overview

The endocrine glands include the pituitary, thyroid, parathyroids, adrenals, pancreatic islets, ovaries, and testes. These glands, which secrete their products directly into the bloodstream, are clearly differentiated from exocrine glands, such as sweat glands, which secrete through ducts onto epithelial surfaces. The hypothalamus provides the link between the nervous system and the endocrine system.

The chemical substances secreted by the endocrine glands are called **hormones.** Hormones help to regulate organ function in concert with the nervous system. This dual regulatory system, in which rapid action by the nervous system is balanced by slower hormonal action, permits precise control of body functions in response to varied changes within and outside the body.

A schematic diagram of the important endocrine glands is shown in Figure 40-1. Table 40-1 lists the important hormones, their target tissue, and some of their properties.

Certain anatomic features are common to the endocrine glands. The glands are composed of secretory cells arranged in minute clusters (acini). No ducts are present, but the glands have a rich blood supply, so that the chemicals they produce can rapidly enter the bloodstream.

Feedback Control. The concentration in the bloodstream of most hormones is maintained at a relatively constant level. If the hormone concentration rises, further production of that hormone is inhibited. When the hormone concentration falls, the rate of production of that hormone increases. This mechanism for regulation of hormone concentration in the bloodstream is called **feedback control.** The principle of feedback control is important in the regulation of many biologic processes.

Mechanism of Hormone Action. Hormones are classified as steroid hormones (such as hydrocortisone), peptide or protein hormones (such as insulin), and amine hormones (such as epinephrine). These different classes of hormones act on the target tissues by different mechanisms. Hormones can alter the function of the target tissue by inter-

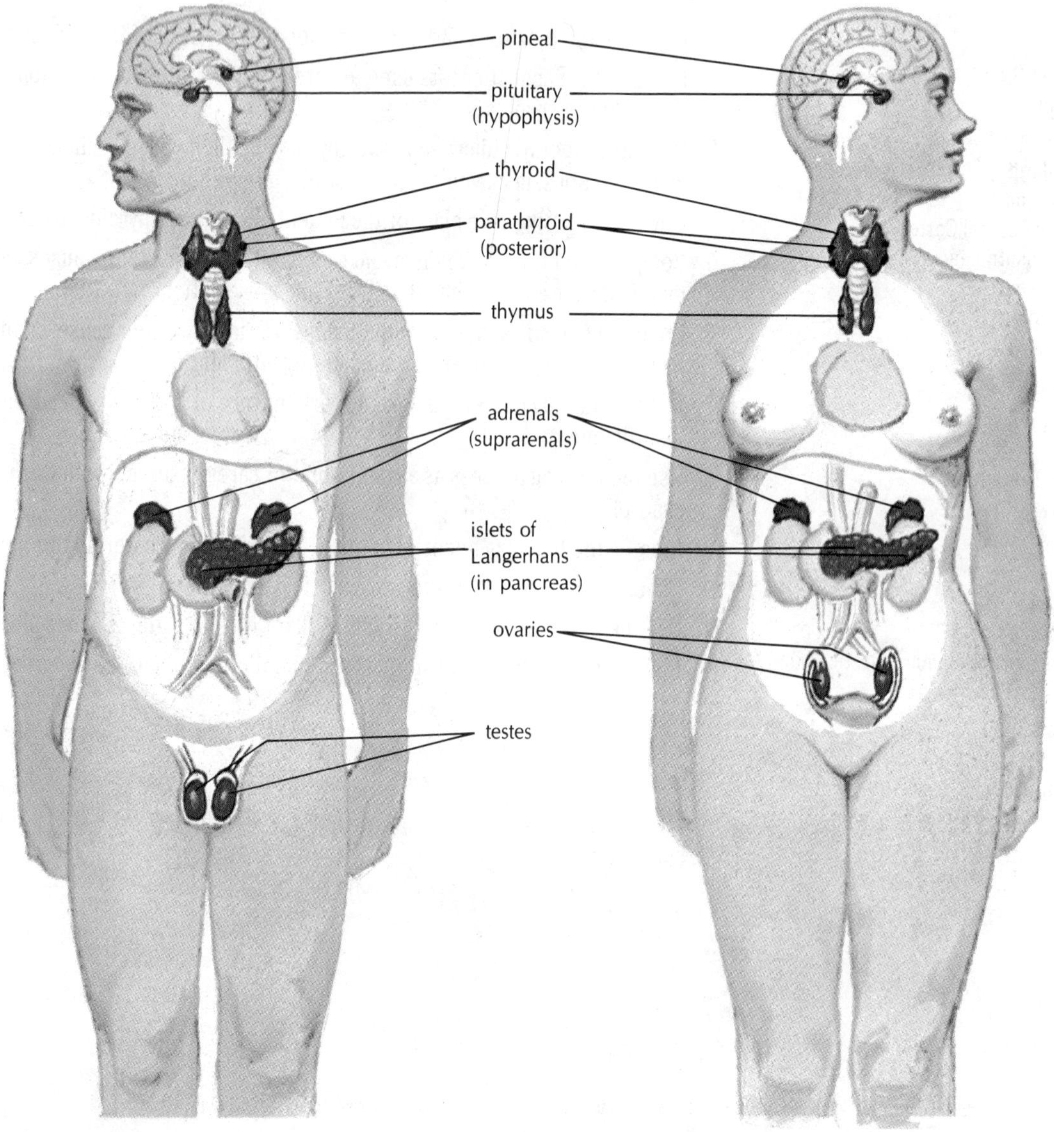

FIGURE 40-1. Major hormone-secreting glands of the endocrine system.

TABLE 40-1 Endocrine System in Summary

Endocrine Gland and Hormone	Principal Site of Action	Principal Processes Affected
Pituitary Gland		
Anterior Lobe		
Growth hormone (somatotropin)	General	Growth of bones, muscles, and other organs
Thyroid-stimulating (TSH)	Thyroid	Growth and secretory activity of thyroid gland
Adrenocorticotropin (ACTH)	Adrenal cortex	Growth and secretory activity of adrenal cortex
Follicle-stimulating (FSH)	Ovaries	Development of follicles and secretion of estrogen
	Testes	Development of seminiferous tubules, spermatogenesis
Luteinizing (LH) or interstitial cell stimulating	Ovaries	Ovulation, formation of corpus luteum, secretion of progesterone
	Testes	Secretion of testosterone
Prolactin or lactogenic (luteotropin)	Mammary glands and ovaries	Secretion of milk; maintenance of corpus luteum
Melanocyte-stimulating	Skin	Pigmentation
Beta lipotropin		
Posterior Lobe		
Antidiuretic (vasopressin)	Kidney	Reabsorption of water; water balance
	Arterioles	Blood pressure
Oxytocin	Uterus	Contraction
	Breast	Expression of milk
Pineal Gland		
Melatonin	Gonads	Sexual maturation
Thyroid Gland		
Thyroxine and triiodothyronine	General	Metabolic rate; growth and development; intermediate metabolism
Calcitonin	Bone	Inhibits bone resorption; lowers blood level of calcium
Parathyroid Glands		
Parathormone	Bone, kidney, intestine	Promotes bone resorption; increases absorption of calcium; raises blood calcium level
Adrenal Glands		
Cortex		
Mineralocorticoids (*e.g.*, aldosterone)	Kidney	Reabsorption of sodium; elimination of potassium
Glucocorticoids (*e.g.*, cortisol)	General	Metabolism of carbohydrate, protein, and fat; response to stress; anti-inflammatory
Sex hormones	General	Preadolescent growth spurt
Medulla		
Epinephrine	Cardiac muscle, smooth muscle, glands	Emergency functions: same as stimulation of sympathetic nervous system
Norepinephrine	Organs innervated by sympathetic nervous system	Chemical transmitter substance; increases peripheral resistance
Islet Cells of Pancreas		
Insulin	General	Lowers blood sugar; utilization and storage of carbohydrate; decreased gluconeogenesis
Glucagon	Liver	Raises blood glucose; glycogenolysis
Somatostatin	General	Lowers blood glucose by interfering with release of growth hormone and glucagon
Testes		
Testosterone	General	Development of secondary sex characteristics
	Reproductive organs	Development and maintenance; normal function

(continued)

TABLE 40-1 *(continued)*

Endocrine Gland and Hormone	Principal Site of Action	Principal Processes Affected
Ovaries		
Estrogens	General	Development of secondary sex characteristics
	Mammary glands	Development of duct system
	Reproductive organs	Maturation and normal cyclic function
Progesterone	Mammary glands	Development of secretory tissue
	Uterus	Preparation for implantation; maintenance of pregnancy
Gastrointestinal Tract		
Gastrin	Stomach	Production of gastric juice
Enterogastrone	Stomach	Inhibits secretion and motility
Secretin	Liver and pancreas	Production of bile; production of watery pancreatic juice (rich in $NaHCO_3$)
Pancreozymin	Pancreas	Production of pancreatic juice rich in enzymes
Cholecystokinin	Gallbladder	Contraction and emptying

(Adapted from Chaffee EE and Lytle IM. Basic Physiology and Anatomy, 4th ed. Philadelphia, JB Lippincott.)

acting with chemical receptors located either on the cell membrane or in the interior of the cell.

Peptide and protein hormones interact with receptor sites on the cell surface, which results in the stimulation of the intracellular enzyme adenyl cyclase. This in turn results in increased production of cyclic 3', 5'-adenosine monophosphate (cyclic AMP). The cyclic AMP inside the cell alters enzyme activity. Thus, cyclic AMP is the "second messenger" that links the peptide hormone at the cell surface to a change in the intracellular environment. Some of the protein and peptide hormones may also act by changing membrane permeability. These hormones act relatively rapidly, within seconds or minutes. The mechanism of action for **amine hormones** is similar to that for peptide hormones.

Steroid hormones, because of their smaller size and higher lipid solubility, penetrate the cell membranes and interact with intracellular receptors. This steroid–receptor complex modifies cell metabolism and formation of messenger ribonucleic acid (RNA) from deoxyribonucleic acid (DNA). The messenger RNA then stimulates protein synthesis within the cell. Steroid hormones, because they exert their action by the modification of protein synthesis, require several hours to exert their effects.

The Pituitary Gland

The pituitary gland, or the hypophysis, has been referred to as the master gland of the endocrine system. It secretes hormones that, in turn, control the secretion of hormones by other endocrine glands (Fig. 40-2). The pituitary itself is controlled in large part by the hypothalamus, an adjacent area of the brain.

The pituitary gland is a round structure approximately 1.27 cm (½ inch) in diameter located on the inferior aspect of the brain and connected to the hypothalamus by the pituitary stalk. The pituitary gland is divided into anterior, intermediate, and posterior lobes.

Posterior Pituitary. The important hormones secreted by the posterior lobe of the pituitary gland are **vasopressin** (antidiuretic hormone [ADH]) and **oxytocin.** These hormones are synthesized in the hypothalamus and travel down the nerve cells that connect the hypothalamus to the posterior pituitary gland, where they are stored.

Vasopressin secretion is stimulated by an increase in the osmolality of the blood or by a decrease in blood pressure. The primary function of vasopressin is to control the excretion of water by the kidney.

Oxytocin secretion is stimulated during pregnancy and at the time of childbirth. The primary functions of oxytocin are to facilitate milk ejection during lactation and to increase the force of uterine contractions during labor and delivery. Exogenous oxytocin is used therapeutically to initiate labor.

Anterior Pituitary. The major hormones of the anterior pituitary gland are follicle-stimulating hormone (FSH), luteinizing hormone (LH), prolactin, adrenocorticotropic hormone (ACTH), thyroid-stimulating hormone (TSH), and growth hormone. The secretion of each of these major hormones is controlled by releasing factors (RF) that are secreted by the hypothalamus. These releasing factors reach the anterior pituitary by way of the bloodstream in a special circulation called the pituitary portal blood system. Other hormones include melanocyte-stimulating hormone and beta lipotropin; the function of lipotropin is poorly understood.

The hormones released by the anterior pituitary enter the general circulation and are transported to their target organs. TSH, ACTH, FSH, and LH have as their main function the release of hormones from other endocrine glands. Prolactin acts on the breast to stimulate milk production. Growth hormone has widespread effects on many target tissues and is discussed below. The other trophic hormones are discussed in conjunction with their target organs.

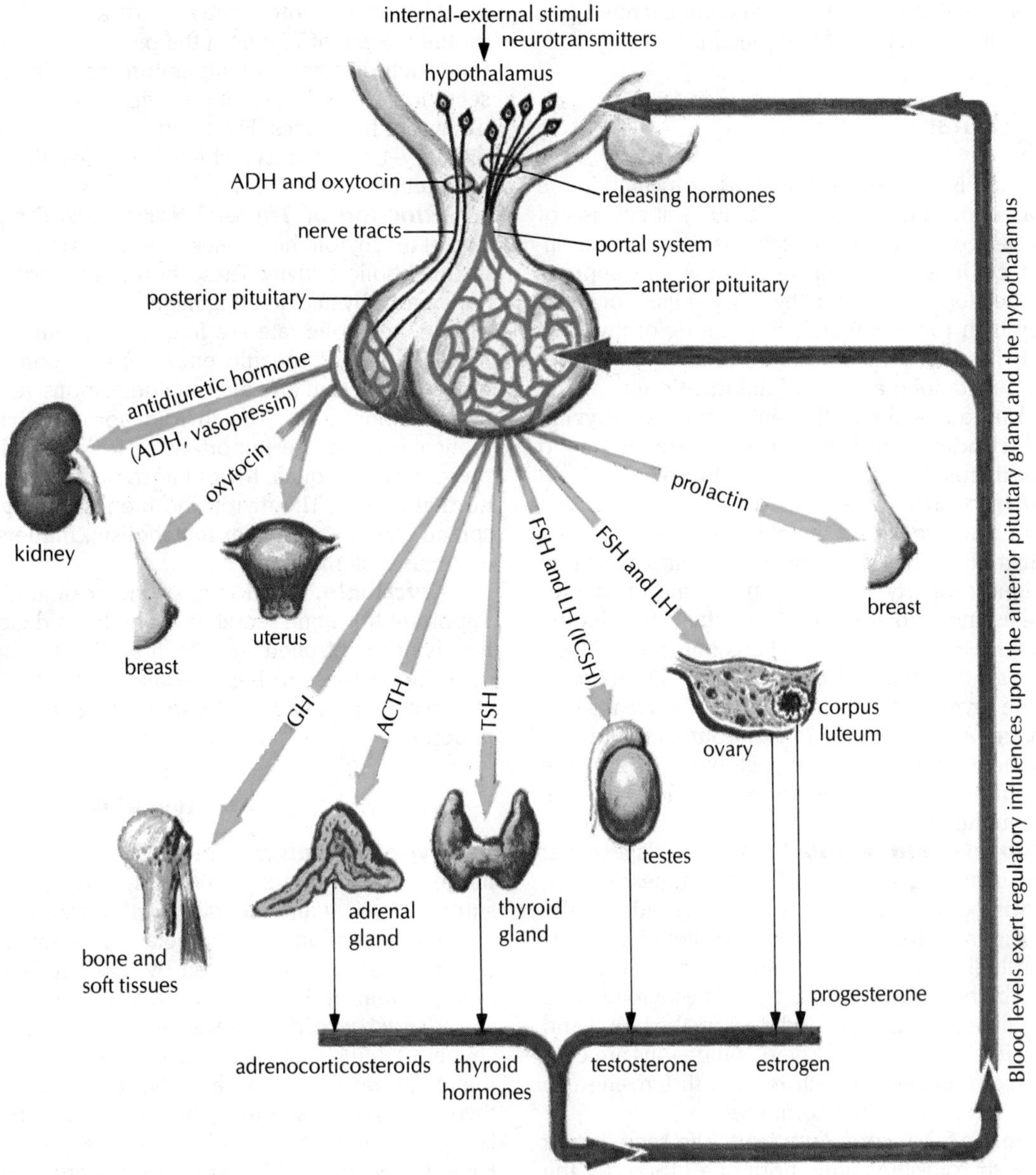

FIGURE 40-2. The pituitary gland, the relationship of the brain to pituitary action, and the hormones secreted by the anterior pituitary and the posterior pituitary.

Growth Hormone. Growth hormone, also referred to as somatotropin, is a protein hormone that increases protein synthesis in many tissues, increases the breakdown of fatty acids in adipose tissue, and increases the glucose level in the blood. These actions of somatotropin are essential for normal growth, although other hormones, such as thyroid hormone and insulin, are required as well. The secretion of growth hormone is increased by stress, exercise, and low blood glucose. The half-life of growth hormone activity in the blood is 20 to 30 minutes. It is largely inactivated in the liver.

Insufficient secretion of growth hormone during childhood results in generalized limited growth and dwarfism. Conversely, oversecretion during childhood results in gigantism, with a person reaching 7 or even 8 feet in height. Excess growth hormone in adults results in deformities of bone and soft tissue and enlargement of viscera but no increase in height. This condition is known as acromegaly.

Abnormal Pituitary Function. Abnormalities of pituitary function are caused by oversecretion or undersecretion of any of the hormones produced or released by the gland. Abnormalities of the anterior and posterior portions of the gland may occur independently. Oversecretion (hypersecretion) most commonly involves ACTH or growth hormone, resulting in the conditions known as Cushing's disease or acromegaly, respectively.

Undersecretion (hyposecretion) commonly involves all of the anterior pituitary hormones and is termed panhypopituitarism. In this condition, the thyroid gland, the adrenal cortex, and the gonads atrophy because of loss of the trophic hormones.

The most common disorder related to posterior lobe dysfunction is diabetes insipidus, a condition in which abnormally large volumes of dilute urine are excreted as a result of deficient production of vasopressin.

The Thyroid Gland

The thyroid gland is a butterfly-shaped organ located in the lower neck anterior to the trachea (Fig. 40-3). It consists of two lateral lobes connected by an isthmus. The gland is approximately 5 cm long and 3 cm wide and weighs approximately 30 g. The blood flow to the thyroid, per gram of gland tissue, is very high (approximately 5 ml/min/g of thyroid), approximately five times the blood flow to the liver. This reflects the high metabolic activity of the thyroid gland. The thyroid gland produces three different hormones: **thyroxine (T_4)** and **triiodothyronine (T_3)**, which are referred to collectively as thyroid hormone, and **calcitonin.**

Thyroid Hormone. Two separate hormones produced by the thyroid gland make up thyroid hormone: thyroxine and triiodothyronine. These hormones are amino acids that have the unique property of containing iodine molecules bound to the amino acid structure. T_4 contains four iodine atoms in each molecule, and T_3 contains only three. These hormones are synthesized and stored bound to proteins in the cells of the thyroid gland until needed for release into the bloodstream. Approximately 75% of bound thyroid hormone is bound to thyroxin-binding globulin (TBG); the remaining bound thyroid hormone is bound to thyroid-binding prealbumin and albumin.

Iodine Uptake and Metabolism. Iodine is essential to the thyroid gland for synthesis of its hormones. In fact, the major use of iodine in the body is by the thyroid, and the major derangement in iodine deficiency is alteration of thyroid function. Iodide is ingested in the diet and absorbed into the blood in the gastrointestinal tract. The thyroid gland is extremely efficient in taking up iodide from the blood and concentrating it within the cells. There, iodide ions are converted to iodine molecules, which react with tyrosine (an amino acid) to form the thyroid hormones.

Regulation of Thyroid Function. The secretion of thyrotropin, or thyroid-stimulating hormone (TSH), by the pituitary gland controls the rate of thyroid hormone release. In turn, the release of TSH is determined by the level of thyroid hormones in the blood. If thyroid hormone concentration in the blood decreases, release of TSH increases, which causes increased output of T_3 and T_4. This is an example of feedback control. Thyrotropin-releasing hormone (TRH), secreted by the hypothalamus, exerts a modulating influence on the release of TSH from the pituitary. Environmental factors, such as a fall in temperature, may lead to increased secretion of TRH and thereby result in elevated secretion of thyroid hormones. Figure 40-4 shows the hypothalamic–pituitary–thyroid axis, which regulates thyroid hormone production.

Function of Thyroid Hormones. The primary function of the thyroid hormones T_3 and T_4 is to control the cellular metabolic activity. These hormones serve as a general pacemaker by accelerating metabolic processes. The effects on the metabolic rate are frequently produced by increasing the level of specific enzymes that contribute to oxygen consumption and altering the responsiveness of tissues to other hormones. The thyroid hormones influence cell replication and are important in brain development. The presence of adequate thyroid hormone is also necessary for normal growth. The thyroid hormones, through their widespread effects on cellular metabolism, influence every major organ system.

Calcitonin. Calcitonin, or thyrocalcitonin, is another important hormone secreted by the thyroid gland. Its secretion is not controlled by TSH. It is secreted by the thyroid gland in response to high plasma levels of calcium, and it reduces the plasma level by increasing calcium deposition in bone.

Abnormalities of Thyroid Function

Hypothyroidism. Inadequate secretion of thyroid hormone during fetal and neonatal development results in stunted physical and mental growth (cretinism) because of general depression of body metabolic activity. In the adult, hypothyroidism is manifested by lethargy, slow mentation, and generalized slowing of body functions.

Hyperthyroidism. Oversecretion of thyroid hormones (hyperthyroidism) is manifested by a greatly increased metabolic rate. Many of the other characteristics of hyperthyroid patients result from the increased response to circulating catecholamines (epinephrine and norepinephrine). Hypothyroidism and hyperthyroidism are discussed in detail in a later section of this chapter.

Goiter. Oversecretion of thyroid hormones is usually associated with an enlarged thyroid gland (goiter). Goiter also commonly occurs in the presence of iodide deficiency. In this latter condition, lack of iodide results in low levels of circulating thyroid hormones, which causes increased re-

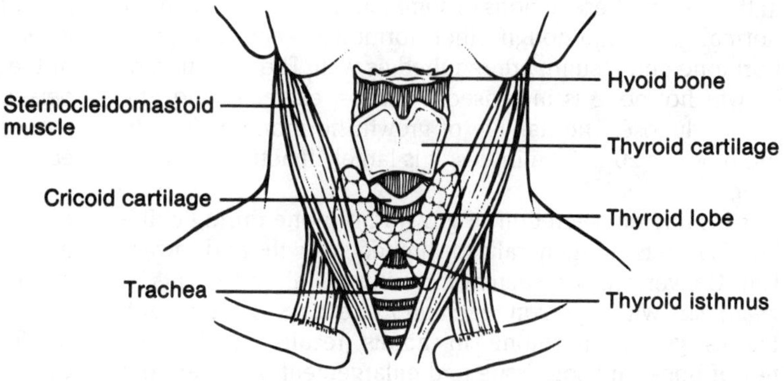

FIGURE 40-3. The thyroid gland and surrounding structures. (Fuller J and Schaller-Ayers J. Health Assessment: A Nursing Approach, 2nd ed. Philadelphia, JB Lippincott, 1994.)

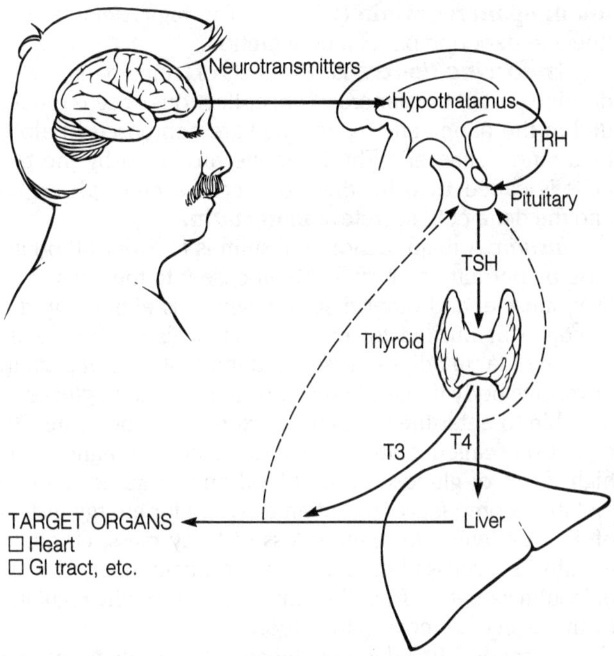

FIGURE 40-4. The hypothalamic–pituitary–thyroid axis. Thyroid-releasing hormone (TRH) from the hypothalamus stimulates the pituitary gland to secrete thyroid-stimulating hormone (TSH). TSH stimulates the thyroid to produce thyroid hormone (T3 and T4). High circulating levels of T3 and T4 inhibit further TSH secretion and thyroid hormone production through a negative feedback mechanism *(dashed lines)*.

lease of TSH; the elevated TSH causes overproduction of thyroglobulin and hypertrophy of the thyroid gland.

Euthyroid refers to thyroid hormone production that is within normal limits.

The Adrenal Glands

There are two adrenal glands in the human, each attached to the upper portion of a kidney. Each adrenal gland is, in reality, two endocrine glands with separate, independent functions. The adrenal medulla at the center of the gland secretes catecholamines, and the outer portion of the gland, the adrenal cortex, secretes corticosteroids.

Adrenal Medulla. The adrenal medulla functions as part of the autonomic nervous system. Stimulation of preganglionic sympathetic nerve fibers, which travel directly to the cells of the adrenal medulla, causes release of the catecholamine hormones epinephrine and norepinephrine. Approximately 90% of the secretion of the human adrenal medulla is epinephrine (also called adrenalin). Catecholamines regulate metabolic pathways to promote catabolism of stored fuels to meet caloric needs from endogenous sources.

The major effects of epinephrine release are involved in preparation to meet a challenge (fight-or-flight response). Secretion of epinephrine causes decreased blood flow to tissues that are not needed in emergency situations, such as the gastrointestinal tract, and causes increased blood flow to those tissues that are important for effective fight or flight, such as cardiac and skeletal muscle. Catecholamines also induce release of free fatty acids, increase the basal metabolic rate, and elevate the level of blood glucose.

Adrenal Cortex. The three kinds of steroid hormones produced by the adrenal cortex are glucocorticoids, the prototype of which is hydrocortisone; mineralocorticoids, mainly aldosterone; and sex hormones, mainly androgens (male sex hormones).

Glucocorticoids. The glucocorticoids are given their name because they have an important influence on glucose metabolism; increased hydrocortisone secretion results in elevated blood glucose levels. However, the glucocorticoids have major effects on the metabolism of almost all organs of the body.

Glucocorticoids are secreted from the adrenal cortex in response to the release of ACTH from the anterior lobe of the pituitary gland. This system represents an example of **negative feedback.** The presence of glucocorticoids in the blood inhibits the release of corticotropin-releasing factor (CRF) from the hypothalamus and also inhibits ACTH secretion from the pituitary. The resultant decrease in ACTH secretion causes diminished release of glucocorticoids from the adrenal cortex.

A functioning adrenal cortex is necessary for life, although survival is possible by appropriate replacement with exogenous adrenocortical hormones.

The glucocorticoids are frequently administered to inhibit the inflammatory response to tissue injury and suppress allergic manifestations. Side effects of glucocorticoids include possible development of diabetes mellitus, osteoporosis, peptic ulcer, increased protein breakdown resulting in muscle wasting and poor wound healing, and redistribution of body fat.

The presence of large amounts of exogenously administered glucocorticoids in the blood inhibits release of ACTH and endogenous glucocorticoids. Because of this, the adrenal cortex can atrophy. If exogenous glucocorticoid administration is suddenly discontinued, adrenal insufficiency results because of the inability of the atrophied cortex to respond adequately.

Mineralocorticoids. Mineralocorticoids exert their major effects on electrolyte metabolism. They act principally on renal tubular and gastrointestinal epithelium to cause increased sodium ion absorption in exchange for excretion of potassium or hydrogen ions. Aldosterone secretion is only minimally influenced by ACTH. It is primarily secreted in response to the presence of angiotensin II in the bloodstream. Angiotensin II is a substance that elevates the blood pressure by constricting arterioles. Its concentration is increased when renin is released from the kidney in response to decreased perfusion pressure. The resultant increased aldosterone levels promote sodium reabsorption by the kidney and the gastrointestinal tract, which tends to restore blood pressure to normal. The release of aldosterone is also increased by hyperkalemia. Aldosterone is the primary hormone for the long-term regulation of sodium balance.

Adrenal Sex Hormones (Androgens). Androgens, the third major type of steroid hormones produced by the adrenal cortex, exert effects similar to those of male sex hormones. The adrenal gland may also secrete small amounts of some estrogens, or female sex hormones. Secretion of adrenal androgens is controlled by ACTH. When secreted in normal amounts, the adrenal androgens probably have little effect, but when secreted excessively, in certain inborn enzyme deficiencies, masculinization may result. This is termed the **adrenogenital syndrome.**

The Parathyroid Gland

The parathyroid glands, normally four in number, are situated in the neck, embedded in the posterior aspect of the thyroid gland. These small glands are easily overlooked and can be removed accidentally at the time of thyroid surgery. Inadvertent surgical removal is the most common cause of hypoparathyroidism.

Parathormone, the protein hormone from the parathyroid glands, regulates calcium and phosphorus metabolism. Increased secretion of parathormone results in increased calcium absorption from the kidney, the intestine, and bones, thereby raising the blood calcium level. Some actions of this hormone are increased by the presence of vitamin D. Parathormone also tends to lower the blood phosphorus level.

Excess parathormone can result in markedly elevated levels of serum calcium, a potentially life-threatening situation. When the product of serum calcium and serum phosphorus (calcium × phosphorus) becomes high, calcium phosphate may precipitate in various organs of the body and cause tissue calcification.

The output of parathormone is regulated by the serum level of ionized calcium. Increased serum calcium results in decreased parathormone secretion, forming a feedback system.

The Pancreas

The pancreas, located in the upper abdomen, has both exocrine (digestive enzymes) and endocrine gland function. In contrast to endocrine glands, an exocrine gland is one whose secretions travel through a duct to their site of utilization and are not secreted into the bloodstream.

Exocrine Pancreas. The secretions of the exocrine portion of the pancreas are collected in the pancreatic duct, which joins the common bile duct and enters the duodenum at the ampulla of Vater. Surrounding the ampulla is the sphincter of Oddi, which partially controls the rate at which the secretions from both the pancreas and the gallbladder enter the duodenum.

The secretions of the exocrine pancreas are digestive enzymes high in protein content and an electrolyte-rich fluid. The secretions are very alkaline because of their high concentration of sodium bicarbonate and are capable of neutralizing the highly acid gastric juice that enters the duodenum. The enzyme secretions include **amylase,** which aids in the digestion of carbohydrates; **trypsin,** which aids in the digestion of proteins; and **lipase,** which aids in the digestion of fats. Other enzymes that promote the breakdown of more complex foodstuffs are also secreted.

The secretion of these exocrine pancreatic juices is stimulated by hormones originating in the gastrointestinal tract. **Secretin** is the major stimulus for increased bicarbonate secretion from the pancreas, and the major stimulus for digestive enzyme secretion is the hormone **cholecystokinin-pancreozymin** (CCK-PZ). The vagus nerve also influences exocrine pancreatic secretion.

Endocrine Pancreas. The islets of Langerhans, the endocrine part of the pancreas, are collections of cells embedded in the pancreatic tissue. They are composed of alpha, beta, and delta cells. The hormone produced by the beta cells is called **insulin,** the alpha cells secrete **glucagon,** and the delta cells secrete **somatostatin.**

Insulin. A major action of insulin is to lower blood glucose by permitting entry of the glucose into the cells of the liver, muscle, and other tissues, where it is either stored as glycogen or burned for energy. Insulin also promotes the storage of fat in adipose tissue and the synthesis of proteins in various body tissues. In the absence of insulin, glucose is not able to enter the cells and is excreted in the urine. This condition, called diabetes mellitus, can be diagnosed by high levels of glucose in the blood and urine. In diabetes mellitus, stored fats and protein are used for energy instead of glucose, with consequent loss of body mass. (Diabetes mellitus is discussed in more detail in Chapter 39.) The rate of insulin secretion from the pancreas is normally regulated by the level of glucose in the blood.

Glucagon. The effects of glucagon (opposite to those of insulin) are chiefly to raise the blood glucose by converting glycogen to glucose in the liver. Glucagon is secreted by the pancreas in response to a fall in the level of blood glucose.

Somatostatin. Somatostatin exerts a hypoglycemic effect by interfering with release of growth hormone from the pituitary and glucagon from the pancreas, both of which tend to raise blood glucose levels.

Endocrine Control of Carbohydrate Metabolism. Glucose for body energy needs is derived by metabolism of ingested carbohydrates and also from proteins by the process of gluconeogenesis. Glucose can be stored temporarily in the liver, muscles, and other tissues in the form of glycogen. The endocrine system controls the level of blood glucose by regulating the rate at which glucose is synthesized, stored, and moved to and from the bloodstream. Through the action of hormones, blood glucose is normally maintained at approximately 100 mg/dl (5.5 mmol/L). Insulin is the primary hormone that leads to a lowering of the blood glucose level. Hormones that act to raise the blood glucose level are glucagon, epinephrine, adrenocorticosteroids, growth hormone, and thyroid hormone.

The Thyroid Gland

Assessment: Tests of Thyroid Function

Several thyroid tests are available and may be necessary to give a complete and accurate picture of thyroid function. In addition, clinical signs and symptoms are evaluated and provide useful information about the function of the thyroid gland.

The stimulating effect of the thyroid gland is exerted through the production and distribution of two hormones: thyroxine (T_4), which maintains body metabolism in a steady state, and triiodothyronine (T_3), which is approximately five times as potent as T_4 and has a more rapid metabolic action. Measurement of the levels of thyroid hormones in the blood is used to assess thyroid function.

Serum T_4. The test most commonly used is the determination of serum T_4 by radioimmunoassay or competitive binding techniques. The range of T_4 in serum is normally between 4.5 and 11.5 μg/dl (58.5 to 150 nmol/L); T_4 is bound mainly to TBG and prealbumin; T_3 is bound less firmly. T_4 is normally bound to proteins. Any factor that alters these binding proteins also changes the T_4 levels. Serious systemic illnesses, medications (*i.e.*, oral contraceptives, steroids, phenytoin, salicylates), and protein wasting as a result of nephrosis and use of androgens may interfere with accurate test results.

Serum T_3. The serum T_3 test measures free and bound, or total, serum content of T_3. Its secretion occurs in response to TSH secretion, as does that of T_4. Although T_3 and T_4 serum levels generally increase or decrease together, the T_3 level appears to be a more accurate indicator of hyperthyroidism, which causes a greater rise in T_3 than T_4 levels. The normal range for serum T_3 is 70 to 220 ng/dl (1.15 to 3.10 nmol/L).

T_3 Resin Uptake Test. The T_3 resin uptake test is an indirect measure of unsaturated TBG. Its purpose is to determine the amount of thyroid hormone bound to TBG and the number of available binding sites. This provides an index of the amount of thyroid hormone already present in the patient's circulation. Normally, TBG is not fully saturated with thyroid hormone, and additional binding sites are available to combine with radioiodine-labeled T_3 added to the patient's blood specimen. The normal T_3 uptake value is 25% to 35% (relative uptake fraction: 0.25 to 0.35), which indicates that approximately one third of the available sites of TBG are occupied by thyroid hormone. If the number of free or unoccupied binding sites is low, as in hyperthyroidism, the T_3 uptake is greater than 35% (0.35). If the number of available sites is high, as occurs in hypothyroidism, the test results are less than 25% (0.25).

T_3 uptake is useful in the evaluation of thyroid hormone levels in patients who have received diagnostic or therapeutic doses of iodine. The test results may be altered by the use of estrogens, androgens, salicylates, phenytoin, anticoagulants, or steroids.

Tests of Thyroid-Stimulating Hormone. The secretion of T_3 and T_4 by the thyroid gland is under the control of thyroid-stimulating hormone (TSH or thyrotropin) from the anterior pituitary gland. Measurement of serum TSH concentration is valuable in the diagnosis and management of thyroid disorders and in differentiating between disorders caused by disease of the thyroid gland itself and disorders caused by disease of the pituitary or hypothalamus.

TSH Radioimmunoassay. The level of TSH in the serum can be measured by radioimmunoassay. It is increased in patients with primary hypothyroidism. Immunoradiometric assay with labeled monoclonal antibody to TSH is a test with high specificity and sensitivity in the measurement of TSH.

Thyrotropin-Releasing Hormone Test. The TRH stimulation test provides a direct means of testing pituitary reserve for TSH and is useful when T_3 and T_4 test results are inconclusive. The patient fasts overnight. Just before and 30 minutes after intravenous administration of TRH, blood samples are drawn for TSH levels. In hypothyroidism caused by primary disease of the thyroid gland, there is an increased serum TSH level; in hypothyroidism caused by disease of the pituitary or hypothalamus, there is an absent or delayed response to TRH. Before the test, the patient is warned that the intravenous administration of TRH may cause temporary facial flushing, nausea, or a desire to urinate. This test is used less frequently today because of the increased specificity and sensitivity of TSH tests.

Thyroglobulin. Thyroglobulin, a precursor for T_3 and T_4, can be measured reliably in the serum by radioimmunoassay. Those factors that increase or decrease thyroid gland activity and the secretion of T_3 and T_4 have a similar effect on thyroglobulin synthesis and secretion. Thyroglobulin levels are increased in thyroid carcinoma, hyperthyroidism, and subacute thyroiditis. They may be high in normal physiologic conditions such as pregnancy. They may be increased or decreased by medications or by diagnostic and therapeutic procedures that temporarily increase the serum levels of thyroglobulin. Measuring the thyroglobulin level is useful in the follow-up and management of patients with thyroid carcinoma and metastatic thyroid disease.

Radioactive Iodine Uptake. The radioactive iodine uptake test measures the rate of iodine uptake by the thyroid gland. The patient is administered a tracer dose of ^{131}I or another radionuclide and a count is made over the thyroid with use of a scintillation counter, which detects and counts the gamma rays released from the breakdown of ^{131}I in the thyroid. It measures the proportion of the administered dose present in the thyroid gland at a specific time after its administration. It is a simple test and provides reliable results. It is affected by the patient's intake of iodide or thyroid hormone; therefore, a careful preliminary clinical history is essential in evaluating results. Normal values vary from one geographic region to another and with the intake of iodine. Patients with hyperthyroidism accumulate a high proportion of the ^{131}I (in some patients up to 90%), whereas patients with hypothyroidism exhibit a very low uptake. This test is also used to determine what dose of ^{131}I should be administered to treat a patient with hyperthyroidism.

Thyroid Scan, Radioscan, or Scintiscan. Similar to the radioactive iodine uptake test, in a thyroid scan a highly focused scintillation detector moves back and forth across the area to be studied in a series of parallel tracks that move progressively downward. At the same time, a printing device records a mark whenever a predetermined number of counts has been received. This produces a visual representation of the localization of radioactivity in the area being scanned. Although ^{131}I has been the most commonly used isotope, several other iodine isotopes, including ^{9m}Tc (sodium pertechnetate), and other radioactive isotopes (thallium and americium), are used in some laboratories because of their physical and biochemical properties, which allow a lower radiation dose to be administered to the patient.

Scans are helpful in determining location, size, shape, and anatomic function of the thyroid gland, particularly when thyroid tissue is substernal or large. Identifying areas of increased function ("hot" areas) or decreased function ("cold" areas) can assist in diagnosis. Although most areas of decreased function are not malignancies, lack of function increases the likelihood of malignancy, particularly if only one nonfunctioning area is present. Scanning of the

TABLE 40-2 Partial List of Medications That May Alter Thyroid Test Results

Estrogens	Opiates
Sulfonylureas	Androgens
Corticosteroids	Salicylates
Iodine	Lithium
Propranolol	Amiodarone
Cimetidine	Clofibrate
5-Fluorouracil	Furosemide
Diphenylhydantoin	Diazepam
Heparin	Danazol
Chloral hydrate	Dopamine antagonists
X-ray contrast agents	Propylthiouracil

entire body, to obtain the total body profile, may be carried out in a search for a functioning thyroid metastasis.

Nursing Implications of Thyroid Tests. When a patient is scheduled for thyroid tests, it is necessary to determine if he has taken medications or agents that contain iodine, because these substances alter the results of some of the scheduled tests. Iodide-containing medications include contrast media and those used in the treatment of thyroid disorders. Other less obvious sources of iodine are topical antiseptics, multivitamin preparations, and food supplements frequently found in health food stores, cough syrups, and amiodarone, an antidysrhythmic agent. Other medications that may affect thyroid function test values are estrogens, salicylates, amphetamines, chemotherapeutic agents, antibiotics, steroids, and mercurial diuretics. The patient should be questioned about the use of these medications, and their use should be noted on the laboratory requisition for thyroid function tests. Table 40-2 gives a partial list of agents that may interfere with accurate testing of thyroid gland function.

Other Tests of Thyroid Function. Other diagnostic tests and assessment procedures that are useful in the detection and diagnosis of thyroid disorders or effects of thyroid disease include the Achilles tendon reflex time (measures period of contraction and relaxation of Achilles tendon reflex), serum cholesterol levels, electrocardiogram (ECG), muscle enzyme studies (alanine transaminase [ALT] or serum glutamic-pyruvic transaminase [SGPT], lactic acid dehydrogenase [LDH], and creatine kinase [CK]). Ultrasound, computed tomography (CT) scanning, and magnetic resonance imaging (MRI) may be used to clarify or confirm results of other diagnostic studies.

Examination of the Thyroid Gland

The thyroid gland is inspected and palpated routinely on all patients. The identification of specific anatomic landmarks is required to ensure an accurate assessment. The lower neck region between the sternocleidomastoid muscles is inspected for anterior swelling or asymmetry. The patient is instructed to extend the neck slightly and swallow. Thyroid tissue rises normally with swallowing. The thyroid is then palpated for size, shape, consistency, symmetry, and the presence of tenderness.

The examiner may perform this portion of the examination from an anterior or a posterior position. The thyroid can be effectively palpated from a position behind the patient, with both hands encircling the patient's neck (see Fig. 40-4). The thumbs are rested on the nape of the patient's neck, while the index and middle fingers palpate for the thyroid isthmus and the anterior surfaces of the lateral lobes. When palpable, the isthmus is perceived as firm and of a rubber band consistency.

The left lobe is examined by positioning the patient with the neck flexed slightly forward and to the left. The thyroid cartilage is then displaced to the left with the fingers of the right hand. This maneuver displaces the left lobe deep into the sternocleidomastoid muscle, where it can be more easily palpated. The left lobe is then palpated by placing the left thumb deep into the posterior area of the sternocleidomastoid muscle, while the index and middle fingers exert opposite pressure in the anterior portion of the muscle. Having the patient swallow during the maneuver may assist the examiner to locate the thyroid as it ascends in the neck. The procedure is reversed for an examination of the right lobe. The isthmus is the only portion of the thyroid that is normally palpable. If a patient has a very thin neck, occasionally two thin, smooth, nontender lobes may also be palpable.

If the thyroid gland is enlarged on palpation, auscultation over both lobes with the diaphragm of the stethoscope is performed. Auscultation will identify the localized audible vibration of a bruit. This is an abnormal finding indicative of increased blood flow through the thyroid gland and necessitates referral to a physician. The presence of tenderness, enlargement, or nodularity within the thyroid also requires referral for additional evaluation (Table 40-3).

Hypothyroidism

Hypothyroidism is a condition in which there is a slow progression of thyroid hypofunction, followed by symptoms indicating thyroid failure. It results from suboptimal levels of thyroid hormone.

Types

More than 95% of patients with hypothyroidism have **primary** or thyroidal hypothyroidism, which refers to dysfunction of the thyroid gland itself (Braverman & Utiger, 1991). When the thyroid dysfunction is caused by failure of the pituitary gland, the hypothalamus, or both, it is known as **central hypothyroidism.** It may be referred to as **pituitary or secondary hypothyroidism** if caused entirely by pituitary disorder, and **hypothalamic or tertiary hypothyroidism** if attributable to a disorder of the hypothalamus resulting in inadequate secretion of TSH because of decreased stimulation by TRH. When thyroid deficiency is present at birth, the condition is known as **cretinism.** In such instances, the mother may also suffer from thyroid deficiency.

The term **myxedema** refers to the accumulation of mucopolysaccharides in subcutaneous and other interstitial

TABLE 40-3 Summary of Findings on Physical Examination of the Thyroid Gland

Physical Finding	Differential Diagnosis	Special Features
Single nodule	Autonomously functioning adenoma	Opposite lobe not palpable
	Adenoma or adenomatous nodule	Rubbery, firm; tenderness suggests recent hemorrhage or infarction
	Cancer	Usually hard; may have associated lymph node enlargement or vocal cord palsy
	Hyperplasia secondary to unilobar agenesis	Opposite lobe not palpable
Multiple nodules	Multinodular goiter	
	Hashimoto's thyroiditis	Firm lobes or irregular surface misinterpreted as multiple nodules
Diffuse goiter	Graves' disease	Bruit or thrill; pyramidal lobe
	Hashimoto's thyroiditis	Irregular surface; pyramidal lobe; rubbery or firm; occasionally tender; fibrous variant may be hard
	Subacute thyroiditis	Unilateral or bilateral tenderness; often hard
	Painless (silent) thyroiditis	Small to medium size; no bruit
	Thyroid lymphoma	Rapidly growing goiter, particularly in setting of preexisting Hashimoto's thyroiditis
	Multinodular goiter	Nodules may be hidden within gland, and may become apparent with thyroid hormone suppression
Tenderness	Subacute thyroiditis	Unilateral or bilateral; tenderness often severe
	Hemorrhagic or infarcted adenoma	Discrete nodule with tenderness
	Hashimoto's thyroiditis	See above; mild tenderness
	Cancer	Irregular, firm thyroid nodule with chronic tenderness

(Braverman LE and Utiger RD. Werner and Ingbar's The Thyroid. A Fundamental and Clinical Text. Philadelphia, JB Lippincott, 1991.)

tissue; although myxedema occurs in long-standing or severe hypothyroidism, the term is used appropriately only to describe the extreme symptoms of severe hypothyroidism.

Causes

The most common cause of hypothyroidism in adults is autoimmune thyroiditis (**Hashimoto's thyroiditis**), in which the immune system attacks the thyroid gland (Tonner & Schlechte, 1993). Symptoms of hyperthyroidism (see p. 1085) may later be followed by those of hypothyroidism and myxedema.

Hypothyroidism also commonly occurs in patients with previous hyperthyroidism who have been treated with radioiodine, surgery, or antithyroid medications. It occurs most frequently in older women. Radiation therapy for treatment of head and neck cancer is becoming a common cause of hypothyroidism in older men; therefore, testing of thyroid function is recommended for all patients who receive such treatment. Other causes of hypothyroidism are presented in Chart 40-1.

Clinical Manifestations

Early symptoms of hypothyroidism are nonspecific, but extreme fatigue makes it difficult for the person to complete a full day's work or participate in usual activities. Reports of hair loss, brittle nails, and dry skin are common, and numbness and tingling of the fingers may occur. On occasion, the voice may become husky, and the patient may complain of hoarseness. Menstrual disturbances such as menorrhagia or amenorrhea occur, in addition to loss of libido. Hypothyroidism affects women five times more frequently than men and occurs most often between 30 and 60 years of age.

Severe hypothyroidism results in a subnormal temperature and pulse rate. The patient usually begins to gain weight even without an increase in food intake, although severely hypothyroid patients may be cachectic. The skin becomes thickened because of an accumulation of mucopolysaccharides in the subcutaneous tissues (the origin of the term **myxedema**). The hair thins and falls out; the face becomes expressionless and masklike. The patient often complains of being cold even in a warm environment.

At first the patient may be irritable and may complain of fatigue, but as the condition progresses, the emotional responses are subdued. The mental process becomes dulled, and the patient appears apathetic. Speech is slow, the tongue enlarges, and hands and feet increase in size. The patient frequently complains of constipation. Deafness also may occur.

Advanced hypothyroidism may produce personality and cognitive changes characteristic of dementia. Inadequate ventilation and sleep apnea can occur with severe hypothyroidism. Pleural effusion, pericardial effusion, and respiratory muscle weakness may also occur.

Severe hypothyroidism is associated with an elevated serum cholesterol level, atherosclerosis, coronary heart

CHART 40-1
Causes of Hypothyroidism

Chronic lymphocytic thyroiditis (Hashimoto's thyroiditis)
Atrophy of thyroid gland with aging
Therapy for hyperthyroidism
- Radioactive iodine (^{131}I)
- Thyroidectomy

Medications
- Lithium
- Iodine compounds
- Antithyroid medications

Radiation to head and neck for treatment of head and neck cancers, lymphoma
Infiltrative diseases of the thyroid (amyloidosis, scleroderma)
Iodine deficiency and iodine excess

disease, and poor left ventricular function. The patient with advanced hypothyroidism is hypothermic and abnormally sensitive to sedatives, opioids, and anesthetic agents. Therefore, these medications are administered only with extreme caution.

Patients with unrecognized hypothyroidism who are undergoing surgery are at increased risk for intraoperative hypotension and postoperative congestive heart failure and altered mental status.

Myxedema coma describes the most extreme, severe stage of hypothyroidism, in which the patient is hypothermic and unconscious. Myxedema coma may follow increasing lethargy, progressing to stupor and then coma. Undiagnosed hypothyroidism may be precipitated by infection or other systemic disease or by use of sedatives or opioid analgesics. The patient's respiratory drive is depressed, resulting in alveolar hypoventilation, progressive CO_2 retention, narcosis, and coma. These symptoms along with cardiovascular collapse and shock will require aggressive and intensive therapy if the patient is to survive. However, even with early vigorous therapy, mortality is high.

Management

The primary objective in management of hypothyroidism is to restore a normal metabolic state by replacing the missing hormone. Synthetic levothyroxine (Synthroid or Levothroid) is the preferred preparation for treating hypothyroidism and suppressing nontoxic goiters. The dosage for hormone replacement is based on the patient's serum TSH concentration. Desiccated thyroid is used less frequently because it often results in transient elevated serum concentrations of T_3, with occasional symptoms of hyperthyroidism. If replacement therapy is adequate, the symptoms of myxedema disappear, and normal metabolic activity is resumed.

In severe hypothyroidism and myxedema coma, management includes maintaining vital functions. Arterial blood gases may be measured to determine carbon dioxide retention and to guide the use of assisted ventilation to combat hypoventilation. Pulse oximetry may also be helpful in monitoring oxygen saturation levels. Fluids are administered cautiously because of the danger of water intoxication. Application of external heat (*i.e.*, heating pads) is avoided because it will increase oxygen requirements and may lead to vascular collapse. If hypoglycemia is evident, concentrated glucose may be prescribed to provide glucose without precipitating fluid overload. Thyroid hormone (usually Synthroid) is administered intravenously until consciousness is restored if myxedema has progressed to myxedema coma. Then the patient is continued on oral thyroid hormone therapy. Because of an associated adrenocortical insufficiency, corticosteroid therapy may be necessary.

Cardiac. Any patient who has had hypothyroidism for a long period is almost certain to have elevated serum cholesterol levels, atherosclerosis, and coronary artery disease. As long as metabolism is subnormal and the tissues, including the myocardium, require relatively little oxygen, a reduction in blood supply is tolerated without overt symptoms of coronary artery disease. However, when thyroid hormone is administered, the oxygen demand increases but oxygen delivery cannot be increased unless, or until, the atherosclerosis improves. This will occur very slowly, if at all. The occurrence of angina is the signal that the oxygen needs of the myocardium exceed its blood supply. Angina or dysrhythmias may occur when thyroid replacement is initiated, because thyroid hormones enhance the cardiovascular effects of catecholamines.

- Myocardial ischemia or infarction may occur in response to therapy in patients with severe, long-standing hypothyroidism or myxedema coma.

The nurse must be alert for signs of angina, especially during the early phase of treatment, and if detected, it must be reported and treated at once to avoid a fatal myocardial infarction. Obviously, the administration of thyroid hormone must be discontinued immediately, and later, when it can be resumed safely, thyroid hormone replacement should be prescribed cautiously at a lower dosage and under the close observation of the physician and the nurse.

Medication Interactions. Precautions must be taken during the course of therapy because of the interaction of thyroid hormones with other medications. Thyroid hormones may increase blood glucose levels, which may necessitate adjustment in doses of insulin or oral hypoglycemic agents. The effects of thyroid hormone may be increased by phenytoin and tricyclic antidepressants. Thyroid hormones may also increase the pharmacologic effects of digitalis glycosides, anticoagulants, and indomethacin, requiring careful observation and assessment by the nurse for side effects of these agents. Bone loss may also occur with thyroid therapy.

- Severe untreated hypothyroidism is characterized by an increased susceptibility to all hypnotic and sedative agents.

Hypnotic and sedative medications, even in small doses, may induce profound somnolence, lasting far longer than anticipated. Moreover, they are likely to cause respiratory depression, which could easily be fatal because of the decreased respiratory reserve and alveolar hypoventilation that occur in severe hypothyroidism and myxedema coma.

Sedatives and hypnotic agents are rarely used in severe hypothyroidism. However, if their use is necessary the dose is one- half or one-third that ordinarily prescribed in patients of similar age and weight with normal thyroid function. If these agents must be used, the patient must be monitored closely for signs of impending narcosis (stuporlike condition) or respiratory failure.

Nursing Management

Activity Modifications. The patient with hypothyroidism experiences decreased energy and moderate to severe lethargy. As a result, the risk for the complications from immobility increases. The patient's ability to exercise and participate in activities is further limited by the changes in cardiovascular and pulmonary status secondary to hypothyroidism. A major role of the nurse is assisting with care and hygiene while encouraging the patient to participate in activities within established tolerance levels to prevent complications of immobility.

Ongoing Monitoring. The patient's vital signs and cognitive level are monitored closely during diagnostic workup and initiation of treatment to detect (1) deterioration of physical and mental status, (2) signs and symptoms indicating that treatment has resulted in the metabolic rate exceeding the ability of the cardiovascular and pulmonary systems to respond, and (3) continued limitations or complications of myxedema.

- Medications are administered to the patient with hypothyroidism *very* cautiously because of altered metabolism and excretion and depressed metabolic rate and respiratory status.

Temperature Regulation. The patient often experiences chilling and extreme intolerance to cold even if the room temperature feels comfortable or hot to others. Extra clothing and blankets are provided, and the patient is protected from drafts. If the patient asks for a heating pad or electric blanket to decrease chilling and discomfort, these measures are avoided because of the risk of peripheral vasodilation, further loss of body heat, and vascular collapse. Additionally, the patient could be burned by using these items without being aware of it because of delayed responses and decreased mental status.

Emotional Support. The patient with moderate to severe hypothyroidism may experience severe emotional reactions to changes in appearance and body image and the frequent delay in diagnosis of the disorder, The nonspecific, early symptoms may produce negative reactions by family members and friends and the patient may have been labeled by family and friends as mentally unstable, uncooperative, or unwilling to participate in self-care activities.

As hypothyroidism is treated successfully and symptoms subside, the patient may experience depression and guilt as a result of the progression and severity of symptoms that occurred. The patient and family are informed that the symptoms and inability to recognize them are common and part of the disorder itself. The patient and family may require assistance and counseling to deal with the emotional concerns and reactions that result.

Patient Education and Home Care Considerations. The patient and family are often very concerned about the changes they have observed as a result of the hypothyroid state. It is often reassuring to the patient and family to be informed that many of the symptoms will disappear as treatment becomes effective. The patient is instructed to continue to use medications as prescribed even after symptoms improve. Dietary instruction is provided to promote weight loss once medication has been initiated and to promote return of normal bowel patterns. Because of the slowed mental processes that occur with hypothyroidism, it is important that a family member also be informed and instructed about treatment goals, medication schedules, and side effects that are to be reported to the physician. Additionally, these instructions and guidelines are provided in writing for the patient, family, and community health nurse to refer to once the patient returns home.

The patient with hypothyroidism and myxedema coma, usually an older woman, is in need of considerable follow-up, teaching, and health care. Before hospital discharge, arrangements are made to ensure that the patient returns to an environment that will promote adherence to the prescribed treatment plan. The patient will require encouragement and assistance in the daily administration of medications. Assistance in devising a schedule or record ensures accurate and complete administration of medications. The importance of continued thyroid hormone replacement and periodic follow-up testing is reinforced, and the patient and family members are instructed about the signs of overmedication and undermedication.

If indicated, a referral to a home care nurse is arranged for assessment of the patient's recovery and ability to cope with the recent changes. The home care nurse assesses the patient's physical and cognitive status, the patient's and family's understanding of the importance of long-term medication therapy as prescribed, and compliance with the medication schedule and recommended follow-up tests and appointments. Subtle signs and symptoms that may indicate either inadequate or excessive thyroxine hormone are documented and reported to the patient's primary health care provider.

Nursing care of the patient with hypothyroidism and myxedema is summarized in Nursing Care Plan 40-1.

Gerontologic Considerations

Most patients with primary hypothyroidism are 40 to 70 years of age and present with long-standing mild to moderate hypothyroidism. Ninety-eight percent to 99% of cases of hypothyroidism in older adults are primary or thyroidal hypothyroidism (Braverman & Utiger, 1991). The higher prevalence of hypothyroidism in the elderly may be related to alterations in immune function with age. However, despite the high incidence of thyroid dysfunction in the elderly, the incidence of undiagnosed or misdiagnosed thyroid disease is far greater in the elderly than in younger patients (Sawin,

(text continues on page 1084)

NURSING CARE PLAN 40–1
Care of the Patient With Hypothyroidism

Nursing Interventions	Rationale	Expected Outcomes
NURSING DIAGNOSIS: Activity intolerance related to fatigue and depressed cognitive process		
GOAL: Increased participation in activities and increased independence		
1. Promote independence in self-care activities.		• Participates in self-care activities. • Reports decreased level of fatigue.
a. Space activities to promote rest and exercise as tolerated.	a. Encourages activities while allowing time for adequate rest.	• Displays interest and awareness in environment.
b. Assist with self-care activities when patient is fatigued.	b. Permits patient to participate to the extent possible in self-care activities.	• Participates in activities and events in environment. • Participates in family events and activities.
c. Provide stimulation through conversation and nonstressful activities.	c. Promotes interest without overly stressing the patient.	• Reports no chest pain, increased fatigue, or breathlessness with increased level of activity.
d. Monitor patient's response to increasing activities.	d. Guards against over- and underexertion by the patient.	
NURSING DIAGNOSIS: Altered body temperature		
GOAL: Maintenance of normal body temperature		
1. Provide extra layer of clothing or extra blanket.	1. Minimizes heat loss.	• Experiences relief of discomfort and cold intolerance.
2. Avoid and discourage use of external heat source (*e.g.,* heating pads, electric or warming blankets)	2. Reduces risk of peripheral vasodilatation and vascular collapse.	• Maintains baseline body temperature. • Reports adequate feeling of warmth and lack of chilling.
3. Monitor patient's body temperature and report decreases from patient's baseline value.	3. Detects decreased body temperature and onset of myxedema coma.	• Uses extra layer of clothing or extra blanket. • Explains rationale for avoiding external heat source.
4. Protect from exposure to cold and drafts.	4. Increases patient's level of comfort and decreases further heat loss.	
NURSING DIAGNOSIS: Constipation related to depressed gastrointestinal function		
GOAL: Return of normal bowel function		
1. Encourage increased fluid intake within limits of fluid restriction.	1. Promotes passage of soft stools.	• Attains return of normal bowel function. • Reports normal bowel function.
2. Provide foods high in fiber.	2. Increases bulk of stools and more frequent bowel movements.	• Identifies and consumes foods high in fiber.
3. Instruct patient about foods with high water content.	3. Provides rationale for patient to increase fluid intake.	• Drinks recommended amount of fluid each day.
4. Monitor bowel function.	4. Permits detection of constipation and return to normal bowel pattern.	• Participates in gradually increasing exercises.
5. Encourage increased mobility within patient's exercise tolerance.	5. Promotes evacuation of the bowel.	• Uses laxatives as prescribed and avoids excessive dependence on laxatives and enemas.
6. Encourage patient to use laxatives and enemas sparingly.	6. Minimizes patient's dependence on laxatives and enemas and encourages normal pattern of bowel evacuation.	

(*continued*)

NURSING CARE PLAN 40–1 *(continued)*
Care of the Patient With Hypothyroidism

Nursing Interventions	Rationale	Expected Outcomes
NURSING DIAGNOSIS: Knowledge deficit about the therapeutic regimen for lifelong thyroid replacement therapy		
GOAL: Knowledge and acceptance of the prescribed therapeutic regimen		
1. Explain rationale for thyroid hormone replacement	1. Provides rationale for patient to use thyroid hormone replacement as prescribed.	• Describes therapeutic regimen correctly. • Explains rationale for thyroid hormone replacement.
2. Describe desired effects of medication to patient.	2. Provides encouragement to patient by identifying improved physical status and well-being that will occur with thyroid hormone therapy.	• Identifies positive outcomes of thyroid hormone replacement. • Administers medication to self as prescribed.
3. Assist patient to develop schedule and checklist to ensure self-administration of thyroid replacement.	3. Increases assurance that medication will be taken as prescribed.	• Identifies adverse side effects that should be reported promptly to physician: recurrence of symptoms of hypothyroidism and occurrence of symptoms of hyperthyroidism.
4. Describe signs and symptoms of over- and underdose of medication.	4. Serves as check for patient to determine if therapeutic goals are met.	
5. Explain the necessity for long-term follow-up to patient and family	5. Increases likelihood that hypo- or hyperthyroidism will be detected and treated.	• Restates need for periodic/long-term follow-up visits to physician.
NURSING DIAGNOSIS: Ineffective breathing pattern related to depressed ventilation		
GOAL: Improved respiratory status and maintenance of normal breathing pattern		
1. Monitor respiratory rate, depth, pattern; pulse oximetry and arterial blood gases.	1. Identifies patient's baseline to monitor further changes and evaluate effectiveness of interventions.	• Shows improved respiratory status and maintenance of normal breathing pattern.
2. Encourage deep breathing and coughing.	2. Prevents atelectasis and promotes adequate ventilation.	• Demonstrates normal respiratory rate, depth, and pattern.
3. Administer medications (hypnotics and sedatives) with caution.	3. Patients with hypothyroidism are *very* susceptible to respiratory depression because of use of hypnotics and sedatives.	• Takes deep breaths and coughs when encouraged. • Demonstrates normal breath sounds without adventitious sounds on auscultation.
4. Maintain patent airway through suction and ventilatory support if indicated (see Chap. 25 for care of patients requiring mechanical ventilation).	4. Use of an artificial airway and ventilatory support may be necessary with respiratory depression.	• Explains rationale for cautious use of medications. • Cooperates with suction procedure and ventilator when necessary.
NURSING DIAGNOSIS: Altered thought processes related to depressed metabolism and altered cardiovascular and respiratory status		
GOAL: Improved thought processes		
1. Orient patient to time, place, date, and events around him or her.	1. Provides reality orientation to patient.	• Shows improved cognitive functioning. • Identifies time, place, date, and events correctly.
2. Provide stimulation through conversation and nonthreatening activities.	2. Provides stimulation within patient's level of tolerance for stress.	• Responds when stimulated.
3. Explain to patient and family that change in cognitive and mental functioning is a result of disease process.	3. Reassures patient and family about the cause of the cognitive changes and that a positive outcome is possible with appropriate treatment.	• Responds spontaneously as treatment becomes effective. • Interacts spontaneously with family and environment.

(continued)

NURSING CARE PLAN 40–1 *(continued)*
Care of the Patient With Hypothyroidism

Nursing Interventions	Rationale	Expected Outcomes
4. Monitor cognitive and mental processes and response of these to medication and other therapy.	4. Permits evaluation of the effectiveness of treatment	• Explains that change in mental and cognitive processes is a result of disease processes. • Takes medications as prescribed to prevent decrease in cognitive processes.
COLLABORATIVE PROBLEM: Myxedema and myxedema coma **GOAL:** Absence of complications		
1. Monitor patient for increasing severity of signs and symptoms of hypothyroidism: a. Decreased level of consciousness; dementia b. Decreased vital signs (blood pressure, respiratory rate, temperature, pulse rate) c. Increasing difficulty in awakening or arousing patient	1. Extreme hypothyroidism may lead to myxedema, myxedema coma and slowing of all body systems if untreated.	• Exhibits reversal of myxedema and myxedema coma • Responds appropriately to questions and surroundings • Vital signs return to normal or near normal ranges • Respiratory status improves with adequate spontaneous ventilatory effort • Reports no episodes of angina or other indicators of cardiac insufficiency • Experiences minimal or no complications caused by immobility
2. Assist in ventilatory support if respiratory depression and failure occur.	2. Ventilatory support is necessary to maintain adequate oxygenation and maintenance of an airway.	
3. Administer prescribed medications (*e.g.,* thyroxine) with extreme caution.	3. The slow metabolism and atherosclerosis of myxedema may result in angina with administration of thyroxine.	
4. Turn and reposition patient at intervals.	4. Minimizes risks associated with immobility.	
5. Avoid use of hypnotic, sedative, and analgesic agents	5. Altered metabolism of these agents greatly increases the risks of their use in myxedema.	

1991). Even the slightest suspicion of hypothyroidism in an older person is reason for testing of serum TSH and probably of T_4.

Altered Signs and Symptoms. The signs and symptoms of hypothyroidism are often atypical in the elderly; the elderly patient may have few or no symptoms until the dysfunction is severe. Depression, apathy, or decreased mobility or activity may be the major initial symptom. In all patients with hypothyroidism, the effects of analgesics, sedatives, and anesthetic agents are prolonged; particular caution is necessary in administration of these agents to the elderly because of concurrent changes in liver and renal function.

Precautions. In the elderly patient with mild-to-moderate hypothyroidism, thyroid hormone replacement must be started with low doses and increased very gradually to prevent serious cardiovascular and neurologic side effects. Angina, for example, may occur because of rapid thyroid replacement in the presence of coronary disease secondary to the hypothyroid state. Congestive heart failure and tachydysrhythmias may worsen during the transition from the hypothyroid state to the normal metabolic state. Dementia may become more apparent during early thyroid hormone replacement in the elderly patient.

Elderly patients with severe hypothyroidism and atherosclerosis may also become confused and agitated if their metabolic rates are raised too quickly in myxedema. Marked clinical improvement follows the administration of hormone replacement; such medication must be continued for life, even though signs of hypothyroidism disappear over a 3- to 12-week period.

Myxedema and **myxedema coma** generally occur exclusively in patients older than 50 years of age. The high mortality of myxedema coma mandates immediate intravenous administration of high doses of thyroid hormone as well as supportive care.

Follow-Up Care. Periodic follow-up monitoring of serum TSH levels is recommended. Because poor compliance with therapy may occur or the patient may take the medications erratically, a careful history may identify the need for further teaching about the importance of the medication. Because of the prevalence of hypothyroidism, testing of serum TSH levels in the elderly every 5 years has been recommended (Sawin, 1991).

Hyperthyroidism

Hyperthyroidism, the second most prevalent endocrine disorder after diabetes mellitus, constitutes a well-defined disease entity, with **Graves' disease** the most common cause. An excessive output of thyroid hormones is thought to be caused by abnormal stimulation of the thyroid gland by circulating immunoglobulins. Long-acting thyroid stimulator (LATS) is found in significant concentration in the serum of many of these patients and may be related to a defect in the patient's immune surveillance system.

Hyperthyroidism affects women five times more frequently than men and peaks in incidence in the third and fourth decades (Schimke, 1992); it may appear after an emotional shock, stress, or an infection, but the exact significance of these relationships is not understood. Other common causes of hyperthyroidism include thyroiditis (see p. 1090) and excessive ingestion of thyroid hormone.

Clinical Manifestations

Thyrotoxicosis. Patients with well-developed hyperthyroidism exhibit a characteristic group of symptoms and signs (sometimes referred to as **thyrotoxicosis**). Their presenting symptom is often nervousness. They are often emotionally hyperexcitable, irritable, and apprehensive; they cannot sit quietly; they suffer from palpitations; and their pulse is abnormally rapid at rest as well as on exertion. They tolerate heat poorly and perspire unusually freely; the skin is flushed continuously, with a characteristic salmon color, and is likely to be warm, soft, and moist. Elderly patients, however, may report dry skin and diffuse pruritus. A fine tremor of the hands may be observed. Patients may exhibit **exophthalmos** (bulging eyes), which produces a startled facial expression.

Other Signs and Symptoms. Other manifestations include an increased appetite and dietary intake, progressive loss of weight, abnormal muscular fatigability and weakness, amenorrhea, and changes in bowel function, with constipation or diarrhea. The pulse rate of these patients ranges constantly between 90 and 160 beats/min; the systolic, but characteristically not the diastolic, blood pressure is elevated; atrial fibrillation may occur; and cardiac decompensation in the form of congestive heart failure is common, especially in elderly patients. Osteoporosis and fracture are also associated with hyperthyroidism.

Cardiac effects may include sinus tachycardia or dysrhythmias, increased pulse pressure, and palpitations; it has been suggested that these changes may be related to increased sensitivity to catecholamines or to changes in neurotransmitter turnover. Myocardial hypertrophy and heart failure may occur if the hyperthyroidism is severe and untreated.

Symptoms of hyperthyroidism may occur with release of excessive amounts of thyroid hormone as a result of inflammation after irradiation of the thyroid or destruction of thyroid tissue by tumor. Such symptoms may also occur with excessive administration of thyroid hormone for treatment of hypothyroidism. Long-standing use of thyroid hormone in the absence of close monitoring may be a cause of symptoms of hyperthyroidism. It is likely to result in premature osteoporosis, particularly in women.

Diagnostic Evaluation

The thyroid gland invariably is enlarged to some extent. It is soft and may pulsate; a thrill often can be felt, and a bruit is heard over the thyroid arteries, which are signs of greatly increased blood flow through the organ.

In advanced cases, the diagnosis is made on the basis of the symptoms and the tests described previously: an increase in serum T_4 and an increased ^{131}I uptake by the thyroid, in excess of 50%.

The course of the disease may be mild, characterized by remissions and exacerbations and terminating with spontaneous recovery in the course of a few months or years. Conversely, it may progress relentlessly, with the untreated person becoming emaciated, intensely nervous, delirious, even disoriented, and the heart eventually fails.

Management

No treatment directed toward the cause of hyperthyroidism is available. However, reducing thyroid hyperactivity provides effective symptomatic relief and removes the principal source of its most important complications.

Three forms of treatment are available for treating hyperthyroidism and controlling excessive thyroid activity: (1) pharmacotherapy, employing antithyroid medications that interfere with the synthesis of thyroid hormones and other agents that control manifestations of hyperthyroidism; (2) irradiation, involving the administration of the radioisotope ^{131}I or ^{125}I for destructive effects on the thyroid gland; and (3) surgery, with removal of most of the thyroid gland. Treatment depends on the cause of the hyperthyroidism and may require a combination of therapeutic approaches.

Pharmacotherapy. The objective of pharmacotherapy is to inhibit one or more stages in hormone synthesis or hormone release; another goal may be to reduce the amount of thyroid tissue, with resulting decreased thyroid hormone production.

Antithyroid agents effectively block the utilization of iodine by interfering with the iodination of thyrosine and the coupling of iodothyrosines in the synthesis of thyroid hormones. This prevents the synthesis of thyroid hormone. The most commonly used medications are propylthiouracil (Propacil, PTU) or methimazole (Tapazole), until the patient is euthyroid (*i.e.*, neither hyperthyroid nor hypothyroid). These medications block extrathyroidal conversion of T_4 to T_3. Because antithyroid medications do not interfere with release or activity of previously formed thyroid hormones, it may take several weeks for relief of symptoms, at which time the maintenance dose is established, followed by a gradual withdrawal of the medication over the next several months.

Therapy is determined on the basis of clinical criteria, including changes in pulse rate, pulse pressure, body weight, size of the goiter, and results of laboratory studies of thyroid function.

Toxic complications of antithyroid medications are relatively uncommon; nevertheless, the importance of periodic follow-up is emphasized because medication sensitization, fever, rash, urticaria, or even agranulocytosis and thrombocytopenia (decrease in granulocytes and platelets) may develop. With any sign of infection, especially pharyngitis and fever or the occurrence of mouth ulcers, the patient is advised to stop the medication, notify the physician immediately, and undergo hematologic studies. Rash, arthralgias, and fever occur in 5% of patients. Agranulocytosis is the most serious toxic side effect and occurs in 1 in every 200 patients. Its incidence is higher in those patients older than 40 years of age. It generally occurs within the first 3 months of therapy but may occur up 1 year after it is started.

Patients on antithyroid medications are instructed not to use decongestants for nasal stuffiness because they are poorly tolerated. Antithyroid medications are contraindicated in late pregnancy because they may produce goiter and cretinism in the fetus.

Thyroid hormone may occasionally be administered with antithyroid medications to put the thyroid gland at rest. In this approach, hypothyroidism from excess antithyroid medication is avoided, as is stimulation of the thyroid gland by TSH. Thyroid hormone is available as desiccated thyroid, thyroglobulin (Proloid), and levothyroxine sodium (Synthroid). These are slow-acting preparations that take about 10 days to achieve their full effect. Liothyronine sodium (Cytomel) has a more rapid onset, and its action is of short duration.

Adjunctive Therapy. *Iodine or iodide compounds,* once the only therapy available for patients with hyperthyroidism, are no longer used as the sole method of treatment. Such compounds decrease the release of thyroid hormones from the thyroid gland and reduce the vascularity and size of the thyroid. Compounds such as potassium iodide, Lugol's solution, and saturated solution of potassium iodide (SSKI) may be used in combination with antithyroid agents or β-adrenergic blockers to prepare the patient with hyperthyroidism for surgery. These agents reduce the activity of the thyroid hormone and the vascularity of the thyroid gland, making the surgical procedure safer.

Solutions of iodine and iodide compounds are more palatable in milk or fruit juice and are administered through a straw to prevent staining of the teeth. These compounds reduce the metabolic rate more rapidly than antithyroid medications, but their action does not last as long.

- Patients receiving these medications should be observed for the development of goiter and should be cautioned against use of over-the-counter medications that contain iodides and can increase the response to iodide therapy. Cough medications, expectorants, bronchodilators, and salt substitutes may contain iodide and should be avoided by the patient receiving iodide therapy.

Beta-adrenergic blocking agents have become an important part of management of hyperthyroidism to control the sympathetic nervous system effects. For example, propranolol is useful in controlling nervousness, tachycardia, tremor, anxiety, and heat intolerance.

Radioactive Iodine. The goal of treatment with radioactive iodine (^{131}I) is to destroy the overactive thyroid cells. Use of ^{131}I is the most common treatment in the elderly. Almost all the iodine that enters and is retained in the body becomes concentrated in the thyroid gland. Therefore, radioactive isotope of iodine is concentrated in the thyroid gland, where it destroys thyroid cells without jeopardizing other radiosensitive tissues. Over a period of weeks or months, those thyroid cells exposed to the radioactive iodine are destroyed, resulting in reduction of the hyperthyroid state and inevitably hypothyroidism.

Use of ablative doses of radioactive iodine causes an acute release of thyroid hormone from the thyroid gland and may cause an increase of symptoms. Therefore, antithyroid agents may be used for several months before treatment with ^{131}I is initiated.

The patient is instructed as to what to expect of this tasteless, colorless radioiodine, which is administered by the physician. If the patient is hospitalized during administration of ^{131}I, radiation safety precautions identified by the hospital's radiation safety committee are followed.

A single dose of the agent is administered by mouth, based on 80 to 160 μCi/g estimated thyroid weight. The patient is observed for signs of thyroid storm (see p. 1087). Seventy percent to 85% of patients are cured by one dose of ^{131}I. An additional 10% to 20% require two doses; rarely is a third dose necessary.

After treatment with ^{131}I, the patient is discharged and is usually followed closely until the euthyroid state is reached. In 3 to 4 weeks, symptoms of hyperthyroidism subside. Because the incidence of hypothyroidism after this form of treatment is very high (*i.e.*, over 90% at 10 years), close follow-up is required to evaluate thyroid function. Thyroid hormone replacement is necessary.

Uses and Contraindications. Radioactive iodine has been used in toxic adenomas or multinodular goiter and in most varieties of thyrotoxicosis (rarely permanently successful) and is preferred for the treatment of patients beyond the childbearing years with diffuse toxic goiter. It is contraindicated in pregnancy and in nursing mothers because radioiodine crosses the placenta and is secreted in breast milk.

Patient Education. Patients often fear medications that are radioactive and require special follow-up and precautions; therefore, they and their family need information and reassurance about the treatment.

Surgical Intervention. Surgery to remove thyroid tissue was once the primary method of treating hyperthyroidism; today surgery is reserved for special circumstances, for example, in pregnant women allergic to antithyroid medications, patients with large goiters, or in patients who are unable to take antithyroid agents.

The surgical removal of about five-sixths of the thyroid tissue (**subtotal thyroidectomy**) practically assures a prolonged remission in most patients with exophthalmic goiter. Before surgery, propylthiouracil is administered until signs of hyperthyroidism have disappeared. Alternatively, a beta-adrenergic blocking agent (propranolol) may be used to reduce the heart rate; however, use of these medications does not create a euthyroid state. Iodine (Lugol's solution or potassium iodide) may be prescribed in an effort to reduce blood loss; however, the effectiveness of this is unknown.

- Patients receiving iodine medication must be monitored for evidence of iodine toxicity (iodism), the appearance of which is the signal for immediate withdrawal of the medication. Symptoms of iodism include swelling of the buccal mucosa, excessive salivation, coryza, and skin eruptions.

Thyroidectomy for treatment of hyperthyroidism usually is scheduled soon after the patient's thyroid function has returned to normal (4 to 6 weeks). Management of the patient undergoing thyroidectomy is discussed on p. 1092.

Relapse Rate and Risk of Hyperthyroidism After Treatment. None of the treatments for thyrotoxicosis is without side effects, and all three forms of treatment (*i.e.*, antithyroid medications, surgery, and radioactive iodine therapy) share the same complications: relapse or recurrent hyperthyroidism and permanent hypothyroidism. The rate of relapse is increased in patients who initially had very severe disease, a long history of dysfunction, ocular and cardiac symptoms, large goiter, and relapse after previous treatment.

Although reports of rate of relapse and the occurrence of hypothyroidism vary among studies, relapse with antithyroid medications is approximately 45% 1 year after completion of therapy and almost 75% 5 years later. Discontinuation of antithyroid medications before therapy is complete usually results in relapse within 6 months in most patients.

The relapse rate after radioactive iodine therapy approaches 26% at 1 year; hypothyroidism occurs in almost 28% of patients at 1 year and in 90% to 100% by 5 years.

The incidence of relapse with subtotal thyroidectomy is 19% at 18 months; an incidence of hypothyroidism of 25% has been reported at 18 months after surgery.

The risk of these complications illustrates the necessity for long-term follow-up of patients undergoing treatment of hyperthyroidism.

Gerontologic Considerations

Although hyperthyroidism is much less common in the elderly than hypothyroidism, patients older than 60 years of age account for 10% to 20% of the cases of thyrotoxicosis (Braverman & Utinger, 1991). Although some older patients develop typical signs and symptoms of thyrotoxicosis, in most, an atypical picture is present and it is often subclinical in nature.

Signs and Symptoms. The major symptoms of the elderly patient with hyperthyroidism may be depression and apathy, often accompanied by significant weight loss; one fourth of the affected elderly experience constipation. In addition, the patient may report cardiovascular symptoms and difficulty climbing stairs or rising from a chair because of muscle weakness. New or worsening congestive heart failure or angina is more likely to occur in the elderly than younger patient. The elderly patient may experience a single manifestation such as atrial fibrillation, anorexia, or weight loss. These signs and symptoms may mask the underlying thyroid disease.

Spontaneous remission of hyperthyroidism is rare in the elderly. Measurement of T_4 and T_3 uptake is indicated in elderly patients with unexplained physical or mental deterioration. Measurement of serum TSH assists in identifying the cause of hypothyroidism.

Treatment. The use of ^{131}I is generally recommended for treatment of thyrotoxicosis in the elderly unless an enlarged thyroid gland is pressing on the airway. However, the hypermetabolic state of thyrotoxicosis must be controlled by antithyroid medications before ^{131}I is used because radiation may precipitate thyroid storm by increasing the release of hormone from the thyroid gland. Thyroid storm, if it occurs, has a mortality rate of 10% in the elderly.

The use of β-blockers may be indicated to decrease the cardiovascular and neurologic signs and symptoms of thyrotoxicosis. However, these agents must be used with extreme caution to minimize adverse effects on cardiac function that may produce congestive heart failure.

If antithyroid agents are used, the patient must be monitored closely because the elderly patient is more likely to develop granulocytopenia.

The dosage of other medications to treat other chronic illnesses in the elderly patient may need modification because of the altered rate of metabolism in hyperthyroidism.

Thyroid Storm (Thyrotoxic Crisis)

Thyroid storm (thyrotoxic crisis) is a form of severe hyperthyroidism, usually of abrupt onset and characterized by high fever (hyperpyrexia), extreme tachycardia, and altered mental state, which frequently appears as delirium. Thyroid storm is a life-threatening condition and is usually precipitated by stress such as injury, infection, nonthyroid surgery, thyroidectomy, tooth extraction, insulin reaction, diabetic acidosis, pregnancy, digitalis intoxication, abrupt withdrawal of antithyroid medications, extreme emotional stress, or vigorous palpation of the thyroid. These factors will precipitate thyroid storm in the partially controlled or completely untreated hyperthyroid patient. Patients who are maintained in a euthyroid state through the proper adjustment of an antithyroid medication may experience stressful conditions uneventfully and without thyrotoxic crisis.

Although thyroid crisis may be difficult to identify, the following signs are suggestive: (1) tachycardia (over 130 beats/min), (2) temperature above 37.7°C (100°F), (3) exaggerated symptoms of hyperthyroidism, and (4) disturbances of a major system, for example, gastrointestinal (weight loss, diarrhea, abdominal pain), neurologic (psychosis, somnolence, coma), or cardiovascular (edema, chest pain, dyspnea, palpitations).

Untreated thyroid storm is almost always fatal, but with proper treatment the mortality rate can be reduced substantially.

Management. The immediate objective is to reduce body temperature and heart rate and prevent vascular collapse. Measures to reduce the temperature include a hypothermia mattress or blanket, ice packs, a cool environment, hydrocortisone, and acetaminophen (Tylenol).

- Salicylates are not used because they displace thyroid hormone from binding proteins and worsen the hypermetabolism.

Humidified oxygen is administered to improve tissue oxygenation and meet the high metabolic demands. Arterial blood gases or pulse oximetry may be used to monitor respiratory status. Intravenous fluids containing dextrose are administered to replace liver glycogen stores that have been decreased in the hyperthyroid patient. Propylthiouracil

(PTU) or methimazole is administered to impede formation of thyroid hormone and block conversion of T_4 to T_3, the more active form of thyroid hormone. Hydrocortisone is prescribed to treat shock or adrenal insufficiency. Iodine is administered to decrease output of T_4 from the thyroid gland. For cardiac problems such as atrial fibrillation, dysrhythmias, and congestive heart failure, sympatholytic agents may be administered. Propranolol in combination with digitalis has been effective in reducing severe cardiac symptoms.

- The patient with thyroid storm or crisis is critically ill and requires astute observation and aggressive and supportive nursing care during and after the acute stage of illness. Care of the patient with hyperthyroidism is the basis of nursing management of the critically ill patient with thyroid storm or crisis.

❑ NURSING PROCESS
The Patient With Hyperthyroidism

Assessment

The health history and examination focus on the occurrence of symptoms related to accelerated or exaggerated metabolism. These include the patient's and family's report of irritability and increased emotional reaction. It is also important to determine the impact that these changes have had on the patient's interaction with family, friends, and coworkers. The history includes other stressors and the patient's ability to cope with stress.

Nutritional status and the presence of symptoms are assessed. The occurrence of symptoms related to excessive output of the nervous system and changes in vision and the appearance of the eyes are noted. The patient's cardiac status is assessed and monitored periodically. The heart rate, blood pressure, heart sounds, and peripheral pulses are assessed.

Because of the likelihood of emotional changes related to hyperthyroidism, the patient's emotional state and psychological status are evaluated. The patient is assessed for irritability, anxiety, sleep disturbances, apathy and lethargy, all of which may occur with hyperthyroidism. The patient's family may provide information about recent changes in the patient's emotional status.

Diagnosis

Nursing Diagnoses

Based on all the assessment data, the major nursing diagnoses of the patient with hyperthyroidism include the following:

- ❑ Altered nutrition related to exaggerated metabolic rate, excessive appetite, and increased gastrointestinal activity
- ❑ Ineffective coping related to irritability, hyperexcitability, apprehension, and emotional instability
- ❑ Disturbance in self-esteem related to changes in appearance, excessive appetite, and weight loss
- ❑ Altered body temperature

Collaborative Problems/ Potential Complications

Based on assessment data, potential complications that may occur include:

- ❑ Thyrotoxicosis or thyroid storm
- ❑ Hypothyroidism

Planning and Implementation

Goals. The goals for the patient may be improved nutritional status, improved coping ability, improved self-esteem, maintenance of normal body temperature, and absence of complications.

Nursing Interventions

Monitoring and Managing Potential Complications

Thyroid Storm. The patient with hyperthyroidism is monitored closely for signs and symptoms that may be indicative of thyroid storm (see p. 1085). Cardiac and respiratory function are assessed by measuring vital signs and cardiac output, ECG monitoring, arterial blood gases, and pulse oximetry. Assessment continues when treatment is initiated because of the potential side effects treatment has on cardiac function. Oxygen is administered to prevent hypoxia, to improve tissue oxygenation, and to meet the high metabolic demands. Intravenous fluids may be necessary to maintain blood glucose levels and to replace lost fluids.

Antithyroid medications (propylthiouracil [PTU] or methimazole) may be prescribed to reduce thyroid hormone levels. In addition, propranolol and digitalis may be prescribed to treat cardiac symptoms. If shock develops, strategies to treat shock must be implemented (see Chapter 15).

Hypothyroidism. Hypothyroidism is likely to occur with any one of the treatments used to treat hyperthyroidism. Therefore, the patient must be monitored periodically. Most patients feel a greatly improved sense of well-being after treatment of hyperthyroidism and often fail to continue to take prescribed thyroxine therapy. Therefore, an important part of patient and family teaching is instruction about the importance of continued therapy after discharge and a discussion of the consequences of failing to take medication.

Improving Nutritional Status. Hyperthyroidism affects all body systems, including the gastrointestinal system. The patient's appetite is increased but may be satisfied by several well-balanced meals of small size, even up to six meals a day. Foods and fluids are selected to replace fluid lost through diarrhea and diaphoresis and to control diarrhea that results from increased peristalsis. Rapid movement of food through the gastrointestinal tract may result in nutritional imbalance and further weight loss. To reduce diarrhea, highly seasoned foods and stimulants such as coffee, tea, cola, and alcohol are discouraged. High-calorie, high-protein foods are encouraged. A quiet atmosphere during mealtime may aid digestion. The patient's weight and dietary intake are recorded to monitor nutritional status.

Enhancing Coping Measures. The patient with hyperthyroidism needs assurance that the emotional reactions being experienced are a result of the disorder and that with effective treatment those symptoms will be controlled. Because of the negative effect these symptoms have on family and friends, they too need reassurance that these symptoms are expected to disappear with treatment.

It is important to use a calm, unhurried approach with the patient. Additionally, stressful experiences are minimized; therefore, the patient is not placed in a hospital room with very ill or talkative patients. The environment is kept quiet and uncluttered. Noises, such as loud music, conversation, and equipment alarms, are minimized. Relaxing activities are encouraged if they do not overstimulate the patient.

If thyroidectomy is planned, the patient is likely to be apprehensive and anxious about the surgery. The patient is informed that while surgery is planned, treatment is necessary to prepare the patient and the thyroid gland for surgical treatment. The patient is assisted by the nurse to take the medications as prescribed and to develop a plan to encourage adherence to the therapeutic regimen. The patient's hyperexcitability and shortened attention span may necessitate repetition of this information and written instructions.

Improving Self-Esteem. The hyperthyroid patient is likely to experience changes in appearance, appetite, and weight. These factors, along with the patient's inability to cope well with family and the illness, may result in loss of self-esteem. The nurse conveys an understanding of the patient's concern about these problems and expresses willingness to assist in developing effective coping strategies. The patient and family are informed that these changes are a result of the dysfunction of the thyroid gland and are in fact out of the person's control.

If changes in appearance are very disturbing to the patient, mirrors may be removed from the room. In addition, family members and personnel are reminded to avoid bringing these changes to the patient's attention. The nurse explains to the patient and family that most of these changes are expected to disappear after effective treatment.

If the patient experiences eye changes secondary to hyperthyroidism, eye care and protection may become necessary. The patient may need instructions about correct instillation of eye drops or ointment prescribed to soothe the eyes and protect the exposed cornea.

The patient may be embarrassed by the need to eat large meals. Therefore, the nurse arranges the setting so that the patient eats alone if desired and avoids commenting on the large dietary intake of the patient, at the same time making sure that the patient receives sufficient food.

Maintaining Normal Body Temperature. The patient with hyperthyroidism frequently finds a normal room temperature uncomfortably warm because of an exaggerated metabolic rate and heat production. The room should be maintained at a cool, comfortable temperature and fresh bedding and clothing provided as needed. Giving cool baths, providing cool or cold fluids, and monitoring body temperature are important in providing relief. The reason for the patient's discomfort and the importance of providing a cool environment are explained to the family and staff.

Patient Education and Home Care Considerations. The patient with hyperthyroidism is instructed about how and when to take prescribed medication. Additionally, the patient needs to know how the medication regimen fits in with the broader therapeutic plan. Because of the patient's hyperexcitability and decreased attention span, a written plan is provided for the patient to use at home. The type and amount of information given to the patient are individualized because of the resulting stress and possible emotional reactions. The patient and family members receive verbal and written information about the desired effects as well as possible side effects of the medications. The patient is instructed about which adverse effects should be reported if they occur. The importance of long-term follow-up is stressed because of the possibility of hypothyroidism after thyroidectomy or treatment with antithyroid medications or ^{131}I.

If a total or subtotal thyroidectomy is anticipated, the patient is informed about what to expect. This information, however, is repeated to the patient as the time of surgery approaches. The patient is also instructed to avoid those situations that have the potential to stimulate the life-threatening occurrence of thyroid storm.

Referral for home care, if indicated, may allow assessment of the home and family environment. In addition, a home care nurse may assess the patient's and family's understanding of the importance of the therapeutic regimen and compliance with it and the recommended follow-up monitoring. The patient may also be assessed for changes indicating return to normal thyroid function as well as physical signs of hyperthyroidism and hypothyroidism.

Evaluation

Expected Outcomes

1. Improves nutritional status.
   a. Reports adequate dietary intake and decreased feelings of hunger.
   b. Identifies high-calorie, high-protein foods and foods to be avoided.
   c. Avoids use of alcohol and other stimulants.
   d. Reports decreased episodes of diarrhea.
2. Demonstrates effective coping methods in dealing with family, friends, and co-workers.
   a. Explains reasons for irritability and emotional instability.
   b. Avoids stressful situations, events, and people.
   c. Participates in relaxing, nonstressful activities.
3. Achieves increased self-esteem.
   a. Verbalizes feelings about self and illness.
   b. Describes feelings of frustration and loss of control to others.
   c. Describes reasons for increased appetite.
4. Maintains normal body temperature.
5. Absence of complications.
   a. Serum thyroid hormone levels are within normal limits.
   b. States signs and symptoms of thyroid storm and hypothyroidism.
   c. Vital signs and results of ECG, arterial blood gases, and pulse oximetry within normal limits.
   d. States importance of regular follow-up and lifelong maintenance of prescribed therapy.

Thyroiditis

Thyroiditis is inflammation of the thyroid gland; it can be acute, subacute, or chronic in nature. Each type of thyroiditis is characterized by inflammation, fibrosis, or lymphocytic infiltration of the thyroid gland.

Acute Thyroiditis. Acute thyroiditis is a rare disorder caused by infection of the thyroid gland by bacteria, fungi, mycobacteria, or parasites. *Staphylococcus aureus* or other staphylococci are the most common causes. It typically causes anterior neck pain and swelling, fever, dysphagia, and dysphonia. Pharyngitis or pharyngeal pain is often present. Examination may reveal warmth, erythema (redness), and tenderness of the thyroid gland. Treatment of acute thyroiditis includes antimicrobial agents and fluid replacement. Surgical incision and drainage may be needed if an abscess is present.

Subacute Thyroiditis. Subacute thyroiditis may be subacute granulomatous thyroiditis (deQuervain's thyroiditis) or painless thyroiditis (silent thyroiditis or subacute lymphocytic thyroiditis).

Subacute granulomatous thyroiditis is an inflammatory disorder of the thyroid gland that predominantly affects women 40 to 50 years of age (Sakiyama, 1993), presents as a painful swelling in the anterior neck that lasts 1 or 2 months and then disappears spontaneously without residual effect. It often follows a respiratory infection. The thyroid enlarges symmetrically and occasionally is painful. The overlying skin is often reddened and warm. Swallowing may be difficult and uncomfortable. Irritability, nervousness, insomnia, and weight loss—manifestations of hyperthyroidism—are common, and many patients experience chills and fever as well.

The purpose of treatment is to control the inflammation. In general, nonsteroidal anti-inflammatory agents (NSAIDs) are used to relieve neck pain. Acetylsalicylic acid (aspirin) is avoided if symptoms of hyperthyroidism occur, because it displaces thyroid hormone from its binding sites and increases the amount of circulating hormone. Beta-blocking agents may be used to control symptoms of hyperthyroidism; antithyroid agents, which block the synthesis of T_4 and T_3, are *not* effective in thyroiditis because the associated thyrotoxicosis results from the release of stored thyroid hormones rather than from their increased synthesis. In more severe cases, oral corticosteroids may be prescribed on occasion to relieve pain and reduce swelling; however, they do not usually affect the underlying cause. In some cases a temporary state of hypothyroidism may develop and may necessitate use of thyroid hormone replacement therapy. Follow-up monitoring is necessary to document the patient's return to a euthyroid state.

Painless thyroiditis (subacute lymphocytic thyroiditis) often occurs in the postpartum period and is thought to be an autoimmune process. Symptoms of hyperthyroidism or hypothyroidism are possible. Treatment is directed at symptoms, and yearly follow-up is recommended to determine the patient's need for treatment of subsequent hypothyroidism.

Chronic Thyroiditis (Hashimoto's Thyroiditis). Chronic thyroiditis, which occurs most frequently in women 30 to 50 years of age, has been termed **Hashimoto's disease,** or **chronic lympocytic thyroiditis;** its diagnosis is based on the histologic appearance of the inflamed gland. In contrast to acute thyroiditis, the chronic forms are usually not accompanied by pain, pressure symptoms, or fever, and thyroid activity is usually normal or low, rather than increased.

Cell-mediated immunity may play a significant role in the pathogenesis of thyroiditis. A genetic predisposition also seems to be significant in its etiology. If untreated, the disease runs a slow, progressive course, leading eventually to hypothyroidism.

The objective of treatment is to reduce the size of the thyroid gland and prevent hypothyroidism. Thyroid hormone therapy is prescribed to reduce thyroid activity and the production of thyroglobulin. If hypothyroid symptoms are present, thyroid hormone is prescribed. Surgery may be required if pressure symptoms persist.

Thyroid Tumors

Tumors of the thyroid gland are classified on the basis of being benign or malignant, as well as on the presence or absence of associated thyrotoxicosis and the diffuse or irregular quality of the glandular enlargement. If the enlargement is sufficient to cause a visible swelling in the neck, the tumor is referred to as a **goiter.**

Goiter

All grades of goiter are encountered, from those that are barely visible to those producing disfigurement. Some are symmetrical and diffuse; others are nodular. Some are accompanied by hyperthyroidism, in which case they are described as **toxic;** others are associated with a euthyroid state and are called **nontoxic** goiters.

Endemic (Iodine-Deficient) Goiter. The most common type of goiter, encountered chiefly in geographic regions where the natural supply of iodine is deficient (*e.g.*, the Great Lakes areas of the United States), is the so-called simple or colloid goiter. Aside from being caused by an iodine deficiency, simple goiter may also be caused by an intake of large quantities of goitrogenic substances in patients with unusually susceptible glands. These substances include excessive amounts of iodine or lithium, which is used in the treatment of manic depressive states.

Simple goiter represents a compensatory hypertrophy of the thyroid gland, presumably caused by stimulation by the pituitary gland. The pituitary gland produces thyrotropin or TSH, a hormone that controls the release of thyroid hormone from the thyroid gland. Its production increases if there is subnormal thyroid activity, as when insufficient iodine is available for production of the thyroid hormone. Such goiters usually cause no symptoms except for the swelling in the neck, which may result in tracheal compression when excessive.

Management. Many goiters of this type recede after iodine imbalance is corrected. Supplementary iodine such as saturated solution of potassium iodide (SSKI) is prescribed to suppress the pituitary's thyroid-stimulating activity.

When surgery is recommended, postoperative complications can be minimized by a preoperative euthyroid state resulting from treatment with antithyroid medications and preoperative iodide administration to reduce the size and vascularity of the goiter.

Prevention. Simple or endemic goiter can be prevented by providing children in iodine-poor regions with iodine compounds. If the mean iodine intake is less than 40 μg/day, the thyroid gland hypertrophies. The World Health Organization recommends that salt be iodized to a concentration of 1 part in 100,000, which is adequate for the prevention of endemic goiter. In the United States, salt is iodized to 1 part in 10,000. The introduction of iodized salt has been the single most effective means of preventing goiter in susceptible populations.

Nodular Goiter. Certain thyroid glands are nodular because of the presence of one or several areas of hyperplasia (overgrowth) that appear to develop under conditions similar to those responsible for the simple goiter. No symptoms may arise as a result of this condition, but, not uncommonly, these nodules slowly increase in size, with some descending into the thorax, where they cause local pressure symptoms. Some nodules become malignant and some become associated with a hyperthyroid state. Thus, the patient with many thyroid nodules may eventually require surgery.

Thyroid Cancer

Cancer of the thyroid is much less prevalent than other forms of cancer; however, it accounts for 90% of endocrine malignancies. Approximately 13,000 new cases of thyroid cancer develop each year. According to the American Cancer Society (1994), approximately 1025 patients die annually of this malignancy.

Causes. External radiation of the head, neck, or chest in infancy and childhood increases the risk of thyroid carcinoma. Between 1940 and 1960, radiation therapy was occasionally used to shrink enlarged tonsillar and adenoid tissue, to treat acne, or to reduce an enlarged thymus. For people exposed to external radiation in childhood, there appears to be an increased incidence in thyroid cancer 5 to 40 years after irradiation. Consequently, people who underwent such treatment should consult a physician, request an isotope thyroid scan as part of the evaluation, follow recommended treatment of abnormalities of the gland, and continue with annual checkups if all is normal.

Types. There are several types of cancer of the thyroid gland; the type determines the course and prognosis.

Papillary adenocarcinoma is the most common type of thyroid cancer, accounting for over half of thyroid malignancies. This neoplasm starts in childhood or early adult life, remains localized, and eventually metastasizes along the lymphatics and lymph nodes if untreated. It appears as an asymptomatic nodule in a normal gland. If papillary adenocarcinoma occurs in the elderly, it is generally more aggressive, as are other types of thyroid cancer when they occur in the elderly. The risk of malignancy increases with family history of thyroid cancer.

Follicular adenocarcinoma appears in later life, usually after age 40, and accounts for 20% to 25% of thyroid neoplasms. It is encapsulated and feels elastic or rubbery on palpation. This tumor eventually spreads by hematogenous routes to bone, liver, and lung. The prognosis is not as favorable as for papillary adenocarcinoma.

Lesions that are single and hard and fixed on palpation or associated with cervical lymphadenopathy suggest malignancy.

Other types of thyroid cancer are **medullary** (5%), which presents as solid, hard nodular tumors, and **anaplastic** (5%), which is hard, irregular masses that grow quickly and may be painful and tender. Almost 50% of anaplastic thyroid carcinomas are found in patients older than 60 years of age. These tumors have an extremely poor prognosis.

Diagnostic Evaluation. The tests of thyroid function may be helpful in evaluating thyroid nodules and masses. However, their results are rarely conclusive.

Needle biopsy of the thyroid gland is used as an outpatient procedure to make a diagnosis of thyroid cancer, to differentiate cancerous thyroid nodules from noncancerous nodules, and to stage the cancer if detected. The procedure is safe and usually requires only a local anesthetic. However, patients who undergo the procedure are followed closely because cancerous tissues may be missed during the procedure. A second type of aspiration or biopsy uses a large-bore needle rather than the fine needle used in standard biopsy; it may be used when the results of the standard biopsy are inconclusive or with rapidly growing tumors. Additional diagnostic studies include ultrasound, MRI, CT scans, thyroid scans, radioactive iodine uptake studies, and thyroid suppression tests.

Management. The treatment of choice of thyroid carcinoma is surgical removal. Total or near-total thyroidectomy is performed when possible.

Modified neck dissection or more extensive radical neck dissection is performed if there is lymph node involvement. Efforts are made to spare parathyroid tissue to reduce risk of postoperative hypocalcemia and tetany. After surgery, ablation procedures are carried out with ^{131}I to eradicate residual thyroid tissue if the tumor is radiosensitive. Radioactive iodine also maximizes the chance of discovering thyroid metastasis at a later date if total body scans are carried out.

After surgery, thyroid hormone is administered in suppressive doses to lower the levels of TSH to a euthyroid state. If remaining thyroid tissue is inadequate to produce sufficient thyroid hormone, thyroxine is required permanently.

Radiation to the thyroid or tissues of the neck may be administered by several routes: oral administration of ^{131}I and through external administration of radiation therapy. The patient who receives external sources of radiation therapy is at risk for mucositis, dryness of the mouth, dysphagia, redness of the skin, anorexia, and fatigue (see Chapter 16 for discussion of these side effects of radiation.) Chemotherapy is only occasionally used in treatment of thyroid cancer.

Patient Education and Follow-Up Care. Postoperatively, the patient needs instructions about the need to take exogenous thyroid hormone to prevent the occurrence of hypothyroidism. Later follow-up includes clinical assessment for recurrence of nodules or masses in the neck and signs of hoarseness, dysphagia, or dyspnea. Chest x-rays are performed as recommended. Total body scans are advised annually for the first 3 postoperative years and less frequently thereafter. Before planned total body scans, thyroid hormones are stopped for about a month before the tests.

T_4, TSH, serum calcium, and phosphorus levels are monitored to determine if the thyroid hormone supplementation is adequate and to note whether calcium balance is maintained.

Although local and systemic reactions to radiation may occur and may include neutropenia or thrombocytopenia (see p. 799), these complications are rare when ^{131}I is used. Surgery combined with radioiodine produces a higher survival rate than does surgery alone.

Patient teaching emphasizes the importance of taking prescribed medications and following recommendations for follow-up monitoring. The patient who is undergoing radiation therapy is also instructed in assessment and management of side effects of treatment.

Patients whose thyroid cancer is detected early and appropriately treated usually do very well. Continued thyroid hormone therapy and periodic follow-up, however, are important to assure the patient's well-being.

Radiation-Induced Thyroid Damage and Cancer

The thyroid gland has a very efficient mechanism to remove iodine from the bloodstream and concentrate or "trap" it for subsequent synthesis of thyroid hormone. The effectiveness of this mechanism to concentrate iodide is reflected in a concentration of iodide 20 to 40 times the concentration of iodide in the plasma.

If milk and other food sources become contaminated with radioactivity as a result of a nuclear detonation or a nuclear power plant accident, the radioactive iodide would become concentrated in the thyroid gland at this very high concentration and would irradiate the thyroid gland, increasing the risk of thyroid gland cancer. Therefore, in communities exposed to increased radioactivity, attempts have been made to block the uptake of radioactive iodide by flooding or saturating the thyroid gland with nonradioactive iodide.

Administration of saturated solutions of potassium iodide (SSKI) or other iodide preparations as soon as possible after exposure occurs almost completely inhibits thyroid absorption of the radioactive iodide and promotes rapid excretion of any that is absorbed.

Thyroidectomy

Partial or complete thyroidectomy may be carried out as primary treatment of thyroid carcinoma, hyperthyroidism, or hyperparathyroidism. The type and extent of the surgery depend on the diagnosis, goal of surgery, and prognosis.

Preoperative Management

Pharmacotherapy. Before undergoing surgery for treatment of hyperthyroidism (see p. 1085), the patient is treated with appropriate medication therapy to return the thyroid hormone levels and metabolic rate to normal and to reduce the risk of thyroid storm and hemorrhage during the postoperative period. Medications that may prolong clotting (*e.g.*, aspirin) are stopped several weeks before surgery to minimize the risk of postoperative bleeding.

Anxiety Reduction. One important approach in the preoperative period is to gain the confidence of the patient and lessen anxiety.

Often the patient's home has been made tense by the patient's restlessness, irritability, and nervousness secondary to hyperthyroidism. It is necessary to protect the patient from such tension and stress to avoid precipitating thyroid storm. If there is evidence of increased stress when family or friends visit, it may be advisable to limit visiting privileges during the preoperative period. Some forms of occupational therapy are recommended if they are quieting and relaxing.

Nutritional Support. Nutritional intake is modified to include adequate carbohydrate and protein foods. A high daily caloric intake is necessary because of the increased metabolic activity and rapid depletion of glycogen reserves. Supplementary vitamins, particularly thiamine and ascorbic acid, are provided. Tea, coffee, cola, and other stimulants are avoided.

Preoperative Preparation. If diagnostic testing is performed before surgery, the patient is informed of the purpose of the test and the preoperative preparations that can be expected to reduce anxiety. In addition, special efforts are made to ensure a good night's rest preceding surgery, although many patients are admitted to the hospital on the day of surgery.

Patient Education. Preoperative teaching includes demonstrating to the patient how to support the neck with the hands after surgery to prevent stress on the incision; that is, raising the elbows and placing the hands behind the neck will provide support and reduce strain and tension on the neck muscles and the surgical incision.

Postoperative Management

The patient is moved and turned carefully to support the head and avoid tension on the sutures. The most comfortable position is the semi-Fowler's position with the head elevated and supported by pillows. Analgesics are administered as prescribed for pain. The patient may receive humidified oxygen to facilitate breathing. The nurse should anticipate apprehension in the patient and inform him or her that oxygen will assist breathing and provide humidity.

Intravenous fluids are administered during the immediate postoperative period; water may be given by mouth as soon as nausea subsides. Usually, there is a little difficulty in swallowing; initially, cold fluids and ice may be taken better than other fluids. Often patients prefer a soft diet to a liquid diet in the immediate postoperative period.

The surgical dressings are assessed periodically and reinforced when necessary. When the patient is in a recumbent position, the sides and the back of the neck as well as the anterior dressing must be observed for bleeding. In addition to monitoring the pulse and the blood pressure for any indication of internal bleeding, it is also important to be alert for complaints of sensation of pressure or fullness at the incision site. Such symptoms may indicate hemorrhage and hematoma formation subcutaneously and should be reported.

Difficulty in respiration occurs as a result of edema of the glottis, hematoma formation, or an injury to the recurrent laryngeal nerve. This complication requires that an airway be inserted. Therefore, a tracheostomy set is kept at the patient's bedside at all times, and the surgeon is summoned at the first indication of respiratory distress.

The patient is advised to talk as little as possible, but when the patient does speak, any voice changes are noted because they might indicate injury to the recurrent laryngeal nerve, which lies just behind the thyroid next to the trachea.

An over-bed table may be used to provide easy access to those materials and items that are needed frequently, such as paper tissues, water pitcher and glass, and a small emesis basin. These are kept within easy reach so that the patient will not need to turn the head to look for them. It is also convenient to use this table when vapor-mist inhalations are prescribed for the relief of excessive mucus secretions.

The patient usually is permitted out of bed as soon as possible and is encouraged to eat foods that are easily eaten. A well-balanced, high-calorie diet is prescribed to promote weight gain. Sutures or skin clips usually are removed on the second day. The patient may be discharged from the hospital the day of surgery or soon afterward if the postoperative course is uncomplicated.

Complications. Hemorrhage, hematoma formation, edema of the glottis, and injury to the recurrent laryngeal nerve are complications that have been reviewed previously (see p. 1092). Occasionally, in thyroid surgery, the parathyroid glands may be injured or removed, producing a disturbance of the calcium metabolism of the body. As the blood calcium level falls, hyperirritability of the nerves, with spasms of the hands and feet and muscular twitchings, occurs. This group of symptoms is termed **tetany,** and its appearance should be reported at once because laryngospasm, although rare, may occur and obstruct the patient's airway. Tetany of this type is usually treated by the intravenous administration of calcium gluconate. This calcium abnormality may be temporary after thyroidectomy.

Patient Education and Home Care Considerations. The necessity for rest, relaxation, and nutrition is explained to both the patient and the family. Specific instructions are given regarding follow-up visits to the physician or the clinic, which are important for monitoring the patient's thyroid status. The patient is permitted to resume former activities and responsibilities completely once recovered from surgery. The patient may be discharged the evening of surgery or within a day of two. Therefore, the patient and family need to be knowledgeable about the signs and symptoms of complications that may occur and those that should be reported.

If indicated, a referral to home care is made; a visit by the home care nurse enables assessment of the patient's recovery from surgery. Additionally, the surgical incision is assessed, and activities to minimize strain on the incision and sutures are reinforced. Family responsibilities and factors relating to the home environment that produce emotional tension often have been implicated as precipitating causes of thyrotoxicosis. A home care visit provides an opportunity to evaluate these factors and possibly alter the environmental situation.

The Parathyroid Glands

Hyperparathyroidism

Hyperparathyroidism, which is caused by overproduction of parathyroid hormone by the parathyroid glands, is characterized by bone decalcification and the development of renal stones containing calcium.

Primary hyperparathyroidism occurs two to four times more often in women than in men and is most frequently seen in patients between 60 and 70 years of age. Approximately 100,000 new cases of hyperparathyroidism occur each year in the United States (NIH Consensus Statement, 1990). Half of the patients currently diagnosed with hyperparathyroidism are asymptomatic.

Secondary hyperparathyroidism with similar manifestations occurs in patients with chronic renal failure and so-called renal rickets as a result of phosphorus retention, increased stimulation of the parathyroid glands, and increased parathyroid hormone secretion.

Clinical Manifestations. The patient may have no symptoms or may experience signs and symptoms resulting from involvement of several body systems. Apathy, fatigue, muscular weakness, nausea, vomiting, constipation, hypertension, and cardiac dysrhythmias, may occur—all attributable to an increased concentration of calcium in the blood. Psychologic manifestations may vary from emotional irritability and neurosis to psychoses caused by the direct effect of calcium on the brain and nervous system. An increase in calcium produces a decrease in the excitation potential of nerve and muscle tissue.

The formation of stones in one or both kidneys, related to the increased urinary excretion of calcium and phosphorus, is one of the important complications of hyperparathyroidism and occurs in 55% of patients with primary hyperparathyroidism. Renal damage results from the precipitation of calcium phosphate in the renal pelvis and parenchyma, resulting in renal calculi (kidney stones), obstruction, pyelonephritis, and renal failure.

Musculoskeletal symptoms accompanying hyperparathyroidism may result from demineralization of the bones or bone tumors composed of benign giant cells resulting from overgrowth of osteoclasts. The patient may develop skeletal pain and tenderness, especially of the back and joints; pain on weight bearing; pathologic fractures; deformities; and shortening of body stature. Bone loss attributable to hyperparathyroidism is a risk factor for fracture.

The incidence of peptic ulcer and pancreatitis is increased with hyperparathyroidism and may be responsible for many of the gastrointestinal symptoms that occur.

Diagnostic Evaluation. The diagnosis of primary hyperparathyroidism is established on the basis of persistent elevation of serum calcium levels and an elevated level of parathormone. Radioimmunoassays for parathormone are very sensitive and differentiate primary hyperparathyroidism from other causes of hypercalcemia in more than 90% of patients with elevated serum calcium levels. An elevated serum calcium level alone is a nonspecific finding because serum levels may be altered by diet, medications, and renal and bone changes. Bone changes may be detected on x-ray or bone scan in advanced cases of the disease. The double antibody parathyroid hormone test is used to distinguish between primary hyperparathyroidism and malignancy as a cause of hypercalcemia. Ultrasound, MRI, thallium scan, and fine-needle biopsy have been used to evaluate the function of the parathyroids and to localize parathyroid cysts, adenomas, or hyperplasia.

Management. The insidious onset and chronic nature of hyperparathyroidism and its diverse and often vague symptoms may result in depression and frustration. The family may have considered the patient's illness to be psychosomatic. An awareness of the course of the disorder and an understanding approach by the nurse may help the patient and family to deal with their reactions and feelings.

The recommended treatment of primary hyperparathyroidism is the surgical removal of abnormal parathyroid tissue. However, in some carefully selected asymptomatic patients with only mildly elevated serum calcium levels and normal renal function, surgery may delayed and the patient followed closely for worsening of hypercalcemia, the deterioration of bone, renal impairment, or the development of kidney stones (renal calculi).

Hydration. Because kidney involvement is possible, patients with hyperparathyroidism are subject to renal calculi. Therefore, a fluid intake of 2000 ml or more is encouraged to help prevent calculus formation. Cranberry juice is suggested because there is some evidence that it may lower urinary *p*H. It can be added to juices and ginger ale for variety. The patient is instructed to report other manifestations of renal calculi, such as abdominal pain and hematuria. Thiazide diuretics are avoided in the patient with hyperparathyroidism because they decrease the renal excretion of calcium and cause further elevations in serum calcium levels. Additionally, the patient should take measures to avoid dehydration. Because of the risk of hypercalcemic crisis, the patient is instructed to seek immediate health care if conditions that commonly produce dehydration (*i.e.*, vomiting, diarrhea) occur.

Mobility. Mobility of the patient, with walking or use of a rocking chair, is encouraged as much as possible because bones subjected to normal stress give up less calcium. Bed rest, increases calcium excretion and predisposes the patient to formation of renal calculi.

Oral phosphate lowers the serum calcium level in some patients. Long-term use is not recommended because of ectopic calcium phosphate deposits in soft tissues.

Diet and Medications. Nutritional needs are met, but the patient is advised to avoid a diet with restricted or excess calcium. If the patient has a coexisting peptic ulcer, specifically prescribed antacids and protein feedings are necessary. Because anorexia is common, efforts are made to improve the patient's appetite. Prune juice, stool softeners, and physical activity, along with increased fluid intake, help to offset constipation, which is a common postoperative problem for these patients.

Nursing Interventions. The nursing management of the patient undergoing parathyroidectomy is essentially the same as that for a patient undergoing thyroidectomy (see p. 1092). However, the previously described precautions about dehydration, immobility, and diet are particularly important in the patient awaiting and recovering from parathyroidectomy. Although not all parathyroid tissue is removed during surgery in an effort to maintain control of calcium–phosphorus balance, the patient must be monitored closely to detect symptoms of tetany, which may be an early postoperative complication. Most patients quickly regain function of the remaining parathyroid tissue and experience only mild, transient postoperative hypocalcemia. In patients with significant bone disease or bone changes, a more prolonged period of hypocalcemia should be anticipated. The patient and family are reminded about the importance of follow-up to ensure return of serum calcium levels to normal.

Hypercalcemic Crisis. Acute hypercalcemic crisis can occur in hyperparathyroidism. This occurs with extreme elevation of serum calcium levels. Serum calcium levels higher than 15 mg/dl (3.7 mmol/L) result in neurologic, cardiovascular, and renal symptoms that can be life-threatening.

Treatment includes rehydration with large volumes of intravenous fluids, diuretic agents to promote renal excretion of excess calcium, and phosphate therapy to correct hypophosphatemia and decrease serum calcium levels by promoting calcium deposit in bone and decreasing gastrointestinal absorption of calcium. Cytotoxic agents (mithramycin), calcitonin, and dialysis may be used in emergency situations to decrease serum calcium levels quickly. The patient in acute hypercalcemic crisis requires close monitoring for life-threatening complications and reversal of serum calcium levels.

A combination of calcitonin and corticosteroids has been administered in emergencies to reduce the serum calcium level by increasing calcium deposition in bone. Other agents that may be administered to decrease serum calcium levels include bisphosphonates (*e.g.*, etidronate [Didronel], pamidronate); these are discussed on p. 226.

The patient requires expert assessment and care to minimize complications and reverse the life-threatening hypercalcemia. Medications are administered with care, and attention is given to fluid balance to promote return of normal fluid and electrolyte balance. Supportive measures are necessary for the patient and family.

Hypoparathyroidism

The most common cause of hypoparathyroidism is inadequate secretion of parathyroid hormone after interruption of the blood supply or surgical removal of parathyroid gland tissue during thyroidectomy, parathyroidectomy, or radical neck dissection. Atrophy of the parathyroid glands of unknown cause is a less common cause of hypoparathyroidism.

Pathophysiology. Symptoms of hypoparathyroidism are caused by a deficiency of parathormone that results in an elevation of blood phosphate (hyperphosphatemia) and a decrease in the concentration of blood calcium (hypocalcemia). In the absence of parathormone there is decreased intestinal absorption of dietary calcium and decreased resorption of calcium from bone and through the renal tubules. Decreased renal excretion of phosphate causes hypophosphaturia, and low serum calcium levels result in hypocalciuria.

Clinical Manifestations. Hypocalcemia causes irritability of the neuromuscular system and contributes to the chief symptom of hypoparathyroidism, **tetany**—a general muscular hypertonia, with tremor and spasmodic or uncoordinated contractions occurring with or without efforts to make voluntary movements. In latent tetany there is numbness, tingling, and cramps in the extremities, with the patient complaining of stiffness in the hands and feet. In overt tetany the signs include bronchospasm, laryngeal spasm, carpopedal spasm (flexion of the elbows and wrists and extension of the carpophalangeal joints, dysphagia, photophobia, cardiac dysrhythmias, and convulsions. Other symptoms include anxiety, irritability, depression, and even delirium. ECG changes and hypotension may also occur.

Diagnostic Evaluation. Latent tetany is suggested by a positive Trousseau's sign or a positive Chvostek's sign. **Trousseau's sign** is positive when carpopedal spasm is induced by occluding the blood flow to the arm for 3 minutes with use of a blood pressure cuff. **Chvostek's sign** is positive when a sharp tapping over the facial nerve just in front of the parotid gland and anterior to the ear causes spasm or twitching of the mouth, nose, and eye (see p. 224).

The diagnosis is often difficult because of vague symptoms, such as aches and pains. Therefore, laboratory studies are especially helpful. Tetany develops at serum calcium levels of 5 to 6 mg/dl (1.2 to 1.5 mmol/L) or lower. Serum phosphate levels are increased, and x-ray studies of bone show increased density. Calcification is detected on x-ray films of subcutaneous or paraspinal basal ganglia of the brain.

Management. The objective of therapy is to raise the serum calcium level to 9 to 10 mg/dl (2.2 to 2.5 mmol/L) and to eliminate the symptoms of hypoparathyroidism and hypocalcemia. When hypocalcemia and tetany occur after a thyroidectomy, the immediate treatment is to administer calcium gluconate intravenously. If this does not decrease neuromuscular irritability and seizure activity immediately, sedatives such as pentobarbital may be administered.

Parenteral parathormone can be administered to treat acute hypoparathyroidism with tetany. However, the high incidence of allergic reactions to injections of parathormone limits its use to acute episodes of hypocalcemia. The patient receiving parathormone is monitored closely for changes in serum calcium levels and allergic reactions.

Because of neuromuscular irritability, the patient with hypocalcemia and tetany requires an environment that is free of noise, sudden drafts, bright lights, or sudden movement. Tracheostomy or mechanical ventilation may become necessary, along with bronchodilating medications, if the patient develops respiratory distress.

Therapy for the patient with **chronic hypoparathyroidism** is determined after serum calcium levels are obtained. A diet high in calcium and low in phosphorus is prescribed. Although milk, milk products, and egg yolk are high in calcium, they are restricted because they also contain high levels of phosphorus. Spinach is also avoided because it contains oxalate, which would form insoluble calcium substances. Oral tablets of calcium salts, such as calcium gluconate, may supplement the diet. Aluminum hydroxide gel or aluminum carbonate (Gelusil, Amphojel) is also administered after meals to bind phosphate and promote its excretion through the gastrointestinal tract.

Variable dosages of a vitamin D preparation—dihydrotachysterol (AT 10 or Hytakerol) or ergocalciferol (vitamin D_2) or cholecalciferol (vitamin D_3)—are usually required and enhance calcium absorption from the gastrointestinal tract.

Nursing Interventions. Nursing management of the patient with possible *acute* hypoparathyroidism includes the following:

- Care of postoperative patients having thyroidectomy, parathyroidectomy, and radical neck dissection is directed toward detecting early signs of hypocalcemia and anticipating signs of tetany, seizures, and respiratory difficulties.
- Calcium gluconate is kept at the bedside with equipment necessary for intravenous administration. If the patient has cardiac problems, is subject to dysrhythmias, or is receiving digitalis, then calcium gluconate is administered slowly and cautiously.
- Calcium and digitalis increase systolic contraction, and, furthermore, they potentiate each other. This may produce potentially fatal dysrhythmias. Consequently, the cardiac patient requires continuous cardiac monitoring and careful assessment.

An important aspect of nursing care is teaching about medications and diet therapy. The patient needs to know the reason for a high calcium and low phosphate intake and the symptoms of hypocalcemia and hypercalcemia and to immediately contact the physician if these symptoms occur.

The Adrenal Gland

Pheochromocytoma

Pheochromocytoma is a tumor that usually is benign and originates from the chromaffin cells of the adrenal medulla. In 80% to 90% of patients, the tumor arises in the medulla; in the remaining patients it occurs in the extra-adrenal chromaffin tissue located in or near the aorta, ovaries, spleen, or other organs. Pheochromocytoma may occur at any age, but its peak incidence is between ages 25 and 50 years (Whalen, Althausen & Daniels, 1992). It affects men and women equally. Because of the high incidence of pheochromocytoma in family members, the patient's family should be alerted and screened for this tumor. Ten percent of the tumors are bilateral, and 10% are malignant.

Pheochromocytoma is the cause of high blood pressure in 0.1% to 0.5% of patients with hypertension (Bravo, 1991). Although it is uncommon, it is one form of hypertension that is usually cured by surgery; without detection and treatment, it is usually fatal.

Pheochromocytoma may occur in the familial form as part of multiple endocrine neoplasia, type II (MEN-II); therefore, it should be considered a possibility in patients with medullary thyroid carcinoma and parathyroid hyperplasia or tumor.

Clinical Manifestations

The nature and severity of symptoms of functioning tumors of the adrenal medulla depend on the relative proportions of epinephrine and norepinephrine secretion. The typical triad of symptoms includes headache, diaphoresis, and palpitations. Hypertension and other cardiovascular disturbances are common. The hypertension may be intermittent or persistent. However, only 50% of patients with pheochromocytoma have sustained or persistent hypertension. If the hypertension is sustained, it may be difficult to distinguish from other causes of hypertension. Other symptoms may include tremor, headache, flushing, and anxiety. Hyperglycemia may result from conversion of liver and muscle glycogen to glucose by epinephrine secretion; insulin may be required to maintain normal blood glucose levels.

The clinical picture in the paroxysmal form of pheochromocytoma usually is characterized by acute, unpredictable attacks, lasting seconds or several hours; during these attacks, the patient is extremely anxious, tremulous, and weak. The patient may experience headache, vertigo, blurring of vision, tinnitus, air hunger, and dyspnea. Other symptoms include polyuria, nausea, vomiting, diarrhea, abdominal pain, and a feeling of impending doom. Palpitations and tachycardia are common.

Blood pressures as high as 350/200 mm Hg have been recorded. Such blood pressure elevations are life threatening and may cause severe complications, such as cardiac dysrhythmias, dissecting aneurysm, stroke, and acute renal failure. Postural hypotension occurs in 70% of patients with untreated pheochromocytoma.

Diagnostic Evaluation

Pheochromocytoma is suspected if signs of sympathetic nervous system overactivity occur in association with marked elevation of blood pressure. However, determination of urine and plasma levels of catecholamines offers the most direct and conclusive test for overactivity of the adrenal medulla.

Total plasma catecholamine (norepinephrine and epinephrine) concentration is measured with the patient supine and at rest for 30 minutes. To prevent elevation of catecholamine levels by the stress of venipuncture, a butterfly needle, scalp vein needle, or venous catheter may be inserted 30 minutes before the blood specimen is obtained.

Factors that may elevate catecholamine levels must be controlled to obtain valid results; these factors include consumption of coffee or tea, use of tobacco, emotional and physical stress, and use of many prescription and over-the-counter medications (*i.e.*, amphetamines, nose drops or sprays, decongestants, and bronchodilators).

Normal plasma values of epinephrine are 100 pg/ml (SI: 590 pmol/L); normal values of norepinephrine are generally less than 100 to 550 pg/ml (SI: 590 to 3240 pmol/L). Values of epinephrine greater than 400 pg/ml (SI: 2180 pmol/L) or norepinephrine values greater than 2000 pg/ml (SI: 11,800 pmol/L) are considered diagnostic of pheochromocytoma; values that fall between normal values and those diagnostic of pheochromocytoma indicate the need for further testing.

Measurement of urinary catecholamine metabolites (metanephrines [MN] and vanillylmandelic acid [VMA]) or free catecholamines are the standard diagnostic tests used in the diagnosis of pheochromocytoma. A 24-hour specimen of urine may be collected for determining free catecholamines, MN, and VMA; the use of combined tests increases the diagnostic accuracy of testing. A number of medications and foods (*e.g.*, coffee, tea, bananas, chocolate, vanilla, aspirin) may alter the results of these tests; therefore, careful instructions to eliminate restricted items must be followed by the patient. Urine collected over a 2- or 3-hour period after an attack of hypertension can be assayed for catecholamine content.

Provocative tests and most suppression tests are used infrequently in the diagnostic evaluation because of the occurrence of false-positive and false-negative test results and because of the risks of hypertensive and hypotensive episodes that may occur.

A **clonidine suppression test** may be performed if the results of plasma and urine tests of catecholamines are inconclusive. Clonidine (Catapres) is a centrally acting, antiadrenergic medication that suppresses the release of neurogenically mediated catecholamines. The suppression test is based on the principle that catecholamine levels are normally increased through the activity of the sympathetic nervous system; in pheochromocytoma, increased catecholamines result from diffusion of excess catecholamines into the circulation, bypassing normal storage and release mechanisms. Therefore, in pheochromocytoma, clonidine will not suppress release of catecholamines.

The results of the test are considered normal if 2 to 3 hours after a single oral dose of clonidine the total plasma catecholamine value decreases at least 40% from the patient's baseline and the absolute value falls below 500 pg/ml. Patients with pheochromocytoma exhibit no change in catecholamine levels. False-positive results, however, may occur in patients with essential hypertension.

Imaging studies, such as CT scans, MRI, and ultrasound, may also be carried out to localize the pheochromocytoma and to determine if more than one tumor is present. MIBG scintigraph uses ^{131}I-metaiodobenzylguanidine (MIBG) to determine the location of the pheochromocytoma and detect metastatic sites outside the adrenal gland. MIBG is a radioactive compound that is taken up by adrenergic cells. It has been helpful in identifying tumors not detected by other tests or procedures. MIBG scintigraphy is a noninvasive, safe procedure that has increased the accuracy of diagnosis of adrenal tumors.

Other diagnostic studies may focus on evaluation of function of other endocrine glands because of the association of pheochromocytoma in some patients with other endocrine tumors.

Management

During an episode or attack of hypertension, tachycardia, anxiety, and the other symptoms of pheochromocytoma, the patient is placed on bed rest with the head of the bed elevated to promote an orthostatic decrease in blood pressure.

Pharmacotherapy. The patient may be moved to the intensive care unit for close monitoring of ECG changes and careful administration of α-adrenergic blocking agents such as phentolamine (Regitine) or smooth muscle relaxants (sodium nitroprusside [Nipride]) to quickly lower the blood pressure.

Phenoxybenzamine (Dibenzyline), a long-acting α-blocker, may be used after the patient's blood pressure is stable to prepare the patient for surgery. β-Adrenergic blocking agents, such as propranolol (Inderal) may be used for patients with cardiac dysrhythmias or those not responsive to α-adrenergic blocking agents. α-Adrenergic and β-adrenergic blocking agents must be used with caution, because patients with pheochromocytoma may have increased sensitivity to them. Still another group of medications that may be used preoperatively are catecholamine synthesis inhibitors such as α-methyl-*p*-tyrosine (metyrosine). These are occasionally used when the effects of catecholamines are not reduced by adrenergic blocking agents.

Surgery. The definitive treatment of pheochromocytoma is surgical removal of the tumor, usually with adrenalectomy. Bilateral adrenalectomy may be necessary if tumors of both adrenal glands are present. Preliminary patient preparation includes effective control of blood pressure and blood volumes. Usually, this is carried out over 10 days to 2 weeks. Phentolamine or phenoxybenzamine (Dibenzyline) may be used safely without causing undue hypotension. Other medications (metyrosine [Demser] and prazosin [Minipress]) have been used to treat pheochromocytoma. The patient needs to be well hydrated before, during, and after surgery to prevent hypotension.

Manipulation of the tumor during surgical excision may cause release of stored epinephrine and norepinephrine with marked increases in blood pressure and changes in heart rate. Therefore, use of sodium nitroprusside (Nipride) and α-adrenergic blocking agents may be required during and after surgery. Exploration of other possible sites of tumor is frequently undertaken to ensure removal of all tumor. As a result, the patient is subject to the stress and effects of a long surgical procedure, which may increase the risk of hypertension postoperatively.

Corticosteroid replacement is required if bilateral adrenalectomy has been necessary. Corticosteroids may also be necessary for the first few days or weeks after removal of a single adrenal gland. Intravenous administration of corticosteroids (methylprednisolone sodium succinate [Solu-Medrol]) may begin the evening before surgery and continue during the early postoperative period to prevent adrenal insufficiency. Oral preparations of corticosteroids (prednisone) will be prescribed after the acute stress of surgery diminishes.

Postoperative Care. The patient will be monitored for several days in the intensive care unit with special attention given to electrocardiographic changes, arterial pressures, fluid and electrolyte balance, and blood glucose levels. Several intravenous lines will be inserted for administration of fluids and medications. Hypotension and hypoglycemia may occur in the postoperative period because of the sudden withdrawal of excessive amounts of catecholamines. Therefore, careful attention is directed toward monitoring and treating these changes.

Hypertension is expected to disappear with treatment; however, approximately 40% of patients may continue to be hypertensive after surgery. This may result if all pheochromocytoma tissue has not been removed, if pheochromocytoma recurs, or if the blood vessels have been damaged by severe and prolonged hypertension.

Several days after surgery, urine and plasma levels of catecholamines and their metabolites are measured to determine whether surgery has been successful. When levels have returned to normal, the patient may be discharged. Thereafter, periodic checkups are required, especially in young patients or in patients whose families have a history of pheochromocytoma.

Nursing Interventions/Patient Teaching

The patient who has undergone surgery to treat pheochromocytoma has experienced a stressful preoperative and postoperative course and may remain fearful of repeated attacks. Although it is usually expected that all pheochromocytoma tissue has been removed, there is a possibility that other sites were undetected and that attacks may recur.

The patient is scheduled for periodic follow-up appointments to observe for return of normal blood pressure and plasma and urine levels of catecholamines. The patient may be required to collect urine specimens for 24 hours before follow-up visits to the clinic or physician's office and is given verbal and written instructions about the procedure. If long-term steroid replacement is necessary, the patient is given instructions on the correct schedule to follow (see p. 1103 for care of patients on long-term corticosteroid therapy).

A follow-up visit from a community or home health nurse may be useful to assess the patient's compliance with the medication schedule and to assist the patient in preventing or dealing with problems that may result from long-term use of corticosteroids.

Disorders of the Adrenal Cortex

The adrenal cortex is necessary for life. Adrenocortical secretions make it possible for the body to adapt to stress of all kinds. Without the adrenal cortex, severe stress causes peripheral circulatory failure, shock, and prostration. Life would be maintained only with nutritional, electrolyte, and fluid replacement and replacement of adrenocortical hormones.

Adrenocortical hormones are classified into three groups: mineralocorticoids, glucocorticoids, and sex hormones.

Mineralocorticoids are concerned with sodium and water retention and potassium excretion. Examples are aldosterone and desoxycorticosterone, a natural precursor of aldosterone.

Glucocorticoids are concerned with metabolic effects, including carbohydrate metabolism. Examples are cortisol and corticosterone. Glucocorticoids enhance the metabolic breakdown of body proteins and fat to provide a source of energy during periods of fasting. They antagonize the action of insulin, enhance protein catabolism, and inhibit protein synthesis. They affect defense mechanisms of the body and influence emotional functioning either directly or indirectly. They also suppress inflammation and inhibit scar tissue formation. In adrenal insufficiency, patients may be depressed or anxious, whereas with excessive replacement they tend to become euphoric.

Sex hormones secreted by the adrenal cortex are androgens and estrogens.

Disorders of the adrenal cortex develop as a result of hyposecretion or hypersecretion of the adrenocortical hormones. Adrenal insufficiency may result from disease, atrophy, hemorrhage, or surgical removal of the adrenal gland or glands.

Adrenocortical Insufficiency (Addison's Disease)

Pathophysiology

Addison's disease, or adrenocortical insufficiency, results when adrenal cortex function is inadequate to meet the patient's need for cortical hormones. Autoimmune or idiopathic atrophy of the adrenal glands is responsible for 75% of cases of Addison's disease (Stern & Tuck, 1994). Other causes include surgical removal of both adrenal glands or infection of the adrenal glands. Tuberculosis (TB) and histoplasmosis are the most common infections that destroy adrenal gland tissue. Although autoimmune destruction has replaced TB as the principal cause of Addison's disease, the increasing incidence of TB should lead to consideration of this in the diagnostic workup. Inadequate secretion of ACTH from the pituitary gland also results in adrenal insufficiency because of decreased stimulation of the adrenal cortex.

The symptoms of adrenocortical insufficiency may also result from the sudden cessation of exogenous adrenocortical hormonal therapy, which suppresses the body's normal response to stress and interferes with normal feedback mechanisms. Treatment with daily administration of corticosteroids for 2 to 4 weeks may suppress function of the adrenal cortex; therefore, Addison's disease should be considered in any patient who has been treated with corticosteroids.

Clinical Manifestations

Addison's disease is characterized by muscular weakness, anorexia, gastrointestinal symptoms, fatigue, emaciation, dark pigmentation of the skin, knuckles, knees, elbows, and mucous membranes, hypotension, low blood glucose, low serum sodium, and high serum potassium. In severe cases the disturbance of sodium and potassium metabolism may be marked by depletion of the sodium and water and severe, chronic dehydration.

As the disease progresses, with acute hypotension developing as a result of hypocorticism, the patient develops **addisonian crisis,** which is characterized by cyanosis, fever, and the classic signs of shock: pallor, apprehension, rapid and weak pulse, rapid respirations, and low blood pressure. In addition, the patient may complain of headache, nausea, abdominal pain, and diarrhea and show signs of confusion and restlessness. Even slight overexertion, exposure to cold, acute infections, or a decrease in salt intake may lead to circulatory collapse, shock, and death if untreated. The stress of surgery or dehydration resulting from preparation for diagnostic tests or surgery may precipitate an addisonian or hypotensive crisis.

Diagnostic Evaluation

Although the clinical manifestations presented appear specific, the onset of Addison's disease usually occurs with nonspecific symptoms. The diagnosis of Addison's disease is confirmed by laboratory test results. Laboratory findings include a decrease in the concentrations of blood glucose and sodium (hypoglycemia and hyponatremia), an increased concentration of serum potassium (hyperkalemia), and an increased white blood cell count (leukocytosis).

The definitive diagnosis is confirmed by low levels of adrenocortical hormones in the blood or urine. Serum cortisol levels are decreased in adrenal insufficiency. If the adrenal cortex is destroyed, baseline values are low, and ACTH injection fails to cause the normal rise in plasma cortisol and urinary 17-hydroxycorticosteroids. If the adrenal gland is normal but not stimulated properly by the pituitary, a normal response to repeated dosages of exogenous ACTH is seen, but no response follows the administration of metyrapone, which stimulates endogenous ACTH.

Management

Immediate treatment is directed toward combating shock: restoring blood circulation, administering fluids, administering corticosteroid replacement, monitoring vital signs, and placing the patient in a recumbent position with legs elevated. Hydrocortisone (Solu-Cortef) is administered intravenously and followed with 5% dextrose in normal saline. Vasopressor amines may be required if hypotension persists.

Antibiotics may be administered if infection has precipitated adrenal crisis in a patient with chronic adrenal insufficiency. Additionally, the patient is assessed closely to identify other factors, stressors, or illnesses that led to the acute episode.

Oral intake may be initiated as soon as tolerated by the patient. Gradually, intravenous fluids are decreased when oral fluid intake is adequate to prevent hypovolemia.

If the adrenal gland does not regain function, the patient needs life-long replacement of corticosteroids and mineralocorticoids to prevent recurrence of adrenal insufficiency and to prevent addisonian crisis in times of stress and illness. Additionally, the patient will probably need to supplement dietary intake with added salt during times of gastrointestinal losses of fluids through vomiting and diarrhea.

Nursing Assessment

The health history and examination focus on the presence of symptoms of fluid imbalance and on the patient's level of stress. The blood pressure and pulse rate are obtained as the patient moves from a lying to a standing position to detect inadequate fluid volume. Additionally, the patient's skin color and turgor are assessed for changes related to chronic adrenal insufficiency and hypovolemia. A history of weight changes, the presence of muscle weakness, and the level of fatigue are obtained. The patient and family members are asked about the onset of illness or increased stress that may have precipitated the acute crisis.

Nursing Interventions

Addisonian Crisis. An important part of nursing management is monitoring the patient for signs and symptoms indicative of addisonian crisis. These symptoms are often the manifestations of shock and may include hypotension, rapid, weak pulse, rapid respiratory rate, pallor, and extreme weakness. The patient with addisonian crisis is at risk for circulatory collapse and shock (see Chapter 15 for management of the patient in shock); therefore, physical and psychologic stress must be avoided. These would include exposure to cold, overexertion, infection, and emotional distress.

The patient with addisonian crisis requires immediate treatment with intravenous administration of fluid, glucose, and electrolytes, especially sodium; replacement of missing corticosteroids; and vasopressors. During acute addisonian crisis, exertion on the patient's part is avoided; therefore, it is important for the nurse to anticipate the patient's needs and take measures to assure that those needs are met.

Careful monitoring of the patient's report of symptoms, and vital signs, weight, fluid and electrolyte balance is essential to monitor the patient's progress and return to a pre-crisis state. To reduce risk of future episodes of addisonian crisis, an effort is made to identify factors that may have led to the episode of crisis.

Restoring Fluid Balance. The patient's skin turgor and mucous membranes are assessed to provide information about fluid balance. Weight changes are recorded daily because they provide information about the adequacy of the patient's fluid and hormone replacement. The patient is instructed to report increased thirst, which may indicate impending fluid imbalance. Frequent monitoring of lying, sitting, and standing blood pressures also provides a useful indicator of fluid balance. A decrease of systolic pressure (20 mm Hg or more) may be indicative of depletion of fluid volume, especially if accompanied by symptoms.

The patient is encouraged to consume foods and fluids that will assist in restoring and maintaining fluid and electrolyte balance. With the assistance of the dietitian, the nurse can provide guidance to the patient to select foods high in sodium during gastrointestinal disturbances and very hot weather.

The nurse instructs the patient and a family member to administer hormone replacement as prescribed and to modify the dosage during illness and other stressful occasions. Written and verbal instructions are provided about the administration of mineralocorticoid (Florinef) or glucocorticoid (prednisone) as prescribed (see p. 1103 for care of patient receiving corticosteroid therapy).

Improving Activity Tolerance. Until the patient's condition is stabilized, precautions are taken to avoid unnecessary activity and events that might be stressful and could precipitate another hypotensive episode. Efforts are made to detect signs of infection or the presence of other stressors that may have triggered the crisis in the first place. Even minor events or stressors that ordinarily would go unnoticed may be excessive in the presence of adrenal insufficiency. During the acute crisis, a quiet, nonstressful environment is maintained. All activities (*e.g.*, bathing, turning) are carried out *for* the patient. All procedures are explained to the patient to reduce anxiety. The nurse explains to the family the rationale for minimizing stress during the acute crisis and the measures for helping the patient reduce or avoid stress. The patient is assisted to increase activity gradually.

Patient Education and Home Care Considerations. Because of the need for life-long replacement of adrenal cortex hormones to prevent adrenal insufficiency and acute adrenal crises with vascular collapse, the patient and family members receive explicit verbal and written instructions about the rationale for replacement therapy and proper dosage. Additionally, they are instructed about how to modify the medication dosage and increase salt intake in times of illness, very hot weather, and other stressful situations. The patient is also instructed about modifying diet and fluid intake to help maintain fluid and electrolyte balance.

The patient and family are frequently provided with a syringe and a vial of injectable steroid, such as Solu-Cortef, for use in emergencies, and are given careful instruction about how and when to use it. The patient is instructed to inform other health care providers, such as dentists, about the use of steroids, to wear a Medic Alert bracelet, and to carry information about the need for steroids at all times. If surgery is needed in the patient with Addison's disease, careful administration of fluids and corticosteroids is necessary before, during, and after surgery to prevent addisonian crisis.

The patient and family need to know the signs of excessive or insufficient hormone replacement. The development of edema or weight gain may signify *too high* a dose of hormone; postural hypotension (fall in systolic blood pressure, lightheadedness, dizziness on standing, and weight loss) frequently signifies *too low* a dose.

Although most patients are able to return to job and family responsibilities soon after hospital discharge, others are unable to do so because of concurrent illnesses or incomplete recovery from the episode of adrenal insufficiency. In these circumstances, it is useful for the nurse to make a referral to the community health or home health nurse who will visit the patient at home, assess recovery, monitor hormone replacement, and assess stress in the home. Additionally, the nurse will have the opportunity to assess the knowledge the patient and family have about medication therapy and dietary modifications. A home visit also provides the opportunity to assess the patient's plans for follow-up visits to the clinic or physician's office.

Cushing's Syndrome

Cushing's syndrome results from excessive, rather than deficient, adrenocortical activity. The syndrome may result from excessive administration of corticosteroids or ACTH or from hyperplasia of the adrenal cortex.

Pathophysiology

Cushing's syndrome may be caused by several mechanisms, including a tumor of the pituitary gland that produces ACTH and stimulates the adrenal cortex to increase its hormone secretion despite adequate amounts being produced. Primary hyperplasia of the adrenal glands in the absence of a pituitary tumor is less common. Administration of corticosteroids or ACTH may also produce Cushing's syndrome. Another less common cause of Cushing's syndrome is the ectopic production of ACTH by malignancies; bronchogenic carcinoma is the most common type of these malignancies. Regardless of the cause, the normal feedback mechanisms that control the function of the adrenal cortex become ineffective, and the usual diurnal pattern of cortisol is lost. The signs and symptoms of Cushing's syndrome are primarily a result of oversecretion of glucocorticoids and androgens (sex hormones), although mineralocorticoid secretion may also be affected.

Clinical Manifestations

When overproduction of the adrenal cortical hormone occurs, arrest of growth, obesity, and musculoskeletal changes occur along with glucose intolerance.

The classic picture of Cushing's syndrome in the adult is that of central type obesity, with a fatty "buffalo hump" in the neck and supraclavicular areas, a heavy trunk, and relatively thin extremities. The skin is thin, fragile, and easily traumatized; ecchymoses (bruises) and striae develop. The patient complains of weakness and lassitude. Sleep is disturbed because of altered diurnal secretion of cortisol.

Excessive protein catabolism occurs, producing muscle wasting and osteoporosis. Kyphosis, backache, and compression fractures of the vertebrae may result. Retention of sodium and water occurs as a result of increased mineralocorticoid activity, producing hypertension and congestive heart failure.

The patient develops a "moon-faced" appearance and may experience increased oiliness of the skin and acne. There is increased susceptibility to infection. Hyperglycemia or overt diabetes may develop. The patient may also report weight gain, slow healing of minor cuts, and bruises.

In females of all ages, virilization may occur as a result of excess androgens. Virilization is characterized by the appearance of masculine traits and the recession of feminine traits. There is an excessive growth of hair on the face (hirsutism), the breasts atrophy, menses cease, the clitoris enlarges, and the patient's voice deepens. Libido is lost in males and females.

Changes occur in mood and mental activity; psychosis may develop on occasion. Distress and depression are common and are increased by the severity of the physical changes that occur with this syndrome. If Cushing's syndrome is a consequence of pituitary tumor, visual disturbances may occur because of pressure of the growing tumor on the optic chiasm. Chart 40-2 summarizes the changes associated with Cushing's syndrome.

CHART 40-2
Clinical Manifestations of Cushing's Syndrome

Ophthalmic
Cataracts
Glaucoma

Cardiovascular
Hypertension
Congestive heart failure

Endocrine/Metabolic
Truncal obesity
Moon face
Buffalo hump
Sodium retention
Hypokalemia
Metabolic alkalosis
Hyperglycemia
Menstrual irregularities
Impotence
Negative nitrogen balance
Altered calcium metabolism
Adrenal suppression

Immune Function
Decreased inflammatory responses
Impaired wound healing
Increased susceptibility to infections

Skeletal
Osteoporosis
Spontaneous fractures
Aseptic necrosis of femur
Vertebral compression fractures

Gastrointestinal
Peptic ulcer
Pancreatitis

Muscular
Myopathy
Muscle weakness

Dermatologic
Thinning of skin
Petechiae
Ecchymoses
Striae
Acne

Psychiatric
Mood alterations
Psychoses

Diagnostic Evaluation

Indicators of Cushing's syndrome include an increase in serum sodium and blood glucose levels and a decreased serum concentration of potassium, a reduction in the number of blood eosinophils, and a disappearance of lymphoid tissue. Measurements of plasma and urinary cortisol levels are obtained. Several blood samples may be collected to determine if the normal diurnal variation in plasma levels is present. This variation is frequently absent in adrenal dysfunction. If several blood samples are required, it is essential that they be collected at the times specified and that the time of collection be noted on the requisition slip.

Dexamethasone suppression tests may be performed to assist in diagnosis of pituitary and adrenal causes of Cushing's syndrome. Varying doses (high or low doses) of dexamethasone, a potent synthetic glucocorticoid, are administered, and plasma cortisol and urine 17-hydroxycorticosteroid levels are obtained. An overnight dexamethasone suppression test can be performed on an outpatient basis and is used as a screening test. Dexamethasone is administered at 11:00 PM, and a plasma cortisol level is obtained at 8:00 AM the next morning.

Other diagnostic studies include a 24-hour urinary free cortisol level and 24-hour urine collection for levels of 17-hydroxycorticosteroids and 17-ketosteroids, the urinary metabolites of cortisol and androgens. In Cushing's syndrome, these levels and plasma cortisol levels are elevated.

The corticotropin-releasing factor (CRF) stimulation test may be used to distinguish pituitary tumors from ectopic sites of ACTH production as the cause of Cushing's syndrome. Radioimmunoassay of plasma ACTH is useful in identifying the cause of Cushing's syndrome. Several of these tests are likely to be performed to screen the symptomatic patient for Cushing's syndrome and to confirm the results of other tests.

A CT scan, ultrasound, or MRI may be performed to localize adrenal tissue and detect tumors of the adrenal gland.

Management

Because many cases of Cushing's syndrome are caused by pituitary tumors rather than tumors of the adrenal cortex, treatment is often directed at the pituitary gland. Surgical removal of the tumor by transsphenoidal hypophysectomy (p. 1106) is the primary treatment of choice and has a very high rate of success (90%) when performed by a skilled surgical team. Radiation of the pituitary gland has also been successful, although it may take several months for control of symptoms. Adrenalectomy (see p. 1103) is the treatment of choice in patients with primary adrenal hypertrophy.

Postoperatively, symptoms of adrenal insufficiency may begin to appear 12 to 48 hours after surgery because of reduction of the high levels of circulating adrenal hormones. Temporary replacement therapy with hydrocortisone may be necessary for several months until the adrenal glands begin to respond normally to the body's needs. If both adrenal glands have been removed (bilateral adrenalectomy), lifetime replacement of adrenal cortex hormones is necessary.

Adrenal enzyme inhibitors (*i.e.*, metyrapone, aminoglutethimide, mitotane, ketoconazole) may be used to reduce hyperadrenalism if the syndrome is caused by ectopic ACTH secretion by a tumor that cannot be totally eradicated. Close monitoring is necessary because symptoms of inadequate adrenal function may result and because of possible side effects of these medications.

If the Cushing's syndrome is a result of externally administered (exogenous) corticosteroids, an attempt is made to reduce or taper the medication dose to the minimum level adequate to treat the underlying disease process (*e.g.*, autoimmune and allergic diseases and rejection of transplanted organs). Frequently, alternate-day therapy decreases the symptoms of Cushing's syndrome and allows recovery of the adrenal glands' responsiveness to ACTH.

❑ NURSING PROCESS
The Patient With Cushing's Syndrome

Assessment

The health history and examination focus on the effects on the body of high concentrations of adrenal cortex hormones and on the inability of the adrenal cortex to respond to changes in cortisol and aldosterone levels. The history includes information about the patient's level of activity and ability to carry out routine and self-care activities. The patient's skin is observed and assessed for trauma, infection, breakdown, bruising, and edema. Changes in physical appearance are noted, and the patient's responses to these changes are elicited. Throughout the interview and examination, the nurse assesses the patient's mental function, including mood, responses to questions, awareness of environment, and level of depression. The patient's family is often a good source of information about gradual or subtle changes in the patient's physical appearance as well as emotional status.

Diagnosis

Nursing Diagnoses

Based on all the assessment data, the major nursing diagnoses of the patient with Cushing's syndrome include the following:

- Risk for injury and infection related to weakness and altered protein metabolism and inflammatory response
- Self-care deficit related to weakness, fatigue, muscle wasting, and altered sleep patterns
- Impaired skin integrity related to edema, impaired healing, and thin and fragile skin
- Body image disturbance related to altered physical appearance, impaired sexual functioning, and decrease in activity level
- Altered thought processes related to mood swings, irritability, and depression

Collaborative Problems/ Potential Complications

Based on assessment data, potential complications may include:

- Addisonian crisis
- Adverse effects of adrenocortical activity

Planning and Implementation

Goals. The patient's major goals include decreased risk of injury and infection, increased ability to carry out self-care activities, improved skin integrity, improved body image, improved mental function, and absence of complications.

Nursing Interventions

Monitoring and Managing Potential Complications

Addisonian Crisis. The patient with Cushing's syndrome whose symptoms are treated by withdrawing corticosteroids or by adrenalectomy or removing a pituitary tumor is at risk for adrenal hypofunction and **addisonian crisis.** If the function of the adrenal cortex has been suppressed by high levels of circulating adrenal hormones, atrophy of the adrenal cortex is likely. If the circulating hormone level is decreased rapidly because of surgery or by abruptly stopping steroid treatment, manifestations of adrenal hypofunction and addisonian crisis may develop.

Additionally, the patient with Cushing's syndrome who experiences highly stressful events such as trauma or emergency surgery is at risk for addisonian crisis because of long-term suppression of the adrenal cortex. Therefore, the patient with Cushing's syndrome is monitored closely for hypotension, rapid, weak pulse, rapid respiratory rate, pallor, and extreme weakness. The patient may require intravenous administration of fluid and electrolytes and corticosteroids.

The patient who experiences trauma or requires emergency surgery will require additional levels of corticosteroids before, during, and after treatment or surgery. If addisonian crisis occurs, the patient is treated for circulatory collapse and shock (see Chapter 15 for management of the patient in shock). Efforts are made to identify factors that may have led to the episode of crisis.

Fluid and Electrolyte Imbalance. Fluid and electrolyte status is monitored by obtaining the patient's daily weight. Because of the increased risk for glucose intolerance and hyperglycemia, blood glucose monitoring is initiated and elevated blood glucose levels are reported to the physician so that treatment can be prescribed if indicated.

Decreasing Risk of Injury and Infection. A protective environment must be established to prevent falls, fractures, and other injuries to bones and soft tissues. The patient who is very weak may require assistance in ambulating to prevent falls or bumping into sharp corners of furniture.

Unnecessary exposure to visitors, staff, or patients with infections is avoided. The patient is assessed frequently for subtle signs of infection because the anti-inflammatory effects of corticosteroids may mask the common signs of inflammation and infection. Foods high in protein, calcium, and vitamin D are recommended to minimize muscle wasting and osteoporosis.

Referral to a dietician may assist the patient in selecting appropriate foods that are also low in sodium and calories.

Preoperative Preparation. The patient is prepared for adrenalectomy, if indicated, and postoperative care (see below). If Cushing's syndrome is a result of a pituitary tumor, a transsphenoidal hypophecestomy may be performed. Diabetes mellitus and peptic ulcer are common in the patient with Cushing's syndrome; therefore, management includes blood glucose monitoring and assessment of stools for blood and appropriate intervention if indicated.

Encouraging Rest and Activity. Weakness, fatigue, and muscle wasting make it difficult for the patient with Cushing's syndrome to carry out normal activities. Yet moderate activity should be encouraged to prevent complications of immobility and promote increased self-esteem. Insomnia often contributes to the patient's fatigue. Rest periods are planned and spaced throughout the day. Efforts are made to promote a relaxing, quiet environment for rest and sleep.

Promoting Skin Care. Meticulous skin care is necessary to avoid traumatizing the patient's fragile skin. Use of adhesive tape is avoided because it can irritate the skin and tear the fragile skin when the tape is removed. The skin and bony prominences are assessed frequently, and the patient is encouraged and assisted to change positions frequently to prevent skin breakdown.

Improving Body Image. If the cause of Cushing's syndrome can be treated successfully, the major physical changes disappear in time. However, the patient may benefit from discussion of the impact the changes have had on self-concept and relationships with others. The weight gain and edema seen with Cushing's syndrome may be modified by a low-carbohydrate, low-sodium diet. A high-protein intake may reduce some of the other bothersome symptoms.

Improving Thought Processes. Explanations to the patient and family members about the cause of emotional instability are important in helping them cope with the mood swings, irritability, and depression that may occur. Psychotic behavior may occur in a few patients and should be reported. The patient and family members are encouraged to verbalize their feelings.

Evaluation

Expected Outcomes

1. Decreases risk of injury and infection.
   a. Is free of fractures or soft-tissue injuries.
   b. Is free of ecchymotic areas.
   c. Experiences no temperature elevation, redness, pain, or other signs of infection and inflammation.
2. Increases participation in self-care activities.
   a. Plans activities and exercises to allow alternating periods of rest and activity.
   b. Reports improved well-being.
   c. Is free of complications of immobility.
3. Attains/maintains skin integrity.
   a. Has intact skin, without evidence of breakdown or infection.
   b. Shows evidence of decreased edema in extremities and trunk.
   c. Changes position frequently and inspects bony prominences daily.
4. Achieves improved body image.
   a. Verbalizes feelings about changes in appearance, sexual function, and activity level.
   b. States awareness that physical changes are a result of excessive corticosteroids.
5. Exhibits improved mental functioning.
6. Absence of complications.
   a. Exhibits normal vital signs and weight and is free of symptoms of addisonian crisis.
   b. Identifies signs and symptoms of adrenocortical hypofunction that should be reported and states measures to take in case of severe illness and stress.
   c. Identifies strategies to minimize complications of Cushing's syndrome.
   d. Complies with recommendations for follow-up appointments.

Primary Aldosteronism

The principal action of aldosterone is to conserve body sodium. Under the influence of this hormone, the kidneys excrete less sodium and more potassium and hydrogen.

Excessive production of aldosterone, which occurs in some patients with functioning tumors of the adrenal gland, causes a distinctive pattern of biochemical changes and a corresponding set of clinical manifestations that are diagnostic of this condition.

Clinical Manifestations. Patients with aldosteronism exhibit a profound decline in the serum levels of potassium (hypokalemia) and hydrogen ions (alkalosis), as demonstrated by an increase in *p*H and carbon dioxide combining power. The serum sodium level is normal or elevated depending on the amount of water reabsorbed with the sodium. Hypertension is the most prominent and almost universal sign of aldosteronism although it is the primary cause of fewer than 3% of cases of hypertension (Stern & Tuck, 1994).

Hypokalemia is responsible for the variable muscle weakness, cramping, and fatigue in patients with aldosteronism, as well as an inability on the part of the kidneys to acidify or concentrate the urine. Accordingly, the urine volume is excessive, leading to polyuria. Serum, by contrast, becomes abnormally concentrated, contributing to excessive thirst (polydipsia) and arterial hypertension. A secondary increase in blood volume and possible direct effects of aldosterone on nerve receptors such as the carotid sinus are other factors producing the hypertension.

Hypokalemic alkalosis may decrease the ionized serum calcium level and predispose the patient to tetany and paresthesias. Trousseau's and Chvostek's signs can be used to assess neuromuscular irritability before overt paresthesia and tetany occur (see p. 224). Glucose intolerance may occur because hypokalemia interferes with insulin secretion from the pancreas.

Diagnostic Evaluation. In addition to a high or normal serum sodium level and low serum potassium level, diagnostic studies indicate, high serum aldosterone levels and low serum renin levels. The measurement of aldosterone excretion rate after salt loading by IV infusions of saline for 3 days or the addition of 10 to 12 g sodium chloride to the patient's diet for 5 to 7 days is a useful diagnostic test for primary aldosteronism.

Management. Treatment of primary aldosteronism usually involves surgical removal of the adrenal tumor through adrenalectomy. Spironolactone may be prescribed to control hypertension.

Adrenalectomy

Adrenalectomy may be used in the treatment of adrenal tumors, primary Cushing's syndrome and aldosteronism. It has largely been replaced by ablative therapy in the treatment of malignancy of the breast and prostate gland to suppress hormone function.

For adrenal tumors all of the endocrine disturbances associated with a hypersecreting tumor of the adrenal cortex or medulla can be relieved completely, and the patient improved dramatically, by surgical removal of the involved gland.

Postoperative Considerations. Adrenalectomy is performed through an incision in the loin or the abdomen. In general, the postoperative care resembles that given for other abdominal surgery; however, the patient is susceptible to fluctuations in adrenocortical hormones and will require administration of corticosteroids, fluids, and other agents to maintain blood pressure and prevent acute complications. If the adrenalectomy is bilateral, replacement of corticosteroids will be life-long; if one adrenal gland is removed, replacement therapy may be necessary temporarily because of suppression of the remaining adrenal gland by high levels of adrenal hormones. Attention is also directed toward maintenance of a normal serum glucose level with insulin and appropriate intravenous fluids and dietary modifications.

Nursing management in the postoperative period includes frequent assessment of vital signs to detect early signs and symptoms of adrenal insufficiency and crisis or hemorrhage. The patient's stress and anxiety level can be minimized by explaining all treatments and procedures, providing comfort measures, establishing priorities of care, and providing rest periods.

Corticosteroid Therapy

Corticosteroids are used extensively for adrenal insufficiency and are also widely used in suppressing inflammation and autoimmune reactions, controlling allergic reactions, and reducing the rejection process in transplantation. Commonly used corticosteroids are listed in Table 40-4. Their **anti-inflammatory** and **antiallergy** actions make corticosteroids effective in treating rheumatic or connective tissue diseases such as rheumatoid arthritis and systemic lupus erythematosus. They are also frequently used in treatment of asthma, multiple sclerosis, and other autoimmune disorders.

TABLE 40-4 Commonly Used Corticosteroid Preparations

Generic Names	Trade Names
Hydrocortisone	Cortisol, Cortef, Hydrocortone, Solu-Cortef
Cortisone	Cortone, Cortate, Cortogen
Dexamethasone	Decadron, Dexameth, Deronil, Delalone, Dexasone, Dexone, Hexadrol
Prednisone	Meticorten, Deltasone, Orasone, Panasol, Novo-prednisone
Prenisolone	Meticortelone, Delta-Cortef, Prelone, Predalone
Methylprednisolone	Medrol, Solu-medrol, Meprolone
Triamcinolone	Aristocort, Kenacort, Kenalog, Cenocort, Azmacort, Aristospan
Beclomethasone	Beconase, Beclovent, Vanceril, Vancenase, Propaderm
Betamethasone	Celestone, Betameth, Betnesol, Betnelan

High doses seem to allow patients to tolerate high degrees of stress. Such **antistress** action may be caused by the ability of corticosteroids to aid circulating vasopressor substances in keeping the blood pressure elevated, or it may be caused by other effects, such as the maintenance of the plasma glucose level.

Side Effects. Although the synthetic corticosteroids are safer for some patients because of relative freedom from mineralocorticoid activity, most natural and synthetic corticosteroids produce similar kinds of side effects. The size of the dose required to bring about desired anti-inflammatory and antiallergy effects also causes metabolic effects, pituitary and adrenal gland suppression, and changes in the function of the central nervous system.

In view of these possible side effects, it is obvious that while corticosteroids are highly effective therapeutically, they may also be very dangerous. Dosages of these medications are frequently altered to allow high concentrations when absolutely necessary and then tapered in an attempt to avoid undesirable effects. This requires that patients be closely observed for side effects and that the dose be reduced when high doses are no longer required. Suppression of the adrenal cortex may persist up to a year after a course of corticosteroids of only 2 weeks' duration.

Therapeutic Uses and Side Effects of Corticosteroids

The dosage of corticosteroids is determined by the nature and chronicity of the illness as well as by any other medical problem the patient has. Rheumatoid arthritis, bronchial asthma, and multiple sclerosis are chronic disorders that corticosteroids do not cure; however, these medications may be useful when other measures do not provide adequate control of symptoms or to treat acute exacerbations.

In such a situation, the adverse effects of corticosteroids are weighed against the current problems of the patient. These medications may be used for a period but then should be gradually reduced as the patient's symptoms subside.

The nurse plays an important role in providing encouragement and understanding during the times the patient may experience recurrence of symptoms and apprehension about these while taking smaller doses.

Acute Conditions. Acute flare-ups and crises are treated with large doses of corticosteroids, as in emergency treatment for bronchial obstruction in status asthmaticus and shock from septicemia caused by gram-negative bacteria. Other measures, such as anti-infective agents or medications, are also used with corticosteroids to treat shock and other major symptoms.

At times corticosteroids are continued past the acute flare-up stage for the purpose of combating possible complications that are deemed worse than the side effects of corticosteroids. Systemic lupus erythematosus is an example of such a condition.

Eye Treatment. A different problem exists when corticosteroids are used in treating eye infections. Outer eye infection can be treated by topical application of eye drops, because these do not cause systemic toxicity. However, long-term application may cause an increase in intraocular pressure, which may lead to glaucoma in some patients. In other patients, prolonged use of corticosteroids may lead to cataract formation.

Dermatologic Disorders. Topical administration of corticosteroids in the form of creams, ointments, lotions, and aerosols is especially effective in many dermatologic disorders. It may be more effective in some conditions to use occlusive dressings around the affected part so that maximum absorption of the medication is achieved. Penetration and absorption are also increased if the medication is applied when the skin is hydrated or moist (*e.g.*, immediately after bathing).

Absorption of topical agents varies with body location. For example, absorption is greater through the layers of skin on the scalp, face, and genital area than on the forearm, and as a result these sites are more susceptible to the side effects of the medication than other sites.

The availability of over-the-counter topical corticosteroids increases the risk of side effects in patients who are unaware of the potential risks of these medications or use them indiscriminately. Excessive use of these agents, especially on large surface areas of inflamed skin, can lead to decreased therapeutic effects and increased side effects.

Dosage Schedule. Attempts have been made to determine the best time to administer pharmacologic doses of steroids. Once the patient's symptoms have been controlled on a 6-hour or 8-hour program, a once-daily or every-other-day schedule may be implemented. In keeping with the natural secretion of cortisol, the best time of the day for the total steroid dose is in the early morning from 7:00 to 8:00 AM. Large-dose therapy at 8:00 AM, when the gland is most active, produces maximal suppression of the gland. A large 8:00 AM dose is more physiologic, because it allows the body to escape effects of the steroids from 4:00 PM to 6:00 AM, when serum levels are normally low, hence minimizing cushingoid effects. If symptoms of the disease being treated are successfully suppressed, alternate-day therapy is helpful in reducing pituitary–adrenal suppression in patients requiring prolonged therapy. Some patients report discomfort associated with symptoms of their primary illness on the second day; therefore, it is important to explain to patients that this regimen is necessary to minimize side effects and suppression of adrenal function.

Tapering of Corticosteroids. Corticosteroid dosages are reduced gradually (tapered) to allow normal adrenal function to return and to prevent steroid-induced adrenal insufficiency. Up to 1 year or more after use of corticosteroids, the patient is at risk of adrenal insufficiency in times of stress. For example, if surgery for any reason is necessary, the patient is likely to require intravenous corticosteroids during and after surgery to prevent the occurrence of acute adrenal crisis. Patients receiving corticosteroids must have an adequate supply of medication on hand so that they do not miss a scheduled dose and increase their risk of adrenal insufficiency.

Chart 40-3 provides an overview of the management of the patient on corticosteroid therapy.

The Pituitary Gland

Hypopituitarism

Hypofunction of the pituitary gland (hypopituitarism) can result from disease of the pituitary gland itself or of the hypothalamus; however, the result is essentially the same. Hypopituitarism may result from destruction of the anterior lobe of the pituitary gland. *Panhypopituitarism* (Simmonds' disease) is total absence of all pituitary secretions and is rare. Postpartum pituitary necrosis (Sheehan's syndrome) is another uncommon cause of failure of the anterior pituitary. It is more likely to occur in women with severe blood loss, hypovolemia, and hypotension at the time of delivery.

Hypopituitarism is also a complication of radiation therapy to the head and neck area. The total destruction of the pituitary gland by trauma, tumor, or vascular lesion removes all stimuli that are normally received by the thyroid, the gonads, and the adrenal glands. The result is extreme weight loss, emaciation, atrophy of all endocrine glands and organs, hair loss, impotence, amenorrhea, hypometabolism, and hypoglycemia. Coma and death will occur without replacement of the missing hormones.

Pituitary Tumors

Pituitary tumors are usually not malignant although their location and effects on hormone production by target organs can cause life-threatening effects. Tumors of the pituitary gland are three principal types, representing an overgrowth of (1) eosinophilic cells, (2) basophilic cells, or (3) chromophobic cells (*i.e.*, cells with no affinity for either eosinophilic or basophilic stains).

Eosinophilic tumors, if they develop early enough in life, result in *gigantism*. The person thus affected may be

CHART 40-3
Side Effects of Corticosteroid Therapy and Implications

Side Effects	Collaborative Interventions
Cardiovascular Effects	
Hypertension Thrombophlebitis Thromboembolism Accelerated artherosclerosis	Monitor for elevated blood pressure Assess for positive Homans' signs Remind patient to avoid positions/situations that restrict blood flow (*e.g.*, crossing legs, prolonged sitting in same position, prolonged trips by car or plane without moving or changing position) Encourage foot and leg exercises when recumbent Encourage low sodium intake Encourage limited intake of fat
Immunologic Effects	
Increased risk of infection and masking of signs of infection	Assess for subtle signs of infection and inflammation Encourage patient to avoid exposure to others with upper respiratory infection Monitor patient for fungal infections Encourage handwashing
Eye Changes	
Glaucoma Corneal lesions	Encourage frequent eye examinations Refer patient to ophthalmologist if changes in visual acuity are detected
Musculoskeletal Effects	
Muscle wasting Poor wound healing Osteoporosis with vertebral compression fractures, pathologic fractures of long bones, aseptic necrosis of head of the femur	Encourage high protein intake Encourage diet high in calcium and vitamin D or calcium and vitamin D supplementation if indicated Take measures to avoid falls and other trauma Use caution in moving and turning patient Encourage postmenopausal women on corticosteroids to consider hormone-replacement therapy Instruct patient to rise slowly from bed or chair to avoid falling due to postural hypotension
Metabolic Effects	
Alterations in glucose metabolism Steroid withdrawal syndrome	Monitor blood glucose levels at periodic intervals Instruct patient about medications, diet, and exercise prescribed to control blood glucose level Report signs of adrenal insufficiency Administer corticosteroids and mineralocorticoids as prescribed Monitor fluid and electrolyte balance Administer fluids and electrolytes as prescribed Instruct patient about importance of taking corticosteroids as prescribed without abruptly stopping therapy Encourage patient to obtain and wear Medic-Alert bracelet Advise patient to notify all health care providers (*e.g.*, dentists, etc.) about need for corticosteroid therapy.
Changes in Appearance	
Moon face Weight gain Acne	Encourage caloric restriction Assure patient that most changes in appearance are temporary and will disappear if and when corticosteroid therapy is no longer necessary.

over 7 feet tall and large in all proportions, yet so weak and lethargic that he can hardly stand. If the disorder begins during adult life, the excessive skeletal growth occurs only in the feet, the hands, the superciliary ridge, the molar eminences, the nose, and the chin, giving rise to the clinical picture called *acromegaly.* Enlargement, moreover, is not confined to the skeleton but involves all tissues and organs of the body. Many of these patients suffer from severe headaches and visual disturbances because the tumors exert pressure on the optic nerves. Assessment of central vision and visual fields may indicate loss of color discrimination, diplopia (double vision), or blindness of a portion of a field of vision. Decalcification of the skeleton, muscular weakness, and endocrine disturbances, similar to those occurring in patients with hyperthyroidism, also are associated with tumors of this type.

Basophilic tumors give rise to **Cushing's syndrome** (see p. 1099) with features largely attributable to hyperadrenalism, including masculinization and amenorrhea in females, truncal obesity, hypertension, osteoporosis, and polycythemia.

Chromophobic tumors, which constitute 90% of pituitary tumors, usually produce no hormones but destroy the rest of the pituitary gland, causing hypopituitarism. Patients with this disease are often obese and somnolent, exhibiting fine, scanty hair; dry, soft skin; pasty complexion; and small bones. They also experience headaches, loss of libido, and visual defects progressing to blindness. Other symptoms include polyuria, polyphagia, a lowering of the basal metabolic rate, and a subnormal body temperature.

Diagnostic Evaluation. Diagnostic evaluation may include careful history and physical examination, including assessment of visual acuity and visual fields. CT scan and MRI are used to diagnose the presence and extent of pituitary tumors. Serum levels of pituitary hormones may be obtained along with measurements of hormones of target organs (*e.g.,* thyroid, adrenal) to assist in diagnosis if other information is inconclusive.

Management of Acromegaly or Pituitary Tumors. Surgical removal of the pituitary tumor through a transsphenoidal approach is considered the treatment of choice (see Chapter 59). Stereotactic radiation therapy, which requires use of a neurosurgical-type stereotactic frame to immobilize the patient, has been used in some patients to guide delivery of external beam radiation therapy precisely to the pituitary tumor with minimal effect on normal tissue. Other treatments include conventional radiation therapy, bromocriptine (dopamine antagonist), and octreotide (synthetic analogue of somatostatin). These medications inhibit production or release of growth hormone and may bring about marked improvement of symptoms. Octreotide may also be used preoperatively to improve the patient's clinical condition and to shrink the tumor.

Hypophysectomy

Hypophysectomy, or removal of the pituitary gland, may be performed for several reasons, including treatment of primary tumors of the pituitary gland. It is the treatment of choice in patients with Cushing's syndrome due to excessive production of ACTH by a tumor of the pituitary gland. In diabetic retinopathy, it is used to halt the progress of hemorrhagic retinopathy and avoid blindness. Hypophysectomy may also be performed on occasion as a palliative measure to relieve bone pain secondary to metastasis of malignant lesions of the breast and prostate.

Several methods can be used to remove or destroy the pituitary. It can be surgically removed through the transfrontal, subcranial, or oronasal–transsphenoidal approaches. Or it can be destroyed by irradiation or cryosurgery. (See Chapter 59 for the transsphenoidal approach to the removal of a pituitary tumor and for the nursing management of a patient undergoing cranial surgery.)

The absence of the pituitary gland alters the function of many parts of the body. Menstruation ceases and infertility occurs after total or nearly total ablation of the pituitary gland. Replacement therapy with corticosteroids and thyroid hormone will be necessary.

Diabetes Insipidus

Diabetes insipidus is a disorder of the posterior lobe of the pituitary gland due to a deficiency of vasopressin, the antidiuretic hormone (ADH). It is characterized by great thirst (polydipsia) and large volumes of dilute urine. It may be secondary to head trauma, brain tumor, or surgical ablation or irradiation of the pituitary gland. It may also occur with infections of the central nervous system (meningitis, encephalitis) or tumors (*e.g.,* metastatic disease, lymphoma of the breast or lung). Another cause of diabetes insipidus is failure of the renal tubules to respond to ADH; this nephrogenic form of diabetes insipidus may be related to hypokalemia, hypercalcemia, and a variety of medications (*e.g.,* lithium, demeclocyclin).

Clinical Manifestations. Without the action of vasopressin on the distal nephron of the kidney, an enormous daily output of very dilute, waterlike urine with a specific gravity of 1.001 to 1.005 occurs. The urine contains no abnormal substances, such as glucose and albumin. Because of the intense thirst, the patient tends to drink 4 to 40 liters of fluid daily, with a special craving for cold water.

In the hereditary form of diabetes insipidus, the primary symptoms may begin at birth. When it occurs in adults, the polyuria usually has an abrupt onset or it may have an insidious onset.

The disease cannot be controlled by limiting the intake of fluids, because loss of high volumes of urine continues even without fluid replacement. Attempts to restrict fluids cause the patient to experience an insatiable craving for fluid and to develop hypernatremia and severe dehydration.

Diagnostic Evaluation. The fluid deprivation test is carried out in which fluids are withheld for 8 to 12 hours or until 3% to 5% of the body weight is lost. The patient is weighed frequently during the time fluid is withheld. Plasma and urine osmolality studies are performed at the beginning and end of the test. The inability to increase specific gravity and osmolality of the urine is characteristic of diabetes insipidus. The patient with diabetes insipidus continues to excrete large volumes of urine with low specific gravity and will experience weight loss, rising serum osmolality, and elevated serum sodium levels. The patient's condition needs to be monitored frequently during the test, and the test is terminated if the patient develops problems such as tachycardia, excessive weight loss, or hypotension.

Other diagnostic procedures include concurrent measurements of plasma levels of vasopressin and plasma and urine osmolality; a trial of desmopressin (synthetic vasopressin); and intravenous infusion of hypertonic saline.

When the diagnosis of diabetes insipidus is confirmed and the cause is not obvious (*e.g.*, head injury), the patient is carefully assessed for the presence of tumors that may be responsible for the disorder.

Management. The objectives of therapy are (1) to assure adequate fluid replacement, (2) to replace vasopressin (which is usually a long-term therapeutic program), and (3) to search for and correct the underlying intracranial pathology. Nephrogenic causes require different management approaches.

Vasopressin Replacement. Desmopressin (DDAVP), synthetic vasopressin without the vascular effects of natural ADH, is particularly valuable because it has a longer duration of action and fewer adverse effects than other preparations previously used to treat the disease. It is administered intranasally with the patient spraying the solution into his or her nose through a flexible calibrated plastic tube. Two to four administrations daily appear to control the symptoms. The agent lypressin (Diapid) is a short-acting agent that is absorbed through the nasal mucosa into the blood; however, its duration may be too short for patients with severe disease. The patient should be observed for chronic rhinopharyngitis if the intranasal route of administration is used.

Another form of therapy is the intramuscular administration of ADH, vasopressin tannate in oil, used when intranasal route is not possible. It is administered every 24 to 96 hours. The vial of medication should be warmed or shaken vigorously before administration. The injection is administered in the evening so that maximum results are obtained during sleep. Abdominal cramps are a side effect of this medication. Rotation of injection sites is necessary to prevent lipodystrophy.

Fluid Conservation. Clofibrate, a hypolipidemic agent, has been found to have an antidiuretic effect on patients with diabetes insipidus who have some residual hypothalamic vasopressin. Chlorpropamide (Diabinese) and thiazide diuretics are also used in mild forms of the disease, because they potentiate the action of vasopressin. The patient receiving chlorpropamide should be warned of the possibility of hypoglycemic reactions.

Nephrogenic Causes. If the diabetes insipidus is renal in origin, these treatments are ineffective. Thiazide diuretics, mild salt depletion, and prostaglandin inhibitors (ibuprofen, indomethacin, and aspirin) are used to treat the nephrogenic form of diabetes insipidus.

Nursing Implications. The patient with possible diabetes insipidus needs encouragement and support if undergoing studies of a possible cranial lesion. The patient and family members are instructed about follow-up care and emergency measures. The patient is also advised to wear a Medic Alert bracelet and to carry medication and information about this disorder at all times. Caution must be used with administration of vasopressin if coronary artery disease is present because it causes vasoconstriction.

Syndrome of Inappropriate Antidiuretic Hormone Secretion

The syndrome of inappropriate antidiuretic hormone secretion (SIADH) refers to excessive ADH secretion from the pituitary gland even in the face of subnormal serum osmolality. Patients with this disorder cannot excrete a dilute urine. They retain fluids and develop a sodium deficiency (**dilutional hyponatremia**). SIADH is often of nonendocrine origin. That is, the syndrome may occur in patients with bronchogenic carcinoma in which malignant lung cells synthesize and release ADH. SIADH has also occurred with severe pneumonia, pneumothorax, and other disorders of the lungs in addition to malignant tumors that affect other organs.

Disorders of the central nervous system, such as head injury, brain surgery or tumor, or infection, are thought to produce SIADH by direct stimulation of the pituitary gland. Some medications (vincristine, phenothiazines, tricyclic antidepressants, thiazide diuretics, and others) and nicotine have been implicated in SIADH; they either directly stimulate the pituitary gland or increase the sensitivity of renal tubules to circulating ADH.

Management. This syndrome is generally managed by eliminating the underlying cause if possible and restricting the patient's fluid intake. Because retained water is slowly excreted through the kidneys, the extracellular fluid volume contracts, and the serum sodium concentration gradually increases toward normal. Diuretics (*e.g.*, furosemide [Lasix]) may be used along with fluid restriction if severe hyponatremia is present.

Nursing Implications. Close monitoring of fluid intake and output, daily weight, urine and blood chemistries, and neurologic status is indicated for the patient at risk for SIADH. Supportive measures and explanations of procedures and treatments assist the patient to deal with this disorder.

The Pancreas

The pancreas has both endocrine and exocrine functions, and these functions are interrelated. The major exocrine function is to facilitate digestion through secretion of enzymes into the proximal duodenum. Secretin and cholecystokinin-pancreozymin (CCK-PZ) are hormones from the gastrointestinal tract that aid in the digestion of food substances by controlling the secretions of the pancreas. Additionally, neural factors also influence pancreatic enzyme secretion. Considerable dysfunction of the pancreas must occur before enzyme secretion decreases and protein and fat digestion becomes impaired. Pancreatic enzyme secretion is normally 1500 to 2500 ml/day.

Gerontologic Considerations. There is little change in the size of the pancreas with age. There is, however, an increase in fibrous material and some fatty deposition in the normal pancreas in patients older than age 70. Additionally, some localized arteriosclerotic changes occur with age. Studies have suggested a decreased pancreatic secretion rate (decreased lipase, amylase, and trypsin) and bicarbonate output in older patients. Some impairment of normal fat absorption occurs with increasing age, possibly because of delayed gastric emptying and pancreatic insufficiency. Decreased calcium absorption also may occur. These changes require care in interpreting diagnostic tests in the normal elderly person and in providing dietary counseling.

Pancreatitis

Pancreatitis (inflammation of the pancreas) is a serious disorder of the pancreas that can range in severity from a relatively mild self-limiting disorder to a rapidly fatal disease that does not respond to any treatment.

Several theories exist about the cause and mechanism of pancreatitis, which is generally described as the autodigestion of the pancreas. Generally, these theories state that the pancreatic duct becomes obstructed, accompanied by hypersecretion of the exocrine enzymes of the pancreas. These enzymes enter the bile duct, where they are activated and, together with bile, back up (reflux) into the pancreatic duct, causing pancreatitis.

Several classification systems are used to describe or categorize the various stages and forms of pancreatitis. The most basic system divides pancreatitis into acute or chronic forms.

Acute Pancreatitis

Pathophysiology and Etiology

Acute pancreatitis, or inflammation of the pancreas, is brought about by the digestion of this organ by its own enzymes, principally trypsin. Eighty percent of patients with acute pancreatitis have biliary tract disease; however, only 5% of patients with gallstones develop pancreatitis. Gallstones enter the common bile duct and lodge at the ampulla of Vater, obstructing the flow of pancreatic juice or causing a reflux of bile from the common bile duct into the pancreatic duct, thus activating the powerful enzymes within the pancreas. Normally, these remain in an inactive form until the pancreatic juice reaches the lumen of the duodenum. Spasm and edema of the ampulla of Vater, resulting from duodenitis, can probably produce pancreatitis.

Long-term alcohol use is a common cause of acute episodes of pancreatitis, but the patient usually has had undiagnosed chronic pancreatitis before the first episode of acute pancreatitis occurs. Other less common causes of pancreatitis include bacterial or viral infection, with pancreatitis a complication of mumps virus. Blunt abdominal trauma, peptic ulcer disease, ischemic vascular disease, hyperlipidemia, hypercalcemia, and the use of corticosteroids, thiazide diuretics, and oral contraceptives have been associated with an increased incidence of pancreatitis. Acute pancreatitis may follow surgery on or near the pancreas or after instrumentation of the pancreatic duct. Acute idiopathic pancreatitis may be responsible for 10 to 30 percent of cases of acute pancreatitis (Steinberg, 1992). In addition, there is a small incidence of hereditary pancreatitis.

Mortality of acute pancreatitis is high (10%) because of shock, anoxia, hypotension, or fluid and electrolyte imbalances. Attacks of acute pancreatitis may result in complete recovery, may recur without permanent damage, or may progress to chronic pancreatitis. The patient admitted to the hospital with a diagnosis of pancreatitis is acutely ill and needs expert nursing and medical care.

Classification. Acute pancreatitis ranges in severity from a relatively mild, self-limiting disorder to a rapidly fatal disease that does not respond to any treatment. Edema and inflammation confined to the pancreas are the major events in the more mild form of pancreatitis, which is termed **interstitial** or **edematous pancreatitis.** Although this is considered the more mild form of pancreatitis, the patient is acutely ill and at risk of developing shock, fluid and electrolyte disturbances, and sepsis.

Acute hemorrhagic pancreatitis represents a more advanced form of acute interstitial pancreatitis. Enzymatic digestion of the gland is more widespread and complete. The tissue becomes necrotic, and the damage extends to the vasculature, so that blood escapes into the substance of the pancreas and into the retroperitoneal tissues. Late complications consist of pancreatic cysts or abscesses. The mortality rate of acute hemorrhagic pancreatitis is 30%.

Clinical Manifestations

Severe abdominal pain is the major symptom of pancreatitis that brings the patient to medical care. Abdominal pain and tenderness, along with back pain, result from irritation and edema of the inflamed pancreas that stimulate the nerve endings. Increased tension on the pancreatic capsule and obstruction of the pancreatic ducts also contribute to the pain. Typically, the pain occurs in the midepigastrium. Pain is frequently acute in onset, occurring 24 to 48 hours after a very heavy meal or alcohol ingestion, and it may be diffuse and difficult to locate. It is generally more severe after meals and is unrelieved by antacids. Pain may be accompanied by abdominal distention, a poorly defined palpable abdominal mass, and decreased peristalsis. Pain caused by pancreatitis is often accompanied by vomiting.

The patient appears acutely ill. Abdominal guarding is present. A rigid or boardlike abdomen may occur and is generally an ominous sign. The abdomen may, however, remain soft in the absence of peritonitis. Ecchymosis (bruising) in the flank or around the umbilicus may indicate severe, hemorrhagic pancreatitis.

Nausea and vomiting are common in acute pancreatitis. The emesis is usually gastric in origin but may also be bile stained. Fever, jaundice, mental confusion, and agitation also may occur.

Hypotension is typical and reflects hypovolemia and shock caused by loss of large amounts of protein-rich fluid into the tissues and peritoneal cavity. The patient may develop tachycardia, cyanosis, and cold, clammy skin in addition to hypotension. Acute renal failure is common.

Respiratory distress and hypoxia are common, and the patient may develop diffuse pulmonary infiltrates, dyspnea, tachypnea, and abnormal blood gas values. Myocardial depression, hypocalcemia, hyperglycemia, and disseminated intravascular coagulopathy may also occur with acute pancreatitis.

Diagnostic Evaluation

The diagnosis of acute pancreatitis is based on a history of abdominal pain, the presence of known risk factors, physical examination findings, and selected diagnostic findings.

Serum amylase and lipase levels are used in making the diagnosis of acute pancreatitis. Peak levels of serum amylase are reached in 24 hours, with a rapid fall to normal levels within 48 to 72 hours; serum lipase rises after 48 hours and remains elevated for 5 to 7 days. Urinary amylase levels also become elevated and remain elevated longer than serum amylase levels. The white blood cell count is usually elevated; hypocalcemia is present in many patients and appears to be correlated with the severity of pancreatitis. Transient hyperglycemia and glucosuria and elevated serum bilirubin levels occur in some patients with acute pancreatitis.

Other laboratory results that may be elevated in acute pancreatitis and used to determine its severity include fibrinogen, C-reactive protein, trypsinogen activation peptide, and polymorphonuclear (PMN) elastase.

X-ray films of the abdomen and chest are obtained to differentiate pancreatitis from other disorders that may cause similar symptoms and to detect the development of pleural effusions. Ultrasound and contrast-enhanced CT scans are used to identify an increase in the diameter of the pancreas and to detect pancreatic cysts, abscesses, or pseudocysts.

Hematocrit and hemoglobin levels are used to monitor the patient for bleeding. Peritoneal fluid that may be obtained through paracentesis or peritoneal lavage may contain increased levels of pancreatic enzymes.

The stools of patients suffering with pancreatic disease are often bulky, pale, and foul smelling. Fat content varies between 50% and 90% in pancreatic disease; normally, the fat content is 20%.

Endoscopic retrograde cholangiopancreatography (ERCP) is rarely used in the diagnostic workup for acute pancreatitis, but it may be valuable in treatment of gallstone pancreatitis.

Several predictors of the severity of pancreatitis and its prognosis have been identified and are listed in Chart 40-4.

Management

Management of the patient with acute pancreatitis is symptomatic and is directed toward preventing or treating complications. All oral intake is withheld to inhibit pancreatic stimulation and secretion of pancreatic enzymes. Total parenteral nutrition (TPN) in acute pancreatitis is usually an important part of therapy, particularly in debilitated patients, because of the metabolic stress associated with acute pancreatitis. Nasogastric suction may be used to relieve nausea and vomiting, to decrease painful abdominal distention and paralytic ileus, and to remove hydrochloric acid so that it does not enter the duodenum and stimulate the pancreas. Cimetidine (Tagamet) is also used to decrease hydrochloric acid secretion.

CHART 40-4
Criteria for Predicting Severity of Pancreatitis

Criteria on Admission

Age > 55 years
WBC > 16,000 mm^3
Serum glucose > 200 mg/dl (SI: > 11.1 mmol/L)
Serum LDH > 350 IU/L (SI: > 350 U/L)
SGOT (AST) > 250 U/ml (SI: 120 U/L)

Criteria Within 48 Hours

Fall in hematocrit > 10% (SI: > 0.10)
BUN increase > 5 mg/dl (SI: > 1.7 mmol/L)
Serum calcium < 8 mg/dl (SI: < 2.0 mmol/L)
Base deficit > 4 mEq/l (SI: > 4 mmol/L)
Fluid retention or sequestration > 6 L
pO_2< 60 mm Hg

2 or fewer signs: 1% mortality
Presence of 3 or more = severe pancreatitis
3–4 signs: 15% mortality
5–6 signs: 40% mortality
> 6 signs: 100% mortality

(Adapted from Wilson C and Imrie CW. Current concepts in the management of pancreatitis. Drug 1991; 41(3):360.)

Pain Management. Adequate pain medication is essential during the course of acute pancreatitis to provide sufficient pain relief and minimize the patient's restlessness, which may stimulate pancreatic secretion further. Morphine and morphine derivatives are avoided because they cause spasm of the sphincter of Oddi. Antiemetics may be prescribed to prevent vomiting.

Intensive Care. Correction of fluid and blood loss and low albumin levels is necessary to maintain fluid volume and prevent renal failure. The patient is usually acutely ill and is monitored in the intensive care unit. Hemodynamic monitoring and monitoring of arterial blood gases are initiated to detect early signs of complications. Antibiotics may be prescribed if infection is present; insulin may be required if significant hyperglycemia occurs. Peritoneal lavage has been effective in some patients with severe pancreatitis, although its use is controversial.

Respiratory Care. Aggressive respiratory care is indicated because of the high risk for elevation of the diaphragm, pulmonary infiltrates and effusion, and atelectasis. Hypoxemia occurs in a significant number of patients with acute pancreatitis even without abnormalities present on x-ray. Respiratory care may range from close monitoring of arterial blood gases to use of humidified oxygen to intubation and mechanical ventilation.

Biliary Drainage. Placement of biliary drains (for external drainage) and stents (indwelling tubes) in the pancreatic duct through endoscopy has been performed with some success. This treatment reestablishes drainage of the pancreas and has resulted in decreased pain and increased weight gain.

Surgical Intervention. Although often risky because the acutely ill patient is a poor surgical risk, surgery may be performed to assist in the diagnosis of pancreatitis (diagnostic laparotomy), to establish pancreatic drainage, or to resect or debride a necrotic pancreas. The patient who undergoes pancreatic surgery may have multiple drains in place postoperatively as well as a surgical incision that is left open and is irrigated and repacked every 2 to 3 days to remove necrotic debris (Fig. 40-5).

Postacute Management. Antacids may be used when the acute episode of pancreatitis begins to resolve. Oral feedings that are low in fat and protein content are initiated very gradually. Caffeine and alcohol are eliminated from the diet. If the episode of pancreatitis occurred during treatment with thiazide diuretics, glucocorticoids, or oral contraceptives, these medications are discontinued. Follow-up of the patient may include ultrasound, x-ray studies, or ERCP to determine if the pancreatitis is resolving and to assess for abscesses and pseudocysts. ERCP may also be used to identify the cause of acute pancreatitis if it is in question and for endoscopic sphincterotomy and removal of gallstones from the common bile duct.

Gerontologic Considerations. Acute pancreatitis affects people of all ages; however, the mortality from acute pancreatitis increases with advancing age. In addition, the pattern of complications changes with age. Younger patients tend to develop local complications, and the incidence of multiple organ failure increases with age, possibly as a result of progressive decreases in physiologic function of major organs with increasing age. Close observation of major organ function (*i.e.,* lungs, kidneys) is indicated, and aggressive treatment is necessary to reduce mortality from acute pancreatitis in the elderly.

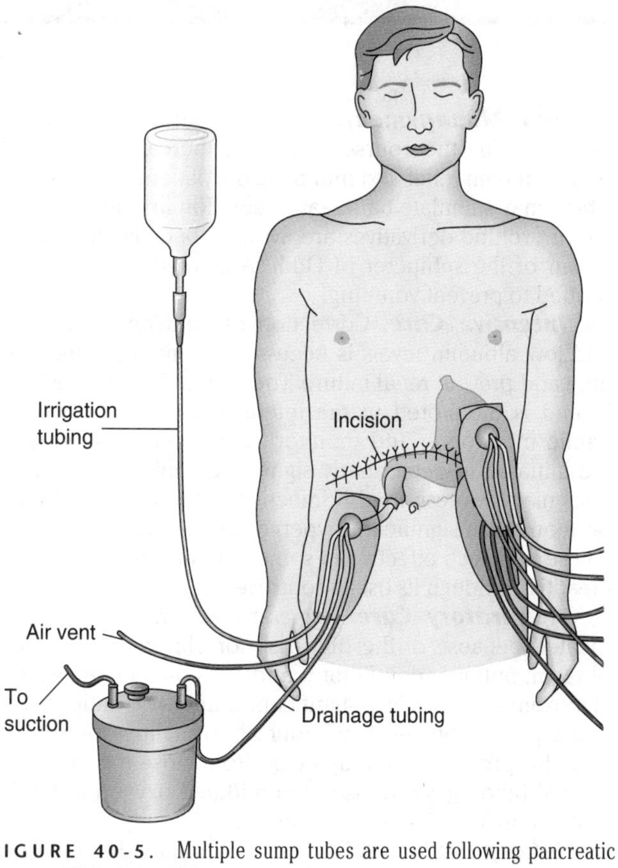

FIGURE 40-5. Multiple sump tubes are used following pancreatic surgery. Triple-lumen tubes consist of ports that provide tubing for irrigation, air venting, and drainage.

❑ NURSING PROCESS
The Patient With Acute Pancreatitis

Assessment

The health history focuses on the presence and character of the patient's abdominal pain and discomfort. The presence of pain, its location, its relationship to eating and to alcohol consumption, and the effect of the patient's efforts to obtain pain relief are noted. The patient's nutritional and fluid status and history of gallbladder attacks and alcohol use are assessed. A history of gastrointestinal problems, including nausea, vomiting, diarrhea, and passage of stools containing fat, is elicited. The abdomen is assessed for pain, tenderness, guarding, and bowel sounds; the presence of a board-like or soft abdomen is noted. Respiratory status, respiratory rate and pattern, and breath sounds are assessed. Normal and adventitious breath sounds and abnormal findings on chest percussion, including dullness at the bases of the lungs and abnormal tactile fremitus (see Chapter 22), are documented.

The emotional and psychological status of the patient and family and their coping are assessed because they are often frightened and anxious because of the severity of the patient's symptoms and the acuity of illness.

Diagnosis

Nursing Diagnoses

Based on all the assessment data, the major nursing diagnoses of the patient with acute pancreatitis include the following:

- ❑ Severe pain related to inflammation, edema, distention of the pancreas, and peritoneal irritation
- ❑ Ineffective breathing pattern related to severe pain, pulmonary infiltrates, pleural effusion, and atelectasis
- ❑ Altered nutritional status related to reduced food intake and increased metabolic demands
- ❑ Impaired skin integrity related to poor nutritional status, bed rest, and multiple drains and surgical wound

Collaborative Problems/ Potential Complications

Based on assessment data, potential complications that may occur include:

- ❑ Fluid and electrolyte disturbances
- ❑ Necrosis of the pancreas
- ❑ Shock and multiple organ failure

Planning and Implementation

Goals. The major goals for the patient include relief of pain and discomfort, improved respiratory function, improved nutritional status, maintenance of skin integrity, and absence of complications.

Nursing Interventions

Relieving Pain and Discomfort. Because the pathologic process responsible for pain is autodigestion of the pancreas, the objectives of therapy are to relieve pain and to decrease secretion of the enzymes of the pancreas. The pain of acute pancreatitis is often very severe, necessitating the liberal use of analgesics. Meperidine (Demerol) is the medication of choice; morphine sulfate is avoided because it causes spasm of the sphincter of Oddi. Oral feedings are withheld to decrease the formation and secretion of secretin. The patient is maintained on parenteral fluids and electrolytes to restore and maintain fluid balance. Nasogastric suction is used to remove gastric secretions and to relieve abdominal distention. The nurse provides frequent oral hygiene and care to decrease discomfort from the nasogastric tube and relieve dryness of the mouth; dryness of the mucous membranes will be increased if the patient is receiving anticholinergic medications to decrease pancreatic secretions.

The acutely ill patient is maintained on bed rest to decrease the metabolic rate and reduce the secretion of pancreatic and gastric enzymes. If the patient experiences increasing severity of pain, this is reported to the physician, because the patient may be experiencing hemorrhage of the pancreas, or the dose of analgesic may be inadequate.

The patient with acute pancreatitis often has a clouded sensorium because of severe pain, fluid and electrolyte disturbances, and hypoxemia. Therefore, frequent and repeated but simple explanations are offered about the need for withholding fluid intake and about maintenance of gastric suction and bed rest.

Improving Breathing Pattern. The patient is maintained in a semi-Fowler's position to decrease pressure on the diaphragm by a distended abdomen and to increase respiratory expansion. Frequent changes of position are necessary to prevent atelectasis and pooling of respiratory secretions. Anticholinergic medications, if prescribed to decrease gastric and pancreatic secretions, also dry the secretions of the respiratory tract, predisposing the patient to obstruction and infection. Pulmonary assessment is essential to observe for any changes in respiratory status. Pulse oximetry or arterial blood gases are monitored to detect changes in respiratory status and to enable their early treatment. The patient is instructed in techniques of coughing and deep breathing to improve respiratory function and is encouraged and assisted to cough and deep breathe every 2 hours.

Improving Nutritional Status. During the attack of acute pancreatitis, the patient is not permitted food and oral fluid intake; however, it is important for the nurse to assess the patient's nutritional status and to note factors that alter the patient's nutritional requirements (*e.g.*, temperature elevation, surgery, drainage). Laboratory test results, daily weights, and anthropometric measures will assist in monitoring the patient's nutritional status.

Total parenteral nutrition (TPN) may be prescribed. In addition to cautious administration of TPN, the nurse monitors the patient's physiologic response by assessing serum glucose levels every 4 to 6 hours. As the patient's acute symptoms subside, oral feedings are reintroduced gradually. Between acute attacks, the patient receives a diet high in carbohydrates and low in fat and proteins. Heavy meals are avoided, as are alcoholic beverages.

Monitoring and Managing Potential Complications. **Fluid and electrolyte disturbances** are common complications because of nausea, vomiting, gastric suction, movement of fluid from the vascular compartment to the peritoneal cavity, and diaphoresis and fever. The patient's fluid and electrolyte status is assessed by noting skin turgor and moistness of mucous membranes. The patient is weighed daily, and fluid intake and output are carefully measured, including urine output, nasogastric secretions, and diarrhea. In addition, the patient is assessed for factors that may affect the patient's fluid and electrolyte status; these may include increased body temperature, fluid loss through diarrhea, vomiting, nasogastric suction, or wound drainage. The nurse observes the patient for the presence of ascites and measures abdominal girth if ascites is suspected. Intravenous fluids are administered and may be accompanied by transfusion of blood and albumin to maintain the patient's blood volume and to prevent or treat shock. Emergency medications are kept readily available because of the risk of circulatory collapse and shock. Decreased blood pressure and reduced urine output are reported promptly because they may indicate hypovolemia and shock or renal failure. Low serum calcium and magnesium levels may occur and require prompt treatment.

Pancreatic necrosis is a major cause of morbidity and mortality in patients with acute pancreatitis. The patient who develops necrosis is at risk for hemorrhage, septic shock, and multiple organ failure. The patient may undergo diagnostic procedures to confirm pancreatic necrosis; surgical debridement or insertion of multiple drains may be performed. The patient with pancreatic necrosis is usually critically ill and requires expert medical and nursing management. The patient is often transferred to the intensive care unit so that close monitoring can be provided.

In addition to careful monitoring of the patient's vital signs and other signs and symptoms, the nurse is responsible for administering prescribed fluids, medications, and blood products; assisting with supportive management such as use of a ventilator; preventing additional complications, and attending to the patient's physical and psychological care.

Shock and multiple organ failure may occur with acute pancreatitis. Hypovolemic shock may occur as a result of hypovolemia and sequestering of fluid in the peritoneal cavity. Hemorrhagic shock may occur with hemorrhagic pancreatitis. Septic shock may occur with bacterial infection of the pancreas. Cardiac dysfunction may occur as a result of fluid and electrolyte disturbances, acid–base imbalances, and release of toxic substances into the circulation.

The patient must be monitored closely for early signs of neurologic, cardiovascular, renal, and respiratory dysfunction. The nurse must be prepared for rapid changes in the patient's status and must be able to respond quickly to rapid and frequent changes in treatments and therapies required to care for this patient. Additionally, the patient's family needs to be kept informed about the status and progress of the patient and must be allowed some time to spend with the patient. (Management of the patient in shock is discussed in detail in Chapter 15).

Improving Skin Integrity. The patient is at risk for skin breakdown because of poor nutritional status, enforced bed rest, and restlessness, which may result in pressure ulcers and breaks in tissue integrity. In addition, the patient who has undergone surgery, has had multiple drains inserted, or has an open surgical incision is at risk for skin breakdown and infection. The wound, drain sites, and skin are assessed carefully for signs of infection, inflammation, and breakdown. Wound care is carried out as prescribed, and precautions are taken to protect intact skin from contact with drainage. Consultation with an enterostomal therapist is often helpful in identifying the most appropriate skin care devices and protocols to use. The patient is turned every 2 hours; use of specialty beds may be indicated to prevent skin breakdown.

Patient Education and Home Care Considerations. The patient who has experienced and survived an episode of acute pancreatitis has been acutely ill. A prolonged period is needed to regain strength and return to previous level of activity. Because of the severity of the acute illness, the patient may not recall many of the facts and explanations given during the acute phase. As a result, this patient often requires repetition and reinforcement of information and instructions. If acute pancreatitis is a result of biliary tract disease such as gallstones and gallbladder disease, additional explanations are needed about the need for a low-fat diet and avoidance of heavy meals. If the pancreatitis is a result of alcohol abuse, the patient needs to be reminded of the importance of eliminating *all* alcohol. When the acute attack has subsided some patients may be inclined to return to their previous drinking habits. Specific information about resources and support groups that may be of assistance in avoiding alcohol in the future is provided to the patient and his family. Referral to Alcoholics Anonymous or other appropriate support groups is essential.

A referral to the community health nurse is often indicated to permit the nurse to assess the patient's home situation, reinforce instructions about fluid and nutrition intake and avoidance of alcohol, and permit the patient and family members to discuss their questions and concerns.

A summary of nursing management of the patient with acute pancreatitis is provided in Nursing Care Plan 40-2.

Evaluation

Expected Outcomes

1. Reports relief of pain and discomfort.
   a. Uses analgesics and anticholinergics as prescribed, without overuse.
   b. Maintains bed rest as prescribed.
   c. Avoids alcohol to decrease abdominal pain.
2. Experiences improved respiratory function.
   a. Changes position in bed frequently.
   b. Coughs and takes deep breaths at least every hour.
   c. Demonstrates normal respiratory rate and pattern, full lung expansion, normal breath sounds.
   d. Demonstrates normal body temperature and absence of respiratory infection.
3. Achieves nutritional and fluid and electrolyte balance.
   a. Reports decrease in number of episodes of diarrhea.
   b. Identifies and consumes high-carbohydrate, low-protein foods.
   c. Explains rationale for eliminating alcohol intake.
   d. Maintains adequate fluid intake within prescribed guidelines.
   e. Exhibits adequate urine output.
4. Exhibits intact skin.
   a. Skin is without breakdown or infection.
   b. Drainage is adequately contained.
5. Absence of complications.
   a. Demonstrates normal skin turgor, moist mucous membranes, normal serum electrolyte levels.
   b. Exhibits stabilization of weight, with no increase in abdominal girth.
   c. Exhibits normal neurologic, cardiovascular, renal, and respiratory function.

Chronic Pancreatitis

Chronic pancreatitis is an inflammatory disorder characterized by progressive anatomic and functional destruction of the pancreas. As cells are replaced by fibrous tissue with repeated attacks of pancreatitis, pressure within the pancreas increases. The end result is mechanical obstruction of the pancreatic and common bile ducts and the duodenum. Additionally, there is atrophy of the epithelium of the ducts, inflammation, and destruction of the secreting cells of the pancreas.

Causes

Alcohol consumption in Western societies and malnutrition worldwide are the major causes of chronic pancreatitis. Excessive and prolonged consumption of alcohol accounts for 75% of all cases in Western society (Holt, 1993). In *alcoholism,* the incidence of pancreatitis is 50 times greater than the rate in the nondrinking population. Long-term alcohol consumption produces hypersecretion of protein in pancreatic secretions. The result is protein plugs and calculi within the pancreatic ducts. Alcohol also has a direct toxic effect on the cells of the pancreas. Damage to these cells is more likely to occur and to be more severe in patients whose diets are poor in protein content and either very high or very low in fat.

Clinical Manifestations

The incidence of chronic pancreatitis is increased in adult men and is characterized by recurring attacks of severe upper abdominal and back pain, accompanied by vomiting. Attacks often are so painful that narcotics, even in large doses, do not provide relief. As the disease progresses, recurring attacks of pain are more severe, more frequent, and of longer duration. Some patients complain of continuous

NURSING CARE PLAN 40–2
Care of the Patient With Acute Pancreatitis

NURSING DIAGNOSIS: Severe pain and discomfort related to edema, distention of the pancreas, and peritoneal irritation

GOAL: Relief of pain and discomfort

Nursing Interventions	Rationale	Expected Outcomes
1. Administer meperidine (Demerol) frequently, as prescribed, based on patient's level of pain and discomfort.	1. Meperidine acts by depressing the central nervous system and thereby increasing the patient's pain threshold. Morphine is avoided because it produces spasm of the sphincter of Oddi.	• Reports relief of pain. • Moves and turns without increasing pain and discomfort. • Rests comfortably and sleeps for increasing periods. • Reports less frequent episodes of pain, discomfort, and cramping.
2. Assess pain level before and after administration of analgesic.	2. Assessment and control of pain are important because restlessness increases body metabolism, which stimulates the secretion of pancreatic and gastric enzymes.	
3. Report unrelieved pain or increasing intensity of pain.	3. Pain may increase pancreatic enzymes and may also indicate pancreatic hemorrhage.	
4. Assist the patient to assume positions of comfort; turn and reposition q2h.	4. Frequent turning relieves pressure and assists in preventing pulmonary and vascular complications.	

GOAL: Reduction of stimulation of the pancreas

Nursing Interventions	Rationale	Expected Outcomes
1. Administer anticholinergic drugs as prescribed.	1. Anticholinergic drugs reduce gastric and pancreatic secretion.	• Reports relief of pain, discomfort, and abdominal cramping. • Takes no fluid and food during acute phase. • Maintains bed rest. • Explains rationale for fluid and dietary restrictions and use of nasogastric drainage.
2. Withhold oral intake.	2. Pancreatic secretion is increased by food and fluid intake.	
3. Maintain the patient on bed rest.	3. Bed rest decreases body metabolism and thus reduces pancreatic and gastric secretions.	
4. Use continuous nasogastric suction. a. Measure gastric secretions at specified intervals. b. Observe and record color and viscosity of gastric secretions. c. Ensure that the nasogastric tube is patent to permit free drainage.	4. Nasogastric suction removes gastric contents and prevents gastric secretions from entering the duodenum and stimulating the secretin mechanism. Decompression of the intestines (if intestinal intubation is used) also assists in relieving respiratory distress.	

GOAL: Relief of discomfort associated with nasogastric drainage

Nursing Interventions	Rationale	Expected Outcomes
1. Use water-soluble lubricant around external nares. 2. Turn patient at intervals; avoid pressure or tension on NG tube 3. Give oral hygiene and gargling solutions without alcohol. 4. Explain rationale for use of nasogastric drainage.	1. Prevents irritation of nares. 2. Relieves pressure of tube on esophageal and gastric mucosa. 3. Relieves dryness and irritation of oropharynx. 4. Assists patient to cope with the drainage, nasogastric tube, and suction.	• Exhibits intact skin and tissue of nares at site of nasogastric tube insertion. • Reports no pain or irritation of nares or oropharynx. • Exhibits moist, clean mucous membranes of mouth and nasopharynx. • States that thirst is relieved by oral hygiene. • States rationale for nasogastric tube and suction.

(continued)

Care of the Patient With Acute Pancreatitis

NURSING DIAGNOSIS: Altered nutrition: Less than body requirements related to inadequate dietary intake, impaired pancreatic secretions, increased nutritional needs secondary to acute illness, and increased body temperature

GOAL: Improvement in nutritional status

Nursing Interventions	Rationale	Expected Outcomes
1. Assess current nutritional status and increased metabolic requirements.	1. Alteration in pancreatic secretions interferes with normal digestive processes. Acute illness, infection, and fever increase metabolic needs.	• Maintains normal body weight. • Demonstrates no additional weight loss. • Maintains normal serum glucose levels. • Reports decreasing episodes of vomiting and diarrhea. • Reports return of normal stool characteristics and bowel pattern. • Consumes foods high in carbohydrate, low in fat and protein. • Explains rationale for high-carbohydrate, low-fat, low-protein diet. • Eliminates alcohol from diet. • Explains rationale for limiting coffee intake and avoiding spicy foods. • Participates in Alcoholics Anonymous or other counseling approach.
2. Monitor serum glucose levels and give insulin as prescribed.	2. Impairment of endocrine function of the pancreas leads to increased serum glucose levels.	
3. Administer intravenous fluid and electrolytes and parenteral nutrition as prescribed.	3. Parenteral administration of fluids, electrolytes, and nutrients is essential to provide fluids, calories, electrolytes, and nutrients when oral intake is prohibited.	
4. Provide high-carbohydrate, low-protein, low-fat diet when tolerated.	4. These foods increase caloric intake without stimulating pancreatic secretions beyond the ability of the pancreas to respond.	
5. Instruct patient to eliminate alcohol and refer to Alcoholics Anonymous if indicated.	5. Alcohol intake produces further damage to pancreas and precipitates attacks of acute pancreatitis.	
6. Counsel patient to avoid excessive use of coffee and spicy foods.	6. Coffee and spicy foods increase pancreatic and gastric secretions.	

NURSING DIAGNOSIS: Ineffective breathing pattern related to splinting from severe pain, pulmonary infiltrates, pleural effusion, and atelectasis

GOAL: Improvement in respiratory function

Nursing Interventions	Rationale	Expected Outcomes
1. Assess respiratory status (rate, pattern, breath sounds) pulse oximetry, and arterial blood gases.	1. Acute pancreatitis produces retroperitoneal edema, elevation of the diaphragm, pleural effusion, and inadequate lung ventilation. Intra-abdominal infection and labored breathing increase the body's metabolic demands, which further decreases pulmonary reserve and leads to respiratory failure.	• Demonstrates normal respiratory rate and pattern and full lung expansion. • Demonstrates normal breath sounds and absence of adventitious breath sounds. • Demonstrates normal arterial blood gases and pulse oximetry. • Maintains semi-Fowler's position when in bed. • Changes position in bed frequently. • Coughs and takes deep breaths at least every hour. • Demonstrates normal body temperature. • Exhibits no signs or symptoms of respiratory infection or impairment. • Is alert and responsive to environment.
2. Maintain semi-Fowler's position.	2. Decreases pressure on diaphragm and allows greater lung expansion.	
3. Instruct and encourage patient to take deep breaths and to cough every hour.	3. Taking deep breaths and coughing will clear the airways and reduce atelectasis.	
4. Assist patient to turn and change position every 2 hours.	4. Changing position frequently assists aeration and drainage of all lobes of the lungs.	
5. Reduce the excessive metabolism of the body. a. Administer antibiotics as prescribed. b. Place patient in an air-conditioned room. c. Administer nasal oxygen as required for hypoxia.	5. Pancreatitis produces a severe peritoneal and retroperitoneal reaction that causes fever, tachycardia, and accelerated respirations. Placing the patient in an air-conditioned room and supporting	

(continued)

NURSING CARE PLAN 40–2 *(continued)*
Care of the Patient With Acute Pancreatitis

Nursing Interventions	Rationale	Expected Outcomes
d. Use a hypothermia blanket if necessary.	the patient with oxygen therapy decrease the workload of the respiratory system and the tissue utilization of oxygen. Reduction of fever and pulse rate decreases the metabolic demands on the body.	

COLLABORATIVE PROBLEM: Fluid and electrolyte disturbances, hypovolemia, shock

GOAL: Improvement in fluid and electrolyte status, prevention of hypovolemia and shock

Nursing Interventions	Rationale	Expected Outcomes
1. Assess fluid and electrolyte status (skin turgor, mucous membranes, urine output, vital signs, hemodynamic parameters)	1. The amount and type of fluid and electrolyte replacement are determined by the status of the blood pressure, the laboratory evaluations of serum electrolyte and blood urea nitrogen levels, the urinary volume, and the assessment of the patient's condition.	• Exhibits moist mucous membranes and normal skin turgor. • Exhibits normal blood pressure without evidence of postural (orthostatic) hypotension. • Excretes adequate urine output. • Exhibits normal, not excessive, thirst. • Maintains normal pulse and respiratory rate. • Remains alert and responsive. • Exhibits normal arterial pressures and blood gases. • Exhibits normal electrolyte levels. • Exhibits no signs or symptoms of calcium deficit (*e.g.,* tetany, carpopedal spasm). • Exhibits no additional losses of fluids and electrolytes through vomiting, diarrhea, or diaphoresis. • Reports stabilization of weight. • Demonstrates no increase in abdominal girth. • Demonstrates no fluid wave on palpation of the abdomen. • Demonstrates stable organ function without manifestations of failure.
2. Assess sources of fluid and electrolyte loss (vomiting, diarrhea, nasogastric drainage, excessive diaphoresis).	2. Electrolyte losses occur from nasogastric suctioning, severe diaphoresis, emesis, and as a result of the patient's being in a fasting state.	
3. Combat shock if present. a. Administer corticosteroids as prescribed to those who do not respond to conventional treatment. b. Evaluate the amount of urinary output. Attempt to maintain this at 50 ml/hr.	3. Extensive acute pancreatitis may cause peripheral vascular collapse and shock. Blood and plasma may be lost into the abdominal cavity, and, therefore, there is a decreased blood and plasma volume. The toxins from the bacteria of a necrotic pancreas may cause shock.	
4. Administer intravenous electrolytes (sodium, potassium, chloride) as prescribed.	4. Patients with hemorrhagic pancreatitis lose large amounts of blood and plasma, which decreases effective circulation and blood volume.	
5. Administer plasma, albumin, and blood products as prescribed.	5. Replacement with blood, plasma or albumin, assists in ensuring effective circulating blood volume.	
6. Keep a supply of intravenous calcium gluconate readily available.	6. Calcium may be prescribed to prevent or treat tetany.	
7. Assess abdomen for ascites formation: a. Measure abdominal girth daily. b. Weight patient daily. c. Palpate abdomen for fluid wave (p. 974)	7. During acute pancreatitis, plasma may be lost into the abdominal cavity, which diminishes the blood volume.	
8. Monitor for manifestations indicating multiple organ failure: neurologic, cardiovascular, renal, and respiratory dysfunction.	8. All body systems may fail if pancreatitis is severe and treatment is ineffective.	

severe pain; others have a dull, nagging constant pain. The risk of dependence on opiates is increased in pancreatitis because of the chronic nature and severity of the pain.

Weight loss is a major problem in chronic pancreatitis; over 75% of patients experience significant weight loss, usually caused by decreased dietary intake secondary to anorexia or fear that eating will precipitate another attack. Malabsorption occurs late in the disease when as little as 10% of pancreatic function remains. As a result, the digestion of foodstuffs, especially proteins and fats, is impaired. The stools become frequent, frothy, and foul smelling because of the impairment of fat digestion, which results in stool with a high fat content. This condition is referred to as **steatorrhea.** As the disease progresses, calcification of the gland may occur and calcium stones may form within the ducts.

Diagnostic Evaluation

Endoscopic retrograde cholangiopancreatography (ERCP) is the most useful study in the diagnosis of chronic pancreatitis. It provides detail about the anatomy of the pancreas and of the pancreatic and biliary ducts. It is also helpful in obtaining tissue for analysis and in differentiating pancreatitis from other conditions such as carcinoma. A CT scan or ultrasound is helpful to detect the presence of pancreatic cyst formation.

A glucose tolerance test evaluates pancreatic islet cell function, information necessary for making decisions about surgical resection of the pancreas. An abnormal glucose tolerance test indicative of diabetes may be present. In contrast to the patient with acute pancreatitis, serum amylase levels and the white blood cell count may not be significantly elevated.

Management

The management of chronic pancreatitis depends on its probable cause in each patient. Nonsurgical approaches may be indicated for the patient who refuses surgery, is a poor surgical risk, or whose disease and symptoms do not warrant surgical intervention. Treatment is directed toward prevention and management of acute attacks, the relief of pain and discomfort, and management of exocrine and endocrine insufficiency of pancreatitis.

Abdominal pain and discomfort are treated and prevented in a manner similar to those used in acute pancreatitis; however, the focus is usually on the use of nonopioid methods to manage pain. The physician as well as the nurse and dietitian emphasize to the patient and family the importance of avoiding alcohol and other foods that the patient has found tend to produce abdominal pain and discomfort. The fact that no other treatment is likely to relieve pain if the patient continues to consume alcohol is stressed to the patient.

Diabetes mellitus resulting from dysfunction of the pancreatic islet cells is treated with diet, insulin, or oral hypoglycemic agents. The hazard of severe hypoglycemia with alcohol use is stressed to the patient and family members. Pancreatic enzyme replacement is indicated in the patient with malabsorption and steatorrhea.

Surgery is generally carried out to relieve abdominal pain and discomfort, to restore drainage of pancreatic secretions, and to reduce the frequency of acute attacks of pancreatitis. The surgical procedure to be performed depends on the anatomic and functional abnormalities of the pancreas, including the location of disease within the pancreas, the presence of diabetes, exocrine insufficiency, biliary stenosis, and pseudocysts of the pancreas. Other factors taken into consideration in determining if surgery is to be performed and what procedure is indicated include continued use of alcohol and the ability of the patient to manage the endocrine or exocrine changes that are expected from surgical alterations.

Pancreaticojejunostomy with a side-to-side anastomosis or joining of the pancreatic duct to the jejunum allows drainage of the pancreatic secretions into the jejunum. Pain relief occurs by 6 months in over 80% of the patients who undergo this procedure, but pain returns in a substantial number of patients as the disease itself progresses.

Patients who undergo surgery may experience increased weight gain and improved nutritional status; this may result from reduction in pain associated with eating rather than from correction of malabsorption. **Other surgical procedures** may be performed for different degrees and types of disease, ranging from revision of the sphincter of the ampulla of Vater, to internal drainage of a pancreatic cyst into the stomach, to insertion of a stent, to wide resection or removal of the pancreas.

Autotransplantation or implantation of the patient's pancreatic islet cells has been attempted to preserve the endocrine function of the pancreas. Testing and refinement of this procedure continue in an effort to improve the results. Morbidity and mortality after these surgical procedures are high because of the poor physical condition of the patient before surgery and the concomitant occurrence of cirrhosis.

Despite these surgical procedures, the patient is likely to continue having pain and digestive difficulties from the pancreatitis unless he or she abstains completely from the use of alcohol.

Pancreatic Cysts

As a result of the local necrosis that occurs at the time of acute pancreatitis, collections of fluid may form in the vicinity of the pancreas. These become walled off by fibrous tissue and are called pancreatic cysts. They are the most common type of pancreatic cysts; other types develop as a result of congenital anomalies or secondary to chronic pancreatitis or trauma to the pancreas.

Diagnosis of pancreatic cysts is made by ultrasound, CT scan, and ERCP. ERCP may be used to define the anatomy of the pancreas and to evaluate the patency of pancreatic drainage. Pancreatic cysts may attain considerable size. Because of their location behind the posterior peritoneum, when they enlarge, they impinge on and displace the stomach or the colon, which are adjacent. Eventually, through pressure or secondary infection, they produce symptoms, requiring that they be drained.

Management

Drainage. Drainage into the gastrointestinal tract or through the skin surface of the abdominal wall may be established. In the latter instance, the drainage is likely to be profuse and destructive to tissue because of the enzyme contents. Hence, steps must be taken to protect the skin in areas adjacent to the drainage site to prevent excoriation. Ointments protect the skin, provided that they are applied before excoriation takes place. Another method involves the constant aspiration of digestive juice from the drainage tract by means of a suction apparatus, so that skin contact with the digestive enzymes is avoided. This method requires expert nursing attention to be sure that the suction tube does not become dislodged from the drainage tract and that the entire apparatus functions properly without interruption.

Consultation with an enterostomal therapist is advised to identify appropriate strategies to maintain drainage while protecting the patient's skin.

Surgery. When chronic pancreatitis develops in association with gallbladder disease, efforts are made to relieve the obstruction by surgically exploring the common duct and removing the stones; usually, the gallbladder is removed at the same time. In addition, an attempt is made to improve the drainage of the common bile duct and the pancreatic duct by dividing the sphincter of Oddi, a muscle that is located at the ampulla of Vater (this surgical procedure is known as a **sphincterotomy**). Nursing care after such surgery is the same as that indicated for all patients undergoing biliary tract surgery. A T tube usually is placed in the common bile duct, requiring a drainage system to collect the bile postoperatively.

Pancreatic Tumors

The incidence of pancreatic cancer has been steadily increasing for the past 20 to 30 years, especially in nonwhite men. It is the fourth leading cause of cancer deaths in the United States and occurs most frequently in the sixth and seventh decades of life. Cigarette smoking, exposure to industrial chemicals or toxins in the environment, and a diet high in fat, meat, or both, are associated with an increased incidence of pancreatic cancer, although their role in the cause is not completely clear. The risk of pancreatic cancer increases as the extent of cigarette smoking increases. Diabetes mellitus, chronic pancreatitis, and hereditary pancreatitis are also associated with pancreatic cancer. The pancreas can also be the site of metastasis from other tumors (Warshaw & Fernandez-del Castillo, 1992).

Cancer may arise in any portion of the pancreas (in the head, the body, or the tail), producing clinical manifestations that vary, depending on the location of the lesion and whether functioning, insulin-secreting pancreatic islet cells are involved. Tumors that originate in the head of the pancreas, the most common location, give rise to a distinctive clinical picture. Functioning islet cell tumors, whether benign (adenoma) or malignant (carcinoma), are responsible for the syndrome of hyperinsulinism (see p. 1119). With these exceptions, the symptoms are nonspecific, and patients usually do not seek medical attention until late in the course of their illness; 80% to 85% of patients have advanced, unresectable disease when the tumor is first detected. In fact, pancreatic carcinoma has the lowest 5-year survival rate of 60 cancer sites surveyed (Warshaw & Fernandez-del Castillo, 1992).

Clinical Manifestations

Pain, jaundice, or both are present in over 90% of patients and along with weight loss are considered classic signs of pancreatic carcinoma. These manifestations may not appear until the disease is far advanced. Other signs include rapid, profound, and progressive weight loss as well as vague upper or midabdominal pain or discomfort that is unrelated to any gastrointestinal function and difficult to describe.

Such discomfort radiates as a boring pain in the midback and is unrelated to posture or activity. Patients with pancreatic carcinoma often find that they get some relief from pain by sitting hunched forward; pain is often accentuated by lying supine. Pain is often progressive and severe, requiring the use of narcotic analgesics. It is often more severe at night.

Malignant cells from pancreatic cancer are often shed into the peritoneal cavity increasing the likelihood of metastasis. The formation of ascites is common.

A very important sign, when present, is the onset of symptoms of insulin deficiency: glucosuria, hyperglycemia, and abnormal glucose tolerance. Diabetes may be an early sign of carcinoma of the pancreas. Meals often aggravate epigastric pain, which usually occurs weeks before the appearance of jaundice and pruritus. A gastrointestinal x-ray series may demonstrate deformities in adjacent viscera caused by the impinging pancreatic mass.

Diagnostic Evaluation

Ultrasound and CT scan are used to identify the presence of pancreatic tumors. ERCP has become a major diagnostic procedure used in making a diagnosis of pancreatic carcinoma. Cells obtained during ERCP are sent to the laboratory for examination.

Percutaneous fine-needle aspiration biopsy of the pancreas is used to diagnose pancreatic tumors and to confirm the diagnosis in patients whose tumors are not resectable, eliminating the stress and postoperative pain of ineffective surgery. In this procedure, a needle is inserted through the anterior abdominal wall into the pancreatic mass under the guidance of CT scan, ultrasound, ERCP, or other imaging techniques. The aspirated material is examined for malignant cells. Although percutaneous biopsy is a valuable diagnostic tool, it has some drawbacks. A false-negative result if small tumors are missed and seeding of cancer cells along the needle track may occur. Low radiation to the site may be used before the biopsy to reduce the risk of seeding.

A percutaneous transhepatic cholangiography (PTC) is another procedure that may be performed to identify obstructions of the biliary tract by a pancreatic tumor.

Several tumor markers (*e.g.*, CA 19-9, CEA, ratio of testosterone to dihydrotestosterone) are being considered in the diagnostic workup; however, no reliable tumor marker for pancreatic carcinoma has been identified.

Angiography, CT scan, and laparoscopy may be performed to determine if the tumor can be successfully removed surgically.

Management

The surgical procedure is usually extensive if carried out to remove resectable localized tumors. However, definitive surgical treatment (*i.e.*, total excision of the lesion) often is not possible because of the extensive growth when the tumor is finally diagnosed and the probable widespread metastases—especially to the liver, lungs, and bones. More often, treatment is limited to palliative measures.

Although pancreatic tumors may be resistant to standard radiation therapy, the patient may be treated with radiation and chemotherapy (Fluorouacil [5-FU]). If the patient undergoes surgery, intraoperative radiation therapy (IORT) may be used to deliver a high dose of radiation to the tumor with minimal injury to other tissues. IORT may also be helpful in relief of pain. Interstitial implantation of radioactive sources has also been used although the rate of complications is high. A large biliary stent inserted percutaneously or through endoscopy may be used to relieve jaundice.

Studies are underway to assess the effects of antiestrogen and antiandrogen agents on pancreatic cancer.

Nursing Interventions. Pain management and attention to nutritional requirements are important nursing measures to improve the patient's level of comfort. Skin care and nursing measures are directed toward relief of pain and discomfort associated with jaundice, anorexia, and profound weight loss. A full-length foam-rubber pad placed under the patient has been beneficial and protects the bony prominences from pressure. Pain associated with pancreatic cancer may be severe and require liberal use of opioids; patient-controlled analgesia (PCA) should be considered in the patient with severe, escalating pain.

Tumors of the Head of the Pancreas

Assessment. Tumors in this region of the pancreas cause obstruction of the common bile duct where it passes through the head of the pancreas to join the pancreatic duct and empty at the ampulla of Vater into the duodenum. Obstruction to the flow of bile produces jaundice, clay-colored stools, and dark urine.

Malabsorption of nutrients and fat-soluble vitamins may result from the obstruction and from the absence of bile from the gastrointestinal tract. Some degree of abdominal discomfort or pain and pruritus may be noted. Nonspecific symptoms such as anorexia, weight loss, and malaise may be present. If these signs and symptoms are present, cancer of this part of the pancreas is suspected.

The jaundice of this disease must be differentiated from the jaundice attributable to a biliary obstruction caused by a gallstone in the common duct, which usually is intermittent and appears typically in obese patients, most often women, who have had previous symptoms of gallbladder disease. The tumors producing the obstruction may arise from the pancreas, from the common bile duct, or from the ampulla of Vater.

Diagnostic Evaluation. Diagnostic studies may include duodenography, angiography by hepatic or celiac artery catheterization, pancreatic scanning, percutaneous transhepatic cholangiography, ERCP, and percutaneous needle biopsy of the pancreas. Biopsy of the pancreas may be performed to aid diagnosis.

Management. Before extensive surgery can be performed, a fairly long period of preparation is often necessary because the patient is often in such a poor nutritional and physical state. Various liver and pancreatic function studies are performed, vitamin K is prescribed to restore the prothrombin activity, and a diet high in protein is often prescribed with pancreatic enzymes. TPN may be administered. Blood transfusions frequently are required as well.

A biliary-enteric shunt may be performed to relieve the jaundice and, perhaps, provide time for a thorough diagnostic evaluation. Total pancreatectomy (removal of the pancreas) may be performed. A pancreatoduodenectomy (Whipple's procedure or resection) is used for potentially curable cancer of the head of the pancreas (Fig. 40-6). It involves removal of the gallbladder, distal portion of the stomach, duodenum, and head of the pancreas, and anastomosis of the remaining pancreas, stomach, and common duct to the jejunum. The result is removal of the tumor, allowing flow of bile into the jejunum. When excision of the tumor cannot be performed, the jaundice may be relieved by diverting the bile flow into the jejunum by anastomosing the jejunum to the gallbladder, a procedure known as cholecystojejunostomy. (Whipple's resection has also been carried out to relieve the pain of chronic pancreatitis.)

Nursing Interventions. Preoperative preparation includes adequate hydration and nutrition, correction of prothrombin deficiency with vitamin K, and treatment of anemia to minimize postoperative complications.

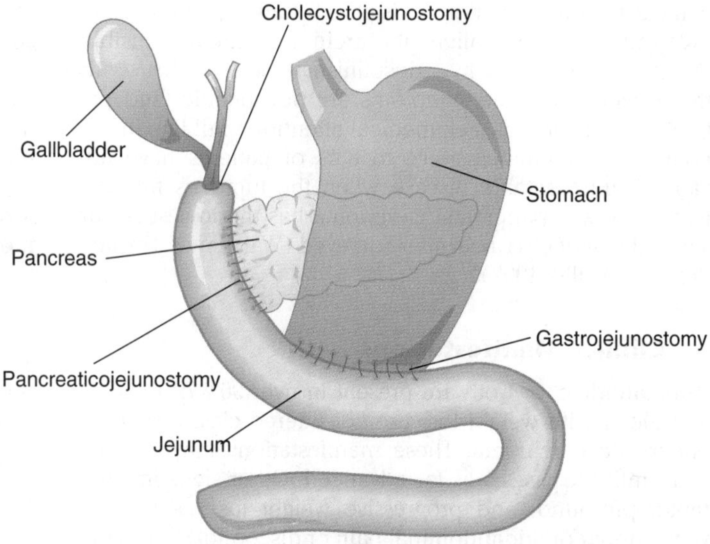

FIGURE 40-6. Pancreatoduodenectomy (Whipple's procedure or resection). End result of the resection of the carcinoma of the head of the pancreas or the ampulla of Vater. The common duct is sutured to the end of the jejunum, and the remaining portion of the pancreas and the end of the stomach are sutured to the side of the jejunum.

The postoperative management of patients who have undergone a pancreatectomy or a pancreatoduodenectomy is similar to the management of patients after extensive gastrointestinal and biliary surgery. The patient's physical status is often less than optimal, increasing the risk of postoperative complications. The psychosocial considerations are based on the fact that the patient has undergone major and risky surgery and is severely ill; thus, anxiety and depression may affect the patient's recovery.

The mortality rate after these procedures has improved because of advances in nutritional support and improved surgical techniques. Preoperatively and postoperatively, the nursing care is directed toward promoting patient comfort, preventing complications, and assisting the patient to return to and maintain as normal and comfortable a life as possible.

Hemorrhage, vascular collapse, and hepatorenal failure remain the major complications of these extensive surgical procedures. The patient is monitored closely in the intensive care unit after surgery, has multiple intravenous and arterial lines in place for fluid and blood replacement as well as for monitoring arterial pressures, and is on a mechanical ventilator in the immediate postoperative period. Careful attention is given to changes in the patient's vital signs, arterial blood gases and pressures, laboratory values, and urine output.

Although the patient's physiologic status is the focus of the health care team in the immediate postoperative period, the patient's psychologic and emotional state must be considered along with that of the family. The immediate and long-term outcome of this extensive surgical resection is uncertain, and the patient and family require emotional support and understanding in the critical and stressful preoperative and postoperative periods.

Pancreatic Islet Tumors

The pancreas contains the islets (islands) of Langerhans—small nests of cells that secrete directly into the bloodstream and, therefore, are part of the endocrine system. The secretion, insulin, is essential for metabolism of glucose. Diabetes mellitus (see Chapter 39) is the result of deficient secretion of insulin.

At least two types of tumors of the pancreatic islet cells are known: those that secrete insulin and those in which insulin secretion is not increased, known as "nonfunctioning" islet cell cancer.

The tumor that produces hypersecretion of insulin causes an excessive rate of glucose metabolism. The resulting hypoglycemia may produce symptoms of weakness, mental confusion, and seizures. These symptoms may be relieved almost immediately by oral or intravenous administration of glucose. The 5-hour glucose tolerance test is helpful in diagnosing insulinoma, the tumor of the pancreatic islet cells that produces excessive insulin, and in distinguishing it from other causes of hypoglycemia.

Surgical Management. Once the diagnosis of a tumor of the islet cells has been made, surgical treatment with removal of the tumor usually is recommended. The tumors may be benign adenomas or they may be malignant. Complete removal usually results in a dramatic cure. In some patients, such symptoms may not be produced by an actual tumor of the islet cells but by a simple hypertrophy of this tissue. In such cases a **partial pancreatectomy**—removal of the tail and part of the body of the pancreas—is performed.

Nursing Interventions. In preparing these patients for surgery, the nurse must be alert for symptoms of hypoglycemia and be ready to administer glucose as prescribed, should symptoms occur. Postoperatively, the nursing management is the same as that after other upper abdominal surgical procedures, with special emphasis on observation of serum glucose levels.

Hyperinsulinism

Hyperinsulinism results from the overproduction of insulin by the pancreatic islets. Symptoms resemble those of excessive doses of insulin and are attributable to the same mechanism—an abnormal reduction in blood glucose levels. Clinically, it is characterized by episodes during which the patient experiences unusual hunger, nervousness, sweating, headache, and faintness; in severe cases, seizures and episodes of unconsciousness may occur. The findings at the time of surgery or at autopsy may indicate hyperplasia (overgrowth) of the islets of Langerhans or a benign or malignant tumor involving the islets and capable of producing large amounts of insulin (see preceding discussion). Occasionally, tumors of nonpancreatic origin produce an insulin-like material that can cause hypoglycemia. This condition occasionally is responsible for seizures coinciding with decreases in the blood glucose to levels that are inadequate to sustain normal brain function (*i.e.,* below 30 mg/dl [1.6 mmol/L]).

All the symptoms that accompany spontaneous hypoglycemia are relieved by the oral or parenteral administration of glucose. Surgical removal of the hyperplastic or neoplastic tissue from the pancreas offers the only successful method of treatment. Approximately 15% of patients with spontaneous or functional hypoglycemia eventually develop diabetes mellitus.

Ulcerogenic (Zollinger–Ellison) Tumors

Some tumors of the islets of Langerhans are associated with a hypersecretion of gastric acid that produces ulcers in the stomach, the duodenum, and even the jejunum. The hypersecretion is so great that even after partial gastric resection enough acid to produce further ulceration may remain. When a marked tendency to develop gastric and duodenal ulcers is noted, an ulcerogenic tumor of the islets of Langerhans is suspected.

These tumors, which may be benign or malignant, are treated, when possible, by excision. Frequently, however, because of extension beyond the pancreas, removal is not possible. In many patients, a total gastrectomy may be necessary to reduce the secretion of gastric acid sufficiently to prevent further ulceration.

BIBLIOGRAPHY

Books

American Cancer Society. Cancer Facts and Figures. Atlanta, American Cancer Society, 1994.

CRITICAL THINKING EXERCISES

1. During a home visit to a patient with recently diagnosed diabetes mellitus, you observe that the patient's grandmother is slow to respond to others, seems depressed and lethargic, and is wearing a heavy coat in the warm house. You suspect that she might have a severe hypothyroid condition. Describe how you would proceed in this situation, how you would determine what actions to take, and how you would prioritize your actions.
2. Your patient is beginning antithyroid medication to control her hyperthyroidism. Her husband has been very concerend about her irritability, rapid mood swings, and weight loss. How would you explain to him the reasons for his wife's symptoms and the rationale for the medication being prescribed?
3. Your patient has been receiving corticosteroids for the treatment of a chronic disease. She has been admitted for an emergency hysterectomy. Based on your knowledge of the effects of the long-term use of corticosteroids, how would you focus your assessment and management strategies of this patient in the postoperative period?
4. Corticosteroids have been prescribed for your patient, and it is expected that she will take them for at least 1 month. How would you instruct her to minimize complications of corticosteroid use?

Becker KL (ed). Principles and Practice of Endocrinology and Metabolism. Philadelphia, JB Lippincott, 1990.

Besser GM and Thorner MO. Clinical Endocrinology. London, Mosby-Wolfe, 1994.

Bradley EL. Acute Pancreatitis: Diagnosis and Therapy. New York, Raven Press, 1994.

Braverman LE and Utiger RD. Werner and Ingbar's The Thyroid: A Fundamental and Clinical Test. Philadelphia, JB Lippincott, 1991.

Burch WM. Endocrinology for the House Officer. Baltimore, Williams & Wilkins, 1988.

DeGroot LJ. Endocrinology. Philadelphia, WB Saunders, 1995.

Diagnosis and Management of Asymptomatic Primary Hyperparathyroidism. NIH Consensus Development Conference Statement. 1990 Oct 29–31; 8(7):1–15.

Fischbach F. Manual of Laboratory Diagnostic Tests. Philadelphia, JB Lippincott, 1992.

Go VLE et al. The Pancreas: Biology, Pathobiology, and Disease. New York, Raven Press, 1993.

Goodman HM. Basic Medical Endocrinology. New York, Raven Press, 1994.

Greenspan FS and Baxter JD. Basic and Clinical Endocrinology. Norwalk, CT, Appleton & Lange, 1994.

Howard JM, Jordan GL Jr, and Reber HA. Surgical Diseases of the Pancreas. Philadelphia, Lea & Febiger, 1987.

Lavin N. Manual of Endocrinology and Metabolism. Boston, Little, Brown, 1994.

Lynn J and Bloom SR. Surgical Endocrinology. Oxford, Butterworth Heinemann, 1993.

National Cancer Institute. Cancer of the Pancreas. Research Report. U.S. Department of Health and Human Services, National Institutes of Health, Washington, DC, October 1987.

Samols E. (ed). The Endocrine Pancreas. New York, Raven Press, 1991.

Stern N and Tuck M. The adrenal cortex and mineralocorticoid hypertension. In Lavin N (ed). Manual of Endocrinology and Metabolism. Boston, Little, Brown, 1994.

Wilson JD and Foster DW. Williams' Textbook of Endocrinology. Philadelphia, WB Saunders, 1992.

Journals

General

Baker JR Jr. Immunologic aspects of endocrine diseases. J Am Med Assoc 1992 Nov 25; 268(20):2899–2903.

Coffland FI. Endocrine disorders affecting the cardiovascular system. Crit Care Nurs Clin North Am 1994 Dec; 6(4):735–745.

Kessler CA. An overview of endocrine function and dysfunction. AACN Clin Iss Crit Care Nurs 1992 May; 3(2):289–299.

Klein I and Ojamaa K. Cardiovascular manifestations of endocrine disease. J Clin Endocrinol Metab 1992 Aug; 75(2):339–342.

McGuire JL. The endocrine system and connective tissue disorders. Bulletin on the Rheumatic Diseases 1990; 39(4):1–8.

Miller M and Gold GC. Acute endocrine emergencies. Clin Geriatr Med 1994 Feb; 10(1):161–184.

Rolih CA and Ober KP. The endocrine response to critical illness. Med Clin North Am 1995 Jan; 79(1):211–224.

Shepherd JJ. The natural history of multiple endocrine neoplasia Type I: Highly uncommon or highly unrecognized? Arch Surg 1991 Aug; 126:935–952.

Siconolfi LA. The forgotten system: Endocrine dysfunction during multiple system organ dysfunction. Crit Care Nurs Q 1994 Feb; 16(4):16–26.

Sikes PJ. Endocrine responses to the stress of critical illness. AACN Clin Iss Crit Care Nur 1992 May; 3(2):379–391.

Snow K et al. Biochemical evaluation of adrenal dysfunction: The laboratory perspective. Mayo Clin Proc. 1992 Nov; 67:1055–1065.

Toto KH. Endocrine physiology: A comprehensive review. Crit Care Nurs Clin North Am 1994 Dec; 6(4):637–653.

Thyroid Disorders

Baker KH and Feldman JE. Thyroid cancer: A review. Oncol Nurs Forum 1993; 20(1):95–104.

Coffland FI. Thyroid-induced cardiac disorders. Crit Care Nurse 1993 Jun; 13(3):25–30.

Corsetti A and Buhl B. Managing thyroid storm. Am J Nurs 1994 Nov; 94(11):39.

Cushing GW. Subclinical hypothyroidism: Understanding is the key to decision making. Postgrad Med 1993 Jul; 94(1):95–97, 100, 102, 106–107.

Harris SC. Thyroid and parathyroid surgical complications. Am J Surg 1992 May; 163(5):476-478.

Herranz-Gonzalez J et al. Complications following thyroid surgery. Arch Otolaryngol Head Neck Surg 1991 May; 117:516–518.

Jordan RM. Myxedema coma. Pathophysiology, therapy, and factors affecting prognosis. Med Clin North Am 1995 Jan; 79(1): 185–194.

Kahky MP and Weber RS. Complications of surgery of the thyroid and parathyroid islands. Surg Clin North Am 1993 Apr; 73(2):307–321.

Kaplan MM. Thyroid hormone therapy: What, when, and how much. Postgrad Med 1993 Jan; 93(1):249–252, 255–256, 260, 262.
Kaye TB. Thyroid function tests. Postgrad Med 1993 Jul; 94(1): 81–83, 87–88, 90.
Sakiyama R. Thyroiditis: A clinical review. Am Fam Physician 1993 Sep; 68(4):615–621.
Sawin CT. Thyroid dysfunction in older persons. Adv Intern Med 1991; 37:223–248.
Schimke RN. Hyperthyroidism: The clinical spectrum. Postgrad Med 1992 Apr; 91(5):229–236.
Tietgens ST and Leinung MC. Thyroid storm. Med Clin North Am 1995 Jan; 79(1):169–184.
Tonner DR and Schlechte JA. Neurologic complications of thyroid and parathyroid disease. Med Clin North Am 1993 Jan; 77(1):251–263.
Wool MS. Thyroid nodules: The place of fine-needle aspiration biopsy in management. Postgrad Med 1993 Jul; 94(1):111, 112, 115, 116, 118, 120, 121.
Yeatts RP. Graves' ophthalmopathy. Med Clin North Am 1995 Jan; 79(1):195–209.

Parathyroid Disorders

Edelson GW and Kleerekoper M. Hypercalcemic crisis. Med Clin North Am 1995 Jan; 79(1):79–92.
Kaplan EL, Yashiro T, and Salti G. Primary hyperparathyroidism in the 1990s: Choice of surgical procedures for this disease. Ann Surg 1992 Apr; 215(4):300–317.
Kahky MP and Weber RS. Complications of surgery of the thyroid and parathyroid slands. Surg Clin North Am 1993 Apr; 73(2):307–321.
Goris ML, Basso LV, and Keeling C. Parathyroid imaging. J Nucl Med 1991 May; 32(5):887–889.
Prinz RA. Parathyroidectomy and more. Mayo Clin Proc 1991 Jul; 66(7):756–759.
Reber PM and Heath H III. Hypocalcemic emergencies. Med Clin North Am 1995 Jan; 79(1):93–106.
Salti GO et al. Continuing evolution in the operative management of primary hyperparathyroidism. Arch Surg 1992 Jul; 127(7): 831–837.

Adrenal Medulla Disorders

Agana-Defensor R and Proch M. Pheochromocytoma: A clinical review. AACN Clin Iss Crit Care Nur 1992 May; 3(2):309–318.
Howard DC. Pheochromocytoma in the pregnant patient: A case study. Am J Crit Care 1992; 1(2):111–114.
Stein PP and Black HR. A simplified diagnostic approach to pheochromocytoma. Medicine 1991 Jan; 70(1):46–66.
Yucha C and Blakeman N. Pheochromocytoma: The great mimic. Cancer Nurs 1991 Jun; 14(3):136–140.
Werbel SS and Ober KP. Pheochromocytoma. Update on diagnosis, localization, and management. Med Clin North Am 1995 Jan; 79(1):131–153.
Whalen RK, Althausen AF, and Daniels GH. Extra-renal pheochromocytoma. J Urol 1992 Jan; 147(1):1–10.

Adrenal Cortex Disorders

Biglieri EG. Spectrum of mineralocorticoid hypertension. Hypertension 1991 Feb; 17(2):251–261.
Davenport J et al. Addison's disease. Am Fam Physician 1991 Apr; 43(4):1338–1342.
Francis IR et al. Integrated imaging of adrenal disease. Radiology 1992 Jul; 184(1):1–13.
Frederick R et al. Addisonian crisis: Emergency presentation of primary adrenal insufficiency. Ann Emerg Med 1991 Jul; 20:802–806.
Grondal S and Hamberger B. Primary aldosteronism. Br J Surg 1992 Jun; 79:484–485.
Mulloy AL and Caruana RJ. Hyponatremic emergencies. Med Clin North Am 1995 Jan; 79(1):155–168.
Peterson A and Drass J. How to keep adrenal insufficiency in check. Am J Nurs 1993 Oct; 93(10):36–39.
Rao RH. Bilateral massive adrenal hemorrhage. Med Clin North Am 1995 Jan; 79(1):107–129.
Stoffer SS. Addison's disease: How to improve patient's quality of life. Postgrad Med 1993 Mar; 93(4):265–266, 271–278.
Werbel SS and Ober KP. Acute adrenal insufficiency. Endocrinol Metab Clin North Am 1993 Jun; 22(2):303–328.
Wilson BA and Malseed RT. Understanding corticosteroids: Pharmacologic and adverse effects. MedSurg Nurs 1993 Aug; 2(4): 322–325.

Pituitary Disorders

Baxter MA. Acromegaly and transsphenoidal hypophysectomy: A case report. AANA J 1994 Apr; 62(2):182–185.
Bell TN. Diabetes insipidus. Crit Care Nurs Clin North Am 1994 Dec; 6(4):675–685.
Chipps E. Transsphenoidal surgery for pituitary tumors. Crit Care Nurse 1992 Jan; 12(1):30–39.
Closson BL, Beck LA and Swift MA. Diabetes insipidus and spinal cord injury: A challenging combination. Rehabil Nurs 1993 Nov–Dec; 18(6)368–374.
Elster AD. Modern imaging of the pituitary. Radiology 1993 Apr; 187(1):1–14.
Klibanski A and Zervas NT. Diagnosis and management of hormone-secreting pituitary adenomas. N Eng J Med 1991 Mar 21; 324(12):822–830.
Nalbach DA and Carson MA. Prolactinoma: A review and case study. Crit Care Nurs 1991 Oct; 11(9):48–49, 52–57.
Rolih CA and Ober KP. Pituitary apoplexy. Endocrinol Metab Clin North Am 1993 Jun: 22(2):291–302.
Smith-Rooker JL, Garret A, and Hodges LC. Case management of the patient with pituitary tumor. Medsurg Nurs 1993 Aug; 2(4): 265–274.

Pancreatic Disorders

Bohnen JMA et al. Guidelines for clinical care: Anti-infective agents for intra-abdominal infection. Arch Surg 1992 Jan; 127(1): 83–89.
Broderick RL. Preventing complications in acute pancreatitis. Dimens Crit Care Nurs 1991 Sep-Oct; 10(6):262–270.
Frey CF. Management of necrotizing pancreatitis. West J Med 1993 Dec; 159(6):675–680.
Holt S. Chronic pancreatitis. South Med J 1993 Feb; 86(2):201–207.
Jalleh RP and Williamson RCN. Pancreatic exocrine and endocrine function after operations for chronic pancreatitis. Ann Surg 1992 Dec; 216(6):656–662.
Kohn CL, Brozenec S, and Foster PF. Nutritional support for the patient with pancreatobiliary disease. Crit Care Nurs Clin North Am 1993 Mar; 5(1):37–45.
Krumberger JM. Acute pancreatitis. Crit Care Nurs Clin North Am 1993 Mar; 5(1):185–202.
Leach SD, Gorelick FS, and Modlin IM. New perspectives on acute pancreatitis. Scand J Gastroenterol 1992; 27(Suppl 192):29–38.
Lillemoe KD. Pancreatic disease in the elderly patients. Surg Clin North Am 1994 Apr; 74(2):317–344.
Marulendra S and Kirby DF. Nutrition support in pancreatitis. Nutr Clin Pract 1995 Apr; 10(2):45–53.
McConnell E and Lewis LW. Managing the patient with pancreatitis. Nursing 1991 Nov; 21(11):98–102.
Peterson KJ and Solie CJ. Interpreting lab values in pancreatitis. Am J Nurs 1994 Nov; 94(11):45 A–B, 56 F.
Ranson JHC. The role of surgery in the management of acute pancreatitis. Ann Surg 1990 Apr; 211(4):382–393.
Sidhu SS and Tandon RK. The pathogenesis of chronic pancreatitis. Postgrad Med J 1995 Feb; 71(832):67–70.

Siegel JH and Cohen SA. Therapeutic pancreaticobiliary endoscopy. Gastroenterologist 1995 Mar; 3(1):28–40.
Smith A. When the pancreas self-destructs. Am J Nurs 1991 Sep; 91(9):38–48.
Steinberg WM. Acute pancreatitis: Never leave a stone unturned. (Editorial). N Engl J Med 1992 Feb 27; 326(9):635–637.
Thompson C. Managing acute pancreatitis. RN 1992 Mar; 55(3): 52–56.
Warshaw AL and Fernandez-del Castillo C. Pancreatic carcinoma. N Engl J Med 1992 Feb 13; 326(7):455–465.
Wilson C and Imrie CW. Current concepts in the management of pancreatitis. Drugs 1991 Mar; 41(3):358–366.

Nursing Research Profile for Unit 9

Metabolic and Endocrine Function

Overview

Nursing research studies in the area of metabolic and endocrine function continue to focus on issues associated with diabetes and factors affecting its management.

Tu K-S, McDaniel G, and Gay JT. Diabetes self-care knowledge, behaviors and metabolic control of older adults. The effect of a posteducational follow-up program. Diabetes Educator 1993 Jan/Feb; 19(1):25–29.

This study was designed to evaluate the impact of postteaching telephone follow-up on patient self-care behaviors and knowledge. A convenience sample of 31 elderly patients with diabetes mellitus participated in the study. The subjects were randomly assigned to an experimental or a control group. Subjects in the experimental group were contacted by telephone within 24 to 48 hours after discharge from the hospital. The calls were repeated at weekly intervals for 3 weeks. Each phone call consisted of assessing the subject's self-care knowledge and practice in self-care activities or behaviors. Supplemental instructions were provided when indicated. Subjects in the control group did not receive a phone call after discharge from the hospital. Diabetes self-care knowledge was assessed in both groups with a diabetes knowledge scale approximately 5 to 6 weeks following hospital discharge, and a telephone intervention checklist was used to assess the effect of the intervention on self-care behaviors such as compliance with home blood glucose monitoring, drug therapy, exercise and diet. Glycosylated hemoglobin (HbA_{1c}) was used to measure the postintervention blood glucose level 3 months after discharge.

Results indicated that the experimental group had higher scores on the knowlege test than the control group, but the difference was not statistically significant. Blood glucose control as measured by HbA_{1c} was also not significantly different in the two groups. However, significantly more individuals in the control group had deficient behaviors related to prevention of hypoglycemia and dietary compliance. The control group members were less likely to report symptoms and seek assistance from health care providers.

Nursing Implications. The findings of this study support the value of follow-up telephone calls to elderly patients with diabetes in promoting compliance with the therapeutic regimen, clarifying information and instructions, and motivating patients to continue to follow the recommendations given to them to control their diabetes.

Schwab T, Meyer J, and Merrell R. Measuring attitudes and health beliefs among Mexican Americans with diabetes. Diabetes Educator 1994 May/Jun; 20(3):221–227.

Non–insulin dependent diabetes (NIDDM) is a major health problem among Mexican-Americans, who are three to five times more likely to suffer the effects of NIDDM than non-Hispanic whites. The risk for vascular complications is also greater, with a six-times greater incidence of end-stage renal disease and a two- to three-times greater incidence of retinopathy. Because of the importance of adherence to diabetes therapy in preventing complications, strategies are needed to assess the attitudes and health beliefs that affect adherence of this group so that effective and realistic intervention strategies can be initiated.

The Health Belief Model (HBM) was used as the theoretical framework for this study of the attitudes and beliefs of low-income Mexican Americans with diabetes. The sample consisted of 199 subjects. Individual interviews were conducted with subjects using a 65-item questionnaire designed to assess the factors identified in the HBM as influences on health behaviors and to address the cultural aspects of the population. The HBM factors included perceived susceptibility, severity, benefits, and barriers. The cultural portion of the questionnaire addressed acculturation and fatalism.

Analysis of the subjects' responses to the questionnaire revealed that the HBM does not explain health beliefs among low-income Mexican Americans. Other factors, such as poverty or daily struggles, may have a greater impact on perceptions of health than do those factors identified in the HBM.

Nursing Implications. The importance of considering cultural factors and beliefs is emphasized by the results of this study. The need for culturally sensitive assessment tools and strategies along with interventions is apparent. Furthermore, the nurse must be nonjudgmental when interacting with patients from other cultures.

Zaldivar A and Smolowitz J. Perceptions of the importance placed on religion and folk medicine by non-Mexican-American Hispanic adults with diabetes. Diabetes Educator 1994 Jul/Aug; 20(4):303–306.

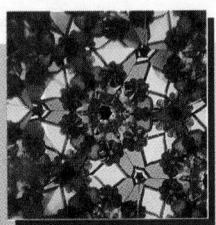

Hispanic adults have a higher incidence of diabetes than African-Americans and non-Hispanic whites and a higher incidence of severe retinopathy and end-stage renal disease. Despite this, there is underutilization of screening and treatment centers by Hispanic adults and a high rate of noncompliance with therapeutic regimens among Hispanics. In an effort to explore factors related to these issues, these researchers examined the views of adult Hispanics toward diabetes and the relationship between those views and motivation to seek medical attention.

A sample of 104 non–Mexican-American Hispanic adults with diabetes were surveyed via a questionnaire developed by the researchers for this study. The questionnaire addressed religious, spiritual, and folk medicine beliefs found in the Hispanic population and beliefs about susceptibility to diabetes and its complications. Analysis of the subjects' responses on the questionnaire revealed that they were knowledgeable about the potential complications of diabetes but believed them to be inevitable. Responses indicated a fatalistic acceptance of diabetes and a sense of hopelessness about their ability to control or prevent long-term complications. Many subjects indicated that control of their diabetes was in God's hands.

Nursing Implications. The results of this study indicate that knowledge about complications is not necessarily a good predictor of one's attitudes toward control of those complications. When teaching about diabetes and its management, the nurse must consider the patient's cultural background and beliefs. Strong beliefs in spiritual influences on diabetes control may be addressed by involving the patient's spiritual advisor in the educational efforts.

Leggett-Frazier N, Turner MS, and Vincent PA. Measuring the diabetes knowledge of nurses in long-term care facilities. Diabetes Educator 1994 Jul/Aug; 20(4):307–310.

As the elderly population grows, the incidence of diabetes in older adults is increasing. Inevitably this will result in a greater number of persons with diabetes in nursing homes. This study was undertaken to assess the knowledge of nurses (RNs and LPNs) in long-term-care facilities about diabetes and its management. A 36-item diabetes knowledge test was developed for use in this study and administered to nurses employed in four long-term-care facilities. The test assessed knowledge about blood glucose and ketone monitoring, medications, illness care, foot care, exercise, diet, hypoglycemia, hyperglycemia, and patient/family education. Of 128 nurses eligible to participate, 59 (46%) completed the test.

The respondents attained a mean score of 67% of the items correct, less than the 70% cutoff score considered to be a passing score by the researchers. The sample scored highest (mean scores > 70%) on foot care and patient/family education and lowest (mean scores < 40%) on illness care, blood glucose monitoring, medications, and hypoglycemia.

Nursing Implications. The results of this study support the need for further education and periodic reinforcement of teaching about diabetes and its management to *all* nurses, including those in long-term-care facilities. Advances in diabetes management make it essential that nurses have a strong foundation in diabetes care regardless of the practice setting.

LeMone P. Human sexuality in adults with insulin-dependent diabetes mellitus. Image: J Nurs Scholarship 1993 Summer; 25(2):101–105.

This qualitative study explored human sexuality in adults with insulin-dependent (Type I) diabetes mellitus. The grounded theory method was used to collect and analyze data. Personal, unstructured interviews were conducted with each participant. The interviews began with a general question about the participant's experiences with sexual function since being diagnosed with insulin-dependent diabetes. Interviews were audiotaped for later analysis. Several coding systems were used to analyze and categorize themes emerging from the interview data. Established methods were used to ensure credibility and verification of the theory that emerged from the study.

Eleven adult men ($n = 6$) and women ($n = 5$) participated in the study. They ranged in age from 27 to 70 years of age and had been diagnosed with insulin-dependent diabetes as adults. The range of years since diagnosis was from 1 year to 28 years. All subjects were Caucasian; nine subjects were married.

The core phenomonon that emerged was described by the researcher as "transforming," reflecting the constant adjustment to the effects of diabetes mellitus and its treatment on sexuality. This process of transforming was dependent on a variety of factors, including control of symptoms, side effects of treatment, duration and severity of illness, and the participants' age and gender.

Subcategories of transforming identified by the researcher included "valuing self" and "meeting intimacy needs." Valuing self reflected integration of new values associated with the diagnosis of diabetes and included accepting oneself as diabetic, feeling different and experiencing loss, and maintaining control over the illness and oneself. Meeting intimacy needs reflected the basic human need for love and belonging and described relationships with others as well as sexual intimacy. Meeting intimacy needs was described as having two conditions: experiencing a change in sexual function because of diabetes and maintaining the relationship.

Nursing Implications. Because of the importance of human sexuality to quality of life, it is important for nurses to recognize the potential impact of diabetes and its treatment on sexuality and sexual function. It is clear from the findings of this study that sexuality extends beyond the physical aspects of sexual function. Although physical sexual function may be affected by diabetes, other aspects of sexuality such as self esteem may also be affected. The results of this study emphasize the importance of assessment and open discussion of these aspects with any patient with diabetes mellitus.

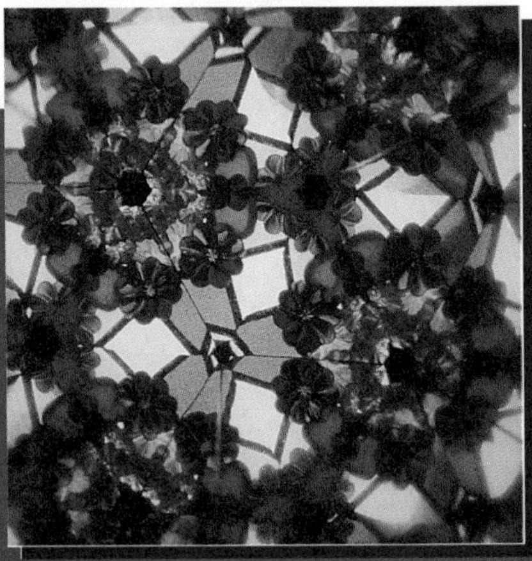

UNIT 10
Urinary and Renal Function

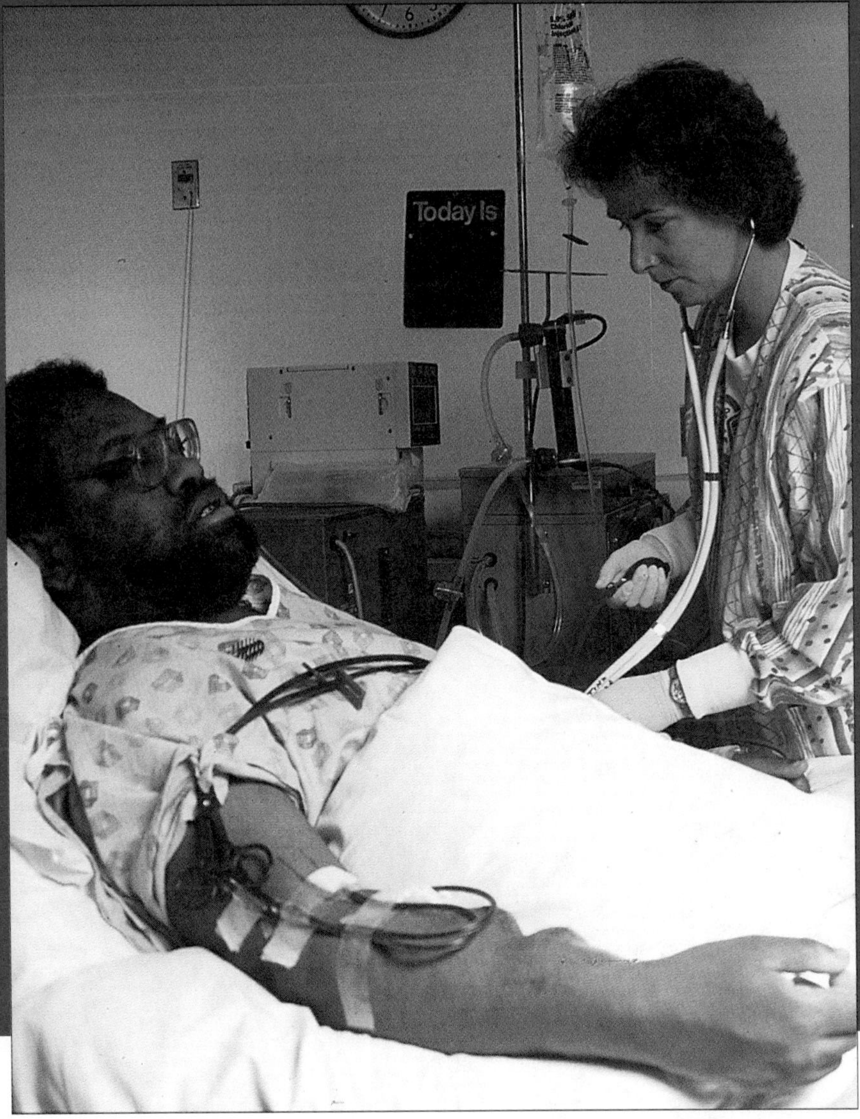

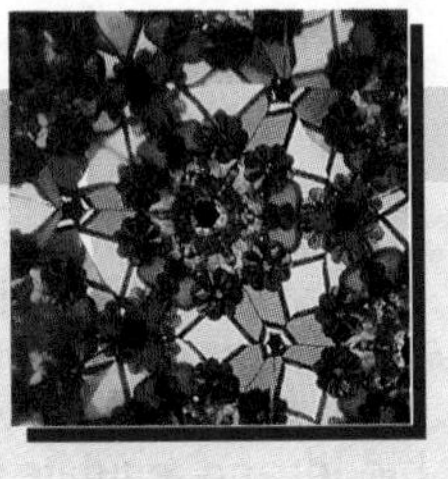

41

Assessment of Urinary and Renal Function

CHAPTER OUTLINE

Physiologic Overview
Anatomy of the Urinary System
Urine Composition
Functions of the Kidney
Storage of Urine and Voiding
Assessment
Clinical Manifestations of Urinary and Renal Dysfunction
Health History
Physical Assessment
Diagnostic Evaluation
Urinalysis
Renal Function Tests
Ultrasound
X-ray and Other Imaging Studies
Endourology (Urologic Endoscopic Procedures)
Biopsy of the Kidney
Radioisotope Studies
Urodynamic Measurements
Nursing Care of Patients Undergoing Assessment of the Urinary/Renal System
Nursing Diagnoses
Planning, Implementation, and Evaluation
Gerontologic Considerations
Critical Thinking Exercises

LEARNING OBJECTIVES

On completion of this chapter, the learner will be able to:

1. Describe the role of the kidney in the regulation of fluid and electrolyte balance, acid–base balance, and blood pressure
2. Use assessment parameters for determining the status of renal and urinary function
3. Describe diagnostic tests used to determine renal and urinary function
4. Use the nursing process to formulate a plan of care for patients undergoing assessment of the urinary/renal system

Physiologic Overview

The kidneys, ureters, bladder, and urethra compose the urinary system. The kidneys' main functions are to regulate fluids and electrolytes and the acid–base composition of body fluids; remove metabolic end products from the blood; and regulate blood pressure. The urine that is formed as a result of these processes is transported from the kidneys through the ureters to the urinary bladder, where it is temporarily stored. During urination, the bladder contracts and the urine is excreted from the body through the urethra.

Although fluid and electrolytes can be lost by other routes and other organs participate in acid–base balance, it is the kidneys that precisely regulate the internal chemical environment of the body. This renal excretory function is necessary to maintain life. However, unlike the cardiovascular and respiratory systems, complete malfunction of the kidneys may not cause immediate death. Dialysis ("artificial kidney") and other treatment modalities can be used as substitutes for certain functions of the kidneys.

An important feature of the renal system is its ability to adapt to wide variations in fluid load based on individual habits and patterns. The kidneys must be able to excrete dietary and metabolic waste products in the amounts that are taken in and not eliminated by other organs. On a daily basis, this usually amounts to 1 to 2 liters of water, 6 to 8 g of salt (sodium chloride), 6 to 8 g of potassium chloride, and 70 mg of acid equivalents per day. In addition, urea, an end product of protein metabolism, and other waste products are excreted in the urine. The amount of the substances taken in may differ if intravenous fluids, total parenteral nutrition, or nasogastric tube feedings are administered.

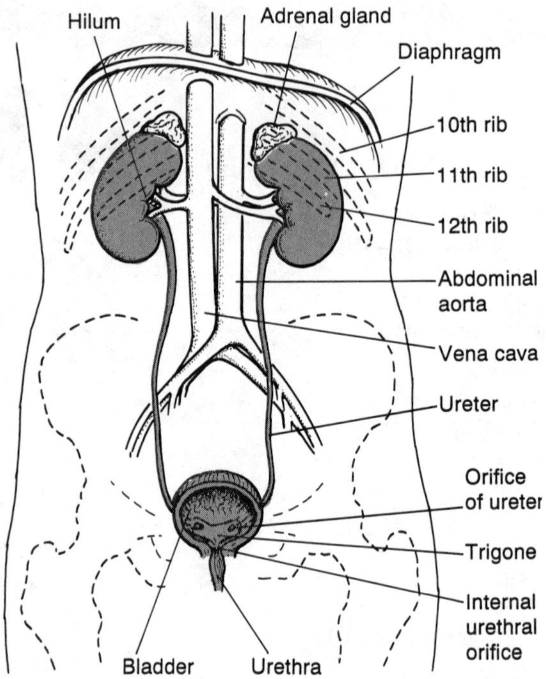

FIGURE 41-1. The urinary tract, showing the location of the kidneys, ureters, and bladder.

Anatomy of the Urinary System

The kidneys are paired organs, each weighing approximately 125 g, located in a position lateral to the lower thoracic vertebrae, a few centimeters to the right and left of the midline (Fig. 41-1). They are surrounded by a thin, fibrous tissue known as the renal capsule. Anteriorly, the kidneys are separated from the abdominal cavity and its contents by layers of peritoneum. Posteriorly, they are shielded by the lower thoracic wall. Blood is supplied to each kidney through the renal artery and is drained through the renal vein. The renal arteries arise from the abdominal aorta, and the renal veins carry blood back into the inferior vena cava. The kidneys can efficiently clear the blood of waste materials, in part because blood flow through the kidneys is great and represents 25% of cardiac output.

Urine is formed within the functional units of the kidneys, known as **nephrons.** The urine formed within these nephrons passes into collecting ducts, the tubules, that join to form the pelvis of each kidney. Each kidney pelvis gives rise to a ureter. The ureter is a long tube with a wall composed largely of smooth muscle. It connects each kidney to the bladder and functions as a conduit for urine.

The urinary bladder is a hollow organ that is situated anteriorly just behind the pubic bone. It acts as a temporary storage reservoir for the urine. The walls of the bladder consist largely of smooth muscle called the detrusor muscle. Contraction of this muscle is mainly responsible for emptying the bladder during urination. The urethra arises from the bladder; in the male it passes through the penis, and in the female opens just anterior to the vagina. In the male, the prostate gland, which lies just below the bladder neck, surrounds the urethra posteriorly and laterally. The external urinary sphincter is a round, voluntary muscle that controls the initiation of urination.

The Nephron. The kidney is divided into an outer portion called the cortex and an inner portion known as the medulla (Fig. 41-2). In the human, each kidney is composed of approximately 1 million nephrons. The nephron, considered the functional unit of the kidney, consists of a glomerulus and a tubule (Fig. 41-3). Like capillaries in general, the walls of the glomerular capillaries are composed of a layer of endothelial cells and a basement membrane. Epithelial cells are located on one side of the basement membrane, and endothelial cells are located on the other. The glomerulus extends to form the tubule, which is divided into three parts: a proximal tubule, the loop of Henle, and a distal tubule. The distal tubules coalesce to form collecting ducts. The ducts pass through the renal cortex and the medulla to empty into the pelvis of the kidney.

Function of the Nephron. The process of urine formation begins as blood flows through the glomerulus. The glomerulus, the beginning of the nephron, is composed of tufts of capillaries that are supplied with blood by an afferent arteriole and drained by an efferent arteriole. The blood pressure determines how fast and under what pressure blood passes through the glomerulus. As the blood passes through this structure, filtering occurs. Water and small molecules are allowed to pass and larger molecules stay in the

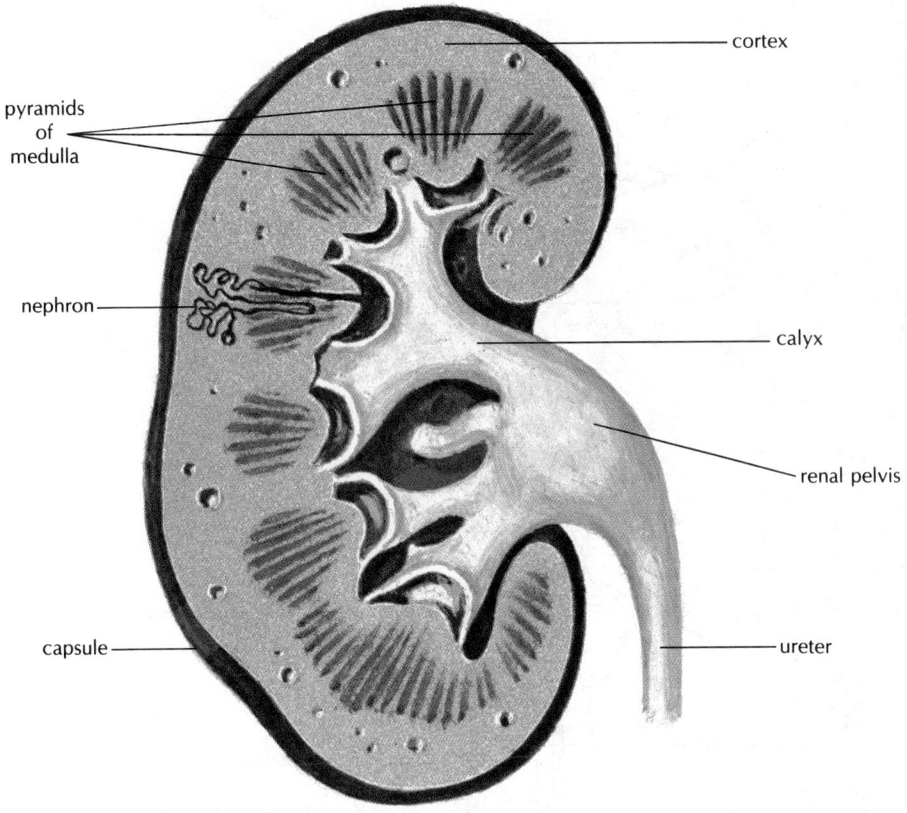

FIGURE 41-2. Section through the kidney, showing its internal structure and an enlarged diagram of the nephron. More than 1 million nephrons are located in the kidney.

blood stream. Fluid is filtered through the walls of the glomerular capillary tufts and enters the tubules. This fluid is known as "filtrate."

Under normal conditions, approximately 20% of the plasma passing through the glomeruli is filtered into the nephron, amounting to about 180 liters of filtrate per day. The filtrate, very similar to blood plasma without its larger molecules (proteins, red cells, white cells, and platelets) consists essentially of water, electrolytes, and other small molecules. Within the tubule, some of these substances are selectively reabsorbed into the blood. Other substances are secreted from the blood into the filtrate as it travels down the tubule. Filtrate becomes concentrated in the distal tubule and collecting ducts and becomes the urine that reaches the pelvis of the kidney. Some substances, such as glucose, are normally completely reabsorbed in the tubule and do not appear in the urine.

The processes of reabsorption and secretion in the tubule frequently involve active transport and require the utilization of energy. The various substances normally filtered by the glomerulus, reabsorbed by the tubules, and excreted in the urine include sodium, chloride, bicarbonate, potassium, glucose, urea, creatinine, and uric acid. The amounts involved are shown in Table 41-1.

Urine Composition

The kidney functions as the main excretory organ of the body. It disposes of end products of the body's metabolism. When the kidneys are functioning normally, the amounts of these materials excreted per day are exactly equal to the amounts ingested and formed, so that over a period of time there is no net change in the total body composition.

Urine is composed primarily of *water.* A normal person ingests approximately 1 to 2 liters of water per day, and normally all but 400 to 500 ml of this fluid intake is excreted in the urine. The remainder is lost from the skin, from the lungs during breathing, and in the feces. *Electrolytes,* including sodium, potassium, chloride, bicarbonate, and other less abundant ions, are also excreted by the kidneys (Table 41-1). The average American diet contains about 6 to 8 g each of sodium chloride (salt) and potassium chloride per day, and nearly all of this is excreted in the urine.

The third group of substances appearing in the urine is made up of the end products of protein metabolism. The major end product is *urea,* of which about 25 g is produced and excreted per day. Other products of protein metabolism that must be excreted are creatinine, phosphates, and sulfates. Uric acid, formed as a product of nucleic acid metabolism, is also eliminated in the urine.

It is important to recognize that some substances that are present in high concentrations in the blood are ordinarily completely reabsorbed by active transport in the renal tubule. Amino acids and glucose, for example, are usually filtered at the glomerulus and reabsorbed so that neither is excreted in the urine. *Glucose,* however, will appear in the urine if its blood level is so high that its concentration in the glomerular filtrate exceeds the capacity of the tubules to reabsorb it. Normally, the glucose is completely reabsorbed when its concentration in the blood is less than 200 mg/dl (11 mmol/L). In diabetes, where the blood glucose levels exceed the kidney's reabsorption capacity, glucose will appear in the urine. *Protein* is also not normally found in the

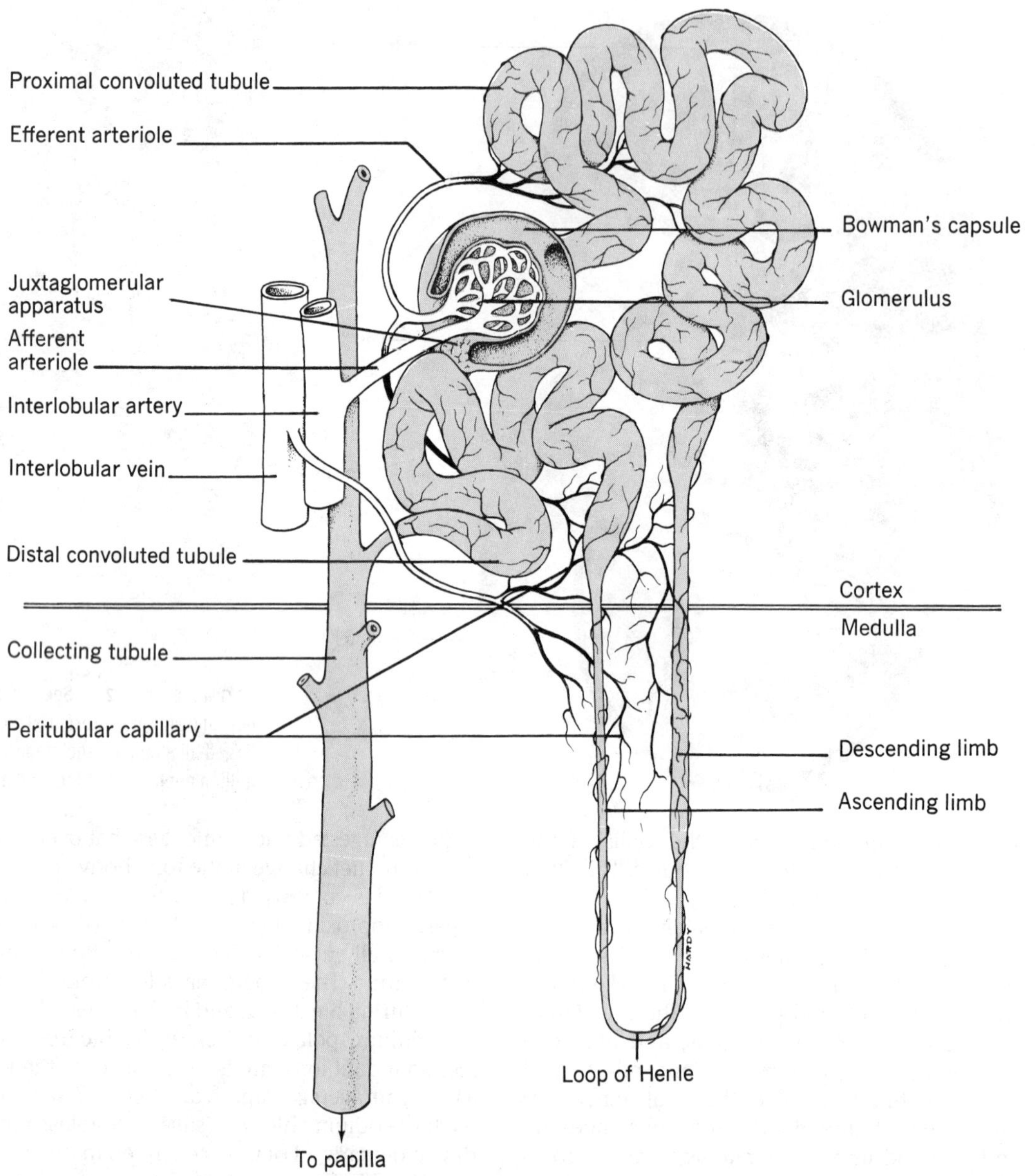

FIGURE 41-3. Diagram of a nephron showing the glomerular and tubular structures.

TABLE 41-1 Filtration, Reabsorption, and Excretion of Certain Normal Constituents of Plasma

	Filtered 24 Hr	Reabsorbed 24 Hr	Excreted 24 Hr*
Sodium	540.0 g	537.0 g	3.3 g
Chloride	630.0 g	625.0 g	5.3 g
Bicarbonate	300.0 g	300.0 g	0.3 g
Potassium	28.0 g	24.0 g	3.9 g
Glucose	140.0 g	140.0 g	0.0 g
Urea	53.0 g	28.0 g	25.0 g
Creatinine	1.4 g	0.0 g	1.4 g
Uric acid	8.5 g	7.7 g	0.8 g

*These are typical normal values. Wide variation is found, depending on diet.

urine. These molecules are not filtered at the glomerulus because of their large size. The appearance of protein in the urine usually signifies damage to the glomeruli that causes them to become porous and leak larger molecules.

Functions of the Kidney

Regulation of Acid Excretion

The catabolism or breakdown of proteins involves the production of acid compounds, in particular phosphoric and sulfuric acids. In addition, a certain amount of acid material is ingested daily. Unlike CO_2, these are nonvolatile acids and cannot be eliminated by the lung. Because accumulation of these acids in the blood would lower its *p*H, (more acidic) and inhibit cell function, they must be excreted in the urine. A person whose kidney function is normal excretes approximately 70 mEq of acid each day. The kidney is able to excrete some of this acid directly into the urine to the extent of lowering urine *p*H to 4.5, 1000 times more acidic than blood.

More acid usually needs to be eliminated from the body than can be excreted directly as free acid in the urine. This is accomplished by the renal excretion of acid that is bound to chemical buffers. The acid (H^+) is secreted by the renal tubular cells into the filtrate, where it is buffered chiefly by phosphate ions and ammonia (when buffered with acid, ammonia becomes ammonium). Phosphate is present in the glomerular filtrate, and ammonia is produced by the cells of the renal tubules and secreted into the tubular fluid. Through the buffering process, the kidney is able to excrete large quantities of acid in a bound form without further lowering the *p*H of the urine.

Regulation of Electrolyte Excretion

Sodium. The amount of electrolytes and water that must be excreted by the kidney each day varies greatly, depending on the amounts ingested. The 180 liters of filtrate formed by the glomeruli each day contain about 1100 g of sodium chloride. All but 2 liters of water and 6 to 8 g of sodium chloride are normally reabsorbed by the kidneys. Water from the filtrate follows the reabsorbed sodium in order to maintain osmotic balance. The remaining water, sodium chloride, other electrolytes, and waste products are then excreted as urine. Thus, more than 99% of the water and sodium filtered at the glomeruli is reabsorbed into the blood by the time the urine leaves the body. By regulating the amount of sodium (and therefore water) reabsorbed, the kidney can regulate the volume of body fluids.

- If sodium is excreted in excess of the amount ingested, the patient will become dehydrated.
- If less sodium is excreted than is ingested, the patient will retain fluid.

The regulation of the amount of sodium excreted depends on **aldosterone,** a hormone synthesized and released from the adrenal cortex. In the presence of increased aldosterone in the blood, less sodium is excreted in the urine since aldosterone fosters renal reabsorption of sodium.

Release of aldosterone from the adrenal cortex is largely under the control of angiotensin, a peptide hormone manufactured in the liver and activated in the lung. Angiotensin levels are in turn controlled by renin, a hormone that is released from cells in the kidneys. This complex system is activated when pressure in the renal arterioles falls below normal levels, as occurs with shock and dehydration. The effect of activation of this system is to increase the retention of water and expansion of intravascular fluid volume. Adrenocorticotropic hormone (ACTH) also stimulates aldosterone secretion independent of fluid volume changes (Fig. 41-4).

Potassium. Another electrolyte whose concentration in the body fluids is regulated by the kidney is potassium, the most abundant intracellular ion. The excretion of potassium by the kidney is increased by elevated aldosterone levels, in contrast to the effects of aldosterone on sodium excretion.

- Retention of potassium is the most life-threatening effect of renal failure.

Regulation of Water Excretion

Regulation of the amount of water excreted is also an important function of the kidney. With a large intake of water or fluid, a large volume of dilute urine must be excreted. Conversely, with a low fluid intake, the urine that is excreted is concentrated.

Osmolality. The relative degree of dilution or concentration of the urine can be measured in terms of its **osmolality.** This term reflects the number of particles (electrolytes and other molecules) dissolved in the urine. The filtrate in the glomerular capillary normally has the same osmolality as the blood, with a value of approximately 300 mOsm/L (300 mmol/L). As the filtrate passes through the tubules and collecting ducts, the osmolality may vary from 50 to 1200 mOsm/L, reflecting the maximal diluting and concentrating abilities of the kidney.

The osmolality of the urine specimen can be measured. In measurement of urine osmolality, the solution is the water component of the urine and the particles are electrolytes and end products of metabolism. When an individual is either dehydrated or retaining fluid there is usually less water and proportionately more particles present (indicating high osmolality), giving the urine its concentrated appearance. When an individual excretes a large volume of water the particles are diluted (indicating low osmolality) and the urine appears dilute.

Certain substances can alter the volume of water excreted and are described as osmotically active. When these substances are filtered they will pull water across the glomerulus and tubules and increase the volume of urine. Glucose and proteins are two examples of osmotically active molecules.

Normal urine osmolality of a normal urine sample is 300 to 1100 mOsm/kg; after a 12-hour fluid restriction urine osmolality normally ranges from 500 to 850 mOsm/kg. This wide range of normal makes the test valuable only in situations where the kidneys' concentrating and diluting abilities are questioned.

Urine Specific Gravity. Urine specific gravity is less precise than urine osmolality and reflects both the quantity and the nature of particles. Therefore, protein, glucose, and intravenous contrast agents affect specific gravity more than osmolality. *Normal specific gravity is 1.015 to 1.025* (when fluid intake is normal).

Antidiuretic Hormone (ADH). Regulation of water excretion and urine concentration is carried out in the tubule by varying the amount of water that is reabsorbed in relation to electrolyte reabsorption. The glomerular filtrate has essentially the same electrolyte composition as the blood plasma without the proteins. The amount of water that is reabsorbed is under the control of antidiuretic hormone (ADH or vasopressin).

ADH is a hormone that is secreted by the posterior part of the pituitary gland in response to changes in osmolality of the blood. With decreased water intake, blood osmolality tends to rise and stimulate ADH release. ADH then acts on the kidney in order to increase reabsorption of water, thereby returning the osmolality of the blood to normal. With excess water intake, the secretion of ADH by the pituitary is suppressed and, therefore, less water is reabsorbed by the kidney tubule. This latter situation leads to increased urine volume (**diuresis**).

- Loss of the ability to concentrate and dilute the urine is the most common early manifestation of kidney disease. A dilute urine of fixed specific gravity (approximately 1.010) or fixed osmolality (approximately 300 mOsm/L) is excreted.

Autoregulation of Blood Pressure

Regulation of blood pressure is also a function of the renal system. A hormone known as **renin** is secreted by the juxtaglomerular cells when blood pressure decreases. An enzyme converts renin to angiotensin I which is then converted to angiotensin II, the most powerful vasoconstrictor known. The vasoconstriction causes the blood pressure to increase. Aldosterone is secreted by the adrenal cortex in response to stimulation by the pituitary gland and release of ACTH in response to poor perfusion or increasing serum osmolality. The result is an increase in blood pressure (Fig. 41-4).

Renal Clearance

The test most commonly used to evaluate how well the kidney performs its excretory function is termed **clearance.** Clearance of substance A is shown by the following equation: clearance equals the urine concentration of A times the urine volume in a given time, divided by the plasma concentration of A.

$$\text{Clearance} = \frac{(\text{urine concentration of A}) \times (\text{urine volume in a given time})}{\text{plasma concentration of A}}$$

For example, if the arterial plasma concentration of a substance is 0.1 mg/ml, the urine concentration of the same substance is 50 mg/ml, and the urine volume is 1.0 ml/min,

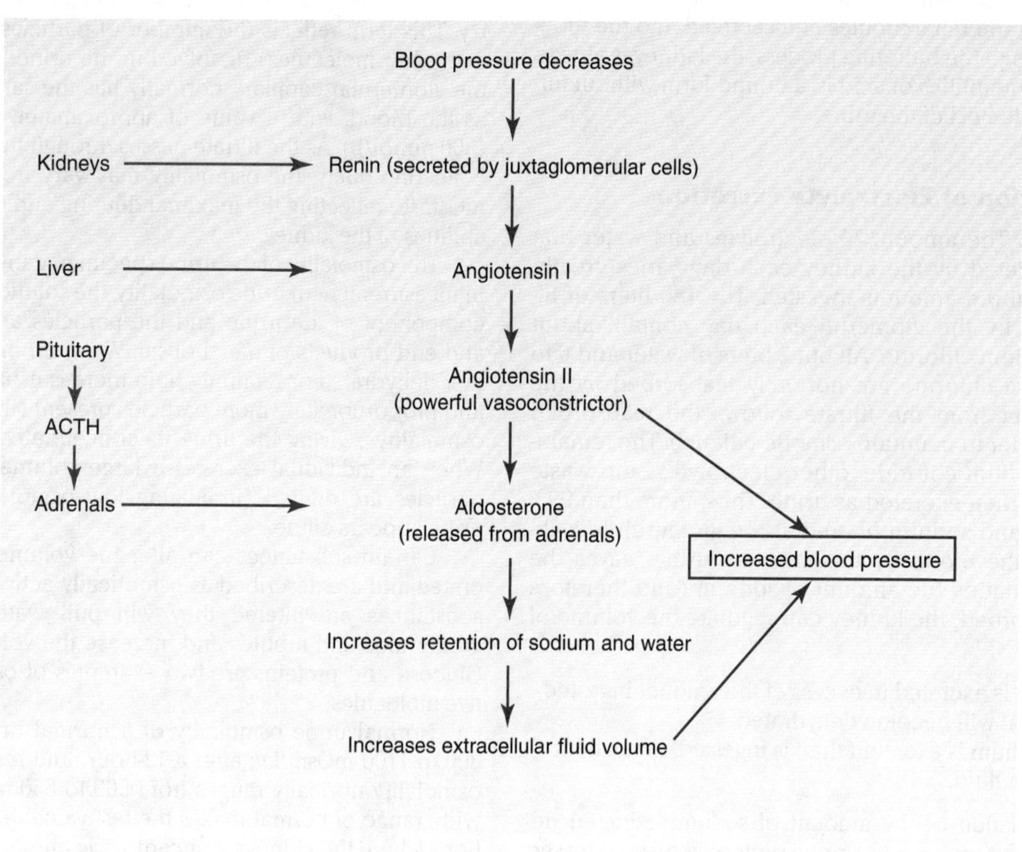

FIGURE 41-4. Regulation of blood pressure.

the clearance of that substance according to the above equation is 500 ml/min. This means that 500 ml of blood are completely cleared of that substance in one minute. In the body, few substances are actually completely cleared from the blood during a single pass through the kidney. In the example given above, if the blood is cleared of only 50% of the substance, urine concentration of the substance would be 25 mg/ml and the calculated renal clearance would be 250 ml/min.

Creatinine. It is possible to measure the renal clearance of any substance, but the one measure that has proved particularly useful is the creatinine clearance. **Creatinine** is an endogenous waste product of skeletal muscle that is excreted by glomerular filtration and is not appreciably reabsorbed or secreted by the renal tubules. Therefore, creatinine clearance is a good measure of the glomerular filtration rate (GFR). *The normal adult GFR is about 100 to 120 ml/min (1.67 to 2.00 ml/sec).*

Storage of Urine and Voiding

Urine formed by the kidney is transported from the renal pelvis through the ureters and into the bladder. This movement is facilitated by peristaltic waves occurring about one to five times per minute and generated by the smooth muscle in the ureter wall. There are no sphincters between the bladder and the ureters, although reflux of urine from the bladder is normally prevented by the unidirectional nature of the peristaltic waves and because each ureter enters the bladder at an oblique angle. However, with overdistention of the bladder due to disease, the elevated pressure in the bladder can be transmitted back through the ureters, leading to ureteral distention and possible reflux or back-up of urine. This can lead to kidney infection (pyelonephritis) and kidney damage from the elevated pressure (hydronephrosis).

Bladder Pressure. The pressure in the bladder is normally very low, even as the urine accumulates, because the bladder's smooth muscle adapts to the increased stretch as the bladder is slowly filled. The first sensations of bladder filling ordinarily occur when about 100 to 150 ml of urine are present in the bladder. In most cases, a desire to void occurs when the bladder contains approximately 200 to 300 ml of urine. With 400 ml, a marked feeling of fullness is usually present.

Muscle Control. Voiding of urine is controlled by contraction of the **external urethral sphincter.** This muscle is under voluntary control and is innervated by nerves from the sacral area of the spinal cord. Voluntary control is a learned behavior and is not present at birth. When there is a desire to urinate, the external urethral sphincter is relaxed, and the **detrusor muscle** (bladder smooth muscle) contracts and expels the urine from the bladder through the urethra. The pressure generated in the bladder during urination (micturition) is approximately 50 to 150 cm of water. Urine remaining in the urethra drains by gravity in the female and is expelled by voluntary muscle contractions in the male.

Neural Control. The contraction of the detrusor muscle is regulated by a reflex involving the parasympathetic nervous system. The reflex is integrated in the sacral portion of the spinal tract. The sympathetic nervous system plays no essential part in micturition but does prevent semen from entering the bladder during ejaculation.

If the pelvic nerves to the bladder and sphincter are destroyed, voluntary control and reflex urination are abolished and the bladder becomes overdistended with urine. If the spinal pathways from the brain to the urinary system are destroyed (for example, after a spinal cord injury), reflex contraction of the bladder is maintained but voluntary control over the process is lost. In both of these situations, the muscle of the bladder can contract and expel urine but the contractions are generally insufficient to empty the bladder completely, and **residual urine** (urine left in the bladder after voiding) remains.

Catheterization. Catheterization—passage of a catheter through the urethra into the bladder—can be used to assess bladder function by permitting the volume of residual urine to be measured. Normally, residual urine amounts to no more than 50 ml. However, catheterization is avoided whenever possible (and strict asepsis is used whenever it is necessary) because it increases the risk of infection. Another test for bladder dysfunction is to measure the pressure in the bladder after instillation of various volumes of saline. This latter procedure is called a **cystometrogram**.

Assessment

Clinical Manifestations of Urinary and Renal Dysfunction

The following signs and symptoms are suggestive of urinary tract disease: pain, changes in voiding, and gastrointestinal symptoms. When renal disease occurs, symptoms may occur in every system of the body.

Pain

Genitourinary pain is not always present in renal disease but it generally occurs in the more acute conditions. Pain from renal disease is usually caused by obstruction and subsequent sudden distention of the renal capsule. Its severity is related to how quickly the distention develops.

Kidney pain may be felt as a dull ache in the costovertebral angle (the area formed by the rib cage and vertebral column) and may extend to the umbilicus. Ureteral disorders produce pain in the back that radiates to the abdomen, upper thigh, testis, or labium. Pain in the flank (the region between the ribs and ilium), radiating to the lower abdomen or epigastrium and often associated with nausea, vomiting, and paralytic ileus, may indicate renal colic. Bladder pain (low abdominal pain or pain over the suprapubic area) can be due to an overdistended bladder or bladder infection. Urgency, tenesmus (painful straining), and terminal dysuria (pain at the end of voiding) are usually present. Pain at the urethral meatus occurs with irritation of the bladder neck or urethra due to infection (urethritis), trauma, or a foreign body in the lower urinary tract.

Severe pain in the scrotal region results from inflammation and edema of the epididymis or testicle or from torsion of the testicle, while perineal and rectal fullness and pain signal acute prostatitis or prostatic abscess. Back and leg pain may be due to metastasis of cancer of the prostate to the pelvic bones. Pain in the penile shaft may originate from urethral problems, while pain in the glans penis is usually due to prostatitis.

It should be noted that many times kidney disease is not accompanied by pain, and it is often diagnosed because of other symptoms that cause a patient to seek help. Examples of these symptoms include pedal edema, shortness of breath, and changes in urinary elimination.

Changes in Voiding (Micturition)

Voiding or micturition is normally a painless function occurring five to six times daily and occasionally once at night. The average person forms and voids 1200 to 1500 ml of urine in 24 hours. The amount is modified by fluid intake, sweating, environmental temperature, vomiting, or diarrhea. Common problems associated with voiding include frequency, urgency, dysuria, hesitancy, incontinence, enuresis, polyuria, oliguria, and hematuria. These problems and others are described in Chart 41-1.

Gastrointestinal Symptoms

Gastrointestinal symptoms may occur with urologic conditions because the gastrointestinal and urinary tracts have common autonomic and sensory innervation and because of renointestinal reflexes. The anatomic relation of the right kidney to the colon, duodenum, head of the pancreas, common bile duct, liver, and gallbladder may cause gastrointestinal disturbances. The proximity of the left kidney to the colon (splenic flexure), stomach, pancreas, and spleen may also result in intestinal symptoms. These may include nausea, vomiting, diarrhea, abdominal discomfort, and paralytic ileus. Appendicitis also may be accompanied by urinary symptoms.

Health History

When obtaining a health history, it is essential to use language and terms that the patient can understand and to be aware of the embarrassment or discomfort people feel in

CHART 41-1
Glossary

- *Urinary frequency* is voiding that occurs more often than usual when compared with the person's usual pattern or the generally accepted norm of once every 3 to 6 hours. It may result from a variety of conditions: infection, diseases of the urinary tract, metabolic disease, hypertension, and certain medications such as diuretics.
- *Urgency* (strong desire to void) may be due to inflammatory lesions in the bladder, prostate, or urethra; acute bacterial infections or chronic prostatitis in men; or chronic posterior urethrotrigonitis (inflammation of the urethra and trigone of the bladder) in women.
- *Burning on urination* is seen in patients with urethral irritation or bladder infection. Urethritis frequently causes burning during the act of voiding, whereas cystitis may produce burning both during and after urination.
- *Dysuria* (painful or difficult voiding) stems from a wide variety of pathologic conditions.
- *Hesitancy* (undue delay and difficulty in initiating voiding) may indicate compression of the urethra, neurogenic bladder, or outlet obstruction.
- *Nocturia* (excessive urination at night) suggests decreased renal concentrating ability, heart failure, diabetes mellitus, or incomplete bladder emptying.
- *Urinary incontinence* (involuntary loss of urine) may result from injury of the external urinary sphincter, acquired neurogenic disease, or severe urgency that results from infection.
- *Stress incontinence* (intermittent leakage of urine due to sudden strain) results from weakness of the sphincteric mechanism.
- *Enuresis* (involuntary voiding during sleep) is physiologic to the age of 3 years. After that time, it may be functional or symptomatic of obstructive disease of the lower urinary tract.
- *Polyuria* (a large volume of urine voided in a given time) may be due to diabetes mellitus, diabetes insipidus, chronic renal disease, diuretics, or excessive fluid intake.
- *Oliguria* (a small volume of urine; output between 100 and 500 ml/24 hr) and *anuria* (absence of urine in the bladder; output less than 100 ml/24 hours) indicate a serious renal dysfunction requiring immediate medical intervention. These conditions may result from such causes as shock, trauma, incompatible blood transfusion, and medication toxicity. Complete absence of urine (absolute anuria) is usually indicative of complete obstruction of the urinary tract.
- *Hematuria* (red blood cells in the urine) is considered a serious sign because it may indicate cancer of the genitourinary tract, acute glomerulonephritis, or renal tuberculosis. The color of bloody urine depends on the *p*H of the urine and the amount of blood present; acid urine is a dark, smoky color, while alkaline urine is red. Hematuria may also be due to systemic causes such as blood dyscrasias (abnormalities of clotting), anticoagulant therapy, neoplasms, trauma, and extreme exercise.
- *Proteinuria (albuminuria)* (abnormal amounts of protein in the urine) is characteristically seen in all forms of acute and chronic renal disease. Normal urine does not contain persistent protein in significant quantities.

discussing genitourinary functions and symptoms. The patient may "forget" or deny symptoms because of anxiety or embarrassment. Renal disease must be distinguished from urinary disease. Urinary tract diseases or disorders involve any of the structures in the urinary system. Renal disease occurs when the kidney is affected. Dysfunction of the kidney can produce a complex array of symptoms noted throughout the body. The history should include the following information related to urinary and renal function:

- The patient's chief concern or reason for seeking health care
- Presence of pain; its location, character, duration, and relationship to voiding; factors that precipitate it and those that relieve it
- History of urinary tract infections
  - Past treatment or hospitalization for urinary tract infection
  - Presence of fever or chills
  - Previous cystoscopy, use of indwelling urinary catheters, and renal or urinary diagnostic tests
- Symptoms of disorders of voiding
  - Dysuria; when it occurs during voiding (at initiation or termination of voiding)
  - Hesitancy; straining; pain during or after urination
  - Incontinence (stress incontinence; urge incontinence; overflow incontinence; functional incontinence)
- A history of any of the following:
  - Hematuria, change in color or volume of urine
  - Nocturia and its date of onset
  - Childhood diseases ("strep throat," impetigo, nephrotic syndrome)
  - Renal calculi (kidney stones), passage of stones or gravel in urine
  - Disorders that affect kidney function or urinary tract function (diabetes mellitus, hypertension, abdominal trauma, spinal cord injury, other neurologic condition)
- For the female patient: number and type (vaginal vs. cesarean) of deliveries; use of forceps; vaginal infection, discharge, or irritation; contraceptive practices
- Any exposure (occupational, environmental, or recreational) to toxins relevant to urinary tract (*e.g.*, chemicals, plastics, pitch, tar, rubber, smoking exposure)
- Presence or history of genital lesions or sexually transmitted diseases
- Any prescription and over-the-counter medications (including those prescribed for renal or urinary problems)
- History of smoking
- History of drug or alcohol abuse

The nurse not only elicits information about the patient's physical complaints but also assesses psychosocial status, such as anxiety, perceived threats to body image, support systems, and sociocultural patterns. Compiling this information during the initial and subsequent nursing assessments enables the nurse to uncover misunderstandings, lack of knowledge, and need for patient teaching.

Physical Assessment

Because renal dysfunction affects all body systems, a general assessment is indicated. Additionally, the assessment focuses on the urinary tract specifically.

Direct palpation may help determine the size and mobility of the kidneys.

- With the patient in a supine position, the examiner places one hand under the patient's back with the fingers clear of the lower ribs. The other hand (palm down) is placed anterior to the kidney, with the fingers just above the level of the umbilicus (Fig. 41-5).
- The patient is instructed to inhale deeply and the examiner's anterior hand is pushed forward.

It may be possible to feel the smooth, rounded lower pole of the kidney between the hands; the right kidney is felt more easily than the left kidney because it is somewhat lower than the left one.

Renal disease may produce tenderness over the costovertebral angle, which lies where the twelfth or bottom rib joins the spine. Auscultation of the upper quadrants of the abdomen is performed to assess for **bruits** (vascular sounds that might indicate stenosis of the renal arteries).

In a rectal examination in the male, the prostate gland is palpated digitally as a part of the study of urinary difficulty that occurs when there is hyperplasia of the prostate in older men (see Chapter 47).

The inguinal area is examined for enlarged nodes, an inguinal or femoral hernia, and a varicocele. In women, the vulva, urethra, and vagina are examined.

During physical assessment, the patient is assessed for edema, which would indicate fluid retention; the face and dependent parts of the body are specifically assessed.

Diagnostic Evaluation

Urinalysis

Urinalysis may provide important clinical information. Although urinalysis is usually performed routinely on admission and in preoperative screening of patients undergoing elective surgery, it has become controversial because it generally produces few positive findings, considering its cost. However, it remains a routine test in most clinical settings. Urine examination includes evaluating the following:

1. Observation of urine color and clarity
2. Assessment of urine odor
3. Measurement of urine acidity and specific gravity
4. Tests for the presence of protein, glucose, and ketone bodies in the urine (proteinuria, glucosuria, and ketonuria, respectively)
5. Microscopic examination of the urine sediment after centrifuging for the detection of red blood cells (hematuria), white blood cells, casts (cylindruria), crystals (crystalluria), pus (pyuria), and bacteria (bacteriuria)

Indications for performing a urinalysis on admission, if it is not a procedure routinely carried out, are presented in

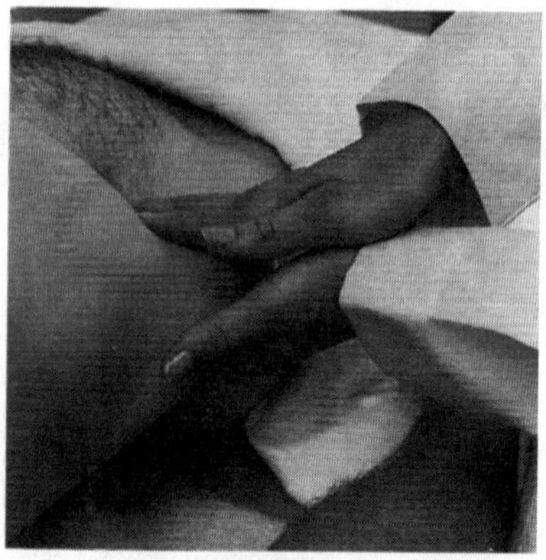

FIGURE 41-5. Technique for palpating the right kidney. One hand is placed under the patient's back with the fingers under the lower rib. The palm of the other hand is placed anterior to the kidney with fingers above the umbilicus. The hand on top is pushed forward as the patient inhales deeply.

Table 41-2. Dipstick urinalysis tests provide a rapid method of screening symptomatic patients for certain substances, including hemoglobin, ketones, protein, and leukocytes (pyuria). Numerous additional tests are applicable in special situations.

Collection of Urine Samples

All urine tests are ideally performed on fresh specimens, preferably the first voiding of the day because this specimen is most concentrated and more likely to reveal abnormalities. Random specimens are satisfactory for most analyses, provided that they have been collected in clean containers and have been adequately protected against bacterial contamination and chemical deterioration. All specimens should be refrigerated as soon as they are obtained. If left standing at room temperature, the urine becomes alkaline because of contamination of urea-splitting bacteria from the environment. Microscopic examination should be performed within a half hour of collection; delay allows cellular elements to disintegrate and bacteria to proliferate in nonsterile specimens. Urine cultures should be processed immediately. If this is not possible, they should be stored at 4°C (39°F).

24-Hour Urine Collection. Many quantitative analytic tests are carried out on specimens of urine collected over a 24-hour period. For this procedure, the patient is instructed to empty the bladder at a specified time (such as 8:00 AM). This urine is discarded. All urine voided during the next 24 hours is collected. The last specimen is collected and saved 24 hours after the collection began (*i.e.*, 8:00 AM).

The patient's bladder should be empty when the test starts and empty when it ends. The urine is collected in a clean container. Depending on the test to be performed, a preservative may be added or the urine may need to be refrigerated. Discarding even one specimen voided during the test period invalidates the test. A successful collection requires understanding and cooperation on the part of the patient and of all involved in the patient's care.

Clean-Catch Midstream Urine Specimens. Urine specimens voided in the usual manner are practically useless for bacteriologic study because of inevitable contamination by organisms residing in the vicinity of the urethral meatus. Such contamination can be avoided by catheterizing the urinary bladder. However, because of the risk of infection, catheterization is not recommended to obtain urine specimens except for specific indications. The clean-catch midstream technique provides the means for reliable bacteriologic studies without catheterization. The instructions for collecting a clean-catch midstream urine specimen are presented in Chart 41-2.

TABLE 41-2 Indications for Diagnostic Admission Urinalysis

History of Following Symptoms	
Dysuria	Frequency
Hesitancy	Urethral discharge
Flank pain	
History of Disorders That Can Affect Renal Function	
Renal disease	Diabetes mellitus
Collagen vascular disease	Exposure to nephrotoxins
Physical Assessment Findings	
Fever of unknown origin	Tenderness at costovertebral angle
Generalized edema	Prostate gland abnormalities
Jaundice	

Renal Function Tests

Renal function tests are used to evaluate the severity of kidney disease and to follow the patient's clinical progress. These tests also provide information about the kidneys' effectiveness in carrying out their excretory function. Results of function tests may be within normal limits until renal function is reduced to less than 50% of normal. Renal function can be assessed most accurately if several tests are performed and their results analyzed together. Common tests of renal function include renal concentration, creatinine clearance, serum creatinine, and blood urea nitrogen (BUN). Table 41-3 explains the purpose and protocol for each of these tests. Because of the important role the kidneys play in maintaining fluid and electrolyte balance, serum electrolyte levels also are assessed.

Ultrasound

Ultrasound uses sound waves that are passed into the body to detect abnormalities. Organs in the urinary system create characteristic ultrasonic images. Abnormalities such as fluid accumulation, masses, malformations, changes in organ size, or obstructions can be identified. Ultrasound is a noninvasive technique, and no special preparation is required except to explain the procedure and its purpose to the patient. Because of its sensitivity, ultrasound has replaced many other diagnostic procedures as the initial diagnostic procedure.

CHART 41-2
Patient Education: Collecting a Clean-Catch Midstream Urine Specimen

Instructions to the Male Patient

- Expose the glans and cleanse the area around the meatus with soap. Remove all soap with water-soaked pledgets.
- Do not collect the first portion of the voiding; discard it.
- Collect the next portion by voiding into a sterile, wide-mouthed bottle or large-caliber tube that is protected by a sterile closure.
- Do not collect the last few drops of urine because prostatic secretions may be introduced into the urine at the end of the urinary stream.

Instructions to the Female Patient

- Separate the labia to expose the urethral orifice.
- Cleanse around the urinary meatus with sponges soaked in liquid soap.
- Wipe the perineum from the front to the back.
- Remove all soap with water-soaked pledgets, wiping from front to back.
- Keep the labia separated and void forcibly, but do not collect the first portion of the voiding. (The distal portion of the urethral orifice is colonized by bacteria; the initial voiding washes away the urethral contaminants.)
- Collect the midstream portion of the urinary flow, making sure that the container does not come in contact with the genitalia.

X-ray and Other Imaging Studies

Kidney, Ureter, and Bladder (KUB) X-ray. An x-ray of the abdomen or KUB (kidney, ureters, and bladder) may be performed to delineate the size, shape, and position of the kidneys and to reveal any abnormalities, such as calculi (stones) in the kidneys or urinary tract, hydronephrosis (distention of the pelvis of the kidney), cysts, tumors, or kidney displacement by abnormalities in the surrounding tissues.

Computed Tomography and Magnetic Resonance Imaging. Computed tomography (CT scan) and magnetic resonance imaging (MRI) are noninvasive techniques that provide excellent cross-sectional views of the kidney and urinary tract. They provide information about the extension of invasive lesions of the kidney.

Intravenous Urography (Excretory Urogram or Intravenous Pyelogram). An intravenous urogram (IVU), also called an intravenous pyelogram (IVP), permits visualization of the kidneys, ureter, and bladder. A radiopaque contrast medium is administered intravenously and is cleared from the bloodstream and concentrated by the kidneys. A **nephrotomogram** may be carried out as part of the study to visualize different layers of the kidney and the diffuse structures within each layer and to differentiate solid masses or lesions from cysts in the kidneys or urinary tract.

Intravenous urography is conducted as part of the initial assessment of any suspected urologic problem, especially in the diagnosis of lesions in the kidneys and ureters. It also provides a rough estimate of renal function. After the contrast agent (sodium diatrizoate or meglumine diatrizoate) is administered intravenously, multiple serial x-rays are obtained to visualize drainage structures.

The key considerations in preparing the patient for this procedure are presented in Chart 41-3.

If the patient has a history of allergies, a test dose of the contrast agent may be injected intradermally. If no skin reaction occurs in 15 minutes, the regular intravenous test dose of contrast material is administered. Although rare, as with the administration of any intravenous medication, an anaphylactic reaction may occur. (This reaction may occur even if the skin sensitivity test has been negative.)

- All IV urogram rooms should have emergency medications (epinephrine, corticosteroids, vasopressors), as well as oxygen, tracheostomy, and other equipment ready for immediate use in case an anaphylactic reaction occurs.

Retrograde Pyelography. In retrograde pyelography, ureteral catheters are passed up through the ureters into the renal pelvis by means of cystoscopy. A contrast agent is then introduced by gravity or injection through the catheter. Retrograde pyelography is usually performed if intravenous urography provides inadequate visualization of the collecting systems. It is used less frequently because of improved techniques in excretory urography.

Infusion Drip Pyelography. Infusion drip pyelography is an intravenous infusion of a large volume of dilute solution of a contrast agent to opacify the renal parenchyma and to completely fill the urinary tract. This method of examination is useful when regular urographic techniques fail to show the drainage structures satisfactorily (*e.g.*, in a patient with an elevated blood urea nitrogen) or when prolonged opacification of the drainage structures is desired so that **tomograms** (body section radiography) can be made. Images are obtained at specified intervals after the start of the infusion to examine the filled and distended collecting system. The patient preparation is the same as for excretory urography (see Chart 41-3), except that fluids are not restricted.

Cystogram. A catheter is inserted into the bladder and contrast material is instilled to outline the bladder wall and to aid in evaluating **vesicoureteral reflux** (backflow of urine from the bladder into one or both ureters). Cystograms are also performed in conjunction with simultaneous pressure recordings inside the bladder.

Cystourethrogram. A cystourethrogram provides visualization of the urethra and bladder either by retrograde injection of contrast agent into the urethra and bladder or by x-ray while the patient excretes the contrast material. The **voiding cystourethrogram** is described in the section on "Urodynamic Measurements" below.

Renal Angiography. This procedure permits visualization of the renal arteries. The femoral (or axillary) artery is pierced with a needle and a catheter is threaded up through the femoral and iliac arteries into the aorta or renal artery. A contrast agent is injected to opacify the renal arterial supply. Angiography enables blood flow dynamics to be evaluated, demonstrates abnormal vasculature, and helps to differentiate renal cysts from renal tumors.

TABLE 41-3 Tests of Renal Function

Test	Purpose/Rationale	Test Protocol
Renal Concentration Test		
Specific gravity Osmolality of urine	Tests the ability to concentrate solutes in the urine. Concentrating ability is lost early in kidney disease; hence, this test shows early defects in renal function.	Fluids may be withheld for 12 to 24 hours to assess the concentrating ability of the tubules under controlled conditions. Specific gravity measurements of urine are taken at specific times to determine urine concentration.
Creatinine Clearance* (Endogenous Creatinine Clearance) Test		
	Provides an approximation of rate of glomerular filtration Measures volume of blood cleared of creatinine in 1 minute A sensitive indicator of early renal disease Useful to follow progress of patient's renal status	All urine is collected over 24-hour period. Draw one sample of blood within the 24-hour period.
Serum Creatinine Test		
	A test of renal function reflecting the balance between production and filtration by renal glomerulus A sensitive indicator of renal function	Test is performed on serum.
Serum Urea Nitrogen (Blood Urea Nitrogen [BUN]) Test		
	Serves as index of renal excretory capacity Serum urea nitrogen is dependent on the body's urea production and on urine flow. Urea is the nitrogenous end product of protein metabolism. BUN levels are also affected by protein intake, tissue breakdown	Test is performed on serum.

*Clearance is the amount of blood cleared of a constituent per unit of time.

Nursing Interventions. Before the procedure, a laxative may be prescribed to evacuate the colon so that unobstructed x-rays can be obtained. The proposed injection sites (groin for femoral approach or axilla for axillary approach) may be shaved. The peripheral pulse sites (radial, femoral, dorsalis pedis) are marked for easy access in postprocedural assessment. The patient is informed that there may be a brief sensation of heat along the course of the vessel when the contrast agent is injected.

Following the procedure, the patient's vital signs are monitored until stable. If the axillary artery was the site of the injection, blood pressure measurements are taken on the opposite arm. The injection or puncture site is examined for swelling and hematoma formation. The peripheral pulses are palpated. The color and temperature of the involved extremity are noted and compared with those of the uninvolved extremity. Cold compresses may be applied to the injection site to decrease edema and pain.

Endourology (Urologic Endoscopic Procedures)

Cystoscopic Examination

The cystoscopic examination (**cystoscopy** or **"cysto"**) is a method for directly visualizing the urethra and bladder. The cystoscope, which is inserted through the urethra into the bladder, has a self-contained optical lens system that provides a magnified, illuminated view of the bladder (Fig. 41-6). The cystoscope is manipulated to allow complete visualization of the urethra and bladder as well as the ureteral orifices and prostatic urethra. Small ureteral catheters can be passed through the cystoscope, allowing assessment of the ureters and the pelvis of each kidney. The cystoscope also permits the urologist to obtain a urine specimen from each kidney to evaluate its function. Cup forceps can be inserted through the cystoscope for biopsy. Calculi may be removed from the urethra, bladder, and ureter via cystoscopy.

The endoscope is passed under direct visualization. The urethra and the bladder are inspected. Sterile irrigating solution is instilled to distend the bladder and wash away blood clots, thereby allowing better visualization. The use of a high-intensity light and interchangeable lenses allows excellent visualization and permits still and motion pictures to be taken of these structures.

Prior to the procedure, a sedative may be administered. A local topical anesthetic is instilled into the urethra by the urologist before the cystoscope is inserted. Intravenous diazepam (Valium) in combination with topical urethral anesthesia may be administered. Alternatively, spinal or general anesthesia may be used.

Nursing Interventions. As with any diagnostic procedure, the nurse describes the procedure in order to prepare the patient and allay fears. Additional preprocedure preparation may include having the patient drink one or two glasses of water.

CHART 41-3
Patient Preparation for an Intravenous Urogram or Pyelogram

1. The patient's history is obtained to identify allergies that might cause an adverse reaction to the contrast agent. The physician and the radiologist are notified of allergy (especially to iodine or shellfish) or suspicion of allergy so that appropriate measures are taken to prevent serious allergic reactions. The suspected allergy is also noted prominently in the patient's record.
2. A laxative may be prescribed the night before the scheduled examination to eliminate feces and gas from the intestinal tract.
3. Liquids may be restricted 8 to 10 hours before the test to promote a concentrated urine. However, elderly patients with marginal renal reserve or function, patients with multiple myeloma, and those with uncontrolled diabetes mellitus may not tolerate dehydration. After consulting with the physician, the nurse may give such patients water to drink during the hours before the test. The patient should not be overhydrated, because this may dilute the contrast agent and thus cause inadequate visualization of the urinary tract.
4. The procedure itself and the sensations produced by injection of the contrast agent and during the procedure (*e.g.*, a temporary feeling of warmth and flushing of the face) are described to the patient.

Postprocedure management is directed at relieving any possible discomfort resulting from the examination. Some burning upon voiding, blood-tinged urine, and urinary frequency from trauma to the mucous membrane may occur after cystoscopic examination. Moist heat to the lower abdomen or warm sitz baths are helpful in relieving pain and promoting muscle relaxation.

Occasionally, following cystoscopic examination the patient with obstructive pathology experiences urinary retention as a result of edema caused by the instrumentation. The patient with prostatic hyperplasia is carefully monitored for urinary retention. Warm sitz baths and relaxant medications are helpful for relieving retention; catheterization, however, may be necessary.

The patient who has undergone instrumentation of the urinary tract (*i.e.*, cystoscopy) is monitored for signs and symptoms of urinary tract infection. Edema of the urethra secondary to local trauma may obstruct urine flow; therefore, the patient is also monitored for signs and symptoms of obstruction.

Renal and Ureteral Brush Biopsy

Brush biopsy techniques provide specific information when abnormal x-ray findings of the ureter or renal pelvis raise uncertainty as to whether the defect is a tumor, a stone, a blood clot, or an artifact. First, a cystoscopic examination is conducted. Then a ureteral catheter is introduced, followed by a biopsy brush that is passed through the catheter. The suspected lesion is brushed back and forth in order to obtain cells and surface tissue fragments for histologic analysis.

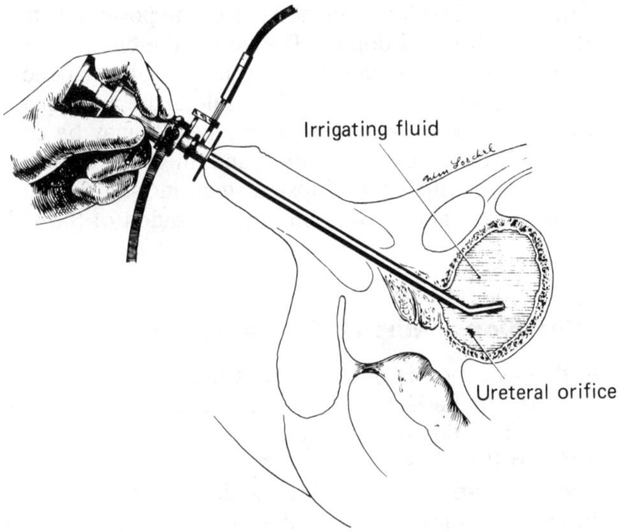

FIGURE 41-6. Cystoscopic examination. A cystoscope is introduced into the bladder. The upper cord is an electric line for the distal end of the cystoscope. The lower tubing leads from a reservoir of sterile irrigating fluid that is used to inflate the bladder.

Following the procedure, intravenous fluids may be administered to help clear the kidneys and prevent clot formation. Urine may contain blood (usually clearing in 24–48 hours) from oozing at the brushing site. Postoperative renal colic occasionally occurs and responds to analgesics.

Renal Endoscopy (Nephroscopy)

Renal endoscopy (nephroscopy) is the introduction of a fiberscope into the pelvis of the kidney, through an incision (pyelotomy) or percutaneously, to view the interior of the renal pelvis, remove calculi, biopsy small lesions, and aid in the diagnosis of renal hematuria and selected renal tumors.

Biopsy of the Kidney

Biopsy of the kidney is performed by inserting a needle through the skin and into the renal tissue or by open biopsy through a small flank incision. It is useful in evaluating the course of renal disease and in obtaining specimens for electron and immunofluorescent microscopy, particularly for glomerular disease. Before the biopsy is carried out, coagulation studies are conducted to identify any risk for postbiopsy bleeding.

Procedure. The patient may be placed on a fasting regimen 6 to 8 hours before the test. An intravenous line is established. A urine specimen is obtained and saved for comparison with the postbiopsy specimen. If a needle biopsy is to be performed, the patient is informed that it will be necessary to hold his or her breath (to prevent movement of the kidney) while the renal biopsy needle is being inserted.

The sedated patient is placed in a prone position with a sandbag under the abdomen. The skin at the biopsy site is infiltrated with a local anesthetic agent. The biopsy needle is introduced just inside the renal capsule of the outer quadrant of the kidney. The location of the needle may be confirmed by fluoroscopy or by ultrasound, in which a special probe is used. With open biopsy, a small incision is made over the kidney and allows direct visualization of the kidney.

Postbiopsy Nursing Management

After the specimen is obtained, pressure is applied to the biopsy site. The patient may be kept in a prone position immediately following biopsy and on bed rest for 24 hours to minimize risk of bleeding.

Hematuria. The patient is monitored closely for hematuria, which may appear soon after biopsy. The kidney is a highly vascular organ, and approximately one fourth of the entire cardiac output circulates through it in about 1 minute. The passage of the biopsy needle punctures the kidney capsule, and bleeding can occur in the perirenal space. Usually, the bleeding subsides on its own, but a large amount of blood can accumulate in this space in a short period of time without noticeable signs until cardiovascular collapse is evident.

- To detect early signs of bleeding, it is important that the vital signs be monitored every 5 to 15 minutes for the first hour and then with decreasing frequency as indicated.
- Signs and symptoms suggestive of bleeding include a rise or fall in blood pressure, tachycardia, anorexia, vomiting, and the development of a dull, aching discomfort in the abdomen.
- Any symptoms of backache, shoulder pain, or dysuria are reported immediately.

Flank pain may occur but usually represents bleeding into the muscle rather than around the kidney. Colicky pain similar to that of ureteral colic may develop when a clot is present in the ureter and may cause excruciating, sharp flank pain that radiates to the groin.

All urine voided by the patient is inspected for evidence of bleeding and compared with the prebiopsy specimen and subsequent voiding samples. If bleeding persists, as indicated by an enlarging hematoma, palpating or manipulating the abdomen is avoided.

Hematocrit and hemoglobin levels are obtained within 8 hours to assess for changes; decreasing levels may indicate bleeding. Usually, the fluid intake is maintained at 3000 ml daily unless the patient has renal insufficiency. If bleeding occurs, the patient is prepared for blood component therapy and surgical intervention to control the hemorrhage, which may necessitate surgical drainage or rarely nephrectomy (removal of kidney).

Patient Education. Delayed hemorrhage can occur several days after biopsy. Therefore, the patient is instructed to avoid strenuous activity, sports, and heavy lifting for at least 2 weeks. The physician or clinic is to be notified if any of the following occurs: flank pain, hematuria, lightheadedness and fainting, rapid pulse, or any other signs and symptoms of bleeding.

Radioisotope Studies

Radioisotope studies are noninvasive procedures that do not interfere with normal physiologic processes and require no specific patient preparation. Radiopharmaceuticals (^{99}Tc-labeled compound or ^{131}I-hippurate) are injected intravenously. Studies are obtained with a scintillation camera placed posterior to the kidney, with the patient in a supine, prone, or sitting position. The resultant image (called a **scan**) indicates the distribution of the radiopharmaceutical within the kidney.

The **Tc scan** provides information about kidney perfusion and is useful when renal function is poor. The **hippurate scan** provides information about kidney function.

Urodynamic Measurements

Urodynamic measurements provide physiologic and structural tests to evaluate bladder and urethral function by measuring the (1) rate of urine flow, (2) bladder pressures during voiding and at rest, (3) internal urethral resistance, and (4) bladder contraction and relaxation. Abdominal, bladder, and detrusor pressures, sphincter activity, bladder innervation, muscle tone, and sacral reflex are assessed.

The following are the urodynamic measurements most frequently performed.

Uroflowmetry (flow rate) is the record of the volume of urine passing through the urethra per time unit (ml/sec).

A **cystometrogram** is a graphic recording of the pressures in the bladder (intravesical) at various phases of filling and emptying of the urinary bladder to assess its function. During the procedure, the amount of fluid instilled into the bladder and voided, as well as the patient's sensations of bladder fullness and urge to void, are recorded. These are then compared with the pressures measured in the bladder during bladder filling and voiding. The patient is first asked to void, and the physician observes the time it takes to initiate voiding; the size, force, and continuity of the urinary stream; and the degree of straining and hesitancy. A retention catheter is passed through the urethra into the bladder. The residual volume is measured and the catheter is left in place. The urethral catheter is connected to a water manometer, and sterile solution is allowed to flow into the bladder, usually at the rate of 1 ml/sec. The patient informs the examiner when the first desire to void is felt, and again when the bladder feels full. The degree of bladder filling at these points is recorded. The pressures above the zero level at the symphysis pubis are measured, and the pressures and volumes within the bladder are plotted and recorded.

The **urethral pressure profile** measures urethral resistance along the length of the urethra. Gas and fluid are instilled through a catheter that is withdrawn while the pressures along the urethral wall are obtained.

A **cystourethrogram** permits visualization of the urethra and bladder either by retrograde injection or by voiding of the contrast agent.

In a **voiding cystourethrogram,** the bladder is filled with a contrast agent, and the patient voids while rapid spot films are taken. The presence or absence of vesicoureteral reflux or congenital abnormalities in the lower urinary tract

NURSING CARE PLAN 41–1
Care of the Patient Undergoing Assessment for Urinary/Renal Dysfunction

NURSING DIAGNOSIS: Knowledge deficit about procedures and diagnostic tests

GOAL: Patient acquires knowledge and understanding of the procedure and tests and expected behaviors

Nursing Interventions	Rationale	Expected Outcomes
1. Assess patient's current level of understanding of planned tests and procedures.	1. Provides basis for further explanations and teaching and gives indication of patient's perception of procedures.	• States rationale for planned diagnostic procedures and tasks and behaviors expected during the procedures.
2. Provide factual description of tests in language and terms the patient understands.	2. Understanding what is expected enhances patient's compliance and cooperation.	• Complies with urine collection, fluid modifications, or other procedures required for diagnostic evaluation.
3. Assess patient's understanding of test results following their completion.	3. Apprehension may interfere with patient's ability to understand information and results provided by physician and other health care providers.	• Restates in own words results of diagnostic assessment. • Asks for clarification of terms and procedures.
4. Reinforce information provided to patient about test results and implications for follow-up care.	4. Provides opportunity for patient to clarify points and anticipate follow-up care.	• Explains rationale for follow-up care. • Participates in follow-up care.

NURSING DIAGNOSIS: Pain and discomfort related to infection, edema, obstruction, or bleeding along urinary tract or invasive diagnostic tests

GOAL: Relief of pain and discomfort

Nursing Interventions	Rationale	Expected Outcomes
1. Assess level of pain and discomfort a. Dysuria b. Burning on urination c. Abdominal pain and discomfort d. Flank pain e. Bladder spasm	1. Provides baseline for evaluating success of interventions and progression of dysfunction.	• Reports decreasing levels of pain and discomfort. • Uses sitz bath as indicated. • Consumes increased fluid intake if indicated. • Reports absence of local symptoms (urgency, frequency, dysuria, and burning on urination).
2. Encourage fluid intake (unless contraindicated).	2. Promotes dilute urine and flushing of lower urinary tract.	
3. Encourage warm sitz baths.	3. Relieves local discomfort and promotes relaxation.	• States ability to start and stop urinary stream without discomfort.
4. Report increased pain to physician.	4. May indicate progression of dysfunction, recurrence of dysfunction, or untoward signs (*e.g.,* bleeding, calculi).	• Identifies signs and symptoms to be reported to health care provider. • Takes medications as prescribed.
5. Administer analgesics and antispasmodics for pain and spasm as prescribed.	5. May be prescribed for pain and spasm.	• Does not delay in emptying bladder. • Uses appropriate hygienic practices: Avoids use of bubble bath. Uses appropriate hygiene after bowel movements.
6. Assess voiding patterns and practices of hygiene and provide instructions about recommended voiding patterns and hygienic practices.	6. Delayed emptying of the bladder and some poor practices of hygiene contribute to discomfort and pain secondary to renal or urinary tract dysfunction.	

NURSING DIAGNOSIS: Fear related to potential alteration in renal function and body part and embarrassment secondary to discussion of urinary function and invasion of genitalia

GOAL: Reduced fear

Nursing Interventions	Rationale	Expected Outcomes
1. Assess patient's level of fear and apprehension.	1. A high level of fear or apprehension can interfere with learning and cooperation.	• Appears relaxed with low level of fear and apprehension.

(*continued*)

NURSING CARE PLAN 41-1 *(continued)*
Care of the Patient Undergoing Assessment for Urinary/Renal Dysfunction

Nursing Interventions	Rationale	Expected Outcomes
2. Explain all procedures and tests to patient.	2. Knowledge about what is expected helps to reduce fear and apprehension.	• States rationale for tests and procedures in a calm, relaxed manner.
3. Provide privacy and respect patient's modesty by closing doors and keeping patient covered and clothed. Keep urinal and bedpan covered and out of sight.	3. Communicates that you are aware of and accept patient's need for privacy and modesty.	• Maintains usual privacy and modesty. • Discusses own urinary tract dysfunction in correct terminology without overt indications of embarrassment or discomfort.
4. Use correct terminology in factual manner when questioning patient about urinary tract dysfunction.	4. Conveys that nurse is comfortable discussing patient's urinary dysfunction and symptoms with patient.	• Is able to relate fears and concerns. • Shows correct understanding of procedures and possible outcomes.
5. Assess patient's fears about perceived changes associated with tests and other procedures.	5. May reveal unfounded fears and misperceptions that can be alleviated by correct understanding.	
6. Instruct patient in relaxation exercises	6. May promote relaxation and assist the patient in coping with uncertainty about outcomes.	

can be demonstrated. The voiding cystourethrogram is also used to investigate difficulty in bladder emptying and incontinence.

Electromyography involves the placement of electrodes in the pelvic floor musculature or anal sphincter to evaluate neuromuscular function of the lower tract.

Nursing Care of Patients Undergoing Assessment of the Urinary/Renal System

All patients, regardless of the extent or type of renal or urinary tract dysfunction, undergo tests to assess the function of the renal and urinary tract. Even those who have had these tests repeatedly in the past are apprehensive about the procedures and the results. Additionally, they frequently feel discomfort and embarrassment about a previously private and personal function: voiding. Although this is a function that health care providers deal with frequently in the course of providing care, it is important to remember that these assessments are not routine to patients.

Nursing Diagnoses

Potential nursing diagnoses for the patient undergoing assessment of urinary or renal function include the following:

- Knowledge deficit about the procedures and diagnostic tests
- Pain and discomfort related to renal infection, edema, obstruction, or bleeding along the urinary tract or invasive diagnostic procedures
- Fear related to possible diagnoses of serious illness and alteration in renal function
- Fear related to embarrassment secondary to discussion of urinary function and invasion of genitalia
- Fluid volume excess related to inability to eliminate fluids

Planning, Implementation, and Evaluation

The goals, nursing interventions, rationales for interventions, and expected outcomes are discussed in more detail in Nursing Care Plan 41-1, Care of the Patient Undergoing Assessment for Urinary/Renal Dysfunction. The diagnostic procedures are often performed in the outpatient laboratory setting or short procedure unit. Therefore, patient and family teaching and monitoring by the patient's family are often indicated. Follow-up telephone calls to the patient by the nurse are often reassuring to the patient and family and provide an opportunity for their questions to be answered.

Gerontologic Considerations

Renal and urinary tract function changes with age. After age 40, there is a progressive decline in the glomerular filtration rate to approximately 50% of normal by age 70. Tubular function, including reabsorption and concentrating ability, is also reduced with increasing age. Although renal function usually remains adequate despite these changes, renal reserve is decreased and may reduce the kidneys' ability to respond effectively to drastic or sudden physiologic changes. At the same time, changes in other body systems often alter the patient's response to illness, resulting in signs and symptoms of illness or infection that are atypical or different from those that commonly occur in younger patients.

Structural or functional abnormalities that occur with aging may prevent complete emptying of the bladder and increase the risk of urinary tract infection, the most common cause of sepsis in patients over 65 years of age. In addition to changes in renal function, there are changes in function of the ureters, bladder, and urethra with aging. The likelihood of prostatic enlargement in the elderly male patient makes assessment of urinary patterns extremely important, because undetected urethral obstruction can result in renal failure and urinary tract infections in elderly men. Elderly women often have incomplete emptying of the bladder and urinary stasis.

The increased occurrence of chronic illness in the elderly and the increased use of prescription and over-the-counter medications indicate the need for a complete health history to identify predisposing conditions, the use of medications, or interactions of several medications that could compromise renal function further. Preparation of the elderly patient for diagnostic tests must be managed carefully to prevent dehydration that might precipitate renal failure in a patient with marginal renal reserve. Limitations in mobility often imposed on or experienced by elderly patients may affect their ability to void adequately or to consume adequate fluids. Patients may limit their own fluid intake to minimize the frequency of voiding or the risk of incontinence; teaching the patient and family about the dangers of an inadequate fluid intake is an important role of the nurse caring for the elderly patient.

CRITICAL THINKING EXERCISES

1. Your patient is scheduled to be discharged in 8 hours after having a renal biopsy. What instructions would you give to the patient and family about precautions and care after discharge in the following situations: (1) the patient lives alone; (2) the patient is a teenager; (3) the patient is in a high-pressure job and wants to return to work as soon as possible; (4) the patient and family are of foreign origins and do not speak English well?
2. Your patient refuses to drink an adequate volume of fluid following an IVP because of her fear of urinary incontinence. Describe the additional assessment data you would need to collect and how you would analyze these data to determine your course of action to ensure that your patient receives an adequate fluid intake without becoming incontinent.

BIBLIOGRAPHY

Books

Agency for Health Care Policy and Research, Public Health Service, U. S. Department of Health and Human Services. Urinary Incontinence in Adults: Clinical Practice Guideline (AHCPR Pub. No. 92-0038). Washington, DC, US Government Printing Office, March 1992.

Alspach JG. Core Curriculum for Critical Care Nursing, 4th ed. Philadelphia, WB Saunders, 1991.

Bates BA. A Guide to Physical Examination and History Taking, 6th ed. Philadelphia, JB Lippincott, 1995.

Carrieri-Kohlman V, Lindsey A, and West C. Pathophysiological Phenomena in Nursing, 2nd ed. Philadelphia, WB Saunders, 1993.

Funk SG. Key Aspects of Elder Care: Managing Falls, Incontinence, and Cognitive Impairment. New York, Springer, 1992.

Gaffney J and Zirker W. Empirical validation of urge incontinence in a sample of elderly women. In Carroll-Johnson R and Paquette M (eds). Classification of Nursing Diagnoses: Proceedings of the Tenth Conference, North American Nursing Diagnosis Association. Philadelphia, JB Lippincott, 1994, 286–287.

Illustrated Manual of Nursing Practice, 2nd ed. Springhouse, PA, Springhouse Corp., 1994.

King BD and Harke J. Coping with Bowel and Bladder Problems. San Diego, Singular Publishing Group, 1994.

Kursh ED and McGuire EJ. Female Urology. Philadelphia, JB Lippincott, 1994.

Mastering Advanced Assessment. Springhouse Advanced Skills Series. Springhouse, PA, Springhouse Corp., 1993.

McCance K and Huether S. Pathophysiology: The Biologic Basis for Disease in Adults and Children, 2nd ed. St. Louis, Mosby, 1994.

Methany N. Fluid and Electrolyte Balance: Nursing Considerations, 2nd ed. Philadelphia, JB Lippincott, 1992.

Price S and Wilson L. Pathophysiology: Clinical Concepts of Disease Processes, 4th ed. St. Louis, Mosby, 1992.

Providing Expert Care for the Acutely Ill. Springhouse Advanced Skill Series. Springhouse, PA, Springhouse Corp., 1994.

Walters MD and Karram MM. Clinical Urogynecology. St. Louis, CV Mosby, 1993.

Woodtli M and Yocum K. Urge incontinence: Identification and clinical validation of defining characteristics. In Carroll-Johnson R and Paquette M (eds). Classification of Nursing Diagnoses: Proceedings of the Tenth Conference, North American Nursing Diagnosis Association. Philadelphia, JB Lippincott, 1994, 182–185.

Journals

Bakris GL and Talbert R. Drug dosing in patients with renal insufficiency. A simplified approach. Postgrad Med 1993 Dec; 94(8):153–156, 159–160, 163–164.

Canzanello VJ and Textor SC. Noninvasive diagnosis of renovascular disease. Mayo Clin Proc 1994 Dec; 69(12):1172–1181.

Childs SJ et al. Asymptomatic bacteriuria: When to worry. Patient Care 1993 Feb 15; 27(3):63–66, 72–73.

Chmielewski C. Renal anatomy and overview of nephron function. ANNA J 1992 Feb; 19(1):34–38.

Cooper C. What color is that urine specimen? Am J Nurs 1993 Aug; 93(8):37.

Fihn SD. Lower urinary tract infection in women. Curr Opin Obstet Gynecol 1992 Aug; 4(4):571–578.

Geyer SJ. Urinalysis and urinary sediment in patients with renal disease. Clin Lab Med 1993 Mar; 13(1):13–20.

Gleckman RA. Urinary tract infection. Clin Geriatr Med 1992 Nov; 8(4):793–803.

Goldfarb DA. The renin–angiotensin system. New concepts in regulation of blood pressure and renal function. Urol Clin North Am 1994 May; 21(2):187–194.

Holechek MJ. Glomerular Filtration and Renal Hemodynamics. ANNA J 1992 June; 19(3):237–245.

Kellen M et al. Predictive and diagnostic tests of renal failure: A review. Anesth Analg 1994 Jun; 78(1):134–142.

Larson TS. Evaluation of proteinuria. Mayo Clin Proc 1994 Dec; 69(12):1154–1158.

Leiner S. Recurrent urinary tract infections in otherwise healthy adult women. Rational strategies for work-up and management. Nurse Pract 1995 Feb; 20(2):48, 51–52, 54–56.

Linday LA. Developmental changes in renal tubular function. J Adolesc Health 1994 Dec; 15(8):648–653.
Lindeman RD. Assessment of renal function in the old. Special considerations. Clin Lab Med 1993 Mar; 13(1):269–277.
Linsenmayer TA. Urologic anatomy and physiology. Phys Med Rehabil Clin North Am 1993 May; 4(2):221-247.
McIntosh LJ and Richardson DA. 30-minute evaluation of incontinence in the older woman. Geriatrics 1994 Feb; 49(2):35–38, 43–44.
Nielsen B. Evaluation of micturition. J Wound Ostomy Continence Nurs 1995 Jun; 22(1):44–50.
Preisig P. Renal physiology series: Part 3 of 8 Urinary concentration and dilution. ANNA J 1992 Aug; (19)4:351–354.
Radke KJ. Renal physiology series: Part 6 of 8. The aging kidney: Structure, function, and nursing practice implications. ANNA J 1994 Jun; 21(4):181–190.
Roehrborn CG. The assessment of patient complains. Prog Clin Biol Res 1994; 386:73–96.
Rousseau P. and Fuentevilla-Clifton A. Urinary incontinence in the aged, Part I. Patient evaluation. Geriatrics 1992 Jun; 47(6): 22–26, 33–34.
Schrier RW and Niederberger M. Paradoxes of body fluid volume regulation in health and disease. A unifying hypothesis. West J Med 1994 Oct; 161(4):393–408.
Summitt RL Jr. Investigative techniques, assessment of incontinence, and urodynamics. Curr Opin Obstet Gynecol 1992 Aug; 4(4):548–553.
Taylor M. Cystometrogram through an indwelling suprapubic catheter. Urol Nurs 1992 Mar; 12(1):26.
Walser M. Assessment of renal function and progression of disease. Curr Opin Nephrol Hypertens 1994 Sep; 3(5):564–567.
Winslow EH. Myth of the clean catch. Am J Nurs 1993 Aug; 93(8): 20.
Wozniak-Petrofsky J. Basics of urodynamics. J Urol Nurs 1993 Apr–June; 12(2):434–463.
Wozniak-Petrofsky J. Fundamental urodynamics: Normal bladder function and patient assessment, Part 1. Urol Nurs 1993 Sep; 13(3):88–92.
Yucha CB. Renal physiology series: Part 5a of 8. Renal control of calcium. ANNA J 1993 Aug; 20(4):440–444.
Zaloga GP. Reagent testing: Rapid, accurate urine testing at the bedside, Part 1. Consultant 1993 June; 33(6):90–92, 95–98.

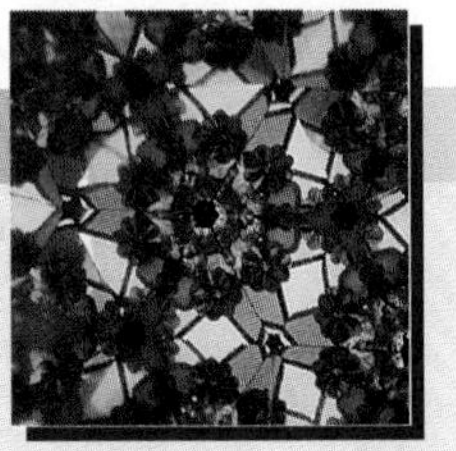

42

Management of Patients With Urinary and Renal Dysfunction

CHAPTER OUTLINE

Fluid and Electrolyte Imbalances

Maintaining Adequate Urinary Drainage
Catheterization
Suprapubic Bladder Drainage

Alterations in Voiding Patterns
Urinary Retention
Urinary Incontinence
Neurogenic Bladder

Dialysis
Hemodialysis
Peritoneal Dialysis
Care of the Hospitalized Dialysis Patient

The Patient Undergoing Kidney Surgery
Preoperative Considerations
Perioperative Concerns
Postoperative Management
NURSING PROCESS: The Patient Undergoing Kidney Surgery

Critical Thinking Exercises

LEARNING OBJECTIVES

On completion of this chapter, the learner will be able to:

1. Describe the sequence of events leading to urinary tract infection in a patient with an indwelling urinary catheter
2. Outline the principles of management of a patient with an indwelling urinary catheter
3. Compare and contrast urinary retention and urinary incontinence: their causes, clinical manifestations, complications, and management
4. Use the nursing process as a framework for the care of patients with urinary retention
5. Discuss strategies for the management of urinary incontinence in the elderly patient
6. Compare and contrast hemodialysis and peritoneal dialysis in terms of underlying principles, procedures, complications, and nursing considerations
7. Describe nursing management of the hospitalized dialysis patient
8. Use the nursing process as a framework for care of patients undergoing kidney surgery

Disorders of the urinary tract may be renal or urologic in origin. Renal disorders are disorders of the kidney. Because the kidney helps regulate body metabolism, the symptoms affect every body system. Urologic disorders, on the other hand, are those disorders affecting the bladder, ureter, urethra, and prostate gland, as well as structural disorders of the kidney.

Fluid and Electrolyte Imbalances

Patients with renal disorders frequently experience fluid and electrolyte imbalances and require close monitoring to detect any signs of impending problems. A fluid intake–output chart is kept to monitor and record important fluid parameters, including the amount of fluid that is ingested or administered parenterally, the volume of urine excreted, other fluid losses, and any change in weight.

These records are essential in determining the patient's fluid allowance and in indicating signs of fluid overload or deficit. The patient whose fluid intake is excessive and exceeds the ability of the kidneys to excrete fluid is said to have a fluid overload and may show symptoms of congestive heart failure (CHF). If fluid intake is inadequate, the patient is said to be underhydrated and may show signs and symptoms of fluid volume deficit. If the patient is receiving intravenous therapy, the flow rate must be adjusted as prescribed to meet the patient's fluid requirements. Repeated blood samples are obtained to evaluate electrolyte balance.

- The most accurate indicator of fluid loss or gain in an acutely ill patient is weight; therefore, daily weight must be obtained and recorded.

The signs of fluid and electrolyte disturbances that may occur in patients with renal disease are listed in Chart 42-1. These signs should be monitored, documented, and reported to other members of the health care team. (See also Chapter 14 on fluid and electrolyte disturbances.)

CHART 42-1
Signs of Fluid and Electrolyte Disturbances in Renal Disorder

1. Acute weight gain (in excess of 5%), edema, moist crackles in lungs, puffy eyelids, and shortness of breath—could indicate fluid volume excess.
2. Acute weight loss (in excess of 5%), a decrease in body temperature, dryness of skin and mucous membranes, longitudinal wrinkles or furrows of the tongue, and oliguria or anuria—could indicate fluid volume deficit.
3. Abdominal cramps, apprehension, seizures, and oliguria or anuria—could indicate sodium deficit or water loss.
4. Dry, sticky mucous membranes, flushed skin, oliguria or anuria, thirst, and rough and dry tongue—could indicate sodium excess.
5. Anorexia, abdominal distention, silent intestinal ileus, weakness, and soft, flabby muscles—could indicate potassium deficit.
6. Diarrhea, intestinal colic, irritability, and nausea—could indicate potassium excess.
7. Abdominal cramps, carpopedal spasm, muscle cramps, tetany, and tingling of ends of fingers—could indicate calcium deficit.
8. Deep bone pain, flank pain, and muscle hypotonicity—could indicate calcium excess.
9. Deep, rapid breathing (Kussmaul), shortness of breath on exertion, stupor, and weakness—could indicate primary base bicarbonate deficit.
10. Depressed respiration, muscle hypertonicity, and tetany—could indicate primary base bicarbonate excess.
11. Chronic weight loss, emotional depression, pallor, fatigue, and soft, flabby muscles—could indicate protein deficit.
12. Positive Chvostek's or Trosseau's sign, seizures, disorientation, hyperactive deep reflexes, and tremor—could indicate calcium or magnesium alteration.
13. Cardiac dysrhythmias—may be present in potassium imbalances.
14. Muscle twitching, paresthesias, cramping, and weakness—may indicate electrolyte imbalances in general.

Maintaining Adequate Urinary Drainage

As indicated in the description of renal function in the preceding chapter, urinary and renal excretion of waste materials is necessary for life. The composition of the body fluids is determined not so much by what a person ingests as by what the kidneys retain. In health, the kidneys are very efficient, excreting the substances that are not needed and retaining those that are. In the patient with a urologic disorder or one with marginal kidney function, care must be taken to assure that urinary drainage is adequate and that kidney function is preserved.

When urine cannot be eliminated naturally and must be drained artificially, catheters may be inserted directly into the bladder, the ureter, or the kidney pelvis. Catheters vary in size, shape, length, material, and configuration. The type of catheter chosen depends on its purpose.

Catheterization

Catheterization can be a life-saving measure, especially when the urinary tract is obstructed or the patient is unable to void. Catheterization may also be used for other reasons: to determine the amount of residual urine in the bladder after the patient has voided; to bypass an obstruction that blocks the flow of urine; to provide postoperative drainage following surgery on the bladder, vaginal area, or prostate; or to provide a means to monitor hourly urinary output in critically ill patients.

- A patient should be catheterized only if absolutely necessary because catheterization commonly leads to urinary tract infection.

Closed Drainage Systems. When an indwelling catheter cannot be avoided, a closed drainage system is essential. This drainage system should be designed to prevent the tubing from being disconnected so as to reduce the risk of contamination. Such a system may consist of an indwelling catheter, a connecting tube, and a collecting bag emptied by drainage valve; or a triple-lumen indwelling urethral catheter attached to a closed sterile drainage system. With the triple-lumen catheter, urinary drainage occurs through one channel; the retention balloon is inflated with water or air through the second channel; and the bladder is continually irrigated with antibacterial solution through the third channel.

Infection Risks

The presence of an indwelling catheter can lead to infection. Bacterial colonization (bacteriuria) will occur within 2 weeks in half of catheterized patients, and in almost all patients within 4 to 6 weeks following insertion of a catheter—even if recommendations for infection control and catheter care are followed carefully.

Urinary tract infections are responsible for over a third of all hospital-acquired infections. Most of these (at least 80%) follow some type of invasive procedure or instrumentation of the urinary tract, usually catheterization. The pathogens responsible for catheter-associated urinary tract infections include *Escherichia coli, Klebsiella, Proteus, Pseudomonas, Enterobacter, Serratia,* and *Candida.* Many of these organisms are part of the patient's endogenous or normal bowel flora or are acquired through cross-contamination by patients or hospital personnel or through exposure to nonsterile equipment.

Catheters impede most of the natural defenses of the lower urinary tract by obstructing the periurethral ducts, by irritating the bladder mucosa, and by providing an artificial route of entry for organisms to enter the bladder.

When catheters are used, microorganisms may gain access to the urinary tract by three main pathways: (1) by being introduced from the urethra into the bladder during catheterization; (2) by finding their way into the thin film of urethral fluid that is located outside of the catheter where the catheter and mucous membrane meet; and (3) the most common way, by migrating to the bladder along the internal lumen of the catheter after the catheter has become contaminated.

Assessment

The patient with an indwelling catheter is observed for signs and symptoms of urinary tract infection: cloudy urine, hematuria, fever, chills, anorexia, and malaise. The area around the urethral orifice is observed for drainage and excoriation. Urine cultures provide the most accurate means of assessing for infection. The color, odor, and volume of urine are also monitored.

The drainage system is assessed to ensure that it provides adequate drainage of urine. The catheter itself is observed to make sure that it is properly anchored to prevent pressure on the urethra at the penoscrotal junction in the male patient, and tension and traction on the bladder in both male and female patients. An accurate record of the patient's fluid intake and urine output provides additional information about the adequacy of renal function and urinary drainage.

Patients at risk for urinary tract infection from catheterization need to be identified, including the elderly and those who are debilitated, chronically ill, immunosuppressed, or diabetic.

The elderly patient with an indwelling catheter to manage incontinence may not exhibit the usual or typical signs and symptoms of infection. Therefore, any subtle change in the patient's physical condition or mental status must be considered a possible indication of infection and must be promptly investigated because the patient may become septic before the infection is diagnosed.

Figure 42-1 summarizes the sequence of events that often follows long-term use of an indwelling catheter in the elderly patient leading to infection and leakage of urine.

Preventing Infection

Certain principles of care are essential to prevent infection in a patient with a closed urinary drainage system. These principles and procedures are listed in Chart 42-2 and should be reviewed carefully.

The catheter is a foreign body in the urethra and produces a reaction in the urethral mucosa with some urethral discharge. However, cleaning the meatus while the catheter is in place is discouraged because the cleansing action can move the catheter to and fro, resulting in an increased risk of infection. To remove obvious encrustations from the external catheter surface, the area can be gently washed with soap during the daily bath. The catheter is anchored as securely as possible to prevent it from moving in the urethra. Encrustations arising from urinary salts may serve as a nucleus for stone formation; however, silicone catheters result in significantly less crust formation.

A liberal fluid intake and an increased urine output must be assured to flush the catheter and to dilute urinary substances that might form encrustations. (The intake must be within limits of the patient's cardiac reserve.)

Measures must be taken to prevent cross-contamination because many urinary tract infections are due to extrinsically acquired organisms. Patients at risk are women, elderly debilitated patients, and those who are critically ill.

- Hand washing is essential when going from one patient to another to provide care and before and after handling any part of the catheter or drainage system.

Urine cultures are obtained as prescribed or indicated in monitoring for infection; many catheters have an aspiration (puncture) port from which a specimen can be obtained.

Controversy exists about the usefulness of taking cultures and treating bacteriuria in patients with indwelling catheters who are asymptomatic because bacteriuria is considered to be inevitable and overtreatment may lead to resistant strains of bacteria.

Minimizing Trauma

Trauma to the urethra can be minimized by using a catheter of the appropriate size. The catheter is lubricated adequately so that it can be inserted easily and gently. It is inserted far enough into the bladder to prevent trauma to the urethral tissues when the retention balloon of the catheter is inflated. Manipulation of the catheter is most often the cause of damage to the bladder mucosa in the catheterized patient. Infection then inevitably occurs when urine invades

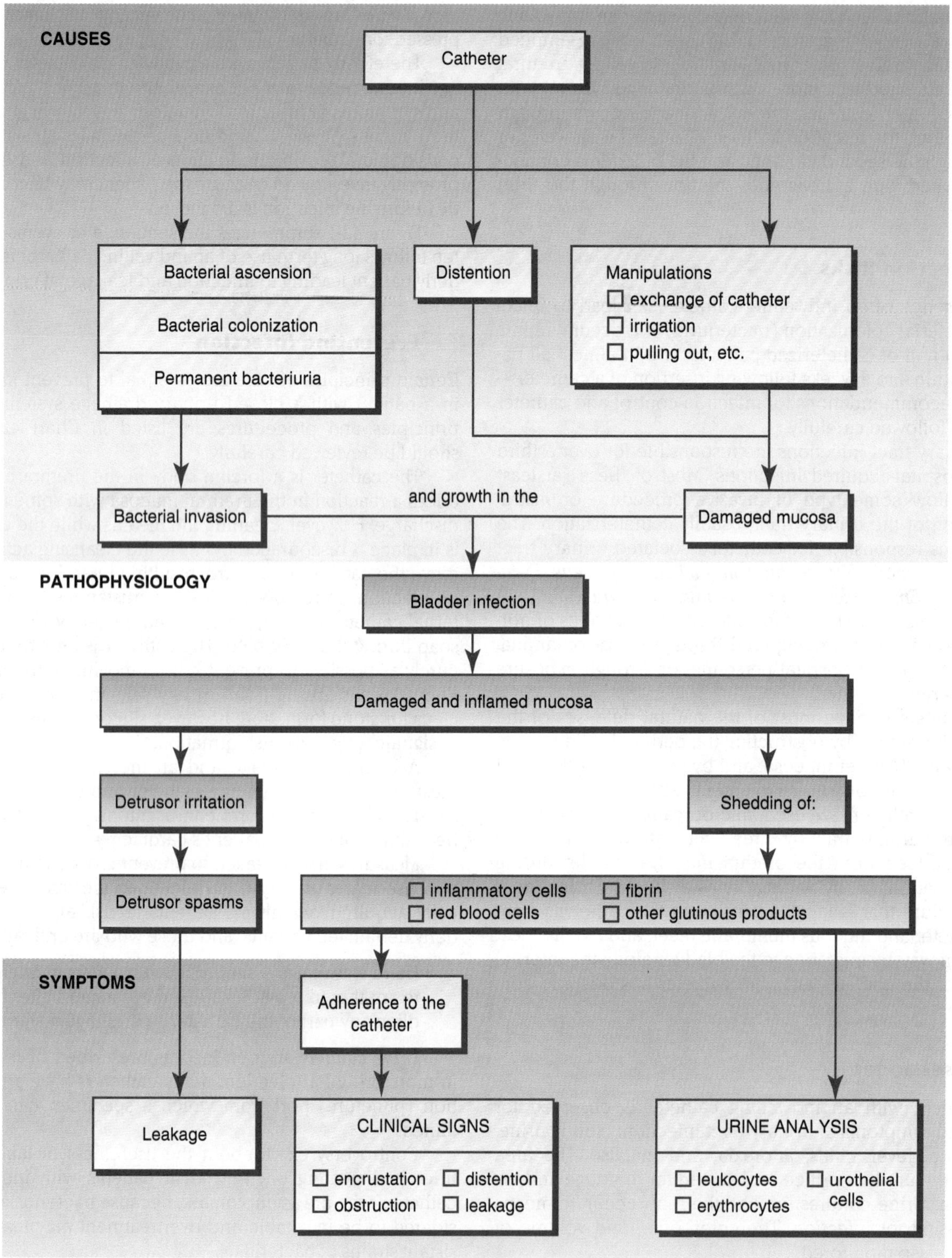

FIGURE 42-1. Pathophysiology and symptoms of bladder infection in long-term catheterized elderly. (Redrawn from Seiler WO and Stahelin HB. Practical management of catheter-associated UTIs. Geriatrics 1988 Aug; 43 [8]:44.)

CHART 42-2

Preventing Infection in the Catheterized Patient

- Strict asepsis is necessary during insertion of the catheter.
- A preassembled and sterile closed urinary drainage system is necessary and should not be disconnected before, during, or after insertion of the catheter.
- To prevent contamination of a closed system, the tubing is *never* disconnected. No part of the collection bag or drainage tube should ever be contaminated.
- The bag is never raised above the level of the patient's bladder because this will cause flow of contaminated urine by gravity into the patient's bladder from the bag.
- Urine should not be allowed to collect in the tubing because a free flow of urine must be maintained to prevent infection. Improper drainage occurs when the tubing is kinked or twisted, allowing pools of urine to collect in the loops of the tubing.
- The drainage bag must *never* touch the floor. The bag and collecting tubing are changed if contamination occurs, if the urine flow becomes obstructed, or if the tubing junctions start to leak at the connections.
- The bag is emptied at least every 8 hours through the drainage valve, and more frequently if there is a large volume of urine, to lessen the risk of bacterial proliferation.
- Care is taken to see that the drainage tube (valve/spout) is not contaminated. A receptacle in which to empty the bag is provided for each patient.
- Irrigation of the catheter is *never* carried out routinely.
- The catheter is *never* disconnected from the tubing to obtain urine samples, irrigate the catheter, or ambulate or transport the patient.
- The catheter should never be left in place longer than necessary.
- If a catheter is left in for days or weeks, then it should be changed periodically, about once each week, and never discontinued without bladder training.
- Inadvertent handling or manipulation of the catheter by the patient or staff is avoided.
- Hand washing is *mandatory* before and after handling of the catheter, tubing, and drainage bag.
- The catheter is washed with soap and water at least twice a day; to-and-fro motion is avoided.
- When the catheter is removed, the patient must void within 8 hours; if the patient is unable to void, the patient is catheterized with a straight catheter.
- If signs of infection (see p. 1182) occur, a urine specimen is obtained immediately for culture.

the damaged mucosa. The catheter is secured properly to prevent it from moving, causing traction on the urethra, or being accidentally removed. Care is taken to ensure that any patient who is confused does not accidentally remove the catheter with the retention balloon still inflated, because such an action would cause bleeding and considerable trauma to the urethra.

In the male patient, the drainage tube (not the catheter) is taped laterally to the thigh to prevent pressure on the urethra at the penoscrotal junction, which can eventually lead to the formation of a urethrocutaneous fistula.

In the female patient, the drainage tubing attached to the catheter is taped to the thigh to prevent tension and traction on the bladder.

Bladder Atony and Retraining

When preparing to discontinue a catheter that has been in for a prolonged period, bladder training should be initiated to develop bladder tone and thus prevent retention.

When a catheter is in place, the bladder does not fill and contract. Therefore, the bladder eventually loses some of its tone (atony). When this occurs and the catheter is removed, the individual may be unable to contract the detrusor muscle and eliminate urine. Bladder training can prevent this. Prior to discontinuing the catheter, it is alternately clamped and unclamped; every few hours, the catheter is clamped for 20 minutes then released. This should allow the bladder to fill and contract the muscle. Release of the clamp allows the bladder to empty. Prolonged use of an indwelling catheter is avoided; bladder atony may be avoided if intermittent catheterization is used in place of an indwelling catheter for an extended period.

Intermittent Self-Catheterization

Intermittent self-catheterization provides periodic drainage of urine from the bladder. It is the treatment of choice following spinal cord injury and other neurologic disorders in which the ability to empty the bladder is impaired. Aseptic techniques are required during the patient's in-hospital training because of the risk of cross-contamination. The patient may use a "clean" (nonsterile) technique at home, where the risk of cross-contamination is reduced.

Self-catheterization promotes independence, results in few complications, and permits more normal sexual relations. The objectives are to decrease the morbidity associated with the long-term use of an indwelling catheter and to achieve catheter-free status if possible.

Teaching emphasizes the importance of frequent catheterization and emptying of the bladder at the prescribed time irrespective of the circumstances. (If the bladder becomes overdistended, blood flow through the bladder wall is decreased and the risk of infection is increased.)

The female patient requires a mirror to help locate the urinary meatus. She is taught to catheterize herself by inserting a catheter 7.5 cm (3 in) into the urethra in a downward and backward direction. The male patient is taught to lubricate the catheter and retract the foreskin of the penis with one hand while grasping the penis and holding it at a right angle to the body. (This maneuver straightens the urethra and makes it easier to insert the catheter.) The catheter is inserted 15 to 25 cm (6–10 in) until the urine begins to flow. After the catheter is removed, it is washed in soapy water, rinsed, and wrapped in a paper towel, or placed in a plastic bag or case. A patient following this routine should be seen by a urologist at regular intervals to assess urinary function and the occurrence of complications.

If the patient is unable to perform intermittent self catheterization, frequently a family member is taught to carry out the procedure at regular intervals during the day.

Suprapubic Bladder Drainage

Suprapubic bladder aspiration is a method of establishing drainage from the bladder by inserting a catheter or tube into the bladder through a suprapubic ("above the pubis") incision or puncture (Fig. 42-2). It is used as a temporary measure to divert the flow of urine from the urethra when the urethral route is impassable (because of injuries, strictures, prostatic obstruction), after gynecologic surgery when bladder dysfunction is likely to occur (vaginal hysterectomy, vaginal repair surgery), and after pelvic fractures.

To facilitate insertion of the suprapubic catheter, the patient is placed in a supine position and the bladder is distended by administering oral or intravenous fluids or by instilling sterile saline into the bladder via a urethral catheter. These measures make it easier to locate the bladder.

The suprapubic area is surgically prepared and the puncture site located approximately 5 cm (2 in) above the symphysis pubis. The bladder may be entered through an incision in the bladder or through a puncture made by a small trocar. The catheter or suprapubic drainage tube is threaded into the bladder and secured with sutures or tape.

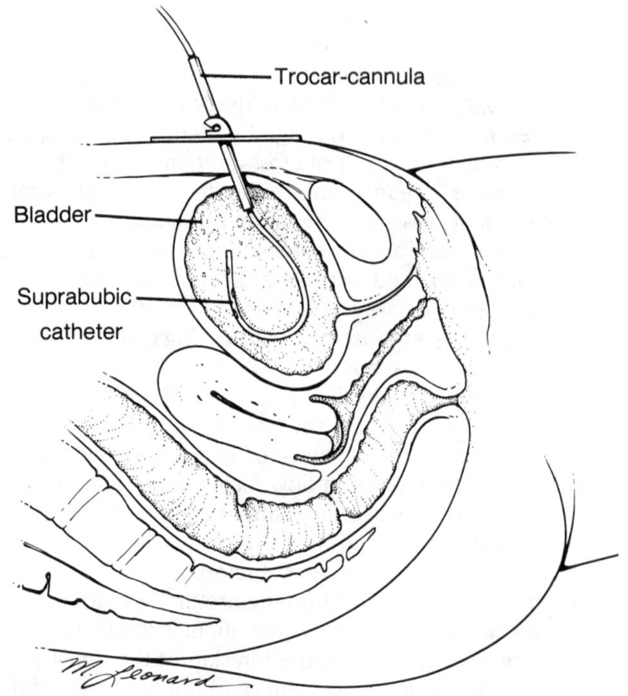

FIGURE 42-2. Suprapubic bladder drainage. A trocar-cannula is used to puncture the abdominal and bladder walls. The catheter is threaded through the trocar-cannula, which is then removed, leaving the catheter in place. The catheter is secured by tape or sutures to prevent accidental removal.

The area around the catheter is covered with a sterile dressing. The catheter is connected to a sterile closed drainage system, and the tubing is secured to prevent tension on the catheter.

Suprapubic bladder drainage may be maintained continuously for several weeks. When the patient's ability to void is to be tested, the catheter is clamped for 4 hours, during which time the patient attempts to void. After the patient voids, the catheter is unclamped and the residual urine is measured. If the amount of residual urine is less than 100 ml on two separate occasions (morning and evening), the catheter is usually removed. However, if the patient complains of pain or discomfort, the suprapubic catheter is usually left in place until the patient is able to void successfully.

Suprapubic drainage offers certain advantages. Patients with suprapubic drainage are usually able to void sooner after surgery than those with urethral catheters. Suprapubic drainage may also be more comfortable than an indwelling catheter. It also provides greater patient mobility, allows measurement of residual volume without urethral instrumentation, and presents less of a risk for bladder infection. The suprapubic catheter is removed when it is no longer necessary, and a sterile dressing is placed over the site.

Alterations in Voiding Patterns

Urinary Retention

Urinary retention (both acute and chronic) refers to the inability to urinate despite the urge or desire to do so. Chronic retention will often lead to overflow incontinence (due to pressure of retained urine in the bladder) or residual urine. **Residual urine** refers to urine that remains in the bladder after voiding.

Retention may occur in any postoperative patient, particularly in those who have undergone surgery on the perineal or anal regions that resulted in reflex spasm of the sphincters. General anesthesia reduces bladder muscle innervation, and thus the urge to void is suppressed. It may also occur in the acutely ill, the elderly, or the bedridden.

Urinary retention may be due to anxiety, prostatic enlargement, urethral pathology (infection, tumor, calculus), trauma, neurogenic bladder dysfunction, and other conditions. Some medications cause urinary retention, including anticholinergics–antispasmodics, such as atropine; antidepressant–antipsychotic agents, such as phenothiazines; antihistamine preparations, such as pseudoephedrine hydrochloride (Sudafed); β-adrenergic blockers, such as propranolol; and antihypertensive agents, such as hydralazine.

Urinary retention may lead to infection, which may develop as a result of overdistention of the bladder, compromised blood supply to the bladder wall, and proliferation of bacteria. Impaired renal function may also occur, particularly if obstruction of the urinary tract is present.

Management

Measures are instituted to prevent overdistention of the bladder and to treat infection or obstruction. Many problems, however, can be prevented by careful nursing assessment and appropriate nursing interventions.

Nursing Assessment

The signs and symptoms of urinary retention may easily be overlooked unless the nurse consciously assesses for them. Therefore, nursing assessment must address the following questions:

- What were the time and volume of the last voiding?
- Is the patient passing small amounts of urine frequently?
- Is the patient dribbling?
- Is the patient complaining of pain or discomfort in the lower abdomen? (Discomfort may be relatively mild if the bladder distends slowly.)
- Is there a rounded swelling arising out of the pelvis (which could indicate retention and a distended bladder)?
- Is there dullness on percussion in the suprapubic region (possibly indicating retention and a distended bladder)?
- Are there other indicators of urinary retention, such as restlessness and agitation?

Nursing Interventions

Promoting Urinary Elimination. Nursing measures to encourage voiding include providing privacy, assisting the patient to the bathroom or commode in order to provide a more natural setting for voiding, or allowing the male patient to stand beside the bed while using the urinal (because most men find this position more comfortable and natural for voiding). Additional measures include providing warmth to relax the sphincters (*i.e.*, sitz baths, warm compresses to the perineum, showers), giving the patient hot tea to drink, and offering encouragement and reassurance.

Following surgical procedures, the prescribed analgesic should be administered because pain in the incisional area can make voiding difficult. When the patient cannot void, careful catheterization is used to prevent overdistention of the bladder. In the case of prostatic obstruction, attempts at catheterization (by the urologist) may not be successful, requiring that a suprapubic catheter be inserted.

Relieving Pain and Discomfort. Relief of urinary retention generally brings relief of abdominal distention, pain, and discomfort. Treatment of the cause (*e.g.*, obstruction) usually relieves the patient's fear that the problem will recur.

Managing Complications. The patient may experience urinary retention with overflow; this indicates the need for catheterization. In addition to immediate catheterization, the patient also needs explanation as to why normal voiding is not occurring. Following restoration of urinary drainage, bladder retraining is initiated for the patient who is unable to void spontaneously. Strategies are implemented to assure an environment and a position that are conducive to voiding. Urine output is monitored closely and reassurance is provided about the temporary nature of retention and successful management strategies.

Urinary Incontinence

Urinary incontinence is the involuntary or uncontrolled loss of urine from the bladder. If urinary incontinence results from an inflammatory condition (cystitis), it will probably be temporary in nature. However, if it results from a serious neurologic condition (paraplegia), it is likely to be permanent.

Over 10 million adults in the United States suffer from urinary incontinence (AHCPR, 1992). It affects persons from all age groups but is particularly common in the elderly. It has been reported that over half of all nursing home residents have urinary incontinence. Although urinary incontinence is *not* a normal consequence of aging, age-related changes in the urinary tract predispose the older person to incontinence.

Age, gender, and number of previous vaginal deliveries are established risk factors and explain, in part, the increased incidence in women. Other suggested risk factors include urinary tract infection, menopause, genitourinary surgery, chronic illness, and various medications. Rashes, pressure ulcers, skin and urinary tract infections, and restrictions of activity are consequences of urinary incontinence.

The costs of care for patients with urinary incontinence are estimated to be over $10.3 billion annually (AHCPR, 1992). The psychosocial costs of urinary incontinence are enormous: embarrassment, loss of self-esteem, and social isolation are common outcomes. Urinary incontinence in the elderly often leads to their institutionalization.

Types of Urinary Incontinence

Stress incontinence is the involuntary loss of urine through an intact urethra as a result of a sudden increase in intra-abdominal pressure. It is seen mostly in women and can be due to obstetric injury, lesions of the bladder neck, extrinsic pelvic disease, fistulas, detrusor dysfunction, and a variety of other conditions. In addition, it may result from congenital conditions (extrophy of the bladder, ectopic ureter).

Urge incontinence occurs when the patient senses the urge to void but is unable to inhibit voiding long enough to reach the toilet. In many cases, uninhibited contraction of the bladder is a concomitant factor; this may occur in the patient with neurologic dysfunction that impairs inhibition of bladder contraction, or in the patient with local symptoms of irritation due to urinary tract infection or bladder tumors.

Overflow incontinence is characterized by frequent, sometimes almost constant, loss of urine from the bladder. The bladder cannot empty normally and becomes overdistended. Despite frequent urine loss, the bladder never empties. Overflow incontinence may be caused by neurologic abnormalities (*i.e.*, spinal cord lesions) or by factors that obstruct the outflow of urine (*i.e.*, medications, tumors, strictures, and prostatic hyperplasia). Neurogenic bladder is discussed separately in the next section.

Functional incontinence refers to those instances in which the function of the lower urinary tract is intact but other factors, such as severe cognitive impairment, make it difficult for the patient to identify the need to void (*e.g.*, Alzheimer's dementia), or physical impairments make it difficult or impossible for the patient to reach the toilet in time for voiding.

Mixed forms of urinary incontinence, which include characteristics of those just described, may also occur. Additionally, urinary incontinence can be a result of the interaction of many factors.

Only with appropriate recognition of the problem, assessment, and referral for diagnostic evaluation and treatment can the outcome of incontinence be determined. *All* persons with incontinence should be considered for evaluation and treatment.

Diagnostic Evaluation

Once the presence of incontinence is recognized, a thorough history is necessary. This will include a detailed description of the problem and a history of medication use. Voiding history, voiding log or diary, and bedside tests (*i.e.*, postvoiding residual urine volume, stress maneuvers) may be used to aid in determining the type of urinary incontinence. A more extensive urodynamic diagnostic evaluation may be performed.

Management

Treatment for urinary incontinence depends on the underlying causative factors. However, before appropriate treatment can be initiated, the presence of the problem must be identified and the possibility of successful treatment recognized. If nurses and other health care workers accept incontinence as an inevitable part of aging and illness or consider it irreversible and untreatable at any age, it cannot be successfully treated. Collaborative, interdisciplinary efforts are often essential in assessing and effectively treating urinary incontinence.

Successful management depends on the type of urinary incontinence and on the causative factors. Urinary incontinence may be transient or reversible; once the underlying cause is successfully treated, the patient's voiding pattern reverts to normal.

Those causes that are reversible and often transient can be recalled by the acronym *DIAPPERS.* These causes include the following: *d*elirium, *i*nfection of the urinary tract, *a*trophic vaginitis or urethritis, *p*harmacologic agents (anticholinergics, sedatives, alcohol, analgesics, diuretics, muscle relaxants, adrenergic agents), *p*sychologic factors (depression, regression), *e*xcessive urine production (excess fluid intake, endocrine disorders that cause diuresis), *r*estricted activity, and *s*tool impaction (AHCPR, 1992). Once these are successfully treated, the patient's voiding pattern often reverts to normal.

Nursing Interventions

Depending on the results of the evaluation, nursing management and/or medical management may be indicated. Nursing measures that are often effective may be simple ones that include assuring an environment that promotes easy access to the bathroom; placing a bedpan or urinal within easy reach; suggesting that the patient leave a light on in the darkened bedroom; and advising the patient to select clothing that is easy to remove when using the toilet.

The patient may also be instructed and encouraged to practice Kegel exercises (see Chart 45-4 in Chapter 45), which may help women of all ages to control incontinence. These exercises strengthen the muscles of the pelvic floor, which improves urethral resistance and urinary control.

Other measures the nurse may use to help the patient manage incontinence include initiating a program of prompted voiding or habit retraining and encouraging the patient to increase fluid intake to prevent constipation and stool impaction, which are frequent factors in urinary incontinence in a sedentary patient. Bladder training (see p. 1154), which may involve the use of biofeedback or behavioral strategies, may also be successful.

Surgical Management

Surgical correction may be indicated for stress incontinence. A wide range of surgical procedures can be used: vaginal repair, abdominal suspension of the bladder, and elevation of the bladder neck. A modified artificial sphincter that uses a silicone-rubber balloon as a self-regulating pressure mechanism is being used to close the urethra (Fig. 42-3). Another method of controlling stress incontinence is the application of electronic stimulation to the pelvic floor by means of a miniature pulse generator with electrodes mounted on an intra-anal plug.

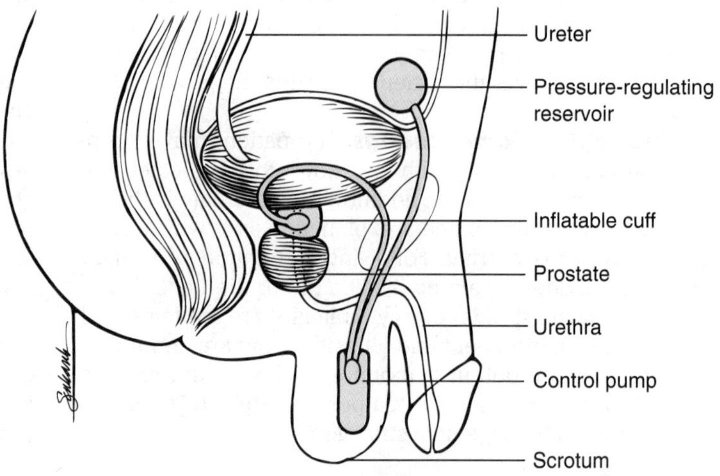

FIGURE 42-3. Artificial urinary sphincter. An inflatable cuff is inserted surgically around the urethra or neck of the bladder. To empty the bladder, the cuff is deflated by squeezing the control pump located in the scrotum.

For other types of incontinence, those nursing measures described above are often more appropriate.

Neurogenic Bladder

Neurogenic bladder refers to a bladder disturbance that results from a lesion of the nervous system. It may be caused by spinal cord injury or tumor, certain neurologic diseases (multiple sclerosis), congenital anomalies (spina bifida, myelomeningocele), infection, and certain systemic disorders (diabetes mellitus).

There are two types of neurogenic bladder: (1) **spastic** or **hypertonic** bladder, characterized by automatic, reflex, or uncontrolled expulsion of urine from the bladder with incomplete emptying, and (2) **flaccid** bladder, with loss of sensation of bladder fullness and thus overfilling and distention of the bladder.

Complications. The major complication of neurogenic bladder is *infection* that results from stasis of urine and subsequent catheterization. *Hypertrophy* of the bladder walls also results, ultimately leading to *vesicoureteral reflux* (backing up of urine from the bladder to the ureters) and *hydronephrosis* (dilation of the internal structures of the kidney by increased pressure of the backed-up urine). *Urolithiasis* (stones in the urinary tract) may develop from urinary stasis and infection and from demineralization of bone due to prolonged bed rest. *Renal failure* is the major cause of death of patients with neurologic impairment of the bladder.

Diagnostic Evaluation

As soon as the patient's condition permits, evaluation studies are performed to assess for bladder and bladder neck problems. The initial studies provide a baseline against which later changes can be measured. Serial studies of BUN, creatinine clearance, and serum creatinine are performed to determine the status of renal function. A cystogram is performed to identify the presence of vesicoureteral reflux. A urethrogram may be performed to detect the presence of urethral complications. Pressure and flow studies and an IV urogram are also performed. A cystoscopic examination may be performed to assess loss of muscle fibers and elastic tissues and to provide an opportunity for biopsy if necessary.

The problems of patients with neurogenic bladder disease vary considerably from patient to patient. It may be difficult initially to assess the long-term rehabilitation potential and eventual urologic disability.

Nursing Interventions

The care of the patient with neurogenic bladder is a major challenge to the health care team. There are several long-term objectives appropriate for patients with all types of neurogenic bladders: (1) to prevent overdistention of the bladder, (2) to empty the bladder regularly and completely, (3) to maintain urine sterility with no stone formation, and (4) to maintain adequate bladder capacity without vesicoureteral reflux.

Emptying the Bladder. The immediate management of the patient with a neurogenic bladder consists of catheterizing the patient intermittently or inserting a three-way catheter with closed drainage to avoid overdistention.

In *intermittent catheterization,* the bladder is catheterized at designated intervals (4, 6, or 8 hours) with a small-diameter catheter. This intermittent emptying approximates physiologic bladder function and avoids complications usually encountered with an indwelling catheter. An hourly fluid intake and output record is maintained to assess the patient's voiding patterns.

If *continuous catheterization* and drainage are used in a male patient, the drainage tube of the catheter is taped laterally to the thigh to avoid the sharp angulation of the catheter and prevent pressure at the penoscrotal angle.

Preventing Infection and Calculi. With the use of either intermittent or continuous catheterization, efforts are made to prevent infection. In addition, a liberal fluid intake is encouraged to reduce the urinary bacterial count, reduce stasis, decrease the concentration of calcium in the urine, and minimize the precipitation of urinary crystals and subsequent stone formation. The patient is kept as mobile as possible, through early ambulation if feasible, or through use of a wheelchair or tilt table. A diet low in calcium is recommended to prevent calculi.

Spastic Bladder

A spastic (reflex, automatic, or hypertonic) bladder is caused by any lesion of the spinal cord above the voiding reflex arc (upper motor neuron lesion). The result is a loss of conscious sensation and cerebral motor control. Reduced bladder capacity and marked hypertrophy of the bladder wall occur. As a result, the bladder empties on reflex, with minimal or no controlling influence to regulate its activity.

Bladder Training Program. The objective of the bladder program is to develop effective spontaneous reflex voiding. The steps of the bladder program are listed in Chart 42-3.

Flaccid Bladder

The flaccid (atonic, nonreflex, or autonomous) neurogenic bladder is caused by a lower motor neuron lesion, most commonly due to trauma. This form of neurogenic bladder has increasingly been recognized as a problem in patients with diabetes mellitus. The bladder continues to fill and becomes greatly distended. The bladder muscle does not contract forcefully at any time. Sensory loss may accompany a flaccid bladder, so the patient feels no discomfort. Overdistention causes damage to the bladder musculature, infection due to stagnant urine, and damage to the kidneys as a result of pressure from the urine.

Management. A patient with a flaccid bladder may be placed on the type of bladder routine outlined in Chart 42-3. A 2-hour voiding schedule is established to prevent overdistention. Parasympathomimetic medications (bethanechol [Urecholine]) may help to increase the contraction of the detrusor muscle. This approach may be very effective, especially for a hypotonic bladder in which there is no significant obstruction of the bladder outlet.

CHART 42-3
Bladder Retraining Guidelines

- The patient drinks a measured amount of fluid from 8 AM to 10 PM; to avoid bladder overdistention, no fluids (except sips) are taken after 10 PM.
- At a specific time, the patient attempts to void by applying pressure over the bladder, tapping the abdomen, or stretching the anal sphincter with a finger to trigger the bladder.
- Immediately following the voiding attempt, the patient is catheterized to determine the amount of residual urine.
- The volumes of urine voided and obtained by catheterization are measured.
- The bladder is palpated at repeated intervals to determine whether distention of the bladder occurs.
- The patient without usual sensation is instructed to be alert for any signs that indicate a full bladder, such as perspiration, coldness of hands or feet, and feelings of anxiety.
- The intervals between catheterizations are lengthened and the patient's program progresses as the volume of residual urine decreases. Catheterization is usually discontinued when the volume of residual urine is at an acceptable level.

Patients can also be taught to perform *self-catheterization* at intervals until spontaneous, complete emptying of the bladder is achieved. Although intermittent catheterization may have to be carried out for a prolonged period of time, it is a safe and successful method of managing patients who have neurogenic bladders.

It is not always possible for the patient to achieve reflex bladder control or self-catheterization. The male patient then may use an *external (condom catheter) collecting device* if the bladder empties well and no residual urine remains. The female patient may need to wear pads or waterproof pants. However, these strategies should be resorted to only after thorough evaluation and attempts at other modes of management.

Surgical intervention may be carried out to correct bladder neck contractures or vesicoureteral reflux or to perform some type of urinary diversion procedure (see Chapter 43).

Dialysis

Dialysis is a process used to remove fluid and waste products from the body when the kidneys are unable to do so.

The purposes are to maintain the life and well-being of the patient until kidney function is restored. Methods of therapy include hemodialysis, hemofiltration, and peritoneal dialysis.

In dialysis, solute molecules diffuse through a semipermeable membrane, passing from the side of higher concentration to that of lower concentration. Fluids pass through the semipermeable membrane by means of osmosis or ultrafiltration (application of external pressure to the membrane). In **hemodialysis**, the membrane is part of the dialyzer or "artificial kidney." In **peritoneal dialysis,** the surface of the peritoneum, or lining of the abdominal wall, serves as the semipermeable membrane.

Hemodialysis may be used when toxins or poisons must be removed immediately to prevent permanent or life-threatening damage. **Hemofiltration** is used to remove excess fluid. Peritoneal dialysis removes fluids more slowly than other forms of dialysis.

Dialysis is used in renal failure to remove toxic substances and body wastes normally excreted by healthy kidneys and in the management of patients with intractable (not responsive to treatment) edema, hepatic coma, hyperkalemia, hypercalcemia, hypertension, and uremia.

Acute dialysis is indicated when there is a high and rising level of serum potassium, fluid overload or impending pulmonary edema, increasing acidosis, pericarditis, and severe confusion. It may also be used to remove certain medications or other toxins (poisoning or medication overdose).

Chronic or **maintenance dialysis** is indicated in chronic renal failure (end-stage renal disease) in the following instances: the occurrence of uremic signs and symptoms affecting all body systems (nausea and vomiting, severe anorexia, increasing lethargy, mental confusion), elevated serum potassium level, fluid overload not responsive to diuretics and fluid restriction, and a general lack of well-being. In addition, the occurrence of a pericardial friction rub is an urgent indication for dialysis in the patient with chronic renal failure.

The decision to initiate dialysis is one that should be reached after thoughtful discussion between the patient, family, and physician. Overwhelming issues are associated with the need for dialysis and often require drastic changes in lifestyle. The nurse can assist the patient and family by answering their questions, clarifying information, and supporting their decision (see the Ethical Question display).

Hemodialysis

It is estimated that more than 100,000 patients currently receive hemodialysis. Hemodialysis is a process used for patients who are acutely ill and require short-term dialysis (days to weeks) or for patients with end-stage renal disease (ESRD) who require long-term or permanent therapy. A synthetic, semipermeable membrane replaces the renal glomeruli and tubules and acts as the filter for the impaired kidneys.

For patients with chronic renal failure, hemodialysis prevents death. However, hemodialysis does not cure or reverse renal disease and is not able to compensate for losses of the kidneys' endocrine or metabolic activities and the impact that renal failure and its treatment have on the patients' quality of life. These patients must undergo dialysis treatment for the rest of their lives (usually three times a week for at least 3 to 4 hours per treatment) or until they receive a successful kidney transplant. Patients are placed on chronic dialysis when they require dialysis therapy for survival and for control of uremic symptoms.

ETHICAL QUESTION:

Should There Be Limits on the Use of Dialysis?

Situation

Hemodialysis is an expensive life-saving procedure that is currently used for more than 100,000 Americans. Hemodialysis allows some people to live near-normal lives despite kidney failure that would otherwise be fatal. Other patients have a less optimistic outlook; for example, patients with multiple system organ failure are treated with hemodialysis that serves to merely prolong their dying process. Dialysis is an expensive medical procedure in an age of ever-increasing scrutiny of health care costs. Is it reasonable to ask for rationing of dialysis? Rationing dialysis by age, HIV status, quality of life, and ability to pay have been suggested as possible options.

Dilemma

The demand of the patient for life-saving treatment conflicts with the public's need to provide and pay for the most cost-effective treatment for all (autonomy versus justice).

Discussion

- What arguments would you offer to support the view that there *should* be limits on the use of dialysis?
- What arguments would you offer to support the view that there *should not* be dialysis rationing?

Principles Underlying Hemodialysis

The objectives of hemodialysis are to extract toxic nitrogenous substances from the blood and to remove excess water. In hemodialysis, the blood, ladened with toxins and nitrogenous wastes, is diverted from the person to a dialyzer, where the blood is cleansed and then returned to the person.

Most dialyzers are either flat plate dialyzers or hollow-fiber artificial kidneys that contain thousands of tiny cellophane tubules that act as semipermeable membranes. The blood flows through the tubules while a dialysate circulates around the tubules. The exchange of wastes from the blood to the dialysate occurs through the semipermeable membrane of the tubules (Fig. 42-4).

Three principles underlie the action of hemodialysis: diffusion, osmosis, and ultrafiltration. The toxins and wastes in the blood are removed by **diffusion,** moving from an area of greater concentration in the blood to an area of lesser concentration in the dialysate. The dialysate is composed of all the important electrolytes in their ideal extracellular concentrations. The electrolyte level in the blood can be brought under control by properly adjusting the dialysate bath. (Small pores in the semipermeable membrane do not allow the loss of red blood cells and proteins.)

Excess water is removed from the blood by **osmosis.** The removal of water can be controlled by creating a pressure gradient; that is, water moves from an area of higher pressure (the patient) to lower pressure (the dialysate). This gradient can be increased by adding negative pressure, known as **ultrafiltration,** to the machine. Negative pressure is an actual suctioning force applied to the membrane and facilitates water removal. Since these patients cannot excrete water, this force is necessary to remove fluid to achieve isovolemia (fluid balance).

The body's buffer system is maintained by the addition of acetate, which diffuses from the dialysate to the patient's blood and is metabolized to form bicarbonate. Purified blood is returned to the body through the patient's vein.

By the end of the dialysis treatment, many waste products have been removed, electrolyte balance has been restored, and the buffer system has been replenished.

During dialysis, the patient, the dialyzer, and the dialysate bath require constant monitoring to detect the numerous complications that can arise (*e.g.*, air embolism, inadequate or excessive ultrafiltration [hypotension, cramping, vomiting], blood leaks, contamination, and shunt or fistula complications). The nurse in the dialysis unit has an important role in monitoring and supporting the patient and in carrying out a continuing program of patient assessment and education.

Dialyzers have undergone changes in technology, and advances have been made in the treatment of end-stage renal disease. As stated earlier, most dialyzers are either flat plate dialyzers or hollow fiber dialyzers. The difference lies in performance and biocompatability. Biocompatability refers to the ability of the dialyzer to accomplish its objectives without causing hypersensitive, allergic, or adverse reactions.

Some dialyzers will remove middle-weight molecules at a faster rate, as well as ultrafiltrate at higher rates. This is thought to reduce neuropathy of the lower extremities, a complication of prolonged hemodialysis. In general, the more efficient the dialyzer, the higher the cost.

Access to the Patient's Circulation

Subclavian and Femoral Catheters. Immediate access to the patient's circulation for emergency hemodialysis is achieved through subclavian catheterization for temporary use. A double-lumen or multi-lumen catheter is inserted into a subclavian vein. Although this method of vascular access is not without risks (*e.g.*, vascular injury such as hematoma, pneumothorax, infection, thrombosis of the subclavian vein, and inadequate flow), it can often be used for several weeks. Femoral catheters can be inserted in the femoral vessels as well for immediate and temporary use. The catheters are removed when no longer needed because the patient's condition has improved or another type of access has been established. It is failure of the permanent access that accounts for the majority of hospital admissions in patients on long-term hemodialysis, making protection of the access one of the priorities of care.

Fistula. A more permanent fistula is created surgically (usually in forearm) by connecting or joining (anastomo-

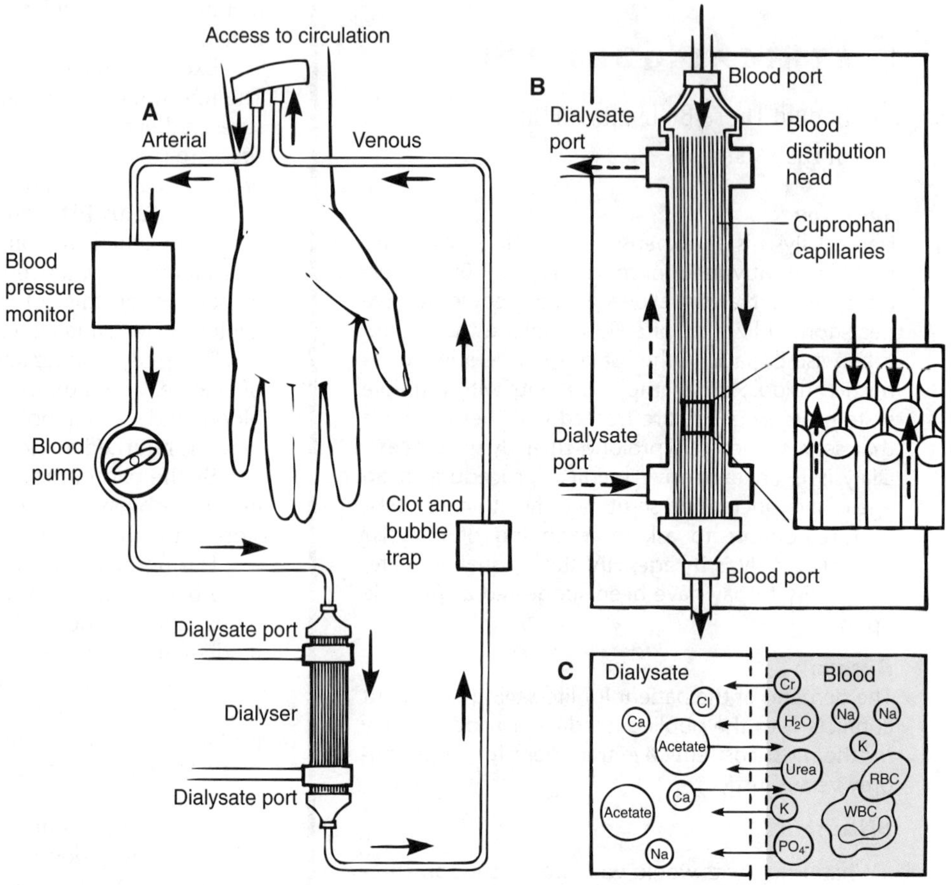

FIGURE 42-4. Schematic drawing of hemodialysis system. Blood from an artery is pumped into a dialyzer, where it flows through the cellophane tubes, which act as the semipermeable membrane (*inset*). The dialysate solution, which has the same chemical composition as the blood except for urea and waste products, flows in around the tubules. The waste products in the blood diffuse through the semipermeable membrane into the dialysate solution (*inset*).

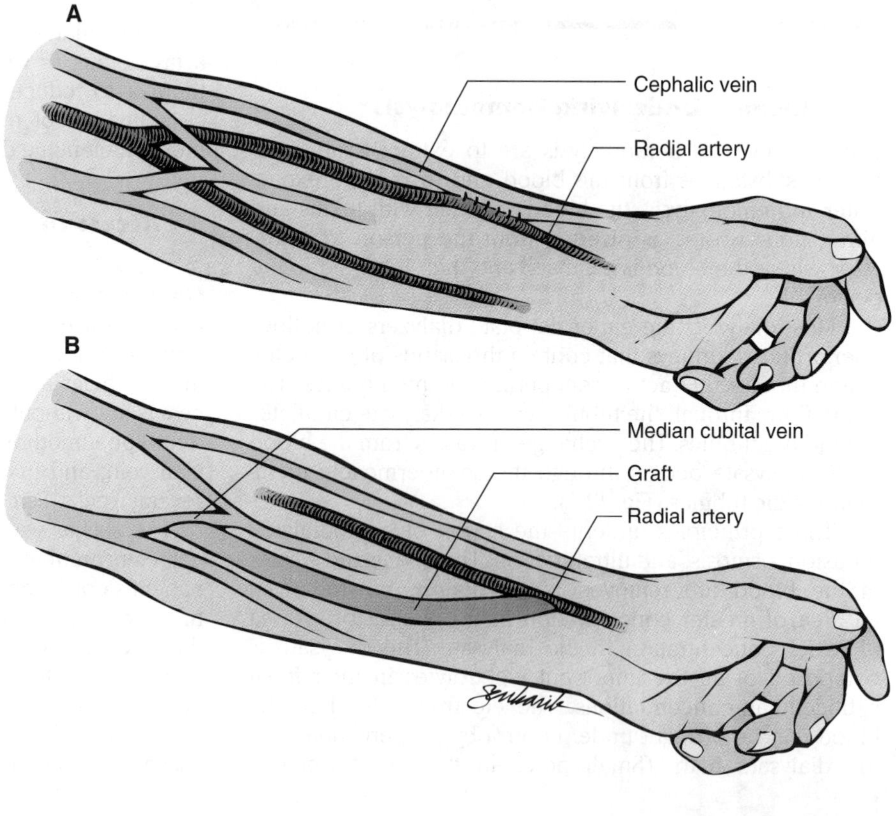

FIGURE 42-5. (**A**) An internal arteriovenous fistula is created by a side-to-side anastomosis of the artry and vein. (**B**) A graft can also be established between the artery and vein.

sis) an artery to a vein, either side to side or end to side (Fig. 42-5*A*). The fistula takes 4 to 6 weeks to "mature" before it is ready for use. This gives time for healing to take place and for the venous segment of the fistula to dilate in order to accommodate two large-bore (14- or 16-gauge) needles. The needles are inserted into the vessel to obtain blood flow adequate to pass through the dialyzer. The arterial segment of the fistula is used for arterial flow and the venous segment for reinfusion of the dialyzed blood. In order to accommodate this blood flow, the arterial and venous segments of the fistula must be larger than normal blood vessels; the patient is encouraged to perform exercises to increase the size of these vessels (*i.e.*, squeezing a rubber ball for forearm fistulas) and thereby accommodate the large-bore needles used in hemodialysis.

Graft. To provide an available segment in which to place dialysis needles, a graft can be created by suturing a piece of bovine artery or vein, Gore-Tex material (heterograft), or saphenous vein graft to the patient's own vessel (Fig. 42-5*B*). Usually, a graft is created when the patient's own vessels are not suitable for a fistula. Grafts are usually placed in the forearm, upper arm, or upper thigh. Patients with compromised vascular systems, such as those with diabetes, often need to have a graft in order to undergo hemodialysis. Because the graft is an artificial vessel, the risk of infection is increased.

Management of the Patient on Long-Term Hemodialysis

Diet and Fluid Considerations. Diet is an important factor for patients on hemodialysis because of the effects of uremia. When damaged kidneys are unable to excrete end products of metabolism, these acidic substances accumulate in the patient's serum and act as poisons or toxins. The symptoms that result from their accumulation are collectively known as **uremic symptoms** and affect every body system. The more toxins that accumulate, the more severe the symptoms. Dietary restriction of protein will reduce the accumulation of nitrogenous wastes and thus minimize the symptoms. Fluid accumulation also occurs and can lead to congestive heart failure and pulmonary edema. Restriction of fluid is then also part of the dietary prescription.

With the effective use of hemodialysis, the patient's dietary intake can be improved but usually requires some adjustment or restriction of protein, sodium, potassium, and fluid intake. In view of the protein restriction, dietary protein must be of high biologic quality and composed of the essential amino acids to prevent poor protein utilization and maintain a positive nitrogen balance. Examples of high biologic protein foods include eggs, meat, milk, and fish.

Impact of Dietary Restrictions. The dietary restriction is a very disturbing and unwelcome change in lifestyle for many patients with chronic renal failure. Since food and drink are important aspects of socialization, patients often feel stigmatized when in the company of others since many times there may be few food options for them. If the restrictions are ignored, life-threatening complications such as hyperkalemia and pulmonary edema may result. Thus, the patient may feel "punished" for responding to basic human drives to eat and drink. If the nurse encounters a patient with symptoms or complications resulting from dietary indiscretion, it is very important to avoid speaking to the patient in harsh, judgmental, and punitive tones.

Medication Considerations. Many medications are excreted wholly or in part by the kidneys. Patients requiring medications (cardiac glycosides, antibiotics, antidysrhythmic agents, antihypertensive agents) are monitored closely to ensure that blood and tissue levels of these medications are maintained without toxic accumulation. Risk of toxic effects of medications must be considered when a patient asks, "Is it safe to take this medicine for a headache?"

Some medications are removed from the blood during dialysis; therefore, adjustment of the dosage by the physician may be required. Medications that are bound to protein will not be removed during dialysis. Removal of other medication metabolites depends on the weight and size of the molecule.

When a patient is receiving dialysis, all medications and their dosages must be evaluated carefully. Antihypertensive therapy, often part of the dialysis patient's regimen, is one example in which communication, teaching, and evaluation can make a difference in patient outcomes. The patient must know when to take and when to withhold the medication. For example, if antihypertensive medications are taken on a dialysis day, a hypotensive effect may occur during dialysis causing dangerously low blood pressure.

Complications

Although hemodialysis can prolong life indefinitely, it does not alter the natural course of the underlying kidney disease, nor does it completely replace kidney function. The patient is subject to a number of problems and complications. One leading cause of death among patients undergoing chronic hemodialysis is arteriosclerotic cardiovascular disease. Disturbances of lipid metabolism (**hypertriglyceridemia**) appear to be accentuated by hemodialysis. Congestive heart failure, coronary heart disease and anginal pain, stroke, and peripheral vascular insufficiency may occur and may incapacitate the patient. Anemia and fatigue contribute to diminished physical and emotional well-being, lack of energy and drive, and loss of interest. Gastric ulcers and other gastrointestinal problems occur from the physiologic stress of chronic illness, medication, and related problems. Disturbed calcium metabolism leads to renal osteodystrophy that produces bone pain and fractures. Other problems include fluid overload associated with congestive heart failure, malnutrition, infection, neuropathy, and pruritus.

Patients with no renal function have been maintained for a number of years by hemodialysis or peritoneal dialysis. Successful kidney transplantation eliminates the need for dialysis treatment. Although the costs of dialysis are reimbursed by Medicare, limitations on the patient's ability to work imposed by illness and dialysis result in a great deal of concern about finances on the part of patients and their families.

Complications of the dialysis treatment itself may include the following:

- *Hypotension* may occur during the treatment as fluid is removed.

- *Air embolism* is rare but can occur if air enters the patient's vascular system.
- *Chest pain* may occur because p O_2 decreases with extracorporeal circulation of blood.
- *Pruritus* may occur during the treatment as the end products of metabolism leave the skin.
- *Dialysis disequilibrium* results from cerebral fluid shifts and is seen as seizures; it is more likely to occur if uremic symptoms are severe.
- *Painful muscle cramping* occurs as fluid and electrolytes rapidly leave the extracellular space.
- *Nausea and vomiting* are common occurrences.

Patient Education

The task of preparing a dialysis patient for discharge from the hospital is often challenging. The disease and its treatment affect every aspect of the patient's life. Often the patient does not fully comprehend the impact of dialysis, and learning needs may go unrecognized until long after discharge. For this reason, good communication between the dialysis nurse, hospital, and home care nurses is essential for providing sound, continuous care.

An assessment is conducted to identify the learning needs of the patient and family members. A patient starting dialysis will receive teaching about the following topics: the purpose of the treatment, medications, side effects of treatment, care of the vascular access, diet and fluid restrictions, fluid overload, prevention and management of complications, psychosocial concerns, and financial considerations. Chart 42-4 presents a list of teaching points for the patient undergoing dialysis.

Once an assessment of learning needs is conducted by the nurse, teaching can begin; however, often there is inadequate time to thoroughly evaluate the patient's learning. Therefore, dialysis staff should be consulted and included because they will be providing the follow-up teaching.

Because the diagnosis of chronic renal failure and the need for dialysis are often overwhelming to the patient and family, teaching must be provided in small increments and time provided for clarification, repetition, and reinforcement. Time must be provided for the patient and family to ask questions and receive clarification. A nonjudgemental attitude is essential to enable the patient and family to discuss options and their feelings about those options. Team conferences are helpful for sharing information and providing every team member the opportunity to discuss the needs of the patient and family.

Psychosocial Considerations

Persons requiring long-term hemodialysis are often concerned about the unpredictability of the illness and the disruption of their lives. They often have financial problems, difficulty in holding a job, waning sexual desires and impotence, depression from being chronically ill, and fear of dying. Younger persons worry about marriage, having children, and the burden that they bring to their families. A regimented lifestyle necessitated by the frequent dialysis treatments and restrictions in food and fluid intake is often demoralizing to the patient and family.

CHART 42-4
Patient Education for the Hemodialysis Patient

Key points in the teaching program include the following:

- The rationale and goals of dialysis treatment
- The relationship of prescribed medications and dialysis
- Side effects of medication and guidelines about when to notify the physician about side effects
- The care of the vascular access; prevention, detection, and management of complications associated with the vascular access
- Rationale for dietary and fluid restrictions; consequences of failure to follow these restrictions
- Guidelines for prevention and detection of fluid overload
- Strategies for detection, management, and relief of pruritus, neuropathy, and other symptoms
- Management of other complications of dialysis and side effects of treatments (dialysis, dietary restrictions, medications)
- Strategies to manage or reduce own anxiety and dependency and those of family members
- Other options available to the patient
- Financial arrangements for dialysis; strategies to identify and obtain resources
- Strategies to maintain independence and to deal with anxious family members

Dialysis imposes an altered lifestyle on the family. The amount of time required for dialysis decreases the time available for social activities and can create conflict, frustration, guilt, and depression in the family. The patient's family and friends may regard the patient as a "marginal person" with a limited life expectancy. It may be difficult for the patient, spouse, and family to express anger and negative feelings. Although normal in this situation, these feelings are often profound and overwhelming, and counseling and psychotherapy may be necessary. Depression may occur and may require treatment with antidepressive agents. It also helps to direct the patient and family to resources that are available for assistance and support. The family should be involved in treatment decisions as much as possible.

The patient should be given the opportunity to express any feelings of anger and concern over the limitations imposed by the disease and treatment, as well as possible financial problems, job insecurity, pain, and discomfort. The sense of loss faced by the patient cannot be underestimated, since every aspect of what once was a "normal life" is disrupted. If anger is not expressed, it may be directed inward and lead to depression, despair, and attempts at suicide; the incidence of suicide is increased in dialysis patients. If the anger is projected outward to other people, it may destroy already threatened family relationships. The patient needs a close relationship with someone to turn to in times of stress and discouragement. Some patients use denial to deal with the overwhelming array of medical problems (*e.g.*, infections, hypertension, anemia, neuropathy). Staff who are tempted to label the patient as noncompliant must consider the impact of renal failure and its treatment on the patient and family and coping strategies that they may use. The nurse can support the patient in identifying effective and safe coping strategies to deal with these ever-present problems and fears.

There are times when a psychiatrist may be needed, since depression may require use of antidepressants. It may also be helpful to refer the patient to a health provider with specific expertise in care of patients receiving dialysis. Clinical nurse specialists, psychologists, and social workers may be helpful in assisting the patient and family deal with the changes brought about by renal failure and its treatment.

Home Dialysis

While most patients needing hemodialysis will undergo the procedure in an outpatient satellite setting, home dialysis is an option for some. However, not all patients are candidates because this procedure requires a highly motivated patient who is willing to take responsibility for the dialysis procedure and is able to adjust each treatment to meet the body's changing needs. It also requires the commitment and cooperation of a partner; often, the patient is not comfortable consuming the time of another.

The decision for home dialysis should never be forced on the patient by the health care team. This endeavor requires many significant changes in the home and family. There are many patients who do not wish to subject their family to home dialysis and often refer to this as "turning my home into a clinic." Whether to perform home hemodialysis must be the patient's and family's decision.

The patient undergoing home hemodialysis and the family member who will serve as assistant must undergo a training program to learn how to prepare, operate, and disassemble the dialysis machine; maintain and clean the equipment; administer medications (heparin) into the machine lines; and handle emergency problems (hemodialysis dialyzer rupture, electrical or mechanical problems, hypotension, shock, and seizures). The patient's home is surveyed to see if electrical outlets and plumbing facilities are adequate. The emphasis is on the patient's assuming primary responsibility for the treatment and a more normal lifestyle.

Other Hemodialysis Methods

High-Flux Dialysis. High-flux dialysis refers to dialysis with newer membranes that increase the clearance of small– and middle–molecular-weight molecules. These membranes are used in conjunction with higher-than-traditional rates of flow for the blood entering and exiting the dialyzer (500–800 ml/min), and for rapid dialysate flow (800 ml). High-flux dialysis increases the efficiency of treatments while shortening their duration and reducing the need for heparin. Not every dialysis unit has the capability of performing high-flux, so it is not a routine method.

Continuous Arteriovenous Hemofiltration. Hemofiltration, or continuous arteriovenous hemofiltration (CAVH), is another method for temporarily replacing kidney function. It is used at the bedside in the intensive care unit for patients with fluid overload secondary to oliguric (low urinary output) renal failure or for patients whose kidneys are unable to handle their acute high metabolic or nutritional needs.

The blood is circulated through a small-volume, low-resistance filter by the patient's own arterial pressure rather than that of the blood pump used in hemodialysis (Fig. 42-6). Blood flows from an artery (via an arteriovenous shunt or arterial catheter) to a hemofilter. Here excess fluids, electrolytes, and nitrogenous waste products are removed by ultrafiltration. The blood then returns to the patient's circulation via the venous arm of the arteriovenous shunt or a venous catheter. The resulting ultrafiltrate contains unwanted solutes and is discarded. Intravenous fluids may be administered to replace fluid removed by the procedure.

The process of hemofiltration is continuous and slow, making it particularly suitable for patients with unstable cardiovascular systems. There is no concentration gradient, so only filtration of fluid occurs. Electrolytes are eliminated only as they are pulled along and removed with the fluid.

Continuous Arteriovenous Hemodialysis. Continuous arteriovenous hemodialysis (CAVHD) has many of the characteristics of CAVH but offers the advantage of a concentration gradient to facilitate more rapid clearance of

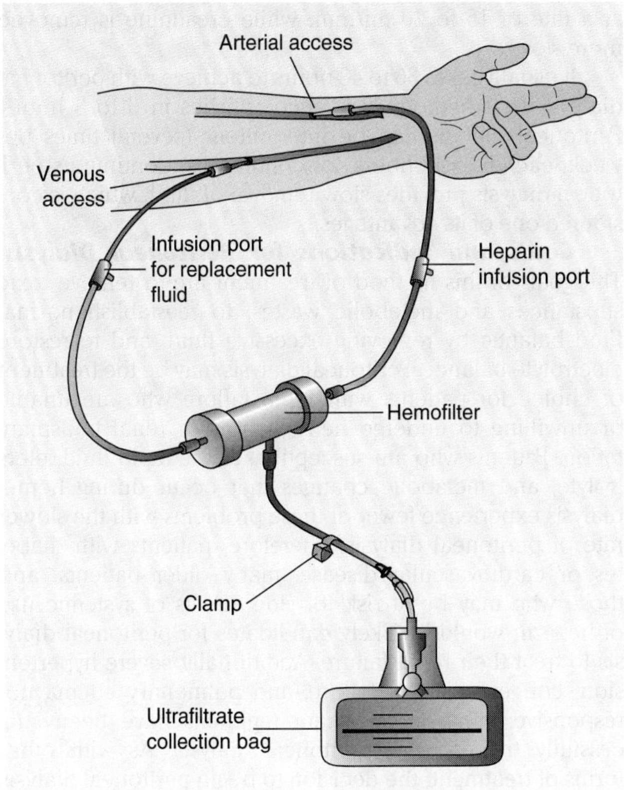

FIGURE 42-6. A schematic representation of a continuous arteriovenous hemofiltration (CAVH) system.

urea. This is accomplished by the circulation of dialysate on one side of a semipermeable membrane. The blood flow through the system is dependent on the patient's arterial pressure, as it is in CAVH; a blood pump is not used as it is in standard hemodialysis.

Major advantages of CAVH and CAVHD are that they do not produce rapid fluid shifts, do not require dialysis machines or dialysis personnel to carry out the procedures, and can be initiated quickly in hospitals without dialysis facilities. Access to the vascular system for these procedures may be through a previously established internal fistula (as used for hemodialysis) or by cannulation of the femoral or radial blood vessels. A pressure gradiant is necessary for optimal filtration; therefore, cannulation of the femoral artery and vein provides the necessary gradiant (difference) in arterial and venous pressures.

Peritoneal Dialysis

In peritoneal dialysis, the surface of the peritoneum, which amounts to approximately 22,000 cm^2, acts as the diffusing surface. An appropriate sterile dialyzing fluid (dialysate) is introduced into the peritoneal cavity through an abdominal catheter at intervals (Fig. 42-7). Urea and creatinine, both metabolic end products normally excreted by the kidneys, are removed (cleared) from the blood by diffusion and osmosis as waste products move from an area of higher concentration (the peritoneal blood supply) to an area of lower concentration (the peritoneal cavity) across a semipermeable membrane (the peritoneal membrane). Urea is cleared at a rate of 15 to 20 ml/min, while creatinine is removed more slowly.

It usually takes 36 to 48 hours to achieve with peritoneal dialysis what hemodialysis accomplishes in 6 to 8 hours. Peritoneal dialysis can be intermittent (several times per week, each 6 to 48 hours) or continuous. Continuous peritoneal dialysis provides slow removal of fluid, which is considered one of its advantages.

Goals and Indications for Peritoneal Dialysis. The goals of this method of treatment are to remove toxic substances and metabolic wastes, to reestablish normal fluid balance by removing excessive fluid, and to restore electrolyte balance. Peritoneal dialysis may be the treatment of choice for patients with renal failure who are unable or unwilling to undergo hemodialysis or renal transplantation. Patients who are susceptible to the rapid fluid, electrolyte, and metabolic changes that occur during hemodialysis experience fewer of these problems with the slower rate of peritoneal dialysis. Therefore, patients with diabetes or cardiovascular disease, many older patients, and those who may be at risk for side effects of systemic use of heparin would be likely candidates for peritoneal dialysis to treat their renal failure. Additionally, severe hypertension, congestive heart failure, and pulmonary edema not responsive to usual treatment regimens have been successfully treated with peritoneal dialysis. As with other forms of treatment, the decision to begin peritoneal dialysis is made by the patient and family in consultation with the physician.

Preparation of the Patient for Peritoneal Dialysis. The patient about to undergo peritoneal dialysis may be

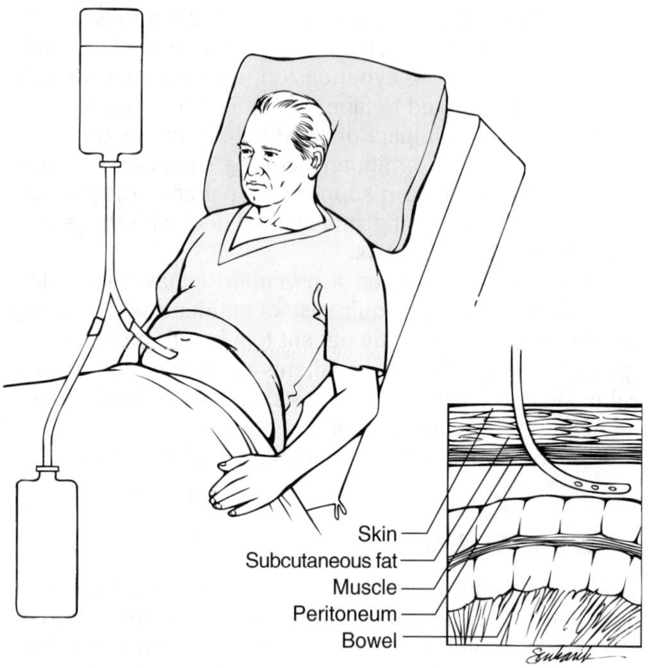

FIGURE 42-7. Peritoneal dialysis. Dialysis fluid is infused into the peritoneal cavity by gravity. After a dwell time of about 20 to 30 minutes (when the fluid is in the peritoneal cavity), the drainage tube is unclamped and the fluid is drained from the peritoneal cavity by gravity (10 to 30 minutes). A new container of fluid is infused immediately.

acutely ill, thus requiring short-term treatment to correct severe disturbances in fluid and electrolyte status, or may be undergoing one of many treatments, as in continuous peritoneal dialysis to treat chronic renal failure. Therefore, the nurse's preparation of the patient and family for peritoneal dialysis is dependent on the patient's physical and psychologic status, level of alertness, previous experience with dialysis, and understanding of and familiarity with the procedure.

The procedure is explained to the patient and a signed consent is obtained. Baseline vital signs, weight, and serum electrolyte levels are recorded. Emptying of the bladder and bowel is indicated to minimize the risk of puncture of internal organs. The nurse also assesses the patient's anxiety about the procedure and provides support and instruction. The catheter is often inserted in the operating room; this is explained to the patient and family.

Preparation of the Equipment for Peritoneal Dialysis. In addition to assembling the equipment for peritoneal dialysis, the nurse consults with the physician to determine the concentration of dialyzing solution to be used and the medications to be added to the dialysate. Heparin may be added to prevent fibrin clot formation and resultant occlusion of the peritoneal catheter. Potassium chloride may be prescribed to prevent hypokalemia. Antibiotics may be added to treat peritonitis.

Prior to the addition of these medications, the dialysate is warmed to body temperature to prevent patient discomfort and abdominal pain and to increase urea clearance by dilation of the vessels of the peritoneum. Solutions that are too cold will cause pain and vasoconstriction and reduce clearance. Solutions that are too hot will burn the peritoneum. Equipment used to heat the solution should be monitored carefully to assure that the desired temperature is obtained.

Immediately prior to initiation of dialysis, the administration set and tubing are assembled. The tubing is filled with the prepared dialysate fluid to reduce the amount of air entering the catheter and peritoneal cavity, which could increase abdominal discomfort and interfere with instillation and drainage of the fluid.

Insertion of the Catheter for Peritoneal Dialysis. Ideally, the peritoneal catheter is inserted in the operating room to maintain surgical asepsis and minimize risk of contamination; however, in some circumstances, the catheter is inserted by the physician at the patient's bedside under strict asepsis. A stylet catheter may be used if it is expected that the peritoneal dialysis will be performed for a very limited period of time. Prior to the procedure, the skin is prepared with a local antiseptic to reduce skin bacteria and reduce the risk of contamination and infection of the catheter site. The physician infiltrates the patient's skin and subcutaneous tissues with a local anesthetic prior to the procedure. A small incision or stab wound is made in the lower abdomen, 3 to 5 cm below the umbilicus; this area is relatively free of large blood vessels and little bleeding should occur. A **trocar** (sharp pointed instrument) is used to puncture the peritoneum as the patient tightens the abdominal muscles by raising his or her head. The catheter is threaded through the trocar and positioned. Dialysis fluid that has been previously prepared is infused into the peritoneal cavity, pushing the **omentum** (peritoneal lining extending from the abdominal organs) away from the catheter. A purse-string suture may be used to secure the catheter in place.

Procedure. For intermittent peritoneal dialysis, the dialyzing solution is allowed to flow freely into the peritoneal cavity. Five to ten minutes are usually required for infusion of 2 liters of fluid. The fluid is allowed to remain in the peritoneal cavity for the prescribed **dwell** or **equilibration time** to allow diffusion and osmosis to occur. Diffusion of small molecules such as urea and creatinine takes place maximally in the first 5 to 10 minutes of the dwell time. At the end of the dwell time, the drainage tube is unclamped and the solution is drained from peritoneal cavity by gravity through a closed system. Drainage is normally completed in 10 to 30 minutes, and the drainage fluid is normally colorless or straw-colored. It should not be cloudy; bloody drainage should not appear after the first few exchanges. A new container of fluid is added, infused, and drained. An exchange (infusion, dwell time, and drainage) may take less than an hour (as may be indicated in acutely ill patients). The number of cycles or exchanges and their frequency are prescribed by the physician based on the patient's physical status and acuity of illness. Care of the patient during peritoneal dialysis is summarized in Guideline 42-1.

Continuous Ambulatory Peritoneal Dialysis

Continuous ambulatory peritoneal dialysis (CAPD) is a form of dialysis used for many patients with end-stage renal disease. Traditional peritoneal dialysis requires skilled nurses and technicians to perform the procedure. Treatments are intermittent, necessitating repeated sessions usually lasting from 6 to 48 hours, during which the patient is relatively immobile. In contrast, CAPD is continuous and usually self-administered. It is performed at home by the patient. Sometimes a family member is trained to perform the exchanges for the patient. The technique is adjusted to the patient's physiologic requirements for dialysis and ability to learn the procedure. This method of treatment must be acceptable to the patient and family and adequate instruction given to assure that they are comfortable and confident in performing the procedure correctly.

The dialysate is delivered from flexible plastic containers through a permanent peritoneal catheter known as a Tenckhoff catheter. This is inserted in the operating room, and is tunnelled through the abdominal cavity and anchored in place by dacron cuffs attached to the catheter. Growth of tissue around the cuff provides a bacteria-resistant seal. A subcutaneous tunnel (5–10 cm in length) provides further protection against bacterial infection (Fig. 42-8).

After the dialysate has infused into the peritoneal cavity through the catheter, the bag is folded and tucked underneath the clothing during the dwell or equilibration time. This provides the patient with some freedom and reduces the number of connections and disconnections necessary at the catheter end of the tubing, thereby reducing the accompanying risk of contamination and peritonitis. At the end of the dwell time, the dialysate is drained from the peritoneal cavity by unfolding the empty bag, opening the clamp, and placing the bag lower than the abdomen near the floor. This allows the peritoneal fluid to drain out by gravity. Following completion of drainage, fresh solution is infused into the peritoneal cavity and the procedure is repeated.

One set of tubing connects the dialysis solution to the catheter. Some tubing systems, known as disconnect sets, allow the catheter to be clamped and disconnected from the long tubing and seem to be better for the patient's body image. Long-life tubing that extends from the dialysate bag to the catheter needs to be changed infrequently.

To reduce the risk of peritonitis, meticulous care is taken to prevent contamination of the catheter, fluid, or tubing and accidental disconnection of the catheter from the tubing. The catheter is protected from manipulation and the catheter entry site is meticulously cared for according to a standardized protocol.

The success of CAPD depends upon the maintenance of the permanent peritoneal catheter. Catheter problems that can arise include one-way obstruction, dislodgment from the pelvis, omental wrapping, dialysate leak, exit-site infection, fibrin-clot formation, and bacterial/fungal contamination.

Principles of CAPD

CAPD works on the same principles involved in other forms of peritoneal dialysis: diffusion and osmosis. However, because CAPD is a continuous treatment, a steady state of serum values of the nitrogenous waste products results. The precise values depend on the residual kidney function, the daily dialysate volume, and the rate at which waste products are produced. Less extreme fluctuations in the patient's laboratory results occur with CAPD than with intermittent

GUIDELINE 42–1
Nursing Care of the Patient During Intermittent Peritoneal Dialysis

Nursing Action	Rationale
I. Promote patient comfort during procedure.	
A. Provide physical comfort measures. 1. Provide frequent back care and massage of pressure areas. 2. Assist patient to turn from side to side. 3. Elevate head of bed at intervals. 4. Allow patient to sit in chair for brief periods if condition permits (only with surgically implanted catheter; with trocar, patient is on bed rest).	The dialysis period is lengthy, and the patient becomes fatigued.
B. Keep patient informed of progress and results. 1. Reinforce teaching about the procedure and its goals. 2. Give patient information about progress (*e.g.,* fluid loss, weight loss, return of electrolyte balance).	Being informed helps the patient to cope and cooperate with the lengthy procedure.
C. Provide care of the whole patient. 1. Provide physiologic and psychologic care throughout procedure, remembering patient's predialysis needs, reactions, concerns, and health problems. 2. Keep family informed about the patient's status and progress.	Focus on the dialysis procedure, rather than on the patient, threatens the patient's psychologic well-being and may result in failure to detect physiologic and emotional problems.
II. Maintain peritoneal dialysis fluid infusion and drainage.	
A. If the fluid is not draining properly, turn the patient from side to side to facilitate the removal of peritoneal drainage. The head of the bed may also be elevated. *Never push in the catheter.* Assess the patency of the catheter. Check for closed clamp, kinked tubing, or air lock.	If the drainage stops, or slows to a drip before the dialyzing fluid has been adequately drained, the catheter tip may be buried in the omentum. Turning the patient may be helpful (or it may be necessary for the physician to reposition the catheter). Pushing in the catheter is contraindicated because it introduces bacteria into the peritoneal cavity.
B. Use strict aseptic technique when adding exchanges or emptying drainage containers.	Minimizes risk of infection.
C. Monitor blood pressure and pulse every 15 minutes during the first exchange, and every hour thereafter. Monitor cardiac rhythm for signs of dysrhythmia.	A drop in blood pressure may indicate excessive fluid loss due to the glucose concentrations of the dialyzing solutions. Changes in vital signs may indicate impending shock or overhydration.
D. Monitor the patient's temperature every 4 hours (especially after catheter removal).	An infection may become evident after dialysis has been discontinued.
E. The procedure is repeated until the serum laboratory values improve. The usual time is 36 to 48 hours; the patient will receive 24 to 48 exchanges (the number dependent on patient's condition). In acute conditions, the catheter is usually removed within 48 to 72 hours. A new trocar is inserted for the next treatment.	The duration of the dialysis depends on the severity of the condition and on the size and weight of the patient.
III. Monitor changes in fluid and electrolyte status, weight changes, vital signs, and intake and output records.	
A. Maintain an exact record of the patient's fluid balance during the treatment. 1. Calculate the status of the patient's loss or gain of fluid at the end of each exchange; check dressing for leakage, and weigh on gram scale if leakage is significant. 2. The fluid balance should be about even or should show *slight* fluid loss or gain, depending on the patient's fluid status. 3. Assure that the record includes the following: a. Exact time of beginning and end of each exchange; starting and finishing time of drainage	Complications (dehydration, circulatory collapse, hypotension, shock, and death) may occur if the patient loses too much fluid through peritoneal drainage. Large fluid losses around the catheter may be missed unless the dressings are checked carefully.

(continued)

GUIDELINE 42–1 *(continued)*
Nursing Care of the Patient During Intermittent Peritoneal Dialysis

Nursing Action	Rationale
b. Amount and type of solution infused and drained c. Fluid balance (cumulative) d. Number of exchanges e. Medications added to dialyzing solution f. Pre- and postdialysis weight, plus daily weight g. Level of responsiveness at beginning, throughout, and at end of treatment h. Assessment of vital signs and patient's condition	
IV. Monitor for complications.	
A. Peritonitis 1. Observe for nausea and vomiting, anorexia, abdominal pain, tenderness, rigidity, and cloudy dialysate drainage. 2. Send specimen of dialysate for WBC and cultures.	Peritonitis is the most common complication. Antibiotics may be added to the dialysate or administered systemically.
B. Bleeding 1. Observe catheter site and drainage for bleeding. 2. Monitor vital signs. 3. Monitor serum hemoglobin and hematocrit.	A small amount of bleeding around a newly inserted catheter is not significant if it does not persist. During the first few exchanges, blood-tinged fluid from subcutaneous bleeding is not uncommon. Small amounts of heparin may be added to inflow solution to prevent the catheter from becoming obstructed or occluded. A hematocrit of the drainage fluid may be obtained to assess the amount of bleeding.
C. Respiratory difficulty 1. Slow the inflow rate. 2. Make sure tubing is not kinked and is draining properly. 3. Prevent air from entering the peritoneal cavity by keeping the drip chamber of the tubing three-fourths full of fluid. 4. Elevate head of bed; encourage coughing and breathing exercises. 5. Turn patient from side to side.	Respiratory difficulty is caused by pressure from the fluid in the peritoneal cavity and the upward displacement of the diaphragm, producing shallow respirations. In severe respiratory difficulty, the fluid from the peritoneal cavity should be drained immediately and the physician notified.
D. Abdominal pain Encourage patient to move about.	Pain may be caused by the dialyzing solution's not being at body temperature, incomplete drainage of the solution, chemical irritation, irritation by the catheter, peritonitis, or air pressing on the diaphragm and causing referred shoulder pain.
E. Leakage 1. Change the dressings frequently around the trocar; use care not to dislodge the catheter. 2. Use sterile, plastic drapes to prevent contamination.	Leakage around the catheter predisposes to peritonitis.
F. Constipation 1. Assist patient to move about in bed. 2. Provide high-fiber foods and fluid within dietary restrictions.	Inactivity, decreased nutrition, use of phosphate binders, and the presence of fluid in the abdomen tend to cause constipation.
G. Low serum albumin 1. Monitor serum protein levels. 2. Assess for edema, hypotension, weight changes.	Small amounts of albumin are lost with each exchange, resulting in a lowered serum albumin. Edema may occur with possible hypotension.

peritoneal dialysis because the dialysis is constantly in progress. The serum electrolytes usually remain in the normal range.

The longer the dwell time, the better the clearance of middle-sized molecules. It is thought that these molecules may be significant uremic toxins. Their clearance is greatly enhanced by CAPD. Low-molecular-weight substances, such as urea, diffuse more rapidly than middle-sized molecules in dialysis, but they are removed more slowly during CAPD than during hemodialysis.

The removal of excess water during peritoneal dialysis is achieved by the use of hypertonic dialyzing solutions that have a high glucose concentration, creating an osmotic gradient. Glucose solutions of 1.5%, 2.5%, and 4.25% are available in several sizes, from 500 ml to 3000 ml, thus allowing the dialysate selection to fit the patient's tolerance, size, and physiologic needs. The higher the glucose concentration, the greater the osmotic gradient and the more water removed. Patients are taught how to select the appropriate solution based on their dietary intake.

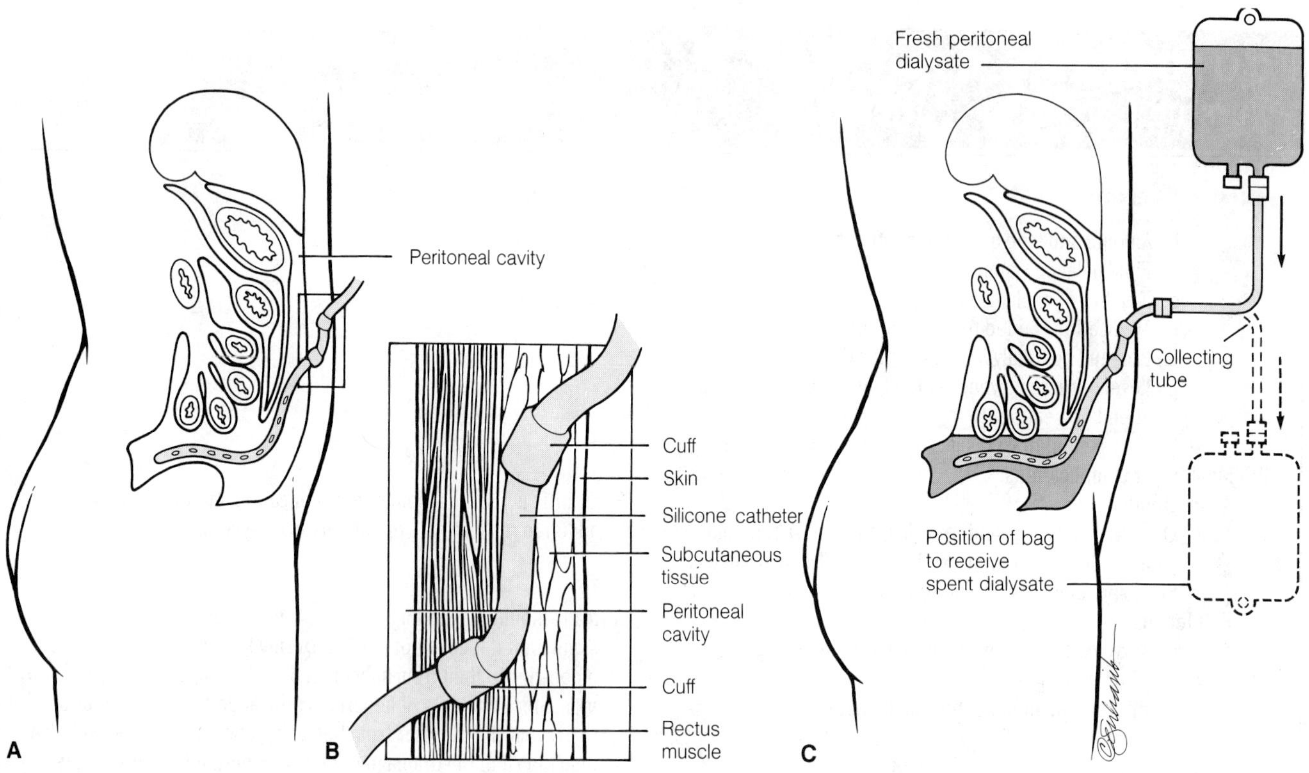

FIGURE 42-8. Continuous ambulatory peritoneal dialysis. (**A**) The peritoneal catheter is implanted through the abdominal wall. (**B**) Dacron cuffs and a subcutaneous tunnel provide protection against bacterial infection. (**C**) Dialysate fluid flows by gravity to the peritoneal catheter into the peritoneal cavity. The fluid is removed by gravity and then discarded. More solution is then infused into the peritoneal cavity until the next drainage period. Dialysis is thus continuous on a 24-hour basis. The patient is free to move around and engage in normal activities.

Exchanges are usually performed four times a day. This technique is continuous, 24 hours a day, 7 days a week. The patient performs the exchanges at intervals spread throughout the day (*e.g.*, at 8 AM, noon, 5 PM, and 10 PM) and sleeps during the night. Each exchange usually takes 30 to 60 minutes or longer to perform; its duration depends on the length of the prescribed dwell time. This consists of a 5- or 10-minute period of infusion, a 20-minute drain period, and a 10-minute, 30-minute, or longer dwell time.

Indications

CAPD is the treatment of choice for most patients who want to perform their own dialysis at home. CAPD is indicated for those patients on maintenance or chronic hemodialysis who have problems with their present treatment modality, such as dysfunction or failure of the vascular access device, excessive thirst, severe hypertension, postdialysis headaches, and severe anemia requiring frequent transfusion.

Patients awaiting a kidney transplant can be safely maintained on CAPD. End-stage renal disease secondary to diabetes is often considered an indication for CAPD as hypertension, uremia, and hyperglycemia are easier to manage with CAPD than with hemodialysis.

Older patients generally do well on CAPD if family or community supports are available. Patients who are able to take an active part in their treatment, want more freedom, and are motivated and willing to carry out the required treatment also do well on CAPD. The patient's family support system, as well as ability to perform CAPD, is considered when the mode of treatment is selected. Support is essential for the treatment to succeed.

Patients choose CAPD to gain freedom from a machine, to achieve control over their daily activities, to avoid dietary restrictions, to increase fluid intake, to elevate the serum hematocrit, to improve control over blood pressure, to be freed from venipuncture, and to gain a general feeling of well-being. Although CAPD gives the appearance of freedom, the treatment is *continuous,* so that the patient is dialyzing 24 hours a day, seven days a week. Some patients find this to be restricting as well and opt for the more intermittent hemodialysis.

Contraindications

Contraindications for CAPD include adhesions from previous surgery or systemic inflammatory disease. Adhesions will reduce clearance of solutes. Another contraindication is recurrent chronic backache with preexisting disc disease, which could be aggravated by the continuous pressure of dialysis fluid in the abdomen. The presence of a colostomy, ileostomy, nephrostomy, or ileal conduit may increase the risk of peritonitis, but is not an absolute contraindication to CAPD. Patients receiving immunosuppressive medications have increased complications because of poor healing of the catheter site. Also, diverticulitis may be a contraindication as CAPD has been associated with rupture of the diverticulum.

Patients with arthritis or poor hand strength may require assistance in performing the exchange. However, blind or partially blind patients and those with other physical limitations have been successful in learning to perform CAPD.

Complications

CAPD is not without complications. Most complications are minor in nature, but several, if left unattended, can have serious consequences for the patient.

Peritonitis. Peritonitis is the most common complication and also the most serious; it occurs in 60% to 80% of patients on peritoneal dialysis. Most peritonitis episodes are due to accidental contamination caused by *Staphylococcus epidermidis.* These episodes result in mild symptoms and have a good prognosis; however, peritonitis due to *Staphylococcus aureus* produces a higher morbidity rate, has a more serious prognosis, and runs a longer course. Gram-negative organisms may originate in the bowel, particularly when there is more than one organism in the peritoneal fluid and when the organisms are anaerobic.

Manifestations of peritonitis include cloudiness of the peritoneal dialysis effluent (drainage) and diffuse abdominal pain. Hypotension and other signs of shock may occur if *S. aureus* is the responsible organism. Drainage fluid is examined for cell count and gram stain and cultured to identify the organism and guide treatment.

Peritonitis is treated in the hospital if the patient is too ill to perform the exchanges. The patient is usually put on intermittent peritoneal dialysis for 48 hours or more or it is stopped entirely while the patient is receiving parenteral antibiotic therapy. Stopping dialysis for several days also promotes phagocytosis by the patient's macrophages; there is evidence that the presence of dialysate in the peritoneal cavity may hamper the response of macrophages to infection.

If the symptoms are mild, the patient is treated as an outpatient. Antibiotics are usually added to the dialysate and also taken orally for 10 days. The infection usually clears in 2 to 4 days. To preserve the patient's remaining renal function, care must be taken in determining the dosage of antibiotics that may be nephrotoxic. Surgical intervention may be necessary if the peritonitis is a result of leakage from the bowel.

With a persistent catheter exit-site infection (usually *S. aureus*), removal of the permanent catheter may be necessary to prevent the development of peritonitis. In patients with fungal peritonitis, the peritoneal catheter should be removed in order to clear the infection. Peritonitis with three positive peritoneal fluid cultures also necessitates catheter removal. The patient is maintained on hemodialysis for about 1 month before a new catheter is inserted.

Regardless of the organism responsible, the patient with peritonitis loses large amounts of protein through the peritoneum; acute malnutrition and delayed healing may result. Therefore, attention must be given to assessment and prompt treatment of these infections.

Leakage. Leakage of dialysate through the incision/insertion site may be noted immediately after the catheter is inserted. Usually, the leak stops spontaneously if dialysis is withheld for several days to give the incision and exit site enough time to heal. During this period, it is important to reduce factors that might delay healing, such as undue abdominal muscle activity and straining during bowel movement. Leakage through the exit site or into the abdominal wall can occur spontaneously months or years after catheter placement. Leakage can often be avoided by beginning with small volumes (100–200 ml) and gradually increasing the volume until a volume of 2000 ml is reached.

Bleeding. A bloody effluent (drainage) may be observed occasionally, especially in young, menstruating females. (The hypertonic fluid pulls blood from the uterus through the opening in the fallopian tubes into the peritoneal cavity.) It is common during the first few exchanges, as some blood exists in the abdominal cavity from the procedure. In many cases, no cause can be found for the bleeding. Catheter displacement from the pelvis has occasionally been associated with the bleeding. Some patients have had bloody effluent following an enema or from minor trauma. Invariably, bleeding stops after a day or two and requires no specific intervention. More frequent exchanges during this time may be necessary to prevent obstruction of the catheter by blood clots.

Other Complications. Other complications include abdominal hernias, probably resulting from the continuously increased intra-abdominal pressure. The types of hernias that have developed include incisional, inguinal, diaphragmatic, and umbilical. The persistently raised intra-abdominal pressure also aggravates symptoms of hiatal hernia and those of hemorrhoids.

Hypertriglyceridemia is frequently found in patients on CAPD, suggesting that this therapy may accelerate atherogenesis. Cardiovascular disease remains a major cause of death in this population of patients.

Low back pain and anorexia due to the presence of fluid in the abdomen and a constant sweet taste related to absorption of glucose may also occur with CAPD.

Mechanical problems may also occur and may interfere with instillation or drainage of the dialysate fluid. Formation of clots in the peritoneal catheter and constipation are factors that may contribute to these problems.

Altered Body Image and Sexuality. Although CAPD has given end-stage renal disease patients more freedom and control over their treatment, it is not without its problems. The patients often experience an altered body image because of the abdominal catheter and the presence of the bag and tubing. Waist size increases from 1 to 2 in (or more) with the presence of fluid in the abdomen, and this affects patients' clothing selection as well as their feeling of "being fat." Body image may be so altered that the patient does not want to look at or care for the catheter for days or weeks. Talking with other patients who have a positive attitude may help. Some patients seem to have no psychologic problems with the catheter; they think of it as their lifeline and as a life-sustaining device. Patients sometimes feel they are doing exchanges all day long and have no free time, particularly in the beginning. They may experience depression because they feel overwhelmed with the responsibility of self-care.

Sexuality and sexual function can be altered; the patient and partner may be reluctant to engage in sexual activities, partly because of the catheter being psychologically "in the way" of sexual performance. The presence of 2 L of dialysate, a peritoneal catheter, and drainage bag may interfere with the sexual function and body image of these patients.

Patient Teaching

Patients are taught to perform CAPD once they are medically stable. They may be taught as inpatients or outpatients. The training usually takes 5 days to 2 weeks (Chart 42-5).

Training Program. During the training period, patients are taught about the basic anatomy and physiology of the kidney; the disease process; the exchange procedure; possible complications and appropriate responses to them; the measurement of vital signs; catheter care; proper hand washing techniques; and, most important, when and whom to call with a problem. Because of the consequences of peritonitis, the patient and family are thoroughly instructed about indicators of peritonitis, preventive measures, and early treatment strategies.

Dietary Measures. The nurse, dietitian and social worker meet with the patient and the family during the training period and at intervals thereafter. Information and instruction about diet are provided. Although the diet of CAPD patients can be liberal, some recommendations are necessary. Because of protein loss with continuous peritoneal dialysis, patients are instructed to eat a high-protein, well-balanced diet. They are also encouraged to increase their fiber intake daily to help prevent constipation, which can impede flow of dialysate into or out of the peritoneal cavity. Often patients gain from 3 to 5 pounds within a month of initiation of CAPD, so they may be asked to limit their carbohydrate intake to avoid an excessive amount of weight gain. Potassium, sodium, and fluid restrictions are not usually needed.

Fluid Intake. Patients usually lose about 2 L of fluid over and above the 8 L of dialysate infused into the abdomen during a 24-hour period, allowing a normal fluid intake even in an anephric patient (a patient without kidneys).

Follow-Up Care. Patients are taught according to their own learning ability and knowledge level, and only as much at one time as they can handle without feeling uncomfortable or becoming overwhelmed. Follow-up care through phone calls, patient visits to the outpatient department, and continuing home care, assist patients in the transition to the home and to the role of active participants in their own health care.

Patients often depend on being able to check with the nurse to see if they are making the right choices as to dialysate or control of blood pressure, or simply to discuss a problem. They may be seen by the CAPD team as outpatients once a month or more if needed. The patient's exchange procedure is evaluated at that time to see that strict aseptic technique is being used. The tubing used to instill the dialysate fluid may be changed by the CAPD nurse every 4 to 8 weeks. Long-life tubing now allows up to six months before tubing changes are necessary. Infrequent tubing changes decrease the risk of possible contamination. Blood chemistry levels are followed closely to make certain the therapy is adequate for the patient.

CHART 42-5
Patient Education for CAPD

- Provide basic information about CAPD
  - Anatomy and physiology
  - The disease process
  - Exchange procedure
  - Potential complications
  - Vital signs measurement techniques
  - Catheter care
  - Contact person for problems
- Describe dietary measures
  - Eat high-protein diet
  - Increase fiber intake to avoid constipation (can interfere with fluid drainage)
  - Limit carbohydrate intake to avoid excessive weight gain
  - No restrictions are usually necessary on potassium, sodium, or fluid intake
- Explain importance of follow-up care to
  - Reinforce aseptic techniques to avoid infection
  - Change tubing when necessary
  - Evaluate blood chemistry levels
  - Provide feedback
  - Allow for questions and additional teaching
- Encourage patient opportunity to express concerns, doubts, and anxieties.

Psychologic Considerations

CAPD is not suitable for all patients with end-stage renal disease, but it is a viable form of therapy for those who want to do self-care and experience a feeling of independence from a machine and its accompanying rigid schedule. If patients are willing to do the exchange as taught, and are able to fit the therapy into their own routines, they can live relatively normal lives and feel a measure of accomplishment and success with CAPD. Often patients report that they feel better on CAPD, have more energy, and feel more normal and healthier. It would be wrong to encourage all patients to seek CAPD. Instead, patients should be helped to find the therapy most suitable for their particular lifestyle and with which they can best reach an optimal state of well-being.

Continuous Cycler Peritoneal Dialysis

Continuous cycler peritoneal dialysis (CCPD) is a combination of overnight intermittent peritoneal dialysis with a prolonged dwell time during the day. The peritoneal catheter is connected to a cycler machine every evening and the patient receives three to five 2-L exchanges during the night. In the morning, the patient caps off the catheter after infusing 1 to 2 L of fresh dialysate. This dialysate remains in the abdominal cavity until the tubing is reattached to the cycler machine at bedtime. The patient is able to sleep because the machine is very quiet, and extra-long tubing allows the patient to move and turn normally during sleep.

This technique decreases the infection rate because of fewer opportunities for contamination with bag changes and tubing disconnections and permits the patient to be free of exchanges throughout the day, making it possible to work more freely and carry out activities of daily living.

Care of the Hospitalized Dialysis Patient

The patient who receives hemodialysis or peritoneal dialysis may be hospitalized for treatment of complications related to the underlying renal abnormality or the dialysis treatment itself. In addition, the patient may be hospitalized for health problems not related to renal dysfunction or its treatment.

Protecting the Vascular Access. When the hemodialysis patient is hospitalized for any reason, care must be taken to protect the vascular access from damage. Therefore, the vascular access is assessed for patency, and precautions are taken to ensure that the extremity with the vascular access is not used for blood pressure measurements or for obtaining blood specimens. The bruit or "thrill" over the venous access site must be evaluated at least every 8 hours. If the thrill is not palpable or the bruit not audible it could indicate clotting of the access. Clotting can occur if the patient has an infection anywhere in the body, since serum viscosity is increased, or if the blood pressure has dropped. When blood flow is reduced through the access for any reason (hypotension, application of blood pressure cuff or tourniquet), blood is then stagnant and clots in the access. The access site can become infected, so it must be washed and when necessary a sterile dressing applied. The renal patient is more prone to infection, so infection control measures must be used for *all* procedures.

IV Therapy Precautions. When intravenous solutions are necessary, the rate of administration must be as slow as possible and should be strictly controlled by a volumetric infusion pump. Since this patient cannot excrete water, indiscriminate use of intravenous therapies can result in pulmonary edema.

Uremic Symptoms. As metabolic end products accumulate, uremic symptoms worsen. Patients whose metabolic rate is accelerated (those on steroid medications, those with infections or bleeding disorders, those undergoing surgery) will accumulate wastes more quickly and may require daily dialysis. These same patients are likely to experience complications sooner rather than later.

Cardiac and Respiratory Complications. Cardiac and respiratory assessment must be conducted frequently. As fluid buildup progresses, *congestive heart failure* and *pulmonary edema* develop. Crackles in the bases of the lungs may indicate pulmonary edema.

Pericarditis may result from the accumulation of uremic toxins. If not detected and treated promptly, this serious complication may progress to pericardial effusion and cardiac tamponade. Pericarditis is detected by patient's report of substernal chest pain (if the patient is able to communicate), low-grade fever (often overlooked), and pericardial friction rub. A pulsus paradoxus (a decrease in blood pressure of more than 10 mm Hg during inspiration) is often present. When pericarditis progresses to effusion, the friction rub disappears, heart sounds become distant and muffled, ECG waves show very low voltage, and the pulsus worsens.

The effusion may progress to life-threatening *cardiac tamponade,* noted by narrowing of the pulse pressure in addition to muffled or inaudible heart sounds, crushing chest pain, dyspnea, and hypotension. Although pericarditis, pericardial effusion, and cardiac tamponade can be detected by chest x-ray, they should also be detected through astute nursing assessment. Because of their clinical significance, assessment of the patient at risk for the development of cardiac complications becomes a priority.

Electrolyte and Dietary Concern. Electrolyte alterations are common, with potassium changes being the most deadly. All intravenous solutions to be administered are evaluated for their electrolyte content and serum laboratory values are assessed daily. The patient's dietary intake must also be monitored for foods that exceed the dietary restriction. The patient's frustrations related to dietary restrictions are often increased if the hospital food is unappetizing; this may lead to dietary indiscretion and hyperkalemia.

Discomfort and Pain. Complications such as pruritus and pain secondary to neuropathy must be managed. Antihistamines and analgesic medications may be prescribed. However, because elimination of metabolites of medications occurs through dialysis rather than through renal excretion, dosages of medications often require adjustment.

Hypertension. Hypertension in renal failure is common and results in part from oversecretion of renin. Many dialysis patients receive some form of antihypertensive therapy and require intense teaching about its purpose and side effects. The trial-and-error approach that may be necessary to identify the most effective agent and dose may be confusing or alarming to the patient if no explanation is provided. Antihypertensive medication must be withheld on dialysis days to avoid hypotension due to the combined effect of the dialysis and the medication.

Infection Risks. Patients with end-stage renal failure often have low white blood cell counts (and decreased phagocytic ability), low red cell counts (anemia), and impaired platelet function. Together these lead to high risk for infection and potential for bleeding following even minor trauma. Infection control is essential since the incidence of infection is high. Infection of the vascular access site and pneumonia are common.

Catheter Site Care. The patient receiving CAPD (continuous ambulatory peritoneal dialysis) is usually well versed in care of the catheter site; however, it is important to use the patient's hospital stay as an opportunity to assess compliance with recommended catheter care and to correct any misperceptions or deviations from correct technique.

Medication Considerations. The medications prescribed for any dialysis patient must be closely monitored to avoid those that are toxic to the kidneys and that may threaten any remaining renal function. All medications must be monitored and alterations in dosages may be necessary to prevent either toxic effects on the kidney or overdosage because of impaired renal excretion. Care must be taken to evaluate all problems and symptoms reported by the patient without attributing them to renal failure or to the fact that the patient is on dialysis.

Psychologic Considerations. The patient who has been receiving dialysis for a while may begin to reevaluate his or her status, the treatment modality, satisfaction with life, and the impact of these factors on his or her family. Opportunity must be provided for the patient to verbalize feelings and reactions and to explore possible options.

It is not uncommon for a patient to consider discontinuing dialysis treatment. These feelings and reactions must be taken seriously, and opportunity provided to discuss them with the dialysis team as well as with a psychologist, psychiatrist, psychiatric nurse, trusted friend, or member of the clergy. The decision of the patient to begin dialysis does not require that dialysis be continued indefinitely. The patient's informed decision about discontinuing treatment, after thoughtful deliberation, should be respected.

The Patient Undergoing Kidney Surgery

A patient may undergo surgery of the kidney to remove obstructions (tumors or calculi); to insert a tube for drainage of the kidney (nephrostomy, ureterostomy); or to remove the kidney itself in treating unilateral kidney disease or renal carcinoma, or managing the patient undergoing renal transplantation.

Preoperative Considerations

Surgery of the kidney is performed only after a period of evaluation and preparation to ensure optimal renal function. Fluids are encouraged to promote increased excretion of waste products before surgery, unless contraindicated because of preexisting renal or cardiac dysfunction. If kidney infection is present preoperatively, wide-spectrum antimicrobial agents may be prescribed to prevent bacteremia. Antibiotics must be administered with extreme care because many of them are toxic to the kidneys. Coagulation studies (prothrombin time, partial thromboplastin time, platelet count) may be indicated if the patient has a history of bruising and bleeding. The general preoperative preparation is similar to that described in Chapter 19.

Patients facing kidney surgery are often apprehensive. They may enter the hospital with pain, fever, and hematuria. Thus, the nurse encourages the patient to recognize and express any feelings of anxiety. Confidence is reinforced by establishing a relationship of trust and by providing expert care. Patients faced with the prospect of losing a kidney may think that they will be dependent on dialysis for the rest of their lives. However, normal function may be maintained by a single healthy kidney.

Perioperative Concerns

The operative incisions for renal surgery include flank, intercostal, lumbodorsal, and transverse abdominal or thoracoabdominal incisions (Fig. 42-9). The difficulties in renal surgery are related to the difficulty in obtaining access to the kidney. Plans are made at this time for managing altered urinary drainage and drainage systems.

Postoperative Management

Because the kidney is a highly vascular organ, hemorrhage and shock are the chief complications following renal surgery. Fluid and blood replacement is frequently necessary in the immediate postoperative period to treat intraoperative blood loss.

Abdominal distention and paralytic ileus are fairly common following surgery on the kidney and ureter and are thought to be due to a reflex paralysis of intestinal peristalsis and manipulation of the colon or duodenum during surgery. Abdominal distention is relieved by decompression via a nasogastric tube. (See p. 400 for treatment of paralytic ileus.) Oral fluids are permitted when the passage of flatus is noted.

If infection occurs, antibiotics are prescribed as necessary on the basis of identification of the causative organism by culture. The toxic effects these agents have on the kidneys must be kept in mind when assessing the patient. Low-dose heparin therapy may be initiated postoperatively to prevent thromboembolism in urologic patients.

Management may also include insertion of a nephrostomy or other drainage tube or the use of ureteral stents (see p. 1169).

Management of Drainage Tubes

Almost all patients undergoing kidney and urologic surgery and many patients with other kidney and urologic disturbances have drains, tubes, or catheters in place. Following surgical procedures such as nephrostomy, pyelotomy, and ureterotomy, drainage tubes may be placed directly in the kidney, pelvis, or ureter in order to divert or drain the urine and keep the surgical incision dry. All catheters and tubes must be kept patent (*e.g.*, draining) to prevent obstruction by blood clots, which can cause infection and eventually kidney damage. Pain caused by the passage of blood clots down the ureter is similar to renal colic.

Nephrostomy Drainage. A nephrostomy tube is inserted directly into the kidney for temporary or permanent urinary diversion either percutaneously or through a surgical incision. A single tube or a self-retaining U-loop or circular nephrostomy tube may be used (see p. 1218). Nephrostomy drainage may be required to provide drainage from the kidney after surgery, conserve or restore drainage, serve to bypass obstruction in the ureter or lower urinary tract, or restore drainage. The nephrostomy tube is attached to a closed drainage system or to a urostomy appliance.

Percutaneous nephrostomy is the insertion of a tube through the skin into the pelvis of the kidney. It is performed to provide external drainage of urine from an obstructed ureter, to provide a route for inserting a ureteral stent (see following discussion), to dissolve renal calculi, to dilate strictures, to close fistulas, to administer medications, to al-

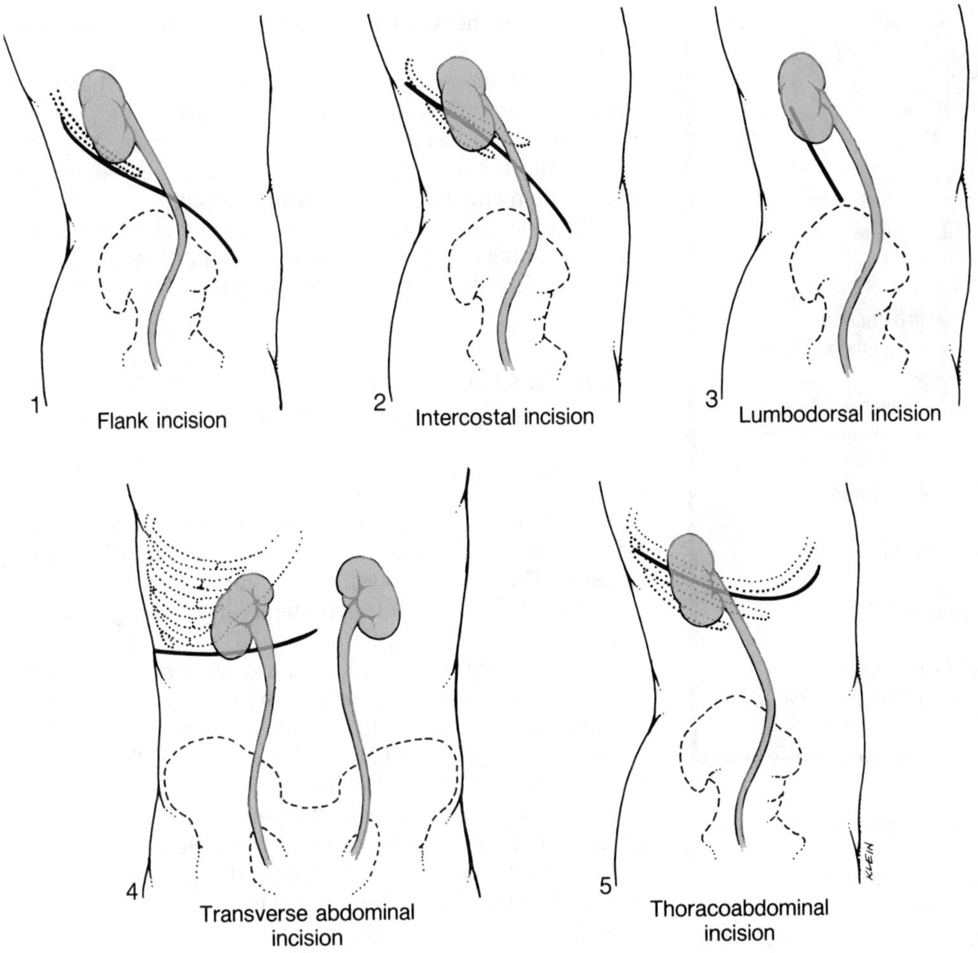

FIGURE 42-9. Standard incisions for urologic surgical procedures.

low insertion of a brush biopsy instrument and nephroscope, or to perform selected surgical procedures.

The skin site is prepared and anesthetized, and the patient is asked to inhale and hold his or her breath while a spinal needle is advanced into the renal pelvis. Urine is aspirated for culture, and a contrast agent may be injected into the pyelocalyceal system. An angiographic catheter guide wire is introduced through the needle to the kidney. The needle is withdrawn and the tract dilated by the passage of tubes or guidewires. The nephrostomy tube is introduced and positioned within the kidney or ureter, fixed by skin sutures, and connected to a closed drainage system.

The patient and tubing are observed for signs of bleeding (immediate or delayed), urinary stones or debris, fistula formation, and infection, and the nephrostomy tube is assessed for adequate drainage. Obstruction of the tube produces pain, trauma, pressure and stress on the suture lines, and infection. If the tube is dislodged inadvertently, it must be immediately replaced by the surgeon because the nephrostomy opening will contract, making it difficult to reinsert the tube.

A *nephrostomy tube is never clamped,* because such an action will cause acute pyelonephritis, nor is the nephrostomy tube ever irrigated. If irrigation is necessary, it is performed by the surgeon. Only 10 ml of warm, sterile saline is used because of the small size of the renal pelvis and the risk of mechanical damage to the kidney or infection from pyelorenal backflow.

Fluid intake is encouraged to produce good mechanical flushing and to dilute urinary particles that cause calculus formation. The urine is kept acidic to prevent the tube from becoming encrusted with urinary sediments. If the patient has a nephrostomy tube in each kidney, output for each catheter is measured and recorded separately. The catheters may be attached to leg collection bags when the patient becomes ambulatory. (See Chart 42-6 for a summary of care of the patient following a nephrostomy.)

Ureteral Stents

A ureteral stent is a tubular device designed to be placed within the ureter. Stents are used to maintain urine flow in patients with ureteral obstruction (from edema, stricture, fibrosis, advanced malignancy), to restore kidney function, to divert urine, to promote healing, and to maintain the caliber/patency of the ureter after surgery (Fig. 42-10).

The stent, usually of soft, flexible silicone, may be temporary or permanent. It may be inserted through a cytoscope or nephrostomy tube or by open surgery. Complications include infection, inflammation secondary to the presence of a foreign body in the genitourinary tract, tube encrustation, bleeding or clot obstruction within the stent, and dislodgment of the stent.

CHART 42-6
Care of the Patient Following a Nephrostomy

1. Assess for possible complications:
   a. Bleeding at nephrostomy site (main complication)
   b. Fistula formation
   c. Infection
2. Assure unobstructed drainage of nephrostomy tube or catheter. (Obstruction will cause pain, trauma, pressure, infection, and stress on suture lines.)
3. If tube becomes dislodged, report immediately. (Surgeon must replace tube immediately to prevent nephrostomy opening from contracting.)
4. Never clamp a nephrostomy tube; this will cause pyelonephritis.
5. Never irrigate a nephrostomy tube. (Irrigation will be performed by surgeon if necessary.)
6. Encourage fluid intake to promote natural flushing of kidney and tube.
7. Measure urine output from tube. If both kidneys have a tube in place, measure output from each tube separately.

Newer stent designs avoid some of these problems. The double-J ureteral stent has a J-shaped curve molded into each end, which prevents upward or downward migration. This stent can be used in place of a nephrostomy or pyelostomy for short- or long-term urinary drainage. The double-pigtail ureteral stent has a pigtail coil at each end, which permits placement of the upper coil (pigtail) in the renal pelvis, with the lower coil at the ureteral orifice. The

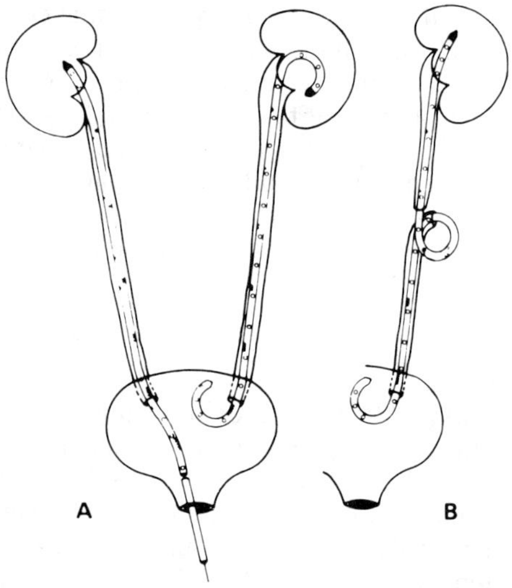

FIGURE 42-10. Ureteral stents. (**A**) Retrograde passage of ureteral stent. The double-J ureteral stent is shaped to resist migration. The proximal J hooks into the lower calix or renal pelvis, and the distal J curves into the bladder. (**B**) Open surgical placement of double-J stent prior to a ureteral anastomosis. (Courtesy of Medical Engineering Corporation, Racine, WI.)

coils prevent the stent from moving and allow free body movement.

Nursing interventions include monitoring for bleeding, observing and measuring output, assessing for purulent drainage at the insertion site or in the drainage bag, and monitoring for stent displacement, which is evidenced by colicky pain and a decrease in urine output.

An indwelling stent usually induces local ureteral reaction, including mucosal edema, which can cause temporary obstruction of the ureter and intense pain.

❑ NURSING PROCESS
The Patient Undergoing Kidney Surgery

Assessment

Immediate care of the postoperative patient who has undergone surgery of the kidney includes assessment of all body systems. The patient's respiratory and circulatory status, pain level, fluid and electrolyte status, and patency and adequacy of urinary drainage are assessed.

Respiratory Status. As with any surgery, use of anesthesia increases the risk of respiratory complications. Therefore, the patient's respiratory status is assessed by monitoring the rate, depth, and pattern of respirations. The location of the surgical incision frequently causes pain on inspiration and coughing. Therefore, the patient tends to splint the chest wall and respirations tend to be shallow. Auscultation is performed to assess for normal and adventitious breath sounds. The location of the surgical incision assists in anticipating respiratory problems and pain.

Circulatory Status and Blood Loss. The vital signs and arterial or central venous pressure are monitored. Skin color and temperature and urine output will also provide information about the adequacy of circulatory status. The surgical incision and drainage tubes are observed frequently to aid in the detection of unexpected blood loss and hemorrhage.

Pain. Pain is a major problem for the patient postoperatively because of the location of the surgical incision and the patient's position on the operating table to permit adequate access to the kidney. The location and severity of pain are assessed before and after administration of analgesics. Abdominal distention, which increases the patient's discomfort, is also noted.

Urinary Drainage. The patient's urinary output and drainage from tubes inserted during surgery are monitored for amount, color, and type of output and drainage. Decreased or absent drainage is reported promptly to the physician, because it may indicate obstruction that could cause pain, infection, and disruption of the suture lines.

Diagnosis

Nursing Diagnoses

Based on the history and assessment data and the type of surgical procedure performed, major nursing diagnoses for the patient include the following:

- ❑ Risk for ineffective airway clearance related to the location of the surgical incision

- ❑ Risk for ineffective breathing pattern related to surgical incision and anesthesia
- ❑ Pain and discomfort related to the location of the surgical incision, the position assumed on the operating table during surgery, and abdominal distention
- ❑ Alteration in urinary elimination related to urinary drainage

Collaborative Problems/ Potential Complications

Based on assessment data, potential complications that may develop include:

- ❑ Bleeding
- ❑ Pneumonia
- ❑ Infection
- ❑ Fluid disturbances (deficit or excess)
- ❑ Deep vein thrombosis

Planning and Implementation

Goals. The major goals for the patient may include maintenance of effective airway clearance and breathing pattern, maintenance of cardiac output, relief of pain and discomfort, maintenance of urinary elimination, maintenance of fluid balance, and absence of complications.

Nursing Interventions

Maintaining Airway Clearance and Breathing Patterns. The surgical approaches to the kidney predispose the patient to respiratory complications and paralytic ileus. Also, with a subcostal or posterior incision, the patient may have severe pain on breathing and coughing. If the pleural cavity has been entered during surgery, pneumothorax may occur, necessitating insertion of a chest tube. The incision is generally close to the diaphragm and, with a substernal incision, the nerves may be stretched and bruised. These factors can lead to pain and limited chest movement during inspiration; breathing patterns are altered or ineffective when the chest cannot fully expand. If the patient cannot generate an effective cough, either because of incisional pain and restriction or from anesthesia, ineffective airway clearance may result.

Adequate use of analgesic medications is necessary to relieve pain so that the patient is able to take deep breaths and cough. If the analgesia is administered at regular, frequent intervals, the patient will be able to perform deep-breathing and coughing exercises more effectively. The incentive spirometer may be used to help maximize lung inflation. The patient is encouraged to cough after each deep breath to loosen secretions.

Relieving Pain. In addition to incisional pain, the patient may experience pain and discomfort from distention of the renal capsule (by tumor or blood clot), ischemia (from occlusion of blood vessels), and stretching of the intrarenal blood vessels. Adequate pain relief is necessary to permit the patient to take deep breaths, cough, turn, and move about. The patient also frequently experiences muscular aches and pains resulting from the position assumed on the operating table, which places anatomic and physiologic stresses on the body. Massage, moist heat, and analgesic medications provide relief. Patient-controlled analgesia (PCA) may be effective in assuring pain control and ability of the patient to ambulate, cough, and deep breathe (see Chapter 13 for discussion of PCA).

Promoting Urinary Elimination. Attention to the patient's urinary output and drainage is essential to preserve and protect the patient's remaining kidney function. Therefore, adequate drainage is critical to prevent obstruction and infection. The output from each urinary drainage tube is recorded separately; very accurate output measurements are essential in monitoring renal function and assuring the patency of the urinary drainage system.

Strict asepsis is used during manipulation of the drainage catheter and tube. Hand washing is mandatory before and after touching any parts of the system. Use of closed drainage systems is essential to avoid contamination of the system and infection. The urinary drainage is monitored closely for changes in volume, color, odor, and constituents. Urinalysis and urine cultures are indicated to follow the patient's progress. Care is taken to be sure that the collection bag is suspended below the patient's bladder to prevent reflux of urine into the urinary tract. However, the bag must be kept off the floor to prevent contamination.

Most urinary drainage systems do not require routine irrigation. If irrigation is necessary and prescribed, however, it should be performed carefully, with the use of sterile solution; with minimal pressure, consistent with the physician's instructions; and with strict asepsis without interruption of the closed drainage system.

Monitoring and Managing Potential Complications. *Bleeding* is a major complication of kidney surgery. If undetected and untreated, bleeding may result in hypovolemia and hemorrhagic shock. The nurse's role is to observe for these complications, to report their signs and symptoms, and to administer prescribed parenteral fluids and blood and blood components if complications occur. Monitoring of the patient's vital signs, skin condition, urinary drainage system, surgical incision, and level of consciousness is necessary to detect evidence of bleeding, decreased circulating blood, and fluid volume and cardiac output. Frequent monitoring of vital signs (initially monitored at least at hourly intervals), arterial blood gases, and urinary output is necessary for early detection of these complications.

If bleeding goes undetected or is late in being detected, the patient may have lost significant amounts of blood and may experience hypoxia. In addition to hypovolemic (hemorrhagic) shock, this type of blood loss may precipitate a myocardial infarction or transient ischemic attack. Bleeding may be suspected when the patient experiences fatigue and when urine output is less than 30 ml per hour. As bleeding persists, late signs of hypovolemia such as cool skin, flat neck veins, and change in level of consciousness or responsiveness will occur. Transfusions of blood component products are indicated along with surgical repair of the bleeding vessel.

Pneumonia may be prevented through use of an incentive spirometer, adequate pain control, and early ambulation. Early signs of pneumonia include fever, increased heart and respiratory rates, and the development of adventitious breath sounds.

Prevention of infection is the rationale for use of asepsis when changing dressings and meticulous care of catheters, other drainage tubes, central venous catheters, and

(text continues on page 1174)

NURSING CARE PLAN 42–1
Care for the Patient Undergoing Surgery of the Kidney

Nursing Interventions	Rationale	Expected Outcomes
NURSING DIAGNOSIS: Risk for ineffective airway clearance related to pain of high abdominal or flank incision, abdominal discomfort, and immobility; risk for ineffective breathing pattern related to high abdominal incision **GOAL:** Adequate airway clearance; normal breathing pattern		
1. Administer analgesics as prescribed.	1. Pain relief enables patient to take deep breaths and cough.	• Takes deep breaths and coughs adequately when encouraged and assisted. • Exhibits respiratory rate of 12–18/min. • Exhibits normal breath sounds without adventitious sounds. • Exhibits full thoracic excursion without shallow respirations. • Uses incentive spirometer with encouragement. • Splints own incision while taking deep breaths and coughing. • Reports progressively less pain and discomfort with coughing and deep breaths. • Exhibits normal blood gases and chest x-ray. • Exhibits normal body temperature with no signs of atelectasis or pneumonia on assessment.
2. Splint patient's incision with hands or pillow to assist patient in coughing.	2. Splints incision and promotes adequate cough and prevention of atelectasis.	
3. Assist patient to change positions frequently.	3. Promotes drainage and inflation of all lobes of the lungs.	
4. Encourage use of incentive spirometer if indicated or prescribed.	4. Encourages adequate deep breaths.	
5. Assist with and encourage early ambulation.	5. Mobilizes pulmonary secretions.	
NURSING DIAGNOSIS: Pain and discomfort related to surgical incision, positioning, and stretching of muscles during kidney surgery **GOAL:** Relief of pain and discomfort		
1. Assess patient's level of pain.	1. Provides baseline for later assessment of pain-relief strategies.	• Reports relief of severe pain and discomfort. • Takes analgesia as prescribed. • States rationale for use of moist heat and massage. • Exercises aching muscles within recommendations. • Gradually increases physical activity and exercise. • Uses distraction, relaxation exercises, and imagery for pain relief. • Exhibits absence of behavioral manifestations of pain and discomfort (*e.g.,* restlessness, perspiration, verbal expressions of pain). • Participates in deep-breathing and coughing exercises.
2. Administer analgesics are prescribed.	2. Promotes pain relief.	
3. Apply moist heat and massage to areas with muscular aches and discomfort.	3. Promotes relaxation and relief of muscle pain and discomfort.	
4. Splint patient's incision with hands or pillow during movement or deep breathing and coughing exercises.	4. Minimizes sensation of pulling or tension on incision and provides sense of support to the patient.	
5. Assist and encourage early ambulation.	5. Promotes resumption of muscle activity exercise.	
NURSING DIAGNOSIS: Fear and anxiety related to diagnosis, outcome of surgery, and alteration in urinary function **GOAL:** Reduction of fear and anxiety		
1. Assess patient's anxiety and fear prior to surgery if possible.	1. Provides a baseline for postoperative assessment.	• Verbalizes reactions and feelings to staff.

(*continued*)

NURSING CARE PLAN 42–1 *(continued)*
Care for the Patient Undergoing Surgery of the Kidney

Nursing Interventions	Rationale	Expected Outcomes
2. Assess patient's knowledge about procedure and expected surgical outcome preoperatively.	2. Provides a basis for further teaching.	• Shares reactions and feelings with family or partner. • Grieves appropriately for self and for changes in role and function.
3. Evaluate the meaning alterations have for patient and family or partner.	3. Enables understanding of patient's reactions/responses to expected and unexpected results of surgery.	• Identifies information needed to promote own adaptation and coping.
4. Encourage patient to verbalize reactions, feelings, and fears.	4. Verbalization of responses is often necessary for patient's understanding of them and ultimate resolution.	• Participates in activities and events in immediate environment. • Accepts visit from support person or participates in support group.
5. Encourage patient to share feelings with spouse or partner.	5. Enables patient and partner to receive mutual support and reduces sense of isolation from each other.	• Identifies support person from own experience and peer group.
6. Offer and arrange for visit from member of support group (*e.g.*, ostomy group, if indicated).	6. Provides support from another person who has encountered the same or a similar surgical procedure and an example of how others have coped with the alteration.	

NURSING DIAGNOSIS: Altered patterns of urinary elimination related to urinary drainage; high risk for infection related to urinary drainage

GOAL: Maintenance of urinary elimination; infection-free urinary tract

Nursing Interventions	Rationale	Expected Outcomes
1. Assess urinary drainage system immediately.	1. Provides basis for further assessment and action.	• Exhibits adequate urinary output and patent drainage system.
2. Assess adequacy of urinary output and patency of drainage system.	2. Provides baseline.	• Exhibits urine output consistent with fluid intake.
3. Use asepsis and hand washing when providing care and manipulating drainage system.	3. Prevents or reduces risk of contamination of urinary drainage system.	• Demonstrates normal laboratory values: BUN, creatinine, urine specific gravity and osmolality.
4. Maintain closed urinary drainage system.	4. Reduces risk of bacterial contamination and infection.	• Exhibits sterile urine on urine culture. • Exhibits clear, dilute urine without debris or encrustation in the drainage system.
5. If irrigation of the drainage system is necessary, use gloves and sterile irrigating solution, and a closed drainage and irrigation system.	5. Permits irrigation when necessary while maintaining closed drainage system, minimizing risk of infection.	• States rationale for avoiding manipulation of catheter, drainage, or irrigation system.
6. If irrigation is necessary and prescribed, it is carried out gently with sterile saline and the prescribed amount of irrigating fluid.	6. Maintains patency of the catheter or drainage system and prevents sudden increases in pressure in the urinary tract that may cause trauma, pressure on sutures or urinary tract structures, and pain.	• Exhibits normal placement of urinary stent or ureteral catheters until removed by physician. • Maintains closed urinary drainage system.
7. Assist patient in turning and moving in bed and when ambulating to prevent displacement or accidental removal of urinary stent or ureteral catheters if in place.	7. Prevents trauma from accidental displacement of urinary stent or ureteral catheter, necessitating repeated instrumentation of the urinary tract (*e.g.*, cystoscopy) to replace them.	• Exhibits normal body temperature without signs or symptoms of urinary tract infection. • Cleans catheter with soap and water.
8. Observe urine color, volume, odor, and constituents.	8. Provides information about adequacy of urine output, condition and patency of drainage system, and debris in urine.	• Consumes adequate fluid intake (6–8 glasses of water or more per day unless contraindicated).
9. Minimize trauma and manipulation of catheter, drainage system, and urethra.	9. Reduces risk of contamination of drainage system and eliminates site of bacterial invasion.	• Urinary drainage system remains in place until removed or discontinued by physician.
10. Clean catheter gently with soap during bath; avoid to-and-fro movement of catheter.	10. Removes debris and encrustations without causing trauma or contamination of urethra.	

(continued)

NURSING CARE PLAN 42–1 *(continued)*
Care for the Patient Undergoing Surgery of the Kidney

Nursing Interventions	Rationale	Expected Outcomes
11. Anchor drainage tube.	11. Prevents movement or slipping of drainage tube, minimizing trauma and contamination of urethra or catheter.	• Maintains urinary drainage system without infection or obstruction. • Maintains urinary diversion as instructed. • Maintains self-care so that environment is odor-free. • States rationale for close follow-up and maintains recommended schedule of appointments with health care providers.
12. Maintain adequate fluid intake.	12. Promotes adequate urinary output and prevents urinary stasis.	
13. Assist with and encourage early ambulation while ensuring placement of urinary drainage system.	13. Minimizes cardiovascular and pulmonary complications while preventing loss, dislodging, or disruption of drainage system.	
14. If patient is to be discharged with urinary drainage system (catheter) in place or a urinary diversion, instruct patient and family member in care.	14. Knowledge and understanding of the drainage system or urinary diversion are essential to prevent infection and other complications.	

NURSING DIAGNOSIS: Risk for fluid volume excess or deficit related to surgical fluid loss, altered urinary output, parenteral fluid administration

GOAL: Normal fluid balance will be maintained

Nursing Interventions	Rationale	Expected Outcomes
1. Weigh patient daily.	1. Daily weight is the most sensitive indicator of fluid loss or gain.	• Patient's weight will be within 2–3 pounds of normal.
2. Take accurate intake and output measurements.	2. Detects fluid retention from poor cardiac or renal output.	• Intake that exceeds output will be detected early.
3. Place all parenteral therapy on an infusion pump.	3. Assures that the patient does not accidentally receive excess or insufficient intravenous fluids.	• The exact amount of solution is infused with no adverse effects resulting from over or under infusion.
4. Monitor amount and characteristics of urine.	4. Assists in detection of possible complications of surgery or tube insertion early.	• Urine is clear and absent of blood, pus, or any foreign substances.
5. Monitor vital signs: temperature, pulse, respiration, and blood pressure.	5. When fluid volume or cardiac output is altered, vital signs will be affected.	• Temperature, pulse, respiration and blood pressure are normal.
6. Auscultate heart and lungs every shift.	6. When fluid volume is increased from either poor cardiac or renal output, fluid will accumulate in the lungs. Also, heart sounds will change as congestive heart failure develops. Frequent auscultation will assure early detection.	• Presence of normal heart and lung sounds.

intravenous catheters for administration of fluids. Insertion sites are monitored closely for signs of inflammation: redness, drainage, heat, and pain. Special care must be taken to prevent urinary infection, which is associated with use of indwelling urinary catheters. Catheters and other invasive tubes are removed as soon they are no longer needed.

Coughing, deep breathing, use of incentive spirometers, early ambulation, and pain management are important to minimize the risk of pneumonia. Antibiotic agents are often administered postoperatively to prevent infection. If antibiotic agents are prescribed, the patient's serum creatinine and blood urea nitrogen (BUN) levels must be monitored closely because many antibiotics may be toxic to the kidney or may accumulate to toxic levels if renal function is decreased.

Prevention of fluid imbalance is a critical component of care for the patient undergoing kidney surgery. Both fluid loss and fluid excess are possible following surgery on the kidney.

Fluid loss may occur during surgery, as a result of excessive urinary drainage that occurs with removal of obstruction, or if diuretics are used for any reason. It can also occur with gastrointestinal losses: with diarrhea resulting from antibiotic use or with nasogastric drainage. If postoperative intravenous therapy is inadequate to match the output or fluids lost, a fluid deficit will result.

Fluid excess or overload may result from cardiac effects of anesthesia, if excessive amounts of fluids are administered, or if the patient is unable to excrete fluid because of changes in renal function. Decreased urine output must be recognized as a risk factor for fluid excess.

Astute assessment skills must be used to detect early signs of fluid excess (such as weight gain, pedal edema, urinary output below 30 ml/h, slightly elevated pulmonary wedge pressure, if available) before those symptoms become severe (appearance of adventitious breath sounds, shortness of breath).

Fluid excess may be treated with fluid restriction and administration of furosemide (Lasix) or other diuretics. If renal insufficiency is present, these medications may not result in removal of excess fluid; therefore, dialysis may be necessary to prevent congestive heart failure and pulmonary edema.

Deep vein thrombosis (DVT) may occur postoperatively because of surgical manipulation of the iliac vessels during surgery. Elastic stockings are applied and the patient is monitored closely for signs and symptoms of DVT and encouraged to exercise the legs. Heparin may be administered postoperatively to reduce the risk of DVT.

Specific nursing interventions for the patient undergoing kidney surgery are presented in Nursing Care Plan 42-1.

Patient Education and Home Care Considerations. If the patient is to be discharged from the hospital with the drainage system in place, measures are taken to be sure that both patient and family understand the importance of maintaining the system correctly and preventing infection. Verbal and written instructions and guidelines are provided to the patient prior to discharge. Specific indications that necessitate notifying the nurse or physician are identified.

Arrangements are made to have the patient visited at home by a home care nurse. The specific instructions and guidelines given to the patient are shared with the home care nurse prior to the home visit. The nurse will assess the patient's ability to carry out the instructions and guidelines in the home and answer questions the patient or family may have about the procedure. Additionally, the nurse assesses the patient for infection and obstruction of the urinary tract, encourages an adequate fluid intake, and assesses the patient's compliance with recommendations. Those signs, symptoms, problems, and questions that should be referred to the physician or other primary health care provider are reviewed by the nurse with the patient and family.

Evaluation

Expected Outcomes

1. Achieves effective airway clearance
   a. Exhibits clear and normal breath sounds, normal respiratory rate, and unrestricted thoracic excursion
   b. Performs deep-breathing exercises, coughs every 2 hours, and uses the incentive spirometer as directed
   c. Demonstrates normal temperature and vital signs
2. Reports progressive decrease in pain
   a. Requires analgesics at less frequent intervals
   b. Turns, coughs, and takes deep breaths as suggested
   c. Ambulates progressively
3. Maintains urinary elimination
   a. Demonstrates unobstructed urine flow from drainage tubes
   b. Exhibits normal fluid and electrolyte balance (normal skin turgor, serum electrolytes within normal range, absence of symptoms of imbalances)
   c. Reports no increase in pain, tenderness, or pressure at drainage site
   d. Exhibits cautious handling of own drainage system
   e. Washes hands before and after handling drainage system and handles it only when necessary
   f. States rationale for use and maintenance of a closed drainage system
4. Participates in self care activities
5. Absence of complications
   a. Demonstrates normal vital signs and arterial and central venous pressures; normal skin turgor, temperature, and color
   b. Exhibits no signs or symptoms of bleeding, shock, or hypovolemia (*e.g.*, decreased urine output, restlessness, rapid pulse)
   c. Exhibits no signs of infection (such as fever and pain) or evidence of deep vein thrombosis (tenderness or redness of calves)
   d. Normal fluid balance is maintained; no rapid weight gain or loss
   e. Breath sounds are clear, no shortness of breath
   f. Urinary output is at least 30 ml per hour

CRITICAL THINKING EXERCISES

1. Your patient has been informed that he has renal insufficiency and is likely to require dialysis. He knows little about dialysis and the different types of dialysis available. Describe how you would develop a teaching plan to explain the different types of dialysis, their goals, and the level of involvement on the part of the patient and family. How might you modify your approach if the patient does not have health insurance? Is so distraught that he cannot seem to hear what you are saying? Tells you that he thinks his life is over and "why bother"?
2. A patient with a neurogenic bladder requires instruction on self-catheterization. How would you conduct your teaching sessions to instruct the patient in the correct procedure? How would you modify your instruction if the patient has a hand tremor? Comes from a culture that is highly sensitive about exposing one's body to others, especially women?
3. A dialysis patient is admitted to the hospital for surgery unrelated to her kidney disorder. How would your preoperative and postoperative care be modified by the patient's renal failure and her need for dialysis?

BIBLIOGRAPHY

Books

Agency for Health Care Policy and Research, Public Health Service, Department of Health and Human Services. Urinary Incontinence in Adults. Clinical Practice Guideline (AHCPR 92-0038). Washington, DC, US Government Printing Office, 1992.

Alspach JG. Core Curriculum for Critical Care Nursing, 4th ed. Philadelphia, WB Saunders, 1991.
Bates BA. A Guide to Physical Examination and History Taking, 6th ed. Philadelphia, JB Lippincott, 1995.
Carrieri-Kohlman V, Lindsey A, and West C. Pathophysiological Phenomena in Nursing, 2nd ed. Philadelphia, WB Saunders, 1993.
Funk SG. Key Aspects of Elder Care: Managing Falls, Incontinence, and Cognitive Impairment. New York, Springer, 1992.
Gaffney J and Zirker W. Empirical validation of urge incontinence in a sample of elderly women. In Carroll-Johnson R and Paquette M (eds). Classification of Nursing Diagnoses: Proceedings of the Tenth Conference, North American Nursing Diagnosis Association. Philadelphia, JB Lippincott, 1994, 286–287.
Groer M and Shekleton M. Basic Pathophysiology: A Holistic Approach, 3rd ed. St. Louis, CV Mosby, 1989.
Illustrated Manual of Nursing Practice, 2nd ed. Springhouse, PA, Springhouse Corp., 1994.
King BD and Harke J. Coping With Bowel and Bladder Problems. San Diego, CA, Singular Publishing Group, 1994.
Kursh ED and McGuire EJ. Female Urology. Philadelphia, JB Lippincott, 1994.
Mastering Advanced Assessment. Springhouse Advanced Skills Series. Springhouse, PA, Springhouse Corp., 1993.
McCance K and Huether S. Pathophysiology: The Biologic Basis for Disease in Adults and Children, 2nd ed. St. Louis, Mosby, 1994.
Methany N. Fluid and Electrolyte Balance: Nursing Considerations, 2nd ed. Philadelphia, JB Lippincott, 1992.
Morbidity and Mortality of Dialysis. NIH Consensus Statement 1995 Nov 1-3:1-33.
Price S and Wilson L. Pathophysiology: Clinical Concepts of Disease Processes, 4th ed. St. Louis, CV Mosby, 1992.
Providing Expert Care for the Acutely Ill. Springhouse Advanced Skill Series. Springhouse, PA, Springhouse Corp., 1994.
Walters MD and Karram MM. Clinical Urogynecology. St. Louis, CV Mosby, 1993.
Woodtli M and Yocum K. Urge incontinence: Identification and clinical validation of defining characteristics. In Carroll-Johnson R and Paquette M (eds). Classification of Nursing Diagnoses: Proceedings of the Tenth Conference, North American Nursing Diagnosis Association. Philadelphia, JB Lippincott, 1994, 182–185.

Journals

General

Asterisks indicate nursing research articles.

Andriole GL Jr. et al. New options in urology. Patient Care 1993 Jan 30; 27(2): 12–18, 21–22, 24.
*Flanerty MJ Sr and O'Brien ME. Family styles of coping in end stage renal disease. ANNA J 1992 Aug:19(4): 345–349.
Kopp J. Psychosocial correlates of diabetes and renal dysfunction. ANNA J 1992 Sep/Oct; (19)5:432–437.
Linday LA. Developmental changes in renal tubular function. J Adolesc Health 1994 Dec;15(8):648–653.
Lindeman RD. Assessment of renal function in the old. Special considerations. Clin Lab Med 1993 Mar; 13(1):269–277.
McIntosh LJ and Richardson DA. 30-minute evaluation of incontinence in the older woman. Geriatrics 1994 Feb; 49(2):35–38, 43–44.
Nielsen B. Evaluation of micturition. J Wound Ostomy Continence Nurs 1995 Jun; 22(1):44–50.
Paterson NE et al. Treating acute anuria or oliguria. Patient Care 1993 Jan 15; 27(1):162–166, 168, 171.
Radke KJ. Renal physiology series: Part 6 of 8. The aging kidney: structure, function, and nursing practice implications. ANNA J 1994 Jun; 21(4):181–190.
*Rittman M et al. Living with renal failure. ANNA J 1993 June; 20(3):327–331.
Schneck DN et al. Lower urinary tract infections in women: A pragmatic approach. Hospital Medicine 1993 May; 29(5):48, 51–52, 53–55.
Varella L. Nutritional support for the patient with renal failure. Crit Care Nurs Clin North Am 1993 Mar; 5(1):79–96.
Yucha CB. Renal physiology series: Part 5a of 8. Renal control of calcium. ANNA J 1993 Aug; 20(4):440–444.

Urinary Incontinence and Bladder Management

Ashworth PD et al. Some social consequences of non-compliance with pelvic floor exercises. Physiotherapy 1993 July; 79(7): 465–471.
Faller NA. Clean intermittent catheterization: An intervention for overflow voiding or overflow incontinence. Ostomy Wound Manage 1992 Sep; 38(7):29–30, 34–37.
Grinspun D. Bladder management for adults following head injury. Rehab Nurs 1993 Sep/Oct; 18(5):300–305.
*Harke JM et al. Barriers to implementing a continence program in nursing homes. Clin Nurs Res 1992 May; 1(2):158–168.
Jackson AB. Bladder management in women. Phys Med Rehabil Clin North Am 1993 May; 4(2):321–328.
Maynard FM. Long term management of neurogenic bladder: Intermittent catheterization. Phys Med Rehabil Clin North Am 1992 May; 4(2):299–310.
Mylotte JM et al. Staying on top of hospital infections. Patient Care 1993 Feb 15; 27(3):116–120, 122–123, 127–128.
Ouslander JG and Schnelle JF. Incontinence in the nursing home. Ann Intern Med 1995 Mar 15; 122(6):438–449.
Ouslander J et al. The dark side of incontinence: Nighttime incontinence in nursing home residents. J Am Geriatr Soc 1993 Apr; 41(4):371–376.
Pearson BD. Liquidate a myth: Reducing liquid intake is not advisable for elderly with urine control problems. Urol Nurs 1993 Sep; 13(3):86 87.
Pieper B and Cleland V. An external urine-collective device for women: A clinical trial. J ET Nurs 1993 Mar–Apr; 20(2):51–55.
Resnick NM. Urinary incontinence in older adults. Hosp Pract 1992 Oct 15; 27(10):139–142, 147, 150.
Rousseau P and Fuentevilla-Clifton A. Urinary incontinence in the aged, Part II. Management strategies. Geriatrics 1992 Jun; 47(6):37–40, 45, 58.
*Sampselle C and DeLancey J. The urine stream interruption test and pelvic muscle function. Nurs Res 1992 Mar/Apr; 41(2): 73–77.
*Skoner MM, Thompson WD and Caron VA. Factors associated with risk of stress urinary incontinence in women. Nurs Res 1994 Sep/Oct; 43(5):301–306.
Summitt RL Jr. Investigative techniques, assessment of incontinence, and urodynamics. Curr Obstet Gynecol 1992 Aug; 4(4): 548–553.
Taylor M. Cystometrogram through an indwelling suprapubic catheter. Urol Nurs 1992 Mar; 12(1):26.
Thayer D. How to assess and control urinary incontinence. Am J Nurs 1994 Oct 94(10):42–47.
Woodtli M. Assessing urge incontinence in elderly women. Geriatr Nurs 1993 Jan–Feb; 14(1):19–22.
Wozniak-Petrofsky J. Urinary incontinence in the elderly: Not a normal part of aging. Urol Nurs 1993 Mar; 13(1):12–16.
*Wyman J et al. Influence of functional, urological and environmental characteristics on urinary incontinence in community dwelling older women. Nurs Res 1993 Sep/Oct; 42(5):270–275.

Urinary Catheters

Culbertson L. A comparison of Foley catheter types in home care use. Home Healthcare Nurse 1992 Nov–Dec; 10(6):45–47.
Fiers S. Indwelling catheters and devices: Avoid the problems. Urology Nurse 1994 Sep; 14(3):141–144.
Gould D. Keeping on tract . . . an overview of recent research on the management of indwelling urethral catheters, indicating

areas where further work is needed. Nurs Times 1994 Oct 5–11; 90(40):58–62.

Fuselier HA. Etiology and management of acute urinary retention Compr Ther 1993 Jan; 19(1):31–36.

Moore K et al. Bacteriuria in intermittent catheterization users: The effect of sterile versus clean reused catheters. Rehabilitation Nursing 1993 Sep/Oct; 18(5):306–310.

Nickel JC. Catheter associated urinary tract infection. New perspectives on old problems. Can J Infect Control 1991 Summer; 6(2):38–42.

Pinkerman M. Indwelling urinary catheters: Reducing infection risks. Nursing 1994 Sep; 24(9):66–68.

Stover SL. Management of bacteriuria and infection in neurogenic bladder. Phys Med Rehabil Clin North Am 1993 May; 4(2): 343–362.

Warren J et al. Long-term urethral catheterization increases risk of chronic pyelonephritis and renal inflammation. J Am Geriatr Soc 1994 Dec; 42(12):1286–1290.

Dialysis

Berkoben M and Schwab S. Maintenance of permanent hemodialysis vascular access patency. ANNA J 1995 Feb; 22(1):17–24.

Brunier GM and Graydon J. The influence of physical activity on fatigue in patients with ESRD on hemodialysis. ANNA J 1993 Aug; 20(4):457–461.

Brunier GM and McKeever PT. The impact of home dialysis on the family: Literature review. ANNA J 1993 Dec; 20(6):653–659.

Dirkes S. How to use the new CVVH renal replacement systems. Am J Nurs 1994 May; 94(5):67–73.

*Dunetz P. Perceptions by medical/surgical nurses of hospitalized dialysis patients. ANNA J 1991 Dec; 18(6):561–564.

Dunetz PS. If your med/surg patient is on dialysis. RN 1992 Sep; 55(9):46–48, 50, 52–53.

Dunn SA. How to care for the dialysis patient. Am J Nurs 1993 Jun; 93(6):26–33.

*Dunn S et al. Quality of life for spouses of C.A.P.D. patients. ANNA J 1994 Aug; 21(5):237–246.

Ferrans CE and Powers MJ. Quality of life of hemodialysis patients. ANNA J 1993 Oct; 20(5):575–581.

Forseter G et al. Hepatitis C in the health care setting II: Seroprevalence among hemodialysis staff and patients in suburban New York City. Am J Infect Control 1993 Feb; 21(1):1, 5–8.

Haas L. Chronic complications of diabetes mellitus: Peritoneal dialysis. ANNA J 1992 Sep/Oct; (19)5:439–445.

Hampton JK. Long term effects of hemodialysis on diabetic patients with ESRD. ANNA J 1992 Sep/Oct; 19(5):455–456.

Jensen S et al. Clinical experience with erythroparetin in continuous ambulatory peritoneal dialysis. ANNA J 1992 Nov/Dec; 19(6):542–545.

*Korniewicz DM and O'Brien ME. Evaluation of a hemodialysis patient education and support program. ANNA J 1994 Feb; 21(1):33–38.

*Montemuro M et al. Participatory control in chronic hospital-based hemodialysis patients. ANNA J 1994 Dec; 21(7) 429–438.

Moss AH, Rettig RA and Cassel CK. A proposal for guidelines for patient acceptance to and withdrawal from dialysis: A follow-up to the ION report. ANNA J 1993 Oct; 29(5):557–561.

Northsea C. Using urokinase to restore patency in double lumen catheters. ANNA J 1994 Aug; 21(5):261–264, 273.

Peters VJ et al. Rehabilitation experiences of patients receiving dialysis. ANNA J 1994 Dec; 21(7):419–426, 457.

INFORMATION/RESOURCES

Agencies

American Association of Kidney Patients
1 Davis Blvd., Suite LL1,
Tampa, FL 33606;
(813) 251-0725

American Society for Artificial Internal Organs
P.O. Box C,
Boca Raton, FL 33429;
(407) 391-8589

National Institute of Diabetes and Digestive and Kidney Diseases
National Institutes of Health,
Bethesda, MD 20892

National Kidney Foundation
30 East 33rd St.,
New York, NY 10016;
(212) 889-2210

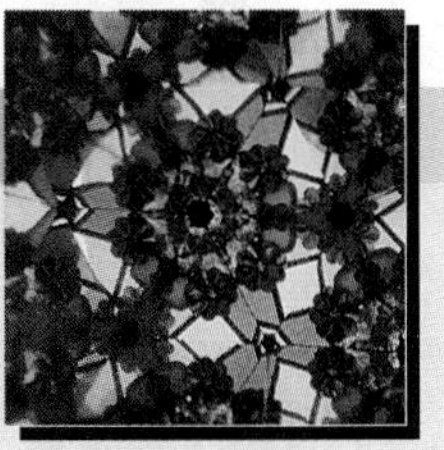

43 Management of Patients With Urinary and Renal Disorders

CHAPTER OUTLINE

Infections and Inflammations of the Urinary Tract
Overview of Urinary Tract Infections
Cystitis (Lower Urinary Tract Infection)
NURSING PROCESS: The Patient With Lower Urinary Tract Infection
Interstitial Cystitis
Urethritis
Pyelonephritis (Upper Urinary Tract Infection)
Perinephric Abscess
Renal Abscess (Renal Carbuncle)
Tuberculosis of the Kidney and Genitourinary Tract
Acute Glomerulonephritis
Chronic Glomerulonephritis
Nephrotic Syndrome
Nephrosclerosis
Hydronephrosis
Renal Failure
Acute Renal Failure
Chronic Renal Failure (End-Stage Renal Disease)
Gerontologic Considerations
Kidney Transplantation
Preoperative Management
Postoperative Management
Urolithiasis
Clinical Manifestations
Diagnostic Evaluation
Management
NURSING PROCESS: The Patient With Renal Stones
Urethral Strictures
Renal Trauma
Bladder Injuries
Renal Cysts
Congenital Anomalies
Renal Tumors
Clinical Manifestations
Management
Nursing Interventions
Cancer of the Bladder
Urinary Diversion
Ileal Conduit Urinary Diversion (Ileal Loop)
Continent Ileal Urinary Reservoir (Kock Pouch)
Ureterosigmoidostomy
Cutaneous Ureterostomy
Cystostomy
Other Urinary Diversion Procedures
NURSING PROCESS: The Patient Undergoing Urinary Diversion
Critical Thinking Exercises

LEARNING OBJECTIVES

On completion of this chapter, the learner will be able to:

1. Identify factors contributing to urinary tract infections
2. Develop a teaching plan for the patient with urinary tract infection
3. Compare and contrast pyelonephritis, glomerulonephritis, and the nephrotic syndrome: causes, pathophysiologic changes, clinical manifestations, and management
4. Describe causes of acute renal failure and chronic renal failure
5. Use the nursing process as a framework for the care of patients with acute renal failure
6. Use the nursing process as a framework for the care of patients with chronic renal failure
7. Develop a postoperative nursing care plan and teaching plan for the patient undergoing kidney transplantation
8. Describe modalities for management of renal calculi (kidney stones)
9. Develop a teaching plan for the patient undergoing treatment for renal calculi (kidney stones)
10. Formulate preoperative and postoperative nursing diagnoses for the patient undergoing surgery for urinary diversion
11. Describe interstitial cystitis and its physical and psychologic impact on the patient

Disorders of the urinary tract and kidneys range from easily treated infections to life-threatening disorders that necessitate organ replacement or long-term treatment with dialysis. Recent advances in pharmacotherapeutics and technology have improved the diagnostic and treatment possibilities for these disorders. Additionally, those disorders that once required surgical intervention and prolonged recuperation can be treated today with noninvasive, nonsurgical techniques.

Infections and Inflammations of the Urinary Tract

Urinary tract infections (UTIs) are caused by the presence of pathogenic microorganisms in the urinary tract, with or without signs and symptoms. The most common site of infection is the bladder (cystitis), but the urethra (urethritis), prostate (prostatitis), and kidney (pyelonephritis) may also be affected. The normal urinary tract is sterile above the urethra.

General risk factors for UTI include inability or failure to empty the bladder completely, decreased natural host defenses, and instrumentation of the urinary tract, including catheterization and cystoscopic procedures. Certain populations of patients are more prone to UTIs than others. Patients with diabetes are at risk because increased urinary glucose levels create an infection-prone environment in the urinary tract. Pregnancy and neurologic disorders also increase the risk of UTI because they result in incomplete emptying of the bladder and stasis of urine.

Bacteriuria refers to the presence of bacteria in the urine. Infections in any part of the urinary tract may persist for months or even years without symptoms. Approximately 900,000 hospitalized patients develop a nosocomial UTI each year. In at least 80% of these hospital-acquired urinary tract infections, instrumentation of the urinary tract or catheterization is the precipitating cause. Two to four percent of these patients will go on to develop a gram-negative sepsis. Over 250,000 cases of acute pyelonephritis occur in the United States each year, with 100,000 of these patients requiring hospitalization.

Overview of Urinary Tract Infections

Contributing Factors

The sterility of the bladder is maintained through several mechanisms: the physical barrier of the urethra, urine flow, ureterovesical junction competence, various antibacterial enzymes and antibodies, and anti-adherence effects mediated by the mucosal cells of the bladder. The normal bladder is capable of clearing itself of even large numbers of bacteria within two days of introduction into the bladder. For infection to occur, bacteria must gain access to the bladder, attach to and colonize the epithelium of the urinary tract to avoid being washed out with voiding, evade host defense mechanisms, and initiate inflammation. The majority of urinary tract infections result from fecal organisms that ascend from the perineum to the urethra and the bladder, adhering to the mucosal surfaces.

An anti-adherence factor, glycosaminoglycan (GAG), normally exerts a nonspecific protective effect against various bacteria. The GAG molecule attracts water molecules, forming a water barrier that serves as a defensive layer between the bladder and the urine. GAG may be impaired by certain agents (cyclamate, saccharin, aspartame, and tryptophan metabolites). Research is under way to identify agents that may enhance anti-adherence activity.

Inflammation, abrasion of the urethral mucosa, incomplete emptying of the bladder, altered metabolic states (diabetes, pregnancy, gout), and immunosuppression increase the risk of UTI by interfering with these normal mechanisms.

Urethrovesical reflux refers to the reflux (backward flow) of urine from the urethra into the bladder (Fig. 43-1*A*). With coughing, sneezing, or straining, the bladder pressure rises, which may force urine from the bladder into the urethra. When the pressure returns to normal, the urine flows back into the bladder, bringing into the bladder bacteria from the anterior portions of the urethra. Urethrovesical reflux is also caused by dysfunction of the bladder neck or urethra. The urethrovesical angle and urethral closure pressure may be altered with menopause, increasing the incidence of infection in postmenopausal women.

Ureterovesical or **vesicoureteral reflux** refers to the flowing back of urine from the bladder into one or both ureters (Fig. 43-1*B*). Normally, the ureterovesical junction prevents urine from traveling back into the ureter. The ureters are tunneled into the bladder wall so that a small portion of the ureter is compressed by the bladder musculature during normal voiding. When the ureterovesical valve is impaired because of congenital causes or ureteral abnormalities, the bacteria may reach and eventually destroy the kidneys.

Fecal contamination of the urethral meatus is a common route of entry of bacteria into the urinary tract. *Sexual intercourse* plays a role in the ascent of organisms from the perineum into the bladder in women. *Instrumentation of the urinary tract* (with catheterization or cystoscopic examinations) is also a major factor in urinary tract infections. *Stasis of urine* in the bladder may lead to infection, which may ultimately spread through the entire urinary system.

Any *obstruction* to urinary flow increases the urinary tract's susceptibility to infection. Common causes of urinary tract obstruction are congenital anomalies, urethral strictures, contracture of the bladder neck, bladder tumors, calculi (stones) in the ureters or kidneys, compression of the ureters, and neurologic abnormalities. In addition, infections may spread to the urinary tract by way of the blood (*hematogenous spread*) or the lymphatic system (*lymphogenous spread*).

The significance and treatment of UTI differ considerably in women and men, as indicated in the following discussion.

Urinary Tract Infections in Women

Urinary tract infections are one of the most common problems seen by primary health care providers, accounting for 6 to 7 million office visits per year. Women make up the vast majority of cases. One of every five women in the United States develops a UTI sometime during her lifetime. Al-

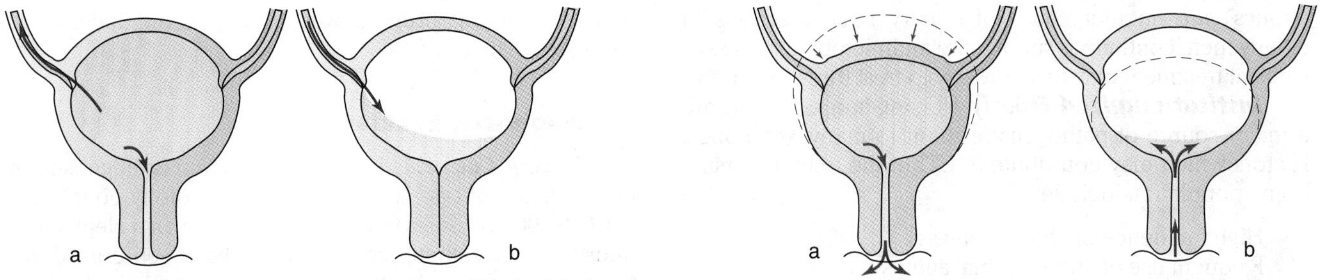

With failure of the ureterovesical valve action, urine moves up the ureters during voiding (*a*) and flows into the bladder when voiding has stopped (*b*). This prevents complete emptying of the bladder, stasis, and contamination of the ureters with bacteria-laden urine.

With coughing and straining, the bladder pressure rises, which may force urine from the bladder into the urethera (*a*). When bladder pressure returns to normal, the urine flows back to the bladder (*b*), which introduces bacteria from the urethra to the bladder.

FIGURE 43-1. Mechanisms of ureterovesical and urethrovesical reflux as causes of urinary tract infection.

though most episodes of UTI in women are simple, uncomplicated infections (90%), such infections during pregnancy must be treated promptly even in the absence of symptoms because there is an increased risk of acute pyelonephritis and premature delivery.

Women are more prone to develop bladder infections because of the short female urethra and its anatomic proximity to the vagina, periurethral glands, and rectum. The organisms most frequently responsible for UTIs in women are those normally found in the gastrointestinal tract: *Escherichia coli, Staphylococcus saprophyticus,* and *Streptococcus faecalis.* Other organisms responsible for urinary tract infections include *Proteus mirabilis,* one or more species of *Klebsiella, Enterobacter,* and *Pseudomonas.*

The critical first step in the pathogenesis of UTIs in women is bacterial colonization of the distal urethra and vagina with one of the above organisms. Flora then ascend to the bladder, where the microorganisms adhere to the epithelium of the urinary tract. Adherence of bacteria tends to be higher during the early, estrogen-dependent phase of the menstrual cycle, following total hysterectomy, and with aging, suggesting that hormonal status has a role. Additionally, atrophy of the urethral epithelium with aging may reduce the force of the urinary stream and, therefore, the effectiveness of the washing out of bacteria with voiding.

Most women with uncomplicated urinary tract infections respond to a single course of treatment with an appropriate antimicrobial agent.

Urinary Tract Infections in Men

Urinary tract infections in men result from ascending infection from the urethra, just as they do in women. However, the length of the urethra, its distance from the rectum in men, and the bactericidal properties of prostatic fluid generally protect men from urinary tract infections. As a result, UTIs in men are much less frequent; when they do occur, they usually indicate a functional or structural abnormality of the genitourinary tract. It has been recommended that men who experience even a single episode of UTI should undergo a urologic workup and be examined for urinary obstruction, prostatic infection, renal stones, or systemic disease.

E. coli is the major organism responsible for UTIs in men. Many other gram-negative bacteria, particularly the *Proteus* species, are responsible for the remaining infections. Relapses are usually caused by the same offending organisms as the initial infection and may be due to failure of the treatment to eradicate the bacteria or the presence of structural or functional abnormalities of the urinary tract. Bacteriuria is unlikely to be eradicated until the cause is treated.

Urinary tract infections in men generally do not respond to short-term (3–4 days) therapy; therefore a 10- to 14-day-course of antibiotics is recommended.

Gerontologic Considerations

The incidence of bacteriuria increases with age and disability, with women affected more frequently than men. Urinary tract infection is the most common cause of acute bacterial sepsis in patients over 65 years of age. Gram-negative sepsis resulting from UTI in the elderly is associated with a mortality rate exceeding 50%.

Structural abnormalities and neurogenic bladder secondary to strokes or autonomic neuropathy of diabetes may prevent complete emptying of the bladder and lead to an increased risk of UTI. When indwelling catheters are used, the risk of UTI rises dramatically as two populations of bacteria can be found in urine of catheterized patients, in the urine itself and on the surface of the catheter.

Women. Elderly women often have incomplete emptying of the bladder and urinary stasis. Postmenopausal women are susceptible to colonization and increased adherence of bacteria to the vagina and urethra in the absence of estrogen. Oral or topical estrogen is effective in some postmenopausal women with recurrent cystitis to restore the glycogen content of vaginal epithelial cells and an acidic *p*H.

Men. The antibacterial activity of prostatic secretions that protects men from bacterial colonization of the urethra and bladder decreases with aging. Although UTIs are rare in men, the prevalence of infection in men over 50 years of age approaches that of women in the same age group.

The dramatic rise in UTI in men as they get older is due largely to prostatic hyperplasia or carcinoma, strictures of the urethra, and neuropathic bladder. The use of catheterization or cystoscopy in the evaluation or treatment may contribute further to UTI. Renal calculi, the use of indwelling urinary catheters, and debilitating illness are other contributing factors. Bacteriuria is increased in men with confusion or dementia and those with bowel or bladder incontinence. The most common cause of recurrent UTI in the male elderly patient is chronic bacterial prostatitis. Transurethral resection (TUR) of the prostate gland may help to reduce its incidence. Infected prostatic calculi (stones) are another cause of urinary tract infections in elderly men; continuous suppressive antimicrobial therapy or surgical treatment may be necessary to treat these infections.

Institutionalized Elderly. Nursing home patients are a major source of pathogens resistant to many antibiotics. Factors which may contribute to UTI in the elderly nursing home population include:

- High incidence of chronic illness
- Frequent use of antimicrobial agents
- Presence of infected pressure ulcers
- Immobility and incomplete emptying of bladder
- Use of a bedpan rather than a commode or toilet

Diligence in hand washing, careful perineal care, and frequent toileting may decrease the incidence of urinary tract infections in nursing home patients.

The organisms responsible for urinary tract infections in the institutionalized elderly may differ from those found in patients residing in the community; this is thought to be due in part to the frequent use of antibiotics by patients in nursing homes. *Escherichia coli* is the most common organism seen in the elderly in the community or hospital. However, patients with indwelling catheters are more likely to be infected with *Proteus, Klebsiella, Pseudomonas,* or *Staphylococci. Enterococci* may be seen in patients who have been previously treated with numerous antibiotics.

Manifestations. Elderly patients often lack the typical symptoms of UTI and sepsis. Although frequency, urgency, and dysuria may occur, nonspecific symptoms such as altered sensorium, lethargy, anorexia, hyperventilation, and low-grade fever may be the only clues to the presence of a UTI. Frequent reinfections are common in the elderly.

Treatment Protocols. Patients in nursing homes may require 7 to 10 days of medication for the treatment to be effective. Controversy exists about the need for treatment of asymptomatic bacteriuria in the institutionalized elderly patient because of the possibility that antibiotic-resistant organisms produced by treatment may be of greater threat to the patient if sepsis occurs.

Treatment must be initiated as soon as infection is detected because of the high mortality associated with sepsis in the elderly. Age-related changes in intestinal absorption of medications and decreased renal function and hepatic flow may necessitate alterations in the antimicrobial regimen used to treat urinary tract infections. Renal function must be monitored and the dose of medications altered accordingly.

Clinical Manifestations

A variety of signs and symptoms are associated with UTI. About one half of all patients found to have bacteria in the urine (bacteriuria) have no symptoms. Signs and symptoms of lower UTI (cystitis) include frequent pain and burning on urination, sometimes accompanied by spasms in the region of the bladder and suprapubic area. Hematuria and back pain may also be present. Signs and symptoms of upper UTI (pyelonephritis) include fever, chills, flank pain, and painful urination. Physical examination reveals pain and tenderness in the area of the costovertebral angle (CVA).

If extensive damage to the kidneys has occurred, manifestations of renal failure may be present and may include nausea, vomiting, pruritus, weight loss, edema, fatigue and shortness of breath.

Diagnostic Evaluation

Colony Count. Urinary tract infection is diagnosed by the presence of bacteria in the urine. A colony count of at least 100,000 colonies per milliliter of urine on a clean-catch midstream or catheterized specimen has been considered the major criterion for the presence of infection. However, UTI and subsequent sepsis have occurred with lower bacterial colony counts. Approximately one third of women with symptoms of acute infections will have negative midstream urine cultures and may go untreated if 100,000 CFU (colony-forming units)/ml is used as the criterion for infection. The presence of *any* bacteria in specimens obtained by suprapubic needle aspiration of the urinary bladder or catheterization is considered indicative of infection.

Cellular Findings. Microscopic hematuria is present in approximately 50% of patients with acute infection. White blood cells are also detected in urinary tract infections; a large number of these cells may be associated with upper rather than lower UTI.

Urine Cultures. Urine cultures may be obtained to identify the specific organism present. However, because of the high probability that the organism in young women with a first or occasional UTI is *Escherichia coli,* cultures are often omitted. It has been suggested that the following groups of patients should have urine cultures obtained when bacteriuria is present:

All men (because of likelihood of structural or functional abnormalities)
All children
Women with history of compromised immune function or renal problems
Patients with diabetes mellitus
Patients who have undergone recent instrumentation (including catheterization) of the urinary tract
Patients who have been hospitalized recently
Patients with prolonged or persistent symptoms
Patients who have had 3 or more UTIs in past year
Pregnant women

Testing Methods. Multistrip dipstick testing for WBCs (leukocyte esterase test) and nitrites (Griess nitrate reduction test) is a common practice, especially in the outpatient setting. If the leukocyte esterase test is positive, it is assumed that the patient has pyuria (WBCs in the urine) and should be treated. The Griess nitrate reduction test is considered positive if bacteria that reduce normal urinary nitrates to nitrites are present.

Tests for Sexually Transmitted Diseases (STDs). Acute urethritis due to sexually transmitted organisms (*i.e., Chlamydia trachomatis, Neisseria gonorrhoeae,* and herpes simplex) or acute vaginitis infections (caused by *Trichomonas* or *Candida*) may be responsible for symptoms similar to those of UTI. Therefore, evaluation for STDs may be performed (see Chapter 65).

Additional Tests. In persons at high risk for complicated or recurring infection, diagnostic studies such as intravenous urogram (IVU) or pyelography (IVP), cystography, and ultrasonography may be carried out following treatment to determine if the infection is secondary to abnormalities of the urinary tract, calculi, a renal mass or abscess, hydronephrosis, or prostatic hyperplasia (hypertrophy). An IV urogram or ultrasonic evaluation, cystoscopy, and urodynamic studies may be indicted to identify the cause of recurrent infection that is resistant to treatment.

Cystitis (Lower Urinary Tract Infection)

Cystitis is an inflammation of the urinary bladder that is most often caused by an ascending infection from the urethra. It may be caused by urine flowing back from the urethra into the bladder (urethrovesical reflux), fecal contamination, or the use of a catheter or cystoscope. (Interstitial cystitis, a noninfectious, inflammatory disorder of the bladder characterized by symptoms similar to those of lower urinary tract infection, is discussed on p. 1185.)

Cystitis occurs more often in women than men. The distal portion of the urethra is frequently colonized with bacteria following colonization from the vagina. A defect of the mucosa of the urethra, vagina, or external genitalia may allow organisms to adhere and colonize at periurethral sites and invade the bladder. Acute cystitis in women is usually caused by *Escherichia coli.* Sexual intercourse is related to UTI, especially in women who fail to void after intercourse. It is thought voiding may wash bacteria from the bladder. Infection is also associated with diaphragm–spermicide contraception because it may cause a partial urethral obstruction and prevent complete emptying of the bladder. Additionally, it has been shown to alter *p*H and normal vaginal flora.

Cystitis in men is secondary to some other factor (*i.e.*, infected prostate, epididymitis, or bladder stones). Consequently, men will undergo a diagnostic workup after the first episode of cystitis to identify and treat the cause.

Clinical Manifestations. The patient with cystitis experiences urgency, frequency, burning and pain on urination, nocturia, and pain or spasm in the region of the bladder and suprapubic area. **Pyuria** (white blood cells in the urine), bacteria, and often red blood cells (**hematuria**) are found on examination of the urine. Office culturing kits provide general qualitative information about the bacterial colony count and identify the organism as gram positive or gram negative.

Management

The ideal treatment for UTI is an antibacterial agent that effectively eradicates bacteria from the urinary tract with minimal effects on fecal and vaginal flora, thereby minimizing the incidence of vaginal yeast infections. (*Yeast vaginitis* occurs in as many as 25% of patients treated with antimicrobial agents that affect vaginal flora; it often causes more symptoms and is more difficult and costly to treat than the original UTI.) Additionally, the antibacterial agent should be low in cost and should produce few side effects and low resistance. Because the organism in initial, uncomplicated urinary tract infections in women is most likely *Escherichia coli* or other fecal flora, the agent should be effective against these organisms.

Various *treatment regimens* have been used successfully to treat uncomplicated lower urinary tract infections in women; from single-dose administration, short-course (3–4 days) medication regimens, or 7- to 10-day courses. The trend is toward a shortened course of antibiotic therapy for uncomplicated UTIs, as about 80% of patients will be cured with three days of treatment (Childs et al., 1993).

Commonly used *medications* include sulfisoxazole (Gantrisin), trimethoprim/sulfamethoxazole (TMP/SMZ, Bactrim, Septra), and nitrofurantoin (Macrodantin). Occasionally, medications such as ampicillin or amoxicillin are used, but *Escherichia coli* has developed resistance to these agents. Pyridium, a urinary analgesic, may also be prescribed to relieve the discomfort associated with the infection.

Regardless of the regimen prescribed, the patient is instructed to take *all* the doses prescribed, even if relief of symptoms occurs promptly. Longer medication courses are indicated for men, pregnant women, and women with pyelonephritis and with other types of complicated urinary tract infections. In pregnant women, cephalexin is the preferred antimicrobial agent, although ampicillin may also be used.

Recurrence. Although treatment of UTI for 3 days is usually adequate in women, recurrence of infection occurs in about 20% of women treated for uncomplicated UTI (Elder, 1992). It has been suggested that infections that recur within two weeks after therapy do so because organisms of the original offending strain remain in the vagina. As persistence of the initial bacteria is relatively rare in women, patients should be referred to a urologist to investigate and correct abnormalities. Recurrence may also occasionally occur if initial treatment was inadequate or administered for too short a period of time. Recurrent infections in men are usually due to persistence of the same organism; further evaluation and treatment are indicated.

Reinfection of the female patient with new bacteria is more common than persistence of the initial bacteria. If the diagnostic evaluation reveals no structural abnormalities in the urinary tract, the woman with recurrent UTI may be instructed to begin treatment on her own whenever symptoms occur and to contact the health care provider only when symptoms persist, fever occurs, or the number of treatment episodes exceeds four in a 6-month period. This patient is instructed in the use of dip-slide culture devices to detect the presence of bacteria.

Long-term use of antimicrobial agents decreases the risk of reinfection and may be indicated in patients with recurrent infections. If recurrence is caused by persistent bacteria from preceding infections, the causative factor (*i.e.*, stone, abscess), if one is present, must be treated. Following treatment and sterilization of the urine, low-dose preventive therapy (nitrofurantoin macrocrystals) each night at bedtime is often used.

If recurrence occurs after completion of antimicrobials, another short course (3–4 days) of full-dose antimicrobial therapy followed by a regular bedtime dose of antimicrobials may be prescribed. If there is no recurrence, medication is taken every other night for 6 to 7 months. Other options include a dose of an antimicrobial agent following sexual intercourse, a dose of the antimicrobial at bedtime, or a dose of the prescribed antimicrobial every other night or three times per week. Guidelines for instructions for patients with recurrent UTI are included in Chart 43-1.

CHART 43-1
Patient Education: Preventing Recurrent Urinary Tract Infections

Hygiene
- Shower rather than bathe in tub.
- Cleanse perineum after each bowel movement with a front-to-back motion.

Fluid Intake
- Drink liberal amounts of fluids.
- Avoid coffee, tea, colas, and alcohol.

Voiding Habits
- Void every 2–3 hours during the day.
- Empty bladder completely with each voiding.
- Void immediately after sexual intercourse.

Medical Therapy
- Take medication *exactly* as prescribed.
- If prescribed, test urine for bacteria with dip-slides.

❑ NURSING PROCESS
The Patient With Lower Urinary Tract Infection

Assessment

A history of urinary signs and symptoms is obtained from the patient with a suspected urinary tract infection. The presence of pain, frequency, urgency, and hesitancy and changes in urine are assessed, documented, and reported. The patient's usual pattern of voiding is assessed to detect factors that may predispose the patient to urinary tract infection. Infrequent emptying of the bladder, the association of symptoms of urinary tract infection with sexual intercourse, contraceptive practices, and personal hygiene are assessed. The patient's knowledge about prescribed antimicrobial medications and preventive health care measures is also assessed. Additionally, the patient's urine is assessed for volume, color, concentration, cloudiness, and odor, all of which are altered by bacteria in the urinary tract.

Diagnosis

Nursing Diagnoses

Based on the assessment data, the nursing diagnoses may include the following:

- ❑ Pain and discomfort related to inflammation and infection of the urethra, bladder, and other urinary tract structures
- ❑ Altered patterns of elimination related to frequency, urgency, and hesitancy
- ❑ Knowledge deficit regarding factors predisposing to infection and recurrence, detection and prevention of recurrence, and pharmacologic therapy

Collaborative Problems/ Potential Complications

Based on assessment data, potential complications may include:

- ❑ Renal failure due to extensive damage of kidney
- ❑ Sepsis

Planning and Implementation

Goals. The major goals for the patient may include relief of pain and discomfort; relief from frequency, urgency, and hesitancy; increased knowledge of preventive measures and treatment modalities; and absence of potential complications.

Nursing Interventions

Relieving Pain and Discomfort. Pain and discomfort associated with urinary tract infection are quickly relieved once antimicrobial therapy is initiated. Antispasmodic agents may be useful in relieving bladder irritability and pain. Aspirin, heat to the perineum, and hot tub baths help relieve discomfort and spasm.

Relieving Frequency, Urgency, and Hesitancy. The patient is encouraged to drink liberal amounts of fluids (water is the best choice) to promote renal blood flow and to flush the bacteria from the urinary tract. Fluids that may be irritating to the bladder (*e.g.*, coffee, tea, colas, alcohol) are avoided. Frequent voiding (every 2–3 h) is encouraged to empty the bladder completely, because this can significantly lower urine bacterial counts, reduce urinary stasis, and prevent reinfection.

Patient Education. Women who have repeated urinary tract infections should receive detailed instructions on the following points:

1. Reduce concentrations of pathogens at the vaginal opening by hygienic measures.
   a. Shower rather than bathe in a tub, because bacteria in the bath water may enter the urethra.
   b. Cleanse around the perineum and urethral meatus after each bowel movement (with a back to front motion).
2. Drink liberal amounts of fluid during the day to flush out bacteria, avoiding coffee, tea, colas, and alcohol.
3. Void every 2 to 3 hours during the day and completely empty the bladder. This prevents overdistention of the bladder and compromised blood supply to the bladder wall, which predispose the patient to UTI.
4. If sexual intercourse is the initiating event for development of bacteriuria:
   a. Void immediately after sexual intercourse.
   b. Take the prescribed single dose of an oral antimicrobial agent following sexual intercourse.
5. If bacteria continue to appear in the urine, long-term antimicrobial therapy may be required to prevent colonization of the periurethral area and recurrence of infection. The medication should be taken after emptying the bladder just before going to bed to ensure adequate concentration of the medication during the overnight period.
6. If prescribed, monitor and test the urine for bacteria with dip-slides (Microstix) as follows:

a. Wash around the urethral meatus several times, using different washcloths.
b. Collect a midstream urine specimen.
c. Remove a slide from its container, dip it into the urine sample, and return it to the container.
d. Incubate the slide at room temperature according to product directions.
e. Read the results by comparing the slide with the colony density chart that comes with the product.
f. Initiate therapy as prescribed and complete the full prescribed course of medication.
g. Notify health care provider if fever occurs or if signs and symptoms persist.

7. Consult health care provider regularly for follow-up, recurrence of symptoms, or infections nonresponsive to treatment.

Monitoring and Managing Complications. Early recognition of UTI and prompt treatment are essential to prevent recurrent infection and the possibility of complications such as *renal failure* and *sepsis*. The goal of treatment is to prevent infection from progressing and causing permanent renal damage and renal failure. Appropriate antimicrobial therapy, liberalization of fluids, frequent voiding, and hygienic measures are commonly prescribed in the management of UTI. The patient is instructed to notify the physician if fatigue, nausea, vomiting, or pruritus occurs. Periodic monitoring of renal function (creatinine clearance, BUN, serum creatinine level) may be indicated for patients with repeated UTI. If extensive renal damage does occur, dialysis may be necessary.

Patients with UTI, especially catheter-associated infection, are at increased risk for gram-negative sepsis. Indwelling catheters should be avoided if at all possible and removed at the earliest opportunity. However, if an indwelling catheter is necessary, specific nursing interventions are initiated to prevent infection. These include strict aseptic technique during insertion using the smallest catheter possible; securing the catheter with tape to prevent movement; frequent inspection of urine for color, odor, and consistency; daily, meticulous perineal care with soap and water; and maintenance of a closed system using the sample port to obtain specimens (see Chapter 42).

Careful assessment of vital signs and level of consciousness may warn of impending sepsis. Positive blood cultures and elevated WBC counts are reported to the physician. Appropriate antimicrobial therapy and liberalization of fluids are prescribed (intravenous antimicrobial therapy and fluids may be required). Prevention of sepsis is key as the mortality rate for gram-negative sepsis is significant, especially in the elderly patient.

Evaluation

Expected Outcomes

1. Experiences relief of pain and discomfort.
   a. Reports absence of pain, urgency, dysuria, or hesitancy on voiding.
   b. Takes analgesics and antimicrobial agents as prescribed.
   c. Drinks 8 to 10 glasses of fluids daily.
   d. Voids every 2 to 3 hours.
   e. Voids urine that is clear and free of odor.
2. Increases knowledge of preventive measures and prescribed treatment modalities as described in Chart 43-1.
3. Is free of complications
   a. Reports no symptoms of infection or renal failure (nausea, vomiting, fatigue, pruritus).
   b. Has normal BUN and serum creatinine levels, negative urine and blood cultures.
   c. Exhibits normal vital signs and temperature; no signs of sepsis.
   d. Maintains adequate urine output (>30 ml/h).

Interstitial Cystitis

Interstitial cystitis (chronic inflammation of the bladder) is not caused by bacteria and does not respond to antibiotics. It occurs mostly in women (age 40–50), but can affect any age, race, or sex. It has been estimated that there are over 450,000 people in the United States affected by the disease. It is characterized by severe, irritable voiding symptoms (urinary frequency, nocturia, urgency, suprapubic pressure, pain with bladder filling) and a markedly diminished bladder capacity. Pain may occur in the abdomen or perineum or radiate to the groin.

The cause of interstitial cystitis is unknown although there is some suggestion of an inflammatory or autoimmune basis. Suggested causes include penetration of urinary irritants into the urothelium or suburothelial tissues due to a defect in the barrier between the urine and bladder wall mucosa.

The urine contains both red and white blood cells even though it is uninfected, and cytology is benign. An increased number of mast cells in the urine is suggestive of interstitial cystitis. The presence of Hunner's ulcers (superficial erosions of the bladder wall) is considered diagnostic; however, these do not occur in all patients.

Interstitial cystitis is a diagnosis made by the process of exclusion because there are no definitive diagnostic criteria. As a result, several years may pass before a definitive diagnosis is made. The lack of more specific diagnostic criteria does not mean that this is a psychologically based disease; rather, it is a physical disorder with psychologic consequences.

Interstitial cystitis is a progressive disease if not treated, and early diagnosis may improve the response to treatment. It is a chronic and disabling condition of the bladder; the pain and frequency may hamper the patient's ability to work or participate in social activities. Many patients have difficulty in coping with the lack of a diagnosis, the inability of health care professionals to provide an explanation for their symptoms, and the persistence of symptoms.

Diagnostic Evaluation

The diagnosis of interstitial cystitis is made by eliminating other causes of these symptoms and on the basis of history, symptoms, signs, cystoscopy, urodynamic studies, histology, and laboratory tests. A micturition chart or diary with recordings of the frequency of voiding and the volume of each voiding over at least 48 to 72 hours may aid in the diagnostic process. Biopsy and radiographic studies such as urography, cystography, skeletal and pelvic x-ray films, ultrasound, and CT scan are obtained to exclude other conditions that could cause similar symptoms. The only abnormal x-ray finding characteristic of interstitial cystitis is a small bladder; however, this may not be present. Urinalysis, culture, residual volume, and flow rate are usually normal in patients with interstitial cystitis.

Interstitial cystitis is characterized by pinpoint petechial hemorrhages that develop throughout the mucosa of the bladder. These areas often coalesce to become hemorrhagic spots on the bladder mucosa that bleed when the bladder is distended under general anesthesia (an important diagnostic criterion). Unlike other causes of painful bladder syndrome, interstitial cystitis may progress to contraction of the bladder with diminished bladder volume.

Cystoscopy is performed and fluid is instilled in the bladder to 80 cm of water pressure for 1 minute with the patient under anesthesia. The bladder is distended to its maximum capacity and the fluid is then drained; the bladder appears normal during this first filling, though a few pinpoint hemorrhages may be noted. In addition, the final portion of drainage may be blood-tinged. The bladder is distended a second time. Again, as soon as bladder capacity is reached and the irrigating fluid is drained, the last portion of the fluid drained is usually blood-tinged. Fissures and scars of the bladder mucosa tend to split as the bladder capacity is reached, thus producing the characteristic appearance of a Hunner ulcer. Re-examination reveals splotchy hemorrhages throughout the bladder, although their distribution may be patchy. The cystoscopic picture does not necessarily correlate with severity of symptoms or response to therapy.

Management

Treatment strategies have included the use of tricyclic antidepressants that through their central and peripheral anticholinergic actions may decrease the excitability of smooth muscle in the bladder. Bladder instillation of various compounds (*i.e.,* silver nitrate, dimethyl sulfoxide, chlorpactin), has been used to try to provide relief. Other treatment has ranged from destruction of ulcers with laser photoirradiation, TENS (transcutaneous electrical nerve stimulation), and bladder removal and urinary diversion, for severe cases.

Clinical trials are under way to identify treatments that will relieve symptoms. Agents currently undergoing clinical trial include subcutaneous heparin (stabilizes mast cells; antagonizes histamine, bradykinin, and prostaglandin E; and inhibits the complement system and action of inflammatory agents); sodium pentasanpolysulfate, or elmirone (thought to coat bladder wall with protective lining); and nalmefene (stops release of histamine which may be released from bladder wall by mast cells).

Nursing Interventions

The patient who presents with the symptoms of interstitial cystitis has often experienced symptoms for a prolonged period of time and has been unable to carry out normal activities of daily living due to these symptoms. The patient has usually been treated by a number of health care providers, often with little relief of symptoms. Consequently, the patient may be depressed and anxious, as well as distrustful and skeptical of proposed treatments, particularly if these have been tried before and have been unsuccessful. The nurse assesses the effectiveness of the patient's ability to cope with the disorder and provides psychologic support. It is crucial that the nurse convey a sense of acceptance to the patient and an appreciation of the severity of the symptoms and their effect on lifestyle. The nurse also provides explanations about diagnostic tests and treatment modalities.

Urethritis

Urethritis, inflammation of the urethra, is usually an ascending infection and may be classified as gonorrheal (see Chapter 65) or nongonorrheal. However, both conditions may be present in the same patient.

Gonorrheal Urethritis. Gonorrheal urethritis is caused by *Neisseria gonorrhoeae* and is transmitted by sexual contact. In the male, inflammation of the meatal orifice occurs with burning on urination. A purulent urethral discharge appears 3 to 14 days (or longer) after sexual exposure. However, the disease may be asymptomatic. In the female, a urethral discharge is not always present and the disease may also be asymptomatic. Therefore, gonorrhea in the female is frequently not diagnosed and reported. In the male, the infection involves the tissues around the urethra, causing periurethritis, prostatitis, epididymitis, and urethral stricture. Sterility may occur as a result of vasoepididymal obstruction. Treatment of gonorrhea is discussed and patient education information is provided in Chapter 65.

Nongonorrheal Urethritis. Urethritis not associated with *Neisseria gonorrhoeae* is usually caused by *Chlamydia trachomatis* or *Ureaplasma urealyticum.* If the male patient is symptomatic, he will complain of mild to severe dysuria and a scanty to moderate urethral discharge. Nongonorrheal urethritis requires prompt antimicrobial treatment with tetracycline or doxycycline; in those patients who do not respond or are allergic to the tetracyclines, erythromycin may be substituted. Follow-up care is necessary to make certain that a cure is achieved. All persons who are sexual partners of patients with nongonorrheal urethritis should be examined for sexually transmitted disease and treated.

Pyelonephritis (Upper Urinary Tract Infection)

Pyelonephritis is a bacterial infection of the renal pelvis, tubules, and interstitial tissue of one or both kidneys. Bacteria reach the bladder via the urethra and ascend to the kidney. Although the kidneys receive 20% to 25% of the cardiac output, bacteria rarely reach the kidney from the blood; less than 3% of cases are due to hematogenous spread.

Pyelonephritis is frequently secondary to ureterovesical reflux, in which an incompetent ureterovesical valve allows the urine to back up (reflux) into the ureters (see Fig. 43-1). Urinary tract obstruction (which increases the susceptibility of the kidneys to infection), bladder tumors, strictures, benign prostatic hyperplasia, and urinary stones are among other causes. Pyelonephritis may be acute or chronic.

Acute Pyelonephritis

Clinical Manifestations. The patient with acute pyelonephritis presents with chills and fever, flank pain, costovertebral angle (CVA) tenderness, leukocytosis, and bacteria and white blood cells in the urine. In addition, symptoms of lower urinary tract involvement, such as dysuria and frequency, are common. Upper urinary tract infection is associated with antibody coating of the bacteria in the urine. (Antibodies coat the bacteria in the renal medulla; when the bacteria are excreted in the urine, the immunofluorescent test can detect the antibody coating.)

Kidneys of patients with acute pyelonephritis are usually enlarged with interstitial infiltrations of inflammatory cells. Abscesses may be noted on the renal capsule and at the corticomedullary junction. Eventually, atrophy and destruction of tubules and the glomeruli may result. When pyelonephritis becomes chronic, the kidneys become scarred, contracted, and nonfunctioning.

Diagnostic Evaluation. An intravenous urogram and ultrasound may be performed to locate any obstruction in the urinary tract; relief of obstruction is essential to save the kidney from destruction. Urine culture and sensitivity tests are obtained to determine the causative organism so that appropriate antimicrobial agents can be prescribed.

Management. Patients with acute pyelonephritis are at risk for bacteremia and warrant intensive antimicrobial therapy. Parenteral therapy is preferred until the patient has been afebrile 24 to 48 hours. At that time, oral agents may be substituted. Less critically ill patients have been effectively treated with oral agents only. To prevent reseeding of residual bacteria, the course of treatment for acute pyelonephritis is usually longer than treatment for cystitis.

A possible problem in treatment is a chronic or recurring infection persisting for months or years without symptoms. After the initial antimicrobial regimen, the patient is maintained on continuous antimicrobial treatment until there is no evidence of infection, all causative factors have been treated or controlled, and kidney function is stabilized. The patient's serum creatinine levels and blood counts are monitored for the duration of the long-term therapy.

Chronic Pyelonephritis

Repeated bouts of acute pyelonephritis may lead to chronic pyelonephritis. However, evidence suggests that chronic pyelonephritis is less frequently a cause of chronic renal failure than previously thought.

Clinical Manifestations. The patient with chronic pyelonephritis usually has no symptoms of infection unless an acute exacerbation occurs. Noticeable signs may include fatigue, headache, poor appetite, polyuria, excessive thirst, and weight loss. Persistent and recurring infection may produce progressive scarring of the kidney, with renal failure the end result.

Diagnostic Evaluation. The extent of the disease is assessed by intravenous urogram and measurements of BUN, creatinine levels, and creatinine clearance. Eradication of bacteria from the urine is undertaken if present.

Management. The choice of an antimicrobial agent is based on identifying the pathogen through urine culture. If the urine cannot be made bacteria-free, nitrofurantoin or a combination of sulfamethoxazole and trimethoprim may be used to suppress bacterial growth. Compromised renal function alters the excretion of antimicrobial agents and necessitates careful monitoring of renal function, especially if the medications are potentially toxic to the kidneys.

Complications. Complications of chronic pyelonephritis include end-stage renal disease (from progressive loss of nephrons secondary to chronic inflammation and scarring), hypertension, and formation of kidney stones (from chronic infection with urea-splitting organisms, resulting in stone formation).

Perinephric Abscess

Perinephric abscess is a renal abscess that extends into the fatty tissue around the kidney. It may be caused by an infection of the kidney, such as pyelonephritis, or may occur as a hematogenous (spread through the bloodstream) infection originating elsewhere in the body. Offending organisms include *Staphylococcus, Proteus* and *E. coli.* Occasionally infection may spread from adjacent areas, such as from diverticulitis or appendicitis.

The *manifestations* often are acute in onset, with chills, fever, leukocytosis, dull ache or palpable mass in the flank, abdominal pain with guarding and costovertebral angle tenderness on palpation. The patient usually appears seriously ill.

Management. The abscess is incised and drained and culture and sensitivity are obtained on all drainage. Appropriate antimicrobial therapy is prescribed. Drains are usually inserted and left in the perinephric space until all significant drainage has ceased. Because the drainage is often profuse, frequent changes of the outer dressings may be necessary. As in the treatment of an abscess in any site, the patient is monitored for sepsis, fluid intake and output, and general response to treatment.

Renal Abscess (Renal Carbuncle)

A renal abscess is a localized infection in the cortex of the kidney. It is often seen in association with pyelonephritis or UTI due to *Enterobactiaceaeu*, or it may be of hematogenous origin (usually *Staphylococcus*). Patients may give a recent history of a cutaneous boil or carbuncle. Signs and symptoms include fever, malaise, dull pain in the region of the kidney, weakness, anorexia, and weight loss. Leukocytosis and sterile urine (no microorganisms seen because infection does not extend into the urinary collection system) are present. Aggressive antibiotic therapy is usually successful. Occasionally, incision and drainage of the abscess may be necessary.

Tuberculosis of the Kidney and Genitourinary Tract

Pathophysiology. Tuberculosis of the kidney and urinary tract is caused by the organism *Mycobacterium tubercu-*

losis. The organism usually travels from the lungs via the bloodstream to the kidneys. Upon arrival in the kidney the microorganism may become dormant for years. The process of tuberculosis generally starts in the glomeruli and then spreads throughout the rest of the nephron, causing progressive renal destruction. Once the renal pelvis is infected, the organism spreads downward to the bladder and may also infect the prostrate, epididymis, and testicles in males.

Clinical Manifestations. At first the symptoms of renal tuberculosis are mild; there is usually a slight afternoon fever, weight loss, night sweats, loss of appetite, and general malaise. Hematuria (microscopic or gross) and pyuria may be present. Pain, dysuria, and urinary frequency, when they occur, are due to bladder involvement. Cavity formations and calcifications may be noted on an intravenous urogram.

Diagnostic Evaluation. A search for tuberculosis elsewhere in the body is conducted when tuberculosis of the kidney or urinary tract is found. The patient is asked about possible exposure to tuberculosis. Three or more clean-voided, first-morning urine specimens are obtained for culture for *M. tuberculosis.*

Management. The objective of treatment is to eradicate the offending organism. Combinations of ethambutol, isoniazid, and rifampin are used to delay the emergence of resistant organisms. Shorter-course chemotherapy (4 months) has been effective in eradicating the organism and in penetrating renal tissue. Surgical intervention may be necessary to treat obstruction and to remove an extensively diseased kidney. Because renal tuberculosis is a manifestation of a systemic disease, all measures to promote the general health of the person are used.

Patient Education and Home Care Considerations. Home care follow-up is initiated to reinforce the importance of taking the prescribed medications exactly as ordered; many patients do not take their medication correctly. The patient is counseled about the need for follow-up examinations (urine cultures, IV urograms), usually for a period of a year. Treatment will be reinstituted if a relapse occurs and the tubercle bacilli again invade the genitourinary tract. Ureteral stenosis or bladder contractures are complications that may develop during the healing process; therefore, the patient is monitored for changes that may indicate the development of these complications.

Acute Glomerulonephritis

Acute glomerulonephritis is a broad term which refers to a group of kidney diseases in which there is an inflammatory reaction in the glomeruli. In most types of glomerulonephritis, IgG, the major immunoglobulin (antibody) found in the serum of humans, can be detected in the glomerular capillary walls. As a result of an antigen–antibody reaction, aggregates of molecules (complexes) are formed and circulate throughout the body. Some of these complexes lodge in the glomeruli, the filtering portion of the kidney, and induce an inflammatory response.

In most cases, the stimulus of the reaction is group A streptococcal infection of the throat, which ordinarily precedes the onset of glomerulonephritis by an interval of 2 to 3 weeks. The streptococcal product, acting as an antigen, stimulates circulating antibodies and results in deposit of the complexes in the glomeruli, producing injury to the kidney. Glomerulonephritis may also follow scarlet fever and impetigo (infection of the skin) and acute viral infections (upper respiratory infections, mumps, varicella, Epstein–Barr, hepatitis B, and HIV infections).

The many forms of glomerulonephritis include proliferative, membranous, membranoproliferative, focal proliferative, and rapidly progressive. Glomerulonephritis can be classified as primary or secondary glomerular injury; primary disorders are due to direct insult while secondary disorders are the result of a systemic illness. Acute glomerulonephritis is predominantly a disease of youth, however viral forms of glomerulonephritis occur across the age spectrum.

Pathophysiology. Cellular proliferation (increased production of endothelial cells lining the glomerulus), infiltration of the glomerulus by leukocytes, and thickening of the glomerular filtration membrane or basement membrane results in scarring and loss of filtering surface. In acute glomerulonephritis, the kidneys become large, swollen, and congested. All renal tissues—glomeruli, tubules, and blood vessels—are affected to varying degrees no matter what type of acute glomerulonephritis is present. In some patients, antigens outside the body (*e.g.*, medications, foreign serum) initiate the process, resulting in the complexes being deposited in the glomeruli. In other patients, the kidney tissue itself serves as the inciting antigen. Electron-microscopy and immunofluorescent analysis of the immune mechanism help identify the nature of the lesion. A kidney biopsy may be needed to differentiate among the various kinds of acute glomerulonephritis.

Clinical Manifestations. Glomerulonephritis may be so mild that it is discovered incidentally through a routine urinalysis, or the history may reveal a preceding episode of pharyngitis or tonsillitis with fever. In the more severe form of the disease, the patient complains of headache, malaise, facial edema, and flank pain. Mild to severe hypertension is seen, and tenderness over the costovertebral angle (CVA) is common. (The costovertebral angles, used as landmarks, are the angles formed on each side of the body by the bottom rib of the rib cage and the vertebral column) (Fig. 43-2).

Diagnostic Evaluation. The primary presenting feature of acute glomerulonephritis is microscopic or macroscopic (gross) hematuria (blood in the urine). The urine may appear cola-colored due to red blood cells and protein plugs or casts. (RBC casts indicate glomerular injury.) Proteinuria, primarily albumin, is also present due to increased permeability of the glomerular membrane. A large percentage of patients have an increased antistreptolysin O titer as a result of a reaction to the streptococcal organism. BUN and serum creatinine levels rise as urine output drops. The patient may be anemic because of loss of red blood cells in the urine and changes in the hematopoietic mechanism of the body.

Serial determinations of antistreptolysin O (ASO) or anti-Dnase B (ADB) titers are often elevated in poststreptococcal glomerulonephritis. Serum complement levels may be decreased but generally return to normal within 2 to 8 weeks. However, over 50% of patients with IgA nephropathy (the most common type of primary glomerulonephritis) will

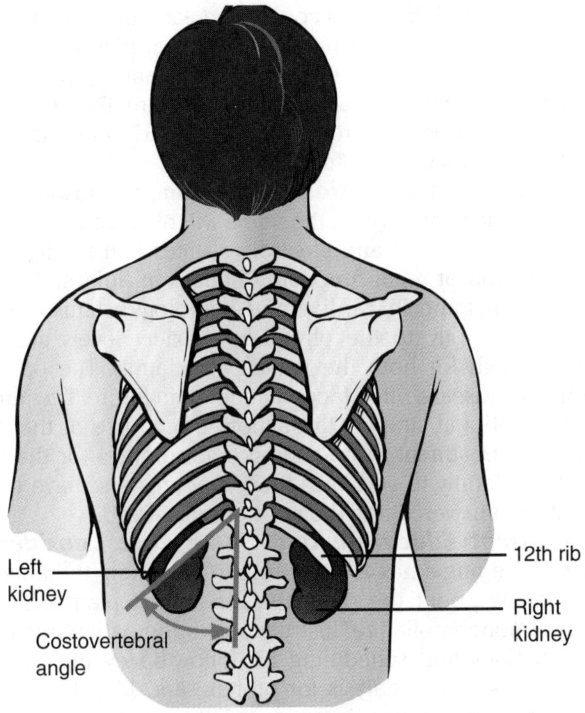

FIGURE 43-2. Location of the costovertebral angle.

have an elevated serum IgA and a normal complement level.

As the patient improves, the amount of urine increases, while the urinary protein and sediment diminish. Usually, more than 90% of children recover. The percentage of recovery for adults is not well established but is probably about 70%. Some patients become severely uremic within weeks and require dialysis for survival. Others, after a period of apparent recovery, insidiously develop chronic glomerulonephritis.

Management. The goals of management of acute glomerulonephritis are to preserve kidney function and to treat complications promptly. If residual streptococcal infection is suspected, penicillin is prescribed. Bed rest is encouraged during the acute phase until the urine clears and the BUN, creatinine, and blood pressure return to normal. The duration of bed rest can be determined by assessing the patient's urine; excessive activity may increase proteinuria and hematuria.

Dietary protein is restricted when renal insufficiency and nitrogen retention (elevated BUN) develop. Sodium is restricted when hypertension, edema, and congestive heart failure are present. Diuretics and antihypertensive agents may be prescribed to control hypertension. Carbohydrates are given liberally to provide energy and reduce the catabolism of protein.

Intake and output are carefully measured and recorded if the patient is hospitalized. Fluids are given according to the patient's fluid losses and daily body weight. Insensible fluid loss through the respiratory and gastrointestinal tracts (500–1000 ml) is considered in estimating fluid loss. Diuresis begins 1 to 2 weeks after the onset of symptoms. Edema decreases and hypertension lessens. However, proteinuria and microscopic hematuria may persist for many months. In some patients, the disease may progress to chronic glomerulonephritis.

Complications include hypertensive encephalopathy, congestive heart failure, and pulmonary edema. Hypertensive encephalopathy is considered a medical emergency, and therapy is directed toward reducing the blood pressure without impairing renal function.

In **rapid progressive glomerulonephritis,** plasma exchange (plasmapheresis) and treatment with steroids and cytotoxic agents have been used to reduce the inflammatory response. In this form of glomerulonephritis, the risk of progression to end-stage renal disease is high without aggressive treatment. Dialysis is initiated in acute glomerulonephritis if manifestations of uremia are severe.

Patient Education and Home Care Considerations. Instructions to the patient include explanations and scheduling for follow-up evaluations of blood pressure, urinalysis for protein, and BUN and creatinine levels to determine if the disease has progressed. The patient is instructed to notify the physician if symptoms of renal failure occur (*e.g.*, fatigue, nausea, vomiting, diminishing urinary output). Any infection must be treated promptly.

A referral to the community health nurse may be indicated to provide an opportunity for careful assessment of the patient's progress and to detect the onset of early symptoms of renal insufficiency. If steroids or cytotoxic agents are prescribed, verbal and written instructions about dosage, desired actions, side effects, and precautions to be followed are provided to the patient and family.

Chronic Glomerulonephritis

Pathophysiology. Chronic glomerulonephritis may have its onset as acute glomerulonephritis or may represent a milder type of antigen–antibody reaction, one so mild that it is overlooked. After repeated occurrences of these reactions, the kidneys are reduced to as little as one-fifth their normal size, consisting largely of fibrous tissue. The cortex shrinks to a layer of 1 to 2 mm in thickness or less. Bands of scar tissue distort the remaining cortex, making the surface of the kidney rough and irregular. Numerous glomeruli and their tubules become scarred, and the branches of the renal artery are thickened. The result is severe glomerular damage that results in end-stage renal disease (ESRD).

Clinical Manifestations. The symptoms of chronic glomerulonephritis are variable. Some patients with severe disease have no symptoms at all for many years. Their condition may accidentally be discovered when hypertension or elevated BUN and serum creatinine levels are discovered. The diagnosis may be suggested during a routine eye examination when vascular changes or retinal hemorrhages are found. The first indication of disease may be a sudden, severe nosebleed, a stroke, or a seizure. Many patients merely notice that their feet are slightly swollen at night. The majority of patients also have general symptoms such as loss of weight and strength, increasing irritability, and an increased need to urinate at night (nocturia). Headaches, dizziness, and digestive disturbances are common.

As chronic glomerulonephritis progresses, signs and symptoms of renal insufficiency and chronic renal failure may develop. The patient appears poorly nourished with a yellow-gray pigmentation of the skin and periorbital and peripheral (dependent) edema. Blood pressure may be normal or severely elevated. Retinal findings include hemorrhage, exudate, narrowed tortuous arterioles, and papilledema. Mucous membranes are pale because of anemia. The neck veins may be distended as a result of fluid overload. Cardiomegaly, a gallop rhythm, and other signs of congestive heart failure may be present. Crackles can be heard in the lungs.

Peripheral neuropathy with diminished deep tendon reflexes and neurosensory changes occurs late in the illness. The patient becomes confused and demonstrates a limited attention span. An additional late finding includes evidence of pericarditis with a pericardial friction rub and pulsus paradoxus (difference in blood pressure during inspiration and expiration of greater than 10 mm Hg).

Diagnostic Evaluation. A number of laboratory abnormalities occur. Urinalysis reveals a fixed specific gravity of approximately 1.010, variable proteinuria, and urinary casts (protein plugs secreted by damaged kidney tubules). As renal failure progresses and the glomerular filtration falls below 50 ml/minute, the following changes are seen:

- Hyperkalemia due to decreased excretion, intake from food and medications, acidosis, and catabolism
- Metabolic acidosis from decreased acid secretion by the kidney and inability to regenerate bicarbonate
- Anemia secondary to decreased erythropoiesis (production of red blood cells)
- Hypoalbuminemia with edema secondary to protein loss through damaged glomerular membrane
- Increased serum phosphorus due to decreased renal excretion
- Decreased serum calcium (calcium binds to phosphorus to compensate for elevated serum phosphorus levels)
- Hypermagnesemia from decreased excretion and ingestion of antacids containing magnesium
- Impaired nerve conduction due to electrolyte abnormalities and uremia

Chest x-rays may show cardiac enlargement and pulmonary edema. The electrocardiogram may be normal but may also reflect hypertension with left ventricular hypertrophy and electrolyte disturbances, such as hyperkalemia and tall, tented (or peaked) T waves.

Management. Patient symptoms will guide the course of treatment for the ambulatory patient with chronic glomerulonephritis. If hypertension is present, the blood pressure is reduced with sodium and water restriction. Proteins of high biologic value (dairy products, eggs, meats) are provided to promote good nutritional status in the patient. Adequate calories are also important to spare protein for tissue growth and repair. Urinary tract infections must be treated promptly to prevent further renal damage.

If severe edema develops, the patient is placed on bed rest. The head of the bed is elevated to promote comfort and diuresis. Weight is monitored daily, and diuretics are used to reduce fluid overload. Sodium intake and fluid intake are adjusted according to the ability of the patient's kidneys to excrete water and sodium.

Initiation of dialysis is considered early in the course of the disease to keep the patient in optimal physical condition, prevent fluid and electrolyte imbalances, and minimize the risk of complications of renal failure. The course of dialysis is smoother if treatment is initiated before the patient develops significant complications.

Nursing Interventions. If the patient is hospitalized or eligible for home visits, the nurse will observe the patient for changes in fluid and electrolyte status and for signs of deterioration of renal function. Changes in fluid and electrolyte status and in cardiac and neurologic status are reported promptly to the physician. Anxiety levels are extremely high for both the patient and family. The patient with renal disease often faces an uncertain future. The nurse gives emotional support throughout the course of the disease and treatment by providing opportunities for the patient and family to verbalize their concerns and have their questions answered and their options discussed.

Patient Education and Home Care Considerations. The nurse has a major role in educating the patient and family about the prescribed treatment plan and the risks of noncompliance. Instructions to the patient include explanations and scheduling for follow-up evaluations of blood pressure, urinalysis for protein, and blood for BUN and creatinine levels to determine if there is progression of disease activity, as well as urinalysis for protein and casts to assess renal function.

A referral to the community health or home care nurse may be indicated to provide an opportunity for careful assessment of the patient's progress and to provide continued education about problems to report to the health care provider (*i.e.*, worsening signs of renal failure such as nausea, vomiting, diminished urine output); recommended diet and fluid modifications; and medication teaching (purpose, side effects, desired effects, dosage, administration schedule). If dialysis is initiated, the patient and family will require considerable assistance and support in dealing with the need for this therapy and its long-term implications. See Chapter 42 for a discussion of dialysis and pp. 1204–1206 for a discussion of kidney transplantation.

Nephrotic Syndrome

Nephrotic syndrome is a clinical disorder characterized by (1) a marked increase in protein in the urine (proteinuria), (2) a decrease in albumin in the blood (hypoalbuminemia), (3) edema, and (4) high serum cholesterol and low density lipoproteins (hyperlipidemia). It is seen in any condition that seriously damages the glomerular capillary membrane and results in increased glomerular permeability.

Pathophysiology. The primary manifestation of nephrotic syndrome is the loss of plasma protein, particularly albumin, in the urine. Although the liver is capable of increasing the production of albumin, it is unable to keep up with the daily loss of albumin through the kidneys. Thus hypoalbuminemia results.

The resultant decreased oncotic pressure leads to generalized edema as fluid moves from the vascular system into the extracellular fluid spaces. A decreased circulating blood volume activates the renin–angiotensin system, leading to retention of sodium and further edema. The diminished protein in the serum stimulates synthesis of lipoproteins in the liver and an elevated lipid concentration in the blood (hyperlipidemia).

The nephrotic syndrome can occur with almost any intrinsic renal disease or systemic disease that affects the glomerulus. Although generally considered a disorder of childhood, nephrotic syndrome does occur in adults, including the elderly. *Causes* include chronic glomerulonephritis, diabetes mellitus with intercapillary glomerulosclerosis, amyloidosis of the kidney, systemic lupus erythematosus, and renal vein thrombosis.

Clinical Manifestations. The major manifestation of nephrotic syndrome is edema. It is usually soft and pitting, and is most commonly found around the eyes (periorbital), in dependent areas (sacrum, ankles, and hands), and in the abdomen (ascites). Other symptoms such as malaise, headache, irritability, and fatigue are common.

Diagnostic Evaluation. Urinalysis shows microscopic hematuria, urinary casts, and other abnormalities. Needle biopsy of the kidney may be performed for histologic examination of renal tissue to confirm the diagnosis.

Complications of nephrotic syndrome include infection (due to a deficient immune response), thromboembolism (especially of the renal vein), pulmonary emboli, and accelerated atherosclerosis.

Management. The objective of management is to preserve renal function. It may be necessary to keep the patient on bed rest for a few days to promote diuresis to reduce the edema. Protein intake is increased to replace urinary losses and restore body proteins. If the edema is severe, the patient is placed on a low-sodium diet. Diuretics are prescribed for the patient with severe edema, and adrenocorticosteroids (prednisone) may be used to reduce proteinuria.

Other medications used in the treatment of nephrotic syndrome include antineoplastic agents (Cytoxan) or immunosuppressive agents (Imuran, Leukeran, or cyclosporine). It may be necessary to repeat treatment with corticosteroids if relapse occurs.

Nursing Interventions. In the early stages, the nursing management is similar to that of the patient with acute glomerulonephritis, but as the disease worsens, management is similar to that of the patient with chronic renal failure (see pp. 1197–1204). The patient who is receiving steroids or cyclosporine requires instructions about the medications and signs and symptoms that warrant reporting to the physician. Assistance with selecting a high-protein diet while restricting cholesterol and fat intake may be necessary.

Nephrosclerosis

Nephrosclerosis is hardening, or sclerosis, of the arteries of the kidney due to prolonged hypertension. This causes decreased blood flow to the kidney and patchy necrosis of the renal parenchyma. Eventually, fibrosis occurs and glomeruli are destroyed.

There are two forms of nephrosclerosis: malignant (accelerated) and benign. **Malignant nephrosclerosis** is often associated with malignant hypertension (diastolic blood pressure > 130 mm Hg). It usually occurs in young adults, with men affected twice as often as women. The disease process progresses rapidly and over 50% of patients die from uremia in a matter of a few years.

Benign nephrosclerosis is usually found in older adults. It is often associated with atherosclerosis as well as hypertension. These patients rarely complain of renal symptoms, even though the urine usually contains protein and occasional casts. Renal insufficiency and associated signs and symptoms occur late in the disease.

Treatment for nephrosclerosis is aggressive antihypertensive therapy.

Hydronephrosis

Hydronephrosis is dilation of the renal pelvis and calyces of one or both kidneys due to an obstruction. Obstruction to the normal flow of urine causes the urine to back up, resulting in increased pressure in the kidney. If the obstruction is in the urethra or the bladder, the back-pressure affects both kidneys, but if the obstruction is in one of the ureters because of a stone or kink, only one kidney is damaged.

Partial or intermittent obstruction may be caused by a renal stone that has formed in the renal pelvis but has moved into the ureter and blocked it. The obstruction may be due to a tumor pressing on the ureter or to bands of scar tissue resulting from an abscess or inflammation near the ureter that pinches it. The disorder may be due to an odd angle of the ureter as it leaves the renal pelvis or to an unusual position of the kidney, favoring a ureteral twist or kink. In elderly males, the most common cause is urethral obstruction at the bladder outlet caused by an enlarged prostate gland. Hydronephrosis can also occur in pregnancy due to the enlarged uterus.

Whatever the cause, as the urine accumulates in the renal pelvis, it distends the pelvis and its calyces. In time, atrophy of the kidney results. As one kidney undergoes gradual destruction, the contralateral kidney gradually enlarges (compensatory hypertrophy). Ultimately, renal function is impaired.

Clinical Manifestations. The patient may be asymptomatic if the onset is gradual. Acute obstruction may produce aching in the flank and back. If infection is present, dysuria, chills, fever, tenderness, and pyuria may occur. Hematuria and pyuria may be present. If both kidneys are affected, signs and symptoms of chronic renal failure may develop.

Management. The goals of management are to identify and correct the cause of the obstruction, to treat infection, and to restore and conserve renal function.

To relieve the obstruction, the urine may have to be diverted by nephrostomy (see Chapter 42) or other types of diversion. The infection is treated with antimicrobial agents because residual urine in the calyces produces infection and pyelonephritis. The patient is prepared for surgical removal of obstructive lesions (calculus, tumor, obstruction of the ureter). If one kidney is severely damaged and its function is destroyed, nephrectomy (removal of the kidney) may be performed.

Renal Failure

Renal failure results when the kidneys are unable to remove the body's metabolic wastes or perform their regulatory functions. The substances normally eliminated in the urine accumulate in the body fluids as a result of impaired renal excretion and lead to a disruption in endocrine and metabolic functions as well as fluid, electrolyte, and acid–base disturbances. Renal failure is a systemic disease and is a final common pathway of many different kidney and urinary tract diseases. Each year an estimated 50,000 Americans die of irreversible kidney failure.

Acute Renal Failure

Pathophysiology

Acute renal failure is a sudden and almost complete loss of kidney function caused by failure of the renal circulation or by glomerular or tubular dysfunction. It is manifested by either anuria, oliguria, or normal urine volume. **Anuria** (less than 50 ml urine per day) and normal urine output are not as common as oliguria. **Oliguria** (less than 400 ml urine per day) is the most common clinical situation seen in acute renal failure.

Regardless of the volume of urine excreted, the patient with acute renal failure experiences rising serum creatinine and blood urea nitrogen (BUN) levels and retention of other metabolic waste products normally excreted by the kidneys.

Causes. Three major categories of conditions cause acute renal failure:

- Prerenal (hypoperfusion of kidney)
- Intrarenal (actual damage to kidney tissue)
- Postrenal (obstruction to urine flow)

Prerenal conditions occur due to a blood flow problem which leads to hypoperfusion of the kidney and a drop in the glomerular filtration rate. Common clinical situations are volume depletion states (hemorrhage or gastrointestinal losses), vasodilation (sepsis or anaphylaxis), and impaired cardiac performance (myocardial infarction, congestive heart failure, or cardiogenic shock).

Intrarenal causes of acute renal failure are the result of structural damage to the glomeruli or kidney tubules. Conditions such as burns, crush injuries, and infections, as well as nephrotoxic agents, may lead to acute tubular necrosis (ATN) and cessation of renal function. With burns and crush injuries, myoglobin (a protein released from muscle when injury occurs) and hemoglobin are liberated, causing renal toxicity, ischemia, or both. Severe transfusion reactions may also cause intrarenal failure; hemoglobin released through hemolysis filters through the glomeruli and becomes concentrated in the kidney tubules to such a degree that precipitation of hemoglobin occurs. Another causative factor is the use of nonsteroidal anti-inflammatory drugs (NSAIDs), especially in elderly patients. These medications interfere with prostaglandins that normally protect renal blood flow, thus leading to ischemia of the kidneys.

Postrenal causes of acute renal failure are usually the result of an obstruction somewhere distal to the kidney. Pressure rises in the kidney tubules; eventually the glomerular filtration rate decreases. Common causes of acute renal failure are summarized in Chart 43-2.

Although the exact pathogenesis of acute renal failure and oliguria is not always known, many times there is a clear-cut underlying problem. Some of these factors may be reversible if identified and treated promptly, before kidney function is impaired. This is true of the following conditions that reduce blood flow to the kidney and impair kidney function: (1) hypovolemia; (2) hypotension; (3) reduced cardiac output and congestive heart failure; (4) obstruction of the kidney or lower urinary tract by tumor, blood clot, or kidney stone; and (5) bilateral obstruction of the renal ar-

CHART 43-2

Causes of Acute Renal Failure

Prerenal

Volume Depletion
Hemorrhage
Renal losses (diuretics, osmotic diuresis)
GI losses (vomiting, diarrhea, nasogastric tubes)

Impaired Cardiac Efficiency
Myocardial infarction
Congestive heart failure
Dysrhythmias
Cardiogenic shock

Vasodilation
Sepsis
Anaphylaxis
Antihypertensive medications or other medications that cause vasodilation

Intrarenal

Prolonged Renal Ischemia

"Pigment Nephropathy"
Myoglobinuria (trauma, crush injuries, burns)
Hemoglobinuria (transfusion reaction, hemolytic anemia)

Nephrotoxic Agents
Aminoglycoside antibiotics (gentamycin, tobramycin)
Radiopaque contrast agents
Heavy metals (lead, mercury)
Solvents and chemicals (ethylene glycol, carbon tetrachloride, arsenic)
Non-steroidal anti-inflammatory drugs (NSAIDs)

Infectious Processes
Acute pyelonephritis
Acute glomerulonephritis

Postrenal

Urinary Tract Obstruction
Calculi
Tumors
Benign prostatic hyperplasia
Strictures
Blood clots

teries or veins. If these conditions are treated and corrected before the kidneys are permanently damaged, the increased BUN, oliguria, and other signs associated with acute renal failure may be reversed.

Phases. There are four clinical phases of acute renal failure: the initiation period, the period of oliguria, a period of diuresis, and a period of recovery.

The **initiation period** begins with the initial insult and ends when oliguria develops.

The **period of oliguria** (urinary volume less than 400 ml/24 h) is accompanied by a rise in the serum concentration of substances usually excreted by the kidneys (urea, creatinine, uric acid, organic acids, and the intracellular cations—potassium and magnesium). The minimum amount of urine needed to rid the body of normal metabolic waste products is 400 ml. It is in this phase that uremic symptoms first appear, and when life-threatening conditions such as hyperkalemia develop.

In some patients there can be a decrease in renal function with increasing nitrogen retention, yet the patient is actually excreting 2 or more liters of urine daily. This is the nonoliguric form of renal failure and occurs predominantly after nephrotoxic antibiotics are administered to the patient; it may occur with burns, traumatic injury, and use of halogenated anesthesia.

In the **period of diuresis**, the third phase, the patient experiences a gradually increasing urinary output, which signals that glomerular filtration has started to recover. Laboratory values stop rising and eventually begin a downward trend. Although the volume of urinary output may reach normal or elevated levels, renal function may still be markedly abnormal. Uremic symptoms may still be present. Therefore, expert medical and nursing management is still required. The patient must be observed closely for dehydration during this phase; if dehydration occurs, the uremic symptoms are likely to increase.

The **period of recovery** signals the improvement of renal function and may take from 3 to 12 months. Laboratory values will return to a normal level for the patient. Although there is a permanent 1% to 3% reduction in the glomerular filtration rate, it is not clinically significant.

Clinical Manifestations and Laboratory Abnormalities

Almost every system of the body is affected when there is failure of the normal renal regulatory mechanisms. The patient appears critically ill and is lethargic with persistent nausea, vomiting, and diarrhea. The skin and mucous membranes are dry from dehydration, and the breath may have the odor of urine (uremic fetor). Central nervous system manifestations include drowsiness, headache, muscle twitching, and seizures.

Changes in Urine Output. The urinary output is scanty, may be bloody, and has a low specific gravity (1.010 compared with a normal value of 1.015–1.025).

Increased BUN and Creatinine Levels. There is a steady rise in the BUN, with the rate of rise dependent on the degree of catabolism (breakdown of protein), renal perfusion, and protein intake. Serum creatinine rises in conjunction with glomerular damage. Serum creatinine levels are useful in monitoring kidney function and disease progression.

Hyperkalemia. A patient with renal disease in which the glomerular filtration rate is reduced is unable to excrete potassium. Protein catabolism results in the release of cellular potassium into the body fluids, causing severe hyperkalemia (high serum K^+ levels). Hyperkalemia may lead to dysrhythmias and cardiac arrest. Sources of potassium include normal tissue catabolism; dietary intake; blood in the gastrointestinal tract; or blood transfusion and other sources (intravenous infusions, potassium penicillin, and extracellular shift in response to metabolic acidosis).

Metabolic Acidosis. Patients with acute oliguria cannot eliminate the daily metabolic load of acid-type substances produced by the normal metabolic processes. In addition, normal renal buffering mechanisms fail. This is reflected by a fall in the blood carbon dioxide combining power and blood *p*H. Thus, progressive metabolic acidosis accompanies renal failure.

Ca^{++} and PO_4^- Abnormalities. There may be an increase in serum phosphate concentrations; serum calcium levels may be low in response to decreased absorption of calcium from the intestine and as a compensatory mechanism for the elevated serum phosphate levels.

Anemia. Anemia inevitably accompanies acute renal failure due to reduced erythropoietin production, uremic gastrointestinal lesions, reduced red cell life span, and blood loss, usually from the GI tract. With the parenteral form of erythropoietin (Epogen) now available, anemia does not present the major problem it once did.

Prevention

A careful history is indicated to determine if the patient has been taking potentially nephrotoxic antimicrobial agents or has been exposed to environmental toxins. The kidneys are especially susceptible to the adverse effects of medications because they receive such a large blood flow (25% of the cardiac output at rest).

The nephrons are exposed to high concentrations of antimicrobial medications as a result of glomerular filtration and tubular secretion and reabsorption and thus are more likely to suffer toxic effects of these medications. Therefore, in patients taking potentially nephrotoxic medications (aminoglycosides, gentamicin, tobramycin, colistimethate, polymyxin B, amphotericin B, vancomycin, amikacin, capreomycin, cyclosporine), renal function should be monitored by evaluating BUN and serum creatinine levels within 24 hours of initiation of medication therapy and at least twice a week while the patient is receiving therapy. Any agent that reduces renal blood flow (*e.g.*, chronic analgesic use) may cause renal insufficiency. Chronic analgesic use, particularly with NSAIDs, causes interstitial nephritis and papillary necrosis. Patients with congestive heart failure or cirrhosis with ascites are at particular risk for NSAID-induced renal failure. Increased age, existing renal disease, and the administration of several nephrotoxic agents simultaneously increase the risk of kidney damage.

Other precautionary measures taken to avoid renal complications include adequate hydration for patients at risk; prompt recognition and treatment of shock, hypotension, and infection; careful monitoring of renal function, urinary output, and central venous and arterial pressures when indicated; and meticulous attention to catheter care,

CHART 43-3
Prevention: Avoiding Acute Renal Failure

- Provide adequate hydration to patients at risk for dehydration:
  - Surgical patients: before, during and after surgery.
  - Patients undergoing intensive diagnostic studies requiring fluid restriction and contrast agents (*e.g.*, barium enema, intravenous pyelograms), especially elderly patients who may not have adequate renal reserve.
  - Patients with neoplastic disorders or disorders of metabolism (*i.e.*, gout) and those receiving chemotherapy.
- Prevent and treat shock promptly with blood and fluid replacement.
- Monitor critically ill patients for central venous and arterial pressures and hourly urine output to detect the onset of renal failure as early as possible.
- Manage hypotension promptly.
- Continually assess renal function (urine output, laboratory values) when appropriate.
- Take precautions to ensure that the appropriate blood is administered to the correct patient in order to avoid severe transfusion reactions, which can precipitate renal complications.
- Prevent and treat infections promptly. Infections can produce progressive renal damage.
- Pay special attention to wounds, burns, and other causes of sepsis.
- Give meticulous care to patients with indwelling catheters to prevent infections from ascending urinary tract. Remove catheters as soon as possible.
- Closely monitor all medications metabolized or excreted by the kidneys for dosage, duration, and blood levels to prevent toxic effects.

wound care, and proper blood transfusion protocols (to avoid severe transfusion reactions). Chart 43-3 presents an overview of preventive measures for acute renal failure.

Management

The kidney has a remarkable ability to recover from insult. Therefore, the objective of treatment of acute renal failure is to restore normal chemical balance and prevent complications so that repair of renal tissue and restoration of renal function can take place. A search is made to identify, treat, and eliminate any possible cause of damage.

Dialysis. Dialysis may be initiated to prevent serious complications of acute renal failure, such as hyperkalemia, pericarditis, and seizures. Dialysis corrects many biochemical abnormalities; allows for liberalization of fluid, protein, and sodium intake; diminishes bleeding tendencies; and may help wound healing. Hemodialysis, hemofiltration, or peritoneal dialysis may be performed. These forms of dialysis are discussed in Chapter 42, which presents treatment modalities for patients with renal dysfunction.

Treatment of Hyperkalemia. Fluid and electrolyte imbalances are a major problem in acute renal failure; hyperkalemia is the most life-threatening of these disturbances. Thus, the patient is monitored for hyperkalemia through serial serum electrolyte levels (potassium value > 5.5 mEq/L; SI: 5.5 mmol/L), ECG changes (tall tented or peaked T waves), and changes in clinical status.

The elevated potassium levels may be reduced by administering ion exchange resins (sodium polystyrene sulfonate [Kayexalate]) orally or by retention enema. Kayexalate works by exchanging a sodium ion for a potassium ion in the intestinal tract. Sorbitol is often administered in combination with Kayexalate to induce a diarrhea-type effect (it induces water loss in the gastrointestinal tract).

If a retention enema is administered (the colon is the major site for potassium exchange), a rectal catheter with a balloon may be prescribed to facilitate retention if necessary. The patient should retain the resin 30 to 45 minutes to promote potassium removal. Afterwards, a cleansing enema may be prescribed to remove the Kayexalate resin as a precaution against fecal impaction.

- A patient with a high and rising level of serum potassium requires immediate hemodialysis, peritoneal dialysis, or hemofiltration.
- Intravenous glucose and insulin or calcium gluconate may be used as an emergency and temporary measure to treat hyperkalemia. Glucose and insulin drive potassium into the cells, thereby lowering serum potassium levels temporarily until potassium is removed by dialysis. Potassium will move out of the cells and rise again to a dangerous level unless removed by dialysis. Calcium gluconate helps protect the heart from the effects of the high potassium levels.
- Sodium bicarbonate may be administered to promote an elevation of plasma *p*H. Sodium bicarbonate increases the *p*H, which causes potassium to move into the cell, and the result is lowering of the patient's serum potassium level. This is short-term therapy and is used with other long-term measures, such as dietary restriction and dialysis.
- All external sources of potassium are eliminated or reduced.

Maintenance of Fluid Balance. Management of fluid balance is based on daily body weight, serial measurements of central venous pressure, serum and urine concentrations, fluid losses, blood pressure, and the clinical status of the patient. The parenteral and oral intake and the output of urine, gastric drainage, stools, wound drainage, and perspiration are calculated and are used as the basis for fluid replacement. The insensible fluid lost through the skin and lungs and produced through the normal metabolic processes is also considered in fluid management.

Acute renal failure causes severe nutritional imbalances due to inadequate intake (from nausea and vomiting), impaired glucose utilization and protein synthesis, and increased tissue catabolism. The patient is weighed daily and can be expected to lose 0.2 to 0.5 kg (½–1 lb) daily if the nitrogen balance is negative (*i.e.*, receiving caloric intake that is less than caloric requirements). If the patient does not lose weight or develops hypertension, fluid retention should be suspected.

Fluid excesses can be detected by the clinical findings of dyspnea, tachycardia, and distended neck veins. The lungs are auscultated for signs of moist crackles. Because pulmonary edema may be caused by excessive administration of parenteral fluids, extreme caution must be used to prevent fluid overload. The development of generalized edema is assessed by examining the presacral and pretibial areas several times daily.

Nutritional Considerations. Dietary proteins are limited to approximately 1 g/kg during the oliguric phase to minimize protein breakdown and to prevent accumulation of toxic end products. Caloric requirements are met with high-carbohydrate feedings, because carbohydrates have a protein-sparing effect (in a high-carbohydrate diet, protein is not used for meeting energy requirements but is "spared" for growth and tissue healing). Foods and fluids containing potassium and phosphorus (bananas, citrus fruits and juices, coffee) are restricted. Potassium intake is usually restricted to 40 to 60 mEq/day, and sodium is usually restricted to 2 g/day. The patient may require total parenteral nutrition (see Chapter 35).

IV Fluids and Diuretics. Adequate blood flow to the kidneys in some patients may be restored by intravenous fluids and medications. Mannitol, furosemide, or ethacrynic acid may be prescribed to initiate a diuresis and prevent or minimize subsequent renal failure. If acute renal failure is caused by hypovolemia secondary to hypoproteinemia, an infusion of albumin may be prescribed. Shock and infection, if present, are treated.

Correction of Acidosis and Elevated Phosphate Levels. When severe acidosis is present, the arterial blood gases must be monitored; appropriate ventilatory measures must be instituted if respiratory problems develop. The patient may require sodium bicarbonate therapy or dialysis.

The patient's elevated serum phosphate concentration may be controlled with phosphate-binding agents (aluminum hydroxide); these help prevent a continuing rise in serum phosphate levels by decreasing absorption of phosphate from the intestinal tract.

Continued Monitoring During Recovery Phase. The oliguric phase of acute renal failure may last from 10 to 20 days and is followed by the diuretic phase, at which time urinary output begins to increase, signaling that kidney function is returning. Blood chemistry evaluations are made to determine the amounts of sodium, potassium, and water needed for replacement, along with assessment for overhydration or underhydration.

After the diuretic phase, the patient is placed on a high-protein, high-calorie diet and is encouraged to resume activities gradually.

Nursing Interventions

General Approach. The nurse has an important role in managing the patient with acute renal failure. In addition to directing attention to the patient's primary disorder, which may be a factor in the development of acute renal failure, the nurse monitors the patient for complications, participates in emergency treatment of fluid and electrolyte imbalances, assesses the patient's progress and response to treatment, and provides physical and emotional support. Additionally, the nurse keeps the family informed about the patient's condition, assists them in understanding the treatments, and provides psychologic support. Although the development of acute renal failure may be the most life-threatening problem, the nurse must continue to include in the plan of care those nursing measures indicated for the patient's primary disorder (*e.g.*, burns, shock, trauma, obstruction of the urinary tract).

Monitoring Fluid and Electrolyte Balance. The serious fluid and electrolyte imbalances that can occur with acute renal failure require the nurse to monitor closely the patient's serum electrolyte levels and physical indicators of these complications during all phases of the disorder.

Hyperkalemia is the most immediate life-threatening imbalance seen in acute renal failure. Parenteral fluids, all oral intake, and all medications are screened carefully to ensure that hidden sources of potassium are not inadvertently administered or consumed. Intravenous solutions must be carefully selected according to the patient's fluid and electrolyte status. The patient's cardiac function and musculoskeletal status are monitored closely for changes suggestive of hyperkalemia.

The patient's *fluid status* is monitored by careful attention to fluid intake, urine output, changes in body weight, the presence of edema, distention of the jugular veins, alterations in heart sounds and breath sounds, and increasing difficulty in breathing.

Indicators of deterioration of fluid and electrolyte status are reported immediately to the physician, and preparation is made for emergency treatment, including the use of glucose and insulin, calcium gluconate, or cation-exchange resins (Kayexalate) to treat hyperkalemia, and the initiation of hemodialysis, peritoneal dialysis, or hemofiltration to correct fluid and electrolyte disturbances.

Reducing Metabolic Rate. The nurse also directs attention to reducing the patient's metabolic rate during the acute stage of renal failure to reduce catabolism and the subsequent release of potassium and accumulation of endogenous waste products (urea and creatinine). Bed rest may be indicated to reduce exertion and the metabolic rate during the most acute stage of the disorder. Fever and infection, both of which increase metabolic rate and catabolism, are prevented or treated promptly.

Promoting Pulmonary Function. Attention is given to pulmonary function, and the patient is assisted to turn, cough, and take deep breaths frequently to prevent atelectasis and respiratory infection. Drowsiness and lethargy may prevent the patient from moving and turning without encouragement and assistance.

Avoiding Infection. Asepsis is essential with invasive lines and catheters to minimize the risk of infection and increased metabolism. An indwelling catheter is avoided if possible because of the high risk of urinary tract infection associated with its use.

Providing Skin Care. The patient's skin may be dry or susceptible to breakdown as a result of edema; therefore, meticulous skin care is important. Additionally, excoriation and itching of the skin may result from the deposit of irritating toxins in the patient's tissues. Massaging bony prominences, turning the patient frequently, and bathing with cool water are often comforting and prevent skin breakdown.

Dialysis Support. The patient with acute renal failure will require treatment with hemodialysis, peritoneal dialysis, or hemofiltration to prevent serious complications; the length of time that these treatments will be necessary varies with the cause and extent of damage to the kidneys. The patient and family will need assistance, explanation, and support during this time. The purpose and rationale of the treatments will be explained to the patient and family by the physician. However, high levels of anxiety and fear may necessitate repeated explanation and clarification by the nurse. The family members may initially be afraid to touch and talk to the patient during the procedure but should be encouraged and assisted to do so.

Although many of the nurse's functions will be devoted to the technical aspects of the procedure, the psychologic needs and concerns of the patient and family cannot be ignored. Continued assessment of the patient for complications of acute renal failure and of its precipitating cause is essential.

Chronic Renal Failure (End-Stage Renal Disease)

Chronic renal failure or end-stage renal disease (ESRD) is a progressive, irreversible deterioration in renal function in which the body's ability to maintain metabolic and fluid and electrolyte balance fails, resulting in uremia (retention of urea and other nitrogenous wastes in the blood). It may be caused by systemic diseases such as diabetes mellitus; chronic glomerulonephritis; pyelonephritis; uncontrolled hypertension; obstruction of the urinary tract; hereditary lesions, such as in polycystic kidney disease; vascular disorders; infections; medications; or toxic agents. Environmental and occupational agents that have been implicated in chronic renal failure include lead, cadmium, mercury, and chromium. Dialysis or kidney transplantation eventually becomes necessary for patient survival.

Pathophysiology

As renal function declines, the end products of protein metabolism (which are normally excreted in urine) accumulate in the blood. Uremia develops and adversely affects every system in the body. The greater the buildup of waste products, the more severe the symptoms. Many of the symptoms of uremia are reversible with dialysis.

Impaired Renal Clearance. Many of the problems seen in renal failure are due to a reduction in the number of functioning glomeruli, leading to decreased clearance from the blood of substances normally cleared by the kidney.

Decreased glomerular filtration rates (GFR) can be detected by obtaining a 24-hour urine for creatinine clearance. As glomerular filtration decreases (due to nonfunctioning glomeruli) the creatinine clearance will decrease and the serum creatinine level will rise. In addition, the blood urea nitrogen (BUN) level is usually elevated. Serum creatinine is the more sensitive indicator of renal function because of its constant production in the body. The BUN is affected not only by renal disease, but by protein intake in the diet, catabolism (tissue and RBC breakdown), and medications such as steroids.

Sodium and Water Retention. The kidney is also unable to concentrate or dilute the urine normally in end-stage renal disease; appropriate responses by the kidney to changes in the daily intake of water and electrolytes, therefore, do not occur. The patient often retains sodium and water, increasing the risk of edema formation, congestive heart failure, and hypertension. Hypertension may also result from activation of the renin–angiotensin axis and the concomitant increased aldosterone secretion. Other patients have a tendency to lose salt; they run the risk of hypotension and hypovolemia. Episodes of vomiting and diarrhea may produce sodium and water depletion, which worsens the uremic state.

Acidosis. With advanced renal disease, metabolic acidosis occurs as the kidney is unable to excrete increased loads of acid (H^+). Decreased acid secretion primarily results from inability of the kidney tubules to secrete ammonia (NH_3^-) and to reabsorb sodium bicarbonate (HCO_3^-). There is also decreased excretion of phosphates and other organic acids.

Anemia. Anemia develops as a result of inadequate erythropoietin production, the shortened life span of red blood cells, nutritional deficiencies, and the uremic patient's tendency to bleed, particularly from the gastrointestinal tract. Erythropoietin, a substance normally produced by the kidney, stimulates bone marrow to produce red blood cells. In renal failure, erthyropoietin production decreases and profound anemia results, producing fatigue, angina, and shortness of breath.

Calcium and Phosphorus Imbalance. Another major abnormality seen in chronic renal failure is a disorder in calcium and phosphorus metabolism. The body's serum calcium and phosphate levels have a reciprocal relationship in the body; as one rises, the other decreases. With decreased filtration through the kidney's glomerulus, there is an increase in the serum phosphate level and a reciprocal or corresponding decrease in the serum calcium level. The decreased serum calcium level causes increased secretion of parathormone from the parathyroid glands. However, in renal failure, the body does not respond normally to the increased secretion of parathormone, and, as a result, calcium leaves the bone, often producing bone changes and bone disease. In addition, the active metabolite of vitamin D (1,25-dihydroxycholecalciferol) normally manufactured by the kidney decreases as renal failure progresses.

Uremic bone disease, often called **renal osteodystrophy,** develops from the complex changes in calcium, phosphate, and parathormone balance.

The rate of decline in renal function and progression of chronic renal failure is related to the underlying disorder, to the urinary excretion of protein, and to the presence of hypertension. Patients who excrete significant amounts of protein or have elevated blood pressure tend to progress more rapidly than those without these conditions.

Clinical Manifestations

As virtually every body system is affected by the uremia of chronic renal failure, patients will exhibit a number of signs and symptoms. The severity of these signs and symptoms is dependent in part on the degree of renal impairment, other underlying conditions, and the patient's age.

Cardiovascular manifestations of chronic renal failure include hypertension (due to sodium and water retention or from activation of the renin–angiotensin–aldosterone system), congestive heart failure and pulmonary edema (due to fluid overload), and pericarditis (due to irritation of the pericardial lining by uremic toxins).

Dermatologic symptoms, including severe itching (pruritis) are common. Uremic frost, the deposit of urea crystals on the skin, is uncommon today because of early and aggressive treatment for end-stage renal disease. *Gastrointestinal symptoms* are also very common and include anorexia, nausea, vomiting, and hiccups. *Neuromuscular* changes including altered levels of consciousness, inability to concentrate, muscle twitching, and seizures have all been observed.

The precise mechanisms for many of these diverse manifestations have not been identified. However, it is generally thought that the accumulation of uremic waste products is the probable cause. Chart 43-4 summarizes the signs and symptoms often seen in chronic renal failure.

CHART 43-4 Signs and Symptoms of Chronic Renal Failure

Cardiovascular
- Hypertension
- Pitting edema (feet, hands, sacrum)
- Periorbital edema
- Pericardial friction rub
- Engorged neck veins

Integumentary
- Gray-bronze skin color
- Dry, flaky skin
- Pruritus
- Ecchymosis
- Thin, brittle nails
- Coarse, thinning hair

Pulmonary
- Crackles
- Thick, tenacious sputum
- Shortness of breath
- Kussmaul-type respirations

Gastrointestinal
- Ammonia odor to breath
- Mouth ulcerations and bleeding
- Anorexia, nausea, and vomiting
- Constipation or diarrhea
- Bleeding from GI tract

Neurologic
- Weakness and fatigue
- Confusion
- Disorientation
- Seizures
- Restlessness of legs
- Burning of soles of feet
- Behavior changes

Musculoskeletal
- Muscle cramps
- Loss of muscle strength
- Bone fractures
- Foot drop

Reproductive
- Amenorrhea
- Testicular atrophy

Management

The goal of management is to maintain kidney function and homeostasis for as long as possible. All factors that contribute to end-stage renal failure and those that are reversible (*e.g.,* obstruction) are identified and treated.

Potential complications of chronic renal failure which necessitate a collaborative approach to care include: (1) *hyperkalemia* due to decreased excretion, metabolic acidosis, catabolism, and excessive dietary intake; (2) *pericarditis,* pericardial effusion, and pericardial tamponade due to retention of uremic waste products and inadequate dialysis; (3) *hypertension* due to sodium and water retention and malfunction of the renin–angiotensin–aldosterone system; (4) *anemia* due to decreased erythropoietin, decreased RBC life span, bleeding in the gastrointestinal tract from irritating toxins, and blood loss during hemodialysis, and (5) *bone disease* and metastatic calcifications due to retention of phosphorus, low serum calcium levels, abnormal vitamin D metabolism, and elevated aluminum levels.

Complications can be prevented or delayed by administering prescribed antihypertensives, erythropoietin, iron supplements, phosphate binding agents, and calcium supplements. It is also essential that the patient receive adequate dialysis treatments to decrease the level of uremic waste products in the blood.

Dietary intervention is necessary with deterioration of renal function and includes careful regulation of protein intake, fluid intake to balance fluid losses, sodium intake to balance sodium losses, and some restriction of potassium. At the same time, adequate calorie intake and vitamin supplementation must be ensured. Protein will be restricted because urea, uric acid, and organic acids—the breakdown products of dietary and tissue proteins—will accumulate rapidly in the blood when there is impaired renal clearance. The allowed protein must be of high biologic value (dairy products, eggs, meats). High-biologic-value proteins are those that are complete proteins and supply the essential amino acids necessary for growth and cell repair. Usually, the fluid allowance is 500 to 600 ml more than the previous day's 24-hour urine output. Calories are supplied by carbohydrates and fat to prevent wasting. Vitamin supplementation is necessary because a protein-restricted diet does not give the necessary complement of vitamins. Additionally, the patient on dialysis may lose water-soluble vitamins from the blood during the dialysis treatment.

Hyperphosphatemia and *hypocalcemia* are treated with aluminum-based antacids that bind dietary phosphorus in the gastrointestinal tract. However, concern about the potential long-term toxicity of aluminum and the association of high aluminum levels with neurologic symptoms and osteomalacia have led some physicians to prescribe calcium carbonate in place of high doses of aluminum-based antacids. This medication also binds dietary phosphorus in the intestinal tract and permits the use of smaller doses of antacids. Both calcium carbonate and phosphorus-binding antacids must be administered with food to be effective. Magnesium-based antacids must be avoided to prevent magnesium toxicity.

Hypertension is managed by intravascular volume control and a variety of antihypertensive medications. *Congestive heart failure* and *pulmonary edema* may also require treatment with fluid restriction, low sodium diets, diuretics, inotropic agents such as digitalis or dobutamine, and dialysis. The *metabolic acidosis* of chronic renal failure usually produces no symptoms and requires no treatment; however, sodium bicarbonate supplements or dialysis may be needed to correct the acidosis if it causes symptoms.

Hyperkalemia is usually prevented by ensuring adequate dialysis treatments with potassium removal and careful monitoring of all medications, both oral and intravenous, for their potassium content. The patient is placed on a potassium-restricted diet. Occasionally Kayexelate, administered orally, may be needed.

Neurologic abnormalities may occur and require that the patient be observed for early evidence of slight twitching, headache, delirium, or seizure activity. The patient is protected from injury by padding the side rails of the bed. The onset of seizures is recorded along with the type, duration, and general effect on the patient. The physician is notified immediately. Intravenous diazepam (Valium) or phenytoin (Dilantin) is usually administered to control seizures. The nursing management of the patient with seizures is discussed in Chapter 60.

Anemia associated with chronic renal failure is treated with Epogen (recombinant human erythropoietin). Anemic patients (hematocrit less than 30%) present with nonspecific symptoms such as malaise, general fatigability, and decreased activity tolerance. Epogen therapy is initiated to achieve a hematocrit of 33% to 38%, which generally alleviates the symptoms of anemia. Epogen is administered either intravenously or subcutaneously three times a week. It may take 2 to 6 weeks for the hematocrit to rise, therefore Epogen is not indicated for patients who need immediate correction of severe anemia. Adverse effects seen with Epogen therapy include hypertension (especially during early stages of treatment), increased clotting of vascular access sites, seizures, and depletion of body iron stores.

The patient receiving Epogen may experience flu-like symptoms with initiation of therapy; these tend to subside with repeated doses. Management involves adjustment of heparin to prevent clotting of the dialysis lines during hemodialysis treatments, frequent monitoring of hematocrit, and periodic assessment of serum iron and transferrin levels. Because adequate stores of iron are necessary for an adequate response to erythropoietin, supplementary iron may be prescribed. In addition, the patient's blood pressure and serum potassium are monitored to detect hypertension and rising serum potassium levels, which may occur with therapy and the increasing red cell mass. The occurrence of *hypertension* requires initiation or adjustment of the patient's antihypertensive therapy. Hypertension that cannot be controlled is a contraindication for recombinant erythropoietin therapy.

Patients who have received Epogen have reported decreased levels of fatigue, an increased feeling of well-being, better tolerance of dialysis, higher energy levels, and improved exercise tolerance. Additionally, this therapy has decreased the need for transfusion and its associated risks (infectious disease, antibody formation, and iron overload).

The patient with increasing symptoms of chronic renal failure is referred to a dialysis and transplantation center early in the course of progressive renal disease. *Dialysis* is usually initiated when the patient cannot maintain a reasonable lifestyle with conservative treatment. The details of dialysis treatment can be found in Chapter 42.

Nursing Interventions

The patient with chronic renal failure requires astute nursing care to avoid the complications of reduced renal function and the stresses and anxieties of dealing with a life-threatening illness.

Potential nursing diagnoses for these patients include the following:

- Fluid volume excess related to decreased urine output, dietary excesses and retention of sodium and water
- Altered nutrition: less than body requirements related to anorexia, nausea and vomiting, dietary restrictions, and altered oral mucous membranes
- Knowledge deficit regarding condition and treatment regimen
- Activity intolerance related to fatigue, anemia, retention of waste products and dialysis procedure
- Self-esteem disturbance related to dependency, role changes, changes in body image and sexual dysfunction

Nursing care is directed toward assessing fluid status and identifying potential sources of imbalance, implementing a dietary program to ensure proper nutritional intake within the limits of the treatment regimen, and promoting positive feelings by encouraging increased self-care and greater independence. It is extremely important to provide explanations and information to the patient and family concerning end-stage renal disease, treatment options, and potential complications. A great deal of emotional support is needed by the patient and family because of the numerous changes experienced. Specific interventions, along with rationale and evaluation criteria, are presented in more detail in Nursing Care Plan 43-1 for a patient with chronic renal failure.

Patient Teaching and Home Care Considerations. The nurse plays an extremely important role in teaching the patient with end-stage renal disease. There is a vast amount of information the patient and family need to understand about renal failure in order to maintain health and avoid complications associated with renal failure. Because of the extensive teaching needed by these patients, the community health nurse and dialysis nurse provide ongoing education and reinforcement of previous teaching, while mon-

(text continues on page 1203)

NURSING CARE PLAN 43–1
Care of the Patient With Chronic Renal Failure

NURSING DIAGNOSIS: Fluid volume excess related to decreased urine output, dietary excesses and retention of sodium and water

GOAL: Maintenance of ideal body weight without excess fluid

Nursing Interventions	Rationale	Expected Outcomes
1. Assess fluid status: a. Daily weight. b. Intake and output balance. c. Skin turgor and presence of edema. d. Distention of neck veins. e. Blood pressure, pulse rate, and rhythm. f. Respiratory rate and effort.	1. Assessment provides baseline and ongoing data base for monitoring changes and evaluating interventions.	• Demonstrates no rapid weight changes. • Maintains dietary and fluid restrictions. • Exhibits normal skin turgor without edema. • Exhibits normal vital signs. • Exhibits no neck vein distention. • Reports no difficulty breathing or shortness of breath. • Performs oral hygiene frequently. • Reports decreased thirst. • Reports decreased dryness of oral mucous membranes.
2. Limit fluid intake to prescribed limit.	2. Fluid restriction will be determined on basis of weight, urine output, and response to therapy.	
3. Identify potential sources of fluid: a. Medications and fluids used to take medications: oral and intravenous. b. Foods.	3. Unrecognized sources of excess fluids may be identified.	
4. Explain to patient and family rationale for restriction.	4. Understanding promotes patient and family cooperation with fluid restriction.	
5. Assist patient to cope with the discomforts resulting from fluid restriction.	5. Increasing patient comfort promotes compliance with dietary restrictions.	
6. Provide or encourage frequent oral hygiene.	6. Oral hygiene minimizes dryness of oral mucous membranes.	

NURSING DIAGNOSIS: Altered nutrition; less than body requirements related to anorexia, nausea, vomiting, dietary restrictions and altered oral mucous membranes

GOAL: Maintenance of adequate nutritional intake

Nursing Interventions	Rationale	Expected Outcomes
1. Assess nutritional status: a. Weight changes. b. Anthropometric measures. c. Laboratory values (serum electrolyte, BUN, creatinine, protein, transferrin, and iron levels).	1. Baseline data allow for monitoring of changes and evaluating interventions.	• Consumes protein of high biologic value. • Chooses foods within dietary restrictions that are appealing. • Consumes high-calorie foods within dietary restrictions. • Takes medications on schedule that does not produce anorexia or feeling of fullness. • Explains in own words rationale for dietary restrictions and relationship to urea and creatinine levels. • Consults written lists of acceptable foods. • Reports increased appetite at meals. • Exhibits no rapid increases or decreases in weight. • Demonstrates normal skin turgor without edema; healing and acceptable plasma albumin levels.
2. Assess patient's nutritional dietary patterns: a. Diet history. b. Food preferences. c. Calorie counts.	2. Past and present dietary patterns can be considered in planning meals.	
3. Assess for factors contributing to altered nutritional intake: a. Anorexia, nausea, or vomiting. b. Diet unpalatable to patient. c. Depression. d. Lack of understanding of dietary restrictions. e. Stomatitis.	3. Information about other factors that may be altered or eliminated to promote adequate dietary intake is provided.	
4. Provide patient's food preferences within dietary restrictions.	4. Increased dietary intake is encouraged.	

(*continued*)

NURSING CARE PLAN 43–1 *(continued)*
Care of the Patient With Chronic Renal Failure

Nursing Interventions	Rationale	Expected Outcomes
5. Promote intake of high biologic value protein foods: eggs, dairy products, meats.	5. Complete proteins are provided for positive nitrogen balance needed for growth and healing.	
6. Encourage high calorie, low-protein, low-sodium, and low-potassium snacks between meals.	6. Reduces source of restricted foods and proteins and provides calories for energy, sparing protein for tissue growth and healing.	
7. Alter schedule of medications so that they are not given immediately before meals.	7. Ingestion of medications just before meals may produce anorexia and feeling of fullness.	
8. Explain rationale for dietary restrictions and relationship to kidney disease and increased urea and creatinine levels.	8. Promotes patient understanding of relationships between diet and urea and creatinine levels to renal disease.	
9. Provide written lists of foods allowed and suggestions for improving their taste without use of sodium or potassium.	9. Lists provide a positive approach to dietary restrictions and a reference for patient and family to use when at home.	
10. Provide pleasant surroundings at mealtimes.	10. Unpleasant factors that contribute to patient's anorexia are eliminated.	
11. Weigh patient daily.	11. Allows monitoring of fluid and nutritional status.	
12. Assess for evidence of inadequate protein intake: a. Edema formation. b. Delayed healing. c. Decreased serum albumin levels.	12. Inadequate protein intake can lead to decreased albumin and other proteins, edema formation, and delay in healing.	

NURSING DIAGNOSIS: Knowledge deficit regarding condition and treatment

GOAL: Increased knowledge about condition and related treatment

Nursing Interventions	Rationale	Expected Outcomes
1. Assess understanding of cause of renal failure, consequences of renal failure, and its treatment: a. Cause of patient's renal failure. b. Meaning of renal failure. c. Understanding of renal function. d. Relationship of fluid and dietary restrictions to renal failure. e. Rationale for treatment (hemodialysis, peritoneal dialysis, transplant).	1. Baseline instruction is provided for further explanations and teaching.	• Verbalizes relationship of cause of renal failure to consequences. • Explains fluid and dietary restrictions as they relate to failure of kidney's regulatory functions. • States relationship of renal failure and need for treatment in own words. • Asks questions about treatment options, indicating readiness to learn. • Verbalizes plans to continue as normal a life as possible. • Uses written information and instructions to clarify questions and seek additional information.
2. Provide explanation of renal function and consequences of renal failure at patient's level of understanding and guided by patient's readiness to learn.	2. Patient can learn about renal failure and treatment as he or she becomes ready to understand and accept the diagnosis and consequences.	
3. Assist patient to identify ways to incorporate changes related to illness and its treatment into life.	3. Patient can see that his or her life does not have to revolve around the disease.	
4. Provide oral and written information as appropriate about: a. Renal function and failure. b. Fluid and dietary restrictions.	4. Patient has information that can be used for further clarification at home.	

(continued)

NURSING CARE PLAN 43–1 *(continued)*
Care of the Patient With Chronic Renal Failure

Nursing Interventions	Rationale	Expected Outcomes
c. Medications. d. Reportable problems, signs, and symptoms. e. Follow-up schedule. f. Community resources. g. Treatment options.		

NURSING DIAGNOSIS: Activity intolerance related to fatigue, anemia, retention of waste products and dialysis procedure

GOAL: Participation in activity within tolerance

Nursing Interventions	Rationale	Expected Outcomes
1. Assess factors contributing to fatigue: a. Anemia. b. Fluid and electrolyte imbalances. c. Retention of waste products. d. Depression.	1. Indications of severity of fatigue are provided.	• Participates in increasing levels of activity and exercise. • Reports increased sense of well being. • Alternates rest and activity. • Participates in selected self-care activities.
2. Promote independence in self-care activities as tolerated; assist if fatigued.	2. Mild/moderate activity and improved self-esteem are promoted.	
3. Encourage alternating activity with rest.	3. Activity and exercise within limits are promoted and adequate rest is encouraged.	
4. Encourage patient to rest after dialysis treatments.	4. Adequate rest is encouraged after dialysis treatments, which are exhausting to many patients.	

NURSING DIAGNOSIS: Self-esteem disturbance related to dependency, role changes, change in body image and changes in sexual function

GOAL: Improved self-concept

Nursing Interventions	Rationale	Expected Outcomes
1. Assess patient's and family's responses and reactions to illness and treatment.	1. Provides data about problems encountered by patient and family in coping with changes in life.	• Identifies previously used coping styles that have been effective and those no longer possible due to disease and treatment (alcohol or drug use; extreme physical exertion). • Patient and family identify and verbalize feelings and reactions to disease and necessary changes in their life. • Seeks professional counseling, if necessary to cope with changes resulting from renal failure. • Reports satisfaction with method of sexual expression.
2. Assess relationship of patient and significant family members.	2. Strengths and supports of patient and family are identified.	
3. Assess usual coping patterns of patient and family members.	3. Coping patterns that may have been effective in past may be potentially destructive in view of restrictions imposed by disease and treatment.	
4. Encourage open discussion of concerns about changes produced by disease and treatment: a. Role changes. b. Changes in life-style. c. Changes in occupation. d. Sexual changes. e. Dependence on health care team.	4. Patient can identify concerns and steps necessary to deal with them.	
5. Explore alternate ways of sexual expression other than sexual intercourse.	5. Alternative forms of sexual expression may be acceptable.	
6. Discuss role of giving and receiving love, warmth, and affection.	6. Sexuality means different things to different people, depending on stage of maturity.	

(continued)

NURSING CARE PLAN 43–1 *(continued)*
Care of the Patient With Chronic Renal Failure

COLLABORATIVE PROBLEMS: Hyperkalemia; pericarditis, pericardial effusion and pericardial tamponade; hypertension; anemia; bone disease and metastatic calcifications

GOAL: Patient experiences an absence of complications

Nursing Interventions	Rationale	Expected Outcomes
Hyperkalemia		
1. Monitor serum potassium levels and notify physician if level greater than 5.5 mEq/L. 2. Assess patient for muscle weakness, diarrhea, ECG changes (tall-tented T waves and widened QRS).	1. Hyperkalemia causes detrimental and potentially life-threatening changes in the body. 2. Cardiovascular signs and symptoms are characteristic of hyperkalemia.	• Patient has normal potassium level. • Experiences no muscle weakness or diarrhea. • Exhibits normal ECG pattern. • Vital signs within normal limits.
Pericarditis, pericardial effusion, and pericardial tamponade		
1. Assess patient for fever, chest pain, and a pericardial friction rub (signs of pericarditis) and if present notify physician. 2. If patient has pericarditis, assess for the following every 4 hours: a. Paradoxical pulse >10 mm Hg. b. Extreme hypotension. c. Weak or absent peripheral pulses. d. Altered level of consciousness. e. Bulging neck veins. 3. Prepare patient for cardiac ultrasound to aid in diagnosis of an effusion and tamponade. 4. If cardiac tamponade develops, prepare patient for emergency pericardiocentesis	1. Approximately 30%–50% of chronic renal failure patients develop pericarditis due to uremia; fever, chest pain, and a pericardial friction rub are classic signs. 2. Pericardial effusion is a common fatal sequelae of pericarditis. Signs of an effusion include a paradoxical pulse (>10 mm Hg drop in blood pressure during inspiration) and signs of shock due to compression of the heart by a large effusion. Cardiac tamponade exists when the patient is severely compromised hemodynamically. 3. Cardiac ultrasound is useful in visualizing pericardial effusions and cardiac tamponade. 4. Cardiac tamponade is a life-threatening condition, with a high mortality rate. Immediate aspiration of fluid from the pericardial space is essential.	• Has strong and equal peripheral pulses. • Absence of a paradoxical pulse. • Absence of pericardial effusion or tamponade on cardiac ultrasound. • Patient has normal heart sounds.
Hypertension		
1. Monitor and record blood pressure as indicated. 2. Administer antihypertensive medications as ordered. 3. Encourage compliance with dietary and fluid restriction therapy. 4. Teach patient to report signs of fluid overload, vision changes, headaches, edema, or seizures.	1. Blood pressure measurements provide objective data for monitoring. Elevated levels may indicate noncompliance. 2. Antihypertensive medications play a key role in treatment of hypertension associated with chronic renal failure. 3. Adherence to diet/fluid restrictions and dialysis schedule will prevent excess fluid and sodium accumulation. 4. These are indications of inadequate control of hypertension and need to alter.	• Blood pressure within normal limits. • Reports no headaches, visual problems, or seizures. • Absence of edema. • Demonstrates compliance with dietary and fluid restrictions.

(continued)

NURSING CARE PLAN 43–1 *(continued)*
Care of the Patient With Chronic Renal Failure

Nursing Interventions	Rationale	Expected Outcomes
Anemia		
1. Monitor RBC count, hemoglobin, and hematocrit levels as indicated. 2. Administer medications as prescribed including iron and folic acid supplements, Epogen, and multivitamins. 3. Avoid drawing unnecessary blood specimens. 4. Instruct patient how to prevent bleeding: avoid vigorous nose blowing and contact sports, and encourage use of a soft toothbrush. 5. Administer blood component therapy as indicated.	1. Provides assessment of degree of anemia. 2. Red blood cells need iron, folic acid, and vitamins to be produced. Epogen stimulates the bone marrow to produce RBC. 3. Anemia is aggravated by drawing numerous specimens. 4. Bleeding from anywhere in the body worsens anemia. 5. Blood component therapy may be needed if the patient is symptomatic.	• Patient has a normal color. • Exhibits hematology values within acceptable limits. • Experiences no bleeding from any site.
Bone disease and metastatic calcifications		
1. Administer the following medications as prescribed: phosphate binders, calcium supplements, Vitamin D supplements. 2. Monitor serum lab values as indicated (calcium, phosphorus, aluminum levels) and report abnormal findings to physician. 3. Assist patient with an exercise program.	1. Chronic renal failure causes numerous physiologic changes affecting calcium, phosphorus, and Vitamin D metabolism. 2. Hyperphosphatemia, hypocalcemia, and excess aluminum accumulation are common in chronic renal failure. 3. Bone demineralization is increased with immobility.	• Exhibits serum calcium, phosphorus, and aluminum levels within acceptable ranges. • Exhibits no symptoms of hypocalcemia. • Has no bone demineralization on bone scan. • Discusses importance of maintaining activity level and exercise program.

itoring the patient's progress and compliance with the treatment regimen. A nutritional referral is helpful because of the numerous dietary changes required.

The patient and family need to know what problems to report to the health care provider: (1) worsening signs of renal failure (nausea, vomiting, decreasing urine output, ammonia odor on breath), and (2) signs of hyperkalemia (muscle weakness, diarrhea, abdominal cramps). The above signs of worsening renal failure, in addition to increasing BUN and serum creatinine levels, may be indicative of a need to alter the dialysis prescription.

Medication teaching (purpose, side effects, desired effects, dosage, and administration schedule) is extremely important because of the large number of medications required. The patient is taught how to assess the vascular access for patency, as well as such precautions as not having venipunctures or blood pressure taken on the access arm. The patient and family will require considerable assistance and support in dealing with the need for dialysis and its long-term implications.

Gerontologic Considerations

Changes in Renal Function. Changes in kidney function with normal aging increase the susceptibility of the elderly to kidney dysfunction and renal failure. Alterations in renal blood flow, glomerular filtration, and renal clearance increase the risk of medication-associated changes in renal function. Precautions are indicated with the administration of all medications because of the frequent use of multiple prescription and over-the-counter medications in the elderly. The incidence of systemic diseases such as atherosclerosis, hypertension, cardiac failure, diabetes, and malignancy increases with advancing age, predisposing the elderly to renal disease associated with these disorders.

With age, the kidney is less able to respond to acute fluid and electrolyte changes. Therefore, acute problems need to be prevented if possible or recognized and treated quickly to avoid kidney damage. When the elderly patient must undergo extensive diagnostic tests, or when new medications (*e.g.*, diuretics) are added, precautions must be taken to prevent dehydration, which can compromise marginal renal function and lead to acute renal failure.

The elderly patient may develop atypical and nonspecific signs of disturbed renal function and fluid and electrolyte imbalances. Recognition of these problems is further hampered by their association with previously existing disorders and the misconception that they are normal changes of aging.

Acute Renal Failure in the Elderly. The incidence of acute renal failure is increasing in older, hospitalized patients. Approximately 50% of those patients who develop acute renal failure during hospitalization for a medical or surgical problem are over 60 years of age. In addition, the mortality rate is slightly higher for acute renal failure in the elderly than for their younger counterparts.

The etiology of acute renal failure in the elderly includes prerenal causes such as dehydration and intrarenal causes such as nephrotoxic agents (medications, contrast agents or media). Diabetes mellitus increases the risk of contrast agent-induced renal failure in the elderly patient because of pre-existing renal insufficiency and the imposed fluid restriction needed for many tests. Multiple prescriptions and the increased use of over-the-counter medications also increase the risk of medication-induced renal damage. Suppression of thirst, enforced bed rest, unavailable water to drink, and confusion all contribute to the older patient's failure to consume adequate fluids, leading to subsequent dehydration and compromising the already decreased renal function.

Chronic Renal Failure in the Elderly. End-stage renal disease has increased at a rate of almost 8% per year for the past 5 years. The elderly (between ages 55–65) are the fastest-growing group developing end-stage renal disease. In the past, rapidly progressive glomerulonephritis, membranous glomerulonephritis, and nephrosclerosis have been the most common causes of chronic renal failure in the elderly. Today, however, diabetes mellitus and hypertension are the leading causes of chronic renal failure. Other common causes of chronic renal failure in the elderly population are interstitial nephritis and urinary tract obstruction.

Clinical Manifestations. The signs and symptoms of renal disease in the elderly are often nonspecific; the occurrence of symptoms of other disorders (congestive heart failure, dementia) can mask the symptoms of renal disease and delay or prevent diagnosis and treatment. The patient often presents with signs and symptoms of nephrotic syndrome, such as edema and proteinuria.

Management of the Older Patient With Renal Failure. Hemodialysis and peritoneal dialysis have been used effectively in the treatment of elderly patients. Although there is no single age limitation for renal transplantation, concomitant disorders (*i.e.*, coronary artery disease, peripheral vascular disease) have made it less common as a form of treatment for the elderly. The outcome has been shown to be comparable to that of younger patients. Some elderly patients elect not to participate in these management strategies. Conservative management including nutritional therapy, fluid control, and medications such as phosphate binders may be considered in those patients who are not suitable for or elect not to participate in dialysis or transplantation.

Kidney Transplantation

Kidney transplantation has become the treatment of choice for the majority of patients with end-stage renal disease. Patients choose kidney transplantation for a variety of reasons, such as the desire to avoid dialysis or to improve their sense of well being, and the wish to lead a more normal life. Additionally, the cost of maintaining a successful transplant is one third that of a dialysis patient.

Kidney transplantation involves transplanting a kidney from a living donor or human cadaver to a recipient who has end-stage renal disease. Kidney transplants from well-matched living donors who are related to the patient (those with compatible ABO and HLA antigens) are slightly more successful than those from cadaver donors. A nephrectomy of the patient's own native kidneys may be performed prior to transplantation. The transplanted kidney is placed in the patient's iliac fossa anterior to the iliac crest. The ureter of the newly transplanted kidney is transplanted into the bladder or anastomosed to the ureter of the recipient (Fig. 43-3).

Preoperative Management

The preoperative goal is to bring the patient's metabolic state to a level as close to normal as possible. A complete physical examination is performed to detect and treat any conditions that could cause possible complications following transplantation. Tissue typing, blood typing and antibody screening are performed to determine compatibility of the tissues and cells of the donor and recipient. Other numerous diagnostic tests must be completed to identify conditions requiring treatment prior to transplant. The lower urinary tract is studied to assess bladder neck function and to detect ureteral reflux.

The patient must be free of infection at the time of renal transplantation because of immunosuppression and the risk of infection. Therefore, the patient is evaluated and treated for gingival disease and dental caries.

A psychosocial evaluation is conducted to assess the patient's ability to adjust to the transplant, coping styles, social history, social support available, and financial resources. A history of psychiatric illness is important to ascertain, because psychiatric conditions are often aggravated by the corticosteroids needed for immunosuppression following transplantation.

Hemodialysis is often performed the day before the scheduled transplantation procedure to optimize the patient's physical status.

Nursing Interventions. The nursing aspects of preoperative management are similar to those for patients undergoing other elective abdominal surgery. Preoperative teaching should include information about postoperative pulmonary hygiene, pain management options, dietary restrictions, intravenous and arterial lines, tubes (indwelling catheter and possibly a nasogastric tube) and early ambulation. The patient who receives a kidney from a living related donor may be concerned about the donor and how the donor will tolerate the surgical procedure.

Most patients have been on dialysis for months or years prior to transplantation. Many have waited months to years for a kidney transplant and will be very anxious about the surgery, possible rejection, and the need to return to dialysis. Helping the patient to deal with these concerns is part of the nurse's role in preoperative management.

Postoperative Management

The goal of care following kidney transplantation is to maintain homeostasis until the transplanted kidney is functioning well. A kidney that functions immediately carries a more favorable prognosis than one that does not.

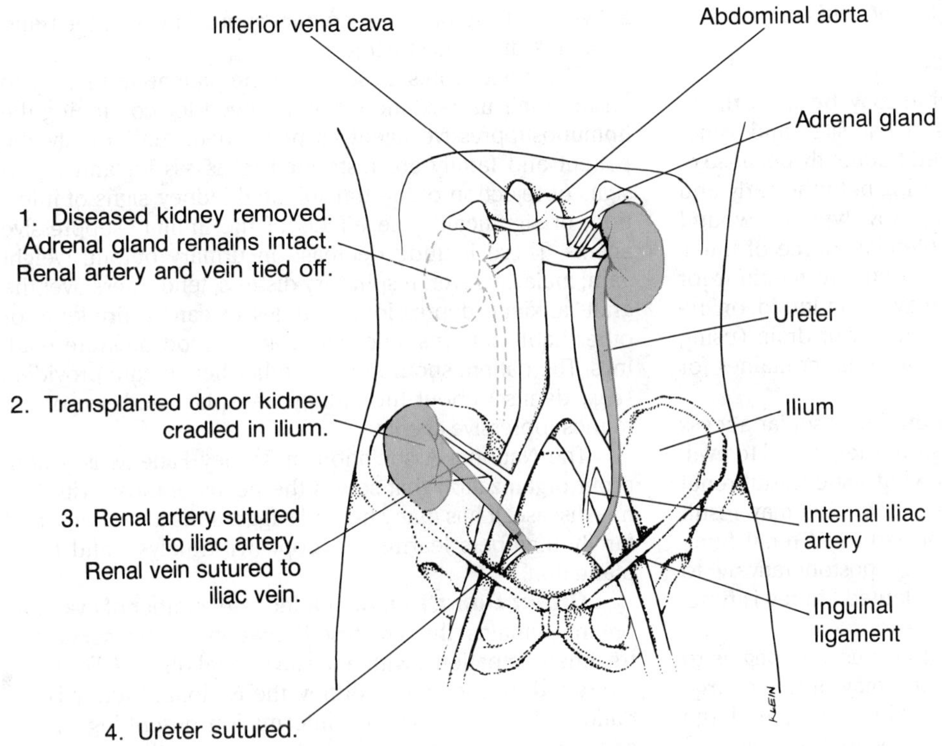

FIGURE 43-3. Renal transplantation: (1) The diseased kidney may be removed and the renal artery and vein tied off. (2) The transplanted kidney is placed in the iliac fossa. (3) The renal artery of the donated kidney is sutured to the iliac artery, and the renal vein is sutured to the iliac vein. (4) The ureter of the donated kidney is sutured to the bladder or to the patient's ureter.

Immunosuppressive Therapy. The survival of a transplanted kidney depends on the ability to block the body's immune response to the transplanted kidney. In order to overcome or minimize the body's defense mechanism, immunosuppressive medications such as azathioprine (Imuran), corticosteroids (prednisone), cyclosporine, and OKT-3 (a monoclonal antibody) are administered. FK-506 (Prograf) was approved by the FDA in April 1994, making it the newest immunosuppressive agent on the market. FK-506 is similar to cyclosporine and approximately 100 times more potent. Antilymphocyte globulin (ALG) is occasionally used to modify the immune response. Plasmaleukapheresis (PLP), lymph drainage, and cyclophosphamide (Cytoxan) are other methods of immunosuppression that are rarely used.

Doses of immunosuppressive agents are gradually tapered over a period of several weeks, depending on the patient's immunologic response to the transplant. The patient will however, take some form of anti-rejection medication for the entire time he or she has the transplanted kidney.

Graft Rejection. Renal graft rejection and failure may occur within 24 hours (hyperacute), within 3 to 14 days (acute), or after many years (chronic). It is not uncommon for acute rejection to occur anytime during the first year following transplantation. Ultrasound may be used to detect enlargement of the kidney, while renal biopsy and radiographic techniques are used to evaluate transplant rejection. If the transplant is rejected the patient will need to return to dialysis. The rejected kidney may or may not be removed depending on when the rejection occurs (acute vs. chronic) and the risk of infection if the kidney is left in place.

Postoperative Nursing Interventions

Assessing for Rejection and Infection. Following a kidney transplant, the patient is assessed for signs and symptoms of transplant rejection: oliguria, edema, fever, increasing blood pressure, weight gain, and swelling or tenderness over the transplanted kidney or graft. Results of blood chemistry tests (BUN and creatinine) and leukocyte and platelet counts are monitored closely, because immunosuppression depresses the formation of leukocytes and platelets. The patient is closely monitored for infection because of susceptibility to impaired healing and infection due to immunosuppressive therapy and complications of renal failure.

- A distinction must be made between infection and rejection because impaired renal function and fever are evidence of both infection and rejection, and treatment differs.

Immunosuppressive medications of the past made the transplant patient more vulnerable to opportunistic infections (candidiasis, cytomegalovirus, *Pneumocystis carinii* pneumonia) and infection with other relatively nonpathogenic viruses, fungi, and protozoa, which can be a major hazard. With use of cyclosporine, the incidence of opportunistic infections has decreased, since it selectively exerts its effect, sparing T cells that protect the patient from life-threatening infections.

The patient is protected from exposure to hospital staff, visitors, and other patients who have active infections. Careful hand washing is imperative; face masks may be worn by hospital staff and visitors to reduce the risk of transmitting infectious agents while the patient is receiving high doses of immunosuppressives.

Septicemia (bacteremia or fungemia) is responsible for a significant number of the deaths associated with renal transplantation.

- Clinical manifestations of septicemia include shaking chills, fever, rapid heartbeat and respirations (tachycardia and tachypnea), and either an increase or a decrease in white blood cells (leukocytosis or leukopenia).

The portal of entry for infection may be the urinary tract, the respiratory tract, the surgical site, and other sources. Urine cultures are performed frequently because of the high incidence of bacteriuria during both the early and the late stages of transplantation. Any type of wound drainage should be viewed as a potential source of infection because drainage is an excellent culture medium for bacteria. Catheter and drain tips may be cultured on removal by cutting off the tip of the catheter or drain (using aseptic technique) and placing it in a sterile container for laboratory culture.

Monitoring Urinary Function. The vascular access for hemodialysis is monitored to ensure patency and to evaluate for evidence of infection. Following a successful renal transplant, the vascular access often clots. This may result from improved coagulation with the return of renal function. Hemodialysis may be necessary postoperatively to maintain homeostasis until the transplanted kidney is functioning well.

A kidney from a living related donor usually begins to function immediately after surgery and may produce large quantities of dilute urine. A cadaver kidney may undergo acute tubular necrosis and therefore may not function for 2 or 3 weeks. Anuria, oliguria, or polyuria may be present. During this stage, the patient may experience significant changes in fluid and electrolyte status; therefore, careful monitoring is indicated. The output from the urinary catheter (connected to a closed drainage system) is measured every hour. Intravenous fluids are administered in accordance with urine volume and serum electrolyte levels and as prescribed by the physician. Hemodialysis may be required if fluid overload and hyperkalemia are present.

Other Potential Complications. Gastrointestinal ulceration and steroid-induced bleeding may occur. Fungal colonization of the gastrointestinal tract (especially the mouth) and urinary bladder may occur secondary to corticosteroid and antibiotic administration. Cardiovascular disease is emerging as an important cause of death following transplantation, due in part to the increasing age of transplantation patients. An additional problem is possible tumor growth, because patients on long-term immunosuppressive therapy have been found to develop malignancies more frequently than the general population.

Psychologic Considerations. The rejection of a transplanted kidney remains a matter of great concern to the patient, the patient's family, and the supporting health care team for many months. The fears of kidney rejection and the complications of immunosuppressive therapy (Cushing's syndrome, diabetes, capillary fragility, osteoporosis, glaucoma, cataracts, acne) place tremendous psychologic stresses on the patient. Anxiety and uncertainty about the future and difficult post-transplant adjustment are often sources of stress for the patient and family.

Patient Education and Home Care Considerations. The patient is advised that follow-up care after transplantation is a lifelong necessity. Individual and written instructions are provided concerning diet, medication, fluids, daily weight, daily measurement of urine, management of intake and output, prevention of infection, resumption of activity, and avoidance of contact sports in which the transplanted kidney may be injured.

The nurse works closely with the patient and family to ensure their understanding of the need for continuing the immunosuppressive agent as prescribed. Additionally, the patient and family are instructed to assess for and report signs of rejection of the transplanted kidney, signs of infection, or significant side effects of the immunosuppressive agents. These include decrease in urinary output; weight gain; malaise; fever; respiratory distress; tenderness over the graft; anxiety; depression; changes in eating, drinking, or other habit patterns; and changes in blood pressure readings. The patient should inform other health care providers (*e.g.*, dentist) about the kidney transplant and use of immunosuppressive agents.

The National Association of Kidney Patients is a nonprofit organization that serves the needs of those with kidney disease. It has many helpful suggestions for patients and family members learning to cope with dialysis and transplantation.

Organ Donation. An inadequate number of available organs remains the greatest limitation to the successful treatment of patients with end-stage renal disease. For those interested in donating a kidney, the National Kidney Foundation will provide written information describing the organ donation program and a card specifying the organ to be donated in the event of death. The card is signed by the donor and two witnesses and is to be carried by the donor at all times. Procurement of an adequate number of kidneys for potential recipients is still a major problem, despite national legislation that requires relatives of deceased patients or patients declared brain-dead to be asked if they would consider organ donation. Nurses are often called on by family members to explain or clarify donation and the possible outcomes.

An example of a critical pathway for renal transplantation is presented on page 1208. The medium length of stay described in this pathway is 8 days.

Urolithiasis

Urolithiasis refers to the presence of stone (calculi) in the urinary tract. Stones are formed in the urinary tract when urinary concentrations of substances such as calcium oxalate, calcium phosphate, and uric acid increase. Stones can also form when there is a deficiency of substances that normally prevent crystallization in the urine, such as citrate. Other conditions which affect the rate of stone formation include the *p*H of the urine and the fluid volume status of the patient (stones tend to occur more often in dehydrated states).

Calculi may be found anywhere from the kidney to the bladder and vary in size from minute granular deposits, called sand or gravel, to bladder stones the size of an orange. The different sites of calculus formation in the urinary tract are shown in Figure 43-4.

Certain factors favor the formation of stones, including infection, urinary stasis, and periods of immobility (slows renal drainage and alters calcium metabolism).

Hypercalcemia (high serum calcium) and **hypercalcuria** (high urine calcium) may be caused by:

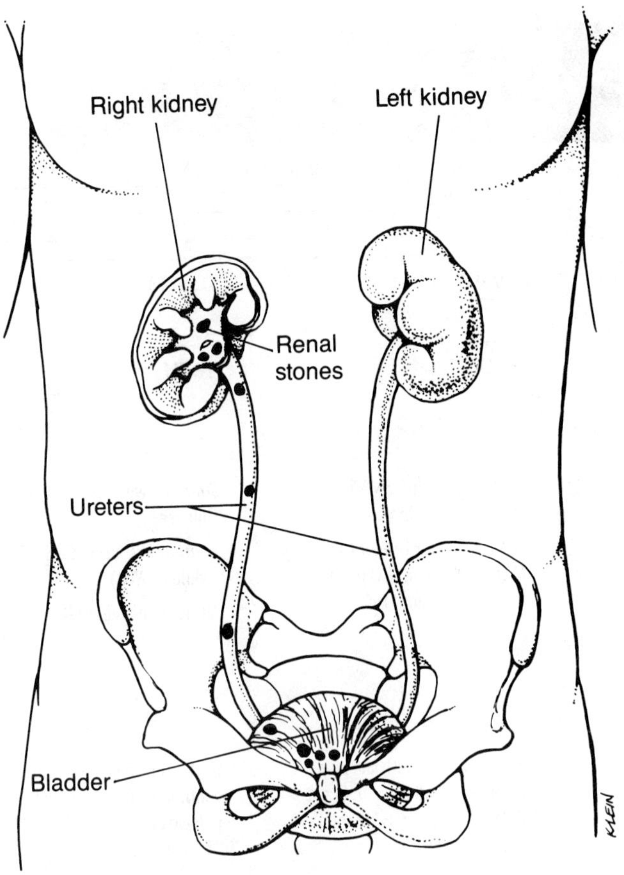

FIGURE 43-4. Various sites of calculous disease of the urinary tract (urolithiasis).

- Hyperparathyroidism
- Renal tubular acidosis
- Malignancy
- Granulomatous diseases (sarcoidosis, tuberculosis), which may cause increased vitamin D production by the granulomatous tissue
- Excessive intake of vitamin D
- Excessive intake of milk and alkali
- Myeloproliferative diseases (leukemia, polycythemia vera, multiple myeloma), which produce an unusual proliferation of blood cells from the bone marrow

These factors promote increased calcium concentrations in blood and urine, causing precipitation of calcium and formation of stones.

For stones containing uric acid, struvite, or cystine, a thorough physical examination and metabolic workup are indicated because of associated disturbances contributing to the stone formation. *Uric acid stones* may be seen in patients with gout. *Struvite stones,* commonly referred to as infection stones, form in persistently alkaline, ammonia-rich urine caused by chronic UTI. *Cystine* stones occur exclusively in patients with a rare inherited defect in renal absorption of cystine (an amino acid).

Urinary stone formation may also occur with inflammatory bowel disease and in individuals with an ileostomy or bowel resection, because these persons absorb more oxalate. Some medications that are known to cause stones in some persons include antacids, Diamox, vitamin D, laxatives, and high doses of aspirin. In many patients, however, no cause may be found.

Renal stones occur predominantly in the third to fifth decades of life and affect men more than women. Approximately 50% of patients with a single renal stone will have another episode within 10 years. The majority of stones contain calcium or magnesium in combination with phosphorus or oxalate. Most stones are radiopaque and can be detected by x-ray.

Clinical Manifestations

The clinical manifestations of stones in the urinary tract depend on the presence of obstruction, infection, and edema. When the stones block the flow of urine, obstruction develops, producing an increase in hydrostatic pressure and distending the renal pelvis and proximal ureter. Infection (pyelonephritis and cystitis with chills, fever, and dysuria) can occur from constant irritation by the stone. Some stones cause few, if any, symptoms while slowly destroying the functional units (nephrons) of the kidney; others cause excruciating pain and discomfort.

Stones in the renal pelvis may be associated with an intense, deep ache in the costovertebral region. Hematuria and pyuria may be noted. Pain originating in the renal area radiates anteriorly and downward toward the bladder in the female and toward the testis in the male. If the pain suddenly becomes acute, with tenderness over the costovertebral area, and nausea and vomiting appear, the patient is having an episode of **renal colic.** Diarrhea and abdominal discomfort may occur. These gastrointestinal symptoms are due to renointestinal reflexes and the anatomic proximity of the kidneys to the stomach, pancreas, and large intestines.

Stones lodged in the ureter cause acute, excruciating, colicky, wave-like pain, radiating down the thigh and to the genitalia. Often the patient has a desire to void, but very little urine is passed, and it usually contains blood because of the abrasive action of the stone. This group of symptoms is called **ureteral colic.** In general, the patient will spontaneously pass stones 0.5 to 1 cm in diameter. Those over 1 cm in diameter usually must be removed or fragmented so that they can be removed or passed spontaneously.

Stones lodged in the bladder usually produce symptoms of irritation and may be associated with urinary tract infection and hematuria. If the stone obstructs the bladder neck, there will be urinary retention. If infection is associated with the presence of a stone, the condition is far more serious, with sepsis threatening the patient's life.

Diagnostic Evaluation

The diagnosis is confirmed by kidneys, ureter, bladder (KUB) studies, intravenous urography, or retrograde pyelography. Blood chemistries and a 24-hour urine test for measurement of calcium, uric acid, creatinine, sodium, *p*H, and total volume are part of the diagnostic workup. Dietary and medication history and family history of renal stones are obtained to identify factors predisposing the patient to the formation of stones.

CRITICAL PATHWAY
Cadaver Renal Transplant

Hahnemann University Hospital
Broad and Vine Streets
Philadelphia, PA

DRG: 302 - Cadaver Renal Transplant
Surgeon:
MLOS: 8 days

Day	Day #1	Day #2	Day #3
POD#	0	1	2
Location	18TU/OR	18TU	18TU
Consults	Anesthesia, Nephrology, Social Service, Endocrine (if Diabetic), Cardiology (if indicated)		
Tests	**PRE-OP:** *Stat:* CBC with diff, PT/PTT, SMA7, Glucose, Amylase, HLA crossmatch, PD fluid cell count, ATG skin test, CXR pre and post CVC insertion *Routine:* SMA 12, T&C 2 units P RBCs **POST-OP:** CXR, CBC with diff and SMA7 with glucose q 12 hrs × 4, 24hr urine collection, SMA 12, amylase, ECG and pulse ox monitoring, TEDs	*Stat:* CBC with diff, SMA 7 with glucose every 12hrs × 2, U/A *Routine:* 24 hour U/A for CrCl, SMA12, CD3 (if on ATG test) Alternate days until D/C	*Stat:* CBC with diff, SMA7 with Glucose *Routine:* U/A, urine C&S, CD3 (while on ATG) Alternate days until D/C
Procedures/ Treatments	Enemas, routine VS, pre and post-op weight, CVC insertion, IS, HD (if indicated)	Continuous CVP, ECG, and pulse ox monitoring, I&O q 1 hr, O_2 via NC, TEDs, VS q 1 hr × 12 then q 2hrs, weigh OD	I&O q 1hr, VS every 2–4 hrs, continuous ECG, CVP, and pulse ox monitoring O_2 via N/C, TEDs, weigh OD
Meds/IVs	Meds as ordered, pre/intra/post op immunosuppression as per protocol, volume replacement as per protocol	Meds/IV replacement as per protocol, and immunosuppression as per protocol	IV replacement as per protocol, po meds, and immunosuppression as per protocol
Activity	Pre op: up and lib Post op: lie on back/operative side, no hip flexion, HOB > 30°	Turn to operative side	OOB
Diet	NPO 8 hours pre-op	Clear liquids	Advance as tolerated
D/C Planning/ Teaching	Pre-op transplant teaching, provide learning manual, orient patient and family to 18TU and explain all procedures.	C&DB, IS, incision splinting, transplant teaching continues	Reinforce pulmonary toilet, transplant teaching continues

Management

The basic goals of management are to eradicate the stone, to determine the stone type, to prevent nephron destruction, to control infection, and to relieve any obstruction that may be present.

Pain Relief. The immediate objective of treatment of renal or ureteral colic is to relieve the pain until its cause can be eliminated; morphine or meperidine is administered to prevent shock and syncope that may result from the excruciating pain. Hot baths or moist heat to the flank areas may also be useful. Unless the patient is vomiting or suffering from congestive heart failure or any other condition requiring fluid restriction, fluids are encouraged. This increases the hydrostatic pressure behind the stone and thus assists it in its downward passage. A high, round-the-clock fluid intake reduces the concentration of urinary crystalloids, dilutes the urine, and ensures a high urinary output.

Stone Removal. Cystoscopic examination and passage of a small ureteral catheter to dislodge the obstructing stone (when possible) immediately relieves back-pressure on the kidney and alleviates the intense pain.

When stones are recovered, chemical analysis is carried out to determine their composition. Stone analysis can provide a clear indication of the underlying disorder. For example, calcium oxalate or calcium phosphate stones usually indicate disorders of oxalate or calcium metabolism, while urate stones suggest a disturbance in uric acid metab-

CRITICAL PATHWAY
Cadaver Renal Transplant

Date of Surgery: ________	Discharge		CMV A B C DR
Clinical Path LOS: 9 days ________	PRA:	Donor Age:	Donor: _ _ _ _
	CIT:	HLA	Recip: _ _ _ _

Day #4	Day #5	Day #6	Day #7 until D/C
3	4	5	6 until D/C
18TU	18TU	18TU	18TU until D/C
→	→	→	→
VS and I&O q 4hrs, weigh OD, monitors dc'd, N/C dc'd	→	→	→
po meds/immunosuppression as per protocol	→	→	→
OOB/Walking	→	→	→
CRF diet	Advance to reg, no caffeine, no conc sweets	→	→
Transplant teaching, visiting nurse referral	Transplant teaching, encourage involvement of significant other(s)	Notify social worker of D/C needs, transplant teaching	Advise pt. of possible D/C date, day 8–10 clinical instructions

olism. Struvite stones (infection stones) account for 15% of urinary calculi. Specific antibacterial agents are administered if infection is present.

Nutrition and Medication Therapy. Nutritional therapy plays an important role in preventing renal stones. An adequate fluid intake and avoidance of certain foods in the diet that make up the main ingredient of the stone (*e.g.*, calcium) may be effective in preventing the development of stones or further increase in the size of existing stones. Unless contraindicated, any patient with renal stones should drink at least eight glasses of water daily to keep the urine dilute.

Calcium Stones. Most stones contain calcium combined with phosphate or other substances. For patients with such stones, reduction of dietary calcium and phosphorus content may help to prevent further stone formation (Chart 43-5). The urine may be acidified by using medications such as ammonium chloride or acetohydroxamic acid (Lithostat).

Sodium cellulose phosphate has been reported to be effective in preventing calcium stones. It binds calcium from food in the intestinal tract, reducing the amount of calcium absorbed into the circulation. If increased parathormone production (resulting in increased serum calcium levels in blood and urine) is a factor in the formation of stones, therapy with thiazide diuretics may be beneficial in reducing the calcium loss in the urine and lowering the elevated parathormone levels. It is also helpful to reduce sodium intake.

Phosphate Stones. A diet low in phosphorus may be prescribed for patients who develop phosphatic calculi (see

CHART 43-5
Prevention of Kidney Stones: Foods to Limit or Avoid

The majority of kidney stones contain calcium, phosphorus, and/or oxalate.

- Vitamin D-enriched foods should be avoided. (Vitamin D increases calcium reabsorption.)
- Table salt and high sodium foods should be reduced. (Sodium competes with calcium for reabsorption in the kidneys.)
- The foods listed below should be avoided.

Dairy: All cheeses (except cottage and pot cheese); milk and milk products (in excess of ½ cup daily); sour cream.
Meat, Fish, Fowl: Brain, heart, liver, kidney, sweetbreads, sardines, fish roe, game (pheasant, rabbit, deer, grouse).
Vegetables: Beet greens, beets, chard, collards, mustard greens, spinach, turnip greens, dried beans, peas, lentils, soybeans, celery, endive.
Fruits: Rhubarb, all berries, currants, figs, concord grapes.
Breads, Cereals, Pastas: Whole grain breads, cereals, crackers, rye bread, all breads made with self-rising flour, oatmeal, brown and wild rice, bran, bran flakes, wheat germ, grits, all dry cereals (except corn flakes, rice krispies, puffed rice).
Beverages: Tea, cocoa, carbonated drinks, draft beer, all beverages made with milk and milk products.
Miscellaneous: Nuts, peanut butter, chocolate, soups made with milk or milk products, all creams, desserts made with milk or milk products (including cakes, cookies, pies).

Chart 43-5). To offset excess phosphorus, aluminum hydroxide gel often is prescribed because it combines with the excess phosphorus, causing it to be excreted through the intestinal tract rather than in the urinary system.

Uric Stones. For uric acid stones, the patient is placed on a low-purine diet to reduce the excretion of uric acid in the urine. Foods high in purine (shellfish, anchovies, asparagus, mushrooms, and organ meats) are avoided, and other proteins may be limited. Allopurinol (Zyloprim) may be prescribed to reduce serum uric acid levels and urinary uric acid excretion. The urine is alkalinized. For cystine stones, a low-protein diet is prescribed, the urine is alkalinized, and penicillamine is administered to reduce the amount of cystine in the urine.

Oxalate Stones. For oxalate stones, a dilute urine is maintained and the intake of oxalate is limited. Foods to avoid include green, leafy vegetables; beans; celery; beets; blackberries; rhubarb; chocolate; tea; coffee; and peanuts.

If the stone is not passed spontaneously or if complications occur, treatment modalities may include extracorporeal shock wave therapy, percutaneous stone removal, or ureteroscopy.

Extracorporeal Shock Wave Lithotripsy. Extracorporeal shock wave lithotripsy (ESWL; Fig. 43-5) is a noninvasive procedure used to break up stones in the calyx of the kidney. After the stones are reduced to small fragments the size of grains of sand, the remnants of the stones are spontaneously voided.

In ESWL, or lithotripsy, a high-energy amplitude of pressure, or shock wave, is generated by the abrupt release of energy and transmitted through water and soft tissues. When the shock wave encounters a substance of different intensity (a renal stone), a compression wave causes the surface of the stone to fragment. Repeated shock waves focused on the stone eventually reduce it to many small pieces. These small pieces are excreted in the urine, usually without difficulty.

The need for anesthesia for the procedure depends on the type of lithotriptor used, which determines the number and intensity of shock waves delivered. An average treatment is between 1000 and 3000 shocks. The first-generation lithotriptors required use of either regional or general anesthesia. However, lithotriptor manufacturers claim that the majority of patients treated with their newer machine require little or no anesthesia.

Although the shock waves usually do not damage other tissue, discomfort from the multiple shocks may occur. The patient is observed for obstruction and infection resulting from blockage of the urinary tract by stone fragments. All urine is strained following the procedure; voided gravel or sand is sent to the laboratory for chemical analysis. Several treatments may be necessary to ensure disintegration of stones.

Although lithotripsy is a costly treatment, it has decreased length of stay and expense because an invasive surgical procedure to remove the renal stone is avoided.

Patient Education. ESWL has been used effectively on an outpatient basis; therefore, the nurse must provide instructions for home care and necessary follow-up. The patient is encouraged to increase fluid intake to assist in the passage of stone fragments, which may occur for 6 weeks to several months after the procedure. The patient and family are instructed about signs and symptoms that indicate the occurrence of complications, such as fever, decreasing urinary output, and pain. It is also important to tell the patient to expect hematuria (it is anticipated in all patients), but it should disappear within 24 hours. The patient is followed closely by the physician to ensure that treatment has been effective and that no complications, such as obstruction, infection, renal hematoma, or hypertension, have developed.

Because the risk of recurring renal stones is high, the nurse provides education about the causes of kidney stones and ways to prevent their recurrence. Appropriate dietary instructions about calcium, uric acid, and oxalate are provided, depending on the composition of the stone.

Endourologic Methods of Stone Removal. The field of endourology integrates the skills of the radiologist and urologist to extract renal calculi without major surgery. A percutaneous nephrostomy (or percutaneous nephrolithotomy) is performed (see Chapter 42), and a nephroscope is introduced through the dilated percutaneous tract into the renal parenchyma. Depending on its size, the stone may be extracted with forceps or by a stone basket. Alternatively, an ultrasound probe may be introduced through the nephrostomy tube with ultrasonic waves used to pulverize

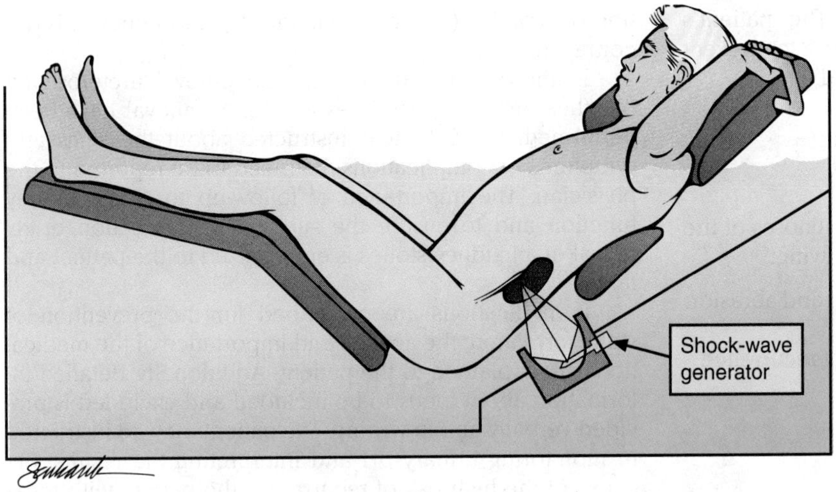

FIGURE 43-5. Extracorporeal shock wave lithotripsy (ESWL). Shock waves are generated in the ellipsoid reflector (shock wave generator). Fluoroscopy is used to position the patient, who is partially immersed in water, so that the shock waves are focused directly at the stone. The shock waves travel through the water to the stone and reduce it to sand-like particles, which are then eliminated in the urine.

the stone. Small stone fragments and stone dust are irrigated and suctioned out of the collecting system. Larger stones may be further reduced by ultrasonic disintegration and then removed with forceps or a stone retrieval basket.

In a similar method, an electrical discharge is used to create a hydraulic shock wave to break up the stone (electrohydraulic lithotripsy). A probe is passed through the cystoscope, and the tip of the lithotriptor is placed near the stone. The strength of the discharge and pulse frequency can be varied. This procedure is performed under topical anesthesia.

After the stone is extracted, the percutaneous nephrostomy tube is left in place for a time to ensure that the ureter is not obstructed by edema or blood clots. The most common complications are hemorrhage, infection, and urinary extravasation. After the tube is removed, the nephrostomy tract closes spontaneously.

Ureteroscopy. Ureteroscopy involves visualization and access to the ureter by inserting instruments through a ureteroscope via cystoscopy. Stones can be fragmented with the use of laser, electrohydraulic lithotripsy, or ultrasound and then removed. A stent may be inserted and left in place for 48 hours or more after the procedure to keep the ureter patent. Hospital stays are generally very short, and some patients can be successfully treated as outpatients.

Stone Dissolution. Infusions of chemolytic solutions (*e.g.*, alkylating agents, acidifying agents) for the purpose of dissolving the stone may be performed as an alternative treatment for patients who are poor risks for other therapy, who refuse other methods, or who have easily dissolved (struvite) stones. A percutaneous nephrostomy is performed, and the warm irrigating solution is allowed to flow continuously onto the stone. The irrigating solution exits the renal collecting system via the ureter or the nephrostomy tube. The pressure inside the renal pelvis is monitored during the procedure.

Several of these treatment modalities may be used in combination to ensure successful removal of the stones.

Surgical Removal. Before the advent of lithotripsy, surgical removal of kidney stones was the major mode of therapy. Today however, surgery is performed only on 1% to 2% of patients. Surgical intervention is indicated if the stone does not respond to other forms of treatment. It may also be performed to correct any anatomic abnormalities within the kidney to improve urinary drainage.

If the stone is in the kidney, the surgery performed may be a **nephrolithotomy** (incision into the kidney with removal of the stone) or a **nephrectomy,** if the kidney is nonfunctional secondary to infection or hydronephrosis. Stones in the kidney pelvis are removed by a **pyelolithotomy,** those in the ureter by **ureterolithotomy,** and those in the bladder by **cystotomy.** If the stone is in the bladder, an instrument may be inserted through the urethra into the bladder; the stone is crushed in the jaws of this instrument. Such a procedure is called a **cystolitholapaxy.** The postoperative nursing management following kidney surgery is discussed in Chapter 42.

❑ NURSING PROCESS
The Patient With Renal Stones

Assessment

The patient with suspected renal stones is assessed for pain and discomfort. The severity and location of pain are determined along with any radiation of the pain. The patient is also assessed for the presence of associated symptoms, such as nausea, vomiting, diarrhea, and abdominal distention. Nursing assessment includes observing for signs of urinary tract infection (chills, fever, dysuria, frequency, and hesitancy) and obstruction (frequent urination of small amounts, oliguria, or anuria). Additionally, the urine is observed for the presence of blood and is strained for stones or gravel.

The history focuses on factors that predispose the patient to urinary tract stones or that may have precipitated the current episode of renal or ureteral colic. Factors that predispose the patient to stone formation may include family history of stones, the presence of cancer or bone marrow disorders or the use of chemotherapeutic agents, inflammatory bowel disease, or a diet high in calcium or purines. Factors that may precipitate stone formation in the patient predisposed to renal calculi include episodes of dehydration, prolonged immobilization, and infection. The patient's knowledge about renal stones and measures to prevent their occurrence or recurrence is also assessed.

Diagnosis

Nursing Diagnoses

Based on the assessment data, the nursing diagnoses of the patient with renal stones may include the following:

- Pain related to inflammation, obstruction, and abrasion of the urinary tract
- Knowledge deficit regarding prevention of recurrence of renal stones

Collaborative Problems/ Potential Complications

Based on assessment data, potential complications may include:

- Infection and sepsis (from UTI and pyelonephritis)
- Obstruction of the urinary tract by a stone or edema with subsequent acute renal failure

Planning and Implementation

Goals. The major goals for the patient may include relief of pain and discomfort, prevention of recurrence of renal stones, and prevention of complications.

Nursing Interventions

Relieving Pain. Immediate relief of severe pain from renal or ureteral colic is accomplished with narcotic analgesics. Intravenous or intramuscular administration may be prescribed to provide rapid relief. The patient is encouraged and assisted to assume a position of comfort. If activity brings some pain relief, the patient is assisted to ambulate. The patient's pain is monitored closely, and increases in severity are reported promptly to the physician so that relief can be provided and additional treatment initiated. The patient is prepared for other treatment (*e.g.*, lithotripsy, percutaneous stone removal, ureteroscopy, or surgery) if severe pain is unrelieved and the stone is not passed spontaneously.

Patient Education. Because it is known that urinary calculi may recur after the first stone forms, the patient is encouraged to follow a regimen to avoid further stone formation. One facet of prevention is to *maintain a high fluid intake,* because stones form more readily in concentrated urine. A patient who has shown a tendency to form stones should drink enough fluid to excrete 3000 to 4000 ml of urine every 24 hours, should adhere to the prescribed diet, and should avoid sudden increases in environmental temperatures, which may cause a fall in urinary volume. Occupations and activities that produce excessive sweating can lead to severe temporary dehydration; therefore, fluid intake should be increased. Sufficient fluids should be taken in the evening to prevent urine from becoming too concentrated at night. Urine cultures may be performed every 1 to 2 months the first year and periodically thereafter. Recurrent urinary tract infection is treated vigorously.

Because prolonged immobilization slows renal drainage and alters calcium metabolism, increased mobility is encouraged whenever possible. In addition, excessive ingestion of vitamins (especially vitamin D) and minerals is discouraged.

If lithotripsy, percutaneous stone removal, ureteroscopy, or other surgical procedures for stone removal have been performed, the patient is instructed about the signs and symptoms of complications that need to be reported to the physician. The importance of follow-up to assess kidney function and to ensure the successful eradication or removal of all kidney stones is emphasized to the patient and family.

If medications are prescribed for the prevention of stone formation, the actions and importance of the medications are explained to the patient. Additionally, detailed information about foods to be included and excluded is provided verbally and in writing. The patient may be instructed in monitoring urinary *p*H and interpreting the results. Because of the high risk of recurrence, the patient with renal stones is taught the signs and symptoms of stone formation, obstruction, and infection and the importance of reporting these signs promptly.

Guidelines for patient teaching for the patient with recurrent renal stones are presented in Chart 43-6.

Monitoring and Managing Potential Complications

Infection and Obstruction. Because renal stones increase the risk for *infection, sepsis,* and *obstruction* of the urinary tract, the patient is instructed to report decreased urine volume and bloody or cloudy urine. The total urine output and patterns of voiding are monitored. Increased fluid intake is encouraged to prevent dehydration and increase hydrostatic pressure within the urinary tract to promote passage of the stone. If the patient is unable to take adequate fluids orally, intravenous fluids will be prescribed. Ambulation is encouraged as a means of moving the stone through the urinary tract.

The nursing care of patients with calculi requires constant observation to detect the spontaneous passage of a stone. All urine is strained through gauze, because uric acid stones may crumble. Any blood clots passed in the urine should be crushed and the sides of the urinal and bedpan

CHART 43-6

Patient Education: The Patient with Recurrent Renal Stones

1. Follow prescribed diet closely.
2. Maintain adequate fluid intake of at least 3000–4000 ml a day.
3. Drink sufficient fluids in the evening to prevent urine from becoming too concentrated during the night.
4. Avoid activities which cause excessive sweating and dehydration.
5. Avoid sudden increases in environmental temperatures which may cause excessive sweating and dehydration.
6. Seek medical attention at first sign of a urinary tract infection.

inspected for clinging stones. The patient is instructed to report any sudden increases in pain immediately due to the possibility of a stone fragment obstructing a ureter. Analgesic medications are administered as prescribed for the relief of pain and discomfort.

The patient's vital signs, including temperature, are monitored closely to detect early signs of infection. Urinary tract infections may be associated with renal stones due to an obstruction from the stone or from the stone itself. All infections should be treated with the appropriate antimicrobial agents prior to stone dissolution.

Evaluation

Expected Outcomes

1. Experiences relief of pain.
2. Exhibits increased knowledge of health behaviors to prevent recurrence.
   a. Consumes high fluid intake (10–12 glasses of fluid per day).
   b. Engages in appropriate activity.
   c. Consumes diet prescribed to reduce dietary factors predisposing to stone formation.
   d. Identifies symptoms to be reported to health care provider (fever, chills, flank pain, hematuria).
   e. Monitors urinary *p*H as directed.
   f. Takes prescribed medication as directed to reduce stone formation.
3. Absence of complications.
   a. Exhibits no signs of sepsis and infection.
   b. Voids 200 to 400 ml of clear urine without red blood cells per voiding.
   c. Reports absence of dysuria, frequency, and hesitancy.
   d. Exhibits normal body temperature.

Urethral Strictures

A urethral stricture is a narrowing of the lumen of the urethra due to scar tissue and contraction. Common causes of strictures are urethral injury (caused by insertion of surgical instruments during transurethral surgery, indwelling catheters, or cystoscopic procedures), straddle injuries and injuries associated with automobile accidents, untreated gonorrheal urethritis, and congenital abnormalities.

The force and size of the urinary stream is diminished and symptoms of urinary infection and retention occur. Stricture causes urine to back up, resulting in cystitis, prostatitis, and pyelonephritis.

Prevention. An important element of prevention is to treat all urethral infections promptly. Prolonged urethral catheter drainage is to be avoided and utmost care should be taken in any type of instrumentation involving the urethra, including catheterization.

Management. Treatment may include gradual dilation of the narrowed area (with metal sounds or bougies) or surgery (internal urethrotomy). If the stricture prevents the passage of a catheter, the urologist uses several small filiform bougies in search of the opening. When one bougie passes beyond the stricture into the bladder, it is fixed in place, and urine will drain from the bladder. The opening then can be dilated by the passage of a larger sound (a dilating instrument) following behind the filiform as a guide. Following dilation, hot sitz baths and non-narcotic analgesics are administered to control the pain. Antimicrobial medications are prescribed for several days after dilation to prevent infection.

Surgical excision or urethroplasty may be necessary for severe cases. A suprapubic cystostomy may be necessary in some patients. The postoperative treatment for cystostomy is described on p. 1222.

Renal Trauma

Various types of injuries of the flank, back, or upper abdomen may result in bruising, lacerations, or actual rupture of the kidney. Normally, the kidneys are protected by the rib cage and musculature of the back posteriorly, and by a cushion of abdominal wall and viscera anteriorly. They are highly mobile and are "fixed" only at the renal pedicle (stem of renal blood vessels and the ureter). With traumatic injury, the kidney can be thrust against the lower ribs, resulting in contusion and rupture. Rib fractures or fractures of the transverse process of the upper lumbar vertebrae may be associated with renal contusion or laceration. Injuries may be blunt (auto and motorcycle accidents, falls, athletic injuries, assaults) or penetrating (gunshot wounds, stabbings). Failure to wear seat belts contributes to the incidence of renal trauma in motor vehicle crashes. Renal trauma is frequently associated with other injuries; up to 80% of patients with renal trauma have associated injuries of other internal organs.

The most common renal injuries are contusions, laceration, rupture, and renal pedicle injuries or small internal laceration of the kidney (Fig. 43-6). The kidneys receive half of the blood flow from the abdominal aorta; therefore, even a fairly small renal laceration can produce massive bleeding.

Clinical Manifestations. Clinical manifestations include pain, renal colic (due to clots/fragments obstructing the collecting system), hematuria, mass in the flank, ecchymoses, and lacerations or wounds of the lateral abdomen and flank. Signs and symptoms of hypovolemia and shock are likely with significant hemorrhage.

Management. The goals of management are to control hemorrhage, pain, and infection; to preserve and restore renal function; and to maintain urinary drainage.

Hematuria is the most common manifestation of renal trauma; therefore, the appearance of blood in the urine following an injury suggests the possibility of renal injury. There is no relationship between the degree of hematuria and the degree of injury. However, hematuria may be absent or detectable only on microscopic examination. All urine is saved and sent to the laboratory for analysis to detect the presence of red blood cells and to follow the course of bleeding. Hematocrit and hemoglobin levels are monitored closely; decreasing values indicate hemorrhage.

The patient is monitored for oliguria and signs of hemorrhagic shock, because a pedicle injury or shattered kidney can lead to rapid exsanguination (lethal blood loss). An expanding hematoma may cause rupture of the kidney capsule. To detect the presence of hematoma, the area around the lower ribs, upper lumbar vertebrae, flank, and abdomen

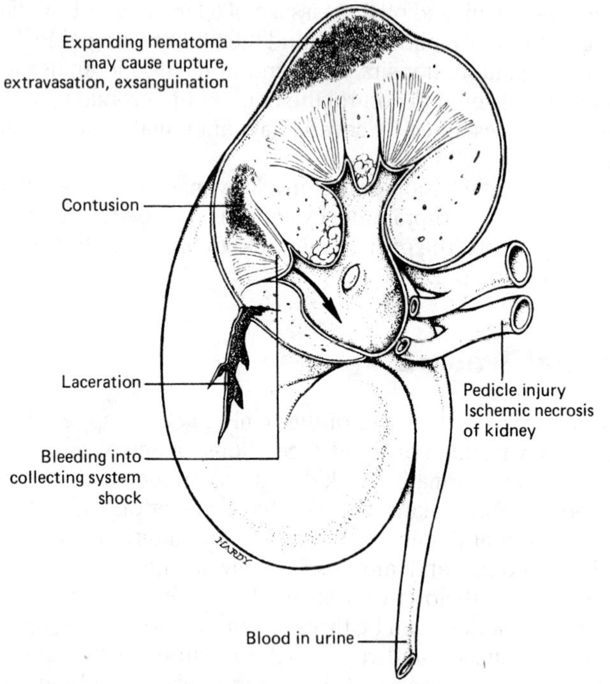

FIGURE 43-6. Types and pathophysiologic effects of renal injuries: contusions, lacerations, rupture, and pedicle injury.

is palpated for tenderness. A palpable flank or abdominal mass with local tenderness, swelling, and ecchymosis suggests renal hemorrhage. The area of the original mass can be outlined with a marking pencil so that the examiner can evaluate the area for change.

Renal trauma is often associated with other injuries to the abdominal organs (liver, colon, small intestines); therefore, the patient is assessed for skin abrasions, lacerations, and entry and exit wounds of the upper abdomen and lower thorax, because these may be associated with renal injury.

Mechanism and Severity of Injury. Renal trauma may be classified on the basis of the mechanism of injury (blunt versus penetrating injuries), the anatomic location, or the severity of the injury.

- *Minor* renal trauma includes contusions, hematomas, and some lacerations of the cortex of the kidney.
- *Major* renal injuries include major lacerations with rupture of the capsule of the kidney.
- *Critical* renal trauma involves multiple and severe lacerations of the kidney with injury to the vascular supply of the kidney.

In *minor injuries* to the kidney, healing may take place with conservative measures. The patient is kept on bed rest until hematuria clears. Intravenous infusions may be necessary, as retroperitoneal bleeding may produce a reflex paralytic ileus. Antimicrobial medications may be prescribed to prevent infection from perirenal hematoma or urinoma (a cyst containing urine). Patients with retroperitoneal hematomas may develop low-grade fever as absorption of the clot takes place.

The patient should be evaluated frequently during the first few days following injury in order to detect flank and abdominal pain, muscle spasm, and swelling over the flank.

- Any *sudden* change in the patient's condition may indicate hemorrhage and requires surgical intervention. The patient's vital signs, urine output, and level of consciousness are monitored to detect evidence of bleeding and shock. Opioid analgesia is avoided because this may mask accompanying abdominal symptoms.
- The patient is prepared for surgical exploration if increasing pulse rate, hypotension, and impending shock occur.

Major renal injuries may be treated conservatively (bed rest, no surgery) or through surgical intervention, depending on the patient's condition and the nature of the injury.

Critical renal injuries and most penetrating injuries require exploratory surgery because of the high incidence of involvement of other organ systems and the serious complications that may result if these injuries are untreated. The damaged kidney may have to be removed (nephrectomy).

Early postoperative complications (within 6 months) include rebleeding, abscess, sepsis, urine extravasation, and fistula formation. Other complications include stone formation, infection, cysts, vascular aneurysms, and loss of renal function.

Patient Teaching. Follow-up care includes monitoring the blood pressure to detect hypertension. Activity is usually restricted for 1 month following trauma to minimize the incidence of delayed or secondary bleeding. The patient is instructed about changes that should be reported to the physician, such as fever, hematuria, flank pain, or any signs of decreasing kidney function. Guidelines for increasing activity gradually are also provided.

Bladder Injuries

Injury to the bladder may occur with pelvic fractures and multiple trauma or from a blow to the lower abdomen when the bladder is full. Blunt trauma may result in contusion (an ecchymosis or large, discolored bruise resulting from escape of blood into the tissues and involving a segment of the bladder wall) or in rupture of the bladder extraperitoneally, intraperitoneally, or a combination of both. Complications from these injuries (hemorrhage, shock, sepsis, and extravasation of blood into the tissues) must be treated promptly.

A retrograde urethrogram is performed first to evaluate for urethral injury. The patient is catheterized *after* the urethrogram is performed to minimize the risk of urethral disruption and extensive, long-term complications, such as stricture, incontinence, and impotence.

Management. Treatment for traumatic rupture of the bladder involves immediate exploratory surgery and repair of the laceration, with suprapubic drainage of the bladder and the perivesical space (around the bladder) along with insertion of an indwelling urinary catheter.

In addition to the usual postoperative care following urologic surgery, the drainage systems (suprapubic, indwelling urethral catheter, and perivesical drains) are closely monitored to ensure adequate drainage until healing takes place. The patient with a ruptured bladder may have gross bleeding for several days after repair.

Renal Cysts

Renal cysts are abnormal, fluid-filled sacs that arise from the kidney tissue. They may be hereditary, acquired, or associated with a host of unrelated conditions. Cysts of the kidney may be single or multiple (polycystic), involving one or both kidneys. Polycystic disease of the adult is inherited as an autosomal dominant trait which equally affects men and women. The kidney gradually grows in size; signs and symptoms become apparent in the fourth or fifth decade of life.

The patient presents with abdominal or lumbar pain, hematuria, hypertension, palpable renal masses, and recurrent urinary tract infections. Renal insufficiency and failure usually develop in the end stages.

Polycystic renal disease is also associated with cystic diseases of other organs (liver, pancreas, spleen) and aneurysms of the cerebral arteries. It has long been recognized that patients on long-term dialysis (both hemodialysis and peritoneal dialysis) develop multiple cysts on their nonfunctioning kidneys. Many of these cysts have also been found to contain cancer cells. Diagnosis of renal cysts is confirmed either by intravenous urography or CT scan.

Management. Because there is no specific treatment for polycystic renal disease, care of the patient is directed toward relief of pain, symptoms, and complications. Hypertension and urinary tract infections are treated aggressively. Dialysis (Chapter 42) is initiated when signs of renal insufficiency and failure occur. Genetic counseling is part of management, because polycystic kidney disease is a hereditary disease. The patient is advised to avoid sports and occupations that present a risk of trauma to the kidney.

Simple cysts of the kidney usually occur unilaterally and differ clinically and pathophysiologically from polycystic kidney disease. The cyst may be drained percutaneously.

Congenital Anomalies

Congenital anomalies of the kidney are not uncommon. Occasionally there is fusion of the two kidneys, forming what is called a **horseshoe kidney.** One kidney may be small and deformed and often is nonfunctioning. Occasionally there may be a double ureter or congenital stricture of the ureter. The treatment of these anomalies is necessary only if they cause symptoms, but it is essential to determine that the other kidney is present and functioning before surgery is undertaken.

Renal Tumors

Cancer of the kidney accounts for 2% of all cancers in adults in the United States; it affects almost twice as many men as women. Risk factors include tobacco use, occupational exposure to industrial chemicals, obesity, and dialysis (the incidence of renal cysts and renal tumors is increased in patients on long-term dialysis). The most common type of renal tumor is renal cell or renal adenocarcinoma, accounting for more than 85% of all tumors of the kidney. These tumors may metastasize early to the lungs, bone, liver, brain, and contralateral kidney. One-fourth to one-half of patients will have metastatic disease at the time of diagnosis.

Clinical Manifestations

Many renal tumors produce no symptoms and are discovered on a routine physical examination as a palpable abdominal mass. The classic triad, occurring late in the course of the disease, is hematuria, pain, and a mass in the flank. *The usual sign that first calls attention to the tumor is painless hematuria,* which may be either intermittent and microscopic or continuous and gross. There may be a dull pain in the back from back-pressure produced by compression of the ureter, extension of the tumor into the perirenal area, or hemorrhage into the kidney tissue. Colicky pains occur if a clot or mass of tumor cells passes down the ureter. Symptoms from metastasis may be the first manifestation of renal tumor and may include unexplained weight loss, increasing weakness, and anemia.

The diagnosis of a renal tumor may require intravenous urography, cystoscopic examination, nephrotomograms, renal angiograms, ultrasonography, or computed tomography (CT scan). These tests may be exhausting for a patient already debilitated by the systemic effects of a tumor, for the elderly patient, and for one anxious about the diagnosis and outcome. The nurse assists the patient physically and psychologically in preparing for these procedures and monitors carefully for signs of dehydration and exhaustion.

Management

The goal of management is to eradicate the tumor before metastasis occurs. A radical nephrectomy is the preferred treatment if the tumor can be removed. This includes removal of the kidney (and tumor), adrenal gland, surrounding perinephric fat and Gerota's fascia, and lymph nodes. Radiation therapy, hormonal therapy, or chemotherapy may be used along with surgery. Immunotherapy may also be helpful.

Renal Artery Embolization. In patients with metastatic renal carcinoma, embolization of the renal artery is performed to occlude the blood supply to the tumor and thus kill the tumor cells. Several days after completion of angiographic studies, a catheter is advanced into the renal artery, and embolizing materials (Gelfoam, autologous blood clot, steel coils) are injected into the artery and carried with the arterial blood flow to occlude the tumor vessels mechanically. This decreases the local blood supply, making removal of the kidney (nephrectomy) easier. It also stimulates an immune response, because infarction of the renal cell carcinoma will release tumor-associated antigens that enhance the patient's response to metastatic lesions. The procedure may also reduce the number of tumor cells entering the venous circulation during surgical manipulation.

Following renal artery embolization and tumor infarction, a characteristic symptom complex labeled "postinfarction syndrome" occurs, lasting 2 to 3 days. The patient has pain localized to the flank and abdomen, elevated temperature, and gastrointestinal complaints. Pain is treated with parenteral analgesics, while aspirin is administered to control fever. Antiemetics, restriction of oral intake, and maintenance with intravenous fluids are used to treat the gastrointestinal complaints.

Biologic Therapy. Success in treating renal tumors with biologic response modifiers has been reported. Patients may be treated with interleukin-2 (IL-2), a protein that regulates cell growth. This may be used alone or in combination with lymphokine-activated killer (LAK) cells, which are white blood cells that have been stimulated by IL-2 to increase their ability to kill cancer cells. Interferon, another biologic response modifier, is also under investigation as a mode of therapy for treating advanced renal cancer.

Nursing Interventions

The patient with a renal tumor may undergo extensive diagnostic and therapeutic procedures, including surgery, radiation therapy, and chemotherapy. Following surgery, the patient usually has catheters and drains in place to maintain a patent urinary tract, to remove drainage, and to permit very accurate measurement of urine output. Because of the location of the surgical incision and the position of the patient during the surgical procedure, pain and muscle soreness are common. The patient requires frequent analgesia during the postoperative period and assistance with turning. Turning, coughing, and taking deep breaths are encouraged to prevent atelectasis and other pulmonary complications. The patient and family require assistance and support to cope with the diagnosis and uncertainties about the prognosis. (See Chapter 42 for postoperative care of the patient undergoing surgery of the kidney and Chapter 16 for care of the oncology patient.)

Follow-up care is essential to detect signs of metastases as well as to reassure the patient and family about the patient's continued well-being. The patient who has had surgery for renal carcinoma should have a yearly physical examination and chest x-ray, because late metastases are not uncommon. All subsequent symptoms should be evaluated with possible metastases in mind.

Cancer of the Bladder

Cancer of the urinary bladder is seen more frequently in persons from age 50 onward and affects men more than women (3:1). Statistics indicate that these tumors account for nearly 1 in 25 cancers diagnosed in the United States. There are two forms of bladder cancer: superficial (which tends to recur) and invasive. About 80% to 90% of all bladder cancers are transitional cell (which means they arise from the transitional cells of the bladder), while the remaining types of tumors are squamous cell and adenocarcinoma.

Risk factors for cancer of the bladder include carcinogens in the work environment, such as dyes, rubber, leather, ink, or paint. Other risk factors include recurrent or chronic bacterial infection of the urinary tract and smoking. Bladder cancer is two times more likely to occur in smokers than nonsmokers. In addition, there may be a relationship between coffee drinking and bladder cancer. Chronic schistosomiasis (parasitic infection that irritates the bladder) is also a risk factor. Cancers arising from the prostate, colon, and rectum in males and from the lower gynecologic tract in females may metastasize to the bladder.

Clinical Manifestations. These tumors usually arise at the base of the bladder and involve the ureteral orifices and bladder neck. *Gross, painless hematuria* is the most common symptom of cancer of the bladder. Infection of the urinary tract is a common complication, producing frequency, urgency, and dysuria. However, any alteration in voiding or change in the urine may indicate cancer of the bladder. Pelvic or back pain may occur with metastasis.

Diagnostic Evaluation. Diagnostic evaluation includes excretory urography, CT scan, ultrasonography, cystoscopy, and bimanual examination under anesthesia. Biopsies of the tumor and adjacent mucosa are the definitive diagnostic procedures.

Transitional cell carcinomas and carcinomas *in situ* shed recognizable cancer cells. Cytologic examination of fresh urine and saline bladder washings provide information about the patient's prognosis, especially for those at high risk for recurrence of primary bladder tumors.

Management. Treatment of bladder cancer depends on the grade of the tumor (based on the degree of cellular differentiation), the stage of tumor growth (the degree of local invasion and the presence or absence of metastasis), and the multicentricity (having many centers) of the tumor. The patient's age and physical, mental, and emotional status are considered in determining treatment modalities.

Transurethral resection or *fulguration* (cauterization) may be performed for simple papillomas (benign epithelial tumors). These procedures eradicate the tumors through surgical incision or electrical current with the use of instruments inserted through the urethra.

The management of superficial bladder cancers presents a challenge because there are usually widespread abnormalities in the bladder mucosa. The entire lining of the urinary tract, or urothelium, is at risk, because carcinomatous changes are found not only in the mucosa of the bladder but also in the mucosa of the renal pelvis, ureter, and urethra. Recurrences are a serious problem; approximately 25% to 40% of superficial tumors recur after transurethral resection or fulguration. Persons with benign papillomas should be followed with cytology and cystoscopy periodically for the rest of their lives because aggressive malignancies may develop from these tumors.

Chemotherapy with use of a combination of methotrexate, vinblastine, doxorubicin (Adriamycin), and cisplatin (M-VAC) has been effective in producing partial remission of transitional cell carcinoma of the bladder in some patients. Intravenous chemotherapy may or may not be accompanied by radiation therapy.

Topical chemotherapy (intravesical chemotherapy or instillation of antineoplastic agents into the bladder resulting in contact of the agent with the bladder wall) is considered when there is high risk of recurrence, when cancer *in situ* is present, or when tumor resection has been incomplete. Topical chemotherapy delivers a high concentration of medication (thiotepa, doxorubicin, mitomycin, ethoglucid, and Bacillus Calmette-Guérin or BCG) to the tumor to promote tumor destruction. BCG is now considered the most effective intravesical agent for recurrent bladder cancer because it enhances the body's immune response to cancer. The patient is allowed to eat and drink prior to the instillation procedure, but once the bladder is full, the patient must retain the intravesical solution for 2 hours before voiding. At the end of the procedure, the patient is encouraged to void and to drink liberal amounts of fluid to flush the medication from the bladder.

Radiation of the tumor may be performed preoperatively to reduce microextension of the neoplasm and viability of tumor cells, thus reducing the chances that the cancer may recur in the immediate area or spread through the circulatory or lymphatic systems. Radiation therapy is also used in combination with surgery or to control the disease in the patient with an inoperable tumor.

A simple *cystectomy* (removal of the bladder) or a radical cystectomy is performed for invasive or multifocal bladder cancer. Radical cystectomy in the male involves removal of the bladder, prostate, and seminal vesicles and immediate adjacent perivesical tissues. In the female, radical cystectomy involves removal of the bladder, lower ureter, uterus, Fallopian tubes, ovaries, anterior vagina, and urethra. It may or may not include a pelvic lymphadenectomy (removal of lymph nodes). Removal of the bladder requires a urinary diversion procedure (see below).

The transitional cell variety of bladder cancer responds poorly to chemotherapy. Cisplatin, doxorubicin, and cyclophosphamide have been administered in various doses and schedules and appear most effective.

Bladder cancer may also be treated by direct infusion of the cytotoxic agent through the arterial supply of the involved organ, achieving a higher concentration of the chemotherapeutic agent with less systemic toxic effects. For more advanced bladder cancer or for patients with intractable hematuria (especially following radiation therapy), a large, water-filled balloon placed within the bladder produces tumor necrosis by reducing the blood supply of the bladder wall (*hydrostatic therapy*). The instillation of formalin, phenol, or silver nitrate has achieved relief of hematuria and strangury (slow and painful discharge of urine) in some patients.

Urinary Diversion

Urinary diversion procedures are performed to divert urine away from the bladder to a new exit site, usually through a surgically created opening in the skin (stoma). These procedures are primarily performed when a bladder tumor requires removal of the entire bladder (cystectomy). Urinary diversion has also been used in the management of pelvic malignancy, birth defects, strictures and trauma to ureters and urethra, neurogenic bladder, chronic infection causing severe ureteral and renal damage, and intractable interstitial cystitis.

Controversy exists concerning the best method of establishing permanent diversion of the urinary tract. New techniques are frequently introduced in an effort to improve patient outcomes and quality of life. The age of the patient, condition of the bladder, body build, degree of obesity, degree of ureteral dilation, state of renal function, and the patient's learning ability and willingness to participate in postoperative care are all taken into consideration in determining the appropriate surgical procedure.

The extent to which the patient accepts urinary diversion depends to a large degree on the location or position of the stoma, whether the drainage pouch/bag establishes a water-tight seal to the skin, and the patient's ability to manage the pouch and drainage apparatus. Therefore, attention must be given to these considerations to promote a positive outcome.

There are two categories of urinary diversion: ureteroenterocutaneous diversions (a portion of the intestines is used to create a new reservoir for urine) and cutaneous diversions (urine drains through an opening created in the abdominal wall and skin). The most common methods of urinary diversion are described below and depicted in Figure 43-7.

Ureteroenterocutaneous Diversions

1. *Conventional conduit:* transplanting the ureters to an isolated section of the terminal ileum (ileal conduit), and bringing one end to the abdominal wall (Fig. 43-7*A*). The ureter may also be transplanted into the transverse sigmoid colon (colon conduit) or proximal jejunum (jejunal conduit).
2. *Continent ileal urinary reservoir (Kock pouch):* transplanting the ureters to an isolated segment of ileum (pouch) with a nipple-like, one-way valve; urine is drained by catheter (Fig. 43-9).
3. *Ureterosigmoidostomy:* introducing the ureters into the sigmoid, thereby allowing urine to flow through the colon and out of the rectum (see Fig. 43-7*B*).

Cutaneous Urinary Diversions

4. *Cutaneous ureterostomy:* bringing the detached ureter through the abdominal wall and attaching it to an opening in the skin (see Fig. 43-7*C*).
5. *Vesicostomy:* suturing the bladder to the abdominal wall and creating an opening (stoma) through the abdominal and bladder walls for urinary drainage (see Fig. 43-7*D*).
6. *Nephrostomy:* inserting a catheter into the renal pelvis via an incision into the flank or by percutaneous catheter placement into the kidney (see Fig. 43-7*E*).

Ileal Conduit Urinary Diversion (Ileal Loop)

The ileal conduit, the oldest of the urinary diversion procedures, is considered the "gold standard" because of the low number of complications and the surgeon's familiarity with the procedure. In an ileal conduit, the urine is diverted by implanting the ureter into a loop of ileum that is led out through the abdominal wall. This loop of ileum is a simple conduit (passageway) for urine from the ureters to the surface. A loop of the sigmoid colon may also be used. An ileostomy bag is used to collect the urine. The resected (cut) ends of the remaining intestine are anastomosed (connected) to provide an intact bowel.

Stents, usually made of thin, pliable tubing, are placed in the ureters to prevent occlusion secondary to postsurgical edema. The ureteral stents allow urine to drain from the kidney to the stoma and provide a method for accurate measurement of urine output. They may be left in place 5 to 15 days postoperatively. To compensate for the space of the

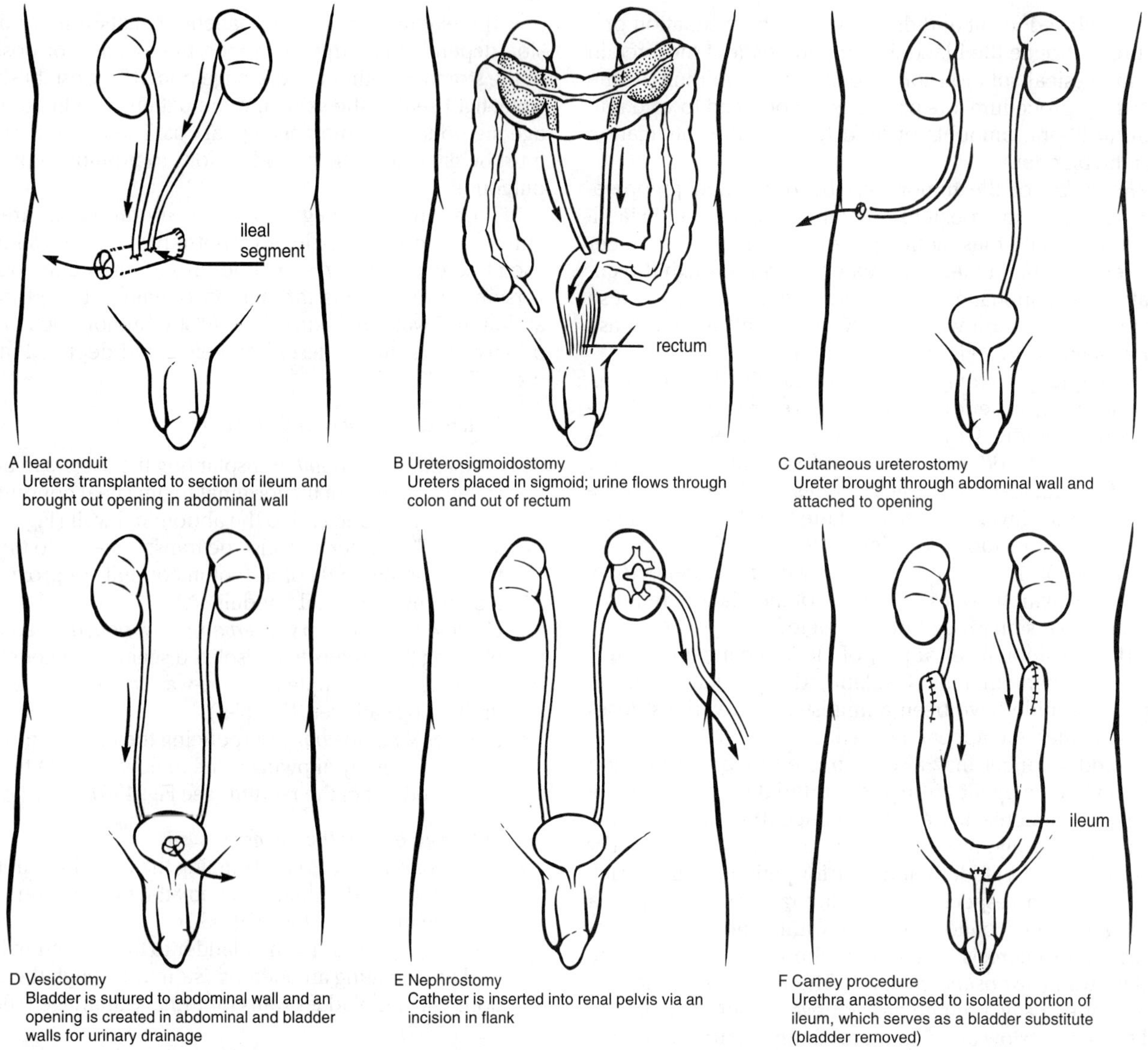
ileal
segment
rectum
A Ileal conduit
Ureters transplanted to section of ileum and brought out opening in abdominal wall
B Ureterosigmoidostomy
Ureters placed in sigmoid; urine flows through colon and out of rectum
C Cutaneous ureterostomy
Ureter brought through abdominal wall and attached to opening
ileum
D Vesicotomy
Bladder is sutured to abdominal wall and an opening is created in abdominal and bladder walls for urinary drainage
E Nephrostomy
Catheter is inserted into renal pelvis via an incision in flank
F Camey procedure
Urethra anastomosed to isolated portion of ileum, which serves as a bladder substitute (bladder removed)

FIGURE 43-7. Methods of urinary diversion.

removed bladder, Jackson-Pratt tubes or other types of drains are inserted to prevent the accumulation of fluid.

After surgery, a skin barrier and a transparent, disposable urinary drainage bag are applied around the conduit and connected to drainage. A custom-cut appliance is used until the edema subsides and the stoma shrinks to normal size. The clear bag allows the stoma to be visualized and the patency of the stent and the urinary output to be better monitored. The ileal bag drains urine constantly (not feces). The appliance (bag) usually remains in place as long as it is watertight; it is changed when necessary to prevent leakage of urine.

Nursing Interventions. Because this patient requires specialized care, a consultation is initiated with an enterostomal therapist or clinical nurse specialist in skin care. In the immediate postoperative period, urine volumes are monitored hourly. An output below 30 ml/h may indicate dehydration or an obstruction in the ileal conduit with possible backflow or leakage from the ureteroileal anastomosis. A catheter may be inserted through the urinary conduit if prescribed to monitor for possible stasis or residual urine from a constricted stoma. Nursing management of the patient with a ureteral stent may include, if prescribed, irrigation with normal saline every 6 to 8 hours. It is important to avoid any tension on the stents because this may dislodge them.

Stoma and Skin Care. The stoma is inspected frequently for bleeding. Minimal bleeding may be seen and implies good blood supply. A change in color of the stoma from a normal pink or red color to a dark purplish color suggests that the vascular supply may be compromised. If cyanosis and compromised blood supply persist, surgical intervention is often necessary.

The stoma is not sensitive to touch, but the skin around the stoma becomes very sensitive if it becomes irritated by urine or by the appliance. The skin is inspected for (1) signs of irritation and bleeding of the stomal mucosa; (2) encrustation and skin irritation around the stoma (from alkaline urine coming in contact with exposed skin); and (3) wound infections.

Urine Testing and Appliance Considerations. Moisture in bed linens or clothing or the odor of urine around the patient should alert the nursing personnel to the possibility of leakage from the appliance, the presence of an infection, or a problem in hygienic management. Because severe alkaline encrustation can accumulate rapidly around the stoma, the urine *p*H is kept below 6.5. Urine *p*H can be determined by testing the urine draining from the stoma, not from the collecting appliance. A properly fitted appliance is essential to prevent exposure of the peristomal skin (skin around the stoma) to urine. If the urine is foul smelling, the stoma is catheterized, if prescribed, in order to obtain a specimen for culture and sensitivity.

Fluids are encouraged in order to flush the ileal conduit and decrease the accumulation of mucus. The patient may excrete a large amount of mucus mixed with urine because of the use of a mucous membrane in formation of the conduit. To relieve anxiety, the patient is reassured that this is a normal occurrence following an ileal conduit.

Complications. Complications following an ileal conduit include wound infection or wound dehiscence, urinary leakage, ureteral obstruction, hyperchloremic acidosis, small bowel obstruction, and stomal gangrene. Delayed complications include ureteral obstruction, contraction or narrowing of the stoma (stomal stenosis), pyelonephritis, and renal calculi.

Patient Teaching

Appliance Selection. The urinary appliance may consist of one or two pieces and may be disposable (usually used once and discarded) or reusable. The choice of appliance is determined by the location of the stoma and the patient's normal activity, body build, and economic resources. A reusable appliance has a faceplate that is attached to the skin surface with cement or adhesive. Either reusable pouches or disposable pouches may be used with the reusable faceplate. Disposable appliances have the advantage of having a surface that is already prepared for application to the skin and of being lightweight and easy to conceal. A skin barrier must be used to protect the skin from excoriation due to exposure to the urine. See Figure 43-8 for examples of appliances.

Determining the Stoma Size. As the postoperative edema subsides, the stoma opening is recalibrated every 3 to 6 weeks for the first few months postoperatively. The correct appliance size is determined by measuring the widest part of the stoma with a ruler. The permanent appliance should be no more than 1.6 mm (1/8 in) larger than the diameter of the stoma and the same shape as the stoma to prevent contact of the skin with drainage.

Changing the Appliance. The appliance is changed at a time that will be most convenient to the patient. Many patients find early morning most convenient because the urine output is reduced. The collecting appliance usually lasts 3 to 5 days before leakage occurs.

Instructions for Applying the Appliance. The appliance system is ideally changed before the system leaks. A variety of appliances are available; regardless of the type of appliance used, a skin barrier is essential to protect the skin from irritation and excoriation. To maintain peristomal skin integrity, a skin barrier or leaking pouch is never patched with tape to prevent accumulation of urine under the skin barrier or faceplate. Because the degree to which the stoma protrudes is not the same in all patients, there are various accessories and custom-made appliances to solve individual problems.

Guidelines for applying reusable and disposable systems are presented in Chart 43-7.

Odor Control. The patient should be advised to avoid foods that give the urine a strong odor (*e.g.*, asparagus, cheese, eggs). A few drops of liquid deodorizer or diluted white vinegar may be introduced through the drain spout into the bottom of the pouch with a syringe or eyedropper. Ascorbic acid by mouth helps acidify the urine and

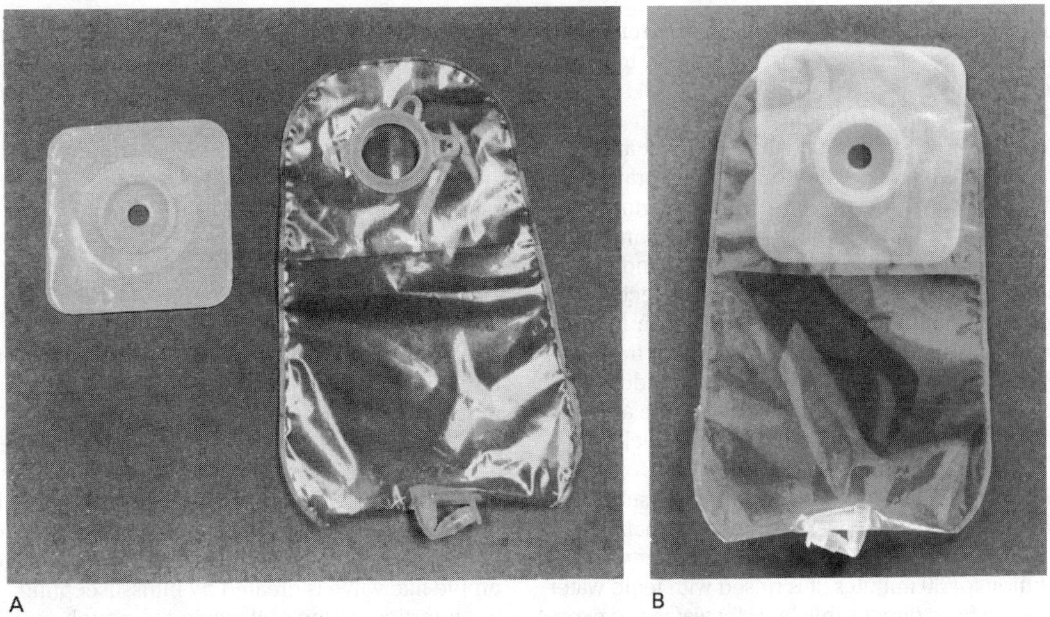

A B

FIGURE 43-8. Skin-protective barrier used with urostomy pouch. (**A**) Squibb Stomahesive wafer (*left*) and Sur-Fit urostomy pouch (*right*). (**B**) Stomahesive wafer with pouch attached.

CHART 43-7
Patient Education: Applying Pouch System in Urinary Diversion

Applying a Reusable Pouch System

1. Gather all necessary supplies.
2. Prepare new appliance according to the manufacturer's directions.
   a. Apply double-faced adhesive disk which has been properly sized to fit the reusable pouch faceplate. Remove paper backing and lay pouch aside.

   or

   b. Apply thin layer of contact cement to one side of the reusable pouch faceplate. Lay pouch aside.
3. Remove soiled pouch gently. Lay aside to clean later.
4. Cleanse peristomal skin with small amount of soap and water. Rinse thoroughly and dry. If a film of soap remains on skin and the site is not allowed to dry, the appliance will not adhere adequately.
5. Use a wick (rolled gauze pad or tampon) on top of stoma opening to absorb urine and keep skin dry throughout appliance change.
6. Inspect peristomal skin (skin around stoma) for irritation.
7. A skin protector wipe or barrier ring may be applied prior to centering the faceplate opening directly over stoma.
8. Position appliance over stoma and press gently into place.
9. A pouch cover can be used or cornstarch applied under the pouch to prevent perspiration and skin irritation.
10. Cleanse soiled pouch and prepare for repeat use.

Applying a Disposable Pouch System

1. Gather all necessary supplies.
2. Measure stoma and prepare an opening in the skin barrier ⅛-inch larger than the stoma and the same shape as the stoma.
3. Remove paper backing from skin barrier and set aside.
4. Gently remove old appliance and set aside.
5. Cleanse peristomal skin with warm water and dry thoroughly.
6. Inspect peristomal skin (skin around stoma) for irritation.
7. Use a wick (rolled gauze pad or tampon) on top of the stoma to absorb urine and keep the skin dry during the appliance change.
8. Center opening of skin barrier over stoma and apply with firm, gentle pressure to attain a watertight seal.
9. If using a two-piece system, snap pouch onto the flanged wafer that adheres to skin.
10. Close drainage tap/spout at bottom of pouch.
11. A pouch cover can be used or cornstarch applied under pouch to prevent perspiration and skin irritation.
12. Apply hypoallergenic tape around the skin barrier in a picture frame manner.
13. Dispose of soiled appliance.

suppress urine odor. Also, the patient should be reminded that the pouch will develop an odor if it is worn too long and not cared for properly.

Managing the Ostomy Appliance. The pouch is emptied via a drain valve when it is one-third full, because the weight of the urine will cause the pouch to separate from the skin if filled more. Some patients prefer wearing a leg bag attached with an adapter to the drainage apparatus. To promote uninterrupted sleep, a collecting bottle and tubing (one unit) are snapped onto an adaptor that connects to the ileal appliance. A small amount of urine is left in the bag when the adaptor is attached to prevent the bag from collapsing against itself. The tubing may be threaded down the pajama leg to prevent kinking. The collecting bottle and tubing are rinsed daily with cool water and once a week with a 3:1 solution of water and white vinegar.

Cleaning and Deodorizing the Appliance. Usually the reusable appliance is rinsed in warm water and soaked in a 3:1 solution of water and white vinegar or a commercial deodorizing solution for 30 minutes. It is rinsed with tepid water and air dried away from direct sunlight. (Hot water and exposure to direct sunlight will dry out the pouch and increase the incidence of cracking.) After drying, the appliance may be powdered with cornstarch and stored. Two appliances are necessary—one to be worn while the other is air drying. The patient is encouraged to contact the local ostomy association for visits, reassurance, and practical information.

Continent Ileal Urinary Reservoir (Kock Pouch)

The continent ileal urinary reservoir is another type of urinary diversion created for patients whose bladder is removed or can no longer function (neurogenic bladder). In this procedure, a segment of the small intestine is surgically isolated from the intestine and serves as a reservoir for urine (Fig. 43-9). The ureters are implanted in the isolated segment and an opening is created connecting the new "bladder" to the abdominal wall. To prevent leakage of urine, a nipple-like valve is created by intussuscepting (telescoping) the intestine. Urine collects in the pouch until a catheter is inserted into the nipple valve and the urine is drained. The

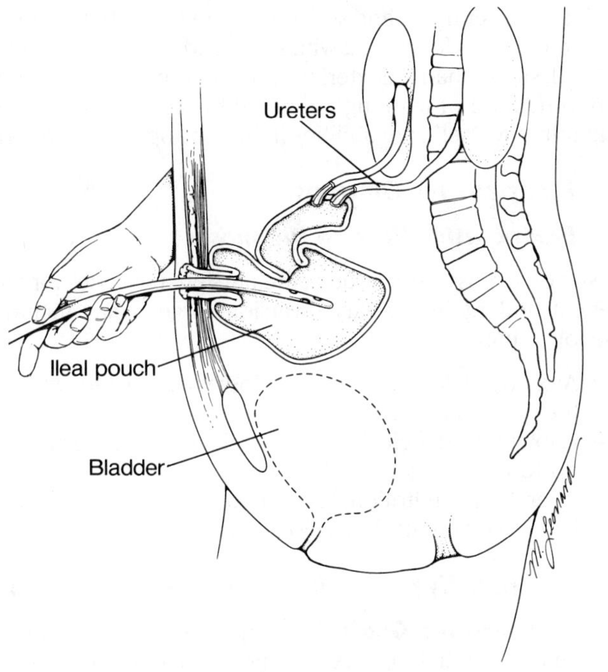

FIGURE 43-9. Continent ileal urinary reservoir (Kock pouch). Urine collects in the pouch and is drained by inserting a catheter through the valve.

advantage of this urinary diversion is that the valve prevents leakage of urine and the drainage of urine is under the control of the patient. The reservoir must be drained at regular intervals by a catheter to prevent absorption of metabolic waste products from the urine, reflux of urine to the ureters, and urinary tract infections.

Ureterosigmoidostomy

Ureterosigmoidostomy is an implantation of the ureters into the sigmoid colon (see Fig. 43-7*B*). It is usually performed for the patient who has had extensive pelvic radiation, previous small bowel resection, or coexisting small bowel disease.

The patient is informed that, following surgery, voiding will occur from the rectum for the rest of his or her life and that an adjustment in lifestyle will be necessary because of urinary frequency (as often as every 2 hours); drainage will have a consistency equivalent to a watery diarrhea. There will be some degree of nocturia. Activities will have to be planned around the frequent need to urinate, which in turn may affect the patient's social life. However, the patient has the advantage of urinary control without having to wear an external appliance.

Preoperative Management. In addition to the usual preoperative regimen, the patient may be placed on a liquid diet for several days preoperatively to reduce residue in the colon. Antimicrobial agents (neomycin, kanamycin) are administered for bowel disinfection. Ureterosigmoidostomy requires a competent anal sphincter, adequate renal function, and active renal peristalsis. The degree of anal sphincter control may be determined by assessing the patient's ability to retain enemas.

Postoperative Management. Postoperatively, a catheter is placed in the rectum to drain the urine and prevent reflux of urine into the ureters and kidneys. The tube is taped to the buttocks and special skin care is given around the anus to prevent excoriation. Irrigations of the rectal tube may be prescribed, but force is never used because of the danger of introducing bacteria into the newly implanted ureters.

Fluid and Electrolyte Concerns. In this procedure, larger areas of the bowel mucosa are exposed to urine and electrolyte reabsorption; as a result, electrolyte imbalance and acidosis may occur. Potassium and magnesium in the urine may cause diarrhea. Fluid and electrolyte balance is maintained in the immediate postoperative period by closely monitoring the patient's serum electrolyte levels and administering appropriate intravenous infusions. Acidosis may be prevented by placing the patient on a low-chloride diet supplemented with sodium potassium citrate.

The patient should be instructed never to wait longer than 2 to 3 hours before emptying urine from the intestine in order to keep rectal pressure low and to minimize the absorption of urinary constituents from the colon. It is essential to teach the patient about the symptoms of urinary tract infection: fever, flank pain, and frequency.

Anal Sphincter Training. After the rectal catheter is removed, the patient learns to control the anal sphincter through special sphincteric exercises. At first, urination is frequent. With reassurance and encouragement and the passage of time, the patient will gain greater control and will learn to differentiate between the need to void and the need to defecate.

Dietary Measures. Specific dietary instructions include avoidance of gas-forming foods (flatus can cause stress incontinence and offensive odors). Other ways to avoid gas are to avoid chewing gum, smoking, and any other activity that involves swallowing air. Salt intake may be restricted to prevent hyperchloremic acidosis. Potassium intake is increased through foods and medication because potassium may be lost in acidosis.

Possible Complications. Pyelonephritis (upper urinary tract infection) due to reflux of bacteria from the colon is fairly common. Long-term antimicrobial therapy may be prescribed to prevent infection. A late complication is adenocarcinoma of the sigmoid colon, possibly due to the exposure of colonic mucosa to urine, leading to cellular changes.

Cutaneous Ureterostomy

A cutaneous ureterostomy (see Fig. 43-7*C*) is accomplished by bringing the detached ureters through the abdominal wall and attaching them to an opening in the skin. This procedure is used for selected patients with ureteral obstruction (advanced pelvic cancer); for poor-risk patients, because it requires less extensive surgery than other urinary diversion procedures; and for patients who have had previous abdominal radiation.

A urinary appliance is fitted immediately following surgery. The management of the patient with a cutaneous ureterostomy is very similar to the care of the patient with an ileal conduit (see p. 1217), although the stomas are usually flush with the skin or retracted.

Cystostomy

An infrequently used method of urinary diversion is the suprapubic cystostomy. A special catheter is usually inserted under local anesthesia through the abdomen into the bladder through either an incision in the lower abdominal wall or a puncture made by a trocar. Generally, a cystostomy is performed on the patient with an obstruction below the bladder (prostatic obstruction) when it is not possible to insert a urethral catheter. A cystostomy may be temporary (until corrective surgery can be performed) or permanent.

The patient with a cystostomy requires liberal amounts of fluid to prevent encrustation around the catheter. Other problems encountered include the formation of bladder stones, acute and chronic infections, and problems in collecting urine. The advice and assistance of an enterostomal therapist are needed in choosing the most suitable urine collection bag and educating and assisting the patient in its use.

Other Urinary Diversion Procedures

Variations on these procedures and innovations in surgical procedures are devised frequently in an effort to identify and perfect procedures that will improve patient outcomes and reduce the incidence of postoperative problems. These include cecal, patched cecal, Mainz reservoirs, and Indiana pouches. These techniques involve isolating a part of the large intestine to form a reservoir for urine and creating an abdominal stoma. Another surgical procedure, the Camey procedure (see Fig. 43-5*F*), uses a portion of the ileum as a bladder substitute. In this procedure, the isolated ileum serves as the reservoir for urine; it is anastomosed directly to the portion of the remaining urethra following cystectomy. This procedure permits emptying of the bladder through the urethra. The Camey procedure, however, applies only to men because the entire urethra is removed when a cystectomy is performed on women.

❑ NURSING PROCESS
The Patient Undergoing Urinary Diversion

Preoperative Nursing Assessment

The patient admitted to the hospital for a urinary diversion surgical procedure is thoroughly assessed. A careful preoperative assessment of cardiopulmonary function is performed because patients undergoing cystectomy (excision of the urinary bladder) are usually older people who may not be able to tolerate a lengthy, complex surgical procedure. Assessment of nutritional status is also important because of possible poor nutritional intake related to the patient's underlying health problems.

Assessment also focuses on the patient and family's understanding of the procedure and the changes in physical structure and function that will result from the surgery. The patient's self-concept and self-esteem are evaluated, in addition to methods for coping with stress and loss. The patient's mental status, hand dexterity and coordination, and preferred method of learning are noted because these factors will influence self-care abilities in the postoperative period.

Preoperative Diagnosis

Preoperative Nursing Diagnoses

Based on the assessment data, the nursing diagnoses for the patient undergoing urinary diversion surgery may include the following:

- ❑ Anxiety related to anticipated losses associated with the surgical procedure
- ❑ Knowledge deficit about the surgical procedure and postoperative care
- ❑ Alteration in nutrition, less than body requirements related to inadequate nutritional intake

Preoperative Planning and Implementation

Preoperative Goals. The major goals for the patient may include relief of anxiety and increased knowledge about the surgical procedure, expected outcomes, and postoperative care; and improved nutritional status in preparation for surgery.

Preoperative Nursing Interventions

Relieving Anxiety. The threat of cancer and removal of the bladder creates a fear related to losses—loss of affection, body image, and security. The patient faces problems in adapting to an external appliance, a stoma, a scar, and altered toileting habits. The male patient must also adapt to sexual impotency. (A penile implant is considered if the patient is a candidate for the procedure.) Women also fear the threats to appearance, body image, and self esteem. A supportive approach, both physical and psychosocial, is needed and includes assessing the patient's self concept and manner of coping with stress and loss; helping the patient identify ways to maintain a typical lifestyle and independence with as few changes as possible; and encouraging the patient to express fears and anxieties about the ramifications of the upcoming surgery. A visitor from the Ostomy Visitation Program of the American Cancer Society can provide emotional support and make adaptation easier both before and after surgery.

Patient Teaching. An enterostomal therapist is invaluable in preoperative teaching and in planning postoperative care. Explanations of the surgical procedure, the appearance of the stoma, the rationale for preoperative bowel preparation, the reasons for wearing a collection device, and the effects of the surgery on sexual functioning (for the male patient) are provided as part of patient teaching.

The placement of the stoma site is planned preoperatively with the patient standing, sitting, or lying down in order to locate the stoma away from bony prominences, skin creases, and fat folds. The stoma should also be placed away from old scars, the umbilicus, and the belt line. *For ease of self care, the patient must be able to see and reach the site comfortably.* The site is marked with indelible ink so that it can be located easily during surgery. The patient is assessed for allergies or sensitivity to tape or adhesives. (Patch testing of certain appliances may be necessary before the ostomy equipment is selected.) It may be helpful to have the patient practice wearing an appliance partially filled with water before surgery.

Improving Nutritional Status. The patient undergoing a urinary diversion procedure for cancer may be severely malnourished because of the tumor, radiation enteritis, and anorexia. Enteral or total parenteral nutrition may be prescribed to support the patient, promote healing, and improve response to treatment.

Preoperative Management. As part of preoperative management, the bowel is cleansed to minimize fecal stasis, decompress the bowel, and minimize postoperative ileus. A low-residue diet is prescribed and antimicrobial medications are administered to reduce pathogenic flora in the bowel and to reduce the risk of infection. Adequate preoperative hydration is imperative to ensure urine flow during surgery and to prevent hypovolemia during the prolonged operative procedure.

Postoperative Management

Postoperative management focuses on maintaining urinary function, preventing postoperative complications (respiratory complications, fluid and electrolyte imbalances, sepsis, fistula formation, and urine leakage), and promoting patient comfort.

Catheters or drainage systems are observed and urine output is monitored carefully. A nasogastric tube is inserted during surgery to decompress the gastrointestinal tract and to relieve pressure on the intestinal anastomosis. It is usually kept in place for several days following surgery. As soon as bowel function resumes, as manifested by bowel sounds, the passage of flatus, and a soft abdomen, oral fluids are permitted. Until that time, intravenous fluids and electrolytes are administered. The patient is assisted to ambulate as soon as possible.

Postoperative Nursing Assessment

The role of the nurse in the immediate postoperative period is to prevent complications and to assess the patient carefully for any signs and symptoms of such complications. The catheters and any drainage devices are monitored closely. Urine volume, patency of the drainage system, and color of the drainage are noted. A sudden decrease in urine volume or increase in drainage is reported promptly to the physician because this development may indicate obstruction of the urinary tract, inadequate blood volume, or bleeding.

Analgesia is administered as prescribed to promote patient comfort and enable the patient to turn, cough, and take deep breaths without excessive pain and discomfort.

Postoperative Diagnosis

Postoperative Nursing Diagnoses

- Risk for impaired skin integrity related to problems in managing the appliance
- Body image disturbance related to urinary diversion
- Potential for sexual dysfunction related to structural and physiologic alterations
- Knowledge deficit about management of urinary function

Collaborative Problems/ Potential Complications

Based on assessment data, potential complications may include:

- Peritonitis due to disruption of anastomosis
- Stomal ischemia and necrosis due to compromise of blood supply to stoma
- Stoma retraction and separation of mucocutaneous border due to tension or trauma

Postoperative Planning and Implementation

Postoperative Goals. The major goals for the patient may include maintenance of peristomal skin integrity, increased self-esteem, appropriate coping mechanisms to accept and deal with altered urinary function and sexuality, increased knowledge about management of urinary function, and prevention of potential complications.

Postoperative Complications.

Complications are not unusual because of the complexity of the surgery, the underlying reason (cancer, trauma) for urinary diversion procedures, and the frequently less-than-optimal nutritional status. Complications may include the usual postoperative complications (*e.g.*, atelectasis, fluid and electrolyte imbalances) as well as breakdown of the anastomoses, sepsis, fistula formation, fecal or urine leakage, and skin irritation. If these occur, the patient will remain hospitalized for an extended length of time and will probably require total parenteral nutrition, gastrointestinal decompression via nasogastric suction, and further surgery. The goals of management will be to establish drainage, provide adequate nutrition for healing to occur, and prevent sepsis.

Postoperative Nursing Interventions

Monitoring and Managing Potential Complications

Peritonitis. Peritonitis can occur postoperatively if there is leakage of urine at the anastomosis. Signs and symptoms include abdominal pain and distention, muscle rigidity with guarding, nausea and vomiting, paralytic ileus (absence of bowel sounds), fever, and leukocytosis. The urine output must be monitored closely, as a sudden decrease in amount with a corresponding increase in drainage from the incision or drains may indicate urine leakage. In addition, the urine drainage device is observed for leakage. The pouch is changed if a leak is observed. Small leaks in the anastomosis may seal themselves, but surgery may be needed for larger leaks.

Vital signs (blood pressure, pulse, temperature) are monitored. Changes in vital signs as well as increasing pain, nausea and vomiting, and abdominal distention are reported to the physician as they may indicate peritonitis.

Stomal Ischemia and Necrosis. A necrotic stoma can result from tension on the mesentery blood vessels, twisting of the bowel segment (conduit) during surgery, or arterial insufficiency. The new stoma must be inspected at least every 4 hours to assess the adequacy of its blood supply. The stoma should be red or pink in color. If the blood supply to the stoma is compromised the color will change to purple, brown, or black. These changes are reported immediately to the physician. The physician or enterostomal therapist may insert a small, lubricated tube into the stoma and shine a flashlight into the lumen of the tube to assess for superficial ischemia versus necrosis. A necrotic stoma requires surgical intervention. If the ischemia is superficial, the dusky stoma will be observed and may slough its outer layer in several days.

Stoma Retraction and Separation. Stoma retraction and mucocutaneous border separation occur due to trauma or tension on the internal bowel segment utilized for creation of the stoma. In addition, mucocutaneous separation can occur if the stoma is not allowed to heal due to accumulation of urine on the stoma and mucocutaneous border. Using a collection drainage pouch with an antireflux valve is helpful because the valve prevents urine from pooling on the stoma and mucocutaneous border. Meticulous skin care and waterproofing of the skin around the stoma promote healing.

If a separation of the mucocutaneous border occurs, surgery is not usually needed. The separated area is protected by applying karaya powder, stoma adhesive paste, and a properly fitted skin barrier and pouch. By protecting the separation, healing is promoted. If the stoma retracts back into the peritoneum, surgical intervention is mandatory.

If surgery is needed as part of management of these complications, the nurse provides explanations to the patient and family. The need for additional surgery is usually perceived as a setback by the patient and family. Therefore, emotional support of the patient and family is provided along with physical preparation of the patient for surgery.

Maintaining Peristomal Skin Integrity. Strategies to promote skin integrity begin with reducing and controlling those factors that increase the patient's risk for poor nutrition and poor healing. As indicated above, meticulous skin care and management of the drainage system are provided by the nurse until the patient is able to manage them and is comfortable doing so. Care is taken to assure an intact drainage system to protect the skin from exposure to drainage. Supplies must be readily available to manage the drainage in the immediate postoperative period. Consistency in implementing the skin care program throughout the postoperative period will result in maintenance of skin integrity and patient comfort. Additionally, maintenance of skin integrity around the stoma will enable the patient and family to adjust more easily to the alterations in urinary function and will help them learn skin care techniques.

Adequate supplies and complete instruction are necessary to enable the patient and a family member to develop competence and confidence in their skills. Written and verbal instructions are provided, and the patient is encouraged to contact the nurse or physician for follow-up questions. Follow-up phone calls from the nurse to the patient and family after the patient's discharge may provide added support. Follow-up visits and reinforcement of correct skin care and appliance management techniques also promote skin integrity. Specific techniques for managing the appliance are described on pp. 1219–1220.

Improving Body Image. The patient's ability to cope with the changes associated with the surgery depends to some degree on body image and self-esteem before the surgery and the support and reaction of others. Allowing the patient to express concerns and anxious feelings can help the coping process begin, especially in adjusting to the changes in toileting habits. The nurse can also help improve the patient's self-concept by teaching the skills needed to be independent in managing the urinary drainage devices. When instructing about ostomy care, privacy is provided to allow the patient an opportunity to ask questions without fear of embarrassment. Explaining why the nurse must wear gloves when performing ostomy care can prevent the patient misinterpreting the use of gloves as a sign of aversion to the stoma.

Exploring Sexuality Issues. Patients who experiences altered sexual function as a result of the surgical procedure may mourn this loss and its meaning to them and their partners. Encouraging the patient and partner to share their feelings about this loss with each other and acknowledging the importance of sexual function and expression may assist the patient and partner to seek sexual counseling if necessary and to explore alternative ways of expressing sexuality. A visit from another "ostomate" who is functioning fully in society and family life may also assist the patient and family in recognizing that full recovery is possible.

Patient Education and Home Care Considerations. A major postoperative objective is to assist the patient to achieve the highest level of independence and self-care possible. The primary nurse and enterostomal therapist work closely with the patient and family to instruct and assist them in all phases of managing the ostomy. The patient is encouraged to participate in decisions regarding the type of collecting appliance and the time of day to change the appliance. The patient is assisted and encouraged to look at and touch the stoma early in order to overcome any fears.

The patient and family need to know the following information about a normal stoma: (1) it should be pink and moist like the inside of the mouth, (2) it is insensitive to pain because it has no nerve endings, and (3) it is vascular and may bleed when cleaned. Additionally, if a segment of the gastrointestinal tract was used to create the urinary diversion, mucus may be visible in the urine. By learning what is normal, the patient and family will become familiar with signs and symptoms to report to the physician or nurse and the problems that they can handle themselves.

Information provided to the patient and the degree of self-care involved are based on the patient's physical recovery from surgery and ability to accept and acquire the knowledge and skill needed for independence. Verbal and written instructions are provided, and the patient is given the opportunity to practice and demonstrate the skills need to manage urinary drainage. Visits from a home care nurse are important to assess the patient's adaptation to the home setting and management of the ostomy. Teaching and reinforcement may assist the patient and family to cope with altered urinary function.

Evaluation

Expected Outcomes

1. Increases knowledge about managing urinary function.
   a. Participates in managing urinary system and in skin care.
   b. Describes anatomic alteration due to surgery
   c. Revises daily routine to accommodate urinary drainage management.

   d. Identifies potential problems and measures to take and reportable signs and symptoms.
2. Exhibits improved self-concept.
   a. Verbalizes acceptance of urinary diversion, stoma, and appliance.
   b. Demonstrates increasing independence in self care, including hygiene and grooming.
   c. Verbalizes acceptance of support and assistance from family members, health care providers, and other "ostomates."
3. Deals with sexuality issues.
   a. Verbalizes concerns about possible alterations in sexuality and sexual function.
   b. Discusses sexual concerns with partner and appropriate counselor.
4. Maintains skin integrity.
   a. Demonstrates intact peristomal skin and skill in managing drainage system and appliance.
   b. Reports no pain or discomfort in peristomal area.
   c. Verbalizes action to take if skin excoriation occurs.
5. Absence of complications.
   a. Reports no pain or tenderness in abdomen.
   b. Demonstrates temperature within normal range.
   c. Demonstrates no leakage of urine from incision or drains.
   d. Urine output is stable and within desired volume limits.
   e. Stoma is red or pink in color, moist in appearance, and appropriately "budded."
   f. Border surrounding stoma is intact and healed.

CRITICAL THINKING EXERCISES

1. Your patient tells you that she is very discouraged because she has had repeated episodes of urinary tract infection over the last 3 years. How would you focus your assessment to assist in uncovering factors associated with these infections? Describe the teaching program you would devise to help the patient reduce the incidence of infection.
2. Your patient is scheduled for extracorporeal lithotripsy to treat kidney stones. Describe how you might explain this procedure in the following situations: (1) the patient is elderly and hard of hearing; (2) the patient is terrified of water and afraid of being electrocuted during the procedure; (3) the patient tells you that the pain is God's way of punishing him; (4) the patient inquires about possible problems that may develop after he goes home.
3. Your patient has cancer of the bladder and is scheduled for a cystectomy and urinary diversion. Describe the types of complications that may arise in the postoperative period and how you would conduct your assessment and management plan to prevent them.

BIBLIOGRAPHY

Books

Allen RD and Chapman JR. A Manual of Renal Transplantation. Boston, Little, Brown, 1994.

Bellomo R and Ronco C (eds). Acute Renal Failure in the Critically Ill. New York, Springer-Verlag, 1995.

Brundage D. Renal Disorders. St. Louis, Mosby Year Book, 1992.

El Nahas AM, Mallick NP and Anderson S. Prevention of Progressive Chronic Renal Failure. New York, Oxford University Press, 1993.

Hampton B and Bryant R. Ostomies and Continent Diversions: Nursing Management. St. Louis, Mosby Year Book, 1992.

Holloway N. Medical Surgical Care Planning. Springhouse, PA, Springhouse Corp., 1993.

King BD and Harke J. Coping with Bowel and Bladder Problems. San Diego, Singular Publ. Group, 1994.

Lazarus JM and Brenner BM. Acute Renal Failure. New York, Churchill Livingstone, 1993.

Nolan MT and Augustine SM. Transplantation Nursing: Acute and Long-Term Management Norwalk, CT, Appleton & Lange, 1995.

Schrier R. Renal and Electrolyte Disorders, 4th ed. Boston, Little, Brown and Co., 1992.

Schrier R and Gottschalk C. Diseases of the Kidney, 5th ed. Boston, Little, Brown and Co., 1993.

Walsh P et al. Campbell's Urology. Philadelphia, WB Saunders, 1992.

Windhager E. Handbook of Physiology and Renal Physiology. New York, Oxford University Press, 1992.

Wyngaarden J. Cecil Textbook of Medicine, Vol. 1, 19th ed. Philadelphia, WB Saunders, 1992.

Journals

Asterisks indicate nursing research articles.

General

Bakris GL and Talbert R. Drug dosing in patients with renal insufficiency. A simplified approach. Postgrad Med 1993 Dec; 94(8):153–156, 159–160, 163–164.

Byers J and Goshorn J. How to manage diuretic therapy. Am J Nurs 1995 February; 95(2):38–44.

Chambers JK. Renal insufficiency: Implications for care of the medical-surgical patient. Medsurg Nurs 1993 Feb; 2(1):33–40.

Ludlow M. Renal handling of potassium. ANNA J 1993 Feb; 20(1): 52–58.

Moore S et al. How to irrigate a nephrosotomy tube. Am J Nurs 1993 July; 93(7):63–67.

Mylotte J et al. Staying on top of hospital infections. Patient Care 1993 Feb 15; 27(3):116–130.

Oldrizzi L, Rugiu C, and Maschio G. Nutrition and the kidney: How to manage patients with renal failure. Nutrition Clin Practice 1994 February; 9(1):3–10.

Oberly ET and Compton A. Nursing interventions for rehabilitating renal patients. ANNA J 1994 Dec; 21(7):407–411.

Solomon R. Strategies to delay renal deterioration. Patient Care 1995 February 15; 29(3):50–57.

Stark J. Interpreting BUN/creatinine levels: It's not as simple as you think. Nursing 1994 September: 24(9):58–61.

*Stevens D and Kohlenberg E. Quality of life in elderly renovascular hypertensive patients. ANNA J 1993 Aug; 20(4):453–456.

Yucha C. Renal control of calcium. ANNA J 1993 Aug; 20(4): 440–445.

Yucha C. Renal control of phosphorus and magnesium. ANNA J 1993 Aug; 20(4):447–451.

Urinary Tract Infections

Bergeron MG. Treatment of pyelonephritis in adults. Med Clin North Am 1995 May; 79(3):619–649.
Childs S et al. Asymptomatic bacteriuria: When to worry. Patient Care 1993 Feb 15; 27(3):63–88.
Colling J et al. Urinary tract infection rates among incontinent nursing home and community dwelling elderly. Urology Nurse 1994 Sep; 14(3):117–119.
Evans P et al. Urine culture in the elderly. Lancet 1994 Dec 24–31; 344(8939):1778–1780.
Hooton T. A simplified approach to urinary tract infection. Hosp Prac 1995 Feb 15; 30(2):23–30.
*Kovach CR, Puetzer M and Gretzinger P. A descriptive study of nosocomial urinary tract infection in a rehabilitation patient population. Rehabil Nurs Res 1993 Fall; 2(2):81–86.
Leiner S. Recurrent urinary tract infections in otherwise healthy adult women. Rational strategies for work-up and management. Nurse Pract 1995 Feb; 20(2):48, 51–52, 54–56.
*Lewis, S. The effect of surveillance definitions on nosocomial urinary tract infection rates in a rehabilitation hospital. Infect Control Hosp Epidemiol 1995 Jan; 16(1):43–48.
Naber K. Urinary tract infections in men, including prostatis, epididymitis, non-specific urethritis and Reiter's syndrome. Curr Opin Infect Dis 1994 Feb; 7(1):9–19, 117–118.
Nicolle L. Urinary tract infection in adult women. Curr Opin Infect Dis 1994 Feb; 7(1):3–8, 115–117.
*Raz R and Stamm W. A controlled trial of intravaginal estriol in postmenopausal women with recurrent urinary tract infections. N Engl J Med 1993 Sep 3; 329(11):753–756.
Walser M. Assessment of renal function and progression of disease. Curr Opin Nephrol Hypertens 1994 Sep; 3(5):564–567.

Disorders of the Kidney

Anderson RJ. Prevention and management of acute renal failure. Hosp Prac 1993 Aug 15; 28(8):61–65, 68–72, 74–75.
Bakris GL and Stein JH. Diabetic nephropathy. Dis Mon 1993 Aug; 39(8):573–611.
Carella MJ, Gossain VV and Rovner DR. Early diabetic nephropathy. Emerging treatment options. Arch Intern Med 1994 Mar 28; 154(6):625–630.
Erickson P. Idiopathic glomerulonephritis: Is it IgA nephropathy? ANNA J 1993 Apr; 20(2):127–134.
King LR. Hydronephrisis. When is obstruction not obstruction? Urol Clin North Am 1995 Feb; 22(1):31–42.
Leondike MR and Shattuck MA. Intravenous cyclophosphamide in lupus nephritis. J IV Nurs 1993 Jan–Feb; 16(1):23–27.
Montseny JJ et al. The current spectrum of infectious glomerulonephritis. Experience with 76 patients and review of the literature. Medicine 1995 Mar; 74(2):63–73.
Neumann M. Severe exacerbation of lupus nephritis and its management. ANNA J 1994 Apr; 21(2):158–160.
Pepe J et al. Abdominal trauma in the elderly. Top Emerg Med 1993 June: 15(2):48–54.
Walker WG. Importance of blood pressure control in the preservation of renal function. South Med J 1994 Oct; 87(10): 1038–1042.
Wiseman K. Nephrotic syndrome: Pathophysiology and treatment. ANNA J 1991 Oct; 18(5):469–478.

Acute Renal Failure

Baer C and Lancaster L. Acute renal failure. Crit Care Nurs Q 1992 Feb; 14(4):1–21.
Dolleris P. Diuretic and vasopressor usage in acute renal failure: A synopsis. Crit Care Nurs Q 1992 Feb; 14(4):28–31.
Douglas S. Acute tubular necrosis: Diagnosis, treatment and nursing implications. AACN Clin Issues Crit Care 1992 Aug; 3(3): 688–697.
Hagland M. The management of acute renal failure in the intensive therapy unit. Intensive Crit Care 1993 Dec; 9(4):237–241.
Stark J. Acute renal failure in trauma: Current perspectives. Crit Care Nurs Q 1994 Feb; 16(4):49–60.
Toto K. Acute renal failure: A question of location. Am J Nurs 1992 Nov; 92(11):44–53.
Vidt DG. Recognition and management of reversible renal failure. South Med J 1994 Oct; 87(10):1018–1027.
Wood J et al. Acute postrenal failure: Reversing the problem. Nursing 1995 March; 25(3):48–50.

Chronic Renal Failure

Binkley L and Whittaker A. Erythropoietin use in the critical care setting. AACN Clin Issues Crit Care 1992 Aug; 3(3):640–649.
Brundage DJ and Swearengen PA. Chronic renal failure: Evaluation and teaching tool. ANNA J 1994 Aug; 21(5):265–270.
*Brunier G et al. The influence of physical activity on fatigue with end stage renal disease on dialysis. ANNA J 1993 Aug; 20(4): 457–462.
Brunier GM. Calcium/phosphate imbalances, aluminum toxicity, and renal osteodystrophy. ANNA J 1994 Jun; 21(4):171–179.
Buckalew VM Jr. End-stage renal disease: Can dietary protein restriction prevent it? South Med J 1994 Oct; 87(10):1034–1037.
Calkins M. Ethical issues in the elderly ESRD patient. ANNA J 1993 Oct; 20(5):569–571.
Chambers J. Renal insufficiency: Implications for care of the medical-surgical patient. Medsurg Nurs 1993 Feb; 2(1):33–40.
*Kutner N et al. Rehabilitation, aging and chronic renal disease. Am J Phys Med Rehabil 1992 Apr; 71(2):97–101.
McCormick T. Ethical issues in caring for patients with renal failure. ANNA J 1993 Oct: 20(5):549–555.
Rittman M et al. Living with renal failure. ANNA J 1993 June; 20(3):327–332.
Rosenberg M. Role of transferrin measurement in monitoring iron status during recombinant human erythropoietin therapy. Dialysis and Transpl 1992 Feb; 21(2):81–90.
Shoop KL. Pruritus in end stage renal disease. ANNA J 1994 Apr; 21(2):147–153.
Smith S. Uremic pericarditis in chronic renal failure: Nursing implications. ANNA J 1993 Aug; 30(4):432–437.

Kidney Transplantation

Beckman N et al. Kidney transplantation: A therapy option. AACN Clin Issues Crit Care 1992 Aug; 3(3):570–583.
Blanford N. Renal transplantation: A case study of the ideal. Crit Care Nurse 1993 Feb; 15(4):46–57.
Duffy MM and Nestor A. Nursing guidelines for cyclosporine. ANNA J 1993 Aug; 20(4):509–511, 514.
Dunne D. Understanding urologic stents. Nursing 1994 November; 24(11):32C–32F.
Fallon L and Lerner L. Renal transplantation. Med-Surg Nurs Q 1993 Winter; 1(3):27–37.
Hilton BA and Starzomski RC. Family decision making about living related kidney donation. ANNA J 1994 Oct; 21(6):346–355, 381.
Juneau B. Psychologic and psychosocial aspects of renal transplantation. Crit Care Nurs Qu. 1995 February; 17(4):62–66.
Lancaster L. Immunogenetic basis of tissue and organ transplantation and rejection. Crit Care Nurs Clin North Am 1992 Mar; 4(1):1–24.
Lange S. Psychosocial, legal, ethical, and cultural aspects of organ donation and transplantation. Crit Care Nurs Clin North Am 1992 Mar; 4(1):25–42.
Winsett RP. Age factors in transplantation. ANNA J 1994 Oct; 21(6):372.

Renal Calculi

Cass A. Comparison of first generation and second generation lithotriptors: Treatment results with 13,864 renal and ureteral calculi. J Urol 1995 Mar; 153(3):588–592.

Gault M et al. Bacteriology or urinary tract stones. J Urol 1995 April; 153(4):1164–1170.

Herrman E and Cockett A. Extracorporeal shock wave lithotripsy for distal ureteral stones. J Urol 1993 June; 149(6):1425–1426.

Ikari O et al. Percutaneous treatment of bladder stones. J Urol 1993 June; 140(6):1499–1500.

Kupin W. A practical approach to nephrolithiasis. Hosp Pract 1995 March 15; 30(3):37–44.

Lowe A et al. Laser lithotripsy: Patient care, staff education. AORN J 1993 Nov; 58(5):961–964, 968–969.

Mobley T et al. Low energy lithotripsy with lithostar: Treatment results with 19,962 renal and ureteral calculi. J Urol 1993 June; 149(6):1419–1423.

Ovenstein R et al. Risk factors for urinary lithotripsy associated sepsis. Infect Control Hosp Epidemiol 1993 Aug; 14(8):469–472.

Shellenbarger T and Krouse A. Treating and preventing kidney stones. Medsurg Nurs 1994 October; 3(5):389–394.

Swanson SK, Heilman RL and Eversman WG. Urinary tract stones in pregnancy. Surg Clin North Am 1995 Feb; 75(1):123–142.

Thomas R et al. An innovative approach to management of lower third ureteral calculi. J Urol 1993 June; 149(6):1427–1429.

Renal Trauma

Hughes C et al. Renal cyst rupture following blunt abdominal trauma: Case report. J Trauma: Injury, Infect Crit Care 1995 Jan; 38(1):28–29.

Nash P, Bruce J and McAninch J. Nephrectomy for traumatic renal injuries. J Urol 1995 Mar; 153(3):609–611.

Ryan CV. Genitourinary trauma and emergencies: Three common aspects. Urol Nurse 1994 Sep; 14(3):100–101.

Tumors of the Urinary Tract and Urinary Diversion

Bissada N. Urinary diversion and bladder substitution: Methods, choices and techniques. J Urol Nurs 1993 Jan–Mar; 12(1): 345–366.

Davis M. Renal cell carcinoma. Semin Oncol Nurs 1993 Nov; 9(4):267–271.

Foster R. What's new in urological cancer. J Urol Nurs 1992 June; 11(2):77–82.

Guinan et al. Renal cell carcinoma: Tumor size, stage and survival. J Urol 1995 March; 153(3):901–903.

Hanson K et al. Endourologic diagnosis and conservative management of upper tract urothelial cancer. Urol Nurse 1994 December; 14(4):159–163.

Klein E. Options in the surgical treatment of bladder cancer. J ET Nurs 1992 July/Aug; 19(4):122–125.

Moore S et al. Treating bladder cancer: New methods, new management. Am J Nurs 1993 May; 93(5):32–39.

Navan J et al. Continent urinary diversion using a modified Indiana pouch in elderly patients. Am J Surg 1994 Oct; 60(10):786–788.

Ofman U. Psychosocial and sexual implications of genitourinary cancers. Semin Oncol Nurs 1993 Nov; 9(4):286–292.

Pack R. Descriptive epidemiology of genitourinary tumors. Semin Oncol Nurs 1993 Nov; 9(4):218–223.

Ponterieri-Lewis V and Vates T. Postoperative management of patients undergoing radical cystectomy and urinary diversion. MedSurg Nurs 1993 Oct; 2(5):369–374.

*Raleigh ED et al. A comparison of adjustment to urinary diversions: A pilot study. J Wound, Ostomy Continent Nurs 1995 Jan; 22(1):58–63.

Razor B. Continent urinary reservoirs. Semin Oncol Nurs 1993 Nov; 9(4):272–285.

Stein, RG. Continent urinary diversion and the ileal cecal pouch with appendostomy: A review of nursing care. J Wound Ostomy Continent Nurs 1995 Jan; 22(1):58–63.

Theyer G et al. Role of multidrug resistance in tumors of the genitourinary tract. Urology 1994 Dec; 44(6):942–950.

*Tsukada K et al. Cranberry juice and its impact on peristomal skin conditions for urostomy patients. Ostomy Wound Manage 1994 Nov–Dec; 40(9):60–67.

Interstitial Cystitis

Czarapata B. Clinical highlights: Management of interstitial cystitis. Urology Nurse 1994 September; 14(3):145–148.

Frye K. Understanding interstitial cystitis. J Urol Nurs 1993 Jan/Mar; 12(1):367–371.

Melson G. Interstitial cystitis: Supporting and education the person with interstitial cystitis. Ostomy Wound Manage 1993 Jan/Feb; 39(1):52–54, 56, 58.

Webster D. Sex and interstitial cystitis: Explaining the pain and planning self-care. Urol Nurs 1993 Mar; 13(1):4–11.

INFORMATION/RESOURCES

Agencies

American Association of Kidney Patients
100 South Ashley Drive, Suite 280,
Tampa, FL 33602;
(813) 223-7099

American Cancer Society
1599 Clifton Rd. NE,
Atlanta, GA 30329;
(404) 320-3333

Cancer Information Service
1-800-4-CANCER

Interstitial Cystitis Association
PO Box 1553, Madison Square Garden Station,
New York, NY 10159;
(212) 979-6057

National Institute of Diabetes and Digestive and Kidney Diseases
National Institutes of Health,
Bethesda, MD 20892

National Kidney Foundation
30 East 33rd St.,
New York, NY 10016;
(212) 889-2210

National Kidney and Urologic Disorders Information Clearinghouse
Box NKUDIC, 9000 Rockville Pike,
Bethesda, MD, 20892;
(301) 468-6345

United Ostomy Association
36 Executive Park, Suite 120,
Irvine, CA 92714-6744;
(714) 660-8624

Wound, Ostomy and Continent Nurses Society (WOCN)
2755 Bristol Street, Suite 110,
Costa Mesa, CA 92626;
(714) 476-0268

Nursing Research Profile for Unit 10

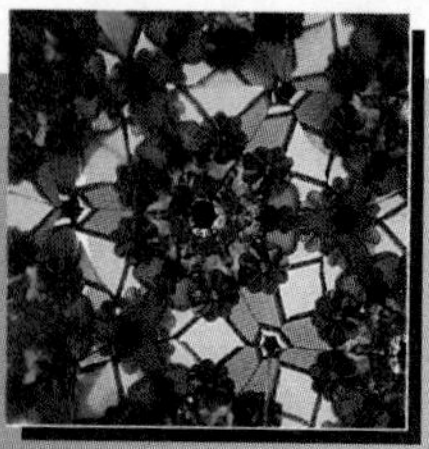

Overview

Topics that have recently received increased attention by nurse researchers have included the psychologic effects of end-stage renal disease (ESRD) and its treatment on patients and their families and their quality of life and fatigue and exercise capacity in dialysis and transplant patients.

Rittman M, et al. Living with renal failure. ANNA J 1993 Jun; 20(3):327–331.

This qualitative study addressed the meaning of living with chronic renal failure as described by the patients. Questions and statements used to guide the interviews were: (1) What is it like to live with renal failure? (2) What things stand out for you as you have learned how to live with renal failure and dialysis treatments? (3) Tell me about a time you will never forget because it taught you something about living with renal failure or being on dialysis.

Six dialysis patients, five men and one woman, were included in the study; they had been on dialysis from 3 to 14 years. Each patient was interviewed for approximately 1 hour while receiving dialysis. Interviews were audio taped, transcribed, and analyzed using methods adapted from hermeneutics, an interpretive approach to analysis.

Three common themes were uncovered. The first theme identified was "Taking on a New Understanding of Being" and addressed early responses to illness. The second theme was "Maintaining Hope" and reflected the importance of seeing possibilities in coping with chronic illness. The last of the three themes was "Dwelling in Dialysis," which relates to the feeling of being "at home" in the dialysis unit. This pattern helped the patients achieve some measure of control in an environment where there is little control. A constitutive pattern, which describes the relationship among the themes, was identified as "Control: The Meaning of Technology." This describes how technology controls bodily function and sustains life. Patients may experience a changed relationship with themselves and a detached and scientific view of themselves along with a reliance on technology.

Nursing Implications. In order to adequately care for patients, nurses must understand the lived experiences of patients who require dialysis for suvival. Recognizing and appreciating the initial experience of many patients of "Taking on a New Understanding of Being" enables the nurse to see the patient's failure to adhere to the therapeutic regimen as a natural part of the process the patient goes though rather than as noncompliance. This view suggests that different approaches to patient education are appropriate at this time. Realizing that "Maintaining Hope" will change with time, the nurse's role changes as illness progresses and the patient's hopes change. An important role of the dialysis nurse is to provide an atmosphere that facilitates hope. "Dwelling in Dialysis" points to the need for nurses to respect the patient's need for space and to incorporate this into the care plan as well as to eliminate references and inferences that dehumanize the patient.

Flaherty MJ Sr and O'Brien ME. Family styles of coping in end stage renal disease. ANNA J 1992 Aug; 19(4):345–349, 366.

The study examined the impact of dialysis on family functioning. Family members included in the study were those identified as significant by patients who were receiving in-center hemodialysis, home hemodialysis, continuous ambulatory peritoneal dialysis (CAPD), and continuous cyclic peritoneal dialysis (CCPD). The Dialysis Family Focused Interview Guide was used to collect qualitative data on 50 family members; the interview guide consisted of 17 open-ended topics related to the impact of dialysis on family functioning. The items were based on previous research and submitted to a panel of experts to establish the interview guide's content validity. Open-ended interviews, using the interview guide, were conducted and audiotaped in the family members' homes. The first interviews were conducted 6 to 8 months after patients began dialysis and were repeated at 12, 16, and 24 months.

Because some of the original 50 clients lost interest, only 20 participated in the full study of four interviews; 9 were interviewed three times and 16 interviewed twice. The sample consisted of 27 spouses, 4 parents (mothers), 10 children, 7 siblings, a niece, and a friend.

Data analysis revealed five categories of coping styles: (1) *Remote Family Style*—this style is present when respondents suggest that ESRD has not affected family members. (2) *Enfolded Family Style*—this style is encountered when family members state that ESRD has strengthened bonds among family members. (3) *Altered Family Style*—this occurs when it is reported that major changes in the families' ADL have occurred and that the patient is more dependent on the family. (4) *Distressed Family Style*—this is identified by responses of grief over ESRD and concern about the patient. (5) *Receptive Family Style*—this style occurs when there is some degree of acceptance of the situation with some adjustment to it. Few differences were found in family coping style by type of dialysis treatment.

The CCPD and CAPD groups were combined because of the small number of patients in the sample receiving CCPD. The preliminary findings of this study indicate that the remote style was the most frequent family style. This could represent denial or that the full impact of dialysis has not been felt as of yet. Some of the families in this group indicated that ESRD was the patient's and not the family's problem. The CAPD/CCPD group was the only group that demonstrated increased distress over time (from the first interview to the fourth). The enfolded family style is typified by the group of patients who dialyze at home.

Nursing Implications. Nurses must be able to identify when an individual *or* a family needs supportive services. Efforts must be made to assess the family's needs as well as those of the patient. When a family is in distress, the nurse must make the appropriate referral. When an individual or family is in distress, as would be the case in the remote family style, support from nursing and other sources may be needed. Because family stress may influence the physical well-being of the patient, family members' success at coping needs to be assessed and the plan of care changed appropriately.

Brunier G and Graydon J. The influence of physical activity on fatigue in patients with ESRD on hemodialysis. ANNA J 1993 Aug; 20(4):457–461.

Fatigue is a common complaint of patients on long-term hemodialysis. The purpose of this descriptive correlational study was to determine the contribution of inactivity to fatigue, as well as the relative influence of anemia on fatigue in patients with end-stage renal disease on dialysis. Determining whether inactivity contributes to fatigue over and above anemia would assist nurses to plan specific interventions to reduce fatigue in these patients.

Fatigue was measured by the fatigue subscale of the Profile of Mood States (POMS). Fatigue level was obtained by summing the subjects' responses (from 0 = not at all to 4 = extremely) to the five adjectives from the POMS fatigue subcale. The possible range of scores was 0 to 20 with a high score indicating a high level of fatigue. The Physical Activity Questionnaire (PAQ) was developed by the researchers to assess physical activities related to housework, work outside the home, and leisure. The energy requirements for activities assessed by the PAQ were calculated in METS (one MET equals the amount of energy needed, or oxygen taken in at rest). Examples include washing dishes (MET value of 2.1), vacuuming (MET value of 3.3), and brisk walking (MET value of 5.0). The Nonspecific Symptoms Questionnaire (NSQ) was developed by the investigators to obtain patients' rating of the frequency of 10 of the most common symptoms reported for dialysis patients. Patients were asked to rate the frequency of symptoms during the previous week using a scale of 1 (never) to 5 (always). Hematocrit levels used in the study were the most recent values obtained through regularly scheduled monthly or biweekly testing.

The sample consisted of 43 patients on hemodialysis, 22 men and 21 women. Their ages ranged from 20 to 92 years with a mean age of 52.3 years. The length of their time on hemodialysis ranged from 1.5 months to 242 months with a mean of 45.4 months. Over one-third of the sample were employed; most of these were employed full-time.

Results of the study revealed a mean score of fatigue of 6.67 (range 0–20). Men reported significantly more fatigue than did women. No relationship was found between fatigue level and length of time on hemodialysis. Most patients (75%) participated only in activities considered light household chores. There was a weak negative relationship between age and MET scores, suggesting that activity levels decline as age increases. Of the 10 symptoms identified on the NSQ, sleep disturbance was reported more frequently than any of the others.

The mean hematocrit level for the sample was 28%, with a range of 19% to 46%. About 50% of the subjects were receiving recombinant erythropoietin (Epogen) therapy; however, there were no significant relationships between level of fatigue and hematocrit level. There were significant relationships between NSQ scores and physical activity, indicating that a high level of fatigue was associated with frequent symptoms. Additionally, there was a significant relationship between fatigue scores and activity level. Subjects who had high levels of fatigue also had low levels of physical activity.

When those factors that were significantly related to fatigue were entered into multiple regression analysis to determine the contribution of each to fatigue scores, level of physical activity, symptoms, and gender together accounted for 57% of the variance in the fatigue scores.

Nursing Implications. It is important for nurses working with hemodialysis patients to carefully assess each patient for level of fatigue and amount of activity being performed. The wide range of scores obtained in this study demonstrate that not all hemodialysis patients experience the same amount of fatigue and that fatigue is an individual experience. Study results seem to indicate that anemia is not a good measure of the degree of fatigue. Inactivity, on the other hand, was found to have an influence on fatigue. Nurses can encourage hemodialysis patients to increase their activity level, either through an exercise program or by increasing household activities and activities of daily living. Relief or management of symptoms, such as sleeplessness, may help to reduce the effects of fatigue.

Dunn S, Lewis S, Bonner P, and Grochowski RM. Quality of life for spouses of CAPD patients. ANNA J 1994 Aug; 21(5):237–246.

The effect of end-stage renal disease and its treatment on patients' quality of life (QOL) is widely recognized.; however, less attention has been given to the quality of life of patients' families. Although patients are taught to perform continuous ambulatory peritoneal dialysis (CAPD) in an effort to promote their independence, the reality is that family members often assume most if not all of the management of CAPD and the care of the patient.

This descriptive correlational study was conducted to (1) describe the QOL for spouses of CAPD patients, (2) determine if there is a relationship between QOL and severity of illness, socioeconomic status, marital adjustment, and coping ability, and (3) determine which of the following was the best predictor of QOL: severity of illness, socioeconomic status, marital adjustment, and coping ability.

Spouses of CAPD patients were asked to complete the instruments. The 68-item Quality of Life Index (QLI) developed by Ferrans and Powers was used to measure QOL. This 6-point Likert Scale measures the individual's satisfaction with various domains of life and the importance of that domain to the individual. The Dyadic Adjustment Scale (DAS), a 32-item scale, was used to measure overall marital adjustment. This scale provides a total score and 4 subscale scores indicating consensus, satisfaction, affection, and cohesion. The Jalowiec Coping Scale was employed to measure coping strategies used by individuals. Forty coping strategies are identified on the questionnaire and are presented in a Likert format. The End Stage Renal Disease Severity Index was completed by nurses to categorize the disease severity of patients whose spouses agreed to participate in the study. Reliability and validity of all scales were described by the investigators. Demographic data were also collected using an instrument developed by the investigators.

Forty-one patients from two dialysis units met the criteria for eligibility; one couple refused to participate. Thirty-eight of the remaining 40 spouses of CAPD patients completed and returned the questionnaires. The mean length of time married was 29.6 years (SD = 16.1). The mean length of time on CAPD was 2.6 years (SD = 2.08). The End Stage Renal Disease Severity Index scores ranged from 1 to 49, with 96 being the highest possible score that could be achieved. The mean score for this sample was 22.3 (SD = 14.6).

An overall QLI score and four subscale scores (psychologic/spiritual, socioeconomic, health/functioning, family) were obtained, with higher scores indicating better QOL. Overall scores were categorized as good, moderate, fair, and poor quality of life. When compared with QLI scores obtained in a study of CAPD patients, QLI scores were lower in the present study. Only 28% of the spouses in the present sample scored above average on the DAS, with 38% and 34% scoring below average and average, respectively. The Jalowiec Coping Scale scores indicated that spouses used more problem-oriented than affective-oriented coping strategies.

Correlation analyses were performed on all of the total scores and subscale scores of each instrument and on selected demographic variables. There was a moderate to strong correlation between total scores of the QLI and DAS. Scores on the psychologic/spiritual subscale of the QLI and the affection subscale of the DAS were the only subscores that were not significantly correlated.

The consensus and affection subscales of the DAS were negatively correlated with the scores on the affective-oriented coping scale of the JCS; that is, the higher the affective-oriented coping scale, the lower the marital adjustment scale. High marital adjustment scores were associated with low use of affective-oriented coping strategies. Years of dialysis had a positive correlation with the affective-oriented coping scale. The ESRD severity index score correlated positively with age.

Data analysis (stepwise multiple regression) indicated that DAS score, indicating overall marital adjustment, was the best predictor of QOL, with income being the second-best predictor. Severity of illness and coping strategies were not found to be predictors of QOL.

Nursing Implications. Quality-of-life issues have received considerable attention when medical treatments for individuals with chronic illness are determined. Because of the effects of end-stage renal disease and its treatment on the quality of life of patients' spouses, the effects on spouses must also be considered. Since nurses have an important role in teaching patients and families how to care for a person with end-stage renal disease, it is important for them to be aware of the impact of illness and its treatment on the patient's family and spouse as well.

Gallagher-Lepak S. Functional capacity and activity level before and after renal transplantation. ANNA J 1991 Aug; 18(4):378–382.

Renal transplantation has traditionally been studied in terms of patient survival and self-report of activity levels and functional impairment. Few studies have addressed rehabilitation of renal transplant patients and measured activity and exercise capacity. The purpose of this study was to evaluate functional capacity and activity levels of renal transplant recipients before transplantation, 6 weeks and 16 weeks after transplantation. A descriptive study design was used to measure functional capacity during treadmill testing and self-reported activity level using the Human Activity Profile (HAP).

The sample consisted of nine renal transplant recipients, ages 23 to 60 years (mean 37.2 years). Six of the subjects were female; three were male. The treadmill portion of the exercise testing utilized a modified Naughton protocol, which is suitable for less physically fit persons. Exercise heart rate and perceived exertion ratings were recorded every 2 minutes. Peak oxygen consumption was also calculated throughout the procedure. All treadmill testing procedures followed American Heart Association standards for exercise testing.

The activity portion of the research study consisted of a paper-and-pencil test (Human Activity Profile) to measure activity level. The tool consisted of 95 activities that ranged from low to high energy demanding. Subjects were asked whether they currently perform the activity, do not perform the activity, or never performed the activity. Activity scores were then compared with age- and gender-matched normative data.

Results of the treadmill testing demonstrated a 24% improvement in functional capacity within the first 6 weeks post-transplantation and an additional 5% improvement during the 6- to 16-week period. Functional capacity was measured utilizing peak oxygen consumption and hematocrit levels. There was minimal improvement in activity level as documented on the Human Activity Profile test at the 6-week mark and greater improvement after 16 weeks. However, the activity level of most of the sample after 4 months was still extremely low (lowest tenth percentile) when compared with normative age-matched data from healthy subjects.

Nursing Implications. The results of this study, despite the small sample size, can assist nurses working with renal transplant patients. There is a need for education and exercise programs to promote increased activity for these patients. It may be necessary to reteach these long-term chronically ill patients how to be more active as part of their daily activities. Further study of functional outcomes and rehabilitation of renal transplant patients, including high-risk patients, is needed.

UNIT 11
Reproductive Function

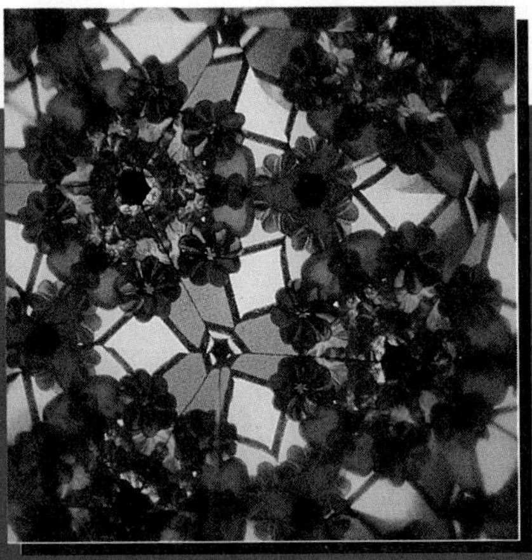

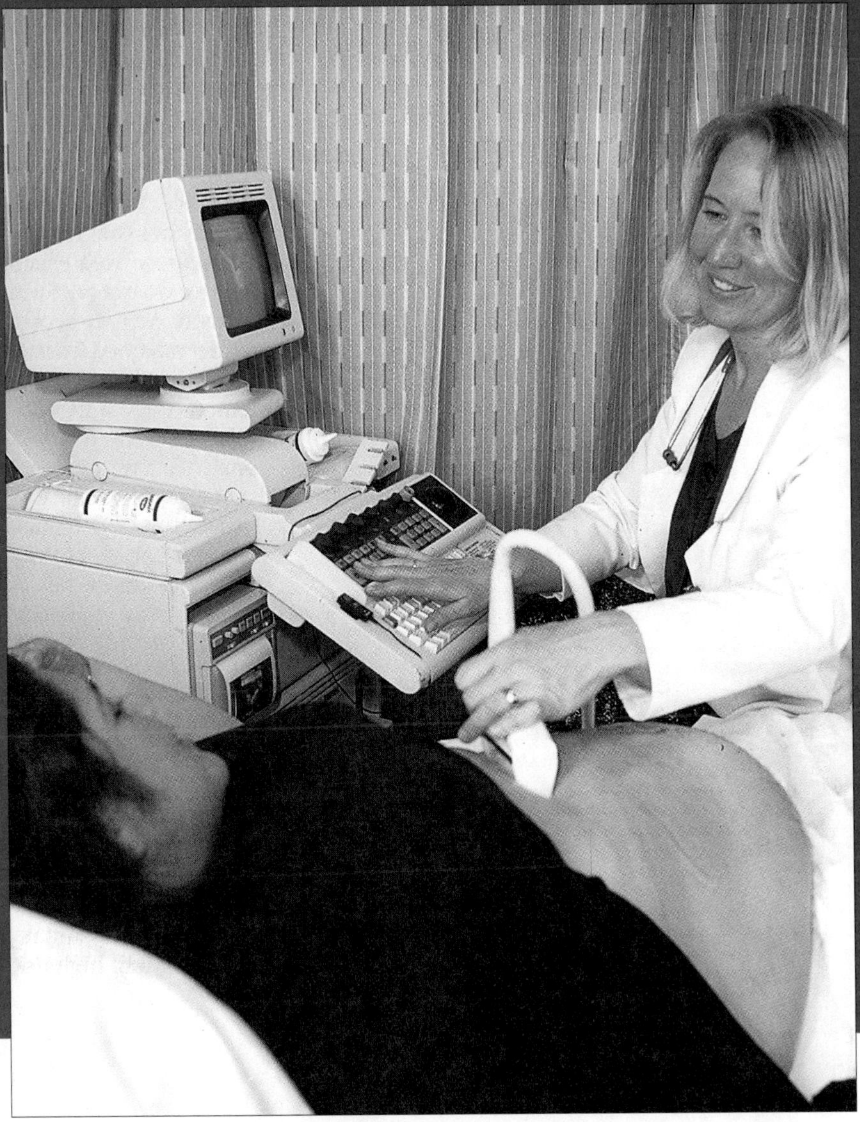

44

Assessment and Management of Patients With Problems Related to Female Physiologic Processes

CHAPTER OUTLINE

LEARNING OBJECTIVES

On completion of this chapter, the learner will be able to:

1. Describe female reproductive function
2. Describe approaches to effective sexual assessment
3. Describe indictors of domestic violence and abuse of women and methods of identification and treatment for a women who is a survivor of abuse
4. Identify the diagnostic examinations and tests used to determine alteration in female reproductive function and describe the nurse's role during these examinations and procedures
5. Describe uses of vaginal and vulvar irrigations and vaginal creams and principles that guide their use
6. Identify factors that cause disturbances of menstruation and related nursing implications
7. Use the nursing process to plan for care of patients with premenstrual syndrome
8. Develop a teaching plan for women experiencing menopause
9. Describe methods of contraception and implications for health care and education
10. Describe the nursing management of the patient having an abortion
11. Describe the causes and management of infertility
12. Use the nursing process to plan for the care of patients with ectopic pregnancies

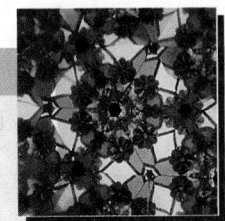

Anatomic and Physiologic Overview

The female reproductive system consists of external and internal structures.

External Genitalia

The external genitalia (the *vulva*) include two thick folds of tissue called the *labia majora* and two smaller lips of delicate tissue called *labia minora,* which lie within the labia majora. The upper portions of the labia minora unite, forming a partial covering for the *clitoris,* a highly sensitive organ composed of erectile tissue. Between the labia minora, below and posterior to the clitoris, is the urinary meatus, the external opening of the female urethra which is about 3 cm (1.5 inches) long. Below this orifice is a larger opening; the vaginal orifice or introitus (Fig. 44-1). On each side of the vaginal orifice is a *vestibular (Bartholin's) gland,* a bean-sized structure that empties its mucous secretion through a small duct. The opening of the duct lies within the labia minora, external to the hymen. The tissue between the external genitalia and the anus is the fourchette, and all of the tissue that makes up the external female genitalia is called the *perineum.*

Internal Reproductive Organs

The internal structures consist of the vagina, uterus, ovaries, and fallopian or uterine tubes (Fig. 44-2).

Vagina. The *vagina,* a canal lined with mucous membrane is 7.5 to 10 cm (3 to 4 inches) long and extends upward and backward from the vulva to the cervix. Anterior to it are the bladder and the urethra, and posterior to it lies the rectum. The anterior and posterior walls of the vagina normally touch each other. The upper part of the vagina, the *fornix,* surrounds the *cervix* (the narrow neck of the uterus).

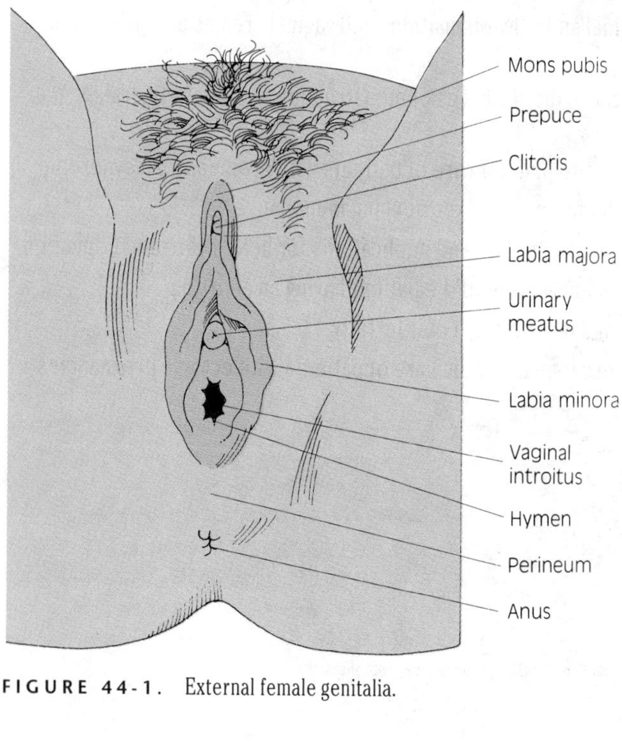

FIGURE 44-1. External female genitalia.

Uterus. The *uterus,* a pear-shaped muscular organ, is about 7.5 cm (3 inches) long and 5 cm (2 inches) wide at its upper part. Its walls are about 1.25 cm (0.5 inch) thick. The size of this organ varies depending on parity (number of viable births) and uterine abnormalities, such as fibroids, a type of tumor that may distort the uterus. A *nulliparous* woman (one who has not completed a pregnancy to the stage of fetal viability) usually has a smaller uterus than a multiparous woman (one who has completed two or more pregnancies to the stage of fetal viability).

The uterus has two parts: the *cervix,* which projects into the vagina, and a larger upper part, the *fundus* or body, which is covered posteriorly and partly anteriorly by peritoneum. The uterus lies posterior to the bladder and is held in position in the pelvic cavity by several ligaments. The *round ligaments* extend anteriorly and laterally to the internal inguinal ring and down the inguinal canal, where they blend with the tissues of the labia majora. The *broad ligaments* are folds of peritoneum extending from the lateral pelvic walls and enveloping the fallopian tubes. The *uterosacral ligaments* extend posteriorly to the sacrum.

The triangular inner portion of the fundus narrows to a small canal in the cervix that has constrictions at each end, referred to as the external os and internal os. The upper lateral parts of the uterus are called the *cornua.* From here the oviducts or *fallopian* (or *uterine*) *tubes* extend outward, their lumina continuous internally with the uterine cavity.

Ovaries. The *ovaries* lie behind the broad ligaments, behind and below the fallopian tubes. They are oval bodies about 3 cm (1.2 inches) long. At birth they contain thousands of tiny egg cells or ova. The ovaries and the fallopian tubes are called the **adnexa.**

At puberty (usually between the 12th and 14th years), the ova begin to ripen or mature. During a period known as the follicular phase, an ovum enlarges as a type of cyst known as a *graafian follicle* until it reaches the surface of the ovary, where rupture occurs. The ovum (or oocyte) is discharged into the peritoneal cavity. This periodic discharge of matured ovum is referred to as *ovulation.* The ovum usually finds its way into the fallopian tube, where it is carried to the uterus. If it meets a spermatozoon, the male reproductive cell, a union occurs and *conception* takes place. After the discharge of the ovum, the cells of the graafian follicle undergo a rapid change. Gradually they become yellow (*corpus luteum*) and produce progesterone, a hormone that prepares the uterus for receiving the fertilized ovum.

Menstruation. If conception does not occur, the ovum disintegrates and the mucous membrane lining the uterus (*endometrium*), which has become thickened and congested, becomes hemorrhagic. The upper layer of lining cells and the blood that appears in the uterine cavity are discharged through the cervix and the vagina (*menstruation*) approximately every 28 days during the reproductive years. After the menstrual flow stops, the endometrium proliferates and thickens from estrogenic stimulation, ovulation recurs, and the cycle begins again. Ovulation usually occurs

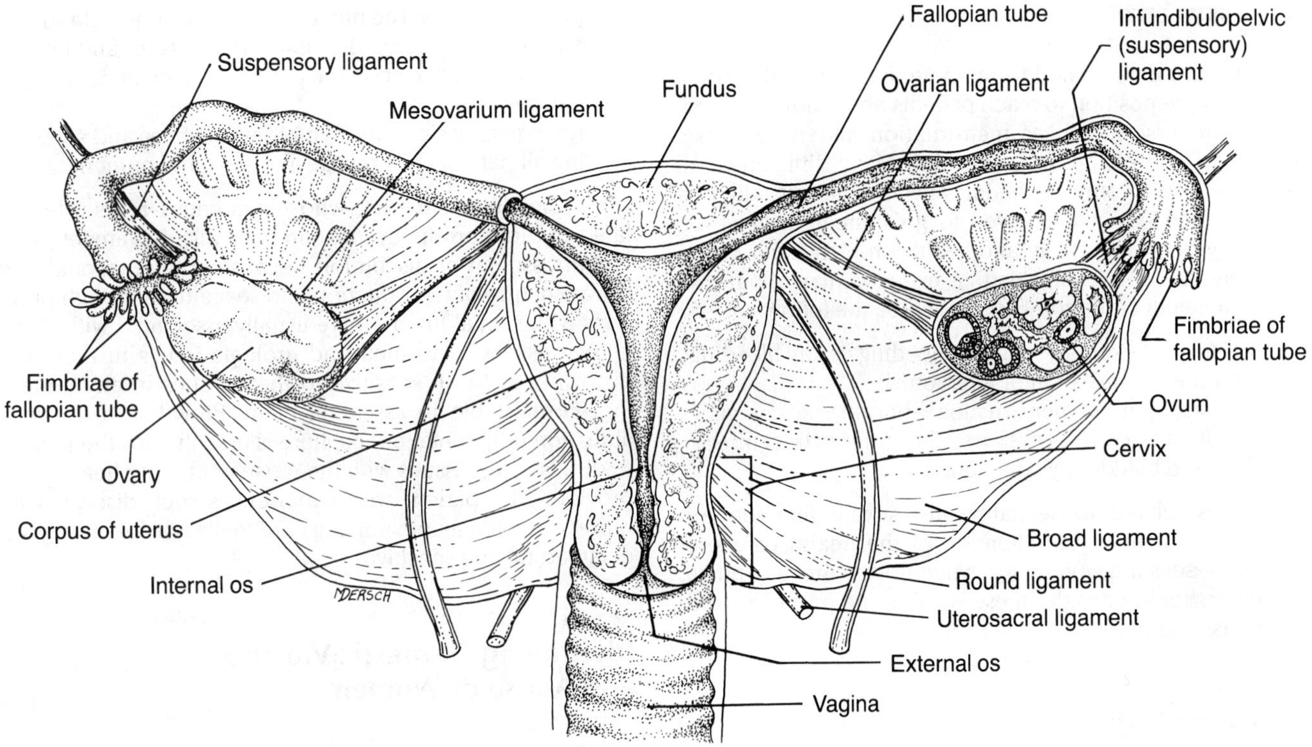

FIGURE 44-2. View of the uterus and related structures.

midway between menstrual periods. The menstrual cycle and menstrual changes are described more fully on p. 1245.

Health Maintenance

As women have increased their presence in the labor market, they have faced key changes in their roles, life-style, and family patterns. Moverover, they have encountered environmental hazards and stress prompting them to focus greater attention on health and health promoting practices. As a result, women are taking greater interest in and responsibility for their own health care. Physical exercise and competitive sports, once considered nonfeminine, are now considered therapeutic.

Other changes over the years include delaying pregnancy and childbearing until well after a career is established. Various methods of contraception have made this option possible.

As women exercise greater control of their health care options, nurses are becoming more knowledgeable about preventive care for women, particularly with regard to their unique needs. The nurse encourages female patients to determine their own health goals and behaviors, teaches about health and illness, offers interventional strategies, and provides support, counseling, and ongoing monitoring. Areas of special interest in health promotion include personal hygiene; strategies for detecting and preventing disease, especially sexually transmitted diseases (STDs), including human immunodeficiency virus (HIV) infection; and issues related to sexuality and sexual function, such as contraception; preconceptional, prenatal, and postnatal care; and menopause.

Hygiene: Patient Education

Concepts of feminine hygiene vary depending on culture. What may be considered appropriate hygiene for a European woman may be viewed differently by an American or Japanese woman. In some societies, an emphasis on cleanliness and neatness may be considered unnecessary, whereas in others climate and local customs may affect the habits practiced. Even members of the same family may have different opinions about personal habits.

Nurses need to understand the variations in attitudes and hygienic practices. Because many methods of feminine hygiene are based on traditional practices, it is necessary to apply common health sense. In some cultures, vaginal douching is viewed as a traditional practice. Modern studies of vaginal physiology, however, show no health benefit from douching; indeed, douches decease normal resistance to infection and may introduce bacteria upward, thereby increasing the likelihood of pelvic infection.

Some women may express concern about genital odor. Such odor infrequently originates from the vagina. Rather, it typically originates externally, arising from the interaction of surface bacteria and oil secreted by the vulvar skin. Significant malodor from the vagina can result from vaginitis or from a retained tampon or other foreign body, and requires examination and treatment. The nurse needs to inform female patients that the vagina is self-cleaning and that a small amount of odor or discharge is normal, although a new or different kind of discharge should be evaluated particularly if the woman has sexual intercourse with multiple partners, a new partner, or a partner who does not use condoms.

Assessment

In collecting data related to reproductive health, the nurse is in a unique position to teach patients about normal physiologic processes, such as menstruation and menopause, and to assess possible abnormalities. Many difficulties encountered by a young or middle-aged woman usually can be corrected easily. If allowed to go untreated, however, they may result in anxiety and health problems. For example, potential danger signals that every woman should report to a health care professional include the following:

- Irregular or excessive vaginal bleeding or any bleeding after menopause or after intercourse
- Persistent painful menstruation, abnormal discharge, painful intercourse (dyspareunia), urinary tract infection, and bladder dysfunction.

Issues related to sexuality and sexual function are typically brought to the attention of the health care provider who sees the woman for gynecologic care; any nurse, however, should consider these issues to be part of routine health assessment.

Sexual History

A sexual assessment is initiated by collecting both subjective and objective data. Essential information from health and sexual histories, physical examination, and laboratory findings all make significant contributions to the data base.

The purpose of a sexual history is to determine the impact of an illness on the patient's sexual health. The sexual history enables the nurse to discuss sexual matters openly and conveys to the patient the nurse's willingness to discuss sexual concerns. Additionally, it gives the patient the opportunity to express sexual concerns to an informed professional. This information can be obtained with the health history after the gynecologic/obstetric or genitourinary history is completed. By incorporating the sexual history into the general health history, the nurse can move from areas of lesser sensitivity to areas of greater sensitivity after establishing initial rapport.

Sexual history taking becomes a dynamic process reflecting an exchange of information between the patient and the nurse and providing the opportunity to clarify myths and explore areas of concern that the patient may not have felt comfortable discussing in the past.

Health Promotion

An important role of the nurse is promoting positive practices and behaviors related to the reproductive and sexual health of each patient. This includes:

- Providing information about scheduling regular examinations to promote health, detect health problems at an early stage, assess problems related to gynecologic and reproductive function, and discuss questions or concerns related to sexual function and sexuality.
- Providing an open, nonjudgmental environment that is crucial if the patient is to feel comfortable discussing personal issues. The nurse must convey understanding and sensitivity when discussing these issues and must assess their impact on the patient and the patient's partner.
- Recognizing signs and symptoms of abuse and screening all patients in a private and safe environment.

Typically, the patient who experiences a disorder related to the reproductive system feels distress, anxiety, and embarrassment or discomfort because of the personal and private nature of reproduction and sexuality. Although problems with sexual function are usually associated with gynecologic issues in women and urologic issues in men, the nurse needs to be sensitive to these issues in any patient and comfortable in assessing them. Providing a comfortable, nonjudgmental atmosphere is essential for the patient to discuss these issues with the nurse or another health care provider. The patient who experiences such disorders requires knowledgeable nursing care that always includes understanding and sensitivity.

Identifying Domestic Violence and Abuse of Women

Nurses need to be aware of the prevalence of abuse and violence directed against women in our society. Abuse can be physical, emotional-psychological, or sexual. It can involve threats or harm to children, pets, or property. Battering is related to the need to maintain control of the relationship and involves fear of one partner by another and control by threats, intimidation, and physical abuse. Because more than 6 million women experience domestic violence each year, battered women are encountered daily in nursing practice. By knowing about this major public health problem, being alert to abuse-related problems, and learning how to elicit information from women about abuse in their lives, nurses can offer intervention for a problem that might otherwise go undetected.

Some women are reluctant to disclose their involvement in an abusive relationship, which some see as their fault because the abuser has convinced them that it is. Many hope that someone will ask them about abuse and provide assistance and support. If they are not directly questioned by health professionals about abuse, women may not disclose the cause of their health problem or injuries or their true reason for seeking health care. Direct questioning is an important part of the nursing assessment. Simply asking a woman whether anyone, including her partner, is hurting her or whether she is ever afraid of her partner may encourage a woman to share her dilemma.

No specific signs or symptoms are diagnostic of battering. Nurses may see an injury that does not fit the account of how it happened; for example, a bruise on the side of the upper arm from "walking into a door." Manifestations of abuse may involve suicide attempts, drug and alcohol abuse, frequent emergency department visits, vague pelvic pain, and depression, or there may be no obvious signs or symptoms.

Violence is rarely a one-time occurrence in a relationship. It usually continues and escalates in severity. This is an important point to emphasize when a woman states that her partner has hurt her but has promised to change. Batterers can change but not without extensive counseling and motivation.

All nurses need to be familiar with local services for battered women. Once nurses ask about domestic violence, they must be prepared to offer appropriate services and referrals. After assuring the patient that she is not alone and stating the belief that no one deserves to be harmed, the nurse should document the incident and refer the patient to the appropriate resources and services.

The National Coalition Against Domestic Violence has information on local shelters in all states and is listed at the end of this chapter. Nurses can also call local shelters for pamphlets describing their services. Placing these pamphlets in waiting rooms, rest rooms, pamphlet racks, and other public areas ensures that the information is widely available. Every health care setting should have a pamphlet rack with information about abuse and appropriate resources and services. Some nurses have found that by leaving literature on domestic violence in the rest room, patients are more likely to take it home to read than to read it in a waiting room with other patients.

Incest and Childhood Sexual Abuse

Many women have survived incest or other sexual abuse as children. Some suffer posttraumatic stress syndrome as a result. Because they are typically told by a family member to keep the abuse a secret, and because many fear family breakup as a result of disclosure, incest and other childhood sexual abuse may remain a secret until adulthood.

It has been reported that female victims of incest have more health problems and undergo more surgery than women who were never victimized. Victims of childhood sexual abuse are reported to experience more chronic depression, morbid obesity, marital instability, gastrointestinal (GI) problems, headaches, and greater use of health care services than do nonvictims. Because more than one in five women are incest survivors, nurses must be aware that many women with health problems may have experienced childhood sexual abuse. Nurses should be prepared to offer support and referral to psychologists, community resources and self-help groups.

Pelvic Examination

An annual breast and pelvic examination is important for all women who are 18 years of age or older and those who are sexually active, regardless of age. The patient deserves empathy and understanding because of the emotional and physical considerations associated with gynecologic examinations. Women may be sensitive about or embarrassed by the usual questions asked by a gynecologic health care provider. Because gynecologic conditions are of a personal and private nature to most women such information is shared only with those directly involved in patient care (as is true with all patient information). Nursing ethics, patient trust, and legal liability demand confidentiality. Whereas many women are apprehensive about gynecologic examinations, women who have been abused, raped, or victimized by incest may be intensely apprehensive and nervous about them. The nurse can provide anxiety-reducing reassurance and support. Women who seem more apprehensive than usual should be asked about a history of abuse.

Throughout the examination, procedures to be performed are explained. This not only encourages the woman to relax but also provides an opportunity for her to ask questions and minimizes the negative reactions that many women associate with gynecologic examinations.

The pelvic examination is a facet of physical assessment that may be performed by the advanced practice nurse. Competency can be attained with proper training and supervision.

Before the examination begins, the patient is instructed to void. This ensures patient comfort and eases the examination. A full bladder can make palpating pelvic organs uncomfortable for the patient and difficult for the examiner. At this time, the nurse may obtain a urine specimen if such tests are part of the total assessment.

Positioning

Although several positions may be used for the pelvic examination, the supine lithotomy position is used most commonly, although the upright lithotomy position in which the woman assumes a semisitting posture may also be used. This position offers several advantages: (1) it is more comfortable; (2) it allows better eye contact between patient and examiner; (3) it may provide an easier means for the examiner to carry out the bimanual examination; and (4) it enables the woman to use a mirror to see her anatomy (if she chooses) to visualize any conditions that require treatment or to learn about using certain types of contraceptive methods.

If the patient is too ill, disabled, or neurologically impaired to lie on a table with stirrups, the Simms's position may be used. In the Simms's position, the patient lies on her left side with her right leg bent at a 90-degree angle. The right labia may be retracted for adequate access to the vagina.

In the supine lithotomy position, the patient lies on the table with her feet on foot rests; she is encouraged to relax so that her buttocks are positioned at the edge of the examination table, and she is asked to relax and spread her thighs as widely apart as possible. Most patients, despite appropriate draping, feel embarrassed. The following equipment is obtained and readily available: a good light source, a vaginal speculum; clean examination gloves; lubricant, spatula, cytobrush, glass slides, fixative solution or spray, and diagnostic testing supplies for screening for occult rectal blood if the woman is over age 40.

Inspection and Findings

When the patient is prepared, the examiner inspects the labia majora and minora; noting epidermal tissue of the labia majora, with hair follicles characteristic of skin that fades to the pink mucous membrane of the vaginal introitus. In the nulliparous woman, the labia minora come together at the opening of the vagina. In women who have delivered children vaginally, the labia minora may gape, and vaginal tissue may protrude.

To identify such protrusions, the examiner asks the patient to "bear down." Trauma to the anterior vaginal wall during childbirth may have resulted in incompetency of musculature, so that a bulge caused by the bladder intruding into the submucosa of the anterior vaginal wall may be seen. This is called a **cystocele.** Childbirth trauma also may have affected the posterior vaginal wall, so that a bulge caused by rectal cavity protrusion may be seen. This is called a **rectocele.** Moreover, the cervix may descend under pressure through the vaginal canal and be seen at the introitus. This is called **uterine prolapse** (see Chapter 45 for a discussion of these structural changes).

The introitus should be free of superficial mucosal lesions. The labia minora may be separated by the fingers of the gloved hand and the lower part of the vagina palpated. In virginal women, a **hymen** of variable thickness may be felt circumferentially within 1 or 2 cm of the vaginal opening. The hymenal ring usually permits the insertion of two fingers but occasionally is sufficiently restricting so that only one finger may enter the vagina. Rarely, the hymen totally occludes the vaginal entrance (imperforate hymen.)

In nonvirginal women, a rim of scar tissue representing the remnants of the hymenal ring may be felt circumferentially around the vagina near its opening. The greater vestibular glands (Bartholin's glands) lie between the labia minora and the remnants of the hymenal ring. In some patients, one of these glands may be abscessed, which can cause discomfort and require incision and drainage.

Speculum Examination and Findings

Assorted sizes of the bivalved speculum are available in metal and plastic. Either should be warmed with a heating pad or warm water to make insertion more comfortable for the patient. The speculum is not lubricated because commercial lubricants may interfere with cervical cytology (Papanicolaou [Pap] smear) findings. The metal speculum has two setscrews. One is along the handle and holds the two valves of the speculum together; this one is tightened. The setscrew that holds the thumb rest in place is loosened. The speculum is grasped in the dominant hand, with the thumb against the back of the thumb rest to keep the tips of the valves closed.

The speculum is rotated slightly counterclockwise and the vaginal orifice is held open by the thumb and the forefinger of the gloved nondominant hand by some examiners. Other examiners find that straight insertion of a speculum with downward pressure on the vagina is more comfortable for the patient.

The speculum is gently inserted into the posterior portion of the introitus and slowly advanced to the top of the vagina; this should not be painful or uncomfortable for the woman. The tip of the speculum may then be elevated and the speculum rotated to a transverse position. The speculum is then slowly opened and the setscrew of the thumb rest tightened to hold the speculum open (Fig. 44-3).

Cervix. The cervix is inspected. In nulliparous women, the cervical os is 2 to 3 cm wide and smooth. Women who have borne children may have a laceration, usually transverse, giving the cervical os a "fishmouth" appearance. Moreover, epithelium from the endocervical canal may have grown onto the surface of the cervix, appearing as beefy red surface epithelium circumferentially around the os.

Abnormal Growth. Malignant changes may not be obviously differentiated from the rest of the cervical mucosa. Small, benign cysts may appear on the cervical surface. These are usually bluish or white and are called **nabothian cysts.** A **polyp** of endocervical mucosa may protrude through the os and usually is dark red. Polyps can cause irregular bleeding; they are rarely malignant and usually are removed easily in an office or clinic setting. A **carcinoma**

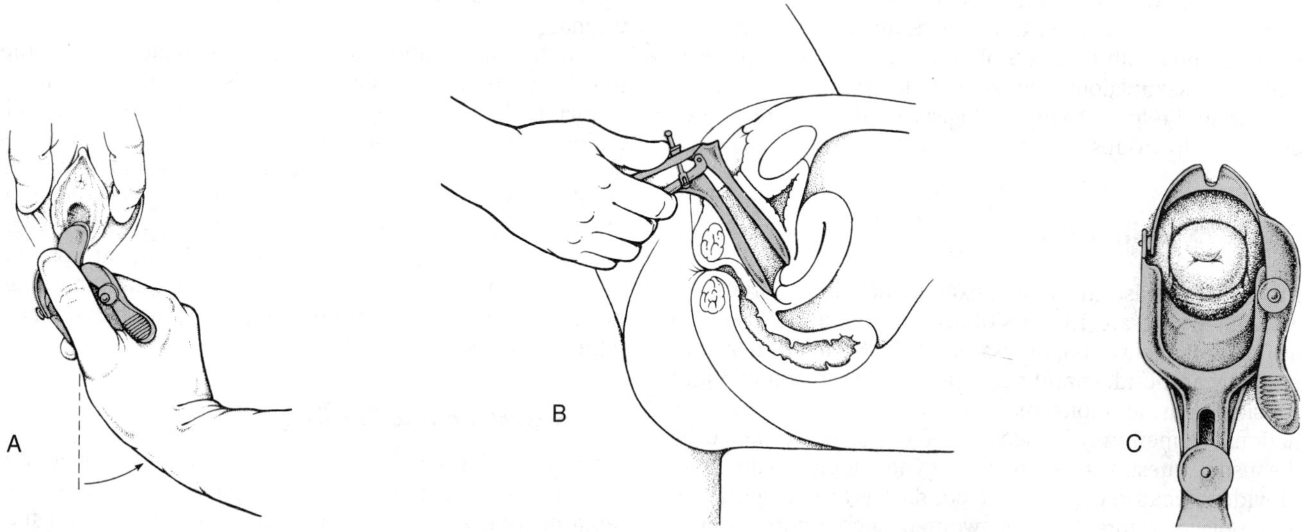

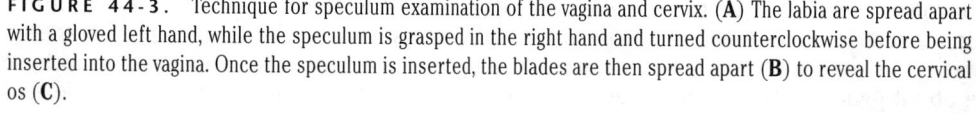

FIGURE 44-3. Technique for speculum examination of the vagina and cervix. (**A**) The labia are spread apart with a gloved left hand, while the speculum is grasped in the right hand and turned counterclockwise before being inserted into the vagina. Once the speculum is inserted, the blades are then spread apart (**B**) to reveal the cervical os (**C**).

may appear as a cauliflower-like growth that bleeds easily when touched. Blueness of the cervix is a sign of early pregnancy (Chadwick's sign).

DES Influences. From 1940 to 1971, diethylstilbestrol (DES) was given orally to prevent miscarriage in some women experiencing bleeding in pregnancy. Although this medication was effective in many cases, it has been associated with genital abnormalities in both female and male offspring. One of every thousand females exposed to DES *in utero* may develop vaginal or cervical clear cell adenocarcinoma. In assessing female patients born during this period, the nurse should ask the patient about this possibility.

Occasionally, the cervix of a woman whose mother took DES has a hooded appearance (a peaked aspect superiorly or a ridge of tissue surrounding it) and is evaluated by colposcopy when identified. DES exposure also has resulted in cryptorchidism (undescended testicles), testicular hypoplasia, and increased incidence of epididymal cysts in male offspring. Women who took DES to preserve a threatened pregnancy may be at greater risk for breast cancer and should be advised to consult their health care provider regarding appropriate breast screening.

Pap Smear. During the pelvic examination, a Pap smear is obtained by rotating a small wooden spatula at the os, followed by a cervical brush rotated in the os. The tissue obtained is spread on a glass slide and sprayed or fixed immediately.

A specimen of any purulent material appearing at the cervical os is obtained for culture. The examiner uses a sterile cotton-tipped applicator to obtain the specimen, which is immediately placed in an appropriate medium for transfer to a laboratory. In patients at high-risk for infection, routine cultures for gonococcal and chlamydial organisms are advocated because of the high incidence of both diseases and the high risk for pelvic infection, fallopian tube damage, and subsequent infertility.

Vaginal Discharge. Vaginal discharge, which may be normal or a result of vaginitis, may be present. Discharge caused by bacteria (bacterial vaginosis, or BV) usually appears gray and purulent. Discharge caused by *Trichomonas* is usually frothy, copious, and malodorous. Discharge caused by *Candida* is thick and white-yellow and has a cottage-cheese appearance.

The vagina is inspected as the examiner withdraws the speculum. It is smooth in young girls and thickens after puberty, with many rugae (folds) and redundancy in the epithelium. In menopausal women, the vagina thins and has fewer rugae because of decreased estrogen.

Bimanual Examination and Findings

To complete the pelvic examination, the examiner performs a bimanual examination from a standing position. The examination is performed with the forefinger and middle finger of the gloved and lubricated hand. These fingers are placed in the vaginal orifice, while the other fingers are held tightly out of the way, with the thumb completely adducted. The fingers are advanced vertically along the vaginal canal and the vaginal wall is palpated. Any firm part of the vaginal wall may represent old scar tissue from childbirth trauma but may also require further evaluation.

Cervical Palpation. The cervix is palpated and assessed for its consistency, mobility, size, and position. The normal cervix is uniformly firm but not hard. Softening of the cervix is a finding in early pregnancy. Hardness may reflect invasion by a neoplasm. Normally, the cervix and uterus are freely movable.

Pain on gentle movement of the cervix is called a positive **chandelier sign** or positive cervical motion tenderness (+ CMT) and usually indicates a pelvic infection. Fixation of the uterus in the pelvis may be a sign of endometriosis or malignancy. The body of the uterus is normally twice the diameter and twice the length of the cervix, curving anteriorly toward the abdominal wall. Some women have a retroverted or retroflexed uterus, which tips posteriorly toward the sacrum, while others have a uterus that is neither anterior or posterior but is midline.

Uterine Palpation. To palpate the uterus, the examiner places the opposite hand halfway between the patient's umbilicus and the pubis and presses firmly toward the vagina (Fig. 44-4). Movement of the abdominal wall causes the body of the uterus to descend, and the pear-shaped organ becomes freely movable between the abdominal examining hand and the examining fingers of the pelvic examining hand.

An accurate impression can be gained of uterine size, mobility, and contour through palpation. Nurse practitioners, nurse midwives, and physicians obtain this skill after performing many examinations with supervision.

Adnexal Palpation. Next, the right and left adnexal areas are palpated to evaluate the fallopian tubes and ovaries. The fingers of the hand examining the pelvis are moved first to one side, then to the other, while the hand palpating the abdominal area is moved correspondingly to either side of the abdomen and downward. The adnexa (ovaries and fallopian tubes) are trapped between the two hands and palpated for an obvious mass, tenderness, and mobility.

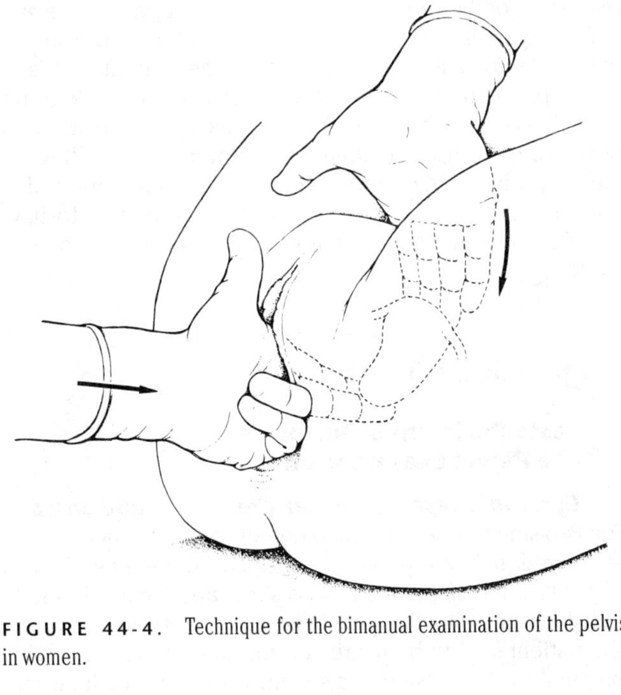

FIGURE 44-4. Technique for the bimanual examination of the pelvis in women.

Commonly the ovaries are slightly tender and the patient needs to be assured that slight discomfort on palpation is normal.

Vaginal and Rectal Palpation. Bimanual palpation of the vagina and cul-de-sac is accomplished by placing the index finger in the vagina and the middle finger in the rectum. To prevent cross-contamination between the vaginal and rectal orifices the examiner puts on new gloves. A gentle movement of these fingers toward each other compresses the posterior vaginal wall and the anterior rectal wall and assists the examiner in identifying the integrity of these structures. In this procedure the patient may sense an urge to defecate. The nurse needs to assure the patient that this will not occur. Ongoing explanations are reassuring, comforting, and educational.

Gerontologic Considerations

Frequent examinations can help in preventing problems of the reproductive tract in the aging female. Often, older women do not have regular gynecologic examinations; and some who have delivered their children at home have never had a pelvic examination. Some regard it as an embarrassing and unpleasant procedure. The role of the nurse in emphasizing an annual pelvic examination for *all* women is of major health teaching significance. The nurse can make the examination a time for education and reassurance, rather than a time of embarrassment.

Perineal pruritus is not an uncommon symptom in the older woman and should be evaluated as it may indicate a possible disease process (diabetes or malignancy). It may also indicate vulvar dystrophy. Dystrophies appear as thickened or whitish discoloration of perineal tissue and need biopsy to rule out abnormal cells suggesting cancer. Topical cortisone and testosterone creams may be prescribed for symptomatic relief.

With relaxing pelvic musculature, uterine prolapse and relaxation of the vaginal walls can occur. Appropriate evaluation and surgical repair can provide relief if the patient is a candidate for surgery. After surgery, the patient needs to know that tissue repair and healing may require additional time. Pessaries, which are latex devices that provide support, are often used if surgery is contraindicated. They are fitted by a health care provider and may reduce discomfort and pressure. Using a pessary requires the patient to have routine gynecologic checkups to monitor for irritation or infection.

Diagnostic Evaluation

Tests Performed During the Pelvic Examination

Cytologic Test for Cancer (Papanicolaou Smear). The Pap smear is performed to detect cervical cancer. Cervical secretions are aspirated or scraped from the cervical os (Fig. 44-5), transferred to a glass slide, and "fixed" immediately by immersing the slide in or spraying it with a fixative. The patient should be instructed not to douche before this examination because doing so can wash away cellular material. The Pap smear should be performed when the patient is not menstruating because blood usually interferes with an accurate interpretation. Guideline 44-1 describes the proper technique for obtaining a cervical specimen for cytologic smear.

Traditionally the Papanicolaou classification of cytologic findings was a numerical range from Class I to Class V, with I being normal and V being malignant. A more descriptive classification system, without number, has been developed, using the following terms: normal; inflammation; atypia (not typical); koilocytosis (a change in cells affected by human papillomavirus [HPV]); mild, moderate, or severe dysplasia; and invasive carcinoma.

Other terminology includes the following categories: *low-grade squamous intraepithelial lesion (LGSIL),* which is equivalent to cervical intraepithelial neoplasia (CIN) type I and to changes related to exposure to HPV. *High-grade squamous intraepithelial lesion* (HGSIL) equates to CIN III and carcinoma *in situ* (CIS). These new terms are seen on Pap smear findings and encompass all precursors to invasive carcinoma of the cervix. These diagnostic terms are described more fully in Table 44-1.

Pap smears that reveal mild inflammation or atypical squamous cells are usually repeated in 3 to 6 months, with findings often returning to normal. Patients are apprehensive, because most women incorrectly assume that an abnormal Pap smear means cancer.

Colposcopy and Cervical Biopsy. All suspicious Pap smears should be evaluated by colposcopy. The *colposcope* is an optical instrument, a portable microscope (magnification from 10 to 25 times), that allows the examiner to visualize the cervix and obtain a sample of abnormal tissue for analysis. Nurse practitioners and gynecologists require special training in this diagnostic technique.

After inserting a speculum and visualizing the cervix and vaginal walls, the examiner applies acetic acid to the cervix. Subsequent abnormal findings that indicate the need for biopsy include leukoplakia (white plaque visible before applying acetic acid), aceto-white tissue (white epithelium after applying acetic acid), punctation (dilated capillaries occurring in a dotted or stippled pattern), mosaicism (a tilelike pattern), and atypical vascular patterns.

An *endocervical currettage (ECC)* is also performed. This analysis of tissue from the cervical canal is performed to determine whether abnormal changes have occurred in the cervical canal. If these biopsy specimens show premalignant cells or cervical intraepithelial neoplasia, the patient usually needs cryotherapy or a cone biopsy (excision of an inverted tissue cone from the cervix).

Cryotherapy. Cryotherapy (freezing cervical tissue with nitrous oxide) and laser treatment are used in the outpatient setting. Cryotherapy may result in cramping and occasional feelings of faintness (vasovagal response). A watery discharge is normal for a few weeks after the procedure.

Cone Biopsy. If the ECC findings indicate abnormal changes or if the lesion extends into the canal, The patient may undergo a cone biopsy. This can be performed surgically or with a procedure called LEEP (loop electrosurgical excision procedure), which uses a laser beam.

Usually performed in the outpatient setting, LEEP is associated with a high success rate in removal of abnormal

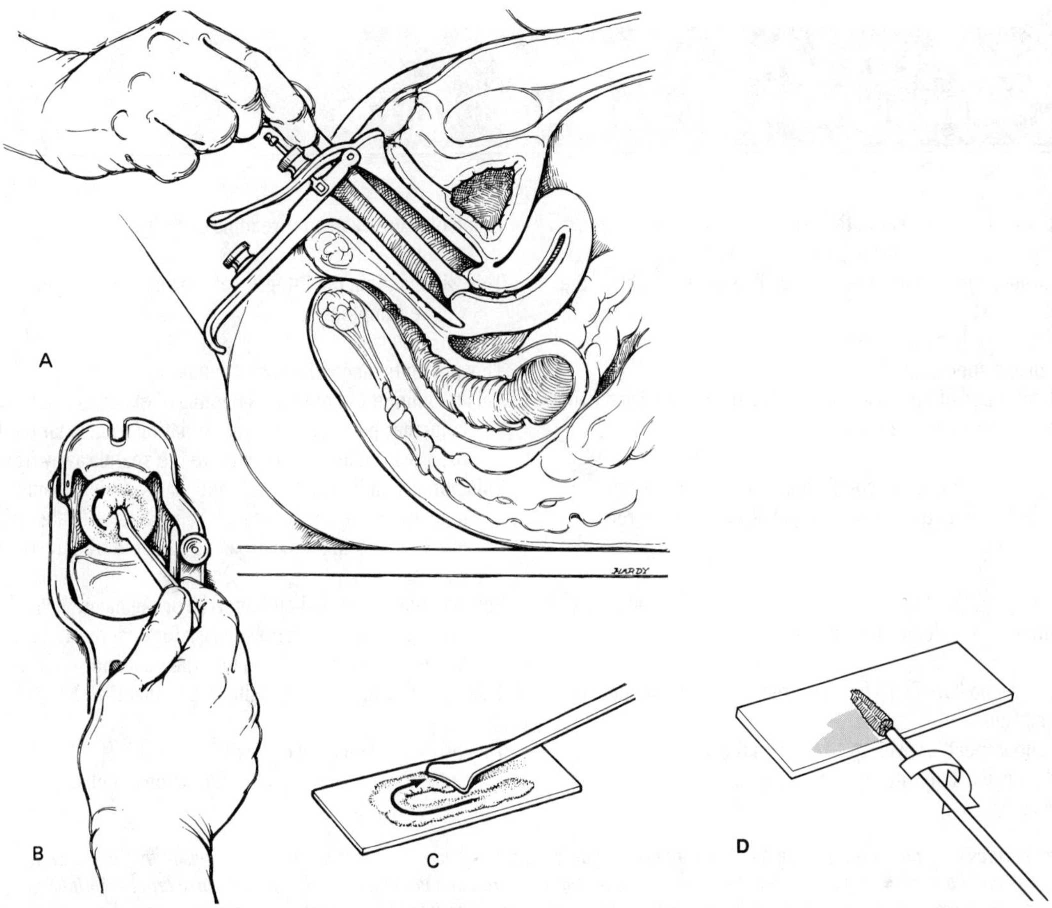

FIGURE 44-5. Method of using a wooden Ayre spatula to obtain cervical secretions for cytology. (**A**) Speculum in place and the Ayre spatula in position at the cervical os. (**B**) The tip of the spatula is placed in the cervical os and the spatula rotated 360 degrees, firmly but nontraumatically. (**C**) Cellular material clinging to the spatula is then smeared smoothly on a glass slide, which is promptly placed in a fixative solution. (**D**) Cytobrush is rotated in the cervical os and rolled onto a glass slide.

cervical tissue and low incidence of complications. The surgeon excises a small porition of the cervix and the pathologist examines the borders of the specimen to determine if they are free of disease. A patient anesthetized for a surgical cone biopsy is advised to rest for 24 hours after the procedure and to leave any vaginal packing in place until the physician removes it (usually the next day). The patient should report any excessive bleeding to the health care provider.

Additional treatment options are discussed and relate to the extent of the lesion, the preferences of the patient, and the skills of the physician. Guidelines regarding postoperative sexual activity, bathing, and other activities are provided by the nurse or the physician. Because open tissue may be potentially exposed to HIV and other pathogens, the patient is usually cautioned to use condoms when resuming sexual activity until healing is complete and verified at follow-up.

Endometrial (Aspiration) Smears and Biopsy. A tissue sample obtained and analyzed directly from the endometrium is an accurate method of diagnosing cellular changes in the endometrium.

Endometrial biopsy, a common method of obtaining endometrial tissue, is performed during the gynecologic pelvic examination as an outpatient procedure. Usually it can be performed without anesthesia; however, a paracervical block is effective if required. In this procedure, the examiner may apply a tenaculum (a clamplike instrument that stabilizes the uterus) after the pelvic examination and then inserts a thin, hollow, flexible tube (pipette) through the cervix into the uterus.

Suction also may be used for retrieving endometrial tissue for laboratory analysis. This procedure is a tolerable and accurate outpatient method for evaluating the endometrium and is usually indicated in cases of midlife irregular bleeding, postmenopausal bleeding, infertility (to identify changes in the uterine lining after ovulation), and in some women on hormone replacement therapy.

Dilatation and Curettage

During a dilatation and curettage (D&C), which may be both diagnostic and therapeutic, the cervical canal is widened with a dilator and the uterine endometrium is scraped with a curette. The purpose of the procedure is to secure endometrial or endocervical tissue for cytologic examination, to control abnormal uterine bleeding, and as a therapeutic measure for incomplete abortion.

GUIDELINE 44–1
Method for Obtaining an Optimal Pap Smear

Technique	Rationale
1. Do not obtain a Pap smear in the presence of menses or frank bleeding (exception: high suspicion of neoplasia).	Blood obscures a proper reading of cells.
2. If performing more than one test (*e.g.*, Pap and GC), obtain the Pap smear first.	This will maintain the integrity of the superficial layer of cells that will be sampled.
3. Label frosted end of slide with pencil.	Ink rubs off glass.
4. Gently insert speculum.	This prevents discomfort and trauma.
5. Place longer end of the Ayre spatula* in cervical canal and firmly scrape the exocervix in a full circle.	This technique will obtain a sampling of exocervix and squamocolumnar junction. (If transformation zone is far out from the os, it may be necessary to move the spatula away from the os.)
6. Insert a saline-moistened cotton-tipped applicator or cytobrush† 2–3 cm into endocervical canal. Rotate 180 degrees and roll out onto a slide.	This obtains endocervical cells and may sample squamocolumnar junction in the cervical canal. Saline prevents absorption of cells into the cotton, thus increasing the yield transferred to the slide.
7. Obtain a vaginal pool sample from the posterior vaginal fornix. (Essential if a suspicious lesion is present.)	This sample may reveal endometrial or vaginal wall cancer. Women over age 45 are at increased risk for endometrial cancer, and these cells might be shed into the posterior fornix.
8. For women who have had a hysterectomy, obtain a sample from the vaginal cuff.	This sampling may detect vaginal wall cancer.
9. Do not rub, repeat, or overlap strokes on the slide.	This prevents damaging or destroying cells.
10. Immediately fix slide with cytologic fixative or place in a jar of 95% alcohol.	Exposure to air or light causes distortion of cells.

**An Ayre spatula is a small wooden spatula with a forked end that is universally available in gynecologic settings in the United States. (Fullerton JT and Barger MK. Papanicolaou smear: An update on classification and management. J Am Acad Nurse Pract 1989 Jul/Sep; 1[3]:86.)*
†Some care providers recommend use of the spatula before the use of the cytobrush to obtain a better sample, as the cytobrush often causes slight bleeding. The spatula obtains cells at the squamocolumnar junction, whereas the brush or swab collects endocervical cells. Both components are necessary for an adequate sampling.

TABLE 44-1 Comparison of Five Classifications of the Pap Smear

Interpretation of Result	Numerical System	Dysplasia Cytologic Classification	Cervical Intraepithelial Neoplasia Classification	Dyskariosis Classification	Bethesda Classification
Negative	Class I	Negative; squamous metaplasia	No designation	Negative	Negative
	Class II	Atypical squamous metaplasia			Atypical squamous cells
Suspicious		Mild dysplasia	CIN I	Borderline	Low-grade squamous intraepithelial lesion*
	Class III	Moderate dysplasia	CIN II	Mild Moderate	
Probable	Class IV	Severe dysplasia Carcinoma *in situ*	CIN III	Severe	High-grade squamous intraepithelial lesion*
Positive	Class V	←------Invasive carcinoma------→			

*The Bethesda working group (1989) suggests that "these two terms encompass the spectrum of terms currently used to delineate the squamous cell precursors to invasive squamous carcinoma, including the grades of CIN, the degrees of dysplasia, and carcinoma in situ."
(Fullerton JT and Barger MK. Papanicolaou smear: An update on classification and management. J Am Acad Nurs Pract 1989 Jul/Sep; 1[3]:87.)

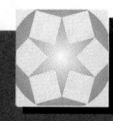

Because this procedure is usually carried out under anesthesia and requires surgical asepsis, it is usually performed in the operating room. However, it may also take place in the outpatient setting with the patient receiving a local anesthetic, supplemented with diazepam (Valium), midazolam (Versed), or meperidine (Demerol).

The nurse usually provides an explanation of the procedure as well as physical and psychological preparation, informing the patient about what the procedure involves and what to expect in the way of postoperative discomfort and bleeding. The perineum is not shaved, but the patient void is instructed prior to the procedure.

The patient is placed in the lithotomy position, the cervix is dilated with an instrument, and endometrial scrapings are obtained by a curette. A perineal pad is placed over the perineum after the procedure and evidence of excessive bleeding is reported. No restrictions are placed on dietary intake. If pelvic discomfort or low back pain occurs, mild analgesics usually provide relief. The physician indicates when sexual intercourse may be safely resumed. To reduce the risk of infection and bleeding, most physicians advise no vaginal penetration for 2 weeks.

Endoscopic Examinations

Laparoscopy (Pelvic Peritoneoscopy). A laparoscopy involves inserting a laparoscope (a tube about 10 mm wide and similar to a small periscope) into the peritoneal cavity through a 2-cm (0.75 inch) incision below the umbilicus to allow visualization of the pelvic structures (Fig. 44-6) Indications for laparoscopy are diagnostic (*e.g.*, in cases of pelvic pain when no cause can be found). Laparoscopy also facilitates minor operative procedures, such as tubal sterilization, ovarian biopsy, and lysing adhesions (scar tissue that can cause pelvic discomfort). A surgical instrument (intrauterine sound or cannula) may be positioned inside the uterus to permit manipulation or movement of the uterus during laparoscopy, affording better visualization.

A better view of the pelvic, lower abdominal, and visceral contents is obtained by injecting a prescribed amount of carbon dioxide intraperitoneally into the cavity. Called *insufflation,* this technique separates the intestines from the pelvic organs. If the patient has requested sterilization, the fallopian or uterine tubes may be electrocoagulated and a segment removed for histologic verification. (Clips are an alternative device for occluding tubes.) Once the laparoscopy is completed, the laparoscope is withdrawn, carbon dioxide is allowed to escape through the outer cannula, the small skin incision is closed with sutures or a clip, and the incision is covered with an adhesive bandage.

The patient is carefully observed for several hours to detect any untoward signs indicating bleeding, injury, or possible burns from the coagulator. These complications rarely occur, however, making laparoscopy a cost-effective and safe outpatient procedure.

Hysteroscopy. Hysteroscopy (transcervical intrauterine endoscopy) allows direct visualization of all parts of the uterine cavity by means of a lighted optical instrument. The procedure is best performed about 5 days after menstruation stops in the estrogenic phase of the menstrual cycle. The vagina and vulva are cleaned and a paracervical anesthetic block is performed. The instrument used for the procedure, a hysteroscope, is passed into the cervical canal and advanced 1 or 2 cm under direct vision. Uterine-distending fluid (normal saline solution or 5% dextrose in water) is infused through the instrument to dilate the uterine cavity and enhance visibility.

Hysteroscopy is most commonly indicated as an adjunct to a D&C and laparoscopy in cases of infertility, unexplained bleeding, retained intrauterine device (IUD), and recurrent early pregnancy loss. Treatment for some conditions (*e.g.*, fibroid tumors) can be accomplished during

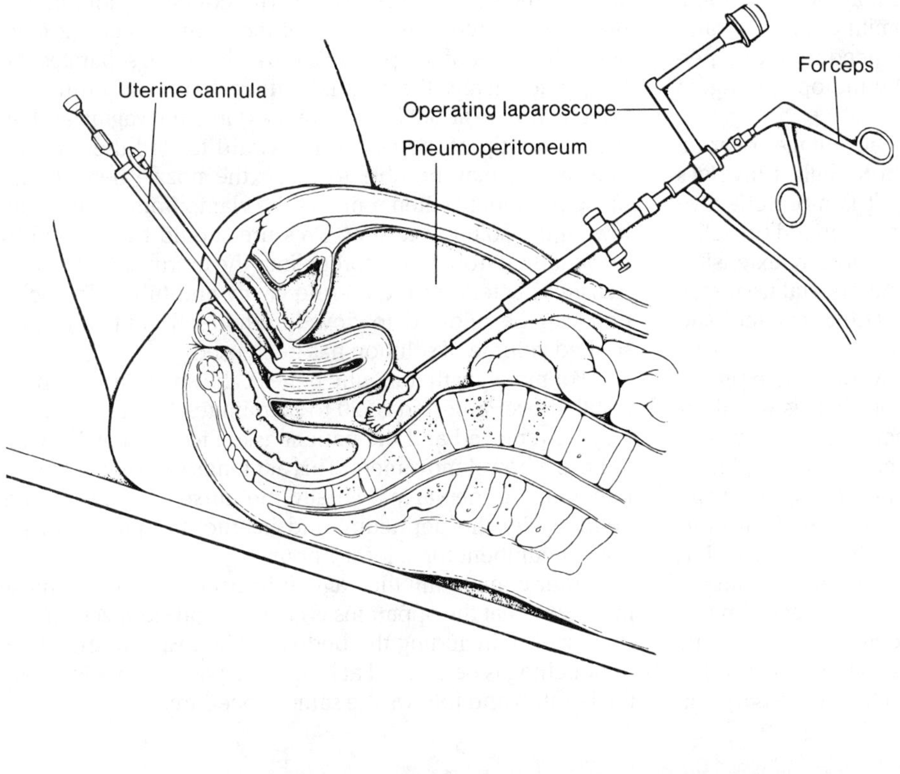

FIGURE 44-6. Laparoscopy. The laparoscope (**right**) is inserted through a small incision in the abdomen. A forceps is inserted through the scope to grasp the fallopian tube. To improve the view, a uterine cannula (**left**) is inserted into the vagina to push the uterus upward. Insufflation of gas creates an air pocket (pneumoperitoneum), and the pelvis is elevated (note the angle), which forces the intestines higher in the abdomen.

this procedure. Hysteroscopy is containdicated in patients with cervical or endometrial carcinoma or acute pelvic inflammation. Endometrial ablation (destruction of the uterine lining) is performed with a hysteroscope and laser beam in cases of severe bleeding that do not respond to other therapies. Performed in an outpatient setting, this rapid procedure is an alternative to hysterectomy for some patients.

Diagnostic Procedures

Many diagnostic procedures are helpful in evaluating pelvic conditions. These may include x-ray, barium enemas, gastrointestinal x-ray series, intravenous urography, and cystography studies. Additionally, because the uterus, ovaries, and fallopian tubes are near the kidneys, ureters, and bladder, urologic diagnostic studies, such as the KUB (kidney, ureter, and bladder) and pyelogram are used, as are angiography and radioisotope scanning, if needed. Other diagnostic procedures include hysterosalpingography and computed tomography (CT) scan.

Hysterosalpingography or Uterotubography. Hysterosalpingography (HSP) is an x-ray study of the uterus and the fallopian tubes after injection of a radiographic contrast agent. The diagnostic procedure is performed to evaluate infertility or tubal patency and to detect any abnormal condition in the uterine cavity. Sometimes the procedure may be therapeutic as the flowing contrast agent flushes debris or loosens adhesions.

The procedure requires placing the patient in the lithotomy position and exposing the cervix with a bivalved speculum. Then a cannula is inserted into the cervix and the contrast agent is injected into the uterine cavity and the fallopian tubes. X-rays are taken to show the path and the distribution of the contrast agent.

In preparation for HSP, the intestinal tract is cleansed with cathartics and an enema so that gas shadows do not distort the x-ray findings. An analgesic may be prescribed. Some patients experience nausea, vomiting, cramps, and faintness. After the test, the patient may need to wear a perineal pad for several hours because the radiopaque agent may stain clothing.

CT Scan. CT scanning has several advantages over ultrasonography (described below), even though it involves radiation exposure and is more costly. It is more effective with an obese patient or a patient with a distended bowel. A CT scan also can demonstrate a tumor and any extension into the retroperitoneal lymph nodes and skeletal tissue, although it has limited value in diagnosing other gynecologic abnormalies.

Ultrasonography. Ultrasonography is a simple procedure based on sound wave transmission that uses pulsed ultrasonic waves at frequencies exceeding 20,000 Hz (formerly cycles per second). The transducer, which is placed in contact with the abdomen (abdominal scan), or a vaginal probe (vaginal ultrasound), which is inserted into the vagina, converts mechanical energy into electrical impulses, which in turn are amplified and recorded on an oscilloscope screen while a photograph or video recording of the patterns is recorded. The entire procedure takes about 10 minutes and involves no ionizing radiation and no discomfort other than a full bladder, which is necessary for good visualization during an abdominal scan. (A vaginal ultrasound or sonogram does not require a full bladder.)

The findings of this test combined with other test results are useful adjuncts to the physical examination, particularly in the obstetrical patient or the patient with abnormal pelvic examination findings.

Magnetic Resonance Imaging. Magnetic resonance imaging (MRI) produces patterns that are finer and more definitive than other x-ray processes without exposing the patient to radiation. It is more costly, however.

Nursing Interventions for Patients With Gynecologic Conditions

Various local treatments may be prescribed to treat gynecologic conditions; these include vaginal irrigations, (douches), vulvar irrigations, and insertion of vaginal medication. **Irrigations** are therapeutic measures used in treating patients with gynecologic diseases. They are used both before and after surgery and are of two types: vulvar and vaginal. Vaginal irrigations are used therapeutically to clean or disinfect the vagina, both before and after surgery. They also soothe inflamed tissues.

Vaginal Irrigations

To administer a **vaginal irrigation**, the nurse positions the patient as comfortably as possible on the bedpan in the dorsal position with the knees apart and the labia separated. Undue exposure of the patient is avoided and the bed is protected by placing an absorbent pad under the bedpan. Commonly used solutions include sterile water, normal saline, and antiseptic solutions.

Vaginal irrigations should be given at a temperature of 43.3°C (100°F) or as prescribed. The container holding the prescribed solution is raised not more than 60 cm (2 feet) above the level of the patient's hips. The nurse separates the labia and cleans the vaginal orifice before inserting the douche nozzle about 5 cm (2 inches) into the vagina and directing the tip of the nozzle backward toward the sacrum. The patient may be able to insert the nozzle herself. The nurse (or patient) then removes the clamp from the tube, allowing the solution to flow. Pressure should be avoided to prevent fluid from being forced into the uterus, which could transmit bacteria to the uterine cavity and tubes. The solution can be allowed to flow intermittently until the prescribed volume of solution has been used.

For maximal therapeutic benefit, the solution should be instilled over a period of 20 to 30 minutes. Then the nozzle may be removed and the patient asked to strain as if trying to have a bowel movement. This act tends to expel any fluid remaining in the vagina. Finally, the nurse can remove the bedpan, dry the perineum, and instruct the patient to remain recumbent for at least 1 hour.

After completing the vaginal irrigation, the nurse must make sure that the apparatus is cleaned and sterilized (if not disposable), including the bedpan. When vaginal irrigation or douching is performed at home, the patient usually lies in the bathtub and follows the same procedure.

Vulvar Irrigations

Vulvar irrigations are indicated chiefly after surgery on the perineum. They should be given after each voiding or bowel movement to keep the incision free from infection. The patient is prepared for a vulvar irrigation in the same way as for a vaginal douche. Warm, sterile water is poured gently over the vulva from a sterile container. The area is dried with sterile gauze or cotton and a sterile dressing or pad is applied and secured with a T-binder, or a self-adhesive pad may be used.

Medications

Vaginal medication (which may be inserted by the patient using an applicator) can be used before and after surgery. In many instances, this procedure may be substituted for therapeutic and cleansing vaginal irrigations or prescribed to treat vaginitis. After inserting the medication, the patient may use a perineal pad to prevent staining the underwear.

Menstrual Cycle

Physiologic Overview

The menstrual cycle is a complex process involving the reproductive and endocrine systems. The ovaries produce steroid hormones, predominantly estrogens and progesterone.

Several different **estrogens** are produced by the ovarian follicle, which consists of the developing ovum and its surrounding cells. The most potent of the ovarian estrogens is *estradiol.* Estrogens are responsible for developing and maintaining the female reproductive organs and the secondary sexual charactertics associated with the adult female. Estrogens play an important role in breast development and in monthly cyclic changes in the uterus.

Progesterone is also important in regulating the changes that occur in the uterus during the menstrual cycle. It is secreted by the *corpus luteum,* which is the ovarian follicle after the ovum has been released. Progesterone is the most important hormone for conditioning the endometrium (the mucous membrane lining the uterus) in preparation for implantation of the fertilized ovum. If pregnancy occurs, the progesterone secretion becomes largely a function of the placenta and is essential for maintaining a normal pregnancy. In addition, progesterone, working with estrogen, prepares the breast for producing and secreting milk.

Androgens are also produced by the ovaries, but only in small amounts. These hormones are involved in the early development of the follicle and also affect the female libido.

Regulation of Ovarian Hormone Secretion

Two gonadotropic hormones are released by the pituitary gland: FSH and LH. *Follicle-stimulating hormones* (FSH) is primarily responsible for stimulating the ovaries to secrete estrogen. *Luteinizing hormone* (LH), is primarily responsible for stimulating the progesterone production. Feedback mechanisms, in part, regulate FSH and LH secretion. For example, elevated estrogen levels in the blood inhibit FSH secretion but promote LH secretion, whereas elevated progesterone levels inhibit LH secretion. In addition, *gondotropin-releasing hormone* (GnRH) from the hypothalamus affects the rate of FSH and LH release.

Menstruation

Secretion of ovarian hormones follows a cyclic pattern that results in changes of the uterine endomentrium and in menstruation (Fig. 44-7 and Table 44-2). At the beginning of the cycle (just after menstruation), FSH output increases, stimulating estrogen secretion. This causes the endometrium to thicken and become more vascular (proliferative phase). Near the middle portion of the cycle, LH output increases, stimulating secretion. At this time, ovulation occurs. Under the combined stimulus of estrogen and progesterone, the endometrium reaches the peak of its thickening and vascularization (secretory phase).

If the ovum has been fertilized, estrogen and progesterone levels remain high and the complex hormonal changes of pregnancy follow. If the ovum has not been fertilized FSH and LH output diminishes; estrogen and progesterone secretion falls rapidly; the ovum disintegrates, and the endometrium, which has become thick and congested, becomes hemorrhagic. The product consisting of old blood, mucus, and endometrial tissue is discharged through the cervix and into the vagina.

This flow of blood, **menstruation**, occurs approximately every 28 days during the reproductive years, although normal cycles can vary from 21 to 42 days. The flow period usually lasts from 4 to 5 days, during which time 50 to 60 ml of blood are lost. After the menstrual flow stops, the endometrium proliferates and thickens from estrogenic stimulation, ovulation recurs, and the cycle repeats. Ovulation usually occurs midway between menstrual periods, or 14 days before the next menstrual period.

A perineal pad is generally used to absorb menstrual discharge; deodorant-treated pads are available, but some women are allergic or sensitive to the deodorants, so their use is discouraged. Tampons are also used extensively; there is no significant evidence of untoward effects from their use, providing there is no difficulty in inserting them. Tampons should not be used for more than 4 hours nor should super-absorbent tampons be used because of their association with toxic shock syndrome (see Chapter 45 for more about this syndrome). If the string breaks or retracts, a woman can be instructed to squat in a comfortable position, insert one finger in the vagina, try to locate the tampon, and remove it. If the woman feels uncomfortable attempting this maneuver or if she cannot remove the tampon, she should consult a health care provider.

Psychosocial Considerations

Girls who are approaching the **menarche** (the onset of menstruation) should be instructed about the normal process of the menstrual cycle before it occurs. Psychologically, it is healthier to refer to this event as a "period" rather than as "being sick" or "having the curse." With adequate

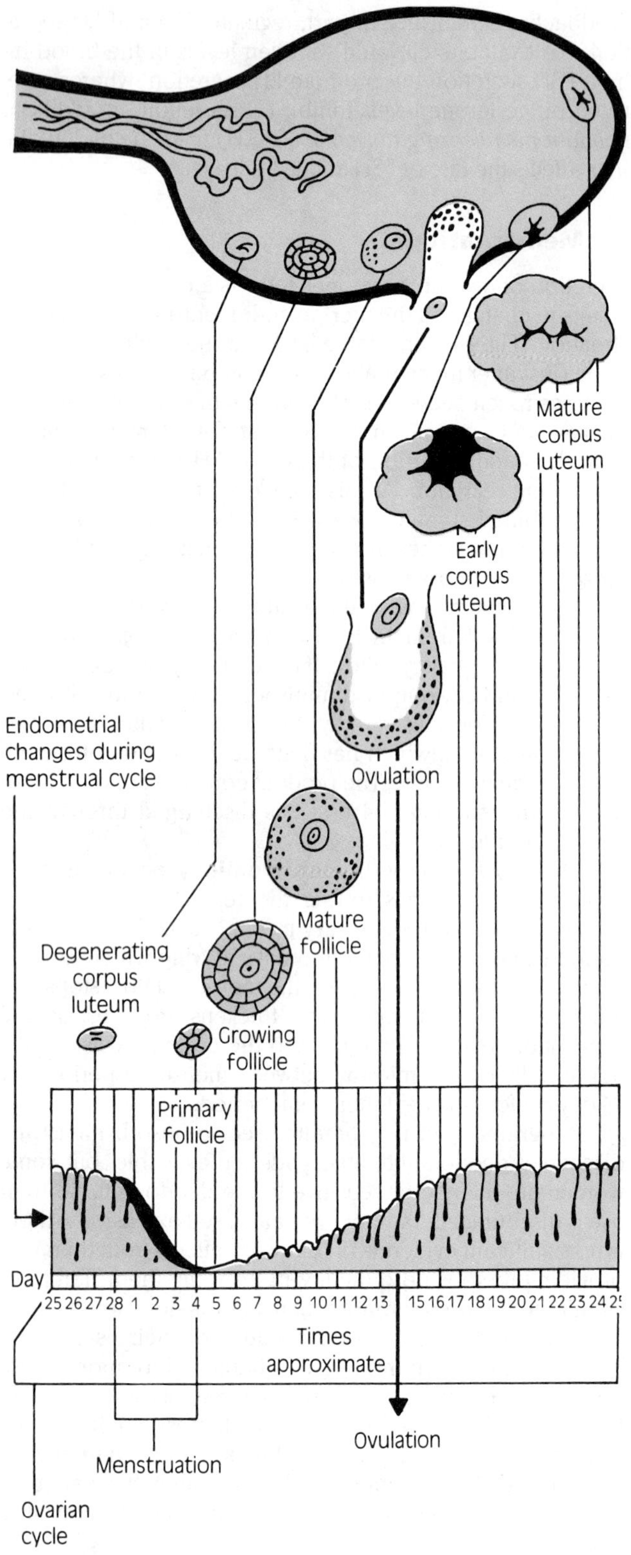

FIGURE 44-7. Schematic representation of one ovarian cycle and the corresponding changes in the endometrium.

nutrition, rest, and exercise, most women feel little discomfort, although occasionally some report breast tenderness and a feeling of fullness 1 or 2 days before menstruation begins. Others report fatigue and some discomfort in the lower back, legs, and pelvis on the first day and temperament or mood changes. Slight deviations from a usual healthful pattern of daily living are considered normal, but signs of excessive deviation may require evaluation.

Cultural Considerations

Menstruation may be viewed and managed differently in different cultures. Some women believe that it is detrimental to change a pad or tampon too frequently; they believe that allowing the discharge to accumulate increases the flow, which is considered desirable. Other beliefs influenced by culture also deserve consideration. For example, some women believe they are vulnerable to illness during menstruation. Some women believe that it is harmful to swim, shower, receive a hair permanent, get teeth filled, or eat certain foods during menstruation. They may also avoid using contraception.

In such situations, the nurse is in a position to provide women with accurate information in an accepting and culturally sensitive manner. The objective is to be sensitive to these unexpressed, deep-rooted beliefs and to provide correct information with sensitivity. Aspects of gynecologic problems cannot always be expressed easily. The nurse needs to convey confidence and openness as well as offer sound advice to facilitate communication.

Premenstrual Syndrome

Premenstrual syndrome (PMS) is a combination of symptoms that occur before the menses and subside with the onset of menstrual flow (Chart 44-1) and is experienced by many women before the onset of each menstrual cycle. The cause is unknown, but several theories suggest estrogen excess or progesterone deficit in the luteal phase of the menstrual cycle. Another theory holds that unidentified hormones cause symptoms at the time of menstrual changes. Other theories point to beta-endorphin activity, serotonin deficiency, progesterone withdrawal, fluid retention, elevated prolactin levels, abnormal prostaglandin metabolism, and disturbance of the hypothalamic-pituitary-ovarian axis.

Major symptoms include headache, fatigue, low back pain, engorged or painful breasts, and a feeling of abdominal fullness. General irritability, mood swings, fear of losing control, binge eating, and crying spells may also occur. Symptoms vary widely from one woman to another and from one cycle to the next in the same person. Great variability is found in the degree of symptoms. Many women are not bothered at all, whereas some experience severe and disabling symptoms.

A generally stressful life and problematic relationships may be related to the intensity of physical symptoms. Some women report moderate to severe life disruption secondary to PMS that negatively affects their interpersonal relationships. PMS may also be a factor in reduced productivity, work-related accidents, and absenteeism.

Identifying the *time* when these symptoms occur helps in determining the diagnosis. Symptoms recur regularly at the same phase of each menstrual cycle, usually 1 week to a few days before menses, and subside once the menstrual flow starts.

TABLE 44-2 Hormonal Changes During Menstrual Cycle

(Times approximate) Phase	Menstrual	Follicular	Ovulation	Luteal	Premenstrual
Days	1 2 3 4 5 6 7 8 9 10 11 12 13 14 15 16 17 18 19 20 21 22 23 24 25 26 27 28 1 2				
Ovary	Degenerating corpus luteum; beginning follicular development	Growth and maturation of follicle	Ovulation	Active corpus luteum	Degenerating corpus luteum
Estrogen Production	Low	Increasing	High	Declining, then a secondary rise	Decreasing
Progesterone Production	None	Low	Low	Increasing	Decreasing
FSH Production	Increasing	High, then declining	Low	Low	Increasing
LH Production	Low	Low, then increasing	High	High	Decreasing
Endometrium	Degeneration and shedding of superficial layer. Coiled arteries dilate, then constrict again	Reorganization and proliferation of superficial layer	Continued growth	Active secretion and glandular dilatation; highly vascular; edematous	Vasoconstriction of coiled arteries; beginning degeneration

Management. With no single treatment or known cure for PMS, women are encouraged to chart their own symptoms, so that they can possibly anticipate and, therefore, cope with them. Some clinicians prescribe analgesics, diuretics, and natural and synthetic progesterones, although long-term risks of progesterone use are unknown. Postaglandin inhibitors (*e.g.*, ibuprofen and anaprox) are also used, as are antidepressants and tranquilizers, such as Zanax and Prozac.

❑ NURSING PROCESS
The Patient With Premenstrual Syndrome

Assessment

The nurse should establish rapport with the patient while obtaining a health history, noting the time when symptoms began and their nature and intensity. The nurse then can determine whether the onset of symptoms occurs before or shortly after the menstrual flow begins. Additionally, the nurse can show the patient how to develop a chart recording the timing and intensity of symptoms (Fig. 44-8). To be meaningful the record should be maintained over at least three cycles. A nutritional history is also elicited to determine if the diet is high in salt or caffeine or a diet low in essential nutrients and alcohol intake.

Diagnosis

Nursing Diagnoses

Based on the health and nutritional history and other assessment data, the major diagnoses for the patient may include the following:

- ❑ Anxiety related to the effects of PMS
- ❑ Ineffective coping of both patient and family related to effects of PMS
- ❑ Knowledge deficit about the cause and management of PMS

Collaborative Problems/ Potential Complications

Based on assessment data, the major complications for the patient may include the following:

CHART 44-1
Cause, Manifestations, and Treatment of Premenstrual Syndrome

Cause

Unknown; may be related to hormonal changes combined with other factors (diet, stress, and lack of exercise)

Physical symptoms

Fluid retention (*e.g.*, bloating, breast tenderness)
Weight gain
Sleep disturbances
Migraine headaches with menstruation
Backache
Vertigo
Nausea, vomiting, or diarrhea
Acne
Food cravings
Constipation

Emotional symptoms

Irritability, mood changes, emotional lability
Hostility
Depression
Anxiety
Lethargy

Treatment

Use of social support and family resources
Nutritious diet consisting of whole grains, fruit, and vegetables; increased water intake
Decreased intake of caffeine, salt, sweets, and alcohol
Multivitamins, B complex, and vitamin B_6
Increased or initiated exercise program
Stress reduction techniques
Progesterone
Antidepressants

- Potential for suicidal and violent, uncontrollable behavior

Planning and Implementation

Goals. The patient's goals may include reduction of anxiety (mood swings, crying, binge eating, fear of losing control), ability to cope with day-to-day stressors and relationships with family and co-workers, increased knowledge about PMS with improved use of control measures, and absence of complications.

Nursing Interventions

Reducing Anxiety. General support and counseling are provided. The patient is asked to participate in her care by keeping a chart of her symptoms. She is encouraged to plan activities around symptomatic times. Her partner and children are included in discussing her problem, if desired. Sharing this information can lead to mutual understanding and lessened tension for the patient. Analgesics, mild tranquilizers, and occasionally, antidepressants may be prescribed.

Promoting Coping. Positive coping measures are facilitated. Partners can be advised to assist by offering support and increased involvement with child care. The patient can try to plan her working time to accommodate the days she will be less productive because of PMS.

Exercise, meditation, imagery, and creative activities to reduce stress should be encouraged. It may also help the patient to know that others recognize and understand what she is experiencing.

Patient Teaching. The nurse can suggest that the patient keep a 3-month record of symptoms and consult with a health care professional in determining the specific diagnosis. The patient should assume responsibility for following a healthful dietary plan or eating small meals and eliminating or restricting sugar, salt, alcohol, caffeine, and nicotine. Supplements of vitamin B_6, calcium, and magnesium may be prescribed. Exercise and relaxation are taught and the patient is encouraged to participate in various health promotion strategies. The patient is encouraged to take medications as prescribed and is instructed about the desired effects of the medications. In some cases, the patient may be able to arrange a flexible monthly work schedule to accommodate PMS symptoms. Enrolling in a PMS group that meets to discuss problems may also help.

Monitoring and Managing Potential Complications. The patient is assessed for suicidal and uncontrollable and violent behavior. Any suggestions of suicidal tendencies must be evaluated by psychiatric consultation immediately. Uncontrollable behavior may lead to violence toward family members. If abuse of children or other members of the patient's family is suspected, reporting protocols are implemented and followed. Referral is made for immediate psychiatric or psychologic care and counseling.

Evaluation

Expected Outcomes

1. Experiences reduction in anxiety
2. Demonstrates adequate coping mechanisms
   a. Keeps a monthly calendar of PMS symptoms
   b. Schedules activities around her symptomatic days
   c. Reports reduced level of stress
3. Follows recommended dietary practices
4. Reports no suicidal ideas or abusive behavior toward family members

Dysmenorrhea

Primary dysmenorrhea is painful menstruation, with no identifiable pelvic pathology. It occurs at the time of menarche or shortly thereafter. It is characterized by crampy pain that begins before or shortly after onset of menstrual flow and continues for 48 to 72 hours. Pelvic examination reflects normal findings. Dysmenorrhea is thought to result from excessive, prostaglandin production, which causes the uterus

Diagnostic Diary A: Evaluation of PMS Symptoms

NAME ____________________

YEAR ____________________

Grading of Symptoms:
0—No Symptoms *2—Moderate Symptoms*
1—Mild Symptoms *3—Severe Symptoms (i.e., Disabling)*

DAY OF CYCLE	1	2	3	4	5	6	7	8	9	10	11	12	13	14	15	16	17	18	19	20	21	22	23	24	25	26	27	28	29	30	31
DATE																															
MENSES																															

PSYCHOLOGICAL SYMPTOMS

Depression																															
Anxiety																															
Irritability																															
Lethargy																															
Insomnia																															
Forgetfulness																															
Confusion																															

PHYSICAL SYMPTOMS

Swelling																															
Breast Tenderness																															
Abdominal bloating																															
Palpitations																															
Weight gain																															
Constipation																															
Headache																															
Rhinitis																															

PAIN SYMPTOMS (Usually NOT associated with PMS)

Menstrual cramps																															
Painful intercourse																															
Pelvic pain																															
Backache																															

Morning weight (lb)																															

FIGURE 44-8. Example of a diary kept by the patient for tracking premenstrual symptoms. (Chihal HJ. Premenstrual Syndrome: A Clinic Manual, 2nd ed. Dallas, Essential Medical Information Systems, 1990, pp 80–81.)

to contract excessively and also results in arteriolar vasospasm. Psychological factors such as anxiety and tension may also contribute to dysmenorrhea. As women grow older, pain tends to decrease and completely resolve after childbirth.

In *secondary dysmenorrhea,* pelvic pathology exists, such as endometriosis, tumor, or pelvic inflammatory disease (PID). These conditions are discussed in Chapter 45. Patients with secondary dysmenorrhea frequently have pain that occurs several days prior to menses, with ovulation and occasionally with intercourse. (See Table 44-3 for a comparison of primary and secondary dysmenorrhea.)

Assessment. A complete physical examination is performed to rule out possible abnormalities, such as strictures of the cervix or vagina, an imperforate hymen, or other conditions, such as endometriosis, PID, adenomyosis, and fibroid uterus. A laparoscopy is usually required to identify organic causes.

Management and Nursing Interventions. In *primary dysmenorrhea,* the reason for the discomfort is explained and the patient is assured that menstruation is a normal function of the reproductive system. If the patient is young and accompanied by her mother, the mother may also need reassurance. Many daughters expect to have painful periods if their mothers did. The discomfort of cramps can be treated once worry and concern over its possible significance are dispelled by adequate explanation. Symptoms usually subside with appropriate medication.

The patient is encouraged to continue her usual activities and to increase physical exercise because exercise provides a neurophysiologic basis for relief. Taking analgesics before cramps start, in anticipation of discomfort, is advised. Aspirin, a mild prostaglandin inhibitor, may be taken at recommended doses every 4 hours. Other useful prostaglandin antagonists include ibuprofen (Motrin), naproxen, Alleve, Anaprox, Naprosyn, and mefenamic acid (Ponstel). If one inhibitor does not provide relief, another may be prescribed. Usually these medications are well tolerated, but some women experience gastrointestinal side effects. Contraindications include allergy, peptic ulcer history, sensitivity to aspirin-like medications, asthma, and pregnancy. Low-dose oral contraceptives provide relief in more than 90% of patients and are indicated in woman with dysmenorrhea who are sexually active but not desirous of pregnancy.

Management of *secondary dysmenorrhea* is directed at diagnosing and treating the underlying cause (*e.g.,* endometriosis or PID).

TABLE 44-3 Comparison of Primary and Secondary Dysmenorrhea

	Primary Dysmenorrhea	Secondary Dysmenorrhea
Symptoms	Cramps, combined with systemic symptoms in some women before onset of flow and for 2 to 3 days after onset	Pain, occurring several days before onset of flow, at ovulation, and with sexual intercourse
Cause	Excess prostaglandin production	Various disease entities
Treatment	Antiprostaglandins, exercise, oral contraceptives	Evaluation and treatment for specific cause (e.g., endometriosis)

Amenorrhea (Absence of Menstrual Flow)

Primary amenorrhea (delayed menarche) refers to those instances when a young woman over age 16 has not begun to menstruate but otherwise shows evidence of sexual maturation, or menstruation may not occur by age 14 in the absence of secondary sex characteristics. Amenorrhea may be of considerable concern but is more than likely due to minor variations in body build, heredity, and environment, as well as in physical, mental, and emotional development.

The nurse provides an opportunity for the patient to express her concerns and anxiety about this problem because the patient may feel that she is different from her peers. A complete physical examination, careful health history, and simple laboratory studies help to rule out possible causes, such as physiologic disorders, metabolic or endocrine difficulties, and systemic diseases. Treatment is directed toward correcting any abnormalities.

Secondary amenorrhea, an absence of menses for 3 cycles or 6 months after a normal menarche in an adolescent, is usually caused by minor emotional upset related to being away from home, attending college, tension from schoolwork, or interpersonal problems. The second most common cause, however, is pregnancy, so a pregnancy test is performed.

Secondary nutritional disturbances may also be factors and may appear as weight loss or gain. Obesity can result in anovulation and subsequent amenorrhea. Anorexia is characterized by lack of menses. The lack of body fat and caloric intake in anorexic individuals affects hormonal function; this is not completely understood. Competitive and serious female athletes typically experience amenorrhea and are frequently placed on hormone replacement therapy to prevent bone loss related to low estrogen levels. On occasion a pituitary or thyroid dysfunction may be detected and treated successfully by appropriate measures. Consultation with a health care provider is necessary.

Abnormal Uterine Bleeding

Menorrhagia. Menorrhagia (also called hypermenorrhea) is defined as prolonged or excessive bleeding at the time of the regular menstrual flow. In early life, the cause is usually related to endocrine disturbance, whereas in later life it usually results from inflammatory disturbances, tumors of the uterus, or hormonal imbalance. Emotional disturbances may also affect bleeding.

The nurse encourages a woman with menorrhagia to see her health care provider and specifically describe the amount of bleeding by pad count and saturation, (*i.e.*, absorbency of personal pad or tampon and number saturated hourly).

Metrorrhagia. Metrorrhagia, vaginal bleeding between regular menstrual periods is probably the most significant form of menstrual dysfunction because it may signal cancer, benign tumors of the uterus, or other gynecologic problems. This condition merits early diagnosis and treatment. Although bleeding between menstrual periods by a woman taking oral contraceptives is usually not serious, irregular bleeding by a woman on hormone replacement therapy should be evaluated.

Postmenopausal Bleeding. Bleeding 1 year after menses cease at menopause must be investigated and a malignant condition must be considered unless proved otherwise. An endometrial biopsy or a D&C is commonly indicated.

Perimenopause

Perimenopause is the period extending from the first signs of menopause—usually hot flashes, vaginal dryness, and irregular menses—to beyond the complete cessation of menses (1 year from last menstrual period). The following facts about perimenopause must be considered by the nurse:

- Sexuality, fertility, contraception, and STDs may be of concern to perimenopausal women.
- Unintended pregnancy is possible because about one third of perimenopausal women use a contraceptive method other than sterilization.
- Perimenopausal women who do not smoke may receive some protection from oral contraceptives against uterine cancer.
- About 16% of breast cancer occurs in this group of women, so breast self-examinations (BSE), routine physical examinations, and mammograms are essen-

tial. Benign breast cysts are common findings. Fine needle aspiration may be used to evaluate most breast masses, avoiding the need for hospitalization and surgery (see Chapter 46).

Because cardiovascular disease is the leading cause of death in older women, diet and exercise are important topics of patient education as is hormone replacement therapy (HRT). Clinicians believe that HRT protects women from heart disease and osteoporosis. The nurse needs to point out various health options to female patients before menopause.

Menopause

Menopause (climacteric or "change of life") is described as the physiologic cessation of menses associated with failing ovarian function, during which reproductive function diminishes and ends. Postmenopause is the period beginning from about 1 year after menses cease and beyond. Menopause is associated with some atrophy of breast tissue and genital organs, losses in bone density, and vascular changes.

Physiologic Overview

The menopausal period marks the end of a woman's reproductive capacity. It usually occurs between the ages of 45 and 52, but may occur in some women as early as 42 or as late as 55. The median age is 51.

Menopause is not a pathologic phenomenon but is a normal part of aging and maturation. Menstruation ceases and because the ovaries are no longer active, the reproductive organs become smaller. No more ova mature; therefore, no ovarian hormones (estrogen) are produced. (An artificial menopause may occur earlier if the ovaries are surgically removed or are destroyed by radiation.) Besides changes in the reproductive system that reduce estrogen levels, multifaceted changes occur throughout the woman's body. These changes include neuroendocrinologic, biochemical, and metabolic alterations related to aging.

Clinical Manifestations

Menopause starts gradually and is usually recognized by changes in menstruation. The monthly flow may increase, decrease, become irregular, and finally cease. Often, the interval between periods lasts longer—a lapse of several months between periods is not uncommon.

Many women are unaware that changes signaling menopause begin to occur as early as the late 30s when ovulation occurs less frequently, estrogen levels decrease, and FSH levels rise in an attempt to stimulate estrogen production. Because of these changes, some women notice irregular menses, breast tenderness, and mood changes long before menopause occurs.

The hot or warm flashes and night sweats reported by some women are directly attributable to hormonal changes. Hot flashes, which denote vasomotor instability, may vary in intensity from a barely perceptible warm feeling to a sensation of extreme warmth accompanied by profuse sweating, causing discomfort, sleep disturbances, and embarrassment.

Other physical manifestations may include possible atrophic changes, dry skin, weight gain, and decreased bone density (osteoporosis) resulting in decreased stature and bone fractures. About 1.2 million new fractures due to osteoporosis occur yearly in the United States. The entire genitourinary system is affected by the reduced estrogen level. Changes in the vulvovaginal area may include a gradual thinning of pubic hair and a slow shrinkage of the labia. Vaginal secretions decrease and the woman may report dyspareunia (discomfort during intercourse), which may be avoided by added lubrication with a water soluble lubricant, such as K-Y jelly, or contraceptive foam. Vaginal cream containing estrogen is often prescribed. The vaginal *p*H rises in menopause, predisposing the woman to bacterial infections (atrophic vaginitis). Discharge, itching, and a sensation of vulvar burning may result. All symptoms require evaluation.

The loss of reproductive capacity may mean disappointment for some women and relief for others. For a woman with a grown family and traditional values, menopause may result in feelings ranging from role confusion to feelings of sexual and personal freedom. Individual circumstances affect the response of each woman and must be considered on an individual basis. Nurses need to be aware and sensitive to all possibilities and take their cues from the patient.

Nurses can encourage women to view menopause as a natural change resulting in freedom from menses and symptoms related to hormonal changes. No relationship exists between menopause and mental health problems; social changes that usually coincide with menopause (*e.g.*, adolescent or grown children, ill partners, and dependent or ill parents) may produce stress.

Management

Hormone Replacement Therapy (HRT). The changes in lipid metabolism that occur during menopause have adverse effects on women, placing them at increased risk for atherosclerosis, angina, coronary artery disease, and osteoporosis. In many cases, HRT reduces the risk of these conditions and of myocardial infarction as well. Additionally, HRT reduces or eliminates persistent and severe hot flashes. Preliminary results of the Postmenopausal Estrogen/Progestin Interventions (PEPI) trial reveal that estrogen alone or in combination with a progestin improves lipoproteins and lowers fibrinogen levels. Unopposed estrogen, however, is not recommended for women who have not had a hysterectomy, as it is associated with endometrial hyperplasia (Writing Group of PEPI Trial, 1995). In addition to its use in preventing heart disease, HRT may help prevent osteoporosis. Factors that increase a women's risk for osteoporosis include a thin body frame, race (Caucasian or Asian), family history of osteoporosis, nulliparity, early menopause, moderate to heavy alcohol ingestion, smoking, caffeine use, sedentary lifestyle, and a diet low in calcium. Women should be advised to remain active or to begin an exercise program of weight-bearing activity, such as walking, to take a calcium supplement, to decrease or stop smoking, and to discuss the appropriateness of HRT with their health care provider.

Contraindications. Current HRT usually consists of estrogen and progesterone. In the past, however, treatment with estrogen alone increased the incidence of uterine cancer. Adding progestin, a synthetic form of progesterone, to the regimen reduced this risk. A woman who has had her uterus removed is usually not given progestins.

Because the risk of breast cancer is increased in women on HRT, a woman with a hormonally dependent breast lesion identified by mammography probably would not be given HRT (although a woman with a breast cancer history may be given therapy if she has very bothersome symptoms). The decision to take HRT is often a difficult one, especially because the research studies needed for the woman to make a well-informed decision are still incomplete.

Hormone replacement therapy also is contraindicated in women with a recent vascular thrombosis, active liver disease or chronically impaired liver function, uterine cancer, and undiagnosed abnormal vaginal bleeding.

Regular follow-up care, including a yearly physical examination and mammogram, is recommended for women on HRT. An endometrial biopsy is indicated for women with persistent irregular bleeding as well.

HRT Regimen. The woman takes both estrogen and progestins daily or estrogen for the first 25 days of the month. She takes a progestin for the last 12 days of the 25-day period to prevent proliferation of the uterine lining, which can result in a malignancy. Estrogen patches, which are replaced twice weekly, are another option but require oral progestin along with them.

Alternative Treatments. Some women feel apprehensive about HRT and the lack of complete data about its long-term effects. These women will benefit from learning about alternatives to HRT (including diet, vitamins, and exercise). However, they need to know that these approaches to menopause have not been examined by researchers. Vitamin B_6 in doses less than 200 mg has been found to relieve some distressing symptoms. Vitamin E has been effective in decreasing hot flashes.

Regular physical exercise, including weight-bearing exercise, raises the heart rate, increases high density lipoprotein levels (HDL), preserves bone content, and helps to maintain bone mass. It may also reduce stress, enhance well-being, and improve self-image. Loss of muscle tissue is mediated by exercise. Women should also be encouraged to decrease caloric intake, decrease fat, and increase whole grains, fiber, fruit, and vegetables. Calcium supplementation (1500 mg/day) may be helpful in preventing bone loss.

Currently, the Women's Health Initiative, a large study on hormone replacement, is being conducted at several sites across the country and should provide important findings regarding the effects of hormone replacement, vitamin therapy, and preventive health measures on women in midlife and older.

Nursing Interventions

Measures should be taken to promote general health. The nurse can explain to the patient that cessation of menses is a physiologic function that is rarely accompanied by nervous symptoms or illness.

The current expected life span after menopause for the average woman is 30 to 35 years, which may encompass as many years as the childbearing phase of her life. The menopause is not a complete change of life, however. Normal sexual urges remain and women retain their usual response to sex long after menopause. Many women enjoy better health after the menopause than before; this is especially true for those who have experienced dysmenorrhea. The individual woman's evaluation of herself and her worth, now and in the future, is likely to affect her emotional reaction to menopause.

An overview of patient teaching points for the menopausal woman is presented in Chart 44-2.

Contraception

Control of human reproduction has been practiced since ancient times. Many methods exist, and acceptance of the concept varies. No perfect method has been developed; all have advantages and disadvantages. Most methods apply to women. Research has addressed contraception methods for men, but for varying reasons few of these methods seem close to being marketable, although several are being explored.

More than half of the 6 million yearly pregnancies in the United States are unintended. More than 1 million occur in teenagers. More than 1 million abortions are performed and more than 400,000 of these are performed on adolescents. Many women who are sexually active or considering becoming sexually activite can benefit from learning about contraception or ways to avoid unwanted pregnancy. Fewer unwanted pregnancies may reduce the number of abortions, abused children, stressed family units, and the consequences of infant mortality and morbidity. It is important that women receive unbiased and nonjudgemental information, understand the benefits and risks of each method, learn about alternatives and how to use them, and receive positive reinforcement and acceptance of their own individual choice. Methods and practices to prevent unwanted or unplanned pregnancies and births are described below.

Abstinence

Abstinence or *celibacy* is the only completely effective means of preventing pregnancy. This may not be a desired or available option for many women because of their own and their partner's values and sexual needs, as well as cultural expectations.

Sterilization: Permanent Conception Control

Sterilization by bilateral *tubal occlusion* or *vasectomy* is the most effective means of contraception after abstinence. Both procedures must be considered permanent because neither method is easily reversable. Woman and men who choose these methods should be certain that they have completed their childbearing, no matter how the circumstances in their life may change. See Chapter 47 for a discussion of vasectomy (male sterilization).

Tubal Ligation. Female sterilization is performed during same-day surgery. The procedure is carried out by laparoscopy with the patient receiving a general or local anesthetic. The laparoscope, a small periscope-like optical instrument, is inserted through a small umbilical incision. Carbon dioxide is introduced to lift other abdominal organs away from the tubal area. The fallopian tubes are visualized and ligated, thereby disrupting their patency. Despite a 99% effectiveness rate and despite sterilization, any woman who has missed a period should be tested for pregnancy because ectopic and intrauterine pregnancies, although rare, may occur. Ovulatory and menstrual function is not affected by sterilization, although some women report heavier menstrual bleeding and more cramping after tubal ligation.

Sterilization by vasectomy and laproscopic tubal ligation are compared in Chart 44-3.

Patient Education. Before sterilization surgery, the patient should be informed that an intrauterine device (IUD), if present, will be removed. If the patient is taking oral contraceptives, she usually continues up to the time of the procedure. Postoperatively, women may experience some abdominal discomfort for a few days, related to the carbon dioxide gas and the manipulation of organs. The woman is instructed to report any of the following: bleeding, pain that persists or increases, and fever. The patient also needs to be informed that for 2 weeks, she is to avoid intercourse, strenuous exercise, and lifting. Risks with the procedure are minimal and are more often related to anesthesia than the surgery itself.

Oral Contraceptives

Physiologic Basis. Oral contraceptive preparations of synthetic estrogen and progesterone block ovarian stimulation by preventing the release of follicle-stimulating hormone (FSH) from the anterior pituitary gland. In the absence of FSH, a follicle does not ripen and ovulation does not occur. This is the mechanism of action of oral contraceptives. Progestins (synthetic forms of progesterone) suppress the luteinizing-hormone surge, prevent ovulation, and also render the cervical mucus impenetrable to sperm. Synthetic estrogens and progestin, found in the many oral contraceptive variations available, differ in androgenic activity.

Types of Oral Contraceptives. There are two kinds of oral contraceptives: "combined" and "progestin only." The difference lies in the presence of estrogen. *Combined preparations* contain estrogen and progestin in every pill; estrogen is not contained in a progestin-only pill. Most women using oral contraceptives take the combination pill. Progestin interferes with cervical mucus production and prevents the uterine endometrium from fully developing. The result of both types of pills is a lighter than normal menstrual flow after pills are taken for 21 days and then stopped for 7 days. The flow is actually withdrawal bleeding from discontinuing hormones because a normal period occurs only with ovulation.

Combined pills now include biphasic preparations that contain a constant amount of estrogen with an increase in

CHART 44-2
Patient Education: The Woman Facing Menopause

General Points

- The climacteric period is normal and self-limiting.
- Fatigue and stress may exaggerate the symptoms.
- A nutritious diet and weight control will improve physical conditioning.
- An exercise program in keeping with your needs promotes well-being.
- Interest and participation in outside activities help to reduce anxiety and tension.
- Changes in former support networks are expected in midlife. These changes include departure of children, aging and increasing dependence of parents, and death of loved ones.
- This is an excellent time for intellectual growth, personal accomplishment, and for initiating new activities and experiences.
- Menopause does not mean terminating sexual functioning.
- An annual physical examination is essential to maintain continuing good health.

To Manage or Prevent Physical Annoyances

- For itching or burning vulvar areas, confer with your health care provider to rule out dermatologic abnormalities and if appropriate to obtain a prescription for a lubricating or hormonal cream.
- To prevent dyspareunia (painful intercourse), use a water-soluble lubricant, such as K–Y Jelly, Replens, hormone cream, or contraceptive foam.
- Improve perineal muscle tone and bladder control by practicing Kegel's exercises daily: Contract the perineal muscles as though stopping urination; hold for 5–10 seconds and release. Repeat frequently during the day.
- Use "bland" skin cream and lotions to prevent dry skin.
- Join a weight-reduction support group such as *Weight Watchers* or a similar group if appropriate. As age increases so does the tendency to gain weight, particulary around the hips, thighs, and abdomen.
- Observe recommended calcium intake because dairy products and calcium supplements may help slow the process of osteoporosis.
- Drink six to eight glasses of water daily and vitamin C (500 mg) as a way to reduce the incidence of urinary tract infection (UTI) related to atrophic changes of the urethra.
- Consider the following points about sexual activity:
  - Frequent sexual activity helps to maintain the elasticity of the vagina.
  - Contraception is advised until 1 year passes without menses.
  - Safer sex is important at any age.

CHART 44-3
Sterilization Methods

Vasectomy

Advantages
- Highly effective
- Relieves the female of the contraceptive burden
- Inexpensive in the long run
- Permanent
- Highly acceptable procedure to most clients
- Very safe
- Quickly performed

Disadvantages
- Protection for the male (It is the female who is at risk for pregnancy)
- A surgical procedure requiring surgical training, aseptic conditions, medications, and technical assistance
- Expensive in the short term
- Serious long-term effects suggested (although currently unproved)
- Permanent (although reversal is possible, it is expensive, requires a highly technical and major surgery, and its results cannot be guaranteed.
- Regret in 5%–10% of patients
- No protection against STDs, including HIV
- Not effective until sperm remaining in the reproductive system are ejaculated

Laparoscopic Tubal Sterilization

Advantages
- Low incidence of complications
- Short recovery
- Leaves small scar
- Quickly performed

Disadvantages
- Permanent
- Reversibility difficult and expensive
- Sterilization procedures technically difficult
- Requires surgeon, operating room (aseptic conditions), trained assistants, medications, surgical equipment
- Expensive at the time performed
- Morbidity and mortality high when considered for 1 year
- If failure, high probability of ectopic pregnancy
- No protection against STDs, including HIV

(Adapted from Hatcher R et al. Contraceptive Technology. Irvington, NY, Irvington Publishers, 1994.)

the progestin on day 10 and triphasic preparations that provide varying low doses of estrogen along with progesterone during the 21-day cycle. The intent of this variation is to provide an effective contraceptive that mimics the normal cycle and has enough progesterone to prevent ovulation and spotting.

Progestin-only "mini" pills contain a progestin and are less protective against pregnancy than combined pills. About 40% of women have ovulatory cycles on this pill. These pills are useful for women who have had estrogen-related side effects on combination pills (*e.g.*, headaches, hypertension, leg pain, chloasma or skin discoloration, weight gain, or nausea). Some health care providers recommend this pill for lactating women who need a hormonal contraceptive method. The risks and benefits of using oral contraceptives are presented in Chart 44-4.

Regimen. To begin using either type of oral contraceptive (depending on the package insert instructions), one pill is taken on the Sunday after a period starts or the first day of a period. Pills are taken for 21 days followed by 7 hormone-free days. The pills come in a package containing all the pills needed for 1 month. Some packages include inactive pills for the 7 days that are hormone-free as some women find it easier to stay in the habit of taking one pill every day. Some women prefer 7 days without pills. After 7 days off or 7 inactive pills, a new package is started.

Side Effects. A few patients experience side effects such as nausea, depression, headache, weight gain, leg

CHART 44-4
Benefits and Risks of Oral Contraceptives

Benefits
- Decreased cramps and bleeding
- Regular bleeding cycle
- Decrease in incidence of anemia
- Possible decrease in acne
- Protection from uterine and ovarian cancer
- Decreased incidence of ectopic pregnancy
- Protection from benign breast disease
- Decreased incidence of pelvic infection

Risks
- Rare in healthy women
- Bothersome side effects (*e.g.*, breakthrough bleeding, breast tenderness)
- Nausea, weight gain, mood changes
- Small increased risk of developing blood clots, stroke, or heart attack, related more to smoking than to oral contraceptive use alone
- Increased incidence of benign liver tumors
- No protection from STDs (possible increased risk with unsafe sex)

cramps, and breast soreness. Usually, these symptoms subside after 3 or 4 months. Because such symptoms are sometimes related to sodium and water retention caused by estrogen, a smaller dose of the hormone or a different hormonal combination, along with salt reduction in the diet, may alleviate the problem. Many patients experience spotting in the first month on the pill or if they take their pill irregularly, so they need to be reassured and advised to take a pill every 24 hours.

Some women with infrequent periods (*i.e.*, less than 6 periods per year) are advised to use another method of contraception. If they use oral contraceptives, it may take a while for their ovaries to resume functioning after they stop using the contraceptive. With respect to how soon fertility resumes after using oral contraceptives, the patient should be told that resumption of normal menses is delayed 2 to 3 months in approximately 20% of users. Most health care providers recommend that the woman use a barrier contraceptive method for 1 to 2 months after stopping the pill before becoming pregnant so that the accurate date of the last menstrual period is available to date the pregnancy.

Using oral contraceptives reduces the incidence of benign breast disease, uterine and ovarian cancers, anemia, and pelvic infection. These health implications are important teaching points for the nurse to convey to potential and actual users of oral contraceptives. Some patients who take oral contraceptives seem to be at increased risk for contracting chlamydia, a common sexually transmitted disease (STD). This is another important point for nurses to emphasize.

- Patients need to be aware that oral contraceptives protect them from pregnancy but not from STDs, including HIV infection.

Sex with multiple partners or sex without a condom may result in chlamydial and other infections including HIV infection.

In general, no definite long-term undesirable effects have been observed with prolonged oral contraceptive use. Fetal anomalies do not appear to be a concern and normal reproductive tract function and fertility are restored after oral contraceptives are discontinued.

Contraindications. *Absolute contraindications* include current or past thromboembolic disorder, cerebrovascular disease, or artery disease; known or suspected breast cancer, known or suspected current or past estrogen-dependent neoplasia; pregnancy; current or past benign or malignant liver tumor; impaired liver function; congenital hyperlipidemia; and undiagnosed abnormal vaginal bleeding.

Relative contraindications include hypertension, bile-induced jaundice, acute phase of mononucleosis, and sickle cell disease. Smoking is also a consideration. Women over age 35 who smoke are at risk for heart problems and should use another method of contraception. Occasionally, neuro-ocular complications arise, but a cause-and-effect relationship has not been established. If visual disturbances occur, oral contraceptives should be discontinued.

Some gynecologists will allow patients with migraine headaches to take oral contraceptives as long as the headaches do not worsen with use or as long as the patient has no neurologic symptoms. (A young woman who has blurred vision with a migraine will probably be discouraged from taking oral contraceptives.) Diabetes is also problematic, although some diabetes specialists allow their patients to use oral contraceptives with careful glucose monitoring. Leiomyomas (fibroid tumors) of the uterus can enlarge with oral contraceptive use. Patients with this condition are advised and monitored carefully, or they discontinue oral contraceptives if fibroids enlarge and choose other contraceptive methods. Guidelines for patient teaching about oral contraceptive use are presented in Chart 44-5.

Implant Contraceptive

The Norplant System is a reversible, low-dose progestin-only contraceptive device consisting of six soft Silastic capsules that are implanted under the skin of the woman's upper arm. The implant releases the progestin levonorgestrel over 5 years thereby inhibiting ovulation.

Contraindications to using this system are acute liver disease or liver tumors, pregnancy, unexplained vaginal bleeding, breast cancer, or a history of thrombophlebitis or pulmonary embolism.

Common side effects include irregular bleeding, weight gain, acne, hair growth, and hair loss. If patients are aware of these disadvantages and side effects, they are more likely to tolerate the implant and continue using it.

Insertion is performed under aseptic conditions in an outpatient setting such as an office or clinic. A small incision is made in the upper arm after the patient receives a local anesthetic. The Norplant capsules are inserted within the first 7 days of the menstrual cycle to avoid the possibility of a preexisting pregnancy. The contraceptive effect occurs within 24 hours. The device can be removed at any time but is effective for 5 years. Insertion usually takes about 15 minutes; removal can be a lengthier and more difficult procedure as tissue encapsulates the implants.

Other concerns must also be considered. The patient should report headaches or visual symptoms to a health care provider because rare instances of intracranial hypertension have been associated with the implant. Papilledema must be ruled out if headaches occur. If pregnancy is desired, previous fertility levels are expected to resume shortly

CHART 44-5
Patient Education: Oral Contraceptives

- Use condoms to protect against infection.
- Take pill at exactly the same time every day.
- Stop smoking or cut down on smoking.
- Report the following symptoms immediately:
  - A – abdominal pains
  - C – chest pains
  - H – headaches
  - E – eye problems (blurred vision or spots)
  - S – severe leg pains

(Adapted from Hatcher R et al. Contraceptive Technology, 16th ed. Irvington, NY, Irvington Publishers, 1993.)

after removal of the Norplant system. The risks of smoking and using this implant are unknown. Women who smoke should be assisted with methods to stop or decrease smoking.

Depo-Provera

An intramuscular injection of Depo-provera, a long-acting progestin, every 3 months effectively inhibits ovulation and provides reliable and convenient contraceptive method. It can be used by lactating women and those with hypertension, liver disease, migraine headaches, heart disease, and hemoglobinopathies. Women who use this method must be prepared for irregular or no bleeding. With continued use, irregular bleeding episodes and spotting decrease and usually, amenorrhea occurs.

Potential disadvantages include irregular or heavy menstrual bleeding, bloating, headaches, hair loss, decreased sex drive, weight loss, or weight gain. In women discontinuing this method, fertility may be delayed; therefore, other methods of contraception may be more appropriate for the woman who wishes to conceive within a year of discontinuing contraception.

Depo-provera is contraindicated in pregnancy, abnormal vaginal bleeding of unknown cause, breast or pelvic cancer, or sensitivity to synthetic progestin. The long-term effects on the infant of a nursing mother who uses depo-provera are unknown but are thought to be negligible; breast cancer and osteoporosis risks are being studied; and the endometrial cancer risk is decreased. Depo-provera does not protect against STDs.

Intrauterine Device

An intrauterine device (IUD) is a small plastic device, usually T-shaped, that is inserted into the endometrial cavity to prevent pregnancy. A string attached to the IUD is visible and palpable at the cervical os. Clinicians think that an IUD prevents conception by causing a local inflammatory reaction, which is toxic to spermatozoa and blastocysts. The IUD does not destroy fertilized eggs, as some people believe.

One type of IUD, the Progestasert, releases progestin and is replaced each year. The progestin may decrease cramping during menses, but patients using this type of IUD have a slightly higher pregnancy rate than those using copper-bearing IUDs. Another available IUD is the Paraguard, a copper-bearing IUD that is effective for 8 years. Copper has an antispermatic effect.

The IUD method is effective over a long time, appears to have no systemic effects and reduces the possibility of patient error. This reversible method of birth control is as effective as oral contraceptives and more effective than barrier methods.

Disadvantages include possible excessive bleeding, cramps, and backaches and a slight risk of tubal pregnancy, pelvic infection, displacement, and rarely, perforation of the cervix and uterus. If a pregnancy occurs with an IUD in place, the device is removed immediately to avoid infection. Spontaneous abortion (miscarriage) may occur on removal.

An IUD method is not usually used in women who have not had children because the nulliparous uterus may be too small to tolerate it. Women with multiple partners, women with heavy or crampy periods, or those with a history of ectopic pregnancy or pelvic infection are encouraged to use other methods. Some practitioners prescribe antibiotics after inserting an IUD to prevent possible infection.

Mechanical Barriers

Diaphragm. The diaphragm is an effective contraceptive device, consisting of a round, flexible spring (50 to 90 mm wide) covered with a domelike latex rubber cup. A spermicidal jelly or cream is used to coat the concavity of the diaphragm before it is inserted deep into the vagina, covering the cervix. The diaphragm combined with a spermicide prevents spermatozoa from entering the cervical canal. The diaphragm is not felt by the user or her partner when properly fitted and inserted. Because women vary in size, diaphragms are designed to fit the individual, making it necessary for the woman's diaphragm to be properly sized and fitted by an experienced health care provider. The woman is instructed in using and caring for the device. A return demonstration ensures that the woman can insert the diaphragm correctly and that it covers the cervix.

Each time that the woman uses the diaphragm she must examine it carefully for flaws. Holding it up to a bright light and scrutinizing it ensures that no pinpoint holes, cracks, or tears have occurred. Contraceptive jelly or cream is applied in a prescribed manner to the concave surface of the diaphragm. If the jelly or cream is applied more than 6 hours before intercourse, it must be reapplied. The diaphragm is then positioned to cover the cervix completely. The diaphragm should remain in place at least 6 hours (but no more than 12 hours) after coitus. Each act of intercourse requires additional spermicide. On removal, the diaphragm is cleansed thoroughly with mild soap and water, rinsed, and dried before it is stored in its original container.

Disadvantages include allergic reactions in those who are sensitive to latex and an association with urinary tract infections. Toxic shock syndrome has been reported in some women who have used diaphragms.

Cervical Cap. The cervical cap is much smaller (22 to 35 mm) than the diaphragm and covers only the cervix, it is used with a spermicide. If a woman can feel her cervix, she can usually learn to use a cervical cap. The chief advantage is that the cap may be left in place for 2 days.

Although convenient to use, the cervical cap may cause cervical irritation; so before fitting a cap, most clinicians obtain a Pap smear and repeat the smear after 3 months. The cap can stay in place for 48 hours and does not require additional spermicide for repeated acts of intercourse.

Female Condom. An innovative contraceptive method for women, the female condom theoretically provides women with control over STDs and HIV as well as pregnancy. A recently introduced version, known as Reality, consists of a cylinder of polyurethane enclosed at one end by a

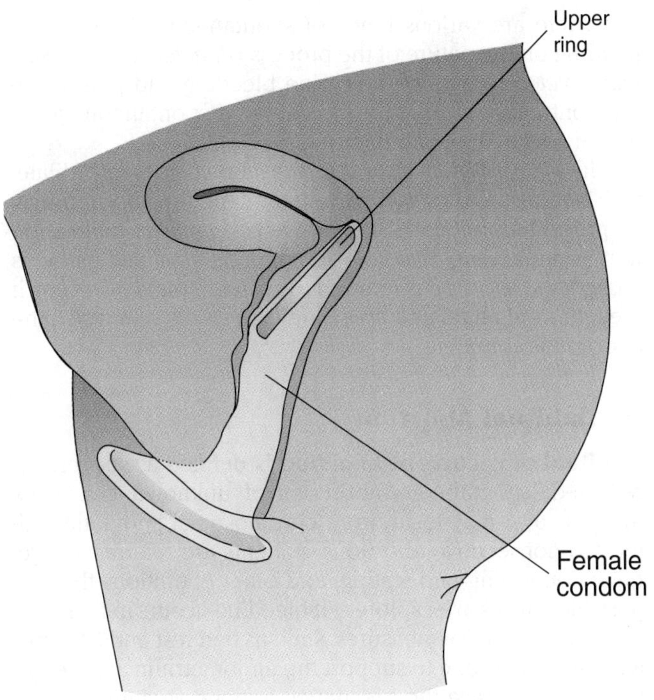

FIGURE 44-9. Female condom. The upper ring keeps the condom in place.

closed ring that covers the cervix and at the other end by an open ring that covers the perineum (Fig. 44-9). Advantages include some degree of protection from STDs (*i.e.*, human papilloma virus, herpes simplex, and HIV). Disadvantages include the inability to use with some coital positions (*i.e.*, standing).

Spermicides. Spermicides are available over-the-counter in foams, inserts, and on condoms. Spermicides are effective contraceptives when used with condoms. When used alone, spermicide are better than no contraception and may provide protection from some STDs.

Male Condom. The male condom is an impermeable, snug-fitting latex cover applied to the erect penis before it enters the vaginal canal. The tip of the condom is pinched while being applied to leave space for ejaculate. If no space is left, ejaculation may cause a tear or hole in the condom and reduce its effectiveness. The penis, with the condom held in place, is removed from the vagina while still erect to prevent the ejaculate from leaking.

The condom is an effective method when used with contraceptive foam. The latex condom also creates a barrier against transmission of STDs, especially gonorrhea, chlamydia infection, and HIV. It is recommended for reducing the risk of HIV infection. However, natural condoms (those made from animal tissue) do not protect against HIV infection. The nurse needs to reassure women that they have a right to insist on their male partner using a condom and a right to refuse having sex without condoms. Nurses should be familiar and comfortable with instructions about using a condom, as many women need to know about this way of protecting themselves from HIV and other STDs.

Coitus Interruptus. Coitus interruptus, withdrawing the penis from the vagina before ejaculation, requires careful control by the male and is a frequently used contraceptive method. Much of the uncertainty and unreliability of this method results from the possible presence of sperm in prejaculatory fluid. Men and women are usually unaware of this fact and need to be informed that withdrawal may be an ineffective contraceptive method.

Rhythm and Natural Methods. The advantages of natural contraceptive methods include the following: (1) they are not hazardous to a person's health, (2) they are inexpensive, and (3) they are approved by some religions. The disadvantages are that they require discipline by the couple who must monitor the menstrual cycle and abstain from sex during the fertile phase. The **rhythm method** of contraception can be difficult to use because it relies on the woman determining her time of ovulation and on avoiding intercourse during the fertile period. The fertile phase (which requires sexual abstinence) is estimated to occur about 14 days before menstruation, although it may occur between the 10th and 17th days. Spermatozoa can fertilize an ovum up to 72 hours after intercourse and the ovum can be fertilized for 24 hours after leaving the ovary. The pregnancy rate with the rhythm method is approximately 40% yearly.

According to some researchers, a woman who carefully determines her "safe period," based on a precise recording of menstrual dates for at least 1 year, and who follows a carefully worked out formula may achieve 80% protection. A long abstinence period during each cycle is required. These prerequisites require more time and control than many women and couples have.

Courses in natural family planning are offered at many Catholic hospitals and some family planning clinics. Chart 44-6 presents guidelines for teaching patients about the natural family planning.

Ovulation detection methods (*e.g.* Ovulindex) are available in most pharmacies. The presence of the enzyme, guaiacol peroxidase, in cervical mucus signals ovulation 6 days beforehand and also affects mucal viscosity.

Test kits are available over the counter and are easy to use and reliable but can be expensive. Ovulation prediction kits are more effective for planning conception than for avoiding it.

CHART 44-6
Patient Education: Natural Rhythm Method of Family Planning

- Keep a daily chart recording the nature of cervical mucus and vaginal wetness (changes as the menstrual cycle progresses).
- Measure basal body temperature at waking (temperature rises for a few days after ovulation).
- Estimate when ovulation will occur based on data and past experience.
- Take a course in this method with sexual partner to increase cooperation and understanding of periods requiring abstinence.

Postcoital Conception Control (Emergency Contraception). A properly timed, adequate dosage of *estrogen* after intercourse can prevent pregnancy. Nurses should be aware of this option and the indications for its use. This method obviously is not suitable for long-term contraception but is valuable in emergency situations such as rape, a defective or torn condom or diaphragm, or other "mishaps" that may occur during intercourse.

This estrogen preparation, administered after intercourse and before ovum implantation, is very effective. Usually, a small dose of oral contraceptives (*i.e.*, levonorgestrol and ethinyl estradiol) is given and repeated in 12 hours. As a side effect, nausea is common and can be minimized by taking the medication with meals and with an antiemetic medication. Other side effects, such as breast soreness and irregular bleeding, may occur but are transient. Any patient using this method should be advised of the 1.6% failure rate and counseled about other contraceptive methods. Morning-after contraception is related to luteal phase dysfunction, producing an endometrium that is out of phase.

Postcoital IUD insertion within 5 days of exposure has been used with a copper-bearing IUD in women who want this method of contraception; however, it may be inappropriate for some women or if other contraindications exist.

Investigational Control. Researchers recognize that the perfect method of conception control does not exist. Barring abstinence, every method has some risk, so research on new methods continues. New methods must undergo extensive and expensive evaluation prior to availability. One method under investigation is the use of vaginal rings that are placed around the cervix and release progestin. The rings may be effective for 3 months. Other methods under investigation include patches, sublingual medications, and disposable diaphragms. Methods under investigation for men include hormonal approaches to block sperm production, vaccines that interrupt sperm transport, hormone analogues, and vasectomies accomplished without the use of a scalpel.

Abortion

Interruption of pregnancy or expulsion of the product of conception before the fetus is viable is called **abortion.**

The fetus is generally considered to be viable any time after the fifth to sixth month of gestation. The term *premature labor* is used when a woman experiences labor at this point in the pregnancy.

Spontaneous Abortion

It is estimated that 1 of every 5 to 10 conceptions results in spontaneous abortion. Most of these occur because of an abnormality in the fetus that makes survival impossible. Other causes may include systemic diseases, hormonal imbalance, or anatomic abnormalities. If a pregnant woman experiences bleeding and cramping, a threatened abortion is diagnosed because an actual abortion is usually imminent. Spontaneous abortion occurs most commonly in the second or third month of gestation.

There are various kinds of spontaneous abortion, depending on the nature of the process (*threatened, inevitable, incomplete* or *complete*). Uterine bleeding and pain (uterine contractions) may be indicative of spontaneous abortion in a woman of childbearing age.

In a threatened abortion, the cervix does not dilate; with bed rest and conservative treatment, the abortion may be prevented. If it cannot be prevented, an inevitable abortion is imminent. If some—but not all—of the tissue is passed, the abortion is referred to as incomplete; however, if the fetus and all related tissue are expressed (removed), the abortion is complete.

Habitual Abortion

Habitual or **recurrent abortion** is defined as successive, repeated, spontaneous abortions of unknown cause. As many as 60% may result from chromosomal anomalies. After two consecutive abortions, patients are referred for genetic counseling and testing, and other conditions that are possible causes are explored. If bleeding occurs in these patients, conservative measures, such as bed rest and administering progesterone to support the endometrium are tried in an attempt to save the pregnancy. Supportive counseling is crucial in this stressful condition.

In the condition known as **incompetent** or **dysfunctional cervix,** the cervix dilates painlessly in the second trimester of pregnancy, often resulting in a spontaneous abortion. In such cases, a surgical procedure called the *cervical cerclage* may be used to prevent the cervix from dilating prematurely. The procedure involves placing a purse-string suture around the cervix at the level of the internal os. Bed rest is usually advised to keep the weight of the uterus off the cervix.

The patient and her health care providers, including those in community health agencies, must be informed that such a suture is in place in this high-risk pregnancy. About 2 to 3 weeks before term or the onset of labor, the suture is cut. Delivery is usually by cesarean section.

Management of Patients Undergoing Spontaneous Abortion. Signs of a threatened abortion are vaginal bleeding and abdominal cramps in a woman who has a delayed period and who has had a positive pregnancy test. The woman is encouraged to see a health care provider, who may recommend bed rest, sexual abstinence, a light diet, and no straining on defecation. If infection is suspected, antibiotics may be prescribed.

Nursing Interventions. Following a spontaneous abortion, all tissue passed vaginally is saved for examination. The patient and all personnel caring for her are alerted to save any discharged material. In the rare case of heavy bleeding, the patient may require transfusions and fluid replacement. An estimate of the bleeding volume can be determined by recording the number of perineal pads and the degree of saturation over 24 hours. When an incomplete abortion occurs, oxytocin may be prescribed to cause uterine contractions before dilatation and evacuation (D&E) or uterine suctioning. This patient having a D&E requires the same nursing care as any woman having a D&C (see p. 1241.)

Because patients experience loss and anxiety, emotional support and understanding are important aspects of nursing care. The response of the woman who desperately wants a baby is very different from that of the woman who does not want to be pregnant but may be frightened by the possible consequences of an abortion.

The nurse must be aware the woman having a spontaneous abortion often will experience a grieving period. The grieving may be delayed or unresolved and may cause other problems until the grief reaction has been resolved. The many reasons for a delayed grief reaction include the following: friends may not have known the woman was pregnant; the woman may not have seen the lost fetus and can only imagine the sex, size, and characteristics of the child who never developed; there is usually no burial service; those who know about the loss (family friends, caregivers) may encourage denial by rarely encouraging crying and talking about the loss.

In any event, providing opportunities for the patient to talk and vent her emotions not only helps but also provides clues for the nurse in planning more specific care. The persons closest to the woman are encouraged to hug her and allow her to talk and freely express her grief. Unresolved grief may manifest itself in persistent vivid memories of the events surrounding the loss, persistent sadness or anger, and episodes of overwhelming emotion when recalling the loss. Dysfunctional grief may require the assistance of a skilled therapist.

Elective Abortion

A voluntary termination of pregnancy (TOP) is called an *elective abortion* and is usually performed by skilled health care providers. In 1973, the Supreme Court ruled that decisions about abortion reside with a woman and her physician in the first trimester. The ruling stated that during the second trimester, the state may regulate practice in the interest of a woman's health, and during the final weeks of pregnancy the state may choose to protect the life of the fetus, except when necessary to preserve the life or health of the woman. Legislation has been passed to increase access to clinics, and to prevent violence toward those who work in abortion facilities.

Approximately 1.6 million abortions are performed every year in the United States. The rate of abortion has decreased slightly. Despite this decrease, not all groups are part of this decline. Pregnancy termination has increased in the following groups: unmarried Caucasian females under age 15, unmarried non-Caucasian adolescents between ages 15 and 19, and married non-Caucasian women between ages 20 and 24. These numbers point out the need for nurses to provide family planning education and counseling.

Legal abortions may be carried out in the following ways, usually in an outpatient setting:

Dilatation and Evacuation or Suction Curettage. The cervix is dilated manually with instrumentation or by a laminaria, and a uterine aspirator is introduced. Suction is applied and tissue is removed from the uterus.

Hypertonic Saline Injection. A small amount of amniotic fluid is removed and replaced by hypertonic saline. Augmentation with oxytocin speeds the process. This method is contraindicated in those with cardiac disease. Although rare, serious complications can occur, including cardiovascular collapse, cerebral edema, pulmonary edema, renal failure, and disseminated intravascular coagulopathy (DIC). Hyperosmolar urea also is used but has a high failure rate.

Prostaglandins. These substances can be introduced into amniotic fluid or by vaginal suppository or intramuscular injection in later pregnancy. Strong uterine contractions ensue within 4 hours, usually resulting in abortion. Oxytocin is not needed. This method prevents the DIC associated with saline-based abortions. Gastrointestinal symptoms (*e.g.*, nausea, vomiting, diarrhea, and abdominal cramping) and fever can occur.

Laminaria. Laminaria tents are made from a species of seaweed or from synthetic material. They are shaped into tampon-like forms with a string on one end. When placed in a moist environment, the tent, which is highly hygroscopic, swells three to five times its original diameter, causing dilatation. The greatest swelling occurs in 4 or 5 hours; however, additional dilatation may occur over the next few hours.

Advantages of laminaria over mechanical dilators include less trauma and more acceptance and tolerance by patients. Disadvantages include discomfort and slight cramping. This method also requires one visit for insertion and a return visit 4 to 6 hours later. There is a risk of low-grade endometritis (inflammation of the endometrium) even though the laminaria is sterilized by radiation or gas. Occasionally, removal is difficult and, rarely, the laminaria may slip into the uterus. An alternative is Lamicel, a synthetic polyethylene sponge impregnated with magnesium sulfate and compressed into a rod. It works more rapidly than Laminaria tents.

RU-486. **RU-486** (Mifepristone) is a progesterone antagonist that prevents ovum implantation. Administered orally within 10 days of an expected period, RU-486 produces a medical abortion in most patients. Prolonged bleeding may occur. Combined with a prostaglandin suppository, it causes an abortion in up to 95% of patients after conception. Other uses for this medication include treating breast cancer, endometriosis, and ectopic pregnancy. Political and religious opposition has slowed its use in the United States.

Methotrexate. **Methotrexate** has also been studied as a means of causing miscarriage. It has been found to have minimal risk and few side effects. Its low cost may provide an alternative for women in the future.

Hysterotomy. A hysterotomy is a miniature cesarean section. This surgical procedure is infrequently used as a method for terminating pregnancy.

Septic Abortion. When unskilled attempts are made to end a pregnancy, the methods usually include administering large amounts of various toxic agents (effects are toxic and the uterus is never fully evacuated) or performing a curettage, entailing associated risks of rupturing the uterus, hemorrhage, or infection. Although this was a major problem in the past, the dissemination of birth control information and liberalized abortion laws have led to a decline in septic abortion.

If a woman who has had a septic abortion receives proper medical attention early enough and is treated with broad-spectrum antibiotics, the prognosis is excellent. Fluid and blood component replacement may be required before careful attempts are made to evacuate the uterus. For the treatment of septic abortion complicated by shock, see the discussions of shock (Chapter 15) and PID (Chapter 45).

Management of the Patient Undergoing Elective Abortion. Before the procedure is performed, the patient's fears, feelings, and options are explored with her by a nurse or counselor trained in pregnancy counseling. After the patient's choice is identified (*i.e.*, continuing pregnancy and parenthood; continuing pregnancy followed by adoption; or terminating pregnancy by abortion), a pelvic examination is performed to determine uterine size. Laboratory studies before an abortion must include a pregnancy test to confirm the pregnancy, the hematocrit value to rule out anemia, an Rh determination, and an STD screen. A patient with anemia may need iron supplement, and an Rh-negative patient may require RhoGam to prevent isoimmunization. Before the procedure, all patients should be screened for STDs to prevent introducing pathogens upward through the cervix during the procedure.

Available contraceptive methods for postponing or preventing pregnancy are reviewed with the patient at this time. Effectiveness depends on the method used and the extent to which the correct instructions for use are followed by the woman and her partner. The woman who has used any method of birth control should be assessed for her understanding of the method and its potential side effects and her satisfaction with the method. If the patient was not using contraception, the nurse explains all methods, benefits, and risks and assists the patient in choosing a contraceptive choice after abortion. An increasingly important related teaching issue is the need to use barrier contraceptive devices (*i.e.*, condoms) for protection against transmission of STDs and HIV infection. The patient is also scheduled for a follow-up appointment 2 weeks after the procedure and is instructed in recognizing and reporting signs of complications (*i.e.*, fever, heavy bleeding, or pain).

Infertility

Infertility is defined as a couple's inability to achieve pregnancy after 1 year of unprotected intercourse. **Primary infertility** refers to a couple who has never had a child. **Secondary infertility** means that at least one conception has occurred but currently the couple cannot achieve a pregnancy. In the United States, infertility is a major medical and social problem affecting 10% to 15% of the population.

Pathophysiology

Possible causes of infertility include uterine displacement by tumors, congenital anomalies, and inflammation. For an ovum to become fertilized, the vagina, fallopian tubes, cervix, and uterus must be patent and the mucosal secretions must be receptive to the sperm. Semen is alkaline, as are cervical secretions, whereas normal vaginal secretion is acidic. Often, more than one factor may be responsible for the problem. Identifying the possible causes may require the services of a gynecologist, urologist, and endocrinologist.

Diagnostic Evaluation

Careful evaluation includes not only physical examination and endocrinologic investigation but also consideration of psychosocial factors. A complete history, physical examination, and laboratory studies are performed on both partners to rule out such causative factors as a previous STD, anomalies, injuries, tuberculosis, mumps orchitis, impaired sperm production, endometriosis, DES, or antisperm antibodies. Induced abortions are not a factor in the ability to conceive, unless they are complicated by infection. Three histories need to be obtained: one of each partner and one of the couple.

Five factors are considered basic to infertility; for the woman, (1) ovarian, (2) tubal, (3) cervical, or (4) uterine conditions; and for the man, (5) seminal conditions. A composite estimate of the relative frequency of the causes of infertility follows:

- Unexplained—28%
- Sperm problem—21%
- Ovulatory failure—18%
- Tubal damage—14%
- Endometriosis—6%
- Coital problem—5%
- Cervical mucus—3%
- Other male problems—2%

Ovarian Factor. Studies performed to determine whether there is regular ovulation and a progestational endometrium adequate for implantation include a basal body temperature chart for at least four cycles, an endometrial biopsy, and serum progesterone level.

Tubal Factor. Hysterosalpingography (see p. 1244) is an x-ray study used to rule out uterine or tubal abnormalities.

Laparoscopy (see p. 1243) permits direct visualization of the tubes and other pelvic structures and can assist in diagnosing conditions that may interfere with fertility (*e.g.*, endometriosis).

Cervical Factor. Cervical mucus can be examined at ovulation and after intercourse to determine whether proper changes occur that promote sperm penetration and survival.

A postcoital cervical mucus test (Sims-Huhner test) is performed between 2 and 8 hours after intercourse. Cervical mucus is aspirated with a medicine dropper–like instrument. Aspirated material is placed on a slide and examined under the microscope for the presence and viability of sperm cells. The woman is instructed not to bathe or douche between coitus and the examination.

Uterine Factor. Fibroids, polyps, and congenital malformations are possible problems in this category. Their presence may be determined by pelvic examination, hysteroscopy, and hysterosalpingography.

Seminal Factor. After 2 to 3 days of sexual abstinence, a specimen of ejaculate is collected in a clean container, kept warm, and examined within 1 hour for the number of sperm (density), percentage of moving forms, quality of forward movement (forward progression), and morphology (shape and form). From 2 to 6 ml of watery alkaline semen is normal; a normal count is 60 million to 100 million sperm/ml, although the incidence of impregnation is lessened only when the count drops below 20 million/ml. A normal semen analysis should show:

- Volume—1.5–5 ml
- Density— >20 million/ml
- Motility—60%
- Forward progression— >2 (scale 1–4)
- Morphology— >60% normal forms
- No sperm clumping, significant red or white blood cells, or thickening of seminal fluid (hyperviscosity)

Males are also affected by varicoceles, varicose veins around the testicle, which are found in 40% of men evaluated for possible infertility. Retrograde ejaculation or ejaculation into the bladder is assessed by urinalysis after ejaculation.

Blood tests for male partners may include measuring testosterone, FSH, LH, (both involved in maintaining testicular function), and prolactin levels and antisperm antibodies (treated with corticosteroids) as well. Other tests may include sperm penetration assay (which measures the ability of sperm to penetrate hamster ova) and testicular biopsy. Nurses need to keep in mind that infertility evaluations are threatening to both women and men alike, but men may equate fertility with masculinity.

Miscellaneous Factors. Miscellaneous factors, including immunologic factors, are being investigated. Some cases of recurrent early pregnancy loss or recurrent natural abortion are due to an abnormal response by the woman to antigens on fetal or placental tissues. Some women have been treated with infusions of their partner's lymphocytes with some success, but this treatment remains experimental, and the long-term effects are unknown.

Management

Infertility is often difficult to treat because it frequently results from a combination of factors. Statistics show that many couples undergoing an infertility evaluation conceive without the cause of infertility coming to light. Likewise, although some couples undergo all tests, the cause of the problem may remain undiscovered. Between these extremes, many problems, both simple and complex, can be discovered and corrected.

Therapy may require surgery to correct a malfunction or anomaly, hormonal supplements, attention to proper timing, and recognition and correction of psychologic or emotional factors.

Nursing interventions to keep in mind when working with couples during infertility evaluations include the following: assist in reducing stress in the relationship, encourage cooperation, protect privacy, foster understanding, and refer the couple to appropriate resources when necessary. Because infertility work-ups are expensive, invasive, stressful, and not always successful, couples need support in working together to grow from this endeavor.

Reproductive Technologies

Numerous technologies have been developed to help in reproduction and to assist in the basic right of procreation. Mechanisms already exist under U.S. law (*e.g.*, institutional review boards and procedures) to foster safe medical procedures while safeguarding the integrity of the participants in these procedures.

Inducing Ovulation With Medication. Inducing ovulation is undertaken when women do not ovulate on their own or ovulate irregularly. Various medications are used depending on the primary cause of infertility. An increased risk of ovarian cancer is possible in women who take fertility drugs; therefore, this risk must be considered.

- *Clomid* is used when the hypothalamus is not stimulating the pituitary gland to release FSH and LH. This medication stimulates follicles in the ovary. It is usually taken on the fifth day of the menstrual cycle for 5 days. Ovulation should occur 4 to 8 days after the last dose. Patients receive instructions about timing intercourse to facilitate fertilization.
- *Pergonal,* a combination of FSH and LH, is used for those with deficiencies in these hormones. Pergonal stimulates the ovaries, so monitoring by ultrasound and hormone levels is essential because overstimulation may occur.
- *Metrodin,* containing FSH with a small amount of LH, is used in some disorders (*i.e.*, polycystic ovarian syndrome) to stimulate follicle growth. Clomid is then used to stimulate ovulation.
- *Chorionic gonadotropin* is used to stimulate release of the egg from the ovary and may be used in combination with the above medications.

Artificial Insemination. Depositing or introducing semen into the female genital tract by artificial means is called **artificial insemination.** If the sperm cannot penetrate the cervical canal normally, artificial insemination, using the partner's semen (AIH, or artificial insemination with sperm from the husband or partner) may be considered. In azoospermia (lack of sperm in the semen), semen from carefully selected donors may be used (AID, or artificial insemination with sperm from donor). Because artificial insemination is likely to be a stressful and difficult situation for couples, nursing support and strategies to promote coping are crucial.

Indications for using artificial insemination include: (1) the male's inability to deposit semen in the vagina, which may be due to premature ejaculation, pronounced hypospadias (a displaced male urethra), or dyspareunia (painful intercourse experienced by the woman); and (2) inability of semen to be transported from the vagina to the uterine cavity, which is usually due to faulty chemical conditions and which may occur with an abnormal cervical discharge. Another indication for artificial insemination is a single woman's desire to have a child.

Partner's Semen. Certain conditions need to be established before semen is transferred to the vagina. The woman must have no abnormalities of the genital system, the tubes must be patent, and ova must be available. In the male, sperm need to be normal in shape, amount, motility, and endurance. The time of ovulation in the woman should be determined as accurately as possible, so that the 2 or 3 days during which fertilization is possible each month can be used. Fertilization seldom occurs from a single insemination. Usually, insemination is attempted between the 10th and 17th days of the cycle; three different attempts may be made during one cycle. Semen is collected by masturbation. Withdrawal and using condoms for sperm collection are considered unsatisfactory by many infertility specialists because some sperm may be lost or adversely affected.

Donor's Semen. When the sperm of the woman's partner are defective or absent or when there is a risk of transmitting a genetic disease, donor sperm may be used. Safeguards are put in place to prevent legal, ethical, emotional, and religious problems. Written consent is obtained to protect all parties involved, including the woman, the donor, and the resulting child.

The donor, selected on the basis of close resemblance to the husband both physically and intellectually, should have no family history of epilepsy, diabetes, or known genetic defects. He should also have negative test results for syphilis and HIV. Preferably, precautions should be taken so that the donor is not known to the recipient and vice versa.

Insemination Procedure. The woman may have been given Clomid and Pergonal to stimulate ovulation before insemination. Sonograms and blood studies of varying hormone levels are used to pinpoint the best time for insemination.

The recipient is placed in the lithotomy position on the examination table, a speculum is inserted, and the vagina and cervix are swabbed with a cotton-tipped applicator to remove any excess secretions. Semen is drawn into a sterile syringe, and a cannula is attached. The semen is then directed to the external os. If this is contraindicated, the semen may be inserted directly into the uterus (intrauterine insemination). In this procedure, the sperm are washed before insertion to remove biochemicals and to select the most active sperm. This is indicated when mucus is inadequate, when antibodies are present, or when sperm count is low. After the careful withdrawal of the syringe, the patient remains in a supine position for 30 minutes.

The success rate for artificial insemination varies. From three to six inseminations may be required over 2 to 4 months. Because this procedure is opposed by the Roman Catholic Church, patients may choose to consult their priest or spiritual advisor.

In Vitro Fertilization (IVF). This procedure is accomplished by first stimulating the ovary to produce multiple eggs or ova, usually with medications such as Pergonal or Clomid, because pregnancy success rates are greater with more than one early embryo. Many different protocols exist for inducing ovulation with one or more agents. Patients are carefully selected and evaluated and cycles are carefully monitored by using ultrasound and assessing estradiol levels. At the appropriate time, the ova are recovered by transvaginal ultrasound retrieval. Sperm and eggs are coincubated for up to 36 hours and the embryos are transferred approximately 48 to 80 hours after retrieval. Implantation should occur in 2 to 3 days. Gamete intrafallopian transfer (GIFT) is a variation of IVF in which oocytes are removed and drawn into a catheter with sperm and then inserted into the fallopian tube, where fertilization occurs. Success rates vary from 20% to 30% The most common indications for these procedures are irreparable tubal damage, endometriosis, immunologic problems, unexplained infertility, inadequate sperm, and exposure to diethylstilbestrol (DES).

Although IVF produced mixed public reactions initially, it is now a standard form of infertility treatment, with hundreds of programs in the United States.

Other Reproductive Technologies. Two other techniques that are utilized in infertility are zygote intrafallopian transfer (ZIFT) and intracytoplasmic sperm injection (ICSI). In ZIFT, an egg is retrieved vaginally, guided by ultrasound while the patient is under light anesthesia. The egg is fertilized *in vitro* and transferred to the fallopian tube at the pronuclear stage prior to cell division the following day. In intracytoplasmic sperm injection (ICSI), an ovum is retrieved as above and a sperm is injected through the zona pellucida, through the egg membrane, and into the egg. The fertilized egg is then transferred back to the donor. These techniques are used when couples have not achieved fertilization in previous IVF cycles or when men have very few motile sperm in their ejaculate. These micromanipulation techniques have the potential of damaging the egg or the sperm and are used only when indicated.

Psychological Issues. Couples involved in infertility and reproductive technology require education and support to cope with anxiety because these procedures are stressful, time consuming, and expensive. RESOLVE, an organization that provides information and group support for infertile patients is a nonprofit self-help group originated by a nurse who experienced difficulty conceiving. The literature on infertility that is produced by this group is an important resource for patients and professionals. Most areas across the country have local support groups. More information can be obtained by writing to RESOLVE, Inc. (see the address at the end of this chapter).

Ectopic Pregnancy

Ectopic pregnancy occurs in about 1 of 79 to 100 pregnancies, when a fertilized ovum (a blastocyst) becomes implanted on any tissue other than the uterine lining such as the fallopian tube, ovary, abdomen, or the cervix (Fig. 44-10.) The highest incidence of ectopic implantation occurs in the fallopian tube.

Possible precipitating factors include salpingitis, peritubal adhesions (following pelvic infection, endometriosis, appendicitis), abnormalities of the fallopian tube (rare and usually related to DES exposure), previous ectopic pregnancy (after one ectopic pregnancy, the risk of recurrence is 7% to 15%), previous tubal surgery, multiple previous induced abortions (particularly if followed by infection), tumors that distort the tube, and IUD and progestin-only contraceptives. Pelvic inflammatory disease (PID) seems to be the major risk factor for ectopic pregnancy. Improved antibiotic therapy for PID usually prevents total tubal closure, but may leave a stricture or narrowing, predisposing the woman to ectopic implantation.

The rate of tubal pregnancies has increased in disproportion to population growth. Ectopic pregnancies are being diagnosed sooner because of advanced diagnostic techniques. Moreover, they are being treated conservatively before emergency rupture and hemorrhage occurs. It may be that the increased numbers result from better diagnostic

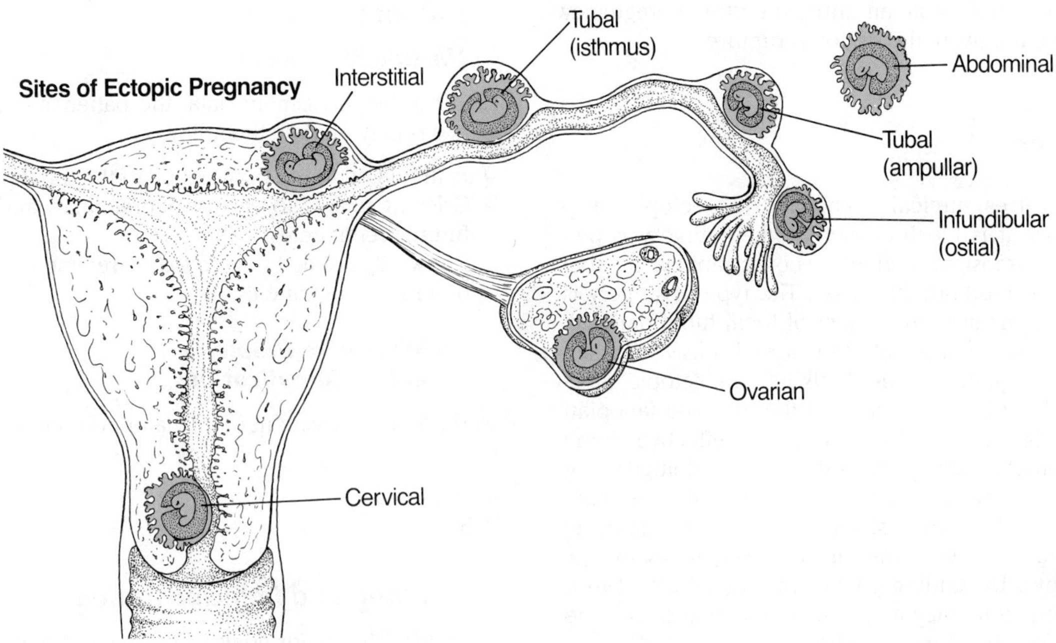

FIGURE 44-10. Sites of ectopic pregnancy.

techniques. Conservative treatment makes ectopic pregnancy less life-threatening than previously, but this condition persists as the second leading cause of maternal mortality in the United States.

Clinical Manifestations

Signs and symptoms vary depending on whether tubal rupture has occurred. Delay in menstruation from 1 to 2 weeks followed by slight bleeding (spotting) or a description of a slightly abnormal period suggests the possibility of an ectopic pregnancy. Symptoms may begin late with vague soreness on the affected side, probably due to uterine contractions and distention of the tube. Typically the patient experiences sharp, colicky pain. Most patients experience pelvic or abdominal pain and some spotting or bleeding. Gastrointestinal symptoms, dizziness, or lightheadedness are common. The patient frequently thinks the abnormal bleeding is a menstrual period, especially if a recent period occurred and was normal. However, even in such circumstances an ectopic pregnancy is possible. Some form of bleeding occurs in more than half of ectopic pregnancies, so most health care providers and patients do not immediately suspect a tubal pregnancy.

If implantation occurs in the fallopian tube, the tube becomes more and more distended. The tube can rupture if the ectopic pregnancy remains undetected for 4 to 6 weeks after conception or longer. When the tube ruptures, the ovum is discharged into the abdominal cavity.

When tubal rupture occurs, the woman experiences agonizing pain, dizziness, faintness, and nausea and vomiting, which are important symptoms to document and report. These symptoms are related to peritoneal reaction to blood escaping from the tube. Air hunger and symptoms of shock may occur and the signs of hemorrhage—rapid, thready pulse; decreased blood pressure; subnormal temperature; restlessness; pallor and sweating—are in evidence. Later the pain becomes generalized in the abdomen and radiates to the shoulder and neck because of accumulating intraperitoneal blood that irritates the diaphragm. During vaginal examination, a large mass of clotted blood that has collected in the pelvis behind the uterus or a tender adnexal mass may be palpable.

Diagnostic Evaluation

Some amount of human chorionic gonadotropin (HCG), the diagnostic hormone of pregnancy, can be detected in all woman who are pregnant. HCG levels double in normal pregnancies every 3 days, but are reduced in abnormal or ectopic pregnancy. Patients typically undergo a blood test to assess HCG. The test is usually repeated in 2 or 3 days. A less than normal increase is cause for suspicion. Urine tests for pregnancy vary in reliability and are not helpful in ectopic pregnancies.

Ultrasound can detect a pregnancy between 5 and 6 weeks from the last menstrual period. Detectable fetal heart movement outside of the uterus on ultrasound is firm evidence of an ectopic pregnancy. On occasion, an ultrasound study is not definitive and diagnosis must be made with combined diagnostic aids (HCG level, ultrasound, pelvic examination, and clinical judgement). Ultrasound with Doppler flow studies, in which color indicates perfusion, are helpful.

Occasionally, the clinical picture makes the diagnosis relatively easy. However, when clinical signs and symptoms are questionable, which is often the case, other aid have value. Laparoscopy is used most often because ...e physician can visually note an unruptured tubal pregnancy and, thereby, circumvent the risk of its rupture.

Management

Treatment involves surgically removing the ectopic pregnancy, because it is life-threatening. When surgery is performed early, almost all patients recover rapidly; if tubal rupture occurs, mortality increases. The type of surgery is determined by the size and extent of local tubal damage; surgery ranges from conservative to more extensive. Conservative surgery would include "milking" an ectopic pregnancy from the tube. A resection of the involved fallopian tube with end-to-end anastomosis may be effective. Some surgeons attempt to salvage the tube with a salpingostomy, which involves opening and evacuating the tube and controlling bleeding. More extensive surgery includes removing the tube alone (salpingectomy) or with the ovary (salpingo-oophorectomy). Depending on the amount of blood lost, blood component therapy and treatment for shock may be necessary before and during surgery.

Methotrexate, a chemotherapeutic agent, is used after surgery to treat any remaining tissue, as indicated by a persistent or rising beta-HCG level. The beta-HCG study is repeated 2 weeks after surgery to assure a falling level.

Another option is using methotrexate without surgery. Because this drug stops the pregnancy from progressing, it interrupts early, small unruptured tubal pregnancies. Side effects include stomatitis and diarrhea, bone marrow suppression, impaired liver function, dermatitis, and pleuritis. Doses are based on the patient's beta-HCG level. Citrovorum factor (leucovorin) has been used to reduce methotrexate's toxic effects. Liver enzymes and serum creatinine levels are monitored. The patient is also monitored by frequent ultrasounds and by assessing serum HCG levels.

Prognosis. Patients should be advised that ectopic pregnancies may recur. Reviewing signs and symptoms with the patient and instructing her to promptly report an abnormal menstrual period are important.

❑ NURSING PROCESS
The Patient With an Ectopic Pregnancy

Assessment

The health history includes the menstrual pattern and any (even slight) bleeding since the patient's last menstrual period (LMP). The patient's description of pains and their location is elicited. She is asked if any sharp, colicky pains have occurred. Then the nurse notes whether pain radiates to the shoulder and neck, possibly caused by rupture and pressure on the diaphragm. Signs and symptoms of rupture are prominent and suggest hemorrhage and shock.

Vital signs, level of consciousness, and nature and amount of vaginal bleeding are monitored. The meaning of the pregnancy to the patient is assessed, if possible, to determine how the woman is coping with the likely loss of the pregnancy.

Diagnosis

Nursing Diagnoses

Based on the assessment data, the patient's major nursing diagnoses may include the following:

- ❑ Pain related to the progression of the tubal pregnancy
- ❑ Grieving related to the loss of pregnancy and effect on future pregnancies
- ❑ Knowledge deficit related to the treatment and impact on future pregnancies

Collaborative Problems/ Potential Complications

Based on the assessment data, major complications may include:

- ❑ Hemorrhage
- ❑ Shock

Planning and Implementation

Goals. The major goals of the patient may include relief of pain, acceptance and resolution of grief and pregnancy loss, understanding the ectopic pregnancy, its treatment and its outcome, and prevention of complications.

Nursing Interventions

Relieving Pain. The abdominal pain associated with ectopic pregnancy may be described as cramping or severe continuous pain. If the patient is to have surgery, preanesthetic medications also may provide pain relief. Postoperatively, analgesic agents are administered liberally; this promotes early ambulation and enables the patient to cough and take deep breaths.

Supporting the Grieving Process. Patients' distress levels vary. If the pregnancy is wanted, loss may or may not be expressed verbally by the patient and her partner. The impact may not be fully realized until much later. The nurse should be available to listen and provide support. The patient's partner, if appropriate, should participate in this process. Even if the pregnancy was unplanned, a loss has been experienced and a grief reaction may follow. Severe and persistent psychologic distress may require psychologic assessment and consultation by a psychotherapist or spiritual advisor.

Patient Teaching. If the patient has experienced life-threatening hemorrhage and shock, these complications must be addressed and treated before in-depth teaching can begin. At this time the patient's attention is focused on the crisis and not on learning. Therefore, it may be later that the patient begins to ask questions about what has happened and why certain procedures were performed. Procedures are explained in terms that a distressed and apprehensive patient can understand. The patient's partner is included in teaching and explanations when possible. After the patient recovers from postoperative discomforts, it may be more appropriate to address any questions and concerns that the patient and her partner may have, including the effect of this pregnancy on future pregnancies. Patient teaching is based on the needs of the patient and her partner and must take into consideration their distress and grief.

Monitoring and Managing Potential Complications. Potential complications of ectopic pregnancy are hemorrhage and shock. Careful assessment is essential to detect the development of these complications. Continuous monitoring of vital signs, level of consciousness, amount of bleeding, and the patient's intake and output provides information about the possibility of hemorrhage and the need to prepare for intravenous therapy. Bed rest is indicated. Hematocrit, hemoglobin, and blood gas levels are monitored to assess hematologic status and adequacy of tissue perfusion. Significant deviations in these laboratory values are reported immediately and the patient is prepared for possible surgery. Blood component therapy may be required if blood loss has been rapid and extensive. If hypovolemic shock occurs, the treatment is directed toward reestablishing tissue perfusion and adequate blood volume. See Chapter 15 for a discussion of the intravenous fluids and medications used in treating hypovolemic shock.

Evaluation

Expected Outcomes

1. Experiences relief of pain
   a. Reports a decrease in pain and discomfort
   b. Ambulates as prescribed, performs therapeutic coughing and deep-breathing
2. Begins to accept loss of pregnancy and expresses grief by verbalizing feelings and reactions to loss
3. Demonstrates an understanding of the causes of ectopic pregnancy
4. Experiences no complications
   a. Exhibits no signs of bleeding hemorrhage or shock
   b. Has decreased amounts of discharge (on perineal pad)
   c. Has normal skin color and turgor
   d. Exhibits stable vital signs and adequate urine output
   e. HCG levels return to normal

CRITICAL THINKING EXERCISES

1. A 38-year-old woman tells you that she has never had a Pap smear done and does not believe it is necessary since she is not sexually active. She also says that she would be afraid that the procedure might detect abnormalities and she is very afraid of having cancer. How would you respond to her?
2. You are a nurse practitioner in a neighborhood clinic. Upon performing a pelvic examination on a 16-year-old, you discover that she is pregnant. Her mother, who has brought her for the examination because she has missed two menstrual periods, asks you the results of the examination. How would you respond to the patient's mother if she insists that her daughter is not sexually active? Has expressed concern that her daughter is pregnant? How would you discuss the results of the examination with the patient?
3. A 47-year-old woman friend tells you that she believes she is perimenopausal. She has read a great deal about menopause, its effect on women's health, and the risks associated with hormone replacement therapy. She asks you for your advice and recommendations about the use of hormone therapy. How would you respond to her request?
4. A 20-year-old college student reports to the student health clinic. She believes she is very early in pregnancy and reports to you that for the last 12 hours she has had sharp abdominal pain, some vaginal bleeding, and dizziness. Analyze the data presented and describe the aspects of assessment you would consider important at this time and the actions you would take and why.
5. During a checkup at the clinic where you work, a 35-year-old divorced patient tells you that she has met a man who has had a number of sexual partners in the last 10 years. She anticipates that she and her friend will become sexual partners but states that she wishes to avoid pregnancy. How would you address the educational and counseling needs of your patient?

BIBLIOGRAPHY

Books

Campbell J and Humphreys J. Nursing Care of Survivors of Family Violence. Reston, VA, Reston Publishing, 1993.

Cunningham F et al. Obstetrics, 19th ed. Norwalk, CT, Appleton & Lange, 1993.

Dickey R. Managing Contraceptive Pill Patients, 8th ed. Durant, OK, Creative Infomatics, 1993.

Dutton M. Empowering and Healing the Battered Woman: A Model for Assessment and Intervention. New York, Springer-Verlag, 1993.

Gascoigne B and Irwin J. Smart ways to stay young and healthy. Berkeley, CA, Ronin Publishing, 1993.

Hatcher R et al. Contraceptive Technology, 16th ed. Irvington, NY, Irvington Publishers, 1993.

Hawkins J et al. Protocols for Nurse Practitioners in Gynecologic Settings, 5th ed. New York, Tiresias Press, 1995.

Horton J (ed). The Women's Health Data Book. Washington, DC, Elsevier, 1992.

Jensen M and Bobak I. Maternity and Gynecologic Care: The Nurse and The Family, 5th ed. St Louis, CV Mosby, 1993.

Pillitteri A. Maternal and Child Health Nursing. Philadelphia, JB Lippincott, 1992.

Sampselle C (ed). Violence Against Women: Nursing Research, Education and Practice Issues. New York, Hemisphere Publishing Company, 1992.

Speroff L et al. Clinical Gynecologic Endocrinology and Infertility. Baltimore, Williams & Wilkins, 1994.

Journals

Asterisks indicate nursing research articles.

General

Andrist LC. Taking a sexual history and educating clients about safe sex. Nurs Clin North Am 1988 Dec; 23(4):959–973.

Brundage J and Pacholski C. Guiding young women's health. NAACOG Clinical Issues in Perinatal Health 1991; 2(2): 271–277.

Colton T, Greenberg E, Noller K. Breast cancer in mothers prescribed diethlstilbestrol in pregnancy. JAMA 1993; 269: 2096–2100.

Dannull V. Exercise, diet and menstrual dysfunction. Nurse Pract [Dialogue] 1992; 3(1):1–3.

Dimond D. Ob-Gyn problems of adolescents are universal. Contemp Ob/Gyn 1993; 38(1):37–51.

*Hitchcock J and Wilson H. Personal risking: Lesbian self-disclosure of sexual orientation to professional health care providers. Nurs Res 1992; 41(3):178–183.

Jennings C. Corner on issues: Raising consciousness about women's health issues. J Am Acad Nurse Pract 1991 Apr/Jun; 3(2):92–94.

Krahn D, Demitrack M, Kurth C, et al. Dieting and menstrual irregularity. J Women's Health 1992; 1(4):289–291.

Stevens-Simon C. Clinical applications of adolescent female sexual development. Nurs Pract 1993 Dec; 18(12):18–29.

Welner S. Gynecologic care of the disabled woman. Contemp Ob/Gyn 1993; 38(1):55–67.

Woods N and Shaver J. The evolutionary spiral of a specialized center for women's health research. Image: Journal of Nursing Scholarship 1992 Mar; 24(3):223–228.

Assessment of Function and Dysfunction of Female Reproductive Function

Appleby J. Management of the abnormal Papanicolaou smear. Med Clin North Am 1995 Mar; 72(2):345–360.

Boyce J and Fruchter R. Deciding on the interval between pap smears. Contemp Ob/Gyn NP 1993 Apr; 1(1):13–21.

Crum C. Koilocytosis in pap smears: How useful a finding? Contemp Ob/Gyn 1993 July; 38(7):66–77.

Herbst A et al. Interpreting the new Bethesda classification system. Contemp Ob/Gyn 1993 Aug; 38(8):86–107.

*Lauver D and Rubin M. Women's concerns about abnormal papanicolau test results. J Obstet Gynecol Neonatal Nurs 1991; 20(2):154–159.

Monty F et al. Abnormal pap smears. Obstet Gynecol 1992; 80(2):385–388.

Schaffer S and Philput C. Predictors of abnormal cervical cytology: Statistical analysis of human papilloma virus and cofactors. Nurse Pract 1993; 17(3):46–50.

Stewart D, Lickrish G and Sierra S. The effect of educational brochures on knowledge and emotional distress in women with abnormal Papanicolaou smears. Obstet Gynecol 1993; 81:280–282.

Wathen PI, Henderson MC and Witz CA. Abnormal uterine bleeding. Med Clin North Am 1995 Mar; 79(2):329–342.

Domestic Violence

Furniss K. Screening for abuse in the clinical setting. AWHONN Clin Iss Perinatal and Wom Health Nurs 1993; 4(3):402–406.

Landenberger, K. Exploration of women's identity: Clinical approaches with abused women. AWHONN Clin Iss in Perinatal and Wom Health Nurs 1993; 4(3)378–384.

*McFarlane J, Parker B, Soeken K and Bullock L. Assessing for abuse during pregnancy. JAMA 1992 June 17; 267(23):3176–3178.

Samselle C. The role of nursing in preventing violence against women. J Obstet Gynecol Neonatal Nurs 1991 Nov/Dec; 20(6):481–487.

Smith M and Martin F. Domestic violence: Recognition, intervention and treatment. Medsurg Nurs 1995 Feb; 4(1):21–25.

Incest

Doob D. Female sexual abuse survivors as patients:Avoiding retraumatization. Arch Psychiatr Nurs 1992 Apr; 6(4):245–251.

Kriedler M. Use of an interactional model with survivors of incest. Iss Ment Health Nurs 1992 Mar–Apr; 13(2):149–158.

Walter K. That was then: Elderly survivors of incest. J Psychosoc Nurs Ment Health Serv 1992 Jan; 30(1):14–16.

Premenstrual Syndrome

Anderson M. You make the diagnosis. Nurs Diag 1992 Oct–Dec; 3(4):147–163.

Chuong C, Otey L and Rosenfeld B. Revising treatments for premenstrual syndrome. Contemp Ob/Gyn 1994 Jan; 39(1):66–76.

Ornitz A and Brown M. Family coping and premenstrual symptomatology. J Obstet Gynecol Neonatal Nurs 1993 Jan/Feb; 22(1): 49–55.

Pirie M et al. Coping with PMS: A women's health center has success with life skills model. Cancer Nurs 1992 Dec; 88(11): 24–46.

Rossignol A and Phillips M. Obstetricians' and gynecologists' beliefs and preferred modes of treatment for women diagnosed with premenstrual symptoms. Womens Health Issues 1992 Spring; 2(1):26–31.

Rubinow D. The premenstrual syndrome. JAMA 1992 Oct 14; 268(14):1908–1912.

Menstruation, Perimenopause, and Menopause

Bernhard L and Sheppard L. Health, symptoms, self-care and dyadic adjustment in menopausal women. J Obstet Gynecol Neonatal Nurs 1993 Sept/Oct; 22(5):456–461.

*Bishop K et al. Effects of age, parity and adherence on pelvic muscle response to exercise. J Obstet Gynecol Neonatal Nurs 1992 Sep/Oct; 21(5):401–406.

Colditz GA et al. The use of estrogens and progestins and the risk of breast cancer in postmenopausal women. N Engl J Med 1995 June 15; 332(24):1589–1593.

Cook M. Perimenopause: An opportunity for health promotion. J Obstet Gynecol Neonatal Nurs 1993 May/June; 22(3):223–228.

*Estok P, Rudy E, Kerr M and Menzel L. Menstrual response to running: Nursing implications. Nurs Res 1993 May/June; 42(3): 158–165.

Fishbein E. Women at midlife: The transition to menopause. Nurs Clin North Am 1992 Dec; 27(4):951–957.

Gambrell R. Estrogen replacement therapy and breast cancer risk. Female Pt 1993 April; 18(4):50–62.

Lichtman R. Perimenopausal hormone replacement therapy. J Nurse Midwifery 1991 Jan; 36(1):30–43.

Legato M. Managing coronary heart disease risk in postmenopausal women. Female Pt 1993 April; 18(4):33–43.

Maddox M. Contraceptive choices for perimenopausal women. Journ Amer Acad Nurs Pract 1993 July/Aug; 5(4):181–184.

Maddox M. Women at midlife: Hormone replacement therapy. Nurs Clin North Am 1992 Dec; 27(4):959–969.

Marten S. Complications of menopause and the risks and benefits of estrogen replacement therapy. Journ Amer Acad Nurs Pract 1993 Mar/Apr; 5(2):55–61.

McMahon M, Peterson C and Schlike J. Osteoporosis: Identifying high-risk persons. Journ Geront Nurs 1992 Oct; 18(10):19–26.

Ravnikar V. Compliance with hormone replacement therapy: Are women receiving the full impact of hormone replacement therapy preventive health benefits? Wom Health Iss 1992 Summer; 2(2):75–82.

Schnare S. Hormone therapy. Contemp Ob/Gyn NP 1993 Sept; 1(3):3–5.
Session D, Kelly A and Jewelewicz R. Current concepts in estrogen replacement therapy in the menopause. Fertil Steril 1993; 59(2):277–284.
Speroff L. HRT for the woman who has had breast Cancer? Contemp Ob Gyn 1993 July; 38(7):33–64.
Speroff L et al. Treating the perimenopausal patient. Contemp Ob/Gyn 1993 May; 38(5):124–142.
Writing Group of the PEPI Trial. Effects of estrogen or estrogen/progestin regimens on heart disease risk factors in postmenopausal women. JAMA 1995 Jan 18; 273(3):199–207.

Conception Control

Cheng T, Savageau J and Sattler A. Confidentiality in health care: A survey of knowledge, perceptions and attitudes among high school students. JAMA 1993 Mar 17; 269:1404–1407.
Farley T et al. Intrauterine devices and pelvic inflammatory disease: An international perspective. Lancet 1992 Mar 28; 339:785–788.
Glasier A et al. Mifepristone (RU 486) compared with high dose estrogen and progestogen for emergency postcoital contraception. New Engl J Med 1992; 327(15):1041–1044.
Gollub E, Stein Z. Commentary: The new female condom-Item 1 on a Woman's AIDS Prevention Agenda. Am J Pub Health 1993 Apr; 83(4):498–500.
Kaunitz A. DMPA: A new contraceptive option. Contemp Ob/Gyn NP 1993 Apr; 1(1):5–12.
King J. Helping patients choose an appropriate method of birth control. Matern Child Nurs 1992 Mar/Apr; 17(2):91–95.
Kobovitch L and Bonovich L. Adolescent pregnancy strategies used by school nurses. J Sch Health 1992 Oct; 62(10):11–14.
Maddox M. Contraceptive choices for perimenopausal women. Journ Amer Acad Nurs Pract 1993 July/Aug; 5(4):181–184.
Norris A and Ford K. Urban low-income African-American and Hispanic youths' negative experiences with condoms: Implications for nursing intervention. Nurse Pract 1993 May; 18(5): 40–48.
Pollack A. Long-term consequences of female and male sterilization. Contemp Ob/Gyn 1993 Aug; 38(8):41–54.
Roth B. Fertility awareness as a component of sexuality education: Prliminary research findings with adolescents. Nurs Pract 1993 Mar; 18(3):40–54.
Rosenfeld J, Zahorik P and Murphy G. Tubal ligation and women's health. Female Pt 1993 Sept; 18(9):63–70.
Rowlands S and Chez R. Emergency postcoital contraception. Contemp Ob/Gyn 1994 Jan;9(1):78–88.
Schnare S. Postcoital contraception. Contemp Ob/Gyn NP 1993 Apr; 1(1):3–4.
Trussel J et al. Condom slippage and breakage rates. Fam Plann Perspect 1992 Jan; 24(1):20–23.
Trussel J et al. Emergency contraceptive pills: A simple proposal to reduce unintended pregnancies. Fam Plann Perspect 1992 June; 24(6):269–273.

Infertility

DeMaio C. Infertility work-up: Clues to watch for during the first visit. Contemp Ob/Gyn NP 1993 Sept; 1(3):6–14.
Gennaro S, Klein A and Miranda L. Health policy dilemmas related to high technology infertility services. Image: J Nurs Scholar Fall 1992, 24(3):191–199.
Goode C and Hahn S. Oocyte donation and in vitro fertilization: The nurse's role with ethical and legal issues. J Obstet Gynecol Neonatal Nurs 1993 Mar/Apr; 22(2):106–111.
Infertility. Contemp Ob/Gyn 1993 Sept 15; 38(special issue):6–58.
Loriaux T. Male infertility: A challenge for primary health care providers. Nurs Pract 1991 March; 16(3):38–46.
Marshak L. The role of the female doctorally prepared nurse in caring for infertile women. Clin Nurs Spec 1993 Jan; 7(1):8–11.
*Prattke T and Gass-Sternas K. Appraisal, coping, and emotional health of infertile couples undergoing donor artificial insemination. J Obstet Gynecol Neonatal Nurs 1993 Nov/Dec; 22(6): 516–527.
Sherrod R. Helping infertile couples explore the option of adoption. J Obstet Gynecol Neonatal Nurs 1992 Nov/Dec; 21(6): 465–470.
Saulsberry S and Pohlhaus M. Assessment and initial management of infertility. J Amer Acad Nurs Pract 1992 Jan–Mar; 4(2):53–57
Wu C and Winkel C. Androgen excess in infertile women. Am J Gyn Health 1993 Mar/Apr; 7(2):18–25.

Abortion

Armstrong B, McDonald A and Sloan M. Cigarette, alcohol and coffee consumption and spontaneous abortion. Am J Pub Health 1992; 82(1):85–87.
Creinin M and Grimes D. Medical options for early abortion. Contemp Ob/Gyn 1994 April; 39(4):85–91.
Forrest J and Henshaw S. Providing controversial health care: Abortion services since 1973. Womens Health Issues 1993 Fall; 3(3):152–157.
Frye B. Abortion. AWHONN Clin Iss in Perinatal and Wom Health Nurs 1993; 4(2):265–271.
Greenslade F et al. Technology introduction and quality of abortion care. J Wom Health 1993 Jan/Feb; 2(1):27–30.
King C. Abortion in nineteenth century America: A conflict between women and their physicians. Womens Health Issues 1992 Spring; 2(1):32–39.
Mandelson M, Maden C and Daling J. Low birth weight in relation to multiple induced abortions. Am J Pub Health 1992 Mar; 82(3):391–394.
McFarlane D. Induced abortion: An historical overview. Am J Gyn Health 1993 May/June; VII(3):77–81.
Overview of Mifepristone and its potential applications. Contracept Report 1993 May; IV(2):7–9.
Polk-Walker G. Counseling implications in a client's choice of anesthesia during a first or repeat abortion. Nurs Forum 1993 Jan–Mar; 28(1):22–27.

Ectopic Pregnancy

Jackson D. Ectopic pregnancy: A case study. J Post Anesth Nurs 1992 Apr; 7(2):115–118.
Montgomery-Rice V and Leach R. New options for the diagnosis and treatment of ectopic pregnancy. Female Pt 1993 May; 18(5):31–44.
Oppenheim E. A sterilized woman who did not feel right. Hosp Pract 1992 Feb 15; 27(2):55–56.
Reinhardt M. Ectopic pregnancy rupture. Am J Nurs 1994 Jul; 94(7):41.
Schwayder J et al. Unilateral twin ectopic pregnancy managed by operative laparoscopy. J Reprod Med 1993 Apr; 38(4):314–316.
Stoval T and Ling F. Single dose methotrexate: An expanded clinical trial. Am J Obstet Gynecol 1993 June; 168(6):1759–1765.

INFORMATION/RESOURCES

Agencies

American College of Obstetricians and Gynecologists (ACOG)
600 Maryland Avenue SW
Washington, DC 20024-2588

American Infertility Society
2131 Magnolia Ave Suite 201
Birmingham, AL

Association for Voluntary Sterilization
708 Third Ave
New York, NY

Association of Women's Health, Obstetrical and Neonatal Nurses-AWHONN (formerly NAACOG)
409 12th St SW Suite 300
Washington, DC 20005

D.E.S. Action
Long Island Jewish Medical Center
New Hyde Park, New York 11040.

National Abortion Rights Action League
825 15th St NW
Washington, DC 2005

National Coalition Against Domestic Violence
P.O. Box 18749
Denver, Colorado 80218-0749

National Association of Nurse Practitioners in Reproductive Health (NANPRH) and Association of Reproductive Health Professionals (ARHP)
2401 Pennsylvania Avenue NW #350
Washington, DC 20037-1718

Nursing Network on Violence Against Women
c/o Dan Sheridan
14980 SW 103rd Avenue
Tigard, Oregon 97224

Planned Parenthood Federation of America
810 Seventh Ave
New York, NY 10019

Resolve National Headquarters
5 Water Street
Arlington, MA 02174

Serono Symposia (Clinical information on infertility)
100 Longwater Circle
Norwell, MA 02061

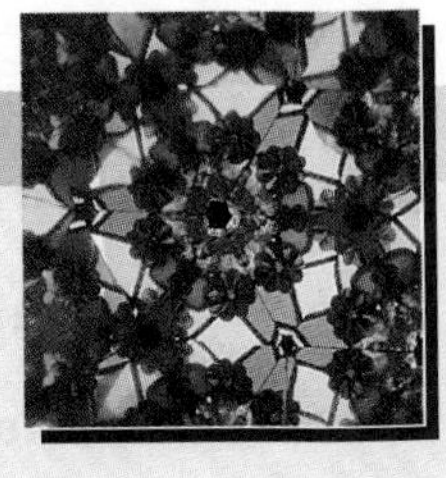

45

Management of Patients With Disorders of the Female Reproductive System

CHAPTER OUTLINE

LEARNING OBJECTIVES

On completion of this chapter, the learner will be able to:

1. Compare the various types of vaginal infections and the risk factors associated with each type
2. Develop an educational program for the patient with a vaginal infection
3. Use the nursing process as a framework for care of the patient with a vulvovaginal infection
4. Use the nursing process as a framework for care of the patient with genital herpes
5. Describe nursing implications for preventing and managing toxic shock syndrome and the rationale for each intervention
6. Use the nursing process as a framework for caring for the patient with toxic shock syndrome
7. Compare the signs and symptoms, management, and nursing care implications of malignant disorders of the female reproductive tract
8. Use the nursing process as a framework for care of the patient undergoing hysterectomy
9. Describe indications for a wide excision of the vulva, or vulvectomy, and the preoperative and postoperative nursing interventions
10. Use the nursing process as a framework for care of the patient undergoing wide excision of the vulva or vulvectomy
11. Compare nursing interventions indicated for the patient undergoing radiation therapy and chemotherapy for cancer of the female reproductive tract

Infections of the Female Reproductive System

Vulvovaginal Infections

Overview and Prevention

The vagina is protected against infection by its normally low *p*H (3.5 to 4.5), which is maintained by the actions of Döderlein's bacili (a part of the normal vaginal flora) and the hormone estrogen. The risk of infection rises if a woman's resistance is lowered by stress or illness, if the *p*H is altered, or if the number of invading organisms increases.

Vulvovaginal infections are common problems and nurses have an important role in providing information that will prevent many of these conditions. To guard against these infections, women of all ages need to understand their own anatomy and the hygienic measures that promote health. These disorders are one of the most common reasons that women consult their health care provider. Continued research into causes and cures is needed, along with better ways to encourage growth of Döderlein's bacillus.

The epithelium of the vagina is highly responsive to estrogen, which induces glycogen formation. The subsequent breakdown of glycogen into lactic acid produces a low vaginal *p*H. (Normal vaginal *p*H value is about 4.) When estrogen decreases, during lactation and menopause, glycogen decreases as well. In adolescents or young women who take oral contraceptives, the normal vaginal flora and glycogen formation are reduced. When patients are treated with antibiotics, the problem may be compounded as these medications further destroy the normal vaginal flora that are needed to maintain the lower *p*H that inhibits the growth of most organisms. With reduced glycogen formation, infections may occur and require careful diagnosis for appropriate treatment.

As the vaginal epithelium matures during the reproductive years, other potential factors may initiate infections, such as sexual intercourse with an infected partner; poor hygiene; and wearing tight, nonabsorbent, and heat-retaining clothing.

During the peri- and postmenopausal periods as estrogen production ceases, the vagina and labia may atrophy (shrink), making the perineal area more susceptible to infection. Risk factors for vulvovaginal infections are summarized in Chart 45-1.

Vulvitis, Leukorrhea, and Nonspecific Vaginitis

Vulvitis (inflammation of the vulva) may occur with other disorders, such as diabetes, dermatologic problems, poor hygiene, or sexually transmitted diseases (STDs), or it may be secondary to a specific vaginitis.

Vulvodynia, or intense burning and inflammation of the vulva, is a puzzling disorder that typically disrupts the lives of the women who are affected. It seems to be related to a high level of calcium oxalate crystals in the urine. With proper diet, symptoms usually abate. This condition can coexist with chronic interstitial cystitis, an irritation of the bladder (see Chapter 43). Trycyclic antidepressants have been effective for some patients with this disorder.

Vaginitis (inflammation of the vagina) occurs when *Candida, Trichomonas,* or bacterial vaginosis, formerly called *Gardnerella vaginalis* and nonspecific or bacterial vaginitis, invade the vagina. The normal whitish vaginal discharge, which occurs in slight amounts during ovulation or just before the onset of menstruation, becomes more profuse when vaginitis occurs. Urethritis may accompany vaginitis because of the proximity of the urethra to the vagina. The discharge may cause itching, odor, redness, burning, and edema, which may be aggravated by voiding and defecation.

Once the causative organism has been identified, appropriate treatment is prescribed. Oral medication may be prescribed or local intravaginal applications of appropriate medication may be dispensed from a tube with an applicator. The applicator is inserted into the vagina, and medication is expressed in the desired amount. Hydrocortisone ointment or cream may be applied externally, as prescribed, for symptomatic relief of itching or perineal irritation.

Specific Vaginal Infections

Specific vaginal infections include candidiasis, bacterial vaginosis, and trichomoniasis (Table 45-1). Chlamydial infections usually affect the cervix.

Candidiasis

Candidiasis is a fungal or yeast infection caused by strains of *Candida.* This organism is usually a normal inhabitant of

CHART 45-1
Risk Factors for Vulvovaginal Infections

- Premenarche
- Pregnancy
- Perimenopause
- Poor personal hygiene
- Tight undergarments
- Synthetic clothing
- Frequent douching
- Allergies
- Oral contraceptives
- Broad-spectrum antibiotics
- Diabetes mellitus
- Low estrogen levels
- Intercourse with infected partner
- Oral–genital contact (yeast can inhabit the mouth and intestinal tract)
- HIV infection

TABLE 45-1 Vaginal Infections

Infection	Cause	Clinical Manifestations	Management Goals
Candidiasis	*Candida albicans, glabrata,* or *tropicalis*	Inflammation of vaginal epithelium producing itching, reddish irritation White, cheeselike discharge clinging to epithelium	Eradicate the fungus by administering an antifungal agent. Frequently used brand names of vaginal creams and suppositories are Monistat, Femstat, Terazol, and Gyne-Lotrimin Review other causative factors (*i.e.,* antibiotic therapy, nylon underwear, tight clothing, pregnancy, oral contraceptives) Assess for diabetes and HIV infection in those with recurrent monilia
Gardnerella-associated bacterial vaginosis or nonspecific vaginitis	*Gardnerella vaginalis* and vaginal anaerobes	Usually no edema or erythema of vulva or vagina Grayish white to yellow-white discharge clinging to external vulva and vaginal walls	Administer metronidazole, with instructions about avoiding alcohol while taking this medication If infection is recurrent, treat partner
Trichomonas vaginalis vaginitis (STD)	*Trichomonas vaginalis*	Inflammation of vaginal epithelium, producing burning and itching Frothy yellowish white or yellowish brown vaginal discharge	Remove exudate, relieve inflammation, restore acidity, and reestablish normal bacterial flora: provide oral metronidazole for patient and partner
Bartholinitis (infection of greater vestibular gland)	*Escherichia coli* *Trichomonas vaginalis* *Staphylococcus* *Streptococcus* Gonococcus	Erythema around vestibular gland Swelling and edema Abscessed vestibular gland	Drain the abscess; provide antibiotic therapy; excise gland of patients with chronic bartholinitis
Cervicitis: acute and chronic	Chlamydia Gonorrhea *Streptococcus* Many pathogenic bacteria	Profuse purulent vaginal discharge Backache Urinary frequency and urgency	Determine the cause: perform cytologic examination of cervical smear and appropriate cultures Eradicate the gonococcus, if present: penicillin (as directed) or spectinomycin or tetracycline, if patient is allergic to penicillin Tetracycline, doxycycline (Vibramycin) to eradicate chlamydia Eradicate other causes: cervical cauterization
Atrophic vaginitis	Lack of estrogen; glycogen deficiency	Discharge and irritation with alkaline *p*H of vaginal secretions	Provide estrogen therapy for vaginal epithelialization; provide topical vaginal estrogen therapy; improve nutrition if necessary; relieve dryness through use of Replens

the mouth, throat, large intestine, and vagina; it propagates in areas that are moist and warm, such as mucous membranes and tissue folds. *C. albicans* is also found in patients who have been on antibiotic therapy, because these medications decrease bacteria, thereby altering natural protective organisms usually present in the vaginal tract. Clinical infection may occur during pregnancy, or with a systemic condition such as diabetes mellitus, or in a patient taking steroids or oral contraceptives. Other varieties of yeast (*e.g., C. globrata*) have also been implicated as causative organisms.

Clinical manifestations include a vaginal discharge that causes itching (pruritus) and possible irritation; appears watery, or thick and tenacious; and may contain white, cheese-like particles. A burning sensation, which may follow urination, may result from excoriation from scratching or other irritants. Symptoms are usually more severe just before menstruation and are usually less responsive to treatment during pregnancy. Diagnosis is made by microscopic identification of spores and hyphae on a glass slide prepared from a discharge specimen and potassium hydroxide.

Management. The goal of management is to eliminate symptoms. Possible medications include antifungal agents such as miconazole (Monistat), nystatin (Mycostatin), clotrimazole (Gyne-Lotrimin) and terconazole (Terazol) cream; these agents are inserted into the vagina with an applicator at bedtime and may be applied to the vulvar area for pruritus. Treatment continues through a menstrual cycle if necessary. Medications are prescribed in a three-dose or seven-night treatment course.

Vaginal creams, effective in eliminating candidiasis or yeast infections, are also available without a prescription. However, patients are cautioned to use these creams only if they are certain that they have a yeast or monilial infection. If they are uncertain about the cause of their symptoms or if they have not obtained relief after using these creams, they are instructed to seek health care promptly.

If chronic, recurrent yeast infections occur, the patient's sexual partner may need to be treated also. Diabetes and HIV infection often result in frequent monilial vaginitis. Women with recurrent vaginal infections should be evaluated by their health care provider. In healthy women, yeast infections are an annoying condition that usually is not recurrent. Women need to be reassured that a vaginal yeast infection is a minor nuisance and not a serious illness.

Bacterial Vaginosis

Bacterial vaginosis has also been called *Gardnerella,* nonspecific, and bacterial vaginitis. It is characterized by an overgrowth of normal vaginal bacteria and an odor that patients describe as fishlike. It is usually accompanied by a heavier-than-normal discharge and is particularly noticeable after sexual intercourse.

It can occur throughout the menstrual cycle and does not produce any local discomfort or pain. More than half of women with bacterial vaginosis do not notice any symptoms. Discharge, if noticed, is gray to yellowish white. The fishlike odor can be detected readily by adding a drop of potassium hydroxide to a sample of vaginal discharge on a glass slide. It is also noted after intercourse when seminal fluid alkalinizes vaginal secretions and produces amines. Under the microscope, vaginal cells are coated with bacteria and are described as "clue cells." The *p*H of the discharge is usually above 4.7 because of the amines that result from enzymes from anaerobes. Lactobacilli, a natural host defense, are usually absent.

Management. Metronidazole, administered twice a day for 1 week, is effective orally; a vaginal gel is also available. Clindamycin (Cleocin) vaginal cream is equally effective. If the infection recurs, most practitioners treat the woman's sexual partner. Bacterial vaginosis usually causes no serious problems but has been associated with premature labor, endometritis, and recurrent urinary tract infection.

Trichomoniasis

Trichomonas vaginalis is a flagellated protozoan that causes a common, usually sexually transmitted vaginitis. A partner may be an asymptomatic carrier who harbors the organism in the urogenital tract and transmits the infection to the other partner.

Clinical manifestations include a vaginal discharge that is thin (sometimes frothy), yellow to yellow-brown, malodorous, and very irritating. An accompanying vulvitis may result, with intense vulvovaginal burning and itching. Diagnosis is made by microscopic detection of the pear-shaped, mobile, flagellate organisms. Inspection with a speculum reveals vaginal and cervical erythema (redness) with multiple small petechiae ("strawberry spots").

Management. The most effective treatment for trichomoniasis is metronidazole (Flagyl). Both partners receive a one-time loading dose or a smaller dose three times a day for 1 week. The one-time dose is more convenient; consequently compliance tends to be greater. The week-long treatment has occasionally been noted to be more effective. Some patients complain of an unpleasant but transient metallic taste when taking metronidazole. Nausea and vomiting, as well as a hot, flushed feeling occur when this medication is taken with an alcoholic beverage. In view of these possible side effects, the patient is strongly advised not to drink alcohol while taking the medication.

Additionally, intercourse should be avoided unless a condom is used. Metronidazole therapy is contraindicated in patients with some blood dyscrasias or central nervous system diseases and in women who are breast-feeding. Because metronidazole may diminish white blood cell production, it is not prescribed without examination, and many health care providers will not prescribe it more than once within a year without first obtaining a complete blood count.

Both trichomoniasis and bacterial vaginosis have been implicated in premature labor if not detected and treated during pregnancy. Nursing implications include implementing a diagnostic evaluation for any abnormal vaginal discharge in a pregnant patient, although most pregnant patients report increased vaginal discharge (due to high estrogen levels).

Chlamydial Infections

Sexually transmitted infection with *Chlamydia trachomatis,* a bacterium, is increasing (see Chapter 65) and is estimated to affect about 4 million patients yearly. Untreated, the infection may lead to pelvic inflammatory disease (PID) and infertility. Clinical manifestations in women resemble those of gonorrhea (cervicitis and mucopurulent discharge) and are typically minor or absent. In males, urethritis and epididymitis may occur. Chlamydia affects the genitourinary tract and can cause pain on urination (dysuria). Diagnosis can be confirmed by culture, smear, or other methods.

The Centers for Disease Control and Prevention (CDC) recommends treatment with doxycycline for 1 week or a single dose of azithromycin. Pregnant women are cautioned not to take tetracycline because of potential adverse effects on the fetus, and erythromycin may be prescribed. Treatment results are usually good if treatment begins early. Possible complications from delayed treatment are tubal disease, PID, and infertility.

Gerontologic Considerations

After menopause, the vaginal mucosa may thin (or atrophy). This condition may be complicated by infection from pyogenic bacteria, resulting in **atrophic vaginitis.** An annoying leukorrhea (vaginal discharge) may cause itching and burning. Management is similar to that for nonspecific bacterial vaginitis. In addition, estrogenic hormones, either taken orally or applied locally as an ointment, are effective in restoring the epithelium.

❑ NURSING PROCESS
The Patient With a Vulvovaginal Infection

Assessment

The woman with vulvovaginal symptoms should be examined soon after their onset. She is instructed not to douche, because doing so removes the vaginal discharge needed to make the diagnosis. The area is observed for erythema, edema, excoriation, and discharge. Each of the infection-producing organisms produces its own characteristic discharge and effect (see Table 45-1). The patient is asked to describe her discharge, if present, and other symptoms such as odor, itching, or burning. Dysuria often occurs as a result of local irritation of the urinary meatus. A urinary tract infection may need to be ruled out by obtaining a urine specimen for culture and sensitivity testing.

Factors contributing to infection include (1) physical and chemical phenomena such as increased perspiration but decreased evaporation (from tight or synthetic clothing), perfumes and powders, soaps, bubble bath, a soiled perineal area, or suppositories and feminine hygiene products; (2) psychogenic factors; and (3) medical conditions or endocrine factors such as a predisposition for vulvar involvement in a patient who has diabetes, is elderly, or is chronically ill. Any medications the patient has been taking are noted, because some hormones and antibiotics may alter the vaginal flora, resulting in an overgrowth of *C. albicans.*

The nurse may prepare a vaginal smear (wet mount) to assist in diagnosing and identifying the infection. A common method for preparing the smear is to collect vaginal secretions with a cotton-tipped applicator and place the secretions on separate glass slides. A drop of saline solution is added to one slide, and a drop of 10% potassium hydroxide is added to another slide for examination under a microscope. If *Gardnerella* or bacterial vaginitis is present, the slide with normal saline solution added shows epithelial cells dotted with bacteria. These are referred to as clue cells. If *Trichomonas* is present, small motile cells are seen. In the presence of yeast, the potassium hydroxide slide reveals the characteristics that are typical of monilia. *Gardnerella* produces a strong odor when mixed with potassium hydroxide. This is called a positive "whiff test" and is indicative of bacterial vaginosis.

Diagnosis

Nursing Diagnoses

Based on the nursing assessment and other data, the patient's major nursing diagnoses may include the following:

- Pain, discomfort, and distress related to burning, odor, or itching from the infectious process
- Anxiety related to stressful symptoms
- Risk for reinfection or spread of infection
- Knowledge deficit about proper hygiene and preventive measures

Planning and Implementation

Goals. The major goals for the patient may include relief of pain and discomfort; reduction of anxiety related to stress symptoms; prevention of reinfection or infection of sexual partner; and acquisition of knowledge about methods for preventing vulvovaginal infections and managing self-care.

Nursing Interventions

Relieving Discomfort and Pain. Vulvovaginal conditions are usually treated on an outpatient basis, unless the patient has other medical problems. Patient education, tact, reassurance, and gentleness are important nursing contributions. Women may express embarrassment, guilt, or anger if they are concerned that the infection may be serious or may have been acquired from a sex partner. In some instances, treatment plans may include the partner.

The nurse may need to reinforce instructions for warm perineal irrigations that can provide comfort and also clean the infected area if indicated. Irrigations may be recommended after each voiding and defecation. Additionally, a sitz bath may be taken either in a tub or by using a small disposable unit that fits over the toilet seat. If the patient's upper thighs are chafed, a dusting of cornstarch powder may alleviate discomfort.

Sexual intercourse is discouraged until relief is achieved. Using a condom is then suggested to prevent reinfection and irritation of sensitive tissues.

Reducing Anxiety. Although vulvovaginal infections are very disturbing and require effective treatment, they are not life-threatening. However, the patient who experiences such an infection may be very anxious and fearful about the significance of symptoms and possible causes. Explaining the cause of symptoms may reduce anxiety related to fear of more serious illness; and discussing strategies that help prevent vulvovaginal infections may help the patient adopt specific strategies to decrease infection and the related symptoms.

Preventing Reinfection or Spread of Infection. One of the basic goals is to reduce tissue irritation caused by scratching or wearing tight clothing. The area needs to be kept clean by daily bathing and adequate cleaning after voiding and defecation. When teaching the patient about medications, such as suppositories, and devices, such as applicators to dispense cream or ointment, the nurse may demonstrate the procedure by using a plastic model of the pelvis and vagina. The nurse should also stress the importance of handwashing before and after each administration of medication. To prevent the medication from escaping from the vagina, the patient should recline for 30 minutes after the medication is inserted. If some seepage of medication occurs, a perineal pad may be worn. To avoid reinfection, the patient and her sexual partner are counseled to avoid sexual intercourse until effective treatment has been completed.

When medications such as antibiotics are prescribed for any infection, the nurse instructs the patient about precautions related to using these agents. In general, long-term use of antibiotics is avoided when possible to prevent candidiasis, which can result from the antibiotics destroying normal flora.

Patient Education and Health Maintenance. In addition to reviewing ways of relieving discomfort and preventing reinfection, the nurse assesses each patient's learning needs relative to the immediate problem. The patient needs to know the characteristics of normal as opposed to abnormal discharge. Questions often arise about douching. Normally, douching is unnecessary because daily bathing or showers and proper cleaning after voiding and defecation keep the perineal area clean. Many patients are misinformed about the presumed necessity for douching or using feminine hygiene products. Douching has a tendency to eliminate normal flora, reducing the body's ability to ward off infection. Repeated douching may result in vaginal epithelial breakdown and chemical irritation.

Therapeutic douching may be recommended and prescribed, however, to reduce unpleasant, abnormal odors; to remove excessive discharge; to change the *p*H (such as vinegar douches); and to serve as an antiseptic irrigating solution (see Chapter 44). The procedure is reviewed with the patient, as is the care and cleaning of equipment so that it is properly disinfected. In the case of recurrent monilia, the perineum should be kept dry. (A hair dryer on a low setting is an effective aid after showering. The patient should be cautioned to use electrical appliances safely and to avoid using them in and around water.) Loose-fitting cotton underwear instead of tight-fitting synthetic, nonabsorbent, heat-retaining garments is recommended. It is also recommended that the woman avoid wearing damp swimsuits for long periods.

Evaluation

Expected Outcomes

1. Experiences reduced pain and discomfort
   a. Cleans the perineum as prescribed
   b. Reports that itching is relieved
   c. Maintains urine output within normal limits and without dysuria
2. Experiences relief of anxiety
3. Remains free from infection
   a. Has no signs of inflammation, pruritus, odors, or dysuria
   b. Notes vaginal discharge appears normal (thin, clear, nonfrothy)
4. Participates in self-care
   a. Takes medication as prescribed
   b. Wears absorbent underwear
   c. Avoids unprotected sexual intercourse
   d. Douches only as prescribed

Human Papillomavirus

Human papillomavirus (HPV) infection is a sexually transmitted disease that may result in small, warty growths on the vulva, labia, cervix, vaginal walls, or rectum. Labial and perineal warts are usually visible and palpable. The virus may also affect the cervix. Cervical changes are not always visible but may show up on Pap smears as koilocytosis. Some strains of the virus are associated with cervical cancer. Other strains are rarely, if ever, associated with cancer. Treatment usually eradicates perineal warts, although they may resolve spontaneously without treatment. Treatment modalities include trichloroacetic acid, podophyllin, interferon, chemotherapeutic agents, electrocautery, and laser treatment. A treatment applied by the patient, consisting of a medication called Condylox, may be an option for use on external lesions.

Patients with HPV should have Pap smears every 6 months for several years because of the propensity of HPV to cause koilocytosis and dysplasia (changes in cervical cells). Male partners may be evaluated by a urologist, because HPV lesions may be difficult to visualize. Urologists may use a colposcope or an application of acetic acid, followed by magnified inspection to aid diagnosis.

Herpesvirus Type-2 Infection (Herpes Genitalis, Herpes Simplex Virus)

Herpes genitalis is a viral infection that causes herpetic lesions (blisters) on the cervix, vagina, and external genitalia. It is a sexually transmitted disease but also may be transmitted asexually from wet surfaces or by self-transmission (*i.e.*, by touching a cold sore and then touching the genital area). The initial infection is very painful and lasts about 1 week. Recurrences are less painful and usually produce minor itching and burning. Some patients have few or no recurrences whereas others may have frequent bouts. Symptoms may occur with stress, sunburn, dental work, or inadequate rest and nutrition.

Etiology and Pathophysiology. Of the known herpesviruses, six affect humans: (1) herpes simplex type 1 (HSV-1), which usually causes "cold sores" of the lips; (2) herpes simplex type 2 (HSV-2), or genital herpes; (3) varicella zoster or shingles; (4) Epstein-Barr virus; (5) cytomegalovirus; and (6) human B-lymphotropic virus (HBLV). HSV-2 appears to be the cause of about 80% of genital and perineal lesions; HSV-1 may cause about 20%.

There is considerable overlap between HSV-1 and HSV-2, which are clinically indistinguishable. Close human contact by mouth, oropharynx, mucosal surface, vagina, and cervix seems necessary to acquire the infection. Other susceptible sites are skin lacerations and conjunctivae. Usually the virus is killed at room temperature by drying. When viral replication diminishes, the virus ascends the peripheral sensory nerves and remains inactive in the nerve ganglia. Another outbreak occurs when the host is subjected to stress. In pregnant women with active herpes, babies delivered vaginally may become infected with the virus. There is a risk of fetal morbidity and mortality if this occurs; therefore, a cesarean section may be performed if the virus recurs near the time of delivery.

Clinical Manifestations. Itching and pain accompany the process as the area becomes red and swollen (edematous). The vesicular state often appears as a blister, which later coalesces, ulcerates, and encrusts. In the female, the labia is the usual primary site, although the cervix, vagina, and perianal skin may be affected. In the male the glans penis, foreskin, or penile shaft are usually affected. Flulike symptoms may occur 3 or 4 days after the lesions appear. Inguinal lymphadenopathy (swollen lymph nodes in the groin), minor temperature elevation, malaise, headache, myalgia (achy muscles), and dysuria (pain on urination) are often noted. In the female, a purulent discharge may develop from a secondary bacterial infection. Pain is evident during the first week and then decreases. The lesions subside in about 2 weeks unless they become secondarily infected.

Rarely, complications may arise from extragenital spread, such as to the buttocks, upper thighs, or even to the eyes as a result of touching lesions. Patients should be advised to wash their hands after contact with lesions. Other potential problems are aseptic meningitis and severe emotional stress related to the diagnosis.

Management. There is no cure for HSV-2 infection, but treatment is aimed at relieving the symptoms. The goals of management are to prevent the spread of infection, make the patient comfortable, decrease potential health risks, and initiate a counseling and education program. Acyclovir (Zovirax), an antiviral agent that can alter the course of the infection, is available for topical, oral, and intravenous use. In general, acyclovir reduces the duration of the infection and is effective in treating and often preventing recurrences. Resistance and long-term side effects do not seem to be major problems. Recurrent episodes are much milder than the initial episode.

❑ NURSING PROCESS
The Patient With a Genital Herpesvirus Infection

Assessment

The health history, a physical and pelvic examination, and collaboration with other health care personnel taking care of the patient establish the nature of the infectious condition. Additionally, the patient is assessed for risk of sexually transmitted diseases (STDs). The perineum is inspected for painful lesions and the patient is assessed for enlarged inguinal lymph nodes.

Diagnosis

Nursing Diagnoses

Based on the assessment data, the patient's major nursing diagnoses may include the following:

- ❑ Pain related to the presence of genital lesions
- ❑ Risk for recurrence of infection or spread of infection
- ❑ Anxiety and distress related to embarrassment over the presence of the disease
- ❑ Knowledge deficit about the disease process and about methods of avoiding spread and preventing recurrences.

Planning and Implementation

Goals. The major goals for the patient may include relief of pain and discomfort, control of infection and its spread, relief of anxiety, knowledge of and adherence to the treatment regimen, and self-care and knowledge about implications for the future.

Nursing Interventions

Relieving Pain. The lesions are to be kept clean, and proper hygienic practices are advocated. Sitz baths ease discomfort and voiding. The patient's clothing should be clean, loose, soft, and absorbent. Aspirin and other analgesics are usually effective in controlling pain. Occlusive ointments and powders are avoided because they prevent the lesions from drying, which in turn helps to kill the virus.

If there is considerable pain and malaise, bed rest may be required. The patient is encouraged to increase fluid intake, to be alert for possible bladder distention, and to note the frequency of voiding. Contact of urine with the herpes lesions usually produces pain and patients often become reluctant to void because of the pain. Voiding can be assisted by pouring warm water over the vulva or by sitz baths. When oral acyclovir is prescribed, the patient is instructed as to when to take the medication and what side effects to note, such as rash and headache. Rest and an appropriate diet are recommended.

Patient Education and Health Maintenance. The problems of genital herpes are both physical and psychologic. Usually, the patient experiences a great deal of stress on learning the diagnosis, and this in itself aggravates the problem. Therefore, when counseling the patient, the nurse should explain the causes of the condition and the manner in which it progresses. Questions are encouraged because they indicate that the patient is receptive to learning.

To prevent transmission, the patient is advised to avoid intercourse until the lesions heal. The nurse can provide reassurance that soon the patient will be able to function normally both socially and sexually. Self-care measures for the person with genital herpes are listed in Chart 45-2.

Evaluation

Expected Outcomes

1. Experiences a reduction in pain and discomfort
2. Keeps infection under control by practicing proper hygienic techniques and taking medication as prescribed
3. Acquires knowledge about genital herpes and how to control and avoid further infection

Toxic Shock Syndrome

Toxic shock syndrome (TSS), a condition first identified in the late 1970s, is caused by a toxin produced by strains of the bacterium *Staphylococcus aureus* in susceptible patients. This condition occurs in menstruating women (although about 45% of TSS cases are not related to menstruation). Risk factors that may predispose a woman to TSS include menstruation, chronic vaginal infection, pelvic infection, lung abscess, surgical wound infection, soft tissue infection, postpartum and gynecologic infections, and use of IV drugs and super-absorbent tampons. TSS has occurred after various clinical infections and may be missed initially if diagnosticians associate it only with menstruation. Using barrier methods of contraception (*e.g.*, diaphragm) has also been implicated, whereas using oral contraceptives seems to reduce the risk. The incidence of TSS is 6 to 7 per 100,000 menstruating women.

Clinical Manifestations. In an otherwise healthy person, the onset of TSS occurs with a sudden fever (up to 38.9°C [102°F]), chills, malaise, and muscle pain. Vomiting, diarrhea, hypotension, headache, a red rash on the palms of the hand,

CHART 45-2
Patient Education: Self-Care for Genital Herpes

- Herpes in transmitted mainly by direct contact; abstinence is required for a brief period.
- Control of the condition will not require a major lifestyle change. Intercourse is avoided during treatment, but hand-holding and kissing are permissible.
- Women can be reassured that they can have children; their obstetricians need to know that they have the condition so they can be monitored appropriately.
- Conscientious hygienic practices of cleanliness (hand washing, perineal cleanliness) must be practiced. The patient should wear loose, comfortable clothing, eat a balanced diet, and get adequate rest and relaxation.
- Lesions should be washed gently with mild soap and running water and lightly dried.
- Prolonged exposure to the sun should be avoided, as it seems to cause recurrences (and skin cancer).
- Occlusive ointments, strong perfumed soaps, or bubble bath should be avoided.
- Medications must be taken as prescribed; follow-up appointments with health care personnel should be kept, and recurrences, which are not as severe as the initial episode, reported.
- The patient is encouraged to join a group to share solutions and experiences and hear about newer treatments. Information can be obtained from HELP (Herpetics Engaged in Living Productively), 260 Sheridan Avenue, Palo Alto, CA 94306.
- Usually precautions are unnecessary in the absence of active lesions.
- Lesions away from the mouth or perineum can be covered with a dressing and an impermeable cover during intercourse; such lesions are infrequent.
- For a partner with no history of genital herpes, a condom should be used.

and signs suggesting early septic shock may develop. A red, macular rash similar to a sunburn often occurs. In some patients, this rash appears first on the torso; in others, it appears first on the hands (palms and fingers) and feet (soles and toes). Inflammation of mucous membranes also may occur. In 7 to 10 days, it may desquamate (become scaly or peel). Myalgia and dizziness are common. Recurrence rate is 30%. Most recurrences develop in the first 2 months after the initial illness and commonly during menstruation.

Urine output decreases and the blood urea nitrogen (BUN) level increases, often resulting in disorientation. Results of laboratory studies also reveal leukocytosis and elevated bilirubin. Uncontrollable hypotension and disseminated intravascular coagulopathy (DIC) may also occur. The clinical picture of shock (described in Chapter 15) results. Respiratory distress may develop as a result of pulmonary edema. If adult respiratory distress syndrome (ARDS) occurs, the outlook becomes grave. About 2% to 3% of patients with TSS die of complications.

Diagnostic Evaluation. Blood and urine specimens are obtained for culture. Additional specimens from the throat and vagina and, possibly, the cervix are cultured as well.

Management. The patient is placed on bed rest, and the treatment plan is directed primarily at controlling the infection with antibiotics and restoring circulating blood volume. In cases of respiratory distress, oxygen therapy is instituted; if signs of acidosis appear, sodium bicarbonate is administered. Calcium is prescribed for hypocalcemia. A Swan-Ganz catheter (for monitoring pulmonary artery pressure), intravenous dopamine, and military antishock trousers (MAST) may be used to manage shock. The entire treatment plan, including strategies directed toward emotional and psychologic concerns, is adjusted according to each patient's condition, which may vary from mild to acute.

❑ NURSING PROCESS
The Patient With Toxic Shock Syndrome

Assessment

Because TSS has been associated most often with menstruation, the health history is directed toward determining whether the patient used tampons recently, which kind she used, how long she retained a single tampon before changing it, and whether she noted any problems when inserting the tampon, which may have injured the vaginal tissue. Because contraceptive sponges and diaphragms have also been implicated in TSS, their use is also assessed.

Diagnosis

Nursing Diagnoses

Based on the assessment data, the patient's major nursing diagnoses may include the following:

- ❑ Anxiety related to the severity and suddenness of the symptoms and to concerns about recovery
- ❑ Fluid volume deficit related to vomiting and diarrhea
- ❑ Fatigue related to severity of illness and of shock, prolonged immobility, excessive nutritional demands and stress
- ❑ Knowledge deficit about risk factors and behaviors

Collaborative Problems/ Potential Complications

Based on assessment data, potential complications may include the following:

- ❑ Disseminated intravascular coagulopathy (DIC)
- ❑ Septic shock

Planning and Implementation

Goals. The major goals for the patient may include reduction of anxiety and emotional stress, absence of vomiting and diarrhea, acquisition of relevant knowledge, and prevention of complications.

Nursing Interventions

Relieving Anxiety. The patient who experiences TSS is usually frightened by the severity and suddenness of the symptoms. Additionally, she feels apprehensive about her own survival and recovery. Providing emotional support and reassurance usually reduces anxiety and apprehension. During the early phases of TSS, the patient is kept informed about diagnostic procedures and treatments. As the patient begins to recover, she is provided with the opportunity to participate in her own care when possible and to take an active role in decision making. Extending that support to the family often helps to alleviate the patient's anxiety as well.

Improving Fluid Volume Status. Because of vomiting and diarrhea, the patient is at risk for fluid volume deficit. Therefore, the nurse closely monitors the patient's fluid intake and output and assesses the patient for clinical manifestations of fluid deficit (rapid pulse, decreased blood pressure, decreased skin turgor, dry mucous membranes). The nurse administers intravenous and oral fluids as prescribed, and carefully documents changes in fluid status, body weight, intake, and output. If vomiting and diarrhea persist, the nurse collaborates with the physician about administering antiemetics and antidiarrheal agents.

The patient with a fluid volume deficit is often thirsty and uncomfortable. Comfort measures (frequent oral hygiene) are important for the patient's sense of well being, as is administering therapy to restore fluid balance.

Decreasing Fatigue. Because the patient with TSS has been seriously ill and may have experienced shock, prolonged immobility, and excessive nutritional demands and stress, recovery may be slow and prolonged. The patient may report extreme fatigue, generalized fatigue, or lack of stamina. Nursing interventions include efforts to assist the patient with self-care and to gradually increase stamina and resume usual activities. Attention to nutritious dietary intake is important to counteract weight loss. The patient's weight and caloric intake are monitored and dietary supplements are provided if necessary. An exercise and activity program to build stamina is planned in collaboration with the patient and the physical therapist.

Patient Education and Health Maintenance. Because use of tampons during menstruation has been linked with TSS, it is recommended that super-absorbent tampons not be used. If tampons are used, they should be changed frequently (every 4 hours) and inserted carefully to avoid abrasions (applicators with rough edges should be avoided). If a diaphragm is used, it should not be left in place longer than 8 to 10 hours. Using tampons is discouraged altogether if the patient has had TSS, as is using the diaphragm or cervical cap during menses or in the first 3 months postpartum. The risk of developing TSS increases any time a woman bleeds vaginally (*i.e.*, during menses and postpartum).

Monitoring and Managing Potential Complications. Closely monitoring and documenting vital signs and arterial blood gas levels provide valuable information about the patient's physical status. Cultures of all body excretions including nose, throat, vagina, and cervix are performed in order to determine the appropriate antibiotic therapy. The nurse notes skin changes as well as fluid intake and loss; these data assist in evaluating hydration and kidney function. The patient is often critically ill, and is cared for in the intensive care unit to facilitate constant monitoring and an immediate response to the onset of complications.

Disseminated intravascular coagulopathy (DIC) has been observed in patients with TSS, making it essential for the nurse to observe the patient for hematomas, petechiae, oozing from needle and infusion sites, cyanosis, and coolness of the nose, fingertips, and toes. Additionally, the patient must be observed for and protected from injury. The nurse also assists in managing DIC by promptly administering prescribed medications.

Because of the likelihood of severe shock, the patient must be monitored closely for changes in vital signs, level of consciousness, and laboratory values. Additionally, the patient's response to prescribed medications and fluids is evaluated. See Chapter 15 for further description of management of shock.

Evaluation

Expected Outcomes

1. Exhibits reduced anxiety and emotional stress
2. Is free of fluid loss and imbalance
   a. Does not experience vomiting and diarrhea
   b. Takes adequate fluids
   c. Maintains blood pressure and pulse rate within normal limits
   d. Exhibits normal skin turgor
3. Experiences decreased fatigue level
4. Demonstrates knowledge of risk factors for TSS and avoids using tampons
5. Absence of complications
   a. Has normal arterial blood gas and coagulation studies
   b. Exhibits no manifestations of infection, sepsis, or shock
   c. Exhibits normal vital signs (blood pressure, pulse, and temperature)

Endocervicitis/Cervicitis

Endocervicitis is an inflammation of the mucosa and the glands of the cervix that may occur when organisms gain access to the cervical glands after intercourse, abortion, intrauterine manipulation, or delivery. If untreated, the infection may extend into the uterus, fallopian tubes, and pelvic cavity.

Inflammation can erode the cervical tissue, resulting in spotting or bleeding. The chief symptom is a whitish discharge from the vagina, at times associated with sacral backache, low abdominal pain, and urinary and menstrual disturbances.

Mucopurulent cervicitis is frequently caused by Chlamydia, with between 3 and 10 million cases occurrir yearly in the United States. The disease is most commonly found in young, sexually active patients with more than one partner and is transmitted through sexual intercourse. It can cause pelvic infections and sterility. Chlamydial infections of the cervix often produce no symptoms, although cervical discharge, dyspareunia, dysuria, and bleeding may occur. Other complications include conjunctivitis and perihepatitis. If a pregnant woman is infected, stillbirth, neonatal death, and premature labor may occur. Chlamydial infection and gonorrhea often coexist. As many as 25% of females who have chlamydial infections also have gonorrhea.

Management. Treatment should be preventive as well as curative. Preventing gonorrhea and chlamydial infection by using condoms and spermicides and by avoiding sexual intercourse with a nonmonogamous partner, or one who has a penile discharge, reduces the incidence of endocervicitis and sexually transmitted diseases.

Treatment is aimed at eradicating both organisms, usually with amoxicillin followed by tetracycline therapy. If chlamydia alone is being treated, therapy usually includes tetracycline, doxycycline, or azithromycin.

Pelvic Infection (Pelvic Inflammatory Disease)

Pelvic inflammatory disease (PID) is an inflammatory condition of the pelvic cavity that may involve the uterus (endometritis), fallopian tubes (salpingitis), ovaries (oophoritis), pelvic peritoneum, or the pelvic vascular system. Infection, which may be acute, subacute, recurrent, or chronic and localized or widespread, is usually caused by bacteria but may be caused by a virus, fungus, or parasite. Gonorrheal and chlamydial organisms are the most likely causes. This condition can result in ectopic pregnancy, infertility, recurrent pelvic pain, and recurrent disease.

Etiology. Pathogenic organisms usually enter the body through the vagina, passing through the cervical canal and into the uterus. Under various conditions the organisms may proceed to one or both fallopian tubes and ovaries and into the pelvis. In bacterial infections that occur after childbirth or abortion, and in some infections related to intrauterine devices, pathogens are disseminated directly through the tissues that support the uterus by way of the lymphatics and blood vessels (Fig. 45-1 A). The increased blood supply required by the placenta provides more pathways for infection. These postpartum and postabortion infections tend to be unilateral.

In gonorrheal infections, the gonococci pass through the cervical canal and into the uterus, where the environment, especially during menstruation, allows them to multiply rapidly and spread to the fallopian tubes and into the pelvis (see Fig. 45-1B). The infection is usually bilateral. In rare instances, some diseases (*e.g.*, tuberculosis) gain access to the reproductive organs by way of the bloodstream from the lungs (see Fig. 45-1C).

One of the most frequent causes of salpingitis (inflammation of the fallopian tube) is chlamydia, possibly accompanied by gonorrhea. Chlamydial infection first involves the cervix and then extends upward, infecting the fallopi-

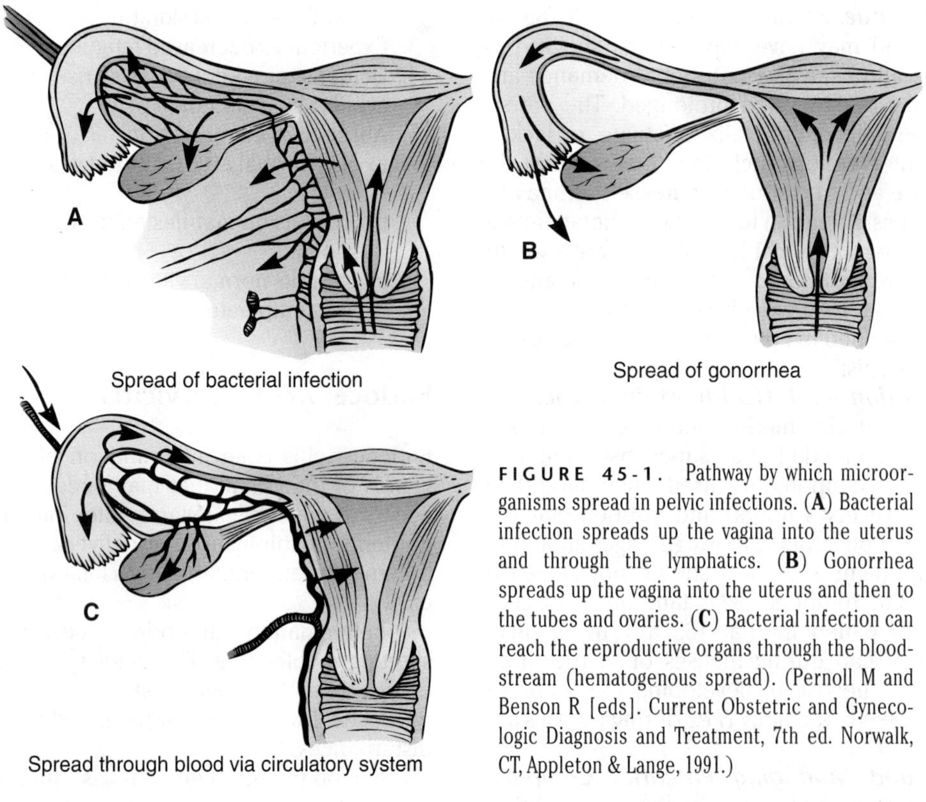

FIGURE 45-1. Pathway by which microorganisms spread in pelvic infections. (**A**) Bacterial infection spreads up the vagina into the uterus and through the lymphatics. (**B**) Gonorrhea spreads up the vagina into the uterus and then to the tubes and ovaries. (**C**) Bacterial infection can reach the reproductive organs through the bloodstream (hematogenous spread). (Pernoll M and Benson R [eds]. Current Obstetric and Gynecologic Diagnosis and Treatment, 7th ed. Norwalk, CT, Appleton & Lange, 1991.)

an tubes or the uterus. It is estimated that about 4 million chlamydial infections occur annually and symptoms may be absent or minor. Prevalence is highest in sexually active young women, those in inner cities, and those of low socioeconomic status. PID is commonly the result of infection with chlamydia. Males may occasionally have symptoms of urethritis but rarely have serious related problems, aside from infecting a partner. Education, awareness, condoms, safer sex practices, and prompt treatment would decrease the incidence of this infection. All patients who are victims of sexual assault should be cultured for chlamydia when they first seek medical attention and treated prophylactically. Cultures should then be repeated in 2 weeks.

Clinical Manifestations. Pelvic infection symptoms usually begin with a vaginal discharge, lower abdominal pelvic pain, and tenderness that occurs after the menses. Pain usually increases during voiding or defecating. Other symptoms include fever, general malaise, anorexia, nausea, headache, and possibly vomiting. On pelvic examination, intense tenderness may be noted on palpation of the uterus or movement of the cervix (cervical motion tenderness, or CMT). Symptoms may be acute and severe or low grade and subtle.

Management. The patient is placed on broad-spectrum antibiotic therapy. Women with mild infections may be treated as outpatients, but hospitalization may be necessary at times. Intensive therapy includes bed rest, intravenous fluids to correct dehydration and acidosis, and intravenous antibiotic therapy. If the patient has abdominal distention or ileus, nasogastric intubation and suction are initiated. Carefully monitoring vital signs and symptoms assists in evaluating the status of the infection. Treating sexual partners is necessary to prevent reinfection.

Complications. Pelvic or generalized peritonitis, abscesses, strictures, and fallopian tube obstruction may develop. Obstruction may cause an ectopic pregnancy in the future if a fertilized egg cannot pass a tubal stricture; or scar tissue may occlude the tubes, resulting in sterility. Adhesions are common and often result in chronic pelvic pain and eventually may require removal of the uterus, fallopian tubes, and ovaries. Other complications include bacteremia with septic shock and thrombophlebitis with possible embolization.

Nursing Interventions. Infection takes its toll, both physically and emotionally. The patient may feel well one day and experience vague symptoms and discomfort the next. She may suffer from constipation and menstrual difficulties as well.

The hospitalized patient is maintained on bed rest and is usually placed in semi-Fowler's position to facilitate dependent drainage. For comfort, heat (heating pad) can be applied to the abdomen externally and warm douches may be prescribed to improve local circulation. In addition, the patient is supported nutritionally and with selective antibiotic therapy as prescribed.

Accurate recording of vital signs and the characteristics and amount of vaginal discharge is necessary as a guide to therapy.

The transmission of infection to others can be minimized in many ways:

- Perineal pads are handled carefully with an instrument or gloves, and the soiled pad is discarded according to hospital guidelines for disposal of biohazardous material.
- Hands are washed carefully with a germicidal soap.

The patient must be informed of the need for precautions and encouraged to take part in procedures to prevent contaminating others as well as protecting herself from reinfection. If reinfection occurs or if the infection spreads, symptoms may include abdominal pain, nausea and vomiting, fever, malaise, malodorous purulent vaginal discharge, and leukocytosis.

Patient teaching consists of explaining how pelvic infections occur and how they can be controlled and avoided. Guidelines and instructions provided to the patient are summarized in Chart 45-3.

If a partner is not well known or has had other sexual partners recently, using a condom may prevent life-threatening infection and its sequelae. All patients who have had PID need to be informed of the signs and symptoms of ectopic pregnancy—pain, abnormal bleeding, faintness, dizziness, and shoulder pain—as they are prone to this complication. (See Chapter 44 for a discussion of ectopic pregnancy.)

HIV Infection and AIDS

Any discussion of vulvovaginal disorders must include the diagnosis of human immunodeficiency virus (HIV) and

CHART 45-3

Patient Education: Controlling and Avoiding PID

- Any pelvic pain and/or abnormal discharge, particularly after sexual exposure, childbirth, or pelvic surgery, should be evaluated as soon as possible.
- Because intrauterine devices (IUDs) may increase the risk for infections, their use should be avoided by women who have multiple sexual partners.
- Proper perineal care procedures must be followed, including wiping from front to back.
- Douching reduces the natural flora that combat infecting organisms and may introduce bacteria upward.
- A health care provider should be consulted if unusual vaginal discharge or odor is noted.
- Important optimal health practices include proper nutrition, exercise, weight control, and safer sex practices (*i.e.,* using condoms; avoiding multiple sexual partners).
- A gynecologic examination should be performed at least once a year.
- Before intercourse, a partner should wear a condom if there is any chance of transmitting infection. (Unless a relationship has always been mutually monogamous, risk of HIV and other STD infection exists.)

acquired immunodeficiency syndrome (AIDS), described in Chapter 50.

Women accounted for almost 18% of new cases of AIDS in 1994, compared with 8% in 1987. Most are in the reproductive age group, and more than 70% are African-American or Hispanic. Over half are IV drug users, whereas the other half have been exposed through sexual contact with HIV-infected partners.

Any break in skin integrity increases the risk of infection (*e.g.*, a herpetic lesion or syphilitic chancre could provide a portal of entry). Syphilis seems to accelerate in HIV-positive patients and proceeds directly from primary to tertiary in some patients. Chlamydia is associated with a higher rate of HIV (which may be related to inflammatory changes of the cervix, providing entry sites). HIV-positive women have a higher rate of human papillomavirus and also seem to have larger and more painful herpes lesions with more recurrences, probably related to immunosuppression from their disease. Acyclovir is appropriate for such patients. Candidiasis occurs frequently in this population, and oral candidiasis may signal a rapidly advancing disease.

Women with HIV must be counseled about contraception and safer sex. Because there is a 25% to 30% chance of perinatal transmission, decisions to conceive or to use contraception must be informed by adequate education and care. (The use of AZT by pregnant women has been shown to significantly decrease perinatal transmission of HIV infection. Therefore, the use of this agent during pregnancy must also be discussed.) For those who choose to avoid conception, condoms and a spermicidal agent or a condom with oral contraceptives are possible choices. The risk of transmitting the virus to or from a partner will decrease with either choice, along with protection from unwanted pregnancies.

Structural Disorders

Fistulas of the Vagina

A fistula is an abnormal, tortuous opening between two internal hollow organs or between an internal hollow organ and the exterior of the body. The name of the fistula indicates the two areas that are connected abnormally: a **vesicovaginal fistula** is an opening between the bladder and the vagina, and a **rectovaginal fistula** is an opening between the rectum and the vagina (Fig. 45-2).

Etiology. Fistulas may occur congenitally; in adults, however, breakdown usually occurs because of tissue damage resulting from injury sustained during surgery, delivery, radiation therapy, or disease processes such as carcinoma.

Clinical Manifestations. Symptoms are dependent on the specific defect. For example, in the patient with a vesicovaginal fistula, urine trickles continuously into the vagina. With a rectovaginal fistula, there is fecal incontinence, and flatus is discharged through the vagina. The combination of such a discharge with a leukorrhea results in a malodorous condition that is difficult to control.

Methylene blue dye helps delineate the course of the fistula. In vesicovaginal fistula, the dye is instilled into the

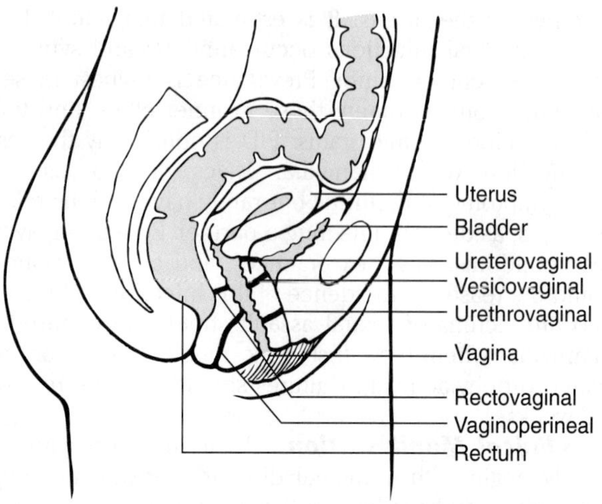

FIGURE 45-2. Common sites for vaginal fistulas: *Vesicovaginal*—bladder and vagina. *Urethrovaginal*—urethra and vagina. *Vaginoperineal*—vagina and perineal area. *Ureterovaginal*—ureter and vagina. *Rectovaginal*—rectum and vagina.

bladder and appears in the vagina. After a negative methylene blue test result, indigo carmine is injected intravenously; the appearance of the dye in the vagina indicates a ureterovaginal fistula. Cystoscopy may then be used to determine the exact location.

Management. The goal is to eliminate the fistula, infection, and excoriation. Frequently, a fistula will heal without surgical intervention. Otherwise surgery is indicated. Usually, the vaginal approach is used for vesicovaginal and urethrovaginal fistulas, and the abdominal approach for fistulas higher in the abdomen. Fistulas that are difficult to repair or very large fistulas may require surgical repair with a urinary or fecal diversion.

Because fistulas usually are related to obstetric or surgical trauma, occurrence in a nulligravid patient or a patient without a history of surgery must be evaluated carefully. Crohn's disease or lymphogranuloma venereum (LGV) may be causes.

Nursing Interventions. Nursing measures are planned to relieve discomfort, prevent infection, and improve the patient's self-concept and self-care abilities.

Healing is promoted by proper nutrition, which includes increasing vitamin C and protein intake; by local cleanliness, achieved by douching and enemas; by rest; and by administering prescribed intestinal antibiotics. A rectovaginal fistula will heal faster if the patient follows a low-residue diet and if the affected tissue drains properly. Warm perineal irrigations and controlled heat-lamp treatments are effective in promoting healing.

For the patient undergoing repair of a vesicovaginal fistula, an indwelling catheter is usually inserted during surgery. Postoperatively, the nurse needs to observe drainage from the catheter and take care to ensure that the catheter functions properly. If the catheter does not drain properly, urine may collect in the bladder, causing pressure that may damage the repaired tissue. If prescribed, bladder irrigation and vaginal irrigations are performed gently, with minimal pressure.

Effective measures to assist the woman whose fistula cannot be repaired must be planned and implemented on an individual basis. Cleanliness, frequent sitz baths, and deodorizing douches are required, as are perineal pads and protective undergarments. Meticulous skin care is necessary to prevent excoriation. Applying bland creams or a light dusting of cornstarch may be soothing. Additionally, attending to the patient's social and psychologic needs are essential components of effective care.

Despite the best surgical intervention, fistulas may recur. Preoperative treatment of any existing vaginitis is important to ensure successful surgery. After surgery, medical follow up continues for at least 2 years to monitor for a possible recurrence.

Cystocele, Rectocele, Enterocele, and Lacerations of the Perineum

Cystocele is a downward displacement of the bladder toward the vaginal orifice (Fig. 45-3). It usually results from injury and strain during childbirth. The condition usually appears some years later when genital atrophy associated with aging occurs, but younger, multiparous, premenopausal women are also affected.

Rectocele and perineal lacerations may affect the muscles and tissues of the pelvic floor and may occur during childbirth. Because of muscle tears below the vagina, the rectum may pouch upward, thereby pushing the posterior wall of the vagina forward. This structural abnormality is called a **rectocele.** At times, the lacerations may extend, completely severing the fibers of the anal sphincter (complete tear). An **enterocele** is a protrusion of intestinal wall into the vagina.

Clinical Manifestations. Because a *cystocele* causes the anterior vaginal wall to bulge downward, the patient usually reports a sense of pelvic pressure, fatigue, and urinary problems such as incontinence, frequency, and urgency. Back pain and pelvic pain may occur as well.

The symptoms of *rectocele* resemble those of cystocele, with one exception—instead of urinary symptoms, the patient may experience rectal pressure. Constipation, uncontrollable gas, and fecal incontinence may occur in patients with complete tears.

Nonsurgical Management. Perineal, or Kegel, exercises are prescribed and often help to strengthen the weakened muscles. These exercises are more effective in the early stages of a cystocele. Kegel exercises involve contracting or tightening the vaginal muscles. The exercises are easy to do and are recommended for all women, including those with a strong vaginal wall. These exercises are described in Chart 45-4.

If surgery is contraindicated or refused, a **pessary** may be prescribed, especially for mild problems. This device is inserted into the vagina and positioned to keep an organ, such as the bladder, uterus, or intestine, properly aligned when a cystocele, rectocele, or prolapse has occurred. Pessaries are usually ring-shaped or doughnut-shaped and are made of various materials, such as rubber or plastic. The size and type are selected and fitted by a gynecologic health care provider. The patient can be taught to remove it at bedtime and reinsert it in upon waking. If it remains in place, the patient should have it removed, examined, and cleaned by her health care provider at prescribed intervals. At this checkup, the internal tissues are examined for pressure points or signs of irritation. Normally, the patient experiences no pain, discomfort, or discharge with a pessary, but if chronic irritation occurs, alternative measures may be needed to prevent injury and malignancy (Fig. 45-4).

Surgical Management. In many cases, surgery helps to correct structural abnormalities. The procedure to repair the anterior vaginal wall is called **anterior colporrhaphy,** repair of a rectocele is called a **posterior colporrhaphy,** and repair of perineal lacerations is called a **perineorrhaphy.**

Displacements of the Uterus

Usually, the uterus and the cervix lie at right angles to the long axis of the vagina and with the body of the uterus inclined slightly forward. The uterus is freely movable

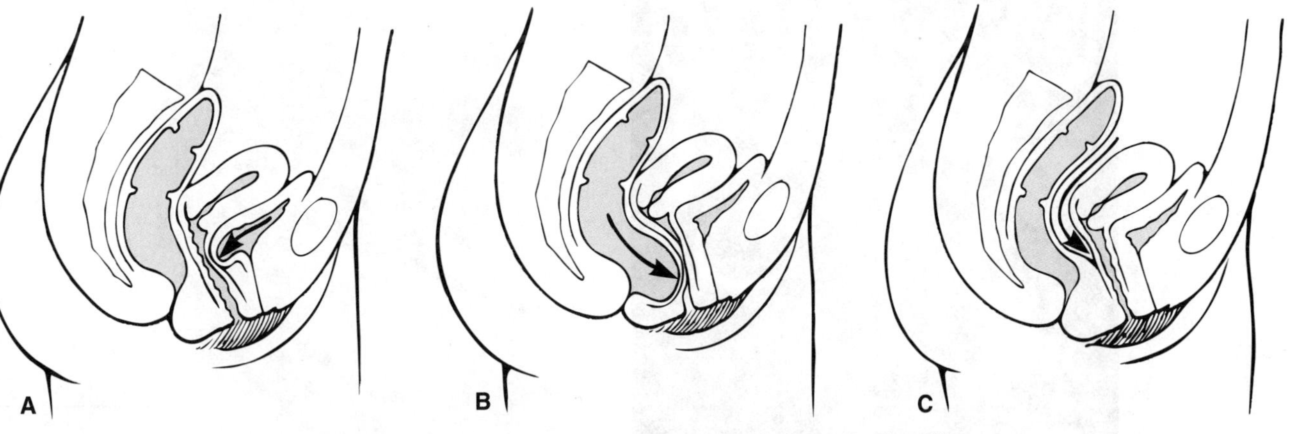

FIGURE 45-3. Diagrammatic representation of the three most common types of pelvic floor relaxation: (**A**) cystocele, (**B**) rectocele, and (**C**) enterocele. *Arrows* depict sites of maximum protrusion.

CHART 45-4
Patient Education: Kegel or Pelvic Muscle Exercises

Purpose: To strengthen and maintain the tone of the pubococcygeal muscle which supports the pelvic organs. Regular performance of these toning exercises may reduce or prevent stress incontinence and uterine prolapse, enhance sensation during sexual intercourse, and hasten postpartum healing.

1. Establish awareness of pelvic muscle function by instructing the woman to "draw in" the perivaginal muscles and anal sphincter as if to control urine or defecation, but without contracting the abdominal, buttock, or inner thigh muscles.
2. Instruct the woman to sustain contraction of the muscles for a period up to 10 seconds, followed by at least 10 seconds of relaxation.
3. Advise the woman to perform these exercises 30–80 times a day.

Note: The training and exercise should be individualized for each patient.

(Urinary Incontinence in Adults: Clinical Practice Guideline. Agency for Health Care Policy and Research. Public Health Service, U.S. Department of Health and Human Services, Rockville, MD, March 1992. AHCPR Pub. No. 92-0038.)

because of the requirements of pregnancy; but the strain of pregnancy, which may involve the formation of adhesions or a weakening of natural uterine supports (or individual variations), may produce changes in the normal position of the uterus. Usually these changes cause no severe problems, but they may produce troublesome symptoms.

Backward Displacements. Backward displacements (known as **retroversion** and **retroflexion**) of the uterus may give rise to such symptoms as backache or pelvic pressure (Fig. 45-5). Most retrograde displacements, however, cause no symptoms. Asymptomatic retroversion of the uterus occurs in approximately 20% of women and is a variant of normal. Women need to be reassured that a uterus that "tips back" is not a problem.

Prolapse and Procidentia. If the structures that support the uterus weaken (typically from childbirth), the uterus may work its way down the vaginal canal (prolapse) and even appear outside the vaginal orifice (procidentia) (Fig. 45-6).

As the uterus descends, it pulls the vaginal walls and even the bladder and rectum with it. Symptoms include pressure and urinary problems (incontinence or retention) from displacement of the bladder. The problems are aggravated when the woman coughs, lifts a heavy object, or stands for a long time. Normal activities, even walking up stairs, may aggravate the problem. The woman with such symptoms is encouraged to seek medical attention, because time will not correct the problem.

Management. Surgery is the treatment of choice. The uterus is sutured back into place and repaired to strengthen and tighten muscle bands. In postmenopausal women, the uterus may be removed (hysterectomy). For elderly women or those who are too ill to withstand the strain of surgery, pessaries may be the treatment of choice.

Nursing Interventions

Patient Education and Health Maintenance. Some problems related to "relaxed" pelvic muscles (cystocele, rectocele, and uterine prolapse) may be prevented. During pregnancy, early visits to the health care provider permit early detection of potential problems. During the postpartum period, perineal exercises to strengthen the muscles can be taught. The woman is instructed to tighten

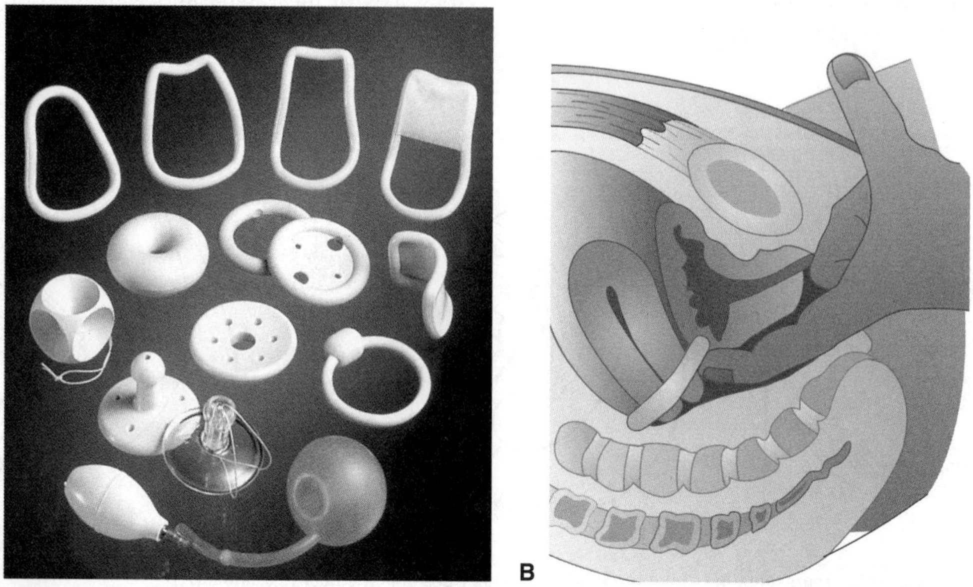

A B

FIGURE 45-4. Examples of pessaries. (**A**) Various shapes and sizes of pessaries available. (**B**) Insertion of one type of pessary.

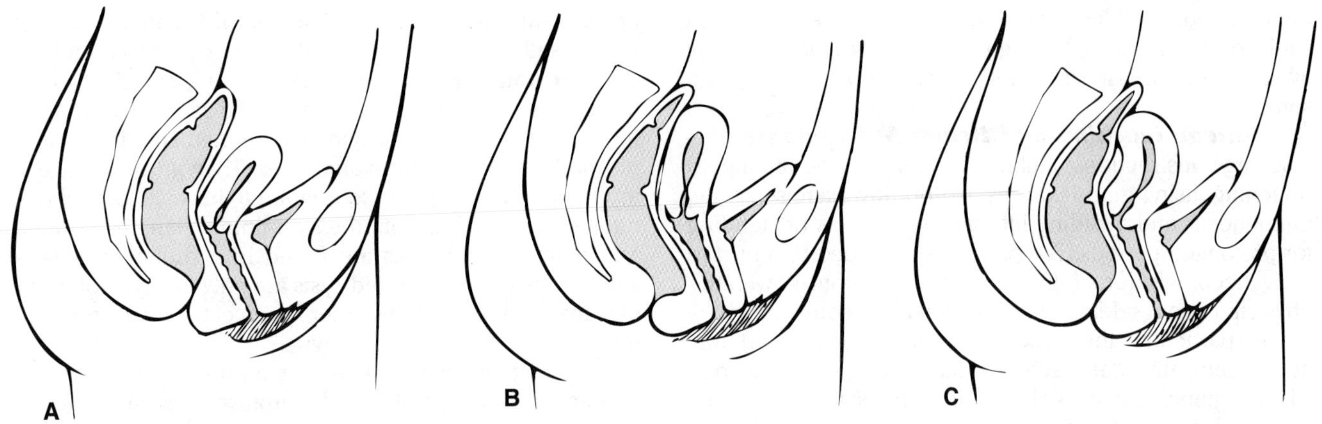

FIGURE 45-5. Retrodisplacements of the uterus. (**A**) The normal position of the uterus detected on palpation. (**B**) In *retroversion* the uterus turns posteriorly as a whole unit. (**C**) In *retroflexion* the fundus bends posteriorly above the cervical end.

and relax gluteal and perineal floor muscles in much the same way she would start and stop the urinary stream. This toning exercise (Kegel's exercise) can be performed at any time.

Delays in obtaining evaluation and treatment may result in complications such as infection, cervical ulceration, cystitis, and hemorrhoids. Therefore, the nurse encourages the patient to obtain prompt treatment for these structural disorders.

Patients who need pessaries may be taught to remove, clean, and reinsert the device. Some pessaries are left in place and examined periodically by a health care provider. Patients using a pessary should not have abnormal discharge, bleeding, or pain and the nurse needs to assess the patient for these symptoms.

Preoperative Nursing Management. Before surgery, the patient needs to know the extent of the proposed surgery, the expectations for the postoperative period, and the effect of surgery on future sexual function. In addition, the patient having a rectocele repair needs to know that before surgery a laxative and a cleansing enema may be prescribed. A perineal shave may be ordered as well.

The patient is usually placed in a lithotomy position for surgery, with special attention given to placing both of her legs in and out of the stirrups simultaneously to prevent muscle strain and excess pressure on the legs and thighs. Other preoperative interventions are similar to those described in Chapter 19.

Postoperative Nursing Management and Rehabilitation. Immediate postoperative goals include preventing infection and pressure on the suture line. This requires perineal care and may preclude using dressings. The patient is always urged to void within a few hours after surgery for cystocele and complete tear. If the patient does not void within this period and reports discomfort or pain in the bladder region after 6 hours, she will need to be catheterized. Some physicians prefer to leave an indwelling catheter in place for 2 to 4 days. Various other bladder care methods are described in Chapter 43. After each voiding or bowel movement, the perineum is cleansed with warm, sterile saline solution (see p. 1245) and dried with sterile absorbent material.

Several methods are used in caring for the sutures. In one method, the sutures are left alone until healing occurs (in 5–10 days). Thereafter, daily vaginal douches with sterile saline solution may be administered during recovery. In another method—the wet method—small, sterile saline douches are administered twice daily, beginning on the day after surgery and continuing throughout recovery.

After an external perineal repair, a heat lamp or hair dryer may be used to help dry the area and promote healing. Commercially available sprays containing combined antiseptic and anesthetic solutions are soothing and effective, and an ice pack applied locally may relieve discomfort. However, the weight of the ice bag must rest on the bed and not on the patient.

Routine postoperative care is similar to that given after abdominal surgery. The patient is positioned in bed, with the head and knees elevated slightly. A liquid diet is given on the first day, and then a full diet is begun as soon as desired.

After surgery for a complete perineal laceration (through the rectal sphincter), special care and attent

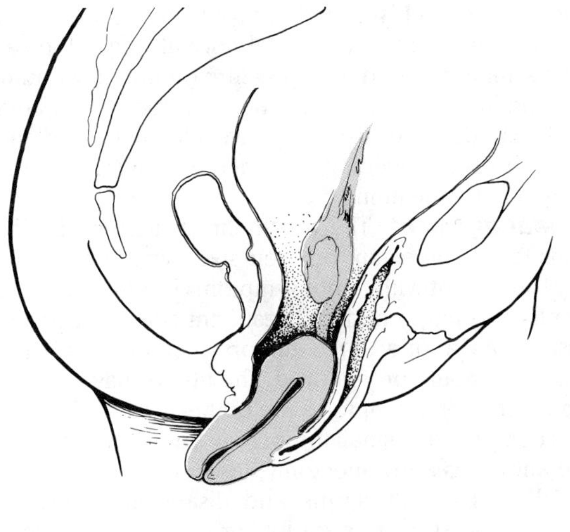

Complete prolapse

FIGURE 45-6. Complete prolapse of the uterus through the introitus.

are required. The bladder is drained via catheter to prevent strain on the sutures. Throughout recovery, stool-softening agents are administered nightly after the patient begins a soft diet.

Patient Teaching and Health Maintenance. Predischarge instructions include information pertaining to douching, using mild laxatives, performing exercise as recommended, and avoiding lifting heavy objects or standing for prolonged periods. The patient is reminded to return to the gynecologist for a follow-up visit and to consult with the physician about safely resuming sexual intercourse.

In particular, the patient is instructed to report any pelvic pain, unusual discharge, inability to carry out personal hygiene, and vaginal bleeding. She is advised to continue with perineal exercises, which are recommended for muscle strength and tone (as described in Chart 45-4).

Benign Tumors and Conditions

Vulvar Cysts

A Bartholin's cyst results from obstruction of a duct in one of the paired vestibular glands located in the posterior third of the vulva, near the vestibule. This cyst is the most common of vulvar tumors. A simple cyst may be asymptomatic, but an infected cyst may cause discomfort. Infection may be due to a *Gonococcus* organism, *Escherichia coli,* or *Staphylococcus aureus* and can cause an abscess with or without involving the inguinal lymph nodes. The usual treatment is incision and drainage followed by antibiotic therapy. If a cyst is asymptomatic, treatment is unnecessary. Moist heat or sitz baths may promote drainage and resolution. If surgery is necessary, laser vaporization may be used.

Vulvar Dystrophy

Vulvar dystrophy is a condition found in older women, causing dry, thickened skin on the vulva or slightly raised, whitish papules or macules. Symptoms usually consist of varying degrees of itching, but some patients have no symptoms. A few patients with vulvar cancer have associated dystrophy. Biopsy and careful follow-up is the standard intervention. If malignant cells are detected, local excision, laser therapy, local chemotherapy, and immunologic treatment are used. Vulvectomy is avoided, if possible, to spare the patient from the stress of disfigurement and possible sexual dysfunction. If the biopsy does not detect cancer, testosterone, estrogen, or cortisone creams are prescribed, depending on the type of dystrophy, to minimize symptoms. By encouraging all patients to perform genital self-examinations regularly and have any itching, lesions, or unusual symptoms assessed by a health care provider, nurses can help prevent complications and progression of vulvar lesions.

Ovarian Cysts

Pathophysiology. The ovary is a common site for cysts, which may be simple enlargements of normal ovarian constituents, the graafian follicle, or corpus luteum, or they may arise from abnormal growth of the ovarian epithelium.

Dermoid cysts are tumors that are thought to arise from parts of the ovum that normally disappear with ripening (maturation). Their origin is undefined and they consist of undifferentiated embryonal cells. They grow slowly and are found during surgery to contain a thick, yellow, sebaceous material arising from the skin lining. Hair, teeth, bone, and many other tissues are found in a rudimentary state within these cysts. Dermoid cysts are only one type of lesion that may develop. Many other types can occur and treatment usually depends on the type.

The patient may or may not report acute or chronic abdominal pain. Symptoms of a ruptured cyst simulate various acute abdominal emergencies, such as appendicitis or ectopic pregnancy. Larger cysts may produce abdominal swelling and exert pressure on adjacent abdominal organs.

The treatment of large ovarian cysts is usually surgical removal. However, if cysts are less than 5 cm wide and appear to be fluid-filled or physiologic in a young, healthy patient, oral contraceptives may be used to suppress ovarian activity and resolve the cyst. About 98% of lesions that occur in women aged 29 and younger are benign. After age 50, only 50% are benign. The postoperative nursing care after surgery to remove an ovarian cyst is similar to that after abdominal surgery, with one exception. The marked decrease in intra-abdominal pressure resulting from removal of a large cyst usually leads to considerable abdominal distention. This complication may be prevented to some extent by applying a snug-fitting abdominal binder.

Benign Tumors of the Uterus: Leiomyomas (Fibroids, Myomas, and Fibromyomas)

Myomatous or fibroid tumors of the uterus are almost always benign (99.5%) and arise from the muscle tissue of the uterus. They are common, occurring in about 20% of white women and 40% to 50% of African-American women. They develop slowly between the ages of 25 and 40 and typically grow large after this period. Fibroids may cause no symptoms or they may produce abnormal vaginal bleeding. Other symptoms are due to pressure on the surrounding organs and include pain, backache, constipation, and urinary problems. Menorrhagia (excessive bleeding) and metrorrhagia (irregular bleeding) may occur because fibroids may distort the uterine lining.

Management. The treatment of uterine fibroids depends to a large extent on their size, symptoms, and location. The patient with minor symptoms is observed closely. If she plans to have children, treatment is as conservative as possible. As a rule, large tumors that produce pressure symptoms should be removed. The uterus may be removed (hysterectomy) if symptoms are bothersome and childbearing is completed. A small tumor may be removed in a procedure known as a myomectomy; laser surgery is often used.

Fibroids usually shrink and disappear during menopause when estrogen is no longer produced. Medications (*e.g.*, luprolide) that induce medical menopause may be prescribed to shrink the tumors. This medical treatment consists of monthly injections which may cause hot flashes and vaginal dryness.

Nursing care for a patient having a hysterectomy is discussed below.

Endometriosis

In endometriosis, a benign lesion or lesions with cells similar to those lining the uterus grow aberrantly in the pelvic cavity outside the uterus. Extensive endometriosis may cause few symptoms, whereas an isolated lesion may produce severe symptoms. Between 3 and 5 million women in the United States are affected by this disorder.

Pathophysiology. In order of frequency, pelvic endometriosis involves the ovary, uterosacral ligaments, cul-de-sac, rectovaginal septum, uterovesical peritoneum, cervix, outer surface of the uterus, umbilicus, laparotomy scar tissue, hernial sacs, and appendix. The misplaced endometrium responds to and depends on ovarian hormonal stimulation. During menstruation, this ectopic tissue bleeds—mostly into areas having no outlet—which causes pain and adhesions. The lesions are typically small, puckered, and brown or blue-black, indicating concealed bleeding.

Endometrial tissue contained within an ovarian cyst has no outlet for the bleeding; this formation is referred to as a **pseudocyst** (chocolate cyst). Adhesions, cysts, and scar tissue may result, causing not only pain, but also infertility.

Incidence. Endometriosis has been diagnosed more frequently as a result of the increased use of laparoscopy. Before laparoscopy, major surgery was necessary before a diagnosis could be made. There is a high incidence among patients who bear children late or those who have fewer children. In countries where tradition favors early marriage and early childbearing, endometriosis is rare. There also appears to be a familial predisposition to endometriosis; it is more common in women whose close female relatives are affected.

Characteristically, endometriosis is found in the young, nulliparous woman between ages 25 and 35. A similar condition affecting the uterine lining in older, multiparous patients is referred to as **adenomyosis.** At one time, these two conditions were thought to be related but are now considered separate entities, although symptoms may be similar and both conditions may be present.

Etiology. The more popular theories regarding the origin of endometrial lesions are the transplantation theory and the metaplasia theory. The transplantation theory suggests that a backflow of menses (retrograde menstruation) transports endometrial tissue to ectopic sites through the fallopian tubes. Transplantation of tissue can also occur during surgery if endometrial tissue is transferred inadvertently by way of surgical instruments. Endometrial tissue can be spread also by lymphatic or venous channels. The metaplasia theory relates to retained remnants of embryonic epithelial tissue, which during growth may be transformed into endometrial tissue by means of outside stimuli. The true cause of endometriosis may be a combination of factors.

Clinical Manifestations. Symptoms vary with the location of endometrial tissue. Usually the chief symptom is a type of dysmenorrhea, unlike typical uterine cramps. The patient complains of a deep-seated aching in the lower abdomen, vagina, posterior pelvis, and back that occurs 1 or 2 days before the menstrual cycle and lasts 2 or 3 days. Some patients, however, have no pain. Abnormal uterine bleeding and dyspareunia (painful intercourse) also may be evident in sexually active women. Excess prostaglandin released from the cells that are shed may contribute to nausea and diarrhea.

Diagnostic Evaluation. A health history, including an account of the menstrual pattern, is necessary to elicit specific symptoms. On bimanual pelvic examination, fixed tender nodules may be detected and uterine mobility may be limited, indicating adhesions. Laparoscopic examination confirms the diagnosis and helps to stage the disease. In Stage 1, the patient has superficial or minimal lesions; Stage 2, mild involvement; Stage 3, moderate involvement; and Stage 4, deep involvement and dense adhesions, with obliteration of the cul-de-sac.

Management. Treatment depends on the patient's symptoms, desire for pregnancy, and the extent of the disease. If the woman is asymptomatic, observation every 6 months may be all that is required. Other therapy for varying degrees of symptoms may be palliation, hormone administration, or surgery. Surgery may involve the use of the laser laparoscope or electrocautery to destroy ectopic endometrial tissue. Palliative measures involve medications (analgesics, prostaglandin inhibitors) and pregnancy, which alleviates symptoms because no menstruation occurs during gestation.

Hormonal therapy, in which oral contraceptives are administered for 6 to 9 months, suppresses menstruation and relieves menstrual pain (dysmenorrhea). Side effects that may occur with oral contraceptives include fluid retention, weight gain, or nausea, which can usually be managed by changing brands or formulations. Depo-Provera, the injectable progesterone contraceptive, may also be used.

Other types of hormonal therapy are also available. A synthetic androgen, danazol (Danocrine), causes atrophy of the endometrium and subsequent amenorrhea. The medication inhibits the release of gonadotropin with minimal overt sex hormone stimulation. The drawbacks of this medication are that it is expensive and may cause troublesome side effects, such as fatigue, depression, weight gain, oily skin, decreased breast size, mild acne, hot flashes, and vaginal atrophy. Another gonadotropin-releasing hormone (GnRH) agonist or GnRH blocker, known as Synarel, decreases estrogen production and causes subsequent amenorrhea. It is administered by nasal spray twice a day for 6 months. Side effects are related to low estrogen levels (*e.g.*, hot flashes and vaginal dryness). Another agent, luprolide (Lupron) is also used and is injected monthly to suppress hormones, induce an artificial menopause, and, thereby, avoid menstrual effects and relieve endometriosis. Some health care providers are prescribing a combination of therapies. Most women continue treatment despite side effects, and symptoms diminish for 80% to 90% of women with mild to moderate endometriosis.

Hormonal medications are not used, however, in patients with a history of abnormal vaginal bleeding, liver, heart, or kidney disease. Possible bone loss from the antiestrogen effects of some of these treatment methods is being studied.

If conservative measures are not helpful, surgery may be necessary. The procedure selected depends on the individual patient's needs. Laparoscopy may be used to fulgurate (cut with high-frequency current) endometrial implants and to lyse (cut) adhesions. Laser surgery is another option made possible by laparoscopy. Lasers can vaporize or coagulate the endometrial implants, thereby destroying this tissue. Depending on circumstances, other surgical possibilities include laparotomy, abdominal hysterectomy, bilateral salpingo-oophorectomy, and appendectomy.

Prognosis. In mild to moderate endometriosis, hormonal or surgical treatment relieves pain and enhances the possibility for pregnancy. For women over age 35 or those willing to sacrifice reproductive capability, definitive surgery (total hysterectomy) provides another alternative.

Nursing Interventions. The health history and physical examination concentrate on identifying specific symptoms, determining when and how long they have been bothersome, and identifying the woman's reproductive desires. This information helps in determining the treatment plan.

Patient goals include relief of pain, dysmenorrhea, and dyspareunia and avoidance of infertility. Nursing interventions include assessing pain and evaluating the techniques and prescribed medications that provide relief. Explaining the various diagnostic procedures helps to alleviate the patient's anxiety.

The nurse also needs to provide emotional support to the woman and her partner who wish to have children. As the treatment plan progresses, the couple may find that pregnancy is not easily possible, and the psychosocial impact of this realization must be recognized and addressed. Alternatives such as *in vitro* fertilization (IVF) or adoption may be discussed at an appropriate time and referrals offered.

The nurse's role in patient education is to dispel myths and encourage the patient to seek care if dysmenorrhea or abnormal bleeding patterns occur. The Endometriosis Association (listed at the end of this chapter) is a helpful resource for patients seeking further information and support for this condition, which can cause disabling pain and severe emotional distress. Patients with endometriosis need access to knowledgeable health care providers and empathetic, supportive treatment.

Adenomyosis. In adenomyosis, the tissue that lines the endometrium invades the uterine wall. The incidence is highest in women from 40 to 50 years of age. Symptoms include hypermenorrhea (excessive and prolonged bleeding), acquired dysmenorrhea, polymenorrhea (abnormally frequent bleeding), and premenstrual staining. Physical examination findings on palpation include an enlarged, firm, and tender uterus. Treatment depends on the severity of bleeding and pain. Hysterectomy, which offers greater relief than more conservative therapies, is currently the treatment of choice.

Malignant Conditions

Malignant tumors of the female reproductive system (excluding breast cancer) are estimated to kill more than 26,400 women in the United States each year. Of these cancers, about 15,800 are new cases of invasive cervical cancer which will result in about 4800 deaths. (These estimates do not include *in situ* cancers.) About 32,800 new cases of uterine cancer are estimated, from which about 5900 deaths will occur yearly. For ovarian cancer, 26,600 new cases will be diagnosed and 14,500 deaths will result. Approximately 5700 other genital cancers will be diagnosed and will cause another 1200 deaths annually (Wingo et al., 1995). Carcinoma *in situ* accounts for approximately 55,000 new cases annually.

Although some cancers are difficult to detect or prevent, yearly pelvic examinations with a Pap smear is a painless and relatively inexpensive method of early detection. Health care providers can encourage women to follow this health practice by providing nonstressful examinations that are educational and supportive and offer an opportunity for the patient to ask questions and clarify misinformation. If more women understood that the pelvic examination and Pap smear do not have to be uncomfortable or embarrassing, early detection rates would undoubtedly improve and lives would be saved.

Cancer of the Cervix

There are two main types of primary uterine cancer: carcinoma of the cervix, which is predominantly epidermoid cancer, and carcinoma of the endometrium, which involves the corpus and body of the uterus.

Cancer of the cervix is less common than it once was because of early detection by Pap smear. Over the last 40 years, invasive cervical cancer has decreased from 45 cases per 100,000 to 15 cases per 100,000 women. However, it is still the third most common female reproductive cancer, excluding breast cancer. It occurs most commonly between ages 30 and 45, but it can occur as early as age 18. Sexual activity has a relationship to the incidence of cervical cancer: in women under age 25, it is more prevalent in those with a history of multiple sexual partners and several early pregnancies. Studies suggest that this type of cancer may be sexually transmitted. Invasive cervical cancer has been identified as an HIV-defining condition. (See Chapter 50 for a discussion of HIV infection and AIDS.)

Risk factors, aside from early age at first intercourse, early childbearing, and multiple partners, include exposure to human papillomavirus (HPV), HIV infection, smoking, and exposure to diethylstilbestrol (DES) *in utero*.

Diagnosis may follow abnormal Pap smear results with dysplasia, or persistent atypical cells, followed by biopsy results identifying cervical intraepithelial neoplasia (CIN) or a high-grade squamous intraepithelial lesion (HGSIL). These terms are used in classifying premalignant cervical lesions. HPV infections are usually implicated in these conditions.

Biopsy findings may also identify cancer *in situ*. Cervical cancer may be detected when a patient complains of discharge, irregular bleeding, or bleeding after sexual intercourse, but the disease usually produces no symptoms.

The vaginal discharge in advanced cervical cancer increases gradually and becomes watery and, finally, dark and foul smelling from necrosis and infection of the tumor. The bleeding, which occurs at irregular intervals, between periods (metrorrhagia), or after menopause, may be slight (just enough to spot the undergarments), and occurs usually after mild trauma (such as intercourse, douching, or defecation). As the disease continues, the bleeding may persist and increase.

Chronic cervical infections seem to play a significant part in cervical cancer. Clinical signs of the disease include a large, reddish growth or a deep, ulcerating crater before the patient notices any symptoms.

As the cancer advances, it may invade the tissues outside the cervix, including the lymph glands anterior to the sacrum. In one third of patients with invasive cervical cancer, the disease involves the fundus. The nerves in this region may be affected, producing excruciating pain in the back and the legs that is relieved only by large doses of opioid analgesia. The final stage, when the disease is untreated, produces extreme emaciation and anemia, usually accompanied by fever due to secondary infection and abscesses in the ulcerating mass, and fistula formation.

Diagnostic Evaluation. Clinical staging estimates the extent of the disease so that treatment can be planned more specifically and prognosis reasonably predicted. The International Classification adopted by the International Federation of Gynecology and Obstetrics (Table 45-2) is the most widely used staging system; the TNM (tumor, nodes, and metastases) classification is also used in describing malignancies (see Table 16-5). In this system, *T* refers to the extent of the primary tumor, *N* to lymph node involvement, and *M* to metastasis, or spread of the disease.

Signs and symptoms are evaluated, and x-rays, laboratory studies, and special examinations such as punch biopsy and colposcopy are performed. Depending on the stage of the cancer, other tests may be performed to determine the extent of disease and appropriate treatment. These tests include dilatation and curettage (D&C), computed tomography (CT) scan, magnetic resonance imaging (MRI), intravenous urogram (IVU), cystogram, and barium x-ray studies.

Management. When precursor lesions such as low-grade squamous intraepithelial lesions (LGSIL) or high-grade squamous intraepithelial lesions (HGSIL) are found by colposcopy and biopsy, conservative nonsurgical removal is possible. Cryotherapy (freezing with nitrous oxide) or laser therapy is effective. Conization (removing a cone-shaped portion of the cervix) is performed when biopsy findings demonstrate CIN III or HGSIL, equivalent to severe dysplasia and carcinoma *in situ.* CIN I and II are consistent with mild to moderate dysplasia or LGSIL (the Bethesda classification).

To clarify current terminology, see Table 44-1, which describes changes in Pap smear terminology. (The Bethesda classification is the most current.) Table 45-3 describes other terms used in cytologic descriptions. (Also see Guideline 44-1, which describes the proper technique for obtaining a cervical tissue specimen for cytologic examination.)

TABLE 45-2 International Classification of Carcinoma of the Uterine Cervix

Stage of Lesion	Location	Description
Stage 0	Carcinoma *in situ*	Cancer limited to epithelial layer; no evidence of invasion
Stage I	Carcinoma strictly confined to cervix	Size is not a criterion
Stage IA		Microinvasive
Stage IB		Clinically obvious stage I
Stage II	Vaginal cancer	Lesion has spread beyond cervix to involve vagina (not lower third) or paracervical region on one or both sides
Stage IIA		Vaginal extension only
Stage IIB		Paracervical extension with or without vaginal involvement
Stage III	Cancer involves lower third of vagina or has extended to one or both pelvic walls	Unequivocal palpable lymph node disease on the pelvic wall IV urogram shows one or both ureters obstructed by the tumor
Stage IIIA		Extends to lower third of vagina only
Stage IIIB		Isolated carcinomatous metastases are palpable on the pelvic wall
Stage IV	Bladder extension	Evidence that carcinoma involves the bladder seen on cystoscopic examination or by presence of vesicovaginal fistula
	Rectal extension Distant spread	Carcinoma spreads outside true pelvis to other organs

TABLE 45-3 Descriptive Terms Used in Cervical Cytology

Atypical squamous metaplasia	Metaplastic squamous cells that contain nuclear features of active inflammation.
Chronic cervicitis	Inflammatory exudate associated with epithelial changes.
Dyskeratocytes	Mature, squamous cells with dense and refringent cytoplasm indicative of human papilloma virus (HPV). May be falsely read as dysplasia.
Giant cells	Large multinucleated cells that may be indicative of herpes.
Koilocytotic atypia (warty atypia)	Hollow squamous cells indicative of HPV.
Parakeratosis	Indicative of estrogen-deficient states.
Regeneration and repair	Features of inflammation and repair seen in squamous and columnar cells.

(Fullerton JT and Barger MK. Papanicolaou smear: An update on classification and management. J Am Acad Nurse Pract 1989 Jul/Sep; 1[3]: 87.)

Patients who have precursor or premalignant lesions (*i.e.*, dysplasia or low-grade SIL), need reassurance that they do not have cancer although the condition, if untreated for a long time, would progress to cancer. Patients with cervical cancer *in situ* also need to know that this is usually a slow-growing and nonaggressive type of cancer that is not expected to recur following appropriate treatment.

If preinvasive cervical cancer occurs when a woman has completed childbearing, a simple hysterectomy is usually recommended. Frequent subsequent periodic examinations are performed to monitor for recurrence.

When the patient has invasive cervical cancer, radiation or radical hysterectomy or both may be performed. The method selected depends on the stage of the lesion and on the judgment and experience of the physician. Some authorities advocate radical surgery, especially when a patient cannot withstand the effects of radiation or has a radiation-resistant cancer. Surgical procedures that may be carried out include the following:

Total hysterectomy—removal of the uterus, and cervix
Radical hysterectomy (Wertheim)—removal of the uterus, adnexa, proximal vagina, and bilateral lymph nodes through an abdominal incision
Radical vaginal hysterectomy (Schauta)—vaginal removal of the uterus, adnexa, and proximal vagina. (*Note:* "Radical" indicates that an extensive area of the paravaginal, paracervical, parametrial, and uterosacral tissues is removed with the uterus.)
Bilateral pelvic lymphadenectomy—removal of the common iliac, external iliac, hypogastric, and obturator lymphatic vessels and nodes
Pelvic exenteration—removal of the pelvic organs, including the bladder or rectum and pelvic lymph nodes and construction of diversional conduit, colostomy, and vagina
Salpingo-oophorectomy (bilateral)—removal of the fallopian tubes and ovaries.

Frequent follow-up by gynecologic oncologists is imperative, because the risk of recurrence is 35% after treatment for invasive cervical cancer. Recurrence usually occurs within the first 2 years. Radiation is often part of treatment to reduce recurrent disease and may be delivered by an external beam or by brachytherapy (method by which the radiation source is placed near the tumor).

Pelvic Exenteration. Some patients with recurrences of cervical cancer are considered for pelvic exenteration, in which a large portion of the pelvic contents is removed. Unilateral leg edema, sciatica, and ureteral obstruction indicate likely disease progression. Patients with these symptoms are not considered for this major surgical procedure. Complications are considerable and include pulmonary emboli, pulmonary edema, myocardial infarction, cerebral vascular accident, hemorrhage, sepsis, small bowel obstruction, fistula formation, urinary obstruction of ileal conduit, and pyelonephritis. Nursing care of these patients is complex and requires coordination and care by experienced health care professionals.

Cancer of the Endometrium

Cancer of the uterine endometrium (fundus or corpus) has increased in incidence, partly because people are living longer and reporting is more accurate. About 32,000 cases are estimated to occur annually with 5900 deaths (Wingo et al., 1995). All women should be encouraged to have annual checkups, including a gynecologic examination. After breast, colorectal, and lung cancer, endometrial cancer is the fourth most common cancer in women and the most common pelvic neoplasm. Treatment consists of total hysterectomy and bilateral salpingo-oophorectomy. Depending on the stage, preoperative and postoperative treatments may include intracavitary radiation or external pelvic radiation.

One third of women with postmenopausal bleeding have cancer of the uterus. The median age is 61, and most patients are at least age 55. Obese women have a slightly higher risk because of increased levels of estrone related to excess weight. This results from conversion of androstenedione to estrone in body fat, which exposes the uterus to unopposed estrogen.

Unopposed estrogen administered in hormone replacement therapy (HRT) is also a potential risk factor. Currently, progesterone is added to the HRT regimen to offset this risk. Women who have been treated with estrogen alone are at increased risk (PEPI, 1995).

Women who received HRT without progesterone can be monitored by regular endometrial aspiration or biopsy to rule out hyperplasia, a precursor of endometrial cancer. Ultrasonography can also measure the thickness of the endometrium. A biopsy or aspiration is diagnostic.

Other risk factors include nulliparity and late menopause (*i.e.*, after age 52). Most uterine cancers are adenocarcinomas originating in the lining of the uterus. Treatment is based on the stage of the disease but almost always begins with a total abdominal hysterectomy along with bilateral salpingo-oophorectomy. External radiation and brachytherapy may follow, depending on results of staging for those patients at high risk for recurrence.

Recurrent cancer usually occurs inside the vaginal vault or in the upper vagina. Recurrent lesions in the vagina are usually treated with surgery and radiation. Recurrent lesions beyond the vagina are treated with hormonal therapy or chemotherapy. Progestin therapy is used frequently. Patients should be prepared for such side effects as nausea, depression, rash, or mild fluid retention with this therapy.

Hysterectomy

A total hysterectomy involves removing the uterus and the cervix. This procedure is performed for many conditions other than cancer, including dysfunctional uterine bleeding; endometriosis; nonmalignant growths on the uterus, cervix, and adnexa; problems of pelvic relaxation and prolapse; and irreparable injury to the uterus. Malignant conditions require a total abdominal hysterectomy and bilateral salpingo-oophorectomy (removal of fallopian tubes and ovaries).

Laparoscopic-assisted hysterectomy is performed by some physicians with excellent results and prompt recovery. This method is used only for vaginal hysterectomy and is performed as a short-stay procedure or ambulatory surgery in carefully selected patients. Patients have a shorter hospital stay and a reduced incidence of postoperative infection.

Preoperative Management. The physical preparation for a patient undergoing a hysterectomy differs little from that for a patient undergoing a laparotomy. Usually, the lower half of the abdomen and the pubic and perineal regions are carefully shaved and cleaned with soap and water (some surgeons do not require that the patient be shaved). The intestinal tract and the bladder need to be empty before the patient is taken to the operating room to prevent contamination and accidental injury to the bladder or intestinal tract. An enema and antiseptic douche are usually prescribed the evening before surgery. The patient receives a sedative to ensure a restful night. Preoperative medications administered the morning of surgery will help the patient relax.

Postoperative Management. The principles of general postoperative care for abdominal surgery apply, with particular attention given to peripheral circulation to prevent thrombophlebitis and DVT (noting varicosities, promoting circulation with leg exercises, and using elastic stockings). Major risks are infection and hemorrhage. In addition, because the surgical site is close to the bladder, voiding problems may occur, particularly after a vaginal hysterectomy.

Edema or nerve trauma may cause temporary loss of bladder tone (bladder atony), and an indwelling catheter may be used. During surgery, the handling of the bowel may cause ileus and interfere with bowel functioning.

❑ NURSING PROCESS
The Patient Undergoing a Hysterectomy

Assessment

The health history, physical and pelvic examination, and laboratory studies are performed. Additional assessment data include the patient's psychosocial responses, as the need for a hysterectomy may elicit strong emotional reactions and fears. If the hysterectomy is performed to remove a malignant tumor, anxiety related to fear of cancer and death adds to the stress of the patient and her family.

Diagnosis

Nursing Diagnoses

Based on all the assessment data, the patient's major nursing diagnoses may include the following:

- Anxiety related to the diagnosis of cancer, fear of pain, perceived loss of femininity, and disfigurement
- Body image disturbance related to altered sexuality, fertility, and relationships with partner and family
- Pain related to surgery and other adjuvant therapy
- Knowledge deficit of the perioperative aspects of hysterectomy and self-care

Collaborative Problems/ Potential Complications

Based on assessment data, potential complications may include:

- Hemorrhage
- Deep vein thrombosis
- Bladder dysfunction

Planning and Implementation

Goals. The major goals for the patient may include relief of anxiety, self-acceptance after loss of the uterus, absence of pain or discomfort, increased knowledge of self-care requirements, and prevention of complications.

Nursing Interventions

Relieving Anxiety. Anxiety stems from several factors: unfamiliar environment, effects of surgery on body image and reproductive ability, fear of pain and other discomfort, and sensitivity and, possibly, feelings of embarrassment about exposure of the genital area in the perioperative period. Conflicts between medical treatment and religious beliefs may be troubling as well. In such cases the nurse needs to determine what the experience means to the patient and how to assist her in expressing her feelings to someone who can understand and help. Throughout the preoperative period, explanations are given about the physical preparations.

Improving Body Image. The patient often has strong emotional reactions to having a hysterectomy, which usually evokes strong personal feelings related to the diagnosis, significant others who may be involved (family, partner), religious beliefs, and the prognosis. Concerns may surface (such as the inability to have children and the effect on femininity), as may questions about the impact of surgery on sexual relationships and satisfaction. The patient needs reassurance that she will still have a vagina and that she can experience sexual intercourse after a temporary postoperative abstinence while tissues heal.

Information that sexual satisfaction and orgasm arise from clitoral stimulation rather than from a uterus reassures many women. Most women note some change in sexual feelings after hysterectomy, but they vary in intensity. In some cases, the vagina is shortened by surgery, and this may affect sensitivity or comfort.

Moreover, when hormonal balances are upset, as usually occurs in reproductive system disturbances, the patient may experience depression and heightened emotional sensitivity to people and situations. The nurse needs to approach and evaluate each patient individually, in light of these factors. The nurse who exhibits interest, concern, and willingness to listen to the patient's fears will assist the patient's progress throughout the surgical experience.

Relieving Pain. A hysterectomy may be performed abdominally or vaginally. The surgeon makes this decision based on the diagnosis and size of the uterus. An abdominal incision is used when the patient has cancer and when the uterus is enlarged. Resultant pain and abdominal discomfort are common. Analgesics are administered as prescribed to relieve pain and promote movement and ambulation.

To relieve discomfort from abdominal distention, a nasogastric tube may be inserted before the patient leaves the operating room, especially if the surgeon handled the viscera excessively, or if a large tumor was removed. Its excision could cause edema because of the sudden release of pressure. In the postoperative period, fluids and food may be restricted for 1 or 2 days. If the patient has abdominal distention or flatus, a rectal tube may be prescribed, as well as applications of heat to the abdomen. When abdominal auscultation detects resumption of bowel sounds signaling peristalsis, the patient can receive additional fluids and a soft diet. Ambulation facilitates the return of normal peristalsis.

Patient Education and Health Maintenance. Information provided to the patient is tailored according to her needs. She must know, however, what limitations or restrictions, if any, to expect. For example, she can expect not to menstruate. Symptoms of menopause will not result if her ovaries are intact, but if they have been removed, hormonal replacement therapy may be considered. A hysterectomy typically causes fatigue and weakness for a few weeks (as major surgery often does). This is to be expected and should gradually improve.

The patient should resume activities gradually. This does not mean sitting for long periods because doing so may cause blood to pool in the pelvis and increase the risk of thromboembolism. The nurse can explain that showers are preferable to tub baths to reduce the possibility of infection and to avoid the dangers of injury from getting in and out of the bathtub from a sitting position. The patient is instructed to avoid straining, lifting, sexual intercourse, or driving until her physician permits her to resume these activities. Vaginal discharge, foul odor, excessive bleeding, any leg redness or pain, or an elevated temperature should be reported to her health care provider promptly. The nurse should be familiar with information given to the patient by the surgeon regarding resumption of sexual intercourse.

Monitoring and Managing Potential Complications

Hemorrhage. Vaginal bleeding and hemorrhage may occur after hysterectomy. To detect these complications early, the nurse counts the perineal pads used, assesses the extent of saturation with blood, and monitors the patient's vital signs. Abdominal dressings are monitored for drainage if an abdominal surgical approach was used. In preparation for hospital discharge, the nurse gives guidelines for restricting activity to promote healing and to prevent postoperative bleeding.

Deep Vein Thrombosis. Because of positioning during surgery, postoperative edema, and immobility, the patient is at risk for deep vein thrombosis and pulmonary embolus. To minimize the risk, elastic stockings are applied. Additionally, the patient is encouraged and assisted to change positions frequently, although pressure under the knees is avoided. The nurse assists the patient to ambulate early in the postoperative period, and the patient is encouraged to exercise her legs and feet while in bed. Additionally the nurse assesses for deep vein thrombosis (leg pain, positive Homans' sign) and pulmonary embolism (chest pain, tachycardia, dyspnea). Because the patient may be discharged within 1 or 2 days of surgery, she is instructed to avoid prolonged sitting in a chair with pressure at the knees, sitting with crossed legs, and immobility.

Bladder Dysfunction. Because of possible difficulty in voiding postoperatively, an indwelling catheter may be inserted before or during surgery and left in place in the immediate postoperative period. If a catheter is in place, it is usually removed shortly after the patient begins to ambulate. After the catheter is removed, the patient's urinary output is monitored; additionally, the abdomen is assessed for distention. If the patient does not void within a prescribed time, measures are initiated to encourage voiding (*e.g.*, assisting the patient up to the bathroom, pouring warm water over the perineum). If the patient cannot void, catheterization may be necessary.

Evaluation

Expected Outcomes

1. Experiences decreased anxiety
2. Accepts changes related to surgery
   a. Discusses changes resulting from surgery with her partner
   b. Verbalizes understanding of her disorder and the treatment plan
   c. Displays minimal depression or sadness
3. Experiences minimal pain and discomfort
   a. Reports relief of abdominal pain and discomfort
   b. Ambulates without pain
4. Verbalizes knowledge and understanding of self-care
   a. Practices deep-breathing, turning, and leg exercises as instructed
   b. Increases activity and ambulation daily
   c. Reports adequate fluid intake and adequate urinary output
   d. Identifies reportable symptoms
   e. Schedules and keeps follow-up appointments
5. Experiences no complications
   a. Has minimal vaginal bleeding and exhibits normal vital signs
   b. Ambulates early
   c. Notes no chest or calf pain and no redness, tenderness, or swelling in the extremities
   d. Reports no urinary problems or abdominal distention

Cancer of the Vulva

Primary cancer of the vulva represents 3% to 5% of all gynecologic malignancies and is seen mostly in postmenopausal women although its incidence in younger women is increasing. More whites than nonwhites are afflicted. Squamous cell carcinoma accounts for most primary vulvar tumors. Less common are Bartholin's gland cancer, basal cell carcinoma, and malignant melanoma. Little is known about what causes this disease.

The median age for cancer limited to the vulva is 44 years, whereas the median age for invasive vulvar cancer is 61 years. The incidence is higher in women with hypertension, obesity, and diabetes. Less radical treatment approaches than vulvectomy (discussed below) are being used.

Clinical Manifestations and Diagnostic Evaluation. Long-standing pruritus is the most common symptom of vulvar cancer. Bleeding, foul-smelling discharge, and pain also may be present, and are usually signs of advanced disease. Early lesions appear as a chronic dermatitis; later the patient may note a lump that continues to grow and becomes a hard, ulcerated, cauliflower-like growth. Biopsy should be performed on any vulvar lesion that persists, ulcerates, or fails to heal quickly with proper therapy.

The nurse is in an ideal position to encourage a woman with these signs and symptoms to seek health care, because this is one of the most curable of all malignant conditions. The lesion is visible and accessible and grows relatively slowly. It begins on the skin surface and is easily noticed as a small ulcer that becomes irritated or itchy or increases in size. Possible increased risk may be related to chronic vulvar irritation and vulvar dystrophy.

Nurses can teach patients about the signs and symptoms of possible vulvar cancer; these include unusual discharge, itching, or bleeding. During a routine gynecologic examination, the patient can also be instructed to perform genital self-examination at the same time that she performs her monthly breast self-examination. Using a mirror, the patient can see what constitutes normal female anatomy and learn about changes that should be reported (*e.g.*, lesions, ulcers, masses, and persistent itching).

Management. Vulvar intraepithelial lesions are preinvasive and are also called vulvar carcinoma *in situ*. They may be treated by local excision, laser vaporization, chemotherapeutic creams (*i.e.*, 5-fluorouracil), or cryosurgery.

When invasive vulvar carcinoma exists, primary treatment may include wide excision or removal of the vulva (vulvectomy). A wide excision is performed only if lymph nodes are normal. Nursing care for a wide excision and vulvectomy are similar.

Radiation is used to treat unresectable tumors. If a widespread area is involved or the disease is advanced, a radical vulvectomy with bilateral groin dissection may be performed. A radical vulvectomy is reserved for patients with metastases involving the lymph nodes. After radical vulvectomy, skin grafting may be required. The need for this surgery is determined on an individual basis. Pelvic exenteration may also be a treatment option.

Preoperative Physical Preparation. In addition to the nursing interventions described in Chapter 19 to prepare the patient physically and psychologically for surgery, skin preparation may include cleansing the lower abdomen, inguinal areas, upper thighs, and vulva with a detergent germicide for several days before the surgical procedure. The extent of surgery depends on the extent of the disease, with more extensive lesions requiring deep pelvic node dissection. Antibiotic and heparin prophylaxis may be prescribed preoperatively and continued postoperatively to prevent infection and pulmonary emboli.

Postoperative Surgical Wound Care. When the patient returns from the operating room, perineal dressings are more likely to remain in place and be comfortable if a T-binder is used. A skin graft from the buttocks may have to be performed if the edges of the excision could not be approximated, and drains may be in place as well. A pressure stent may be applied to the grafted site to promote adhesion. Nursing care includes monitoring for suppuration (accumulation of purulent material) under the graft and assisting the patient to keep the perineal area clean and dry.

The wound is cleansed daily with warm, normal saline irrigations or other antiseptic solutions as prescribed. A transparent dressing or Xeroform gauze may be in place over the wound to minimize exposure to the air and subsequent pain. Heat lamp treatments may be prescribed.

NURSING PROCESS
The Patient Undergoing a Wide Excision of the Vulva or Vulvectomy

Assessment

In addition to the physical assessment findings, the health history is a valuable tool for establishing rapport with the patient. The reason for the patient seeking health care is apparent. What the nurse can tactfully elicit is the reason a delay, if any, occurred, in seeking health care, for example, because of modesty, economics, denial, neglect, or fear (abusive partners sometimes prevent women from seeking care). The patient's health habits are identified and her receptivity to learning evaluated. Psychosocial factors are also assessed. Preoperative preparation and psychologic encouragement begin at this time.

Diagnosis

Nursing Diagnoses

Based on all the assessment and other data, the patient's major nursing diagnoses may include the following:

- Anxiety related to the diagnosis and surgery
- Alternation in skin integrity related to the wound and drainage
- Pain related to surgical incision and subsequent wound care
- Sexual dysfunction related to change in body part
- Self-care deficit related to lack of understanding of perineal care and general health status

Collaborative Problems/ Potential Complications

Based on assessment data, potential complications may include:

- Wound infection and sepsis
- Deep vein thrombosis
- Hemorrhage

Planning and Implementation

Goals. The major goals for the patient may include acceptance of and preparation for surgical intervention, recovery of optimal sexual function, ability to perform adequate and appropriate self-care, and prevention of complications.

Nursing Interventions

Preoperative

Relieving Anxiety. The patient must be allowed time to talk and ask questions. Fear often decreases when a woman of childbearing age who is to undergo wide excision of the vulva or vulvectomy learns that the possibility for subsequent sexual relations is good and that pregnancy is possible after a wide excision. The nurse must know what information the physician has given to the patient about the surgery to reinforce that information and address the patient's questions and concerns.

Postoperative

Relieving Pain and Discomfort. Because of the wide excision, the patient may experience severe pain and discomfort even with minimal movement. Inadequate pain relief will inhibit the patient's mobility and increase the likelihood of complications. Therefore, analgesics are administered preventively to relieve pain and increase the patient's comfort level. Careful positioning using pillows usually increases comfort, as do soothing backrubs. A low Fowler's position or, occasionally, a pillow placed under the knees will reduce pain by relieving tension on the incision; however, efforts must be made to avoid pressure behind the knees which will increase the risk of deep vein thrombosis. Positioning the patient on her side, with pillows between her legs and against the lumbar region provides comfort and reduces tension on the wound.

Improving Skin Integrity. The patient may be confined to bed for several days to promote healing of the surgical and donor sites (if skin grafts were used). An air mattress or ("egg crate") convoluted foam pad or mattress can assist in distributing weight and relieving pressure. Moving from one position to another requires time and patience on the part of both patient and nurse. Installing an overbed trapeze bar may help the patient to move herself. Ambulation may be attempted on the second day.

The extent of the surgical incision and the type of dressing are considered when choosing strategies to promote skin integrity. Intact skin needs to be protected from drainage and moisture, and dressings must be changed as needed to ensure patient comfort and to perform wound care and irrigation (if prescribed), and permit observation of the surgical site. The appearance of the surgical site and the characteristics of drainage are assessed and documented. Once the dressings are removed, a bed cradle may be used to keep the bed linens away from the surgical site. The nurse must prevent the patient from exposure when visitors arrive or someone else enters the room.

Supporting Positive Sexuality and Sexual Function. The patient who undergoes vulvar surgery usually experiences concerns about the impact of the surgery on her sexual attractiveness and functioning. Establishing a trusting nurse–patient relationship is important for the patient to feel comfortable expressing her concerns and fears. The patient is encouraged to share and discuss her concerns with her sexual partner.

Because alterations in sexual sensation and functioning depend on the extent of surgery, the nurse needs to know about any structural–functional changes resulting from the surgery. Consulting with the surgeon will clarify which changes to expect, and referring the patient and her partner to a sex counselor may help them address these changes and resume satisfying sexual activity.

Patient Education and Home Care Considerations. Preparing the patient for hospital discharge begins with her hospital admission. She is encouraged to share her concerns as she recovers and to assume increasing responsibility for her own care. She is encouraged and assisted in caring for the surgical site and in increasing activities gradually. Words of encouragement are particularly reassuring.

Posthospital care requires giving complete instructions to a family member who will help care for the patient at home and to the community health or home care nurse who will provide follow-up care. Depending on the changes resulting from the surgery, the patient and her family may need assistance performing wound care and urinary catheterization, and detecting complications. Follow-up phone calls by the nurse to the patient are usually reassuring to the patient and family, who may be responsible for performing complex care procedures at home during the immediate posthospital period. Consulting with the nurse who will provide home follow-up care after discharge is essential to ensure continuity of care.

Monitoring and Managing Potential Complications

Preventing Infection. The location and extent of the incision put the patient at risk for infection and sepsis. The patient is monitored closely for local and systemic signs and symptoms of infection: purulent drainage, redness, increased pain, fever, and an increased white blood cell count. The nurse will assist in obtaining tissue specimens for culture, if infection is suspected, and will administer antibiotics as prescribed. Hand washing, always an important infection-preventing measure, is of particular importance whenever there is an extensive area of exposed tissue. Catheters, drains, and dressings are handled carefully and with gloves to avoid cross-contamination. A low-residue diet will prevent straining on defecation and wound contamination. Sitz baths are discouraged after a wide excision because of the risk of infection.

Deep Vein Thrombosis. The patient is at risk for deep vein thrombosis (DVT) because of the positioning required during surgery, postoperative edema, and the usually prolonged immobility needed to promote healing. Elastic stockings are applied and the patient is encouraged to perform ankle exercises to minimize venous pooling which leads to deep vein thrombosis. The patient is encouraged and assisted to change position by using the overhead trapeze. Pressure behind the knees is avoided when positioning the patient because this may increase venous pooling. The patient is assessed for signs and symptoms of DVT (leg pain, positive Homans' sign) and pulmonary embolism (chest pain, tachycardia, dyspnea). Fluid intake is encouraged to prevent dehydration, which also increases the risk for DVT.

Hemorrhage. The extent of the surgical incision and possibly wide excision of tissue increase the risk of postoperative bleeding and hemorrhage. Although the pressure dressings that are applied after surgery minimize the risk, the patient must be monitored closely for signs of hemorrhage and resulting hypovolemic shock. These signs may include decreased blood pressure, increased pulse rate, decrease urine output, decreased mental status, and cold, clammy skin.

If hemorrhage and shock occur, treatment interventions include fluid replacement, blood component therapy, and vasopressor medications. Laboratory results (*e.g.*, hematocrit and hemoglobin levels) and hemodynamic monitoring will be used to assess the patient's response to treatment. Depending on the specific cause of hemorrhage, the patient may be returned to the operating room. The patient who experiences hemorrhage will be anxious and apprehensive. Providing brief explanations of the procedures being performed and offering reassurance that the problem has been identified and is being taken care of contribute to reducing the anxiety and fears of the patient and her family.

Evaluation

Expected Outcomes

1. Adjusts to the trauma of the surgical experience
   a. Uses available resources in coping with and alleviating emotional stress
   b. Asks questions related to postoperative expectations
   c. Demonstrates willingness to discuss alternative approaches to sexual expression
2. Obtains pain relief
   a. Reports progressive decline in pain and discomfort
   b. Assumes position of comfort
3. Maintains skin integrity
   a. States reason for using a special air mattress or other device
   b. Uses overhead trapeze to change position frequently
   c. Exhibits healing of surgical site without excoriated skin
   d. Cares for incision and surgical site as instructed
4. Exhibits positive outlook about sexuality and sexual functioning
   a. Verbalizes concerns and anxieties about sexual functioning
   b. Discusses options and alternative approaches to sexual intercourse
5. Increases participation in self-care activities
   a. Demonstrates self-care activities as instructed
   b. Identifies signs and symptoms of complications that should be reported to the nurse or physician
   c. Properly cleans the surgical site after voiding and defecation
6. Experiences no complications
   a. Is free of any signs and symptoms of infection: has normal vital signs (temperature, blood pressure, pulse rate), has no purulent discharge
   b. Identifies activities to prevent deep vein thrombosis: avoids crossing legs or sitting with pressure against knees; exercises ankles and legs
   c. Exhibits no signs or symptoms of DVT (leg pain, redness, edematous, or swollen, extremities)
   d. Demonstrates no signs or symptoms of hemorrhage

Cancer of the Vagina

Cancer of the vagina usually results from metastasized choriocarcinoma or from cancer of the cervix or adjacent organs (such as the uterus, vulva, bladder, or rectum). Primary cancer of the vagina is uncommon.

Risk factors include previous cervical cancer, *in utero* exposure to DES, previous vaginal or vulvar cancer, previous radiation therapy, history of HPV (human papillomavirus), or pessary use. Any patient with previous cervical cancer should be examined regularly for vaginal lesions.

Before 1970, vaginal cancer was considered to occur predominantly in postmenopausal women. In the 1970s, it was shown that maternal ingestion of DES affected female offspring who were exposed *in utero*. Benign genital tract abnormalities have occurred in some of these young women. Vaginal adenosis (abnormal tissue growth) may also occur. The risk of clear cell tumor related to DES exposure is 0.14 to 1.4 in 1000 women. Colposcopy is indicated for all women exposed to this medication. If colposcopic examination discloses adenosis or a significant cervical lesion, follow-up is essential.

Vaginal pessaries, used to support prolapsed tissues, have been associated with vaginal cancer only if the devices were not cared for properly (*i.e.*, regularly cleaned and the vagina examined by a health care professional), because pessaries can be a source of chronic irritation. Symptoms of vaginal cancer are spontaneous bleeding, vaginal discharge, pain, and urinary or rectal symptoms (or both).

Management. Laser therapy is becoming a common treatment option in early vaginal and vulvar cancer. Radiation is another type of treatment and is delivered by external beam to the pelvis, by vaginal intracavitary radiation using a tandem and colpostats, or by interstitial vaginal implants using an obturator and vaginal template. For a tumor located in the lower third of the vagina, radical node dissection is followed by radiation.

Encouraging close cooperation with the health care personnel is the prime focus of nursing interventions with young women who were exposed to DES *in utero* and who are at an age when sexuality and all its ramifications, including pregnancy, are significant. Emotional support for mothers and daughters is essential. For young women who have had vaginal reconstructive surgery, specific vaginal dilating procedures may be initiated and taught. Water-soluble lubricants are helpful in reducing painful intercourse (dyspareunia). If a lesion requiring treatment develops, all aspects and effects of radiation therapy, chemotherapy, or surgery need to be explored on an individual basis.

Cancer of the Fallopian Tubes

Malignancies of the fallopian tube are rare and the least common type of genital cancer. Symptoms include a profuse, watery discharge and a colicky lower abdominal pain or abnormal vaginal bleeding. An enlarged fallopian tube may be found on examination. Surgery followed by radiation therapy is the usual treatment.

Cancer of the Ovary

Ovarian cancer is a frustrating disease to patients and health care providers because its silent onset and lack of warning symptoms usually result in advanced disease by the time of diagnosis. It is the leading cause of death among gynecologic malignancies. This disease has an annual incidence of about 13.8 women per 100,000. Unfortunately, about 75% of cases are detected at a late stage. It is difficult to diagnose and is unique in that it may give rise to many primary cancers and may be the site of metastases from other cancers. It carries an annual mortality rate of 14,500 deaths and is the sixth most prevalent cause of cancer deaths in women (Wingo et al., 1995). Most cases affect women between ages 50 and 59. Its incidence is highest in industrialized countries, except for Japan, where its incidence is low.

A woman with ovarian cancer has a threefold to fourfold increased risk of breast cancer and women with breast cancer have an increased risk of ovarian cancer. No definitive causative factors have been determined, but oral contraceptives seem to provide a protective effect. Heredity may play a part, and many physicians advocate biannual pelvic examinations for women having one or two relatives with ovarian cancer. Despite careful examination, ovarian tumors are usually deep in the pelvis and difficult to detect. No early screening mechanism exists at present, although tumor markers are being explored. Transvaginal sonograms and Ca-125 antigen testing are helpful in those at high risk for developing this condition. Currently, tumor-associated antigens are helpful in follow-up care after diagnosis and treatment, but not in early general screening.

Risk factors include a high-fat diet; smoking; alcohol; using talcum powder perineally; a history of breast, colon, or endometrial cancer; and a family history of breast or ovarian cancer. Nulliparity, infertility, and anovulation are additional risk factors. Survival rates depends on the stage of the cancer at diagnosis.

Clinical Manifestations. Signs and symptoms include irregular menses, increasing premenstrual tension, heavy menstrual flow (menorrhagia) with breast tenderness, early menopause, abdominal discomfort, dyspepsia, pelvic pressure, and urinary frequency. These symptoms are typically vague, but any woman with gastrointestinal symptoms and without a known diagnosis must be evaluated with ovarian cancer in mind. Flatulence, fullness after a light meal, and increasing abdominal girth are significant symptoms.

The combination of two major clues—a long history of ovarian dysfunction and vague, undiagnosed, persistent gastrointestinal symptoms—should alert the nurse to the possibility of early ovarian malignancy. Any palpable ovary in a woman who has gone through menopause is usually investigated because ovaries shrink after menopause.

Diagnosis. Any enlarged ovary must be investigated. Pelvic examination will not detect early ovarian cancer and pelvic imaging techniques are not always definitive. About 75% of ovarian cancers have metastasized by the time of diagnosis; about 60% have spread beyond the pelvis.

Of the many different ovarian cancer cell types, epithelial tumors constitute 90%. Germ cell tumors and stromal tumors make up the other 10%.

Management. Surgical removal is the treatment of choice, with the preoperative workup including barium enema, proctosigmoidoscopy, upper GI series, chest x-ray, and intravenous urography (IVU). Staging the tumor is an important activity used to direct treatment (Table 45-4 summarizes ovarian cancer stages). A total abdominal hysterectomy with removal of the fallopian tubes and ovaries and the omentum (bilateral salpingo-oophorectomy and omentectomy) is the standard procedure for early disease. Then, ra-

TABLE 45-4 Stages of Cancer of the Ovary

I—Growth limited to the ovaries
II—Growth involves one or both ovaries with pelvic extension
III—Growth involves one or both ovaries with metastases outside the pelvis or positive retroperitoneal or inguinal nodes
IV—Growth involves one or both ovaries with distant metastases

diation therapy and intraperitoneal implantation of phosphorus 32 (^{32}P), a radioactive isotope, may follow surgery. Chemotherapy, with single or multiple agents—but usually including cisplatin, cyclophosphamide, or carboplatin—is also used.

Paclitaxel (Taxol), a promising agent derived from the Pacific yew tree, works by causing microtubules within the cells to gather and preventing the breakdown of these threadlike structures. In general, cells cannot function when they are clogged with microtubules and they cannot divide. Because this medication often causes leukopenia, the patient may need to take G-CSF (granulocyte colony-stimulating factor) as well. Taxol is contraindicated in patients with hypersensitivity to medications formulated in polyoxyethylated castor oil and in patients with baseline neutropenia. Adverse cardiac effects are also associated with Taxol, so the agent is not used in patients with cardiac disorders. Hypotension, dyspnea, angioedema, and urticaria indicate severe reactions which usually occur soon after the first and second doses are administered. The nurse must be prepared to treat anaphylaxis. The patient should be prepared for inevitable hair loss.

Two agents also undergoing clinical trials are G-CSF, which allows ultra-high-dose chemotherapy, and camptothecins, which inhibit DNA replication. Other medications include hexamethylmelamine (being studied for use alone and in combination with other agents), sulofenur, progestins, tamoxifen, and GnRh analogues. Genetic engineering and identification of cancer genes may make gene therapy a future possibility.

After adjunct therapies are completed, a second-look laparotomy may be performed in some clinical centers to evaluate the treatment results and to obtain multiple tissue samples for biopsy. Occasionally, catheters are left in place if radioactive agents are to be used postoperatively. Chemotherapy is the most common form of treatment in advanced disease. Intraperitoneal infusions of cisplatin may be administered by a Port-a-cath or a Tenckoff catheter.

Nursing Management. After other data are assessed and evaluated, nursing measures include those related to the patient's various treatment plan, be it surgery, radiation, chemotherapy, or palliation. Emotional support, comfort measures, and information, plus attentiveness and caring are meaningful aids to this patient and her family.

Patients who have pelvic surgery to remove the tumor are observed and treated as other patients having abdominal surgery. If ovarian cancer occurs in a young woman and the tumor is unilateral, it is removed. Childbearing, if desired, is encouraged in the near future. After childbirth, surgical re-exploration may be performed and the remaining ovary may be removed. If both ovaries are involved, surgery is performed and chemotherapy follows.

If the patient's treatment includes intraperitoneal instillation of ^{32}P and other chemotherapeutic agents, the nurse will need to turn the patient frequently to ensure distribution throughout the peritoneal cavity. The catheter insertion site, if present, must be observed for infection, as must the site of the implanted port used for administering these agents.

Cisplatin is used frequently in chemotherapeutic treatment of ovarian cancer, both alone and in combination with other agents, and in intraperitoneal applications. Patients may require bone marrow transplantation to treat ovarian cancer. Care for these patients is described in Chapter 16.

Patients with advanced ovarian cancer may develop ascites and pleural effusion. Nursing care may include administering IV therapy to alleviate fluid and electrolyte imbalances, initiating total parenteral nutrition (TPN) to provide adequate nutrition, providing postoperative care after intestinal bypass to alleviate an obstruction, and managing tubes. These conditions are complex and often require assistance and support from an oncology nurse specialist.

Radiation Therapy

Radiation is usually the treatment of choice for squamous cell carcinoma of the cervix, depending on the stage of the cancer. However, in uterine and ovarian cancers, radiation is usually an adjunct to surgery. When radiation is the definitive treatment of cervical cancer, a combination of external pelvic radiation and internal (intracavitary) irradiation may be used. Only in the earliest microinvasive carcinomas of the cervix is intracavitary irradiation used alone. Cure rates exceeding 85% can be expected with cervical cancer limited to the cervix alone. As the disease extends into the parametrium, the cure rate drops to about 65%. Once the disease extends to the pelvic sidewalls, however, perhaps only one third of the patients will be cured, although many more will benefit from the palliative effects of radiation (*i.e.*, reduction in tumor bulk and control of infection, pain, and bleeding).

The cervix and uterus lend themselves naturally to internal irradiation because they can serve as a receptacle for radioactive sources. Isotopes of radium and cesium are used for intracavitary irradiation. Intraoperative radiation is a technique that allows radiation to be applied directly to the affected area during surgery.

Intraoperative radiation therapy (IORT) uses an electron beam directed at the disease site. This direct-view irradiation may be used when para-aortic nodes are involved or for unresectable (inoperable) or partially resectable neoplasms. Benefits include accurate beam direction (which precisely limits the radiation to the tumor) and the ability during treatment to block sensitive organs from radiation. IORT is usually combined with external beam radiation preoperatively or postoperatively.

Radiation Side Effects. Radiation side effects are cumulative and tend to appear when the total dose exceeds the body's natural capacity to repair the damage caused by radiation. Radiation enteritis, resulting in diarrhea and abdominal cramping, and radiation cystitis, manifested by urinary frequency, urgency, and dysuria, may occur. These effects are manifestations of the normal tissues' response to radiation therapy. Occasionally, severe reactions will require interrupting treatment until normal tissue repair occurs.

The radiation oncologist and nurse must carefully inform the patient in advance of possible side effects and implement management strategies when they occur. Such measures include dietary control (restricting the amount of fiber, roughage, and lactose) and the use of antispasmodic agents. The goal of a low-residue diet is to prevent frequent bowel movements and to avoid blockage resultir from possible constriction of the gastrointestinal tract. The following guidelines may be helpful:

- Limit dairy products to two servings daily.
- Avoid raw fruits, beans, peas, and popcorn.
- Eat white or refined breads and cereals only.
- Eat ground or well-cooked, tender meats, eggs, and cheese.
- Consume juices without pulp, canned fruit, and cooked vegetables.

Evaluating the patient's (and family's) physical, emotional, and learning needs are part of the nursing assessment before and during treatment. Information overload, along with anxiety that impairs learning, must be anticipated.

Any method of therapy requires adequate preparation, education, and emotional support. The patient who has been adequately prepared, supported, and educated before treatment through expert nursing care will find it easier to cope with the rigors and stress of cancer.

Internal (Intracavitary) Irradiation. In the operating room, the patient receives an anesthetic and is examined, after which specially prepared applicators are inserted into the endometrial cavity and vagina. These devices are not loaded with radioactive material until the patient returns to her room. X-ray films are obtained to verify the precise relationship of the applicator to the normal pelvic anatomy and to the tumor. Only when this study is completed does the radiation oncologist load the applicators with predetermined amounts of radioactive material. This procedure, called **afterloading**, allows for precise control of the radiation exposure received by the patient, with minimal exposure of the physician, nurse, and other health care personnel. A patient undergoing internal radiation treatment remains isolated in a private room until the application is completed. Adjacent rooms may need to be evacuated and a lead shield placed at the doorway to the patient's room.

Of the various applicators developed for intracavitary treatment, some are inserted into the endometrial cavity and endocervical canal as multiple small irradiators (*e.g.*, Heyman's capsules). Others consist of a central tube (a tandem or intrauterine "stem") placed through the dilated endocervical canal into the uterine cavity, which remains in fixed relationship with the irradiators placed in the upper vagina on each side of the cervix (vaginal ovoids) (Fig. 45-7).

When the applicator is inserted, an indwelling urinary catheter is also inserted. Vaginal packing is inserted to keep the applicator in place and to keep other organs such as the bladder and rectum as far from the radioactive source as possible. The objective of the internal treatment is to maintain the distribution of internal radiation at a fixed dosage throughout the application. Such applications usually last 24 to 72 hours, depending on dose calculations made by the radiation physicist.

Intracavitary Brachytherapy. Automated high-dose-rate intracavitary brachytherapy systems have been developed that allow outpatient radiation therapy. Treatment time is shorter, thereby decreasing patient discomfort. Staff exposure to radiation is also avoided.

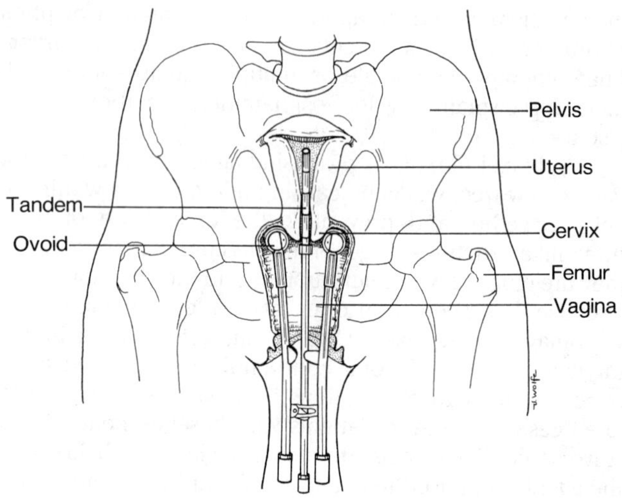

FIGURE 45-7. Placement of tandem and ovoids for internal radiation therapy. (Copyright J. Wolfe.)

Nursing Management During Intracavitary Radiation Therapy

The radioactive elements used in intracavitary therapy are radium, cesium, iridium, and cobalt, the latter two being used most frequently. Cesium has a long half-life and no gaseous by-products. During the treatment, diligent nursing care must be given. The patient is carefully observed and care is provided; however, the nursing staff must minimize radiation exposure to themselves as much as possible by applying the principles of time, distance, and shielding as follows:

- Minimize amount of time near a radioactive source.
- Maximize distance from radioactive source.
- Use required shielding to minimize exposure

Nurses who are or may be pregnant should not be involved in the immediate care of such patients. Visits to the patient should have a specific purpose; nurse–patient contacts provide a good opportunity for the patient to talk about her anxiety and fear. To minimize radiation exposure, the nurse remains as far away from the radiation source as possible (*i.e.*, at the entrance to the room) but makes special efforts to provide some time for discussing the patient's anxieties and fears.

The nurse needs to explain that during the treatment, the patient must stay on absolute bed rest. She may move from side to side with her back supported by a pillow, and the head of the bed may be raised to 15 degrees. She should be encouraged to practice deep-breathing and coughing exercises and to flex and extend the feet to stretch the calf muscles, promoting circulation and venous return. Elastic stockings are important. Back care, though appreciated by the patient, needs to be performed within the minimal time allowed at the bedside.

Usually, the patient receives a low-residue diet to prevent frequent bowel movements. Of the many nursing concerns, primary concerns involve not dislodging the applicator and providing the patients with emotional support and physical comfort. A urinary catheter will be in place and must be inspected frequently to ensure that it drains properly. The chief hazard of improper drainage is that the bladder may become distended and its walls exposed to radiation. Although perineal care is not performed at this time, any profuse discharge should be reported immediately to the radiation oncologist or gynecologic surgeon.

Additional nursing interventions include observing the patient for temperature elevation, nausea, and vomiting. These symptoms should be reported, because they may indicate such complications as infection or perforation. Finally, the radiation oncologist takes steps to secure the internal applicator in place. Nursing personnel need not be preoccupied with the fear that the applicator will be prematurely extruded, but should monitor from time to time to see that the applicator or the radioactive sources have not been dislodged. Should this happen, the staff should avoid touching the radioactive object and notify the Radiation Safety Department at once.

Patient teaching includes informing the patient that abdominal fullness, cramping, backache, and the urge to void are normal feelings during therapy. Severe pain should not be experienced. Administering mild opioids may be helpful.

The Radiation Safety Department will give specific safety precautions to those who will be in contact with the patient, including health care providers and family. Nurses caring for the patient will receive directions about safe times and distances related to care provisions to ensure that their occupational exposure is *As Low As Reasonably Achievable* (ALARA). Other instructions vary but may include the following:

- Film badges or pocket ion chambers are worn to monitor exposure.
- Rubber gloves are needed to dispose of any soiled matter that may be contaminated. (These gloves, however, do not provide protection from sealed radiation sources.)
- Specific laundry and housekeeping directions will be provided.
- The patient will be restricted to her room and allowed no visitors who are or may be pregnant or who are younger than age 18.
- A discharge survey is usually performed by Radiation Safety personnel before the patient leaves the room to ensure that all sources of radiation have been removed.

Applicator Removal. The radiation oncologist calculates precisely the radiation dose. At the end of the prescribed period, the nurse may be requested to assist the physician in removing the applicator. Because the sources are "afterloaded," they can be removed by the physician in the same manner as they were inserted. This does not require local or general anesthesia and is performed in the patient's room. Medicating the patient with a mild sedative may be required, however, before removing the applicator.

Post-Treatment Care. Progressive ambulation is recommended after any period of enforced bed rest. Diet may be offered as tolerated. The patient may shower as soon as she wishes but should be instructed not to douche after removal of the applicator. Because the cervix may have been dilated, any chance of bacterial contamination should be minimized.

CRITICAL THINKING EXERCISES

1. Your patient has received a diagnosis of genital herpesvirus infection and becomes very upset, stating that her boyfriend lied to her when he told her that she was his first sexual partner. What approach would you take to assist her in learning about herpes infection and in dealing with it?
2. Your patient has been admitted to the hospital with possible toxic shock syndrome. Describe the type of emergency management strategies you would anticipate and the nursing measures you would plan for the patient's hospital stay and long-term recovery. Include the rationale for your decisions.
3. How would you explain Kegel exercises to a woman? How would your explanation differ if the woman understands little English?
4. Your 57-year-old patient is scheduled for surgery to treat cancer of the vulva. In discussing with her the strategies to prevent postoperative complications, you realize that her husband believes that they will never be able to have sexual relations again. How would you handle this situation? Describe the approach you would take in discussing this with the patient's husband.
5. Your patient has had an intracavitary device inserted to deliver radiation directly to the uterus. During a restless night, the device has become dislodged. Indicate the immediate actions you would take and explain the rationale for them. What further actions would you take?

Nurses caring for patients undergoing radiation therapy need to assess any possible misconceptions about this mode of treatment that the patient and family may have both before and after treatment. The oncology clinical nurse specialist may be an invaluable resource for information and problem-solving assistance, if necessary. Resources for further clinical and patient information are listed at the end of Chapter 16 on oncology.

BIBLIOGRAPHY

Books

American Cancer Society. Cancer Facts and Figures, 1994. Atlanta, American Cancer Society, 1994.

Ashwanden P et al. Oncology Nursing: Advances, Treatments and Trends into the 21st Century. Rockville, MD, Aspen Systems, 1990.

Baird S, McCorkle R, and Grant R. Cancer Nursing: A Comprehensive Textbook. Philadelphia, WB Saunders, 1991.

Bobak IM and Jensen MD. Maternity and Gynecologic Care: The Nurse and the Family. St. Louis, Mosby Year Book, 1993.
DiSaia P and Creasman W. Clinical Gynecological Oncology. St. Louis, CV Mosby, 1993.
Dow K and Hilderley L. Nursing Care in Radiation Oncology. Philadelphia, WB Saunders, 1991.
Dunnihoo D. Fundamentals of Gynecology and Obstetrics. Philadelphia, JB Lippincott, 1990.
Emans J and Goldstein D. Pediatric and Adolescent Gynecology, 3rd ed. Boston, Little, Brown, 1990.
Fogel C and Lauver D. Sexual Health Promotion. Philadelphia, WB Saunders, 1990.
Greenwald P, Kramer BS and Weed DL. Cancer prevention and control. New York, Marcel Dekker, 1995.
Holleb A, Fink D, and Murphy G. American Cancer Society Textbook of Clinical Oncology. Atlanta, Ga, American Cancer Society, 1991.
Lichtman R and Papera S. Gynecology Well-Woman Care. Norwalk, CT, Appleton and Lange, 1990.
Miaskowsi C (ed). Oncology Nursing. Albany, Delmar Publishers, 1995.
Nichols DH and Sweeney PJ. Ambulatory Gynecology. Philadelphia, JB Lippincott, 1995.
O'Hara MW. Psychological Aspects of Women's Reproductive Health. New York, Springer, 1995.
Quilligan E and Zuspan F (eds). Current Therapy in Obstetrics and Gynecology 3. Philadelphia, WB Saunders, 1990.
Sweet R and Gibbs R. Infectious Diseases of the Female Genital Tract. Baltimore, Williams and Wilkins, 1990.
Wittes R (ed). Manual of Oncologic Therapeutics 1991–1992. Philadelphia, JB Lippincott, 1991.

Journals

Asterisks indicate nursing research articles.

General

Barber H, Creasman W, and Knapp R. A rational approach to ovarian masses. Patient Care 1993 Jan; 27(1):50–72.
Bayer SR and DeCherney AH. Clinical manifestations and treatment of dysfunctional uterine bleeding. JAMA 1993 Apr 4; 269(14):1823–1828.
Butler RN et al. Love and sex after 60: How to evaluate and treat the sexually active woman. Geriatrics 1994 Nov; 49(11):33–34, 37–38, 41–42.
Centers for Disease Control: 1989 sexually transmitted diseases treatment guidelines. MMWR 1989; 38(S-8):1–43.
Garner C. Uses of GnRH anonists. J Obstet Gynecol Neonatal Nurs 1994 Sep; 23(7):563–570.
Garry R. Various approaches to laparoscopic hysterectomy. Curr Opin Obstet Gynecol 1994 Jun; 6(3):215–222.
*Griffin C. Pelvic muscles during rest: Responses to pelvic muscle exercise. Nurs Res 1994 May/Jun; 43(3):164–167.
Lawhead R. Vulvar self-examination: What your patient should know. Female Patient 1990 Jan; 15(1):33–38.
Lichtman R. Perimenopausal hormone replacement therapy: Review of the literature. J Nurse Midwifery 1991 Jan/Feb; 36(1): 30–48.
Summitt RL Jr. et al. Outpatient hysterectomy: Determinants of discharge and rehospitalization in 133 patients. Am J Obstet Gynecol 1994 Dec; 171(6):1480–1484.
Wathen PI, Henderson MC and Witz CA. Abnormal uterine bleeding. Med Clin North Am 1995 Mar; 79(2):329–344.

Gerontologic Considerations

Blesch K and Prohaska T. Cervical cancer screening in older women: Issues and interventions. Cancer Nurs 1991 June; 14(3):141–147.
Dickson G. A feminist poststructuralist analysis of the knowledge of menopause. ANS Adv Nurs Sci 1990 Mar; 12(3):15–31.
Wood N. The use of vaginal pessaries for uterine prolapse. Nurse Pract 1992 July; 17(7):31–38.

Vulvovaginal Infections

Burnhill M. Clinician's guide to counseling patients with chronic vaginitis. Contemp Ob Gyn 1990 Jan; 35(1):37–44.
Goode MA, Grauer K, and Gums JG. Infectious vaginitis. Selecting therapy and preventing recurrence. Postgrad Med 1994 Nov 1; 96(6):85–88, 91–98.
Havens C et al. Diagnosing gynecologic infections. Patient Care 1990 Apr 30; 24(8):74–89.
Neri A, Rabinerson D and Kaplan B. Bacterial vaginosis: Drug versus alternative treatment. Obstet Gynecol Surv 1994 Dec; 49(12):809–813.
Overman B. The vagina as an ecologic system. J Nurse Midwifery 1993 May/June; 38(3):146–151.
Reed BD and Eyler A. Vaginal infections: Diagnosis and management. Am Fam Physician 1993 Jun; 47(8):1805–1818.
Thomason J and Scaglione N. Basics of managing bacterial vaginosis. Contemp ObGyn-NP 1993 Sep; 1(3):15–17.
Sobel JD et al. Single oral dose fluconazole compared with conventional clotrimazole topical therapy of *Candida vaginitis*. Fluconazole Vaginitis Study Group. Am J Obstet Gynecol 1995 Apr; 172(4 Pt 1):1263–1268.
Sobel JD. Controversial aspects in the management of vulvovaginal candidiasis. J Am Acad Dermatol 1994 Sep; 31(3 Pt 2): S10–S13.
Sobel JD. Candial vulvovaginitis. Clin Obstet Gynecol 1993 Mar; 36(1):153–165.

Sexually Transmitted Diseases

Bowie WR. Antibiotics and sexually transmitted diseases. Infect Dis Clin North Am 1994 Dec; 8(4):841–857.
Centers for Disease Control and Prevention. 1993 sexually transmitted diseases treatment guidelines. MMWR: Morb Mortal Wkly Rep 1993 Sep 24; 42(RR-14):1–102.
Centers for Disease Control and Prevention. Recommendations for the prevention and management of *Chlamydia trachomatis* infections, 1993. MMWR: Morb Mortal Wkly Rep 1993 Aug 6; 42(RR-12):1–39.
Centers for Disease Control and Prevention. Update: AIDS among women—United States, 1994. MMWR: Morb Mortal Wkly Rep 1995 Feb 10, 44(5):81–84.
Cohen MS, Hook EW III and Hitchcock PJ. Sexually transmitted diseases in the AIDS era: Part II. Infect Dis Clin North Am 1994 Dec; 8(4):751–925.
Corcoran GD and Ridgway GL. Antibiotic chemotherapy of bacterial sexually transmitted diseases in adults: A review. Int J STD AIDS 1994 May–Jun; 5(3):165–171.
Sipes C. Guidelines for assessing HIV in women. MCN: Am J Maternal Child Nurs 1995 Jan–Feb; 20(1):29–33.
Westrom LV. Sexually transmitted diseases and infertility. Sex Transm Dis 1994 Mar–Apr; 21(2 Suppl):S32–S37.

Toxic Shock Syndrome

Colbry S. A review of toxic shock syndrome: The need for education still exists. Nurse Pract 1992 Sep; 17(9):39–46.
Hanrahan SN. Historical review of menstrual shock syndrome. Women Health 1994; 21 (2–3):141–165.
Stegbauer C. The human immunodeficiency virus and nonmenstrual toxic shock syndrome: A female case presentation. Nurse Pract 1994 Jan; 19(1):68–71.
Strausbaugh LJ. Toxic shock syndrome. Are you recognizing its changing presentations? Postgrad Med 1993 Nov 1; 94(6):107–108, 111–113, 117–118.

Woods SL and Jackson B. The human immunodeficiency virus and nonmenstrual toxic shock syndrome: A female case presentation. Nurse Pract 1994 Jan; 19(1):68–71.

Herpes Simplex Type 2

Brock B et al. Frequency of asymptomatic shedding of herpes simplex virus in women with genital herpes. JAMA 1990 Jan 19; 263(3):418–420.

Catotti DN, Clarke P, Catoe KE. Herpes revisited: Still a cause of concern. Sex Transm Dis 1993 Mar–Apr; 20(2):77–80.

Davies K. Genital herpes: An overview. J Obstet Gynecol Neonatal Nurs 1990 Sep/Oct; 19(5):401–406.

Pelvic Disorders

Apuzzio J and Joegsberg B. PID: Hard to find, but essential to treat. Contemp ObGyn-NP 1993 June; 1(2):6–11.

DeCherney A, Dawoofd M, and Chestnut C. Endometriosis therapy: What impact on bone mass? Contemp Ob Gyn 1993 Oct; 38(10):62–74.

Padian NS and Washington AE. Pelvic inflammatory disease. A brief overview. Ann Epidemiol 1994 Mar; 4(2):128–132.

Quan M. Pelvic inflammatory disease: Diagnosis and management. J Am Board Fam Pract 1994 Mar–Apr; 7(2):110–123.

Soper DE. Pelvic inflammatory disease. Infect Dis Clin North Am 1994 Dec; 8(4):821–840.

Treybig M. Primary dysmenorrhea or endometriosis. Nurse Pract 1989 May; 14(5):8–18.

Structural Disorders

Holley RL. Enterocele: A review. Obstet Gynecol Surv 1994 Apr; 49(4):284–293.

Nichols DH and Genadry RR. Pelvic relaxation of the posterior compartment. Curr Opin Obstet Gynecol 1993 Aug; 5(4):458–464.

Benign Tumors and Pelvic Conditions

Adamson GD. Treatment of uterine fibroids: Current findings with gonadotropin-releasing hormone agonists. Am J Obstet Gynecol 1992 Feb; 166(2):746–751.

Christiansen JK. The facts about fibroids. Presentation and latest management options. Postgrad Med 1993 Sep 1; 94(3):129–134, 137.

Damewood MD. Pathophysiology and management of endometriosis. J Fam Pract 1993 Jul; 37(1):68–75.

Dawood MY. Considerations in selecting appropriate medical therapy for endometriosis. Int J Gyneacol Obstet 1993 40 Suppl: S29–S42.

Demario MA and Rock JA. New considerations for the classification of endometriosis. Int J Gynaecol Obstet 1993 40 Suppl:S9–S20.

Olive DL and Schwartz LB. Endometriosis. N Engl J Med 1993 Jun 17; 328(24):1759–1769.

Condyloma Acuminata: Human Papillomavirus

Carlone J (ed). Human papillomavirus: A growing epidemic. Nurs Pract Forum 1990 June; 1(1):10–62.

Deitch K. Symptoms of chronic vaginal infection and microscopic condyloma in women. J Obstet Gynecol Neonatal Nurs 1990 Mar/Apr; 19(2):133–138.

Lehr S and Lee M. The psychosocial and sexual trauma of a genital HPV infection. Nurs Pract Forum 1990 June; 1(1):25–30.

Moscicki A. HPV infection in teenage girls. Med Aspects Hum Sexuality 1990 July; 24(7):2227.

Nettina S and Kauffman F. Diagnosis and management of sexually transmitted genital lesions. Nurs Pract 1990 Jan; 15(1):20–39.

Schiffman M. Latest HPV findings: Some clinical implications. Contemp Ob Gyn 1993 Oct; 38(10):27–41.

Toole K et al. Cervical dysplasia and condyloma as risks for carcinoma: Two case studies. MCN Am J Matern Child Nurs 1990 May/June; 15(3):170–175.

Hysterectomy

Bachman G. Psychosexual aspects of hysterectomy. Wom Health Iss 1990 Fall; 1(1):41–49.

Bernhard L. Men's views about hysterectomies and women who have them. Image: J Nurs Scholarship 1992 Fall; 24(3):177–181.

Bernstein S et al. The appropriateness of hysterectomy. JAMA 1993 May 12; 269(18):2398–2400.

Dulaney P et al. A comprehensive education and support program for women experiencing hysterectomies. J Obstet Gynecol Neonatal Nurs 1990 July/Aug; 19(4):319–325.

Hysterectomy and its alternatives. Consumer Report 1990 Sep; 55(9):603–607.

Patient guide. Female Patient 1990 Jan; 15(1):62–63.

Rose B. Informed consent and hysterectomy: Enhancing the right to know. Am J Public Health 1991; 82(4):609–610.

Symposium: Laparoscopic-assisted vaginal hysterectomy. Contemp Ob Gyn 1993 (Technology Issue):71–100.

Thomas J et al. Home visiting for a posthysterectomy population. Home Healthcare Nurs 1992 June; 10(3):47–51.

Williamson M. Sexual adjustment after hysterectomy. J Obstet Gynecol Neonatal Nurs 1992 Jan/Feb; 21(1):42–47.

AIDS in Women

*Jacob J. Self-assessed learning needs of oncology nurses caring for individuals with HIV related disorders: A national survey. Cancer Nurs 1990 Aug; 13(4):246–255.

Moroso G and Holman S. Counseling and testing women for HIV. NAACOG's Clinical Issues in Perinatal and Women's Health Nursing 1990; 1(1):10–19.

Sinclair B. Epidemiology and transmission of infection by human immunodeficiency virus. NAACOG's Clinical Issues in Perinatal and Women's Health Nursing 1990; 1(1):1–9.

Smeltzer SC and Whipple B. Women and HIV infection: Review of research and literature. Image: J Nurs Scholarship 1991 Winter; 23(4):249–256.

Fistulas

Grogan J et al. A nursing intervention for intractable incontinence. J Ent Nurs 1993 Sep/Oct; 20(5):228–229.

Guidos B et al. Perineal skin protection with an enterovaginal fistula. J ET Nurs 1993 Sep/Oct; 20(5):220–221.

Reproductive Malignancy

Barakat RR and Benjamin I. Surgery for malignant gynecologic disease. Curr Opin Obstet Gynecol 1993 Jun; 5(3):311–317.

Berek J. Monoclonal antibodies role in combating gyn malignancies. Contemp Ob Gyn 1990 Feb; 35(2):109–120.

Blesch K and Prohaska T. Cervical cancer screening in older women. Cancer Nurs 1991; 14(3):141–147.

Campion M and Reid R. Screening for gynecological cancer. Obstet Gynecol Clin North Am 1990 Dec; 17(4):695–727.

Chamorro T. Cancer of the vulva and vagina. Semin Oncol Nurs 1990 Aug; 6(3):198–205.

*Christman N. Uncertainty and adjustment during radiotherapy. Nurs Res 1990 Jan/Feb; 39(1):17–20.

Classification and staging of gynecologic malignancies. ACOG Technical Bulletin 1991 May; 155.

Graham C. Cervix cancer prevention and detection update. Semin Oncol Nurs 1993 Aug; 9(3):155–162.

Gribbin M. Could you detect these oncological crises? RN 1990 June; 53(6):36–42.

Grimes DA and Economy KE. Primary prevention of gynecologic cancers. Am J Obstet Gynecol 1995 Jan; 172 (1 Pt 1):227–235.

Keys H. Gynecologic Oncology Group randomized trials of combined technique therapy for vulvar cancer. Cancer 1993 Feb 15; 71(4 Suppl):1691–1696.

Levenback C. Gynecologic oncology: A review for ET nurses. J Wound Ostomy Continence Nurs 1994 Jul; 21(4)141–148.

McMullin M. Holistic care of the patient with cervical cancer. Nurs Clin North Am 1992 Dec; 27(4):847–857.
*Mishel M and Sorenson D. Uncertainty in gynecological cancer. A test of mediating functions of mastery and coping. Nurs Res 1991 May/June; 40(3):167–171.
Nail L. Coping with intracavitary radiation treatment for gynecologic cancer. Cancer Pract 1993 Sep/Oct; 1(3):218–224.
Nezhat C et al. The role of laparoscopy in the management of gynecologic malignancy. Semin Surg Oncol 1994 Nov–Dec; 10(6): 431–439.
Northouse L and Peters-Golden H. Cancer and the family: Strategies to assist spouses. Semin Oncol Nurs 1993 May; 9(2):74–83.
*Picard H. Fatigue in cancer patients: A descriptive study. Cancer Nurs 1991 Feb; 14(1):13–19.
Rostad ME. The radical vulvectomy patient: Preventing complications. Dimens Crit Care Nurs 1988 Sep/Oct; 7(5):289–294.
Rubin M and Lauver D. Assessment and management of cervical intraepithelial neoplasia. Nurse Pract 1990 Oct; 15(10): 23–31.
Wender R. Cancer screening in primary care. Female Patient 1993 June; 18(6):33–39.
Wilson S and Morse J. Living with a wife undergoing chemotherapy. Image: J Nurs Scholarship 1991 Summer; 23(2):78–84.
Wingo PA et al. Cancer statistics. CA Cancer J Clin 1995 Jan 45(1):8–30.
Woodward J. The triple C approach to the detection of cervical cancer. Nurs Pract Forum 1990 June; 1(1):31–39.
Wright V (ed). Contemporary colposcopy. Obstet Gynecol Clin North Am 1993 Mar; 20(1):1–260.
Writing group of the PEPI Trial. Effects of estrogen or estrogen/progestin regimens on heart disease risk factors in postmenopausal women. JAMA Jan 18; 273(3):199–207.
Yarbro C (ed). Effects of cancer on women. Semin Oncol Nurs 1995 May; 11(2):78–147.

Ovarian Cancer

Bookman M and Ozols R. Future directions for Paclitaxel in the treatment of ovarian cancer. Semin Oncol Nurs 1993 Nov; 9(4) Supplement 2:21–29.
Brucks J. Ovarian cancer: The most lethal gynecological malignancy. Nurs Clin North Am 1992 Dec; 27(4):835–845.
Carlson KJ, Skates SJ and Singer DE. Screening for ovarian cancer. Ann Intern Med 1994 Jul 15; 121(2):124–132.
Farias-Eisner R, Kim YB, Berek JS. Surgical management of ovarian cancer. Semin Surg Oncol 1994 Jul–Aug; 10(4):268–275.
Hankinson S et al. Tubal ligation, hysterectomy, and risk of ovarian cancer. JAMA 1993 Dec 15; 270(23):2813–2818.
Lilley L and Scott H. What you need to know about taxol. Am J Nurs 1993 Dec; 93(12):46–50.
Mackey SE and Creasman WT. Ovarian cancer screening. J Clin Oncol 1995 Mar; 13(3):783–793.
Moore D. New therapies for ovarian cancer. Female Patient 1993 Sep; 18(9):29–32.
Ovarian Cancer: Screening, Treatment, and Follow-up. NIH Consensus Statement 1994 Apr 5–7; 12(3):1–30.
Qazi F and McGuire WP. The treatment of epithelial ovarian cancer. CA Cancer J Clin. 1995 Mar–Apr; 45(2):88–101.
Schapira M et al. The effectiveness of ovarian cancer screening. Ann Intern Med 1993 June; 118:838–843.
Teneriello MG and Park RC. Early detection of ovarian cancer. CA Cancer J Clin 1995 Mar–Apr; 45(2):71–87.

Cervical Cancer

Appleby J. Management of the abnormal Papanicolaou smear. Med Clin North Am 1995 Mar; 79(2):345–360.
Kerr J. Cervical cancer: Improving the service. Nurs Stand 1995 25–31; 9(18):26–29.
Lovjoy NC and Anastasi JK. Squamous cell cervical lesions in women with and without AIDS. Biochemical risk factors, prevention, and policy. Cancer Nurs 1994 Aug; 17(4)294–307.
Shepherd JC and Fried RA. Perventing cervical cancer: The role of the Bethesda system. Am Fam Physician 1995 Feb 1; 51(2): 434–440, 443–444.

Vulvar Cancer

Perez CA et al. Radiation therapy in management of carcinoma of the vulva with emphasis on conservative therapy. Cancer 1993 Jun 1; 71(11):3707–3716.

Uterine Cancer

Dunton C. Treatment of early invasive (1A) and advanced stage (IIB–IVA) cervical carcinoma. Am J Gynecol Health 1990 Nov/Dec; 4(6):192–194.
Hubbard J et al. Cancer of the endometrium. Semin Oncol Nurs 1990 Aug; 6(3):206–213.
Mettlin C et al. Defining and updating the American Cancer Society guidelines for the cancer-related checkup: Prostate and endometrial cancers. CA Cancer J Clin 1993 Jan/Feb; 43(1): 42–46.

INFORMATION/RESOURCES

Agencies

American Cancer Society
1599 Clifton Rd NE,
Atlanta, GA 30329
(800) ACS-2345

American Social Health Association
PO Box 13827,
Research Triangle Park, NC 27709

Endometriosis Association
8585 N. 76th Place,
Milwaukee, WI 53223
(800) 992-3636

Herpetics Engaged in Living Productively (HELP)
260 Sheridan Avenue,
Palo Alto, CA 94306

Resolve Inc (Infertility)
5 Water Street,
Arlington, MA 02174
(617) 643-2424

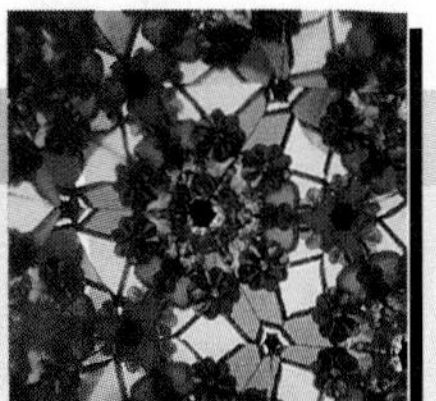

46

Assessment and Management of Patients With Breast Disorders

CHAPTER OUTLINE

Anatomic Overview
Psychosocial Implications
Incidence of Breast Disease and Changes
Assessment: Breast Examination
Female Breast
Male Breast
Self-Examination of the Breast
Diagnostic Screening Techniques
Mammography
Ultrasonography
Fine-Needle Aspiration and Surgical Biopsy
Conditions Affecting the Nipple
Breast Infections
Benign Cysts and Tumors of the Breast
Breast Discharge
Other Conditions
Breast Cancer
Etiology
Risk Factors
Clinical Manifestations
Diagnosis
Breast Cancer Staging
Types of Breast Cancer
Prognosis
Changing Approach to Breast Cancer Management
Treatment of Breast Cancer
Quality of Life and Breast Cancer
Pregnancy and Breast Cancer
NURSING PROCESS: The Patient With Breast Cancer
Nursing Management of the Patient With Advanced Breast Cancer
Reconstructive Breast Surgery
Hypertrophy of the Breast
Surgery to Enlarge or Uplift the Breasts
Reconstructive Procedures
Prophylactic Mastectomy
Diseases of the Male Breast
Gynecomastia
Male Breast Cancer
Critical Thinking Exercises

LEARNING OBJECTIVES

On completion of this chapter, the learner will be able to:

1. Develop a teaching plan for breast self-examination for the hospitalized patient and for consumer groups
2. Describe diagnostic tests used to detect breast disorders
3. Use the nursing process as a framework for care of the patient with cancer of the breast
4. Compare the therapeutic usefulness of chemotherapy, surgery, and radiation in treating breast cancer
5. Describe the physical, psychosocial, and rehabilitative needs of the patient who has had a mastectomy

Suzanne C. Smeltzer and Brenda G. Bare: Brunner and Suddarth's Textbook of Medical-Surgical Nursing, 8th Edition. © 1996 Lippincott-Raven Publishers.

Anatomic Overview

In males and females the breasts are the same until puberty, when estrogen and other hormones initiate breast development in females. This development usually occurs about the age of 10 and continues until about age 16, although the range is wide and can vary from 9 to 18 years. Stages of breast development are described as Tanner stages 1 through 5 after the physician who initiated the classification of adolescent breast changes. Stage 1 describes a prepubertal breast. Stage 2 is breast budding, the first sign of puberty in a female. Stage 3 involves further enlargement of breast tissue and the areola (a darker tissue ring around the nipple) and stage 4 occurs when the nipple and areola form a secondary mound on top of breast tissue. Stage 5 is a larger breast with a single contour.

Figure 46-1 shows the anatomy of the fully developed breast. The breast contains glandular (parenchyma) and ductal tissue, along with fibrous tissue that binds the lobes together and fatty tissue in and between the lobes. These paired mammary glands are located between the second and sixth ribs over the pectoralis major muscle from the sternum to the midaxillary line; each extends into the axilla, an area of breast tissue called the **tail of Spence.** Cooper's ligaments, which are fascial bands, support the breast on the chest wall.

Each breast consists of 12 to 20 cone-shaped lobes that are made up of lobules containing clusters of acini, small structures ending in a duct. All of the ducts in each lobule empty into an ampulla, which then opens onto the nipple after narrowing. About 85% of breast tissue is fat.

Psychosocial Implications

In Western culture, the breast plays a significant role in a woman's sexuality. A woman's reaction to any actual or suspected disease may include fear of disfigurement, fear of loss of sexual attractiveness, and fear of death. These fears may cause a woman to delay getting any possible breast problem evaluated.

All health care providers, aware of these implications, should encourage a woman to examine her own breasts and teach her to recognize early changes that may indicate problems. The nurse plays a pivotal role in preventive education. Almost all settings lend themselves to teaching, providing information, and encouraging appropriate care for prevention, detection, and treatment of breast problems.

Incidence of Breast Disease and Changes

Although many disorders of the female breast are benign, nearly 184,000 new cases of breast cancer are expected to be diagnosed in 1996. About 1% of these cancers occur in men. Benign breast disease also occurs frequently in women and arouses a great deal of concern. Because of the variations in breast tissue that occur during the menstrual cycle, pregnancy, and menopause, normal changes must be distinguished from those that may signal disease. Most women notice increased tenderness and lumpiness before their menstrual period; therefore, breast self-examination (BSE) is

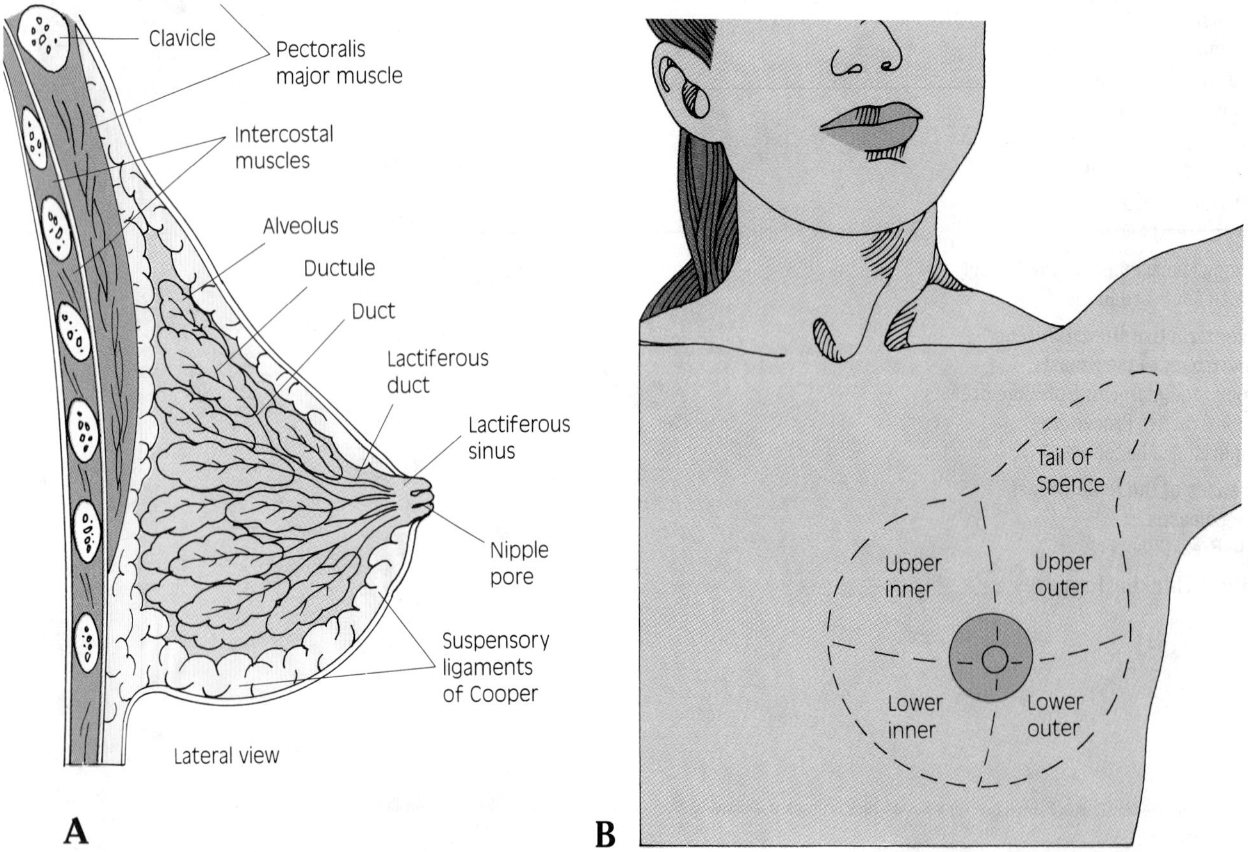

FIGURE 46-1. (A) Anatomy of the breast. (B) Areas of breast, including the tail of Spence.

encouraged after menses (day 5 to day 10, counting the first day of menses as day 1) when less fluid is retained. Many women have grainy-textured breast tissue, but these areas are usually less nodular after menses. Benign lesions include, among others, fibrocystic changes, fibroadenomas, and cysts.

Assessment: Breast Examination

Female Breast

Examination of the female breast is conducted during any general physical or gynecologic examination or whenever the patient suspects, complains of, or fears breast disease. A clinical breast examination is recommended at least every 3 years for women between ages 20 and 40, and then annually. A complete and thorough breast examination including instruction in breast self-examination takes at least 5 minutes or more.

Inspection. Examination begins with inspection. The patient disrobes to the waist and sits in a comfortable position facing the examiner. The breasts are inspected for size and symmetry. A slight difference in size is common and is generally a normal finding. The skin is inspected for color, venous pattern, and thickening or edema. Erythema (redness) may indicate benign local inflammation or superficial lymphatic invasion by a neoplasm. A prominent venous pattern can signal increased blood supply demanded by a tumor. Edema and pitting of the skin may result from a neoplasm blocking lymphatic drainage and giving the skin an orange-peel appearance (peau d'orange), a classic sign of advanced breast cancer. (Examples of abnormal breast findings can be found in Chart 46-1.)

Nipples, though different in each patient, are normally similar in size and shape. A slight inversion of one or both nipples is not uncommon and is a significant finding only when of recent origin. Ulceration, rashes, or nipple discharge requires evaluation. To elicit a dimpling or retraction that may otherwise go undetected, the examiner instructs the patient to raise both arms overhead. This maneuver normally elevates both breasts equally. Next, the patient is instructed to place her hands at her waist and push in. These movements, causing contraction of the pectoral muscles, do not normally alter the breast contour or nipple direction. Any dimpling or retraction during these position changes suggests a potential malignancy. The clavicular and axillary regions are inspected and palpated for swelling, discoloration, lesions, or enlarged lymph nodes.

Palpation. Palpation of the axillary and clavicular areas is easily performed with the patient seated. To examine the axillary lymph nodes, the examiner gently abducts the patient's arm from the thorax. The patient's left forearm is grasped gently and supported with the examiner's left hand. The right hand is then free to palpate the axilla and note any lymph nodes that may be lying against the thoracic wall. The flat parts of the fingertips are used to gently palpate the areas of the central, lateral, subscapular, and pectoral nodes (Fig. 46-2). Normally, these lymph nodes are not palpable but if they are enlarged, their size, location, mobility, consistency, and tenderness are noted.

The patient is then assisted to a supine position. Before the breast is palpated, the patient's shoulder is elevated by a small pillow to balance the breast on the chest wall (Fig. 46-3). Failure to do this allows the breast tissue to slip laterally, and a breast mass may be missed in this thickened tissue. Light, systematic palpation includes the entire surface of the breast, and the axillary tail. The examiner may choose to proceed in a clockwise direction following imaginary concentric circles from the outer limits of the breast toward the nipple. Other acceptable methods are to palpate from each number on the face of the clock toward the nipple in a clockwise fashion or along imaginary vertical lines on the breast.

During palpation, the examiner notes tissue consistency, tenderness, and/or masses. If a mass is detected, it is described by its location (*e.g.*, left breast, 2 cm from the nipple at the 2 o'clock position). Size, shape, consistency, border delineation, and mobility are included in the description. Finally, the areola around the nipple is gently compressed to detect any discharge or secretion.

The breast tissue of the adolescent is usually firm and lobular, whereas that of postmenopausal women is more likely to feel thinner and more granular. During pregnancy and lactation, the breasts are firmer and larger, with lobules that are more distinct. Hormonal changes cause the areolae to darken. Cysts are commonly found in menstruating women and are usually well defined and freely movable. Premenstrually, cysts may be larger and more tender. Malignant tumors, on the other hand, tend to be hard, of pencil-eraser consistency, poorly defined, fixed to the skin or underlying tissue, and usually nontender. Any abnormalities detected during inspection and palpation should be evaluated by a physician (see Chart 46-1).

Male Breast

Because breast cancer can occur in men, examination of the male breast and axillae is an important part of physical assessment. The nipple and areola are inspected for masses, lesions, or discharge. The areola is palpated for masses. Gynecomastia (overdeveloped mammary glands in the male) is differentiated from the soft, fatty enlargement of obesity by the firm enlargement of glandular tissue beneath and immediately surrounding the areola. The same procedure for palpating the female axillae is used when assessing the male axillae. Treatment of breast cancer in males is similar as well.

Most cancers in men are found at a later stage, possibly because men are not as conscious about breast lumps as are women.

Self-Examination of the Breast

Because many breast cancers are detected by women themselves, priority is given to teaching all women how and when to examine their breasts. It is estimated that only 25% to 30% of women perform breast self-examination proficiently and regularly each month. Younger women, who may have normal lumps in their breast, find it particularly difficult to perform BSE. Even women who perform BSE may delay seeking medical attention because of fear, economic factors, lack of education, reluctance to act if no pain is involved, psychologic factors, and modesty.

Proponents of breast self-examination argue that most le- sions are self-detected, making BSE important for detec

CHART 46-1
Abnormal Breast Findings

Retraction Signs
- Signs include skin dimpling, creasing, or changes in the contour of the breast or nipple
- Secondary to fibrosis or scar tissue formation in the breast
- Retraction signs may appear only with position changes or with breast palpation.

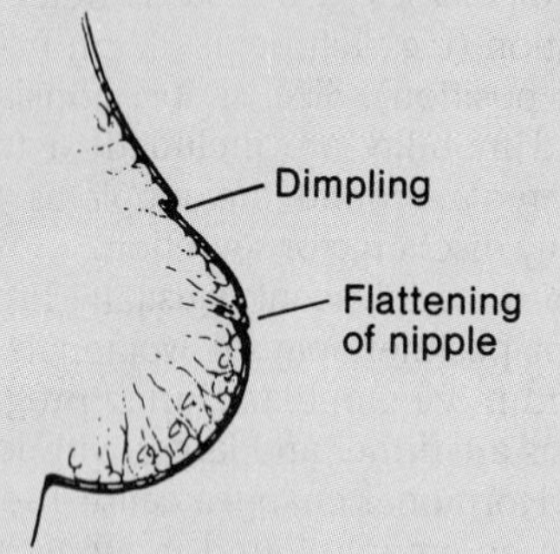

Retraction signs

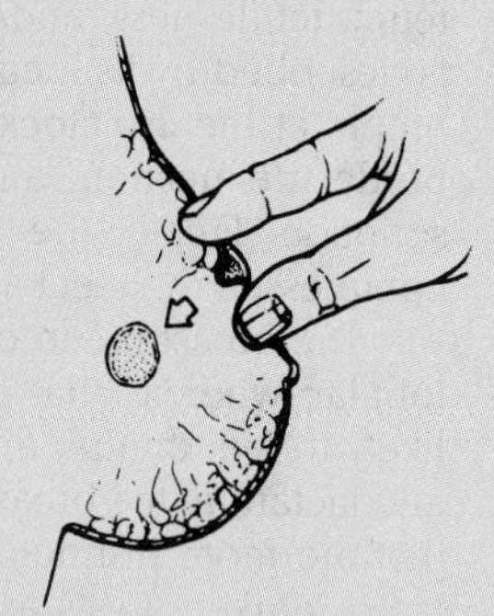
Retraction with compression

Breast Cancer Mass (Malignant Tumor)
- Usually occurs as a single mass (lump) in one breast
- Usually nontender
- Irregular shape
- Firm, hard, embedded in surrounding tissue
- Referral and biopsy indicated for definitive diagnosis

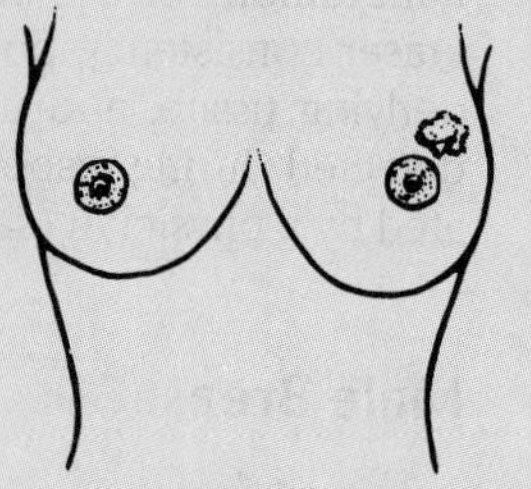
Breast cancer mass

Breast Cyst (Benign Mass of Fibrocystic Disease)
- Occur as single or multiple lumps in one or both breasts
- Usually tender (omitting caffeine reduces tenderness); tenderness increases during premenstrual period
- Round shape
- Soft or firm, mobile
- Referral and biopsy indicated for definitive diagnosis, especially for first mass; later masses may be evaluated over time by a specialist

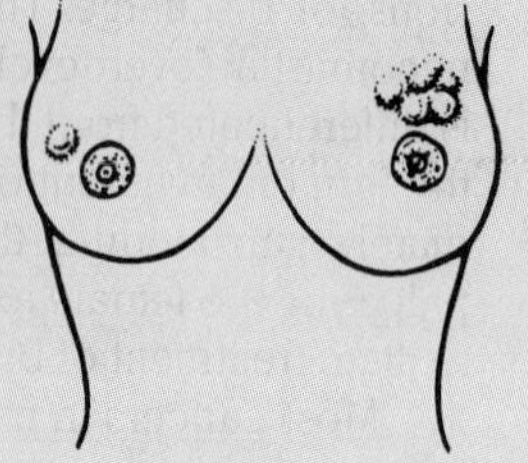
Breast cysts

Fibroadenoma (Benign Breast Lump)
- Usually occurs as a single mass in women aged 15–35 years
- Usually nontender
- May be round or lobular
- Firm, mobile, and not fixed to breast tissue or chest wall
- No premenstrual changes
- Referral and biopsy indicated for definitive diagnosis

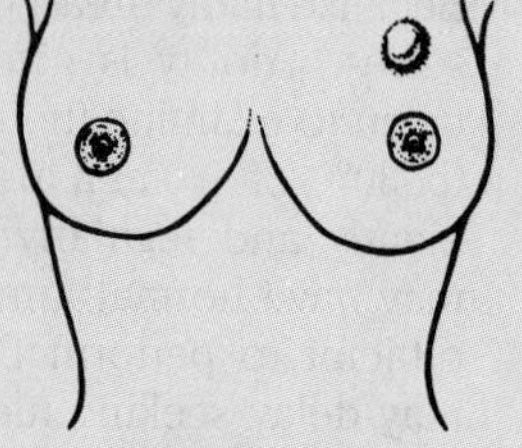
Fibroadenoma

Increased Venous Prominence
- Associated with breast cancer if unilateral
- Unilateral localized increase in venous pattern associated with malignant tumors
- Normal with breast enlargement associated with pregnancy and lactation if bilateral and bilateral symmetry

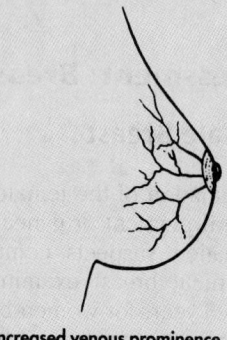

Increased venous prominence

Peau d'Orange (Edema)
- Associated with breast cancer
- Caused by interference with lymphatic drainage
- Breast skin has "orange peel" appearance
- Skin pores enlarge
- May be noted on the areola
- Skin becomes thick, hard, immobile
- Skin discoloration may occur

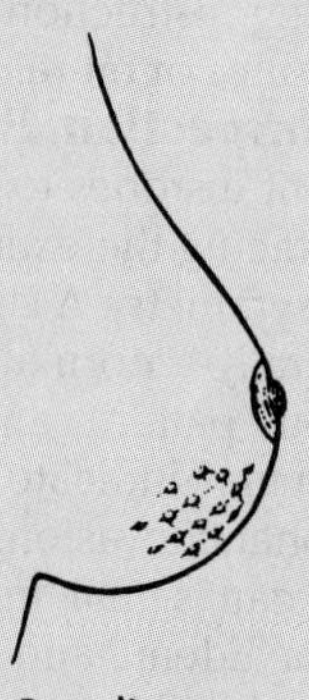
Peau d'orange

Nipple Inversion
- Considered normal if longstanding
- Associated with fibrosis and malignancy if recent development

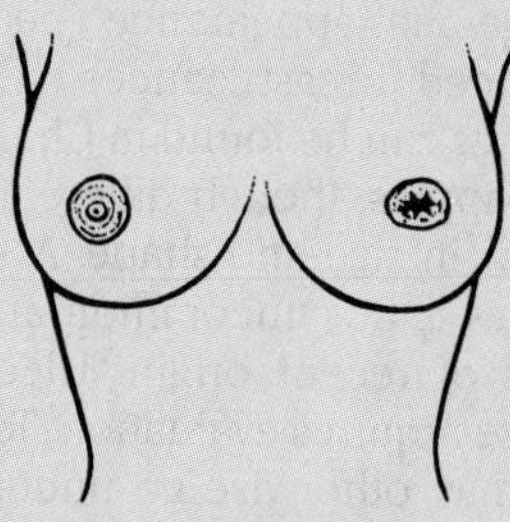
Nipple inversion

Acute Mastitis (Inflammation of the Breasts)
- Associated with lactation but may occur at any age
- Nipple cracks or abrasions noted
- Breast skin reddened and warm to touch
- Tenderness
- Systemic signs include fever and increased pulse

Paget's Disease (Malignancy of Mammary Ducts)
- Early signs: Erythema of nipple and areola
- Late signs: Thickening, scaling, and erosion of the nipple and areola

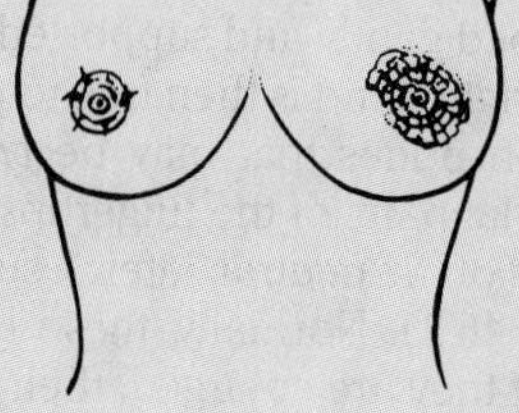
Paget's disease

(From Fuller, J. and Schaller-Ayers, J.: Health Assessment: A Nursing Approach, 2nd ed. JB Lippincott, Philadelphia, 1994.)

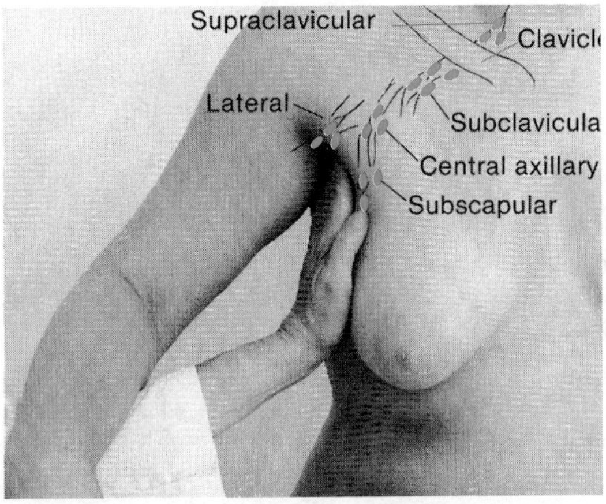

FIGURE 46-2. Palpating axillary nodes in breast examination. (Fuller J and Schaller-Ayers J. Health Assessment: A Nursing Approach, 2nd ed. Philadelphia: JB Lippincott, 1994.)

breast cancer early. On the other hand, others believe that lumps detected by BSE are an incidental finding, and that no studies conclusively demonstrate that BSE decreases overall mortality from breast cancer. Nevertheless, BSE continues to be an important part of health promotion. It can be taught to and practiced by all women. The nurse is in a unique position to inform and educate all women about the benefits of regular BSE and the importance of seeking prompt medical attention when lumps are found.

Resources for BSE Education. Several nursing strategies that may increase motivation to perform BSE have been identified. A personal commitment to this practice on the part of the nurse is one of these strategies. Films about BSE can be obtained from local chapters of the American Cancer Society. Patient teaching of BSE is presented in Chart 46-2. The BSE in-hospital program of the National Cancer Institute in Bethesda, Maryland, offers information and teaching aids to assist nurses in teaching patients about BSE and breast cancer. The National Alliance for Breast Cancer Organizations (NABCO), a clearinghouse for lay materials on breast cancer education, is another resource.

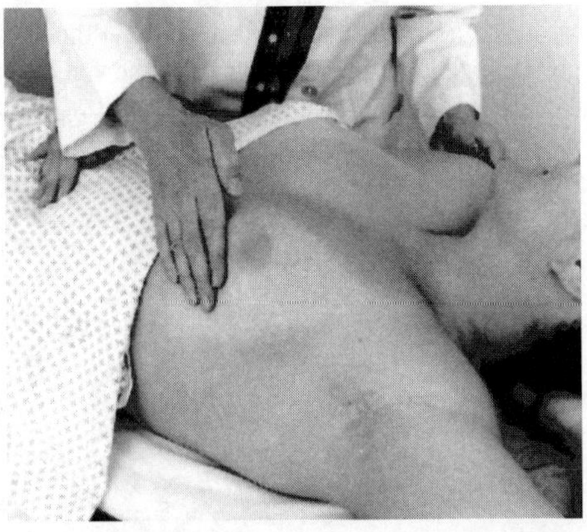

FIGURE 46-3. Breast examination with the woman in a supine position. The entire surface of the breast is palpated from the outer edge of the breast to the nipple. (Fuller J and Schaller-Ayers J. Health Assessment: A Nursing Approach, 2nd ed. Philadelphia, JB Lippincott, 1994.)

The optimal time for BSE is between days 5 and 10 of the menstrual cycle, counting the first day of menses as day 1. A postmenopausal woman is encouraged to examine her breasts on the first day of every month to promote a regular BSE routine.

All patients who have had a mastectomy are carefully instructed in how to examine the remaining breast and the incisional site to detect any nodules, which may indicate recurrent disease.

Diagnostic Screening Techniques

Mammography

Mammography is a breast imaging technique that can detect nonpalpable lesions. The procedure takes about 20 minutes and can be performed in a hospital x-ray department or an independent imaging center. Two views are taken of each breast: a craniocaudal view and a mediolateral view. For these views, the breast is mechanically compressed from top to bottom and side to side. Women may experience some fleeting discomfort because maximum compression is necessary for proper visualization. Current mammograms are compared with previous mammograms. Any changes are a cause for concern and follow-up. Mammography may detect a breast tumor before it is clinically palpable (*i.e.*, smaller than 1 cm); however, it has limitations and is not foolproof. A false-negative rate ranging between 5% and 10% applies.

Patients scheduled for a mammogram may voice concern about exposure to radiation. The radiation exposure is equivalent to about 1 hour of exposure to sunlight, so patients would have to have many mammograms in a year to increase their cancer risk. The benefits of this test outweigh the risks. Because quality of mammography varies widely from one setting to the next, it is important for women to find accredited breast care centers that produce reliable mammograms.

Current mammographic screening guidelines from the American Cancer Society (ACS) recommend a mammogram every 1 to 2 years for women between ages 40 and 50 and a yearly mammogram after age 50. Baseline mammograms for women between the ages of 35 and 40 are not currently suggested. However, younger women at high risk may still want to have baseline studies. Nurses need to alert women to these guidelines and their implications so that they can make informed choices.

Screening mammography combined with physical examination and breast self-examination have demonstrated effectiveness in reducing overall mortality from breast cancer by 30% among women between ages 50 and 69. However, studies of the effectiveness of screening mammography in women between ages 40 and 49 are inconclusive, mainly because no clinical trials have been conducted on the effects of mammography on younger women. Because breast cancer is the leading cause of death among women between ages 35 and 50, regular mammographic screening may offer similar benefit to women under age 50.

Despite the decreased mortality associated with mammographic screening, it has not been used equitably acro

CHART 46-2
Patient Education: Breast Self-Examination (BSE)

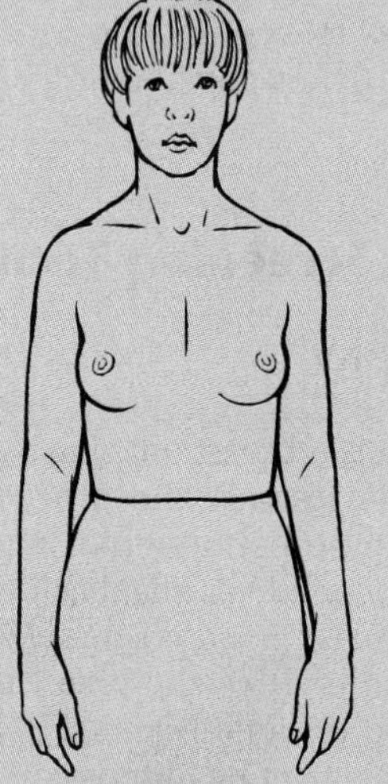

Step 1

1. Stand before a mirror.
2. Check both breasts for anything unusual.
3. Look for discharge from the nipple, puckering, dimpling, or scaling of the skin.

The next two steps are done to check for any changes in the contour of your breasts. As you do them, you should be able to feel your muscles tighten.

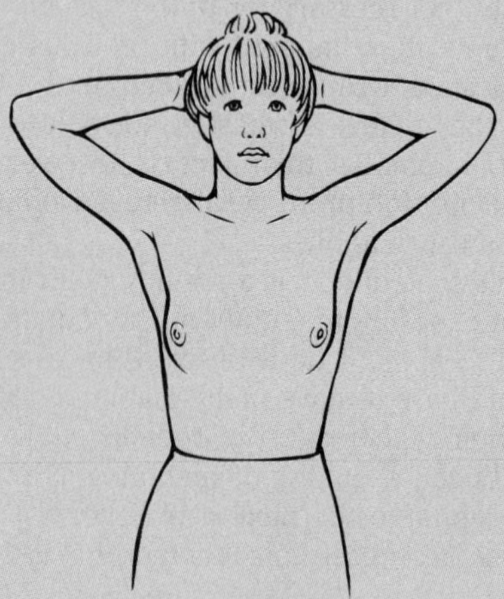

Step 2

1. Watch closely in the mirror as you clasp your hands behind your head and press your hands forward.
2. Note any change in the contour of your breasts.

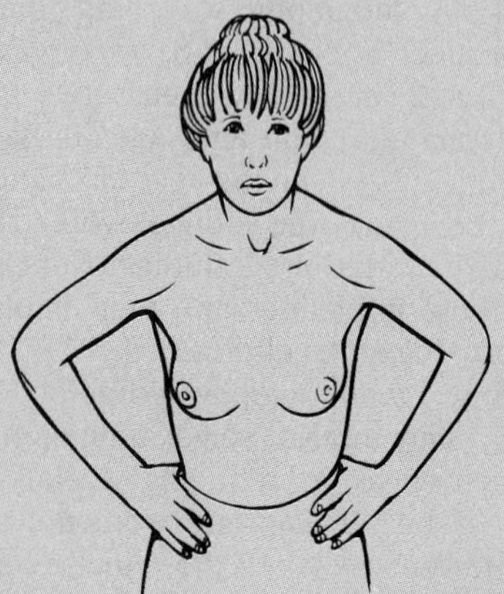

Step 3

1. Next, press your hands firmly on your hips and bow slightly toward the mirror as you pull your shoulders and elbows forward.
2. Note any change in the contour of your breasts.

Some women do the next part of the examination in the shower. Your fingers will glide easily over soapy skin, so you can concentrate on feeling for changes inside the breast.

(continued)

CHART 46-2 *(continued)*

Patient Education: Breast Self-Examination (BSE)

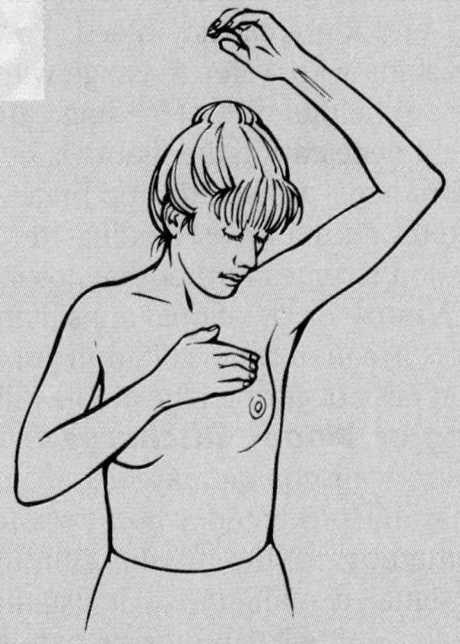

Step 4

1. Raise your left arm.
2. Use 3 or 4 fingers of your right hand to feel your left breast firmly, carefully, and thoroughly.
3. Beginning at the outer edge, press the flat part of your fingers in small circles, moving the circles slowly around the breast.
4. Gradually work toward the nipple.
5. Be sure to cover the whole breast.
6. Pay special attention to the area between the breast and the underarm, including the underarm itself.
7. Feel for any unusual lumps or masses under the skin.

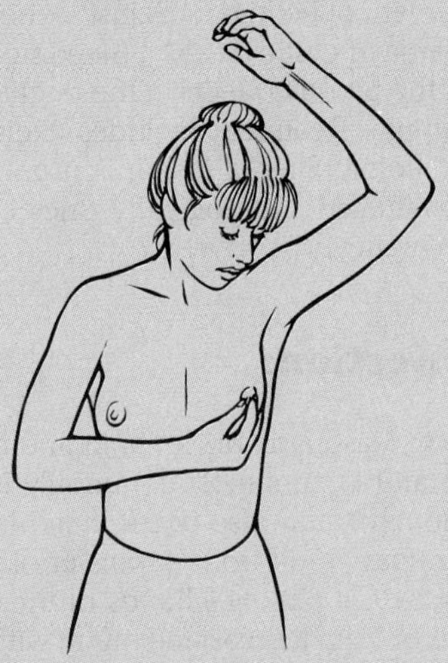

Step 5

1. Gently squeeze the nipple and look for a discharge.
2. If you have any discharge during the month—whether or not it is during your BSE—see your doctor.
3. Repeat the examination on your right breast.

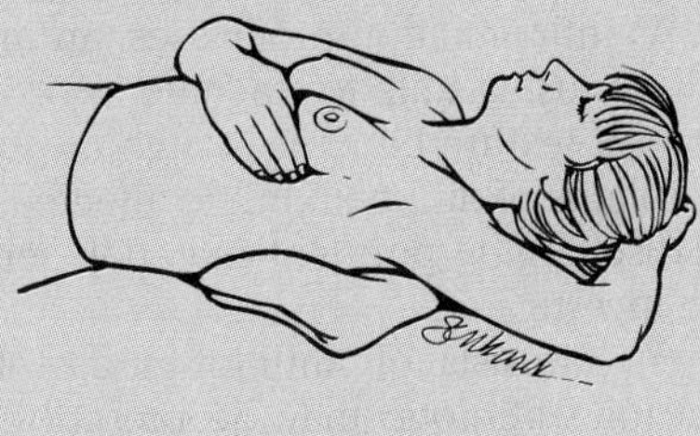

Step 6

1. Steps 4 and 5 should be repeated lying down.
2. Lie flat on your back with your left arm over your head and a pillow or folded towel under your left shoulder. (This position flattens your breast and makes it easier to check.)
3. Use the same circular motion described above.
4. Repeat on your right breast.

(What you need to know about breast cancer. U.S. Department of Health and Human Services, Public Health Service, National Institutes of Health, Bethesda, MD, 1989.)

the U.S. population. Some studies (Zapka et al., 1989; Zapka, Breen & Kessler, 1994; Kiefe et al., 1994; Perez-Stable et al., 1994) indicate that nearly 75% of women have had a mammogram during their lifetime, yet only 40% continue to follow current screening guidelines. Older women, poor women, minority women, and those without health insurance seldom have the means to undergo mammography or the resources for follow-up treatment when positive lesions are detected. In addition, failure of physicians and other health care providers to recommend routine mammograms has contributed to the problem. Many nurses direct their efforts to educating women about the benefits of mammography, working to overcome barriers to screening mammography, especially among the elderly, and assisting in developing educational materials targeted to specific literacy levels and ethnic groups.

Galactography, injection of less than 1 ml of radiopaque material through a cannula into a ductal opening on the areola followed by a mammogram, is performed when the patient has a bloody nipple discharge or when a solitary dilated duct is noted on mammography. These symptoms may be indicative of a benign lesion or a cancerous one.

Ultrasonography

Ultrasonography (ultrasound) is used with mammography to distinguish fluid-filled cysts from other lesions. A transducer is used to transmit high-frequency sound waves through the skin and into the breast. The echo of the sound waves in contact with the breast tissues varies with their density. The echoing waves are interpreted electronically and then displayed on a screen. This technique is 95% to 99% accurate in diagnosing cysts but does not definitively rule out a malignant lesion.

Fine-Needle Aspiration and Surgical Biopsy

Fine-needle aspiration is performed on an outpatient basis and is usually initiated when a lesion is detected by mammography or palpation. After the injection of a local anesthetic (if used), a fine needle at the end of a syringe is directed into the site to be sampled. Then the syringe is used to draw tissue or fluid into the needle. This cytologic material is spread on a slide and sent to the laboratory for analysis. The procedure can be performed less expensively than other diagnostic methods and results are usually available quickly.

Surgical biopsies are usually performed in an outpatient setting under local anesthesia. The biopsy involves excising a lesion and sending it to the laboratory for pathologic examination.

Excisional biopsy is the usual procedure for any palpable breast mass. The entire lesion with a margin of surrounding tissue is removed. In cases of possible cancer, proper handling of the tissue specimen is needed to assess accurately estrogen and progesterone hormone receptors.

To perform a *tru-cut core biopsy,* the surgeon uses a special needle with a large lumen to remove a core of tissue. This procedure is used when a tumor is relatively large and close to the skin surface. If cancer is diagnosed, this tissue is also tested for estrogen and progesterone receptors. Hormonal therapy (described below) may then be used in patients found to have these receptors.

Wire needle localization is a technique used when mammography detects minute, pinpoint calcifications (indicating a potential malignancy) or nonpalpable lesions. A small needle is inserted, usually painlessly, followed by another mammogram to ensure that the needle designates the area to undergo biopsy. A small guide wire remains after the needle is withdrawn to ensure a precise biopsy. Follow-up mammograms verify that the precise area was located and the tumor excised.

In a *stereotactic biopsy,* mammograms are obtained with the patient in a prone position in which the breasts are accessible for mammography. A computer calculates the exact position of the lesion. A device inserts a needle into the breast tissue at the position identified by the computer and removes a few cells from the lesion. Several passes may be needed to make sure that the lesion is adequately sampled.

Conditions Affecting the Nipple

Fissure. A fissure is a longitudinal ulcer that tends to develop in breast-feeding women. If the nipple becomes irritated from the infant sucking on it, a raw area can become painful and infected, and the area may bleed. Prevention is important. Daily washing with water, massage with lanolin, and exposure to air are helpful. Breast-feeding can continue with a nipple shield, if necessary. If the fissure is severe or extremely painful, the woman is advised to stop breast-feeding; a breast pump can be used until breast-feeding can be resumed. Persistent ulceration requires further diagnostic and therapeutic approaches. A nurse or lactational consultant may be helpful because nipple irritation can result from improper positioning (*i.e.,* the infant has not grasped the areola fully).

Bleeding or Bloody Discharge from the Nipple. At times, a bloody discharge may seep from the nipple. This discharge may be produced when pressure is placed on one area at the edge of the areola. Although a bloody discharge can signal a malignancy, it usually results from a wartlike, benign epithelial tumor or papilloma growing in one of the larger collecting ducts just at the edge of the areola or in an area of cystic disease. Bleeding occurs with any trauma, and the blood collects in the duct until it is pressed out at the nipple. Treatment includes excision of the duct with the papilloma. Such a lesion is usually benign, but it should be evaluated histologically once it is removed to rule out malignancy.

Breast Infections

Mastitis. Mastitis is an inflammation or infection of breast tissue and occurs most commonly in breast-feeding women, although it may also occur in nonlactating women. The infection may result from a transfer of microorganisms to the breast by the patient's hands or the hands of others caring for her or from a breast-fed infant with an oral, eye, or skin infection. Mastitis may also be caused by blood-borne organisms. As inflammation progresses, an infection of the ducts results, causing milk to stagnate in one or more lobules. The breast texture becomes tough or doughy, and the patient complains of dull pain in the affected region. A nipple that is discharging purulent material, serum, or blood needs to be investigated.

Treatment consists of antibiotics and local heat. A broad-spectrum antibiotic may be prescribed for 7 to 10 days. The patient should wear a snug bra and perform personal hygiene carefully. Adequate rest and hydration are important aspects of management.

Lactational Abscess. A breast abscess may develop as a consequence of acute mastitis. In such a case, the area affected becomes tender and red. Purulent matter can usually be expressed from the nipple, and incision and drainage is usually required. At the time of drainage specimens are obtained for cultures.

Benign Cysts and Tumors of the Breast

Fibrocystic Breast Changes. Fibrocystic changes of the breast occur as ducts dilate and cysts form. This condition occurs most commonly in women between the ages of

30 to 50 years. Although the cause is unknown, estrogen seems to be a factor because cysts usually disappear after menopause. Cystic areas often fluctuate in size, depending on the menstrual cycle. They are usually larger premenstrually and smaller postmenstrually because of the retention of fluid in the days preceding the menstrual period. The cysts may be painless or may become very tender premenstrually. Occasionally, a patient may report shooting pains. A supportive bra, decreased salt and caffeine intake, and vitamin E supplements may be helpful; however, some women note no change with this regimen. Diuretics and analgesics may be prescribed. Occasionally, oral contraceptives are prescribed, but symptoms usually recur once the pills are discontinued.

A biopsy is occasionally performed to differentiate cystic changes from a true mass. If a specimen of a fibrocystic tissue shows atypical hyperplasia, the patient is at increased risk for developing breast cancer.

If pain and tenderness are severe, danazol (Danocrine) may be prescribed; this agent has an antiestrogenic effect and, therefore, decreases breast pain and nodularity. Danazol is used only in severe cases because of its potential side effects, which include flushing, vaginitis, and androgenic changes (virilization).

Breast Discharge

Breast discharge in a woman who is not lactating may be related to many causes. Carcinoma, papilloma, pituitary adenomas, cystic breasts, and many medications can result in a discharge of fluid from the nipple. Oral contraceptives, pregnancy, estrogen replacement therapy, chlorpromazine-type medications, and frequent breast stimulation may be contributing factors. In some athletic women, breast discharge may result from the movement of breast tissue during running or aerobic exercises. Breast discharge should be evaluated by the patient's health care provider but it is not often a cause for alarm. The discharge is examined for fat globules to determine if it is breast milk. It is also tested for occult blood, as malignancy must be considered.

Other Conditions

Fat necrosis is a rare condition of the breast that is often related to trauma from a blow, but it may be indistinguishable from carcinoma. The entire mass is usually excised.

Gigantomastia or **macromastia** (overly large breasts) is a problem for some women. Weight loss and various medications have been tried to little avail. Reduction mammoplasty (discussed later in this chapter) is an elective procedure for the patient who is physically or emotionally distressed.

Fibroadenomas are firm, round, movable, benign tumors of the breast that usually affect women in their late teens to late thirties. These masses are nontender and are sometimes removed for diagnostic certainty.

Cystosarcoma phyllodes is a fibroepithelial lesion that tends to grow rapidly. It is rarely malignant and is surgically excised. If it is malignant, mastectomy follows. (Variations in breast masses are described in Table 46-1.)

Superficial thrombophlebitis or **Mondor's disease** is an uncommon condition that is usually associated with pregnancy, trauma, or breast surgery. Pain and redness occur as a result of a superficial thrombophlebitis in the vein that drains the outer part of the breast. The mass is usually

TABLE 46-1 Variations in Breast Masses

The most common breast masses are due to fibrocystic changes, fibroadenomas, or malignancy. Biopsy is usually needed for confirmation, but the following characteristics are diagnostic clues.

Characteristics	Fibrocystic Changes	Fibroadenomas	Malignancy
(Illustrations show how the lump may feel, because it is usually not visible.)	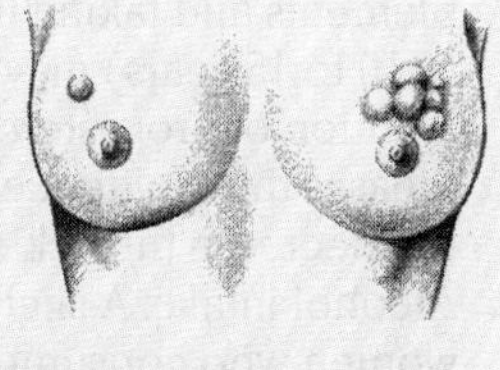	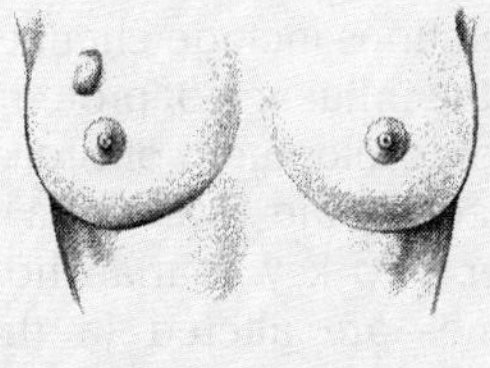	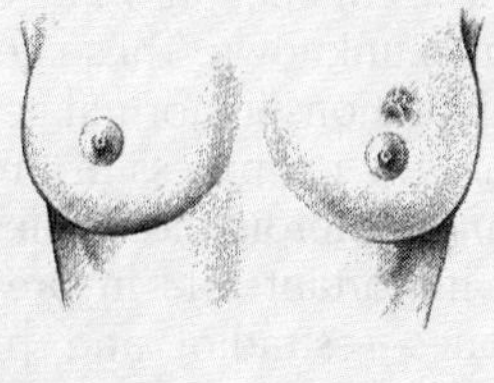
Age	30–60, regress after menopause except with estrogen therapy	Puberty to menopause	30–90 years; most common, 40–80 years
Number	Single or multiple	Usually single	Usually single
Shape	Round	Round, disc, or lobular	Irregular or stellate
Consistency	Soft to firm, usually elastic	Usually firm	Firm or hard
Mobility	Mobile	Mobile	May be fixed to skin or underlying tissues
Tenderness	Usually tender	Usually nontender	Usually nontender
Retraction signs	Absent	Absent	May be present

(Adapted from Bates BA. A Guide to Physical Examination, 6th edition. Phildelphia, JB Lippincott, 1995.)

linear, tender, and red (erythematous). Treatment consists of analgesics and heat.

Breast Cancer

Breast cancer is a major health problem in the United States. Its overall incidence rose by 54% in the 40 years between 1950 and 1989. The incidence rate rose constantly by 1% yearly until the 1980s, when it jumped by 4%. During the 1970s and 1980s, the overall incidence of breast cancer rose by 21% among all women with the incidence increasing by 49% among older women. Mortality rates from breast cancer have remained unchanged for 40 years, suggesting that current treatment with surgery, radiation therapy, and chemotherapy have produced only modest improvements in overall survival.

At present, there is no cure for breast cancer. Because of the rising incidence, unchanged mortality rates, and lack of cure, breast cancer survivors, advocates, and activists have brought social and political attention to this disease and put it in the national spotlight. Activists have demanded and obtained increased federal funding for a national breast cancer program aimed at finding a cure.

Current statistics indicate that the lifetime risk of developing breast cancer is 1 in 8 women. This risk is not the same for all age groups. For example, the risk of developing breast cancer by age 35 is 1 in 622; the risk of developing breast cancer by age 60 is 1 in 24. According to the American Cancer Society, 183,400 new cases of breast cancer were diagnosed in 1995, with an estimated 46,240 deaths. Women who are diagnosed with early stage breast cancer have a 5-year survival rate of 93%. By the year 2000, nearly 2 million women in the United States will have been affected by breast cancer, with more than 460,000 dying of the disease in the 1990s.

Etiology

There is no single, specific cause of breast cancer; rather a series of genetic, hormonal, and, possibly, environmental events may contribute to its development. Growing evidence indicates that genetic alterations are associated with breast cancer, yet what causes the genetic alterations remains unknown. These genetic alterations include changes or mutations in normal genes, and the influence of proteins that either suppress or promote the development of breast cancer. Steroid hormones produced by the ovaries have an important role in breast cancer. Two key ovarian hormones—estradiol and progesterone—are altered in the cellular environment, which can affect growth factors for breast cancer.

Risk Factors

Although there are no specific known causes of breast cancer, researchers have identified a cluster of risk factors. These factors are important in helping to develop prevention programs. One must bear in mind, however, that nearly 60% of women diagnosed with breast cancer have no identifiable risk factors other than their hormonal environment. Thus, all women are considered at risk for developing breast cancer during their lifetime. Nonetheless, identifying risk factors provides a means for identifying women who may benefit from increased surveillance and early treatment. In addition, further research into risk factors will help in developing effective strategies to prevent or modify breast cancer in the future.

Risk factors include:

1. A personal history of breast cancer. The risk of developing breast cancer in the other breast increases approximately 1% each year.
2. Daughters or sisters (first-degree relatives) of women with breast cancer. The risk increases two times if the mother was affected with cancer before age 60; the risk increases 4 to 6 times if breast cancer occurred in two first-degree relatives.
3. Early menarche. The breast cancer risk increases in women in whom menses began before age 12.
4. Nulliparity and late maternal age at first birth. Women having their first child after age 30 have twice the risk of developing breast cancer as women having their first child before age 20.
5. Late menopause. Menopause after age 50 increases the risk of developing breast cancer. In comparison, women who have bilateral oophorectomy before age 35 have one third the risk.
6. History of benign breast disease. Women having breast tumors with proliferative epithelial changes have a double risk of breast cancer; women with atypical hyperplasia have a quadruple risk of developing the disease.
7. Exposure to ionizing radiation after puberty and before age 30 nearly doubles the risk.
8. Obesity—a weak risk factor among postmenopausal women. However, obese women diagnosed with the disease have a higher mortality rate, which is most often related to delayed diagnosis.
9. Oral contraceptives. Women who take oral contraceptives have an increased risk of developing breast cancer. However, this excess risk declines rapidly after discontinuing the medication.
10. Hormone replacement therapy. There are conflicting reports on the risk of breast cancer with hormone replacement therapy. Older women taking estrogen supplements and taking them for a long time (over a range of 10 to 15 years) may have an increased risk. While the addition of progesterone to estrogen replacement decreases the incidence of endometrial cancer, it does not decrease the risk of breast cancer.
11. Alcohol intake. A slightly increased risk is found in women who consume even one drink daily. The risk doubles among women drinking three drinks daily. In countries where wine is consumed regularly (*e.g.,* France and Italy), the rate is slightly higher. Some research findings suggest that young women who drink alcohol are more vulnerable in later years.

A high-fat diet was once thought to increase the risk of breast cancer. Epidemiologic studies of American and Japanese women showed a fivefold difference in the rate of breast cancer between the two groups, with American women having the greater incidence. Japanese women who

CHART 46-3
Risk Factors in Breast Cancer

1. Personal history of breast cancer
2. Sisters or daughters who have had breast cancer
3. Early menarche—before age 12
4. No children or having had first child after 30
5. Menopause occurring after age 50
6. History of benign breast disease
7. Exposure to radiation after puberty and before age 30
8. Obesity
9. Oral contraceptives
10. Hormone replacement therapy
11. Daily intake of alcohol

migrated to the United States were shown to have breast cancer rates similar to their Caucasian counterparts. Recent cohort studies show only weak or inconclusive relationships between high-fat diet and breast cancer. However, because fat is implicated in colon cancer and heart disease, women may benefit from teaching efforts focused on lowering overall caloric intake of fat.

Silicone breast implants have recently been associated with fibrous capsular contraction and certain immune disorders. However, there is no evidence that breast implants are associated with an increased risk of breast cancer.

A summary of risk factors for breast cancer is presented in Chart 46-3.

Clinical Manifestations

Breast cancers can occur anywhere in the breast, but the majority occur in the upper outer quadrant where most breast tissue is located. Breast cancers are more common in the left breast. Generally, the lesions are nontender rather than painful, fixed rather than mobile, and hard with irregular borders rather than encapsulated and smooth. Complaints of diffuse breast pain and tenderness occurring at the time of menstruation are usually associated with benign breast disease. However, marked pain at presentation may be associated with breast cancer in the later stages.

With the increased use of mammography, more women are seeking treatment at an earlier stage of disease. These women may have no symptoms and no palpable lump, but abnormal lesions are detected on mammography. Unfortunately, many women with advanced disease seek initial treatment only after ignoring symptoms. For example, they may seek attention for dimpling or for a peau d'orange (orange-peel) appearance of the skin—a condition caused by swelling which results from obstructed lymphatic circulation in the dermal layer. Nipple retraction and lesions fixed to the chest wall may also be evident. Metastasis to the skin is manifested by ulcerating and fungating lesions. Certainly these classic signs and symptoms characterize breast cancer in the late stages. However, a high index of suspicion should be maintained with any breast abnormality and prompt evaluation should be performed.

Diagnosis

Techniques to determine the histologic and tissue diagnosis of breast cancer include fine-needle aspiration, excisional (or open) biopsy, core biopsy, and needle localization (described above).

Breast Cancer Staging

Staging involves classifying breast cancer according to the extent of disease (Fig. 46-4). Staging of any cancer is important because it helps the health care team recommend the best treatment available, offer a prognosis, and compare the results of alternative treatment regimens. Several blood tests and diagnostic procedures are performed in staging the disease. These include chest x-rays, bone scans, and liver function tests. The clinical staging most used for breast cancer is the TNM system which evaluates the size of *t*umor, number of involved *n*odes, and evidence of distant *m*etastasis. The TNM classification system was adopted by the American Joint Committee on Cancer Staging and End Results Reporting (see Table 46-2).

Pathologic staging based on histology provides a more accurate prognosis. Essential stages are summarized below:

Stage I consists of tumors less than 2 cm, no involved lymph nodes, and no detectable metastases.
Stage II consists of tumors greater than 2 cm but less than 5 cm, with negative or positive unfixed lymph nodes, and no detectable metastases.
Stage III consists of tumors greater than 5 cm, or a tumor of any size that invades the skin or chest wall, with positive fixed lymph nodes in the clavicular area, and without evidence of metastases.
Stage IV consists of tumors of any size, with either cancerous or normal lymph nodes, and distant metastases.

Types of Breast Cancer

Aside from the staging criteria, other pathologic features and prognostic tests are used to identify different patient groups who may benefit from adjuvant treatment. Histologic examination of the cancer cells helps determine the prognosis and leads to a better understanding of how the disease progresses.

Infiltrating ductal carcinomas are the most common histologic type and account for 75% of all breast cancers. These tumors are notable because of their hardness on palpation. They usually metastasize to the axillary nodes. Prognosis is poorer than for other cancer types.

Infiltrating lobular carcinoma is rare and accounts for 5% to 10% of breast cancers. These tumors typically occur as an area of ill-defined thickening in the breast as compared with the infiltrating ductal types. They are most often multicentric, that is, several areas of thickening may occur in one or both breasts. Infiltrating ductal and infiltrating lobular carcinomas have similar axillary node involvement, however, the sites of distant metastases will differ. Ductal carcinomas usually spread to bone, lung, liver or brain,

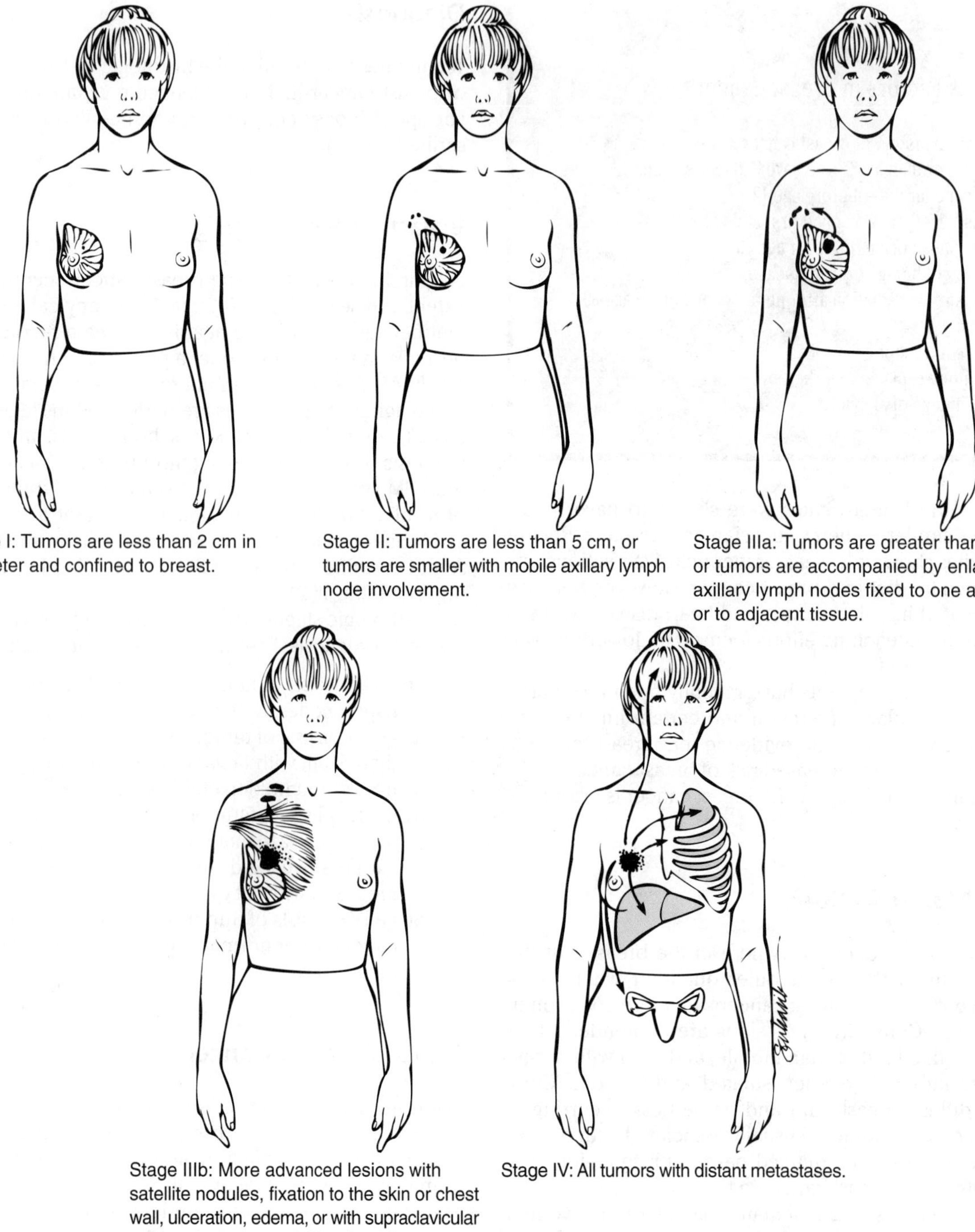

Stage I: Tumors are less than 2 cm in diameter and confined to breast.

Stage II: Tumors are less than 5 cm, or tumors are smaller with mobile axillary lymph node involvement.

Stage IIIa: Tumors are greater than 5 cm, or tumors are accompanied by enlarged axillary lymph nodes fixed to one another or to adjacent tissue.

Stage IIIb: More advanced lesions with satellite nodules, fixation to the skin or chest wall, ulceration, edema, or with supraclavicular or intraclavicular nodal involvement.

Stage IV: All tumors with distant metastases.

FIGURE 46-4. Stages of breast cancer.

while lobular carcinomas usually metastasize to meningeal surfaces or other unusual sites.

Medullary carcinoma constitutes about 6% of breast cancers and grows in a capsule inside a duct. This type of tumor can become large but is slow to expand, so the prognosis is often favorable.

Mucinous cancer accounts for about 3% of breast cancers. A mucus producer, it is also slow-growing; thus, it has a more favorable prognosis than many other types.

Tubular ductal cancer is rare, accounting for only 2% of cancers. Because axillary metastasis is uncommon with this histology, prognosis is excellent.

Inflammatory carcinoma is a rare type of breast cancer (1% to 2%) that produces symptoms that are different from those of other breast cancers. The localized tumor is tender and painful; the breast is abnormally firm and enlarged. The skin over it is red and dusky. Often, edema and nipple retraction occur. These symptoms rapidly grow more severe and usually prompt the woman to seek health care sooner than the woman with a small breast mass. The disease can spread to other parts of the body rapidly; chemotherapeutic agents play a major role in attempting to control the progression of this disease. Radiation and surgery are also used to control spread.

TABLE 46-2 Breast Cancer Staging by Tumor, Nodes, and Metastasis (TNM staging)

Stage 0	Tis	N0	M0
Stage I	T1	N0	M0
Stage IIA	T0	N1	M0
	T1	N1	M0
	T2	N0	M0
Stage IIB	T2	N1	M0
	T3	N0	M0
Stage IIIA	T0	N2	M0
	T1	N2	M0
	T2	N2	M0
	T3	N1	M0
	T3	N2	M0
Stage IIIB	T4	Any N	M0
	Any T	N3	M0
Stage IV	Any T	Any N	M1

Primary Tumor (T)

T0	No evidence of primary tumor
Tis	Carcinoma *in situ:* intraductal carcinoma, lobular carcinoma *in situ,* or Paget's disease of the nipple with no tumor
T1	Tumor ≤ 2 cm in greatest dimension
T2	Tumor > 2 cm but not > 5 cm in greatest dimension
T3	Tumor > 5 cm in greatest dimension
T4	Tumor of any size with direct extension to chest wall or skin

Regional Lymph Nodes (N)

N0	No regional lymph node metastasis
N1	Metastasis to movable ipsilateral axillary lymph node(s)
N2	Metastasis to ipsilateral axillary lymph node(s) fixed to one another or to other structures
N3	Metastasis to ipsilateral internal mammary lymph node(s)

Distant Metastasis (M)

M0	No distance metastasis
M1	Distant metastasis (includes metastasis to ipsilateral supraclavicular lymph node(s))

(Adapted from American Joint Committee on Cancer. Manual for Staging of Cancer, 4th ed. Philadelphia, JB Lippincott, 1992, pp. 151–152.)

Paget's disease of the breast is a less common type of breast cancer. Burning and itching are frequent symptoms. The tumor itself may be ductal or invasive. Often, a tumor mass cannot be palpated underneath the nipple where this disease arises. Mammography may be the only diagnostic study that detects the tumor.

In Situ Breast Carcinoma

In situ carcinoma of the breast is being detected more frequently with the widespread use of screening mammography. This disease is characterized by the proliferation of malignant cells within the ducts and lobules, without invasion into the surrounding tissue. There are two types of *in situ* carcinoma: ductal and lobular.

Ductal carcinoma in situ (DCIS) is divided histologically into two major subtypes: comedo and noncomedo. Because there are many questions about whether DCIS progresses to invasive cancer, the most common treatment is mastectomy with cure rates of 98% or 99%. However, breast conservation therapy (limited surgery and radiation therapy) is a reasonable option that may be considered for localized lesions.

Lobular carcinoma in situ (LCIS) is characterized by proliferation of cells within breast lobules. LCIS is usually an incidental finding, is commonly located in areas of multicentric disease, and is rarely associated with invasive cancer. This disease occurs more frequently in younger women and may be a considered a **premalignant marker** (rather than a malignancy) for the development of breast cancer.

Prognosis

Several features of breast tumors contribute to the prognosis. Generally, the smaller the tumor, the better the prognosis. Carcinoma of the breast is not a pathologic entity that develops overnight. It starts with a genetic alteration in a single cell. It can take approximately 16 doubling times for a carcinoma to become 1 cm or larger, at which point it becomes clinically apparent. Assuming that it takes 30 days for each doubling time, it would take a minimum of 2´ years for a carcinoma to become palpable. If the doubling time were 210 days, it would take up to 17 years before that carcinoma would be palpable.

At diagnosis, approximately 45% of patients have evidence of regional or distant spread or metastasis. The most frequent route of regional spread is to the axillary lymph nodes. Survival is associated with regional spread of disease. For example, the overall 5-year survival rate is greater than 90% if the tumor is confined to the breast. However, when cancer cells have spread to the regional nodes, the overall 5-year survival rate falls under 60%. Other sites of lymphatic spread include the internal mammary and supraclavicular nodes (lymphatic drainage of the breast is illustrated in Fig. 46-5). Distant metastasis can affect any organ, but the most common sites are the bone (71%), lungs (69%), liver (65%), pleura (51%), adrenals (49%), skin (30%), and brain (20%).

In addition to tumor size, nodal involvement, evidence of metastasis, and histologic type, other measures help in determining the prognosis. The presence of estrogen and progesterone receptor proteins indicates a retention of the regulatory controls of the mammary epithelium. Presence of both receptor proteins is associated with an improved prognosis; their absence with a poorer prognosis. Similarly, a tumor with a high degree of differentiation is associated with a better prognosis than is a poorly differentiated, anaplastic tumor. Assessment of a tumor's proliferative rate (S-phase fraction) and DNA content (ploidy) by laboratory assay help to determine prognosis. Tumors classified as diploid (normal DNA content) are associated with a better prognosis than are tumors classified as aneuploid (abnormal DNA content).

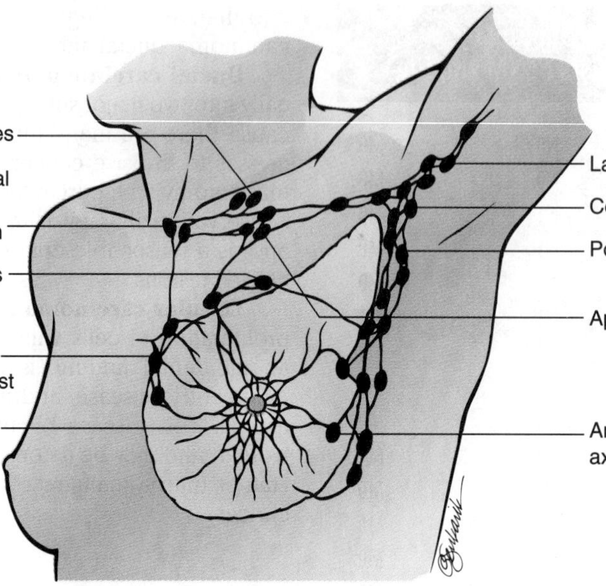

FIGURE 46-5. Lymphatic drainage of the breast.

Changing Approach to Breast Cancer Management

Changes in the local management of breast cancer reflect current understanding of the disease process and have gone from the classic surgical approach of Halsted to management approaches consistent with micrometastasis at the time of diagnosis. The Halsted approach assumed that breast cancer spread in an orderly and centrifugal fashion and that tumors grew locally, infiltrated regional lymph nodes directly, and then spread distantly. Regional lymph nodes were thought to serve as a barrier for the spread of tumor cells and the bloodstream was considered of little significance as a route of tumor spread. The surgical management of breast cancer developed by Halsted in 1893 reflected these beliefs. Halsted implemented radical mastectomy—removal of both the pectoralis major and pectoralis minor muscles and thorough axillary node dissection. Unfortunately, morbidity and mortality rates did not improve with this procedure.

Recently, clinical and biologic observations suggest that metastasis may be present in some women at the time of diagnosis so that survival is less affected by local treatment. This approach proposes that there is no orderly pattern of tumor spread, regional lymph nodes are ineffective barriers, and the bloodstream is an important metastatic route. This change in approach to breast cancer management stresses the importance of systemic chemotherapy to help improve overall survival.

In 1990, the National Institutes of Health Consensus Development Conference on Breast Cancer issued its third statement on the management of breast cancer. Based on results of worldwide data, surgery that conserved the breast (such as a lumpectomy) along with radiation therapy was found to be as effective in controlling the cancer locally as modified radical mastectomy. In addition, recommendations for systemic treatment with chemotherapy were based on the patient's menopausal status and the presence of hormone receptors. For a premenopausal woman without involvement of the lymph nodes, adjuvant chemotherapy was recommended if the woman is at high risk for recurrence. For a postmenopausal woman without involvement of the lymph nodes adjuvant chemotherapy was not recommended regardless of hormone receptor status. For premenopausal women with involvement of the nodes, adjuvant chemotherapy was recommended. In a postmenopausal woman, hormone therapy was recommended if the woman had estrogen-receptor (ER) positive tumors. See page 1318 for more information.

In 1991, the National Cancer Institute issued a clinical alert that altered the recommendations of the 1990 Consensus Development Conference Statement. This alert suggested that *all* premenopausal, node-negative women at high risk for recurrent disease should be given adjuvant chemotherapy. This clinical alert was issued before results of clinical trials were published, thus creating some confusion among clinicians and patients alike. Nevertheless, the current management of breast cancer is based on local or systemic treatment and on the individual characteristics of the patient and the disease.

Decisions regarding local treatment with either mastectomy or breast-conserving surgery with radiation vary widely. Mastectomy is still performed in most cases. Women have not routinely been presented with the option for breast-conserving surgery by their physicians, and in many instances, insurance reimbursement patterns favor mastectomy. Thus, women have not uniformly had the opportunity to exercise informed choice in their options for local treatment.

Treatment of Breast Cancer

Local Treatment of Breast Cancer

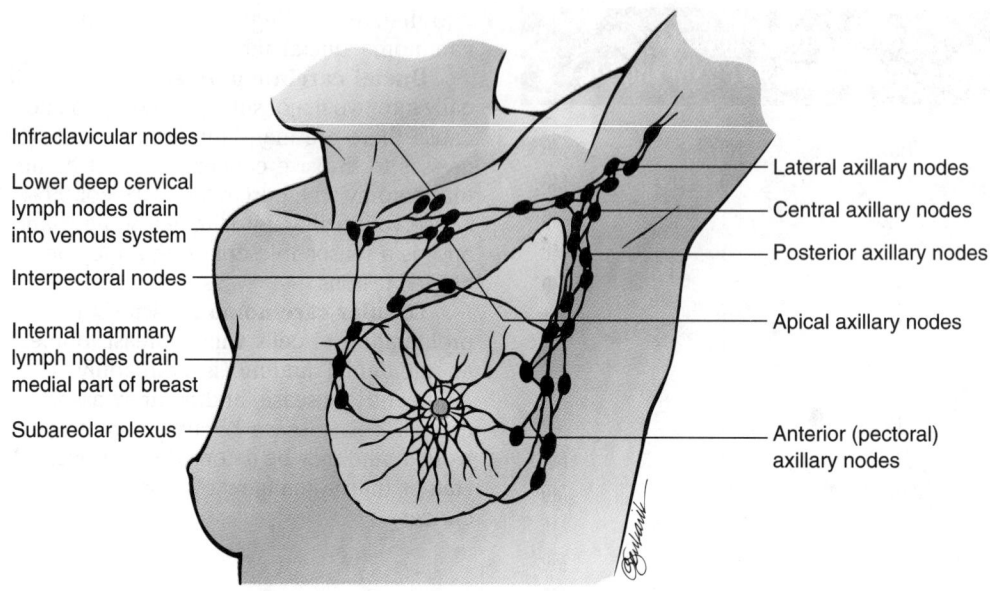

The main goal of local therapy is eradicating the local presence of the cancer. The procedures most often used for the local management of breast cancer are mastectomy with or without reconstruction and breast-conserving surgery combined with radiation therapy.

1. *Modified radical mastectomy:* removal of the entire breast tissue, along with axillary lymph nodes. The pectoralis major and pectoralis minor muscles remain intact.
2. *Breast-conserving surgery*: lumpectomy; segmental mastectomy; or quadrantectomy, a resection of the involved breast quadrant, and removal of the axillary nodes (axillary node dissection) to remove the tumor, followed by a course of radiation therapy to remove residual, microscopic disease.

Mastectomy

Before surgery, the surgeon plans an incision that will provide maximum opportunity to remove the tumor and the affected nodes. At the same time, efforts are made to avoid a scar that will be visible and restrictive. An objective of treatment is to maintain or restore normal function to the hand, arm, and shoulder girdle on the affected side after surgery. Skin flaps and tissue are handled meticulously to ensure proper viability, hemostasis, and drainage. If reconstructive surgery is planned, a consultation is made with a plastic surgeon before the mastectomy.

After the tumor is removed, bleeding points are ligated and the skin is closed over the chest wall. Skin grafting is performed if the skin flaps are too small to close the wound. A nonadherent dressing (Adaptic) may be applied and covered by a pressure dressing. Two drainage tubes may be placed in the axilla and beneath the superior skin flap and portable suction devices may be used. The dressing may be held in place by wide elastic bandages.

Postoperative Issues. Postoperatively, the patient may experience both physical and psychologic effects. Infection or an accumulation of serosanguineous fluid (seroma) and blood (hematoma) may occur at the incisional site. In addition, nerve trauma with resultant phantom breast sensations can occur during recovery and for several years after mastectomy. Impaired arm and shoulder mobility and chest wall tightness can result from disrupted lymphatic and venous drainage. Psychologically, the loss of a breast may result in altered body image and self-concept. Other major psychosocial concerns include uncertainty about the future, fear of recurrence, and the impact of breast cancer and its treatment on family and work activities.

Radiation Therapy

With breast-conserving surgery, a course of external beam radiation therapy usually follows excision of the tumor mass to decrease the chance of recurrence and to eradicate residual cancer. Postoperative radiation is rare after mastectomy today. In the past, however, interstitial iridium implants, requiring a 2-day hospitalization, were used to provide added radiation to the site of the original tumor. Today, external, electron beam treatments have largely replaced interstitial implantation. External beam radiation provided by a linear accelerator using photons is delivered on a daily basis over 4.5 weeks to the entire breast region. In addition, a concentrated radiation dose or "boost" is administered to the primary tumor site via electrons. Before radiation is delivered, patients undergo a planning session for radiation treatment that will serve as the model for daily treatments. Small permanent ink markings are used to identify the breast tissue to be irradiated. Patients need reassurance about the procedure and specific self-care instructions related to side effects and their management.

Postradiation Reaction. Generally, radiation therapy is well tolerated. Side effects are temporary and usually consist of a mild to moderate skin reaction and fatigue. The fatigue that occurs with radiation usually begins about 2 weeks after treatment and may last for several weeks after the treatments are completed. Fatigue can be depressing, as can the frequent trips to the oncology unit. The patient needs to be reassured that the fatigue is normal and not a sign of recurrence. Rare complications of radiation therapy to the breast include pneumonitis, rib fracture, and breast fibrosis.

Patient Teaching. Self-care instructions for patients receiving radiation are based on maintaining skin integrity and include the following points: using mild soap with minimal rubbing, avoiding perfumed soaps or deodorants, using hydrophilic lotions (Lubriderm, Eucerin, Aquaphor) for dryness, using Aveeno soap if pruritus occurs, and avoiding tight clothes, underwire bras, and excessive temperatures or ultraviolet light.

The general skin care guidelines used for radiation should continue to be followed. Patients may note increased redness and, rarely, skin breakdown in the "booster site." Important aspects of follow-up care include teaching patients to minimize exposure of the treated area to the sun for 1 year and reassuring them that minor twinges and shooting pain in the breast are normal reactions after radiation treatment.

Reconstruction

After mastectomy, some women may elect to have reconstructive surgery, which provides considerable psychologic benefit. Support groups provide education and peer support for those patients who are candidates for and interested in breast reconstruction. Some concerns that women may have about reconstructive surgery are cost, safety, and timing—whether to undergo reconstruction immediately (at the time of mastectomy) or delay it (6 months to 1 year after surgery). Cost to the patient may vary depending on her health insurance, but because reconstruction is considered rehabilitative surgery, it is often covered.

In regard to safety, there are the usual surgical risks of infection, potential reaction to anesthesia, and the potential risk of a cosmetically unsatisfactory result. Reconstructive surgery is contraindicated if a woman has locally advanced metastatic or inflammatory breast cancer. Currently, criteria for selecting cancer patients for reconstruction are being developed to reduce the risk of recurrent cancer. For now, some clinicians recommend delaying reconstruction 1 to 2 years after completing chemotherapy or radiation therapy or 6 months after surgery.

If a woman decides to have reconstructive surgery at the time of the mastectomy, she avoids future surgery, although the total operative time increases. Some women find that immediate reconstruction lessens the feelings of loss and disfigurement. Occasionally, reconstruction cannot be performed because skin and muscles are too tight. Loose, supple skin and subcutaneous tissue with a sufficient blood supply contribute to reconstructive success. Some women benefit by waiting until later because initially they are not sure about their choice.

Reconstructive surgery is discussed later in this chapter; surgical treatment options are summarized in Table 46-3.

Not all women desire reconstruction, nor are all women candidates for reconstructive surgery. In these instances, patients may need information about available external prostheses and the names of medical supply shops where they can be fitted for these devices.

Systemic Treatment of Breast Cancer

Chemotherapy is administered to eradicate the micrometastatic spread of the disease. An overview of chemotherapy is presented in Chapter 16. Although chemotherapy is generally initiated after mastectomy, there is no single standard means for setting up the sequence for chemotherapy sessions when patients have undergone breast-conserving surgery and radiation therapy. In some instances, chemotherapy is administered for several cycles, then radiation therapy is initiated, and the final cycles of chemotherapy are administered after radiation. In other instances, chemotherapy is not initiated until the course of radiation therapy is completed. Ongoing clinical trials may help to determine which treatment produces the best outcomes.

Chemotherapy regimens for breast cancer combine several agents to increase the tumor cell destruction and to minimize medication resistance. The chemotherapeutic agents used most often in combination are cytoxan (C), methotrexate (M), fluorouracil (F), and adriamycin (A). A CMF or CAF regimen is a common treatment protocol. In less common use are CMFVP (cytoxan, methotrexate, fluorouracil, vincristine, and prednisone) or AC (adriamycin and cytoxan). Decisions regarding the chemotherapeutic protocol are based on the individual patient's age, physical status, disease status, and whether she is participating in a clinical trial. Systemic treatment modalities are summarized in Table 46-4.

Reactions to Chemotherapy. Anticipatory anxiety is a common response among patients facing chemotherapy. Today, however, side effects can be managed very well, with many women continuing their daily work and routine schedules. This has occurred in large measure because of the meticulous educational and psychologic preparation provided to patients and their families by their oncology nurses, oncologists, social workers, and other members of the health care team.

Common physical side effects of chemotherapy for breast cancer include nausea, vomiting, taste changes, alopecia (hair loss), mucositis, dermatitis, fatigue, weight gain, and bone marrow depression. In addition, premenopausal women receiving chemotherapy may experience temporary or permanent amenorrhea leading to sterility.

Less common side effects include hemorrhagic cystitis and conjunctivitis. Although the cause is unknown, weight gain of more than 10 lb occurs in about half of all patients. Aerobic exercise during chemotherapy treatment has been shown to minimize weight gain. The sense of well-being that comes from exercise and its anxiety-alleviating effects may also be helpful.

Side effects may vary with the chemotherapeutic agent used. Adriamycin can be toxic to tissue if it infiltrates out of the vein, so it is usually diluted and infused through a large vein. Nausea and vomiting can occur. Antiemetics and tranquilizers may provide relief, as may visual imagery and relaxation exercises. Adriamycin may cause alopecia. Obtaining a wig before hair loss occurs may prevent some of the associated emotional trauma. The patient needs reassurance that new hair will grow when treatment is completed, although the color and texture of the hair may differ. The American Cancer Society offers a program known as "Look Good, Feel Better" that provides useful tips for applying cosmetics during chemotherapy.

Teaching points that should be emphasized to minimize hair loss include:

1. Avoid shampooing daily.
2. Use a mild, protein-based shampoo with conditioner every 4 to 7 days; rinse thoroughly and pat dry.
3. Let hair dry naturally; electric hair dryers, curlers, and curling irons can increase hair loss. Hair clips, barrettes, bobby pins, hair sprays and dyes should be avoided.
4. Do not brush hair; use a wide-toothed comb.
   Use of an eyebrow pencil or false eyelashes may be suggested if hair loss affects eye areas.

Nurses working with patients receiving chemotherapy play an important role in assisting those who have difficulty with the side effects of treatment. Encouraging the use of medications to limit nausea, vomiting, and mouth sores reduces the trauma of the patient's experience during chemotherapy. It is helpful to provide a list of wig suppliers in the patient's geographic region and become familiar

TABLE 46-3 Surgical Treatment of Breast Cancer

Surgical Procedure	Description
Partial mastectomy Lumpectomy Wide excision Segmental mastectomy	Relatively synonymous terms to describe removal of varying amounts of breast tissue, including the malignant tissue and some surrounding tissue. Axillary nodes are dissected.
Quadrantectomy	A type of partial mastectomy in which a quadrant of tissue may be removed.
Axillary node dissection	Removal of some fat-enmeshed axillary nodes for biopsy
Modified radical mastectomy	Removal of all breast tissue and axillary node dissection
Radical mastectomy	Removal of entire breast along with pectoralis major and minor muscles in conjunction with axillary node dissection

TABLE 46-4 Selected Systemic Treatment Modalities for Cancer of the Breast

Type of Treatment	Goals of Therapy	Possible Side Effects	Nursing Interventions
Chemotherapy	Destroy neoplastic cells Decrease or prevent metastasis		
Adriamycin (A)		ECG changes, tachycardia, nausea, vomiting, stomatitis, hair loss, severe cellulitis if infiltration occurs	*Nausea & vomiting:* Administer antiemetics as prescribed. Encourage high fluid intake. Monitor fluid intake and output.
Cytoxan (C)		Nausea, vomiting, anorexia, menstrual abnormalities, hemorrhagic cystitis	*Anorexia:* Assist patient and family to identify appetizing foods. Provide frequent small meals if better tolerated than 3 regular meals. Refer to dietician for assistance in planning palatable, nutritious meals.
Methotrexate (M)		Stomatitis, CNS changes, hair loss	
5-Fluorouracil (F)		CNS changes, weakness and malaise, somatitis	
Vinblastine (Velban)		CNS changes, neurotoxicity, nausea, vomiting, constipation, stomatitis	*Stomatitis:* Avoid commercial mouth washes; use baking soda, salt and water rinses, or oral anesthetic agents.
Vincristine (V)		Hair loss; neurotoxicity with sensory loss (numbness, tingling), depressed reflexes, weakness	*Hair loss:* Avoid brushing, blow drying, frequent shampooing. Encourage use of turbans and scarves. Encourage patient to obtain wig before hair loss occurs.
Combination therapy: CMF CAF CMFVP (prednisone added)			*CNS changes:* Monitor for weakness, malaise, fatigue, seizures, change in cognitive status. Assist with ADL if fatigue and malaise occur.
			Neurotoxicity: Monitor deep tendon reflexes, assess gait and muscle strength, monitor for changes in sensory function.
			Fluid retention: Monitor weight, fluid intake and output, skin turgor.
			Cardiac changes: Monitor ECG, cardiac rate and rhythm; notify physician of dysrhythmias.
			Hypercalcemia: Monitor serum calcium levels, monitor cardiac rate and rhythm.
			Constipation: Monitor bowel function. Consider that constipation may be indicative of neurotoxicity. Administer stool softeners, laxatives as prescribed. Encourage adequate intake of fluids and fiber.

(continued)

TABLE 46-4 *(continued)*

Type of Treatment	Goals of Therapy	Possible Side Effects	Nursing Interventions
			Anxiety: Administer tranquilizers as prescribed. Encourage use of strategies to minimize anxiety (imagery, relaxation)
Hormonal Therapy			
Androgens fluxoymesterone (Halotestin)	Suppress estrogens	Masculinization, fluid retention, cholestatic jaundice, hypercalcemia	*Hormonal instability:* Observe for changes (hot flashes, vaginal bleeding, flare); facial hirsutism, deepening of voice; fluid retention, Cushing's syndrome (fullness of face, lower extremity edema; weight gain); increased blood pressure. Assess for thrombophlebitis. Monitor serum calcium levels. Assure patient that most changes are temporary.
Estrogens (diethylstilbesterol/ DES)	Suppress FSH and LH	Nausea, vomiting, anorexia, dizziness, headache	
Corticosteroids (prednisone)	Suppress estrogen production by the adrenals and decrease urinary estrogen metabolites	Cushing's syndrome: fullness of face, weight gain, edema of lower extremities	
Antihormonal agents Aminogluethimide (Cytadren)	Enzyme antagonist that inhibits estrogen synthesis	CNS changes: dizziness, clumsiness, drowsiness, depression, headache	
Megestrol acetate (Megace)	Progestational agent; may decrease number of estrogen receptors in breast tissue	Weight gain, hot flashes, vaginal bleeding, increased blood pressure, edema, depression, flare	
Tamoxifen (Nolvadex)	Estrogen antagonist; effective in palliative treatment in postmenopausal women with positive assays for estrogen receptors	Anorexia, hot flashes, lethargy	

FSH, follicle-stimulating hormone; LH, luteinizing hormone.
This listing of medications, side effects, and nursing interventions is not meant to be exhaustive but is rather a sample of frequently used chemotherapeutic agents for breast cancer.

with the use of creative scarves and turbans to minimize patient discomfort with hair loss. Taking time to explain side effects and possible solutions may alleviate some of the anxiety of women who feel uncomfortable asking questions. Because many women are distressed by financial concerns and time spent away from the family, nursing support and teaching can avert serious emotional distress during treatment.

Chemotherapy may have a negative effect on the patient's self-esteem, sexuality, and well-being. Combined with the stress of a potentially life-threatening diagnosis, changes in self-esteem, sexuality, and well-being can be overwhelming. However, most women with breast cancer today are treated in a multidisciplinary environment. In addition, numerous community support and advocacy groups are available to these patients and their families. Important aspects of nursing care include communication, facilitating support groups, encouraging patients to ask questions, and promoting the patient's trust and faith in health care providers. Adequate time for patient discussion must be built into clinical visits. The more informed a patient is about the side effects of chemotherapy and how to manage them, the better she can anticipate and deal with them.

Hormonal Therapy

Decisions about hormonal therapy for breast cancer are based on the index of estrogen and progesterone receptors derived from an assay of tumor tissue taken during the original biopsy. The tissue requires special handling by laboratory technicians with expertise in proper assessment techniques. Normal breast tissue contains receptor sites for estrogen. However, only about one third of breast cancers are estrogen dependent, or ER-positive (ER+). An ER+ assay indicates that tumor growth depends on estrogen supply; therefore, measures that reduce hormone production may limit the progression of the disease. ER+ tumors may grow more slowly than those that do not depend on estrogen, or are ER-negative (ER–). Less than 3 fmol/mg is considered negative. Values of 3 to 10 are questionable, and values greater than 10 are considered positive. The greater the value, the more beneficial the anticipated effect from hormone suppression. Patients with both estrogen- and progesterone-positive receptors (PR+) generally have a more favorable prognosis than patients with ER– and PR– tumors. Most positive progesterone receptive tumors also have a positive estrogen receptor status, so this factor becomes a prognostic indicator. The loss of progesterone receptors can be a sign of advancing disease. Premenopausal women and perimenopausal women are more likely to have non–hormone-dependent lesions. Postmenopausal women (more than 5 years) are likely to have hormone-dependent lesions.

Hormonal therapy may include surgery to remove endocrine glands (*i.e.*, the ovaries, pituitary, or adrenal glands) with the goal of suppressing hormone secretion. Oophorectomy (removal of the ovaries) is one treatment option for premenopausal women with estrogen-dependent tumors.

Tamoxifen is the primary hormonal treatment used in breast cancer today. Megace, diethylstilbestrol (DES), fluoxymesterone (Halotestin), and aminoglutethimide (Cytadren) are other hormonal agents used to suppress hormone-dependent tumors. Each is described below:

1. *Tamoxifen*. This agent is considered to be as effective as oophorectomy and is the most commonly used method of hormonal manipulation. It was initially indicated for treating postmenopausal patients with positive estrogen receptor and positive axillary nodes. Some treatment centers across the country are increasing use of tamoxifen in high-risk, premenopausal women after adjuvant chemotherapy. Current chemoprevention clinical trials are also under way using tamoxifen in premenopausal and postmenopausal women at high risk for developing breast cancer. This antiestrogenic agent has few side effects, but some patients may experience nausea, vomiting, hot flashes, fluid retention, and depression.
2. *Diethylstilbestrol* (DES). This agent suppresses the release of follicle-stimulating hormone (FSH) and luteinizing hormone (LH), thereby decreasing ovarian production of estrogen and estrogen binding. This medication is used less frequently than tamoxifen because side effects are more common (*i.e.*, weight gain, fluid retention, nausea).
3. *Megestrol* (Megace). How megestrol works is unknown. It may decrease the number of estrogen receptors. Increased appetite and weight gain are possible side effects.
4. *Fluoxymesterone* (Halotestin). This testosterone derivative suppresses estrogen by suppressing FSH and LH. Side effects include virilization (*i.e.*, increased facial hair, deepened voice, clitoral hypertrophy, and increased libido).
5. *Aminoglutethimide* (Cytadren). This medication inhibits aromatase, the enzyme responsible for converting androgens to estrogens. Its effects are similar to surgical removal of the adrenal glands. Side effects include a rash that may cause itching. Because adrenal function may be suppressed, the patient is monitored for signs of adrenal cortical hypofunction; hydrocortisone is administered to prevent these undesired effects.

These medications may be associated with menopausal symptoms such as vasomotor changes. Hypercalcemia may also occur and may necessitate discontinuing the medication. Patient education about medication and possible reactions is an important issue for nurses providing care for patients receiving hormonal therapy.

Bone Marrow Transplantation

Because chemotherapy and radiation therapy dosage are limited by the degree of their toxicity to the bone marrow, bone marrow transplant (BMT) is increasingly being used. Studies have indicated that autologous BMT induces a response in 50% to 80% of women, 30% of whom have a complete response for several years (Antman & Gale, 1988). Initially, mortality rates were high with autologous BMT, due to sepsis. However, the current use of growth factors to stimulate the bone marrow have led to an overall decline in mortality. The procedure involves removing bone marrow from the patient and then providing high-dose chemotherapy. The patient's bone marrow, spared from the effects of chemotherapy, is then reinfused intravenously. This highly specialized procedure is usually performed in specialized transplantation centers, and specific patient preparation, education, and support must be given throughout the treatment course. BMT is described more fully on p. 285.

Future Treatment Modalities

Research studies are in progress to develop chemotherapeutic agents that modify multidrug resistance and agents that enhance or modify standard chemotherapy. Research in breast cancer treatment and prevention includes the following areas: oncogenes (tumor genes that control cell growth), growth factors (substances released by cancer cells to make the environment more conducive to growth), and monoclonal antibodies (synthetic antibodies that fight cancer cells). Biologic response modifiers (*e.g.*, interferon or other substances that help increase the body's immune system response) may become a method of treatment.

Quality of Life and Breast Cancer

Despite current treatment, there has been only a slight overall improvement in survival for breast cancer patients. Consequently, quality of life considerations have become important issues in treatment and recovery. Quality of life is a multidimensional construct that includes functional (self-care) status, psychologic well-being, social and family functioning, and spiritual well-being. These parameters are important indicators of how well an individual is functioning after diagnosis and treatment.

Breast cancer is the most frequently investigated cancer in quality of life studies (Kiebert, de Haes, & van de Velde, 1991). Early psychosocial studies emphasized that the loss of the breast was the single most important factor in women's adjustment, especially in Western cultures. Thus, it is not surprising that studies of women's adjustment to breast cancer found similar results (Kiebert, de Haes, & van de Velde, 1991). However, a growing body of research indicates that concerns related to uncertainty about one's future, day-to-day issues occurring in work and family relationships, and demands of illness are more important factors in adjusting to having breast cancer than the loss of the breast alone (Schag et al., 1993; Loveys & Klaich, 1991). For example, younger women are more vulnerable to issues of psychosocial adjustment than older women. They worry about their jobs and whether they will be able to keep important health care benefits. They are concerned about their work productivity and career advancement. They face many family concerns related to whether they can have children, whether they will live to see their children grow up, and whether their disease will recur and incapacitate them. Middle-aged women worry about their disease in relation to their family and work. However, they also worry about their aging parents and whether they will be able to care for them in the future. They are increasingly concerned about their daughters' risk for breast cancer. Older women are more vulnerable to chronic health problems. Living an average of 16 years longer than men, older women face loss of their social circles, deal with the potential for other diseases, and worry about whether they will have the resources to pay for medications (Vinokur et al., 1990; Fink, 1987).

These concerns are intertwined with the impact of breast cancer on the family. Studies indicate that up to 35% of families of women with breast cancer experience significant changes in family functioning. More than 25% of children also experience problems related to their mothers' breast cancer. In addition, families shoulder substantial costs in caring for family members with advanced breast cancer (Stommel, Given, & Given, 1991). These out-of-pocket, unreimbursed expenses include lost wages and salaries and lost opportunities.

When faced with any life-threatening illness, spiritual and existential concerns usually surface. Patients with breast cancer often express the need to talk about the uncertainties of their future, and their hope and faith that they will be able to manage whatever crisis or challenge comes their way.

Pregnancy and Breast Cancer

From 2% to 5% of breast cancers occur in pregnant women. Detecting lumps, changes in breast tissue, and masses is more difficult during pregnancy because of the normal physiologic changes that occur during gestation. Because many women discontinue breast self-examination during pregnancy, an important aspect of health promotion is to encourage this examination throughout pregnancy.

If a mass is found during pregnancy, mammography with appropriate shielding, needle aspiration, and biopsy are indicated. Treatment is basically the same as in other women, although radiation is contraindicated in pregnancy. Some oncologists begin chemotherapy as early as the 16th week of pregnancy because fetal organs are already formed at this point. If systemic treatment is necessary, a cesarean section is performed as soon as safety of the fetus allows. If a mass is found while a woman is breast-feeding, she is urged to stop breast-feeding to allow the breast to involute (return to its baseline state) before surgery. If aggressive disease is detected early in pregnancy and chemotherapy is advised, termination of the pregnancy is a choice that some patients may consider.

After treatment is complete, younger women may consider having children, in which case many individual issues must be addressed: the patient and her partner's desire for children and family; disease and prognostic concerns; age; fertility and infertility issues; and social, financial, ethical, and quality-of-life issues. Although waiting times vary, most women are advised to wait 2 years before becoming pregnant. Most retrospective studies (Danforth, 1991) indicate that pregnancy after treatment for breast cancer does not seem to increase the risk of the disease recurring. Counseling, providing accurate information, and active listening and caring are important nursing interventions when patients are involved in making difficult personal decisions about treatment options, childbearing, or terminating pregnancy.

❑ NURSING PROCESS
The Patient With Breast Cancer

Assessment

The health history includes an assessment of the patient's reaction to the diagnosis and her ability to cope with it. Pertinent questions include the following:

- How is the patient responding to the diagnosis?
- What coping mechanisms does she find most helpful?
- What psychologic or emotional supports does she use?
- Is there a partner, family member, or friend available to assist her in making treatment choices?
- What are the most important areas of information she needs?
- Is the patient having any discomfort?

Patients who have lost close relatives to breast cancer may have difficulty coping with the possible diagnosis of breast cancer, because memories of loss and death can emerge during their own crisis.

Diagnosis

Nursing Diagnoses

Based on the health history and other assessment data, the patient's major nursing diagnoses may include the following:

Preoperative

- Knowledge deficit about breast cancer and treatment options
- Fear and ineffective coping related to the diagnosis of cancer, its treatment, and the prognosis

Postoperative

- Pain and discomfort
- Impaired skin integrity due to surgical incision
- Body image disturbance related to mastectomy and the side effects of radiation and chemotherapy
- Self-care deficit related to partial immobility of upper arm on the operative side
- Potential sexual dysfunction related to the loss of a body part, change in self-image, and fear of partner's reaction to this loss

Collaborative Problems/ Potential Complications

Based on assessment data, potential complications may include:

- Lymphedema

Planning and Implementation

Goals. The major goals for the patient may include increased knowledge about disease and its treatment, reduction of preoperative and postoperative fear, emotional stress, and anxiety; pain relief, maintenance of skin integrity; improved self-concept; improved self-care; improved sexual function, and absence of complications.

Nursing Interventions

Preoperative

Patient Teaching About Breast Cancer and Treatment Options. The patient confronting the diagnosis of breast cancer typically reacts with feelings of fear, dread, and anxiety. In view of the usually overwhelming emotional reactions to the diagnosis, the patient must be given time to absorb the significance of the diagnosis and any information that will help her to evaluate available treatment options.

The nurse caring for the woman who has just received a diagnosis of breast cancer needs to be knowledgeable about current treatment options and able to discuss them with the patient. The nurse should be aware of the information that has been given to the patient by the physician in order to answer specific questions the patient may have.

Information about the surgery, including the location and extent of the tumor and postoperative treatments involving radiation therapy and chemotherapy, are details that the patient needs to help her make decisions. As appropriate, the nurse discusses the extent and side effects of treatment, frequency and duration of treatment, and goals with the patient. Methods to compensate for physical changes related to mastectomy are also discussed and planned (*i.e.,* prostheses and plastic surgery). The amount and timing of the information provided are based on the patient's responses, coping ability, and readiness to learn.

Reducing Fear and Improving Coping Ability. The patient's emotional preparation begins when the tentative diagnosis of cancer is made. The patient may have the diagnostic procedure performed in the surgeon's office or in the hospital when she is admitted for ambulatory or same-day surgery for a biopsy. Fears and concerns are common and are discussed with the patient. If she will undergo a mastectomy, information about various resources and options are made available. Such services include prostheses, reconstructive surgery, and groups such as Reach to Recovery.

The nurse provides anticipatory teaching and counseling at each stage of the process and details information about which sensations can be expected during additional diagnostic procedures. The patient is introduced to other members of the oncology team—radiation oncologist, medical oncologist, oncology nurse, and social worker—and acquainted with the role that each of these health care providers will assume in her care.

Once the treatment plan has been established, the nurse needs to promote the best preoperative physical, psychologic, social, and nutritional well-being possible. The patient usually prefers to be active in her care and decision making.

Postoperative

Relieving Pain and Discomfort. Regular nursing assessments of pain and discomfort are important because patients experience differing degrees of pain intensity. Some women may have severe incisional pain whereas others may have more generalized pain and discomfort of the chest wall and in the affected arm. Moderate elevation of the involved extremity is one means of relieving pain. Patient-controlled analgesia (PCA) may be of considerable assistance in assuring adequate pain relief and comfort (see Chapter 13 for a discussion of PCA).

Maintaining Skin Integrity. In the immediate postoperative period, the patient will have a snug but not tight dressing over the surgical site and one or more drainage tubes in place. A particular concern is preventing fluid from accumulating under the chest wall incision by maintaining the patency of the surgical drain. The dressing and drain are inspected for bleeding and the extent of drainage is monitored regularly. Initially the drainage will appear bloody but will become serous within 1 or 2 days. The drain is usually left in place for a week or until the output is less than 30 ml in 24 hours. Usually, the patient is discharged with a drain in place; she will, therefore, need to learn how to empty the reservoir and measure the drainage.

Dressing changes present opportunities for the nurse and patient to discuss the incision, particularly how it looks and feels and progressive changes in its appearance. The patient needs to know that sensation is decreased in the operative area because the nerves were disrupted during surgery and that gentle care is needed to avoid injury. Teaching the patient to recognize signs of infection or irritation is important. Using the term *incision* rather than *scar* reduces the feelings of deformity and disfigurement that may accompany physical alteration. After the surgical site heals appropriately, the patient may massage the area gently with vitamin E or other lotions to promote circulation and increase skin elasticity.

Reducing Stress and Improving Coping Skills. Patients may initially be uncomfortable looking at the surgical incision. No matter how prepared an individual may be, the actual site of one's own incision may still be difficult to view. Exploring this sensitive area must be a careful nursing action, and cues provided by the patient must be respected and sensitively handled.

Ongoing assessment of the patient's support systems is important, and the patient's spouse or partner, if any, may need guidance, support, and education as well. In addition, the patient may benefit from a wide network of available community resources including Reach to Recovery, advocacy groups, and her spiritual advisor.

Another important aspect of nursing care includes answering the patient's questions and addressing her concerns about treatment options that may follow surgery. Being knowledgeable about the plan of care and encouraging the patient to ask questions of the appropriate members of the health care team will promote coping during recovery.

Promoting Self-Care. Patients need information about the possibility of postoperative surgical edema and strategies to prevent it. Cuts, bruises, and infections on the operative side increase the likelihood of developing lymphedema. Careful patient teaching and reinforcement of teaching can help the patient absorb this information. Pamphlets, books, and support groups may also be helpful supplements (see the list of resources at the end of this chapter).

Ambulation is encouraged once the patient is free of postanesthesia nausea and is tolerating fluids. The nurse supports the patient on the nonoperative side. Once drainage tubes are removed, passive range-of-motion exercises are initiated to increase circulation and muscle strength and to prevent joint stiffness. Hand exercises are also important. Self-care activities, including brushing the teeth, washing the face, and combing and fixing the hair are physically and emotionally therapeutic. Exercises such as "climbing the

CHART 46-4
Patient Education: Postmastectomy Exercises

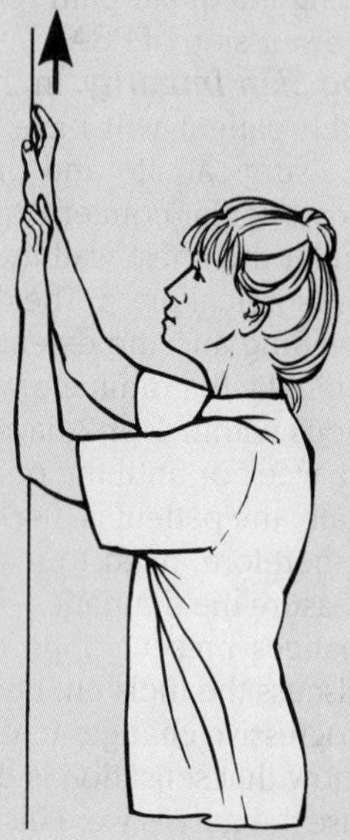

1. *Wall handclimbing.* Stand facing the wall with feet apart and toes as close to the wall as possible. With elbows slightly bent, place the palms of the hand on the wall at shoulder level. By flexing the fingers, work the hands up the wall until arms are fully extended. Then reverse the process, working the hands down to the starting point.

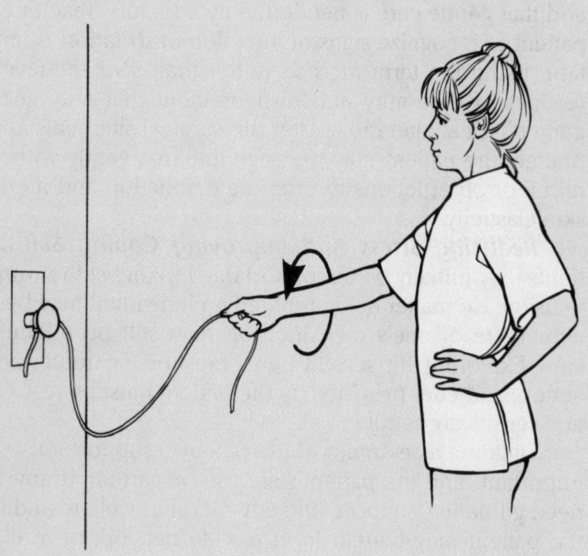

2. *Rope turning.* Tie a light rope to a doorknob. Stand facing the door. Take the free end of the rope in the hand on the side of surgery. Place the other hand on the hip. With the rope-holding arm extended and held away from the body (nearly parallel with the floor), turn the rope, making as wide swings as possible. Begin slowly at first; speed up later.

(continued)

wall" with the fingers encourage the patient to use her arm and prevent contractures from developing. Pain should not accompany therapeutic exercise; mild discomfort, effort, and anxiety, however, may occur initially. If the patient has skin grafts or a tense, tight surgical incision, exercises must be introduced gradually by the health care members working as a team. Range-of-motion, muscle-training exercises are described in Chart 46-4. Using the muscles in both arms as well as proper posture is encouraged. If a patient is favoring the affected side, or splinting the surgical site, or not standing up straight, any exercise will be ineffective.

Normal household and work-related arm activities are promoted to maintain muscle tone. Moving the arms actively during walking, keeping the operative site clean, avoiding injury to the hand and arm, and wearing loose, nonconstrictive clothing are all important aspects of patient education.

Improving Sexual Function. Any change in the patient's body image and self-esteem or the partner's response may increase the couple's anxiety level and are factors that may alter sexual function. Some partners have difficulty looking at the incision, whereas others seem to be unaffected and comfortable. Either response affects the patient's

CHART 46-4 *(continued)*

Patient Education: Postmastectomy Exercises

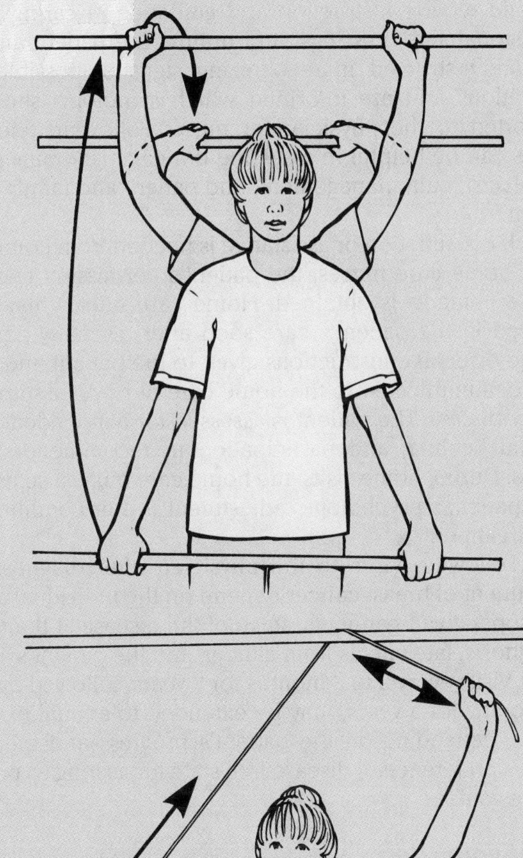

3. *Rod or broomstick lifting.* Grasp a rod with both hands, held about 2 feet apart. Keeping the arms straight, raise the rod over the head. Bend elbows to lower the rod behind the head. Reverse maneuver, raising the rod above the head, then return to the starting position.

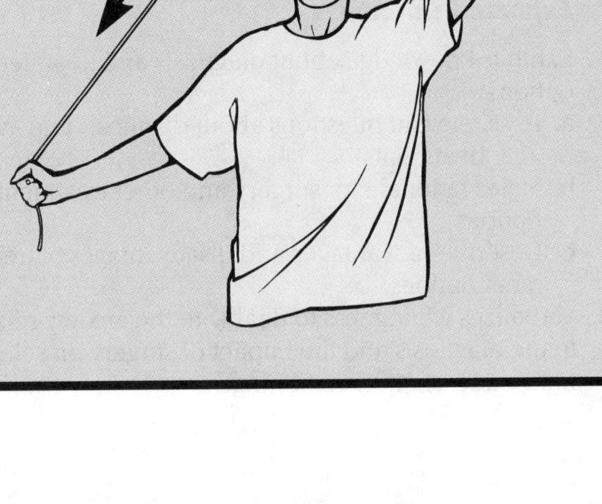

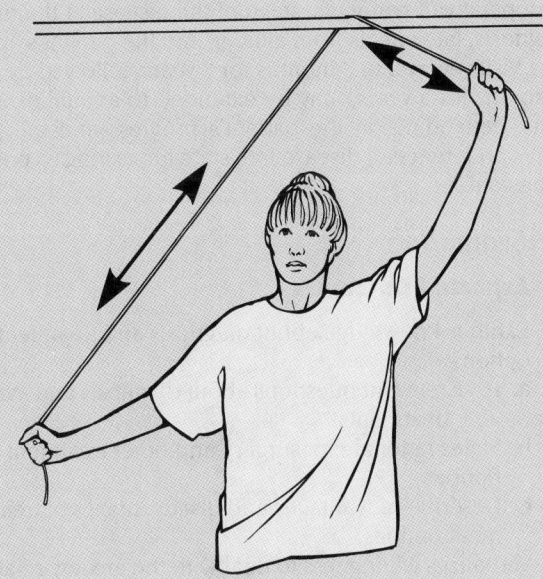

4. *Pulley tugging.* Toss a light rope over a shower curtain rod or doorway curtain rod. Stand as nearly under the rope as possible. Grasp an end in each hand. Extend the arms straight and away from the body. Pull the left arm up by tugging down with the right arm, then the right arm up and the left down in a see-sawing motion.

self-image, sexuality, and acceptance. Discussion about how the patient sees herself and about possible decreased libido related to fatigue, nausea, or anxiety may help clarify issues for her and her partner. Clarifying misconceptions (*i.e.*, that cancer can be transmitted sexually or by fondling) is important. Encouraging open discussion about fears, needs, and desires may reduce the couple's stress. Suggestions regarding varying the time of day for sexual activity (when the patient is least tired) or assuming positions that are most comfortable can be helpful, as are alternative options (*i.e.*, hugging, kissing, manual stimulation) for expressing affection.

Monitoring and Managing Potential Complications

Lymphedema. Lymphedema results if functioning lymphatic channels are inadequate to ensure a return flow of lymph to the general circulation. If axillary nodes and the lymph system were removed, a collateral or auxiliary system must take over their function. This usually occurs within a month's time and is facilitated by moving and exercising the arm. Postoperative education emphasizes the need to continue the exercise. Most patients do not develop massive lymphedema, especially if they are carefully instructed in and encouraged to elevate, massage, and exercise the affected arm for 3 to 4 months. Doing so will help prevent this disfiguring and possibly disabling swelling from developing. Patient education guidelines to avoid this problem are presented in Chart 46-5.

Positioning will help to promote venous lymphatic drainage. The affected arm is elevated to promote fluid drainage via the lymphatic and venous pathways. Lymphedema is usually prevented by each joint being positioned higher than the more proximal joint. If lymphedema occurs, its extent is usually related to the amount of collateral lymphatic channels removed during surgery. Functional recovery of arm and shoulder motion is promoted by performing limited exercise for the first 24 hours. Active range of motion exercise can usually begin on the third postoperative day.

CHART 46-5

Patient Education: Avoiding Lymphedema

Avoid burns while cooking or smoking (and avoid smoking, if possible).
Avoid sunburns.
Use an electric razor with a narrow head for underarm shaving to reduce the risk of nicking or scratching the skin.
Wash cuts promptly, treat them with antibacterial medication, and cover them with a sterile dressing; check often for redness, soreness, or other signs of infection.
Never cut cuticles; rather, use hand cream or lotion.
Wear protective gloves when gardening and when using strong detergents.
Use a thimble when sewing.
Avoid contact with harsh chemicals and abrasive compounds.
Use insect repellent to avoid bites and stings.
Avoid elastic cuffs and other restrictive devices on clothing.

If marked lymphedema occurs, the arm is elevated on a pillow so that the elbow is higher than the shoulder. The hand is elevated further to facilitate drainage. Elastic bandages and other constrictions are avoided because these may hinder formation of collateral lymphatic pathways. Some patients wear custom-made elastic sleeves from wrist to shoulder during active hours if necessary in cases of persistent swelling. Studies indicate that marked lymphedema occurs more commonly when a radical mastectomy is performed.

Patient Education and Home Care Considerations. The patient is often discharged within days of surgery and with drains still in place. In preparation for hospital discharge, the nurse needs to assess the patient's physical readiness to resume self-care. Additionally, the patient's psychologic status and emotional readiness for returning home and resuming previous activities and roles are evaluated. The patient and family caregiver, if available, should receive instruction and guidance in caring for the incisional site, dressings, and drains. The patient and family are instructed in recognizing signs of possible complications and are informed which symptoms should be reported to the physician or nurse. Follow-up telephone calls can be helpful in assessing drainage (if drains remain in place), pain management, and patient and family adjustment.

If consultation or assistance is needed from community and home care nurses, the patient's permission to initiate these contacts is obtained. Home care nurses may be involved in the patient's care soon after discharge; and the same discharge instructions given to the patient and family are communicated to the home care nurse to assure continuity of care. The patient is assessed for lymphedema, incisional healing, and participation in recommended exercises. During home visits, the home care nurse also assesses the patient's psychologic adjustment to her condition and the treatment.

Follow-up visits to the physician after diagnosis and treatment of breast cancer depend on the individual and on postoperative treatments, stage of the disease at the time of diagnosis, late effects from cancer, and the patient's adaptation. Visits every 2 to 3 months for 2 years, followed by every 6 months for 5 years, may be extended to annual examinations, depending on the patient's progress and the physician's preference. A disease-free state for as long as possible is the goal.

Evaluation

Expected Outcomes

1. Exhibits knowledge about diagnosis and treatment options
   a. Asks relevant questions about diagnosis and available treatments
   b. States rationale for surgery and other treatment options
   c. Describes advantages and disadvantages of treatment options
2. Verbalizes willingness to deal with the anxiety related to the diagnosis and the impact of surgery on self-image and sexual functioning

3. Reports that pain has decreased
4. Exhibits clean, dry, and intact surgical incision, without signs of inflammation
5. Participates actively in self-care activities
   a. Performs exercises as prescribed
   b. Participates in self-care activities within recommended limits
6. Discusses issues of sexuality and resumption of sexual function
7. Demonstrates knowledge of postdischarge recommendations and restrictions
   a. Describes follow-up care and activities
   b. Demonstrates appropriate care of incision and drains
8. Experiences no complications
   a. Identifies signs and symptoms of reportable complications (*i.e.*, redness, heat, pain, edema)
   b. Describes side effects of chemotherapy and strategies or measures to cope with such effects if they occur
   c. Takes care to avoid cuts, bruises, infection, and stress on hand and arm on affected side
   d. Explains how to contact appropriate care providers in case of complications

Care of the patient with breast cancer is summarized in Nursing Care Plan 46-1.

Nursing Management of the Patient With Advanced Breast Cancer

The patient with advanced breast cancer is monitored closely for signs that the tumor has recurred or that metastasis has occurred. The following studies are conducted in instances of inoperable breast cancer or extensive spread of the disease: metastatic x-ray series (chest, skull, long bones, and pelvis); liver function tests; mammogram of remaining breast tissue; and bone, liver, and brain imaging. In half of all patients with recurrent disease the cancer reappears in the local or regional lymph nodes, and in one fourth, other organs become involved. Bone involvement of the hips, spine, ribs, and pelvis may also occur.

Regression or relief of symptoms is the goal of nursing and medical management, with the quality of survival time an important focus of nursing intervention. Assessing the patient's physical and psychosocial status is a challenge for the nurse. Information from family members and significant others is valuable.

Palliative treatment, if necessary, is also an important aspect of care. Comfort and a pain-free existence, even if the disease cannot be eradicated, enhance the quality of remaining life. In patients with bone metastases that cause pain and decreased mobility, hospice and home health care may be indicated. Specific arrangements for these services may be planned and discussed early, before the actual need arises to decrease patient distress. Severe anxiety and depression may occur. Treatment modes vary and depend on the patient's condition and the modalities available. Chapter 16 provides more information on the general care of the patient with advanced cancer, including hospice care.

Reconstructive Breast Surgery

Hypertrophy of the Breast

Because breasts play such an important part in the self-image of many women, any perceived abnormality may lead to a request for surgical intervention. Variations in the size of the breasts are the most common reason for women to seek information about procedures to alter breast size. Breasts that are too large are called hypertrophied. If the enlargement occurs early in life, it is called virginal breast hypertrophy. The condition is usually bilateral, but may affect just one breast, also causing distress. Hypertrophy in later life almost always affects both breasts.

Symptoms of Breast Hypertrophy. Tenderness, diffuse pains, and fatigue are common complaints of women with this condition. Premenstrual tenderness and pain are marked. The weight of an enlarged breast causes a dragging sensation in the shoulder, and support is commonly futile, despite use of the most supportive bra. Many women have deep grooves in their shoulders from the weight borne by bra straps.

Discomfort and embarrassment when wearing bathing suits and participating in athletic events may be limiting and posture can also be affected. Social life can become restricted, with insecurity developing from poor self-image.

Mammoplasty

After a surgical or plastic surgery consultation, a **reduction mammoplasty** may be performed under general anesthesia. One approach is an incision beneath the breast and a similar curved incision in the skin of the anterior breast. The surgeon then removes excess tissue and transplants the nipple to a new location. Skin edges are approximated with sutures, and the nipple is secured with sutures. Drains are placed in the incision where they remain for 1 to 2 days. Simple gauze dressings are applied, without pressure.

Postoperative Nursing Interventions. After mammoplasty, usual postoperative nursing care is indicated. Patients are ambulatory fairly quickly and usually describe their surgery as nontraumatic, possibly because of the relief that they experience. Hypertrophy will not recur, but if the patient gains weight the breasts may enlarge. The newly transplanted nipple most likely will turn black and become scab-covered. As the nipple regains a new blood supply, the scab falls off and the appearance approximates normal. Lactation may be impossible after this type of surgery, although half of women who have this surgery can breast-feed successfully. Feelings postoperatively may be a mixture of euphoria, relief, sorrow over the loss of a body part, and anxiety over these feelings. Providing reassurance is an important nursing measure.

Surgery to Enlarge or Uplift the Breasts

Augmentation mammoplasty is requested fairly frequently and is performed through an incision along the undermargin

(text continues on page 1328)

NURSING CARE PLAN 46–1
Care of the Patient With Breast Cancer

NURSING DIAGNOSIS: Fear and ineffective coping related to the diagnosis of breast cancer, its treatment, and prognosis

GOAL: Reduction of emotional stress, fear, and anxiety

Nursing Interventions	Rationale	Expected Outcomes
1. Begin emotional preparation of the patient (and partner) as soon as she is informed of tentative diagnosis.	1. This enables the patient to initiate coping responses.	• Displays reduced emotional stress and anxiety and exhibits an ability to cope with the problem. • Participates in the treatment plan and asks questions relating to the best choice for her particular needs. • States that anger, anxiety, depression, denial, and withdrawal are normal reactions. • Responds positively to the information she has received. • Describes her appreciation of social support of family, friends, and women who have had breast surgery as a significant aid in coping with a stressful experience. • Is aware that partner has been advised and prepared with regard to supportive role. • Reads literature provided.
2. Assess a. Personal experience with and knowledge about breast cancer b. Coping mechanisms in crisis c. Support systems d. Affective state re: diagnosis	2. These factors strongly affect the patient's behavior and ability to deal with the diagnosis, surgery, and follow-up treatment. If a patient has lost close relatives or friends to breast cancer, she will probably react differently from a patient who has friends surviving with an excellent quality of life.	
3. Inform the patient of recent research and new treatment modalities for breast cancer.	3. Increasing options and improved results both statistically and cosmetically greatly reduce the fear and promote acceptance of the treatment plan.	
4. Describe the experiences the patient will face and encourage her questions.	4. Fear of the unknown decreases.	
5. Acquaint her with available resources to facilitate her recovery.	5. The information about new prosthetics, reconstruction specialists, and other resources confirms that a great deal of attention is being given to newer treatment methods for breast cancer.	

NURSING DIAGNOSIS: Disturbance in self-concept related to nature of surgery and side effects of radiation and/or chemotherapy

GOAL: Realistic adaptation to changes that will occur relative to treatment modalities

Nursing Interventions	Rationale	Expected Outcomes
1. Confirm with the physician the nature of the treatment anticipated.	1. This sets the basis for a cooperative therapeutic plan that will prevent conflicting information from reaching the patient.	• Decides on the treatment plan after discussing with physician and family. • Verbalizes that grief must run its course. • Uses her support system effectively; plans future activities with them. • Eventually looks at her incision site and participates in dressing changes. • Expresses an understanding of the long-term benefits of chemotherapy/radiation (if prescribed) even though there may be uncomfortable side effects.
2. Explain that it is normal to experience grief at the loss of a body part.	2. With this understanding, the patient can then be free to move to the next level of coping.	
3. Encourage visits by loved ones and understanding friends.	3. Support systems that are meaningful to the patient are more endurable than those from relative strangers.	
4. Explain that it is normal not to want herself or partner to view the incision (do not refer to this as a "scar"); further reinforce the fact that each day the site will look better.	4. This reduces the feeling that she will never be able to accept her altered body.	
5. Discuss the use of prosthesis, reconstruction possibilities, and clothing adjustment as realistic and attainable expectations.	5. The emphasis on the positive and the availability of adaptations will enhance her self-concept and promote positive acceptance of the treatment plan.	

(continued)

NURSING CARE PLAN 46–1 *(continued)*
Care of the Patient With Breast Cancer

NURSING DIAGNOSIS: Pain related to tissue trauma from incision(s)

GOAL: Absence of pain and discomfort

Nursing Interventions	Rationale	Expected Outcomes
1. Assess intensity, nature, and location of pain.	1. Provides baseline to assess effectiveness of pain-relief measures.	• Reports when pain is worsening and accepts prescribed pain medication.
2. Administer analgesia by IM, oral, or IV route as prescribed.	2. Promotes pain relief.	• Adjusts her position to relieve discomfort; uses small pillows effectively.
3. Collaborate with physician about use of patient-controlled analgesia (PCA).	3. Patient-controlled analgesia results in pain relief and increased comfort and maintains patient's sense of control.	• Exercises frequently; moves affected arm gently and shows progress in moving from passive to active exercises.
4. Explain that analgesics are available for pain relief.	4. Analgesics and narcotics can interrupt nerve pathways to the brain and spinal cord.	• Describes home-related activities that will provide the required range of motion of the affected arm.
5. Proper body positioning will promote comfort, such as semi-Fowler's position and elevation of the arm of the affected side.	5. Stress on the incision site is reduced; gravity reduces fluid accumulation in the arm. (Squeezing ball and wrist flexion begin in first 24 hours.)	• Relates procedures to follow if accidental injury is sustained.
6. Promote passive and then active exercises of the hand, arm, and shoulder of the affected side.	6. This will stimulate circulation, promote neurovascular competence, and prevent stasis and subsequent stiffening of the shoulder girdle.	• Orders medical identification tags when arm lymphedema is diagnosed.
7. Encourage protection and the avoidance of anything that can break through the skin barrier to impose stress on the arm and shoulder (cuts, burns, strong detergents, infections, carrying a heavy bag or purse).	7. Impaired circulation and weakened nerves are vulnerable to sudden or prolonged stress.	
8. Suggest application of an effective cream several times a day.	8. This practice will keep the skin healthy, intact, pliable, and resistant to breakdown.	
9. Instruct patient to contact the physician if the arm or incision site becomes painful, swollen, or red.	9. Early treatment of possible infection or injury will avoid further discomfort and complications.	
10. Suggest wearing a medical identification tag if there is a potential for injury or edema.	10. A recognized medical identification tag will serve as a precaution against injury to the affected arm.	

NURSING DIAGNOSIS: Self-care deficit related to partial immobility of upper extremity on side of breast surgery

GOAL: Avoidance of impaired mobility and achievement of self-care to the fullest possible level

Nursing Interventions	Rationale	Expected Outcomes
1. Encourage patient's active participation in postoperative care.	1. Patient involvement enhances and facilitates the recovery process.	• Participates in dressing change; expresses interest in working with rehabilitative team including physical therapist.
2. Encourage patient's socialization, particularly with others who have successfully recovered in similar circumstances.	2. Humans thrive more effectively and happily when they are able to relate to others socially.	• Shows concern about her appearance and accepts suggestions from rehabilitation support groups.
3. Make progressive modifications in the patient's exercise program as dictated by comfort and tolerance levels.	3. There is lessened strain on tissues; improvement is consistent.	• Participates in self-care (*i.e.,* dressing, bathing, grooming).
4. Commend the patient when ingenuity and creativity are in evidence, such as an attractive hair style or make-up application.	4. Psychologic well-being complements the effects of optimal physical good health.	• Verbalizes anticipation and enjoyment of partner's visits and relates her progress.

(*continued*)

NURSING CARE PLAN 46–1 *(continued)*
Care of the Patient With Breast Cancer

NURSING DIAGNOSIS: Possible sexual dysfunction related to loss of body part and fear of partner's reaction to this loss

GOAL: Identification of alternative satisfying/acceptable sexual experiences

Nursing Interventions	Rationale	Expected Outcomes
1. Become comfortable in discussing sexuality; display a caring, nonjudgmental, supportive attitude.	1. The patient will easily sense insincerity, insecurity, lack of knowledge, and inexperience. Nurses new to this area can obtain assistance from the oncology clinical nurse specialist.	• Responds by conveying trust and a desire to obtain assistance; asks appropriate questions. • Includes partner in aspects of the medical problem that concern both.
2. Encourage, at the appropriate time, both partners to discuss their concerns; this can be done before and after major treatment.	2. The patient will not feel that she is alone in facing problems that may concern both partners.	• Accepts the incision site as evidenced by assisting with dressings and using an appropriate prescribed emollient such as cocoa butter.
3. Arrange for privacy when discussing personal problems with the patient.	3. Sensitive personal problems are not revealed when people not close to the patient are present.	• Expresses awareness that any adjustments take time but that with patience and understanding, the desired goals can be approached and possibly reached.
4. Describe the incision site and its appearance to the partner before partner actually sees it.	4. Partner will know what to expect and not likely register shock in front of the patient.	
5. Emphasize that behavioral changes take time and should not be interpreted as rejection.	5. The very nature of undergoing any surgery takes time for acceptance, recuperation, and perhaps altered lifestyle.	

COLLABORATIVE PROBLEM: Infection, injury, lymphedema, neurovascular deficits

GOAL: Avoidance of complications

Nursing Interventions	Rationale	Expected Outcomes
1. Encourage the elevation of the arm, if not contraindicated, with each joint positioned higher than the more proximal joint.	1. Edema is reduced and there is less pressure on the nerves and blood vessels; pain and discomfort are reduced.	• Demonstrates how to place pillows so that proper elevation of arm is maintained. • Describes strategies for avoiding injury and infection.
2. Inform patient to avoid injury, strenuous activity, or infection.	2. These can stimulate fluid accumulation and compromise the neurovasculature of the arm.	• Gradually moves the arm freely so that hair combing and "climbing the wall" can be achieved with no discomfort. Avoids the discomfort of a frozen shoulder.
3. Describe and demonstrate exercises in a step-up fashion from simple to more involved.	3. A graduated exercise program will improve muscle tone and hasten full range of activities with avoidance of impairment such as a frozen shoulder.	• Acquires good health habits and avoids complications.
4. Recommend physical therapy and a weight-reduction program if indicated.	4. Properly prescribed activities and exercise plus diet modification are general health measures that enhance well-being and thwart complications.	

of the breast, in the axilla, or at the border of the areola. The breast is then elevated and a pocket is formed between the breast and the chest wall into which various types of synthetic materials are inserted to enlarge and uplift the breast. These procedures may be performed on an outpatient basis with local anesthesia by an experienced plastic surgeon. Complications that may occur (*e.g.*, infection) may require subsequent removal of the implant.

Silicone implants have been used in the past; however, because of reported systemic complications associated with their use, they have been removed from the market. They are now available only to women enrolled in controlled clinical trials designed to study specific safety questions. Long-term risks associated with their use are also being studied. Saline implants may be utilized. Women need to be aware that accurate mammograms are particularly difficult with implants because the implants obscure breast tissue.

Reconstructive Procedures

The choice of surgical procedure for reconstruction is based on the condition of the overlying skin and underlying muscle. Nipple reconstruction may be performed separately. Surgical procedures are described in Figs. 46-6 and 46-7.

Tissue expanders may be used. An empty Silastic bag is inserted during surgery and a small tube remains outside the breast. Small amounts of normal saline solution are injected over several weeks; the tissue expander then is replaced by a permanent implant. Long-term effects of these implants are also unknown.

Flap surgery is another option. The transrectus abdominal muscle is cut to form a flap, which will accommodate a large breast reconstruction. The loss of abdominal muscle is a potential problem. If the latissimus dorsi is used, the amount of muscle used is smaller, and so it is less likely to be troublesome. A gluteal flap from the buttocks is another option. All choices involve the risk imposed by any surgery, including bleeding and infection.

Postoperative Nursing Management. Suction tubes are inserted and connected to closed drainage. Measures to reduce tension on the incisions include elevating the head of the bed by 30 degrees and flexing the patient's knees to reduce tension on an abdominal incision. Antiemetics are administered to control nausea and vomiting; and analgesics are administered to reduce pain and discomfort. Assessing circulation by observing the color and temperature of the newly reconstructed breast area is an important nursing function. Mottling or an obvious decrease in skin temperature is reported to the surgeon immediately. Drainage of more than 50 ml should also be reported.

During ambulation on the first postoperative day, the patient will usually protect the surgical incision by splinting. Gradually, she will achieve a more upright position. The patient will be advised to avoid bras and breast massage until the physician indicates that no injury will result. Elevating the arms above the shoulder and lifting more than 5 lb are avoided for 1 month postoperatively to avoid stress on the incision.

Prophylactic Mastectomy

Some women who are at high risk for breast cancer may elect to undergo prophylactic mastectomy. Possible candidates are women who have a strong family history and very cystic breasts, previous cancer in one breast and progressive nodularity in the other, lumpy breasts and a suspicious mammogram, atypical hyperplasia discovered on a previous biopsy, cystic breast changes requiring several biopsies, or extreme fear of breast cancer.

Diseases of the Male Breast

Gynecomastia

Gynecomastia or overdeveloped breast tissue in the male is the most common male breast condition. Adolescent males can be affected by this condition because of hormones secreted by the testes. Gynecomastia usually

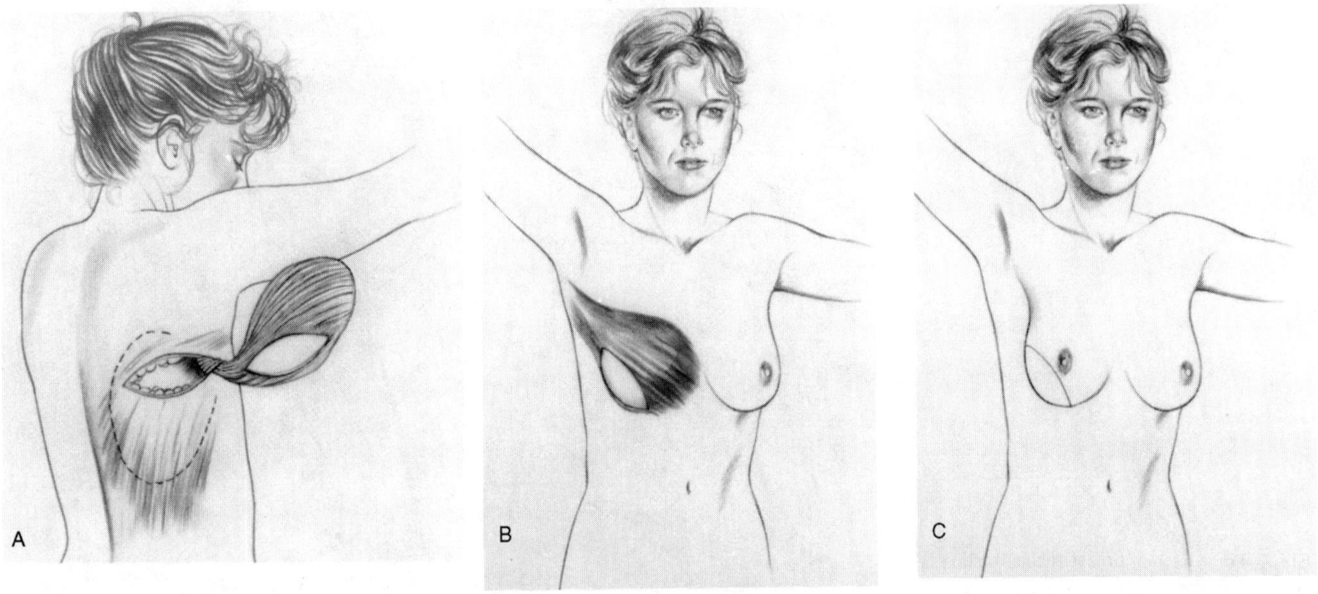

An elliptical incision identifies the skin tissue (island) that will be attached to dissected latissimus dorsi muscle (dissected underneath skin in area of dotted line). This muscle and skin flap are then threaded through a tunnel under the skin (subaxillary) and brought out at the breast site.

Flap in place after being tunneled from back to front of the chest.

Flap is in place re-creating breast contour with reconstructed nipple and areola.

FIGURE 46-6. Breast reconstruction: myocutaneous flap procedure using the latissimus dorsi muscle. (Adapted from The Breast Cancer Digest, 2nd ed. Bethesda, MD, U.S. Department of Health and Human Services, Public Health Service.)

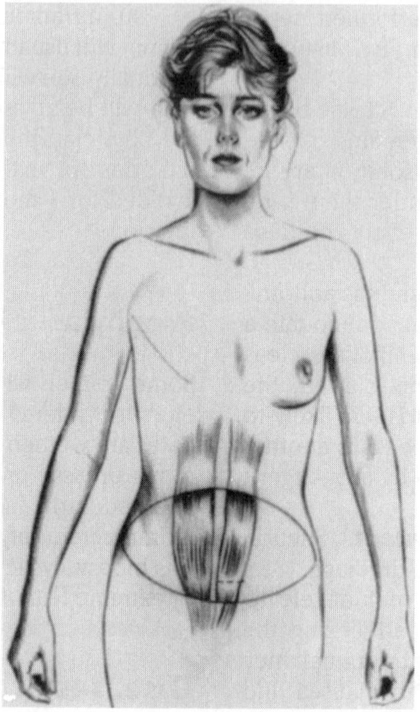

An elliptical lower abdominal incision is made, and one of two vertical abdominal muscles is cut.

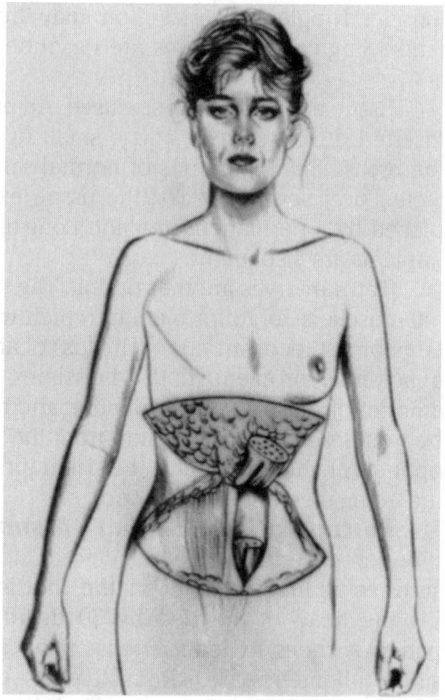

The skin flap including muscle and fat is tunneled under the skin of the upper abdominal area and lower chest to the breast site.

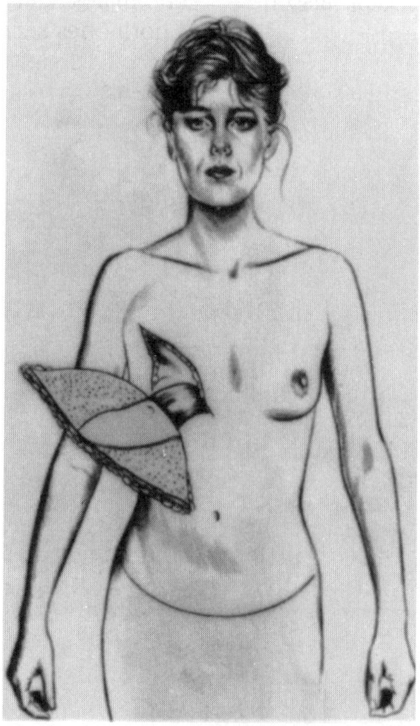

The flap will be positioned and molded to the contour of the breast. Blood supply continues with the flap.

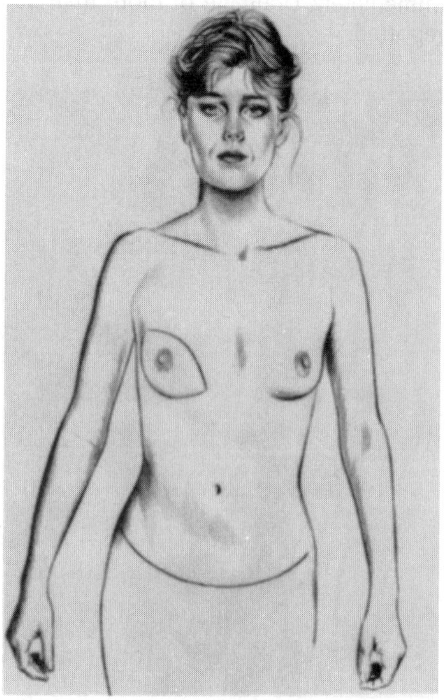

With the flap and a reconstructed nipple and areola in place, the breast contour is recreated.

FIGURE 46-7. Breast reconstruction: Myocutaneous flap procedure using the abdominis rectus muscle. (Adapted from The Breast Cancer Digest, 2nd ed. Bethesda, MD, U.S. Department of Health and Human Services, Public Health Service.)

CRITICAL THINKING EXERCISES

1. Your 35-year-old patient has just been diagnosed with breast cancer. Her mother, aunt, and one of her sisters have all had breast cancer. She is very worried about her own children's well-being and future. Describe the teaching proigram you feel is indicated for this patient and her children.
2. A 52-year-old woman reports to you that she has never had a mammogram and is afraid to have one done. How would you respond to her and what teaching would you provide?
3. You are assigned to two patients undergoing surgery for the treatment of breast cancer. One is scheduled for a lumpectomy; the other is to have a modified radical mastectomy. How would your nursing assessment and management differ for these two patients?

subsides in 1 or 2 years, but it can occur before or after puberty. It is usually unilateral and presents as a firm, tender mass beneath the areola. In adult males, gynecomastia may be diffuse and related to medications (*i.e.*, digitalis, reserpine, ergotamine, and phenytoin). Pain and tenderness are initial symptoms.

Male Breast Cancer

Cancer of the male breast accounts for 1% of all breast cancers. Symptoms can include a painless lump beneath the areola, nipple retraction, and skin ulceration. Average age at the time of diagnosis is 60 years. Diagnostic and treatment modalities are similar to those used for women. Risk factors may include history of mumps orchitis, radiation exposure, and Klinefelter's syndrome (a chromosomal condition reflecting decreased testosterone levels).

Because detection usually occurs well into the disease, treatment generally consists of a radical mastectomy because the pectoral muscles are involved. Radiation therapy may be used postoperatively. Prognosis varies depending on stage of disease at the time of detection. Bone and soft tissue are usually the most common sites of advanced disease and metastasis. Orchidectomy (removal of the testes), adrenalectomy (removal of an adrenal gland) and hypophysectomy (removal of the pituitary gland) may be used in advanced disease.

BIBLIOGRAPHY

Books

American Cancer Society. Cancer Facts and Figures 1994. Atlanta, American Cancer Society, 1994.

Bates B. A Guide to Physical Examination, 6th ed. Philadelphia, JB Lippincott, 1995.

Baum M, Saunders C and Meredith S. Breast Cancer: A Guide for Every Woman. New York, Oxford University Press, 1994.

Berger KJ and Bostwick J III. A Woman's Decision: Breast Care, Treatment and Reconstruction. St. Louis, Quality Medical Publisher, 1994.

Cancer Statistics 1995. Atlanta, GA, American Cancer Society.

Drukker B. The Evaluation of Conditions of the Breast. Woodbury, CT, Cine-Med Inc., for American College of Obstetricians and Gynecologists, 1993.

Fogel C and Lauver D. Sexual Health Promotion. Philadelphia, WB Saunders, 1990.

Greenwald P, Kramer BS and Weed DL. Cancer Prevention and Control. New York, Marcel Dekker, 1995.

Groenwald S. Cancer Nursing: Principles and Practices. Boston, Jones and Bartlett, 1993.

Holland J and Rowland J. Handbook of Psychooncology. New York, Oxford University Press, 1989.

Love SM. Dr. Susan Love's Breast Book. Reading, MA, Addison-Wesley, 1995.

Mansel RE (ed). Recent Developments in the Study of Benign Breast Disease: The Proceedings of the 5th International Symposium on Benign Breast Disease. New York, Parthenon, 1994.

Miaskowsi C (ed). Oncology Nursing. Albany, Delmar Publishers, 1995.

O'Grady LF. A Practical Approach to Breast Disease. Boston, Little, Brown, 1995.

Packer SH and Jobe WE. Percutaneous Breast Biopsy. New York, Raven Press, 1993.

Powell DE and Stelling CB. The Diagnosis and Detection of Breast Disease. St. Louis, Mosby, 1994.

Wise L and Johnson H Jr (eds). Breast Cancer: Controversies in Management. Armonk, NY, Futura Pub. 1994.

Journals

Asterisks indicate nursing research articles.

General

Baird S. Benign breast disease: Meeting women's needs. Innovations in Oncol Nurs 1993; 9(3):1–19.

*Benedict S, Williams RD and Baron PL. Recalled anxiety: From discovery to diagnosis of a benign breast mass. Oncol Nurs Forum 1994 Nov–Dec; 21(10):1723–1727.

*Benedict S, Williams RD and Baron PL. The effect of benign breast biopsy on subsequent breast cancer detection practices. Oncol Nurs Forum 1994 Oct; 21(9):1467–1475.

Berkell H, Birdsel DL, and Jenkins H. Breast augmentation: A risk factor for breast cancer? N Engl J Med 1992; 326(25):1623–1649.

Conry C. Evaluation of a breast complaint: Is it cancer? Am Fam Physician 1994 Feb 1; 49(2):445–450.

Edge D and Segatore M. Assessment and management of galactorrhea. Nurse Pract 1993 June; 18(6):35–49.

*Henquin N, Trostler N and Horn Y. Nutritional risk factors and breast cancer in Jewish and Arab women. Cancer Nurs 1994 Aug; 17(4):326–333.

Link JS. Benign breast disease. Nurse Practitioner Forum 1993 Jun; 4(2):96–99.

Marchant DJ (ed). Contemporary management of breast disease I: Benign disease. 1994 Sep; 21(3):421–554.

Merkatz B. Gel-filled breast implants: an update. Contemp Ob Gyn 1992 July; 37(7):31–41.

National Conference on Gynecologic Cancers. Cancer 1993; Suppl 71(4).

Schumann D. Health risks for women with breast implants. Nurse Practitioner: Am J Primary Health Care 1994 Jul; 19(7):19–20, 23–25, 29–30.

Prevention, Breast Self-Examination, and Mammography

Brown LW and Williams RD. Culturally sensitive breast cancer screening programs for older Black women. Nurse Practitioner: Am J Primary Health Care 1994 Mar; 21, 25–26, 31.

*Champion VL. Beliefs about breast cancer and mammography by behavioral stage. Oncol Nurs Forum 1994 Jul; 21(6): 1009–1014.

Champion V and Scott C. Effects of a procedural/belief intervention on breast self-examination performance. Res Nurs Health 1993; 16:163–170.

Harris R and Leininger L. Clinical strategies for breast cancer screening: Weighing and using the evidence. Ann Intern Med 1995 Apr 1; 122(7):539–547.

Houldin A and Lowery B. Emotional distress in breast cancer patients. Med-Surg Nurs Q 1992 Fall; 1(2):1–26.

Kuhrik NS et al. Evaluating women with fibrocystic breast condition. Am J Nurs 1994 Jul; 94(7):16 A–D.

Lauver D. Identifying women's descriptions of breast tissue for the promotion of breast self examination. Health Care Women Int 1991 Jan/Mar; 12(1):73–83.

Lauver D. Psychosocial variables, race and intention to seek care for breast cancer syptoms. Nurs Res 1992 Jul–Aug; 41(4): 236–241.

*Lauver D. Care-seeking behavior with breast cancer symptoms in Caucasian and African-American women. Res Nurs Health 1994 Dec; 17(6):421–431.

Leslie NS et al. Evaluation of a breast examination facilitation device. J Adv Nurs 1995 Jan; 21(1):28–33.

*Lierman LM et al. Effects of education and support on breast self-examination in older women. Nurs Res 1994 May/Jun; 43(3): 158–163.

*Lierman LM et al. Using social support to promote breast self-examination performance. Oncol Nurs Forum 1994 Jul; 21(6):1051–1057.

Mettlin C and Smart CR. Breast cancer detection guidelines for women aged 40 to 49 years: Rationale for the American Cancer Society reaffirmation of recommendations. CA Cancer J Clin 1994 Jul–Aug; 44(4):249–255.

*Shaw CR, Wilson SA and O'Brien ME. Information needs prior to breast biopsy. Clin Nurs Res 1994 May; 3(2):119–131.

Stratton B et al. Breast self exam proficiency. J Woman's Health 1994 Jun; 3(3):185–195.

Vogel V. Mammographic screening in younger women. Female Patient 1993 May; 18(5):21–27.

*Walcott-McQuigg JA, Logan B and Smith E. Prevention health practices of African American women. J Nat Black Nurses Assoc 1994; 7(1):25–35.

Zapka JG et al. Effect of a community health center intervention on breast cancer screening among Hispanic American women. Health Serv Res 1993 Jun; 28(2):223–235.

Zapka JG et al. Impact of a breast cancer screening community intervention. Prev Med 1993 Jun; 22(1):34–53.

Cancer

Baron RH and Walsh A. Nine facts everyone should know about breast cancer. Am J Nurs 1995 Jul; 95(7):29–33.

Boothe VA et al. Tamoxifen in the treatment and prevention of breast cancer. Cancer Pract 1994 Sep–Oct; 2(5):335–342.

Breen N and Kessler L. Changes in the use of screening mammography: Evidence from the 1987 and 1990 National Health Interview Surveys. Am J Public Health 1994 Jan; 84(1): 62–67.

Danforth D. How subsequent pregnancy affects women with a prior history of breast cancer. Oncology 1991; 5(11):23–30.

*Dow KH, Harris JR, and Roy C. Pregnancy after breast-conserving surgery and radiation therapy for breast cancer. J Natl Cancer Inst 1994; 16:131–137.

Dow KH. Having children after breast cancer. Cancer Pract 1994 Nov–Dec; 2(6):407–413.

Eberlin TJ. Current management of carcinoma of the breast. Ann Surg 1994 Aug; 220(2):121–136.

Ganz PA. Advocating for the woman with breast cancer. CA Cancer J Clin 1995 Mar–Apr; 45(2):114–126.

Harris J et al. Breast cancer, Part 1. N Engl J Med 1992 Jul 30; 327(5): 319–327. Part 2. 1992 Aug 6; 327(6): 390–397. Part 3. 1992 Aug 13; 327(7): 473–480.

Jaiyesimi I et al. Carcinoma of the male breast. Ann Intern Med 1992 Nov; 117(9):771–777.

Johnson JR. Caring for the woman who's had a mastectomy. Am J Nurs 1994 May; 94(5):25–31.

Kiefe CI et al. Is cost a barrier to screening mammography for low income women receiving Medicare benefits? A randomized trial. Arch Intern Med 1994 June 13; 154(11):1217–1224.

Knobf MT. Treatment options for early stage breast cancer. Medsurg Nurs 1994 Aug; 3(4):249–259, 328.

Knobf MT. Decision-making for primary breast cancer treatment. Medsurg Nurs 1994 Jun; 3(3):169–175, 180.

Lauver D and Tak Y. Optimism and coping with a breast cancer symptom. Nurs Res 1995 Jul/Aug; 44(4):202–207.

Marchant DJ (ed). Contemporary management of breast disease II: Breast cancer. 1994 Dec; 21(4):555–804.

Morrow M. Breast disease in elderly women. Surg Clin North Am 1994 Feb; 74(1):145–161.

Nielsen B and East D. Advances in breast cancer: Implications for care. Nurs Clin North Am 1990 June; 25(2):365–375.

*Northouse LL et al. Emotional distress reported by women and husbands prior to a breast biopsy. Nurs Res 1995 Jul/Aug; 44(4):196–201.

Perez-Stable EJ et al. Self-reported use of cancer screening tests among Latinos and Anglos in a prepaid health plan. Arch Intern Med 1994 May; 154(11):1217–1224.

*Pierce P. Deciding on breast cancer treatment: A description of decision behavior. Nurs Res 1993 Jan–Feb; 42(1):22–28.

Speroff L. The risk of breast cancer associated with oral contraception and hormone replacement therapy. Women Health Iss 1992 Summer; 2(2):63–74.

Stommel M, Given CW, and Given B. The cost of cancer home care to families. Cancer 1991 Mar; 71(5):1867–1874.

Vinokur A et al. The process of recovery from breast cancer for younger and older patients: Changes during the first year. Cancer 1990 Mar; 65:1242–1254.

Zapka JG et al. Breast cancer screening by mammography: Utilization and associated factors. Am J Public Health 1989 Nov; 79(11):1499–1502.

Surgical Treatment of Breast Cancer

Carlson GW. Breast reconstruction. Surgical options and patient selection. Cancer. 1994 Jul 1; 74(1 Suppl):436–439.

Giomuso CB and Suster V. Free flap breast reconstruction. Medsurg Nurs 1994 Feb; 3(1):9–24.

Granda C. Nursing management of patients with lymphedema associated with breast cancer therapy. Cancer Nurs 1994 Jun; 17(3):229–235.

Harden JT and Girard N. Breast reconstruction using an innovative flap procedure. AORN J 1994 Aug; 60(2):184–192.

Kiebert GM, de Haes JC, and van de Velde CJ. The impact of breast-conserving treatment and mastectomy on the quality of life of early-stage breast cancer patients: A review. J Clin Oncol 1991; 1059–1070.

Love S. Breast removal and reconstruction. Harvard Medical School Health Letter 1990 Feb; 15(4):3–6.

Chemotherapy

Gould K, Gates ML and Miaskowski C. Breast cancer prevention: A summary of chemoprevention trial with tamoxifen. Oncol Nurs Forum 1994 Jun; 21(5):835–840.

Jaiyesimi IA et al. Use of tamoxifen for breast cancer: Twenty-eight years later. J Clin Oncol 1995 Feb; 13(2):513–529.

*Mock V et al. A nursing rehabilitation program for women with breast cancer receiving adjuvant chemotherapy. Oncol Nurs Forum 1994 Jun; 21(5):899–908.

Rogers BB. Taxol: A promising new drug of the '90s. Oncol Nurs Forum 1993 Nov–Dec; 20(10):1483–1489.

*Ward S et al. Patient's reactions to completion of adjuvant breast cancer therapy. Nurs Res 1992; 41(6):362–366.

Radiation Therapy

*Christman N. Uncertainty and adjustment during radiotherapy. Nurs Res 1990 Jan/Feb; 39(1):17–47.

*Harrison-Woermke DE and Graydon JE. Perceived informational needs of breast cancer patients receiving radiation therapy after excisional biopsy and axillary node dissection. Cancer Nurs 1993 Dec; 16(6):449–455.

Mast D and Wood D. Preparing patients with breast cancer for brachytherapy. Oncol Nurs Forum 1990 Feb; 17(2):267–270.

Pierce S and Harris J. The role of radiation therapy in the management of primary breast cancer. Ca 1991 Mar/Apr; 41(2):85–96.

Strohl R. Radiation therapy: Recent advances and nursing implications. Nurs Clin North Am 1990 June; 25(2):309–328.

Pregnancy and Breast Cancer

Baron RH. Dispelling the myths of pregnancy-associated breast cancer. Oncol Nurs Forum 1994 Apr; 21(3):507–512.

Dow KH. Breast cancer and fertility. NAACOG's Clinical Issues in Perinatal and Women's Health Nursing 1990; 1(4):444–452.

Larkin K. Cancer and pregnancy. NAACOG's Clinical Issues in Perinatal and Women's Health Nursing 1990;1(2):255–261.

Petrek JA. Breast cancer during pregnancy. Cancer 1994 Jul 1; 74(1 suppl):518–527.

Petrek JA. Pregnancy safety after breast cancer. Cancer. 1994 Jul 1; 74(1 suppl):528–531.

Preftakes DK. Breast cancer and pregnancy: Implications for perinatal care and fetal outcomes. J Perinatal Neonatal Nurs 1994 Mar; 7(4):31–41.

Geriatric Considerations

Castiglione M, Gelber R, and Goldhirsch A. Adjuvant systemic therapy for breast cancer in the elderly. J Clin Oncol 1990 Mar; 8(3):519–526

Fanciosa D and Shaw SLJ. Breast cancer and benign breast disease in men. Nurse Practitioner Forum 1994 Mar; 5(1):56–58.

Hecht JR and Winchester DJ. Male breast cancer. Am J Clin Pathol 1994 Oct; 102(4 Suppl 1):S25–S30.

Wagner JL et al. Carcinoma of the male breast: Update 1994. Med Pediatr Oncol 1995 Feb; 24(2):123–132.

Psychologic Aspects of Breast Cancer and Its Treatment

Carlsson M and Hamrin E. Psychological and psychosocial aspects of breast cancer and breast cancer treatment: A literature review. Cancer Nurs 1994 Oct; 17(5):418–428.

Ferrans CE. Quality of life through the eyes of survivors of breast cancer. Oncol Nurs Forum 1994 Nov–Dec; 21(10):1645–1651.

*Graydon JE. Women with breast cancer: Their quality of life following a course of radiation therapy. J Advanced Nurs 1994 Apr; 19(4):617–622.

*Freedman TG. Social and cultural dimensions of hair loss in women treated for breast cancer. Cancer Nurs 1994 Aug; 17(4):334–341.

*Halstead MT and Fernsler JI. Coping strategies of long-term cancer survivors. Cancer Nurs 1994 Apr; 17(2):94–100.

*Hilton BA. Family communication patterns in coping with early breast cancer. West J Nurs Res 1994 Aug; 16(4):366–391.

Loveys BJ and Klaich K. Breast cancer: Demands of illness. Oncol Nurs Forum 1991 Jan–Feb; 18(1):75–80.

Schag CA et al. Characteristics of women at risk for psychosocial distress in the year after breast cancer. J Clin Oncol 1993 Apr; 11(4):783–793.

*Wyatt G, Kurtz ME and Liken M. Breast cancer survivors: An exploration of quality of life issues. Cancer Nurs 1993 Dec; 16(6):440–448.

Breast Surgery

Fowler ME. Body contouring surgery. Nurs Clin North Am 1994 Dec; 29(4):753–761.

Mangan MA. Current concepts in breast reconstruction. Nurs Clin North Am 1994 Dec; 29(4):763–776.

Oberle K and Allen M. Breast augmentation surgery: A woman's health issue. J Adv Nurs 1994 Nov; 20(5):844–852.

INFORMATION/RESOURCES

Agencies

American Cancer Society
1599 Clifton Road, NE,
Atlanta, GA 30329-4251
(404) 320-3333
(Extensive professional and patient literature is available, including booklets on reconstruction, radiation, and chemotherapy.)

National Alliance of Breast Cancer Organizations
1180 Avenue of the Americas, 2nd Floor,
New York, NY 10036
(212) 719-0154

National Breast Cancer Coalition
P.O. Box 98114,
Washington, DC 20007-7374
(An activist group that has raised funds and consciousness levels regarding breast cancer and was instrumental in obtaining funds for research on prevention.)

National Cancer Institute
Public Inquiry Section, Office of Cancer Communications, National Cancer Institute, Building 31, Room 10 A 24,
Bethesda, MD 20892
(Patient materials can be ordered on the following topics: biopsies, treatment options, mastectomy, radiation, chemotherapy, reconstruction, diet, and clinical trials.)

Reach to Recovery Program—I Can Cope Program
(Information available through local American Cancer Society chapters.)

Y-ME Breast Cancer Support Program
1757 Ridge Road,
Homewood, IL 60430

47

Assessment and Management of Patients With Disorders of the Male Reproductive System

CHAPTER OUTLINE

LEARNING OBJECTIVES

On completion of this chapter, the learner will be able to:

1. Describe anatomy and function of the male reproductive system
2. Discuss nursing assessment of the male reproductive system and identify diagnostic tests that complement assessment
3. Discuss the causes and management of male sexual dysfunction
4. Compare the four types of prostatectomy with regard to advantages and disadvantages
5. Use the nursing process as a framework for care of the patient undergoing prostatectomy
6. Describe the nursing management of patients with cancer of the male reproductive organs
7. Describe the various conditions affecting the testes and penis, their pathophysiology, clinical manifestations, and management

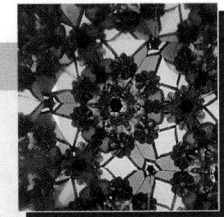

Anatomy and Physiology

In the male, several organs serve as parts of both the urinary tract and the reproductive system.

Disorder in the male reproductive organs may interfere with the functions of either or both systems. As a result, diseases of the male reproductive system are usually treated by a urologist. The structures in the male reproductive system are the testes, the vas deferens (ductus deferens) and the seminal vesicles, the penis, and certain accessory glands, such as the prostate gland and Cowper's gland (bulbourethral gland) (Fig. 47-1).

Testicular Development. The **testes** are formed in the embryo within the abdominal cavity near the kidney. During the last month of fetal life, they descend posterior to the peritoneum, to pierce the abdominal wall in the groin. Later they progress along the inguinal canal into the scrotum. In this descent they are accompanied by blood vessels, lymphatics, nerves, and ducts, which support the tissue and make up the spermatic cord. This cord extends from the internal inguinal ring through the abdominal wall and the inguinal canal to the scrotum. As the testes descend into the scrotum, a tubular extension of peritoneum accompanies them. Normally this tissue is obliterated, the only remaining portion being that which covers the testes, the **tunica vaginalis.** (When this peritoneal process is not obliterated but remains open into the abdominal cavity, a potential sac remains, into which abdominal contents may enter to form an indirect inguinal hernia.)

The testes are encased in the scrotum, which keeps them at a slightly lower temperature than the rest of the body to facilitate **spermatogenesis** (production of sperm). The testes consist of numerous seminiferous tubules in which the spermatozoa form. Collecting tubules transmit the spermatozoa into the epididymis, a hoodlike structure lying on the testes and containing winding ducts that lead into the vas deferens. This firm, tubular structure passes upward through the inguinal canal to enter the abdominal cavity behind the peritoneum and then extends downward toward the base of the bladder. An outpouching from this structure is the **seminal vesicle,** which acts as a reservoir for testicular secretions. The tract is continued as the ejaculatory duct, which then passes through the prostate gland to enter the **urethra.** Testicular secretions take this pathway as they exit the penis in the reproductive act.

Glandular Function. The testes have a dual function: the formation of spermatozoa from the germinal cells of the seminiferous tubules and the secretion of male sex hormone, **testosterone,** which induces and preserves the male sex characteristics.

The **prostate gland** lies just below the neck of the bladder. It surrounds the urethra and is traversed by the ejaculatory duct, a continuation of the vas deferens. This gland produces a secretion that is chemically and physiologically suitable to the needs of the spermatozoa in their passage from the testes.

The **Cowper's gland** lies below the prostate within the posterior aspect of the urethra. This gland empties its secretions into the urethra at the time of ejaculation, providing lubrication.

The **penis** has a dual function: it is the organ for copulation and for urination. Anatomically, it consists of a glans penis, a body, and a root. The glans penis is the soft, rounded portion at the distal end of the penis. The urethra, the tube that carries urine, opens at the tip of the glans. Normally, the glans is covered or protected by elongated penile skin—the foreskin—which may be retracted to expose the glans. The body of the penis is composed of erectile tissues containing numerous blood vessels that become distended, leading to an erection during sexual excitement. The **urethra,** which passes through the penis, extends from the bladder through the prostate to the distal end of the penis.

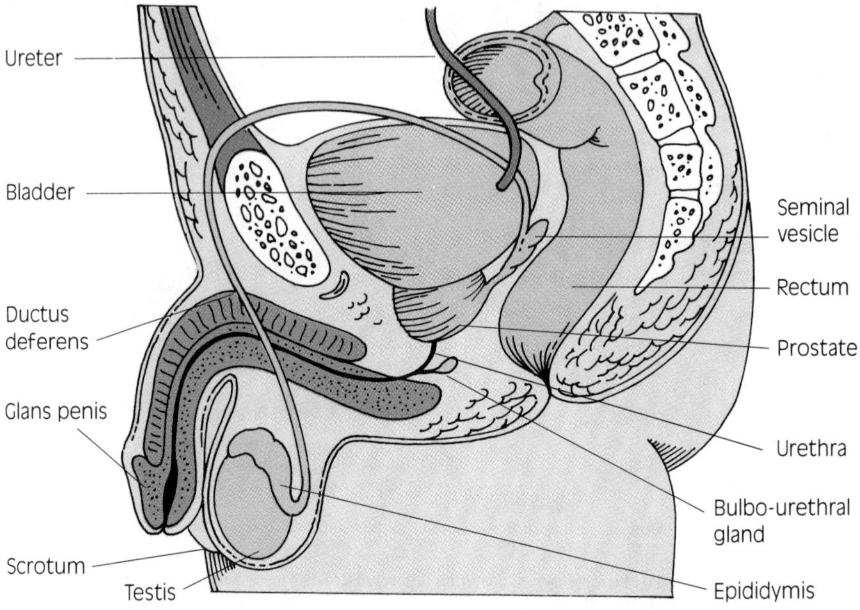

FIGURE 47-1. Organs of the male reproductive system.

Assessment of Male Reproductive Function

Health History

To assess sexual function in the male, the health history focuses on sexual function as well as manifestations of sexual dysfunction. In addition, the patient is asked about changes in urinary function and symptoms that may occur with an obstruction caused by an enlarged prostate gland. The patient is asked about his usual state of health and any recent changes in general physical activity as well as sexual activity. Any symptoms or changes in function are explored fully and described in detail. Factors that may affect sexual functioning (*i.e.*, stress; physical disease; use of medications, drugs, or alcohol) are identified.

Physical Examination

In addition to the customary aspects of the physical examination, two essential components address disorders of the male genital or reproductive system: the digital rectal examination and the testicular examination.

Digital Rectal Examination. The digital rectal examination (DRE) is recommended as part of the regular health checkup for every man over age 40; it is invaluable in screening for cancer of the prostate gland. The DRE enables the examiner to assess the size, shape, and consistency of the prostate gland (Fig. 47-2). Tenderness of the prostate gland upon palpation and the presence and consistency of any nodules are noted. Although having this examination may be embarrassing for the patient, it is a most important screening tool that should be part of every physical examination.

Testicular Examination. The male genitalia are inspected for abnormalities and palpated for masses. The scrotum is palpated carefully for nodules, masses, or inflammation. Examining the scrotum can reveal such disorders as hydrocele, hernia, or tumor of the testis. The penis is inspected and palpated for ulcerations, nodules, signs of inflammation, and discharge. The testicular examination provides an excellent opportunity to instruct the patient about techniques for testicular self-examination and its importance in early detection of testicular cancer (discussed later in this chapter).

Diagnostic Studies

Diagnostic studies that relate to the male reproductive organs and to the ability to participate in sexual activity may be performed. They include the following.

Prostate-Specific Antigen. The prostate gland produces a substance known as prostate-specific antigen (PSA), which may be measured in a blood specimen and which increases with prostate cancer. The PSA test and DRE are used to detect prostate cancer. PSA increases with prostate cancer.

Ultrasound. Transrectal ultrasound studies (TRUS) may be performed in patients with abnormalities detected by DRE or those with elevated PSA levels. TRUS may be used in detecting nonpalpable prostate cancers and in staging localized prostate cancer. Needle biopsies of the prostate are commonly guided by ultrasound.

Prostate Fluid or Tissue Analysis. Specimens of prostatic fluid or tissue may be obtained for culture when disease or inflammation of the prostate gland is suspected. A biopsy of the prostate gland may be necessary to obtain tissue for histologic examination. This may be performed at the time of prostatectomy or via a perineal or transrectal needle biopsy.

Tests of Male Sexual Function. If the patient is unable to engage satisfactorily in sexual intercourse, a detailed history is obtained. Nocturnal penile tumescence tests may be conducted in a sleep laboratory to monitor changes in penile circumference (using a mercury strain gauge placed around the penis) during sleep. Test results help to determine the cause of erectile impotence. Arterial blood flow to the penis is measured with the Doppler probe. Nerve conduction tests and psychologic evaluations are also part of the diagnostic workup and are usually conducted by a specialized team of health care providers.

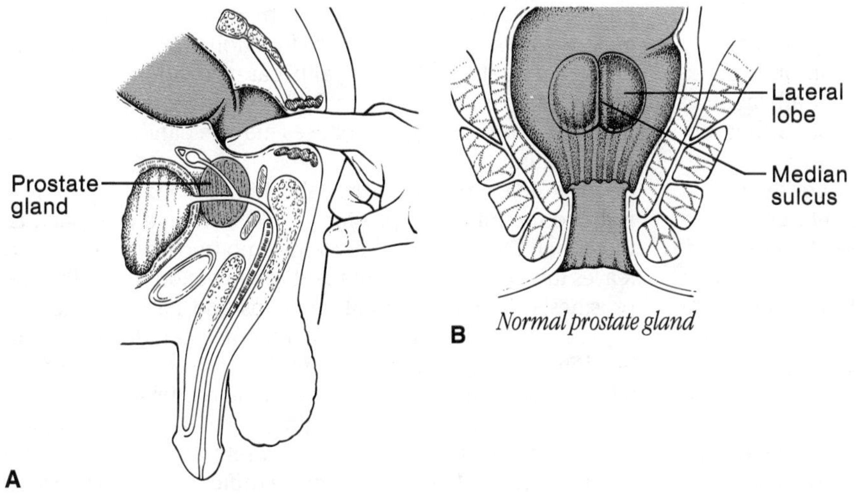

FIGURE 47-2. (**A**) Palpation of the prostate gland during digital rectal examination (DRE) enables the examiner to assess the size, shape, and texture of the gland. (**B**) The prostate is round, with a palpable median sulcus or groove separating the two lobes. It should feel firm and be free of nodules and masses. (Fuller J and Schaller-Ayers J. Health Assessment: A Nursing Approach, 2nd ed. Philadelphia, JB Lippincott, 1994.)

Congenital Malformations

Congenital malformations of the male reproductive system include cryptorchidism, hypospadias, and epispadias. **Cryptorchidism** is the most common congenital defect and is a failure of the testes to descend into the scrotum.

Hypospadias and **epispadias** are congenital anomalies of the urethral opening. In hypospadias the urethral opening is a groove on the underside of the penis. In epispadias the urethral opening is on the dorsum of the penis.

These anatomic abnormalities may be repaired by various types of plastic surgery, usually when the boy is very young.

Disorders of Male Sexual Function

Erectile Dysfunction

Erectile dysfunction, also called **impotence,** is the inability to either achieve or maintain an erection sufficient to accomplish intercourse. The man may report decreased frequency of erections, inability to achieve a firm erection, or rapid detumescence (subsiding of erection). Incidence ranges from 25% to 50% in men over 65 years of age. The physiology of erection and ejaculation is complex and involves sympathetic and parasympathetic components. At the time of erection, pelvic nerves carry parasympathetic impulses that dilate the smaller blood vessels of the region and increase blood flow to the penis, expanding the corpora cavernosa.

Erectile dysfunction has both psychogenic and organic causes. Psychogenic causes include anxiety, fatigue, depression, and cultural pressure to perform sexually. Research suggests, however, that organic impotence may account for more impotence than previously realized. Organic causes include occlusive vascular disease, endocrine disease (diabetes, pituitary tumors, hypogonadism with testosterone deficiency, hyperthyroidism, and hypothyroidism), cirrhosis, chronic renal failure, genitourinary conditions (radical pelvic surgery), hematologic conditions (Hodgkin's disease, leukemia), neurologic disorders (neuropathies, Parkinsonism), trauma to the pelvic or genital area, drugs (alcohol, psychoactive agents, anticholinergics) and drug abuse. Table 47-1 lists medications that are commonly associated with erectile dysfunction.

Diagnosis of erectile dysfunction requires a sexual and medical history; an analysis of presenting symptoms; physical examination; and detailed assessment of all medications taken and alcohol and drug use; as well as various laboratory studies.

Nocturnal penile tumescence tests are conducted in sleep laboratories to monitor changes in penile circumference. In healthy men, nocturnal penile erections closely parallel rapid eye movement (REM) sleep in occurrence and duration. Organically impotent men show inadequate sleep-related erections that correspond to their waking performance. The nocturnal penile tumescence test can help to determine whether erectile impotence has an organic or psychologic cause.

Arterial blood flow to the penis is measured by means of a Doppler probe. Additionally, nerve conduction tests and extensive psychologic evaluation are carried out.

TABLE 47-1 Medications Associated With Erectile Dysfunction

Methyldopa (Aldomet)
Guanethidine (Ismelin)
Clonidine (Catapres)
Reserpine (Serpasil)
Spironolactone (Aldactone)
Diuretics (*e.g.,* Diuril)
Chlorthalidone (Hygroton)
Prazosin (Minipress)
Clofibrate (Atromid-S)
Methantheline (Banthine)
Cimetidine (Tagamet)
Propranolol (Inderal)
Methadone (Dolophine)
Baclofen (Lioresal)
Ethionamide (Trecator)
Perhexiline (Pexid)
Hexamethonium (Methium Cl)
Mecamylamine HCl (Inversine)
Trimethaphan camsylate (Arfonad)
Propantheline (Pro-Banthine)
Disulfiram (Antabuse)
Digoxin (Lanoxin)
Cancer chemotherapy agents

(Leiblum SR and Segraves RT. Sex therapy with aging adults. In Leiblum SR and Rosen RC [eds]. Principles and Practice of Sex Therapy: Update for the 1990s, 2nd ed. New York, Guilford Press, 1989, p. 365.)

Management. Treatment, which depends to some extent on the cause, can be medical, surgical, or both. Nonsurgical therapy includes treating associated conditions such as alcoholism and readjusting hypertensive agents or other medications. Endocrine therapy may be instituted for erectile dysfunction secondary to hypothalamic–pituitary–gonadal dysfunction and may reverse the condition. Insufficient penile blood flow may be treated with vascular surgery. Patients with erectile dysfunction from psychogenic causes are referred to a health care provider or therapist specializing in sex therapy. Patients with erectile dysfunction secondary to organic causes may be candidates for penile implants.

Penile implants are available in two types: the semirigid rod and the inflatable prosthesis. The semirigid rod (such as the Small-Carrion prosthesis) has no movable parts and leaves the man with a permanent semierection. The inflatable prosthesis simulates natural erections and natural flaccidity.

Complications after implantation include infection, erosion of the prosthesis through the skin (more common with the semirigid rod than the inflatable prosthesis), and persistent pain, which may require removal of the implant. Cystoscopic surgery such as transurethral resection of the prostate (TUR, also TURP) is more difficult with a semirigid rod than with the inflatable prosthesis. Factors to consider in choosing a prosthesis are the patient's activities of daily living, social activities, and expectations of the patient and his partner. Ongoing counseling for the patient and his partner is usually necessary to help them in adapting to the prosthesis.

Negative-pressure (vacuum) devices may also be used to induce an erection. A plastic cylinder is placed over the flaccid penis and negative pressure is applied. When an erection is attained, a constriction band is placed around the base of the penis to maintain the erection. Although many men find this method satisfactory, others experience premature loss of penile rigidity or pain when applying suction or during intercourse.

Pharmacologic measures to induce erections can involve injecting vasoactive agents such as papaverine and phentolamine directly into the penis. Complications include priapism (a persistent abnormal erection) and development of fibrotic plaques at the injection sites.

Ejaculation Problems

Premature Ejaculation. Premature ejaculation occurs when a man cannot voluntarily control the ejaculatory reflex and, once aroused, reaches orgasm before or shortly after intromission. It is the most common dysfunction in men.

Retarded Ejaculation. Retarded ejaculation is the involuntary inhibition of the ejaculatory reflex. The varying responses include occasional ejaculation through intercourse or self-stimulation or the complete inability to ejaculate under any circumstances.

Effects of Illness and Disability on Sexual Function

Effects of trauma, chronic illness, and physical disability on sexual function can be profound. In addition to the effect of psychogenic factors, physical changes associated with illness and injury can potentially impair sexual function. White et al. (1992) studied the sexual activities, concerns, and interests of 79 men with spinal cord injuries. Of 11 items listed, sex ranked lowest in terms of satisfaction and fifth in terms of importance. Areas of sexual activity about which the men were most concerned included not satisfying a partner, getting or giving a sexual disease, urinary accidents, and not getting enough personal satisfaction. The men were highly interested in learning methods and techniques to achieve sexual satisfaction and helping a partner cope emotionally with the limitations on sexual activity and the ability to have children.

Persons with illness and disabilities may need the assistance of a sex counselor to find, implement, and integrate their sexual beliefs and behaviors into a healthy and satisfying lifestyle.

Gerontologic Considerations

As men age, the prostate gland enlarges, prostate secretion decreases, the scrotum hangs lower, the testes become smaller and more firm, and pubic hair becomes sparser and stiffer. Changes in gonadal function include a decline in plasma testosterone levels and reduced production of progesterone. Other changes include decreasing sexual function, slower sexual responses, increased incidence of genitourinary tract cancer, and urinary incontinence for various reasons.

Male reproductive capability is maintained with advancing age. Although degenerative changes occur in the seminiferous tubules, spermatogenesis (production of sperm) continues. Sexual function, however, involving libido (desire) and potency, decreases (Morley & Kaiser, 1989). Vascular problems cause approximately one half of the cases of impotence in males over 50 years of age.

Hypogonadism occurs in up to one fourth of older men. The relationship of hypogonadism to impotence is uncertain. This decline is more evident in men over age 70 but is also noted in men in their 60s.

In older men the sexual response slows. Erection takes longer in men over 50 years of age and full erections may not be attained until orgasm. Sexual function is affected by several factors, such as psychologic problems, illnesses, and medications. In general, the sexual act takes longer. In older men, ejaculatory control increases; however, if erection is partially lost, there may be difficulty in attaining a full erection again, and resolution may occur without orgasm. Sexual activity is closely correlated with the man's sexual activity of his earlier years; if he was more active than average as a young man, he will most likely continue to be more active than average in his later years.

Cancers of the kidney, bladder, and prostate all have increased incidence in men over age 50. Screening tests for hematuria and digital rectal examinations may uncover a higher percentage of malignancies at earlier stages.

Urinary incontinence in the elderly male may have many causes including medications and age-related conditions, such as neurologic diseases or benign prostatic hyperplasia (also referred to hypertrophy and called an enlarged prostate by the lay public). Routine laboratory tests are performed to exclude reversible causes of urinary incontinence. For some patients with severe incontinence, augmentation cystoplasty (repair of the bladder) with the placement of an artificial genitourinary sphincter may help alleviate this problem.

Infections of the Male Genitourinary Tract

Acute uncomplicated cystitis in adult men is uncommon, but is occasionally noted in men whose sexual partners have vaginal infection with *E. coli.* **Asymptomatic bacteriuria** may also occur from genitourinary manipulation, catheterization, or instrumentation.

Sexually transmitted diseases (STDs) involving the male genitourinary tract commonly include gonorrhea and syphilis. Controversy surrounds the role of sexually transmitted diseases in male infertility (Moskowitz & Mellinger, 1992). Refer to Chapter 65 for the management of patients with infectious diseases.

Infection of the genital tract with human papillomavirus (HPV) is increasing in prevalence. This infection manifests itself as genital condylomas, or genital warts. The risk for developing genitourinary cancers not only increases for the man with HPV infection, but also for his sex partner. From 50% to 80% of male partners of women with abnormal cervical cells have evidence of HPV infection. Currently the incidence of HPV infection in sexually active populations is estimated to range from 2% to 10%. Therefore, diagnosing and treating the man with an HPV infection, such as condyloma acuminatum, is important to minimize cancer risks as well as to decrease disease transmission.

Examining the genitals after an acetic acid solution (vinegar) has been applied to the skin in that area is important for all men at risk for HPV. The acetic acid solution causes the affected epithelium to whiten. Additional strategies for diagnosing and treating HPV infection vary depending on the anatomic location and the degree of cellular change.

Treatment methods for condyloma acuminatum include topical chemicals, cryosurgery with liquid nitrogen, and laser therapy. Recurring HPV infection is common due to latent HPV infection in normal-appearing skin. To be most effective, treatment needs to include both partners.

Health care providers need to identify and screen those at high risk for HPV infection and teach strategies to prevent its transmission. Sexual abstinence during treatment and recovery is advised to minimize spread of the disease. Using condoms and spermicides containing nonoxynol-9 for at least 6 months after treatment is also recommended to decrease HPV transmission (Lilley & Schaffer, 1990) and transmission of other STDs as well, including HIV infection.

Recent studies suggest that trichomoniasis enhances susceptibility to HIV infection. Trichomoniasis is associated with nonchlamydial, nongonococcal urethritis. Other risk factors include sexual contact with an infected partner or prior treatment for trichomoniasis or nongonococcal urethritis.

Use of condoms can help minimize the risk of acquiring STDs. Group counseling about condom use has been studied in men being treated at a clinic for an STD. In one study (Cohen et al., 1992), men who received group counseling had a lower rate of STD reinfection than those who did not. The strongest predictor of reinfection was a history of STD infection prior to the infection that was being treated at the time of the counseling.

Conditions of the Prostate

Prostatitis

Prostatitis is an inflammation of the prostate gland caused by infectious agents (bacteria, fungi, mycoplasma) or by various other problems (*e.g.*, urethral stricture, prostatic hyperplasia). Microorganisms usually are carried to the prostate from the urethra. Prostatitis may be classified as bacterial or abacterial, depending on the presence or absence of microorganisms in the prostatic fluid.

Clinical Manifestations. The symptoms of prostatitis may include perineal discomfort, burning, urgency, frequency, and pain with or after ejaculation. **Prostatodynia** (pain in the prostate) is manifested by pain on voiding or perineal pain without evidence of inflammation or bacterial growth in the prostatic fluid.

Acute bacterial prostatitis may produce sudden fever and chills and perineal, rectal, or low back pain. Urinary symptoms such as dysuria, frequency, urgency, and nocturia may occur. Some patients, however, are asymptomatic.

Chronic bacterial prostatitis is a major cause of relapsing urinary tract infection in men. Symptoms are usually mild, consisting of frequency, dysuria, and occasionally urethral discharge. High fever and chills are uncommon.

Diagnosis. Diagnosis of prostatitis requires a careful history, culture of prostatic fluid or tissue, and, occasionally, a histologic examination of the tissue. To locate the source of a lower genitourinary infection (bladder neck, urethra, prostate), it is necessary to collect a divided urinary specimen for segmental urine culture. After cleaning the glans penis and retracting the foreskin (if present), the patient voids 10 to 15 ml of urine into a container. This represents urethral urine. Without interrupting the urinary stream, he collects 50 to 75 ml of urine in a second container; this represents bladder urine.

If the patient does not have acute prostatitis, the physician immediately performs a prostatic massage and collects any prostatic fluid that is expressed into a third container. If it is not possible to collect prostatic fluid, the patient voids a small quantity of urine. The specimen may contain the bacteria present in the prostatic fluid. Urinalysis after prostate examination commonly reveals many white blood cells.

Management. The goal of therapy for acute bacterial prostatitis is to avoid the complications of abscess formation and septicemia. A broad-spectrum antibiotic agent (to which the causative organism is sensitive) is administered for 10 to 14 days. Intravenous administration of the agent may be necessary to achieve high serum and tissue levels. The patient is encouraged to remain on bed rest to alleviate symptoms quickly. Comfort is promoted with analgesics (to relieve pain), antispasmodics and bladder sedatives (to relieve bladder irritability), sitz baths (to relieve pain and spasm), and stool softeners (to prevent pain from straining at stool).

Swelling of the prostate gland may produce urinary retention. Other complications include epididymitis, bacteremia, and pyelonephritis.

Chronic bacterial prostatitis is difficult to treat because most antibiotics diffuse poorly from the plasma into the prostatic fluid. Nevertheless, antibiotics may be prescribed, including trimethoprim-sulfamethoxazole, tetracycline, minocycline, and doxycycline. Continuous therapy with low-dose antibiotics to suppress the infection may also be indicated. Additionally, the patient is advised that the urinary tract infection may recur and is instructed in recognizing its symptoms.

As with acute bacterial prostatitis, comfort measures involve antispasmodics, sitz baths, stool softeners, and evaluation of any sexual partner to reduce the possibility of cross-infection.

Similarly, the treatment of **nonbacterial prostatitis** is directed toward relieving symptoms.

Patient Education and Health Maintenance. The patient is instructed to complete the prescribed course of antibiotics. Hot sitz baths (10–20 minutes) may be taken several times daily. Fluids are encouraged to satisfy thirst, but fluids are not "forced" because an effective medication level must be maintained in the urine. Foods and liquids that have diuretic action or that increase prostatic secretions should be avoided. They include alcohol, coffee, tea, chocolate, cola, and spices. During periods of *acute* inflammation, sexual arousal and intercourse should be avoided.

Treatment for *chronic* prostatitis may include reducing the retention of prostatic fluid by ejaculation through sexual intercourse or masturbation. To minimize discomfort, the patient should avoid sitting for long periods. Medical follow-up is necessary for at least 6 months to 1 year, since prostatitis caused by the same or different organisms can occur.

Benign Prostatic Hyperplasia (Enlarged Prostate)

In many patients more than 50 years of age, the prostate gland enlarges, extending upward into the bladder and obstructing the outflow of urine by encroaching on the vesical orifice. This condition is known as benign prostatic hyperplasia (BPH), the enlargement, or hypertrophy, of the prostate. BPH is the most common pathologic condition in older men and the second most common cause of surgical intervention in men over age 60.

Examination reveals a prostate that is large, rubbery, and nontender. The cause is uncertain, but evidence suggests that hormones initiate hyperplasia of the supporting stromal tissue and the glandular elements in the prostate.

The hypertrophied lobes may obstruct the vesical neck or prostatic urethra, thereby causing incomplete emptying and urinary retention. As a result, a gradual dilation of the ureters (hydroureter) and kidneys (hydronephrosis) can occur. Urinary tract infections may result from urinary stasis, whereby some urine remains in the urinary tract and serves as a medium for infective organisms.

Clinical Manifestations and Diagnostic Evaluation. The obstructive and irritative symptom complex (referred to as **prostatism**) includes increased frequency of urination, nocturia, urgency, hesitancy in starting urination, abdominal straining, a decrease in the volume and force the urinary stream, interruption of the urinary stream, dribbling (in which urine dribbles out after urination), a sensation that the bladder has not emptied completely, acute urinary retention (when more than 60 ml of urine remains in the bladder after urination), and recurrent urinary tract infections. Ultimately, azotemia (accumulation of nitrogenous waste products) and renal failure can occur with chronic urinary retention and large residual volumes. Generalized symptoms also may be noted, including fatigue, anorexia, nausea and vomiting, and epigastric discomfort.

A physical examination that includes a digital rectal examination and a battery of diagnostic tests may be performed to determine the degree to which the prostate is enlarged, the presence of any changes in the bladder wall, and the efficiency of renal function. These tests may include urinalysis and urodynamic studies to assess any obstruction in urine flow patterns. Renal function studies including serum creatinine studies may be performed to determine if there is renal impairment from prostatic back-pressure and to evaluate renal reserve. Complete blood studies are performed. Because hemorrhage is a major postoperative complication, all clotting defects must be corrected. A high percentage of patients with BPH have cardiac or respiratory complications, or both, because of their age; therefore, cardiac and respiratory function are also assessed. Other diseases producing similar symptoms include urethral stricture, prostate cancer, neurogenic bladder, and urinary bladder stones.

Management. The treatment plan depends on the cause, the severity of the obstruction, and the condition of the patient. If a patient is admitted as an emergency because he cannot void, he is immediately catheterized. The ordinary catheter may be too soft and pliable to advance through the urethra into the bladder. In such cases, a thin wire called a stylet is introduced (by a urologist) into the catheter to prevent the catheter from collapsing when it encounters resistance. In severe cases, metal catheters with a pronounced prostatic curve may be used. Sometimes an incision is made into the bladder (a suprapubic cystostomy) to provide adequate drainage.

Although prostatectomy (described below) to remove the hyperplastic prostatic tissue is frequently performed, other treatment options are available. These include "watchful waiting," transurethral incision of the prostate (TUIP), balloon dilation, alpha blockers, and 5-α-reductase inhibitors (AHCPR, 1994). "Watchful waiting" is the appropriate treatment for many patients because the likelihood of progression of the disease or the development of complications is unknown. Patients are monitored periodically for severity of symptoms, physical findings, laboratory testing, and diagnostic urologic tests (AHCPR, 1994).

Alpha-1-adrenergic receptor blockers (*e.g.*, terazosin) relax smooth muscle of the bladder neck and prostate. Although the long-term efficacy of these agents is not known, they do reduce symptoms in many patients. Research into the long-term usefulness of these agents is ongoing (AHCPR, 1994).

Because the hormonal component of benign prostatic hyperplasia has been identified, one method of treatment involves hormonal manipulation with antiandrogen agents such as finasteride (Proscar). In clinical studies, 5 α-reductase inhibitors such as finasteride have been effective in preventing the conversion of testosterone to dihydrotestosterone. With decreased levels of dihydrotestosterone, suppression of glandular cell activity and decreases in prostate size have been demonstrated. Side effects of these medications include gynecomastia (breast enlargement), erectile dysfunction, and flushing.

The Patient Undergoing Prostate Surgery

The preoperative objectives before prostate surgery are to assess the patient's general health status and to establish optimum renal function. Prostate surgery should be performed before acute urinary retention develops and damages the upper urinary tract and collecting system.

Surgical Procedures

Several approaches are used to remove the hypertrophied portion of the prostate gland: transurethral resection of the prostate, suprapubic prostatectomy, perineal prostatectomy, and retropubic prostatectomy (Table 47-2). In these approaches, the surgeon removes all hyperplastic tissue, leaving behind only the capsule of the prostate. The transurethral approach is a closed procedure; the other three are open procedures (*i.e.*, a surgical incision is required).

A **transurethral resection** of the prostate (TUR or TURP) is the most common procedure and can be carried out through endoscopy. The surgical and optical instrument is introduced directly through the urethra to the prostate, which

TABLE 47-2 Comparison of Surgical Approaches for Prostatectomy

The surgical approach of choice depends on (1) the size of the gland, (2) the severity of the obstruction, (3) the age of the patient, (4) the condition of patient, and (5) the presence of associated diseases.

Surgical Approach	Advantages	Disadvantages	Nursing Implications
Transurethral Resection (TUR or TURP) (removal of prostatic tissue by instrument introduced through urethra)	Avoids abdominal incision Safer for surgical-risk patient Shorter hospitalization and recovery periods Lower morbidity rate Causes less pain	Requires highly skilled surgeon Recurrent obstruction, urethral trauma, and stricture may develop. Delayed bleeding may occur.	Monitor for hemorrhage. Observe for symptoms of urethral stricture (dysuria, straining, weak urinary stream).
Open Surgical Removal			
Suprapubic approach	Technically simple Offers wide area of exploration Permits exploration for cancerous lymph nodes Allows more complete removal of obstructing gland Permits treatment of associated bladder lesions	Requires surgical approach through the bladder Control of hemorrhage difficult Urine may leak around the suprapubic tube Recovery may be prolonged and uncomfortable	Monitor for indications of hemorrhage and shock. Give meticulous aseptic care to the area around suprapubic tube.
Perineal approach	Offers direct anatomic approach Permits gravity drainage Particularly effective for radical cancer therapy Allows hemostasis under direct vision Low mortality rate Lower incidence of shock Ideal for very old, frail, and poor-surgical-risk patient with large prostate	Higher postoperative incidence of impotence and urinary incontinence Possible damage to rectum and external sphincter Restricted operative field Greater potential for infection	Avoid using rectal tubes or thermometers and enemas after perineal surgery. Use drainage pads to absorb excess urinary drainage. Provide foam rubber ring for patient comfort in sitting. Anticipate urinary leakage around the wound for several days after the catheter is removed.
Retropubic approach	Avoids incision into the bladder Permits surgeon to see and control bleeders Shorter recovery period Less bladder sphincter damage	Cannot treat associated bladder disease Increased incidence of hemorrhage from prostatic venous plexus; pubic osteitis	Monitor for hemorrhage. Anticipate posturinary leakage for several days after removing the catheter.

can then be viewed directly. The gland is removed in small chips with an electrical cutting loop (Fig. 47-3*A*). This procedure, which requires no incision, may be used for glands of varying size and is ideal for patients who have small glands and who are considered poor surgical risks.

This approach means a shorter hospital stay; however, strictures are more frequent, and repeated procedures may be necessary. A transurethral prostatectomy rarely causes erectile dysfunction but may cause retrograde ejaculation because removing the prostatic tissue at the bladder neck can cause the seminal fluid to flow backward into the bladder rather forward through the urethra.

Suprapubic prostatectomy is one method of removing the gland through an abdominal incision. An incision is made into the bladder, and the prostate gland is removed from above (see Fig. 47-3*B*). Such an approach can be used for a gland of any size, and few complications occur, although blood loss may be greater than with other methods. Another disadvantage is the need for an abdominal incision, with the concomitant hazards of any major abdominal surgical procedure.

Perineal prostatectomy involves removing the gland through an incision in the perineum (see Fig. 47-3*C*). This approach is practical when other approaches are not possible, and is useful for an open biopsy. Postoperatively, the wound may easily become contaminated because the incision is near the rectum. Moreover, incontinence, impotence, or rectal injury are more likely complications of this surgery.

Retropubic prostatectomy is another technique and is more common than the suprapubic approach. The surgeon makes a low abdominal incision and approaches the prostate gland between the pubic arch and the bladder without entering the bladder (see Fig. 47-3*D*). This proce-

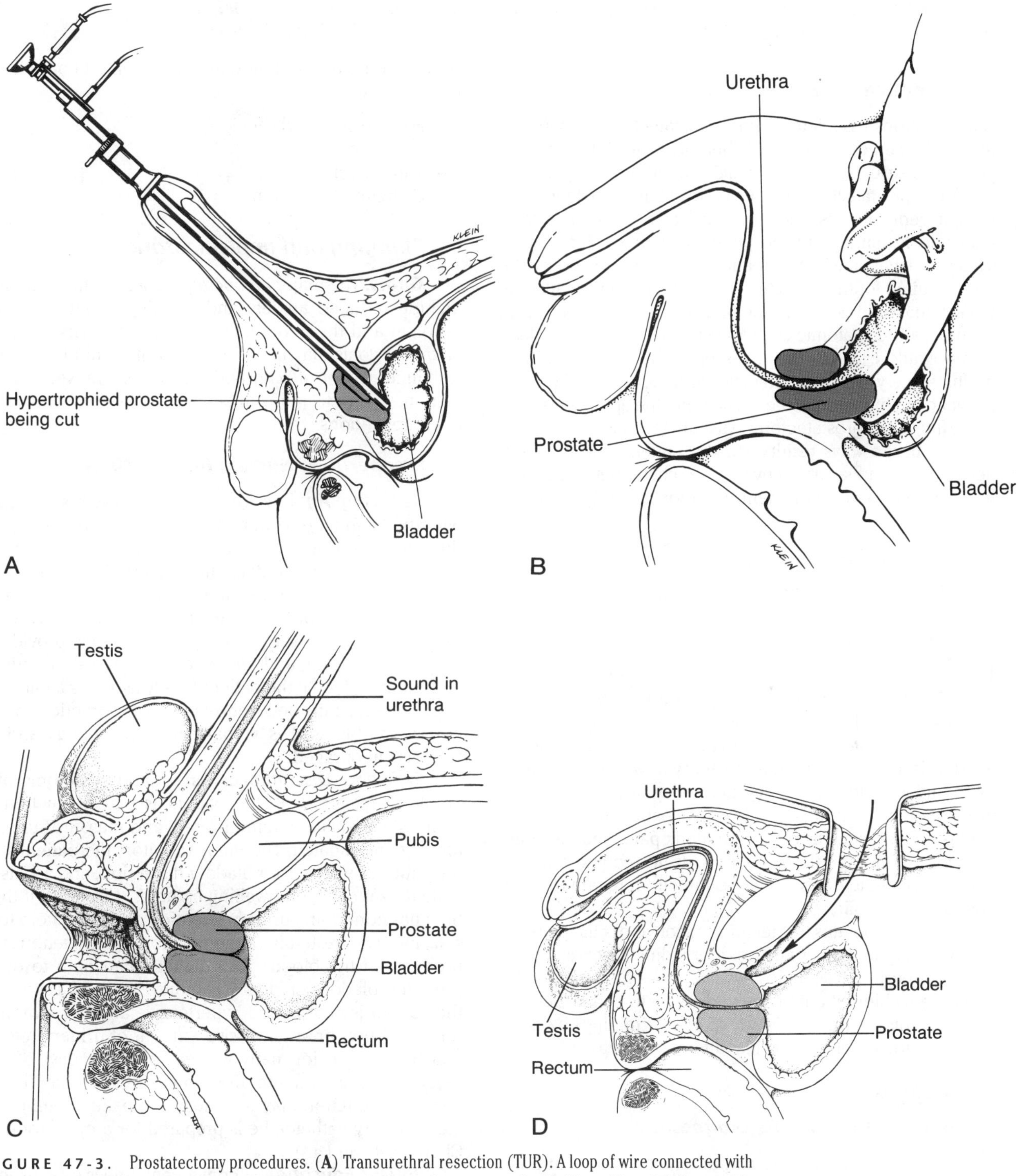

FIGURE 47-3. Prostatectomy procedures. (**A**) Transurethral resection (TUR). A loop of wire connected with a cutting current is rotated in the cystoscope to remove shavings of prostate at the bladder orifice. (**B**) Suprapubic prostatectomy. With an abdominal approach, the prostate is shelled out of its bed. (**C**) Perineal prostatectomy. Two retractors on the left spread the perineal incision to provide a view of the prostate. (**D**) Retropubic prostatectomy is performed through a low abdominal incision. Note two abdominal retractors and *arrow* pointing to the prostate gland.

dure is suitable for large glands located high in the pelvis. Although blood loss can be better controlled and the surgical site is easier to visualize, infections can readily start in the retropubic space.

Transurethral incision of the prostate (TUIP) is another procedure used in the treatment of BPH in which an instrument is passed through the urethra. One or two incisions are made in the prostate and prostate capsule to reduce the prostate's pressure on the urethra and reduce urethral constriction. TUIP is indicated when the prostate gland is small (30 gm or less) and would be effective in treatment in many cases of BPH. It can be performed on an outpatient basis and has a lower complication rate than other prostate surgical procedures (AHCPR, 1994).

Complications

Complications associated with a prostatectomy depend on the type of surgery and include hemorrhage, clot formation, catheter obstruction, and sexual dysfunction.

Most prostatectomies do not result in impotence (although perineal prostatectomy may cause impotence from unavoidable damage to the pudendal nerves). In most instances, sexual activity may be resumed in 6 to 8 weeks, the time required for the prostatic fossa to heal. After ejaculation, the seminal fluid goes into the bladder and is excreted with the urine. (The anatomic changes in the posterior urethra lead to retrograde ejaculation.) A vasectomy may be performed during surgery to prevent infection from spreading from the prostatic urethra through the vas and into the epididymis.

After total prostatectomy (usually for cancer), impotence almost always results. For the patient who does not desire to give up sexual activity, a prosthetic penile implant may be used to make the penis rigid for sexual intercourse.

❑ NURSING PROCESS
The Patient Undergoing Prostatectomy

Assessment

The nurse assesses how benign prostatic hyperplasia (BPH) has affected the patient's lifestyle during the past few months. Has he been reasonably active for his age? What is his presenting urinary problem (described in the patient's words)? Is it decreased force of urinary flow, decreased ability to initiate voiding, urgency, frequency, nocturia, dysuria, urinary retention, hematuria? Does the patient report associated problems, such as back pain, flank pain, and lower abdominal or suprapubic discomfort? If he reports such discomfort, possible causes may be infection, retention, and, possibly, renal colic.

The nurse obtains further information about the patient's family history of cancer and heart or kidney disease, including hypertension. Has he lost weight? Does he appear pale? Can he raise himself out of bed and return to bed without assistance? This information may help in determining how soon he will return to normal activities after prostatectomy.

Diagnosis

Preoperative Nursing Diagnoses

Based on the health history and all other assessment data, the patient's major nursing diagnoses may include the following:

- ❑ Anxiety related to the inability to void
- ❑ Pain related to bladder distention
- ❑ Knowledge deficit about factors related to the problem and the treatment protocol

Postoperative Nursing Diagnoses

- ❑ Pain related to the surgical incision, catheter placement, and bladder spasms
- ❑ Knowledge deficit about postoperative and convalescent management

Collaborative Problems/ Potential Complications

Based on the assessment data, the potential complications may include:

- ❑ Hemorrhage and shock
- ❑ Infection
- ❑ Thrombosis
- ❑ Catheter obstruction

Planning and Implementation

Goals. The major *preoperative* goals for the patient may include reduced anxiety and learning about his prostate problem and the perioperative experience. His major *postoperative* goals may include correction of fluid volume disturbances, relief of pain and discomfort, prevention of infection, ability to perform self-care activities, and absence of complications.

Preoperative Nursing Interventions

Reducing Anxiety. The nurse familiarizes the patient with the hospital environment and initiates measures to reduce anxiety. Communication is established regarding the degree to which he understands his problem and what the physician has already told him. Because the patient may be sensitive and embarrassed to discuss problems related to the genitalia and issues of sexuality, the nurse provides privacy and a trusting and professional relationship. Guilt feelings often surface if the patient falsely assumes a cause-and-effect relationship between early sexual practices and his current problems. His verbalization of feelings and concerns is encouraged.

Relieving Discomfort. If signs and symptoms of discomfort are apparent, the patient is placed on bed rest, analgesic agents are administered, and measures to relieve anxiety are initiated. The nurse monitors the patient's voiding patterns, watches for bladder distention, and assists with catheterization. An indwelling catheter is inserted if the patient has continuing urinary retention or if laboratory test results indicate azotemia (accumulation of nitrogenous waste products in the blood). The catheter can help to decompress the bladder gradually over several days, especially if the patient is elderly and hypertensive and has diminished renal function or an excessive amount of urinary retention that has existed for many weeks. For a few days after the bladder begins draining, the blood pressure may fluctuate and renal function may decline. If the patient cannot tolerate a urinary catheter, he is prepared for a cystostomy (see Chapters 42 and 43).

Patient Education. A convenient time is established for the patient (ensuring his privacy) to review the anatomy of the affected parts and how they function in relation to the urinary and reproductive systems. Using diagrams and other teaching aids may be effective. The nurse explains what will take place as the patient is prepared for diagnostic tests and then for surgery (depending on the kind of prostatectomy planned). The nurse describes the type of incision, which varies with the type of surgical approach (directly over the bladder, low on the abdomen, or in the perineal area; in the case of a transurethral procedure, no incision will be made). The patient is informed about the type of drainage system that is expected, the type of anesthesia, and the recovery room procedure. The amount of information is individualized based on the patient's needs and questions. Procedures expected during the immediate perioperative period are explained, questions are answered, and support is provided.

Preoperative Preparation. When the patient is scheduled for a prostatectomy, the preparation described in Chapter 19 is provided. Elastic stockings are applied before surgery and are particularly important if the patient is placed in a lithotomy position during surgery. A preoperative enema may prevent postoperative straining, which can induce postoperative bleeding.

Postoperative Nursing Interventions

Relieving Pain. After a prostatectomy, the patient remains on bed rest for the first 24 hours. If pain occurs, the cause and location must be determined. It may be related to the incision; it may be the result of excoriation of the skin at the catheter site; it may be in the flank area, indicating a kidney problem; or it may be due to bladder spasms. Bladder irritability can initiate bleeding and result in clot formation, leading to urinary retention.

When patients are experiencing bladder spasms, they may note an urgency to void, a feeling of pressure or fullness in the bladder, and bleeding from the urethra around the catheter. Medications that relax the smooth muscles can help to ease the spasms, which can be intermittent and severe. Warm compresses to the pubis or sitz baths may relieve the spasms.

The nurse monitors the drainage tubing and irrigates the system as prescribed to relieve any obstruction that may cause discomfort. Usually, the catheter is irrigated with 50 ml of irrigating fluid at a time. It is important to make sure that the same amount is recovered in the drainage receptacle. Securing the catheter to the leg or abdomen can help to decrease tension on the catheter and prevent bladder irritation.

Discomfort may be caused by dressings that are too snug, too saturated with drainage, or improperly placed. Pain medications are administered as prescribed.

Patient Education and Health Maintenance. When the patient is ambulatory, he is encouraged to walk but not to sit for prolonged periods, as this increases intra-abdominal pressure and the possibility of discomfort and bleeding. Prune juice and stool softeners are provided to ease bowel movements and to prevent excessive straining. If an enema is prescribed, it is administered with caution to avoid possible rectal perforation.

As the patient recovers and drainage tubes are removed, he may show signs of discouragement and depression because he cannot regain bladder control immediately. Moreover, urinary frequency and burning may occur after the catheter is removed. Teaching the following exercises may help the patient in regaining urinary control.

- Tense the perineal muscles by pressing the buttocks together; hold this position; relax. This exercise can be performed 10 to 20 times each hour while sitting or standing.
- Try to interrupt the urinary stream after starting to void; wait a few seconds and then continue to void.

Perineal exercises should continue until the patient gains full urinary control. The patient is instructed to urinate as soon as he feels the *first* urge to do so. It is important for the patient to know that regaining urinary control is a gradual process, that he may continue to "dribble" after being discharged from the hospital, but that the dribbling should gradually diminish (up to 1 year). The urine may be cloudy for several weeks after surgery but should clear as the prostate area heals.

While the prostatic fossa heals (6–8 weeks), the patient should try not to engage in any activities that produce Valsalva effects (straining at stool, heavy lifting), as this increases venous pressure and may produce hematuria. He should avoid long motor trips and strenuous exercise, which increase the tendency to bleed. He also should know that spicy foods, alcohol, and coffee may cause discomfort. The patient is cautioned to drink enough fluids to avoid dehydration, which increases the tendency for a blood clot to form and obstruct the flow of urine. Signs of complications, such as bleeding, passage of blood clots, a decrease in the urinary stream, urinary retention, or urinary tract infection symptoms, are to be reported to the physician.

Because many patients who undergo prostatectomy are elderly and may have other health problems, the patient may benefit from a visit by the home care nurse who assesses physical status, including healing of the surgical incision, catheter care if indicated, and adherence of the patient to discharge instructions. The patient may need to be reminded that return of bladder control may take some time.

Monitoring and Managing Potential Complications. After prostatectomy, it is important to observe the patient for major complications such as hemorrhage, infection, thrombosis, and catheter obstruction.

Hemorrhage. Because a hyperplastic prostate gland is very vascular, the immediate dangers after a prostatectomy are bleeding and shock. Bleeding may occur from the bed of the prostate. Bleeding may also result in the formation of clots, which then obstruct the flow of urine. The drainage begins as reddish pink and then clears to a light pink within 24 hours after surgery.

- Bright red bleeding with increased viscosity and numerous clots usually indicates arterial bleeding. Venous blood appears darker and less viscous.
- Arterial hemorrhage usually requires surgical intervention (*e.g.*, suturing of bleeders or transurethral coagulation of bleeding vessels), whereas venous bleeding may be controlled by applying prescribed traction to the catheter so that the balloon holding the catheter in place applies pressure to the prostatic fossa.

Infection. After perineal prostatectomy, the surgeon usually changes the dressing on the first postoperative day. Further dressing changes may become the nurse's responsibility. Careful aseptic technique is used, because the possibility for infection is great. Dressings can be held in place by a double-tailed, T-binder bandage or a padded athletic supporter. The tails cross over the incision to give double thickness, and then each tail is drawn up on either side of the scrotum to the waistline and fastened.

Rectal thermometers, rectal tubes, and enemas are avoided because of the risk of injury to and bleeding in the prostatic fossa. After the perineal sutures are removed, the perineum is cleansed as indicated. A heat lamp may be directed to the perineal area to promote healing. The scrotum is protected with a towel while the heat lamp is in use. Sitz baths are also used to promote healing.

Urinary tract infections and epididymitis are possible complications after prostatectomy. The patient is assessed for their occurrence; if they occur, the nurse administers antibiotics as prescribed. Management of epididymitis is discussed in more detail below.

Thrombosis. Patients undergoing prostatectomy have a high incidence of deep vein thrombosis (DVT) and pulmonary embolism. In such cases the physician may prescribe prophylactic (preventive) low-dose heparin therapy. The nurse assesses the patient frequently after surgery for manifestations of DVT and applies elastic stockings to reduce the risk of DVT and pulmonary embolism. Nursing and medical management of DVT and pulmonary embolism are detailed in Chapters 21 and 24, respectively. The patient who is receiving heparin must be closely monitored for excessive bleeding.

Obstructed Catheter. After a transurethral prostatic resection, *the catheter must drain well;* an obstructed catheter produces distention of the prostatic capsule and resultant hemorrhage. Furosemide (Lasix) may be prescribed to promote urination and initiate postoperative diuresis, thereby helping to keep the catheter patent.

- ❏ The lower abdomen is observed to ensure that the catheter has not become blocked. An overdistended bladder presents a distinct, rounded swelling above the pubis.
- ❏ The drainage bag, dressings, and incisional site are examined for bleeding. The color of the urine is noted and documented; a change in color from pink to amber indicates reduced bleeding.
- ❏ Blood pressure, pulse, and respirations are monitored and compared with baseline preoperative vital signs to detect hypotension. The nurse also observes the patient for restlessness, cold sweats, pallor, any drop in blood pressure, and an increasing pulse rate.

Drainage of the bladder may be accomplished by gravity through a closed sterile drainage system. A three-way drainage system is useful in cleansing the bladder and preventing clot formation (Fig. 47-4). Some urologists leave an indwelling catheter attached to a dependent drainage system. Gentle irrigation of the catheter may be prescribed to remove any obstructing clots.

- ❏ If the patient complains of pain, the tubing is examined. The drainage system is irrigated, if indicated and prescribed, to clear any obstruction before an analgesic is administered. Usually, the catheter is irrigated with 50 ml of irrigating fluid at a time. The amount of fluid recovered in the drainage bag must equal the amount of fluid injected.
- ❏ Overdistention of the bladder is avoided because it can induce secondary hemorrhage by stretching the coagulated blood vessels in the prostatic capsule.
- ❏ An intake and output record is maintained, including the amount of fluid used for irrigation.

The drainage tube (not the catheter) is taped to the shaved inner thigh to prevent traction on the bladder. If a cystostomy catheter is in place, it is taped to the abdomen. The nurse explains the purpose of the catheter to the patient and assures him that the urge to void results from the presence of the catheter and from bladder spasms. He is cautioned not to pull on the catheter, because this causes bleeding and subsequent catheter blockage, which leads to urinary retention.

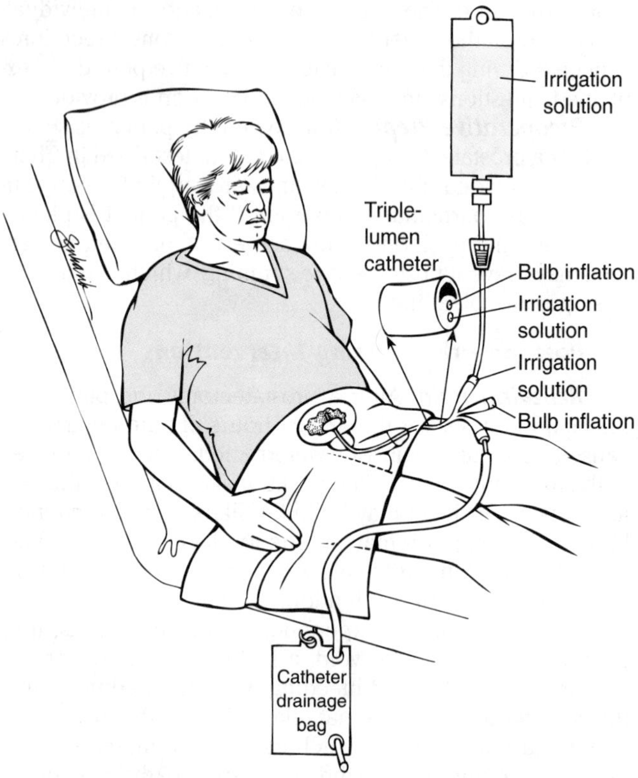

FIGURE 47-4. A three-way system for bladder irrigation.

Catheter Removal. After the catheter is removed (usually when the urine appears clear), urine may leak around the wound for several days in patients who have undergone perineal, suprapubic, and retropubic surgery. The cystostomy tube may be removed before or after the urethral catheter is removed. Some urinary incontinence may occur following catheter removal and the patient is informed that this will probably subside in time.

Evaluation

Expected Preoperative Outcomes

1. Demonstrates reduced anxiety
2. States that pain and discomfort are decreased.
3. Relates understanding of the surgical procedure and postoperative course and practices perineal muscle exercises and other techniques useful in facilitating bladder control

Expected Postoperative Outcomes

1. Relates relief of discomfort
2. Responds positively to self-care measures
   a. Increases activity and ambulation daily
   b. Produces urine output within normal ranges and consistent with intake
   c. Performs perineal exercises and interrupts urinary stream to promote bladder control
   d. Avoids straining and lifting heavy objects
4. Is free of complications
   a. Maintains vital signs within normal limits

b. Exhibits wound healing, without signs of inflammation or hemorrhage
c. Maintains acceptable level of urinary elimination
d. Maintains optimal drainage of catheter and other drainage tubes

Cancer of the Prostate

Cancer of the prostate is the most common cancer in men (other than nonmelanoma skin cancer) and the second most common cause of cancer deaths in American men older than age 55. In African-American men, prostate cancer is the most prevalent cancer overall; its incidence is almost twice that of the general population and the death rate is about three times greater. About 1 in 11 men in the United States will develop prostate cancer. Approximately 125,000 new cases of prostate cancer are diagnosed each year and 32,000 men who already have it die of it each year. The growth of the prostate gland is dependent on the presence of androgenic hormones such as testosterone. Because dihydrotestosterone is an important promoter of prostate cancer, medications such as finasteride are being advocated as a means of inhibiting prostatic cell proliferation and killing prostatic cancer cells.

Clinical Manifestations. Cancer of the prostate in its early stages rarely produces symptoms. The symptoms that develop from urinary obstruction occur late in the disease. This cancer tends to vary in its course. If the neoplasm is large enough to encroach on the bladder neck, symptoms and signs of urinary obstruction occur, namely, difficulty and frequency of urination, urinary retention, and decreased size and force of the urinary stream. Prostatic cancer commonly metastasizes to bone and lymph nodes. Symptoms related to metastases include backache, hip pain, perineal and rectal discomfort, anemia, weight loss, weakness, nausea, and oliguria (decreased urine output). Hematuria may result from the cancer invading the urethra or bladder, or both. Unfortunately, these may be the first overt indications of prostate cancer.

Early Detection. When prostate cancer is detected at an early stage, the likelihood of cure is high. Every man over age 40 should have a digital rectal examination (DRE) as part of his regular health checkup. Routine repeated rectal palpation of the gland (preferably by the same examiner) is important because early cancer may be felt as a nodule within the substance of the gland or as an extensive hardening in the posterior lobe. The more advanced lesion is "stony hard" and fixed. Digital rectal examination also provides useful clinical information about the rectum, anal sphincter, and quality of stool.

Diagnostic Evaluation. The diagnosis of prostate cancer is confirmed by a histologic examination of tissue removed surgically by transurethral resection, open prostatectomy, or needle biopsy (perineal or transrectal). Fine-needle aspiration is a quick, painless method of obtaining prostate cells for cytologic examination. The procedure is helpful for determining the stage of disease as well.

Most prostate cancers are diagnosed when a man seeks medical attention for symptoms of a urinary obstruction or after abnormalities are found by digital rectal examination. Incidentally detected cancer with transurethral resection of the prostate for clinically benign disease and prostatism occurs in 10% to 20% of patients. Rarely do patients have other signs and symptoms such as azotemia (nitrogen compounds in the blood), weakness, anemia, or bone pain.

The **prostate-specific antigen (PSA),** a neutral serine protease, is produced by the normal and neoplastic ductal epithelium of the prostate and secreted into the glandular lumen. A simple blood test can detect and measure PSA levels. The concentration of PSA in the blood is proportional to the total prostatic mass. Although the PSA level indicates the presence of prostate tissue, it does not necessarily indicate malignancy. PSA testing is routinely used to monitor the patient's response to cancer therapy and to detect local progression and early recurrence of prostate cancer. The combination of digital rectal examination and PSA testing appears to be a cost-effective, early method for detecting prostate cancer.

Transrectal ultrasound (TRUS) studies are used for men who have elevated PSA levels and abnormal DRE findings. TRUS studies help in detecting nonpalpable prostate cancers and assist with staging localized prostate cancer. Needle biopsies of the prostate are commonly guided by ultrasound.

Other tests include bone scans to detect metastatic bone disease, skeletal x-ray studies to show osteoblastic metastases, excretory urography to detect changes caused by ureteral obstruction, renal function tests, and lymphangiography to find metastases in the pelvic nodes.

Management

Treatment selections are based on the stage of the disease and the patient's age and symptoms. Table 47-3 summarizes the treatment options for the various stages of prostate cancer.

Surgery. A radical prostatectomy (removal of the prostate and seminal vesicles) still remains the standard surgical procedure for patients who have potentially curable disease and a life expectancy of 10 years or more. This procedure may be followed by bilateral orchiectomy (removal of the testes). Sexual impotence follows radical prostatectomy, and 5% to 10% of patients have various degrees of urinary incontinence. (See the Nursing Process on p. 1344 for care of the patient after prostatectomy.)

Radiation. If prostate cancer is detected in its early stage, the treatment may be curative radiation therapy—either teletherapy with a linear accelerator or interstitial irradiation (implantation of radioactive iodine or gold combined with pelvic lymphadenectomy). Side effects, which usually are transitory, include inflammations of the rectum, bowel, and bladder (proctitis, enteritis, and cystitis) due to the radiation doses and the proximity of the rectum, bowel, and bladder. Irritation of the bladder and urethra from radiation therapy can cause pain during ejaculation. There is a greater preservation of sexual potency, however, with radiation therapy than with surgery.

Because approximately half of the patients have locally advanced tumors or evidence of metastatic disease at the time they first seek treatment, palliative measures are indicated. Although cures are unlikely with advanced prostate cancer, many men survive for long intervals apparently free of metastatic disease.

TABLE 47-3 Staging System for Cancer of the Prostate

	Tumor	Nodes	Metastasis	Histopathologic Grade
Stage I	T1	N0	M0	G2, 3–4
Stage II	T2	N0	M0	Any G
Stage III	T3	N0	M0	Any G
Stage IV	T4 or any T	N0–N3	M0 or M1	Any G

Primary Tumor (T)

T0 = No evidence of primary tumor

T1 = Clinically inapparent tumor not palpable or visible by imaging

T2 = Tumor confined within the prostate

T3 = Tumor extends through the prostatic capsule

T4 = Tumor is fixed or invades adjacent structures other than the seminal vesicles

Regional Lymph Nodes (N)

N0 = No regional lymph node metastatis

N1 = Metastasis in a single lymph node ≤ 2 cm in greatest dimension

N2 = Metastasis in a single lymph node > 2 cm but not > 5 cm in greatest dimension or multiple lymph node metastasis, none > 5 cm

N3 = Metastatis in a lymph node > 5 cm greatest dimension

Distant Metastasis (M)

M0 = No distant metastasis

M1 = Distant metastasis

Histopathologic Grade (G)

G1 = Well differentiated

G2 = Moderately differentiated

G3–4 = Poorly differentiated or undifferentiated

(Adapted from American Joint Committee on Cancer. Manual for Staging of Cancer, 4th edition. Philadelphia, JB Lippincott, 1992.)

Hormonal Therapy. Hormonal therapy is one method used to control rather than cure prostate cancer. In the early 1940s, it was determined that most prostate cancers were androgen-dependent and could be controlled by androgen withdrawal. Hormonal therapy for advanced prostate cancer suppresses all androgenic stimuli to the prostate by decreasing the circulating plasma testosterone levels or interrupting the conversion to and/or binding of dihydrotestosterone. As a result, the prostatic epithelium atrophies (decreases). Hormonal therapy is accomplished either by orchiectomy (removal of the testes) or by administering medications.

Orchiectomy effectively lowers plasma testosterone levels because about 93% of circulating testosterone is of testicular origin. As a result, the testicular stimulus required for continued prostatic growth is completely removed and results in prostatic atrophy. Although orchiectomy does not cause the side effects associated with other hormonal therapies, it carries a significant emotional impact.

Estrogen therapy, usually in the form of diethylstilbestrol (DES), has long been used to inhibit the gonadotropins responsible for testicular androgenic activity, thereby removing the androgenic hormone that promotes the growth of the malignancy.

DES relieves symptoms, reduces tumor size, decreases pain from metastatic nodules, and promotes an improved sense of well-being. However, DES significantly increases the risk of thromboembolism, pulmonary embolism, myocardial infarction, and stroke. Other side effects of estrogen therapy include impotence, decreased libido, difficulties in achieving orgasm, decreased sperm production, and gynecomastia (enlargement of breasts in men).

Newer hormonal therapies include the luteinizing hormone releasing hormone (LHRH) agonists and antiandrogen agents such as flutamide. Flutamide causes adrenal androgen suppression, whereas LHRH suppresses testicular androgen. Cyproterone acetate is a synthetic progesterone derivative that provides effective, competitive inhibition of androgens at the target cells. In contrast to estrogen, the newer hormonal agents have a lower incidence of cardiovascular side effects, gynecomastia, and decreased sexual function. Hot flushing can occur with orchiectomy or LHRH agonist therapy because these agents increase activity which releases norepinephrine and stimulates the thermoregulatory centers of the body.

Other Therapies. Cryosurgery of the prostate gland is a newer attempt to ablate prostate cancer in patients who could not physically tolerate surgery or in those whom prostate cancer has recurred. Chemotherapy such as doxorubicin, cisplatin, and cyclophosphamide may also be used.

To keep the urethral passage patent may require repeated transurethral resections. When this is impractical, catheter drainage is instituted by way of the suprapubic or transurethral route.

With advanced prostate cancer, blood transfusions are administered to maintain adequate hemoglobin levels when bone marrow is replaced by tumor. Radiation therapy to skeletal lesions can relieve bone pain. Pain may also be controlled by estrogens and narcotics and, if necessary, by severing spinal cord pain fibers through neurosurgery.

Sexual Dysfunction Associated With Prostate Cancer

Men with prostate cancer commonly experience sexual dysfunction before the diagnosis is made. Each treatment for prostate cancer further increases the incidence of sexual problems.

With nerve-sparing radical prostatectomy, the chance of recovering erections is better for men who are younger and in whom both neurovascular bundles are spared. Hormonal therapy also affects the central nervous system mechanisms that mediate sexual desire and arousability.

The prevalence rate of erectile dysfunction after definitive radiation therapy is approximately 25%. Researchers have found that men with borderline function before radiation therapy were more likely to experience impotence after therapy than men who had full erections and engaged in intercourse several times a month (Banker, 1988; Zinreich et al., 1990).

Care of the patient with cancer of the prostate is summarized in Nursing Care Plan 47-1.

Conditions Affecting the Testes and Adjacent Structures

Undescended Testis (Cryptorchidism)

Cryptorchidism is the absence of one or both testes from the scrotum. The testes may be located in the abdominal cavity or inguinal canal. If the testis does not descend, a surgical procedure known as **orchiopexy** is performed to position it properly.

In orchiopexy, an incision is made over the inguinal canal, and the testis is brought down and placed in the scrotum. To maintain the proper position of the testis, traction may be applied to the thigh by means of a suture drawn from the lower end of the scrotum.

Orchitis

Orchitis is an inflammation of the testes (testicular congestion), usually caused by pyogenic, viral, spirochetal, parasitic, traumatic, chemical, or unknown factors.

Mumps is one such factor. When postpubertal men contract mumps, about one in five develops some form of orchitis 4 to 7 days after the jaw and neck swell. The testis may show some atrophy. In past years, sterility and impotence often resulted. Today, a man who has never had mumps and who is exposed to the disease receives gamma globulin immediately; the disease is likely to be less severe, with minimal or no complications.

Management. If the cause of orchitis is bacterial, viral, or fungal, therapy is directed at the specific infecting organism. Rest, elevation of the scrotum, ice packs to reduce scrotal edema, antibiotics, analgesics, and anti-inflammatory medications are recommended.

Epididymitis

Epididymitis is an infection of the epididymis that usually descends from an infected prostate or urinary tract. It also may develop as a complication of gonorrhea. In men under 35 years of age, the major cause of epididymitis is *Chlamydia trachomatis.* The infection passes upward through the urethra and the ejaculatory duct, and then along the vas deferens to the epididymis.

The patient complains of unilateral pain and soreness in the inguinal canal along the course of the vas deferens, and then develops pain and swelling in the scrotum and the groin. The epididymis becomes swollen and extremely painful; the patient's temperature is elevated. The urine may contain pus (pyuria) and bacteria (bacteriuria), and the patient may experience chills and fever.

Management. If the patient is seen within the first 24 hours after onset of pain, the spermatic cord may be infiltrated with a local anesthetic agent to relieve pain. If the epididymitis is from a chlamydial infection, the patient and his sexual partner must be treated with antibiotics. The patient is observed for abscess formation as well. If no improvement occurs within 2 weeks, an underlying testicular tumor should be considered. An epididymectomy (excision of the epididymis from the testis) may be performed for patients with recurrent, incapacitating episodes of epididymitis or for those with chronic, painful conditions. With long-term epididymitis, the passage of sperm may be obstructed. If the obstruction is bilateral, infertility may result.

Nursing Interventions/Patient Education. The patient is placed on bed rest and the scrotum is elevated with a scrotal bridge or folded towel to prevent traction on the spermatic cord and to promote venous drainage and relieve pain. Antimicrobials are administered as prescribed until the acute inflammation subsides.

Intermittent cold compresses to the scrotum may help ease the pain. Later, local heat or sitz baths may help resolve the inflammation. Analgesics are administered for pain relief as prescribed.

The patient should be instructed to avoid straining, lifting, and sexual excitement until the infection is under control. He should continue taking analgesics and antibiotics as prescribed and using ice packs if necessary to relieve discomfort. He needs to know that it may take 4 weeks or longer for the epididymis to return to normal.

Vasectomy

Vasectomy, or male sterilization, is the ligation and transection of part of the vas deferens, with or without removal of a segment of the vas. To prevent the passage of the sperm from the testes, the vas deferens is exposed through a surgical opening in the scrotum or by use of a sharp, curved hemostat (Fig. 47-5). The severed ends are occluded with ligatures or clips, or the lumen of each vas is sealed by cautery. The spermatozoa, which are manufactured in the testes, cannot travel up the vas deferens after this surgery.

Because seminal fluid is manufactured predominantly in the seminal vesicles and prostate gland, which are unaffected by vasectomy, no noticeable decrease occurs in the amount of ejaculate, but it contains no spermatozoa. Because the sperm cells have no exit, they are reabsorbed into the body. The procedure has no effect on sexual potency, erection, ejaculation, or production of male hormones. The procedure provides no protection against sexually transmitted diseases.

Couples who worry about pregnancy resulting from contraceptive failure often report a decrease in concern and an increase in spontaneous sexual arousal after vasectomy. Concise and factual preoperative explanations may minimize or relieve the patient's concerns related to masculinity. Although a relationship between vasectomy and autoimmune disorders and prostatic cancer has been suggested, there is no clinical evidence of either.

The patient is advised that he will be sterile but that potency will not be altered after a bilateral vasectomy. On rare occasions, a spontaneous reanastomosis of the vas deferens occurs, which may result in the partner becoming pregnant. As with any surgical procedure, an informed legal

(text continues on page 1354)

NURSING CARE PLAN 47–1
Care of the Patient With Prostate Cancer

NURSING DIAGNOSIS: Anxiety related to concern and lack of knowledge about the diagnosis, treatment plan, and prognosis

GOAL: Reduced stress and improved ability to cope

Nursing Interventions	Rationale	Expected Outcomes
1. Obtain health history to determine the following: a. Patient's concerns b. His level of understanding of his health problem c. His past experience with cancer d. Whether he knows his diagnosis of malignancy and its prognosis e. His support systems and coping methods	1. Nurse clarifies information and facilitates patient's understanding and coping.	• Appears relaxed. • States that anxiety has been reduced or relieved. • Demonstrates understanding of illness and treatment when questioned. • Engages in open communication with others.
2. Provide education about diagnosis and treatment plan: a. Explain in simple terms what diagnostic tests to expect; how long they will take, and what will be experienced during each test. b. Review treatment plan and allow patient to ask questions.	2. Helping the patient to understand the diagnostic tests and treatment plan will help decrease his anxiety and promote cooperation.	
3. Assess his psychologic reaction to his diagnosis/prognosis and how he has coped with past stresses.	3. This information provides clues in determining appropriate measures to facilitate coping.	

NURSING DIAGNOSIS: Altered urinary elimination related to urethral obstruction secondary to prostatic enlargement or tumor and loss of bladder tone due to prolonged distention/retention

GOAL: Improved pattern of urinary elimination

Nursing Interventions	Rationale	Expected Outcomes
1. Determine patient's usual pattern of urinary function.	1. Provides a baseline for comparison and goal to work toward.	• Voids at normal intervals. • Reports absence of frequency, urgency, or bladder fullness. • Displays no palpable suprapubic distention after voiding. • Maintains balanced intake and output.
2. Assess for signs and symptoms of urinary retention: amount and frequency of urination, suprapubic distention, complaints of urgency and discomfort.	2. Voiding 20 to 30 ml frequently and output less than intake suggests retention.	
3. Catheterize patient to determine amount of residual urine.	3. Determines amount of urine remaining.	
4. Initiate measures to treat retention: a. Encourage assuming normal position for voiding. b. Recommend using Valsalva maneuver. c. Administer prescribed cholinergic agent. d. Monitor effects of medication.	a. Usual position provides relaxed conditions conducive for voiding. b. Exerting pressure tends to force urine out of bladder. c. Stimulates bladder contraction. d. If unsuccessful, another measure may be required.	
5. Consult with physician regarding intermittent or indwelling catheterization; assist with procedure as required.	5. Catheterization will relieve urinary retention until the specific cause is determined; it may be an obstruction that can be corrected only surgically.	

(continued)

NURSING CARE PLAN 47–1 *(continued)*
Care of the Patient With Cancer of the Prostate

Nursing Interventions	Rationale	Expected Outcomes
6. Monitor catheter function; maintain sterility of closed system; irrigate as required.	6. Adequate functioning of catheter is to be ensured to achieve purpose and to prevent infection.	
7. Prepare patient for surgery if indicated.	7. Surgical removal of obstruction may be necessary.	

NURSING DIAGNOSIS: Knowledge deficit related to new health problem: cancer, urinary difficulties, and treatment modalities

GOAL: Understanding of health problem and ability to care for self

Nursing Interventions	Rationale	Expected Outcomes
1. Encourage communication with the patient.	1. This is designed to establish rapport and trust	• Discusses his concerns and problems freely.
2. Review the anatomy of the involved area.	2. Orientation to one's anatomy is basic to understanding its function.	• Asks questions and shows interest in his condition.
3. Be specific in selecting information that is relevant to the patient's particular treatment plan.	3. This is based on the treatment plan, as it varies with each patient; individualization is desirable.	• Describes activities that help or hinder recovery. • Identifies ways of attaining/maintaining bladder control.
4. Identify ways to reduce pressure on the operative area after prostatectomy. a. Avoid prolonged sitting (in a chair, long automobile rides), standing, walking. b. Avoid straining, such as during exercises, bowel movement, lifting, and sexual intercourse.	4. This is to prevent bleeding; such precautions are in order for 6 to 8 weeks postoperatively.	• Demonstrates satisfactory technique and understanding of catheter care. • Lists signs and symptoms that must be reported should they occur.
5. Familiarize patient with ways of attaining/maintaining bladder control.	5. These measures will help control frequency and dribbling, and aid in preventing retention.	
a. Encourage urination every 2 to 3 hours; discourage voiding when supine.	a. By sitting or standing, patient is more likely to empty his bladder.	
b. Avoid drinking cola and caffeine beverages; urge a cut-off time in the evening for drinking fluids to minimize frequent voiding during the night.	b. Spacing the kind and amount of liquid intake will help to prevent frequency.	
c. Describe perineal exercises to be performed every hour.	c. Exercises will assist him in starting and stopping the urinary stream.	
d. Develop a schedule with patient so that it will fit into his routine.	d. A schedule will assist in developing a workable pattern of normal activities.	
6. Demonstrate catheter care; encourage his questions; stress the importance of position of urinary receptacle.	6. By requiring a return demonstration of care, collection, and emptying of his device, he will become more independent and also can prevent backflow of urine, which can lead to infection.	

NURSING DIAGNOSIS: Altered nutrition: Less than body requirements related to decreased oral intake because of anorexia, nausea, and vomiting brought on by cancer or its treatment

GOAL: Maintain optimal nutritional status

Nursing Interventions	Rationale	Expected Outcomes
1. Assess the amount of food eaten.	1. This assessment will help determine nutrient intake.	• Responds positively to his favoite foods.

(continued)

Nursing Interventions	Rationale	Expected Outcomes
2. Routinely weigh patient.	2. Weighing the patient on the same scale under similar conditions can help monitor changes in weight.	• Assumes responsibility for his oral hygiene. • Notes increase in weight after improved appetite.
3. Listen to patient's explanation of why he is unable to eat more.	3. His explanation may present easily corrected practices.	
4. Cater to his individual food preferences (*e.g.*, avoiding foods that are too spicy or too cold).	4. He will be more likely to consume larger servings if food is palatable and appealing.	
5. Recognize effect of medication or radiation therapy on appetite.	5. Many chemotherapeutic agents and radiation therapy promote anorexia.	
6. Inform patient that alterations in taste can occur.	6. Aging and the disease process can reduce taste sensitivity. In addition, smell and taste can be altered as a result of the body's absorption of by-products of cellular destruction (brought on by malignancy and its treatment).	
7. Use measures to control nausea and vomiting. a. Administer prescribed antiemetics; around the clock if necessary. b. Provide oral hygiene after vomiting episodes. c. Provide rest periods after meals.	7. Vomiting can decrease appetite.	
8. Provide frequent small meals, and a comfortable and pleasant environment.	8. Smaller portions of food are less overwhelming to the patient.	
9. Assess patient's ability to obtain and prepare foods.	9. Disability or lack of social support can hinder the patient's ability to obtain and prepare foods.	

NURSING DIAGNOSIS: Sexual dysfunction related to effects of therapy: chemotherapy, hormonal therapy, radiation therapy, surgery

GOAL: Ability to resume/enjoy modified sexual functioning

Nursing Interventions	Rationale	Expected Outcomes
1. Determine from nursing history what effect patient's medical condition is having on his sexual functioning.	1. Usually decreased libido and, later, impotence may be experienced.	• Describes the reasons for changes in sexual functioning. • Discusses with appropriate health care personnel alternative approaches and methods of sexual expression.
2. Inform patient of the effects of prostate surgery, orchiectomy (when applicable), chemotherapy, irradiation, and hormonal therapy on sexual function.	2. Treatment modalities may alter sexual function, but each is evaluated separately with regard to its effect on a particular patient.	
3. Include his partner in developing understanding and in discovering alternative, satisfying close relations with each other.	3. Often the bonds between a couple are strengthened with new appreciation and support that had not been evident before the current illness.	

NURSING DIAGNOSIS: Pain related to progression of disease and treatment modalities

GOAL: Relief of pain

Nursing Interventions	Rationale	Expected Outcomes
1. Evaluate nature of patient's pain and its location and intensity using pain scale.	1. Determining nature and causes of pain and its intensity helps to select proper relief modality and provide baseline for later comparison.	• Reports relief of pain. • Expects exacerbations, reports their quality or intensity, and obtains relief.

(continued)

NURSING CARE PLAN 47–1 *(continued)*
Care of the Patient With Cancer of the Prostate

Nursing Interventions	Rationale	Expected Outcomes
2. Avoid activities that aggravate or worsen pain.	2. Bumping the bed is an example of an action that can intensify the patient's pain.	
3. Because pain usually is related to bone metastasis, ensure that patient's bed has a bed board on a firm mattress. Also protect the patient from falls/injuries.	3. This will provide added support and is more comfortable. Protecting the patient from injury protects him from additional pain.	
4. Provide support for affected extremities.	4. More support coupled with reduced movement of the part helps in pain control.	
5. Prepare patient for radiation therapy if prescribed.	5. Radiation therapy may be effective in controlling pain.	
6. Administer analgesics or opioids at regularly scheduled intervals as prescribed.	6. Analgesics alter perception of pain and provide comfort. Regularly scheduled analgesics around the clock rather than prn provide more consistent pain relief.	
NURSING DIAGNOSIS: Impaired physical mobility and activity intolerance related to tissue hypoxia, malnutrition, and exhaustion and to spinal cord or nerve compression from metastases		
GOAL: Improved physical mobility		
1. Assess for factors causing limited mobility (*e.g.*, pain, hypercalcemia, limited exercise tolerance).	1. This information offers clues to the cause; if possible, cause is treated.	• Achieves improved physical mobility. • Relates that short-term goals are encouraging him because they are attainable.
2. Provide pain relief by administering prescribed medications.	2. Analgesics/opioids allow the patient to increase his activity more comfortably.	
3. Encourage use of assistive devices: cane, walker.	3. Support may offer the security needed to become mobile.	
4. Involve significant others in helping patient with range of motion exercises, positioning, and walking.	4. Assistance from partner or others encourages patient to repeat activities and achieve goals.	
5. Praise the patient for achieving small gains.	5. Encouragement stimulates improvement of performance.	
6. Assess nutritional status.	6. See Nursing Diagnosis: Alterated nutrition: Less than body requirements.	
COLLABORATIVE PROBLEMS: Hemorrhage, infection, bladder neck obstruction		
GOAL: Absence of complications		
1. Alert the patient to changes that may occur (after discharge) and that need to be reported:	1. Certain changes signal beginning complications, which call for nursing and medical interventions.	• Experiences no bleeding or passage of blood clots. • Reports no pain around the catheter. • Experiences normal frequency of urination. • Reports normal urinary output. • Maintains bladder control.
a. Continued bloody urine; passing blood clots	a. Hematuria with or without blood clot formation may occur postoperatively.	
b. Pain; burning around the catheter	b. Indwelling urinary catheters may be a source of infections.	
c. Frequency of urination	c. Urinary frequency may be caused by urinary tract infections or by bladder neck obstruction, resulting in incomplete voiding	
d. Diminished urinary output	d. Bladder neck obstruction decreases the amount of urine that is voided.	
e. Increasing loss of bladder control	e. Urinary incontinence may be a result of urinary retention.	

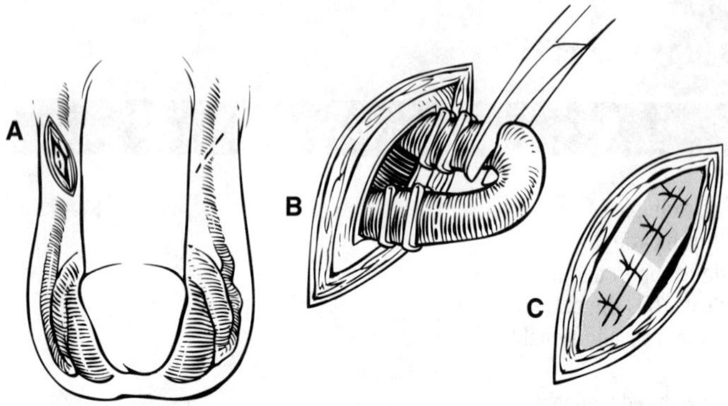

FIGURE 47-5. A vasectomy is a surgical resection of the vas deferens to prevent passage of sperm from the testes to the urethra during ejaculation.

consent form must be completed before the procedure is performed.

Complications of vasectomy include scrotal ecchymoses and swelling, superficial wound infection, vasitis (inflammation of the vas deferens), epididymitis or epididymo-orchitis, hematomas, and spermatic granuloma. A spermatic granuloma is an inflammatory response to the collection of sperm leaking into the scrotum from the severed end of the proximal vas. This can initiate recanalization of the vas, possibly resulting in pregnancy of the partner.

Nursing Interventions/Patient Education. Ice bags are applied intermittently to the scrotum for several hours after surgery to reduce swelling and to relieve discomfort. The patient is advised to wear cotton, jockey-type briefs for added comfort and support. He may become greatly concerned about the discoloration of the scrotal skin and superficial swelling. These are temporary conditions that occur frequently after vasectomy, and may be relieved by sitz baths.

Sexual intercourse may be resumed as desired, although fertility remains for a varying time after vasectomy until the spermatozoa stored distal to the severed vas have been evacuated. Other methods of contraception should be used until infertility is confirmed by an examination of ejaculate. Some physicians examine a specimen 4 weeks after the vasectomy to determine sterility; others examine two consecutive specimens 1 month apart, and still others consider a patient sterile after 36 ejaculations.

Vasovasostomy (Sterilization Reversal). Microsurgical techniques are being used in an attempt to reverse vasectomies (**vasovasostomy**), which restores patency to the vas deferens. Many men will have sperm in their ejaculate after a reversal, and 40% to 75% can impregnate a partner.

Banking Sperm. Storing fertile semen in a sperm bank *before* a vasectomy is an option for men who face an unforeseen life event that may cause them to want to father a child. The success rate in achieving pregnancy with frozen sperm is uncertain, and legal problems related to using stored sperm make this an ongoing issue.

Tumors of the Testes

Testicular cancer, which ranks first in cancer deaths among men in the 20- to 35-year age group, is the most common cancer in men from age 15 to 35 years and the second most common malignancy from age 35 to 39. Such cancers are classified as germinal or nongerminal. **Germinal tumors** arise from the germinal cells of the testes (seminomas, teratocarcinomas, and embryonal carcinomas); **nongerminal tumors** arise from epithelium. Most neoplasms are germinal, with about 40% of these being seminomas. Seminomas tend to remain localized, whereas nonseminomatous tumors are fast-growing. The cause of testicular tumors is unknown, but cryptorchidism, infections, and genetic and endocrine factors appear to play a part in their development.

The risk of testicular cancer is 35 times greater for men with any type of undescended testis than for the general population. Testicular tumors are usually malignant and tend to metastasize early, spreading from the testis to the lymph nodes in the retroperitoneum and to the lungs.

Clinical Manifestations. The symptoms appear very gradually with a mass or lump on the testicle and generally painless enlargement of the testis. The patient may complain of heaviness in the scrotum, inguinal area, or lower abdomen. Backache (from retroperitoneal node extension), pain in the abdomen, loss of weight, and general weakness may result from metastasis.

- The enlargement of the testis without pain is a significant diagnostic finding.

One effective early detection method is testicular self-examination. An essential part of health promotion practices for men should include testicular self-examination. Teaching men to perform self-examination as depicted in Chart 47-1 is an important intervention for early detection of this disease.

Diagnostic Evaluation. Human chorionic gonadotropin and α-fetoprotein are tumor markers that may be elevated in patients with testicular cancer. (Tumor markers are substances synthesized by the tumor cells and released into the circulation in abnormal amounts.) Newer immunocytochemical techniques can help identify the cells that apparently produce these markers. Tumor marker levels in the blood are used for diagnosis, staging, and monitoring the response to treatment. Other diagnostic tests include intravenous urography to detect any ureteral deviation caused by a tumor mass; lymphangiography to assess the extent of tumor spread to the lymphatic system; and computed tomography (CT scan) of the chest and abdomen to determine the extent of the disease in the lungs and retroperitoneum.

Management. Testicular cancer is one of the most curable solid tumors. The goals of management are to eradicate the disease and achieve a cure. Treatment selection is based on the cell type and the anatomic extent of the disease. The testis is removed by orchiectomy through an inguinal incision with a high ligation of the spermatic cord. A gel-filled prosthesis can be implanted to offset the absence of one testis. After unilateral orchiectomy for testicular cancer, most patients experience no impairment of endocrine function. However, other patients have decreased hormonal levels, suggesting that the unaffected testis is not functioning at normal levels. Retroperitoneal lymph node dissection (RPLND) to prevent lymphatic spread of the cancer may be performed after orchiectomy. Although normal

CHART 47-1

Patient Education: Testicular Self-Examination (TSE)

Testicular self-examination (TSE) is to be performed once a month; it is neither difficult nor time consuming. A convenient time is often after a warm bath or shower when the scrotum is more relaxed.

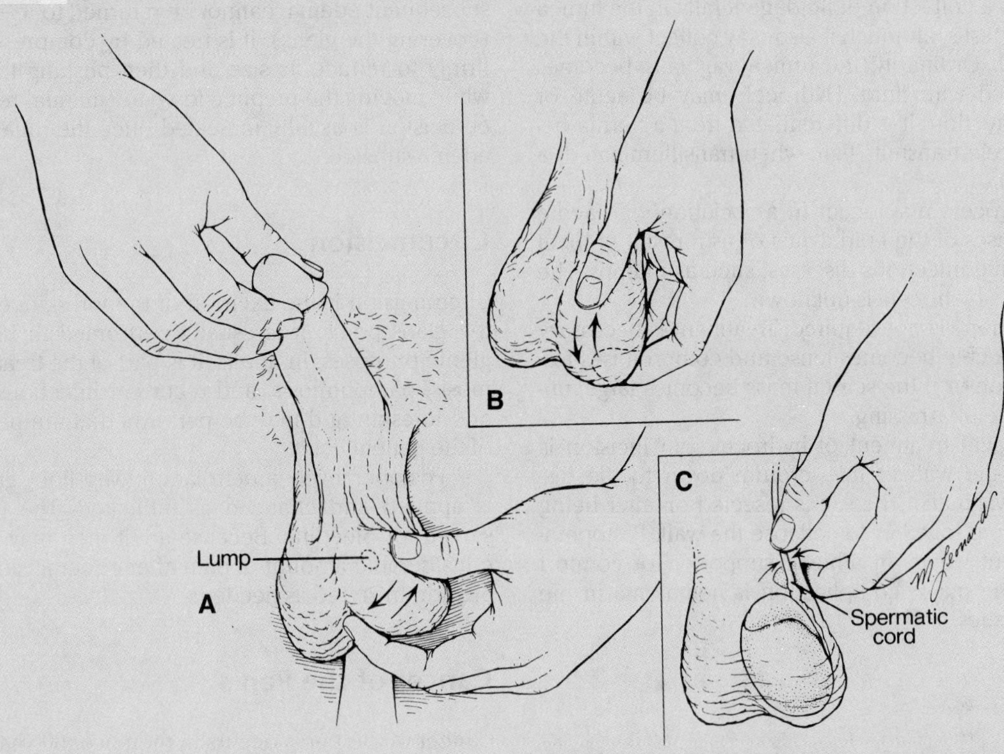

1. Use both hands to palpate the testis; the normal testicle is smooth and uniform in consistency.
2. With the index and middle fingers under the testis and the thumb on top, roll the testis gently in a horizontal plane between the thumb and fingers (*A*).
3. Feel for any evidence of a small lump or abnormality.
4. Follow the same procedure and palpate upward along the testis (*B*).
5. Locate the epididymis (*C*), a cordlike structure on the top and back of the testicle that stores and transports sperm.
6. Repeat the examination for the other testis. It is normal to find that one testis is larger than the other.
7. If you find any evidence of a small, pealike lump, consult your physician. It may be due to an infection or a tumor growth.

libido and orgasm are usually unimpaired after RPLND, the patient may develop ejaculatory dysfunction with resultant infertility. Sperm banking before surgery may be considered.

Postoperative irradiation of the lymph nodes from the diaphragm to the iliac region is used in treating seminomas and is only delivered to the side of the tumor. The other testis is shielded from radiation to preserve fertility. Radiation is also used for patients who do not respond to chemotherapy or for whom lymph node surgery is not recommended.

Testicular carcinomas are highly responsive to medication therapy. Multiple chemotherapy with cisplatin and other agents such as vinblastine, bleomycin, dactinomycin, and cyclophosphamide gives a high percentage of complete remission. Good results may be obtained by combining different types of treatment, including surgery, radiation therapy, and chemotherapy. Even with disseminated testicular cancer, the prognosis is favorable, and the disease probably curable because of advances in diagnosis and treatment.

Nursing Interventions/Patient Education. Because the patient may have difficulty in accepting his condition, issues related to body image and sexuality should be addressed. He needs encouragement to maintain a positive attitude during what may be a long course of therapy. He also needs to know that radiation therapy will not necessarily prevent the patient from fathering children, nor does unilateral excision of a tumor necessarily decrease virility.

A patient with a history of one testicular tumor has a greater chance of developing subsequent tumors. Follow-up studies include chest x-rays, excretory urography, radioimmunoassay of human chorionic gonadotropins and α-fetoprotein levels, and examination of lymph nodes to detect recurrent malignancy.

Hydrocele

A **hydrocele** is a collection of fluid, generally in the tunica vaginalis of the testis, although it also may collect within the spermatic cord. Ordinarily, the tunica vaginalis becomes widely distended with fluid. Hydrocele may be acute or chronic. On detection, it is differentiated from a hernia because a hydrocele transmits light when transilluminated; a hernia does not.

Acute hydrocele may occur in association with acute infectious diseases of the epididymis or as a result of local injury or systemic infectious diseases, such as mumps. The cause of chronic hydrocele is unknown.

Usually, therapy is not required. Treatment is necessary only if the hydrocele becomes tense and compromises testicular circulation or if the scrotal mass becomes large, uncomfortable, or embarrassing.

In the surgical treatment of hydrocele, an incision is made through the wall of the scrotum down to the distended tunica vaginalis. The sac is resected or, after being opened, is sutured together to collapse the wall. Postoperatively, the patient wears an athletic supporter for comfort and support. The major complication is hematoma in the loose scrotal tissues.

Varicocele

A **varicocele** is an abnormal dilation of the veins of the pampiniform venous plexus in the scrotum (the network of veins from the testis and the epididymis which constitute part of the spermatic cord). Varicoceles usually occur in the veins on the upper portion of the left testicle in adults. In some men, a varicocele has been associated with infertility. Few, if any, subjective symptoms may be produced by the enlarged spermatic vein, and no treatment is required unless fertility is a concern. Symptomatic varicocele (pain, tenderness, and discomfort in the inguinal region) is corrected surgically by ligating the external spermatic vein at the inguinal area. An ice pack may be applied to the scrotum for the first few hours after surgery to relieve edema. The patient then wears a scrotal supporter.

Conditions Affecting the Penis

Phimosis

Phimosis, a condition in which the foreskin is constricted so that it cannot be retracted over the glans, can occur congenitally or from inflammation and edema. With the trend away from routine circumcision of newborns, the child and adult require early instruction in cleansing the prepuce. In adults who do not clean the preputial area, normal secretions accumulate, causing subsequent inflammation (**balanitis**), which can lead to adhesions and fibrosis. The thickened secretions become encrusted with urinary salts and calcify, forming calculi in the prepuce. In elderly men, penile carcinoma may develop. Phimosis is corrected by circumcision (see below). The patient is instructed in proper hygienic care of the foreskin.

Paraphimosis is a condition in which the foreskin is retracted behind the glans and, because of narrowness and subsequent edema, cannot be returned to its usual position (covering the glans). It is treated by compressing the glans firmly to reduce its size and then pushing the glans back while moving the prepuce forward (manual reduction). Circumcision is usually indicated once the inflammation and edema subside.

Circumcision

Circumcision is the excision of the foreskin, or prepuce, of the glans penis. It is usually performed in infancy for hygienic purposes. In adults, it is part of the treatment for phimosis, paraphimosis, and recurrent infections of the glans and foreskin and may be performed at the personal desire of the patient.

Postoperatively a petrolatum (Vaseline) gauze dressing is applied and changed as indicated. The patient is observed for bleeding. Because adult men may experience a considerable amount of pain after circumcision, analgesics are administered as needed.

Cancer of the Penis

Cancer of the penis occurs in men over 60 years of age and represents about 0.5% of malignancies in men in the United States. In some countries, however, the incidence is 10%. Cancer of the penis rarely occurs in circumcised males. It appears on the skin of the penis as a painless, wartlike growth or ulcer. Cancer of the penis can involve the glans, the coronal sulcus under the prepuce, the corporal bodies, the urethra, and regional or distant lymph nodes. Bowen's disease is a form of squamous cell carcinoma *in situ* of the penile shaft. Typically, a man delays seeking treatment for more than a year, probably because of guilt, embarrassment, or ignorance.

Management. Smaller lesions involving only the skin may be controlled by excisional biopsy. Topical chemotherapy with 5-fluorouracil cream may be one option in selected patients. Radiation therapy is used to treat small squamous cell carcinomas of the penis or for palliation in advanced tumors or lymph node metastasis. Partial penectomy (removal of the penis) is preferred to total penectomy if possible; about 40% of patients can then participate in sexual intercourse and stand for urination. The shaft of the penis can still respond to sexual arousal with an erection and has the sensory capacity for orgasm and ejaculation. Total penectomy is indicated when the tumor is not amenable to conservative treatment. After a total penectomy, the patient may still experience orgasm with stimulation of the perineum and scrotal area.

Patient Education. Circumcision in infancy almost eliminates the possibility of penile cancer, because chronic irritation and inflammation of the glans penis predispose to penile tumors. In uncircumcised men, personal hygiene is an important preventive measure.

Priapism

Priapism is an uncontrolled, persistent erection of the penis that causes the penis to become large, hard, and painful. It occurs from either neural or vascular causes, including sickle cell thrombosis, leukemic cell infiltration, spinal cord tumors, and tumor invasion of the penis or its vessels. This condition may result in gangrene and often results in impotence, whether treated or not.

Priapism is a urologic emergency. The goal of therapy is to improve venous drainage of the corpora cavernosa to prevent ischemia, fibrosis, and impotence. The initial treatment is directed at relieving the erection and includes bed rest and sedation. The corpora may be irrigated with an anticoagulant, which allows stagnant blood to be aspirated. Shunting procedures to divert the blood from the turgid corpora cavernosa to the venous system (corpora cavernosa–saphenous vein shunt) or into the corpus spongiosum–glans penis compartment may be attempted.

Peyronie's Disease

Peyronie's disease involves the buildup of fibrous plaques in the sheath of the corpus cavernosum. These plaques are not visible when the penis is relaxed. When erect, however, curvature of the penis occurs that can be painful and can make sexual intercourse difficult or impossible. Peyronie's disease primarily occurs in middle-aged and older men. Although the plaques may shrink over time, surgical removal of the plaques may be necessary.

Urethral Stricture

Urethral stricture is a condition in which a section of the urethra is narrowed. It can occur congenitally or from a scar along the urethra. Traumatic injury to the urethra, for example, from instrumentation or infections, can result in strictures. Treatment involves dilation of the urethra or, in severe cases, urethrotomy (surgical removal of the stricture).

CRITICAL THINKING EXERCISES

1. A 47-year-old man tells you that he is uncertain about the meaning of an elevated prostate-specific antigen (PSA) level and asks you for an explanation and for advice about what action to take. How would you respond to his request? Describe the factors you would consider in formulating your response.
2. You are assigned to care for two patients who have undergone prostatectomy. One has had a transurethral resection (TURP); the other has undergone an open surgical approach to remove the prostate. How would your care differ for these two patients? How would your assessment be directed to detect possible complications?
3. A 28-year-old man is seeking treatment for his sixth episode of sexually transmitted disease (STD). In addition to assisting with medical management and follow-up, describe other interventions you would consider for this patient.

BIBLIOGRAPHY

Books

Agency for Health Care Policy and Research. Benign Prostatic Hyperplasia: Diagnosis and Treatment. Clinical Practice Guidelines. Number 8. U.S. Department of Health and Human Services. AHCPR Publication No. 94-0582. Bethesda MD, 1994.

Bennett AH (ed). Impotence: Diagnosis and Management of Erectile Dysfunction. Philadelphia, WB Saunders, 1994.

Das S and Crawford ED (eds). Cancer of the Prostate. New York, Marcel Dekker, 1993.

Fitzpatrick JM and Kane RJ (eds). The Prostate. New York, Churchill Livingstone, 1989.

Glenn JF. Urologic Surgery, 4th ed. Philadelphia, JB Lippincott, 1991.

Gray M. Genitourinary Disorders. St. Louis, Mosby Year Book, 1992.

Hanks GE, Myers CE, and Scardino PT. Cancer of the prostate. In DeVita VT, Hellman S and Rosenberg SA (eds). Principles and Practice of Oncology, 3rd ed. Philadelphia, JB Lippincott, 1993, 1073–1113.

Hill GS. Uropathology, Vols. 1 and 2. New York, Churchill Livingstone, 1989.

Leiblum SR and Rosen RC (eds). Principles and Practice of Sex Therapy: Update for the 1990s, 2nd ed. New York, Guilford Press, 1989.

Perez CA et al. Carcinoma of the prostate. In DeVita VT, Hellman S, and Rosenberg SA (eds). Principles and Practice of Oncology, 3rd ed. Philadelphia, JB Lippincott, 1989, 1023–1058.

Schover LR. Sexuality and Cancer: For the Man Who Has Cancer, and His Partner. Atlanta, American Cancer Society, Inc, 1988.

Tanagho EA and McAninch JW (eds). Smith's General Urology, 13th ed. Nowalk, CT, Appleton and Lange, 1992.

Walsh PC et al. Campbell's Urology, Vols. 1–3, 6th ed. Philadelphia, WB Saunders, 1992.

Journals

Asterisks indicate nursing research articles.

General

Aikey C. Erectile dysfunction. Urol Nurs 1992 Sep; 12(3):96–103.

*Berry DL. Return-to-work experiences of people with cancer. Oncol Nurs Forum 1993; 20(6):905–911.

Buczny B. Impotence in older men: A newly recognized problem. J Gerontol Nurs 1992 May; 18(5):25–30.

Cohen DA et al. Group counseling at STD clinics to promote use of condoms. Public Health Report 1992 Nov–Dec; 107(6):727–731.

Feldman HA et al. Impotence and its medical and psychological correlates: Results of the Massachusetts male aging study. J Urol 1994 Jan; 151(1):54–61.
Kurgan A, Nunnelee JD and Zilberman M. The importance of early detection of variocele in adolescent males. Nurse Practitioner 1994 Oct; 19(10):36–37.
Lewis JH. Nursing management for patients using external vacuum devices: A unique opportunity. Urol Nurs 1993 Sep; 13(3):80–85.
*Millon-Underwood S and Sanders E. Factors contributing to health promotion behaviors among African-American men. Oncol Nurs Forum 1990 Sep/Oct; 17(5):707–712.
Morley JE. Management of impotence: Diagnostic considerations and therapeutic options. Postgrad Med 1993 Feb 15; 93(3): 65–67, 71–72, 149–151.
Moskowitz MD and Mellinger BC. Sexually transmitted diseases and their relation to male infertility. Urol Clin North Am 1992 Feb; 19(1):35–45.
Mulholland SG and Stefanelli JL. Genitourinary cancer in the elderly. Am J Kidney Dis 1990 Oct; 16(4):324–328.
Orr DP et al. Factors associated with condom use among sexually active female adolescents. J Pediatr 1992 Feb; 120(2 Pt 1): 311–317.
Pack R. Descriptive epidemiology of genitourinary cancers. Semin Oncol Nurs 1993 Nov; 9(4):218–223.
*Post-White J, Carter M, Anglim MA. Cancer prevention and early detection: Nursing students' knowledge, attitudes, personal practices, and teaching. Oncol Nurs Forum 1993; 20(5): 743–749.
Rosen RC and Leiblum SR. Treatment of male erectile disorder: Current options and dilemmas. J Sex Marital Ther 1993; 8(1): 5–8.
Smith DB and Babaian RJ. The effects of treatment for cancer on male fertility and sexuality. Cancer Nurs 1992; 15(4):271–275.
White MJ et al. Sexual activities, concerns and interests of men with spinal cord injury. Am J Phys Med Rehabil 1992 Aug; 71(4):225–231.
Wilson W. The effect of drugs on male sexual function and fertility. Nurse Pract 1991; 16(9):12–24.

Male Contraception

Comhaire FH. Male contraception: Hormonal, mechanical and other. Hum Reprod 1994 Apr; 9(4):586–590.
Raspa RF. Complications of vasectomy. Am Fam Physician 1993 Nov 15; 48(7):1264–1268.

Assessment of Function and Dysfunction of Male Reproductive Function

Aikey C. Erectile dysfunction. Urol Nurs 1992 Sep; 12(3):96–103.
Crawford ED et al. The effect of digital rectal examination on prostate-specific antigen levels. JAMA 1992 Apr 22–29; 267(16):2227–2228.
DuBeau CE and Resnick NM. Evaluation of the causes and severity of geriatric incontinence. A critical appraisal. Urol Clin North Am 1991 May; 18(2):243–256.
Kemp ED. Prostate cancer. Finding and managing it. Postgrad Med 1992 Jul; 92(1):67–74, 77–84, 89.
Lakin M. The evaluation and nonsurgical management of impotence. Semin Nephrol 1994 Nov; 14(6):544–550.
Littrup PJ et al. Prostate cancer screening: Current trends and future implications. CA Cancer J Clin 1992 July–Aug; 42(4):198–211.
*Martin JP. Male cancer awareness: Impact of an employee education program. Oncol Nurs Forum 1990 Jan/Feb; 17(1):59–64.
Mettlin C et al. Defining and updating the American Cancer Society guidelines for the cancer-related checkup: Prostate and endometrial cancers. CA Cancer J Clin 1993 Jan–Feb; 43(1): 42–46.
Morley JE. Management of impotence. Diagnostic considerations and therapeutic options. Postgrad Med 1993 Feb 15. 93(3): 65–67, 71–72.
Morley JE and Kaiser FE. Sexual function with advancing age. Med Clin North Am 1989 Nov; 73(6):1483–1495.
NIH Consensus Conference. Impotence. NIH Consensus Development Panel on Impotence. JAMA 1993 Jul 7; 270(1):83–90.
O'Keefe M and Hunt DK. Assessment and treatment of impotence. Med Clin North Am 1995 Mar; 79(2):415–434.
Richie JP. Detection and treatment of testicular cancer. CA Cancer J Clin 1993 Mar/Apr; 43(3):151–175.
*Rudolf VM et al. The practice of TSE among college men: Effectiveness of an educational program. Oncol Nurs Forum 1988 Jan/Feb; 15(1):45–48.
White MJ et al. Sexual activities, concerns and interests of men with spinal cord injury. Am J Phys Med Rehabil 1992 Aug; 71(4):225–231.
Wilson W. The effect of drugs on male sexual function and fertility. Nurse Pract 1991; 16(9):12–24.

Infertility

Baker HW. Male infertility. Endocrinol Metab Clin North Am 1994 Dec; 23(4):783–793.
Gilbaugh JH III and Lipshultz LI. Nonsurgical treatment of male infertility. An update. Urol Clin North Am 1994 Aug; 21(3): 531–548.
Honig SC. New diagnostic techniques in the evaluation of anatomic abnormalities of the infertile male. Urol Clin North Am 1994 Aug; 21(3):417–432.
Howards SS. Treatment of male infertility. N Engl J Med 1995 Feb 2; 332(5):312–317.
Sigman M. Assisted reproductive techniques and male infertility. Urol Clin North Am 1994 Aug; 21(3):505–515.
Thompson ST. Prevention of male infertility: An update. Urol Clin North Am 1994 Aug; 21(3):365–376.

Benign Prostatic Hyperplasia

Gerber GS. Lasers in the treatment of benign prostatic hyperplasia. Urology 1995 Feb; 45(2):193–199.
Hill SJ, Lawrence SL and Lepor H. New use for alpha blockers: Benign prostatic hyperplasia. Am Fam Physician 1994 Jun; 49(8):1885–1888, 1893–1894.
Jonler M et al. Benign prostatic hyperplasia. Endocrinol Metab Clin North Am 1994 Dec; 23(4):795–807.
Monda JM and Oesterling JE. Medical management of prostatic obstruction. J Urol Nurs 1994 Apr–Jun; 13(2):717–738.
Moul JW. Benign prostatic hyperplasia. New concepts in the 1990s. Postgrad Med 1993 Nov 1; 94(6):141–146, 151–156.
Schlegel PN. Medical management of prostatic diseases. Adv Intern Med 1994; 39:569–601.

Prostate Cancer

Berger NS. Prostate cancer: Screening and early detection update. Semin Oncol Nurs 1993 Aug; 9(3):180–183.
Brawer MK. The diagnosis of prostate carcinoma. Cancer 1993 Feb 1; 71(3 Suppl):899–905.
Brenner ZR and Krenzer ME. Update on cyrosurgical ablation for prostate cancer. Am J Nurs 1995 Apr; 95(4):44–48.
Cher ML and Carroll PR. Screening for prostate cancer. West J Med 1995 Mar; 162(3):235–242.
Crawford ED et al. The effect of digital rectal examination on prostate-specific antigen levels. JAMA 1992 Apr 22–29; 267(16):2227–2228.
D'Elia FL and Fomella LG. Prostate cancer update 1995. Compr Ther 1995; 21(1):35–40.
Ellis WJ and Lange PH. Prostate cancer. Endocrinol Metab Clin North Am 1994 Dec; 23(4):809–824.

Epstein BE and Hanks GE. Prostate cancer: Evaluation and radiotherapeutic management. CA Cancer J Clin 1992 July–Aug; 42(4):223–240.

Fleming C et al. A decision analysis of alternative treatment strategies for clinically localized prostate cancer. JAMA 1993 May 26; 269(20):2650–2658.

Garnick MB. Prostate cancer: Screening, diagnosis, and management. Ann Intern Med 1993 May 15; 118(10):804–818.

Geller J. Basis for hormonal management of advanced prostate cancer. Cancer 1993 Feb 1; 71(3 Suppl):1039–1045.

Geller J and Sionit L. Castration-like effects on the human prostate of a 5α-reductase inhibitor, finasteride. J Cell Biochem 1992; 16H(Suppl):109–112.

Gormley GJ. Chemoprevention strategies for prostate cancer: The role of 5α-reductase inhibitors. J Cell Biochem 1992; 16H(Suppl):113–117.

Gormley GJ et al. The effect of finesteride in men with benign prostatic hyperplasia. N Engl J Med 1992 Oct 22; 327(17): 1185–1191.

Greco KE and Kulawiak L. Prostate cancer prevention: Risk reduction through life-style, diet, and chemoprevention. Oncol Nurs Forum 1994 Oct; 21(9):1504–1511.

Held JL et al. Cancer of the prostate: Treatment and nursing implications. Oncol Nurs Forum 1994 Oct; 21(9):1517–1529.

Kemp ED. Prostate cancer. Finding and managing it. Postgrad Med 1992 July; 92(1):67–74, 77–84, 89.

Lee WR, Giantonio B, and Hanks GE. Prostate cancer. Curr Probl Cancer 1994 Nov–Dec; 18(6):295–357.

Littrup PJ et al. Prostate cancer screening: Current trends and future implications. CA Cancer J Clin 1992 July–Aug; 42(4):198–211.

Littrup PJ et al. The benefit and cost of prostate cancer early detection. CA Cancer J Clin 1993 Mar/Apr; 43(3):134–149.

Mahon SM and Casperson DS. Focus on oncology: Mass screening for prostate cancer—a community hospital's experience. J Urol Nurs 1993 Jan–Mar; 12(1):372–378.

Maxwell MB. Cancer of the prostate. Semin Oncol Nurs 1993 Nov; 9(4):237–251.

*McKee JM. Cues to action in prostate cancer screening. Oncol Nurs Forum 1994 Aug; 21(7):1171–1176.

Mettlin C et al. Defining and updating the American Cancer Society guidelines for the cancer-related checkup: Prostate and endometrial cancers. CA Cancer J Clin 1993 Jan–Feb; 43(1):42–46.

Mettlin C et al. American Cancer Society–National Prostate Cancer Detection Project. Results from multiple examinations using transrectal ultrasound, digital rectal examination, and prostate specific antigen. Cancer 1993 Feb 1; 71(3 Suppl):891–898.

Moore S et al. Nerve-sparing prostatectomy. Am J Nurs 1992 Apr; 92(4):59–64.

Travis M and Gwozdz DT. Nursing case management for patients with TURP. Urol Nurs 1993 June; 13(2):48–54.

Waldman AR and Osborne DM. Screening for prostate cancer. Oncol Nurs Forum 1994 Oct; 21(9):1513–1517.

Waxman ES. Sexual dysfunction following treatment for prostate cancer: Nursing assessment and interventions. Oncol Nurs Forum 1993; 20(10):1567–1571.

Testicular Cancer

Brock D et al. Testicular cancer. Semin Oncol Nurs 1993 Nov; 9(4):224–236.

Brodsky MS. Testicular cancer survivors' impressions of the impact of the disease on their lives. Qualitative Health Res 1995 Feb; 5(1):78–96.

Clore ER. A guide for the testicular self-examination. J Pediatr Health Care 1993 Nov–Dec; 7(6):264–268.

Heinrich-Rynning T. Prostatic cancer treatments and their effects on sexual functioning. Oncol Nurs Forum 1987; 14(6): 37–41.

Higgs DJ. The patient with testicular cancer: Nursing management of chemotherapy. Oncol Nurs Forum 1990 Mar/Apr; 17(2): 243–249.

*Martin JP. Male cancer awareness: Impact of an employee education program. Oncol Nurs Forum 1990 Jan/Feb; 17(1): 59–64.

*Reno DR. Men's knowledge and health beliefs about testicular cancer and testicular self-examination. Cancer Nurs 1988 Apr; 11(2):112–117.

Richie JP. Detection and treatment of testicular cancer. CA Cancer J Clin 1993 Mar/Apr; 43(3):151–175.

Rosella JD. Testicular cancer health education: An integrative review. J Adv Nurs 1994 Oct; 20(4):666–671.

*Rudolf VM et al. The practice of TSE among college men: Effectiveness of an educational program. Oncol Nurs Forum 1988 Jan/Feb; 15(1):45–48.

Schover LR. Sexual rehabilitation after treatment for prostate cancer. Cancer 1993 Feb 1; 71(3 Suppl):1024–1030.

Turner D. Testicular cancer and the value of self-examination. Nurs Times 1995 Jan 4–11; 30(1):30–31.

Zinreich ES et al. Pre and posttreatment evaluation of sexual function in patients with adenocarcinoma of the prostate. Int J Radiat Oncol Biol Phys 1990 Sep; 19(3):729–732.

Nursing Research Profile for Unit 11

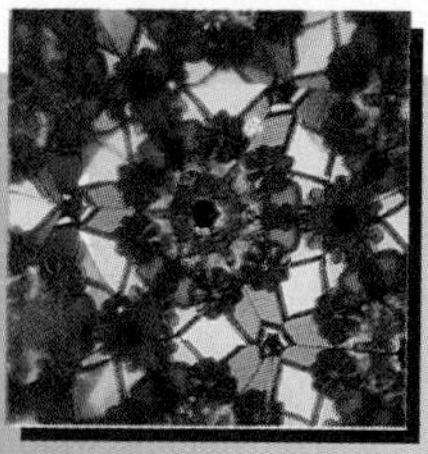

Reproductive Function

Overview

Nursing research studies reviewed here focus on the development of a typology of perimenstrual symptoms, factors influencing early detection of prostate cancer, and women's reactions to completion of adjuvant therapy for treatment of breast cancer.

Mitchell ES, Woods NF, and Lentz MJ. Differentiation of women with three perimenstrual symptom patterns. Nurs Research 1994 Jan/Feb; 43(1):25–30.

The purpose of this study was to develop a typology of premenstrual symptoms by describing and differentiating three perimenstrual symptom severity patterns in women: premenstrual syndrome (PMS), premenstrual magnification (PMM), and low symptom (LS). PMS is characterized by low symptom severity postmenses and higher severity premenses, whereas women with PMM experience a pattern of medium to high symptom severity postmenses and a higher level of severity premenses. LS is characterized by low severity of symptoms and little change from postmenses to premenses.

A community-based sample of women was recruited for the study. To be eligible for the study, women had to be between the ages of 18 and 45, not currently pregnant, not being treated for a gynecologic problem, having menstrual periods, not taking oral contraceptives, and able to write and understand English. Eligible subjects were asked to complete an in-home interview and keep a health diary during at least one menstrual cycle; 142 women who met inclusion criteria, returned a completed health diary, and fell into one of the three categories being examined in this study were included in the final sample.

Data collected during the in-home interview addressed social demands (measured by a life events survey), menstrual socialization (subjects' expectations about menarche, mothers' premenstrual symptoms), feminine socialization (Attitudes Toward Women Scale), parity (self-report of number of confirmed pregnancies), personal health habits (health habits questionnaire), and psychologic distress level (Center for Epidemiologic Studies Depression Scale). Three two-way discriminant analyses were performed to differentiate variables associated with the three patterns of symptom severity.

The women with PMS (n = 26) had more psychologic distress, more years of education, and a mother with more premenstrual symptoms than the women in the LS group (n = 91). When women in the PMM group (n = 25) were compared with the LS group, those with PMM were similar to those with PMS in psychologic distress and mother's premenstrual symptoms. However, the women with PMM had more negative effects from stressful life events and were younger than those with low symptoms. When women in the PMS group were compared with the PMM group, those with PMS were found to be older, had more education, engaged in healthier behavior, and held more nontraditional roles about the roles of women when compared with the PMM group. Women in the PMM group had more stress in their lives than women in the PMS group. Psychologic distress was the strongest factor differentiating women with PMM and PMS from those in the LS group.

Nursing Implications. The results of this study indicate that a number of factors are associated with PMS. Further, the findings indicate that there are several distinct subgroups among women who report premenstrual symptoms. Further research is needed to describe these differences further and to identify specific interventions for these subgroups.

Million-Underwood S. Factors influencing early detection of prostate cancer. Appl Nurs Res 1992 Feb; 5(1):30–31.

Although cancer of the prostate gland is a leading cause of death of American men, few men participate in early detection programs for this disease. This study was conducted to determine the attitudes and beliefs of men about prostate cancer susceptibility, screening procedures, and the efficacy of early detection and treatment. In addition, the effect of these attitudes and beliefs on participation in prostate cancer screening programs was investigated. A 33-item questionnaire developed by the investigator included questions that addressed prostate cancer screening and treatment, perceived risk for developing prostate cancer, and actual use of prostate cancer screening procedures. Content validity of the instrument was obtained by a panel of clinical experts prior to its use.

The convenience sample comprised 90 men whose ages ranged from 39 to 78 years; the mean age was 43.75 (SD = 7.3). Analysis of data revealed that although 88% of the subjects believed that if more men participated in prostate screening there would be fewer deaths from prostate cancer, only 42% of the sample indicated that they had ever had a screening digital rectal examination (DRE). Subjects who believed that a routine DRE was an essential part of health maintenance were more likely to have had a DRE. Sixty-one percent of the subjects indicated that DRE was "too embarrassing." The majority of subjects (77%) indicated that the occurrence of prostate cancer in a friend or relative caused them to consider the possibility of prostte cancer in themselves.

Nursing Implications. The findings of this study demonstrated that attitudes and beliefs greatly influence participation in prostate cancer screening. Although many men were concerned about the possibility of developing prostate cancer and perceived themselves to be at risk, most were reluctant to undergo screening procedures. Therefore, it is important to integrate men's knowledge of personal risks and their understanding of the importance of screening procedures when teaching and counseling about health maintenance and measures to reduce prostate cancer.

Ward SE, et al. Patients' reactions to completion of adjuvant breast cancer therapy. Nurs Res 1992 Nov/Dec; 41(6): 362–366.

Chemotherapy treatment regimens following surgery or radiation in women with breast cancer are both physically and emotionally stressful. It is often assumed that women would feel relief and experience lower levels of stress when treatment cycles were completed. In the study, 38 women with early-stage breast cancer were examined to determine the psychologic distress experienced with the completion of therapy. Data collection occurred at three points: (1) the first day of adjuvant therapy, (2) 1 week following chemotherapy completion, and (3) following completion of a course of radiation therapy. Information was gathered using several scales as well as by specific questioning. Scales used included the Center for Epidemiologic Studies Depression Scale (CDES), the Problems Checklist (PC), and a Side Effects Checklist (SEC). Participants were specifically questioned about a feeling of loss of a "safety net" after treatment completion, their perceived illness timeline, and their perceptions of treatment efficacy.

Results of the study showed that 30% of women felt that a safety net was removed when treatment was completed. Overall, depression scores decreased from the first measurement to the last. Those individuals with the highest depression scores at the end of treatment also displayed a more chronic perception of their illness and had experienced more side effects of therapy. Several participants also noted that they found it beneficial to be asked if they were upset after treatment was over, since this reassured them that this was not an unusual reaction.

Nursing Implications. This study alerts nurses to an often overlooked crisis point in cancer treatment–the completion of therapy. Patients may feel vulnerable as treatment ends, especially if side effects continue. Nurses must be aware of stressful times for patients and be prepared to assist them to cope during these times. Continued follow-up after treatment has been completed is useful to assess for continued side effects as well as to assess patients' coping and reintegration of emotional equilibrium.

Swanson JL, Dibble SL and Chenitz WC. Clinical features and psychosocial factors in young adults with genital herpes. Image: J Nurs Scholarship 1995 Spring 27(1):16–22.

This study was undertaken to increase our knowledge of genital herpes with the goal of assisting health care providers in the education and counseling of persons with genital herpes. The specific purpose of the study was to identify clinical characteristics and psychosocial factors in young adults with genital herpes. The psychosocial factors were then compared with a normative data population. There were 70 participants in the study, recruited through newspaper advertisements and offices of health care professionals. To be eligible for the study, participants had to have written confirmation of genital herpes; be between the ages of 18 and 35; be English speaking; report a history of at least one genital herpes lesion in the previous 12 months; have had one or more recurrence; and have no history of hospitalization for treatment of psychiatric, drug, or alcohol problems.

The following instruments were administered to participants: the Genital Herpes Questionnaire and a semi-structured interview guide, both developed by the investigators; the Beck Depression Inventory; the Symptom Checklist-90-Revised; the Daily Hassles and Uplists Scale; and the Tennessee Self-Concept Scale. Specific information about the experience of having genital herpes (duration of diagnosis and general health history) was obtained through the interview.

Length of time that participants reported having genital herpes ranged from 1 to 15 years (mean = 5.01 years; SD = 3.31 years). They reported an average time lapse of 14 months (SD = 20.89 months) from onset of symptoms to diagnosis. The mean number of recurrences in the past year was 5.37 (SD = 4.79), and the most frequent causes of recurrence reported by participants were stress (93%), menstruation (69% of women), sexual intercourse (68%), and overexertion (59%). Other causes reported included sleeplessness, colds, fever, masturbation, and sunlight. Treatments used for relief of symptoms included oral medications (acyclovir), dietary changes, support groups, and a variety of topical and oral therapies and other strategies. Analysis of the scales revealed that participants with genital herpes scored significantly (p = .005–.031) lower on self concept (social self, physical self, and family self) than did the normative sample. Although 66% of the sample had normal scores on the depression scale, 29% were mild to moderately depressed and 6% were moderately to severely depressed; there were no differences when these scores were compared with those of the normative group. Although the frequency of hassles was greater (p = .0001) in the genital herpes sample than in the normative group, the intensity of hassles was comparable.

Nursing Implications. Although the authors acknowledge that their findings may be affected by recruitment strategies used in this study, they identify several implications for nursing practice. Because of the frequent recurrence of genital herpes in this group and the participants' perceived relationship of recurrence to stress, stress management techniques may be important in teaching persons with this disorder. Because of the stigma of this disorder, counseling is warranted.

UNIT 12

Immunologic Function

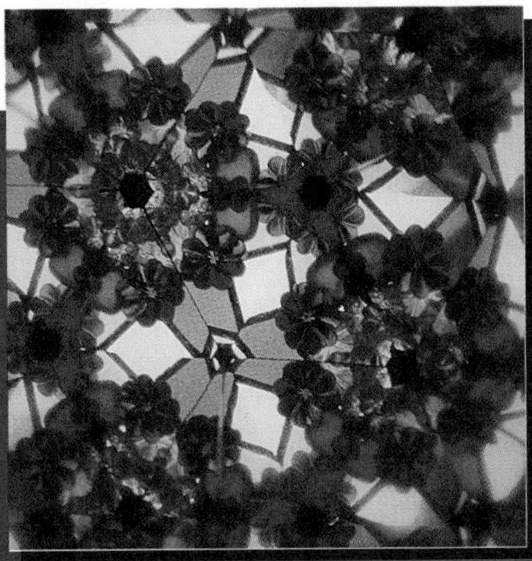

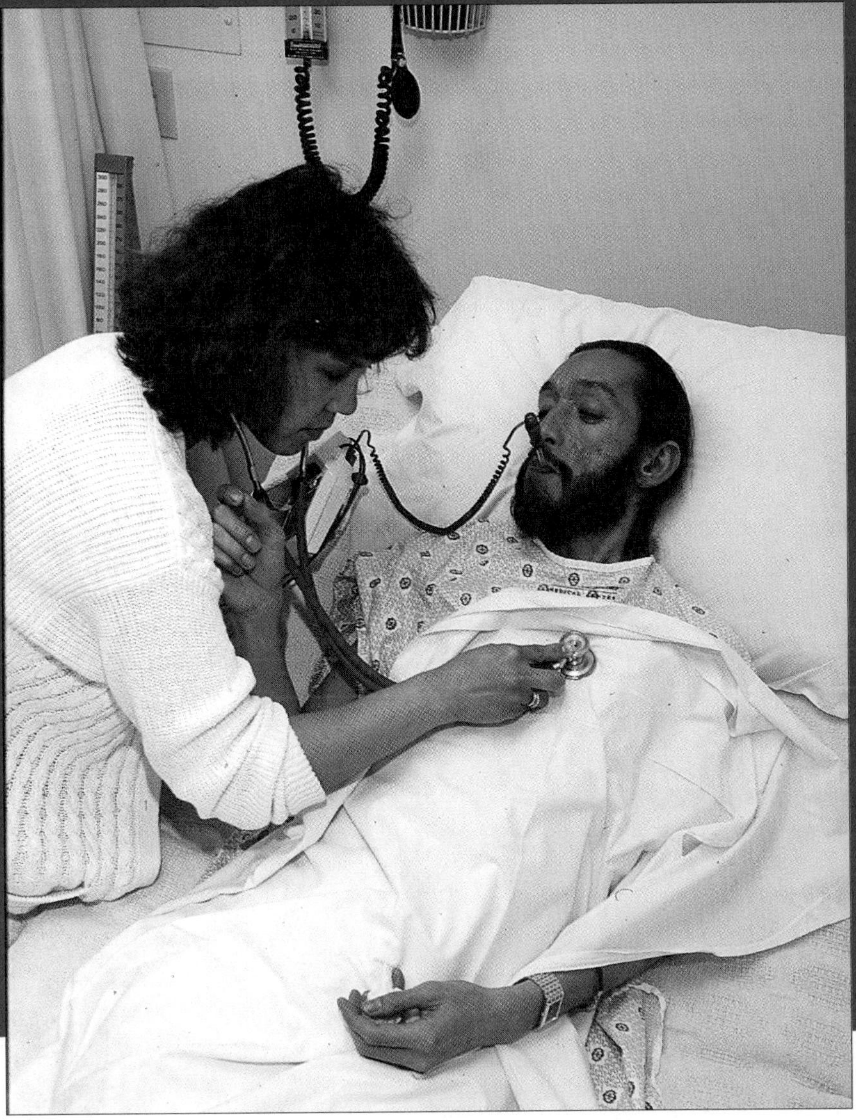

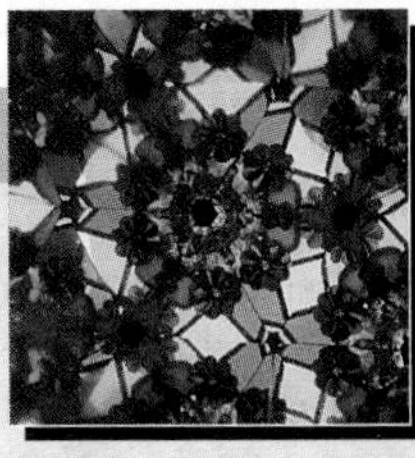

48

Assessment of Immune Function

CHAPTER OUTLINE

LEARNING OBJECTIVES

On completion of this chapter, the learner will be able to:

1. Describe the body's general immune responses and the stages of the immune system response
2. Differentiate between cellular and humoral immune responses
3. Describe the effects of the following variables on function of the immune system: age, gender, nutrition, psychoneuroimmunologic, concurrent illness, cancer, medications, and radiation
4. Use assessment parameters for determining the status of immune function

Suzanne C. Smeltzer and Brenda G. Bare: Brunner and Suddarth's Textbook of Medical-Surgical Nursing, 8th Edition. © 1996 Lippincott-Raven Publishers.

Overview

Before performing an assessment of the immune system, it is first necessary to understand its components and general function. Essentially, the system is made up of the white blood cells, the bone marrow, and the lymphoid tissues, which include the thymus gland, the lymph nodes, the spleen, and tonsils and adenoids and similar tissues (Fig. 48-1).

Among the white blood cells involved in immunity are the B lymphocytes (B cells) and the T lymphocytes (T cells). Both kinds of cells arise from lymphoblasts manufactured in the bone marrow (Fig. 48-2). B lymphocytes mature in the bone marrow and then enter circulation; T lymphocytes move from the bone marrow to the thymus where they mature into several kinds of cells capable of different functions.

Other significant structures are the lymph nodes, spleen, tonsils, and adenoids. Located throughout the body, the lymph nodes remove foreign material from the lymph before it enters the bloodstream and also serve as centers for immune cell proliferation. The spleen, composed of red and white pulp, acts somewhat like a filter. The red pulp is the site where old and injured red blood cells are destroyed. The white pulp contains concentrations of lymphocytes. The remaining lymphoid tissues, such as the tonsils and adenoids and other mucoid lymphatic tissues, defend the body against microorganisms.

Whereas the term **immunity** refers to the body's specific protective response to an invading foreign agent or organism, the term **immunopathology** refers to the study of diseases resulting from dysfunctions within the immune system. Disorders of the immune system may stem from excesses or deficiencies of immunocompetent cells, alterations in the function of these cells, immunologic attack on self-antigens, or inappropriate or exaggerated responses to specific antigens. Disorders related to autoimmunity are those diseases in which the normally protective immune response paradoxically turns against or attacks the body itself, leading to tissue damage. Disorders related to hypersensitivity are those conditions in which the body produces inappropriate or exaggerated responses to specific antigens. Disorders related to gammopathies are those that result from overproduction of immunoglobulins. Disorders related to immunodeficiencies can be categorized as either primary disorders, in which the deficiency results from improper development of the immune cells or tissues and is usually genetic, or secondary disorders, in which the deficiency results from some interference with an already developed immune system. These disorders are discussed in other chapters of this textbook. To understand immunopathology, one must first understand how the body's immune system functions normally.

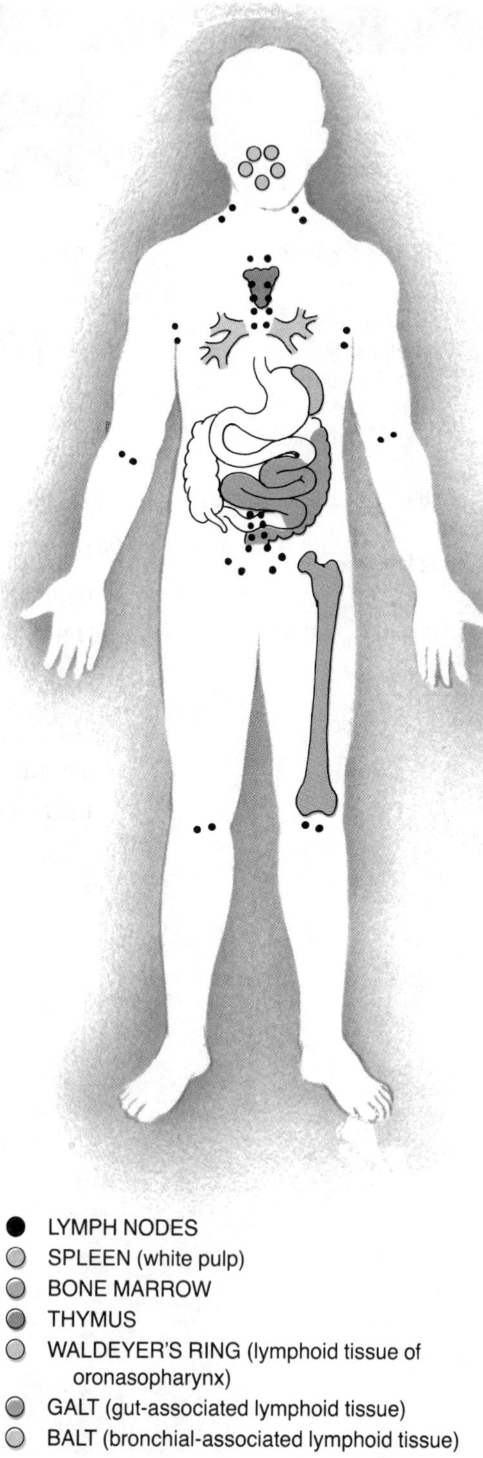

FIGURE 48-1. Structures of the normal immune system. (Rubin E and Farber JL. Pathology, 2nd ed. Philadelphia, JB Lippincott, 1994.)

Immunity: Natural and Acquired

There are two general types of immunity: natural and acquired. Natural immunity, which is a nonspecific immunity, is present at birth, whereas acquired or specific immunity develops after birth. Although each type of immunity plays a distinct role in defending the body against harmful invaders, the various components usually act in an interdependent manner.

Natural Immunity

Natural immunity provides a nonspecific response to any foreign invader, regardless of the composition of the in-

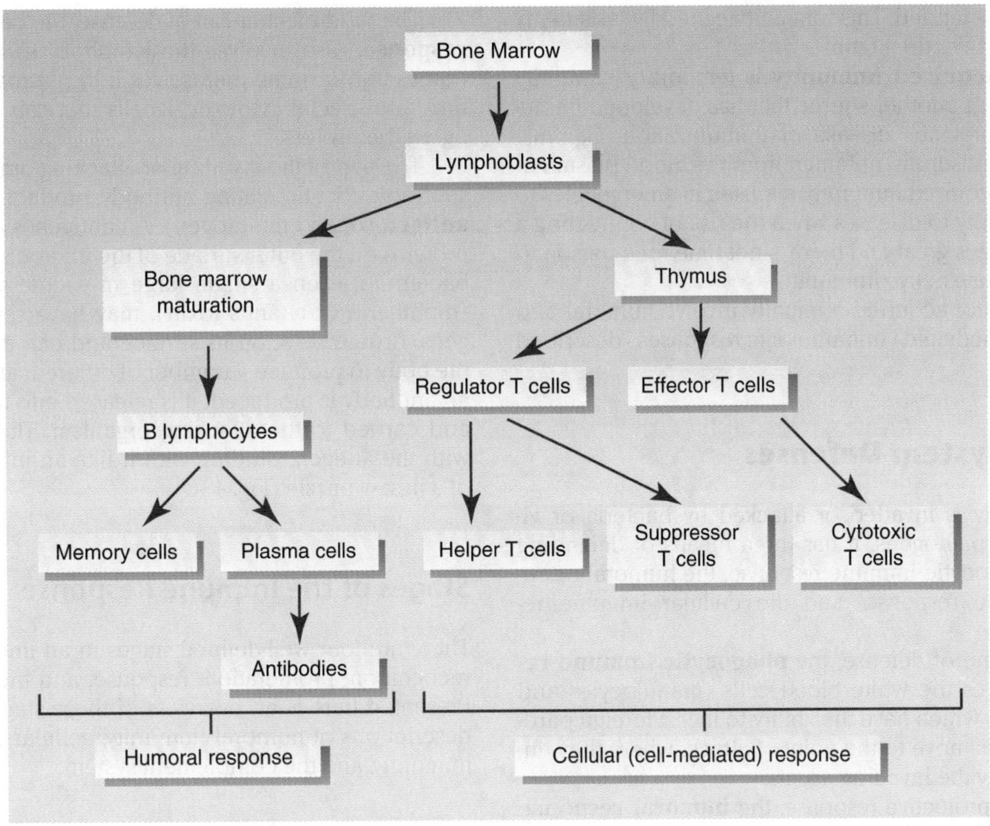

FIGURE 48-2. Development of immune cells.

vader. The basis of natural defense mechanisms is merely the ability to distinguish between friend and foe or "self" and "nonself." Such natural mechanisms include physical and chemical barriers, the action of white blood cells, and inflammatory responses.

Physical barriers include intact skin and mucous membranes, which prevent pathogens from gaining access to the body, and the cilia of the respiratory tract along with coughing and sneezing responses, which act to filter and clear pathogens from the upper respiratory tract before they can invade the body further. Chemical barriers such as acidic gastric juices, enzymes in tears and saliva, and substances in sebaceous and sweat secretions act in a nonspecific way to destroy invading bacteria and fungi. Viruses are countered by other means, such as interferon. **Interferon** is one type of biologic response modifier, which is a nonspecific viricidal substance naturally produced by the body and capable of activating other components of the immune system.

White blood cells, or leukocytes, participate in both the natural and the acquired immune responses. Granular leukocytes, or granulocytes (so called because of granules in their cytoplasm), include neutrophils, eosinophils, and basophils. **Neutrophils** (also called polymorphonuclear leukocytes or PMNs because their nuclei have multiple lobes) are the first cells to arrive at the site where inflammation occurs. **Eosinophils** and **basophils,** other types of granulocytes, increase in number during allergic reactions and stress responses. **Granulocytes** fight invasion by foreign bodies or toxins by releasing cell mediators, such as histamine, bradykinin, and prostaglandins, and engulfing the foreign bodies or toxins. **Nongranular leukocytes** include monocytes or macrophages (referred to as histiocytes when they enter tissue spaces) and lymphocytes. **Monocytes** also function as **phagocytic cells,** which means that they can engulf, ingest, and destroy greater numbers and quantities of foreign bodies or toxins than granulocytes. **Lymphocytes,** consisting of B cells and T cells, play major roles in humoral and cell-mediated immunity, as will be discussed later.

The **inflammatory response** is a major function of the natural (nonspecific) immune system elicited in response to tissue injury or invading organisms. Chemical mediators assist in the inflammatory response to minimize blood loss, wall off the invading organism, activate phagocytes, and promote fibrous scar formation and regeneration of injured tissue. (The inflammatory response is discussed in detail later.)

Acquired Immunity

Acquired immunity consists of immunologic responses that are not present at birth but that are acquired during life. Acquired immunity usually develops as a result of contracting a disease or generating a protective immune response through immunization. Weeks or months after exposure to the disease or immunization, an immune response develops sufficiently to prevent development of the disease on reexposure to it. There are two types of acquired immunity: active and passive. In **active acquired immunity** the immunologic defenses are developed by the body of the person being defended. This immunity generally lasts many years or even the entire lifetime.

Passive acquired immunity is temporary immunity transmitted from another source that has developed immunity through previous disease or immunization. Gammaglobulin and antiserum, obtained from the blood plasma of persons with acquired immunity, are used in emergencies to provide immunity to diseases when the risk of contracting a specific disease is great and there is not time for a person to develop adequate active immunity.

Both types of acquired immunity involve humoral and cellular (cell-mediated) immunologic responses (described later).

Immune System Defenses

When the body is invaded or attacked by bacteria or viruses or other pathogens, it has three means of defending itself: the phagocytic immune response, the humoral or antibody immune response, and the cellular immune response.

The first line of defense, the **phagocytic immune response,** involves the white blood cells (granulocytes and macrophages), which have the ability to ingest foreign particles. These cells move to the point of attack, where they engulf and destroy the invading agents.

A second protective response, the **humoral response** (sometimes called antibody response), begins with the lymphocytes, which can transform themselves into plasma cells that manufacture antibodies. These antibodies, which are highly specific proteins, are transported in the bloodstream and have the ability to disable the invaders.

The third mechanism of defense, the **cellular immune response,** also involves the lymphocytes, which, in addition to transforming themselves into plasma cells, can also turn into special cytotoxic T cells that can attack the pathogens themselves.

The part of the invading or attacking organism that is responsible for stimulating antibody production is called an **antigen** (or an immunogen). An antigen is a small patch of proteins on the outer surface of the microorganism. A single bacterium, even a single large molecule such as a toxin (diphtheria or tetanus toxin), may have several such antigens, or **markers,** on its surface and can therefore induce the body to produce a number of different antibodies. Once an antibody is produced, it is released into the bloodstream and carried to the attacking organism. There it combines with the antigen, binding with it like an interlocking piece of a jigsaw puzzle (Fig. 48-3).

Stages of the Immune Response

There are four well-defined stages in an immune response: recognition, proliferation, response, and the effector stage. Presented here is an overview of these stages, followed by descriptions of humoral immunity, cellular (cell-mediated) immunity, and the complement system.

Recognition Stage

The basis of any immune reaction is, first and foremost, **recognition.** It is the immune system's ability to recognize antigens as foreign, or nonself, that is the initiating event in

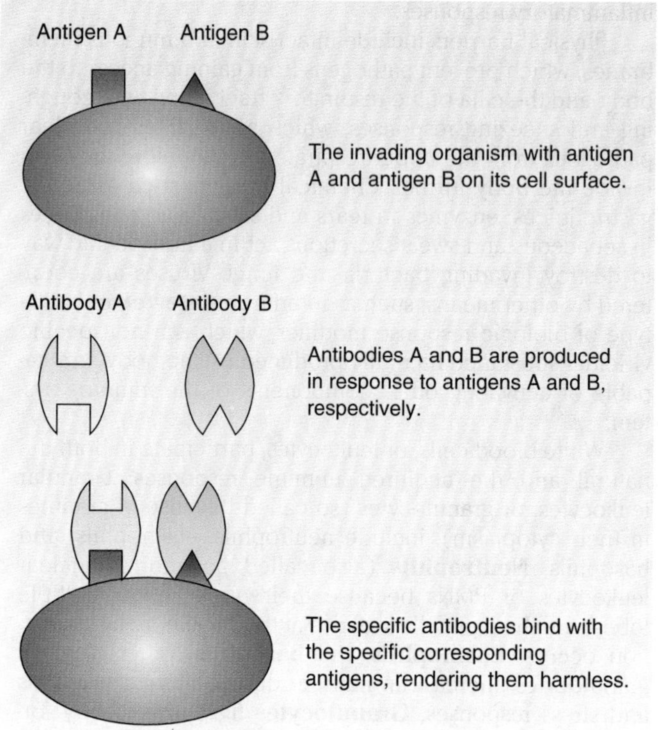

FIGURE 48-3. Antibody specificity. Antibodies are produced by B-cell lymphocytes to bind with specific antigens.

any immune reaction. The body must first recognize invaders as foreign before it can react to them.

Surveillance by Lymph Nodes and Lymphocytes. The body accomplishes recognition using lymph nodes and lymphocytes for surveillance. Lymph nodes, which are widely dispersed, are distributed close to all of the body's surfaces, internal as well as external. They continuously discharge small lymphocytes into the bloodstream. These lymphocytes patrol the tissues and vessels that drain the areas served by that node. Basically, the lymph nodes and lymphocytes make up the immune system.

Circulating Lymphocytes. There are lymphocytes in the lymph nodes themselves and lymphocytes that circulate in the blood. The total lymphocytes in the body add up to a mass of cells of impressive number. These lymphocytes recirculate from the blood to lymph nodes and from the lymph nodes back into the bloodstream, in a never-ending series of patrols. Some circulating lymphocytes can survive for decades. Some of these small, hardy cells maintain their solitary circuits for the lifetime of the person.

The exact way in which circulating lymphocytes recognize antigens on foreign surfaces is not known. At present, it is thought that recognition depends on specific receptor sites on the surface of the lymphocytes. It appears that macrophages, a type of nongranular leukocyte found in body tissues, play an important role in helping these circulating lymphocytes to process the antigens. Foreign materials enter the body, and a circulating lymphocyte comes into physical contact with the surfaces of these materials. Upon contact, the lymphocyte, with the help of macrophages, either removes the antigen from the surface or in some way picks up an imprint of its structure. For example, in a streptococcal throat infection, the streptococcal organism gains access to the mucous membranes of the throat, and a circulating lymphocyte moving through the tissues of the neck comes in contact with the organism. The lymphocyte, familiar with the surface markers on the cells of its own body, recognizes the antigens on the microbe as different (nonself) and the streptococcal organism as antigenic (foreign). This triggers the second stage of the immune response—proliferation.

Proliferation Stage

The circulating lymphocyte containing the antigenic message returns to the nearest lymph node. Once in the node, the sensitized lymphocyte stimulates some of the resident dormant lymphocytes to enlarge, divide, proliferate, and differentiate into either T lymphocytes or B lymphocytes. Enlargement of the lymph nodes in the neck in conjunction with a sore throat is one example of the immune response.

Response Stage

In the response stage, the changed lymphocytes will function in either a humoral or a cellular fashion.

Initial Humoral Responses. The production of antibodies by the B lymphocytes in response to a specific antigen begins the humoral response. *Humoral* refers to the fact that the antibodies are released into the bloodstream and so reside in the plasma or fluid fraction of the blood.

Initial Cellular Responses. The returning sensitized lymphocytes migrate to areas of the lymph node (other than those areas containing lymphocytes programmed to become plasma cells), where they stimulate the residing lymphocytes to become cells that will attack microbes directly rather than through the action of antibodies. These transformed lymphocytes are known as **cytotoxic T cells.** The T stands for *thymus,* denoting the fact that during the embryologic development of the immune system, these lymphocytes spent some time in the thymus of the developing fetus, at which time they were genetically programmed to become T cells rather than the antibody-producing B lymphocytes. Viral rather than bacterial antigens induce a cellular response. This response is manifested by the increasing number of lymphocytes (lymphocytosis) seen in the blood smears of people with viral illnesses, such as infectious mononucleosis. (Cellular immunity is discussed in detail later.)

Most immune responses to antigens involve both humoral and cellular responses, though one usually predominates. During transplantation rejection, the cellular response predominates, whereas in the bacterial pneumonias and sepsis, the humoral response plays the dominant protective role (Chart 48-1).

Effector Stage

In the effector stage, either the antibody of the humoral response or the cytotoxic T cell of the cellular response reaches and couples with the antigen on the surface of the foreign object. The coupling initiates a series of events that

CHART 48-1
Role of Cellular and Humoral Immune Responses

Whereas B-cell antibodies are distinctive components of the humoral immune response, cytotoxic T cells are distinguishing components of the cellular immune response. Some specific roles of B cells and T cells follow:

Humoral Responses

- Bacterial phagocytosis and lysis
- Anaphylaxis
- Allergic hay fever and asthma
- Immune complex disease
- Bacterial and some viral infections

Cellular Responses

- Transplant rejection
- Delayed hypersensitivity (tuberculin reaction)
- Graft-versus-host disease
- Tumor surveillance or destruction
- Intracellular infections
- Viral, fungal, and parasitic infection

in most instances results in the total destruction of the invading microbes or the complete neutralization of the toxin. The events involve an interplay of antibodies (humoral immunity), complement, and action by the cytotoxic T cells (cellular immunity). Figure 48-4 summarizes the phases of the immune response.

Humoral Immune Response

The humoral response is characterized by production of antibodies by the B lymphocytes in response to a specific antigen. Although the B lymphocyte is ultimately responsible for the production of antibodies, both the macrophages of natural immunity and the special T-cell lymphocytes of cellular immunity are involved in recognizing the foreign substance and in producing antibodies.

Antigen Recognition

Several theories exist about the mechanisms by which the B lymphocytes recognize the invading antigen and produce appropriate antibodies in response—probably because there are several different methods by which the B

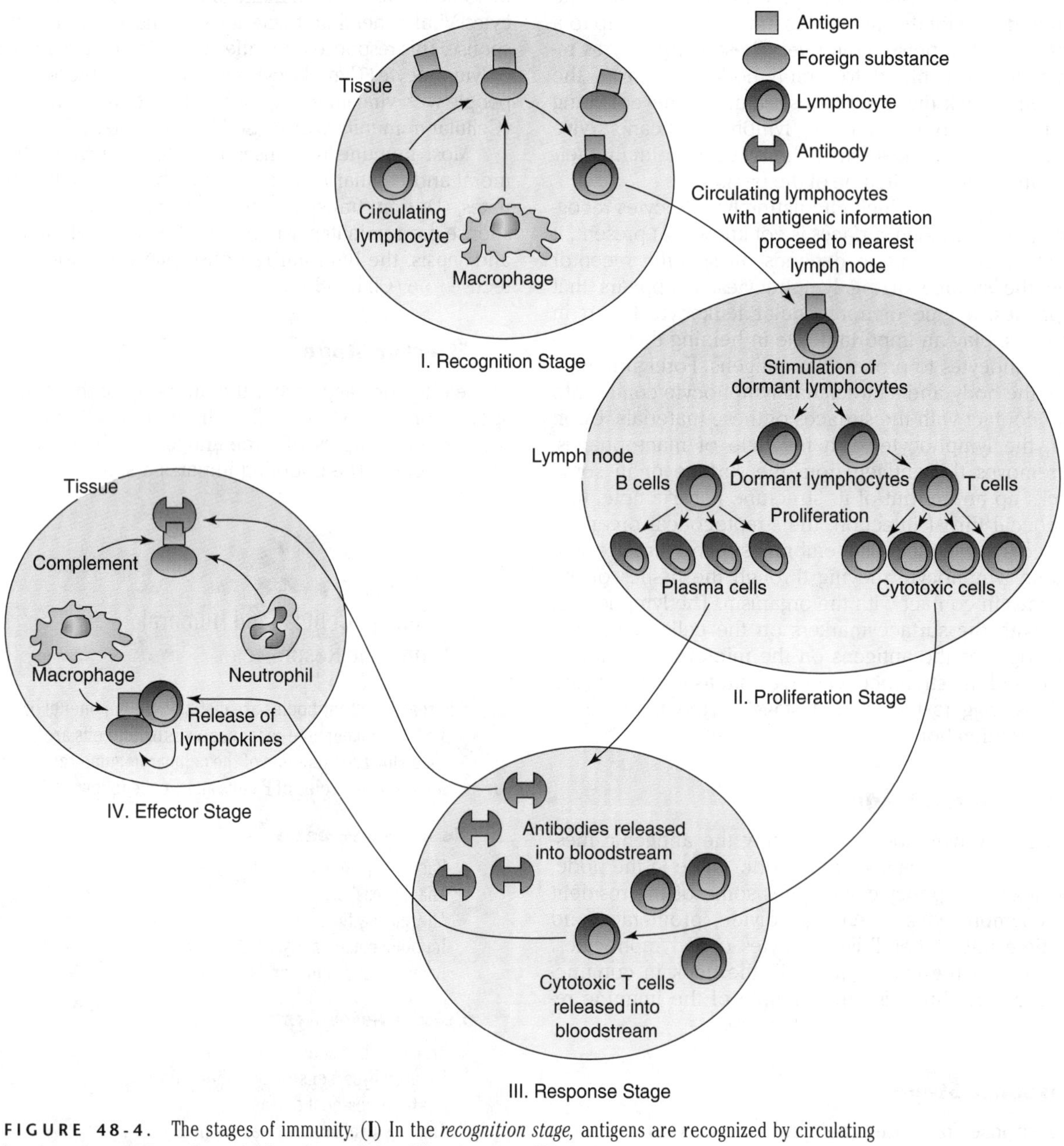

FIGURE 48-4. The stages of immunity. (**I**) In the *recognition stage,* antigens are recognized by circulating lymphocytes and macrophages, giving rise to the *proliferation stage* (**II**). In this stage, the dormant lymphocytes (T cells) proliferate and differentiate into cytotoxic T cells or B cells responsible for formation and release of antibodies. (**III**) In the *response stage,* the cytotoxic T cells and the B cells perform cellular and humoral functions, respectively. (**IV**) In the *effector stage,* antigens are destroyed or neutralized through the action of antibodies, complement, macrophages, and cytotoxic T cells.

lymphocyte recognizes antigens. These different means of antigen recognition may also be responsible for different types of antibody response. Some antigens seem to have the ability to trigger antibody formation by the B lymphocytes directly, whereas others require the assistance of T cells.

T cells (or T lymphocytes) are part of a surveillance system dispersed throughout the body. These lymphocytes recycle through the general circulation, tissues, and lymphatic system. It is thought that, with the assistance of macrophages, the T lymphocyte recognizes the antigen of a foreign invader. The T lymphocyte picks up the antigenic message or "blueprint" of the antigen and returns to the nearest lymph node with that message.

Antibodies: Production, Structure, Function

Production

B lymphocytes, which are stored in the lymph nodes, are subdivided into thousands of clones, each responsive to a single group of antigens having almost identical characteristics. Carrying the antigenic message back to the lymph node stimulates specific clones of the B lymphocyte to enlarge, divide, proliferate, and differentiate into plasma cells capable of producing specific antibodies to the antigen. Other B lymphocytes differentiate into B lymphocyte clones with a memory for the antigen. These memory cells are responsible for the more exaggerated and rapid immune response in a person who is repeatedly exposed to the same antigen.

Structure

Antibodies are large proteins that are called **immunoglobulins** because they are found in the globulin fraction of the plasma proteins. Each antibody molecule consists of two subunits, each of which contains a light and a heavy peptide chain (Fig. 48-5). The subunits are held together by a chemical link composed of disulfide bonds. Each subunit has a portion that serves as a binding site for a specific antigen. This site, referred to as the **Fab fragment,** provides the "lock" portion that is highly specific for an antigen. An additional portion, known as the **Fc fragment,** allows the antibody molecule to take part in the complement system.

The body can produce five different types of immunoglobulins. Immunoglobulins in general are designated by the symbol Ig, and each of the five types, or classes, is identified by a specific letter of the alphabet (IgA, IgD, IgE, IgG, and IgM). Classification is based on the chemical structure and biologic role of the individual immunoglobulin. Some of the outstanding characteristics of the immunoglobulins may be summarized as follows:

IgG (75% of Total Immunoglobulin)

- Appears in serum and tissues (interstitial fluid)
- Assumes major role in blood-borne and tissue infections
- Activates complement system
- Enhances phagocytosis
- Crosses placenta

IgA (15% of Total Immunoglobulin)

- Appears in body fluids (blood, saliva, tears, breast milk, and pulmonary, gastrointestinal, prostatic, and vaginal secretions)
- Protects against respiratory, gastrointestinal, and genitourinary infections
- Prevents absorption of antigens from food
- Passes to neonate in breast milk for protection

IgM (10% of Total Immunoglobulin)

- Appears mostly in intravascular serum

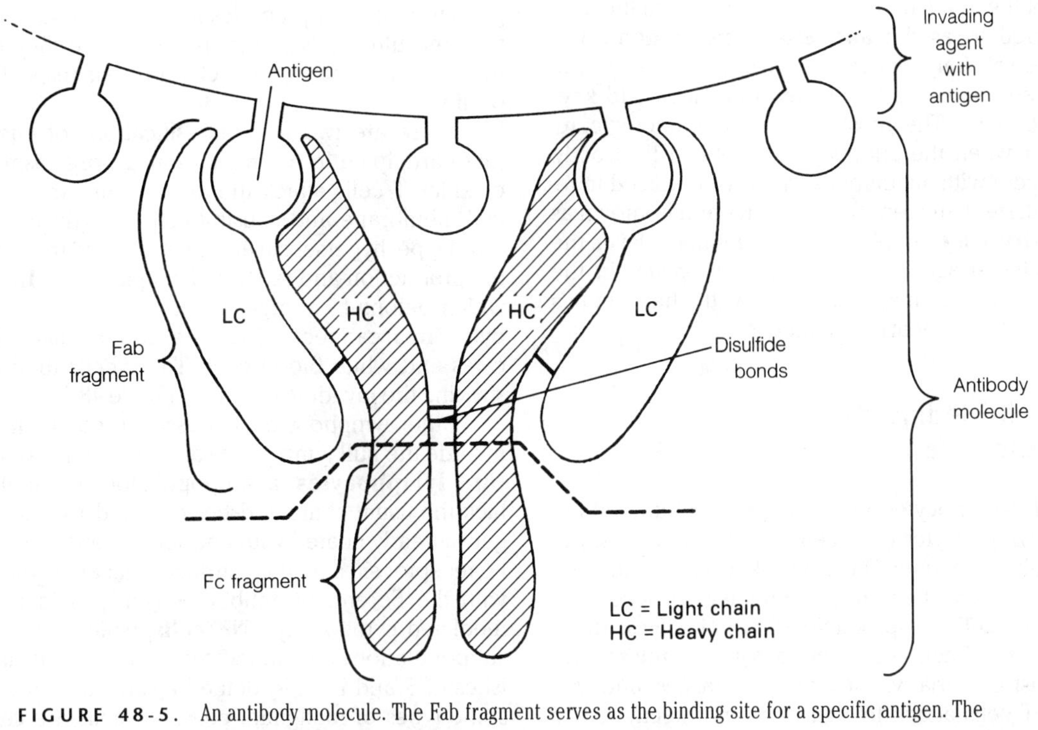

FIGURE 48-5. An antibody molecule. The Fab fragment serves as the binding site for a specific antigen. The Fc fragment initiates classical complement activation.

- Appears as the first immunoglobulin produced in response to bacterial and viral infections
- Activates complement system

IgD (0.2% of Total Immunoglobulin)
- Appears in small amounts in serum
- Possibly influences B-lymphocyte differentiation, but role unclear

IgE (0.004% of Total Immunoglobulin)
- Appears in serum
- Takes part in allergic and hypersensitivity reactions
- Possibly helps in defense against parasites

Function

Antibodies defend against foreign invaders in several ways, and the type of defense employed depends on the structure and composition of both the antigen and the immunoglobulin. As discussed above, the antibody molecule has at least two combining sites known as the Fab fragments. One antibody can act as a cross-link between two antigens, causing them to bind or clump together. This clumping effect, referred to as **agglutination,** helps in clearing the body of the invading organism by facilitating phagocytosis. Some antibodies have the ability to assist in removing offending organisms through the process of **opsonization.** In this process, the antigen–antibody molecule is coated with a sticky substance that also facilitates phagocytosis.

Antibodies also promote the release of vasoactive substances, such as **histamine** and **slow-reacting substance (SRS)**, two of the chemical mediators of the inflammatory response. In addition, antibodies are involved in activating the complement system.

Antigen–Antibody Binding

The portion of the antigen involved in binding with the antibody is referred to as the **antigenic determinant.** The binding of the Fab fragment (antibody binding site) to the antigenic determinant can be likened to a "lock and key" situation (Fig. 48-6). The most efficient immunologic responses occur when the antibody and antigen fit exactly. Poor fit can occur with an antibody that was produced in response to a different antigen. This phenomenon is known as **cross-reactivity.** For example, in acute rheumatic fever, the antibody produced against *Streptococcus pyogenes* in the upper respiratory tract may cross-react with the patient's heart tissue, leading to heart valve damage.

Cellular (Cell-Mediated) Immune Response

Whereas the B lymphocytes are the soldiers of humoral immunity, the T lymphocytes (or T cells) are primarily responsible for cellular immunity. These lymphocytes spend time in the thymus, where they are programmed to become T cells rather than antibody-producing B lymphocytes. There are several types of T cells, each with designated roles in the defense against bacteria, viruses, fungi, parasites, and malignant cells. T cells attack foreign invaders directly rather than by producing antibodies.

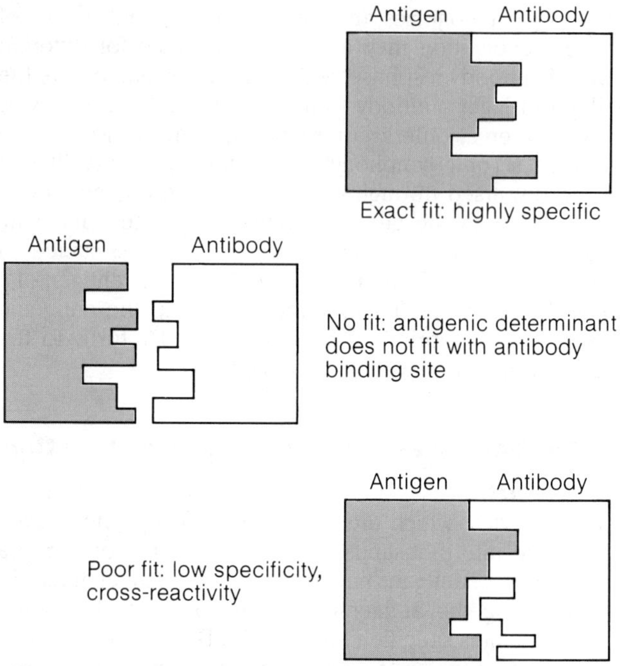

FIGURE 48-6. Antigen–antibody binding. (**Top**) A highly specific antigen–antibody complex. (**Middle**) No match and therefore no immune response. (**Bottom**) Poor fit or match with low specificity; antibody reacts to antigen with *similar* characteristics, producing cross-reactivity.

Cellular reactions are initiated by the binding of an antigen with an antigen receptor located on the surface of a T cell. This may occur with or without the assistance of macrophages. The T cells then carry the antigenic message, or blueprint, to the lymph nodes, where the production of other T cells is stimulated. Some T cells remain in the lymph nodes and retain a memory for the antigen. Other T cells migrate from the lymph nodes into the general circulatory system and ultimately to the tissues, where they remain until they either come in contact with their respective antigens or die.

There are two main classifications of effector T cells that participate in destroying foreign organisms. Cytotoxic, or killer, T cells attack the antigen directly by altering the cell membrane and causing cell lysis (disintegration). Delayed-type hypersensitivity cells protect the body through the production and release of lymphokines. **Lymphokines**, which belong to a larger group of glycoproteins known as **cytokines**, can recruit, activate, and regulate other lymphocytes and white blood cells. These cells then assist in destroying the invading organism (Table 48-1).

Other lymphocytes that assist in combating organisms include the null lymphocyte and the natural killer (NK) cell. **Null lymphocytes**, a subpopulation of lymphocytes that lack the usual characteristics of B and T cells, destroy antigens already coated with antibody. These cells have special Fc receptor sites on their surfaces that allow them to couple with the Fc end of antibodies (antibody-dependent, cell-mediated cytotoxicity). **NK cells**, which represent another subpopulation of lymphocytes without the usual characteristics of T and B cells, defend against microorganisms and some types of malignant cells. NK cells are capable of directly killing invading organisms and producing cytokines.

TABLE 48-1 Cytokines and Their Biologic Effects

Cytokine*	Action
Interleukin-1	Promotes differentiation of T and B cells, natural killer (NK) and null cells
Interleukin-2	Stimulates growth of T cells and special activated killer lymphocytes (known as lymphocyte-activated killer cells—LAK cells)
Interleukin-3	Stimulates growth of mast cells and other blood cells
Interleukin-4	Stimulates growth of T and B cells, mast cells, and macrophages
Interleukin-5	Stimulates antibody responses
Interleukin-6	Stimulates growth and function of B cells and antibodies
Permeability factor	Increases vascular permeability, allowing white cells into area
Interferon	Interferes with viral growth, stopping the spread of viral infection
Migration inhibitory factor	Suppresses movement of macrophages, keeping macrophage in area of foreign cells
Skin reactive factor	Induces inflammatory response
Cytotoxic factor (lymphotoxin)	Kills certain antigenic cells
Macrophage chemotactic factor	Attracts macrophages into the area
Lymphocyte blastogenic factor	Stimulates more lymphocytes, recruiting additional lymphocytes into the area
Macrophage aggregation factor	Causes clumping of macrophages and lymphocytes
Macrophage activation factor	Allows macrophages to adhere to surfaces more readily
Proliferation inhibitor factor	Inhibits growth of certain antigenic cells
Cytophilic antibody	Binds to an Fc receptor on macrophages thereby permitting macrophages to bind to antigens
Tumor necrosis factor (alpha)	Stimulates inflammation, wound healing, and tissue remodeling
Tumor necrosis factor (beta)	Mediates inflammation and graft rejection

*Cytokines are biologically active substances released by cells to regulate growth and function of other cells within the immune system. Lymphocytes produce lymphokines, and monocytes and macrophages produce monokines. The table above lists some of the cytokines that play a role in immune system functioning.

The discovery of additional T lymphocytes known as helper and suppressor cells has contributed to the understanding that humoral and cellular immune responses are not separate, unrelated processes but branches of the immune response that can and do affect each other. Upon contact with the antigen, helper T cells (also referred to as T4 cells) release cytokines known as interleukins, interferon-γ, and tumor necrosis factor, which stimulate growth and functioning of white blood cells and T and B cells.

Helper T cells (T4) are subdivided into two populations depending on the type of cell that they help. Helper T_1 cells produce lymphokines that activate other T cells (interleukin-2, or IL-2), natural and cytotoxic T killer cells (interferon-γ), and other inflammatory cells (tumor necrosis factor). Helper T_2 cells produce lymphokines (interleukin-4 and interleukin-5), which activate B cells to grow and differentiate.

In addition, helper T cells contribute to the differentiation of null and NK cells. Suppressor T cells have the ability to decrease B-cell production, thereby keeping the immune response at a level that is compatible with health (*e.g.*, sufficient to fight infection adequately without attacking the body's healthy tissues); see Table 48-2.

Complement System

Circulating plasma proteins, which are made in the liver and activated when an antibody couples with its antigen, are known as **complement.** These proteins interact sequentially with one another in a cascade or "falling domino" effect. This complement cascade alters the cell membranes on which antigen and antibody complex form, permitting fluid to enter the cell and leading eventually to cell lysis and death. In addition, activated complement molecules attract macrophages and granulocytes to areas of antigen–antibody reactions. These cells continue the body's defense by devouring the antibody-coated microbes and by releasing bacterial agents.

Complement plays a very important role in the immune response. Destruction of an invading or attacking organism or toxin is not achieved merely by the binding of the antibody and antigens; it also requires activation of complement, the arrival of killer T cells, or the attraction of macrophages.

Classical Pathway of Complement Activation. There are two ways to activate the complement system. One, the **classical pathway** (the first method discovered), involves the reaction of the first of the circulating comple-

TABLE 48-2 Lymphocytes Involved in Immune Responses

Cell Type	Function	Type of Immune Response
B Cell	Produces antibodies or immunoglobulins (IgA, IgD, IgE, IgG, IgM)	Humoral
T Cell		Cellular
Helper T4	Attacks foreign invaders (antigens) directly Initiates and augments inflammatory response	
Helper T_1	Increases B-cell antibody production	
Helper T_2	Increases activated cytotoxic T cells	
Suppressor T	Suppresses the immune response	
Memory T	Remembers contact with an antigen on subsequent exposures mount an immune response	
Cytotoxic T (killer T)	Lyses cells infected with virus; plays role in graft rejection	
Non-T or -B Lymphocytes		
Null cells	Destroys antigens already coated with antibody	Nonspecific
Natural killer (NK) (granular lymphocyte)	Defends against microorganisms and some types of malignant cells; produces cytokines	

ment proteins (C_1) with the receptor site of the Fc portion of an antibody molecule after formation of an antigen–antibody complex. The activation of the first complement component then activates all the other components in the following sequence: C_4, C_2, C_3, C_5, C_6, C_7, C_8, and C_9. (The components are named in the sequence in which they were discovered.)

Alternate Pathway of Complement Activation. The alternative method of complement activation occurs without the formation of antigen–antibody complexes. This alternate pathway can be initiated by the release of bacterial products such as endotoxins. When complement is activated through this pathway, the process bypasses the first three components (C_1, C_4, and C_2) and begins with C_3. Whatever the method of activation, however, once activated, the complement can and does destroy cells by altering or damaging the cell membrane of the antigen, by chemically attracting phagocytes to the antigen (chemotaxis), and by rendering the antigen more vulnerable to phagocytosis (opsonization). The complement system enhances the inflammatory response by releasing vasoactive substances.

This response is usually therapeutic and can be lifesaving if the cell attacked by the complement system is a true foreign invader, such as a streptococcal or staphylococcal organism. However, if that cell is, in reality, part of the person—a cell of the brain or liver, the tissue lining the blood vessels, or the cells of a transplanted organ or skin graft—the result can be devastating disease and even death. The result of the immune response—the vigorous attack on any material identified as foreign, the deadliness of the struggle—is obvious in the purulent material, or pus (the remains of microbes, granulocytes, and macrophages, T-cell lymphocytes, plasma proteins, complement, and antibodies) that accumulates in wound infections and abscesses.

Role of Interferons

Biologic response modifiers (BRM), such as the interferons, are currently under investigation to determine their roles in the immune system and their potential therapeutic effects in disorders characterized by disturbed immune responses. Interferons have antiviral and antitumor properties. In addition to responding to viral infection, they are produced by T lymphocytes, B lymphocytes, and macrophages in response to antigens. They are thought to modify the immune response by suppressing antibody production and cellular immunity. They also facilitate the cytolytic role of macrophages and NK cells. Interferons are undergoing extensive testing to evaluate their effectiveness in treating tumors, AIDS, and multiple sclerosis; some interferons are already used to treat immune-related disorders.

Factors Affecting Immune System Function

Like any other body system, the immune system functions at desired levels depending on the function of other body systems and related factors, such as age, gender, nutrition, disease, and external influences.

Age. Persons at the extremes of the life span are more likely to develop problems related to immune system functioning than are those in their middle years. Frequency and severity of infections are increased in elderly persons, possibly from a decreased ability to respond adequately to invading organisms. Both the production and the function of T and B lymphocytes may be impaired. The incidence of autoimmune diseases also increases with aging, possibly from a decreased ability of antibodies to differentiate between self and nonself. Failure of the surveillance system to recognize mutant, or abnormal, cells may be responsible for the high incidence of cancer associated with increasing age.

Declining function of various organ systems associated with increasing age also contributes to impaired immunity. Decreased gastric secretions and motility allow normal intestinal flora to proliferate and produce infection, causing gastroenteritis and diarrhea. Decreased renal circulation, filtration, absorption, and excretion contribute to urinary tract infections. Moreover, prostatic enlargement and neurogenic bladder can impede urine passage and subsequently bacterial clearance through the urinary system. Urinary stasis, common in the elderly, permits the growth of organisms.

Exposure to tobacco and environmental toxins will impair pulmonary function. Prolonged exposure to these agents decreases the elasticity of lung tissue, the effectiveness of cilia, and the ability to cough effectively. These impairments hinder the removal of infectious organisms and toxins, increasing the elderly person's susceptibility to pulmonary infections and cancers.

Finally, with aging the skin becomes thinner and less elastic. Peripheral neuropathy and the accompanying decreased sensation and circulation may lead to stasis ulcers, pressure ulcers, abrasions, and burns. Impaired skin integrity predisposes the aging person to infection from organisms that are part of normal skin flora.

Gender. The ability of sex hormones to modulate immunity has been well established. There is evidence that estrogen modulates the activity of T lymphocytes (especially suppressor cells) whereas androgens act to preserve interleukin-2 (IL-2) production and suppressor cell activity. The effects of sex hormones on B cells are less pronounced. Estrogen activates the autoimmune-associated B cell population that expresses the CD5 marker (an antigenic marker on the B cell). Estrogen tends to be immunoenhancing whereas androgen is immunosuppressive. In general, autoimmune diseases are more common in females than in males.

Nutrition. Adequate nutrition is essential for optimal functioning of the immune system. Impaired immune function due to protein-calorie deficiency may result from lack of adequate vitamins, which are essential in the synthesis of DNA and proteins. Vitamins also help in the regulation of cell proliferation and maturation of immune cells. Excess or deficiency of trace elements (*i.e.,* copper, iron, manganese, selenium, or zinc) in the diet generally suppresses immune function. Fatty acids are the building blocks that make up the structural components of cell membranes. Lipids are precursors of vitamins A, D, E, and K as well as cholesterol. Both excess and deficiency of fatty acids have been found to suppress immune function.

Depletion of protein reserves results in atrophy of lymphoid tissues, depression of antibody response, reduction in the number of circulating T cells, and impaired phagocytic function. As a result, susceptibility to infection is greatly increased. During periods of infection and serious illness, nutritional requirements may be exaggerated further, potentially contributing to depletion of protein, fatty acid, vitamin, and trace elements and an even greater risk of impaired immune response and sepsis.

Psychoneuro-immunologic Factors. Evidence from clinical observations and studies in humans and animals indicates that the immune response is regulated and modulated in part by neuroendocrine influences (Terr, 1991). Lymphocytes and macrophages have receptors capable of responding to neurotransmitters and endocrine hormones. Lymphocytes can produce and secrete ACTH and endorphin-like compounds. Neurons in the brain, especially in the hypothalamus, can recognize prostaglandins, interferons, and interleukins as well as histamine and sertonin, which are released during the inflammatory process. Like all other biologic systems functioning in the interest of homeostasis, the immune system is integrated with other psychophysiologic processes and is subject to regulation and modulation by the brain.

Conversely, the immune processes can affect neural and endocrine function, including behavior. Thus, the interaction of the nervous system and immune system appears to be bidirectional. Growing evidence indicates that measurable immune system parameters can be influenced by biobehavioral strategies involving self-regulation. Examples of these strategies are relaxation and imagery techniques, biofeedback, humor, hypnosis, and conditioning.

Other Organ Diseases. Conditions such as burns or other forms of injury, infection, and cancer may contribute to altered immune system function. Major burns or other factors cause impaired skin integrity and compromise the body's first line of defense. Loss of large amounts of serum with burn injuries depletes the body of essential proteins, including immunoglobulins. The physiologic and psychologic stressors associated with surgery or injury stimulate cortisol release from the adrenal cortex; increased serum cortisol also contributes to suppression of normal immune responses.

Chronic illness may contribute to immune system impairments in a variety of ways. Renal failure is associated with a deficiency in circulating lymphocytes. In addition, immune defenses may be altered by acidosis and uremic toxins. An increased incidence of infection in diabetes has been associated with vascular insufficiency, neuropathy, and poor control of serum glucose levels. Recurrent respiratory tract infections are associated with chronic obstructive pulmonary disease as a result of altered inspiratory and expiratory function and ineffective airway clearance.

Cancer. Immunosuppression contributes to the development of cancers. However, cancer itself is immunosuppressive. Large tumors can release antigens into the blood; these antigens combine with circulating antibodies and prevent them from attacking the tumor cells. Furthermore, tumor cells may possess special blocking factors that coat tumor cells and prevent destruction by killer T lymphocytes. During the early development of tumors, the body may fail to recognize the tumor antigens as foreign and subsequently fail to initiate destruction of the malignant cells. Hematologic cancers such as leukemia and lymphoma are

TABLE 48-3 Selected Medications and Effects on the Immune System

Drug Classification (and Examples)	Effects on the Immune System
Antibiotics (in large doses)	**Bone marrow suppression**
Chloramphenicol (Chloromycetin)	Leukopenia, aplastic anemia
Dactinomycin (Cosmogen)	Agranulocytosis, neutropenia
Gentamycin sulfate (Garamycin)	Agranulocytosis, granulocytosis
Penicillins	Agranulocytosis
Streptomycin	Leukopenia, neutropenia, pancytopenia
Vancomycin	Transient leukopenia
Antithyroid Drugs	
Propylthiouracil	Agranulocytosis, leukopenia
Nonsteroidal anti-inflammatory drugs (NSAIDs) in large doses	**Inhibits prostaglandin synthesis or release**
Aspirin	Agranulocytosis
Ibuprofen	Neutropenia, leukopenia
Indomethacin	Agranulocytosis, leukopenia,
Phenylbutazone	Pancytopenia, agranulocytosis, aplastic anemia
Adrenal Corticosteroids	**Immunosuppression**
Prednisone	
Antineoplastic Agents (Cytotoxic Agents)	**Immunosuppression**
Alkylating agents:	
Cyclophosphamide (Cytoxan)	Leukopenia, neutropenia
Mechlorethamine HCl (Mustargen)	Agranulocytosis, neutropenia
Cyclosporine	Leukopenia, inhibits T-cell function
Antimetabolites	**Immunosuppression**
Fluorouracil (pyrimidine antagonist)	Leukopenia, eosinophilia
Methotrexate (folic acid antagonist)	Leukopenia, aplastic bone marrow
Mercaptopurine (6-MP) (purine antagonist)	Leukopenia, pancytopenia

associated with altered production and function of white blood cells and lymphocytes.

Medications. Certain medications can cause both desirable and undesirable alterations in immune system functioning. Four major classifications of medications have the potential for causing immunosuppression: antibiotics, corticosteroids, nonsteroidal anti-inflammatory drugs (NSAIDs), and cytotoxic agents (Table 48-3). Therapeutic use of these agents requires striking a delicate balance between therapeutic benefit and dangerous suppression of host defense mechanisms.

Radiation. Radiation therapy may be used in treating cancer or in preventing allograft rejection. Radiation destroys lymphocytes and decreases the population of cells required to replace them. The size or extent of the irradiated area determines the extent of immunosuppression. Whole-body radiation may leave the individual totally immunosuppressed.

Assessment of Immune Function

An assessment of immune function begins with a health history and physical examination. The history should contain detailed information regarding past and present factors and events providing clues to the status of the immune system, as well as factors and events that may affect function of the immune system. These may include infections, allergies, autoimmune disorders, neoplastic disease, chronic illness, previous surgery, immunizations, medications, blood transfusions, other factors that affect immune function, and laboratory and diagnostic test results. Physical assessment includes palpation of the lymph nodes and examination of the skin, mucous membranes, and respiratory, gastrointestinal, genitourinary, cardiovascular, and neurosensory systems.

Health History

Infection and Immunization

The patient is asked about his immunization status (*i.e.*, immunizations received recently and as a child) and the usual childhood diseases. Known past or present exposure to tuberculosis is assessed, and the dates and results of any tuberculin tests (tine test or purified protein derivative [PPD]) and chest x-ray examinations are obtained. Recent exposure of the patient to any infections and the exposure dates are elicited. A history of past and present infections and the dates and types of treatments that were used are obtained along with a history of multiple persistent infections, fevers of unknown origin, lesions or sores, or any type of drainage.

Allergy

The patient is asked about history of any allergies, including types of allergens (pollens, dust, plants, cosmetics, food, medications, vaccines), the symptoms experienced, and seasonal variations in occurrence or severity in the symptoms. A history of testing and treatments that the patient has received or is currently receiving for these allergies and the effectiveness of the treatments is obtained. All medication and food allergies are listed on an allergy alert sticker and placed on the front of the patient's health record or chart to alert others to the possibility of these allergies. Continued assessment for potential allergic reactions in this patient is vital.

Autoimmune Disorders

The patient is asked about any autoimmune disorders such as lupus erythematosis, rheumatoid arthritis, or psoriasis. The onset, severity, remissions and exacerbations, functional limitations, treatments that the patient has received or is currently receiving, and the effectiveness of the treatments are described.

Neoplastic Disease

A family history of cancer is obtained. If there is a family history of cancer, the type of cancer, age of onset, and relationship (maternal or paternal) of the patient to the affected family member is noted. A history of cancer in the patient is also obtained, along with the type of cancer and date of diagnosis. All treatments that the patient has received or is currently receiving are recorded; treatment modalities such as radiation and chemotherapy suppress immune function and place the patient at risk for infection. Dates and results of any cancer screening tests that were performed are obtained.

Chronic Illness and Surgery

The health assessment includes a history of chronic illnesses such as diabetes mellitus, renal disease, or chronic obstructive pulmonary disease. A history of onset and severity of illnesses as well as treatment that the patient is

CHART 48-2
Selected Tests for Evaluating Immunologic Status

Various laboratory tests may be ordered to assess immune system activity or dysfunction. The studies may detect evidence of leukocytes and lymphocytes, humoral immunity, cellular immunity, phagocytic cell function, complement activity, hypersensitivity reactions, specific antigen-antibodies, or HIV infection.

Leukocytes and Lymphocyte Tests
- White blood cell (WBC) count and differential
- Bone marrow biopsy

Humoral Immunity (Antibody-Mediated) Tests
- B-cell quantification with monoclonal antibody
- *In vivo* immunoglobulin synthesis with T-cell subsets
- Specific antibody response
- Total serum globulins and individual immunoglobulins (by electrophoresis, immunoelectrophoresis, single radial immunodiffusion, nephelometry, isohemaglutin techniques)

Cellular (Cell-Mediated) Immunity Tests
- Total lymphocyte count
- T-cell and T-cell subset quantification with monoclonal antibody
- Delayed hypersensitivity skin test
- Cytokine production
- Lymphocyte response to mitogens, antigens, and allogenic cells
- Helper and suppressor T-cell functions

Phagocytic Cell Function Tests
- Nitroblue tetrazolium reductase assay

Complement Component Tests
- Total serum hemolytic complement
- Individual complement component titrations
- Radial immunodiffusion
- Electroimmunoassay
- Radioimmunoassay
- Immunonephelometric assay
- Immunoelectrophoresis

Hypersensitivity Tests
- Scratch test
- Patch test
- Intradermal test
- Radioallergosorbent test (RAST)

Specific Antigen-antibody Tests
- Radioimmunoassay
- Immunoflorescence
- Agglutination
- Complement fixation test

HIV Infection Tests
- Enzyme linked immunosorbent assay (ELISA)
- Western blot
- CD4 and CD8 cell counts
- P24 antigen test
- Polymerase chain reaction (PCR)

receiving for his illness is obtained. Additionally, a history of surgical removal of the spleen, lymph nodes, or thymus or a history of organ transplant is noted as these conditions may place the patient at risk for impaired immune function.

Medications and Blood Transfusions

A history of past and present medications is obtained. In large doses, antibiotics, corticosteroids, cytotoxic agents, salicylates, and NSAIDs as well as anesthetics can cause immune suppression (see Table 48-3). A history of single or multiple blood transfusions is obtained, as previous exposure to foreign antigens through transfusion may be associated with abnormal immune function. Additionally, although the risk of exposure to the human immunodeficiency virus (HIV) is extremely low for patients who report having had a blood transfusion after 1985, the year testing of blood for HIV was initiated in the United States, a risk still exists.

Factors That Affect the Immune System

A detailed history of smoking, alcohol consumption, dietary intake, amount of perceived stress, and occupational or residential exposure to radiation or pollutants is obtained. Poor nutritional status, smoking, stress, excessive consumption of alcohol, and exposure to radiation and pollutants have been associated with impaired immune function and are assessed in the history.

Physical Examination

On physical examination, the patient's skin and mucous membranes are assessed for lesions, dermatitis, purpura (subcutaneous bleeding), urticaria, inflammation, or any discharge. Additionally, signs of infection are noted. The patient's temperature is recorded and the patient is observed for chills and sweating. The anterior and posterior cervical, axillary, and inguinal lymph nodes are palpated for enlargement; if palpable nodes are detected, the location, size, consistency, and complaints of tenderness upon palpation are noted. Joints are assessed for tenderness and swelling and for limited range of motion. The patient's respiratory status is evaluated by monitoring the respiratory rate and assessing for the presence of cough (dry or productive) and any abnormal lung sounds (wheezing, crackles, ronchi). The patient is assessed for rhinitis, hyperventilation, and bronchospasm.

The patient's cardiovascular status is evaluated by assessing for hypotension, tachycardia, dysrhythmia, vasculitis, and anemia. The patient's gastrointestinal status is assessed by checking for hepatosplenomegaly, colitis, and vomiting and diarrhea. Genitourinary status is assessed by observing the patient for signs of infection (frequency and burning on urination, hematuria, and discharge). The patient is assessed for neurosensory status changes (i.e., cognitive dysfunction, hearing loss, visual changes, headaches and migraines, ataxia, and tetany). The patient's nutritional status, level of stress, and coping ability are also assessed, along with his or her age and any functional limitations (fatigue and endurance).

CRITICAL THINKING EXERCISES

1. A young, sexually active woman asks if you think it is a good idea for her to be tested for HIV infection. How would you respond to her, and what recommendations would you give and why?
2. Your patient is a 74-year-old man hospitalized with a fractured hip. His long-standing arthritis and inflammatory bowel disease have been treated with anti-inflammatory medications for the last 20 years. Describe the parameters you would consider in assessing his immune function and explain how the altered immune function would affect your care.

Laboratory and Diagnostic Evaluations

A series of blood tests, skin tests, and a bone marrow biopsy may be performed to evaluate the patient's immune competence. Specific laboratory and diagnostic tests will be discussed in greater detail along with specific disease processes. Laboratory and diagnostic tests used to evaluate immune competence are summarized in Chart 48-2.

REFERENCES AND SELECTED READINGS

Books

Barrett JT. Medical Immunology Text and Review. Philadelphia, FA Davis, 1991.

Chapel H and Haeney M. Essentials of Clinical Immunology. Oxford, Blackwell Scientific Publications, 1993.

Cohen N, Moynihan JA, and Ader R. Behavioral Regulation of Immunity. In IM Roitt and PJ Delves (eds). Encyclopedia of Immunology. London, Academic Press, 1992.

Dubey DP and Yunis EJ. Physiologic and environmental influences on the immune system: Aging and nutritional effects on immune functions in humans. In DP Sites and AI Terr (eds). Basic and Clinical Immunology, 7th ed. Norwalk CT, Appleton & Lange, 1991.

Jackson GH and Proctor SJ. Disorders of blood cells and haemostasis. In IM Danes (ed). Textbook of Adverse Drug Reactions. Oxford, Oxford University Press, 1991.

Kuby J. Immunology. New York, WH Freeman, 1992.

Lehne RA. Pharmacology for Nursing Care. Philadelphia, WB Saunders, 1994.

Roitt I. Essential Immunology, 8th ed. Cambridge MA, Blackwell Scientific Publishing, 1994.

Roitt I, Brostoff J, and Male D. Immunology, 3rd ed. St. Louis, Mosby Year Book, 1993.

Ruddle NH. Tumor necrosis factor beta. In IM Roitt and PJ Delves (eds). Encyclopedia of Immunology. London, Academic Press, 1992.

Sites DP and Terr AI (eds). Basic and Clinical Immunology. Norwalk CT, Appleton & Lange, 1991.

Talal N. Sex hormones and immunity. In IM Roitt and PJ Delves (eds). Encyclopedia of Immunology. London, Academic Press, 1992.

Terr AI. Physiologic and environmental influences on the immune system: Psychoneuroimmunology. In DP Sites and AI Terr (Eds). Basic and Clinical Immunology, 7th ed. Norwalk CT, Appleton & Lange, 1991.
Tracey KJ and Cerami A. Tumor necrosis factor alpha. In IM Roitt and PJ Delves (eds). Encyclopedia of Immunology. London, Academic Press, 1992.
Virella G, Goust JM, and Fudenberg HH (eds). Introduction to Medical Immunology, 2nd ed. New York, Marcel Dekker, 1990.

Journals

Immunology (General)

Adler WH. Immune function in the elderly. Geriatrics 1989 Aug; 44(suppl A): 7–10.
Epersen S. Nursing support of host defences. Critical Care Quarterly 1986 June; 51–56.
Halley FM. Self-regulation of the immune system through biobehavioral strategies. Biofeedback and Self Regulation 1991 Mar; 16(1):55–74.
Lehmann S. Immune function and nutrition. The role of the intravenous nurse. Journal of Intravenous Nursing 1991 Nov-Dec; 14(6):406–420.
Lopez M, Fleisher T, and deShazo RD. Use and interpretation of diagnostic immunologic laboratory tests. JAMA 1992 Nov 25; 268(20):2970–2990.
Weigle WO. The effects of aging on the immune system. Hosp Pract 1989 Dec; 24(12):112–116, 118, 119.

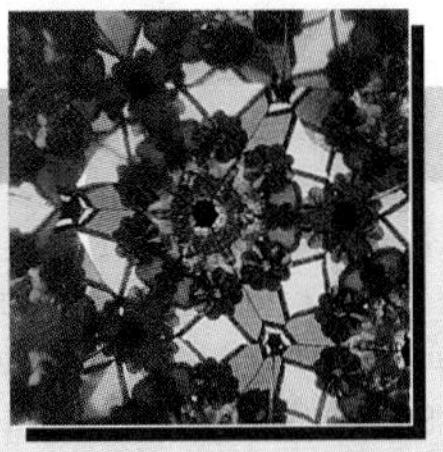

49

Management of Patients With Immunodeficiency Disorders

CHAPTER OUTLINE

LEARNING OBJECTIVES

On completion of this chapter, the learner will be able to:

1. Compare the various immunodeficiency disorders with regard to causes, clinical manifestations, medical and nursing management, complications and available treatments
2. Discuss nursing diagnoses that commonly occur with immunodeficiency disorders
3. Discuss nursing and medical management of patients with immunodeficiency disorders
4. Describe the management and nursing care of the patient receiving IV gamma globulin

Immunodeficiency Disorders

Immunodeficiency disorders may be caused by a defect or deficiency in phagocytic cells, B lymphocytes, T lymphocytes, or complement. The specific symptoms and their severity, age of onset, and prognosis depend on which components of the immune system are affected and the degree to which their functions are impaired. Regardless of the underlying cause of immunodeficiency, the cardinal symptoms include chronic or recurrent severe infections, infections caused by unusual organisms or organisms that are normal body flora, poor response to treatment of infections, and chronic diarrhea. Immunodeficiencies may be classified as either primary or secondary and by the components of the immune system that are affected.

Primary Immunodeficiencies

Primary immunodeficiencies are rare disorders with genetic origins that are seen primarily in infants and young children. Symptoms usually develop early in life once protection from maternal antibodies decreases. Without treatment, infants and children with these disorders seldom survive to adulthood. These disorders may involve one or more components of the immune system. Symptoms of immune deficiency diseases are related to the role that the deficient component normally plays (Table 49-1).

Phagocytic Dysfunction

Clinical Manifestations

Phagocytic cell disorders are manifested by an increased incidence of bacterial infections. In addition to bacterial infections, persons with hyperimmunoglobulinemia E (HIE) syndrome, formerly known as Job's syndrome, develop fungal infections from *Candida* organisms and viral infections from herpes simplex or herpes zoster. These individuals are afflicted with recurrent furunculosis, cutaneous abscesses, chronic eczematoid dermatitis, bronchitis, pneumonia, chronic otitis media, and sinusitis. White blood cells are unable to produce an inflammatory response to the skin infections; this results in deep-seated cold abscesses, which lack the classic signs and symptoms of inflammation (redness, heat, and pain).

Diagnostic Evaluation

Diagnosis is made from the history, signs and symptoms, and an indirect examination of the cytocidal activity of the phagocytic cells by the nitroblue tetrazolium (NTB) reductase test.

Management

Treatment for these disorders includes managing bacterial infections with prophylactic antibiotic therapy. In persons with HIE syndrome, treatment may be needed for fungal as well as viral infections. Granulocytic transfusions have been used but have often been unsuccessful because of the short half-life of the cells. Treatment with granulocyte-macrophage colony-stimulating factor (GM-CSF) or granulocyte CSF (G-CSF) may prove to be successful because these proteins draw cells from the bone marrow and hasten their maturation.

B-cell Deficiencies

There are two types of inherited B-cell deficiencies. The first type results from lack of differentiation of B-cell precursors into mature B cells, with a resultant lack of plasma cells and the disappearance of germinal centers from all lymphatic tissues. This phenomenon leads to a complete lack of antibody production against invading bacteria, viruses, and other pathogens. Infants born with this disorder suffer from severe infections starting soon after birth. This syndrome is called **sex-linked agammaglobulinemia (Bruton's disease)** because all antibodies disappear from the patient's plasma.

The second type of B-cell deficiency results from a lack of differentiation of B-cells into plasma cells. Only diminished antibody production occurs with this disorder. Although plasma cells are the most vigorous producers of antibodies, the individual has normal lymph follicles and many B lymphocytes that produce some antibodies. This syndrome is called **hypogammaglobulinemia.** This is a frequently occurring immunodeficiency and thus it is called **common variable immunodeficiency (CVID).** This term encompasses a variety of defects ranging from IgA deficiency, in which only the plasma cells that produce IgA are lacking, to the other extreme in which there is a severe panhypoglobulinemia (general lack of immunoglobulins in the blood).

Clinical Manifestations

CVID is the most common primary immunodeficiency seen in adulthood. Men and women are equally affected. Although the onset of this disease can occur at any age, it occurs most often in the second decade of life. More than 50% of individuals with CVID develop pernicious anemia. Common findings on examination include lymphoid hyperplasia of the small intestine and spleen as well as gastric atrophy detected by biopsy of the stomach. Frequently, individuals with CVID also develop other autoimmune diseases such as arthritis and hypothyroidism. CVID must be distinguished from secondary immunodeficiency diseases caused by protein-losing enteropathy, nephrotic syndrome, or burns.

Individuals with CVID are susceptible to infections with encapsulated bacteria such as *Haemophilus influenza, Streptococcus pneumoniae,* and *Staphylococcus aureus.* Frequent respiratory tract infections typically lead to chronic progressive bronchiectasis and pulmonary failure. Infection with *Giardia lamblia* occurs commonly in these individuals. Opportunistic infections with *Pneumocystis carinii* are seen only in individuals who have a concomitant deficiency in T-cell immunity.

Diagnostic Evaluation

The diagnosis of CVID is made from the history of bacterial infections, quantification of B-cell activity, and reported signs and symptoms. Laboratory tests are performed to assess the number of B lymphocytes and to measure total as well as specific immunoglobulin levels. Total serum glob-

TABLE 49-1 Selected Primary Immunodeficiency Disorders

Immune Component	Disorder	Major Symptoms	Treatment
Phagocytic cells	Hyperimmunoglobulinemia E (HIE) syndrome	Bacterial, fungal, and viral infections; deep-seated cold abcesses	Antibiotic therapy and treatment for viral and fungal infections Granulocyte-macrophage colony-stimulating factor (GM-CSF Granulocyte CSF)
B-lymphocytes	Sex-linked (agammaglobulinemia (Bruton's disease)	Severe infections soon after birth	Passive pooled plasma or gamma-globulin
	Common variable immunodeficiency (CVID)	Bacterial infections, infection with *Giardia lamblia*	IV gamma globulin Metronidazole (Flagyl) Quinacrine HCl (Atabrine)
		Pernicious anemia	Vitamin B_{12}
		Chronic respiratory infections	Antimicrobial therapy
	IgA deficiency	Predisposition to recurrent infections, adverse reactions to blood transfusions or gammaglobulin, autoimmune diseases, hypothyroidism	None
	IgG_2deficiency	Heightened incidence of infectious diseases	Pooled gamma globulin
T-lymphocytes	DiGeorge's syndrome thymic hypoplasia	Recurrent infections; hypoparathyroidism; hypoeakemia, tetany, convulsions; congenital heart disease; possible renal abnormalities; abnormal facies	Thymus graft
	Chronic mucotaneous candidiasis	*Candida albicans* infections of mucous membrane, skin, and nails, endocrine abnormalities (hypoparathyroidism, Addison's disease)	Topical antifungal miconozole IV amphotericin B Oral antifungals Clotrimazole Ketoconazole
B and T lymphocytes	Ataxia-telangiectasia	Ataxia with progressive neurologic deterioration, telangiectasia (vascular lesions), recurrent infections, malignancies	Antimicrobial therapy, management of presenting symptoms, fetal thymus transplant, IV gamma globulin
	Nezelof's syndrome	Severe infections, malignancies	Antimicrobial therapy, IV gamma globulin, bone marrow transplant, thymus transplant, thymus factors
	Wiscott-Aldrich syndrome	Thrombocytopenia resulting in bleeding, infections, malignancies	Antimicrobial therapy, splenectomy with continuous antibiotic prophylaxis, IV gamma globulin, bone marrow transplant
	Severe combined immunodeficiency disease (SCID)	Overwhelming severe fatal infections soon after birth (also includes opportunistic infections)	Antimicrobial therapy, IV gamma globulin, fetal liver and/or thymus transplant, bone marrow transplant (has replaced liver and thymus transplants)
	Angioneurotic edema	Episodes of edema in various parts of the body including respiratory tract and bowels	Pooled plasma, androgen therapy
Complement system	Paroxysmal nocturnal hemoglobinuria (PNH)	Lysis of erythrocytes due to lack of decay-accelerating factor (DAF) on erythrocytes	None

ulin level alone is an inadequate measure since there may be a compensatory overproduction of one globulin; this masks the loss of a missing globulin or one that is present in very low amounts. Antibody titers to confirm successful childhood vaccination are determined by specific serologic tests. Previous successful childhood immunization indicates that B cells were functioning adequately earlier in life. Hemoglobin and hematocrit levels are obtained if signs and symptoms suggesting pernicious anemia are present.

Management

Individuals with CVID may need replacement therapy with IV gamma globulin. Individuals who are receiving adequate treatment with IV gamma globulin do not usually require prophylactic antibiotics unless they also have chronic respiratory disease. Antimicrobial therapy is prescribed for respiratory infections to prevent complications such as pneumonia, sinusitis, or otitis media. Intestinal infestation with *Giardia lamblia* is treated with a 7-day course of metronidazole (Flagyl) or a 7-day course of quinacrine hydrochloride (Atabrine). Individuals who have pernicious anemia will receive parenteral injections of vitamin B_{12} at monthly intervals.

T-cell Deficiencies

Pathophysiology and Management

The loss of T-cell function is usually accompanied by some loss of B-cell activity because of the regulatory role that T-cells play in the immune system. The status of T cells can be evaluated by peripheral blood lymphocyte counts. Lymphopenia may signify a T-cell deficit. T cells constitute 65% to 85% of peripheral blood lymphocytes. It is also important to evaluate whether the T cells are capable of producing the expected T-cell responses. This can be done through dermal sensitization of the individual or by stimulating the individual's T cells *in vitro*.

DiGeorge's syndrome or **thymic hypoplasia** is a T-cell deficiency that occurs when the thymus gland fails to develop normally during embryogenesis. Infants born with DiGeorge's syndrome have hypoparathyroidism with resultant hypocalcemia that is resistant to standard therapy, congenital heart disease, abnormal facies and, possibly, renal abnormalities. These infants are susceptible to yeast, fungal, protozoan, and viral infections. They are particularly susceptible to childhood diseases (chickenpox, measles, and rubella), which are usually severe and may be fatal.

Chronic mucocutaneous candidiasis with or without endocrinopathy is a disorder associated with a selective defect in T-cell immunity thought to be caused by an autosomal recessive inheritance. It is considered an autoimmune disorder in which the thymus and other endocrine glands are involved in the autoimmune process. The initial presentation of chronic mucocutaneous candidiasis may be either chronic candidial infection or idiopathic endocrinopathy. It affects both males and females. Individuals may survive to the second or third decade of life. The disease causes extensive morbidity resulting from endocrine dysfunction. Problems may include hypocalcemia and tetany secondary to hypofunction of the parathyroid glands. Hypofunction of the adrenal cortex (Addison's disease) is the major cause of death in these individuals, and it may develop suddenly and without any history of previous symptoms.

Chronic skin and mucous membrane candidial infections are difficult to treat, although systemic infections with *Candida* do not usually occur. Individuals with severe candidial infection of the skin and mucous membranes often develop severe psychologic problems. Topical treatment with various antifungal agents has been tried but with little success. Topical miconozole therapy has been reported to have provided control in some individuals. Courses of IV amphotericin B have been beneficial in some individuals, but its use is limited because of its renal toxicity. Oral clotrimazole and ketoconozole have been reported to be beneficial.

B- and T-cell Deficiencies

Pathophysiology and Management

Ataxia-telangiectasia is a disorder affecting both T- and B-cell immunity. It is inherited in an autosomal recessive manner. There is a selective IgA deficiency in 40% of individuals with this disease. IgA and IgG subclass deficiencies as well as IgE deficiencies have been identified. Variable degrees of T-cell deficiencies are observed and become more severe with advancing age. The disease involves the neurologic, vascular, endocrine, and immune systems. The onset of ataxia (uncoordinated muscle movement) and telangiectasia (vascular lesions caused by dilated blood vessels) usually occurs in the first 4 years of life, but many individuals may remain symptom free for 10 or more years. Morbidity with chronic lung disease, mental retardation, neurologic symptoms, and physical disability becomes severe as individuals approach the second decade of life. Long-term survivors develop progressive deterioration of immunologic and neurologic functions. Some affected individuals have reached the fifth decade of life. The primary causes of death in these individuals are overwhelming infection and lymphoreticular or epithelial cancer. Treatment includes early management of infections with antimicrobial therapy, management of chronic lung disease with postural drainage and physical therapy, and management of other presenting symptoms. Other treatments include transplantation of fetal thymus tissue and IV gamma globulin.

Nezelof's syndrome is thought to be caused by a genetic recessive characteristic. Infants born with Nezelof's syndrome do not have a thymus gland and have various degrees of B-cell immunodeficiency associated with various combinations of increased, decreased, or normal immunoglobulin levels. These infants are highly susceptible to viral, bacterial, fungal, and protozoan infection; they also have a high incidence of malignant disease.

Both B and T cells are missing in **severe combined immunodeficiency disease (SCID)**. There is a complete absence of humoral as well as cellular immunity caused by an X-linked or autosomal genetic abnormality. In some instances sporadic forms of the disease occur. **Wiscott-Aldrich syndrome** is a variant of SCID with thrombocytopenia (loss of platelets) in addition to the absence of T and B cells.

Prognosis is generally poor because most affected infants develop overwhelming fatal infections. Treatment options under investigation include bone marrow transplantation, IV immunoglobulin replacement, thymus-derived factors, and thymus gland transplantation. As treatment becomes successful, an increased number of those who previously would have died in infancy may live to adulthood.

Deficiencies of the Complement System

As techniques to identify the individual complement components have improved, a steady increase in the identification of deficiencies of the complement system has occurred. C_2 and C_3 component deficiencies result in diminished resistance to bacterial infections. **Angioneurotic edema** is caused by an inherited deficiency of the inhibitor of C_1 esterase, which opposes the release of mediators of inflammation. A deficiency of this inhibitor results in frequent episodes of edema in various parts of the body.

Individuals with **paroxysmal nocturnal hemoglobinuria (PNH)** lack decay-accelerating factor (DAF), found on erythrocytes (red blood cells). DAF normally protects the erythrocytes from lysis (disintegration). In PNH, the complement component C_{3b} accumulates on the CR_1 molecule on the erythrocyte, acts as a binding site for the late-acting component, and allows lysis to occur.

Secondary Immunodeficiencies

Secondary immunodeficiencies are more common than primary deficiencies and frequently occur as a result of underlying disease processes or from the treatment of these diseases. Common causes of secondary immunodeficiencies are malnutrition, chronic stress, burns, uremia, diabetes mellitus, certain autoimmune disorders, certain viruses, exposure to immunotoxic medications and chemicals, and self-administration of recreational drugs and alcohol. Acquired immunodeficiency syndrome (AIDS) is the most common secondary immunodeficiency disorder; it is discussed in detail in Chapter 50. Individuals with secondary immunodeficiencies suffer with immunosuppression and are often referred to as **immunocompromised hosts.** Interventions for secondary immunodeficiencies include eliminating the contributing factors, treating the underlying condition, and using sound principles of infection control.

Medical Management

Medical management for *primary immunodeficiencies* may include replacement therapy with IV gamma globulin and reconstitution therapy with self-renewing precursor cells through fetal thymus transplants and bone marrow transplants. Individuals with phagocytic deficiencies may be treated with GM-CSF or G-CSF. Treatment of viral, bacterial, fungal, and protozoan infections may include antiviral, antibiotic, antifungal, and antiprotozoal therapy. Individuals with pernicious anemia may need injections of vitamin B_{12}. Management is directed toward treating underlying disease processes and controling symptoms. Management of *secondary immunodeficiencies* includes diagnosing and treating underlying disease processes.

Nursing Considerations

Nursing management of immunocompromised individuals includes a careful assessment of the individual's immune status. Because the immunocompromised patient is at high risk for infection, assessment focuses on history of past infections, particularly the type and frequency of infection; signs and symptoms of any current skin, respiratory, gastrointestinal, or genitourinary infection; and level of knowledge of the disease and measures that prevent infection. Assessment also focuses on nutritional status, stress level and coping skills, use of alcohol, drugs, or tobacco, and general hygiene; all of these factors affect immune function.

Nursing care is directed toward reducing the patient's risk for infection, assisting with medical measures aimed at treating infection, improving the patient's nutritional status, and maintaining bowel and bladder function. Other aspects of nursing care include assisting the patient in stress management and in adopting a lifestyle that enhances immune system function.

The nurse monitors the patient for signs and symptoms of infection: fever; chills; cough with or without sputum; shortness of breath; difficulty breathing; difficulty swallowing; white patches in the oral cavity; swollen lymph glands; nausea; vomiting; persistent diarrhea; frequency, urgency, or pain on urination; redness, swelling, or drainage from skin wounds; lesions on the face, lips, or perianal area; persistent vaginal discharge with or without perianal itching; and persistent abdominal pain.

The nurse also monitors laboratory values indicating infection, such as white blood cell count and differential cell count. Culture and sensitivity reports from wound drainage, lesions, sputum, stool, urine, and blood are monitored to identify pathogenic organisms and appropriate antimicrobial therapy.

Interventions are initiated to reduce the risk of preventable infections. They include washing hands carefully, encouraging the patient to cough and perform deep-breathing exercises at regular intervals, and protecting the integrity of the skin and mucous membranes. All health care personnel must use strict aseptic technique when performing invasive procedures such as dressing changes, venipunctures, and bladder catheterizations. Changes in laboratory results and subtle changes in clinical status are reported to the physician because the immunocompromised patient may not develop typical signs and symptoms of infection.

Patient Education and Home Care Considerations

The patient and the caregivers are instructed about signs and symptoms indicative of infection. They are also alerted to actions to take if they occur—for example, contact the health care provider and initiate prescribed therapy. The patient and caregiver need instruction about any prophylactic medication regimen, including dosage, indications times, actions, and side effects. They also need to learn about other ways to prevent infection (Chart 49-1).

CHART 49-1

Patient Education: Guidelines for Avoiding Infection

The following measures may help prevent infection:

- Report the following signs and symptoms of infection to the health care provider: fever; chills; wet or dry cough; breathing problems; swallowing problems; white patches in the mouth; swollen glands; nausea; vomiting; persistent abdominal pain; persistent diarrhea; problems with urination; red, swollen, or draining wounds; sores or lesions anywhere on the body; and persistent vaginal discharge with or without itching.
- Wash hands frequently and thoroughly especially before eating, after using the bathroom, and before and after performing health care procedures.
- Use cream and emollients to protect dry skin from chafing and cracking and allowing organisms to enter the body.
- As directed, perform recommended personal hygiene procedures–for example, foot care to prevent fungal infection.
- Avoid persons who have known illnesses or who have recently been vaccinated.
- Maintain a well-balanced diet with adequate calories. Avoid raw fruits and vegetables, thoroughly cook all food, and immediately refrigerate all leftover food.
- Clean kitchen and bathroom surfaces with disinfectant to prevent bacterial and fungal growth.
- Avoid alcohol, tobacco, and unprescribed medications.
- Take prescribed medications exactly as directed.
- Develop ways to cope with stress successfully, exercise regularly, and obtain adequate rest.

Management of Patients Receiving IV Gamma Globulin

During the past decade, gamma globulin has become suitable for IV use. Previously, immunoglobulin was available only for intramuscular injection. However, IV gamma globulin can now be administered in greater, more effective doses without painful side effects. Replacement therapy is indicated in primary and secondary immunodeficiency disorders in which the patient has insufficient amounts of gamma globulin.

IV gamma globulin is supplied in a 5% solution or as a lyophilized powder with a reconstituting diluent. It is prepared from Cohn fraction II that is obtained from pools of 1,000 to 10,000 donors. Currently, seven different IV preparations are approved for use by the Food and Drug Administration. All seven contain comparable amounts of desired antibodies and have been shown through extensive clinical testing to be effective and safe. The risk of transmitting hepatitis, HIV, or other known viruses is *extremely* small.

Dosage. The optimal dose for a person is determined by that person's response. In most instances the recommended IV dose is 350 to 500 mg per kilogram of body weight given once monthly or 150 to 250 mg every 2 weeks. When patients receive gamma globulin less frequently, they may develop fatigue, malaise, and other symptoms before their next treatment. Subsequently they comply readily with weekly or biweekly administration. To prevent unpleasant side effects, administration of IV gamma globulin should be performed at a slow rate not to exceed 3 ml/minute. Self-infusion in the home can decrease the cost and inconvenience of frequent hospitalization for infusions.

Adverse Effects. Reactions to intramuscular gamma globulin have included complaints of flank pain, shaking chills, and tightness in the chest. The reaction terminates with a slight rise in body temperature. Moreover, hypotension may develop with severe reactions. Reactions to IV gamma globulin are generally less severe and can be controlled by slowing the infusion rate. Patients with low gamma globulin levels have more severe reactions than those with normal levels (for example, patients who receive gamma globulin for thrombocytopenia or Kawasaki disease). Reactions can be prevented or minimized by administering aspirin before the infusion or by IV administration of an antihistamine such as diphehydramine (Benadryl) before the infusion. In some instances a patient receives prednisone to avoid a reaction, but this is usually not necessary.

In rare instances, systemic anaphylactic reactions have been observed after administering gamma globulin or whole plasma. Patients who are IgA deficient have IgE antibodies to IgA and require the administration of plasma or immunoglobulin replacement from IgA-deficient individuals. Because all IV gamma globulin preparations contain some IgA, they carry the risk of causing an anaphylactic reaction in patients with IgE anti-IgA antibodies.

Special Nursing Considerations. Nursing management includes assessing the patient's understanding of the treatment and possible adverse reactions. The patient will need information about expected benefits and outcomes of the treatment and expected adverse reactions and their management. Patients who can perform self-infusion at home are instructed in sterile technique, medication dosages, administration rate, and detection and management of adverse re-

CRITICAL THINKING EXERCISES

1. Gamma globulin infusions have been prescribed for your patient who has an immunodeficiency. He tells you that he is very fearful that he may contract HIV infection or AIDS from the infusion. How would you respond to these fears and concerns?
2. During a visit to evaluate the home environment of a patient who is immunocompromised, you note spoiled food in the kitchen, dirty dishes and countertops, an unclean bathroom, and the presence of several cats and dogs. Explain the course of action you would take to assure a safe environment for your patient.

actions. Referral for home care nursing and infusion therapy may be necessary.

The patient is weighed before treatment and vital signs are obtained before, during, and after treatment. The nurse then administers the prescribed pretreatment prophylactic aspirin and antihistamine. Next the nurse administers and monitors the IV infusion of gamma globulin and assesses for adverse reactions, including anaphylactic shock.

BIBLIOGRAPHY

Books

Ammann AJ. Antibody (B Cell) Immunodeficiency Disorders. In Sites DP and Terr AI (eds). Basic and Clinical Immunology. Norwalk CT, Appleton & Lange, 1991.

Ammann AJ. Combined antibody (B cell) and cellular (T cell) immunodeficiency disorders. In Sites DP and Terr AI (eds). Basic and Clinical Immunology. Norwalk CT, Appleton & Lange, 1991.

Amman AJ. T Cell immunodeficiency disorders. In Sites DP and Terr AI (eds). Basic and Clinical Immunology. Norwalk CT, Appleton & Lange, 1991.

Barrett JT. Medical Immunology Text and Review. Philadelphia, FA Davis, 1991.

Chapel H and Haney M. Essentials of Immunology. Oxford, Blackwell Scientific Publications, 1993.

Clark WR. The Experimental Foundations of Modern Immunology. New York, John Wiley & Sons, 1991.

Conley ME. Congenital immunodeficiency diseases. In Lichtenstein LM and Fauci AS (eds). Current Therapy In Allergy And Rheumatology. Philadelphia, BC Decker, 1992.

Constantinides P. General Pathobiology. Norwalk CT, Appleton & Lange, 1994.

Croenenberger JH and Jennette JC. Immunology: Basic Concepts, Diseases and Laboratory Methods. Norwalk CT, Appleton and Lange, 1988.

Geha RS. Severe combined immunodeficiency disease. In Lichtenstein LM and Fauci AS (eds). Current Therapy In Allergy, Immunology, and Rheumatology. Philadelphia, BC Decker, 1992.

Lachmann, PJ. Complement deficiencies—genetic and acquired. In Lachmann PJ, Peters K, Rosen FS, and Walport MJ (eds). Clinical Aspects of Immunology. Boston, Blackwell Scientific Publications, 1993.

Rosen FS. Common variable immunodeficiency. In Lichtenstein LM and Fauci AS (eds). Current Therapy In Allergy, Immunology, and Rheumatology. Philadelphia, BC Decker, 1992.

Rosen FS. The primary specific immunodeficiencies. In Lachmann PJ, Peters K, Rosen FS, and Walport MJ (eds). Boston, Blackwell Scientific Publications, 1993.

Shyur SD and Hull HR. Job's syndrome of hyperimmunoclobulin E and recurrent infections. In Lichtenstein LM and Fauci AS (eds). Current Therapy In Allergy, Immunology, And Rheumatology. Philadelphia, BC Decker, 1992.

Virella G, Goust JM, and Fudenberg HH (eds). Introduction to Medical Immunology. New York, Marcel Dekker, 1990.

Journals

Immunology (General)

Ballow M, Levinson AI, Gelfand E, and Schwartz SA. Future directions of immunoglobulin therapy: Forward. J Clin Immunol 1990 Nov Supp; 10(6):3S-4S.

Berkman SA, Lee ML, and Gale RP. Clinical uses of intravenous immunoglobulins. Ann Intern Med 1990; 112:278–292.

Buckley RH. Immunodeficiency diseases. JAMA 1987 Nov; 258(20): 2841–2850.

Coffman RL. T-helper heterogeneity and immune response patterns. Hosp Pract 1989 Aug; 24(8):101–133.

DiJulio J. Hematopoiesis: An overview. Oncol Nurs Forum 1991 Mar; 18(2):3–6.

Eperson S. Nursing support of host defenses. Crit Care Q 1986 June; 51–55.

Griffin JP. nursing care of the critically ill immunocompromised patient. Crit Care Q 1986 June; 25–33.

Heinzel FP. Infections in patients with humoral immunodeficiency. Hosp Pract 1989 Sep; 24(9):99–130.

Nossal GJV. Current concepts: Immunology—the basic components of the immune system. N Engl J Med 1987 May 21; 316(21):1320–1325.

Young LS. Infections in patients with cellular immunodeficiency. Hosp Pract 1989 Aug; 24(8):191–212.

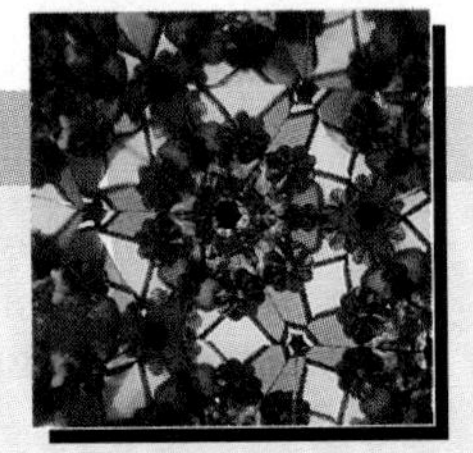

50

Acquired Immunodeficiency Syndrome

CHAPTER OUTLINE

Overview
Pathophysiology
Incidence
Transmission
Prevention of Transmission
Clinical Manifestations
Diagnostic Evaluation
Management
Supportive Care
NURSING PROCESS: The Patient With AIDS
Critical Thinking Exercises

LEARNING OBJECTIVES

On completion of this chapter, the learner will be able to:

1. Describe the pathophysiology of HIV infection
2. Describe the modes of transmission of HIV infection
3. Explain the physiology underlying the clinical manifestations of HIV infection
4. Describe the management and nursing care of patients with HIV infection
5. Describe nursing diagnoses common to patients with AIDS
6. Use the nursing process as a framework for care of the patient with AIDS

Overview

Acquired immunodeficiency syndrome (AIDS) is defined as the most severe form of a continuum of illnesses associated with **human immunodeficiency virus** (HIV) infection. Over the years, HIV has been referred to as human T-cell lymphotropic virus type III (HTLV III) and lymphadenopathy associated virus (LAV). Manifestations of HIV infection range from mild abnormalities in the immune response without overt signs and symptoms to profound immunosuppression associated with various life-threatening infections and rare malignancies. In the fall of 1982 the Centers for Disease Control and Prevention (CDC) issued a case definition of AIDS after the first 100 cases were reported. Since then the CDC has revised the case definition twice (in 1987 and 1993), thereby increasing the number of reportable AIDS cases.

Pathophysiology

HIV belongs to a group of viruses known as **retroviruses,** which indicates that the virus carries its genetic material in ribonucleic acid (RNA) rather than deoxyribonucleic acid (DNA). The HIV virion (a complete virus particle surrounded by a protective coat) contains RNA in a truncated bullet-shaped core of which p24 is the major structural component. Knobs that protrude through the viral wall consist of the protein gp120 anchored to the protein gp41. It is the gp120 portion of the HIV that selectively binds to CD4-positive (CD4+) cells.

CD4+ cells include monocytes, macrophages, and **helper T4 lymphocytes** (called CD4+ cells when referring to HIV infection), the most numerous of these cells. After binding to the helper T4 cell membrane, the HIV injects two identical strands of RNA into the helper T4 cell. Using an enzyme known as **reverse transcriptase,** HIV reprograms the genetic materials of the infected T4 cell to make double-stranded DNA. This DNA is incorporated into the T4 cell nucleus as a provirus and permanent infection is established.

The HIV replication cycle is restricted to this stage until the infected cell is activated. Activation of the infected cell may be achieved by antigens, mitogens, select cytokines (tumor necrosis factor alpha or interleukin 1), or virus gene products of such viruses as cytomegalovirus (CMV), Epstein-Barr, herpes simplex, and hepatitis. Consequently, whenever the infected T4 cell is activated, HIV replication and budding occur and the T4 cell is destroyed. Newly formed HIV is then released into the blood plasma and infects other CD4+ cells.

Infection of monocytes and macrophages appears to be persistent and does not result in significant cell death, but these cells serve as reservoirs for HIV, allowing the virus to hide from the immune system and to be transported throughout the system to infect a variety of body tissues. Most of these tissues either contain the CD4+ molecule or have the ability to produce it. Studies show that after the initial infection, approximately 25% of lymph node cells are infected with HIV as well. Viral replication is ongoing throughout the course of HIV infection; the primary site is lymphoid tissue. When the immune system is stimulated, HIV replication occurs and the virus is disseminated into the blood plasma, with subsequent infection of other CD4+ cells. More recent studies suggest that the immune system in HIV infection is more active than previously thought, as evidenced by the production of as many as 2 billion CD+4 lymphocytes daily. The entire population of peripheral CD4+ cells turns over every 15 days (Ho et al., 1995).

The rate of HIV production is thought to be associated with the health status of the infected individual. If that person is not fighting another infection, HIV reproduction may proceed slowly. HIV reproduction appears to accelerate, however, when the person is combating another infection or when the immune system is stimulated. This may explain the latent period exhibited by some persons after infection with HIV. For example, one person may remain symptom-free for many years; however, a large portion of infected persons (up to 65%) go on to develop symptomatic HIV disease or AIDS within 10 years of infection (Pinching, 1992).

In the immune response, several important roles are played by the T4 lymphocyte: recognition of foreign antigens, activation of antibody-producing B lymphocytes, stimulation of cytotoxic T lymphocytes, production of lymphokines, and defense against parasitic infections. When T4 lymphocyte function is impaired, organisms that do not usually cause disease have the opportunity to invade and cause serious illness. Infections and malignancies that develop as a result of immune system impairment are referred to as **opportunistic infections.**

Incidence

As of December 1994, there were 441,528 reported cases of AIDS and 270,870 deaths from AIDS in adults, adolescents, and children in the United States. In January 1993, the surveillance definition for AIDS was expanded to include conditions that occur earlier in the course of HIV infection, resulting in an increase in the number of cases of AIDS reported. Surveillance reports also indicate a substantial increase of HIV infection in the heterosexual population, especially on the East Coast.

In the United States, most persons with AIDS have engaged in high-risk behaviors, such as male homosexual relations, IV drug use, and heterosexual relations with an HIV-infected partner or one at risk for infection. Also at risk are persons who received blood or blood products contaminated with HIV (especially before blood screening was instituted in 1985) and children born to mothers with HIV infection.

Analysis of the sociodemographic and exposure categories indicates that in 1994, African-American and Hispanics accounted for 49.9% of all cases of AIDS; non-Hispanic whites accounted for 48.9%; and Asians, Pacific Islanders, Native Americans, and Alaskan natives accounted for 0.02%. This was the first year that African-Americans and Hispanics accounted for the greatest number of cases of AIDS. African-Americans and Hispanics account for approximately 46% of cases in men, 75% of cases in women, and 80% of cases in children. It has been suggested that this disproportionate representation may be related to IV drug use, having sex with an IV drug user, and a lack of access to health care and education.

Large urban areas continue to report more cases of AIDS than rural areas because of a higher incidence of IV drug use and high-risk sexual practices. HIV is predominantly an infection of young people, with most cases involving persons between ages 17 and 55. However, it has also been reported in elderly men and women. Moreover, according to the CDC, from 1991 to 1992 the largest proportionate increase (9.8%) in reported cases of AIDS occurred in women, especially those from ages 20 to 29. These women acquired the disease through heterosexual contact while they were adolescents. An increase of AIDS in this child-bearing age group is expected to result in an increase in the number of children with HIV infection. AIDS has reached epidemic proportions in other parts of the world as well.

Transmission

The routes of transmission of HIV are similar to those of hepatitis B. In male homosexuals, *anal intercourse* or manipulation increases chances of trauma to the rectal mucosa and subsequently increases chances of exposure to the virus through body secretions. Increased frequency of these practices and sex with multiple partners also contributes to the spread of this disease. *Heterosexual intercourse* with individuals who have HIV infection is also a mode of transmission that is growing significantly.

Transmission by *intravenous drug use* occurs through direct blood exposure to contaminated needles and syringes. Although the amount of blood in a syringe is relatively small, the cumulative effect of repeatedly sharing contaminated equipment leads to an increased risk of transmission.

Blood and blood products, including those used by hemophiliacs, can transmit HIV to recipients. However, the risk associated with transfusions has been reduced as a result of voluntary self-deferral, serologic testing, heat treating of clotting factor concentrates, and more effective virus inactivation methods (Donegan, 1990). The incidence for health care workers who are exposed to HIV through needle-stick injury is estimated to be less than 1%. Large-scale studies of exposed health care workers are being conducted by the CDC and other groups. The virus may also be transmitted *in utero* from mother to child and later through breast milk.

Prevention of Transmission

Until an effective vaccine is developed, preventing the transmission of HIV by eliminating or reducing risk behaviors is essential. Primary prevention efforts through effective educational programs are vital for control and prevention. AIDS is not transmitted by casual contact. Epidemiologic evidence indicates that HIV is transmitted only through intimate sexual contact, parenteral exposure to infected blood or blood products, and perinatal transmission from mother to neonate. Studies of nonsexual household contacts of AIDS patients as well as nonsexual person-to-person contact that generally occurs in the workplace have not demonstrated any increased risk for transmission of AIDS through such contact.

In the interest of public health, the CDC and the Surgeon General of the United States have issued recommendations for preventing the transmission of HIV (Guideline 50-1). These guidelines apply to health care workers in all settings as well as families and friends providing care in the home. The guidelines entitled "Universal Blood

GUIDELINE 50–1
Universal Precautions to Prevent Transmission of HIV

1. Consider sharp items (*e.g.,* needles, scalpel blades) potentially infective and handle with extraordinary care to prevent accidental injuries.
2. Place disposable syringes and needles, scalpel blades, and other sharp items in puncture-resistant containers located as near as is practical to the area in which they were used. Needles should not be recapped, purposely bent, broken, removed from disposable syringes, or otherwise manipulated by hand.
3. Wear protective barriers (gloves, gowns, masks, and protective eyewear) to prevent exposure to blood, body fluids containing visible blood, and other fluids to which universal precautions apply. The type of protective barrier should be appropriate for the procedure being performed and the type of exposure anticipated.
4. Immediately and thoroughly wash hands and other skin surfaces that are contaminated with blood, body fluids containing visible blood, or other body fluids to which universal precautions apply.
5. Minimize the need for emergency mouth-to-mouth resuscitation, by keeping mouth pieces, resuscitation bags, or other ventilation devices easily available for use in areas where the need for resuscitation is predictable.
6. During pregnancy, be especially careful and maintain proper precautions. Health care workers who are pregnant are not known to be at greater risk of contracting HIV infection than those who are not pregnant; however, if a health-care worker develops HIV infection during pregnancy, the infant is at increased risk of infection resulting from perinatal transmission.
7. In the home setting, flush blood and body fluids down the toilet.
8. Wrap contaminated items that cannot be flushed down the toilet securely in a plastic bag and place in a second bag before discarding in a manner consistent with local regulations for solid waste disposal.
9. Clean spills of blood or other body fluids with soap and water or a household detergent. Freshly prepared solutions of sodium hypochlorite (household bleach) in concentrations of 1:10 dilution are effective disinfectants. Persons cleaning spills should wear gloves.

(U.S. Department of Health and Human Services. Update: Universal precautions for prevention of transmission of human immunodeficiency virus, hepatitis B virus and other bloodborne pathogens in health care settings. MMWR 1988 June; 37[24]:377–382.)

and Body Fluid Precautions" are intended to prevent parenteral, mucous membrane, and nonintact skin exposures of health care providers to blood-borne pathogens of all patients regardless of HIV status. Although HIV has been isolated from all types of body fluids, the risk of transmission to health care providers is less likely from contact with feces, nasal secretions, sputum, sweat, breast milk, tears, urine, and vomitus unless they contain visible blood. The CDC suggests that universal precautions be applied to blood; cerebrospinal, synovial, pleural, peritoneal, pericardial, amniotic, and vaginal fluids; and semen. In emergency circumstances when differentiation between fluid types is difficult, all body fluids are considered potentially hazardous.

Another isolation system, the Body Substance Isolation System, is used by some institutions as an alternative to Universal Blood and Body Fluid Precautions. This system offers an even broader isolation strategy to reduce the risk of disease transmission to patients and health care workers alike, and eliminates the need for health care workers to identify particular body fluids. The elements of body substance isolation are listed in Guideline 50-2.

Clinical Manifestations

The clinical manifestations of AIDS are widespread and may affect virtually any organ system. Diseases associated with HIV infection and AIDS result from infections, malignancies, and/or the direct effect of HIV on body tissues. The following discussion is limited to the most common clinical manifestations and effects of severe HIV infection.

Respiratory

***Pneumocystis carinii* Pneumonia.** Shortness of breath, dyspnea (labored breathing), cough, chest pain, and fever are associated with various opportunistic infections, such as those caused by *Mycobacterium avium-intracellulare* (MAI), cytomegaloviruses (CMV), and *Legionella*. However, the most common infection in persons with AIDS is **Pneumocystis carinii pneumonia (PCP),** which was one of the first opportunistic diseases described in association with AIDS. It is the initial manifestation of AIDS in 60% of patients. Without prophylactic therapy, PCP will develop in 80% of all HIV-infected individuals. *P. carinii*

GUIDELINE 50-2
Infection Prevention Measures: Body Substance Isolation System

The following guidelines were developed to prevent infection transmission during patient care:

Handwashing
- Wash hands for 10 seconds with soap, running water, and friction before touching patients and any time the hands have been soiled.

Gloves
- Put on clean gloves just before contact with mucous membranes and nonintact skin.
- Wear appropriate gloves any time hands are likely to have contact with moist body substances.
- Remove gloves immediately after task is completed.

Gowns or Plastic Aprons
- Wear any time it is likely that clothing or skin will be soiled.

Masks
- Wear when working directly over large areas of open skin.
- Wear when it is likely that nasal and oral mucous membranes will be spattered with moist body substances.

Needles and Sharps
- Discard in rigid, puncture-resistant containers.
- Do not recap used needles by hand.
- Be particularly careful when manipulating small devices such as heparin locks.

Roommate Selection
- Avoid roommate combinations in which one patient is likely to have contact with the other patient's moist body substances.
- Assign patients with airborne communicable diseases to private rooms or rooms with immunocompetent roommates.

Trash and Linen
- Bag all soiled trash and linen securely.
- Discard according to facility policy.
- Wear gloves and protective garments when handling soiled linen and trash.

Housekeeping
- Clean all rooms on a regular schedule.
- Clean articles, equipment, and furniture soiled with moist body substances immediately. Wear gloves.

Laboratory Specimens
- Handle all laboratory specimens with equal care. No special precautionary labels are required.

Signs and Labels
- Avoid signs and labels identifying patients known to have infectious diseases. These are unnecessary and may encourage a double standard of care.
- Identify rooms of patients with airborne communicable diseases so that susceptibility of care providers can be assessed.

Compliance of Care Providers
- Develop a program to ensure that health care workers comply with the infection precautions system.

(Adapted from Jackson M and Lynch P. Infection prevention and control in the era of the AIDS/HIV epidemic. Semin Oncol Nurs 1989 Nov; 5(4):240.)

was originally classified as a protozoan; however, studies and analysis of its ribosomal RNA structure suggest that it is a fungus. However, its structure and antimicrobial sensitivity are very different from other disease-causing fungi. It causes disease only in immunocompromised hosts. It invades and proliferates within the pulmonary alveoli, resulting in consolidation of the pulmonary parenchyma.

The clinical presentation of PCP in the AIDS patient is generally less acute than in persons who are immunosuppressed as a result of other conditions. The time between the onset of symptoms and the actual documentation of disease may be weeks to months. Patients with AIDS initially develop nonspecific signs and symptoms such as fevers, chills, nonproductive cough, shortness of breath, dyspnea, and occasionally chest pain. PCP may be present despite the absence of crackles. Arterial oxygen concentrations in patients breathing room air may be mildly decreased, indicating minimal hypoxemia.

Untreated, PCP will eventually progress to cause significant pulmonary impairment and, ultimately, respiratory failure. A few patients have a dramatic onset and fulminant course involving severe hypoxemia, cyanosis, tachypnea, and altered mental status. Respiratory failure can develop within 2 to 3 days of initial symptoms.

PCP can be diagnosed definitively by identifying the organism in lung tissue or bronchial secretions. This is accomplished by such procedures as sputum induction, bronchial-alveolar lavage, and transbronchial biopsy (by fiberoptic bronchoscopy).

Mycobacterium avium *Complex.* *Mycobacterium avium* complex (MAC) disease is emerging as a leading cause of bacterial infections in persons with AIDS. Organisms belonging to MAC include *M. avium, M. intracellulare,* and *M. scrofulaceum.* MAC, a group of acid-fast bacilli, usually cause respiratory infection but are also commonly found in the gastrointestinal tract, lymph nodes, and bone marrow. Most patients with AIDS have widespread disease at the time of diagnosis and are usually debilitated. MAC infections are associated with rising mortality rates.

HIV-associated *M. tuberculosis* tends to occur in IV drug users and other groups with a preexisting high prevalence of tuberculosis infection. Unlike other opportunistic infections, tuberculosis (TB) tends to occur early in the course of HIV infection and usually precedes a diagnosis of AIDS. This early occurrence is associated with the development of caseating granulomas, which should raise the suspicion of a diagnosis of TB. At this stage, TB responds well to antituberculosis therapy. TB that occurs late in HIV infection is characterized by absence of a tuberculin skin test response because the compromised immune system can no longer respond to the TB antigen. In the later stages of HIV infection, TB is associated with dissemination to extrapulmonary sites such as the central nervous system, bone, pericardium, stomach, peritoneum, and scrotum. Multiple drug-resistant strains of the bacillus have now emerged and are often associated with noncompliance with antituberculosis therapy.

Gastrointestinal

The gastrointestinal manifestations of AIDS include loss of appetite, nausea, vomiting, oral and esophageal candidiasis, and chronic diarrhea. Diarrhea is a problem for 50% to 90% of all AIDS patients. In some instances, gastrointestinal symptoms may be related to the direct effect of HIV on the cells lining the intestines. Some of the enteric pathogens that occur most frequently, which are identified by stool cultures or intestinal biopsy, include *Cryptosporidium muris, Salmonella,* CMV, *Clostridium difficile,* and *M. avium-intracellulare.* For patients with AIDS, the effects of diarrhea can be devastating in terms of profound weight loss (more than 10% of body weight), fluid and electrolyte imbalances, perianal skin excoriation, weakness, and inability to perform the usual activities of daily living.

Oral candidiasis, a fungal infection, is nearly universal in all patients with AIDS and AIDS-related conditions and commonly precedes other life-threatening infections. It is characterized by creamy white patches in the oral cavity. When untreated, oral candidiasis will progress to involve the esophagus and stomach. Associated signs and symptoms include difficult and painful swallowing and retrosternal pain. Some patients also develop ulcerating oral lesions and are particularly susceptible to dissemination of candidiasis to other body systems.

Wasting Syndrome. Wasting syndrome is now included in the revised case definition for AIDS. Diagnostic criteria include profound involuntary weight loss exceeding 10% of baseline body weight and either chronic diarrhea for more than 30 days or chronic weakness and documented intermittent or constant fever in the absence of any concurrent illness that could explain these findings. This protein–energy malnutrition is multifactorial. In some AIDS-associated illnesses patients experience a hypermetabolic state in which excessive calories are burned and lean body mass is lost. This state is similar to that seen in stress states such as sepsis and trauma and can lead to organ failure. A distinction between cachexia (wasting) and malnutrition or between cachexia and simple weight loss is important because the metabolic derangement seen in wasting syndrome may not be modified by nutritional support alone.

Anorexia, diarrhea, gastrointestinal malabsorption, and lack of nutrition in chronic disease all contribute to wasting syndrome. However, progressive tissue wasting has been seen in several persons with only modest gastrointestinal involvement and without diarrhea (Medynski, 1993). Tumor necrosis factor (TNF) and interleukin-1 (IL-1) are cytokines that play important roles in AIDS-related wasting syndrome. Both act directly on the hypothalamus to cause anorexia. Cytokine-induced fever accelerates the body's metabolism by 14% for every 1°F increase in temperature. TNF causes inefficient use of lipids by reducing enzymes that are needed for fat metabolism, whereas IL-1 triggers the release of amino acids from muscle tissue. Persons with AIDS generally experience increased protein metabolism in relation to fat metabolism, which results in significant decreases in lean body mass due to muscle and protein breakdown.

Hypertriglyceridemia seen in persons with AIDS is attributed to chronically elevated cytokine levels and can persist in persons with AIDS for months without tissue wasting and loss of lean body mass. It is believed that infections and sepsis lead to transient rises in TNF, IL-1, and other cell mediators above the chronically elevated levels generally seen, and it is these transient rises in TNF and IL-1 that trigger muscle wasting.

Cancer

Individuals with AIDS have a higher than usual incidence of cancer. This may be related to HIV stimulation of developing cancer cells or to the immune deficiency allowing cancer-causing substances, such as viruses, to transform susceptible cells into malignant cells. Kaposi's sarcoma, certain types of B-cell lymphomas, and invasive cervical carcinoma are included in the CDC classification of AIDS-related malignancies. Carcinomas of the skin, stomach, pancreas, rectum, and bladder also occur more frequently than expected in persons with AIDS.

Kaposi's Sarcoma. Kaposi's sarcoma (KS; pronounced KA-po-sheez), the most common HIV-related malignancy, is a disease involving the endothelial layer of blood and lymphatic vessels. When first noted in 1872 by Dr. Moritz Kaposi, KS characteristically presented as lower-extremity skin lesions in elderly men of Eastern European ancestry. The disease was slow to progress and easily treated; this form is often referred to as *classic* KS. An *endemic* form of KS, found in children and young men in equatorial Africa, is more virulent than the classic form.

Acquired KS occurs in individuals who are treated with immunosuppressive agents and commonly occurs in patients who have undergone organ transplantation. In such patients, acquired KS usually resolves once the dose of the immunosuppressive medication is decreased or discontinued. In persons with AIDS, *epidemic* KS is most often seen in male homosexuals and bisexuals. Although the histopathology of all forms of KS is virtually identical, the clinical manifestations differ with AIDS-related KS, which exhibits a more variable and aggressive disease course ranging from localized cutaneous lesions to disseminated disease involving multiple organ systems.

Cutaneous lesions appearing anywhere on the body are usually brownish pink to deep purple. They may be flat or raised and surrounded by ecchymoses (hemorrhagic patches) and edema (Fig. 50-1). Rapid development of lesions involving large areas of skin is associated with extensive disfigurement.

The location and size of some lesions can lead to venous stasis, lymphedema, and pain. Ulcerative lesions disrupt skin integrity and increase patient discomfort and susceptibility to infection. The most common sites of visceral involvement include the lymph nodes, gastrointestinal tract, and lungs. Involvement of internal organs may eventually lead to organ failure, hemorrhage, infection, and death. Diagnosis of KS is confirmed by biopsy of suspected lesions. Prognosis depends on the extent of the tumor, presence of constitutional symptoms, and the CD4+ count. Death may result from tumor progression, but more often it results from other complications of HIV disease.

B-cell Lymphomas. B-cell lymphomas are the second most common malignancy occurring in persons with AIDS. Lymphomas associated with AIDS usually differ from those occurring in the general population. Patients with AIDS are generally much younger than the usual population affected by non-Hodgkin's lymphoma (NHL). In addition, AIDS-related lymphomas tend to develop outside the lymph nodes, most commonly in the brain, bone marrow, and gastrointestinal tract. These types of lymphomas are characteristically of a higher grade, indicating aggressive growth and resistance to treatment. The course of AIDS-related lymphomas includes multiple sites of organ involvement and complications related to developing opportunistic infections. Although aggressive combination chemotherapy is frequently successful in NHL not associated with HIV infection, it is less successful in persons with HIV because of the severe hematologic toxicity and complications of opportunistic infections that occur from treatment.

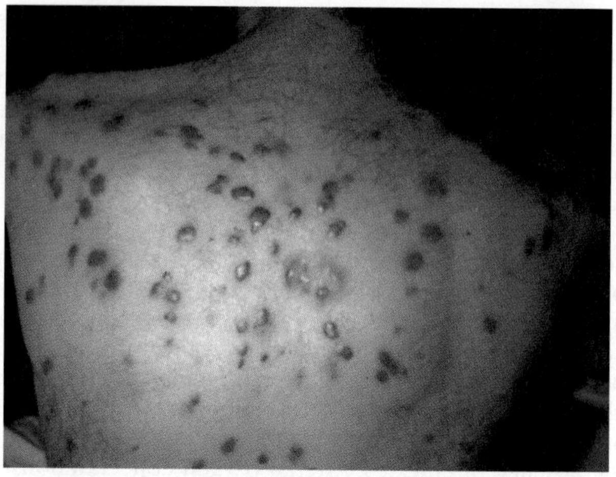

FIGURE 50-1. Lesions of AIDS-related Kaposi's sarcoma. Whereas some patients may have lesions that remain flat, others may experience extensively disseminated, raised lesions with edema. (From DeVita VT Jr, Hellman S, and Rosenberg SA (eds). AIDS: Etiology, Diagnosis, Treatment and Prevention, 3rd ed. Philadelphia, JB Lippincott, 1992.)

Neurologic

An estimated 80% of all patients with AIDS experience some form of neurologic involvement during the course of HIV infection. Many neuropathologic disorders are underreported because patients may have neurologic involvement without overt signs or symptoms. Neurologic complications involve central, peripheral, and autonomic functions. Neurologic dysfunction results from the direct effects of HIV on nervous system tissue, opportunistic infections, primary or metastatic neoplasms, cerebrovascular changes, metabolic encephalopathies, or complications that are secondary to therapy. Immune system response to HIV infection in the central nervous system includes inflammation, atrophy, demyelination, degeneration, and necrosis.

HIV Encephalopathy. Also referred to as **AIDS dementia complex (ADC),** HIV encephalopathy occurs in at least two thirds of patients with AIDS, and substantial evidence exists that ADC is a direct result of HIV infection. HIV has been found in large amounts in both the brain and CSF of patients with ADC. The brain cells that are infected by HIV are predominantly the CD4+ cells of monocyte/macrophage lineage. It is believed that HIV infection triggers the release of toxins or lymphokines that result in cellular dysfunction or interfere with neurotransmitter function rather than cause cellular damage. It is a clinical syndrome characterized by a progressive decline in cognitive, behavioral, and motor functions. Signs and symptoms may be subtle and difficult to distinguish from fatigue, depression, or the adverse effects of treatments for infections and malignancies.

Early manifestations include memory deficits, headache, difficulty with concentration, progressive confusion, psychomotor slowing, apathy, and ataxia. Later stages include global cognitive impairments, delay in verbal responses, a vacant stare–like affect, spastic paraparesis, hyperreflexia, psychosis, hallucinations, tremor, incontinence, seizures, mutism, and death. Confirming the diagnosis of HIV encephalopathy may be difficult. Extensive neurologic evaluation includes a computed tomography (CT) scan, which may indicate diffuse cerebral atrophy and ventricular enlargement. Other tests that may detect abnormalities include magnetic resonance imaging (MRI), analysis of CSF through lumbar puncture, and brain biopsy.

Cryptococcus neoformans. A fungal infection, *Cryptococcus neoformans* is the fourth most common opportunistic infection among patients with AIDS and the third most common infectious agent causing neurologic disease. Cryptococcal meningitis is characterized by symptoms such as fever, headache, malaise, stiff neck, nausea, vomiting, mental status changes, and seizures. Diagnosis is confirmed by CSF analysis.

Progressive Multifocal Leukoencephalopathy. Progressive multifocal leukoencephalopathy (PML) is a demyelinating central nervous system disorder caused by a J.C. virus (named for the patient whose cultures grew the virus) that infects the oligodendroglia. PML affects approximately 3% of AIDS patients. Clinical manifestations may begin with mental confusion and rapidly progress to include blindness, aphasia, paresis (slight paralysis), and death. Other common infections involving the nervous system include *Toxoplasma gondii*, CMV, and *M. tuberculosis*.

Other Neurologic Disorders. Other neurologic manifestations include both central and peripheral neuropathies. **Vascular myelopathy** is a degenerative disorder affecting lateral and posterior columns of the spinal cord, resulting in progressive spastic paraparesis, ataxia, and incontinence. **HIV-related peripheral neuropathy** is thought to be a demyelinating disorder associated with pain and numbness in the extremities, weakness, diminished deep tendon reflexes, orthostatic hypotension, and impotence.

Integumentary

Cutaneous manifestations are associated with HIV infection and the accompanying opportunistic infections and malignancies. KS is described on p. 1394. Opportunistic infections such as herpes zoster and herpes simplex are associated with painful vesicles that disrupt skin integrity. Molluscum contagiosum is a viral infection characterized by deforming plaque formation. Seborrheic dermatitis is associated with an indurated, diffuse, scaly rash involving the scalp and face. Patients with AIDS may also exhibit a generalized folliculitis associated with dry, flaking skin or atopic dermatitis such as eczema or psoriasis. Up to 60% of patients treated with trimethoprim-sulfamethoxazole (TMP/SMZ) for PCP develop a drug-related rash that is pruritic with pinkish red macules and papules. Regardless of the origin of these rashes, patients experience discomfort and are at increased risk for additional infection from disrupted skin integrity.

Clinical Manifestations Specific to Women

Persistent, recurrent vaginal **candidiasis** may be the first sign of HIV infection in women. Past or present genital ulcer disease is a risk factor for the transmission of HIV infection. Women with HIV infection are more susceptible to and have increased rates and recurrence of genital ulcer disease and venereal warts. Ulcerative sexually transmitted diseases (STDs) such as chancroid, syphilis, and herpes are more severe in these women. **Human papillomavirus (HPV)** causes venereal warts and is a risk factor for **cervical intraepithelial neoplasia** (CIN), a precursor to cervical cancer. It is now becoming increasingly clear that women with HIV are more than ten times as likely to develop CIN than those not infected with HIV. There is a strong association between abnormal Papanicolaou smears and HIV seropositivity. HIV-seropositive women with cervical carcinoma present with a more advanced stage of disease and have more persistent and recurrent disease and a shorter interval to recurrence and death than women who do not have HIV infection (Gibbs & Zeeman, 1993).

A significant percentage of women who require hospitalization for pelvic inflammatory disease (PID) have HIV infection. These women are at increased risk for PID, and the inflammation associated with PID may potentiate the transmission of HIV infection. Moreover, women with HIV appear to have a higher incidence of menstrual abnormalities, including amenorrhea or bleeding between periods, than women without HIV infection.

The failure of health care providers to consider HIV infection in women may lead to a later diagnosis, thereby denying women appropriate treatment. Disorders of the female reproductive system are discussed in Chapter 45.

Patient Education

Because HIV in women usually occurs during the childbearing years, family planning issues need to be addressed. Attempts to achieve pregnancy by couples in which one partner has HIV and one does not expose the unaffected partner to the virus. Although HIV transmission through artificial insemination with washed semen from an HIV-infected partner has been documented, preliminary results using processed semen have been encouraging. However, HIV has been found in the spermatozoa of patients with AIDS, and HIV may even replicate in the male germ cell. Women planning to become pregnant need to have adequate information about the risks of transmitting HIV infection to themselves, their partner, and their future children.

Gerontologic Considerations

More than 10% of all AIDS cases in the United States have occurred in persons age 50 or older. Of this percentage, 25% are age 60 or older. HIV infection in the elderly may be underreported and underdiagnosed because health care professionals erroneously believe that older persons are not at risk for HIV infection. Many older adults are sexually active but do not use condoms, viewing them only as a means of unneeded birth control and not considering themselves at risk for HIV infection. Sexual expression in the elderly population is not limited to heterosexual partners. Many older homosexual men who grew up and lived in an era when disclosure of their sexual orientation was not acceptable have lost long-time partners and may now turn to younger males for sexual gratification. Older adults may also be IV drug users or may have received HIV-infected blood via transfusions before 1985; as a result they may be at risk for HIV infection.

Normal age-related changes include a reduction in immune system function similar to that of HIV infection. Older adults are normally at greater risk for infections, cancer, and autoimmune disorders. Many older adults also experience the loss of loved ones, resulting in depression and bereavement, factors that are also associated with depressed immune function. HIV-related dementia in the older adult may imitate Alzheimer's disease and may be misdiagnosed. As with anyone at risk for HIV infection, the elderly patient needs educational programs that address HIV infection prevention.

HIV as a Chronic Illness

Earlier diagnosis and treatment of opportunistic infections and antiviral therapy are thought to be responsible for a dramatic improvement in survival of persons with AIDS since the early years of the epidemic; thus, HIV infection is now being described as a chronic disorder. Persons with chronic disability resulting from HIV infection frequently experience fatigue, decreased endurance, weight loss, edema, blindness, and swallowing difficulties leading to various degrees of functional impairment. Many persons with HIV infection experience neurologic involvement resulting in dementia, hemiplegia, spastic paraparesis, painful neuropathies, and proximal and distal muscle weakness. In addition to medical and nursing management, many persons with chronic HIV infection need the rehabilitation services of occupational, physical, and speech therapists.

Almost all AIDS patients develop at least one opportunistic infection during the course of their disease. Although many infections are successfully treated, some persons never fully recover and are at increased risk for a second infection or cancer. Treatment is often complicated by the debilitating signs and symptoms of HIV infection/AIDS, which include unexplained fatigue, headache, profuse night sweats, unexplained weight loss, dry cough, shortness of breath, extreme weakness, diarrhea, and persistent lymphadenopathy. Chronic illness develops when opportunistic diseases and the symptoms of HIV infection/AIDS do not resolve.

The effects of chronic illness—decreased energy, increased expenses, change in lifestyle, repeated and prolonged hospitalizations—can be devastating. Persons who progress to the terminal phases of HIV infection/AIDS are usually severely immunocompromised. Multiple local and disseminated infections involving several organ systems are common. Many persons become profoundly malnourished as a result of impaired oral intake, gastrointestinal malabsorption, and the effects of opportunistic diseases. Pulmonary, renal, and hepatic failure may develop as a result of infection or malignancy. Skin breakdown related to immobility, profuse diarrhea, and progression of KS is common. Neurologic impairments may progress to coma and eventually death.

Patients in the advanced stages of HIV infection/AIDS usually cannot work, maintain current roles or relationships, or care for themselves independently. Death occurs because there is no known effective treatment for the opportunistic diseases or the patient no longer responds to standard therapy.

Diagnostic Evaluation

Laboratory Tests

Since the discovery of HIV in 1983, scientists have learned much about its characteristics and pathogenicity. Based on this knowledge, diagnostic tests, some still investigational, have been developed. Laboratory tests are now used to diagnose HIV and to monitor disease progression and response to treatment in the HIV-infected person. Table 50-1 summarizes laboratory tests used to diagnose and track progression of HIV infection.

HIV Antibody Tests

When an individual is infected with HIV, the immune system responds by producing antibodies against the virus. Antibodies generally develop within 3 to 12 weeks of exposure but may take as long as 6 to 14 months, which explains why a person may be infected but may not test positive initially. Unfortunately, the antibodies for HIV are ineffective and cannot halt the development of HIV infection. The ability to document HIV antibodies in the blood has permitted screening of blood products and has facilitated diagnostic evaluations of individuals with HIV infection. In 1985, the Food and Drug Administration (FDA) licensed an HIV antibody assay for all blood and plasma donations.

Three tests are used to confirm the presence of antibody to HIV and to assist in diagnosing HIV infection. The **enzyme-linked immunosorbent assay (ELISA)** test identifies antibodies directed specifically against HIV. The ELISA test does not establish a diagnosis of AIDS but rather indicates that the individual has been exposed to or infected with HIV. Persons whose blood contains antibodies for HIV are said to be **seropositive.** The **Western blot assay** is another test that can identify HIV antibodies and is used to confirm seropositivity as identified by the ELISA procedure. **Indirect immunofluorescence assay (IFA)** is now being used by some physicians instead of the Western blot to confirm seropositivity. Another test, the **radioimmunoprecipitation assay (RIPA),** detects HIV protein rather than antibody.

Implications of Testing for Nurses

Before any HIV test is performed, the meaning of the test and possible test results are explained, and informed consent for the test is obtained from the patient. The results of the HIV antibody testing are carefully explained to the patient. All test results are kept confidential. The implications of antibody test results are summarized in Chart 50-1. Education and counseling about the test results and disease transmission are essential whenever HIV antibody testing is performed.

Patients who test seronegative may develop a false sense of security, which may result in continued high-risk

TABLE 50-1 Selected Laboratory Tests for Diagnosing and Tracking HIV and Assessing Immune Status

Test	Findings in HIV Infection
HIV Antibody Tests	
ELISA	• Positive test result confirmed by Western blot
Western blot	• Positive
Indirect immunofluorescence assay (IFA)	• Positive test result confirmed by Western blot
Radioimmunoprecipitation assay (RIPA)	• Positive, more sensitive and specific than Western blot
HIV Tracking	
p24 antigen	• Positive for free viral protein
Polymerase chain reaction (PCR)	• Detection of HIV RNA or DNA
Peripheral blood mononuclear cell (PBMC) culture for HIV-1	• Positive when two consecutive assays detect reverse transcriptase or p24 antigen in increasing magnitude
Quantitative cell culture	• Measures viral load within cells
Quantitative plasma culture	• Measures viral load via free infectious virus in the plasma
B2 microglobulin	• Protein is increased with disease progression.
Serum neopterin	• Increased levels seen with disease progression.
Immune Status	
#CD4+ cells	• Decreased
%CD4+ cells	• Decreased
CD4:CD8 ratio	• Decreased ratio of CD4:CD8
WBC count	• Normal to decreased
Immunoglobulin levels	• Increased
CD4 cell function tests	• T4 cells have decreased ability to respond to antigen
Skin test sensitivity reaction	• Decreased to absent

behaviors or feelings that they are immune to the virus. They may need ongoing counseling to help them modify high-risk behaviors and to return for repeated testing. Other patients may experience anxiety regarding the uncertainty of their status.

Patients' psychologic responses to seropositive test results may include feelings of panic, depression, and hopelessness. The social and interpersonal consequences of a positive test result can be devastating. Individuals may lose their sexual partners or their health insurance because of disclosure; they may experience discrimination in employment and housing, as well as social ostracism. Patients who test positive may need ongoing counseling as well as referrals for social, financial, medical, and psychologic support services.

HIV Tracking

Direct determination of HIV presence and activity is used to track the progression of the disease as well as response to treatment. The viral core protein is referred to as p24. The **p24 antigen capture assay** is highly specific for HIV-1. However, the levels of p24 in asymptomatic HIV-infected persons are very low. Persons with measurable titers of p24 progress to AIDS much sooner. The p24 antigen capture assay has been used along with other tests, such as the CD4+, to evaluate the treatment effects of antiviral agents. It is being replaced in clinical drug trials by a process known as the **polymerase chain reaction (PCR).** The PCR, also called gene amplification, is used to detect HIV RNA or proviral DNA. One disadvantage is that false-positive test results can occur if the reagents used in the test are contaminated. Currently PCR is being used to detect HIV in high-risk HIV seronegative persons before the development of antibodies, to confirm a positive ELISA, to monitor viral burden over time, to screen neonates, and to determine the exact strain of virus that is present. **HIV culture** or **quantitative plasma culture** and **plasma viremia** are additional tests that measure viral burden.

Other tests may be performed to monitor immune status or to monitor the progression of HIV disease (see Table 50-1).

AIDS Diagnosis

The manifestations of HIV infection vary. Diagnosis is based on clinical history, identification of risk factors, physical examination, laboratory evidence of immune dysfunction, identification of HIV antibodies, signs and symptoms, and infections and/or malignancies included in the CDC classification system for HIV infection. This classification system

CHART 50-1
Patient Education: Interpretation of HIV Test Results

HIV antibody is produced in response to HIV infection. Because seropositivity does not diagnose or confirm AIDS or project future illness, HIV test results must be interpreted cautiously. Some considerations for patients follow.

Interpretation of Positive Test Results

- Antibodies to the AIDS virus are present in your blood.
- You have been infected with the AIDS virus and your body has produced antibodies.
- You probably have active HIV in your body and should assume that you can pass the virus to others.
- You do not necessarily have AIDS.
- You may not necessarily get AIDS in the future.
- You are not immune to AIDS.

Interpretation of Negative Test Results

- Antibodies to the AIDS virus are not present in your blood at this time, which can mean that you have not been infected with HIV or if you have been infected, your body has not produced antibodies (which takes from 3 weeks to 6 months or longer).
- Continue to take precautions. The test result does not mean you are immune to the virus, nor does it mean that you are not infected (it just means that your body may not have produced antibodies yet).

categorizes HIV infection and AIDS in adults and adolescents on the basis of clinical conditions associated with HIV infection and CD4+ T-cell counts. The revised classification system is presented in Table 50-2.

The expanded AIDS surveillance case definition has led to the identification and earlier diagnosis of more persons with AIDS. The clinical conditions are grouped into three categories listing clinical conditions for each category. The CD4+ T-cell counts cover three ranges, which guide clinical and therapeutic management of HIV-infected persons. Although the revised classification emphazises CD4+ T-cell counts, it allows for CD4+ percentages (percentage of CD4+ T cells of total lymphocytes). The CD4+ percentage is less subject to variation on repeated measurements than is the absolute CD4+ T-cell count; however, data correlating the natural history of HIV infection with the CD4+ percentage have not been as consistently available as data on absolute CD4+ T-cell counts.

Clinical Categories

Clinical **Category A** consists of one or more listed conditions without any of the conditions listed in Categories B or C. **Category B** consists of symptomatic conditions in HIV-infected persons that are not included in the conditions listed in Category C. These conditions must also meet one of the following criteria: (1) the condition is due to HIV infection or a defect in cellular immunity; and (2) the condition must be considered to have a clinical course or require management that is complicated by HIV infection. If an individual was once treated for a Category B condition and has not developed a Category C disease but is now asymptomatic, that person's illness would be considered Category B. **Category C** includes clinical conditions listed in the AIDS surveillance case definition. Once a person has had a Category C condition, the person will remain in Category C. A listing of the CD4+ T-cell ranges and clinical conditions for categories A, B, and C are presented in Table 50-2. This current system, although more inclusive of clinical conditions experienced by persons with HIV infection, does not include recurrent and persistent vaginal candida (yeast) infections frequently seen in women with HIV infection.

Management

Medical management includes several approaches, including treatment of HIV-associated infections and malignancies, arresting HIV replication through antiviral agents, and augmentation and restoration of the immune system through the use of immunomodulators. Supportive care is important because of the debilitating effects of HIV infection and AIDS, including malnutrition, skin breakdown, weakness, immobility, and altered mental status.

Medications for HIV-Related Infections

General Infections. **Trimethoprim-sulfamethoxazole,** called TMP-SMZ (Bactrim, Septra), is an antibacterial agent for treating various organisms causing infection. AIDS patients who are treated with TMP-SMZ experience an unusually high incidence of adverse effects, such as fevers, rashes, leukopenia, thrombocytopenia, and renal dysfunction. Recently, desensitization for TMP-SMZ drug-related reactions has been successful.

Pneumocystis carinii *Pneumonia.* In the last several years, there have been many advances in the treatment of PCP. The drug of choice for PCP in patients with AIDS as well as immunocompromised patients without HIV infection, TMP-SMZ is available in both IV as well as oral preparations. There is no advantage to IV administration for patients who have normal gastrointestinal function.

Pentamidine, an antiprotozoal medication, is used as an alternative agent for combating PCP. If adverse effects develop or if patients do not improve clinically when treated with TMP-SMZ, the health care provider may recommend pentamidine. Intramuscular administration is avoided because of the potential for painful sterile abscess formation. IV pentamidine may cause severe hypotension if it is administered too rapidly. Adverse effects of pentamidine also include impaired glucose metabolism (with frank diabetes mellitus), renal damage, hepatic dysfunction, and neutropenia. The initial success of aerosolized pentamidine (AP) led to its use as a treatment for mild to moderate PCP; however, it has proved to be less effective and more costly than TMP-SMZ, and early relapses are common. Because of these limitations, the inhalant form of pentamidine is usually reserved for patients with mild to moderate PCP who are intolerant to other treatments. The combination of TMP-SMZ and pen-

TABLE 50-2 Classification System for HIV Infection and Expanded AIDS Surveillance Case Definition for Adolescents and Adults

Diagnostic Categories: CD4+ T-cell categories	Clinical Categories: A Asymptomatic, acute (primary) HIV or PGL	B Symptomatic, not (A) or (C) conditions	C AIDS-indicator conditions
(1) ≥500/μL	A1	B1	C1
(2) 200–499/μL	A2	B2	C2
(3) <200/μL AIDS-indicator T-cell count	A3	B3	C3

As of January 1, 1993, persons with AIDS-indicator conditions (clinical category C) and those in categories A3 or B3 were considered to have AIDS.

Clinical Category A

Includes one or more of the following in an adult or adolescent with confirmed HIV infection and without conditions in clinical categories B and C:

- Asymptomatic HIV infection
- Persistent generalized lymphadenopathy (PGL)
- Acute (primary) HIV infection with accompanying illness or history of acute HIV infection

Clinical Category B

Examples of conditions in clinical Category B include, but are not limited to:

- Bacillary angiomatosis
- Candidiasis, oropharyngeal (thrush), or vulvovaginal (persistent, frequent, or poorly responsive to therapy)
- Cervical dysplasia (moderate or severe)/cervical carcinoma *in situ*
- Constitutional symptoms, such as fever (38.5°C) or diarrhea exceeding 1 month in duration
- Hairy leukoplakia, oral
- Herpes zoster (shingles), involving at least two distinct episodes or more than one dermatome
- Idiopathic thrombocytopenic purpura
- Listeriosis
- Pelvic inflammatory disease, particularly if complicated by tubo-ovarian abscess
- Peripheral neuropathy

Clinical Category C

Examples of conditions in adults and adolescents include:

- Candidiasis of bronchi, trachea, or lungs; esophagus
- Cervical cancer, invasive
- Coccidioidomycosis, disseminated or extrapulmonary
- Cryptococcosis, extrapulmonary
- Cryptosporidiosis, chronic intestinal (exceeding 1 month's duration)
- Cytomegalovirus disease (other than liver, spleen, or lymph nodes)
- Cytomegalovirus retinitis (with loss of vision)
- Encephalopathy, HIV-related
- Herpes simplex: chronic ulcer(s) (exceeding 1 month's duration); or bronchitis, pneumonitis, or esophagitis
- Histoplasmosis, disseminated or extrapulmonary
- Isosporiasis, chronic intestinal (exceeding 1 month's duration)
- Kaposi's sarcoma
- Lymphoma, Burkitt's (or equivalent term); immunoblastic (or equivalent term); primary, of brain
- *Mycobacterium-avium* complex or *M. kansasii*, disseminated or extrapulmonary
- *Mycobacterium tuberculosis*, any site (pulmonary or extrapulmonary)
- *Mycobacterium*, other species or unidentified species, disseminated or extrapulmonary
- *Pneumocystis carinii* pneumonia
- Pneumonia, recurrent
- Progressive multifocal leukoencephalopathy
- *Salmonella* septicemia, recurrent
- Toxoplasmosis of brain
- Wasting syndrome due to HIV

(Adapted from Centers for Disease Control, U.S. Department of Health and Human Services. 1993 revised classification system for HIV infection and expanded surveillance case definition for AIDS among adolescents and adults. MMWR 1992; 41(RR 17):1–19.)

tamidine has shown no additional benefit and is avoided because of the cumulative toxic effects that may result.

The combination of oral **trimethoprim** (Proloprim, Trimpex) and **dapsone** (Avlosulfon, DDS) has proved highly effective for mild to moderate PCP. Other medications being evaluated as rescue therapy for patients who fail to improve or respond to conventional therapy include IV **clindamycin** (Cleosin HCl), oral **primaquine, trimetrexate, hydroxynapthoquinone**, and **atovaquone** (Mepron). Some patients with moderate to severe PCP benefit from systemic corticosteroids; however, there are no data to justify the use of corticosteroids for mild PCP or rescue therapy.

Mycobacterium avium *Complex*. Treatment for MAC infections has not been clearly established and involves multidrug regimens administered over a prolonged period. Combination therapy with **ethambutal, rifampin, clofazimine** (Lamprene), and **ciprofloxacin** (Cipro) with or without **amikacin** has been associated with drug toxicity, no bacterial cure, and poor prognosis. **Clarithromycin** (Biaxin) and **azithromycin** (Zithromax), newer antibiotics used in multidrug regimens, are being evaluated for effectiveness in treating MAC. Rifabutin has been shown to be effective in preventing MAC in persons with HIV infection who have CD4+ cell counts of 200/mm^2 or lower.

Meningitis. Current primary therapy for cryptococcal meningitis is IV **amphotericin B** with or without oral **flucytosine** or **fluconozole** (Diflucan). The patient is monitored for serious potential adverse effects of amphotericin B, including anaphylaxis, renal and hepatic impairment, electrolyte imbalances, anemia, fevers, and rigors. Intrathecal administration of amphoteracin B has been used in place of or in combination with IV administration in patients who have failed to respond to the latter. Until fluconazole, a new antifungal agent, was approved and used for lifelong suppressive therapy, frequent relapses and high mortality rates often necessitated prolonged therapy with IV amphotericin B. In some instances, the patient continues to receive IV amphotericin in the home setting. Oral fluconazole is used as suppressive therapy when the CSF is negative for the organism. This medication is less toxic and better tolerated than amphotericin B.

Cytomegalovirus Retinitis. Retinitis caused by cytomegalovirus (CMV) is a leading cause of blindness in individuals with AIDS. In 1989, the FDA approved the use of **ganciclovir** for treating CMV retinitis. Because ganciclovir does not kill the virus but rather controls its growth, it must be given for the remainder of the patient's life. Discontinuation of the medication is associated with the relapse of retinitis within 1 month. Initially, ganciclovir is given IV every 8 to 12 hours for 2 to 3 weeks. Maintenance therapy is given once a day for 5 to 7 days each week. In some patients, CMV retinitis progresses despite treatment. Adverse effects that necessitate patient teaching and outpatient monitoring include bone marrow suppression (producing a decrease in white blood cell and platelet counts), oral candidiasis, and liver and renal impairments.

Long-term venous access is established and the patient and caregiver are taught the technique for home administration of ganciclovir. A common adverse reaction to ganciclovir is severe neutropenia, which limits the concomitant use of **zidovudine** (ZDV, AZT). For patients who cannot tolerate systemic ganciclovir because of severe neutropenia, infection at the venous access site, or the need to take zidovudine, intravitreal injections of ganciclovir have been effective.

Foscarnet (Foscavir), another agent used to treat CMV retinitis, is administered intravenously every 8 hours for 2 to 3 weeks. Maintenance therapy is given over 2 to 3 hours five times a week. This agent can be given with zidovudine. Common adverse reactions to foscarnet are nephrotoxicity, including acute renal failure, and electrolyte imbalances, including hypocalcemia, hyperphosphatemia, and hypomagnesemia; these can be life threatening. Other common adverse effects include seizures, gastrointestinal disturbances, anemia, phlebitis at the infusion site, and low back pain. Other medications being evaluated for the treatment of CMV retinitis include **acyclovir** (Zovirax), **alpha-interferon,** and combination therapy with ganciclovir (Cytovene) and **immune globulin.**

Other Conditions. Acyclovir and foscarnate are being used to treat encephalitis caused by herpes simplex or herpes zoster. **Pyrimethamine** (Daraprim) and **sulfadiazine** or **clindamycin** (Cleosin HCl) are used both for treatment and for lifelong suppressive therapy for *Toxoplasmosis gondii.* Esophageal or oral candidiasis is treated topically with **clotrimazole** (Mycelex) oral troches or **nystatin** suspension. Chronic refractory infection with candidiasis (thrush) or esophageal involvement is treated with **ketoconazole** or **fluconazole.**

Management of Chronic Diarrhea

Although many forms of infectious diarrhea respond to treatment, it is not unusual for the infections to recur and become a chronic problem. Therapy with **octreotide acetate** (Sandostatin), a synthetic analogue of somatostatin, has been shown to be effective in managing chronic severe diarrhea. High concentrations of somatostatin receptors have been found in the gastrointestinal tract as well as other tissues. Somatostatin inhibits many physiologic functions, including gastrointestinal motility and intestinal secretion of water and electrolytes.

Management of Wasting Syndrome

Management of wasting syndrome includes treating the underlying causes of both systemic and gastrointestinal tract opportunistic infections. Malnutrition itself increases the risk of infection and may also increase the incidence of opportunistic infections. Nutrition therapy should be integrated into the overall management plan and should be tailored to meet the nutritional needs of the patient, from oral diet to enteral tube feedings through parenteral nutritional support if needed. As with all patients, a balanced diet is essential for the person with HIV infection. Calorie counts should be obtained for all AIDS patients with unexplained weight loss to evaluate nutritional status and to initiate appropriate therapy. The goal is to maintain the patient's ideal weight and, when necessary, to increase weight. The following guidelines are useful for calculating needed calories and protein intake (Hoyt & Staats, 1991):

- Calories: 35 to 44 kilocalories/kilogram of body weight/day
- Protein: 2 to 2.5 grams of protein/kilogram of body weight/day

Oral supplements may be used to supplement diets deficient in calories and protein. Ideally, oral supplements should be lactose free (many persons with HIV infection are lactose intolerant), high in calories and easily digestable protein, low in fat with the fat easily digestable, palatable, inexpensive, and tolerated without causing diarrhea. **Advera** is a nutritional supplement that has been developed specifically for persons with HIV infection and AIDS. Parenteral nutrition is the final option because of the costs and associated risks, including infections.

Appetite stimulants have been successfully used in patients with AIDS-related anorexia. **Megestrol acetate** (Megace), a synthetic oral progesterone preparation used to treat breast cancer, promotes significant weight gain and inhibits cytokine IL-1 synthesis. It has been used in patients with HIV infection; it increases body weight primarily by increasing body fat stores. **Dronabinol** (Marinol) is synthetic **tetrahydrocannabinol** (THC), which is the active ingredient in marijuana. It has been used to relieve nausea and vomiting associated with cancer chemotherapy. Preliminary results show that after beginning Marinol therapy, almost all patients with HIV infection experience a modest weight gain (Gorter, 1991; Medynski, 1993). The effects on body composition are unknown.

Treatment of Malignancies

Management of KS is usually difficult because of the variability of symptoms and the organ systems involved. KS is rarely life threatening except when there is pulmonary or gastrointestinal involvement. The treatment goal is reduction of symptoms by decreasing the size of the skin lesions, reducing discomfort associated with edema and ulcerations, and controlling symptoms associated with mucosal or visceral involvement. No one systemic treatment has been shown to increase survival. Localized treatment includes surgical excision of the lesions or application of liquid nitrogen to local skin lesions and injections of intraoral lesions with dilute **vinblastine.** Injection of intraoral lesions has been associated with local pain and skin irritation. To date the most effective chemotherapy regimen appears to be **ABV (adriamycin, bleomycin**, and **vincristine).** Significant myelosupression occurs in 40% to 50% of patients on this regimen, with a 30% increase in the incidence of opportunistic infections. Radiation therapy is effective as a palliative measure to relieve localized pain due to tumor mass (especially in the legs) or for KS lesions that are disfiguring or anatomically inconvenient.

Alpha-interferon for Kaposi's Sarcoma. Interferon is known for its antiviral and antitumor effects. Patients treated with alpha-interferon for cutaneous KS have experienced tumor regression and improved immune system function. Positive responses have been observed in 30% to 50% of patients, with the best responses seen in those with limited disease and no opportunistic infections. Alpha-interferon is administered by either the intravenous, intramuscular, or subcutaneous route. Patients may self-administer interferon at home or receive it in an outpatient setting. Teaching about its correct administration and management of adverse effects is provided by the nurse.

Lymphomas. The success of treatment of AIDS-related lymphomas has been limited because of the rapid progression of these malignancies. Combination chemotherapy and radiation therapy regimens have achieved approximately a 50% response rate with markedly short durations. Because standard regimens for non-AIDS lymphomas have been ineffective, many clinicians suggest that AIDS-related lymphomas be studied as a separate group in clinical trials.

Antiretroviral Therapy

Currently four antiretroviral agents are approved by the FDA for treating HIV infection: **zidovudine** (ZDV; formerly called azidothymidine [AZT] or Retrovir), **dideoxyinosine** or **didanosine** (ddI [Videx]), **dideoxycytidine** (ddC [Hivid]), and **stavudine** (d4T, Zerit). These medications inhibit viral reverse transcriptase and prevent reproduction of HIV by mimicking one of the molecular substances used by HIV to build DNA for new virus particles. By altering the structural components of the DNA chain, new virus production is inhibited.

Zidovudine. The discovery of zidovudine has been significant in the fight against AIDS. In 1987, the FDA approved zidovudine for severe HIV infection/AIDS. In 1990, zidovudine was approved for use earlier in the course of infection before profound immunosuppression occurs. In 1994, it was approved for use in pregnant women who are HIV positive to reduce the risk of perinatal transmission of the infection.

Measurement of the CD4+ count is an important parameter used to determine the level of immunosuppression. The CD4+ count reflects the number of circulating helper T-cell lymphocytes. Normal CD4+ counts range from 700 to 1200/mm^3. Currently, therapy with zidovudine has been approved for all HIV-infected persons whose CD4+ counts are below 500/mm^3. Studies show that zidovudine delays progression to AIDS or symptomatic disease in persons who are HIV positive without symptoms but with CD4+ cell counts below 500 mm^3 (Volberding et al, 1990) or in those with mild symptoms and CD4+ cell counts below 200 mm^3 (Fischl et al, 1990). Zidovudine decreases p24 antigen and increases T4 cell counts.

Zidovudine can be quite toxic to the bone marrow, producing dose-limiting anemia and neutropenia that may require the drug to be discontinued. Zidovudine may need to be discontinued if the patient requires treatment for opportunistic infections, lymphomas, and other malignancies because the treatments for these conditions may also cause hematologic toxicity. Granulocyte colony-stimulating factor (G-CSF) and epoetin alpha (human recombinant erythropoietin [Epogen, Procrit]) have proved effective in treating anemia and neutropenia associated with using zidovudine. Colony-stimulating factors are substances naturally produced by the body to stimulate growth and production of both red and white blood cells.

Other adverse effects of zidovudine include nausea, abdominal discomfort, fevers, chills, myalgias, and headache; less common adverse effects include confusion, somnolence, and seizures. Patient teaching about the importance of regular medical examinations and the assessment and management of adverse effects is indicated. Referrals for financial counseling are often needed because of the high cost of the medication.

Dideoxyinosine. For many patients, dideoxyinosine (didanosine [ddI]) has had promising results as an alternative to zidovudine. The major dose-limiting toxicities associated with ddI are pancreatitis, which can be fatal, and peripheral neuropathy. Other toxicities include diarrhea, restlessness, and increased serum uric acid levels (when ddI is given in high doses).

Dideoxycytidine. Dideoxycytidine (ddC) does not penetrate the spinal fluid so is not as effective as zidovudine in treating AIDS-related encephalopathy. Severe peripheral neuropathy has been noted with treatment with high doses. Other toxicities include gastrointestinal intolerance and mucosal ulcerations. Because the HIV virus mutates rapidly, drug resistance occurs; therefore, combination antiviral therapy may offer the best hope for controlling HIV infection.

Stavudine. Stavudine may be prescribed for patients with advanced HIV infection who are unresponsive to other antiviral agents or who cannot tolerate their side effects. Major adverse reactions include peripheral neuropathy, suppression of bone marrow, myalgia, and hepatotoxicity. Peripheral neuropathy is the major dose-limiting side effect; patients are instructed to report the occurrence of pain, burning, aching, weakness, or other changes in sensation.

Protease Inhibitors

Protease inhibitors (PI) are medications that inhibit the function of protease, an enzyme needed for HIV replication and the production of infectious virions. Inhibition of HIV-1 protease results in noninfectious virus particles with reduced reverse transcriptase activity. Because these agents inhibit virus replication in a different way than reverse transcriptase inhibitors such as zidovudine, they show promise when used with reverse transcriptase inhibitors. L-524 and RO 31-8959 are two investigational protease inhibitors. Side effects include headache and gastrointestinal upset.

Some medications interfere with the HIV affinity for T4 lymphocytes. Others alter the viral membrane and prevent the virus from entering host cells. Inhibition of viral reproduction is another mechanism of action. Most of the agents are in various phases of clinical trials in which they are being evaluated for toxicity and maximal tolerated doses (phase I clinical trial), activity against HIV (phase II), and effectiveness as compared with other drugs (phase III). For a listing of antiretroviral agents, see Table 50-3.

Immunomodulators

Combating AIDS requires not only agents that will inhibit viral growth but also agents that will restore or augment the damaged immune system. Low-dose oral alpha-interferon (IFN-alfa) is being studied for its antiviral properties as well as its ability to stimulate macrophages and T-cell lymphocytes. As discussed earlier in this chapter, parenteral alpha-interferon is also being used to treat cutaneous KS. Other substances being evaluated for their role in macrophage and lymphocyte stimulation include interleukin 2, isoprinosine, diethyldithiocarbamate (DTC), lentinan, and granulocyte macrophage colony-stimulating factor (G-CSF). As discussed earlier, G-CSF along with erythropoietin is being used to reverse anemia and neutropenia caused by zidovudine therapy.

Many of these substances cause a flulike reaction including fevers, chills, arthralgias, myalgias, and headache. In addition, some agents cause nausea, vomiting, elevated liver enzymes, neutropenia, confusion, and behavioral changes. The nurse plays an important role in this treatment modality by participating in assessment and management of adverse effects, providing patients with appropriate support and education, and participating in collection of data for clinical trials.

Vaccines

A vaccine is a substance that triggers the production of antibodies in an effort to destroy the offending organism. Researchers have been working to develop a vaccine for HIV since the virus was discovered. Several vaccine trials are under way in seronegative human volunteers. Because of the complex nature and behavior of HIV, most scientists agree that a vaccine for HIV will not be available for many years. In the absence of guidelines for developing long-term protection from HIV infection, it is unknown which type of immune response (*i.e.*, neutralizing antibodies, cytotoxic T lymphocytes, or both) is necessary for full protection. Another issue to be considered in developing and testing a vaccine is identification of an appropriate study population. For example, it may be difficult to determine whether a decline in infection rate in male homosexuals results from a vaccine or from a change in sexual practices as a result of massive educational efforts. Studying IV drug users for several years in vaccine trials is likely to be difficult because these individuals often have unstable home situations and are involved in illicit activities. Finally, several legal and ethical concerns are likely, including liability of vaccine manufactures, potential development of seropositivity or AIDS in the test subjects, and emergence of serious adverse effects.

TABLE 50-3 Antiviral Agents

Medication	Side Effects
Nucleoside Analogs–Reverse Transcriptase Inhibitors	
Zidovudine (ZDV) (Retrovir) (Formerly called AZT)	Anemia, granulocytopenia, nausea, GI discomfort, headache, confusion, hepatitis, nail discoloration, seizures, myositis, fevers, chills
Didanosine (ddI) (Videx)	Pancreatitis, peripheral neuropathy, nausea, diarrhea, confusion, seizures, headaches, electrolyte abnormalities, cardiac dysrhythmias
Zalcitabine, dideoxycytidine (ddC) (HIVID)	Esophageal ulcers, peripheral neuropathy, stomatitis, pancreatitis, fever, rash, oral aphthous ulcers, hyperglycemia
Stavudine (d_4T) (Zerit)	Peripheral neuropathy, headaches, hepatotoxicity, anemia, nausea
Non-nucleoside Reverse Transcriptase Inhibitors	
Foscarnet (Foscavir)	Increased thirst, nausea, anorexia, headaches, flank pain, muscle twitching, renal failure, elevated creatinine, mild proteinuria, tremors, seizures, genital ulcers
Nevirapine	Rash, fever, thrombocytopenia
Protease Inhibitors	
L-drug (L524) and R031-8985	Headache, GI upset

Supportive Care

Persons who become weak and debilitated as a result of chronic illness associated with HIV infection typically require many kinds of supportive care. Nutritional support may be as simple as providing assistance for obtaining or preparing meals. For persons with more advanced nutritional impairment that results from decreased intake, wasting syndrome, or gastrointestinal malabsorption associated with diarrhea, parenteral feedings such as total parenteral nutrition may be required. Imbalances that result from nausea, vomiting, and profuse diarrhea often necessitate intravenous fluid and electrolyte replacement. Skin breakdown associated with KS, perianal skin excoriation, and immobility is managed with thorough and meticulous skin care involving regular turning, cleansing, and applying medicated ointments and dressings.

Pulmonary symptoms such as dyspnea and shortness of breath may be related to infection, KS, or fatigue. For these patients, oxygen therapy, relaxation training, and energy conservation techniques may be helpful. Patients with severe respiratory dysfunction may require mechanical ventilation. Pain associated with skin breakdown, abdominal cramping, peripheral neuropathy, or KS is managed by analgesics given at regular intervals around the clock. Relaxation and guided imagery may be helpful in reducing pain and anxiety in some patients.

Alternative Therapies

Traditional Western medicine focuses on the treatment of disease. These treatments or interventions are taught in medical schools and are used by physicians in the care of patients. Alternative therapies are viewed as unconventional and unorthodox treatments or interventions not traditionally taught in medical schools. Alternative therapy stresses the need to treat the whole person and recognizes the interaction of the body, mind, and spirit. What is considered to be an alternative therapy in one culture may actually be a traditional therapy in another. The use of alternative therapy in HIV infection and AIDS has resulted from disillusionment with standard medical treatment, which to date has provided no cure. Used with traditional therapies, alternative therapies may improve the patient's overall wellbeing.

Alternative therapies can be divided into four categories. (1) **Spiritual or psychologic** therapies may include humor, hypnosis, faith healing, guided imagery, and positive affirmations. (2) **Nutritional** therapies may include vegetarian or macrobiotic diets, vitamin C or beta-carotene supplements, and turmeric, which contains curcumin, a food spice supplement. Chinese herbs such as traditional herbal mixtures as well as compound Q (a Chinese cucumber extract) and Monmordica charantia (bitter melon), which is given as an enema, are also used. (3) **Drug and biologic** therapies include medicines not approved by the FDA. Examples of these include N-acetylcysteine (NAC), pentoxifylline (Trental), and 1-chloro-2, 4-dinitrobenzene (DNCB). Also included in this category are oxygen therapy, ozone therapy, and urine therapy. (4) Treatment with **physical forces** and **devices** may include acupuncture, accupressure, massage therapy, reflexology, therapeutic touch, yoga, and crystals.

Many patients who use these alternative therapies do not always report their use to their health care providers. To obtain a complete health history, the nurse should ask questions about using alternative therapies. Patients may need to be encouraged to report their use to their primary health care provider. Problems may arise when patients are using alternative therapies while they are participating in clinical drug trials. They may have significant adverse side effects, making it difficult to assess the effects of the medications in the clinical trial. The nurse needs to become familiar with the potential adverse side effects of alternative therapies. The nurse who suspects that the alternative therapy is causing a side effect needs to discuss this with the patient, the alternative therapy provider, and the primary health care provider. It is very important for the nurse to view alternative therapies with an open mind and to try to understand the importance of this treatment to the patient. Doing so will improve communication with the patient and reduce conflict so that all involved in care can meet the patient's needs.

❑ *NURSING PROCESS*
The Patient With AIDS

The nursing care of persons with AIDS is challenging because of the potential for any organ system to be the target of infections or cancers. In addition, this disease is complicated by many emotional, social, and ethical issues. The plan of care for the patient with AIDS is individualized to meet the needs of the patient.

Assessment

Nursing assessment includes identification of potential risk factors, including a history of risky sexual practices and IV drug use. The patient's physical status and psychologic status are assessed. All factors affecting immune system functioning are thoroughly explored.

Nutritional status is assessed by obtaining a dietary history and identifying factors that may interfere with oral intake, such as anorexia, nausea, vomiting, oral pain, or difficulty swallowing. In addition, the patient's ability to purchase and prepare food is assessed. Weight, anthropometric measurements, and blood urea nitrogen (BUN), serum protein, albumin, and transferrin levels provide objective measurements of nutritional status.

The **skin and mucous membranes** are inspected daily for evidence of breakdown, ulceration, or infection. The oral cavity is monitored for redness, ulcerations, and the presence of white creamy patches indicative of candidiasis. It is especially important to assess the perianal area for excoriation and infection in those patients with profuse diarrhea. Wound cultures are ordered to identify infectious organisms.

Respiratory status is assessed by monitoring the patient for cough, sputum production, shortness of breath, orthopnea, tachypnea, and chest pain. The presence and quality of breath sounds are also investigated. Other measures of pulmonary function include chest x-ray findings, arterial blood gas values, and pulmonary function test results.

Neurologic status is determined by assessing the patient's level of consciousness, orientation to person, place, and time, and the occurrence of memory lapses. The patient is also assessed for sensory deficits (visual changes, headache, numbness and tingling in the extremities) and motor involvement (altered gait, paresis, or paralysis) and seizure activity.

Fluid and electrolyte status is assessed by examining the skin and mucous membranes for turgor and dryness. Increased thirst, decreased urine output, low blood pressure or a decrease in systolic blood pressure between 10 and 15 mm Hg with a concurrent rise in pulse rate when the patient sits up, weak and rapid pulse, and urine specific gravity of 1.025 or more may indicate dehydration. Electrolyte imbalances such as decreased serum sodium, potassium, calcium, magnesium, and chloride typically result from profuse diarrhea. The patient is assessed for signs and symptoms of electrolyte depletion; these may include decreased mental status, muscle twitching, muscle cramps, irregular pulse, nausea and vomiting, and shallow respirations.

The patient's **level of knowledge** about the disease and the means of disease transmission is evaluated. In addition, the level of knowledge of family and friends is assessed. The patient's psychologic reaction to the AIDS diagnosis is important to explore. Reactions vary among individuals and may include denial, anger, fear, shame, withdrawal from social interactions, and depression. It is often helpful to gain an understanding of how the patient has dealt with illness and major life stress in the past. The patient's resources for support are also identified.

Diagnosis

Nursing Diagnoses

The list of potential nursing diagnoses is extensive because of the complex nature of this disease. However, based on assessment data, major nursing diagnoses for the patient may include the following:

- Impaired skin integrity related to cutaneous manifestations of HIV infection, excoriation, and diarrhea
- Diarrhea related to enteric pathogens and/or HIV infection
- Risk for infection related to immunodeficiency
- Activity intolerance related to weakness, fatigue, malnutrition, impaired fluid and electrolyte balance, and hypoxia associated with pulmonary infections
- Altered thought processes related to shortened attention span, impaired memory, confusion, and disorientation associated with HIV encephalopathy
- Ineffective airway clearance related to *Pneumocystis carinii* pneumonia (PCP), increased bronchial secretions, and decreased ability to cough related to weakness and fatigue
- Pain related to impaired perianal skin integrity secondary to diarrhea, Kaposi's sarcoma, and peripheral neuropathy
- Altered nutrition: Less than body requirements, related to decreased oral intake
- Social isolation related to stigma of the disease, withdrawal of support systems, isolation procedures, and fear of infecting others
- Anticipatory grieving related to changes in life-style and roles and to unfavorable prognosis
- Knowledge deficit related to means of preventing HIV transmission and self-care

Collaborative Problems/ Potential Complications

Based on the assessment data, possible complications may include

- Opportunistic infections
- Impaired breathing or respiratory failure
- Wasting syndrome and fluid and electrolyte imbalance
- Adverse reaction to medications

Planning and Implementation

Goals. Goals for the patient may include achievement and maintenance of skin integrity, resumption of usual bowel habits, absence of infection, improved activity tolerance, improved thought processes, improved airway clearance, increased comfort, improved nutritional status, increased socialization, expression of grief, increased knowledge regarding disease prevention and self-care, and absence of complications.

Nursing Interventions

Promoting Skin Integrity. Skin and oral mucosa are assessed routinely for changes in appearance, location and size of lesions, and evidence of infection and breakdown. The patient is encouraged to maintain a balance between rest and mobility whenever possible. Patients who are immobile are assisted to change position every 2 hours. Devices such as alternating-pressure mattresses and low- and high-air loss beds are used to prevent skin breakdown. Patients are encouraged to avoid scratching, to use nonabrasive, nondrying soaps, and to apply nonperfumed skin moisturizers to dry skin surfaces. Routine oral care is also encouraged.

Medicated lotions, ointments, and dressings are applied to affected skin surfaces as prescribed. Adhesive tape is avoided. Skin surfaces are protected from friction and rubbing by keeping bed linens free of wrinkles and avoiding tight or restrictive clothing. Patients with foot lesions are advised to wear white cotton socks and shoes that do not cause the feet to perspire. Antipruritics, antibiotics, and analgesics are administered as prescribed.

The patient's perianal region is assessed frequently for impairment of skin integrity and infection. The patient is instructed to keep the area as clean as possible. The perianal area is cleaned after each bowel movement with nonabrasive soap and water to prevent further excoriation and breakdown of the skin and infection. If the area is very painful, soft cloths or cotton sponges may prove to be less irritating than washcloths. In addition, sitz baths or gentle irrigation may facilitate cleaning and promote comfort. The area is dried thoroughly after cleaning. Topical lotions or ointments may be prescribed to promote healing. Wounds are cultured if infection is suspected so that the appropriate antimicrobial treatment can be initiated. Debilitated patients may require assistance in maintaining hygienic practices.

Promoting Usual Bowel Habits. The patient's bowel patterns are assessed for the occurrence of diarrhea. The nurse monitors frequency and consistency of stools and reports of abdominal pain or cramping associated with bowel movements. Factors that exacerbate frequent diarrhea are also assessed. The quantity and volume of liquid stools are measured to document fluid volume losses. Stool cultures are obtained to identify pathogenic organisms.

The patient is counseled about ways to decrease diarrhea. The physician may recommend restriction of oral intake to rest the bowel during periods of acute inflammation associated with severe enteric infections. As the patient's dietary intake is increased, foods that act as bowel irritants, such as raw fruits and vegetables, popcorn, carbonated beverages, spicy foods, and foods of extreme temperatures, should be avoided. Small, frequent meals help to prevent abdominal distention. The physician may prescribe medications such as anticholinergic antispasmodics or opioids, which decrease diarrhea by decreasing intestinal spasms and motility; administration of antidiarrheal agents on a regular schedule may be more effective than their administration as needed. Antibiotics and antifungal agents may also be prescribed to combat pathogens identified by stool cultures.

Preventing Infection. The patient and caregivers are instructed to monitor for signs and symptoms of infection. These include fever; chills; night sweats; cough with or without sputum production; shortness of breath; difficulty breathing; oral pain or difficulty swallowing; creamy white patches in the oral cavity; unexplained weight loss; swollen lymph nodes; nausea; vomiting; persistent diarrhea; frequency, urgency, or pain on urination; headache; visual changes or memory lapses; redness, swelling, or drainage from skin wounds; and vesicular lesions on the face, lips, or perianal area. The nurse also monitors laboratory values that indicate infection, such as the white blood cell count and differential. The physician may decide to culture specimens of wound drainage, skin lesions, urine, stool, sputum, mouth, and blood to identify pathogenic organisms and the most appropriate antimicrobial therapy.

Patient teaching includes strategies to avoid infection. The importance of personal hygiene is emphasized. Kitchen and bathroom surfaces should be cleaned regularly with disinfectants to prevent fungal and bacterial growth. Patients with pets are instructed to have another person clean areas soiled by animals, such as bird cages and litter boxes. If this is not possible, the patient should use gloves to clean up after pets. Patients are advised to avoid exposure to others who are sick or who have been recently vaccinated. Patients with AIDS and their sexual partners are *strongly* urged to avoid exposure to body fluids during sexual activities and to use condoms for any form of sexual intercourse. IV drug use is *strongly* discouraged because of the risk to the patient of other infections and transmission of HIV infection to others. Patients who are already infected by HIV are also urged to avoid exposure to bodily fluids (through sexual activity or IV drug use) in order to prevent reinfection with other HIV strains. The importance of avoiding smoking and maintaining a balance between diet, rest, and exercise is also emphasized. All health care professionals must remember to maintain strict aseptic technique when performing invasive procedures such as venipunctures and bladder catheterizations and to observe universal precautions in all patient care.

Improving Activity Tolerance. Activity tolerance is assessed by monitoring the patient's ability to ambulate and perform activities of daily living. Patients may be unable to maintain usual levels of activity because of weakness, fatigue, shortness of breath, dizziness, and neurologic involvement. Assistance in planning daily routines that maintain a balance between activity and rest may be necessary. In addition, patients benefit from instructions about energy conservation techniques, such as sitting while washing or while preparing meals. Personal items that are frequently used should be kept within the patient's reach. Measures such as relaxation and guided imagery may be beneficial because they decrease anxiety that contributes to weakness and fatigue.

Collaboration with other members of the health care team may uncover other factors associated with increasing fatigue and strategies to address them. For example, if fatigue is related to anemia, the administration of Epogen as prescribed may relieve some of the fatigue and increase the patient's activity tolerance.

Improving Thought Processes. The patient is assessed for alterations in mental status that may be related to neurologic involvement, metabolic abnormalities, infection, side effects of treatment, and/or coping mechanisms. Mental status is assessed as early as possible to provide a baseline for monitoring changes in behavior (Table 50-4). Manifestations of neurologic impairment may be difficult to distinguish from psychologic reactions to HIV infection, such as anger and depression.

The patient and family are helped to understand and cope with changes in thought processes. The patient is reoriented to person, place, and time whenever necessary; it is usually helpful to keep a clock and calendar within the patient's view. The patient's family and friends are encouraged to bring favorite objects from home to provide a familiar and less threatening environment if the patient is hospitalized. All instructions given to the patient are delivered in simple and clear language. Measures to protect the patient from injury are instituted; these may include placing the call bell within easy reach, keeping the bed side rails up and the bed in a low position, instructing the patient to wear shoes and slippers with nonskid soles, and monitoring the patient during shaving.

Strategies for improving or maintaining functional abilities and for providing a safe environment are used for patients with HIV encephalopathy (Chart 50-2).

Improving Airway Clearance. Respiratory status, including rate, rhythm, use of accessory muscles, and breath sounds; mental status; and skin color must be assessed at least daily. Any cough and the quantity and characteristics of sputum are documented. Sputum specimens are analyzed for infectious organisms. Pulmonary therapy (coughing, deep breathing, postural drainage, percussion, and vibration) is provided as often as every 2 hours to prevent stasis of secretions and to promote airway clearance. Because of weakness and fatigue, many patients may require assistance in attaining a position (such as a high or semi-Fowler's) that will facilitate breathing and airway clearance. The provision of adequate rest periods is essential to maximize the patient's energy expenditure and prevent excessive fatigue. The patient's fluid volume status is evaluated so that adequate hydration can be maintained as well. Unless contraindicated by renal or cardiac disease, intake of 3 L of fluid daily is encouraged. Humidified oxygen may be prescribed, nasopharyngeal or tracheal suctioning, intubation,

TABLE 50-4 Mental Status Assessment and Observations in HIV Infection

Assessment	Function	Selected Descriptors
Appearance	Physical characteristics, grooming, dress	Obese, cachectic, emaciated, poor eye contact, clean, disheveled, inappropriate dress for weather, slumped posture
Behavior	Motor activity	Restless, agitated, lethargic, hyperactive, rigid, repetitive
Speech	Verbal communication	Intelligible, clear, slurred, rapid, slowed, pressured, repetitive, perseveration, mute
Mood	General feeling tone	Friendly, fearful, hostile, euphoric, despondent, labile
Affect	Emotional expression	Appropriate, bizarre, flat, blunted, apathetic, overly dramatic
Cognition	Memory and orientation	Oriented to time, place, person, confused, disoriented, distractible, short attention span, intact remote and immediate memory, forgetful
Comprehension	Intellectual functioning	Able to abstract, concrete, poor judgment, lacks insight, unable to compute, lacks general knowledge, able to learn
Thought process	Expression of thoughts	Goal oriented, tangential, delusional, looseness of associations, delusional, confabulation, obsessive, ritualistic
Perception	Perspective of world	Presence of auditory, visual, olfactory, or kinesthetic hallucinations

and mechanical ventilation may be necessary to maintain adequate ventilation.

Relieving Pain and Discomfort. The patient is assessed for the quality and quantity of pain associated with impaired perianal skin integrity, the lesions of KS, and peripheral neuropathy. In addition, the effects of pain on elimination, nutrition, sleep, affect, and communication are explored, along with exacerbating and relieving factors. Cleaning the perianal area as previously described can promote comfort. Topical anesthetics or ointments may be prescribed. Soft cushions or foam pads may be used to increase comfort while sitting. The patient is instructed to avoid foods that act as bowel irritants. Antispasmodics and antidiarrheal preparations may be prescribed to reduce discomfort and frequency of bowel movements. If necessary, systemic analgesics may also be prescribed.

Pain from KS is frequently described as a sharp, throbbing pressure and heaviness if lymphedema is present. Pain management may include using nonsteroidal anti-inflammatory agents (NSAIDs) and opioids as well as such nonpharmacologic approaches as relaxation techniques. When NSAIDs are used in patients receiving zidovudine, hepatic and hemotologic status needs to be monitored. The patient with pain related to peripheral neuropathy frequently describes it as burning, numbness, and "pins and needles." Pain management measures may include opioids, tricyclic antidepressants, and elastic stockings to equalize pressure. Tricyclic antidepressants have been found helpful in controlling the symptoms of neuropathic pain. They also potentiate the actions of opioids and can be used to relieve pain without increasing the dose of the opioid.

Improving Nutritional Status. Nutritional status is assessed by monitoring weight; dietary intake; anthropometric measurements; and serum albumin, BUN, protein, and transferrin levels. The patient is also assessed for factors that interfere with oral intake, such as anorexia, oral and esophageal candida infection, nausea, pain, weakness, and fatigue, and for lactose intolerance. Based on the results of assessment, the nurse can implement specific measures to facilitate oral intake.

Control of nausea and vomiting with antiemetic medications administered on a regular basis may increase the patient's dietary intake. Inadequate food intake resulting from pain caused by mouth sores or a sore throat may be managed by administering prescribed opioids and viscous lidocaine (rinse the mouth and swallow). Additionally, the patient is encouraged to eat foods that are easy to swallow and to avoid rough, spicy, or sticky food items and foods that are excessively hot or cold. Oral hygiene before and after meals is encouraged.

When fatigue and weakness interfere with intake, the patient is encouraged to rest before meals. In addition, meals should be scheduled so that they do not occur immediately after painful or unpleasant procedures. The patient with diarrhea and abdominal cramping is encouraged to avoid foods that stimulate intestinal motility and abdominal

CHART 50-2
Nursing Interventions for Nursing Diagnoses in HIV Encephalopathy

Altered Thought Processes

- Assess mental status and neurologic functioning.
- Monitor for drug interactions, infections, electrolyte imbalance, and depression.
- Frequently orient the patient to time, place, person, reality, and the environment.
- Use simple explanations.
- Teach the patient to perform tasks in incremental steps.
- Provide memory aids (clocks and calendars).
- Provide memory aids for medication administration.
- Post activity schedule.
- Give positive feedback for appropriate behavior.
- Teach caretakers how to orient patient to time, place, person, reality, and the environment.
- Encourage the patient to designate a responsible person to assume power of attorney.

Sensory Perceptual Alterations

- Assess sensory impairment.
- Decrease amount of stimuli in the patient's environment.
- Correct inaccurate perceptions.
- Provide reassurance and safety if the patient displays fear.
- Provide a feeling of security and stability in the patient's environment.
- Teach caregivers how to recognize inaccurate sensory perceptions.
- Teach caregivers techniques to correct inaccurate perceptions.
- Teach the patient and caregivers to report any changes in the patient's vision to the patient's health care provider.

Risk for Injury

- Assess the patient's level of anxiety, confusion, or disorientation.
- Assess the patient for delusions or hallucinations.
- Remove potentially dangerous objects from the patient's environment.
- Structure the environment for safety (ensure adequate lighting, avoid clutter, provide bed rails if needed).
- Supervise smoking.
- Do not let the patient drive a car if confusion is present.
- Instruct the patient and caregiver in home safety.
- Provide assistance as needed for ambulation and in getting in and out of bed.
- Pad headboard and side rails if the patient has seizures.

Self-Care Deficit

- Encourage performing activities of daily living within the patient's level of ability.
- Encourage independence but intervene if the patient cannot perform an activity.
- Show or demonstrate how to perform any activity that the patient is having difficulty accomplishing.
- Keep strict records of food and fluid intake.
- Weigh patient weekly.
- Encourage the patient to eat, and offer nutritious meals, snacks, and adequate fluids.
- If patient is incontinent, establish a routine toileting schedule.
- Teach caregivers how to meet the patient's self-care needs.

distention, for example, fiber-rich food or lactose if the patient is lactose intolerant. The dietitian is consulted to determine the patient's nutritional requirements. The patient is instructed about ways in which to enhance the nutritional value of meals. The addition of eggs, butter, margarine, and fortified milk (powdered skim milk is added to milk to increase the caloric content) to gravies, soups, or milkshakes can provide additional calories and protein. Using commercial supplements such as puddings, powders, milkshakes, and Advera (a nutritional product specifically designed for people with HIV infection or AIDS) may be advised. Patients who cannot maintain nutritional status through oral intake may require enteral or parenteral feedings. Instruction is provided to patients and families about how to administer such feedings when patients return home. Community health and home care nurses provide additional teaching and support for the patient after discharge from the hospital. A social worker may be consulted to identify sources of financial support for patients who cannot purchase or prepare meals. Referral to community resources may be indicated if the patient cannot shop for or prepare meals. These resources may provide volunteers who can assist patients in the home and community.

Decreasing the Sense of Social Isolation. AIDS patients are at risk for double stigmatization. They have what society refers to as "a dread disease," and they may have a life-style that differs from what is considered acceptable by many people. Most persons with AIDS are young adults at a developmental stage usually associated with establishing intimate relationships and personal and career goals and having and raising children. Their focus changes as they are faced with a disease that has no cure and a limited life expectancy. In addition, they may be forced to reveal hidden life-styles or behaviors to family, friends, coworkers, and health care providers. As a result, persons with HIV infection may be overwhelmed with emotions such as anxiety, guilt, shame, and fear. They also may be faced with multiple losses, such as rejection by family and friends and loss of sexual partners, family and friends; financial security; normal roles and functions; self-esteem; privacy; ability to control bodily functions; ability to interact meaningfully with the environment; and sexual functioning. Some patients may harbor feelings of guilt because of their chosen life-style or because of the possibility of having infected others in current or previous relationships. Other patients may feel anger toward sexual partners who transmitted the virus.

Infection-control measures used in the hospital or at home may further contribute to the patient's emotional isolation. Any or all of these stressors may cause the patient with AIDS to withdraw both physically and emotionally from social contact.

Nurses are in a key position to provide an atmosphere of acceptance and understanding of persons with AIDS and their families and partners. A patient's usual level of social interaction is assessed as early as possible to provide a baseline for monitoring changes in behavior indicative of social isolation (*e.g.*, decreased interaction with staff or family, hostility, noncompliance). Patients are encouraged to express feelings of isolation and loneliness and are assured that these feelings are not unique or abnormal.

Providing information about how to protect themselves and others may help patients avoid social contact. Patients, family, and friends must be assured that AIDS is not spread through casual contact. Educating ancillary personnel, nurses, and physicians will help to reduce factors that might contribute to patients' feelings of isolation. Patient care conferences that address the psychosocial considerations regarding patients with AIDS may help sensitize nurses to patients' needs.

Coping With Grief. The nurse can help patients verbalize feelings and explore and identify resources for support and mechanisms for coping, especially when the patient is grieving through anticipated losses. Patients are encouraged to maintain contact with family and friends and to use local or national AIDS support groups and hotlines. If at all possible, losses are identified and dealt with. Interaction with and support of family, friends, or coworkers is encouraged. Patients are also encouraged to engage in their usual activities whenever possible.

Patient Education and Home Care Considerations. Patients, families, and friends are instructed about the routes of transmission of AIDS. All fears and misconceptions are thoroughly discussed. In addition, the nurse discusses precautions necessary to prevent transmitting HIV, including using condoms during vaginal or anal intercourse; avoiding oral contact with the penis, vagina, or rectum; avoiding sexual practices that might cut or tear the lining of the rectum, vagina, or penis; and avoiding sexual contact with multiple partners, individuals known to be HIV infected, persons who use illicit IV drugs, and sexual partners of persons who use IV drugs (Guideline 50-3). Patients who are HIV positive or who use IV drugs are instructed not to donate blood. IV drug users who are unwilling to stop using drugs are advised to avoid sharing drug equipment with others.

Many persons with AIDS can return to the community and resume their usual daily activities. Others who return home cannot continue employment or maintain their preexisting level of independence. Families or caregivers may need assistance in providing supportive care. They must receive instructions about how to prevent disease transmission. They need instruction in handwashing techniques and in methods for safely handling items soiled with body fluids. Caregivers in the home are taught how to administer medications, including IV preparations. Guidelines about infection, follow-up care, diet, rest, and activity are also necessary. Both the patient and the caregivers require support and guidance in coping with AIDS.

Community health nurses, home care nurses, and hospice nurses are in an excellent position to provide the support and guidance so often needed in the home setting. As hospital costs continue to rise and insurance coverage continues to decline, the complexity of home care continues to increase. Community health and home care nurses are key in the administration of parenteral antibiotics, chemotherapy, and nutrition in the home.

In addition, complicated wound care or respiratory care is often required in the home. Patients and families are seldom able to meet these skilled care needs without the assistance of nurses. Hospice nurses are increasingly called upon to provide physical and emotional support to patients and families as AIDS patients enter the terminal stages of disease. This support takes on special meaning when AIDS patients lose friends and family members who fear the disease or feel anger concerning their life-style.

GUIDELINE 50-3
Safer Sex and Behaviors

- Practice abstinence.
- Reduce the number of sexual partners to one.
- Always use latex condoms with a water-soluble lubricant containing the spermicide nonoxynol-9.
- Do not reuse condoms.
- Do not use cervical caps or diaphragms without using a condom as well.
- Always use dental dams for oral female genital or anal stimulation.
- Avoid anal intercourse because this practice may injure tissues.
- Avoid manual–anal intercourse (fisting).
- Do not ingest urine or semen.
- Avoid having sex with persons who are injecting drug users.
- Engage in nonpenetrative sex such as body massage, social kissing (dry), mutual masturbation, fantasy, and sex films.
- If female, avoid pregnancy if you or your sexual partner is HIV seropositive.
- Inform prospective sexual partners of your HIV-positive status.
- Notify previous and present sexual partners if you learn that you are HIV seropositive.
- If HIV seropositive, do not have unprotected sex with another HIV-seropositive person because cross-infection with another HIV strain can increase the severity of the disease.
- Do not share needles, razors, toothbrushes, sexual toys, or other blood-contaminated articles.
- If HIV seropositive, do not donate blood, plasma, body organs, or sperm.

Nurses may also refer patients to many community programs located in towns and cities throughout the country. These programs offer a range of services for patients, friends, and families, including help with housekeeping, grooming, and meals; transportation and shopping; individual and group therapy; support for caregivers; telephone networks for the homebound; and legal and financial assistance. These services are typically provided by both professional and nonprofessional volunteers.

Monitoring and Managing Potential Complications. Patients who are immunosuppressed are at risk for **opportunistic infections.** Therefore, anti-infective agents may be prescribed and laboratory specimens obtained and analyzed periodically to monitor their effectiveness. The patient and the caregiver need to learn which signs and symptoms of opportunistic infections should be immediately reported to the health care provider; these include fever, malaise, difficulty breathing, nausea or vomiting, diarrhea, difficulty swallowing, and any occurrences of swelling or discharge.

Impaired breathing is a major complication that increases the patient's discomfort and anxiety and may lead to **respiratory failure** and cardiac failure. The patient's respiratory rate and pattern are monitored and the lungs auscultated for abnormal sounds. The patient is asked to report shortness of breath and increasing difficulty in carrying out usual activities. The pulse rate and rhythm and blood pressure are monitored. Blood tests are performed to monitor oxygen saturation, cholesterol, and triglyceride levels. Suctioning and oxygen therapy may be prescribed to assure an adequate airway and to prevent hypoxia. Mechanical ventilation may be necessary for a patient who cannot maintain adequate ventilation as a result of pulmonary infection, fluid and electrolyte imbalance, or respiratory muscle weakness. Arterial blood gas values are used to guide ventilator settings. If the patient is intubated, a method must be established to allow communication with the nurse and others. Attention must be given to assisting the patient on mechanical ventilation to cope with the stress associated with intubation and ventilator assistance. The possible need for mechanical ventilation in the future should be discussed early in the course of the disease, when the patient is able to make his or her desires about treatment known. (See the discussion of mechanical ventilation in Chapter 25).

Wasting syndrome and **fluid and electrolyte disturbances,** including dehydration, are common complications of HIV infection and AIDS. The patient's nutritional and electrolyte status is evaluated by monitoring weight gains or losses, skin turgor, ferritin levels, hemoglobin and hematocrit values, and electrolyte levels. Fluid and electrolyte status is monitored on an ongoing basis; fluid intake and output and urine specific gravity may be monitored daily if the patient is hospitalized with complications. The patient's skin is assessed for dryness and adequate turgor. Vital signs are monitored for decreases in systolic blood pressure or increases in pulse rate upon sitting or standing. Signs and symptoms of electrolyte disturbances such as muscle cramping, weakness, irregular pulse, decreased mental status, nausea, and vomiting are documented and reported to the physician. Serum electrolyte values are monitored and abnormalities reported when indicated.

The nurse helps the patient select foods that will replenish electrolytes, such as oranges and bananas (potassium) and cheese and soups (sodium). A fluid intake of 3 L or more, unless contraindicated, is encouraged to replace fluid lost from diarrhea. In addition, measures to control diarrhea are initiated. If fluid and electrolyte imbalances persist, the nurse may administer IV fluids and electrolytes as prescribed. Therapeutic and potentially adverse effects of parenteral therapy are monitored.

Adverse reactions to medications are of concern in patients who often receive many medications to treat HIV infection or its complications. Many medications can cause severe toxic effects. Patient education includes information about the purpose of the medications; their correct administration; side effects, including those that should be brought to the immediate attention of the patient's physician or nurse practitioner; and strategies to manage or prevent side effects. Signs and symptoms of antiviral agents that should be reported immediately include the following: for zidovudine (ZDV, AZT, Retrovir)—headache, fever, fatigue, rash, muscle pain, severe upper abdominal pain, and shortness of breath; for didanosine (ddI, Videx)—diarrhea, upper abdominal pain, persistent nausea and vomiting, pain, tingling, or numbness, difficulties breathing, and mental confusion; for dideoxycytidine (ddC, Hivid)—mouth sores, rashes, itching, upper abdominal pain, persistent nausea and vomiting, numbness or tingling, mental confusion, and convulsion; and for stavudine—numbness, pain, or tingling of the extremities.

Other medications that may be required include but are not limited to opioids, tricyclics, and NSAIDs for pain relief; medications for treatment of opportunistic infections; antihistamines (diphenhydramine) for relief of pruritus (itching); acetaminophen or aspirin for management of fever; and antiemetics for control of nausea and vomiting. Use of many of these medications concurrently with zidovudine may cause hepatic and hematologic abnormalities; careful laboratory monitoring for these abnormalities is warranted.

Evaluation

Expected Outcomes

1. Maintains skin integrity
2. Resumes usual bowel habits
3. Experiences no infections
4. Maintains adequate level of activity tolerance
5. Maintains usual level of thought processes
6. Maintains effective airway clearance
7. Experiences increased sense of comfort, less pain
8. Maintains adequate nutritional status
9. Experiences decreased sense of social isolation
10. Progresses through grieving process
11. Reports increased understanding of AIDS and participates in self-care activities as possible
12. Absence of complications

Selected interventions and outcomes are discussed in Nursing Care Plan 50-1.

Emotional and Ethical Concerns for Nurses

Nurses in all settings may be called upon to provide care for patients with HIV infection. In doing so, they encounter not

(text continues on page 1415)

NURSING CARE PLAN 50–1
Care of the Patient With Acquired Immunodeficiency Syndrome (AIDS)

Nursing Interventions	Rationale	Expected Outcomes
NURSING DIAGNOSIS: Diarrhea related to enteric pathogens and/or HIV infection		
GOAL: Resumption of usual bowel habits		
1. Assess patient's normal bowel habits.	1. Provides baseline for evaluation.	• Bowel habits return to normal.
2. Assess for diarrhea: frequent, loose stools; abdominal pain or cramping, volume of liquid stools, and exacerbating and alleviating factors.	2. Detects changes in status, quantifies loss of fluid, and provides basis for nursing measures.	• Reports decreasing episodes of diarrhea and abdominal cramping. • Identifies and avoids foods that irritate the gastrointestinal tract.
3. Obtain stool cultures and administer antimicrobial therapy as prescribed.	3. Identifies pathogenic organism.	• Appropriate therapy is initiated as prescribed.
4. Initiate measures to reduce hyperactivity of bowel:	4. Bowel rest may decrease acute episodes.	• Exhibits normal stool cultures. • Maintains adequate fluid intake.
a. Maintain food and fluid restrictions as prescribed by physician.	a. Reduces stimulation of bowel.	• Maintains body weight and reports no additional weight loss.
b. Discourage smoking.	b. Nicotine acts as bowel stimulant.	• States rationale for avoiding smoking.
c. Avoid bowel irritants such as fatty or fried foods, raw vegetables, and nuts. Offer small, frequent meals.	c. Prevents stimulation of bowel and abdominal distention and promotes adequate nutrition.	• Enrolls in program to stop smoking. • Uses medication as prescribed. • Maintains adequate fluid status.
5. Administer anticholinergic antispasmodics and opioids or like medications as prescribed.	5. Decreases intestinal spasms and motility.	• Exhibits normal skin turgor, moist mucous membranes, adequate urine output, and no excessive thirst.
6. Maintain fluid intake of at least 3 L unless contraindicated.	6. Prevents hypovolemia.	
NURSING DIAGNOSIS: Risk for infection related to immunodeficiency		
GOAL: Absence of infection		
1. Monitor for infection: fever, chills, and diaphoresis; cough; shortness of breath; oral pain or painful swallowing; creamy white patches in oral cavity; urinary frequency, urgency, or dysuria; redness, swelling, or drainage from wounds; vesicular lesions on face, lips, or perianal area.	1. Early detection of infection is essential for prompt initiation of treatment. Repeated and prolonged infections contribute to patient's debilitation.	• Identifies reportable signs and symptoms of infection. • Reports signs and symptoms of infection if present. • Exhibits and reports absence of fever, chills, and diaphoresis. • Exhibits normal (clear) breath sounds without adventitious breath sounds.
2. Teach patient or caregiver about need to report possible infection.	2. Allows early detection of infection.	• Maintains weight.
3. Monitor white blood cell count and differential	3. Elevated WBC is associated with infection.	• Reports adequate energy level without excessive fatigue.
4. Obtain cultures of wound drainage, skin lesions, urine, stool, sputum, mouth, and blood as prescribed. Administer antimicrobial therapy as prescribed.	4. Offending organism must be identified in order to initiate appropriate treatment.	• Reports absence of shortness of breath and cough. • Exhibits pink, moist oral mucous membranes without fissures or lesions.
5. Instruct patient in ways to prevent infection:	5. Minimizes exposure to infection and transmission of HIV infection to others.	• Appropriate therapy is administered. • Infection is prevented. • States rationale for strategies to avoid infection.
a. Clean kitchen and bathroom surfaces with disinfectants.		• Modifies activities to reduce exposure to infection or infectious persons.
b. Clean hands thoroughly after exposure to body fluids.		• Practices "safer sex."
c. Avoid exposure to others' body fluids or sharing eating utensils.		• Avoids sharing eating utensils and toothbrush.

(continued)

NURSING CARE PLAN 50–1 *(continued)*
Care of the Patient With Acquired Immunodeficiency Syndrome (AIDS)

Nursing Interventions	Rationale	Expected Outcomes
d. Turn, cough, and deep breathe, especially when activity is decreased. e. Maintain cleanliness of perianal area. f. Avoid handling pet excreta or cleaning litter boxes, bird cages, or aquariums. g. Cook meat and eggs thoroughly.		• Exhibits normal body temperature. • Uses recommended techniques to maintain cleanliness of skin, skin lesions, and perianal area. • Have others handle pet excreta and cleanup. • Uses recommended cooking techniques.
6. Maintain aseptic technique when performing invasive procedures such as venipunctures, bladder catheterizations, and injections.	6. Prevents hospital-acquired infections.	

NURSING DIAGNOSIS: Ineffective airway clearance related to Pneumocystis pneumonia, increased bronchial secretions, and decreased ability to cough related to weakness and fatigue

GOAL: Improved airway clearance

Nursing Interventions	Rationale	Expected Outcomes
1. Assess and report signs and symptoms of altered respiratory status: tachypnea, use of accessory muscles, cough, color and amount of sputum, abnormal breath sounds, dusky or cyanotic skin color, restlessness, confusion, or somnolence.	1. Indicates abnormal respiratory function.	• Maintains normal airway clearance: Respiratory rate <20/minute Unlabored breathing without using accessory muscles and flaring nares (nostrils) Skin color pink (without cyanosis) Alert and aware of surroundings Arterial blood gas values normal Normal breath sounds without adventitious breath sounds
2. Obtain sputum sample for culture prescribed by physician. Administer antimicrobial therapy as prescribed.	2. Aids in identification of pathogenic organisms.	• Begins appropriate therapy. • Takes medication as prescribed.
3. Provide pulmonary care (cough, deep breathing, postural drainage, and vibration) every 2 to 4 hours.	3. Prevents stasis of secretions and promotes airway clearance.	• Reports improved breathing. • Maintains clear airway.
4. Assist patient in attaining semi- or high Fowler's position.	4. Facilitates breathing and airway clearance.	• Coughs and takes deep breaths every 2–4 hours as recommended.
5. Encourage adequate rest periods.	5. Maximizes energy expenditure and prevents excessive fatigue.	• Demonstrates appropriate positions and practices postural drainage every 2–4 hours.
6. Initiate measures to decrease viscosity of secretions: a. Maintain fluid intake of at least 3 L per day unless contraindicated. b. Humidify inspired air as prescribed by physician. c. Consult with physician concerning use of mucolytic agents delivered through nebulizer or IPPB treatment.	6. Facilitates expectoration of secretions; prevents stasis of secretions.	• Reports reduced breathing difficulty when in semi- or high-Fowler's position. • Practices energy-conserving strategies and alternates rest with activity. • Demonstrates reduction in thickness (viscosity) of pulmonary secretions.
7. Perform tracheal suctioning as needed.	7. Removes secretions if patient is unable to do so.	• Reports increased ease in coughing up sputum.
8. Administer oxygen therapy as prescribed.	8. Increases availability of oxygen.	• Uses humidified air or oxygen as prescribed and indicated.
9. Assist with endotracheal intubation; maintain ventilator settings as prescribed.	9. Maintains ventilation.	• Indicates need for assistance with removal of pulmonary secretions. • Understands need for and cooperates with endotracheal intubation and use of a mechanical ventilator. • Verbalizes concerns about respiratory difficulty, intubation, and mechanical ventilation.

(continued)

NURSING CARE PLAN 50–1 *(continued)*
Care of the Patient With Acquired Immunodeficiency Syndrome (AIDS)

NURSING DIAGNOSIS: Altered nutrition, less than body requirement, related to decreased oral intake

GOAL: Improvement of nutritional status

Nursing Interventions

1. Assess for malnutrition with height, weight, age, BUN, serum protein, albumin, transferrin levels, hemoglobin, hematocrit, cutaneous anergy, and anthropometric measurements.
2. Obtain dietary history, including likes and dislikes and food intolerances.
3. Assess factors that interfere with oral intake.
4. Consult with dietitian to determine patient's nutritional needs.
5. Reduce factors limiting oral intake:
   a. Encourage patient to rest prior to meals.
   b. Plan meals so that they do not occur immediately after painful or unpleasant procedures.
   c. Encourage patient to eat meals with visitors or others when possible.
   d. Encourage patient to prepare simple meals or to obtain assistance with meal preparation if possible.
   e. Serve small, frequent meals: 6 per day.
   f. Limit fluids 1 hour prior to meals and with meals.
6. Instruct patient in ways to supplement nutrition: consume protein-rich foods (meat, poultry, fish) and carbohydrates (pasta, fruit, breads).
7. Consult with physician about alternative feeding (enteral or parenteral nutrition)
8. Consult with social worker or community liaison about financial assistance if patient cannot afford food.

Rationale

1. Provides objective measurement of nutritional status.
2. Defines need for nutritional education; helps individualize interventions.
3. Provides basis and directions for interventions.
4. Facilitates meal planning.
5. (Reduce factors limiting oral intake)
   a. Minimizes fatigue, which can decrease appetite.
   b. Decreases noxious stimuli.
   c. Limits social isolation.
   d. Limits energy expenditure.
   e. Prevents overwhelming patient.
   f. Reduces satiety.
6. Provides additional proteins and calories.
7. Provides nutritional support if patient is unable to take sufficient amounts by mouth.
8. Increases availability of resources and nutrition.

Expected Outcomes

- Identifies factors limiting oral intake and uses resources to promote adequate dietary intake.
- Reports increased appetite.
- States understanding of nutritional needs.
- Identifies ways to minimize factors limiting oral intake.
- Rests before meals.
- Eats in pleasant, odor-free environment.
- Arranges meals to coincide with visitors' visits.
- Reports increased dietary intake.
- Uses oral hygiene prior to meals.
- Takes pain medication prior to meals as prescribed.
- States ways to increase protein and caloric intake.
- Identifies foods high in protein and calories.
- Consumes foods high in protein and calories.
- Reports decreased rate of weight loss.
- Maintains adequate intake.
- States rationale for enteral or parenteral nutrition if needed.
- Demonstrates skill in preparing alternate sources of nutrition.

NURSING DIAGNOSIS: Knowledge deficit related to means of preventing HIV transmission

GOAL: Increased knowledge concerning means of preventing disease transmission

Nursing Interventions

1. Instruct patient, family, and friends about routes of transmission of HIV.
2. Instruct patient, family, and friends about means of preventing transmission of HIV:
   a. Avoid sexual contact with multiple partners, and use precautions if sexual partner's HIV status is not certain.

Rationale

1. Knowledge about disease transmission can help prevent spread of disease; may also alleviate fears.
2. (Means of preventing transmission of HIV)
   a. The risk of infection increases with the number of sexual partners, male or female, and sexual contact with those who engage in high-risk behaviors.

Expected Outcomes

- Patient, family, and friends state means of transmission.
- Reports and demonstrates practices to reduce exposure of others to HIV.
- Avoids intravenous drug use.
- Demonstrates safe sexual practices.
- Identifies means of preventing disease transmission.

(continued)

NURSING CARE PLAN 50–1 *(continued)*
Care of the Patient With Acquired Immunodeficiency Syndrome (AIDS)

Nursing Interventions	Rationale	Expected Outcomes
b. Use condoms during sexual intercourse (vaginal, anal, oral-genital); avoid mouth contact with the penis, vagina, or rectum; avoid sexual practices that can cause cuts or tears in the lining of the rectum, vagina, or penis.	b. Reduces risk of transmission of HIV.	• States that sexual partners are informed about positive HIV antibodies in blood. • Avoids IV drug use and sharing of drug equipment with others.
d. Avoid sex with prostitutes and others at high risk.	d. Many prostitutes are infected with HIV through sexual contact with multiple partners or intravenous drug use.	
e. Do not use intravenous drugs; if addicted and unable or unwilling to change behavior, use clean needles and syringes.	e. Clean needles and syringes are the only way to prevent HIV transmission for those who continue to use drugs. Taking precautions is important for those who are antibody-positive to prevent transmitting HIV.	
f. Women who may have been exposed to AIDS through sexual or drug practices should consult with a physician prior to becoming pregnant; consider use of ZDV if pregnant.	f. AIDS can be transmitted from mother to child in utero; ZDV during pregnancy significantly reduces perinatal transmission of HIV.	

NURSING DIAGNOSIS: Social isolation related to stigma of the disease, withdrawal of support systems, isolation procedures, and fear of infecting others

GOAL: Decreased sense of social isolation

Nursing Interventions	Rationale	Expected Outcomes
1. Assess patient's usual patterns of social interaction.	1. Establishes basis for individualized interventions.	• Shares with others the need for valued social interaction.
2. Observe for behaviors indicative of social isolation, such as decreased interaction with others, hostility, noncompliance, sad affect, and stated feelings of rejection or loneliness.	2. Social isolation may be manifested in several ways.	• Demonstrates interest in events, activities, and communication. • Verbalizes feelings and reactions to diagnosis, prognosis, and life changes. • Identifies means of transmission of AIDS.
3. Provide instruction concerning means of transmission of HIV.	3. Provision of accurate information corrects misconceptions and alleviates anxiety.	• States ways of preventing transmission of AIDS virus to others while maintaining contact with valued friends and relatives.
4. Assist patient to identify and explore resources for support and positive mechanisms for coping (*e.g.*, contact with family, friends, AIDS task force).		• Reveals AIDS diagnosis to others when appropriate.
5. Allow time to be with patient other than for medications and procedures.	5. Promotes feelings of self-worth and provides social interaction.	• Identifies resources (*i.e.*, family, friends, and support groups).
6. Encourage participation in diversional activities such as reading, television, or hand crafts.	6. Provides distraction.	• Uses resources when appropriate. • Accepts offers of assistance and support. • Reports decreased sense of isolation. • Maintains contacts with those of importance to him or her. • Develops or continues hobbies that effectively serve as diversion or distraction.

(continued)

NURSING CARE PLAN 50–1 *(continued)*
Care of the Patient With Acquired Immunodeficiency Syndrome (AIDS)

Nursing Interventions	Rationale	Expected Outcomes
COLLABORATIVE PROBLEMS: Opportunistic infections; impaired breathing; wasting syndrome and fluid and electrolyte imbalances; adverse reaction to medications		
GOAL: Absence of complications		
Opportunistic Infections		
1. Monitor vital signs.	1. Changes in vital signs. Increases in pulse rate, respirations, blood pressure, and temperature may indicate infection.	• Exhibits stable vital signs • Experiences control of infection. • Identifies signs and symptoms correctly, and experiences no complications.
2. Collect laboratory specimens and monitor test results.	2. Smears and cultures can identify causative agents such as bacteria, fungi and protozoa and sensitivity studies can identify antibiotics or other medications effective against the causative agent.	
3. Instruct the patient and caregiver about signs and symptoms of infection and the need to report them early.	3. Early recognition of symptoms facilitates prompt treatment and avoids extra complications.	
Impaired Breathing		
1. Monitor respiratory rate and pattern.	1. Rapid shallow breathing, diminished breath sounds and shortness of breath may indicate respiratory failure resulting in hypoxia.	• Maintains stable respiratory rate and pattern within the normal limits. • Exhibits no adventitious lung sounds; normal breath sounds. • Has stable pulse rate and blood pressure within normal limits, and exhibits no evidence of hypoxia.
2. Auscultate the chest for breath sounds and abnormal lung sounds.	2. Crackles and wheezes may indicate fluid in the lungs which disrupts respiratory function and alters the blood's oxygen-carrying capacity.	
3. Monitor pulse rate, blood pressure, and oxygen saturation levels.	3. Changes in pulse rate, blood pressure, and oxygen levels may indicate the development of respiratory or cardiac failure.	
Wasting Syndrome and Fluid and Electrolyte Disturbances		
1. Monitor weight and laboratory values for nutritional status.	1. Weight loss, malnutrition, and anemia are common in HIV infection and increase risk for super infection.	• Maintains stable weight. • Hemoglobin, hematocrit and ferritin levels stabilize within normal limits. • Sustains fluid-electrolytes balance within normal limits. • Exhibits no signs and symptoms of dehydration.
2. Monitor intake and output and laboratory values for fluid and electrolyte imbalance (potassium, sodium, calcium, phosphorus, magnesium and zinc).	2. Chronic diarrhea, inadequate oral intake, vomiting and profuse sweating deplete electrolytes. Small intestine inflammation may impair the absorption of fluids and electrolytes.	
3. Monitor for and report signs and symptoms of dehydration.	3. Fluid loss results in decreased circulating volume leading to tachycardia, dry skin and mucous membranes, poor skin turgor, elevated urine specific gravity, and thirst. Early detection allows early treatment.	

(continued)

NURSING CARE PLAN 50-1 *(continued)*
Care of the Patient With Acquired Immunodeficiency Syndrome (AIDS)

Nursing Interventions	Rationale	Expected Outcomes
Reactions to Medications		
1. Monitor for drug interactions.	1. Persons with HIV infection receive many medications for HIV and for disease complications. Using medications concurrently with zidovudine may cause hepatic and hematologic abnormalities. Early detection of drug interaction is necessary to prevent complications.	• Experiences no serious side effects or complications from medications. • Correctly describes medication regimen and complies with therapy.
2. Monitor for and report side effects from antiretroviral agents promptly.	2. Side effects from antiretroviral agents can be life-threatening. Serious side effects include anemia, pancreatitis, peripheral neuropathy, mental confusion, and persistent nausea and vomiting. Corrective measures need to be instituted.	
3. Instruct the patient and caregiver in the medication regimen.	3. Knowledge of the medication purpose, (correct administration, side effects, and strategies to manage or prevent side effects) promotes safety and greater compliance with treatment.	

only the physical challenges of this epidemic but also emotional and ethical concerns. The concerns raised by health care professionals involve issues such as fear of contagion, responsibility for giving care, values clarification, confidentiality, developmental stages of patients and caregivers, and poor prognostic outcomes.

Many patients with HIV infection have engaged in "stigmatized" behaviors. Because these behaviors challenge some traditional religious and moral values, nurses may feel reluctant to provide nursing care for these patients. In addition, health care providers may still have fear and anxiety about disease transmission despite education concerning infection control and the low incidence of transmission to health care providers (see the Ethical Question display). Nurses are encouraged to examine their personal beliefs and use the values clarification process to approach controversial issues. The American Nurses Association's Code for Nurses can also be used to help resolve ethical dilemmas that might affect the quality of care given to HIV-infected patients.

Nurses are responsible for protecting the patient's right to privacy by safeguarding confidential information. Inadvertent disclosure of confidential patient information may result in personal, financial, and emotional hardships for HIV-infected individuals. The controversy surrounding confidentiality concerns identifying the circumstances when information can be disclosed to others. Health care team members need accurate patient information to conduct assessment, planning, implementation, and evaluation of patient care. Failure to disclose HIV status could compromise the quality of patient care. Sexual partners of HIV-infected patients should know about the potential for infection and the need to engage in safer sex practices as well as the potential need for testing and medical care. Nurses are advised to discuss concerns about confidentiality with nurse administrators and physicians to identify the most appropriate courses of action.

AIDS has a high mortality rate. Most nurses have never faced an epidemic in which almost all patients will experience serious illness and die within a relatively short time. Nurses may struggle with the value and meaning of their professional roles as they witness repeated instances of deterioration. Exposure to so many deaths in a population that is at the same developmental stage as many nurses can create feelings of stress. Contributing to this stress are personal fears of contagion or disapproval of the patient's life-style and behaviors. Unlike cancer or other diseases, AIDS is associated with controversies challenging our legal and political systems as well as religious and personal beliefs. Nurses who feel stressed and overburdened may experience physical and mental distress in the form of fatigue, headache, changes in appetite and sleep patterns, helplessness, irritability, apathy, negativity, and anger.

Many strategies have been used by nurses to cope with stress associated with caring for AIDS patients. Education and provision of up-to-date information help to alleviate apprehension and prepare nurses to deliver safe, high-quality patient care. Interdisciplinary meetings allow participants to support one another and still provide comprehensive patient care. Staff support groups give nurses an opportunity to problem-solve and explore values and feelings about caring for AIDS patients and their families; they also provide a forum for grieving. Other sources of support include nursing administrators, peers, and spiritual leaders.

ETHICAL QUESTION

Should All Patients Be Screened For HIV Upon Hospital Admission?

Situation

The human immunodeficiency virus (HIV) causes AIDS, an incurable and ultimately fatal disease. Many HIV-positive people are unaware that they carry the virus and thus spread the virus unknowingly through blood and body fluid contact. Because health care workers are at risk for infection, would a policy that screened all patients for HIV upon admission to the hospital infringe on the liberty and privacy of patients?

Dilemma

The patient's right to privacy conflicts with health care worker's rights to protection from HIV infection (autonomy versus integrity of the professions). The patient's right to privacy conflicts with society's need to contain the deadly virus and stem a deadly epidemic (autonomy versus justice).

Discussion

- What arguments would you offer in *favor* of screening all patients for HIV upon admission to the hospital?
- What arguments would you offer *against* screening all patients for HIV upon admission to the hospital?

CRITICAL THINKING EXERCISES

1. Laboratory reports indicate that the pneumonia in a 32-year-old hospitalized patient is *Pneumocystis carinii* pneumonia (PCP) and that the patient is HIV positive. The patient, who is recently married, does not want his wife informed of his HIV status and has stated that he does not plan to tell her himself. What issues would you consider in caring for this patient, in maintaining his privacy and confidentiality, and in protecting his wife? Describe how you would handle this situation and explain how you reached this decision.
2. You are making a home visit to a patient with HIV encephalopathy. Describe the aspects of the home environment you would assess to ensure safety and adequate care.
3. A coworker accidentally sticks herself with a needle but states that she is too frightened to report it to the employee health office. Compare the pros and cons of reporting the incident yourself. What actions would you take and why?
4. The wife of a patient hospitalized with AIDS asks you directly, "Does my husband have AIDS?" Explain how you would respond to her and why you decided on this course of action.
5. You are caring for an HIV-positive patient who tells you that she and her husband are considering having a child. She asks you what you think of this idea. How would you respond to her? Explain the information you would consider in your response.

BIBLIOGRAPHY

Books

Afdhal N. Gastrointestinal manifestations. In Libman H and Witzburg RA (eds). HIV Infection: A Clinical Manual, 2nd ed. Boston, Little, Brown and Company, 1993.

Agency for Health Care Policy and Research. Evaluation and Management of Early HIV Infection. Clinical Practice Guideline No. 7. U.S. Department of Health and Human Services (Pub. No. 94-0572). Washington DC, 1994.

American Nurses Association. Nursing and HIV/AIDS. Washington DC, American Nurses Association, 1994.

Barat LM and Craven DE. Cyromegalovirus infection. In Libman H and Witzburg RA (eds). HIV Infection: A Clinical Manual, 2nd ed. Boston, Little, Brown and Company, 1993.

Battinelli DL and Peters ES. Oral manifestations. In Libman H and Witzburg RA (eds). HIV Infection: A Clinical Manual, 2nd ed. Boston, Little, Brown and Company, 1993.

Cohen FL and Durham JD. Women, Children, and HIV/AIDS. New York, Springer Publishing Company, 1993.

Cooley TP. Kaposi's sarcoma. In Libman H and Witzburg RA (eds). HIV Infection: A Clinical Manual, 2nd ed. Boston, Little, Brown, and Company, 1993.

Cooley TP. AIDS-related lymphoma. In Libman H and Witzburg RA (eds). HIV Infection: A Clinical Manual, 2nd ed. Boston, Little, Brown and Company, 1993.

Gibbs G and Zeeman B. HIV infection in women. In Libman H and Witzburg RA (eds). HIV Infection: A Clinical Manual, 2nd ed. Boston, Little, Brown and Company, 1993.

Donegan E. Transmission of HIV in blood products. In Cohen PT, Sand MA and Volberding PA (eds). The AIDS Knowledge Base. Waltham MA, Medical Publishing Group, 1990.

Durham JD and Cohen FL. The Person with AIDS: Nursing Perspectives. New York, Springer Publishing Company, 1991.

Fallon J and Masusr H. Acquired immunodeficiency syndrome: Treatment of opportunistic diseases. In Lichtenstein LM and Fauci AS (eds). Current Therapy in Allergy, Immunology, and Rheumatology, 4th ed. St. Louis, BC Decker/Mosby Year Book, 1992.

Fishbein MC and Qiao JH. Cardiovascular system. In Nash G and Said JW (eds). Pathology of AIDS and HIV Infection. Philadelpha, WB Saunders, 1993.

Flaskerud JH and Ungvarski PJ. HIV/AIDS: A Guide to Nursing Care, 3rd ed. Philadelphia, WB Saunders, 1995.

Galantino ML. Clinical Assessment and Treatment of HIV: Rehabilitation of a Chronic Illness. Thorofare NJ, Slack Incorporated, 1992.

Girolami UD, Henin D and Hauw JJ. Ocular pathology. In Nash G and Said JW (eds). Pathology of AIDS and HIV Infection. Philadelpha, WB Saunders, 1992.

Grady C. HIV disease: Pathogenesis and treatment. In Faskerud JH and Ungvarski PJ (eds). HIV/AIDS: A Guide to Nursing Care, 2nd ed. Philadelphia, WB Saunders, 1992.

Grimes DE and Grimes RM. AIDS and HIV Infection. St. Louis, CV Mosby, 1994.

Hartshorn KL. Antiretroviral therapy. In Libman H and Witzburg RA (eds). HIV Infection: A Clinical Manual, 2nd ed. Boston and Company, 1993.

Johnson MA and Johnstone FD. HIV Infection In Women. New York, Churchill Livingstone, 1993.

Kwan TH and Hood A. Associated cutaneous diseases. In Nash G and Said JW (eds). Pathology of AIDS and HIV Infection. Philadelphia, WB Saunders, 1992.

Land H. A Complete Guide to Psychosocial Intervention. Milwaukee, WI, Family Service America, 1992.

Leahne, RAL. Pharmocology for Nursing Care, 2nd ed. Philadelphia, WB Saunders, 1994.

Libman H and Witzburg RA. HIV Infection: A Clinical Manual, 2nd ed. Boston, Little, Brown and Company, 1993.

Mitsuyasu RT. Acquired immunodeficiency syndrome: Therapy for neoplastic complications. In Lichtenstein LM and Fauci AS (eds). Current Therapy In Allergy, Immunology, And Rheumatology, 4th ed. St Louis, BC Decker/Mosby Year Book, 1992.

Nash G and Said JW. Pathology of AIDS and HIV Infection. Philadelphia, WB Saunders, 1992.

Nash S. Gastrointestinal and hepatobiliary disease. In Nash G and Said JW (eds). Pathology of AIDS and HIV Infection. Philadelphia, WB Saunders, 1992.

National Association of People with AIDS. HIV in America: A Profile of the Challenges Facing Americans Living With HIV. Washington DC, National Association of People with AIDS, 1992.

National Research Council. AIDS: The Second Decade. Washington, DC, National Academy Press, 1990.

Pinching AJ. Acquired immune deficiency syndrome (AIDS). In Roitt IM and Delves PJ (eds). Encyclopedia of Immunology (Vol 1). New York, Academic Press, 1992.

Scura KW and Whipple B. HIV infection and AIDS and the elderly. In Stanley M and Beare PG (eds). Gerontological Nursing. Philadelphia, FA Davis Company, 1995.

Schochetman G and George JR. AIDS Testing Methodology and Management Issues. New York, Springer-Verlag, 1992.

Siano N and Lipsett S. No Time to Wait: A Complete Guide to Treating, Managing and Living with HIV infection. New York, Bantam Books, 1993.

Sonigo P and Girard M. AIDS vaccines: Concepts and first trials. In Rosen FS and Seligmann M (eds). Immunodeficiencies. Newark NJ, Gordon and Breach, 1993.

Tizard IR. Immunology: An Introduction, 3rd ed. Philadelphia, Saunders College Publishing, 1992.

Venna N. Neurologic manifestations. In Libman H and Wirtzburg RA (eds). HIV Infection: A Clinical Manual, 2nd ed. Boston, Little, Brown and Company, 1993.

Viner BL. Pneumocystis pneumonia. In Libman H and Witzburg RA (eds). HIV Infection: A Clinical Manual, 2nd ed. Boston, Little, Brown and Company, 1993.

Virella G, Goust JM, and Fudenberg HH (eds). Introduction to Medical Immunology, 2nd ed. New York, Marcel Dekker, 1990.

Wagner RP and Farber HW. Pulmonary manifestations. In Libman H and Witzburg RA (eds). HIV Infection: A Clinical Manual, 2nd ed. Boston, Little, Brown and Company, 1993.

Watstein SB and Laurich RN. Source Book: AIDS and Women. Phoenix, Oryx Press, 1991.

Workman ML, Ellerhorst-Ryan J and Hargrave-Koertge V Nursing Care of the Immunocompromised Patient. Philadelphia, WB Saunders, 1993.

Journals

Asterisks indicate nursing research articles.

*Anderson R, Grady C and Ropka M. A comparison of calculated energy requirements to measured resting energy expenditure in HIV-1–infected subjects. JANAC 1994 Nov–Dec; 5(6):30–34.

*Baigis-Smith J, Coombs VJ and Larson E. HIV infection, exercise and immune function. Image J Nurs Scholarship 1994 Winter; 26(4):277–281.

*Beaman ML and Strader MK. STD patients' knowledge about AIDS and attitudes toward condom use. J Community Health Nurs 1989; 6(3):155–164.

Benedict S and Colagreco J. Fungal infections associated with malignancies, treatments, and AIDS. Cancer Nurs 1994 Oct; 17(5):411–417.

Bornstein J, Rahat MA and Abramovici H. Etiology of cervical cancer: Current concepts. Obstet Gynecol Surv 1995 Feb; 50(2):146–154.

Bradley-Springer LA. Reproductive decision-making in the age of AIDS. Image J Nurs Scholarship 1994 Fall; 26(3):241–246.

Centers for Disease Control, U.S. Department of Health and Human Services. 1993 revised classification system for HIV infection and expanded surveillance case definition for AIDS among adolescents and adults. MMWR 1992; 41(RR 17):1–19.

Chlebowshi RT et al. Long term effects of early nutritional support with new enterotropic peptide-based formulas vs. standard enteral formula in HIV-infected patients: Randomized propsective trial. Nutrition 1993 Nov/Dec; 9(6):507–512.

Cole FL and Slocumb EM. Mode of acquiring AIDS and nurses' intention to provide care. Res Nurs Health 1994 Aug; 17(4): 303–309.

Durham JD. The changing HIV/AIDS epidemic: Emerging psychosocial challenges for nurses. Nurs Clin North Am 1994 Mar; 29(1):9–18.

Dwyer JT et al. The use of unconventional remedies among HIV-positive men living in California. JANAC 1995 Jan–Feb; 6(1): 17–28.

*Elderidge AD et al. Prevalence and characteristics of pain in persons with terminal-stage AIDS. J Adv Nurs 1994 Aug; 20(2): 260–268.

Grady C and Vogel S. Laboratory methods for diagnosing and monitoring HIV infection. JANAC 1993 Apr–Jun; 4(2):11–21.

Hall BA. Ways of maintaining hope in HIV disease. Res Nurs Health 1994 Aug; 17(4):283–293.

Hamilton JD et al. A controlled trial of early versis late treatment with zidovudine in symptomatic human immunodeficiency virus infection: Results of the Veterans Affairs Cooperative Study. N Engl J Med 1992; 326:437–443.

Harvath TA et al. Dementia-related behaviors in Alzheimer's disease and AIDS. J Psychosoc Nurs Mental Health Services 1995 Jan; 33(1):35–39.

Hedges CB. Recognizing the patient at risk for opportunistic infections. Medsurg Nurs 1994 Dec; 3(6):445–452.

Ho DD et al. Rapid removal of plasma virons and CD4 lymphocytes in HIV infection. Nature 1995 Jan 12; 373(6510):123–126.

Hoover DR. The effects of long-term zidovudine therapy and *Pneumocystis carinii* prophylaxis on HIV disease. A review of the literature. Drugs 1995 Jan; 49(1):20–36.

*Hoyt MJ et al. The effect of chemical dependency on pain perceptions in persons with AIDS. JANAC 1994 May–Jun; 5(3):33–38.

*Hurley PM and Ungvarski PJ. Home healthcare needs of adults living with HIV disease/AIDS in New York City. JANAC 1994 Mar–Apr; 5(2):33–40.

*Janson-Bjerklie S, Holzemer W and Henry SB. Patients' perceptions of pulmonary problems and nursing interventions during hospitalization for *Pneumocystis carinii* pneumonia. Am J Crit Care 1992 July; 1(1):114–121.

Klaus BD. Late manifestations of HIV infection and AIDS. Nurse Practitioner: Am J Primary Health Care 1994 Jun; 19(6):4–5.
Kulwicki A and Cass PS. An assessment of Arab American knowledge, attitudes, and beliefs about AIDS. Image J Nurs Scholarship. 1994 Spring; 26(1):13–17.
*Lauver D et al. HIV risk status and preventive behaviors among 17,619 women. J Obstet Gynecol Neonatal Nurs 1995 Jun; 24(1):33–39.
Lovejoy NC and Anastasi JK. Squamous cell cervical lesions in women with and without AIDS: Biochemical risk factors, prevention, and policy. Cancer Nurs 1994 Aug; 17(4):294–307.
Masur H et al. Public Health Service Task Force recommendations for antipneumocystis prophylaxis for patients infected with HIV. AIDS Patient Care 1990 Apr; 4(2):5–14.
McCann TV. The global epidemic of human immunodeficiency virus infection: Past reflections, future directions. Holistic Nurs Practice 1995 Jan; 9(2):18–29.
Merrill A. AIDS and malnutrition: Dual assaults on the body. Home Healthcare Nurs 1995 Jan–Feb; 13(1):56–63.
Mosdell KW and Viscounti JA. Emerging indications for octreoide therapy, part 1. Am J Hosp Pharm 1994 May 1; 519:1184–1193.
Mosier L. The stigmatized patient with AIDS in the intensive care unit: The role of the advanced practice nurse. AACN Clin Iss Crit Care Nurs 1994 Nov; 5(4):495–500.
*Newshan GT and Wainapel SF. Pain characteristics and their management in persons with AIDS. JANAC 1993 April–June; 4(2): 53–59.
Newton HB. Common neurologic complications of HIV-1 infection and AIDS. Am Fam Physician 1995 Feb 1; 51(2):387–398.
*Nokes KM, Wheeler K and Kendrew J. Development of an HIV assessment tool. Image J Nurs Scholarship. 1994 Summer; 26(2): 133–138.
Norr KF et al. AIDS prevention for women: A community-based approach. Nurs Outlook 1992 Nov/Dec; 40(6):250–256.
O'Dell M and Dillon ME. Rehabilitation in adults with human immunodeficiency virus-related diseases. Am J Med Rehabil 1992 June; 71(3):183–190.
*Powell-Cope GM. Family caregivers of people with AIDS: Negotiating partnerships with professional health care providers. Nurs Res 1994 Nov–Dec; 43(6):324–330.
Schuerman DA. Clinical concerns: AIDS in the elderly. J Gerontol Nurs 1994 Jul; 20(7):11–17.
Smeltzer SC. Women and AIDS: Sociopolitical issues. Nursing Outlook 1992 July/August; 40(4):152–157.
Smeltzer SC and Whipple. Women and HIV infection. Image: J Nurs Scholarship 1991 Winter; 23(4):249–256.
Tierney AJ. HIV/AIDS—Knowledge, attitudes and education of nurses: A review of the research. J Clin Nurs 1995 Jan; 4(1): 13–21.
Ungvarski PJ. Comorbidities of HIV-1/AIDS in adults. JANAC 1994 Nov–Dec; 5(6):35–44.
Ungvarski PJ, Schmidt J, and Neville S. Planning home care services for people living with AIDS. Home Healthcare Nurse 1994 Mar–Apr; 12(2):17–23.
U.S. Department of Health and Human Services. Guidelines for prevention of transmission of HIV and hepatitis B virus to health-care and public safety workers. MMWR 1989 Jun; 38 (S-6):3–37.
U.S. Department of Health and Human Services. HIV/AIDS Surveillance Report 1994 December; 6(2):1–39.
Van Wissen K and Wooden K. Nurses' attitudes and concerns to HIV/AIDS: A focus group approach. J Adv Nurs 1994 Dec; 20(6):1141–1147.
Wei X et al. Viral dynamics in human immunodeficiency virus type I infection. Nature 1995 Jan 12; 373(6510):117–122.
Wyness MA. AIDS demenia complex: Guidelines for nursing care. AXON 1994 Dec; 16(2):37–46.
Zelewsky MG and Birchfield M. Women living with the human immunodeficiency virus: Home-care needs. J Obstet Gynecol Neonatal Nurs 1995 Feb; 24(2):165–172.

INFORMATION/RESOURCES

Agencies

AIDS Action Council
729 Eighth St. SE, Suite 200,
Washington, DC 20003,
(202) 547-3101

AIDS Clinical Trials Information Service
P.O. Box 6003
Rockville, MD 20849-6003
800-874-2572 (800-TRIALS-A),
800-243-7012,
301-738-6616 (FAX)

AIDS Program
Centers for Infectious Diseases, CDC
1600 Clifton Rd.,
Atlanta, GA 30333,
(800) 342-AIDS

American Foundation for AIDS Research
733 Third Avenue, 12th Floor
New York, NY 10017
212-682-7440,
212-682-9812 (FAX)

American Red Cross
AIDS Education Office, 431 18th St NW,
Washington, DC 20006,
(202) 737-8300 (or local Red Cross)

CDC National AIDS Clearinghouse
P.O. Box 6003
Rockville, MD 20849-6003,
800-458-5231,
800-243-7012,
301-738-65616 (FAX)

CDC National AIDS Hotline
P.O. Box 12827 Research Triangle Park,
NC 27709
800-342-AIDS,
800-344-7432 (Spanish),
800-243-7889

Gay Men's Health Crisis Network
P.O. Box 274, 132 West 24th St.,
New York, NY 10011,
(212) 807-6655

Hemophilia and AIDS/HIV Network for the Dissemination of Information The National Hemophilia Foundation
110 Greene Street, Suite 303
New York, NY 10012
212-431-8541,
800-42-HANDI,
212-431-0906 (FAX)

Hispanic AIDS Committee for Education and Resources
1139 W Hildebrant, Suite B,
San Antonio, TX 78201,
(512) 732-3108

Hispanic AIDS Forum
c/o APRED, 853 Broadway Suite 2007,
New York, NY 10003,
(212) 870-1902 or 870-1864
HIV Telephone Consultation Service from San Francisco General Hospital 800-933-3413

Minority Task Force on AIDS
c/o New York City Council of Churches,
475 Riverside Dr., Room 456,
New York, NY 10115,
(212) 749-1214

Mothers of AIDS Patients (MAP)
c/o Barbara Peabody,
3403 E St., San Diego, CA 92102,
(619) 234-3432

National Association of People with AIDS
1413 K Street, N.W., Eighth Floor
Washington, D.C. 20005
202-898-0414,
202-898-0435 (FAX),
703-998-3144 (BBS)

National AIDS Information Clearinghouse (NAIC)
P.O. Box 6003,
Rockville, MD 20850,
(301) 762-5111

National Coalition of Gay Sexually Transmitted Disease Services
c/o Mark Behar,
P.O. Box 239,
Milwaukee, WI 53201-0239,
(414) 277-7671

National Council of Churches/AIDS Task Force
475 Riverside Dr., Room 572,
New York, NY 10115,
(212) 870-2421

National Lawyers Guild AIDS Network
211 Gough St., 3rd Floor,
San Francisco, CA 94102
293-2437

National Library of Medicine
8600 Rockville Pike
Bethesda, MD 20894
301-496-6308 (Public Information)

New York City Department of Health Division of AIDS Program Service
125 W orth St., Box A/1,
New York, NY 10013,
(212) 566-7103,
Hotline: (718)485-8111

Project Inform
1965 Market Street, Suite 220
San Francisco, CA 94103
415-558-8669,
800-882-7422,
415-558-0684 (FAX)

Public Affairs Office
Hubert H. Humphrey Bldg., Room 725-H,
200 Independence Ave. SW,
Washington, DC 20201,
(202) 245-6867

AIDS Education and Training Centers (ETCs)

Central Office

AIDS ETC Program
5600 Fishers Lane, Room 4C-03
Rockville, MD 20857
301-443-6364,
301-433-8890 (FAX)
Contact for information about local ETC.

AIDS Hotlines

English: (800) 342-AIDS (2437)
Spanish: (800) 344-7432
TDD Service for the Deaf: (800) 243-7889
HIV Telephone Consultation Service: (800) 933-3413
American Foundation for AIDS Research: (800) 39AMFAR (392-6327)
AIDS Treatment Data Network: (212) 268-4196
AIDS Treatment News: (800) TREAT 1-2 (873-2812)
AIDS Clinical Trials Information Service (ACTIS): (800) TRIALS-A (874-2572)
Drug Abuse Hotline (800) 662-HELP (4357)
Pediatric and Pregnancy AIDS Hotline (212) 430-3333
National Hemophilia Foundation (212) 219-8180
Hemophilia and AIDS/HIV Network for Dissemination of Information (HANDI) (800) 42-HANDI (424-2634)
National Pediatric HIV Resource Center (800) 362-0071
National Association of People with AIDS (202) 898-0414
Teens Teaching AIDS Prevention Program (TTAAPP) National Hotline(800) 234-TEEN (8336)
National Gay Task Force AIDS Information Hotline: (800) 221-7044; (212) 807-6016 (NY State)
National Sexually Transmitted Disease Hotline/American Social Health Association: (800) 227-8922
PHS AIDS Hotline: (800) 342-AIDS; (800) 342-2437

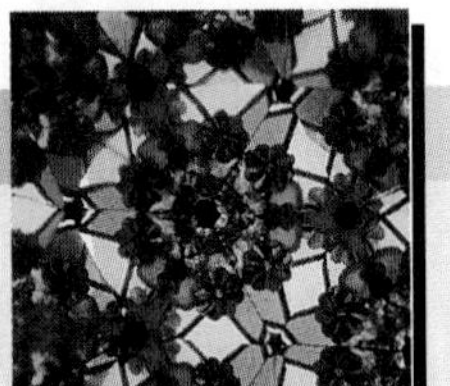

51

Management of Patients With Allergic Disorders

CHAPTER OUTLINE

LEARNING OBJECTIVES

On completion of this chapter, the learner will be able to:

1. Describe the types of hypersensitivity
2. Explain the physiology underlying allergic reactions
3. Describe the management and nursing care of patients with allergic disorders
4. Use the nursing process as a framework for care of the patient with allergic rhinitis
5. Describe the prevention and management of anaphylaxis

The human body is menaced by a host of potential invaders—allergens as well as microbial organisms—that constantly threaten its surface defenses. After penetrating those defenses, agents compete with the body for its nutrients and, if allowed to flourish unimpeded, disrupt its enzyme systems and destroy its vital tissues. To protect against these agents, the body is equipped with an elaborate defense system. The first line of defense consists of the epithelial cells that coat the skin and make up the lining of the respiratory, gastrointestinal, and genitourinary tracts. The structure and continuity of these surfaces and the resistance to penetration are initial deterrents to invaders.

One of the most effective body defense mechanisms is its capacity to equip itself rapidly with weapons (*antibodies*) individually designed to meet each new invader, namely, specific protein *antigens*. Antibodies react with antigens in a variety of ways: (1) by coating their surface if they are particular substances, (2) by neutralizing them if they are toxic, and (3) by precipitating them out of solution if they are dissolved. The antibodies prepare the antigen for action by the phagocytic cells of the blood and the tissues.

If the antigen is truly foreign, the body is protected against it; if not, *immunopathology* may occur. When this happens, the normally protective immune response results in dysfunctions within the immune system. *Hypersensitivity* (allergy) disorders are those diseases in which the body produces inappropriate or exaggerated responses to specific antigens.

Allergic Reaction: Physiologic Overview

Antibody Production

B Cells and Immunoglobulins

The *B cell*, or *B lymphocyte*, is programmed to produce one specific antibody. When a B cell encounters a specific antigen, it stimulates production of plasma cells. The plasma cell is the site of antibody production. The response of this mechanism to an antigen is the outpouring of antibody for the purpose of destroying and removing the antigen.

Antibodies that are formed by lymphocytes and plasma cells in response to an immunogenic stimulus constitute a group of serum proteins called *immunoglobulins*. These can be found in the lymph nodes, tonsils, appendix, and Peyer's patches of the intestinal tract or circulating in the blood and lymph.

Classes of Immunoglobulins. There are five classes of immunoglobulins, designated as follows: IgE, IgD, IgG, IgM, and IgA. Antibodies of the IgM, IgG, and IgA classes have definite and well-established protective functions. These include neutralization of toxins and viruses, and precipitation, agglutination, and lysis of bacteria and other foreign cellular material. (See Chapter 48 for further discussion of these functions.)

IgE levels are elevated in allergic disorders and some parasitic infections. IgE-producing cells are located in the respiratory and intestinal mucosa. Two or more IgE molecules bind together to an allergen and trigger mast cells or basophils to release histamine, serotonin, kinins, slow-reacting substance of anaphylaxis (SRS-A), and the neutrophil factor. These mediators produce allergic skin reaction, asthma, and hay fever. The remaining immunoglobulins are discussed in Chapter 48.

Antibody/Antigen Combination. Antibodies combine with antigens in a very special way, which has been likened to keys fitting into a lock. Antigens (keys) only fit certain antibodies (locks); hence, the term *specificity* has been coined in relation to the specific reaction of an antibody to an antigen. There are many variations and complexities in these patterns.

Antibody molecules are *bivalent,* that is, they have two combining sites. Because of this, the antibody easily becomes a cross-link between two antigen groups, causing them to clump together (*agglutination*). By this action, foreign invaders in the bloodstream are cleared. Agglutination is the means of determining blood group in laboratory tests.

T Cells

The *T cell,* or *T lymphocyte,* a second type of lymphocyte with a major role in the immune system, assists the B cells or lymphocytes in the production of antibodies. T cells work by secreting substances known as *lymphokines,* which assist the immune response by encouraging cell growth, promoting cell activation, directing the flow of cell activity, destroying target cells, and stimulating the macrophages. Macrophages digest antigens and present the antigen to the T cells; they initiate the immune response and assist in removal of cells and other debris.

Antigens that are important in immediate hypersensitivity are divided into two groups: complete protein antigens and low-molecular-weight substances.

Complete Protein Antigens. Complete protein antigens, such as animal dander, pollen, and horse serum, stimulate a complete humoral response. (*Humoral immunity* refers to substances, including antibodies, that circulate primarily in the serum and lymph.)

Low-Molecular-Weight Substances. Low-molecular-weight substances, such as medications, function as haptens (incomplete antigens) binding to tissue or serum proteins to produce a carrier complex that initiates an antibody response. The production of antigen-specific IgE antibodies requires active communication between macrophages, T cells, and B cells. Allergen sensitization begins when the allergen is absorbed through the respiratory tract, gastrointestinal tract, or skin. The macrophage processes the antigen and presents it to the appropriate T cell. B cells that are influenced by the T cell mature into an allergen-specific IgE immunoglobulin—secreting plasma cell that synthesizes and secretes antigen-specific IgE antibody (Fig. 51-1).

Chemical Mediators

When mast cells are stimulated by antigens, powerful chemical mediators are released that cause a sequence of physiologic events resulting in symptoms of immediate hypersensitivity. There are two types of chemical mediators: primary, which are preformed and found in mast cells or basophils, and secondary, which are inactive precursors formed or re-

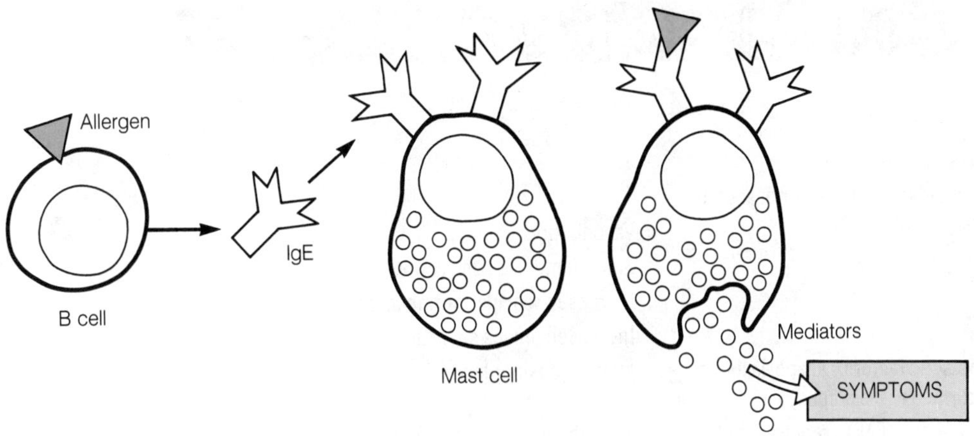

FIGURE 51-1. Allergen triggers B cell to make IgE antibody, which attaches to mast cell. When that allergen reappears, it binds to the IgE and triggers the mast cell to release its chemicals. (U.S. Dept. of Health and Human Services. Understanding the Immune System. NIH Publication No. 88-529, July 1988, p 19.)

leased in response to primary mediators. The most prevalent known primary and secondary mediators are described below. (See Table 51-1 for a summary of the actions of primary and secondary chemical mediators.)

Primary Mediators

Histamine. Histamine plays an important role in regulating the immune response. Physiologic effects of histamine upon major organs include (1) contraction of bronchial smooth muscle resulting in wheezing and bronchospasm, (2) dilation of small venules and constriction of larger vessels, causing erythema, edema, and urticaria, and (3) an increase in secretion of gastric and mucosal cells, resulting in diarrhea. Histamine acts on many target organs through two types of receptors: H_1 and H_2 receptors. Histamine receptors appear on different types of lymphocytes, particularly T-lymphocyte suppressor cells and basophils. H_1 receptors are found predominantly on bronchiolar and vascular smooth muscle cells. H_2 receptors are found on gastric parietal cells. Antihistamines are categorized by these receptors. Diphenhydramine (Benadryl) is an example of an antihistamine medication displaying an affinity for H_1 receptors, whereas cimetidine, another pharmacologic agent, targets H_2 receptors to inhibit gastric secretions in peptic ulcer disease.

Eosinophil Chemotactic Factor of Anaphylaxis (ECF-A). This chemotactic factor is preformed in mast cells and released upon degranulation to inhibit the action of leukotrienes and histamine.

Platelet-Activating Factor (PAF). This factor is responsible for initiating platelet aggregation at sites of immediate hypersensitivity reactions. PAF also causes bronchoconstriction and increased vascular permeability. It also activates factor XII or Hageman factor, which induces the formation of bradykinin.

Leukotrienes. Leukotrienes are chemical mediators that initiate the inflammatory response. One of these substances, slow-reacting substance of anaphylaxis (SRS-A), has long been known to produce sustained spasm of the bronchioles. Compared with histamine, leukotrienes are 100 to 1000 times more potent in causing bronchospasm. Many manifestations of inflammation can be attributed, in part, to leukotrienes.

Bradykinin. Bradykinin contracts smooth muscles of the bronchi and blood vessels. It causes increased permeability of the capillaries resulting in edema. Bradykinin stimulates nerve cell fibers and produces pain.

Serotonin. Serotonin is released during platelet aggregation, causing contraction of bronchial smooth muscle.

Prostaglandins. Prostaglandins produce smooth muscle contraction as well as vasodilation and increased capillary permeability. The fever and pain that occur with inflammation are due, in part, to the prostaglandins.

Allergy

Allergy is an inappropriate and often harmful response of the immune system to normally harmless substances. An *allergic reaction* is a manifestation of tissue injury resulting from interaction between an antigen and an antibody. When the body is invaded by an antigen, usually a protein that is recognized as foreign, a series of events takes place with the goal of making the invader harmless, destroying it, and ridding the body of it. When lymphocytes respond to the antigen, antibodies are often produced. Common allergic reactions occur when the immune system of a susceptible person responds aggressively to a substance that is normally harmless (*e.g.*, dust, weed pollen). The production of chemical mediators in allergic reactions may produce symptoms that range from mild to life threatening.

The immune system is composed of many cells and organs and substances that are secreted by these cells and organs. These parts of the immune system must work together to assure adequate defense against invaders (*i.e.*, virus, bacteria, other foreign substances) without destruction of the body's own tissues by an overly aggressive reaction.

Hypersensitivity

A hypersensitivity reaction usually does not occur after the first exposure to an allergen. The reaction follows a reexposure after sensitization in a predisposed individual. Sensitization initiates the humoral response or buildup of antibodies. To promote understanding of the immunopathogenesis of disease, hypersensitivity reactions have been classified by

TABLE 51-1 Chemical Mediators of Hypersensitivity

Mediators	Action
Primary Mediators	
(Preformed and found in mast cells or basophils)	
Histamine (preformed in mast cells)	Vasodilation Smooth muscle contraction Increased vascular permeability Increased mucus secretions
Eosinophil chemotactic factor of anaphylaxis (ECF-A) (preformed in mast cells)	Attracts eosinophils
Platelet-activating factor (PAF) (requires synthesis by mast cells, neutrophils, and macrophages)	Smooth muscle contraction Incites platelets to aggregate and release serotonin and histamine
Prostaglandins (chemically derived from arachidonic acid; require synthesis by cells)	D and F series → bronchoconstriction E series → bronchodilation D, E, and F series → vasodilation
Basophil kallikrein (preformed in mast cells)	Frees bradykinin, which causes: a. Bronchoconstriction b. Vasodilation c. Nerve stimulation
Secondary Mediators	
(Inactive precursors formed or released in response to primary mediators)	
Bradykinin (derived from precursor kininogen)	Smooth muscle contraction Increased vascular permeability Stimulates pain receptors Increased mucus production
Serotonin (preformed in platelets)	Smooth mucle contraction Increased vascular permeability
Heparin (preformed in mast cells)	Anticoagulant
Leukotrienes (derived from arachidonic acid and activated by mast cell degranulation) C, D, and E or slow-reacting substance of anaphylaxis (SRS-A)	Smooth muscle contraction Increased vascular permeability

Gell and Coombs into four specific types of reactions (Fig. 51-2). Most allergies are identified as either type I or type IV hypersensitivity reactions.

Anaphylactic (Type I) Hypersensitivity

This is an immediate anaphylactic hypersensitivity with reaction beginning within minutes of exposure to an antigen. When chemical mediators continue to be released, a delayed reaction may continue for up to 24 hours. This reaction is mediated by IgE antibodies (reagins) rather than IgG or IgM antibodies. Type I hypersensitivity requires previous exposure to the specific antigen, which results in the production of IgE antibodies by plasma cells. This takes place in the lymph nodes where helper T cells aid in promoting this reaction. The IgE antibodies bind to membrane receptors on mast cells found in connective tissue and basophils. During reexposure, the antigen binds to adjacent IgE antibodies, activating a cellular reaction that triggers degranulation and the release of chemical mediators (histamine, leukotrienes, and eosinophil chemotactic factor of anaphylaxis [ECF-A]).

Primary chemical mediators are responsible for the symptoms of type I hypersensitivity because of their effects on the skin, lungs, and gastrointestinal tract. Clinical symptoms are determined by the amount of the allergen, the amount of mediator released, the sensitivity of the target organ, and the route of allergen entry. Type I hypersensitivity reactions may include both local and systemic anaphylaxis.

Atopic Diseases

A type I hypersensitivity response results in atopic (allergic) diseases, which affect 10% to 20% of the U.S. population. Genetic factors play a role in susceptibility to these diseases. Disorders characterized as atopic are anaphylaxis, allergic rhinoconjunctivitis, atopic dermatis, urticaria and angioedema,

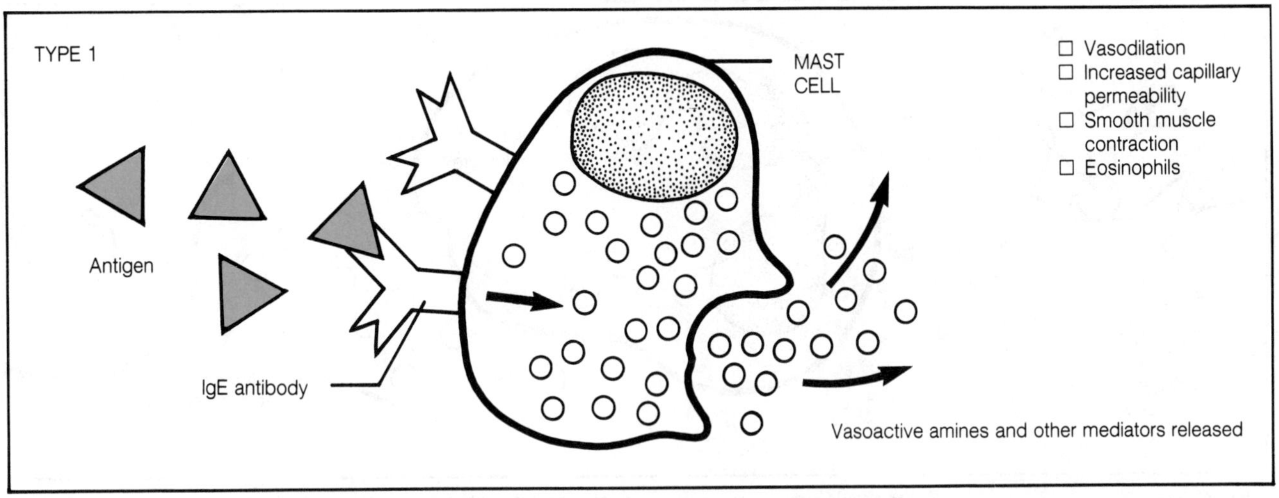

Reactions	Pathophysiology	Signs and symptoms	Clinical examples
Anaphylactic (immediate, atopic, IgE-mediated, reaginic)	IgE antibodies bind to certain cells; antigen binding causes release of vasoactive amines and other mediators, resulting in vasodilation, increased capillary permeability, smooth-muscle contraction, and eosinophilia.	Systemic: angioedema; hypotension; bronchial, GI, or uterine spasm; stridor Local: urticaria	Extrinsic asthma, seasonal allergic rhinitis, systemic anaphylaxis, reactions to stinging insects, some food and drug reactions, some cases of urticaria, infantile eczema

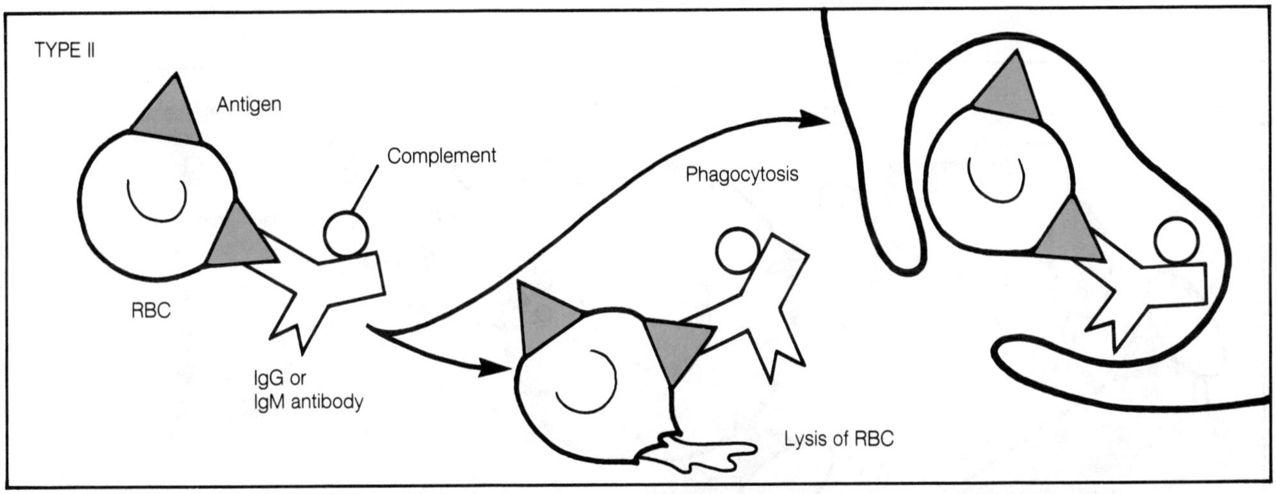

Reactions	Pathophysiology	Signs and symptoms	Clinical examples
Cytotoxic (cytolytic, complement-dependent cytotoxicity, cell-stimulating)	IgG or IgM antibodies bind to cellular or exogenous antigens. This can result in activation of complement components through C3 with phagocytosis or opsonization of the cell or activation of the full complement system with cytolysis or tissue damage.	Varies with disease; can include dyspnea, hemoptysis, fever	Goodpasture's syndrome, autoimmune hemolytic anemia, thrombocytopenia, pemphigus, pemphigoid, pernicious anemia, hyperacute graft rejection of transplanted kidney, transfusion reaction, hemolytic disease of the newborn, some drug reactions

FIGURE 51-2. Four types of hypersensitivity reactions. (Text of figure from Nurse's Clinical Library: Immune Disorders. Copyright 1985, Springhouse Corp.) *(continued)*

gastrointestinal allergy, and asthma. These atopic diseases are discussed under Common Allergic Disorders on p. 1430.

Cytotoxic (Type II) Hypersensitivity

A cytotoxic hypersensitivity occurs when the system mistakenly identifies a normal constituent of the body as foreign. This reaction may be a result of a cross-reacting antibody and could eventually lead to cell and tissue damage. Type II hypersensitivity involves the binding of either IgG or IgM antibody to the cell-bound antigen. The result of antigen-antibody binding is activation of the complement cascade (see Chapter 48) and destruction of the cell to which the antigen is bound.

A type II hypersensitivity reaction is involved in myasthenia gravis, in which the body mistakenly generates antibodies against normal receptors of nerve endings. Another example is Goodpasture's syndrome, in which antibodies

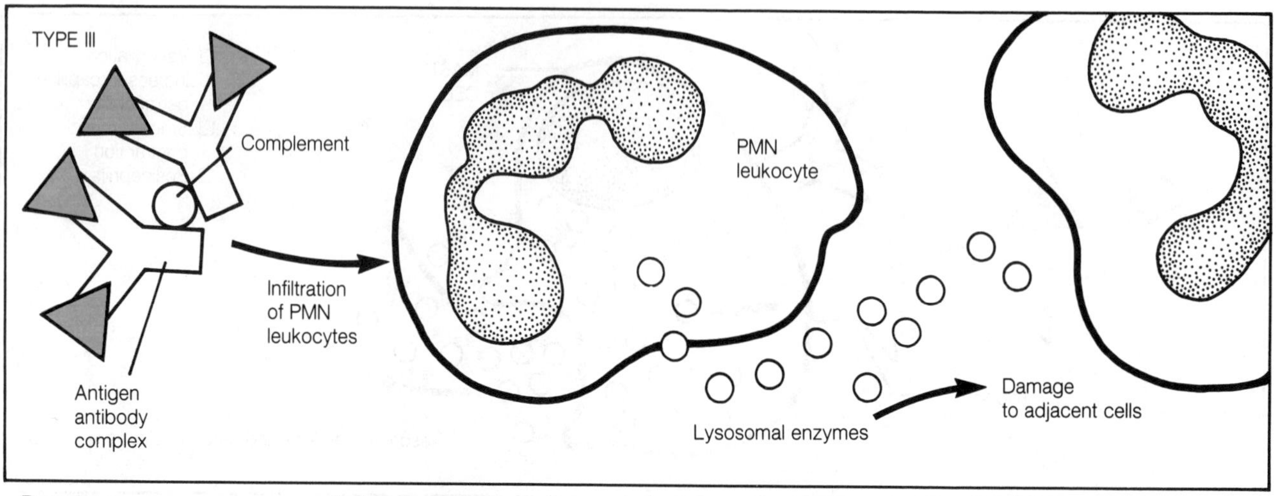

Reactions	Pathophysiology	Signs and symptoms	Clinical examples
Immune complex (soluble complex, toxic complex)	IgG or IgM antigen-antibody complexes are deposited in tissue where they activate complement. This reaction is marked by infiltration of polymorphonuclear leukocytes and by release of lysosomal proteolytic enzymes and permeability factors in tissues, which produce an acute, inflammatory reaction.	Urticaria; multiform, scarlatiniform, or morbilliform rash; adenopathy; joint pain; fever; serum sickness-like syndrome	Systemic: serum sickness due to serum, drugs, or viral hepatitis antigen; acute glomerulonephritis; systemic lupus erythematosus; rheumatoid arthritis; polyarteritis; cryoglobulinemia Local: Arthus reaction

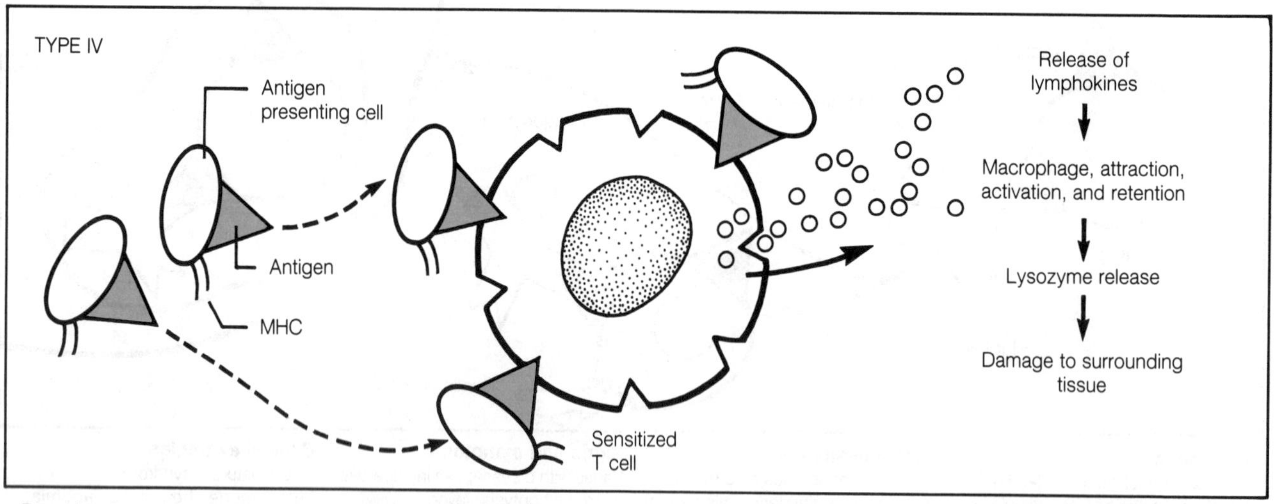

Reactions	Pathophysiology	Signs and symptoms	Clinical examples
Delayed (cellular, cell-mediated, tuberculin-type)	An antigen-presenting cell presents antigen to T cells in presence of MHC. The sensitized T cells release lymphokines, which stimulate macrophages; lysozymes are released; and surrounding tissue is damaged.	Varies with disease; can include fever, erythema, and itching.	Contact dermatitis, graft-versus-host disease, allograft rejection, granuloma due to intracellular organisms, some drug sensitivities, Hashimoto's thyroiditis, tuberculosis, sarcoidosis

FIGURE 51-2. *(continued)*

against lung and renal tissue are generated, producing lung damage and renal failure. Drug-induced immune hemolytic anemia, Rh-hemolytic disease of the newborn, and incompatible blood transfusion reactions are examples of type II hypersensitivities that result in red blood cell destruction.

Immune Complex (Type III) Hypersensitivity

Immune complexes are formed when antigens bind to antibodies and are cleared from the circulation by phagocytic action. When these complexes are deposited in tissues or vascular endothelium, two factors contribute to injury: the increased amount of circulating complexes and the presence of vasoactive amines. As a result, there is an increase in vascular permeability and tissue injury. The joints and kidneys are particularly susceptible to this type of injury. Type III hypersensitivity is associated with systemic lupus erythematosus, rheumatoid arthritis, serum sickness, certain types of nephritis, and some types of bacterial endocarditis.

Delayed-Type (Type IV) Hypersensitivity

This reaction, also known as cellular hypersensitivity, occurs 24 to 72 hours after exposure to an allergen. It is mediated by sensitized T cells and macrophages. An example of this reaction is the effect of an intradermal injection of tuberculin antigen or purified protein derivative (PPD). Sensitized T cells react with the antigen at or near the injection site. Release of lymphokines attracts, activates, and retains macrophages at the site. Lysozymes are released by macrophages, resulting in tissue damage. Edema and fibrin are responsible for the positive tuberculin reaction. Contact dermatitis is a type IV hypersensitivity that results from exposure to allergens such as cosmetics, adhesive tape, topical medications, medication additives, and plant toxins. The primary exposure results in sensitization; reexposure causes a hypersensitivity reaction composed of low-molecular-weight molecules or haptens that bind with proteins or carriers and are then processed by the Langerhans cells in the skin. The symptoms that occur include itching, erythema, and raised lesions.

Assessment and Diagnosis of Allergic Disorders

History and Physical Examination

A comprehensive allergy history and a thorough physical examination provide useful data for the diagnosis and management of patients with allergic disorders. An assessment sheet is useful for obtaining and organizing this information (Chart 51-1).

The degree of difficulty and discomfort experienced by the patient because of allergic symptoms and the degree of improvement in those symptoms with and without treatment are assessed and documented. The relationship of symptoms to exposure to possible allergens is noted.

Diagnostic Tests

Assessment of the patient with allergic disorders commonly includes blood tests, smears of body secretions, skin tests, and the RAST (radioallergosorbent test). Results of laboratory blood studies provide supportive data for various diagnostic possibilities; however, they are not the major criteria for the diagnosis of allergic disease. Initial studies may include the following:

Complete Blood Count With Differential. The white blood cell (WBC) count is usually normal except during infective states. Eosinophils normally make up 1% to 3% of the total number of WBC. A level between 5% and 15% is nonspecific but does suggest allergic reaction.

Moderate eosinophilia—15% to 40% of blood leukocytes as eosinophils are found in patients with allergic disorders as well as in patients with malignancy, immunodeficiencies, parasitic infections, congenital heart disease, and those receiving peritoneal dialysis.

Severe eosinophilia—50% to 90% of blood leukocytes as eosinophils are found in the idiopathic hypereosinophilic syndrome.

Total Eosinophil Count. Accurate counts of eosinophils can be obtained by using special diluting fluids that hemolyze erythrocytes and stain the eosinophils.

Smears for Eosinophils. During symptomatic episodes, nasal secretions, conjunctival secretions, and sputum of atopic patients usually reveal eosinophils, which indicate an active allergic response.

Total Serum IgE Levels. High total serum IgE levels support the diagnosis of atopic disease; however, a normal IgE level does not exclude the diagnosis of an allergic disorder. IgE levels are not as sensitive as the paper radioimmunosorbent test (PRIST) and the enzyme-linked immunosorbent assay (ELISA). Indications for determining IgE levels include:

- Evaluation of immunodeficiency
- Evaluation of drug reactions
- Initial laboratory screening for allergic bronchopulmonary aspergillosis
- Evaluation of allergy among children with bronchiolitis
- Differentiation of atopic and nonatopic eczema
- Differentiation of atopic and nonatopic asthma and rhinitis

Skin Tests. Skin testing entails the simultaneous intradermal injection or superficial application (epicutaneous), at separate sites, of several solutions. These contain individual antigens representing an assortment of allergens, including pollen, most likely to be implicated in the patient's disease. The clinical significance of positive reactions (wheal and flare) depends on correlation with the history, physical findings, and results of other laboratory tests.

Skin tests lend importance to other evidence obtained from the patient's history. They indicate which of several antigens are most likely to provoke symptoms, and they provide some clue to the intensity of the patient's sensitization.

The dosage of the pollen injected is also important. Most patients are hypersensitive to more than one pollen; under testing conditions, they may not react (although they usually do) to the specific pollens that induce their attacks.

If there is any doubt about the validity of the skin tests, a RAST (see p. 1430) or a provocative challenge test may be performed. In the provocative challenge test, the suspected antigen is applied to the sensitive tissue (such as the conjunctiva, nasal or bronchial mucosa, or to the gastrointestinal tract by ingestion of allergens) and the response is observed.

If a skin test is indicated, there is a reasonable suspicion that a specific allergen is producing symptoms in an allergic patient. Several precautionary steps, however, must be observed prior to skin testing:

- Testing is not performed during periods of bronchospasm.
- Epicutaneous tests (scratch or prick tests) are performed prior to other testing methods in an effort to minimize the risk of systemic reaction.
- Emergency equipment must be available to treat anaphylaxis (see pp. 1431–1432).

CHART 51-1
Allergy Assessment Sheet

Name ______ Age ______ Sex ______ Date ______

I. Chief complaint: ______

II. Present illness: ______

III. Collateral allergic symptoms: ______

Eyes: Pruritus ______ Burning ______ Lacrimation ______
Swelling ______ Injection ______ Discharge ______

Ears: Pruritus ______ Fullness ______ Popping ______
Frequent infections ______

Nose: Sneezing ______ Rhinorrhea ______ Obstruction ______
Pruritus ______ Mouth-breathing ______
Purulent discharge ______

Throat: Soreness ______ Postnasal discharge ______
Palatal pruritus ______ Mucus in the morning ______

Chest: Cough ______ Pain ______ Wheezing ______
Sputum ______ Dyspnea ______
Color ______ Rest ______
Amount ______ Exertion ______

Skin: Dermatitis ______ Eczema ______ Urticaria ______

IV. Family allergies

V. Previous allergic treatment or testing: ______
Prior skin testing: ______
Medications: Antihistamines Improved ______ Unimproved ______
Bronchodilators Improved ______ Unimproved ______
Nose drops Improved ______ Unimproved ______
Hyposensitization Improved ______ Unimproved ______
Duration ______
Antigens ______
Reactions ______
Antibiotics Improved ______ Unimproved ______
Corticosteroids Improved ______ Unimproved ______

VI. Physical agents and habits: ______

Bothered by:

Tobacco for ______ years
Cigarettes ______ packs/day
Cigars ______ per day
Pipes ______ per day
Never smoked ______
Bothered by smoke ______

Alcohol ______ Air cond. ______
Heat ______ Muggy weather ______
Cold ______ Weather changes ______
Perfumes ______ Chemicals ______
Paints ______ Hair spray ______
Insecticides ______ Newspapers ______
Cosmetics ______

VII. When symptoms occur: ______
Time and circumstances of 1st episode: ______
Prior health: ______
Course of illness over decades: progressing ______ regressing ______
Time of year: ______ Exact dates: ______
Perennial ______
Seasonal ______
Seasonally exacerbated ______
Monthly variations (menses, occupation): ______
Time of week (weekends vs. weekdays): ______
Time of day or night: ______
After insect stings: ______

VIII. Where symptoms occur: ______
Living where at onset: ______
Living where since onset: ______

(continued)

CHART 51-1 *(continued)*

Allergy Assessment Sheet

Effect of vacation or major geographic change: ____
Symptoms better indoors or outdoors: ____
Effect of school or work: ____
Effect of staying elsewhere nearby: ____
Effect of hospitalization: ____
Effect of specific environments: ____
Do symptoms occur around: ____
old leaves ____ hay ____ lakeside ____ barns ____
summer homes ____ damp basement ____ dry attic ____
lawnmowing ____ animals ____ other ____
Do symptoms occur after eating:
cheese ____ mushrooms ____ beer ____ melons ____
bananas ____ fish ____ nuts ____ citrus fruits ____
other foods (list) ____
Home: city ____ rural ____
house ____ age ____
apartment ____ basement ____ damp ____ dry ____
heating system ____
pets (how long) ____ dog ____ cat ____ other ____

Bedroom:	Type	Age	*Living room:*	Type	Age
Pillow	____	____	Rug	____	____
Mattress	____	____	Matting	____	____
Blankets	____	____	Furniture	____	____
Quilts	____	____			
Furniture	____	____			

Anywhere in home symptoms are worse: ____
IX. What does patient think makes symptoms worse? ____
X. Under what circumstances is patient free of symptoms? ____
XI. Summary and additional comments: ____

- The methods of skin testing include prick skin tests, scratch tests, and intradermal skin testing (Fig. 51-3). Following prick skin or scratch tests, intradermal skin testing is performed with allergens that did not elicit positive reactions. Since a larger antigen challenge is being used, local or systemic reactions could occur if the same antigens that produced positive skin or scratch reactions are used. The patient's back is the most suitable area of the body for skin testing because it permits the performance of many tests.

The Multi-Test applicator (Lincoln Labs) is a commercially available device with multiple test heads that allows simultaneous administration of antigens by multiple punctures at different sites.

Interpretation of Skin Tests. Familiarity with and consistent use of a chosen grading system are essential. The grading system used should be identified on a skin test sheet for later interpretation. A positive reaction, evidenced by the appearance of an urticarial wheal (Fig. 51-4) or by localized erythema (redness) in the area of inoculation or contact, is considered indicative of sensitivity to the corresponding antigen.

There may be false-negative results due to improper technique, outdated allergen solutions, and prior use of medications that suppress skin reactivity. Corticosteroids and antihistamines suppress skin test reactivity and should be withheld 48 to 96 hours before testing, depending on the duration of their activity. False-positive skin tests may result from improper preparation or administration of allergen solutions.

Interpretation of positive or negative skin tests must be based on the patient's history, physical examination, and other laboratory results. The following guidelines are used for the interpretation of skin test results:

1. Skin tests are more reliable for diagnosing atopic sensitivity in patients with allergic rhinoconjunctivitis than in patients with asthma.
2. Positive skin tests correlate highly with food allergy.
3. The use of skin tests to diagnose immediate hypersensitivity to medications is limited because metabolites of medications, not the medications themselves, are usually responsible for causing hypersensitivity.

Provocative Testing. Provocative testing involves the direct administration of an allergen to the respiratory mucosa with observation of target organ response. This type of testing is helpful in identifying clinically significant allergens in patients with a large number of positive tests. Major disadvantages of this type of testing are the limitation of one

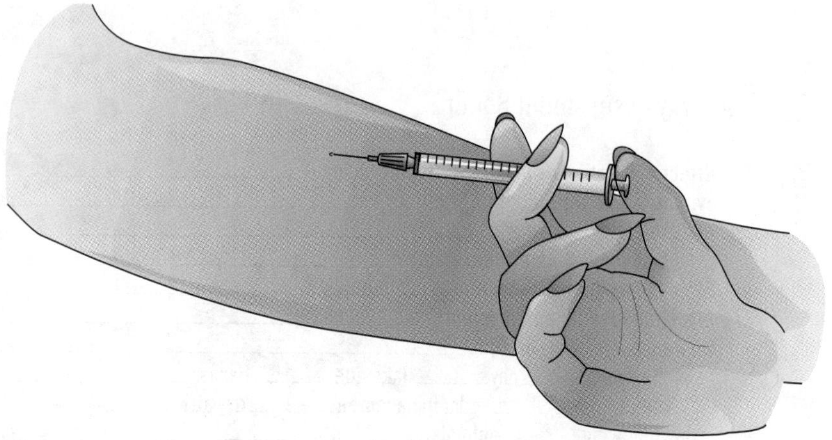

FIGURE 51-3. Intradermal testing. A 0.5-ml or 1-ml sterile syringe with a 26/27 gauge intradermal needle is used to inject 0.02 to 0.03 ml of intradermal allergen. The needle is inserted with the bevel facing upward and the syringe at a slight angle. The skin is penetrated superficially, and a small amount of the allergen solution is injected to create a bleb (raised area) approximately 5 mm in diameter. A separate sterile syringe and needle are used for each injection.

antigen per session and the risk of producing severe symptoms, particularly bronchospasm, in patients with asthma.

Radioallergosorbent Test. The radioallergosorbent test (RAST) is a radioimmunoassay that measures allergen-specific IgE. A sample of the patient's serum is exposed to a variety of suspected allergen particle complexes. If antibodies are present, they will combine with radio-labeled allergens. After the patient's serum is centrifuged, radioimmunoassay detects the allergen-specific IgE antibody. Test results are then compared with control values. In addition to detecting an allergen, RAST also indicates the quantity of allergen necessary to evoke an allergic reaction. Values are reported on a scale from 0 to 5; 2+ or greater is considered significant. The major advantages of RAST over other tests include (1) decreased risk of systemic reaction, (2) stability of antigens, and (3) lack of dependence on skin reactivity modified by medications. The major disadvantages include (1) the limited allergen selection, (2) reduced sensitivity as compared with intradermal skin tests, (3) lack of immediately available results, and (4) cost.

Allergic Disorders

Anaphylaxis

Anaphylaxis is a clinical response to an immediate (type I hypersensitivity) immunologic reaction between a specific antigen and an antibody. The reaction results from IgE antibody in the following manner: (1) An antigen attaches to the IgE antibody fixed to the surface membrane of mast cells and basophils, causing these target cells to become activated. (2) Mast cells and basophils then release mediators, causing vascular changes; activation of platelets, eosinophils, and neutrophils; and activation of the coagulation cascade. An anaphylactoid (anaphylaxis-like) reaction is clinically similar to anaphylaxis. However, it is not mediated by antigen—antibody interactions but rather as a result of substances that act directly on the mast cells or tissues causing the release of mediators. This reaction may occur with medications, food, exercise, and cytotoxic antibody transfusions.

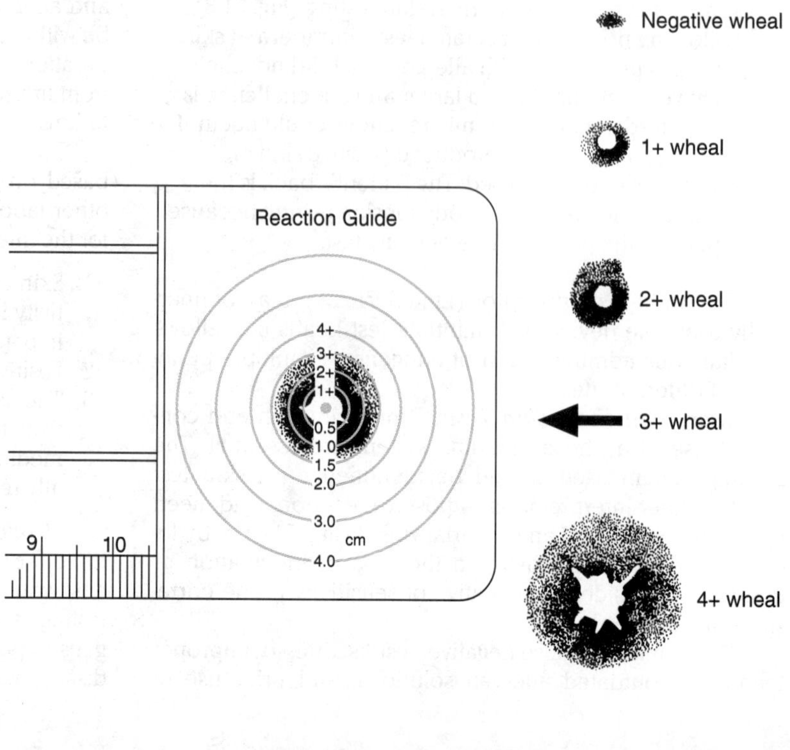

FIGURE 51-4. Interpretation of skin reactions following intradermal injection. Negative = wheal soft with minimal erythema. 1+ = wheal present (5–8 mm) with associated erythema. 2+ = wheal (7–10 mm) with associated erythema. 3+ = wheal (9–15 mm) slight pseudopodia possible with associated erythema. 4+ = wheal (12 mm+) with pseudopodia and diffuse erythema. (Courtesy of Center Laboratories, Port Washington, NY.)

Types of Analphylactic Reactions

Local. Local anaphylactic reactions usually involve urticaria and angioedema at the site of the antigen exposure and can be severe but are rarely fatal.

Systemic. Systemic reactions occur within approximately 30 minutes of exposure in the following organ systems: cardiovascular, respiratory, gastrointestinal, and integumentary.

Clinical Manifestations

The major signs and symptoms of anaphylactic reactions may be categorized as mild, moderate, and severe systemic reactions.

Mild. Mild systemic reactions consist of peripheral tingling and a warm sensation and may be accompanied by a fullness in the mouth and throat. Nasal congestion, periorbital swelling, pruritus, sneezing, and tearing of the eyes can also be expected. Onset of symptoms begins within the first 2 hours of exposure.

Moderate. Moderate systemic reactions may include any of the above symptoms in addition to flushing, warmth, anxiety, and itching. More serious reactions include bronchospasm and edema of the airways or larynx with dyspnea, cough, and wheezing. The onset of symptoms is the same as for a mild reaction.

Severe. Severe systemic reactions have an abrupt onset with the same signs and symptoms described above and progress rapidly to bronchospasm, laryngeal edema, severe dyspnea, and cyanosis. Dysphagia (difficulty swallowing), abdominal cramping, vomiting, diarrhea, and seizures can also occur. Rarely, cardiac arrest and coma result.

Treatment

Specific treatment depends on the severity of the reaction. Initially, respiratory and cardiovascular function are evaluated. If the patient is in cardiac arrest, cardiopulmonary resuscitation is instituted. Oxygen is provided in high concentrations during cardiopulmonary resuscitation or when a patient is cyanotic, dyspneic, or wheezing. Epinephrine, in a solution of 1:1000 dilution, is given subcutaneously in the upper extremity or thigh and may be followed by a continuous infusion. Antihistamines and corticosteroids may also be given to prevent recurrences of the reaction and for urticaria and angioedema. To maintain blood pressure and normal hemodynamic status, volume expanders and vasopressor agents are given. In persons with episodes of bronchospasm or a history of bronchial asthma or chronic obstructive pulmonary disease, aminophylline and corticosteroids may also be administered to improve airway patency and function. In instances where hypotension is unresponsive to vasopressors, intravenous administration of glucagon may be used for its acute inotropic and chronotropic effects. Patients with severe reactions are observed closely for 12 to 14 hours. Because of the potential for recurrences, patients with even mild reactions must be educated concerning this risk.

Patient Education: Prevention

Prevention is the single most important aspect of the management of anaphylaxis. Individuals sensitive to insect bites and stings, those who have experienced food or medication reactions, and those who have experienced idiopathic or exercise-induced anaphylactic reactions should always carry an emergency kit that contains epinephrine. The Epipen from Center Laboratories is a commercially available first-aid device that delivers premeasured doses of 0.3 mg (Epipen) and 0.15 mg (Epipen Jr.) of epinephrine (Fig. 51-5). The autoinjection system requires no preparation and the self-administration technique is uncomplicated (Guideline 51-1). The nurse provides instruction to all patients at risk for potentially fatal anaphylactic reactions. It is important that the patient be given an opportunity to demonstrate the correct technique for use; an Epipen training device is available to assist in this effort. The patient is provided with oral and written information about the emergency kit as well as strategies to avoid exposure to threatening allergens.

It is essential that a careful history of any sensitivity to suspected antigens be obtained before administering any medication, particularly in parenteral form, to a patient because this route is associated with the most severe anaphylaxis.

Patients who are predisposed to anaphylaxis should wear some form of identification related to drug allergies. One example is the Medic-Alert bracelet.

Persons who are allergic to insect venom may require venom immunotherapy, which is used as a control measure and not a cure. Insulin-allergic diabetic patients and penicillin-sensitive patients may require desensitization. Desensitization is based on controlled anaphylaxis with a gradual release of mediators. Patients who undergo desentization are cautioned that there should be no lapses in therapy since this may lead to the reappearance of an allergic reaction when the medication is reinstitued.

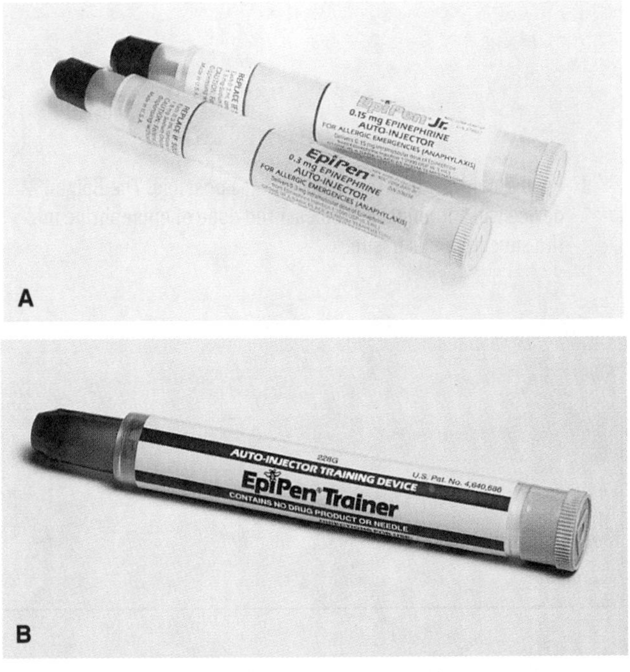

FIGURE 51-5. (**A**) The Epipen and Epipen Jr. Autoinjectors are commercially available first-aid devices that administer premeasured doses of epinephrine. (**B**) An Epipen training device is available for patients to practice correct self-injection technique. (Courtesy of Center Laboratories, Port Washington, NY.)

GUIDELINE 51-1
Self-Administration of Epinephrine

The patient is taught how to inject epinephrine in the event of an anaphylactic reaction. The patient should be encouraged to practice this technique using a training device.

1. Carefully uncap the Epipen® device, holding it so that the injecting end is upright.

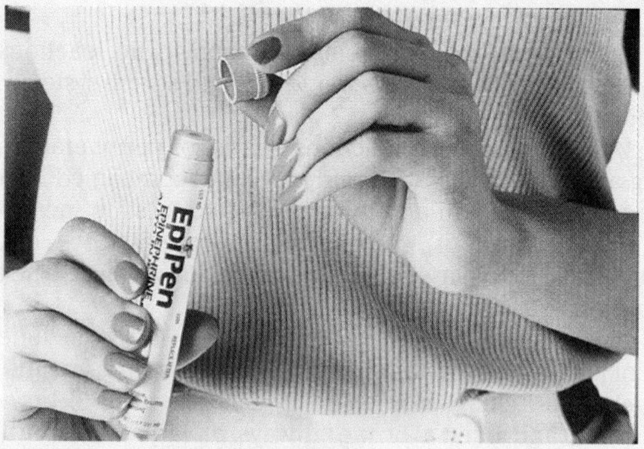

2. Position the device at the mid portion of the thigh.

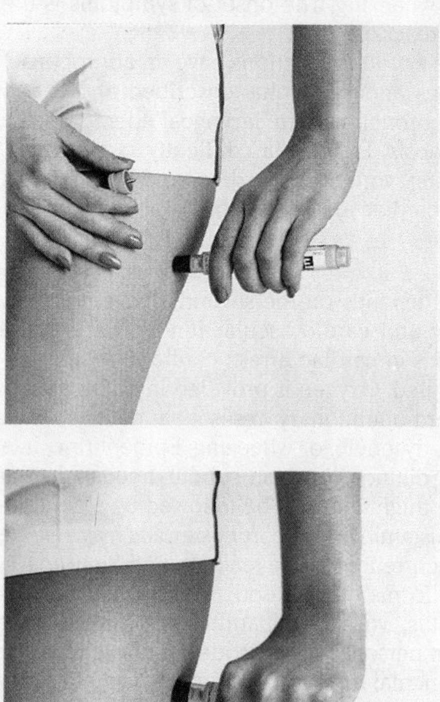

3. Push the device into the thigh as far as possible. The Epipen® device will autoinject a premeasured dose of epinephrine into the subcutaneous tissue.

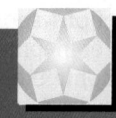

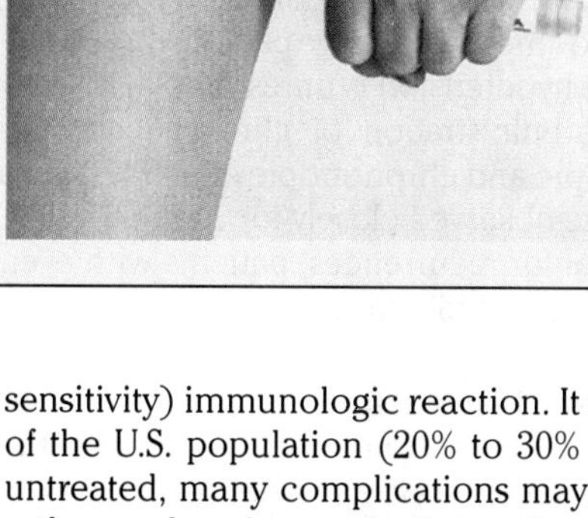

Allergic Rhinitis

Allergic rhinitis (hay fever, chronic allergic rhinitis, pollinosis) is the most common form of respiratory allergy presumed to be mediated by an immediate (type I hypersensitivity) immunologic reaction. It affects about 8% to 10% of the U.S. population (20% to 30% of adolescents). When untreated, many complications may result, such as allergic asthma, chronic nasal obstruction, chronic otitis media with hearing loss, anosmia (absence of the sense of smell), and, in children, orofacial dental deformities. Early diagnosis and adequate treatment are essential.

Because allergic rhinitis is induced by airborne pollens or molds, it is characterized by the following seasonal occurrences:

Early spring—tree pollen (oak, elm, poplar)
Early summer (rose fever)—grass pollen (Timothy, red-top)
Early fall—weed pollen (ragweed)

Each year, attacks begin and end at approximately the same time. Airborne mold spores require warm, damp weather. Although there is no rigid seasonal pattern, these spores appear in early spring, are rampant during the summer, and taper off and disappear by the first frost.

Pathophysiology

Sensitization begins by ingestion or inhalation of an antigen. On reexposure, the nasal mucosa reacts by the slowing of ciliary action, edema formation, and leukocyte (primarily eosinophil) infiltration. Histamine is the major mediator of allergic reactions in the nasal mucosa. Tissue edema is a result of vasodilation and increased capillary permeability.

Clinical Manifestations

Typical findings of allergic rhinitis include nasal congestion, clear, watery discharge, intermittent sneezing, and nasal itching. Itching of the throat and soft palate are common. Drainage of nasal mucus into the pharynx initiates multiple attempts to clear the throat and results in a dry cough or hoarseness. Headache, pain over the paranasal sinuses, and epistaxis can accompany allergic rhinitis. It is a chronic condition, and symptoms depend upon environmental exposure and intrinsic host responsiveness.

Diagnostic Evaluation

In most cases of seasonal allergic rhinitis, early diagnosis by history and physical examination is necessary. Diagnostic studies that may be performed include nasal smears, peripheral blood counts, total serum IgE, epicutaneous testing, intradermal testing, RAST, food elimination and challenge, and nasal provocation tests.

Management

The goal of therapy is to provide relief from symptoms. Therapy may include one or all of the following interventions: avoidance therapy, pharmacotherapy, or immunotherapy. It is essential that oral instruction be reinforced by written information to provide the patient with permanent reminders. A knowledge of general concepts regarding assessment and therapy in allergic diseases is important. The nurse has an active role in the management of patients with these disorders and may be in a position to advise patients who are potential candidates for one or another of these procedures.

Avoidance Therapy (Avoidance of Allergens)

In avoidance therapy, every attempt is made to remove those allergens that act as precipitating factors. Simple measures and environmental controls are often effective in decreasing symptoms. Examples of these include use of air conditioners, air cleaners, humidifiers/dehumidifiers, and smoke-free environments.

Pharmacotherapy

Antihistamines. Antihistamines are now classified as H_1-receptor antagonists or H_1-blockers, which are used in the management of mild allergic disorders, and H_2-receptor antagonists, which are used to treat gastric and duodenal ulcers. H_1-blockers bind selectively to H_1 receptors, preventing the actions of histamines at these sites. They do not prevent the release of histamine from mast cells or basophils. The H_1-antagonists have no effect on H_2-receptors, but they do have the ability to bind to nonhistaminic receptors. The ability of certain antihistamines to bind to and block muscarinic receptors underlies several of the prominent anticholingergic side effects of these medications.

Oral antihistamines are readily absorbed. They are most effective when given at the first occurrence of symptoms because they prevent the development of new symptoms by blocking the actions of histamine at the H_1-receptors. The effectiveness of these medications is limited to certain patients with hay fever, vasomotor rhinitis, urticaria (hives), and mild asthma. They are rarely effective in other conditions or in severe conditions of any sort.

Antihistamines are the major class of medications prescribed for the symptomatic relief of allergic rhinitis. The major side effect of this group of medications is sedation. Additional side effects include nervousness, tremors, dizziness, dryness of mouth, palpitations, anorexia, nausea, and vomiting. They are contraindicated during the third trimester of pregnancy, for nursing mothers and newborns, in children, the elderly, and in patients whose conditions can be aggravated by muscarinic blockade (*i.e.*, asthma, urinary retention, open-angle glaucoma, hypertension, and prostatic hypertrophy).

Newer antihistamines are called second-generation or nonsedative H_1-receptor antagonists. Unlike first-generation H_1-receptor antagonists, they do not cross the blood–brain barrier and do not bind to cholinergic, serotonin, or alpha adrenergic receptors. They bind to peripheral rather than central nervous system H_1-receptors, causing less sedation. Although they are no more potent than their predecessors and are more expensive than traditional antihistamines, they are gradually replacing the older H_1-receptor antagonists in the treatment of allergic rhinoconjunctivitis. They are generally well tolerated; however, two of them (terfenadine and astemizole) have been associated with fatal cardiac dysrhythmias, usually as a result of overdosage or concomitant use with any one of three antibiotics: erythomycin, itraconozole, or ketoconozole. Table 51-2 lists the chemical classes of first- and second-generation H_1 antihistamines, the side effects, and nursing implications.

Adrenergic Agents. Adrenergic agents are vasoconstrictors of mucosal vessels and are used topically (nasal and ophthalmic) in addition to the oral route. The topical route (drops and sprays) causes fewer side effects than oral administration; however, it is recommended that their use be limited to a few days to avoid rebound congestion. Adrenergic nasal decongestants are used for the relief of nasal congestion when applied topically to the nasal mucosa. They

TABLE 51-2 Chemical Classes of H_1 Antihistamines

Classification and Example	Major Side Effects	Nursing Implications
Sedating		
1. Ethanolamines Ex: diphenhydramine (Benadryl)	A. Drowsiness, confusion	A. Teach patient to avoid alcohol, driving, or engaging in any hazardous activities until CNS response to drug treatment is stabilized.
	B. Dry mouth, nausea, vomiting	B. Suggest sucking on hard candy or ice chips for relief of dry mouth.
	C. Photosensitivity	C. Encourage use of sunscreen and hat while outdoors.
	D. Urinary retention	D. Assess for urinary retention; monitor urinary output.
2. Piperazines Ex: hydroxyzine (Atarax)	A. Dulls mental alertness; drowsiness	A. Teach patient to avoid alcohol, driving, or engaging in any hazardous activities until CNS response to drug treatment is stabilized.
	B. Dry mouth	B. Suggest sucking on hard candy or ice chips for relief of dry mouth.
3. Alkylamines Ex: chlorpheniramine (Chlor-trimeton)	A. Causes less CNS depression than other groups. Best class for daytime use.	A. Teach patient to avoid alcohol, driving, or engaging in any hazardous activities until CNS response to drug treatment is stabilized.
4. Ethylenediamines Ex: tripelennamine (PBZ)	A. Produces GI upset	A. Administer medication with food or milk to decrease GI distress. Increase fluid intake.
	B. Drowsiness	B. Teach patient to avoid alcohol, driving, or engaging in any hazardous activities until CNS response to drug treatment is stabilized.
	C. Palpitations	C. Instruct patient to sit and relax a few minutes before activity.
5. Phenothiazines Ex: promethazine (Phenergan)	A. Produces heavy sedation and drowsiness	A. Teach patient to avoid alcohol, driving, or engaging in any hazardous activities until CNS response to drug treatment is stabilized.
	B. Nasal congestion	B. Encourage use of humidification at home.
	C. Hypotension	C. Instruct patient to rise from a sitting position slowly.
Non-sedating		
1. Astemizole (Hismanal)	A. Cardiac dysrhythmias, potential cardiac arrest	A. Teach patient not to exceed the prescribed dose; teach him to notify all physicians that he is on hismanal and is unable to take the antibiotics erythromycin, itraconazole, or ketoconaxole.
	B. Nausea, diarrhea, and abdominal pain	B. Teach patient to take medication at least 2 hours after a meal or have no food for 1 hour after taking the medication because of decreased or poor medication absorption.
	C. Increased appetite and weight gain	C. Counsel patient to monitor weight and report increase in appetite and weight to physician.
	D. Dizziness	D. Teach patient to avoid hazardous activity, stop medication, and notify physician. Dizziness may signal impending cardiac dysrhythmia.
2. Loratadine (Claritin)	A. Gastrointestinal upset	A. Counsel patient to take the medication on an empty stomach.
3. Terfenadine (Seldane, Teldane)	A. Cardiac dysrhythmias	A. Teach patient not to exceed the prescribed dose.
	B. Headache, dizziness	B. Teach patient to avoid hazardous activity. Stop medication if dizzy and notify physician; dizziness may signal impending cardiac dysrhythmia.
	C. Gastrointestinal upset	C. Teach patient to take medication with food.
	D. Drug interaction with antibiotics (erythromycin, itraconazole, and ketoconazole)	D. Teach patient to notify all physicians that he or she is on Seldane or Teldane and is unable to take certain antibiotics.

activate the alpha-adrenergic receptor sites on the smooth muscle of the nasal mucosal blood vessels; this reduces local blood flow, fluid exudation, and mucosal edema. Topical ophthalmic drops are used for symptomatic relief of eye irritations due to allergies. Potential side effects include hypertension, dysrhythmias, palpitations, CNS stimulation, irritability, tremor, and tachyphylaxis (acceleration of hemodynamic status).

Examples of adrenergic decongestants and their routes of administration are found in Table 51-3.

Intranasal Cromolyn Sodium. Intranasal cromolyn sodium (Nasalcrom) is a spray that acts by stabilizing the

TABLE 51-3 Adrenergic Decongestants and Their Routes of Administration

Adrenergic Decongestant	Generic Name	Route of Administration
Naphazoline hydrochloride	Privine	Topical
Oxymetazoline hydrochloride	Afrin, Dristan long-lasting, Neo-Synepherine 12 hour, Sinex long-lasting	Topical
Phenylephrine hydrochloride	Neo-Synepherine	Topical
Phenylpropanolamine hydrochloride	Propagest	Oral
Pseudoephedrine hydrochloride	Sudafed	Oral
Tetrahydrozoline hydrochloride	Collyrium, Murine Plus, Visine	Topical ophthalmic and nasal preparations
Xylometazoline hydrochloride	Neo-Synephrine II, Otrivin	Topical

mast cell membrane and inhibiting the release of histamine and other mediators of the allergic response. It is used prophylactically before exposure to allergens or therapeutically in chronic allergic rhinitis. It is as effective as antihistamines but less effective than intranasal steroids (see below) in the treatment of seasonal allergic rhinitis. It is important that patients be informed that the beneficial effects of the medication may take a week or so to develop. The medication is of no benefit in the treatment of nonallergic rhinitis. Adverse effects are usually mild (*i.e.*, sneezing, local stinging, and burning sensations).

Corticosteroids. Intranasal corticosteroids are indicated for more severe cases of allergic and perennial rhinitis that cannot be controlled by more conventional medications such as decongestants, antihistamines, and intranasal cromolyn. Currently, four preparations are available:

- Beclomethasone (Beconase, Vancenase)
- Dexamethasone (Decadron Phosphate Turbinaire)
- Flunisolide (Nasalide)
- Triamcinolone (Nasacort)

Owing to their anti-inflammatory actions, all four are equally effective in preventing or suppressing all of the major symptoms of allergic rhinitis. They are administered via metered spray devices. If the nasal passages are blocked, a topical decongestant can be used to clear the passages prior to the administration of the intranasal corticosteroid. It is important that patients be informed that full benefit may not be achieved for several days to 2 weeks.

Adverse effects of intranasal corticosteroids are mild and include drying of the nasal mucosa and burning and itching sensations. These effects are thought to be caused by the vehicle used to administer the medication and not by the medications themselves. Systemic effects are more likely with dexamethosone; it is recommended that use of this medication be limited to 30 days. Beclomethasone, flunisolide, and triamcinolone are deactivated rapidly after absorption so that they do not achieve significant blood levels. Since they can suppress host defenses, they must be used with caution in persons with tuberculosis or untreated bacterial infections of the lungs.

Oral and parenteral corticosteroids are used when conventional therapy has failed and symptoms are severe and of short duration. They can control symptoms of allergic reactions such as hay fever, medication-induced allergies, and allergic reactions to insect stings. Since the response to corticosteroids is delayed, they have little or no value in acute therapy for severe reactions such as anaphylaxis. Patients who receive corticosteroids must be cautioned not to stop taking the medication suddenly or without specific instructions from the physician. The patient is also instructed about side effects, which include fluid retention, weight gain, hypertension, gastric irritation, glucose intolerance, and adrenal suppression (see p. 1105).

Immunotherapy

Immunotherapy is indicated only when IgE hypersensitivity (type I hypersensitivity) is demonstrated to specific inhalant allergens that the patient is unable to avoid (house dust, pollens). Goals of immunotherapy include reducing the level of circulating IgE, increasing the level of blocking antibody IgG, and reducing mediator cell sensitivity. Immunotherapy has been most effective for ragweed pollen; however, treatment for grass, tree pollen, cat, and house dust mite allergens has also been effective.

Correlation of a positive skin test with a positive allergic history is an indication for immunotherapy if the allergen cannot be avoided. The value has been fairly well established in instances of allergic rhinitis and bronchial asthma that are clearly due to sensitivity to one of the common pollens, molds, or house dust. Although immunotherapy is referred to as a "hypersensitization" procedure, the effects are most likely attributable to the opposite process (*i.e.*, immunization). This procedure appears to stimulate the production of a new antibody with the capacity to neutralize the allergy-provoking properties of the responsible allergen.

Although helpful in most patients, immunotherapy does not cure the condition. Before immunotherapy is initiated, the patient must understand what to expect and the importance of continuing therapy for several years. When skin tests are performed, the results are correlated with clinical manifestations; treatment is based on the patient's needs rather than on skin tests.

The most common method of treatment is the serial injection of one or more antigens that are selected in each particular case on the basis of skin tests. This method provides a simple and efficient technique for identifying IgE antibodies to specific antigens. Specific treatment consists of injecting extracts of the pollens or mold spores that cause symptoms in a particular patient. Injections begin with very small amounts and are gradually increased, usually at weekly intervals, until a maximum tolerated dose is attained. Maintenance "booster" injections are given at 2- to 4-week intervals, frequently for a period of several years, before maximum benefit is achieved.

There are three methods of injection therapy: coseasonal, preseasonal, and perennial. When treatment is given on a **coseasonal basis,** it is initiated during the season in which the patient experiences symptoms. This method has been used less frequently in recent years because it has been found to be ineffective and there is increased risk of systemic reactions. **Preseasonal therapy** injections are given 2 to 3 months before symptoms appear, allowing time for hyposensitization to occur. This treatment is discontinued after the season begins. **Perennial therapy** is administered all year round, usually on a monthly basis, and is the preferred method owing to more effective, longer-lasting results.

Precautions. Because there is a possibility that the injection of an allergen may induce systemic reactions, it is given only in a physician's office or the clinic where epinephrine is immediately available. Because of the dangers involved, injections should not be given by a lay person or by the patient. The patient remains in the office or clinic for a minimum of 30 minutes and is observed for possible development of systemic symptoms. If a large, local swelling develops at the injection site, the next dose should *not* be increased, because this may be a warning of a possible systemic reaction. Therapeutic failure is evident when a patient does *not* (1) experience a decrease of symptoms within 12 to 24 months, (2) develop an increase in tolerance to known allergens, and (3) decrease the use of medications to reduce symptoms. Potential causes of treatment failure include misdiagnosis of allergies, inadequate doses of allergen, newly developed allergies, and inadequate environmental controls.

NURSING PROCESS
The Patient With Allergic Rhinitis

Assessment

The examination and history of the patient reveal sneezing, often in paroxysms, thin and watery nasal discharge, itching eyes and nose, lacrimation, and occasionally headache. The nursing history includes a personal or family history of allergy. The allergy assessment will identify the nature of antigens, seasonal changes in symptoms, and medication history. The nurse also obtains subjective data about how the patient feels just before symptoms become obvious, such as the occurrence of pruritus, breathing problems, and tingling sensations. In addition to these symptoms, hoarseness, wheezing, hives, rash, erythema, or edema is noted. Any relationship between emotional problems or stress and the triggering of allergy symptoms is assessed.

Diagnosis

Nursing Diagnoses

Based on the data collected from the patient history and assessment, the patient's major nursing diagnoses may include:

- Ineffective breathing pattern related to allergic reaction
- Knowledge deficit about allergy and the recommended modifications in life-style and self-care practices
- Impaired coping with chronicity of condition and need for environmental modifications

Collaborative Problems/ Potential Complications

Based on assessment data, potential complications may include:

- Anaphylaxis
- Impaired breathing
- Adverse reactions to medications
- Noncompliance with medical regimen

Planning and Implementation

Goals. The goals for the patient may include restoration of normal breathing pattern, knowledge about the causes and control of allergic symptoms, improved coping with alterations and modifications, and absence of complications.

Nursing Interventions

Improving Breathing Pattern. The patient is instructed and assisted to modify his environment to reduce the severity of allergic symptoms or prevent their occurrence. Additionally, he is instructed to maintain normal breathing patterns by reducing exposure to persons with upper respiratory infections (URIs). If URI occurs, the patient is encouraged to take deep breaths and cough frequently to assure adequate gas exchange and prevent atelectasis. The patient is instructed to seek medical attention, because allergy symptoms along with URI may compromise adequate lung function. Compliance with medications and other treatment regimens is encouraged and reinforced.

Increasing Knowledge About Allergy and Strategies to Control Symptoms. Instruction for the patient includes discussion of strategies to minimize exposure to allergens, desensitization procedures, and correct use of medications.

Instruction about other strategies to control allergic symptoms is based on the individual needs of the patient as determined by the results of tests, the severity of symptoms, and the motivation of the patient and family to deal with the condition. Some general suggestions for those sensitive to dust and mold in the home include the following:

1. Try to maintain a dust-free environment, particularly in the bedroom:
   a. Reduce contents to barest minimum; remove drapes, curtains, and venetian blinds and replace with pull shades.
   b. Remove carpets; wash woodwork and floor and thereafter dust and vacuum daily. Wood flooring or linoleum is preferable to rugs.
   c. Replace stuffed furniture with wood pieces that can be dusted easily.
   d. Avoid tufted bedspreads, stuffed toys, feather pillows; replace them with easily washable cotton material.
   e. Cover the mattress with a hypoallergenic cover that can be zippered to fit snugly.

f. Avoid wearing fabrics that cause itching.

2. Within the house as a whole, reduce dust by the following practices:
   a. Use steam or hot water for heating rather than hot air.
   b. Use air filters or air conditioning.
   c. Wear a mask if cleaning is being done.
3. For patients sensitive to pollen or mold, reduce exposure to them:
   a. Determine times of the year when pollen count is highest; reduce exposure at these times.
   b. Avoid barns, weeds, dry leaves, and freshly cut grass.
   c. Wear a mask at times of increased exposure (*e.g.*, windy days, when grass is being cut).
   d. Seek air-conditioned areas at the height of the allergy season.
   e. Take antihistamines as prescribed.
   f. Avoid sprays and perfumes; use hypoallergenic cosmetics.
4. Determine specific foods that may be a problem. Avoid what appears to be troublesome food for a period of time. By trial, one can develop a list of foods that are to be avoided. Examples include fish, nuts, eggs, and chocolate.

If the patient is to undergo desensitization, the nurse reinforces the physician's explanation regarding the purpose and procedure. It is necessary to follow instructions thereafter regarding the subsequent series of inoculations, usually given every 2 weeks or every month. These include (1) remaining in the physician's office at least 30 minutes after the injection so that emergency treatment may be given if the patient has a reaction, (2) avoiding rubbing or scratching the injection site, and (3) continuing with the series for the period of time required.

In addition to avoiding situations that bring on allergic symptoms, the patient needs to understand the rationale, actions, and side effects of all medications prescribed to control the allergy and the correct methods of administration.

Because antihistamines often produce drowsiness, the patient is cautioned about this and other side effects of the particular medication. Operating machinery, driving a car, and activities requiring intense concentration should be postponed. The patient is also informed about the dangers of drinking alcohol when taking these medications as they tend to exaggerate the effects of alcohol.

The patient must be aware of the effects caused by *overuse* of the sympathomimetic agents in nose drops or sprays. A condition referred to as *rhinitis medicamentosa* may result (Fig. 51-6). After topical application of the drug, a rebound period may occur in which the nasal mucous membranes become more edematous and congested than they were before the medication was used. Such a reaction encourages the use of more drug. A cyclical pattern of activity results. The topical agent must be discontinued immediately and completely to correct this problem.

Adjusting to Chronic Disorder. Although allergic reactions are infrequently life threatening, they require constant vigilance for allergens and modification of the patient's life-style or environment to prevent recurrence of symptoms. Allergic symptoms are often present year-round and create discomfort and inconvenience for the patient. Although he may not feel ill during allergy seasons, he often does not feel well either. The necessity of being alert for possible allergens in the environment and their presence throughout the environment may be tiresome for the patient and place extra burdens on his ability to lead a normal life. Stress related to these difficulties may in turn increase the frequency or severity of symptoms.

To assist the patient in adjusting to these modifications, the nurse must have an appreciation of the difficulties encountered by the patient. The patient is encouraged to verbalize his feelings and concerns in a supportive environment and to identify strategies to deal with them effectively.

Monitoring and Managing Potential Complications

Anaphylaxis and Impaired Breathing. Respiratory and cardiovascular functioning can be dangerously altered during allergic reactions due to the reaction itself or to medications used to treat it. Therefore, the patient's respiratory and cardiovascular status is evaluated by monitoring the respiratory rate, assessing for the presence of breathing difficulties or abnormal lung sounds, monitoring the pulse rate and rhythm, and blood pressure. Vital signs are monitored and recorded regularly or any time the patient complains of any symptoms such as itching or difficulty breathing. In the event of signs and symptoms indicative of anaphylaxis, emergency medications and equipment must be available for immediate use.

Adverse Reactions to Medications. Excessive doses of astemizole or terfenadine can lead to death from dysrhythmias or cardiac arrest. Adverse signs and symptoms should

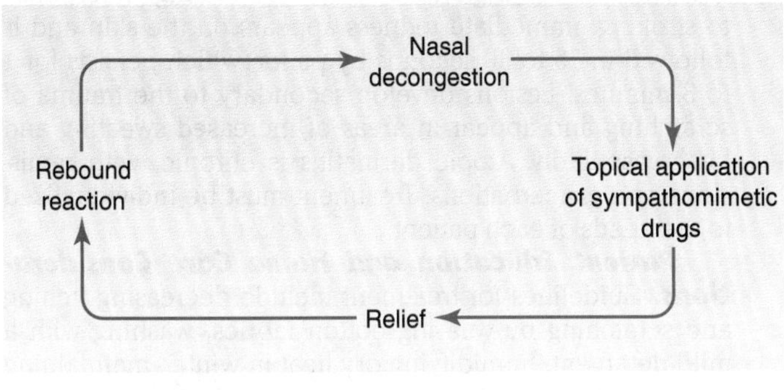

FIGURE 51-6. Rhinitis medicamentosa. This cyclic pattern results from overuse of sympathomimetic nose drops or sprays.

be immediately reported to the physician (*i.e.*, urticaria, difficulty breathing, dry mouth, palpitations, headaches, or dizziness). The patient should know the names, dose, frequency, actions, and side effects of all medications taken.

Noncompliance With Medical Regimen. Knowledge of the treatment regimen does not necessarily insure compliance. Having the patient identify potential barriers and explore acceptable solutions for lifestyle changes needed for effective management of the condition can increase compliance with the treatment regimen.

Evaluation

Expected Outcomes

1. Exhibits normal breathing patterns
   a. Lungs clear to auscultation
   b. Exhibits absence of adventitious breath sounds (crackles, rhonchi, wheezing)
   c. Demonstrates an effective respiratory rate
   d. Reports no respiratory distress (shortness of breath, difficulty on inspiration or expiration)
2. Demonstrates knowledge about allergy and strategies to control symptoms
   a. Identifies causative allergens, if known
   b. States methods of avoiding allergen and how to control for indoor and outdoor precipitating factors
   c. Describes name, purpose, side effects, and method of administration of prescribed medications
   d. Identifies when to seek immediate medical attention for severe allergic responses
   e. Describes activities that are possible and how involvement in them can be maximized without activating the allergies
3. Experiences relief of discomfort and adapts to the inconveniences of an allergy
   a. Relates the emotional aspects of the allergic response
   b. Removes from the environment those items that retain dust
   c. Wears a dampened mask if dust or mold may be a problem
   d. Avoids smoke-filled rooms and dust-filled or freshly sprayed areas
   e. Uses air-conditioned areas for a major part of the day
   f. Takes antihistamines as prescribed; participates in hyposensitization program, if applicable
4. Absence of complications
   a. Vital signs remain within normal limits
   b. Reports no symptoms or episodes of anaphylaxis (urticaria, itching, peripheral tingling, fullness in the mouth and throat, flushing, or difficulty swallowing) or coughing, wheezing, or difficulty breathing
   c. Demonstrates *correct* procedure to self-administer emergency medications to treat severe allergic reaction
   d. Correctly states untoward signs and symptoms to report to physician
   e. Correctly states medication names, dose and frequency of administration, medication actions and side effects, and signs and symptoms to report to physician
   f. Discusses acceptable lifestyle changes and solutions for identified potential barriers for compliance with treatment and medication regimen

Contact Dermatitis

Contact dermatitis (dermatitis venenata) is a type IV delayed hypersensitivity reaction response. It is an inflammatory, often eczematous condition caused by a skin reaction to a variety of irritating or allergenic materials. There are four basic types: *allergic, irritant, phototoxic,* and *photoallergic* (Table 51-4). Almost any substance can produce contact dermatitis. Poison ivy is probably the most common example; cosmetics, soaps, detergents, and industrial chemicals are frequent offenders. The skin sensitivity may develop after brief or prolonged periods of exposure, and the clinical picture may appear hours or weeks after the sensitized skin has been exposed.

Clinical Manifestations. Symptoms include itching, burning, erythema, skin lesions (vesicles), and edema, followed by weeping, crusting, and finally drying and peeling of the skin. In severe responses, hemorrhagic bullae may develop. Repeated reactions may be accompanied by thickening of the skin and pigmentary changes. Secondary invasion by bacteria may develop in skin abraded by rubbing or scratching. Usually, there are no systemic symptoms unless the eruption is widespread.

Diagnosis. Diagnosis may be made on the basis of the location of the eruption and history of exposure. However, in cases of obscure irritants or an unobservant patient, diagnosis may be extremely difficult and many trial-and-error procedures may be involved before the cause is correctly determined. Patch tests on the skin with suspected offending agents may clarify the diagnosis. Treatment modalities for each type of contact dermatitis are outlined in Table 51-4.

Atopic Dermatitis

Atopic dermatitis is a type I immediate hypersensitivity disorder. A family history is common. Incidence of atopic dermatitis is highest in infants and children. Most patients have significant elevations of serum IgE and peripheral eosinophilia. Pruritus and hyperirritability of the skin are the most consistent features of atopic dermatitis and are related to large amounts of histamine in the skin. Excessive dryness of the skin with resultant itching is related to changes in lipid content, sebaceous gland activity, and sweating. In response to stroking, immediate redness appears on the skin and is followed in 15 to 30 seconds by pallor, which persists for 1 to 3 minutes. Lesions develop secondary to the trauma of scratching and appear in areas of increased sweating and hypervascularity. Atopic dermatitis is chronic, with remissions and exacerbations. Treatment must be individualized to the needs of each patient.

Patient Education and Home Care Considerations. Guidelines for treatment include decreasing itching and scratching by wearing cotton fabrics, washing with a mild detergent, humidifying dry heat in winter, maintaining

TABLE 51-4 Summary of Characteristics, Diagnostic Testing, and Treatment of Types of Contact Dermatitis

Type	Etiology	Clinical Presentation	Diagnostic Testing	Treatment
Allergic	A type IV hypersensitivity reaction that results from contact of skin and allergenic substance. It has a sensitization period of 10–14 days.	Vasodilation and perivascular infiltrates on the dermis Intracellular edema Usually seen on dorsal aspects of hand	Patch testing (contraindicated in acute, widespread dermatitis)	Avoid offending material Burow's solution or cool water compress Systemic corticosteroids (prednisone) for 7–10 days Topical corticosteroids for mild cases Oral antihistamines to relieve pruritus
Irritant	Results from contact with a substance that chemically or physically damages the skin on a nonimmunologic basis. Occurs after first exposure to irritant or repeated exposures to milder irritants over an extended time.	Dryness lasting days to months Vesiculation, fissures, cracks Hands and lower arms most common areas	Clinical picture Appropriate negative patch tests	Identification and removal of source of irritation Application of hydrophilic cream or petrolatum to soothe and protect Topical corticosteroids and compresses for weeping lesions Antibiotics for infection and oral antihistamines for pruritus
Phototoxic	Resembles the irritant type but requires sun and a chemical in combination to damage the epidermis.	Similar to irritant dermatitis	Photopatch test	Same as for allergic and irritant dermatitis
Photoallergic	Resembles allergic dermatitis but requires light exposure in addition to allergen contact to produce immunologic reactivity	Similar to allergic dermatitis	Photopatch test	Same as for allergic and irritant dermatitis

room temperature at 68°F to 72°F (20°C to 22.2°C), using antihistamines such as diphenhydramine (Benadryl) or terfenadine (Seldane), and avoiding animals, dust, sprays, and perfumes. The patient is encouraged to keep skin moisturized by taking daily baths to hydrate the skin and by using topical skin moisturizers. Topical corticosteroids are used on the skin to prevent inflammation, and any infection is treated with antibiotics to eliminate *Staphylococcus aureus* when indicated.

Dermatitis Medicamentosa (Medication or Drug Reactions)

Dermatitis medicamentosa, a type I hypersensitivity disorder, is the term applied to skin rashes induced by the internal administration of certain drugs or medications. Certain medications tend to induce eruptions of similar types, although individuals react differently to each medication.

In general, drug reactions appear suddenly, have a particularly vivid color, present characteristics that are more spectacular than the somewhat similar eruptions of infectious origin, and, with the exception of bromide and the iodide rashes, disappear rapidly after the medication is withdrawn. Rashes may be accompanied by systemic or generalized symptoms. Upon discovery of a medication allergy, patients are warned that they have a hypersensitivity to a particular medication and are advised not to take it again.

Skin eruptions related to medication therapy suggest more serious hypersensitivities. The nurse should assess the patient and report any appearance of eruptions so that early treatment can be initiated.

Urticaria and Angioneurotic Edema

Urticaria (hives) is a type I hypersensitive allergic reaction of the skin characterized by the sudden appearance of pinkish, edematous elevations that vary in size and shape, itch, and cause local discomfort. They may involve any part of the body, including the mucous membranes (especially those of the mouth), the larynx (occasionally with serious respiratory complications), and the gastrointestinal tract.

Each hive remains for a period of time varying from a few minutes to several hours before disappearing. For hours or days, clusters of these lesions may come, go, and return episodically. If this sequence continues indefinitely, the condition is called *chronic urticaria*.

Angioneurotic edema involves the deeper layers of the skin, resulting in more diffuse swelling rather than the discrete lesions characteristic of hives. Occasionally one may be seen that covers the entire back. The skin over it may appear normal but often has a reddish hue. It does not pit on pressure, as ordinary edema does. The regions most often involved are the lips, eyelids, cheeks, hands, feet, genitalia, and tongue; the mucous membranes of the larynx, the bronchi, and the gastrointestinal canal may also be affected, particularly in cases of the hereditary type. Swellings may appear suddenly, in a few seconds or minutes, or slowly, in 1 or 2 hours. In the latter case, their appearance often is preceded by itching or burning sensations. Seldom does more than a single swelling appear at one time, although one may develop while another is disappearing. Infrequently they recur in the same region. Individual lesions usually last from 24 to 36 hours. On rare occasions, they recur with remarkable regularity at intervals of 3 to 4 weeks.

Hereditary Angioedema

Hereditary angioedema, although not an immunologic disorder in the usual sense, is included in this section because of its resemblance to allergic angioedema and because of the seriousness of this condition. Symptoms are due to edema of the skin, the respiratory tract, or the digestive tract. Attacks may be precipitated by trauma or may seem to occur spontaneously.

When skin is involved, the swelling is usually diffuse, does not itch, and is usually not accompanied by urticaria. Gastrointestinal edema may cause abdominal pain severe enough to suggest the need for surgery. Edema of the upper respiratory tract may cause marked swelling of the uvula and of the larynx, resulting in suffocation. Acute laryngeal edema is the most serious manifestation of this disorder and has resulted in death due to asphyxiation in nearly 20% of these patients. Attacks usually subside within 3 to 4 days, but during this time the patient should be observed carefully for signs of laryngeal obstruction, which may necessitate tracheostomy as a life-saving measure. Epinephrine, antihistamines, and corticosteroids are usually used in treatment, but the success of these agents is limited.

Food Allergy

Estimates of the incidence of type I hypersensitivity, IgE-mediated food allergy range from 0.1% to 7.0% of the population. Clinical symptoms are classic allergic symptoms (urticaria, atopic dermatitis, wheezing, cough, laryngeal edema, angioedema) and gastrointestinal symptoms (itching; swelling of lips, tongue, and palate; abdominal pain; nausea; cramps; vomiting; and diarrhea). Almost any food can cause allergic symptoms. The most common offenders are nuts, peanuts, eggs, milk, soy, wheat, and chocolate. A careful diagnostic workup is required for any patient with a suspected food hypersensitivity; included in this is a detailed allergy history, a physical examination, and pertinent diagnostic tests. When testing for allergy, skin testing is used for identifying the source of symptoms and is useful in identifying specific foods as causative agents.

Therapy for food hypersensitivity includes elimination or reduction of the sensitive food. Pharmacologic therapy is necessary in patients with uncontrolled exposure to offending foods or patients with multiple food sensitivities not responsive to elimination measures. Medication therapy involves the use of H_1 and H_2 antihistamines, adrenergic agents, corticosteroids, and cromolyn sodium.

Many food allergies disappear with time, particularly in children. About a third of proven allergies disappear in 1 to 2 years if the patient carefully avoids the offending food.

Serum Sickness

The illness known as serum sickness is an example of an immune complex type III hypersensitivity. It has traditionally resulted from the administration of therapeutic antisera of animal sources for the treatment or prevention of infectious diseases such as tetanus, pneumonia, rabies, diphtheria, botulism, and venomous snake and black widow spider bites. With the advent of human anti-tetanus serum and antibiotics, classic serum sickness is much less common now than in previous years. However, various medications (pri-

CRITICAL THINKING EXERCISES

1. During a patient's hospital admission procedure, you inquire about allergies. The patient reports that he is allergic "to everything." Describe the additional information you would obtain from him and how you would document this information on the patient's medical record.
2. Your patient has had a skin test done prior to receiving contrast media because of the possibility that she is allergic to the contrast agent. She reports pruritus, tightness in the throat and chest, and a feeling of anxiety. How would you respond to this situation? Describe the medical management you would anticipate and the nursing strategies you expect to carry out.
3. A patient is undergoing extensive diagnostic studies to identify the allergens that are causing her allergic symptoms. What recommendations would you give to her about her home environment? How might you modify those instructions if the patient lives near an industrial area? On a farm? Has small children, each of whom has a favorite pet?

marily penicillin) may cause a serum sickness–like reaction similar to that caused by foreign sera.

Clinical Manifestations

Symptoms are due to a reaction and immunologic attack upon the serum or medication. Antibodies appear to be of the IgE and IgM classes. Early manifestations, beginning 6 to 10 days after the administration of the medication, include an inflammatory reaction at the site of injection of the medication, followed by regional and generalized lymphadenopathy. There is usually a skin rash, which may be urticarial or purpuric, and the joints are frequently tender and swollen. Vasculitis may occur in any organ but is most commonly observed in the kidney, resulting in proteinuria and, occasionally, casts in the urine. There may be mild to severe cardiac involvement. Peripheral neuritis may cause temporary paralysis of the upper extremities or may be widespread, causing Guillain-Barré syndrome.

Management

The usual course lasts for several days to a few weeks if untreated, but the patient responds promptly and completely if treated with antihistamines and corticosteroids. Aggressive therapy, including ventilator support, may be necessary if peripheral neuritis and Guillain-Barré syndrome occur.

BIBLIOGRAPHY

Books

Barrett JT. Medical Immunology Text and Review. Philadelphia, FA Davis, 1991.

Bouchner BS. Systemic anaphylaxis. In Lichtenstein LM and Fauci AS (eds). Current Therapy in Allergy, Immunology, and Rheumatology, 4th ed. St Louis, BC Decker/Mosby Year Book, 1992.

Chapel H and Haney M. Essentials of Clinical Immunology, 3rd ed. Boston, Blackwell Scientific Publications, 1993.

Czarnetzki BM. Chronic urticaria. In Lichtenstein LM and Fauci AS (eds). Current Therapy in Allergy, Immunology, and Rheumatology, 4th ed. St. Louis, BC Decker/Mosby Year Book, 1992.

Frank MM (ed). Samter's Immunologic Diseases. Boston, Little, Brown, 1995.

Frank MM. Hereditary angioedema. In Lichtenstein LM and Fauci AS (eds). Current Therapy in Allergy, Immunology and Rheumatology, 4th ed. St. Louis, BC Decker/Mosby Year Book, 1992.

Haney M. Allergy. In Gooi HG and Chapel H (eds). Clinical Immunology: A Practical Approach. New York, Oxford University Press, 1990.

Hanifen JM. Atopic dermatitis. In Lichtenstein LM and Fauci AS (eds). Current Therapy in Allergy, Immunology, and Rheumatology, 4th ed. St. Louis, BC Decker/Mosby Year Book, 1992.

Holgate ST and Church MK. Allergy. New York, Gower Medical Publishing, 1993.

Lehne RA. Pharmacology for Nursing Care, 2nd ed. Philadelphia, WB Saunders Company, 1994.

McGrath KG. Anaphylaxis. In Patterson R (ed). Allergic Diseases: Diagnosis and Management. Philadelphia, JB Lippincott, 1993.

Middleton E Jr. Allergy: Principles and Practice. St. Louis, Mosby, 1993.

Mygind N. Allergic rhinitis. In Lichtenstein LM and Fauci AS (eds). Current Therapy in Allergy, Immunology, and Rheumatology, 4th ed. St Louis, BC Decker/Mosby Year Book, 1992.

Ormerod, AD and Greaves MS. Physical urticaria and angioedema. In Lichtenstein LM and Fauci AS (eds). Current Therapy in Allergy, Immunology, and Rheumatology, 4th ed. St. Louis, BC Decker/Mosby Year Book, 1992

Shatz GS. Anaphylaxis. In Korenblat PE and Wedner HJ (eds). Allergy Theory and Practice. Philadelphia, WB Saunders, 1992.

Simons FER and Simons KJ. Use of nonsedative antihistamines. In Lichtenstein LM and Fauci AS (eds). Current Therapy in Allergy, Immunology, and Rheumatology, 4th ed. St. Louis, BC Decker/Mosby Year Book, 1992

Terr AI. Mechanisms of hypersensitivity and anaphylaxis and urticaria. In Sites DP and Terr AI (eds). Basic and Clinical Immunology. Norwalk CT, Appleton & Lange, 1991.

Tizard IR. Immunology. New York, Saunders College Publishing, 1992.

Weiler JM and Maves KK. Drug reactions. In Lichtenstein LM and Fauci AS (eds). Current Therapy in Allergy, Immunology, and Rheumatology, 4th ed. St Louis, BC Decker/Mosby Year Book, 1992.

Journals

Abel EA. Contact dermatitis: Recognition and management. Hospital Medicine 1992 Nov; 28(11):101–2, 105, 107–8.

Atkinson TP and Kaliner MA. Anaphylaxis. Med Clin North Am 1992 Jul; 76(4):841–855.

Badhwar AK and Druce HM. Allergic rhinitis. Med Clin North Am 1992 Jul; 76(4):789–903.

Barton EC. Latex allergy: Recognition and management of a modern problem. Nurse Pract 1993 Nov; 18(11):54–58.

Bernstein DI. Occupational asthma. Med Clin North Am 1992 Jul; 76(4):917–934.

Bjornsdottir US and Busse WW. Respiratory infections and asthma. Med Clin North Am 1992 Jul; 76(4):895–915.

Borish L and Joseph BZ. Inflammation and the allergic response. Med Clin North Am 1992 Jul; 76(4):765–787.

Carroll P. Speed: The essential response to anaphylaxis. RN 1994 Jun; 57(6):26–31.

Chang BL, Vredevoe D and Hirsch M. Allergy as a risk factor for nursing care problems in the elderly cancer patient. Cancer Nurs 1995 Apr; 18(2):83–88.

Fernandez-Caldas E and Fox RW. Environmental control of indoor air pollution. Med Clin North Am 1992 Jul; 76(4): 935–952.

Gordon BR. Prevention and management of office allergy emergencies. Otolaryngol Clin North Am 1992 Feb; 25(1):119–134.

Horan RF, Sheffer AL and Briner WW Jr. Physical allergies. Med Sci Sports Exerc 1992 Aug; 24(8):845–848.

Hough DO and Dec KL. Exercise induced asthma and anaphylaxis. Sports Med 1994 Sep; 18(3):162–172.

Huston DP and Bressler RB. Urticaria and angioedema. Med Clin North Am 1992 Jul; 76(4):805–840.

Jackson D. Latex allergy and anaphylaxis—what to do? J Intraven Nurs 1995 Jan–Feb; 18(1):33–52.

Kirkevold M. Toward a practice theory of caring for patients with chronic skin disease. Scholarly Inquiry for Nursing Practice: An International Journal 1993; 7(1):37–52.

Long K and Long R. Treatment considerations for allergic rhinitis. Nurse Practioner Forum 1993 March; 4(1):6–8.

Marks DR and Marks LM. Food allergy. Manifestations, evaluation, and management. Postgrad Med 1993 Feb; 93(2): 191–196, 201.

Meeropol EV and Leger RR. Latex allergy: Collaborative nursing research using a consortium model. Clin Nurse Specialist 1993 Sep; 7(5):254–257.

Moeser LC. Anaphylaxis: A preventable complication of home infusion therapy. J Intraven Nurs 1991 Mar–Apr; 14(2):108–112.

Norman PS. Allergic rhinitis: Combined therapy improves control. Consultant 1991 August; 31(8): 25–29.

Ohman JL Jr. Allergen immunotherapy: Review of efficacy and current practice. Med Clin North Am 1992 Jul; 76(4):977–991.

Opper FH and Burakoff R. Food allergy and intolerance. Gastroenterologist 1993 Sep; 1(3):211–220.

Patten BC and Holt JA. When your patient is allergic. Am J Nurs 1992 Sep; 92(9):58–61.

Reisman RE. Stinging insect allergy. Med Clin North Am 1992 Jul; 76(4):883–894.

Reisman RE. Insect stings. N Engl J Med 1994 Aug 25; 331(8): 523–527.

Roth R. Allergic response. Emergency 1990 June; 22(6):28–32.

Szefler SJ. Anti-inflammatory drugs in the treatment of allergic disease. Med Clin North Am 1992 Jul; 76(4):953–975.

Simms J. Latex allergy alert. Canadian Nurse 1995 Feb; 91(2):27–30.

Smith DL and deShazo RD. Allergy and immunology. JAMA 1994 Jun 1; 271(21):1653–1654.

Sussman GL and Beezhold DH. Allergy to latex rubber. Ann Intern Med 1995 Jan 1; 122(1):43–46.

Weiss ME. Drug allergy. Med Clin North Am 1992 Jul; 76(4):857–882.

Winbourn M. Food allergy, the hidden culprit. J Am Acad Nurse Practitioners 1994 Nov; 6(11):515–522.

Workman ML. The immune system: Your defensive partner and offensive foe. AACN Clin Iss Crit Care Nurs 1993 Aug; 4(3):453–470.

Yunginger JW. Anaphylaxis. Ann Allergy 1992 Aug; 69(2):87–96.

INFORMATION/RESOURCES

Agencies

American Academy of Allergy and Immunology
611 E. Wells St.,
Milwaukee, WI 53202
(For a series of patient-oriented pamphlets, Tips to Remember)

The Asthma and Allergy Foundation of America
1125 15th St. NW Suite 502,
Washington, DC 20005,
(202) 466-7643.Center Laboratories

Division of EM Pharmaceuticals, Inc.,
35 Channel Dr., Port
Washington, NY 11050
Manufacture allergy medications.

National Institute of Allergy and Infectious Diseases
National Institute of Health,
Bldg 31. Room 7A50,
9000 Rockville Pike,
Bethesda, MD 20892,
(301) 496-5717.
Provide public education through pamphlets.

Medic Alert Foundation International
PO Box 1009,
Turlock, CA 95380
Provides emergency medical identification in either necklace or bracelet style that includes hidden medical condition and membership number, which can be called collect. A wallet card is provided with additional emergency information.

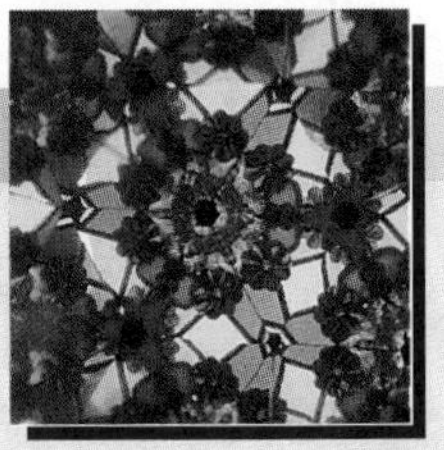

52

Management of Patients With Rheumatic Disorders

CHAPTER OUTLINE

LEARNING OBJECTIVES

On completion of this chapter, the learner will be able to:

1. Explain the inflammatory and degenerative components of the rheumatic diseases and their relationship
2. Describe the assessment and diagnostic evaluation for patients with suspected diagnosis of rheumatic disease
3. Discuss nursing diagnoses and collaborative problems that commonly occur with rheumatic disorders and describe appropriate nursing interventions for each
4. Use the nursing process as a framework for the care of the patient with a rheumatic disease, such as connective tissue disease or osteoarthritis
5. Describe the systemic effects of a connective tissue disease
6. Devise a teaching plan for the patient with newly diagnosed rheumatic disease

Overview of the Rheumatic Diseases

Commonly called arthritis (inflammation of a joint) and thought of as one condition, the rheumatic diseases are actually more than 100 different types of disorders. They primarily affect skeletal muscles, bones, ligaments, tendons, and joints of males and females of *all* ages. Some disorders are more likely to occur at a particular time of life or to affect one gender more than the other. The impact of these conditions can be life-threatening or merely an inconvenience, and the problems caused by the rheumatic diseases are not only the obvious limitations in mobility and activities of daily living but also the subtle systemic effects that can lead to organ failure and death or result in problems such as pain, fatigue, altered self-image, and sleep disturbances.

Moreover, the onset of these conditions may be acute or insidious, and the course may be marked by periods of remission (a period when disease symptoms are reduced or absent) and exacerbation (a period when symptoms occur or increase). Treatment can be very simple and aimed at localized relief, or it can be complex and directed toward relieving systemic effects. Permanent changes may result from the disease.

The rheumatic diseases are classified into ten categories (Chart 52-1) demonstrating the wide variety of the multisystem disorders composing the rheumatic diseases. The inclusion of conditions that secondarily may affect the musculoskeletal structure emphasizes the diversity of the rheumatic diseases.

This chapter describes the rheumatic diseases and presents common concepts of pathophysiology, assessment and diagnosis, disease management, and nursing process. Two of the ten categories are addressed in detail; the diffuse connective tissue diseases (which include rheumatoid arthritis [also called rheumatoid disease], systemic lupus erythematosus, scleroderma, polymyositis, and polymyalgia rheumatica) are examples of the **inflammatory rheumatic diseases;** and osteoarthritis is an example of a **degenerative rheumatic disease.** Disorders in the other categories are summarized.

Pathophysiology

Understanding the normal anatomy and physiology of the diarthrodial or synovial joints is key to understanding the pathophysiology of the rheumatic diseases. The function of the synovial joints is movement. Each synovial joint has a

CHART 52-1
Classification of the Rheumatic Diseases

1. Diffuse connective tissue diseases
   - Rheumatoid arthritis
   - Juvenile arthritis
   - Lupus erythematosus (*discoid, systemic, drug-related)
   - Scleroderma (localized, systemic sclerosis)
   - Polymyositis (dermatomyositis)
   - Sjögren's syndrome
   - Overlap syndromes (mixed connective tissue disease)
   - Others (polymyalgia rheumatica, erythema nodosum)
2. Arthritis associated with spondylitis (Spondyloarthropathies)
   - Ankylosing spondylitis
   - Reiter's syndrome
   - Psoriatic arthritis
   - Arthritis associated with inflammatory bowel disease
3. Osteoarthritis (i.e., osteoarthrosis, degenerative joint disease)
   - Primary
   - Secondary
4. Rheumatic syndromes associated with infectious agents
   - Direct (bacterial, viral, fungal, parasitic)
   - Reactive (bacterial, viral, postimmunization)
5. Metabolic and endocrine diseases associated with rheumatic states
   - Crystal-associated conditions (gout, pseudogout)
   - Biochemical abnormalities (amyloidosis, hemophilia)
   - Endocrine diseases (diabetes mellitus, acromegaly)
   - Immunodeficiency diseases
   - Hereditary disorders (hypermobility syndromes)
6. Neoplasms
   - Primary
   - Secondary (metastatic, multiple myeloma, leukemia)
7. Neurovascular disorders
   - Charcot joints
   - Compression syndrome (carpal tunnel syndrome, radiculopathy, spinal stenosis)
   - Reflex sympathetic dystrophy
   - Raynaud's phenomenon or disease
8. Bone, periosteal, and cartilage disorders
   - Osteoporosis
   - Osteomalacia
   - Hypertrophic osteoarthropathy
   - Diffuse idiopathic skeletal hyperostosis
   - Paget's disease of bone
9. Extra-articular disorders
   - Juxtaarticular lesions (bursitis, de Quervain tendon lesion, epicondylitis, popliteal [Baker]cyst
   - Low back pain
   - Intervertebral disc disorders
   - Regional pain syndromes (metatarsalgia, cervical pain
10. Miscellaneous disorders associated with articular manifestations
    - Palindromic rheumatism
    - Intermittent hydrarthrosis
    - Sarcoidosis
    - Chronic active hepatitis

*Examples in parentheses are not all inclusive.
(Modified from Schumacher HR [ed]. Primer on the Rheumatic Diseases, 10th ed. Atlanta, Arthritis Foundation, 1993.)

given range of motion, although each person does not have the same range of motion in the movable joints.

In a normal synovial joint, **articular cartilage** covers the bone end of the joint and provides a smooth, resilient surface for movement. **Synovial membrane** lines the inner surface of the fibrous capsule and secretes fluid into the space between the bones. This **synovial fluid** functions as a shock absorber and a lubricant, allowing the joint to move freely in the appropriate direction.

The joint is the area most commonly affected by the **inflammation** and degeneration seen in rheumatic diseases. Despite the diversity of rheumatic diseases, from localized involvement of one joint to systemic, multisystem disorders, they all involve some degree of inflammation and degeneration, which may occur simultaneously. Inflammation is demonstrated in the joints as synovitis. In inflammatory rheumatic diseases, inflammation is the primary process and the degeneration that occurs is secondary, resulting from the effect of **pannus** (proliferation of synovial tissue). The inflammation is a result of the immune response.

Conversely, in degenerative rheumatic diseases, a secondary inflammatory process occurs. This synovitis is usually milder, representing a reactive process, and is more likely to be seen in advanced disease. The synovitis may be related to the release of free cartilage proteoglycan from the deteriorating articular cartilage, but immunologic factors may also be involved.

Understanding these processes and how they are related is the key to accurate diagnosis, disease management, and nursing interventions for the person with a rheumatic disease.

Inflammation

Inflammation involves a series of related steps. The first step is the triggering event in which the antigen stimulus activates monocytes and T lymphocytes (also called T cells). Next, the immunoglobulin antibodies form immune complexes with antigens (type III reaction—immune complex mediated). Phagocytosis of the immune complexes is initiated, which generates an inflammatory reaction (joint swelling, pain, and edema) (Fig. 52-1).

During the next step, there is a deviation from the normal immune response. Phagocytosis produces chemicals such as leukotrienes and prostaglandins. Leukotrienes contribute to the inflammatory process by attracting other white cells to the area. Prostaglandins act as modifiers to inflammation: in some cases, they increase inflammation; in other cases, they slow it down. Leukotrienes and prostaglandins produce enzymes, such as collagenase, that break down collagen, a vital part of a normal joint. The release of these enzymes in the joint causes edema, proliferation of synovial membrane and pannus formation, destruction of cartilage, and erosion of bone.

The immunologic inflammatory process begins with the presentation of antigens to T cells (T lymphocytes), followed by a proliferation of T and B cells. B cells are a source for antibody-forming cells, or plasma cells. In response to specific antigens, plasma cells produce and release antibodies. Antibodies team up with corresponding antigens to form pairs, or immune complexes. The immune complexes build up and are deposited in synovial tissue or other organs in the body, thereby triggering the inflammatory reaction that can ultimately damage the involved tissue.

The systemic nature of the rheumatic disease category known as the diffuse connective tissue diseases is reflected in the resultant widespread inflammatory process. Although focused in the joints, inflammation also involves other areas. The blood vessels (vasculitis and arteritis), lungs, heart, and kidneys may also be affected by the inflammation. In the joints, this inflammatory response is manifested as pannus extending throughout the joint space and, if persistent, eroding the articular cartilage, causing secondary degenerative changes to the joint.

Degeneration

Degeneration of the articular cartilage is caused by a physiologic imbalance between mechanical stress and the ability of the joint tissues to resist that stress. Either the articular cartilage and bone are normal but excessive load (force from the weight of the body) applied to the joints causes the tissues to fail, or a physiologically reasonable load is applied to the joint but the articular cartilage or bone is defective. Defective cartilage or bone may result from genetic and endocrine factors.

Articular cartilage plays two essential mechanical roles in joint physiology. First, the articular cartilage provides a

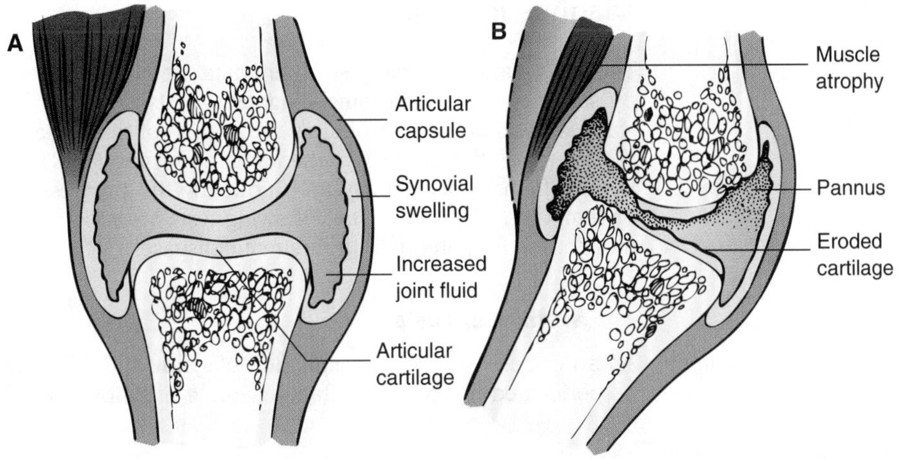

FIGURE 52-1. Inflammatory response in the joint. (**A**) The joint at left sustains synovial swelling and fluid accumulation. (**B**) The joint at right displays pannus (a proliferation of synovial tissue), eroded articular cartilage, and joint space narrowing—all of which contribute to muscle atrophy and ankylosis (joint rigidity and immobility).

remarkably smooth weight-bearing surface and, with synovial fluid, provides extremely low friction during movement. Secondly, the cartilage transmits load or pressure to the bone, dissipating the mechanical stress.

Mechanical Stress. Articular cartilage is highly resistant to wear under conditions of repeated movement, but repetitive impact loading (velocity at which the force is applied) rapidly leads to joint failure at the cartilage level. When a person walks, three to four times the body weight is transmitted through the knee. A deep knee bend transmits up to nine times the body weight through the patellofemoral joint. As a joint undergoes repeated mechanical stress, the elasticity of the joint capsule, articular cartilage, and ligaments is reduced. The **articular plate** (subchondral bone) thins and its ability to absorb shock decreases. There is narrowing of the joint space and loss of stability. When the articular plate disappears, bony spurs (**osteophytes**) form at the edges of the joint surfaces, and the capsule and synovial membranes thicken. The joint cartilage degenerates and atrophies (shrinks), the bones harden and hypertrophy (thicken) at their articular surfaces, and the ligaments calcify. As a result, sterile joint effusions and secondary synovitis may be present (Fig. 52-2).

Altered Lubrication. In addition to the changes in the articular cartilage and subchondral bone, lubrication of the joint is also a factor in joint degeneration. With joint loading (forces carried through the joint), lubrication depends on a film of interstitial fluid squeezed out of the cartilage upon compression of the opposing surfaces of the joint. The mechanisms that normally operate under high-weight loads to produce this lubricating film may be affected.

Immobility. Immobilization of a joint is another factor that can produce degenerative changes in articular cartilage. These changes are more marked and appear earlier in areas of contact but also occur in areas not subject to mechanical compression. Cartilage degeneration due to joint immobility may result from loss of the pumping action of lubrication that occurs with joint movement. By 3 weeks after remobilization of the joint, the cartilage abnormalities are reversed. However, impact exercising (activities such as running) prevent reversal of the atrophy. Instead, slow, gradual range of motion is thought to be very important in preventing cartilage injury.

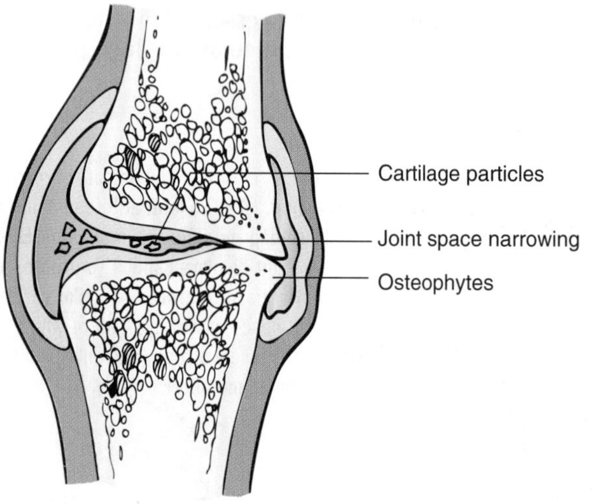

FIGURE 52-2. Joint space narrowing and osteophytes (bone spurs) are characteristic of degenerative changes in joints.

Clinical Manifestations

Pain is the symptom of a rheumatic disease that most commonly causes a person to seek medical attention. Other common symptoms include joint swelling, limited movement, stiffness, weakness, and fatigue.

Assessment

Assessment begins with a general health history, which includes the onset of symptoms and how they evolved, family history, and any other contributing factors. This is followed by a complete physical assessment. Because many of the rheumatic diseases are chronic conditions, the health history should also include information about the patient's perception of the problem, previous treatments and their effectiveness, the patient's support systems, and the patient's current knowledge base and the source of that information.

Assessment for rheumatic diseases combines the physical examination with a functional assessment. Inspection of the patient's general appearance occurs during initial contact. Gait, posture, and general musculoskeletal size and structure are observed. Gross deformities and abnormalities in movement are noted. The symmetry, size, and contour of other connective tissues, such as the skin and adipose tissue, are also noted and recorded. Chart 52-2 outlines the important areas for consideration during the physical assessment.

The functional assessment is a combination of history (what the patient reports that he or she can and cannot do) and examination (observation of activities the patient demonstrates what he or she can and cannot do, such as dressing and getting in and out of a chair). Observation also includes the adaptations and adjustments the patient may have made (sometimes without awareness), for example, lowering the mouth to the fork rather than raising the fork to the mouth. In the hospital or home setting, the nurse can often identify functional changes.

Diagnostic Evaluation

The history and physical assessment data are supplemented by supportive or confirming diagnostic tests. In some instances, tests are used to follow the course of the disease. For example, the erythrocyte sedimentation rate (ESR) reflects inflammatory activity and indirectly the progression or remission of disease. The following tests are most commonly used for patients with rheumatic diseases.

Arthrocentesis

An arthrocentesis (needle aspiration of synovial fluid) may be performed not only to obtain a sample of synovial fluid

CHART 52-2

Physical Assessment: Significant Aspects in Rheumatic Diseases

In addition to the head-to-toe assessment or systems review, the following are important areas of consideration to be noted when performing the complete physical assessment for a patient with a known or suspected rheumatic disease.

Manifestation	Significance
Skin (inspect and inquire)	
1. Rash/lesions	1. Associated with lupus erythematosus (LE), vasculitides, adverse effect of medication
2. Increased bruising	2. Associated with several rheumatic diseases and adverse effect of medication
3. Erythema	3. Sign of inflammation
4. Thinning	4. Adverse effect of medication
5. Warmth	5. Sign of inflammation
6. Photosensitivity	6. Associated with systemic lupus erythematosus (SLE), dermatomyositis, adverse effect of medication
Hair (inspect and inquire)	
1. Alopecia or thinning	1. Associated with rheumatic diseases or adverse effect of medication
Eye (inspect and inquire)	
1. Dryness, grittiness	1. Associated with Sjögren's syndrome (commonly occurring with rheumatoid arthritis [RA] and LE)
2. Decreased acuity or blindness	2. Associated with temporal arteritis, drug complications
3. Cataracts	3. Adverse effect of medication
4. Decreased peripheral vision	4. Adverse effect of medication
5. Conjunctivitis/uveitis	5. Associated with ankylosing spondylitis and Reiter's syndrome
Ear (inquire)	
1. Tinnitus	1. Adverse effect of medication
2. Decreased acuity	2. Adverse effect of medication
Mouth (inspect and inquire)	
1. Buccal/sublingual lesions	1. Associated with vasculitis, dermatomyositis, adverse effect of medication
2. Altered sense of taste	2. Adverse effect of medication
3. Dryness	3. Associated with Sjögren's syndrome
4. Dysphagia	4. Associated with myositis
5. Difficulty chewing	5. Associated with decreased range of motion in jaw
Chest (inspect and inquire)	
1. Pleuritic pain	1. Associated with RA and SLE
2. Decreased chest expansion	2. Associated with ankylosing spondylitis (AS)
3. Activity intolerance (dyspnea)	3. Associated with pulmonary hypertension in scleroderma
Cardiovascular System (inspect, inquire, palpate)	
1. Blanching of fingers on exposure to cold	1. Associated with Raynaud's phenomenon
2. Peripheral pulses	2. Deficit may indicate vascular involvement or edema associated with medication effect or rheumatic diseases, especially SLE or scleroderma
Abdomen (inquire and palpate)	
1. Altered bowel habits	1. Associated with scleroderma, spondylosis, ulcerative colitis, decreased physical mobility, medication effect
2. Nausea/vomiting/bloating/pain	2. Adverse effect of medication
3. Weight change	3. Associated with RA (decreased), adverse effect of medication (increased or decreased)

(continued)

CHART 52-2 *(continued)*

Physical Assessment: Significant Aspects in Rheumatic Diseases

Manifestation	Significance
Genitalia (inspect and inquire)	
1. Dryness/itching	1. Associated with Sjögren's syndrome
2. Abnormal menses	2. Adverse effect of medication
3. Altered sexual performance	3. Fear of pain (or of pain caused by partner) and limitation of motion may affect sexual mobility
4. Hygiene	4. Poor hygiene may be related to limitations in activities of daily living
5. Urethritis, dysuria	5. Associated with AS and Reiter's syndrome
6. Lesions	6. Associated with vasculitis
Neurologic (inspect and inquire)	
1. Paresthesias of extremities 2. Abnormal reflex pattern	1 & 2. Nerve compressions associated with carpal tunnel syndrome, spinal stenosis, etc.
3. Headaches	3. Associated with temporal arteritis, adverse effect of medication
Musculoskeletal (inspect and palpate)	
1. Joint redness/warmth/swelling/tenderness/deformity—location of first joint involved, pattern of progression, symmetry, acute vs chronic nature	1. Signs of inflammation
2. Joint range of motion	2. Decreased ROM may indicate severity or progression of disease
3. Surrounding tissue findings Muscle atrophy, subcutaneous nodules, popliteal cyst	3. Extra-articular manifestations
4. Muscle strength (grip)	4. Muscle strength decreases with increased disease activity
Lab Values	
1. Erythrocyte sedimentation rate (ESR)	1. Indicator of inflammation
2. Complete blood count (CBC)	2. Anemia often associated with systemic disease
3. Platelet count	3. Drug complications (decreased) or associated with SLE
4. Salicylate level	4. Measure of therapeutic level to decrease inflammation

for analysis but also to relieve pain—usually in the knee or shoulder. The joint is anesthetized locally, and a large-bore needle is inserted into the joint space to obtain a fluid specimen. Because this procedure has the potential for introducing bacteria into the joint, the assisting nurse shares responsibility in ensuring that aseptic technique is followed. Following the procedure, the patient is observed and should be instructed about signs of infection and **hemarthrosis** (bleeding into the joint). Synovial fluid is usually analyzed in cases such as suspected joint infection; to determine the presence of inflammatory cells; and to identify crystals or the presence of blood indicating trauma.

Normally, synovial fluid is clear, viscous, straw-colored, and scanty in volume with few cells. In inflammatory joint disease, however, the fluid may become cloudy, milky, or dark yellow and may contain numerous inflammatory cells, such as leukocytes (white blood cells) and complement (a plasma protein associated with immunologic reactions). The viscosity is reduced in inflammatory disease, and copious amounts of fluid may be present. Diagnostically, this is a valuable test. However, it may be difficult to obtain joint fluid in small joints such as the fingers or wrist.

X-ray Studies

X-rays are often used in evaluating patients with a rheumatic disease. The timing of the studies influences their usefulness. It is unlikely that a patient with a 2-month history of joint inflammation will have demonstrable changes on x-ray; however, someone with knee crepitus (a grating sound heard on movement) will likely show severe joint degeneration. X-ray studies can be used over time to monitor disease activity and progression. X-rays taken over time can demonstrate the loss of cartilage and narrowing of the joint space. X-rays can also demonstrate cartilage abnormalities, joint erosions, abnormal bony growth, and osteopenia (decreased bone mineralization).

Arthrography is a diagnostic x-ray technique used to detect connective tissue disorders. A radiopaque substance or air is injected into the joint cavity, especially of the knee or shoulder, to outline the contour of the joint. Then the joint is put through passive range of motion while a series of x-rays are obtained. The patient is reassured that the radiopaque substance will be absorbed systemically and joint swelling will consequently subside. The patient is instructed to observe for signs of infection and hemarthrosis following the procedure.

Bone and Joint Scans

A bone scan reflects the degree to which the crystal lattice of bone "takes up" or absorbs a bone-seeking radioactive isotope. An area demonstrating increased uptake, such as a joint, is considered abnormal. A **joint scan** allows determination of joint damage throughout the body. It is the most sensitive study for detecting early disease.

Biopsies

A **muscle biopsy** is carried out to examine skeletal muscle. The procedure may be performed in the operating room under local anesthesia. A surgical incision is made, the desired specimen is obtained, and the specimen is sent to the laboratory for microscopic analysis. A pressure dressing is applied, and the affected extremity is immobilized for 12 to 24 hours. Muscle biopsy is useful in diagnosing myositis.

An **arterial biopsy** may be performed to examine a specimen of an arterial wall. Most frequently, the temporal artery is selected, but other arteries may undergo biopsy as indicated. The procedure is similar to that for the incisional muscle biopsy. Arterial biopsy most often confirms inflammation of the vessel wall, or **arteritis,** a type of vasculitis.

A **skin biopsy** may be performed to confirm inflammatory connective tissue diseases, such as lupus erythematosus or scleroderma. A specimen may be lightly scraped from the patient's skin without causing discomfort. Deeper skin biopsies may need to be carried out when scraping is not sufficient.

Blood Tests

In general, **serum laboratory studies** in rheumatology are based on the assumption that most rheumatic diseases are autoimmune disorders. Although many of the tests are highly complex and technical, no one test used in isolation sufficiently supports a diagnosis of a rheumatic disease. In Table 52-1 some of the most common serum studies are listed with corresponding normal value ranges and primary indications. Because many of the tests require special laboratory techniques, they may not be used in every health care facility. The physician determines which tests are necessary, basing this decision on the patient's symptoms, stage of disease, cost, and likely benefit of the test.

Diagnostic Implications

Diagnosis of a specific rheumatic disease may or may not be relatively simple and clear-cut. Commonly, observation of clinical signs and symptoms over time is needed to make the diagnosis. It is the combination of history, assessment and testing, and evolving manifestations of the disease that may require explanation and interpretation to the patient with early disease. This is especially true for those people with a multisystem rheumatic disease, such as one of the connective tissue diseases.

Finding crystals or bacteria in the synovial fluid is specifically diagnostic for gout or infectious arthritis, respectively. Diagnosis may be more presumptive in the case of the older person who is thought to have osteoarthritis based on single joint involvement, supportive x-ray findings, and no evidence of other disease processes.

Many forms of rheumatic disease can be accurately diagnosed by the primary health care provider. Patients with more complicated signs and symptoms may need referral to a **rheumatologist,** a physician who specializes in diagnosing and treating people with rheumatic disease. Patients should know which type of rheumatic disease they have, not just that they have "arthritis" or "arthritis of the knee."

Management

A treatment program involving the multidisciplinary team, including the patient, is the basis for managing the rheumatic diseases. The chronic nature of most of these diseases mandates that the patient understand the disease, have the information necessary to make good self-management decisions, and be presented with a therapeutic program that is compatible with life-style. Table 52-2 outlines the goals and strategies of basic rheumatic disease management.

Medications are used with the rheumatic diseases to control inflammation and, in some instances, to modify the disease. Three basic categories of useful medication include the salicylates, nonsteroidal anti-inflammatory drugs (NSAIDs), and slow-acting anti-rheumatic agents. Table 52-3 reviews the various medications often used.

Controlling the inflammation related to the disease process will help in managing pain, but often this is a delayed response. Non-opioid medications are often used for pain management, especially early in the treatment program until other measures can be instituted effectively.

Nursing Implications

All patients receiving medication as part of disease management are thoroughly instructed regarding medication type, purpose, dosage, side effects, and procedures for monitoring for side effects. Barriers to compliance are assessed and measures are taken to promote adherence with the medication and treatment program.

Nonpharmacologic methods of pain management are important, especially using therapeutic heat or cold and joint protection using devices such as a cane or a wrist splint. Different methods may be needed or may work better at different times.

The ongoing nature of most rheumatic diseases makes it important to maintain and, when possible, improve joint mobility and functional status. The individualized exercise program is crucial to movement. Table 52-4 summarizes the exercises appropriate for patients with rheumatic diseases.

The major challenge for the patient and the care provider is the need to adjust all aspects of treatment

TABLE 52-1 Common Serum Studies for Rheumatic Diseases

Test	Normal Value	Significance
Serum		
Creatinine		
Metabolic waste excreted through the kidneys	0.6–1.2 mg/dl (SI: 50–110 μmol/L)	Increase may indicate renal damage in SLE, scleroderma, and polyarteritis
Erythrocyte Sedimentation Rate (ESR)		
Measures the rate at which red blood cells (RBCs) settle out of unclotted blood in 1 hour	Westergren = *Men* 0–15 mm/hr, *Women* 0–20 mm/hr Wintrobe = *Men* 0–9 mm/hr, *Women* 0–15 mm/hr	Increase usually seen in inflammatory CTD An increase indicates rising inflammation, resulting in clustering of RBCs, which makes them heavier than normal. The higher the ESR, the greater the inflammatory activity
Hematocrit		
Measures the size, capacity, and number of cells present in blood	*Men:* 45–50 vol/dl *Women:* 40–45 vol/dl	Decrease can be seen in chronic inflammation (anemia of chronic disease); also, blood loss through bowel due to medication
Red Blood Cell (RBC) Count		
Measures circulating erythrocytes	*Men:* Average 4.8 million/μl *Women:* Average 4.3 million/μl	Decreased in RA, SLE
White Blood Cell (WBC) Count		
Measures circulating leukocytes	5000–10,000 cells/mm^3	May be decreased in SLE
VDRL (Venereal Disease Research Laboratory)		
Measures antibody to syphilis	Nonreactive	False-positive sometimes found with SLE
Uric Acid		
Measures level of uric acid in serum	2.5–8 mg/dl (SI: 0.15–0.5 mmol/L)	Increase seen with gout
Serum Immunology		
Antinuclear Antibody (ANA)		
Measures antibodies that react with a variety of nuclear antigens If antibodies are present, further testing determines the type of ANA circulating in the blood (anti-DNA, anti-RNP).	Negative A few healthy adults have a positive ANA	Positive test is associated with SLE, RA, scleroderma, Raynaud's disease, Sjögren's syndrome, necrotizing arteritis The higher the titer, the greater the inflammation The pattern of immunofluorescence (speckled, homogeneous, or nucleolar) helps determine the diagnosis
Anti-DNA, DNA binding		
Titer measurement of antibody to double-stranded DNA	Negative	High titer seen in SLE; increases in titer may indicate increase in disease activity
Complement levels—C_3, C_4		
Complement is a protein substance that binds with antigen-antibody complexes for the purpose of lysis. When the number of complexes increases markedly, complement is used for lysis, thus depleting the amount available in the blood.	C_3: 55–120 mg/dl (SI: 550–1200 mg/L) C_4: 11–40 mg/dl (SI: 110–400 mg/L)	Decrease may be seen in RA and SLE Decrease indicates autoimmune and inflammatory activity
C-Reactive Protein Test (CRP)		
Shows presence of abnormal glycoprotein due to inflammatory process	Trace 6 μg/ml	A positive reading indicates active inflammation Often positive for RA, disseminated lupus erythematosus

(continued)

TABLE 52-1 *(continued)*

Test	Normal Value	Significance
Immunoglobulin Electrophoresis Measures the values of immunoglobulins	IgA 50–300 mg/dl (SI: 0.5–3 g/L) IgG 635–1400 mg/dl (SI: 6.35–14 g/L) IgM 40–280 mg/dl (SI: 0.4–2.8 g/L)	Increased levels are found in people who have autoimmune disorders
Rheumatoid Factor (RF) Determines the presence of abnormal antibodies seen in CTD	Negative	Positive titer > 1:80 Present in 80% of those with RA Positive RF may also suggest SLE, Sjögren's syndrome, or mixed CTD. The higher the titer (number at right of colon), the greater the inflammation
Tissue Typing **HLA-B27 Antigen** Measures presence of HLA antigens, which are used for tissue recognition	Negative	Found in 80%–90% of those with ankylosing spondylitis and Reiter's syndrome

SLE, systemic lupus erythematosus; CTD, connective tissue disease; RA, rheumatoid arthritis; RNP, ribonucleic protein.

according to the activity of the disease. Especially for the patient with an active diffuse connective tissue disease, such as rheumatoid arthritis or systemic lupus erythematosus, activity level adjustments may vary from day to day and even within the day itself.

NURSING PROCESS
The Patient With a Rheumatic Disease

Assessment

The depth and focus of the nursing assessment depend on several factors. These factors include the health care setting (clinic or office, home, extended care facility, or hospital), the role of the nurse (home care nurse; nurse practitioner; hospital, clinic or office nurse), and the needs of the patient. The nurse is often the first of the health care team members to come in contact with the patient and is often the care provider in the best position to assist with basic care and hygiene. This may enable the nurse to assess the patient's perceptions of the disorder and situation, actions taken to relieve symptoms, plans for treatment, and expectations. The nurse's assessment may lead to identifying problems that can be addressed by nursing interventions and, through collaboration with other team members, to achieving the expected patient outcomes.

The health history and physical assessment focus on current and past symptoms such as fatigue, weakness, pain, stiffness, fever, or anorexia and the effects of these symptoms on the patient's life-style and self-image. Because the rheumatic diseases affect many body systems, the history and physical assessment include a review and examination of all systems, with particular attention given to those areas most commonly affected, including the musculoskeletal system. Chart 52-2 provides a guide to the physical assessment of the patient with rheumatic disorders. The patient's psychologic and mental status and social support systems are also assessed, as is the patient's ability to participate in daily activities, comply with the treatment regimen, and manage self-care. The information obtained can give insight into the patient's understanding of the medication regimen and may reveal misuse of medications, noncompliance, or use of unproven remedies. Additional areas assessed include the patient's understanding, motivation, knowledge,

TABLE 52-2 Goals and Strategies for Rheumatic Diseases

Major Goals	Management Strategy
Suppress inflammation and the autoimmune response	Administer medications (anti-inflammatory and disease-modifying)
Control pain	Protect joints; ease pain with splints, thermal modalities, relaxation techniques
Maintain or improve joint mobility	Implement exercise programs for joint motion and muscle strengthening
Maintain or improve functional status	Make use of adaptive devices and techniques
Increase patient's knowledge of disease process	Provide and reinforce patient teaching
Promote self-management by patient compatible with the therapeutic regimen	Emphasize compatibility of therapeutic regimen and lifestyle

TABLE 52-3 Medications Used in Rheumatic Diseases

Medication	Actions, Use, and Indications	Nursing Implications and Assessment for Drug Intolerance
Salicylates Aspirin (buffered or enteric-coated) Choline magnesium trisalicylate Choline salicylate Salsalate	*Actions:* Anti-inflammatory, analgesic, and antipyretic Acetylated salicylates are platelet aggregation inhibitors Used in early phase of disease Anti-inflammatory dosage will produce blood salicylate levels of 20–30 mg/dl	Administer with meals to prevent gastric irritation Assess for tinnitus, gastric intolerance, GI bleeding, and purpura
Nonsteroidal Anti-inflammatory Drugs (NSAIDs) **Propionic Acid Derivatives** Ibuprofen (Motrin) Flurbiprofen (Ansaid) Ketopreofen (Orudis, Oruvail) Naproxen (Naprosyn) Oxaprozin (DayPro) **Fenamates** Melclofenamate (Meclomen) **Pyrazoles** Phenylbutazone (Butazolidin) Oxyphenbutazone (Tandearil) **Osicams** Piroxicam (Feldene) **Acetic Acid Derivatives** Diclofenac (Voltaren) **Indene Derivatives:** Indomethacin (Indocin) Sulindac (Clinoril) Tolmetin (Tolectin) **Pyranocarboxyliz acid** Etodolac (Lodine) **Naphthylalkanone** Nabumatone (Relafen)	*Actions:* Anti-inflammatory, analgesic, antipyretic, platelet aggregation inhibitor Anti-inflammatory effect occurs in about 4 weeks All NSAIDs are useful for short-term treatment of an acute gouty attack NSAIDs are used as an alternative to salicylates for a first-line therapy in several rheumatic diseases	With long-term administration, monitor for gastrointestinal, CNS, cardiovascular, renal, hematologic, and skin adverse reactions. Aspirin products should be avoided. Provide acetaminophen for headaches, fever
Slow-Acting Anti-Rheumatic Agents **Gold-Containing Compounds** Aurothioglucose (Solganal) Gold sodium thiomalate (Myochrysine) Auranofin (Ridaura)	*Actions:* Anti-inflammatory, mechanism unknown; suppresses synovitis during active stage of rheumatoid disease IM preparations initially given weekly, then frequency decreases to every 2–4 weeks PO gold given daily in capsule form, dosage remains constant Onset of benefit from drug may be 3–6 months	Administer concurrently with anti-inflammatory agents until benefits from gold therapy are achieved. Assess for signs and symptoms of drug toxicity: stomatitis, dermatitis, diarrhea, proteinuria, hematuria, bone marrow suppression. Anticipate possible nitroid reaction 1–36 hours after injection of gold sodium thiomalate.
Penicillamine	*Action:* Mechanism unknown, may improve lymphocyte function May take 2–3 months before benefits are seen	Monitor blood and urine every other injection. Administer concurrently with anti-inflammatory agents

(continued)

TABLE 52-3 *(continued)*

Medication	Actions, Use, and Indications	Nursing Implications and Assessment for Drug Intolerance
	Taken on empty stomach Useful in RA and SS	Assess for signs and symptoms of toxicity: gastric irritation, decreased taste sensation, skin rash or itching, bone marrow suppression, proteinuria Monitor blood and urine every 2 weeks until stabilized, then monthly
Hydroxychloroquine (Plaquenil) **Chloroquine (Aralen)**	*Action:* Anti-inflammatory, mechanism unknown Useful in RA and SLE May take 2–4 months before benefits are seen	Administer concurrently with anti-inflammatory agents Assess for signs and symptoms of toxicity: changes in vision, GI disturbance, skin rash, sun sensitivity, bleaching of hair, headaches Schedule required ophthalmologic exams every 6 months
Immunosuppressives Methotrexate Azathioprine (Imuran) Cyclophosphamide (Cytoxan)	*Actions:* Used in aggressive RA or SLE that is unresponsive to conventional therapy These drugs have teratogenic potential Action is believed to result from cytotoxic effects of inhibiting lymphocytes or macrophages and thus interfering with joint inflammation	Highly toxic: be alert for bone marrow depression, GI ulcerations, skin rashes, alopecia, bladder toxicity, reduced resistance to infections. Monitor patient with weekly blood evaluation and urinalysis Advise patient of contraceptive measures because of teratogenicity
Corticosteroids Prednisone (Deltasone) Prednisolone (Delta-Cortef) Hydrocortisone (Cortef)	Corticosteroids used in treatment of incapacitating active RA, SLE, scleroderma, necrotizing arteritis Use of corticosteroids for long periods has wide range of adverse effects Used with caution and tapered to minimal maintenance dose if possible Onset of action is rapid, within the first week	Watch for toxic effects with high doses or long-term treatment: osteoporosis, fractures, avascular necrosis; gastric ulcers, psychiatric problems, infection susceptibility, hirsutism, acne, moon facies, abnormal fat deposition, edema, emotional disorders, menstrual disorders; hyperglycemia, hypokalemia, hypertension; cataracts and glaucoma
Corticosteroids **Intra-articular Injections**	Given when arthritic reaction has been suppressed and one or two joints are not responding to treatment Given when only one or two joints are affected Given to patient with extremely painful joints to allow physical therapy Relieves pain. Benefit may last from weeks to months No more than three injections in a single joint should be given	Inform the patient that an inflamed joint may respond to local injection when it has failed to come under control through other general systemic measures, that joints most amenable to corticosteroid injections are ankles, knees, hips, shoulders, and hands, that repeated injections can cause joint damage

coping abilities, past experiences, preconceptions, and fears. The effects of the disease on the patient's self-concept and coping abilities are also assessed. The patient's perception of the condition and its impact will influence the decisions, choices, and actions associated with treatment recommendations.

Diagnosis

Nursing Diagnoses

Although many nursing diagnoses are appropriate for the patient with a rheumatic disease, a few of the most common follow:

TABLE 52-4 Suggested Exercises to Promote Mobility

Inflammatory Process (Pain)	Recommended Exercise	Patient Performance Level
Acute exacerbation; severe pain	Passive range of motion (ROM)	Unable to perform exercises alone
Subacute; moderate or minimal pain	Active assistive or active ROM within pain tolerance	Can perform with help from another person or an assistive mechanical device
Inactive; remission; minimal pain or absence of pain	Active ROM; isometrics	Can perform alone

- Pain related to inflammation and increased disease activity, fatigue, or limited mobility
- Fatigue related to increased disease activity, pain, inadequate sleep/rest, deconditioning, inadequate nutrition, emotional stress/depression
- Impaired physical mobility related to decreased range of motion, muscle weakness, pain on movement, limited endurance, lack of or improper use of ambulatory devices
- Self-care deficits related to contractures, fatigue, or loss of motion
- Body image disturbance related to physical and psychologic changes and dependency caused by disease or treatment
- Ineffective coping related to actual or perceived lifestyle or role changes

Collaborative Problems/ Potential Complications

Based on assessment data, potential complications may include:

- Complications secondary to the effects of medications

Planning and Implementation

Goals. The major goals for the patient may include relief of pain and discomfort, relief of fatigue, increased mobility, maintenance of self-care, improved body image, and absence of complications.

Nursing Interventions

An understanding of the underlying disease process (*i.e.*, degeneration or inflammation, as well as degeneration resulting from inflammation or inflammation resulting from degeneration) guides the nurse's thought processes. In addition, the nurse's knowledge of whether the condition is localized or more widely systemic influences the scope of the nursing activity.

Some rheumatic diseases (*e.g.*, osteoarthritis) are more localized alterations in which control of symptoms such as pain or stiffness is possible. Others (*e.g.*, gout) have a known cause and specific treatment to control the symptoms. The diseases that usually present the greatest challenge are those with systemic manifestations such as the diffuse connective tissue diseases.

Nursing Care Plan 52-1 details the nursing interventions to be considered for each nursing diagnosis.

Relieving Pain and Discomfort. Medications are used in the short term to relieve acute pain. Because the pain may be persistent, non-opioid analgesics such as acetaminophen are also employed. After administering medications, the nurse needs to reassess pain levels at intervals. With persistent pain, assessment findings should be compared with baseline measurements and evaluations. Additional measures include exploring coping skills and strategies that have worked in the past.

The patient needs to understand the importance of taking medications, such as the NSAIDs and disease-modifying drugs, exactly as prescribed to achieve maximum benefits. These benefits include relief of pain as the disease is brought under control. Because disease control and pain relief are delayed, the patient may mistakenly believe the medication is ineffective or may think of the medication as merely "pain pills" and take them only sporadically, failing to achieve control over the disease activity.

A weight reduction program may be recommended to relieve stress on painful joints. Heat applications are also helpful in relieving pain, stiffness, and muscle spasm. Superficial heat may be supplied in the form of warm tub baths or showers and warm moist compresses. Paraffin baths (dips) offer concentrated heat and are helpful to patients with wrist and small-joint involvement. Maximum benefit is achieved within 20 minutes of application. More frequent use for shorter lengths of time is most beneficial. Therapeutic exercises can be carried out more comfortably and effectively after heat has been applied.

In some patients, however, heat may actually increase pain, muscle spasm, and synovial fluid volume. If the inflammatory process is acute, cold applications may be tried in the form of moist packs or an ice bag. Both heat and cold are analgesic to nerve pain receptors and can relax muscle spasms. Safe use of heat and cold must be evaluated and taught, particularly for patients with impaired sensation.

The use of braces, splints, and assistive mobility devices such as canes, crutches, and walkers eases pain by limiting movement or stress from weight bearing on painful joints. Acutely inflamed joints can be rested by applying splints to limit motion. Splints also support the joint to relieve spasm. Canes and crutches can relieve stress from inflamed and painful weight-bearing joints while promoting safe ambulation. Cervical collars may be used to support the weight of the head and limit cervical motion. A metatarsal bar or special pads may be put into shoes if foot pain or deformity is present.

Other strategies for relieving pain and increasing comfort may be introduced to the patient and may include muscle relaxation techniques, imagery, self-hypnosis, and distraction.

Decreasing Fatigue. Fatigue related to rheumatic disease can be both acute (brief and relieved by rest or sleep)

(text continues on page 1458)

NURSING CARE PLAN 52–1
Care of the Patient With a Rheumatic Disease

Nursing Interventions	Rationale	Expected Outcomes
NURSING DIAGNOSIS: Pain related to inflammation and increased disease activity, tissue damage, limited mobility, or lowered tolerance level		
GOAL: Improvement in comfort level; incorporation of pain management techniques into daily life		
1. Provide variety of comfort measures: a. Application of heat or cold b. Massage, position changes, rest c. Foam matress, supportive pillow, splints d. Relaxation techniques, diversional activities	1. Pain may respond to nondrug interventions such as joint protection, exercise, relaxation, and thermal modalities.	• Identifies factors that exacerbate or influence pain response. • Identifies and uses pain management measures. • Verbalizes decrease in pain. • Reports signs and symptoms of side effects in timely manner to prevent additional problems. • Verbalizes that pain is characteristic of rheumatic disease. • Establishes realistic pain-relief goals. • Verbalizes that pain often leads to the use of nontraditional and unproved self-treatment methods. • Identifies changes in quality or intensity of pain.
2. Administer anti-inflammatory, analgesic, and slow-acting anti-rheumatic medications as directed.	2. Pain of rheumatic disease responds to individual or combination drug regimens.	
3. Individualize medication schedule to meet patient's need for pain management.	3. Previous pain experiences and management strategies may be different from those needed for persistent pain.	
4. Encourage verbalization of feelings on pain and chronicity of disease.	4. Verbalization is a necessary step in coping.	
5. Instruct on pathophysiology of pain and rheumatic disease, and assist patient to identify that pain often leads to unproved treatment methods.	5. Knowledge of rheumatic pain and appropriate treatment may help patient avoid unsafe, ineffective therapies.	
6. Assist in identification of pain that leads to use of unproven methods of treatment.	6. The impact of pain on an individual's life often leads to misconceptions about pain and pain management techniques.	
7. Assess for subjective changes in pain.	7. The individual's description of the pain sensation is a more reliable indicator than objective measurements such as change in vital signs, body movement, and facial expression.	
NURSING DIAGNOSIS: Fatigue related to increased disease activity, pain, inadequate sleep/rest, deconditioning, inadequate nutrition, and emotional stress/depression		
GOAL: Incorporates as part of daily activities those measures necessary to modify fatigue		
1. Provide instruction in fatigue	1. The patient's understanding of fatigue will affect his or her actions.	• Self-evaluates and monitors fatigue pattern. • Verbalizes the relationship of fatigue to disease activity. • Uses comfort measures as appropriate. • Practices effective sleep hygiene and routine. • Makes use of various devices (splints, canes) and methods (bed rest, relaxation techniques) to ease different kinds of fatigue. • Incorporates time management strategies in daily activities. • Uses appropriate measures to prevent physical and emotional fatigue.
a. Relationship of disease activity to fatigue.	a. The amout of fatigue is directly related to the activity of the disease.	
b. Describe comfort measures while providing them.	b. Relief of discomfort can relieve fatigue	
c. Develop and maintain a sleep routine (warm bath and relaxation techniques that promote sleep).	c. Effective bedtime routine promotes restorative sleep.	
d. Explain importance of rest for relieving systemic, articular, and emotional stress.	d. Different kinds of rest are needed to relieve fatigue and are based on patient need and response.	
e. Explain how to use energy conservation techniques (pacing, delegating, prioritizing).	e. A variety of measures can be used to conserve energy.	

(continued)

NURSING CARE PLAN 52–1 *(continued)*
Care of the Patient With a Rheumatic Disease

Nursing Interventions	Rationale	Expected Outcomes
f. Identify physical and emotional factors that can cause fatigue.	f. Awareness of the various causes of fatigue provides the basis for measures to modify the fatigue.	• Has an established plan to ensure well-paced, therapeutic activity schedule. • Adheres to therapeutic program. • Follows a planned conditioning program. • Consumes a nutritious diet consisting of appropriate food groups and recommended daily allowance of vitamins and minerals.
2. Facilitate development of appropriate activity/rest schedule.	2. Alternating rest and activity conserves energy while allowing most productivity	
3. Encourage adherence to the treatment program.	3. Overall control of disease activity can decrease the amount of fatigue.	
4. Refer to and encourage a conditioning program.	4. Deconditioning resulting from lack of mobility, understanding, and disease activity contributes to fatigue.	
5. Encourage adequate nutrition, including source of iron from food and supplements.	5. A nutritious diet can help counteract fatigue.	

NURSING DIAGNOSIS: Impaired physical mobility related to decreased range of motion, muscle weakness, pain on movement, limited endurance, lack of or improper use of ambulatory devices

GOAL: Attains and maintains optimal functional mobility

Nursing Interventions	Rationale	Expected Outcomes
1. Encourage verbalization regarding limitations in mobility.	1. Mobility is not necessarily related to deformity. Pain, stiffness, and fatigue may temporarily limit mobility. The degree of mobility is not synonymous with the degree of independence. Decreased mobility may influence a person's self-concept and lead to social isolation.	• Identifies factors that interfere with mobility. • Describes and uses measures to prevent loss of motion. • Identifies environmental (home, school, work, community) barriers to optimal mobility. • Uses appropriate techniques and/or assistive equipment to aid mobility. • Identifies community resources available to assist in managing decreased mobility.
2. Assess need for OT/PT consultation: a. Emphasize ROM of affected joints. b. Promote use of ambulatory devices. c. Explain use of safe footwear. d. Use individual appropriate positioning/posture.	2. Therapeutic exercises, proper footwear, and/or assistive equipment may improve mobility. Correct posture and positioning are necessary for maintaining optimal mobility.	
3. Assist to identify environmental barriers.	3. Furniture and architectural adaptations may enhance mobliity.	
4. Encourage independence in mobility and assist as needed. a. Allow ample time for activity b. Provide rest period after activity. c. Reinforce principles of joint protection and work simplification.	4. Changes in mobility may lead to a decrease in personal safety.	
5. Initiate referral to community health agency.	5. The degree of mobility may be slow to improve or may not improve with intervention.	

NURSING DIAGNOSIS: Self-care deficits

GOAL: Achieves self-care independently or with the use of resources

Nursing Interventions	Rationale	Expected Outcomes
1. Assist patient to identify self-care deficits and factors that interfere with ability to perform self-care activities.	1. The ability to perform self-care activities is influenced by the disease activity and the accompanying pain, stiffness, fatigue, muscle weakness, loss of motion, and depression.	• Identifies factors that interfere with the ability to perform self-care activities. • Identifies alternative methods for meeting self-care needs.

(continued)

NURSING CARE PLAN 52–1 *(continued)*
Care of the Patient With a Rheumatic Disease

Nursing Interventions	Rationale	Expected Outcomes
2. Develop a plan based on the patient's perceptions and priorities on how to establish and achieve goals to meet self-care needs, incorporating joint protection, energy conservation, and work simplification concepts. a. Provide appropriate assistive devices. b. Reinforce proper use of assistive devices. c. Allow patient to control timing of self-care activities. d. Explore with the patient different ways to perform difficult tasks or ways to enlist the help of someone else.	2. Assistive devices may enhance self-care abilities. Effective planning for changes must include the patient who must accept and adopt the plan.	• Uses alternative methods for meeting self-care needs. • Identifies and uses other health care resources for meeting self-care needs.
3. Consult with community health care agencies when individuals have attained a maximum level of self-care yet still have some deficits, especially regarding safety.	3. Individuals differ in ability and willingness to perform self-care activities. Changes in ability to care for self may lead to a decrease in personal safety.	

NURSING DIAGNOSIS: Body image disturbance related to physical and psychological changes and dependency imposed by chronic illness

GOAL: Achieves a reconciliation between self-concept and the physical and psychologic changes imposed by the rheumatic disease

Nursing Interventions	Rationale	Expected Outcomes
1. Help patient identify elements of control over disease symptoms and treatment. 2. Encourage verbalization of feelings, perceptions, and fears. a. Help to assess present situation and identify problems. b. Assist to identify past coping mechanisms. c. Assist to identify effective coping mechanisms.	1. The individual's self-concept may be altered by the disease or its treatment. 2. The individual's coping strategies reflect the strength of his self-concept.	• Verbalizes an awareness that changes taking place in self-concept are normal responses to rheumatic disease and other chronic illnesses. • Identifies strategies to cope with altered self-concept.

NURSING DIAGNOSIS: Ineffective coping related to actual or perceived lifestyle or role changes

GOAL: Use of effective coping behaviors for dealing with actual or perceived limitations and role changes

Nursing Interventions	Rationale	Expected Outcomes
1. Identify areas of life affected by disease. Answer questions and dispel possible myths. 2. Develop plan for managing symptoms and enlisting support of family and friends to promote daily function.	1. The impact of disease may be more or less manageable once identified and explored reasonably. 2. By taking action and involving others appropriately, patient develops or draws on coping skills and community support.	• Names functions and roles affected and not affected by disease process. • Describes therapeutic regimen and states actions to take to improve, change, or accept a particular situation, function, or role.

COLLABORATIVE PROBLEMS: Complications secondary to effects of medications

GOAL: Experiences absence or resolution of complications

Nursing Interventions	Rationale	Expected Outcomes
1. Perform periodic clinical assessment and laboratory evaluation.	1. Skillful assessment helps detect early symptoms of side effects of medications.	• Complies with monitoring procedures and experiences minimal side effects.

(continued)

NURSING CARE PLAN 52–1 *(continued)*
Care of the Patient With a Rheumatic Disease

Nursing Interventions	Rationale	Expected Outcomes
2. Instruct in correct self-administration, side effects, and importance of monitoring, 3. Counsel regarding methods of reducing side effects and symptom management. 4. Administer medications in modified doses as prescribed if complications occur.	2. The patient needs accurate information about medication and side effects to avoid or manage them. 3. Appropriate identification and early intervention may minimize complications. 4. Modifications may help minimize side effects or other complications.	• Takes medication as prescribed, and lists potential side effects. • Identifies strategies to reduce side effects. • Reports that side effects or complications have subsided.

and chronic. Chronic fatigue, related to the disease process, is persistent, cumulative, and not eliminated by rest but is influenced by biologic, psychologic, social, and personal factors.

Disease-related factors that may influence the amount and severity of fatigue include persistent pain, sleep disturbance, impaired physical activity, and disease duration. Pain increases fatigue by requiring additional physical and emotional energy to deal with it. It may also cause the patient to expend more energy to do tasks in a way that causes less pain. Pain also may interfere with sleep, thereby affecting fatigue level.

Nursing interventions are directed at modifying and reducing the fatigue. Efforts to regain energy may be accomplished by utilizing rest periods. Patient needs will determine the type of rest and how much is needed. Naps or night-time sleep can provide systemic rest. Splints can provide articular rest by limiting motion and stress on the joints. Relaxation techniques can provide emotional rest. Stiffness, depression, and medications may also compromise the quality of sleep and increase daytime fatigue. Inactivity of people with arthritis may lead to deconditioning and fatigue; therefore, measures to build endurance should be instituted. These conditioning exercises, such as walking, swimming, or biking, require gradual progression of activity and monitoring of disease activity.

Psychosocial factors with an effect on fatigue include depression, learned helplessness, and perceived social support. These factors affect the patient's perception and evaluation of the fatigue. Improvement of functional status can positively affect mood.

Promoting Restorative Sleep. Good quality of sleep is important in helping the patient cope with pain, prevent physical fatigue, and deal with the changes necessitated by a chronic disease. The sleep of patients whose disease is active (in flare) is frequently reduced in time and fragmented by prolonged awakenings. A sleep-inducing routine, medication, and comfort measures may help improve the quality of sleep.

Increasing Mobility. Proper body positioning is essential to minimize stress on inflamed joints and prevent deformities that limit mobility. All joints should be supported in a position of optimal function. When in bed, the patient should lie flat on a firm mattress, with feet positioned against a footboard, and only one pillow under the head because of the risk of dorsal kyphosis. A pillow should not be placed under the knees, because this promotes flexion contracture. The patient lies on the abdomen several times daily to prevent hip flexion contracture.

Active range-of-motion exercises are encouraged because they prevent joint stiffness. If the patient cannot actively range the joints, passive range of motion should be performed.

Measures to reinforce proper body posture and increase mobility include walking erect and using chairs with straight backs. When seated, the patient should rest the feet flat on the floor and the shoulders and hips against the back of the chair.

Care must be taken that splinting for comfort does not restrict mobility later. The knee is splinted at full extension and the wrist at slight dorsiflexion. Because of the predominant strength of flexor muscles, the joints should not be permitted to "freeze" in positions of flexion. This can be prevented by regularly removing the splint and exercising the joint through a range of motion. Splints may need to be modified when changes occur in joint structure.

Additionally, assistive devices may be necessary for mobility. They should be properly fitted and the patient instructed in their correct and safe use. A cane should be long enough to allow for only a slight bend of the elbow and should be held in the hand *opposite* the affected side. Crutches may need to be of the forearm-trough style to protect the upper extremities if the disease involves the patient's hands and wrists. This is especially important for the patient undergoing rehabilitation after any lower extremity joint reconstructive surgery. Assistive devices can mean the difference between dependence and independence in mobility; however, they may also alter the patient's body image, which may become a barrier to compliance with treatment.

Facilitating Self-Care. Adaptive equipment may increase the patient's independence. When introducing adaptive equipment, however, the nurse should be sensitive to the patient's feelings and demonstrate acceptance and positive attitudes about using these devices. The nurse needs to keep in mind that a patient's deformity need not equate with disability. For example, swollen hands may be more limiting than deformed hands. The hospital-based and extended care facility nurse can help preserve the patient's independence in these settings by making adaptive equipment for eating, toileting, bathing, and dressing available for use. In the home, the nurse can encourage using these devices. Again, by relieving pain, stiffness, and fatigue, the nurse may increase the patient's ability to perform self care.

Improving Body Image. All aspects of the patient's life, including the patient's perception of self, work role, social life, sexual function, and financial status, may be altered because of the unpredictability and uncertainty of the course of a rheumatic disease. Body-image changes may cause social isolation and depression. The nurse and the family need to empathize with the patient's emotional reactions to the disease. Communication should be encouraged so that the patient and family verbalize feelings, perceptions, and fears related to the disease. The nurse helps the patient and family identify areas in which they have some control over disease symptoms and treatment. The nurse also encourages commitment to the treatment program, which is a key to positive outcomes.

Monitoring and Managing Potential Complications

Avoiding Drug-Induced Complications. Medications used for treating rheumatic diseases have the potential for serious and adverse effects. The physician bases the prescribed medication regimen on clinical findings and past medical history, then monitors for side effects with periodic clinical assessments and laboratory monitoring. The nurse has a major role in working with the physician and pharmacist to help the patient recognize and deal with side effects from medications. These side effects may include gastrointestinal bleeding or irritation, bone marrow suppression, kidney or liver toxicity, increased incidence of infection, mouth sores, rashes, and changes in vision. Other signs and symptoms include bruising, breathing problems, dizziness, jaundice, dark urine, black or bloody stools, diarrhea, nausea and vomiting, and headaches. Systemic and local infections, which often can be masked by high doses of corticosteroids, need to be monitored closely. (Refer to Table 52-3 for further side effects of drugs used in treating rheumatic diseases.) Patient instruction also includes teaching techniques of correct self-administration, methods of reducing side effects, and measures to ensure regular monitoring. The nurse can be available for consultation between physician visits. If side effects occur, the medication may need to be stopped or the dose reduced. The patient may experience an increase in symptoms while the complication is being resolved or a new medication is being initiated. In such cases, the nurse's counseling regarding symptom management may relieve potential anxiety and distress.

Avoiding Infection and Organ Failure. The patient's vital signs, level of consciousness, and symptoms of infection are monitored closely to detect systemic and local infections, which often can be masked by high doses of corticosteroids. The patient's vital signs, intake and output, edema, respiratory status, and skin color are monitored for signs of toxicity and other complications, including organ failure. Renal failure, not uncommon in systemic lupus erythematosus, may require intravenous chemotherapy, dialysis, or (in extreme cases) renal transplantion. Because treatment of complications often requires hospitalization, patient education and emotional support are required to help the patient cope with the unexpected complications of an already serious disease. Family support and involvement in care are encouraged.

Evaluation

Expected Outcomes

1. Experiences relief of pain or improved comfort level
   a. Identifies factors that cause or increase pain
   b. Uses pain management strategies effectively
   c. Identifies realistic goals for pain relief
   d. Reports decreased pain and increased comfort level
2. Experiences reduction in level of fatigue
   a. Identifies factors that contribute to fatigue
   b. Verbalizes the relationship of fatigue to disease activity
   c. Schedules periodic rest periods and identifies and uses other measures to prevent or modify fatigue
   d. Reports decreased level of fatigue
3. Increases or maintains level of mobility
   a. Identifies factors that impede mobility
   b. Participates in activities and exercises that promote or maintain mobility
   c. Uses assistive devices appropriately and safely
   d. Demonstrates good body alignment and posture
4. Maintains self-care activities
   a. Participates in self-care activities within capabilities
   b. Uses adaptive equipment and alternative methods to increase participation in self-care activities
   c. Maintains self-care at highest possible level
5. Experiences improved body image
   a. Verbalizes concerns about the impact of rheumatic disease on appearance and function
   b. Reconciles body image and changes caused by disease
   c. States acceptance of self-worth
   d. Sets and achieves meaningful goals
6. Experiences absence of complications
   a. Takes medications as prescribed
   b. States potential side effects of medications and names reportable side effects
   c. Understands rationale for monitoring
   d. Identifies strategies to reduce risks of side effects

Patient Education and Home Care Considerations

Patients may be unfamiliar with their disease process and treatment regimen. They need to verbalize their concerns and ask questions. They need answers that will be meaningful when they are at home and managing their own care. Pain, fatigue, and depression can interfere with the patient's ability to learn and should be addressed before initiating an educational program. Various educational strategies may then be used, depending on the patient's previous knowledge base, interest level, degree of comfort, social or cultural influences, and readiness to learn. The nurse instructs the patient about basic disease management, medications, and necessary adaptations in life-style.

Persistent inflammation and autoimmune activity lead to joint and tissue damage. Because suppression of those responses requires the use of anti-inflammatory, slow-acting anti-rheumatic and immunosuppressive agents, the patient is taught about prescribed medications, including rationale, side effects, self-administration, and required monitoring procedures.

The nurse assesses for barriers to compliance and makes appropriate referrals. Because many of the medications to suppress inflammation are injectable, the nurse may administer the medication to the patient or teach self-injection procedure. These frequent contacts allow the nurse to reinforce other disease management techniques.

If hospitalized, the patient is encouraged to practice new self-management skills with support from caregivers and significant others. The nurse then reinforces disease management skills during each patient contact.

Diffuse Connective Tissue Diseases

Diffuse connective tissue disease (CTD) is a term that refers to a group of disorders, chronic in nature, characterized by diffuse inflammation and degeneration in the connective tissues. These disorders share similar clinical features and may affect some of the same organs. The characteristic clinical course is one of exacerbations and remissions. The diffuse CTDs have unknown etiologies but are thought to be the result of immunologic abnormalities. The CTDs include rheumatoid arthritis, systemic lupus erythematosus, scleroderma, polymyositis, and polymyalgia rheumatica.

Rheumatoid Arthritis

Pathophysiology

In rheumatoid arthritis (RA), the autoimmune reaction (described earlier) primarily occurs in the synovial tissue. Phagocytosis produces enzymes within the joint. The enzymes break down collagen, causing edema, proliferation of the synovial membrane, and ultimately pannus formation. Pannus destroys cartilage and erodes the bone (see Fig. 52-1). The consequence is loss of articular surfaces and joint motion. The muscles are affected as the muscle fibers undergo degenerative changes, with loss of muscle elasticity and contractile power.

Clinical Manifestations

Clinical manifestations of RA vary and usually reflect the stage and severity of the disease. Joint pain, swelling, warmth, erythema, and lack of function are classic clinical features of RA. Palpation of the joints reveals spongy or boggy tissue. Fluid can often be aspirated from the inflamed joint.

The characteristic pattern of joint involvement begins with the small joints in the hands, wrists, and feet. As the disease progresses, knees, shoulders, hips, elbows, ankles, cervical spine, and temporomandibular joints are involved. The onset of symptoms is usually acute; symptoms are usually bilateral and symmetric. In addition to joint pain and swelling, another classic sign of RA is joint stiffness, especially in the morning, lasting for more than 30 minutes.

Limitation in function can occur even in the early stages of disease before bony changes occur and when there is active inflammation in the joints. Joints that are hot, swollen, and painful are not easily moved, and the patient tends to guard or protect these joints through immobilization. Immobilization for extended periods can lead to contractures, creating soft-tissue deformity.

Deformities of the hands and feet are common in RA. The deformity may be caused by misalignment resulting from swelling, progressive joint destruction, or the subluxation (partial dislocation) that occurs when a bone slips over another and eliminates the joint space.

RA is a systemic disease with multiple extra-articular features. Most common are fever, weight loss, fatigue, anemia, lymph node enlargement, and Raynaud's phenomenon (cold- and stress-induced vasospasm causing episodes of digital blanching or cyanosis). Rheumatoid nodules may be noted in patients who have more advanced RA; they are present in 20% to 25% of patients. These nodules are usually nontender and movable in the subcutaneous tissue; they usually appear over bony prominences such as the elbow, are varied in size, and can disappear spontaneously. Nodules occur only in individuals who have rheumatoid factor (RF). The nodules often are associated with rapidly progressive and destructive disease. Other extra-articular features include arteritis, neuropathy, scleritis, pericarditis, splenomegaly, and Sjögren's syndrome (dry eyes and dry mucous membranes).

Diagnostic Evaluation

Several factors can contribute to an RA diagnosis: rheumatoid nodules, joint inflammation detected on palpation, and certain laboratory findings. Rheumatoid factor is present in more than 80% of patients with rheumatoid arthritis; however, its presence alone is not diagnostic of RA. The erythrocyte sedimentation rate (ESR) is significantly elevated with RA. The red blood cell (RBC) count and C_4 complement component are decreased. The C-reactive protein (CRP) and antinuclear antibody (ANA) test results may also be positive. An arthrocentesis shows synovial fluid that is cloudy, milky, or dark yellow and contains numerous inflammatory cells, such as leukocytes and complement.

X-ray studies are performed to help diagnose and monitor the progression of disease. The x-ray films will show characteristic bony erosions and narrowed joint spaces occurring later in the disease.

Management

For **early RA,** treatment begins with education, a balance of rest and exercise, and referral to community agencies for support. Medical management begins with therapeutic doses of salicylates or NSAIDs. When used in full therapeutic dosages, these medications provide both anti-inflammatory and analgesic effects. Patients are instructed to take medications as prescribed to maintain a consistent blood level to optimize the effectiveness of the anti-inflammatory drug.

The trend in management is toward a more aggressive pharmacologic approach earlier in the disease. A window of opportunity for symptom control and improved disease management occurs within the first 2 years of disease onset. Unless inflammation can be totally controlled with anti-inflammatory drugs, the slow-acting anti-rheumatic agents (antimalarials, gold, penicillamine, or sulfasalazine) will be initiated early in treatment. If symptoms appear to be aggressive (*i.e.*, early bony erosions at the joint), methotrexate may be considered. The goal is to prevent destruction of the joint.

Additional analgesia may be prescribed for periods of extreme pain. Narcotic analgesics are avoided because of the potential for continuing need for pain relief. Nonpharmacologic pain management techniques should be taught (*i.e.*, relaxation techniques, heat and cold applications). Table 52-3 provides more information on the drugs used in the treatment of RA.

For **moderate, erosive RA,** a formal program with occupational and physical therapy is prescribed to educate the patient about principles of joint protection, pacing activities, work simplification, range of motion, and muscle-strengthening exercises. The patient is encouraged to participate actively in the management program. The medication program is reevaluated periodically, and appropriate changes are made if indicated.

For **persistent, erosive RA,** reconstructive surgery and corticosteroids are often prescribed. Reconstructive surgery is indicated when pain cannot be relieved by conservative measures. Surgical procedures include synovectomy (excision of the synovial membrane), tenorrhaphy (suturing a tendon), arthrodesis (surgical fusion of the joint), and arthroplasty (surgical repair of the joint). However, surgery is not performed during disease flares.

Systemic corticosteroids are used when the patient has unremitting inflammation and pain and/or needs a "bridging" medication while waiting for the slow-acting anti-rheumatic agent (*e.g.*, gold) to begin working. Low-dose corticosteroid therapy is recommended for the shortest time necessary (to minimize side effects). Joints that are severely inflamed and fail to respond promptly to the measures outlined above may be treated by local injection of a corticosteroid.

For **advanced, unremitting RA,** immunosuppressive drugs are prescribed because of their ability to affect the production of antibodies at the cellular level. These include high-dose methotrexate, cyclophosphamide, and azathioprine. However, these drugs are highly toxic and can produce bone marrow depression, anemia, gastrointestinal disturbances, and rashes. Plasmapheresis, lymphopheresis, and total lymphoid irradiation are experimental procedures introduced in the 1970s that are now thought to have little or no role in managing rheumatic diseases except in instances of acute life-threatening situations that have failed to respond to conventional, aggressive therapies.

Through all stages of RA, depression and sleep deprivation may require the short-term use of low-dose antidepressant medications such as amitriptyline to reestablish an adequate sleep pattern and better manage chronic pain.

Patients with RA frequently experience anorexia, weight loss, and anemia. A dietary history will identify usual eating habits and food preferences. The patient is then taught how to select foods that include the daily requirements from the basic food groups, with emphasis on foods high in vitamins, protein, and iron for tissue building and repair. For the extremely anorexic patient, small, frequent feedings with increased protein supplements may be prescribed. Some medications (*i.e.*, oral corticosteroids) used in RA treatment stimulate the appetite and, when combined with decreased activity, may lead to weight gain.

Nursing Considerations. The nursing care of the patient with RA follows the basic care plan (see Nursing Care Plan 52-1). The most common problems of the RA patient are pain, sleep disturbance, fatigue, and limited motion. The patient with newly diagnosed RA will need information about the disease to make daily self-management decisions and to cope with having a chronic disease.

Systemic Lupus Erythematosus

Pathophysiology

Systemic lupus erythematosus (SLE) seems to result from disturbed immune regulation that causes an exaggerated production of autoantibodies. This immunoregulatory disturbance is brought about by some combination of genetic, hormonal (as evidenced by the usual onset during the child-bearing years), and environmental factors (sunlight, thermal burns). Certain drugs, such as hydralazine (Apresoline), procainamide (Pronestyl), isoniazid, chlorpromazine, and some anticonvulsants, have been implicated in chemical or drug-induced SLE, as have foods such as alfalfa sprouts.

In SLE, the increase in autoantibody production is thought to result from abnormal suppressor T-cell function, which results in immune complex deposition and ensuing tissue damage. Inflammation stimulates antigens, which in turn stimulate additional antibodies, and the cycle repeats.

Clinical Manifestations

The onset of SLE may be insidious or acute. For this reason, the patient with SLE may remain undiagnosed for many years. Clinical features of SLE involve multiple body systems. The musculoskeletal system is involved with arthralgias and arthritis (synovitis), which are common presenting features of SLE. Joint swelling, tenderness, and pain on movement are common and are accompanied by morning stiffness.

Several different types of skin manifestations may occur in patients with SLE; these include subacute cutaneous lupus erythematosus (SCLE) and discoid lupus erythematosus (DLE). The most familiar (but occurring in fewer than 50% of patients) skin manifestation is an acute cutaneous lesion consisting of a butterfly-shaped rash across the bridge of the nose and cheeks (Fig. 52-3). There may be only skin involvement in some cases of lupus erythematosus (discoid). In some patients, the initial skin involvement may be the precursor to more systemic involvement. The lesions often worsen during exacerbations (flares) of the systemic disease and may be provoked by sunlight or artificial ultraviolet light.

Oral ulcers may involve the buccal mucosa or the hard palate. They occur in crops, are often associated with exacerbations, and may accompany skin lesions. Pericarditis is the most common cardiac manifestation and occurs in up to 30% of patients. It may be asymptomatic and is often accompanied by pleural effusions. Lung and pleural involvement occurs in 20% to 40% of patients; this is most often manifested by pleuritis or pleural effusions.

The vascular system can be involved, with inflammation of the terminal arterioles producing papular, erythematous, and purpuric lesions. These lesions may develop on the fingertips, elbows, toes, and extensor surfaces of the forearms or lateral sides of the hand and may progress to necrosis.

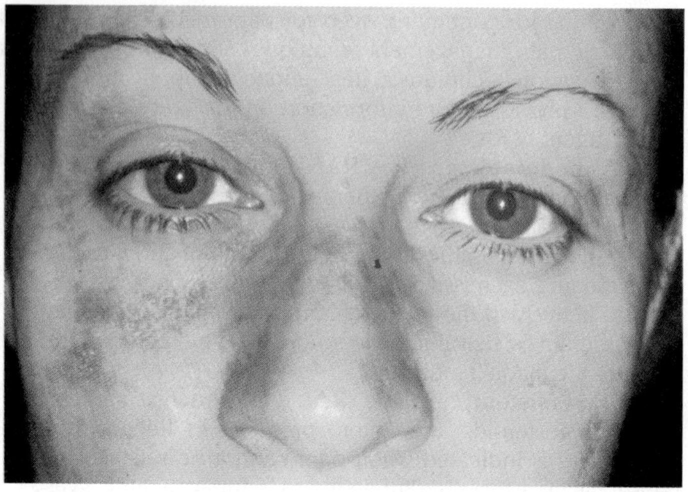

FIGURE 52-3. The characteristic butterfly rash of systemic lupus erythematosus. (Drs. S. Wilson and W. Larson, SmithKline Beecham.)

Lymphadenopathy occurs in 50% of all SLE patients at some time during the course of illness. Renal involvement occurs in about 32% of patients with SLE, and the glomeruli of the kidneys are usually affected. The extent of kidney damage indicates whether renal involvement will be reversible.

The varied and frequent neuropsychiatric presentations of SLE are now more widely recognized. These are generally demonstrated by subtle changes in behavior patterns or cognitive ability. The spectrum of central nervous system involvement is wide and encompasses the entire range of neurologic disease. Depression and psychosis are frequent.

Diagnostic Evaluation

Diagnosis of SLE is based on a complete history and blood tests. Classic symptoms include fever, fatigue, and weight loss and possibly arthritis, pleurisy, and pericarditis. No single laboratory test confirms SLE; rather, serum testing reveals moderate to severe anemia, thrombocytopenia, leukocytosis, or leukopenia and positive anti-nuclear antibodies. Other diagnostic immunologic tests support but do not confirm the diagnosis. (See Table 52-1 for more detailed information regarding these tests.)

Management

Treatment for SLE includes management of acute and chronic disease. Acute disease requires interventions directed at controlling increased disease activity or exacerbations that may involve any organ system. Disease activity is a composite of clinical and laboratory features that reflect active inflammation secondary to SLE. Management of the more chronic condition involves periodic monitoring and recognition of meaningful clinical changes requiring adjustments in therapy. Patient education is extremely important.

The goals of treatment include preventing progressive loss of organ function, reducing the likelihood of acute disease, minimizing disease-related disabilities, and preventing complications from therapy. Management of SLE involves regular monitoring to assess disease activity and therapeutic effectiveness.

Medication therapy for SLE is based on the concept that local tissue inflammation is mediated by exaggerated or heightened immune responses, which can vary widely in intensity and require different therapies at different times. The NSAIDs are used for minor clinical manifestations and are often used along with corticosteroids in an effort to minimize corticosteroid requirements.

Corticosteroids are the single most important medication available for treatment. They are used topically for cutaneous manifestations, in low oral doses for minor disease activity, and in high doses for major disease activity. Bolus IV administration is regarded as an alternative to traditional high-dose oral use. Antimalarial drugs are effective for managing cutaneous, musculoskeletal, and mild systemic features of SLE. Immunosuppressive agents (alkylating agents and purine analogs) are used because of their effect on immune function. These drugs are regarded as experimental and are generally reserved for patients who have serious forms of SLE and who have not responded to conservative therapies. Table 52-2 contains more information about these medications.

Nursing Considerations. In addition to the general assessment performed for a patient with a rheumatic disease, assessment for known or suspected SLE has special features. The skin is inspected for erythematous rashes. Cutaneous erythematous plaques with an adherent scale may be observed on the scalp, face, or neck. Areas of hyperpigmentation or depigmentation may be noted depending on the phase and type of the disease. The patient should be questioned about skin changes (because these may be transitory) and specifically about sensitivity to sunlight or artificial ultraviolet light. The scalp should be inspected for alopecia and the mouth and throat for ulcerations reflecting gastrointestinal involvement.

Cardiovascular assessment includes auscultation for pericardial friction rub, which may be associated with myocarditis and may accompany pleural effusions. The pleural effusions and infiltrations reflect respiratory insufficiency and are demonstrated by abnormal lung sounds. Papular, erythematous, and purpuric lesions that may become necrotic suggest vascular involvement. These lesions may develop on the fingertips, elbows, toes, and extensor surfaces of the forearms or lateral sides of the hand.

Joint swelling, tenderness, warmth, pain on movement, and stiffness are signs of musculoskeletal involvement. The joint involvement is often symmetric and similar to that found in rheumatoid arthritis. Edema and hematuria indicate renal involvement. In addition to the physical assessment, confirming evidence of systemic involvement can be found in laboratory findings. Interactions with the patient and family may provide further evidence of systemic involvement. The neurologic assessment is directed at identifying and describing any central nervous system problems. The patient and family members can be asked about any behavioral changes, neuroses, or psychosis. Signs of depression should be noted, as well as reports of seizures, chorea, or other CNS manifestations.

The nursing care of the patient with SLE is based on the basic care plan (see Nursing Care Plan 52-1) for a patient with rheumatic disease. The patient's most frequent problems are fatigue, impaired skin integrity, body image disturbance, and lack of knowledge for self-management decisions. The disease or its treatment may produce dramatic changes in appearance and considerable distress for the patient. The changes and the unpredicatable course of SLE necessitate expert assessment skills and nursing care and sensitivity to the psychologic reactions of the patient.

Scleroderma

Pathophysiology

Like other diffuse CTDs, scleroderma has a variable course with remissions and exacerbations; its prognosis, however, is not as optimistic as that of lupus. The disease commonly begins with skin involvement. Mononuclear cells cluster on the skin and stimulate lymphokines to stimulate procollagen. Insoluble collagen is formed and accumulates excessively in the tissues. Initially, the inflammatory response causes edema formation, with a resulting taut, smooth, and shiny skin appearance. The skin then undergoes fibrotic changes leading to loss of elasticity and movement. Eventually the tissue degenerates and becomes nonfunctional. This chain of events, from inflammation to degeneration, also occurs in blood vessels, major organs, and body systems, potentially resulting in death.

Clinical Manifestations

Scleroderma starts insidiously with Raynaud's phenomenon and swelling in the hands. The skin and the subcutaneous tissues become increasingly hard and rigid and cannot be pinched up from the underlying structures. Wrinkles and lines are obliterated. The skin is dry because sweat secretion over the involved region is suppressed. The extremities stiffen and lose mobility. The condition spreads slowly. For years, these changes may remain localized in the hands and the feet (scleroderma). The face appears masklike, immobile, and expressionless, and the mouth becomes rigid.

The changes within the body, although not visible directly, are vastly more important than the visible changes. The left ventricle of the heart is involved, resulting in congestive heart failure; the esophagus hardens, interfering with swallowing; the lungs sustain scarring, impeding respiration; digestive disturbances occur because of hardening (sclerosing) of the intestinal mucosa; and progressive renal failure may occur.

The patient may manifest a variety of symptoms referred to as the *CREST syndrome.* The letters CREST stand for calcinosis (*c*alcium deposits in the tissues), *R*aynaud's phenomenon, *e*sophageal hardening and dysfunctioning, *s*clerodactyly (scleroderma of the digits), and *t*elangiectasis (capillary dilation that forms a vascular lesion).

Diagnostic Evaluation

There is no one conclusive test to diagnose scleroderma. A complete history and physical examination are performed to note any fibrotic changes in the skin, lungs, heart, or esophagus. A skin biopsy is performed to identify cellular changes specific to scleroderma. Pulmonary studies will show ventilation perfusion abnormalities. An ECG will identify pericardial effusion (often present with cardiac involvement). Esophageal studies demonstrate decreased motility in 75% of patients with scleroderma. Blood tests may detect antinuclear antibodies (ANAs), indicating a connective tissue disorder and possibly distinguishing the subgroup of scleroderma. A positive ANA test result is common with scleroderma. An ANA finding that demonstrates the anticentromere pattern is associated with the CREST syndrome.

Management

Treatment of scleroderma depends on the clinical manifestations. All patients require personal counseling during which realistic individual goals may be determined. Currently no drug regimen has proved effective in controlling scleroderma; however, various drugs can be used to treat the symptoms. Penicillamine has been the most promising medication in decreasing skin thickening, reducing the rate of new visceral organ involvement, and prolonging life. Captopril and other potent antihypertensive agents are effective in controlling hypertensive crises. Anti-inflammatory medications can be used to control arthralgia, stiffness, and general musculoskeletal discomfort. Vasodilators have not proved effective for vascular abnormalities. Supportive easures include decreasing pain and limiting disability. A moderate exercise program is encouraged to prevent joint contractures. Patients are advised to avoid extreme temperatures and to use lotions to minimize skin dryness.

Nursing Considerations. The nursing assessment may focus on the sclerotic changes in the skin, contractures in the fingers, and color changes or lesions in the fingertips. Assessment of systemic involvement requires a systems review with special attention to gastrointestinal, pulmonary, renal, and cardiac symptoms. Limitations in mobility and self-care activities should be assessed along with the impact the disease has had (or will have) on body image. Refer to Chart 52-2 for a guide to assessment of multisystem problems.

The nursing care of the patient with SS is based on the basic care plan (see Nursing Care Plan 52-1) for patients with a rheumatic disease. The most frequent problems of the patient with SS include impaired skin integrity; self-care deficits; altered nutrition, less than body requirements; and body image disturbance. The patient with advanced disease may also have problems with impaired gas exchange, decreased cardiac output, impaired swallowing, and constipation.

Polymyositis

Pathophysiology

The pathogenesis of polymyositis (PM) is multifactorial. A genetic predisposition is likely. Drug-induced disease is rare but has been reported. Some evidence suggests a viral link. PM is classified as autoimmune because autoantibodies are present; however, these antibodies do not cause damage to muscle cells, indicating only an indirect role in tissue damage.

Clinical Manifestations

The onset of PM varies from sudden with rapid progression to a very slow, insidious onset. Proximal muscle weakness is typically a first symptom. Muscle weakness is usually symmetric and diffuse. Dermatomyositis, a related condition, is most commonly identified by an erythematous smooth or scaly lesion found over the joint surface.

Diagnostic Evaluation

As with other diffuse connective tissue disorders, no one test confirms PM. A complete history and physical examination will help to exclude other muscle-related disorders. An electromyogram (EMG) is performed to rule out degenerative muscle disease. Muscle biopsy may reveal inflammatory infiltrate in the tissue. Serum studies indicate increased muscle enzyme activity.

Management

Treatment of PM involves corticosteroid therapy, with high doses initially and gradual dosage reduction over several months as muscle enzyme activity decreases. Patients who do not respond to corticosteroids require the addition of an immunosuppressive agent (see Table 52-3). For those patients who are unresponsive to corticosteroids and immunosuppressive medications (up to 10% of patients), plasmapheresis may be tried. Skin rashes may respond to hydroxychloroquine. Physical therapy is initiated slowly with ROM exercises to maintain joint mobility, followed by gradual strengthening exercises.

Nursing Considerations. The nursing care of the patient with PM is based on the basic care plan (see Nursing Care Plan 52-1) for a patient with rheumatic disease. The most frequent problems of the PM patient are impaired physical mobility; fatigue; self-care deficit; and insufficient knowledge of self-management techniques.

Polymyalgia Rheumatica

Pathophysiology

The cause of polymyalgia rheumatica (PMR) is unknown. The disease is predominant in Caucasians—often in first-degree relatives—and an association with the genetic marker (HLA-DR4) suggests a familial predisposition. Immunoglobulin deposits in the walls of inflamed temporal arteries also suggest an autoimmune process.

Clinical Manifestations

PMR is characterized by severe proximal muscle discomfort with mild joint swelling. Complaints of severe aching in the neck, shoulder, and pelvic muscles are common. Stiffness is noticeable most often in the morning and after periods of inactivity. Systemic features include low-grade fever, weight loss, malaise, anorexia, and depression. Because PMR generally occurs in people 50 years of age and older, it may be confused with, or disregarded as, an inevitable consequence of aging.

Giant cell arteritis (GSA) is sometimes associated with PMR and may cause headaches, changes in vision, and jaw claudication. These symptoms should be heeded immediately because of the potential for a sudden and permanent loss of vision. Both of these conditions generally run a self-limited course lasting several months to several years.

Diagnostic Evaluation

Diagnosis is difficult because of the lack of specificity of tests. A markedly high erythrocyte sedimentation rate is a screening test but is not definitive. Diagnosis is more likely to be made by eliminating other potential diagnoses and is highly dependent upon the skills and experience of the diagnostician. The dramatic and immediate response to treatment with corticosteroids is considered by some to be diagnostic.

Management

PMR (without GSA) is treated with moderate doses of corticosteroids. NSAIDs are sometimes used for mild disease. For patients with GSA, rapid initiation and strict adherence to a regimen of corticosteroids is essential to avoid the complication of blindness.

Nursing Considerations. Nursing assessment focuses on musculoskeletal tenderness, weakness, and decreased function. Careful attention should be directed toward assessing the head (vision, headaches, and jaw claudication).

The nursing care of the patient with PMR is based on the basic care plan (see Nursing Care Plan 52-1) for a patient with rheumatic disease. The most common problems of the patient with PMR are pain and insufficient knowledge of the medication regimen.

Degenerative Joint Disease (Osteoarthritis)

Osteoarthritis (OA), also known as degenerative joint disease or osteoarthrosis (even though inflammation may be present), is the most common and frequently disabling of the joint disorders. OA is both overdiagnosed and trivialized; it is frequently overtreated or undertreated. The functional impact of OA on quality of life, especially for elderly patients, is often ignored.

OA has been classified as primary (idiopathic), with no prior event or disease related to the OA, and secondary. The distinction between primary and secondary OA, however, is not always clear.

Increasing age directly relates to the degenerative process in the joint as the ability of the articular cartilage to resist microfracture with repetitive low loads diminishes. OA often begins in the third decade of life and peaks between the fifth and sixth decades. By age 75, 85% of the population will have either x-ray or clinical evidence of OA. However, only 15% to 25% of this number experience significant symptoms.

Pathophysiology

OA may be thought of as the end result of many pathologies combining in a generalized predisposition to the disease. OA affects the articular cartilage, subchondral bone (the bony plate that supports the articular cartilage), and synovium and causes a mixture of degradation, inflammation, and repair. The basic degenerative process in the joint was described earlier in this chapter and is exemplified in OA. Understanding of OA has been greatly expanded beyond what previously was thought of as simply "wear and tear" related to aging. Risk factors for OA include age, female gender, genetic predisposition, obesity, mechanical joint stress, joint trauma, previous bone or joint disorders, and a history of inflammatory, endocrine, or metabolic disease.

A hereditary subset of OA known as nodal generalized OA (involving three or more joint groups) has been confirmed. This type of OA involves a primary inflammatory process. Postmenopausal women in the same family have been observed to have a type of OA of the hands characterized by the presence of nodes at the distal interphalangeal joint and at the proximal interphalangeal joint in the hand.

Congenital and developmental disorders of the hip are well known for predisposing a person to OA of the hip. These include congenital subluxation–dislocation of the hip, acetabular dysplasia, Legg-Calvé-Perthes disease, and slipped capital femoral epiphysis.

Obesity has been associated with OA of the knee in women. Although this may be as a result of additional mechanical stress and misalignment of the knee joint in relationship to the rest of the body because of the diameter of the thighs, obesity may have a direct metabolic effect on cartilage. Mechanically, it is thought that obesity increases the force across the joint and, therefore, causes cartilage degeneration. The metabolic factor theory suggests that there is a hormone or biologic mediator linked with obesity that causes OA. Obesity is associated with increased subchondral bone mass, which may lead to bony stiffness that makes subchondral bone less flexible upon impact loading, transmitting more force to overlying articular cartilage, thus making it more susceptible to injury.

Obese women have been shown to have an incidence of OA of the knee nearly four times that of women of average weight. The question has been raised as to whether obesity precedes OA or is the result of a sedentary life-style adopted by symptomatic patients; recent studies suggest the former. It has also been shown that obesity during young adulthood, when OA is extremely rare, increases the risk of later OA of the knee. Weight loss in the mid or later years appears to reduce the risk for later OA of the knee. These findings appear to apply more to women than to men, in whom knee injury may be a more important causal agent. Thus, preventing or reducing obesity may be important in preventing OA of the knee.

Mechanical factors such as joint trauma, sports activities, and occupation have also been implicated. These factors include cruciate ligament damage and meniscal tears, heavy physical activity, and frequent knee bending.

Clinical Manifestations

The primary clinical manifestations of OA are pain, stiffness, and functional impairment. The pain in OA is due to an inflamed synovium, stretching of the joint capsule or ligaments, irritation of nerve endings in the periosteum over osteophytes, trabecular microfracture, intraosseous hypertension, bursitis, tendinitis, and muscle spasm. Stiffness, which is most commonly experienced in the morning or after awakening, usually lasts less than 30 minutes and decreases with movement. Functional impairment is due to pain on movement and limited motion caused by structural changes in the joints.

Although OA occurs most often in weight-bearing joints (hips, knees, cervical and lumbar spine), the middle and end finger joints are also often involved. Characteristic bony nodes may be present; on inspection and palpation these are usually painless, unless inflammation is present.

Diagnostic Evaluation

Defining who has OA is complicated in that only 30% to 50% of patients with changes seen on x-ray films report symptoms. A physical assessment of the musculoskeletal system will show tender and enlarged joints. Inflammation, when present, is not the destructive type seen in the connective tissue diseases such as RA. OA is characterized by a progressive loss of the joint cartilage, which appears on x-ray films as a narrowing of joint space (since cartilage is not radiographic). In addition, reactive changes occur at the joint margins and on the subchondral bone in the form of osteophytes (or spurs) as the cartilage attempts to regenerate. Neither the presence of osteophytes nor joint space narrowing alone is specific for OA; combined, however, they are sensitive and specific findings. In early or mild OA the correlation between joint pain and synovitis is weak. Serum studies are not useful in the diagnosis of this disorder.

Management

Although no treatment stops the degenerative process, certain preventive measures can slow the progress if undertaken early enough. These include weight reduction, preventing injuries, perinatal screening for congenital hip disease, and ergonomic approaches to job stress modification. Therapeutic management consists of pharmacotherapy, supportive measures, and surgical intervention when pain is intractable and function has been lost.

The pharmacologic regimen is based on newer understanding of the damage from OA caused by the metabolic active remodeling process and is directed at improving cartilage repair and retarding breakdown. Some studies have raised the possibility that salicylates and some of the NSAIDs may accelerate the progression of cartilage breakdown in OA. Acetaminophen may be as effective as an NSAID in the symptomatic treatment of OA. Initially, high daily doses of acetaminophen are prescribed along with nonpharmacologic measures of pain relief. Side effects and cost of NSAIDs are greater than acetaminophen. If control of joint symptoms is not achieved within a reasonable period, an NSAID is then prescribed. Ongoing reassessment is directed at reducing the dosage or using the NSAID only intermittently at times of joint pain exacerbation. Intra-articular injections of corticosteroids are used cautiously for an immediate, short-term effect when a joint is acutely inflamed.

Conservative treatment measures include the use of heat, weight reduction, joint rest and avoidance of joint overuse, orthotic devices to support inflamed joints (splints, braces), and isometric and postural exercises. Occupational and physical therapy can help the patient adopt self-management strategies.

Tidal irrigation (washing debris from the joint space), arthroscopic debridement, drilling of osteochondral defects, or abrasion arthroplasty (to smooth the joint surface) may reduce pain in knees with OA, but studies show a high percentage of placebo effect. For patients with end-stage disease, joint **arthroplasty** (replacement) can relieve pain and restore loss of function. OA of the knee accounts for most knee surgery, including most total knee replacements.

Spondyloarthropathies

The seronegative spondyloarthropathies are another category of systemic inflammatory disorders of the skeleton. The spondyloarthropathies include ankylosing spondylitis, reactive arthritis, and psoriatic arthritis. Spondyloarthritis is also associated with inflammatory bowel diseases such as regional enteritis (Crohn's disease) and ulcerative colitis.

This group of rheumatic diseases has several clinical features in common. The inflammation in these diseases tends to occur peripherally at the sites of attachment, at tendons, joint capsules, and ligaments. Periosteal inflammation may be present. Many of these patients have arthritis of the sacroiliac joints. There is a strong tendency for these conditions to occur in families. Onset tends to occur during young adulthood, and the disease affects men more often than women. The human leukocyte antigen (HLA) B27 genetic marker is found frequently.

Ankylosing spondylitis (AS) affects the cartilaginous joints of the spine and surrounding tissues. Occasionally the large synovial joints such as hips, knees, or shoulders may be involved. The characteristic feature of AS is back pain. As the disease progresses, the entire spine may become ankylosed (fixed), causing respiratory compromise and complications. AS is usually diagnosed around the second or third decade of life. The disease is not usually as severe in females as in males, in whom the disease is more prevalent and likely to include significant systemic involvement

Reiter's syndrome affects young adult males and is characterized primarily by urethritis, arthritis, and conjunctivitis. Dermatitis and ulcerations of the mouth and penis may also be present. Low back pain is common.

Psoriatic arthritis (PA) is characterized by synovitis, polyarthritis, and spondylitis. One third of patients with psoriasis also have arthritis, making the incidence of PA similar to that of rheumatoid arthritis. As many as 20% of patients with PA have a severe course of disease, leading to deformity and joint damage. Early treatment is important as most of the damage appears to occur early in the course of the disease.

Medical management of the spondyloarthropathies focuses on treating pain and maintaining mobility by suppressing inflammation. For the patient with AS, good body positioning and posture are essential so that ankylosis, if it does occur, is in the most functional position. Patient education directed at maintaining range of motion with a regular exercise and muscle-strengthening program is especially important. Surgical management may include total hip replacement.

Salicylates, NSAIDs, and corticosteroids often produce marked improvement in back, skin, and joint symptoms. Methotrexate is also used to control psoriasis as well as joint inflammation.

Metabolic and Endocrine Diseases Associated With Rheumatic States

Metabolic and endocrine diseases are also associated with rheumatic states. These include biochemical abnormalities (amyloidosis and scurvy), endocrine diseases (diabetes mellitus and acromegaly), immunodeficiency diseases (AIDS), and other hereditary disorders (hypermobility syndromes). The most common conditions of this category, however, are the crystal-induced arthropathies in which crystals, such as monosodium urate (gout) or calcium pyrophosphate (calcium pyrophosphate dihydrate disease [*CPPD*] or pseudogout), are deposited within joints.

Gout

Gout is a heterogeneous group of conditions related to a genetic defect of purine metabolism (hyperuricemia). There is either oversecretion of uric acid or a renal defect resulting in decreased excretion of uric acid, or a combination of both.

In primary hyperuricemia, elevated serum urate levels or manifestations of urate deposition appear to be consequences of faulty uric acid metabolism. Primary hyperuricemia may be due to severe dieting or starvation, excessive intake of foods that are high in purines (shellfish, organ meats), or heredity. In secondary hyperuricemia, the gout is a minor clinical feature secondary to any of a number of genetic or acquired processes, including conditions in which there is an increase in cell turnover (leukemia, multiple myeloma, some types of anemias, psoriasis) and an increase in cell breakdown. Altered renal tubular function, either as a major action or as an unintended side effect of certain pharmacologic agents (diuretics such as thiazides and furosemide, low-dose salicylates) and ethanol, can contribute to uric acid underexcretion.

Pathophysiology

Hyperuricemia (serum concentration greater than 7.0 mg/dl [SI: 0.4 μmol/L]) can (but does not always) cause monosodium urate crystal deposition. Attacks of gout seem to be related to sudden increases or decreases of serum uric acid levels. When the urate crystals precipitate within a joint, an inflammatory response occurs and an attack of gout begins. With repeated attacks, accumulations of sodium urate crystals, called tophi, are deposited in peripheral areas of the body, such as the great toe, the hands, and the ear. Renal urate lithiasis (kidney stones) with chronic renal disease secondary to urate deposition may develop.

The finding of urate crystals in the synovial fluid of asymptomatic joints suggests that factors other than crystals may be related to the inflammatory reaction. Recovered monosodium urate crystals are coated with immunoglobulins that are mainly IgG. IgG enhances crystal phagocytosis, thereby demonstrating immunologic activity.

Clinical Manifestations

Manifestations of the gout syndrome include acute gouty arthritis (recurrent attacks of severe articular and periarticular inflammation), tophi (crystalline deposits accumulating in articular tissue, osseous tissue, soft tissue, and cartilage), gouty nephropathy (renal impairment), and uric acid urinary calculi. Four stages of gout can be identified: asymptomatic hyperuricemia, acute gouty arthritis, intercritical gout, and chronic tophaceous gout.

Fewer than one in five hyperuricemic individuals will at any point develop clinically apparent urate crystal deposition. The subsequent development of gout is directly related to the duration and magnitude of the hyperuricemia. Therefore, the commitment to lifelong pharmacologic treatment of hyperuricemia is deferred until there is an initial attack of gout.

For those hyperuricemic individuals who are going to develop gout, acute arthritis is the most common early clinical manifestation. The metatarsophalangeal (MTP) joint of the big toe is the most common (75% of patients) joint affected, but the tarsal area, ankle, or knee may also be targeted. The acute attack may be triggered by trauma, alcohol ingestion, dieting, drugs, surgical stress, or illness. The abrupt onset often occurs at night, awakening the patient with severe pain, redness, swelling, and warmth of the affected joint. Early attacks tend to subside spontaneously over 3 to 10 days even without treatment. The attack is followed by a symptom-free period—the intercritical stage—until the next attack, which may not come for months or years. However, with time, attacks tend to occur more frequently, involve more joints, and last longer.

Tophi are generally first noted an average of 10 years after the onset of gout. About 50% of inadequately treated patients eventually develop tophaceous deposits. Tophi are generally associated with more frequent and severe inflammatory episodes. Higher serum concentrations of uric acid are also associated with more extensive tophus formation. Tophi most commonly occur in the synovium, olecranon bursa, subchondral bone, infrapatellar and Achilles tendons, subcutaneous tissue on the extensor surface of the forearms, and overlying joints. They have also been found in the aortic walls, heart valves, nasal and ear cartilage, eyelids, cornea, and sclerae. Joint enlargement may cause a loss of motion.

Parenchymal compromise and renal stones may occur in patients with gout. The risk of urolithiasis is increased in patients with gout. The incidence of renal stones is two times higher for patients with secondary gout than for those with primary gout. Stone formation is related to the increase in serum uric acid, acidity of the urine, and urinary concentration.

Management

Colchicine (oral or parenteral) or an NSAID, such as indomethacin, is used to relieve an acute attack of gout. Medical management of hyperuricemia, tophi, joint destruction, and renal problems is usually initiated after the acute inflammatory process has subsided. Uricosuric agents, such as probenecid, correct hyperuricemia and dissolve deposited urate. Allopurinol is also an effective medication, but its use is limited because of the risk of toxicity. When reduction of the serum urate level is indicated, the uricosuric agents are the medications of choice. When the patient has, or is at risk for, renal insufficiency or renal calculi (kidney stones), allopurinol is the medication of choice (Table 52-5).

Arthritis Associated With Infectious Agents

Arthritis, tenosynovitis, and bursitis can be associated with infectious agents. Some inflammation of joints, tendons, and bursa is directly related to infection caused by bacterial, viral, fungal, or parastic agents. Bacterial arthritis is the most rapidly destructive form of infectious arthritis. There are two major classes of bacterial arthritis: arthritis caused by *Neisseria gonorrhea* and non-gonococcal bacterium. Most prevalent of the non-gonococcal agents are *Staphylococcus aureus* and the various streptococcal variants. Less common pathogens are related to syphilis, tuberculosis, leprosy, fungus (particularly coccidiomycosis), mycoplasmas, and viral agents such as rubella, parvovirus, and hepatitis B.

The characteristic symptom is an acute onset of a warm, swollen joint. The diagnosis is made by culture of the bacterium from the synovial fluid. This condition is a medical emergency necessitating early diagnosis and appropriate treatment to eliminate the causative organism, otherwise the joint may be destroyed relatively quickly.

Neoplasms and Neurovascular, Bone, and Extra-articular Disorders

Primary **neoplasms** of joints, tendon sheaths, and bursae are rare. Most arise from the synovium and are benign. These benign tumors include neoplasm and tumoral conditions such as lipoma, hemangioma, and fibroma and tumor-like lesions such as ganglion, bursitis, and synovial cyst. The malignant tumors include primary tumors such as synovial and bone sarcomas and secondary involvement as manifestations of joint invasion by leukemia, lymphoma, and myeloma or carcinomatous metastasis. Neoplasms may be reported as back or neck pain.

Neurovascular disorders include the compression syndromes such as those with peripheral entrapment

TABLE 52-5 Medications Used in Gout

Medication	Actions and Use	Nursing Implications
Colchicine	Lowers the deposition of uric acid and interferes with leukocytes and kinin formation, thus reducing inflammation. Does not alter serum or urine levels of uric acid. Used in acute and chronic management.	*Acute management:* Administer when attack first begins. Dosage is increased until pain is relieved or diarrhea develops. *Chronic management:* Prolonged use may decrease vitamin B12 absorption. Causes gastrointestinal upset in the majority of patients.
Probenecid (Benemid)	Uricosuric agent. Inhibits renal reabsorption of urates and increases the urinary excretion of uric acid. Prevents tophi formation.	Be alert for nausea, rash, and constipation.
Allopurinol (Zyloprim)	Xanthine oxidase inhibitor. Interrupts the breakdown of purines before uric acid is formed. Inhibits xanthinoxidase because it blocks uric acid formation.	Be alert for side effects, including bone marrow depression, vomiting, and abdominal pain.

(carpal tunnel syndrome), radiculopathy, and spinal stenosis. Raynaud's phenomenon or disease and erythromelalgia are also included in this category.

Bone and cartilage disorders include osteoporosis, osteomalacia, hypertrophic osteoarthropathy, diffuse idiopathic skeletal hyperostosis (DISH), Paget's disease, osteonecrosis, avascular necrosis, costochondritis, osteolysis or chondrolysis, and biomechanical or anatomic abnormalities. Notably these conditions involve destruction, infection, or remodeling of bone.

Extra-articular rheumatism is a descriptive term for a group of conditions affecting structures other than the joints. Included are general and regional pain syndromes, low back pain and intervertebral disc disorders, tendonitis and/or bursitis, and ganglion cysts.

Fibromyalgia, a generalized pain syndrome sometimes called fibrositis (a misnomer because inflammation is not present), is a poorly understood chronic condition characterized by diffuse musculoskeletal aching and pain, fatigue, morning stiffness, and disturbed sleep. Although many patients complain of joint pain and may have some mild joint tenderness, there is no evidence of joint swelling or an inflammatory or degenerative process. Patients do, however, have multiple tender points in specific areas. Disturbances of non-REM sleep, mechanical stresses on the lumbar and cervical spine, emotional distress, and disturbance of CNS endorphins and enkephalins are among the hypothesized causes of this disorder. Fibromyalgia is not progressive. The difficulty in diagnosis and the chronic nature of the pain make the nursing care of these patients especially important. Support includes reassurance that although the pain can be severe at times, fibromyalgia is neither deforming nor crippling, and control of the pain is possible. Tricyclic antidepressants are used at bedtime to increase the amount of non-REM sleep. The focus is on maintaining activity and helping patients learn to "work through" the pain (continue activity despite discomfort). A regular conditioning program, such as walking, keeps muscles toned. Relaxation and stress-management techniques are important treatment modalities.

Miscellaneous Disorders

The last category in the classification of the rheumatic diseases is aptly labeled **miscellaneous disorders** because it contains a mix of disorders frequently associated with arthritis and other conditions. These disorders include the direct result of trauma (including internal derangement and loose bodies of joints), pancreatic disease (related to avascular necrosis or osteonecrosis), sarcoidosis (a multisystem disorder particularly of the lymph nodes and lungs), and palindromic rheumatism (an uncommon variety of recurring and acute arthritis and periarthritis with symptom-free periods of days to months that in some may progress to rheumatoid arthritis). Other conditions include villonodular synovitis, chronic active hepatitis, and drug-related rheumatic syndromes. The nursing interventions related to these varied conditions are specific to the multisystem problems experienced by the patient, but the musculoskeletal components should not be neglected or overlooked.

Gerontologic Considerations

Although the rheumatic diseases affect people of all ages, from infancy through childhood, adolescence, and maturity, arthritis is commonly thought of as an inevitable consequence of aging by the patient, family, and society as a whole. Many older people expect and accept the immobility and self-care problems related to the rheumatic diseases and do not seek help, thinking that nothing can be done. Careful diagnosis and appropriate treatment can improve the quality of life for older persons with arthritis. However, the rheumatic diseases do have some special implications for the older adult.

In elderly patients, other medical conditions may take precedence; arthritis is commonly a secondary diagnosis and concern. In such cases, the nurse can play a significant role in identifying the impact of the arthritis on the individual's life-style, independence, and other chronic or acute conditions.

The frequency, pattern of onset, clinical features, severity, and impact on function of the rheumatic disease in elderly patients may be different in very old patients. Some of the rheumatic diseases are more prevalent with advancing age (OA); one is exclusive to the older person (polymyalgia rheumatica); and some may be less severe for the elderly than for the younger patient. However, OA, the most prevalent activity-limiting condition among older persons, may account for more total disability among elderly patients than many diseases that are considered more serious (*e.g.*, stroke or cancer).

In some instances, the age of the patient and coexisting health problems may make diagnosis difficult. A missed diagnosis of RA or PMR is not unusual because of the assumption that most older people with joint problems have OA. It may be difficult to differentiate problems associated with aging from those caused by a rheumatic disease.

RA that begins in the later years has been shown to differ prognostically and therapeutically from RA that begins earlier. In the elderly patient with initial RA, onset is more likely to be abrupt; however, the clinical course does not seem to differ from that of RA with an insidious onset. Moreover, patients with elderly-onset RA are less likely to have subcutaneous nodules or rheumatoid factor at disease onset.

Other conditions (soft tissue problems such as bursitis) are not in themselves impairing but, when combined with the physiologic processes of aging, may have significant effects on the quality of life. In fact, the effects of most forms of arthritis may lead to considerable changes in the life-style of the individual and may threaten independence. Decreased vision and altered balance in the elderly patient may be problematic for the person whose arthritis in the lower extremities affects locomotion. The combination of poor hearing, diminished vision, forgetfulness, and depression contribute to nonadherence to the treatment regimen in elderly patients as well. Special techniques for promoting patient safety and self-management may need to be employed. Strategies that include memory aids for medications may be necessary.

Partly because of the more frequent contact of the elderly with the health care system, overtreatment or inappropriate treatment is a distinct possibility. Effective exercise programs are not instituted because of inadequate teaching time and follow-up by a therapist. Complaints of pain may be met with a prescription for an opioid analgesic rather than instructions of rest, use of an assistive device, and local comfort measures such as heat or cold. Acetaminophen may be appropriate and worth trying before using an NSAID that poses a greater chance of side effects. Intra-articular corticosteroid injections, with their usual rapid relief of symptoms, may be requested by the patient who is unaware of the consequences of too frequent use.

Pharmacologic treatment of rheumatic disease in the older patient is more difficult than for younger patients. If the medications used have an effect on the senses (hearing, cognition), this effect is intensified in the elderly. The cumulative effect of medications is accentuated because of the physiologic changes of aging. For example, decreased renal function in the elderly alters the metabolism of certain medications, such as the NSAIDs. Elderly patients are more prone to such side effects as gastroduodenal ulceration or bleeding, and they are more likely to use nonprescription remedies, to try many different medications (polypharmacy), and to be more susceptible to unproven treatment methods.

Elderly patients with some form of arthritis may unnecessarily accept or endure pain, loss of ambulation, and difficulty with activities of daily living. The need to view oneself as capable of managing life independently despite increasing age may take considerable energy. The body image and self-esteem of the elderly person with arthritis, combined with underlying depression, may interfere with the use of assistive devices such as canes. Use of adaptive equipment such as long-handled reachers or tongs may be viewed as evidence of aging rather than as a means of increased independence.

The elderly person usually has a life-long pattern of dealing with stress. Depending on the success of that pattern, the elderly person can often maintain a positive attitude and self-esteem when faced with a rheumatic disease—especially with the support of a skillful nurse.

Patient Education and Home Care Considerations

The impact of rheumatic disease on everyday life is not always evident when the patient is seen in the hospital or an ambulatory care setting. The increased frequency with which nurses see patients in the home provides opportunities for recognizing problems and implementing interventions aimed at improving the quality of life of patients with rheumatic disorders.

The patient encountered in the home setting will typically have a rheumatic disease that is secondary to the primary reason for the visit. In such cases, the problems caused by the rheumatic disease may interfere with the treatment of the primary condition. For example, the patient who is recovering from coronary artery surgery may have been instructed to exercise but is unable or only partially able to do so because of the rheumatic disease. Conversely, treatment of the primary condition may cause or increase problems related to the rheumatic disease. For example, the cardiac patient who has been instructed to walk long distances every day may find that doing so increases the symptoms of osteoarthritis in the knees.

Compliance with the therapeutic treatment program can be more easily monitored in the home setting where physical and social barriers to adherence are more readily identified. The newly diagnosed insulin-dependent diabetic or a diabetic patient who is converting to insulin therapy may find that he or she is unable to accurately fill the syringe or administer the injection because of impaired joint mobility. Appropriate adaptive equipment needed to increase independence in care and function is usually identified more readily when the nurse sees how the patient functions in the home.

The home care nurse is in the position to instruct and advise the patient about signs of disease exacerbation and the need to contact or see the physician for reevaluation. Otherwise, patients are likely to wait until the next appointment.

Home-based self-management of the chronic rheumatic diseases may be particularly challenging for older people, and the home care nurse can help these patients manage medications, secure adaptive equipment for self-care, and identify community resources such as Meals-on-Wheels.

For patients at risk for impaired skin integrity, the home care nurse can closely monitor skin status and also instruct, provide, or supervise the patient and family in preventive skin care measures.

The home care nurse assesses the patient's need for assistance in the home and supervises home health aides who may meet many of the needs of the patient with a rheumatic disease. Referrals to physical and occupational therapists may be made as problems are identified and limitations increase.

A community-based nurse can visit the home to make sure the patient can function as independently as possible despite mobility problems and can safely manage treatments and pharmacotherapy. The patient and family should be alerted to support services such as local Arthritis Foundation chapters.

CRITICAL THINKING EXERCISES

1. You are caring for a 46-year-old woman following a second knee replacement because of rheumatoid arthritis. She depends on other family members for assistance with most activities because her hands, hips, and knees are severely affected. She tells you that she does not want to be a burden on her family any longer. Explore possible strategies you could suggest she try during her hospitalization and when she is recovering at home.
2. As a nurse in an immunology clinic, you receive a call from a young woman who has just been informed that her sister has been diagnosed with systemic lupus erythematosus (SLE). She is very concerned about her own risks and those of her children for developing this disorder. How would you respond to her concerns and fears?
3. An elderly woman is admitted for surgery to treat suspected cancer of the colon. She has a history of osteoarthritis. How would you modify your care of this patient because of the osteoarthritis?
4. A nonsteroidal anti-inflammatory drug (NSAID) has been prescribed for your patient because of rheumatoid arthritis. What instructions and recommendations would you give to the patient to ensure safe administration of this medication? If the patient tells you that she has a hard time remembering whether she has taken her medication, how would you modify or focus your instructions?

BIBLIOGRAPHY

Books

American Nurses Association, Arthritis Health Professions Association. Outcome Standards for Rheumatology Nursing Practice. Kansas City, MO, American Nurses Association, 1983.

Banwell BF and Gall V (eds). Physical Therapy Management of Arthritis. New York, Churchill Livingstone, 1988.

Ehrlich GE (ed). Rehabilitation Management of Rheumatic Conditions, 2nd ed. Baltimore, Williams & Wilkins, 1986.

Fries JF. Arthritis: A Take Care of Yourself Health Guide for Understanding Your Arthritis. Reading, MA, Addison-Wesley, 1995.

Kelley WN. Textbook of Rheumatology. Philadelphia, WB Saunders, 1993.

Madison PJ et al (eds). Oxford Textbook of Rheumatology. New York, Oxford Medical Publications, 1993.

Pigg JS, Driscoll PW, and Caniff R. Rheumatology Nursing: A Problem-Oriented Approach. Albany, Delmar, 1985.

Schumacher HR (ed). Primer of Rheumatic Diseases, 10th ed. Atlanta, Arthritis Foundation, 1993.

Sledge CB et al (eds). Arthritis Surgery. Philadelphia, WB Saunders, 1994.

Journals

Asterisk indicates nursing research article.

Affleck G et al. Coping with rheumatoid arthritis pain from day to day: patterns and correlates. Arthritis Care Res 1991; 4:S21.

Agarwal AK. Gout and pseudogout. Prim Care 1993 Dec; 20(4): 839–855.

*Ailinger RL and Dear MR. Self-care agency in persons with rheumatoid arthritis. Arthritis Care Res 1993 Sep; 6(3):134–140.

*Ailinger RL and Schweitzer E. Patients' explanations of rheumatoid arthritis. West J Nurs Res 1993 Jun; 15(3):340–351.

*Albrecht M et al. The Albrecht nursing model for home healthcare: Predictors of satisfaction with a self-care intervention program. J Nurs Adm 1993 Jan; 23(1):51–54.

*Allaire SH et al. The impact of rheumatoid arthritis on the household work performance of women. Arth Rheum 1991 Jun; 34(6):669–678.

*Bailey JM and Nielsen BI. Uncertainty and appraisal of uncertainty in women with rheumatoid arthritis. Orth Nurs 1993 Mar/Apr; 12(2):63–67.

*Belza B. The impact of fatigue on exercise performance. Arth Care Res 1994 Dec; 7(4):176–189.

*Belza BL et al. Correlates of fatigue in older adults with rheumatoid arthritis. Nurs Res 1993 Mar/Apr; 42(2):93–99.
Brandt KD. NSAIDs in the treatment of osteoarthritis. Friends or foes? Bull Rheum Dis 1993 Oct; 42(6):1–4.
*Braden CJ. Patterns of change over time in learned response to chronic illness among participants in a systemic lupus erythematosus self-help course. Arthritis Care Res 1991 Dec; 4(4): 158–167.
*Burckhardt CS et al. A comparison of pain perceptions in women with fibromyalgia and rheumatoid arthritis; Relationship to depression and pain extent. Arthritis Care Res 1992 Dec; 5(4): 216–222.
*Burke M and Flaherty MJ. Coping strategies and health status of elderly arthritic women. J Adv Nurs 1993 Jan; 18(1):7–13.
Calkins E. Arthritis in the elderly. Bull Rheum Dis 1991;40(3): 1–9.
Carpenter DR and Hudacek S. Polymyalgia rheumatica: a comprehensive review of this debilitating disease. Nurs Pract 1994 June; 19(6):50–58.
Cash JM and Wilder RL. Refractory rheumatoid arthritis. Therapeutic options. Rheum Dis Clin North Am 1995 Feb; 21(1): 1–18.
Chan KA et al. The lag time between onset of symptoms and diagnosis of rheumatoid arthritis. Arth Rheum 1994 Jun; 37(6): 814–820.
*Clough DH. The effects of cognitive distortion and depression on disability in rheumatoid arthritis. Res Nursing and Health 1991; 14(6):439–446.
*Collier IC. Assessing functional status of the elderly. Arthritis Care Res 1988 Mar; 1(1):45–52.
Collo MCB et al. Evaluating arthritic complaints. Nurs Pract 1991 Feb; 16(2):9–10, 12–14, 17–18.
Cronan TA, Kaplan RM, and Kozin F. Factors affecting unprescribed remedy use among people with self-reported arthritis. Arthritis Care Res 1993 Sep; 6(3):149–155.
*Crosby LJ. Factors which contribute to fatigue associated with rheumatoid arthritis. J Adv Nurs 1991 Aug; 16(8):974–981.
Daltroy LH, et al. Does musculoskeletal function deteriorate in a predictable sequence in the elderly? Arthritis Care Res 1992 Sep; 5(3):146–150.
Davis GC, Cortez C, and Rubin BR. Pain management in the older adult with rheumatoid arthritis or osteoarthritis. Arthritis Care Res 1990; 3:127–131.
Dexter PA. Joint exercise in elderly persons with symptomatic osteoarthritis of the hip or knee. Arthritis Care Res 1992; 5:36–41.
*Downe-Wamboldt B. Coping and life satisfaction in elderly women with osteoarthritis. J Adv Nursing 1991; 16:1328–1335.
Duna GF and Cash JM. Treatment of refractory cutaneous lupus erythematosus. Rheum Dis Clin North Am 1995 Feb; 21(1): 99–115.
Fessler BJ and Boumpas DT. Severe major organ involvement in systemic lupus erythematosus. Diagnosis and management. Rheum Dis Clin North Am 1995 Feb; 21(1):81–98.
Furst DE. Predictors of worsening clinical variables and outcomes in rheumatoid arthritis. Rheum Dis Clin North Am 1994 May; 20(2):309–319.
Gerber LH and Hicks JE. Surgical and rehabilitation options in the treatment of the rheumatoid arthritis patient resistant to pharmacologic agents. Rheum Dis Clin North Am 1995 Feb; 21(1): 19–39.
Grindel CG. Fatigue and nutrition. Medsurg Nurs 1994 Dec; 3(6):475–481, 195.
Halverson PB and Holmes SB. Systemic lupus erythematosus: medical and nursing treatments. Orth Nurs 1993 Nov/Dec; 11(6): 17–25.
Hampson SE et al. Self-management of osteoarthritis. Arthritis Care Res 1993 Mar; 6(1):17–22.
Harris ED Jr. Rheumatoid arthritis: Pathophysiology and implications for therapy. N Engl J Med 1990 May 3; 322(18):1277–1289.
*Hawley DJ and Wolfe F. Sensitivity to change of the health assessment questionnaire (HAQ) and other clinical and health status measures in rheumatoid arthritis: Results of short-term clinical trials and observational studies versus long-term observational studies. Arthritis Care Res 1992 Sep; 5(3): 130–136.
Hayes KW. Heat and cold in the management of rheumatoid arthritis. Arthritis Care Res 1993 Sep; 6(3):156–166.
Hill J. Caring and curing. Nurs Times 1991 Nov 6; 87(45):29–31.
Hill J. Assessing rheumatic disease. Nurs Times 1991 Jan 23; 87(4): 33–35.
Hochberg MC. Epidemiologic considerations in the primary prevention of osteoarthritis. J Rheumatol 1991; 18:1438–1440.
Hooker RS. Clinical characteristics of the seronegative spondyloarthropathies. J Amer Acad Phys Assist 1992 Feb; 5(2): 110–120.
Katz PR and Yelin EH. Life activities of persons with rheumatoid arthritis with and without depressive symptoms. Arthritis Care Res 1994 Jun; 7(2):69–77.
Kennedy LG, Edmunds L, and Calin A. The natural history of ankylosing spondylitis. Does it burn out? J Rheumatol 1993; 20(4): 688–692.
Klippel JH. Systemic lupus erythematosus: Treatment-related complications superimposed on chronic disease. JAMA 1990 Apr 4; 263(13):1812–1815.
Kuper BC and Failla S. Shedding new light on lupus. 1994 Am J Nurs 1994 Nov; 94(11):26–32.
Lambert VA. Arthritis. Ann Rev Nurs Research 1991; 9:3–18.
Lash AA. Why so many women? Part 1. Systemic lupus erythematosus. Medsurg Nurs 1993 Aug; 2(4):259–264.
Lash AA. Systemic lupus erythematosus. Part 2. Diagnosis, Treatment Modalities, and Nursing Management. Medsurg Nurs 1993 Oct; 2(5):375–385.
*Lee HJ. Comparison of selected health behavior variables in elderly women with osteoarthritis in different environments. Arthritis Care Res 1993 Mar; 6(1):31–37.
Legerton CW III, Smith EA and Silver RM. Systemic sclerosis (scleroderma). Clinical management of its major complications. Rheum Dis Clin North Am 1995 Feb; 21(1):203–216.
Liang MH and Fortin P. Management of osteoarthritis of the hip and knee. N Engl J Med 1991 Jul 11; 325(2):125–127.
Mandell BF and Lipani J. Refractory osteoarthritis. Differential diagnosis and therapy. Rheum Dis Clin North Am 1995 Feb; 21(1): 163–178.
Minor MA and Sanford MK. Physical interventions in the management of pain in arthritis. Arthritis Care Res 1993 Dec: 6(4): 197–206.
Michet CJ. Osteoarthritis. Prim Care 1993 Dec; 20(4):815–826.
*Neuberger GB et al. Promoting self-care in clients with arthritis. Arthritis Care Res 1993 Sep; 6(3):141–148.
*Orr PM and Bratton GN. The effect of an inpatient arthritis rehabilitation program on self-assessed functional ability. Rehab Nurs 1992 Nov/Dec; 17(6):306–310.
Osial TA Jr, Cash JM and Eisenbeis CH Jr. Arthritis-associated syndromes. Rheum Dis Clin North Am 1993 Dec; 20(4): 857–882.
Panush RS. Is there a role for diet or other questionable therapies in managing rheumatic diseases? Bull Rheum Dis 1993 Jun; 42(4):1–4.
Perry E. Living with rheumatoid arthritis. Heart and Lung 1991 Jul; 20(4):416–418.

Petri M. Systemic lupus erythematosus and pregnancy. Rheum Dis Clin North Am 1994 May; 20(2):87–118.

Pigg JS and Schroeder PM. Frequently occurring problems of patients with rheumatic disease: The ANA outcome standards for rheumatology nursing practice. Nurs Clin North Am 1984 Dec; 19(4):697–708.

Pigg JS. Rheumatology nursing: Evolution of the role and functions of a subspecialty. Arthritis Care Res 1990 Sep; 3(3):109–115.

Powell MA. Polymyalgia rheumatica. J Am Acad Nurs Pract 1991 Oct-Dec; 3(4):188–189.

Refern S. Sexuality and arthritis. Nursing (Oxford) 1991 Oct 24–Nov 6; 4(44):17–19.

Rheinard JD and Calkins E. Geriatric issues in the diagnosis and management of patients with rheumatic disorders. Prim Care 1993 Dec; 20(4):911–923.

Richardson A. Rheumatoid arthritis in pregnancy. Nursing Standard 1992 July 29; 6(45):25–28.

Shmerling RH. Rheumatic fluid analysis. A critical appraisal. Rheum Dis Clin North Am 1994 May; 20(2):503–512.

*Sotosky JR et al. Arthritis problem indicator: Preliminary report on a new tool for use in the primary care setting. Arthritis Care Res 1992 Sep; 5(3):157–162.

St Clair EW, Haynes BF. The future of rheumatoid arthritis treatment. Bull Rheum Dis 1993 Apr; 42(2):1–4.

Steven MB. The clinical spectrum of SLE. Maryland Med J 1991 Oct; 40(10):875–885.

Sutton JD. SLE: Management overview. Maryland Med J 1991 Oct; 40(10):935–938.

Ulak LJ. Special considerations for SLE patients. Medsurg Nurs 1995 Apr; 4(2):146–148.

Verbrugge LM. Disability transitions for older persons with arthritis. J Aging Health 1992; 4:212–243.

Wetherbee L. Caring for clients with arthritis. Home Healthcare Nurse. 1994 Jan/Feb; 12(1):13–18.

Wilke WS and Hoffman GS. Treatment of corticosteroid-resistant giant cell arteritis. Rheum Dis Clin North Am 1995 Feb; 21(1): 59–71.

Wood J and Redfern S. Arthritis and the individual. Nursing (Oxford) 1991 Sep 26–Oct 9; 4(42):9–11.

Yeomans AC. Assessment and management of gouty arthritis. Nurse Pract 1991 Apr; 16(4):18, 21, 25–26.

INFORMATION/RESOURCES

Agencies

American Lupus Society
23751 Madison St.,
Torrance, CA 90505,
(213) 542-8891

Ankylosing Spondylitis Association
511 N. La Cienge, Suite 216,
Los Angeles, CA 90048,
(800) 777-8189

The Arthritis Foundation
1314 Spring St.,
Atlanta, GA 30309,
(404) 872-7100 or 1-800-933-0032 (information line)

Lupus Foundation of America, Inc.
1717 Massachusettes Ave. NW, Suite 203,
Washington, DC 20036,
(703) 660-6523

National Institute of Arthritis and Musculoskeletal and Skin Diseases
National Institutes of Health, Information Clearinghouse,
P.O. Box AMS, 9000 Rockville Pike,
Bethesda, MD 20892

Scleroderma International Foundation
1725 York Ave. #29F,
New York, NY 10128,
(212) 427-7040

Sjögren's Syndrome Foundation, Inc.
382 Main St., Port
Washington, NY 11050,
(516) 767-2866

United Scleroderma Foundation, Inc.
P.O. Box 399,
Watsonville, CA 95077,
(408) 728-2202

Nursing Research Profile for Unit 12

Overview

Nursing research studies related to immune dysfunction have focused on HIV infection/AIDS and rheumatic disorders.

Nokes KM, Wheeler K and Kendrew J. Development of an assessment tool. Image: J Nurs Scholarship 1994 Summer; 26(2):133–138.

The purpose of this study was to establish the validity and reliability of a visual analog scale that rates HIV-related symptom severity and general well-being. The HIV Assessment Tool (HAT) measures the client's perception of the severity of HIV-related symptoms and their effect on self-care activities and general well-being.

The sample consisted of 156 volunteer subjects who were categorized into three groups: hospitalized or ambulatory HIV positive (n = 60); hospitalized or outpatients with CDC-defined AIDS according to the 1987 classification system (n = 43); and healthy college students who were HIV-antibody negative (n = 53). All subjects were 18 years or older and were able to read English.

Quality of life (QOL) was measured with a modified Karnofsky scale. Most of the subjects with HIV disease (n = 43) reported that their performance status was fully active, asymptomatic on the QOL measure. Subjects with CDC-defined disease reported that their performance status was restricted but they were able to be ambulatory and to carry out light work (n = 16) or able to be up more than 50% of their waking hours and were capable of self-care but were unable to work (n = 14). In this study, no subject was completely bedridden. Subjects completed a personal information sheet and the HAT, which took 10 to 15 minutes.

Test-retest reliability was assessed by administering the HAT twice to subjects, although the timing of the retest ranged from 1 to 2 hours to 1 week later. Discriminant validity was assessed by comparing scores of HIV-positive subjects, those with AIDS, and healthy control subjects. The mean scores of healthy control subjects (college students) on the HAT differed significantly from the means of those who were HIV-positive and those with AIDS, although the scores of the latter two groups did not differ. Concurrent validity was supported by a correlation of .51 (p <.001) of scores on the HAT and the QOL measure. Factor analysis revealed three factors within the HAT: general well-being, general symptoms, and HIV-specific symptoms. Internal consistency reliability coefficients of the factors supported the reliability of the HAT.

Although the results of this study support the reliability and validity of the HAT, the investigators recommend that reliability estimates be calculated whenever this tool is used with different samples. Additional symptoms reported by subjects (raspy or sore throat, dry mouth, altered taste, depression, emotional upsets, chills, sweating, severe itchiness, hair loss, ringing in the ears, fingernail changes, and bone aches) will be included in future versions of the HAT.

Nursing Implications. After further refinement of the tool, nurses can use it to assess the self-care needs of persons with HIV infection and to evaluate the effectiveness of nursing interventions. However, a neurologic assessment may be indicated before the administration of the HAT if HIV-related dementia is suspected. Community health nurses may be able to use the HAT to note symptom changes and to address each individual's unique and changing health care needs. This information can help clients understand what measures may relieve their symptoms and increase their sense of control.

Williams AB. Women at risk: An AIDS educational needs assessment. Image: J Nurs Scholarship 1991 Winter; 23(4):208–213.

This study was a qualitative exploratory needs assessment of 21 women at risk for HIV infection or who were already HIV-antibody positive with or without symptoms. They were at risk for HIV infection from their own injecting drug use (IDU) or they were heterosexual partners of drug users. Purposive sampling was used. The Health Belief Model (HBM) served as the study's framework for understanding the dynamics of behavior change in response to health care recommendations. Perceived self-efficacy was also examined since it has emerged as an important predictor of sexual risk-taking behaviors in the context of AIDS risk–reduction programs.

Subjects and/or their significant others were clients from an outpatient methadone treatment program for opiate addicts in a Northeastern city. The majority of reported AIDS cases in this city have been associated with IDU, and a quarter of the cases are women. A semistructured interview schedule with open-ended questions was utilized and interviews were audiotaped. All subjects spoke English so that no verbal communication problems existed. The researcher individually approached each subject and obtained verbal consent. Bias factors were addressed by a review of the interview schedule by four professional nurses with clinical expertise in HIV/AIDS and substance abuse and through field testing of the questions and interview schedule.

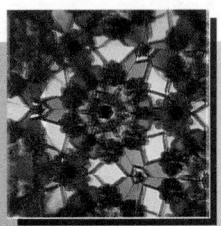

The results revealed that women had an understanding of AIDS transmission and "safer sex" and "safe drug use" recommendations. They had little information about new therapies and early interventions for HIV disease. They perceived AIDS as a very serious health threat and were aware of their personal vulnerability to the disease; however, their perceptions of personal vulnerability were compromised when there was a perceived threat of loss of or damage to valuable relationships with others. The subjects were aware that abstinence was more effective than the use of condoms and that not sharing drug equipment was better than cleaning this equipment. Women perceived themselves as capable of taking action to protect themselves from AIDS in some situations but not in others. The situations in which they thought they might be less capable were those that involved the immediate need for drugs and those that involved significant relationships with others.

The women were very concerned about their personal relationships with significant male partners, children, family members, friends, professionals, and others in the community. They had concerns regarding whether they could trust others to take recommended protective actions. They also expressed concern about whether professionals and persons in the community would treat them with respect and concern. They feared being labeled as persons with AIDS, and this fear inhibited their ability to participate in AIDS education and support activities. The impact of AIDS was perceived by them to further heighten the isolation and mistrust characteristic of the drug-using community.

Nursing Implications. Many persons with HIV infection have heard public health messages about the seriousness of the disease and the pessimistic view of the prognosis. Nurses need to share messages of hope and to educate women about early interventions that are available to them that can improve both the quality and quantity of life. Many women with AIDS or HIV infection have a personal history of drug use. Thus, more awareness is needed about resources to help women to stop using drugs and to assist women to obtain clean drug equipment until they and their partners can get into drug rehabilitation programs. Nurses can help decrease the public stigma of AIDS through role modeling and advocacy. Involvement in the development of public health policy and education regarding the inclusion of women's concerns is important.

Ailinger RL and Schweitzer E. Patient's explanations of rheumatoid arthritis. West J Nurs Res 1993 June; 15(3):340–351.

The investigators examined the social and cultural meanings that patients give to their illness experience. Their assumption was that these meanings are important factors in choice and perceived efficacy of care, self-care practices, and adherence with regimens. A self-explanatory model was used by asking the convenience sample group of 59 patients with rheumatoid arthritis seven questions: What do you think has caused your problem? Why do you think it started when it did? What does your sickness do to you? How severe is it? What do you fear most about your sickness? What are the chief problems your sickness has caused for you? What are the important results you hope to receive from treatment?

In this study, nontraditional beliefs did not compose the main category of response to etiology and onset. Sixty-four percent of the respondents (including all the males in the study) stated that they did not know the cause of their disease. Thirty-one percent of the study participants felt that stress was the causative factor.

The major problems were identified as functional loss (80%), role change (67%), pain (53%), fatigue (43%), and psychologic effects (25%). Expectations of respondents were the same for relief from pain (25%) and improved function (25%); 10%, showing little realistic knowledge of their condition, hoped the disease would go away (cure). The most common fear was incapacity (68%), which included dependence on others and wheelchair confinement.

Nursing Implications. Nurses may be unaware of the differences between their views and those of their patients. The authors urge focusing on the patients' perception of the illness experience and not just on the physiologic processes.

The findings demonstrate that although finding a cause is important to health professionals, it is less relevant to patients who are primarily interested in immediate treatment improvements. The expectations of the patients about treatment were practical and included improvement of function and stabilization of the condition. The information provided by this study can help nurses better understand their patients and communicate with them.

Belza BL, et al. Correlates of fatigue in older adults with rheumatoid arthritis. Nurs Research 1993 Mar/Apr; 42(2):93–99.

The purposes of this study were to describe the prevalence of fatigue, examine the association between fatigue and doctor visits, and identify correlates of fatigue in rheumatoid arthritis. One hundred and thirty-three patients participated in this study, which used multiple instruments to address the study's variables. On the average, a high degree of fatigue was reported to occur every day, to remain constant during the course of a week, and to most often affect walking and household chores. When controlling for disease severity and insurance coverage, respondents who reported more fatigue made more visits to the rheumatologist than those reporting less fatigue. The following variables explained a significant amount of variance in rating of fatigue: pain rating, functional status, sleep quality, female gender, co-morbid conditions, and duration of disease. Limitations of this study include the lack of controlling for fatigue associated with completion of the questionnaires. Fatigue could have increased while completing the questionnaires, thereby being a confounding factor for the measures completed last. No normative data are available.

Nursing Implications. Owing to the multidimensionality of fatigue, nursing assessment needs to incorporate inquiry into fatigue severity, distress, impact, and timing. Problems of pain, sleep, other medical conditions, psychologic status, physical inactivity, and other factors thought by the patient to influence fatigue should also be explored. Strategies to reduce fatigue include management of pain, enhanced sleep, a program of physical activity and exercise, and improvement of functional status. Resolution or amelioration of one problem may lead to improvement of other parameters.

UNIT 13

Integumentary Function

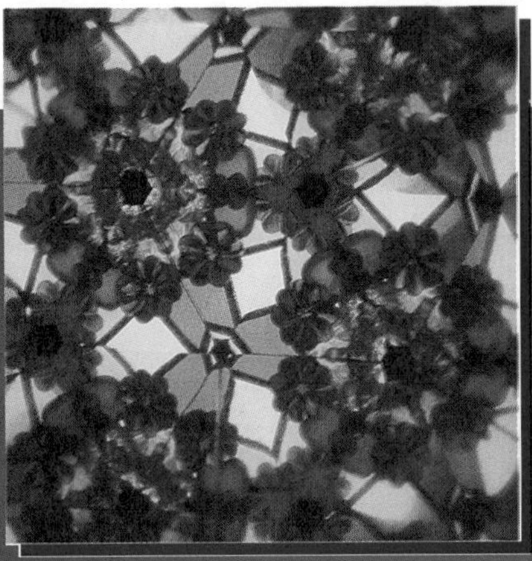

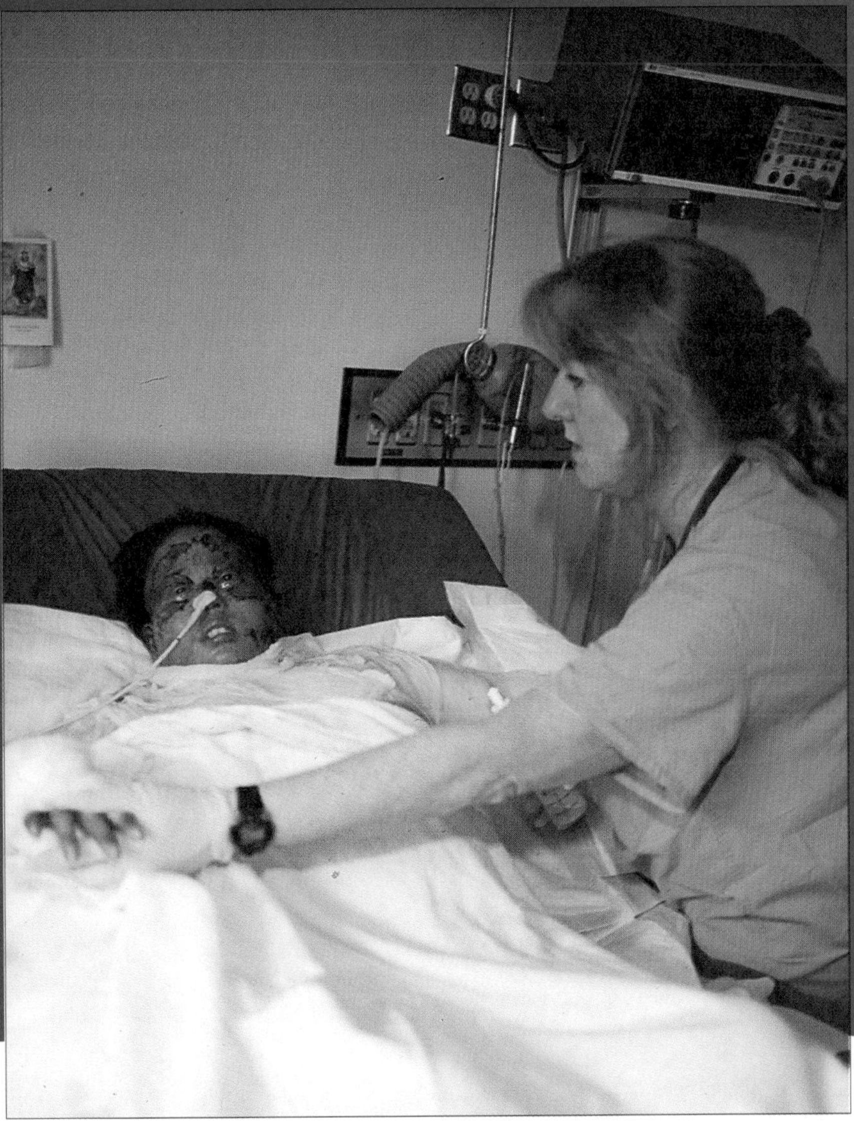

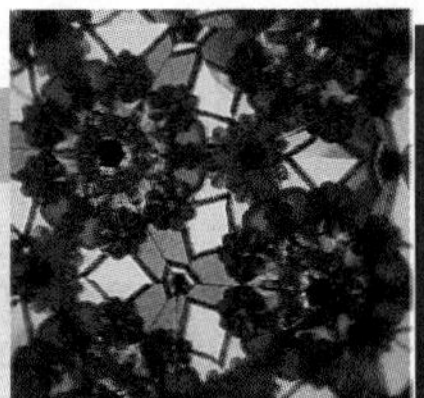

53

Assessment of Integumentary Function

CHAPTER OUTLINE

LEARNING OBJECTIVES

On completion of this chapter, the learner will be able to:

1. Identify the structures and functions of the skin
2. Differentiate the composition and function of each skin layer: epidermis, dermis, and subcutaneous tissue
3. Identify and describe primary and secondary skin lesions, and their pattern and distribution
4. Recognize common skin eruptions and manifestations associated with systemic disease
5. Describe the normal aging process of the skin and skin changes common to the elderly
6. List appropriate questions that will help elicit information during an assessment of the skin
7. Describe the components of physical assessment most useful when examining the skin, hair, and nails
8. Discuss common skin tests and procedures used in diagnosing skin and related disorders

Skin problems are encountered frequently in nursing practice. Skin-related complaints account for up to 10% of all ambulatory patient visits in this country. Because the skin mirrors the general condition of the patient, many systemic conditions may be accompanied by dermatologic manifestations.

The psychologic stress of illness or various personal and family problems are commonly exhibited outwardly as dermatologic problems. Any hospitalized patient may suddenly develop itching and a rash secondary to the treatment regimen. In certain systemic conditions, such as hepatitis and cancer, dermatologic manifestations may be the first sign of the disorder.

Anatomic and Physiologic Overview

The largest organ system of the body, the skin is indispensable for human life. Skin forms a barrier between the internal organs and the external environment and participates in many vital functions of the body. The skin is continuous with the mucous membrane at the external openings of the digestive, respiratory, and urogenital systems. Because skin disorders are readily visible, dermatologic complaints are commonly the primary reason for a patient to seek health care.

Anatomy of the Skin

The skin is composed of three layers: the **epidermis,** the **dermis,** and the **subcutaneous tissue** (Fig. 53-1). Each layer becomes more differentiated (mature and with more specific functions) as it rises from the basal stratum germinativum layer to the outermost stratum corneum layer. The epidermis comprises the outermost layer, with a thickness of about 0.1 mm on the eyelids to about 1 mm on the palms of the hands and soles of the feet (Morton, 1993). This external layer of stratified epithelial cells is composed predominantly of **keratinocytes.**

The epidermis, which is contiguous with the mucous membranes and the lining of the ear canals, consists of live, continuously dividing cells covered on the surface by dead cells that were originally deeper in the dermis but were pushed upward by the newly developing, more differentiated cells underneath. This external layer is almost completely replaced every 3 to 4 weeks. The dead cells contain large amounts of **keratin,** an insoluble, fibrous protein that

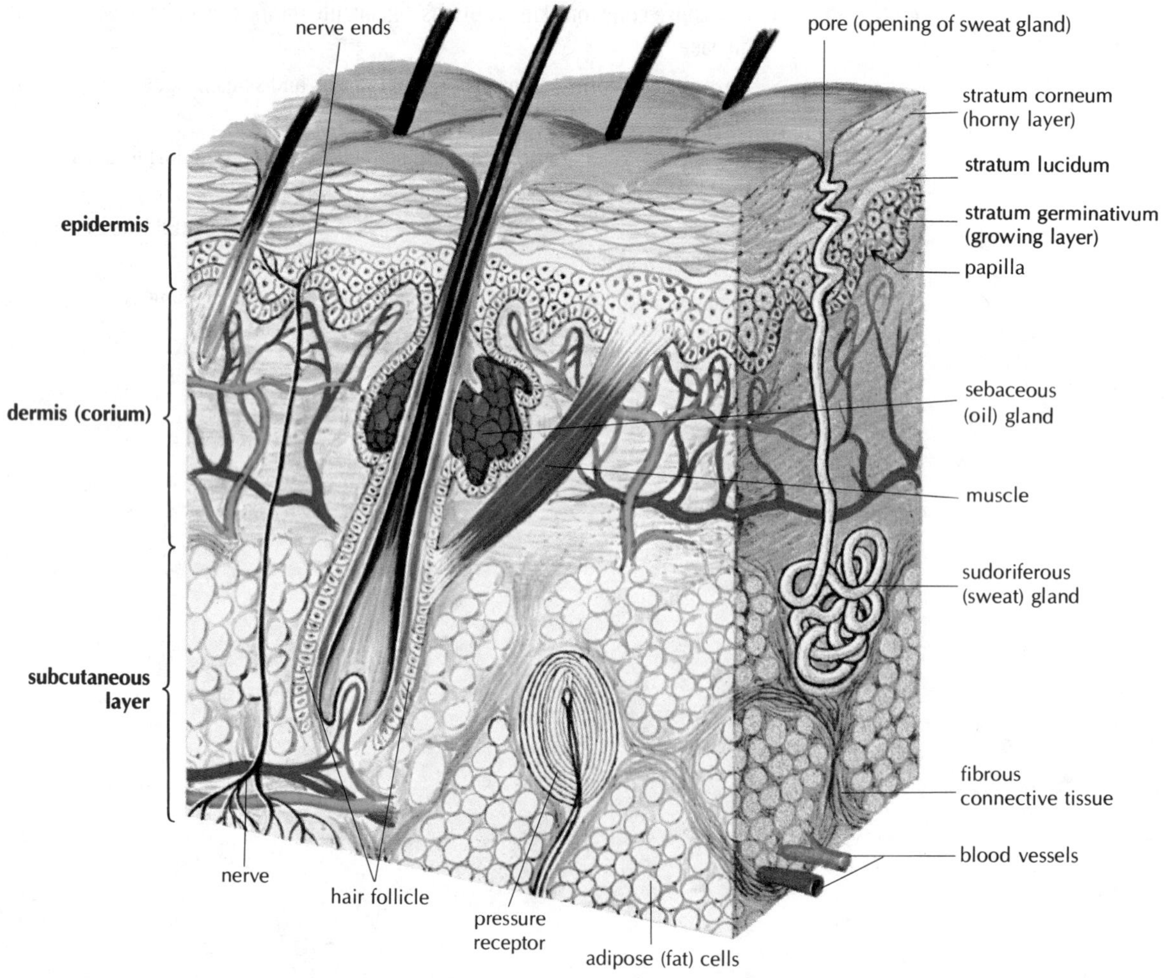

FIGURE 53-1. Anatomic structures of the skin.

forms the outer barrier of the skin and has the capacity to repel pathogens and prevent excessive fluid loss from the body (Holbrook, 1991). Keratin is the principal hardening ingredient of the hair and nails.

Melanocytes are the special cells of the epidermis that are primarily involved in producing the pigment **melanin,** which colors the skin and hair. The more melanin, the darker the color. Most of the skin of dark-skinned persons and the darker areas of the skin on light-skinned persons (*e.g.,* the nipple) contain larger amounts of this pigment. Normal skin color depends on race and varies from light pink to brown. Systemic disease will affect skin color as well. For example, the skin appears bluish when there is insufficient oxygenation of the blood, yellow-green in persons with jaundice, or red or flushed when there is inflammation or fever. Table 53-1 summarizes some common skin manifestations of systemic diseases.

Production of melanin is controlled by a hormone secreted from the hypothalamus of the brain, called melanocyte-stimulating hormone (MSH). It is believed that melanin can absorb ultraviolet light and thus protect the individual from the harmful effects of the ultraviolet rays in sunlight.

Two other cells are common to the epidermis: Merkel and Langerhans cells. **Merkel cell** function is not clearly understood, but is thought to have a role in the neuroendocrine pathway of the epidermis (Holbrook, 1991). **Langerhans cells** are believed to play a significant role in cutaneous antigen–antigen response (Elmets, 1992).

The epidermis is modified in different areas of the body. It is thickest over the palms of the hands and soles of the feet and contains increased amounts of keratin. The thickness of the epidermis can increase with use and can result in calluses forming on the hands or corns forming on the feet.

The junction of the epidermis and dermis is an area of many undulations and furrows called **rete ridges.** This junction anchors the epidermis to the dermis and permits the free exchange of essential nutrients between the two layers. This interlocking between the dermis and epidermis produces ripples on the surface of the skin. On the fingertips these ripples are called **fingerprints.** They are perhaps a person's most individual characteristic and they almost never change.

The dermis makes up the largest portion of the skin, providing strength and structure (Eckert, 1992). It is composed of two layers: papillary and reticular. The **papillary** dermis lies directly beneath the epidermis and is composed primarily of fibroblast cells capable of producing one form of collagen, a component of connective tissue. The **reticular** layer lies beneath the papillary layer and also produces collagen and elastic bundles. The dermis is also made up of blood and lymph vessels, nerves, sweat and sebaceous glands, and hair roots. The dermis is often referred to as the "true skin."

The **subcutaneous tissue** or **hypodermis** is the innermost layer of the skin. It is primarily adipose tissue, which provides a cushion between the skin layers and such internal structures as the muscles and the bone. It permits skin mobility, molds body contours, and insulates the body (Holbrook, 1991). Fat is deposited and distributed according to the person's gender, and in part accounts for the difference in body shape between men and women. Overeating results in increased deposition of fat beneath the skin. The subcutaneous tissues and amount of fat deposited are important factors in body temperature regulation.

Hair. An outgrowth of the skin, hair is present over the entire body except for the palms of the hands and soles of the feet. The hair consists of a root formed in the dermis and a hair shaft that projects beyond the skin. It grows in a cavity called a hair follicle. The proliferation of cells in the bulb of the hair causes the hair to form (Fig. 53-1).

Hair follicles undergo cycles of growth and rest. The rate of growth varies; beard growth is the most rapid, followed by hair on the scalp, axillae, thighs, and eyebrows. The growing phase, **anagen,** may last up to 6 years for scalp hair, whereas the **telogen** or resting phase is approximately 4 months (Baden, 1991). During telogen, hair sheds from the body. The hair follicle will recycle into the growing phase spontaneously, or it can be induced by plucking out hairs. Growing and resting hair can be found side by side on all parts of the body. About 90% of the 100,000 hair follicles on a normal scalp are in the growing phase at any one time. From 50 to 100 scalp hairs are shed each day (Baden, 1991).

Hairs in different parts of the body serve different functions. The hairs of the eyes (eyebrows and lashes), nose, and ears filter out dust, bugs, and airborne debris. Hair of the skin provides thermal insulation in lower animals. This function is enhanced during cold or fright by the piloerection (hairs "standing on end") caused by contraction of the tiny arrector muscles attached to the hair follicle. The piloerector response that occurs in humans is probably vestigial.

Hair color is supplied by varying amounts of melanin within the hair shaft. Gray or white hair reflects the loss of pigment. In certain locations on the body, hair growth is controlled by sex hormones. The most vivid examples are the hair on the face (beard and mustache) and the hair on the chest and back that are controlled by the male hormones known as androgens.

Hair quantity and distribution can be affected by endocrine conditions. For example, Cushing's syndrome causes hirsutism (excessive hair growth, especially in women); hypothyroidism (underactive thyroid) causes changes in hair texture. In many cases, cancer chemotherapy and radiation therapy will cause hair thinning or weakening of the hair shaft, resulting in partial or complete **alopecia** (hair loss) from the scalp as well as from other parts of the body.

Nails. On the dorsal surface of the fingers and toes, a hard, transparent plate of keratin, called the **nail,** overlies the skin. The nail grows from its root, which lies under a thin fold of skin called the **cuticle.** The nail protects the fingers and toes by preserving their highly developed sensory function, which promotes certain fine functions, such as picking up small objects.

Nail growth is continuous throughout life, with an average growth of 0.1 mm daily. (Kvedar & Baden, 1991). Growth is faster in fingernails than toenails and tends to slow with aging. Complete renewal of a fingernail takes about 170 days, whereas toenail renewal takes from 12 to 18 months.

Glands of the Skin. The **sebaceous glands** are associated with hair follicles. The ducts of the sebaceous glands empty an oily secretion onto the space between the hair follicle and the hair shaft. For each hair there is a sebaceous

TABLE 53-1 Selected Cutaneous Manifestations of Systemic Diseases

Common cutaneous manifestations of systemic diseases include *pruritus* (itching), which may result from chronic renal disease, scabies, pediculosis (lice), obstructive biliary disease with jaundice, Hodgkin's and non-Hodgkin's lymphoma, or medication reactions; *pallor,* which suggests anemia or a cardiopulmonary disorder; and *skin thickening and hardening,* such as that which occurs with scleroderma and dermatomyositis.

	Manifestation	Systemic Disease
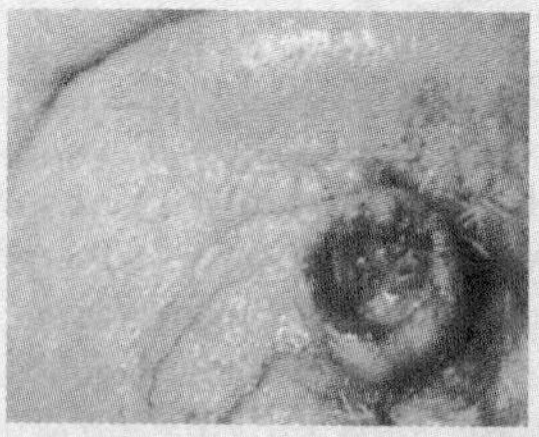	Plaques and scales on the nose, chin, ears, scalp, malar (cheek) area; telangiectasis (red spidery lines)	Connective tissue disorder (such as systemic lupus erythematosis)
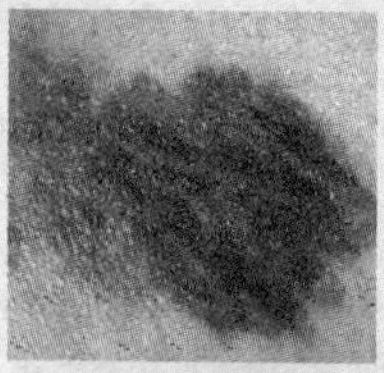 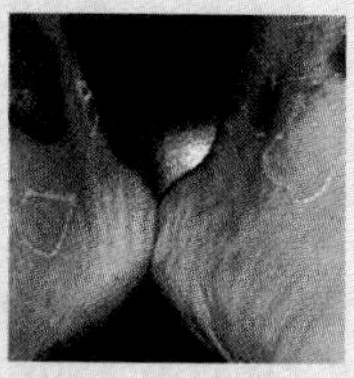	Ecchymosis (bruise) and purpura (bleeding into the skin)	Platelet disorder, vessel fragility
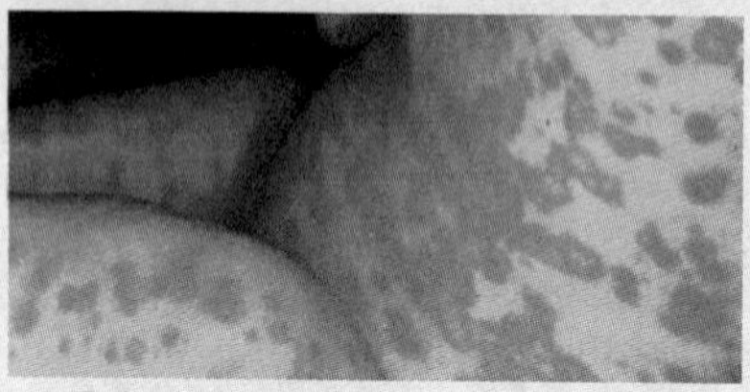	Urticaria (wheals or hives)	Infections, allergic reactions
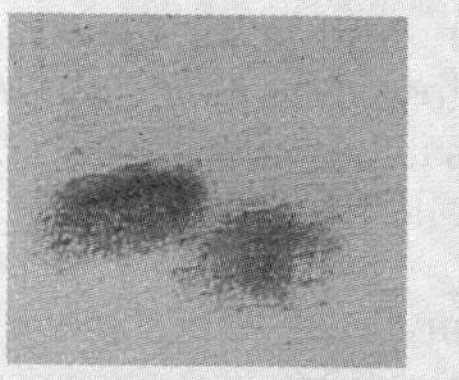 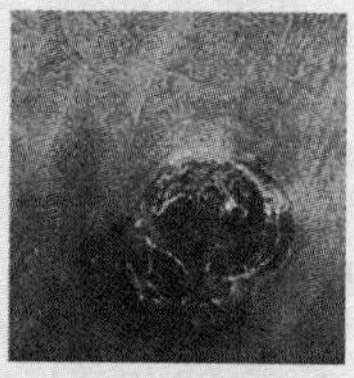	Cutaneous lesions: blue-red or dark brown plaques and nodules	Kaposi's sarcoma
	Macular, tan café-au-lait spots	Neurocutaneous disorders, such as neurofibromatosis (von Recklinghausen's disease)
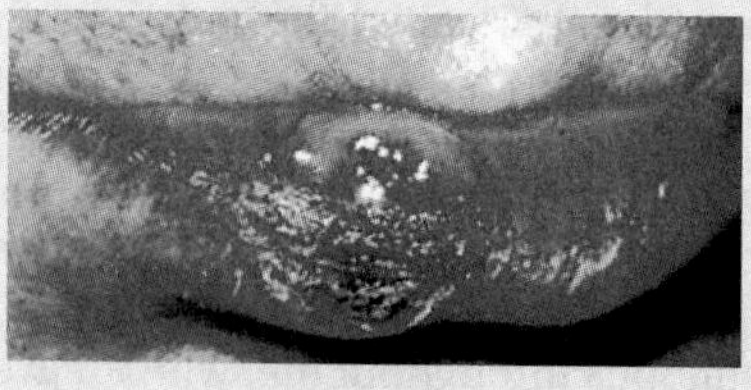	Painless chancre or ulcerated lesion	Syphilis

Note: The examples cited above include some, but not all, cutaneous manifestations of systemic disease.
(Source of photos: Bates BA. A Guide to Physical Examination and History Taking, 6th ed. Philadelphia, JB Lippincott, 1995.)

gland, the secretions of which lubricate the hair and render the skin soft and pliable (see Fig. 53-1).

Sweat glands are found in the skin over most of the body surface. They are heavily concentrated on the palms of the hands and soles of the feet. Only the glans penis, the margins of the lips, the external ear, and the nail bed are devoid of sweat glands. Sweat glands are subclassified into two categories: eccrine and apocrine.

The **eccrine** sweat glands are found in all areas of the skin. Their ducts open directly onto the skin surface. The

apocrine sweat glands are larger, and, in contrast to that of the eccrine glands, their secretion contains parts of the secretory cells. They are located in the axillae, anal region, scrotum, and labia majora. Their ducts generally open onto hair follicles. The apocrine glands become active at puberty. In the female, they enlarge and recede with each menstrual cycle.

Apocrine glands produce a milky sweat that is broken down by bacteria to produce the characteristic underarm odor. Specialized apocrine glands called **ceruminous glands** are found in the external ear, where they produce **cerumen** (wax).

The thin, watery secretion called **sweat** is produced in the basal coiled portion of the eccrine gland and is released into its narrow duct. Sweat is composed predominantly of water and contains about half of the salt content of the blood plasma. Sweat is released from eccrine glands in response to elevated ambient temperature and elevated body temperature. The rate of sweat secretion is under the control of the sympathetic nervous system. Excessive sweating of the palms and soles, axillae, forehead, and other areas may occur in response to pain and stress.

Functions of the Skin

Protection

The skin covering most of the body is only about 1 or 2 mm thick, yet it provides very effective protection against invasion by bacteria and other foreign matter. The thickened skin of the palms and soles protects against the effects of the constant trauma that occurs in these areas.

The **stratum corneum** (SC) portion of the epidermis provides the most effective barrier to environmental factors, such as chemicals, sunlight, viruses, fungi, insect bites, wind burn, and trauma. It can prevent penetration from harmful external substances or loss of fluids and other substances vital to body homeostasis (see the "Water Balance" discussion below). Various lipids (fatty substances) may be absorbed through the stratum corneum, including fat-soluble vitamins (A and D) and steroid hormones. Medications and other substances may enter the skin through the epidermis via the transepidermal route or through the openings of the follicles.

The dermal skin layer provides mechanical strength and toughness, through its fibrous connective tissue and collagen fibers. The intertwining of the elastic fibers and collagen with the epidermis allows the skin to behave as one unit. The dermis is made of a vascular network, roots of body hairs, and the sweat and sebaceous glands. Because the epidermis is avascular, the dermis provides an efficient transport barrier to substances that can penetrate the stratum corneum and the epidermis (Russel et al., 1992). Other factors that affect the protective function of the skin include skin age, area of skin involved, and vascular status.

Sensation

The receptor endings of nerves in the skin allow the body to constantly monitor the conditions of the immediate environment. The primary functions of the receptors in the skin are to sense temperature, pain, light touch, and pressure (or heavy touch). Different nerve endings are responsible for responding to each of the different stimuli. Although the nerve endings are distributed over the entire body, they are more concentrated in some areas than in others. For example, the fingertips are much more densely innervated than the skin of the back.

Water Balance

The stratum corneum has the capacity to absorb water, thereby preventing an excessive loss of water and electrolytes from the internal body and retaining moisture in the subcutaneous tissues. When skin is damaged, as occurs with a severe burn, for example, large quantities of fluids and electrolytes may be lost rapidly, possibly leading to circulatory collapse, shock, and death.

On the other hand, the skin is not completely impermeable to water. Small amounts of water continuously evaporate from the skin surface. This evaporation, called **insensible perspiration,** amounts to approximately 600 ml daily for a normal adult. Insensible water loss varies with the body temperature. In a person with a fever, this loss can increase. During immersion in water, the skin can accumulate water up to three or four times its normal weight. A common example of this is the swelling of the skin after prolonged bathing.

Temperature Regulation

The body continuously produces heat as a result of the metabolism of food, which produces energy. This heat is dissipated primarily through the skin. Three major physical processes are involved in loss of heat from the body to the environment. The first process, **radiation,** is the transfer of heat to another object of lower temperature situated at a distance. The second process, **conduction,** is the transfer of heat from the body to a cooler object in contact with it. Heat transferred by conduction to the air surrounding the body is removed by the third process, **convection,** which consists of bulk movement of warm air molecules away from the body.

Evaporation from the skin aids heat loss by conduction. Heat is conducted through the skin into water molecules on its surface, causing the water to evaporate. The water on the skin surface may be from insensible perspiration, sweat, or the environment.

Normally, all of these mechanisms for heat loss are utilized. When the ambient temperature is very high, however, radiation and convection are ineffective, and evaporation becomes the only means for heat loss.

Under normal conditions, metabolic heat production is exactly balanced by heat loss, and the internal temperature of the body is maintained constant at approximately 37°C (98.6°F). The rate of heat loss depends primarily on the surface temperature of the skin, which is a function of the skin blood flow. Under normal conditions, the total blood circulated through the skin is approximately 450 ml/min, or between 10 and 20 times the amount of blood required to provide necessary metabolites and oxygen (Scheuplein, 1991). Blood flow through these skin vessels is controlled primarily by the sympathetic nervous system. Increased blood flow to the skin results in more heat delivered to the skin and a greater rate of heat loss from the body. On the other hand, decreased skin blood flow decreases the skin temperature and helps conserve heat for the body. When the temperature of the body begins to fall, as occurs on a cold day, the blood vessels of the skin constrict, thereby reducing heat loss from the body.

Sweating is another process by which the body can regulate the rate of heat loss. Sweating will not occur until the core body temperature exceeds 37°C regardless of skin temperature (Scheuplein, 1991). In extremely hot environments, the rate of sweat production may be as high as 1 L/hr. Under some circumstances, for example with emotional stress, sweating may occur as a reflex and may be unrelated to the necessity to lose heat from the body.

Vitamin Production

Skin exposed to ultraviolet light can convert substances necessary for synthesizing vitamin D (cholecalciferol). Vitamin D is essential for preventing **rickets,** a condition that results from a deficiency of vitamin D, calcium, and phosphorus and that causes bone deformities (Morton, 1993).

Immune Response Function

Recent findings (Nickoloff, 1993) indicate that several dermal cells (Langerhans cells, interleukin-1 producing keratinocytes, and subsets of T-lymphocytes) are important components of the immune system. Ongoing research should more clearly define the role of these dermal cells in immune function.

Gerontologic Considerations

Before conducting a skin assessment, the nurse needs to be aware of significant changes that occur with aging. The major changes in the skin of older people include dryness, wrinkling, uneven pigmentation, and various proliferative lesions. Cellular changes associated with aging include a thinning at the junction of the dermis and epidermis. This results in fewer anchoring sites between the two skin layers so that even minor injury or stress to the epidermis can cause it to shear away from the dermis. This phenomenon of aging may account for the increased vulnerability of aged skin to trauma (Webster & Uitto, 1992). With increasing age, the epidermis and dermis thin and flatten, causing wrinkles, sags, and overlapping skin folds (Fig. 53-2).

Loss of the subcutaneous tissue substances of elastin, collagen, and subcutaneous fat diminish the protection and cushioning of underlying tissues and organs and decrease muscle tone.

Cellular replacement slows as a result of aging. As the dermal layers thin, the skin becomes fragile and transparent. The blood supply to the skin also changes with age. Vessels, especially the capillary loops, decrease in number and in size (Webster and Uitto, 1992). These vascular changes contribute to delayed wound healing commonly seen in the elderly patient. In addition, both sweat and sebaceous glands decrease in number and functional capacity, leading to dry and scaly skin. Reduced hormonal levels of androgens are thought to contribute to declining sebaceous gland function.

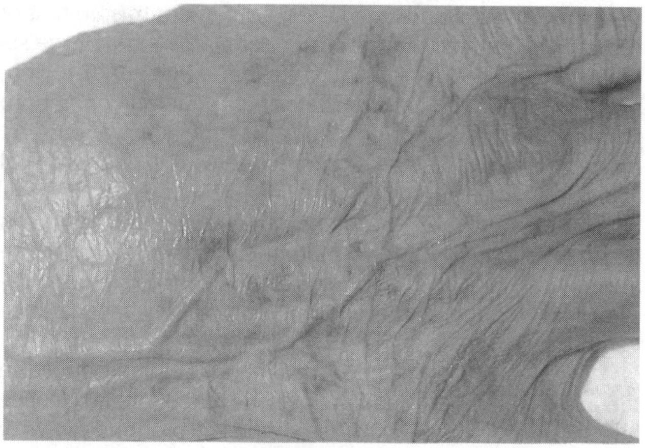

FIGURE 53-2. Close-up of the dorsum of a 90-year-old person's hand shows the wrinkling and overlapping folds common to aging skin.

Hair growth gradually diminishes, especially over the lower legs and dorsum of the feet. Thinning is common to the scalp, axilla, and pubic hair. Other functions affected with normal aging include the barrier function, sensory perception, and thermoregulation (Morton, 1993).

Photoaging, or damage from excessive sun exposure, has detrimental effects on the normal aging of skin. A lifetime of outdoor work or outdoor activities (construction workers, lifeguards, or sunbathers) without prudent use of sunscreens can lead to profound wrinkling, increased loss of elasticity, mottled pigmented areas, cutaneous atrophy, and benign or malignant lesions. Figure 53-3 demonstrates the effects of excessive lifetime sun exposure and aging.

In summary, the elderly skin undergoes many physiologic changes associated with the normal aging process. A lifetime of excessive sun exposure, systemic diseases, poor nutrition, and medications can enhance the range of skin problems and the rapidity with which skin problems appear. The outcome is an increasing vulnerability to injury and to certain diseases. Skin problems are common among older people.

Assessment of the Skin

Health History

When caring for patients with dermatologic disorders, the nurse obtains important information through the health history and direct observations. In many cases, the patient or family feels more comfortable talking with the nurse and supplies pertinent information they may have withheld or forgotten to divulge to the physician or other health care providers. The nurse's skill in physical assessment and an understanding of the anatomy and function of the skin can ensure that deviations from normal are recognized, reported, and documented.

During the health history interview, the patient should be asked about any family and personal history of skin allergies, allergic reactions to food, medications, chemicals, previous skin problems, and skin cancer. The names of cosmet-

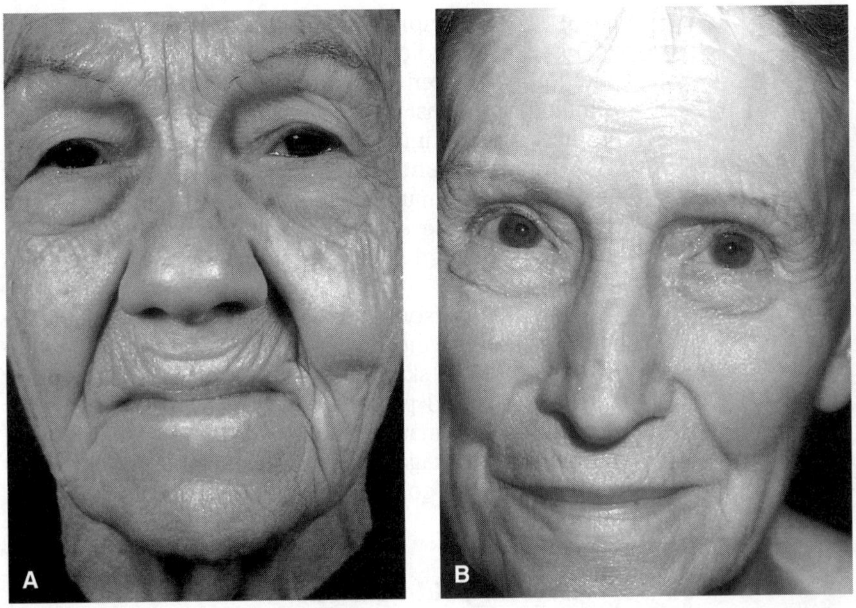

FIGURE 53-3. The effects of sun exposure and related aging. (**A**) The face of a 70-year-old woman who was exposed to sun throughout her life shows mottled hyperpigmentation, fine wrinkles, and deep furrows. (**B**) The face of a 90-year-old woman who avoided sun exposure throughout her life is blemish free, with marked elasticity and minor deepening of expression lines. (Patterson JA. Aging and Clinical Practice Skin Disorders: Diagnosis and Treatment. New York, Igaku-Shoin Medical Publishers, 1989.)

ics, soaps, shampoos or other personal hygiene products are obtained if there have been any recent skin problems noted with the use of these products. The health history will contain specific information about the onset, signs and symptoms, location, and duration of any pain, itching, rashes, or other discomfort experienced by the patient. Chart 53-1 provides a list of selected questions typically used in obtaining appropriate information.

Physical Examination

Assessment of the skin involves the entire skin area, including the mucous membranes, scalp, and nails. The skin is a reflection of a person's overall health, and alterations commonly correspond to disease in other organ systems.

Inspection and **palpation** are the chief procedures used in examining the skin and require that the room be well lighted and warm. A penlight may be used to highlight lesions. The patient completely disrobes and is adequately draped. Gloves are always worn during skin examination.

The general appearance of the skin is assessed by observing color, temperature, moisture, dryness, skin texture (rough or smooth), lesions, vascularity, mobility, and the condition of the hair and nails. Skin turgor, possible edema, and elasticity are assessed by palpation.

Skin color varies from person to person and ranges from ivory to deep brown. The skin of exposed portions of the body, especially in sunny, warm climates, tends to be more pigmented than that of the rest of the body. The vasodilative effects of fever, sunburn, and inflammation produce a pink or reddish hue to the skin. Pallor is an absence of or decrease in normal skin tones and vascularity and is best observed in the conjunctivae.

The bluish hue of **cyanosis** indicates cellular hypoxia and is easily observed in the extremities, nail beds, lips, and mucous membranes. **Jaundice,** a yellowing of the skin, is directly related to elevations in serum bilirubin and is often noted in the sclerae and mucous membranes (Fig. 53-4).

Assessing Patients With Dark Skin

The color gradations that occur in dark-skinned persons are largely determined by genetic transmission; they may be described as light, medium, or dark. In dark-skinned persons, melanin is produced at a faster rate and in larger quantities than in lighter-skinned persons. Healthy, dark skin has a reddish base or undertone. The buccal mucosa, tongue, lips, and nails normally appear pink.

In examining the dark-skinned patient, it is important to have good lighting and to examine the skin and the nail beds, as well as the mouth. All suspicious areas are palpated.

The degree of pigmentation of the dark-skinned patient's skin may affect the appearance of a lesion. Lesions may be black, purple, or gray instead of the tan or red color seen in light-skinned patients.

Erythema. Because there is a tendency for dark skin to assume a purplish-grayish cast when an inflammatory process is present, it may be difficult to detect **erythema** (redness of the skin caused by congestion of the capillaries). To determine possible inflammation, the skin is palpated for increased warmth or for smoothness (edema) or hardness. The adjacent lymph nodes are also palpated.

Rash. In instances of pruritus (itching), the patient should be asked to indicate which areas of the body are involved. The skin is then stretched gently to decrease the reddish tone and make the rash stand out. The differences in skin texture are then assessed by running the tips of the fingers lightly over the skin. Usually, the borders of the rash can be felt. The patient's mouth and ears are included in the examination. (Sometimes rubeola, or measles, will cause a red cast to appear on the tip of the ears.) Finally, the patient's temperature is assessed and the lymph nodes are palpated.

Cyanosis. When a person with dark skin is in shock, the skin usually assumes a grayish cast. To detect cyanosis, the areas around the mouth and lips and over the cheekbones and earlobes should be observed. Other indications include cold, clammy skin; a rapid, thready pulse; and

CHART 53-1
Patient History: Skin Disorders

Patient history relevant to skin disorders may be obtained by asking the following questions:

- When did you first notice this skin problem (also investigate duration and intensity)?
- Has it occurred previously?
- Are there any other symptoms?
- What site was first affected?
- What did the rash or lesion look like when it first appeared?
- Where and how fast did it spread?
- Are there itching, burning, tingling, or crawling sensations?
- Is there any loss of sensation?
- Is the problem worse at a particular time or season?
- Do you have any idea how it started?
- Do you have a history of hay fever, asthma, hives, eczema, or allergies?
- Does anyone in your family have skin problems or rashes?
- Did the eruptions appear after certain foods were eaten?
- Had there been recent intake of alcohol?
- Was there a relation between a specific event and the outbreak of the rash or lesion?
- What medications are you taking?
- What topical medication (ointment, cream, salve) have you put on the lesion (include over-the-counter medications)?
- What skin products or cosmetics do you use?
- What is your occupation?
- What in your immediate environment (plants, animals, chemicals, infections) might be precipitating this problem? Is there anything new or are there any changes in the environment?
- Does anything touching your skin cause a rash?
- Is there anything else you wish to talk about in regard to this problem?

rapid, shallow respirations. When the conjunctivae of the eyelids are examined for **petechiae** (small, red spots due to escape of blood), it is important not to mistake them for normal melanin deposits.

Color Changes. Changes in skin color in dark-skinned persons are noticeable and usually cause distress to the patient. For example, **hypopigmentation** (loss of or decrease in skin color), which may be due to **vitiligo** (a condition characterized by destruction of melanocytes in limited or extensive skin areas), may cause more concern in the dark-skinned person because it is so readily visible. **Hyperpigmentation** (increase in color) may occur after disease or injury to the skin. A pigmented nasal crease below the eye may be an external sign of allergy. However, pigmented streaks in the nails are considered to be normal.

In general, persons with dark skin suffer from the same skin conditions as those with light skin, although they are less likely to have skin cancer and scabies. On the other hand, dark-skinned persons have a greater propensity for keloid or scar formation and for disorders resulting from occlusion or blockage of hair follicles. Table 53-2 provides an overall view of color changes in light and dark-skinned persons.

Assessing Skin Lesions

Skin lesions are the most prominent characteristics of dermatologic conditions. They vary in size, shape, and cause and are classified according to their appearance and origin.

Skin lesions can be described as primary or secondary. **Primary lesions** are the initial lesions and are characteristic of the disease itself. **Secondary lesions** result from external causes, such as scratching, trauma, infections, or changes caused by wound healing. Depending on the stage of development, skin lesions are further categorized according to type and appearance (Chart 53-2).

A preliminary assessment of the eruption or lesion should help to identify the type of dermatosis (abnormal skin condition) and indicate whether the lesion is primary or secondary. At the same time, the anatomic distribution of the eruption should be noted because certain diseases tend to affect certain sites of the body and are distributed in characteristic patterns and shapes (Figs. 53-5 and 53-6). To determine the extent of the regional distribution, the left and right sides of the body should be compared while the color and shape of the lesions are noted. Following observation, the lesions are palpated to determine their texture, shape, and border and to see if they are soft or filled with fluid, or hard and fixed to the surrounding tissue.

A metric ruler is used to measure the size of the lesions so that any further extension can be compared with this initial baseline measurement. The dermatosis is then documented on the patient's health record; it should be described clearly and in detail, with precise terminology.

(text continues on page 1488)

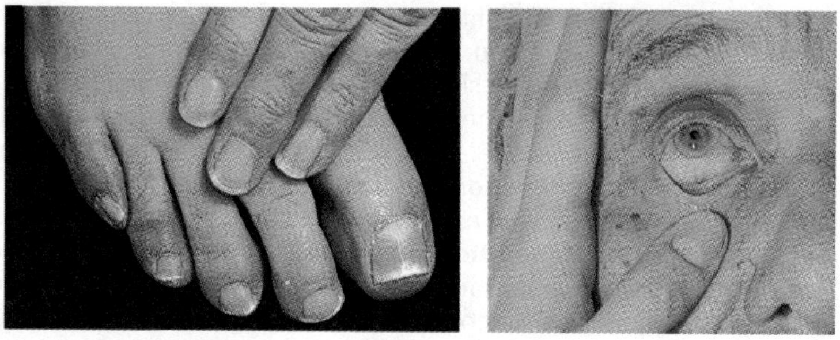

FIGURE 53-4. Examples of skin color changes: the bluish tint of cyanosis (**left**) and the yellow hue of jaundice (**right**).

TABLE 53-2 Color Changes in Light and Dark Skin

Etiology	Light Skin	Dark Skin
Pallor		
Anemia—decreased hematocrit Shock—decreased perfusion, vasoconstriction	Generalized pallor	Brown skin appears yellow-brown, dull; black skin appears ashen gray, dull (observe areas with least pigmentation: conjunctivae, mucous membranes)
Local arterial insufficiency	Marked localized pallor (lower extremities, especially when elevated)	Ashen gray, dull; cool to palpation
Albinism—total absence of pigment melanin	Whitish pink	Tan, cream, white
Vitiligo—patchy depigmentation caused by the destruction of melanocytes	Patchy, milky white spots, often symmetric bilaterally	Same
Cyanosis		
Increased amount of unoxygenated hemoglobin: Central—chronic heart and lung disease cause arterial desaturation	Dusky blue	Dark but dull, lifeless. Only severe cyanosis is apparent in skin (observe conjunctiva, oral mucosa, nail beds)
Peripheral—exposure to cold, anxiety	Nail beds dusky	
Erythema		
Hyperemia—increased blood flow through engorged arterial vessels, such as in inflammation, fever, alcohol intake, blushing	Red, bright pink	Purplish tinge, but difficult to see (palpate for increased warmth with inflammation, taut skin, and hardening of deep tissues)
Polycythemia—increased red blood cells, capillary stasis	Ruddy blue in face, oral mucosa, conjunctiva, hands and feet	Well concealed by pigment (observe for redness in lips)
Carbon monoxide poisoning	Bright, cherry red in face and upper torso	Cherry red nail beds, lips, and oral mucosa
Venous stasis—decreased blood flow from area, engorged venules	Dusky rubor of dependent extremities (a prelude to necrosis with pressure ulcer)	Easily masked (use palpation to identify warmth or edema)
Jaundice		
Increased serum bilirubin level, over 2–3 mg/100 ml due to liver inflammation or hemolytic disease as occurs after severe burns or some infections	Yellow first in sclera, hard palate, mucous membranes and then over skin	Check sclera for yellow near limbus. Do not mistake normal yellowish fatty deposits in the periphery under eyelids for jaundice. Jaundice best noted in junction of hard and soft palate; also palms
Carotenemia—increased level of serum carotene from ingestion of large amounts of carotene-rich foods	Yellow-orange tinge in forehead, palms and soles, nasolabial folds; but no yellowing in sclera or mucous membranes	Yellow-orange tinge in palms and soles
Uremia—renal failure causes retained urochrome pigments in the blood	Orange-green or gray overlaying pallor of anemia. May also have ecchymoses and purpura	Easily masked (rely on laboratory and clinical findings)
Brown-Tan		
Addison's disease—cortisol deficiency stimulates increased melanin production	Bronzed appearance, an "external tan," most apparent around nipples, perineum, genitalia, and pressure points (inner thighs, buttocks, elbows, axillae)	Easily masked (rely on laboratory and clinical findings)
Café au lait spots—due to increased melanin pigment in basal cell layer	Tan to light brown, irregularly shaped, oval patch with well-defined borders	

(Jarvis, C. Physical Examination and Health Assessment. Philadelphia, WB Saunders 1992, 254–255, with permission.)

CHART 53-2
Primary and Secondary Skin Lesions

Primary Skin Lesions

Primary skin lesions are original lesions arising from previously normal skin. Secondary lesions can originate from primary lesions.

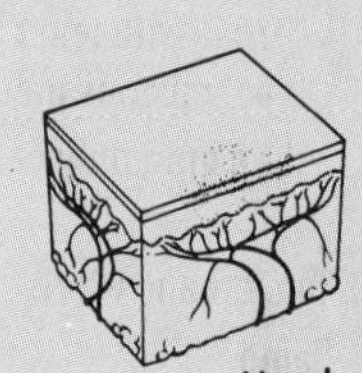
Macule

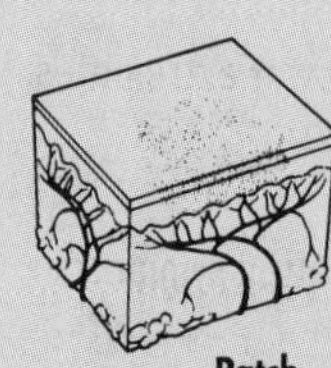
Patch

Macule, Patch

- *Macule:* <1 cm, circumscribed border
- *Patch:* >1 cm, may have irregular border
- Flat, nonpalpable skin color change (color may be brown, white, tan, purple, red)

Examples:
Freckles, flat moles, petechia, rubella, vitiligo, port wine stains, ecchymosis

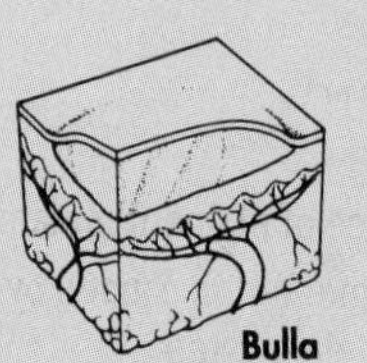
Bulla

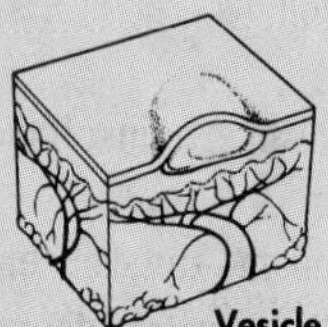
Vesicle

Vesicle, Bulla

- *Vesicle:* <0.5 cm
- *Bulla:* >0.5 cm
- Circumscribed, elevated, palpable mass containing serous fluid

Examples:
Vesicles: Herpes simplex/zoster, chickenpox, poison ivy, second degree burn (blister)
Bulla: Pemphigus, contact dermatitis, large burn blisters, poison ivy, bullous impetigo

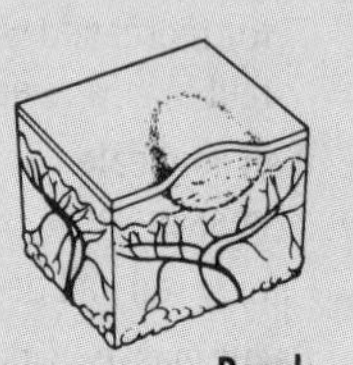
Papule

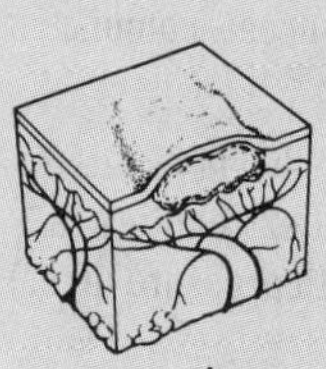
Plaque

Papule, Plaque

- *Papule:* <0.5 cm
- *Plaque:* >0.5 cm
- Elevated, palpable, solid mass
- Circumscribed border
- Plaque may be coalesced papules with flat top

Examples:
Papules: Elevated nevi, warts, lichen planus
Plaques: Psoriasis, actinic keratosis

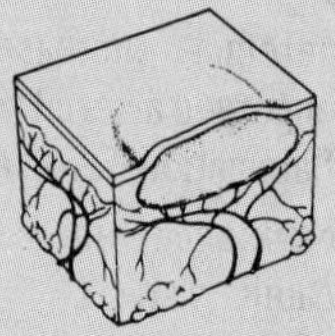
Wheal

Wheal

- Elevated mass with transient borders
- Often irregular
- Size, color varies
- Caused by movement of serous fluid into the dermis
- Does not contain free fluid in a cavity as, for example, a vesicle

Examples:
Urticaria (hives), insect bites

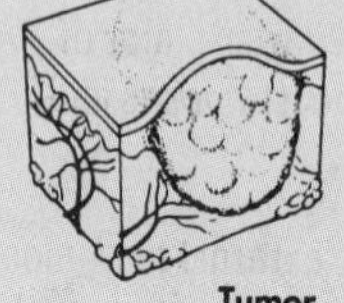
Tumor

Nodule, Tumor

- *Nodule:* 0.5–2 cm
- *Tumor:* >1–2 cm
- Elevated, palpable, solid mass
- Extends deeper into the dermis than a papule
- Nodules circumscribed
- Tumors do not always have sharp borders

Examples:
Nodules: Lipoma, squamous cell carcinoma, poorly absorbed injection, dermatofibroma
Tumors: Larger lipoma, carcinoma

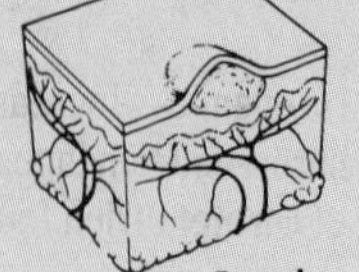
Pustule

Pustule

- Pus-filled vesicle or bulla

Examples:
Acne, impetigo, furuncles, carbuncles

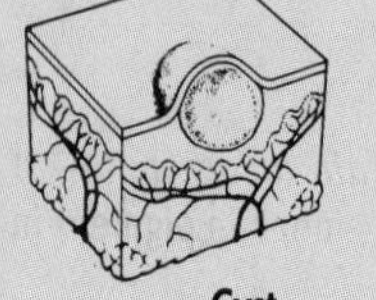
Cyst

Cyst

- Encapsulated fluid-filled or semisolid mass
- In the subcutaneous tissue or dermis

Examples:
Sebaceous cyst, epidermoid cyst

(continued)

CHART 53-2 (continued)

Primary and Secondary Skin Lesions

Secondary Skin Lesions

Secondary skin lesions result from changes in primary lesions.

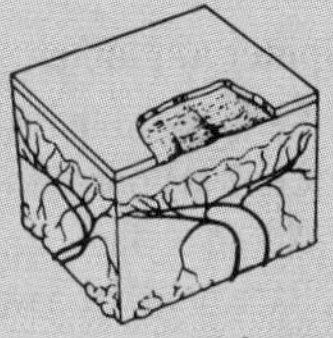

Erosion

Erosion

- Loss of superficial epidermis
- Does not extend to dermis
- Depressed, moist area

Examples:
Ruptured vesicles, scratch marks

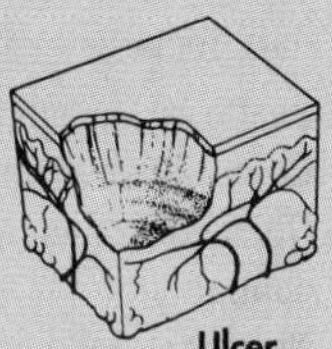

Ulcer

Ulcer

- Skin loss extending past epidermis
- Necrotic tissue loss
- Bleeding and scarring possible

Examples:
Stasis ulcer of venous insufficiency, pressure ulcer

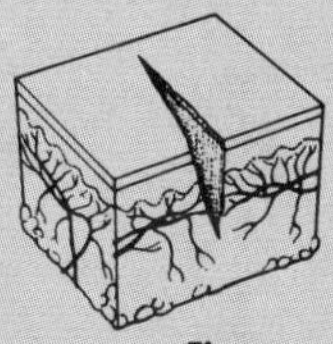

Fissure

Fissure

- Linear crack in the skin
- May extend to dermis

Examples:
Chapped lips or hands, athlete's foot

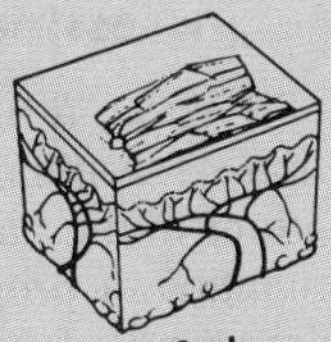

Scales

Scales

- Flakes secondary to desquamated, dead epithelium
- Flakes may adhere to skin surface
- Color varies (silvery, white)
- Texture varies (thick, fine)

Examples:
Dandruff, psoriasis, dry skin, pityriasis rosea

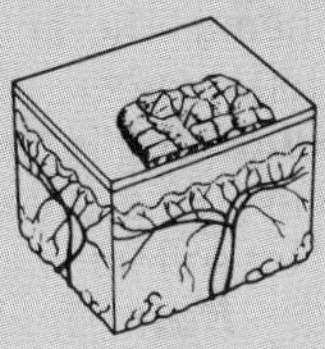

Crust

Crust

- Dried residue of serum, blood or pus on skin surface
- Large adherent crust is a scab

Examples:
Residue left following vesicle rupture: impetigo, herpes, eczema

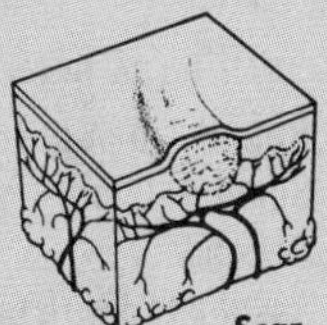

Scar

Scar (Cicatrix)

- Skin mark left after healing of a wound or lesion
- Represents replacement by connective tissue of the injured tissue
- Young scars: red or purple
- Mature scars: white or glistening

Examples:
Healed wound or surgical incision

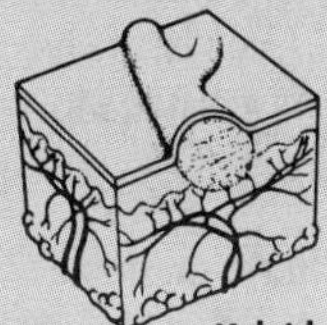

Keloid

Keloid

- Hypertrophied scar tissue
- Secondary to excessive collagen formation during healing
- Elevated, irregular, red
- Greater incidence in African-Americans

Example:
Keloid of ear piercing or surgical incision

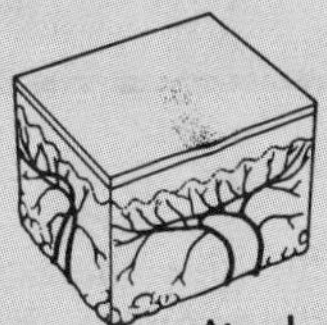

Atrophy

Atrophy

- Thin, dry, transparent appearance of epidermis
- Loss of surface markings
- Secondary to loss of collagen and elastin
- Underlying vessels may be visible

Example:
Aged skin, arterial insufficiency

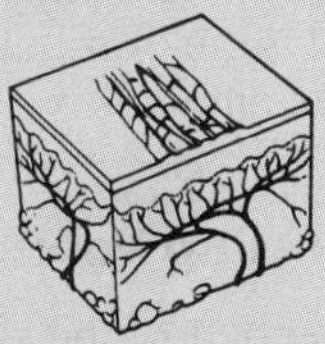

Lichenification

Lichenification

- Thickening and roughening of the skin
- Accentuated skin markings
- May be secondary to repeated rubbing, irritation, scratching

Example:
Contact dermatitis

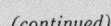

(continued)

CHART 53-2 (continued)
Primary and Secondary Skin Lesions

Vascular Skin Lesions

Petechia (*pl.* petechiae)
- Round red or purple macule
- Small: 1–2 mm
- Secondary to blood extravasation
- Associated with bleeding tendencies or emboli to skin

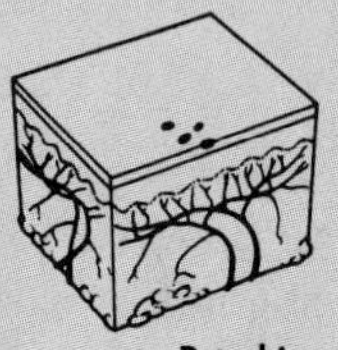
Petechiae

Ecchymosis (*pl.* ecchymoses)
- Round or irregular macular lesion
- Larger than petechia
- Color varies and changes: black, yellow, and green hues
- Secondary to blood extravasation
- Associated with trauma, bleeding tendencies

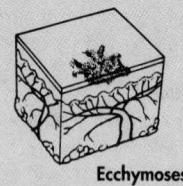
Ecchymoses

Cherry Angioma
- Papular and round
- Red or purple
- Noted on trunk, extremities
- May blanch with pressure
- Normal age-related skin alteration
- Usually not clinically significant

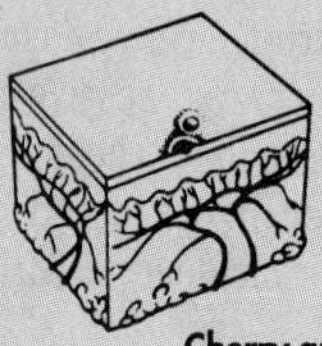
Cherry angioma

Spider Angioma
- Red, arteriole lesion
- Central body with radiating branches
- Noted on face, neck, arms, trunk
- Rare below the waist
- May blanch with pressure
- Associated with liver disease, pregnancy, vitamin B deficiency

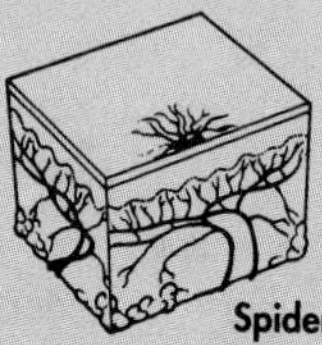
Spider angioma

Telangiectasis (Venous Star)
- Shape varies: spider-like or linear
- Color bluish or red
- Does not blanch when pressure is applied
- Noted on legs, anterior chest
- Secondary to superficial dilation of venous vessels and capillaries
- Associated with increased venous pressure states (varicosities)

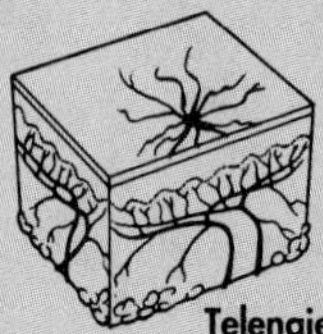
Telengiectasis

After the characteristic distribution of the lesions has been determined, the following information should be obtained and described clearly and in detail:

- What is the color of the lesion?
- Is there redness, heat, pain, or swelling?
- How large an area is involved? Where is it?
- Is the eruption macular, papular, scaling, oozing, discrete, confluent?
- What is the distribution of the lesion—symmetric, linear, circular?

Assessing Vascularity and Hydration

Once the color of the skin has been inspected and lesions have been noted, an assessment of vascular changes in the skin is performed. A description of vascular changes includes location, distribution, color, size, and the presence of pulsations. Common vascular changes include petechiae, ecchymoses, telangiectases, angiomas, and venous stars.

Skin moisture, temperature, and texture are assessed primarily by palpation. The elasticity (turgor) of the skin, which decreases in normal aging, may be a factor in assessing the hydration status of a patient.

Assessing the Nails and Hair

Nails. A brief inspection of the nails includes observation of configuration, color, and consistency. Many alterations in the nail or nailbed reflect local or systemic abnormalities in progress or result from past events (Fig. 53-7). Transverse depressions known as **Beau's lines** in the nails may reflect retarded growth of the nail matrix secondary to severe illness or, more commonly, local trauma. Ridging, hypertrophy, and other changes may also be visible with local trauma. **Paronychia,** an inflammation of the skin around the nail, is usually accompanied by tenderness and erythema. The angle between the normal nail and its base is 160 degrees. When palpated, the nail base is usually firm. **Clubbing** is manifested by a straightening of the normal angle (180 degrees or greater) and a softening of the nail base. This softening is perceived as spongelike when palpated.

Hair. The hair assessment is carried out by inspecting and palpating. Gloves are worn and the examination room should be well lighted. Separating the hair so that the condition of the skin underneath can be easily seen, the nurse notes color, texture, and distribution. Any abnormal lesions, evidence of itching, inflammation, or signs of infestation (lice or mites) are documented.

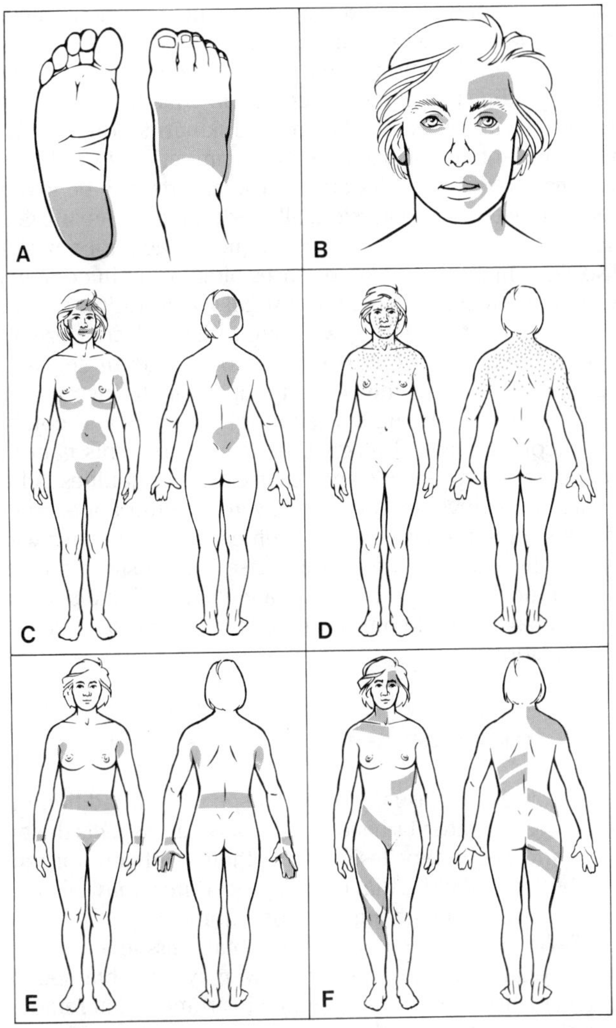

FIGURE 53-5. Anatomic distribution of common skin disorders: (**A**) contact dermatitis (shoes); (**B**) contact dermatitis (cosmetics, perfumes, earrings); (**C**) seborrheic dermatitis; (**D**) acne; (**E**) scabies; (**F**) herpes zoster (shingles).

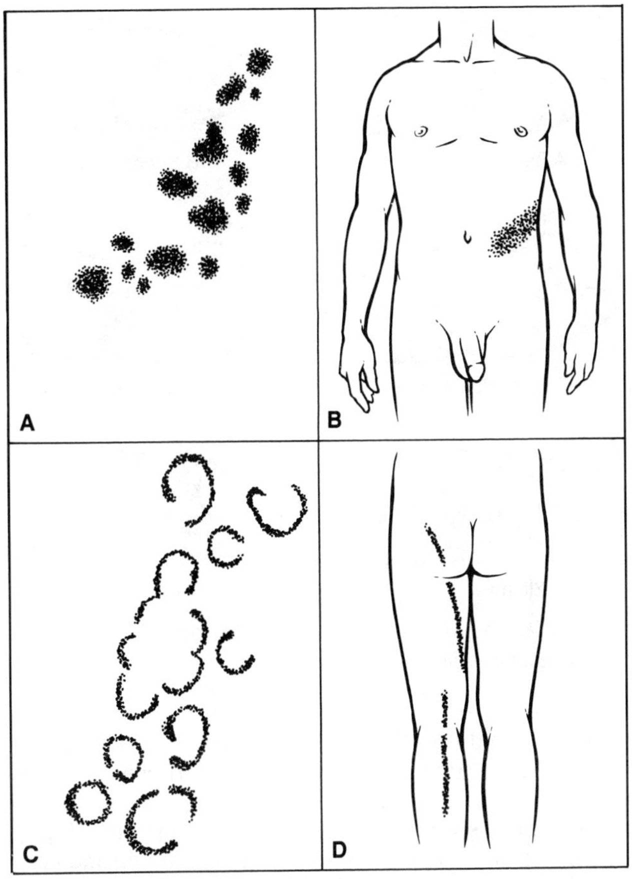

FIGURE 53-6. Examples of different configurations of skin lesions: (**A**) grouped; (**B**) zosteriform; (**C**) annular (circular) and arciform (arc); (**D**) linear.

Color and Texture. Natural hair color ranges from white to black. Hair color begins to gray as one ages, initially appearing during the third decade of life when the loss of melanin begins to become apparent. However, it is not unusual for the hair of younger persons to turn gray due to family hereditary traits. The person with **albinism** (partial or complete absence of pigmentation) is genetically predispositioned to white hair from birth. The natural state of the hair can be altered by using hair dyes, bleaches, and curling or relaxing products. The type of products used should be identified during the assessment.

The texture of scalp hair ranges from fine to thick; silky to brittle; oily to dry; shiny to dull; and straight, curly, or kinky. Dry, brittle hair may result from overuse of hair dyes, hair dryers, and curling irons or from thyroid dysfunction. Oily hair is usually due to increased secretion from the sebaceous glands close to the scalp (Grimes & Burns, 1992). If the patient indicates that there has been a recent change in hair texture, the underlying reason should be pursued. The alteration may arise simply from the overuse of commercial hair products or from changing to a new shampoo.

Distribution. Body hair distribution varies with location. Hair over most of the body is fine, except in the axillae and pubic areas, where it is coarse and develops at puberty. Pubic hair distribution in males forms a diamond shape extending up to the umbilicus. Female pubic hair resembles an inverted triangle. If the pattern found is more characteristic of the opposite sex, further investigation is in order since this may indicate an endocrine problem. Racial differences in hair are expected, such as straight hair in Asians and curly, coarser hair in African-Americans.

Men tend to have more body and facial hair than women. Loss of hair, **alopecia,** can occur over the entire body or be confined to a specific area. Scalp hair loss may be localized to patchy areas or may range from generalized thinning to total baldness. When assessing scalp hair loss, it is important to investigate the underlying cause with the patient. Patchy hair loss may be from habitual "hair pulling" or from excess traction on the hair (braiding too tightly); excessive use of dyes, straighteners, and oils; chemotherapeutic agents (doxorubicin or cyclophosphamide); fungus infection; or moles or cancer on the scalp. Regrowth may be erratic and distribution may never attain previous thickness.

Hair Loss. The most common cause of hair loss is male pattern baldness, which affects more than half of the male

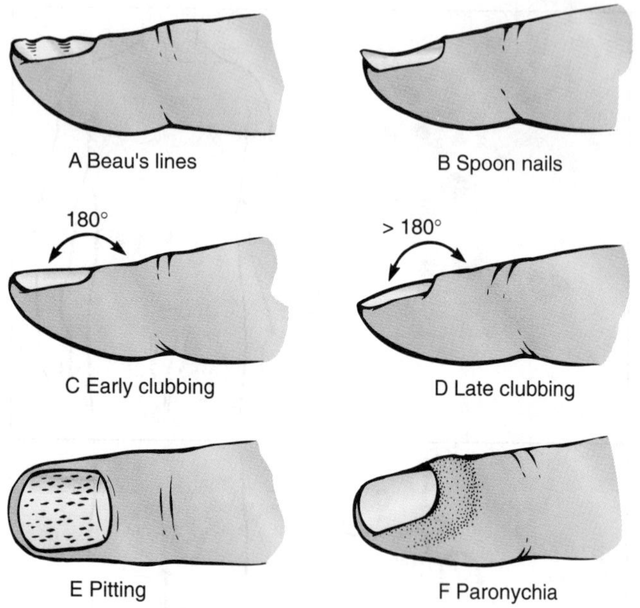

FIGURE 53-7. Common nail disorders: (**A**) Beau's lines; (**B**) spoon nails; (**C**) early clubbing; (**D**) late clubbing; (**E**) pitting; (**F**) paronychia.

population and is believed to be related to heredity, aging, and androgen (male hormone) levels. Androgen is necessary for male pattern baldness to develop. The pattern of hair loss begins with receding of the hairline in the frontal-temporal area and progresses to gradual thinning and complete loss of hair over the top of the scalp and crown. Figure 53-8 shows the usual male pattern hair loss.

Other Changes. Male pattern hair distribution called **hirsutism** (increased body hair) may be seen in some women at the time of menopause, when the hormone estrogen is no longer produced by the ovaries. In women with hirsutism, excessive hair may grow on the face, chest, shoulders, and pubic area. When menopause is ruled out as the underlying etiology, hormonal abnormalities related to pituitary or adrenal dysfunction must be pursued.

Assessment of Psychosocial Concerns

Because patients with skin conditions (1 in 20 persons) can see and feel their problems, they are more likely to be disturbed by their ailments than are patients with other conditions. Skin conditions can lead to cosmetic disfigurement, social isolation, job loss, and economic hardship.

Some conditions may subject the patient to a protracted illness, leading to feelings of depression, frustration, self-consciousness, and rejection. Itching and skin irritation also may be a constant annoyance and are common features of most skin diseases. The result of these discomforts may be loss of sleep, anxiety, and depression, all of which reinforce the general distress and fatigue that so frequently accompany skin disorders. In addition, skin diseases often result in concerns related to self-image and interpersonal relationships.

For patients suffering with such physical and psychologic discomforts, the nurse needs to provide understanding, explanations of the problem, appropriate instructions related to treatment, nursing support, patience, and continual encouragement. It takes time to help patients gain insight into their problems and resolve their difficulties. It becomes imperative, therefore, to overcome the appearance of aversion that might be felt when caring for patients with unattractive skin disorders. The nurse should show no sign of hesitancy when approaching patients with skin disorders. Such behavior would only reinforce the psychologic trauma of the disorder.

Diagnostic Evaluation

Dermatology is a visually oriented specialty. In addition to obtaining the patient's history, the examiner inspects the primary and secondary lesions and their configuration and distribution. Certain diagnostic procedures may also be used to help in identifying skin conditions.

Skin Biopsy. Performed to obtain tissue for microscopic examination, a skin biopsy may be obtained by scalpel excision or by a skin punch instrument that removes a small core of tissue. Biopsies are performed on skin nodules of uncertain origin to rule out malignancy, on plaques of unusual shapes and colors, and to secure an exact diagnosis in blistering and other disorders.

Immunofluorescence (IF). Designed to identify the site of an immune reaction, IF testing combines an antigen or antibody with a fluorochrome dye (antibodies can be made fluorescent by attaching them to a dye). IF tests on skin (**direct IF test**) are techniques to detect autoantibodies directed against portions of the skin. The **indirect IF test** detects specific antibodies in the patient's serum.

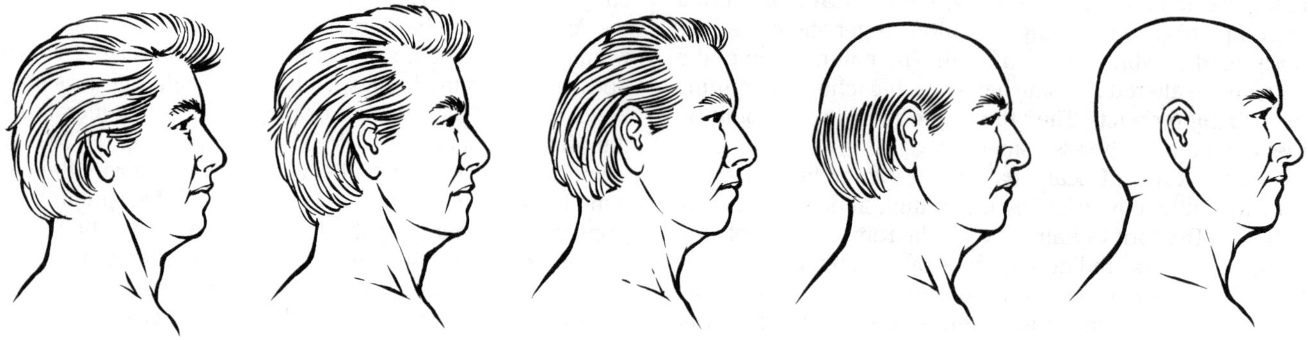

FIGURE 53-8. The progression of male pattern hair loss from normal full hair to receding frontal hairline and balding tonsure to male baldness and, finally, full baldness.

Patch Testing. Performed to identify substances to which the patient has developed an allergy, patch testing involves applying the suspected allergens to normal skin under occlusive patches. If dermatitis develops, redness, fine bumps, or itching are considered a *weak* positive reaction; fine blisters, papules, and severe itching indicate a *moderate* positive reaction; and blisters, pain, and ulceration indicate a *strong* positive reaction.

Explanations to the patient before and during the patch test usually include the following:

1. Do not use any cortisone-type medication for 1 week before the test date.
2. Small samples of each test material will be applied to a disc. The discs are then taped to the upper back (unless contraindicated). The number of test samples applied will vary (20 to 30).
3. The procedure usually takes about 30 minutes.
4. Keep the test area (back) dry while the tape is in place. Showers and swimming are not permitted.
5. Return on the date specified (2 to 3 days) to have the discs removed and the test site examined and evaluated.

Skin Scrapings. Tissue samples are scraped from suspected fungal lesions. This is performed with a scalpel blade moistened with oil so that the scraped skin adheres to the blade. The scraped material is transferred to a glass slide, covered with a cover slip, and examined microscopically.

Tzanck Smear. This test is used to examine cells from blistering skin conditions, such as herpes zoster, varicella, herpes simplex, and all forms of pemphigus. The secretions from a suspected lesion are applied to a glass slide, stained, and examined.

Wood's Light Examination. This test relies on a special lamp for producing long-wave ultraviolet rays (black light) that result in a characteristic dark purple fluorescence. The color of the fluorescent light is best seen in a darkened room, where it is possible to differentiate epidermal from dermal lesions and hypo-pigmented and hyperpigmented lesions from normal skin. The patient is reassured that the light is not harmful to skin or eyes.

Clinical Photographs. These photographs are taken to show the nature and extent of the skin condition and are used to determine progress or improvement resulting from treatment.

CRITICAL THINKING EXERCISES

1. An elderly, debilitated patient is to be discharged home to be cared for by her daughter. You know that skin trauma and pressure ulcers can occur if proper care is not carried out. How would you instruct the daughter in preventing these skin problems, especially in someone as elderly as her mother?
2. You are caring for a young man who has had surgery. You notice that his face, arms, and torso are very tan. He states that he does yard work during summer breaks from school and spends time at the beach whenever he can. Describe the type of precautions you would suggest in view of the harmful effects ultraviolet rays can have on the skin.

BIBLIOGRAPHY

Books

Baden HP. Hair follicles and pathophysiology of certain hair disorders. In Soter NA and Baden HP. Pathophysiology of Dermatologic Diseases. New York, McGraw-Hill, 1991.

Eckert RL. Structure and function of skin. In Mukhtar H (ed). Pharmacology of the Skin. Boca Raton, CRC Press, 1992.

Elmets CA. Cutaneous photocarcinogenesis. In Mukhtar H (ed). Pharmacology of the Skin. Boca Raton, CRC Press, 1992.

Grimes J and Burns E. Health Assessment in Nursing Practice. Boston, Jones & Bartlett Publishers, 1992.

Holbrook KA. Structure and development of the skin. In Soter NA and Baden HP. Pathophysiology of Dermatologic Diseases. New York, McGraw-Hill, Inc., 1991.

Jarvis C. Physical Examination and Health Assessment. Philadelphia, WB Saunders, 1992.

Kvedar JC and Baden HP. Pathophysiology of nails. In Soter NA and Baden HP. Pathophysiology of Dermatologic Diseases. New York, McGraw-Hill, 1991.

Leveque JL and Agache PG (eds). Aging Skin: Properties and Functional Changes. New York, Dekker, 1993.

Montagna W, Prota G, and Kenney JA. Black Skin: Structure and Function. San Diego, Academic Press, Inc., 1993.

Morton PG. Health Assessment in Nursing. Springhouse, PA, Springhouse Corp., 1993.

Mukhtar H (ed). Pharmacology of the Skin. Boca Raton, CRC Press, 1992.

Nickoloff BJ (ed). Dermal Immune System. Boca Raton, CRC Press, 1993.

Rook A and Dawber R (eds). Diseases of the Hair and Scalp. Boston, Blackwell Scientific, 1991.

Russell O et al. Percutaneous absorption. In Mukhtar H (ed). Pharmacology of the Skin. Boca Raton, CRC Press, 1992.

Scheuplein RJ. Temperature regulation in the skin. In Soter NA and Baden HP. Pathophysiology of Dermatologic Diseases. New York, McGraw-Hill, 1991.

Webster GF and Uitto J. Pharmacology of the aging skin. In Mukhtar H (ed). Pharmacology of the Skin. Boca Raton, CRC Press, 1992.

Journals

Flory C. Skin assessment. RN 1992 June; 55(6):22–26.

Halpern AC. Pigmented lesions in the elderly. Hosp Pract Sep 30 1993; 28(9A):74–78.

Knight A. Skin changes in systemic disease. Practitioner 1993; 237:144–149.

Lazar AP. Cutaneous manifestations of systemic disease. Compr Ther 1992; 18(9):5–9.

McGovern M and Kuhn K. Skin assessment of the elderly client. J Gerontol Nurs 1992 Apr; 18(4):39–43.

Poorman SG and Webb CA. Sexuality and self-concept: Issues in skin diseases. Dermatology Nursing 1992 Aug; 4(4):279–284.

Sher TH. Clinical evaluation of generalized pruritus. Compr Ther 1992 Sep; 18(9):14–19.

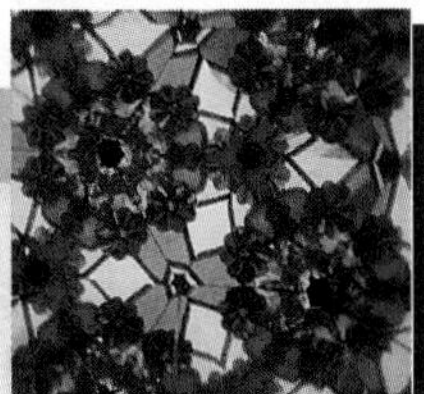

54 Management of Patients With Dermatologic Problems

CHAPTER OUTLINE

Management of Patients With Skin Disorders
Dressings for Skin Conditions
Therapeutic Baths (Balneotherapy)
Pharmacotherapy
NURSING PROCESS: The Patient With an Abnormal Skin Condition

Pruritus
Management
Perianal Itching

Secretory Disorders
Seborrheic Dermatoses
Acne Vulgaris
NURSING PROCESS: The Patient With Acne

Infections and Infestations of the Skin
Bacterial Infections (Pyodermas)
Viral Infections
Mycotic (Fungal) Infections

Parasitic Skin Diseases
Pediculosis (Infestation by Lice)
Scabies

Contact Dermatitis

Noninfectious Inflammatory Dermatoses
Psoriasis
NURSING PROCESS: The Patient With Psoriasis
Exfoliative Dermatitis
Pemphigus Vulgaris
NURSING PROCESS: The Patient With Pemphigus Vulgaris
Toxic Epidermal Necrolysis
NURSING PROCESS: The Patient With Toxic Epidermal Necrolysis

Ulcers and Benign Tumors of the Skin
Ulcerations
Tumors of the Skin

Cancer of the Skin
Causes and Prevention
Types of Skin Cancer
Malignant Melanoma
NURSING PROCESS: The Patient With Malignant Melanoma
Metastatic Skin Tumors

Other Malignancies of the Skin
Kaposi's Sarcoma

Dermatologic and Plastic Reconstructive Surgery
Wound Coverage: Grafts and Flaps
Chemical Face Peeling
Dermabrasion
Management of the Patient With Facial Reconstructive Surgery
NURSING PROCESS: The Patient With Facial Reconstructive Surgery
Face Lift
Laser Treatment of Cutaneous Lesions

Hair Disorders
Androgenetic Alopecia

Critical Thinking Exercises

LEARNING OBJECTIVES

On completion of this chapter, the learner will be able to:

1. Describe the general management of the patient with an abnormal skin condition
2. Use the nursing process as a framework for care of the patient with acne
3. Describe the health education needs of the patient with infections of the skin and parasitic skin diseases
4. Use the nursing process as a framework for care of patients with noninfectious inflammatory dermatoses
5. Describe the management and nursing care of the patient with cancer of the skin
6. Use the nursing process as a framework for care of the patient with malignant melanoma
7. Describe characteristics of the various types of Kaposi's sarcoma
8. Compare the various types of dermatologic and plastic reconstructive surgeries
9. Compare chemical and surgical planing and the related nursing needs of the patient
10. Use the nursing process as a framework for care of the patient undergoing facial reconstructive surgery

Management of Patients With Skin Disorders

Nursing care for patients with dermatologic problems includes topical and systemic medications, wet dressings, other special dressings, and therapeutic baths.

The major objectives of therapy are to (1) prevent damage to healthy skin, (2) prevent secondary infection, (3) reverse the inflammatory process, and (4) relieve the symptoms.

Preventing Damage to Healthy Skin. Some skin problems are markedly aggravated by soap and water. Therefore, bathing routines are modified according to the condition.

- Denuded skin, whether the area of desquamation is large or small, is excessively prone to damage by chemicals and trauma.

The friction of a towel, if applied with vigor, is sufficient to excite a brisk inflammatory response that causes any existing lesion to flare up and extend. Thus, the essence of skin care and protection in bathing a patient with skin abnormalities is to use a mild, superfatted soap or soap substitute and to ensure the complete removal of the soap by rinsing before blotting the area dry with a soft cloth. Deodorant soaps should be avoided in these patients.

Special care needs to be given when changing dressings. Pledgets saturated with oil will help loosen crusts, remove exudates, or free an adherent dry dressing. The dressing may also be saturated with sterile saline or another prescribed solution, which softens it and permits it to be pulled away gently.

Preventing Secondary Infection. Potentially infectious skin lesions should be regarded strictly as such, and proper precautions should be observed until the diagnosis is established. Some lesions with pus contain infectious material. Although some genital lesions are infectious, most are minor irritations.

- The nurse and physician must adhere to universal precautions and wear either clean or sterile gloves when inspecting or changing the dressing. Proper disposal of any contaminated dressing is carried out according to agency protocol.

Reversing the Inflammatory Process. The type of skin lesion (oozing, infected, or dry) usually determines which local medication or treatment is prescribed. As a rule, if the skin is acutely inflamed (hot, red, and swollen) and is oozing, it is best to apply wet dressings and soothing lotions. In chronic conditions in which the skin surface is dry and scaly, water-soluble emulsions, creams, ointments, and pastes are used. The therapy must be changed as the response indicates. The patient is instructed to contact the physician if the medication or compresses seem to irritate the disorder. Success or failure of skin therapy usually depends on adequate instruction and motivation of the patient and the interest and support of the health personnel.

Dressings for Skin Conditions

Wet Dressings

Wet dressings (wet compresses applied to the skin) are usually used for acute, weeping, inflammatory lesions. They may be sterile or nonsterile (clean), depending on the condition. Wet dressings (1) reduce inflammation by producing constriction of the blood vessels (thereby decreasing vasodilation and local blood flow in inflammation); (2) clean the skin of exudates, crusts, and scales; (3) maintain drainage of infected areas; and (4) promote healing by facilitating the free movement of epidermal cells across the involved skin so that new granulation tissue forms. Wet dressings are used for vesicular, bullous, pustular, and ulcerative disorders, as well as for inflammatory conditions. Before these dressings are applied, the hands are washed and sterile or clean gloves are put on.

Wet compresses generally contain room-temperature tap water or a saline solution. Other agents used may include silver nitrate, aluminum acetate (Burow's solution), potassium permanganate, 5% acetic acid, and sodium hypochlorite (Dakin's solution). While some wet dressings must be covered to prevent evaporation, most are allowed to remain open to the air. The **open dressing** requires frequent changes because evaporation is rapid. The **closed dressing** is changed less frequently. However, there is always a danger that it will cause not only softening but actual maceration of the underlying skin. **Wet-to-dry dressings** are used to remove exudate from erosions or ulcers. The dressing remains in place until it dries. It is then removed without soaking so that crusts, exudate, or pus from the skin lesion will adhere to the dressing and be removed with it.

New, commercially produced **moisture-retentive dressings** can perform the same functions as the wet compresses but are more efficient at removing exudate because of their higher moisture-vapor transmission rate; some have reservoirs that can hold excessive exudate (Eaglestein, 1993). A number of moisture-retentive dressings are already impregnated with saline solution, petrolatum, zinc-saline solution, hydrogel, and antimicrobials, thereby eliminating the need to coat the skin to avoid maceration. The main advantage of moisture-retentive dressings over wet compresses is the decreased frequency of dressing change required. Depending on the product used and the type of dermatologic problem encountered, most moisture-retentive dressings may remain in place from 8 to 12 hours; some can remain in place as long as a week.

When wet compresses are chosen instead of moisture-retentive dressings, they can be made using smooth muslin or cotton materials that are cut and folded to make dressings two to four layers thick, or commercially available dressings can be used. The dressing is saturated with the prescribed solution, wrung out, and applied. Usually wet compresses are kept cool or at room temperature. Compresses are reapplied every 5 to 10 minutes to ensure continuing wetness. Wet compresses are usually applied for about 20 minutes, three to four times daily during the acute phase, unless another schedule is prescribed. Medications applied to moist skin immediately after removal of wet compresses are absorbed better than when applied to dry skin. If extensive skin areas are to be treated, the patient must be kept warm; not more than one-third of the body should be treated at one time.

When warm, wet compresses are prescribed, the area must be observed carefully to avoid burning the skin. If a closed dressing is used, it may be covered with sterile towels to hold the dressing in place and further protected with a plastic film. In this way, the temperature can be maintained for a longer period.

Dressing materials are discarded after use according to agency policy. Usually, the acute stage of dermatitis subsides within 48 to 72 hours of treatment. Wet compresses continued beyond this point can lead to dry skin.

Occlusive Dressings

Occlusive dressings may be commercially produced or made, less expensively, from sterile or nonsterile gauze squares or wrap. Occlusive dressings cover topical medication that is applied to the dermatoses (abnormal skin lesions). The area is kept airtight by using plastic film (such as plastic wrap). Plastic film is thin and readily adapts to all sizes, body shapes, and skin surfaces. Plastic surgical tape containing a corticosteroid in the adhesive layer can be cut to size and applied to individual lesions. Generally, plastic wrap should be used no more than 12 hours a day.

Home Care. To apply the dressing at home, the patient receives the following instructions: (1) wash the area, then pat dry; (2) rub medication into the lesion while the skin is moist; (3) cover with plastic (*e.g.*, plastic wrap, vinyl gloves, plastic bags); and (4) cover with an elastic bandage, dressing, or paper tape to seal the edges. Dressings should be removed for 12 of every 24 hours to prevent skin thinning (atrophy), **striae** (bandlike streaks), **telangiectasia** (small, red lesions caused by dilation of blood vessels), and maceration.

Other forms of dressings used to cover topical medications include soft cotton cloth and stretchable cotton dressings (Surgitube, Tubergauze), which can be used for fingers, toes, hands, and feet. The hands can be covered with disposable polyethylene or vinyl gloves sealed at the wrists; the feet can be wrapped in plastic bags covered by cotton socks. When large areas of the body must be covered, cotton cloth topped by expandable stockinette can be used. Disposable diapers or cloths folded diaper-fashion are useful for dressing the groin and the perineal areas. Axillary dressings can be made of cotton cloth or a commercially prepared dressing may be used and taped in place or held by dress shields. A turban or plastic shower cap is useful for holding dressings on the scalp. A face mask, made from gauze with holes cut out for the eyes, nose, and mouth, may be held in place with gauze ties looped through holes cut in the four corners of the mask.

Therapeutic Baths (Balneotherapy)

Baths or soaks, known as **balneotherapy,** are useful when large areas are involved to remove crusts, scales, and old medications and to relieve the inflammation and itching that accompany acute dermatoses. The water temperature should be comfortable, and the bath should not exceed 20 to 30 minutes because of the tendency of baths and soaks to produce skin maceration. For the different types of therapeutic baths and their uses, see Table 54-1.

Pharmacotherapy

Topical Medications

Because skin is easily accessible and, therefore, easy to treat, topical medications can often be used. High concentrations of some medications can be applied directly to the affected site with little systemic absorption and, therefore, few systemic side effects. However, some medications are readily absorbed through the skin and can produce systemic effects. Because topical preparations may induce allergic contact dermatitis in sensitive persons, any untoward response should be reported immediately and the medication discontinued.

Medicated lotions, creams, ointments, and powders are frequently used to treat skin lesions. In general, wet dressings, with or without medication, are used in the acute stage; lotions and creams are reserved for the subacute stage; and ointments are used when inflammation has become chronic and the skin is dry with scaling and **lichenification** (leathery thickening).

Lotions are of two types: **suspensions,** consisting of a powder in water that requires shaking before application,

TABLE 54-1 Types of Therapeutic Baths

Bath Solution and Medication	Uses	Nursing Interventions
Water	Same effects as wet dressings	• Fill the tub half full. • Keep the water at a comfortable temperature. • Do not allow the water to cool excessively. • Use a bath mat—*medications may cause tub to be slippery.* • Apply a lubricating agent to wet skin after bath if emollient action is desired—increases hydration. Because tars are volatile, the bath area should be well ventilated. • Dry by blotting with a towel. • Keep room warm to minimize temperature fluctuations. • Encourage patient to wear light, loose clothing after the bath.
Saline	Used for widely disseminated lesions	
Colloidal (Aveeno, oatmeal)	Antipruritic; soothing	
Sodium bicarbonate	Cooling	
Starch	Soothing	
Medicated tars (Alma-Tar, Balnetar)	Psoriasis and chronic eczematous conditions.	
Bath oils (Alpha-Keri, Lubath, Domol)	Antipruritic and emollient actions; acute and subacute eczematous eruptions	

and **clear solutions,** containing completely dissolved active ingredients. Lotions are usually applied directly to the skin but a dressing soaked in the lotion can be placed on the affected area. A suspension such as **calamine** provides a rapid cooling and drying effect as it evaporates, leaving a thin medicinal layer of powder on the affected skin. Lotions are frequently used to replenish lost skin oils or to relieve pruritus. Lotions must be applied every 3 or 4 hours for sustained therapeutic effect. If left in place for a longer period of time they may crust and cake on the skin. **Linaments,** lotions with oil added, prevent crusting and may be used for this purpose (MacKie, 1991). Because lotions are easy to use, compliance is generally high.

Powders usually have a talc, zinc oxide, bentonite, or cornstarch base and are dusted on the skin with a shaker or with cotton sponges. Although their medical action is brief, powders act as hygroscopic agents, which absorb and retain moisture and reduce friction between skin surfaces and the bedding.

Creams may be suspensions of oil in water or emulsions of water in oil with ingredients to prevent bacterial and fungal growth (MacKie, 1991). Both may cause an allergic reaction such as contact dermatitis. Oil-in-water creams are easily applied and usually are the most cosmetically acceptable to the patient. Although they can be used on the face, they tend to have a drying effect. Water-in-oil emulsions are greasier and are preferred for drying and flaking dermatoses. Creams are generally rubbed into the skin by hand. They are used for their moisturizing and emollient effects.

Gels are semisolid emulsions that become liquid when applied to the skin or scalp. They are cosmetically acceptable to the patient because they are not visible after application, and they are greaseless and nonstaining. Most topical steroids are prescribed in gel form because the gel appears to penetrate more effectively than other skin preparations.

Pastes are mixtures of powders and ointments and are used in inflammatory conditions. They adhere to the skin, but may be difficult to remove without using an oil, such as olive oil or mineral oil.

Ointments retard water loss and lubricate and protect the skin, and are preferred for chronic or localized skin conditions. Both pastes and ointments are applied with a wooden tongue depressor or by hand, with gloves.

Spray and **aerosol** preparations may be used on extensive lesions. These evaporate on contact and are used infrequently.

With all types of topical medication, the patient is taught to apply the medication gently but thoroughly and, when necessary, to cover these medications with a dressing to protect clothing. Table 54-2 lists some commonly used topical preparations.

TABLE 54-2 Common Topical Preparations and Medications

Bath preparations	Alpha-Keri bath oil
	Neutrogena bath oil
	Aveeno oatmeal bath powder
	Oilated Aveeno bath powder
	Balnetar
	Lubath
Creams	Aquacare
	Acid Mantle Creme
	Curel
	Eucerin
	Moisturel
	Nutraderm
Lotions	Alpha-Keri lotion
	Dermassage
	Lubriderm
Ointments	Aquaphor
	Hydrophilic petrolatum
	Vaseline Petroleum Jelly
	White or yellow petrolatum
Topical anesthetics	Xylocaine (lidocaine) of various strengths in the form of sprays, ointments, lotions
Topical antibiotics	Bacitracin ointment
	Bacitracin and polymyxin B ointment (Polysporin)
	1% Clindamycin phosphate (Cleocin T)
	2% Erythromycin solution (Eryderm, Erymax, T-Stat)
	1% Gentamicin sulfate cream or ointment (Garamycin)
	2% Mupirocin
	1% Silver sulfadiazine cream (Silvadene)

Corticosteroids are widely used in treating dermatologic conditions to provide anti-inflammatory, antipruritic and vasoconstrictive effects (Litt, 1993). The patient is taught to apply this medication according to strict guidelines, using it sparingly, yet rubbing it into the prescribed area thoroughly. Absorption of topical corticosteroid is enhanced when the skin is hydrated or the affected area is covered by an occlusive or moisture-retentive dressing. Inappropriate use of topical corticosteroids can result in both local and systemic side effects, especially when the medication is absorbed through inflamed and excoriated skin, under occlusive dressings, or when used for long periods on sensitive areas (Litt, 1993; MacKie, 1991). Local side effects may include skin atrophy and thinning, **striae** (bandlike streaks), and **telangiectases** (small, red lesions caused by dilation of blood vessels). Thinning of the skin results from the ability of corticosteroids to inhibit skin collagen synthesis (Litt, 1993). The thinning process can be reversed by discontinuing the medication, but striae and telangiectasia are permanent (MacKie, 1991). Systemic side effects may include hyperglycemia and symptoms of Cushing's syndrome (Litt, 1993). Caution is required when applying corticosteroid around the eyes because long-term use may cause such disorders as glaucoma or cataracts. In addition, the antiinflammatory effect of corticosteroid may mask existing viral or fungal infections.

Strong (fluorinated) corticosteroids are applied cautiously to the face, because they may produce acne-like dermatitis, known as **perioral dermatitis,** steroid-induced

rosacea (characterized by lesions around the nose and cheeks), and **hypertrichosis** (excessive hair growth). Table 54-3 lists topical corticosteroid preparations according to potency. Because some topical corticosteroid preparations are available without prescription, patient instruction about prolonged and inappropriate use is essential.

Intralesional Therapy

Intralesional therapy consists of injecting a sterile suspension of medication (usually a corticosteroid) into or just below a lesion. Although this treatment may have an anti-inflammatory effect, local atrophy may result if the medication is injected into subcutaneous fat. Skin lesions treated with intralesional therapy include psoriasis, keloids, and cystic acne. Occasionally, immunotherapeutic and antifungal agents are administered by intralesional therapy.

TABLE 54-3 Potency of Common Topical Corticosteroid Preparations

Potency	Topical Corticosteroid Preparation
Lowest	0.1% Dexamethasone (Decaderm)
	0.25–2.5% Hydrocortisone (Hytone, Nutraderm, Penecort, Synacort, Cortef)
	0.25 or 1.0% Methylprednisolone acetate (Medrol)
Low	0.01% Betamethasone valerate (Valisone)
	0.1% Clocortolone (Cloderm)
	0.05% Desonide (Tridesilon)
	0.01% Fluocinolone acetonide (Synalar)
	0.025% Flurandrenolide (Cordran)
	0.2% Hydrocortisone valerate (Westcort)
	0.025% Triamcinolone acetonide (Aristocort, Kenalog)
Intermediate	0.025% Betamethasone benzoate (Benisone, Uticort)
	0.1% Betamethasone valerate (Valisone)
	0.05% Desoximetasone (Topicort)
	0.025% Fluocinolone acetonide (Fluonid)
	0.05% Flurandrenolide (Cordran)
	0.025% Halacinonide (Halog)
	0.1% Triamcinolone acetonide (Aristocort, Kenalog)
High	0.1% Amcinonide (Cyclocort)
	0.05% Betamethasone dipropionate (Diprosone)
	0.25% Desoximetasone (Topicort)
	0.2% Fluocinolone (Synalar)
	0.05% Fluocinonide (Lidex)
	0.1% Halcinonide (Halog)
	0.5% Triamcinolone acetonide (Aristocort, Kenalog)
	0.05% Diflorasone diacetate (Florone, Maxiflor)
Highest	0.05% Betamethasone dipropionate (Diprolene)
	0.05% Clobetasol propionate (Temovate)

(Patterson JAK. Aging and Clinical Practice Skin Disorders: Diagnosis and Treatment. New York, Igaku-Shoin Medical Publishers.)

Systemic Medications

Systemic medications are also prescribed for skin conditions. These include the corticosteroids for short-term therapy for contact dermatitis or for long-term treatment of a chronic dermatosis, such as pemphigus vulgaris. Other frequently used systemic medications include antibiotics, antifungals, antihistamines, sedatives and tranquilizers, analgesics, and cytotoxic agents.

❑ NURSING PROCESS
The Patient With an Abnormal Skin Condition

Assessment

The skin is the most visible organ of the body. When a dermatologic condition arises, it is difficult for the patient to ignore it or to conceal it from others. A disease of the skin may arise as a distinct entity unto itself or be the outward manifestation of an unrelated systemic disease.

The health history and direct observation provide information about the patient's perception of the dermatosis, how it began, what may have precipitated the condition, what relieves the symptoms, and other physical or emotional problems the patient is experiencing. A complete physical examination should be performed. (See Chapter 53 to review the assessment of the integumentary system.)

Diagnosis

Nursing Diagnoses

Based on the assessment data, major nursing diagnoses may include:

- ❑ Risk for impaired skin integrity related to changes in the barrier function of the skin
- ❑ Pain and itching related to skin lesions
- ❑ Sleep pattern disturbance related to pruritis
- ❑ Body image disturbance related to unsightly appearance of the skin
- ❑ Knowledge deficit about the treatment regimen

Collaborative Problems/ PotentialComplications

Based on the assessment data, a potential complication may include the following:

- ❑ Infection

Planning and Implementation

Goals. The major goals of the patient may include maintenance of skin integrity, relief of discomfort, achieving restful sleep, development of self-acceptance, acquiring knowledge of skin care, and absence of complications.

Nursing Interventions

Maintaining Skin Integrity. Many persons have dry and sensitive skin that is easily irritated. This is especially true of elderly patients. Too much or too vigorous washing and scrubbing can increase the problem. Soaps are also irritating. Persons with sensitive skin should bathe or be bathed with tepid water with minimal soap, taking care to rinse well and dry by gently patting the skin with a towel. An emollient can be applied to damp skin to trap moisture. Dry air is irritating because it reduces skin moisture; therefore, keeping the environment humidified is also helpful.

Skin problems of the hands are a common complaint. The skin of the back of the hand is thin, accounting for its sensitivity and dryness and its poor tolerance of soaps and detergents. Persons with this problem should protect the hands from contact with soaps, solvents, detergents, and other chemicals by wearing cotton-lined, heavy-duty vinyl gloves when handling these agents. Persons with irritations of the hands can be advised to wear white cotton gloves (cosmetic gloves) for dry housework and to minimize contact with water.

In patients with diagnosed skin conditions, the skin should be protected from maceration (excessive hydration of the stratum corneum) when applying wet dressings. Thermal injuries must be prevented as well.

The patient with a compromised immune system is at increased risk for cutaneous infection. Nursing Care Plan 54-1 summarizes nursing interventions for persons with skin problems related to trauma and infection.

Relieving Discomfort. A rash that seems trivial to the observer may be causing extreme discomfort to the patient. Cystic lesions, for example, may be tender and painful. Many skin disorders produce itching, making the patient irritable and unable to sleep. Pruritus is a significant symptom that scratching does not relieve. The patient is advised to keep cool, especially at night, and to avoid taking hot baths and wearing woolen clothing. If itching persists, the patient is advised to see the physician, who may prescribe a topical agent.

In providing care for a patient with itching skin lesions, the nurse attempts to discover the cause of discomfort. A *sudden* onset of generalized rash may indicate a medication allergy. Other causes are discussed in the section below on pruritus.

Nursing interventions appropriate for relieving itching include humidifying the environment with a room humidifier, maintaining a cool temperature, removing excess bedding and clothing, and limiting soaps to those made for sensitive skin. The nails are trimmed to decrease skin damage from scratching. Every effort should be made to keep the skin hydrated and moistened to avoid skin breakdown. The patient is advised to avoid using over-the-counter preparations to relieve itching because the skin problem may be increased by irritation or sensitization from self-medication.

Gradual evaporation of water from dressings cools the skin and relieves pruritus. The nurse reinforces this teaching, and makes sure that the patient understands that normal skin should be protected during the application of wet dressings. The patient is taught to moisten an adherent dressing before removal to relieve discomfort. When taking therapeutic baths (a form of wet dressing), the patient is advised to limit bathing time to 20 to 30 minutes to prevent skin maceration. Generally, therapeutic baths may be taken twice daily.

Achieving Restful Sleep. Irritation and itching interfere with normal sleep. The following measures to promote sleep are discussed with the patient:

- Keep a regular schedule for sleeping; go to bed at the same time and get up at the same time.
- Avoid caffeinated beverages late in the evening.
- Use a bedtime routine or ritual to ease the transition from wakefulness to sleep.
- Exercise regularly.

In addition, the bedroom should be well ventilated and humidified. Other measures to promote skin comfort and aid relaxation are found in Nursing Care Plan 54-1.

Increasing Self-Acceptance. Physical appearance exerts profound influence in society and in the way people are treated. Preferential treatment is often bestowed on someone who is perceived as being attractive. Clean and healthy skin is intimately correlated with "attractiveness" and, thereby, one's self-esteem.

Skin diseases can cause emotional suffering and can affect social and business relationships and recreational activities. For example, persons with eczema often have difficulty convincing others that their disease is not contagious. Those with flaking and scaling conditions may be wary of meeting new people. Comments from strangers may be difficult to deal with. Diminishing self-confidence, excessive fixation on skin defects, and worry about scarring are frequently found in persons with acne. All of these factors can generate negative emotions in the patient.

The nurse understands that body image is a complex psychologic concept that is related to the mental concept of self and self-esteem. Allowing patients to express their feelings freely gives them a sense of support and acceptance. Mutual trust and respect between patient and nurse are necessary to promote communication.

Understanding Skin Care. Informed patients are usually less anxious and more cooperative. Thus, teaching them about their condition and its treatment may make them more hopeful, which may reinforce their ability to use their resources effectively.

Self-care, particularly hair and skin care, can make a difference in the way others perceive the patient. Appropriate cosmetics can bring substantial benefits to a person with a chronic skin condition or disfigurement. A referral to an expert cosmetologist to camouflage birthmarks, mottled skin, scars, and chronic dermatitis can be advantageous. Persons who remain depressed over their condition may benefit from psychologic counseling.

Patient Education and Home Care Considerations. Healthy skin reflects one's general health. Principles of good nutrition, exercise, rest, and sleep are emphasized in any teaching program focused on skin care. In addition, preprinted materials are available. They describe common dermatologic conditions ranging from acne and warts to postoperative measures including care of an open wound, suture care, or applying soaks or topical medications (Epstein, 1991).

(text continues on page 1502)

NURSING CARE PLAN 54–1
Care of Patients With Dermatoses (Abnormal Skin Conditions)

NURSING DIAGNOSIS: Impaired skin integrity related to changes in the barrier function of the skin

GOAL: Maintenance of skin integrity

Nursing Interventions	Rationale	Expected Outcomes
1. Protect healthy skin from maceration (excessive hydration of stratum corneum) when applying wet dressings.	1. Maceration of healthy skin can cause skin breakdown and extension of the primary condition.	• Maintains skin integrity. • Absence of maceration. • No signs of thermal injury. • Absence of infection. • Applies prescribed topical medication. • Takes prescribed medication on schedule.
2. Remove moisture from skin by blotting gently and avoiding friction.	2. Friction and maceration play a major role in some skin diseases.	
3. Guard carefully against risks of thermal injuries from excessively hot wet dressings and from subtle heat injuries (heating pads, radiators).	3. Patients with dermatoses may have decreased sensitivity to heat.	
4. Advise patient to use sunscreening agents.	4. Many cosmetic problems and virtually all cutaneous malignancies can be attributed to chronic skin damage.	

NURSING DIAGNOSIS: Pain and itching related to skin lesions

GOAL: Relief of discomfort

Nursing Interventions	Rationale	Expected Outcomes
1. Examine area of involvement.	1. Understanding the extent and characteristics of the skin involved helps in planning interventions.	• Achieves relief of discomfort. • Verbalizes that itching has been relieved. • Demonstrates absence of skin excoriation from scratching. • Complies with prescribed treatment. • Keeps skin hydrated and lubricated. • Demonstrates intact skin; skin regaining healthy appearance.
a. Attempt to discover cause of discomfort.	a. Helps to identify appropriate comfort measures.	
b. Record observations in detail, using descriptive terminology.	b. An accurate description of a cutaneous eruption is necessary for diagnosis and treatment. Many skin conditions appear similar but have different etiologies. Cutaneous inflammatory response may be muted in elderly patients.	
c. Anticipate possible allergic reaction; obtain a medication history.	c. A generalized rash, particularly of sudden onset, may indicate a medication allergy.	
2. Control environmental and physical factors.	2. Itching is aggravated by heat, chemicals, and physical irritants.	
a. Keep humidity about 60%; use a humidifier.	a. At low humidity, the skin loses water.	
b. Maintain a cool environment.	b. Coolness deters itching.	
c. Use mild soap (Dove) or soap made for sensitive skin (Neutrogena, Aveeno).	c. These contain no detergents, dyes, or hardening agents.	
d. Remove excess clothing or bedding.	d. Promotes cool environment.	
e. Wash bed linens and clothing with mild soap.	e. Strong soaps can cause skin irritation.	
f. Stop repeated exposures to detergents, cleansers, and solvents.	f. Any substance that removes water, lipids, or protein from the epidermis alters the barrier function of the skin.	

(continued)

NURSING CARE PLAN 54–1 *(continued)*
Care of Patients With Dermatoses (Abnormal Skin Conditions)

Nursing Interventions	Rationale	Expected Outcomes
3. Use skin-care measures to maintain skin integrity and promote comfort.	3. The skin is an important barrier that must be maintained intact in order to function properly.	
a. Provide tepid cooling baths or cool dressings for itching.	a. Gradual evaporation of water from dressings cools the skin and relieves pruritus.	
b. Treat dryness (xerosis) as prescribed.	b. Dry skin can produce areas of dermatitis with redness, itching, scaling, and, in more severe forms, swelling, blistering, cracking, and weeping.	
c. Apply skin lotion or cream immediately after bathing.	c. Effective hydration of the stratum corneum prevents compromise of the barrier layer of the skin.	
d. Keep nails trimmed.	d. Trimming decreases skin damage from scratching.	
e. Apply prescribed topical therapy.	e. This helps to relieve symptoms.	
f. Help the patient accept the prolonged treatment that some conditions require.	f. Effective coping measures usually promote comfort.	
g. Advise the patient to refrain from using salves or lotions that are commercially available.	g. The patient's problem may be caused by irritation or sensitization from self-medication.	

NURSING DIAGNOSIS: Sleep pattern disturbance related to pruritus

GOAL: Achievement of restful sleep

Nursing Interventions	Rationale	Expected Outcomes
1. Prevent and treat dry skin.	1. Nocturnal pruritus interferes with normal sleep.	• Achieves restful sleep. • Reports relief of itching. • Maintains appropriate environmental conditions. • Avoids caffeine in late afternoon and evening. • Identifies measures to promote sleep. • Experiences satisfactory rest/sleep pattern.
a. Advise patient to keep bedroom well ventilated and humidified.	a. Dry air will make skin feel itchy. A comfortable environment promotes relaxation.	
b. Keep skin moisturized.	b. This prevents water loss. Dry, itchy skin can usually be controlled but not cured.	
c. Bathe/shower only as absolutely necessary if skin is excessively dry. Use no soap or only mild soap. Apply skin lotion/cream immediately after bathing while skin is damp.	c. These measures preserve skin moisture.	
2. Advise patient of the following measures that may be helpful in promoting sleep:		
a. Keep a regular schedule for sleeping. Go to bed at the same time; get up at same time.	a. Regularity of sleep schedule is important in maintaining sleep.	
b. Avoid caffeinated drinks late in the evening.	b. Caffeine has peak effect 2–4 hours after being consumed.	
c. Exercise regularly.	c. Exercise appears to have beneficial sleep effect if performed in late afternoon.	
d. Use a bedtime routine or ritual.	d. This eases transition from wakefulness to sleep.	

(continued)

NURSING CARE PLAN 54–1 *(continued)*
Care of Patients With Dermatoses (Abnormal Skin Conditions)

NURSING DIAGNOSIS: Body image disturbance related to unsightly skin appearance

GOAL: Development of increasing self-acceptance

Nursing Interventions	Rationale	Expected Outcomes
1. Assess patient for disturbance of self-image (avoidance of eye contact, self-negating verbalizations, expression of disgust about skin condition).	1. Disturbance of body image may accompany any disease or condition that is apparent to the patient. An impression of one's own body has an effect on self-concept.	• Develops increasing acceptance of own body. • Follows through and participates in self-care measures. • Reports feeling in control of situation. • Gives self positive reinforcement. • Verbalizes a more healthful self-regard. • Appears less self-conscious; is not afraid to socialize and be seen by others. • Uses concealing and highlighting techniques to enhance appearance.
2. Identify psychosocial stage of development.	2. There is a relationship between development stage, self-image, and the patient's reaction to and understanding of skin condition.	
3. Provide opportunity for expression. Listen (in an open, nonjudgmental way) to expressions of grief/anxiety about changes in body image.	3. The patient needs the experience of being heard and understood.	
4. Assess the patient's concerns and fears. Assist anxious patient to develop insight and identify and cope with problems.	4. This gives health care personnel opportunity to neutralize undue anxiety and restore reality to the situation. Fear is an element destructive to adaptation.	
5. Support patient's efforts to improve body image (participation in skin treatments; grooming). 6. Help patient toward self-acceptance. 7. Encourage socialization with others. 8. Advise patient of available cosmetic measures to conceal disfiguring conditions.	5–8. A positive approach and suggestions of cosmetic techniques are often helpful in promoting self-acceptance and socialization.	

NURSING DIAGNOSIS: Knowledge deficit about skin care and methods of treating skin ailment

GOAL: Understanding of skin care

Nursing Interventions	Rationale	Expected Outcomes
1. Determine what the patient knows (understands and misunderstands) about the condition.	1. Provides baseline data for developing the teaching plan.	• Acquires understanding of skin care. • Follows treatment as prescribed and can verbalize rationale for measures taken. • Carries out prescribed baths, soaks, wet dressings. • Uses topical medication appropriately. • Understands importance of nutrition to skin health.
2. Keep the patient informed; correct misconceptions/misinformation.	2. Patients need to have a sense that there is something they can do. Most patients benefit from explanations and reassurance.	
3. Demonstrate application of prescribed therapy (wet compresses; topical medication).	3. Allows patient the opportunity to visualize the correct way to perform therapies.	
4. Advise the patient to keep skin moist and flexible with hydration and application of skin cream and lotion.	4. The stratum corneum needs water to stay flexible. Application of skin cream or lotion to damp skin prevents dry, rough, cracked, and scaly skin.	
5. Encourage the patient to attain a healthy nutritional status.	5. The appearance of the skin reflects a person's general health. Skin changes may be a feature of abnormal nutrition.	

(continued)

NURSING CARE PLAN 54-1 *(continued)*
Care of Patients With Dermatoses (Abnormal Skin Conditions)

Nursing Interventions	Rationale	Expected Outcomes
COLLABORATIVE PROBLEMS: Infection		
GOAL: Absence of complications		
1. Have a high index of suspicion for an infection in patients with compromised immune systems.	1. Any condition that compromises the immune status increases the risk of cutaneous infection.	• Remains free of infection. • Verbalizes skin care measures that promote cleanliness and prevent breakdown. • Identifies signs and symptoms of infection to report. • Identifies adverse effects of medications that should be reported to health care personnel. • Participates in skin care measures (*e.g.*, dressing changes, soaks).
2. Instruct the patient clearly and in detail about the therapeutic regimen.	2. Effective patient education is dependent on the interpersonal skills of the health professionals and on giving clear instructions reinforced through written instructions.	
3. Apply intermittent wet dressings as prescribed to reduce intensity of inflammation.	3. A wet dressing produces evaporative cooling, causing constriction of superficial cutaneous vessels and thereby decreasing erythema and serum production. Wet dressings help in debridement of vesicles and crusts and control inflammatory processes.	
4. Provide tub baths and soaks as prescribed.	4. Loosens exudates and scales.	
5. Administer prescribed antimicrobial agents.	5. Kills or prevents the growth of the infectious organism.	
6. Use topical medications containing corticosteroids as prescribed and as indicated. a. Observe lesion periodically for changes in response to therapy. b. Instruct the patient about possible adverse effects of long-term use of fluorinated topical corticosteroids.	6. Corticosteroids have an anti-inflammatory action, resulting in part from their ability to induce vasoconstriction of the small vessels in the upper dermis. Extensive prolonged use of topical corticosteroids can lead to antiproliferative effects on epidermal cells (loss of hair in area used).	
7. Advise patient to stop using any skin agent that makes the problem worse.	7. A contact dermatitis or allergic reaction may develop from any ingredient in the medication.	

A patient who is receiving treatment for a skin condition is usually informed by the physician what the skin condition is, its source or cause, and what to expect from treatment. Some patients hear or understand only part of what is being said. Many patients find it helpful to have a relative or friend present, not only for emotional support, but also to listen to treatment instructions which may be lengthy and complex. Printed information sheets are helpful to reinforce instructions. They can be taken home and referred to as needed, and they can answer questions about the condition or incidental queries about such things as skin cancer, sunscreens, or office hours, fees, billing policies, and emergency contact information (Baker, 1991). Information sheets can be individualized by writing specific or additional information directly on the sheet, for example how to apply a topical medication, the amount to apply, the size of the area to be treated, and the frequency of application.

Potential side effects may be identified and highlighted on the sheet to emphasize their importance. A major problem encountered in using printed information is the readability level. Information must be written at or near a fifth grade reading level so that most patients can understand and comply with the instructions. To ensure a general reading level, information should be presented in short sentences, using familiar or common words and large type. Only essential information should be included, without unnecessary detail. This is especially important for elderly patients or those with visual deficits (Baker, 1991).

Monitoring and Managing Complications: Infection. Potentially infectious skin lesions should be treated with proper precautions until the diagnosis is established and the infecting organism identified. Keeping the affected area clean and administering medications as prescribed are primary defenses against infection, as is adequate nutrition. The patient should be instructed how to perform daily skin care (including dressing changes, if appropriate) and how to recognize and report general signs and symptoms of infection, such as redness, swelling, pain, pus, and fever.

Evaluation

Expected Outcomes

1. Maintains skin integrity
   a. Indicates absence of skin cracking
   b. Protects skin from contact with irritating substances
   c. Applies emollient to skin as prescribed
2. Achieves relief of discomfort
   a. Uses topical medication and treatments as prescribed
   b. Reports relief of itching
3. Achieves more restful sleep
   a. States is "sleeping better"
   b. Reports an increased feeling of well-being
4. Demonstrates increasing self-acceptance
   a. Voices fewer self-deprecating remarks
   b. Pays attention to appearance
5. Acquires understanding of skin care
   a. Verbalizes rationale of prescribed treatment
   b. Demonstrates ability to perform treatments

Pruritus

Pruritus (itching) is one of the most common complaints in dermatologic disorders, causing alterations in comfort and leading to changes in the integrity of the skin if the patient responds by scratching. Itch receptors are unmyelinated, penicillate (brushlike) nerve endings that are found exclusively in the skin, mucous membranes, and cornea (Sher, 1992). Scratching causes the inflamed cells and nerve endings to release histamine, which produces more pruritus and in turn a vicious itch-scratch cycle. Although pruritus usually is due to primary skin disease with resultant rash or lesions, it may occur without any skin manifestations. This is referred to as **essential pruritus** which generally has a rapid onset, may be severe, and interferes with the person's normal daily activities.

Pruritus may be the first indication of systemic internal disease such as diabetes mellitus, blood disorders, or cancer. Itching may also accompany renal, hepatic, and thyroid diseases. Chart 54-1 lists some of the systemic disorders associated with generalized pruritus. Some common oral medications such as aspirin, antibiotic therapy, hormones (estrogens, testosterone, or oral contraceptives), and opioids (morphine or cocaine) may cause pruritus as well (Sher, 1992). Certain soaps and chemicals, treatment with radiation therapy, prickly heat (miliaria), and contact with woolen garments are also associated with pruritus. Pruritus may occur in elderly persons as a result of dry skin. Itching may also be caused by psychologic factors such as excessive stress in family or work situations. The person with pruritus may or may not have a rash.

Pruritus typically leads to scratching, which usually is more severe at night. Pruritus is reported less frequently during waking hours, probably because the person is distracted by daily activities. At nighttime when there are few distractions, the slightest pruritus cannot be easily ignored. The secondary effects include excoriations, redness, raised areas on the skin (wheals), infections, and changes in pigmentation. Severe itching is debilitating.

CHART 54-1
Systemic Disorders Associated With Generalized Pruritus

Renal
- Chronic renal disease

Obstructive biliary disease
- Primary biliary cirrhosis
- Extrahepatic biliary obstruction
- Intrahepatic cholestasis of pregnancy
- Drug-induced cholestasis

Endocrine
- Thyrotoxicosis
- Hypothyroidism
- Diabetes mellitus
- Carciniod syndrome

Hematopoietic
- Iron deficiency anemia
- Polycthemia vera

Psychiatric Disorders
- Emotional stress

Myeloproliferative Disorders
- Hodgkin's disease
- Lymphoma
- Leukemia
- Multiple myeloma
- Mycosis fungoides

Visceral Malignancies
- Breast carcinoma
- Gastric carcinoma
- Lung carcinoma

Neurologic Disorders
- Multiple sclerosis
- Brain abscess
- Brain tumor

Infestations
- Scabies
- Trichinosis
- Pediculosis corporis
- Onchocerciasis

Miscellaneous
- Xerosis

Sher, TH. Clinical Evaluation of Generalized Pruritus. Comprehensive Therapy 1992; 18(9): 15, with permission.

Management

A thorough history and physical examination will usually provide clues to the underlying cause of the pruritus (hay fever, allergy, recent ingestion of a new medication, change of cosmetics). Once the cause has been identified and removed, treatment of the condition should relieve the pruritus. Signs of infection and environmental clues, such as warm, dry air or irritating bed linens, should be identified. In general, washing with soap and hot water is avoided, although a warm bath with a mild soap followed by applying a bland emollient to moist skin can control **xerosis** (dry skin). Applying a cold compress, ice cube, or cool agents that contain soothing menthol and camphor that constrict blood vessels may also help. If pruritus continues, further investigation of a systemic problem is advised.

Bath oils (Lubath, Alpha-Keri) containing a surfactant that makes the oil mix with bath water may be sufficient for cleaning. However, an elderly patient or a patient with unsteady balance should avoid adding oil as it increases the danger of slipping in the bathtub.

Topical corticosteroids may be beneficial as anti-inflammatory agents to decrease itching. Oral antihistamines are even more effective because they can overcome the effects of histamine release from damaged mast cells. An antihistamine, such as **diphenhydramine** (Benadryl), prescribed in a sedating dose at bedtime is effective in producing a restful and comfortable sleep. Nonsedating antihistamine medications such as terfenadine (Seldane) should be used to relieve daytime pruritus. Tricyclic antidepressants, such as **doxepin** (Sinequan), may be prescribed for pruritus of neuropsychogenic origin.

Nursing Interventions. The nurse reinforces the reasons for the prescribed therapeutic regimen and counsels the patient on specific points of care. If baths have been prescribed, the patient is reminded to use tepid (not hot) water and to shake off the excess water and blot between intertriginous (body fold) areas with a towel. Rubbing vigorously with the towel is avoided because this overstimulates the skin and causes more itching. It also removes water from the stratum corneum. Immediately after bathing, the skin should be lubricated with an emollient that traps moisture.

The patient is instructed to avoid situations that cause vasodilation (expansion of the blood vessels). Examples include exposure to an overly warm environment and ingestion of alcohol and hot foods and liquids. All will induce or intensify itching (Sher, 1992). Using a humidifier is helpful if ambient environmental air is dry and provokes pruritus. Activities that result in perspiration should be limited; body sweat may be irritating and promote general itching. If the patient is troubled at nighttime with itching that interferes with sleep, the nurse can advise wearing cotton clothing next to the skin rather than synthetic materials. The room should be kept cool and humidified. Vigorous scratching is to be avoided and nails kept trimmed to prevent skin damage and infection. When the underlying cause of pruritus is not known and further testing is required, the nurse explains each test and the expected outcome.

Perianal Itching

Pruritus of the anal and genital regions may be caused by small particles of fecal material lodged in the perianal crevices or attached to anal hairs, or by perianal skin damage caused by scratching, moisture, and decreased skin resistance as a result of corticosteroid or antibiotic therapy. Other possible causes of perianal itching include local irritants such as scabies and lice, local lesions such as hemorrhoids, fungal or yeast infections, and pinworm infestation. Conditions such as diabetes mellitus, anemias, hyperthyroidism, and pregnancy may also result in perianal pruritus.

Patient Education and Home Care Considerations. The patient is instructed to follow proper hygienic measures and to discontinue home and over-the-counter remedies. The perianal area should be rinsed with lukewarm water and the area blotted dry with cotton balls. Premoistened tissues may be used after defecation.

As part of health teaching, the patient is instructed to avoid bathing in water that is too hot and to avoid using bubble baths, sodium bicarbonate, or detergent soaps, all of which aggravate dryness. To keep the perianal skin as dry as possible, patients should avoid wearing underwear made of synthetic fabrics. Local anesthetic agents should not be used because of possible allergenic effects. The patient should also avoid vasodilating agents or stimulants (alcohol, coffee) and mechanical irritants such as rough or woolen clothing.

Secretory Disorders

The main secretory function of the skin is performed by the sweat glands, which help to regulate body temperature. These glands excrete a fluid, perspiration, which evaporates, thereby cooling the body. The sweat glands are located in various parts of the body and respond to different stimuli. Those on the trunk generally respond to thermal stimulation; those on the palms and soles respond to nervous stimulation; and those in the axillae and on the forehead respond to both kinds of stimulation.

As a rule, moist skin is warm, and dry skin is likely to be cool. However, this is not a hard and fast rule. It is not unusual to observe cold sweats; warm, dry skin in a dehydrated patient; and very hot, dry skin peculiar to some febrile states.

Seborrheic Dermatoses

Seborrhea is excessive production of sebum (secretion of sebaceous glands) in those areas where glands are normally found in large numbers (face, scalp, eyebrows, eyelids, at the sides of the nose and upper lip, malar [cheek] regions, ears, axillae, under the breasts, groin, and gluteal crease of the buttocks). **Seborrheic dermatitis** is a chronic inflammatory disease of the skin with a predilection for areas that are well supplied with sebaceous glands or lie between skin folds, where the bacterial count is high.

Clinical Manifestations

Two forms of seborrheic dermatoses can occur: an oily form and a dry form. Either form may start in childhood with fine scaling of the scalp or other areas and may continue throughout life. The oily form appears moist or greasy. There may be patches of sallow, greasy skin, with or without scaling, and slight erythema (redness), predominantly on the forehead, nasolabial fold, beard area, and scalp, and between adjacent skin surfaces in the regions of the axillae, groin, and breasts. Small pustules or papulopustules resembling acne may appear on the trunk. The dry form, consisting of flaky desquamation of the scalp with a profuse amount of fine, powdery scales, is commonly called **dandruff.**

The mild forms of the disease are asymptomatic. When scaling occurs, it is often accompanied by pruritis, which may lead to scratching and secondary complications, such as infection and excoriation.

Seborrheic dermatitis has a genetic predisposition, and hormones, nutritional status, infection, and emotional stress influence its course. The remissions and exacerbations of this condition should be explained to the patient.

Management

Because there is no known cure for seborrhea, the objective of therapy is to control the disorder and allow the skin to repair itself. Seborrheic dermatitis of the body and face may respond to a topically applied corticosteroid cream, which allays the secondary inflammatory response. However, this medication should be used with caution near the eyelids, because it can induce glaucoma and cataracts in predisposed persons. Patients with seborrheic dermatitis may develop a secondary *Candida* (yeast) infection in body creases or folds. To avoid this, patients should be advised to ensure maximum aeration of the skin and to clean carefully areas where there are creases or folds in the skin. Patients with persistent candidiasis should be evaluated for diabetes.

The mainstay of dandruff treatment is proper shampooing, which should be done frequently (daily or at least three times weekly) with medicated shampoos. Two or three different types of shampoo should be used in rotation to prevent the seborrhea from becoming resistant to a particular shampoo. The shampoo is left on at least 5 to 10 minutes. As the condition of the scalp improves, the treatment can be less intense. Antiseborrheic shampoos include those containing selenium sulfide suspension, zinc pyrithione shampoos, salicylic acid–sulfur shampoos, and tar shampoos that contain sulfur and salicylic acid.

Nursing Interventions

A person with seborrheic dermatitis is advised to remove external irritants and to avoid excess heat and perspiration; rubbing and scratching prolong the disorder. To avoid secondary infections, the patient should air the skin and keep skin folds clean and dry.

Instructions for using medicated shampoos are reinforced for those with dandruff that requires treatment.

The patient is cautioned that seborrheic dermatitis is a chronic problem that tends to wax and wane. The goal is to keep it under control. Patients need to be encouraged to adhere to the treatment program. Those who become discouraged and disheartened by the effect on body image should be treated with sensitivity and an awareness of their need to express their feelings.

Acne Vulgaris

Acne vulgaris is a common follicular disorder affecting susceptible pilosebaceous follicles (hair follicles) most commonly found on the face, neck, and upper trunk. It is characterized by closed comedones (whiteheads), open comedones (blackheads), papules, pustules, nodules, and cysts.

Acne is the most commonly encountered skin condition in adolescents and young adults between ages 12 and 35. Both sexes are affected equally, with the highest incidence between ages 14 and 17 for girls, and 16 and 19 for boys (Clark, 1993). It becomes more marked at puberty and during adolescence, perhaps because at this age certain endocrine glands that influence the secretions of the sebaceous glands are functioning at peak activity. Acne appears to stem from an interplay of genetic, hormonal, and bacterial factors. In most cases there is a family history of acne (Stawiski, 1992).

Pathogenesis

During childhood, the sebaceous glands are small and virtually nonfunctioning. These glands are under endocrine control, especially the androgens. During puberty, androgens stimulate the sebaceous glands, causing them to enlarge and to secrete a natural oil, **sebum,** which rises to the top of the hair follicle and flows out onto the skin surface. In adolescents who develop acne, androgenic stimulation produces a heightened response in the sebaceous glands so that acne occurs when the pilosebaceous ducts become plugged with an accumulation of sebum. This accumulated material forms comedones.

Clinical Manifestations

The initial lesions of acne are comedones. **Closed comedones (whiteheads)** are obstructive lesions formed from impacted lipids or oils and keratin that plug the dilated follicle. Whiteheads are small, whitish papules with minute follicular openings that generally cannot be seen. These closed comedones may evolve into **open comedones,** in which the contents of the ducts are in open communication with the external environment. Open comedones are termed **blackheads.** The color of the blackhead results not from dirt but from an accumulation of lipid, bacterial, and epithelial debris.

Although the exact cause is not known, some closed comedones may rupture and result in an inflammatory reaction caused by leakage of follicular contents (sebum, keratin, bacteria) into the dermis. This inflammatory response may result from the action of certain skin bacteria, such as *Propionibacterium acnes,* that live in the hair follicles and break down the triglycerides of the sebum into free fatty acids and glycerine. The resultant inflammation is seen clinically as erythematous papules, inflammatory pustules, and inflammatory cysts. Mild papules and cysts drain and heal on their own without treatment. Deeper papules and cysts may result in scarring of the skin (Stawiski, 1992). Acne is numerically graded. A person with grade I acne has fewer than 10 comedones, papules, or pustules on one side of the face; a person with grade II, 10 to 20 comedones, papules, or pustules; grade III, 25 to 50; and grade IV, more than 50 (Stawiski, 1992).

Diagnostic Evaluation

The diagnosis of acne is based on the individual's history and physical examination, evidence of lesions characteristic of acne, and age. Acne does not occur until puberty. The presence of the typical comedones (whiteheads and blackheads), along with excessively oily skin is characteristic. Oiliness is more prominent in the midfacial area, while other parts of the face may appear dry. When there are numerous lesions, some of which are open, the person may exude a distinct sebaceous odor. Females may report a history of flare-ups a few days before menses. Biopsy of lesions is seldom necessary for a definitive diagnosis.

Management

The goals of management are to reduce bacterial colonies, decrease sebaceous gland activity, prevent the follicles from becoming plugged, reduce inflammation, combat secondary infection, minimize scarring, and eliminate factors that predispose the person to acne. The therapeutic regimen depends on the type of lesion (comedonal, papular, pustular, cystic).

There is no predictable cure for the disease, but combinations of therapies are available that can control its activity effectively. Topical treatment may be all that is needed to treat mild to moderate lesions as well as superficial inflammatory lesions (papular or pustular).

Dietary Therapy. Although food restrictions have been recommended from time to time in treating acne, diet does not play a major role in therapy. The elimination of a specific food or food product associated with a flare-up of acne, such as chocolate, cola, fried food, or milk products, should be promoted.

Skin Hygiene. In mild cases of acne, washing at least two times daily with a cleansing soap, such as Lava, Dial, or Neutrogena, may be all that is required. These soaps can remove the excessive skin oil and the comedone in most cases. Another effective method to dislodge comedones is with an abrasive sponge such as a Buf-Puf (Clark, 1993). Providing positive reassurance, listening attentively, and being sensitive to the feelings of the patient with acne are essential contributors to the patient's psychologic well-being and understanding of the disease and treatment plan.

Using oil-based cosmetics or creams is discouraged. Many over-the-counter commercial preparations claim to be effective in managing acne. However, their therapeutic effectiveness is questionable; in some cases, they may make acne worse. The patient should be encouraged to discontinue using these self-remedies and to adhere to the prescribed therapy. The duration of treatment will depend on the extent and severity of the acne. In severe cases, treatment may extend over months or even years.

Topical Pharmacotherapy

Benzoyl Peroxide. Benzoyl peroxide preparations are widely used because they produce a rapid and sustained reduction of inflammatory lesions. They depress sebum production and lead to the breakdown of the comedone plugs. They also produce an antibacterial effect by suppressing *Propionibacterium acnes.* Initially, benzoyl peroxide causes redness and scaling, but generally the skin adjusts quickly to its use. Usually the patient applies a gel of benzoyl peroxide once daily. In many instances this will be the only treatment needed. Benzoyl peroxide, benzoyl erythromycin, and benzoyl sulfur combinations are available over the counter and by prescription.

Vitamin A Acid. Topically applied vitamin A acid (tretinoin) is used to clear the keratin plugs from the pilosebaceous ducts. Vitamin A acid speeds up the cellular turnover, forces out the comedones, and prevents new comedones. Thus, it is effective in the treatment of comedonal acne.

The patient should be informed that symptoms may worsen during early weeks of therapy because inflammation may occur during the process. Erythema and peeling are also a frequent result. Improvement may take from 8 to 12 weeks. Some patients cannot tolerate this therapy. The patient is cautioned against sun exposure while using this topical medication because it may cause an exaggerated sunburn. Package insert directions are to be followed carefully.

Topical Antibiotics. Applying topical antibiotics in treating acne has become widespread. Topical antibiotics suppress the growth of *P. acnes;* reduce skin-surface free fatty acid levels; decrease comedones, papules, and pustules; and have no systemic side effects. Topical preparations containing tetracycline, clindamycin, erythromycin, or meclocycline are frequently used.

Systemic Therapy

Systemic Antibiotics. Oral antibiotics, such as tetracycline, administered in small doses over a long period are very effective in treating patients with moderate and severe acne, especially when the acne is inflammatory and results in pustules, abscesses, and scarring. Therapy may continue for months to years. The patient is advised to take tetracycline at least 1 hour before or 2 hours after meals, because the medication is poorly absorbed with food. Tetracycline is contraindicated in children under age 12 and in pregnant women. Although this medication is considered safe for long-term use in most cases, administration during pregnancy can affect the developing teeth, causing enamel hypoplasia and permanent discoloration of teeth in infants (Stawiski, 1992). Side effects of tetracyclines include photosensitivity, nausea, diarrhea, vaginitis in women, and cutaneous infection in either gender. (In some women, broad-spectrum antibiotics may suppress normal vaginal bacteria and predispose the patient to candidiasis, a fungal infection.)

Oral Retinoids. Synthetic vitamin A compounds **(retinoids)** are being used with dramatic results in patients with nodular cystic acne that is unresponsive to conventional therapy. One compound is **isotretinoin** (Accutane), which is also used for active inflammatory papular pustular acne that has a tendency to scar. Isotretinoin reduces sebaceous gland size and inhibits sebum production. It also causes the epidermis to shed **(epidermal desquamation),** thereby unseating and expelling existing comedones.

The most common side effect, experienced by almost all patients, is **cheilitis** (inflammation of the lips). Drying and chapping of the skin and mucous membranes are also frequently encountered. These changes are reversible with the withdrawal of the medication. Most important, isotretinoin is teratogenic in humans, meaning that it can have an adverse effect on a fetus, causing central nervous system and cardiovascular defects and structural abnormalities of the face. Therefore, contraceptive measures for women of childbearing age are obligatory during treatment and for about 4 to 8 weeks thereafter. Patients are also cautioned not to take vitamin A supplements while on this medication, to avoid additive toxic effects.

Hormone Therapy. Estrogen therapy (progesterone–estrogen preparations) has been found to suppress sebum production and reduce skin oiliness. It is usually reserved for young women when the acne begins somewhat later than usual and tends to flare at certain times in the menstrual cycle, which is often irregular. Estrogen in the form of estrogen-dominant oral contraceptive compounds may be administered on a prescribed cyclic regimen. Estrogen is not administered to males because of undesirable side effects. Table 54-4 summarizes current commonly prescribed treatment modalities for acne vulgaris.

Surgical Treatment

Surgical treatment of acne consists of comedo extraction, injections of corticosteroids into the inflamed lesions, and incision and drainage of large, fluctuant, nodular cystic lesions. **Cryosurgery** (freezing with liquid nitrogen) may be used for nodular and cystic forms of acne. Patients with deep scars may be treated with deep abrasive therapy **(dermabrasion),** in which the epidermis and some superficial dermis are removed down to the level of the scars.

Comedo Extraction. Comedones may be removed with a comedo extractor. The site is first cleaned with an alcohol sponge. The comedo is nicked with an 18-gauge needle or scalpel blade to incise the follicular opening, widen the port, and facilitate the removal of the comedo. The opening of the extractor is then placed over the lesion, and direct pressure is applied to cause extrusion of the plug through the expressor.

Removal of comedones will leave areas of erythema, which may take several weeks to subside. Recurrence of comedones after extraction is common because part of the comedo frequently remains in the pilosebaceous canal.

TABLE 54-4 Commonly Prescribed Treatments for Acne Vulgaris*

Kind of Therapy	Prescribed Treatment Agent
Topical	Benzoyl peroxide
	Benzoyl-erythromycin
	Benzoyl-sulfur
	Topical antibiotics:
	Clindamycin lotion and gel
	Erythromycin lotion, gel, and swabs
	Meclocycline cream
	Tetracycline lotion
	Resorcinol
	Salicylic acid
	Sulfur
	Tretinoin
	Various soaps, cleansers, and astringents
Systemic	Oral antibiotics:
	Tetracycline
	Erythromycin
	Minocycline
	Trimethoprim-sulfamethoxazole
	Accutane (isotretinoin)
	Hormones:
	Corticosteroids
	High dose for anti-inflammatory action
	Low dose to suppress androgen action
	Sex hormones (women only)
	Estrogen
	Antiandrogens
Surgical	Extraction of comedonal contents
	Drainage of pustules and cysts
	Excision of sinus tracts and cysts
	Intralesional corticosteroids
	Cryotherapy
	Dermabrasion for scars

*Treatments listed are commonly used but do not include all available forms of therapy.

❑ NURSING PROCESS
The Patient With Acne

Assessment

Almost all persons have an occasional blemish or lesion during adolescence. The nurse, through observation and listening, finds out how patients perceive their skin condition. One young person will view a small blemish as intolerable, while another teenager will regard more extensive involvement as "normal." Adolescents, who are in their formative years of development, are vulnerable and need to be approached with empathy and compassion as they attempt to deal with acne. The nurse keeps this in mind during assessment and other contacts with adolescents.

Teenage and young women in the childbearing years who are being treated for acne should be assessed regarding their sexual activity and contraceptive methods, especially if treatment involves using isotretinoin (Accutane), known to have teratogenic properties. Its use mandates using birth control measures for 2 months before therapy begins, during therapy, and for the 2 months after completing therapy.

A complete list of the cosmetics, creams, skin moisturizers, and over-the-counter acne preparations currently used by the patient should be obtained. In addition, it is helpful to assess the patient's perception of factors that seem to precipitate flare-ups of acne or make the lesions worse, for example foods and beverages; friction or pressure from clothing, such as shirt collars, football helmets, chin straps, or head bands; or trauma from trying to express a comedo manually.

The skin is stretched gently and the lesions are inspected during the physical assessment. Closed comedones (which are precursors of larger inflammatory lesions) appear as slightly elevated small papules. Open comedones appear flat or slightly raised with a central follicular impaction. The characteristics of inflammatory lesions (papules, pustules, nodules, or cysts) are documented.

Diagnosis

Nursing Diagnoses

Based on the assessment data, the patient's major nursing diagnoses may include:

- Ineffective management of therapeutic regimen related to insufficient knowledge about the condition (its causes, course, prevention, treatment, and skin care)
- Body image disturbance related to embarrassment and frustration over appearance

Collaborative Problems/ Potential Complications

Based on the assessment data, potential complications that may develop include:

- Scarring
- Infection

Planning and Implementation

Goals. The major goals of the patient may include understanding the condition to enhance compliance with prescribed therapy, development of self-acceptance, and absence of complications.

Nursing Interventions

Increasing Treatment Compliance and Understanding. Before treatment begins, patients are counseled and assured that the problem is not related to uncleanliness, dietary indiscretions, masturbation, sexual activity, or any of the other common misconceptions. It is important to reinforce the concept that acne arises from a combination of factors, including heredity, large sebaceous glands, and large numbers of *P. acnes* bacteria, all of which are beyond the control of the patient. It is also important to stress that it usually takes 4 to 6 weeks or more of careful compliance with the recommended treatment for results to be seen.

Teaching the rationale for using oral and topical medications and explaining their actions and potential side effects will promote patient understanding, encourage personal involvement and commitment to care, and enhance compliance. It is important that the patient be informed that medications such as topical tetracycline may discolor the skin, that benzoyl peroxide will bleach clothing that it touches, and that frequent blood tests (to monitor white blood cell, red blood cell, platelet, alkaline phosphatase, serum glutamic-oxalocetic and pyruvic transaminases [SGOT and SGPT], and lactic acid dehydrogenase [LDH] levels) are needed if the patient takes isotretinoin (Clark, 1993).

Patients are counseled that acne is unlikely to clear up in a short time and that they must persist with consistent treatment *every day.* If topical medications are provided, they must be applied to all lesions, not just those that are inflamed.

Patients are instructed to use the prescribed cleaning product. It is helpful to reassure them that most acne medications cause some drying and peeling, although the sudden appearance of diffuse redness and vesicles suggests contact allergy. Misconceptions must be corrected because understanding promotes compliance and a better chance of success.

Promoting Self-Acceptance. The patient is enrolled as a partner in therapy. It is essential to take the patient's problems seriously and to provide understanding, reassurance, and support. All facets of the emotional factors involved must be taken into account, including the possibility that acne can become a power struggle between teenager and parents when stressful situations (*e.g.,* final exams) cause exacerbations. Stress reduction techniques may be helpful.

Patient Education and Home Care Considerations. In addition to receiving instructions for taking prescribed medications, patients are instructed to wash the face and other affected areas with mild soap and water twice a day to remove surface oils and prevent obstruction of the oil glands. They are cautioned to avoid scrubbing the face constantly because acne is not caused by dirt and cannot be washed away.

Mild abrasive soaps and drying agents are prescribed to eliminate the oily feeling that troubles many patients. At the same time, they are cautioned to avoid excessive abrasion because it makes acne worse. It is also important to realize that soap itself can irritate the skin. Using a polyester sponge pad (Buf-Puf) promotes the mechanical removal of superficial skin cells **(epidermabrasion)** and may help some patients. Hair should be kept off the face and shampooed daily if necessary.

All forms of friction and trauma are to be avoided: propping the hands against the face, rubbing the face, and wearing tight collars and helmets. Patients are instructed to keep hands away from the face and not to squeeze pimples or blackheads. Squeezing merely worsens the problem, because a portion of the blackhead is pushed down into the skin, which may cause the follicle to rupture. Because cosmetics, shaving creams, and lotions can aggravate acne, these substances are best avoided unless the patient is advised otherwise. There is no evidence that a particular food can cause or aggravate acne. In general, a nutritious diet is followed.

Monitoring and Managing Potential Complications

Scarring. Prevention of scarring is the ultimate goal of therapy. The chance of scarring increases as the grade of acne increases. Grades III–IV (25 to > 50 comedones, papules, or pustules) usually require longer-term therapy with systemic antibiotics or isotretinoin (Accutane). Patients should be warned that discontinuing these medications can exacerbate acne, lead to more flare-ups, and increase the chance of deep scarring. Moreover, manipulation of the comedones, papules, and pustules increases the potential for increased scarring.

When acne surgery is prescribed to extract deep-seated comedones or inflamed lesions, or to incise and drain cystic lesions, the intervention itself may result in further scarring. Dermabrasion, which levels existing scar tissue, has the potential for increasing scar formation as well. In addition, hyper- or hypo-pigmentation may affect the tissue involved. The patient should be informed of these potential outcomes before electing surgical intervention for acne.

Infection. Female patients on long-term antibiotic therapy with tetracycline should be advised to watch for and report signs and symptoms of oral or vaginal candidiasis, a yeastlike fungal infection (Clark, 1993).

Evaluation

Expected Outcomes

1. Develops increasing understanding of the skin problem
   a. Reviews drawings of obstructive and inflammatory lesions of acne
   b. Reads patient education brochures
   c. Reads product information brochure and written instructions of the prescribed medication
2. Adheres to the prescribed therapy
   a. Verbalizes a major commitment to required treatment that may take months or years
   b. Expresses that the treatment must continue when the skin clears
   c. Follows cleansing program
3. Develops self-acceptance
   a. Identifies someone with whom to talk over problems
   b. Expresses optimism about outcome of treatment
4. Demonstrates no complications
   a. Reports no signs of infection
   b. Verbalizes that picking and squeezing blemishes/lesions will aggravate the condition and may cause scarring
   c. Reports no scarring or flare-ups
   d. Complies with therapy

Infections and Infestations of the Skin

Bacterial Infections (Pyodermas)

Bacterial infections of the skin may be primary or secondary. Primary skin infections originate in previously normal-appearing skin and are usually caused by a single organism. Secondary skin infections arise from a pre-existing skin disorder or from disruption of the skin integrity resulting from injury or surgery. In either case, several microorganisms may be implicated, for example *Staphylococcus aureus,* or group A streptococci.

The most common primary bacterial skin infections are impetigo and folliculitis. Folliculitis may lead to furuncles or carbuncles.

Impetigo

Impetigo is a superficial infection of the skin caused by staphylococci, streptococci, or multiple bacteria.

The exposed areas of the body, face, hands, neck, and extremities are most frequently involved. Impetigo is contagious and may spread to other parts of the patient's skin or to other members of the family who touch the patient or use towels or combs that are soiled with the exudate of the lesions.

Although impetigo is seen at all ages, it is particularly common among children living in poor hygienic conditions. Often it appears secondary to pediculosis capitis (head lice), scabies (itch mites), herpes simplex, insect bites, poison ivy, or eczema. Ill health, poor hygiene, and malnutrition may predispose an adult to impetigo.

Bullous impetigo, a superficial infection of the skin caused by *Staphylococcus aureus,* is characterized by the formation of bullae from original vesicles. The bullae rupture, leaving a raw, red area.

Clinical Manifestations. The lesions begin as small, red macules, which quickly become discrete, thin-walled vesicles that soon rupture and become covered with a loosely adherent honey-yellow crust (Fig. 54-1). These crusts are easily removed and reveal smooth, red, moist surfaces on which new crusts soon develop. If the scalp is involved, the hair is matted, distinguishing the condition from ringworm.

Management. Systemic antibiotic therapy is the usual treatment. It reduces contagious spread, treats deep infection, and prevents acute glomerulonephritis (kidney infection), which may occur as an aftermath of streptococcal skin diseases. In nonbullous impetigo, benzathine penicillin or oral penicillin may be prescribed. Bullous impetigo is treated with a penicillinase-resistant penicillin (cloxacillin, dicloxacillin).

Topical antibacterial therapy (*e.g.*, mupirocin) may be prescribed when the disease is limited to a small area. However, topical therapy requires that the medication be applied to the lesions several times daily for a week, in which case it may be impossible for some patients or their caregivers to comply completely with therapy. In addition, topical antibiotics generally are not as effective as systemic therapy in eradicating or preventing the spread of streptococci from the respiratory tract. Therefore the risk of developing glomerulonephritis increases.

When topical therapy is prescribed, lesions are soaked or washed with soap solution to remove the central site of bacterial growth, thus giving the topical antibiotic an opportunity to reach the infected site. After the crusts are removed, a topical medication (*e.g.*, neomycin, bacitracin) may be applied. Gloves are worn when providing patient care.

An antiseptic solution, such as povidone–iodine (Betadine) or chlorhexidine (Hibiclens), may be used to clean

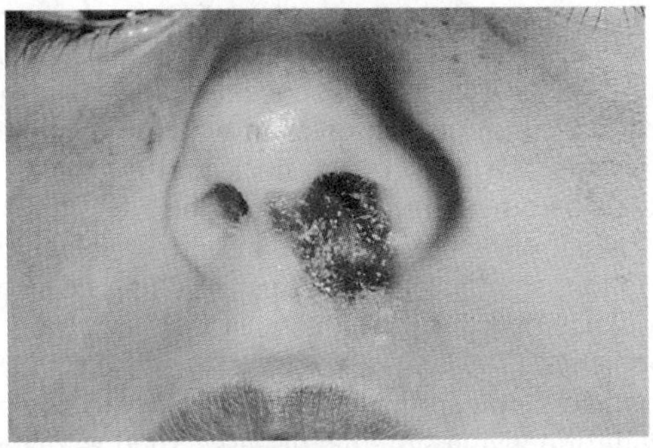

FIGURE 54-1. Impetigo of the nostril.

the skin, reduce bacterial content in the infected area, and prevent spread.

Patient Education and Home Care Considerations. The patient and family should be instructed to bathe at least once daily with bactericidal soap. Cleanliness and good hygienic practices help prevent the spread of the lesions from one skin area to another and from one person to another. Each person should have a separate towel and washcloth. Because impetigo is a contagious disorder, an infected child should be kept away from other children until the lesions have healed.

Folliculitis, Furuncles, and Carbuncles

Folliculitis is a staphylococcal infection that arises within the hair follicles. Lesions may be superficial or deep. Single or multiple papules or pustules appear close to the hair follicles. Folliculitis is commonly seen in the beard area of men who shave and on women's legs. Other areas include the axillae, trunk, and buttocks.

Pseudofolliculitis barbae ("shaving bumps") is an inflammatory reaction on the face of curly-haired men caused by ingrowing hairs that pierce the skin and provoke an irritative reaction. Curly hair has a curved root that grows at a more acute angle. This is a common problem in African-American men but may also occur in others. The initial treatment is to avoid shaving and grow a beard. If this is not possible, a handbrush may be used over the facial area to dislodge the hairs mechanically. If the patient must remove facial hair, a depilatory cream may be useful.

A **furuncle (boil)** is an acute inflammation arising *deep* in one or more hair follicles and spreading into the surrounding dermis. It is a deeper form of folliculitis. (**Furunculosis** refers to multiple or recurrent lesions.) Furuncles may occur anywhere on the body but are more prevalent in areas subjected to irritation, pressure, friction, and excessive perspiration, such as the back of the neck, the axillae, or the buttocks.

A furuncle may start as a small, red, raised, painful "pimple." Frequently, the infection progresses and involves the skin and subcutaneous fatty tissue, causing tenderness, pain, and surrounding cellulitis. The area of redness and induration represents an effort of the body to keep the infection localized. The bacteria (usually staphylococci) produce necrosis of the invaded tissue. The characteristic pointing of a boil follows in a few days. When this occurs, the center becomes yellow or black, and the boil is said popularly to have "come to a head."

A **carbuncle** is an abscess of the skin and subcutaneous tissue representing an extension of a furuncle that has invaded several follicles and is large and deep-seated. It is usually caused by a staphylococcal infection. Carbuncles appear most commonly in areas in which the skin is thick and inelastic. The back of the neck and the buttocks are common sites. In carbuncles, the extensive inflammation frequently is not associated with a complete walling off of the infection, so absorption occurs, resulting in high fever, pain, leukocytosis, and even extension of the infection to the bloodstream.

Furuncles and carbuncles are more likely to occur in patients with underlying systemic diseases, such as diabetes or hematologic malignancies, and those receiving immunosuppressive therapy for other diseases. Both are more prevalent in hot climates, especially on skin beneath occlusive clothing.

Management. In treating staphylococcal infections, it is important not to rupture or destroy the protective wall of induration that localizes the infection. Therefore, the boil or pimple should never be squeezed.

The follicular disorders (folliculitis, furuncles, carbuncles) are usually caused by staphylococci, although if the immune system is impaired, the causative organisms may be gram-negative bacilli.

Systemic antibiotic therapy, selected by sensitivity study, is generally indicated. Oral cloxacillin, dicloxacillin, and flucloxacillin are first-line medications. Cephalosporins and erythromycin are also effective.

Supportive Care. Intravenous fluids, fever sponges, and other supportive treatments are indicated for patients who are very ill or suffering with toxicity. Warm, moist compresses increase vascularization and hasten resolution of the furuncle or carbuncle. The surrounding skin may be cleaned gently with antibacterial soap and an antibacterial ointment may be applied.

Extraction. When the pus has localized and is fluctuant (moving in palpable waves), a small incision with a scalpel will speed resolution by relieving the tension and ensuring direct evacuation of the pus and slough. The patient is instructed to keep the draining lesion covered with a dressing.

Anti-infective Measures. Soiled dressings are handled according to universal precautions. Nursing personnel should carefully follow isolation precautions to avoid becoming staphylococcus carriers. Disposable gloves are worn when caring for these patients.

- Special precautions must be taken with boils on the face because the skin area drains directly into the cranial venous sinuses. Sinus thrombosis, with fatal pyemia, has been known to develop after manipulation of a boil in this location.

Bed rest is advised for patients who have boils on the perineum or in the anal region, and a course of systemic antibiotic therapy is indicated to control the spread of the infection.

Patient Education and Home Care Considerations. To prevent and control staphylococcal skin infections (boils, carbuncles), the staphylococcus must be eliminated from the skin and environment. Efforts must be made to increase the patient's resistance and provide a hygienic environment.

If lesions are actively draining, the mattress and pillow should be covered with plastic material and wiped off with disinfectant daily; the bed linens, towels, and clothing should be laundered after each use; and the patient should shower and shampoo with an antibacterial soap and shampoo for an indefinite period, commonly for several months.

Prevention of recurrent infection has been achieved by prescribed antibiotics such as a daily dose of oral clindamycin to be taken continuously for about 3 months. It is essential that the patient take the full dose for the time prescribed. The purulent exudate (pus) is a source of reinfection or transmission of infection to caregivers.

When the patient has a history of recurrent infections, a carrier state may exist, which should be investigated and treated with an antibacterial cream such as mupirocin.

Viral Infections

Herpes Zoster (Shingles)

Herpes zoster (shingles) is an inflammatory viral condition in which the virus produces a painful vesicular eruption along the area of distribution of the sensory nerves from one or more posterior ganglia. It is caused by the varicella virus, commonly known as varicella zoster virus, which is a member of a group of DNA viruses. (The viruses of chickenpox and herpes zoster are indistinguishable; hence the name varicella zoster.) It is assumed that herpes zoster represents a reactivation of latent varicella (chickenpox) virus and reflects lowered immunity. After a case of chickenpox runs its course, it is believed that the varicella zoster viruses responsible for the outbreak lie dormant inside nerve cells near the brain and spinal cord. Later, when these latent viruses are reactivated, they travel by way of the peripheral nerves to the skin. There, the viruses multiply, creating a red rash of small, fluid-filled blisters. About 10% of adults get shingles during their lifetime, usually after age 50. There is an increased frequency of herpes zoster in patients with weakened immune systems and malignancies, especially the leukemias and the lymphomas.

Clinical Manifestations. The eruption is usually accompanied or preceded by pain, which may radiate over the entire region supplied by the nerves. The pain may be burning, lancinating (tearing, sharply cutting), stabbing, or aching. Some patients have no pain, but itching and tenderness may occur over the area. At times, malaise and gastrointestinal disturbances precede the eruption.

The patches of grouped vesicles appear on the red and swollen skin. The early vesicles contain serum and later become purulent, rupture, and form crusts. The inflammation is usually unilateral, involving the thoracic, cervical, or cranial nerves in a bandlike configuration. The blisters are usually confined to a narrow region of the face or trunk. The clinical course varies from 1 to 3 weeks. If an ophthalmic nerve is involved, the patient may have a painful eye. Inflammation and a rash on the trunk may cause pain at the slightest touch. The healing time varies between 7 and 26 days.

Herpes zoster in healthy adults is usually localized and benign. However, in immunosuppressed patients, the disease may be severe and the clinical course acutely disabling.

Management. The goals of management are to relieve the pain and to reduce or avoid complications. These include infection, scarring, and postherpetic neuralgia and eye complications.

The pain is controlled with analgesics, because adequate pain control during the acute phase will help prevent persistent pain patterns.

Systemic corticosteroids are prescribed for patients over age 50 to reduce the incidence and duration of postherpetic neuralgia (persistent pain of the affected nerve after healing). Healing usually occurs sooner in those who have been treated with steroids. Triamcinolone (Aristocort, Kenacort, Kenalog) injected subcutaneously under painful areas is effective as an anti-inflammatory agent.

There is some evidence that infection is arrested if oral acyclovir is administered within 24 hours of the initial eruption. Intravenous acyclovir, if started early, is effective in significantly reducing the pain and halting the progression of the disease. Another antiviral medication, vidarabine, may also be tried. In older persons, the pain from herpes zoster may persist as postherpetic neuralgia for months after the skin lesions disappear.

If the eye is involved, the patient is referred to an ophthalmologist, because keratitis, uveitis, ulceration, and blindness may occur. This is referred to as ophthalmic herpes zoster.

A susceptible person can acquire chicken pox through contact with the infective vesicular fluid of a patient with herpes zoster. A person with a previous history of chicken pox is immune and, therefore, not at risk of infection after exposure to patients with herpes zoster.

Patient Education and Home Care Considerations. The nurse assesses the patient's discomfort and response to medication and collaborates with the physician to make necessary adjustments to the treatment regimen. The patient is taught how to apply wet dressings or medication to the lesions and to follow proper hand-washing techniques to avoid spreading the virus.

Diversionary activities and relaxation techniques are encouraged to assure restful sleep—all of which help to alleviate discomfort.

A caregiver may be required to assist with dressings, particularly if the patient is elderly and unable to apply them. Relatives, neighbors, or a community health nurse may need to help with dressing changes and food preparation for patients who cannot care for themselves or prepare nourishing meals.

Mycotic (Fungal) Infections

The fungi, tiny representatives of the plant kingdom that feed on organic matter, are responsible for various common skin infections. In some cases, they affect only the skin and its appendages (*i.e.*, hair and nails), but in others, the internal organs are involved. In the latter instance, fungal disease may be life-threatening. Superficial infections, on the other hand, rarely cause even temporary disability and respond readily to treatment. Secondary infection with bacteria or *Candida* or both may occur.

The most common fungal skin disorder is known as **tinea** or "**ringworm.**" Tinea infections affect the head, body, groin, feet, and nails. Table 54-5 summarizes the tinea infections.

To obtain material for diagnosis, the lesion is cleaned and a scalpel is used to remove scales from the margin of the lesion. The scales are dropped onto a slide to which potassium hydroxide has been added. The diagnosis is made by examining the infected scales microscopically and by isolating the organism in culture.

Under **Wood's light** a specimen of infected hair appears fluorescent, which may be helpful in diagnosing some cases of tinea capitis.

Tinea Pedis (Ringworm of the Feet; Athlete's Foot)

Tinea pedis is the most common fungal infection. It commonly affects teenagers and young adults, although it can

TABLE 54-5 Tinea (Ringworm) Infections

Type and Location	Clinical Manifestations	Treatment
Tinea capitis (ringworm of scalp)	Contagious fungal infection of the hair shaft. Common in children. Round patches of redness and scaling. Small pustules or papules at edges. Hair brittle; breaks easily at scalp.	Griseofulvin. Shampoo hair 2–3 times a week (Exsel, Selsun shampoos)
Tinea corporis (ringworm of body)	Begins with erythematous macule advancing to rings of papules or vesicles with central clearing. Lesions found in clusters—may extend to scalp, hair, or nails. Pruritic. (Infected pet may be the source.)	Ketoconazole Griseofulvin
Tinea cruris (ringworm of groin—"jock itch")	Pruritus with small, red, scaly patches extending to circular plaques with elevated scaly or vesicular borders.	*Mild conditions:* Topical medications, such as clotrimazole, ketoconazole, miconazole, haloprogin *Severe conditions:* Oral griseofulvin
Tinea pedis (ringworm of feet—"athlete's foot")	Pruritus—soles of feet, spaces between toes affected. Inflamed vesicles (acute) or scaly, dusky, or red rash (chronic).	*Acute infections:* Soak with Burow's saline or potassium permanganate solutions Topical antifungals: miconazole (Lotrimin AF, Mycelex, Micatin), clotrimazole *Resistant infections:* terbinafine, griseofulvin
Tinea unguium (ringworm of nails)	More common in toenails. Associated with long-time fungal infection of feet. Nails thicken, crumble easily, and lack luster. Whole nail may be destroyed.	*Long-term therapy* (6 mo–1 yr): Griseofulvin (for fingernails) Amphotericin B lotion; miconazole; clotrimazole Nystatin (if caused by *Candida albicans*)

occur in any age group or either gender. It is especially prevalent in those who use communal showers or swimming pools (MacKie, 1991).

Clinical Manifestations. Tinea pedis may appear as an acute or chronic infection on the soles of the feet or between the toes. The toenail may also be involved if the infection is chronic. Lymphangitis and cellulitis may occur occasionally when bacterial superinfection occurs. Sometimes a mixed, fungal–bacterial–yeast infection occurs.

Management. During the acute (vesicular) phase, soaks of Burow's saline, or potassium permanganate solutions are used to remove the crusts, scales, and debris and to reduce the inflammation. Topical antifungals (miconazole; clotrimazole) are applied to the infected areas. Topical therapy is continued for several weeks because of the high rate of recurrence.

Patient Education and Home Care Considerations. Footwear provides a favorable environment for fungi; thus, the causative fungi may be in the shoes or socks. Because moisture encourages the growth of fungi, the patient is instructed to keep the feet as dry as possible, including the areas between the toes. Small pieces of cotton can be placed between the toes at night to absorb moisture. Socks should be made of absorbent cotton, and hosiery should have cotton feet, because synthetic material does not absorb perspiration as well as cotton.

For persons whose feet perspire excessively, perforated shoes permit better aeration of the feet. Plastic- or rubber-soled footwear should be avoided. Talcum powder or antifungal powder applied twice daily helps to keep the feet dry. Several pairs of shoes should be alternated so that they can dry completely before being worn again.

Tinea Corporis (Ringworm of the Body)

Tinea corporis affects the face, neck, trunk, and extremities on which the typical ringed lesion appears (Fig. 54-2). Animal varieties (nonhuman variety) are known to cause an intense inflammatory reaction in humans because they are not normally adapted to living on human hosts. Humans make contact with animal varieties through contact with pets or through contact with objects that have been in contact with an animal.

Management. Topical antifungal medication may be applied to small areas. Oral griseofulvin is used in extensive cases. Side effects of griseofulvin include photosensitivity, skin rashes, headache, and nausea. Ketoconazole, an antifungal agent, shows real promise in patients with chronic fungal (dermatophyte) infections, including those resistant to griseofulvin.

Patient Education and Home Care Considerations. The patient is instructed to use a clean towel and

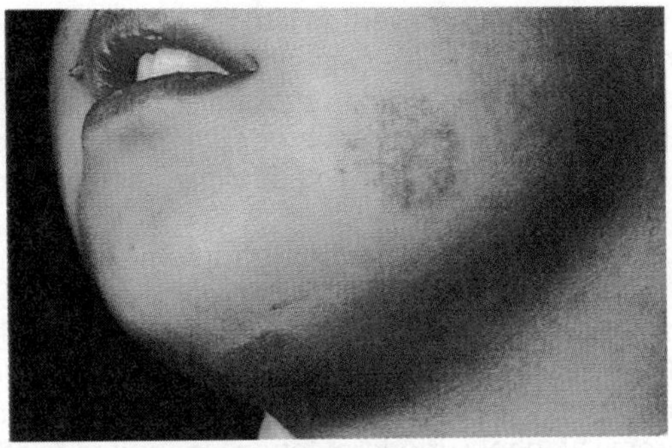

FIGURE 54-2. Tinea corporis (ringworm) of the face.

washcloth daily. All skin areas and skin folds that retain moisture must be dried thoroughly because fungal infections thrive in heat and moisture. Clean cotton clothing should be worn next to the skin.

Tinea Capitis (Ringworm of the Scalp)

Ringworm of the scalp is a contagious fungal infection of the hair shafts and a common cause of hair loss in children. Clinically, one or several round, red, scaling patches are present. Small pustules or papules may be seen at the edges of such patches. As the hairs in the affected areas are invaded by the fungi, they become brittle and break off at or near the surface of the scalp, leaving bald patches. Most cases of tinea capitis heal without scarring, so the hair loss is only temporary.

Management. Griseofulvin, an antifungal agent, is prescribed for patients with tinea capitis. Topical agents do not provide an effective cure because the infection occurs within the hair shaft and below the surface of the scalp. However, topical agents can be used to inactivate organisms already on the hair. This minimizes contagion and eliminates the need to clip the hair. Infected hairs break off anyway, and noninfected ones may remain in place. The hair should be shampooed two to three times weekly, and a topical antifungal preparation should be applied to reduce dissemination of the organisms.

Patient Education and Home Care Considerations. Because tinea capitis is contagious, the patient and family should be advised to set up a hygienic regimen for home use. Each person should have a separate comb and brush and should avoid exchanging hats and other headgear. All infected members of the family and household pets must be examined because familial infections are relatively common.

Tinea Cruris (Ringworm of the Groin)

Tinea cruris ("jock itch") is ringworm infection of the groin, which may extend to the inner thighs and buttock area. It is commonly associated with tinea pedis. It occurs most frequently in young joggers, obese persons, and those who wear tight underclothing.

Management. Mild infections may be treated with topical medication such as clotrimazole, miconazole, or haloprogin for at least 3 to 4 weeks to ensure complete eradication of the infection. Oral griseofulvin may be required for more severe infections.

Patient Education and Home Care Considerations. Heat, friction, and maceration (from sweating) predispose the patient to the infection. As much as possible, the patient is instructed to avoid excessive heat and humidity and wearing nylon underwear, tight-fitting clothing, and a wet bathing suit. The groin area should be cleaned, dried thoroughly, and dusted with a topical antifungal agent, such as tolnaftate (Tinactin) as a preventive measure, because the infection is apt to recur.

Tinea Unguium (Onychomycosis)

Tinea unguium (ringworm of the nails) is a chronic fungal infection of the toenails or, less commonly, the fingernails. It is usually caused by *Trichophyton* species (*T. rubrum, T. mentagrophytes*) or *Candida albicans*. It is usually associated with longtime fungal infection of the feet. The nails become thickened, friable (easily crumbled), and lusterless. In time, debris accumulates under the free edge of the nail, and, ultimately, the nail plate separates. Because of the chronicity of this infection, the entire nail may be destroyed.

Management. Griseofulvin is usually prescribed orally for 6 months to 1 year when the fingernails are involved, but griseofulvin is not of value in treating candidal infections; these must be treated topically with amphotericin-B lotion, miconazole, clotrimazole, nystatin, or other preparations. In general, these products penetrate poorly, and the infections are difficult to treat. Response to griseofulvin in fungal infections of the toenails is poor at best. Frequently, when the treatment is stopped the infection returns.

Parasitic Skin Diseases

Pediculosis (Infection by Lice)

Lice infestation affects persons of all ages. Three varieties of lice infest humans: **Pediculus humanus capitis** (head louse); **Pediculus humanus corporis** (body louse); and **Phthirus pubis** (pubic, or "crab," louse). Lice are termed **ectoparasites** because they live on the outside of the host's body. They depend on the host for their nourishment, feeding on human blood approximately five times a day. They inject their digestive juices and excrement into the skin, which causes severe itching.

Pediculosis Capitis

Pediculosis capitis is an infestation of the scalp by the head louse, *Pediculus humanus capitis.* The female head louse lays her eggs (nits) close to the scalp. The nits become firmly attached to the hair shafts with a tenacious substance. The young lice hatch in about 10 days and reach maturity in 2 weeks.

Clinical Manifestations. Head lice are found most commonly along the back of the head and behind the ears. The eggs are visible to the naked eye as silvery, glistening oval bodies that are difficult to remove from the hair. The bite of the insect causes intense itching, and the resultant scratching often leads to secondary bacterial infection, such as impetigo or furunculosis. The infestation is more common in children and people with long hair. Head lice may be transmitted directly by physical contact or indirectly by infested combs, brushes, wigs, hats, and bedding.

Management. Treatment involves washing the hair with a shampoo containing lindane (Kwell) or pyrethrin compounds with piperonyl butoxide (RID or R&C Shampoo). The patient is instructed to shampoo the scalp and hair according to the product directives. After the hair is rinsed thoroughly, it is combed with a fine-toothed comb that is dipped in vinegar to remove any remaining nits or nit shells freed from the hair shafts. These are extremely difficult to remove and may have to be picked off with the fingernails, one by one (hence the expression *nit picking*).

All articles, clothing, towels, and bedding that might have lice or nits should be washed in hot water—at least 54°C (130°F)—or dry-cleaned to prevent reinfestation. Upholstered furniture, rugs, and floors should be vacuumed frequently. Combs and brushes are also disinfected with the shampoo. All family members and close contacts are treated.

Complications such as severe pruritus, pyoderma (pus-forming infection of the skin), and dermatitis are treated with antipruritics, systemic antibiotics, and topical corticosteroids.

Patient Education and Home Care Considerations. The patient is reassured that head lice may infest anyone and are not a sign of uncleanliness. This condition spreads rapidly, so treatment must be started immediately. School epidemics may be managed by having all of the students shampoo their hair on the same night. Students should be warned not to share combs, brushes, or hats. Each family member should be inspected for head lice daily for at least 2 weeks. The patient should be instructed that lindane may be toxic when not used properly.

Pediculosis Corporis and Pediculosis Pubis

Pediculosis corporis is an infestation of the body by the body louse, *Pediculus humanus corporis*. This is a disease of unwashed persons or those who live in close quarters and do not change their clothing.

Clinical Manifestations. The areas of the skin chiefly involved are those that come in closest contact with the underclothing (*i.e.*, the neck, trunk, and thighs). The body louse lives chiefly in the seams of underwear and clothing, to which it clings as it pierces the skin with its proboscis. Its bites cause characteristic minute hemorrhagic points. Widespread excoriation may appear as a result of intense itching and scratching, especially on the trunk and neck. Among the secondary lesions produced are parallel linear scratches and a slight degree of eczema. In long-standing cases, the skin may become thick, dry, and scaly, with dark pigmented areas.

Pediculosis pubis, infestation by *Phthirus pubis* (crab louse), is extremely common. The infestation is generally localized in the genital region and transmitted chiefly by sexual contact.

Reddish brown "dust" (the excretions of the insects) may be found in underclothing. Lice may also infest the hairs of the chest, axillary hair, beard, and eyelashes. Gray-blue macules may sometimes be seen on the trunk, thighs, and axillae as a result of either the reaction of the insects' saliva with bilirubin (converting it to biliverdin) or an excretion produced by the salivary glands of the louse.

The pubic crease should be examined with a magnifying glass to detect the presence of *Phthirus pubis* crawling down a hair shaft or nits cemented to the hair or at the junction with the skin.

Itching is the most common symptom, particularly at night. Infestation by pubic lice may coexist with sexually transmitted diseases (gonorrhea, candidiasis, syphilis).

Management. The patient is instructed to bathe with soap and water. Then, either lindane (Kwell) or malathion in isopropyl alcohol (Prioderm lotion) is applied to affected areas of the skin and to hairy areas, according to the product information directives. An alternative topical therapy is a pyrethrin-based pediculicide (RID, which is an over-the-counter preparation) or 0.03% copper oleate (Cuprex). If the eyelashes are involved, petrolatum may be thickly applied twice daily for 8 days, followed by mechanical removal of any remaining nits.

Complications, such as severe pruritus, pyoderma (pus-forming infection of the skin), and dermatitis, are treated with antipruritics, systemic antibiotics, and topical corticosteroids. It is important to remember that body lice are capable of transmitting epidemic disease in humans, namely, rickettsial disease (epidemic typhus, relapsing fever, and trench fever). The causative organism may be in the gastrointestinal tract of the insect and may be excreted on the skin surface of the infested person.

Patient Education and Home Care Considerations. All family members and sexual contacts must be treated and educated in personal hygiene and methods to prevent or control infestation. The patient and partner must also be scheduled for a diagnostic workup for coexisting sexually transmitted disease. All clothing and bedding should be machine-washed or dry-cleaned.

Scabies

Scabies is an infestation of the skin by the itch mite, *Sarcoptes scabiei*. The disease may be found in poor persons living under substandard hygienic conditions, but it is also common in very clean individuals. It is commonly found among the sexually active. However, infestations are not dependent on sexual activity because the mites frequently involve the fingers, and hand contact may produce infection. In children, overnight stays with friends or the exchange of clothes may be a source of infection. Health care personnel who have prolonged "hands on" physical contact with an infected patient may likewise become infected.

The adult female burrows into the superficial layer of the skin and remains there for the rest of her life. With her jaws and the sharp edges of the joints of her forelegs, the mite extends the burrow, laying two to three eggs daily for up to 2 months. She then dies. The larvae (eggs) hatch in 3 to 4 days and progress through larval and nymphal states to form adult mites in about 10 days.

Clinical Manifestations. It takes approximately 4 weeks from the time of contact for the patient's symptoms to appear. The patient complains of severe itching caused by a delayed type of immunologic reaction to the mite or its fecal pellets. During examination, the patient is asked where the itch is most severe. A magnifying glass and a penlight are held at an oblique angle to the skin while a search is made for the small, raised burrows. The burrows may be multiple, straight or wavy, brown or black, threadlike lesions, most commonly observed between the fingers and on the wrists.

Other sites are the extensor surfaces of the elbows, the knees, the edges of the feet, the points of the elbows, around the nipples, in the axillary folds, under pendulous breasts, and in or near the groin or gluteal fold, penis, or scrotum. Red pruritic eruptions usually appear between adjacent skin areas. The burrow, however, is not always visible. Any patient with a rash may have scabies.

One classic sign of scabies is the increased itching that occurs at night, perhaps because the increased warmth of the skin has a stimulating effect on the parasite. Also, hypersensitivity to the organism and its products of excretion may contribute to the itching. If the infection has spread, other members of the family and close friends will also complain of itching about a month later.

Secondary lesions are quite common and include vesicles, papules, excoriations, and crusts. Bacterial superinfection may result from constant excoriation of the burrows and papules.

Diagnostic Evaluation. The diagnosis is confirmed by recovering *Sarcoptes scabiei* or the mites' by-products from the skin. A sample of superficial epidermis is scraped off the top of the burrows or papules with a small scalpel blade. The scrapings are placed on a microscope slide and examined through a low-powered microscope to demonstrate the mite at any stage (adult, eggs, egg casings, larva, nymph) and fecal pellets.

Management. The patient is instructed to take a warm, soapy bath or shower to remove the scaling debris from the crusts and then to dry thoroughly and allow the skin to cool.

A scabicide, such as lindane (Kwell) or crotamiton (Eurax cream and lotion), is applied thinly to the entire skin from the neck down, sparing only the face and scalp (which are not affected in scabies). The medication is left on for 12 to 24 hours, after which the patient is instructed to wash thoroughly. One application may be curative, but it is advisable to repeat the treatment in 1 week.

- It is important that the patient understand these directions because application of a scabicide immediately after bathing and before the skin dries and cools increases percutaneous absorption of the scabicide and the potential for such central nervous system abnormalities as seizures.

Patient Education and Home Care Considerations. The patient should wear clean clothing and sleep between freshly laundered bed linens. All bedding and clothing should be washed in very hot water and dried on the hot dryer cycle because the mites are known to survive up to 36 hours in linens. If bed linens or clothing cannot be washed in hot water, it is advised that they be dry-cleaned.

After the treatment is completed, the patient should apply an ointment, such as a topical corticosteroid, to skin lesions because the scabicide may irritate the skin. The patient's hypersensitivity does not cease upon destruction of the mites. Itching may continue for a few days or weeks as a manifestation of hypersensitivity, particularly in atopic (allergic) persons. This is not a sign that the treatment has failed. The patient is instructed *not* to apply more scabicide (because this will cause more irritation and increased itching) and *not* to take frequent hot showers (because this dries the skin and produces itching).

All family members and close contacts should be treated simultaneously to eliminate the mites. If scabies is sexually transmitted, the patient may require treatment for coexisting sexually transmitted disease. Scabies may also coexist with pediculosis.

Gerontologic Considerations. Although the older patient itches severely, the vivid inflammatory reaction seen in younger people seldom occurs. Scabies may not be recognized in the elderly person and the itching may erroneously be attributed to the dry skin of old age or to anxiety.

Health care personnel in extended care facilities should wear gloves when providing hands-on care for a patient suspected of having scabies until the diagnosis is confirmed and treatment accomplished. It is advisable to treat all residents, staff, and families of patients at the same time to prevent reinfection.

Contact Dermatitis

Contact dermatitis (dermatitis venenata) is an inflammatory reaction of the skin to physical, chemical, or biologic agents. The epidermis is damaged by repeated physical and chemical irritations. Contact dermatitis may be of the primary irritant type, in which a nonallergic reaction results from exposure to an irritating substance, or it may be allergic (**allergic contact dermatitis**), resulting from exposure of sensitized persons to contact allergens. (Allergic dermatoses are discussed in Chapter 51.) Common causes of **irritant contact dermatitis** are soaps, detergents, scouring compounds, and industrial chemicals. Predisposing factors include extremes of heat and cold, frequent contact with soap and water, and a preexisting skin disease.

Clinical Manifestations. The eruptions begin when the causative agent contacts the skin. The first reactions include itching, burning, and erythema, followed soon by edema, papules, vesicles, and oozing or weeping. In the subacute phase, these vesicular changes are less marked, and they alternate with crusting, drying, fissuring, and peeling. If repeated reactions occur, or if the patient continually scratches the skin, thickening of the skin (**lichenification**) and **pigmentation** (coloration) occur. Secondary bacterial invasion may follow.

Management. The objectives of management are to rest the involved skin and protect it from further damage. The distribution pattern of the reaction is determined to differentiate between allergic and irritant contact dermatitis. A detailed history is obtained. Then, the offending irritant is identified and removed. Local irritation should be avoided, and soap is not generally used until healing occurs.

Many preparations are advocated for relieving dermatitis. In general, a bland, unmedicated lotion is used for small patches of erythema (inflamed skin). Cool, wet dressings also are applied over small areas of vesicular dermatitis. Finely cracked ice added to the water often enhances its antipruritic effect.

CHART 54-2
Patient Education: Strategies for Avoiding Contact Dermatitis

The following precautions may help you avoid a repeated case of contact dermatitis. Follow these instructions for at least 4 months after your skin appears to be completely healed.

- Study the pattern and location of your dermatitis and think about which things have touched your skin and which things may have caused the problem.
- Try to avoid contact with these materials.
- Avoid heat, soap, and rubbing—all of which are external irritants.
- Avoid topical medications, lotions or ointments, except those that are specifically prescribed for your condition.
- Wash your skin thoroughly immediately after exposure to possible irritants.
- When wearing rubber gloves, for example, for washing dishes or general cleaning, be sure to wear cotton-lined rubber gloves, and do not wear them more than 15 or 20 minutes at a time.

Wet dressings usually help clear the oozing eczematous lesions. Then, a thin layer of cream or ointment containing one of the corticosteroids may be used. Medicated baths at room temperature are prescribed for larger areas of dermatitis. In widespread conditions, a short course of systemic corticosteroids may be prescribed. (See Chart 54-2 for patient education–home care guidelines.)

Noninfectious Inflammatory Dermatoses

Psoriasis

Psoriasis is a chronic, noninfectious, inflammatory disease of the skin in which the production of epidermal cells occurs at a rate that is approximately six to nine times faster than normal. The cells in the basal layer of the skin divide too quickly, and the newly formed cells move so rapidly to the skin surface that they become evident as profuse scales or plaques of epidermal tissue. The psoriatic epidermal cell may travel from the basal cell layer of the epidermis to the stratum corneum (skin surface) and be cast off in 3 to 4 days, which is in sharp contrast to the normal 26 to 28 days. As a result of the increased number of basal cells and rapid cell passage, the normal events of cell maturation and growth cannot take place. This abnormal process does not allow the normal protective layers of the skin to form.

One of the most common skin diseases, psoriasis affects approximately 2% of the population (Camp, 1992). It is thought that the condition stems from a hereditary defect that causes overproduction of keratin. Although the primary cause is unknown, a combination of specific genetic make-up and environmental stimuli may trigger the onset of disease. There is some evidence that the cell proliferation is mediated by the immune system. Periods of emotional stress and anxiety aggravate the condition, and trauma, infections, and seasonal and hormonal changes are trigger factors. The onset may occur at any age but is most common between the ages of 10 and 30 years (Stiller, 1994). Psoriasis has a tendency to improve and then recur periodically throughout life.

Clinical Manifestations

The lesions appear as red, raised patches of skin covered with silvery scales. The scaly patches are formed by the buildup of living and dead skin that results from the vast increase in rate of skin-cell growth and turnover (Fig. 54-3). If the scales are scraped away, the dark red base of the lesion is exposed, producing multiple bleeding points. These patches are not moist and may or may not itch.

The lesions may remain small, giving rise to the term **guttate psoriasis.** Usually, the lesions enlarge slowly, but after many months they coalesce, forming extensive, irregularly shaped patches. Psoriasis may range from a cosmetic source of annoyance to a physically disabling and disfiguring affliction.

Particular sites of the body tend to be affected by this ailment; they include the scalp, the area over the elbows and knees, the lower part of the back, and the genitalia. Psoriasis also appears on the extensor surfaces of the arms and

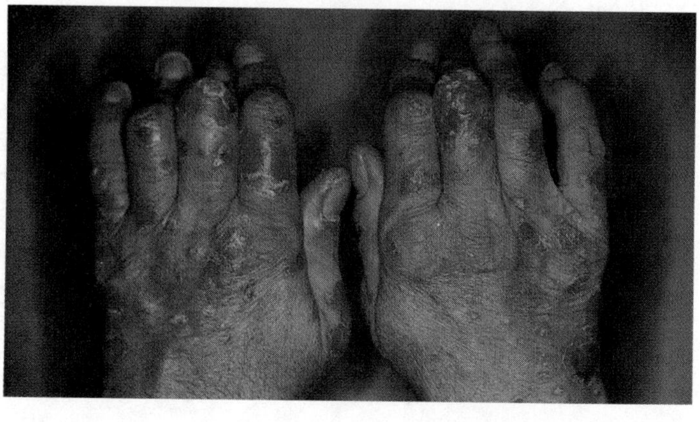

FIGURE 54-3. Psoriasis of the hand. (Sauer GC, Manual of Skin Diseases, 6th ed. Philadelphia, JB Lippincott, 1991.)

legs, on the scalp and ears, and over the sacrum and the intergluteal fold. Bilateral symmetry is a feature of psoriasis. In approximately one quarter to one half of the patients, the nails are involved, with pitting, discoloration, crumbling beneath the free edges, and separation of the nail plate. When psoriasis occurs on the palms and soles, it can cause pustular lesions.

Complications

The disease may be associated with asymmetric rheumatoid factor-negative arthritis of multiple joints. The arthritic development can occur either before or after the skin lesions appear. The relationship between arthritis and psoriasis is not understood. Another complication is an exfoliative psoriatic state in which the disease progresses to involve the total body surface.

Psychologic Considerations. Psoriasis may cause despair and frustration for the patient; observers may stare, comment, ask embarrassing questions, or even avoid the person. The disease can eventually exhaust the patient's resources, interfere with his or her job, and make life miserable in general. Teenagers are especially vulnerable to the psychologic effects of this ailment. The family, too, is affected, because time-consuming treatments, messy salves, and constant shedding of scales may disrupt home life and cause resentment. The patient's frustrations may be expressed through hostility directed at health care personnel and others.

Diagnostic Evaluation

The presence of the classic plaque-type lesions generally confirms the diagnosis of psoriasis. Lesions tend to change histologically as they progress from early to chronic plaques. Therefore, biopsy of the skin is of little value in diagnosis, and there are no specific blood tests helpful in diagnosing the condition. When in doubt, the physician should assess for signs of nail and scalp involvement, as well as a positive family history.

Management

The goals of management are to slow the rapid turnover of epidermis, to promote resolution of the psoriatic lesions, and to control the disease because there is no known cure.

The therapeutic approach should be one that the patient understands; it should be cosmetically acceptable and not too disruptive of lifestyle. It will involve the commitment of time and effort by the patient and possibly the family.

First, any precipitating or aggravating factors are removed. Then an assessment is made of lifestyle, because psoriasis is significantly affected by stress. The patient must also be advised that treatment of severe psoriasis can be time-consuming, expensive, and aesthetically unappealing at times.

Three types of therapy are standard: topical, intralesional, and systemic.

Topical Therapy. Topically applied agents are used to slow down the overactive epidermis without affecting other tissues. Medications include tar preparations, anthralin, salicylic acid, and corticosteroids. Treatment with these agents tends to suppress **epidermopoiesis** (creation of epidermal cells).

Tar formulations include lotions, ointments, pastes, creams, and shampoos. Tar baths or tar preparations may retard and inhibit the rapid growth of psoriatic tissue. Coal tar preparations are photosensitizing agents, so patients should be warned not to expose treated skin to the sun. Tar therapy may be combined with carefully graded doses of ultraviolet-B light, which produces radiation in wavelengths between 280 and 320 nanometers (nm). Ultraviolet-B light seems to potentiate the action of tar. The tar is partially removed before ultraviolet light exposure to allow maximum transmission of light. During this phase of treatment, the patient is advised to wear goggles and to protect the eyes. Using a timer will prevent the danger of severe burns from overexposure to the light rays. A daily tar shampoo followed by an application of steroid lotion may be used for scalp lesions. The patient is also taught to remove excess scales by scrubbing with a soft brush while bathing.

Anthralin preparations (Anthra-Derm, Dritho-Creme, Lasan) are useful for thick psoriatic plaques that are resistant to other coal tar or corticosteroid preparations. The patient is instructed to apply anthralin medication with a tongue blade or gloved fingers, taking special care not to cover normal skin. The hands must be washed after handling anthralin, because a chemical conjunctivitis can result from touching the eyes while medication is still on the hands. The preparation is left on the skin from 8 to 12 hours.

Topical corticosteroids may be applied for their anti-inflammatory effect. Once the medication is applied, the area is covered with an occlusive plastic film dressing to enhance medication penetration and to soften the scaly plaques. Tape that is impregnated with corticosteroid medication may be used in patients who have relatively few but resistant psoriatic plaques. However, after the corticosteroid treatment stops, the psoriasis may quickly reappear (rebound phenomenon) and, in some instances, be more extensive.

When psoriasis involves large areas of the body, topical corticosteroid treatment can become expensive. In this event, other treatment modalities (coal tar, ultraviolet light) may be used in combination. As with anthralin, hand washing is stressed following application.

Occlusive dressings may be applied on a few areas or more extensively. Some patients will require a hydrocolloid (Duoderm) occlusive dressing over the entire body. For the hospitalized patient, large plastic bags may be used—one for the upper body (with holes cut out for the head and arms) and one for the lower body (with holes for the legs). This leaves only the extremities to wrap. In some dermatologic units, large rolls of tubular plastic are used (such as the kind used by dry-cleaners to cover clean clothes).

- When these substances are used, it is important to check for flammability. Some thin, plastic films will burn slowly (if touched by a lighted cigarette), whereas others will burst rapidly into flame. The patient should be cautioned not to smoke while wrapped in these dressings.

For patients being treated at home, a plastic vinyl jogging suit may be purchased. The medication is applied and the suit simply put over it. The hands can be wrapped in gloves, the feet in plastic bags, and the head in a shower cap.

Intralesional Therapy. Intralesional injections of triamcinolone acetonide (Aristocort, Kenalog-10, Trymex) can be administered directly into highly visible or isolated patches of psoriasis that are resistant to other forms of therapy. Care must be taken to ensure that normal skin is not injected with the medication.

Systemic Therapy. Systemic cytotoxic preparations, such as methotrexate, have been used in treating extensive psoriasis that fails to respond to other forms of therapy. Other systemic medications in current use include hydroxyurea (Hydrea) and cyclosporine A (CyA).

Methotrexate appears to function by inhibiting DNA synthesis in epidermal cells, thereby reducing the turnover time of the psoriatic epidermis. However, the medication can be very toxic, especially to the liver, which can suffer irreversible damage. Thus, laboratory studies must be monitored to ensure that the hepatic, hematopoietic, and renal systems are functioning adequately.

The patient should avoid drinking alcohol while on methotrexate, because this increases the possibility of liver damage. The medication is teratogenic (producing physical defects in the fetus) in pregnant women.

Hydroxyurea inhibits cell replication by affecting DNA synthesis. The patient is monitored for signs and symptoms of bone marrow depression.

Cyclosporine A, a cyclic peptide used to prevent rejection of transplanted organs, has shown some success in treating severe therapy-resistant cases of psoriasis. Its use, however, is limited by its side effects of hypertension and nephrotoxicity (Stiller, 1994).

Oral retinoids (synthetic derivatives of vitamin A and its metabolite, vitamin A acid) modulate the growth and differentiation of epithelial tissue and thus show great promise in treating the patient with severe psoriasis.

Photochemotherapy. A treatment for severely debilitating psoriasis is psoralen and ultraviolet-A (PUVA) light therapy, which involves the patient taking a photosensitizing medication (usually 8-methoxypsoralen) in a standard dose with subsequent exposure to long-wave ultraviolet light when medication plasma levels peak. Although the mechanism of action is not completely understood, it is thought that when psoralen-treated skin is exposed to ultraviolet-A light, the psoralen binds with DNA and decreases cellular proliferation. PUVA is not without its hazards; it has been associated with long-term risks of skin cancer, cataracts, and premature aging of the skin.

PUVA therapy requires that psoralen be taken orally and followed in 2 hours by irradiation with high-intensity, long-wave ultraviolet light. (Ultraviolet light is the portion of the electromagnetic spectrum containing wavelengths ranging from 180 to 400 nm.)

The PUVA unit consists of a light chamber containing high-output blacklight lamps and an external reflectance system. The exposure time is calibrated according to the specific unit in use and the anticipated tolerance of the patient's skin. The patient is usually treated two or three times a week until the psoriasis clears. An interim period of 48 hours between treatments is necessary, because it takes this long for any burns resulting from PUVA therapy to become evident.

After the psoriasis clears, the patient begins a maintenance program. Once little or no disease is active, less potent therapies are used to keep minor flare-ups under control.

Ultraviolet B (UVB) light therapy is also used to treat generalized plaque. It is combined with topical coal tar (Goeckerman therapy). Side effects are similar to those of PUVA therapy.

❑ NURSING PROCESS
The Patient With Psoriasis

Assessment

The nursing assessment focuses on how the patient is coping with the psoriatic skin condition, the appearance of the "normal" skin, and the appearance of the skin lesions (see "Clinical Manifestations," above). The major notable manifestations are red, scaling papules that coalesce to form oval, well-defined plaques. Silvery white scales are also present. Adjacent skin areas reveal red, smooth plaques with a macerated surface. It is important to examine the areas especially prone to psoriasis: elbows, knees, scalp, gluteal cleft, fingers, and toenails (for small pits).

The nurse should assess the impact of the disease on the patient and the coping strategies used for conducting normal activities and interactions with family and friends. Many patients need reassurance that the condition is not infectious, not a reflection of poor personal hygiene, and not a skin cancer.

Diagnosis

Nursing Diagnoses

Based on the nursing assessment data, the patient's major nursing diagnoses may include:

- ❑ Knowledge deficit of the disease process and treatment
- ❑ Impaired skin integrity related to lesions and inflammatory response
- ❑ Body image disturbance related to embarrassment over appearance and self-perception of uncleanliness

Collaborative Problems/ Potential Complications

Based on the assessment data, potential complications include:

- ❑ Psoriatic arthritis

Planning and Implementation

Goals. Major goals for the patient may include increased understanding of psoriasis and the treatment regimen, achievement of smoother skin with control of lesions, development of self-acceptance, and absence of complications

Nursing Interventions

Promoting Understanding. The nurse explains with sensitivity that currently there is no cure for psoriasis, that lifetime management is necessary, and that the condition can usually be cleared and controlled. The pathophysiology of psoriasis is reviewed as are the factors that provoke it: any irritation or injury to the skin (cut, abrasion, sunburn), any current illness (*e.g.*, pharyngeal streptococcal infection), and emotional stress. It is emphasized that repeated trauma to the skin as well as an unfavorable environment (*e.g.*, cold) or a specific medication (*e.g.*, lithium, beta blockers, indomethacin) may exacerbate psoriasis. The patient is cautioned about taking any nonprescribed medications because some may aggravate a mild psoriasis.

Reviewing and explaining the treatment regimen are essential to ensure compliance. For example, if the patient has a mild condition confined to localized areas, such as the elbows or knees, the application of an emollient to maintain softness and minimize sealing may be all that is required. On the other hand, if the patient uses anthralin, the dosage schedule, possible side effects, and problems to report to the nurse or physician need to be explained.

Most patients will need a more comprehensive plan of care that will range from using topical medications and shampoos to more complex and lengthy treatment with systemic medications and photochemotherapy, such as psoralens and ultraviolet-A (PUVA) therapy. Patient education sheets that include a description of the therapy and specific guidelines are helpful, but cannot replace the face-to-face discussion of the treatment plan. Table 54-6 summarizes current treatments.

Increasing Skin Integrity. To avoid injuring the skin, the patient should be advised not to pick or scratch the affected areas. Measures to prevent dry skin are encouraged since dry skin causes psoriasis to worsen. Too-frequent washing produces more soreness and scaling. Water should be warm, not hot, and the skin should be dried by patting with a towel rather than by vigorous rubbing. Emollients have a moisturizing effect, providing an occlusive body film on the skin surface so that normal water loss through the skin is halted, allowing the trapped water to hydrate the stratum corneum. A bath oil or emollient cleansing agent can give comfort to sore and scaling skin. Softening the skin can prevent fissures (see also Nursing Care Plan 54-1).

Improving Self-Concept and Body Image. A therapeutic relationship between health care professionals and the patient with psoriasis is one that includes both education and support. Once established, the patient should begin to feel more confident and empowered in carrying out the therapeutic regimen and in using coping strategies that help deal with the altered self-concept and body image brought about by the disease.

Introduction to successful coping strategies used by others with psoriasis and suggestions for reducing or coping with stressful situations at home, school, or work will facilitate a more positive outlook and acceptance of the chronic nature of the disease.

Patient Education and Home Care Considerations. Printed patient education materials may be provided to reinforce face-to-face discussions with the patient about treatment guidelines and other considerations. For example, the patient and the family caregiver may need to know that the topical agent anthralin will leave a brownish purple stain on the skin but that the discoloration will subside when anthralin treatment stops. Additionally they should be instructed to cover lesions treated with anthralin (with gauze, stockinette, or other soft coverings) to avoid staining clothing, furniture, or bed linens.

TABLE 54-6 Summary of Current Treatments for Psoriasis

Topical Agents	Use	Selected Agents
Coal tar products	Mild to moderate lesions	Coal tar and salicylic acid ointment, Aquatar, Estar gel, Fototar, anthralin (Anthra-Derm, Dritho-Creme), Neutrogena T/Derm, Psori Gel
Topical corticosteroids	Mild to moderate lesions	Aristocort, Kenalog, Trymex, betamethasone valerate (Betatrex, Beta-Val, Valisone)
	Lesions on face, groin, axillae	DesOwen, Tridesilon, Aclovate
Coal tar shampoos	Scalp lesions	Neutrogena T/Gel, Polytar, Zetar, Lasan (pomade), Danex, Head & Shoulders, Zincon, Selsun Blue, Capitrol, Bakers P&S (emulsifying agent with phenol, saline solution, and mineral oil)
Occlusive dressings	Body and limb lesions	Hydrocolloid occlusive dressings (Duoderm), Restore, plastic wrap over corticosteroids, Cordran (tape impregnated with corticosteroid flurandrenolide)
Intralesional therapy	Thick plaques	Kenalog-10 (only when other therapies fail), Cordran impregnated tape, Fluoroplex
	Nails	
Systemic therapy	Extensive lesions and nails	Methotrexate, methotrexate sodium (Folex, Mexate); hydroxyurea (Hydrea); retinoic acid, such as etretinate (Tegison) (not used for pregnant women or during childbearing age)
	Psoriatic arthritis	Oral gold (auranofin), etretinate, methotrexate
Phototherapy	Severe disease	UVA or UVB light with topical coal tar preparations (Goeckerman therapy); UVB light therapy with topical coal tar (Estar gel) (modified Goeckerman therapy); UVB light therapy and anthralin (Ingram therapy); photochemotherapy (PUVA) (combines UVA light and oral psoralen tablets or topical tripsoralen or methoxsalen)

Patients using topical corticosteroid preparations repeatedly on the face and around the eyes should be aware that cataract development is possible. Strict guidelines for applying these medications should be emphasized, because overuse can result in skin atrophy, striae (streaks), and medication resistance.

Tar preparations can be extremely messy and difficult to apply and are therefore not well accepted by most patients. As much as 2 hours or more may be needed to apply medications and carry out cosmetic efforts. Providing helpful tips on application and the expected outcome of the therapy will go a long way to ensuring compliance.

Photochemotherapy (PUVA), which is reserved for moderate to severe psoriasis, produces photosensitization, which means that the skin is sensitive to the sun until methoxsalen has been excreted from the body (in about 6 to 8 hours). Therefore, patients undergoing PUVA treatments should avoid exposure to the sun. If exposure is unavoidable, the skin must be protected with sunscreen and clothing. Gray or green tinted wraparound sunglasses should be worn to protect the eyes during and after treatment and ophthalmologic examinations should be performed on a regular basis. Nausea, which may be a problem in some patients, is lessened when methoxsalen is taken with food. Lubricants and bath oils may be used to help remove scales and prevent excess dryness. No other creams or oils are to be used except on areas that have been shielded from ultraviolet light. Contraceptives should be used by sexually active women of reproductive age, because the teratogenic effect of PUVA has not been established. The patient is kept under constant and careful supervision and is encouraged to recognize unusual changes in the skin.

If desired, patients may be referred to a mental health professional who can ease emotional strain and give support. Belonging to a support group may also help patients acknowledge that they are not alone in experiencing life adjustments in response to a visible, chronic disease. The National Psoriasis Foundation publishes periodic bulletins and reports about new and relevant developments in this condition (see Bibliography under "Agencies").

Monitoring and Managing Potential Complications

Psoriatic Arthritis. The diagnosis of psoriasis, especially when it is accompanied by the complication of arthritis, is usually difficult to make. Psoriatic arthritis involving the sacroiliac and distal joints of the fingers may be overlooked, especially if the patient presents with the typical psoriatic lesions well established (MacKie, 1991). On the other hand, patients who complain of mild joint discomfort and some pitting of their fingernails may not be diagnosed with psoriasis until the more obvious cutaneous lesions appear.

The complaint of joint discomfort in the patient with psoriasis should be noted and evaluated further. The symptoms of psoriatic arthritis can mimic the symptoms of Reiter's disease and ankylosing spondylitis. Therefore, a definitive diagnosis must be made. Treatment of the condition usually involves joint rest, application of heat, and salicylates (MacKie, 1991).

The patient will require education about the care and treatment of the involved joints and the need for compliance with therapy. The incidence of psoriatic arthropathy is not known since the symptoms are so variable. It is believed, however, that when the psoriasis is extensive and a family history of inflammatory arthritis is elicited, the chance of the patient developing psoriatic arthritis increases substantially. It is recommended that a rheumatologist be consulted and assist in the diagnosis and treatment of the arthropathy.

Evaluation

Expected Outcomes

1. Acquires knowledge and understanding of disease process and its treatment
   a. Describes psoriasis and the prescribed therapy
   b. Verbalizes that trauma, infection, and emotional stress may be trigger factors
   c. Maintains control with appropriate therapy
   d. Demonstrates proper application of topical therapy
2. Achieves smoother skin and control of lesions
   a. No new lesions appear
   b. Keeps skin lubricated and soft
3. Develops self-acceptance
   a. Identifies someone with whom to discuss feelings and concerns
   b. Expresses optimism about outcomes of treatment
4. Experiences no psoriatic arthritis
   a. No joint discomfort experienced
   b. Cutaneous lesions controlled with no extension of disease

Exfoliative Dermatitis

Exfoliative dermatitis is a serious condition characterized by a progressive inflammation in which erythema and scaling occur in a more or less generalized distribution. It may be associated with chills, fever, prostration, severe toxicity, and an itchy scaling of the skin. There is a profound loss of stratum corneum (outermost layer of the skin), which causes capillary leakage, hypoproteinemia, and negative nitrogen balance. Because of widespread dilation of cutaneous vessels, large amounts of body heat are lost. Thus, exfoliative dermatitis has a marked effect on the entire body.

Exfoliative dermatitis has a variety of causes. It is considered to be a secondary or reactive process to an underlying skin or systemic disease. It may appear as a part of the lymphoma group of diseases and may actually precede the appearance of lymphoma. Preexisting skin disorders that have been implicated as a cause include psoriasis, atopic dermatitis, and contact dermatitis. It also appears as a severe reaction to many medications, including penicillin and phenylbutazone. The etiology is unknown in approximately 25% of cases.

Clinical Manifestations

This condition starts acutely as either a patchy or a generalized erythematous eruption accompanied by fever, malaise, and, occasionally, gastrointestinal symptoms. The skin color changes from pink to dark red. After a week, the characteristic exfoliation (scaling) begins, usually in the form of thin flakes that leave the underlying skin smooth and red, with new scales forming as the older ones come off. Hair loss may accompany this disorder. Relapses are common. The systemic effects include high-output congestive heart failure, intestinal disturbances, breast enlargement, elevated levels of uric acid in the blood (hyperuricemia), and temperature disturbances.

Management

The objectives of management are to maintain fluid and electrolyte balance and to prevent infection. The treatment is individualized and supportive and should be initiated as soon as the condition is diagnosed.

The patient is hospitalized and placed on bed rest. All medications that may be implicated are discontinued. A comfortable room temperature should be maintained because the patient does not have normal thermoregulatory control as a result of temperature fluctuations caused by vasodilation and evaporative water loss. Fluid and electrolyte balance must be maintained because there is considerable water and protein loss from the skin surface. Plasma volume expanders may be indicated.

Continual nursing assessment is carried out to detect infection. The disrupted, erythematous, moist skin is susceptible to infection and becomes colonized with pathogenic organisms, which produce more inflammation. Antibiotics, prescribed if infection is present, are selected on the basis of culture and sensitivity.

- The patient is observed for signs and symptoms of congestive heart failure because hyperemia and increased cutaneous blood flow can produce cardiac failure of high-output origin.

Hypothermia may also occur because increased blood flow in the skin, coupled with increased water loss through the skin leads to heat loss by radiation, conduction, and evaporation. Changes in vital signs are closely monitored and reported.

As in any acute dermatitis, topical therapy is used to give symptomatic relief. Soothing baths, compresses, and lubrication with emollients are used to treat the extensive dermatitis. The patient is likely to be extremely irritable because of the severe itching. Oral or parenteral corticosteroids may be prescribed when the disease is not controlled by more conservative therapy. When a specific cause is known, more specific therapy may be used. The patient is advised to avoid all irritants in the future, particularly medications.

Pemphigus Vulgaris

Pemphigus vulgaris is a serious disease of the skin characterized by the appearance of bullae (blisters) of various sizes (*e.g.*, 1–10 cm) on apparently normal skin (Fig. 54-4) and mucous membranes (*e.g.*, mouth, vagina).

Available evidence indicates that pemphigus is an autoimmune disease involving IgG, an immunoglobulin. It is thought that the pemphigus antibody is directed against a specific cell-surface antigen in epidermal cells. A blister forms from the antigen-antibody reaction. The level of serum antibody is predictive of disease severity. Genetic factors may also play a role in its development, with the highest incidence in those of Jewish descent. This disorder usually occurs in men and women in middle and late adulthood.

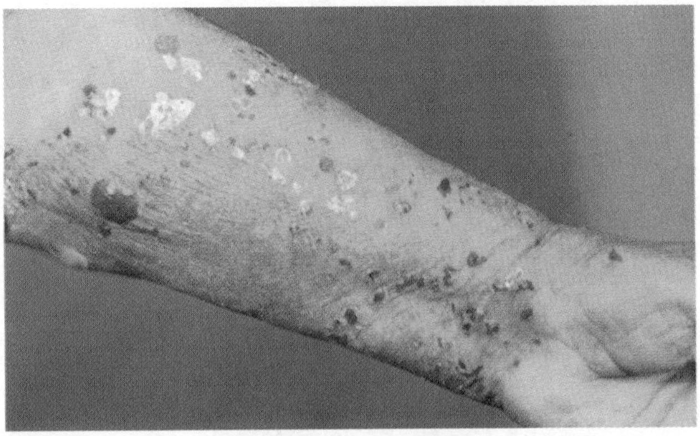

FIGURE 54-4. Pemphigus vulgaris blisters on the forearm. (Sauer GC. Manual of Skin Diseases, Philadelphia, JB Lippincott, 1991.)

Clinical Manifestations

Most patients initially present with oral lesions appearing as irregularly shaped erosions that are painful, bleed easily, and heal slowly. The skin bullae enlarge, rupture, and leave large, painful eroded areas that are accompanied by crusting and oozing. A characteristic offensive odor emanates from the bullae and the exuding serum. There is blistering or sloughing of uninvolved skin when minimal pressure is applied (Nikolsky's sign). The eroded skin heals slowly, so that eventually huge areas of the body are involved (Fig. 54-5). Bacterial superinfection is common.

Complications. The most common complications of pemphigus vulgaris arise when the disease process is widespread. Prior to the advent of corticosteroid and immunosuppressive therapy, the patient was very susceptible to secondary bacterial infection. Skin bacteria have relatively easy access to the bullae as they ooze, rupture, and leave denuded areas that are open to the environment.

Fluid and electrolyte imbalance results from the loss of both fluid and protein as the bullae rupture. Hypoalbuminemia is common when the disease process includes extensive areas of the body skin surface and mucous membranes.

Diagnostic Evaluation

A specimen from the blister and surrounding skin will demonstrate **acantholysis** (separation of epidermal cells from each other because of damage to or an abnormality of the intracellular substance). Circulating antibodies (pemphigus antibodies) may be detected by immunofluorescent studies of the patient's serum.

Management

The goals of therapy are to bring the disease under control as rapidly as possible, to prevent loss of serum and the development of secondary infection, and to promote reepithelialization of the skin (renewal of epithelial tissue).

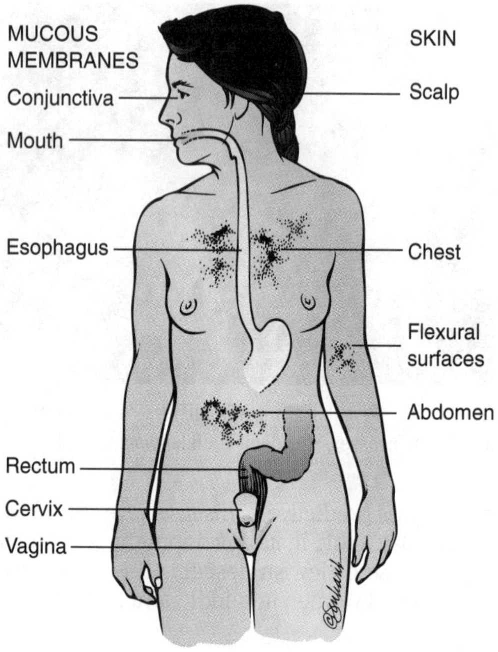

FIGURE 54-5. Distribution of lesions in pemphigus vulgaris.

Corticosteroids are administered in high doses to control the disease and keep the skin free of blisters. The high dosage level is maintained until remission is apparent. In some cases the corticosteroid therapy must be maintained for the lifetime of the individual.

Corticosteroids are administered with or immediately after a meal and may be accompanied by an antacid as prophylaxis against gastric complications. Essential to therapeutic management are daily evaluations of body weight, blood pressure, blood glucose levels, and fluid balance. (High-dosage corticosteroid therapy has its own serious toxic effects; see Chapter 40.)

Immunosuppressive agents (azathioprine, cyclophosphamide, gold) may be prescribed to help control the disease and reduce the corticosteroid dose. **Plasmapheresis** (plasma exchange) temporarily decreases the serum antibody level and has been used with variable success, although it is generally reserved for life-threatening cases.

❑ NURSING PROCESS
The Patient With Pemphigus Vulgaris

Assessment

Because patients with pemphigus vulgaris are usually hospitalized at one time or another during exacerbations of the disease, the nurse soon discovers that pemphigus may be a cause of significant disability. The constant discomfort and distress of the patient and foul odor of the lesions make effective assessment and nursing management a challenge.

Disease activity is monitored clinically by examining the skin for the appearance of new blisters, which are usually tense and not easily broken. The scalp, chest, and adjacent skin areas are examined for blistering. Areas where healing has occurred may show signs of hyperpigmentation. Particular attention is given to assessing for signs and symptoms of infection.

Diagnosis

Nursing Diagnoses

Based on nursing assessment data, the patient's major nursing diagnoses may include:

- Pain of oral cavity and skin related to blistering and erosions
- Impaired skin integrity related to ruptured bullae and denuded areas of the skin
- Anxiety and ineffective coping related to the appearance of the skin and no hope of a cure

Collaborative Problems/ Potential Complications

Based on the assessment data, potential complications include:

- Infection and sepsis related to loss of protective barrier of skin and mucous membranes
- Fluid volume deficit and electrolyte imbalance related to loss of tissue fluids

Planning and Implementation

Goals. The major goals of the patient may include relief of discomfort from lesions, skin healing, reduced anxiety and improve coping capacity, and absence of complications.

Nursing Interventions

Relieving Oral Discomfort. The patient's entire oral cavity may be affected with erosions and denuded surfaces. A necrotic slough may develop over these areas, adding to the patient's misery and interfering with food intake. Weight loss and hypoproteinemia may result. Meticulous oral hygiene is important to keep the oral mucosa clean and allow the epithelium to regenerate. Frequent mouth washes are prescribed to rinse the mouth of debris and to soothe ulcerative areas. Commercial mouth washes are avoided. The lips are kept moist with lanolin, petrolatum, or lip balm. Cool mist therapy is helpful to humidify environmental air.

Enhancing Skin Integrity. Cool, wet dressings or baths are protective and soothing. The patient with painful and extensive lesions should be premedicated with analgesics before skin care is initiated. Patients with large areas of blistering have a characteristic odor that decreases when secondary infection is controlled. After the patient's skin is bathed, it is dried carefully and dusted liberally with nonirritating powder, which enables the patient to move freely in bed. Fairly large amounts are necessary to keep the patient from sticking to the sheets. Tape should never be used on the skin because it may produce more blisters. Hypothermia is common, and measures to keep the patient warm and comfortable are priority nursing activities.

The nursing management of patients with bullous skin conditions is similar to that of patients with extensive burns (see Chapter 55).

Reducing Anxiety. Critical to the nursing management of the patient with pemphigus is the development of a trusting relationship. This encompasses the way the nurse listens, interacts, and demonstrates a warm and caring manner. The patient has legitimate concerns that may be reduced when the health team responds appropriately. The patient is encouraged to express anxieties, discomfort, and feelings of hopelessness freely. This is necessary for specific reassurance to be most effective.

Attention to the psychologic needs of the patient requires being available, giving expert nursing care, and educating the patient and the family. Arranging for a family member or a close friend to spend more time with the patient can be supportive. When patients receive information about the disease and its treatment, uncertainty and anxiety are reduced and the patient's capacity to act on his or her own behalf is enhanced.

A referral for psychologic counseling may be helpful to assist the patient in dealing with fears, anxiety, and depression.

Monitoring and Managing Potential Complications

Infection and Sepsis. The patient is susceptible to infection because the barrier function of the skin is compromised. Bullae are also susceptible to infection, and sepsis may follow. The skin is kept clean to eliminate debris and dead skin and to prevent infection.

Secondary infection may be accompanied by offensive odor from oral lesions. *Candida albicans* of the mouth is commonly seen in patients on high-dose corticosteroid therapy. The oral cavity should be inspected daily and any changes noted and reported. Oral lesions are slow to heal.

Infection is the leading cause of death. Particular attention is given to assessing the patient for signs and symptoms of local and systemic infection. "Trivial" complaints or minimal changes are investigated because corticosteroids mask or alter typical signs and symptoms of infection. The patient's vital signs are taken and temperature fluctuations monitored. The patient is observed for chills, and all secretions and excretions are monitored for changes suggestive of infection. Results of culture and sensitivity tests are followed. Antimicrobials are administered as prescribed, and response to treatment is noted. Health care personnel perform effective hand-washing techniques and use gloves.

Environmental contamination is avoided as much as possible by having the housecleaning personnel dust with a damp cloth and wash the floor with a wet mop. Protective isolation measures may be implemented, and universal precautions are used.

Fluid and Electrolyte Imbalance. Extensive denudation of the skin leads to fluid and electrolyte imbalance. There is significant loss of fluids and of sodium chloride from the skin. This sodium chloride loss is responsible for many of the systemic symptoms associated with the disease and is treated with administration of intravenous saline infusions.

A large amount of protein and blood is lost from the denuded skin areas. Blood component therapy may be prescribed to maintain the blood volume as well as the hemoglobin and plasma protein concentrations. Serum albumin, protein, hemoglobin, and hematocrit values are monitored.

The patient is encouraged to maintain adequate oral fluid intake. Cool, nonirritating fluids (*e.g.*, grape or apple juice) are encouraged to maintain hydration. Small, frequent meals or snacks of high-protein, high-calorie foods (Ensure, Sustacal, eggnogs, milkshakes) will help maintain nutritional status. Total parenteral nutrition is considered if the patient cannot eat an adequate diet.

Evaluation

Expected Outcomes

1. Achieves relief from pain of oral lesions
   a. Identifies therapies that reduce pain
   b. Uses mouth washes and anesthetic-antiseptic aerosol mouth spray
   c. Drinks chilled fluids at 2-hour intervals
2. Achieves skin healing
   a. States purpose of therapeutic regimen
   b. Cooperates with soaks/bath regimen
   c. Reminds personnel to use liberal amounts of nonirritating powder on bed linens
3. Experiences decreased anxiety and increased ability to cope
   a. Verbalizes concerns about condition, self, and relationships with others
   b. Participates in self-care
4. Experiences no infection
   a. Cultures from bullae, skin, and orifices are negative for pathogenic organisms
   b. Has no purulent drainage
   c. Shows signs that skin is clearing
   d. Has normal temperature
5. Attains fluid and electrolyte balance
   a. Keeps intake record to assure adequate fluid intake and normal fluid and electrolyte balance.
   b. Verbalizes an understanding of the necessity for intravenous infusion therapy
   c. Urine output within normal limits
   d. Has serum chemistry and hemoglobin and hematocrit values within normal limits

Toxic Epidermal Necrolysis

Toxic epidermal necrolysis (TEN) is a severe, potentially fatal skin disease and the most severe form of **erythema multiforme.** Mortality from TEN approaches 30% (Schopf et al., 1991). Its etiology is unknown, but it is probably linked to the immune system and may be a reaction to medications, or secondary to a viral infection. Antibiotics, anticonvulsants, butazones, and sulfonamides are the medications most frequently implicated in TEN.

Clinical Manifestations

TEN is characterized by initial signs of conjunctival burning or itching, cutaneous tenderness, fever, cough, sore throat, headache, extreme malaise, and myalgias (aches and pains). These signs are followed by a rapid onset of erythema (reddening of the skin), involving much of the skin surface and mucous membranes (oral mucosa, conjunctiva, and genitalia). In severe cases of mucosal involvement, there may be danger of damage to the larynx, bronchi, or esophagus from ulcerations (Stampien & Schwartz, 1992). Large, flaccid bullae develop in some areas; in other areas, large sheets of epidermis are shed, exposing the underlying dermis. Fingernails, toenails, eyebrows, and eyelashes may all be shed along with the surrounding epidermis. The skin is excruciatingly tender, and the loss of skin leaves a weeping surface similar to that of a total body second-degree burn; thus, the condition is also referred to as **scalded skin syndrome.**

Complications. Sepsis and keratoconjunctivitis are complications of TEN. Unrecognized and untreated sepsis can be life-threatening. Keratoconjunctivitis can impair vision and result in conjunctival retraction, scarring, and corneal lesions (Haus, Pacquet, & Marechal-Courtois, 1993).

Diagnostic Evaluation

Histologic studies of frozen skin cells from a fresh lesion and cytodiagnosis of collections of cellular material from a freshly denuded area are conducted. A history of ingestion of medications known to be implicated in precipitating TEN may verify medication reaction as the underlying cause.

Immunofluorescent studies may be performed to detect atypical epidermal autoantibodies. A genetic predisposition to erythema multiforme has been suggested, but is not confirmed for all cases (Stampien & Schwartz, 1992).

Management

The goals of treatment include control of fluid and electrolyte balance, prevention of sepsis, and prevention of ophthalmic complications. Supportive care is the mainstay of treatment.

All nonessential medications are discontinued immediately. If possible, the patient is treated in a regional burn center because aggressive treatment similar to that given for a severe burn is required. Skin loss may approximate 100% of the total body surface area. Surgical debridement or hydrotherapy in a Hubbard tank (a large steel tub) may be performed initially to remove involved skin.

Tissue samples are obtained from the nasopharynx, eyes, ears, blood, urine, skin, and unruptured blisters and cultured to identify the pathogenic organisms. Intravenous fluids are prescribed to maintain fluid and electrolyte balance, especially in the patient who has severe mucosal involvement and who cannot easily swallow nourishment. However, because an indwelling intravenous catheter may be the site of infection, fluid replacement is carried out by nasogastric tube and then orally as soon as possible.

Initial treatment with systemic corticosteroids is controversial. In some instances, experts think that early corticosteroid treatment will prevent cutaneous extension, whereas in other situations corticosteroids may cause significant systemic side effects and delay recovery (Stampien & Schwartz, 1992). In patients with TEN thought to result from a medication reaction, corticosteroids may be administered.

Protecting the skin with topical agents is crucial. Various topical antibacterial and anesthetic agents are used to prevent wound sepsis and to assist with pain management. Systemic antibiotic therapy is employed with extreme caution. Temporary biologic dressings (*e.g.*, pigskin, amniotic membrane) or plastic semipermeable dressings (Vigilon) may be used to reduce pain, decrease evaporation, and prevent secondary infection until the epithelium is renewed. Meticulous oropharyngeal and eye care is essential when there is severe involvement of the mucous membranes and the eye.

❑ NURSING PROCESS
The Patient With Toxic Epidermal Necrolysis

Assessment

A careful inspection of the skin is made, and its appearance and the extent of involvement of toxic epidermal necrolysis is noted. The normal skin is closely observed to determine if new areas of blisters are developing. Seepage from blisters is monitored for amount, color, and odor. Inspection of the oral cavity for blistering and erosive lesions is performed daily; the patient is assessed daily for itching, burning, and dryness of the eyes. The patient's ability to swallow and drink fluids, as well as speak normally, is determined.

The patient's vital signs are monitored and special attention is given to the presence and character of fever and the respiratory rate, depth, rhythm, and cough. The characteristics and amount of respiratory secretions are noted. Assessment for high fever, tachycardia, and extreme weakness and fatigue is essential, because these indicate the process of epidermal necrosis, increased metabolic needs, and possible gastrointestinal and respiratory mucosal sloughing. Urine volume, specific gravity, and color are monitored. The insertion sites of intravenous lines are inspected for signs of local infection. The patient's daily weights are recorded.

The patient is asked to describe fatigue and pain levels. An attempt is made to evaluate the patient's level of anxiety. The patient's basic coping mechanisms are assessed and effective coping strategies are identified.

Diagnosis

Nursing Diagnoses

Based on the assessment data, the patient's major nursing diagnoses may include:

- ❑ Impaired tissue integrity (oral, eye, and skin) related to epidermal shedding
- ❑ Fluid volume deficit and electrolyte losses related to loss of fluids from denuded skin
- ❑ Risk for altered body temperature (hypothermia) related to heat loss secondary to skin loss
- ❑ Pain related to denuded skin, oral lesions, and possible infection
- ❑ Anxiety related to the physical appearance of the skin and prognosis

Collaborative Problems/ Potential Complications

Based on the assessment data, potential complications that may develop include:

- ❑ Sepsis
- ❑ Conjunctival retraction, scars, and corneal lesions

Planning and Implementation

Goals. The major goals of the patient may include achievement of skin and oral tissue healing, attainment of fluid balance, prevention of heat loss, relief of pain, reduction of anxiety, and absence of complications.

Nursing Interventions

Maintaining Skin and Mucous Membrane Integrity. The local care of the skin is an important area of nursing management. The skin denudes easily, even when the patient is lifted and turned. It may be necessary to place the patient on a circular turning frame. The nurse applies the prescribed topical agents that reduce the bacterial population of the wound surface. Warm compresses, if prescribed, should be applied *gently* to denuded areas. The topical antibacterial agent may be used in conjunction with hydrotherapy in a tank, bathtub, or shower. The nurse monitors the patient's condition during the treatment and encourages the patient to exercise the extremities during the hydrotherapy.

The painful oral lesions make oral hygiene difficult. Careful oral hygiene is performed to keep the oral mucosa clean. Prescribed mouth washes, anesthetics, or coating agents are used frequently to rid the mouth of debris, soothe ulcerative areas, and control foul mouth odor. The oral cavity is inspected several times a day, and any changes are documented and reported. Petrolatum (or prescribed ointment) is applied to the lips.

Attaining Fluid Balance. The vital signs, urine output, and sensorium are observed for indications of hypovolemia. Mental changes from fluid and electrolyte imbalance, sensory overload, or sensory deprivation may occur. Laboratory test results are evaluated, and abnormal results are reported. The patient is weighed daily (with a bed scale if necessary).

The nurse regulates intravenous fluids at prescribed infusion rates and assesses for systemic (overinfusion or underinfusion) and local (infection) complications. Oral lesions may result in dysphagia, making tube feeding or total parenteral nutrition necessary. Prescribed enteral nourishment or enteral supplements can be administered by tube feeding until oral ingestion can be tolerated. Daily calorie count and accurate recording of all intake and output are essential.

Preventing Hypothermia. A patient with TEN is prone to chilling. Dehydration may be made worse by exposing the denuded skin to a continuous current of warm air. The patient is usually sensitive to room temperature changes. Measures implemented for a burn patient, such as cotton blankets, ceiling-mounted heat lamps, or heat shields, are useful in maintaining the patient's comfort and body temperature. To minimize shivering and heat loss, the nurse should work rapidly and efficiently when large wounds are exposed for wound care. The patient's temperature is carefully monitored.

Relieving Pain. The nurse assesses the patient's pain, its characteristics, any factors that influence the pain, and the patient's behavioral responses. Prescribed analgesics are administered, and the nurse observes and documents pain relief and any side effects. Analgesics are administered before performing painful treatments. Thorough explanations and speaking soothingly to the patient during treatments can allay the anxiety that may intensify pain. Emotional support and reassurance and implementing measures that promote rest and sleep are basic in achieving pain control. As the pain diminishes and the patient has more physical and emotional energy, self-management techniques for pain relief, such as progressive muscle relaxation and imagery, may be taught.

Reducing Anxiety. Because the lifestyle of patients with TEN has been abruptly changed to one of complete dependence, an assessment of their emotional state may reveal anxiety, depression, and fear of dying. Patients can be reassured that these reactions are normal. Then they need nursing support, honest communication, and hope that their situation can improve. They are encouraged to express their feelings to someone they trust. Listening to their concerns and being readily available with skillful and compassionate care are important anxiety-relieving interventions.

Emotional support by a psychiatric nurse, chaplain, psychologist, or psychiatrist may be invaluable for promoting coping during the long recovery period.

Monitoring and Managing Potential Complications

Sepsis. The major cause of death from TEN is infection, and the most common sites of infection are the skin and mucosal surfaces, lungs, and blood. The organisms most involved are *Staphylococcus aureus, Pseudomonas, Klebsiella, Escherichia coli, Serratia, and Candida.* Close monitoring of vital signs and noting any adverse changes in respiratory, renal, or gastrointestinal function may quickly detect the beginning of an infection. Strict asepsis is always maintained during the performance of routine skin care measures. Hand washing and wearing sterile gloves when carrying out procedures are necessary at all times. When the condition involves a large portion of the body, the patient should be in a private room to prevent possible cross-infection from other patients. Visitors should wear protective garments and wash their hands before coming into contact with the patient. Persons with any infectious disease should not visit the patient until they are no longer a danger to the patient.

Conjunctival Retraction, Scars, and Corneal Lesions. The eyes are inspected daily for signs of itching, burning, and dryness which may indicate progression of TEN to keratoconjunctivitis, the principal eye complication. Applying a cool, damp cloth over the eyes may relieve burning sensations. The eyes are kept clean and observed for signs of discharge or discomfort and the progression of symptoms is documented and reported. Administering an eye lubricant, when prescribed, may alleviate dryness and prevent corneal abrasion. Using eye patches or reminding the patient periodically to blink may also counteract dryness. The patient is instructed to avoid rubbing the eyes or putting any medication into the eyes that has not been prescribed or approved by the physician.

Evaluation

Expected Outcomes

1. Achieves increasing skin and oral tissue healing
   a. Demonstrates areas of healing skin
   b. Swallows fluids and speaks clearly

2. Attains fluid balance
   a. Demonstrates laboratory values within normal ranges
   b. Maintains urine volume and specific gravity within acceptable range
   c. Shows stable vital signs
   d. Increases intake of oral fluids without discomfort
   e. Gains weight, if appropriate
3. Attains thermoregulation
   a. Body temperature within normal range
   b. Reports no chills
4. Reports lessening of pain intensity
   a. Uses analgesics as prescribed
   b. Uses self-management techniques for relief of pain
5. Appears less anxious
   a. Discusses concerns freely
   b. Sleeps for progressively longer periods
6. Experiences no complication, such as sepsis and impaired vision
   a. Body temperature within normal range
   b. Laboratory values within normal ranges
   c. Has no abnormal discharges or signs of infection
   d. Continues to see objects at baseline acuity level
   e. Shows no signs of keratoconjunctivitis

Ulcers and Benign Tumors of the Skin

Ulcerations

The superficial loss of surface tissue due to death of the cells is called an ulceration. A simple ulcer, such as the kind found in a small, superficial, second-degree burn, tends to heal by **granulation** (new tissue granules) if kept clean and protected from injury. If it is exposed to the air, the serum that escapes will dry and form a scab, under which the epithelial cells will grow and cover the surface completely. Certain diseases cause characteristic ulcers—tuberculous ulcers and syphilitic ulcers are examples.

Ulcers Caused by Deficient Arterial Circulation. Ulcers related to problems with arterial circulation are seen in patients with peripheral vascular disease, arteriosclerosis, Raynaud's disease, and frostbite. In these patients, the treatment of the ulceration must be carried out in conjunction with the treatment of the arterial disease. The danger is from secondary infection. Frequently, amputation of the part is the only effective therapy. (For further detail about problems of arterial circulation see Chapter 31.)

Pressure Ulcers. Pressure ulcers result from continuous pressure on a particular area of the skin (see Chapter 18).

Tumors of the Skin

Cysts

Cysts of the skin are epithelium-lined cavities containing fluid or solid material.

Epidermal cysts (epidermoid) occur frequently and may be described as slow-growing, firm, elevated tumors found most frequently on the face, neck, upper chest, and back. Removal of the cysts provides cure.

Pilar cysts (trichilemmal cysts), originally called sebaceous cysts, are most frequently found on the scalp. They apparently originate from the middle portion of the hair follicle and from the cells of the outer hair root sheath. The treatment is surgical removal.

Benign Tumors

Seborrheic Keratoses. These tumors are benign, wartlike lesions of varying size and color, ranging from light tan to black. They are usually located on the face, shoulders, chest, and back and are the most common skin tumors seen in middle-aged and elderly persons. They may be cosmetically unacceptable to the patient, and a black keratosis may be erroneously diagnosed as malignant melanoma. The treatment is removal of the tumor tissue by excision, by electrodesiccation, and curettage, or by applying carbon dioxide or liquid nitrogen.

Actinic keratoses are premalignant skin lesions that develop in chronically sun-exposed areas of the body. They appear as rough, scaly patches with underlying erythema. These lesions may gradually transform into cutaneous squamous cell carcinoma.

Verrucae (Warts). Warts are common benign skin tumors caused by infection with the human papilloma virus that belongs to the DNA virus group. All age groups may be affected, but the condition occurs most frequently between ages 12 and 16 years. There are many types of warts.

As a rule, warts are asymptomatic, except when they occur on weight-bearing areas, such as the soles of the feet. They may be treated with locally applied laser therapy, liquid nitrogen, salicylic acid plasters, electrodesiccation, or cantharidin.

Venereal Warts. Warts occurring on the genitalia and perianal areas are known as *condyloma acuminata* and have been shown to be sexually transmitted. These are treated with podophyllin in tincture of benzoin, which is applied to the wart and washed off later. Other treatment modalities include liquid nitrogen, cryosurgery, electrosurgery, and curettage.

Angiomas (Birthmarks). Birthmarks are benign vascular tumors involving the skin and the subcutaneous tissues. They may occur as flat, violet-red patches (port-wine angiomas) or as raised, bright red, nodular lesions (strawberry angiomas). The latter have a tendency to involute spontaneously. Port-wine angiomas, on the other hand, usually persist indefinitely. Most patients use masking cosmetics (Covermark or Dermablend) to camouflage the defect. The argon laser is being used on various angiomas with some success.

Pigmented Nevi (Moles). Moles are common skin tumors of various sizes and shades, ranging from yellowish brown to black. They may be flat, macular lesions or elevated papules or nodules that occasionally contain hair. The great majority of pigmented nevi are harmless lesions. However, in rare cases, malignant changes supervene and a melanoma develops at the site of the nevus. Some authorities feel that all congenital moles should be removed, because these may have a higher incidence of malignant change. Nevi that show a change in color or size or become symptomatic (itch) or develop irregular borders should be removed to determine if malignant changes have occurred. Moles that occur in unusual places should be examined carefully for any irregularity and for notching of the border and variation in color. (Early melanomas may frequently show some redness and irritation and areas of bluish pigmentation where the pigment-containing cells have become deeper in the skin.) Nevi larger than 1 cm should be examined carefully. Excised nevi should be examined histologically.

Keloids. Keloids are benign overgrowths of fibrous tissue at the site of a scar or trauma. They appear to be more common among dark-skinned persons. Keloids are asymptomatic but may cause disfigurement and cosmetic concern. The treatment, which is not always satisfactory, consists of surgical excision, intralesional corticosteroid therapy, and radiation.

Dermatofibroma. A dermatofibroma is a common benign tumor of connective tissue that occurs predominantly on the extremities. It is a firm, dome-shaped papule or nodule that may be skin-colored or have a pinkish brown hue. Excisional biopsy is the recommended method of treatment.

Neurofibromatosis (von Recklinghausen's Disease). Neurofibromatosis is a hereditary condition manifested by pigmented patches (café-au-lait macules), axillary freckling, and cutaneous neurofibromas that vary in size. Developmental changes may occur also in the nervous system, muscles, and bone. Malignant degeneration of the neurofibromas may occur in some patients.

Cancer of the Skin

Skin cancer is the most common form of cancer in the United States. If it continues at the present rate, an estimated one of eight fair-skinned Americans may develop skin cancer, especially basal cell carcinoma. Because the skin is easily inspected, skin cancer is readily seen and detected and is the most successfully treated type of cancer.

Causes and Prevention

Exposure to the sun is the leading cause of skin cancer; incidence is related to the total amount of exposure to the sun. Sun damage is cumulative, and harmful effects may be severe by age 20. The increase in skin cancer is probably due to changing lifestyles and the emphasis on sunbathing and related activities. Protective measures should be used throughout life.

Persons who do not produce sufficient melanin (pigment) in the skin to protect underlying tissue are very susceptible to sun damage. Those at greatest risk are fair, blue-eyed, red-haired persons of Celtic ancestry, or persons with ruddy or light complexions, as well as those who suffer prolonged sunburn and do not tan.

Others at risk are outdoor workers (such as farmers, sailors, fishermen) and people who are exposed to the sun over a period of time. Elderly persons with sun-damaged skin are also at risk, as are persons who have had a history of x-ray treatment for acne or benign skin lesions.

Workers exposed to certain chemical agents (arsenic, nitrates, coal, tar and pitch, oils and paraffins) are also included in the risk group. People who have scars from severe burns may develop skin cancer 20 to 40 years later. Squamous cell cancer can develop in areas of chronically draining osteomyelitis because neoplastic changes can develop in the fistulae. Longtime ulcers of the lower extremity may be the site of origin of skin cancer. In fact, any condition causing scarring or chronic irritation may lead to cancer. Immunosuppressed patients have an increased incidence of malignant skin tumors. Genetic factors are also involved.

Environmental Factors. Changes in the ozone layer from the effects of worldwide industrial air pollutants, such as chlorofluorocarbons, have prompted concern that skin cancers, especially malignant melanoma, will increase in incidence. The ozone is a thin and variable stratospheric layer of bluish, explosive gas formed by the sun's ultraviolet radiation on an allotropic form of oxygen. The ozone layer is known to vary in depth with the seasons and is thickest at the North and South Poles and thinnest at the equator. It is believed that it helps protect the earth from the effects of solar ultraviolet radiation. Proponents of this theory predict an increase in skin cancers as a consequence of changes in the ozone layer. Further research should disclose whether ozone destruction is a viable concern and a potential health hazard.

Types of Skin Cancer

The most common types of skin cancer are basal cell carcinoma, squamous cell (epidermoid) carcinoma, and malignant melanoma.

Clinical Manifestations

Basal cell carcinoma (BCC) arises from the basal cell layer of the epidermis or the hair follicles. This is the most common type of skin cancer. It generally appears on the sun-exposed areas of the body and is more prevalent in regions where the population is subjected to intense and extensive exposure to the sun. The incidence is proportional to the age of the patient (average age 60) and the total amount of sun exposure and is inversely proportional to the amount of melanin pigment in the skin. (See Chart 54-3 for skin cancer prevention guidelines.)

BCC usually begins as a small, waxy nodule with rolled, translucent, pearly borders; telangiectatic vessels may be present. As it grows, it undergoes central ulceration and sometimes crusting (Fig. 54-6). The tumors appear most frequently on the face. Basal cell carcinoma is characterized by invasion and erosion of contiguous (adjoining) tissues. It rarely metastasizes, but recurrence is common. However, a neglected lesion can account for the loss of a nose, an ear, or a lip. Other lesions of this disease may appear as shiny, flat, gray, or yellowish plaques.

Squamous cell carcinoma (SCC) is a malignant proliferation arising from the epidermis. Although it usually appears on sun-damaged skin, it may arise from normal skin or from preexisting skin lesions. It is of greater concern than basal cell carcinoma because it is a truly invasive

CHART 54-3
Patient Education: Preventing Skin Cancer

Because skin cancer rates are rising, taking preventive measures such as the ones outlined below may help individuals avoid increasing their skin cancer risk.

- Do not try to tan if your skin burns easily, never tans, or tans poorly.
- Avoid unnecessary exposure to the sun, especially during times when ultraviolet radiation (sunlight) is most intense (10 AM to 3 PM).
- *Do not become sunburned.*
- Apply a protective sunscreen if you must be in the sun; sunscreens block out harmful sun rays.
- Use a sunscreen with an SPF of 15 or higher. Sunscreens are rated in strengths from 4 (weakest) to above 15 (ultra sun protection). This is called SPF (solar protection factor) and is printed on the bottle.
- Reapply water-resistant sunscreens after swimming or during prolonged sun exposure.
- Avoid oils. Applied before or during sun exposure, oils do *not* protect against sunburn or sun damage.
- Use a lip balm that contains a sunscreen with the highest SPF number.
- Wear appropriate protective clothing (*e.g.*, broad-brimmed hat, long-sleeved clothing). However, clothing does not provide complete protection, because up to 50% of the sun's damaging rays can go through clothes. Ultraviolet rays also penetrate clouds.
- Do not use sun lamps for indoor tanning; avoid commercial tanning booths.
- Caution children, especially those with fair skin, to avoid excessive exposure to the sun and to use a sunscreen to prevent later skin cancers.

carcinoma metastasizing by the blood or lymphatic system. Metastases account for 75% of deaths from SCC. The lesions may be primary, arising on both the skin and mucous membranes, or may develop from a precancerous condition, such as actinic keratosis (lesions occurring in sun-exposed areas), leukoplakia (premalignant lesion of the mucous membrane), or scarred or ulcerated lesions. It appears as a rough, thickened, scaly tumor that may be asymptomatic or may involve bleeding (Fig. 54-7). The border of the lesion may be wider, more infiltrated, and more inflammatory than that of basal cell carcinoma. Secondary infection can occur. Exposed areas, especially of the upper extremities and of the face, lower lip, ears, nose, and forehead, are common sites.

Skin cancer is diagnosed by biopsy and histologic evaluation.

Metastases. The incidence of metastases is related to the histologic type and the level or depth of invasion. Usually, tumors arising in sun-damaged areas are less invasive and rarely cause death, whereas SCC arising without a history of sun or arsenic exposure or scar formation appears to have a greater chance of metastatic spread. The patient should be evaluated subsequently for regional lymph node metastases.

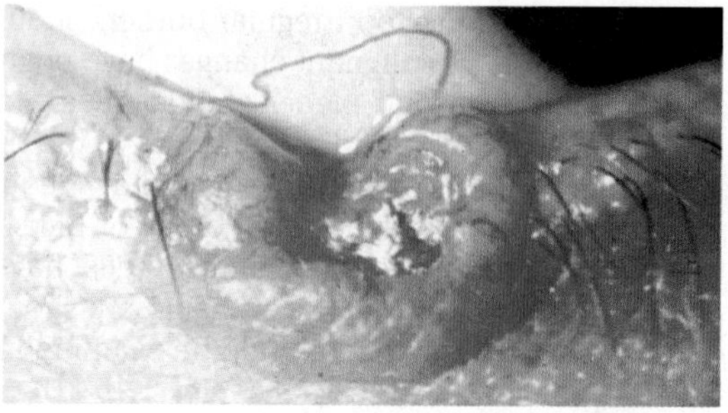

FIGURE 54-6. Basal cell carcinoma. (Bates B. A Guide to Physical Examination and History Taking, 6th ed. Philadelphia, JB Lippincott, 1995.)

Management

The goal of treatment is to eradicate or completely destroy all the tumor. The method of treatment depends on the tumor location, the cell type (location and depth), the cosmetic desires of the patient, the history of previous treatment, whether or not the tumor is invasive, and the presence or absence of metastatic nodes.

The management of basal cell and squamous cell carcinomas includes surgical excision, Mohs' micrographic surgery, electrosurgery, cryosurgery, and radiation therapy.

Surgical Excision. The primary goal is to remove the tumor entirely. The best way to maintain cosmetic appearance is to properly place the incision along natural skin tension lines and natural anatomic body lines. In this way, scars are less noticeable. The size of the incision will depend on tumor size and location but usually involves a length-to-width ratio of 3:1.

The adequacy of the surgical excision is verified by microscopic evaluation of sections of the specimen. When the tumor is large, reconstructive surgery with use of a skin flap or skin grafting may be required. The incision is closed in layers to enhance cosmetic effect. A pressure dressing applied over the wound provides support. Infection following a simple excision is uncommon if proper surgical asepsis is maintained during and after the procedure.

Moh's Micrographic Surgery. Mohs' micrographic surgery (MMS) is the most accurate and the most conserving of normal tissue for removing malignant cutaneous lesions. When the surgical technique was first introduced,

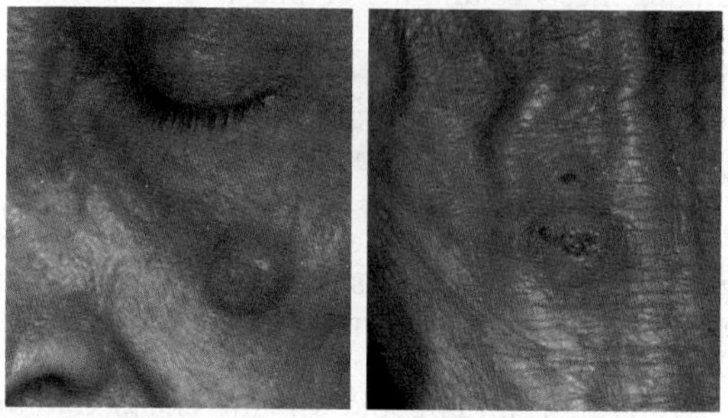

FIGURE 54-7. Squamous cell carcinoma on the face and back of the hand. (Bates B. A Guide to Physical Examination and History Taking, 6th ed. Philadelphia, JB Lippincott, 1995.)

the excision followed an application of zinc chloride paste to the tumor (chemosurgery). Currently, MMS is performed without the initial chemosurgery component. The procedure requires that the tumor be removed layer by layer. The first layer excised includes all evident tumor and a small margin of normal-appearing tissue. The specimen is frozen and analyzed by section to determine if all the tumor has been removed. It not, additional layers of tissue are removed and examined until all tissue margins are tumor-free.

In this manner, only tumor and a safe normal-tissue margin are removed; thus, MMS is the recommended tissue-sparing procedure. Cure rates for both basal cell carcinoma and squamous cell carcinoma with MMS approach 99%; thus, it is the treatment of choice. This surgical technique is also the most effective for tumors that occur around the eyes, nose, upper lip, and auricular and periauricular areas.

Electrosurgery. Electrosurgery is the destruction or removal of tissue by electrical energy. The current is converted to heat, which then passes to the tissue from a cold electrode. Electrosurgery may be preceded by curettage, which is carried out by excising the skin tumor by scraping its surface with a curette. Electrodesiccation is then implemented to achieve hemostasis and to destroy any viable malignant cells at the base of the wound or along its edges. Electrodesiccation is useful for small lesions (smaller than 1–2 cm [0.4–0.8 in] wide).

This method takes advantage of the fact that the tumor in each instance is softer than surrounding skin and therefore can be outlined by a curette, which "feels" the extent of the tumor. The tumor is removed and the base cauterized. The process is repeated three times. Usually, healing occurs within a month.

Cryosurgery. Cryosurgery destroys the tumor by deep-freezing. A thermocouple needle apparatus is inserted into the skin, and liquid nitrogen is directed to the center of the tumor until a temperature of –40°C to –60°C is reached at the tumor base. Liquid nitrogen has the advantage of having the lowest boiling point of all cryogens tried, is inexpensive, and is easy to obtain.

The tumor tissue is frozen, allowed to thaw, and then refrozen. The site thaws naturally and then becomes gelatinous and heals spontaneously. Swelling and edema follow the freezing. The appearance of the lesion varies. Normal healing, which may take 4 to 6 weeks, occurs faster in areas with a good blood supply.

Radiation Therapy. Radiation therapy is frequently performed for cancer of the eyelid, the tip of the nose, and areas in or near vital structures (*e.g.*, facial nerve). It is reserved for older patients, because x-ray changes may be seen after 5 to 10 years and malignant changes in scars may be induced by x-rays 15 to 30 years later.

The patient should be informed that the skin may become red and blistered. A bland skin ointment (prescribed by the physician) may be applied to relieve discomfort. The patient should also be cautioned against exposure to the sun.

Nursing Interventions

Because many skin cancers are removed by excision, patients are usually treated in outpatient surgical units. The role of the nurse is that of teaching the patient postoperative self-care activities.

The wound is usually (but not always) covered with a dressing to protect the site from physical trauma, external irritants, and contaminants. The patient is advised when to report for a dressing change or is given written and verbal information on how to change dressings—including what type of dressing to purchase, how to remove dressings and apply fresh ones, and the importance of hand washing before and after the procedure.

The patient is advised to watch for excessive bleeding and tight dressings that compromise circulation. If the lesion is in the perioral area, the patient is instructed to drink liquids through a straw and limit excess talking and facial movement.

After the sutures are removed, an emollient cream may be used to help reduce dryness. Applying a sunscreen over the wound is advised to prevent postoperative hyperpigmentation if the patient spends time outdoors.

Patient Education. The follow-up treatment should be regular, including palpation of the adjacent lymph nodes. Additionally, the patient should be instructed to seek treatment for any moles that are subject to repeated friction and irritation and to watch for indications of potential malignancy in moles (such as increase in size, ulceration, bleeding, or exudation). Another point to emphasize is the importance of follow-up evaluations throughout the lifetime.

Malignant Melanoma

A malignant melanoma is a malignant neoplasm in which atypical **melanocytes** (pigment cells) are present in both the epidermis and the dermis (and sometimes the subcutaneous cells). It is the most lethal of all the skin cancers and is responsible for about 2% of all cancer deaths.

It can occur in one of several forms: superficial spreading melanoma, lentigo-maligna melanoma, nodular melanoma, and acral-lentiginous melanoma. These types have certain clinical and histologic features as well as different biologic behaviors. Most melanomas derive from cutaneous epidermal melanocytes, but some appear in preexisting nevi (moles) in the skin or develop in the uveal tract of the eye. Melanomas frequently appear simultaneously with cancer of other organs.

The incidence of melanoma doubles every 10 years, a rise that is probably related to increased recreational sun exposure and better methods of early detection. Peak incidence occurs between ages 20 and 45. The incidence of melanoma is increasing faster than that of almost any other cancer, and the mortality rate is increasing faster than that of any other cancer except lung cancer.

Etiology and Risk Factors

The etiology is unknown, but ultraviolet rays are a strongly suspected cause. In general, at greatest risk are persons with fair complexions, blue eyes, red or blonde hair, and freckles. These persons synthesize melanin more slowly. Persons of Celtic or Scandinavian origin are at greater risk as well as persons who burn and do not tan. In areas where sunlight is intense, there is a disproportionate increase in incidence. Older Americans retiring to the southwestern United States appear to have a higher incidence. Others at risk have had a melanoma in the past, have a family history of melanoma, have giant congenital nevi, or have a significant history of severe sunburn.

Up to 10% of melanoma patients are members of melanoma-prone families who have multiple changing moles (dysplastic nevi) that are susceptible to malignant transformation. Persons with **dysplastic nevus syndrome** have been found to have unusual moles, larger and more numerous moles, lesions with irregular outlines, and pigmentation located all over the skin. Microscopic examination of dysplastic moles shows disordered, faulty growth.

Clinical Manifestations

The **superficial spreading melanoma** occurs anywhere on the body and is the most common form of melanoma. It usually affects persons of middle age and occurs most frequently on the trunk and lower extremities. The lesion tends to be circular with irregular outer portions. The margins of the lesion may be flat or elevated and palpable (Fig. 54-8, left). This type of melanoma may appear in a combination of colors, with hues of tan, brown, and black mixed with gray, bluish black, or white. Sometimes there is a dull pink rose color in a small area within the lesion.

The **lentigo-maligna melanomas** are slowly evolving, pigmented lesions that occur on exposed skin areas, especially the dorsum of the hand, the head, and neck in elderly people. Often the lesions are present for many years before they are examined by the physician. They first appear as tan, flat lesions and in time undergo changes in size and color.

The **nodular melanoma,** the second most common type, is a spherical, blueberry-like nodule with a relatively smooth surface and relatively uniform, blue-black color (Fig. 54-8, right). It may be dome-shaped with a smooth surface. It may have other shadings of red, gray, or purple. Sometimes nodular melanomas appear as irregularly shaped plaques. The patient may describe this as a blood blister that fails to resolve. A nodular melanoma invades directly into adjacent dermis (vertical growth) and hence has a poorer prognosis.

Acral-lentiginous melanoma is a form of melanoma that occurs in areas not excessively exposed to sunlight and where hair follicles are absent. It is found on the palms of the hands, on the soles, in the nail beds, and in the mucous membranes in dark-skinned persons. These melanomas appear as irregular, pigmented macules that develop nodules. They may become invasive early.

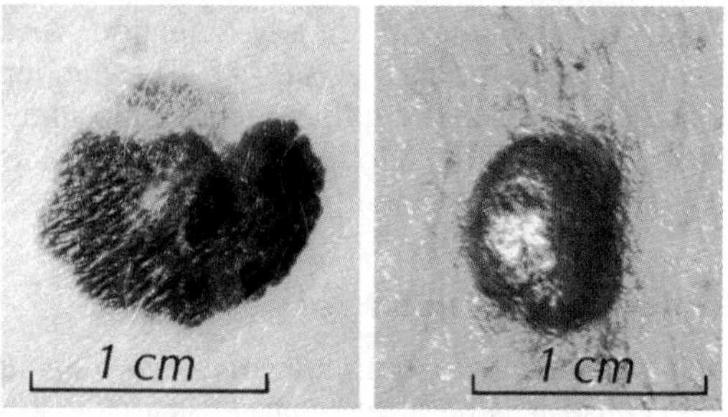

FIGURE 54-8. Two forms of malignant melanoma: superficial spreading (**left**) and nodular (**right**). (Bates B. A Guide to Physical Examination and History Taking, 6th ed. Philadelphia, JB Lippincott, 1995.)

Diagnostic Evaluation

Biopsy results confirm the diagnosis of melanoma. An excisional biopsy specimen reveals histologic information on the type, level of invasion, and thickness of the lesion. An excisional biopsy specimen that includes a 1-cm margin of normal tissue and a portion of underlying subcutaneous fatty tissue is sufficient for staging either a melanoma in situ or an early, noninvasive melanoma. Incisional biopsy should be performed when the suspicious lesion is too large to safely remove without extensive scarring (Runkle & Zalonznik, 1994). Biopsy specimens obtained by shaving, curettage, or needle aspiration are not considered reliable histologic proof of disease.

A thorough history and physical examination is very important in the diagnostic process. The examination should include not only a thorough skin examination, but also palpation of regional lymph nodes that drain the lesional area. Because melanoma occurs in families, a positive family history of melanoma is investigated so that first-degree relatives, who may be at high risk of developing melanoma, can be evaluated for atypical lesions. A chest x-ray, complete blood count (CBC), liver function tests, and radionuclide or computed tomography (CT) scans are usually ordered when metastatic disease is suspected.

Prognosis. The prognosis for long-term (5-year) survival is considered poor when the lesion exceeds 4 mm in thickness. The prognosis for patients with melanoma on the hand, foot, or scalp is bleak as well. These patients have an increased chance of metastasis. Metastases from a melanoma tend to occur in bone, liver, lungs, spleen, central nervous system, and lymph nodes (Runkle & Zalonznik, 1994). Men and elderly patients with melanoma tend to have a poorer prognosis.

Management

The therapeutic approach to malignant melanoma depends on the level of invasion and the depth of the lesion. Surgical excision is the treatment of choice for small, superficial lesions. Deeper lesions require wide local excision, after which skin grafting may be needed. A regional lymph node dissection is commonly performed to rule out metastasis.

❑ NURSING PROCESS
The Patient With Malignant Melanoma

Assessment

An assessment of the patient with malignant melanoma is based on the patient's history and symptoms. The patient is asked specifically about pruritus, tenderness, and pain, which are *not* features of a benign nevus. The patient is also questioned about changes in preexisting moles or the development of new, pigmented lesions. Persons at risk are assessed carefully.

A magnifying lens and good lighting are needed for inspecting the skin for **irregularity** and **changes** in the mole. Signs that suggest malignant changes include the following:

1. *Variegated color*
   a. Colors that may indicate malignancy in a brown or black lesion are shades of red, white, and blue; shades of blue are considered ominous.
   b. White areas within a pigmented lesion are suspicious.
   c. Some malignant melanomas are not variegated but instead are uniformly colored (bluish black, bluish gray, bluish red).
2. *Irregular border*
   a. Angular indentation or notch in the border of the mole is noted.
3. *Irregular surface*
   a. Uneven elevations of the surface (irregular topography) may be palpable or visible. The change in the surface may be from smooth to scaly.
   b. Some nodular melanomas have a smooth surface.

The common sites of melanomas are the skin of the back, the legs (especially in women), between toes and on the feet, face, scalp, fingernails, and backs of hands. In dark-skinned persons, melanomas are most likely to occur in the less pigmented sites: palms, soles, subungual areas, and mucous membranes.

The diameter of the mole is measured, because melanomas are commonly larger than 6 mm. Satellite lesions (those situated near the mole) are noted.

Diagnosis

Nursing Diagnoses

Based on the nursing assessment data, the patient's major nursing diagnoses may include:

- Pain related to surgical excision and grafting
- Anxiety and depression related to possible life-threatening consequences of melanoma and disfigurement
- Knowledge deficit about early signs of melanoma

Collaborative Problems/ Potential Complications

Based on the assessment data, potential complications that may develop include:

- Metastasis

Planning and Implementation

Goals. The major goals of the patient may include relief of pain and discomfort, reduction of anxiety, knowledge of early signs of melanoma, and absence of complications.

Nursing Interventions

Relieving Pain and Discomfort. Surgical removal of melanoma in different locations (head and neck, eye, trunk, abdomen, extremities, central nervous system) presents different challenges, taking into consideration the removal of the primary melanoma, the intervening lymphatic vessels, and the lymph nodes to which metastases may spread. Nursing management of the patient having surgery in these regions is discussed in the appropriate chapters.

Nursing intervention following surgery for a malignant melanoma centers on promoting comfort, because wide excision surgery may be necessary. A split-thickness or full-thickness skin graft may be necessary when large defects are created by surgical removal of a melanoma. Anticipating the need for and administering appropriate analgesic medication are important.

Reducing Anxiety. Psychologic support is essential when disfiguring surgery is performed. Support includes allowing patients to express feelings about the seriousness of this cutaneous neoplasm, understanding their anger and depression, and conveying understanding of these feelings. During the diagnostic workup and staging of the depth, type, and extent of the tumor, the nurse answers questions, clarifies information, and helps clear up misconceptions. Learning that they have a melanoma can cause patients considerable fear and anguish. Pointing out patients' resources, past effective coping mechanisms, and social support systems helps them to cope with the problems associated with diagnosis, treatment, and continuing follow-up.

Patient Education and Home Care Considerations. The best hope of controlling the disease lies in educating patients regarding the *early* signs of melanoma. Patients at risk are taught to examine their skin and scalp monthly in an orderly manner (Chart 54-4).

- A key factor in the development of malignant melanoma is exposure to sunlight.

Monitoring and Managing Potential Complications

Metastasis. The prognosis of malignant melanoma is related to the depth of dermal invasion and the thickness of the lesion. The deeper and thicker (>4 mm) the melanoma, the greater the likelihood of metastasis. If the melanoma is growing radially (horizontally) and is characterized by peripheral growth with minimal or no dermal invasion, the prognosis is favorable. When the melanoma progresses to the vertical growth phase (decimal invasion), the prognosis is poor. Lesions with ulceration correlate with a poor prognosis. Malignant melanoma can spread via both the bloodstream and the lymphatic system and can metastasize to any organ of the body, but especially to the lungs, liver, and bones. Melanomas of the trunk appear to have a poorer prognosis than those of other sites, perhaps because the network of lymphatics in the trunk permits metastasis to regional lymph nodes.

Managing Metastases. The present treatment for metastatic melanoma is largely unsuccessful and cure is generally not possible. Further surgical intervention may be performed to debulk the tumor or to remove part of the organ involved (such as the lung, liver, or colon). The rationale for more extensive surgery, however, is for relief of symptoms, not for cure.

Chemotherapy for metastatic melanoma may be used; however, few agents (dacarbazine, nitrosureas, and cisplatin) have been effective in controlling the disease

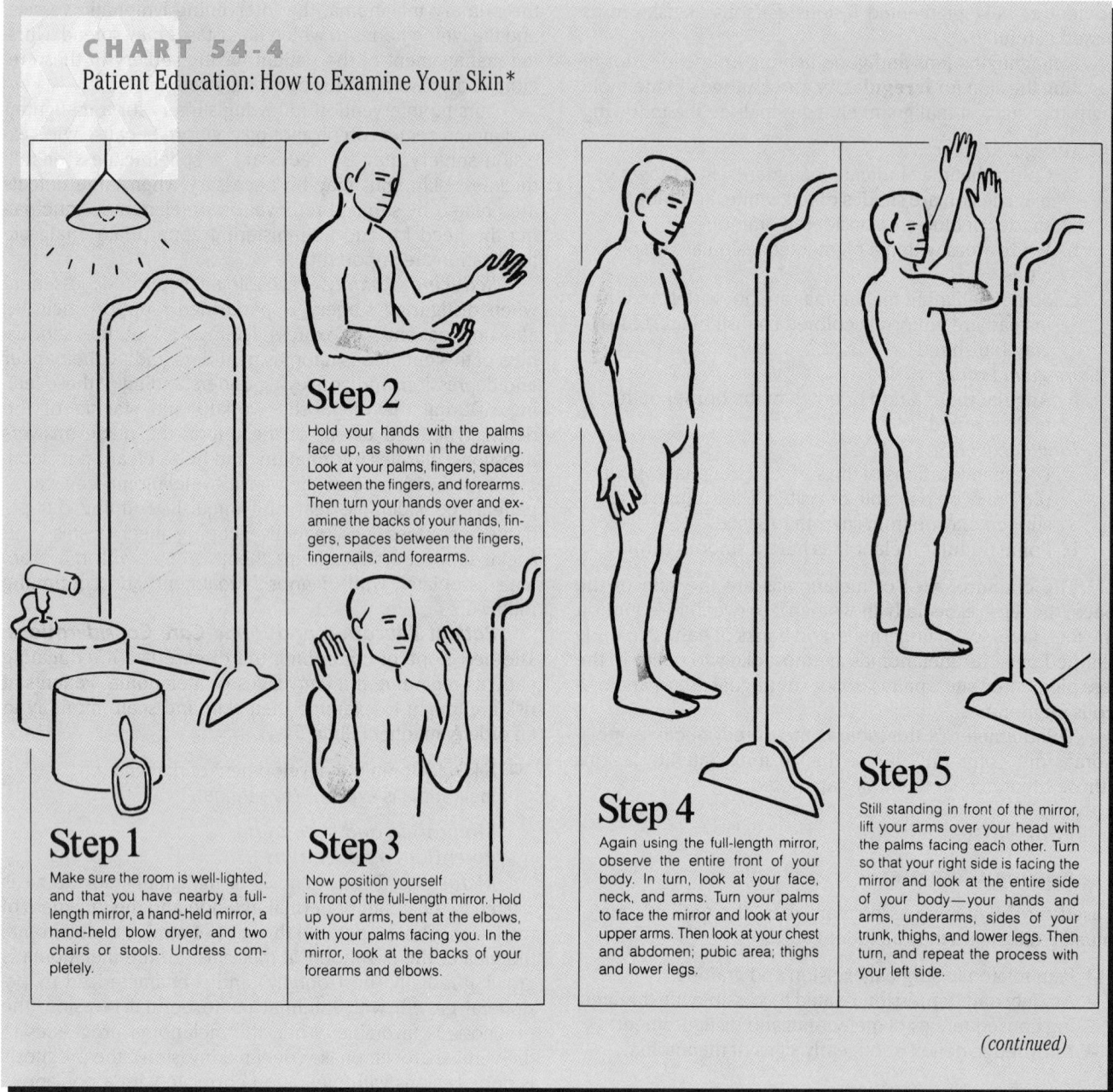

CHART 54-4
Patient Education: How to Examine Your Skin*

Step 1

Make sure the room is well-lighted, and that you have nearby a full-length mirror, a hand-held mirror, a hand-held blow dryer, and two chairs or stools. Undress completely.

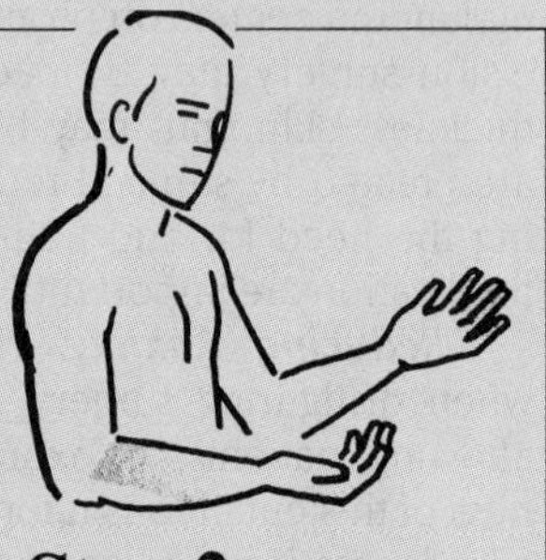

Step 2

Hold your hands with the palms face up, as shown in the drawing. Look at your palms, fingers, spaces between the fingers, and forearms. Then turn your hands over and examine the backs of your hands, fingers, spaces between the fingers, fingernails, and forearms.

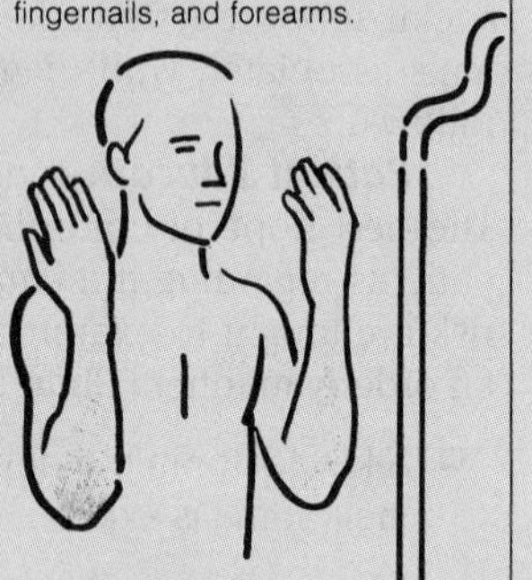

Step 3

Now position yourself in front of the full-length mirror. Hold up your arms, bent at the elbows, with your palms facing you. In the mirror, look at the backs of your forearms and elbows.

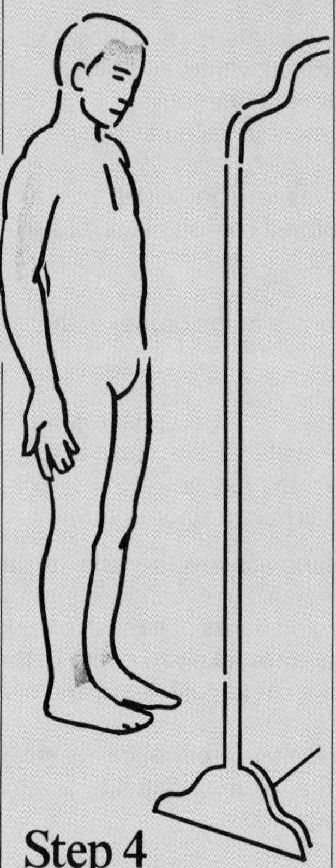

Step 4

Again using the full-length mirror, observe the entire front of your body. In turn, look at your face, neck, and arms. Turn your palms to face the mirror and look at your upper arms. Then look at your chest and abdomen; pubic area; thighs and lower legs.

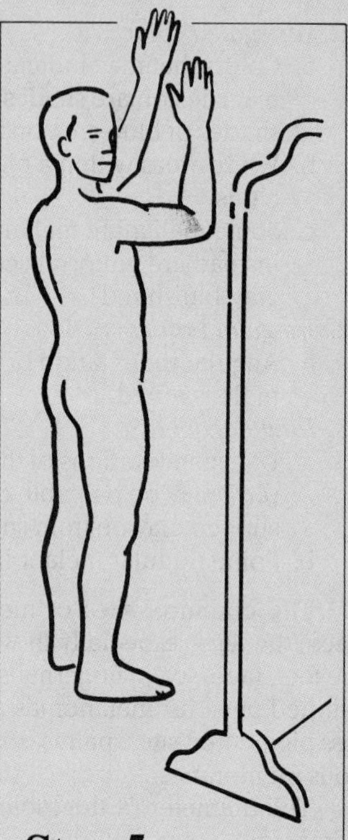

Step 5

Still standing in front of the mirror, lift your arms over your head with the palms facing each other. Turn so that your right side is facing the mirror and look at the entire side of your body—your hands and arms, underarms, sides of your trunk, thighs, and lower legs. Then turn, and repeat the process with your left side.

(continued)

(Runkle & Zalonznik, 1994). When the melanoma is located in an extremity, regional perfusion may be utilized. The chemotherapeutic agent is perfused directly into the area that contains the melanoma. This approach delivers a high concentration of cytotoxic agents yet avoids systemic, toxic side effects. The limb is perfused for 1 hour with high concentrations of the medication at temperatures of 39°C to 40°C (102.2°F to 104°F) with a perfusion pump. Inducing hyperthermia enhances the effect of the chemotherapy so that a smaller total dose can be used. It is hoped that regional perfusion can control the metastasis, especially if it is used in combination with surgical excision of the primary lesion and with regional lymph node dissection.

Immunotherapy has been tried for metastatic melanoma with varied success. Immunotherapy encompasses treatment methods that modify not only immune function but also other biologic responses to cancer. There have been some encouraging results from several forms of immunotherapy (bacillus Calmette Guérin [BCG] vaccine, *Cornebacterium paravum*, levamisole). Research is currently under way to investigate the effects of biologic response modifiers (alpha interferon, interleukin-2), adaptive immunotherapy (lymphokine-actived killer cells), and monoclonal antibodies directed at melanoma antigens.

The role of the nurse in caring for the patient with malignant melanoma is holistic. It is imperative that the nurse knows about the most effective current therapies, delivers supportive care, provides and clarifies information about the therapy and the rationale for its use, identifies potential side effects of therapy and ways to manage them,

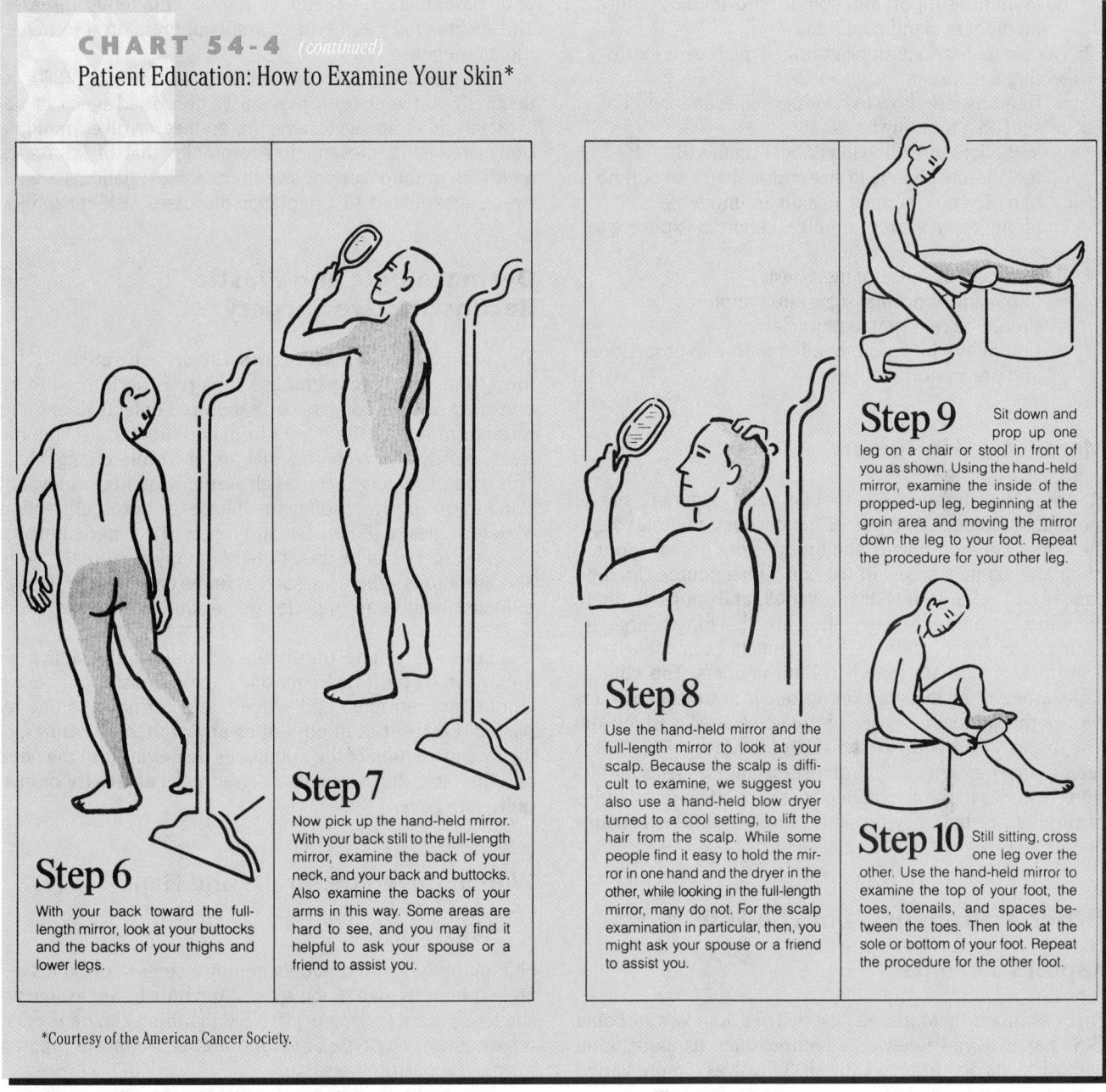

CHART 54-4 *(continued)*

Patient Education: How to Examine Your Skin*

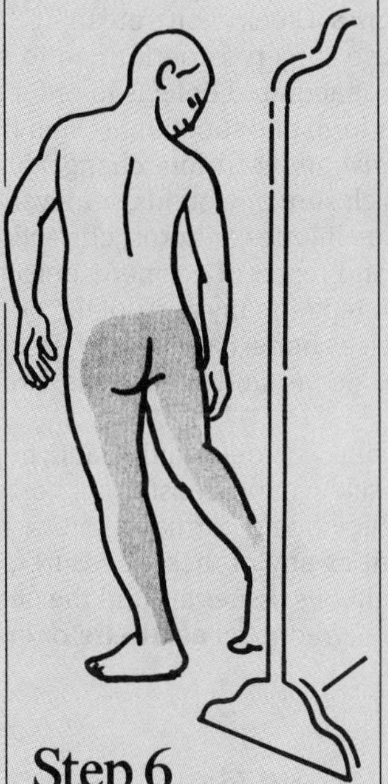

Step 6

With your back toward the full-length mirror, look at your buttocks and the backs of your thighs and lower legs.

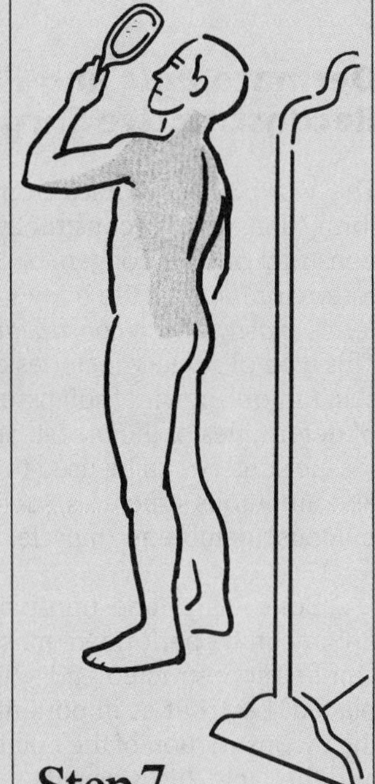

Step 7

Now pick up the hand-held mirror. With your back still to the full-length mirror, examine the back of your neck, and your back and buttocks. Also examine the backs of your arms in this way. Some areas are hard to see, and you may find it helpful to ask your spouse or a friend to assist you.

Step 8

Use the hand-held mirror and the full-length mirror to look at your scalp. Because the scalp is difficult to examine, we suggest you also use a hand-held blow dryer turned to a cool setting, to lift the hair from the scalp. While some people find it easy to hold the mirror in one hand and the dryer in the other, while looking in the full-length mirror, many do not. For the scalp examination in particular, then, you might ask your spouse or a friend to assist you.

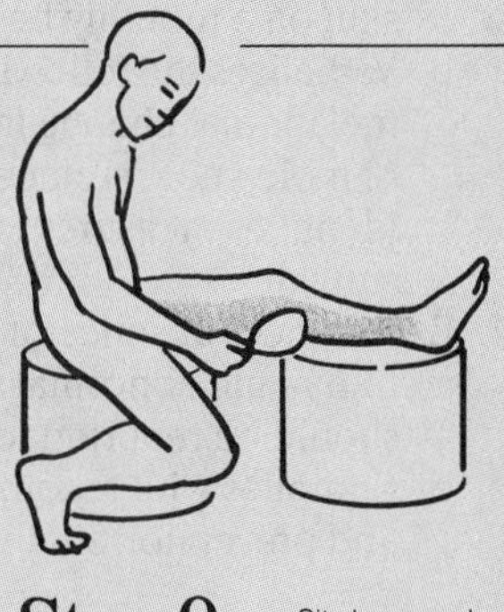

Step 9

Sit down and prop up one leg on a chair or stool in front of you as shown. Using the hand-held mirror, examine the inside of the propped-up leg, beginning at the groin area and moving the mirror down the leg to your foot. Repeat the procedure for your other leg.

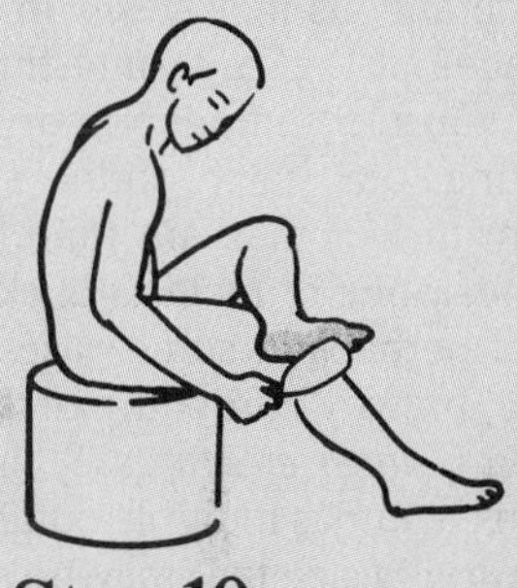

Step 10

Still sitting, cross one leg over the other. Use the hand-held mirror to examine the top of your foot, the toes, toenails, and spaces between the toes. Then look at the sole or bottom of your foot. Repeat the procedure for the other foot.

*Courtesy of the American Cancer Society.

and instructs the patient and family about the expected outcomes of treatment. The nurse monitors and documents symptoms that may indicate metastasis: lung (difficulty breathing, shortness of breath, increasing cough); bone (pain, decrease in mobility and function, pathologic fractures); liver (change in liver enzyme levels, pain, jaundice). Nursing care is planned according to the patient's symptoms.

While the chance of a cure for malignant melanoma is dismal, the nurse encourages the patient to have hope in the therapy employed while maintaining a realistic perspective about the disease process and ultimate outcome. Moreover, the nurse provides time for the patient to express fears and concerns regarding future activities and relationships; offers information about support groups and contact persons, and arranges hospice/palliative care services. (See Chapter 16 for more information on the care of the patient with cancer.)

Evaluation

Expected Outcomes

1. Experiences relief of pain and discomfort
   a. States pain has lessened and is diminishing
   b. Exhibits healing of surgical scar without heat, redness, or swelling
2. Achieves reduction of anxiety
   a. Expresses fears and fantasies
   b. Asks questions about medical condition
   c. Requests repetition of facts about melanoma

   d. Identifies support and comfort provided by family member or significant other
3. Demonstrates an understanding of the means for detecting melanoma
   a. Demonstrates how to conduct self-examination of skin on a monthly basis
   b. Verbalizes the following danger signals of melanoma: change in size, color, shape, or outline of mole, mole surface, or skin around mole
   c. Identifies measures to protect self from exposure to sunlight
4. Experiences absence of metastasis
   a. Can name abnormal signs and symptoms that should be reported to physician
   b. Complies with recommended follow-up procedures and prevention strategies

Metastatic Skin Tumors

The skin is an important, although not a common, site of metastatic cancer. All types of cancer may metastasize to the skin, but carcinoma of the breast is the primary source of cutaneous metastases in women. Other sources include cancer of the large intestine, ovaries, and lungs. In men, the most common primary sites are the lungs, large intestine, oral cavity, kidneys, or stomach. Skin metastases from melanomas are found in both genders. The clinical appearance of metastatic skin lesions is not distinctive, except perhaps in some cases of breast cancer in which diffuse, brawny hardening of the skin of the involved breast is seen (*cancer en cuirasse*). In most instances, metastatic lesions occur as multiple cutaneous or subcutaneous nodules of varying size that may be skin-colored or different shades of red.

Other Malignancies of the Skin

Kaposi's Sarcoma

First described by Moritz Kaposi in 1872, Kaposi's sarcoma (KS) has received renewed attention since its association with AIDS. Its occurrence with AIDS involves a more varied and aggressive form of KS than was seen previously.

Before the AIDS epidemic, Kaposi's sarcoma (KS) was considered a rare type of malignancy. It was subdivided into three categories: classic KS, African (endemic) KS, and KS associated with immunosuppressant therapy.

Classic KS occurs predominantly in men of Mediterranean or Jewish ancestry between ages 40 and 70. Most patients have nodules or plaques on the lower extremities that rarely metastasize beyond the lower extremities. This type of KS is characterized as chronic, relatively benign, and rarely fatal.

African KS affects persons predominantly in the eastern half of Africa near the equator. Men are affected more often than women, and children can be affected as well. The disease may resemble classic KS or it may become infiltrative and progress to lymphadenopathic forms.

KS associated with immunosuppressive therapy, as in transplant patients, is characterized by local skin lesions and disseminated visceral and mucocutaneous diseases. The greater the degree of immunosuppression, the higher the incidence of KS.

AIDS-related KS was identified in the early 1980s as distinctly different from previously described types of KS. Typically it is an aggressive tumor that involves multiple body organs. Its presentation resembles that of KS associated with immunosuppressive therapy. Most patients are between ages 20 and 40. Chapter 50 discusses AIDS-related KS.

Dermatologic and Plastic Reconstructive Surgery

The word *plastic* comes from a Greek word meaning "to form." Plastic or reconstructive surgery is performed to reconstruct or alter congenital or acquired defects in order to restore or improve the body's form and function. (Often the terms *plastic* and *reconstructive* are used interchangeably.) This type of surgery includes closure of wounds, removal of skin tumors, repair of soft-tissue injuries or burns, correction of deformities of the breast, and repair of cosmetic defects. Plastic surgery can be used to repair many parts of the body and numerous structures, such as bone, cartilage, fat, fascia, mucous membrane, muscle, nerve, and cutaneous structures.

Bone inlays and transplants for deformities and nonunion can be performed; muscle can be transferred; nerves can be reconstructed and spliced; and cartilage can be replaced. Last, but as important as any of these measures, is the reconstruction of the cutaneous tissues around the neck and the face; this is usually referred to as **aesthetic** or **cosmetic surgery.**

Wound Coverage: Grafts and Flaps

Skin Grafts

Skin grafting is a technique whereby a section of skin is detached from its own blood supply and transferred as free tissue to a distant (recipient) site. Skin grafting can be used to repair almost any type of wound and is the most common form of reconstructive surgery.

Skin grafts are commonly used to repair defects that result from excision of skin tumors, to cover areas denuded of skin, and to cover wounds in which insufficient skin is available to permit wound closure. They are also used when primary closure of the wound increases the risk of complications or when primary wound closure will interfere with function.

Skin grafts may be classified as autografts, allografts, or xenografts. An **autograft** is tissue obtained from the patient's own skin. An **allograft** is tissue obtained from a donor of the same species. These grafts are also called **allogeneic** or **homograft.** A **xenograft** or **heterograft** is tissue from another species.

Grafts are also referred to by their thickness. A skin graft may be split-thickness (thin, intermediate, or thick) or full-thickness, depending on the amount of dermis included in the specimen. A split-thickness graft can be cut at varying thicknesses and is commonly used to cover large wounds or

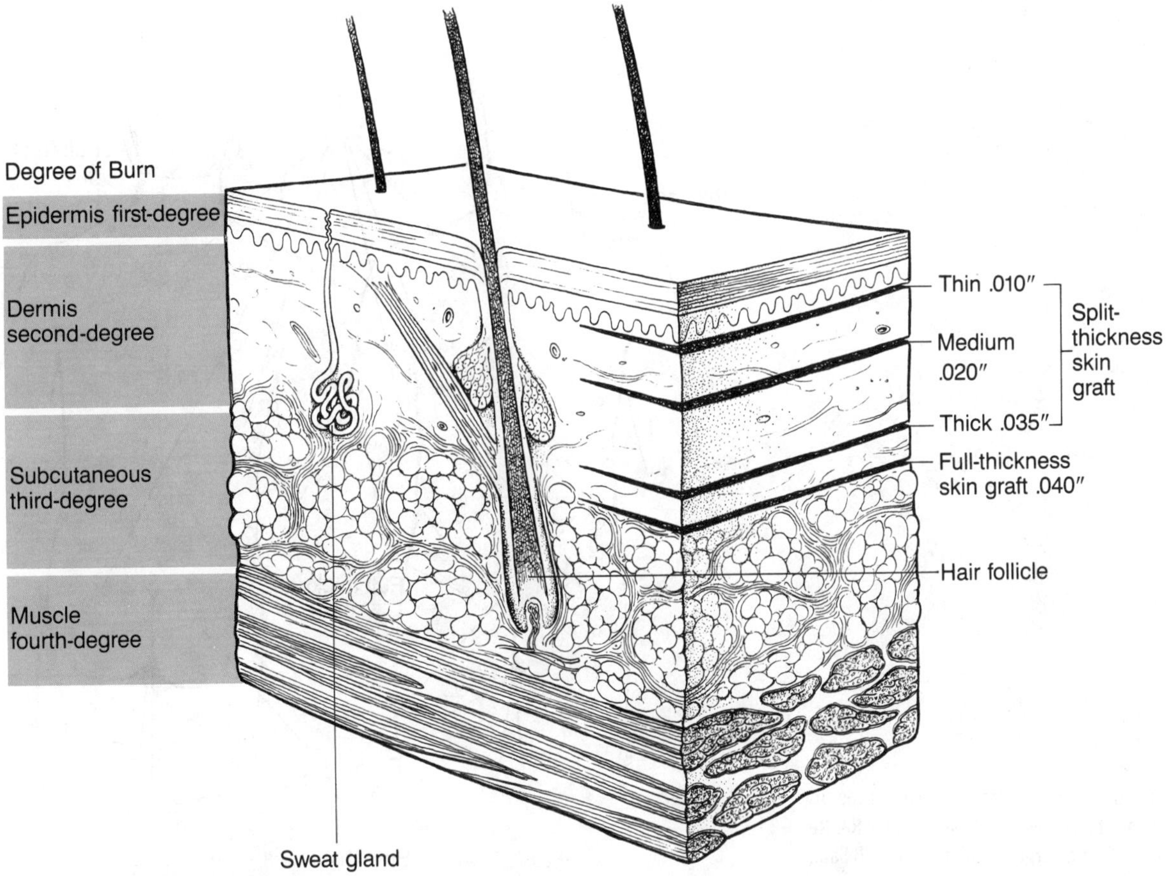

FIGURE 54-9. Layers of skin appropriate for split-thickness and full-thickness grafts.

defects for which a full-thickness graft or flap is impractical (Fig. 54-9). A full-thickness graft consists of epidermis and the entire dermis without the underlying fat. It is used to cover wounds that are too large to be closed directly.

Application of the Graft. A graft is obtained by a variety of instruments: razor blades, skin-grafting knives, electric- or air-powered dermatomes, or drum dermatomes. The skin graft is taken from the "donor" or "host" site and applied to the desired site, called the "recipient" site or "graft bed."

For a graft to survive and be effective, certain conditions must be met: (1) the recipient site must have an adequate blood supply so that normal physiologic function can resume; (2) the graft must be in close contact with its bed (to avoid accumulation of blood or fluid); (3) the graft must be fixed firmly (immobilized) so that it remains in place on the recipient site; and (4) the area must be free of infection.

The graft, when applied to the recipient site, may or may not be sutured in place. It may be slit and spread apart to cover a greater area. The process of revascularization (establishing the blood supply) and reattachment of a skin graft to a recipient bed is referred to as a "take."

After a skin graft is put in place, it may be left exposed (in areas that are impossible to immobilize) or covered with a light dressing or a pressure dressing, depending on the area.

Patient Education and Home Care Considerations. The patient is instructed to keep the affected part immobilized as much as possible. For a facial graft, strenuous activity must be avoided. A graft on the hand or arm may be immobilized with a splint. When a graft is placed on a lower extremity, the part is kept elevated because the new capillary connections are fragile and excess venous pressure may cause rupture. When ambulation is permitted, the patient wears an elastic stocking to counterbalance venous pressure.

The patient, family member, or other caregiver is instructed to inspect the dressing daily. Unusual drainage or an inflammatory reaction around the wound margin suggests infection and should be reported to the physician. Any fluid, purulent drainage, blood, or serum that has collected will be gently evacuated by the surgeon, because accumulation of this material would cause the graft to separate from its bed.

When the graft appears pink, it apparently is vascularized. After 2 to 3 weeks, mineral oil or a lanolin cream is massaged into the wound to moisten the graft and stimulate circulation. Because there may be loss of feeling or sensation in the grafted area for a prolonged period, the application of heating pads and exposure to sun are avoided to prevent burns and further skin trauma.

Donor Site for Skin Grafting

Selection Criteria. The donor site is selected with several criteria in mind: (1) achieving the closest possible color match in keeping with the amount of skin graft required; (2) matching the texture and hair-bearing qualities; (3) obtaining the thickest possible skin graft without jeopardizing the healing of the donor site (Fig. 54-10); and

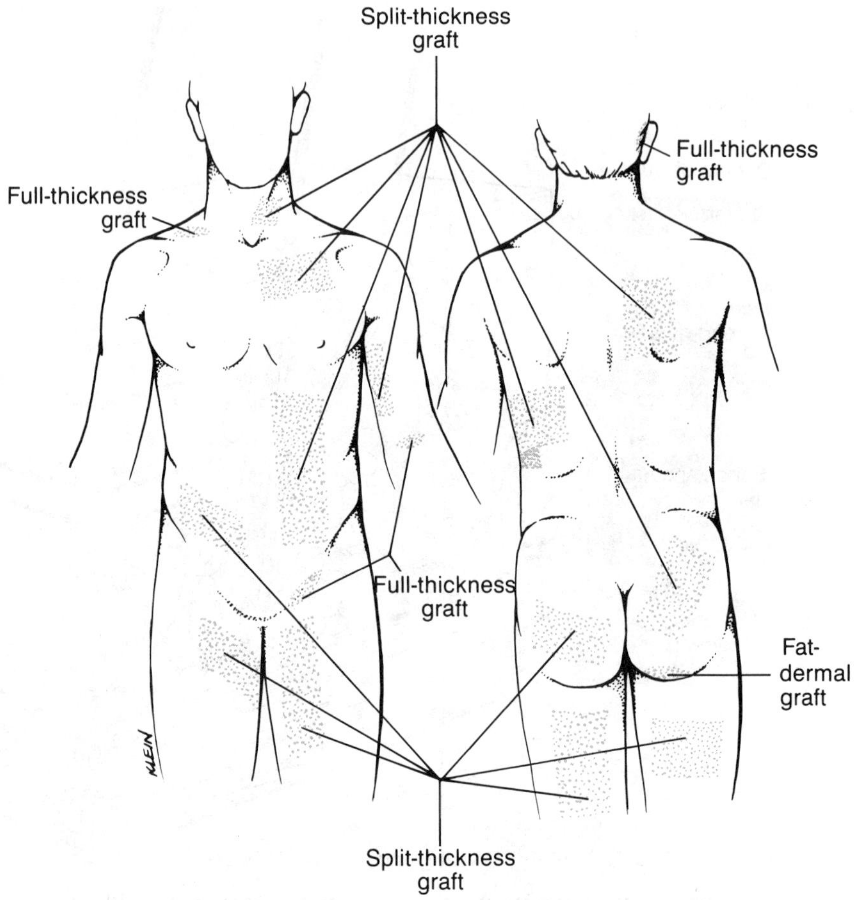

FIGURE 54-10. Commonly used sites for donor skin grafts. (Converse JM and Brauer RA. Reconstructive Plastic Surgery. Philadelphia, WB Saunders.)

(4) considering the cosmetic effects of the donor site after healing, so that it is in an inconspicuous location.

Donor Site Care. Detailed attention to the donor site is just as important as the care of the recipient area. The donor site heals by reepithelialization of the raw, exposed dermis. Usually a single layer of nonadherent, fine-mesh gauze is placed directly over the donor site. Absorbent gauze dressings are then placed on top to absorb blood or serum from the wound. A membrane dressing (such as Op-Site) may be used and provides certain advantages: it is transparent and allows the wound to be observed without disturbing the dressing, and it permits the patient to shower without fear of saturating the dressing with water.

After healing, the patient is instructed to keep the donor site soft and pliable with cream (lanolin, olive oil). Extremes in temperature, external trauma, and sunlight are to be avoided both for donor sites and grafted areas because these areas are sensitive, especially to thermal injuries.

Flaps

Another form of wound coverage may be provided by flaps. A **flap** is a segment of tissue that remains attached at one end (called a **base** or **pedicle**) while the other end is moved to a recipient area. Its survival depends on functioning arterial and venous blood supplies and lymphatic drainage in its pedicle or base. A flap differs from a graft in that a portion of the tissue is attached to its original site and retains its blood supply. (An exception is the free flap, described below.)

Flaps may consist of skin, mucosa, muscle, adipose tissue, omentum, and bone. They are used for wound coverage and provide bulk, especially when bone, tendon, blood vessels, or nerve tissue is exposed. Flaps are used to repair defects caused by congenital deformity, trauma, or tumor ablation (removal, usually by excision) in an adjacent part of the body.

Flaps offer an aesthetic solution, because a flap retains the color and texture of the donor area, is more likely to survive than a graft, and can be used to cover nerves, tendons, and blood vessels. However, several surgical procedures are usually required to advance a flap. The major complication is necrosis of the pedicle or base due to failure of the blood supply.

Free Flaps. A striking advance in reconstructive surgery is the use of **free flaps** or **free-tissue transfer,** achieved by means of microvascular techniques. A free flap is completely severed from the body and transferred to another site, and it receives early vascular supply from microvascular anastomosis (attachment) with vessels at the recipient site. Thus, the procedure is generally completed in one step, eliminating the need for a series of surgical procedures to move the flap. Microvascular surgery allows surgeons to use a variety of donor sites for tissue reconstruction.

Chemical Face Peeling

Chemical face peeling is a skin planing technique that involves the application of a chemical mixture to the face for the purpose of causing superficial destruction of the epidermis and the upper layers of the dermis. It is used to treat fine wrinkles, keratoses, and pigment problems. It is especially useful for wrinkles at the upper and lower lip, forehead, and periorbital areas (Kotler, 1994).

Pretreatment may consist of cleansing the face and hair for several days before the intended procedure with a hexachlorophene detergent. Pretreatment medication (analgesic and tranquilizer) may be prescribed to alleviate apprehension and control pain. This permits the patient to be sedated yet conscious during the procedure. Some patients prefer not to be awake during therapy and request general anesthesia.

The type of chemical used depends on the planned depth of the peel. A phenol-based chemical in an oil–water emulsion is commonly used in the procedure because it causes a controlled, predictable chemical burn. The chemical is carefully applied in a systematic manner to the face with cotton-tipped applicators. The conscious patient will feel a burning sensation at this time. A mask of waterproof adhesive may then be applied directly to the skin and molded closely to the contours of the face, thereby acting as an occlusive dressing that increases the chemical penetration and action. (Some surgeons think that equally good results can be obtained with occlusive tape.) After the tape mask is applied the burning sensation continues. The tape mask remains in place for 12 to 24 hours. Frequent small doses of analgesics and tranquilizers are prescribed to keep the patient comfortable.

Complications. Complications may arise when control of the chemically induced burn cannot be sustained. Complications include pigment changes, infection, milia (small inclusion cysts that disappear after several months), scarring, atrophy, sensitivity changes, and long-term erythema (4 to 5 months) and pruritus.

Patient Education and Home Care Considerations. Because chemical face peeling is performed in the physician's office or in an outpatient surgical department, the majority of care takes place in the home setting. After 6 to 8 hours, the face becomes edematous and the eyelids often swell shut. The patient should be reassured that this reaction is expected and normal. The patient is cautioned to move the mouth as little as possible so that the tape continues to adhere to the skin. The head of the bed is elevated, and liquids are administered through a straw. Most of the burning sensation and discomfort subside after the first 12 to 24 hours.

By the second day, the patient may feel moisture under the dressings as serous exudate seeps from the chemically exfoliated skin. Dressings are usually removed 24 to 48 hours after treatment, exposing skin resembling a second-degree burn. The patient may be alarmed by the appearance of the skin and should be reassured. After the tape mask is removed, some surgeons dust the treated skin surface with thymol-iodine powder for its drying and bacteriostatic effects. Application of triple antibiotic ointment may be substituted in some cases. The skin surface is left uncovered to dry. The patient may be permitted to wash the face with lukewarm water or advised to shower several times daily to help remove any remaining crust from the face (Kotler, 1994). An ointment is prescribed to cover the face and soften and loosen the crust between washings.

The nurse reinforces the physician's explanation that the redness of the skin will gradually subside over the next 4 to 12 weeks. Although a line between treated and untreated skin may be noted, makeup is usually permitted after the first few weeks. The patient is cautioned to avoid direct or reflected sunlight, because the treatment reduces the natural protection of the skin from sun. The skin will probably never tan evenly again. Blotchy pigmentation can occur with exposure to the sun.

Dermabrasion

Dermabrasion (skin planing) is a form of skin abrasion used to correct acne scarring, aging, and sun-damaged skin. A special instrument (motor-driven wire brush, diamond-impregnated disk, serrated wheel) is used in the procedure. The epidermis and some superficial dermis is removed, while enough of the dermis is preserved to allow reepithelialization of the treated areas. Results are best in the face because it is rich in intradermal epithelial elements.

Preparation and Procedure. The primary reason for undergoing dermabrasion is to improve appearance. The surgeon explains to the patient what can be expected from dermabrasion. The patient should also be informed about the nature of the postoperative dressing, what discomfort may be experienced, and how long it will be before the tissues look normal.

Dermabrasion may be performed in the physician's office, the operating room, or an outpatient setting. It is performed under local or general anesthesia. During the procedure, some dermatologic surgeons use refrigerant anesthetics to turn the skin into a numb, solid mass of rigid tissue and to provide a momentarily bloodless surgical field. During and after planing, the area is irrigated with copious amounts of saline solution to remove debris and allow the surgeon to see the area. A dressing impregnated with ointment is usually applied to the abraded surface.

Patient Education and Home Care Considerations. The nurse instructs the patient about the after-effects of the surgery. Edema occurs during the first 48 hours and may cause the eyelids to close. The head of the bed is elevated to hasten fluid drainage. Erythema occurs and can last for weeks or months. After 24 hours, the dressing may be removed (upon physician directives). When the serum oozing from the skin begins to gel, the patient applies the prescribed ointment to the face several times a day to prevent hard crusting and to keep the abraded areas soft and flexible. Clear water cleansing or soaking of the face is started with physician approval to remove crusts from the healing skin.

The patient is advised to avoid extreme cold and heat and excessive straining or lifting, which may bruise delicate new capillaries. Direct or reflected sunlight is avoided for 3 to 6 months, and a sunscreen should be used.

Management of the Patient With Facial Reconstructive Surgery

Reconstructive procedures on the face are individualized to the patient's needs and desired outcomes. They are performed to repair deformities or restore normal function as much as possible. They may vary from closure of small defects to complicated procedures involving implantation of prosthetic devices to conceal a large defect or reconstruct a lost part of the face (*e.g.*, nose, ear, jaw). Each surgical procedure is custom-tailored and involves a variety of incisions, flaps, and grafts.

In correcting a primary defect, the surgeon may have to create a secondary defect. Although the procedure may restore some function, such as eating or talking, the cosmetic or aesthetic results may be limited. The original appearance of a patient who has severe damage to soft tissue and bone structure can seldom be restored. Multiple surgical procedures may be required. The process of facial reconstruction is usually slow and tedious.

❑ NURSING PROCESS
The Patient With Facial Reconstructive Surgery

Assessment

The face is a part of the body that every person desires to keep at its best or improve because most human interactions involve the face. When the face loses its appearance and function (*e.g.*, by accident or cancer), significant emotional reactions often occur. Changes in appearance frequently cause anxiety and depression. Patients with facial changes frequently mourn for the lost part, suffer a loss of self-esteem due to reactions or rejection by others, and withdraw and isolate themselves. Health care personnel can acknowledge that anxiety and depression are appropriate for what the patient is experiencing.

In addition, the nurse assesses the patient's emotional responses, and identifies strengths as well as usual coping mechanisms to determine how the patient will handle the surgical procedure. Any area in which the patient and family will need extra support is also identified.

The preoperative assessment will determine the extent of disfigurement and improvement that can be anticipated, as well as the patient's understanding and acceptance of these limitations. The nurse is in a better position to reinforce factual information and clarify misconceptions when the surgeon has fully informed the patient about the procedure, the functional defects that may result, the possible need for a tracheostomy and/or other prosthesis, and the probability of additional surgery. The nurse instructs the patient about various postoperative measures: intravenous feedings, the use of a nasogastric tube to allow gastric decompression and prevent vomiting, and the frequent and lengthy dressing periods that may be required to care for wounds, flaps, and skin grafts. Extra time is needed when presenting this information to anxious patients because they may not hear, concentrate, or comprehend what is being said.

Diagnosis

Nursing Diagnoses

Based on the nursing assessment data, the patient's major nursing diagnoses may include:

- ❑ Ineffective airway clearance related to tracheobronchial secretions
- ❑ Pain related to facial edema and effects of the procedure
- ❑ Altered nutrition: Less than body requirements related to changed physiology of oral cavity, drooling, impaired chewing and swallowing, or excision surgery affecting the tongue
- ❑ Impaired verbal communication related to trauma/surgery producing anatomic and physiologic abnormalities of speech
- ❑ Body image disturbance related to disfigurement
- ❑ Altered family processes related to grief reaction and disruption of family life

Collaborative Problems/ Potential Complications

Based on the assessment data, potential complications that may develop include:

- ❑ Infection

Planning and Implementation

Goals. The major goals of the patient may include maintenance of a patent airway and pulmonary function, achievement of increased comfort, attainment and maintenance of adequate nutritional status, development of an effective communication method, reinforcement of positive self-concept, achievement of effective family coping, and absence of infection.

Nursing Interventions

Maintaining Airway and Pulmonary Function. The immediate postoperative concern following facial reconstruction is maintenance of an adequate airway. If the patient has regained consciousness, mental confusion with combative, anxious behavior is a sign of anoxia (reduced oxygen supply to tissues). Sedatives or opioids are not prescribed in this situation because they may impair oxygenation. If the patient shows signs of restlessness, the airway is carefully inspected to detect laryngeal edema or accumulation of tracheobronchial mucus. Secretions are suctioned as necessary until the patient can manage the secretions without help. If the patient has a tracheostomy, suctioning is performed with sterile technique to prevent infection and cross-contamination. (See Chapter 25 for care of the patient with a tracheostomy.)

Achieving Comfort and Relieving Pain. Edema of the face is uncomfortable and is a consequence of facial reconstructive surgery. The patient's head and upper torso are kept slightly elevated (if the blood pressure is stable) to help reduce facial edema. Suction catheters attached to closed drainage may be in place to keep the tissue in close apposition and to remove serous discharge. If extensive reconstruction has been performed, the patient's head should be properly aligned and supported so that minimal stress is placed on the suture line.

Mild doses of analgesics are prescribed to control pain. If bone grafts have been used for reconstruction, there is usually considerable pain in the donor area.

If the patient has head and neck cancer and increasing levels of pain, more sophisticated nursing management will be required (see Chapter 13.)

Maintaining Adequate Nutrition. After oral and pharyngeal edema have diminished, the incisional areas and flaps are healed, and the patient is able to swallow saliva, fluids may be offered, followed gradually by soft foods. If the patient cannot meet nutritional needs by the oral route, total parenteral nutrition (infusion of nutrients, water, and vitamins into the stomach or proximal small intestine via tube) is initiated.

The formula strength and feeding rate are gradually increased until the desired daily caloric level is attained. (See Chapter 35 for nursing management of the patient requiring enteral feedings.) Patients who have had radical surgery for large, encroaching neoplasms may experience difficulty resuming oral intake of food. Positive nutrition is reflected in weight gain, and nutritional status is monitored by daily checks of weight and periodic assessments of serum protein and electrolyte levels.

Enhancing Communication. Communication problems may be a major difficulty and may range from little or no problem to loss of oral speech. Some tumors and injuries require extensive surgical treatment that involves the larynx, tongue, and mandible. Paper, pen or pencil, and a firm writing surface should be provided. If the patient cannot write, a pictograph board may be used. Referral to a speech therapist may be necessary for the patient who has undergone structural changes.

The family may become frustrated by the patient's inability to communicate. The patient soon senses this, and both parties may withdraw. Allowing the family to vent their feelings and fears (away from the patient) is important.

Improving Self-Concept. Success in rehabilitation of the patient undergoing reconstructive surgery depends on the relationships among the patient and the nurse, the physician, and other health care personnel. Mutual trust, respect, and clear lines of communication are essential. Unhurried care provides emotional reassurance and support.

Often the kinds of dressings that must be worn, the unusual positions that have to be maintained, and the temporary incapacities that must be experienced can be upsetting to the most stable person. Honest reinforcement of the patient's coping improves self-esteem. If prosthetic devices are to be used, the patient is taught how to use and care for them in order to gain a sense of greater independence. Once involved in self-care activities, the patient may feel some control over what was previously an overwhelming situation.

Patients with severe disfigurement are encouraged to socialize in the hospital to experience the reactions of others in a more protected environment. Gradually they can widen their sphere of contact. Every effort is made to cover or mask defects. Patients may require support by members of the mental health team to accept their changed appearance.

Promoting Family Coping. The family is informed about the patient's appearance following surgery, the presence of supportive equipment, and ways that the equipment aids in recovery. It is helpful to join the family for a few minutes during their first postoperative visit to help them cope with the changes they will see.

A major nursing task is to support the family in their decision to participate (or not to participate) in the patient's treatment. Nursing interventions also include helping the family members communicate by suggesting techniques for reducing anxiety and stress and promoting problem solving and decision making. These activities encourage family members and promote growth.

Monitoring and Managing Potential Complications

Infection. Secondary infection is a primary concern after reconstructive surgery. The source of infection will depend on the location and extent of the procedure, the suture line, and the pedicle flap.

The mouth is inspected to note the location of sutures so that they are not accidentally disturbed during the cleaning process. The mouth is cleaned according to protocol several times daily. Loose blood clots may be removed by gentle swabbing. The patient is advised not to loosen clots with the tongue because this may cause fresh bleeding. The patient is instructed not to use fingers to clean or remove blood clots as this may introduce organisms that cause infection.

The suture line will be under stress for several days after surgery because of edema, increased drainage, and hematoma formation. The nurse assesses the suture line carefully for signs of increased tension and infection (elevated temperature, increasing edema, redness, bleeding, and increased pain) with each dressing change. Dressings may need to be changed many times a day until the drainage begins to dissipate. Drainage and edema are expected following reconstructive surgery; however, both should lessen and the process will be hastened by using properly placed, functioning suction devices and keeping the head of the bed elevated about 45 degrees. The nurse inspects each suction device, empties them promptly, and documents the amount and consistency of drainage, as well as any unusual odor. When drainage is not removed or if saturated dressings are left unchanged for long periods, infection is likely to occur. Strict asepsis must always be carried out during wound care.

If a pedicle flap is used in reconstruction, it may become a source of infection if its circulation becomes compromised. Poor circulation may result from a hematoma forming beneath the flap and causing increased pressure on the underlying vasculature. The nurse inspects the flap for change in color and temperature indicative of poor circulation. Signs of necrosis, increased drainage, and an odor may be a further forewarning of an infection and should be reported promptly.

Reinforcing preoperative teaching about wound healing, the need for strict sterile technique, good personal hygiene, and the need to restrict movement and stress on the operative site is an important part of the nurse's role in postoperative care and in the prevention of secondary infection.

Evaluation

Expected Outcomes

1. Maintains patent airway
   a. Demonstrates respiratory rate within normal limits
   b. Exhibits normal breath sounds
   c. Demonstrates no signs of choking or aspiration
2. Achieves increasing comfort
   a. Reports decreasing pain
   b. Follows instructions on proper positioning

   c. Avoids movements that add stress to the operative site
3. Attains adequate nutrition
   a. Consumes adequate amounts of food and fluids
   b. Progressively gains weight, with gradual approach toward normal weight range
   c. Maintains serum protein and electrolyte levels within normal range
4. Communicates effectively
   a. Uses appropriate aids to enhance communication
   b. Interacts with health care team members, family, and other support persons using new communication strategies
5. Develops positive self-image
   a. Expresses positive feelings about surgical changes
   b. Demonstrates increasing independence in self-care activities
   c. Uses prosthetic devices independently (when appropriate)
   d. Verbalizes plans for resuming usual activities (*e.g.*, work, recreation)
6. Family members cope with situation
   a. Demonstrate decreasing anxiety and conflict
   b. Verbalize what to expect
7. Experiences no postoperative infection
   a. Demonstrates vital signs within normal limits
   b. Undergoes normal wound healing without signs of infection or sepsis
   c. Lists signs of infection that should be reported
   d. Understands the need for asepsis (sterile procedures) and good personal hygiene

Face Lift

Rhytidectomy (face lift) is a surgical procedure on the face to remove soft tissue folds and minimize cutaneous wrinkles. It is performed to improve and create a more youthful appearance.

Psychologic preparation requires that the person recognize the limitations of surgery and the fact that miraculous rejuvenation will not occur. The patient is informed that the face may appear bruised and swollen after the dressings are removed and that several weeks may pass before the edema subsides.

The procedure is performed under local or general anesthesia; the outpatient setting has become an increasingly popular site for the surgery. The incisions are placed in areas of concealment (natural skin folds and creases and areas hidden by hair). The loose skin, separated from underlying muscle, is pulled upward and backward. Excess skin that overlaps the incision line is removed. More recently, liposuction-assisted rhytidectomy is being performed. In this procedure, fat is suctioned from the body via a cannula through a small incision.

Patient Education and Home Care Considerations. The patient is encouraged to rest quietly for the first 2 postoperative days until the dressings are removed. The head of the bed is elevated and neck flexion is discouraged to avoid compromising the circulation and the suture line. The patient may feel some degree of tightness of the face and neck due to pressure created by the newly tightened muscles, fascia, and skin. Analgesics may be prescribed to relieve discomfort. A liquid diet may be given by means of straws, and a soft diet is permitted if chewing is not too uncomfortable.

When the dressings are removed, the skin is gently cleaned of crusting and oozing and coated with the prescribed topical ointment. Any hair matted with drainage may be combed with warm water and a wide-toothed comb.

The patient is advised not to lift or bend for 7 to 10 days because this activity may increase edema and provoke bleeding. Activities are gradually resumed. When all sutures are removed, the hair may be shampooed and blown dry with *warm*, not hot, air to avoid burning the ears, which may be numb for a while.

The patient needs to know that a face lift will not stop the aging process and that with time, the tissues will resume the downward drift. Some patients have two or more face lifts.

Sudden pain indicates that blood is accumulating underneath the skin flaps, and it should be reported to the surgeon immediately. Complications include sloughing of the skin, deformities of the face and neck, and partial facial paralysis. Cigarette smoking has been implicated as a cause of skin slough in some patients.

Laser Treatment of Cutaneous Lesions

Lasers are devices that amplify or generate highly specialized light energy. They are capable of mobilizing immense heat and power when focused at close range and are valuable tools in surgical procedures. Several types of lasers (the argon laser, carbon dioxide laser, and tunable pulse-dye laser) are used in dermatologic surgery. Each type of laser emits its own unique wavelength with color spectrum.

Argon Laser

The **argon laser** produces a blue-green visible light that is absorbed by vascular tissue and hence is useful in treating vascular lesions: port-wine stains, telangiectases, vascular tumors, and pigmented lesions. The argon beam is capable of penetrating approximately 1 mm of skin and reaches the pigmented layer, causing protein coagulation in this area. An immediate effect is that tiny blood vessels under the skin are coagulated, causing the area to turn a much lighter color. A crust forms within a few days.

During the procedure, the patient may require local anesthesia (lidocaine) only if the lesion, such as a port-wine stain, is greater than 0.5 cm wide. Laser beams, regardless of type, are reflected and scattered in all directions during the treatment. Laser radiation is known to be hazardous to the human eye. Therefore, the eyes of the patient and all personnel involved in the surgical procedure and those who are within the immediate surgical environment must be protected by wearing orange, argon light-absorbing safety goggles.

Patient Education and Home Care Considerations. Cold compresses are usually applied over the treatment area for approximately 6 hours to minimize edema, exudate, and loss of capillary permeability. The patient is advised that swelling will subside in 1 to 2 days to be followed by a crust that will last 7 to 10 days. The patient should avoid picking at the crust. An antibacterial ointment is applied sparingly until the crust separates. Makeup is not applied until the wound has healed. Sun exposure of the treated area is avoided to prevent hypopigmentation. Sunscreen is to be used when exposure is unavoidable.

Carbon Dioxide Laser

The **carbon dioxide** (CO_2) laser emits invisible light in the infrared spectrum that is absorbed at the skin surface because of the high water content of the skin and the long wavelength of the CO_2 light.

As the laser beam strikes human tissue, it is absorbed by the intracellular and extracellular water, which vaporizes, destroying the tissue. The CO_2 laser is a precise surgical instrument for use in vaporizing and excising tissue with minimal tissue damage. Because the beam can seal blood and lymphatic vessels, it creates a dry surgical field that makes many procedures easier and quicker. It is therefore safe to use on patients with bleeding disorders or those receiving anticoagulant therapy. It is useful for removing epidermal nevi, tattoos, certain warts, skin cancer, ingrown toenails, and keloids. Incisions made with the laser heal and scar much like those made by a scalpel.

During laser use, eye safety for patient and personnel is maintained by wearing clear safety goggles. In addition, it is advisable that all persons involved wear a laser-grade surgical mask to avoid inhaling by-product smoke, referred to as a **plume** (Sliney, 1992).

Patient Education and Home Care Considerations. Immediately after CO_2 laser treatment, the treated area turns a charcoal color. The wound is covered with antibacterial ointment and a nonadhesive dressing. The patient is instructed to keep the wound dry between gentle cleanings with mild soap several times a day. After the skin is cleaned, a prescribed ointment and light dressing are applied.

Because nerve endings and lymphatic vessels are sealed by the laser, less edema and pain follow the laser procedure than conventional surgery. A mild analgesic is sufficient to maintain patient comfort. Wound healing occurs by secondary intention with granulation tissue appearing within a week; complete healing occurs in several weeks. Sun exposure to the area should be avoided for approximately 6 months.

Application of a sunscreen with a solar protection factor (SPF) of at least 15 is recommended. Persons who are known to be at high risk for skin cancer from sun exposure (fair complexion, red-haired, history of skin cancer, history of prolonged sunburn, and those who do not tan easily) may be advised to use sunscreens of SPF 15 or greater that can block out ultraviolet B as well as ultraviolet A light.

Pulse-Dye Laser

The tunable pulse-dye laser (having varying wavelengths) is the latest laser available for dermatologic surgery. It is especially useful in treating cutaneous vascular lesions (port-wine stains, telangiectasia). Eye protection used for the argon and CO_2 lasers is not sufficient when the pulse-dye laser is in use. Special eyeglasses, such as those made of didymium glass, are required for the patient and all personnel. The procedure itself is generally painless. For those requiring anesthesia, lidocaine without epinephrine is sufficient because local vasoconstriction (which epinephrine induces) is not necessary.

Patient Education and Home Care Considerations. After treatment, there may be a sensation of "stinging" in the treated area for several hours. Applying ice to the area and a light antibacterial ointment followed by a nonstick dressing (Telfa) usually eases any discomfort.

If crusting occurs, the patient is advised to wash the area gently with soap and water and reapply the antibacterial cream twice daily until the crust disappears.

Makeup should not be applied until all crust is removed. Sun exposure should be avoided. Sunscreens with an SPF of 15 or higher should be used for 3 to 4 months after the treatment. Complete removal of the lesion, especially a port-wine stain, is not anticipated. The patient should be informed that several treatments may be necessary.

Hair Disorders

Androgenetic Alopecia

Alopecia, or hair loss, can result from many conditions: infection of the scalp, hair dyes, increasing age, medications, and change in androgen (hormone) levels. Androgenetic alopecia occurs in men and women. While male pattern baldness is more familiar, women too can lose hair in much the same pattern. Because hair is so visible and so much a part of body image and self-esteem, hair loss can create devastating emotional and social problems for both genders.

Clinical Manifestations

Male androgenetic alopecia is frequently noted for the first time after puberty when the androgen level changes. Hair loss is seen initially as a "receding hairline" in the bitemporal area in white men between ages 20 and 50. This may be the extent of hair loss or it may continue to progress. When hair loss begins during the 20s, it appears to be a more progressive and intensive loss (Olsen, 1994). Hair loss may extend over the entire vertex of the scalp. There are cultural differences in the pattern of male hair loss: Asians and Native Americans generally do not lose their frontal hairline and usually hair loss occurs later in life. African-American men tend to have less baldness compared with men of other races (Olsen, 1994).

Women with androgenetic alopecia begin to notice hair loss in the third and fourth decades of life. Bitemporal hairline recession is similar to that found in men but is generally not as prominent. Women appear to develop diffuse hair loss involving the entire scalp. In both male and female androgenetic alopecia, there is a family history of male pattern baldness in first-degree relatives.

Management

There are literally hundreds of over-the-counter products claiming to promote hair growth or retard hair loss. Many of these products are expensive and time consuming to use, yet seldom do they provide an effective remedy for regaining lost hair. This can result in overwhelming emotional distress, disappointment, and expense.

Topical minoxidil 2% (Rogaine) is the only medication approved by the Food and Drug Administration (FDA) for androgenetic alopecia. The preparation is applied to the scalp twice daily. It takes at least a year of constant treatment before any evidence of hair regrowth can be observed. Side effects of therapy include allergic contact dermatitis and folliculitis (Olsen, 1994). Hair growth is maintained only while treatment continues; therefore, long-term use of minoxidil can become very expensive.

Topical tretinoin, used as a single agent or in combination with minoxidil, has been studied for its effects on hair regrowth. Combination therapy appears to have more potential benefits than tretinoin used alone. The side effects of scalp irritation and photosensitivity, however, would appear to be limiting factors in its acceptance.

Natural-looking hairpieces have been developed that allow the wearer to feel more attractive.

CRITICAL THINKING EXERCISES

1. A corticosteroid cream has been prescribed for a patient at a dermatology clinic. The patient expresses relief that he now has a medicine that he can use to relieve his symptoms whenever they occur. How would you caution this patient about the use of this medication, and how would you explain the reasons for these precautions?
2. An elderly patient complains of very dry, itchy skin. Based on your knowledge of the skin changes that occur in the elderly, how would you proceed to instruct and guide this patient? What if the patient were a 30-year-old mother of two small children? How would you assess this situation, and what factors might you surmise could be causing the dry, itchy skin in a person of this age?
3. A teenage patient requests a diet to control his acne. Describe how you would explain to this patient the nutritional and dietary considerations associated with acne. Consider other factors that might need to be assessed in counseling this patient.
4. A patient in a home for senior citizens has several red vesicular areas on her right breast, under the breast, and on her back. She tells you that the areas are painful and that she has been applying a hydrocortisone cream to them. How would you assess this situation to determine what course of action to take? Explain your reasoning for deciding how to proceed.

Hair Transplantation Surgery. Hair transplantation surgery (hair replacement surgery) involves transplanting hair-bearing skin from the sides and posterior portions of the scalp to recipient spaces in the bald areas. This redistributes the patient's remaining hair as naturally and evenly as possible over the bald scalp area and is accomplished by a process called **punch grafting,** by **scalp reduction,** or by using flaps of various kinds.

Punch grafting is performed in four or more sessions on an outpatient basis; the number of sessions depends on the extent of baldness. Hairpieces and hats should not be worn for at least a week after the transplant.

Scalp reduction is a surgical procedure in which the bald portion of the scalp is reduced by staged surgical excisions. It is usually the procedure of choice for baldness of the vertex (top of head) and anterior vertex regions.

Hair-bearing flaps can be transposed from adjacent areas into bald areas. This procedure may be performed in several stages over several months. With the use of flaps, 200 to 250 hairs per square centimeter, about normal density, can be transferred. Thus, hair is obtained instantly as soon as the flap is rotated over the bald area. Infection and bone necrosis can complicate scalp surgery.

BIBLIOGRAPHY

Books

Abel EA (ed). Photochemotherapy in Dermatology. New York, Igaku-Shoin Medical Publishers, Inc., 1992.

Achauer BM, VanderKam VM, and Berns MW. Lasers in Plastic Surgery and Dermatology. New York, Thieme Medical Publishers, Inc., 1992.

Camp RDR. Psoriasis. In Champion RH, Burton JL, and Ebling FGH (eds). Textbook of Dermatology. Oxford, Blackwell Scientific Publications, 1992.

Gee G and Moran TA. AIDS: Concepts in Nursing Practice. Baltimore, Williams & Wilkins, 1988.

Gilchrest BA. Retinoid pharmacology and skin. In Mukhtar H (ed). Pharmacology of the Skin. Boca Raton, CRC Press, 1992.

Kotler R. Facial peeling: Phenol. In Parish LC and Lask GP. Aesthetic Dermatology. New York, McGraw-Hill, Inc. Health Professions Division, 1994.

MacKie RM. Clinical Dermatology: An Illustrated Textbook. Oxford, Oxford University Press, 1991.

Marks JG and DeLeo VA. Contact and Occupational Dermatology. St. Louis, Mosby-Year Book, 1992.

Marzulli FN and Maibach HI (eds). Dermato-Toxicology. New York, Hemisphere Publishing Corporation, 1991.

Mukhtar H. (ed). Pharmacology of the Skin. Boca Raton, CRC Press, 1992.

Olsen EA (ed). Disorders of Hair Growth: Diagnosis and Treatment. New York, McGraw-Hill, Inc. Health Professions Division, 1994.

Parish LC and Lask GP. Aesthetic Dermatology. New York, McGraw-Hill, Inc. Health Professions Division, 1991.

Roenigk HH and Maibach HI (eds). Psoriasis. New York, Marcel Dekker, Inc., 1991.

Shelley WB and Shelley ED. Advanced Dermatologic Diagnosis. Philadelphia, WB Saunders, 1992.

Sliney DH. Laser safety for plastic surgery and dermatology. In Achauer et al. Lasers in Plastic Surgery and Dermatology. New York, Thieme Medical Publishers, Inc., 1992.

Soter NA and Baden HP (eds). Pathophysiology of Dermatologic Diseases. New York, McGraw-Hill, Inc., 1991.

Stawiski MA. Acne and related conditions. In Price SA and Wilson LM. Pathophysiology: Clinical Concepts of Disease Processes. St. Louis, Mosby-Year Book, 1992.

Journals

Baker G. Writing easily read patient education handouts: A computerized approach. Semin Dermatol 1991 June; 10(2):102–106.
Beacham BE. Common dermatoses in the elderly. Am Fam Physician 1993 May; 47(6):1145–1450.
Berwick M et al. The role of the nurse in skin cancer prevention, screening, and early detection. Semin Oncol Nurs 1991 Feb; 7(1):64–71.
Brown CD and Zitelli JA. A review of topical agents for wounds and methods of wounding. Guidelines for wound management. J Dermatol Surg Oncol 1993; 19:732–737.
Buller DB and Buller MK. Approaches to communicating preventive behaviors. Semin Oncol Nurs 1991 Feb; 7(1):53–56.
Clark C. Acne—general practice management. Practitioner 1993 Feb; 237:160–164.
Eaglestein WH. Occlusive dressings. J Dermatol Surg Oncol 1993; 19:716–720.
Epstein E. Strategies for using patient instruction sheets. Semin Dermatol 1991 June; 10(2):98–101.
Estes SA and Estes J. Therapy of scabies: Nursing homes, hospitals, and the homeless. Semin Dermatol 1993 March; 1:26–33.
Evans C. Skin Surgery. Practitioner 1993 Feb; 237:139–142.
Feingold DS. Staphylococcal and streptococcal pyodermas. Semin Dermatol 1993 Dec; 12(4):331–335.
Flory C. Skin assessment. RN 1992 June; 55(6):22–26.
Fraser MC, Hartge P, and Tucker MA. Melonoma and non-melanoma skin cancer: Epidemiology and risk factors. Semin Oncol Nurs 1991; 7(1):2–12.
Friedman LC et al. Skin self-examination in a population at increased risk for skin cancer. Am J Prev Med 1993; 9(6):359–364.
Friedman RJ et al. Malignant melanoma in the 1990's: The continued importance of early detection and the role of physician examination and self-examination of the skin. CA Cancer J Clinicians 1991 July/Aug; 41(4):201–226.
Gawkrodger D. Atopic eczema. Practitioner 1993 Feb; 237:166–171.
Goldstein SM. Advances in the treatment of superficial candida infections. Semin Dermatol 1993 Dec; 12(4):315–330.
Haus C, Paquet P, and Marechal-Courtois C. Long-term corneal involvement following drug-induced toxic epidermal necrolysis (Lyell's disease). Ophthalmologica 1993; 206(3):115–118.
Kirkevold M. Toward a practice theory of caring for patients with chronic skin disease. Scholarly Inquiry for Nursing Practice: An International Journal 1993; 7(19):37–52.
Klaus MV and Wieslthier JS. Contact dermatitis. Am Fam Physician 1993 Sep; 48(4):629–632.
Kligman AM. Tretinoin (Retin-A) therapy of photoaged skin. Compr Ther 1992; 18(9):10–13.
Lawler PE. Cutaneous malignant melanoma. Semin Oncol Nurs 1991 Feb; 7(1):26–35.
Leffell DJ, Berwick M, and Bolognia J. The effect of pre-education on patient compliance with full body examination in a public skin cancer screening. J Dermatol Surg Oncol 1993; 19:660–663.
Lesher J, Levine N, and Treadwell P. Fungal skin infections: Common but stubborn. Patient Care 1994 Jan;16–44.
Levine AM. AIDS-related malignancies: The emerging epidemic. J Natl Cancer Inst 1993; 85(17):1382–1397.
Leyden JJ and Aly R. Tinea pedis. Semin Dermatol 1993 Dec; 12(4):280–284.
Litt JZ. Steroid-induced rosacea. Am Fam Physician 1993 May; 47(1):67–71.
Loescher LJ and Meyskens FL. Chemoprevention of human skin cancers. Semin Oncol Nurs 1991; 7(1):45–52.
Mawn VB and Fleischer AB. A survey of attitudes, beliefs, and behavior regarding tanning bed use, sunbathing, and sunscreen use. Journal of the Academy of Dermatology 1993; 29:959–962.
McKeown A. Pulsed-dye laser treatment of vascular lesions. Dermatology Nurs 1991; 3(5):330–334.
McPherson ML. The use of topical corticosteroids. Journal of Home Health Care Practice 1993 May; 5(3):50–55.
Motta GL. How moisture-retentive dressings promote healing. RN 1993 Dec; 23(12):26–33.
Myskowski PL. Editorial. Kaposi's sarcoma: Where do we go from here? Arch Dermatol 1993 Oct; 129:1320–1323.
Orkin M and Maibach HI. Scabies therapy—1993. Semin Dermatol 1993 Mar; 1:22–25.
Rapaport MJ. Choosing a broad-spectrum sunscreen with UVA protection. Dermatology Nurs 1991 Apr: 3(2):83–102.
Roberts D and Evans G. Management of superficial fungal infections. Practitioner 1993 Feb; 237:153–157.
Runkle GP and Zalonznik AJ. Malignant melanoma. Am Fam Physician 1994 Jan; 49(1):91–100.
Safai B, Diaz B, and Schwartz J. Malignant neoplasms associated with human immunodeficiency virus infection. CA Cancer J Clin 1992 Mar–Apr; 42(2):74–95.
Schleper JR. Teaching skin self-examination. Dermatology Nurs 1991 June; 3(3):174–176.
Schlnitz LS and Garden JM. Applications of lasers for skin disorders. Compr Ther 1992; 18(9):28–31.
Schopf E et al. Toxic epidermal necrolysis and Steven-Johnson syndrome: An epidemiologic study from West Germany. Arch Dermatol 1991 Jan; 127(6):839–842.
Sher TH. Clinical evaluation of generalized pruritus. Compr Ther 1992; 18(9):14–19.
Stampien TM and Schwartz RA. Erythema multiforme. Am Fam Physician 1992 Oct; 46(4):1171–1176.
Sterling GB et al. Scabies. Am Fam Physician 1992 Oct; 46(4): 1237–1241.
Stiller MJ. A management update on psoriasis. Hospital Medicine 1994 Jan; 30(1):28–35.
Vargo NL. Basal and squamous cell carcinomas: An overview. Semin Oncol Nurs 1991 Feb; 7(1):13–25.

INFORMATION/RESOURCES

Agencies

American Cancer Society, Inc.
1599 Clifton Rd NE
Atlanta, GA
800 (ACS-2345)

National Institute of Arthritis and Musculoskeletal and Skin Diseases
National Institutes of Health,
Bethesda, MD 20892

National Psoriasis Foundation
6415 SW Canyon Court,
Suite 200,
Portland, OR 97221

Skin Cancer Foundation
575 Park Ave S,
New York, NY 10016

55

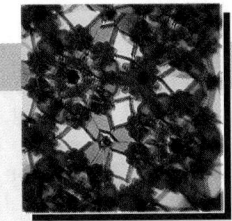

Management of Patients With Burn Injury

CHAPTER OUTLINE

Pathophysiology of Burns
Systemic Response
Local Response and Extent of Burns

Emergent/Resuscitative Phase of Burn Care
On-the-Scene Care
Emergency Medical Management
Management of Fluid Loss and Shock
NURSING PROCESS: Burn Care During the Emergent/Resuscitative Phase

Acute or Intermediate Phase of Burn Care
The Burn Wound
Threat of Infection
General Wound Care
Wound Cleaning
Topical Antibacterial Therapy
Dressing Changes
Debridement
Grafting the Burn Wound
Pain Management
Nutritional Support

Disorders of Wound Healing
NURSING PROCESS: Burn Care During the Acute Phase

Rehabilitation Phase of Burn Care
Home Care and Follow-Up
NURSING PROCESS: Burn Care During the Rehabilitation Phase

Patient Education and Home Care Considerations

Gerontologic Considerations

Critical Thinking Exercises

LEARNING OBJECTIVES

On completion of this chapter, the learner will be able to:

1. Describe the local and systemic effects of a major burn injury
2. Describe on-the-scene care for the person who experiences a burn injury
3. Describe the three phases of burn care and the priorities of care for each phase
4. Compare and contrast the potential fluid and electrolyte alterations of the emergent/resuscitative and acute phases of burn management
5. Describe the nurse's role in the following areas of management: pain management, restrictions of activity and joint motion, psychologic support of the patient and family, nutritional support, pulmonary care, patient and family education
6. Describe the goals of the following aspects of burn wound care and the nurse's role in each of the following: wound cleansing, dressing changes, grafting of burn wound, topical antibacterial therapy, debridement
7. Use the nursing process as a framework for care of the patient during the emergent/resuscitative phase, the acute phase, and the rehabilitation phase of burn care
8. Identify community services and resources that may be used by the patient discharged from the hospital with a major burn injury

Suzanne C. Smeltzer and Brenda G. Bare: Brunner and Suddarth's Textbook of Medical-Surgical Nursing, 8th Edition. © 1996 Lippincott-Raven Publishers.

Approximately 2.5 million people experience burn injury in the United States each year. Of this group, 200,000 require outpatient treatment and 100,000 are hospitalized. About 12,000 people die from burns and related inhalation injuries annually. One million work days are lost each year by burn injury. More than half of burn injuries leading to hospital admissions could have been prevented. Nurses can play an active role in preventing fires and burns by teaching prevention concepts and promoting legislation related to fire safety.

Young children and elderly persons are at particularly high risk for burn injury. Adolescent males and men of working age also are burned more frequently than would be expected by their representation in the total population. Most burn injuries occur in the home. Cooking, heating, or using electrical appliances are usually involved. Industrial accidents also account for many burn injuries.

The National Institute for Burn Medicine, which collects statistical data from burn centers throughout the United States, notes that most patients (75%) are victims of their own actions. Scalds in toddlers; playing with matches in school-age children; electrical injury in adolescent males; and drug, alcohol, and cigarette use in adults all contribute to the statistics. Cobb, Maxwell and Silverstein (1992) found that about 13% of hospitalized burn patients or their family members had previously been hospitalized for burn injury. Nurses must be instrumental in intervening to break this cycle of burn injury.

There are four major goals relating to burns:

1. Prevention
2. Institution of life-saving measures for the severely burned person
3. Prevention of disability and disfigurement through early, specialized, individualized treatment
4. Rehabilitation of the individual through reconstructive surgery and rehabilitative programs

Survival Prediction. Very young and very old persons have a high risk of mortality following burn injuries. The chances of survival are greater in children over age 5 and in young adults age 40 or younger. Inhalation injuries in addition to cutaneous burns worsen the patient's prognosis. Outcome depends on the depth and extent of the burn as well as on the preinjury health status and age of the patient.

Pathophysiology of Burns

Burns are caused by a transfer of energy from a heat source to the body. Heat may be transferred through conduction or electromagnetic radiation. Burns are categorized as thermal, radiation, or chemical. Tissue destruction results from coagulation, protein denaturation, or ionization of cellular contents. The skin and the mucosa of the upper airways are the sites of tissue destruction. Deep tissues, including the viscera, can be damaged by electrical burns or through prolonged contact with the burning agent. Organ necrosis and failure can result.

The depth of the injury depends on the temperature of the burning agent and the duration of contact with the agent. For example, in the case of scald burns in adults, 1 second of contact with hot tap water at 68.9°C (156°F) may result in a burn that destroys both the epidermis and the dermis, causing a full-thickness (third-degree) injury. Fifteen seconds of exposure to hot water at 56.1°C (133°F) results in a similar full-thickness injury. Temperatures less than 111°F are tolerated for long periods without injury.

Burn care must be planned according to the extent and depth of the injury and then proceeds through the three phases of burn care: the emergent/resuscitative phase, the acute or intermediate phase, and the rehabilitative phase.

Systemic Response

Pathophysiologic changes resulting from major burns during the initial burn-shock period include tissue hypoperfusion and organ hypofunction secondary to decreased cardiac output, followed by a hyperdynamic and hypermetabolic phase. Patients whose burns do not exceed 20% of their body surface area (BSA) primarily have a localized response. The incidence, magnitude, and duration of pathophysiologic changes in burns are proportional to the extent of burn injury, with a maximum response seen in burns covering 60% or greater of the patient's BSA. The initial systemic event following a major burn injury is hemodynamic instability, resulting from loss of capillary integrity and a subsequent shift of fluid, sodium, and protein from the intravascular space into the interstitial spaces. Figure 55-1 illustrates pathophysiologic processes in acute major burns. Hemodynamic instability involves not only cardiovascular but also fluid and electrolyte, blood volume, pulmonary, and other mechanisms.

Cardiovascular Response

Cardiac output decreases before any significant change in blood volume is evident. As fluid loss continues and vascular volume decreases, cardiac output continues to fall and blood pressure drops. This is the onset of burn shock. In response, the sympathetic nervous system releases catecholamines, which results in an increase in peripheral resistance (vasoconstriction) and an increase in pulse rate. The peripheral vascular vasoconstriction further decreases cardiac output.

Prompt fluid resuscitation allows the blood pressure to stay in the low normal range and the cardiac output to improve. Despite adequate fluid resuscitation, cardiac filling pressures—central venous pressure, pulmonary artery pressure, and pulmonary artery wedge pressure—remain low during the burn-shock period. If inadequate fluid resuscitation occurs, distributive shock will occur (discussed in Chapter 15.)

Generally, the greatest volume of fluid leak occurs in the first 24 to 36 hours after the burn, peaking by 6 to 8 hours. As the capillaries begin to regain their integrity, burn shock resolves and fluid returns to the vascular compartment. As fluid is reabsorbed from the interstitial tissue into the vascular compartment, blood volume increases. If renal and cardiac function are adequate, urinary output increases. Diuresis continues for several days to 2 weeks.

As previously noted, in burns involving less than 30% of the total BSA, the loss of capillary integrity and shift of fluid are localized to the burn itself, resulting in blister formation

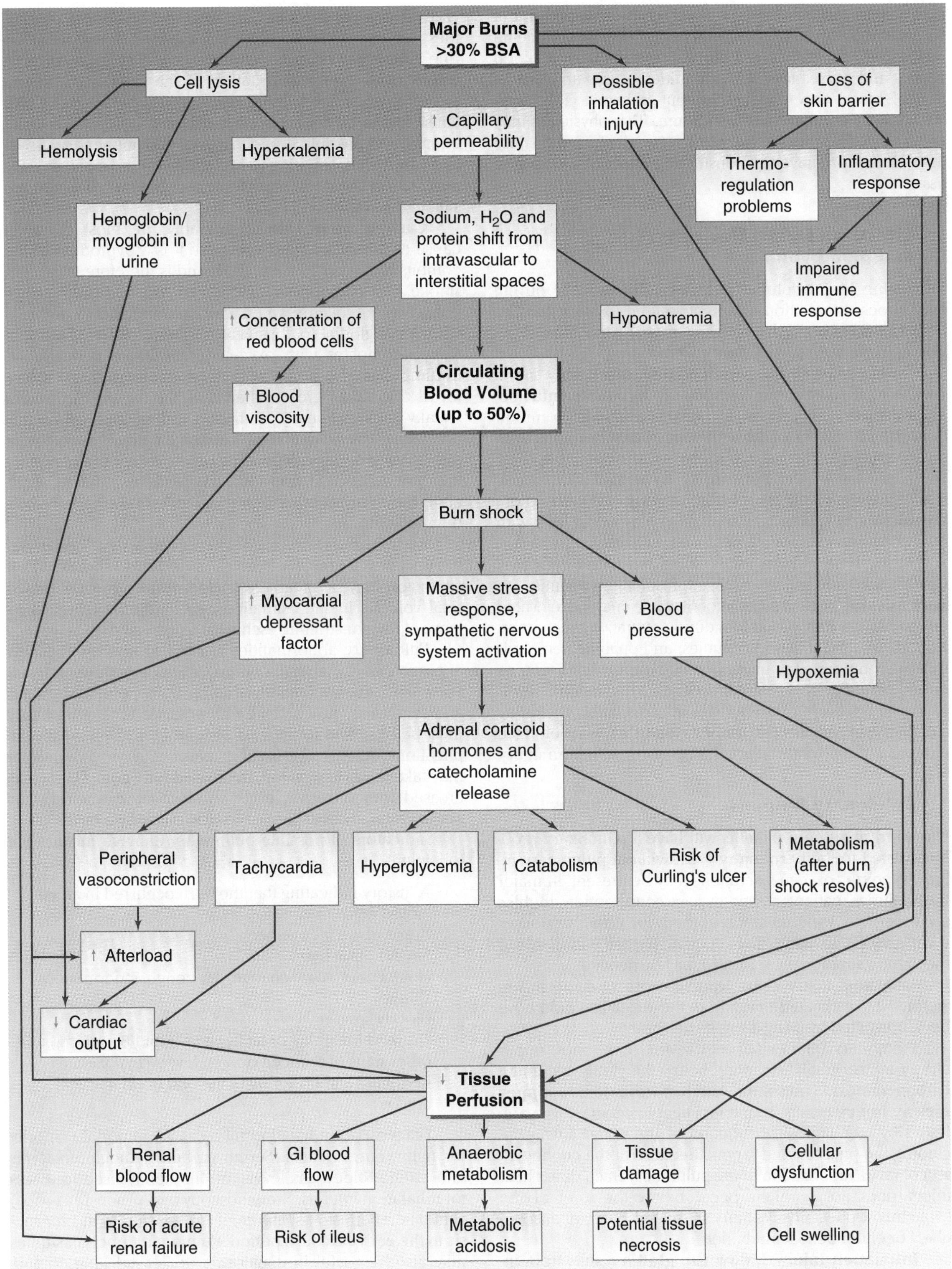

FIGURE 55-1. Overview of physiologic changes that occur after acute burn injury.

and edema only in the area of injury. Patients with more severe burns develop massive systemic edema. As edema increases in circumferential burns, pressure on small blood vessels and nerves in distal extremities causes an obstruction of blood flow and consequent ischemia. This complication is compartment syndrome. The physician may need to perform an **escharotomy** (surgical incision into the eschar) to relieve the constricting effect of the burned tissue.

Effects on Fluids, Electrolytes, and Blood Volume

Circulating blood volume decreases dramatically during burn shock. In addition, evaporative fluid loss through the burn wound may reach 3 to 5 L or more over a 24-hour period until the burn surfaces are covered.

During burn shock, serum sodium levels vary in response to fluid resuscitation. Usually **hyponatremia** (sodium depletion) is present. Hyponatremia is also common during the first week of the acute phase, as water shifts from the interstitial to the vascular space.

Immediately after burn injury, **hyperkalemia** (excessive potassium level) results from massive cell destruction. **Hypokalemia** (potassium depletion) may occur later with fluid shifts and inadequate potassium intake.

At the time of burn injury, some red blood cells may be destroyed and others damaged, resulting in anemia. Despite this, the patient's hematocrit value may be elevated due to plasma loss. Blood loss during operative procedures, wound care and diagnostic studies, and ongoing hemolysis further contribute to anemia. Blood transfusions are required periodically to maintain adequate hemoglobin levels for oxygen delivery. Abnormalities in coagulation, including a decrease in platelets (**thrombocytopenia**) and prolonged clotting and prothrombin times, also occur with burn injury.

Pulmonary Response

One third of all burn patients will have a pulmonary problem related to the burn injury. Even without pulmonary injury, **hypoxia** (oxygen starvation) may be present. In major burn injuries, patients' tissue oxygen consumption doubles secondary to hypermetabolism and localized responses (White, 1993). To assure that adequate oxygen is available to the tissues, supplemental oxygen may be needed.

Inhalation injury is the leading cause of death in fire victims. It is estimated that half of these deaths could have been prevented by using a smoke detector.

Pulmonary injuries fall into several categories: upper airway injury; inhalation injury below the glottis, including carbon monoxide poisoning; and restrictive defects. **Upper airway injury** results from direct heat or edema. It is manifested by mechanical obstruction of the upper airway, including the pharynx and larynx. Because of the cooling effect of rapid vaporization in the pulmonary tract, direct heat injury does not normally occur below the level of the bronchus. Upper airway injury is treated by *early* nasotracheal or endotracheal intubation.

Inhalation injury below the glottis results from inhaling the products of incomplete combustion or noxious gases. These products include carbon monoxide, sulfur oxides, nitrogen oxides, aldehydes, cyanide, ammonia, chlorine, phosgene, benzene, and halogens. The injury directly results from chemical irritation of the pulmonary tissues at the alveolar level. Inhalation injuries below the glottis cause loss of ciliary action, hypersecretion, severe mucosal edema, and possibly, bronchospasm. The pulmonary surfactant is reduced, resulting in **atelectasis** (lung collapse). Expectoration of carbon particles in the sputum is the cardinal sign of this injury.

Carbon monoxide is probably the most common cause of inhalation injury because it is a byproduct of the combustion of organic materials and is therefore present in smoke. The pathophysiologic effects are due to tissue hypoxia, which occurs when carbon monoxide combines with hemoglobin to form carboxyhemoglobin. This substance competes with oxygen for available hemoglobin-binding sites. The affinity of hemoglobin for carbon monoxide is 200 times greater than that for oxygen. Treatment usually consists of early intubation and mechanical ventilation with 100% oxygen. However, some patients may require only oxygen therapy, depending on the extent of pulmonary injury and edema. Using 100% oxygen is essential to accelerate the removal of carbon monoxide from the hemoglobin molecule.

Restrictive defects arise when edema develops under full-thickness burns encircling the neck and thorax. Chest excursion may be greatly restricted, resulting in decreased tidal volume. In such situations, escharotomy (surgical release of the constricting eschar) is a necessity.

Pulmonary abnormalities are not always immediately apparent. More than half of burn victims with pulmonary involvement do not initially demonstrate pulmonary signs and symptoms. Any patient with possible inhalation injury must be observed for at least 24 hours for respiratory complications. Airway obstruction may occur very rapidly or may take hours to develop. Decreased lung compliance, decreased arterial oxygen levels, and respiratory acidosis may occur gradually over the first 5 days following a burn.

Indicators of possible pulmonary damage include the following:

- A history indicating that the burn occurred in an enclosed area
- Burns of the face or neck
- Singed nasal hair
- Hoarseness, voice change, dry cough, stridor, sooty sputum
- Bloody sputum
- Labored breathing or tachypnea (rapid breathing) and other signs of reduced oxygen levels (hypoxemia)
- Erythema and blistering of the oral or pharyngeal mucosa

Diagnosis of inhalation injury is an important priority for many burn victims. Serum carboxyhemoglobin levels and arterial blood gas levels are frequently used to assess for inhalation injuries. Bronchoscopy and xenon-133 (^{133}Xe) ventilation-perfusion scans can also be used to aid diagnosis in the early postburn period. Pulmonary function studies may also be useful in diagnosing decreased lung compliance or obstructed air flow.

Pulmonary complications that can occur secondary to inhalation injuries include acute respiratory failure and adult respiratory distress syndrome (ARDS). Respiratory failure occurs when the extent of ventilation and gas exchange impairment is life threatening for the patient. The immediate intervention is intubation and mechanical ventilation. If independent ventilation is impaired by restricted chest excursion, immediate escharotomy is needed. ARDS may develop in the first few days after the burn injury secondary to systemic and pulmonary responses to the burn and inhalation injury. Respiratory failure and ARDS are discussed in Chapter 24.

Other Systemic Responses

Renal function may be altered as a result of decreased blood volume. Destruction of red blood cells at the injury site results in free hemoglobin in the urine. If muscle damage occurs (for example, from electrical burns), myoglobin will be released from the muscle cells and excreted by the kidney. Adequate fluid volume replacement restores renal blood flow, increasing glomerular filtration rate and urine volume. If there is inadequate blood flow through the kidney, the hemoglobin and myoglobin occlude the renal tubules, resulting in the complication of acute tubular necrosis and renal failure (see Chapter 43).

The immunologic defenses of the body are greatly altered by a burn injury. All levels of immune response are adversely affected. The loss of skin integrity is compounded by the release of abnormal inflammatory factors, altered levels of immunoglobulins and serum complement, impaired neutrophil function, and a reduction in lymphocytes (**lymphocytopenia**). Immunosuppression places the burn patient at high risk for sepsis.

Loss of skin also results in an inability to regulate body temperature. Burn patients may therefore manifest low body temperatures in the early hours postburn, but as hypermetabolism resets core temperatures, burn patients become hyperthermic for much of the postburn period, even in the absence of infection.

Two potential gastrointestinal complications may occur: **paralytic ileus** (absence of intestinal peristalsis) and **Curling's ulcer.** Decreased peristalsis and bowel sounds are manifestations of paralytic ileus resulting from burn trauma. Gastric distention and nausea may lead to vomiting unless gastric decompression is initiated. Gastric bleeding secondary to the massive physiologic stress may be signaled by occult blood in the stool, regurgitation of coffee ground–like material from the stomach, or bloody vomitus. These signs suggest gastric or duodenal erosion (Curling's ulcer).

Local Response and Extent of Burns

Burn Depth

Burns are classified according to the depth of tissue destruction and are identified as **superficial partial-thickness** injuries, **deep partial-thickness** injuries, or **full-thickness** injuries. Corresponding descriptive terms are first-, second-, and third-degree burns. (See Chapter 54, Fig. 54-9 for a diagram of skin layers.) The local response to burn injury depends on the depth of tissue destruction.

- In a **superficial partial-thickness (first-degree) injury,** the epidermis is destroyed or injured and a portion of the dermis may be injured. The wound may be painful and may appear red and dry, as in sunburn, or it may be blistered.
- A **deep partial-thickness (second-degree) injury** involves destruction of the epidermis and upper layers of the dermis and injury to deeper portions of the dermis. The wound is painful, appears red, and exudes fluid. Blanching of the burned tissue is followed by capillary refill; hair follicles remain intact.
- A **full-thickness (third-degree) injury** involves total destruction of epidermis and dermis and, in some cases, underlying tissues as well. The color of the wound varies widely from white to red, brown, or black. The burned area is painless because nerve fibers are destroyed. The wound has a leathery appearance. Hair follicles and sweat glands are destroyed.

Table 55-1 describes these wounds in detail. Generally, the burn wound is not of uniform depth. When assessed, the wound usually includes areas of superficial injury at the periphery with increasing depth proximally (near the core). Each burned area has three zones of injury. The inner area is the most damaged, and the outer zone the least. These zones are illustrated in Figure 55-2. The inner area is known as the zone of coagulation, where cellular death occurs. The middle area is the zone of stasis, where there is compromised blood supply, inflammation, and tissue injury. This area can be salvaged to some extent with successful fluid resuscitation. Research into additional methods to reverse the capillary stasis in the zone of stasis is in progress (Rockwell & Ehrlich, 1992; Wong & Munster, 1993). The outer area is the zone of hyperemia. This zone is essentially a first-degree burn, which should heal within a week and which is more characteristic of flame and electrical injuries than of injuries caused by hot liquids.

In determining the depth of a burn, it is important to consider the following factors:

- A history of how the injury occurred
- The causative agent, such as flame or a scalding liquid
- The temperature of the burning agent
- The duration of contact with the agent
- The thickness of the skin

Extent of Body Surface Area Burned

Rule of Nines. An estimation of the total body surface area (BSA) involved in a burn is simplified by using the Rule of Nines (Fig. 55-3). The Rule of Nines is a quick way to calculate the extent of burns. The system assigns percentages in multiples of nine to major body surfaces.

Lund and Browder Method. A more precise method of estimating the extent of burned BSA is the Lund and Browder method, which recognizes that the percentage of BSA of various anatomic parts, especially the head and legs, changes with growth. By dividing the body into very small areas and providing an estimate of the proportion of

TABLE 55-1 Characteristics of Burns According to Depth

Depth of Burn and Causes	Skin Involvement	Symptoms	Wound Appearance	Recuperative Course
Superficial (First-Degree)				
Sunburn Low-intensity flash	Epidermis	Tingling Hyperesthesia (super sensitivity) Pain that is soothed by cooling	Reddened; blanches with pressure Minimal or no edema	Complete recovery within a week Peeling
Partial-Thickness (Second-Degree)				
Scalds Flash flame	Epidermis and part of dermis	Pain Hyperesthesia Sensitive to cold air	Blistered, mottled red base; broken epidermis; weeping surface Edema	Recovery in 2 to 3 weeks Some scarring and depigmentation Infection may convert it to third-degree
Full-Thickness (Third-Degree)				
Flame Prolonged exposure to hot liquids Electric current	Epidermis, entire dermis, and sometimes subcutaneous tissue	Pain free Shock Hematuria (blood in the urine) and possibly, hemolysis (blood cell destruction) Possible entrance and exit wounds (electrical burn)	Dry; pale white, leathery, or charred Broken skin with fat exposed Edema	Eschar sloughs Grafting necessary Scarring and loss of contour and function Loss of digits or extremity possible

BSA accounted for by such body parts, one can obtain a reliable estimate of the total BSA burned. The initial evaluation is made upon arrival at the hospital and is revised on the second and third postburn days, because the demarcation usually is not clear until then.

Palm Method. In patients with scattered burns, a method to estimate the percentage of burn is the palm method. The size of the patient's palm is approximately 1% of the body surface area (BSA). The size of the palm can be used for assessing the extent of burn injury.

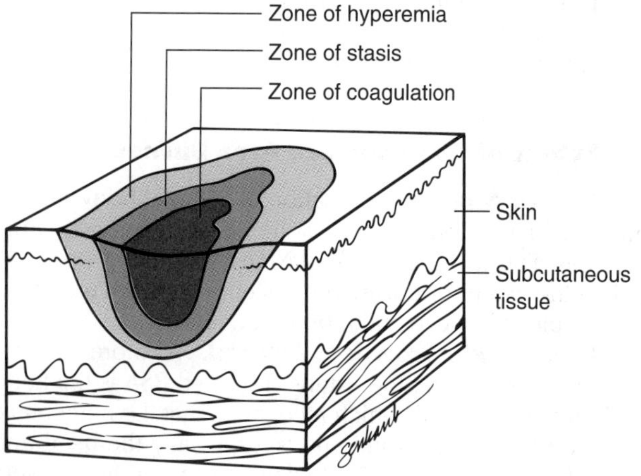

FIGURE 55-2. Zones of burn injury.

Emergent/Resuscitative Phase of Burn Care

As noted previously, the pathophysiology and management of a burn can be divided into three phases. Although priorities exist for each of the phases, it is imperative to remember that these phases overlap and that assessment and management of specific problems and complications are *not* limited to these phases but take place throughout the course of burn care. The three phases and the priorities for care are summarized in Table 55-2.

On-the-Scene Care

The first priority in on-the-scene care for a burn victim is to prevent injury to the rescuer. If needed, fire and emergency medical services should be requested at the first opportunity. Additional emergency procedures follow:

- **Extinguish the flames.** When clothes catch on fire, the flames can be extinguished if the victim falls to the floor or ground and rolls ("drop and roll"); anything available to smother the flames, such as a blanket, rug, or coat, may be used. Standing still forces the victim to breathe flames and smoke, and running fans the flames. If the burn source is electrical, the electrical source must be disconnected.

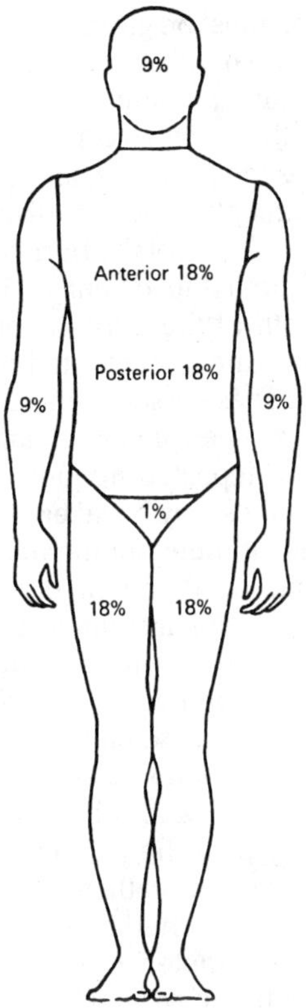

FIGURE 55-3. The Rule of Nines: Estimated percentage of body surface area (BSA) in the adult.

- **Cool the burn.** After the flames are extinguished, the burned area and adherent clothing are soaked with cold water, briefly, to cool the wound and halt the burning process. Once a burn has been sustained, the application of cold is the best first-aid measure. Soaking the burn area intermittently in cool water or applying cold towels gives immediate and striking relief from pain and restricts local tissue edema and damage. However, one should *never* apply ice directly to the burn or use cold soaks or dressings for longer than several minutes; such a procedure may worsen the tissue damage and lead to hypothermia in patients with large burns.
- **Remove restrictive objects.** Although adherent clothing may be left in place, other clothing and all jewelry should be removed to allow for assessment and to prevent constriction secondary to rapidly developing edema.
- **Cover the wound.** The burn should also be covered as quickly as possible to minimize bacterial contamination and decrease pain by preventing air from coming into contact with the injured surface. Sterile dressings are best, but any clean, dry cloth can be used as an emergency dressing. Ointments and salves are *not* used. In fact, other than the dressing, no medication or material should be applied to the burn wound.
- **Irrigate chemical burns.** Chemical burns resulting from contact with a corrosive material are irrigated immediately. Most chemical laboratories have a high-pressure shower for such emergencies; if such an injury occurs at home, clothes should be removed immediately, and all areas of the body that have come in contact with the chemical should be rinsed in a shower or other source of continuously running water. If a chemical gets in or near the eyes, the eyes should be flushed with cool, clean water immediately. Outcomes for the patient with chemical burns are significantly improved by rapid, sustained flushing of the injury at the scene.

Airway, Breathing, Circulation. Although the local effects of a burn are the most evident, the systemic effects pose a greater threat to life. Therefore, it is important to remember the ABCs of all trauma care during the early postburn period:

- **A**irway
- **B**reathing
- **C**irculation (and *C*ervical-spine immobilization if indicated)

TABLE 55-2 Phases of Burn Care

Phase	Duration	Priorities
Emergent or immediate resuscitative phase	From onset of injury to completion of fluid resuscitation	· First aid · Prevention of shock · Prevention of respiratory distress · Detection and treatment of concomitant injuries · Wound assessment and initial care
Acute phase	From beginning of diuresis to near completion of wound closure	· Wound care and closure · Prevention or treatment of complications, including infection · Nutritional support
Rehabilitation phase	From major wound closure to return to individual's optimal level of physical and psychosocial adjustment	· Prevention of scars and contractures · Physical, occupational, and vocational rehabilitation · Functional and cosmetic reconstruction · Psychosocial counseling

Breathing must be assessed and a patent airway established immediately during the initial minutes of emergency care. Many burn victims sustain some degree of concomitant pulmonary dysfunction, as previously described.

- Immediate therapy is directed toward establishing an airway and administering *humidified* 100% oxygen. If such a high concentration of oxygen is not available under emergency conditions, oxygen by mask or nasal cannula is given initially. If qualified personnel and equipment are present and if the victim has severe respiratory distress or airway edema, the rescuers can insert an endotracheal tube and initiate manual ventilation.

The circulatory system must also be assessed quickly. Apical pulse and blood pressure are monitored frequently. Tachycardia (abnormally rapid heart rate) and slight hypotension are expected in the untreated patient soon after the burn. At the same time, a secondary head-to-toe survey of the patient for other potentially life-threatening injuries should be performed.

Prevention of Shock. Preventing shock in a person with a major burn is imperative. Therefore, intravenous fluid therapy is initiated as soon as available.

- No food or fluid is given by mouth, and the patient is placed in a position that will prevent aspiration of vomitus, because nausea and vomiting typically occur as a result of paralytic ileus, which results from the stress of injury.

Usually rescue workers will cool the wound, establish an airway, supply oxygen, and start an intravenous line.

Emergency Medical Management

The patient is transported to the nearest emergency department. The hospital and physician are alerted that the patient is en route to the emergency department so that life-saving measures can be initiated immediately by a trained team.

Initial priorities in the emergency department remain airway, breathing, and circulation. For mild pulmonary injury, inspired air is humidified and the patient is encouraged to cough so that secretions can be removed by suctioning. For more severe situations, it is necessary to remove secretions by bronchial suctioning and to administer bronchodilators and mucolytic agents. If edema of the airway occurs, endotracheal intubation may be indicated. Continuous positive airway pressure and mechanical ventilation may also be required to achieve adequate oxygenation.

After adequate respiratory and circulatory status has been established, attention is directed to the burn wound itself. All clothing and jewelry are removed. Flushing of chemical burns with water is continued. The patient is checked for contact lenses; these are removed immediately if chemicals have contacted the eyes or if facial burns have occurred. It is important to validate an account of the burn scenario provided by the patient, witnesses at the scene, and paramedics and to assess for cervical spinal injuries or head injury if the patient was involved in an explosion, a fall, a jump, or an electrical injury.

Careful attention must be given to aseptic technique. Attending personnel wear masks, caps, and gowns; sterile gloves are worn when attending the burn wounds. The physician evaluates the patient's general condition, assesses the burn, determines the priorities, and directs the individualized plan of treatment, which is divided into systemic management and local care of the burned area.

Assessment of both the extent of body surface area burned and the depth of the burn is completed. Full- and partial-thickness burns are documented on burn assessment diagrams (Fig. 55-4). These assessments are performed after soot and debris have been gently cleaned from the burn wound. Assessment is repeated frequently throughout burn wound care. Photographs may be taken of the burn areas initially and periodically throughout the treatment. In this way, healing progress may be determined quickly. Such documentation is invaluable for insurance claims and legal issues. Sterile or pathogen-free (freshly laundered) sheets are placed under and over the patient to protect the area from contamination and to decrease pain caused by air currents.

A history of preexisting diseases, allergies, medications and use of drugs, alcohol, and tobacco is obtained at this point to appropriately plan the patient's care. A large-bore (16 or 18 gauge) intravenous catheter should be inserted in a nonburned area if not inserted earlier. Some patients may have a central venous catheter so that large amounts of intravenous fluids can be given quickly and central venous pressures can be monitored. If the patient's burn exceeds 20% BSA or if the patient is nauseated, a nasogastric tube should be inserted and connected to suction to prevent paralytic ileus (lack of peristalsis).

An indwelling urinary catheter is inserted to permit more accurate monitoring of urinary output and renal function. Baseline height; weight; arterial blood gases, hematocrit, and electrolyte values; blood typing and cross matching; urinalysis; and chest x-ray films are obtained. If the patient has an electrical burn, a baseline electrocardiogram is performed. Because burns are contaminated wounds, tetanus prophylaxis is administered if the patient's immunization status is not current.

Although the major focus of care during the emergent phase is physical stabilization, the nurse must also attend to the patient's and family's psychologic needs. Burn injury is a crisis, causing variable emotional responses. The patient's and family's coping abilities and available supports should be assessed along with assessment of physical status and provision of care. Circumstances surrounding the burn injury should be considered when providing care. Individualized psychosocial support must be given to the patient and his family. Because the emergent burn patient is usually anxious and in pain, those in attendance should provide reassurance and support, explanations of procedures, and adequate pain medication. Because poor tissue perfusion accompanies burn injuries, only intravenous pain medication (usually morphine) is given. If the patient wishes to see a spiritual advisor, one is notified.

Transfer to a Burn Center

The depth and extent of the burn are considered in determining whether the patient should be transferred to a burn

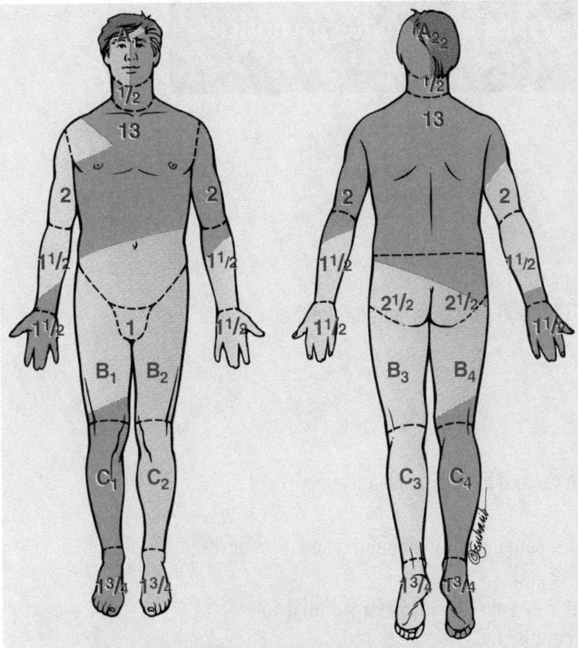

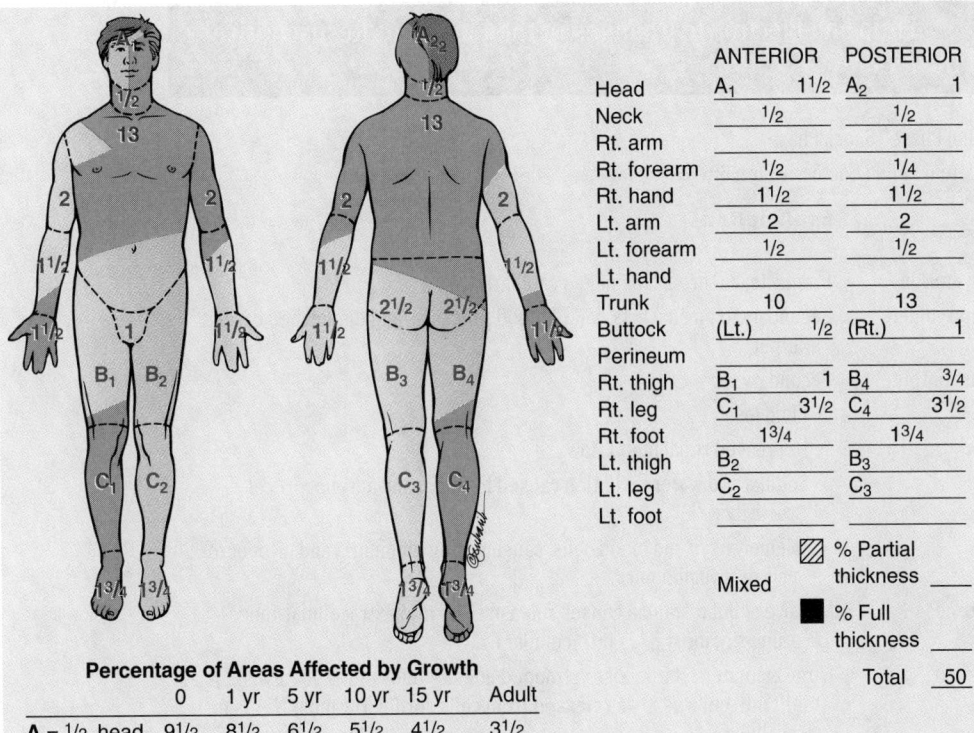

	ANTERIOR	POSTERIOR
Head	A_1 $1^1/_2$	A_2 1
Neck	1/2	1/2
Rt. arm		1
Rt. forearm	1/2	1/4
Rt. hand	$1^1/_2$	$1^1/_2$
Lt. arm	2	2
Lt. forearm	1/2	1/2
Lt. hand		
Trunk	10	13
Buttock	(Lt.) 1/2	(Rt.) 1
Perineum		
Rt. thigh	B_1 1	B_4 3/4
Rt. leg	C_1 $3^1/_2$	C_4 $3^1/_2$
Rt. foot	$1^3/_4$	$1^3/_4$
Lt. thigh	B_2	B_3
Lt. leg	C_2	C_3
Lt. foot		

Mixed ▨ % Partial thickness ____

■ % Full thickness ____

Total 50

Percentage of Areas Affected by Growth

	0	1 yr	5 yr	10 yr	15 yr	Adult
A = 1/2 head	$9^1/_2$	$8^1/_2$	$6^1/_2$	$5^1/_2$	$4^1/_2$	$3^1/_2$
B = 1 thigh	$2^3/_4$	$3^1/_4$	4	$4^1/_4$	$4^1/_2$	$4^3/_4$
C = 1/2 leg	$2^1/_2$	$2^1/_2$	$2^3/_4$	3	$3^1/_4$	$3^1/_2$

FIGURE 55-4. Sample chart for estimating percentage of body surface area burned (indicated by *shading*). (Courtesy of Crozer-Chester Medical Center, Upland, PA.)

center. Chart 55-1 lists the American Burn Association's criteria for burn center referral after initial assessment and management.

If the patient is to be transported to a burn center, the following measures are instituted before transfer: a secure intravenous line is placed with fluid infusing at the rate required to attain urine output of at least 30 ml per hour; a patent airway is ensured; adequate pain relief is attained; and adequate peripheral circulation is established in any burned extremity. Wounds are covered with sterile, dry dressings and the patient is kept comfortably warm. Assessments and treatments are documented, and this information is provided to the burn center personnel.

Management of Fluid Loss and Shock

Next to handling respiratory difficulties, the most urgent need is preventing irreversible shock by replacing lost fluids and electrolytes. Table 55-3 summarizes the fluid and electrolyte changes in the emergent phase of burn care. Intravenous lines and an indwelling catheter must be in place before implementing fluid resuscitation. Baseline weight and laboratory test results are obtained as well. These parameters must be monitored closely in the immediate postburn (resuscitation) period.

Fluid Replacement

There is no known way to stop fluid from moving into the interstitial spaces, but fluid replacement is possible. The

CHART 55-1

American Burn Association Criteria for Referral to a Burn Center

- Third-degree burns exceeding 5% body surface area (BSA) in any age group
- Second- and third-degree (partial- and full-thickness) burns exceeding 10% BSA in patients under age 10 or over age 50.
- Second- and third-degree burns exceeding 20% BSA in all other age groups
- Second- and third-degree burns that affect the face, hands, feet, genitalia, perineum, and major joints
- Electrical burns including lightning injury
- Chemical burns with serious threat of functional or cosmetic impairment
- Inhalation injury with burn injury
- Circumferential burns of the extremity and chest
- Burn injury in patients with preexisting illnesses that could complicate management
- Burn injury with trauma in which burn injury poses the greatest risk

(Data adapted from Nebraska Burn Institute, *Advanced Burn Life Support Manual*, Lincoln, NE, 1990.)

TABLE 55-3 Fluid and Electrolyte Changes in the Emergent/Resuscitative Phase of Burn Care

Fluid Accumulation Phase (Shock Phase)
Plasma → Interstitial Fluid (Edema at Burn Site)

Observation	Explanation
Generalized dehydration	Plasma leaks through damaged capillaries.
Reduction of blood volume	Secondary to plasma loss, fall of blood pressure, and diminished cardiac output
Decreased urinary output	Secondary to: Fluid loss; Decreased renal blood flow; Sodium and water retention caused by increased adrenocortical activity; (Hemolysis of red blood cells, causing hemoglobinuria and myonecrosis or myoglobinuria)
Potassium (K^+) excess	Massive cellular trauma causes release of K^+ into extracellular fluid (ordinarily, most K^+ is intracellular).
Sodium (Na^+) deficit	Large amount of Na^+ is lost in trapped edemat fluid and exudate and by shift into cells as K^+ is released from cells (ordinarily most Na^+ is extracellular).
Metabolic acidosis (base-bicarbonate deficit)	Loss of bicarbonate ions accompanies sodium loss.
Hemoconcentration (elevated hematocrit)	Liquid blood component is lost into extravascular space.

(Adapted from Metheny NM and Snively WD. Nurses' Handbook of Fluid Balance. Philadelphia, JB Lippincott.)

projected fluid requirements for the first 24 hours are calculated by the physician based on the extent of the patient's burn injury. Some combination of fluid categories may be used: (1) **colloids**—whole blood, plasma, and plasma expanders and (2) **crystalloids/electrolytes**—physiologic sodium chloride or lactated Ringer's solution. Adequate fluid resuscitation results in slightly decreased blood volume levels during the first 24 postburn hours and restores plasma levels to normal by the end of 48 hours.

Formulas have been developed for estimating fluid loss based on the estimated percentage of burned BSA and the weight of the patient. These are individualized to meet the requirements of each patient. The various formulas are discussed below and summarized in Chart 55-2.

The Consensus Formula. As early as 1978, the NIH Consensus Development Conference on Supportive Therapy in Burn Care established that salt and water are essential requirements of burn patients but that colloid may or may not be useful during the first 24 to 48 postburn hours.

The consensus formula provides for the volume of balanced salt solution to be administered in the first 24 hours in a range of 2 to 4 ml per kilogram per percent (ml/kg/%) burn. Generally, 2 ml/kg/% burn of lactated Ringer's solution may be used initially for adults. This is the most common fluid replacement formula in use today. As with the other formulas, half of the calculated total should be given over the first 8 postburn hours, and the other half should be given over the next 16 hours. The rate and volume of the infusion must be regulated according to the patient's response.

Studies have demonstrated that with large burns there is a failure of the sodium–potassium pump (a physiologic mechanism involved in fluid–electrolyte balance) at the cellular level. Thus, persons with very large burns may need proportionately more milliliters of fluid per percent of burn than those with smaller burns. Additionally, patients with electrical injury, pulmonary injury, and delayed fluid resuscitation and those who were burned while intoxicated may need additional fluids.

Fluid Replacement Example: 70-kg (About 168 lb) Patient With 50% Body Surface Area (BSA) Burn

1. Consensus formula: 2 to 4 ml/kg/% BSA
2. Calculate $2 \times 70 \times 50 = 7000$ ml/24 hours
3. Plan to administer: First 8 hours = 3500 ml, or 437 ml/hr; next 16 hours = 3500 ml, or 219 ml/hr

Most of the fluid replacement formulas use isotonic electrolyte solutions. Regardless of which standard replacement formula is used, the patient receives approximately the same fluid volume and sodium replacement during the first 48 hours. Another fluid replacement method requires hypertonic electrolyte solutions. This method uses concentrated solutions of sodium chloride and lactate (a balanced salt solution) so that the resulting fluid has a concentration of 250–300 mEq of sodium. The rationale for this replacement method is that by increasing serum osmolality, fluid

CHART 55-2
Guidelines and Formulas for Fluid Replacement in Burn Patients

Consensus Formula

Lactated Ringer's solution (or other balanced saline solution): 2–4 ml × kg body weight × % body surface area (BSA) burned. Half to be given in first 8 hours; remaining half to be given over next 16 hours.

Evans Formula

1. Colloids: 1 ml × kg body weight × % BSA burned
2. Electrolytes (saline): 1 ml × kg body weight × % BSA burned
3. Glucose (5% in water): 2000 ml for insensible loss
   Day 1: Half to be given in first 8 hours; remaining half over next 16 hours.
   Day 2: Half of previous day's colloids and electrolytes; all of insensible fluid replacement.

Maximum of 10,000 ml over 24 hours. Second- and third-degree burns exceeding 50% BSA are calculated on the basis of 50% BSA.

Brooke Army Formula

1. Colloids: 0.5 ml × kg body weight × % BSA burned
2. Electrolytes (lactated Ringer's solution): 1.5 ml × kg body weight × % BSA burned
3. Glucose (5% in water): 2000 ml for insensible loss
   Day 1: Half to be given in first 8 hours; remaining half over next 16 hours.
   Day 2: Half of colloids; half of electrolytes; all of insensible fluid replacement.

Second- and third-degree burns exceeding 50% BSA are calculated on the basis of 50% BSA.

Parkland/Baxter Formula

Lactated Ringers' solution: 4 ml × kg body weight × % BSA burned.
   Day 1: Half to be given in first 8 hours; half to be given over next 16 hours.
   Day 2: Varies. Colloid is added.

Hypertonic Saline Solution

Concentrated solutions of sodium chloride (NaCl) and lactate with concentration of 250–300 mEq of sodium per liter, administered at a rate sufficient to maintain a desired volume of urinary output. Do not increase the infusion rate during the first 8 postburn hours. Serum sodium levels must be monitored closely. Goal: Increase serum sodium level and osmolality to reduce edema and prevent pulmonary complications.

will be "pulled" back into the vascular space from the interstitial space. Reduced systemic and pulmonary edema have been reported after administering hypertonic solutions.

- *Note:* Formulas are only a guide. Patient response—evidenced by heart rate, blood pressure, and urine output—is the primary determinant of actual fluid therapy and must be assessed at least hourly. Patient outcomes are improved by optimal fluid resuscitation.

Goals of Fluid Replacement Therapy

The total volume and rate of intravenous fluid replacement are gauged by the burn patient's response. Goals of fluid replacement are a systolic blood pressure exceeding 100 mm Hg, pulse rate less than 110/minute, and urine output of 30 to 50 ml/hour.

- *These parameters are far more important in resuscitation than any formula.* Indeed, the patient's individual response *is* the formula.

Additional gauges of fluid requirements and response to fluid resuscitation include hematocrit, hemoglobin, and serum sodium levels. If the hematocrit and hemoglobin levels decrease or if the urinary output is greater than 50 ml/hour, the rate of intravenous fluid administration may be decreased. The goal is to maintain serum sodium levels in the normal range during fluid replacement.

❑ NURSING PROCESS
Burn Care During the Emergent/Resuscitative Phase

Assessment

Assessment data obtained by prehospital providers (rescuers, such as emergency medical technicians) are shared with the physician and nurse in the emergency department. Nursing assessment in the emergent phase of burn injury focuses on the major priorities for any trauma patient, with the wound as a secondary consideration. Aseptic management of the burn wounds and invasive lines continues.

Vital signs are checked frequently. Respiratory status is monitored closely. Apical, carotid, and femoral pulses are evaluated. Cardiac monitoring is indicated if the patient has a history of cardiac disease, electrical injury, or respiratory problems, or if the pulse is dysrhythmic or the rate is abnormally slow or rapid.

If all extremities are burned, determining blood pressure may be difficult. A sterile dressing applied under the blood pressure cuff will protect the wound from contamination. Because increasing edema makes blood pressure difficult to auscultate, a Doppler (ultrasound) device or a noninvasive electronic blood pressure device may be helpful. In severe burns, an arterial catheter is used for blood pressure measurement and for collecting blood specimens. Peripheral pulses on burned extremities are checked hourly. The Doppler instrument is also useful for monitoring peripheral pulses.

Large-bore intravenous lines and an indwelling urinary catheter are inserted, and the nurse's assessment includes monitoring fluid intake and output. Urine output, an excellent indicator of circulatory status, is monitored carefully and measured hourly. The amount of urine first obtained when the urinary catheter was inserted is recorded, because it may assist in determining the extent of preburn renal function and fluid status. Urine specific gravity; *p*H; and glucose, acetone, protein, and hemoglobin levels are assessed frequently.

Burgundy-colored urine suggests the presence of hemochromogen and myoglobin resulting from muscle damage from deep burns associated with electrical injury or prolonged contact with flames. Glucosuria is a common finding in the early postburn hours and results from the release of stored glucose from the liver in response to stress.

Although not responsible for calculating the patient's fluid requirements, the nurse needs to know the maximal volume of fluid the patient should receive. Infusion pumps and rate controllers are useful devices for correctly delivering a complex regimen of prescribed intravenous fluids. Monitoring intravenous therapy is a major nursing responsibility.

Body temperature, body weight, history of preburn weight, allergies, tetanus immunization, past medical and surgical problems, current illnesses, and use of medication are assessed. A head-to-toe assessment is performed, focusing on signs and symptoms of concomitant illness, injury, or developing complications.

Assessing the extent of the burn wound continues and is facilitated by using anatomic diagrams (described previously). In addition, the nurse works with the physician to assess the depth of the wound and identify areas of full- and partial-thickness injury.

The neurologic assessment focuses on the patient's level of consciousness, psychologic status, pain and anxiety levels, and behavior. The patient's and family's understanding of the injury and treatment is assessed as well.

Diagnosis

Nursing Diagnoses

Based on the assessment data, *priority* nursing diagnoses in the emergent/resuscitative phase of burn care may include the following:

- Impaired gas exchange related to carbon monoxide poisoning, smoke inhalation, and upper airway obstruction
- Ineffective airway clearance related to edema and the effects of smoke inhalation
- Fluid volume deficit related to increased capillary permeability and evaporative fluid loss from the burn wound
- Hypothermia related to loss of skin microcirculation and open wounds
- Pain related to tissue and nerve injury and emotional impact of injury
- Anxiety related to fear and the emotional impact of injury

Collaborative Problems/ Potential Complications

Based on the assessment data, potential complications in the emergent/resuscitative phase of burn care include:

- Acute respiratory failure
- Distributive shock
- Acute renal failure
- Compartment syndrome
- Paralytic ileus
- Curling's ulcer

Planning and Implementation

Goals. The major goals for the emergent/resuscitative phase of burn care include maintenance of a patent airway, ventilation, and tissue oxygenation; attainment of optimal fluid and electrolyte balance and perfusion of vital organs; maintenance of normal body temperature; minimal pain and anxiety; and absence of potential complications.

Nursing Interventions

Promoting Gas Exchange and Airway Clearance. Assessing for adequate gas exchange and airway clearance is an essential nursing activity. The patient's respiratory rate, quality, and depth are noted. The lungs are auscultated for adventitious (abnormal) sounds. In addition to ongoing nursing assessment of respiratory status, a pulse oximeter can be used to monitor oxygen levels in arterial blood. Drawbacks to using a pulse oximeter in burn patients are that poor tissue perfusion and edema may make it difficult to get an accurate signal, and the oximeter cannot differentiate carboxyhemoglobin from oxyhemoglobin. However, Barillo and coauthors (1990) reported a moderate to high correlation ($r = 0.82$) between pulse oximetry readings and oxygen saturations obtained by arterial blood gas analysis in burn patients. Pulse oximetry readings are useful for monitoring trends and changes in oxygenation status in the burn patient.

Aggressive pulmonary care measures, including turning the patient, encouraging coughing and deep breathing, initiating periodic forceful inspiration with incentive spirometry, and removing accumulated secretions by tracheal suctioning, as needed, are particularly important in the burn patient with an inhalation injury. Positioning the patient to decrease the work of breathing and promote optimal chest expansion and administering humidified oxygen or initiating mechanical ventilation may further decrease metabolic stress and ensure adequate tissue oxygenation. Asepsis is maintained throughout care to avoid contaminating the respiratory tract and to prevent infection, which increases metabolic oxygen requirements.

Restoring Fluid and Electrolyte Balance. Rapid fluid shifts and losses during the early postburn period require that nurses frequently assess vital signs and urinary output, as well as central venous pressure, pulmonary artery pressure, and cardiac output in the critically ill burn patient. Intravenous fluids are provided as prescribed. The volume infused should be comparable to the volume of urinary output. Meticulous documentation of intake and output and daily weight is required. Serum electrolyte levels are monitored. The nurse will usually be the first caregiver to recognize developing fluid and electrolyte imbalances. (See Chapter 14 for a detailed discussion of fluid and electrolyte disturbances.)

Maintaining Normal Body Temperature. Burn patients are prone to chilling and hypothermia because a loss of the skin decreases the patient's ability to retain body heat. The room temperature is adjusted according to the patient's needs. An environment that is too warm may cause fluid loss through perspiration and may promote bacterial growth. Overcooling of a room, which can easily occur when staff members regulate the temperature to keep themselves comfortable, will chill the patient. Subsequent shivering will increase metabolic demands. A patient who is allowed to control environmental room temperature will usually select a temperature of 32.2° to 32.8°C (90° to 91°F). Cotton blankets, ceiling-mounted heat lamps, and aluminum-insulated blankets help maintain the patient's comfort. Heat shields with sensors and blanket-draped bed cradles to deflect drafts are also useful. Efficiently and rapidly removing dressings and performing wound care also shorten the time that the patient is exposed to ambient temperature, which thereby reduces shivering and metabolic stress.

Minimizing Pain and Anxiety. The burn patient is frequently in intense pain and highly anxious from the onset of the burn injury.

- ❑ Symptoms of restlessness and anxiety, often attributed to pain, may actually stem from hypoxia. Therefore, a careful respiratory assessment is essential before administering analgesics, which may depress the respiratory system, in the early postburn period.

Pain. Intravenous morphine or other opioid analgesics are usually prescribed to relieve pain. However, high doses are avoided in the emergent phase because of the danger of respiratory depression in the nonmechanically ventilated patient and the possibility of masking other symptoms. Subcutaneous and intramuscular routes of administration are not used because the impaired circulation in the injured tissue makes absorption unpredictable. Intravenous sedatives may also be needed. It is vital to provide adequate pain-relieving medication in patients with acute burns not only to ensure comfort but also to decrease the tissue oxygen demand resulting from the physiologic pain response. Because of its intensity, burn-related pain may be impossible to eliminate altogether.

Anxiety. Normally, the patient and family experience severe emotional stress and anxiety. However, high anxiety levels must be avoided in the emergent burn patient for two reasons: (1) anxiety increases the physical and psychologic pain associated with the burn injury and (2) high anxiety levels further increase physiologic stress, which is detrimental to the patient. Vigilant assessment of family dynamics, coping strategies, and anxiety levels can facilitate planning of individualized interventions.

During the emergent period, emotional support and simple explanations about procedures and care should be provided. Because physical stabilization is the priority in this period, however, psychosocial interventions are limited to supporting the patient and family through the initial shock of injury. Adequate pain relief helps to reduce anxiety levels and increase coping abilities. If the patient remains highly anxious and agitated after psychologic interventions, antianxiety medications may be considered by the health care team.

Monitoring and Managing Potential Complications

Acute Respiratory Failure. If the patient has a patent airway and spontaneous respirations, the nurse assesses further for signs of inhalation injury, such as increased hoarseness, stridor (audible, shrill breathing), abnormal respiratory rate and depth, or mental changes caused by hypoxia. Nursing assessment includes reviewing results of laboratory and x-ray studies. Although chest x-ray and arterial blood gas findings may be normal initially, changes will often occur over time with the progression of an inhalation injury. The nurse reports promptly to the physician any signs of respiratory compromise resulting from edema and prepares to assist with intubation (to open the airway) or escharotomy as required.

Authorities no longer recommend using prophylactic antibiotics or corticosteroids in inhalation injury. If an actual infection exists, antibiotic therapy will be guided by results of Gram stains and culture and sensitivity tests of the sputum.

Distributive Shock. The patient must be monitored for early signs of hypovolemic shock or fluid overload secondary to adequate fluid resuscitation. Most commonly, fluid deficit occurs, which may develop into distributive shock. Signs of distributive shock include altered mental status; change in respiratory status; decreased urine output, blood pressure, central venous and pulmonary capillary wedge pressure and cardiac output; and increased pulse rate. Distributive shock is managed by increasing intravenous fluids and closely monitoring fluid status. (Shock is described in further detail in Chapter 15.)

Acute Renal Failure. Inadequate urine output may indicate inadequate fluid resuscitation or the onset of acute renal failure, particularly if hemoglobin or myoglobin is detected in the urine. Such patients require larger amounts of fluid to increase the urine output, thereby flushing the renal tubules and preventing acute tubular necrosis, which may lead to renal failure. Urine output, urine quality, and blood urea nitrogen (BUN) and creatinine levels must be monitored closely. (See Chapter 43 for further discussion of acute renal failure.)

Compartment Syndrome. The neurovascular status of the extremities is assessed carefully, particularly if burns are circumferential. This assessment helps detect compromised circulation resulting from increased edema from constriction caused by eschar formation in full-thickness burns. Peripheral pulses are checked hourly with an ultrasound Doppler device. Elevating the affected extremities may be indicated to help reduce edema. Any extremity pain, loss of peripheral pulses, or loss of sensation must be reported immediately to the physician so that escharotomies can be performed if needed.

Paralytic Ileus. Gastric dilation and paralytic ileus frequently occur in the early postburn period. Nausea and abdominal distention (bloating) are symptoms. A nasogastric tube is inserted early in treatment to prevent vomiting and aspiration of gastric contents into the lungs. The tube is connected to low intermittent suction until bowel sounds resume. The abdominal area should be assessed regularly for distention and bowel sounds. As burn shock resolves and bowel sounds and activity return, oral feedings should begin as soon as possible.

Curling's Ulcer. Severely burned patients are prone to gastric and duodenal ulcers because of hypersecretion of gastric acid, and the consequent erosion of the gastric mucosa, in response to the stress of the burn injury. Gastric *p*H should be assessed regularly in the patient who has a nasogastric tube. The *p*H should be maintained at a level less acidic than usual through antacid therapy. Histamine blockers, such as cimetidine (Tagamet) or ranitidine (Zantac), are administered as prescribed to prevent gastric erosion and bleeding ulcers. Nasogastric aspirate and stools should be checked for occult blood. A sudden drop in hemoglobin should alert the nurse to potential gastrointestinal bleeding, which must be reported to the physician. Gastric surgery may be indicated if the bleeding cannot be controlled medically.

Evaluation

Expected Outcomes

1. Maintains gas exchange and airway clearance
   a. Experiences no dyspnea
   b. Exhibits respiratory rate between 12 and 20 breaths/minute
   c. Has clear lungs sounds on auscultation
   d. Demonstrates arterial oxygen saturation level exceeding 96% (by pulse oximetry)
   e. Has minimal, colorless, and thin respiratory secretions
2. Regains optimal fluid and electrolyte balance and perfusion of vital organs
   a. Maintains serum electrolyte levels within normal limits
   b. Demonstrates heart rate and blood pressure within normal limits
   c. Has clear sensorium
   d. Shows normal reflexes and muscle tone indicative of electrolyte balance
   e. Voids clear, yellow urine; protein, sugar, acetone, *p*H, and specific gravity values are within normal limits
   f. Has normal hemoglobin and hematocrit values
3. Demonstrates acceptable body temperature
   a. Maintains body temperature within range of 37.2° to 38.3°C (98.6° to 101°F)
   b. Reports comfort without chills or shivering
4. States that pain is controlled
   a. Reports lower pain level
   b. Shows no nonverbal cues (grimaces, irritability) of pain
5. Patient and family experience minimal anxiety
   a. Patient and family verbalize understanding of emergent burn care
   b. Patient can answer simple questions
6. Experiences no complications
   a. Breathes spontaneously with adequate tidal volume
   b. Has arterial blood gas values within normal limits
   c. Demonstrates normal chest x-ray findings
   d. Has no signs of cerebral hypoxia
   e. Voids between 0.5 and 1.0 ml/kg urine hourly
   f. Maintains blood pressure within patient's normal range (usually higher than 90/60 mm Hg)
   g. Has heart rate within normal range (usually below 110 beats/min)
   h. Has normal BUN and creatinine levels
   i. Reports no paresthesias (numbness or tingling) or symptoms of ischemia of nerves and muscles (compartment syndrome)
   j. Has peripheral pulses detectable by Doppler
   k. Shows no abdominal distention on palpation
   l. Exhibits no blood in gastric aspirate and stools

Nursing care of the patient during the emergent/resuscitative phase of burn injury is described in Nursing Care Plan 55-1.

Acute or Intermediate Phase of Burn Care

The acute or intermediate phase of burn care follows the emergent/resuscitative phase of burn care and begins 48 to 72 hours after the burn injury. During this phase, attention is directed toward continued assessment and maintenance of respiratory and circulatory status, fluid and electrolyte balance, and gastrointestinal function. Burn wound care and pain control are priorities at this stage.

Airway obstruction caused by upper airway edema can take as long as 48 hours to develop. Changes detected by x-ray and blood gas studies may occur as the effects of resuscitative fluid and the chemical reaction of smoke ingredients with lung tissues become apparent. The patient's arterial blood gas level and other parameters guide the need for intubation or mechanical ventilation.

As capillaries regain integrity, at 48 or more postburn hours, fluid moves from the interstitial to the intravascular compartment, and diuresis begins (Table 55-4). If cardiac or renal function is inadequate, for instance in the elderly patient or the patient with preexisting cardiac disease, fluid overload occurs and symptoms of congestive heart failure may result (see Chapter 28). Detection of early signs allows for early intervention and carefully calculated fluid intake. Vasoactive drugs, diuretics, and fluid restriction may be used to support circulatory function and prevent the complications of congestive heart failure and pulmonary edema.

Cautious administration of fluids and electrolytes continues during this phase of burn care because of the shifts in fluid from interstitial to intravascular compartments, losses of fluid from large burn wounds, and the patient's physiologic responses to the burn injury. Blood transfusions are given if necessary to treat blood loss and anemia.

Fever is common in burn patients after burn shock resolves. A resetting of core body temperature in severely burned persons results in a body temperature a few degrees higher than normal for several weeks postburn. Bacteremia and septicemia also cause fever in many patients. Acetaminophen (Tylenol) and hypothermia blankets may be required to maintain body temperature in a range of 37.2° to 39.4°C (99° to 103°F) to reduce metabolic stress and tissue oxygen demand.

Central venous, peripheral arterial, or pulmonary artery thermodilution catheters may be required for monitoring venous and arterial pressures, pulmonary artery, pulmonary capillary wedge pressures, or cardiac output. Generally, however, invasive vascular lines are avoided unless absolutely necessary because they provide an additional port for infection in this already greatly compromised patient.

Infection progressing to septic shock is the major cause of death in patients who have survived the first few days following extensive burns. The immunosuppression that accompanies extensive burn injury places the patient at high

(text continues on page 1563)

NURSING CARE PLAN 55–1
Care of the Patient During the Emergent/Resuscitative Phase of Burn Care

Nursing Interventions	Rationale	Expected Outcomes
NURSING DIAGNOSIS: Impaired gas exchange related to carbon monoxide poisoning, smoke inhalation, and upper airway obstruction		
GOAL: Maintenance of adequate tissue oxygenation		
1. Provide humidified oxygen.	1. Humidified oxygen provides moisture to injured tissues; supplemental oxygen increases alveolar oxygenation	• Absence of dyspnea • Respiratory rate between 12 and 20 breaths/min
2. Assess breath sounds, respiratory rate, rhythm, depth, and symmetry. Monitor patient for signs of hypoxia.	2 These provide baseline for further assessment and evidence of increasing respiratory compromise	• Lungs clear on auscultation • Arterial oxygen saturation >96% by pulse oximetry
3. Observe for the following: a. Erythema or blistering of lips or buccal mucosa b. Singed nostrils c. Burns of face, neck, or chest d. Increasing hoarseness e. Soot in sputum or tracheal tissue in respiratory secretions	3. These signs indicate possible inhalation injury and risk of respiratory dysfunction	• Arterial blood gas levels within normal limits
4. Monitor arterial blood gas values, pulse oximetry readings, and carboxyhemoglobin levels.	4. Increasing pCO_2 and decreasing pO_2 and O_2 saturation may indicate need for mechanical ventilation.	
5. Report labored respirations, decreased depth of respirations, or signs of hypoxia to physician immediately.	5. Immediate intervention is indicated for respiratory difficulty	
6. Prepare to assist with intubation and escharotomies.	6. Intubation allows mechanical ventilation. Escharotomy enables chest excursion in circumferential chest burns	
7. Monitor mechanically ventilated patient closely (refer to Chapter 25).	7. Monitoring allows early detection of decreasing respiratory status or complications of mechanical ventilation	
NURSING DIAGNOSIS: Ineffective airway clearance related to edema and effects of smoke inhalation		
GOAL: Maintain patent airway and adequate airway clearance		
1. Maintain patent airway through proper patient positioning, removal of secretions, and artificial airway if needed.	1. A patent airway is crucial to respiration	• Patent airway • Respiratory secretions are minimal, colorless, and thin
2. Provide humidified oxygen.	2. Humidity liquefies secretions and facilitates expectoration	• Respiratory rate, pattern, and breath sounds normal
3. Encourage patient to turn, cough, and deep breathe. Encourage patient to use incentive spirometry. Suction as needed.	3. These activities promote mobilization and removal of secretions	
NURSING DIAGNOSIS: Fluid volume deficit related to increased capillary permeability and evaporative losses from the burn wound		
GOAL: Restoration of optimal fluid and electrolyte balance and perfusion of vital organs		
1. Observe vital signs (including central venous pressure or pulmonary artery pressure, if indicated), urine output,	1. Hypovolemia is a major risk immediately after the burn injury. Overresuscitation might cause fluid overload	• Serum electrolytes within normal limits • Urine output between 0.5 and 1.0 ml/kg/hr • Blood pressure higher than 90/60 mm Hg

(continued)

NURSING CARE PLAN 55–1 *(continued)*
Care of the Patient During the Emergent/Resuscitative Phase of Burn Care

Nursing Interventions	Rationale	Expected Outcomes
and be alert for signs of hypovolemia or fluid overload.		• Heart rate less than 120 beats/min • Exhibits clear sensorium • Voids clear yellow urine with specific gravity within normal limits
2. Monitor urine output at least hourly and weigh patient daily.	2. Output and weight provide information about renal perfusion, adequacy of fluid replacement, and fluid requirement and fluid status	
3. Maintain IV lines and regulate fluids at appropriate rates, as prescribed.	3. Adequate fluids are necessary to maintain fluid and electrolyte balance and adequate perfusion of vital organs	
4. Observe for symptoms of deficiency or excess of serum sodium, potassium, calcium, phosphorus, and bicarbonate.	4. Rapid shifts in fluid and electrolyte status are possible in the postburn period	
5. Elevate head of patient's bed and elevate burned extremities.	5. Elevation promotes venous return	
6. Notify physician immediately of decreased urine output, blood pressure, CVP, PA, PAWP or increased pulse rate	6. Because of the rapid fluid shifts in burn shock, fluid deficit must be detected early so that distributive shock does not occur	

NURSING DIAGNOSIS: Hypothermia related to loss of skin microcirculation and open wounds

GOAL: Maintenance of adequate body temperature

Nursing Interventions	Rationale	Expected Outcomes
1. Provide a warm environment through use of heat shield, space blanket, heat lights or blankets.	1. A stable environment minimizes evaporative heat loss	• Body temperature remains in 36.1 to 38.3° C (97° to 101° F) range • Absence of chills or shivering
2. Work quickly when wounds must be exposed	2. Minimal exposure minimizes heat loss from wound	
3. Assess core body temperature frequently.	3. Frequent temperature assessments help detect developing hypothermia	

NURSING DIAGNOSIS: Pain related to tissue and nerve injury and emotional impact of injury

GOAL: Control of pain

Nursing Interventions	Rationale	Expected Outcomes
1. Use pain scale to assess pain level (*i.e.,* 1 to 10) Differentiate from hypoxia.	1. Pain level provides baseline for evaluating effectiveness of pain-relief measures. Hypoxia can cause similar signs and must be ruled out before pain medication is administered	• States pain level is decreased. • Absence of nonverbal cues of pain.
2. Administer intravenous opioid analgesics as prescribed. Observe for respiratory depression in the nonmechanically ventilated patient. Assess response to analgesic.	2. Intravenous administration is necessary because of altered tissue perfusion from burn injury	
3. Provide emotional support and reassurance.	3. Emotional support is essential to reduce fear and anxiety resulting from burn injury. Fear and anxiety increase the perception of pain	

(continued)

NURSING CARE PLAN 55–1 *(continued)*
Care of the Patient During the Emergent/Resuscitative Phase of Burn Care

Nursing Interventions	Rationale	Expected Outcomes
NURSING DIAGNOSIS: Anxiety related to fear and the emotional impact of burn injury		
GOAL: Minimization of patient's and family's anxiety		
1. Assess patient's and family's understanding of burn injury, of coping skills and family dynamics.	1. Previous successful coping strategies can be fostered for use in the present crisis. Assessment allows planning of individualized interventions	• Patient and family verbalize understanding of emergent burn care • Able to answer simple questions
2. Individualize responses to the patient's and family's coping level.	2. Reactions to burn injury are extremely variable. Interventions must be appropriate to the patient's and family's present level of coping	
3. Explain all procedures to the patient and the family in clear, simple terms.	3. Increased understanding alleviates fear of the unknown. High levels of anxiety may interfere with understanding of complex explanations	
4. Maintain adequate pain relief.	4. Pain increases anxiety	
5. Consider administering prescribed antianxiety medications if the patient remains extremely anxious despite nonpharmacologic interventions.	5. Anxiety levels during the emergent phase may exceed the patient's coping abilities. Medication decreases physiologic and psychologic anxiety responses	
COLLABORATIVE PROBLEMS: Acute respiratory failure, distributive shock, acute renal failure, compartment syndrome, paralytic ileus, Curling's ulcer.		
GOAL: Absence of complications		
Acute Respiratory Failure		
1. Assess for increasing dypsnea, stridor, changes in respiratory patterns.	1. Such signs reflect deteriorating respiratory status	• Arterial blood gas values within acceptable limits: pO_2 >80 mm Hg, PCO_2 <50 mm Hg • Breathes spontaneously with adequate tidal volume • Chest x-ray findings normal • Absence of cerebral signs of hypoxia
2. Monitor pulse oximetry, arterial blood gas (ABG) values for decreasing pO_2, oxygen saturation and increasing pCO_2.	2. Such signs reflect decreased oxygenation status	
3. Monitor chest x-ray results.	3. X-ray may disclose pulmonary injury	
4. Assess for restlessness, confusion, difficulty attending to questions, or decreasing level of consciousness.	4. Such manifestations may indicate cerebral hypoxia	
5. Report deteriorating respiratory status immediately to physician.	5. Acute respiratory failure is life threatening and immediate intervention is required	
6. Prepare to assist with intubation or escharotomies as indicated.	6. Intubation allows mechanical ventilation. Escharotomies allow improved chest excursion with respirations	
Distributive Shock		
1. Assess for decreasing urine output, PAP, PCWP, blood pressure, cardiac output or increasing pulse.	1. Such signs and symptoms may indicate distributive shock and inadequate intravascular volume	• Urine output between 0.5 ml/kg/hr and 1.0 ml/kg/hr

(continued)

NURSING CARE PLAN 55–1 *(continued)*
Care of the Patient During the Emergent/Resuscitative Phase of Burn Care

Nursing Interventions	Rationale	Expected Outcomes
2. Assess for progressive edema as fluid shifts occur. 3. Adjust fluid resuscitation in collaboration with the physician in response to physiologic findings.	2. As fluid shifts into the interstitial spaces in burn shock, edema occurs and may compromise tissue perfusion 3. Optimal fluid resuscitation prevents distributive shock and improves patient outcomes	• Blood pressure within patient's normal range (usually >90/60 mm Hg) • Heart rate within patient's normal range (usually <110/min.) • PAP, PCWP, CO remain within normal limits
Acute Renal Failure		
1. Monitor urine output, blood urea nitrogen (BUN) and creatinine levels. 2. Report decreased urine output or increased BUN and creatinine values to physician. 3. Assess urine for hemoglobin or myoglobin. 4. Administer increased fluids as prescribed.	1. These values reflect renal function 2. These laboratory values indicate possible renal failure 3. Hemoglobin or myoglobin in the urine points to an increased risk of renal failure 4. Fluids help to flush out hemoglobin and myoglobin from renal tubules and decreases the potential for renal failure	• Adequate urine output • BUN and creatinine values remain normal
Compartment Syndrome		
1. Assess peripheral pulses hourly with Doppler ultrasound device. 2. Assess warmth, capillary refill, sensation and movement of extremity hourly. Compare affected with unaffected extremity. 3. Remove blood pressure cuff after each reading. 4. Elevate burned extremities. 5. Report loss of pulse or sensation or presence of pain to physician immediately. 6. Prepare to assist with escharotomies.	1. Assessment with Doppler device substitutes for auscultation and indicates characteristics of arterial blood flow 2. These assessments indicate characteristics of peripheral perfusion 3. Cuff may act as a tourniquet as extremities swell 4. Elevation reduces edema formation 5. These signs and symptoms may indicate inadequate tissue perfusion 6. Escharotomies relieve the constriction caused by swelling under circumferential burns and improve tissue perfusion	• Absence of parasthesias or symptoms of ischemia of nerves and muscles • Peripheral pulses detectable by Doppler
Paralytic Ileus		
1. Maintain nasogastric tube on low intermittent suction until bowel sounds resume. 2. Auscultate for bowel sounds, abdominal distention	1. This measure relieves gastric and abdominal distention, also prevents vomiting 2. As bowel sounds resume, feeding may be slowly initiated. Abdominal distention reflects inadequate decompression	• Absence of abdominal distention • Normal bowel sounds within 48 hours

(continued)

NURSING CARE PLAN 55–1 *(continued)*

Care of the Patient During the Emergent/Resuscitative Phase of Burn Care

Nursing Interventions	Rationale	Expected Outcomes
Curling's Ulcer		
1. Assess gastric aspirate for *p*H and blood.	1. Acidic *p*H indicates need for antacids or histamine blockers. Blood indicates possible gastric bleeding	• Absence of abdominal distention • Normal bowel sounds within 48 hours • Gastric aspirate and stools do not contain blood.
2. Assess stools for occult blood.	2. Blood in stools may indicate gastric or duodenal ulcer	
3. Administer histamine blockers and antacids as prescribed.	3. Such medications reduce gastric acidity and risk of ulceration	

risk for sepsis. The infection that begins within the burn site may spread to the bloodstream.

The Burn Wound

The burn wound is unique among wounds because it involves a large amount of dead tissue (eschar) that remains in place for a prolonged time. It is rapidly colonized by pathogenic bacteria; exudes large quantities of water, protein, and electrolytes; and frequently requires that tissue be moved through skin grafting from another part of the body to achieve permanent closure.

Threat of Infection

Despite aseptic precautions and the use of topical antimicrobial agents, the burn wound is an excellent medium for bacterial growth and proliferation. Bacteria such as *Staphylococcus, Proteus, Pseudomonas, Escherichia coli,* and *Klebsiella* enterobacteria find optimal conditions for growth within the burn wound. The burn eschar is a nonviable crust with no blood supply, so neither polymorphonuclear leukocytes or antibodies nor systemic antibiotics can reach the area. Phenomenal numbers of bacteria—more than one billion per gram of tissue—may appear and subsequently spread to the bloodstream or release their toxins, which reach distant sites. Fungi such as *Candida albicans* also grow easily in burn wounds.

When the burn wound is healing through spontaneous reepithelialization or is being prepared for skin grafting, it must be protected from burn wound sepsis. Burn wound sepsis has these characteristics:

- 10^5 bacteria per gram of tissue
- Inflammation
- Sludging and thrombosis of dermal blood vessels

TABLE 55-4 Fluid and Electrolyte Changes in the Acute Phase of Burn Care

Fluid Remobilization Phase (State of Diuresis)
Interstitial Fluid → Plasma

Observation	Explanation
Hemodilution (decreased hematocrit)	Blood cell concentration is diluted as fluid enters the intravascular compartment; loss of red blood cells destroyed at burn site.
Increased urinary output	Fluid shift into intravascular compartment increases renal blood flow and causes increased urine formation.
Sodium (Na^+) deficit	With diuresis, sodium is lost with water; existing serum sodium is diluted by water influx.
Potassium (K^+) deficit (occurs occasionally in this phase)	Beginning on the fourth or fifth postburn day, K^+ shifts from extracellular fluid into cells.
Metabolic acidosis	Loss of sodium depletes fixed base; relative carbon dioxide content increases.

(Adapted from Metheny NM and Snively WD. Nurses' Handbook of Fluid Balance. Philadelphia, JB Lippincott.)

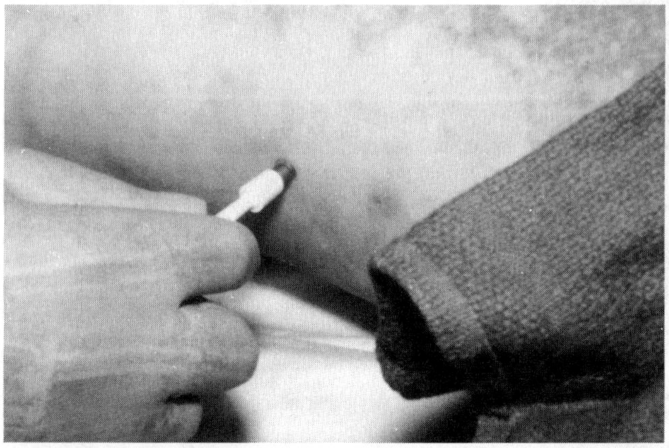

FIGURE 55-5. Punch biopsy. This technique permits tissue analysis for evidence of infection.

The primary source of bacterial infection appears to be the patient's own intestinal tract. A major secondary source is the environment. Cap, gown, mask, and gloves are worn while caring for the patient with open burn wounds to prevent infection. Sterile technique is used when caring directly for burn wounds.

Antibiotics are seldom given prophylactically because of the risk of promoting resistant strains of bacteria. Tissue specimens are taken for culture regularly to monitor colonization of the wound by microbial organisms. These may be swab, surface, or tissue biopsy cultures. Swab or surface cultures are noninvasive, simple, and painless, but data obtained from such cultures apply only to the area sampled; therefore, invasive wound biopsy cultures may be required (Fig. 55-5). Systemic antibiotics are administered when there is documentation of burn wound sepsis or other positive cultures such as urine, sputum, or blood. Sensitivity of the organisms to the prescribed antibiotics should be determined prior to administration. Several parenteral antimicrobial agents may be given together to fight the infection.

General Wound Care

Wound care includes cleaning and debridement, application of topical antimicrobial agents, and dressings. Gauze, biologic, biosynthetic, and synthetic materials may be used. Split-thickness skin grafts are required to close full-thickness and deep partial-thickness wounds. Special procedures must be followed for burns of the face, ears, eyes, and genitalia. The use of hyperbaric oxygen therapy to facilitate wound healing is controversial and is not a routine component of burn wound care.

Wound Cleaning

Various measures can be taken to clean the burn wound. Total immersion hydrotherapy is performed in some settings; bedside baths are performed as well. In other settings, the patient is suspended on a vinyl stretcher over a tub and showered. A walk-in bath, a tub, or a whirlpool may be used. The agitation in the whirlpool promotes cleaning and gently massages the tissues. Because of the high risk of infection and sepsis, either plastic liners or thorough decontamination of hydrotherapy equipment is necessary to prevent cross-contamination. Tap water alone, saline, or antiseptic solutions, such as dilute iodine or bleach preparations, may be used. The temperature of the bath is maintained at 37.8°C (100°F), and the temperature of the room should be maintained between 26.6° and 29.4°C (80° to 85°F). Hydrotherapy should be limited to a 20- to 30-minute period to prevent chilling and additional metabolic stress.

During the bath, the patient is encouraged to be as active as possible. Hydrotherapy provides an excellent medium for exercising the extremities and cleaning the entire body. When the patient is removed from the tub after the bath, any residue adhering to the body is washed away with a clear water spray or shower.

Unburned areas, including the hair, must be washed regularly as well. At the time of wound cleaning, all skin is inspected for any hints of redness, breakdown, or local infection. Hair in and around the burn area except the eyebrows should be clipped short. Intact blisters may be left, but the fluid should be aspirated with a needle and syringe and discarded.

Conscientious management of the burn wound is essential. When nonviable loose skin is removed, aseptic conditions must be established. Skin near the burned area is shaved to prevent possible contamination from hair follicles.

Wound cleaning is usually performed at least daily in wound areas that are not undergoing surgical intervention. When the eschar begins to separate from the viable tissue beneath, approximately between 1½ and 2 postburn weeks, more frequent cleaning and debridement may be in order.

After a tub bath, the patient's wounds are gently patted dry with sterile towels and the prescribed method of wound care is performed. Physician preferences, the skill level of the nursing staff, and resources in terms of number of personnel, supplies, and time must be considered in choosing the best method for a given patient. Whatever the method, the goal is to protect the wound from overwhelming proliferation of pathogenic organisms and invasion of deeper tissues until either spontaneous healing or skin grafting can be achieved. Patient comfort and ability to participate in the prescribed treatment are also important considerations.

Topical Antibacterial Therapy

There is general agreement that some form of antimicrobial therapy applied to the burn wound is the best method of local care in extensive burn injury. Topical antibacterial therapy does not sterilize the burn wound but simply reduces the number of bacteria so that the overall microbial population can be controlled by the body's host defense mechanisms. Topical therapy promotes efforts to convert the open, dirty wound to a closed, clean one.

No single agent is universally effective. Using different agents at different times in the postburn period may be necessary. Bacteriologic cultures are required to monitor the effect of topical medications.

Before the topical agent is reapplied, the previously applied topical agent must be thoroughly removed. The number of times the dressings are changed and soaked is planned to promote optimal therapeutic use of the topical agent.

Criteria for topical agents include the following: (1) it is effective against gram-negative organisms, *Pseudomonas aeruginosa, Staphylococcus aureus,* and even fungi; (2) it is clinically effective; (3) it penetrates the eschar but is not systemically toxic; (4) it does not lose its effectiveness, thereby permitting another infection to develop; (5) it is cost effective, available, and acceptable to the patient; and (6) it is easy to apply, minimizing nursing care time. The three most commonly used topical agents are **silver sulfadiazine** (Silvadene), **silver nitrate,** and **mafenide acetate** (Sulfamylon). These agents are detailed in Table 55-5.

Many other topical agents are available, including **povidone-iodine ointment (10%), gentamicin sulfate, nitrofurazone (Furacin), Dakin's solution, acetic acid, miconazole,** and **chlortrimazole.** All topical agents must be used with consideration given to the microbial population found in the burn wound. Prudent use and alternation of antimicrobial agents results in less-resistant strains of bacteria, greater effectiveness of the agents, and a decreased risk of sepsis for the patient.

Dressing Changes

Dressings are changed in the patient's unit, hydrotherapy room, or treatment area approximately 20 minutes after administering an analgesic. They may also be changed in the operating room after the patient is anesthetized. A mask, hair cover, disposable plastic apron or cover gown, and gloves are worn by health care personnel when removing the dressings. The outer dressings are slit with blunt scissors, and the soiled dressings are removed and disposed of following established procedures for contaminated materials.

Dressings that adhere to the wound can be removed more comfortably if they are moistened with saline solution or if the patient is allowed to soak for a few moments in the tub. The remaining dressings are *carefully* and *gently* removed with forceps or gloved hands. The patient may participate in removing the dressings, providing some degree of control over this painful procedure. The wounds are then cleaned and debrided to remove debris, any remaining topical agent, exudate, and dead skin. Sterile scissors and forceps may be used to trim loose eschar and encourage separation of devitalized skin. During this procedure, the wound and surrounding skin are carefully inspected. The color, odor, size, exudate, signs of reepithelialization, and other characteristics of the wound and the eschar and any changes from the previous dressing change are noted. Because wound care procedures, particularly tub baths, are metabolically stressful, the patient is assessed for signs of chilling, fatigue, changes in hemodynamic status, and pain unrelieved by analgesics or relaxation techniques.

When the wound is clean, the burned areas are patted dry and the prescribed topical agent is applied. The wound

TABLE 55-5 Overview of Topical Antibacterial Agents Used for Burn Wounds

Agent	Indication	Application	Nursing Implications
Silver sulfadiazine 1% (Silvadene) water-soluble cream	• Most bactericidal agent • Minimal penetration of eschar	Apply 1/16-inch layer of cream with a sterile glove 1 to 3 times daily.	• Watch for leukopenia 2 to 3 days after initiation of therapy. (Leukopenia usually resolves within 2 or 3 days.) • Anticipate formation of psuedo-eschar (proteinaceous gel), which is removed easily after 72 hours.
Silver nitrate 0.5% aqueous solution	• Bacteriostatic and fungicidal • Does *not* penetrate eschar	Apply solution to gauze dressing and place over wound. Keep the dressing wet but covered with dry gauze and dry blankets to decrease vaporization.	• Monitor serum sodium (Na^+) and potassium (K^+) levels and replace as prescribed. Silver nitrate solution is hypotonic and acts like a wick for sodium and potassium.
Mafenide acetate 5% to 10% (Sulfamylon) hydrophilic-based cream	• Effective against gram-negative and gram-positive organisms. • Diffuses rapidly through eschar. • In 10% strength, it is the agent of choice for electrical burns because of its ability to penetrate thick eschar.	Remoistened every 2 hours and redress wound twice a day. Apply thin layer with sterile glove twice a day and leave open as prescribed. Or if the wound is dressed, change the dressing every 6 hours as prescribed.	• Protect bed linen and clothing from contact with silver nitrate, which stains everything it touches black. • Monitor arterial blood gas levels and discontinue as prescribed, if acidosis occurs. Mafenide acetate is a strong carbonic anhydrase inhibitor that may reduce renal buffering and cause metabolic acidosis. • Premedicate the patient with an analgesic before applying mafenide acetate because this agent causes severe burning pain for up to 20 minutes after application.

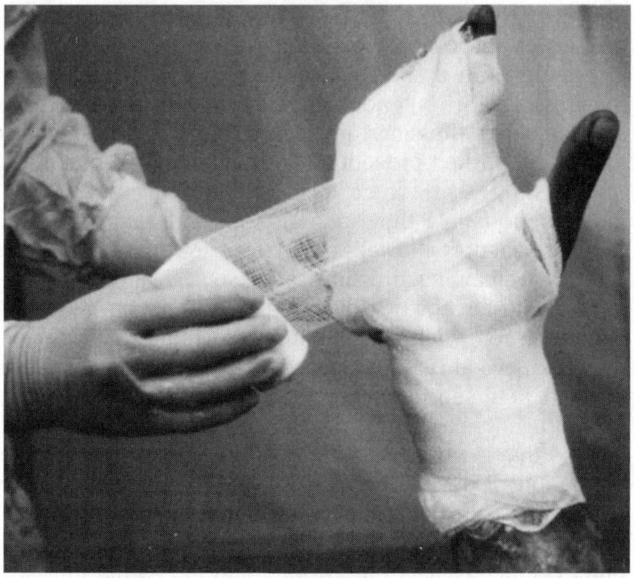

FIGURE 55-6. Application of dressing to a hand burn.

is then covered with several layers of dressings (Fig. 55-6). A light dressing is used over joint areas to allow for motion (unless the area has a graft there and motion is contraindicated). A light dressing is also applied over areas for which a splint has been designed to conform to the body contour for proper positioning. Circumferential dressings should be applied distally to proximally.

Close communication and cooperation among the patient, surgeon, nurse, and other health care team members are essential for optimal burn wound care. Different wound areas on a given patient may require a variety of wound care techniques. Diagrams posted at the bedside are useful to inform staff of the current prescription for wound care, splints to be applied over dressings, and the exercise regimen to be followed before dressings are reapplied.

Exposure Versus Occlusive Dressing

Exposure Method. Occasionally a wound is treated by exposing it to air. Wound care proceeds in the described manner, a topical agent is applied (mafenide most frequently), but no dressings are applied. The success of the exposure method depends on keeping the immediate environment free of organisms. Some practitioners maintain that everything coming in contact with the patient must be sterile. Linens are sterile; those who come in direct contact with the patient wear masks, caps, sterile gowns, and gloves; and visitors are instructed to wear protective garb and not to touch the bed or hand the patient anything. Other practitioners maintain a clean environment and rely on the efficiency of the topical antibacterial agents to limit burn wound infection.

The patient's room must be maintained at a comfortably warm temperature with 40% to 50% humidity to prevent excessive evaporative fluid losses as well as to maintain the patient's body temperature. A cradle may be placed over the patient to prevent sheets from coming in contact with the burn area, to minimize the effects of air currents to which a burn patient is unusually sensitive, and to provide some covering.

Generally small areas such as the face, neck, or perineum may also be effectively treated with the exposure method, while other areas of the wound may be dressed.

Occlusive Dressings. There is a role for occlusive dressings in treating specific wounds. Occlusive dressings are a thin gauze that is either preimpregnated with a topical antimicrobial or applied after topical antimicrobial application. Occlusive dressings are most often seen over areas with new skin grafts. These dressings are applied under sterile conditions in the operating room. Their purpose is to protect the graft, promoting an optimal condition for its adherence to the recipient site. Ideally, these dressings remain in place for 3 to 5 days, at which time they are removed by the physician for examination of the graft.

When these dressings are applied, precautions are taken to prevent two body surfaces from touching, such as fingers or toes, ear and scalp, the areas under the breasts, any point of flexion, or between the genital folds. Functional body alignment positions are maintained by using splints or by careful positioning of the patient.

Debridement

Debridement is another facet of burn wound care. This technique has two goals:

- To remove tissue contaminated by bacteria and foreign bodies, thereby protecting the patient from invasion of bacteria
- To remove devitalized tissue or burn eschar in preparation for grafting and wound healing

After partial- and full-thickness burns occur, bacteria that are present at the interface of the burned tissue and the viable tissue underneath gradually liquefy the collagen fibrils that hold the eschar in place for the first or second postburn week. Proteolytic and other natural enzymes cause this phenomenon.

Natural Debridement. With natural debridement, the dead tissue separates from the underlying viable tissue spontaneously. Using antibacterial topical agents, however, tends to slow down this natural process of eschar separation. It is advantageous to the patient to speed this process through other means, such as mechanical or surgical debridement, thereby reducing the time during which bacterial invasion and other iatrogenic problems may arise.

Mechanical Debridement. Mechanical debridement involves using surgical scissors and forceps to separate and remove the eschar. This technique can be performed by physicians, experienced nurses, or physical therapists and is usually done with daily dressing changes and wound cleaning procedures. Debridement by these means is carried out to the point of pain and bleeding. Hemostatic agents or pressure can be used to stop bleeding from small vessels.

Dressings are also helpful debriding agents. Coarse-mesh dressings applied dry or wet-to-dry (applied wet and allowed to dry) will slowly debride the wound of exudate and eschar when they are removed. Topical enzymatic debridement agents such as sutilains (Travase), a proteolytic enzyme derived from *Bacillus subtilis* and supplied in a petrolatum base, can also be helpful in debriding wounds. Because such agents are not antibacterial in themselves, they should be used with topical antibacterial therapy to protect the patient from bacterial invasion.

Surgical Debridement. Surgical debridement is an operative procedure involving either primary excision of the full thickness of the skin down to the fascia (tangential excision) or shaving the burned skin layers gradually down to freely bleeding, viable tissue. This may be initiated a few days postburn or as soon as the patient is hemodynamically stable and edema has decreased. The wound is then covered immediately by a skin graft or dressing. A temporary biologic dressing or biosynthetic dressing may be used until a skin graft can be applied during a subsequent operation.

Using excision is selective, particularly with large burns, for the following reasons: The procedure carries with it a high risk of extensive blood loss (as much as 100 to 125 ml of blood per percent of body surface area excised) and lengthy operating and anesthesia time. However, when used, excision offers shorter hospital stays and, possibly, decreased potential complications from invasive burn wound sepsis.

Grafting the Burn Wound

If wounds are deep (full-thickness) or extensive, spontaneous reepithelialization is not possible. Therefore, a skin transplant or a graft of the patient's own skin (autograft) is required. Main areas for skin grafting include the face, for cosmetic and psychologic reasons; the hands and other functional areas such as the feet; and areas that involve joints. Grafting permits earlier functional ability and reduces contractures. When burns are very extensive, the chest and abdomen may be grafted first to reduce the burn surface.

During wound healing, granulation tissue develops. It fills the space created by the wound, creates a barrier to bacteria, and serves as a bed for epithelial cell growth.

Richly vascular granulation tissue is pink, firm, shiny, and free of exudate and debris. It should have a bacterial count of less than 100,000 per gram of tissue to optimize graft take. A preoperative culture is mandatory before autografting, because enzymes of bacteria can dissolve a graft and lead to its failure. Beta-hemolytic *Streptococcus* is of particular significance in terms of graft failure.

Autografts

Autografts come from the patient's own skin. They can be split-thickness, full-thickness, pedicle flaps, or cultured epithelium. Full-thickness and pedicle flaps are more commonly used for reconstructive surgery, months or years after the initial injury.

Use of cultured epithelium is in the experimental stages at several burn centers. Basically the procedure involves a biopsy of the patient's skin in an unburned area. Keratinocytes are then isolated and epithelial cells are cultured in a laboratory. The original epithelial cell sample can multiply to 10,000 times its original size over 30 days. These cells are then attached to the burn wound. Varying degrees of success have been reported, but results are encouraging (Wong & Munster, 1993).

Split-thickness autografts can be applied in sheets or in postage stamp–like pieces, or they can be expanded by meshing so that they can cover 1½ to 9 times more than a given donor site area. Skin meshers enable the surgeon to cut tiny slits into a sheet of donor skin, making it possible to cover large areas of total body surface area with smaller amounts of donor skin. These expanded grafts cling to the recipient site more easily than sheet grafts and prevent the accumulation of blood, serum, air, or purulent material under the graft. However, any kind of graft other than a sheet graft will contribute to scar formation as it heals. Using expanded grafts is commonly necessary in large wounds but should always be viewed as a compromise in terms of cosmetic effects.

If blood, serum, air, fat, or necrotic tissue lies between the recipient site and the graft, there may be partial or total loss of the graft. Infection and mishandling of the graft, as well as trauma during dressing changes, account for most other instances of graft loss.

Using split-thickness grafts allows the remaining donor site to retain sweat glands and hair follicles. Healing time of the donor site is minimized.

Care of Patients With Autografts. Occlusive dressings are commonly used initially after grafting to immobilize the grafts. Homografts, heterografts, or synthetic dressings may also be used to protect the grafts (see below). The graft may be left open, with skin staples to immobilize it, which allows close observation of the graft progress.

The first dressing change is usually performed by the surgeon 3 to 5 days postoperatively, or earlier in case of purulent drainage or a foul odor. If the graft is dislodged, sterile saline compresses will help prevent drying of the graft until the physician reapplies it. The patient begins exercising the grafted area 5 to 7 days after grafting.

Care of Donor Site. A moist gauze dressing is applied during the operative period to maintain pressure and to stop any oozing. A thrombostatic agent such as thrombin or epinephrine may be applied directly to the site as well. The donor site may be treated in several ways, from single-layer gauze impregnated with petrolatum, scarlet red, or bismuth to new biosynthetic dressings. Donor sites must remain clean, dry, and free from pressure. Ultimately, because a donor site is a partial-thickness wound, it will heal spontaneously within 7 to 14 days with proper care.

Biologic Dressings (Homografts and Heterografts)

Biologic dressings consist of homografts (or allografts) and heterografts (or xenografts). **Homografts** are skin obtained from living or recently deceased humans. The amniotic membrane (**amnion**) from the human placenta may also be used as a biologic dressing. **Heterografts** consist of skin taken from animals (usually pigs).

Homografts tend to be the most expensive biologic dressings. They are available from several skin banks in various regions of the country in fresh and cryo-preserved (frozen) forms. Homografts are thought to provide the best infection control of all the biologic or biosynthetic dressings available. Revascularization occurs within 48 hours, and the graft may be left in place for several weeks.

Amnion is low in cost and is available in hospitals with burn centers and specialized tissue-banks, which obtain and process it in cooperation with obstetric services. However, amnion grafts do not become vascularized by the patient's vessels and can be left in place only briefly.

Pigskin is available from commercial suppliers. It is available fresh, frozen, or lyophilized (freeze-dried) for longer shelf life. Pigskin impregnated with a topical antibacterial such as silver nitrate is also available.

Biologic dressings have several uses. In extensive burns, they can be life saving by providing temporary wound closure and protecting the granulation tissue until autografting is complete. This is common in patients with large areas of burn and little remaining normal skin donor sites.

Biologic dressings are used to debride untidy wounds after eschar separation as well. With each biologic dressing change, debridement occurs. Once the biologic dressing appears to be "taking," or adhering to the granulating surface with minimal underlying exudation, the patient is ready for an autograft.

Biologic dressings provide immediate coverage for clean, superficial burns and decrease the wound's evaporative water and protein loss. They decrease pain by protecting nerve endings and are an effective barrier against water and bacteria. When applied to superficial partial-thickness wounds, they appear to speed healing.

Biologic materials can be left open or covered. They stay in place for varying lengths of time but are removed in instances of infection or rejection.

Biosynthetic and Synthetic Wound Coverings

Problems with availability, sterility, and cost have prompted the search for biosynthetic and synthetic skin substitutes, which may eventually replace biologic dressings as temporary wound coverings. Currently, the most widely used synthetic dressing is Biobrane, which is composed of a nylon, Silastic membrane combined with a collagen derivative. The material is semitransparent and sterile. It has an indefinite shelf life and is less costly than homograft or pigskin. Like biologic dressings, Biobrane protects the wound from fluid loss and bacterial invasion.

Biobrane adheres to the wound fibrin, which binds to the nylon-collagen material. Within 5 days, cells migrate into the nylon mesh. Generally, adherence to the wound surface correlates directly with low bacterial counts. When the Biobrane dressing adheres to the wound, the wound remains stable and the Biobrane can remain in place for 3 to 4 weeks. Biobrane II dressings (Fig. 55-7) readily adhere to donor sites and meticulously clean debrided partial-thickness wounds; they will remain until spontaneous epithelialization and wound healing occur. Biobrane can be laid on top of a wide-meshed autograft to protect the wound until the autograft epithelium grows out to close the interstices. As the Biobrane gradually separates, it is trimmed, leaving a healed wound.

Biobrane is also useful for intermediate or long-term closure of a surgically excised wound until an autograft becomes available. Like biologic dressings, Biobrane should not be used over grossly contaminated or necrotic wounds. Removal of Biobrane after several weeks is similar to but easier than removal of a vascularized allograft and leaves a bleeding granulation bed that readily accepts an autograft.

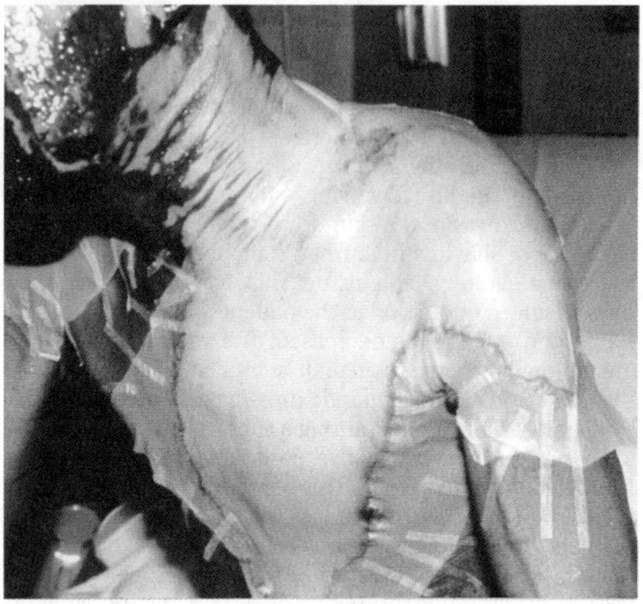

FIGURE 55-7. Biobrane II immediately after its application to a superficial to partial-thickness burn injury of the clavicular, pectoral, and supraclavicular areas. (Used with permission of Winthrop Pharmaceuticals Wound Care Division, New York.)

Several other synthetic dressing are available for burn wound care. Op-Site, a thin, transparent, polyurethane elastic film, can be used to cover clean partial-thickness wounds and donor sites. This dressing is occlusive and waterproof yet permeable to water vapor and air; this permeability not only provides protection from microbial contamination but also allows for the exchange of gases that occurs much more quickly in a moist environment. Other synthetic dressings used for burn wounds include Tegaderm, N-Terface, and Duo-Derm.

Artificial skin is available under the trade name Integra. This is the newest type of synthetic dressing. A dermal analogue, Integra is composed of two main layers. The epidermal layer, consisting of Silastic, acts as a bacterial barrier and prevents water loss from the dermis. The dermal layer is composed of animal collagen. It interfaces with the open wound surface and allows migration of fibroblasts and capillaries into the material. This "neodermis" becomes a permanent structure. The artificial dermis is biodegraded and resorbed. The epidermal layer is removed 2 to 3 weeks after application and is replaced with the patient's own skin. Contracture has been reported to be minimal with no hypertrophic scarring. The appearance resembles normal skin.

Pain Management

The outstanding features of burn pain are its intensity and long duration. Further, necessary wound care carries with it the anticipation of pain and anxiety; the pain experienced is often severe.

Over a typical burn pain course, there are many peaks and valleys. The primary pain from the burn itself is intense in the initial acute postburn phase. This primary pain gradually subsides, but for weeks thereafter, until the skin heals or skin grafts are applied and take, the pain level remains high because of treatment-induced pain. Wound cleaning, dressing change, debridement, and physical therapy are often performed simultaneously or serially, inflicting intense pain. Even when grafts are applied, making the burn site more comfortable, donor sites are created; these may be intensely painful for several days. Discomfort related to tissue healing, such as itching, tingling, and tightness of contracting skin and joints, further adds to the duration if not the intensity of pain over weeks or months.

Because pain cannot be eliminated short of complete anesthesia, the goal is to minimize the pain with analgesics before the patient faces wound care procedures. With adequate staff working gently, swiftly, and skillfully, the duration of pain from wound care can be shortened. Bolus doses of morphine or meperidine (Demerol) are often provided. Ketamine anesthesia administered intravenously is also used for some wound care procedures in burn units. Sedation with antianxiety mediations such as lorazepam (Ativan) or midazolam (Versed) may be indicated in addition to analgesia.

Patient-controlled analgesia (PCA), continuous morphine infusions at 2 to 3 mg/hr, and sustained-release oral morphine, given every 12 hours with an additional dose before wound care, have helped burn patients. Self-administered nitrous oxide also helps to make dressing changes more tolerable for patients who have sufficient hand function to hold a mask to their faces intermittently during dressing changes.

Early surgical excision with grafting under anesthesia may be the best way to reduce the overall pain experience for burn patients.

Nutritional Support

Hypermetabolism persists after burn injury until wounds are closed, thereby increasing the basal metabolic need by as much as 100%. The goal of nutritional support is to promote a state of positive nitrogen balance. The nutritional support required is based on the patient's preburn status and the extent of total BSA burned.

Several formulas exist for estimating the daily metabolic expenditure and caloric requirements of burn patients. Protein requirements may range from 1.5 to 4.0 gm of protein per kilogram of body weight every 24 hours. Lipids are included in the nutritional support of every burn patient because of their importance for wound healing, cellular integrity, and absorption of fat-soluble vitamins. Carbohydrates are included to meet caloric goals as high as 5000 calories daily and to spare protein, which is essential for wound healing. The patient also needs adequate vitamins and minerals.

Current research findings are bringing about rapid changes in specific guidelines for estimating energy expenditure during various phases of postburn recovery. The proportions of fat, protein, and carbohydrate are carefully planned for maximal use. Overfeeding can also be detrimental. Therefore, a dietitian familiar with current concepts in nutrition for burn patients should be consulted for all patients with major burns.

Patients lose a great deal of weight during recovery from severe burns. Reserve fat deposits are catabolized, fluids are lost, and caloric intake may be limited. Because burns lower the patient's resistance to infection and disease, the nutritional status must be improved even though the patient has a poor appetite and is weak.

As soon as gastrointestinal function resumes after the patient's condition stabilizes, nutritional support begins. The enteral route is preferred, and many burn patients will tolerate oral fluids and food. In patients with extensive burns, tube feeding may be initiated to ensure a certain number of daily calories. In this case, high-protein, high-caloric snacks and fluids may be offered as supplements to the essential tube feedings. A diet containing semisolid or solid food is usually begun toward the end of the first week when the patient's tolerance for food improves.

Indications for total parenteral nutrition (TPN) include weight loss greater than 10% of normal body weight, inadequate intake of enteral nutrition due to clinical status, prolonged wound exposure, and malnutrition or debilitated condition before injury. The risk of infection at the site of the central venous catheter required for TPN must be considered. Moreover, the risk of Curling's ulcer continues in the acute phase. Management as discussed in the emergent phase continues.

Disorders of Wound Healing

Disorders of wound healing in the burn patient result from excessive abnormal healing or inadequate new tissue formation. Hypertrophic scarring and keloid formation result from excessive, abnormal healing.

Scars. Hypertrophic scars and wound contractures are more likely to occur if the initial burn injury extends below the level of the deep dermis. Healing of these deep wounds results in the replacement of normal integument with highly metabolically active tissues that lack the normal architecture of the skin. In the collagen layer beneath the epithelium, many fibroblasts proliferate gradually. Myofibroblasts, cells that have the ability to contract, are also present in immature wounds. As these elements contract, the collagen fibers, which normally lie in flat bundles, tend to form a wavy pattern. Eventually the collagen bundles take on a supercoiled appearance and collagen nodules develop. The scar becomes very red (because of its hypervascular nature), raised, and hard. Scar management occurs mainly in the rehabilitative phase, after the wounds are closed. Hypertrophic scarring may cause severe contracture across involved joints. However, these scars are limited to the area of injury and gradually regress over time.

Keloids. In other patients, a large, heaped-up mass of scar tissue develops and may extend beyond the wound surface. This is called a **keloid.** Keloids tend to be found in darkly pigmented persons, grow outside of wound margins, and are more likely to recur after surgical excision.

Failure to Heal. Failure of the wound to heal may relate to many factors, including infection and inadequate nutrition. A serum albumin level below 2 g/dl is usually a factor in impaired healing in the burn patient.

Contractures. Contractures are another concern as wounds heal. The burn wound tissue will shorten because of the force exerted by the fibroblasts and the flexion of muscles in natural wound healing. An opposing force provided by splints, traction, and purposeful movement and positioning must be used to counteract deformity in burns affecting joints.

❑ NURSING PROCESS
Burn Care During the Acute Phase

Assessment

Continued assessment of the burn patient during the early weeks following the burn focuses on hemodynamic alterations, wound healing, pain and psychosocial responses and early detection of complications. Assessment of respiratory and fluid status remains the highest priority for detection of potential complications.

Vital signs are measured frequently. Continued assessment of peripheral pulses is essential for the first few postburn days while edema continues to increase, potentially damaging peripheral nerves and restricting blood flow. Observation of the electrocardiogram (ECG) may give clues to cardiac dysrhythmias resulting from potassium imbalance, preexisting cardiac disease, or the effects of electrical injury or burn shock.

Assessment of residual gastric volumes and *p*H in the patient with a nasogastric tube is also important and gives clues to early sepsis or the need for antacid therapy. Blood in the gastric fluid or the stools must also be noted and reported.

Assessment of the burn wound requires an experienced eye, hand, and sense of smell. Important wound assessment features include size, color, odor, eschar, exudate, abscess formation under the eschar, epithelial buds (small pearl-like clusters of cells on the wound surface), bleeding, granulation tissue appearance, progress of grafts and donor sites, and quality of surrounding skin. Any significant changes in the wound are reported to the physician, because they usually indicate burn wound or systemic sepsis and require immediate intervention.

Other significant and ongoing assessments focus on pain and psychosocial responses, daily body weights, caloric intake, general hydration, and serum electrolyte, hemoglobin, and hematocrit levels. Assessment for excessive bleeding from blood vessels adjacent to areas of surgical exploration and debridement is necessary as well.

Diagnosis

Nursing Diagnoses

Based on the assessment data, *priority* nursing diagnoses in the acute phase of burn care may include the following:

- ❑ Fluid volume excess related to resumption of capillary integrity and fluid shift from interstitial to intravascular compartment
- ❑ Risk for infection related to loss of skin barrier and impaired immune response
- ❑ Altered nutrition: less than body requirements related to hypermetabolism and wound healing needs
- ❑ Impaired skin integrity related to open burn wounds
- ❑ Pain related to exposed nerves, wound healing, and treatments
- ❑ Impaired physical mobility related to burn wound edema, pain, and joint contractures
- ❑ Ineffective individual coping related to fear and anxiety, grieving, and forced dependence on health care providers
- ❑ Altered family processes related to burn injury
- ❑ Knowledge deficit about the course of burn treatment

Collaborative Problems/ Potential Complications

Based on the assessment data, potential complications that may develop in the acute phase of burn care may include:

- ❑ Congestive heart failure and pulmonary edema
- ❑ Sepsis
- ❑ Acute respiratory failure
- ❑ Adult respiratory distress syndrome
- ❑ Visceral damage (electrical burns)

Planning and Implementation

Goals. The major goals for the patient may include restoration of normal fluid balance; absence of infection; attainment of anabolic state and normal weight; improved skin integrity; reduction of pain and discomfort; optimal physical mobility; adequate patient and family coping; adequate patient and family knowledge of burn treatment, and absence of complications. Achievement of these goals requires a collaborative interdisciplinary approach to patient management.

Nursing Interventions

Restoring Normal Fluid Balance. To reduce the risk of fluid overload and consequent congestive heart failure, the nurse closely monitors the patient's intravenous and oral fluid intake, using intravenous infusion pumps to minimize the risk of rapid fluid infusion. To monitor changes in fluid status, careful intake and output records and daily weights are measured. Changes in pulmonary arterial, wedge, and central venous pressures, as well as in blood pressure and pulse rate, are reported to the physician. Low-dose dopamine to increase renal perfusion and diuretics may be prescribed to promote increased urine output. The nurse's role is to administer these medications as prescribed and to monitor the patient's response.

Preventing Infection. A major part of the nurse's role during the acute and other phases of burn care is detecting and preventing infection. The nurse is responsible for providing a clean and safe environment and for closely scrutinizing the burn wound to detect early signs of infection. Culture results and white blood cell counts are monitored.

Aseptic technique is used for wound care procedures and for any invasive procedures such as insertion of intravenous lines and urinary catheters or tracheal suctioning. Meticulous handwashing before and after each patient contact is also an essential component of preventing infection.

The nurse protects the patient from sources of contamination, including other patients, staff members, visitors, and equipment. Invasive lines and tubings must be routinely changed according to the Centers for Disease Control and

Prevention (CDC) recommendations. Tube feeding reservoirs, ventilator circuits, and drainage containers are replaced regularly. Fresh flowers or plants are not permitted in the patient's room because of the risk of microorganism growth. Visitors are screened to avoid exposing the immunocompromised burn patient to pathogens.

Patients can inadvertently promote migration of microorganisms from one burned area to another by touching their wounds or dressings. Bed linens also can spread infection through either colonization with wound microorganisms or fecal contamination. Regularly bathing unburned areas and changing linens can help prevent infection.

Maintaining Adequate Nutrition. Oral fluids should be initiated slowly when bowel sounds resume. The patient's tolerance is noted. If vomiting and distention do not occur, fluids may be increased gradually and the patient may advance to a normal diet or to tube feedings.

The nurse collaborates with the dietitian to plan a protein- and calorie-rich diet that is acceptable to the patient. Family members may be encouraged to bring nutritious and favored foods to the hospital. Milkshakes and sandwiches made with peanut butter, meat, or cheese may be offered as snacks between meals and late in the evening. Nutritional supplements such as Ensure or Resource may be offered. Caloric intake must be documented. Vitamin and mineral supplements may be given.

If caloric goals cannot be met by oral feeding, a nasogastric tube is inserted and used for continuous or bolus feedings of specific formulas. The volume of residual gastric secretions should be checked to ensure absorption. Total parenteral nutrition (TPN) may also be required (see Chapter 35).

Patients should be weighed each day and their weights graphed. This can be used to help them set goals for their own nutritional intake and to monitor weight loss and gain. Ideally, the patient will lose no more than 5% of preburn weight if aggressive nutritional management is implemented.

The patient who is experiencing anorexia requires encouragement and support from the nurse to increase food intake. The patient's surroundings should be as pleasant as possible at mealtime. Catering to food preferences and offering snacks high in protein and vitamins are ways of encouraging the patient to gradually increase intake.

Improving Skin Integrity Through Wound Care. Wound care is usually the single most time-consuming element of burn care after the emergent phase. The physician will prescribe the desired topical antibacterial agents and specific biologic, biosynthetic, or synthetic wound coverings and will plan for surgical excision and grafting. The nurse has an opportunity to make astute assessments of wound status, to use creative approaches to wound dressing, and to support the patient during the emotionally distressing and very painful experience of wound care.

The nurse serves as the coordinator of the complex aspects of wound care and dressing changes for the patient. The nurse must be aware of the rationale and nursing implications for the various wound management approaches. Nursing functions include assessing and recording any changes or progress in wound healing and keeping all members of the health care team informed of changes in the wound or treatment. Using a diagram, updated daily by the nurse responsible for the patient's care, helps to inform all those concerned about the latest wound care procedures in use for the patient.

The nurse also assists the patient and family by instruction, support, and encouragement to take an active part in dressing changes and wound care when appropriate. Discharge planning needs for wound care are anticipated early in the course of burn management, and the strengths of the patient and family are assessed and used in preparing for eventual discharge and home care.

Relieving Pain and Discomfort. Pain is more severe in second-degree burns than in third-degree burns because the nerve endings are not destroyed. Exposed nerve endings are sensitive to cool, moving air; therefore, a sterile covering can help to reduce pain. However, patients with third-degree burns still experience deep pain and pain in the areas surrounding their burns.

Analgesics and antianxiety medications are administered as prescribed. Frequent assessment of pain and discomfort is essential. To increase its effectiveness, pain medication must be provided before the pain becomes too severe.

Nursing interventions such as teaching the patient relaxation techniques, giving the patient some control over wound care and analgesia, and providing frequent reassurance are helpful. Guided imagery may be effective in altering patients' perceptions of and responses to pain. Other pain-relieving approaches include distraction through video programs or video games; hypnosis, biofeedback, and behavioral modification have also been useful for pain management.

The nurse works quickly to complete treatments and dressing changes to reduce pain and discomfort. The patient is encouraged to take analgesic medications before painful procedures. The patient's response to the medication and other interventions is assessed and documented.

Healing burn wounds are typically described by patients as "itchy" and "tight." Oral antipruritic agents, a cool environment, frequent lubrication of the skin with water or a silica-based lotion, exercise and splinting to prevent skin contracture, and diversional activities all help to promote comfort in this phase.

Promoting Physical Mobility. An early priority is to prevent complications resulting from immobility. Deep breathing, turning, and proper repositioning are essential nursing practices to prevent atelectasis and pneumonia, to control edema, and to prevent pressure ulcers and contractures. These interventions are modified to meet the individual patient's needs. Air-fluidized beds and rotation beds may be useful, and early sitting and ambulation are encouraged. Whenever the lower extremities are involved, elastic pressure bandages should be applied before the patient is placed in an upright position. These bandages promote venous return and minimize swelling.

The burn wound is in a dynamic state for a year or more after wound closure. During this time, aggressive efforts must be made to prevent contracture and hypertrophic scarring. Both passive and active range-of-motion exercises are initiated from the day of admission and are continued after grafting within prescribed limitations. Splints or functional devices may be applied to extremities for contracture control. The nurse monitors the splinted areas for signs of vascular insufficiency and nerve compression.

Strengthening Coping Strategies. In the acute phase of burn care, the patient is facing the reality of the burn trauma and is grieving over obvious losses. Depression, regression, and manipulative behavior are common coping mechanisms used by burn patients. Withdrawal from participation in required treatments and regression must be viewed with an understanding that such behavior helps the patient cope with an enormously stressful event. Much energy goes into maintaining vital physical functions and wound healing in the early postburn weeks, leaving little emotional energy for coping in a mature and effective manner. Nurses can assist patients to develop effective coping strategies by setting specific expectations for behavior, promoting truthful communication to build trust, helping patients practice appropriate strategies, and giving positive reinforcement when appropriate. Most importantly, the nurse and all members of the health care team must demonstrate acceptance of the patient.

The patient frequently ventilates feelings of anger. At times the anger may be directed inward because of a sense of guilt—perhaps for causing the fire or even for surviving when loved ones perished—or the anger may reach outward toward those who escaped unharmed or to those who are now providing care. One way to help the patient handle these emotions is to enlist someone to whom the patient can vent feelings without fear of retaliation. A nurse, social worker, or clergy member who is not involved in direct care activities may fill this role successfully.

Burn patients are very dependent on health care team members during the long period of acute illness. However, even when physically unable to contribute much to self-care, they can be included in decisions regarding care and encouraged to assert their individuality in terms of preferences and recognition of their unique identities. As patients improve in mobility and strength, the nurse works with them to set realistic expectations for self-care, including self-feeding, assistance with wound care procedures, exercise, and planning for the future. Many patients respond positively to the use of contractual agreements and other strategies that recognize their independence and their specific role as part of the health care team moving toward the goal of self-care.

Supporting Patient and Family Processes. Family functioning is disrupted with burn injury. One of the nurse's responsibilities is to support the patient and family and to address their verbalized and unverbalized concerns. Family members need to be instructed in ways that they can support the patient as adaptation to burn trauma occurs. The family also needs support by the health care team. The burn injury has tremendous psychologic, economic, and practical impact on the patient and his family. Referrals for social services or psychologic counseling should be made as appropriate. This support continues into the rehabilitation phase.

Patient Education and Home Care Considerations. Burn patients are commonly sent to burn centers far from home. Because burn injuries are not anticipated, family roles are disrupted. Therefore, both the patient and the family need thorough information about the patient's burn care and expected course of treatment. It is important to assess the patient's and family's ability to grasp the educational content and not to provide information to the patient or his family before they can cope with it. To reinforce content, verbal information should be supplemented by videos, models, or printed materials if available. Patient and family education remains a priority in the rehabilitation phase.

Monitoring and Managing Potential Complications

Congestive Heart Failure and Pulmonary Edema. The patient is assessed for fluid overload that may occur as fluid is mobilized from the interstitial compartment back into the intravascular compartment. If the cardiac and renal systems cannot compensate for the excess vascular volume, congestive heart failure and pulmonary edema may result. The patient is assessed for signs of congestive heart failure, including decreased cardiac output, oliguria, jugular vein distention, edema, and the onset of an S_3 or S_4 heart sound. Increasing central venous pressure (CVP), pulmonary artery (PA), and wedge pressures indicate increased fluid volume.

Crackles in the lungs and increased difficulty with respiration may indicate a fluid buildup in the lungs, which is reported promptly to the physician. In the meantime, the patient is positioned comfortably, with the head of the bed raised (if not contraindicated because of other treatments or injuries) to promote lung expansion and gas exchange. Management of this complication includes providing supplemental oxygen, administering intravenous diuretics, carefully assessing the patient's response, and (possibly) providing vasoactive medications.

Sepsis. The signs of early systemic sepsis are subtle and require a high index of suspicion and very close monitoring of changes in the patient's status. Early signs of sepsis may include increased temperature, increased pulse rate, widened pulse pressure, and flushed, dry skin in unburned areas. As with many observations of the burn patient, one needs to look for patterns or trends in the data. (See Chapter 15 for a more detailed discussion of septic shock.)

Wound and blood cultures are performed as prescribed, and results are reported to the physician immediately. The nurse also observes for early signs of septicemia and promptly intervenes, administering prescribed intravenous fluids and antibiotics to prevent septic shock, a complication with a high mortality rate. Antibiotics must be given as scheduled to maintain proper blood concentrations. Serum antibiotic levels are monitored for evidence of maximal effectiveness; the patient is monitored for toxic side effects.

Acute Respiratory Failure and Adult Respiratory Distress Syndrome. The patient's respiratory status is monitored closely for increased difficulty in breathing, change in respiratory pattern, and onset of adventitious (abnormal) sounds. Typically at this stage, signs and symptoms of injury to the respiratory tract become apparent. Respiratory failure may follow. As described previously, signs of hypoxia (oxygen depletion), decreased breath sounds, wheezing, tachypnea, stridor, and sputum tinged with soot (or, in some cases, containing sloughed tracheal tissue) are among the many possible findings that can be auscultated or observed.

Patients on mechanical ventilation must be assessed for a decrease in tidal volume and lung compliance. The hallmark sign of the onset of adult respiratory distress syndrome (ARDS) is hypoxemia on 100% oxygen, decreased lung compliance, and significant shunting. The physician should be notified immediately of deteriorating respiratory status.

Medical management of the patient with acute respiratory failure requires intubation and mechanical ventilation if it is not already in use. If ARDS had developed, higher oxygen levels, positive end-expiratory pressure (PEEP), and pressure support (PS) will be used with mechanical ventilation to promote gas exchange across the alveolar–capillary membrane.

Visceral Damage. The nurse is alert to signs of necrosis of visceral organs injured by electricity. Tissues affected are usually between the entrance and exit wounds of the electrical burn. All patients with electrical burns should undergo ECG monitoring, with dysrhythmias being reported to the physician. Careful attention must also be paid to signs or reports of pain related to deep muscle ischemia in these patients. To minimize the severity of this complication, visceral ischemia must be detected as early as possible. The physician can perform fasciotomies to relieve the swelling and ischemia in the muscles and fascia and to promote oxygenation of the injured tissues. Because of the deep cutting involved with fasciotomies, the patient must be monitored carefully for signs of excessive blood loss and hypovolemia.

Evaluation

Expected Outcomes

1. Achieves optimal fluid balance
   a. Maintains intake, output, and body weight that correlate with expected pattern
   b. Exhibits vital signs, CVP, PA, and wedge pressures that remain within designated limits
   c. Demonstrates increased urine output in response to diuretic and vasoactive medications
   d. Has heart rate lower than 110 beats/minute in normal sinus rhythm
2. Experiences no localized or systemic infection
   a. Has wound culture results showing minimal bacteria
   b. Has normal urine and sputum culture results
3. Demonstrates anabolic nutritional status
   a. Gains weight daily after initial loss secondary to fluid diuresis and no oral intake of food or fluid
   b. Shows no signs of protein, vitamin, or mineral deficiencies
   c. Meets required nutritional needs entirely by oral intake
   d. Participates in selecting diet containing prescribed nutrients
   e. Exhibits normal serum protein levels
4. Demonstrates improved skin integrity
   a. Sustains generally intact skin that remains free of infection, pressure, and injury
   b. Demonstrates remaining open wound areas that are pink, reepithelializing, and free of infection
   c. Demonstrates donor graft sites that are clean and healing
   d. Has healed wounds that are soft and smooth
   e. Demonstrates skin that is lubricated and elastic
5. Experiences minimal pain
   a. Requests analgesics only for specific wound care procedures or physical therapy activities
   b. Reports minimal pain
   c. Gives no physiologic or nonverbal cues that pain is moderate or severe
   d. Uses pain control measures such as nitrous oxide, relaxation, imagery, and distraction techniques to cope with and alleviate discomfort
   e. Can sleep without being disturbed by pain
   f. Reports skin is comfortable, with no itching or tightness
6. Demonstrates optimal physical mobility
   a. Improves range of motion of joints daily
   b. Demonstrates preinjury range of motion of all joints
   c. Experiences no signs of calcification around the joints
   d. Participates in activities of daily living
7. Uses appropriate coping strategies to deal with postburn problems
   a. Verbalizes reactions to burns, therapeutic procedures, losses
   b. Identifies coping strategies used effectively in previous stressful situations
   c. Accepts dependency on health care providers during acute phase
   d. Verbalizes realistic view of problems resulting from burn injury and plans for future
   e. Cooperates with health care providers in required therapy
   f. Participates in decision making regarding care
   g. Resolves grief over losses resulting from burn injury and circumstances surrounding injury (*e.g.*, death of others, damage to home or other property)
   h. States realistic objectives for plastic surgery, further medical intervention, and results
   i. Verbalizes realistic abilities and goals
   j. Displays hopeful attitude toward future
8. Relates appropriately in patient/family processes
   a. Patient and family verbalize feelings regarding change in family interactions
   b. Family emotionally supports the patient during the hospitalization
   c. Family states that own needs are met
9. Patient and family verbalize understanding of the treatment course
   a. State rationale for different aspects of treatment
   b. State realistic time period for recovery
10. Experiences no complications
   a. Has clear-sounding lungs on auscultation
   b. Exhibits no dyspnea or orthopnea and can breathe freely when standing, sitting, and lying down
   c. Exhibits no S_3 or S_4 heart sounds or jugular venous distention
   d. Experiences urine output, CVP, PAP, PCWP and cardiac output within normal limits
   e. Exhibits normal blood, sputum, and urine culture results
   f. Maintains arterial blood gas values within normal limits
   g. Has normal lung compliance
   h. Has no visceral organ damage
   i. Experiences stable cardiac rhythm

Nursing care of the patient in the acute phase of burn care is discussed further in Nursing Care Plan 55-2.

(text continues on page 1579)

NURSING CARE PLAN 55–2
Care of the Patient During the Acute Phase of Burn Care

Nursing Interventions	Rationale	Expected Outcomes
NURSING DIAGNOSIS: Fluid volume excess related to resumption of capillary integrity and fluid shift from interstitial to intravascular compartment		
GOAL: Maintenance of optimal fluid balance		
1. Monitor vital signs, intake and output, weight. Assess for edema, jugular vein distention (JVD), crackles.	1. These signs and symptoms reflect fluid status	• Intake, output, and body weight correlate with expected pattern. • Vital signs, CVP, PAP, PCWP remain within designated limits. • Urine output increases in response to diuretic and vasoactive medications.
2. Notify physician of urine output <30 ml/hr, weight gain, JVD, crackles, increased CVP, PAP, PCWP.	2. These indicate increased fluid volume	
3. Maintain intravenous fluids on pumps or rate controllers.	3. Regulation prevents accidental fluid bolus	
4. Administer diuretics or dopamine as prescribed. Assess response.	4. Dopamine increases renal perfusion, which increases urine output. Diuretics promote increased urine formation and urine output and decrease intravascular volume	
NURSING DIAGNOSIS: Risk for infection related to loss of skin barrier and impaired immune response		
GOAL: Absence of localized or systemic infection		
1. Use asepsis in all aspects of patient care: a. Meticulous handwashing before and after patient care. b. Use clean or sterile gloves for wound care. c. Wear isolation gown or protective plastic apron for patient care. d. Wear mask and hair cover when wounds are exposed and during sterile procedures. e. Change invasive lines and tubings as recommended by CDC.	1. Aseptic techniques minimize risk of cross-contamination and spread of bacterial contamination	• Wound cultures show minimal bacteria • Normal blood, urine and sputum cultures • Absence of signs and symptoms of infection and sepsis
2. Screen visitors for respiratory, gastrointestinal, or integumentary infections. Provide isolation gowns for visitors without active infection and instruct in handwashing.	2. Avoiding known infecting agents prevents introduction of additional microorganisms	
3. Exclude plants and flowers in water from patient's room.	3. Stagnant water is a potential source of bacterial growth	
4. Inspect wound for signs of infection, purulent drainage or discoloration.	4. Such signs indicate localized infection	
5. Monitor white blood cell (WBC) count, culture and sensitivity results.	5. Increased WBC count indicates infection. Culture and sensitivity indicate microorganisms present and appropriate antibiotics to be used.	
6. Administer antibiotics as prescribed.	6. Antibiotics reduce bacteria	
7. Provide regular linen changes and assist patient with personal hygiene.	7. These measures reduce potential bacterial colonization of burn wound	

(*continued*)

NURSING CARE PLAN 55-2 *(continued)*
Care of the Patient During the Acute Phase of Burn Care

Nursing Interventions	Rationale	Expected Outcomes
8. Report to physician decreased bowel sounds, tachycardia, decreased blood pressure, decreased urine output, fever, and flushing.	8. These signs may indicate sepsis	
9. Administer fluids and vasoactive medications as prescribed. Assess response.	9. These agents are used to maintain tissue perfusion in sepsis	

NURSING DIAGNOSIS: **Altered nutrition: less than body requirements related to hypermetabolism and wound healing**

GOAL: **Attainment of anabolic nutritional status**

Nursing Interventions	Rationale	Expected Outcomes
1. Provide high-calorie, high-protein diet; include patient preferences and home-made food. Give nutritional supplements as prescribed.	1. The patient needs sufficient nutrients for wound healing and increased metabolic requirements	• Gains weight daily after initial loss • Exhibits no signs of protein, vitamin or mineral deficiencies • Meets required nutritional needs entirely by oral intake. • Participates in selection of diet with prescribed nutrients • Serum protein levels within acceptable range
2. Monitor patient's daily weight and calorie count.	2. These measures assist in determining whether dietary needs are being met	
3. Administer supplemental vitamins and minerals as prescribed.	3. These help meet additional nutritional needs; adequate vitamins and minerals are necessary for wound healing and cellular function	
4. Administer enteral or total parenteral nutrition per protocol if dietary needs are not met through oral intake.	4. Nutritional techniques ensure nutritional needs are met	
5. Report abdominal distention, large gastric residual volumes, or diarrhea to physician.	5. These signs may indicate intolerance of route or type of feeding	

NURSING DIAGNOSIS: **Impaired skin integrity related to open burn wounds**

GOAL: **Demonstration of improved skin integrity**

Nursing Interventions	Rationale	Expected Outcomes
1. Clean wounds, body and hair daily.	1. Daily cleaning reduces potential bacterial colonization	• Skin is generally intact, and free of signs of infection, pressure and trauma. • Open wounds are pink, reepithelializing, and free of infection. • Donor sites are clean and reepithelializing. • Healed wounds are soft and smooth. • Skin is lubricated and elastic.
2. Provide wound care as prescribed.	2. Care promotes wound healing	
3. Apply topical antibacterial agents and dressing as prescribed.	3. Wound care regimen reduces bacterial colonization and promotes healing	
4. Prevent pressure, infection, and mobilization of autografts.	4. These measures promote graft "take" and healing	
5. Provide donor site care.	5. Care promotes healing of donor site	
6. Provide adequate nutritional support.	6. Adequate nutrition is essential for normal granulation and healing	
7. Assess wound and graft sites. Report signs of poor healing, poor graft take, or trauma to physician.	7. Early intervention for poor wound healing or graft take is essential. Grafted or healed burn wounds are susceptible to trauma	

NURSING DIAGNOSIS: **Pain related to exposed nerves, wound healing and treatments**

GOAL: **Reduction or control of pain**

Nursing Interventions	Rationale	Expected Outcomes
1. Assess pain level using pain scale. Observe for nonverbal indicators of pain: grimacing, tachycardia, clenched fists.	1. Pain assessment data provide baseline for assessing response to interventions	• Requests analgesics for specific wound care procedures or physical therapy activities

(continued)

NURSING CARE PLAN 55–2 *(continued)*
Care of the Patient During the Acute Phase of Burn Care

Nursing Interventions	Rationale	Expected Outcomes
2. Educate the patient about the usual pain trajectory in burn recovery and options for pain control. Allow patient as much control as possible regarding pain management. 3. Offer analgesics approximately 20 minutes before painful procedures. 4. Provide pain medication before pain becomes severe. 5. Instruct and assist patient in relaxation, imagery, distraction techniques. 6. Assess and document the patient's response to interventions. 7. Administer antianxiety and antipruritic agents as indicated. 8. Lubricate healing burn wounds with water- or silica-based lotion.	2. Knowledge reduces fear of the unknown, and provides some measure of control to the patient 3. Premedication allows time for therapeutic response 4. Pain is more easily controlled before it becomes severe 5. Nonpharmacologic pain measures provide multiple interventions to decrease pain sensation 6. Patient's responses assist in ascertaining best pain control techniques for the patient 7. These medications help to increase patient's comfort 8. These preparations decrease sensation of skin tightness	• States pain in minimal • Gives no physiologic or nonverbal cues that pain is moderate or severe • Uses pain control measures such as nitrous oxide, relaxation, imagery, and distraction techniques to assist with coping with pain • Can sleep without being disturbed by pain • Reports skin is comfortable with no itching or tightness

NURSING DIAGNOSIS: Impaired physical mobility related to burn wound edema, pain and joint contractures

GOAL: Achievement of optimal physical mobility

Nursing Interventions	Rationale	Expected Outcomes
1. Position patient carefully to prevent flexed position in burned areas. 2. Implement range of motion (ROM) exercises several times daily. 3. Assist with early sitting and ambulation. 4. Use splints and exercise devices recommended by occupational and physical therapists. 5. Encourage self-care to the extent of the patient's ability.	1. Proper positioning reduces risk of flexion contractures 2. ROM exercises minimize muscle atrophy 3. Early mobility encourages increased use of muscles 4. Such devices encourage activity while maintaining proper position of joints 5. Self-care promotes both independence and increased activity	• Improves range of motion of joints daily • Demonstrates preinjury range of motion of all joints • Absence of signs of periarticular calcification • Participates in activities of daily living

NURSING DIAGNOSIS: Ineffective individual coping related to fear and anxiety, grieving and forced dependence on health care providers

GOAL: Use of appropriate coping strategies to deal with post-burn problems.

Nursing Interventions	Rationale	Expected Outcomes
1. Assess patient for coping abilities and previous successful coping strategies. 2. Demonstrate acceptance of patient. Provide positive feedback and support. 3. Assist patient to set achievable short-term goals for increased independence in activities of daily living. 4. Use multidisciplinary approach to promote mobility and independence. 5. Consult with health care team members for assistance with regressive or maladaptive behaviors.	1. Psychosocial data provide baseline for planning care 2. Acceptance encourages self-esteem and continued progress toward independence 3. Short-term goal-setting leads to pattern of success for patient. Long-term goals may seem unrealistic or unattainable to patient 4. Communication among disciplines provides consistent approach 5. Collaboration utilizes the expertise of others	• Verbalizes reactions to burns, therapeutic procedures, losses • Identifies coping strategies used previously in stressful situations • Accepts dependency on health care providers during acute illness • Resolves grief over losses resulting from burn injury • Participates in decision making regarding care • Has hopeful attitude toward future

(continued)

Care of the Patient During the Acute Phase of Burn Care

Nursing Interventions	Rationale	Expected Outcomes
NURSING DIAGNOSIS: Altered family processes related to burn injury		
GOAL: Achievement of appropriate patient/family processes		
1. Assess patient and family's perception of impact of burn injury on family functioning.	1. Assessment data provide baseline from which to plan care	• Patient verbalizes feelings regarding alteration in family interactions.
2. Demonstrate willingness to listen. Provide realistic support.	2. Empathetic attitude promotes verbalizing of concerns	• Family can emotionally support the patient during hospitalization.
3. Refer family to social services and other resources as needed.	3. Collaboration assists to comprehensively address concerns	• Family states that needs are met.
4. Explain the usual burn patient's coping patterns to family. Discuss ways that they can support the patient.	4. Explanations help decrease anxiety about the unknown and promote appropriate intervention by families towards patient	
NURSING DIAGNOSIS: Knowledge deficit about the course of burn treatment		
GOAL: Verbalization of understanding of the course of burn treatment by patient and family		
1. Assess readiness of patient and family to learn.	1. Limit education to patient's and family's ability to process information	• States rationale for different aspects of treatment
2. Explore patient and family's previous experience with hospitalization and illness.	2. This information provides a baseline for explanations and indication of patient's and family's expectations	• States realistic time period for recovery
3. Review general course of burn treatment with patient and family.	3. Knowing what to expect prepares patient and family for upcoming events	• Patient and family participate in management plans as appropriate
4. Explain importance of patient participation in care for optimal results.	4. This information provides specific direction to patient	
5. Realistically explain length of time involved in burn recovery.	5. Honesty promotes realistic expectations	
COLLABORATIVE PROBLEMS: Congestive heart failure, pulmonary edema, sepsis, acute respiratory failure, adult respiratory distress syndrome, visceral damage (electrical burns)		
GOAL: Absence of complications		
Congestive Heart Failure (CHF) and Pulmonary Edema		
1. Assess for decreased urine output, jugular vein distention (JVD), or an S_3 or S_4 heart sound.	1. These signs may indicate decreased cardiac output and the onset of congestive heart failure	• Lungs clear to auscultation
2. Monitor for increases in CVP, PAP, PCWP, or decrease in cardiac output.	2. Increased pressures indicate increased preload and intravascular volumes. Decreasing cardiac output reflects less oxygen and nutrients available to the tissues and may indicate the onset of CHF	• Absence of dypsnea, orthopnea, JVD, and S_3 or S_4 heart sounds
3. Assess for crackles on lung ausculation, dypsnea, orthopnea, or decreased oxygenation detected by pulse oximetry or ABGs.	3. Such signs may indicate progression of congestive heart failure to pulmonary edema	• Urine output, CVP, PAP, PCWP and CO within normal limits
4. Report the above signs and symptoms to the physician.	4. Medical intervention is needed	

(continued)

NURSING CARE PLAN 55–2 *(continued)*
Care of the Patient During the Acute Phase of Burn Care

Nursing Interventions	Rationale	Expected Outcomes
5. Position patient with the head of bed up 45 to 90 degrees as tolerated.	5. Elevation facilitates gas exchange	
6. Administer diuretics as prescribed. Assess patient's response.	6. Diuretics increase urine output and decrease cardiac preload and intravascular volumes	
Sepsis		
1. Assess for fever, increased pulse, widened pulse pressure, and flushed, dry skin in unburned areas. Watch trends and notify physician if noted.	1. Such signs may indicate impending sepsis	• Normal blood, sputum and urine cultures • Absence of tachycardia, widening pulse pressure, and flushed, dry skin in unburned areas
2. Monitor wound and blood cultures and notify physician of positive cultures	2. Positive cultures indicate infection and possible sepsis	
3. Administer fluids, vasoactive medications and antibiotics as prescribed. Monitor for therapeutic response. Check that infecting organisms are sensitive to prescribed antibiotics.	3. Antibiotics kill susceptible bacteria. Intravenous fluids and vasoactive medications maintain intravascular volume and blood pressure	
4. Monitor for therapeutic serum antibiotic levels.	4. Antibiotics are most effective at therapeutic levels. Excessive levels can cause systemic damage	
Acute Respiratory Failure/Adult Respiratory Distress Syndrome (ARDS)		
1. Assess for respiratory distress, changes in respiratory patterns or onset of adventitious breath sounds. Report to physician.	1. Such problems indicate possible acute respiratory failure. Pulmonary complications may not appear for 24 to 48 hours after the burn injury.	• Arterial blood gases within normal limits • Normal lung compliance • Absence of respiratory distress • Improved pO_2 level
2. Monitor pulse oximetry and ABG levels for decreasing oxygen saturation and pO_2. Report to physician.	2. Decreasing oxygenation indicates deteriorating respiratory status. Medical intervention is needed	
3. Monitor the mechanically ventilated patient for decreased spontaneous tidal volumes and lung compliance.	3. Respiratory problems reflect increased difficulty with ventilation, and may indicate the onset of ARDS	
4. In collaboration with the physician and respiratory therapist, administer positive end-expiratory pressure (PEEP), pressure support (PS). Assess patient's response.	4. PEEP and PS optimize diffusion of oxygen across the alveolar capillary membrane	
Visceral Damage (Electrical Burns)		
1. Assess patient for signs of deep pain. Focus on areas between entrance and exit wounds of burn.	1. Pain may reflect visceral damage	• Absence of visceral organ damage • Stable cardiac rhythm
2. Monitor ECG rhythm.	2. The patient with electrical burns is at risk for dysrhythmias	
3. Report to the physician any complaints of deep pain or dysrhythmias.	3. Visceral damage requires immediate intervention	

Rehabilitation Phase of Burn Care

Although long-term aspects of burn care are discussed last, rehabilitation begins *immediately* after the burn has occurred—as early as the emergent period.

In the aftermath of the acute stages of injury, the burn patient increasingly focuses on the alterations in self-image and life-style that may occur. Wound healing, psychosocial support, and restoring maximum functional activity remain priorities. The focus on maintaining fluid and electrolyte balance and improving nutritional status continues. Reconstructive surgery to improve body appearance and function may be needed.

In a retrospective survey, Cobb, Maxwell, and Silverstein (1990) found that younger and older patients with severe burn injury reported an impaired quality of life. The older burn survivors reported changes in their physical activity and economic status. Younger burn survivors reported impairment of social, psychologic, and employment status. Counseling, both psychologic and vocational, and support groups may be helpful factors in recovery. Family members also need support and guidance in assisting the patient's return to optimal health.

Home Care and Follow-Up

Follow-up care planned by the multidisciplinary burn care team will be necessary. Preparations should begin during the early stages of care. It is a great challenge to the health care team to prepare a person for independent functioning after such a traumatic event.

As the inpatient phase of recovery becomes shorter, the focus of rehabilitative interventions will be directed toward outpatient care or care in a rehabilitation center. In the long term, a good deal of care for the healed burns will be performed by the patient and others at home. Patients commonly leave the hospital with small areas of clean, open wounds that are healing slowly. These areas should be washed daily with mild soap and water, and the prescribed topical agent or dressing should be applied.

Elastic Pressure Devices. The wound is in a dynamic state for 1½ to 2 years after the burn occurs. If appropriate measures are instituted during this active period, the scar tissue loses its redness and softens. Healed areas that are prone to hypertrophic scarring require the patient to wear a pressure garment (Fig. 55-8). These devices are especially useful for partial-thickness wounds that required more than 2 weeks to heal and for the edges of grafted skin. Applying elastic pressure garments loosens collagen bundles and encourages parallel orientation of the collagen to the skin surface with the disappearance of the dermal nodules. As pressure continues over time, there is a restructuring of the collagen and a decrease in vascularity and cellularity.

The physical therapist or a representative of the manufacturer of elastic pressure garments measures the patient for correct fit. While awaiting the arrival of the garment, soft, tubular, knit elastic pressure bandages can be used to help desensitize the patient's skin, protect healing areas, provide pressure, and promote venous return. Patients must be educated regarding the need for lubrication and protection of the healing skin and the necessity of wearing pressure garments for at least a year after the injury. A program including elastic pressure garments, splints, and exercise under the supervision of an experienced physical and occupational therapy team is recommended for optimal functional and cosmetic results.

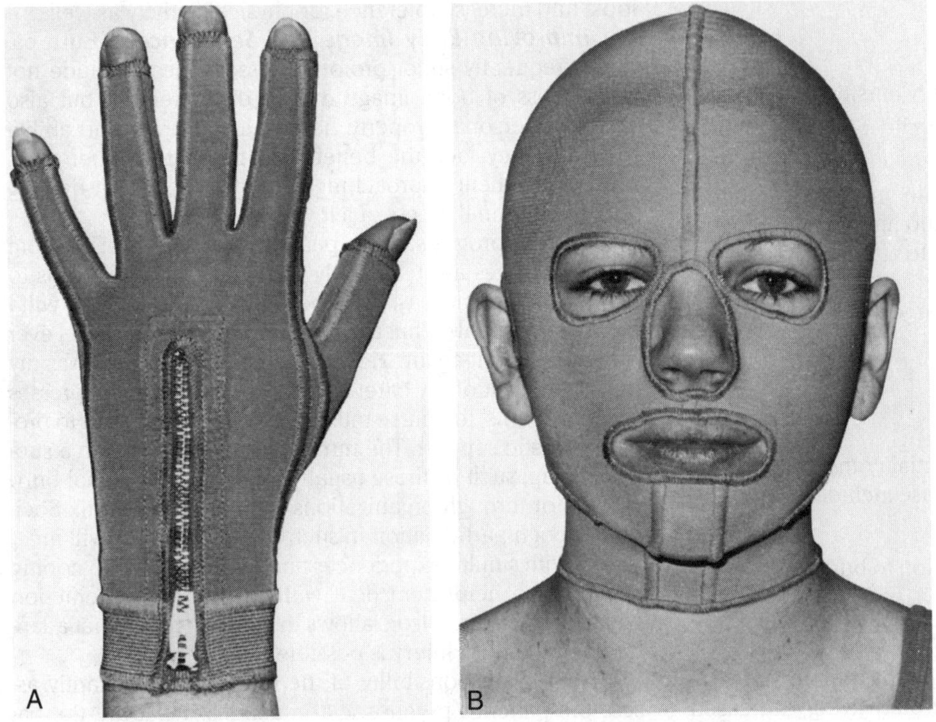

FIGURE 55-8. Elastic pressure garments. Application of pressure garments helps prevent hypertrophic burn scarring. (**A**) Elastic pressure glove. (**B**) Elastic pressure face mask. (Illustrations courtesy of Jobst Institute, Inc, Toledo, OH.)

NURSING PROCESS
Burn Care During the Rehabilitation Phase

Assessment

Information about the patient's educational level, occupation, leisure activities, cultural background, religion, and family interactions is obtained early. The patient's self-concept, mental status, emotional response to the injury and hospitalization, level of intellectual functioning, previous hospitalizations, response to pain and pain relief measures, and sleep pattern are also essential components of a comprehensive assessment. Information about the patient's general self-concept, self-esteem, and coping strategies in the past will be valuable in addressing emotional needs.

Ongoing physical assessments related to rehabilitation goals include range of motion of affected joints, functional abilities in activities of daily living, early signs of skin breakdown from splints or positioning devices, evidence of neuropathies (neurologic damage), activity tolerance, and quality or condition of healing skin. The patient's participation in care and ability to demonstrate self-care in such areas as ambulation, eating, wound cleaning, and applying pressure wraps are documented on a regular basis. In addition to these assessment parameters, specific complications and treatments require additional specific assessments; for example, the patient undergoing primary excision requires postoperative assessment.

Recovery from burn injury involves every system of the body, so assessment of the burn patient must be comprehensive and continuous. Priorities will vary at different points during the rehabilitation phase. Understanding the pathophysiologic responses to burn injury form the framework for detecting early progress or signs and symptoms of complications. Early detection leads to early intervention and enhances the potential for successful rehabilitation.

Diagnosis

Nursing Diagnoses

Based on the assessment data, *priority* nursing diagnoses in the long-term rehabilitation phase of burn care may include the following:

- Activity intolerance related to pain on exercise, limited joint mobility, muscle wasting, and limited endurance
- Body image disturbance related to altered physical appearance and self-concept
- Knowledge deficit of post-discharge home care and follow-up needs

Collaborative Problems/ Potential Complications

Based on the assessment data, potential complications that may develop in the rehabilitation phase include:

- Contractures
- Inadequate psychologic adaptation to burn injury

Planning and Implementation

Goals. The major goals for the patient include increased participation in activities of daily living; increased understanding of the injury, treatment, and planned follow-up care; adaptation and adjustment to alterations in body image, self-concept, and life-style; and absence of complications.

Nursing Interventions

Promoting Activity Tolerance. Nursing interventions that must be carried out according to a strict regimen and the pain that accompanies movement take their toll on a burn patient. The patient may become confused and disoriented and lack the energy to participate optimally in care. The nurse must schedule care in such a way that each patient has periods of uninterrupted sleep. A good time for planned patient rest is after the stress of dressing changes and exercise, while pain interventions and sedatives may still be effective. This plan must be communicated to family members and other care providers. Hypnotics given in the evening, as prescribed, may promote sleep at night. Because burn patients frequently have nightmares related to the burn injury, the nurse listens to and reassures the patient when such nightmares, or other fears and anxieties about the outcome of the injury, cause insomnia.

Reducing metabolic stress by relieving pain, preventing chilling or fever, and promoting physical integrity of all body systems will help the patient conserve energy for therapeutic activities and wound healing.

The nurse incorporates physical therapy exercises in the patient's care to prevent muscle atrophy and to maintain the mobility required for daily activities. The patient's activity tolerance, strength, and endurance will gradually increase if activity occurs over increasingly longer periods. Fatigue, fever, and pain tolerance are monitored and used to determine the amount of activity to be encouraged on a daily basis. Scheduling activities, such as family visits, recreational or play therapy—such as video games, listening to the radio, watching television, or walking to the patient lounge—can provide diversion, improve the patient's outlook, and increase tolerance for physical activity as well.

Improving Body Image and Self-Concept. Burn patients frequently suffer profound losses. These include not only a loss of body image due to disfigurement but also losses of personal property, homes, loved ones, and ability to work. They lack the benefit of anticipatory grief often seen in a patient approaching surgery or a person dealing with the terminal illness of a loved one.

As care progresses, the patient who is recovering from burns becomes aware of daily improvement and begins to exhibit basic concerns: Will I be disfigured? How long will I be in the hospital? What about my job and family? Will I ever be independent again? How can I pay for my care? Was my burn the result of my carelessness? As the patient expresses such concerns, the nurse must take time to listen and to provide realistic support. The nurse can refer patients to a support group, such as those usually available at regional burn centers or through organizations such as the Phoenix Society. Through participation in such groups, patients will meet others with similar experiences and learn to develop coping strategies to help them deal with their losses. Interaction with other burn survivors allows the patient to see that adaptation to the burn injury is possible.

A major responsibility of the nurse is to constantly assess the patient's psychosocial reactions. What are the patient's fears and concerns? Does the patient's fear involve losing control of care, losing independence, or losing sanity itself? Is it fear of rejection by family and loved ones? Is it fear of being unable to cope with pain or physical appearance? Is it concern about sexual function? Being aware of these anxieties and understanding the basis of the patient's fears enables the nurse to provide support and to cooperate with other members of the health care team in developing a plan to help the patient handle these feelings.

When caring for burn patients, the nurse needs to be aware that there are prejudices and misunderstandings in society about those who are "different." Opportunities and accommodations available to others are often denied to those who are disfigured. Such amenities include social participation, employment, prestige, various roles, and status. The health care team must actively promote a healthy body image and self-concept in burn survivors so that they can accept or challenge others' perceptions of the disfigured. Survivors themselves who must show others who they are, how they function, and how they want to be treated.

The nurse can help patients practice their responses to people who may stare or inquire about their injury once they are discharged from the hospital. The nurse can help patients build self-esteem by recognizing their uniqueness—for example, with small gestures such as providing a birthday cake, combing the patient's hair before visiting hours, sharing information on the availability of a cosmetician to enhance appearance, and teaching the patient ways to direct attention away from a disfigured body shell to the self within. Consultants such as psychologists, social workers, vocational counselors, and teachers are valuable participants in assisting burn patients regain their self-esteem.

Patient Education and Home Care Considerations. Patients will be better able to participate in their care if they are aware of the consequences of the injury, the goals of planned treatment, and their role in ongoing care. As discussed earlier, this education begins in the emergency department and continues throughout rehabilitation.

Families are included in planning and carrying out care to the extent allowed by their interest and ability and the patient's needs. In preparation for discharge, the patient and family are instructed in wound care, exercises, using pressure garments, and follow-up care. They are taught to recognize abnormal signs to report to the physician and available resources to help them meet their future needs.

Monitoring and Managing Potential Complications

Contractures. With early and aggressive physical and occupational therapy, contractures are rarely a long-term complication. However, surgical intervention is indicated if a full range of motion in the burn patient is not achieved. (See Chapter 18 for a discussion of contractures.)

Impaired Psychologic Adaptation to the Burn Injury. Some patients, particularly those with limited coping skills or psychologic function or a history of psychiatric problems before the burn injury, may not achieve adequate psychologic adaptation to the burn injury. This problem is beyond the scope of nursing intervention. Psychologic counseling or psychiatric referral should be obtained as soon as evidence of major coping problems appears.

Evaluation

Expected Outcomes

1. Demonstrates activity tolerance required for desired daily activities
   a. Obtains sufficient sleep daily
   b. Reports absence of nightmares or sleep disturbances
   c. Shows gradually increasing tolerance and endurance in physical activities
   d. Can concentrate during conversations
   e. Has energy available to sustain desired daily activities
2. Adapts to altered body image
   a. Verbalizes an accurate description of alterations in body image postburn
   b. Accepts physical appearance
   c. Demonstrates interest in resources that may positively affect body appearance and function
   d. Uses cosmetics, wigs, and prostheses as desired to achieve acceptable appearance
   e. Socializes with significant others, peers, and usual social group
   f. Seeks and achieves return to role in family, school, or community as a contributing member
3. Demonstrates knowledge of required self-care and follow-up care
   a. Describes surgical procedures and treatments accurately
   b. Verbalizes detailed plan for follow-up care
   c. Demonstrates ability to perform wound care and prescribed exercises
   d. Returns for follow-up appointments as scheduled
   e. Identifies resource people and agencies to contact for specific problems
4. Exhibits no complications
   a. Demonstrates full range of motion
   b. Shows no signs of withdrawal or depression
   c. Displays no psychotic behaviors

Patient Education and Home Care Considerations

As hospital stays become shorter, outpatient and home care of burn patients take on increasing importance. Patients and families must gradually be educated during the hospital course to care for the burn wound by active participation as early as possible. Initially, looking at and touching the burn wound may be difficult and even frightening to some family members and patients. However, with encouragement and support, most patients and family members can handle follow-up wound care with little need for professional care on a daily basis.

An additional area that the nurse must address before discharge is burn prevention. As previously cited, one study found that 13% of hospitalized burn patients were family "repeaters" (Cobb, Maxwell, and Silverstein, 1992). Because a large number of burns occur in the home setting, it is imperative that the patient and his family receive and understand burn prevention rules for the home.

Follow-Up Care. Before hospital discharge, follow-up care for the burn patient is carefully planned by members of the interdisciplinary health care team. The nurse is often responsible for coordinating all aspects of care and ensuring that the patient's needs are met. Many patients require outpatient physical and/or occupational therapy, often several times weekly. Information about specific exercises and use of elastic pressure garments and splints is fully reviewed with both the patient and family, and written instructions are provided for reference.

Patients who receive care in a burn center usually return to a burn clinic periodically for evaluation of their status by the burn team, modification of home care instructions, and planning for reconstructive surgery. Other patients receive ongoing care from the general or plastic surgeon who cared for them during hospitalization. Still other patients require the services of a rehabilitation center and may be transferred to such a center for aggressive rehabilitation before going home.

Burn patients who return home but who cannot manage their own burn care will need assistance from home health care personnel. Patients with inadequate support systems are likely to need help after discharge as well. The community or home health nurse can provide assistance with wound care and exercises. Patients with severe or persistent depression or difficulty adjusting to their social and/or occupational roles may require referral to a psychologist, psychiatrist, or vocational counselor.

Community Resources. Several burn patient support groups and other organizations throughout the United States offer services for burn victims. They provide caring persons (often recovered burn victims) who can visit a burn patient in the hospital or home or telephone a patient and family periodically to provide support and counseling about skin care, cosmetics, and problems related to psychosocial adjustment. Such organizations, and many regional burn centers, sponsor group meetings and social functions at which outpatients are welcome. Some also provide school-reentry programs and are active in burn-prevention activities.

Gerontologic Considerations

Reduced mobility, changes in vision, and decreased sensation in the feet and hands place elderly persons at higher risk for burn injury. Turner, Leman, and Jordan (1989) found that cooking injuries accounted for 27% of elderly women's admissions to one burn center. Nurses in community and home settings need to assess an elderly patient's ability to safely perform activities of daily living, assist elderly patients and families to modify the environment to ensure safety, and make referrals as needed. An important goal with all persons, not just elderly ones, is preventing burn injury.

The morbidity and mortality associated with burns are usually greater in elderly than in younger patients. Thinning and loss of elasticity of the skin in the elderly predispose them to a deep injury from a thermal insult that might cause a less severe burn in a younger person. Moreover, chronic illnesses decrease the aged person's ability to withstand the multisystem stresses imposed by burn injury. Decreased function of the cardiovascular, renal, and pulmonary systems increases the need to closely observe elderly patients with even relatively small burns during the emergent and acute phases. Acute renal failure is much more common in elderly patients than in those under age 40. The margin of difference between hypovolemia and fluid overload is very small. Suppressed immunologic response, a high incidence of malnutrition, and an inability to withstand metabolic stressors (such as a cold environment) further compromise the elderly person's ability to heal.

Eschar separation in full-thickness burns is typically delayed in elderly patients, and because older persons are frequently poor risks for surgical excision, prolonged hospitalization and immobilization and associated problems may be common. However, if the elderly patient can tolerate surgery, the physician may prefer to remove the eschar and to cover the wound with biologic dressings or an autograft before infection and other problems cause the patient to deteriorate.

Other Nursing Concerns. Nursing assessment of the elderly burn patient should include particular attention to pulmonary function, response to fluid resuscitation, and signs of mental confusion or disorientation. A careful his-

CRITICAL THINKING EXERCISES

1. A 62-year-old patient is being treated for second- and third-degree burns over 20% of her body. She received these burns in her home 3 days ago. She is becoming confused, is refusing to eat or drink fluids, and is not cooperating with dressing changes. She is afebrile and her vital signs have not changed significantly from her baseline values. Analyze the data at hand and explain why you think these cognitive changes have occurred. Based on your analysis, explain the assessment and management strategies you would implement at this time, and describe the patient outcomes that would indicate that your interventions have been successful.
2. An 18-year-old has experienced severe burns of the head and neck necessitating a tracheostomy. It is expected that the burned areas will require extensive skin grafting. Describe the physical and developmental issues you would consider important in the immediate care of this patient, and explain how you would expect these issues to change during the different phases of burn care.
3. Your patient is expected to be discharged from the hospital after 1 month of treatment for severe burns of the legs. What instructions and recommendations would you give to the patient and family to ensure that his recovery will continue? If this patient lived alone, how would you modify your teaching and discharge planning?

tory of preburn medications and preexisting illnesses is essential.

Nursing care promotes early mobilization, aggressive pulmonary care, and attention to preventing complications. Because of lowered resistance, the danger of burn wound sepsis and lethal systemic septicemia is not only increased but also more likely in elderly patients. Moreover, fever may not be present in the elderly to signal such events. Therefore, surveillance for other signs of infection becomes even more important.

Rehabilitation must take into account preexisting functional abilities and problems such as arthritis and low activity tolerance. Lack of family members available and able to provide home care is common. It is imperative that social services and community nursing services be contacted to provide optimal care and supervision following hospital discharge.

REFERENCES AND SELECTED READINGS

Books

Caine RM and Lefcourt ND. Patients with burns. In Clochesy JM et al (Eds). Critical Care Nursing. Philadelphia, WB Saunders, 1993.

Molter NC et al. Burns. In Hartshorn J, Lamborn M, and Noll ML (Eds). Introduction to Critical Care Nursing. Philadelphia, WB Saunders, 1993.

Nebraska Burn Institute. Advanced Burn Life Support Manual. Lincoln, NE, Nebraska Burn Institute, 1990.

Pruitt BA Jr and Goodwin C. Burn Injury. In EF Moore (Ed). Early Care of the Injured Patient, 4th ed. St. Louis, CV Mosby, 1990.

Richard RL and Staley MJ. Burn Care and Rehabilitation: Principles and Practice. Philadelphia, FA Davis, 1994.

Journals

Arons JA et al. The surgical applications and implications of cultured human epidermis: A comprehensive review. Surgery 1992; 111:4–11.

Barillo DJ et al. How accurate is pulse oximetry in patients with burn injuries? J Burn Care Rehabil 1990 Mar/Apr; 11(2):162–166.

Bayley EW et al. Standards for burn nursing practice. J Burn Care Rehabil 1989 Jul/Aug; 10(4):362–372.

Bayley EW. Wound healing in the patient with burns. Nurs Clin North Am 1990 Mar; 25(1):205–222.

Burgess MC. Initial management of a patient with extensive burn injury. Crit Care Nurs Clin North Am 1991 Jun; 3(2):165–179.

Carrougher GJ. Inhalation Injury. AACN Clin Issues Crit Care Nurs 1993 May; 4(2):367–377.

Cianci P and Sato R. Adjunctive hyperbaric oxygen therapy in the treatment of thermal burns: A review. Burns 1994 Feb; 20(1): 5–14.

Cioffi WG and Rue LW. Diagnosis and treatment of inhalation injuries. Crit Care Nurs Clin North Am 1991 Jun; 3(2):191–198.

Clayton MC and Solem LD. No ice, no butter. Advice on management of burns for primary care physicians. Postgrad Med 1995 May; 97(5):151–155, 159–160, 165.

Cobb N, Maxwell G, and Silverstein P. "Burn repeaters" and injury control. J Burn Care Rehabil 1992 Jul/Aug; 13(4):382–387.

Cobb N, Maxwell G, and Silverstein P. Patient perception of quality of life after burn injury. J Burn Care Rehabil 1990 Jul/Aug; 11(4):330–333.

Cooper DM. Optimizing wound healing: A practice within nursing's domain. Nurs Clin North Am 1990 Mar; 25(1):163–180.

Duncan DJ and Driscoll DM. Burn wound management. Crit Care Nurs Clin North Am 1991 Jun; 3(2):199–220.

Everett JJ et al. Pain assessment from patients with burns and their nurses. J Burn Care Rehabil 1994 Mar–Apr; 15(2):194–198.

Faldmo L and Kravitz M. Management of acute burns and burn shock resuscitation. AACN Clin Issues Crit Care Nurs 1993 May; 4(2):351–366.

Fowler A. Nursing management of a patient with burns. Br J Nurs 1994 Nov 24–Dec 7; 3(21):1105–1106, 1108–1112.

Fratianne RB et al. When is enough enough? Ethical dilemmas on the burn unit. J Burn Care Rehabil 1992 Sept/Oct; 13:600–603.

Hammond J and Ward CG. Decision not to treat/do not resuscitate order for the burn patient in the acute setting. Crit Care Med 1989 Feb; 117(2):136–138.

Harden NG and Luster SH. Rehabilitation considerations in the care of the acute burn patient. Crit Care Nurs Clin North Am 1991 Jun; 3(2):245–253.

Keane A. Survivors of residential fires: Implications for nursing care. Med-Surg Q 1992 Fall; 1(2):88–101.

*Keane A et al. Psychological distress in survivors of residential fires. Soc Sci Med 1994 Apr; 38(8):1055–1060.

Kravitz M. Immune consequences of burn injury. AACN Clin Iss Crit Care Nurs 1993 May; 4(2):399–413.

Lewandowski R et al. Burn injuries in the elderly. Burns 1993 Dec; 19(6):513–515.

Miller AC, Hickman LC and Lemasters GK. A distraction technique for control of burn pain. J Burn Care Rehabil 1992 Sept/Oct; 13:576–580.

Molter NC. When is the burn injury healed? Psychosocial implications of care. AACN Clin Issues Crit Care Nurs 1993 May; 4(2): 424–432.

Orr J and Hain T. Burn wound management: An overview. Professional Nurse 1994 Dec; 10(3):153–156.

Rockwell WB and Ehrlich HP. Reversible burn injury. J Burn Care Rehabil 1992 Jul/Aug; 13(4):403–406.

Rue LW et al. Wound closure and outcome in extensively burned patients treated with cultured autologous keratinocytes. J Trauma 1993 May; 34(5):662–667.

Rue LW and Cioffi WG. Resuscitation of thermally injured patients. Crit Care Nurs Clin North Am 1991 Jun; 3(2):181–189.

Schmidt MA, French L, and Kalil ET. How soon is safe? Ambulation of the patient with burns after lower extremity skin grafting. J Burn Care Rehabil 1991 Jan/Feb; 12(1):33–37.

Slater AL, Slater H, and Goldfarb IW. Effect of aggressive surgical treatment of older patients with burns. J Burn Care Rehabil 1989 Nov/Dec; 10(6):527–530.

Thurston N et al. Emotional responses of hospitalized patients with burns to debridement during the acute phase. J Burn Care Rehabil 1995 May–June; 6(3):269–275.

Turner DG, Leman CJ and Jordan MH. Cooking-related burn injuries in the elderly: Preventing the "Granny Gown" burn. J Burn Care Rehabil 1989 Jul/Aug; 10(4):356–359.

van der Does AJW. Patients' and nurses' ratings of pain and anxiety during burn wound care. Pain 1989 Oct; 39(1):95–101.

Walter PH. Burn Wound Management. AACN Clin Issues Crit Care Nurs 1993 May; 4(2):378–387.

Weber JM and Tompkins DM. Improving survival: infection control and burns. AACN Clin Issues Crit Care Nurs 1993 May; 4(2): 414–423.

White, KM. Using continuous SVO_2 to assess oxygen supply/demand in the critically ill patient. AACN Clin Issues Crit Care Nurs 1993 Feb; 4(1):134–147.

Wong L and Munster AM. New techniques in burn wound management. Surg Clin North Am 1993 Apr; 73(2):363–371.

Note: Also see issues of The Journal of Burn Care and Rehabilitation and BURNS—The Journal of the International Society for Burn Injuries.

INFORMATION/RESOURCES

Agencies

Alisa Ann Ruch Burn Foundation
20944 Sherman Way, Suite 115,
Canoga Park, CA 91303,
(818) 883-7700

American Burn Association
c/o Cleon W. Goodwin, MD, Secretary, American Burn Assn.
New York Hospital—Cornell Medical Center,
525 East 68th St. Room L-706,
New York, NY 10021
(800) 548—BURN

Baltimore Regional Burn Center Foundation, Inc.
4940 Eastern Ave.,
Baltimore, MD 21224
(410) 550-0895

Burn Awareness Coalition
P. O. Box 17840,
Encino, CA 91416
(818) 994-4661

Burn Concerns, Inc., National Consultant Service
7700 Via Napoli,
Burbank, CA 91504
(818) 767-6782

Burn Foundation
1128 Walnut St.,
Philadelphia, PA 19107
(215) 629-9200

Burn Institute
3702 Ruffin Rd. #101,
San Diego, CA 92123-1812
(619) 541-2277

Burn Prevention Foundation
5000 Tilghman St., Suite 110,
Allentown, PA 18104
(215) 481-9810

The David F. Sloan Memorial Burn Foundation
Billings, MT
(406) 657-7228

Fire Fighters Burn Foundation of Westchester-Putnam Counties, N.Y., Inc.
P. O. Box 911,
Yonkers, NY 10703-0911
(914) 375-0540

Firefighters Burn Fund, Inc.
202-666 St. James St.,
Winnepeg, Manitoba, Canada R3G 3J6
(204) 783-1733

Firefighters Pacific Burn Institute
3101 Stockton Blvd.
Sacramento, CA 95820
(916) 739-8525

Greater Cincinnati Burn Victim Foundation
Cincinnati F. D. Local 48,
213 West 9th St,
Cincinnati, OH 45202
(513) 241-3541

International Association of Fire Fighters Burn Foundation
1750 New York Ave, NW,
Washington, DC 20006
(202) 737-8484

Mid-Continent Burn Foundation
P. O. Box 248,
Shawnee Mission, KS 66201

National Burn Institute (previously Nebraska Burn Institute)
770 N. Cotner, Suite 323,
Lincoln, NE 68505
(402) 483-4795

National Institute for Burn Medicine
909 E. Ann St.,
Ann Arbor, MI 48104
(313) 769-9000

Northern California Burn Council
c/o Andrew McGuire, Director, Trauma Foundation,
Trauma Center, Building 1,
San Francisco General Hospital,
San Francisco, CA 94110

Northwest Burn Foundation
958 N. 127th,
Seattle, WA 98133
(206) 361-9844

Orange County Burn Association
1985 So. State College Blvd.,
Anaheim, CA 92806
(714) 634-1199

The Phoenix Society for Burn Survivors
11 Rust Hill Rd.,
Levittown, PA 19056
(215) 946—BURN
(800) 888—BURN for burn survivors

UNIT 14

Sensorineural Function

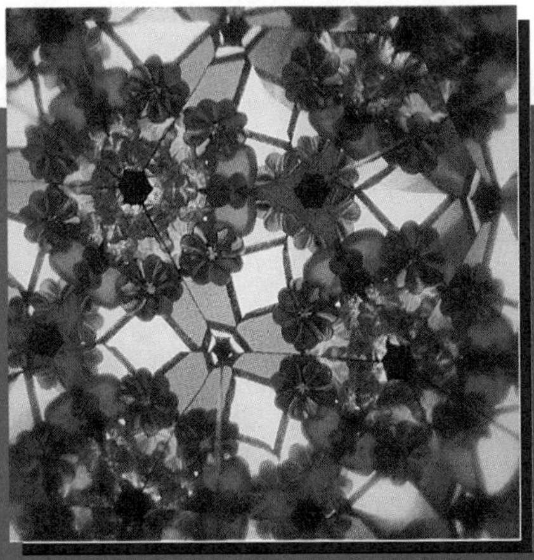

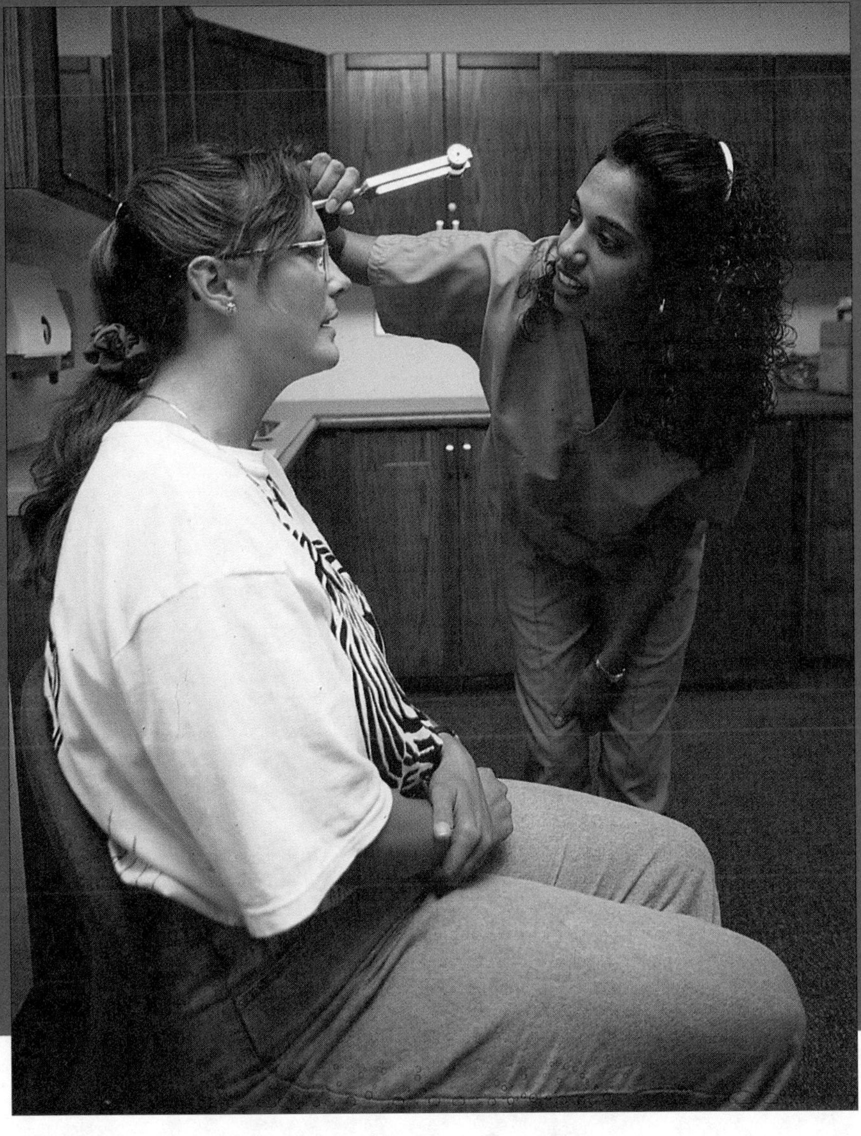

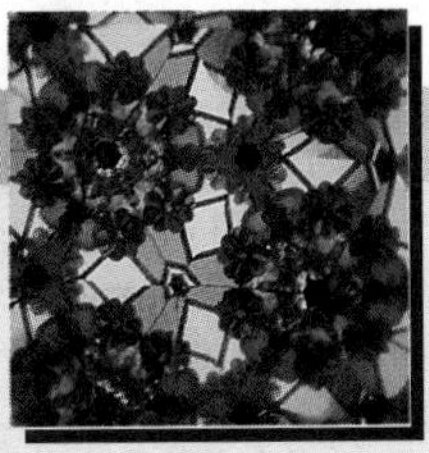

56

Assessment and Management of Patients With Vision Problems and Eye Disorders

CHAPTER OUTLINE

LEARNING OBJECTIVES

On completion of this chapter, the learner will be able to:

1. Identify significant eye structures and describe their functions
2. Describe a systematic approach to ophthalmic assessment from external to internal structures
3. Identify diagnostic tests used for assessment of the eyes and of vision
4. Describe the care and precautions required for contact lenses
5. Describe the nursing care of patients having surgery for corneal disorders and for detached retina
6. Use the nursing process as a framework for care of patients undergoing cataract removal
7. Use the nursing process as a framework for care of patients with glaucoma
8. Describe the emergency care of patients with traumatic eye injury
9. Use the nursing process as a framework for care of patients with eye disorders
10. Specify the care procedures used for patients with eye disorders
11. Describe the health care needs of blind persons
12. Describe the nursing responsibilities related to sensory deprivation from loss of sight
13. Identify the components of health education directed toward preventive eye care

Anatomy and Physiology

The eye (Fig. 56-1) is the organ of vision. A highly specialized and complex structure, it receives and sends visual data to the cerebral cortex. (See Chart 56-1 for a glossary of special ophthalmologic terms.) An entire lobe of the brain, the occipital lobe, is devoted to interpreting visual images. Moreover, seven cranial nerves (CN) have connections to the eyes: for vision (CN II); eye movement (CN III, IV and VI); pupillary reaction (CN III); eyelid elevation (CN III); and eyelid closure (CN VII). Brainstem connections permit coordinated eye movement.

The **eyeballs** and related structures are protected and housed in round bony hollows called the **orbits.** The eyeball, which occupies a small part of the orbit, is protected and cushioned by fat which lies behind the eyeball. Nerves and blood vessels that supply nutrients and transmit impulses to the brain are also present within the orbit. Attached to the external eyeball are organized bands of muscles innervated by CN III, IV, and VI. These extraocular muscles work together to coordinate eye movement.

The orbit is a potential space for fluid, blood, and air to collect because of anatomic proximity to the sinuses and blood vessels. Encroachment of other components into the orbital vault can result in shifting, compression, or protrusion of the eyeball and surrounding structures. Although there are individual differences in a person's eyes, they should be nearly symmetrical in size and position.

Structures of the External Eye

The external structures of the eyes are the eyelids and eyelashes. In front of the eye are the eyelids, two movable musculofibrous folds that open and close to protect and distribute tears over the eye and control the amount of light that enters. The lids are made of skin without subcutaneous fat. In fair individuals, extensive microvascularity may give the lids a bluish tint. Eyelids are elastic and easily stretched, as seen in blunt trauma and orbital edema. The lid margins terminate in tarsal plates, located at the lid borders. These borders contain many small glands, ducts, ciliary shafts, and eyelashes.

The junction of the upper and lower eyelid is known as the **canthus.** The outer, **lateral canthus** is on the lateral-temporal aspect of the eye. The inner, **medial canthus** contains the **puncta,** openings that allow tears to drain into the upper portion of the lacrimal system (Fig. 56-2) The elliptical space between open eyelids is called the palpebral fissure. The undersides of the lids are lined with palpebral conjunctiva, a thin, vascular, transparent mucous membrane that continues over the anterior sclera to the outer margins of the cornea.

Lid position is partially controlled by two cranial nerves: CN III is responsible for opening the lid; CN VII, for closing the lid. When closed, the lids should meet fully. When open, the upper eyelid should rest naturally on the upper portion of the iris, just above the pupil. No white crescent of sclera should be seen above or below the **corneoscleral rim** (limbus, or border).

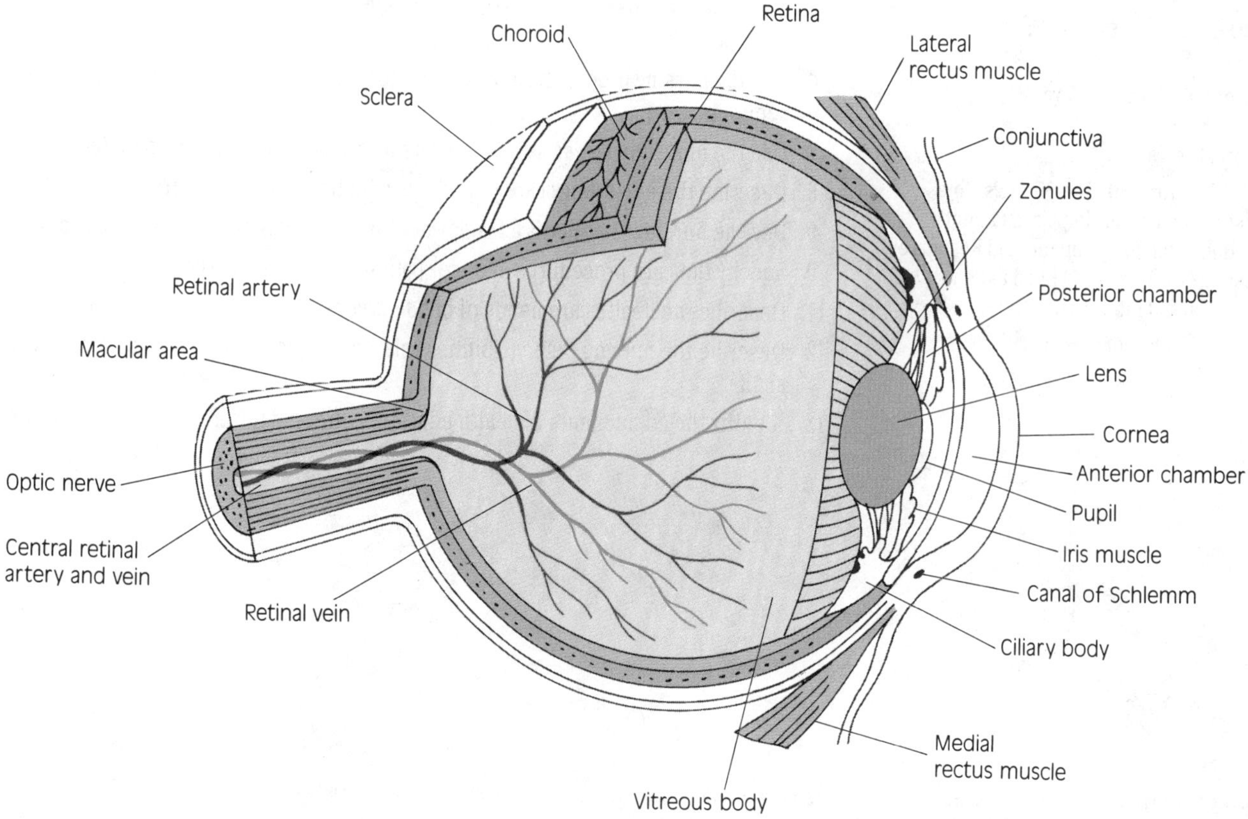

FIGURE 56-1. Cross-section of the eye.

CHART 56-1
Glossary of Ophthalmologic Terms

Ocular Anatomy

anterior chamber space in the eye filled with aqueous humor, bounded in front by the cornea and in back by the iris and anterior portion of the crystalline lens

aqueous humor clear, watery fluid circulating in the anterior and posterior chambers of the eye; produced by the ciliary body

blind spot gap in the visual field that corresponds to the area of the retina devoid of photosensitive cells; point where the optic nerve enters the eye

canal of Schlemm aqueous humor drainage channel encircling the periphery of the anterior chamber and communicating with the trabecular meshwork

canaliculi small tear drainage tubes in the inner aspect of the upper and lower lids leading from the puncta to the common canaliculus and then to the tear sac

canthus the angle at either end of the space between the eyelids

choroid vascular pigmented middle layer of the eye between the retina and sclera

ciliary body portion of uveal tract between base of iris and anterior part of choroid; consists of ciliary processes and ciliary muscle, which encompasses a circular rim behind the iris

cones and rods two types of retinal receptor cells. The functions of cones are visual acuity and color discrimination; rods make peripheral vision possible in decreased light.

conjunctiva mucous membrane that lines the inner eyelids (palpebral) and extends to the corneoscleral rim of the anterior surface of the eyeball (bulbar)

cornea clear, transparent anterior part of the fibrous coat of the eyeball

corneoscleral rim the circular junction of the cornea and the sclera; called the limbus

crystalline lens transparent biconvex structure separating the aqueous from the vitreous humor spaces. Its function is to refract rays of light and bring them to focus on the retina.

epicanthus vertical fold of skin covering the inner canthus of the eye, extending toward the nose

fovea centralis retinae a pit in the middle of the macula lutea adapted for most acute vision; made almost entirely of cones

fundus oculi posterior inner pole of the eye seen through an ophthalmoscope

iris (pl. irides) colored, circular, contractile membrane located between the cornea and crystalline lens and in the center forms the pupil

lacrimal sac dilated proximal pouch of the lacrimal system connecting the two nasolacrimal ducts and canaliculi

lens see crystalline lens

limbus the edge of the cornea where it joins the sclera

macula lutea retinae depression at the center of the retina surrounding the fovea, lateral to and slightly below the optic disc; responsible for acute central vision

optic disc (disk) area in the retina where the optic nerve enters; produces the blind spot; the intraocular position of the optic nerve formed by fibers coming from the sensory retina leading to transmission to the visual cortex

optic nerve second cranial nerve that carries visual impulses from the retina to the brain

palpebral relating to the eyelid

posterior chamber space filled with aqueous humor anterior to the lens and posterior to the iris

puncta tear drainage opening in the medial aspect of the margin of each eyelid allowing flow into the lacrimal duct

pupil circular, contractile opening in the center of the iris that regulates the amount of light entering the eye

retina innermost layer of the eye wall composed of nervous tissue; contains light-sensitive rods and cones that receive images of external objects and transmit visual impulses through the optic nerve to the brain

rods see cones and rods

sclera white part of the eye; tough, fibrous, opaque layer continuous with the cornea, which together form the external protective coat of the eye.

uvea the middle, pigmented, vascular coat of the eye; includes the iris, ciliary body, and the choroid

vitreous transparent, colorless, gelatinous mass filling the rear two thirds of the eye between the crystalline lens and the retina

zonule numerous fine tissue strands that stretch from the ciliary processes to the crystalline lens and hold the lens in position

Eye Disorders

aphakia absence of the crystalline lens of the eye

astigmatism refractive error in which light rays are prevented from coming to a single point of focus on the retina because of an unequal curvature of the cornea or lens

blepharitis inflammation of the edges of the eyelids

cataract loss of transparency of the crystalline lens

chalazion a meibomian cyst

dacryocystitis inflammation of the lacrimal sac

diplopia seeing one object as two (double vision)

ectropion turning out (eversion) of the eyelid

emmetropia normal vision; refractive condition in which parallel rays focus exactly on the retina without the aid of accommodation

endophthalmitis serious, generalized intraocular inflammation predominantly involving the vitreous cavity, but may also involve the anterior chamber of the eye

(continued)

CHART 56-1 *(continued)*
Glossary of Ophthalmologic Terms

entropion turning in (inversion) of the eyelid

epiphoria excessive production of tears

esotropia inward deviation of one eye (crossed eyes)

exophthalmos abnormal protrusion of the eyeballs

exotropia outward deviation of one eye (wall eyes)

glaucoma group of diseases of the eye characterized by increased intraocular pressure, which cause pathologic changes in the optic disc and progressive defects in the field of vision

hemianopsia blindness in half the field of vision

hordeolum, external (sty) infection of the glands of Moll or Zeiss

hordeolum, internal infection of meibomian gland

hyperopia, hypermetropia farsightedness

hypertropia upward deviation of one eye

hyphema blood in the anterior chamber of the eye

hypopyon pus in the anterior chamber of the eye

hypotony abnormally low intraocular pressure

keratitis inflammation of the cornea

keratoconus cone-shaped deformity of the cornea with central noninflammatory thinning

myopia nearsightedness

nystagmus repetitive involuntary rapid movement of the eyeball

optic atrophy degeneration of the optic nerve

papilledema swelling of the optic disc

photophobia abnormal sensitivity to light

presbyopia lessening of the power of accommodation due to the aging process

pterygium thick, triangular growth of tissue of the conjunctiva, which may extend onto the cornea

ptosis drooping of the upper eyelid

retinal detachment separation of the sensory retina from the underlying pigmented epithelial layer

retinitis pigmentosis hereditary progressive bilateral degeneration of the retina

strabismus misalignment of the eyes caused by extraocular muscle imbalance; both eyes do not fixate on the object being observed

sty see hordeolum, external

sympathetic ophthalmia uveitis of the uninjured eye due to sensitization to uveal pigment after a penetrating injury of the other eye

trabeculum meshwork in the anterior chamber angle through which the aqueous humor flows to leave the eye

trachoma severe, chronic bacterial (Chlamydia trachomatis) infection of the conjunctiva and cornea

uveitis inflammation of the iris, ciliary body, or choroid

xerosis abnormal dryness of the conjunctiva and cornea caused by deficiency of tears

Ophthalmic Pharmacologic Agents

cycloplegic an agent that paralyzes the ciliary muscle

miotic an agent that causes pupillary contraction

mydriatic an agent that causes pupillary dilation

Common Abbreviations

D diopter, the unit of measurement of strength or refractive power of lenses (a 1-D lens brings parallel light rays to a focus 1 m from the lens)

ECCE extracapsular cataract extraction

EOM extraocular muscles

HT hypertropia

ICCE intracapsular cataract extraction

IOL intraocular lens

IOP intraocular pressure

OD (oculus dexter) or **RE**—right eye

OS (oculus sinister) or **LE**—left eye

OU (oculi unitas)—both eyes together

PHACO phacoemulsification cataract extraction

PKP penetrating keratoplasty

RK radial keratotomy

ST esotropia

Blinking of the eyelids spreads a film of lubricating and moisturizing tears over the eyeball surface. Reflex blinking protects the eye from debris and foreign particles. The eyelashes complement lid function by sifting out dust and debris, protecting the external eye from injury. The mechanical action of blinking creates suction in the upper nasolacrimal system, facilitating drainage of tears.

Lacrimal System

The lacrimal system maintains a moist environment for the external, anterior eye. The production of tears supplies natural lubrication and dilutes and rinses away foreign particles. Two kinds of tears are normally produced: **lubricating tears,** consisting of oil, water, and mucus, and **aqueous tears** produced in response to emotion or irritation and containing only water. Excessive watery tears do not adhere to the eyes but overflow onto the cheek.

Tears contain several components produced by a number of glands. The **lacrimal glands,** which produce watery tears, are located in the anterior lateral roof of the upper orbit. This location allows tears to wash across the eye diagonally toward the medial canthus. **Accessory lacrimal glands** keep the anterior eye moist. These include the glands of Zeiss (sebaceous) and the Moll's gland (ciliary) located within the lid borders. Additional meibomian (sebaceous) glands are located in a single row across the lid tarsus (the broad framework of the lid) and contribute to the oily component of tears. This oily layer prevents the tear film from evaporating or overflowing. It also ensures airtight closure of the lids, holds the tear film together, and provides a smooth and regular optical surface.

Goblet cells within the conjunctiva add mucin to the tear film, which adheres to the corneal epithelium. Conditions that involve any part of this "tear factory" can alter these important functions. Inadequate tear formation or faulty lid closure can result in drying and eventual damage to the external eye.

Tears, which leave the eye by way of the lacrimal drainage system in the nasal sinuses, exit through the puncta, two small, oval openings in the upper and lower aspects of the medial canthus. From there they pass through the upper and lower **canaliculi,** which join the lacrimal sac and duct, and into the nasal sinuses. During crying, the excess production of aqueous tears exceeds the capacity of the lacrimal "bladder," and the tears spill out onto the cheek. Factors that interfere with proper drainage of tears include trauma to any part of the lacrimal system, inflammation and swelling, accumulation of secretions, and excess tear production.

Eye Muscles

Movement of the eye is controlled by six extraocular muscles (Fig. 56-3), which insert into the sclera and are innervated by CN III, IV, and VI. The lateral rectus muscle abducts and the medial rectus muscle adducts the eye. These two muscles must work together for side-to-side eye movement. The superior rectus muscle elevates and adducts and the inferior rectus muscle depresses and adducts. The superior oblique muscle directs the eye laterally and inferiorly, and the inferior oblique muscle directs it superiorly and laterally.

Blood Supply

The eye's blood supply originates from branches of the internal carotid artery, its ophthalmic artery branch. The central retinal artery and the **choriocapillaris** of the choroidal layer provide blood to the retina; both must be intact to maintain retinal function. Venous circulation essentially follows the arterial pattern. On inspection with an ophthalmoscope, the veins appear larger and darker than their arterial counterparts.

The parts of the eye that should be avascular (bloodless) are the lens and cornea. These structures must remain free of blood vessels so that light may pass through unobstructed and focus sharply on the retina. When the cornea is injured, tiny blood vessels can develop across it, rendering it less transparent. Blood vessels that develop in the cornea, except at the extreme edges, are always pathologic and may be seen with the naked eye. The cornea receives its nutrition from oxygen dissolved in the tears, from the aqueous humor (the fluid in the anterior chamber), and a small amount from tiny vessels surrounding the corneoscleral limbus. The lens is avascular for the same reasons as is the cornea.

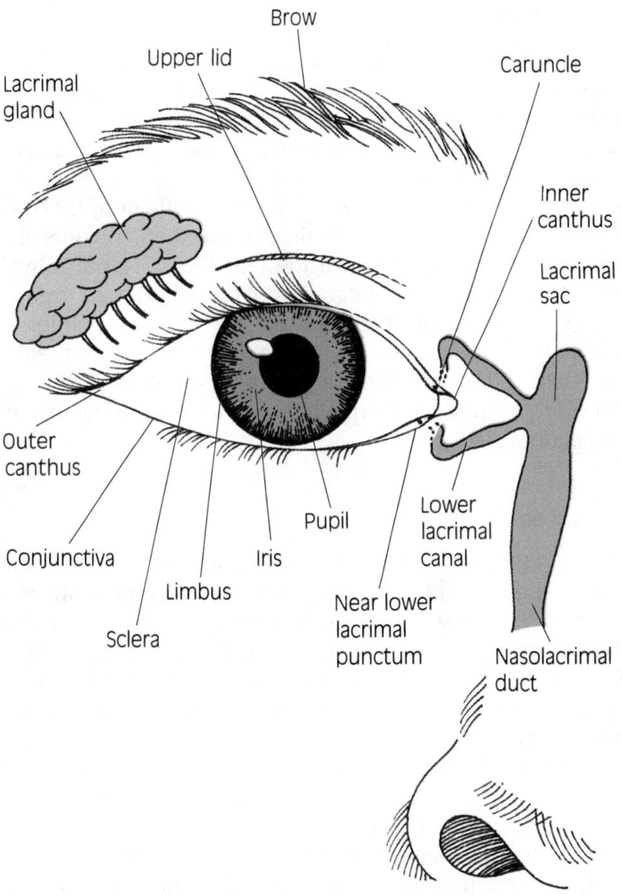

FIGURE 56-2. Structures of the external eye and position of the internal lacrimal structures.

Eyeball

The eyeball is lined with three primary layers: sclera, uvea (which contains the choroid), and retina. Each layer has its own particular structure and function. These layers contribute to the eye's round shape when filled with vitreous humor (the gelatinous substance between the lens and the retina).

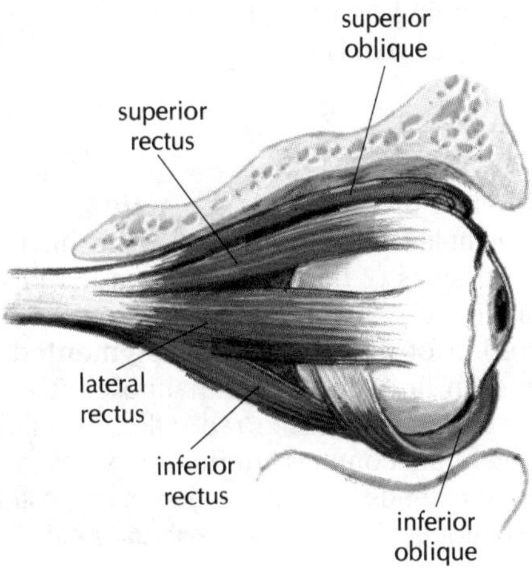

FIGURE 56-3. The extraocular muscles responsible for eye movement. The medial rectus muscle (not shown) is responsible for opposing the movement of the lateral rectus muscle.

Sclera

The tough, outermost layer is the **sclera**—the "white" of the eyes. Thinning of the sclera may give it a blue appearance. Posteriorly, the sclera has an opening through which the optic nerve and the central retinal blood vessels pass. Anteriorly it becomes continuous with the cornea. The anterior scleral surface is covered loosely with **conjunctiva,** a thin, transparent mucous membrane that contains the many glands responsible for the tear film. The **palpebral conjunctiva** lines the undersides of the lids and is continuous with the **bulbar conjunctiva** that covers the anterior sclera. (This is fortunate so that a contact lens cannot really be "lost" in the eye.) The conjunctiva terminates at the corneoscleral limbus. It normally contains a generous blood vessel network.

Uvea

The middle pigmented layer is the uveal tract, which consists of the choroid, iris, and ciliary body. The **choroid** is a vascular layer that provides blood to the pigmented epithelial layer of the retina and peripheral sensory retina. The choroid lines the posterior chamber of the eye and extends from the ciliary body, anteriorly, and the optic nerve, posteriorly.

The **iris** is the pigmented muscular structure that gives the eye its characteristic color. The iris is the anterior aspect of the uveal tract and divides the space between the cornea and the lens into an anterior and posterior chamber. It is a thin, circular, muscular diaphragm that has at its center a round opening, the **pupil**. The pupil changes size as the iris spontaneously adapts to light by dilating or constricting.

These changes control the amount of light entering the eye, thereby facilitating vision in varying degrees of light intensity. Encircling the posterior side of the iris is the ciliary body.

The **ciliary body** contains muscle fibers that contract and relax the lens zonules (the structures that hold the lens in place). The ciliary body plays a role in maintaining intraocular pressure (IOP) by secreting **aqueous humor,** a watery, transparent liquid that fills the anterior and posterior chambers and drains through the canal of Schlemm. The continuous production and drainage of this liquid is responsible for maintaining constant IOP, normally measured in the range of 12 to 21 mm Hg.

Retina

The inner layer of the eyeball is the **retina,** a thin, semitransparent, eight-layered tissue that lines the inner eye wall. The innermost layers of the retina contain the photosensitive and ganglionic cells of the sensory retina. The outer, one-layer portion of the retina is the **pigmented epithelium.** When seen through the ophthalmoscope, the retina demonstrates the characteristic "red reflex," actually an orange glow. The retina contains arteries and veins that supply it with blood. It extends from the optic nerve, posteriorly, to its anterior scalloped fringe (**ora serrata**) near the ciliary body.

Rods and Cones. The retina contains two types of photosensitive cells known as **rods** and **cones.** Rods are responsible for peripheral vision, low-light visibility, and distinguishing the shapes and borders of objects. Rods are located primarily in the peripheral aspects of the retina.

Cones are responsible for color discrimination and acute vision. They are located more centrally with the highest concentrations in the **macula lutea.** The central macula has a slight depression called the **fovea centralis,** which consists entirely of cones. The eye usually attempts to focus light on this area. Seen through an ophthalmoscope, the macula appears darker than the rest of the retina because of its thinness in relation to the rest of the retina. Blood is supplied to the macula exclusively by the choroid.

The retina is loosely attached to the pigmented epithelium and supported by the gel-like vitreous humor that fills the globe. If the vitreous humor shrinks or retracts, as occurs with aging, the sensory retina may pull away from its pigmented epithelium. Development of tiny holes or tears in the retina disrupt this union as well, allowing fluid to leak behind the retina and detach it.

Optic Disc. Located slightly nasally, but centrally, in the retina is the **optic disc.** This is where the sensory retina converges to form the optic nerve. Because the optic disc has no photosensitive cells, it is a blind spot in the visual field. The central retinal artery and vein branch from the center of the optic head.

Seen through an ophthalmoscope, the optic disc has a slight impression, or physiologic cup, which should occupy no more than one third of the disc and which should have a distinct border. In conditions of increased IOP, this disc can become more hollowed out, thereby contributing to destruction of the optic nerve and visual loss. The disc margins may also appear blurred without distinct edges, as occurs in papilledema (swelling of the optic disc) and elevations of intracranial pressure.

The retina is stimulated by light that passes through the cornea, the lens, and vitreous humor. The degree of sharp focus depends on the shape of the eyeball and the clear refraction (pathway) of light, which influences light focusing on the retina. Persons with **myopia,** or nearsightedness, may have elongated eyeballs that focus light in front of the retina, making distant images blurry. Persons with **hyperopia,** or farsightedness, focus light beyond the retina.

Once light impulses reach the retina, a series of chemical and neurologic connections send the impulses to the pigmented epithelium, which transfers them to the optic nerve (CN II). The optic nerve then transmits the impulses across the X-shaped optic chiasm to the visual cortex of the brain's occipital lobe, where the impulses are interpreted.

Anything, such as disease or trauma, that interferes with the passage of light, the visual pathway, the conversion of light impulses, or transmission—from the cornea to the visual cortex—can interfere with vision and diminish or eliminate sight. Fortunately, many pharmacologic, medical, and surgical interventions are available for preserving and, possibly, restoring sight.

Structures of the Anterior Chamber

The anterior portion of the eye is bounded posteriorly by the front surfaces of the iris and lens and anteriorly by the cornea. It is the first step in the pathway of light for vision.

The anterior chamber is fluid filled and bulges slightly, giving it a convex shape. Intraocular pressure (IOP) is maintained by aqueous humor filling the chamber. To maintain a constant pressure in the globe, drainage of aqueous humor through the trabecular meshwork and the canal of Schlemm must match its production by the ciliary body. Normal IOP ranges between 12 and 21 mm Hg.

Cornea

The cornea is the clear, convex structure over the anterior one sixth of the eye. Positioned centrally in front of the iris, the cornea must be kept moist for health of its epithelial surface. To function as an optical lens, it must remain smooth. Tear film, evenly spread by the blinking eyelids, provides both moisture and comfort. The transparency of the cornea results from its uniform structure, its avascularity, and the relative dehydration provided by the endothelial layer and the epithelial barricade to external fluid entering the cornea. The cornea consists of five layers: the epithelium, Bowman's membrane, stroma, Descemet's membrane, and the endothelium.

Epithelium. The epithelium, the outermost layer, has four to six layers of cells endowed with sensitive nerve endings and microvilli. It is the only layer capable of regeneration and is completely replaced about every 7 days. Primary regeneration of the epithelium occurs after 24 hours. This high rate of cellular turnover is important, especially when rapid healing is desired, for example, after surgery, injury, or ulceration.

Stroma. The stroma is the thick bulk of the cornea and is sandwiched between Bowman's membrane, anteriorly, and Descemet's membrane, posteriorly. Injury at the Bowman's membrane level or deeper results in scar formation.

Endothelium. The endothelium is only one layer thick and is in contact with aqueous humor on the interior of the anterior chamber. Its cells have a pumplike mechanism to prevent aqueous humor from entering the cornea, keeping the cornea relatively dry and clear. Health of the endothelium is crucial because it does not regenerate. The epithelium provides a barrier to external water entering the cornea. Decreased oxygenation to the epithelial layer can cause corneal edema. Once fluid leaks into the cornea, the cornea becomes clouded and hazy, which interferes with vision. A cloudy, hazy cornea may occur with acute increases in IOP because the excessive pressure disrupts endothelial function.

Because the cornea is a major refractive structure, it is vitally important to visual acuity. Optimal refraction requires integrity of the corneal surface, smoothness, transparency, and convexity. Small changes in the cornea caused by damage or disease can cause great changes in visual acuity.

The other function of the cornea is protection. The cornea is highly innervated by sensory branches of the trigeminal nerve (CN V) and readily perceives sensory input as painful. This is why even the tiniest of objects in the cornea are poorly tolerated. Threats to the eye initiate a corneal reflex. The cornea safeguards the eye from foreign substances. When the cornea is irritated, tears persist to flood out the irritant, photophobia develops, and almost an irresistible urge to rub the eyes occurs. Intense pain is usually referred to the underside of the upper lid. This sensation may persist even after objects have been removed as long as the cornea is irritated. Persons whose corneal reflex is diminished or whose sensory faculty is impaired may lose this corneal protection. This is particularly true when the cornea is exposed to the air.

Iris

The iris is a highly vascular structure with variable pigment (determined genetically). Eye color depends on the amount of melanin present in the iris; the lighter the color, the greater the amount of light that enters the eye. Some people with very light eyes experience **photophobia** (sensitivity to light). The converse is true of dark-eyed individuals. There are no two irides alike, including fellow eyes in the same individual. The iris is part of the uveal, or pigmented, tract and joins the choroidal layer at its edge and the ciliary body on its underside.

Like the shutter of a camera, the iris constantly adjusts to various conditions, allowing an appropriate amount of light to enter the eye. The pupil is the round opening in the center of the iris. Sympathetic autonomic nervous system innervation to the iris (flight or fight) results in pupillary dilation. Pupillary dilator muscles of the iris pull the iris back like a curtain, opening the pupil. Parasympathetic innervation of the iris from CN III, the oculomotor nerve, activates the circular, pupillary constrictor muscles on the inner aspect of the pupil and draws it closed in a purse string manner. Most of the time, both systems have some input to the iris. Only when one system predominates over the other or when nervous impulses are blocked will pure dilation or constriction occur. Medications and stress responses may cause this phenomenon.

When penetrated, the iris muscle contracts toward the site of injury, giving the pupil and iris a characteristic, teardrop shape. The iris can actually protrude into the anterior chamber and outside the cornea. Being vascular, the iris can bleed rather easily when injured, and hyphema may develop. Dilated blood vessels may be seen on the surface of the iris (rubeosis) in some conditions.

Pupil

The pupil is a space provided by the internal ring of the iris. The pupil is characteristically round, regular, and the same in size and response to light in both eyes. **Anisocoria,** or unequal pupils, is a normal finding in about 20% of the population. In others, unequal pupils may signal central nervous system disease. Pupils are located slightly nasal to the center of the cornea. Pupillary constriction and dilation in reaction to light occurs as a result of several neuronal connections. When light enters the eye, photosensitive cells send messages to the pupillary constrictor muscle by way of CN III. This reduces the amount of distortion and glare produced by excessive light rays. Low light levels activate the pupillary dilator muscles, which retract the iris and open the pupil. Five times more energy enters the eye when the pupil dilates. Destruction of photosensitive cells can reduce pupillary function. Pupillary constriction also occurs when the eyes converge with near vision. Accommodation of the lens should accompany pupillary constriction.

Crystalline Lens

The crystalline lens is a biconvex, avascular, colorless, and transparent structure suspended behind the iris by zonules of the ciliary body. The anterior and posterior capsule surrounds and supports the lens. The lens should be avascular to allow for clear transmission of light.

Ciliary Body

The ciliary body, a ring of tissue contiguous with the iris, follows a 360-degree course on its underside. The ciliary body is a part of the uveal tract, has pigmented cells, and is vascular and muscular. The ciliary body has two functions: it manufactures aqueous humor and adjusts the shape of the lens for accommodation, or focusing.

Aqueous humor is necessary for nourishing the cornea and maintaining intraocular tension.

The ciliary body has suspension ligaments, called zonules, which support the lens and attach it to the ciliary body behind the iris. Muscles of the ciliary body contract and relax to shape the lens for appropriately refracting light.

Accommodation. To facilitate near vision, the ciliary body contracts, relaxing the zonules, and the lens fattens and allows light to be focused on the retina. This process is known as **accommodation.** The lens is suspended behind the iris to refract and bend light to focus it on the retina. The shape of the lens is determined by the traction created from contraction and relaxation of the ciliary zonules. The lens in a young person is highly pliable and shapes easily for accommodation. With aging, the lens may yellow, become rigid, and accommodate less.

Aqueous Humor

Aqueous humor produced in the posterior chamber by the ciliary body circulates around the lens and iris into the anterior chamber. The aqueous fluid delivers essential nutrients to the avascular tissues of the anterior chamber: the cornea, lens, and the trabecular meshwork. It removes metabolites from and provides the proper chemical environment for the eye. Once in the anterior chamber, aqueous humor filters into the trabecular meshwork en route to the canal of Schlemm. The trabecular meshwork encircles the circumference of the anterior chamber and is embedded in the angle formed at the corneoscleral limbus. The trabeculum is encircled by the oval-shaped canal of Schlemm, which communicates with the trabecular meshwork, where aqueous humor is incorporated into the venous drainage of the eye. As long as aqueous humor is produced and drained in equal amounts, constant intraocular pressure (IOP) is maintained in the anterior chamber.

IOP results from the balance between aqueous humor formation and the resistance of aqueous humor outflow. IOP is not constant. It fluctuates over the course of the day and can be affected by the seasons of the year, exercise, postural changes, eyelid movement, foods, and medications. Conditions that increase IOP may result in progressive structural and functional damage to the eye.

Structures of the Posterior Chamber

The posterior chamber is a small segment bounded anteriorly by the posterior side of the lens and posteriorly by the vitreous humor. The ciliary body, the ciliary zonules, the posterior aspect of the lens, and aqueous humor are in the posterior chamber. This area is visible only through special instruments.

When the lens and iris stick together (synechiae), aqueous humor cannot flow from the posterior to the anterior chamber. This pupillary blockage results in aqueous humor becoming trapped in the posterior chamber behind the lens. Consequently, pressure rises and pushes the iris forward, compressing the trabecular meshwork, which further prohibits drainage.

Vitreous Body

The vitreous body is the largest, most posterior chamber of the eye. Bounded anteriorly by the lens and ciliary body and posteriorly by the retina, the vitreous body is made of transparent collagen gel and fluid, which basically molds and shapes the eyeball. In younger individuals, the vitreous is approximately 80% gel. It should be avascular and without particulate matter. Any moving debris in the vitreous casts shadows on the retinal surface, causing the symptom known as "floaters." In contact with and attached to the entire retina, vitreous humor shrinks as an individual ages, and severe states of dehydration and can contribute to retinal detachment.

Gerontologic Considerations

As a person ages, vision becomes less efficient. The pupil becomes less responsive to light because of sclerosis of the pupillary sphincter, which results in decreased pupil size. The lens becomes more opaque, and the visual field decreases, making peripheral vision more difficult. Eyes adapt to darkness less rapidly; therefore, vision at night or in dimly lit areas is less acute in older people. With advancing years, accommodation slows as the lens gradually loses its elastic nature and becomes a relatively solid mass. *Presbyopia* is the loss of visual accommodation because of age-related changes. Ciliary muscles also become less flexible and functional. Because near vision requires the greatest work by the ciliary muscles, near vision is compromised earliest, a condition that requires the individual to wear corrective lenses, such as reading glasses, bifocal lenses, or even trifocal lenses.

With aging, the liquid portion of vitreous humor increases to approximately 50%. With advancing age, collagen materials in of the vitreous body clump together and such clumping produces "floaters," which may be apparent in the field of vision. The retina may show degenerative changes, especially the macula, in which very small sclerotic changes result in impaired vision.

Ophthalmic Assessment

The nurse's role in eye care includes assessment as well as patient education and follow-up care. In this role the nurse collaborates with many health care personnel and eye care specialists (Chart 56-2).

Assessment of the eyes and their supportive structures may be considered a component of the neurologic examination because the eyes are located in the head and are directly connected and structurally a part of the nervous system. Thus, the ophthalmic assessment is the neurovisual component of the sensory examination.

Methods of ophthalmic assessment that may prove useful to the nurse are presented. It is assumed that more specific and detailed assessment skills than those presented here are needed in specialized areas of ophthalmology.

CHART 56-2
Eye Care Specialists

Of the many health care specialists, the functions of those providing ophthalmologic services are often misunderstood.

- An **ophthalmologist** is a physician (M.D. or D.O.) who is licensed to practice medicine and surgery and who specializes in all aspects of eye and vision care. In diagnosis and treatment, the ophthalmologist uses and prescribes medication, eyeglasses, contact lenses, and performs surgery. In addition to the general ophthalmologist, there are those who specialize in specific eye problems such as pediatric conditions, corneal disease, retinal and vitreous disease, glaucoma, oculoplastics, and low vision.
- An **optometrist** is a licensed, independent doctor of optometry (O.D.) who specializes in determining the need for glasses and screening patients for abnormalities of the eye. The optometrist treats visual disturbances with glasses and contact lenses and may also prescribe exercises for muscle imbalances.
- An **optician** is a licensed technician who dispenses glasses and other optical devices according to prescriptions written by optometrists and ophthalmologists.
- An **ocularist** is a technician who makes artificial eyes and other ophthalmic prostheses.
- Other important services are provided by **specialized support technicians.** These are members of the ophthalmic team who assist in examination, diagnostics, and treatment. Ophthalmic technicians usually practice in ophthalmic clinics and physicians' offices and assist in many aspects of examination and diagnostics. Other support technicians specialize in other diagnostic testing, such as ophthalmic ultrasonography, photography, visual fields, and fluorescein angiography.

Ophthalmic assessment may consist of a brief overview as a component of a general physical examination or a selective, careful examination of the eye itself. The degree of potential ophthalmic involvement dictates whether an abbreviated or extensive evaluation is performed.

There are three areas of ophthalmic assessment that are addressed in this chapter: the history taking, physical examination, and special ophthalmic diagnostic and refractive procedures.

Ophthalmic History

Before performing a physical assessment of the eyes, the nurse should obtain the patient's ophthalmic, medical, and treatment history, all of which may contribute to the ophthalmic condition. Information to be obtained includes information about vision changes and safety measures and depends on the reason for performing the ophthalmic examination.

A history of ophthalmic conditions is important when gathering baseline data. One should investigate a history of any eye disorders, such as cataract, glaucoma, retinal detachment, or visual disturbances. Consideration is given to risk factors associated with age. The history should include questions about glaucoma, diabetes, hypertensive disease, eye trauma, eye surgery, and other disorders and diseases that can affect vision. It is important also to identify the dates of onset and treatment of these conditions, and whether the patient has ever had noninvasive ophthalmic procedures, such as laser treatments or photocoagulation.

A history of ophthalmic symptoms, such as photophobia, headaches (including location and frequency), dizziness, ocular or brow pain, itching of the eyes, tearing, floaters, and any eye discharge should be obtained. Pain, if reported, is assessed with regard to location, onset, duration, associated visual changes, circumstances when pain occurs, relief measures, and severity. Changes in visual impairment or visual field loss are identified. It is important also to determine whether conditions or symptoms are unilateral or bilateral.

The patient is asked if he or she has refractive correction and the visual acuity score, if known. Use of corrective lenses for near or far vision, or both, and the effectiveness of refraction should be noted. Care provided by eye care specialists and the frequency of this care is noted. Other important information includes current use of over-the-counter or prescription ophthalmic medications.

An abbreviated ophthalmic history for any patient might include the following questions: Do you have any problems with your eyes or vision? Do you take any eye medications? Do you wear glasses, contact lenses, or other forms of vision correction? Have you ever had any special ophthalmic procedures, such as surgery or laser treatments? Have you ever seen an eye care specialist?

Family history of ophthalmic disorders is also assessed and includes questions about glaucoma, blindness, hypertensive disease, cataracts, and diabetes, as well as response to treatment for these diseases.

Associated Medical History

Many disorders are accompanied or manifested by ocular symptoms and recognizable changes in visual structures and function. Diabetes mellitus and hypertension are common causes of changes in ocular vasculature and are responsible for retinopathies (retinal diseases) and blindness in a significant portion of the affected population. It is important to determine if there is history of embolic diseases, because tiny emboli can travel into the central retinal artery and occlude it, resulting in loss of retinal circulation and vision.

Myasthenia gravis may manifest itself with ocular symptoms, which may present as ptosis (drooping eyelids) early in the onset of this disease. Optic neuritis frequently occurs in patients with multiple sclerosis. Recent head trauma or other severe neurologic illness can produce ophthalmic findings such as papilledema (swelling of optic disk), visual field defects, and pupillary changes. Migraine headaches may be associated with ophthalmic symptoms.

Useful related information includes the patient's current medication regimen. Many medications have ophthalmic effects and may affect visual acuity. For example, sympathomimetic or vagolytic medications may produce persistent pupillary dilation. Other medications, such as morphine sulfate, can cause pupillary constriction. Some medications may affect the extraocular muscles so that the eyes are misaligned. Others may affect the production of aqueous humor by the ciliary body. Medications that influence fluid balance, for example, diuretics, may reduce intraocular tension with fluid loss.

Psychosocial History

Other important assessment areas include psychologic, demographic, and home environmental concerns. This is particularly important to the home health nurse when evaluating the environment of patients who are visually impaired. Environmental considerations might include safety issues within the living area, climate, cleanliness, pests and insects, exposure to external irritants, and other factors that may affect ophthalmic health. Evidence of physical abuse patterns might present in the form of eye contusions.

When asking questions about the patient's history, one should consider the effect that ophthalmic conditions may have on the patient's activities of daily living and employment. Many aspects of daily life depend on visual acuity; safety and successful functioning may be threatened by decreased visual acuity. Driving, caring for children, and other skills used in many peoples' daily lives may be affected by an eye disorder. The patient's life-style—type of work, leisure, and sports activities—should also be evaluated. The patient is asked if the reported ophthalmic problem has affected any usual functions. Then the nurse can assess how the patient has coped with the problem.

The psychologic enjoyment that can be gained through vision may be analogous to the pleasure of hearing music. Deprivation of this form of sensory input can be devastating to many individuals, particularly if they are suddenly deprived of sight. Those with congenital blindness tend to adapt to their world quite well. Those with sudden visual loss have more difficulties adjusting after relying on vision for maneuvering about in the world and using sensory input for human contact. Those who are visually impaired tend to call on other senses such as hearing and touch, which become more acute. It is critical to determine what facilitates communication, understanding, and meaning for them. The sound of someone's voice may be very important to the visually impaired person, whereas others may rely more on touch. It is important to find out what sensory input is meaningful to the individual so that health care personnel can adapt communication of important things, such as orientation to the environment and ophthalmic care.

Gerontologic Considerations

The main causes of visual problems in the United States are disorders that occur mostly in the aged. Assessment of the support and care systems that are available to elderly patients is important. Follow-up appointments and care may involve travel, which can be a major logistical problem as well as a costly one. Safety issues must be considered when the patient has low vision or requires transportation after pharmacologic pupillary dilation and cycloplegia (ciliary paralysis). A thorough ophthalmic examination can take some time to complete. Some elderly people have difficulty in maintaining certain positions for extended periods because of musculoskeletal problems, such as arthritis.

Physical Assessment of Vision and the Eye

Examination of the eye is an essential component of the physical examination, not only because eye health is important to the well-being of the patient but also because the state of the eye reflects the general state of health. The retina, which may be viewed with the ophthalmoscope, is the only site in the human body where the vascular bed may be examined directly. Diseases such as hypertension and diabetes produce changes in the retinal vasculature that are readily observable. The pupil is the window to human microcirculation.

Assessment of Visual Acuity

The eye provides visual stimuli to the occipital cortex. Visual acuity is important to test, because it is the most important function of the eye. It should be performed first so that vision is assessed before actually touching the eye.

Formal testing of visual acuity should be a part of every patient's data base. Visual acuity is tested with an eye chart (Snellen chart) placed 6 meters (20 feet) from the patient or by using a near card. The patient is instructed to cover one eye with a piece of paper or cardboard, to keep both eyes open, and to read each line of the chart until the print can no longer be distinguished. If the patient wears corrective lenses, acuity should be assessed with and without the lenses.

Illiteracy may be circumvented by using charts (the Snellen chart) that display the letter *E* in four different positions. This also enables one to assess the vision of children as young as age 5. Gross examination of visual acuity can be obtained at the bedside using basic techniques. Such assessments as perception of light, hand motion, counting fingers, and reading are easy to perform and give practical information regarding vision of the patient.

Visual acuity is expressed in a ratio that relates what a person with normal vision sees from a distance of 20 feet to what the patient can see from a distance of 20 feet. Acuity of 20/50 means that the patient can see from 20 feet away what is normally visible from 50 feet away; 20/200, the boundary of legal blindness, indicates that the patient can see at 20 feet what the normal eye sees at 200 feet. Such patients can only discern with accuracy the large letter at the top of the Snellen chart. The patient whose visual acuity is less than 20/20 when corrected by his own glasses should be referred to an ophthalmologist or an optometrist.

After age 40, the lens of the eye may become rigid and incapable of accommodating its shape to close-range vision (presbyopia). Having a patient read newsprint at a distance of one foot is the general screening test for presbyopia. Patients who experience difficulty with this examination are referred to a specialist for further evaluation.

Assessment of Eye Movement

The extraocular muscles (see Fig. 56-3) are the six small muscles attached to each eye that move the eyeball. They

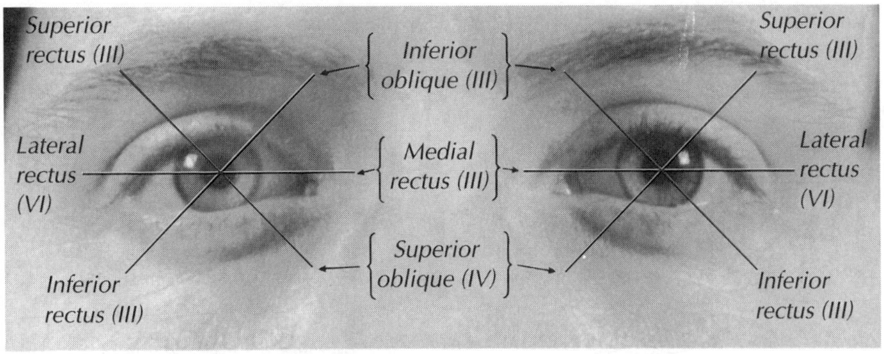

FIGURE 56-4. The six cardinal fields of gaze are governed by the six extraocular muscles. (Bates B: A Guide to Physical Examination and History Taking, 6th ed. Philadelphia, JB Lippincott, 1995.)

are innervated by three of the cranial nerves (CN III, IV, and VI). Synergistic (correlated) action of the extraocular muscles of both eyes results in parallel gaze. The mechanism by which this takes place is highly complex, and an analysis of abnormality requires consultation with a physician.

Parallel alignment of the eyes may be easily detected by shining a light directly into the eyes while the patient stares at the light source. The site of light reflection of the eyes should be identical. Light reflexes that vary from one eye to the other indicate a disturbance in parallel vision.

Cover Test. Despite normal alignment of both eyes when they function together, the tendency of either eye to drift to the nasal side or to the temporal side (and the necessity to involuntarily compensate for this with effort) may be assessed by the **cover test.** One of the patient's eyes is covered by a card or by the hand of the examiner, and the patient is asked to focus the uncovered eye on a stationary object while keeping the covered eye open. The card or hand is abruptly removed from the covered eye, which is then observed for any abnormal movement. If the eye, when covered, has drifted to the temporal side, it will snap back into alignment when the cover is removed. Conversely, if it has drifted to the nasal side, the reverse phenomenon will occur. The tendency of an eye to drift, when covered, to the temporal side is called an **exophoria;** the tendency of an eye to drift to the nasal side is called an **esophoria.**

Coordinated Gaze. Integrity of the nervous control of the muscles of the eye may be assessed by directing the patient, while keeping the head still, to move his eyes in the six cardinal positions of gaze (Fig. 56-4) while following an object. The object is moved laterally to either side along the horizontal axis and then along two oblique axes, each of which makes a 60-degree angle with the horizontal axis. Each of the cardinal positions of gaze represents the function of one of the six extraocular muscles attached to each eye. If **diplopia,** or double vision, develops during the transition to any one of the cardinal positions of gaze, the examiner has an indication that one or more of the extraocular muscles are failing to function properly. This also holds true if one of the eyes fails to move with the other.

When extraocular movements are assessed, the eye is observed for **nystagmus,** an irregular jerking movement of the eyes, as gaze shifts to a lateral position. Nystagmus has two components: a fast component in one or the other direction and a slower subsequent component that brings the eye back to the intended position. Nystagmus on extreme lateral gaze is a normal finding, however, and can be avoided by not placing the object too far laterally. A number of conditions, such as multiple sclerosis and elevated Dilantin (phenytoin) levels, may result in nystagmus. Although many of these conditions are benign, others may reflect severe pathologic processes.

The eyes should move together symmetrically and in the same direction. When the eyes do not move together, the phenomenon is called **strabismus.** This can result in double or blurred vision because the images projected on each respective retina are different. Strabismus is one of the causes of **amblyopia.**

Caloric Examination. When assessing for brain viability, a caloric examination may be performed. This involves instilling either warm or cold water into the ear. In the healthy individual, this provokes rapid nystagmus toward or away from the water injection. Performing caloric tests in healthy people can evoke vomiting and extreme pain. An absence of nystagmus during caloric testing is one clinical sign of brain death.

Assessment of Visual Fields

Along with visual acuity, the visual fields should be assessed. For the most part, humans have a round field of vision, including a blind spot where the optic nerve enters the eye and where there are no photosensitive retinal cells. Although the visual field (Fig. 56-5) can be assessed precisely by an ophthalmologist, a rough estimate may be made in the office or at the patient's bedside when the examiner is concerned with any general disturbance of the visual field, for example, in a patient with a cerebrovascular accident (stroke) or glaucoma. A patient with a stroke may lose one fourth or one half of the visual fields of both eyes. Visual deficits resulting from glaucoma tend to follow a distinctive pattern of progressive loss of peripheral vision (tunnel vision), which unfortunately is a late finding.

A simple and reliable method of testing the fullness of the visual field is direct confrontation and use of finger-count testing. The examiner and patient sit between 1 and 2 feet apart, directly facing each other. The patient is instructed to cover one eye with a card, without applying pressure, while looking directly at the examiner's nose. The examiner in turn covers one eye as a method of comparison. If the patient has covered the left eye, for instance, the examiner covers the right eye. The patient is asked to gaze fixedly on the examiner's nose and to identify the number of fingers present in the superior and inferior fields of gaze temporally and nasally. The examiner's fingers are moved from the farthest position out toward the middle in vertical,

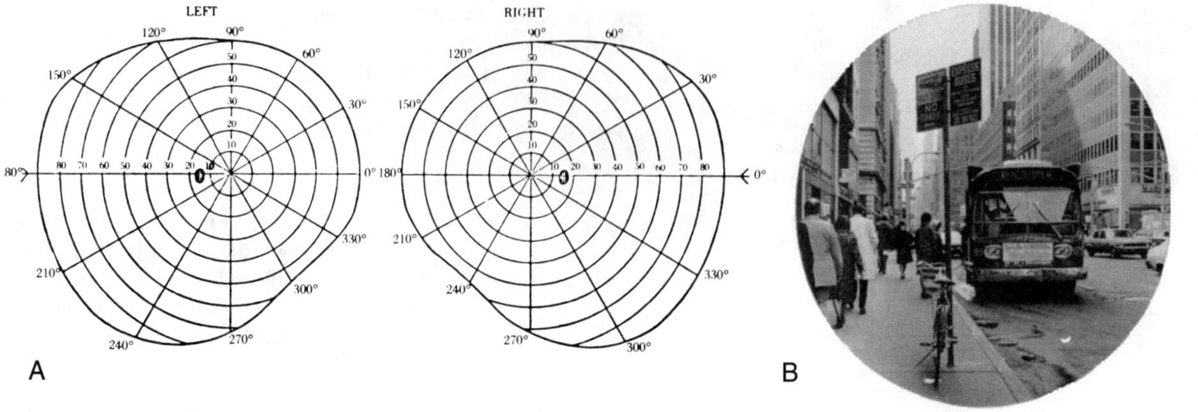

FIGURE 56-5. (**A**) Visual field charts showing peripheral vision of 180 degrees with both eyes. (**B**) Photograph representing what a person with normal (20/20) vision sees. (Photograph courtesy of The Lighthouse, The New York Association for the Blind.)

horizontal, and oblique planes, similar to assessing cardinal fields of gaze. The nasal, temporal, superior, and inferior fields are assessed by bringing the object into view from various peripheral points. During each maneuver, the patient informs the examiner of the moment when the object becomes visible while maintaining a forward gaze.

To test the nasal fields of gaze for the same eye, the examiner switches the object from the right hand to the left hand. The entire procedure is reversed for an assessment of the fields of vision of the other eye. Gross determination of the field of vision can be detected in this way. When confrontation testing shows decreases in visual fields, or blind spots, the patient is referred to an ophthalmologist for further evaluation.

In addition to the bedside testing of visual fields, there are more sophisticated, quantifiable ways to measure visual fields. The Goldmann perimeter or newer automated perimetry testing devices use systematic plotting of perception of light dots projected on a circular bowl with the head located in its center.

Examination of the Eye

Techniques commonly used in ophthalmic examination are inspection and palpation. Visual inspection is accomplished with specialized ophthalmic instruments and lights. Palpation may be used to assess orbital tenderness and deformity and to express discharge from the puncta. Palpation is also used to detect gross (readily apparent) levels of intraocular tension.

As with any kind of physical examination, the nurse uses a systematic approach, usually the "outside-in" approach. External structures of the eye and orbit are evaluated first; then the internal structures are examined.

Physical Examination of the Eye

The external structures of the eye are examined primarily by inspection. These structures include the eyebrow, eyelid, eyelashes, lacrimal apparatus, conjunctiva, cornea, anterior chamber, iris, and pupil.

When conducting the examination from the outside in, the nurse first observes the general appearance of the eyes from a distance, noting general symmetry and the position and alignment of the eyes. Although no one's eyes are exactly identical, they should be basically the same size and configuration. Variation from one side to the other may indicate atrophy or increased dimension, such as occurs with tumors or swelling within the orbital vault. Both eyes should be relatively the same color, although different eye colors are possible. Eye color pales with aging, depigmenting diseases, and certain autoimmune disorders.

The eyebrows are observed for the quantity and distribution of hair. The eyelids are inspected for color, skin condition, and the presence and direction of eyelash growth. The lid margins are examined for lesions such as styes or tumors. Sometimes with anterior fossa basilar skull fractures, blood may seep from torn dura into the orbital space; the resulting hematoma produces a black-eye appearance known as raccoon's eyes. A patient with such a fracture is assessed for an accompanying cerebrospinal fluid leak from the nose (rhinorrhea). The orbital ridge is palpated for defects. Irregularity of the orbital bony rim may be present with orbital blow-out or facial fractures. Subsequent trapping of extraocular muscles or cranial nerve tracts can occur. Also noted are scars, swelling, bruising, lacerations, other injuries, and foreign objects.

Eyelids

The position of the lids in relation to the eyeballs is assessed. Lid position and symmetry are an important part of the cranial nerve (CN) examination. To assess CN III, the nurse instructs the patient to lightly close the eyes to determine whether the eyes close fully. Opening the eyes assesses CN VII.

After the eyes open, the position of the lids is observed to see if they are symmetrical and basically resting on the same part of the irides. No sclera should be visible above or below the cornea. Lid position should be symmetrical, and the upper lid should rest just past the corneal limbus and above the pupil. The lid should not cover the pupil, which would interfere with vision. Full visibility of the iris, cornea, or sclera should not be present in a resting, conversational mode. Seeing more of the eye indicates protrusion, or **exophthalmos,** possibly caused by hyperthyroidism or masses within the orbit.

Classic exopthalmos, such as that seen in Graves' disease (hyperthyroidism), is thought to be from autoimmune processes that result in orbital inflammation and swelling of the muscles and fat. Unilateral protrusion may be associated with masses within the orbit, such as tumors, whereas bilateral protrusion might indicate generalized edema. Lid retraction may simulate the appearance of a protruding eye.

The eyes and eyelids of people who are malnourished or dehydrated have a sunken appearance because the orbital fat stores behind the eyeball and fluids are lost. **Ptosis** (drooping of the lid) may be caused by edema, muscle weakness, a congenital defect, or a neurologic problem (CN III) caused by trauma or disease.

The lids play an important role in eye integrity. They protect the eye from foreign matter with a blink reflex devoted to this purpose. Assessment of an intact blink reflex is part of the cranial nerve examination and determination of the level of consciousness. Involuntary blinking intervals are highly individual and are assessed if present.

Finally, the nurse observes the direction of the eyelid. The lid should rest flatly on the surface of the eye. An eyelid that turns outward is called **ectropion;** this eyelid does not close well and the external eye becomes exposed and dry. An eyelid that turns inward is called **entropion.** The eyelashes of this lid become sharp weapons, and corneal irritation develops from blinking and contact with skin and hair. Chronic diseases of the lids can damage them, producing abnormal lid position and closure. Indeed, many patients with chronic lid infections go on to develop dry eyes and corneal ulcers and abrasions from persistent irritation and loss of lashes.

Eyelashes

The nurse should next examine the eyelashes for their position and distribution. Usually serving a protective function, they may also become irritants to the eyes when they become long and unruly. Long, wild lashes can produce corneal irritation. Persons with abnormal depigmentation and albinism, chronic infections, and autoimmune diseases may develop white lashes, or **poliosis.**

Lacrimal System

The structures and function of tear formation and drainage are assessed. The lacrimal system consists of the secretory and drainage divisions. Aqueous tears are produced by the lacrimal gland located under the upper lateral orbit. If glandular enlargement is suspected, the upper lid is everted to expose and inspect the gland for swelling and inflammation. The tear film is observed generally for moisture or dryness. Performing Schirmer's test is a simple way to detect the amount of tear formation. A slightly folded litmus-like paper is hooked in the lower lid and remains in place for 5 minutes. The paper acts as a wick, absorbing produced tears. This test may be performed with or without local anesthetics. After 5 minutes, the extent of wetness is measured. Test results are considered normal when the range of wetting is $\geq$ 10 mm; greater than 25 mm may suggest excess tear production.

The drainage component of the lacrimal system includes the puncta, canaliculi, lacrimal sacs, and nasolacrimal ducts. Drainage is first assessed by observing the puncta. They are tiny, oval openings in the medial upper and lower canthus that serve to drain tears into the **canaliculi.** They serve as the upper portion of the drainage system for tears to flow into the lacrimal sac and duct. Sometimes the puncta become inflamed and may appear red and "pouting." Edema and exudate can occlude the upper portion of the lacrimal system, causing tears to overflow onto the face. The lacrimal drainage system can become inflamed and obstructed, producing a bulging of the sac on the side of the bridge of the nose. This is common in children. Exudate or other drainage is assessed for its color, location, and approximate amount. Obstruction or inflammation of the nasolacrimal duct can often be identified by palpating the side of the nose near the medial canthus of the eye. The area is assessed for tenderness and enlargement. Any expression of discharge from the puncta is noted and described.

Examination of the Anterior Eye

The sclera and bulbar conjunctiva are inspected concurrently. The lids are separated by placing the index finger on the patient's upper orbital rim and the thumb on the lower rim to avoid soft tissue trauma. As the lids are gently separated, the patient is instructed to look up, down, and to each side. The externally visible bulbar conjunctiva is inspected. Small capillaries are normally visible in the conjunctiva, and the fibrous sclera is normally white.

In dark-skinned persons, however, the sclera is often yellowish; this is a normal finding, not to be confused with jaundice, a yellowing of the sclera found in liver and gallbladder disease. The sclera appears bluish when it is thin. The palpebral conjunctiva of the lower lid is readily inspected by having the patient look upward while the lower lid is gently everted with gentle traction on the lower orbital rim. Similarly, the upper lid must be everted to visualize its palpebral conjunctiva (Guideline 56-1).

The eye is divided into two chambers: anterior and posterior. The location of the anterior segment chamber allows for gross inspection without specialized instruments. The posterior chamber, however, is only visible with lighted, mirrored, or magnified instruments.

Examination of the Cornea

Usually a slit lamp is used to examine the cornea thoroughly; however, the nurse can observe several features using a penlight. The first thing to observe is the general health of the cornea. To inspect the corneal surface, the examiner shines a penlight on the anterior portion. Normally, the cornea is smooth with a singular, symmetrical, bright, mirror-like light reflex. Irregularities are typically detected by defects in the light reflection on the cornea. A scattered light reflex may indicate an irregular surface or corneal edema.

Next, the clarity of the cornea is observed. The cornea should be transparent so that light passes freely through it. When the cornea and anterior chamber are clear, the details of the iris are clearly seen. The cornea is observed for scarring, which usually appears whitish gray. Scars can indicated previous trauma, surgery, or infections. Cloudiness of the cornea is seen in cases of corneal edema, as in acute glaucoma, post-traumatic and surgical events, or any event that disrupts the epithelium. Most of the cornea has

GUIDELINE 56–1
Inspecting the Upper Palpebral Conjunctiva

To examine the upper palpebral conjunctiva, for example to extract a foreign object or to assess scleral color or blood supply, requires eversion of the upper eyelid as follows:

1. Ask the patient to look down. Explain what to expect; then gently grasp the upper eyelashes between the thumb and index finger and pull forward.

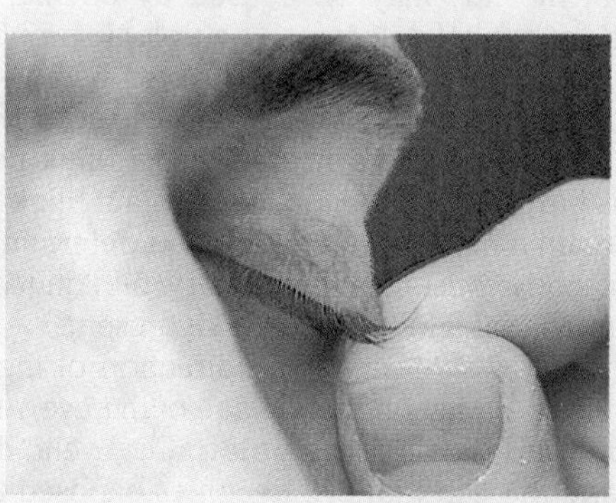

2. Place a small stick, such as a tongue blade or a cotton-tipped applicator, at the tarsal fold. Gently fold the eyelid back while the patient continues looking downward.

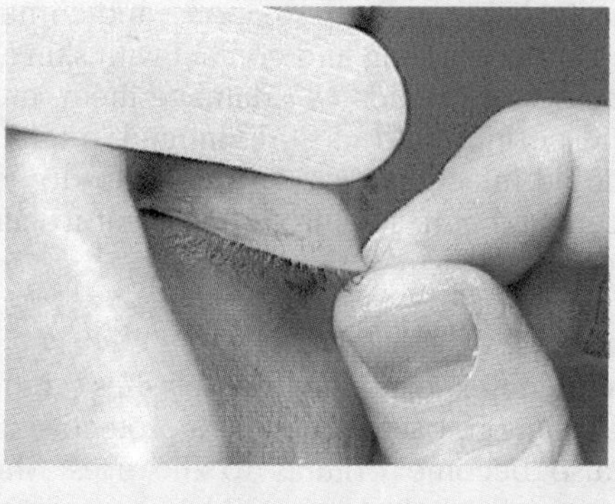

3. Use the thumb to secure the eyelashes against the eyebrow. Then observe for a foreign body, excessive redness, exudates, or hemorrhages (usually located near the corneal limbus and radiating outward). Check vascularity as well, noting whether the vessels move with eye movement. The conjunctiva should move freely over the scleral surface.

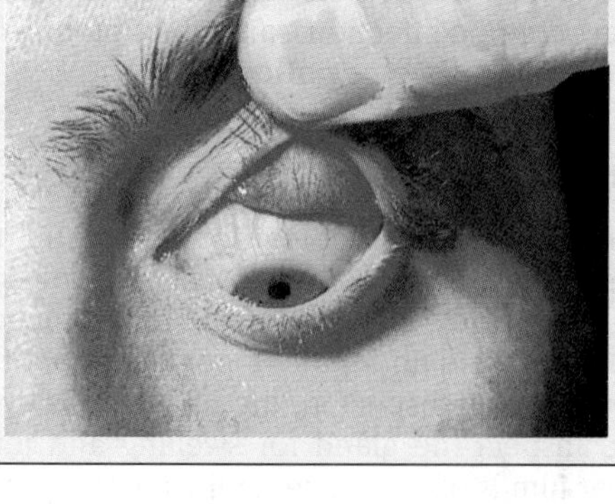

no blood vessels. Development of blood vessels into the cornea or a prominence of vessels around the perimeter is noted. These blood vessels are abnormal and can obstruct vision. Shadows cast on the iris may indicate a corneal lesion or forward displacement of the anterior chamber.

To evaluate the shape of the cornea, and the depth of the anterior chamber, the nurse shines the penlight obliquely from the patient's side. Findings may include **keratoconus,** a bulging, pointed cornea caused by thinning layers or a flattened chamber with decompression, which may result from a ruptured globe or open surgical wound, or increases in intraocular pressure as the iris bulges forward.

The cornea protects the eye by being highly sensitive. When even slightly irritated, such as with a stray eyelash, a corneal reflex is induced. Corneal sensitivity is assessed by sweeping separate wisps of clean cotton against each cornea, taking care not to touch the lids or lashes. This should elicit a prompt and equal blink, bilaterally, and tearing.

In unconscious persons, a corneal reflex can be elicited by lightly tapping the upper lid covering the cornea. If the cornea is intact, the patient will blink. Foreign bodies in the cornea may elicit symptoms of pain, photophobia, and tearing. Corneal trauma may produce severe symptoms and make examination difficult. To examine the cornea and other eye structures, a topical anesthetic may be required. The anesthetic works almost instantly, affords relief to the patient, and promotes ease of examination.

To detect corneal ulcers and foreign bodies, topical fluorescein dye may be administered before examination. Fluorescein dye adheres to denuded epithelium and appears bright green when illuminated with a **slit lamp,** a special light used for examining the eye.

Rose bengal dye stains epithelial defects better than fluorescein, however. It is used to diagnose conjunctival disease, such as **keratoconjunctivitis sicca,** an inflammation of the anterior eye caused by drying. If someone has a ruptured globe, or holes in the cornea, eye drops should never be used, because they may enter the eye and destroy nonregenerative endothelial cells. Moreover, topical dyes stain soft contact lenses; thus, the lenses must be removed before administering dye.

The limbus should be examined for the extension of blood vessels or for a deep red color, which is seen in uveal tract inflammation. Elderly patients sometimes develop **arcus senilis,** a benign grayish ring around the edge of the cornea. However, when this is seen in younger individuals, it may indicate elevated serum lipid levels.

Examination of the Iris and Anterior Chamber

While examining the cornea, the aqueous humor in the anterior chamber is assessed for clarity. Under certain conditions, the presence of cells and clouding (flare) in the aqueous humor may be visible. This clouding is caused by an increase in proteinaceous material produced by an inflammation in the anterior chamber. Severe infectious processes can occur in the anterior chamber, leaving white blood cells and infectious debris. An accumulation of pus in the anterior chamber is called a **hypopyon.** Blood vessels in the structures of the anterior chamber can become injured or fragile and rupture, spilling blood into its cavity. Blood in the anterior chamber is called a **hyphema.** Both of these conditions can be seen more clearly after the patient has been sitting upright so that gravity allows for settling of contents, forming a visible fluid level in the anterior chamber.

The iris is examined for its shape, symmetry, and color. There are no two irides alike, which makes everyone unique. The iris is inspected for continuity and unusual markings. When blood vessels develop or native blood vessels are distended, as with inflammatory processes, they may be visible in the iris. Tortuous blood vessels formed in diabetes are called **rubeosis irides.**

Examination of the Pupil

The pupil is the opening in the center of the iris. When examining the pupils, reaction to light and near vision with convergence are assessed, for example, to evaluate changes in the central nervous system (CNS) or in intracranial pressure. The iris changes size to control the light entering the eye. When photosensitive cells of the retina are subjected to bright light, the normal pupil promptly constricts in a regular, concentric fashion. The reaction should be brisk and symmetrical. There should be a simultaneous, constrictive reaction of the unstimulated, opposite pupil as well.

Constriction of the stimulated pupil is called the **direct light reflex,** whereas constriction of the opposite pupil is termed **consensual,** or **indirect, light reflex.** Consensual reaction is evaluated in both eyes. Exploration of this phenomenon allows one to distinguish between blindness from optic nerve damage or blindness from central disease. In a nerve-damaged eye, direct light stimulation produces no pupillary response, but in the undamaged eye, direct light stimulation elicits a response in the damaged eye. Sluggish or absent reactions may occur in cases of increased intracranial pressure.

If the patient can follow commands, the nurse can test the pupillary reaction to near vision and convergence. The pupils do not react to accommodation accomplished by the lens (adjustments that occur when vision is shifted from far to near). They do, however, constrict when the eyes converge (cross) on nearby objects. This is best observed by asking the patient to focus on an object at a distance and follow the examiner's finger, which moves inward 3 to 5 inches from the patient's nose. In response, the pupil normally constricts as the eyes converge to focus on the examiner's finger. Lens accommodation is not observable but assumed.

Autonomic disease, for example, from syphilis or diabetes, may result in a pupil that cannot respond to light but that can respond to accommodation. Such a pupil is known as an **Argyll Robertson pupil.**

Although pupils should be approximately the same size and shape, procedures such as lens implantation, iridectomy, traumatic and congenital defects, or congenital anisocoria, may cause varying shapes. For example keyhole shape or wedge defects in the iris are usually indicative of **iridectomy,** performed to lower intraocular pressure.

Some patients with increasing intracranial pressure may have pupillary changes that require serial examinations. Patients with purely lateral brain injuries may show distinct unilateral pupillary signs. For example, the pupil may develop an oval shape just before it becomes fully dilated and fixed. This usually localizes the lesion on the side of the affected pupil and is an early, yet subtle, sign of increased intracranial pressure.

When all findings of the pupillary examination are normal, they are commonly documented and abbreviated PERRLA: Pupils equal, round and reactive to light and accommodation, keeping in mind that accommodation is assessed in aware, cooperative patients, and it is the near convergence, not accommodation, of the lens that causes pupillary constriction. Other descriptive findings are documented in detail in a narrative note.

Examination of the Crystalline Lens

Typically, one cannot see the lens, although from an angle looking into a dilated pupil, one might see a slight reflection of the anterior capsule. People with advanced (ripe) cataracts have a hazy lens, and the pupil appears clouded and gray-white. In newborns the pupil is examined as well for evidence of congenital cataracts. A white pupil (**leukocoria**) can indicate a cataract but may also represent an intraocular tumor, such as retinoblastoma. Some call this a "cat's eye." Any opaque material obstructing the pupil can block the passage of light and therefore vision. When present in children younger than 6 years of age, this can result in amblyopia and poor vision.

Direct eye trauma may knock the lens loose into the vitreous or the anterior chamber, or it may dangle crookedly in the pupil. During slit-lamp examination, zonules can sometimes be seen with pieces of the lens suspended from them. Connective tissue disorders, such as those seen in Marfan's syndrome, are commonly associated with lens dislocation.

Examination of the Posterior Segment

Because the posterior structures lie behind the visible anterior structures, they cannot be seen by traditional observation. To examine the posterior segment and the vitreous humor, a clear medium is required. The rule of thumb is "if the patient can see out, one should see in." Examination of the vitreous humor, retina, and other posterior structures requires using an ophthalmoscope, which calls for considerable practice and skill. In some settings, evaluation of the fundus (the inner eye) is not a common nursing function. However, nurses who practice in specialized ophthalmic settings, who conduct physical examinations, or who function in advanced nursing practice may use this skill often.

Ideally the patient's pupil should be dilated to facilitate the examination, and the room should be dark to minimize natural reactions to light and to facilitate the examiner's visualization of distinct structures. Typically, eye drop medications such as phenylephrine or cyclopentate are given to dilate the pupil, which allows for full visualization of the fundus. However, these medications also impair vision for several hours after the examination so the patient will require sunglasses to prevent photophobic reactions and someone to take him or her home.

- In rare circumstances, full dilation of the pupil can precipitate an acute glaucoma attack as the pupil bunches up into the narrowed trebeculum, occluding aqueous humor drainage.

One should keep this in mind when instilling dilating drops in patients with a history of narrow angle glaucoma. Other medications that cause pupillary dilation, such as atropine, can produce the same result in these patients.

Diagnostic Evaluation

Ophthalmoscopy

The internal eye is called the **fundus** and comprises the retina, optic disc, macula, and retinal vessels. It can be visualized through an **ophthalmoscope,** a hand-held instrument that projects light through a prism and bends the light at 90 degrees, allowing the observer to view the retina. The direct ophthalmoscope has several lenses arranged on a wheel. A lens may be chosen by rotating the wheel with the index finger without interrupting the inspection. The small, unfiltered aperture is appropriate and most useful for standard ophthalmoscopy. Indirect ophthalmoscopy involves using a binocular scope with bright illumination, which facilitates a broader view of the ocular fundus.

To avoid a confrontation of noses, the right eye of the patient is examined with the right eye of the examiner, and the left eye of the patient with the left eye of the examiner (Fig. 56-6). The room is darkened to enhance pupillary dilation. The patient is instructed to hold the eyes still and focus on a real or imagined distant object. The ophthalmoscope is gripped firmly in the hand, with the index finger resting on the lens wheel. The head of the ophthalmoscope is braced within the angle made by the eyebrow and the nose. The

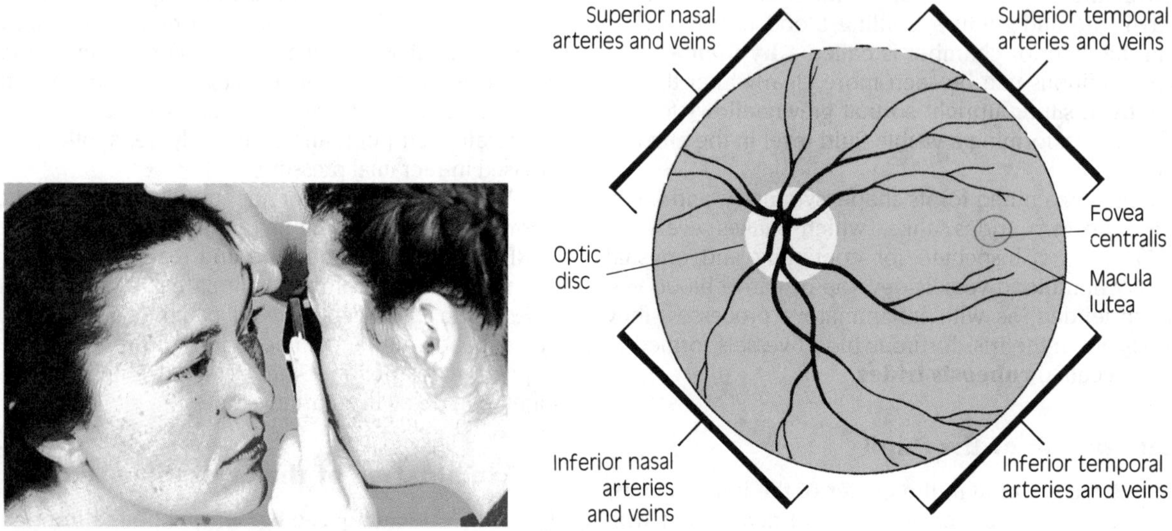

FIGURE 56-6. To examine the fundus of the eye (**right**) with an ophthalmoscope (**left**), the nurse uses her left eye to inspect the patient's left eye, places her right hand on the patient's left forehead, and holds the eyelid open. The fundus at right represents normal findings.

lens chosen for initial inspection should be the one labeled zero unless the examiner is knowingly correcting his own defect in visual acuity. An examiner who wears corrective lenses should become proficient in ophthalmoscopy while wearing the lenses and use the zero lens setting. Provided that the patient has 20/20 vision, the zero lens should enable the examiner to obtain a precise focus on the retina. Otherwise, the lens wheel is rotated until the retina comes into focus. Lenses labeled with a red numeral are for **hyperopic** (farsighted) patients; lenses labeled with a black numeral are for **myopic** (nearsighted) patients.

With the patient appropriately gazing into the distance, and with the ophthalmoscope properly positioned within the cradle of the examiner's orbit, the examiner approaches the patient, standing approximately 37.5 cm (15 inches) away and about 15 degrees to the side of the patient's gaze. When the light is focused on the pupil, the retina glows red (or orange) through the dilated pupil opening. This is known as the **red reflex.** (The red reflex is visible in many photographs where the camera flash reflects off the retina.) The examiner then moves closer to the patient. Placing a hand on the patient's forehead, the examiner rests his or her forehead on the hand and focuses through the ophthalmoscope. The retina should be in focus, and the venules and arterioles that course through it are apparent (see Fig. 56-6). In scanning the surface of the retina, the examiner needs to hold the scope firmly, moving the head rather than the instrument.

Examining the fundus includes evaluating the optic disc, retinal blood vessels, retinal characteristics, macular area, and vitreous humor: the disc, for its physiologic cup and proportional size; the blood vessels, for size, distribution, crossings, and color reflection; the retinal fundus, for general color and hemorrhage, fluid, and attachment; the macula and fovea centralis, for color (darker red) and central reflection. The vitreous humor can be cloudy and contain larvae, foreign bodies, other ocular structures, such as the lens and retinal fragments, and streaks. This may interfere with the transmission of visual impulses or the ability to visualize the retina clearly.

Measurement of Ocular Pressure

Tonometry is a technique for measuring intraocular pressure (IOP). Schiotz tonometry requires using a metal, handheld instrument (the tonometer) that rests on the anesthetized cornea. The results can be variable but are a good estimate of IOP. Another pressure gauge, the Goldmann applanation tonometer, attaches to a slit lamp to measure IOP. It is considered the most accurate form of measuring IOP.

Administration of fluorescein dye and topical anesthesia are required before applanation tonometry. IOP can also be measured with a pneumotonometer, which delivers a small puff of air against the eye to measure the pressure. This method is particularly useful when contact with the cornea is not desired. Assessing IOP is a usual component of a comprehensive eye examination, and the pressure should be closely followed in patients who have glaucoma or who are at high risk for developing intraocular hypertension. An increase in IOP is the cardinal sign of glaucoma, a disease responsible for more than one fifth of the cases of blindness in the United States.

A general determination of IOP can be made by applying gentle finger pressure over the sclera of the closed eye. The tips of both forefingers are placed on the closed upper lid. One finger gently presses inward while the adjacent finger senses the amount of pressure exerted against it. Some examiners then compare the tension felt or perceived in the patient's eye with the pressure in their own. At best, this maneuver provides a general estimation, and it requires practice. However, when accurate measurement is required, tonometry is indicated. Hydration of the patient may be assessed by palpating for intraocular tension. A soft eyeball may signal dehydration.

Slit-Lamp Examination

A slit lamp is an instrument commonly found in an ophthalmologist's office or an area where ophthalmic evaluations occur. During a slit-lamp examination, the patient sits and leans the forehead against the supportive structure of the slit lamp. The examiner turns on the lamp and shines various shapes and colors of light into the frontal surface of the eye. The instrument magnifies the cornea, sclera, and anterior chamber, and provides oblique views into the trabeculum with special lenses. Most slit lamps are equipped with an applanation tonometer.

For the examination the room should be darkened and the patient cooperative. The nurse or technician usually assists by administering eye drops to dilate the pupils before examination. The use of superficial stains and dyes, such as 2% fluorescein solution, may be used to study the exterior corneal surface for regularity and foreign bodies. Irregularities are associated with ulcer formation.

Before slit-lamp examination, the patient should be prepared so that any dressings are removed, the eye is cleaned, and appropriate eye drops, such as topical anesthetics and dyes, are given. The procedure is explained and instructions supplied.

Imaging Procedures

Occasionally it is necessary to view the eye in relation to the skull and other soft tissues. Because the eye sits in the intracranial vault, abnormalities in the skull can affect the orbit and ophthalmic structures. Blowout fractures of the orbit can trap extraocular muscles or nerves and limit free movement of the affected eye. X-ray of the skull can identify cranial abnormalities. Magnetic resonance imaging (MRI) and computerized tomography (CT) scanning can be used to identify intraocular and extraocular growths and anatomic structures.

Ultrasonography

Ultrasound is used to measure ocular dimensions and structures. Ultrasonic scans are used to measure the depth and shape of the eyeball before insertion of intraocular lens implants so that the correct refraction can be achieved.

In ultrasonography high-frequency waves are emitted from a small probelike transducer placed on the eye. After striking the ocular tissues, the sound waves echo and are picked up by the same transducer. They are converted to waveforms and displayed on an oscilloscope. The procedure is painless but requires a local eye anesthetic. After the test, the patient is cautioned not to rub the eyes. Two primary types of ultrasound are used in ophthalmology: A-scan and B-scan.

A-scan—ultrasound is useful for differentiating between benign and malignant tumors, measuring the eye for an intraocular lens (IOL) implant, and monitoring congenital glaucoma.

B-scan—ultrasound is useful for detecting and locating various structures within the eye that may be obscured by hemorrhage, cataract, or other opacities.

Endothelial Cell Count

An endothelial cell counter is a photographic instrument that attaches to a slit lamp and produces high-resolution images detailing endothelial cell morphology: cell size, shape, density, and boundaries, as well as intercellular bodies and pathologic processes. This is a valuable preoperative test for identifying a compromised endothelium, which increases the risk of postoperative complications.

Fluorescein Angiography

An evaluation of the ophthalmic blood vessels can be made with fluorescein angiography. Contrast dye is injected into a peripheral vein, and serial photographs are taken of the fundus. This test helps determine the extent of retinal vascular disorders, such as those related to diabetes and hypertension, papilledema, and central retinal artery occlusion.

Refraction and Accommodation

Minor defects and alignments of the eyes can be seen in almost everyone. Refractive correction is unnecessary for most of these defects. When refractive correction is necessary, however, it is performed to relieve symptoms such as blurred vision, headache, or eye fatigue, and not for improving the health of the eye. Several types of corneal refractive surgery are available to correct myopia, hyperopia, and astigmatism. The procedures may eliminate the need for eyeglasses or reduce the strength of the prescription required to correct vision.

Refractive errors include **myopia** (nearsightedness), **hyperopia** or **hypermetropia** (farsightedness) (Fig. 56-7), **anisometropia** (unequal focus of the two eyes), **astigmatism** (asymmetric focus), and **presbyopia** (inability to change focus).

Refractive errors and their treatment are best understood when related to the process of accommodation. Accommodation occurs when the ciliary muscles contract, relaxing the zonules, and increasing the curvature of the lens. This causes the refractive, "light-bending" power of the eye to increase (accommodation), allowing the eye to focus on near objects. (*Note:* When light passes through various eye structures, such as the pupil and the lens, the shape of those structures bends the light so that it may or may not focus normally on the retina.) When the ciliary muscles relax, the refractive power of the eye is at its lowest possible strength, as typified in paralysis of the ciliary body (cycloplegia).

With aging, the ability of the eye to accommodate gradually decreases because of increased rigidity of the lens (presbyopia). The lens is less able to change shape in response to visual challenge of focusing on near objects. After

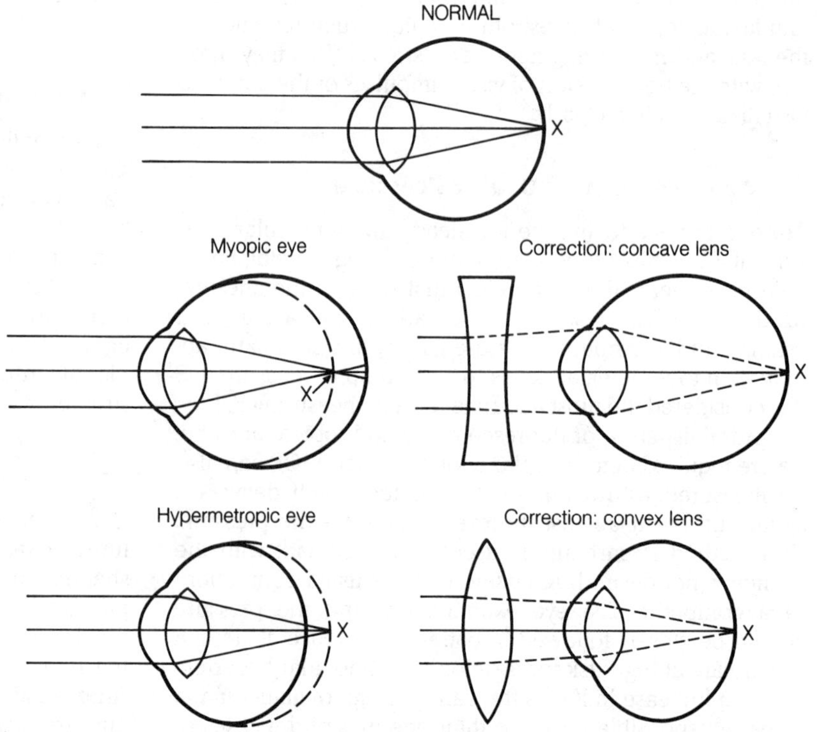

FIGURE 56-7. Normal vision compared with myopia (nearsightedness) and hypermetropia (hyperopia; farsightedness).

age 40 many individuals notice a decreased ability to accommodate, especially with regard to close work.

The condition of a normal eye focused for distance, without accommodation, is known as **emmetropia.** The eye clearly sees objects in the distance without effort and, using accommodation, it can focus on close objects.

With myopia, the eye may have an oblong shape or excessive reactive power and focuses light from distant objects in front of the retina. The myopic eye cannot clearly see objects in the distance because it has no way to reduce this excessive refractive power. Decreased distant vision is the only symptom apparent with myopia.

With hyperopia, the eye has insufficient reactive power to focus light on the retina. Rather, the rays of light entering the eye are focused behind the retina. Impairment of near vision results.

Astigmatism results from unequal curvature of the cornea. Diagnosis of astigmatism is accomplished by keratometry. The focus of light rays is distorted, and the patient cannot focus horizontal and vertical rays on the retina at the same time. Vision is generally blurred, and the patient often complains of eye discomfort. Either hyperopia or myopia may coexist with astigmatism. Astigmatism cannot be eliminated by accommodation but can generally be corrected by glasses ground to neutralize the unequal curvature. Special toric soft contact lenses may also be used to correct for astigmatism.

The strength and type of lens that will overcome refractive errors are determined by means of a **retinoscope.** On the basis of this examination, an appropriate corrective lens is selected and then further refined by having the patient read letters on the Snellen chart through several different lenses. Automated refractors, which rely on photoelectric light-sensitive devices, may also be used. The patient sits in front of the instrument and is instructed to look steadily at a target. An electronic printout indicates the refractive error to be corrected. Other types of automated refractors require the patient to make focusing adjustments by turning a knob.

Refractive Correction

Refractive errors may be corrected with eyeglasses, contact lenses (Table 56-1), intraocular lenses, or other surgery, such as radial keratotomy, by which serial cuts are made in the cornea to flatten it. This allows greater posterior focusing of light on the retina and corrects myopia so that corrective lenses are not needed. Postoperatively some patients may complain of glare or overcorrection or undercorrection. These patients may still need corrective lenses.

Therapeutic Nonrefractive Lenses. Other types of contact lenses include special eye devices to administer medications, to bandage the anterior eye, and to irrigate the eye after a chemical burn. Persons who have had ocular trauma, keratoconus (protruding cornea), scarred and irregular corneas, and who are poor risks for corneal transplantation have been helped by scleral lenses, which make functional, sometimes excellent, visual acuity possible for some.

Removal of Contact Lenses. Contact lenses are designed to be worn while the person is awake and fully conscious (the exception is extended-wear lenses). They should be removed as a safety measure if the wearer is incapacitated because of accident, sickness, or other cause. It is important never to instill fluorescein dye while contact lenses are in place, because the dye may stain the lenses. A conscious or semiconscious patient is asked if he or she is wearing contact lenses. If the patient's condition permits, the patient may remove the lenses alone or with some assistance. If the patient is unconscious, the nurse needs to observe for contact lenses by gently separating the eyelids and shining a light on the eye from the side. A colleague who wears contact lenses may be of help in removing the lenses of these patients.

The nurse removes the patient's contact lenses if the patient cannot. The following procedure is used for hard contact lenses:

- After thorough handwashing, the nurse places one thumb on the upper eyelid and one thumb on the lower eyelid, near the margin of each eyelid.
- The eyelids are separated.
- A visible lens should slide easily with a gentle movement of the eyelids. Then a small suction cup may be used to retrieve the lens.
- If the lens does not drop out easily, the position of the lens is identified.
- If the lens can be seen but cannot be removed, *force should never be used.* Rather the lens is gently slid onto the sclera, where it can remain with relative safety until experienced help is obtained.

If the patient is wearing soft contact lenses, it is best to wait until someone experienced in removing these types of lenses is available to lend assistance. If soft lenses are left in place for many hours, they do little harm.

Conditions of the Eye

The eye is subject to many conditions, some of which are primary and some of which are secondary to disorders of other body organs. Many of these conditions are preventable; others, if detected and treated early, can be controlled, and vision can be preserved. The following sections of this chapter focus on the prevention and management of common ophthalmic disorders. The sequence of the presentation is from the outside in.

Disorders of the Eyelids

The eyelids are particularly vulnerable to infection because they are constantly exposed to objects in the environment, including human hands. They are also moist from tear formation and normal drainage. Warmth, moisture, and opportunistic organisms make an environment conducive to infection. Good general hygiene of the eyes and eyelids usually prevents infections.

Blepharitis

Blepharitis is a chronic inflammation of the eyelid margins. It may be caused by seborrhea (nonulcerative), the most

TABLE 56-1 Features of Corrective Lenses

Durability	Advantages	Disadvantages
Eyeglasses (Spectacles)		
Excellent	Excellent vision correction Easily cared for	Fogging in cool weather Some cosmetic objections Unsuitable for certain activities, and sports, some occupational drawbacks May need to be replaced more frequently than soft contact lenses
Hard Contact Lenses		
With care, may last 15–20 years	Excellent vision correction Usually less costly than other types Effective for persons with astigmatism Lightweight and thin; float on eyeball Lens moves with the eye Gas-permeable variety transports oxygen to cornea	Uncomfortable for some Require period of adaptation Possibility of eventual intolerance May pop out of position Gas-impermeable variety blocks oxygen to cornea; blinking required for oxygen transport
Soft Contact Lenses		
May require more frequent replacement (usually replaced every 1–3 years)	More comfortable than hard lenses Can be worn longer than hard lenses Improved peripheral vision; lens moves with the eye Flexible because lens absorbs water	Require time daily for sanitation Greater risk of eye irritation, infection, and corneal edema and ulcers Not as effective for astigmatism Possibility of eventual intolerance Highest risk of ulcerative keratitis with disposable variety (Schein, 1994)
Extended-Wear Lenses		
Most fragile of all lenses May have to be replaced every 6 months or more often	Provide corrected vision around the clock May be worn for an extended period, but no longer than prescribed by ophthalmologist Benefit elderly and nearsighted individuals	Expensive More frequent visits to eye physician Risk of corneal injury, conjunctivitis, chemical insensitivity May not correct vision as well as other lenses Possibility of eventual intolerance Prone to cloudiness from protein deposits
Progressive Power Lenses		
Same durability as the two kinds of lenses: (eyeglasses and soft contact lenses)	Correct distant, intermediate, near vision without lines common to bifocal and trifocal lenses Safe to wear during sports and stenuous activity	Some prescriptive limitations, optical aberrations, and fitting difficulties

common form, or staphylococcal infection (ulcerative), or both.

Clinical Manifestations. The chief symptoms are irritation, burning, itching of the lid margins, and red-rimmed eyes. Many scales, flakes, or granulations cling to the lashes. Concurrent symptoms include loss of lashes, development of white eyelashes, and dilated blood vessels at the lid margin.

Management. Treatment includes daily meticulous cleaning of the lid margins using a cotton-tipped applicator, a nonirritating shampoo such as "no-tears" baby shampoo, water, and mild friction. Warm compresses may be applied across both eyes. Using aseptic technique, the patient or nurse can remove crusted matter with a washcloth and apply topical antibiotics and steroids. Patient education is an essential element in success of this home-based treatment.

Stye (External Hordeolum)

A stye is an infection of the superficial lid glands of Zeis or Moll. The infection is usually caused by *Staphylococcus aureus*.

Clinical Manifestations. The principle symptoms are subacute pain, redness, and swelling of a localized area of the lid that may rupture. Styes are localized to the lid margins.

Management. Treatment with warm, moist compresses for 10 to 15 minutes, three or four times daily, hastens the healing process. If the condition does not begin to resolve within 48 hours, incision and drainage may be indicated. Application of topical sulfonamides and antibiotics may be prescribed.

Chalazion (Internal Hordeolum)

A chalazion is a chronic granulomatous inflammation of the meibomian gland marked by localized, painless swelling that develops over a period of weeks. Palpation usually indicates a small, painless nodule in the eyelid. Uninfected chalazia usually do not require treatment and disappear spontaneously within a few months. A chalazion may develop secondary infection (internal hordeolum) with suppurative inflammation, usually on the internal, conjunctival eyelid surface.

Management. Treatment may include warm compresses, massage and expression of the glandular secretions, or antibiotic therapy and corticosteroid drops or injections. Excision is indicated if the chalazion grows large enough to distort vision or becomes a cosmetic blemish.

Tumors of the Eyelids

Tumors on the eyelids are similar to other skin tumors. They may be benign or malignant. Exposure to ultraviolet light is thought to be partially responsible for development of some lid carcinomas.

Basal Cell Carcinoma

Basal cell carcinoma is the most common neoplasm of the eyelids.

Clinical Manifestations. These tumors tend to be located on the lid margins, close to the inner canthus. They have an ulcerated appearance and a distinct central aspect and pearly margins.

Management. Treatment for basal cell carcinoma consists of excising superficial lesions and using a freezing probe (cryotherapy) for inner canthus lesions. Treatment should be prompt because neglected basal cell tumors can invade the orbit and cranium. Astute examination by the health care professional in screening situations, and during physical and ophthalmic examinations, is particularly important in early detection and treatment.

Squamous Cell Carcinoma

Squamous cell carcinomas have only one tenth the incidence of basal cell carcinoma.

Clinical Manifestations. Like basal cell carcinomas, squamous cell carcinomas are nodular and elevated. They have irregular surfaces with pearly margins. The centers tend to ulcerate and have more of a pearly appearance than basal cell tumors. They tend to develop around the lid margins near the outer canthus.

Xanthelasmas

Xanthelasmas are deposits of lipid material on the eyelids. They are slightly elevated yellowish lesions. They tend to be located along the lid margin and have sharp, demarcated edges. Xanthelasmas may be a normal finding or they may be associated with disorders of fat metabolism, which requires further evaluation.

Abnormalities of Eyelid Position

Ineffective closure of the eyelids may expose the external eye to air, drying, and invasion by organisms.

Blepharoptosis (**ptosis**) is the term used to describe a condition in which the upper eyelid droops, lying lower than the top of the iris on the eye surface. This condition may result from damage to the cranial nerves that innervate the lid or from trauma, surgery, neurologic disorders such as Bell's palsy and myasthenia gravis, tumors, edema, or a congenital abnormality.

Exophthalmus (or **proptosis**) is a condition in which the eyes seem to bulge from the orbit. It can be caused by retraction of the eyelids or from mechanical alteration of ocular contents from displacement by other components, such as edema, hemorrhage, tumors, or inflammation. Although it appears so, the eye is not actually enlarged; it is just being pushed away from the orbital socket. When both eyes are involved, a metabolic condition, such as hyperthyroidism, may be the cause. Unilateral exophthalmus may be from a tumor. Exophthalmus prevents natural closure of the lids because the palpebral fissure widens.

Entropion and ectropion are other pathologic lid positions. In **entropion** the eyelid, (usually the lower lid) is turned inward. The turned-in lid and its lashes irritate the fragile and sensitive cornea and external eye. Common effects of entropion are tearing, conjunctival injection, and secondary corneal or conjunctival infections. Entropion also prohibits airtight lid closure, thereby increasing the eye's risk of exposure.

In **ectropion** the eyelid margin is turned outward, prohibiting the eye from effectively closing. The lid may sag and droop open, exposing the usually hidden palpebral conjunctiva and cornea. Ectropion can involve both the upper and lower eyelids. When the lower lid is involved, the punctum is drawn away from the lacrimal lake, and tearing occurs. Entropion and ectropion may be caused by injury to the lids, chronic lid infections, aging, spasm, and neurologic defects.

Gerontologic Considerations

With aging, the lids lose elasticity and begin to sag. Sometimes they can sag to excess, obstructing vision. An oculoplastic procedure, known as blepharoplasty, can be performed to provide better function and appearance. This is performed using a local anesthetic. The patient usually has "black eyes" for a week or so.

Disorders of the Lacrimal System

The main problems associated with diseases of the lacrimal system are related to tear production or inflammation of the lacrimal drainage system. Excess tear production can be caused by reflex stimulation of the lacrimal glands and by obstructions in any part of the lacrimal drainage system as a result of edema, trauma, infectious discharge, or inflammation. This problem is managed by correcting the underlying abnormality. Although annoying, excess tearing alone does not result in visual loss.

Dry eyes are usually the result of decreased tear production, commonly caused by scarring secondary to chronic conjunctival infections, tear gland abnormalities, and neurologic disorders. Production of lubricating tears decreases with age and may diminish to the point where the eyes do not have enough moisture for protection and comfort. Symptoms of dry eyes are burning, redness, pain, itchiness, difficulty in moving the lids, and stringy mucus. The eyes respond to dryness by increasing the amount of watery tears, which, ironically, results in tearing but does not help the lubrication problem.

Dry eyes accompanied by a dry mouth and arthritis is known as Sjögren's syndrome.

Management. Treatment of dry eyes includes avoidance of irritants, such as smoke and smog, and humidification of the environment. Placing tiny plugs in the puncta or closing them surgically may be helpful in some individuals, but the procedure must be performed cautiously because a reflex reduction in tears may result.

Dry eyes are usually cared for by instilling artificial tears, preferably those with prolonged wetting action. Meticulous hygiene is important for preventing infection, and ointment at bedtime is often helpful. A new treatment device consists of a pair of eyeglasses equipped with tiny nozzles aimed at the inner corners of the eyes. The nozzles deliver droplets to the eyes at regular intervals or at the push of a button. This device may be useful for administering medications for other eye conditions as well.

Dacryocystitis

Acute dacryocystitis is a suppurative cellulitis of the lacrimal sac secondary to nasolacrimal duct obstruction.

Clinical Manifestations. Symptoms include pain over the lacrimal drainage site and intense swelling at the upper bridge of the nose, which may produce discharge from the puncta when expressed. The puncta become red and swollen, and may actually "pout."

Management. This condition usually responds well to antibiotic therapy and warm compresses. Chronic conditions, however, require probing of the lacrimal system or dacryocystorhinostomy (a surgical procedure that creates an outflow channel into the nasal cavity) to relieve the obstruction.

Disorders of the Conjunctiva

Conjunctivitis

Conjunctivitis is an inflammation of the conjunctiva and is characterized by swelling and exudates. In conjunctivitis the eye has a general pink appearance, thus the common term **pink eye.**

Conjunctivitis has many origins. It may be infectious (bacterial, chlamydial, viral, fungal, parasitic), immunologic (allergic), irritative (chemical, thermal, electrical, radiational, for example from ultraviolet light) or associated with systemic disease.

Most conjunctivitis is bilateral. Unilateral involvement suggests a toxic or chemical origin.

Clinical Manifestations. Signs and symptoms of conjunctivitis may include hyperemia (redness), discharge, edema, tearing, itching, burning, or a "scratching" or foreign body sensation.

Signs and symptoms of gonorrheal conjunctivitis, which can threaten vision, include copious, purulent drainage and lid swelling. This disease may be transmitted to newborns and is treated initially with silver nitrate and systemic antibiotics.

Management. Conjunctivitis is usually self-limiting. However, depending on the causative factor, treatment may include systemic or topical antibiotics, anti-inflammatory agents, eye irrigation, eyelid cleaning, or warm compresses.

When conjunctivitis is caused by microorganisms, the patient should be taught how to avoid contaminating the unaffected eye and other people. The nurse can instruct the patient to avoid rubbing the affected eye and then touching the unaffected eye, to wash hands after touching the affected eye, and to use a fresh, separate washcloth, towel, and handkerchief. Special care must be taken by health care personnel to avoid spreading conjunctivitis among patients.

Trachoma

Trachoma, a chlamydial conjunctivitis, is an infectious disease that affects more than 500 million people world wide. It is the world's leading cause of preventable blindness and primarily affects people in Africa, the Middle East, and Asia. It is rare in the United States, except among Native Americans in the Southwest, and is becoming less prevalent. It is typically bilateral. Without prompt treatment trachoma involves the cornea, resulting in scarring and, often, blindness. It is spread by direct contact, fomites, and, possibly, insect vectors. Trachoma can be prevented by proper sanitation and education.

Clinical Manifestations. The principal symptoms are mild itching and irritation. After an acute inflammatory process, follicles appear on the conjunctiva. Blurring of vision and increasing discomfort occur. The upper palpebral conjunctiva are affected. Consequences of trachoma include scarring of the eyelids with ultimate entropion and **trichiasis** (inversion of eyelashes). This may expose the conjunctiva and cornea and prevent effective closure of the eyelids. In some, this ultimately results in corneal trauma and ulceration, requiring prompt treatment.

Management. Trachoma is particularly contagious and is spread by direct contact and any objects that come in contact with the eye, such as towels and washcloths. Therefore, personal cleanliness is a key prevention factor. Public education is essential in preventing the spread of trachoma. Isolating known cases and initiating antibiotic therapy early may help control the disease. If untreated, it lasts for months or years. Medical treatment consists of a 3- to 4-week course of tetracycline or sulfonamides. The World Health Organization reports great strides in eliminating this curable disease.

Pterygium

Ptergium is a triangular fibrovascular connective tissue overgrowth of the intrapalpebral bulbar conjunctiva with extension to the cornea. It usually advances from the nasal side.

The exact cause is unknown, but it is thought to be an irritative and degenerative phenomenon caused by ultraviolet light because it is common among people who spend a lot of time out of doors, especially in tropical areas. Surgical removal and partial-thickness corneal transplantation is indicated if the pterygium encroaches on the visual axis or causes significant discomfort. In 30% to 50% of patients, pterygia reoccur after surgery. Beta radiation postoperatively reduces the rate of recurrence but is not without complications. Mitomycin eye drops, an antimetabolite-antibiotic agent, have been reported effective in preventing recurrences. Mitomycin-C is an antineoplastic agent that has such side effects as inflammation, photophobia, tearing, and pain.

Conjunctival Hemorrhage

Injection of the conjunctiva is the term used to describe superficial dilation of blood vessels in the fornices that fade toward the corneoscleral limbus. The determination of conjunctival involvement can be made by inspecting for movement of the blood vessels within the movable conjunctiva. Administration of 1:1000 epinephrine solution constricts vessels in the conjunctiva.

Scleral hemorrhages tend to be confined to the corneoscleral limbus, which fades to the fornices; they are nonmovable, unresponsive to epinephrine, and dark scarlet.

Hyperemia of the conjunctiva occurs during dilation of blood vessels by external irritants, medication administration, and ocular infections. Conjunctival hemorrhage is caused by rupture of blood vessels. Conjunctival hemorrhages are usually benign and are caused by anything that produces bleeding in the body. They can result from any upper thoracic straining, such as forceful coughing or vomiting. They also may occur spontaneously. Although the patient may be alarmed about the red eye appearance, conjunctival hemorrhages produce no other symptoms. They also tend to be self-limiting, reabsorbed within about 2 weeks, and do not require treatment.

Disorders of the Cornea

Because of its refractive function, the cornea plays a vital role in visual acuity. Disorders of the cornea can greatly affect and ultimately threaten vision.

The surface of the cornea is convex, and its smooth optical surface contributes to sharpness of vision. Irregularities in the shape of the cornea and variation in its thickness may impair vision.

Trauma, infection, congenital anomalies, tumors, and inherited or acquired disorders of the cornea may impair its function. Scarring, opacifications, and alteration in corneal architecture may result in mild to severe visual loss.

Because there are many nonmyelinated nerve fibers in the cornea, most corneal lesions cause pain, photophobia, and tearing. Pain may be severe, may seem disproportionate to the amount of damage, and may incapacitate the individual. Movement of the eyelids over the cornea increases pain, which usually persists until healing is complete. Although topical anesthetics relieve this discomfort, they also interfere with healing and are contraindicated for long-term use. Because corneal lesions interfere with the cornea's ability to transmit and refract light, the patient usually reports blurred vision.

Corneal edema is a common sign of corneal disorders. The integrity of the endothelium and epithelium is vital to the cornea's function and clear state. The epithelium forms a barrier to external fluids, whereas the endothelium removes stromal fluid. If either function is lost (as in epithelial hypoxia from hard contact lenses, or increases in IOP exceeding 50 mm Hg), the cornea may become edematous. This appears as a dull haziness of the cornea. Some epithelial edemas are effectively treated with topical hyperosmotic agents to "draw" the excess fluid from the epithelium. Corneal thickness can be measured to determine the degree of swelling or thickness. Increased thickness may indicate endothelial cell failure.

Corneal Abrasions

Corneal abrasions are defects in the epithelial layer. They may be caused by trauma, foreign bodies, contact lenses worn for a prolonged time, defects in the tear film, difficulty with eyelid closure, or malposition of the eyelids or eyelashes. Corneal abrasions and foreign bodies are more fully discussed in the section on ocular trauma. Recurrent corneal abrasions, which may result from rubbing the eye, are treated with artificial lubricating ointment at bedtime or a bandage-type soft contact lens (a nonprescription contact lens that is used to protect the cornea from irritation caused by lid movement).

Microbial Keratitis

The cornea is particularly susceptible to infection and injury because of its anterior location and degree of exposure. People who cannot blink effectively, because of neurologic disorders or level of consciousness, are particularly vulnerable to corneal drying and irritation. Infections may cause ulcerations in the corneal surface and ultimately may result in loss of an intact globe (eyeball) and anterior chamber patency.

Microbial keratitis (infection of the cornea) can be caused by a various bacterial, viral, fungal, or parasitic organisms. Even small abrasions are a port for bacteria. Most infections of the cornea occur as a result of trauma or compromised systemic or local defense mechanisms. Moreover, systemic corticosteroid therapy modifies the immune reaction, and long-term use allows opportunistic organisms to invade the cornea.

Corneal ulcers can develop from corneal infections. These ulcers are identified by slit-lamp examination after instilling fluorescein drops to demonstrate the geography or shape and size of the ulcer under a special light. Fluorescein dye adheres to areas denuded of corneal epithelium. Various organisms produce various characteristic designs that are helpful in diagnosis. A small spatula is used to scrape epithelial cells from the cornea for examination and microbial analysis.

Clinical Manifestations. Marked inflammation of the globe, sensation of a foreign body in the eye, mucopurulent discharge with the eyelids stuck together on awakening, epithelial ulceration, and **hypopyon** (pus in the anterior chamber) may indicate corneal infection. In advanced disease, there may be perforation of the cornea, extrusion of the iris, and endophthalmitis. Culture and sensitivity tests are necessary to confirm the diagnosis and to identify the causative pathogen.

Management. Patients with severe corneal infections are usually hospitalized to allow frequent administration (as often as every 30 minutes) of antimicrobial drops and regular examination by the ophthalmologist. Meticulous handwashing is imperative. Gloves are worn whenever nursing interventions involve the eye. The lids are kept clean, and cool compresses may be ordered. The patient is monitored for signs of increased IOP. Acetaminophen may be required for pain management. Cycloplegics and mydriatics may be prescribed to alleviate pain and inflammation. Patching and bandage-type soft contact lenses are avoided until after the infection has been controlled, because they encourage microbial growth. They then may be required to facilitate healing of epithelial defects.

Corneal ulcers that invade down to Bowman's membrane result in scarring. This scar is opaque and interferes with clear passage of light. Chronic corneal infections may also promote the development of new blood vessels (known as **neovascularization**) in the cornea. Neovascularization, along with scarring, renders the cornea irregularly opaque and interferes with visual acuity. Corneal transplantation is a surgical treatment for scarring of the cornea, whether it is from infectious or traumatic causes.

Nursing care of the patient after transplantation involves appropriate follow-up examinations, drop instillation, ophthalmic hygiene, and prevention of postoperative complications. Patient education, in terms of understanding and meticulously following the physician's instructions, is crucial to the successful reception of a donor cornea.

Exposure Keratitis

Exposure keratitis may develop whenever the cornea is inadequately moistened and protected by the eyelids. Corneal drying occurs and may be followed by ulceration and secondary infection. Exposure of the cornea may result from conditions such as exophthalmos, paresis of CN VII (facial nerve), or Bell's palsy, but it also may be of concern in the patient who is comatose or anesthetized.

Management. Taping the lids or light patching of the lubricated eye in those with decreased sensorium protects the cornea. For others, a bandage-type soft contact lens may be indicated.

A bandage-type soft contact lens is fitted to preserve the corneal surface, encourage healing of epithelial defects, and provide comfort. Its use may be indicated in corneal dystrophies, persistent epithelial erosions, complications after corneal surgery, infectious keratitis (after the infection is controlled), dry eyes, and chemical burns.

Contraindications are active infection, immunosuppression, being bedridden, and poor hygienic practices. The patient must be reliable and able to comply with a follow-up examination schedule. Possible complications of bandage-type soft contact lenses include infection, corneal infiltrates, hypopyon (pus in the anterior chamber), corneal edema, corneal neovascularization, and contact lens deposits.

A collagen shield may be used when short-term corneal protection is required. The shield resembles a contact lens in shape but is made from a porcine scleral collagen that has been dehydrated and sterilized. The eye is anesthetized before application. Once the shield is applied, it conforms to the shape of the cornea and absorbs fluid from the tears. It dissolves over 24 to 72 hours, depending on the type. The shield provides lubrication and protection to the cornea without the complications of a contact lens.

The collagen shield may be hydrated initially with an antibiotic solution to provide high, sustained antibiotic levels over a long period. Subsequent topical medications also may be administered. Collagen shields are used to protect the cornea after injury and to deliver medications after cataract extraction and penetrating keratoplasty and to facilitate treatment of severe infection.

Corneal Dystrophies

Corneal dystrophies are inherited, bilateral alterations of the cornea with abnormal deposition of substances. They are of unknown origin. The effects on vision depend on the type of dystrophy, age of the patient, and possible complications such as recurrent erosions.

Fuchs's Dystrophy. Fuchs's dystrophy affects the corneal endothelium and compromises its pump mechanism. The disorder becomes evident during the third or fourth decade and is slowly progressive. Women are more often affected than men. Endothelial decomposition results in corneal edema, opacification, scarring, and visual impairment. This disorder can be successfully treated in its early stages by corneal transplantation, provided all diseased tissue is removed.

Keratoconus

Keratoconus is a noninflammatory, progressive thinning of the cornea, which assumes a conical configuration. It usually becomes evident during puberty and affects women more frequently than men. It is usually bilateral. Blurring and distortion of vision are the earliest symptoms. As the disease progresses, irregular astigmatism and high myopia cannot be corrected with eyeglasses. The patient must wear hard or soft toric contact lenses (special lenses to correct astigmatism) or undergo corneal transplantation. Transplantation of the diseased cornea has a 95% success rate. Patients are advised to avoid rubbing their eyes, because vigorous rubbing can contribute to the disease process.

Management: Corneal Transplantation

Penetrating keratoplasty, or **corneal transplantation,** is the microsurgical, full-thickness replacement of the cornea with tissue from a human donor (Fig. 56-8). Trephines (circular blades) are used to incise both the damaged recipient and the healthy donor cornea in "cookie-cutter" fashion. The new corneal button replaces the native cornea and is secured in the recipient eye with very fine suture material.

This procedure may be combined with cataract extraction or intraocular lens (IOL) insertion. Patients who require corneal transplantation are placed on a computerized eye

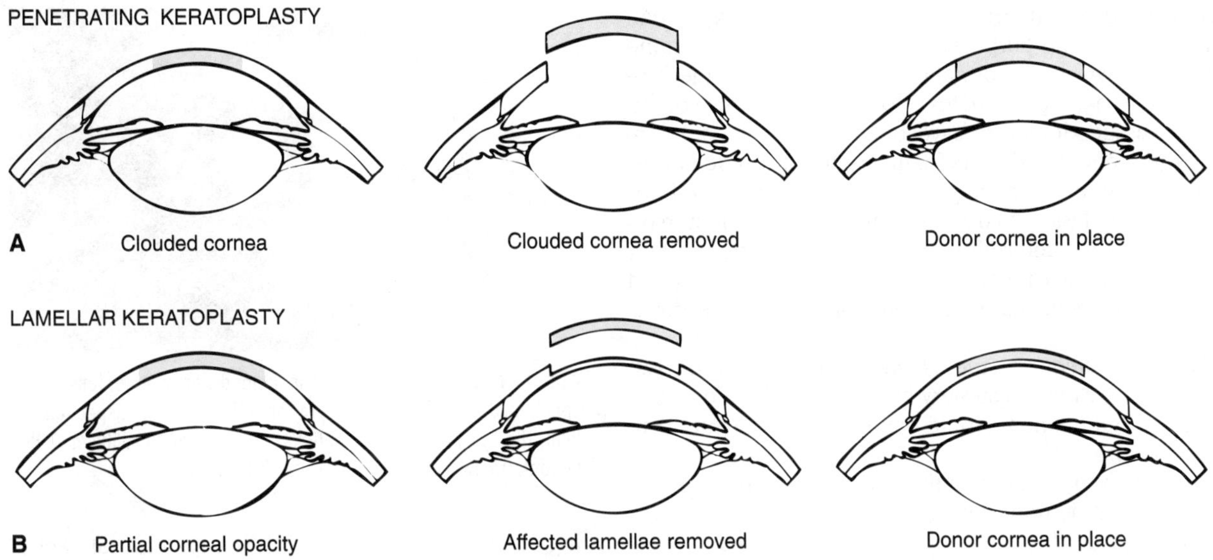

FIGURE 56-8. Full and partial corneal transplantation. (**A**) Penetrating keratoplasty: a full-thickness (7- to 8-mm) disc is removed from the host and replaced with a matching full-thickness button from the donor. (**B**) Lamellar keratoplasty: a thin layer of corneal tissue is excised from the host eye, sparing the stroma and entire endothelium.

bank waiting list. When a suitable cornea becomes available, surgery is scheduled at once. For best results, the donor cornea should be removed from the donor within 8 to 10 hours of death (to prevent softening of the cornea).

Penetrating keratoplasty (PKP) is used to restore vision in patients with corneal dystrophies, corneal degenerations, keratoconus, resolved microbial keratitis, traumatic scarring, corneal pigmentation, and chemical burns.

Possible complications of surgery include hemorrhage, epithelial defects, wound leaks, glaucoma, and graft rejection. Partial-thickness (lamellar), nonpenetrating keratoplasty involves grafting only selected layers of donor cornea to replace diseased tissue. **Epikeratoplasty** is a surgical procedure in which the donor cornea is grafted onto the existing cornea denuded of epithelium. Epikeratoplasty is now possible without the use of sutures, which reduces operative time and surgical trauma. Keratoprostheses are artificial corneal implants. They are used in individuals who experience repeated failure of donor grafts or who have a significant underlying disorder preventing conventional surgery.

Preoperative Nursing Interventions. Because keratoplasty is elective surgery, there is generally ample time for the patient to receive preoperative instruction and to understand the nature of the surgical procedure. Most patients are optimistic about the likelihood of improved vision. The nurse, nevertheless, must allow the patient time to express concerns or ask questions that the patient may still have. Physically, the patient should be free of respiratory or eye infections to promote postoperative healing.

Postoperative Nursing Interventions. Goals for postoperative nursing care are (1) to monitor for and avoid activities that will cause an elevation of IOP as well as pressure on the affected eye, (2) to rest the eye so that healing progresses smoothly, and (3) to institute measures that will prevent infection of the eye.

Elevated IOP reduces the vascular supply and can cause optic nerve atrophy and damage to the graft. To prevent pressure from increasing within the eye, the nurse must be cognizant of those activities that can elevate pressure (sneezing, coughing, straining during defecation, or lifting heavy objects). Loss of aqueous humor through the suture line could cause prolapse of the iris, adhesions of the iris to the cornea, or malformation of the anterior chamber. If IOP is elevated, pharmacologic control can be achieved with such medications as acetazolamide, which inhibits the production of aqueous humor.

Healing is slow because the cornea is avascular, which also increases the possibility of infection. Thus, meticulous sterile technique is followed in dressing changes to protect the susceptible corneal epithelium from infection. Antibiotic ointments or drops or a collagen shield hydrated with antibiotic solution may be used prophylactically.

Rejection of the donor graft is the primary cause of corneal transplant failure. Rejection is more common in younger recipients, in those who receive bilateral or repeated grafts, and in those with corneas that were neovascularized preoperatively. A decrease in vision is the first sign of rejection, which may not be evident for weeks to years. New blood vessels (neovascularization) and precipitates may develop in the graft. Treatment of rejection with corticosteroids carries a good prognosis when initiated early.

Eye Donation

Donation of the eyes is a benevolent gesture at the time of death. Eye donation is considered tissue donation and can be done at almost any age. Harvesting of the eyeball may be accomplished by a trained individual at the bedside or in a medical examiner's office. Usually the entire globe (eyeball) is enucleated, placed in preservative solution, and maintained in a controlled, cool environment. Many parts of the eye, primarily corneal and scleral tissue, can be used for grafting purposes. It is important to determine the patient's wishes for donation on admission to the hospital (required in most states). Required requests for organ and tissue donation have been implemented to increase the umbers of donors for the high existing demands. Significant value is placed on one's eyes, and sometimes it is an motional issue to donate them. It is often the nurse's responsibility to determine the patient's wishes, either by a conversation with the patient or with the designated sur-rogate for health care decisions, or by advance directives.

Patient Education and Home Care Considerations. Corneal transplantation surgery has restored sight for many people, and many more would benefit if donor tissue were available. Nurses can play a vital role, both professionally and personally, by educating the public about the need for eye donation. It is important for people to know that they can make a vital difference by providing the means to restore sight, and that anyone may become an eye donor by completing a donor card or authorizing donation on the back of the driver's license. The decision to become a future donor should be shared with significant others or a designated health care surrogate so that the appropriate action can be taken when needed. If the decision is not made and documented before death, the next of kin may consent to donating the eyes after death. Family members may be reassured by knowing the following:

- There will be no visible sign of disfigurement after procurement.
- The body will be treated with respect.
- The donation will not interfere with funeral arrangements.
- There is no cost to the family.
- The donation will remain confidential.

The following criteria are used for selecting corneal transplant donors.

- Known time of death (eyes should be obtained within 6 hours of death)
- Probable cause of death
- No sepsis or transmissible infectious disease (such as human immunodeficiency virus [HIV], hepatitis B)
- Age over 26 weeks of gestation. No upper age limit, although, because older eyes have lost some endothelium, corneas from younger persons are more desirable.

When patients are pronounced brain dead and their corneas will be donated, it is important to maintain care of the eyes. This eye care includes protecting the surfaces of the eyes and keeping them moist. Saline solution is instilled every 2 to 4 hours, and the lids are taped shut and covered with moist gauze. Using eye ointment is contraindicated. Any eyes not suitable for transplantation can be used in one of many valuable eye research projects.

Disorders of the Lens: Cataracts

A cataract is any opacification of the normally clear, transparent crystalline lens (Fig. 56-9). It is usually a result of aging but may be present at birth (congenital cataract). It may also be associated with blunt or penetrating trauma, long-term corticosteroid use, systemic disease, such as diabetes mellitus or hypoparathyroidism, radiation exposure, exposure to long hours of bright sunlight (ultraviolet light), or other eye disorders such as anterior uveitis.

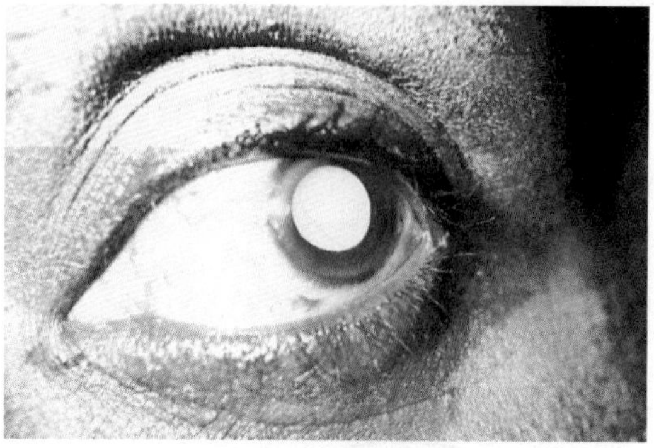

FIGURE 56-9. A cataract is a cloudy, or opaque, lens. On visual inspection, the cataract appears gray or milky white. On inspection with a penlight, the eye lacks the red reflex. (Courtesy of Dr. William C. Byrne, OD, Optometric Eyecare Center, Fairless Hills, PA.)

Pathophysiology

The normal lens is a clear, transparent, button-like structure posterior to the iris; it possesses strong refractive powers. The lens consists of three anatomic components. In the central zone is the **nucleus,** peripherally is the **cortex,** and surrounding both is an anterior and posterior **capsule.** With aging, the nucleus takes on a yellowish brown hue. Surrounding opacities are spokelike white densities occurring anteriorly and posteriorly to the nucleus. Opacity of the posterior capsule is the most significant form of cataract—it has the appearance of frost on a window.

Physical and chemical changes in the lens may produce a loss of transparency. Changes in the multiple fine fibers (zonules) that extend from the ciliary body to the outer circumference of the lens, for example, may cause the person to complain of distorted images. A chemical change in lens protein may cause coagulation, thereby clouding vision by blocking the passage of light to the retina. One theory is that a breakdown in normal lens protein occurs with an influx of water into the lens. This process disrupts the tight lens fibers and interferes with the transmission of light. Another theory poses that an enzyme plays a part in protecting the lens from degeneration. The amount of the enzyme decreases with aging and is absent in many patients with cataracts.

Cataracts usually develop bilaterally, but at differing rates. They can be caused by traumatic or systemic events, such as diabetes, but are typically a consequence of normal aging. Most cataracts develop chronically and "mature" as one approaches the seventh decade. Cataracts may be congenital and should be identified early, because a missed diagnosis may lead to amblyopia and permanent visual loss. The most common factors that contribute to cataract development include ultraviolet-B radiation, medications, alcohol, smoking, diabetes, and inadequate intake over time of antioxidant vitamins.

Clinical Manifestations

Cataracts are diagnosed primarily by subjective symptoms. Typically, patients report diminished visual acuity and glare and some degree of functional impairment caused by this visual loss. Objective findings usually include a grayish, pearly haze of the pupil so that the retina cannot be visualized with an ophthalmoscope.

As the lens becomes opaque, it scatters light instead of transmitting a sharply focused image on the retina. The result is a disabling glare, dimmed or blurred vision with distorted images, and poor night vision (Fig. 56-10). The pupil, which is normally black, may appear yellowish, gray, or white. Cataracts usually develop gradually over a period of years, and as the cataract worsens, stronger corrective lenses no longer improve sight.

People with cataracts typically develop strategies to avoid the disabling glare that is caused by extraneous light. For example, some rearrange the furniture in their homes so that lights do not shine directly in their eyes. Some wear a wide-brimmed hat or sunglasses and lower the visor while driving during the day.

Diagnostic Evaluation

In addition to the usual eye tests, keratometry, and slit-lamp and ophthalmoscopic examinations, A-scan ultrasound (echography) and the endothelial cell count are particularly useful diagnostic tools, especially if surgery is being considered. With an endothelial cell count of 2000 cells/mm^3, the patient is a good candidate for phacoemulsification and implantation of an IOL.

Management

There is no medical treatment for cataracts, and they cannot be removed with laser surgery. However, investigation is in progress with a new laser procedure used to liquefy the lens before suctioning it out through a cannula (Pokalo, 1992).

If vision can be corrected with pupillary dilators and strong refraction to a point that the patient can carry on activities of daily living, then treatment is usually conservative. It is important to assess the effect of a cataract on the patient's daily life. Assessing the degree of impairment of daily functions, such as grooming, ambulation, recreational activities, driving, and ability to work, is essential in deciding which treatment best suits the individual.

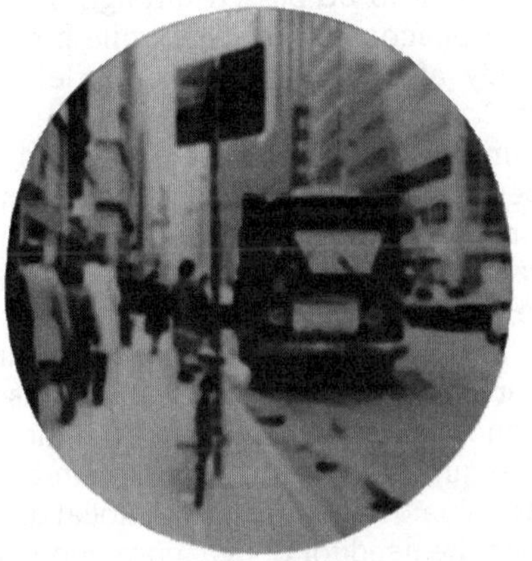

FIGURE 56-10. A person with cataracts experiences diminished acuity because the lens of the eye becomes opaque. The field of vision is unaffected and there is no scotoma (vision loss or depression). What the person sees, however, appears hazy, particularly in glaring light. (Courtesy of The Lighthouse, The New York Association for the Blind.)

Surgery may be indicated for those who require acute vision for work or safety. It is usually indicated when the best corrected vision is 20/50 or worse, if visual acuity interferes with the safety or quality of life, or if visualizing the posterior segment is necessary to evaluate progression of certain diseases of the retina or optic nerve, such as diabetes and glaucoma.

Cataract surgery is the most frequently performed surgery in people older than age 65. Today cataracts are most often removed under local anesthesia on an outpatient basis, although patients may be hospitalized when it is medically indicated. Successful return to useful vision is accomplished in more than 95% of patients.

Decisions to have surgery are highly individualized. Financial and psychosocial support and consequences of surgery should be evaluated, because this is important for postoperative management of the patient.

Most surgeries are performed under local (retrobullar or peribulbar) anesthesia, which immobilizes the eye. Antianxiety medications may be administered to allay claustrophobic feelings related to surgical draping. General anesthesia may be needed for those who cannot take local anesthetics, who cannot cooperate for physical or psychological reasons, or who do not respond to local anesthesia.

Two surgical techniques are available for cataract removal: intracapsular and extracapsular extraction (Fig. 56-11). The indications for surgical intervention are loss of vision that interferes with the patient's normal activities or a cataract that causes glaucoma or interferes with the diagnosis and treatment of other ocular disorders, such as diabetic retinopathy.

Intracapsular Cataract Extraction

Intracapsular cataract extraction (ICCE) is the removal of the entire intact lens as a unit. After the zonules are separated, the lens is removed by a cryoprobe, which is placed directly on the lens capsule. **Cryosurgery** relies on freezing temperatures to remove a lesion or abnormality. The cryosurgical instrument operates on the principle that a cold metal adheres to a moist object. When the cryoprobe is placed directly on the lens capsule, the capsule adheres to the probe. The lens is gently removed. Formerly the primary mode of cataract removal, ICCE is a rare procedure today because of the availability of more sophisticated surgical techniques.

Extracapsular Cataract Extraction

Extracapsular cataract extraction (ECCE) is currently the more preferred technique and accounts for approximately 98% of cataract surgeries. A microscope is used for visualizing the eye structure during the surgery. The procedure involves removing the anterior capsule, expressing the lens nucleus, and aspirating the remaining soft cortical fragments using irrigation and suction. Leaving the posterior capsule and lens zonules intact preserves the architecture

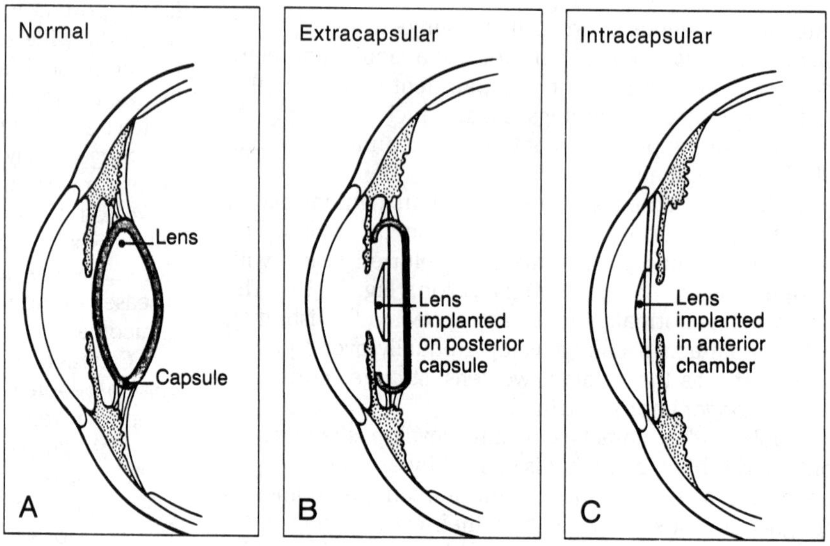

FIGURE 56-11. Cataract extraction surgeries. (**A**) Cross section of normal eye anatomy. (**B**) Extracapsular lens extraction involves removing the lens but leaving the posterior capsule intact to receive a synthetic intraocular lens. (**C**) Intracapsular lens extraction involves removing the lens and lens capsule and implanting a synthetic intraocular lens in the anterior chamber. (Reproduced with permission from Patient Care, Patient Care Communications, Inc, Darien CT. Artist, Paul J. Singh-Roy. All rights reserved.)

of the posterior portion of the eye, thus reducing the incidence of serious complications.

Phacoemulsification is the most recent innovation in extracapsular extraction. It permits the removal of the lens through a smaller incision by using a high-frequency ultrasound device to fragment the lens nucleus and cortex into small particles that are then aspirated through the same hand piece that also provides continuous irrigation. This technique requires less convalescent time and decreases the incidence of postoperative astigmatism. Both the irrigation-aspiration and phacoemulsification techniques preserve the posterior capsule, which is used to support an IOL.

Cataract extraction and IOL implantation also can be performed in conjunction with corneal transplantation or surgery for glaucoma.

Lens Replacement. Because the crystalline lens is responsible for one third of the focusing power of the eye, whenever the lens is removed, the patient requires optical correction. This correction can be provided by one of three methods: aphakic spectacles, contact lenses, or an IOL implant.

Aphakic spectacles provide good central vision. The 25% to 30% magnification, however, results in a corresponding reduction in and distortion of peripheral vision, which causes difficulty in evaluating spatial relations, making objects seem much closer than they really are. These eyeglasses also cause spherical aberrations, turning straight lines into curves. Binocular vision is not possible unless the lens has been removed from both eyes. There is usually a lengthy period of adjustment until the patient can coordinate movements, judge distances, and function safely with a limited visual field. Aphakic glasses are typically thick and cumbersome and make the eyes appear unusually large.

Contact lenses are far less visually disabling than aphakic spectacles. There is no significant magnification (5% to 10%), no spherical aberration, no decrease in visual field, and no false spatial orientation. These lenses provide almost complete visual rehabilitation for those who can master insertion, removal, and maintenance and who can wear them comfortably. Many elderly people have diminished manual dexterity, making hygienic care of daily-wear contact lenses difficult. For some patients, extended-wear lenses may provide a reasonable alternative; however, extended-wear lenses require frequent office visits for removal and cleaning. They are also expensive and often need replacement because of loss or breakage. Another disadvantage is the increased risk of infectious keratitis.

Intraocular lens (IOL) implants offer an alternative to the thick, heavy aphakic glasses used to correct postoperative vision. IOL implants have become the optical correction of choice largely because of refinements in microsurgical techniques and improvements in IOL design. An IOL is a plastic permanent lens that is surgically implanted in the eye. It produces images that are normal in size and shape. Because IOLs eliminate the disabling optical effects of aphakic spectacles and the inconvenience of contact lenses, approximately 97% of cataract surgeries (more than a million each year) are performed with IOL insertion.

A recent development is a lens that can be folded for insertion, allowing it to be passed through the smaller incision made for phacoemulsification while preserving a full-size lens body after implantation. This lens insertion is possible with "no- or one-stitch" surgeries.

Approximately 95% of IOLs are positioned in the posterior chamber, and the remaining 5% in the anterior chamber. Anterior chamber lenses are used for patients who have had an intracapsular extraction or who have had the posterior capsule inadvertently ruptured during an extracapsular procedure. The combination of extracapsular extraction and posterior lens insertion is preferred because it carries a lower incidence of sight-threatening complications. Many patients still require some form of refraction after IOL insertion for near vision. The advent of multifocal diffractive IOLs has decreased the need for optical correction in nearly half its recipients, according to recent FDA reports (Roy & Tindall, 1993).

There are several contraindications for IOL implantation, including recurrent uveitis, proliferative diabetic retinopathy, and neovascular glaucoma.

Complications. Although there is an excellent chance for full visual recovery after cataract extraction or IOL implantation, there is some risk of complications. Corneal endothelial damage, pupillary block, glaucoma, hemorrhage, wound fistula, cystoid macular edema, choroidal detachment, uveitis, and endophthalmitis have been observed. The IOL may become malpositioned. It may be repositioned with the sequential use of dilating drops, head positioning and the use of constricting drops, or the patient may require additional surgery to reposition or remove the IOL.

A common complication of surgery is the formation of secondary membranes, which occurs in about 25% of patients within 3 to 36 months after surgery. The membranes may be erroneously referred to as an opacification of the posterior capsule or as secondary cataracts. These membranes are formed as a result of proliferation of residual lens epithelium. They interfere with vision by impeding the passage of light and increasing glare disability. An opening through the membranes (capsulotomy) can be made with a needle or with laser (Yag laser) surgery to reestablish vision.

Cataract surgery is commonly performed in outpatient surgical settings. If the patient has bilateral cataracts requiring ECCE, only one procedure is performed at one time. Usually a waiting period of 6 to 8 weeks is recommended between the two surgeries.

Patient Education and Home Care Considerations. After a brief postoperative recovery period after cataract extraction or IOL implantation, the patient is discharged with instructions about eye medications, cleaning and protection, activity level and restrictions, diet, pain control, positioning, office appointments, the expected postoperative course, and symptoms that are to be reported immediately to the surgeon (see Chart 56-3). It is preferable that this education be reinforced postoperatively and appropriate arrangements for home care be made. The patient is instructed to make arrangements for transportation home, care during that evening, and transportation for a follow-up visit to the surgeon the next day. Determining the need for home health aides is important before surgery.

Patients usually progress rather quickly to normal daily activities. However, bending and lifting heavy objects are restricted for approximately 1 week, depending on the type of surgery performed. An eye shield worn at night and eyeglasses (sunglasses when outdoors in bright light) during the day are necessary for about 2 weeks to protect the eye from injury. This need for protection must be stressed because many patients who have had cataracts removed are older and at risk for falling; blunt trauma to the eye could rupture the globe, causing loss of vision. Patients are usually given a new prescription for eye glasses within 6 to 8 weeks after surgery. See Nursing Care Plan 56-1 for perioperative care of the eye patient.

Disorders of the Uveal Tract

The uveal tract, consisting of the iris, ciliary body, and choroid, is subject to systemic and infectious diseases. Diabetes contributes to neovascularization of the iris, which may appear visibly as tangled tortuous blood vessels (rubeosis irides). There are congenital disorders of the uveal tract

(text continues on page 1618)

CHART 56-3
Patient Education: Self-care After Cataract Surgery

Note: Review with patient or significant other or caregiver. Print directions in large letters using felt-tipped pen for strong contrast.

Activity Limitations

Permissible

- Watch television; read if necessary but use moderation
- Do usual activities in moderation
- At first, "sponge bath"; later, use tub or shower (with assistance)
- Do not bend over sink or tub; tilt head slightly backward when washing hair
- Sleep with protective perforated metal eye shield at night; wear glasses during the day
- When sleeping, lie on back or side, not abdomen
- Sedentary activities
- Wear sunglasses for comfort
- Kneel or squat when picking up something from the floor

Avoid (for approximately 1 week)

- Sleeping on affected side
- Rubbing eyes; squeezing eyelids shut
- Straining at bowel movements
- Getting soap near eyes
- Lifting anything heavier than 15 pounds
- Sexual relations until ______(date)
- Driving, if possible
- Coughing, sneezing, and vomiting
- Bending head down below waist; bend knees only and keep back straight to pick up something from the floor

Medications and Eye Care

- Use medications as directed.
- Wash hands before and after instilling eye medications.
- Clean around eye with sterile cotton balls or gauze pads moistened with sterile water or normal saline solution; wipe eyelid gently from inner corner to outer corner.
- To instill eye drops, be seated and tilt head back; gently pull down lower eyelid margin.
- Wear protective, perforated metal eye shield at night; wear glasses during the day.
- Take all eye medications exactly as prescribed so that dosages can be checked and adjusted by the physician at the first return visit.

Report Unusual Signs and Symptoms

- Pain in and around eyes, persistent headaches
- Any pain not relieved by prescribed pain medication
- Pain accompanied by ocular redness, swelling, or drainage; inflammation, discharge from eyes
- Sudden onset of brow pain
- Changes in visual acuity, blurring, double vision, a film over visual field, light flashes, showers or spots before eyes, halos around lights

NURSING CARE PLAN 56–1

Perioperative Care of the Eye Patient (Cataract, Retina, Glaucoma, Cornea)

Nursing Interventions	Rationale	Expected Outcomes
NURSING DIAGNOSIS: Fear or anxiety related to sensory impairment and lack of understanding about postoperative care, medication administration		
GOAL: Reduction of emotional stress, fear, and depression; acceptance of surgery and understanding of instructions		
1. Assess degree and duration of visual impairment. Encourage conversation to determine patient's concerns, feelings, and level of understanding. Answer questions, offer support, assist patient to devise methods for coping.	1. Information can replace fear of the unknown. Coping mechanisms can help patients to deal with worry, fear, depression, tension, resentment, anger, and rejection.	• Verbalizes understanding of received information. • Uses methods for coping and is able to relax. • Is able to locate call bell, foods on dinner tray, furnishings, bathroom. • Verbalizes understanding of perioperative events and complies with directions and therapeutic regimen. • Is not startled or frightened by interactions or environment. • Participates in ADL as ability allows. • Recognizes limitations. • Family or significant others assist patient with care as needed. • Participates in social and diversional activities of interest as allowed or able.
2. Orient patient to new surroundings.	2. Familiarity with environment helps to decrease anxiety and increase safety.	
3. Explain perioperative routine. *Preoperative:* Level of activity, dietary restriction, medications. *Intraoperative:* Importance of lying still during surgery or giving surgeon warning of need to cough or change position. Face covered with drapes, and O_2 provided. Unfamiliar noises from equipment. Monitoring, including frequent BP measurements. *Postoperative:* Positioning, patching, level of activity, importance of assistance with ambulation until stable and vision adequate.	3. An informed patient is more likely to accept treatment and comply with instructions.	
4. Explain interventions in detail; announce yourself with each interaction; interpret unfamiliar sounds; use touch to assist with verbal communication.	4. Patients who are visually impaired depend on other sensory input for information.	
5. Encourage to carry out ADL as ability allows. Order finger foods for those who can not see well enough or do not have the coping skills to use utensils.	5. Self-care and independence will promote feelings of well-being.	
6. Encourage participation of family or significant others in patient care.	6. Patient may not be able to perform all tasks related to treatment and self-care.	
7. Encourage participation in social and diversional activities as allowed (visitor, radio, audio tapes, book tapes, TV, crafts, games).	7. Social isolation and prolonged unoccupied time may result in negative feelings.	
NURSING DIAGNOSIS: Risk for injury related to visual impairment or knowledge deficit		
GOAL: Prevention of injury		
1. Assist patient when able to ambulate postoperatively until stable and has adequate vision or coping skills (remember that bilaterally patched patients are unable to see), using the sighted guide technique	1. Reduces risk of falling or injury when gait unsteady or without coping skills for visual impairment.	• Requests assistance with ambulation when indicated. • Able to maneuver safely in environment. • Wears appropriate eye protective device during prescribed timeframe.

(continued)

NURSING CARE PLAN 56–1 *(continued)*
Perioperative Care of the Eye Patient (Cataract, Retina, Glaucoma, Cornea)

Nursing Interventions	Rationale	Expected Outcomes
2. Assist patient in arranging environment. Do not rearrange furnishings without re-orienting patient.	2. Facilitates independence and reduces risk of injury.	• Manipulation of the lids is accomplished by resting fingers only on the bony orbits (see section on eye trauma). • No injury occurs to eye.
3. Orient patient to room.	3. Promotes safe mobility in the environment	
4. Discuss need for wearing metal shield or glasses when ordered.	4. Metal shield or glasses protect the eye from injury.	
5. Apply *no* pressure to the traumatized eye.	5. Pressure on the eye could result in serious further damage.	
6. Use proper procedure to administer eye medications.	6. Injury may result if the medication container is allowed to touch the eye.	

COLLABORATIVE PROBLEMS: Infection of surgical site or other ocular structures, retinal detachment, increased IOP, perforation of surgical site.

GOAL: Complications will be avoided or reported promptly to the physician.

Nursing Interventions	Rationale	Expected Outcomes
1. Maintain rigorous aseptic technique; perform frequent handwashing.	1. Will minimize risk of infection.	• No signs of infection. • Signs and symptoms of complications are recognized early and reported immediately. • Required position is maintained. • Activity limitations are observed. • Avoids restricted actions. • Demonstrates proper technique for administration of eye medications
2. Observe for and report immediately to the physician signs and symptoms of complications, *i.e.,* hemorrhage; increased IOP (sudden brow pain); infection (redness, edema, purulent drainage); pain not relieved by prescribed medication; light flashes; changes or decrease in visual function; changes in eye structure (iris prolapse, pear-shaped pupil, wound dehiscence); adverse reactions to medications.	2. Early recognition of complications may reduce the risk of permanent visual loss.	
3. Explain prescribed position.	3. Head elevation and avoiding lying on the operative side will decrease amount of edema. Maintaining the prescribed position when a gas bubble has been placed in the vitreous body will promote retinal reattachment and reduce the risk of cataract formation or corneal endothelial damage.	
4. Instruct the patient regarding activity limitations—bed rest, with bathroom privileges; increase in activities gradually as tolerated.	4. Activity limitations may be prescribed to facilitate healing and avoid further damage to the eye or injury.	
5. Explain actions to be avoided, as prescribed—coughing, sneezing, vomiting (request medication for), bending, excessive straining at defecation, lifting heavy objects (more than 20 pounds), squeezing eyes shut, rubbing eyes, fast jerky head motions.	5. May produce complications such as vitreal prolapse or wound dehiscence due to increased wound tension on very fine sutures.	

(continued)

NURSING CARE PLAN 56–1 *(continued)*
Perioperative Care of the Eye Patient (Cataract, Retina, Glaucoma, Cornea)

Nursing Interventions	Rationale	Expected Outcomes
6. Administer medications as prescribed, following prescribed technique.	6. Medications administered other than as prescribed may compromise healing or cause complications. If the container is allowed to touch the eye, there is an increased risk for infection from the contaminated medication.	

NURSING DIAGNOSIS: Pain related to trauma, increased IOP, inflammation surgical intervention, or instillation of dilating drops.

GOAL: Reduction of pain and IOP.

Nursing Interventions	Rationale	Expected Outcomes
1. Administer medications for pain and IOP control as prescribed. 2. Apply cold compresses as ordered for blunt trauma. 3. Reduce light levels; light dimmed, shades/drapes drawn. 4. Encourage use of dark glasses in strong light.	1. Use of prescribed medication relieves pain and IOP and increases comfort. 2. Decrease in edema reduces pain. 3. Lower light levels may be more comfortable after surgery. 4. Strong light causes discomfort after the use of dilating drops.	• Verbalizes that pain and IOP are reduced. • Edema relieved. • Verbalizes increase in comfort. • Wears dark glasses after instilling dilating drops.

NURSING DIAGNOSIS: Potential for self-care deficit related to impaired vision.

GOAL: Able to meet self-care needs

Nursing Interventions	Rationale	Expected Outcomes
1. Instruct patient and significant other regarding signs and symptoms of complications to be reported immediately to the physician. 2. Provide verbal and written instructions for patient and significant other on proper technique to administer medications. Discuss indications for use of medication as well as normal and abnormal responses. Suggest methods for identifying containers (red top, green label). 3. Evaluate need for assistance after discharge. Ascertain availability of help by significant others or arrange for appropriate referrals. 4. Teach patient and family sighted-guide technique	1. Early recognition and treatment of complications may reduce the risk for further damage. 2. Use of proper technique will reduce the risk of infection and injury to the eye. Knowledge of normal drug responses may increase compliance. Knowledge of abnormal responses will help in decision regarding reportable changes. Written instructions are used for reenforcement after discharge. 3. Resources are available for home health, escort, and companion services. 4. Allows safe movement in environment	• Verbalizes signs and symptoms to be reported. • Patient and significant other verbalize or demonstrate understanding of correct technique for administering medications and the normal and abnormal drug responses. • Identifies needs for assistance. • Appropriate referrals made. • Patient and caregiver demonstrate safe mobility using the sighted-guide technique

as well: absence of all (aniridia) or part (coloboma) of the iris, absence of portions of the choroidal layer, and differing color of the irides are examples.

Uveitis

Uveitis is the inflammation of one or all structures of the uveal tract. Because the uvea contains many of the blood vessels that nourish the eye and because it borders many other parts of the eye, inflammation of this layer may threaten vision. Causative factors include allergens, bacteria, fungi, viruses, chemicals, trauma, and systemic illness such as sarcoidosis or ulcerative colitis.

Clinical Manifestations and Management. **Acute anterior uveitis** (iritis) is the most common type, and is characterized by a history of pain, photophobia, blurring of vision, and red eye. Dilating drops are instituted immediately to prevent scar formation and adhesion to the lens (synechiae), which may cause glaucoma by impeding aqueous outflow. Local corticosteroids are used to decrease the inflammation, and sunglasses and pain management provide symptomatic relief.

Intermediate uveitis (pars planitis, chronic cyclitis) is characterized by "floating spots" in the field of vision. Topical or injected corticosteroids are used in severe cases.

Posterior uveitis (inflammation affecting the choroid or retina) is usually associated with some form of systemic disease, such as AIDS, herpes simplex or zoster, toxoplasmosis, tuberculosis, or sarcoidosis. The patient complains of decreased or distorted vision. Eye redness and pain may be reported. Systemic corticosteroids are indicated to reduce the inflammation along with treatment of the underlying systemic condition.

Sympathetic Ophthalmia

Sympathetic ophthalmia is a rare but devastating bilateral uveitis that occurs after a latent period of days to years after a penetrating injury to the uveal tract. The cause is unknown, but it is probably related to a hypersensitivity to uveal pigment.

Clinical Manifestations. Initially, the injured eye becomes inflamed, followed by inflammation of the unaffected (sympathetic) eye. If untreated, the disease progresses to bilateral blindness.

Management. Enucleation of the sightless eye within 10 days of an injury is usually recommended to reduce the risk of sympathetic disease in the other eye. Such a drastic step is usually not undertaken the day of injury. Instead, the wounds are closed and the patient is allowed time to give informed consent. In patients whose eyes are not severely injured and for whom there is hope of some useful vision, enucleation is not a consideration. If sympathetic ophthalmia does develop, it is treated with local and systemic corticosteroids and dilating drops. Cytotoxic medications may be required.

Enucleation. Enucleation is the complete surgical removal of the eyeball. Indications for this procedure are blindness after penetrating injury, blindness with recalcitrant (stubbornly resistant) infection, painful blind eyes that are unresponsive to medical treatment, and selected tumors of the eye. The procedure is accomplished by incising the conjunctiva, detaching extraocular muscles, severing the optic nerve, and removing the eye. The muscles are then reapproximated over a ball implant that maintains the volume of the orbit. The conjunctiva is closed, and a plastic conformer is positioned to maintain the fornices of the conjunctival sac during healing. Later the patient is referred to an ocularist for removal of the conformer, prosthesis fitting, and training in its use. There are several types of procedures for eye removal and decisions about the type of surgery depend on the degree of ocular and orbital involvement.

Nursing Implications. A pressure dressing is applied postoperatively for 24 to 48 hours to help reduce the swelling. Ice compresses also may be used to decrease the swelling. Postoperatively, antibiotic and steroid ointments may be prescribed. Mucus that collects over the surface of the conformer may require gentle irrigation. The eyelids are to be kept clean. A long-term complication of enucleation may be a sunken orbit, which can be managed by the ocularist or by reconstructive surgery. Complications of surgery include hemorrhage, infection, and extrusion of the implant.

Patients requiring an enucleation require considerable emotional and psychological support. Because they no longer have binocular vision, they also need assistance in learning how to judge distances with the remaining eye (monocular vision) and how to move forward with a panning motion (moving the head from right to left, scanning the panorama) to see obstacles and objects.

Disorders of Aqueous Humor Circulation: Glaucoma

Glaucoma is one of the leading causes of blindness in Western society. It is estimated that in the United States 2 million people have glaucoma. Of these, almost half are visually impaired, with nearly 70,000 legally blind; 5500 additional people become legally blind each year.

When glaucoma is diagnosed early and managed properly, blindness is almost always preventable. Most cases of glaucoma, however, are asymptomatic until extensive and irreversible damage has already occurred. Therefore, routine eye examinations and screening clinics play a vital role in detecting this disease. It is recommended that all who are at risk for developing glaucoma and those older than age 35 have periodic examinations by an ophthalmologist to assess IOP, visual fields, and the optic nerve head.

Glaucoma affects people of all ages but is more prevalent with increasing age, affecting approximately 2% of those older than age 35. Others at risk are diabetics, African Americans, those with a family history of glaucoma, and people who have had previous eye trauma or surgery or who have received long-term corticosteroid treatment.

The term **glaucoma** refers to a group of diseases that differ in their pathophysiology, clinical presentation, and treatment. They are generally characterized by visual field loss caused by damage to the optic nerve. This damage is related to the level of IOP, which is too high for proper functioning of the optic nerve. The higher the pressure, the more rapidly optic nerve damage progresses. The increased IOP results from pathologic changes that prevent normal circulation of aqueous humor (Fig. 56-12)

Although there is no cure for glaucoma, it may be controlled with medication. Laser or conventional (incisional) surgery may also be required. The goal of treatment is to arrest or slow progression enough to maintain good lifetime vision. This is usually accomplished by reducing the IOP.

Classification of Glaucomas

Glaucoma is classified as two types: open-angle and angle-closure (formerly closed angle). In open-angle glaucoma, the aqueous humor has free access to the trabecular meshwork, and the angle is normal size. In angle-closure glaucoma, the iris blocks the trabecular meshwork and limits the flow of aqueous humor out of the anterior chamber. These categories are further divided into primary (cause

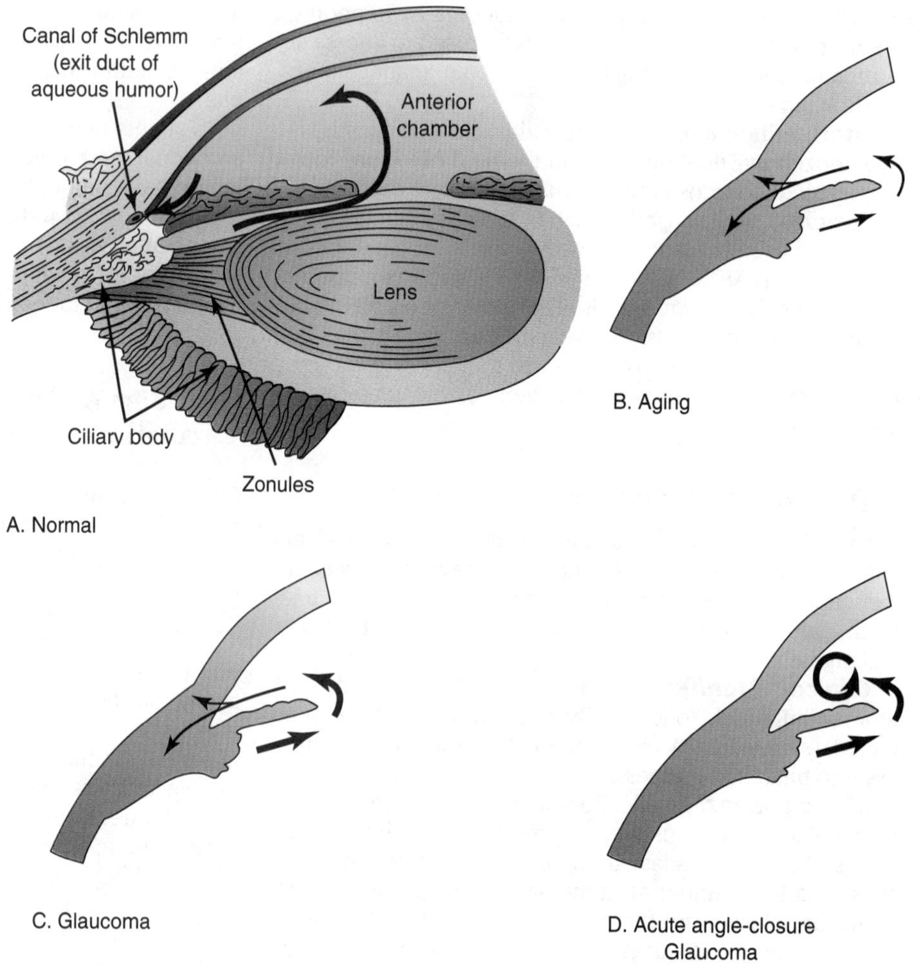

FIGURE 56-12. The flow of aqueous humor and the effects of pathologic changes. (**A**) Normal eye anatomy and flow of aqueous humor fluid from the ciliary body to the posterior chamber, through the pupil, into the anterior chamber, out through the trabecular meshwork to the canal of Schlemm, and into venous circulation. (**B**) In the aging person, *less* aqueous humor (*thin arrows*) follows the same pathway. (**C**) In glaucoma, more aqueous humor flows into the anterior chamber (thick arrows) than leaves it (*thin arrows*), which accounts for increased IOP. (**D**) Obstruction at the canal of Schlemm results in aqueous humor collecting in the anterior chamber and causing a medical emergency known as acute angle-closure glaucoma.

unknown, usually bilateral and possibly hereditary) and secondary (cause known) glaucomas.

Classifications of glaucoma include the following:

I. Open-angle glaucoma
  A. Primary
  B. Normal-tension
  C. Secondary
II. Angle-closure glaucoma
  A. Primary
    1. With pupillary block
      a. Acute
      b. Subacute
      c. Chronic
    2. Without pupillary block
  B. Secondary
    1. With pupillary block
    2. Without pupillary block
III. Combined-mechanism glaucoma
IV. Developmental/congenital glaucoma

Primary Glaucomas

Primary open-angle glaucoma (formerly simple or wide-angle glaucoma) is characterized by atrophy of the optic nerve and cavitation of the physiologic cup and typical visual field defects. Normal-pressure, open-angle glaucoma is characterized by the occurrence of changes when IOP is within normal parameters.

Primary angle-closure glaucoma is the result of an anatomic defect that causes the anterior chamber to be shallow. This produces a narrow drainage angle at the peripheral iris and the trabeculum. Persons with primary angle-closure glaucoma may never experience any problems and may have normal pressure unless there is an acute closure of the angle as the iris dilates, bunches up into the angle, and blocks the outflow of aqueous humor from the trabeculum. Or they may have an episode precipitated by moderate pupillary dilation or marked pupillary miosis.

These events may occur during pupil dilation from being in a dark room or medications that acutely dilate the pupil. Dilation may result from fear or pain, dim illumination, or various topical or systemic medications (vasoconstrictors, bronchodilators, tranquilizers, and anti-Parkinson's agents).

Activities, such as reading, that cause forward movement of the lens and miotic therapy may be precipitating factors as well. A glaucoma episode may occur in anatomically predisposed people who previously had completely normal results of eye examinations or who were totally asymptomatic. Those with a family history of this type of glaucoma should have a slit-lamp examination and gonioscopy to evaluate the anterior chamber angle.

Acute angle-closure glaucoma is a fairly rare medical emergency that can produce significant visual loss. The patient usually complains of severe, generalized ocular pain. Elevated pressures disrupt the dehydrating function of the endothelial surface of the cornea, resulting in corneal edema. The central iris normally overlies the anterior lens surface, which causes slight resistance to aqueous humor flow from the posterior chamber through the pupil to the anterior chamber. When flow through the pupil is blocked (pupillary block) by the lens, however, the resultant increase in pressure in the posterior chamber balloons the peripheral iris forward in contact with the trabecular meshwork, and the iris may appear to be bulging. This finding is called **iris bombé.** This can narrow or completely close the anterior chamber angle and causes elevated IOP (see Fig. 56-12D).

A light shown from the lateral side of the eye may show a shallow (< 3 mm) or flat anterior chamber when the iris bulges forward and touches the inner surface (endothelium) of the cornea. Pupillary block also may be a result of posterior synechiae in which the iris adheres to the lens, which may result from scleral buckling surgery or from a swollen, dislocated, or abnormally shaped lens. The iris and lens may stick together (synechiae), producing an irregular pupil with reduced reactivity to light. Clinically, this appears as a mid-dilated pupil that is not reactive to light. The conjunctiva are typically angry red. The patient may develop nausea and vomiting.

The goal of emergency management of acute angle-closure glaucoma is to decompress (reduce) ocular hypertension. Mannitol may be given intravenously to promote osmotic diuresis and reduction of general eye fluid and IOP. Carbonic anhydrase inhibitors may be given intravenously to reduce aqueous humor production. Direct eyeball massage can lower IOP and may be attempted. It is customary to treat both eyes with laser iridotomy to prevent future attacks. More often than not, a patient seeking treatment for a painful red eye has a foreign body, or conjunctival or corneal disease, and not angle-closure glaucoma.

Secondary Glaucomas

Glaucomas are secondary when the cause is evident and associated with disorders that are responsible for the elevation in IOP. These glaucomas are typically unilateral. They can occur with open or closed angles or combinations of both.

In **secondary open-angle glaucoma,** elevated IOP results from an increased resistance to aqueous humor outflow through the trabecular meshwork, the canal of Schlemm, and the episcleral venous system. The trabecular pores may be blocked with any type of debris, blood, pus, or other matter. This increased resistance may result from long-term corticosteroid use, intraocular tumors, uveitis from diseases such as herpes simplex or herpes zoster, or trabecular meshwork blockage by lens material, viscoelastic substance (used in cataract surgery), blood, or pigment. Elevation in episcleral venous pressure from conditions such as chemical burns, retrobulbar tumors, thyroid disease, arteriovenous fistulas, jugular superior vena cava, or pulmonary venous obstruction can also result in increased IOP. In addition, open-angle glaucoma may occur after cataract extraction, IOL implantation (especially anterior chamber lenses), scleral buckling, vitrectomy, posterior capsulotomy, or trauma.

In **secondary angle-closure glaucoma,** increased resistance to aqueous humor outflow is caused by blockage of the trabecular meshwork by the peripheral iris. The condition is usually caused by changes in the flow of aqueous humor after disease or surgery. Anterior involvement follows development of membranes in neovascular glaucoma, trauma, aniridia, and endothelial disease. Posterior causes occur with pupillary block because the lens or IOL occlude the usual flow of aqueous humor to the anterior chamber.

Normal-Tension Glaucoma and Ocular Hypertension

Normal IOP levels are defined by population statistics. For some people, IOP in the normal range may be too high for continued health of the optic nerve. At the other end of the scale are instances of elevated IOP without evidence of optic nerve damage, in which the optic nerve head seems resistant to higher than normal pressures. Eventually glaucoma-related damage develops in some of these people.

Combined-mechanism glaucoma is a combination of two or more forms of disease. Open-angle glaucoma complicated by angle-closure glaucoma (or narrowing of the angle that impedes outflow of the aqueous humor) is the most common form of combined-mechanism glaucoma.

Assessment and Clinical Manifestations

Ocular and health histories can provide valuable clues to the diagnosing, classifying, and managing glaucoma. Important aspects of the ocular history include symptoms of elevated IOP, uveitis, trauma, surgery, prolonged use of systemic or topical corticosteroids, or a family history of glaucoma.

In a review of systems, special attention is given to the following conditions that can cause, aggravate, or mimic glaucoma: diabetes mellitus; systemic hypertension; a shock episode; and cardiovascular, cerebrovascular, thyroid, respiratory, or demyelinating diseases.

Current medications are recorded, noting those that are associated with glaucoma, for example, tricyclic antidepressants, antihistamines, phenothiazides, monoamine oxidase (MAO) inhibitors, anticholinergic and antispasmodic agents, and anti-Parkinsonian medications.

Diagnostic Evaluation

A glaucoma diagnostic workup includes examination of the eye with an ophthalmoscope to assess damage to the optic nerve, tonometry to measure IOP, perimetry to measure the scope of the field of vision, and ocular and medical histories.

Primary open-angle glaucoma is the most common type of glaucoma, yet it is the most difficult to recognize early because the patient is asymptomatic until late in its course. It is insidious in onset, slowly progressive, and small areas of peripheral vision loss may go unnoticed. By the time visual field loss becomes apparent to the patient, extensive irreversible damage to the optic nerve has usually

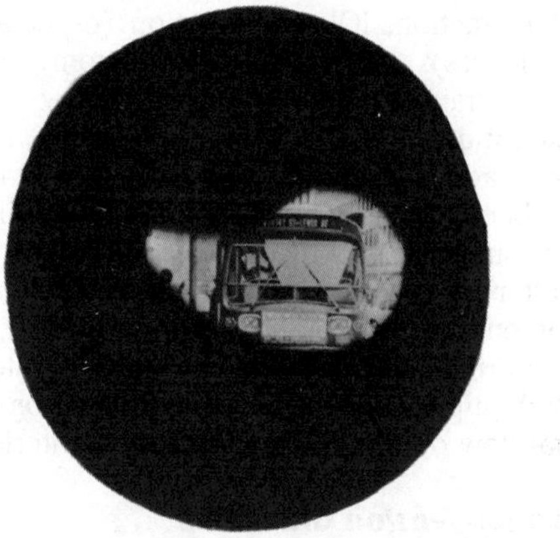

FIGURE 56-13. Advanced glaucoma involves loss of peripheral vision, but the individual still retains most central vision. (Photo courtesy of The Lighthouse, The New York Association for the Blind.)

already occurred (Fig. 56-13). Ophthalmologic examinations are necessary to diagnose the disease early enough to provide appropriate treatment to prevent significant visual loss and blindness.

Primary open-angle glaucoma is so prevalent that glaucoma assessments are warranted as screening examinations in middle age and as a part of general ophthalmic examinations. Primary open-angle glaucoma is a bilateral disease, but damage is often asymmetric. One eye typically is involved earlier and more severely than the other.

Symptoms of acute angle-closure glaucoma include pain, halo vision (seeing halos around lights), blurred vision, redness, and a change in the eye's appearance. Ocular pain may be caused by a rapid rise in IOP, by inflammation, or by medication-induced side effects (*e.g.*, ciliary muscle spasm). Severe ocular pain may be accompanied by nausea, vomiting, sweating, or bradycardia. Redness may be associated with acute iritis, medication reaction, neovascular glaucoma, hyphema, subconjunctival hemorrhage, or elevated episcleral venous pressure. Corneal edema, resulting from a rapid rise in IOP or corneal epithelial decompensation, may produce halo vision. Episodic blurring of vision may also be noted. Some patients notice a change in the appearance of the eye, including haziness of the cornea, ocular displacement, and alteration in pupil position, size, or shape.

Management

The objective of glaucoma treatment is to lower the IOP to a level consistent with retaining vision. The treatment varies depending on the classification of the disease and response to therapy. Medication therapy, laser surgery, and conventional surgery may be used to control progressive damage resulting from glaucoma.

Pharmacotherapy

Medication therapy is the initial and principle treatment for **primary open-angle glaucoma.** Although the regimen may change, therapy usually continues for life. If this therapy fails to adequately decrease the IOP, the next option for most patients is laser trabeculoplasty with continued medication administration. Some patients require trabeculectomy. Laser or incisional surgery, however, is usually an adjunct to, rather than a replacement for, medication therapy.

Acute angle-closure glaucoma with pupillary block is a rare surgical emergency. Medications are used to reduce the IOP as much as possible before laser or incisional iridectomy. In some instances, medications alone may terminate the attack, but there is a high incidence of recurrence. There is a high incidence of later involvement of the other eye as well. Bilateral laser iridotomy is therefore recommended.

Treatment of **secondary glaucomas** is directed at the underlying condition as well as the elevated IOP. For example, glaucomas caused by corticosteroid therapy are managed by discontinuing the corticosteroid medication. Uveitis with glaucoma is treated with anti-inflammatory agents. Antiviral agents, cycloplegics, and topical corticosteroids are prescribed for glaucoma associated with herpes simplex and herpes zoster.

- Use of pupillary dilating (mydriatic) medication is contraindicated for patients with glaucoma.

Most medications have some side effects, which usually subside after 1 to 2 weeks. In some instances, however, a medication may need to be discontinued because the patient cannot tolerate it. Common side effects of topical medications include blurred vision; dim vision, especially at night; and difficulty focusing. Occasionally, the patient's heart rate and breathing are affected.

Systemic agents may cause tingling of fingers or toes, drowsiness, loss of appetite, bowel irregularities, and, occasionally, kidney stones. Patients should be informed about possible side effects. Those who are warned in advance are more likely to cope successfully with the situation.

Beta-adrenergic Antagonists. Topical beta-adrenergic antagonists are now the most widely used hypotensive agents because they are effective in many types of glaucoma and do not produce some of the side effects frequently seen with other medications. Beta-adrenergic antagonists reduce IOP by decreasing aqueous humor formation. Nonselective beta-adrenergic blockers affect both beta-1 and beta-2 receptors. Common beta-blockers are timolol, levobunolol (Betagen), and optipranolol (Metipranolol). Beta-selective agents, such as betaxolol (Betoptic), only affect specific beta-receptor sites. Using these agents reduces some of the cardiopulmonary side effects observed with use of non–beta-selective medications, such as respiratory distress, heart block, and hypotension.

Cholinergic Agents. Topical cholinergic medications (*e.g.*, pilocarpine hydrochloride, 1%–4%, acetylcholine chloride, carbachol) are used in the short-term management of glaucoma with pupillary block because of their direct effect on the parasympathetic receptors in the iris and ciliary body. As a result, the pupillary sphincter constricts, the iris tightens, iris tissue volume in the angle decreases, and the peripheral iris pulls away from the trabecular meshwork. These changes allow aqueous humor to reach the outflow channels and, therefore, reduce IOP.

Adrenergic Agonists. The mechanism of action of adrenergic compounds in glaucoma is not fully understood. They are used with beta-adrenergic blocking agents, having a synergistic rather than an opposing effect. Topical adrenergic agonists reduce IOP by increasing aqueous humor outflow, promoting pupillary dilation, decreasing aqueous humor production, and constricting the conjunctival blood vessels. Examples of adrenergic stimulating agents are epinephrine and phenylephrine hydrochloride (Neo-synephrine). Epinephrine eye drops (0.1% solution) are widely used in treating open-angle glaucoma. Phenylephrine (1%, 2.5%) is commonly used to dilate the eye before examining the ocular fundus and treating uveitis.

Carbonic Anhydrase Inhibitors. Carbonic anhydrase inhibitors, *e.g.*, acetazolamide (Diamox), are administered systemically to lower IOP by decreasing aqueous humor formation. They are used to manage open-angle glaucoma (long-term) and to treat acute angle-closure glaucoma (short-term) and self-limiting glaucomas, such as those that develop after trauma. They also may be required after iridectomy to control residual glaucoma. They may be given orally or intravenously during acute attacks of glaucoma.

Osmotic Diuretics. Oral (*e.g.*, glycerol) or intravenous (*e.g.*, mannitol) hyperosmotic agents reduce IOP by increasing the osmolality of the plasma and drawing water from the eye into the vascular circulation. Hyperosmotic medications are helpful in the short-term treatment of acute glaucoma. They are used to lower IOP preoperatively so that surgery can be performed on a more normotensive eye. They also may prevent the need for surgery in transient glaucoma.

Laser Surgery for Glaucoma

Laser surgery to enhance aqueous humor flow and decrease IOP may be indicated as the primary treatment for glaucoma, or it may be required when medication therapy is poorly tolerated or ineffective in lowering IOP. Lasers can be used to perform many procedures related to treating glaucoma (Chart 56-4).

Conventional Surgery

Conventional surgical procedures are performed when laser techniques are unsuccessful, laser equipment is unavailable, or when the patient is not a good candidate for laser surgery (*e.g.*, a patient who cannot sit still or follow instructions). Routine filtration procedures are associated with successful decrease in IOP in 80% to 90% of patients.

Peripheral or **sector iridectomy** is performed to remove a portion of the iris to allow aqueous humor flow from the posterior chamber to the anterior chamber. It is indicated in the treatment of glaucoma with pupillary block if laser treatment is unsuccessful or unavailable.

Trabeculectomy (filtering procedure) is performed to create a new drainage pathway through the sclera. This is accomplished by dissecting a half-thickness flap of sclera hinged at the limbus. A segment of trabecular tissue is removed, the scleral flap is reattached, and the conjunctiva is securely sutured to prevent leakage of aqueous fluid. Trabeculectomy increases aqueous humor outflow by bypassing the usual drainage structures. As fluid flows through this new channel, a bleb (blister or bubble) forms. It can be observed on examination of the conjunctiva. Complications after filtering procedures include hypotony (abnormally low IOP), hyphema (blood in the anterior chamber of the eye), infection, and failure of the filtration.

Seton procedures involve using various synthetic aqueous shunt devices to maintain a patent drainage fistula. An open tube is implanted in the anterior chamber and connects to an episcleral drainage field. These devices are most often used in patients with high IOP, those who are poor surgical risks, or those whose previous filtration procedures have failed. Possible complications of drainage implants include cataract formation, hypotony, corneal decompensation, and erosion of the apparatus.

CHART 56-4
Laser Procedures for Glaucoma

- **Peripheral iridectomy**—creates a full-thickness hole in the iris to allow aqueous humor to flow from the posterior chamber to the anterior chamber. Indications for this procedure include:
  - Acute primary angle-closure glaucoma with pupillary block
  - Fellow eye of a patient who has had an attack of acute primary angle-closure glaucoma
  - Chronic, subacute, or intermittent primary angle-closure glaucoma
  - Prophylactic treatment of anatomically narrow anterior chamber angle glaucoma
  - Combined-mechanism glaucoma
  - Secondary angle-closure glaucoma, including ciliary block and aphakic (absence of a crystalline lens) pupillary block glaucoma
- **Trabeculoplasty**—modifies the trabecular meshwork to increase aqueous humor outflow. It is used when medication therapy alone is insufficient to control IOP in open-angle glaucoma.
- **Gonioplasty**—contracts the peripheral iris to eliminate contact with the trabecular meshwork. It is performed when iridectomy does not resolve the problem of iris blockage at the angle.
- **Pupilloplasty**—enlarges miotic pupillary area by contracting the iris fibers and stretching the pupillary opening.
- **Synechiolysis**—pulls lightly adherent adhesions away from the angle wall of the cornea.
- **Sphincterotomy**—creates radial cuts in the iris sphincter muscle to allow pupillary enlargment.
- **Cyclophotocoagulation**—destroys some of the ciliary processes to reduce aqueous humor production.
- **Goniophotocoagulation**—eradicates new vessels in anterior chamber neovascularization. It is used with panretinal photocoagulation to treat neovascular glaucoma.

Nursing Implications

The patient may require a short hospital stay after surgery. Progressive ambulation is allowed, depending on the patient's age and physical condition. Vigorous activity and movements that cause the patient to bear down as in Valsalva's maneuver (with resulting increased IOP), such as straining, lifting, and bending, are to be avoided for 1 week. The patient is not permitted to drive for 1 week. The eye is patched for 24 hours or longer if needed, and water should be kept out of the eye.

Broad-spectrum antibiotic drops may be instilled for 4 to 5 days, and a topical corticosteroid may be used for many weeks to reduce inflammation and scarring. Occasionally, more potent antifibrinolytic or anti-inflammatory agents, such as 5-fluorouracil (5-FU) and oral corticosteroids, may be prescribed. Because aspirin may induce bleeding, it is contraindicated, and pain is usually managed with acetaminophen. Reading causes rapid, jerky eye movements; thus it is discouraged until permitted by the physician.

Patient Education and Home Care Considerations

Patients diagnosed with glaucoma are faced with learning how to live with a chronic health condition. Members of the health care team, especially nurses, can help them with this difficult adjustment by providing the information needed to understand the disorder, its treatment, and their responsibilities in its management. An informed patient is more likely to take an active role in his or her own care. Patient participation is imperative because optimum reduction of IOP and control of damage depend on the patient adhering to the medication regimen and attending follow-up examinations.

Patients are given written instructions that identify the name of each medication and describe the containers (*e.g.*, green top, yellow label), and the frequency and times of administration. They should understand the expected action and the possible side effects. The importance of making medication administration a part of the daily routine is stressed so that doses are not missed. Patients need to understand that medications are to be continued even when IOP is under control.

Patients should be aware that their responsibilities include good eye care, maintenance of good physical health, and a life-style consistent with low levels of stress. Eye care involves keeping the eyes clean and free of irritants, avoiding rubbing, using nonallergenic cosmetics, and wearing goggles while swimming and protective glasses while playing sports or working in the yard or other potentially hazardous areas.

Noting how the eyes appear and feel is important as well. Unusual changes that should be reported to the physician include excessive irritation, watering, blurring, cloudy vision, discharge, rainbows around lights at night, flashes of light, and floating objects in the field of vision.

Because treating glaucoma is a matter of control rather than cure, it usually involves life-long management. Follow-up examinations are necessary to determine the effectiveness of therapy, to monitor IOP, and to assess the visual field and optic disc. The frequency of follow-up visits depends on the level and stability of IOP and the extent of damage. Patients who are newly diagnosed, or who have a highly elevated IOP and wide fluctuations from visit to visit, extensive optic nerve head cupping or visual field loss, or only one eye with visual function, require more frequent examination.

An explanation is given regarding the importance of timely follow-up examinations. It may be helpful for patients to know why each diagnostic study is ordered and what the findings mean.

Maintaining good health and limiting stress may have a positive effect on eye pressure. Maintaining proper nutrition and salt restriction, avoiding excessive fluid intake, maintaining an appropriate weight level, exercising, and taking time for fun and relaxation may be helpful. Sharing feelings and concerns with family and friends or talking with other patients with glaucoma may be useful in learning how to live with the condition.

Gerontologic Considerations

Older adults are at high risk for glaucoma and are three to four times more likely to develop glaucoma than younger adults. Often, dimming vision is accepted as part of aging, and medical assistance is not sought. Therefore, as part of the physical examination of anyone over age 35, tonometry should be recommended and eye pressure periodically assessed thereafter.

A major concern of health care providers caring for patients with glaucoma is the tendency of these patients to stop taking their eye drops, claiming that it does not help. They must be helped to understand that the eye drops keep glaucoma from worsening. Discontinuing the medication will allow the glaucoma to continue insidiously until blindness occurs. Other problems often experienced by elderly patients, such as arthritis, loneliness and depression, constipation (straining on defecation), and potential for falling and accidents must be considered when caring for the patient with glaucoma.

Disorders of the Posterior Chamber: Retinal and Vitreous Problems

Retinal Detachment

Retinal detachment occurs when there is a separation of the neurosensory retina from the underlying pigment epithelium layer of the retina. Because the neurosensory retina, the part of the retina containing the rods and cones, is detached from the nourishing retinal pigment epithelium, these photosensitive cells cannot perform their visual function, and loss of sight results.

Retinal detachment may be caused by congenital malformations, metabolic disorders, vascular disease, intraocular inflammation, neoplasms, trauma, or degenerative changes in the vitreous or retina. Most commonly, they are caused by the mechanical forces associated with posterior vitreous detachment and retinal tears. Retinal holes, which affect 5% to 13% of the population, and lattice degeneration, which affects approximately 8% of the population, are asymptomatic retinal degenerative defects that require periodic examinations because they lead to retinal detachment.

Rhegmatogenous (tear-induced) detachments are the most common detachments, with an incidence of 1:10,000 of the population each year, primarily in the 40- to 70-year-old age-group. There is a male preponderance thought to be related to trauma. Predisposing conditions include high (greater than 8 Diopters) myopia (nearsightedness), lattice degeneration, aphakia (surgical removal of part or all of the crystalline lens), and trauma.

Degenerative changes (liquefaction), associated with aging, in the vitreous, causing traction on the retina, are usually responsible for these retinal tears.

The vitreous body is a meshwork of collagen fibers filled with hyaluronic acid and water, and it is attached to the inner retinal surface. Although the vitreous is originally gelatinous, the hyaluronic acid concentration decreases with age, and the vitreous becomes more liquefied. As this occurs, the individual often notices a few clear floaters, a normal finding. Liquefaction deprives the collagen fibers of their support and causes them to collapse and move forward. When the vitreous collapses, it usually separates easily from the posterior retina, but in some cases the vitreous adheres to a portion of the posterior retina and pulls on the retina as it collapses, causing a tear.

If left untreated, rhegmatogenous detachments usually become total and may progress to retinal atrophy, secondary cataract formation, chronic uveitis, hypotony, and phthisis bulbi (atrophy of the eyeball with blindness).

Clinical Manifestations. The patient usually reports a history of floaters or flashing lights or both. The floaters may be perceived as tiny dark spots or cobwebs. These floating particles consist of retinal cells and blood that are released at the time of the tear and cast shadows on the retina as they drift by (see Fig. 56-14). Later the patient may notice a spreading shadow or curtain moving across the field of vision, resulting in blurred vision and loss of visual field as the retina separates from the pigmented epithelium. Decreased central acuity or loss of central vision indicates that the macular area is involved.

A patient with suspected retinal detachment must be referred to a retinal specialist immediately for emergency treatment. The pupil is dilated, and the fundus is examined with an indirect ophthalmoscope and a hand-held condensing lens. This method of examination provides a wide field of view so that the entire retina may be examined and all tears identified.

Management. Inflammatory detachments are usually treated medically. However, some exudative or serous retinal detachments (due to an associated process such as a tumor or inflammation that produces subretinal fluid without a retinal break) respond to laser photocoagulation. Laser procedures form scar tissue on the retina, sealing it to the pigmented epithelium. Diabetic retinopathy or trauma with vitreous hemorrhage may require vitreous surgery to relieve the tractional forces to the retina that they cause. Radiation therapy may be useful in treating retinal detachments associated with intraocular tumors.

Patients with a confirmed diagnosis of retinal detachment are usually admitted to the hospital the same day. Depending on the extent or location of the retinal detachment, the patient may require emergency surgery or ocular rest in preparation for surgery. Ocular rest includes bilateral eye patching and bed rest and is instituted to facilitate retinal settling and to prevent the detachment from spreading. The affected eye is maximally dilated before surgery, permitting the surgeon to see the fundus.

Scleral buckling is the primary surgical procedure performed to reattach the retina. Transscleral cryotherapy is applied around each retinal tear, producing a chorioretinal adhesion that seals the break so that liquid vitreous can no longer pass through into the subretinal space. A piece, or pieces, of silicone (the buckle) are sutured and infolded into the sclera, physically indenting, or buckling, the sclera, choroid, and photosensitive layers up to the pigmented epithelium, supporting the breaks. When the retina thus comes into contact with the underlying, supportive tissue, normal physiologic function is restored. Often, external, syringe drainage of subretinal fluid is necessary to bring the detached retina closer to the buckled area so that the retina can be reattached.

During surgery it may be necessary to inject inert gas (*e.g.*, sulfahexafluoride SF6, octofluroptopane C3F8, or air bubble) into the vitreous body to maintain IOP or to assist in flattening the retina. Depending on which gas is used, the bubble will be reabsorbed and replaced by aqueous fluid in 3 days to 2 months.

Between 90% and 95% of retinal detachments can be reattached and good visual acuity achieved with scleral buckling, although more than one procedure may be needed. Full visual recovery may not be achieved, even with successful reattachment, in patients with chronic retinal detachments or in those with macular involvement. Detachments that cannot be reattached by scleral buckling may require vitreous surgery.

Approximately 25% of patients with complex retinal detachments do not respond to conventional surgical procedures. Instillation of perfluorocarbon liquid as an adjunct to treatment of these patients has improved visual outcome.

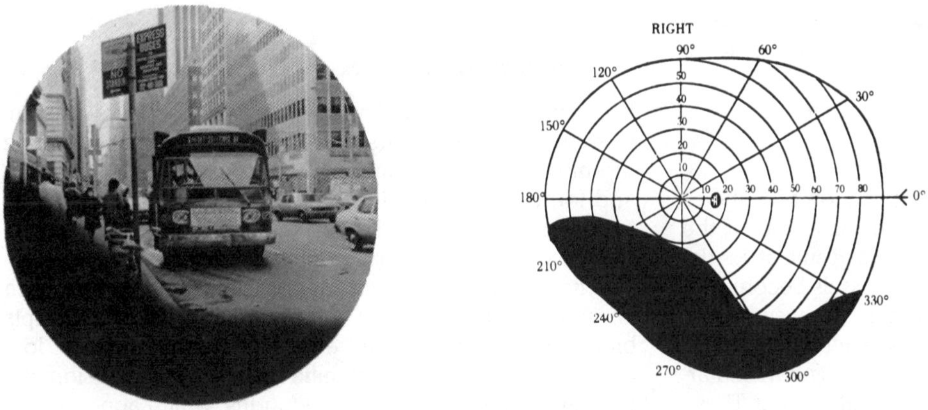

FIGURE 56-14. Retinal detachment causes a field of vision defect. Detachments are usually superior, so the shadow or defect is perceived as inferior. (Photo courtesy of The Lighthouse, The New York Association for the Blind.)

Postoperative Management. Postoperatively the patient's activity may be limited to bed rest with bathroom privileges. If both of the patient's eyes are patched, or if vision in the unaffected eye is low, the patient needs assistance when out of bed to prevent falls and jarring. If there is a gas bubble in the eye, a prescribed position must be maintained so that the gas effectively tamponades the retinal break. The patient must not assume a flat supine position for any length of time because the gas bubble would rise and push the iris forward, causing acute glaucoma in aphakic patients (those who have had the crystalline lens removed). In other patients, the bubble would rest against the crystalline lens, causing cataract formation. Pupillary dilation is maintained to facilitate postoperative examination.

Early complications after retinal surgery may include increased IOP, glaucoma, infection, choroidal detachment, failure of the retina to reattach, or redetachment of the retina. The nurse monitors the patient for the following signs and symptoms, which are reported to the physician: pain that does not respond to medication, purulent or excessive mucoid drainage, severe nausea and vomiting, eye redness and swelling, cloudy vision, halos around lights, or any symptoms of retinal detachment.

Late complications include infection, extrusion of the buckling material through the conjunctiva or erosion though the eyeball, proliferative vitreoretinopathy (scar tissue involving the retina), diplopia, refractive errors, or astigmatism.

Infectious Endophthalmitis

Infectious endophthalmitis is an abscess of the vitreous body. It may occur as a result of endogenous (internal source) infection, such as emboli from endocarditis, or exogenous (external source) seeding from penetrating injuries or surgery. The patient may report eye pain and loss of vision. Clouding of the normally transparent structures of the eye may be seen.

Management. Treatment may include intraocular injection of antibiotics and vitrectomy.

Vitrectomy is the surgical procedure performed to remove part or all of the vitreous gel. Indications for this surgical intervention, in addition to infectious endophthalmitis, include unresolved hemorrhage, traction and giant retinal detachment, failure of the retina to reattach after scleral buckling, epiretinal membranes, diabetic retinopathy, penetrating injury, and intraocular foreign body.

After the vitreous gel is removed, fluid, air, inert gas, or silicone oil is used to replace the vitreous. The postoperative considerations and management are similar to those for scleral buckling.

Diabetic Retinopathy

Diabetic retinopathy is a frequent complication of diabetes mellitus and is caused by damage to or occlusion of the blood vessels that nourish the retina as a result of inadequate blood glucose control. Weakened vessels become hyperpermeable and leak, causing microhemorrhages, retinal swelling, or exudative deposits. Progressive retinal ischemia stimulates the formation of new blood vessels (neovascularization), which may proliferate on the vitreal surface. These new vessels are fragile and may rupture, causing subretinal dot hemorrhages or bleeding into the vitreous body. Also, they may form fibrovascular bands that contract, resulting in traction and subsequent retinal detachment. Exudates may also accumulate within the retina and may be visible on diagnostic evaluation.

Clinical Manifestations. If fluid collects at the macula, the patient notices blurred central vision. Vitreous hemorrhage results in cloudy or hazy vision of sudden onset. Most people with diabetic retinopathy eventually develop vision problems. Diabetic retinopathy is the leading cause of new blindness among adults in the United States.

Management. In some self-limiting cases, treatment is not indicated; in most cases, however, laser photocoagulation surgery is useful. An intense beam of laser light is used to seal off leaking blood vessels and destroy abnormal new ones. The macula area is avoided if at all possible, because diminished central vision can occur from scarring produced by laser therapy. If there is vitreous hemorrhage or traction detachment of the retina, vitrectomy may be required to remove the bloody vitreous, release the traction, or remove membranes.

Patient Education. The risk of developing diabetic retinopathy is greater for patients who have had diabetes for a long time. Diabetes currently affects 7 million Americans, so development of this disorder has the potential to affect many people. Persons with diabetes should be made aware of this risk and encouraged to comply with their diets, medications, and exercise regimens in an effort to control blood glucose levels and hypertension. They also should be directed to seek regular eye examinations because the ophthalmologist may detect signs of diabetic retinopathy long before symptoms are evident to the patient. Early diagnosis and treatment by a retinal specialist can greatly reduce the risk of severe visual loss. For additional discussion of diabetic retinopathy, see Chapter 39.

Hypertensive Retinopathy

Hypertension (see Chapter 31) is responsible for many general vascular changes and can cause changes in ocular blood vessels. The blood vessels take on a copper wire appearance with arteriosclerosis, and arteriovenous (AV) nicking may be visible. Hypertension can result in flame-shaped hemorrhages in the retina, especially near the optic disc. These occur with extreme elevations of blood pressure with development of problems similar to those of diabetic retinopathy.

Central Retinal Artery Occlusion (CRAO)

When the central retinal artery is occluded, a sudden, painless loss of vision occurs. **CRAO** is usually a consequence of embolic disease, commonly seen with atrial fibrillation and formation of mural thrombi that escape into the cerebral circulation, emboli from cardiac valves, and arteriosclerosis-induced emboli. Branches occluded result in visual field deficits in the area supplied by that branch. When an embolus lodges in the small retinal artery, it interrupts blood flow and the retina becomes ischemic. Periodic loss of vision is known as **amaurosis fugax.** Total occlusion can be visualized by examining the fundus, which appears with a pale retina, retinal artery changes (red, thin threads, segmented box-car), and a bright cherry-red spot where the choroid-fed macula shines through.

Management. CRAO is a medical emergency requiring prompt treatment, usually within the hour of onset, to be most effective. The patient usually seeks treatment for a sudden painless loss of vision in one eye. Treatment given after 3 hours or development of a cherry-red spot is associated with poor visual outcomes. Treatment aims include releasing the embolus into a more distal vessel and disrupting vasospasm. Intermittent massage of the globe for 5-second intervals with quick release is indicated immediately. Administration of 95% oxygen for 10 minutes every hour may be helpful. Underlying embolic diseases should be treated, and the cause of emboli is evaluated.

Age-Related Macular Degeneration

Age-related macular degeneration (AMD) is a condition that results in the progressive loss of central vision, leading to legal blindness. It is caused by damage to or deterioration of the photoreceptor cells in the area of the macula. It is thought to be hereditary and is associated with chronic vascular hypertension.

Affecting approximately 1.7 million people, AMD is the leading cause of severe visual loss for people older than age 65. Almost one third of the people older than age 50 have some degree of macular degeneration. If the fovea is damaged, the symptoms are caused by the loss of central vision and include distortion, blurring, or total loss of central vision, loss of contrast sensitivity, increased glare, and dimming of color vision. Peripheral vision is usually retained, and the patient has the potential to remain independent.

Management. There is no treatment available for most types of macular degeneration, but in a few cases early diagnosis and laser treatment may stabilize or improve the condition. Sometimes taking high doses (800 mg) of vitamin E is recommended. Magnifying devices, high-contrast print, and strong illumination may be helpful. Investigation is ongoing into refining and applying retinal cell transplantation to save vision in AMD (Boyd-Monk, 1993c).

Retinitis Pigmentosa

Retinitis pigmentosa refers to a group of hereditary disorders characterized by progressive visual field loss and night blindness caused by degeneration of the retina. The disease affects approximately 100,000 Americans. Onset usually occurs in youth or young adulthood, although it can be seen at any age. The disease course is 30 to 40 years or more from onset and results in total or near-total loss of vision at age 60 or 70 years.

Clinical Manifestations. Night blindness during adolescence is an initial sign of this disease. It progresses with ring scotomas (visual field area losses), which progress peripherally, until tubular, tunnel vision is present. Eventually, the scotoma encroaches on the central vision, and all vision is lost. Approximately 75% of patients are myopic, and 50% develop posterior subcapsular cataracts.

Management. Currently, no treatment is available; however, with recent advances in biotechnology and molecular biology, genetic therapy might someday prove helpful.

Patients should be followed closely by the ophthalmologist because other treatable disorders (such as glaucoma) and myopia may develop. Doses of vitamins A and E may be helpful. (Experimental animals deficient in vitamin A develop degenerative changes in the retina.) Some professionals advise patients to avoid bright light and use pupillary constricting medications. Genetic counseling should be obtained to determine the risk factors to other family members or future offspring. Low-vision aids are usually indicated.

Defective Color Vision

Defective color vision (color blindness) is usually a hereditary disorder. Normally there are three types of cones in the retina: red, green, and blue. They all work together to perceive a wide range of colors. In approximately 8% of men and 0.4% of women, however, there is an abnormal gene that may slightly alter or completely eliminate one, two, or all three types of cones. Red–green defects are the most common. Persons with these defects are insensitive to deep red light and confuse shades of red, green, and yellow. Because the choice of occupation may depend on the ability to correctly perceive color, testing should be performed at an early age.

Defective color vision also may be acquired. It can be caused by retinal disease, poisoning, some medications, or aging. Persons with acquired defective color vision should be referred to an ophthalmologist for diagnosis and management of the causative disorder.

Ocular Emergencies

A few ophthalmic conditions are considered medical emergencies. Time to treatment is a key factor in preserving the eye or sight.

The following is a list of ocular emergencies. Patients with these conditions should be treated immediately by an ophthalmologist. A few hours' delay may lead to permanent damage.

- Trauma: corneal abrasions and foreign bodies, lacerations of the eyeball, intraocular foreign bodies, and ruptured globe
- Corneal ulcer or infection
- Severe conjunctivitis
- Orbital cellulitis
- Chemical burns
- Acute iritis
- Acute glaucoma
- Occlusion of the central retinal artery
- Retinal detachment
- Endophthalmitis

Those conditions that should receive treatment as soon as possible but in which a delay of a few days may not be an immediate threat to sight, include

- Chronic glaucoma
- Vitreous hemorrhage
- Unilateral exophthalmos of recent origin
- Acute dacryocystitis

Ocular tumors
Optic nerve disorders

It is estimated that 90% of all eye injuries are preventable. Chart 56-5 gives recommendations of the American Academy of Ophthalmology for prevention of eye injuries.

Ophthalmic Trauma

Ophthalmic trauma is a common cause of unilateral visual loss in young people. It is often a result of accidents in and around the home, battery explosions, motor vehicle crashes, or sports injuries. Eye trauma concomitant with multiple trauma is not uncommon. Examination of the injured eye should proceed with great caution to avoid further injury.

Situations that suggest physical abuse patterns may appear in the form of ophthalmic trauma and are reportable using appropriate state agency guidelines.

Assessment and Clinical Manifestations. When evaluating a patient with ocular trauma, the first priority is to obtain a history of the injury, how it happened, and associated visual changes. Sometimes immediate treatment, as in chemical burns, should be initiated without further examination. The history is followed by examination and documentation of visual acuity, eye mobility, and visual inspection of the outer structures.

Inspection of the outer structures of the eyes that discloses relatively minor damage does not preclude the possibility of severe injury. The examiner usually has a high index of suspicion for ocular trauma when the external eye structures are injured. The eyelids are thin, and a laceration of the lid could also involve the cornea or sclera. A small painless wound in the lid may be the only external evidence of a penetrating injury. The force sufficient to cause contusion of the eyelid (black eye) may also cause intraocular bleeding, retinal detachment, or global rupture.

Whenever there is reason to suspect laceration, penetrating injury, or rupture of the globe, either by the mechanism of injury or the evidence of external trauma, *no pressure* should ever be directed on the eye. Such pressure could cause extrusion of intraocular contents and irreparable damage. Separation of the lids can be safely accom-

CHART 56-5
Patient Education: Guidelines for Preventing Eye Injuries

In and Around the House

Make sure that all spray nozzles are directed away from you before you press down on the handle.
Read instructions carefully before using cleaning fluids, detergents, ammonia, or harsh chemicals. Wash hands thoroughly after use.
Use grease shields on frying pans to decrease spattering.
Wear special goggles to shield your eyes from fumes and splashes when using powerful chemicals.
Use opaque goggles to avoid burns from sunlamps.

In the Workshop

Protect your eyes from flying fragments, fumes, dust particles, sparks, and splashed chemicals by wearing safety glasses.
Read instructions thoroughly before using tools and chemicals and follow precautions for their use.

Around Children

Pay attention to age and responsibility level of a child when selecting toys and games. Avoid projectile toys such as darts and pellet guns.
Supervise children when they are playing with toys or games that can be dangerous.
Teach children the correct way to handle potentially dangerous items such as scissors and pencils.

In the Garden

Do not let anyone stand on the side or in front of a moving lawn mower.
Pick up rocks and stones before going over them with the lawn mower. These stones can hurl out of the rotary blades and rebound off curbs or walls, causing severe injury to the eye.
Make sure that pesticide spray can nozzles are directed away from your face.
Avoid low-hanging branches.

Around the Car

Before opening the hood of the car, put out all smoking materials and matches. Use a flashlight, not a match or lighter, to look at the battery at night.
Wear goggles when grinding metal or striking metal against metal while performing auto body repair.
When using jumper cables to start the car, wear goggles; make sure the cars are not touching one another; make sure the jumper cable clamps never touch each other; never lean over the battery when attaching cables. *Never* attach a cable to the negative terminal of the dead battery.

In Sports

Wear protective safety glasses, especially for sports such as racquetball, squash, tennis, baseball, and basketball.
Wear protective caps, helmets, or face protectors when appropriate, especially for sports such as ice hockey.

Around Fireworks

Wear eye glasses or safety goggles.
Do not use explosive fireworks.
Never allow children to ignite fireworks.
Do not stand near others when lighting fireworks.
Do not try to relight duds. Douse them in water.

Reprinted with permission of the American Academy of Ophthalmology, revised 1993) plished by resting the thumb and forefinger against the upper and lower orbital margins. In addition, the patient should be warned not to squeeze the lids shut.

Signs of possible severe injury to the globe include:

- Pain (although small penetrating wounds may be painless)
- Subconjunctival hemorrhage
- Conjunctival laceration
- Enophthalmia (abnormal displacement of the eye backward or downward because of loss of contents or orbital fracture)
- Iris defect
- Pupil displacement; may be caused by anterior chamber collapse
- Hyphema (blood in the anterior chamber)
- Lowered IOP (soft eye)—**Do not palpate the eye**
- Extrusion of ocular contents (iris, lens, vitreous, retina)
- Hypopyon (purulent material in the anterior chamber)—a late sign of trauma

Management. If severe injury of the globe is suspected, further manipulation of the eye is avoided until the time of surgery. A light dressing is applied (**no pressure**), and a metal shield that rests on the orbital bones is taped from the forehead to the cheek. Bilateral patching may be helpful because movement of the eyes should be kept to a minimum. Parenteral antibiotics are initiated, and analgesics, antiemetics, and tetanus antitoxin are administered as prescribed.

When rupture of the globe is ruled out, examination of the other structures of the eye can be accomplished. Laceration of the lids may require simple suturing, antibiotic ointment, and a dressing. Depending on the extent and involvement of other structures, surgery may be required.

Foreign Bodies

Patients with foreign bodies in the conjunctiva may complain of a foreign body sensation, especially with eyelid movement, profuse tearing, and conjunctival injection (redness). The inner surface of the lower lid should be inspected, and the upper lid should be everted and examined.

Management. Nonpenetrating foreign bodies under the upper lid may be removed by lifting the upper lid over the lower lid, which allows the lashes of the lower lid to brush the object off the inside of the upper lid.

Alternatively, the object may be removed by irrigation, taking care not to touch the cornea. If the foreign body cannot be removed in this fashion, the eye should be closed and patched and the patient referred to an ophthalmologist. One of the dangers of a conjunctival foreign body is the threat of damage to the cornea.

Superficial foreign bodies of the cornea may only require irrigation to remove them. Embedded foreign bodies, however, require the attention of an ophthalmologist. Fluorescein staining is often used to outline superficial epithelial defects. A topical anesthetic is given before removing the foreign body, which is accomplished with a blunt-tipped instrument. A cotton-tipped applicator is not used because it rubs off too much epithelium. Deeply embedded materials may require surgery.

When the corneal epithelium, which is a natural barrier to microorganisms, is compromised, the eye is vulnerable to infection. A corneal wound, therefore, should be inspected daily for evidence of infection until it heals completely.

Corneal Abrasions

Corneal abrasions are common ocular injuries in which epithelial cells are lost. Abrasions can be caused by scratches from objects such as a mascara brush, a twig, or fingernail. They also may result from a foreign body or contact lenses worn for too long.

Clinical Manifestations. The patient presents seeking treatment for sudden onset of pain, which is often intense, photophobia, foreign body sensation, and tearing. Visual acuity may be normal or decreased, depending on the site of the lesion.

Management. Topical anesthetics are used only during the initial treatment because their prolonged use delays healing and can mask further damage that could lead to permanent corneal scarring. Corticosteroids are also avoided. Topical antibiotics are prescribed prophylactically, and a short-acting cycloplegic (to paralyze the eye) is administered topically to alleviate pain. A pressure eye patch is used to immobilize the lids and promote comfort and healing. Patching of the other eye and bed rest for 24 hours may be indicated for extensive abrasions. If the underlying layers of the cornea are not involved, healing occurs without scarring, usually within 24 to 48 hours. A follow-up visit is required to monitor epithelialization and healing.

Chemical Burns

Chemical burns to the conjunctiva or cornea should be irrigated with copious amounts of physiologic solution or water immediately. The easiest and quickest way to flush the eye is to have the patient hold his or her head under a faucet and allow the water to run gently over the eye and wash it out; alternately, the patient can place his or her face in water and open and close the eyes. It is usually more satisfactory, however, to flush the eye with a syringe, if available, taking care not to contaminate the other eye if it has not already been contaminated. Continuous flushing for at least 20 minutes is imperative. Plain tap water is adequate under such circumstances and should begin at the site of injury and continue until arrival at the treatment facility. There should be no delay in irrigation—not to examine the eye or measure visual acuity. The "first responders," including the victim, are the ones who can make a primary difference in the outcome of chemical burns. Emergent management of chemical burns is important in education of the public.

Irrigation and Management. Administering topical anesthetic drops before irrigating the eye relieves pain. A lid speculum and standard IV tubing and solution are used for irrigation. Neutralizing solutions are avoided because the heat released by their reaction with the chemical could cause further injury. If the irritant is alkaline, irrigation should continue for at least 1 hour; these substances continue to denature protein and continue to work unless removed. It is important that the upper and lower lids are everted and examined to detect lingering particles and then adequately flushed. Acid solutions tend to do initial damage but not persistent damage.

After irrigation, the eye is dilated, and antibiotics are instilled as prescribed. Collagenase inhibitors such as acetylcysteine (Mucomyst) or sodium edetate (EDTA) are prescribed to treat severe alkali burns. A soft contact lens may be used as a bandage-type lens to facilitate healing and decrease the abrasive effect of blinking. This lens is not removed for instilling other medications. Persistent pain may be an indication to discontinue using the contact lens, however.

Bilateral eye patching may provide the patient with more comfort than patching the affected eye alone because both eyes move together; however, this advantage needs to be weighed against the disadvantage of vision loss. Patients with chemical burns are treated by an ophthalmologist because complications such as infection, delayed scarring, neovascularization, and corneal perforation are possible.

Blunt Trauma to the Eye

The orbit is normally sufficient to take the brunt of most threats to the eye. The causes of blunt trauma are usually sports related, for example, collision with balls, bats, and so forth. Other common causes involve motor vehicle crashes and violent trauma. Orbital contusion of the eyelids is common and usually resolves with cold compresses and time. Most blunt trauma can be treated effectively by resting the eye over a few weeks' time.

Hyphema

Hyphema is blood in the anterior chamber. It is often associated with blunt trauma, but it may occur spontaneously, or in ocular vascular pathology. This blood can move around in the anterior chamber, stain the inner surface of the cornea, and blur vision. For this reason, it is recommended that the patient be kept upright and still. If the upright position is maintained, the blood settles and levels off in the anterior chamber. There is a notable incidence of rebleeding between 24 and 48 hours after significant hyphema. In most patients bleeding will seal off, but a small percentage of patients (5%–7%) tend to rebleed in a few days. The incidence warrants bed rest for a few days after detection.

The degree of concern over hyphema depends on the amount of blood present in the anterior chamber. High levels of hyphema increase the risk of secondary glaucoma from blood obstructing the trabeculum.

Management. Besides keeping the patient upright and resting, blood may need to be evacuated surgically from the anterior chamber. The goal of treatment is to allow for gradual reabsorption of the blood by resting the eye. Bed rest at home with pressure patching of the eye is recommended. If the patient can remain at rest and has daily transportation to the ophthalmologist, home care is appropriate. However, if the patient does not have a support system or circumstance that allows for resting of the eye, hospitalization may be required. African-Americans who present with hyphema must be evaluated for sickle cell anemia. Spontaneous hyphema in persons taking anticoagulants requires evaluation of therapeutic medication levels.

Ruptured Globe

Rupture of the globe is a serious ophthalmic disorder in which the integrity of the eyeball is lost. This is a medical emergency and requires immediate surgical intervention. Because situations that are handled promptly offer the patient a greater chance for some, if not all, restored visual function, timely treatment is crucial.

Clinical Manifestations. Recognition of the ruptured globe may be evident by objects in the cornea or other anterior structures, or obvious laceration. Other signs might be a pointed pupil. This indicates that the iris is pulled to the side of injury and often is protruding out the cornea or sclera. The iris is pigmented and appears like a glob on the surface of the eye. Any small cuts in the sclera appear black from the pigmented, vascular choroid. This can be easily overlooked, but recognition of this finding may save a patient's vision. Sometimes there are hidden ruptures, so the entire anterior eye should be inspected if possible, including the area under the lids.

Management. The three cardinal rules of managing a ruptured globe follow:

1. **Do not cause more harm or injury.** When a severe eye injury, such as a ruptured globe, has been sustained, the tendency is for the patient to rub it. The nurse should do whatever is necessary to prevent the patient from further injuring the eye. This can be accomplished by placing a shield or cup over the eye and preventing the hands from reaching for the eye. Health care professionals should also prevent further insult to the eye by avoiding unnecessary manipulation of the eyelids or eyes, especially during examination. When manipulating the lids, the tendency is to push forward against the eye, thereby increasing the possibility of further extrusion of eye contents. If examining the eye is absolutely necessary, a lid speculum should be applied, which applies vertical, rather than forward pressure.

   Once a global rupture has been determined, it is important that an experienced ophthalmologist see the patient as quickly as possible. Ruptured globe requires surgery within 4 hours of onset to prevent infection and loss of eye function. The outcome of a ruptured globe depends on a multidisciplinary approach, because all who come in contact with the patient affect the outcome. The patient is reassured that the ophthalmologist can offer the greatest help. Sedation and analgesia are provided to reduce anxiety and promote the patient's cooperation.
2. **No eye drops!** Because the integrity of the globe is already compromised, it is important not to introduce anything into the eye that could cause more damage. Drop concentration intended for local action can be caustic and irritating to the interior eye. This includes dyes, which may stain the inside of the cornea and obscure vision, if it is restored.
3. **Cover and protect the globe and contact an ophthalmologist.** The eye is protected and covered with a Foxx shield or cup. A moist lubricated cup can be inserted over the eye. If a foreign object is protruding from the globe, stabilization of the object and protection is necessary.

- One should never attempt to remove a penetrating object from the eye no matter how obtrusive it may appear.

Ophthalmic Laser Surgery

Ophthalmic laser surgery is one of the most important developments during the past decade in treating many eye conditions. This procedure is a noninvasive alternative to incisional surgery and results in decreased risk of infection, shorter postoperative course, and less expense. Therapy is usually performed on an outpatient basis with topical anesthetics. This avoids the risks and complications of general or retrobulbar anesthesia required for conventional surgery.

The term **laser** is an acronym for *l*ight *a*mplification by *s*timulated *e*mission of *r*adiation. The laser machine produces energy and emits a narrow, uniform beam of light that can be focused precisely on selected tissue. Depending on the type of laser used, heat coagulation, cutting, or microexplosion can be produced. The laser may be used to treat retinal breaks, diabetic retinopathy, retinal vein occlusion, macular degeneration, glaucoma, some tumors, and opacities of the posterior capsule after cataract surgery with IOL implantation.

The most recent addition to the laser field is the excimer laser, which is still in the investigational phase. It offers the possibility of altering the focusing strength of the eye by computer-controlled recontouring of the cornea, thereby correcting refractive errors, primarily myopia. This is known as photorefractive keratectomy (PRK). Excimer laser removal of corneal scars is known as phototherapeutic keratectomy (PTK).

Possible complications of laser surgery include iritis, cataract formation, hyphema, corneal damage, and retinal burns. There may also be increased IOP, which is usually transient. Patients who are at risk for increased IOP after therapy require monitoring for 1 to 2 hours after the procedure.

Contraindications for laser procedures include target tissue that cannot be visualized, corneal edema, an uncooperative patient, or a patient who cannot sit still.

Patient Education for Laser Surgery

The patient and family members should be prepared for the procedure by informing them about what will be experienced before and after laser surgery. Many people are afraid of lasers, and this anxiety may cause agitation, movement, or syncope during the procedure. Patients should be informed that anesthetic drops will be administered before treatment, that they will be seated comfortably with the head positioned on a headrest, and that the surgeon will stabilize the eye. They need to know to expect a tingling sensation, a flash of light, and a clicking sound with each application. Patients are informed to tell the surgeon immediately if they feel faint.

Postoperatively the patient can expect some blurring of vision for about 1 hour and possibly some discomfort. Therefore, arrangements must be made for transportation home. The patient may experience a dull pain in the eye. Post-treatment headache may be relieved by acetaminophen. There are usually no restrictions on activity or diet.

The patient and family should be told that several treatment sessions may be necessary when the patient's condition requires an extensive number of laser treatments. Excessive treatment at one time can cause uveitis, macular edema, exudative retinal detachment, or narrowing of the anterior chamber with angle closure. Administration of apraclonidine, a relatively selective alpha-antagonist, before laser procedures reduces the degree of increase in IOP.

Laser surgery can be performed to treat ciliary block (malignant) glaucoma, reopen failed filtering sites, sever sutures after trabeculectomy, and rupture cysts of the iris or ciliary body. Laser treatment used in glaucoma achieves IOP reduction in approximately 85% of all patients; however, most continue to require antiglaucoma medications.

❑ *NURSING PROCESS*
The Patient With an Eye Disorder

Assessment

An initial health history is taken to determine the patient's primary problem, such as difficulty in reading, blurred vision, a burning sensation in the eyes, watering of the eyes, double vision, spots before the eyes, or isolated areas of lost vision (scotomas, myopia, or hyperopia). The nurse should determine whether the problem is in one or both eyes and how long the patient has had this difficulty.

It is also important to explore the patient's general ocular condition or status: Does he or she wear glasses or contact lenses? When were they assessed last? Is the patient under the regular care of an ophthalmologist? When was the last eye examination? Was eye pressure assessed? Does the patient have difficulty seeing (focusing) at close range or at a distance? Are problems reading or watching television reported? What about problems differentiating colors, or problems with lateral or peripheral vision? Has the patient had any past eye injuries or eye infections? If so, when? What eye problems exist in the patient's family?

A pertinent eye history is essential. What past illnesses has the patient had?

- ❑ Childhood—strabismus, amblyopia, injuries?
- ❑ Adult—glaucoma, cataract, eye injury or trauma, corrected or uncorrected refractive errors, and how corrected? Any previous eye surgery? Any hypertension, diabetes, thyroid disorders, sexually transmitted diseases, allergies, cardiovascular and collagen diseases, neurologic condition?
- ❑ Family illnesses—Is there a history of eye disorders in first-degree relatives or grandparents?

The patient's understanding of eye care and treatment is elicited to identify misconceptions or misinformation that can be corrected early.

Diagnosis

Nursing Diagnoses

Based on the nursing assessment data, the patient's major nursing diagnoses may include the following:

- Pain related to injury, inflammation, increased IOP, or surgical intervention.
- Fear and anxiety related to impaired vision and loss of autonomy
- Sensory/perceptual alteration (visual), related to ocular trauma, inflammation, infection, tumor, structural diseases, or degeneration of photosensitive cells
- Knowledge deficit about preoperative and postoperative care
- Self-care deficit related to impaired vision
- Social isolation related to limited ability to participate in diversional and social activities secondary to impaired vision

Collaborative Problems/ Potential Complications

Based on assessment data, potential complications that may develop in medical, surgical, or traumatic ophthalmic disorders include:

- Infection of ocular structures
- Retinal detachment
- Intraocular hypertension/Secondary glaucoma
- Secondary cataract formation
- Perforation of the globe

Planning and Implementation

Goals. The major goals of the patient may include relief of pain, control of anxiety, prevention of further visual deterioration, understanding and acceptance of treatment, accomplishment of self-care activities, including medication administration, avoidance of social isolation, and absence of complications.

Nursing Interventions

Relieving Pain. Pain may result from trauma, such as a scratched cornea or increasing pressure within the eye. An eye patch helps to limit eye movement and relieve related pain. The uncovered eye should also rest because the eyes move in synchrony.

Because light causes pain in many eye conditions, and because eye rest facilitates healing after eye surgery, subdued lighting is used. If those assisting the patient need light to carry out their activities, then dim artificial lights may be used. The patient may be instructed to avoid reading for some time after ophthalmic surgery or disease.

Prescribed analgesics and antibiotics may also help to control discomfort. Reducing emotional disturbances and physical stresses promotes relaxation, which in turn helps to relieve the patient's pain.

Alleviating Fear and Anxiety. Sharing the results of the physical examination and diagnostic studies with the patient and explaining the diagnosis and treatment plan are interventions that promote the patient's participation in care. In turn the patient feels a sense of control and autonomy, which helps reduce fear and anxiety.

Decreasing Sensory Deprivation. When the eyes are bandaged, distortions in perception can occur, such as "eye-patch delirium," inappropriate behavior, and loss of position sense. Often these problems are magnified and become frightening and upsetting to the patient. One way to assist the patient in overcoming these unsettling feelings is to reorient him or her periodically to reality and to the environment and to offer reassurance, explanations, and understanding. Anyone entering the patient's room should speak and identify himself or herself to avoid startling the patient.

Teaching the Patient About Perioperative Procedures. Before ophthalmic surgery, preparations must be made with scrupulous care so that complications are minimized, comfort is achieved, delay is minimized, and the patient is informed. If the patient will receive an anesthetic, the nurse can explain that the type of anesthesia usually determines the preparations. For example, if general anesthesia is used, the lower intestinal tract is evacuated the morning of the surgery and only a liquid diet is given after that. Before preparing the eyes for surgery, the nurse covers the patient's hair with a cap and cleans his or her face. Commonly a series of preoperative eye drops is administered before surgery. Then the nurse monitors for systemic absorption of drops, which may affect blood pressure, heart rate, and ventilation. Preoperative antibiotics are usually prescribed. Throughout preparations the nurse explains the activities and encourages the patient to discuss concerns so that they may be addressed before surgery.

After surgery in which both eyes are bandaged, the patient remains in bed in a supine position with a small pillow under the head. Pillows may be placed on each side of the head to keep it still, and siderails are set in place to promote safety and a sense of security. The patient is provided with a call bell or light and instructed to ask for help rather than move or strain in an attempt to be self-sufficient.

If the patient receives a local anesthetic during the surgical procedure, the patient is usually ambulatory in a few hours after surgery.

The ophthalmologist is notified immediately if the patient has excessive pain or if the dressings are disturbed.

- Morphine is never given to ophthalmic patients unless it is certain that vomiting will not injure the eye.

Promoting Self-Care Activities. The patient is encouraged to carry out as much self-care as possible to promote a feeling of self-sufficiency. Nursing assistance is provided as needed. A patient who cannot see is assisted with eating, but if the patient is accustomed to feeding himself or herself, the patient is encouraged to do so. Elimination is promoted by proper diet, stool softeners, or enemas, as prescribed. Patients are not to read, smoke, or shave unless permitted to do so by the physician. The patient must be cautioned against rubbing the eyes or wiping them with a soiled handkerchief. Any patient receiving dilating medications should wear dark glasses.

Medication bottles and instructions should be labeled in large letters and used where there is plenty of light. The patient must learn to wash hands thoroughly before using any medication. The nurse initially supervises the patient who is instilling eye drops, so that the instillation technique becomes effective and specific. For example, the patient may find it convenient to rest the base of the hand holding the eye dropper against the forehead and pinch the lower lid to form a V-trough to catch the eye drop.

The patient's home environment is assessed for safety, and the patient or a family member is encouraged to remedy any safety hazards. In addition, lighting is adapted to the patient's needs so that it is not too bright and not too glaring, yet it is bright enough for adequate vision.

Encouraging Socialization and Coping Skills. The anxiety typically experienced by the patient with an eye condition requires as much consideration as physical needs. A person's dependence on sight is emphasized when one faces a temporary or possibly permanent loss of this vital sense. Anxiety, fear, and depression are common reactions; tension, resentment, anger, rejection, and withdrawal also may occur. By allowing the patient to express these feelings, the nurse can then take steps to help the patient learn to cope and adjust to the situation.

The patient is encouraged to have visitors and to socialize. Depending on the patient's interests and preferences, suggestions can be made for diversional activities. When permissible, a radio or tape player and occupational therapy may be used to keep the patient's mind occupied. Interest, empathy, and understanding on the part of the nurse enhance the patient's sense of well-being. Because of differences of personality, the approaches to addressing the anxiety of individual patients vary. When permanent blindness is apparent, reeducation in activities of daily living may be performed by specially trained personnel or persons with similar conditions and concerns.

Monitoring and Managing Potential Complications. Regardless of the cause of an eye problem, measures can be initiated in an attempt to control as well as to prevent further progression of deterioration. This can be accomplished by resting the eye, restricting activities, using dark glasses, or instilling a prescribed local anesthetic.

Infection. Any time the eyeball is subjected to trauma, surgery, or external organisms, the potential for infection exists. A red, inflamed eye is a common presenting complaint in ophthalmology. It is important to differentiate the cause of redness and to treat it accordingly. The nurse observes for changes in visual acuity, discharge, pain, and inflammation. Prophylactic and therapeutic administration of systemic and topical antimicrobial medications may be prescribed. Meticulous hygiene and care to prevent cross-contamination among patients is crucial in preventing infection. Care is taken to avoid contaminating ophthalmic drops and other solutions by avoiding touching the eye with the container and by using individual minimum doses. These measures are crucial because development of endophthalmitis may lead to the need for enucleation. Observation for infection in those with penetrating injuries and corneal disruption is essential.

Retinal Detachment. Retinal detachment is a potential complication of many ocular procedures, surgery, and traumatic events. Elderly patients, those with history of retinal detachment, or persons with diabetes are particularly prone to retinal detachment. The nurse instructs such patients especially to report any signs of retinal detachment such as floaters and changes in visual fields. After retinal surgery, the nurse reinforces the need to maintain correct positioning to facilitate reattachment of the retinal layers.

Intraocular Hypertension. Intraocular hypertension is a common problem in ophthalmology because so many factors can precipitate increases in IOP. Monitoring IOP before and after eye procedures and surgery promotes early detection of changes in aqueous humor circulation. **Secondary glaucomas** can aggravate and cause other ocular problems, further threatening eye function. Detection of changes in the anterior chamber depth, eye pain, blurred vision, conjunctival injection (redness), and pupillary changes are crucial areas for prompt management to prevent damage to the optic nerve.

Secondary Cataracts. Secondary cataracts may develop after trauma or other metabolic diseases. The patient presents with common symptoms of a cataract. A common occurrence after ECCE, the posterior capsule may become clouded by the development of secondary membranes. The patient is monitored for diminished visual acuity and is prepared for laser capsulotomy (with an Nd-Yag laser) if indicated. This is a long-term complication. Its average onset is 2 years after cataract extraction.

Perforation of the Globe. A perforated globe is probably the most undesirable complication other than panophthalmitis. Surgical procedures, trauma, or corneal ulcers may place the patient at high risk for perforation of the cornea or globe. The patient is monitored for signs indicating loss of anterior chamber integrity (hypotony, a shallow anterior chamber, decreased vision, and prolapsed iris).

Patient Education and Home Care Considerations. Over the years, there has been a shift from hospital-based to outpatient-based eye surgery. This largely results from advanced technology that affords surgical safety and ease, and from high inpatient costs. Moreover, the ability to make smaller surgical incisions coupled with improved preoperative diagnostic testing allows patients to undergo many types of procedures in the outpatient setting. For this reason, patients are usually treated in and discharged from the outpatient centers. Observation for potential complications, transportation and support for follow-up examinations, and administration of ophthalmic solutions and general eye care are all necessary parts of the recuperative process after eye surgery.

The need for patient and family education is stronger than ever, because the burden for postdischarge care rests on caregivers or the patient at home. There are many issues for education, and the time for teaching is relatively short; therefore, determining the understanding and skills of the caregiver or patient is a priority before discharge. Determining who will be the postoperative caregiver is equally important. Then, educational needs are individualized and tailored to particular sensory deficits, age, and educational levels. If at all possible, education is accomplished before the surgical procedure so that time is available for further questions and additional arrangements. Arrangements for home health care may be necessary for individuals with limited support.

Evaluation

Expected Outcomes

1. Experiences less pain.
   a. Takes prescribed medication to counteract irritation, to rest the eyes, and to treat or prevent any infection.
   b. Applies prescribed cold or warm compresses.
   c. Reduces eye activity by applying appropriate eye dressing and resting the eye.

   d. Protects eye from additional injury by using a protective shield.
2. Shows evidence of calmness and absence of anxiety.
3. Copes with limitations in sensory perception.
   a. Exhibits orientation to time, place, and surroundings.
   b. Responds appropriately to others.
4. Accepts treatment regimen and carries out recommendations safely and accurately.
   a. Washes hands before using eye drops and taking medications.
   b. Reports any untoward signs, such as watering eyes and pain.
   c. Reduces eye activity by using an eye patch if prescribed.
   d. Asks appropriate, relevant questions during follow-up visits to the physician.
5. Practices self-care activities effectively.
   a. Demonstrates how to perform ophthalmic treatments such as administration of eye drops/medications, eye hygiene.
   b. Cleans lenses effectively as taught.
   c. Lists safety measures to prevent falls, such as repair or removal of loose carpeting and clutter.
   d. Describes proper lighting for reading and hand crafts.
6. Participates in diversional and social activities.
7. Verbalizes understanding of treatment regimen, follow-up care, and visits to the physician.

Ophthalmic Nursing Care

The eye is such an important organ that its care and protection are major considerations from the day of birth. The nurse, as an important member of the health team and as a teacher and a practitioner of sound health habits, can provide excellent health education in eye care and in the prevention of eye diseases.

Sound principles of safety and care need to be stressed at an early age. Such problems as headache, dizziness, tiredness after close eye work ("the letters run together"), and itchy eyes should be assessed by a health care provider. Also significant are inflamed or watery eyes; red-rimmed, encrusted, or puffy lids; recurring styes; crossed eyes; and unequal pupils. Unusual behavior should be noted, such as holding a book too closely, frowning, blinking, squinting, rubbing the eyes, and failing in school or study work.

The importance of eye care has been recognized by industries that require workers to wear protective eye glasses or faceshields. Safety glasses should be worn when the task warrants it. Eyes should be protected from bright sun, sunlamps, ultraviolet rays, and aerosol products such as hair spray. In the home, ammonia and alkali products, such as lye, present a particularly dangerous hazard for both children and adults and should be stored in safe places out of reach and used with care.

Eyes need to rest after being used for close work for a time. Occasionally glancing out the window or around the room provides relaxation.

The importance of adequate and well-placed light in preventing eyestrain is essentially not a medical problem but one of general, industrial, and social concern.

Medical management of patients with eye conditions has changed drastically in recent years and has resulted in less frequent need for hospitalization. For example, a patient undergoing cataract surgery no longer needs to stay in the hospital. Rather, this surgery and many other ophthalmic surgical procedures are performed in same-day surgery units, on an outpatient basis, thereby allowing the patient to return home on the same day as the surgery. Such brief contact with the patient or family allows the nurse only a short time for observation, assessment, nursing interventions, patient evaluation, and instruction. Therefore, any teaching sessions or demonstrations of self-care procedures must be performed in such a way as to ensure that the patient and family understand their responsibilities for self-care and can recognize those signs and symptoms that may require professional consultation and intervention. Although outpatient surgery is common for some eye disorders, many eye problems do require more prolonged hospital care.

Special Eye Care

When caring for someone who is severely debilitated, who has a lid closure deficit, or who cannot perform self-care (for example, an unconscious patient), the nurse needs to observe for conditions that cause drying of the eyes and then perform general eye hygiene. It is the nurse's responsibility to protect the eyes from excessive exposure and drying. Using lubricating drops and ointments along with light patching of the eyes to maintain a closed position can prevent iatrogenic (accidental, care-induced) complications of corneal scarring and infection. There is no substitute for good eyelash and eyelid hygiene with mild soap or baby shampoo and water.

The lashes and lids can be cleaned from the inner to outer canthus with cotton balls impregnated with irrigation solution. The degree and frequency of eye care depends on the amount and character of drainage present. It is important to demonstrate procedures to caregivers of the patient, when appropriate.

General Eye Care

Eye Patching

Various circumstances necessitate the use of eye patches. Typically, after an ophthalmic procedure, the eye may be patched to protect it and to collect drainage. Accumulation of drainage can be excessive and prolonged and can become an excellent medium for bacterial growth.

Simple patches may be used to gently cover the eyes and close the lids. This is useful in resting the eye, preventing it from exposure and protecting it from light. Patches are also used after trauma to the eye. Many ocular problems render people photophobic (sensitive to light). Sometimes using dark glasses may substitute for patching.

Simple Eye Patch. A simple eye patch is placed over the eye with tape applied diagonally from the top of the forehead to the cheek without pressure on the eye. If further protection is warranted, for example, to avoid a high risk of injury, a metal or plastic cover can be placed over the eye patch and secured in the same fashion. Bilateral patching is sometimes used when both eyes require rest. Because bilateral patching threatens the patient's safety, it is imperative that the patient has readily available assistance and a safe environment.

Pressure Patch. Pressure patches are used when complete immobilization of the eye is preferred. They are also sometimes used to decrease IOP or facilitate drainage of aqueous humor.

Administering Ophthalmic Medication

A wide variety of ophthalmic medications are available for both diagnostic and therapeutic use. Nurses, patients, and their family members must understand the correct techniques for using these medications. The label should be read before each instillation and the appropriate eye identified to verify the correctness of both the medication and the site. The hands are washed immediately before treatment. To avoid injury to the eye, the tip of the bottle or tube should *never* touch the eye or the eyelid. Contaminated medications are discarded.

The puncta should be occluded with a finger after drop administration for 2 minutes to avoid systemic absorption. If more than one medication is to be used, there should be at least 30 seconds between each because the eye is not capable of holding more than one drop at a time. Containers should be tightly capped when not in use. Old medications, as evidenced by the expiration date, color change, or sediment, are discarded.

Eye Drops

Various medication solutions are instilled into the eyes in treating nearly every kind of eye disorder.

Before drops are instilled, it is important to make sure that the correct medication is being given. Some medications (*e.g.*, miotic and mydriatic) act in exactly opposite ways (Table 56-2). Therefore, if one of these medications is indicated in the treatment of a certain eye disease, the other is contraindicated. For this reason, drop containers must be clearly labeled and the labels carefully checked before using the medications. Most eye medications are easily identified by characteristic color labeling. Mydriatics typically come in red-labeled bottles, miotics in green-labeled containers. Yellow and blue labels are used for beta-adrenergic blocking agents.

In addition, the solution should be observed for color changes and sedimentation, which indicate that the solution is deteriorating. If this is the case, the solution is discarded and a fresh one obtained. Patients are especially cautioned against using medication of any kind that has been in the medicine cabinet at home for months or years. Patients should be instructed to note the medication expiration date and discard those medications that are outdated.

Instillation. The eye is not sterile, because it is exposed to the external environment, including the human hands. However, vision is so important that ophthalmic preparations should always be kept sterile to prevent infection. Handwashing before instillation of medication is imperative. If the eye has a dressing, these steps are followed: (1) The hands are washed before the dressing is removed. (2) The dressing is removed. (3) The hands are washed again before instilling the eye drops. Before the medication is instilled into the eyes, the lids and the lashes are cleaned from the inner to outer canthus with a moistened cotton ball. The patient's head then is tilted backward and inclined slightly to the side, so that the solution runs away from the tear duct and the other eye, preventing contamination (Guideline 56-2).

Many people struggle with instillation of eye drops unnecessarily. When something is coming toward the cornea, reflex blinking occurs. It is important to get the cornea out

TABLE 56-2 Comparison of Miotic and Mydriatic Agents

Agent	Indications	Effects
Miotic (green-labeled containers)		
Physostigmine, pilocarpine	To decrease intraocular pressure (IOP), for example, in glaucoma	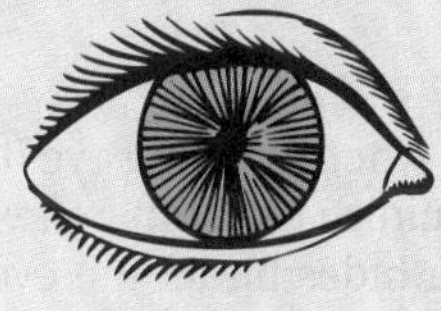 · Pupillary constriction · Spasm of accommodation · Decreased IOP
Mydriatic (red-labeled containers)		
Atropine, scopolamine	· To facilitate examination of retina and optic disc · To rest ciliary body in inflammation · To prevent synechiae in uveitis	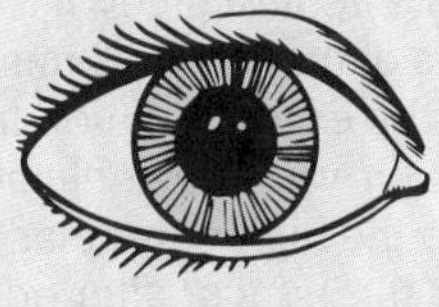 · Pupillary dilation · Paralysis of accommodation · Increased IOP

GUIDELINE 56-2
Administering Eye Drops and Ointment

Instilling Eye Drops

- Instruct the patient to look upward.
- Gently pinch the lower eyelid to form a V-shaped pocket.
- Without touching the eye with the applicator, drop the prescribed amount of medication into the pocket.
- Release the eyelid.
- With a tissue, gently depress the middle canthus or the punctum to prevent the medication from draining into the nasal passages and to sponge away any overflow.
- Instruct the patient to close both eyes *gently* because squeezing the eyelids tightly may expel the medication. Closed eyelids keep the medication in the eye longer.

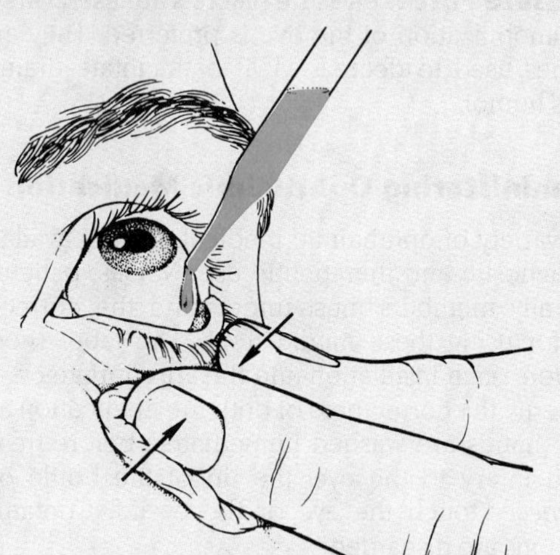

Applying Eye Ointment

- Instruct the patient to look upward.
- Depress the lower eyelid slightly to evert it.
- Beginning near the inner canthus and moving toward the ear, express the ointment along the conjunctiva, filling only the middle third of the lower lid.
- Lightly massage the eyelid to distribute the medication, or ask the patient to roll his or her eyes.

Note: *Before and after administering eye medication, the person instilling the medication must wash his or her hands.*

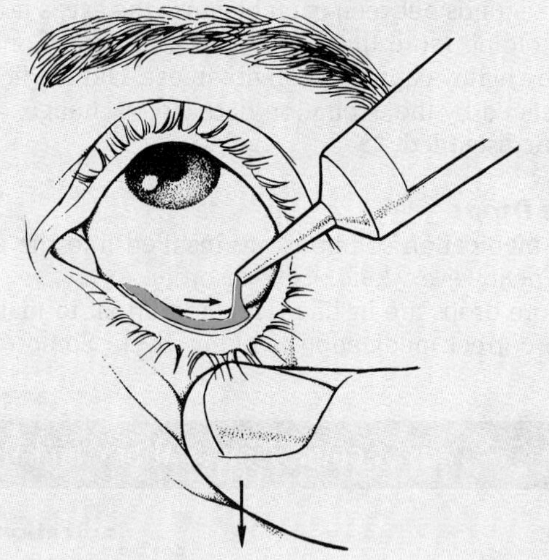

of the way when instilling eye drops to prevent injury to it as well as diminish the blink reflex. When the patient looks up, the cornea hides under the eyelid and does not detect oncoming objects that provoke a blink. Touching the cornea startles the patient; this increases the probability that the patient will jump and contaminate the dispensing tip of the eye dropper and possibly injure the eye.

In most circumstances, it is appropriate to press the middle canthus of the eye for 2 minutes after instilling the drops to prevent the excess solution from entering the nose. Some drops contain vasoactive elements that can be readily absorbed into the highly vascular nasal passages, so pressing a tissue over the puncta after administration of drops is prudent. The nurse should monitor blood pressure and pulse after administration of certain types of vasoactive drops to observe for systemic effects of the medication.

It is also important to demonstrate to the patient and caregiver how to instill the drops so that accurate placement of drops can be performed at home if indicated. It is also important to tell the patient or caregiver not to touch the lid with the dropper because doing so will contaminate the eye dropper. It is for this reason that many ophthalmic preparations come in single-dose droppers (minims), which are disposed of after one use.

Ointments

Ointments of various kinds are used frequently in treating inflammatory diseases of the lids, the conjunctiva, and the cornea. Those prescribed most commonly are antibiotics, anti-inflammatory agents, and various combinations of the two.

Ointments are applied by gently pulling down the lower lid and expressing a small amount of the ointment from the tube onto the conjunctiva (see Guideline 56-2). Care is taken not to touch the eye or the eyelid with the tube. The eye only holds a small amount of ointment, so excessive application should be avoided.

Ointments have a tendency to make the vision blurry, so safety issues regarding visual acuity must be addressed.

Ocular Irrigations

Ocular irrigations are indicated in treating various inflammations of the conjunctiva, in preparing the patient for eye surgery, and in removing inflammatory secretions. They are also used for their antiseptic effect. The irrigant to be used depends on the patient's condition. The irrigating apparatus is simple, consisting of a commercially prepared irrigating bottle containing sterile ophthalmic solution (Blinx, Dacriose) and a small, curved basin, gloves, and cotton for catching the fluid and the secretions. Each patient's solutions should be in a plastic dispenser with a cap and label. Gloves are worn during these procedures.

- The patient lies supine or sits with the head tilted backward and inclined slightly toward the side. If the patient is seated, the basin may be held by the patient. If the patient is lying down, it may be placed so that it will catch the fluid as it runs from the eye. The nurse stands in front of the patient.
- After the lids are carefully cleaned to remove dust, secretions, and crusts, the lids are held open with the thumb and the fingers of one hand, and the eye is flushed gently, directing the stream away from the nose or cornea. The fluid is never directed toward the nose, because of the danger that it may spill over into the other eye. The procedure is continued until the eye is entirely free of secretions.
- It must be remembered that little force or pressure is used, because of the danger of injury. For the same reason, and to prevent contamination, no part of the irrigator should touch the eye, the lid, or the lashes.
- When the irrigation has been completed, the eye and the cheek are dried gently with cotton.

Continuous Irrigation. Continuous irrigation is indicated in chemical burns, resistant corneal ulcers, uveitis, socket infections after enucleation, or conditions that require constant medication or debridement. Before irrigation, a local anesthetic may be instilled (except in the case of chemical burn). The easiest method for continuous irrigation is to direct sterile saline solution through standard IV tubing. Special contact lenses are available that can be attached to the tubing so that the irrigant flows continuously into the eye.

Warm Wet Compresses

Heat relieves pain and increases the circulation, thereby promoting absorption and reducing tension in the eye. It is especially valuable for conjunctivitis accompanied by excessive secretions. Heat is best applied in the form of compresses composed of seven or eight layers of gauze or cotton just large enough to cover the eye as follows:

- The patient is moved to the side of the bed, and a towel is used to cover the chest. A layer of cold cream or petrolatum jelly may be applied to the skin of the eyelid and the adjacent cheek to protect the skin from maceration.
- The compresses then are moistened in a basin of water or other prescribed solution that has been heated.
- The fluid, which should be kept at a temperature between 46° and 49°C (115° to 120°F), is expressed or squeezed from the pad, and the compress, after being tested for temperature, is placed gently over the closed eyelid.
- The pads are changed every 30 to 60 seconds for 10 to 15 minutes, and the application is repeated every 2 or 3 hours.
- At the end of the application period, the lid is dried gently with cotton.
- New pads are used for each application. If the eye has a purulent secretion, the compresses are applied to one eye at a time, the solution and the basin being changed between applications to avoid transferring infection from one eye to the other. Gloves must be worn when carrying out this procedure.

Cold Compresses

Cold causes capillary constriction that tends to reduce the amount of secretion and relieve pain during the early stages of acute inflammatory conditions of the conjunctiva. Cold compresses are also useful in relieving itching caused by allergic conjunctivitis.

The patient is prepared in the same manner as for the application of warm compresses. The pads are moistened in the prescribed solution and placed over the closed eye. Latex gloves or small plastic bags filled with ice can be used to maintain the cold temperature. These are placed on top of the moistened pads. They are applied to the closed lids and are changed every 15 to 30 seconds for a period ranging between 5 and 15 minutes each hour.

- Cold compresses are never used in treating inflammations of the eye (iritis, keratitis), because cold, by constricting the capillaries, interferes with the nutrition of the cornea.

Visual Impairment: The Nurse's Role

Vision allows one to experience the world by taking continuous pictures of what is occurring in the environment. It plays a role in safety, alerting a person to approaching objects and abysses. It allows for committing distinctive characteristics of persons, things, and events, to memory. It affords mobility by promoting body–eye coordination. Vision fosters communication through reading and nonverbal cues, such as facial expressions and body movements. Looking into one's eyes and diverting one's eyes during communication signals messages about feelings of intimacy, self-concept, sharing, honesty, and so forth.

Clearly, visual perception is important for safety and function within the world. Those who must adapt to sightlessness usually compensate in ways that promote communication, safety, and perception of the world by other senses such as hearing and touch.

Assisting the Visually Impaired Patient

Orientation and mobility are important aspects of assisting the patient who is visually impaired. As suggested earlier, sight is particularly important for assurance—in knowing who is around and when imminent dangers lurk about. A hospital is an "inhospitable" place for many and poses potential threats for those with good vision, let alone someone with visual impairment.

It is the nurse's responsibility to determine ways to promote comfort and security and reduce anxiety within the environment of patients who cannot see. It is often helpful for the nurse to put on a blindfold, and assisted by a colleague, simulate activity as a visually impaired person.

Orientation and mobility require an explanation of sounds and the environment and awareness of people who will likely enter the environment. One must use the correct stance to lead the person who is visually impaired. Many people do this incorrectly; patients and significant others may require training in this skill.

To lead the blind or severely impaired person, one stands just in front of the person. The visually impaired person should grasp the elbow of the leader and follow a half gait behind. One should never attempt to drag or pull the person by the arm. This is terribly frightening and leaves the person unprotected and disoriented. The leader should keep the elbow bent at a 90-degree angle and walk at a pace that the person can follow without hesitating. The person can then take cues from the leader. The sighted leader must be aware of the space occupied by both the leader and the visually impaired person.

Another common activity the nurse helps the visually impaired patient do is "negotiate" the room. The patient is taken around the room and bathroom to become familiar with the architecture and furnishings. Some patients can walk without assistance, provided they are sufficiently oriented to the environment. In some situations, the nurse may think that the patient will require assistance. If so, the call bell or light is placed within easy reach of the patient.

Mealtime can be confusing for the patient. The patient is provided with a comfortable sitting arrangement with the tray or table easily accessible. A biblike covering is provided in the event that food is spilled. The arrangement of food on the plate and tray can be explained by taking the patient's hand and locating objects on the tray or by identifying objects on the plate as if the plate were a clock. For example potatoes may be in the 6 o'clock position, the peas at 2 o'clock. All caregivers are trained to assist patients in this way.

The nurse is able to assist the visually impaired patient in several ways: as (1) an educator, (2) a support person, (3) a caregiver, and (4) a liaison with the physician.

By conferring with the physician regarding what has been told to the patient about the diagnosis, anticipated treatment, and prognosis, the nurse is able to reinforce this information, answer questions, provide support, and relay to the physician the patient's and caregiver's reactions and understanding. To augment the patient's adjustment and rehabilitation, honest prognostic information is essential, even if there is little hope for recovery of vision. The nurse is often helpful in determining when the time is right for conveying such information. The nurse may open discussion about feelings and fears about visual impairment and may discover that the patient has misconceptions about the impairment. Frequently, self-imposed limitations are more restricting than actual physical disabilities. Attitudes and beliefs of the nurse can have a direct or indirect effect on the patient. A positive attitude that focuses on abilities rather than disabilities has the potential for affecting the patient's self-esteem and body image in a beneficial way.

It is not unusual for persons with disabilities to experience discrimination. People who are visually impaired do not necessarily have a hearing deficit and should be spoken to in an appropriate fashion. Like most adults, the sight-impaired individual is required to maneuver within the world and be productive. Showing the patient ways to do this safely and supporting the patient's independence promotes independence and autonomy. Expressions of pity are not only embarrassing but can be offensive to many who have managed to progress through rehabilitation. A visually impaired person should always be treated with the dignity accorded any other person. As with any other patient, the nurse determines the patient's desired activities and interests and attempts to facilitate these. Visually impaired people can be easily excluded and abandoned and left to spend much time alone. Ensuring that the patient has a partner for conversation and that he has diversional activities can be helpful. Self-confidence improves with successful functioning within the environment.

The nurse orients the visually impaired person by guiding the patient to survey the room, navigate the walls, doors, obstacles, and touch the furniture. The patient should be informed of any change in the environment. A door is either left open or closed. A half-open door can present a hazard. A patient walking alone should learn to use a lightweight walking stick to intercept obstacles.

Personal appearance is a significant part of the patient's care. The patient is taught to dress without assistance and to perform grooming activities and other hygienic and cosmetic functions. Other activities such as table etiquette and writing are taught during rehabilitation and contribute to successful functioning in society.

Enlisting Community Support and Resources

Familiarity with resources that are available to help the patient is a nursing responsibility. A patient declared legally blind is referred to the state agency for the blind. A directory of agencies serving the visually handicapped in the United States is available from the American Foundation for the Blind. In most states, the only way to obtain rehabilitation training is through a state agency for the blind.

Because of legislative changes to facilitate those with physical disabilities, adaptations in public buildings (such as Braille signs in elevators) assist the visually impaired. Effective aids that "talk," such as clocks, calculators, thermometers, and scales, are available. Also available is an optical scanner that "reads" lines of text and transmits signals to a computer (programmed to recognize letters) that turns the signals into words and pronounces them. A similar device scans words and records the shape of letters, then converts them into vibrations felt by the fingertips of the user. Technology continues to provide devices to expand the world of those with limited vision.

Assisting Low-Vision and Blind Patients

The term **legally blind** refers to those persons whose best corrected vision is 20/200 or worse in the better eye or whose visual field is restricted to 20 degrees. Many of these people have some useful vision, so the term **blind,** meaning the absence of any functional vision, can be misleading. Each individual requires assessment to determine if he or she has any functional vision and, if so, how much.

Low vision and **partially sighted** are terms used to describe visual impairment that cannot be corrected with ordinary eyeglasses, contact lenses, or intraocular implants. It may be a result of birth defects, inherited diseases, glaucoma, cataract, macular degeneration, retinal detachment, or aging. It is estimated that approximately 20 million people in the United States have some type of visual impairment. Of these, approximately 1.4 million have a vision loss that interferes with normal living. More than a million of these 1.4 million are visually impaired rather than totally blind. Approximately 500,000 persons are legally blind.

Low-vision treatment should start at whatever stage the patient experiences difficulty with customary visual tasks. The responsibility of health care providers, however, does not end with the diagnosis, prevention, or treatment of the disorder that results in visual impairment or blindness. Despite this sensory loss, patients can live meaningful and rewarding lives, and it is important that they receive early referral for rehabilitation, counseling, or financial assistance. Health care providers need to know what sources are available and how to use them. Individuals and agencies with expertise in the area of low-vision treatment include:

- Low-vision specialist in ophthalmology
- Local and state agencies for the blind and visually impaired
- Low-vision clinics
- American Foundation for the Blind
- National Association for Visually Handicapped
- National Center for Vision and Aging, *The Lighthouse*
- National Federation of the Blind

Low-vision services include:

- Assessment of visual condition
- Clinical examination
- Orientation and mobility training
- Employment and financial consultation
- Educational, vocational, and psychological counseling
- Vocational rehabilitation
- Adaptive training skills for independent living
- Special education
- Support groups
- Training in the use of low-vision aids

The low-vision aids that follow are designed to make the most of available vision (those in italics can also be used by persons who are blind):

- Magnifying eyeglasses
- Hand and stand magnifiers
- Telescopes
- Large-print books, newspapers, and magazines
- *Talking books*
- *Braille*
- Closed-circuit TV—produces highly magnified image
- *Tactilely marked watches and clocks*
- *Tactilely modified table-top games*
- Enlarged telephone dials
- *Kitchen implements, tools, medication devices*
- *Talking clocks, timers, scales, calculators, and computers*
- *Text scanner—converts text to audio mode or braille*
- *Speech synthesizer*
- Flashlight eye sonar devices
- *Canes, including laser canes*
- *Seeing Eye dogs*

In addition to low-vision devices, adequate lighting is imperative. For greatest visibility, the light source should be close to the work. High-intensity lights with adjustable arms work well for this purpose.

A patient who has marked visual impairment or who is newly blind needs a great deal of help in making a healthy adjustment. For the most part, this help is entrusted to those skilled in such rehabilitation. The nurse, however, can follow certain practices when caring for such a patient, recognizing that there are stages through which this person moves:

1. Denial—a normal response to loss
2. Value changes—a period of adaptation to aids that the person never expected to use
3. Independence–dependence conflict—a period of attempting to accept the condition without becoming completely dependent
4. Coping with stigma—a period of coping with the attitudes and judgments that prevail among the sighted toward the sightless, such as the belief that they are helpless, unemployable, completely dependent, or depressed
5. Learning to communicate in social settings without visual cues

The major goal for the patient is to adjust to sightlessness or near sightlessness by

1. Adapting to the use of auxiliary aids
2. Accepting the new condition without becoming completely dependent
3. Continuing with physical self-care
4. Coping with the social climate and prevailing stigma that are prevalent
5. Learning to communicate without visual cues
6. Adhering to the prescribed therapeutic regimen

Prevention and Education

The nurse, as an important member of the health care team, and as a teacher and a practitioner of sound health habits, can provide education in eye care, eye safety, and the prevention of eye disease. The nurse can help people to learn how to prevent cross-contamination or spread of infectious diseases to others through the practice of good hygiene. The nurse can encourage people to have periodic eye examinations and can recommend ways to prevent eye injury.

When and how often a person's eyes should be examined depends on the person's age, risk factors for disease, and ocular symptoms. Individuals with ocular symptoms should have immediate eye examination. Those who are without symptoms but who are at high risk for ocular disease should have periodic eye examinations. Patients taking medications that can affect the eyes, such as corticosteroids, hydroxychloroquine sulfate, thioridazine HC1, or amiodarone, should also be examined regularly. All others should have a routine glaucoma evaluation at age 35 and periodic reevaluations every 2 to 5 years.

Ocular signs and symptoms requiring examination at any age include:

Loss, dimness, or distortion of vision
Double vision
Pain in or around the eyes
Swelling of the eyelids or protrusion of the eye
Excessive tearing or discharge from the eyes
Floaters or flashes of light
Halos around lights
Sudden crossing or deviation of the eye
Change in the color of the iris

Risk factors for ocular disease and frequency of examination include:

Diabetes—at diagnosis and annually thereafter
Family history of glaucoma, cataracts, retinal detachments, or other hereditary or familial eye conditions—annually
Hypertension: at diagnosis and annually thereafter
Age 65 or older—every 2 years

CRITICAL THINKING EXERCISES

1. An elderly patient tells you that she is having trouble reading the newspaper and seeing the numbers on the telephone. She indicates that she has accepted her vision problems as part of the aging process. Devise a teaching plan for her and explain the reasons for any suggestions you would offer. How would you modify the plan if the patient has the main responsibility of caring for her invalid husband and giving him his medications, or if she is helping to raise her three grandchildren?
2. An unconscious patient who has been in a motor vehicle crash is treated in the emergency department. The patient has contact lenses in place. Describe the actions you would take and explain the rationale for them. How might these actions change if the patient has lacerations around the eyelids and nose?
3. During preoperative assessment of a patient who is to have cataracts removed, you discover that the patient has driven himself to the hospital and has no one to take him home. Explain why this is a problem and how you would handle the situation.
4. A patient who has had laser surgery for glaucoma expresses relief that his glaucoma has been cured and that he will no longer have to worry about it. Explain how this man's reaction might cause you concern, and describe the preventive measures you might take in providing additional helpful information and instruction for him.

BIBLIOGRAPHY

Books

Agency for Health Care Policy and Research (AHCPR). Cataracts in Adults: Management of Functional Impairment. Clinical Practice Guideline No. 4. Rockville MD, Public Health Service, U.S. Department of Health and Human Services, February 1993.

Albert, Jakobiec C (eds). Principles and Practice of Opthamology: Clinical Practice, Volumes 1–5. Philadelphia, WB Saunders, 1994.

Aston SJ, Maino J (eds). Clinical Geriatric Eye Care. Boston, Butterworth Heinemann, 1993.

Blodi Fl, Mackensen G, and Neubauer H (eds). Surgical Ophthalmology. New York, Springer-Verlag, 1991.

Bowers AC and Thompson JM. Clinical Manual of Health Assessment. St. Louis, CV Mosby, 1992.

Brightbill E, Frederick S (eds). Corneal Surgery: Theory, Technique, and Tissue, 2nd ed. St. Louis, CV Mosby, 1993.

Catalano RA (ed). Ocular Emergencies. Philadelphia, WB Saunders, 1992.

Faye EE and Stuen CS (eds). The Aging Eye and Low Vision: A Study Guide for Physicians. New York, The Lighthouse, 1992.

Goldberg S. Ophthalmology Made Ridiculously Simple. Miami, Medmaster, 1991.

Guyton AC. Textbook of Medical Physiology, Philadelphia, WB Saunders, 1991.

Hart WM (ed). Adler's Physiology of the Eye, St. Louis, Mosby Year Book, 1992.

Malasanos L, Barkauskas RV, and Stoltenber-Allen K. Health Assessment. St. Louis, CV Mosby, 1990.

Margo CE, Hamed LM, and Mames RN (eds). Diagnostic Problems in Clinical Ophthalmology, Philadelphia, WB Saunders, 1994.

Miller SJH (ed). Parsons' Diseases of the Eye, New York, Churchill Livingstone, 1990.

Newell FW. Ophthalmology: Principles and Concepts, St. Louis, Mosby–Year Book, 1992.

Noyori K et al. (eds). Ophthalmic Laser Therapy. New York, Mosby, 1992.

Schachat AP et al. (eds). Current Practice in Ophthalmology, St. Louis, Mosby–Year Book, 1992.

Seidel HM et al. Mosby's Guide to Physical Examination. St. Louis, CV Mosby, 1991.

Smolin G, Thoft RA (eds). The Cornea, 3rd ed. Boston, Little, Brown, 1994.

Wilson-Pauwels LW, Akesson EJ, and Stewart PA. Cranial Nerves: Anatomy and Clinical Comments. Toronto, BC Decker, 1988.

Journals

Affel EL. Ophthalmic ultrasonography: A-scans. J Ophthalmic Nurs Technol 1990 Mar/Apr; 11(2):46–56.

Ai E and Kelly MP. Ophthalmic manifestations of AIDS. J Ophthalmic Nurs Technol 1992 Jul/Aug; 11(4):148–156.

Allen M and Birse E. Stigma and blindness. J Ophthalmic Nurs Technol 1991 Jul/Aug; 10(4):147–152.

Allen M. Adjusting to visual impairment. J Ophthalmic Nurs Technol 1990 Mar/Apr; 9(2):47–51.

Allen M. Origins of beliefs and attitudes towards blindness. J Opthalmic Nurs Technol 1994 Nov/ Dec 13(6):278–280.
Allen M and Oberle K. Follow-up of day-surgery cataract patients. J Ophthalmic Nurs Technol 1993 Sep/Oct; 12(5):211–216.
Annand F. A challenge for the 1990's: Patient education. J Ophthalmic Nurs Technol 1992 Sep/Oct; 11(5):206–210.
Bailey KL. Low vision: The forgotten treatment. J Ophthalmic Nurs Technol, 1991 May/Jun; 10(3):103–105.
Bensinger R. Color vision testing. J Ophthalmic Nurs Technol 1992 Jul/Aug; 11(4):161–163.
Beran RF et al. Refractive surgery and the athlete. J Opthalmic Nurs Technol 1995 Jan/Feb 14(1):11–16.
Best SJ. Visual fields in glaucoma and neuro-ophthalmology. J Ophthalmic Nurs Technol 1992 Mar/Apr; 11(2):46–56.
Binder PS. Excimer laser photoablation: Miracle or menace. J Opthalmic Nurs Technol 1994 Mar/April 13(2):61–63
Boltz MM. Troubleshooting ophthalmic nursing problems in the geriatric clinical population. J Ophthalmic Nurs Technol 1993 Sep/Oct; 12(5):229–231.
Boyd-Monk H. Eye trauma in the workplace. J Ophthalmic Nurs Technol 1991a May/Jun; 10(3):117–123.
Boyd-Monk H. How to use a direct ophthalmoscope. J Ophthalmic Nurs Technol 1991b Jan/Feb; 10(1):23–27.
Boyd-Monk H (ed). News and announcements. J Ophthalmic Nurs Technol 1992a Jan/Feb; 11(1):33–35.
Boyd-Monk H (ed). Research highlights. J Ophthalmic Nurs Technol 1992b May/Jun; 11(3):125.
Boyd-Monk H. Acuvue patients report fewer complications than conventional daily lens wearers. J Ophthalmic Nurs Technol 1993a Jul/Aug; 12(4):186.
Boyd-Monk H (ed). News and announcements. J Ophthalmic Nurs Technol 1993b Mar/Apr; 12(2):80–81.
Boyd-Monk H (ed). News and announcements. J Ophthalmic Nurs Technol 1993c Jul/Aug; 12(4):185–187.
Brown GC. Retinal vascular diseases. J Ophthalmic Nurs Technol 1991 Mar/Apr; 10(2):71–75.
Caramella F. Silicone oil as a vitreous substitue in vitreoretinal surgery. J Opthalmic Nurs Technol 1994 Sept/Oct 13(5):241–242.
Colenbrander A and Fletcher DC. Low vision rehabilitation: Visual acuity measurement in the low vision range. J Ophthalmic Nurs Technol 1992 Mar/Apr; 11(2):62–69.
Colenbrander A and Fletcher DC. Low vision rehabilitation: Basic concepts and terms. J Ophthalmic Nurs Technol 1992 Mar/Apr; 11(1):5–9.
Colenbrander A and Fletcher DC. Low vision rehabilitation: Vision requirements for driving. J Ophthalmic Nurs Technol 1992 Mar/Apr; 11(2):111–115.
DHHS/AHCPR. Cataract in adults: Management of functional impairment: A patient's guide. J Ophthalmic Nurs Technol 1993 Jul/Aug; 12(4):159–162.
Edmonds SE. Resources for the visually impaired. J Ophthalmic Nurs Technol 1990 Jan/Feb; 9(1):14–15.
Faherty B. Chronic blepharitis: Easy nursing interventions for a common problem. J Ophthalmic Nurs Technol 1992 Jan/Feb; 11(1):20–22.
Fishbaugh J. Lessons on dilation. Insight 1994a April; 19(1):30–32
Fishbaugh J. Cornea: Confocal microscopy. Insight 1994b June; 19(2):26–27, 32.
Foxall MJ et al. Living arrangements, loneliness and social support of low vision older clients. J Ophthalmic Nurs Technol 1993 Mar/Apr; 12(2):67–74.
Frangie JP and Finne NP. Corneal edema and bullous keratopathy. J Ophthalmic Nurs Technol 1992 Sep/Oct; 11(5):211–214.
Franko-Gazzarari MD. Eye banking in America. J Ophthalmic Nurs Technol 1991 Mar/Apr; 10(2):63–65.
Frederick M. Care of the patient with AIDS and CMV retinitis. J Opthalmic Nurs Technol 1994 July/Aug; 13(4):156–160.
Gerali PS. Lifesight: Growing older with good vision. J Ophthalmic Nurs Technol 1991 Jul/Aug; 10(4):181–182.
Goldblum K. Knowledge deficit in the ophthalmic surgical patient. Nurs Clin North Am 1992 Sep; 27(3):715–725.
Grimes MR, Scardino MA, and Martone JF. Worldwide blindness. Nurs Clin North Am 1992 Sep; 27(3):807–816.
Haefemeyer JW and Knuth JL. Albinism. J Ophthalmic Nurs Technol 1991 Mar/Apr; 10(2):55–62.
Hagan JC and Wyatt B. Preoperative evaluation and workup of the cataract and IOL implant patient. J Ophthalmic Nurs Technol 1993 May/Jun; 12(3):123–128.
Hannon VM. Cataract surgery. J Ophthalmic Nurs Technol 1993 Nov/Dec; 11(6):13–17.
Harrison KW. Disposable contact lens wear systems. J Ophthalmic Nurs Technol 1990 May/Jun; 9(3):96–98.
Holland SP, Chee C, Grimes M. The challenge of eye disease: The patient's perspective. J Ophthalmic Nurs Technol 1991 Mar/Apr; 10(2):52–54.
Hupp SL. Visual fields in neuro-ophthalmology. J Ophthalmic Nurs Technol 1993 Nov/Dec; 12(6):259–265.
Jairath N et al. Effective discharge preparation of elderly cataract day surgery patients. J Ophthalmic Nurs Technol 1990 Jul/Aug; 9(4):157–160.
Judge J. Overview of the red eye. J Ophthalmic Nurs Technol 1992; 11(5):197–202.
Kaye B. The cure for lazy eye. J Ophthalmic Nurs Technol 1990 May/Jun; 9(3):90–93.
Kelly J. Nursing intervention in the treatment of cataracts. Br J Nurs 1994 June/July; 3(12):602–606.
Kelly JS. Topical opthalmic drug administration: Practical guide. Br J Nurs 1994 May 26–June 8;3(10):518–520
Kobari Y et al. Ocular fixation using a baseball catcher's mask for postoperative prone position. J Ophthalmic Nurs Technol 1993 Jul/Aug; 12(4):163–166.
Krupin T. Implanted aqueous shunt devices for glaucoma surgery. J Ophthalmic Nurs Technol 1992 Jan/Feb; 11(1):23–25.
Legro MW. Quality of life and cataracts: A review of patient-centered studies of cataract surgery outcomes. J Ophthalmic Nurs Technol 1991 Nov/Dec; 10(6):260–272.
Long KL and Long R. Treating open-angle glaucoma. Nurse Practitioner 1994 Dec; 5(6):205–206.
McConnell EA. Administering eyedrops. Nursing 1994 May; 24(5): 22.
McManus M. Mobile eye units n the fight against eye disease in east Africa. J Ophthalmic Nurs Technol 1993 Jan/Feb; 12(1):19–21.
Paige BA. The eximer laser: Program implementation and nursing implications. J Ophthalmic Nurs Technol 1992 Nov/Dec; 11(6):251–255.
Plona RP and Schremp PS. Nursing care of patients with ocular manifestations of HIV infection. Nurs Clin North Am 1992 Sep; 27(3):793–205.
Pokalo C. Lasers liquefy cataractous lenses. J Ophthal Nurs Technol 1992 May–June; 11(3):125.
Rakow PL. Innovative uses for disposable lenses. J Ophthalmic Nurs Technol 1992 Mar/Apr; 11(2):184–185.
Rakow PL. Scleral lenses come full cycle. J Ophthalmic Nurs Technol 1993 Nov/Dec; 12(6):287–289.
Rapuano CJ. Topical anesthetic abuse: A case report of bilateral corneal ring infiltrates. J Ophthalmic Nurs Technol 1990 May/Jun; 9(3):94–95.
Raskin P and Arauz-Pacheco C. The treatment of diabetic retinopathy: A view for the internist. Ann Intern Med 1992 Aug; 117(3):226–233.
Romanella A, Abramson DH, and Servodidio CA. Unusual presenting signs of retinoblastoma: A case study. J Ophthalmic Nurs Technol 1991 May/Jun; 10(3):98–102.
Rowell M. Eradication of vitamin A deficiency: With 5 cents and a vegetable garden. J Ophthalmic Nurs Technol 1993 Sep/Oct; 12(5):217–224.

Roy RH and Tindall R. Multifocal IOL technology and clinical applications. J Ophthalmic Nurs Technol 1993 Jul/Aug; 12(4):172–174.

Ruehl CA and Schremp PS. Nursing care of the cataract patient: Today's outpatient approach. Nurs Clin North Am 1992 Sep; 27(3):727–743.

Sandler RL. Clinical snapshot: Glaucoma. Am J Nurs 1995 Mar; 95(3):34–35.

Schein OD et al. The impact of overnight wear on the risk of contact lens-associated ulcerative peratilis. Arch Ophthalmol 1994 Feb; 112(2):186–190.

Shakin EP and Lucier AC. Retinitis pigmentosa. J Ophthalmic Nurs Technol 1990 Jan/Feb; 9(1):6–9.

Smith SC. Diabetic retinopathy. Nurs Clin North Am 1992 Sep; 27(3):745–759.

Smith SC. Impromptu teaching and a collaborative approach: Enhancing the patient's comprehension and satisfaction. J Ophthalmic Nurs Technol 1990 Mar/Apr; 9(2):57–60.

Spires R. Perfluorocarbon liquid in the management of complex retinal detachments. J Ophthalmic Nurs Technol 1992 Jul/Aug; 11(4):157–160.

Spires R. Epikeratoplasty. J Ophthalmic Nurs Technol 1991 Nov/Dec; 10(6):257–259.

Spires R. Postoperative instillation of mitomycin eye drops in the treatment of primary pterygium. J Ophthalmic Nurs Technol 1991 Jan/Feb; 10(1):15–17.

Turrif TW and Gerali PS. Don't play games with your eyes. J Ophthalmic Nurs Technol 1991 Mar/Apr; 10(2):82–83.

Vader LA. Vision and vision loss. Nurs Clin North Am 1992 Sep; 27(3):705–713.

Watson ME and Fine IH. The first assistant's role in managing phacoemulsification complications. J Ophthalmic Nurs Technol 1991 Jul/Aug; 19(4):172–176.

Woods S. Macular degeneration. Nurs Clin North Am 1992 Sep; 27(3):761–775.

Yamada S et al. An eye on comfort: Positioning the patient for ophthalmic surgery. J Ophthalmic Nurs Technol 1993 Mar/Apr; 12(2):75–78.

Yeatts RP and Clontz DM. Graves' ophthalmology. J Ophthalmic Nurs Technol 1990 Jan/Feb; 9(1):16–21.

INFORMATION/RESOURCES

Agencies

American Academy of Ophthalmology
Public Information Program,
PO Box 7424,
San Francisco, CA 94120

American Council of the Blind (ABC)
1010 Vermont Ave, Suite 1100 NW,
Washington, DC 20005

American Foundation for the Blind
15 West 16th St,
New York, NY 10011

American Optometric Association (AOA)
243 Lindbergh Blvd,
St Louis, MO 63141

American Society of Ophthalmic Registered Nurses, Inc (ASORN)
P.O. Box 3030,
San Francisco, CA 94119

Better Vision Institute Inc (BVI)
1800 N Kent St Suite 1220,
Rosslyn, VA 22209

Braille Institute
741 N Vermont Ave,
Los Angeles, CA 90029

Contact Lens Society of America (CLSA)
523 Decatur St, Suite 1,
New Orleans, LA 70130

Eye-Bank Association of America (EBAA)
1725 I St NW,
Washington, DC 20006–2403

Leader Dogs for the Blind
1039 Rochester Rd,
Rochester, MI 48063

Library of Congress, National Library Service for Blind and Physically Handicapped
1291 Taylor St NW
Washington, DC 20542

National Association for Visually Handicapped (NAVH)
22 W. 21st St,
New York, NY 10010

National Braille Association (NBA)
1290 University Ave,
Rochester, NY 14607

National Federation of the Blind (NFB)
1800 Johnson St,
Baltimore, MD 21230

National Society to Prevent Blindness (NSPB)
500 E Remington Rd,
Schaumburg, IL 60173

Recording for the Blind (RFB)
20 Roszel Rd,
Princeton, NJ 08540

Seeing Eye (SE)
P.O. Box 375M,
Washington Valley Rd,
Morristown, NJ 07960

Taping for the Blind (TFTB)
3935 Essex Lane,
Houston, TX 77027

The Lighthouse
111 E. 59th St,
New York, NY 10022

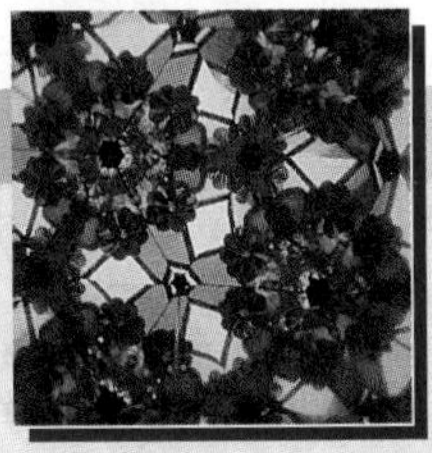

57

Assessment and Management of Patients With Hearing Problems and Ear Disorders

CHAPTER OUTLINE

Anatomy and Physiology of the Ear
External Ear Anatomy
Middle Ear Anatomy
Inner Ear Anatomy
Balance and Dizziness
Physiologic Principles Underlying Sound Conduction
Hearing Loss
Assessment of Hearing Ability
Examination of the Ear
Auditory and Vestibular Diagnostic Procedures
Communicating With the Hearing Impaired
Conditions of the External Ear
Otalgia
Cerumen Impaction
Foreign Bodies
Otitis Externa
Malignant Otitis Externa
Masses of the External Ear
Conditions of the Middle Ear
Tympanic Membrane Perforation
Acute Otitis Media
Serous Otitis Media
Chronic Otitis Media
NURSING PROCESS: The Patient Undergoing Mastoid Surgery
Otosclerosis
Middle Ear Masses
Conditions of the Inner Ear
Motion Sickness
Ménière's Disease
Labyrinthitis
Ototoxicity
Acoustic Neuroma
Aural Rehabilitation
Hearing Aids
Implanted Hearing Devices
Hearing Guide Dogs
Critical Thinking Exercises

LEARNING OBJECTIVES

On completion of this chapter, the learner will be able to:

1. Describe methods used to assess hearing
2. Identify ways to communicate effectively with a person who is hearing impaired
3. Differentiate problems of the external ear from those of the middle ear and inner ear
4. Compare the various types of tympanoplasty procedures and the nursing care of patients undergoing these procedures
5. Describe the patient teaching guidelines for patients undergoing middle ear and mastoid surgery
6. Describe the clinical manifestations, diagnosis, and management of the patient with Ménière's disease

The ear is a sensory organ with dual and complex functions—hearing and balance. Its anatomy is correspondingly intricate; see Chart 57-1 for definitions of the anatomic parts and their functions. The sense of hearing plays a very important role in one's participation in activities of daily living. It is essential for normal development and maintenance of speech, and the ability to communicate with others through speech depends on the ability to hear.

The early detection and the accurate diagnosis of otologic disorders is important. Among those who help diagnose and/or treat otologic disorders are otolaryngologists, pediatricians, internists, nurses, audiologists, speech pathologists, and educators. Nurses involved in the specialty of otolaryngology now can become certified in otorhinolaryngology–head and neck nursing (CORLN). This chapter addresses the assessment and management of otologic disorders common to the adult population. The reader is referred to pediatric otolaryngology literature for otologic disorders pertaining to that population.

Anatomy and Physiology of the Ear

External Ear Anatomy

The external ear, which comprises the auricle (or pinna) and the external auditory canal, is separated from the middle ear by a disclike structure called the tympanic membrane (eardrum). The ears are located on either side of the head at approximately eye level. The auricle is attached to the side of the head by skin and is composed mainly of cartilage, except for the fat and subcutaneous tissue in the earlobe. The auricle aids in the collection of sound waves and their passage into the external auditory canal. Just anterior to the external auditory meatus is the temporomandibular joint. The head of the mandible can be felt by placing a fingertip in the external auditory meatus while opening and closing the mouth. The external auditory canal is approximately 2.5 centimeters in length. The lateral one-third is an elastic cartilaginous and dense fibrous framework to which thin skin is attached. The medial two-thirds is bone lined with thin skin. The external auditory canal ends at the tympanic membrane. The skin of the canal contains specialized glands, ceruminous glands, which secrete a brown, waxlike substance called cerumen (ear wax). The ear's self-cleaning mechanism moves old skin cells and cerumen to the outer part of the ear. The cerumen seems to have antibacterial properties and serves as a protection for the skin.

Middle Ear Anatomy

The middle ear comprises the tympanic membrane (eardrum) laterally and the otic capsule medially; the middle ear cleft lies between the two. The tympanic membrane lies at the end of the external auditory canal and marks the lateral limits of the middle ear. This membrane, which is about 1 cm in diameter and very thin, is normally pearly gray in color and translucent.

The middle ear is an air-filled cavity that houses the ossicles (middle ear bones) and is connected by the eustachian tube to the nasopharynx. It is also contiguous with some air-filled cells in the adjacent mastoid portion of the temporal bone. The middle ear contains the three smallest bones (ossicles) of the body: the malleus, incus, and stapes. The ossicles are held in place by joints, muscles, and ligaments, which assist in the transmission of sound. There are two small fenestrae (the oval and round windows) in the medial wall of the middle ear, which separate the middle ear from the inner ear. The footplate of the stapes sits in the oval window, where sound is transmitted to the inner ear. The round window provides an exit for sound vibrations. The round window is covered by a very fine membrane, and the stapes footplate is secured by a rather tenuous annulus, or ring-shaped structure. Both the round window membrane and the oval window annulus are susceptible to rupture. When this occurs, fluid from the inner ear can leak into the middle ear; this condition is known as a perilymph fistula.

The eustachian tube, which is approximately 1 mm wide and 35 mm long, connects the middle ear to the nasopharynx. Normally, the eustachian tube is closed, but it opens by action of the palate muscles when performing the Valsalva maneuver or by yawning or swallowing. The tube serves as a drainage channel for normal and abnormal secretions of the middle ear and equalizes pressure in the middle ear with that of the atmosphere.

Inner Ear Anatomy

The inner ear is housed deep within the petrous portion of the temporal bone. The organs for hearing (cochlea) and balance (semicircular canals), as well as cranial nerves VII (facial nerve) and VIII (cochleovestibular nerve), are all part of this complex anatomy. The cochlea and semicircular canals together constitute the bony labyrinth. The three semicircular canals—posterior, superior, and lateral—lie at 90-degree angles to one another and contain sensory receptor organs related to equilibrium. These receptor end-organs are stimulated by changes in the rate or direction of an individual's movement.

The cochlea is a snail-shaped, bony tube about 3.5 cm in length with two and a half spiral turns and contains the end-organ for hearing, called the organ of Corti. Within the bony labyrinth, but not completely filling it, lies the membranous labyrinth. The membranous labyrinth is bathed in a fluid called perilymph, which communicates directly with the cerebrospinal fluid of the brain via the cochlear aqueduct. The membranous labyrinth comprises the utricle, the saccule, the semicircular canals, the cochlear duct, and the organ of Corti. The membranous labyrinth holds a fluid called endolymph. There is a delicate balance of perilymph and endolymph in the inner ear; many inner ear disorders occur when their balance is disrupted. Angular acceleration results in movement of the inner ear fluids in the canals and stimulates the hair cells of the membranous labyrinth. This results in electrical activity that travels along the vestibular division of cranial nerve VIII to the brain. Change in head position and linear acceleration stimulate the hair cells of the utricle. This also results in electrical activity being transmitted to the brain by cranial nerve VIII. In the internal auditory canal, the cochlear (acoustic) nerve, arising from the cochlea, joins the vestibular nerve, arising from the semicir-

CHART 57-1
Glossary

Ear Anatomy

Acoustic pertaining to sound or the sense of hearing

Acoustic nerve the division of the eighth cranial (vestibulocochlear) nerve, which goes to the cochlea

Auricle the projected part of the external ear also known as the pinna

Cerumen brown, waxlike secretion found in the external auditory canal

Cochlea the winding, snail-shaped bony tube that forms a portion of the inner ear and contains the organ of Corti, the transducer for hearing

Endolymph the pale transparent fluid within the membranous labyrinth of the inner ear

Eustachian tube the 3- to 4-cm tube that extends from the middle ear to the nasopharynx

External auditory canal the canal leading from the external auditory meatus to the tympanic membrane; about 2.5 cm in length

External ear the portion of the ear that consists of the auricle and external auditory canal; it is separated from the middle ear by the tympanic membrane

Incus the second of the three ossicles in the middle ear; it articulates with the malleus and stapes; the anvil

Inner ear the portion of the ear that consists of the cochlea, vestibule, and semicircular canals

Internal auditory canal a canal in the petrous portion of the temporal bone, which houses the facial and vestibulocochlear nerves (cranial nerves VII and VIII)

Malleus the first (most lateral) and largest of the three ossicles in the middle ear; it is connected to the tympanic membrane laterally and articulates with the incus; the hammer

Middle ear the small air-filled cavity in the temporal bone, which contains the three ossicles

Organ of Corti the end-organ of hearing located in the cochlea

Ossicle a small bone; there are three in the middle ear, the malleus, incus, and stapes

Oval window a fenestra (aperture) between the vestibule of the inner ear and the middle ear occupied by the base of the stapes

Pinna the outer part of the external ear, which collects and directs sound waves into the external auditory canal; the auricle

Round window a fenestra between the middle ear and the inner ear at the base of the cochlea occupied by the round window membrane

Semicircular canals the superior, posterior, and lateral bony tubes that form part of the inner ear; contain the receptor organs for balance

Stapes the third (most medial) ossicle of the middle ear; it articulates with the incus and its footplate fits into the oval window; the stirrup

Temporal bone a bone on both sides of the skull at its base; composed of the squamous, mastoid, and petrous portions

Tympanic membrane the membrane that separates the middle ear from the external auditory canal

Vestibulocochlear nerve cranial nerve VIII; auditory nerve and vestibular nerve

Conditions and Procedures

Acute otitis media inflammation in the middle ear of short duration (less than 6 weeks)

Cholesteatoma a benign tumor of the middle ear and/or mastoid

Conductive hearing loss a loss of hearing in which efficient sound transmission to the inner ear is interrupted by some obstruction or disease process

Endolymphatic hydrops a dilation of the endolymphatic space of the inner ear; it is the pathologic correlate of Ménière's disease

Labyrinthitis inflammation of the labyrinth or inner ear

Ménière's disease a condition of the inner ear characterized by a triad of symptoms: episodic vertigo, tinnitus, and fluctuating sensorineural hearing loss

Middle ear effusion fluid in the middle ear

Myringotomy (tympanotomy) an incision in the tympanic membrane

Ossiculoplasty surgical reconstruction of the middle ear bones

Otalgia pain in the ear

Otitis externa inflammation of the external auditory canal

Otitis media inflammation of the middle ear

Otorrhea inflammation of ear with discharge

Otosclerosis a condition characterized by abnormal spongy bone formation around the stapes

Perilymph fistula a leakage of fluid from the inner ear to the middle ear generally through the oval and/or round window membrane(s)

Sensorineural hearing loss a loss of hearing related to damage of the end-organ for hearing and/or cranial nerve VIII

Tinnitus a subjective perception of sound with internal origin; unwanted noises in the head or ear

Tympanoplasty surgical repair of the tympanic membrane of middle ear cular canals, utricle, and saccule, to become the vestibulocochlear nerve (cranial nerve VIII). Joining this nerve in the internal auditory canal is the facial nerve (cranial nerve VII). The internal auditory canal takes these nerves and their blood supply to the brainstem.

Balance and Dizziness

Disorders of balance and the vestibular system afflict more than 30 million Americans aged 17 or older and account for over 100,000 hip fractures in the elderly population each year. Body balance is maintained by the cooperation of the muscles and joints of the body (proprioceptive system), the eyes (visual system), and the labyrinth (vestibular system). These areas take their information about equilibrium, or balance, to the brain (cerebellar system) for coordination and perception in the cerebral cortex. The brain, of course, obtains its blood supply from the heart and arterial system. A problem in any of these areas, such as arteriosclerosis or impaired vision, can cause a balance disturbance. The vestibular apparatus of the inner ear provides feedback regarding the movements and the position of the head in space, coordinates all body muscles, and positions the eyes during rapid motion or head movement.

The term **dizziness** is used frequently by patients and health care providers to describe any altered sensation of orientation in space; it is, however, a nonspecific and nondescriptive term. Since a balance disorder is something experienced only by the patient, it is important to establish with the patient exactly what symptoms are felt. **Vertigo** is defined as the hallucination or illusion of motion; movement of the individual or the individual's surroundings is experienced. Most people with vertigo describe a spinning sensation or feel as though objects are moving around them. Vertigo is the classic symptom experienced when fairly rapid and asymmetric dysfunction of the peripheral vestibular system (inner ear) occurs. **Ataxia** is the failure of muscular coordination and may be present in patients with vestibular disease. Syncope, fainting, and loss of consciousness are not forms of vertigo, nor are they characteristic of an ear problem; they usually indicate disease in the cardiovascular system.

Physiologic Principles Underlying Sound Conduction

Sound enters the ear through the external auditory canal and causes the tympanic membrane to vibrate (Fig. 57-1). The vibrations transmit sound, in the form of mechanical energy, through the lever action of the ossicles to the oval window. This mechanical energy is then transmitted through the inner ear fluids to the cochlea, where it is converted to electrical energy. The electrical energy travels via the vestibulocochlear nerve to the central nervous system, where it is analyzed and interpreted in its final form as sound. During this transmission process, the sound waves encounter progressively smaller mass, from the large size of the auricle to the small oval window, which results in increasing amplitude (or loudness) of the sound.

The functional physiology of the oval and round windows plays an important role. The oval window is bordered by the flexible annular ligament of the stapes and the membrane of the round window is compliant, allowing for essential, equal, and opposite movement during sound stimulation. The stapedial footplate receives impulses transmitted by the incus and the malleus from the tympanic membrane. The round window, which opens on the opposite side of the cochlear duct, is protected from sound waves by the intact tympanic membrane, thus permitting motion of the inner ear fluids by sound wave stimulation. For example, in the normally intact tympanic membrane, sound waves stimu-

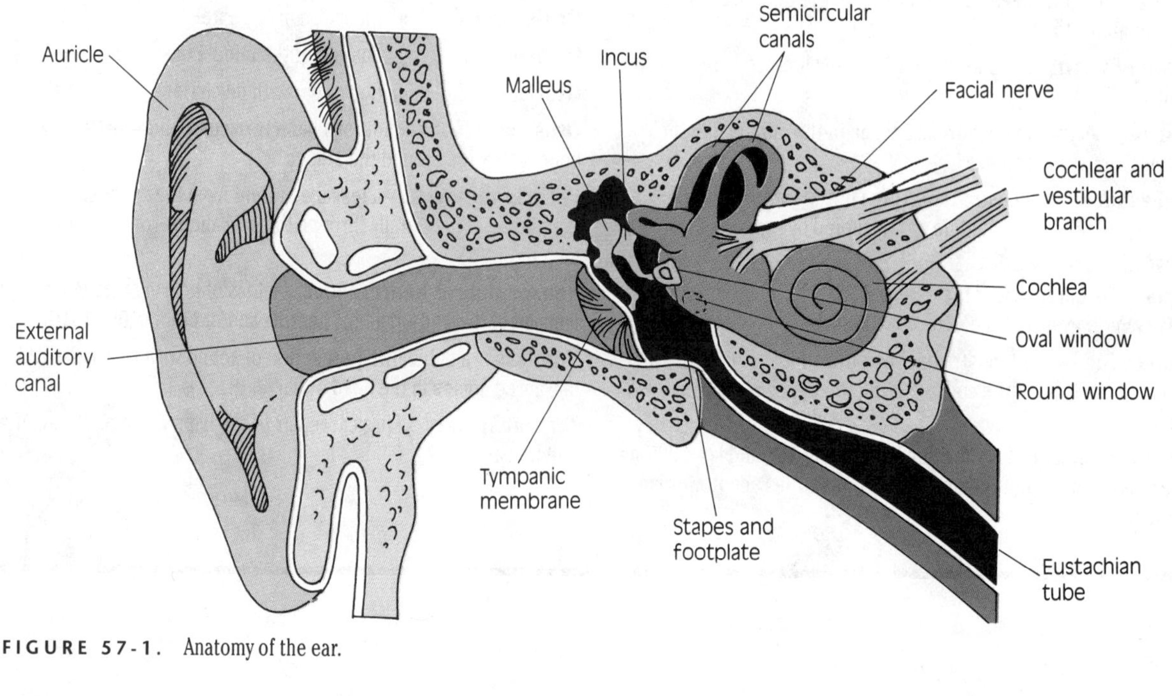

FIGURE 57-1. Anatomy of the ear.

late the oval window first, and a lag occurs before the terminal effect of the stimulus reaches the round window. This lag phase is changed, however, when a perforation of the tympanic membrane is large enough to allow sound waves to impinge on both the oval and round windows simultaneously. This effect cancels the lag and prevents the maximal effect of inner ear fluid motility and its subsequent effect in stimulating the hair cells in the organ of Corti. The result is a reduction in hearing ability.

Sound waves transmitted by the tympanic membrane to the ossicles of the middle ear are transferred to the cochlea, the organ of hearing, which is lodged in the labyrinth of the inner ear. An important ossicle is the stapes, which rocks and sets up vibrations (waves) in fluids contained in the inner ear. These fluid waves, in turn, cause movement of the basilar membrane to occur that then stimulates the hair cells of the organ of Corti, in the cochlea, to move in a wavelike manner. The movements of the membrane set up electrical currents that stimulate the various areas of the cochlea. The hair cells set up neural impulses that are encoded and then transferred to the auditory cortex in the brain, where they are decoded into a sound message.

Hearing may occur over two pathways. Sounds that are transmitted by way of the air-filled external and middle ear travel by way of air conduction. Sounds transmitted through bone directly to the inner ear travel by means of bone conduction. Normally, air conduction is the more efficient pathway; however, defects in the tympanic membrane or interruption of the ossicular chain disrupt normal air conduction and result in a loss of the sound–pressure ratio and a conductive hearing loss.

Hearing Loss

There are two types of hearing loss. Conductive loss usually results from an external ear disorder, such as impacted cerumen, or middle ear disorders, such as otitis media or otosclerosis. In such instances, the efficient transmission of sound by air to the inner ear is interrupted. The second type, sensorineural loss, involves damage to the cochlea or vestibulocochlear nerve.

In addition to conductive loss and sensorineural loss, there can also occur a mixed hearing loss as well as a functional hearing loss. The patient with a mixed hearing loss has both a conductive and sensorineural loss due to a dysfunction of both air and bone conduction. A functional (or psychogenic) hearing loss is nonorganic and unrelated to detectable structural changes in the hearing mechanisms; it is usually a manifestation of an emotional disturbance.

More than 20 million people in the United States suffer from some form of hearing loss. Most of these people can be helped with medical or surgical therapies or with a hearing aid. The nurse and physician play a major role in diagnosing hearing loss and guiding patients toward assistance.

Psychosocial Considerations

Hearing impairment may cause changes in personality and attitude, the ability to communicate, the awareness of surroundings, and even in the ability to protect oneself. In a classroom, a student with impaired hearing may show disinterest, inattention, and failing grades. A person at home may feel isolated because of an inability to hear the clock chime, the refrigerator hum, the birds sing, or the traffic pass. A hearing-impaired pedestrian may attempt to cross the street at the wrong time because of failure to hear an approaching car. The person with a hearing loss may miss parts of a conversation and may believe that people are talking about him or her. Many people are not even aware that their hearing is gradually becoming impaired. Often it is not the person with the hearing loss, but the people with whom he or she is communicating, who recognize the impairment first.

Not infrequently, a person with a hearing loss refuses to seek medical attention. Because of fear that hearing loss is a sign of advancing age, many people refuse to wear a hearing aid. Others feel self-conscious when they wear an aid. Introspective patients will generally ask those with whom they are trying to communicate to let them know if difficulties in communication exist. These attitudes and behaviors should be taken into account when counseling patients who need hearing assistance. The nurse keeps in mind that the decision to wear a hearing aid is a personal one that is affected by these attitudes and behaviors.

Although some hearing difficulty may be due to impacted cerumen, which is readily treated, proper assessment is best performed by an otologist or otolaryngologist. An **otologist** is a physician who specializes in diagnosing and treating problems of the ear. An **otolaryngologist** is a physician who specializes in problems relating to the ear, nose, and throat. An **audiologist,** one who specializes in the nonmedical evaluation and rehabilitation of hearing disorders, may also participate in the evaluation.

Gerontologic Considerations

With aging, changes occur in the ear that may eventually lead to hearing deficits. Few changes occur in the external ear except that cerumen tends to become harder and drier and there is a greater chance of impaction. In the middle ear, the tympanic membrane may atrophy or become sclerotic. The inner ear changes with a degeneration of cells at the base of the cochlea. There seems to be a familial predisposition to sensorineural hearing loss. This is manifested by a loss in the ability to hear high-frequency sounds, followed in time by the loss of middle and lower frequencies. The term **presbycusis** is used to describe this progressive hearing loss. Presbycusis is, however, a diagnosis of exclusion, and other causes of this sensorineural hearing loss should be ruled out.

Early signs of hearing loss may include tinnitus, increasing inability to hear at group meetings, and a need to turn up the volume of the television (Chart 57-2). The literature (Paparella et al., 1991) suggests that 25% of people between ages 65 and 74 years and 50% of people aged 75 years and older experience hearing difficulties. The cause is unknown and linkages to diet, metabolism, arteriosclerosis, stress, and heredity have been inconsistent.

Other factors affect hearing in the elderly population, such as life-long exposure to loud noises (*e.g.*, jets, guns, heavy machinery, circular saws). Certain medications, such as the aminoglycosides and even aspirin, have ototoxic effects because renal changes in the older person result in delayed drug excretion. Many older people take quinine for

CHART 57-2
Symptoms of Hearing Loss

Speech deterioration The person who slurs words or drops word endings, or produces flat-sounding speech, may not be hearing correctly. The ears guide the voice, both in loudness and pronunciation.

Fatigue If a person tires easily when listening to conversation or to a speech, fatigue may be the result of straining to hear. Under these circumstances, the person may become irritable very easily.

Indifference It is easy for the person who cannot hear what others are saying to become depressed and disinterested in life in general.

Social withdrawal Not being able to hear what is going on around him causes the hearing impaired person to withdraw from situations that might prove embarrassing.

Insecurity Lack of self-confidence and fear of mistakes create a feeling of insecurity in many hearing impaired persons. No one likes to say the wrong thing or do anything that might tend to make him look foolish.

Indecision-Procrastination Loss of self-confidence makes it increasingly difficult for a hearing impaired person to make decisions.

Suspiciousness The hearing impaired person, who often hears only part of what is being said, may suspect that others are talking about him or that portions of the conversation relating to him are deliberately spoken softly so that he will not hear them!

False pride The hearing impaired person wants to conceal the hearing loss. Consequently, he often pretends he is hearing when he actually is not.

Loneliness and unhappiness Although everyone wishes for quiet now and then, *enforced* silence can be boring and even somewhat frightening. People with a hearing loss often feel isolated.

Tendency to dominate the conversation Many hearing impaired people tend to dominate the conversation, knowing that as long as it is centered on them and they can control it they are not so likely to be embarrassed by some mistake.

(Courtesy of Maico Hearing Instruments.)

treatment of leg cramps, which can cause a hearing loss. Psychogenic factors and other disease processes (*e.g.*, diabetes) also may be partially responsible for sensorineural hearing loss.

Hearing impairment should not be assumed to be a normal consequence of aging. When a problem occurs, an evaluation by an otologist or otolaryngologist and an audiogram are warranted. Even with the best of medical care, the older person has to learn to adjust to varying degrees of hearing loss. Care of elderly patients includes recognizing emotional reactions related to hearing loss such as (1) suspicion of others because of an inability to hear adequately, (2) frustration and anger, with repeated statements such as "I didn't hear what you said," and (3) feelings of insecurity because of the inability to hear the telephone or alarms.

The nurse who understands the different types of hearing loss will be more successful in adapting a communication style to fit the patient's needs. Trying to speak in a loud voice to a person who cannot adequately hear high-frequency sounds only makes matters worse. On the other hand, strategies such as talking into the least-impaired ear, using gestures, and facial expressions may help.

Noise and Its Effect on Hearing

Noise (unwanted and unavoidable sound) has been identified as one of the environmental hazards of the 20th century. The sheer volume of noise that surrounds us daily has increased from a simple annoyance into a potentially dangerous source of physical and psychologic damage.

In terms of physical impact, loud, persistent noise has been found to cause constriction of peripheral blood vessels, increased blood pressure and heart rate (because of increased secretion of adrenalin), and increased gastrointestinal activity. Additional research is needed to address the overall effects of noise on the human body. It seems certain, however, that a quiet environment is more conducive to peace of mind. A person who is ill feels more at ease when noise is kept to a minimum.

Many environmental factors have an adverse effect on the auditory system and, with time, result in permanent sensorineural hearing loss. The most common mechanism is *noise-induced hearing loss.* This is, fortunately, a preventable disorder. The term noise-induced hearing loss is used to describe hearing loss that follows a long period of exposure to loud noise (*e.g.*, heavy machinery, engines, artillery), whereas acoustic trauma refers to the hearing loss caused by a single exposure to an extremely intense noise, such as an explosion. Usually, noise-induced hearing loss occurs at a high frequency (around 4000 hertz [Hz]), although with continued noise exposure the hearing loss can become more severe and include adjacent frequencies. The minimum noise level known to cause noise-induced hearing loss, regardless of duration, is about 85 to 90 decibels (dB). Noise exposure is inherent in many occupations such as mechanics, printing, aviation, and rock music as well as in hobbies such as woodworking and hunting.

The Occupational Safety and Health Act (OSHA) requires that workers wear ear protection to prevent noise-induced hearing loss when exposed to noise above the legal limits. There are no medications that will protect against noise-induced hearing loss; hearing loss is permanent because the hair cells in the organ of Corti themselves are destroyed. Ear protection against noise is the most effective preventive measure available.

Assessment of Hearing Ability

Examination of the Ear

The external ear is examined by inspection and direct palpation, whereas the tympanic membrane is inspected, as is the middle ear, by otoscope and indirect palpation by using a pneumatic otoscope. It is impossible to inspect the inner ear, but various assessment methods can give a gross assessment of its function. Assessment of auditory acuity is included in every physical examination.

Physical Assessment. Inspection of the external ear is a simple procedure but often overlooked. The auricle and surrounding tissues are inspected for deformities, lesions, and discharge as well as size, symmetry, and angle of attachment to the head. Movement of the auricle does not normally elicit pain. If this maneuver is painful, acute external otitis is suspected. Tenderness upon palpation in the area of the mastoid may indicate acute mastoiditis or inflammation of the posterior auricular node. Occasionally, sebaceous cysts and tophi (subcutaneous mineral deposits) may be present on the pinna. A flaky scaliness on or behind the auricle usually indicates seborrheic dermatitis and may be present on the scalp and facial structures as well.

To examine the external auditory canal and tympanic membrane, the patient's head is tipped away from the examiner. The otoscope is held in one hand while the auricle is grasped with the other hand firmly and pulled upward, backward, and slightly outward (Fig. 57-2). This straightens the canal in the adult, allowing the examiner to better visualize the tympanic membrane. The speculum is gently and slowly inserted into the ear canal, and the eye is held close to the magnifying lens of the otoscope to visualize the canal and tympanic membrane. The largest speculum that the canal can accommodate (usually 5 mm in an adult) is guided gently down into the canal and slightly forward. Because the distal portion of the canal is bony and covered by a sensitive layer of epithelium, only light pressure may be used without causing pain.

Any discharge, inflammation, or foreign body in the external auditory canal is noted. The healthy tympanic membrane is pearly gray and is positioned obliquely at the base of the canal. The landmarks are identified if visible (Fig. 57-3): the pars tensa and cone of light, the umbo, the manubrium of the malleus, and its short process. A slow circular movement of the speculum allows further visualization of the malleolar folds and periphery. The position and color of the membrane as well as any unusual markings or deviation in the cone of light are noted. The presence of fluid, air bubbles, blood, or masses in the middle ear should be noted.

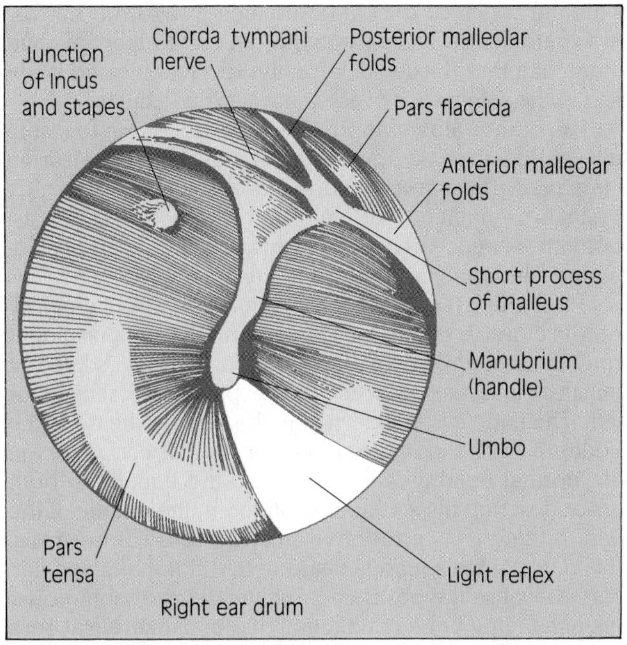

FIGURE 57-3. Illustration of the normal right tympanic membrane as it would be seen through the otoscope.

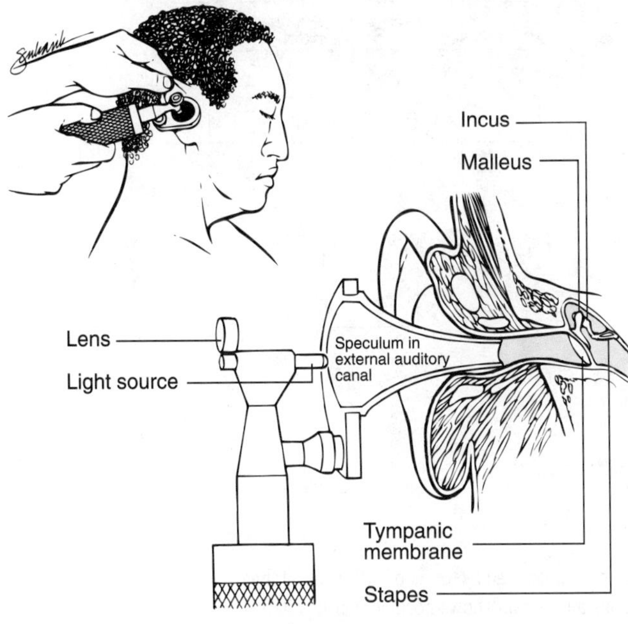

FIGURE 57-2. Technique for using the otoscope.

Proper otoscopic examination of the external auditory canal and tympanic membrane requires that the canal be free of large amounts of cerumen. Cerumen is normally present in the external canal, and small amounts should not interfere with otoscopic examination. If the tympanic membrane cannot be visualized because of cerumen, the external canal may be gently irrigated if there are no contraindications. In the event that adherent cerumen is present, a small amount of mineral oil or over-the-counter cerumen softener may be instilled within the ear canal and the patient instructed to return for subsequent removal of the cerumen and inspection of the ear. The use of instruments such as a cerumen currette for cerumen removal is reserved for otolaryngologists and nurses with specialized training because of the danger of perforating the tympanic membrane and excoriating the external auditory canal. Cerumen buildup is a common cause of hearing loss and of local irritation.

Auditory Acuity. A general estimation of the patient's hearing is effectively screened by assessing the patient's ability to hear a whispered phrase or a ticking watch. A soft whisper is produced by the examiner, who has first made a full exhalation. One ear is tested at a time. To exclude one ear from the testing, the examiner covers the untested ear with the palm of the hand. From a distance of 1 to 2 feet from the unoccluded ear and out of visual range, the patient with normal acuity can correctly repeat what was whispered. If a ticking watch is used, the examiner holds the watch at a distance of 3 inches from his or her own auricle (assuming the examiner has normal hearing) and then holds the watch at the same distance away from the patient's auricle. Because a watch produces a higher-pitched sound than the whispered voice, it is less reliable and is not used as the sole means of assessing auditory acuity.

Use of the Weber and Rinne tests enables one to distinguish conductive loss from sensorineural loss when hearing is impaired. These tests are not part of the usual screening physical examination but are useful if a more discrete assessment is needed, if hearing loss is detected, or if substantiation of audiometric results is desired.

The **Weber test** uses bone conduction to test lateralization of sound. A tuning fork is set in motion by grasping it firmly by its stem and tapping it on the examiner's knee or knuckles. It is then placed on the patient's forehead or teeth. The patient is asked whether the sound is heard in the middle of the head, the right ear, or the left ear. A person with normal hearing will hear the sound equally in both ears or describe the sound as centered in the middle of the head. If there is a **conductive hearing loss** (otosclerosis, otitis media), the sound is heard better in the affected ear. This is because the obstruction obliterates the room noise, thus enhancing bone conduction. If a **sensorineural loss** exists, however, the sound lateralizes to the better-hearing ear. The Weber test is useful in cases of unilateral hearing loss.

In the **Rinne test**, the stem of a vibrating tuning fork is placed behind the auricle on the mastoid bone (bone conduction) until the patient can no longer hear the sound. The tuning fork is then shifted to within 1 inch of the external auditory canal meatus (air conduction). Under normal circumstances the patient continues to hear the sound, demonstrating that air conduction lasts longer than bone conduction. In conductive hearing loss, bone conduction exceeds air conduction; once bone conduction through the temporal bone has subsided, the patient is unable to hear the fork through the usual conductive mechanism. In contrast, sensorineural loss permits sounds to be conducted by air better than by bone, although neither is a good conductor and all sounds may be perceived to be distant and faint.

Auditory and Vestibular Diagnostic Procedures

Many diagnostic procedures are available to measure the auditory and vestibular systems. These tests are usually performed by an audiologist who has earned a master's degree and, after a clinical fellowship, is recognized by the American Speech-Language-Hearing Association with a certificate of clinical competence in audiology (CCC/A).

In the detection of hearing loss, the audiometer is the single most important diagnostic instrument. Audiometric testing is of two kinds: (1) **pure-tone audiometry,** in which the sound stimulus consists of a pure or musical tone (the louder the tone before the patient perceives it, the greater the hearing loss), and (2) **speech audiometry,** in which the spoken word is used to determine the ability to hear and discriminate sounds.

The audiologist performs the testing while the patient wears earphones and signals upon hearing a tone. When the tone is applied directly over the external auditory canal meatus, air conduction is measured. When the stimulus is applied to the mastoid bone, bypassing the conductive mechanism (the ossicles), nerve conduction is tested. For accuracy, audiometric evaluations are performed in a soundproof room. Responses are plotted on a graph known as an audiogram.

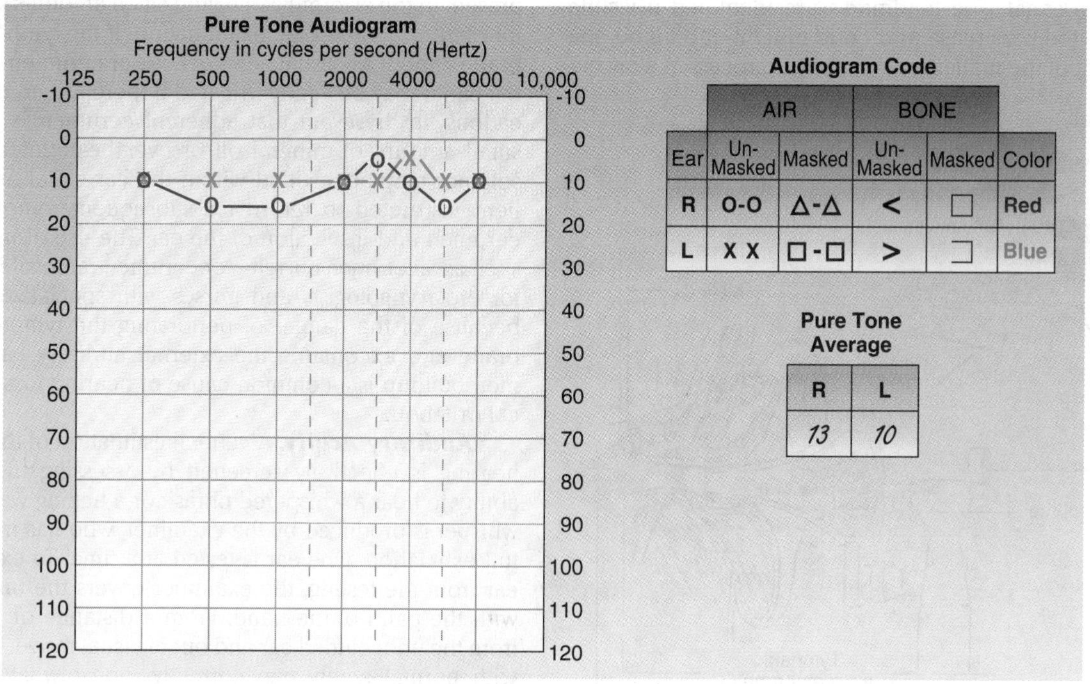

FIGURE 57-4. An audiogram presents a graphic outline of hearing as measured by tones of different pitches ranging from 125 through 8000 cycles per second (cps) or Hertz (Hz). This audiogram shows normal hearing bilaterally. The box on the right indicates the symbols used on an audiogram.

TABLE 57-1 Severity of Hearing Loss

Loss in Decibels	Classification
0–15	Normal hearing
>15–25	Slight hearing loss
>25–40	Mild hearing loss
>40–55	Moderate hearing loss
>55–70	Moderate to severe hearing loss
>70–90	Severe hearing loss
>90	Profound hearing loss

Frequency refers to the number of sound waves emanating from a source per second—cycles per second or hertz (Hz). The normal human ear perceives sounds ranging in frequency from 20 to 20,000 Hz. The frequencies from 500 to 2000 Hz are important in understanding everyday speech (Fig. 57-4); this is referred to as the speech range. **Pitch** is the term used to describe frequency; a tone with 100 Hz is considered of low pitch, and a tone of 10,000 Hz is considered of high pitch. The unit for measuring loudness (intensity of sound) is the decibel (dB), the pressure exerted by sound. Hearing loss is measured in decibels, which is a logarithmic function of intensity and not easily converted into a percentage. The critical level of loudness is approximately 30 dB. Some examples of common sound intensities include the shuffling of papers in quiet surroundings, which occurs at about 15 dB; a low conversation, 40 dB; and a jet plane 100 feet away, which registers at about 150 dB. Sound louder than 80 dB is perceived by the human ear to be harsh. Sound that is perceived as uncomfortable can be damaging to the inner ear. Table 57-1 shows a suggested classification of hearing loss. In treating patients surgically to improve hearing loss, the aim is to improve the hearing level to 30 dB or better within the speech frequencies. An audiogram will differentiate between conductive hearing loss (Fig. 57-5) and sensorineural hearing loss (Fig. 57-6). Speech discrimination is also measured (Fig. 57-7).

A tympanogram, or impedance audiometry, measures middle ear muscle reflex to sound stimulation, as well as compliance of the tympanic membrane, by changing the air pressure in a sealed ear canal (Fig. 57-8). Compliance is impaired with middle ear disease.

The auditory brainstem response (ABR) is a detectable electrical potential from cranial nerve VIII (acoustic) and ascending auditory pathways of the brainstem in response to sound stimulation. It is an objective method of measuring hearing since the patient's active participation is not required as it is in the behavioral audiogram. Electrodes are placed on the patient's forehead and acoustic stimuli, usually in the form of clicks, are made in the ear. The resulting electrophysiologic measurements can determine at which decibel level a patient hears and if there are any impairments along the nerve pathways, such as tumors on cranial nerve VIII.

Electrocochleography (ECoG) is the recording of electrophysiologic potentials of the cochlea and cranial nerve VIII in response to acoustic stimuli. The resulting ratio is used to assist in diagnosing disorders of inner ear fluid balance such as Ménière's disease and perilymph fistula. The procedure is performed by placing an electrode as close as possible to the cochlea, either in the external

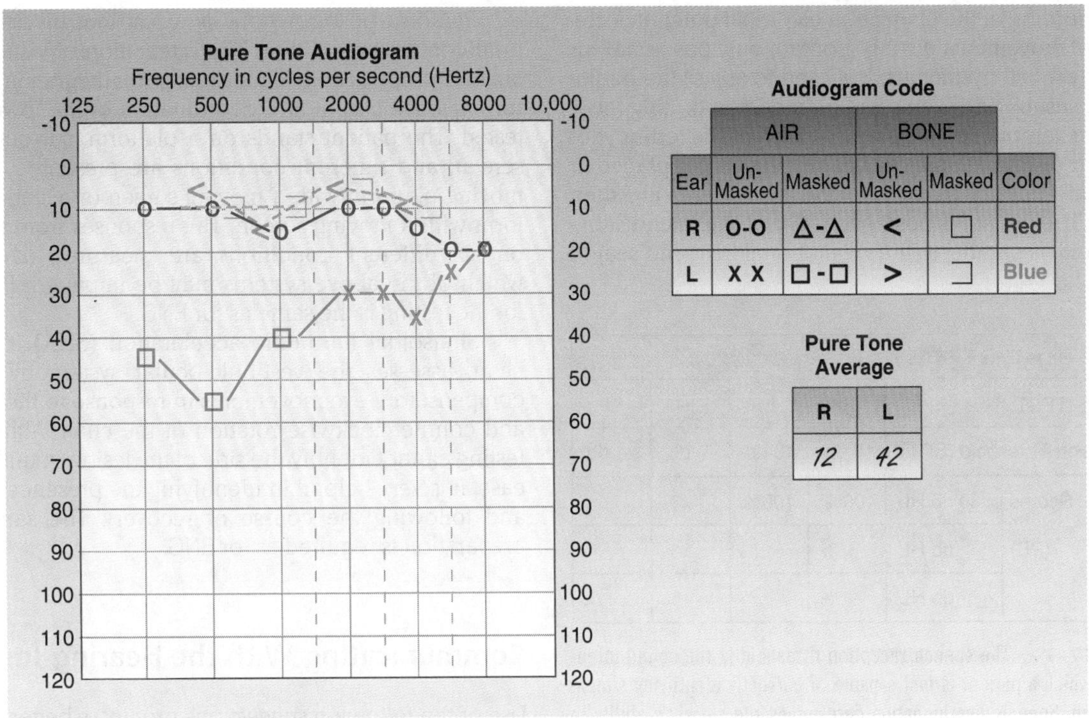

FIGURE 57-5. This audiogram shows a conductive hearing loss in the left ear. Note the difference between the air and bone conduction. This is known as an air–bone gap.

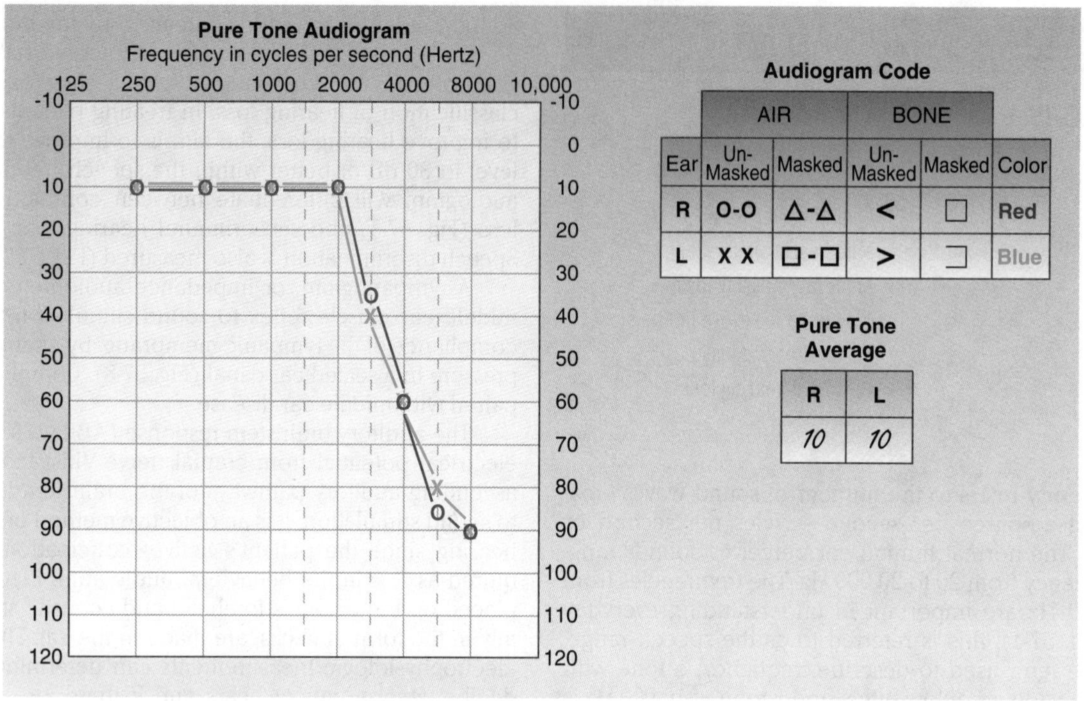

FIGURE 57-6. This audiogram shows a high-frequency sensorineural hearing loss bilaterally. This type of hearing loss is normally symmetric; further evaluation should be made when hearing loss is asymmetric.

auditory canal next to the tympanic membrane or via a transtympanic electrode placed through the tympanic membrane near the round window membrane. In preparation for the testing, patients are asked not to take any diuretics for 48 hours before the test so that fluid balance of the inner ear will not be altered.

Electronystagmography (ENG) is the measurement and graphic recording of the changes in electrical potentials created by eye movements during spontaneous, positional, or calorically evoked nystagmus. It is used to assess the oculomotor and vestibular systems and their corresponding interaction. For example, in the caloric portion of the testing, hot and cold air or water (bithermal caloric testing) is placed in the external auditory canal, and eye movements are then measured. The patient is positioned so that the lateral semicircular canal is parallel to the gravitational field and seated while electrodes are placed on the forehead and near the eyes. Patients are asked not to take any vestibular suppressants, such as sedatives, tranquilizers, antihistamines, or alcohol, as well as vestibular stimulants, such as caffeine, for 24 hours before testing. ENG helps in the diagnosis of conditions such as Ménière's disease and tumors of the internal auditory canal or posterior fossa.

Platform posturography is a test that investigates postural control capabilities. The integration of visual, vestibular, and proprioceptive cues (sensory integration) with motor response output and coordination of the lower limbs is tested. The patient stands on a platform, surrounded by a screen, and different conditions are presented, such as a moving platform with a moving screen or a stationary platform with a moving screen. The responses from the patient on six different conditions are measured and indicate which of the above systems may be impaired. Preparation for the testing is the same as for ENG.

Sinusoidal harmonic acceleration (SHA), or a rotary chair, assesses the vestibulo-ocular system by analyzing compensatory eye movements in response to the clockwise and counterclockwise rotation of the chair. Although SHA testing cannot identify the side of the lesion in unilateral disease, it is very helpful in identifying the presence of disease and following the course of recovery. The same patient preparation is required as for ENG.

SPEECH HEARING TESTS					
TEST		R	L	BIN	SF
Sp. Reception Threshold (SRT)		10 db	10 db	db	db
Sp. Discrim. Scores	80 db HL	100%	100%	%	%
(PB)	___db HL	%	%	%	%
	___db HL	%	%	%	%

FIGURE 57-7. The speech reception threshold is the sound intensity level at which a patient is just capable of correctly identifying simple speech stimuli. Speech discrimination determines the patient's ability to distinguish different sounds, in the form of words, at a decibel level where sound is heard.

Communicating With the Hearing-Impaired

Use of the following suggestions promotes better communication with hearing-impaired persons whose speech is difficult to understand.

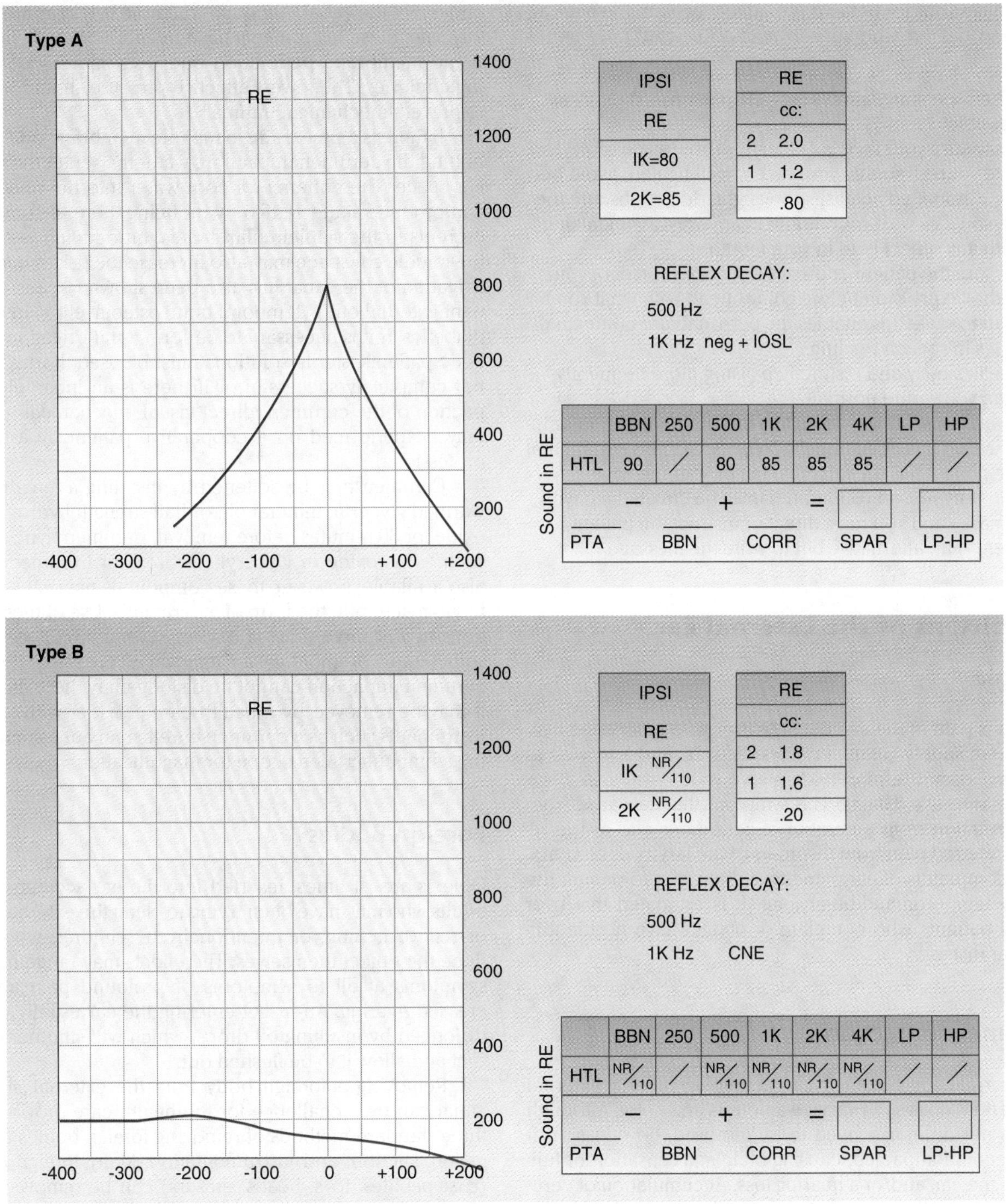

FIGURE 57-8 The typical normal, or type A, tympanogram shows a pressure/compliance curve by changing air pressure in a sealed ear canal. A typical "flat," or type B, tympanogram shows an absence of a pressure/compliance peak and indicates middle ear effusion or massive ossicular fixation.

1. Devote full attention to what the person is saying. Look and listen—do not try to attend to another task while listening.
2. Engage the speaker in conversation when it is possible for you to anticipate the replies. This enables you to become accustomed to any peculiarities in speech patterns.
3. Try to determine the essential context of what is being said; you can often fill in the details from context.
4. Do not try to appear as if you understand if you do not.
5. If you cannot understand at all or have serious doubt about your ability to understand what is being said, have the person write the message rather than risk misunderstanding. Having the person repeat the message in speech, after you know its content, also aids you in becoming accustomed to his pattern of speech.

Suggestions for better communication with the hearing-impaired person who speech reads (lip reads) are as follows:

1. When speaking, always face the person as directly as possible.
2. Make sure your face is as clearly visible as possible; locate yourself so that your face is well lighted; avoid being silhouetted against strong light; do not obscure the person's view of your mouth in any way; avoid talking with any object held in your mouth.
3. Be sure the patient knows the topic or subject of your verbal expression before going ahead with what you plan to say—this enables the person to use contextual clues in speech reading.
4. Speak slowly and distinctly, pausing more frequently than you would normally.
5. If you question whether some important direction or instruction has been understood, check to be certain that the patient has the full meaning of your message.
6. If for any reason your mouth must be covered (as with a mask) and you must direct or instruct the patient, there is no alternative but to write the message.

Conditions of the External Ear

Otalgia

Otalgia is pain in the ear. Because the ear is innervated by a rich nerve supply (cranial nerves V, VII, IX, and X as well as the second and third cervical nerve roots), the skin is extremely sensitive. Otalgia is a symptom that can arise from local irritation from a number of conditions and as the result of referred pain from disorders of the larynx or pharynx. Many complaints of ear pain are actually due to pain in the nearby temporomandibular joint. It is estimated that over 50% of patients who complain of otalgia have no identifiable ear disease.

Cerumen Impaction

It is normal for cerumen to accumulate in the external canal and it does so in varying amounts and color. Although it does not ordinarily need to be removed, on occasion it may become impacted, causing otalgia, a sensation of fullness in the ear, and/or a hearing loss. Accumulation of cerumen is especially significant in the geriatric population as a cause of hearing deficit. Attempts to clear the external auditory canal with matches, hair pins, and other implements are dangerous because trauma to the skin may result in infection or damage to the eardrum.

Management. Cerumen may be removed by irrigation, suction, or instrumentation. Unless there is a history of perforated tympanic membrane or there is inflammation of the external ear (otitis externa), gentle irrigation is an acceptable procedure for removing impacted cerumen. This technique is effective if the cerumen is not tightly packed in the external auditory canal. Successful removal of cerumen by irrigation requires that some of the water stream get behind the obstructing cerumen in order to push it laterally and out of the canal. Although water pic irrigators are generally safe, these instruments have been associated with tympanic membrane perforation and even more serious otologic injuries. The lowest effective pressure should be used to prevent mechanical trauma.

If there is a preexisting tympanic membrane perforation behind the cerumen impaction, water may enter the middle ear space. The entrance of cool water into the middle ear can produce acute vertigo by inducing thermal convection currents in the semicircular canals. Introducing water into the middle ear space may also increase the risk of infection. Irrigation of the canal has also been shown to cause malignant external otitis (temporal bone osteomyelitis) in elderly diabetics. If it is necessary to perform aural irrigation in diabetic patients, sterile solutions must be used. If irrigation is not completely successful or if there is an incomplete impaction of the cerumen, direct visual, mechanical removal may be performed on a cooperative patient by a trained professional.

Cerumen may be softened by instilling a few drops of warmed glycerin, mineral oil, or half-strength hydrogen peroxide for 30 minutes before removal. Cerumenolytic agents, such as peroxide in glyceryl (Debrox) or Cerumenex, are also available; however, these compounds may cause an allergic reaction in the form of a dermatitis. Use of these solutions two or three times a day for several days is generally sufficient to promote easier removal of the impaction. If a cerumen impaction cannot be dislodged by these methods, it may be removed by a health care provider with specific instruments such as a cerumen curette and aural suction using a binocular microscope for magnification.

Foreign Bodies

Objects are, at times, inserted into the ear accidentally by adults who may have been trying to clean the external canal or relieve itching, or intentionally by children who introduce the object themselves. The effects may range from no symptoms at all to symptoms of profound pain and decreased hearing. An insect entering the ear usually can be dislodged by instilling oil drops, which will smother the insect and allow it to be flushed out.

Removing a foreign body from the external auditory canal can be a challenge for the health care provider. The three standard methods of removing foreign bodies are irrigation, suction, and instrumentation. Many foreign bodies (*e.g.*, pebbles, toys, beads, erasers) can be removed by irrigation unless there is a history of tympanic membrane perforation. However, vegetable foreign bodies (*e.g.*, seeds, beans, peas) and insects have a tendency to swell, so irrigation is contraindicated. Many of the foreign bodies that do not lend themselves to irrigation may be removed with suction. If instrumentation is used, direct visualization of the canal is necessary to prevent damage. Attempts to remove any foreign body from the external canal may be dangerous in unskilled hands. The object may be pushed completely into the bony portion of the canal, lacerating the skin and perforating the tympanic membrane. In young children or in cases of difficult extractions in adults, removal of the foreign body may need to be performed under general anesthesia in the operating room.

Otitis Externa

Infections, primarily bacterial or fungal, are among the most common problems encountered in the ear. The many causes of otitis externa (infection of the external ear) include water in the ear canal (swimmer's ear), trauma to the skin of the ear canal permitting entrance of organisms into the tissues, and systemic conditions such as vitamin deficiency and endocrine disorders. The normal ear canal is sterile in some persons; in others, *Staphylococcus albus* and/or other organisms such as diphtheroids are present. The most common pathogens in otitis externa are *Staphylococcus aureus* and *Pseudomonas* species. The most common fungus isolated in both normal and infected ears is *Aspergillus.* External otitis is often due to a dermatosis such as psoriasis, eczema, or seborrheic dermatitis. Even allergic reactions to hair spray, hair dye, and permanent wave lotions can cause dermatitis, which clears when the offending agent is removed.

Clinical Manifestations. The patient usually presents with pain, discharge from the external auditory canal, aural tenderness (usually not present in middle ear infections), and occasionally fever, cellulitis, and lymphadenopathy. Other complaints may include pruritus and hearing loss or a feeling of fullness. Upon otoscopic examination the ear canal is erythematous and edematous. Discharge may be yellow or green and foul smelling. In fungal infections the hairlike black spores may even be visualized.

Management. The principles of therapy are aimed at relieving the discomfort, reducing the swelling of the ear canal, and eradicating the infection. It is not uncommon for patients to require prescription analgesics for the first 48 to 92 hours. If the tissues of the external canal are edematous, it may be necessary to insert a wick to keep the canal open so that liquid medications (*e.g.*, Burow's solution, antibiotic otic preparations) may be introduced. These medications may be administered by dropper at room temperature. Such medications are usually combinations of antibiotics and corticosteroid agents to soothe the inflamed tissues. If there is cellulitis or fever, systemic antibiotics may be required. Antifungal agents may be prescribed when appropriate.

Patients are reminded to avoid self-cleaning of the external auditory canal and not to use cotton-tipped applicators. The patient should also avoid swimming or allowing water to enter the ear when shampooing or showering. A piece of lamb's wool or a cotton ball can be covered in a water-insoluble gel (such as Vaseline) and placed in the ear to prevent water contamination. Patients can prevent infection by using antiseptic otic preparations after swimming, such as Swim Ear or Ear Dry, unless there is a history of tympanic membrane perforation or a current ear infection.

Malignant Otitis Externa

A more serious, although rare, form of external ear infection is malignant otitis externa (temporal bone osteomyelitis). This is a progressive, debilitating, and occasionally fatal infection of the external auditory canal, surrounding tissue, and the base of the skull. It is usually caused by *Pseudomonas aeruginosa* in patients with low resistance to infection, such as diabetics. Successful treatment includes control of the diabetes, administration of antibiotics (usually intravenously), and aggressive local wound care. Standard parenteral antibiotic treatment includes the combination of an antipseudomonal agent and an aminoglycoside, both of which have potentially serious side effects. Since aminoglycosides are nephrotoxic and ototoxic, patients' serum aminoglycoside levels and renal and auditory function must be monitored during therapy. Local wound care includes limited debridement of the infected tissue, including bone and cartilage, depending on the extent of the infection.

Masses of the External Ear

Small, hard, bony protrusions seen in the lower posterior bony portion of the ear canal are called **exostoses.** They most often occur bilaterally. The skin covering the exostosis is normal. Many people feel exostoses are caused by an exposure to cold water, as in scuba divers or surfers.

Malignant tumors also may be found in the external ear. Most common are basal cell carcinomas on the pinna and squamous cell carcinomas in the ear canal. If untreated, squamous cell carcinoma may spread through the temporal bone, causing facial nerve paralysis and hearing loss. Carcinomas must be treated surgically.

Conditions of the Middle Ear

Tympanic Membrane Perforation

A tympanic membrane perforation is usually caused by trauma or infection. Sources of trauma include skull fracture, explosive injury, or a severe blow to the ear. Less frequently, perforation is caused by foreign objects (*e.g.*, cotton-tipped applicators, bobby pins, keys) being pushed too far into the external auditory canal. In addition to tympanic membrane perforation, injury to the ossicles and even the inner ear may result from this type of action; thus, attempts by patients to clear the external auditory canal should be discouraged. During infection, the tympanic membrane may rupture if the pressure in the middle ear is greater than the atmospheric pressure in the external auditory canal.

Management. Most tympanic membrane perforations heal spontaneously within weeks after rupture, although some may take up to several months. During the healing process the ear must be protected from water. Some perforations persist because of the growth of scar tissue over the edges of the perforation, thus preventing extension of the epithelial cells across the margins and final healing. Perforations that do not heal on their own may require surgery. In the case of a head injury or temporal bone fracture, a patient is observed for evidence of cerebrospinal fluid otorrhea or rhinorrhea—a clear, watery drainage from the ear or nose, respectively.

The patient must protect the ear from water when a tympanic membrane perforation occurs. The decision to perform a tympanoplasty (repair of the tympanic membrane) is usually based on the need to prevent potential infection from water entering the ear or the desire to improve the patient's hearing. There are a variety of surgical techniques; all basically involve placing tissue across the perforation to allow healing. Surgery is usually successful in closing the perforation permanently and improving hearing; it is usually performed on an outpatient basis.

Acute Otitis Media

Acute otitis media is an acute infection of the middle ear. The primary cause of acute otitis media is the entrance of pathogenic bacteria into the normally sterile middle ear. This most commonly occurs when there is eustachian tube dysfunction such as obstruction caused by upper respiratory infections, inflammation of surrounding structures (*e.g.*, sinusitis, adenoid hypertrophy), or allergic reactions (*e.g.*, allergic rhinitis). Bacteria commonly found as the causative organisms are *Streptococcus pneumoniae, Hemophilus influenzae,* and *Moraxella catarrhalis.* The mode of entry of the bacteria in most patients is probably through the eustachian tube from contaminated secretions in the nasopharynx. Bacteria may also enter the middle ear in tympanic membrane perforation. A purulent exudate is usually present in the middle ear and results in a conductive hearing loss.

Clinical Manifestations. The symptoms of otitis media may vary with the severity of the infection and may be either very mild and transient or very severe. The condition is usually unilateral in adults, and otalgia may be present. The pain is relieved after spontaneous perforation of the tympanic membrane or after myringotomy (incision of the tympanic membrane). Other symptoms may include drainage from the ear, fever, hearing loss, and tinnitus. Upon otoscopic examination, the external auditory canal is often fairly normal in appearance, and there is no pain with movement of the auricle. The tympanic membrane is erythematous and often bulging. Table 57-2 differentiates acute external otitis from acute otitis media.

Management. The outcome of otitis media depends on the efficacy of therapy (*i.e.*, the prescribed dose of an oral antibiotic and the duration of therapy), the virulence of the bacteria, and the physical status of the patient. With early and appropriate broad-spectrum antibiotic therapy, otitis media may clear up with no serious sequelae. If drainage occurs, an antibiotic otic preparation is usually prescribed. The condition may become subacute (*i.e.*, lasting 3 weeks to 3 months), with persistent purulent discharge from the ear. Rarely does permanent hearing loss occur. Secondary complications involving the mastoid and other serious intracranial complications, such as meningitis or brain abscess, are rare but can occur.

Myringotomy (Tympanotomy). An incision in the tympanic membrane is known as myringotomy or tympanotomy. The tympanic membrane is anesthetized using a local anesthetic such as phenol or by iontophoresis. In iontophoresis an electrical current flows through a lidocaine-and-epinephrine solution to numb the ear canal and tympanic membrane. The procedure is painless and takes less than 15 minutes. Under the microscope an incision is then made through the tympanic membrane to relieve pressure and to drain serous or purulent fluid from the middle ear. Normally, this procedure is not necessary for the treatment of acute otitis media; however, it may be performed if pain persists. Myringotomy also allows for identification of the infecting organism and determination of its sensitivity to antibiotic agents. The incision heals within 24 to 72 hours. If episodes of acute otitis media recur and there is no contraindication, a ventilating, or pressure-equalizing (PE), tube may be inserted. The ventilating tube temporarily takes the place of the eustachian tube in equalizing pressure and is retained for 6 to 18 months. The ventilating tube is then extruded with normal skin migration of the tympanic membrane, and the hole heals in nearly every case. Ventilating tubes are more commonly used to treat recurrent episodes of acute otitis media in children than in adults.

Serous Otitis Media

Serous otitis media (middle ear effusion) implies fluid, without evidence of active infection, in the middle ear. In theory,

TABLE 57-2 Comparison of Clinical Features: Acute Otitis Externa and Acute Otitis Media

Feature	Acute Otitis Externa	Acute Otitis Media
Otorrhea	May or may not be present	Present if tympanic membrane perforates; discharge is profuse
Otalgia	Persistent, may awaken patient at night	Relieved if tympanic membrane ruptures
Aural tenderness	Present on palpation of auricle	Usually absent
Systemic symptoms	Absent	Fever, upper respiratory infection, rhinitis
Edema of external auditory canal	Present	Absent
Tympanic membrane	May appear normal	Erythema, bulging, may be perforated
Hearing loss	Conductive type	Conductive type

this fluid results from a negative pressure in the middle ear caused by eustachian tube obstruction. This condition is found primarily in children; it is important to note that, when it occurs in adults, some other underlying cause for the eustachian tube dysfunction must be sought. A middle ear effusion is frequently seen in patients following radiation therapy and barotrauma (*e.g.*, scuba diving) and in patients with eustachian tube dysfunction from a concurrent upper respiratory infection or allergies. Barotrauma occurs when there are sudden pressure changes in the middle ear due to changes in barometric pressure, such as in scuba diving or airplane descent, and fluid becomes trapped in the middle ear. A carcinoma obstructing the eustachian tube should be ruled out in an adult with persistent unilateral serous otitis media.

Clinical Manifestations. Patients may complain of hearing loss, fullness in the ear or a sensation of congestion, and perhaps even popping and crackling noises, which occur as the eustachian tube attempts to open. The tympanic membrane will appear dull on otoscopy, and air bubbles in the middle ear may be visualized. The audiogram will usually show a conductive hearing loss.

Management. Serous otitis media need not be medically treated unless infection occurs (acute otitis media). If the hearing loss associated with middle ear effusion causes a problem to the patient, a myringotomy can be performed and a tube may be placed to keep the middle ear ventilated. Corticosteroids, in small doses, sometimes decrease the edema of the eustachian tube in cases of barotrauma.

Chronic Otitis Media

Chronic otitis media is a condition associated with irreversible tissue pathology and usually is the result of repeated episodes of acute otitis media. It is often associated with persistent perforation of the tympanic membrane. Chronic infections of the middle ear not only cause damage to the tympanic membrane but also can destroy the ossicles and almost always involve the mastoid. Before the discovery of antibiotics, infections of the mastoid were life-threatening. Now, the judicious use of medications in acute otitis media has made acute coalescent mastoiditis a rare condition. Most cases of **acute mastoditis** today are found in patients who did not receive adequate ear care and had untreated ear infections. Chronic mastoiditis is more common, and some believe this chronic infection can lead to formation of cholesteatoma, which is the ingrowth of skin (squamous epithelium) from the outer layer of the tympanic membrane into the middle ear. The skin from the lateral tympanic membrane forms the outer sac, which fills with degenerated skin and sebaceous material. The sac can be attached to the structures of the middle ear and mastoid. If untreated, cholesteatoma will continue to grow and may cause facial nerve paralysis, sensorineural hearing loss and/or balance disturbance (from erosion of the inner ear), and brain abcess.

Clinical Manifestations. The symptoms may be minimal, with varying degrees of hearing loss and the presence of a persistent or intermittent foul-smelling otorrhea. Pain is not usually present except in cases of acute mastoiditis, when the postauricular area will be tender to the touch and even erythematous and edematous. Cholesteatoma, by itself, usually does not cause pain. Otoscopic evaluation of the tympanic membrane may reveal a perforation, and cholesteatoma may present as a white mass behind the tympanic membrane or coming through to the external canal from a perforation. Cholesteatoma may also not be observable to the examining otoscopist. Audiometric results in cases of cholesteatoma often show a conductive or mixed hearing loss.

Management. Local treatment consists of careful cleansing of the ear using the microscope and suction instruments. Instillation of antibiotic drops or application of antibiotic powder often helps if a purulent discharge is present. Systemic antibiotics are usually not prescribed except in cases of acute infection.

Tympanoplasty. Various surgical procedures may be used after medical treatments are determined to be ineffective. The most common is a tympanoplasty—surgical reconstruction of the tympanic membrane and ossicles. The purpose of a tympanoplasty is to reestablish middle ear function, close the tympanic membrane perforation, prevent recurrent infection, and improve hearing. Historically, there are five types of tympanoplasties. The simplest surgical procedure, type I (myringoplasty), is designed to close a perforation in the tympanic membrane. The other procedures, types II through V, involve more extensive repair of middle ear structures. The structures and the degree of involvement may differ, but part of all tympanoplasty procedures includes restoring the continuity of the sound conduction mechanism.

Tympanoplasty is performed through the external auditory canal, either transcanal or through a postauricular incision. The contents of the middle ear are carefully inspected, and the ossicular chain is evaluated. Ossicular interruption is most frequent in chronic otitis media, but problems of reconstruction may also occur with malformations of the middle ear and ossicular dislocations due to head injuries. Dramatic improvement in hearing can result from closure of a perforation and reestablishment of the ossicles. Surgery is usually performed in an outpatient environment under general anesthesia. Patient teaching guidelines for middle ear and mastoid surgery are presented in Table 57-3.

Mastoidectomy. The objectives of mastoid surgery are to remove the cholesteatoma, gain access to diseased structures, and create a safe, dry, and healthy ear. If possible, the ossicles are reconstructed during the initial surgical procedure. However, on occasion the extent of the disease dictates that this be performed as part of a planned second stage operation. A mastoidectomy is usually completed through a postauricular incision, and infection is eliminated completely by removing the mastoid air cells. The facial nerve runs through the middle ear and mastoid and is put at some risk during mastoid surgery, although it is infrequently injured. As the patient awakens from anesthesia, any evidence of facial paresis should be reported to the physician. If facial weakness is present, the mastoid dressing should be loosened and the patient will be taken back to surgery, the wound opened, and a facial nerve decompression performed to decompress the bony canal surrounding the facial nerve. A second mastoidectomy may be necessary 6 months after the first to check for recurrent cholesteatoma. The hearing mechanism can be reconstructed at this time if cholesteatoma is completely eradicated. The success rate for correcting this conductive hearing loss is approximately 50% to 60%.

TABLE 57-3 Patient Teaching for Middle Ear and/or Mastoid Surgery

Postoperative instructions for middle ear and mastoid surgery vary greatly among otolaryngologists. These patient teaching guidelines may require modification for the individual patient.

1. Antibiotics and other medications are to be taken as prescribed.
2. Nose blowing is to be avoided for a few weeks after surgery.
3. Sneezing and coughing should be done with the mouth open for a few weeks after surgery.
4. Patient can usually return to work 2 to 3 days postoperatively. Heavy (greater than 25 pounds) lifing, straining, and bending over are to be avoided for a few weeks after surgery.
5. It is normal to have popping and crackling in the ear that was operated on for approximately 3 to 5 weeks after surgery.
6. Packing in the operated ear, as well as blood and fluid in the middle ear after surgery, will cause a hearing loss. Patient may also feel that he is talking in a well or hears echoing.
7. Minor ear discomfort is normal and use of the analgesics prescribed is warranted. Excessive ear pain should be reported to the surgeon.
8. Some slightly bloody or serosanguineous drainage from the ear is normal after surgery. Excessive or purulent ear drainage should be reported to the surgeon.
9. The cotton ball in the ear can be changed as needed. The patient is not to touch or remove any packing from the external auditory canal.
10. The postauricular suture line should be cleansed with hydrogen peroxide twice daily and a thin layer of antibiotic ointment (*e.g.,* Bacitracin) applied until sutures are removed.
11. The surgeon should be consulted for instructions regarding air travel.
12. Getting water in the operated ear must be avoided for 2 weeks after surgery. The hair may be shampooed 2 to 3 days postoperatively if the ear is protected from water by saturating a cotton ball with vaseline (or some other water-insoluble substance) and placing it in the ear. If the postauricular suture line becomes wet, the area should be patted dry (not rubbed) and covered with a thin layer of antibiotic ointment.

Surgery is usually performed under general anesthesia and in an outpatient setting. The patient will have a mastoid pressure dressing, which can be removed 24 to 48 hours after surgery. Patient teaching guidelines are detailed in Table 57-3.

❑ NURSING PROCESS
The Patient Undergoing Mastoid Surgery

Although several otologic surgical procedures are performed under local anesthesia, mastoid surgery is done using general anesthesia.

Assessment

The health history includes a complete description of the ear problem, including infection, otalgia, otorrhea, hearing loss, and vertigo. Data are collected about the duration and intensity of the problem, causation, and previous treatments. Information is obtained about other health problems and all medications that the patient is taking. In addition, questions pertaining to drug allergies and family history of ear disease should be asked.

Physical assessment includes observation for erythema, edema, otorrhea, lesions, and odor of discharge. The results of an audiogram should be reviewed.

Diagnosis

Nursing Diagnoses

Based on the assessment data, the patient's major nursing diagnoses may include:

- ❑ Anxiety related to surgical procedure, potential loss of hearing, potential taste disturbance, and potential loss of facial movement
- ❑ Acute pain related to mastoid surgery
- ❑ Risk for infection related to mastoidectomy, placement of grafts, prostheses, and electrodes, surgical trauma to surrounding tissues and structures
- ❑ Altered auditory sensory perception related to ear disorder/ear surgery/ear packing
- ❑ Risk for trauma related to balance difficulties or vertigo during the immediate postoperative period
- ❑ Altered sensory perception related to potential damage to facial nerve (cranial nerve VII) and the chorda tympani nerve
- ❑ Impaired skin integrity related to ear surgery, incisions, and graft sites
- ❑ Knowledge deficit about mastoid disease, surgical procedure, and postoperative care and expectations

Planning and Implementation

Goals. The major goals of caring for a patient undergoing mastoidectomy may include reduction of anxiety; freedom from discomfort; prevention of infection; stabilization, or improvement, of hearing; absence of injury or vertigo; absence of, or adjustment to, altered sensory perception; return of skin integrity; and knowledge regarding the disease process, surgical procedure, and postoperative care.

Nursing Interventions

Reducing Anxiety. The nurse reinforces information that the otologic surgeon has discussed with the patient, including anesthesia, the location of the incision (postauricular), and expected surgical results (hearing, balance, taste, facial movement). The patient is encouraged to discuss any anxieties and concerns about the surgery.

Relieving Pain. Most patients complain very little about incisional pain following mastoid surgery but do experience some ear discomfort. It is desirable for the patient to take the prescribed analgesic for the first 24 hours postoperatively and then only as needed. The patient is instructed in the use of and side effects of the medication. It is common for patients to have a feeling of aural fullness or pressure after surgery due to residual blood or fluid in the middle ear. A tympanoplasty may also be performed at the time of the mastoidectomy. A wick, or some kind of external auditory canal packing, is used after a tympanoplasty to stabilize the tympanic membrane. Patients may experience intermittent sharp, shooting pains in the ear for 2 to 3 weeks postoperatively as the eustachian tube opens and allows air to enter the middle ear.

Preventing Infection. Measures are initiated to prevent infection in the operative ear. The external auditory canal wick, or packing, may be impregnated with an antibiotic solution before instillation. Prophylactic antibiotics are given as prescribed, and the patient is instructed to prevent water from entering the external auditory canal for 2 weeks. A cotton ball or lamb's wool smeared with a water-insoluble substance (*i.e.*, Vaseline) and placed in the ear will usually prevent water contamination. The postauricular incision should be kept dry for 2 weeks. Signs of infection such as an elevated temperature and purulent drainage are observed for and reported. It is normal for some serosanguineous drainage to occur from the external auditory canal postoperatively.

Improving Communication. Hearing in the operative ear may be reduced for several weeks due to edema, accumulation of blood and tissue fluid in the middle ear, and dressings or packing. Thus, measures to improve communication may be initiated, such as reducing environmental noise, facing the patient when speaking, speaking clearly and distinctly without shouting, providing good lighting if the patient relies on speech reading, and using nonverbal clues (*e.g.*, facial expression, pointing, gestures) and other forms of communication. Family members or significant others must be instructed regarding effective practices so they may communicate successfully with the patient. If the patient uses hearing-assistive devices, one may be used in the unoperated ear.

Preventing Injury. Vertigo may occur following mastoid surgery if the semicircular canals or other areas of the inner ear are manipulated. This symptom is relatively uncommon after this type of ear surgery and usually is temporary. Antiemetics or antivertiginous medications (*e.g.*, antihistamines) can be prescribed should a balance disturbance or vertigo occur. The nurse should monitor the patient for effects of the medication to see if the desired results have been obtained or if any untoward reactions occur. The patient should be instructed on the expected effects and potential side effects. Safety measures such as assisted ambulation are carried out to prevent the patient from falling owing to vertigo or balance disturbance.

Preventing Altered Sensory Perception. Facial nerve injury is a potential, although rare, complication of mastoid surgery. The patient should be instructed to report immediately any evidence of facial nerve (cranial nerve VII) weakness, such as drooping of the mouth or the side of the face on the operative side. A more frequent occurrence, however, is a temporary disturbance in the chorda tympani nerve, a small branch of the facial nerve that runs through the middle ear. Patients may experience a taste disturbance and dry mouth on the operative side for several months until the nerve regenerates.

Wound Healing. The head of the bed is usually elevated, or the patient is asked to sleep on two pillows, for a few days postoperatively to prevent edema and promote drainage. The patient is instructed to avoid heavy lifting, straining, and nose blowing for 2 to 3 weeks after surgery to prevent dislodging the tympanic membrane graft or ossicular prosthesis. Also, the patient should avoid putting the head in a dependent position, such as in bending at the waist. These activities increase intracranial pressure, which in turn puts pressure on the ear. Changes in barometric pressure occasioned by activities such as air travel should be avoided for 4 to 6 weeks after surgery.

Improving Knowledge. Information about the surgery and operating room environment is important for the patient to know before surgery. Discussing postoperative expectations helps to decrease anxiety about the unknown. Postoperative instructions for mastoid surgery vary among otologic surgeons; therefore, it is important for the nurse to be aware of the surgeon's preferences when teaching the patient.

Evaluation

Expected Outcomes

1. Anxiety about surgical procedure has lessened
    a. Verbalizes and exhibits less stress, tension, and irritability
    b. Tells nurse he or she can accept results of surgery and adjust to possible hearing impairment
2. Free of discomfort or pain
    a. Shows no signs of facial grimacing, moaning, or crying
    b. Uses analgesics appropriately
3. No signs or symptoms of infection
    a. Vital signs are normal including temperature
    b. No purulent drainage from the external auditory canal
    c. Describes method for preventing water from contaminating packing
4. Hearing has stabilized or improved
    a. Describes surgical goal for hearing and whether that goal has been met
    b. Verbalizes that sounds unable to be heard preoperatively are heard postoperatively
5. Demonstrates no injury or trauma secondary to vertigo
    a. Reports absence of vertigo or balance disturbance
    b. Experiences no injury or fall
    c. Modifies environment to avoid falls (*e.g.*, night light, no clutter on stairs)
6. Does not have, or has adjusted to, altered sensory perception
    a. Reports no taste disturbance, mouth dryness, or facial weakness
7. Demonstrates good skin integrity
    a. Lists ways to prevent dislodging graft or prosthesis
    b. Reiterates limitations in activities and for how long regarding bathing, lifting, and air travel
8. Understands (as confirmed by conversation) the reasons and methods of care or treatment
    a. Shares knowledge with family about treatment protocol
    b. Describes treatment and the time frame for the recovery phase
    c. Discusses the discharge plan formulated with the nurse with regard to rest periods, medication, and activities permitted and restricted
    d. Lists symptoms that should be reported to health care personnel
    e. Keeps follow-up appointments

Ossiculoplasty. Many people use the term tympanoplasty to include ossiculoplasty, which is surgical reconstruction of the middle ear bones to restore hearing. Prostheses are often used to reconnect the ossicles and thus reestablish the sound conduction mechanism. These prostheses are made of many different materials including Teflon, stainless steel, and hydroxyapatite. The greater the damage, the lower the success rate for restoring normal hearing.

Otosclerosis

Otosclerosis involves the stapes and is thought to be caused by the formation of new, abnormal spongy bone, especially around the oval window, with resulting fixation of the stapes. It is more common in females, frequently hereditary, and may be made worse by pregnancy. The efficient transmission of sound is prevented because the stapes is unable to vibrate and carry the sound as conducted from the malleus and incus to the inner ear. The condition can involve one or both ears and presents as a progressive conductive or mixed hearing loss. The patient may or may not complain of tinnitus. Otoscopic examination usually reveals a normal tympanic membrane. Bone conduction is better than air conduction upon Rinne testing. The audiogram confirms a conductive hearing loss or a mixed loss, especially in the low frequencies.

There is no known nonsurgical treatment for otosclerosis, although some people feel the use of Fluorical (a flouride supplement) may retard abnormal spongy bone growth. Auditory rehabilitation of the patient may be accomplished through amplification (hearing aid) or surgery. A stapedectomy is usually performed transcanal and involves removing the entire stapes and inserting a suitable prosthesis (Fig. 57-9). Some surgeons elect to remove only part of the stapes footplate (stapedotomy) in an effort to improve their results. Regardless of the method used, the prosthesis helps bridge the gap between the incus and the inner ear, providing better sound conduction. Patient teaching guidelines are presented in Table 57-3. Balance disturbance or true vertigo, which rarely occurs in other middle ear surgeries, can occur for a short time after stapedectomy. Stapes surgery is very successful in improving hearing.

Middle Ear Masses

Other than cholesteatoma, masses in the middle ear are rare. Glomus jugulare is a tumor that arises from the jugular bulb. A histologically identical tumor that arises from Jacobson's nerve and remains limited to the middle ear is known as a glomus tympanicum. Upon otoscopy, a red blemish on or behind the tympanic membrane is indicative of a glomus tumor. The treatment for glomus tumors is surgical except in poor surgical candidates, in whom radiation therapy is used.

A facial nerve neuroma is a tumor on cranial nerve VII, the facial nerve. These types of tumors are often not visible on otoscopic examination but are suspected when a patient presents with a facial nerve paresis. Radiologic evaluation is necessary to determine the site of the tumor along the facial nerve. The treatment is surgical removal.

Other less frequently encountered problems of the middle ear include cholesterin granuloma and tympanosclerosis. Cholesterin granuloma is an immune system reaction to the by-products of blood (cholesterol crystals) within the middle ear. Tympanosclerosis is a deposit of collagen and calcium within the middle ear that can harden around the ossicles as a result of repeated infection. It can also be found as plaque on the tympanic membrane, in which case it is of little consequence.

Conditions of the Inner Ear

Motion Sickness

Motion sickness is a disturbance of equilibrium caused by constant motion, such as occurs aboard a ship or boat or while riding on a merry-go-round, swing, or even in the back seat of a car. The syndrome manifests itself in sweating, pallor, nausea, and vomiting caused by vestibular overstimulation. These manifestations may persist for several hours after the stimulation stops. Over-the-counter antihistamines used to treat vertigo, such as Dramamine or Bonine, are helpful in providing some relief. Cholinergic medications, such as scopolamine patches, may be helpful and are replaced every few days. Side effects such as dry mouth and drowsiness do occur with these medications and may prove to be more troublesome than helpful. Patients must be warned to avoid potentially hazardous activities such as driving a car or operating heavy machinery if they experience drowsiness.

Ménière's Disease

Ménière's disease is named after a French physician, Prosper Ménière, who in 1861 first described a triad of symptoms (episodic incapacitating vertigo, tinnitus, and fluctuating sensorineural hearing loss) as an ear disease and not a central, or brain, disease. The etiology of Ménière's disease is unknown but many theories exist, including abnormal hormonal and neurochemical influences on the blood flow to the labyrinth, electrolyte disturbance within labyrinthine fluids, allergic reaction, and autoimmune disorders. Some attribute the impairment of the microvasculature of the inner ear to abnormally high levels of metabolites (glucose, insulin, triglycerides, and cholesterol) in the blood.

Ménière's disease is currently thought to represent an abnormal inner ear fluid balance caused by a malabsorption in the endolymphatic sac. However, evidence indicates that many people with Ménière's disease may have a blockage in the endolymphatic duct. Regardless of the cause, endolymphatic hydrops, which is a dilation in the endolymphatic space, develops. Either increased pressure in the system or rupture of the inner ear membranes occurs and produces Ménière's symptoms. There are many problems that may mimic Ménière's disease, such as trauma, infection, allergies, perilymph fistula, and otosclerosis.

It is estimated that 2.4 million people in the United States have Ménière's disease. It is more common in adults, with an average age of onset in the 40s. Symptoms usually begin between the ages of 20 and 60; however, it has been reported in children as early as age 4 and adults of all ages up to the 90s. Ménière's disease appears to be equally common in both genders, and the right and left ears are affected

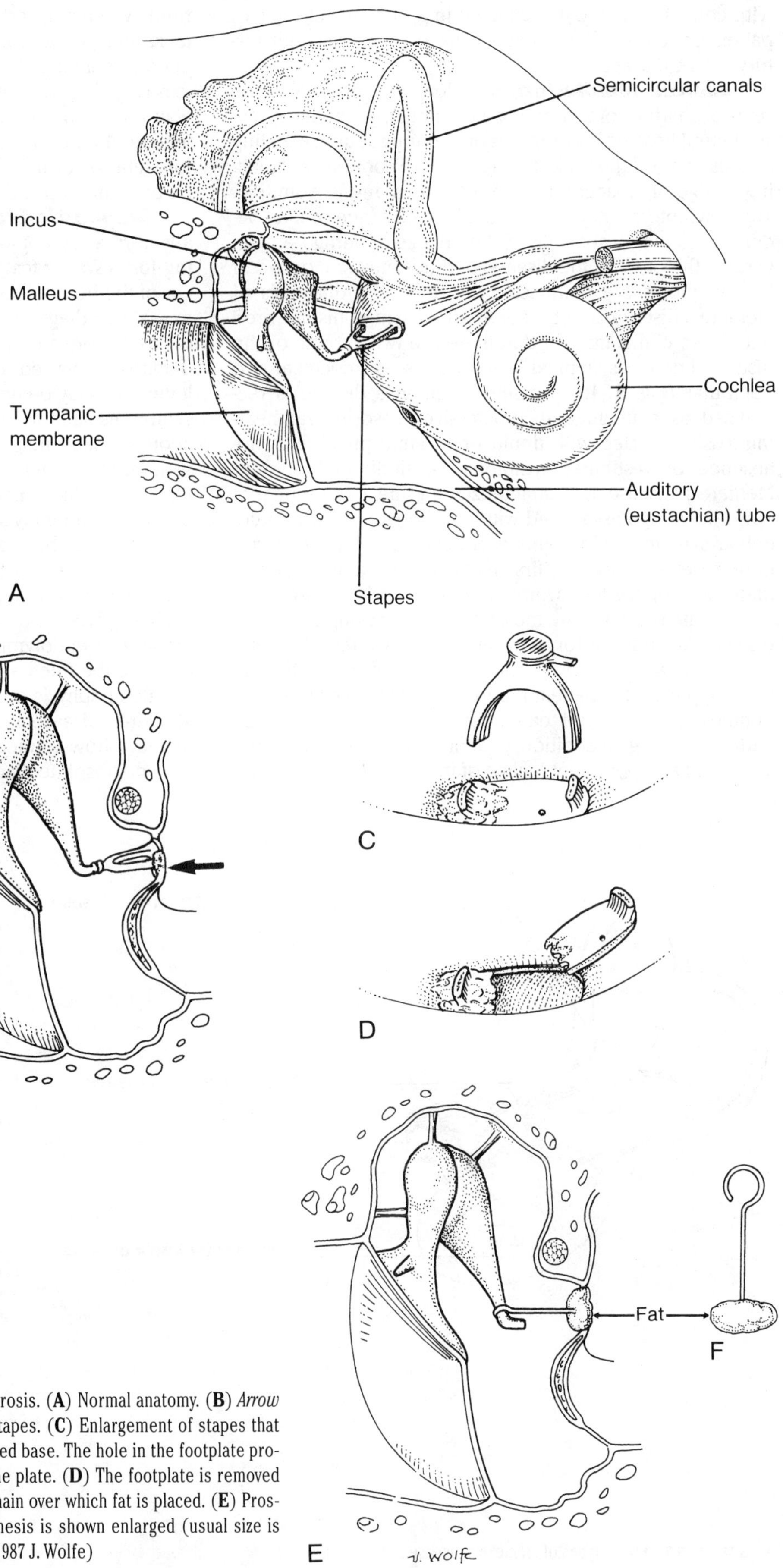

FIGURE 57-9. Stapedectomy for otosclerosis. (**A**) Normal anatomy. (**B**) *Arrow* points to sclerotic process at the foot of the stapes. (**C**) Enlargement of stapes that has been broken away surgically from its diseased base. The hole in the footplate provides an area where an instrument can grasp the plate. (**D**) The footplate is removed from its base. Some otosclerotic focus may remain over which fat is placed. (**E**) Prosthesis of wire and fat is positioned. (**F**) Prosthesis is shown enlarged (usual size is 4 mm) with fat attached to one end. (Copyright 1987 J. Wolfe)

with equal frequency. It is bilateral in approximately 20% of patients, and up to 20% of patients have a positive family history for the disease.

Clinical Manifestations. Ménière's disease represents a quadrad of symptoms: fluctuating, progressive sensorineural hearing loss, tinnitus or a roaring sound, a feeling of pressure or fullness in the ear, and episodic incapacitating vertigo often accompanied by nausea and/or vomiting. These symptoms may be only a minor nuisance or may become disabling, especially if the attacks of vertigo are severe. At the onset of the disease, perhaps only one or two of the symptoms are manifested; however, the diagnosis of Ménière's disease is not made until all symptoms are present. Some clinicians feel that there are two subsets of the disease, known as atypical Ménière's disease: cochlear and vestibular (Fig. 57-10). Cochlear Ménière's disease is recognized as a fluctuating, progressive sensorineural hearing loss associated with tinnitus and aural pressure in the absence of vestibular symptoms or findings. Vestibular Ménière's disease is characterized as the occurrence of episodic vertigo associated with aural pressure with no cochlear symptoms. Some patients develop cochlear or vestibular Ménière's disease first; most patients, however, eventually develop the four symptoms of Ménière's disease.

Vertigo is usually the most troublesome symptom of the disease. A careful history is taken, which will reveal the frequency, duration, severity, and character of the vertigo attacks. Typically, the patient reports that vertigo will last from minutes to hours and can be accompanied by nausea and/or vomiting. In addition, patients complain of diaphoresis as well as a persistent feeling of imbalance or disequilibrium, which may last for days. They may also complain of attacks that awaken them at night, but they usually experience a feeling of well-being between attacks. The hearing loss may fluctuate, and the tinnitus and aural pressure may wax and wane with changes in hearing. The tinnitus and feeling of aural pressure may be present only during or before attacks, or they may be constant. Changes in barometric pressure or position may precipitate an attack.

Diagnostic Evaluation. Physical examination is usually normal except for evaluation of cranial nerve VIII. A tuning fork (Weber test) will usually lateralize to the opposite ear of the hearing loss (the one affected with Ménière's disease). The diagnosis of Ménière's disease is usually based on the history along with results from some audiovestibular diagnostic procedures. Additional laboratory and radiologic tests may be performed to rule out other causes of the symptoms such as syphilis, autoimmune disease, stroke, or acoustic neuroma. An audiogram typically reveals a sensorineural hearing loss in the affected ear. This can be in the form of a "Pike's Peak" pattern, which looks like a hill or mountain, or it may show a sensorineural loss in the low frequencies. As the disease progresses, the hearing loss becomes more severe. Sometimes a dehydration audiogram is performed in which the patient drinks a dehydrating agent, such as glycerol or urea, which theoretically reduces the amount of endolymphatic hydrops. This is useful in documenting the fluctuating nature of the hearing loss. Electrocochleography is abnormal in about 60% of patients with Ménière's disease; the electronystagmogram may be normal or may show reduced vestibular response. There is, however, no absolute diagnostic test for Ménière's disease.

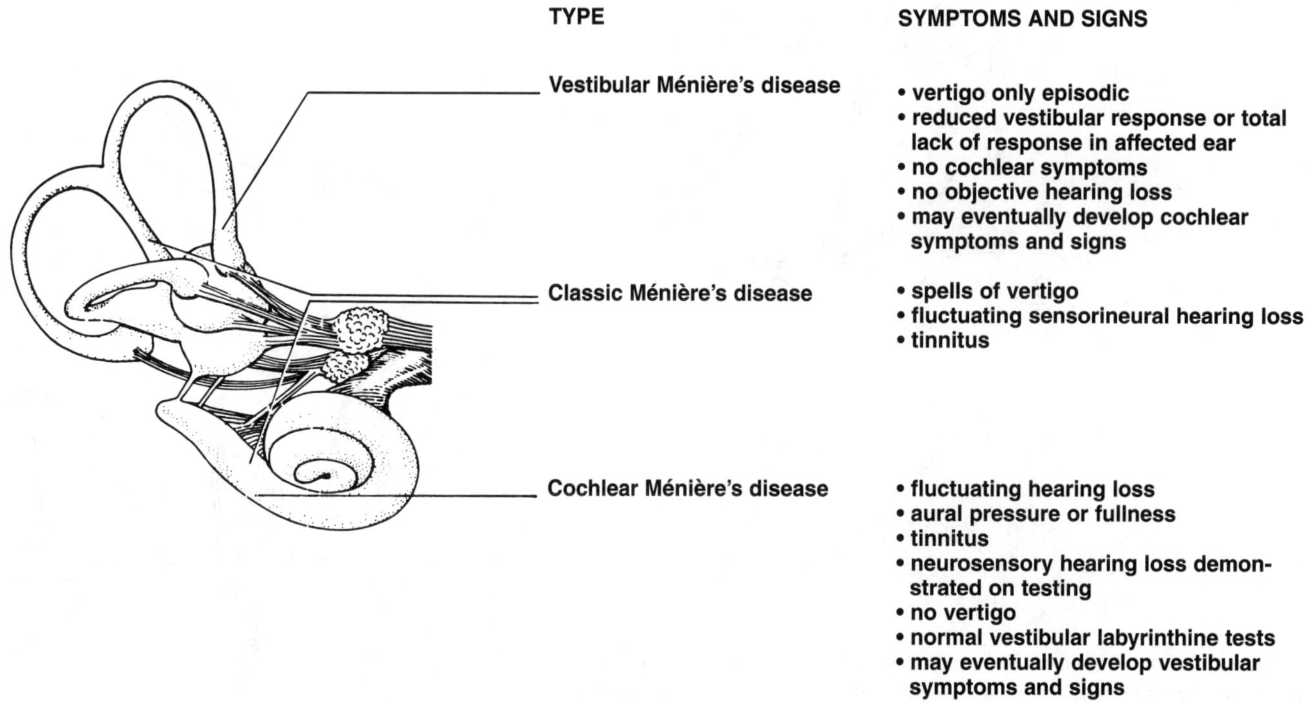

TYPE
SYMPTOMS AND SIGNS
Vestibular Ménière's disease
• vertigo only episodic
• reduced vestibular response or total lack of response in affected ear
• no cochlear symptoms
• no objective hearing loss
• may eventually develop cochlear symptoms and signs
Classic Ménière's disease
• spells of vertigo
• fluctuating sensorineural hearing loss
• tinnitus
Cochlear Ménière's disease
• fluctuating hearing loss
• aural pressure or fullness
• tinnitus
• neurosensory hearing loss demonstrated on testing
• no vertigo
• normal vestibular labyrinthine tests
• may eventually develop vestibular symptoms and signs

FIGURE 57-10. Types of Ménière's disease.

Management. Treatment may include recommending changes in life-style and habits or surgical treatment. However, Ménière's disease is not a life-threatening problem; therefore, a patient may elect to do nothing at any point during the treatment continuum. Some patients improve with time as the disease "burns out." There is no cure for Ménière's disease; treatment is designed to eliminate vertigo or stop the progression of, or stabilize, the disease.

Treatment approaches include rehabilitative and dietary strategies as well as medical and surgical treatment. Many patients can control their symptoms by adhering to a low-sodium (2000 mg/day) diet. The amount of sodium is one of many factors that regulate the balance of fluid within the body. Sodium and fluid retention disrupts the delicate balance between endolymph and perilymph in the inner ear. Caffeine and nicotine are vasoactive stimulants, and avoiding these substances may reduce symptoms. Many patients are told to avoid ingesting alcohol as it may precipitate an attack. There is some belief, however, that the attack of vertigo may be precipitated by an allergic reaction to the yeasts in alcohol rather than caused by the alcohol itself.

Medical treatment for vertigo consists of antihistamines, such as meclizine (Antivert), which suppress the vestibular system. Tranquilizers such as diazepam (Valium) may be used in acute instances to help control vertigo, but because of their addictive nature are not used on a long-term basis. Antiemetics such as promethazine (Phenergan) suppositories help not only the nausea and vomiting but also the vertigo because of their antihistamine effect. Diuretics such as Dyazide or hydrochlorothiazide will sometimes help relieve the symptoms of Ménière's disease by lowering the pressure in the endolymphatic system. Patients should be reminded to eat foods containing potassium, such as bananas, tomatoes, and oranges, if on a diuretic that causes potassium loss. Vasodilators, such as nicotinic acid, papaverine hydrochloride (Pavabid), and methantheline bromide (Banthine), have no proven scientific basis for alleviating the symptoms of Ménière's disease.

Surgical Management. Although the majority of patients are successfully treated with conservative therapy, many continue to have disabling attacks of vertigo. If these attacks adversely affect their quality of life, patients may elect to undergo surgical therapy for relief. However, hearing loss, tinnitus, and aural fullness may continue since the surgical treatment of Ménière's disease is aimed at eliminating the attacks of vertigo.

Endolymphatic sac decompression or shunt theoretically equalizes the pressure in the endolymphatic space. A shunt or drain is inserted in the endolymphatic sac via a postauricular incision. A 75% success rate for eliminating the attacks of vertigo has been reported (Meyerhoff & Rice, 1992). This procedure is favored by many otololaryngologists as a first-line surgical approach to the vertigo of Ménière's disease, because it is relatively simple and safe and can be performed on an outpatient basis.

Ototoxic medications, such as streptomycin or gentamicin, can be given to patients by systemic injections or infusion into the middle and inner ear. The success rate for eliminating vertigo is high, about 85%, but the risk of significant hearing loss is also high. This procedure of inner ear perfusion usually requires an overnight stay in the hospital, and many patients experience a period of imbalance that lasts several weeks.

Labyrinthectomy procedures by transcanal and transmastoid approaches are also about 85% successful in eliminating vertigo, but the auditory function of the inner ear is destroyed. Added morbidity is associated with these procedures, and some otologists feel that if a patient is to be subjected to these risks (*i.e.*, facial nerve, cerebrospinal fluid leak, total hearing loss), a potentially more successful procedure such as a vestibular nerve section (sectioning cranial nerve VIII) should be performed.

The vestibular nerve section gives the most assurance (approximately 98%) of eliminating the attacks of vertigo. It can be performed translabyrinthine (through the hearing mechanism) or in a manner that will conserve hearing (suboccipital or middle cranial fossa), depending on the degree of hearing loss. Most patients with Ménière's disease who are incapacitated by attacks of vertigo have very little or no effective hearing anyway. Cutting the nerve actually prevents the brain from receiving input from the semicircular canals. This procedure requires a few days' stay in the hospital. Nursing care for the patient with vertigo is presented in Nursing Care Plan 57-1.

Labyrinthitis

Labyrinthitis is an inflammation of the inner ear and may be of bacterial or viral origin. Bacterial labyrinthitis, although relatively rare since the introduction of antibiotics, most frequently occurs as a complication of bacterial meningitis. The infection extends to the inner ear through the internal auditory canal or cochlear aqueduct. Bacterial infection caused by otitis media, or cholesteatoma, can enter the inner ear by penetrating the oval or round window membranes. Viral labyrinthitis is a common medical diagnosis, but little is known about this disorder, which affects both hearing and balance. The most commonly identified causative viruses are mumps, rubella, rubeola, and influenza. Viral illnesses of the upper respiratory tract are also known to cause labyrinthitis. Vestibular neuritis can cause the same symptoms as labyrinthitis except that hearing is not affected.

Labyrinthitis is characterized by a sudden onset of incapacitating vertigo, usually with nausea and vomiting, varying degrees of hearing loss, and possibly tinnitus. The first episode is usually the worst; subsequent attacks, which usually occur over a period of several weeks to months, are less severe. Treatment for bacterial labyrinthitis includes intravenous antibiotic therapy, fluid replacement, and administration of a vestibular suppressant as well as antiemetic medications. Treatment of viral labyrinthitis is symptomatic with the use of antiemetics and antivertiginous agents.

Ototoxicity

A variety of medications (Table 57-4) are known to adversely affect the cochlea, vestibular apparatus, or cranial nerve VIII. Only a few, such as aspirin and quinine, cause reversible hearing loss. At high doses, aspirin toxicity also can produce tinnitus. Intravenous medications, especially the aminoglycosides, are the most common cause of ototoxicity and actually destroy the hair cells in the organ of Corti.

(text continues on page 1667)

NURSING CARE PLAN 57–1
Care of the Patient with Vertigo

NURSING DIAGNOSIS: High risk for injury related to altered mobility because of gait disturbance and vertigo

GOAL: Remains free of any injuries associated with imbalance and/or falls

Nursing Interventions	Rationale	Expected Outcomes
1. Assess for vertigo including history, onset, description of attacks, duration, frequency, and any associated ear symptoms (hearing loss, tinnitus, aural fullness).	1. History provides basis for interventions.	• Experiences no falls due to balance disturbance. • Fear and anxiety are reduced. • Performs exercises as prescribed. • Takes prescribed medications appropriately. • Assumes horizontal position when dizzy. • Keeps head still when dizzy. • Indentifies a characteristic fullness or sense of pressure in the ear as occurring before a full-blown attack. • Reports measures that help reduce vertigo.
2. Assess extent of disability in relation to activities of daily livng.	2. Extent of disability indicates risk of falling.	
3. Teach or reinforce vestibular/balance therapy as prescribed.	3. Exercises hasten labyrinthine compensation, which may decrease vertigo and gait disturbance.	
4. Administer, or teach administration of, antivertiginous medications and/or vestibular sedation medication; instruct patient about side effects.	4. Alleviates acute symptoms of vertigo.	
5. Encourage patient to lie down when dizzy; side rails up on bed.	5. Decreases possibility of falling and injury.	
6. Place pillow on each side of head to restrict movement.	6. Movement aggravates vertigo.	
7. Assist patient in identifying aura (presence of aural symptoms) that suggests an attack is impending.	7. Recognition of aura may trigger the need to take medication before an attack occurs, thereby minimizing the severity of effects.	
8. Recommend that the patient keep eyes open and stare straight ahead when lying down and experiencing vertigo.	8. Sensation of vertigo decreases and motion decelerates if eyes are kept in a fixed position.	

NURSING DIAGNOSIS: Impaired adjustment related to disability requiring change in life-style due to unpredictability of vertigo

GOAL: Modifies life-style to decrease disability and exert maximum control and independence within limits posed by chronic vertigo

Nursing Interventions	Rationale	Expected Outcomes
1. Encourage patient to identify personal strengths and roles that can still be fulfilled.	1. Maximizes sense of regaining control and independence.	• Exerts maximum control of environment and independence within limits imposed by vertigo. • Is informed about condition. • Family and significant others are included in rehabilitation process. • Uses strengths and potentials to engage in the most independent and constructive life-style.
2. Provide information about vertigo and what to expect.	2. Reduces fear and anxiety.	
3. Include family and significant others in rehabilitative process.	3. Perceived beliefs of significant others are important for patient's adherence to medical regimen.	
4. Encourage patient to maintain sense of control by making decisions and assuming more responsibility for care.	4. Reinforces positive psychologic and social outcomes.	

NURSING DIAGNOSIS: Risk for fluid volume deficit related to increased fluid output, altered intake, and medications

GOAL: Maintains a normal fluid–electrolyte balance

Nursing Interventions	Rationale	Expected Outcomes
1. Assess, or have patient assess, intake and output (including emesis, liquid stools, urine, and diaphoresis). Monitor laboratory values.	1. Accurate records provide basis for fluid replacement.	• Laboratory values are within normal limits. • Alert and oriented; vital signs are within normal limits, skin turgor is normal; electrolytes are normal.

(continued)

NURSING CARE PLAN 57–1 *(continued)*
Care of the Patient with Vertigo

Nursing Interventions	Rationale	Expected Outcomes
2. Assess indicators of dehydration, including blood pressure (orthostasis), pulse, skin turgor, mucous membranes, and level of consciousness.	2. Prompt recognition of dehydration allows early intervention.	• Mucous membranes are moist. • Vomiting or diarrhea has stopped; usual oral intake has been resumed.
3. Encourage oral fluids as tolerated; discourage beverages containing caffeine (a vestibular stimulant).	3. Oral replacement is begun as soon as possible to replace losses. Caffeine may increase diarrhea.	
4. Administer, or teach administration of, antiemetics and antidiarrheal medication as prescribed and needed. Instruct patient in side effects.	4. Antiemetics reduce nausea and vomiting, reducing fluid losses and improving oral intake. Antidiarrheal medication reduces intestinal motility and fluid losses.	

NURSING DIAGNOSIS: Anxiety related to threat of, or change in, health status and disability effects of vertigo

GOAL: Experiences less or no anxiety

Nursing Interventions	Rationale	Expected Outcomes
1. Assess level of anxiety. Help patient identify coping skills used successfully in the past.	1. Guides therapeutic interventions and participation in self-care. Past coping skills can relieve anxiety.	• Fear and anxiety about vertiginous attacks reduced or eliminated. • Acquires knowledge and skills to deal with vertigo.
2. Provide information about vertigo and its treatment.	2. Increased knowledge helps to decrease anxiety.	• Feels less tension, apprehension, and uncertainty.
3. Encourage patient to discuss anxieties and explore concerns about vertigo attacks.	3. Promotes awareness and understanding of relationship between anxiety level and behavior.	• Utilizes stress management techniques when needed.
4. Teach patient stress management techniques or make appropriate referral.	4. Improved stress management can reduce the frequency and severity of some vertiginous attacks.	• Avoids upsetting encounters. • Repeats instructions given and verbalizes understanding of treatments.
5. Provide comfort measures and avoid stress-producing activities.	5. Stressful situations may exacerbate symptoms of the condition.	
6. Instruct patient in aspects of treatment regimen.	6. Patient knowledge helps to decrease anxiety.	

NURSING DIAGNOSIS: Risk for trauma related to balancing difficulties

GOAL: Reduces the risk of trauma by adapting the home environment and by using rehabilitative devices as necessary

Nursing Interventions	Rationale	Expected Outcomes
1. Assess for balance disturbance and/or vertigo by taking history and by examination for nystagmus, positive Romberg, and inability to perform tandem Romberg.	1. Peripheral vestibular disorders cause these signs and symptoms.	• Has adapted home environment or uses rehabilitative devices to reduce risk of falling. • Ambulates with needed assistance. • Visual and proprioceptive risks are identified.
2. Assist with ambulation when indicated.	2. Abnormal gait can predispose patient to unsteadiness and falls.	• Activity level is increased.
3. Assess for visual acuity and proprioceptive deficits.	3. Balance depends upon visual, vestibular, and proprioceptive systems.	• Home environment is free of hazards.
4. Encourage increased activity level with or without use of assistive devices.	4. Increased activity may help retrain balance system.	
5. Help identify hazards in home environment.	5. Adaptation of home environment can reduce risk of falls during rehabilitative process.	

(continued)

NURSING CARE PLAN 57–1 *(continued)*
Care of the Patient with Vertigo

Nursing Interventions	Rationale	Expected Outcomes
NURSING DIAGNOSIS: Ineffective individual coping related to personal vulnerability and unmet expectations stemming from vertigo		
GOAL: Develops coping skills necessary to decrease vulnerability and unmet needs and demonstrates effective coping		
1. Assess patient's cognitive appraisal of illness and factors that may be contributing to patient's inability to cope. 2. Provide factual information about treatment and future health status. 3. Encourage and help patient participate in decision making about adjustments in life-style. 4. Encourage patient to maintain diversional or recreational activities, exercise, and social events. 5. Help patient identify personal strengths and develop coping strategies based on previous positive experiences in dealing with stress, and situational supports. 6. Refer patient to support groups or counseling as indicated.	1. To improve patient's self-image. To enhance coping process. 2. To clarify any misinformation or confusion. 3. To help patient regain sense of power and control in self-care with activities of daily living. 4. Social isolation and avoiding pleasant activities intensify isolation and reduce ability to cope with vertigo. 5. To enhance patient's strengths that help maintain hope. 6. May help patient feel less alone and isolated.	• Copes effectively with vertigo. • Has acquired knowledge and skills to cope with vertigo. • Verbalizes less threatening appraisal of situation. • Is involved in outside activities. • Identifies specific strategies for coping. • Utilizes support groups or counseling as appropriate.
NURSING DIAGNOSIS: Diversional activity deficit related to environmental lack of such activity		
GOAL: Engages in diversional activities		
1. Assess level and type of diversional activity to plan appropriate activities. 2. Discuss usual pattern of diversional activities with patient. Suggest opportunities to continue meaningful diversional activities.	1. Boredom may be exhibited as well as depression; helps determine tolerances as well as preferences. 2. To provide information about perceived and actual stressors that influence activity level; to support patient's sense of self-worth and productivity.	• Verbalizes decreased feelings of boredom and appears alert and animated. • Seeks realistic opportunities for involvement in diversional activities.
NURSING DIAGNOSIS: Self-care deficit: feeding, bathing/hygiene, dressing/grooming, toileting, related to labyrinth dysfunction and episodes of vertigo		
GOAL: Able to care for self		
1. Administer, or teach administration of, antiemetics and other prescribed medications to relieve nausea and vomiting associated with vertigo. 2. Encourage patient to care for bodily needs when free of vertigo. 3. Review diet with patient and care givers. Offer fluids as necessary.	1. Antiemetics and sedative-type medications depress stimuli in the cerebellum. 2. Spacing activities is important because episodes of vertigo vary in occurrence. 3. Sodium restriction helps improve an inner ear fluid imbalance in some patients thereby decreasing vertigo. Fluids help prevent dehydration.	• Carries out necessary functions during symptom-free periods. Takes medications to relieve nausea or vomiting. • Carries out daily activities. • Accepts dietary plan and reports its effectiveness. Drinks fluids in sufficient amounts.

(continued)

NURSING CARE PLAN 57–1 *(continued)*
Care of the Patient with Vertigo

Nursing Interventions	Rationale	Expected Outcomes
NURSING DIAGNOSIS: Powerlessness related to illness regimen and being helpless in certain situations due to vertigo/balance disturbance		
GOAL: Experiences increased sense of control over life and activities despite vertigo/balance disturbance		
1. Assess patient's needs, values, attitudes, and readiness to initiate activities.	1. Involving patient in planning activities and care enhances potential for mastery.	• Does not restrict activities unnecessarily due to vertigo.
2. Provide opportunities for patient to express feelings (catharsis) about self and illness.	2. Expressing feelings increases understanding of individual coping styles and defense mechanisms.	• Verbalizes positive feelings about own ability to achieve a sense of power and control.
3. Help patient identify previous coping behaviors that were successful.	3. Awareness increases understanding of stressors that trigger feeling of powerlessness. Awareness of past successes enhances self-confidence.	• Previous successful coping behaviors are identified.

To prevent loss of hearing or balance, patients receiving potential ototoxic medications should be appropriately counseled on the signs and symptoms of the side effects of these medications. Patients on intravenous antibiotics should be monitored with an audiogram twice a week while receiving therapy.

Acoustic Neuroma

An acoustic neuroma is a slow-growing, benign tumor of cranial nerve VIII, usually arising from the Schwann cells of the vestibular portion of the nerve. Most acoustic tumors arise within the internal auditory canal and extend into the cerebellopontine angle to press upon the brainstem. Acoustic neuromas account for 5% to 10% of all intracranial tumors and seem to occur with equal frequency in men and women at any age, although most occur during middle age. Most acoustic neuromas are unilateral except in von Recklinghausen's disease (neurofibromatosis or NF-2) in which bilateral tumors occur.

The most common presenting symptoms in patients with an acoustic neuroma are unilateral tinnitus and hearing loss with or without vertigo or balance disturbance. It is important to note asymmetry in audiovestibular test results so that further workup to rule out an acoustic neuroma can be performed. Magnetic resonance imaging (MRI) with a paramagnetic contrast agent (gadolinium or magnevist) is

TABLE 57-4 Examples of Ototoxic Medications

Diuretics	**Aminoglycoside Antibiotics**
Ethacrynic acid	Amikacin
Furosemide	Gentamicin
Acetazolamide	Kanamycin
Chemotherapeutic Agents	Netilmicin
Cisplatin	Neomycin
Nitrogen mustard	Streptomycin
Antimalarials	Tobramycin
Quinine	**Other Antibiotics**
Chloroquine	Erythromycin
Anti-inflammatory Agents	Minocycline
Salicylates (aspirin)	Polymyxin B
Indomethacin	Vancomycin
Chemicals	**Metals**
Alcohol	Gold
Arsenic	Mercury
	Lead

the imaging study of choice. If a patient is claustrophobic, cannot tolerate an MRI, or the scan is unavailable, a computed tomography (CT) scan with contrast dye is performed. An MRI with contrast should identify a 2- to 3-mm tumor, whereas a CT scan with contrast may miss tumors of 2 cm in diameter.

Surgical removal of acoustic tumors is the treatment of choice since they do not respond well to radiation or chemotherapy. Because treatment of acoustic tumors crosses several specialties, a multidisciplinary approach involving both a neurotologist and a neurosurgeon is usually taken. The objective of the surgery is to remove the tumor while preserving facial nerve function. Most acoustic tumors have damaged the cochlear portion of cranial nerve VIII so that no real serviceable hearing exists before surgery. In these patients, the surgery is performed translabyrinthine and the hearing mechanism is destroyed. If hearing is still good preoperatively, the suboccipital or middle cranial fossa approach to removing the tumor may be used, and intraoperative monitoring of cranial nerve VIII will be performed to save the hearing.

Complications of surgery for acoustic neuroma include facial nerve paralysis, cerebrospinal fluid leak, meningitis, and cerebral edema. A 3% mortality rate nationwide has been reported (Paparella et al., 1991). Complication rates decrease significantly with the experience of the surgical team.

Aural Rehabilitation

If a hearing loss is permanent or not amenable to medical or surgical intervention or if the patient elects not to have surgery, aural rehabilitation may be beneficial. The purpose of aural rehabilitation is to maximize the hearing-impaired person's communication skills. Aural rehabilitation includes auditory training, speech reading, speech training, and the use of hearing aids. Auditory training emphasizes listening skills, so the hearing-impaired person concentrates on the speaker. Speech reading (formerly known as lip reading) can help fill in the gaps of words that might be missed, but many words sound and look similar (*e.g.*, words that begin with b, m, and p). Speech training attempts to conserve, develop, and prevent deterioration of current speech skills.

It is important to identify the type of hearing impairment a person has so that rehabilitative efforts can be directed at meeting a particular need. Surgical correction may be all that is necessary to treat and improve a conductive hearing loss (Fig. 57-11). With recent advances in hearing aid technology, amplification for patients with sensor-

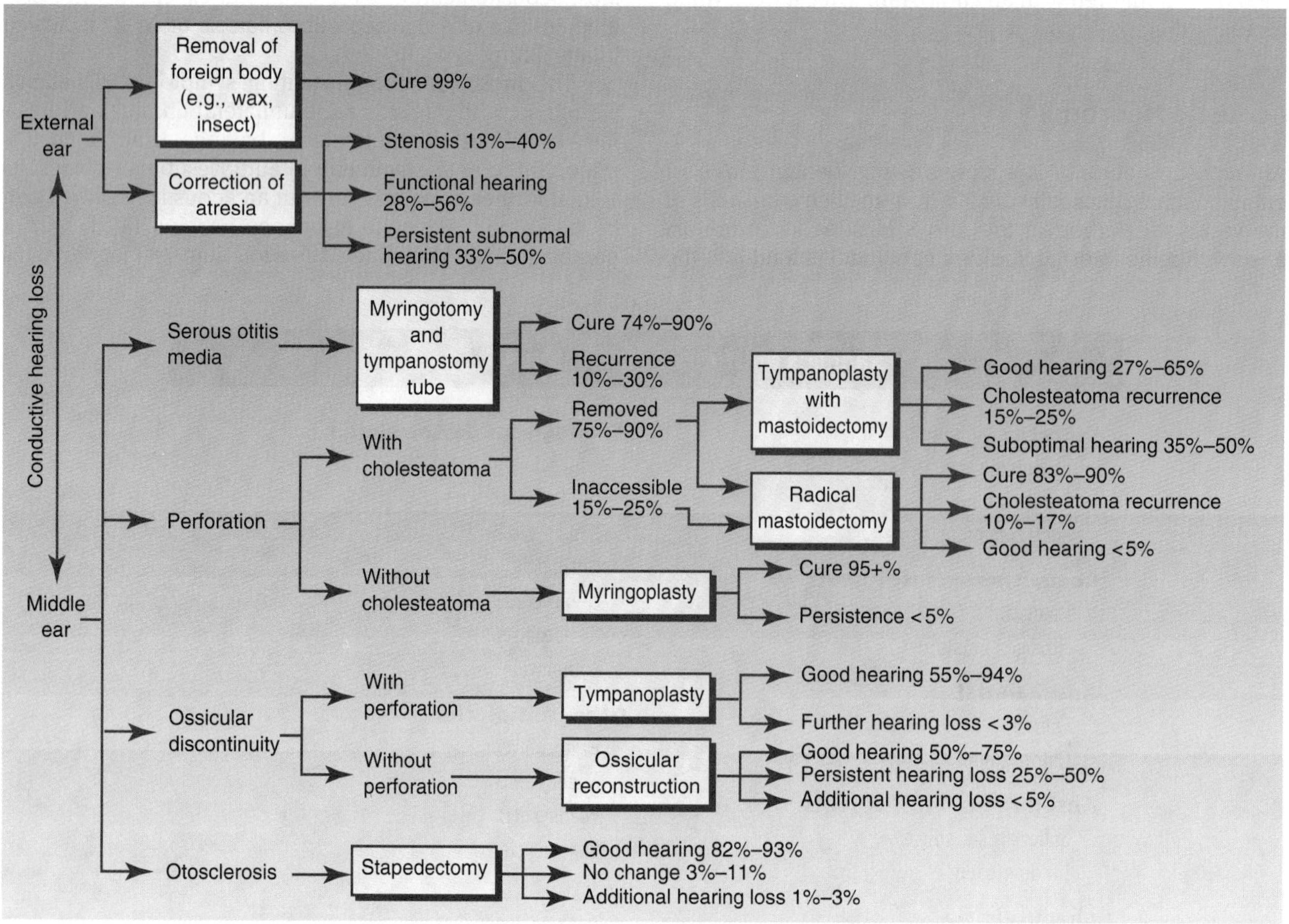

FIGURE 57-11. Conductive hearing loss. When a patient presents with this problem, the above flow chart indicates how the diagnosis determines the management of the patient and further predicts the outcome. (Jafek BW and Balkany TJ. Conductive hearing loss. In Eiseman B. Prognosis of Surgical Disease. Philadelphia, WB Saunders.)

ineural hearing loss is more helpful than it has been in the past. It is imperative that a patient have an audiogram and medical clearance by an otolaryngologist before being fitted for a hearing aid.

Hearing Aids

A hearing aid is an instrument through which sounds, both speech and environmental, are received by a microphone, converted to electrical signals, amplified, and reconverted to acoustic signals. Many aids available for sensorineural hearing loss depress the low frequencies, or tones, and give better hearing for the high frequencies. A helpful, but not critical, guideline is that a hearing aid may be of benefit to a patient when the hearing loss is more than 30 dB in the range of 500 to 2000 Hz in the better-hearing ear. Many types of hearing aids are available with the latest technology, and the aid should be fitted according to the needs of the patient (*e.g.*, type of hearing loss, manual dexterity) rather than by brand names (Table 57-5). It is estimated that 98% of all hearing aids sold today are either behind-the-ear (BTE), in-the-ear (ITE), or in-the-canal (ITC) types. The evolution in hearing aid development has led to smaller and more effective aids. A hearing aid should be fitted by a certified audiologist holding a license to dispense hearing aids. In many states a consumer protection law is applicable, and the hearing aid may be returned after a trial use if the patient is not completely satisfied.

A hearing aid makes sounds louder, but it does not faithfully reproduce the sounds nor does it improve a patient's ability to discriminate words or understand speech. Therefore, people who have low discrimination scores on audiogram (*i.e.*, 20%) may benefit little from a hearing aid. Hearing aids amplify all sounds including background noise, which may be disturbing to the wearer. There are, however, computerized hearing aids available that compensate for background noise or allow amplification at certain programmed frequencies rather than at all frequencies. Occasionally, depending on the type of hearing loss, binaural aids (*i.e.*, one for each ear) may be indicated.

The FDA has established regulations on hearing aids to protect the health and safety of people with hearing impairments:

1. A medical evaluation of the impairment by a licensed physician must be obtained within 6 months before the purchase of a hearing aid.
   a. Such a written statement from a physician, however, may be waived by the client (a fully informed adult 18 years of age or older) on signing a document to this effect.
   b. Children must be evaluated by a physician.
2. Health professionals who dispense hearing aids are required to refer prospective users to a physician if any of the following eight specified otologic conditions are evident:
   a. Visible congenital or traumatic deformity of the ear
   b. Active drainage from the ear within the previous 90 days
   c. Sudden or rapidly progressive hearing loss within the previous 90 days
   d. Complaints of dizziness or tinnitus
   e. Unilateral hearing loss that occurred suddenly or within the previous 90 days

TABLE 57-5 Hearing Aids

Site and Range of Hearing Loss	Advantages	Disadvantages
Body (mild–profound)	Separation of receiver and microphone prevents acoustic feedback, allowing high amplification. Generally used in a school setting.	Bulky; requires long wire, which may be cosmetically displeasing; some loss of high-frequency response.
Behind the ear (mild–profound)	Larger size permits use of larger components that enable the aid to provide more power and features; most versatile due to size; no long wires.	Large size
In the ear (mild–moderately severe)	One-piece custom fit to contour of ear; no tubes or cords; miniature microphone is located in the ear, which is a more natural placement; more cosmetically appealing due to easy concealment.	Smaller size limits output; patients who have arthritis or cannot perform tasks requiring good manual dexterity may have difficulty with the small size of aid and/or battery; can require more repair than the behind-the-ear aid.
In the canal (mild–moderately severe)	Same as in-the-ear aids; less visible, so more cosmetically pleasing.	Even smaller than in-the-ear aids; requires good manual dexterity.

   f. Audiometric air–bone gap equal to or greater than 15 dB at 500, 1000, and 2000 Hz
   g. Significant accumulation of cerumen or a foreign body in the external auditory canal
   h. Pain or discomfort in the ear
3. A *user instruction brochure* is to accompany every hearing aid device. In this brochure, the following information is presented:
   a. Specification that good health practice requires a medical evaluation before purchasing a hearing aid
   b. Notification that any of the eight designated otologic conditions listed above should be investigated by a physician before purchase of a hearing aid
   c. Instructions for proper use, maintenance, and care of the hearing aid as well as instructions for replacing or recharging the batteries
   d. Repair service information
   e. Description of avoidable conditions that could adversely affect or damage the hearing aid
   f. Specification of any known side effects that may warrant physician consultation (*e.g.*, skin irritation, accelerated cerumen accumulation)

Care of the Hearing Aid. A hearing aid must be cared for carefully, and the wearer should know how to do so as well as what to do if the aid fails. The nurse must also have a basic knowledge of the hearing aid to assist a patient who is unable or unwilling to care for the aid when ill. The ear mold, the only part of the instrument that may be washed, is washed frequently (even daily if necessary) in soap and water, and the cannula is cleansed with a small applicator or pipe cleaner. The ear mold must be dry before it is snapped into the receiver. The transmitter is usually worn behind the ear or in the frame of the eyeglasses. Spare parts should be available to the wearer.

Inadequate amplification, a whistling noise, or pain from the mold may occur when a hearing aid is not functioning properly (Chart 57-3). If the hearing aid still does not work after it is checked for malfunctions (*e.g.*, switch is on, batteries are new and positioned correctly), the patient should notify the hearing aid dispenser. If the unit requires extended time for repair, the dispenser may lend the patient a hearing aid until the repair can be accomplished.

When occluded by a hearing aid, the external auditory canal can become moist, as air is trapped in this space. Common medical problems among wearers of hearing aids are otitis externa and pressure ulcers in the external auditory canal or meatus.

CHART 57-3
Hearing Aid Problems

Whistling Noise
Loose Ear Mold
- Improperly made
- Improperly worn
- Worn out

Improper Aid Selection
- Too much power required in aid with inadequate separation between microphone and receiver
- Open mold used inappropriately

Inadequate Amplification
- Dead batteries
- Wax in ear
- Wax or other material in mold
- Wires or tubing disconnected from aid
- Aid turned off or volume too low
- Improper mold
- Improper aid for degree of loss

Pain From Mold
- Improperly fitted mold
- Ear skin or cartilage infection
- Middle ear infection
- Ear tumor
- Unrelated causes:
  - Temporomandibular joint
  - Throat or larynx
  - Other

(Sataloff RT. Choosing the right hearing aid. Hosp Pract 16[5]:32A.)

Implanted Hearing Devices

Three types of implanted hearing devices are either currently available or in the investigational stage: the cochlear implant, the bone conduction device, and the semi-implantable hearing device. Cochlear implants are for patients with little or no hearing. Bone conduction devices (*i.e.*, Audiant) transmit sound through the skull to the inner ear. These are used in patients with a conductive hearing loss in which a hearing aid might be contraindicated (*i.e.*, chronic infection). The device is implanted postauricularly under the skin into the skull and an external device—worn above the ear, not in the canal—transmits the sound through the skin. Semi-implantable hearing aids, although not yet approved by the FDA except in testing sites, will still require the use of an external device.

Cochlear Implant. A cochlear implant is an auditory prosthesis used for people with profound sensorineural hearing loss bilaterally who cannot benefit from conventional hearing aids. The hearing loss may be congenital or acquired. An implant is an inner ear device that helps a person detect medium to loud environmental sounds and perhaps some conversation; it does not restore normal hearing. The implant is designed to provide stimulation directly to the auditory nerve and to bypass the hair cells of the inner ear, which are not functioning. The microphone and signal processor are worn outside the body, like a hearing aid. A transmitter outside the body with a receiver inside is used to provide a direct connection between the signal processor and electrodes of the implant. The electrical stimuli are sent inside the body to the implanted electrodes. The electrical signals stimulate the auditory nerve fibers, and the signals are then sent to the brain where they are interpreted.

Candidates for cochlear implant, who are usually at least 2 years of age, are selected after careful screening by otologic history, physical examination, audiologic testing, and radiographic and psychologic testing. The general criteria for choosing adults who may benefit from a cochlear implant are:

- A profound sensorineural hearing loss in both ears
- Inability to hear and recognize speech through hearing aids
- Deafness after learning oral speech and language (postlinguistically deafened)
- No medical contraindication to a cochlear implant or general anesthesia
- Indications that being able to hear would enhance the patient's life

The surgery involves implanting a small receiver in the temporal bone, through a postauricular incision, and placing electrodes into the inner ear (Fig. 57-12). The microphone and transmitter are worn on an external unit, which is fitted postoperatively. The patient will then undergo extensive cochlear rehabilitation with the multidisciplinary team, which includes an audiologist and speech pathologist, and may need several weeks or months to learn to properly interpret the sounds heard. For example, the patient will learn to differentiate between the sounds made by a doorbell and those made by a telephone. There are wide variations of success with cochlear implants and much controversy about their use, especially among the deaf community.

CRITICAL THINKING EXERCISES

1. An elderly patient in an extended-care facility appears withdrawn and distrustful of others. She does not participate in conversations with other residents. You suspect that she has a hearing loss. Describe the strategies you would use to assess this patient's hearing. What intervention strategies would you implement if your assessment (1) confirms that the woman has a hearing loss? (2) indicates that she does not have a hearing loss?
2. An antiemetic and a tranquilizer have been prescribed for a patient with Ménière's disease. You realize that safety precautions are indicated. Devise a teaching plan for this patient and explain the reasons behind each part of the plan.
3. The daughter of an elderly patient complains that her father refuses to use his hearing aid. How would you focus your assessment to gather other pertinent information in determining a plan of action? Describe the patient outcomes you anticipate your interventions will achieve.

Hearing Guide Dogs

Specially trained dogs are available to assist the person with a hearing loss. Persons who live alone are eligible to apply for a dog trained by International Hearing Dog, Inc. At home the dog reacts to the sound of a telephone, a doorbell, an alarm clock, a baby's cry, a knock at the door, a smoke alarm, or an intruder. The dog does not bark but alerts his master by physical contact; the dog then runs to the source of the noise. In public, the dog positions itself between the hearing-impaired person and any potential hazard that the person cannot hear, such as an oncoming vehicle or a hostile person. In many states, a hearing-impaired person with

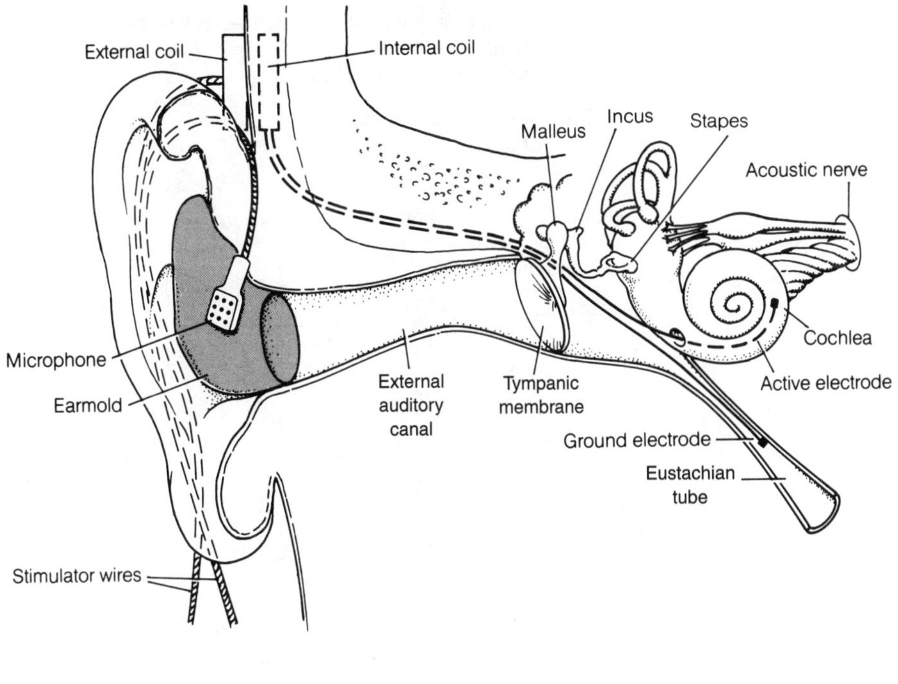

FIGURE 57-12. The cochlear implant. The internal coil has a stranded electrode lead. The electrode is inserted through the round window into the scala tympani of the cochlea. The external coil (the transmitter) is held in alignment with the internal coil (the receiver) by a magnet. The microphone receives the sound. The stimulator wire receives the signal after it has been filtered, adjusted, and modified so that the sound is at a comfortable level for the patient. Sound is passed by the external transmitter to the inner coil receiver by magnetic conduction and is then carried by the electrode to the cochlea.

a certified hearing guide dog is legally permitted access to public transportation, public eating places, and stores, including grocery markets.

BIBLIOGRAPHY

Books

Cummings CW et al. Otolaryngology—Head and Neck Surgery. St. Louis, CV Mosby, 1993.

Glasscock ME and Stambaugh GE. Surgery of the Ear. Philadelphia, WB Saunders, 1990.

Meyerhoff WL and Rice DH. Otolaryngology—Head and Neck Surgery. Philadelphia, WB Saunders, 1992.

Paparella MM et al. Otolaryngology, Volume 2: Otology and Neuro-otology. Philadelphia, WB Saunders, 1991.

Sigler BA and Schuring LT. Ear, Nose, and Throat Disorders—Mosby's Clinical Nursing Series. St. Louis, CV Mosby, 1993.

Society of Otorhinolaryngology–Head and Neck Nurses, Inc. Nursing Practice Guidelines for Care of the Otorhinolaryngology—Head and Neck Patient. New Smyrna Beach, FL, 1994.

Journals

Asterisks indicate nursing research articles.

Chovaz CJ. Communicating with the hearing impaired patient. Axone 1992 March; 13(3):77–80.

Cohen H, Rubin AM, and Gombash L. The team approach to treatment of the dizzy patient. Arch Phys Med & Rehab 1992 Aug; 73(8):703–708.

*Lusk SL et al. Test of the health promotion model as a causal model of workers' use of hearing protection. Nurs Res 1994 May/June; 43(3):151–157.

McConnell EA. How to irrigate the ear. Nursing 1992 Jan; 22(1):66.

NIH Consensus Development Conference Statement. Acoustic neuroma. 1991 Dec 11–13; 9(4).

Pollock KJ. Ménière's disease: A review of the problem. ORL—Head and Neck Nurs 1995; 13(2):10–13.

Ross V, Echevarria KH, and Robinson B. Geriatric tinnitus: Causes, clinical treatment, and prevention. J Geriatr Nurs 1991 Oct; 17(10):6–11.

Webber-Jones J. Doomed to deafness? Am J Nurs 1992 Nov; 92(11):37–39.

INFORMATION/RESOURCES

Agencies

Acoustic Neuroma Association
P.O. Box 398
Carisle, PA 17013

Alexander Graham Bell Association for the Deaf, Inc.
3417 Volta Place, NW
Washington, D. C. 20007

American Academy of Audiology
1735 N. Lynn Street
Arlington, VA 22209

American Academy of Facial Plastic and Reconstructive Surgery
110 Vermont Ave., NW, Suite 220
Washington, D.C. 20005

American Academy of Otolaryngology–Head and Neck Surgery
One Prince Street
Alexandria, VA 22314

American Speech-Language-Hearing Association
10801 Rockville Pike, Department AP
Rockville, MD 20852

American Tinnitus Association
P.O. Box 5
Portland, OR 97207

Council for Better Hearing and Speech Month
3417 Volta Place, NW
Washington, D.C. 20007

International Hearing Dog Inc.
5901 East 89th Ave.
Henderson, CO 80640

National Hearing Aid Society
20361 Middlebelt
Livonia, MI 48152

National Institute on Deafness and
Other Communication Disorders
National Institutes of Health
Building 31, Room 3c35
9000 Rockville Pike
Bethesda, MD 20892

Self Help for Hard of Hearing People
4848 Battery Lane, Dept. E
Bethesda, MD 20814

Society of Otorhinolaryngology and Head–Neck Nurses, Inc.
116-A Canal Street
New Smyrna Beach, FL 32168

The Deafness Research Foundation
55 East 34th St.
New York, NY 10016

Vestibular Disorders Association
P.O. Box 4467
Portland, OR 97208

UNIT 15
Neurologic Function

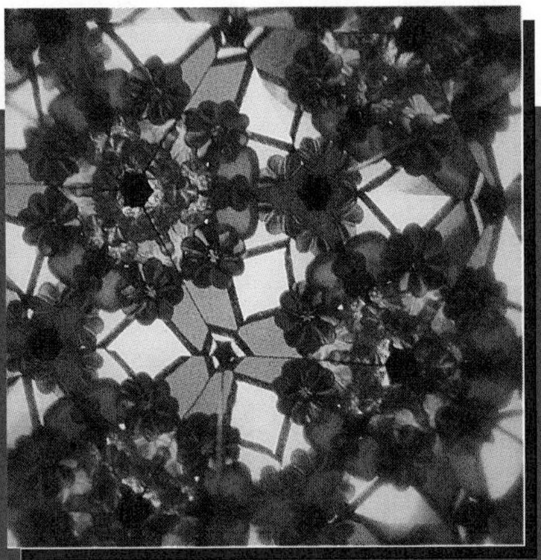

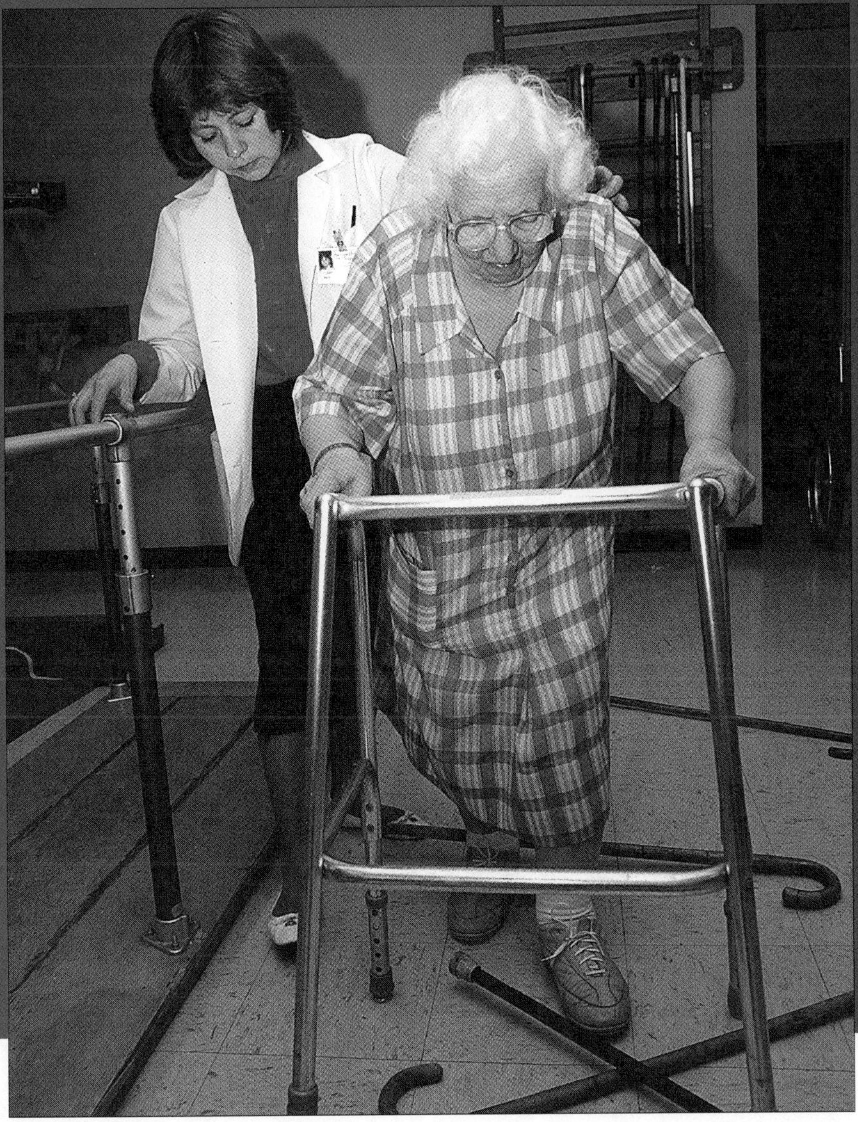

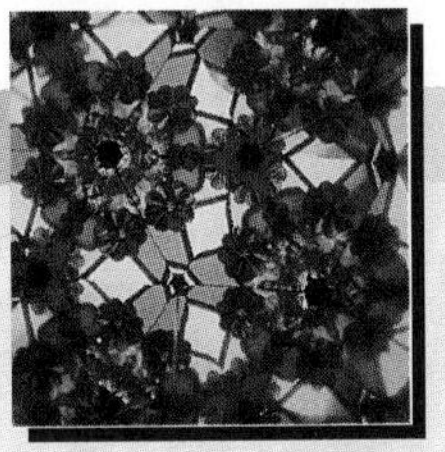

58

Assessment of Neurologic Function

CHAPTER OUTLINE

Overview of Anatomy and Physiology
The Brain
Functions of the Cerebral Cortex
The Spinal Cord

The Neurologic Examination
Cerebral Function
Glasgow Coma Scale
Examination of the Cranial Nerves
Examination of the Motor System
Examination of the Reflexes
Sensory Examination

Gerontologic Considerations
Nursing Implications

Diagnostic Tests and Procedures
Imaging Procedures
Echoencephalography
Air Studies
Electrophysiologic Tests
Special Procedures

Critical Thinking Exercises

LEARNING OBJECTIVES

On completion of this chapter, the learner will be able to:

1. Differentiate between pathologic changes that affect motor control and those that affect sensory pathways
2. Compare the functioning of the sympathetic and parasympathetic nervous systems
3. Describe the significance of physical assessment to the diagnosis of neurologic dysfunction
4. Describe changes in neurologic function with aging and their impact on neurologic assessment findings
5. Describe diagnostic tests used for assessment of neurologic function and the related nursing implications

Overview of Anatomy and Physiology

The nervous system consists of the brain, the spinal cord, and the peripheral nerves. These structures are responsible for control and coordination of cellular activities throughout the body by the transmission of electrical impulses. The impulses travel by way of nerve fibers and pathways, which are direct and continuous. The responses are instantaneous as a result of changes in electrical potential, which transmit the signals.

The Brain

The brain is divided into three major divisions: the cerebrum, the brainstem, and the cerebellum. It is contained in a rigid, bony structure called the skull, which protects the brain from injury. Four bones join together to form the skull: the frontal, parietal, temporal, and occipital bones (Fig. 58-1). At the base of the skull there are three divisions called fossas. The anterior fossa contains the frontal lobes of the cerebral hemispheres; the middle fossa contains the parietal, temporal and occipital lobes; and the posterior fossa contains the brain stem and medulla. (See Chart 58-1 for a glossary of terms used in this chapter.)

The Meninges

Beneath the skull the brain and spinal cord are covered by three membranes or meninges. The meninges are composed of fibrous connective tissue that protects, supports, and provides nourishment to the brain. The meninges are the dura mater, the arachnoid, and the pia mater (Fig. 58-2).

Dura mater—the outermost layer; covers the brain and the spinal cord. It is tough, thick, nonelastic, fibrous, and gray. There are two extensions of the dura: the falx cerebri, which separates the two hemispheres in a longitudinal plane, and the *tentorium,* which is an infolding of the dura that forms a tough membranous shelf. This shelf supports the hemispheres and separates them from the lower part of the brain (the posterior fossa). When excess pressure occurs in the cranial cavity, brain tissue may be compressed against the tentorium or displaced downward, a process called herniation.

Arachnoid—the middle membrane; a flimsy, delicate membrane that closely resembles a spider web, hence the name arachnoid. It is white in color because it has no blood supply. The arachnoid layer contains the choroid plexus, which is responsible for the production of cerebrospinal fluid (CSF). This membrane also has unique finger-like projections, called arachnoid villi, which absorb CSF. In the normal adult, approximately 500 ml of CSF are produced each day; all but 150 ml are absorbed by the villi. Villi absorb CSF; thus when blood enters the system (from trauma, a ruptured aneurysm, stroke, and so forth), they become obstructed. When the arachnoid villi become obstructed, hydrocephalus (increased size of ventricles) can result.

Pia mater—the innermost membrane; a thin, transparent layer that hugs the brain closely and extends into every fold of the brain's surface.

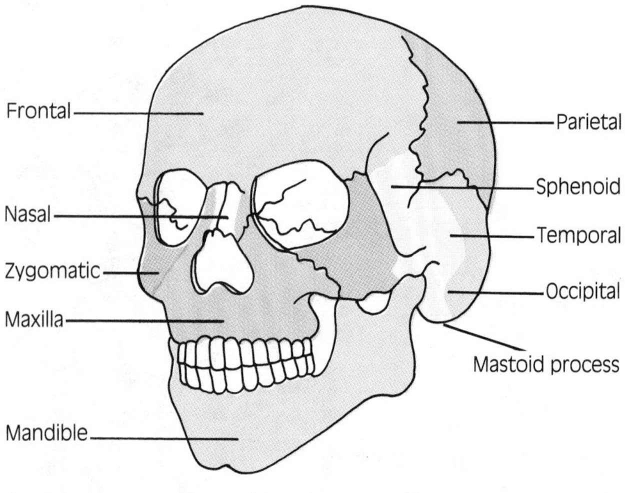

FIGURE 58-1. Bones of the skull.

Cerebrum

The **cerebrum** consists of two hemispheres and four lobes. The *gray matter* is in the external or outer layer of the cerebrum, and the *white matter* makes up the internal layer of the cerebrum. Gray matter is composed principally of nerve cell bodies that are concentrated in the cerebral cortex, nuclei, and basal ganglia. White matter is composed of nerve cell processes, which form tracts or commissures connecting various parts of the brain with one another. The cerebral hemispheres (telencephelon) contain the largest amount of central nervous system (CNS) tissue. This area, which is where control of high motor function occurs, is responsible for an individual's function and intelligence. The four lobes are as follows (Fig. 58-3):

Frontal—the largest lobe; located in the anterior fossa. This area controls an individual's affect, judgment, personality, and inhibitions.

Parietal—a pure sensory lobe. This area allows one to interpret sensation. The only sense that does not interact here is smell. The parietal lobe allows an individual to know the position and space of his body. Patients with damage to this area may experience hemineglect syndrome.

Temporal—integrates the sensations of taste, smell, and hearing. Short-term memory is associated with this area.

Occipital—the posterior lobe of the cerebral hemisphere, responsible for visual interpretation.

The corpus collosum is a thick collection of nerve fibers that connects the two hemispheres of the brain and is responsible for the transmission of information from one side of the brain to the other. Information transferred is sensory, memory, and learned discrimination. Right-handed people and some left-handed people have cerebral dominance on the left side of the brain for verbal, linguistic, arithmetical, calculating, and analytic functions. The nondominant hemisphere is responsible for geometric, spatial, visual, pattern, and musical functions. The basal ganglia,

CHART 58-1
Glossary

Nervous System Characteristics, Reflexes, Conditions, and Disorders

agnosia loss of ability to recognize objects through a particular sensory system. **Visual agnosia** refers to the inability to name an object even though it may be familiar. There are also **auditory** and **tactile agnosias.**

agraphia inability to express thoughts in writing due to a lesion of the CNS

aneurysm a weakening or bulge in an arterial wall

anopsia nonuse or suppression of vision in one eye

aphasia loss of the ability to express oneself or to understand language

apraxia inability to perform purposeful movement when paralysis is not present

ataxia inability to coordinate muscle movements, resulting in difficulty in walking, talking, and performing self-care tasks

Babinski reflex (sign) a reflex action of the toes, indicative of abnormalities in the motor control pathways leading from the cerebral cortex

cerebral hemorrhage a hemorrhage into an area of the brain that results in loss of function for that part of the brain; commonly referred to as a cerebrovascular accident (CVA) or stroke

corneal reflex normal blinking on touching of the cornea

decerebrate posturing abnormal posturing with extension and external rotation of the arms and wrists, extension and plantar flexion and internal rotation of the feet

decorticate posturing abnormal posturing with flexion and internal rotation of the arms and wrists, extension and plantar flexion and internal rotation of the feet

dementia organic loss of intellectual function

diplopia (double vision) seeing two images of a single object

dysarthria difficulty in forming or articulating words. This may be caused by damage to the motor areas of the cerebrum or damage to the brain stem. This term encompasses speech that is slurred, too fast or slow, or of abnormal pitch.

electroencephalography (EEG) a method of recording, in graphic form, the electrical activity of the brain

electromyography (EMG) a method of recording, in graphic form, the electrical activity of the muscle

flaccid limp, floppy, lacking tone

focal arising from, or limited to, one part

hemiplegia or paresis weakness or paralysis of one side of the body, or part of it, due to an injury to the motor areas of the brain

infarction a zone of tissue deprived of blood supply

monoplegic (paresis) paralysis (weakness) of one limb

multiple sclerosis a disorder characterized by demyelination of the white matter of the brain and the spinal cord

myelography (myelogram) a radiologic study of the spinal cord after injection of a contrast medium into the subarachnoid space

myopathy any degenerative disease of a muscle

nuchal rigidity (neck stiffness) a sign of irritation or infection of the meninges

neuralgia pain in a nerve or along the course of one or more nerves

oculomotor concerned with eye movement

otorrhea fluid (usually CSF) drainage from the ear

paraparesis/paraplegia weakness/paralysis of both legs and the lower part of the trunk

photophobia the inability to tolerate light

position (postural) sense knowledge of where each part of the body is without looking at it

ptosis drooping of an eyelid

quadriparesis a weakness that involves all four extremities

quadriplegia paralysis of all four extremities

reflex an automatic response to stimuli

rhinorrhea fluid (usually CSF) draining from the nose

spasticity an abnormal increase in muscle tone, causing the muscles to resist being stretched.

stroke, cerebral see **cerebral hemorrhage**

tetraplegia paralysis of all four extremities; the same as quadriplegia

tinnitus ringing in the ears

tone the tension present in a muscle at rest

xanthochromic yellow in color; used in reference to CSF

comprising a number of nuclei and located deep in the cerebral hemispheres, are responsible for subconcious motor control of fine body movements, including those of the hands and lower extremities.

Diencephalon

The middle fossa or diencephalon contains the thalamus, hypothalamus, and pituitary gland (Fig. 58-4).

The **thalamus** lies on either side of the third ventricle and acts primarily as a relay station for all sensation except for smell. All memory, sensation, and pain impulses pass through this section.

The **hypothalamus** is located anterior and inferior to the thalamus. It controls and regulates the autonomic nervous system. It works with the pituitary to maintain fluid balance, maintains temperature regulation by promoting vasoconstriction or vasodilation, and influences hormonal

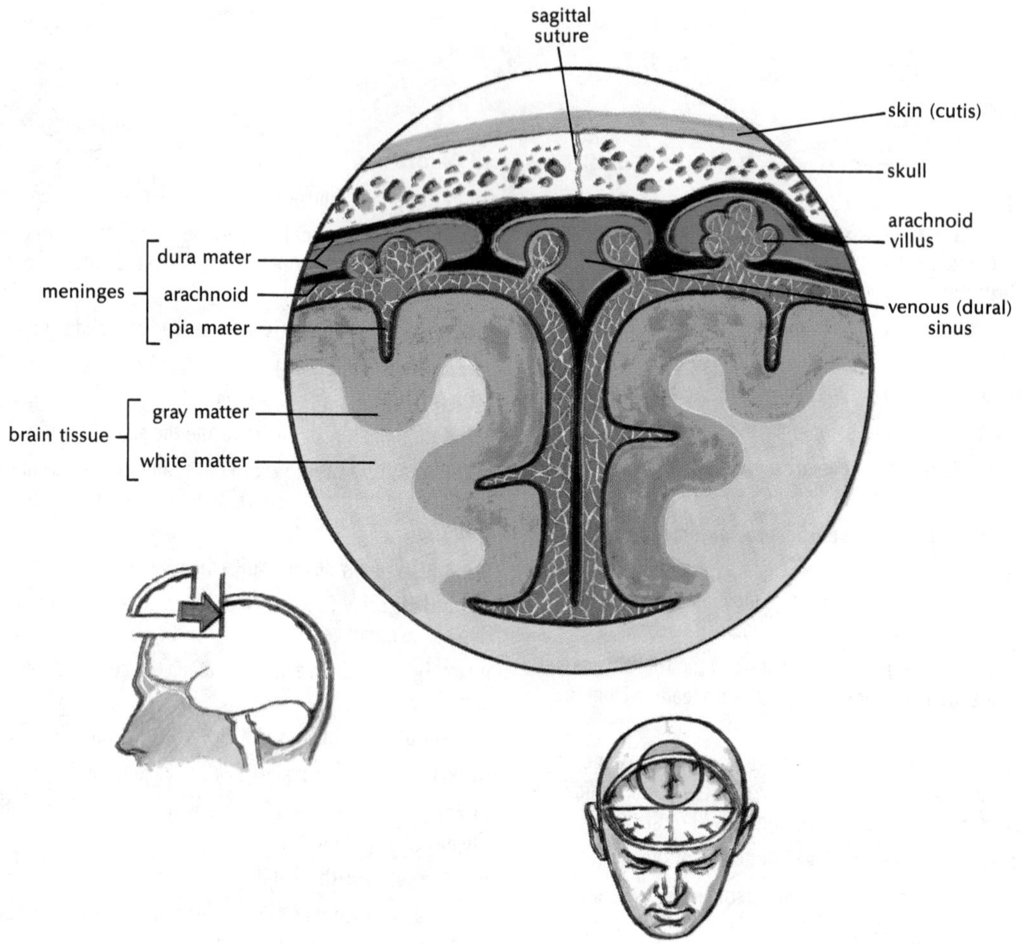

FIGURE 58-2. Meninges and related parts as seen through the frontal section of the top of the head.

secretion by the pituitary gland. The hypothalamus is the site of the hunger center and is involved in weight control. It houses centers that regulate the sleep, blood pressure, and aggressive and sexual behavior, and the center for emotional responses (*i.e.*, blushing, rage, depression, panic, and fear).

The **pituitary** gland is considered the master gland because of the number of hormones and functions it controls. With its hormones the pituitary is able to control the function of the kidneys, pancreas, reproductive organs, thyroid, adrenal cortex, and other organs. The pituitary is the third most common site for brain tumors in adults; frequently they are detected by physical signs and symptoms that can be traced to the pituitary. The anterior lobe of the pituitary produces growth hormone, adrenocorticotropic hormone (ACTH), prolactin, thyroid-stimulating hormone (TSH), follicle-stimulating hormone (FSH), and luteinizing hormone (LH). The posterior lobe stores antidiuretic hormone (ADH), which influences the kidneys' excretion or retention of water. The two most common syndromes associated with ADH abnormalities are diabetes insipidus (DI) and syndrome of inappropriate ADH (SIADH).

Nerve fibers from all portions of the cortex converge in each hemisphere and make their exit in the form of tight bundles known as the **internal capsule**. Having entered the pons and the medulla, each bundle crosses the corresponding bundle from the opposite side. Some of these axons make connections with axons from the cerebellum, basal ganglia, thalamus, and hypothalamus; some connect with the cranial nerve cells. Other fibers from the cortex and the subcortical centers are channeled through the pons and the medulla into the spinal cord.

Functions of the Cerebral Cortex

Although the various cells in the cerebral cortex are quite similar in appearance, their functions vary widely, depending on their locations. The topography of the cortex in relation to certain of its specific functions is shown in Figure 58-5. The posterior portion of each hemisphere (*i.e.*, the occipital lobe) is devoted to all aspects of visual perception. The lateral region, or temporal lobe, incorporates the auditory center. The midcentral zone, or parietal zone, posterior to the fissure of Rolando, is concerned with sensation; the anterior portion is concerned with voluntary muscle movements.

The large area beneath the forehead (*i.e.*, the frontal lobes) contains the association pathways that determine emotional attitudes and responses and contribute to the

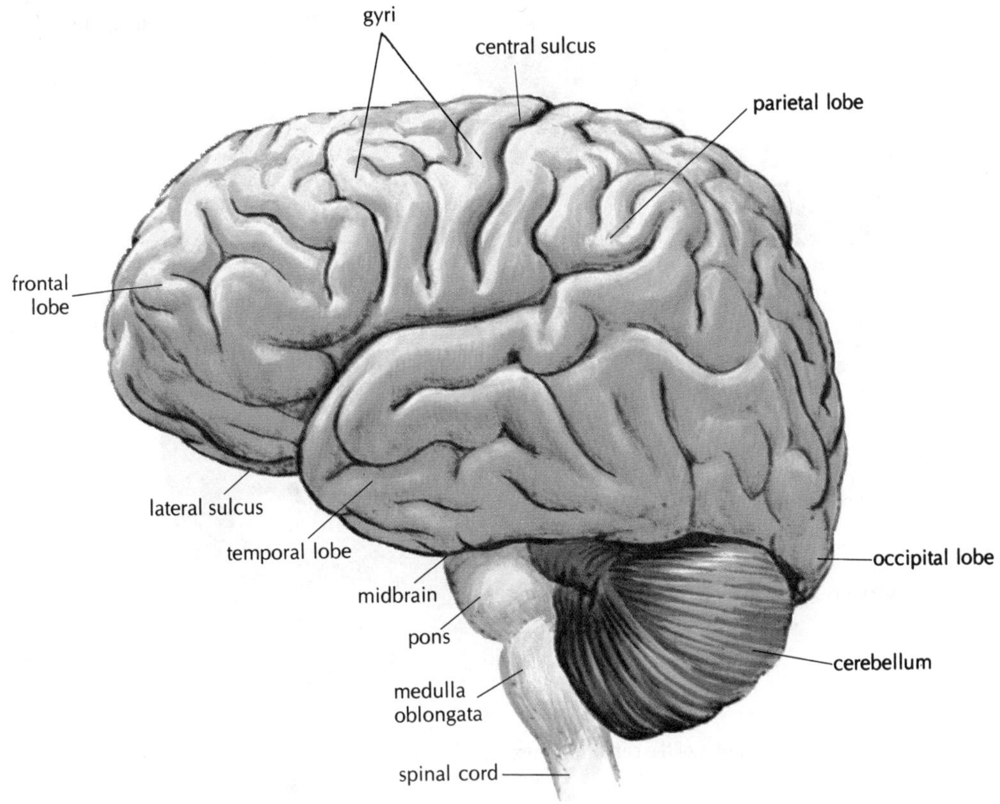

FIGURE 58-3. View of the external surface of the brain showing lobes and key parts.

formation of thought processes. Damage to the frontal lobes as a result of trauma or disease is by no means incapacitating from the standpoint of muscular control or coordination, but it affects a person's personality, as reflected by basic attitudes, sense of humor and propriety, self-restraint, and motivations.

Brain Stem

The **brain stem** is located in the posterior fossa. It consists of the midbrain, pons, and medulla oblongata (see Fig. 58-3). The **midbrain** or mesencephalon connects the pons and the cerebellum with the cerebral hemispheres; it contains sensory and motor pathways and serves as the center for auditory and visual reflexes. The **pons** is situated in front of the cerebellum between the midbrain and the medulla and is a bridge between the two halves of the cerebellum, as well as between the medulla and the cerebrum. The pons also contains motor and sensory pathways.

The **medulla oblongata** transmits motor fibers from the brain to the spinal cord and sensory fibers from the spinal cord to the brain. Most of these fibers cross, or decussate, at this level. The pons also contains important centers controlling heart, respiration, and blood pressure and is the site of origin of the fifth through eighth cranial nerves.

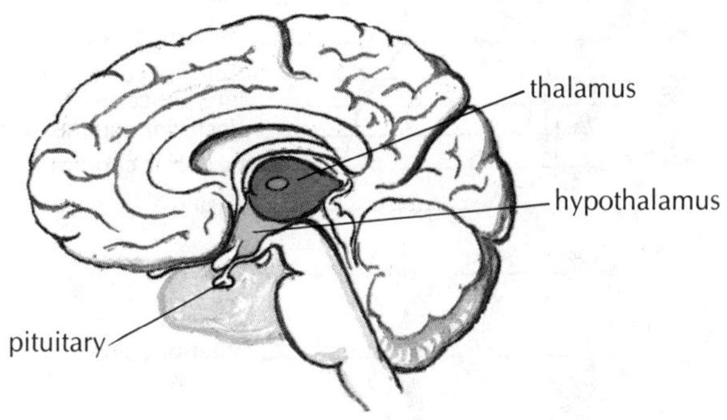

FIGURE 58-4. Diagram showing the thalamus, hypothalamus, and pituitary (hypophysis).

Cerebellum

The cerebellum is located in the posterior fossa and is separated from the cerebral hemispheres by a fold of dura mater, the tentorium cerebelli. The cerebellum has both excitatory and inhibitory actions and is largely responsible for smoothness and coordination of movement. Additionally, it controls fine movement, balance, position sense, and integration of sensory input.

Cerebral Circulation

Cerebral circulation receives approximately 20% of the cardiac output or 750 ml per minute. Since the brain does not store nutrients and has a high metabolic demand, the high flow is a necessity. The brain's blood pathway is unique because it flows against gravity; its arteries fill from below and the veins drain from above. The brain lacks additional collateral blood flow, which may result in irreversible tissue

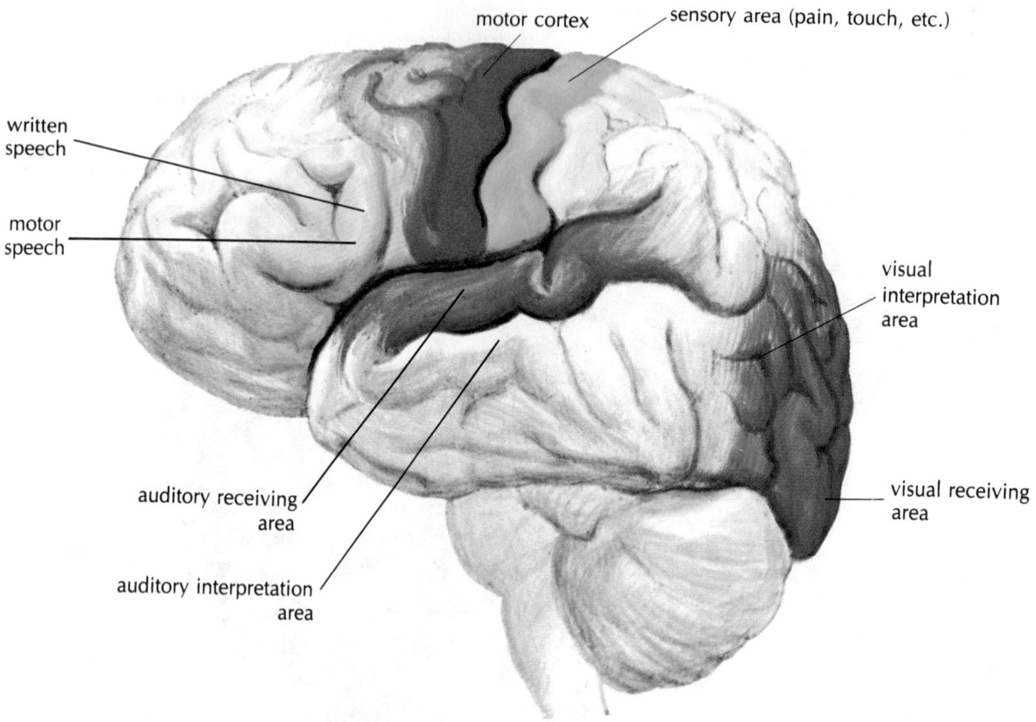

FIGURE 58-5. Functional areas of the cerebral cortex.

damage; this is in contrast to other organs, which may be able to tolerate decreases in blood flow because of their adequate collateral flow.

Arteries. The arterial blood supply to the brain is provided by two internal carotid arteries and two vertebral arteries and their extensive system of branches. The internal carotids arise from the bifurcation of the common carotid and supply much of the anterior circulation of the brain. The vertebral arteries branch from the subclavian arteries, flow back and upward on either side of the cervical vertebrae, and enter the cranium through the foramen magnum. Joining to become the basilar artery at the level of the brain stem, the vertebrobasilar arteries supply most of the posterior circulation of the brain. The basilar artery divides to form the two branches of the posterior cerebral arteries.

Circle of Willis. At the base of the brain surrounding the pituitary gland, a ring of arteries is formed between the vertebral and internal carotid arterial chains. This ring is called the *circle of Willis* and is formed from the branches of the internal carotid arteries, anterior and middle cerebral arteries, and anterior and posterior communicating arteries (Fig. 58-6). Blood flow from the circle of Willis directly affects the anterior and the posterior cerebral circulation. The arteries of the circle of Willis provide alternative routes of blood flow if one of the major arteries leading to it becomes occluded.

FIGURE 58-6. Arterial blood supply of the brain, including the circle of Willis, as viewed from the ventral surface.

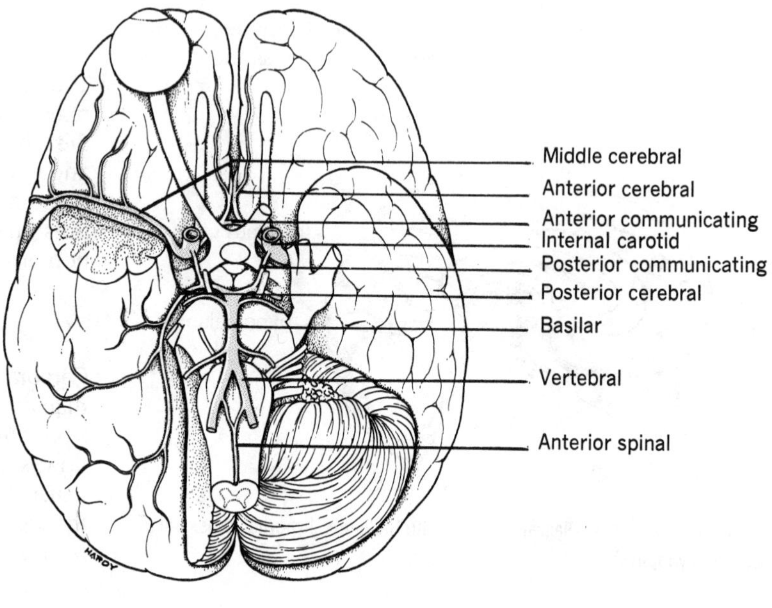

The arterial anastomosis along the circle of Willis is a frequent site of aneurysms, which may be congenital. Aneurysms can be formed when blood pressure at a weakened arterial wall causes the artery to balloon out. An aneurysm can press on adjacent cerebral structures, such as the optic chiasm, causing visual disturbances. If an artery becomes occluded by vasospasm, an embolus, or a thrombus, the neurons distal to the occlusion are deprived of their blood supply and the cells quickly die. The result is a stroke (cerebrovascular accident or infarction). The effects of the occlusion depend on which vessels are involved and which areas of the brain these vessels supply.

Veins. Venous drainage for the brain does not accompany the arterial circulation as in other body structures. The veins of the brain reach the brain's surface and join larger veins. These cross the subarachnoid space and empty into the larger dural sinuses, which are the vascular channels lying within the tough dura meter. The network of the sinuses carries venous outflow for the brain and empties into the internal jugular vein back to the central circulatory system. Cerebral veins are unique because, unlike other veins in the body, they do not have valves to prevent blood from flowing backwards.

Blood–Brain Barrier

The CNS is inaccessible to many substances that circulate in the blood (*i.e.*, dyes, medications, antibiotics). After being injected into the blood, these substances do not reach the neurons of the CNS; this phenomenon is called the *blood–brain barrier.* The endothelial cells of the brain's capillaries form continuous tight junctions, creating a barrier to macromolecules and many compounds. The barrier to the large molecules entering the cerebrospinal fluid (CSF) is the low permeability of the secretory cells of the choroid plexus. All substances entering the CSF must filter through the capillary membranes of the choroid plexus. Often altered by trauma, cerebral edema, and cerebral hypoxemia, the blood–brain barrier has implications in the treatment and medication selection for CNS disease processes.

Cerebrospinal Fluid

Cerebrospinal fluid (CSF), a clear and colorless fluid with a specific gravity of 1.007, is produced in the ventricles and is circulated around the brain and the spinal cord by the ventricular system. There are four ventricles: the right and left lateral, third, and fourth ventricles. The two lateral ventricles open into the third ventricle at the interventricular foramen or the foramen of Monro. The third and fourth ventricles connect via the aqueduct of Sylvius. The fourth ventricle supplies CSF to the subarachnoid space and down the spinal cord on the dorsal surface.

CSF is produced in the choroid plexus of the lateral, third, and fourth ventricles. The ventricular and subarachnoid system contains approximately 150 ml of fluid; 15 to 25 ml of CSF is located in each lateral ventricle.

The organic and inorganic contents of CSF are similar to those of plasma, but their concentration is somewhat different. CSF is analyzed for protein, glucose, and chloride on routine analysis; it may also be tested for immunoglobulins. Normally, CSF has a minimal number of white blood cells and no red blood cells.

CSF is returned to the brain and is then circulated around the brain, where it is absorbed by the arachnoid villi. From the arachnoid villi CSF is mixed with venous blood in the superior sagittal sinus.

The Spinal Cord

The spinal cord and brainstem form a continuous structure extending from the cerebral hemispheres and serving as a connecting link between the brain and the periphery, such as skin and muscles. Approximately 45 cm (18 inches) long and about the thickness of a finger, it extends from the foramen magnum at the base of the skull to the upper level of the body of the second lumbar vertebra, where it terminates in a fibrous band called the conus medullaris. Continuing below the second lumbar space are the nerve roots that extend beyond the conus, which are called the cauda equina since they resemble a horse's tail.

Spinal Nerves. The spinal cord is composed of 33 segments: 7 cervical, 12 thoracic, 5 lumbar, 5 sacral, and 4 to 5 coccygeal segments. The spinal cord has 31 pairs of spinal nerves; each segment has one for each side of the body (Fig. 58-7). Like the brain, the spinal cord consists of grey and white matter. Grey matter in the brain is external and white matter is internal; in the spinal cord, grey matter is in the center and surrounded on all sides by white matter.

Vertebral Column. The vertebral column protects the spinal cord, allows for movement of the head and limbs, and stabilizes bony structures for ambulation. The vertebrae are separated by discs except for the first and second cervical, sacral, and coccygeal vertebrae. Each vertebra has a ventral body and a dorsal or neural arch, which is posterior to the body. Along with the neural arch are two pedicles and laminae. The vertebral body, neural arch, pedicles, and laminae all surround the vertebral canal.

Spinal Cord Structure. The spinal cord is surrounded by the meninges, dura, arachnoid, and pia maters. Between the dura mater and the vertebral canal is the epidural space. The spinal cord is an H-shaped structure with nerve cell bodies (grey matter) surrounded by ascending and descending tracts (white matter) (Fig. 58-8). The lower portion of the H is broader than the upper portion and corresponds to the anterior horns. It is in these horns that the cells lie that have the fibers that form the anterior (motor) root end and are essential for the voluntary and reflex activity of the muscles supplied by them. The thinner posterior (upper horns) portion contains cells with fibers that enter over the posterior (sensory) root end and thus serve as a relay station in the sensory/reflex pathway.

In the thoracic region of the spinal cord is a projection from each side at the crossbar of the H of grey matter called the lateral horn. It contains the cells that give rise to the autonomic fibers of the sympathetic division. The fibers leave the spinal cord through the anterior roots in the thoracic and upper lumbar segments.

Spinal Tracts. The white matter forms the greater part of the spinal cord and can be subdivided into three groups of fibers called tracts or pathways. The *posterior tract* conducts sensation, principally the perception of touch, pressure, vibration, position, and passive motion from the same side of the body. Before reaching the cerebral cortex, these

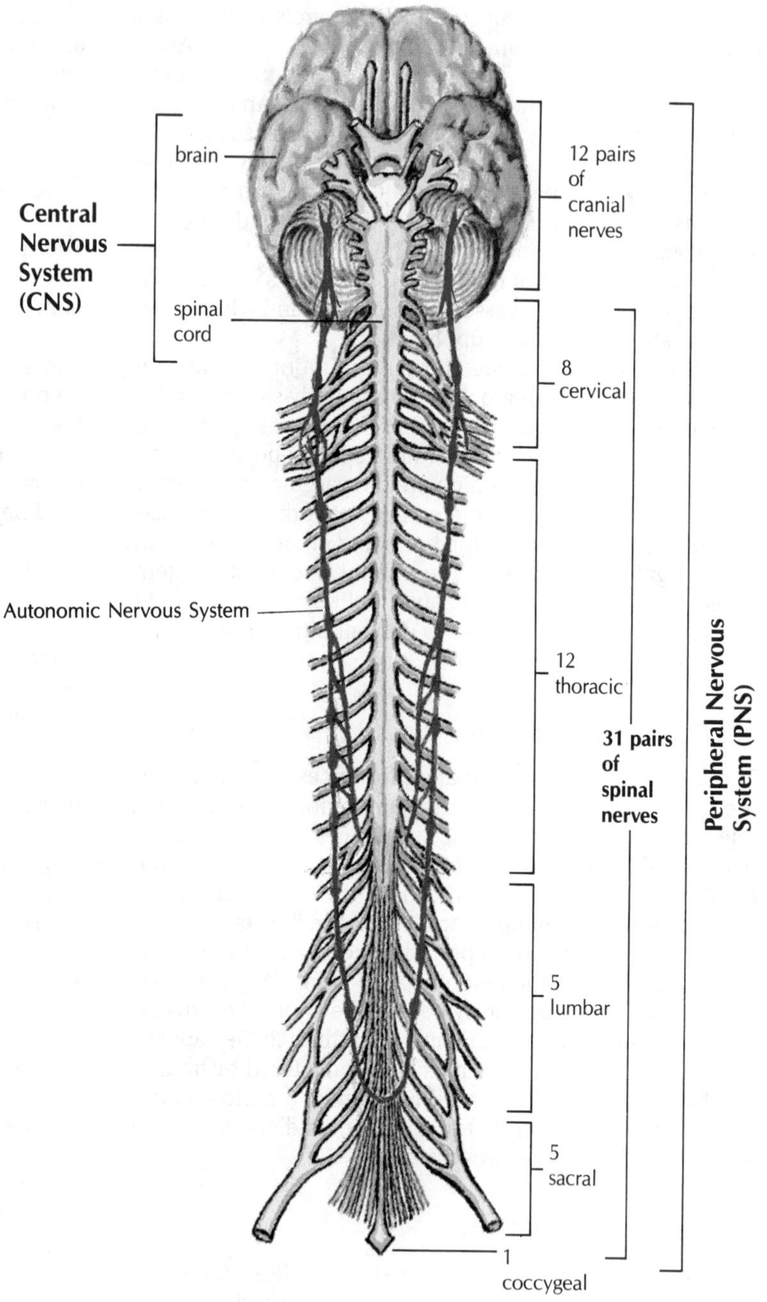

FIGURE 58-7. Parts of the nervous system, including the spinal cord and the spinal nerves.

fibers cross to the opposite side in the medulla oblongata. The *spinothalamic tract* (the fibers that cross to the opposite side immediately after entering the spinal cord and then ascend) transmits pain and temperature impulses to the thalamus and cortex. The *lateral (pyramidal, corticospinal) tract* conducts motor impulses to the anterior horn cells from the opposite side of the brain. These descending fibers, the nerve cells of which are found in the precentral cortex, cross in the medulla oblongata in what is called the decussation of the pyramids.

Visual Pathways

In the rear of each hemisphere the fibers of the corresponding optic nerve end. These receiving cells are responsible for vision. Assessment of a patient's vision is completed by testing visual acuity using a Snellen chart and ordinary newsprint. The patient's vision should be tested with and without corrective lenses.

To conduct the test for visual fields, the patient is asked to cover one eye and look at the examiner's nose. Starting at the periphery of each quadrant of vision, the examiner moves a finger or a cotton-tipped applicator in front of the patient toward the center of vision. The patient is asked to signal as soon as the finger or applicator is seen. The test is performed for each eye. This procedure reveals gross defects. If more information is desired, the patient is referred for more specific testing. Visual extinction may be tested by moving the fingers simultaneously in opposite sides of the visual fields.

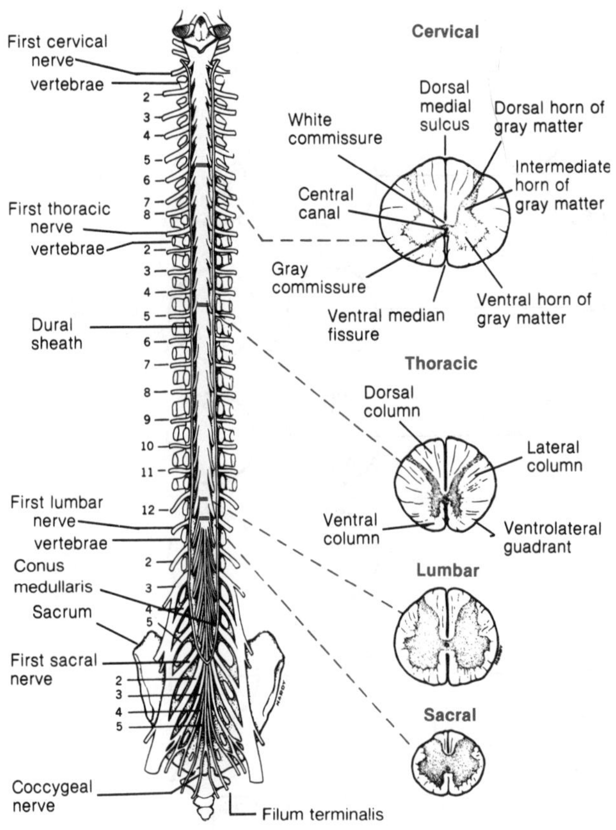

FIGURE 58-8. Cross-sectional diagram of the spinal cord at the cervical, thoracic, lumbar, and sacral levels.

The tests for visual fields may demonstrate disturbances in function along the optic pathways, including sense organs and neurons in the retina, fibers of the optic nerve and tract, and the occipital lobe.

Visual Changes. Damage to cells of the optic nerves in one of the hemispheres will result in the person being half-blind and having cortical blindness. This individual will have no vision on one side of the midline and is said to have hemianopsia (half-blindness). Figure 58-9 illustrates visual pathways and changes in vision resulting from lesions at different locations along the optic tracts.

Cortical blindness of one optic area (*e.g.*, of the posterior tip of one cerebral hemisphere) always affects both eyes equally. *Total blindness* in one eye may be due to a disease of the eye itself, the retina, or its optic nerve. Just behind the two eyes, however, the optic nerves become confluent (the optic chiasm), then separate and continue to the brain as two optic tracts.

In each of these tracts is just half of each optic nerve, so that if one tract is injured, blindness occurs in exactly one half of each eye. For example, if the right tract is injured, the patient is blind on the right half of each retina, so that with that eye he can see nothing to his left but can see perfectly to his right. An optic nerve lesion produces partial or complete blindness in the eye that the nerve serves. A complete lesion of one optic tract results in blindness in the opposite half of both visual fields. An abnormality in the temporal lobe may produce blindness in the upper quadrants of both visual fields on the side opposite the lesion. A lesion in the parietal lobe may produce contralateral blindness in the corresponding lower quadrants of both eyes. In a lesion of the occipital lobe, contralateral blindness may occur in the corresponding half of each visual field, but central vision is intact (see Fig. 58-9).

The pituitary gland is located just beneath the chiasm; a pituitary tumor often disturbs the optic chiasm and produces blindness of both inner halves of the retinas, because it is only the fibers in the nasal halves of the optic nerves that cross. In many cases, visual problems may lead a patient to seek medical attention and, through a thorough eye examination, neurologic diseases are detected.

Motor System

A vertical band of cortex on each cerebral hemisphere governs the voluntary movements of the body. This region, known as the *motor cortex,* can be located accurately. The exact location within the brain in which the voluntary movements of the muscles of the face, the thumb, the hand, the arm, the trunk, and the leg originate are known (Fig. 58-10). Before a person can move a muscle, these particular cells must send the stimulus down along their fibers. If these cells are stimulated with an electric current, the muscles they control contract.

En route to the pons, as described previously, the motor fibers converge into a tight bundle known as the *capsule.* A comparatively small injury to the capsule causes paralysis in more muscles than does a much larger injury to the cortex itself.

Within the medulla, the motor axons from the cortex form two well-defined bands known as the *corticospinal* or *pyramidal tracts.* Here, most of these fibers cross (or decussate) to the opposite side, continuing thereafter as the *crossed* pyramidal tract. The remaining fibers then enter the spinal cord on the original side as the *direct* pyramidal tract. Each fiber in this tract finally crosses to the opposite side of the cord near the point of termination and comes to an end within the gray matter constituting the anterior horn on that side, in proximity to a motor nerve cell. Fibers of the crossed pyramidal tract terminate within the anterior horn and make connections with anterior horn cells on the same side. All of the motor fibers of the spinal nerves represent extensions of these anterior horn cells, with each of these fibers communicating with only one particular muscle fiber.

The motor system is complex, and motor function reflects the integrity of the corticospinal tracts, the extrapyramidal system, and cerebellar function. A motor impulse traverses two neurons.

Several motor nerve tracts, other than the corticospinal, are contained in the spinal cord. Some represent the pathways of the so-called extrapyramidal system, establishing connections between the anterior horn cells and the automatic control centers located in the basal ganglia and the cerebellum. Others are components of reflex arcs, forming synaptic connections between anterior horn cells and sensory fibers that have entered adjacent or neighboring segments of the cord.

Upper and Lower Motor Neurons

Each muscle fiber is under voluntary control through a combination of two nerve cells. One is located in the motor

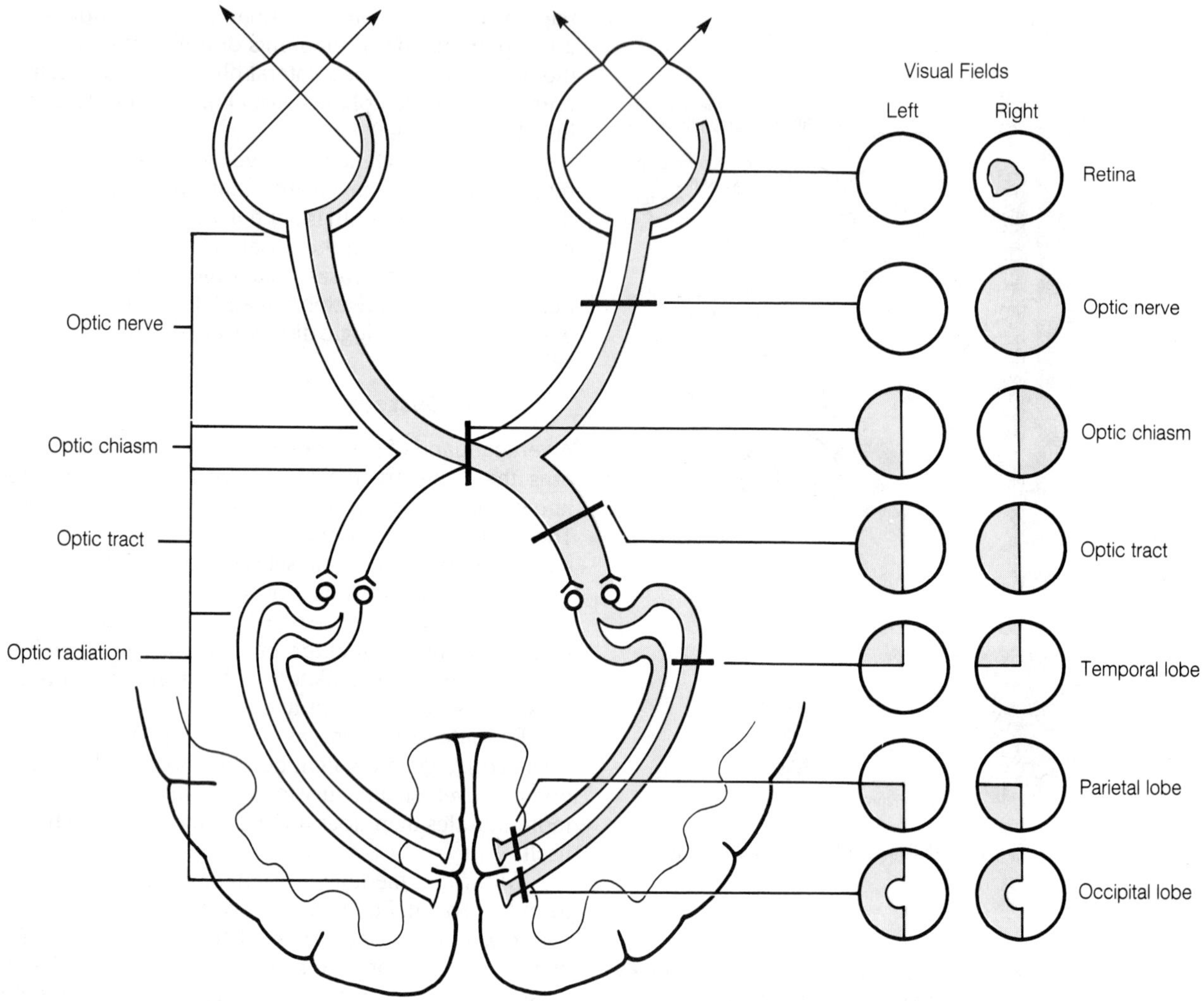

FIGURE 58-9. Visual field defects and sites of lesions. *Shaded areas* indicate areas without vision.

cortex, its fiber in the direct or crossed pyramidal tract, and the other is located in the anterior horn of the spinal cord, its fiber running to the muscle. The former is referred to as the *upper motor neuron (UMN)*, the latter as the *lower motor neuron (LMN)*. Every motor nerve serving a muscle is a bundle composed of several thousand lower motor neurons.

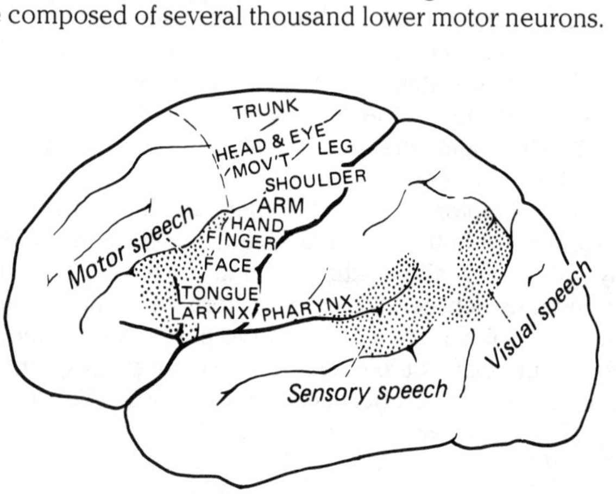

FIGURE 58-10. Diagrammatic representation of the cerebrum, showing locations for motor movements of various portions of the body.

The motor pathways from the brain to the spinal cord as well as from the cerebrum to the brain stem are formed by UMNs. The UMNs begin in the cortex of the opposite side of the brain, descend through the internal capsule, cross to the opposite side in the brain stem, descend through the corticospinal tract, and synapse with the LMNs in the cord. The UMNs are contained entirely within the CNS. The LMN receives the impulse in the posterior part of the cord and runs to the myoneural junction. In contrast to the UMNs, the LMNs terminate in the muscle. The clinical features of lesions of UMNs and LMNs are discussed in the sections that follow and in Table 58-1.

Upper Motor Neuron Lesions. UMN lesions can involve the motor cortex, the internal capsule, the spinal cord, and other structures of the brain through which the corticospinal tract descends. If the UMN is damaged or destroyed, as frequently occurs with stroke, paralysis (loss of voluntary movement) results. However, because inhibitory influences of an intact UMN are now impaired, reflex (involuntary) movements are uninhibited. The result is that the muscle does not atrophy or become limp; on the contrary, it remains permanently more tense than normal and exhibits spastic paralysis. Paralysis associated with UMN lesions usu-

TABLE 58-1 Results of Lesions of Upper Motor Neuron (UMN) Versus Lower Motor Neuron (LMN)

UMN Lesions	LMN Lesions
Loss of voluntary control	Loss of voluntary control
Increased muscle tone	Decreased muscle tone
Muscle spasticity	Flaccid paralysis of muscles
No muscle atrophy	Muscle atrophy
Hyperactive and abnormal reflexes	Absent or decreased reflexes

ally affects a whole extremity, both extremities, or an entire half of the body.

The severe leg spasms that occur in patients with complete spinal cord injury are another example of UMN lesions; the spasms result from the preserved reflex arc along the spinal cord below the level of injury and are a hallmark of UMN disease.

Hemiplegia (paralysis of an arm and leg on the same side of the body) is an example of UMN paralysis. If hemorrhage, an embolus, or a thrombus destroys the fibers from the motor area in the internal capsule, the arm and the leg of the opposite side become stiff and very weak or paralyzed, and the reflexes are exaggerated. When both legs are paralyzed, the condition is called *paraplegia*. Paralysis of all four extremities is *quadriplegia* or *tetraplegia*.

Lower Motor Neuron Lesions. An individual is considered to have LMN damage if a motor nerve is severed between the muscle and the spinal cord, thus destroying the final common pathway to a muscle. The result of LMN damage is that the muscle becomes paralyzed and the person is unable to move that muscle. The nerve takes no part in reflex movements, and the muscle becomes limp and atrophied due to disuse. If the patient has injured the spinal trunk and it is able to heal, he or she may regain the use of the muscles connected to that section of the spinal cord. If the anterior horn motor cells are destroyed, however, the nerves cannot regenerate and the muscles are never useful again. This sequence of events occurs in anterior poliomyelitis. Flaccid paralysis and atrophy of the affected muscles are the principal signs of LMN disease.

Extrapyramidal Motor Controls

The smoothness, the accuracy, and the strength that characterize the muscular movements of a normal person are attributable to the influence of the cerebellum and the basal ganglia.

The cerebellum (see Fig. 58-3), nestled beneath the posterior lobe of the cerebrum, is responsible for coordinating, balancing, timing, and synergizing with precision all muscular movements that originate in the motor centers of the cerebral cortex. Through the action of the cerebellum, the contractions of opposing muscle groups are adjusted in relation to each other to maximal mechanical advantage; muscular contractions can be sustained evenly at the desired tension and without significant fluctuation, and reciprocal movements can be reproduced at high and constant speed, in stereotyped fashion, and with relatively little effort.

The basal ganglia, masses of gray matter in the midbrain beneath the cerebral hemispheres, border or project into the lateral ventricles and lie in proximity to the internal capsule. It is their function to control habitual or automatic acts and to maintain a postural background against which voluntary movements are performed. These ganglia, aided by their connections with the organs of special sense, keep the contractile tone of every muscle in the trunk and the extremities in a constant state of adjustment, so that a person is able to keep his balance regardless of the posture of his body, in darkness as well as in light. Moreover, because of the basal ganglia, the person is equipped to react swiftly, appropriately, and automatically to any smell, sight, or sound that demands an immediate response.

Dyskinesias. Loss of cerebellar function, which may occur as a result of an intracranial injury or some type of an expanding mass (*i.e.,* a hemorrhage, abscess, or tumor), results in a loss of muscle tone, weakness, and fatigue. Depending on the area of the brain affected, the patient will present with different motor symptoms or responses. The patient may demonstrate decorticate, decerebrate, or flaccid posturing, usually due to cerebral trauma.

Decortication (decorticate posturing) is the result of lesions of the internal capsule or cerebral hemispheres, in which the patient presents with flexion and internal rotation of the arms and wrists and extension, internal rotation, and plantar flexion of the feet.

Decerebration (decerebrate posturing) is the result of lesions at the midbrain and is more ominous than decortication. The patient presents with extension and external rotation of the arms and wrists and extension, plantar flexion, and internal rotation of the feet. Flaccid posturing is usually the result of lower brain stem dysfunction. A patient will exhibit no motor function, is limp and floppy, and lacks motor tone. Flaccidity preceded by decerebration in a patient with cerebral injury indicates severe neurologic impairment, which can lead to a declaration of brain death. However, before the declaration of brain death, the patient must have the potential for a spinal cord injury ruled out, the effects of all neuromuscular paralyzing agents must have worn off, and any other possible causes must be investigated.

A patient may present with involuntary tremors that increase in intensity in association with voluntary movements, and inability to control movements accurately or to coordinate muscles efficiently or smoothly; every act is performed in disjointed fashion. The patient is incapable of performing fine, rapidly repeated, coordinated movements with speed or uniformity. The above characteristics, called *adiadochokinesis*, signal that there is a problem with the cerebellum. When the patient walks, he staggers from side to side because his gait is unsteady, like that of an individual who is intoxicated and attempting to walk (*i.e.,* feet wide apart and the steps short).

Destruction or dysfunction of the basal ganglia leads not to paralysis but to muscular rigidity, with consequent disturbances of posture and movement. Such patients are afflicted by a tendency to display involuntary movements.

These may take the form of *coarse tremors,* characterized by approximately six oscillations per second; *athetosis,* movement of a slow, squirming, writhing, twisting type; or *chorea,* marked by spasmodic, purposeless, and grotesque motions of the trunk and the extremities, and facial grimacing. Clinical syndromes based on lesions involving the basal ganglia include parkinsonism and Huntington's disease (see Chapter 60); Wilson's disease, or hepatolenticular degeneration; and spasmodic torticollis.

Sensory Function

The Thalamus. The thalamus, a major receiving and transmitting center for the afferent sensory nerves, is a large structure located in the middle fossa (midbrain). It lies next to the third ventricle, forming its lateral wall, and forms the floor of the lateral ventricle. It is also in proximity to the basal ganglia and adjacent to the internal capsule. The thalamus serves to integrate sensory impulses, as in the recognition of pain or variation in temperature or touch. The thalamus is responsible for the sense of movement and position and the ability to recognize size, shape, and quality of objects. It is also responsible for the routing of all sensory stimuli to their destinations, including the cerebral cortex, which receives them and translates them into appropriate responses.

Sensory Pathways. The transmission of sensory impulses from their points of origin to their cerebral destinations involves three neuron relays; moreover, there are three major pathways by which they may be routed, depending on the type of sensation that is registered. Specific knowledge of these paths is important from the standpoint of neurologic diagnoses, being indispensable for the accurate localization of brain and cord lesions in many patients.

The axon of the nerve in which the sensory impulse originates enters the spinal cord by way of the posterior root. Axons conveying sensations of heat, cold, and pain immediately enter the posterior gray column of the cord, where they make connections with the cells of secondary neurons. Pain and temperature fibers cross immediately to the opposite side of the cord and course upward to the thalamus. Fibers carrying sensations of touch, light pressure, and localization do not connect immediately with the second neuron but ascend the cord for a variable distance before entering the gray matter and completing this connection. The axon of the secondary neuron crosses the cord and proceeds upward to the thalamus.

The third category of sensation, produced by stimuli arising from muscles, joints, and bones, includes position sense and vibratory sense. These stimuli are conveyed, uncrossed, all the way to the brain stem by the axon of the primary neuron. In the medulla, synaptic connections are made with cells of the secondary neurons, whose axons then cross to the opposite side and proceed to the thalamus.

Sensory Losses. Severance of a sensory nerve results in total loss of sensation in its area of distribution. Transection of the spinal cord yields complete anesthesia below the level of injury. Selective destruction or degeneration of the posterior columns of the spinal cord is responsible for a loss of position sense in segments distal to the lesion, unaccompanied by loss of touch, pain, or temperature perception. Persons with such disorders of the posterior columns, unless they look, cannot tell where their feet are or in what direction they are pointing; moreover, they cannot perceive vibrations in the affected area. A lesion, such as a cyst, in the center of the spinal cord causes dissociation of sensation—loss of pain at the level of the lesion. This occurs because the fibers carrying pain and temperature cross the cord immediately on entering; thus, any lesion that divides the cord longitudinally divides these fibers. Other sensory fibers ascend the cord for variable distances, some even to the medulla itself, before crossing, thereby bypassing the lesion and avoiding destruction.

Dysesthesias. Irritative lesions affecting the posterior spinal nerve roots may cause impairment of tactile sensation, including intermittent severe pains that are referred to their areas of distribution. Tingling of the fingers and the toes is a prominent symptom of combined systems disease, presumably due to degenerative changes in the sensory fibers that extend to the thalamus (*i.e.,* belonging to the spinothalamic tract).

Autonomic Nervous System

The contractions of muscles that are not under voluntary control, including the heart muscle, the secretions of all digestive and sweat glands, and the activity of certain endocrine organs, are controlled by a major component of the nervous system known as the autonomic nervous system. The term *autonomic* refers to the fact that the operations of this system are independent of the desires and intentions of the person. The autonomic nervous system is not subject to one's will—that is, it is in a sense autonomous.

To the extent that the autonomic nervous system is not subject to regulation by the cerebral cortex, it resembles the extrapyramidal systems that are centered in the cerebellum and the basal ganglia. However, in other respects it is unique. First, its regulatory effects are exerted not on individual cells but on large expanses of tissue and on entire organs. Second, the responses that it elicits do not appear instantaneously but only after a lag period. These responses are sustained far longer than other neurogenic responses, a type of response that is calculated to ensure maximal functional efficiency on the part of receptor organs, such as the blood vessels and the hollow viscera. The autonomic nervous system regulates visceral effectors to maintain or quickly restore homeostasis.

The quality of these responses is explained by the fact that the autonomic nervous system transmits its impulses only partly by way of nerve pathways, the remainder of the route being serviced by chemical mediators, resembling in this respect the endocrine system. Electrical impulses, conducted through nerve fibers, stimulate the formation of specific chemical agents at strategic locations within the muscle mass, the diffusion of these chemicals being responsible for the contraction.

Hypothalamus. Overall supervision of the autonomic nervous system is considered a function of the hypothalamus. The hypothalamus is a portion of the diencephalon (interbrain) immediately beneath and lateral to the lower portion of the wall of the third ventricle. It includes among its components the optic chiasm; the tuber cinereum; the pituitary stalk, which originates from the latter; and the pituitary gland itself. Large cell groups in adjacent portions of the hypothalamus have the role of autonomic regulation. These centers are richly endowed with connections linking the autonomic system with the thalamus, the cortex, the olfactory apparatus, and the pituitary gland. Here reside the mechanisms for the control of visceral and somatic reactions that were originally important for defense or attack but in humans are associated with emotional states (*i.e.,* fear, anger, anxiety); for the control of metabolic processes, including fat, carbohydrate, and water metabolism; for the regulation of body temperature, arterial pressure, and all muscular and glandular activities of the gastrointestinal tract; for control of genital functions; and for the sleep rhythm. The proximity, histologic similarity, and multiple connections between the pituitary gland, the master endocrine gland, and this portion of the brain suggest that the hypothalamus controls the endocrine and autonomic nervous systems, commanding all vital processes.

Sympathetic and Parasympathetic Nervous Systems

The autonomic nervous system contains two divisions that are anatomically and functionally distinct—the sympathetic and the parasympathetic nervous systems. Most of the tissues and the organs under autonomic control are innervated by both systems. Sympathetic stimuli are mediated by norepinephrine, and parasympathetic impulses are mediated by acetylcholine. These chemicals produce opposing and mutually antagonistic effects.

Sympathetic Nervous System. A unique function of the sympathetic division of the autonomic nervous system is to serve as an emergency preparedness system. Under stress conditions from either physical or emotional causes, sympathetic impulses increase greatly. The body prepares for the "fight or flight" response when threatened. As a result, bronchioles dilate for easier gas exchange; the heart's contractions are stronger and faster; the arteries to the heart and voluntary muscles dilate, carrying more blood to them; peripheral blood vessels constrict, making the skin feel cool but shunting blood to essential active organs; the pupils dilate; the liver releases glucose for quick energy; peristalsis slows down; hair stands on end; and perspiration increases. This sudden increase in sympathetic discharge is the same as if the body has been given an injection of adrenalin, hence the term *adrenergic nervous system* is sometimes used when referring to this condition.

Sympathetic neurons are located in the thoracic and the lumbar segments of the spinal cord; their axons, called *preganglionic fibers,* emerge by way of all anterior nerve roots from the eighth cervical or first thoracic segment to the second or third lumbar segment, inclusive. A short distance from the cord, these fibers diverge to join a chain, composed of 22 linked ganglia, that extends the entire length of the spinal column, flanking the vertebral bodies on both sides. Some form multiple synapses with nerve cells within the chain. Others traverse the chain without making connections or losing continuity to join large "prevertebral" ganglia in the thorax, the abdomen, or the pelvis or one of the "terminal" ganglia in the vicinity of an organ, such as the bladder or the rectum (Fig. 58-11). Postganglionic nerve fibers originating in the sympathetic chain rejoin the spinal nerves that supply the extremities and are distributed to blood vessels, sweat glands, and smooth muscle tissue in the skin. Postganglionic fibers from the prevertebral plexuses (*i.e.,* the cardiac, pulmonary, splanchnic, and pelvic plexuses) supply structures in the head and the neck, the thorax, the abdomen, and the pelvis, respectively, having been joined in these plexuses by fibers from the parasympathetic division.

The adrenal glands, kidneys, liver, spleen, stomach, and duodenum are under the control of the giant celiac plexus, familiarly known as the *solar plexus.* This receives its sympathetic nerve components by way of the three splanchnic nerves, composed of preganglionic fibers from nine segments of the spinal cord (*i.e.,* T4 to L1), and is joined by the vagus nerve, representing the parasympathetic division. From the celiac plexus, fibers of both divisions travel along the course of blood vessels to their target organs.

Parasympathetic Nervous System. The parasympathetic system functions as the dominant controller for most visceral effectors much of the time. During quiet, nonstressful conditions, impulses from parasympathetic fibers (cholinergic) predominate. The fibers of the parasympathetic system are located in two sections, one in the brain stem and the other from spinal segments below L2. Because of the location of these fibers, the parasympathetic system is referred to as the *craniosacral* division, as distinct from the *thoracolumbar* (sympathetic) division of the autonomic nervous system.

The cranial parasympathetics arise from the midbrain and the medulla oblongata. Fibers from cells in the midbrain travel with the third oculomotor nerve to the ciliary ganglia, where postganglionic fibers of this division are joined by those of the sympathetic system other being one of controlled opposition, with a delicate balance maintained between the two at all times.

Sympathetic Syndromes. Certain syndromes are distinctive to diseases of the sympathetic nerve trunks. Among these are dilation of the pupil of the eye on the same side as a penetrating wound of the neck (evidence of disturbance of the cervical sympathetic cord); temporary paralysis of the bowel (indicated by the absence of peristaltic waves and the distention of the intestine by gas) after fracture of any one of the lower dorsal or upper lumbar vertebrae with hemorrhage into the base of the mesentery; and the marked variations in pulse rate and rhythm that often follow compression fractures of the upper six thoracic vertebrae.

The Neurologic Examination

The neurologic examination is a sophisticated and subtle process, comprising a large number of tests of highly specialized function. Although the neurologic examination is often limited to a simple screening, it is necessary for the examiner to be able to conduct a thorough neurologic assessment when the history or other physical findings warrant it.

The brain and spinal cord cannot be inspected, percussed, palpated, and auscultated as directly as other systems of the body. A neurologic assessment is divided into five components: *cerebral function, cranial nerves, motor system, sensory system,* and *reflex status.* As in other facets

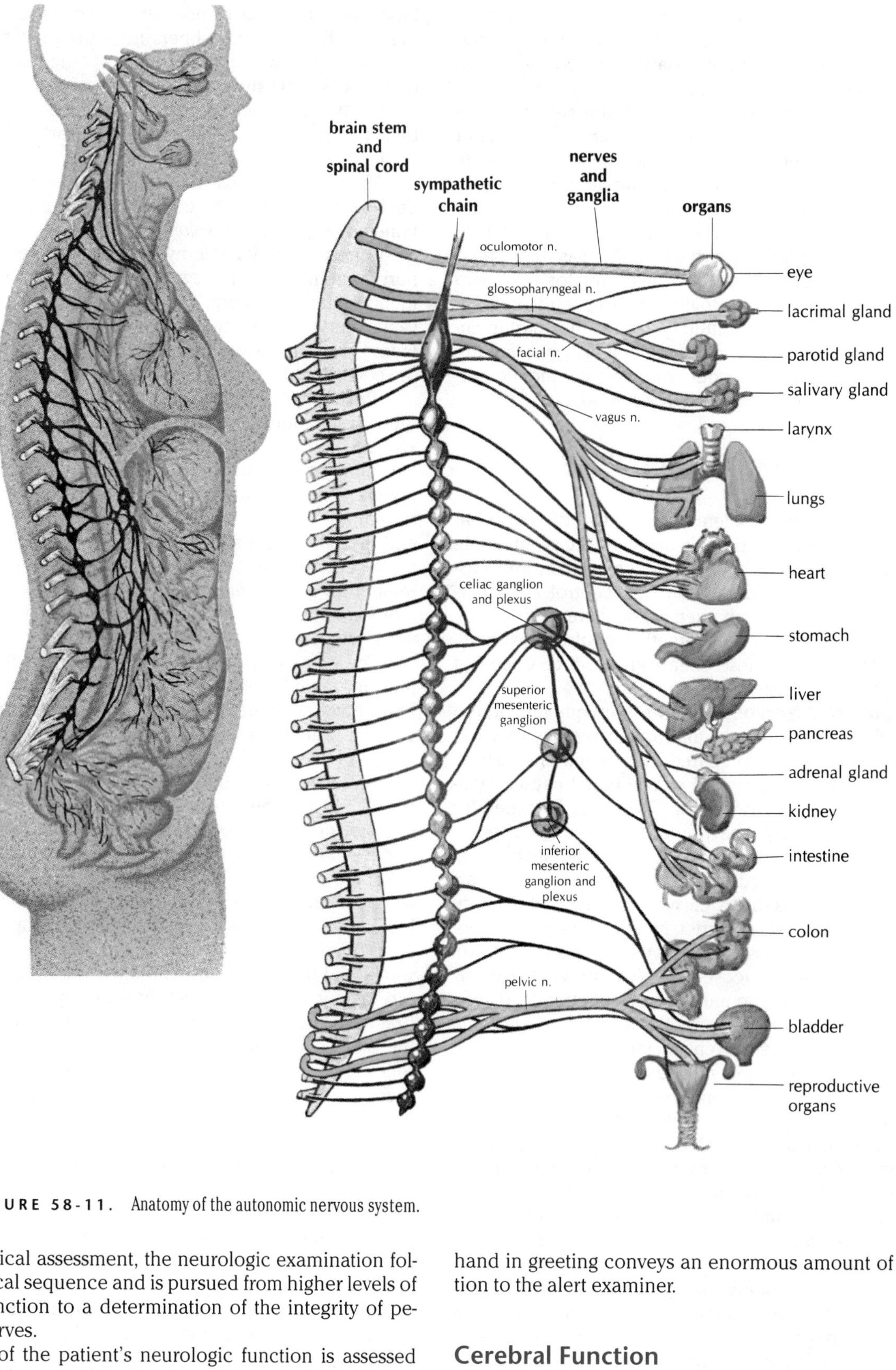

FIGURE 58-11. Anatomy of the autonomic nervous system.

of the physical assessment, the neurologic examination follows a logical sequence and is pursued from higher levels of cortical function to a determination of the integrity of peripheral nerves.

Much of the patient's neurologic function is assessed during the history and during the routine of the earlier parts of the physical examination. One can learn much about speech patterns, mental status, gait, stance, motor power, and coordination. The simple act of shaking a patient's hand in greeting conveys an enormous amount of information to the alert examiner.

Cerebral Function

Cerebral abnormalities may cause disturbances in communication, intellectual functioning, and in patterns of emotional behavior.

Mental Status. Adequate cerebral functioning is determined by assessing the patient's mental status. The examiner observes the patient's appearance and behavior, noting the patient's dress, grooming, and personal hygiene. Observation of posture, gestures, movements, facial expressions, and motor activity often provides important information about the patient. The patient's manner of speech and level of consciousness are also observed. Is the patient's speech clear and coherent? Is the patient alert and responsive or drowsy and stuporous?

Intellectual Function. Intellectual function is tested when doubts exist about the patient's intellectual competence. Often, patients in a toxic state or those who have destruction of the frontal cortex appear superficially normal until or unless one or more tests of integrative capacity are performed.

First, the examiner determines whether the patient is oriented to time, place, and person. Does the patient know what day it is, what year it is, and the name of the president of the United States? Is the patient aware of where he or she is? Is the patient aware of who the examiner is and of his or her purpose for being in the room? Is the capacity for immediate memory intact?

A person with an average IQ is able to repeat seven digits without faltering and is able to recite five digits backward. The examiner might ask the patient to count backward from 100 or to subtract 7 from 100, then 7 from that, and so forth. The capacity to interpret well-known proverbs tests abstract reasoning, which is a higher intellectual function; for example, does the patient know what is meant by "a rolling stone gathers no moss"?

Thought Content. It is important to assess the patient's thought content during the course of the interview. Are the patient's thoughts spontaneous, natural, clear, relevant, and coherent? Does the patient have any fixed ideas, illusions, or preoccupations? What are his or her insights into these thoughts? Preoccupation with death or morbid events, evidence of hallucinations, and paranoid ideation are all important and require further evaluation.

Emotional Status. An assessment of cerebral functioning also includes the patient's emotional status. Is the patient's affect natural and even or irritable and angry, anxious, apathetic, or euphoric? Does his or her mood fluctuate normally, or does he or she unpredictably swing from joy to sadness during the interview? Is affect appropriate to words and thought content? Are verbal communications consistent with nonverbal communications?

Perception. The examiner may now consider more specific areas of higher cortical function. **Agnosia** is the inability to interpret or recognize objects seen through the special senses. The patient may see a pen but not know what it is called or what to do with it. The patient may even be able to describe it but not to interpret its function. The patient may experience auditory or tactile agnosia, as well as visual agnosia. Each of the dysfunctions implicates a different part of the cortex (Chart 58-2).

To screen for agnosia, the examiner tests the patient's cortical sensory interpretation. The patient is shown a familiar object and asked to identify it by name. Next, a familiar sound (bell) is made and the patient is asked to identify its source. Tactile interpretation is easily assessed by placing a familiar object (*e.g.*, key, coin) in the patient's hand and having him or her identify it while both eyes are closed.

CHART 58-2

Types of Agnosia and Corresponding Sites of Lesions

Type of Agnosia	Affected Cerebral Area
Visual	Occipital lobe
Auditory	Temporal lobe (lateral and superior portions)
Tactile	Parietal lobe
Body parts and relationships	Parietal lobe (postero-inferior regions)

Motor Ability. An assessment of cortical motor integration is carried out by asking the patient to perform a skilled act (throw a ball, move a chair). Successful performance hinges on the person's ability to understand the activity desired and on normal motor strength. Failures signal cerebral dysfunction.

Language Ability. Lastly, language function is assessed. The person with normal neurologic function is able to understand and communicate in spoken and written language. Does the patient answer questions relevantly? Can he or she read a sentence from a newspaper and explain its meaning? Can the patient write his or her name or copy a simple figure that the examiner has drawn? A deficiency in language function is called **aphasia**. Different types of aphasia result from injury to different parts of the brain (Chart 58-3). Aphasia is discussed in detail in Chapter 59.

Clinician's Interpretations. Interpretation of neurologic abnormalities is a highly sophisticated and technical process. It is the obligation of the examiner to record and report what is found. Analysis and the conclusions that may be drawn from these findings usually depend on the examiner's extensive knowledge of neuroanatomy, neurophysiology, and neuropathology.

Impact on Life Style. The nurse includes in the assessment of neurologic function the impact the neurologic impairment will have on the individual's current life style. This nursing perspective examines two issues: the

CHART 58-3

Types of Aphasia and Region of Brain Involved

Type of Aphasia	Brain Area Involved
Auditory-receptive	Temporal lobe
Expressive speaking	Inferior posterior frontal areas
Visual-receptive	Parietal-occipital area
Expressive writing	Posterior frontal area

limitations imposed by the neurologic deficit within the context of the patient's role in society and a plan of care that will support adaptation to the neurologic insult within the individual's support system.

Glasgow Coma Scale

The Glasgow Coma Scale (GCS), which addresses three areas of neurologic functioning, gives an overview of the patient's level of responsiveness and has been used extensively to evaluate the neurologic status of patients who have had a head injury. It does not take the place of an in-depth neurologic assessment; rather, it evaluates the patient's motor, verbal and eye-opening responses. These elements are further subdivided into different levels, and the best responses the patient makes to predetermined stimuli are recorded as shown in Chart 58-4. Each response is given a number (high for normal and low for impaired), and the summation of these figures gives an indication of the severity of coma and a prediction of possible outcome. The lowest score is 3 (least responsive); the highest is 15 (most responsive). A score of 7 or less is generally accepted as coma and requires appropriate nursing intervention for the comatose patient.

Figure 58-12 is a neurologic observation chart that incorporates the GCS, vital signs, pupillary size and reactivity, and extremity movement and strength, which provides a comprehensive record of the patient's neurologic status at any given time. This or any other standardized format for obtaining and recording neurologic status is recommended to standardize and facilitate care and communication between caregivers.

CHART 58-4
Glasgow Coma Scale

Eyes Open:	
Spontaneously	4
To speech	3
To pain	2
No response	1
Best Motor Response:	
Obeys	6
Localizes pain	5
Withdraws	4
Abnormal flexion	3
Extends	2
No response	1
Verbal Response	
Oriented	5
Confused conversation	4
Inappropriate words	3
Incomprehensible sounds	2
No response	1
Total:	3–15

Examination of the Cranial Nerves

Twelve pairs of cranial nerves emerge from the undersurface of the brain. They are designated by Roman numerals I to XII, according to the order of their location (see Chapter 60, Fig. 60-14). The cranial nerves are often assessed during a complete head and neck examination. These nerves, their functions, and the tests for their measurement are outlined in Table 58-2.

Examination of the Motor System

A thorough examination of the motor system includes an assessment of muscle size, muscle tone, muscle strength, coordination, and balance. The patient is instructed to walk across the room while the examiner notes his posture and gait. The muscles are inspected, and palpated if necessary, for their size and symmetry. Any evidence of atrophy or involuntary movements (tremors, tics) is noted. Muscle tone is evaluated by palpating various muscle groups at rest and during passive movement. Resistance to these movements is assessed and documented. Abnormalities in tone include spasticity, rigidity, or flaccidity.

Muscle Strength. Muscle strength is tested by assessing the patient's ability to flex or extend the extremities against resistance. The function of an individual muscle or group of muscles is evaluated by placing the muscle at a disadvantage. The quadriceps, for example, is a powerful muscle responsible for straightening the leg. Once the leg is straightened, it is exceedingly difficult for the examiner to flex the knee. Conversely, if the knee is flexed and the patient is asked to straighten the leg against resistance, a more subtle disability can be elicited. It is important to compare the two sides to detect subtle changes in muscle strength.

Many clinicians use a five-point scale to rate muscle strength. A 5 indicates full power of contraction; 4 indicates fair, but not full, strength; 3 indicates just sufficient strength to overcome the force of gravity; 2 indicates the ability to move but not to overcome the force of gravity; 1 indicates minimal contractile power; and 0 indicates no contraction whatsoever.

Assessment of muscle strength can be as detailed as necessary. One may quickly test the strength of the proximal muscles of the upper and lower extremities, comparing both sides. The strength of the finer muscles that control the function of the hand and the foot can then be assessed.

Balance and Coordination. Cerebellar influence on the motor system is reflected in balance control and coordination. Coordination in the hands and upper extremities is tested by having the patient perform *rapid, alternating movements* and *point-to-point testing.* First, the patient is instructed to pat the thigh as fast as possible with one hand. Each hand is tested separately. Then the patient is instructed to turn the hands from a supine to a prone position as rapidly as possible. Lastly, the patient is asked to touch each of the fingers with the thumb in a consecutive motion. Speed, symmetry, and degree of difficulty are noted.

Point-to-point testing is accomplished by having the patient touch the examiner's extended finger and then his or

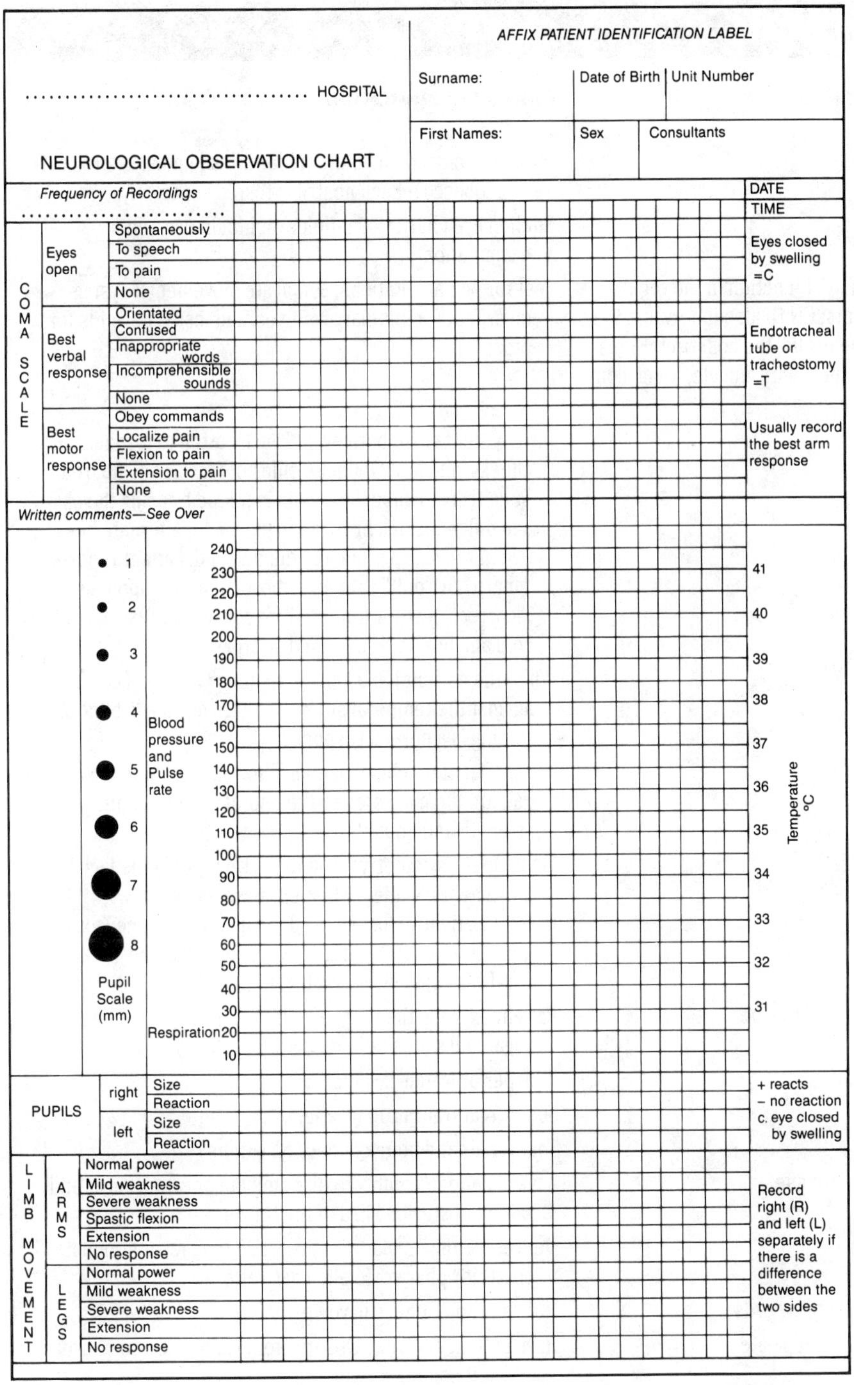

FIGURE 58-12. Example of a neurologic observation chart that includes the Glasgow Coma Scale.

her own nose. This is repeated several times. This assessment is then carried out with the patient's eyes closed.

Coordination in the lower extremities is tested by having the patient run the heel down the anterior surface of the tibia. Each leg is tested in turn. Inability to perform these maneuvers is referred to as **ataxia**. The presence of ataxia or tremors (rhythmic, involuntary movements) during these movements suggests cerebellar disease.

It is not necessary to carry out each of these assessments for coordination. During a routine examination, it is advisable to perform a simple screening of the upper and lower extremities by having the patient perform either rapid, alternating movements or point-to-point testing. When abnormalities are observed, a more thorough examination is indicated.

The **Romberg test** is a screening measurement for balance. The patient stands with feet together and arms at the side, first with eyes open and then with both eyes closed for 20 to 30 seconds. The examiner stands close and reassures the patient that he or she will be supported if he or she begins to fall. Slight swaying is normal. Additional cerebellar tests for balance in the ambulatory patient include hopping in place, alternating knee bends, and heel-to-toe walking.

TABLE 58-2 Cranial Nerves

Cranial Nerve	Function	Clinical Examination
I (olfactory)	Sense of smell	With eyes closed, the patient identifies familiar odors (coffee, tobacco). Each nostril is tested separately.
II (optic)	Visual acuity	Snellen eye chart; visual fields; ophthalmoscopic examination
III (oculomotor) IV (trochlear) VI (abducens)	Cranial nerves III, IV, and VI function in the regulation of eye movements; CN III also innervates the levator muscle of the eyelid, the constrictor muscle of the pupil, and the ciliary muscle, which controls accommodation.	Test for ocular rotations, conjugate movements, nystagmus. Test for pupillary reflexes, and inspect eyelids for ptosis.
V (trigeminal)	Facial sensation	Have patient close both eyes. Touch cotton to forehead, cheeks, and jaw. Opposite sides of face are compared. Sensitivity to superficial pain is tested by using the sharp and dull ends of a broken tongue blade. Alternate between the sharp point and the dull end. Patient reports "sharp" or "dull" with each movement. If responses are incorrect, test for temperature sensation. Test tubes of cold and hot water are used alternately.
	Corneal reflex	While the patient looks up, *lightly* touch a wisp of cotton against the temporal surface of each cornea. A blink and tearing is a normal response.
	Mastication	Have the patient clench jaw and move it from side to side. Palpate the masseter and temporal muscles, noting strength and equality.
VII (facial)	Facial muscle movement Facial expression Tear and saliva secretion	Observe for symmetry while the patient performs facial movements: smiles, whistles, elevates eyebrows, frowns, tightly closes eyelids against resistance (examiner attempts to open them). Observe face for flaccid paralysis (shallow nasolabial folds).
	Taste: anterior two thirds of tongue	Patient extends the tongue. Ability to discriminate between sugar and salt is tested.
VIII (vestibulocochlear)	Hearing and equilibrium	Whisper or watch-tick test Test for lateralization (Weber) Test for air and bone conduction (Rinne)
IX (glossopharyngeal)	Taste: posterior third of tongue	Assess patient's ability to discriminate between sugar and salt on posterior third of the tongue.
X (vagus)	Pharyngeal contraction	Depress a tongue blade on posterior tongue, or stimulate posterior pharynx to elicit gag reflex.
	Symmetric movement of vocal cords	Note any hoarseness in voice.
	Symmetric movement of soft palate	Have patient say "ah." Observe for symmetric rise of uvula and soft palate.
	Movement and secretion of thoracic and abdominal viscera	
XI (spinal accessory)	Movement of sternocleidomastoid and trapezius muscles	Palpate and note the strength of the trapezius muscles while the patient shrugs shoulders against resistance. Palpate and note the strength of each sternocleidomastoid muscle as the patient turns head against opposing pressure of the examiner's hand.
XII (hypoglossal)	Movement of the tongue	While the patient protrudes the tongue, any deviation or tremors are noted. The strength of the tongue is tested by having the patient move the protruded tongue from side to side against a tongue depressor.

Examination of the Reflexes

The motor reflexes are involuntary contractions of muscles or muscle groups in response to abrupt stretching near the site of the muscle's insertion. The tendon is struck directly with a reflex hammer, or indirectly by striking the examiner's thumb, which is placed firmly against the tendon. Testing these reflexes enables the examiner to assess involuntary reflex arcs that depend on the presence of afferent stretch receptors, spinal synapses, efferent motor fibers, and a variety of modifying influences from higher levels. Common reflexes that may be tested include the biceps, brachioradialis, triceps, patellar, and ankle (or Achilles) reflexes (Fig. 58-13).

Technique. A reflex hammer is used to elicit a *deep tendon reflex (DTR)*. The stem of the hammer is held loosely between the thumb and index finger, allowing a full swinging motion. The wrist motion is similar to that used during percussion. The extremity is positioned so that the tendon is slightly stretched. This requires a sound knowledge of the location of muscles and their tendon attachments. The tendon is then struck briskly and the response compared with the corresponding reflex on the opposite side of the body. Wide variation in reflex response may be considered normal. It is more important, however, that the reflexes be symmetrically equivalent. When the comparison is made, both sides should be equivalently relaxed and each tendon struck with equal force.

Valid findings depend on several factors: proper use of the reflex hammer, proper positioning of the extremity, and a relaxed patient. If the reflexes are symmetrically diminished or absent, the examiner may use a technique called **reinforcement** to increase reflex activity. This involves the isometric contraction of other muscle groups. If lower extremity reflexes are diminished or absent, the patient is instructed to lock the fingers together and pull in opposite directions. Having the patient clench the jaw or press the heels against the floor or examining table may similarly elicit more reliable biceps, triceps, or brachioradialis reflexes.

Grading the Reflexes. The absence of reflexes is significant, although ankle jerks (Achilles reflex) may be absent in older people. Reflex responses are often graded on a scale of 0 to 4+:

4+ —hyperactive with sustained clonus
3+ —hyperactive
2+ —normal
1+ —hypoactive
0 —absent

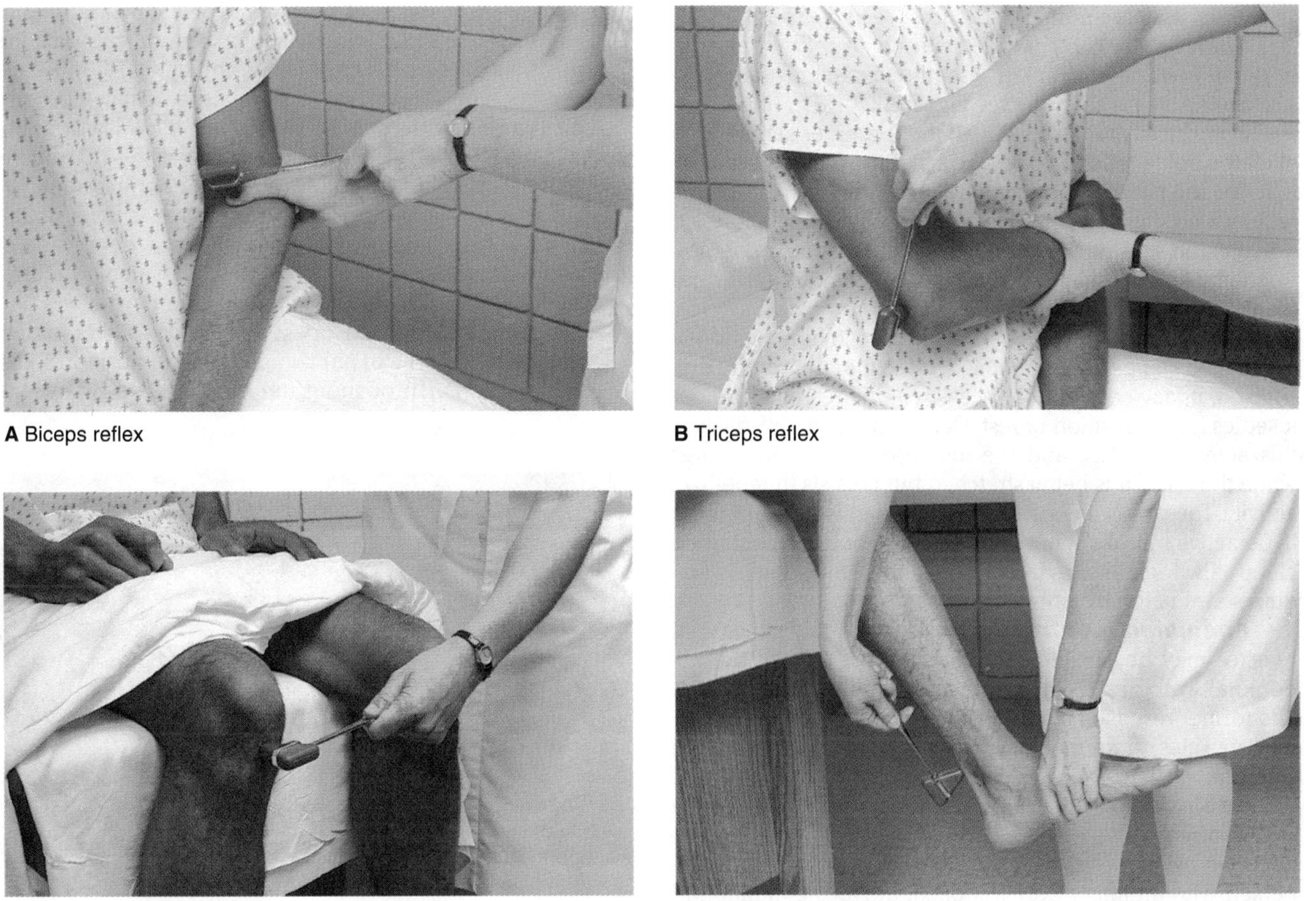

A Biceps reflex
B Triceps reflex
C Patellar reflex
D Ankle or Achilles reflex

FIGURE 58-13. Techniques for eliciting major tendon reflexes.

As was previously mentioned, scale ratings are highly subjective. When used, the findings are recorded as a fraction, indicating the scale range (*e.g.*, 2/4). Some examiners prefer to use the terms *present, absent,* and *diminished* when describing reflexes.

Biceps Reflex. The biceps reflex is elicited by striking the biceps tendon of the flexed elbow. The examiner supports the forearm with one arm while placing the thumb against the tendon and striking the thumb with the reflex hammer. The normal response is flexion at the elbow and contraction of the biceps (see Fig. 58-13*A*).

Triceps Reflex. To elicit a triceps reflex, the patient's arm is flexed at the elbow and positioned in front of the chest. The examiner supports the patient's arm and identifies the triceps tendon by palpating 2.5 to 5 cm (1 to 2 in) above the elbow. A direct blow on the tendon normally produces contraction of the triceps muscle and extension of the elbow (see Fig. 58-13*B*).

Brachioradialis Reflex. With the patient's forearm resting on the lap or across the abdomen, the brachioradialis reflex is assessed. A gentle strike of the hammer 2.5 to 5 cm (1 to 2 in) above the wrist results in flexion and supination of the forearm.

Patellar Reflex. The patellar reflex is elicited by striking the patellar tendon just below the patella. The patient may be in a sitting or a lying position. If the patient is supine, the examiner supports the legs to facilitate relaxation of the muscles. Contraction of the quadriceps and knee extension are normal responses (see Fig. 58-13*C*).

Ankle Reflex. To facilitate an ankle reflex, the foot is dorsiflexed at the ankle and the hammer strikes the stretched Achilles tendon (see Fig. 58-13*D*). This reflex normally produces plantar flexion. If the examiner is unable to elicit the ankle reflex and suspects that the patient is unable to relax, the patient is instructed to kneel on a chair or similar elevated, flat surface. This position places the ankles in dorsiflexion and reduces any muscular tension in the gastrocnemius. The Achilles tendons are struck in turn, and plantar flexion is usually demonstrated.

Clonus. When reflexes are *very* hyperactive, a phenomenon called *clonus* may be elicited. If the foot is abruptly dorsiflexed, it may continue to "beat" two or three times before it settles into a position of rest. Occasionally in CNS disease this activity persists, and the foot does not come to rest while the tendon is being stretched but persists in repetitive activity. The unsustained clonus associated with normal but hyperactive reflexes is not considered pathologic. Sustained clonus always indicates the presence of CNS disease and requires evaluation by a physician.

Abdominal Contraction Reflex. Certain superficial reflexes may be elicited by scratching the skin of the abdominal wall (Fig. 58-14) or the inside of the thigh in men. The former results in involuntary contraction of the abdominal muscles, and the latter results in retraction of the scrotum.

Babinski Response. A well-known reflex, indicative of CNS disease affecting the corticospinal tract, is the *Babinski response.* If the lateral aspect of the sole of the foot of a person with an intact CNS is stroked, the toes contract and are drawn together (Fig. 58-15). In patients who have CNS disease of the motor system, the toes fan out and are drawn back. This is normal in newborns but represents serious abnormality in adults. A variety of other reflexes convey similar information. Many of them are interesting but not particularly informative.

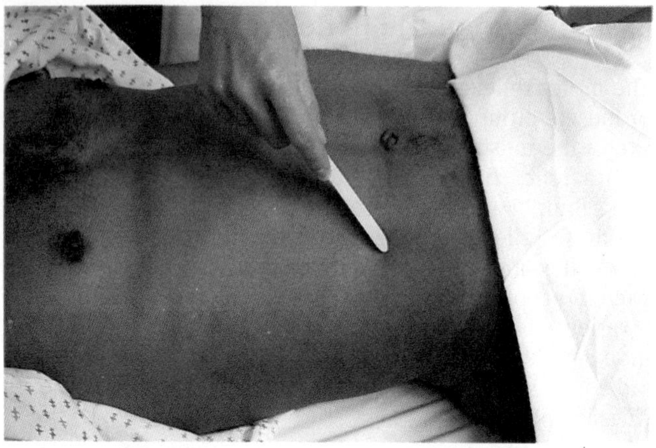

FIGURE 58-14. Testing superficial reflexes by stroking the skin of the abdominal wall.

Sensory Examination

The sensory system is even more complex than the motor system because sensory modalities are carried in different tracts, located in different portions of the spinal cord. The sensory examination is largely subjective and requires the cooperation of the patient. It is recommended that the examiner become familiar with dermatomes that represent the distribution of the peripheral nerves that arise from the spinal cord (Fig. 58-16). Most sensory deficits result from peripheral neuropathy and follow anatomic dermatomes. Exceptions to this include major destructive lesions of the brain; loss of sensation, which may affect an entire side of the body; and the neuropathies associated with alcoholism, which occur in a glove-and-stocking distribution.

Assessment of the sensory system involves tests for tactile sensation, superficial pain, vibration, and position sense (proprioception). Throughout the sensory assessment, the

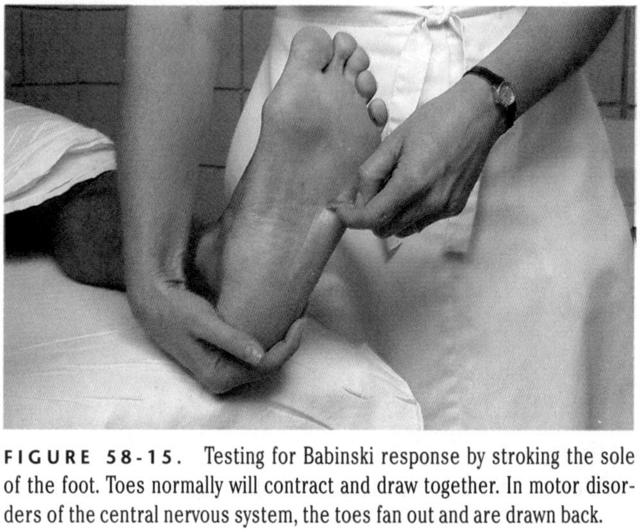

FIGURE 58-15. Testing for Babinski response by stroking the sole of the foot. Toes normally will contract and draw together. In motor disorders of the central nervous system, the toes fan out and are drawn back.

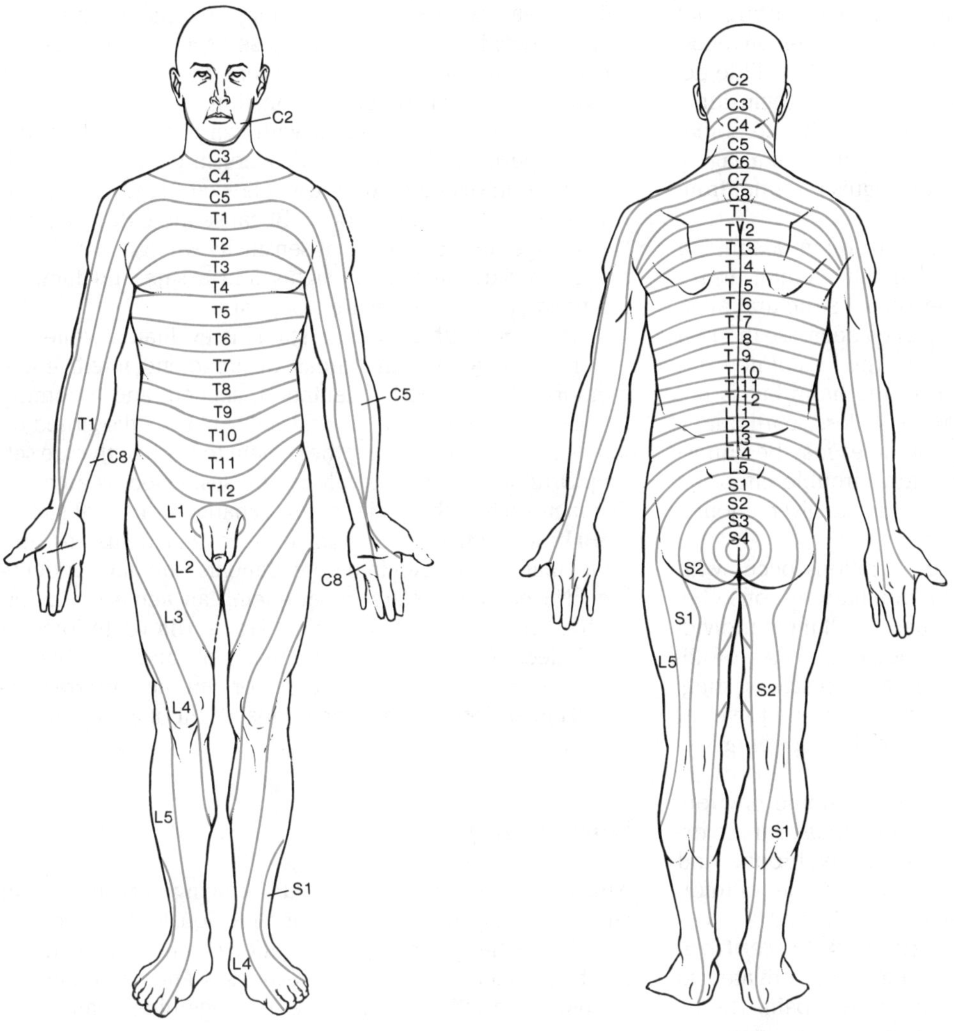

FIGURE 58-16. Dermatome distribution. (Fuller J and Schaller-Ayers J. Health Assessment: A Nursing Approach, 2nd ed. Philadelphia, JB Lippincott, 1994.)

patient's eyes are closed. The cooperation of the patient is encouraged by simple directions and reassurance that the examiner will not hurt or startle the patient.

Tactile sensation is assessed by lightly touching a cotton wisp to corresponding areas on each side of the body. The sensitivity of proximal parts of the extremities is compared with that of distal parts.

Pain and temperature sensations are transmitted together in the lateral part of the cord. Thus, it is not necessary to test for temperature sense in most circumstances. Superficial pain can be assessed by determining the patient's sensitivity to a sharp object. The patient is asked to differentiate between the sharp and dull ends of a broken wooden cotton swab or tongue blade; using a safety pin should be avoided because it breaks the integrity of the skin. Both the sharp and dull sides of the object are applied with equal intensity at all times, and the two sides are tested symmetrically.

Vibration and proprioception (the subjective sense of joint position) are transmitted together in the posterior part of the cord. Vibration may be evaluated through the use of a low-frequency (128- or 256-Hertz) tuning fork. The handle of the vibrating fork is placed against a bony prominence, and the patient is asked whether he or she feels a sensation and instructed to signal the examiner when the sensation ceases. If the patient does not perceive the vibrations at the distal bony prominences, the examiner progresses upward with the tuning fork until the vibrations are perceived by the patient. As with all measurement of sensation, side-to-side comparison is made.

Position sense may be determined by asking the patient to close both eyes and indicate, as the toes are moved, in which direction movement has taken place. Vibration and position sense are often lost together, frequently in circumstances where all others remain intact.

Integration of sensation in the brain must now be evaluated. This may be performed by testing two-point discrimination. That is, if the patient is touched with two sharp objects simultaneously, are they perceived as two or as one? If touched simultaneously on opposite sides of the body, the patient should normally report being touched in two places. If only one site is reported, the one not being recognized is said to demonstrate *extinction.* A good test of higher cortical sensory ability is that of *stereognosis.* The patient is instructed to close both eyes and identify a variety of objects (*e.g.,* keys, coins) that are placed in one hand by the examiner.

Gerontologic Considerations

The nervous system of older adults undergoes many changes from the normal aging process and is extremely vulnerable to general systemic illness. Changes throughout the nervous system vary in degree as the person ages. Nerve fibers that connect directly to muscles show little decline in function with age, as do simple neurologic functions that involve a number of connections in the spinal cord. Disease processes that complicate the normal aging processes often make it difficult to distinguish normal from abnormal changes.

Structural Changes. The elderly often assume a flexed posture and display muscle rigidity, tremor, and a slowness in movements. Among the known structural alterations that occur with increasing age are a decrease in brain weight and in the number of synapses. The loss of neurons occurs in select layers and regions of the brain but is not consistent throughout the CNS. Memory loss, particularly for recent events, and slower reaction times may be annoyances to the elderly, and they may have trouble choosing among several responses to a situation unless given enough time to reach a decision.

A number of other neurologic alterations occur with the aging process. For example, the pupillary response becomes more sluggish or may not appear at all if the individual has cataracts. Other changes include diminished or absent Achilles reflexes, loss of strength, and muscle wasting.

Sensory Alterations. Sensory isolation due to visual and hearing loss causes confusion, anxiety, disorientation, misinterpretation, and a feeling of inadequacy. Sensory alterations may require modification of the home environment and extra orientation to new surroundings. Simple explanations of routines, the location of the bathroom, and how to operate the call bell are just a few examples of information the elderly patient needs when hospitalized.

Temperature Regulation and Pain Perception. Other manifestations of neurologic changes are related to temperature regulation and the ability to feel pain. The elderly patient usually feels cold more easily than heat and may require extra covering when in bed; a room temperature somewhat higher than usual may be desirable. Perception of a reaction to painful stimuli may be decreased with age. Because pain is an important warning signal, the nurse must use caution when applying hot or cold packs or any therapeutic interventions. The geriatric patient may be burned or suffer frostbite before being aware of any discomfort.

More accurate assessment of physical signs and symptoms may be necessary to alleviate conditions underlying complaints of pain, such as abdominal discomfort or chest pain, which may be more serious than the patient's perception might indicate.

Taste and Smell Alterations. The acuity of the taste buds decreases with age, which along with an altered olfactory sense causes a decreased appetite. Extra seasoning often increases food intake, as long as it does not cause gastric irritation. The reduced olfactory sense arises from the atrophy of the olfactory organs.

A decreased sense of smell may present a safety hazard, because elderly persons living alone may be unable to detect household gas leaks or fires if they occur.

Tactile and Visual Alterations. Another neurologic alteration in the elderly patient is the dulling of tactile sensation as a result of a decrease in the number of areas of the body responding to all stimuli and in the number and sensitivity of sensory receptors. There may be difficulty in identifying objects by touch, and because fewer tactile cues are received from the bottom of the feet, the person may get confused as to his position and location.

These factors, combined with sensitivity to glare, decreased peripheral vision, and a constricted visual field, may result in disorientation, especially at night when there is little or no light in the room. Because the elderly person takes longer to recover visual sensitivity when moving from a light to dark area, night lights and a safe and familiar arrangement of furniture are essential.

Mental Status. Mental status is evaluated while the history is obtained, and areas of judgment, intelligence, memory, affect, mood, orientation, speech, and grooming are assessed. Changes in mental status may be discerned by family members who bring the patient to the health care setting. Drug toxicity should always be suspected as a causative factor when the patient has a change in mental status. **Delirium** (mental confusion, usually with delusions and hallucinations) is seen in elderly patients who have underlying CNS damage or are experiencing an acute condition such as infection or dehydration. **Dementia** (deterioration of intellectual function) may be reversible and treatable (as in drug toxicity or thyroid disease) or chronic and irreversible. **Depression** may produce impairment of attention and memory.

Nursing Implications

Nursing care for the patient with an aging nervous system should include the modifications previously described. In addition, patient teaching is also affected because the nurse must understand the altered responses and the changing needs of the elderly patient before beginning health education.

When caring for the elderly patient, the nurse adapts activities such as preoperative teaching, diet therapy, and instruction about new medications, their timing, and doses to the changes in the aging nervous system. The nurse considers the aged person's difficulty with fine motor movement and failing vision. When using visual aids, adequate lighting without glare, contrasting colors, and large print are used to offset visual difficulties caused by rigidity and opacity of the lens in the eye and slower pupillary reaction.

Procedures and preparation needed for diagnostic tests are explained, taking into account the possibility of impaired hearing and slowed responses in the elderly. Even with hearing loss, the elderly patient often hears adequately if the health care provider uses a low-pitched, clear speaking voice; shouting only makes it harder for the patient to understand the spoken voice. Providing auditory and visual cues aids understanding.

Teaching at an unrushed pace and using reinforcement enhances learning and retention. Material should be short, concise, and concrete. Vocabulary is matched to the patient's ability, and terms are clearly defined. The elderly patient requires adequate time to receive and respond to stimuli, to learn, and to react. These measures allow comprehension, memory, and formation of association and concepts.

As more research is carried out on the healthy geriatric population, the effects of normal aging on the nervous system will be distinguished from the effects of disease processes. Identifying the normal aging process may then open avenues for research into the prevention of degenerative nervous system changes that impair motor functions in the elderly.

Diagnostic Tests and Procedures

Imaging Procedures

Computed Tomography Scanning

Computed tomography (CT) makes use of a narrow beam of x-ray to scan the head in successive layers. The images that are produced provide cross-sectional views of the brain, with distinguishing differences in tissue densities of the skull, cortex, subcortical structures, and ventricles. The brightness of each portion, or "slice," of brain in the final image is proportional to the degree to which it absorbs x-ray. The image is displayed on an oscilloscope or TV monitor and is photographed.

Lesions in the brain are seen as variations in tissue density differing from the surrounding normal brain tissue. Abnormalities of tissue indicate possible tumor masses, brain infarction, displacement of the ventricles, and cortical atrophy. Whole-body CT scanners allow sections of the spinal cord to be visualized. The injection of water-soluble iodinated contrast material into the subarachnoid space through lumbar puncture improves the visualization of the spinal and intracranial contents on these images. The CT scan has replaced the myelogram as a diagnostic procedure for the diagnosis of herniated lumbar discs.

CT scanning is usually performed first without contrast material and then with intravenous contrast enhancement. The patient lies on an adjustable table with the head held in a fixed position, while the scanning system rotates around the head. (The patient serves as the axis, and the machine is rotated around the axis, resulting in a cross-sectional image.) The patient must lie with the head held perfectly still and with a careful effort not to talk or move the face, because head motion may cause considerable distortion of the image.

CT scanning is noninvasive, painless, and has a high degree of sensitivity for detecting lesions. As newer versions are developed and physicians become more and more sophisticated at interpreting them, the number of diseases and injuries that are able to be diagnosed is increasing, and the need for invasive diagnostic procedures is decreasing.

Positron Emission Tomography

Positron emission tomography (PET) is a computer-based nuclear imaging technique that can produce images of actual organ functioning. The patient either inhales a radioactive gas or is injected with a radioactive substance that emits positively charged particles. When these positrons combine with negatively charged electrons (normally found in the body's cells), the resultant gamma rays can be detected by a scanning device. In the scanning equipment, detectors are arranged in a ring and produce a series of two-dimensional views at various levels of the brain. This information is integrated by computer and gives a composite picture of the brain at work.

PET permits the measurement of blood flow, tissue composition, and brain metabolism. The brain is one of the most metabolically active organs, consuming 80% of the glucose the body uses. PET measures this activity in specific areas of the brain and is able to detect changes in glucose use.

This test is useful in showing metabolic changes in the brain (Alzheimer's disease), locating lesions (brain tumor, epileptogenic lesions), identifying blood flow and oxygen metabolism in stroke patients, evaluating new therapies for brain tumors, and revealing biochemical abnormalities associated with mental illness.

Patient Preparation. Patient preparation involves explaining the test and teaching the patient about inhalation techniques and the possible sensations (*i.e.*, dizziness, lightheadedness, headache) that may occur. The intravenous injection of the radioactive substance produces similar side effects. Relaxation exercises are used to reduce anxiety during the test.

Single Photon Emission Computed Tomography

Single photon emission computed tomography (SPECT) is a three-dimensional imaging technique using nuclear medicine procedures that employ radionuclides and instruments that emit and detect, respectively, single photons. Gamma photons are emitted from a radiopharmaceutical agent administered to the patient and are detected by a rotating gamma camera or cameras; the image is sent to a minicomputer. This approach allows areas behind overlying structures or background to be viewed, which greatly increases the contrast between normal and abnormal tissue. It is relatively inexpensive, and patient participation time is similar to that of CT scanning.

SPECT is useful in detecting the extent and location of abnormally perfused areas of the brain, thus allowing detection, localization, and sizing of stroke (before it is visible by CT scan), localization of seizure foci in epilepsy, and evaluation of perfusion before and after neurosurgical procedures. Pregnancy and breastfeeding are contraindications to SPECT. Therefore, premenopausal women are advised to practice effective contraception before and for several days after testing, and the woman who is breastfeeding is instructed to stop nursing for the period of time recommended by the nuclear medicine department.

Magnetic Resonance Imaging

Magnetic resonance imaging (MRI) uses a powerful magnetic field to obtain images of different areas of the body. Magnetized photons (hydrogen nuclei) within the body align like small magnets in this magnetic field. After bombardment with radiofrequency pulses, the protons emit signals, which are converted to images. MRI has the potential for identifying cerebral abnormality earlier and more clearly than other diagnostic tests. It can provide information about the chemical changes within cells, thus allowing the clinician to monitor a tumor's response to treatment. It does not require ionizing radiation.

Patient Preparation. Before the patient is taken to the room where the MRI is to be performed, all metallic objects (jewelry, including wedding rings, watches, hair pins) must be removed, as well as credit cards (the magnetic field can erase them). A complete history is also obtained to reveal if any metal objects are inside the patient (*e.g.*, aneurysm clips, orthopedic hardware, pacemakers, artificial heart valves, intrauterine devices). These objects could malfunction, be dislodged, or heat up as they absorb energy.

Procedure. The patient lies on a flat platform that is moved into a tube containing the magnet. The scanning process is painless, but the patient hears the thumping of the magnetic coils as the magnetic field is being pulsed. Because the MRI scanner is a narrow tube, patients may experience claustrophobia; sedation may be prescribed in these circumstances.* Patient preparation should include teaching the patient relaxation techniques and informing him that he will be able to talk to the staff by means of a microphone located inside the scanner.

Cerebral Angiography

Cerebral angiography is an x-ray study of the cerebral circulation after a contrast agent has been injected into a selected artery. Cerebral angiography is a valuable tool for investigating vascular disease, aneurysms, and arteriovenous malformations. It is frequently performed before a patient undergoes a craniotomy so that the cerebral arteries and veins are visualized and to determine the site, size, and nature of the pathologic processes. It is also used to assess the patency and adequacy of the cerebral circulation.

Most cerebral angiograms are performed by threading a catheter through the femoral artery in the groin and up to the desired vessel. The procedure may also be accomplished by direct puncture of the carotid or vertebral artery or by retrograde injection of a contrast agent into the brachial artery.

Patient Preparation. The patient should be well hydrated, and clear liquids are usually permitted up to the time of the study. Before going to the radiology department, the patient is instructed to void. The locations of the appropriate peripheral pulses are marked with a felt-tip pen. The patient is asked to remain immobile during the imaging process and is told to expect a brief feeling of warmth in the face, behind the eyes, or in the jaw, teeth, tongue, and lips, and a metallic taste when the contrast agent is injected.

After the groin is shaved and prepared, a local anesthetic is administered to prevent pain at the insertion site and to reduce arterial spasm. A catheter is introduced into the femoral artery, flushed with heparinized saline, and filled with contrast agent. Fluoroscopy is used to guide the catheter to the appropriate vessels. During injection of the contrast agent, images are made of the arterial and venous phases of circulation through the brain.

Postprocedure Care. In some instances, patients may experience major or minor arterial block due to embolism, thrombosis, or hemorrhage, producing a neurologic deficit. Signs of such an occurrence include alterations in the level of responsiveness and consciousness, weakness on one side of the body, motor or sensory deficits, and speech disturbances. Therefore, it is necessary to observe the patient frequently for these signs and to report them immediately if they occur.

The injection site is observed for hematoma formation (a localized collection of blood), and an ice bag may be applied intermittently to the puncture site to relieve swelling and discomfort. Because a hematoma at the puncture site or embolization to a distant artery affects the peripheral pulses, these pulses are monitored frequently. The color and temperature of the involved extremity are also assessed to detect possible embolism.

Digital Subtraction Angiography

In digital subtraction angiography, x-ray images of the area in question are obtained before and after the injection of a contrast agent. The computer "subtracts" the second set of films and produces an enhanced image of the carotid and vertebral arterial systems. This procedure is less invasive than arteriography because the injection can be given through a peripheral venous access.

Myelography

A myelogram is an x-ray of the spinal subarachnoid space following the injection of a contrast agent or air into the spinal subarachnoid space through a spinal puncture. It outlines the spinal subarachnoid space and shows any distortion of the spinal cord or spinal dural sac caused by tumors, cysts, herniated vertebral discs, or other lesions.

After the contrast agent is injected, the head of the table is tilted down and the course of the contrast medium is observed on x-ray. The contrast agent may be water soluble or oil based. Metrizamide is a water-soluble contrast agent that is absorbed by the body and excreted by the kidneys. It does not have to be removed by the needle route from the spinal canal because it is highly soluble and clears relatively quickly from the CSF. Side effects include headache, which is most probably due to CNS irritation by the metrizamide.

If iophendylate (Pantopaque), an oil-based iodine compound, is used for myelography, the radiologist may remove it by syringe and needle aspiration. The patient may complain of sharp pain down the leg if a nerve root is irritated during aspiration. This is remedied by rotating the needle point or adjusting the depth of the needle.

Patient Preparation. Because many patients have some misconceptions about this procedure, the nurse can answer questions and clarify the explanation offered by the physician. The patient should be aware that the x-ray table may be tilted in varying positions during the study. The meal that would normally be eaten before the procedure is omitted. A sedative may be prescribed to help the patient cope with a rather lengthy test.

Postprocedure Care. After myelography, when a water-soluble agent has been used, the patient lies in bed with the head of the bed elevated 30 to 45 degrees to reduce the rate of upward dispersion of the medium. The patient may be ambulatory or remain in bed as prescribed by the physician.

After a procedure in which an oil-based agent has been used, the patient should lie prone for 2 to 3 hours and in a recumbent position for the amount of time specified by the

*Newer versions of MRI machines are less claustrophobic than the first devices and are available in some locations.

physician (usually 12 to 24 hours) to reduce CSF leakage and decrease the frequency of headache. Usually, the patient is permitted to turn from side to side.

The patient is encouraged to drink liberal amounts of fluid for rehydration and replacement of CSF and to decrease the incidence of post–lumbar puncture headache. The blood pressure, pulse, respiratory rate, and temperature are monitored, as well as the patient's ability to void. Other untoward signs include fever, stiff neck, photophobia (sensitivity to light), and signs of chemical or bacterial meningitis.

Myelography is performed less frequently today because of the sensitivity of CT scanning and MRIs.

Lumbar Epidural Venography

In lumbar epidural venography, a catheter is inserted percutaneously into the femoral vein and guided into the ascending lumbar vein or internal iliac vein. The contrast agent is injected to fill the epidural veins overlying the disc spaces and to opacify the epidural venous plexus. The procedure may be useful in the diagnosis of herniated lumbar discs that are not visualized on myelography. It shows deviation or compression of the epidural veins due to a herniated disc or tumor.

The procedure is relatively easy to perform, well tolerated, fairly painless, and not associated with arachnoiditis. Lumbar epidural venography and myelography may be performed as complementary diagnostic studies. After the test, the site is observed for evidence of hematoma formation.

Radionuclide Imaging Studies (Brain Scan)

Radionuclide imaging is based on the principle that a radiopharmaceutical agent may diffuse through the blood–brain barrier at a point where the barrier has been disrupted and collect in abnormal cerebral tissue. (Normal brain tissue is relatively impermeable.) There is increased uptake of radioactive material at the site of pathology.

In this procedure, a radioactive agent is injected intravenously. The radioactivity subsequently transmitted through the skull is traced by a scanner that prints out an image, or a gamma camera is used to monitor the passage of the radiopharmaceutical agent through the cerebral circulation to gain information about cerebral blood flow.

Brain scanning is particularly useful in evaluating vascular lesions of the brain and meninges and in locating vascular neoplasms and brain tumors. It is useful in the early detection and evaluation of stroke, abscess, and follow-up of surgical or radiation therapy of the brain. Newer techniques permit the evaluation of cerebral circulation during the brain scan. However, CT scanning is replacing traditional radioisotope scanning.

Echoencephalography

Echoencephalography is the recording of sound waves reflected by the structures of the brain in response to ultrasound signals created by a transducer positioned over specific areas of the head. Echoencephalography is a rapid and useful technique to determine the position of midline structures of the brain and the distance from the midline to the lateral ventricular wall or the third ventricular wall. Therefore, it is performed to detect a shift of the cerebral midline structures caused by subdural hematoma, intracerebral hemorrhage, massive cerebral infarction, and neoplasms. It is useful in evaluating hydrocephalus because it can detect dilation of the ventricles.

Noninvasive carotid flow studies use ultrasound imagery and Doppler measurements of arterial blood flow to evaluate carotid and deep orbital circulation. These tests are often obtained before arteriography, which carries combined risks of strokes and death (0.5% to 2%). Carotid Doppler studies, carotid ultrasonography, oculoplethysmography, and ophthalmodynamometry are four common noninvasive vascular studies that analyze the arterial blood flow and detect arterial stenosis, occlusion, and plaques.

Patient Preparation. There are no special preparations for these studies except for patient education. To reduce anxiety, the patient is informed that this is a noninvasive test, that a hand-held transducer will be placed over the neck and orbits of the eyes, and that some type of water-soluble jelly is used on the transducer.

Air Studies

The CSF spaces in and around the brain may be seen on x-ray examination when the fluid is replaced with a gas. This is based on the principle that gas inserted in the ventricular and subarachnoid systems serves as a contrast agent, because air is less dense than fluid to x-rays. The CSF may be partially replaced with air through pneumoencephalography and ventriculography.

Pneumoencephalography is a diagnostic procedure in which air or gas is instilled through a lumbar puncture as a means of demonstrating the ventricular system and subarachnoid space overlying the hemispheres and basal cisterns. A small amount of CSF is removed and an equal amount of air injected. A special chair allows the patient to be rotated in all directions so that air may be placed selectively in the desired cavities. Images are then made and studied.

Ventriculography is an x-ray taken of the lateral ventricles after CSF has been withdrawn and air or gas injected into the lateral ventricles through openings in the skull.

These studies are rarely performed since the advent of CT and MRI scanning.

Electrophysiologic Tests

Electroencephalography

An electroencephalogram (EEG) represents a record of the electrical activity generated in the brain and obtained through electrodes applied on the scalp surface or through microelectrodes placed within the brain tissue. It provides physiologic assessment of cerebral activity.

EEG is a useful test for diagnosing seizure disorders such as the epilepsies and is a screening procedure for coma or organic brain syndrome. It also serves as an indicator of brain death. Tumors, abscesses, brain scars, blood clots, and infection may cause electrical activity to differ from normal patterns of rhythm and rate.

Procedure. Electrodes are arranged on the scalp to record the electrical activity in various regions of the head. The amplified activity of the neurons between any two of these electrodes is recorded on a continuously moving paper sheet; this record is the encephalogram.

For a baseline recording, the patient lies quietly with both eyes closed. The patient may be asked to hyperventilate for 3 to 4 minutes and then look at a bright, flashing light for photic stimulation. These are activation procedures performed to evoke abnormal electrical discharges, especially seizure potentials. A sleep EEG may be recorded after sedation because some abnormal brain waves are seen only when the patient is asleep. If the epileptogenic area is inaccessible to conventional scalp electrodes, nasopharyngeal electrodes may be used.

Depth recording of EEG is performed by introducing electrodes stereotactically into a target area of the brain, as dictated by the patient's seizure pattern and scalp EEG. It is used to identify patients who may benefit from surgical excision of epileptogenic foci.

Special transsphenoidal, mandibular, and nasopharyngeal electrodes can be used, and videorecording combined with EEG monitoring and telemetry is used in hospital settings to capture epileptiform abnormalities and their sequelae. Some epilepsy centers provide long-term ambulatory EEG monitoring with portable cassette recorders.

Patient Preparation. To increase the chances of recording seizure activity, it is sometimes recommended that the patient be deprived of sleep on the night before the EEG. Tranquilizers and stimulants should be withheld 24 to 48 hours before an EEG, because these medications can alter the EEG wave patterns or mask the abnormal wave patterns of seizure disorder. Coffee, tea, chocolate, and cola drinks are omitted in the meal before the test because of their stimulating effect. The meal is not omitted, however, because an altered blood glucose level can also cause changes in the brain wave patterns.

The patient is informed that the standard EEG takes 45 to 60 minutes or longer if a sleep EEG is performed. At the same time, the patient is assured that the procedure does not cause an electric shock and that the EEG is a diagnostic test and not a form of treatment.

Evoked Potential Studies

In evoked potential studies electrodes are placed on the scalp and an external stimulus is applied to peripheral sensory receptors to elicit or evoke changes or responses in the brain waves. Evoked changes are detected with the aid of computerized devices that extract the signal, display it on an oscilloscope, and store the data on magnetic tape or disc.

These studies are based on the concept that any insult or dysfunction that can alter neuronal metabolism or disturb membrane function may change evoked responses in brain waves. In neurologic diagnosis they reflect conduction times in the peripheral nervous system. In clinical practice the visual, auditory, and somatosensory systems are most often tested.

In **visual evoked responses**, the patient looks at a visual stimulus (flashing lights, a checkerboard pattern on a screen). The average of several hundred stimuli is recorded by EEG leads placed over the occiput. The transit time from the retina to the occipital area is measured using computer-averaging methods.

Auditory evoked responses or brain stem evoked responses are measured by applying an auditory stimulus (a repetitive auditory click) and measuring the transit time up the brain stem into the cortex. Specific lesions in the auditory pathway modify or delay the response.

In **somatosensory evoked responses**, the peripheral nerves are stimulated (electrical stimulation through skin electrodes), and the transit time up the spinal cord to the cortex is measured and recorded from scalp electrodes.

This test is used to detect a deficit in spinal cord conduction and to monitor cord function during operative procedures. Because myelinated fibers conduct impulses at a higher rate of speed, nerves with intact myelin sheath record the highest velocity. Demyelination of nerve fibers leads to a decrease in conduction velocity, as found in Guillain-Barré syndrome, multiple sclerosis, and polyneuropathies.

Patient Preparation. There is no specific patient preparation other than to reassure and encourage the patient to relax. The patient is advised to remain perfectly still throughout the recording to prevent artifacts (potentials not generated by the brain) that interfere with the recording and interpretation of the test.

Electromyography

An electromyogram (EMG) is obtained by introducing needle electrodes into the skeletal muscles to measure changes in the electrical potential of the muscles and the nerves leading to them. The electrical potentials are shown on an oscilloscope and amplified by a loudspeaker so that both the sound and appearance of the waves can be analyzed and compared simultaneously.

EMGs are useful in determining the presence of a neuromuscular disorder and myopathies. They help to distinguish weakness due to neuropathy (functional or pathologic changes in the peripheral nervous system) from weakness due to other causes.

Patient Preparation. No special patient preparation is required. The patient is informed that he will experience a sensation similar to that of an intramuscular injection as the needle is inserted into the muscle. The muscles examined may ache for a short time after the procedure.

Nerve Conduction Studies

Nerve conduction studies are performed by stimulating a peripheral nerve at several points along its course and recording the muscle action potential or the sensory action potential that results. Surface or needle electrodes are placed on the skin over the nerve to stimulate the nerve fibers. This test is useful in the study of peripheral nerve neuropathies.

Special Procedures

Lumbar Puncture and Examination of Cerebrospinal Fluid

A lumbar puncture (spinal tap) is carried out by inserting a needle into the lumbar subarachnoid space to withdraw

CSF for diagnostic and therapeutic purposes. The purposes are to obtain CSF for examination, measure and reduce CSF pressure, determine the presence or absence of blood in the CSF, detect spinal subarachnoid block, and administer antibiotics intrathecally—that is, into the spinal canal—in certain cases of infection.

The needle is usually inserted into the subarachnoid space between the third and fourth or fourth and fifth lumbar vertebrae. Because the spinal cord divides into a sheaf of nerves at the first lumbar vertebra, the needle is inserted below the level of the third lumbar vertebra to prevent the spinal cord from being punctured (see Fig. 58-17).

A successful lumbar puncture requires that the patient be relaxed; an anxious patient is tense, and the increased anxiety may cause an increase in the pressure reading. The normal range of spinal fluid pressure with the patient in a lateral recumbent position is 70 to 200 mm H_2O. Pressures over 200 mm H_2O are considered abnormal.

A lumbar puncture may be quite dangerous in the presence of an intracranial mass lesion, because intracranial pressure is decreased by the removal of CSF and the brain may herniate downward through the tentorium and the foramen magnum.

Queckenstedt's Test. A lumbar manometric test (Queckenstedt's test) may be performed by compressing the jugular veins on each side of the neck during the lumbar puncture. The increase in pressure caused by the compression is noted; then the pressure is released and pressure readings are made at 10-second intervals.

Normally, CSF pressure rises rapidly in response to compression of the jugular veins and returns quickly to normal when the compression is released. A slow rise and fall in pressure indicates a partial block due to a lesion compressing the spinal subarachnoid pathways. If there is no pressure change, a complete block is indicated. This test is not performed if an intracranial lesion is suspected.

Procedure for Lumbar Puncture. See Guideline 58-1.

Examination of the Cerebrospinal Fluid. CSF should be clear and colorless. Pink, blood-tinged, or grossly bloody CSF may indicate a cerebral contusion, laceration, or subarachnoid hemorrhage. Sometimes with a difficult

GUIDELINE 58–1
Assisting with a Lumbar Puncture

A needle is inserted into the subarachnoid space through the third and fourth or fourth and fifth lumbar interspace to withdraw spinal fluid (Fig. 58-17).

Preprocedure

1. Assure the patient that inserting the needle into the spine will not cause paralysis.
2. See that the patient's bowel and bladder are emptied.

Procedure (performed by the physician)

1. The patient is positioned as follows:
   a. The patient is placed on one side with back toward the physician.
   b. The thighs and legs are flexed as much as possible to increase the space between the spinous processes of the vertebrae, for easier entry into the subarachnoid space.
   c. A small pillow is placed under the patient's head to maintain the spine in a horizontal position.
   d. A pillow may be placed between the legs to prevent the upper leg from rolling forward.
   e. The nurse may assist the patient to maintain the position to avoid sudden movement, which can produce a traumatic (bloody) tap.
2. The patient is instructed to breathe normally because hyperventilation may lower an elevated pressure.
3. The physician inserts the needle into the subarachnoid space through the third and fourth or fourth and fifth lumbar interspace.

Postprocedure

1. Instruct the patient to lie prone for 2–3 hours to separate the alignment of the dural and arachnoid needle punctures in the meninges, to reduce the leakage of CSF.
2. Encourage increased fluid intake to reduce the risk of postprocedure headache.

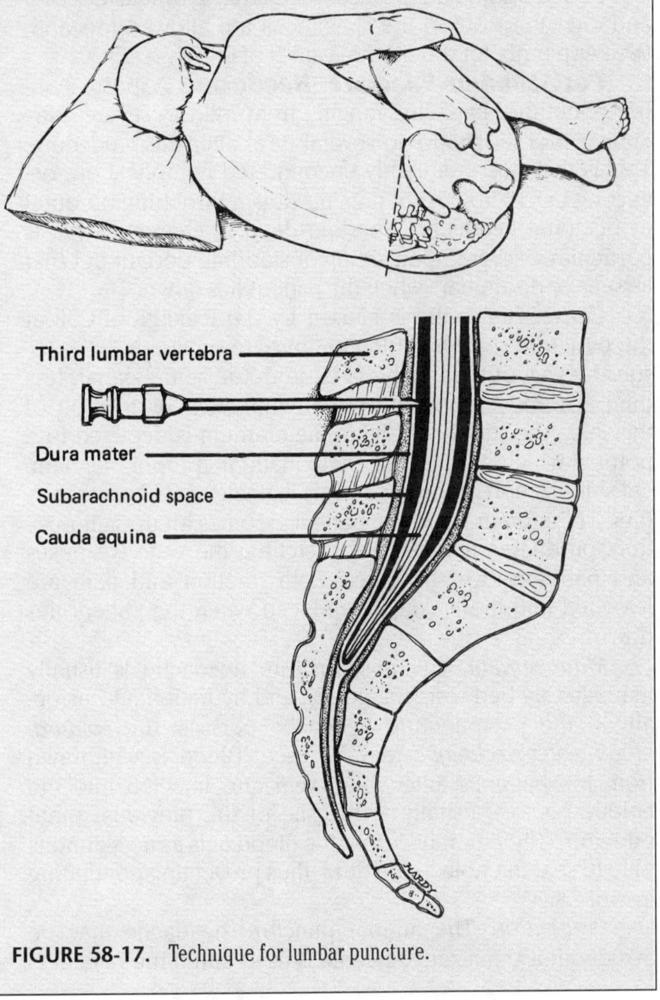

FIGURE 58-17. Technique for lumbar puncture.

CRITICAL THINKING EXERCISES

1. Your patient is scheduled to have a lumbar puncture (spinal tap) and states that she is afraid that she may end up paralyzed as a result of the procedure. Based on your knowledge of the anatomy and physiology of the central nervous system, how would you structure your explanation to reassure the patient and dispel her fears?
2. Your patient is to have magnetic resonance imaging (MRI). How would you explain the test to the patient and the precautions that are needed before the procedure? How would you adjust your approach if the patient has difficulty understanding English? Is elderly and has severe skeletal deformities?

lumbar puncture, the CSF initially is bloody because of local trauma but then becomes clearer.

Usually, specimens are obtained for cell count, culture, glucose, and protein. The specimens should be sent to the laboratory immediately because changes will take place and alter the result if the specimens are allowed to stand. (See Appendix for the normal values of CSF.)

Post–Lumbar-Puncture Headache. A post—lumbar puncture headache, ranging from mild to severe, may appear in a few hours to several days after the procedure. This is the most frequently encountered complication, occurring in 11% to 25% of patients. It is a throbbing bifrontal or occipital headache, dull and deep in character, that is particularly severe upon sitting or standing upright but that lessens or disappears when the patient lies down.

Cause. Headache is caused by the leakage of CSF at the puncture site. The fluid continues to escape into the tissues by way of the needle track from the spinal canal. It is then absorbed promptly by the lymphatics. As a result of this leak, the supply of CSF in the cranium is depleted to a point at which it is insufficient to maintain proper mechanical stabilization of the brain. This leakage of CSF allows settling of the brain when the patient assumes an upright position, producing tension and stretching the venous sinuses and pain-sensitive structures. Both traction and pain are lessened and the leakage is reduced when the patient lies down.

Management. The postpuncture headache is usually managed by bed rest, analgesics, and hydration. Occasionally, if the postpuncture headache persists, the *epidural blood patch technique* may be used. Blood is withdrawn from the patient's antecubital vein and injected into the epidural space, usually at the site of the previous spinal puncture. The rationale is that the blood acts as a gelatinous plug to seal the hole in the dura, thus preventing continuing loss of CSF.

Prevention. The lumbar puncture headache may be avoided if a small-gauge needle is used and if the patient is encouraged to remain prone after the procedure. When a large volume of fluid (> 20 ml) is removed, the patient is positioned prone for 2 hours, then flat in a side-lying position for 2 to 3 hours, and then supine or prone for 6 more hours. Keeping the patient flat overnight may reduce the incidence of headaches.

Other complications of a lumbar puncture include herniation of the intracranial contents, traumatic complications, spinal epidural abscess, spinal epidural hematoma, and meningitis.

BIBLIOGRAPHY

Books

Bernat JL. Ethical Issues in Neurology. Boston, Butterworth-Heinemann, 1994.

Haerer AF. DeJong's The Neurologic Examination. Philadelphia, JB Lippincott, 1992.

Hickey JV. Clinical Practice of Neurological and Neurosurgical Nursing, 3rd ed. Philadelphia, JB Lippincott, 1992.

Strub RL and Black FW. The Mental Status Examination in Neurology. Philadelphia, FA Davis, 1993.

Westmoreland BF et al. Medical Neurosciences: An Approach to Anatomy, Pathology and Physiology by Systems and Levels. Boston, Little, Brown, 1994.

Journals

Baker ND et al. The efficacy of routine head computed tomography (CT scan) prior to lumbar puncture in the emergency department. J Emerg Med 1994 Sep–Oct; 12(5):597–601.

Drislane FW. Migrainous phenomenon precipitated by lumbar puncture headache. Cephalalgia 1994 Oct; 14(5):379–380.

Dykes PC. Minding the five P's of neurovascular assessment. Am J Nurs 1993 Jun; 93(6):38–39.

Guin PR and Freudenberger K. The elderly neuroscience patient: Implications for the critical care nurse. AACN Clin Issues Crit Care Nurs 1992 Feb; 3(1):98–105.

Jeret JS et al. Clinical predictors of abnormality disclosed by computed tomography after mild head trauma. Neurosurgery 1993 Jan; 32(1):9–15.

Hilton G. Review of neurobehavioral assessment tools [review]. Heart Lung 1992 Sep; 20(5 Pt 1):436–442.

Lang SM and Bernardo LM. SCIWORA syndrome: Nursing assessment. Dimensions Crit Care Nurs 1993 Sep–Oct; 15(5): 247–254.

Marciello MA et al. Magnetic resonance imaging related to neurologic outcome in cervical spinal cord injury. Arch Phys Med Rehabil 1993 Sep; 74(9):940–946.

Morewood GH. A rational approach to the cause, prevention and treatment of postdural puncture headache. Can Med Assoc J 1993 Oct 15; 149(8):1087–1093.

Morgenlander JC. Lumbar puncture and CSF examination: Answers to three commonly asked questions [review]. Postgrad Med 1994 Jun; 95(8):125–128.

Muller B et al. Atrumatic needle reduces the incidence of post–lumbar puncture syndrome. J Neurol 1994 May; 241(6): 376–380.

Practice parameters: Lumbar puncture (summary statement). Report of the Quality Standards Subcommittee of the American Academy of Neurology. Neurology 1993 Mar; 43 (3 Pt 1): 625–627.

Silberstein SD and Corbett JJ. The forgotten lumbar puncture. Cephalalgia 1993 Jun; 13(3):212–213.

Steward-Amidei C. Assessing the comatose patient in the intensive care unit. AACN Clin Issues Crit Care Nurs 1991 Nov; 2(4): 613–622.

Tso EL et al. Cranial computed tomography in the emergency department evaluation of HIV-infected patients with neurologic complaints. Ann Emerg Med 1993 Jul; 22(7):1169–1176.

Warshaw G and Tanzer F. The effectiveness of lumbar puncture in the evaluation of delirium and fever in the hospitalized elderly. Arch Fam Med 1993 Mar; 2(3):293–297.

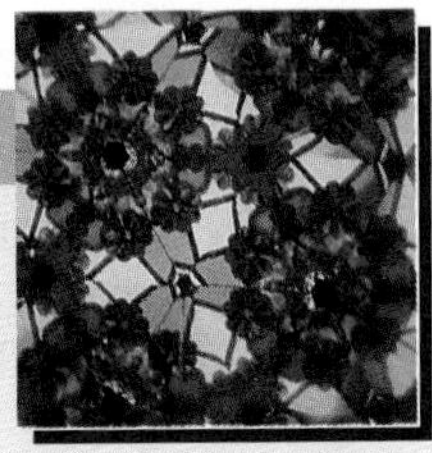

59 Management of Patients With Neurologic Dysfunction

CHAPTER OUTLINE

LEARNING OBJECTIVES

On completion of this chapter, the learner will be able to:

1. Describe the special nursing needs of patients with neurologic dysfunction
2. Use the nursing process as a framework for care of the patient with neurologic dysfunction
3. Identify the early and late clinical manifestations of increased intracranial pressure
4. Use the nursing process as a framework for care of the patient with increased intracranial pressure
5. Describe the multiple needs of the unconscious patient
6. Use the nursing process as a framework for care of the unconscious patient
7. Describe the various types of aphasia and the nursing management of the aphasic patient
8. Identify the risk factors of stroke and related measures for stroke prevention
9. Compare the various types of stroke: their causes, clinical manifestations, and nursing and medical management
10. Use the nursing process as a framework for care of the patient with stroke
11. Use the nursing process as a framework for care of the patient undergoing intracranial surgery
12. Compare the various types of neurosurgical procedures used to treat intractable pain

Neuroscience nursing is a specialty requiring an understanding of neuroanatomy, neurophysiology, neurodiagnostic testing, critical care nursing, and rehabilitation nursing. In addition to ongoing assessment of the patient's neurologic function and health needs, the nurse's role is to help the patient identify problems, set mutual goals, direct a course of action, use appropriate nursing interventions (including teaching, counseling, and coordinating activities), and evaluate the outcomes of care.

Neurologic problems can result in alterations in a person's cognitive, sensory, and neuromuscular functions and can adversely affect self image; however, the nurse and health care team provide essential care, offer a variety of solutions to existing problems, help the patient gain control, and explore the educational and supportive resources available in the community to provide assistance. The goals are to achieve as high a level of function as possible and enhance the quality of life for the patient and family.

❑ NURSING PROCESS
The Patient With Neurologic Dysfunction

Assessment

The patient with a neurologic dysfunction undergoes a thorough neurologic examination (described in Chapter 58). The examination involves tests of several major areas of functioning, including cerebral, cranial nerve, motor system and sensory system function, and reflex responses. Observing the patient's movements and inquiring as to any changes in sensation are part of the initial assessment. When assessing neurologic dysfunction, the nurse observes the patient's level of alertness and determines whether there is a disturbance of consciousness or alteration in mental and emotional status. Cognitive function is tested by determining if the patient is oriented to person, place, and time. Intellectual functions are evaluated by asking questions of general knowledge, ascertaining reasoning ability, and assessing recent and remote memory. An assessment is also made of the person's language abilities. Loss of function and certain alterations in function may indicate neurologic deterioration and must be reported. These indices are described further in the discussions of specific types of neurologic dysfunctions that follow.

Diagnosis

Nursing Diagnoses

There is no known cure for many neurologic illnesses. The nursing goal is to help the patient adapt to the dysfunction and continue with life in as meaningful a way as possible. Nursing interventions include identifying and accepting the patient's self-protective responses, providing information, assisting the patient to set achievable goals, reinforcing positive coping skills, and offering ongoing support.

Many patients with neurologic conditions face a wide range of possible nursing diagnoses, including the following:

- ❑ Ineffective breathing pattern
- ❑ Impaired swallowing
- ❑ Impaired skin integrity
- ❑ Impaired physical mobility
- ❑ Self-care deficits
- ❑ Pain
- ❑ Hyperthermia
- ❑ Altered oral mucous membranes
- ❑ Impaired tissue integrity: cornea
- ❑ Altered nutrition: less than body requirements
- ❑ Altered urinary and bowel elimination
- ❑ Altered thought processes
- ❑ Sexual dysfunction
- ❑ Ineffective individual coping
- ❑ Altered family processes

Collaborative Problems/ Potential Complications

Potential complications that may occur include:

- ❑ Respiratory failure
- ❑ Pneumonia
- ❑ Aspiration
- ❑ Pressure ulcers

Planning and Implementation

Goals. The goals for the patient with neurologic dysfunction include improved respiratory status and swallowing; maintenance of skin integrity and oral hygiene; increased mobility and self care; pain relief; temperature control; enhanced coping, cognitive, and sexual functioning; and absence of complications.

Nursing Interventions

Improving Breathing. Patients with neuromuscular disorders such as Guillain-Barré syndrome and myasthenia gravis and neurologic disorders such as cervical spinal cord injury may have weakness of the diaphragm, intercostal muscles, and accessory muscles of respiration that compromises ventilation. When the diaphragm is paralyzed the patient is in danger while supine, when hypoventilation may be particularly severe. Additionally, the patient's inability to take deep breaths and cough effectively results in retained secretions and atelectasis. The end result may be respiratory insufficiency and failure.

Nursing interventions include monitoring the adequacy of alveolar ventilation by taking frequent measurements of the respiratory rate, vital capacity, and inspiratory force. Measures to promote chest expansion include elevating the head of the bed 30 degrees and working with the respiratory therapist in assessing the effectiveness of incentive spirometry, and providing chest physiotherapy, naso/oral tracheal suctioning, and positive-pressure breathing.

Respiratory Support Measures. If the disorder appears to be progressing (increasing respiratory rate; vital capacity less than 10–15 ml/kg of body weight; or inspiratory force less than –25 cm H_2O), the patient may require insertion of an endotracheal tube or tracheostomy and mechanical ventilation. In many instances, the neuromuscular weakness is reversible, but the patient often requires prolonged ventilatory support.

Maintenance of Airway. In patients with depressed states of consciousness, a common cause of airway obstruction is the posterior displacement of oropharyngeal soft tissue structures; the tongue becomes flaccid and falls back against the posterior pharyngeal wall. An immediate nursing intervention is to extend the patient's head or elevate the mandible. Placing the patient on his side allows the tongue to fall to the side and away from the back of the pharynx. It may be necessary to insert an oropharyngeal tube or airway.

Prolonged placement of the oral airway may result in pressure ulcers forming on the lip and the upper palate; therefore, the tissue under the oral airway should frequently be assessed for pressure ulcer formation.

Promoting Swallowing. Neurologic disorders that impair breathing often cause swallowing problems. Patients with such dysfunction are at risk for aspirating secretions or regurgitated gastric contents. The conscious patient is observed for paroxysms of coughing or nasal regurgitation when swallowing liquids. The patient with impaired swallowing, ineffective laryngeal function, and diminished cough reflexes is placed in a lateral position to avoid aspiration. Respiratory function may be improved by clearing the obstructed airway by suctioning and by instituting mechanical ventilation to correct the hypoxia.

Tube Feedings. Patients with swallowing dysfunctions may require nasogastric tube feedings to prevent aspiration and ensure adequate nutrition. Nursing responsibilities in feeding include placing the patient in an upright position, checking the position of the tube before feeding, ensuring that the cuff of the endotracheal tube (if in place) is inflated, and giving the tube feeding slowly. The feeding tube is aspirated periodically to ensure that the feedings are passing through the gastrointestinal tract. Retained or residual feedings increase the potential risk of aspiration. Patients with retained feedings may benefit from the placement of a gastrostomy tube. In a patient with a nasogastric tube, the feeding tube should be placed in the duodenum to reduce the risk of aspiration.

Maintaining Skin Integrity. Special nursing challenges arise when the patient is paralyzed and has sensory disturbances or altered mental status (confusion, depression, stupor, or coma). Patients with chronic neurologic conditions usually have some physical defect and are at risk for developing pressure ulcers. Prevention is the hallmark of management. For the patient with impaired neurologic function, prevention includes changing position frequently, maintaining alignment, using pressure-reducing mattresses and wheelchair overlays, inspecting the skin for signs of pressure, having properly fitted wheelchair cushions, and wearing a wrist watch with a buzzer alarm (for auditory cuing) as a reminder to the patient to shift position to relieve pressure. Additional discussion of the prevention of pressure ulcers is presented in Chapter 18.

Promoting Physical Mobility. Any paralyzed extremity deserves careful attention. Care must be taken to see that the patient does not lie on the extremity too long and that the circulation to the part is not impeded. To prevent contractures, the nurse ensures that the patient is positioned correctly and that the joints are moved either actively or passively through their range of motion several times daily. Family members are frequently taught active and passive range of motion to enable them to participate in the care of the patient.

Muscle weakness (lack of strength) is seen in clinical conditions that have resulted from lesions of the cortex, brain stem, spinal cord, anterior horn cells, peripheral nerve, neuromuscular junction, or muscle. In general, therapeutic exercises are carried out to increase strength. The patient should not exercise to the point of fatigue because weakness may occur from overuse. Patients with neurologic conditions have increased energy demands resulting from motor involvement, the secondary effects of deconditioning, and the emotional stress of living with a disability.

Preventing Contractures. A patient with neurologic dysfunction is at risk for painful contractures; lying in bed causes the feet to drop into plantar flexion and the knees and hips to flex (if the head of the bed is raised). Fibrous tissue stiffening within muscles occurs, and painful spasticity accentuates the problem. The key to this type of pain is preventing it by positioning the patient properly and using appropriate range-of-motion exercises for each joint several times a day. Encouraging the patient to participate in self-care is important.

Promoting Self-Care. An impairment of neuromuscular function can interfere with self-care activities. The nurse, working collaboratively with other rehabilitation team members, evaluates the patient's joint range of motion, sensation, muscle strength, endurance, and coordination, as well as ability to learn. The patient is taught self-care skills and compensatory techniques to enhance existing abilities (see Chapter 18). Occupational and physical therapists are helpful in identifying alternative approaches to promote self-care.

Relieving Pain. As in any other condition, the nursing assessment of the patient with pain due to neurologic dysfunction focuses on how the patient is functioning. The nurse works with the patient to determine the location of the pain, its distribution, the degree of limitation, its intensity, and its adverse effects on the patient's life. The nurse listens to the patient's description of pain and identifies factors that increase and decrease the pain. Patients with chronic pain from neurologic conditions often become depressed and anxious and experience insomnia. In addition, they may limit their activities because of the pain, which causes a generalized fatigue.

Nursing interventions include establishing a trusting relationship with the patient, teaching the patient about pain and its relief, decreasing noxious stimuli, providing distraction from pain, and using assistance from other professionals. The nurse administers the prescribed analgesic and monitors the patient's response. Nursing interventions also include appropriate reassurance to relieve the anxiety that often occurs with pain. Maximum function within the limitations of the patient's disability is encouraged. Explanations of the deleterious effects of prolonged inactivity are provided.

Specific nursing interventions for the relief of pain and discomfort are found in Chapter 13 and in the discussions of headache, intracranial and spinal surgery, head injuries, and the neurosurgical relief of pain.

Managing Hyperthermia. Because of damage to the heat-regulating center in the brain or severe intracranial infection, neurologic and neurosurgical patients often develop very high temperatures. Such temperature elevations must be controlled, because the increased metabolic demands of the brain will overburden cerebral circulation and oxygenation, resulting in cerebral deterioration. *Persistent hyperthermia is indicative of brain stem damage and indicates a poor prognosis.*

Hyperthermia is also seen in the neurologically impaired patient with CNS, respiratory, urinary, and wound infections, and in drug reactions.

Reducing body temperature is a major goal in treating some cerebral disorders. It has been shown that body temperatures well below normal decrease cerebral edema, reduce the oxygen and metabolic requirements of the brain, and protect the brain from continued ischemia. If body metabolism can be reduced by lowering body temperature, the collateral circulation in the brain may be able to provide an adequate blood supply to the brain.

Inducing and maintaining hypothermia is a major clinical procedure and requires knowledge and skilled nursing observation and management. It is desirable to begin treatment before the patient's temperature gets too high.

- All bedding over the patient should be removed (with the possible exception of a light sheet or small drape).
- Repeated doses of aspirin or acetaminophen are given as prescribed.
- Cool sponge baths and an electric fan blowing over the patient to increase surface cooling may be helpful.
- The use of the hypothermia blanket and equipment is usually effective in controlling neurogenic hyperthermia.

Frequent temperature monitoring is indicated to assess the patient's response to the therapy and to prevent an excessive decrease in temperature and shivering. Shivering may increase cellular oxygen demands and result in cellular hypoxia; it may also increase ICP by isometric muscle contraction. Chlorpromazine (Thorazine) is administered as prescribed to control shivering.

Maintaining Oral Hygiene. The unconscious patient is at risk for parotitis (inflammation of the parotid gland) if the mouth is not kept clean. The condition of the patient's oral mucous membranes is assessed frequently, because buccal structures tend to become exceedingly dry after a short period of mouth breathing. The lips, tongue, and gums are cleansed and lubricated at frequent intervals, and the patient's fluid intake is maintained at an adequate level.

A patient who is intubated requires frequent oral care, suctioning, and repositioning of the endotracheal tube from one side of the mouth to the other to prevent oral ulceration. As stated previously, in patients with oral airways the mucous membranes should be inspected for pressure ulcer formation. The oral airway should be removed and repositioned.

Maintaining Eye Care. When facial paralysis from any cause makes it impossible for the patient to shut his eyes or the patient has an impaired corneal reflex, the cornea is left exposed, which can lead to keratitis and corneal ulceration. Gentle cleansing of the eyelids with sterile warm water or sterile normal saline every few hours removes discharge and debris. Artificial tears or a lubricant may be instilled when prescribed. An eye shield or patch is worn when necessary.

Care should be taken to ensure that the eyelid is closed when the patch is worn, to prevent the cornea from ulcerating further from friction caused by the eye patch. The nurse inspects the eyes regularly for signs of inflammation. Patients who are conscious and able can administer their own eye care with proper instruction and supervision.

Providing Adequate Nutrition. Patients with neurologic dysfunction are at risk for nutritional disorders. Depression, so commonly encountered in patients with neurologic conditions, may suppress the appetite. Nutritional problems also arise if chewing and swallowing are impaired.

Some patients require gastrostomy feedings (see Chapter 35), usually ingesting foods that have been prepared in a food blender. The blenderized meal is tolerated well because the patient's gastrointestinal tract is accustomed to this type of diet. In addition to initiating a referral to the dietitian for nutritional counseling, the nurse works with the occupational therapist to obtain eating utensils that assist the patient to compensate for a physical disability.

Maintaining Urinary and Bowel Elimination. Many patients with CNS disease may experience temporary or permanent urinary and fecal incontinence. The hygienic care of patients with incontinence is an important nursing priority. Some patients benefit from the initiation of a bowel and bladder regimen that may reduce urinary and fecal incontinence. This regimen should begin as soon as the patient is stable and the indwelling urinary catheter is removed.

The management of bladder disturbances due to a lesion of the nervous system is discussed in Chapter 18, as is promotion of a bowel training program. The management of urinary incontinence from other causes is discussed in Chapter 42.

Managing Cognitive Dysfunction. Some patients with certain neurological disorders, such as brain tumors, head injuries, and strokes, experience cognitive impairment characterized by deficits in memory or impaired abstract thinking, judgment, and intellectual performance. Such problems profoundly affect not only the patient but also the caregiver and the family.

In general, the nurse counsels the family to provide a stable, dependable environment, minimize confusion, provide sensory cues, give information simply and in a positive manner, and readjust tasks to fit the patient's level of functioning. When the patient becomes agitated and displays undesirable behavior, providing some type of motor distraction (giving him something to hold) and reducing environmental stimulation (turning off the television) can be effective. Patients may also respond to taped messages from family members. These tapes provide familiar voices to the patient and may reduce aggitation. Managing patients with brain damage involves a combination of psychiatric and neuroscience nursing skills.

Managing Sexual Dysfunction. Sexual dysfunction may be due to a lesion in the neural pathways in which there is loss of erection, lubrication, ejaculation, or emission. The nurse encourages expression of concerns and feelings. The patient and partner need to be assured that their concerns and fears about sexual function are important issues deserving attention. Discussion of these issues and counseling by one skilled in sexual counseling of the disabled can be initiated.

Promoting Effective Coping. Patients with neurologic dysfunctions face multiple stressors: serious and often unpredictable outcomes; assault on self-image; and, in many instances, a long-term illness. The patient and family may respond to the diagnosis and the lengthy treatment with depression, anger, denial, and anxiety.

The family faces the disruption caused by illness, which means an alteration in life-style, role changes, and possible intrafamilial conflicts. Denial or nonacceptance by the family can produce enormous strains on its individual members. The family requires time to deal with their feelings of powerlessness, ambivalence, anger, and guilt. Supportive members of the health care team may assist the family in coping with these feelings. Family members should be included and educated about the patient's therapy, understand the nature of the neurologic dysfunction and the meaning of remissions and exacerbations, and have some awareness of present and future changes.

Monitoring and Managing Potential Complications

Pneumonia. Vigorous chest physiotherapy, suctioning, and frequent monitoring of pulmonary function are essential to prevent respiratory distress or failure and pneumonia. Pneumonia, in turn, can lead to respiratory distress or failure and may necessitate endotracheal intubation. Once intubated, patients with neurologic dysfunction may require a prolonged period of "weaning" from the ventilator due to muscle weakness and dependency on the ventilator. Should pneumonia develop, the patient will require antibiotic therapy. Arterial blood gases should be monitored to assess respiratory function and cultures obtained to identify the presence of infective organisms. Efforts are made to reduce the risk for aspiration and aspiration pneumonia.

Pressure Ulcers. Although preventing pressures is imperative, should ulcers develop, extensive debridement, dressing changes, and skin grafting may be necessary. Pressure ulcers are assessed for drainage, odor, and the presence of granulating tissue. As a result of a sacral pressure ulcer the patient may require a diverting colostomy until the pressure ulcer has healed.

Evaluation

Expected Outcomes

1. Exhibits improved respiratory status
   a. Arterial blood gases within acceptable range
   b. Absence of crackles
2. Handles secretions without aspiration
3. Demonstrates adequate skin integrity
   a. Adheres to turning and positioning schedule
   b. Skin intact without evidence of pressure ulcers
4. Demonstrates improving joint mobility
   a. Participates in range-of-motion exercises
   b. Uses adaptive equipment
   c. Exhibits no contractures
5. Participates in self-care activities within limitations
   a. Compensates for limitations
   b. Identifies goals for self-care
6. Reports no pain
7. Achieves adequate nutritional intake
   a. Maintains weight
   b. Exhibits safe feeding methods
8. Exhibits increasing control of bowel and bladder function
   a. Actively participates in bowel and bladder management program
   b. Experiences infrequent bowel and bladder incontinence
9. Exhibits pre-illness cognitive function
   a. Exhibits insight into cognitive limitations
   b. Uses alternative approaches to compensate for altered cognitive function
10. Verbalizes the ability to participate in satisfactory sexual relationship
11. Demonstrates use of effective coping skills
12. Exhibits no complications
   a. Exhibits no manifestations of pneumonia, respiratory failure, or aspiration
   b. No evidence of pressure ulcers

Increased Intracranial Pressure

Pathophysiology

Intracranial pressure (ICP) is the result of the amount of brain tissue, intracranial blood volume, and cerebrospinal fluid (CSF) within the skull at any one time. The normal ICP varies depending on the position of the patient and is considered to be less than or equal to 15 mm Hg.

The rigid cranial vault contains brain tissue (1400 g), blood (75 ml), and CSF (75 ml). The volume and pressure of these three components are usually in a state of equilibrium. The **Monro-Kellie hypothesis** states that because of the limited space for expansion within the skull, an increase in any one of these components causes a change in the volume of the other, by either displacing or shifting CSF, increasing the absorption of CSF, or decreasing cerebral blood volume. Without such changes, intracranial pressure will begin to rise.

Under normal circumstances, minor changes in blood volume and CSF volume occur constantly when there are changes in intrathoracic pressure (coughing, sneezing, straining), posture, and blood pressure, and fluctuations in arterial blood gas levels. Pathologic conditions such as head injury, stroke, inflammatory lesions, brain tumor, or intracranial surgery alter the relationship between intracranial volume and pressure.

Cerebral Blood Flow. Increased ICP may significantly reduce cerebral blood flow and result in ischemia. If complete ischemia occurs and lasts for more than 3 to 5 minutes, the brain will suffer irreversible damage. In the early stages of cerebral ischemia, the vasomotor centers are stimulated and the systemic pressure rises to maintain cerebral blood flow. Usually this is accompanied by a slow bounding pulse and respiratory irregularities. These changes in blood pressure, pulse, and respiration are of importance clinically because they are clues to the existence of increased ICP.

The concentration of carbon dioxide in the blood and in brain tissues also has a role in the regulation of cerebral blood flow. A rise in carbon dioxide partial pressure ($PaCO_2$) causes the cerebral blood vessels to dilate, leading to increased cerebral blood flow and increased ICP, whereas a fall in $PaCO_2$ has a vasoconstricting effect. Decreased venous outflow may also increase cerebral blood volume, thus raising ICP.

Cerebral Edema. Cerebral edema or swelling occurs when there is an increase in the water content of the CNS. Certain brain tumors are associated with the excessive production of antidiuretic hormone, resulting in fluid retention. Even a small tumor may create a great increase in ICP. Table 59-1 identifies the factors that cause an increase in ICP and the associated physiology and nursing interventions.

Increased ICP as a Secondary Effect. Although an elevated ICP is most commonly associated with head injury, an elevated pressure may be seen as a secondary effect in a variety of other conditions: brain tumors, subarachnoid hemorrhage, and toxic and viral encephalopathies. Thus, increased ICP is the summation of a number of physiologic processes. Increased ICP from any cause affects cerebral perfusion and produces distortion and shifts of brain tissue.

Cerebral Response to Increased ICP. There are two stages of cerebral adjustment to the increase in ICP—compensation and decompensation.

Compensation. During the compensation phase, the brain and its components are able to alter their volume to allow for the expanding volume of brain tissue. The ICP, during this phase, is less than the arterial pressure, thus maintaining cerebral perfusion pressure. The patient in this stage does not demonstrate any changes in neurologic function.

The **cerebral perfusion pressure** (CPP) is calculated by subtracting the value of the ICP from the mean arterial pressure (MAP). The normal CPP is 60 to 150 mm Hg. The autoregulatory mechanism of the brain, once impaired, may cause CPP to be greater than 150 mm Hg or less than 60 mm Hg. Patients with CPP less than 50 mm Hg experience irreversible neurologic dysfunction due to decreased cerebral perfusion resulting in changes at the cellular level and cerebral hypoxia.

Decompensation. At a certain volume, the ability of the brain to compensate for an increase in pressure becomes ineffective and the decompensation phase begins. In this phase, the patient exhibits a change in mental status and in vital signs: bradycardia, widening pulse pressure, and respiratory changes. At this point, herniation of the brain stem occurs and occlusion of the cerebral blood flow ensues if therapeutic intervention is not initiated. **Herniation** occurs when a portion of brain tissue shifts from an area of high pressure to an area of lower pressure (Fig. 59-1). The herniated tissue exerts pressure on the brain area to which it has herniated or shifted and interferes with the blood supply in that area. Cessation of cerebral blood flow results in cerebral hypoxia leading to "brain death."

The term *brain death* is frequently used to identify those patients who lack cerebral function. The term may be misleading because although brain function has ceased, the patient's heart continues to beat, blood pressure is discernible, and breathing continues by mechanical venti-

TABLE 59-1 Increased ICP and Interventions

Factor	Physiology	Interventions	Rationale
Cerebral edema	Can be caused by contusion, tumor, or abscess; water intoxication (hypo-osmolality); alteration in the blood-brain barrier (protein leaks into the tissue causing water to follow)	Administer osmotic diuretics as prescribed (monitor serum osmolality) Maintain head of bed elevated 30 degrees Maintain alignment of the head	Promotes venous return Prevents impairment of venous return through the jugular veins
Hypoxia	A decrease in the PaO_2 causes cerebral vasodilation at less than 60 mm Hg	Maintain PaO_2 greater than 60 mm Hg Maintain oxygen therapy Monitor ABGs Suction the patient when needed Maintain a patent airway	Prevents hypoxia and vasodilation
Hypercapnia (elevated CO_2)	Causes vasodilation	Maintain $PaCO_2$ (normally 25–30 mm Hg), through hyperventilation	Decreased $PaCO_2$ prevents vasodilation and thus reduces the cerebral blood volume
Impaired venous return	Increases the cerebral blood volume	Maintain head alignment Elevate head of bed 30 degrees	Hyperextension, rotation, or hyperflexion of the neck causes a decreased venous return
Increase in intrathoracic or abdominal pressure	Increase in these pressures due to coughing, PEEP, Valsalva maneuver causes a decrease in venous return	Monitor ABGs and keep PEEP as low as possible Provide humidified oxygen Administer laxatives as prescribed.	To keep secretions loose and easy to suction or expectorate Soft bowel movements will prevent straining or Valsalva maneuver

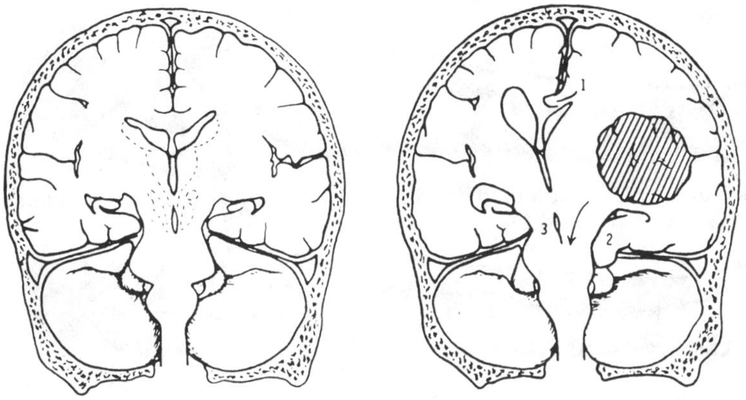

FIGURE 59-1. Cross section of a normal brain (**left**) and a brain with intracranial shifts from supratentorial lesions (**right**). (1) Herniation of the cingulate gyrus under the falx. (2) Herniation of the temporal lobe into the tentorial notch. (3) Downward displacement of the brain stem through the notch. (From Plum F and Posner J, Diagnosis of Stupor and Coma, 2nd ed. Contemporary Neurology Series. Philadelphia, FA Davis, 1972.)

lation. When discussing brain death with family members, it is important to use the word "dead" rather than "brain death," which may confuse them. (See the Ethical Question display.)

Clinical Manifestations

When ICP increases to the point at which the brain's ability to adjust has reached its limits, neural function is impaired; this may be manifested by changes in the level of consciousness and by abnormal respiratory and vasomotor responses.

The level of responsiveness/consciousness is the most important indicator of the patient's condition.

- The earliest sign of increasing ICP is *lethargy.* Slowing of speech and delay in response to verbal suggestions are early indicators.

Any sudden change in the patient's condition, such as becoming restless (without apparent cause), appearing confused, or displaying increasing drowsiness, has neurologic significance. These signs may result from compression of the brain due to either swelling from hemorrhage or edema or an expanding intracranial lesion (hematoma or tumor), or a combination of both.

As pressure increases, the patient may react only to loud auditory or painful stimuli. At this stage, serious impairment of brain circulation is probably taking place, and immediate surgical intervention may be required.

Abnormal motor responses in the form of decortication, decerebration, or flaccidity may occur. The patient may initially respond by assuming a decorticate posture. In **decortication,** there is internal rotation and flexion of the upper extremities and plantar flexion of the lower extremities (Fig. 59-2*A*); this occurs with damage to the cerebral hemispheres. **Decerebration**, the extension and outward rotation of the upper extremities and plantar flexion of the lower extremities (Fig. 59-2*B*), represents damage to the midbrain or pons. If the stupor deepens, the patient responds to painful stimuli by moaning but may not attempt to withdraw.

As the condition worsens, **flaccidity** occurs; the extremities become flaccid and reflexes are absent. The patient has a rag doll appearance. The jaw sags and the tongue becomes flaccid; airway obstruction and inadequate respiratory exchange may occur. When the coma is profound, with the pupils dilated and fixed and respirations impaired, a fatal outcome is usually inevitable.

ETHICAL QUESTION:

When Should Life Support be Discontinued from Brain Dead Patients?

Discussion

Although brain death is legally defined as death in all 50 states, families and health care professionals continue to struggle with this concept. As a result, physicians may offer families of brain dead patients the *option* of discontinuing life support, or they may leave the impression that the brain-dead patient might recover. Brain-dead patients can be left on life-support systems for days or weeks at great monetary expense. Should familes be encouraged to agree to the discontinuation of life support for their brain-dead family member?

Dilemma

The family's desire to act in the best interest of the patient conflicts with current medical practice (beneficence versus integrity of the health professions).

Discussion

- What arguments would you offer *in favor of* discontinuing life support for brain-dead patients within hours of diagnosis regardless of family wishes?
- What arguments would you offer *in favor of* waiting for family consent to discontinue life support?

Management

Increased ICP constitutes a true emergency and must be treated promptly. As pressure rises, the brain substance is compressed. Secondary phenomena caused by circulatory impairment and edema may lead to death.

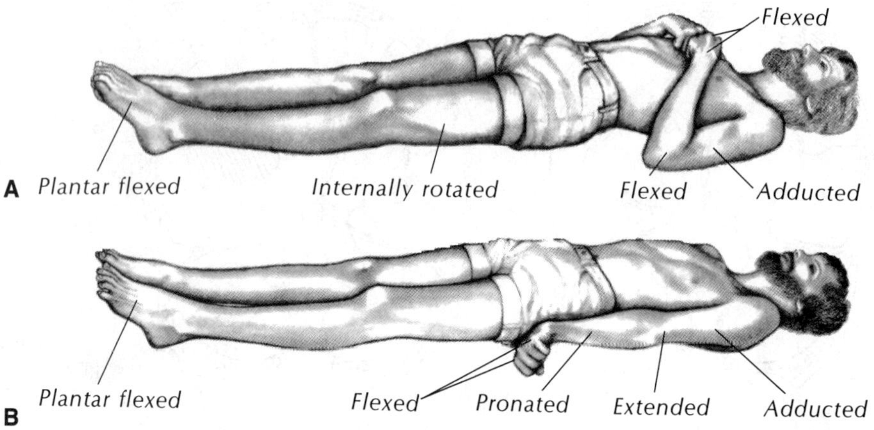

FIGURE 59-2. Abnormal posture responses to stimuli. (**A**) Decorticate posturing involving adduction and flexion of upper extremities, internal rotation of lower extremities, and plantar flexion of the feet. (**B**) Decerebrate posturing involving extension and outward rotation of the upper extremities and plantar flexion of the feet.

The immediate management to relieve increased ICP is based on reducing the size of the brain by decreasing cerebral edema, lowering the volume of CSF, or decreasing blood volume, while maintaining cerebral perfusion. These goals are accomplished by administering osmotic diuretics and corticosteroids, restricting fluids, draining CSF, hyperventilating the patient, controlling fever, and reducing cellular metabolic demands.

Decreasing Cerebral Edema. *Osmotic diuretics* (mannitol, glycerol) may be given to dehydrate the brain and reduce cerebral edema. They act by drawing water across intact membranes, thereby reducing the volume of brain and extracellular fluid. An indwelling urinary catheter is usually inserted to monitor urinary output and to manage the resulting diuresis. When a patient is receiving osmotic diuretics, serum osmolality should be determined to assess hydration status.

Corticosteroids (such as dexamethasone) help reduce edema surrounding brain tumors when a brain tumor is the cause of increased ICP.

Maintaining Cerebral Perfusion. The cardiac output is maintained to provide adequate perfusion to the brain. Improvements in cardiac output are made using fluid volume and inotropic agents, such as dobutamine hydrochloride. The effectiveness of the cardiac output is reflected in the cerebral perfusion pressure (p. 1710).

Reducing CSF and Blood Volume. *CSF drainage* may be frequently employed because the removal of even a small amount of CSF may dramatically reduce ICP and restore cerebral perfusion pressure. Care should be used in draining CSF, since excessive drainage may result in collapse of the ventricles.

Hyperventilation with a volume ventilator or manual resuscitation bag produces respiratory alkalosis, which in turn causes cerebral vasoconstriction. The result of this action is a reduction in cerebral blood volume and lowering of ICP. It is considered a short-term means of control.

Controlling Fever. Temperature control is aimed at preventing an elevation of temperature, because fever increases cerebral metabolism and the rate at which cerebral edema forms. Strategies to reduce temperature include administration of antipyretic medications, as prescribed, and use of a cooling blanket. The patient's temperature is monitored closely, and the patient is observed for shivering, which should be avoided because it increases the patient's ICP. Chlorpromazine (Thorazine) may be prescribed to control shivering.

Reducing Metabolic Demands. Reduction of cellular metabolic demands may also be accomplished through the administration of high doses of *barbiturates* when the patient is not responsive to conventional treatment. The mechanism by which barbiturates decrease ICP and protect the brain is uncertain, but the resultant comatose state is thought to reduce metabolic requirements of the brain, thus providing some protection.

Another method of reducing cellular metabolic demand and improving oxygenation is administration of pharmacologic *paralyzing agents* (muscle relaxants such as pancuronium [Pavulon]). The patient who receives these agents is unable to move; the result is a decreased oxygen demand at the cellular level. Because the patient is unable to respond or report pain, sedation and analgesia must be provided since the paralyzing agents do not provide either.

Patients receiving barbiturates or pharmacologic paralyzing agents are cared for in a critical care unit and require cardiovascular monitoring, endotracheal intubation, mechanical ventilation, intracranial pressure monitoring, and arterial pressure monitoring. Patients who are receiving barbiturates also require monitoring of blood and serum barbiturate levels.

Evaluating Pharmacologic Paralysis. The level of pharmacologic paralysis can be assessed by the **"train of four" procedure** or test. This procedure tests the patient's response to four electrical impulses applied to the ulnar nerve .5 seconds apart. If the receptors in the neuromuscular junction are not totally saturated—that is, some of the receptors are able to accept impulses—the patient will demonstrate a twitching movement of the thumb. A patient whose thumb does not twitch is said to be overparalyzed, and the paralyzing agent should be reduced to a level at which the patient has some twitch response.

In addition to the twitch response, other important parameters that must be assessed include blood pressure, heart rate, respiratory rate, and response to ventilator therapy (*e.g.*, bucking the ventilator). The level of pharmacologic paralysis is adjusted based on the twitch response and the physical assessment parameters.

Complications of Increased ICP

Complications of increased ICP include brain stem herniation, diabetes insipidus, and syndrome of inappropriate anti-diuretic hormone.

Brain stem herniation results from excessive increase in intracranial pressure, when the pressure builds in the cranial vault and the brain tissue presses down on the brain stem. This increasing pressure on the brain stem results in the cessation of blood flow to the brain, causing irreversible brain anoxia and brain death.

Diabetes insipidus (DI) is the result of decreased secretion of anti-diuretic hormone. The patient has excessive urine output. Therapy consists of administration of fluid volume, electrolyte replacement, and vasopressin (Desmopressin, DDAVP) therapy. Diabetes insipidus is discussed in more detail in Chapter 40.

Syndrome of inappropriate anti-diuretic hormone (SIADH) is the result of increased secretion of antidiuretic hormone. The patient becomes volume overloaded and has decreased urine output. Treatment of SIADH includes fluid restriction and administration of phenytoin to decrease ADH release or lithium to increase free water loss. Further discussion of this syndrome is presented in Chapter 40.

❑ *NURSING PROCESS*
The Patient With Increased Intracranial Pressure

Assessment

The patient's level of consciousness is assessed based on the criteria identified in the Glasgow Coma Scale: eye opening, verbal response and motor response. (See p. 1690 for a more detailed discussion of the Glasgow Coma Scale.)

The patient's responses are rated on a scale of from 3 to 15. A 3 indicates a severe impairment of neurologic function; a score of 15 indicates that the patient is responsive to the three criteria.

Eye opening can assist in determining the cause of a neurologic deficit. If the patient is in a coma but has spontaneous eye opening, the problem may be metabolic, whereas if the patient has no eye opening there could be a neurologic problem.

Verbal response must be carefully evaluated. One cannot assume that because the patient responds, he or she is oriented. The examiner needs to further assess the patient's orientation to time, place, and person. When recording the response of a patient who is intubated, the examiner should write down "T" (T for a tracheostomy or endotracheal tube in place) because the patient will be unable to respond verbally.

The **motor response** includes spontaneous movement, movement caused by noxious stimuli such as an injection or pinch, and posturing. The two types of posturing to note are decerebrate and decorticate (see Fig. 59-2). Occasionally, these responses cannot be elicited if the patient has been given pharmacologic paralyzing agents. In this case, the total assessment is not completed and the reason is documented.

Patients with increased ICP demonstrate other changes that may herald a further increase in ICP. These include subtle changes, changes in vital signs, headache, pupillary changes, and vomiting.

Subtle Changes. Restlessness, headache, forced breathing, purposeless movements, and mental cloudiness may be early clinical indications of rising ICP. The first indicator of increasing intracranial pressure is a change in the level of consciousness.

Changes in Vital Signs. Alterations in vital signs may be a late sign of increased ICP. As the ICP increases, the pulse rate and respiratory rate decrease and the blood pressure and temperature rise. Specific signs to observe for include arterial hypertension, bradycardia, and respiratory irregularity; the development of any of these signs warrants further investigation. Respiratory irregularities that are frequently observed include *Cheyne-Stokes breathing* (rhythmic waxing and waning of rate and depth of respirations alternating with brief periods of apnea) and *ataxic breathing* (irregular breathing with a random sequence of deep and shallow breaths).

The vital signs of the patient compensate as long as the circulation of the brain is preserved. If, as a result of brain compression, the major circulation begins to fail, the pulse and respirations become rapid and the temperature usually rises but does not follow a consistent pattern. The pulse pressure (the difference between the systolic and the diastolic pressure) widens; this is considered a serious development. Immediately preceding these changes in clinical responses, there is usually a period when the pulse fluctuates rapidly, varying from a slow rate to a rapid one. Immediate surgical intervention is necessary to prevent death.

The vital signs may not always be altered, even in the event of increased ICP. The patient is assessed for changes in the level of responsiveness and for the presence of shock; these manifestations aid in evaluation.

Headache. The headache is constant, increasing in intensity, and aggravated by movement or straining.

Pupillary and Ocular Changes. Increasing pressure or an expanding clot can displace the brain against the oculomotor or optic nerves, producing pupillary changes.

- ❑ The pupils are periodically inspected with a penlight to evaluate size, configuration, and reaction to light. Both eyes are compared for similarities or differences.
- ❑ Gaze is evaluated as to whether it is conjugate (paired; working together) or dysconjugate.
- ❑ The ability of the eyes to abduct and adduct is assessed to evaluate cranial nerve function.
- ❑ The retina and optic nerve are inspected for hemorrhage and papilledema.

Vomiting. Recurrent or projectile vomiting may occur with increased pressure on the reflex center for vomiting located in the medulla.

Clinical assessment is not always a reliable guide in recognizing increased ICP, especially in comatose patients. In certain situations, ICP monitoring is an essential part of management (see pp. 1715–1718).

Diagnosis

Nursing Diagnoses

Based on the assessment data, the patient's major nursing diagnoses may include the following:

- ❑ Altered cerebral tissue perfusion related to the effects of increased ICP
- ❑ Ineffective breathing patterns related to neurologic dysfunction (brain stem compression, structural displacement)

- Ineffective airway clearance related to accumulation of secretions secondary to depression of level of responsiveness
- Risk for fluid volume deficit related to dehydration procedures
- Altered urinary and bowel elimination related to effects of medication, indwelling urethral catheter, and diminished fluid/food intake
- Risk for infection related to ICP monitoring system (intraventricular catheter)

Other relevant nursing diagnoses could include altered oral mucous membranes related to mouth-breathing, absence of pharyngeal reflex, and inability to ingest fluids; potential for impairment of skin integrity related to immobility and constraints imposed by ICP monitoring system; impaired tissue integrity (cornea) related to diminished or absent corneal reflex; and altered family processes related to crisis situation. (These diagnoses are discussed in the sections on the patient undergoing intracranial surgery, p. 1737, and the patient with a head injury, Chapter 60.)

Collaborative Problems/ Potential Complications

Based on the assessment data, potential complications may include:

- Brain stem herniation
- Diabetes insipidus
- Syndrome of inappropriate antidiuretic hormone (SIADH)

Planning and Implementation

Goals. The goals for the patient may include achievement of cerebral tissue perfusion through reduction in ICP, normalization of respiration, achievement of airway clearance, restoration of fluid balance, normal urinary and bowel function, absence of infection, and absence of complications.

Nursing Interventions

Achieving Cerebral Tissue Perfusion. In addition to ongoing nursing surveillance, the following nursing strategies may be employed to reduce factors contributing to the elevation of ICP:

- The patient is monitored for bradycardia and a rising blood pressure, called Cushing's reflex, which are signs of increasing ICP.
  - The patient's head is kept in a neutral (midline) position, which is maintained with the use of a cervical collar if necessary, to promote venous drainage.
  - Slight elevation of the head is maintained to aid in venous drainage unless otherwise prescribed.
  - Extreme rotation of the neck and flexion of the neck are avoided because compression or distortion of the jugular veins increases ICP.
- Extreme hip flexion is avoided because this position causes an increase in intra-abdominal and intrathoracic pressures, which can produce a rise in ICP.
- The Valsalva maneuver, which can be produced by straining at defecation or even moving in bed, is to be avoided. Stool softeners may be prescribed. If the patient is alert and able to eat, a diet high in fiber may be indicated.
  - The patient can be instructed to exhale (which opens the glottis) while being moved or turned passively.
- Isometric muscle contractions are also contraindicated, because they raise the systemic blood pressure and hence the ICP.
- Relatively minor changes in the patient's position may significantly affect ICP. If monitoring parameters demonstrate that turning the patient raises ICP, rotating beds and turning sheets may be used and the patient's head may be held by the nurse's hands during turning to minimize the stimuli that increase ICP.
- Before suctioning is instituted, the patient should be preoxygenated and hyperventilated using the sigh mode on the ventilator with 100% oxygen. Suction should not last longer than 15 seconds.
- Nursing activities that raise ICP should be avoided if possible. Spacing the occurrence of nursing interventions may prevent transient increases in ICP.
- During nursing interventions the ICP should not rise above 25 mm Hg and should return to baseline levels within 5 minutes.
- Emotional stress and frequent arousal from sleep are to be avoided. A calm atmosphere is maintained. Environmental stimuli (noise, conversation) should be minimal.
- Abdominal distention, which increases intra-abdominal and intrathoracic pressure and ICP, should be noted. Enemas and cathartics are avoided if possible.
- High levels of positive end-expiratory pressure (PEEP) are avoided since PEEP may decrease venous return to the heart and decrease venous drainage from the brain through increased intrathroacic pressure.

Attaining Normal Respiratory Pattern. The patient must be monitored constantly for respiratory irregularities. Increased pressure on the frontal lobes or deep midline structures may result in Cheyne-Stokes respirations, whereas pressure in the midbrain may cause hyperventilation. When there is involvement of the lower portion of the brain stem (the pons and medulla), respirations become irregular and eventually cease.

When hyperventilation therapy is used to reduce ICP (by causing cerebral vasoconstriction and a decrease in cerebral blood volume), the nurse collaborates with the respiratory therapist in monitoring the arterial carbon dioxide pressure ($PaCO_2$), which is usually maintained between 25 and 30 mm Hg.

- A neurologic observation record (see Fig. 58-12) is maintained, and all observations are made in relation to the patient's baseline condition. Repeated assessments of the patient are made (sometimes minute by minute) so that improvement or deterioration may be noted immediately. If the patient's condition deteriorates, preparations are made for surgical intervention.

Achieving Airway Clearance. The patency of the airway is assessed. If secretions are obstructing the airway, they must be suctioned with care, because transient elevations of ICP occur with suctioning. The patient is hyperoxygenated before and after suctioning to maintain adequate oxygenation. Hypoxia caused by poor oxygenation leads to poor cerebral perfusion. Coughing is discouraged because coughing and straining also increase ICP. The lung fields are auscultated at least every 8 hours to determine the presence of adventitious sounds or any areas of congestion. Elevating the head of the bed may aid in clearing secretions as well as improving venous drainage of the brain.

Attaining Fluid Balance. The administration of various dehydrating agents is part of the treatment protocol. Corticosteroids are used to reduce cerebral edema; also, fluids may be restricted. All of these treatment modalities promote the development of dehydration.

The patient's skin turgor, mucous membranes, serum, and urine osmolality are monitored for signs of dehydration. If fluids are given intravenously, the nurse makes sure that they are administered at a slow to moderate rate with an IV infusion pump to prevent too-rapid administration. For the patient receiving mannitol, the nurse observes for the possible development of congestive heart failure and pulmonary edema because mannitol may cause fluid to shift from the intracellular compartment to the intravascular system.

For patients undergoing dehydrating procedures, vital signs, including blood pressure, must be monitored to assess fluid volume status. These patients also need careful oral hygiene because dehydration is associated with mouth dryness. Frequent rinsing of the mouth, lubrication of the lips, and removal of encrustations relieve dryness and promote comfort.

Attaining Normal Urinary and Bowel Elimination. The urine is tested for specific gravity and monitored for glucose. A complication of corticosteroid therapy is hyperglycemia.

An indwelling urinary catheter is usually inserted to permit assessment of renal function and fluid status. The nurse observes for purulent drainage and encrustation at the urinary meatus, maintains the patency of the catheter and an unobstructed flow of urine by proper positioning of the tubing and drainage bag, uses measures to prevent cross-contamination (*e.g.*, handwashing, keeping patients with infections separate from other patients), and monitors urine for the presence of infection (cloudy, bloody, or foul-smelling urine).

During the acute phase the urine output should be monitored every 2 to 4 hours; an output greater than 200 ml/hr for 2 consecutive hours may indicate the onset of diabetes insipidus.

The patient's lower abdomen is assessed for signs of bowel distention, and the area is auscultated for bowel sounds. Usually the stools are tested for blood if the patient is on high doses of corticosteroids because gastrointestinal bleeding is a complication of this therapy. The patient is cautioned to avoid straining while having a bowel movement because the Valsalva maneuver can increase ICP.

Preventing Infection. Infection is the greatest risk when ICP is monitored with an intraventricular catheter (see discussion, next section). Most health care facilities have written protocols for managing these systems and maintaining their sterility, and strict adherence to them is essential.

The dressing over the ventricular catheter must be kept dry because a wet dressing is conducive to bacterial growth. Aseptic technique is used when managing the system and changing the ventricular drainage bag. The drainage system is also checked for loose connections because they cause leakage and contamination of the CSF as well as inaccurate readings of ICP. The patient is monitored for signs and symptoms of meningitis: fever, chills, nuchal (neck) rigidity, and increasing or persisting headache.

Monitoring and Managing Potential Complications. The patient's ICP is monitored closely for continuous elevation or significant increase over baseline. The patient's vital signs are assessed at the time the increase in ICP is noted. Patients with impending brain herniation will exhibit an increase in blood pressure, a decrease in heart rate, and a change in pupillary response. The response of the patient who is not receiving paralyzing agents may change from decerebrate or decorticate posturing to a flaccid or rag doll appearance. The patient requires rapid intervention of mannitol or drainage of CSF if a drainage system (ventriculostomy) is in place.

The patient's urine output should be monitored closely. Diabetes insipidus requires fluid and electrolyte replacement along with the administration of vasopressin (Desmopressin, DDAVP) to replace and slow the urine output. Serum electrolytes should be monitored for replacement.

Syndrome of inappropriate anti-diuretic hormone (SIADH) requires fluid restriction and monitoring of serum electrolytes.

Evaluation

Expected Outcomes

1. Demonstrates improved cerebral tissue perfusion
   a. Becomes increasingly oriented to time, place, and person
   b. Follows verbal commands; answers questions correctly
2. Attains normal respirations
   a. Breathes in a normal pattern
   b. Attains or maintains arterial blood gas values within acceptable range
3. Is free of excessive airway secretions
4. Attains improved fluid balance
   a. Takes fluids orally
   b. Serum and urine osmolality are within acceptable range
5. Attains normal urinary and bowel elimination
6. Has no sign of infection
   a. Has no fever
   b. Dressings and arterial, intravenous, and urinary catheter sites free of signs of infection
   c. Has no purulent drainage from ventricular drainage system
7. Is free of complications
   a. Urine output is within normal limits
   b. Serum electrolytes are within acceptable limits
   c. Intracranial pressure remains within normal limits
   d. Responds to commands appropriately without decerebrate or decorticate posturing

Monitoring Intracranial Pressure

ICP is monitored by measuring CSF pressure within the lateral ventricle, the subarachnoid space, and the epidural space. Waveforms are captured and recorded on an oscilloscope to reflect the pressure exerted within the skull by the brain, cerebral blood, and CSF. The volume of any of these elements can expand as a result of tumor, trauma, edema, bleeding, and cerebral vessel dilatation. ICP monitoring provides a continuous reflection of the intracranial status.

The purposes of ICP monitoring are to (1) identify increased pressure early in its course (before cerebral damage occurs), (2) quantify the degree of abnormality, (3) initiate appropriate treatment, (4) provide access to CSF for sampling and drainage, and (5) evaluate the effectiveness of treatment.

A large number of devices are available to monitor ICP by means of sensors or transducers that are either connected to an intraventricular catheter or implanted in the skull (Fig. 59-3). The standard types are the intraventricular catheter, subarachnoid screw or bolt, and epidural pressure-recording devices. A fiberoptic transducer-tipped catheter is an alternative to these devices.

Ventricular Catheter Monitoring. In ventricular catheter monitoring (see Fig. 59-3*A*) a fine catheter is inserted into a lateral ventricle, by means of either a twist drill or burr hole opening. The catheter is connected by way of a fluid-filled system to a transducer, which records the pressure in the form of an electrical impulse. In addition to obtaining continuous ICP recordings, the ventricular catheter allows CSF to drain, particularly during acute rises in pressure. The ventriculostomy also can be used to drain the ventricle of blood.

This method of monitoring is useful in patients with infratentorial brain tumors and aneurysms. Also, continuous drainage of ventricular fluid under pressure control is an effective method of treating intracranial hypertension. Another advantage of an indwelling ventricular catheter is the route it provides for the intraventricular administration of medications and the instillation of air or a contrast medium for ventriculography (see Chapter 58).

Complications include ventricular infection, meningitis, ventricular collapse, occlusion of the catheter by brain tissue or blood, and problems with the monitoring system.

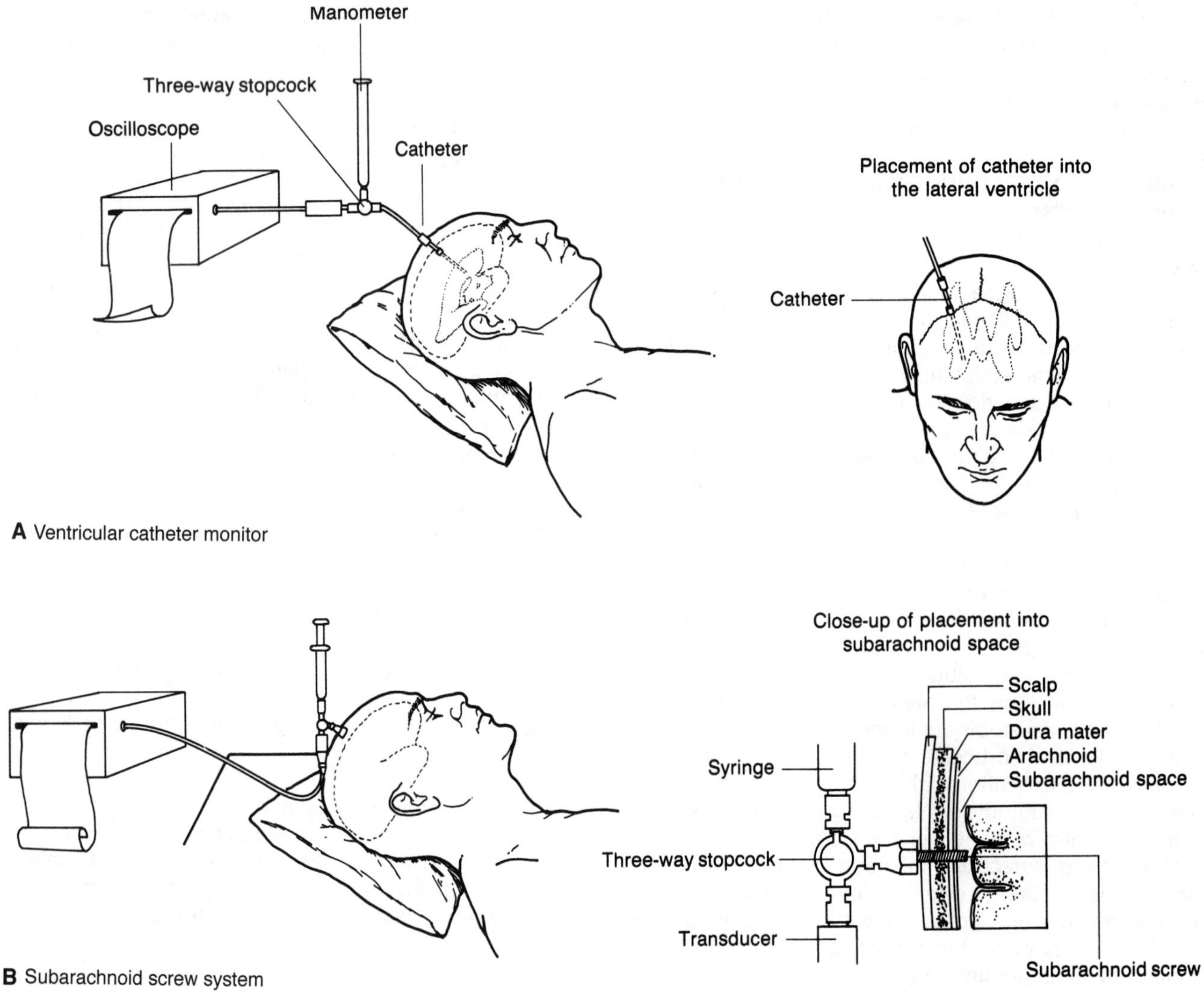

FIGURE 59-3. Intracranial pressure monitoring devices: (**A**) ventricular catheter and (**B**) subarachnoid or hollow screw. These devices are connected to a pressure transducer and display system.

Subarachnoid Screw. The subarachnoid screw (or bolt) is a hollow screw that is inserted through the skull and dura mater to the cranial subarachnoid space (see Fig. 59-3*B*). It has the advantage of not requiring a ventricular puncture. The subarachnoid screw is inserted through a small hole in the skull under local anesthesia; it is attached to a pressure transducer, and the output is recorded on an oscilloscope for continuous monitoring.

The hollow screw technique is useful in patients with head trauma and those with supratentorial brain tumors. It has the additional advantage of avoiding complications from brain shift and small ventricle size. Complications include blockage of the screw by clot or brain tissue, which leads to loss of pressure tracing and a decrease in accuracy at high ICP readings.

A **disposable stopcock network** is used for both the ventricular catheter and hollow screw monitoring systems to connect the patient to a pressure transducer and display system. The network contains a three-way stopcock attached to the screw or ventricular catheter and a nondistensible saline-filled tubing leading from one outlet of the three-way stopcock to a manifold containing the pressure transducer. The pressure transducer transmits a waveform through the electrical circuitry to a display system for continuous monitoring. The system is flushed with sterile saline at prescribed intervals to keep the device patent.

Epidural Monitoring. Another method of ICP monitoring requires implantation of a miniature transducer in the epidural space, usually through a burr hole in the skull. One type of epidural ICP-monitoring mode is the *pneumatic flow sensor*, which functions on a nonelectrical basis. This pneumatic epidural monitoring system has a low incidence of infection and complications and appears to read pressures accurately. Calibration of the system is maintained automatically, and abnormal pressure waves trigger an alarm system. One disadvantage to the epidural catheter is the inability to withdraw CSF for analysis.

Fiberoptic Transducer-Tipped Catheter. A fiberoptic transducer-tipped catheter (FTC) is becoming widely used as an alternative to standard intraventricular, subarachnoid, and subdural systems. The miniature transducer reflects pressure changes, which are converted to electrical signals in an amplifier and displayed on a digital monitor. The FTC can be inserted into the ventricle, subarachnoid space, subdural space, or brain parenchyma or under a bone flap.

ICP Wave Forms

ICP is not in a steady state but fluctuates, as indicated by waves of high pressure and troughs of relatively normal pressure. These waves have been classified as A waves (plateau waves), B waves, and C waves (Fig. 59-4).

The **plateau waves (A waves)** are transient, paroxysmal, recurring elevations of ICP that may last from 5 to 20 minutes and range in amplitude between 50 and 100 mm Hg. Plateau waves have clinical significance and indicate changes in vascular volume within the intracranial compartment that are beginning to compromise cerebral perfusion. A waves may increase in amplitude and frequency, reflecting cerebral ischemia and brain damage that can occur before overt signs and symptoms of raised ICP are seen clinically. This is especially true in the unconscious patient. Rapid variations of pressure waves may also indicate a potentially serious intracranial situation. Therefore, ICP monitoring provides a more objective evaluation of early or changing trends of ICP than other forms of observation.

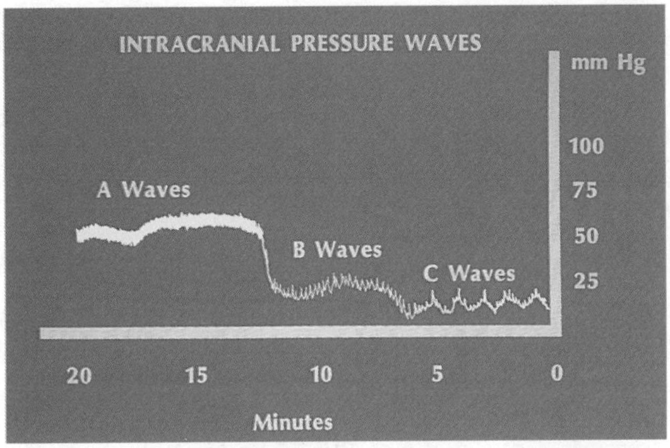

FIGURE 59-4. Intracranial pressure waves. Composite diagram of A (plateau) waves, which indicate changes in vascular volume; B waves, which may indicate intracranial hypertension and variations in the respiratory cycle; and C waves, which relate to variations in systemic arterial blood pressure and respirations.

B waves are of shorter duration (30 seconds to 2 minutes) with smaller amplitude (up to 50 mm Hg). They have less clinical significance but, if seen in runs in a patient with depressed consciousness, may precede the appearance of A waves. B waves may be seen in patients with intracranial hypertension and decreased intracranial compliance.

C waves are small, rhythmic oscillations with frequencies of approximately six per minute. They appear to be related to rhythmic variations of the systemic arterial blood pressure and respirations.

Clinical Implications. ICP is expressed by ventricular fluid pressures that normally fluctuate in the range of 0 to 10 mm Hg (110 to 140 mm H_2O). Sustained elevations above 15 mm Hg (200 mm H_2O) are generally considered abnormal.

Nursing Implications of ICP Monitoring

The trend of ICP measurements over time is an important indication of the underlying state of the patient. The measurement of ICP is only one parameter of patient assessment, however. Repeated neurologic checks and clinical examinations remain important measures.

Strict aseptic technique is used when handling any part of the monitoring system. The insertion site is inspected for signs of infection. The patient's temperature, pulse, and respirations are closely monitored for systemic signs of infection. All connections and stopcocks are checked for leaks because small leaks can distort pressure readings.

When ICP is recorded, the transducer is zeroed at a particular reference point, usually 2.5 cm (1 in) above the ear in the supine patient; this point corresponds to the level of the foramen of Monro (Fig. 59-5). (CSF pressure readings depend on the patient's position.) For subsequent pressure readings, the patient's head should be in the same position relative to the transducer.

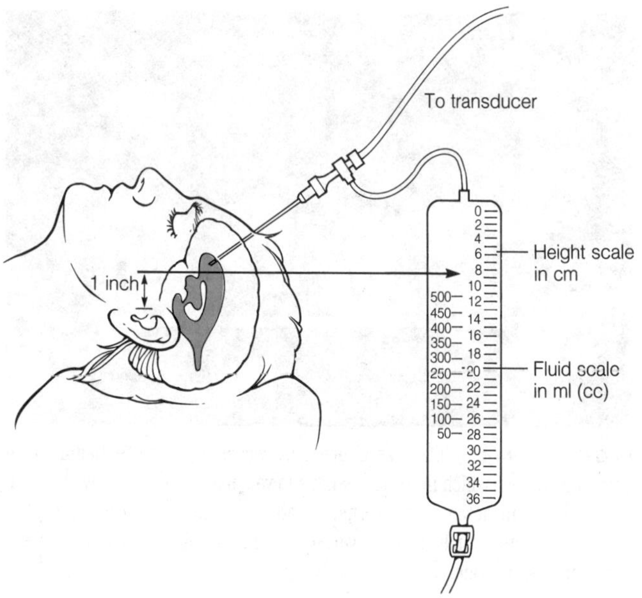

FIGURE 59-5. Location of foramen of Monro for calibration of ICP monitoring system.

Whenever technology is associated with patient management, the nurse must be certain that the technology remains functioning. The most important concern must be the patient who is attached to the technology. Talking in a soothing tone and gently touching the patient's hand or stroking the cheek may be helpful in reducing emotional stress.

The patient with an increase in ICP can initially be alert and oriented without apparent neurologic deficit, or may be unresponsive. Astute observation, comparison of findings with previous observations, and interventions can assist in preventing life-threatening elevations of ICP. Assessment of the patient includes the Glasgow Coma Scale, pupil changes, posture changes, and ICP measurement.

Gerontologic Considerations. Geriatric patients with increased ICP may demonstrate an alteration in their mental status. The altered mental status may be a result of the change in ICP or of the aging process. The nurse needs to involve the patient's family in obtaining a baseline assessment of mental status. Radiologic examination may reveal that the geriatric patient has a chronic or old hematoma; however, the family may be unaware of falls the patient has experienced when alone. The family should be included in the treatment plan as much as possible, because of the possible need for assistance at home or for a long-term care facility.

Electrophysiologic Monitoring

The patient with increased ICP may also undergo electrophysiologic monitoring. *Evoked potential monitoring* is accomplished by measuring the electrical potentials produced by nerve tissue in response to external stimulation. The external stimulation can be either auditory, visual, or sensory. This diagnostic test is useful for following the course of a patient in a drug-induced coma, one receiving muscle relaxants, or in any condition in which clinical examination is unreliable. Special EEG recording devices are used to evaluate some forms of abnormal EEG activity. The major nursing responsibility is ensuring that the electrodes are not displaced during patient care interventions.

The Unconscious Patient

Unconsciousness is a condition in which cerebral function is depressed, ranging from stupor to coma. In **stupor,** the patient shows symptoms of annoyance when stimulated by something unpleasant, such as a pinch or loud clapping of hands, and may draw back or make facial grimaces or unintelligible sounds. **Coma** is a clinical state of unconsciousness in which the patient is unaware of himself or herself and the environment. **Akinetic mutism** is a state of unresponsiveness to the environment in which the patient makes no movement or sound but sometimes opens his or her eyes. A **persistent vegetative state** is one in which the patient is described as wakeful but devoid of conscious content, without cognitive or effective mental function.

The causes of unconsciousness may be neurologic (head injury, stroke), toxicologic (drug overdose, alcohol intoxication), or metabolic (hepatic or renal failure, diabetic ketoacidosis).

Diagnostic Evaluation

Laboratory tests used to identify the cause of unconsciousness include tests for blood glucose, electrolytes, serum ammonia, blood urea nitrogen (BUN), osmolality, calcium, prothrombin time, serum ketones, alcohol, drugs, and arterial blood gases.

Medical Management

The first priority of treatment of the unconscious patient is to obtain and maintain a patent airway. The patient may be either orally or nasally intubated, or a tracheostomy may be performed. Until the determination has been made concerning the patient's ability to breathe on his own, a mechanical ventilator is used to maintain adequate oxygenation. An intravenous catheter is inserted to maintain fluid balance status, and nutritional support by either a feeding tube or gastrostomy tube should be started. The circulatory status of the patient (blood pressure, heart rate) is monitored to ensure that adequate perfusion to the body and brain is being maintained.

Complications

Potential complications for the unconscious patient include respiratory failure, pneumonia, pressure ulcers, and aspiration. **Respiratory failure** may develop shortly after the patient becomes unconscious. If the patient is unable to breathe on his or her own, supportive care is initiated to provide adequate ventilation. **Pneumonia** is commonly seen in patients who are receiving mechanical ventilation or in those who are unable to maintain and clear their airway. The unconscious patient is unable to move or turn, resulting in remaining in a fixed position. This predisposes the patient to **pressure ulcers,** which may become infected and be a source of sepsis. **Aspiration of gastric contents** or feedings may occur, precipitating the development of pneumonia or occluding the airway.

❑ NURSING PROCESS
The Unconscious Patient

Assessment

The level of consciousness (responsiveness) is assessed by evaluating eye-opening responses, verbal responses, and motor responses to a command or painful stimulus. These responses are assessed and scored using the Glasgow Coma Scale (see p. 1690). The pupils are evaluated as to size, equality, and reaction to light. In addition, the movement of the eyes is noted. Facial symmetry, swallowing reflexes, and deep tendon reflexes are noted.

If the patient is not responding to commands, motor response is tested by applying a painful stimulus (firm but *gentle* pressure) on the supraorbital notch or to the nailbed or by squeezing a muscle. If the patient attempts to push away or withdraw, the response is recorded as purposeful or appropriate. An inappropriate or nonpurposeful response is random and aimless.

The unconscious patient with severely impaired cerebral function may respond to a stimulus with *decorticate* or *decerebrate posturing* (see p. 1711). Decerebrate posturing indicates a more severe alteration in responsiveness. The patient with flaccid motor response has the most neurologic involvement; this patient is unable to move any extremity and has no muscle tone in any of the extremities. Paralysis or stroke must be ruled out as a cause of flaccidity.

Body functions (circulation, respiration, elimination, fluid and electrolyte balance) are examined in a systematic manner. If the patient is comatose and localized signs are severe, it is assumed that neurologic disease is present until proved otherwise. If the patient is comatose and a pupillary light reflex is preserved, a toxic or metabolic disorder is suspected.

Important signs to evaluate in assessing the unconscious patient include level of consciousness, respiration, pupil size and reaction to light, eye movement, corneal reflexes, facial symmetry, swallowing reflex, response to noxious stimuli, possible Babinski sign, and abnormal posturing. Chart 59-1 summarizes the assessment signs and clinical significance in each of these areas.

Diagnosis

Nursing Diagnoses

Based on the assessment data, the patient's major nursing diagnoses may include the following:

- ❑ Ineffective airway clearance related to inability to clear respiratory secretions
- ❑ Risk for injury related to altered cognitive status
- ❑ Risk for fluid volume deficit related to inability to ingest fluids
- ❑ Altered oral mucous membranes related to mouth-breathing, absence of pharyngeal reflex, and inability to ingest fluids
- ❑ Risk for impaired skin integrity related to immobility or restlessness
- ❑ Impaired tissue integrity of cornea related to diminished or absent corneal reflex
- ❑ Ineffective thermoregulation related to damage to hypothalamic center
- ❑ Altered urinary elimination (incontinence or retention) related to the unconscious state
- ❑ Altered bowel elimination (diarrhea and/or constipation) related to the unconscious state
- ❑ Altered family processes related to sudden crisis of unconsciousness

Collaborative Problems/ Potential Complications

Based on the assessment data, potential complications may include:

- ❑ Respiratory distress or failure
- ❑ Pneumonia
- ❑ Aspiration
- ❑ Pressure ulcer

Planning and Implementation

Goals. The goals of care of the unconscious patient may include maintenance of a clear airway, protection from injury, attainment of fluid volume balance, achievement of intact oral mucous membranes, maintenance of normal skin integrity, absence of corneal irritation, attainment of thermoregulation, absence of urinary retention and infection, absence of diarrhea or fecal impaction, maintenance of intact family or support system, and absence of complications.

The quality of nursing care provided for an unconscious patient may literally mean the difference between life and death, because the patient's protective reflexes are impaired. The nurse must assume responsibility for the patient until the basic reflexes return (coughing, blinking, and swallowing) and the patient becomes conscious and oriented. Thus, the major nursing goal is to provide these protective reflexes until the patient regains these functions.

Nursing Interventions

Maintaining the Airway. The most important consideration in the management of the unconscious patient is to establish an adequate airway and ensure ventilation. Obstruction of the airway is a risk facing the unconscious patient because the epiglottis and tongue may relax, occluding the oropharynx, or the patient may aspirate vomitus or nasopharyngeal secretions.

- ❑ The patient is positioned in a lateral or semiprone position, which permits the jaw and tongue to fall forward and thus facilitates drainage of secretions.
- ❑ An unconscious patient must not be allowed to remain on the back.
- ❑ The accumulation of secretions in the pharynx presents a serious problem. Because the patient is unable to swallow and lacks pharyngeal reflexes, these secretions must be removed to eliminate the danger of aspiration.
- ❑ Elevating the head of the bed to a 30-degree angle helps prevent aspiration of secretions.
- ❑ The patient requires frequent suctioning and oral hygiene.

CHART 59-1
Nursing Assessment of the Unconscious Patient

Examination	Clinical Assessment	Clinical Significance
Level of responsiveness or consciousness	Eye opening; verbal and motor responses; pupils (size, equality, reaction to light)	Obeying commands is a favorable response and demonstrates a return to consciousness
Pattern of respiration		Disturbances of respiratory center of brain may result in various respiratory patterns
	Cheyne-Stokes respiration	Suggests lesions deep in both hemispheres; area of basal ganglia and upper brain stem
	Hyperventilation	Suggests onset of metabolic problem or brainstem damage
	Ataxic respiration with irregularity in depth/rate	Ominous sign of damage to medullary center
Eyes		
Pupils (size, equality, reaction to light)	Equal, normally reactive pupils	Suggests that coma is toxic or metabolic in origin
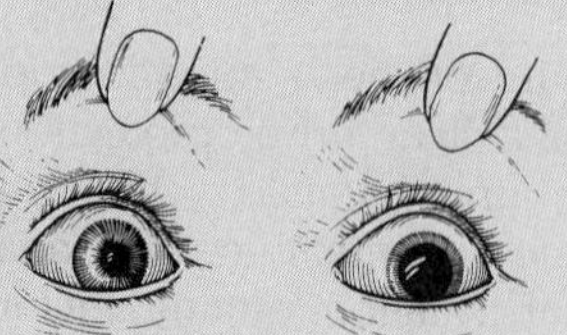	Equal or unequal diameter	Localizing sign
	Progressive dilatation	Indicates increasing intracranial pressure
	Fixed dilated pupils	Indicates injury at level of midbrain
Eye movements	Normally eyes should move from side to side	Functional and structural integrity of brain stem is assessed by inspection of extraocular movements; usually absent in deep coma
Corneal reflex 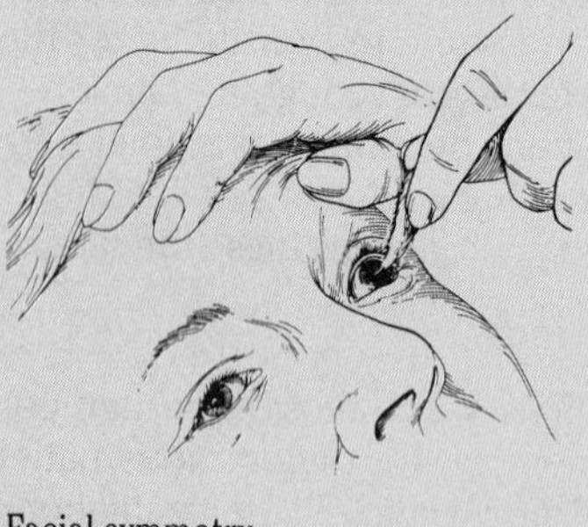	When cornea is touched with a wisp of clean cotton, blink response is normal	Tests cranial nerves V and VII; localizing sign if unilateral; absent in deep coma
Facial symmetry	Asymmetry (sagging, decrease in wrinkles)	Sign of paralysis
Swallowing reflex	Drooling versus spontaneous swallowing	Absent in coma Paralysis of cranial nerves X and XII
Neck	Stiff neck	Subarachnoid hemorrhage, meningitis
	Absence of spontaneous neck movement	Fracture or dislocation of cervical spine
Response of extremity to noxious stimuli 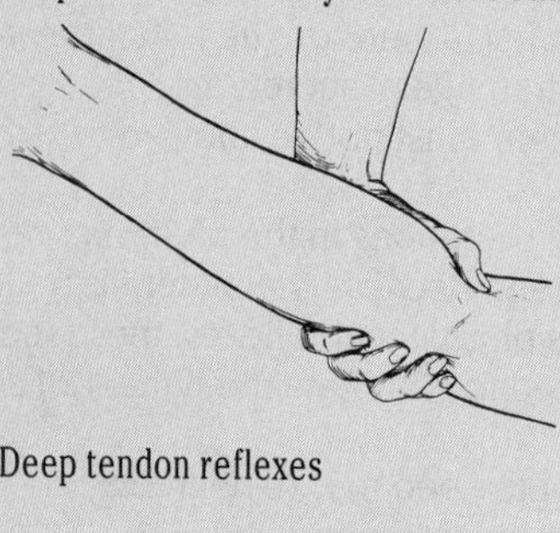	Firm pressure on a joint of the upper and lower extremity Observe spontaneous movements	Asymmetrical response in paralysis Absent in deep coma
Deep tendon reflexes	Tap patellar and biceps tendons	Brisk response may have localizing value Asymmetric response in paralysis Absent in deep coma

(continued)

CHART 59-1 *(continued)*
Nursing Assessment of the Unconscious Patient

Examination	Clinical Assessment	Clinical Significance
Pathologic reflexes 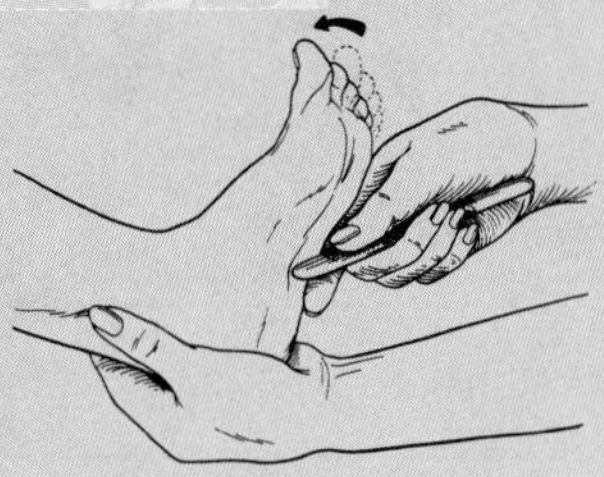	Firm pressure with blunt object on sole of foot moving along lateral margin and crossing to the ball of foot	Flexion of the toes, especially the great toe, is normal except in newborn Dorsiflexion of toes (especially great toe) indicates contralateral pathology of corticospinal tract (Babinski reflex) Localizing signs
Abnormal posture	Observation for posturing (spontaneous or in response to noxious stimuli) Flaccidity with absence of motor response Decorticate posture (flexion and internal rotation of forearms and hands) Decerebrate posture (extension and external rotation)	Deep extensive brain lesion Seen with cerebral hemisphere pathology and in metabolic depression of brain function Decerebrate posturing indicates deeper and more severe dysfunction than does decorticate posturing; implies brain stem pathology; poor prognostic sign

- Suctioning is performed to remove secretions from the posterior pharynx and upper trachea. With the suction turned off, a whistle-tip catheter is lubricated with a water-soluble lubricant and inserted to the desired level. Then the suction is turned on (negative pressure) while the aspirating catheter is withdrawn with a twisting motion of the thumb and forefinger. This twisting maneuver prevents the suctioning end of the catheter from irritating the tracheal or pharyngeal mucosa, because irritation increases secretions and produces mucosal trauma and bleeding. Before and after suctioning, the patient is hyperoxygenated and hyperventilated to prevent hypoxia.
- The chest is auscultated at least every 8 hours for crackles, rhonchi, or absence of breath sounds.
- The patient may require intubation and mechanical ventilation. The nurse must maintain the patency of the endotracheal tube or tracheostomy, provide frequent oral care, monitor arterial blood gases, and maintain ventilator settings.
- Chest physiotherapy and postural drainage are initiated to promote pulmonary hygiene unless contraindicated by the patient's underlying condition.

Maintaining Safety. For the protection of the patient, padded siderails are provided and raised at all times. Every measure that is available and appropriate for calming and quieting a disturbed patient should be carried out. Any form of restraint is likely to be countered by the patient with resistance, leading to self-injury or to a dangerous increase in ICP; therefore, physical restraints should be avoided if possible and a written prescription obtained if their use is essential.

Maintaining Fluid and Nutritional Balance. The patient is assessed for hydration status; the mucous membranes are examined and the skin is assessed for tissue turgor. The fluid needs of this patient are initially met by giving the required fluids intravenously and then by nasogastric or gastrostomy feedings.

- Intravenous solutions and blood transfusions for patients with intracranial conditions must be administered slowly. If given too rapidly, they may increase the ICP. The quantity of fluids administered may be restricted to minimize the possibility of producing cerebral edema.
- Fluids are never given by mouth to the patient who cannot swallow. The ability to swallow without choking may be tested by placing a wet swab in the patient's mouth and observing the ability to swallow the small amount of liquid from the swab.
- A feeding tube, placed in the duodenum, or a gastrostomy tube may be inserted for the administration of enteral feedings.

Maintaining Healthy Oral Mucous Membranes. The patient's mouth is inspected for dryness, inflammation, and the presence of crusting. The unconscious patient requires conscientious oral care because there is a risk of parotitis if the mouth is not kept scrupulously clean. The mouth is cleansed and rinsed carefully to remove secretions and crusts and to keep the mucous membranes moist. A thin coating of petrolatum on the lips prevents drying, cracking, and the formation of encrustations. If the patient has an endotracheal tube, the tube should be moved to the opposite side of the mouth daily to prevent ulceration of the mouth and lips.

Maintaining Skin Integrity. Preventing skin breakdown requires continuing nursing assessment and intervention. Special attention is given to unconscious patients because they are insensitive to external stimuli. This includes a regular schedule of turning to avoid pressure, which can cause breakdown and necrosis of the skin. Turning also provides kinesthetic (sensation of movement), proprioceptive (awareness of position), and vestibular (equilibrium) stimulation. After turning, the patient is carefully repositioned to prevent ischemic necrosis over pressure areas. Dragging the patient up in bed must be avoided because this creates a shearing force and friction on the skin surface.

Maintaining correct body position is important; equally important is passive exercise of the extremities so that contractures are prevented (Fig. 59-6). The use of splints or foam boots aids in the prevention of footdrop and eliminates the pressure of bedding on the toes. Trochanter rolls supporting the hip joints keep the legs in proper alignment. The arms should be in abduction, the fingers lightly flexed, and the hands in a position of slight supination. The patient's heels and feet should be assessed for pressure areas (Fig. 59-7). Specialty beds, such as fluidized or low-air-loss beds, may be used to decrease pressure on bony prominences.

Maintaining Corneal Integrity. Some unconscious patients lie with their eyes open and have inadequate or absent corneal reflexes. The cornea is likely to become irritated or scratched, leading to keratitis and corneal ulcers.

The eyes may be cleansed with cotton balls moistened with sterile normal saline to remove debris and discharge (Fig. 59-8). If artificial tears are prescribed, they may be instilled every 2 hours. Periocular edema (swelling around the eyes) often occurs after cranial surgery. Cold compresses may be prescribed, and care must be exerted to avoid contact with the cornea. Eye patches should be used cautiously because of the potential for corneal abrasion from the cornea coming in contact with the patch.

Attaining Thermoregulation. High fever in the unconscious patient may be caused by infection of the respiratory or urinary tract, drug reactions, or damage to the hypothalamic temperature-regulating center. A slight elevation of temperature may be caused by dehydration. The temperature of the environment is determined by the patient's condition. If body temperature is elevated, a minimum amount of bedding—a sheet or perhaps only a small drape—is used.

The room may be cooled to 18.3°C (65°F). However, if the patient is elderly and does not have an elevated temperature, a warmer environment is needed. Regardless of the temperature, the air should be fresh and free from odors.

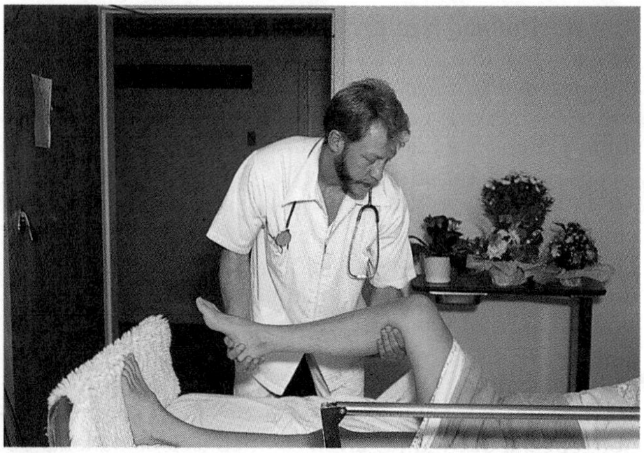

FIGURE 59-6. Passive range-of-motion exercises are carried out frequently to prevent contractures in the unconscious patient.

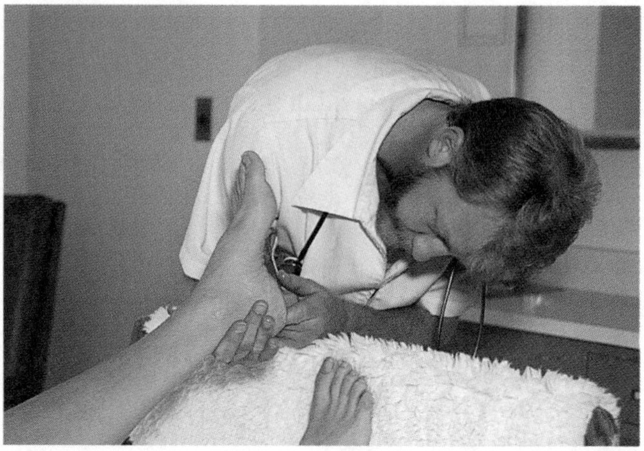

FIGURE 59-7. Maintaining skin integrity in the unconscious patient includes frequent turning, skin care, and assessment of pressure areas such as the back of the foot.

- The body temperature of an unconscious patient is *never* taken by mouth. Rectal temperature is preferred to the less accurate axillary temperature.

Hyperthermia is treated by the measures described on p. 1707. Shivering is avoided.

Preventing Urinary Retention. The unconscious patient is either incontinent or has urinary retention. The patient's bladder is palpated at intervals to determine whether urinary retention is present, because a full bladder may be an overlooked cause of incontinence.

If there are signs of urinary retention, initially an indwelling urinary catheter attached to a closed drainage system is inserted. Because the catheter is a major cause of urinary infection, the patient is observed for fever and cloudy urine. The area around the urethral orifice is inspected for drainage. The urinary catheter is usually removed when the patient has a stable cardiovascular system and if no problems with diuresis, sepsis, or voiding existed before the onset of coma. Although many unconscious patients urinate spontaneously after catheter removal, the patient's bladder should be palpated periodically for urinary retention.

An external catheter (condom catheter) for the male patient and absorbent pads for the female patient can be used for the unconscious patient who can urinate spontaneously although involuntarily. As soon as consciousness is regained, a bladder training program is initiated.

The incontinent patient is monitored frequently for skin irritation and skin breakdown. Appropriate skin care is implemented to prevent these complications.

Promoting Bowel Function. The abdomen is assessed for distention by listening for bowel sounds and measuring the girth of the abdomen with a tape measure. There is a risk of diarrhea from infection, antibiotics, and hyperosmolar fluids. Frequent loose stools may also occur with fecal impaction. Commercial fecal collection bags are available for patients with fecal incontinence.

Immobility and lack of dietary fiber may cause constipation. The nurse monitors the number and consistency of bowel movements and performs a rectal examination for signs of fecal impaction. The patient may require an enema every other day to empty the lower colon. Enemas may be contraindicated, however, if the Valsalva maneuver in-

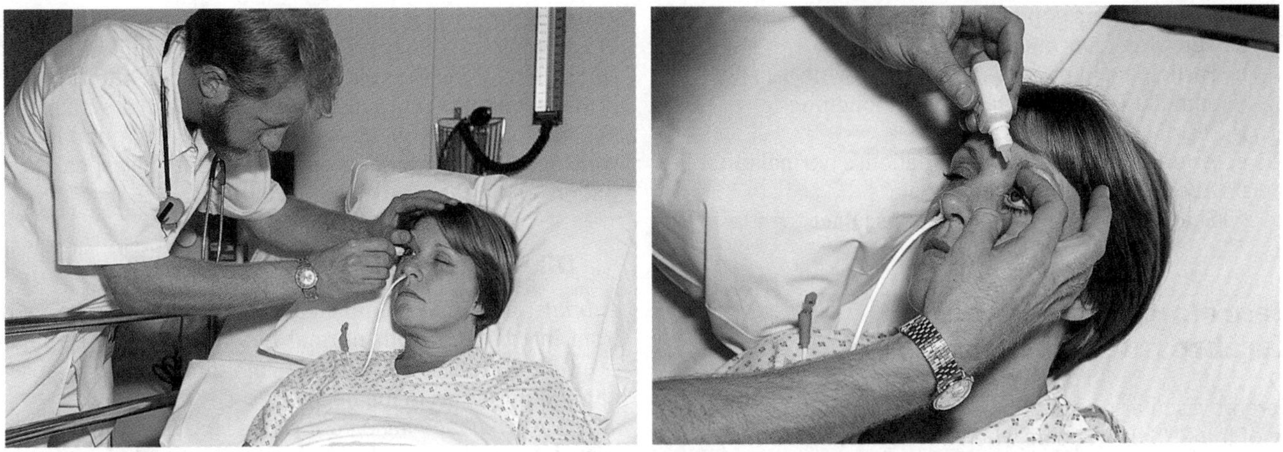

FIGURE 59-8. Eye care of the unconscious patient includes cleansing the eyelids to remove encrustations and instilling eyedrops, if prescribed.

creases a compromised ICP. A glycerin suppository stimulates bowel emptying. Stool softeners may be prescribed and can be administered with tube feedings.

Promoting Sensory Stimulation. Continuing sensory stimulation is provided to help overcome the profound sensory deprivation of the unconscious patient. Efforts are made to maintain the sense of daily rhythm by keeping the usual day and night patterns for activity and sleep. The nurse touches and talks to the patient and encourages family members and friends to do so. Communication is extremely important and includes touching the patient and spending enough time with him or her to become sensitive to his or her needs. It is also important to avoid making any negative comments about status or prognosis in the patient's presence.

The nurse orients the patient to time and place at least once every 8 hours. Sounds from the patient's home and workplace may be introduced by means of a tape recorder. In addition, family members can read to the patient from a favorite book and may suggest radio and television programs that the patient previously enjoyed as a means of enriching the environment and providing familiar input. When the patient has regained consciousness, videotaped family or social events may assist the patient in recognizing family and friends and allow him or her to be a part of missed events.

Supporting the Family. The family of the unconscious patient may be thrown into a sudden state of crisis and go through the process of severe anxiety, denial, anger, remorse, grief, and reconciliation. To assist family members to mobilize their own adaptive capacities, the nursing personnel can reinforce and clarify information about the patient's condition, permit the family to be involved in the care of their loved one, and listen to and encourage ventilation of feelings and concerns while supporting them in their decision-making process concerning posthospitalization management and placement. Families may benefit from participation in support groups offered through the hospital, rehabilitation facility, or community organizations.

Attaining Self-Care. The unconscious patient is dependent on the nursing staff for all activities of daily living (ADLs). As soon as consciousness returns, the nurse begins to teach, support, encourage, and supervise these activities until the patient gains independence. (See Activities of Daily Living in Chapter 18.)

Monitoring and Managing Potential Complications. **Pneumonia, aspiration,** and **respiratory failure** are potential complications in any patient who is unconscious and unable to protect his or her own airway or to turn, cough, and take deep breaths. The longer the period of unconsciousness, the greater the risk that the patient will develop pulmonary complications.

The patient's vital signs and respiratory function are monitored closely to detect any signs of respiratory failure or distress. Total blood count and arterial blood gases are assessed for adequate red blood cells to carry oxygen and the effectiveness of ventilation. Chest physiotherapy and suctioning are initiated to prevent respiratory complications such as pneumonia. If pneumonia develops, cultures are obtained to identify the organism so that appropriate antibiotics can be administered.

The unconscious patient is monitored closely for evidence of impaired skin integrity, and strategies to prevent skin breakdown and **pressure ulcers** are continued through all phases of care, including hospital, rehabilitation, and home care. Those factors that contribute to impaired skin integrity (*e.g.*, incontinence, inadequate dietary intake, pressure on bony prominences, edema) are addressed. If pressure ulcers do develop, strategies to promote healing are undertaken. Additionally, care is taken to prevent bacterial contamination of pressure ulcers, as this may lead to sepsis and septic shock. Assessment and management of pressure ulcers are discussed in detail in Chapter 18.

Evaluation

Expected Outcomes

1. Maintains clear airway and demonstrates appropriate breath sounds
2. Experiences no injuries
3. Attains/maintains adequate fluid status
   a. Has no clinical signs of dehydration
   b. Demonstrates normal range of serum electrolytes
4. Attains/maintains healthy oral mucous membranes
5. Maintains normal skin integrity
6. Has no corneal irritation
7. Attains or maintains thermoregulation
8. Has no urinary retention
9. Has no diarrhea or fecal impaction

10. Family members coping with crisis
    a. Verbalize fears and concerns
    b. Participate in patient's care and provide sensory stimulation through talking and touching
11. Is free of complications:
    a. Arterial blood gases within patient's normal range
    b. Absence of signs of pneumonia
    c. Skin over pressure areas remains intact

Neurologic Deficits Due to Cerebrovascular Disease

Cerebrovascular disease refers to any functional abnormality of the CNS that occurs when the normal blood supply to the brain is disrupted. The pathology may involve an artery, a vein, or both. Cerebral circulation can become impaired as a result of partial or complete occlusion of a blood vessel or hemorrhage resulting from a tear in the vessel wall. The blood vessel most frequently associated with cerebrovascular disease is the internal carotid artery.

Vascular disease of the CNS may be caused by arteriosclerosis (most common), hypertensive changes, arteriovenous malformations, vasospasm, inflammation, arteritis, or embolism. As a result of vascular disease, blood vessels lose their elasticity, become hardened, and develop atheromatous deposits, or plaques, which may be the source of an embolus. The lumen of the vessel may gradually close, causing impairment of cerebral circulation and ischemia of the brain. If cerebral ischemia is transient, as in a transient ischemic attack, there is usually no lasting neurologic deficit. Occlusion of a large vessel, however, produces cerebral infarction. The vessel may rupture and produce hemorrhage.

Transient Ischemic Attacks

A transient ischemic attack (TIA) is a transient or temporary episode of neurologic dysfunction commonly manifested by a sudden loss of motor, sensory, or visual function. It may last a few seconds or minutes but no longer than 24 hours. Complete recovery usually occurs between attacks. A TIA may serve as a warning of impending stroke, which has its greatest incidence in the first month after the first attack.

The cause of this clinical entity is a temporary impairment of blood flow to a specific region of the brain due to a variety of reasons, including atherosclerosis of the vessels supplying the brain, obstruction of cerebral microcirculation by a small embolus, a decrease in cerebral perfusion pressure, cardiac dysrhythmias, and so on.

The most common sites of atherosclerosis in the extracranial arteries are at the bifurcation of the common carotid and at the origin of the vertebral arteries. Among the intracranial arteries, the middle cerebral artery is the most common site of atherosclerosis.

Clinical Manifestations

The classic symptom of carotid artery disease is *amaurosis fugax* (fleeting blindness) occurring without warning, in which there is sudden, painless loss of vision of one eye or dimming or graying out of the field of vision of one eye. This symptom is suggestive of retinal ischemia due to insufficiency of the homolateral ophthalmic or carotid artery. If the ischemia occurs in the vertebral basilar system, vertigo, diplopia, disturbances of consciousness, numbness or weakness in either a hand or leg, and difficulty speaking or understanding speech may be exhibited.

Diagnostic Evaluation

A *bruit* (abnormal sound heard on auscultation resulting from interference with normal blood flow) may be heard over the carotid artery. There are diminished or absent carotid pulsations in the neck.

Carotid phonoangiography may be performed, which provides auscultation, direct visualization, and photographic recording of carotid bruits. *Oculoplethysmography* (OPG) measures pulsation in blood flow through the ophthalmic artery. *Carotid angiography* visualizes intracranial and cervical vessels.

Digital subtraction angiography is used to define carotid artery obstruction and provide information on patterns of cerebral blood flow.

Management

Patients who are not candidates for surgical intervention may be placed on anticoagulant therapy to prevent future attacks and a possible massive cerebral infarction. Platelet-inhibiting drugs (particularly aspirin) are useful in decreasing the occurrence of cerebral infarction in patients who have experienced multiple TIAs. Prevention of future attacks is accomplished through treatment of hypertension and hyperglycemia and cessation of smoking.

Surgical intervention procedures in common use are endarterectomy (see below) and angioplasty, in which a catheter with a balloon is inserted in the artery to break up the plaque and dilate the artery.

Carotid Endarterectomy

A carotid endarterectomy is the removal of an atherosclerotic plaque or thrombus from the carotid artery to prevent stroke in patients with occlusive disease of the extracranial cerebral arteries. (Most ischemic strokes are associated with lesions of the extracranial arteries.)

Postoperative Care. After endarterectomy, a neurologic flow sheet is used to closely monitor and document the patient's neurologic status. The neurosurgeon is notified immediately if the patient develops a neurologic deficit. Formation of a thrombus at the side of endarterectomy can be suspected if there is a sudden increase in neurologic deficits, such as weakness on one side of the body. The patient should be prepared for reoperation.

The *primary complications* of carotid endarterectomy are stroke, cranial nerve injuries, infection or hematoma of the wound, and carotid artery disruption.

It is important to maintain adequate *blood pressure* levels in the immediate postoperative period. *Hypotension* is avoided to prevent cerebral ischemia and thrombosis.

Uncontrolled *hypertension* may precipitate cerebral hemorrhage, edema, hemorrhage in the operative wound, or disruption of the arterial reconstruction. Sodium nitroprusside is commonly used to reduce the blood pressure to previous levels.

Close cardiac monitoring is necessary because these patients have a high incidence of coronary artery disease.

Difficulty in swallowing, hoarseness, or other signs of *cranial nerve dysfunction* must be assessed. Some swelling in the neck after surgery is expected; if large enough, however, swelling and hematoma formation can obstruct the patient's airway. A tracheostomy set must be available.

Lack of treatment and monitoring of a patient who has experienced previous TIAs may result in a stroke and irreversible deficits.

Stroke (Cerebrovascular Accident)

A stroke, or cerebrovascular accident (CVA), is a sudden loss of brain function resulting from disruption of the blood supply to a part of the brain. Frequently it is the culmination of cerebrovascular disease of many years' standing.

Stroke is the primary neurologic problem in the U.S. and in the world. Although preventive efforts have brought about a steady decline in its incidence in the last several years, stroke is the third ranking cause of death, with an overall mortality rate of 18% to 37% for the first stroke and as high as 62% for subsequent strokes. There are approximately 2 million people surviving strokes who have some disability; of these, 40% need assistance with activities of daily living.

Causes of Stroke

A stroke usually results from one of four events: (1) thrombosis (a blood clot within a blood vessel of the brain or neck), (2) cerebral embolism (a blood clot or other material carried to the brain from another part of the body), (3) ischemia (decrease of blood flow to an area of the brain), and (4) cerebral hemorrhage (rupture of a cerebral blood vessel with bleeding into the brain tissue or spaces surrounding the brain). The result is an interruption in the blood supply to the brain, causing temporary or permanent loss of movement, thought, memory, speech, or sensation.

Cerebral Thrombosis. Cerebral arteriosclerosis and slowing of the cerebral circulation are major causes of cerebral thrombosis, which is the most common cause of stroke.

The signs of cerebral thrombosis vary. Headache is rather uncommon at the onset. Some patients may experience dizziness, cognitive changes, or seizures, and some may have an onset indistinguishable from that of intracerebral hemorrhage or cerebral embolism. In general, cerebral thrombosis does not develop abruptly, and a transient loss of speech, hemiplegia, or paresthesias in one half of the body may precede the onset of severe paralysis by a few hours or days.

Cerebral Embolism. Pathologic abnormalities of the left side of the heart, such as infective endocarditis, rheumatic heart disease, and myocardial infarction, as well as pulmonary infections, are the sites where emboli originate. It is possible that the insertion of a prosthetic heart valve may precipitate a stroke, because there is an increased incidence of embolism after this procedure. The risk of stroke following valve replacement can be reduced with postoperative anticoagulant therapy. Pacemaker failure, atrial fibrillation, and cardioversion for atrial fibrillation are other possible causes of cerebral emboli and stroke.

The embolus usually lodges in the middle cerebral artery or its branches, where it disrupts the cerebral circulation.

- Sudden onset of hemiparesis or hemiplegia with or without aphasia or loss of consciousness in a patient with cardiac or pulmonary disease is characteristic of cerebral embolism.

Cerebral Ischemia. Cerebral ischemia (insufficiency of the blood supply to the brain) is due mainly to atheromatous constriction of the arteries supplying the brain. The most common manifestation is a TIA.

Cerebral Hemorrhage. Hemorrhage may occur outside the dura mater (extradural or epidural hemorrhage), beneath the dura mater (subdural hemorrhage), in the subarachnoid space (subarachnoid hemorrhage), or within the brain substance (intracerebral hemorrhage). Figure 59-9 illustrates the locations of epidural, subdural, and intracerebral hematomas.

Extradural Hemorrhage. Extradural hemorrhage (epidural hemorrhage) is a neurosurgical emergency that requires urgent care. It usually follows skull fracture with a tear of the middle artery or other meningeal artery. The patient must be treated within hours of the accident in order to survive (see the section on head injury in Chapter 60.)

Subdural Hemorrhage. Subdural hemorrhage (excluding *acute* subdural hemorrhage) is basically the same as an epidural hemorrhage, except that in subdural hematoma usually a bridging vein is torn. Thus, a longer period (longer lucid interval) is required for the hematoma to form and

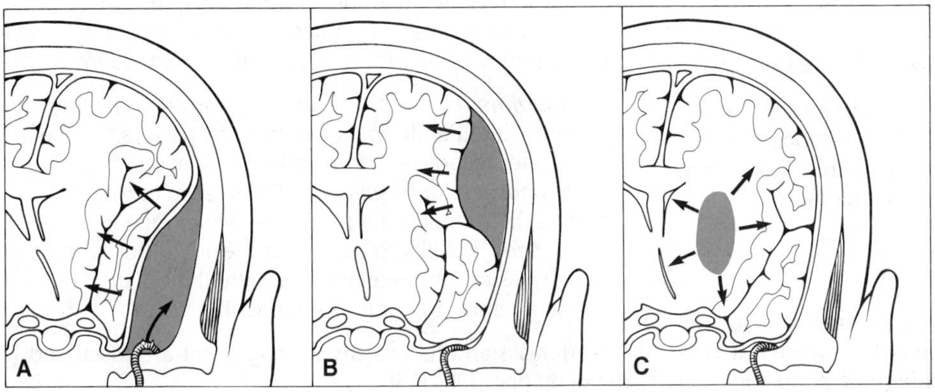

FIGURE 59-9. Cerebral hemorrhage or bleeding. (**A**) Epidural or extradural hematoma—bleeding between the inner skull and the dura, compressing the brain underneath. (**B**) Subdural hematoma—bleeding between the dura mater and arachnoid membrane. (**C**) Intracerebral hemorrhage—bleeding in the brain or the cerebral tissue with displacement of surrounding structures.

cause pressure on the brain. Some patients may have chronic subdural hemorrhages without exhibiting signs or symptoms. (This is also discussed in the section on head injury in Chapter 60.)

Subarachnoid Hemorrhage. Subarachnoid hemorrhage (hemorrhage occurring in the subarachnoid space) may occur as a result of trauma or hypertension, but the most common cause is a leaking aneurysm in the area of the circle of Willis and congenital arteriovenous malformations of the brain. Any artery within the brain can be the site of an aneurysm. (The treatment of intracranial aneurysms is discussed in Chapter 60.)

Intracerebral Hemorrhage. Hemorrhage or bleeding into the brain substance is most common in patients with hypertension and cerebral atherosclerosis, because degenerative changes due to these diseases usually cause rupture of the vessel. Strokes frequently occur in the 40- to 70-year-old age group. In persons younger than 40, intracerebral hemorrhages are usually caused by arteriovenous malformations, hemangioblastomas, and trauma. They also may be due to certain types of arterial pathology, presence of brain tumor, and the use of medications (oral anticoagulants, amphetamines, and a variety of addictive drugs).

The bleeding is usually arterial and occurs particularly around the basal ganglia. The clinical picture and the prognosis depend mainly on the degree of hemorrhage and brain damage. Occasionally, the bleeding ruptures the wall of the lateral ventricle and causes intraventricular hemorrhage, which is frequently fatal.

Usually the onset is abrupt, with severe headache. As the hematoma enlarges, a more pronounced neurologic deficit occurs in the form of decreased alertness and abnormalities in the vital signs. Patients with extensive bleeding and hemorrhage have a pronounced decrease in their level of consciousness and may become stuporous or completely unresponsive. If the bleeding is limited or develops gradually, there may be no significant pressure effects. Conversely, the full deficit may evolve in a matter of hours. A marked reduction in consciousness (stupor/coma) in the early phase of the bleeding episode usually has an ominous prognosis.

The treatment of intracerebral hemorrhage is controversial. If the hemorrhage is small, the patient is treated conservatively and symptomatically.

- The blood pressure is carefully reduced with antihypertensive medications. The patient's neurologic deficit may worsen if the blood pressure is reduced too low or too rapidly. The most effective form of treatment is the prevention of hypertensive vascular disease.

Risk Factors and Prevention of Stroke

Prevention of stroke is the best possible approach. Steps are taken to alter those factors and human conditions that predispose certain people to stroke or increase their risk of having a stroke. Chart 59-2 summarizes those risk factors.

CHART 59-2
Risk Factors in Stroke

- Hypertension—the major risk factor. Controlling hypertension is the key to preventing stroke.
- Cardiovascular disease—cerebral embolisms may originate in the heart.
  - Coronary artery disease
  - Congestive heart failure
  - Left ventricular hypertrophy
  - Rhythm abnormalities (especially atrial fibrillation)
  - Rheumatic heart disease
- High cholesterol
- Obesity
- Elevated hematocrit increases the risk of cerebral infarction
- Diabetes—associated with accelerated atherogenesis
- Oral contraceptives (especially with coexisting hypertension, smoking, and high estrogen levels)
- Smoking
- Drug abuse (especially cocaine)
- Alcohol consumption

Clinical Manifestations

A stroke causes a wide variety of neurologic deficits, depending on the location of the lesion (which vessels are obstructed), the size of the area of inadequate perfusion, and the amount of collateral (secondary or accessory) blood flow. Function of the damaged brain cannot be fully restored.

Motor Loss. Stroke is a disease of the upper motor neurons (see Table 58-1) and results in loss of voluntary control over motor movements. Because the upper motor neurons decussate (cross), a disturbance of voluntary motor control on one side of the body may reflect damage to the upper motor neurons on the opposite side of the brain. The most common motor dysfunction is **hemiplegia** (paralysis of one side of the body) due to a lesion of the opposite side of the brain. **Hemiparesis,** or weakness of one side of the body, is another sign.

In the early stage of stroke, the initial clinical feature may be flaccid paralysis and loss of or decrease in the deep tendon reflexes. When these deep reflexes reappear (usually by 48 hours), increased tone is observed along with spasticity (abnormal increase in muscle tone) of the extremities on the affected side.

Communication Loss. Other brain functions affected by stroke are language and communication. Stroke is the most common cause of aphasia. Dysfunction of language and communication may be manifested by the following:

- *Dysarthria* (difficulty in speaking), as demonstrated by poorly intelligible speech caused by paralysis of the muscles responsible for producing speech
- *Dysphasia* or *aphasia* (defective speech or loss of speech), which is mainly expressive or receptive
- *Apraxia* (inability to perform a previously learned action), as may be seen when a patient picks up a fork and attempts to comb his hair with it

Aphasia and its nursing management are discussed in detail on pp. 1735–1736.

Perceptual Disturbances. Perception is the ability to interpret sensation. Stroke can result in visual perception dysfunctions, disturbances in visual–spatial relationships, and sensory loss.

Visual perceptual dysfunctions are due to disturbances of the primary sensory pathways between the eye and visual cortex. **Homonymous hemianopsia** (loss of half of the visual field) may occur from stroke and may be temporary or permanent. The affected side of vision corresponds to the paralyzed side of the body (see assessment of visual field changes in Chapter 58). The patient's head turns away from the affected side of his body and he tends to neglect that side and the space on that side; this is called **amorphosynthesis**. In such instances, the patient is unable to see food on half of the tray, and only half of the room is visible. It is important for the nurse to constantly remind the patient of the other side of the body, maintain alignment of the extremities and, if possible, place the extremities where the patient is able to see them.

To assess for hemianopsia, the patient is asked to look at the examiner's face. The examiner's finger is placed about 30 cm (12 in) from the patient's ear on the unaffected side and is moved inward toward his field of vision. The patient is asked to indicate when he first detects movement of the examiner's finger. Inability to detect movement on one or both sides suggests visual neglect and hemianopsia.

This decreased field of vision must be kept in mind during all rehabilitation procedures. Personnel should approach the patient on the side where visual perception is intact. All visual stimuli (clock, calendar, television) should be placed on this side. The patient can be taught to turn his or her head in the direction of the defective visual field to compensate for this loss. The nurse should make eye contact with the patient and draw his or her attention to the affected side by encouraging the patient to move his or her head. The nurse may also want to stand at a position that encourages the patient to move or turn in order to visualize who is in the room. Increasing the natural or artificial lighting in the room and providing eyeglasses are important in increasing vision.

Disturbances in visual–spatial relationships (perceiving the relationship of two or more objects in spatial areas) are frequently seen in patients with left hemiplegia. The patient may not be able to dress without assistance because of an inability to match the clothing to the body parts. To assist this patient, the nurse can take steps to keep the environment organized and uncluttered because the patient with a perceptual problem is easily distracted. It is useful to suggest that the patient slow down and to offer some gentle reminders of where an object is located.

Sensory losses from stroke may take the form of slight impairment of touch or may be more severe, with loss of proprioception (ability to perceive position and motion of body parts) as well as difficulty in interpreting visual, tactile, and auditory stimuli.

Impairment of Cognitive Function and Psychologic Effects. If damage has occurred to the frontal lobe, learning capacity, memory, or other higher cortical intellectual functions may be impaired. Such dysfunction may be reflected in a limited attention span, difficulties in comprehension, forgetfulness, and a lack of motivation, which cause these patients to encounter frustrating problems in their rehabilitation programs. Depression is common and may be exaggerated by the patient's natural response to this catastrophic illness. Other psychologic problems are common and are manifested by emotional lability, hostility, frustration, resentment, and lack of cooperation.

Bladder Dysfunction. After a stroke the patient may have transient urinary incontinence due to confusion, inability to communicate needs, and inability to use the urinal/bedpan because of impaired motor and postural controls. Occasionally after a stroke the bladder becomes atonic, with impaired sensation in response to bladder filling. Sometimes control of the external urinary sphincter is lost or diminished. During this period, intermittent catheterization with sterile technique is carried out. When muscle tone increases and deep tendon reflexes return, bladder tone increases and spasticity of the bladder may develop. Because the patient's sense of awareness is clouded, persistent urinary incontinence or urinary retention may be symptomatic of bilateral brain damage. Continuing bladder and bowel incontinence may reflect extensive neurologic damage.

Summary. Table 59-2 reviews the neurologic deficits frequently seen in patients with strokes. Table 59-3 compares the symptoms seen in right hemispheric stroke with those seen in left hemispheric stroke. Approximately 90% of the population have left-hemisphere dominance, which controls the right side of the body. A small number of left-handed people have left- rather than right hemisphere dominance.

Management of the Acute Phase of a Patient With Stroke

A patient who is in deep coma on admission to the hospital is considered to have a poor prognosis. Conversely, a fully conscious patient faces a more favorable outcome. The acute phase usually lasts 48 to 72 hours. Management of the unconscious patient is described on pp. 1718–1722. Maintaining the airway and adequate ventilation are priorities in the acute phase.

- The patient is placed in a lateral or semiprone position with the head of the bed slightly elevated to lower cerebral venous pressure.
- Endotracheal intubation and mechanical ventilation are necessary for patients with massive stroke, because respiratory arrest is usually the life-threatening factor in this situation.
- The patient is monitored for pulmonary complications (aspiration, atelectasis, pneumonia), which may be due to loss of airway reflexes, immobility, or hypoventilation.
- The heart is examined for abnormalities in size and rhythm and signs of congestive heart failure.

Management

Medical treatment of the patient with a stroke may include diuretics to reduce cerebral edema, which reaches maximum levels 3 to 5 days after cerebral infarction. Anticoagulants may be prescribed to prevent further development or propagation of the thrombosis or embolization from

TABLE 59-2 Neurologic Deficits of Stroke: Manifestations and Nursing Implications

Neurologic Deficit	Manifestation	Nursing Implications/ Patient Teaching Applications
Visual Field Deficits		
Homonymous hemianopsia (Loss of half of the visual field)	· Unaware of persons or objects on side of visual loss · Neglect of one side of the body · Difficulty judging distances	Place objects within the patient's intact field of vision. Approach the patient from side of his intact field of vision. Instruct/remind the patient to turn his head in the direction of visual loss to compensate for loss of visual field. Encourage the use of eye glasses if available. When teaching the patient, do so within patient's intact visual field.
Loss of peripheral vision	· Difficulty seeing at night · Unaware of objects or the borders of objects	Place objects in the patient's center of vision Encourage the use of a cane or other object to identify objects in the periphery of the visual field. Avoid night driving or other risky activities in the darkness.
Diplopia	· Double vision	Explain to the patient the location of an object when placing it near the patient. Consistently place patient care items in the same location.
Motor Deficits		
Hemiparesis	· Weakness of the face, arm, and leg on the same side (due to a lesion in the opposite hemisphere)	Place objects within the patient's reach on the nonaffected side. Instruct the patient to exercise and increase the strength on the unaffected side.
Hemiplegia	· Paralysis of the face, arm and leg on the same side (due to a lesion in the opposite hemisphere)	Encourage the patient to provide range-of-motion exercises to the affected side. Provide immobilization as needed to the affected side. Maintain body alignment in functional position. Exercise unaffected limb to increase mobility, strength, and use.
Ataxia	· Staggering, unsteady gait · Unable to keep feet together, needs a broad base to stand	Support patient during the initial ambulation phase. Provide supportive device for ambulation (*i.e.*, walker, crutches, cane). Instruct the patient not to walk without assistance or supportive device.
Dysarthria	· Difficulty in forming words	Provide the patient with alternative methods of communicating. Allow the patient sufficient time to respond to verbal communication. Support patient and family to alleviate frustration related to difficulty in communicating.
Dysphagia	· Difficulty in swallowing	Test the patient's pharyngeal reflexes before offering food or fluids. Assist the patient with meals. Place food on the unaffected side of the mouth. Allow ample time to eat.
Sensory Deficits		
Paresthesia (occurs on the side opposite the lesion)	· Numbness and tingling of body parts · Difficulty with proprioception	Instruct the patient to avoid using this body part as the dominant limb. Provide range of motion to affected areas and apply corrective devices as needed. Place patient care items toward the nonaffected side.

(continued)

TABLE 59-2 (continued)

Neurologic Deficit	Manifestation	Nursing Implications/ Patient Teaching Applications
Verbal Deficits		
Expressive aphasia	• Unable to form words that are understandable; may be able to speak in single-word responses	Encourage patient to repeat sounds of the alphabet.
Receptive aphasia	• Unable to comprehend the spoken word; is able to speak but may not make sense	Speak slowly and clearly to assist the patient in forming the sounds.
Global aphasia	• Combination of both receptive and expressive aphasia	Speak clearly and in simple sentences; use gestures or pictures when able.
Cognitive Deficits	• Short- and long-term memory loss • Decreased attention span • Impaired ability to concentrate • Poor abstract reasoning • Altered judgment	Reorient patient to time, place, and situation frequently. Use verbal and auditory cues to orient patient. Provide familiar objects (family photographs, favorite objects). Use noncomplicated language with the patient. Match visual tasks with a verbal cue: holding a toothbrush, simulate brushing of teeth while saying, "I would like you to brush your teeth now." Minimize distracting noises and views when teaching the patient. Repeat and reinforce instructions frequently.
Emotional Deficits	• Loss of self-control • Emotional lability • Decreased tolerance to stressful situations • Depression • Withdrawal • Fear, hostility, and anger • Feelings of isolation	Support patient during uncontrollable outbursts. Discuss with the patient and family that the outbursts are due to the disease process. Encourage patient to participate in group activity. Provide stimulation for the patient. Control stressful situations, if possible. Provide a safe environment. Encourage patient to express feelings and frustrations related to disease process.

TABLE 59-3 Comparison of Left-Sided and Right-Sided Hemispheric Stroke

Left Hemispheric Stroke	Right Hemispheric Stroke
Paralysis on right side of body	Paralysis on left side of body
Right visual field defects	Left visual field defects
Aphasia (expressive, receptive, or global)	Spacial–perceptual deficits
Altered intellectual ability	Increased distractibility
Slow, cautious behavior	Impulsive behavior and poor judgment
	Lack of awareness of deficits

See Table 59-2 for associated clinical manifestations and interventions.

elsewhere in the cardiovascular system. Antiplatelet medications may be prescribed because platelets play a major role in thrombus formation and embolization.

Complications

Complications of a stroke include cerebral hypoxia, decrease in cerebral blood flow, and extension of the area of injury.

Cerebral hypoxia is minimized by providing adequate oxygenation of blood to the brain. Brain function is dependent upon available oxygen being delivered to the tissues. Administering supplemental oxygen and maintaining the hemoglobin and hematocrit at acceptable levels will assist in maintaining tissue oxygenation.

Cerebral blood flow is dependent upon the blood pressure, cardiac output, and integrity of cerebral blood vessels. Adequate hydration (intravenous fluids) must be ensured to reduce blood viscosity and improve cerebral blood flow. Extremes of hypertension or hypotension need to be avoided to prevent changes in cerebral blood flow and the potential for extending the area of injury.

Cerebral embolism may occur after myocardial infarction or atrial fibrillation or may originate from a prosthetic heart valve. The embolus will decrease blood flow into the brain and further compromise cerebral blood flow. Dysrythmias may result in an inconsistant cardiac output and the disruption of local thrombus. In addition, a dysrhythmia may have caused a cerebral embolus and must be corrected.

❑ NURSING PROCESS
The Patient With a Stroke

Assessment

A neurologic flow sheet is maintained to reflect the following nursing assessment parameters:

1. A change in the level of consciousness or responsiveness as evidenced by movement, resistance to changes of position, and response to stimulation; orientation to time, place, and person
2. Presence or absence of voluntary or involuntary movements of the extremities; the tone of the muscles; the body posture; and the position of the head
3. Stiffness or flaccidity of the neck
4. Eye opening, the comparative size of the pupils and pupillary reactions to light, and ocular position
5. The color of the face and the extremities; the temperature and moisture of the skin
6. The quality and rates of pulse and respiration; arterial blood gases as indicated, body temperature, and arterial pressure
7. Ability to speak
8. Volume of fluids ingested or administered and the volume of urine excreted each 24 hours

When the patient begins to regain consciousness, signs of extreme fatigue and confusion are apparent as a result of the cerebral edema that follows a stroke. To reduce any anxiety, efforts should be made at frequent intervals to orient the patient to time and place and to offer reassurance.

If the lesion occurs in the dominant hemisphere, the patient also is likely to have aphasia. A nondominant hemispheric lesion may result in apraxia (inability to perform previously learned movements).

After the acute phase, the nurse assesses the following functions: mental status (memory, attention span, perception, orientation, affect, speech/language), sensation/perception (usually the patient has decreased awareness of pain and temperature); motor control (upper and lower extremity movement); and bladder function.

Nursing assessment continues to focus on the impairment of function in the patient's daily activities because the quality of life after stroke is closely related to the patient's functional status.

Diagnosis

Nursing Diagnoses

Based on the assessment data, the major nursing diagnoses for a patient with a stroke may include the following:

- ❑ Impaired physical mobility related to hemiparesis, loss of balance and coordination, spasticity, and brain injury
- ❑ Pain (painful shoulder) related to hemiplegia and disuse
- ❑ Self-care deficits (hygiene, toileting, transfers, feeding) related to stroke sequelae
- ❑ Incontinence related to flaccid bladder, detrusor instability, confusion, difficulty in communicating
- ❑ Altered thought processes related to brain damage, confusion, inability to follow instruction
- ❑ Impaired verbal communication related to brain damage
- ❑ Risk for impaired skin integrity related to hemiparesis/hemiplegia, decreased mobility
- ❑ Altered family processes related to catastrophic illness and caregiving burdens

Collaborative Problems/ Potential Complications

Based on the assessment data, potential complications include:

- ❑ Decreased cerebral blood flow
- ❑ Inadequate oxygen delivery to the brain

Planning and Implementation (Rehabilitation Phase)

Although rehabilitation begins on the day the patient has the stroke, the process is intensified during the convalescent phase and requires a coordinated team effort. It is very helpful for the team to know what the patient was like before this catastrophic illness: abilities, mental and emotional state, behavioral characteristics, and activities of daily living.

Goals. The major goals for the patient (and family) may include improvement of mobility, avoidance of shoulder pain, achievement of self-care, attainment of bladder control, improvement of thought processes, achievement of some form of communication, maintenance of skin integrity, restoration of family functioning, and absence of complications.

Nursing Interventions

Improving Mobility and Preventing Deformities. A hemiplegic patient has unilateral paralysis (paralysis on one side). When control of the voluntary muscles is lost, the strong flexor muscles exert control over the extensors. The arm tends to adduct (adductor muscles are stronger than abductors) and to rotate internally. The elbow and the wrist tend to flex, the affected leg tends to rotate externally at the hip joint and flex at the knee, and the foot at the ankle joint supinates and tends toward plantar flexion.

Positioning. Correct positioning is important to prevent contractures; measures are used to relieve pressure, assist in maintaining good body alignment, and prevent compressive neuropathies, especially of the ulnar and peroneal nerves.

Proper Bed Position. A bed board under the mattress provides firm support for the body. The patient should remain flat in bed except when engaged in ADLs. Maintaining the upright position in bed for extended periods contributes to hip flexion deformity and sacral pressure ulcer formation.

A *footboard* may be used at intervals during the flaccid period after a stroke to keep the feet at right angles to the legs when the patient is in a supine (dorsal) position. This prevents footdrop and the heel cords from shortening as a result of contracture of the gastrocnemius muscles. High-top sneakers may also be used for this purpose, but care must be taken to avoid pressure on the heels and ankles.

When spasticity develops, a footboard is generally avoided as it may increase spasticity and cause plantar flexion deformity. If the affected extremity is spastic, a bed cradle is used to keep the bed linens off the extremity.

Because flexor muscles are stronger than extensor muscles, a *posterior splint* applied at night may prevent flexion of the affected extremity and maintain correct positioning during sleep (Fig. 59-10).

Preventing Shoulder Adduction. To prevent adduction of the affected shoulder, a pillow is placed in the axilla when there is limited external rotation; this keeps the arm away from the chest. A pillow is placed under the arm, and the arm is placed in a neutral (slightly flexed) position, with distal joints positioned higher than the more proximal joints (Fig. 59-11). Thus, the elbow is higher than the shoulder and the wrist is higher than the elbow. This helps to prevent edema and the resultant fibrosis that will prevent normal range of motion if the patient regains control of the arm.

Preventing Hip Rotation. A *trochanter roll* extending from the crest of the ilium to the mid-thigh is used to prevent external rotation at the hip joint. A sandbag applied at the side of the leg will not prevent external rotation, because this motion originates in the ball-and-socket joint of the hip. The knee has no such rotating function. The trochanter roll acts as a mechanical wedge under the projection of the greater trochanter and prevents the femur from rolling.

Hand and Finger Position. The fingers are positioned so that they are barely flexed. The hand is placed in slight supination (palm faces upward), which is its most functional (*i.e.*, useful) position. If the upper extremity is flaccid, a volar resting splint can be used to support the wrist and hand in a functional position. If the upper extremity is spastic, a hand roll is *not* used because it stimulates the grasp reflex. In this instance a dorsal wrist splint is useful in allowing the palm to be free of pressure. Every effort is made to prevent hand edema.

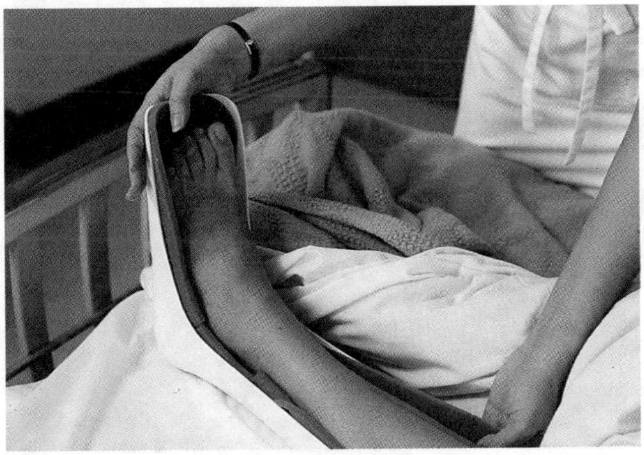

FIGURE 59-10. Foot supports may be used to maintain proper alignment in patients who have suffered a stroke.

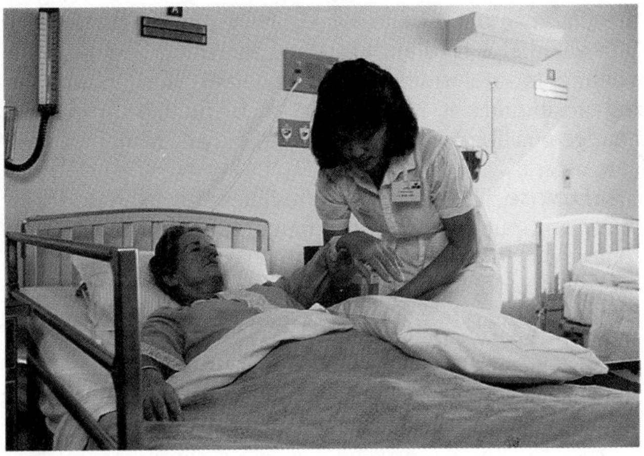

FIGURE 59-11. Pillows are used following a stroke to place the affected arm in an appropriate position.

Changing Positions. The patient's position should be changed every 2 hours. To place a patient in a lateral (side-lying) position (Fig. 59-12*A*), a pillow is placed between the legs before the patient is turned. The upper thigh should not be acutely flexed. The patient may be turned from side to side, but the amount of time spent on the affected side should be limited because of impaired sensation. Lying on the affected side, however, is thought to increase the patient's awareness of the side and allows use of the unaffected hand.

If possible, the patient is placed in a prone position for 15 to 30 minutes several times a day. A small pillow or a support is placed under the pelvis, extending from the level of the umbilicus to the upper third of the thigh (see Fig. 59-12*B*). This helps to promote hyperextension of the hip joints, which is essential for normal gait and helps

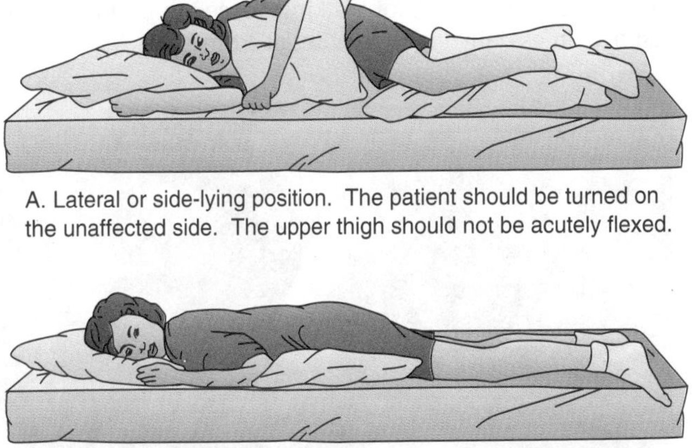

A. Lateral or side-lying position. The patient should be turned on the unaffected side. The upper thigh should not be acutely flexed.

B. Prone position. A pillow is placed under the pelvis to help promote hyperextension of the hip joints, which is essential for normal gait. Note position of arms.

FIGURE 59-12. Methods of positioning a patient who has had a stroke: (**A**) lateral or side-lying position; (**B**) prone position with pillow support.

prevent knee and hip flexion contractures. The prone position also helps to drain bronchial secretions and prevents contractural deformities of the shoulders and knees. During positioning it is important to reduce pressure and change position frequently to prevent the formation of pressure ulcers.

Exercise. The affected extremities are exercised passively and put through a full range of motion four or five times a day to maintain joint mobility, regain motor control, prevent development of a contracture in the paralyzed extremity, prevent further deterioration of the neuromuscular system, and enhance circulation (Fig. 59-13). Exercise is helpful in preventing venous stasis, which may predispose the patient to thrombosis and pulmonary embolus.

Repetition of an activity forms new pathways in the CNS and therefore encourages new patterns of motion. At first, the extremities are usually flaccid. If tightness occurs in any area, the range-of-motion exercises should be performed more frequently. (See Chapter 18 for techniques of range-of-motion exercises.)

The patient is observed for signs and symptoms that may indicate pulmonary embolus or excessive cardiac workload during exercise; these include shortness of breath, chest pain, cyanosis, and increasing pulse rate during the exercise period.

Frequent short periods of exercise always are preferable to longer periods at infrequent intervals. *Regularity* in exercise is most important. Improvement in muscle strength and maintenance of range of motion can be achieved only through daily exercise.

The patient is encouraged and reminded to exercise the unaffected side at intervals throughout the day. It is helpful to work out a written time schedule that can be used to remind the patient of the exercise activities. The nurse has the responsibility of supervising and supporting the patient during these activities. The patient can be taught to put the unaffected leg under the affected one to move it when turning and exercising. Flexibility, strengthening, coordination, endurance, and balancing exercises prepare the patient for ambulation and provide a goal. Quadriceps muscle setting and gluteal setting exercises are started early to improve the muscle strength needed for walking; these are performed at least five times daily for 10 minutes at a time.

Preparing for Ambulation. As soon as possible the patient is assisted out of bed. Usually, when hemiplegia has resulted from a thrombosis, an active rehabilitation program is started as soon as the patient regains consciousness; a patient who has had a cerebral hemorrhage cannot participate actively until all evidence of bleeding is gone.

The patient is first taught to maintain balance while sitting and then to learn to balance while standing. If the patient has difficulty in achieving standing balance, a tilt table, which slowly brings the patient to an upright position, can be used. Tilt tables are especially helpful for those patients who have been on bed rest for prolonged periods and are having orthostatic blood pressure changes.

If the patient needs a wheelchair, the folding type with hand brakes is the most practical because it allows the patient to manipulate the chair. The chair should be low enough to allow the patient to propel it with the uninvolved foot and narrow enough to permit it to be used in the home. When the patient is transferred from the wheelchair, the brakes are applied on both sides of the chair.

The patient is usually ready to walk as soon as standing balance is achieved. Parallel bars are useful in these first efforts. A chair or wheelchair should be readily available in case the patient suddenly becomes fatigued or feels dizzy.

The training periods for ambulation should be short and frequent. As the patient gains in strength and confidence, an adjustable cane can be used for support. Generally, a three- or four-prong cane provides a stable support in the early phases of the training program.

Preventing Shoulder Pain. Up to 70% of stroke patients suffer from severe pain in the shoulder that prevents them from learning new skills, because shoulder function is essential in achieving balance and performing transfers and self-care activities. Three problems can occur: painful shoulder, subluxation of the shoulder, and shoulder–hand syndrome.

A flaccid shoulder joint may be overstretched by the use of excessive force in turning the patient or from overstrenuous arm and shoulder movement. To prevent *shoulder pain,* the nurse should never lift the patient by the flaccid shoulder or pull on the affected arm or shoulder. If the arm is paralyzed, *subluxation* (incomplete dislocation) at the shoulder can occur from overstretching of the joint capsule

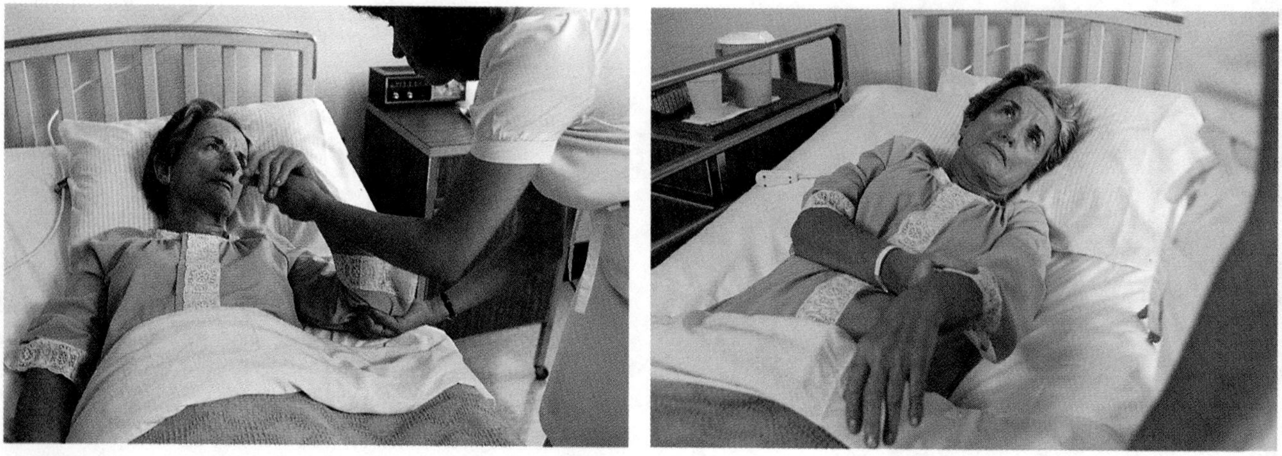

FIGURE 59-13. Range-of-motion exercises are carried out frequently for a stroke patient to prevent contractures. The patient is encouraged to exercise the affected arm.

and musculature by the force of gravity when the patient sits or stands in the early stages after a stroke. This results in severe pain. *Shoulder–hand syndrome* (painful shoulder and generalized swelling of the hand) can cause a frozen shoulder and ultimate atrophy of subcutaneous tissues. When a shoulder becomes stiff, it is usually more painful.

These problems can be prevented by proper patient movement and positioning. The flaccid arm is positioned on a table or pillows while the patient is seated. Some clinicians advocate the use of a properly worn sling when the patient first becomes ambulatory to prevent the paralyzed upper extremity from dangling without support. Range-of-motion exercises are important in preventing painful shoulder. Overstrenuous arm movements are avoided. The patient is instructed to interlace the fingers, place the palms together, and push the clasped hands slowly forward to bring the scapulae forward; he or she then raises both hands above his or her head. This is repeated throughout the day. The patient is instructed to flex the affected wrist at intervals and move all the joints of the affected fingers. He or she is encouraged to touch, stroke, rub, and look at both hands. Pushing the heel of the hand firmly down on a surface is useful. Elevation of the arm and hand is also important in preventing dependent edema of the hand. Patients with continuing pain after movement and positioning have been attempted may require the addition of analgesia to their treatment program.

Achieving Self-Care. As soon as the patient is able to sit up, personal hygiene activities are encouraged. The patient is helped to set realistic goals and, if feasible, a new task is added daily. The first step is to carry out all self-care activities on the unaffected side. Such activities as combing the hair, brushing the teeth, shaving with an electric razor, bathing, and eating can be carried out with one hand and are suitable for self-care. Although the patient may feel awkward at first, the various motor skills can be learned by repetition and the unaffected side will become stronger with use. The nurse must be sure that the patient does not neglect the affected side. Assistive devices will help make up for some of the patient's deficits. A small towel is easier to control while drying after bathing, and boxed paper tissues are easier to use than a roll of toilet tissue.

Dressing Activities. The patient's morale will improve if ambulatory activities are carried out in street clothes. The family is instructed to bring in clothing that is preferably a size larger than that normally worn. Clothing fitted with front or side fasteners or Velcro closures is the most suitable. The patient has better balance if most of the dressing activities are done in a seated position.

The clothing is placed on the patient's affected side in the order in which the garments are to be put on. Using a large mirror while dressing helps make the patient aware of what he or she is putting on the affected side. Each garment is put on the affected side first. The patient has to make many compensatory movements when dressing that can produce fatigue and painful twisting of the intercostal muscles. Support and encouragement are provided to prevent the patient from becoming overly fatigued and discouraged. Even with intensive training, not all patients are able to achieve independence in dressing skills.

Attaining Bladder Control. Most stroke patients have bladder problems in the early stage, but bladder control is usually quickly regained. The patient's voiding pattern is analyzed and the urinal/bedpan offered on this pattern or schedule. The upright posture and standing position is helpful for male patients during this aspect of rehabilitation. (See also Chapter 18 for a bladder retraining program.)

Improving Thought Processes. After a stroke the patient may have problems with cognitive, behavioral, and emotional deficits related to brain damage. In many instances, however, a considerable degree of function can be recovered because not all areas of the brain are equally damaged; some remain more intact and functional than others.

After assessment procedures that delineate and describe the patient's problems, the neuropsychologist, interacting when possible with the primary care physician, psychiatrist, nurse, and other professionals, structures a training program using cognitive-perceptual retraining, visual imagery, reality orientation, and cuing procedures to compensate for losses.

The role of the nurse is supportive. The nurse reviews the results of neuropsychologic testing, observes the patient's performance and progress, gives positive feedback, and, most important, conveys an attitude of confidence and hopefulness. Interventions capitalize on the patient's strengths and remaining abilities while attempting to improve performance of affected functions. Other interventions are similar to those for improving cognitive functioning after a head injury (see pp. 1795–1796).

Achieving Communication. Aphasia impairs the patient's ability to communicate, both in understanding what is being said and in the ability to express oneself. The speech-language therapist assesses the communication needs of the stroke patient, describes the precise deficit, and suggests the best overall method of communication for the patient. There are many language intervention strategies for the adult aphasic person, and the program is individually tailored. Goals are jointly established as the patient is expected to take an active part.

Nursing interventions include doing everything possible to make the atmosphere conducive to communication. This includes being sensitive to the patient's reactions and needs and responding to them in an appropriate manner, always treating the patient as an adult. The nurse lends strong moral support and understanding to allay anxiety. A consistent schedule, routines, and repetitions help the patient to function in spite of significant deficits. A written copy of the daily schedule, a folder of personal information (birth date, address, names of relatives), checklists, and an audiotaped list help the patient's memory and concentration. Surrounding the patient with familiar objects and photographs and caring people is reassuring.

When talking with the patient, it is important to have the patient's attention, speak slowly, and keep the language of instruction consistent. One instruction is given at a time, and time is allowed for the patient to process what has been said. The use of gestures may enhance comprehension. Other nursing strategies for helping the aphasic patient are found on pp. 1735–1736.

Maintaining Skin Integrity. The patient who has a stroke may be at risk for skin and tissue breakdown because of altered sensation and inability to respond to pressure and discomfort by turning and moving. Therefore, preventing skin and tissue breakdown requires frequent assessment of the skin, with particular emphasis on bony areas and dependent parts of the body. During the acute phase a specialty bed (*e.g.*, low air loss bed) may be used until the patient is able to move independently or assist in moving.

A regular turning and positioning schedule must be followed to minimize pressure and prevent skin breakdown. Pressure-relieving devices may be employed but must not be used in place of regular turning and positioning. The turning schedule (at least every 2 hours) must be adhered to even if pressure-relieving devices are used to prevent tissue and skin breakdown. When the patient is positioned or turned, care must be used to minimize shear and friction forces, which cause damage to tissues and predispose the patient's skin to breakdown.

The patient's skin must be kept clean and dry; gentle massage of healthy (non-reddened) skin and maintenance of adequate nutrition are other factors that help to maintain normal skin and tissue integrity.

Improving Family Coping Through Health Teaching. Members of the patient's family play an important role in the patient's recovery. Some type of counseling and support system should be available to them to prevent the care of the patient from taking a significant toll on their health and interfering too radically with their life-style. Respite care—planned short-term care to ease the burden of the family in providing continuous 24-hour care—may be available from an adult day care center. Some hospitals also offer weekend respite care. Family coping is also facilitated by involving others in the patient's care and teaching stress management techniques and methods for maintaining personal health.

The family may have difficulty in accepting the patient's disability and may be unrealistic in their expectations. They are given information about the expected outcomes of the patient's stroke and are counseled to avoid doing for the patient those things that he or she can do. They are assured that their loving and warm interest is part of the patient's therapy.

The family needs to be informed that the rehabilitation of the hemiplegic patient requires many months and that progress may be slow. The gains made by the patient during the time spent in the hospital or rehabilitation unit must be maintained. All should approach the patient with a supportive and optimistic attitude, focusing on the abilities that remain. The rehabilitation team, the medical and nursing team, the patient, and his family all must be involved in developing attainable goals for the patient at home.

Most relatives of stroke patients have problems with the emotional aspects of care. The family should be prepared to expect occasional episodes of emotional lability. The patient may laugh or cry easily, be irritable and demanding or depressed and confused. The nurse can explain to the family that the patient's laughing does not necessarily connote happiness nor does crying reflect sadness, and that emotional lability usually improves with time.

Sexual Dysfunction. Sexual functioning can be profoundly altered by stroke. Often stroke is such a catastrophic illness that the patient experiences loss of self-esteem and value as a sexual being. Although research in this area of stroke management is limited, it appears that post-stroke patients consider sexual function to be important, but most experience sexual dysfunction after stroke. The patient and partner may benefit from sexual counseling about alternative approaches to sexual expression.

Patient Education and Home Care Considerations

Planning Care. The recovery and rehabilitation process following stroke may be prolonged, requiring patience and perseverance on the part of the patient and family. Depending on the specific neurologic deficits resulting from the stroke, the patient at home may require the services of a number of health care professionals. The care of the patient at home is often coordinated by the nurse. The patient's family—often the patient's spouse—will require assistance in planning and providing aspects of care. Simultaneously, the patient's spouse often requires reminding to attend to personal health problems and well-being.

Emotional Aspects. The family is advised that the patient will often tire easily, will become irritable and upset by small events, and is likely to show less interest in things. Because a stroke frequently occurs in the later stages of life, there is the possibility of intellectual decline related to dementia.

Emotional problems associated with stroke are often related to speech dysfunction and frustrations about being unable to communicate effectively. A speech therapist coming to the home allows the family to be involved and gives the family practical instructions to help the patient between speech therapy sessions.

Depression is a common and serious problem in the stroke patient. Antidepressant therapy may help if depression dominates the patient's life. As progress is made in the rehabilitation program, some problems will diminish. The family can help by continuing to support the patient and giving positive reinforcement for the progress that is being made.

Home Modification. An occupational therapist may be helpful in assessing the patient's home environment and recommending modifications designed to assist the patient to become more independent. For example, a shower is more convenient than a tub for the hemiplegic patient, because most patients do not gain sufficient strength to get up and down from a tub. Sitting on a stool of medium height with rubber suction tips permits him to wash with greater ease. A long-handled bath brush with a soap container is helpful to the patient who has only one functional hand. If a shower is not available, a stool may be placed in the tub and a portable shower hose attached to the faucet. Handrails may be attached beside the bathtub and the toilet.

Supportive Resources. Numerous self-help devices are available to assist the patient in ADLs. Community-based stroke clubs allow the patient and family to learn from others with similar problems and to share their experiences. The patient is encouraged to continue with hobbies, recreational and leisure interests, and contact with friends to prevent social isolation.

All nurses coming in contact with the patient should encourage the patient to keep active, adhere to the exercise program, and remain as self-sufficient as possible.

Monitoring and Managing Potential Complications. The patient's vital signs and oxygenation status are assessed to maintain adequate blood flow to the brain and tissue oxygenation. Therapies to improve oxygenation, such as supplemental oxygen, suctioning, and chest physiotherapy are used to improve respiratory gas exchange. An adequate cardiac output is maintained by medications to strengthen the contractility of the heart and decrease the blood pressure (if the patient is hypertensive) and by fluid administration.

Evaluation

Expected Outcomes

1. Achieves improved mobility
   a. Avoids deformities; absence of contractures and footdrop
   b. Participates in prescribed exercise program
   c. Achieves sitting balance
   d. Uses unaffected side to compensate for loss of function of hemiplegic side
2. Has no complaints of shoulder pain
   a. Demonstrates shoulder mobility; exercises shoulder
   b. Elevates arm and hand at intervals
3. Achieves self-care; performs hygienic care and uses adaptive equipment
4. Attains bladder continence
5. Participates in cognitive improvement program
6. Demonstrates improved communication
   a. Maintains intact skin without breakdown; demonstrates normal skin turgor and participates in turning and position activities
7. Family members demonstrate a positive attitude and coping mechanisms
   a. Encourage patient in exercise program
   b. Take an active part in rehabilitation process
8. Absence of complications
   a. Blood pressure and heart rate are within normal limits for the patient
   b. Arterial blood gases are within normal limits

Aphasia

Aphasia is a disturbance of language function resulting from injury or disease of the brain centers. It may involve impairment of the ability to read and write as well as to speak, listen, calculate, comprehend, and understand gestures. Terms used to describe aphasia are presented in Chart 59-3. About 1 to 1.5 million adults in the U.S. have a chronic disabling aphasia.

The major causes of aphasia are stroke, head injury, and brain tumor. An estimated 20% of stroke patients develop aphasia. The number of aphasic patients is growing because more patients are surviving stroke.

Broca's Area. The cortical area that is responsible for integrating the myriad association pathways required for the comprehension and formulation of language measures little more than 1 square inch in size. The principal speech center, called **Broca's area**, is located in a convolution adjoining the middle cerebral artery; this area is responsible for control of the combinations of muscular movements needed to speak each word. The cells that govern the muscles of speech are in the motor area of the cortex. Speaking requires a combination or sequence of combinations of muscular contractions. Not only must the muscles of the vocal cords contract, but also those of the throat, the tongue, the soft palate, the lips, and the chest wall must contract. The cells of Broca's convolution direct the cells of the motor area, which make the muscles contract at the proper time and with the proper force.

Broca's area is so near the left motor area that a disturbance in the motor area often affects the speech area. This

CHART 59-3
Glossary of Selected Terms Relating to Aphasia*

acalculia; dyscalculia difficulty in dealing with mathematical processes or numerical symbols in general

agnosia failure to recognize familiar objects perceived by the senses

- **auditory agnosia** inability to recognize significance of sounds
- **color agnosia** inability to recognize differences in color
- **tactile agnosia** inability to recognize familiar objects by touch or feel
- **visual object agnosia** inability to recognize objects; visual acuity may or may not be intact

agraphia; dysgraphia disturbances in writing intelligible words

alexia; dyslexia difficulty in reading

anomia; dysnomia difficulty in selecting appropriate words, particularly nouns

aphasia loss of the ability to express oneself or to understand language.

- **receptive aphasia** inability to understand what someone else is saying; often associted with damage to the temporal lobe area.
- **expressive aphasia** inability to express oneself; often associated with the left frontal lobe area.

apraxia inability to perform previously learned purposeful motor acts on a voluntary basis

- **verbal apraxia** difficulty in forming and organizing intelligible words although the musculature is intact

dysarthria defects of articulation due to neurologic causes

hemianopsia blindness of one half of the field of vision in one or both eyes

paraphasia a frequently observed characteristic in many aphasic patients; uses wrong words, word substitutions, grammatical errors, faults in word usage; may be observed in both oral and written language

perseveration continued and automatic repetition of an activity or word or phrase that is no longer appropriate

*The prefix *a* means "without" or "absence." The prefix *dys* refers to "difficulty" or "disordered." These prefixes are frequently used interchangeably in these conditions.

is the reason that so many patients paralyzed on the right side (due to damage or injury to the left side of the brain) are unable to speak, whereas in those paralyzed on the left side, speech disturbances are less common. Some patients are not affected, but these usually are left-handed persons whose speech area is located in the right hemisphere.

Assessment

The speech-language therapist, in cooperation with the neurologist, assesses the communication abilities of the patient. Information is obtained regarding the patient's pre-illness speech-language skills and interests. Formalized, standardized tests and observational methods are used to evaluate comprehension, mathematical, reading, and residual language skills.

The nursing assessment of the aphasic patient includes *listening* to him, asking him to follow simple directions (*e.g.*, "Pick up the book"), and observing him cope with his dysfunction.

Management of the Aphasic Patient

Promoting Positive Self-Esteem. A patient with aphasia should be given as much psychologic security as possible. Patience and understanding are essential while the patient learns to speak. At the same time, the patient is treated as an adult. A kind, unhurried manner combined with encouragement, patience, and a willingness to invest time are required. Relearning speech and language skills may take several years.

An aphasic person may become depressed because of the inability to talk to others. Not being able to talk on the telephone or answer a question or being excluded from conversation causes anger, frustration, fear of the future, and a sense of hopelessness.

The nurse must accept the patient's behavior and feelings, relieve his or her embarrassment, and give support and assurance that there is nothing wrong with his or her intelligence. A common pitfall is for the nurse or other health care team member to complete the thoughts or sentences of the patient. This should be avoided since it may cause the patient to feel more frustrated at not being allowed to speak and may deter efforts to practice putting thoughts together and completing the sentence.

The environment should be relaxed and permissive, and the patient should be encouraged to socialize with family and friends. Often the aphasic person has almost an obsession with orderliness; thus, nurses and family members should return items in the room to their proper place.

Improving Communication Abilities. It is essential that aphasic patients be guided in their efforts to improve their communication skills. Listening as well as speaking skills are emphasized in the rehabilitation program. The patient may also benefit from a communication board, which has pictures of commonly requested needs and phrases. The board may be translated into several languages. The patient should be encouraged to verbalize personal needs and to use the board when unable to express these needs.

Increasing Auditory Stimulation. First the patient is encouraged to *listen.* Speaking is thinking out loud, and the emphasis is on *thinking.* The patient must think and sort out incoming messages and formulate a response. Listening requires mental effort, yet the patient must struggle against mental inertia and needs time to organize an answer.

In working with the aphasic patient, the nurse must remember to *talk to* the patient while caring for him or her. This provides social contact for the patient. Chart 59-4 describes points to keep in mind when communicating with the aphasic patient.

Helping the Family Cope. Helping the family cope with irrevocable changes in their life-style is accomplished by talking about the stroke or head injury, acknowledging the changes that have occurred, focusing on the patient's abilities, and informing them of support systems.

The attitude of the family is an important factor in helping the patient adjust to this deficit. Family members are encouraged to act naturally and treat the patient in the same manner as before the illness. They should be aware that the patient's ability to speak may vary from day to day and that fatigue has an adverse effect on speech. They also should be aware that the patient may strike out verbally when emotional controls are lowered. The patient is likely to become frustrated. Tears and laughter may occur without apparent cause, and frequent mood shifts are common.

Support groups such as stroke clubs and group therapy for aphasic patients can help in the socialization and motivation of the patient as well as aid in the relief of anxiety and tension. The strain of the constant adjustment to the patient's illness, demands, and needs, as well as the financial drain and the change in life-style, can produce extreme tension and distress in the family. Members of the family often go through a period of mourning.

In addition to learning as much as possible about the support of the patient with aphasia, family members should also be counseled to continue a life of their own and to seek the aid of a social worker, clergyman, or psychologist if they need additional help in dealing with their frustrations and pressures. (See references at the end of the chapter for resources for patients with aphasia.)

CHART 59-4
Communicating with the Aphasic Patient

- Face the patient and establish eye contact.
- Speak in a normal manner and tone.
- Use short phrases and pause between phrases to allow the patient time to understand what is being said.
- Limit conversation to practical and concrete matters.
- Use gestures, pictures, and objects.
- As the patient uses and handles an object, say what the object is. It helps to match the words with the object or action.
- Be consistent in using the same words and gestures each time you give instructions or ask a question.
- Keep extraneous noises and sounds to a minimum. Too much background noise can distract the patient or make it difficult to sort out the message being spoken.

The Patient Undergoing Intracranial Surgery

Technologic advances and refinement of imaging procedures and surgical techniques have made it possible for neurosurgeons to localize and treat intracranial lesions with greater precision than ever before. Improved imaging techniques, illumination, and magnification have made it possible to obtain a three-dimensional view of the surgical site. Microsurgical instruments allow delicate tissue to be separated without trauma. Ultrasonic dissecting systems permit certain brain and spinal cord tumors to be removed quickly and precisely. Probes can be placed deep into brain tissue to apply interstitial radiation, hyperthermia, or chemotherapy. Suture material smaller than a strand of human hair permits very small nerves and vessels to be sutured and anastomosed.

The use of stereotactic frames and equipment allows precise localization of a specific target point in the brain; stereotactic approaches are used with lasers and the gamma knife. Lasers enable neurosurgeons to remove tumors precisely with minimal trauma to surrounding tissue, an important consideration in neurosurgery. Vessels adjacent to structures can be coagulated without causing injury to the structures themselves. The gamma knife (which is not really a knife) is used to deliver a high level of radiation to intracranial lesions with the purpose of destroying deep and inaccessible lesions in a single treatment session. This approach is referred to as radiosurgery, although it does not involve conventional surgical approaches. For some patients, the craniotomy remains the most appropriate approach and may be combined with other treatment modalities.

Surgical Approaches

A **craniotomy** involves opening the skull surgically to gain access to intracranial structures. This procedure is performed to remove a tumor, relieve ICP, evacuate a blood clot, and control hemorrhage. A bony flap is made into the skull and is replaced after surgery, held in place by periosteal or wire sutures. In general, two approaches through the skull are used: (1) above the tentorium (supratentorial craniotomy) into the supratentorial compartment and (2) below the tentorium into the infratentorial (posterior fossa) compartment. A transsphenoidal approach through the mouth and nasal sinuses is used to gain access to the pituitary gland. Table 59-4 compares the three different surgical approaches: supratentorial, infratentorial, and transsphenoidal.

The intracranial structures may be approached through *burr holes* (Fig. 59-14), which are circular openings made in the skull by either a hand drill or an automatic craniotome (which has a self-controlled system to stop the drill when the bone is penetrated). Burr holes are made for exploration or diagnosis. They may be used to determine the presence of cerebral swelling and injury and the size and position of the ventricles. They are also a means of evacuating an intracranial hematoma or abscess and for making a bone flap in the skull and allowing access to the ventricles for decompression purposes, ventriculography, or shunting procedures.

Other cranial procedures include *craniectomy* (an excision of a portion of the skull) and *cranioplasty* (repair of a cranial defect by means of a plastic or metal plate).

Diagnostic Evaluation

Preoperative diagnostic procedures may include computed tomography (CT scanning) to demonstrate the lesion and show the degree of surrounding brain edema, the ventricular size, and the displacement. Magnetic resonance imaging (MRI) provides information similar to that of the CT scan, with the additional advantage of examining the lesion in other planes. Cerebral angiography may be used to study the tumor blood supply or give information about vascular lesions. Transcranial Doppler flow studies evaluate the blood flow of intracranial blood vessels.

Management

Preoperative Management

Usually patients are placed on anticonvulsant medication (phenytoin) before surgery to reduce the risk of postoperative seizures. Before surgery, steroids (dexamethasone) may be administered to reduce cerebral edema. Fluids may be restricted. A hyperosmotic agent (mannitol) and a diuretic (furosemide) may be given intravenously immediately before and sometimes during surgery if the patient tends to retain water, as do many who have intracranial dysfunction. An indwelling urinary catheter is inserted before the patient is taken to the operating room to drain the bladder during the administration of diuretics and to permit urinary output to be monitored. The patient may be given antibiotics if there is a chance of cerebral contamination or diazepam preoperatively to allay anxiety.

The scalp is shaved immediately before surgery (usually in the operating room) so that any resultant superficial abrasions do not have time to become infected.

Postoperative Management

An arterial line and a central venous pressure (CVP) line may be in place to monitor blood pressure and measure CVP. The patient may or may not be intubated and may receive supplemental oxygen therapy.

Reducing Cerebral Edema. Medication therapy to reduce cerebral edema includes the administration of mannitol, which increases serum osmolality and draws free water from areas of the brain (with an intact blood–brain barrier). The fluid is then excreted by osmotic diuresis. Dexamethasone may be administered intravenously every 6 hours for 24 to 72 hours; subsequently the dosage is tapered.

Relieving Pain and Preventing Seizures. Acetaminophen is usually given for temperature over 99.6°F (37.5°C) and for pain. Frequently the patient will have a headache after a craniotomy, usually as a result of the scalp nerves being stretched and irritated during surgery. Codeine, given parenterally, is usually sufficient to relieve headache. Anticonvulsant medication (phenytoin, diazepam) is prescribed for patients who have undergone supratentorial craniotomy, because of the high risk of epilepsy

TABLE 59-4 Comparison of Cranial Surgical Approaches

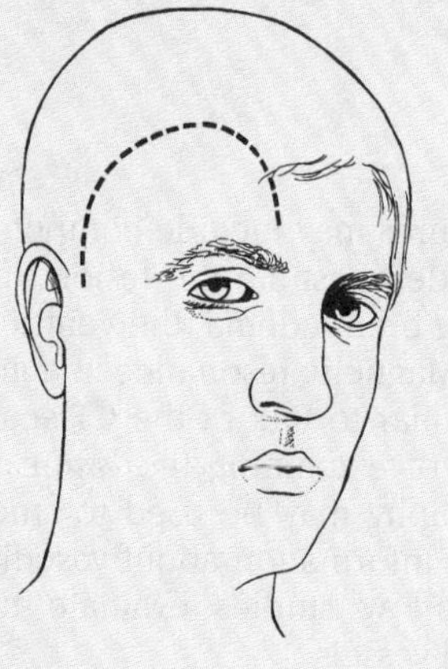

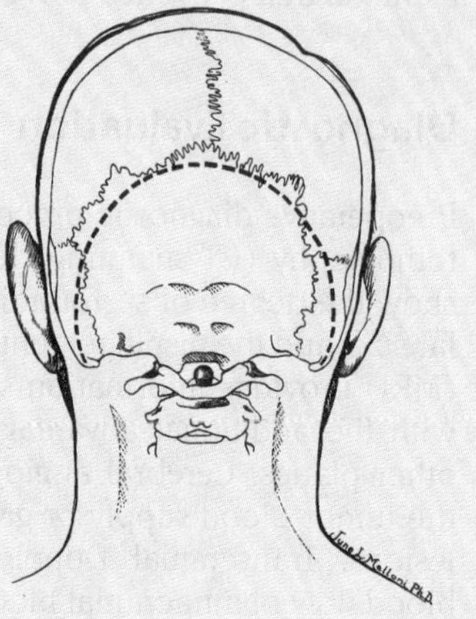

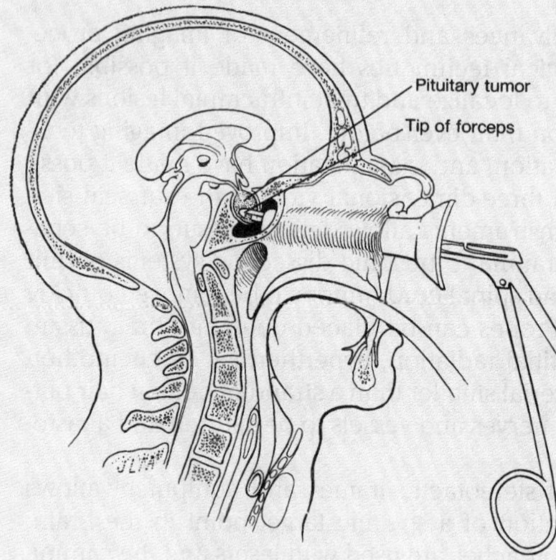

	Supratentorial	Infratentorial	Transsphenoidal
Site of Surgery	Above the tentorium	Below the tentorium, brain stem	Sella turcica and small pituitary tumors
Incision Location	Incision is made above the area to be operated on; is usually located behind the hairline	Incision is made at the nape of the neck, around the occipital lobe	Incision is made beneath the upper lip to gain access into the nasal cavity
Selected Nursing Interventions	Maintain head of bed elevated 30–45 degrees with neck in neutral alignment Position the patient on either side or back. (Avoid positioning patient on operative side if a large tumor has been removed.)	Maintain neck in straight alignment. Avoid flexion of the neck to prevent possible tearing of the suture line. Position the patient on either side. (Check protocol for guidelines for positioning of patient.)	Maintain nasal packing in place and reinforce as needed. Instruct patient to avoid blowing his nose. Provide frequent oral care. Keep head of bed elevated to promote venous drainage and drainage from the surgical site.

after supratentorial neurosurgical procedures. Serum levels are monitored to keep the medications within therapeutic range.

Monitoring ICP. A ventricular catheter, or some type of drainage, is frequently inserted in patients undergoing surgery for tumors of the posterior fossa. The catheter is connected to an external drainage system. The patency of the catheter is noted by the pulsations of the fluid in the tubing. The ICP can be assessed by setting up the system with a stopcock attached to the pressure tubing and transducer. The ICP can be monitored by the turn of the stopcock. Care is required to ensure that the system is tight at all connections and that the stopcock is in the proper position to avoid drainage of CSF fluid, which may result in collapse of the ventricles if excessive fluid is removed. The catheter is removed when the ventricular pressure is normal and stable. The neurosurgeon must be notified if at any time the catheter appears to be obstructed.

Ventricular shunting is sometimes performed before certain surgical procedures to control intracranial hypertension, particularly in patients with posterior fossa tumors.

Complications

Complications of intracranial surgery include increased ICP, infection, and neurologic deficits.

Increased ICP may develop as a result of cerebral edema or swelling and is treated with mannitol, an osmotic diuretic. The patient may also require intubation and use of paralyzing agents.

Infection is possible because of the open incision. The patient should receive antibiotic therapy, and the dressing and wound site should be monitored for signs of infection: increased drainage, foul odor, purulent drainage, and redness and swelling along the incision line.

Neurologic deficits may result from the surgery. Postoperatively the patient's neurologic status is closely monitored for any changes.

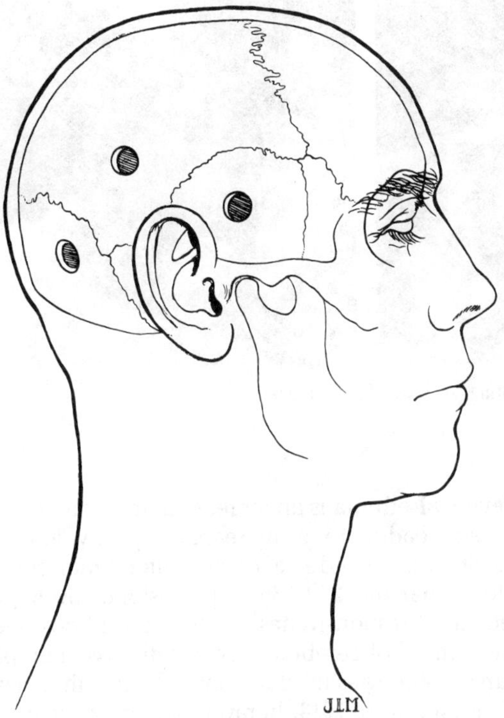

FIGURE 59-14. Burr holes may be used in neurosurgical procedures to make a bone flap in the skull, to aspirate a brain abscess, or to evacuate a hematoma.

❑ NURSING PROCESS The Patient Undergoing Intracranial Surgery

Preoperative Assessment

Proper assessment of the postoperative status of the patient requires an awareness of the patient's preoperative status so that a comparison can be made between the patient's preoperative and postoperative signs and symptoms. This assessment includes evaluating the level of consciousness and responsiveness to stimuli and identifying the presence of any neurologic deficits, such as paralysis, visual dysfunction, alterations in personality or speech, and bladder and bowel disturbances. Motor function of the hands is tested by the strength of the hand grip. Observations of leg movement are noted if the patient is not ambulatory.

The patient's and family's understanding of the anticipated surgical procedure and its possible sequelae is assessed, along with their reactions to the impending surgery. Additionally, the availability of support systems for the patient and family is assessed.

Preoperative Nursing Interventions

In preparation for surgery, the patient's physical and emotional status are brought to an optimal level to reduce the risk of postoperative complications. The patient's physical status is assessed for neurologic deficits and their potential impact following surgery. If the patient's arms or legs are paralyzed, trochanter rolls are applied to the extremities, and the feet are positioned against a footboard. A patient who is able to ambulate is encouraged to do so. If the patient is aphasic, writing materials or picture and word cards showing the bedpan, glass of water, blanket, and other frequently used items may be supplied to help improve communication.

The emotional preparation of the patient includes providing information about what to expect postoperatively. The large head dressing applied after surgery may impair hearing ability temporarily. Vision may be limited if the eyes are swollen shut. If a tracheostomy or endotracheal tube is in place, talking will be impossible; thus, an alternate method of communication must be developed before surgery.

An altered cognitive state may make the patient unaware of the impending surgery. Even so, encouragement and attention to the patient's needs are necessary. Whatever the state of awareness of the patient, the family needs reassurance and support, because they recognize the seriousness of brain surgery.

Postoperative Assessment

The frequency of postoperative monitoring is based on the patient's clinical status. Assessing respiratory function is essential because small degrees of hypoxia can increase cerebral ischemia. The respiratory rate and pattern are monitored, and arterial blood gas values are reviewed. Fluctuations in the patient's vital signs are carefully monitored and documented because they indicate increased ICP. The patient's rectal temperature is measured at intervals to assess for hyperthermia secondary to damage to the hypothalamus.

Neurologic checks are made frequently to detect increased ICP resulting from cerebral edema or bleeding. A change in the patient's level of consciousness or response to stimuli may be the first sign of increasing ICP.

Assessment of neurologic status focuses on the patient's level of consciousness, eye signs, motor response, and vital signs (Fig. 59-15). The patient is observed for subtle signs of neurologic deficit, such as diminished response to stimuli, speech problems, difficulty in swallowing, weakness or paralysis of an extremity, visual changes (diplopia, blurred vision), paresthesias, or seizures. Restlessness may occur as the patient becomes more responsive or may be due to pain, confusion, hypoxia, or other stimuli.

The patient's surgical dressing is inspected for evidence of bleeding and CSF drainage. In patients undergoing transsphenoidal surgery, the nasal packing that was inserted during surgery is checked for blood or CSF drainage. The nurse must be alert to the development of complications (p. 1741), and all assessment is carried out with these problems in mind.

Diagnosis

Nursing Diagnoses

Based on the assessment data, the patient's major nursing diagnoses after intracranial surgery may include the following:

- ❑ Altered cerebral tissue perfusion related to cerebral edema
- ❑ Potential for ineffective thermoregulation related to damage to the hypothalamus, dehydration, and infection

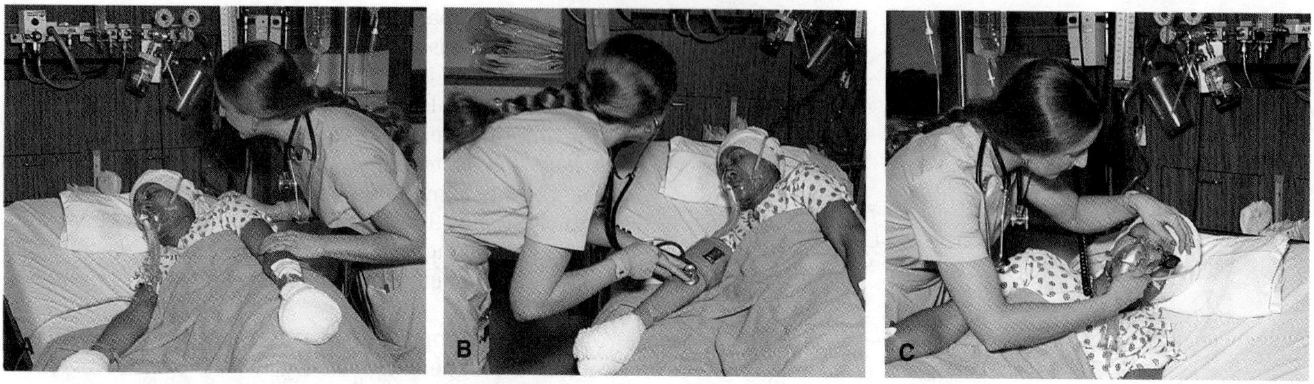

FIGURE 59-15. Postoperative assessment following a craniotomy includes evaluating (**A**) level of consciousness or responsiveness, (**B**) vital signs, and (**C**) eye changes.

- Potential for impaired gas exchange related to hypoventilation, aspiration, and immobility
- Sensory-perceptual alterations (visual, auditory, speech) related to periorbital edema, head dressing, endotracheal tube, and effects of ICP
- Body image disturbance related to change in appearance or physical disabilities

Other nursing diagnoses may include impaired communication (aphasia) related to insult to brain tissue and high risk for impaired skin integrity related to immobility, pressure, and incontinence. There may be impaired physical mobility related to a neurologic deficit secondary to the neurosurgical procedure.

Collaborative Problems/ Potential Complications

Based on the assessment data, potential complications may include:

- Increased intracranial pressure
- Bleeding and hypovolemic shock
- Fluid and electrolyte disturbances
- Infection
- Seizures

Planning and Implementation

Goals. The major goals for the patient may include achievement of neurologic homeostasis to improve cerebral tissue perfusion, achievement of thermoregulation, ability to cope with sensory deprivation, normal ventilation and gas exchange, adaptation to changes in body image, and absence of complications.

Postoperative Nursing Interventions

Achieving Neurologic Homeostasis. Attention to the respiratory status is essential because even slight decreases in the oxygen level (hypoxia) can cause cerebral ischemia and affect the patient's clinical course and outcome. The endotracheal tube is left in place until the patient shows signs of awakening and has adequate spontaneous ventilation, as evaluated clinically and by arterial blood gas analysis. Secondary brain damage can result from impaired cerebral oxygenation.

Cerebral edema is an increase in the water content of brain tissue leading to an increase in brain volume. Some degree of cerebral edema occurs after brain surgery; it tends to be maximal 24 to 36 hours postoperatively, producing decreased responsiveness on the second postoperative day. The control of cerebral edema is discussed on p. 1712. The nursing strategies used to control factors that may raise ICP are found on p. 1714. Intraventricular drainage is carefully monitored, using strict asepsis if any part of the system is handled.

The vital signs and neurologic checks (level of consciousness and responsiveness, pupillary and motor responses) are assessed every 15 minutes to 1 hour. Extreme head rotation is avoided as this raises ICP. After supratentorial surgery, the patient is placed on the back or side (unoperated side if a large lesion was removed) with one pillow under the head. The head of the bed may be elevated 20 to 30 degrees according to the level of the ICP and the neurosurgeon's instructions. After posterior fossa (infratentorial) surgery, the patient is kept flat on one side (off the back) with the head on a small, firm pillow. The patient may be turned on either side, but the head should not be flexed onto the chest. When the patient is being turned, the body should be turned as a unit to prevent placing strain on the incision and possibly tearing the sutures.

The patient's position is changed every 2 hours and skin care is given frequently. During position changes, care is taken to prevent disruption of the ICP monitoring system. A turning sheet from the head to the mid-thigh level makes it easier to move and turn the patient.

Regulating Temperature. Moderate temperature elevation can be expected after intracranial surgery because of reaction to blood at the operative site or in the subarachnoid space. Injury to the hypothalamic centers that regulate body temperature can occur during surgery. High fever is treated vigorously to combat the effect of an elevated increasing temperature on brain metabolism and function.

Nursing interventions include monitoring the temperature and using measures to reduce body temperature: removing blankets, applying ice bags to axilla and groin areas, using a hypothermia blanket as prescribed, and administering prescribed medications to reduce fever.

Conversely, hypothermia may be seen after lengthy neurosurgical procedures. Therefore, frequent measurements of rectal temperature are necessary. Rewarming should occur slowly to prevent shivering and increased cellular oxygen demand.

Improving Gas Exchange. The patient undergoing neurosurgery is at risk for impaired gas exchange and pulmonary infections because of immobility, immunosuppression, decreased levels of consciousness, and fluid restriction. Immobility compromises the respiratory system by causing pooling and stasis of secretions in dependent areas and the development of atelectasis. Patients whose fluid intake is restricted may be more vulnerable to atelectasis as a result of inability to expectorate thickened secretions. Pneumonia is frequently seen in neurosurgical patients, possibly related to aspiration.

The patient is observed for signs of respiratory infection: rise in temperature, increase in pulse rate, and changes in respirations. The lungs are auscultated for decreased breath sounds and adventitious sounds.

The patient is repositioned every 2 hours to mobilize secretions and prevent stasis. When the patient regains consciousness, additional measures are instituted, such as yawning, sighing, deep breathing, use of incentive spirometry, and coughing (unless contraindicated) to expand collapsed alveoli. Suctioning may be needed to remove secretions that cannot be raised by coughing. However, it is important to remember that coughing and suctioning raise ICP. Increasing the humidity may help to loosen secretions. The nurse and the respiratory therapist work together to monitor the effects of chest physical therapy.

Coping With Sensory Deprivation. Periorbital edema is a common consequence of intracranial surgery because fluid drains into the dependent periorbital areas when the patient has been positioned in a prone position during surgery. A hematoma may form under the scalp and spread down to the orbit, producing an area of ecchymosis (black eye). Sometimes the eyes cannot be opened for a few days because of edema of the eyelids.

Preoperatively, the patient and family should be informed that one or both eyes may be edematous temporarily following surgery. Postoperatively, placing the patient in a head-up position and applying cold compresses over the eyes will help reduce the edema. If periorbital edema increases significantly, the surgeon is notified as it may indicate that a postoperative clot is developing or that there is increasing ICP and poor venous drainage. Health care personnel should announce their presence when entering the room to avoid startling the patient whose vision is impaired because of the periorbital edema.

Achieving Self-Acceptance. The patient is encouraged to verbalize feelings and frustrations about any change in appearance. Nursing support is based on the patient's reactions and feelings. Factual information may need to be provided if the patient has misconceptions about puffiness about the face, periorbital bruising, and hair loss. Attention to grooming, the use of personal clothing, and covering the head with a turban (and ultimately a wig until hair growth occurs) are encouraged. Social interaction with close friends, family, and hospital personnel may increase the patient's sense of self-worth.

As the patient assumes more responsibility for self-care and participates in more activities, a sense of control and personal competence will develop. The family and social support system can be of assistance to the patient until adaptation is fully made.

Patient Education and Home Care Considerations. The recovery at home of a neurosurgical patient depends on the extent of the procedure and its success. The patient's strengths as well as limitations are explained to the family, along with their part in promoting his or her recovery. Because administration of anticonvulsant medication is a priority, the patient and family are encouraged to use a check-off system to make sure the medication is taken. The patient may need to be accompanied while walking if sudden attacks of dizziness or seizures occur.

Usually dietary restrictions are not required unless another health problem requiring a special diet exists. Although taking a shower or tub bath is permitted, the scalp should be kept dry until all the sutures have been removed. A clean scarf or cap may be worn until a wig or hairpiece is purchased. If skull bone has been removed, the neurosurgeon may suggest a protective helmet.

After a craniotomy, the patient is usually more sensitive to loud noises. Television noise can be irritating to the convalescing person. If the patient is aphasic, speech therapy may be necessary. This is likely to be a long-term and time-consuming process, requiring patience and continuing encouragement on the part of all who are working with the patient.

When tumor, injury, or disease make the prognosis poor, care is directed toward making the patient as comfortable as possible. With return of the tumor or cerebral compression, the patient becomes less alert and aware. Other possible sequelae include paralysis, blindness, and seizures. The home care nurse, hospice nurse and social worker work with the family to plan for additional home health care or hospice services to place the patient in an extended-care facility. (See also the section on cerebral metastases in Chapter 60.)

Patients who do not develop complications are discharged from the hospital as soon as possible. Patients with motor deficits require management similar to that after a stroke (see p. 1727). Those with postoperative cognitive and speech impairment require psychologic evaluation, speech therapy, and rehabilitation. The nurse works collaboratively with the physician and other health care professionals during hospitalization and home care to achieve as complete a rehabilitation of the patient as possible.

Monitoring and Managing Potential Complications. Complications that may develop within hours after surgery include increased intracranial pressure, bleeding and hypovolemic shock, altered fluid and electrolyte balance (including water intoxication), infection, and seizures. These problems require close collaboration between the nurse and the surgeon.

Increased Intracranial Pressure, Bleeding, and Hypovolemic Shock. Increased ICP, bleeding, and hypovolemic shock are life threatening to the patient who has undergone intracranial neurosurgery. The following must be kept in mind when caring for all patients who undergo such surgery:

- An increase in blood pressure and decrease in pulse with respiratory failure may indicate increased ICP.

- A drop in blood pressure, a rapid pulse and respiration, and a pale and cold body are usually manifestations of hypovolemic shock after lengthy surgical procedures. Its treatment depends on the cause of the hypovolemic shock. Fluid replacement is indicated if hypovolemia is due to fluid loss or diabetes insipidus; blood component therapy is indicated if blood loss is the cause.
- An accumulation of blood under the bone flap (extradural, subdural, intracerebral) may pose a threat to life. A clot must be suspected in any patient who does not awaken as expected or whose condition deteriorates. An intracranial hematoma is suspected if the patient has any new postoperative neurologic deficits (especially a dilated pupil on the operative side). In these events, the patient is returned to the operating room immediately for evacuation of the clot if indicated.
- Cerebral edema, infarction, metabolic disturbances, and hydrocephalus are conditions that may simulate the clinical manifestations of a clot.

The patient is monitored closely for indicators of complications, and early signs and trends in clinical status are reported to the surgeon. Treatments are initiated promptly, and the nurse assists in evaluating the patient's response to treatment. The nurse also provides support to the patient and family.

Should signs and symptoms of increased intracranial pressure occur, efforts to decrease the ICP are initiated: alignment of the head in a neutral position without flexion to promote venous drainage, elevation of the head of the bed to 30°, administration of mannitol (osmotic diuretic), and possible administration of pharmacologic paralyzing agents.

Fluid and Electrolyte Disturbances. Fluid and electrolyte imbalance may occur because of the patient's underlying condition and its management or as complications of surgery. Fluid and electrolyte disturbances can contribute to the development of cerebral edema.

The postoperative fluid regimen depends on the type of neurosurgical procedure and is calculated on an individual basis. The volume and composition of fluids are adjusted according to daily electrolyte determinations and intake and output.

Sodium retention may occur in the immediate postoperative period. Serum and urine electrolytes, blood urea nitrogen (BUN), blood glucose, weight, and clinical status are monitored. The intake and output are measured in view of losses associated with fever, respiration, and CSF drainage. Fluids may have to be restricted in patients with cerebral edema.

Oral fluids are usually resumed in a short period, and the body's own homeostatic mechanisms regulate electrolyte balance. Some patients with posterior fossa tumors may have impaired swallowing, however, and fluids may have to be administered by way of alternate routes.

Patients undergoing surgery for brain tumors may be on large doses of corticosteriods and thus may have a tendency to develop *hyperglycemia*. Therefore, serum glucose levels are measured every 4 hours.

Because these patients are prone to *gastric ulcers*, antacids or H2-receptor blockers may be prescribed to reduce the secretion of gastric acid. The patient is monitored for bleeding and assessed for gastric pain.

After surgery in and around the pituitary gland and hypothalamus, the patient may develop symptoms of *diabetes insipidus* (DI), which is characterized by excessive urinary output. The urine specific gravity is measured hourly, and fluid intake and output charts are monitored. Fluid replacement must compensate for urine output and serum potassium must be monitored.

The *syndrome of inappropriate secretion of antidiuretic hormone* (SIADH), resulting in water retention with hyponatremia and serum hypo-osmolality, occurs in a wide variety of CNS dysfunctions (brain tumor, head trauma) causing fluid disturbances. Nursing management of this syndrome requires careful intake and output measurements, specific gravity determinations of urine, and monitoring of serum and urine electrolyte studies, while following directives for fluid restriction. This syndrome is usually self-limiting.

Infection. The patient undergoing neurosurgery is at risk for infection related to the neurosurgical procedure (brain exposure, bone exposure, wound hematomas) and the presence of intravenous and arterial lines for fluid administration and monitoring. Risk for infection is increased in those patients who undergo lengthy intracranial operations and those with external ventricular drains in place longer than 48 to 72 hours.

The incision site is monitored for evidence of redness, tenderness, bulging, separation, or foul odor. The dressing is often stained with blood in the immediate postoperative period. It is important to reinforce the dressing with sterile pads so that contamination and infection are avoided. (Blood is an excellent culture medium for bacteria.) If the dressing is heavily stained or displaced, it should be reported immediately. (A drain is sometimes placed in the craniotomy wound to facilitate drainage.)

After suboccipital surgical procedures, CSF may leak through the wound. This complication is dangerous because of the possibility of *meningitis*. Any sudden discharge of fluid from a cranial or spinal wound is reported at once because a massive leak requires direct surgical repair. Attention should be paid to the patient complaining of a salty taste because this can be due to CSF trickling down the throat. The patient is advised to avoid coughing, sneezing, or nose blowing, which may cause CSF leakage by creating pressure on the operative site.

Other causes of infection in the patient undergoing intracranial surgery are similar to those in other postoperative patients: phlebitis, deep vein thrombosis, and urinary tract infections.

Aseptic technique is used when handling dressings, drainage systems, and intravenous and arterial lines. The patient is monitored carefully for signs and symptoms of infection, and cultures are obtained from the patient with suspected infection. Appropriate antibiotics are administered as prescribed.

Seizures. Seizures and epilepsy may be complications after any intracranial neurosurgical procedure. Preventing seizures is essential to avoid further cerebral edema. Administering the prescribed anticonvulsant medication before and immediately after surgery may prevent the appearance of seizures in subsequent months and years. Status epilepticus (occurrence of prolonged seizures without recovery of consciousness in the intervals between seizures) may occur after craniotomy and also may be related to the development of complications (hematoma, ischemia). The management of status epilepticus is described in Chapter 60.

Other Complications. Other complications may occur during the first 2 weeks or later and may threaten the patient's recovery. The most important of these are thromboembolic complications (deep vein thrombosis, pulmonary embolism), pulmonary and urinary infection, and pressure ulcers. Most of these complications may be avoided by frequent change of position, adequate suctioning of secretions, assessment for pulmonary complications, observation for urinary complications, and skin care.

Evaluation

Expected Outcomes

1. Achieves neurologic homeostasis/improved cerebral tissue perfusion
   a. Opens eyes on request; uses recognizable words progressing to normal speech
   b. Obeys commands with appropriate motor responses
2. Attains thermoregulation and normal body temperature
3. Copes with sensory deprivation
4. Has normal gas exchange
   a. Arterial blood gases within normal
   b. Breath sounds clear without adventitious sounds
   c. Takes deep breaths and changes position as directed
5. Demonstrates an improving self-concept
   a. Pays attention to grooming
   b. Visits and interacts with others
6. Absence of complications
   a. Intracranial pressure is normal
   b. Bleeding at surgical site is minimal and surgical incision is healing without evidence of infection
   c. Body temperature is normal
   d. Fluid balance and electrolyte levels are within desired ranges.
   e. Exhibits no evidence of seizures

An overview of care of the patient undergoing intracranial surgery is presented in Chart 59-5.

Transsphenoidal Surgery

Tumors located within the sella turcica and small adenomas of the pituitary can be removed by way of the transsphenoidal approach (see Table 59-4).

The incision is made beneath the upper lip, and entry is then gained successively into the nasal cavity, sphenoidal sinus, and sella turcica. Although the initial opening may be made by an otorhinolaryngologist, the neurosurgeon completes the opening into the sphenoidal sinus and exposes the floor of the sella. Microsurgical techniques provide improved illumination, magnification, and visualization so that nearby vital structures can be avoided.

The transsphenoidal approach offers direct access to the sella with minimal risk of trauma and hemorrhage. It avoids many of the risks of craniotomy, and the postoperative discomfort is similar to that of other transnasal surgical procedures. It may also be used for pituitary ablation (removal) in patients with disseminated breast or prostatic cancer.

Preoperative Evaluation

The preoperative workup includes a series of endocrine tests, rhinologic evaluation (to assess the status of the sinuses and nasal cavity), and neuroradiologic studies. Funduscopic examination and visual field determinations are performed, because the most serious effect of pituitary tumor is localized pressure on the optic nerve or chiasm. In addition, the nasopharyngeal secretions are cultured because a sinus infection is a contraindication to an intracranial procedure through this approach. Corticosteroids may be given preoperatively and postoperatively (because the surgery involves removal of the pituitary, the source of adrenocorticotropic hormone [ACTH] is removed). Antibiotics may or may not be administered prophylactically.

Deep breathing is taught preoperatively. The patient is instructed on the technique for avoiding vigorous coughing and sneezing because these actions may cause a CSF leak after surgery. Instructions include applying pressure on the inner aspect of both sides of the nose to control sneezing.

Postoperative Management

Because the procedure disrupts the oral and nasal mucous membranes, management focuses on preventing infection and promoting healing. Medications given to the patient include antimicrobials (which are continued until the nasal packing inserted at the time of surgery is removed), corticosteroids, analgesics for discomfort, and agents for the control of diabetes insipidus, when necessary.

The nasal packing is removed in 24 hours to several days. The area around the nares is cleaned with the prescribed solution to remove crusted blood and moisten the mucous membranes.

Postoperative Nursing Interventions

The vital signs are measured to monitor hemodynamic, cardiac, and ventilatory status. Because of the anatomic proximity of the pituitary gland to the optic chiasm, visual acuity is assessed at regular intervals. One method is to ask the patient to count the number of fingers held up by the nurse. Evidence of decreasing visual acuity suggests an expanding hematoma.

Oral Care. The major discomfort of the patient is related to the nasal packing and to mouth dryness and thirst from mouth-breathing. Oral care is provided every 4 hours or more frequently. Usually, the patient's teeth are not brushed until the incision above the teeth has healed. The use of warm saline mouth rinses and a cool mist vaporizer is helpful. Petrolatum is soothing when applied to the lips. A room humidifier assists in keeping the patient's mucous membranes moist.

Positioning and ICP Precautions. The head of the bed is raised to decrease pressure on the sella turcica and to promote normal drainage. The patient is cautioned

CHART 59-5
Summary: Nursing Management of the Patient Undergoing Intracranial Surgery

Postoperative Interventions

Nursing Diagnosis: Potential for ineffective breathing pattern related to postoperative cerebral edema
Goal: Achievement of adequate respiratory function

1. Establish proper respiratory exchange to eliminate systemic hypercapnia and hypoxia, which increase cerebral edema.
   a. Unless contraindicated, place the patient in a lateral or a semiprone position to facilitate respiratory gas exchange until consciousness returns.
   b. Suction trachea and pharynx *cautiously* to remove secretions; suctioning can raise intracranial pressure.
   c. Maintain patient on controlled ventilation if prescribed to maintain normal ventilatory status; monitor arterial blood gas results to determine respiratory status.
   d. Elevate the head of the bed 30.5 cm (12 in) after patient is conscious to aid venous drainage of the brain.
   e. Administer nothing by mouth until active coughing and swallowing reflexes are demonstrated, to prevent aspiration.

Nursing Diagnosis: Potential alteration in fluid volume related to intracranial pressure or diuretics
Goal: Attainment of fluid and electrolyte balance

1. Monitor for polyuria especially during first postoperative week; diabetes insipidus may develop in patients with lesions around the pituitary or hypothalamus
   a. Measure urinary specific gravity at intervals.
   b. Monitor serum and urinary electrolyte levels.
2. Evaluate patient's electrolyte status; patients may retain water and sodium.
   a. Early postoperative weight gain indicates fluid retention; a greater than estimated weight loss indicates negative water balance.
   b. Loss of sodium and chloride will produce weakness, lethargy, and coma.
   c. Low potassium will cause confusion and decreased level of responsiveness.
3. Weigh patient daily; keep intake and output record.
4. Administer prescribed intravenous fluids cautiously—rate and composition depend on fluid deficit, urine output, and blood loss. Fluid intake and fluid losses should remain relatively equal.

Nursing Diagnosis: Alteration in sensory perceptions (visual/auditory) related to periorbital edema and head dressings
Goal: Compensate for sensory deprivation

1. Perform supportive measures until the patient is able to care for himself or herself.
   a. Change position as indicated; be aware that position changes can increase intracranial pressure.
   b. Administer prescribed analgesics (codeine) that do not mask the level of responsiveness.
2. Use measures prescribed to relieve signs of periocular edema.
   a. Lubricate eyelids and around eyes with petrolatum.
   b. Apply light, cold compresses over eyes at specified intervals.
   c. Observe for signs of keratitis if cornea has no sensation.
3. Put extremities through range of motion exercises.
4. Evaluate and support patient during episodes of restlessness.
   a. Evaluate for airway obstruction, distended bladder, meningeal irritation from bloody cerebrospinal fluid.
   b. Pad patient's hands and bed rails to prevent injury.
5. Reinforce blood-stained dressings with sterile dressing; blood-soaked dressings act as a culture medium for bacteria.
6. Orient patient frequently to time, place, and person.

Monitor and Manage Complications

1. Cerebral edema
   a. Assess patient's level of responsiveness/consciousness; decreased level of consciousness may be the first sign of increased intracranial pressure.
      (1) Eye opening (spontaneous, to sound, to pain); pupillary reactions to light
      (2) Response to commands
      (3) Assessment of spinal motor reflexes (pinch Achilles tendon, arm, or other body site)
      (4) Observation of patient's spontaneous activity
   b. Maintain a neurologic flow sheet to assess and document neurologic status, fluid administration, laboratory data, medications and treatments.
   c. Evaluate for signs and symptoms of increasing intracranial pressure, which can lead to ischemia and further impairment of brain function.
      (1) Assess patient minute by minute, hour by hour, for:
         - Diminished response to stimuli
         - Fluctuations of vital signs
         - Restlessness
         - Weakness and paralysis of extremities
         - Increasing headache
         - Changes or disturbances of vision; pupillary changes
      (2) Modify nursing management to prevent further increases in intracranial pressure.
   d. Control postoperative cerebral edema as prescribed.
      (1) Administer corticosteroids and osmotic diuretics as prescribed to reduce brain swelling.
      (2) Monitor fluid intake; avoid overhydration
      (3) Maintain a normal temperature. Temperature control may be impaired in certain neurologic states, and fever increases the metabolic demands of the brain.
         - Monitor rectal temperature at specified intervals. Assess temperature of extremities, which may be cold and dry due to impaired heat-losing mechanisms (vasodilation and sweating).
         - Employ measures as prescribed to reduce excessive fever: ice bags to axillae and groin; hypothermia blanket. Use ECG monitoring to detect dysrhythmias during hypothermia procedures.
      (4) Employ hyperventilation when prescribed (results in respiratory alkalosis, which causes cerebral vasoconstriction and reduces circulation, and intracranial pressure).

(continued)

CHART 59-5 (continued)

Summary: Nursing Management of the Patient Undergoing Intracranial Surgery

(5) Elevate head of bed to reduce intracranial pressure and facilitate respirations.
(6) Avoid excessive stimuli.
(7) Use intracranial pressure monitoring if patient is at risk for intracranial hypertension.

2. Intracranial hemorrhage
   a. Postoperative bleeding may be intraventricular, intracerebellar, subdural, or extradural.
   b. Observe for progressive impairment of state of consciousness and other signs of increasing intracranial pressure.
   c. Prepare deteriorating patient for return to surgery for evacuation of hematoma.
3. Seizures (There is a greater risk with supratentorial operations.)
   a. Administer prescribed anticonvulsants; monitor anticonvulsant blood levels.
   b. Observe for status epilepticus, which may occur after any intracranial surgery.
4. Infections
   a. Urinary tract infections
   b. Pulmonary infections related to aspiration secondary to depressed level of responsiveness; may result in atelectasis and aspiration pneumonia
   c. CNS infections (postoperative meningitis, cerebrospinal fluid shunt infection)
   d. Wound infections/septicemia
5. Venous thrombosis
   a. Assess Homans' sign.
   b. Apply elastic stockings.
   c. Administer anticoagulant therapy as prescribed.
6. Leakage of cerebrospinal fluid
   a. Differentiate between cerebrospinal fluid and mucus.
      (1) Collect fluid on Dextrostix; if cerebrospinal fluid is present, the indicator will have a positive reaction, as cerebrospinal fluid contains glucose.
      (2) Assess for moderate elevation of temperature and mild neck rigidity.
   b. Caution patient against nose blowing or sniffing.
   c. Elevate head of bed as prescribed.
   d. Assist with insertion of CSF drainage system if inserted to reduce CSF pressure.
      (1) Ventricular catheters may be inserted in the patient undergoing surgery of the posterior fossa (ventriculostomy); the catheter(s) is connected to a closed drainage system.
      (2) Administer antibiotics as prescribed.
7. Gastrointestinal ulceration; monitor for signs and symptoms of hemorrhage, perforation, or both (probably caused by stress response).

Evaluation

Expected Outcomes

1. Demonstrates normal breathing pattern
   a. Absence of crackles
   b. Demonstrates active swallowing and coughing reflexes
2. Attains/maintains fluid balance
   a. Takes fluids orally
   b. Maintains weight within expected range
3. Compensates for sensory deprivation
   a. Makes needs known
   b. Demonstrates improvement of vision
4. Reveals absence of complications
   a. No evidence of increased intracranial pressure
   b. Opens eyes on request
   c. Obeys commands
   d. Has appropriate motor responses
   e. Shows increasing alertness
   f. No evidence of rhinorrhea, otorrhea, or CSF leakage
   g. Absence of fever
   h. No evidence of inflammation or infection around wound
   i. Absence of seizures

against blowing his or her nose or engaging in any activity that raises ICP, such as bending over or straining during urination or defecation.

Fluid and Electrolyte Monitoring. Intake and output are measured as a guide to fluid and electrolyte replacement. The urinary specific gravity is measured after each voiding. The patient's daily weight is monitored. Fluids are generally given when nausea ceases, and the patient then progresses to a regular diet.

Complications

Manipulation of the posterior pituitary gland during surgery may produce transient *diabetes insipidus* of several days' duration that is treated with vasopressin. Occasionally, diabetes insipidus persists. Other complications include CSF leakage, postoperative meningitis, and SIADH.

Home care considerations include advising the patient to use a room humidifier to keep the mucous membranes moist and to soothe irritation. The head of the bed is elevated for at least 2 weeks after surgery.

Neurologic and Neurosurgical Approaches to Pain Management

The management of long-term pain requires a multidisciplinary approach. (See Chapter 13 for a discussion of pain, its assessment, and pharmacologic and noninvasive methods of treatment.)

Intractable pain refers to pain that cannot be relieved satisfactorily by usual approaches, including medications. Such pain usually is the result of malignancy (especially of the cervix, bladder, prostate, and lower bowel), but it may occur in other conditions, such as postherpetic neuralgia, trigeminal neuralgia, spinal cord arachnoiditis, and uncontrollable ischemia and other forms of tissue destruction.

Neurologic and neurosurgical methods available for pain relief include (1) stimulation procedures—intermittent electric stimulation of a tract or center to inhibit the transmission of pain impulses, (2) administration of intraspinal opiates, and (3) interruption of the tracts conducting the pain impulse from the periphery to cerebral integration centers. The latter are destructive or ablative procedures.

Stimulation Procedures

Electrical stimulation, or neuromodulation, is a method of suppressing pain by applying controlled low-voltage electrical pulses to the different parts of the nervous system. Electrical stimulation is thought to relieve pain by blocking painful stimuli or by stimulating the release of endogenous opiates (natural pain-relieving peptides, or endorphins). This pain-modulating technique is administered by many modes. Transcutaneous electrical nerve stimulation and dorsal column stimulation are the most frequent types of electrical stimulation used. In addition, there are also brain-stimulating techniques in which electrodes are implanted in the periventricular area of the posterior third ventricle, allowing the patient to stimulate this area to produce analgesia.

Transcutaneous electric nerve stimulation (TENS) is the passage of small electrical currents through the skin (see Fig. 13-6) for the purpose of controlling localized pain. Electrodes are placed over the site of pain, along the course of the major peripheral nerves innervating the area, or over the peripheral plexus. The patient operates the amplitude control until stimulation, detected by a vibration, buzzing, or tapping sensation, is felt within the deeper tissue. The amplitude is increased slowly until the sensation is perceived at the site or origin of pain or along radiating pathways. The patient controls the amplitude, frequency, and duration of stimulation. TENS has been successful in the well-prepared patient in the early management of acute pain as well as in the patient with chronic pain. It is most effective when used as part of a comprehensive rehabilitation program for relief and elimination of pain.

Dorsal column stimulation (DCS) is a technique used for the relief of chronic, intractable pain in which a surgically implanted device allows the patient to apply pulsed electrical stimulation to the dorsal aspect of the spinal cord to block pain impulses. (The largest accumulation of afferent fibers is found in the dorsal column of the spinal cord.)

The dorsal column stimulation unit consists of a radio-frequency stimulation transmitter, a transmitter antenna, a radio-frequency receiver, and a stimulation electrode. The battery-powered transmitter and antenna are worn externally; the receiver and electrode are implanted.

A laminectomy is performed above the highest level of pain input, and the electrode is placed in the epidural space over the posterior column of the spinal cord. (The placement of the stimulating systems is varied.) A subcutaneous pocket is constructed over the clavicular area or some other site for placement of the receiver. The two are connected by a subcutaneous tunnel.

Percutaneous epidural neurostimulation is a method of neurostimulation in which electrodes are inserted percutaneously into the spinal epidural space. It appears to be effective in treating arachnoiditis and postamputation neuroma.

Deep brain stimulation is performed for special pain problems when the patient does not respond to the usual techniques of pain control. With the patient under local anesthesia, electrodes are introduced through a burr hole in the skull and inserted into a selected site in the brain, depending on the location or type of pain. After the effectiveness of stimulation is confirmed, the implanted electrode is connected to a radio-frequency device or pulse generator system operated by external telemetry.

Nursing Implications

With each of these systems, the patient is provided with written and verbal instructions about its use and side effects. With TENS, the skin is cleansed and electrode gel is applied to the electrodes, which are then placed over the nerves that innervate the painful area. The electrodes are secured with hypoallergenic tape. Skin irritation from the tape, gels, or electrodes is the most common adverse effect of TENS. The patient is instructed to keep a record evaluating the effectiveness of TENS. If there is a progression of pathology (as in advanced cancer), changes in amplitude may be necessary.

Following surgery or percutaneous insertion of electrodes to establish the dorsal column stimulation, epidural neurostimulation, or deep brain stimulation system, the patient is assessed for infection or drainage (*i.e.*, CSF) at the insertion site. Other post-procedure assessments are based on the specific procedure performed; for example, the care for the patient undergoing surgery to insert electrodes for the dorsal column stimulator is similar to that required for a laminectomy. The patient is assessed for evidence of paraplegia, quadriplegia, and urinary incontinence.

Complications include infection, cord trauma, CSF leakage, and pain around the implantation site. Failure of the stimulating system and development of tolerance may occur later.

Nursing interventions include teaching the patient and family about the system, encouraging the patient to keep a record of amplitude and frequency settings and the relief obtained, and monitoring for complications.

Intraspinal Opioids

Opioid receptors exist not only in the brain but also in the substantia gelatinosa of the spinal cord. These receptors can combine with locally administered opioids (morphine) injected epidurally or intrathecally to produce long-lasting pain relief with little or no blunting of the patient's level of responsiveness and no losses of sensory, motor, or sphincter function. (Care of the patient receiving intraspinal opioids for pain relief is discussed in detail in Chapter 13.)

Numerous techniques are employed, but most include placing a catheter in the epidural or subarachnoid space with a spinal needle and inserting the catheter as near as possible to the spinal segment where the pain is projected. Small doses of morphine are injected into the system at regular intervals. If the patient requires long-term management, an implantable programmable pump is used.

After the procedure the patient is evaluated for the degree of pain relief, which ranges from good to excellent. The catheter insertion site is inspected for evidence of infection.

This method allows the patient to be at home. The necessary dose of medication is small; the patient is alert and usually able to function at a relatively high level. He may complain of generalized itching and urinary retention (self-limited) for several days. With long-term use there can be tolerance buildup and mechanical failure (catheter obstructed, dislodged, broken) of the administration system. If the patient has rapid tumor growth, the dosage of morphine is increased, but the doses needed are low in comparison with those required for systemic administration for intractable pain.

Destructive or Ablative Procedures

Pain-conducting fibers can be interrupted at any point from their origin to the cerebral cortex. Some part of the nervous system is destroyed, resulting in varying amounts of neurologic deficit and incapacity. In time, pain usually returns as a result of either regeneration of axonal fibers or the development of alternative pain pathways.

Cordotomy

Cordotomy is the division of certain tracts of the spinal cord. It may be performed percutaneously, by the open method after laminectomy, or by other techniques.

Percutaneous cordotomy uses radio-frequency currents to produce lesions in the anterolateral surface of the spinal cord. With the patient under local anesthesia, a needle is inserted into the neck below and behind the mastoid process. It is guided into the spinal cord under x-ray control, and an electrode is inserted through it. By means of radio-frequency currents, a lesion is made at the desired spinal cord level.

Verification of electrode placement is determined by the patient's response to stimulation. The procedure generally is well tolerated by emaciated and debilitated patients.

Open cordotomy involves the surgical division of the anterolateral columns of the spinal pain fibers high in the thoracic or cervical region. This procedure interrupts or destroys conduction of pain and temperature sensation, while touch and position sense are preserved. The spinal cord is exposed by laminectomy.

Cordotomy is used most frequently in controlling the severe pain of terminal cancer, especially of the thorax, abdomen, or lower extremities. Because a significant percentage of cordotomies lose their effectiveness in 1 to 5 years, the procedure is used for pain associated with conditions in which survival time is limited.

Postoperative Nursing Management. The principles of nursing management after a laminectomy apply to postoperative and rehabilitation care of patients undergoing cordotomy (see Chapter 60). After a cordotomy, the patient may be kept flat for the prescribed time, because there is less tension on the incision in this position. A patient with a thoracic cordotomy may be turned to the prone position. In instances of a cervical incision, pillows should not be used when the patient is in a supine position. Trauma to the surgical site is reduced when the neck is kept in a neutral position. The patient is turned as a unit (log fashion) by two persons using a turning sheet to avoid twisting the body and putting pressure on the incision.

In addition to surgical interventions for intractable pain, nonsurgical techniques may be of some benefit (see Chapter 13 for further discussion of pain management).

Assessment for Complications. The patient is monitored for respiratory complications, as well as for signs of fatigue and weakening of the voice. The patient may ventilate adequately while awake but may experience progressive hypercarbia and hypoxia while asleep. Therefore, arterial blood gases are monitored, and assisted mechanical ventilation is initiated if required.

Because hemorrhage may result in motor and sensory loss, the motion, strength, and sensation of each extremity must be tested every few hours, or more frequently if necessary, during the first 48 hours postoperatively. If hemorrhage is suggested or detected, immediate surgical intervention is imperative. Because the patient has no sense of temperature, the skin should be palpated at intervals to ascertain any changes in temperature. Because pressure ulcers may develop without the patient realizing it, the patient is taught to inspect his skin using a hand mirror to view the hard-to-see areas and to change position frequently. Urinary retention may occur. There is usually a slow return to normal voiding, but this cannot be guaranteed. If there is permanent loss of urinary control from a high cervical procedure, a bladder training program is started.

Rhizotomy

Rhizotomy, the surgical division of the spinal roots, is used for controlling severe chest pain of lung cancer and for pain relief in head and neck malignancies.

Because many patients with metastatic malignancies may not be able to tolerate an open rhizotomy, a **percutaneous rhizotomy** may be performed, in which a radio-frequency current is used to selectively coagulate the pain fibers while the fibers concerned with touch and proprioception are preserved.

In a **chemical rhizotomy**, alcohol, phenol, or a mixture of agents is injected into the subarachnoid space. The medication is maneuvered over the affected nerve roots by tilting the patient to the desired level. This renders the sensory nerve roots functionless. The patient's perception of pain is absent, but the motor nerve roots are usually not affected.

Psychosurgical Approaches

The purpose of psychosurgical procedures is to alter the patient's response to pain. A **thalamotomy** is the destruction (either unilateral or bilateral) of the specific cell groups within the thalamus. Burr holes are made in the skull, electrodes are placed in the target area by stereotaxic techniques, and a radio-frequency current is then directed through the electrodes to create the lesion. This procedure represents the highest level in the CNS in which pain pathways can be interrupted and is usually performed for malignancy of the head and neck.

CRITICAL THINKING EXERCISES

1. Your patient has experienced a severe head injury and is being monitored for increased intracranial pressure (ICP). While changing his linens, you note that the ICP increased and remained increased for 10 minutes. Based on your analysis of these data, how would you determine what actions to take in response to the patient's increased ICP? Explain how you reached this conclusion and what outcomes you are hoping to achieve by your actions.
2. You are caring for two patients who have experienced strokes. One patient has had a left hemispheric stroke, the other a right hemispheric stroke. What different manifestations would you expect to note in each patient, and how would your care differ for them?
3. Following cranial surgery, your patient has developed expressive aphasia. How would this development affect your interaction with the patient? How would you explain the manifestations of expressive aphasia to the patient's family, and what suggestions would you give to them about how to communicate with their loved one?

Cingulotomy is a unilateral or bilateral interruption of the anterior cingulate bundle in the frontal lobe of the brain. It is accomplished by either an open or a stereotaxic approach. It tends to modify the patient's affective reaction to pain.

BIBLIOGRAPHY

Books

Agency for Health Care Policy and Research, Public Health Service. U.S. Department of Health and Human Services. Panel for the Prediction and Prevention of Pressure Ulcers in Adults. Pressure Ulcers in Adults: Prediction and Prevention. Clinical Practice Guideline Number 3. AHCPR Publication No. 92-0047. Rockville, MD, May 1992.

Agency for Health Care Policy and Research, Public Health Service. U.S. Department of Health and Human Services. Urinary Incontinence Guideline Panel. Urinary Incontinence in Adults: Clinical Practice Guideline. AHCPR Publication No. 92-0038. Rockville, MD, March 1992.

Agency for Health Care Policy and Research, Public Health Service. U.S. Department of Health and Human Services. Panel for the Prediction and Prevention of Pressure Ulcers in Adults. Treatment of Pressure Ulcers. Clinical Practical Guideline No. 15. AHCPR Publication No. 94-0652. Rockville, MD, December 1994.

Agency for Health Care Policy and Research, Public Health Service. U.S. Department of Health and Human Services. Post-Stroke Rehabilitation. Clinical Practice Guideline. AHCPR Publication No. 95-0662. Rockville, MD, May 1995.

Barnett H (ed). Stroke: Pathophysiology, Diagnosis, and Management, 2nd ed. New York, Churchill Livingstone, 1992.

Bates B. A Guide to Physical Examination and History Taking, 6th ed. Philadelphia, JB Lippincott, 1995.

Bernat JL. Ethical Issues in Neurology. Boston, Betterworth-Heinemann, 1994.

Boggs R and Wooldridge-King M (ed). AACN Procedure Manual for Critical Care, 3rd ed. Philadelphia, WB Saunders, 1993.

Bonica J. The Management of Pain, 2nd ed. Philadelphia, Lea & Febiger, 1990.

Bornstein R and Brown G (eds). Neurobehavioral Aspects of Cerebrovascular Disease. New York, Oxford University Press, 1991.

Cammermeyer M and Appledorn C. Core Curriculum for Neuroscience Nursing. Chicago, American Association of Neuroscience Nurses, 1990.

Caplan L. Stroke: A Clinical Approach. Boston, Butterworth-Heinemann, 1993.

Gilman S and Winans S. Manter and Gatz's Essentials of Clinical Neuroanatomy and Physiology, 8th ed. Philadelphia, FA Davis, 1992.

Haerer A (ed). DeJong's The Neurologic Examination, 5th ed. Philadelphia, JB Lippincott, 1994.

Hickey JV. The Clinical Practice of Neurologic and Neurosurgical Nursing, 3rd ed. Philadelphia, JB Lippincott, 1992.

Jennett B and Lindsay K. An Introduction to Neurosurgery, 5th ed. Boston, Butterworth-Heinemann, 1994.

Rudy E. Advanced Neurological and Neurosurgical Nursing, 2nd ed. St. Louis, CV Mosby, 1994.

Strub RL and Black FW. The Mental Status Examination in Neurology. Philadelphia, FA Davis, 1993.

Treiger N. Pain Control. St. Louis: CV Mosby, 1994.

Vos H. Neurologic alterations. In Thelan L et al (eds). Critical Care Nursing: Diagnosis and Management, 2nd ed. St. Louis, CV Mosby, 1994.

Wall P and Melzack R (ed). Textbook of Pain, 3rd ed. New York, Churchill Livingstone, 1994.

Weiner W and Goetz CG (ed). Neurology for the Non-Neurologist, 2nd ed. Philadelphia, JB Lippincott, 1989.

Westmoreland BF et al. Medical Neurosciences: An Approach to Anatomy, Pathology and Physiology by Systems and Levels. Boston, Little, Brown, 1994.

Journals

Asterisks indicate nursing research articles.

Bell SD et al. Cerebral hemodynamics: Monitoring arteriojugular oxygen content differences. J Neurosci Nurs. 1994 Oct; 26(5): 270–277.

Counsell CN, Guin PR and Limbaugh B. Coordinated care for the neuroscience patient: Future directions. J Neurosci Nurs 1994 Aug; 26(4):245–250.

Davis M and Lucatorto M. Mannitol revisited. J Neurosci Nurs 1994 Jun; 26(3):170–174.

Furlong TG. Neurologic complications of immunosuppressive cancer therapy. Oncol Nurs Forum 1993 Oct; 20(9):1337–1352.

*Grossman M. Received support and psychological adjustment in critically-injured patients and their family. J Neurosci Nurs 1995 Feb; 27(1):11–23.

*Grossman D et al. Current nursing practices in fever management. Medsurg Nurs 1995 Jun; 4(3):193–198.

Guin PR and Freudenberger K. The elderly neuroscience patient: Implications for the critical care nurse. AACN Clin Iss Crit Care Nurs 1992 Feb; 3(1):98–105.

Hilton G. Secondary brain injury and the role of neuroprotective agents. J Neurosci Nurs 1994 Aug 26(4):251–255.

*Myles GL et al. Quantifying nursing care in barbiturate-induced coma with the therapeutic intervention scoring system. J Neurosci Nurs 1995 Feb; 27(1):35–42.

Wall BM, Philips JP, Howard JC. Validation of increased intracranial pressure and high risk for increased intracranial pressure. Nurs Diagn 1994 Apr–Jun; 5(2):74–81.

*Way C and Segatore M. Development and preliminary testing of the neurological assessment instrument. J Neurosci Nurs 1994 Oct; 26(5):278–287.

Care of the Neurosurgical Patient

*Garcia-Larrea L, Artru F, Bertrand O, Pernier J, and Mauguiere F. The combined monitoring of brain stem auditory evoked potentials and intracranial pressure in coma: A study of 57 patients. J Neurol Neurosurg Psychiatr 1992 Sept: 55(9):792.

Gentilello LM. Advances in the management of hypothermia. Surg Clin North Am 1995 Apr; 75(2):243–256.

Nathadwarawala KM, Nicklin J, and Wiles CM. A timed test of swallowing capacity for neurological patients. J Neurol Neurosurg Psychiatr 1992 Sept: 55(9):822.

Stroke and Transient Ischemic Attacks

Adams RJ. Management issues for patients with ischemic stroke. Neurology 1995 Feb; 45 (2 Suppl 1):S15–S18.

*Boynton DE, Sepulveda LI and Chang B. Effective coping with stroke disability in a community setting: The development of a causal model. J Neurosci Nurs 1994 Aug; 26(4):193–203.

Brass L, Fayad P, and Levine S. Transient ischemic attacks in the elderly: Diagnosis and treatment. Geriatrics 1992 May; 47(5): 36–54.

Camp YG et al. Stop and look: Two approaches to manage stroke patients. J Neurosci Nurs 1995 Feb; 27(1):24–28.

Cochran I et al. Stroke care—Piecing together the long-term picture. Nursing 1994 Jun; 24(6):34–41.

Dobkin B. The economic impact of stroke. Neurology 1995 Feb; 45(2 Suppl 1):S6–S9.

Eliasziw M. et al. Prognosis for patients following a transient ischemic attack with and without a cerebral infarction on brain CT. North American Symptomatic Carotid Endarterectomy Trial (NASCET) Group. Neurology 1995 Mar; 45(3 Pt 1):428–431.

Falconer J et al. Predicting stroke inpatient rehabilitation outcome using a classification tree approach. Arch Phys Med Rehabil 1994 Jun; 75(6):619–625.

Gauvitz DF. How to protect the dysphagic stroke patient. Am J Nurs 1995 Aug; 95(8):34–38.

Goldstein L and Matchar D. Clinical assessment of stroke. JAMA 1994 Apr 13; 271(14):1114–1120.

Hydo B. Designing an effective clinical pathway for stroke patients. Am J Nurs 1995 Mar; 95(3):44–50.

Kelly-Hayes M and Paige C. Assessment and psychologic factors in stroke rehabilitation. Neurology 1995 Feb; 45(2 Suppl 1):S29–S32.

Lugger KE. Dysphagia in the elderly stroke patient. J Neurosci Nurs 1994 Apr; 26(2):78–84.

Pallicino P, Snyder W, and Granger C. The NIH stroke scale and the FIM in stroke rehabilitation. Stroke 1992 June; 23(6):919.

Raps EC and Galetta SL. Stroke prevention therapies and management of patient subgroups. Neurology 1995 Feb; 45(2 Suppl 1):S19–S24.

Sacco RL. Risk factors and outcomes for ischemic stroke. Neurology 1995 Feb; 45(2 Suppl 1):S10–S14.

Whitney F. Drug therapy for acute stroke. J Neurosci Nurs 1994 Apr. 26(2):111–117.

Increased Intracranial Pressure

Arbour R. What you can do to reduce increased I.C.P. Nursing 1993 Nov; 23(11):41–46.

Brucia JJ, Owen DC, and Ruby EB. The effects of lidocaine on intracranial hypertension. J Neurosci Nurs 1992 Aug; 24(4): 205–214.

Chambers K et al. An evaluation of the Camino ventricular bolt system in clinical practice. Neurosurgery 1993 Nov; 33(5): 866–868.

Eddy VA et al. Aggressive use of ICP monitoring is safe and alters patient care. Am Surg 1995 Jan; 61(1):24–29.

*Feldman Z, Kanter MJ, Robertson, et al. Effects of head elevation on increased intracranial pressure, cerebral perfusion pressure and cerebral blood flow in head injured patients. J Neurosurg 1992; 76:207.

Franges E. 16 tips for monitoring ICP. Nursing 1994 Jul; 24(7): 32M–32R.

Germon K. Intracranial pressure monitoring in the 1990s. Crit Care Nurse Q 1994 May; 17(1):21–32.

Lang EW and Chesnut RM. Intracranial pressure. Monitoring and management. Neurosurg Clin North Am 1994 Oct; 5(4):573–605.

Lee MW et al. The efficacy of barbiturate coma in the management of uncontrolled intracranial hypertension following neurosurgical trauma. J Neurotrauma 1994 Jun; 11(3):325–331.

Pickard JC and Czosnyka M. Management of raised intracranial pressure. J Neurol Neurosurg Psychiatr 1993 Aug; 56(8):845–858.

Rauch M, Mitchell P, and Tyler M. Validation of risk factors for the nursing diagnosis decreased intracranial adaptive capacity. J Neurosci Nurs 1993; 22(3):173.

Richmond TS. Intracranial pressure monitoring. AACN Clin Iss Crit Care Nurs 1993 Feb; 4(1):148–160.

Rising CJ. The relationship of selected nursing activities to ICP. J Neurosci Nurs 1993 Oct. 25(5):302–308.

Schickner DJ and Young RF. Intracranial pressure monitoring: Fiberoptic monitor compared with the ventricular catheter. Surg Neurol 1992 Apr; 37(4):251–254.

Schultz M, Moore K, Foote AW. Bacterial ventriculitis and duration of ventriculostomy catheter insertion. J Neurosci Nurs 1993 Jun; 5(3):158–164.

Shpritz DW. Practical points in understanding intracranial pressure. J Post Anesth Nurs 1994 Dec; 9(6):357–359.

Steele ME. Trends in the care and treatment of patients with increased intracranial pressure. Axone 1992 Jun; 13(4):125–128.

Pain

Schickner D and Young R. Intracranial pressure monitoring: Fiberoptic monitor compared with the ventricular catheter. Surg Neurol 1992 Apr; 37(4):251–254.

Tsubokawa T et al. Chronic motor cortex stimulation in patients with thalmic pain. J Neurosurg 1993 Mar; 78(3):393–401.

Unconsciousness and Coma

Ackerman L. Alteration in level of responsiveness. A proposed nursing diagnosis. Nurs Clin North Am 1993 Dec; 28(4):729–745.

*Lawrence M. The unconscious experience. Am J Crit Care 1995 May; 4(3):227–232.

Morris K. Assessment and communication of conscious level: An audit of neurosurgical referrals. Injury 1993 Jul; 24(6):369–372.

Intracranial Surgery

Alexander E III and Loeffler JS. Radiosurgery using a modified linear accelerator. Neurosurg Clin North Am 1992 Jan; 3(1):167–190.

Stephanian E et al. Gamma knife surgery for sellar and suprasellar tumors. Neurosurg Clin North Am 1992 Jan; 3(1):207–218.

Neurological and Neurosurgical Management of Pain

Abbott R. Electrical stimulation in selective dorsal rhizotomy. Adv Neurol 1993; 63:263–270.

Citera JA. The use of local anesthetics in the treatment of chronic pain. Orthop Nurs 1992 Jan–Feb; 11(1):27–33.

Lamer TJ. Treatment of cancer-related pain: When orally administered medications fail. Mayo Clin Proc 1994 May; 69(5):473–480.

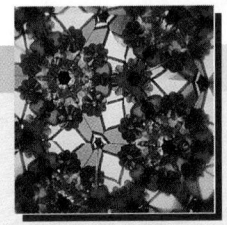

60

Management of Patients With Neurologic Disorders

CHAPTER OUTLINE

Headache
Classification
Assessment
Migraine
Other Vascular Headaches
Tension Headache (Muscle Contraction Headache)
Brain Tumors
Classification
Specific Tumors
Clinical Manifestations
Diagnostic Evaluation
Management
Cerebral Metastases
NURSING PROCESS: The Patient With Cerebral Metastases or Incurable Brain Tumor
Meningitis
Bacterial Meningitis
Intracranial Infection: Brain Abscess
Clinical Manifestations
Diagnostic Evaluations
Management
Intracranial Aneurysm
Pathophysiology
Clinical Manifestations
Diagnostic Evaluation
Management
NURSING PROCESS: The Patient With a Cerebral Aneurysm
Multiple Sclerosis
Pathophysiology
Clinical Manifestations
Diagnostic Evaluation
Management
NURSING PROCESS: The Patient With Multiple Sclerosis
Parkinson's Disease
Pathophysiology
Clinical Manifestations
Diagnostic Evaluation
Management
NURSING PROCESS: The Patient With Parkinson's Disease
Huntington's Disease
Pathophysiology
Clinical Manifestations
Management
Alzheimer's Disease
Neuromuscular Diseases
Myasthenia Gravis
NURSING PROCESS: The Patient With Myasthenia Gravis
Amyotrophic Lateral Sclerosis
The Muscular Dystrophies
Convulsive Disorders
Seizures
The Epilepsies
NURSING PROCESS: The Patient With Epilepsy
Head Injuries
Scalp Injuries
Fractures of the Skull
Brain Injury
Intracranial Hemorrhage
General Approach to Head Injuries
NURSING PROCESS: The Patient With a Head Injury
Spinal Cord Injury
Prevention
Pathophysiology
Emergency Management
Clinical Manifestations
Diagnostic Evaluation
Management of Spinal Cord Injury (Acute Phase)
NURSING PROCESS: The Patient With An Acute Spinal Cord Injury
The Quadriplegic or Paraplegic Patient
Management
NURSING PROCESS: The Patient With Quadriplegia or Paraplegia
Intraspinal Tumors
Preoperative Management
Surgical Management
Herniation of an Intervertebral Disc
Clinical Manifestations
Diagnostic Evaluation
Management
Herniation of a Cervical Intervertebral Disc
Management
NURSING PROCESS: The Patient Undergoing a Cervical Discectomy
Herniation of a Lumbar Disc
Diagnostic Evaluation
Management
Cranial Nerve Disorders
Trigeminal Neuralgia (Tic Douloureux)
Bell's Palsy
Disorders of the Peripheral Nervous System
Peripheral Neuropathies
Guillain-Barré Syndrome (Polyradiculoneuritis)
NURSING PROCESS: The Patient With Guillain-Barré Syndrome
Critical Thinking Exercises

LEARNING OBJECTIVES

On completion of this chapter, the learner will be able to:

1. Compare the various types and causes of headache

2. Use the nursing process as a framework for care of patients with migraine headaches
3. Describe brain tumors: their classification, clinical manifestations, diagnosis, and management
4. Use the nursing process as a framework for care of patients with cerebral metastases or inoperable brain tumors
5. Describe subarachnoid precautions and their application to the patient with a cerebral aneurysm
6. Use the nursing process as a framework for care of patients with multiple sclerosis
7. Use the nursing process as a framework for care of patients with Parkinson's disease
8. Compare myasthenia gravis, amyotrophic lateral sclerosis, and muscular dystrophy: their pathophysiology, clinical manifestations, and nursing and medical management
9. Describe disorders of the cranial nerves, their manifestations, and indicated nursing interventions

Headache

Headache or *cephalgia* is one of the most common of all human physical complaints. Headache is actually a symptom rather than a disease entity and may indicate organic disease (neurologic or other disease), a stress response, vasodilation (migraine), skeletal muscle tension (tension headache), or a combination of the above.

Classification

Headaches are difficult to categorize and define. Little pathophysiologic evidence or diagnostic testing can support the diagnosis of headache. Headaches may manifest themselves differently within individuals over the course of a lifetime, and the same type of headache may have different characteristics among different individuals.

The most current classification of headaches as issued by the Headache Classification Committee of the International Headache Society is as follows:

1. Migraine (with and without aura)
2. Tension-type headache
3. Cluster headache and paroxysmal hemicrania
4. Miscellaneous headaches associated with structural lesion
5. Headache associated with head trauma
6. Headache associated with vascular disorders (*e.g.*, subarachnoid hemorrhage)
7. Headache associated with nonvascular intracranial disorders (*e.g.*, brain tumor)
8. Headache associated with use of chemical substances or their withdrawal
9. Headache associated with noncephalic infection
10. Headache associated with metabolic disorder (*e.g.*, hypoglycemia)
11. Headache or facial pain associated with disorders of the head, neck, or their structures (*e.g.*, acute glaucoma)
12. Cranial neuralgias (persistent pain of cranial nerve origin)

Assessment

The data obtained for the health history should reflect the patient's own words about the headache as described in response to the following questions:

- How old were you when these headaches started? Under what circumstances did they start?
- What is the location? Is it unilateral or bilateral? Does it radiate?
- What is the quality—dull, aching, steady, boring, burning, intermittent, continuous, paroxysmal?
- How many headaches occur during a given time?
- Are there any precipitating factors (environmental, such as sunlight and weather change; foods; exertion; other)?
- What makes the headache worse (coughing, straining)?
- What time (day or night) does it occur?
- Are there any associated symptoms such as facial pain, lacrimation, scotomas (blind spots in the field of vision)?
- What usually relieves the headache (aspirin, ergot preparation, food, heat, rest, neck massage)?
- Does nausea, vomiting, weakness, or numbness in the extremities accompany the headache?
- Does the headache interfere with your daily activities?
- Do you have any allergies?
- Do you have insomnia, poor appetite, loss of energy?
- Is there a family history of headache? "Sick" headache?

- What is the relationship of the headache to lifestyle or physical or emotional stress?
- What medications are you taking?

Migraine

Migraine is a symptom-complex characterized by periodic and recurrent attacks of severe headache. The cause of migraine has not been clearly demonstrated, but it is primarily a vascular disturbance that occurs more commonly in women and has a strong familial tendency.

Pathophysiology

The cerebral signs and symptoms of migraine result from varying degrees of cortical ischemia. The typical attack begins with vasoconstriction affecting the arteries of the scalp and certain cerebral or retinal vessels. Extracranial and intracranial blood vessels then dilate, causing pain and discomfort. Studies suggest that the dilated artery becomes hyperpermeable and that sterile local inflammatory reactions occur in the vicinity of the painful, dilated arteries. It is proposed that vasoactive substances (histamine, serotonin, plasmokinins) participate in this sterile inflammatory reaction.

Certain foods containing tyramine, monosodium glutamate, nitrites, or milk products may trigger headaches. Foods in these categories include aged cheese, chocolate, and many processed foods. Oral contraceptives may increase the frequency and severity of attacks in some women.

Clinical Manifestations

Often the headache begins on awakening, but it can occur at any time. The classic migraine attack can be divided into three phases: the aura, the headache, and the recovery phase.

Aura Phase. When a migraine is accompanied by an aura, the aura may last for up to 30 minutes and may provide enough time for the patient to take the prescribed medication to avert a full-blown attack (described in later section). This period is characterized by sensory manifestations, predominantly visual disturbances (light flashes). Other symptoms that may follow include numbness and tingling of the face or hands, mild confusion, slight weakness of an extremity, and dizziness.

This period of aura corresponds to the painless vasoconstriction that is the initial physiologic change characteristic of classic migraine. Cerebral blood flow studies performed during migraine headaches demonstrate that during all phases of the attack cerebral blood flow is reduced throughout the brain, with subsequent loss of autoregulation and impaired CO_2 responsiveness.

Headache Phase. As the initial symptoms begin to recede, they are followed by a unilateral (in two thirds of patients) and throbbing headache. This headache is severe and incapacitating and is often associated with photophobia, nausea, and vomiting. Its duration varies, ranging from several hours to a day or longer.

Recovery Phase. The recovery phase is a period of muscle contraction in the neck and scalp with associated muscle ache and localized tenderness. Exhaustion is common, and any physical exertion exacerbates the headache pain. During this postheadache phase, patients may sleep for extended periods.

Diagnostic Evaluation

The diagnostic evaluation includes a detailed history, a physical assessment of the head and neck, a neurologic examination including cranial nerve testing, evaluation of the size and reaction of the pupils, a funduscopic examination of the eyes, and testing of motor and sensory functions.

The health history focuses on assessing the headache itself, with particular emphasis on identifying the factors that precipitate or provoke the headache. Patients are encouraged to describe their headaches in their own words. History can be obtained according to the following procedures.

General History. Because headache often can be the presenting symptom of a wide variety of both physiologic and psychological disturbances, a general health history is an essential component of the patient database. General review questions should cover major medical and surgical illness as well as a body systems review. Headache may be a symptom of endocrine, hematologic, gastrointestinal, infectious, renal, cardiovascular, psychiatric, or hemologic disease.

A complete medication review is important. Medication history can provide insight into the patient's overall health status. Antihypertensives, such as hydralazine, diuretics, anti-inflammatory drugs, and monoamine oxidase inhibitors are a few of the categories of drugs that can provoke headaches. Although sometimes exaggerated in importance, emotional factors can play a role in the precipitation or development of many headaches. Stress is thought to be a major initiating factor in migraine headaches; therefore, sleep patterns, level of stress, recreational interests, appetite, emotional problems, and family stressors are relevant.

Family History. There is a strong familial tendency for headache disorders. A positive family history is strongly suggestive of the diagnosis of migraine headache.

Occupational History. A direct relationship may exist between exposure to toxic substances and headache. Careful questioning may be required to identify a comprehensive list of the chemicals to which workers are exposed. Under the Right to Know law, employees should have access to the Material Safety Data Sheets for all the substances with which they come in contact in the workplace. In addition, the occupational history includes assessment of the workplace as a possible source of stress.

Headache History. A complete description of the headache itself is crucial. The patient's age at onset of headache, its frequency, location, duration, type of pain, factors that relieve and precipitate the event, and associated symptoms are reviewed.

Diagnostic Tests. For patients who demonstrate abnormalities on the neurologic examination, computed tomography (CT) or magnetic resonance imaging (MRI) may be used to detect underlying causes such as tumor or aneurysm. Other diagnostic tests may be indicated for patients with persistent or disabling headache pain.

Management

Therapy for migraine headache is divided into abortive (symptomatic) and preventive approaches. The symptomatic or abortive approach is best employed in patients who suffer frequent attacks and is aimed at relieving or limiting a headache at the onset or while it is in progress. The preventive approach is used in patients who experience frequent attacks at regular or predictable intervals and may have medical conditions that preclude the use of abortive therapies.

Management of Acute Attack. Ergotamine preparations (taken orally, sublingually, subcutaneously, intramuscularly, by rectum, or by inhalation) may be effective in aborting the headache if taken *early* in the migraine process. Ergotamine tartrate acts on smooth muscle, causing prolonged constriction of the cranial blood vessels. Each patient's dosage is titrated according to individual needs. Side effects include aching muscles, paresthesias, nausea, and vomiting. Cafergot, a combination of ergotamine and caffeine, can arrest or reduce the severity of the headache in 90% of migraine sufferers, especially if administered early.

Sumatriptan (Imitrex) is a medication used for the treatment of acute migraine and cluster headaches. It has been found to be significantly more effective than oral Cafergot in relieving moderate to severe migraine in a large number of patients. A subcutaneous form is available in an autoinjector for immediate patient use. Careful instructions to patients are important to prevent drug reactions.

During the acute attack, the patient may find relief by lying quietly in a darkened room with the head slightly elevated. Drinking black coffee also may be helpful in some patients. Symptomatic therapy for migraine includes analgesics, sedatives, antianxiety agents, and antiemetics.

Prevention. Preventive medical management of migraine employs the daily use of one or more agents that are thought to block the physiologic events leading to an attack. Drug therapy is carried out at intervals of 3 to 6 months and is gradually tapered because natural remissions of migraine do occur. Treatment regimens vary greatly, as do patient responses; thus, close monitoring is indicated.

The most widely used and important medication for the prevention of migraine is propranolol (Inderal). Beta-blocking agents such as propranolol inhibit the action of beta-receptors—cells in the heart and brain that control the dilation of blood vessels. The ability of beta-blockers to halt the dilation of blood vessels in the brain is believed to be a major reason for their antimigraine action.

Methysergide (Sansert) is an effective prophylactic agent in preventing frequent and severe migraine attacks; before the widespread use of propranolol in migraine prevention, it was the drug of choice. It is thought to inhibit or block the effects of serotonin, a substance possibly involved in the mechanism of vascular headaches. Troublesome side effects include abdominal discomfort, muscle cramps, edema, numbness, tingling of extremities, and depression. There should be a medication-free interval of at least 1 to 2 months after every 6-month course of treatment because of the potential complications of retroperitoneal fibrosis and pleuropulmonary and cardiac fibrosis.

Additional drug therapy includes the use of antidepressants, barbiturates, and tranquilizers. These medications should be used cautiously and only on a short-term basis because of the risk of drug dependence.

Nursing Interventions

When migraine headache has been diagnosed, the goals of nursing management are to treat the acute event of the headache and to prevent recurrent episodes. Prevention involves patient education regarding precipitating factors, possible lifestyle or habit changes that may be helpful and pharmacologic measures.

Relief of Pain. Nursing care is directed toward treatment of the acute episode. A migraine headache in the early phase requires abortive drug therapy instituted as soon as possible. Some headaches actually may be prevented if the appropriate medications are taken before the onset of pain. Nursing care during a fully developed attack includes comfort measures such as a quiet, dark environment and elevation of the head of the bed 30 degrees. In addition, symptomatic treatment such as antiemetics may be indicated.

Patient Education. Although there is a wide variation in the personality types of those who are subject to migraine, there is some evidence that the hard-driving, somewhat compulsive perfectionist is most vulnerable to this condition. Migraine headaches are likely to occur when a person is ill, overtired, or feeling stressed. Stress is believed to be a factor in the precipitation of migraine. Instruction about the importance of proper diet, adequate rest, and coping strategies may help the patient deal with stress. Identifying circumstances that precipitate headaches may assist the patient in the development of alternate means of coping.

Long intervals between meals also should be avoided. The patient is advised to awaken at the same time each day, as disruption in the normal sleeping pattern provokes a migraine in many patients. The possibility that oral contraceptives are a contributing factor should be investigated.

The patient is encouraged to keep a record of the circumstances surrounding the attack (*e.g.*, activities, food, feelings) to determine if there is a pattern to the migraine episodes. If so, a change in the pattern may help avoid the attacks.

Patients can be helped to develop insight into their feelings, behavior, and conflicts and to make the necessary modifications in lifestyle on the basis of these analyses. Regular periods of exercise and relaxation are suggested, and any offending or provoking factors (allergens, fatigue, foods, environmental stresses) are removed or reduced to obtain relief.

The National Headache Foundation (see bibliography) provides a list of clinics in the United States and the names of physicians who specialize in headache and who are members of the American Association for the Study of Headache.

Other Vascular Headaches

Cluster Headache

Cluster headaches are another severe form of vascular headache. They are seen most frequently in men. The attacks come in clusters or groups, with excruciating pain localized in the eye and orbit and radiating to the facial and temporal regions. The pain is accompanied by watering of the eye and nasal congestion. Each attack lasts from 15 minutes to 2 hours and may have a crescendo—decrescendo pattern.

One theory postulates that this type of headache is due to dilatation of orbital and nearby extracranial arteries. Cluster headaches may be precipitated by alcohol, nitrites, vasodilators, and histamines. Eliminating these factors helps in preventing the headaches. Cluster headache responds to vasoconstricting agents (ergotamine tartrate). The serotonin antagonist, methysergide, and the beta-blocker, propranolol, also may provide relief. Chlorpromazine may also be effective.

Cranial Arteritis

Inflammation of the cranial arteries is characterized by a severe headache localized in the region of the temporal arteries. The inflammation may be generalized, in which cranial arteritis is part of a vascular disease, or of a focal type, in which only the cranial arteries are involved. Cranial arteritis is a cause of headache in the older population, reaching its greatest incidence in those over the age of 70.

Often the disease begins with general manifestations, such as fatigue, malaise, weight loss, and fever. Clinical manifestations associated with inflammation (heat, redness, swelling, tenderness, or pain over the involved artery) usually are present. Sometimes a tender, swollen, or nodular temporal artery is visible. Visual problems are caused by ischemia of the involved structures.

Cranial arteritis is thought to represent an immune vasculitis in which immune complexes are deposited within the walls of affected blood vessels, producing vascular injury and inflammation. A biopsy may be performed on the involved artery to confirm or refute the diagnosis.

Treatment consists of early administration of a corticosteroid drug to prevent the possibility of loss of vision due to vascular occlusion or rupture of the involved artery. The patient is instructed not to stop the medication abruptly because this can lead to relapse. Analgesic agents are given for comfort.

Tension Headache (Muscle Contraction Headache)

Emotional or physical stress may cause contraction of the muscles in the neck and scalp, resulting in tension headache. The headache may be characterized by a steady, constant feeling of pressure that usually begins in the forehead, the temple, or the back of the neck. It is often bandlike or may be described as "a weight on top of my head." Tension headaches tend to be more chronic than severe and are probably the most common type of headache. The patient needs reassurance that the headache is not due to a brain tumor. This is a common unspoken fear. Symptomatic relief may be obtained by local heat, massage, analgesics, antidepressants, and muscle relaxants.

Brain Tumors

A brain tumor is a localized intracranial lesion that occupies space within the skull. Tumors usually grow as a spherical mass but can grow diffusely, infiltrating tissue. The effect of neoplasms occurs from compression and infiltration of tissue. A variety of physiologic changes result, causing any or all of the following pathophysiologic events:

- Increased intracranial pressure (ICP) and cerebral edema
- Seizure activity and focal neurologic signs
- Hydrocephalus
- Altered pituitary function

Primary brain tumors represent approximately 20% of all deaths from cancer, whereas 20% to 40% of all cancer patients develop metastasis to the brain from other sites. Brain tumors rarely metastasize outside of the central nervous system but metastatic lesions to the brain occur commonly from the lung, breast, lower gastrointestinal tract, pancreas, kidney, and skin (melanomas).

The highest incidence of brain tumors in adults occurs in the fifth, sixth and seventh decades with a slightly higher incidence in men. In adults, most brain tumors originate from *glial cells* (glial cells make up the structure and support system of the brain and spinal cord) and are *supratentorial* (located above the covering of the cerebellum). Neoplastic lesions in the brain ultimately cause death by impairing vital functions, such as respiration, or by increasing ICP.

Classification

Brain tumors may be classified into several groups: (1) those arising from the coverings of the brain, such as a dural meningioma; (2) those developing in or on the cranial nerves, best exemplified by an acoustic neuroma; (3) those originating within brain tissue, such as the various gliomas; and (4) metastatic lesions originating elsewhere in the body. Tumors of the pituitary and pineal glands and of cerebral blood vessels are also included in the types of brain tumors as indicated in Chart 60-1. Relevant clinical considerations include the location and the histologic character of the tumor. Tumors may be benign or malignant. Because a benign tumor can occur in a vital area, however, it can have effects as serious as those of a malignant tumor.

Specific Tumors

Gliomas. Malignant glioma is the most common brain neoplasm accounting for approximately 45% of all brain tumors. Usually, these tumors cannot be totally removed because they spread by infiltrating into the surrounding neural tissue and therefore are not amenable to resection without causing considerable damage to vital structures.

Pituitary Adenomas. The *pituitary gland,* also called the *hypophysis,* is a relatively small gland located in the sella turcica. It is attached to the hypothalamus by a short stalk (hypophyseal stalk) and is divided into two lobes: the

CHART 60-1
Classification of Brain Tumors

Tumors Originating in the Brain Tissue

Gliomas—infiltrating tumors that may invade any portion of the brain; most common type of brain tumor

Subclassified according to cell type:
- Astrocytomas (grades 1 and 2)
- Glioblastomas (grades 3 and 4 astrocytomas)
- Ependymomas
- Medulloblastomas
- Oligodendrogliomas
- Colloid cysts

Tumors Arising From Covering of Brain

Meningioma—encapsulated, well-defined, growing outside the brain tissue; compresses rather than invades brain

Tumors Developing in or on the Cranial Nerves

Acoustic neuroma—derived from sheath of acoustic nerve
Optic nerve spongioblastoma polare

Metastatic Lesions

Most commonly from lung and breast

Tumors of the Ductless Glands

Pituitary
Pineal

Blood Vessel Tumors

Hemangioblastoma
Angioma

Congenital Tumors

anterior (adenohypophysis) and the posterior (neurohypophysis). The anterior lobe secretes growth hormone, adrenocorticotrophic hormone (ACTH), thyroid-stimulating hormone (TSH), prolactin, the gonadotropic hormones, follicle-stimulating hormone (FSH), and luteinizing hormone (LH). The posterior pituitary stores and releases antidiuretic hormone (vasopressin) and oxytocin.

Pressure Effects. Pituitary tumors represent approximately 8% to 12% of all brain tumors and will cause symptoms owing to pressure on adjacent structures or to hormonal changes (hyperfunction or hypofunction of the pituitary). Pressure from pituitary adenomas may be exerted on the optic nerves, optic chiasm, or optic tracts, or on the hypothalamus or the third ventricle when the tumors invade the cavernous sinuses or expand into the sphenoid bone. These pressure effects produce headache, visual dysfunction, hypothalamic disorders (*e.g.*, disorders of sleep, appetite, temperature, emotions), increased ICP, and enlargement and erosion of the sella turcica.

Hormonal Effects. Functioning pituitary tumors can produce one or more hormones normally produced by the anterior pituitary. These hormones may cause prolactin-secreting pituitary adenomas (prolactinomas), growth hormone-secreting pituitary adenomas that produce acromegaly in adults, and ACTH-producing pituitary adenomas that give rise to Cushing's disease. Adenomas secreting TSH or FSH-LH occur infrequently, whereas adenomas that produce both growth hormone and prolactin are relatively common.

The female patient whose pituitary gland is secreting excessive quantities of prolactin presents with *amenorrhea* or *galactorrhea* (excessive or spontaneous flow of milk). Male patients with prolactinomas may present with impotence and hypogonadism.

Acromegaly, caused by excess growth hormone, produces enlargement of the hands and feet, distortion of the facial features, and pressure on peripheral nerves (entrapment syndromes).

The clinical features of *Cushing's disease,* a condition associated with prolonged overproduction of cortisol, occur with excessive production of ACTH. Manifestations include a form of obesity with redistribution of fat to the facial, supraclavicular, and abdominal areas; hypertension; purple striae and ecchymoses; osteoporosis; glucose intolerance; and emotional disorders.

Treatment. Most pituitary adenomas are treated by transsphenoidal microsurgical removal (see Chapter 59), whereas the remainder of tumors that cannot be removed completely are treated by radiation.

Angiomas. Brain angiomas (masses composed largely of abnormal blood vessels) are found either in or on the surface of the brain. Some persist throughout life without causing symptoms; others give rise to symptoms of brain tumor. Occasionally, the diagnosis is suggested by the presence of another angioma somewhere in the head or by a *bruit* (an abnormal sound) audible over the skull. Because the walls of the blood vessels in angiomas are thin, these patients are at risk for a cerebral vascular accident (stroke). In fact, cerebral hemorrhage in persons under 40 years of age should suggest the possibility of an angioma.

Acoustic Neuroma. An acoustic neuroma is a tumor of the eighth cranial nerve, the nerve for hearing and balance. It usually arises just within the internal auditory meatus, where it frequently expands before filling the cerebellopontine recess.

An acoustic neuroma may grow slowly and attain considerable size before it is correctly diagnosed. The patient usually experiences loss of hearing, tinnitus, and episodes of vertigo and staggering gait. As the tumor becomes larger, painful sensations of the face may occur on the same side as a result of the tumor's compression of the fifth cranial nerve.

With improved x-ray techniques and the use of the operating microscope and microsurgical instrumentation, even large tumors can be removed through a relatively small craniotomy. Some of these tumors may be suitable for stereotactic radiotherapy rather than surgery.

Clinical Manifestations

Brain tumors produce both diffuse clinical manifestations when they cause increased ICP and localized signs and symptoms as a result of the tumor interfering with specific regions of the brain.

Increasing Intracranial Pressure Symptoms. As discussed in Chapter 59, according to the modified Monro-Kellie hypothesis, the skull is a rigid compartment containing essential noncompressible contents: brain matter, intravascular blood, and cerebrospinal fluid. If any one of these components of the skull increases in volume, ICP will increase unless one of the other components decreases in volume. Consequently, any change in volume occupied by the brain—as occurs with disorders such as brain tumor or cerebral edema—will produce signs and symptoms of increased intracranial pressure.

Symptoms of increased ICP are caused by a gradual compression of the brain owing to the growth of the tumor. The effect is to disrupt the equilibrium that exists between the brain, the cerebrospinal fluid, and the cerebral blood—all located within the skull. As the tumor grows, compensatory adjustments may occur through compression of intracranial veins, through reduction of cerebrospinal fluid volume (by increased absorption or decreased production), a modest decrease of cerebral blood flow, and reduction of intracellular and extracellular brain tissue mass. When these compensatory mechanisms fail, the patient develops signs and symptoms of increased ICP.

Symptoms of ICP. The most common symptoms produced by this pressure are headache, vomiting, papilledema ("choked disc" or edema of the optic nerve), personality changes, and a variety of focal deficits including motor, sensory, and cranial nerve dysfunction.

Headache, although not always present, is most common in the early morning and is made worse by coughing, straining, or sudden movement. It is thought to be caused by the tumor invading, compressing, or distorting the pain-sensitive structures or by edema that accompanies the tumor.

Headaches are usually described as deep or expanding or as dull but unrelenting. Frontal tumors usually produce a bilateral frontal headache; pituitary gland tumors produce pain radiating between the two temples (bitemporal); in cerebellar tumors the headache may be located in the suboccipital region at the back of the head.

Vomiting, seldom related to food intake, is usually due to irritation of the vagal centers in the medulla. If the vomiting is of the forceful type, it is described as projectile vomiting.

Papilledema (edema of the optic nerve) is present in 70% to 75% of patients and is associated with visual disturbances such as decreased visual acuity, diplopia, and visual field deficits.

Localized Symptoms. Localized symptoms occur when specific regions of the brain are disrupted, resulting in locally referable signs, such as sensory and motor abnormalities, visual alterations, and seizures.

Because the functions of the different parts of the brain are known, the location of the tumor can be determined, in part, by identifying functions that are affected by the presence of the tumor.

- *A tumor of the motor cortex* manifests itself by causing seizure-like movements localized on one side of the body, called *Jacksonian seizures.*
- *An occipital lobe tumor* produces visual manifestations: contralateral homonymous hemianopsia (visual loss in one half of the visual field on the opposite side of the tumor) and visual hallucinations.
- *Tumors of the cerebellum* cause dizziness, an ataxic or staggering gait with a tendency to fall toward the side of the lesion, marked muscle incoordination, and nystagmus (involuntary rhythmical eye movements) usually in the horizontal direction.
- *Tumors of the frontal lobe* frequently produce personality disorders, changes in emotional state and behavior, and a disinterested mental attitude. The patient often becomes extremely untidy and careless and may use obscene language.
- *Tumors of the cerebellopontine angle* usually originate in the sheath of the acoustic nerve and give rise to a sequence of symptoms that is most characteristic of all brain tumor symptomatology.
  - First, tinnitus and vertigo appear, soon followed by progressive nerve deafness (eighth cranial nerve dysfunction).
  - Next there is numbness and tingling of the face and the tongue (due to involvement of the fifth cranial nerve).
  - Later, weakness or paralysis of the face develops (seventh cranial nerve involvement).
  - Finally, because the enlarging tumor presses on the cerebellum, abnormalities in motor function may be present.
- Intracranial tumors can produce personality changes, confusion, speech dysfunction, and disturbances of gait, especially in elderly patients. The most frequent tumor types in the elderly are meningiomas, glioblastomas, and cerebral metastases from other sites.

Many tumors are not so easily localized, because they lie in the so-called *silent areas* of the brain (*i.e.*, areas in which functions are not definitely determined).

The *progression* of the signs and symptoms is important, because it indicates tumor growth and expansion.

Diagnostic Evaluation

The history of the illness and the manner in which the symptoms evolved are important in diagnosing brain tumors. A neurologic examination indicates the areas of the central nervous system involved. To assist in the precise localization of the lesion, a battery of tests is performed. CT imaging gives specific information concerning the number, size, and density of the lesions and the extent of secondary cerebral edema. It also provides information about the ventricular system. MRI is helpful in the diagnosis of brain tumors. Its use has resulted in the detection of smaller lesions; it is particularly helpful in detecting tumors in the brain stem and pituitary regions, where bone interferes with CT (Fig. 60-1). Computer-assisted stereotactic (three dimensional) biopsy is being used to diagnose deep-seated brain tumors and to provide a basis for treatment and prognostic information. Cerebral angiography provides visualization of cerebral blood vessels and can localize most cerebral tumors.

An electroencephalogram (EEG) can detect abnormal brain waves in regions occupied by a tumor and can enable evaluation of temporal lobe seizures.

Cytologic studies of the cerebrospinal fluid may be performed to detect malignant cells, because tumors of the central nervous system are capable of shedding cells into the cerebrospinal fluid.

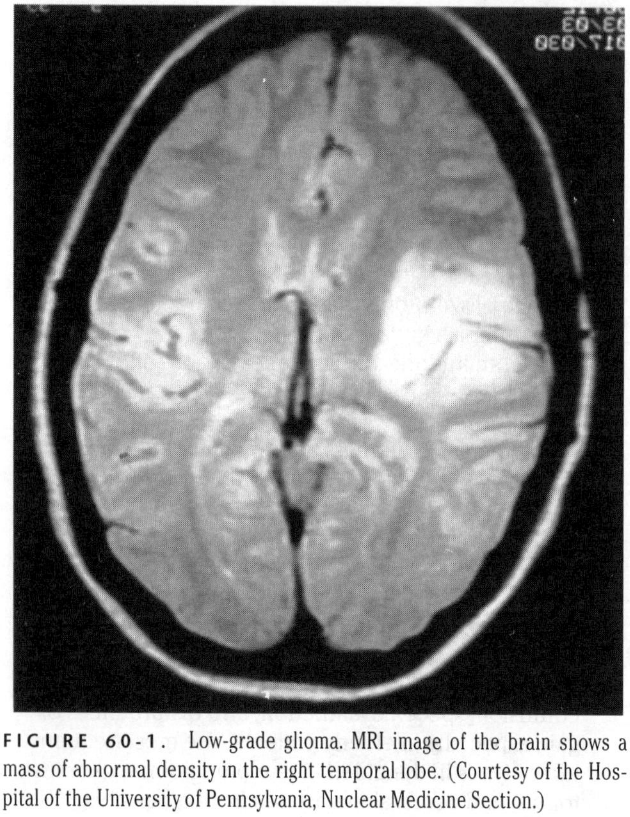

FIGURE 60-1. Low-grade glioma. MRI image of the brain shows a mass of abnormal density in the right temporal lobe. (Courtesy of the Hospital of the University of Pennsylvania, Nuclear Medicine Section.)

Management

An untreated brain tumor ultimately leads to death, either from increasing ICP or from the brain damage it causes. Patients with possible brain tumor should be evaluated and treated as soon as possible before irreversible neurologic damage occurs.

The objective is to remove or destroy all of the tumor or as much as possible without increasing the neurologic deficit (paralysis, blindness) or to achieve relief of symptoms by partial removal (decompression). A variety of treatment modalities may be used; the specific approach depends on the type of tumor, its location, and accessibility. In many patients, combinations of these modalities may be used.

Conventional **surgical approaches** require an incision into the skull (craniotomy). This approach is used in general to cure patients with meningiomas, acoustic neuromas, cystic astrocytomas of the cerebellum, colloid cysts of the third ventricle, congenital tumors such as dermoid cyst, and some of the granulomas. For patients with malignant glioma, complete removal of the tumor and cure are not possible, but the rationale for resection includes relieving intracranial pressure, removing any necrotic tissue, and reducing the bulk of the tumor, which theoretically leaves behind fewer cells to become resistant to radiation or chemotherapy.

Stereotactic approaches involve use of a three-dimensional frame that allows *very* precise localization of the tumor; a stereotactic frame and multiple imaging studies (x-rays, CT) are used to localize the tumor and verify its position. **Lasers** or **radiation** can be delivered with stereotactic approaches. Radioisotopes (^{131}I) can also be implanted directly into the tumor to deliver high doses of radiation to the tumor (brachytherapy) while minimizing effects on surrounding brain tissue.

The use of the **gamma knife** to perform **"radiosurgery"** allows deep, inaccessible tumors to be treated, often in a single session. Precise localization of the tumor is accomplished using the stereotactic approach and by minute measurements and precise positioning of the patient. A very high dose of radiation is then delivered by multiple narrow beams. An advantage of this method is that no surgical incision is needed; a disadvantage is the lag time between treatment and the desired result.

Other treatment modalities include **chemotherapy** and **external beam radiation therapy,** used by themselves or in combination with the approaches described above. Radiation therapy, the cornerstone of treatment for many brain tumors, also decreases recurrences of incompletely resected tumors. **Intravenous autologous bone marrow transplantation** is used in some patients who will receive chemotherapy or radiation therapy because it has the potential to "rescue" the patient from the bone marrow toxicity associated with high doses of chemotherapy and radiation. A fraction of the patient's bone marrow is aspirated, usually from the iliac crest, and stored. The patient receives large doses of chemotherapy or radiation therapy to destroy large numbers of malignant cells. The marrow is then reinfused intravenously after treatment is completed. **Corticosteroids** may be used before treatment to permit a thorough diagnostic evaluation and afterwards to reduce cerebral edema and promote a smoother, more rapid recovery.

Nursing Interventions

The patient with a brain tumor may have problems with aspiration related to cranial nerve dysfunction. Preoperatively, the gag reflex and ability to swallow are evaluated. If there is a diminished gag response, the plan of care includes teaching the patient to direct food and fluids toward the unaffected side, placing the patient upright to eat, offering a semisoft diet, and having suction readily available. Function should be reassessed postoperatively, as changes can occur.

The problems of increased ICP caused by the tumor mass are reviewed in Chapter 59. The nurse performs neurologic checks, monitors vital signs, maintains a neurologic flow chart, spaces nursing interventions to prevent rapid increase in ICP, and reorients the patient when necessary to person, time, and place. Patients with changes in cognition caused by the lesion require frequent reorientation and the use of orienting devices (personal possessions, photographs, lists, clock), supervision of and assistance with self-care, and ongoing monitoring and intervention for prevention of injury. Patients with seizures are carefully monitored.

Motor function is checked at intervals because specific motor deficits may be involved, depending on the tumor's location. Sensory disturbances are assessed. The patient's speech is evaluated. Eye movement and pupillary size and reaction may be affected by cranial nerve involvement.

The nursing process applied to the patient undergoing neurosurgery is found in Chapter 59.

Cerebral Metastases

A significant number of patients suffer central nervous system complications as a result of systemic cancer and neurologic deficits caused by metastases to the brain. Metastatic lesions to the brain comprise 50% of all intracranial tumors. Cerebral metastasis is the most common neurologic complication of systemic cancer. This fact becomes more important clinically as more patients with all forms of cancer live longer as a result of improved therapies.

Neurologic symptoms and signs include headache, gait disturbances, vision deterioration, personality changes, altered mentation (memory loss and confusion), focal weakness, paralysis, aphasia, and seizures. These problems can be devastating to both patient and family.

Management

The treatment of metastatic brain cancer is palliative and involves eliminating or reducing serious symptomatology. Even when palliation is the goal, distressing signs and symptoms can be resolved, thereby improving the quality of life for both the patient and family. Patients with intracerebral metastases who are not treated have a steady downhill course with a very limited survival time, whereas those who are treated may survive for slightly longer periods.

The therapeutic approach includes radiation therapy, which is the foundation of treatment, surgery (usually for a single intracranial metastasis), chemotherapy, or a combination of these methods.

Corticosteroids may be helpful in relieving headache and alterations of consciousness. It is thought that corticosteroids (dexamethasone, prednisone) reduce inflammation around the metastatic deposits and decrease the edema surrounding them.

Other medications include osmotic agents (mannitol, glycerol) to decrease the fluid content of the brain, which leads to a decrease in ICP. Anticonvulsant drugs (phenytoin) are used to prevent and treat seizures. Encouraging results have been seen in the treatment of metastatic lesions with chemotherapeutic agents such as carmustine (BCNU).

If the patient has severe pain, morphine can be infused into the epidural or subarachnoid space via a spinal needle and a catheter as near as possible to the spinal segment where the pain is projected. Small doses of morphine are administered at prescribed intervals (see Chapter 13).

❑ *NURSING PROCESS* *The Patient With Cerebral Metastases or Incurable Brain Tumor*

Assessment

The nursing assessment focuses on how the patient is functioning, moving, and walking; adapting to weakness or paralysis and to visual and speech loss; and dealing with seizures.

A dietary history is taken to assess dietary intake and food intolerances and preferences. Anthropometric measurements confirm the loss of subcutaneous fat and lean body mass. Biochemical measurements (albumin, transferrin, total lymphocyte count, creatinine index, and urinary tests) are reviewed to assess the degree of malnutrition, impaired cellular immunity, and electrolyte balance.

Cachexia (weak and emaciated condition) is seen in patients with metastases and is characterized by anorexia, pain, weight loss, altered metabolism, muscle weakness, malabsorption, and diarrhea. The patient may experience altered taste sensations secondary to dysphagia, weakness, and depression. Distortions and diminution of the sense of smell (*anosmia*) frequently occur among these patients.

Assessment is made for symptoms that cause distress to the patient, including pain, respiratory problems, elimination and urination problems, sleep disturbances, and impairment of skin integrity, fluid balance, and temperature regulation. These problems may be caused by tumor invasion, compression, or obstruction.

The nurse may work with the social worker to assess the impact of the patient's illness on the family in terms of home care, altered relationships, financial problems, time pressures, and intrafamily problems. This information is important in helping family members strengthen their coping skills.

Diagnosis

Nursing Diagnoses

Based on the assessment data, the patient's major problems may include the following:

- Self-care deficits related to loss or impairment of motor and sensory function and decreased cognitive abilities
- Altered nutrition, less than body requirements, related to cachexia due to treatment and tumor effects, decreased nutritional intake, and malabsorption
- Anxiety related to anticipation of death, uncertainty, change in appearance, altered lifestyle
- Potential for altered family processes related to anticipatory grief and the burdens imposed by the care of the person with a terminal illness

Other nursing diagnoses of the patient with cerebral metastases may include pain related to tumor compression; impaired gas exchange related to dyspnea; constipation related to decreased fluid and dietary intake and medications; alteration in urinary elimination related to reduced fluid intake, vomiting, and reactions to medications; sleep pattern disturbances related to discomfort and fear of dying; impairment of skin integrity related to cachexia, poor tissue perfusion, and decreased mobility; potential or actual fluid volume deficit related to fever, vomiting, and low fluid intake; impaired thermal regulation related to hypothalamic involvement, fever, and chills. The reader is referred to Chapter 16 for appropriate assessment and nursing interventions for the patient with cancer.

Planning and Implementation

Goals. The goals of the patient may include compensating for self-care deficits, attaining improved nutrition, reducing anxiety, and enhancing family coping skills.

Nursing Interventions

Compensating for Self-Care Deficits. The patient may have difficulty participating in goal-setting, as the tumor metastasizes and affects cognitive function. It is important to encourage the family to keep the patient mobile and at the highest level of functioning possible. Increasing assistance with self-care activities will be required. The patient with cerebral metastasis and the family live with uncertainty. They are encouraged to plan for each day and make that day count. The tasks and challenges are to assist the patient to find useful coping mechanisms, adaptations, and compensations in solving problems that arise. This helps patients maintain some sense of control. An individualized exercise program helps maintain strength, endurance, and range of motion. Eventually referral for home health care assistance may be necessary.

Improving Nutrition. Patients with nausea, vomiting, breathlessness, and pain are rarely interested in eating. These symptoms must be managed or controlled by assessment, planning, and appropriate nursing and medical interventions.

The nurse teaches the family how to position the patient for comfort during meals. The timing of meals is important. Food is offered when the patient is more rested and in less distress from pain or the effects of treatment. The patient needs to be clean, comfortable, and free of pain, in an environment that is as attractive as possible. This requires planning to minimize offensive sights, sounds, and odors. Oral hygiene helps to improve oral intake. Nursing ingenuity is called on to make food more palatable, provide enough fluids, and increase opportunities for socialization. This involves communication and interaction with the dietician, physician, patient, and family. The family is taught to keep a daily weight chart. It may be necessary to record the quantity of food eaten to determine the daily calorie count.

Dietary supplements, as preferred by the patient, can be encouraged to meet increased caloric needs. If the patient refuses to eat the foods needed, it may be wise to offer whatever foods are acceptable to the patient.

When the patient shows marked deterioration as a result of tumor growth and effects, some other form of nutritional support (tube feeding, total parenteral nutrition) may become necessary. Nursing interventions include assessing the patency of the central and intravenous (IV) line or feeding tube, monitoring the insertion site for infection, checking the infusion rate, monitoring intake and output, and changing the IV tubing and dressing. These techniques can be taught to the caregivers at home. Additionally, total parenteral nutrition can be provided at home.

The quality of life for the patient may serve to guide in the selection, initiation, and maintenance of nutritional support. The patient may become weary with all the urging to eat and the discussions about food, and may not desire aggressive nutritional intervention. The subsequent course of action should take into consideration the wishes of the patient and family.

Relieving Anxiety. Persons with cerebral metastases may be restless, with changing moods that may include intense depression, euphoria, paranoia, and severe anxiety. The response of patients to terminal illness reflects their pattern of reaction to other crisis situations. Serious illness imposes additional strains that often bring other unresolved problems to light. The patient's own coping strategies can help deal with anxious and depressed feelings. Caregivers need to be sensitive to the patient's stated concerns.

Patients need the opportunity to exercise some control over their situation. A sense of mastery can be gained as they learn to understand the disease and its treatment, and how to deal with their feelings. The presence of family, friends, clergy, and health professionals may be supportive. Support groups such as Make Today Count may provide a feeling of support and strength.

Spending time with patients allows them time to talk and to communicate their fears and concerns. Open communication and acknowledging fears are often therapeutic. Touch is also a form of communication. These patients need reassurance that continuing care will be provided and that they will not be abandoned. The situation becomes more endurable when others share in the experience of dying.

If a patient's emotional reactions are very intense or prolonged, additional help from a member of the clergy, social worker, mental health professional, occupational therapist, or recreational therapist may be indicated.

Enhancing Family Coping. The family needs to be reassured that their loved one is receiving optimal care and that attention will be paid to the patient's changing symptoms and to their problems. When the patient can no longer carry out self-care, the family is helped with the essentials of the patient's physical care and assisted in finding support systems (social worker, home health aid, community health and home care nurse, hospice care). The nursing goal is to keep anxiety at a manageable level.

Patient Education and Home Care Considerations. It is important to assess the changing needs of the patient and the family and to inform them about resources and services that may assist family members to deal with changes in the patient's condition. Teaching needs of the patient and family are likely to change as the disease progresses. Home care nursing and hospice services are valuable resources that should be made available to the patient and the family. Anticipating needs before they occur often can assist in smooth initiation of services. Personal and telephone contact by the nurse with the patient and family are helpful approaches.

Hospice Care. The patient and family who elect to care for the patient at home as the disease progresses benefit from the care and support provided through hospice services. Steps to initiate hospice care, including discussion of hospice care as an option, should not be postponed until the patient's death is imminent. Exploration of hospice care as an option should be initiated at a time when hospice care can provide support to the patient and family and can assist in allowing death with dignity.

Evaluation

Expected Outcomes

1. Engages in self-care activities as long as possible
   a. Uses assistive devices or accepts assistance
   b. Schedules periodic rest periods to permit maximal participation in self-care
2. Maintains as optimal a nutritional status as possible
   a. Eats and accepts food within limits of condition
   b. Accepts assistance with meals if indicated
3. Reports being less anxious
   a. Is less restless and is sleeping better
   b. Verbalizes concerns about death
   c. Participates in activities of personal importance as long as feasible
4. Family members seek help as needed
   a. Demonstrate ability to bathe, feed, and care for the patient
   b. Express feelings and concerns to appropriate health professionals
   c. Discuss and seek hospice care as an option

Meningitis

Meningitis is an inflammation of the meninges (membranes surrounding the brain and spinal cord) and is caused by a viral, bacterial, or fungal organism. Meningitis is further classified as aseptic, septic, and tuberculous. *Aseptic meningitis* refers to either viral meningitis or cases of meningial irritation from other causes such as brain abscess, encephalitis, lymphoma, leukemia, or blood in the subarachnoid space. *Septic meningitis* refers to meningitis caused by bacterial organisms such as meningococcus, staphylococcus, or influenza bacillus. *Tuberculous meningitis* is caused by the tubercle bacillus.

Meningeal infections generally originate in one of two ways: either through the bloodstream as a consequence of other infections, such as cellulitis, or by direct extension such as might occur after a traumatic injury to the facial bones. In a small number of cases the cause is iatrogenic or secondary to invasive procedures (*e.g.*, lumbar puncture) or invasive devices (*e.g.*, ICP monitoring devices).

Bacterial Meningitis

By far the most significant form of meningitis is the bacterial type. The bacteria most frequently encountered in acute bacterial meningitis are *Neisseria meningitidis* (meningococcal meningitis), *Streptococcus pneumoniae* (in adults), and *Haemophilus influenzae* (in children and young adults). These three organisms account for about 75% of the cases of bacterial meningitis.

The mode of transmission is by direct contact, including droplets and discharges from the nose and throat of carriers (most often) or infected persons. Of those exposed to it, most do not develop the infection but become carriers. An increased incidence of meningitis caused by enteric gram-negative bacteria has occurred in the elderly, as well as in those who have had neurosurgery or who have a compromised immune response.

Bacterial meningitis is endemic in the United States and throughout the world, and occurs most frequently in the winter and spring months. Overall, the incidence of bacterial meningitis has declined in the Western world owing primarily to sophisticated social and hygienic standards. Outbreaks are most likely to occur among those living in crowded conditions such as in cities, crowded institutions, military installations, or prisons, although the disease also occurs in rural areas. In less-developed countries, meningitis remains a major health problem.

Pathophysiology

Bacterial meningitis starts as an infection of the oropharynx and is followed by septicemia, which extends to the meninges of the brain and upper region of the spinal cord.

Predisposing factors include upper respiratory tract infections, otitis media, mastoiditis, sickle cell anemia and other hemoglobinopathies, recent neurosurgical procedures, head trauma, and immunologic defects. The venous channels serving the posterior nasopharynx, middle ear, and mastoid drain toward the brain and are near the veins draining the meninges; these channels favor bacterial proliferation.

The organism enters the bloodstream and causes an inflammatory reaction in the meninges and underlying cortex, which may result in thromboses and reduced cerebral blood flow. The cerebral tissue is metabolically impaired as a result of meningeal exudate, vasculitis, and hypoperfusion. A purulent exudate may spread over the base of the brain and spinal cord. The inflammation also spreads to the membrane lining the cerebral ventricles. Bacterial meningitis is associated with profound alterations in intracranial physiology, including increased permeability of the blood—brain barrier, cerebral edema, and increased ICP.

In acute infections, however, the patient dies from the toxin of the bacteria before meningitis develops. In these patients the infection is overwhelming, with adrenal damage, circulatory collapse, and associated widespread hemorrhages (Waterhouse-Friderichsen syndrome) occurring as a result of endothelial damage and vascular necrosis caused by the meningococci.

Clinical Manifestations

The symptoms of meningitis result from infection and increased ICP.

Headache and fever are frequently the initial symptoms. The headache associated with meningitis is usually severe and is the result of meningeal irritation. Fever is generally present and remains high throughout the course of the illness.

Changes in level of consciousness are associated with bacterial meningitis. Disorientation and memory impairment are common early in the course of the illness. The changes that occur are dependent on the severity of illness as well as the individual response to the physiologic processes. Behavioral manifestations also are common. As the illness progresses, lethargy, unresponsiveness, and coma may develop.

Meningeal irritation results in a number of well-recognized signs commonly seen in all types of meningitis:

Nuchal rigidity (stiff neck) is an early sign. Any attempts at flexion of the head are difficult because of the presence of spasm in the muscles of the neck. Forceful flexion causes severe pain.

Positive Kernig's sign: When the patient is lying with the thigh flexed on the abdomen, the leg cannot be completely extended.

Positive Brudzinski's sign: When the patient's neck is flexed, flexion of the knees and hips is produced; when passive flexion of the lower extremity of one side is made, a similar movement is seen in the opposite extremity.

Also, for reasons that are unknown, these patients complain of **photophobia** or extreme sensitivity to light.

Seizures and increased ICP also are associated with meningitis. Seizures occur secondary to focal areas of cortical irritability. Signs of increasing ICP secondary to purulent exudate or cerebral edema include the characteristic vital sign changes (widened pulse pressure and bradycardia), respiratory irregularity, headache, vomiting, and depressed levels of consciousness.

A **rash** is one of the striking feature of meningococcal meningitis (neisseria meningitidis). About half of all patients with this type of meningitis develop skin lesions ranging from a petechial rash with purpuric lesions to large areas of ecchymosis.

A **fulminating infection** occurs in about 10% of patients with meningococcal meningitis, with signs of overwhelming septicemia: an abrupt onset of high fever, extensive purpuric lesions (over the face and extremities), shock, and signs of disseminated intravascular coagulopathy (DIC). Death may occur within a few hours of onset of the infection.

The infecting organisms usually can be identified through cultures of the cerebrospinal fluid and blood. Counterimmunoelectrophoresis (CIE) is widely used to detect bacterial antigens in body fluids, particularly cerebrospinal fluid and urine.

Management

Successful management depends on the administration of an antibiotic that crosses the blood—brain barrier into the subarachnoid space in sufficient concentration to halt the multiplication of bacteria. Cerebrospinal fluid (CSF) and blood cultures are obtained, and antimicrobial therapy is started immediately. Penicillin, ampicillin, or chloramphenicol, or one of the cephalosporins, may be used. Other antibiotics may be used if resistant strains of bacteria are identified. The patient is maintained on large IV doses of the appropriate antibiotic.

Dehydration or shock is treated with fluid volume expanders. Seizures, which may occur in the early course of the disease, are controlled with diazepam or phenytoin. An osmotic diuretic (*e.g.*, mannitol) may be used to treat cerebral edema.

Nursing Interventions

The patient's prognosis may depend on the supportive care given. The patient is very ill, and the combination of fever, dehydration, alkalosis, and cerebral edema may predispose to seizures. Airway obstruction, respiratory arrest, or cardiac dysrhythmias may follow. Thus, many of the nursing interventions are collaborative with those of the physician.

- In meningitis of all types, the patient's clinical status and vital signs are constantly assessed as altered consciousness may lead to airway obstruction. Arterial blood gas determinations, insertion of a cuffed endotracheal tube (or tracheostomy), and mechanical ventilation may be prescribed. Oxygen may be given to maintain the arterial partial pressure of oxygen (PO_2) at desired levels.
- Arterial pressures are monitored to assess for incipient shock, which precedes cardiac or respiratory failure. Generalized vasoconstriction, circumoral cyanosis, and cold extremities may be noted. The high fever is reduced to decrease the work load on the heart and the brain's oxygen demand. (See Chapter 65, Nursing Care Plan 65-1, for nursing interventions for the patient with an infectious disease.)
- Rapid intravenous fluid replacement may be prescribed, but care is taken not to overhydrate the patient because of risk of cerebral edema.
- The body weight, serum electrolytes, urine volume and specific gravity, and urine osmolality are closely monitored, especially if inappropriate antidiuretic hormone (ADH) secretion is suspected.
- Continuing nursing management requires ongoing assessment of the patient's clinical status, attention to skin and oral hygiene, promotion of comfort, and protection during seizures (p. 0000) and while comatose.
- Discharge from the nose and mouth is considered infectious. Respiratory isolation is advised until 24 hours following the initiation of antibiotic therapy.

Prevention

Persons in close contact with the patient should be considered candidates for antimicrobial prophylaxis (rifampin). Close contacts are observed and immediately examined if fever or other signs and symptoms of meningitis develop.

Meningococcal vaccine currently licensed in the United States includes the polysaccharides of groups A, C, W135, and Y, and is used primarily in military recruits. The vaccine may be of benefit for some travelers visiting countries that are experiencing epidemic meningococcal disease. Vaccination also should be considered as an adjunct to antibiotic chemoprophylaxis for anyone living with a patient who develops meningococcal infection.

A polysaccharide vaccine (Haemophilus b polysaccharide vaccine) against invasive *Haemophilus influenzae* type b has been licensed in the United States and is now used routinely in pediatrics for the prevention of meningitis.

Meningitis in Other Conditions

Meningitis in AIDS. Aseptic, cryptococcal, and tuberculous meningitis have been reported in patients with AIDS. Acute and chronic forms of aseptic meningitis may occur with AIDS; both are accompanied by headache, but signs of meningeal irritation generally occur with the acute form. Aseptic meningitis with AIDS may be accompanied by cranial nerve palsies. The meningitis is thought to be related to direct infection of the central nervous system by human immunodeficiency virus (HIV), as it can be isolated from the CSF.

Cryptococcal meningitis is the most common fungal infection of the central nervous system in patients with AIDS. Patients may experience headache, nausea, vomiting, seizures, confusion, and lethargy. Some patients develop few if any symptoms because of blunted inflammatory response occurring in the immunocompromised patient; others develop atypical features.

The treatment of crytococcal meningitis is IV administration of amphotericin B, which may be used with or without 5-flucytosine. Maintenance therapy with amphotericin may be necessary to prevent relapse.

Meningitis in Lyme Disease. Lyme disease is a multisystem inflammatory process caused by the tick-transmitted spirochete *Borrelia burgdorferi*. The neurologic abnormalities that are associated with the disease are seen in its later stages (stages 2 or 3). Stage 2 occurs either with the characteristic rash or from 1 to 6 months after it has disappeared. Neurologic abnormalities associated with this stage of Lyme disease include aseptic meningitis, chronic lymphocytic meningitis, and encephalitis. These patients can also experience cranial nerve inflammation including Bell's palsy and other peripheral neuropathies. Stage 3 (the chronic form of the disease) begins years after the initial tick infection and is characterized by arthritis, skin lesions, and further neurologic abnormalities.

Most patients with stage 2 and 3 Lyme disease are treated with IV antibiotics, usually penicillin. Meningeal and systemic symptoms will begin to improve within days although other symptoms such as headache and radicular pain may persist for weeks.

Intracranial Infection: Brain Abscess

A brain abscess is a collection of infectious material within the tissue of the brain. It may occur by *direct invasion of the brain* from intracranial trauma or surgery; by *spread of infection from nearby sites* such as the sinuses, ears, and teeth (paranasal sinus infections, otitis media, dental sepsis); or by *spread of infection from other organs* (lung abscess, infective endocarditis); and can be a complication associated with some forms of meningitis. Brain abscess is a complication encountered increasingly in patients whose immune systems have been suppressed through either therapy or disease. To prevent brain abscesses, otitis media, mastoiditis, sinusitis, dental infections, and systemic infections should be treated promptly.

Clinical Manifestations

The clinical manifestations of a brain abscess result from alterations in intracranial dynamics (edema, brain shift), infection, or the location of the abscess. Headache, usually worse in the morning, is the patient's most continuing symptom. Vomiting is also common. Focal neurologic signs (weakness of an extremity, decreasing vision, seizures) may occur, depending on the site of the abscess. There may be a change in the patient's mental status, as reflected in lethargic, confused, irritable, or disoriented behavior. Fever may or may not be present.

Diagnostic Evaluation

Repeated neurologic examinations and continuing assessment of the patient are necessary to determine accurately the location of the abscess. CT is invaluable in locating the site of the abscess, after the evolution and resolution of suppurative lesions, and in determining the optimal time for surgical intervention.

Management

The goal of management is to eliminate the abscess. Brain abscess is treated with antimicrobial therapy and surgical incision or aspiration. Antimicrobial treatment is given to eliminate the causative organism or reduce its virulence. Large intravenous doses are usually prescribed preoperatively to penetrate brain tissue and the brain abscess. The therapy is continued postoperatively. Corticosteroids may be given to help reduce the inflammatory cerebral edema if the patient shows evidence of an increasing neurologic deficit.

Anticonvulsant medications (phenytoin, phenobarbital) may be given as prophylaxis against seizures. Multiple abscesses may be treated with appropriate antimicrobial therapy alone, with close monitoring by CT scans.

After treatment of brain abscess neurologic deficits may include hemiparesis, seizures, visual defects, and cranial nerve palsies because of possible interference with brain tissue. Relapse is common, with a high mortality rate.

Intracranial Aneurysm

An intracranial (cerebral) aneurysm is a dilation of the walls of a cerebral artery that develops as a result of

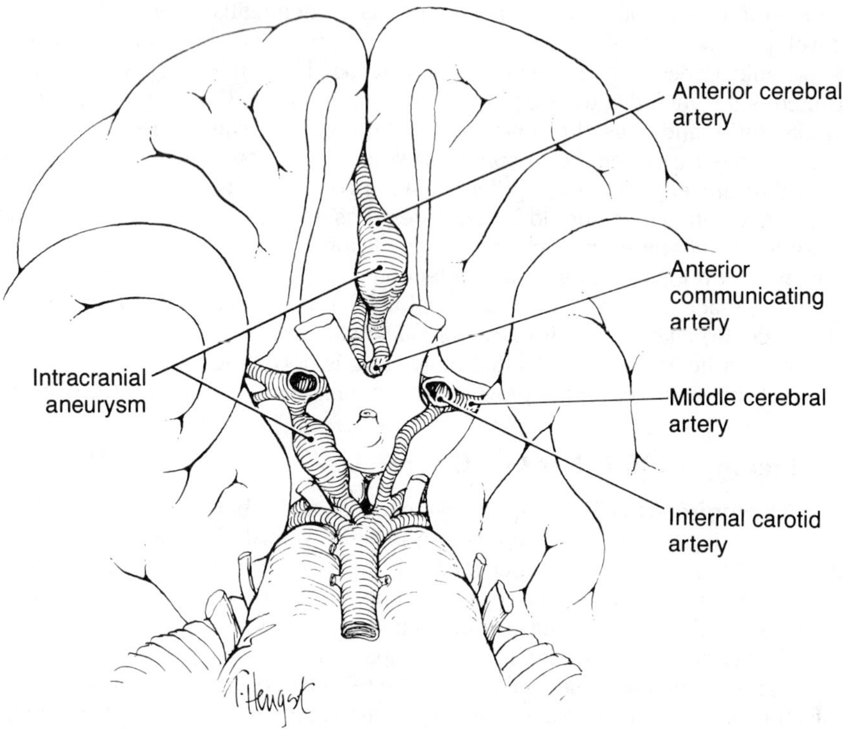

FIGURE 60-2. Intracranial aneurysm.

weakness in the arterial wall (Fig. 60-2). The cause of aneurysms is unknown, although research is ongoing in an attempt to understand this problem.

An aneurysm may be due to atherosclerosis, resulting in a defect in the vessel wall with subsequent weakness of the wall; a congenital defect of the vessel wall; hypertensive vascular disease; head trauma; or advancing age.

The cerebral arteries most commonly affected by an aneurysm are the internal carotid, anterior cerebral, anterior communicating, and middle cerebral arteries. A small percentage develop in the vertebrobasilar area. Multiple cerebral aneurysms are not uncommon.

Pathophysiology

Symptoms are produced when the aneurysm enlarges and presses on nearby cranial nerves or brain substance, or more dramatically, when the aneurysm ruptures, causing *subarachnoid hemorrhage* (hemorrhage into the cranial subarachnoid space). Normal brain metabolism is disrupted by the brain being exposed to blood; by an increase in ICP resulting from the sudden entry of blood into the subarachnoid space, which compresses and injures brain tissue; or by ischemia of the brain resulting from the reduced perfusion, pressure, and vasospasm that frequently accompany subarachnoid hemorrhage.

In addition to aneurysms, other causes of subarachnoid hemorrhage include arteriovenous malformations, tumors, trauma, blood dyscrasias, and unknown factors.

Clinical Manifestations

Rupture of the aneurysm usually produces a sudden, unusually severe headache and often loss of consciousness for a variable period. There may be pain and rigidity of the back of the neck and spine due to meningeal irritation. Visual disturbances (visual loss, diplopia, ptosis) occur when the aneurysm is adjacent to the oculomotor nerve. Tinnitus, dizziness, and hemiparesis also may occur.

At times, an aneurysm "leaks" blood, leading to the formation of a clot that seals the site of rupture. In this instance, the patient may show little neurologic deficit, or there may be severe bleeding, resulting in cerebral damage followed rapidly by coma and death.

Prognosis depends on the neurologic condition of the patient, age, associated diseases, and the extent and location of the aneurysm. Subarachnoid hemorrhage from an aneurysm is a catastrophic event with up to a 50% mortality rate.

Diagnostic Evaluation

The diagnosis is confirmed by CT scan; lumbar puncture, which reveals blood in the cerebrospinal fluid; and cerebral angiography, which shows the location and size of the aneurysm and gives information about the affected artery, adjoining vessels, and vascular branches.

Management

The goals of treatment are to allow the brain to recover from the initial insult (bleeding), to prevent or minimize the risk of rebleeding, and to prevent or treat other complications. Potential complications include rebleeding; cerebral vasospasm resulting in cerebral ischemia; acute hydrocephalus, which results when free blood obstructs the reabsorption of cerebrospinal fluid by the arachnoid villi; seizures; and anxiety. Management consists of bed rest with sedation to prevent agitation and stress, management of the vasospasm, and surgical or medical treatment to prevent rebleeding.

Vasospasm. The development of cerebral vasospasm (narrowing of the lumen of the involved cranial blood vessel) is a serious complication of subarachnoid hemorrhage and accounts for 40% to 50% of the morbidity and mortality of those who survive the initial intracranial bleed. The mechanism responsible for the spasm is not clear, but the occurrence of vasospasm correlates with increasing amounts of blood in the subarachnoid cisterns and cerebral fissures, as visualized by CT scan.

Vasospasm leads to increased vascular resistance, which impedes cerebral blood flow and causes brain ischemia and infarction. The signs and symptoms exhibited by the patient reflect the areas of the brain involved. Vasospasm often is heralded by a worsening headache, a decrease in level of consciousness (confusion, lethargy, disorientation), or the appearance of a new focal neurologic deficit (aphasia, hemiparesis [partial paralysis affecting one side of the body]).

Vasospasm frequently occurs within the 4th to 12th day after initial hemorrhage when the clot undergoes the lytic process (dissolution), increasing the chances of rebleeding.

It is believed that early operation to clip the aneurysm prevents rebleeding, and that removal of blood from the basal cisterns around the major cerebral arteries may prevent development of vasospasm. The intravenous administration of the calcium-blocker nimodipine during the critical time in which vasospasm may develop may protect against delayed ischemic deterioration. Advances in technology have led to the introduction of interventional neuroradiology for the treatment of aneurysms. Endovascular techniques may be used in selected patients to occlude the artery supplying the aneurysm with a balloon or occlude the aneurysm itself. As more studies on these techniques are completed, it is likely that their use will increase.

Management of vasospasm remains difficult and controversial. One explanation is that vasospasm is caused by an increased influx of calcium into the cell; thus medication therapy is designed to block or antagonize this action and may prevent or reverse the action of vasospasm already present. Calcium blockers are approved and available, including verapamil (Isoptin) and nifedipine (Procardia). Other therapy for vasospasm is aimed at minimizing the deleterious effects of the associated cerebral ischemia and includes fluid volume expanders and induced arterial hypertension, normotension, or hemodilution. The use of papaverine and recombinant tissue plasminogen activator is being investigated.

Increased Intracranial Pressure. An increase in ICP almost always follows a subarachnoid hemorrhage, usually because of disturbed circulation of CSF caused by blood in the basal cisterns. If the patient shows evidence of deterioration from increased ICP (due to cerebral edema, herniation, hydrocephalus, or vasospasm), CSF drainage may be instituted by lumbar puncture or ventricular catheter drainage, and mannitol is given to reduce ICP.

When mannitol is used as a long-term measure to control ICP, dehydration and disturbances in electrolyte balance (hyponatremia/hypernatremia; hypokalemia/hyperkalemia) may occur. Mannitol acts by osmotically pulling water out of the brain as well as by reducing total body water through diuresis. The patient is monitored for signs of dehydration and for rebound elevation of ICP.

If surgery is delayed or contraindicated, antifibrinolytic agents (aminocaproic acid; tranexamic acid) may be administered to delay or prevent dissolution of the clot at the site of the aneurysmal rupture.

Systemic Hypertension. Efforts are made to prevent sudden systemic hypertension. If blood pressure is elevated, antihypertensive therapy (nitroprusside) may be prescribed. Hemodynamic monitoring by arterial line is carried out to detect and avoid a precipitous drop in blood pressure, which can produce brain ischemia. Because seizures cause blood pressure elevation, anticonvulsant agents are administered prophylactically. Stool softeners are used to prevent straining, which also can elevate the blood pressure.

Analgesics (codeine, acetaminophen) may be prescribed for head and neck pain. The patient is fitted with graded pressure elastic stockings to prevent deep vein thrombosis, a threat to any patient on bed rest.

Surgical Management

The patient is prepared for surgical intervention as soon as the condition is considered stable. The nursing management of the patient after a craniotomy is discussed in Chapter 59.

The goal of surgery is to prevent further bleeding. This objective is accomplished by isolating the aneurysm from its circulation or by strengthening the arterial wall. An aneurysm may be excluded from the cerebral circulation by means of a ligature or a clip across its neck. If this is not anatomically possible, the aneurysm can be reinforced by wrapping it with plastic, muscle, or some other substance.

An extracranial—intracranial arterial bypass may be performed to establish collateral blood supply to allow surgery on the aneurysm. Alternatively, an extracranial method may be used, whereby the carotid artery is gradually occluded in the neck to reduce pressure within the blood vessel. After ligation of the carotid artery, there is some risk of cerebral ischemia and sudden hemiplegia because during the surgical procedure there is a temporary occlusion of the blood supply to the brain (unless a temporary inlying bypass shunt is used). In anticipation of these complications, measurements of cerebral blood flow and internal carotid pressure may be taken to identify those patients who are at risk for postoperative ischemic episodes.

Other postoperative complications include the appearance of psychological symptoms (disorientation, amnesia, Korsakoff's syndrome, personality impairment), intraoperative embolization, postoperative internal artery occlusion, fluid and electrolyte disturbances (from dysfunction of the neurohypophyseal system), and gastrointestinal bleeding.

❑ *NURSING PROCESS*
The Patient With a Cerebral Aneurysm

Assessment

A complete neurologic assessment is performed initially and should include an evaluation of the following: (1) level of consciousness; (2) pupillary reaction; (3) motor and sensory function; (4) cranial nerve deficits (extraocular eye movements, facial droop, presence of ptosis); and (5) speech difficulties, visual disturbance or other neurologic deficits, and headache.

Neurologic assessment findings are documented and reported as indicated. Frequency of these assessments varies and is determined by the patient's condition. Any changes in the patient's condition require reassessment and thorough documentation; changes should be reported immediately.

Alteration in level of consciousness often is the earliest sign of deterioration in a patient with a cerebral aneurysm. Because nurses have the most frequent contact with patients, it is often the nurse who is the first to detect what may be subtle changes. Mild drowsiness and slight slurring of speech may be early signs that the patient's level of consciousness is deteriorating. Frequent nursing assessment is critical in the patient with known or suspected cerebral aneurysm.

Diagnosis

Nursing Diagnoses

Based on the assessment data, the patient's major nursing diagnoses may include the following:

- Altered cerebral perfusion due to bleeding from the aneurysm
- Sensory or perceptual alteration due to the restrictions of subarachnoid precautions
- Anxiety due to illness or restrictions of subarachnoid precautions

Collaborative Problems/ Potential Complications

Based on the assessment data, potential complications that may develop include the following:

- Seizures
- Vasospasm

Planning and Implementation

Goals. The goals for the patient may include improved cerebral tissue perfusion, relief of sensory and perceptual deprivation, relief of anxiety, and the absence of complications.

Nursing Interventions

Improving Cerebral Tissue Perfusion. The patient is monitored continually for neurologic deterioration occurring from recurrent bleeding, increasing ICP, or vasospasm. A neurologic flow record is kept. The blood pressure, pulse, level of responsiveness (an indicator of cerebral perfusion), pupillary responses, and motor function are checked hourly. The respiratory status is monitored because reduction in PO_2 in brain areas with impaired autoregulation increases the chances of a cerebral infarction. Any changes are reported immediately.

Subarachnoid precautions are implemented to provide a nonstimulating environment and prevent increases in intracranical pressure and further bleeding. The patient is placed on immediate and absolute bed rest in a quiet, nonstressful setting because activity, pain, and anxiety elevate the blood pressure, which increases the risk of bleeding. Visitors, except for family, are restricted.

The head of the bed is elevated moderately to provide venous drainage and decrease ICP. Some neurologists, however, prefer that the patient remain flat to increase cerebral perfusion.

Any activity that suddenly increases the blood pressure or obstructs venous return is avoided. This includes the Valsalva maneuver, straining, forceful sneezing, pulling up in bed, acute flexion or rotation of the head and neck (which compromises the jugular veins), and cigarette smoking. Any activity requiring exertion is contraindicated. The patient is instructed to exhale through the mouth during voiding or defecation to decrease strain. No enemas are permitted but stool softeners and mild laxatives are prescribed. Both prevent constipation, which would cause an increase in ICP, as would enemas. Dim lighting is helpful because photophobia (visual intolerance of light) is common. Coffee and tea, unless decaffeinated, are usually eliminated.

All personal care is administered by the nurse. The patient is fed and bathed to prevent any exertion that might raise the blood pressure. External stimuli are kept to a minimum, including no television, no radio, no reading, and maintenance of visitor restriction. Visitors are restricted in an effort to keep the patient as quiet as possible. This precaution must be individualized based on patient condition and response to visitors. A sign indicating this restriction should be placed on the door of the room, and the restrictions should be discussed with both patient and family.

The purpose of subarachnoid precautions should be thoroughly explained to both the patient (if possible) and family.

Relieving Sensory Deprivation and Anxiety. Sensory stimulation is kept to a minimum. For patients who are awake, alert, and oriented, an explanation of the restrictions helps reduce the patient's sense of isolation. Reality orientation is provided to help maintain orientation.

Keeping the patient well informed of the plan of care provides reassurance and helps minimize anxiety. Appropriate reassurance also helps relieve the patient's fears and anxiety. The family also requires information and support.

Monitoring and Managing Potential Complications.

Seizures. Seizure precautions are maintained for every patient who may be at risk for seizure activity. These include having fully functioning suction equipment at the bedside; suction catheter, a padded tongue blade, and an oral airway. Padded side rails are provided to protect the patient from possible injury. Should a seizure occur, maintaining the patient's airway and preventing injury are the primary goals. Medication therapy is initiated at this time if it has not already been initiated. The medication of choice is phenytoin (Dilantin), as this drug usually provides adequate anticonvulsant action while causing no drowsiness at therapeutic levels.

Vasospasm. The patient must be assessed for signs of possible vasospasm: intensified headaches, a decrease in level of responsiveness (confusion, disorientation, lethargy), or evidence of aphasia or partial paralysis. These signs may develop several days following surgery or on the initiation of treatment and must be reported immediately.

If vasospasm has been diagnosed, prescribed medications such as calcium blockers or fluid volume expanders are administered.

Evaluation

Expected Outcomes

1. Demonstrates intact neurologic status and normal vital signs and respiratory patterns

   a. Is alert and oriented to time, place, and person
   b. Demonstrates normal speech patterns and intact cognitive processes
   c. Demonstrates normal and equal strength, movement, and sensation of all four extremities
   d. Exhibits normal deep tendon reflexes and pupillary responses
2. Demonstrates normal sensory perceptions
   a. States rationale for subarachnoid precautions
   b. Exhibits clear thought processes
3. Exhibits reduced anxiety level
   a. Is less restless
   b. Exhibits absence of physiologic indicators of anxiety (*i.e.*, normal vital signs; normal respiratory rate; absence of excessive, fast speech)
4. Is free of complications
   a. Exhibits normal vital signs and neuromuscular activity without seizures
   b. Verbalizes understanding of seizure precautions
   c. Exhibits absence of vasospasm
   d. Exhibits normal mental status and normal motor and sensory status
   e. Reports no visual changes

Multiple Sclerosis

Multiple sclerosis (MS) is a chronic, degenerative progressive disease of the central nervous system characterized by the occurrence of small patches of demyelination in the brain and spinal cord. **Demyelination** refers to the destruction of myelin, the fatty and protein material that surrounds certain nerve fibers in the brain and spinal cord, which results in impaired transmission of nerve impulses (Fig. 60-3).

The cause of MS is not known. Research evidence suggests that myelin damage is the primary event, and that it results from a viral infection early in life that becomes apparent as an immune process later in life. Although some form of viral infection may be the initiating mechanism, a defective immune response is thought to have a major role in the pathogenesis of MS.

Epidemiologic findings indicate that MS is more common in people living in the northern temperate climate zones. It is one of the most disabling neurologic diseases of young adults (20 to 40 years of age) in the United States, affecting twice as many women as men. Its occurrence in patients who are young increases the medical, psychological, social, and economic problems encountered by both patient and family.

Pathophysiology

In MS, the demyelination is scattered irregularly throughout the central nervous system (Fig. 60-4). Myelin is lost from the axis cylinders and the axons themselves degenerate. The plaques or patches in the involved areas become sclerosed, interrupting the flow of nerve impulses and resulting in a variety of manifestations, depending on which nerves are affected. The areas most frequently affected are the optic nerves, chiasm, tracts, the cerebrum, the brain stem and cerebellum, and the spinal cord.

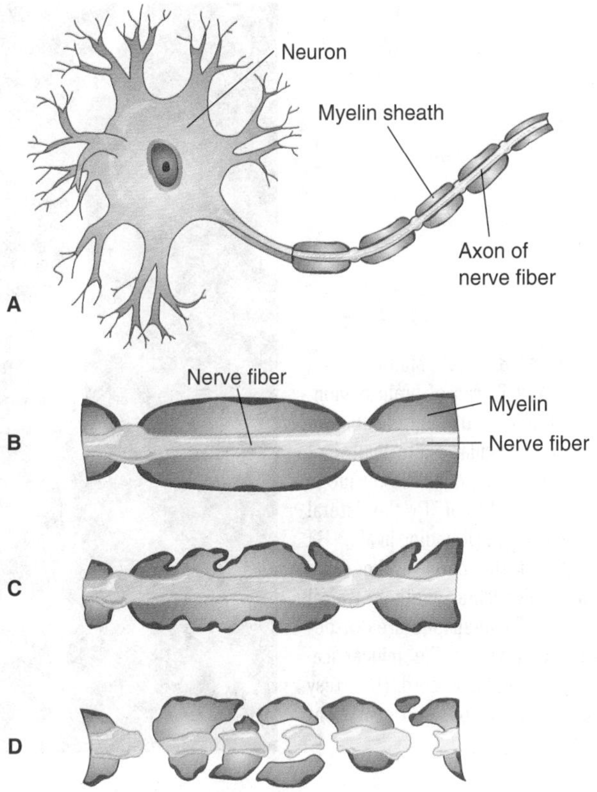

FIGURE 60-3. The process of demyelination. **A** and **B** depict a normal nerve cell and axon with myelin. **C** and **D** show the slow disintegration of myelin, resulting in a disruption in axon function.

Clinical Manifestations

The course of MS may assume many different patterns. Most patients begin with a relapsing–remitting course with complete recovery between relapses. Other patients have a chronic progressive course from the outset with a progressive decline in function. A rapidly progressive course is much less frequent. In other patients, the disease follows a benign course with a normal life span and symptoms so mild that patients do not seek health care and treatment.

The signs and symptoms of MS are varied and multiple, reflecting the location of the lesion (plaque) or combination of lesions. The primary symptoms most commonly reported are fatigue, weakness, numbness, difficulty in coordination, and loss of balance. Visual disturbance due to lesions in the optic nerves or their connections may include blurring of vision, diplopia, patchy blindness (*scotoma*), and total blindness.

Spastic weakness of the extremities and loss of the abdominal reflexes are due to involvement of the main motor pathways (*pyramidal tracts*) of the spinal cord. Disruption of the sensory axons may produce sensory dysfunction. Cognitive and psychosocial problems, including depression, may reflect frontal or parietal lobe involvement; severe cognitive changes with dementia are rare. Involvement of the cerebellum or basal ganglia can produce *ataxia* (impaired coordination of movements) and tremor. Emotional lability and euphoria result from loss of the control connections between the cortex and the basal ganglia and may occur in

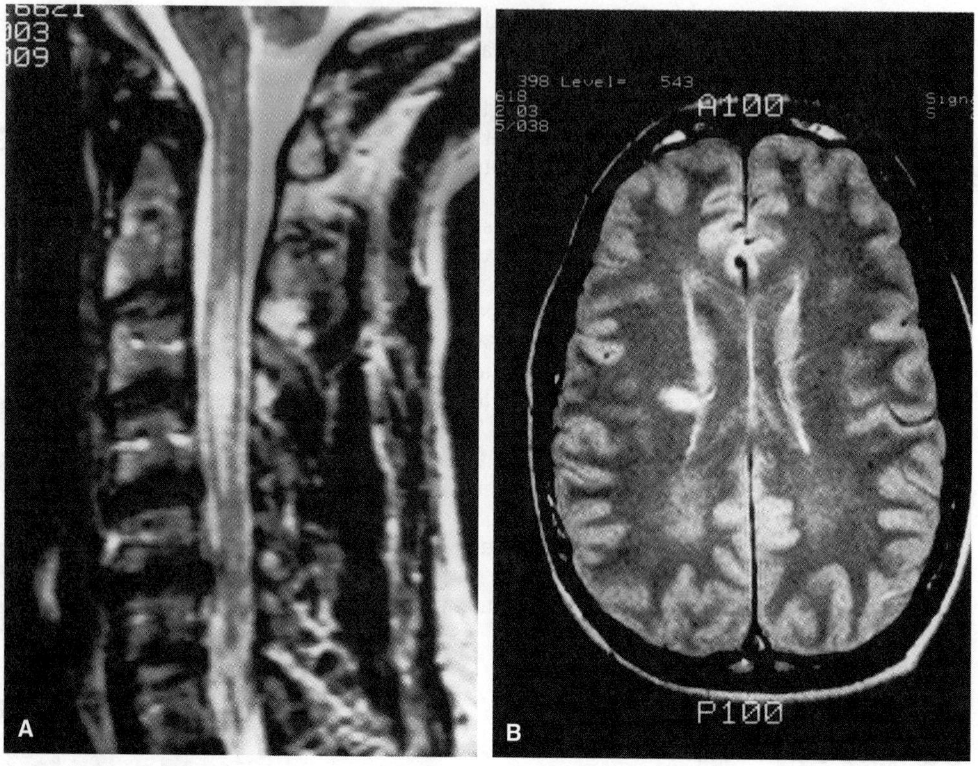

FIGURE 60-4. Multiple sclerosis. (**A**) CT scan of brain demonstrating an area of demyelination in the periventricular white matter of the right frontal lobe. The plaque is seen perpendicular to the lateral ventricle, a typical finding in MS. (**B**) An MRI of the cord in the same patient highlights another typical finding; a flame-shaped area of demyelination within the midcervical region of the spinal cord. (Courtesy of the Danbury Hospital Department of Radiology.)

patients with MS. Bladder, bowel, and sexual problems are common.

Secondary complications of MS include urinary tract infections, constipation, pressure ulcers, contracture deformities, dependent pedal edema, pneumonia, and reactive depressions. Emotional, social, marital, economic, and vocational problems may also be a consequence of the disease.

Exacerbations and remissions are characteristic of MS. During exacerbations new symptoms appear and existing ones worsen; during remissions symptoms decrease or disappear. Relapses may be associated with periods of emotional and physical stress. MRI studies demonstrate that many plaques do not produce serious symptoms, and patients with these plaques are not seriously incapacitated but have long periods of remission between episodes. There is evidence that remyelination actually occurs in some patients.

Diagnostic Evaluation

Electrophoresis study of the CSF usually discloses the presence of *oligoclonal banding* (several bands of gamma G immunoglobulin [IgG]), reflecting immunoglobulin abnormalities. In fact, abnormal IgG antibody appears in the CSF of up to 95% of patients with MS. Evoked potential studies are carried out to help define the extent of the disease process and monitor changes. CT scans may show cerebral atrophy. MRI has become a primary diagnostic tool for visualizing small plaques and for evaluating the course of the disease and effect of the treatment. Underlying bladder dysfunction is diagnosed by urodynamic studies. Neuropsychological testing may be indicated to assess cognitive impairment. A sexual history helps to identify specific areas of concern.

Management

No cure exists for MS. An individualized, organized, and rational treatment program is indicated to relieve the patient's symptoms and provide continuing support. Many patients with MS are in stable condition and require only intermittent treatment aimed at controlling symptoms; others experience steady progression of their disease.

Pharmacotherapy. Corticosteroids and ACTH are used as anti-inflammatory agents that may improve the nerve conduction. Because immune mechanisms may be a factor in the pathogenesis of MS, a number of pharmacologic agents are being tried to modulate the immune response and reduce the rate at which the disease progresses and the frequency and severity of the exacerbations. These medications include azathioprine, cyclophosphamide, and interferon.

Beta interferon (Betaseron) has been approved for use in relapsing-remitting MS patients with a relapsing-remitting course. Betaseron has been found to be effective in significantly reducing the number and severity of acute exacerbations with MRI scanning showing fewer areas of demyelination in brain tissue. This is the first promising new drug to become available for MS treatment, although hundreds have been tried.

Other modalities (*e.g.*, radiation, copolymer 1 and cladribine) are currently under investigation as possible treatments for progressive forms of MS.

Baclofen, an antispasmodic agent, is the current treatment of choice for spasticity. Patients with severe spasticity and contractures may require nerve blocks and surgical intervention to prevent further disability.

Bowel and Bladder Management. Management of bladder and bowel control are among the patient's most difficult problems. Generally, bladder symptoms fall into the following categories: (1) inability to store urine (hyperreflexic; uninhibited); (2) inability to empty the bladder (hyporeflexic; hypotonic); and (3) a mixture of both types. A variety of medications may be used to treat these problems. Intermittent self-catheterization is an effective treatment of bladder dysfunction.

Often urinary tract infection is superimposed on the underlying neurologic dysfunction. Ascorbic acid may be given to acidify the urine, making bacterial growth less likely. Antibiotics are prescribed when appropriate.

❑ *NURSING PROCESS*
The Patient With Multiple Sclerosis

Assessment

Nursing assessment addressess actual and potential problems associated with the disease, including neurologic problems, secondary complications, and the impact of the disease on the patient and family. The patient's movements and walking are observed to determine if there is danger of falling. Assessment of function is carried out both when the patient is well rested and when fatigued. The patient is assessed for weakness, spasticity, visual impairment, and incontinence. Additional areas of assessment include: How has MS affected the patient's lifestyle? How well is the patient coping? What would the patient like to do better?

Diagnosis

Nursing Diagnoses

Based on all the assessment data, the patient's major nursing diagnoses may include the following:

- ❑ Impaired physical mobility related to weakness, muscle paresis, spasticity
- ❑ Risk for injury related to sensory and visual impairment
- ❑ Altered urinary and bowel elimination related to spinal cord dysfunction
- ❑ Altered thought processes (loss of memory, dementia, euphoria) related to cerebral dysfunction
- ❑ Ineffective coping
- ❑ Impaired home maintenance management related to physical, psychological, and social limits imposed by MS
- ❑ Potential for sexual dysfunction related to spinal cord involvement or psychological reactions to condition

Planning and Implementation

Goals. The major goals for the patient may include promotion of physical mobility, avoidance of injury, achievement of bladder and bowel continence, improvement of cognitive function, development of coping strengths, improved self-care, and adaptation to sexual dysfunction.

Nursing Interventions

An individualized program of physical therapy, rehabilitation, and education is combined with emotional support. The nursing interventions include patient education to enable the person with MS to deal with the physiologic, social, and psychological problems that accompany chronic disease.

Promoting Physical Mobility. Relaxation and coordination exercises promote muscle efficiency for the person with MS. Progressive resistive exercises are used to strengthen weak muscles, because diminishing muscle power is a significant problem for these patients.

Activity and Rest. The patient is encouraged to work up to a point just short of fatigue. Vigorous physical exercise is *not* advisable because it raises the body temperature and may aggravate symptoms. Prolonged exercise that tires an extremity may cause paresis, numbness, or incoordination. The patient is advised to take frequent short rest periods, preferably lying down. Extreme fatigue may be a contributing factor in exacerbation of symptoms.

Exercises. Walking exercises improve the gait, particularly when there is loss of position sense of the legs and feet. If certain muscle groups are irreversibly affected, other muscles can be trained to take over their actions.

Minimizing Spasticity and Contractures. Muscle spasticity is common and, in its later stages, is characterized by severe adductor spasm of the hips with flexor spasm of the hips and knees. If this is not relieved, fibrous contractures of these joints with resultant pressure ulcers over the sacrum and hips (due to inability to position the patient properly) occur. Warm packs may be beneficial, but hot baths should be avoided because of risk of burn injury secondary to sensory loss and the risk of increasing symptoms which is associated with an elevation of the body temperature.

Daily exercises for muscle stretching are prescribed to minimize joint contractures. Special attention is given to hamstrings, gastrocnemius muscles, hip adductors, biceps, and wrist and finger flexors. Muscle spasticity is common and interferes with normal function. A stretch-hold-relax routine is helpful for relaxing and treating muscle spasticity. Swimming and stationary bicycling are useful, and progressive weight-bearing can relieve spasticity in the legs. The patient should not be hurried in any of these activities because this often increases spasticity.

Minimizing Effects of Immobility. Because of the decreased physical activity and immobility that often occur with MS, complications associated with immobility, including pressure ulcers and accumulation of bronchial secretions, need to be considered and steps taken to prevent them. Measures to prevent such complications include assessment and maintenance of skin integrity, and coughing and deep breathing exercises.

Preventing Injury. If motor dysfunction causes problems of incoordination and clumsiness, or if ataxia is apparent, the patient is at risk for falling. To overcome this disability, the patient is taught to walk with feet wide apart to widen the base of support and to increase walking stability. If there is loss of position sense, the patient is taught to watch the feet while walking. Gait training may require assistive devices (walker, cane braces, crutches, parallel bars) and physical therapy. If the gait remains inefficient, a wheelchair or motorized scooter may be the solution. The occupational therapist is a valuable resource person in suggesting and securing aids to promote independence. If incoordination is a problem and tremor of the upper extremities occurs when voluntary movement is attempted (*intention tremor*), weighted bracelets or wrist cuffs are helpful. The patient is trained in transfer and activities of daily living.

Because sensory loss may occur in addition to motor loss, pressure ulcers are a continuing threat to skin integrity. Confinement to a wheelchair increases the risk. (See p. 343 for a discussion of the prevention and treatment of pressure ulcers.)

Promoting Bladder and Bowel Control. The patient with urinary frequency, urgency, or incontinence requires special support. The sensation of the need to void must be heeded immediately, so the bedpan or urinal should be readily available. A voiding time schedule is set up (every 1½ to 2 hours initially, with gradual lengthening of the time intervals). The patient is instructed to drink a measured amount of fluid every 2 hours and then attempt to void 30 minutes after drinking. Using a timer or wristwatch with an alarm may be helpful for the patient who does not have enough sensation to signal the need to empty the bladder. The nurse encourages the patient to take the prescribed medications to treat bladder spasticity, as this allows greater independence. Intermittent self-catheterization has been very successful in maintaining bladder control.

If the female patient has permanent urinary incontinence, urinary diversion procedures may be considered. The male patient may wear a condom appliance for urine collection.

Bowel problems include constipation, fecal impaction, and incontinence. Adequate fluids, dietary fiber, and a bowel-training program frequently are effective in solving these problems (see p. 347).

Improving Sensory and Cognitive Function. Measures may be taken if visual and speech defects occur (the cranial nerves relating to sight and speech may be affected by MS).

Vision. An eye patch or an eyeglass occluder may be used to block visual impulses of one eye when the patient has *diplopia* (double vision). Prism glasses may be helpful for the bedridden patient who is having difficulty reading in the supine position. Persons with any physical limitations preventing them from reading regular print materials are eligible for the free talking book services of the Library of Congress (see Bibliography for address) or may wish to obtain large-type books available at most local libraries.

Speech. When the cranial nerves controlling the mechanisms of speech are involved, *dysarthrias* (defects of articulation) marked by slurring, low volume of speech, and difficulties in phonation are seen. There are also problems with shallow breathing. A speech-language therapist teaches the patient, family, and health team members about communication problems and the use of compensatory techniques.

Cognition and Emotional Responses. Cognitive impairment and emotional lability may occur early in MS and may impose numerous stresses on the patient and family. Embarrassing and humiliating symptoms may result in "inappropriate" responses by the patient. As there may be organic changes in the brain, MS patients may be forgetful and easily distracted and may exhibit emotional lability.

Patients adapt to illness in a variety of ways, which may include denial, depression, withdrawal, and hostility. Compassion and significant emotional support are required to help patients adapt to the changes and uncertainties associated with MS and to cope with the disruption in their lives. The patient is assisted to set meaningful and realistic goals to achieve a sense of purpose, to remain as active as possible, and to keep up social interests and activities. Hobbies may help the patient's morale and provide satisfying interests if the disease progresses to the stage in which normal activities cannot be pursued.

The family should be made aware of the nature and degree of cognitive impairment. The environment is kept structured, and lists and other memory aids are used to help the patient maintain a daily routine.

Strengthening Coping Mechanisms. The family may face overwhelming frustrations and problems. MS strikes individuals who are often in a productive stage of life and concerned about career and family responsibilities. Family conflict, disintegration, separation, and divorce are not uncommon. Often very young family members assume the responsibility of caring for a disabled parent. Nursing interventions in this area include alleviating stress and making appropriate referrals for counseling and support to minimize the adverse effects of dealing with chronic illness.

The nurse, mindful of these complex problems, initiates home care and coordinates a network of services, including social services, speech therapy, physical therapy, and homemaker services. To strengthen the patient's coping skills, as much information as possible is provided. People who live with chronic illness need an updated list of assistive devices, services, and resources that are available.

Coping through problem-solving involves helping the patient define the problem and develop alternatives for its management. Careful planning, flexibility, and maintaining a hopeful attitude are useful for psychological and physical adaptation.

Improving Self-Care. MS can affect every facet of daily living. Once certain abilities are lost, they are often impossible to regain. Physical abilities may vary from day to day. Modifications that allow independence in self-care should be implemented (raised toilet seat, bathing aids, telephone modifications, long-handled comb, tongs, modified clothing). Physical and emotional stresses should be avoided as much as possible, because these may worsen symptoms and impair performance. Exposure to heat increases fatigue and muscle weakness. Air-conditioning in at least one room is recommended. Exposure to extreme cold may increase spasticity. Continuing health care and follow-up are recommended.

Adapting to Sexual Dysfunction. Patients with MS and their partners face problems that interfere with sexual activity, arising not only as a direct consequence of nerve damage but also from psychological reactions to the disease. Easy fatigability, conflicts arising from dependency and depression, emotional lability, loss of self-esteem, and feelings of self-worth compound the problem. Erectile and ejaculatory disorders in men and orgasmic dysfunction and adductor spasms of the thigh muscles in women can make sexual intercourse difficult or impossible. Bladder and bowel incontinence and urinary tract infections add to the difficulties.

An experienced sexual counselor helps bring into focus the patient's or partner's sexual resources and suggests relevant information and supportive therapy. Sharing and communicating feelings, planning for sexual activity (to counteract fatigue), exercising different sexual options, and demonstrating a willingness to experiment may open up a wide range of sexual enjoyment and experiences.

Patient Education and Home Care Considerations. Because the diagnosis of MS often is made when the patient is in the most productive years of life, many questions about the disease and the patient's future arise. The patient with MS is encouraged to contact the local chapter of the National Multiple Sclerosis Society for services, publications, and contact with others with MS. Local chapters provide direct services to patients. Through group participation, the patient has an opportunity to meet others with similar problems, to share experiences, and to learn self-help methods in a social environment.

If the disease progresses, the patient and family will require assistance to deal with new disabilities and changes. Teaching of new self-care techniques may be initiated in the clinic setting; reinforcement of these new techniques is often provided in the patient's home by the community health or home care nurse.

The nurse who has continuing contact with the patient and the family is often in an ideal situation to assess changes in the patient's health status and to assess how both the patient and the family are coping with these changes.

Evaluation

Expected Outcomes

1. Adapts to impaired mobility and spasticity
   a. Participates in gait-training and rehabilitation program
   b. Establishes a balanced program of rest and exercise
   c. Uses assistive devices
2. Avoids injury
   a. Uses visual cues to compensate for decreased sense of touch or position
   b. Asks for assistance when necessary
3. Attains or maintains improved bladder and bowel control
   a. Monitors self for urine retention and employs intermittent self-catheterization technique, if indicated
   b. Identifies the signs and symptoms of urinary tract infection
   c. Maintains adequate fluid and fiber intake
4. Compensates for cognitive dysfunction
   a. Uses lists to compensate for memory losses
   b. Discusses problems with trusted advisor or friend
   c. Substitutes new activities for those that have been given up
5. Demonstrates improved coping strategies
   a. Maintains sense of control
   b. Makes plans to modify lifestyle
   c. Verbalizes desire to pursue goals and developmental tasks of adulthood
6. Adapts to changes in sexual function
   a. Is able to discuss problem with partner and appropriate health professional
   b. Identifies alternate means of sexual expression

Parkinson's Disease

Parkinson's disease is a progressive neurologic disorder affecting the brain centers that are responsible for control and regulation of movement. It is characterized by **bradykinesia** (slowness of movement), tremor, and muscle stiffness or rigidity.

Pathophysiology

The major lesion appears to result in a loss of pigmented neurons, particularly those in the substantia nigra of the brain (Fig. 60-5). (The *substantia nigra* is a collection of midbrain nuclei that project fibers to the corpus striatum.) One of the major neurotransmitters in this area of the brain, and in other parts of the central nervous system, is dopamine, which has an important inhibiting function in the central control of movement. Although dopamine normally exists in high concentration in certain parts of the brain, in Parkinson's disease it is depleted in the substantia nigra and the corpus striatum. Depletion of dopamine levels in the basal ganglia is associated with bradykinesia, rigidity, and tremors.

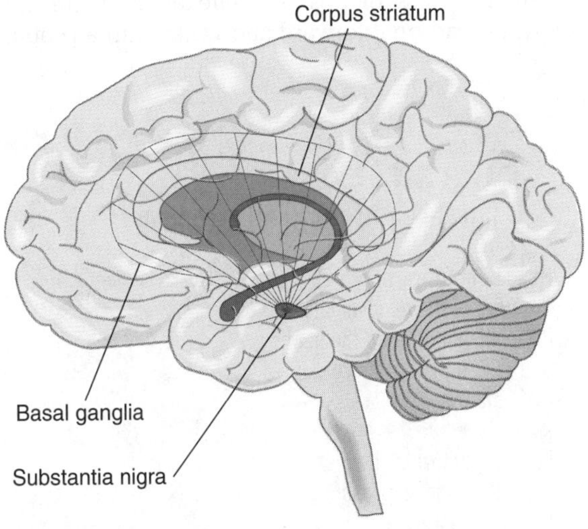

FIGURE 60-5. The nuclei in the substantia nigra project fibers to the corpus striatum. The nerve fibers carry dopamine to the corpus striatum. The loss of dopamine nerve cells from the brain's substantia nigra is thought to be responsible for the symptoms of parkinsonism.

Regional cerebral blood flow is reduced in patients with Parkinson's disease, and there is a high prevalence of dementia. Biochemical and pathologic data suggest that demented patients with Parkinson's disease may have coexistent Alzheimer's disease.

In most patients, the cause of the disease is unknown. Arteriosclerotic parkinsonism is seen more frequently in older age groups. It may follow encephalitis, poisoning or toxicity (manganese, carbon monoxide), hypoxia, or may be drug induced, but in most cases the cause is unknown. The disease is most prevalent among persons in their 60s and is the second most common neurologic disorder of the elderly.

Clinical Manifestations

The chief manifestations of Parkinson's disease are impaired movement, muscular rigidity, resting tremor, muscle weakness, and loss of postural reflexes. Early signs include a stiffening of the extremities and a waxlike rigidity in the performance of all movements. The patient has difficulty in initiating, maintaining, and performing motor activities, and experiences some delay in carrying out normal activity.

As the disease progresses, the tremor begins, frequently in one hand and arm, then the other, and later in the head, although the tremor may remain unilateral. The tremor is characteristic: it is a slow, turning motion (pronation—supination) of the forearm and the hand, and a motion of the thumb against the fingers as if rolling a pill between the fingers. It increases when the patient is concentrating or feeling anxious, and is present while the patient is at rest.

Other characteristics of the disease affect the face, stature, and gait. There is loss of normal arm swing. Eventually, the rigid extremities become definitely weaker. Because there is limited movement in the muscles, the face has so little expression that it is said to be masklike (with infrequency of blinking), a feature that can be recognized at a glance.

There is a loss of postural reflexes, and the patient stands with head bent forward and walks with a propulsive gait. Difficulty in pivoting and loss of balance (either forward or backward) may lead to frequent falls (Chart 60-2).

Frequently these patients show signs of depression, and it has not been established whether the depression is a reaction to the disorder or related to a biochemical abnormality. Mental manifestations may appear in the form of cognitive, perceptual, and memory deficits. A number of psychiatric manifestations (personality changes, psychosis, dementia, acute confusion) are particularly common among the elderly.

Complications from immobility (pneumonia, urinary tract infection) and the consequences of falls and accidents are major causes of death.

CHART 60-2
Clinical Features of Parkinsonism

- Head bent forward
- Tremors of the head and hand
- Pill-rolling motion of the hands
- Shuffling and propulsive gait
- Rigid stance
- Akinesia
- Loss of postural reflexes
- Masklike facial expression
- Stooped posture
- Weight loss
- Drooling

Diagnostic Evaluation

Early diagnosis of Parkinson's disease can be difficult as the patient can rarely pinpoint when symptoms started. Often someone close to the patient notices a change such as stooped posture, a stiff arm, a slight limp, or tremor. Handwriting changes may be an early diagnostic clue. A diagnosis of Parkinson's disease usually can be made with certainty when there is evidence of tremor, rigidity, and bradykinesia (abnormally slow movements). The history of the patient's symptoms and the results of the neurologic examination are carefully evaluated.

Management

The goal of treatment is to enhance dopamine transmission. Medication therapy includes antihistamines, anticholinergics, amantadine, levodopa, monoamine oxidase (MAO) inhibitors, and antidepressants. Many of these agents can cause psychiatric side effects in the elderly.

Antihistamines. Antihistamines have mild central anticholinergic and sedative effects, and may be helpful in allaying tremors.

Anticholinergic Therapy. Anticholinergic agents (trihexyphenidyl, procyclidine, and benztropine mesylate) are effective for controlling the tremor and rigidity of parkinsonism. These medications may be used in combination with levodopa. They counteract the action of acetylcholine in the central nervous system. Side effects include blurred vision, flushing, rash, constipation, urinary retention, and acute confusional states. Intraocular pressure is closely monitored because these drugs are contraindicated in patients with narrow-angle glaucoma. Patients with prostatic hyperplasia are monitored for signs of urinary retention.

Amantadine Hydrochloride. Amantadine hydrochloride (Symmetrel), an antiviral agent, is used early in the treatment of Parkinson's disease to reduce rigidity, tremor, and bradykinesia. It is thought to act by releasing dopamine from neuronal storage sites. Adverse reactions include psychiatric disturbances (mood changes, confusion, hallucinations), nausea, epigastric distress, headache, and visual impairment.

Levodopa Therapy. Levodopa, although not a cure, is currently the most effective agent for the treatment of Parkinson's disease. Levodopa is converted from (MD4)L

(MD4)-dopa to dopamine in the basal ganglia. As stated above, dopamine concentrations normally found in the cells of the substantia nigra are depleted in patients with Parkinson's disease. Presumably symptom relief is obtained secondary to the higher levels of dopamine available with levodopa.

The beneficial effects of levodopa are most pronounced in the first few years of treatment. Benefits to the patient begin to wane and adverse side effects become more severe with the passage of time. Confusion, hallucinations, depression, and sleep alterations are associated with prolonged use. The patient may experience an on–off reaction in which sudden periods of near immobility ("off effect"), lasting minutes to hours, are followed by a sudden return of effectiveness ("on effect").

Dyskinesias (abnormal involuntary movements) are fairly common side effects, and include facial grimacing, rhythmic jerking movements of the hands, head bobbing, chewing and smacking movements, and involuntary movements of the trunk and extremities. This is probably due to the body's failure to readjust properly to the disappearance of dopamine. One method of dealing with on–off fluctuations is to give a "drug holiday" by taking the patient off the drug. This usually requires hospitalization and expert medical and nursing care.

Levodopa usually is given in combination with a decarboxylase inhibitor, carbidopa (Sinemet), which allows a greater concentration of levodopa to reach the brain and decrease the peripheral side effects.

Dopamine-Agonist—Ergot Derivatives. These agents (bromocriptine and pergolide) are thought to be dopamine receptor agonists; they are useful when added to levodopa and in patients experiencing on–off reactions to smooth out clinical fluctuations.

Pergolide (Permax) is the newest of this classification. It is ten times more potent than bromocriptine, although therapeutically this is of no particular advantage. Patient response to these medications is quite individual, and for reasons not well understood response to one agent may be better than to the other.

MAO Inhibitors. Eldepryl (called Deprenyl in Europe, marketed in the United States as Selegilene) is one of the most exciting developments in the pharmacotherapy of Parkinson's disease. This medication inhibits dopamine breakdown; thus increased amounts of dopamine are available. It has been found to smooth out the fluctuations in function that occur in this disease; unlike the other forms of therapy it may actually slow the progression of the disease.

Antidepressants. Tricyclic antidepressants may be given to alleviate the depression that is so common in Parkinson's disease.

Surgical Intervention

Although several different approaches have been the subject of recent research, surgical management of Parkinson's disease remains investigational and controversial. In some patients with disabling tremor or with severe levodopa-induced dyskinesia, surgery may be considered. Although surgery provides some relief in selected patients, it has not been demonstrated to alter the course of the disease or assure permanent improvement. Stereotactic surgical procedures that have been used include **subthalamotomy** and **pallidotomy.**

Other approaches include transplantation of neural tissue into the basal ganglia in an effort to reestablish normal dopamine release. **Neural transplantation** of the patient's adrenal medulla into the basal ganglia has been effective in relieving symptoms in a few patients. Transplantation of neural cells using fetal tissue has also been attempted; however, this procedure is controversial. Research into these and other surgical and nonsurgical approaches continues.

❑ *NURSING PROCESS*
The Patient With Parkinson's Disease

Assessment

The health history and assessment focus on how the disease has affected the patient's activities and functional abilities. Patients are observed for what they can do and what changes in function occur throughout the day. Responses after the administration of medications are also noted. Patients are asked what improvements they would like to see. The following questions may be helpful:

- ❑ Do you have leg or arm stiffness?
- ❑ Have you experienced any irregular jerking of your arms or legs?
- ❑ Have you ever been "frozen" or rooted to the spot and unable to move?
- ❑ Does your mouth water excessively?
- ❑ Have you (or others) noticed yourself grimacing or making faces or chewing movements?
- ❑ What specific activities do you have difficulty doing?

During this assessment, the patient is observed as moving about, walking, or drinking.

Diagnosis

Nursing Diagnoses

Nearly every patient with a movement disorder has some functional alteration and may have some type of behavioral dysfunction. Based on the assessment data, the patient's major nursing diagnoses may include the following:

- ❑ Impaired physical mobility related to muscle rigidity and weakness
- ❑ Self-care deficits (eating, drinking, dressing, hygiene) related to tremor and motor disturbance
- ❑ Constipation related to medication and reduced activity
- ❑ Altered nutrition, less than body requirements, related to tremor, slowness in eating, difficulty in chewing and swallowing
- ❑ Impaired verbal communication related to decreased speech volume, slowness of speech, inability to move facial muscles
- ❑ Ineffective coping related to depression and dysfunction due to disease progression

Other nursing diagnoses may include sleep pattern disturbances, knowledge deficit, alteration in thought processes, and ineffective family coping.

Planning and Implementation

Goals. The patient's goals may include improvement of mobility, attainment of independence in activities of daily living, achievement of adequate bowel elimination, attainment and maintenance of satisfactory nutritional status, achievement of communication, and development of positive coping mechanisms.

Nursing Interventions

Improving Mobility

Exercise. A progressive program of daily exercise will increase muscle strength, improve coordination and dexterity, reduce muscular rigidity, and prevent contractures that occur when muscles are not used. Walking, riding a stationary bicycle, swimming, and gardening are all exercises that help maintain joint mobility. Stretching exercises (stretch-hold-relax) help loosen the joint structures. Postural exercises are important to counter the tendency of the head and neck to be drawn forward and down. Special walking techniques must also be learned to offset the shuffling gait and the tendency to lean forward.

Walking Technique. The patient's balance may also be adversely affected because of the rigidity of the arms. (Arm swinging is necessary in normal walking.) The patient is taught early in the course of the disease to concentrate on walking erect, to watch the horizon, and to use a wide-based gait (*i.e.*, walking with the feet separated). A conscious effort must be made to swing the arms and raise the feet while walking and to use a heel-toe, heel-toe gait in fairly long strides. The patient is advised to practice walking to marching music or to the sound of a ticking metronome, because this provides sensory reinforcement. Breathing exercises while walking help to move the rib cage and transport oxygen to poorly aerated parts of the lungs. Frequent rest periods aid in preventing frustration and fatigue.

Warm baths and massage in addition to passive and active exercises help relax muscles and relieve painful muscle spasms that accompany rigidity.

Enhancing Self-Care Activities. Teaching and support of the patient during activities of daily living promote self-care. (See Chapter 18 for rehabilitation techniques.)

Environmental modifications are necessary to compensate for functional disabilities. These patients have difficulty turning in bed and getting in and out of bed. Bedside rails, an overbed frame with a trapeze if the patient has a hospital bed at home, or a rope tied to the foot of the bed provide assistance in pulling oneself up without help.

Improving Bowel Elimination. A patient with parkinsonism may have severe problems with constipation. Among the factors causing this condition are weakness of the muscles used in defecation, lack of exercise, inadequate fluid intake, and decreased autonomic nervous system activity. The medications used for the treatment of the disease also inhibit normal intestinal secretions. A regular bowel routine may be established by encouraging the patient to follow a regular time pattern, consciously increase fluid intake, and eat foods with a moderate fiber content. A raised toilet seat is a useful device to facilitate toilet activities because the patient has difficulty in moving from a standing to a sitting position.

Improving Nutrition. Patients with parkinsonism have difficulty in maintaining their weight. They become embarrassed by their slowness and untidiness in eating. Their mouths are dry from the medications and they experience difficulty chewing and swallowing. They are at risk for aspiration owing to decreased cough reflexes. They may not be aware that they are aspirating, and may develop bronchopneumonia. Saliva accumulates in some patients because they swallow slowly. Because of problems in eating, these patients may eventually show a considerable weight loss.

Enhancing Swallowing. Swallowing disorders are also due to tongue tremor, hesitancy in initiating swallowing, difficulty in shaping food into a bolus, and disturbances in pharyngeal motility. To offset these problems, the patient should sit in an upright position during mealtime. A semisolid diet with thick liquids is easier to swallow than solids and thin liquids. Thin liquids should be avoided. It is helpful for patients to think through the swallowing sequence. The patient is taught to place the food on the tongue, close lips and teeth, lift the tongue up and then back, and swallow. The patient is encouraged to chew first on one side of the mouth and then on the other. To control the build-up of saliva, the patient is reminded to hold the head upright and make a conscious effort to swallow. Massaging the facial and neck muscles before meals may be beneficial.

Assistive Devices. An electric warming tray keeps food hot and permits the patient to rest during the prolonged time that it takes to eat. Special utensils also assist at mealtime. A plate that is stabilized, a nonspill cup, and eating utensils with built-up handles are useful self-help devices. Supplementary feedings augment caloric intake. Monitoring weight on a weekly basis indicates whether caloric intake is adequate.

Improving Communication. Speech disorders are present in most patients with Parkinson's disease. Their low-pitched, monotonous, soft speech requires that they make a conscious effort to speak slowly, with deliberate attention to what they are saying. Patients are reminded to face the listener, exaggerate the pronunciation of words, speak in short sentences, and take a few deep breaths before speaking.

A speech-language therapist may be helpful in designing speech improvement exercises and assisting health care personnel to develop a method of communication to meet the patient's needs. Having the patient speak into a tape recorder periodically is useful in monitoring the patient's progress. A small electronic amplifier is helpful if the patient has difficulty being heard.

Supporting Coping Abilities. Faithful adherence to an exercise and walking program helps to delay the progress of the disease. Encouragement and reassurance can be given by praising the patient for perseverance and pointing out that activities are being maintained through active participation. A combination of physiotherapy, psychotherapy, medication therapy, and support group participation may help combat the depression that so often accompanies this condition.

Patients with Parkinson's disease often feel embarrassed, apathetic, inadequate, bored, and lonely. These feelings may be due, in part, to physical slowness and the great effort that even small tasks require. Patients are assisted and encouraged to set achievable goals (*e.g.*, improvement of mobility).

Because parkinsonism tends to lead to withdrawal and depression, patients must be **active** participants in their therapeutic program, including social and recreational events. There should be a planned program of activity throughout the day to prevent too much daytime sleeping as well as disinterest and apathy.

Every effort should be made to encourage patients to carry out the tasks involved in coping with their own daily needs and to retain independence. Doing things *for* the patient merely to save time runs contrary to this basic goal of improving coping abilities.

Patient Education and Home Care Considerations. The need for information about Parkinson's disease is ongoing as adaptations and concessions are made to the illness. Every effort is made to explain the nature of the disease and its management to offset anxieties and fears that may be as disabling as the disease itself. The American Parkinson's Disease Foundation publishes booklets and a newsletter for patient education.

The family is under considerable stress from living with and caring for a disabled person. Giving them information about treatment and care prevents many unnecessary problems. The caregiver is included in the plan and may be counseled to learn stress reduction techniques, to include others in the care-giving process, to obtain periodic relief from responsibilities, and to have a yearly health assessment. Giving family members "permission" to express feelings of frustration, anger, and guilt is often helpful to them.

Evaluation

Expected Outcomes

1. Strives toward improved mobility
   a. Participates in exercise program daily
   b. Walks with wide base of support; exaggerates arm swinging when walking
   c. Takes prescribed medications faithfully
2. Progresses toward self-care
   a. Allows time for self-care
   b. Uses self-help devices
3. Maintains bowel function
   a. Consumes adequate fluid intake
   b. Increases dietary intake of fiber
   c. Reports regular pattern of bowel function
4. Attains improved nutritional status
   a. Swallows without choking
   b. Takes time while eating
5. Achieves a method of communication
   a. Communicates needs
   b. Practices speech exercises
6. Copes with effects of Parkinson's disease
   a. Sets realistic goals
   b. Demonstrates persistence in meaningful activities
   c. Verbalizes feelings to appropriate person

Huntington's Disease

Huntington's disease (HD) is a chronic, progressive, hereditary disease of the nervous system that results in progressive involuntary choreiform (dancelike) movement and dementia. It affects men and women of all races. Because it is transmitted as an autosomal dominant genetic disorder, each child of a parent with Huntington's disease has a 50% risk of inheriting the illness.

Pathophysiology

The basic pathology involves premature death of cells in the basal ganglia, the region deep within the brain involved in the control of movement. There is also loss of cells in the cortex, the region of the brain associated with thinking, memory, perception, and judgment. Research suggests that the disease may be related to a lack of important brain chemicals, such as gamma-aminobutyric acid (GABA) and acetylcholine (ACh), that inhibit nerve action. Onset usually occurs between the ages of 35 and 45; the disease progresses slowly with death occurring in 10 to 15 years. About 10% of patients are children.

A genetic marker for HD has been identified through the use of recombinant deoxyribonucleic acid (DNA) technology. As a result, researchers now can identify presymptomatic individuals who will develop this disease. Although this presymptomatic test for HD can remove the uncertainty, it offers no hope of cure or even specific determination of its onset.

Clinical Manifestations

The most prominent clinical features of the disease are abnormal involuntary movements (*chorea*), intellectual decline, and, often, emotional disturbance.

Chorea. As the disease progresses, a constant writhing, twisting, uncontrollable movement may involve the entire body. These motions are devoid of purpose or rhythm, although patients may try to turn them into purposeful movement. All of the body musculature is involved. Facial movements produce tics and grimaces. Speech is affected, becoming slurred, hesitant, often explosive, and eventually unintelligible. Chewing and swallowing are difficult and there is a constant danger of choking and aspiration.

As with speech, the gait becomes disorganized to the point that ambulation eventually is impossible. Although independent ambulation should be encouraged for as long as possible, a wheelchair usually is necessary at some point. (Eventually, the patient is confined to bed, as the chorea interferes with walking, sitting, and all activities.) Control of bladder and bowel is lost.

Cognitive Changes. Cognitive function is usually affected, with dementia usually occurring. Initially, the patient generally is aware that the disease is responsible for the myriad dysfunctions that are occurring.

Emotional Changes. The mental and emotional changes that occur with HD may be more devastating to the patient and family than the abnormal movements. Patients may be nervous, irritable, or impatient. In the early stages of the illness patients are particularly subject to uncontrollable fits of anger; profound, often suicidal depression; apathy; or euphoria. Judgment and memory are impaired and dementia eventually ensues. Hallucinations, delusions, and paranoid thinking may precede the appearance of disjointed movements. Emotional symptoms often become less acute as the disease progresses.

Physical Course. Despite a ravenous appetite, often for sweets, patients usually become emaciated and exhausted. Eventually, patients succumb to heart failure, pneumonia, or infection, or die as a result of a fall or choking.

Management

Although no treatment halts or reverses the underlying process, several methods of management have fairly good palliative results. The phenothiazines, butyrophenones, and thioxanthenes, which predominantly block dopamine receptors, improve the chorea in many patients. Chorea also is lessened by reserpine (depletes presynaptic dopamine) and tetrabenazine (reduces dopaminergic transmission).

The patient's motor signs must be assessed and evaluated on an ongoing basis so that optimal therapeutic drug levels may be reached. **Akathesia** (motor restlessness) in the overmedicated patient is a danger because it may be mistaken for the restless fidgetiness of the illness and consequently be overlooked.

In certain types of the disease in which hypokinetic motor impairment resembles parkinsonism, some benefit may be obtained from antiparkinsonism therapy (see p. 1772).

Patients who have emotional disturbances, particularly depression, may be helped by antidepressant medications. The threat of suicide is always present. Psychotic symptoms usually respond to antipsychotic drugs. Psychotherapy aimed at allaying anxiety and reducing stress may be beneficial. It is imperative that nurses look beyond the disease to focus on the patient's needs and capabilities (Chart 60-3).

Patient Education and Home Care Considerations. A program combining medical, psychologic, social, occupational, speech, and physical rehabilitation services is needed to help the patient and family cope with this severely disabling illness. Huntington's disease exacts enormous emotional, physical, social, and financial tolls on every member of the patient's family. Entire families often live under a heavy burden of uncertainty, anxiety, and guilt.

Individuals of childbearing age may wish information about their risk for Huntington's disease when considering pregnancy and childbearing, or couples who would consider abortion may consider the test at the time of an amniocentesis. For most people the benefits of testing remain questionable and controversial.

Not only is genetic counseling crucial, but patients and their families also require access to long-term psychologic counseling, marriage counseling, and emotional, financial, and legal support. Regular follow-up helps to allay fear of abandonment.

Home care assistance, work and recreation day centers, respite care, and eventually skilled long-term care are necessary to help the patient and family cope with the constant strain of the illness. Although nothing can stop the relentless progression of the disease, families who have had supportive care have benefited tremendously.

Voluntary health organizations are major aids to families and have been largely responsible for bringing the illness to national attention. The Huntington's Disease Foundation of America (see Bibliography for address) is oriented toward helping patients and their families by providing information, referrals, family and public education, and support for research.

Alzheimer's Disease

Alzheimer's disease, or senile dementia of the Alzheimer's type, is a chronic, progressive, and degenerative brain disorder accompanied by profound effects on memory, cognition, and ability for self-care. Approximately 10% of the population over the age of 65 is affected, and the prevalence reaches 47% by age 85. It is one of the most feared disorders of modern times because it has catastrophic consequences for the patient and family, who experience what has been termed an "endless funeral." (See Chapter 12 for a detailed discussion of the manifestations, management, and nursing care of the patient with Alzheimer's disease.)

Neuromuscular Diseases

Myasthenia Gravis

Myasthenia gravis is a disorder affecting the neuromuscular transmission of the voluntary muscles of the body; it is characterized by excessive weakness and fatigability particularly of voluntary muscles and those innervated by cranial nerve function. Although onset can occur at any age, it is seen most often in women between the ages of 15 and 35 and in men over 40.

Pathophysiology

The basic abnormality in myasthenia gravis is a defect in the transmission of impulses from nerve to muscle cells due to loss of available or normal receptors on the postsynaptic membrane of the neuromuscular junction. Studies have shown a 70% to 90% reduction in the number of acetylcholine receptors at individual neuromuscular junctions. Myasthenia gravis is considered an autoimmune disease in which antibodies directed against acetylcholine receptors (AChR) impair neuromuscular transmission.

Clinical Manifestations

The disease is characterized by *extreme muscular weakness* and easy fatigability, which generally is worse after effort and is relieved by rest. Patients with this disease tire on such slight exertion as combing the hair, chewing, and talking, and must stop for rest. Symptoms vary according to the muscles affected. Symmetric muscles are involved, particularly those innervated by cranial nerves. Because of the involvement of the ocular muscles, **diplopia** (double vision) and **ptosis** (drooping of the eyelids) are

CHART 60-3
Care of the Patient with Huntington's Disease

Nursing Diagnosis

Potential for injury from falls and possible skin breakdown (pressure ulcers, abrasions) resulting from constant movement

Nursing Interventions

Pad the sides and head of the bed; ensure that the patient can see over the sides of bed.
Use lamb's wool padding for heel and elbow protection.
Keep the skin meticulously clean.
Apply emollient cleansing agent and skin lotion frequently.
Use *soft* sheets and bedding.
Have patient wear football padding or other forms of padding.
Encourage ambulation with assistance to maintain muscle tone.
Restrain the patient (only if absolutely necessary) in bed or chair with padded protective devices, making sure that they are loosened frequently.

Nursing Diagnosis

Inadequate nutritional intake and dehydration resulting from difficulty in swallowing or chewing and danger of choking or aspirating food

Nursing Interventions

Administer phenothiazines as prescribed before meals (appears to calm some patients)
Use a warming tray.
Talk to the patient before mealtime to promote relaxation; use mealtime for social interaction. Provide undivided attention. Help the patient enjoy the mealtime experience.
Learn the position that is best for *this* patient. Keep patient as close to upright as possible while feeding. Stabilize patient's head gently with one hand while feeding.
Show the food and tell the patient what the foods are (*e.g.,* whether hot or cold).
Encircle the patient with one arm and get as close as possible to provide stability and support. Use pillows and wedges for additional support.
Do not interpret stiffness, turning away, or sudden turning of the head as rejection; these are uncontrollable choreiform movements.
For feeding, use a long-handled spoon (iced-tea spoon). Place spoon on middle of tongue and exert slight pressure.
Place bite-sized food between teeth. Serve stews, casseroles, thick liquids, avoid too many milk drinks (produces mucus).
Disregard messiness. Treat the person with dignity.
Wait for the patient to chew and swallow before introducing another spoonful. Make sure that bite-sized food is small.
Give between-meal feedings. Constant movement uses more calories. Patients are often voracious, particularly for sweets.
Use *blenderized meals* if patient cannot chew; do not repeatedly give the same strained baby foods; gradually introduce increased textures and consistencies to the diet.
For swallowing difficulties:
- Apply gentle deep pressure around the patient's mouth.
- Rub fingers in circles on the patient's cheeks.
- Rub fingers simultaneously down each side of the patient's throat.

Develop skill in Heimlich maneuver (to be used in the event of choking).

Nursing Diagnosis

Pyschologic isolation and ineffective communication from excessive grimacing and unintelligible speech

Nursing Interventions

Read to the patient.
Employ biofeedback and relaxation therapy to reduce stress.
Use speech and language therapy to help maintain and prolong communication abilities.
Try to devise a communication system, perhaps using cards with words or pictures of familiar objects, before verbal communication becomes too difficult. Patients can indicate correct card by hitting it with hand, grunting, or blinking the eyes.
Learn how this particular patient expresses needs and wants—particularly nonverbal messages (widening of eyes, responses).
Patients can understand even if unable to speak. Do not isolate patients by ceasing to communicate with them.

Nursing Diagnosis

Intellectual impairment and emotional disturbance

Nursing Interventions

Have clock, calendar, and wall posters in view.
Interact with the patient in a *creative* manner.
Use every opportunity for one-to-one contact.
Use music for relaxation.
Reorient the patient after awakening.
Have the patient wear an identification bracelet with name, telephone number, and "memory impaired" on it.
Keep the patient in the social mainstream.
Recruit and train volunteers for social interaction. Role model appropriate interactions.
Do not abandon a patient because the disease is eventually terminal. Patients are *living* until the end.

early symptoms. The patient has a sleepy, masklike expression because the facial muscles are affected. Laryngeal involvement produces **dysphonia** (voice impairment) in the form of a nasal sound of the voice or difficulty in articulation. Weakness of the bulbar muscles causes problems with chewing and swallowing and presents a danger of choking and aspiration. Some 15% to 20% of patients complain of weakness of arm and hand muscles and, less commonly, of leg muscle weakness, which makes these patients subject to falls.

- Progressive weakness of the diaphragm and intercostal muscles may produce respiratory distress, which is an acute emergency.

Diagnostic Evaluation

The signs and symptoms of myasthenia gravis are sometimes so striking that a presumptive diagnosis can be made on the basis of the patient's history and physical examination. An injection of edrophonium (Tensilon), a medication that facilitates the transmission of impulses at the myoneural junction, is used to confirm the diagnosis. Within 30 seconds of an intravenous injection of edrophonium, most patients with myasthenia improve substantially but only temporarily. Improvement in muscle strength after administration of this agent represents a positive test and usually confirms the diagnosis.

Demonstration of anti-AChR antibodies in the serum is found in nearly 90% of patients with generalized myasthenia and in about 70% of those with symptoms restricted to the eye muscles (ocular form).

Electromyography (EMG) is used to measure the electrical potential of muscle cells but is not considered specifically diagnostic for myasthenia gravis.

Management

Management of myasthenia gravis is directed at improving function through the administration of anticholinesterase medications and reducing and removing circulating antibodies. Therapy includes anticholinesterase agents and immunosuppressive therapy, including plasmapheresis, and thymectomy.

Anticholinesterase agents act by increasing the relative concentration of available acetylcholine at the neuromuscular junction. They are given to increase the response of the muscles to nerve impulses and to improve strength. However, they provide only symptomatic relief.

Medications in current use include pyridostigmine bromide (Mestinon), ambenonium chloride (Mytelase), and neostigmine bromide (Prostigmin).

Most patients prefer pyridostigmine because it produces fewer side effects. The dosage is increased gradually until maximal benefits are obtained (additional strength, less fatigue), although normal muscle strength may not be achieved and the patient will likely have to adapt to some disability.

Anticholinesterase medications are given with milk, crackers, or other buffering substances. Their *side effects* include abdominal cramps, nausea, vomiting, and diarrhea. Small doses of atropine, given once or twice daily, may reduce or prevent these side effects. Other side effects of anticholinesterase therapy include adverse effects on skeletal muscles, such as fasciculations (fine twitching), spasm, and weakness. The effects on the central nervous system include irritability, anxiety, insomnia, headache, dysarthria, syncope (fainting), seizures, and coma. Increased salivation and lacrimation, increased bronchial secretions, and moist skin may also be noted.

- The nursing (and patient) priority is to give the prescribed medication according to an exact time schedule to control the patient's symptoms. *Any delay in administration of medications may result in the patient's inability to swallow making oral administration problematic.* An increase in muscle strength within 1 hour after the administration of the anticholinesterase drug is expected.

After the initial medication doses have been adjusted, the patient learns to take the medication according to individual needs and time plan. Further adjustments may be necessary in the presence of physical or emotional stress and intercurrent infection.

Immunosuppressive therapy is directed toward reducing the production of antireceptor antibody or removing it directly by plasma exchange (described below). Immunosuppressive therapy includes corticosteroids, plasmapheresis, and thymectomy. Corticosteroid therapy may benefit the patient with severe generalized myasthenia. Corticosteroids exert their effect by suppressing the patient's immune response, thus decreasing the amount of blocking antibody. The anticholinesterase dosage is lowered while the patient's ability to maintain effective respirations and to swallow is monitored. The steroid dosage is gradually increased and the anticholinesterase medication is slowly reduced.

Prednisone, taken on alternate days to lower the incidence of side effects, appears to be successful in suppressing the disease. Sometimes the patient shows a marked decrease in muscle strength right after therapy is started, but this is usually only temporary. If hospitalized, the patient can be given a call bell to use in emergency situations and should be closely monitored for signs of respiratory distress.

Cytotoxic drugs have also been used. Although the precise mechanism of action is not fully understood, drugs such as azathioprine (Imuran) and cyclophosphamide (Cytoxan) reduce the circulating antiacetylcholine receptor antibody titers. Side effects are significant, however, and only patients with severe disease are treated with these agents.

Plasma exchange (plasmapheresis) is a technique that permits selective removal of the patient's plasma and plasma components. The remaining cells are reinfused. Plasma exchange produces a temporary reduction in the titer of circulating antibodies. This process has caused remarkable improvement in some patients but does not treat the underlying abnormality (production of antireceptor antibody) over the long term.

Surgical Management

In myasthenia gravis patients the thymus seems to be involved in the process of AChR antibody production. **Thymectomy** (surgical removal of the thymus) causes substantial remission of the disease, especially in patients with tumor or hyperplasia of the thymus gland. Thymectomy is carried out through the sternum because the entire thymus must be removed.

It is thought that thymectomy *early* in the course of the disease is specific therapy, as it prevents formation of antireceptor antibodies. After surgery, the patient is monitored in an intensive care unit with special attention given to ventilatory function.

Myasthenic Crisis Versus Cholinergic Crisis

Myasthenic crisis is the sudden onset of muscular weakness in patients with myasthenia and usually is the result of undermedication or no cholinergic medication at all. In addition, myasthenic crisis may result from progression of the disease itself, emotional upset, systemic infections, certain medications, surgery, or trauma. It is manifest by the sudden onset of acute respiratory distress and an inability to swallow or speak. Weakness of respiratory, laryngeal, and bulbar musculature can cause respiratory depression and airway obstruction if not treated promptly.

Cholinergic crisis is caused by overmedication with cholinergic or anticholinesterase agents. In addition to the muscle weakness and respiratory depression of myasthenic crisis, these patients experience a variety of gastrointestinal symptoms, including nausea, vomiting, and diarrhea, as well as sweating, increased salivation, and bradycardia.

Medication Precautions. A number of medications aggravate myasthenia gravis, and the patient is advised to consult with the physician before taking any new medications, including antibiotics, cardiovascular drugs, anticonvulsant and psychotrophic drugs, morphine, quinine and related agents, beta-blockers, and nonprescription drugs. Novocain should be avoided, and the patient's dentist so advised.

❑ NURSING PROCESS
The Patient With Myasthenia Gravis

Assessment

The patient with myasthenia gravis usually is managed as an outpatient unless hospitalization is required for diagnostic testing or to manage symptoms or complications. The health history and assessment focus on the patient and family's knowledge about the disease and the treatment program that has been established. The more knowledgeable they are, the less likely the patient is to develop complications. It is important to determine what the patient's medication therapy schedule was while at home, as this same schedule is likely to be the one of choice at the time of discharge. In addition, an assessment of the patient's functional capability and support system assists in determining discharge needs for services.

Diagnosis

Nursing Diagnoses

Based on the assessment data, the patient's potential nursing diagnoses may include the following:

- Ineffective breathing pattern related to respiratory muscle weakness
- Impaired physical mobility due to voluntary muscle weakness
- Risk for aspiration related to weakness of bulbar muscles

Other nursing diagnoses of the patient with myasthenia gravis may include risk for injury related to voluntary muscle weakness; activity intolerance; ineffective airway clearance; anxiety; altered nutrition, less than body requirements; and body image disturbance.

Collaborative Problems/ Potential Complications

Based on the assessment data and knowledge of the disease process, potential complications that may develop include:

- Myasthenic crisis
- Cholinergic crisis

Planning and Implementation

Goals. The patient's major goals may include improved respiratory function, increased physical mobility, avoidance of aspiration, and absence of complications (myasthenic and cholinergic crises).

Nursing Interventions

Improving Respiratory Function. For a patient with diminishing ventilatory capacity, the nurse assesses respiratory rate, depth, and breath sounds, and monitors the results of pulmonary function tests (tidal volume, vital capacity, inspiratory force) at frequent intervals to detect pulmonary problems before changes in arterial blood gas levels occur and before symptoms become clinically apparent.

When there is severe weakness of abdominal, intercostal, and pharyngeal muscles, the patient is unable to cough and breathe deeply or clear secretions. Chest physical therapy, including postural drainage to mobilize secretions and suctioning to remove secretions, may have to be performed frequently.

The patient with insufficient gas exchange experiences anxiety sometimes bordering on panic. This is compounded by an inability to communicate verbally and by a tendency to choke. Acknowledging the patient's fears and addressing the problem promptly can give assurance that the nurse understands the concerns. The patient gains some sense of control through skilled care and the calm support of the nurse.

Increasing Physical Mobility. The patient's goal is improvement of strength and endurance. To be a participant in treatment, the patient must learn the basic facts about anticholinesterase agents—their action, timing, dosage adjustment, symptoms of overdose, and toxic effects. The importance of taking the medication on time is emphasized. The patient is encouraged to keep a diary to determine fluctuation of symptoms and to know when the medication is wearing off.

In addition, it may be helpful to include the following:

- Taking medication 30 minutes before meals for maximal muscle strength
- Planning adequate rest periods throughout the day
- Setting a realistic schedule daily and spacing activities
- Wearing appropriate shoes to minimize weakness and prevent injury

Certain factors may increase weakness and precipitate a myasthenic crisis: emotional upset, infections (particularly respiratory infections), vigorous physical activity, and exposure to heat (hot baths, sun bathing) and cold. These situations should be avoided. To avoid the risk of fatigue, it is best to rest *before* becoming too tired. A cervical collar can be useful for patients with weak neck muscles who are having difficulty supporting the head. Adaptive or self-help devices are available and are useful in helping the patient handle the disease more effectively and live as full a life as possible. The patient also is advised to wear an identification bracelet such as Medic Alert.

Improving Communication. The weakened speech muscles in patients in myasthenia crisis may interfere with communication. Techniques for improving communication include listening to patients; repeating what they have tried to communicate to clarify and verify information; and asking patients to blink their eyes or wiggle their fingers or toes for yes and no answers. After the period of myasthenic crisis has resolved, patients usually are able to make their needs known.

Providing Eye Care. Impaired vision results from ptosis of one or both eyelids, decreased eye movement, or double vision. Nursing interventions to help the patient cope include taping the eyes open for short intervals, instilling artificial tears to prevent corneal damage when eyelids do not close completely, placing a patch over one eye when double vision is a problem, and keeping the patient informed while giving care.

Applying a thin adhesive tape over the upper eyelid helps relieve ptosis. Sunglasses diminish the effects of bright light that frequently increase eye problems.

Preventing Aspiration. Decreased ability to chew and swallow may result in choking and aspiration. The patient is assessed for drooling, regurgitation through the nose, and choking while attempting to swallow. Suction should be immediately available. Rest before meals is encouraged to reduce muscle fatigue. The patient is placed in an upright position with neck slightly flexed to facilitate swallowing. Soft foods in gravy or sauces appear to be swallowed more easily than liquids. If the patient is taking an anticholinesterase agent, the nurse makes sure it is given 1 hour before mealtime to ensure maximal muscle strength. Because muscles of mastication may be stronger in the morning, calorie intake can be increased at breakfast. The patient is encouraged to rest after eating.

Mealtimes should coincide with the peak effects of anticholinesterase if the patient has difficulty swallowing. If choking occurs frequently, blenderized food may be easier to swallow. Again, suction should be available at home as well as during hospitalization and the patient and family instructed in its use. Gastrostomy feedings may be necessary in some patients to ensure adequate nutritional status.

Monitoring and Managing Potential Complications

Myasthenic and Cholinergic Crises. Respiratory distress combined with varying signs of dysphagia (difficulty swallowing), dysarthria (difficulty speaking), eyelid ptosis, diplopia, and prominent muscle weakness are symptoms of myasthenic or cholinergic crisis.

- Providing adequate ventilatory assistance takes precedence in the immediate management of the patient with myasthenic crisis.
- The patient is suctioned, because aspiration is a common problem. Arterial blood is drawn for arterial blood gas analysis. Endotracheal intubation and mechanical ventilation may be needed (see Chapter 25). The patient is placed in an intensive care unit for constant monitoring, as this condition is marked by intense and sudden fluctuations.

Intravenous edrophonium (Tensilon) is used to differentiate the type of crisis. It improves the condition of the patient in myasthenic crisis, temporarily worsens that of the patient in cholinergic crisis, and is unpredictable in brittle crisis. If the patient is in true myasthenic crisis, neostigmine methylsulfate (Prostigmin) is administered intramuscularly or intravenously.

If the edrophonium (Tensilon) test is inconclusive or there is increasing respiratory weakness, all anticholinesterase drugs are withdrawn and atropine sulfate is given to reduce excessive secretions.

Other supportive measures include the following:

- Arterial blood gases, serum electrolytes, input and output, and daily weight are monitored.
- If the patient is unable to swallow, nasogastric tube feedings may be prescribed (200 ml at a time). (Postural drainage should not be performed for half an hour after feeding.)
- Sedatives and tranquilizers are avoided because these agents aggravate hypoxia and hypercapnia and can cause respiratory and cardiac depression.

Evaluation

Expected Outcomes

1. Achieves adequate respiratory function
   a. Exhibits normal respiratory rate and depth and normal muscle strength
   b. Adheres to established medication schedule
   c. States that manual resuscitation bag and portable suction are available for home use
   d. Avoids situations that may predispose to colds and infections, which might exacerbate symptoms
2. Adapts to impaired mobility
   a. Establishes a balanced program of rest and exercise
   b. Identifies measures to conserve energy; paces self
   c. Uses assistive devices
   d. Establishes and adheres to a medication schedule that maximizes muscle strength
3. Experiences no aspiration
   a. Exhibits normal breath sounds
   b. Eats slowly and selects appropriate (soft) diet
   c. Establishes a medication schedule that coincides with mealtime
4. Recovers from myasthenic and cholinergic crises
   a. Lists signs and symptoms of crisis
   b. Adheres to medication regimen
   c. Wears Medic Alert bracelet

The Myasthenia Gravis Foundation has materials written for both lay and professional readers, available on request (see Bibliography for address).

Amyotrophic Lateral Sclerosis

Amyotrophic lateral sclerosis (ALS) is a disease of unknown cause in which there is a loss of motor neurons (nerve cells controlling muscles) in the anterior horns of the spinal cord and the motor nuclei of the lower brain stem. As these cells die, the muscle fibers that they supply undergo atrophic changes. The degeneration of the neurons may occur in both the upper and lower motor neuron systems.

ALS affects more men than women, with onset occurring usually in the fifth or sixth decade. It is often referred to as *Lou Gehrig's disease* after the famous ballplayer who suffered from it.

Clinical Manifestations. The clinical manifestations of ALS depend on the location of the affected motor neurons, because specific neurons activate specific muscle fibers. The chief symptoms are progressive muscle weakness, atrophy, and fasciculations (twitching). Loss of motor neurons in the anterior horns of the spinal cord results in progressive weakness and atrophy of the muscles of the arms, trunk, or legs. Spasticity usually is present, and the stretch reflexes become brisk and overactive. Usually the anal and bladder sphincters are intact because the spinal nerves that control muscles of the rectum and urinary bladder are not affected.

In about 25% of patients, weakness starts in the musculature supplied by the cranial nerves and there is difficulty talking, swallowing, and ultimately breathing. When the patient ingests liquids, soft palate and upper esophageal weakness causes the liquid to be regurgitated through the nose. Weakness of the posterior tongue and palate impairs the ability to laugh, cough, or even blow the nose. When bulbar muscles are impaired, there is progressive difficulty in speaking and swallowing, and aspiration becomes a problem. The voice assumes a nasal sound and speech articulation becomes so disrupted that the patient's speech is unintelligible. Some emotional lability may be present, but intellectual function is not impaired. Eventually respiratory function is compromised.

The prognosis generally is based on the area involved and the speed with which the disease progresses. Death usually occurs as a result of infection, respiratory failure, or aspiration. The average time from onset of the disease to death is approximately 3 years. A small number of patients may survive for longer periods.

Diagnostic Evaluation. ALS is diagnosed on the basis of the signs and symptoms, because no clinical or laboratory tests are specific for this disease. Electromyographic studies of the affected muscles indicate reduction in the number of functioning motor units.

Management. No specific treatment for ALS is available. Symptomatic treatment and rehabilitative measures are employed to support the patient and improve the quality of life. Baclofen or diazepam may be useful for patients troubled by spasticity, because spasticity causes pain and interferes with self-care. Quinine therapy may be prescribed for painful muscle cramps. The effect of high doses of thyrotropin-releasing hormone, a naturally occurring hormone produced by the brain and found in the motor neurons of the spinal cord, on function is under investigation. Interferon, a compound that appears to stimulate the body's defense system, is another investigational drug.

A patient experiencing problems with aspiration and swallowing may require nasogastric feedings. A cervical **esophagostomy** (opening into the esophagus) or a gastrostomy may be performed to bypass the larynx, to prevent aspiration, and to provide for long-term nutritional support.

Mechanical ventilation (using negative-pressure ventilators) is an option when alveolar hypoventilation develops. The decision for the use of life support measures is made by the patient and family and should be based on a thorough understanding of the disease, the prognosis, and the implications of initiating such therapy. Patients are encouraged to complete an advance directive or "living will" to preserve their autonomy in decision making.

The ALS Association has broad programs of research funding, patient and clinical services, patient information and support, and medical and public information (see Bibliography for address). The ALS Association Quarterly Newsletter is filled with practical information.

The Muscular Dystrophies

The muscular dystrophies are a group of chronic muscle disorders characterized by progressive weakening and wasting of the skeletal or voluntary muscles. Most of these diseases are inherited. The pathologic features include degeneration and loss of muscle fibers, variation in muscle fiber size, phagocytosis and regeneration, and replacement of muscle tissue by connective tissue. The common characteristics of these diseases include varying degrees of muscle wasting and weakness; abnormal elevation in serum creatine phosphokinase, indicating a leakage of muscle enzymes; and myopathic findings on EMG and muscle biopsy. The differences center around the pattern of inheritance, the muscles involves, the age of onset, and the rate of progression.

Management

Treatment for the muscular dystrophies at this time focuses on supportive care and prevention of complications.

Supportive management is intended to keep the patient as active and functioning as normally as possible and to minimize functional deterioration. A therapeutic exercise program is prescribed for the individual patient to prevent muscle tightness, contractures, and disuse atrophy. Night splints and stretching exercises are used to delay contracturs of the joints, especially the ankles, knees, and hips. Braces may compensate for muscle weakness.

Spinal deformity is a severe problem. Weakness of trunk muscles and spinal collapse occur almost routinely in patients with severe neuromuscular disease. In the battle against spinal deformity, the patient is fitted with an orthotic jacket to improve sitting stability and reduce trunk deformity. This measure also supports cardiovascular status. In time, spinal fusion is performed to maintain spinal stability. Other procedures may be carried out to correct deformities.

Compromised pulmonary function may be due either to progression of the disease or to deformity of the thorax secondary to severe scoliosis. Intercurrent illnesses, upper respiratory infections, and fractures from falls must be vigorously treated in a way that minimizes immobilization, because joint contractures will become worse if the patient's activities are restricted more than usual.

Other difficulties aside from muscle weakness and contractures, may be manifested in relation to the underlying disease. Dental and speech problems may result from weakness of the facial muscles, which makes it difficult to attend to dental hygiene and to speak coherently. Gastrointestinal tract problems may include gastric dilatation, rectal prolapse, and fecal impaction. Finally, cardiomyopathy appears to be a common complication in all forms of muscular dystrophy.

Genetic counseling is advised for parents and siblings of the patient because of the genetic nature of this disease. The Muscular Dystrophy Association works to combat neuromuscular disease through research, programs of patient services and clinical care, and professional and public education (see Bibliography for address).

Nursing Interventions

The goals of the patient and the nurse are to maintain function at optimal levels and to enhance the quality of life. This is accomplished in part by attending to the patient's physical requirements, which are considerable, without losing sight of emotional and developmental needs. The patient and family are actively involved in decision making.

During hospitalization for treatment of complications, the knowledge and expertise of the patient and family members responsible for caregiving in the home are assessed. Because the patient and family caregivers often have developed caregiving strategies that work effectively for them, these strategies need to be acknowledged and accepted and provisions must be made to assure that they are maintained during hospitalization.

Patient Education and Home Care Considerations. Many of the management goals are addressed in the patient's home and community. Both the neuromuscular disease and the associated deformities may progress in adolescence and adulthood. Self-help and assistive devices can aid in achieving a greater degree of independence. Additional self-help devices become necessary as more muscle groups become affected. The patient is encouraged to continue with range-of-motion exercises to prevent contractures, which are particularly disabling.

Respiratory Support. The family is taught to monitor the patient for respiratory problems. As respiratory difficulties develop, patients and their families need information regarding appropriate respiratory support. Options currently exist that can provide ventilatory support (negative pressure devices, positive-pressure ventilators) while allowing mobility. Patients can remain relatively independent in a wheelchair, for example, while being maintained on a ventilator at home for many years.

Activity Support. Practical adaptations must be made to cope with the effects of chronic neuromuscular disability. To maximize functional independence, the patient at various stages of the disease may require a manual or an electric wheelchair, gait aids, upper and lower extremity and spinal orthoses, seating systems, bathroom equipment, lifts, ramps, and additional ADL assistive devices, all of which require a team approach. The home health nurse assesses how the patient and family are managing, makes referrals, and coordinates the activities of the physical therapist, occupational therapist, and social services.

Emotional Support. Of great concern to the patient are the issues surrounding the threat of increasing disability. The patient is faced with a drawn-out, progressive loss of function, leading eventually to death. Helplessness and powerlessness are common in the course of prolonged illness. Each functional loss involves a period of grieving and mourning. The patient is assessed for signs of depression, anger, bargaining, or denial.

A psychiatric nurse clinician or other mental health professional is invaluable in helping the patient cope and adapt to chronic disease. By understanding and addressing the physical and psychological needs of the patient and family, the nurse can communicate strength to the patient and help provide a hopeful, supportive, and nurturing environment.

Convulsive Disorders

Seizures

Seizures (convulsions) are episodes of abnormal motor, sensory, autonomic, or psychic activity (or a combination of these) as a consequence of sudden excessive discharge from cerebral neurons. A part or all of the brain may be involved. The seizures usually are sudden and transient.

The causes are varied and are classified as idiopathic (genetic, developmental defects) and acquired. Among the causes of acquired seizures are hypoxemia of any cause, including vascular insufficiency, fever (childhood), head injury, hypertension, central nervous system infections, metabolic and toxic conditions (*e.g.*, renal failure, hyponatremia, hypocalcemia, hypoglycemia, pesticides), brain tumor, drug withdrawal, and allergies. Stroke and cerebral metastasis are the leading causes of seizures in the elderly.

Often there is memory loss for the seizure and for a short time thereafter. Brain damage may occur when seizures are severe or prolonged. The patient is at risk for hypoxia, vomiting, and pulmonary aspiration or persistent metabolic abnormalities.

The immediate therapeutic goal is to control the seizure, and the long-term goal is to determine and control the cause.

Nursing Assessment During a Seizure

A major responsibility of the nurse is to observe and to record the sequence of symptoms. The nature of the seizure usually indicates the type of treatment that is indicated. Before and during a seizure the following should be assessed and documented:

1. The circumstances before the seizure (visual, auditory or olfactory stimuli, tactile stimuli, emotional or psychological disturbances, sleep, hyperventilation).
2. The first thing the patient does in a seizure—where the movements or the stiffness starts, conjugate gaze position, and the head at the beginning of the seizure. This information gives clues to the location of the epileptogenic focus in the brain. (In recording, it is important to state whether or not the beginning of the seizure was observed.)
3. The type of movements in the part of the body involved.
4. The areas of the body involved. (Turn back bedding and expose patient.)

5. The size of both pupils. Are the eyes open? Did the eyes or head turn to one side?
6. Whether or not automatisms (involuntary motor activity such as lip smacking or repeated swallowing) were observed.
7. Incontinence of urine or feces.
8. Duration of each phase of the seizure.
9. Unconsciousness, if present, and its duration.
10. Any obvious paralysis or weakness of arms or legs after the seizure.
11. Inability to speak after the seizure.
12. Movements at the end of the seizure.
13. Whether or not the patient sleeps afterward.
14. Whether or not the patient was confused after the seizure.

Nursing Management During a Seizure

During a seizure, the nursing goal is to prevent injury to the patient. This includes not only physical support but psychological support as well. Steps to prevent or minimize injury to the patient are presented in Guideline 60-1.

The Epilepsies

The epilepsies are a symptom—complex of several disorders of brain function characterized by recurring seizures. There may be associated loss of consciousness, excess movement or loss of muscle tone or movement, and disturbances of behavior, mood, sensation, and perception. Thus, epilepsy is not a disease but a symptom.

The basic problem is thought to be an electrical disturbance (dysrhythmia) in the nerve cells in one section of the brain, causing them to emit abnormal, recurring, uncontrolled electrical discharges. The characteristic epileptic seizure is a manifestation of this excessive neuronal discharge.

Incidence. An estimated 1% of the population (more than 2 million people) in the United States have epilepsy, with some 100,000 new patients diagnosed each year. There has been an increasing incidence of this condition, probably due to a number of factors. Improved obstetric and neonatal care saves babies who experience respiratory, circulatory, and other distress during delivery; these infants may be predisposed to intermittent seizures. The improved medical, surgical, and nursing management of patients with head injuries, brain tumors, meningitis, and encephalitis saves those whose conditions may produce cerebral changes with resultant seizures. Also, advances in electroencephalography (EEG) have aided in identifying patients with epilepsy. Education has served to enlighten the general public and has lessened the stigma associated with the condition, so that more persons are willing to acknowledge that they have epilepsy.

Altered Physiology

Messages from the body are carried by the neurons (nerve cells) of the brain by means of discharges of electrochemical energy that sweep along them. These impulses occur in bursts whenever a nerve cell has a task to perform. Sometimes these cells or groups of cells continue firing after a task is finished. During the period of unwanted discharges, parts of the body controlled by the errant cells may perform erratically. Resultant discomfort and dysfunction range from mild to incapacitating, and usually cause unconsciousness. When these uncontrolled, abnormal discharges occur repeatedly, a person is said to have epilepsy. The erratic physical movements are called *seizures*.

GUIDELINE 60-1
Care of the Patient Having a Seizure

During Seizure

- Provide privacy and protect the patient from curious onlookers. (The patient who has an *aura* [warning of an impending seizure] may have time to seek a safe, private place.)
- Ease the patient to the floor, if possible.
- Protect the head with a pad to prevent injury (from stiking a hard surface).
- Loosen constrictive clothing.
- Push aside any furniture that may injure the patient during the seizure.
- If the patient is in bed, remove pillows and raise siderails.
- If an aura precedes the seizure, insert a padded tongue blade between the teeth to reduce the possibility of the tongue or cheek being bitten.
- *Do not attempt to pry open jaws that are clenched in a spasm to insert* anything. Broken teeth and injury to the lips and tongue may result from such an action.
- No attempt should be made to restrain the patient during the seizure, because muscular contractions are strong and restraint can produce injury.
- If possible, place the patient on one side with head flexed forward, which allows the tongue to fall forward and facilitates drainage of saliva and mucus. If suction is available, use it if necessary to clear secretions.

After the Seizure

- Keep the patient on one side to prevent aspiration. Make sure the airway is patent.
- There is usually a period of confusion after a grand mal seizure.
- A short apneic period may occur during or immediately after a generalized seizure.
- The patient, on awakening, should be reoriented to the environment.
- If the patient experiences severe excitement after a seizure (postictal), try to handle the situation with calm persuasion and gentle restraint.

Causes. The cause of seizures in many people is unknown. Scientists have produced seizures in experimental animals through surgical injury or chemical or electrical stimulation. Epilepsies often follow birth trauma, asphyxia neonatorum, head injuries, some infectious diseases (bacterial, viral, parasitic), toxicity (carbon monoxide and lead poisoning), circulatory problems, fever, metabolic and nutritional disorders, and drug or alcohol intoxication. They are also associated with brain tumors, abscesses, and congenital malformations. In most cases of epilepsy, the cause is unknown (idiopathic). There is evidence that susceptibility to some types may be inherited. Epilepsy strikes before the age of 20 in greter than 75% of patients.

The epilepsies have little to do with intelligence in most cases. Persons with epilepsy who do not have other brain or nervous system disabilities fall within the same intelligence ranges as does the overall population. Epilepsy is not synonymous with mental retardation or illness. However, many who are retarded because they have serious neurologic damage often have epilepsy too, thus pulling the mean IQ for all epilepsy victims below that of the so-called normal range.

Prevention

A society-wide effort incorporating a wide range of measures must be mounted for the prevention of epilepsy. Because the infants of mothers who take certain anticonvulsant medications for epilepsy are at risk, these women need careful monitoring, including blood studies to detect the level of anticonvulsant medications taken throughout pregnancy. High-risk mothers (teenagers, women with histories of difficult deliveries, drug use, diabetes, or hypertension) should be identified and monitored closely during pregnancy because a brain lesion or injury that ultimately causes epilepsy may occur to the fetus during pregnancy and delivery.

Childhood infections (measles, mumps, bacterial meningitis) should be controlled with appropriate vaccination. Lead poisoning is another preventable cause of epilepsy. Parents with a child who has had a febrile seizure should be instructed about methods to control fever (cool sponging, antipyretic medications).

Head injury is one of the main causes that can be prevented. Through highway safety programs and occupational safety precautions, not only can lives be saved, but the possible development of epilepsy from head injury can be prevented.

Screening programs to identify children with seizure disorders at an early age, and seizure prevention programs with the judicious use of anticonvulsant medications and modification of lifestyle are part of this prevention plan.

Clinical Manifestations

Depending on the location of the discharging neurons, seizures may range from a simple staring spell to prolonged convulsive movements with loss of consciousness. The variations in seizures have been classified internationally according to the area of the brain involved, and have been identified as partial, generalized, and unclassified. **Partial** seizures are focal in origin and affect only part of the brain. **Generalized** seizures are nonspecific in origin and affect the entire brain simultaneously. **Unclassified** seizures are so termed because of incomplete data. (See Chart 60-4 for the international classification of seizures.)

The initial pattern of the seizures indicates the region of the brain in which the seizure originates. Also it is important to determine if the patient has had an **aura,** a premonitory or warning sensation before an epileptic seizure, which may indicate the origin of the seizure (*e.g.*, seeing a flashing light may indicate the seizure originated in the occipital lobe).

In **simple partial seizures,** only a finger or hand may shake, or the mouth may jerk uncontrollably. The person may talk unintelligibly, may be dizzy, and may experience unusual or unpleasant sights, sounds, odors, or tastes, but without loss of consciousness.

In **complex partial seizures,** the person either remains motionless or moves automatically but inappropriately for time and place, or may experience excessive emotions of fear, anger, elation, or irritability. Whatever the manifestations, the person does not remember the episode when it is over.

Generalized seizures, more commonly referred to as *grand mal seizures,* involve both hemispheres of the brain, causing both sides of the body to react. There may be intense rigidity of the entire body followed by jerky alternations of muscle relaxation and contraction (generalized tonic–clonic contraction). The simultaneous contractions

CHART 60-4
International Classification of Seizures

Partial Seizures (seizures beginning locally)

1. Simple partial seizures (with elementary symptoms, generally without impairment of consciousness)
   a. With motor symptoms
   b. With special sensory or somatosensory symptoms
   c. With autonomic symptoms
   d. Compound forms
2. Complex partial seizures (with complex symptoms, generally with impairment of consciousness)
   a. With impairment of consciousness only
   b. With cognitive symptoms
   c. With affective symptoms
   d. With psychosensory symptoms
   e. With psychomotor symptoms (automatisms)
   f. Compound forms
3. Partial seizures secondarily generalized

Generalized Seizures (bilaterally symmetric, without local onset)

1. Tonic-clonic seizures
2. Tonic seizures
3. Clonic seizures
4. Absence seizures
5. Atonic seizures
6. Myoclonic seizures (bilaterally massive epileptic)
7. Infantile spasms

of the diaphragm and chest muscles may produce a characteristic epileptic cry. Often the tongue is chewed and the patient is incontinent of urine and stool. After 1 or 2 minutes, the convulsive movements begin to subside; the patient relaxes and lies in deep coma, breathing noisily. The respirations at this point are chiefly abdominal. In the postictal state (after the seizure), the patient often is confused and hard to arouse, and may sleep for hours. Many patients complain of headache or sore muscles.

Diagnostic Evaluation

The diagnostic assessment is aimed at determining the *type* of seizures, their frequency and severity, and the factors that precipitate them. A developmental history is taken, including events of pregnancy and childbirth, to seek evidence of pre-existing injury. A search is made for illnesses or head injuries that may have affected the brain. In addition to a physical and neurologic examination, diagnostic examinations include biochemical, hematologic, and serologic studies. CT imaging is used to detect lesions in the brain, focal abnormalities, cerebrovascular abnormalities, and cerebral degenerative changes.

The electroencephalogram (EEG) furnishes diagnostic evidence in a substantial proportion of patients with epilepsy and aids in classifying the type of seizure. Abnormalities in the EEG usually continue to be apparent between seizures, or, if concealed, may be brought out by hyperventilation or during sleep. In addition, microelectrodes can be inserted deep in the brain to probe the action of single brain cells. It should be noted, however, that some persons with seizures may have normal EEGs, whereas persons who have never had seizures may have abnormal EEGs. Telemetry and computerized equipment are used to take and store EEG readings on computer tapes while patients pursue their normal activities. Videorecording of seizures taken simultaneously with EEG telemetry is useful in determining the type of seizure as well as its duration and magnitude. This type of intensive monitoring is revolutionizing the treatment of severe epilepsy in this country.

Management

The management of epilepsy is individualized to meet the special needs of each patient and not just to manage and prevent seizures. Management differs from patient to patient because some forms of epilepsy arise from brain damage and others depend on alterations of brain chemistry.

Pharmacotherapy. Many anticonvulsant medications are available to control seizures, although the mechanisms of their actions are still unknown. The objective is to achieve seizure control with minimal side effects. Medication therapy controls rather than cures seizures. The medication is selected on the basis of the type of seizure being treated and the effectiveness and safety of the medication. If properly prescribed and taken, these medications control seizures in 50% to 60% of patients with recurring seizures, and provide partial control in another 15% to 35%. The condition of some 15% to 35% of patients is not improved by any available medication.

Usually treatment is started with a single medication. The starting dose and the rate at which the dosage is increased depend on whether or not side effects develop. The drug levels are monitored in the blood, because the rate of drug absorption varies among people. Changing to another medication may be necessary if seizure control is not achieved or when toxicity makes it impossible to increase the dosage. The drug may need to be adjusted because of concurrent illness, weight changes, or increases in stress. Sudden withdrawal of anticonvulsant medication can cause seizures to occur with greater frequency or can precipitate the development of status epilepticus (see p. 1788).

Side effects of these medications may be divided into three groups: (1) idiosyncratic or allergic disorders, which present primarily as skin reactions; (2) acute toxicity, which may occur when the medication is initially prescribed; or (3) chronic toxicity, which occurs late in the course of drug therapy.

The manifestations of drug toxicity are variable, and any organ system may be involved. Periodic physical examinations and laboratory tests are performed for patients receiving medications known to have hematopoietic, genitourinary, or hepatic effects.

Thorough oral hygiene after each meal, regular dental care, and regular gum massage are important for the patient taking phenytoin (Dilantin) to prevent or control gingival hyperplasia. Table 60-1 summarizes the anticonvulsant medications in current use. Chart 60-5 includes teaching guidelines for the patient taking anticonvulsant medications.

Surgery for Epilepsy. Surgery is indicated for patients whose epilepsy results from intracranial tumors, abscess, cysts, or vascular anomalies.

Some patients have intractable seizure disorders that do not respond to medication. There may be a focal atrophic process secondary to trauma, inflammation, stroke, or anoxia. If the seizures originate in a reasonably well-circumscribed area of the brain that can be excised without producing significant neurologic deficits, the removal of the epileptogenic focus generating the seizures seems to give long-term control and improvement.

This type of neurosurgery has been aided by several modern advances, including microsurgical techniques, depth electroencephalography, improved illumination and hemostasis, and the introduction of neuroleptanalgesic agents (droperidol and fentanyl). These techniques, combined with local infiltration of scalp incisions, enable the neurosurgeon to perform surgery on an alert and cooperative patient. With special testing devices, electrocortical mapping, and the patient's response to stimulation, the boundaries of the epileptogenic focus are determined. Any abnormal epileptogenic focus (*i.e.*, abnormal area of the brain) is then removed.

❑ NURSING PROCESS
The Patient With Epilepsy

Assessment

The nurse elicits information about the patient's seizure history. The patient is asked about the factors or events that may precipitate the seizures. Alcohol intake is documented. The effects of epilepsy on lifestyle are assessed: What are the

TABLE 60-1 Major Anticonvulsant/Antiepileptic Drugs

Generic Name	Dose-Related Side Effects	Toxic Effects
Carbamazepine	Dizziness; drowsiness Unsteadiness; nausea and vomiting Diplopia; mild leukopenia	Severe skin rash Blood dyscrasias Hepatitis
Primidone	Lethargy; irritability Diplopia; ataxia Sexual impotence	Skin rash
Phenytoin	Visual problems Hirsutism Gingival hyperplasia Dysrhythmias	Severe skin reaction Peripheral neuropathy Ataxia; drowsiness Blood dyscrasias
Phenobarbital	Sedation; irritability Diplopia Ataxia	Skin rash
Ethosuximide	Nausea and vomiting Headache Gastric distress	Skin rash Blood dyscrasias Hepatitis Lupus erythematosus
Valproate	Nausea and vomiting Weight gain Loss of hair	Hepatotoxicity Skin rash Blood dyscrasias Nephritis

limitations imposed by the seizure disorder? Does the patient have a recreational program? Social contacts? Is work a positive experience? What coping mechanisms are used?

Observation and assessment during and after a seizure assist in identifying the type of seizure and its management.

CHART 60-5
Patient Education: Taking Anticonvulsive Medications

1. Take medication daily to keep the blood level constant to prevent seizures.
2. Report to the laboratory for blood sampling before taking morning medication when testing is prescribed.
3. Do not stop taking the medication abruptly; sudden withdrawal of medication may cause seizures.
4. Avoid alcohol; check with physician before taking additional prescription or over-the-counter medications.
5. Avoid activities that require alertness and coordination (*e.g.*, driving, operating machinery) until after the effects of the medication have been evaluated.
6. Maintain oral hygiene and have regular dental care.
7. Carry a personal identification card stating the name of the medication you are taking.

Diagnosis

Nursing Diagnoses

Based on the assessment data, the patient's major nursing diagnoses may include the following:

- Fear related to the ever-present possibility of having seizures
- Ineffective coping related to stresses imposed by epilepsy
- Knowledge deficit about epilepsy and its control

Collaborative Problems/ Potential Complications

The major potential complication of patients with epilepsy is:

- Status epilepticus

Planning and Implementation

Goals. The major goals for the patient may include control of seizures, achievement of a satisfactory psychosocial adjustment, acquisition of knowledge and understanding about the condition, and absence of complications of epilepsy.

Nursing Interventions

Reducing Fear of Seizures. Fear that a seizure may occur unexpectedly can be reduced by the patient's compliance with the prescribed treatment. The complete cooperation of the patient and family is of the utmost importance. They must have confidence in the value of the regimen that is prescribed. It must be emphasized that the prescribed anticonvulsant medication must be taken on a continuing basis and that it is not a habit-forming drug. It may be taken without fear of drug dependence for many years if necessary, if the patient is under health care supervision and follows instructions faithfully.

The control of seizures depends in part on the patient's understanding and cooperation. Lifestyle and environment are assessed to identify factors that may precipitate seizures: emotional disturbances, new environmental stressors, onset of menstruation in female patients, or fever. The patient is encouraged to follow a regular and moderate routine in lifestyle, diet (avoiding excessive stimulants), exercise, and rest. (Sleep deprivation may lower the patient's threshold to seizures.) Moderate activity is good therapy, but excessive expenditure of energy is to be avoided.

Some patients need to avoid photic stimulation (bright flickering lights, television viewing). Wearing dark glasses or covering one eye may help control this problem.

Tension states (anxiety, frustration) induce seizures in some patients. Classes in stress management may be of value. Because seizures are known to occur with alcohol intake, alcoholic beverages are restricted. The best therapy is to follow the treatment plan to avoid stimuli that precipitate seizures.

Improving Coping Mechanisms. It has been noted that the social, psychologic, and behavioral problems frequently accompanying epilepsy can be more of a handicap than the actual seizures. Epilepsy may be accompanied by feelings of fear, alienation, depression, and uncertainty. The patient must cope with the constant fear of a seizure and its embarrassing consequences. Children with epilepsy may be ostracized and excluded from school and peer activities. These problems are compounded during adolescence and add to the challenges of dating, not being able to drive, and feeling different. Adults face all of these problems plus the burden of finding employment; making decisions concerning marriage and childbearing; noninsurability; stigma; and legal barriers. Alcohol abuse may complicate matters. The burden on the family is great, and family problems may run the gamut of outright rejection to overprotection. As a result of all these factors, many persons with epilepsy have psychological and behavioral problems.

Counseling assists the individual and family to understand the condition and the limitations imposed by it. Social and recreational opportunities are necessary for good mental health. Some persons are not able to cope with epilepsy; others have psychologic problems resulting from brain damage. Those with seizures originating in the temporal lobes of the brain (areas controlling thought and emotions) have particular emotional problems. Symptoms of schizophrenia and impulsive or irritable behavior may be due to brain damage associated with temporal lobe seizures. These patients require comprehensive mental health services.

Patient Education. Of all the services that are contributed by the nurse caring for the person with epilepsy, perhaps the most valuable are efforts to modify the attitudes of the patient and family toward the disease itself.

Mental Outlook. For the observer, an epileptic seizure may be a terrifying event; for the person who has seizures, every seizure is potentially a source of humiliation and shame. This results in anxiety, depression, hostility, and secrecy. The reaction of shame and denial may extend to family members as well.

Ongoing encouragement should be given patients to enable them to overcome feelings of inferiority and self-consciousness resulting from seizures. The patient with epilepsy should carry an emergency medical identification card in wallet or purse or wear an identification bracelet around the wrist.

Oral Hygiene. Patient education includes the importance of oral hygiene and dental care to prevent or control gingival hyperplasia in patients receiving phenytoin (Dilantin). The patient is advised about the importance of regular gum massage and regular flossing to prevent hyperplasia. The patient also is counseled to inform all health care providers of the medication being taken because of the possibility of drug interactions when other medications are prescribed.

Financial Considerations. Because epilepsy is a long-term disorder, the regular use of costly medications may present a sizable burden to the patient and family. The Epilepsy Foundation of America offers a mail-order program to provide medications at minimal cost and access to life insurance. This organization serves as a referral source for special services for persons with epilepsy (see Bibliography for address).

Vocational Rehabilitation. For many, employment problems still remain the greatest handicap of epilepsy. Studies have demonstrated that the person with epilepsy who is properly placed in work has a satisfactory job performance. The director of each State Vocational Rehabilitation agency can provide information about vocational rehabilitation. The Epilepsy Foundation of America has developed a training and placement service. If the individual's seizures are not well controlled, information about sheltered workshops or home employment programs may be obtained.

Counseling and job training are provided for qualified persons through the Veterans' Administration. The US Civil Service Commission now grants government jobs to individuals if seizures are controlled and the person is otherwise qualified. The Rehabilitation Act helped to end job discrimination of the handicapped. The Americans With Disabilities Act of July 26, 1992, prohibits employers from discriminating against qualified individuals with a disability. A qualified individual with a disability is an individual who with or without reasonable accommodation can perform the essential functions of the position that such an individual holds or desires. This landmark legislation has resulted in wider knowledge about the rights of persons with disabilities, and the number of employers who knowingly hire persons with epilepsy is increasing.

General Information. The Commission for the Control of Epilepsy and Its Consequences makes recommendations about the social, legal, scientific, economic, and humanitarian aspects of epilepsy in the United States. Epilepsy International sponsors international congresses, publishes *Epilepsia* (the international journal on epilepsy), and has ongoing projects of international significance.

Ongoing Evaluation. Persons who have uncontrollable seizures and psychologic and social maladaptation with other overwhelming problems can be referred to comprehensive epilepsy centers where continuous television and EEG monitoring, specialized treatment, and rehabilitation services are available.

Genetic Counseling. Hereditary transmission of epilepsy has not been proved. Decisions about marriage and childbearing are made on an individual basis, and such options should not be denied to persons with epilepsy. Genetic counseling is advised, however.

Monitoring and Managing Potential Complications. Status epilepticus, the major complication, is described below. Another complication is toxicity of medications. The patient and family are instructed about side effects and are given specific guidelines to use to assess and report signs and symptoms indicating medication overdose.

Evaluation

Expected Outcomes

1. Maintains control of seizures
   a. Complies with treatment regimen and identifies the hazards of stopping the medication
   b. Identifies the side effects of medications
   c. Avoids factors or situations that may precipitate seizures (flickering light, hyperventilation, alcohol)
   d. Follows a healthful lifestyle by getting enough sleep and eating meals at regular times to avoid hypoglycemia
2. Improves psychosocial adjustment by discussing feelings
3. Gains knowledge and understanding of epilepsy
4. Is free of seizures and the complication of status epilepticus

Status Epilepticus

Status epilepticus (acute prolonged seizure activity) is a series of generalized seizures that occur without full recovery of consciousness between attacks. The term has been broadened to include continuous clinical or electrical seizures lasting at least 30 minutes, even without impairment of consciousness. It is considered a major medical emergency. Status epilepticus produces cumulative effects. Vigorous muscular contractions impose a heavy metabolic demand and can interfere with respirations. There is some respiratory arrest at the height of each seizure that produces venous congestion and hypoxia of the brain. Repeated episodes of cerebral anoxia and swelling may lead to irreversible and fatal brain damage. Factors that precipitate status epilepticus include withdrawal of anticonvulsant medication, fever, and intercurrent infection.

Management

The goals of treatment are to stop the seizures as quickly as possible, to ensure adequate cerebral oxygenation, and to maintain the patient in a seizure-free state. Airway and adequate oxygenation are established. If the patient remains deeply unconscious, a cuffed endotracheal tube is inserted. Intravenous diazepam is given slowly in an attempt to halt seizures immediately. Other anticonvulsant medications (phenytoin, phenobarbital) are given after diazepam is administered to maintain a seizure-free state, because the anticonvulsant effect of diazepam is short lived.

An intravenous line is established and blood samples are obtained to monitor serum electrolytes, urea, and glucose levels. EEG monitoring may be useful in determining the nature of epileptogenic activity. Vital signs and neurologic signs are monitored on a continuing basis. An intravenous infusion of dextrose is given if hypoglycemia has caused the seizure. If initial treatment is unsuccessful, general anesthesia with a short-acting barbiturate may be used.

Serum concentration of the anticonvulsant drug is measured, because a low level suggests that the patient was not taking the medication or that the dosage was too low. Cardiac involvement or respiratory depression may be severe and life threatening. There is also the potential for postictal (after a seizure) cerebral swelling.

Nursing Interventions

The nurse initiates ongoing assessment and monitoring of respiratory and cardiac function. There may be delayed depression of respiration and blood pressure as a result of the medications given to halt the seizures. Nursing assessment also includes monitoring and documenting the seizure type and the general condition of the patient.

The patient is turned to the side-lying position if possible, to assist in draining pharyngeal secretions. Suction equipment must be available because there is danger of aspiration. The intravenous line is closely monitored because it may become dislodged during seizures.

A person who has received long-term anticonvulsant therapy has a significant risk of fractures resulting from bone disease (osteoporosis, osteomalacia, and hyperparathyroidism), a side effect of drug treatment. Thus, during seizures the patient should be protected from injury with padded side rails and kept under constant observation. No effort should be made to restrain movements. The patient having seizures can inadvertently injure nearby persons, so nurses should take care to protect themselves. Other nursing interventions for the person having seizures are presented in Guideline 60-1.

Head Injuries

Injuries to the head involve trauma to the scalp, skull, and brain. Head injuries are among the most frequent and serious neurologic disorders, and have reached epidemic proportions as a result of traffic accidents. An estimated 100,000 persons die annually from head injuries, and more than 700,000 have injuries severe enough to require hospitalization. Of this group, between 50,000 and 90,000 people a year are left with intellectual or behavioral deficits that preclude their return to normal life. Two thirds of these are below the age of 30, with males outnumbering females. Detectable blood alcohol levels have been found in more than 50% of head-injured patients treated in emergency departments. At least half of all severely head-injured patients have significant injuries to other parts of the body. Hypovolemic shock in a head-injured patient is usually due to injuries to other parts of the body.

A major risk to the patient who experiences head injury is damage to the brain resulting from bleeding or swelling in response to the injury and resulting increased intracranial pressure (ICP). Increased ICP is described in further detail in Chapter 59.

Scalp Injury

Because of its many blood vessels, the scalp bleeds profusely when injured. Scalp wounds are also a portal of entry for intracranial infections. Trauma may result in an abrasion (brush wound), contusion, laceration, or avulsion. A subcutaneous injection of procaine makes it easier for the wound to be cleaned and treated. The area is irrigated to remove foreign material and minimize the chance of infection before lacerations are closed.

Fractures of the Skull

A skull fracture is a break in the continuity of the skull caused by trauma. It may occur with or without damage to the brain. The presence of a skull fracture usually means that there was considerable force on impact. Skull fractures are classified as open or closed. In an *open* fracture, the dura is torn, and in a *closed* fracture, the dura is not torn.

Clinical Manifestations

The symptoms, aside from those of the local injury, depend on the amount and the distribution of brain injury. Pain, persistent or localized, usually suggests that a fracture is present.

Fractures of the cranial vault produce swelling in the region of the fracture, and for this reason an accurate diagnosis cannot be made without an x-ray study.

Fractures of the base of the skull tend to traverse the paranasal sinus of the frontal bone or the middle ear located in the temporal bone; thus, they frequently produce hemorrhage from the nose, the pharynx, or the ears, and blood may appear under the conjunctive. An area of *ecchymosis,* or bruising, may be seen over the mastoid (Battle's sign). Basal skull fractures are suspected when CSF escapes from the ears (*cerebrospinal fluid otorrhea*) and the nose (*cerebrospinal rhinorrhea*). Drainage of cerebrospinal fluid is a serious problem because infection such as meningitis can occur if organisms gain access to the cranial contents through the nose, ear, or sinus through a tear in the dura.

Brain laceration or contusion is suggested by bloody spinal fluid.

Diagnostic Evaluation

Although a rapid physical examination and evaluation of neurologic status demonstrate the more obvious brain injuries, the less apparent abnormalities found in head injuries may be detected by CT scan of the head, which can differentiate subtle changes in the degree to which the soft tissue absorbs the x-rays. It is accurate and safe in showing the presence, nature, location, and extent of the lesion as well as in disclosing cerebral edema, contusion, intracerebral or extracerebral hematoma, subarachnoid and intraventricular hemorrhage, and late traumatic changes (infarction, hydrocephalus). Where available, MRI also is being used to evaluate patients with head injury.

Cerebral angiography may also be used and demonstrates the presence of supratentorial, extracerebral, and intracerebral hematomas and cerebral contusion. Lateral and anteroposterior views of the skull are obtained.

Management

Nondepressed skull fractures, generally do not require surgical treatment, but close observation of the patient is essential.

Depressed skull fractures require surgical intervention. The scalp is shaved and cleansed with large amounts of saline to remove all debris, and the fracture is exposed. The skull fragments are elevated and the area is debrided. Closure of the dura is carried out if possible, and the wound is closed. Large defects in the skull can be repaired later with metallic or plastic plates if necessary. In instances of a clean wound and an intact dura, the elevated fragments can be replaced at the time of the initial surgery, making a later cranioplasty unnecessary. Penetrating wounds require surgical debridement to remove foreign bodies and devitalized brain tissue and to control hemorrhage. Antibiotic treatment is instituted immediately, and blood component therapy is administered if indicated.

Fractures of the base of the skull are serious because they are usually open (involving the paranasal sinuses or middle or external ear) and may involve leakage of cerebrospinal fluid. A **halo sign**, which is a combination of blood surrounded by a yellowish stain, may be seen on bed linens or the head dressing and is highly suggestive of a *cerebrospinal fluid leak.* The nasopharynx and the external ear should be kept clean, and usually a plug of sterile cotton is placed in the ear or a sterile cotton pad may be taped loosely under the nose or against the ear to collect the draining fluid. The patient who is conscious is cautioned against sneezing or blowing the nose. The head usually is elevated 30 degrees to reduce ICP and promote spontaneous closure of the leak. (Some neurosurgeons prefer that the bed be kept flat.) Persistence of spinal fluid rhinorrhea or otorrhea usually requires surgical intervention.

Brain Injury

The most important consideration in any head injury is whether or not the brain has been injured. Even "minor" injury can cause significant brain damage. The brain is unable to store oxygen and glucose to any significant degree. The cerebral cells need an uninterrupted blood supply for these nutrients. Irreversible brain damage and cell death occur when blood supply is interrupted for only a few minutes because damaged neurons cannot regenerate.

Serious brain injury may occur, with or without fracture of the skull, after blows or injuries to the head that produce contusions, laceration, and hemorrhage of the brain.

Concussion

A cerebral concussion after head injury is a temporary loss of neurologic function with no apparent structural damage. A concussion generally involves a period of unconsciousness lasting from a few seconds to a few minutes. The jarring of the brain may be so slight as to cause only dizziness and spots before the eyes (spoken of as "seeing stars"), or there may be complete loss of consciousness for a time. If the brain tissue in the frontal lobe is affected, the patient may exhibit bizarre irrational behavior, whereas involvement of the temporal lobe can produce temporary amnesia or disorientation.

Treatment of concussion involves observing the patient for headache, dizziness, irritability, and anxiety (*postconcussion syndrome*), which may follow this type of injury. Giving the patient information, explanations, and encouragement may reduce some of the problems of postconcussion syndrome.

The patient may be hospitalized overnight for observation or discharged from the hospital in a relatively short time after a concussion. The family is instructed to observe for the following signs and symptoms and to notify the physician or clinic or bring the patient back to the emergency department if they occur:

- Difficulty in awakening
- Difficulty in speaking
- Confusion
- Severe headache
- Vomiting
- Weakness of one side of the body

The patient is advised to resume normal activities slowly.

A concussion was once considered a minor head injury and was thought to be without significant sequalae. However, studies have demonstrated that there are often disturbing and sometimes residual effects including attention deficits, difficulty with memory, and disruption in work habits. The elderly should be particularly assessed for "minor" head injury. Unrecognized "minor" head trauma may account for behavioral and confusional episodes in some elderly people. A misdiagnosed or untreated episode of confusion in an elderly patient may result in long-term disability that might have otherwise been avoided if detected and treated promptly.

Contusion

A cerebral contusion is a more severe cerebral injury in which the brain is bruised, with possible surface hemorrhage. The patient is unconscious for a considerable period. The symptoms, as would be expected, are more marked. The patient may lie motionless; the pulse is feeble, the respirations shallow, and the skin cold and pale. Often there is involuntary evacuation of the bowels and the bladder. The patient may be aroused with effort but soon slips back into unconsciousness. The blood pressure and the temperature are subnormal, and the picture is somewhat similar to that of shock.

In general, persons with widespread injury who have abnormal motor function, abnormal eye movements, and elevated ICP have a poor outcome. Conversely, the patient may recover consciousness completely and perhaps pass into a stage of cerebral irritability.

In the stage of cerebral irritability, the patient is no longer unconscious but, on the contrary, is easily disturbed by any form of stimulation, noises, light, and voices, and may become hyperactive at times. Gradually, the pulse, respirations, temperature, and other body functions return to normal. However, recovery is often delayed. Residual headache and vertigo are common, and often impaired mental function or seizures occur as a result of irreparable cerebral damage.

Intracranial Hemorrhage

Hematomas (collections of blood) that develop within the cranial vault are the most serious results of brain injury. The hematoma is referred to as *epidural*, *subdural*, or *intracerebral*, depending on its location. The main effects are frequently delayed until the hematoma is large enough to cause distortion and herniation of the brain and increased ICP.

- The signs and symptoms of cerebral ischemia resulting from compression caused by a hematoma are variable and depend on the speed with which vital areas are encroached on or the changes that involve the underlying brain.

In general, a small hematoma that develops rapidly may be fatal, whereas a more massive hematoma that develops slowly may allow the patient to adapt.

Epidural Hematoma (Extradural Hematoma or Hemorrhage)

After a head injury, blood may collect in the epidural (extradural) space between the skull and the dura. This often results from fractures of the skull that cause rupture or laceration of the middle meningeal artery, which runs between the dura and the skull located just inferior to a thin portion of temporal bone; hemorrhage from this artery causes pressure on the brain.

Clinical Manifestations. The symptoms produced are caused by the expanding hematoma. Usually, there is a momentary loss of consciousness at the time of injury, followed by an interval of apparent recovery (lucid interval). It should be noted that although the lucid interval is characteristic of an epidural hematoma, it does not occur in approximately 15% of patients with this lesion. During the lucid interval, compensation for the expanding hematoma takes place by rapid absorption of CSF and decreased intravascular volume, which maintains a normal ICP. When these mechanisms can no longer compensate, even a small increase in the volume of the blood clot produces a marked elevation of ICP. Then, often suddenly, signs of compression appear (usually deterioration of consciousness and signs of focal neurologic deficits such as dilation and fixation of a pupil or paralysis of an extremity), and the patient deteriorates rapidly.

Management. An epidural hematoma is considered an extreme emergency, as marked neurologic deficit or even cessation of breathing may occur within minutes. The treatment consists of making openings through the skull (*burr holes*), removing the clot, and controlling the bleeding point.

Subdural Hematoma

A subdural hematoma is a collection of blood between the dura and the underlying brain, a space normally occupied by a film of fluid. The most common cause is trauma, but it may also occur in various bleeding tendencies and aneurysms. A subdural hemorrhage is more frequently venous in origin and is attributed to the rupture of small vessels that bridge the subdural space.

A subdural hematoma may be acute, subacute, or chronic, depending on the size of the involved vessel and the amount of bleeding present.

Acute subdural hematomas are associated with major head injury involving contusion or laceration. Usually the patient is comatose, and the clinical signs are similar to those of epidural hematoma. A rising blood pressure with slowing of pulse and respirations indicates a rapidly increasing hematoma.

Subacute subdural hematoma is the sequela of less severe contusions and is suspected in patients failing to regain consciousness after head trauma. Signs and symptoms are similar to those of an acute subdural hematoma.

The mortality rate for patients with acute and subacute subdural hematomas is high, because frequently there is associated brain damage.

If the patient can be transported rapidly to the hospital, an immediate craniotomy is performed to open the dura, allowing for the solid subdural clot to be evacuated. Successful outcome also depends on the control of ICP and careful monitoring of respiratory function (see The Patient Undergoing Intracranial Surgery in Chapter 59).

Chronic subdural hematomas can develop from seemingly minor head injuries and are seen most frequently in the elderly. The elderly are prone to this type of head injury secondary to brain atrophy, which is an expected consequence of the aging process. Seemingly minor head trauma may result in enough impact to shift brain contents abnormally with negative sequalae. The time between injury and onset of symptoms may be lengthy (*e.g.*, months), so the actual insult may be forgotten. Symptoms may appear weeks after what seemed to be a minor injury.

A chronic subdural hematoma imitates other conditions and may be mistaken for a stroke. The bleeding is less profuse and there is compression of the intracranial contents. The blood within the brain changes in character in 2 to 4 days, becoming thicker and darker. In a few weeks, the clot breaks down and has the color and consistency of motor oil. Eventually, calcification or ossification of the clot takes place. The brain adapts to this foreign body invasion, and the patient's clinical signs and symptoms fluctuate. There may be severe headache, which tends to come and go; alternating focal neurologic signs; personality changes; mental deterioration; and focal seizures. Unfortunately, the patient may be labeled neurotic or psychotic if the cause of the symptoms is overlooked.

The *treatment* of a chronic subdural hematoma consists of surgical evacuation of the clot by suction or irrigation of the area. The procedure may be carried out through multiple burr holes, or a craniotomy may be performed for a sizable subdural mass lesion that cannot be drained through burr holes.

Intracerebral Hemorrhage and Hematoma

Intracerebral hemorrhage is bleeding into the substance of the brain. It is commonly seen in head injuries in which force is exerted to the head over a small area (missile injuries or bullet wounds; stab injury). These hemorrhages within the brain may also result from systemic hypertension, which causes degeneration and rupture of a vessel; rupture of a saccular aneurysm; vascular anomalies; intracranial tumors; systemic causes, including bleeding disorders such as leukemia, hemophilia, aplastic anemia, and thrombocytopenia; and complications of anticoagulant therapy.

There may be an insidious development with the onset of neurologic deficits followed by headache. Medical therapy involves careful administration of fluids and electrolytes, antihypertensive medications, control of ICP, and supportive care. Surgical intervention by craniotomy or craniectomy permits removal of the blood clot and control of hemorrhage but may not be possible either because of the inaccessible location of the bleeding or the lack of a clearly circumscribed area of blood that can be removed. Physical therapy usually is required for optimal rehabilitation of these and all head injury patients.

General Approach to Head Injuries

Clinical Manifestations

Brain trauma affects every system of the body. The clinical manifestations of brain injury include disturbances of consciousness, confusion, pupillary abnormalities, sudden onset of neurologic deficits, and changes in vital signs. There may be visual and hearing impairment, sensory dysfunction, spasticity, headache, vertigo, movement disorders, seizures, and many other effects. Because CNS injury alone is not likely to produce shock, the presence of hypovolemic shock suggests the possibility of multisystem injury.

Diagnostic Evaluation

The initial physical and neurologic examinations provide the baseline on which all future examination comparisons are made. CT is the primary neuroimaging diagnostic tool, and it is useful in the evaluation of soft-tissue injuries.

Management

A person with a head injury is presumed to have a cervical spine injury until proved otherwise. From the scene of the accident the patient is transported on a board, with head and neck maintained in alignment with the axis of the body. Slight traction should be maintained on the head, and a cervical collar applied and maintained until cervical spine x-rays have been obtained and the absence of cervical spinal cord injury documented.

All therapy is directed toward the preservation of brain homeostasis and prevention of secondary brain damage.

This includes stabilization of cardiovascular and respiratory function to maintain adequate cerebral perfusion. Hemorrhage is controlled, hypovolemia is corrected, and blood gas values are maintained at desired values.

Treatment of Increased ICP. As the damaged brain swells with edema or a collection of blood forms, a rise in ICP occurs and requires aggressive treatment. ICP is monitored closely and, if increased, it is managed by maintaining adequate oxygenation, administering mannitol, which reduces cerebral edema by osmotic dehydration; hyperventilation; the use of steroids; elevation of the head of the bed; and possibly neurosurgical intervention. Surgery is required for evacuation of blood clots, debridement and elevation of depressed fractures of the skull, and suture of severe scalp lacerations. Devices to monitor ICP can be inserted during surgery or at the bedside using aseptic technique. The patient is cared for in the intensive care unit where expert nursing and medical care are readily available.

Other Support Measures. Treatment also includes ventilatory support, prevention of seizures, and maintenance of fluid, electrolyte, and nutritional balance. Patients with severe head injury who are in coma are intubated and mechanically ventilated to control and protect the airway. Controlled hyperventilation also induces hypocapnia, which prevents vasodilation, lowers cerebral blood flow, decreases cerebral blood volume, and thus reduces ICP.

Because seizures are common after head injury and can cause secondary brain damage from hypoxia, anticonvulsant therapy may be started.

If the patient is very agitated, chlorpromazine may be prescribed to quiet the patient without decreasing the level of consciousness. A nasogastric tube may be inserted, as reduced gastric motility and reverse peristalsis are associated with head injury, making regurgitation common in the first few hours.

❑ NURSING PROCESS
The Patient With a Head Injury

Assessment

The health history may include the following questions:

- At what time did the injury occur?
- What caused the injury? A high velocity missile? An object striking the head? A fall?
- What was the direction and force of the blow?
- Was there a loss of consciousness? What was the duration of the unconscious period? Could the patient be aroused? (A history of unconsciousness or amnesia after a head injury indicates a significant degree of brain damage, whereas subsequent changes can reflect recovery or indicate the development of secondary brain damage.)

Areas of Assessment

Level of Consciousness and Responsiveness. The level of consciousness or responsiveness is regularly assessed because an alteration in the level of consciousness precedes all other changes in vital and neurologic signs. The Glasgow coma scale is used to assess level of consciousness based on the three criteria of eye opening, verbal responses, and motor responses to a verbal command or painful stimuli. (See Chapter 59 for more detailed discussion of the Glasgow coma scale.)

Monitoring Vital Signs. Although deterioration of the patient's level of consciousness is the most sensitive neurologic indication of impending danger, vital signs are monitored at frequent intervals to assess the intracranial status. Figure 60-6 depicts the general assessment parameters for the patient with a head injury.

- Signs of increasing ICP include slowing of the pulse, increasing systolic blood pressure, and widening pulse pressure.
- As brain compression increases, the vital signs tend to be reversed—the pulse and respiration become rapid, and the blood pressure may decrease. This is an ominous development, as is a rapid fluctuation of vital signs.
- A rapid rise in body temperature is regarded as unfavorable, because hyperthermia increases the metabolic demands of the brain and may indicate brain stem damage—a poor prognostic indicator. The temperature is maintained below 38°C (100.4°F).
- Tachycardia and arterial hypotension may indicate that bleeding is occurring elsewhere in the body.

Motor Function. Motor function is assessed frequently by observing spontaneous movements, asking the patient to raise and lower the extremities, and comparing the strength and equality of the hand grasp at periodic intervals. The presence or absence of spontaneous movement of each extremity is noted and speech and eye signs are assessed.

- If the patient does not demonstrate spontaneous movement, responses to painful stimuli are assessed. Abnormal responses (lack of motor response; extension responses) carry a poorer prognosis.
- The patient's ability to speak and the quality of speech are also assessed. The capacity to speak indicates a high level of brain function.
- The patient's spontaneous eye opening is evaluated.
- The size and equality of the pupils and their reaction to light are assessed. A unilaterally dilated and poorly responding pupil may indicate a developing hematoma with subsequent pressure on the third cranial nerve due to shifting of the brain. If both pupils become fixed and dilated, overwhelming injury and intrinsic damage to the upper brain stem usually are indicated, another poor prognostic sign.

Complications. Deterioration in the patient's condition may be due to an expanding intracranial hematoma, progressive cerebral edema, and herniation of the brain.

Cerebral Edema and Herniation. Cerebral edema is the most common cause of increased intracranial pressure in the patient who has received a head injury; the peak swelling following head injury occurs approximately 72 hours after injury. The intracrancial pressure increases because of the inability of the intact skull to expand despite the increased volume of its contents with swelling of the

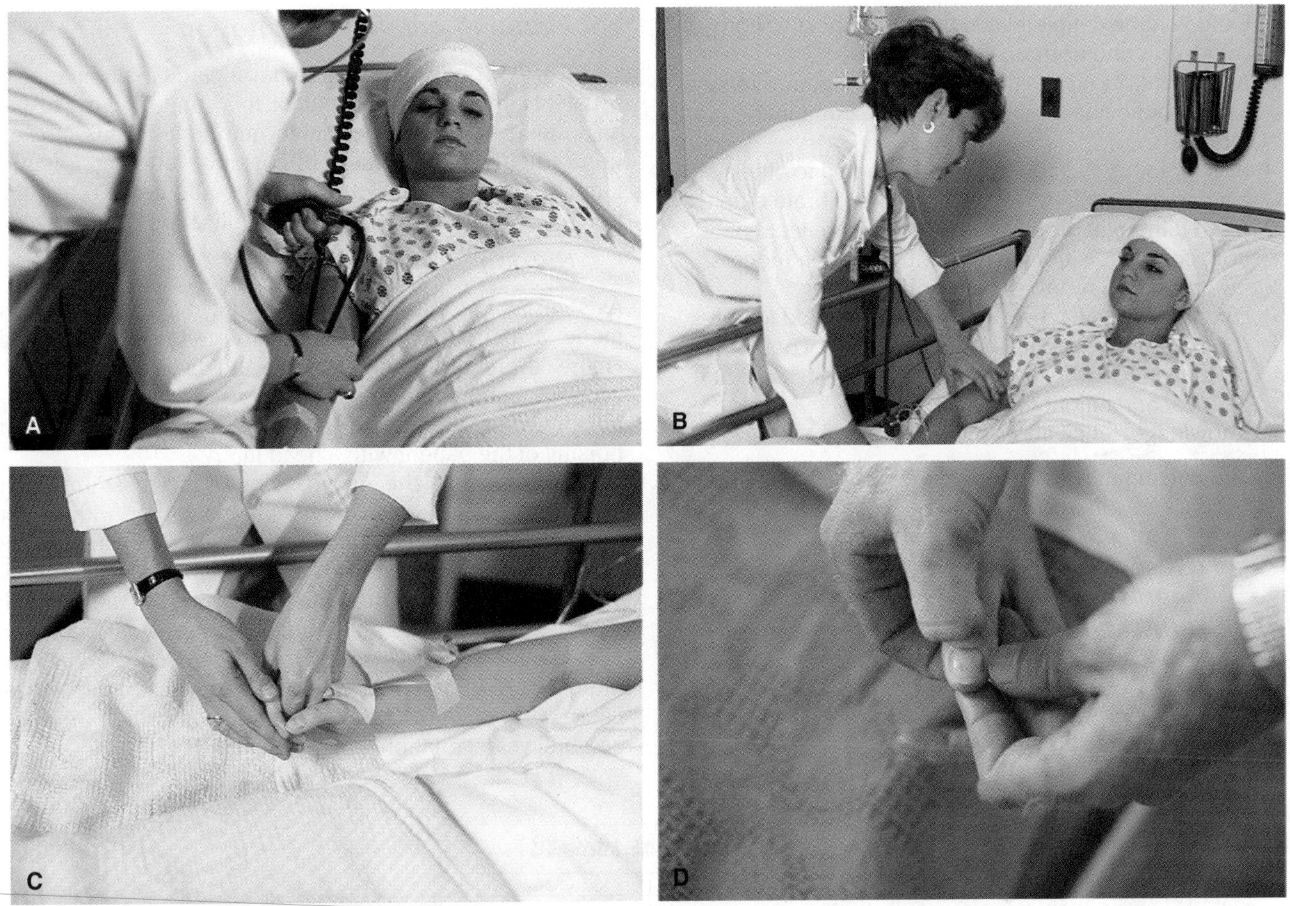

FIGURE 60-6. Assessment parameters for the patient with a head injury include (**A**) vital signs, (**B**) eye opening and responsiveness, and (**C, D**) motor response reflected in hand strength or response to painful stimulus.

brain resulting from trauma. As a result of the edema and increased ICP, pressure is exerted on brain tissue and the rigid internal structures of the skull. Depending on the site of the swelling, downward or lateral displacement (**herniation**) of the brain through or against the rigid structures occurs producing ischemia, infarction, irreversible brain damage, and death. Measures to control ICP are listed in Chart 60-6.

CHART 60-6
Controlling ICP in Head Injury Patient

- Elevate the head of the bed to 30 degrees.
- Maintain the patient's head and neck in neutral alignment (no twisting).
- Initiate measures to prevent the Valsalva maneuver (*i.e.*, stool softeners).
- Administer medications prescribed to decrease ICP (*i.e.*, diuretics, corticosteroids).
- Maintain normal body temperature.
- Hyperventilate the patient on mechanical ventilation; administer oxygen.
- Maintain fluid restriction.
- Avoid noxious stimuli (suctioning, painful procedures).
- Administer sedation to reduce metabolic demands.

Neurologic and Psychologic Deficits. The head-injured patient may develop focal nerve palsies such as *anosmia* (lack of sense of smell) or eye movement abnormalities and focal neurologic deficits such as aphasia, memory defects, and posttraumatic seizures or epilepsy. Patients may be left with residual organic psychologic deficits (impulsiveness, emotional lability, or uninhibited, aggressive behaviors) and, as a consequence of the impairment, lack insight into their emotional responses.

Other complications after traumatic head injuries include systemic infections (pneumonia, urinary tract infection, septicemia), neurosurgical infections (wound infection, osteomyelitis, meningitis, ventriculitis, brain abscess) and heterotrophic ossification (painful bone overgrowth in weight-bearing joints).

Diagnosis

Nursing Diagnoses

Based on all the assessment data, the patient's major nursing diagnoses may include the following:

- Ineffective airway clearance and ventilation related to hypoxia

- ❑ Fluid volume deficit related to disturbances of consciousness and hormonal dysfunction
- ❑ Altered nutrition, less than body requirements, related to metabolic changes, fluid restriction, and inadequate intake
- ❑ Risk for injury (self-directed and directed to others) related to disorientation, restlessness, and brain damage
- ❑ Altered thought processes (deficits in intellectual function, communication, memory, information processing) related to results of brain injury
- ❑ Potential for ineffective family coping related to unresponsiveness of patient, unpredictability of outcome, prolonged recovery period, and the patient's residual physical and emotional deficit
- ❑ Knowledge deficit about rehabilitation process

The nursing diagnoses for the unconscious patient and the patient with increased ICP also apply (both are discussed in Chapter 59).

Collaborative Problems/ Potential Complications

Based on all the assessment data, the major complications include the following:

- ❑ Cerebral edema and herniation

Planning and Implementation

Goals. The patient's goals may include maintenance of a patent airway, achievement of fluid and electrolyte balance, achievement of adequate nutritional status, prevention of injury, improvement of cognitive function, effective family coping, increased knowledge about the rehabilitation process, and prevention of complications.

Nursing Interventions

As soon as the initial assessment and diagnostic tests are made, a neurologic flow chart is started and maintained. Figure 60-7 identifies the extensive and diverse nursing interventions and includes nursing assessments, priorities for nursing interventions, and anticipatory and rehabilitation nursing of the patient with a head injury.

Maintaining the Airway. One of the most important nursing goals in the management of the patient with a head injury is to establish and maintain an adequate airway. The brain is extremely sensitive to hypoxia, and a neurologic deficit can worsen if the patient is hypoxic. Therapy is directed toward maintaining adequately oxygenated circulation so that there is a supply of oxygenated blood to the brain to preserve cerebral function. An obstructed airway causes CO_2 retention and hypoventilation, which produces cerebral vessel dilation and increases ICP.

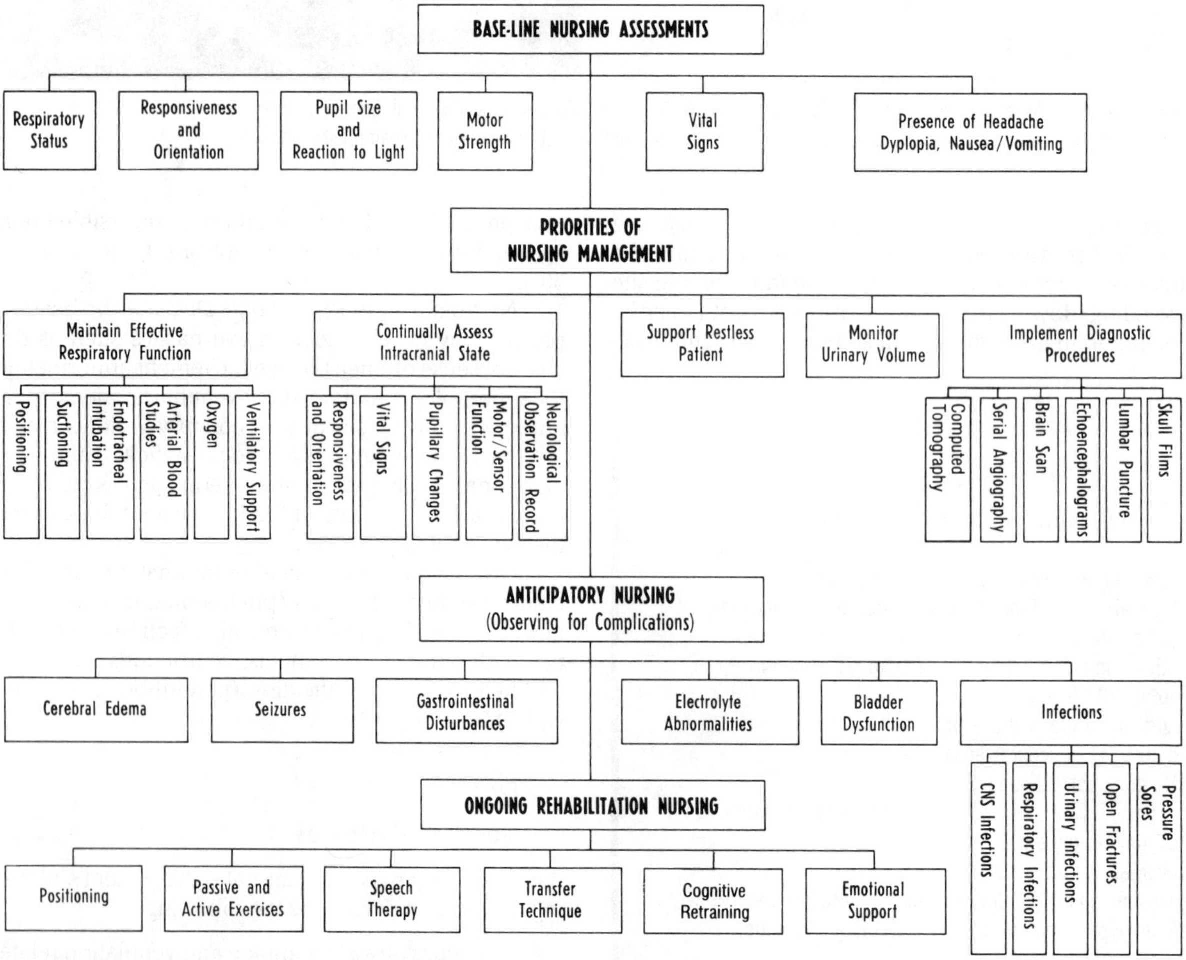

FIGURE 60-7. Nursing interventions for the patient with a head injury.

Therapeutic and nursing activities to ensure an adequate exchange of air are summarized in Chapter 25 and include the following:

- Keep the unconscious patient in a position that facilitates drainage of oral secretions, with the head of the bed elevated about 30 degrees to decrease intracranial venous pressure.
- Establish effective suctioning procedures. (Pulmonary secretions produce coughing and straining, which increase ICP.)
- Guard against aspiration and respiratory insufficiency.
- Monitor arterial blood gases to assess adequacy of ventilation. (The goal is to keep blood gases within normal range to ensure adequate cerebral blood flow.)
- Monitor the patient on mechanical ventilation.

Monitoring Fluid and Electrolyte Balance. Brain damage can produce metabolic and hormonal dysfunctions. The monitoring of serum electrolyte concentrations is important, especially in patients receiving osmotic diuretics, those with inappropriate antidiuretic hormone secretion, and those with post-traumatic diabetes insipidus.

- Serial studies of blood and urine electrolytes and osmolality are carried out because head injuries may be accompanied by disorders of sodium regulation. Sodium retention may last several days, followed by sodium diuresis. Increasing lethargy, confusion, and seizures may be due to electrolyte imbalance.
- Endocrine function is evaluated by monitoring serum electrolytes, glucose values, and intake and output.
- Urine is tested regularly for acetone.
- A record of daily weight is kept, especially if the patient has hypothalamic involvement and is at risk for the development of diabetes insipidus.

Providing Adequate Nutrition. Head injury results in metabolic changes that increase calorie consumption and nitrogen excretion. Steroid therapy also increases the catabolic state. As soon as the patient's condition has stabilized, nasogastric feedings are started unless there is discharge of CSF from the nose (*cerebrospinal rhinorrhea*).

Elevating the head of the bed and aspirating the nasogastric tube before feeding (for evidence of residual feeding in the stomach) are measures used to prevent distention, regurgitation, and aspiration. A continuous-drip infusion or pump may be used to regulate the feeding. The principles and technique of nasogastric feedings are discussed in Chapter 35. The feeding tube usually is kept in place until the swallowing reflex returns.

Preventing Injury. As the patient emerges from coma, there is often a period of lethargy and stupor followed by a period of agitation. Each stage is variable and depends on the individual, the depth and duration of coma, and the patient's age. The patient emerging from a coma may become increasingly agitated toward the end of the day. Restlessness may be due to hypoxia, fever, pain, or a full bladder. It may indicate injury to the brain but may also be a sign that the patient is regaining consciousness. (Some restlessness may be beneficial because the lungs and extremities are exercised.) Agitation may also be due to annoyance from an indwelling urinary catheter, intravenous lines, restraints, and repeated neurologic checks.

- Assess the patient to ensure that the airway is adequate and the bladder is not distended. Check bandages and casts for constriction.
- To protect the patient from self-injury and dislodging of body tubes, use padded side rails or wrap the patient's hands in mitts (Fig. 60-8) Avoid restraints when possible because straining against them can increase ICP or cause other injury.
- Avoid opioids as a means of controlling restlessness because these medications depress respiration, constrict the pupils, and alter the level of the patient's responsiveness.
- Use a floor bed (floor mattresses surrounded by a wall of mattresses) to allow freedom of movement and promote patient safety.
- Minimize environmental stimuli by keeping the room quiet, limiting visitors, speaking calmly, and providing frequent orientation information (*e.g.*, explaining where the patient is and what is being done).
- Provide adequate lighting to prevent visual hallucinations.
- Do not disrupt the patient's sleep–wake cycles.
- Lubricate the skin with oil or emollient lotion to prevent irritation due to rubbing against the sheet.
- If incontinence is a problem, consider using an external sheath catheter on a male patient. Because prolonged use of an indwelling catheter inevitably produces infection, the patient may be placed on an intermittent catheterization schedule.

Improving Cognitive Functioning. Although many brain-damaged patients survive because of resuscitative and supportive technology, they frequently sustain significant cognitive sequelae that may not be detected during the acute phase of injury. Cognitive impairment includes memory deficits, decrease in ability to focus and sustain attention to a task (easily distracted), reduced ability to process information, and slowness in thinking, perceiving, communicating, reading, and writing. An estimated 25% to 38% of these persons develop psychiatric or emotional problems.

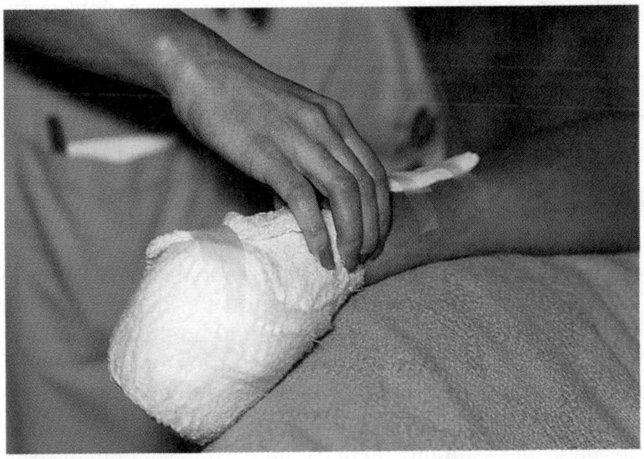

FIGURE 60-8. Hands of a patient with a head injury may be wrapped in mitts to prevent self injury.

Resulting psychosocial, behavioral, emotional, and cognitive impairments are devastating to the family as well as to the patient.

These problems require collaboration among many disciplines. A *neuropsychologist* (specialist in evaluating and treating cognitive problems) plans a program and initiates therapy or counseling that is designed to help the patient reach maximal potential. Cognitive rehabilitation activities are directed at redeveloping the patient's ability to devise new problem-solving strategies. The retraining is carried out over an extended period and may include the use of computer-training programs, video games, sensory stimulation and reinforcement, behavior modification, and reality orientation. Assistance from many disciplines is necessary during this phase of recovery. Intellectual ability may not improve after time, but social and behavioral aspects may.

The nurse needs to be aware that there are fluctuations in the orientation and memory of such patients. They are easily distracted. If they are pushed to a level greater than their impaired cortical functioning allows, symptoms of fatigue and stress (headache, dizziness) may occur.

Supporting Family Coping. Serious head injury can produce a great deal of prolonged stress in the family because of the patient's physical and emotional deficits, the unpredictable outcome, and altered family relationships. Families report difficulties in dealing with changes in temperament, behavior, and personality. These are associated with disruption in family cohesion, loss of leisure pursuits, and loss of work capacity, as well as the social isolation and entrapment of the caretaker. The family may experience anger, grief, guilt, and denial in recurring cycles.

The family is asked how the patient is different at this time. What has been lost? What is most difficult about coping with this situation? Helpful interventions include providing family members with accurate and honest information and encouraging them to continue to set well-defined, mutual, short-term goals. Family counseling helps deal with overwhelming feelings of loss and helplessness and gives guidance to the management of inappropriate behaviors. Support groups are available to provide a forum for sharing problems, developing insight, referring information, networking, and gaining assistance in maintaining realistic expectations and hope.

The National Head Injury Foundation serves as a clearinghouse for information and resources for patients with head injuries and their families, including specific information on coma, rehabilitation, behavioral consequences of head injury, and family issues. This organization can provide names of facilities and professionals who work with persons with head injuries and can assist families in organizing local support groups.

Patient and Family Education and Home Care Considerations. Rehabilitation of the patient with a head injury begins at the time of injury and extends into the home and community. Depending on the degree of brain damage, the patient may be referred to a rehabilitation setting specialized in cognitive restructuring of the brain-injured patient. The patient is encouraged to continue the rehabilitation program after discharge, because improvement in status may continue up to 3 or more years after injury. The effects of changes in the head-injured patient and the need for long-term rehabilitation on the family and their coping abilities need frequent assessment. Teaching and continued support of the patient and family are essential as their needs and the patient's status change.

Because posttraumatic seizures occur frequently, anticonvulsant medications may be prescribed for 1 to 2 years after injury. The patient and family require instruction about the side effects of these medications and about the importance of taking them as prescribed. Depending on the ultimate recovery and rehabilitation of the patient, the patient is encouraged to return to normal activities gradually.

Evaluation

Expected Outcomes

1. Attains or maintains effective airway clearance, ventilation, and brain oxygenation
   a. Achieves normal blood gas values and has normal breath sounds on auscultation
   b. Mobilizes and clears secretions
2. Achieves satisfactory fluid and electrolyte balance
   a. Demonstrates serum electrolytes within normal range
   b. Has no clinical signs of dehydration or overhydration
3. Attains adequate nutritional status
   a. Has less than 50 ml of aspirate in stomach before each tube feeding
   b. Is free of gastric distention and vomiting
   c. Shows minimal weight loss
4. Avoids injury
   a. Shows lessening agitation and restlessness
   b. Is oriented to time, place, and person
5. Shows improvement in cognitive function and improved memory
6. Family members demonstrate adaptive coping mechanisms
   a. Have joined support group
   b. Share their feelings with appropriate health care personnel
7. Patient and family members participate in rehabilitation process as indicated
   a. Take active role in identifying rehabilitation goals and participate in recommended activities
   b. Family prepares for discharge of patient
8. Absence of complications
   a. Exhibits normal ICP, normal vital signs and body temperature, and increasing orientation to time, place and person
   b. Demonstrates desired response to measures to reduce ICP

Spinal Cord Injury

Spinal cord injury is a major health problem affecting 150,000 to 500,000 persons in the United States, with an estimated 10,000 new injuries occurring each year. It is an injury that occurs predominantly in males, with young men accounting for over 75% of all such injury. Half of these injuries result from motor vehicle accidents; most of the others occur from falls, sporting and industrial accidents, and gunshot wounds. Two thirds of the victims are 30 years of age or younger. The estimated total annual cost of these injuries exceeds $2 billion a year. There is a high frequency of associated injuries and medical complications.

The vertebrae most frequently involved in spinal cord injuries are the 5th, 6th, and 7th cervical (neck), the 12th thoracic, and the 1st lumbar vertebrae. These vertebrae are the most susceptible because there is a greater range of mobility in the vertebral column in these areas.

Prevention

The predominant risk factors for spinal cord injury include age, sex, and substance abuse, including alcohol and drug use. The frequency with which these risk factors are associated with spinal cord injuries serves to emphasize the importance of primary prevention. To prevent this devastating and catastrophic injury, the following steps should be taken: (1) reduction in driving speed, (2) use of seat belt and shoulder harness, (3) wearing of helmets by motorcyclists and bikers, (4) educational programs directed against driving while intoxicated, (5) water safety instruction, (6) prevention of falls, and (7) use of protective devices and proper coaching techniques in sports.

Paramedical personnel are taught the importance of properly removing a car-crash victim from a motor vehicle and of following proper methods in transporting the victim to a hospital emergency department to avoid further and possibly permanent damage to the spinal cord.

Pathophysiology

Damage to the spinal cord ranges from transient concussion (from which the patient fully recovers) to contusion, laceration, and compression of the cord substance (either alone or in combination), to complete transection of the cord (which renders the patient paralyzed below the level of the injury).

When hemorrhage occurs in the area of the spinal cord, the blood may seep into the extradural, subdural, or subarachnoid spaces of the spinal canal. Immediately after a contusion or tear injury, the nerve fibers begin to swell and disintegrate. Blood circulation to the gray matter of the spinal cord is impaired. Not only is there injury to the spinal cord vasculature, but a pathogenic process appears to be responsible for the progressive damage of the acute spinal cord injury. A secondary chain of events produces ischemia, hypoxia, edema, and hemorrhagic lesions, which in turn result in destruction of myelin and axons.

These secondary reactions, believed to be the principal causes of spinal cord degeneration at the level of injury, are now thought to be reversible 4 to 6 hours after injury. Therefore, if the cord has not suffered irreparable damage, some method of *early* treatment with corticosteroids and other anti-inflammatory drugs is needed to prevent partial damage from developing into total and permanent damage (see Management Section.)

Emergency Management

The immediate management of the patient at the scene of the accident is critical, because improper handling can cause further damage and loss of neurologic function. Any victim of a motor vehicle or driving accident, a contact sport injury, fall, or any direct trauma to the head and neck must be considered to have a spinal cord injury until such an injury is ruled out.

- At the scene of the accident, the victim must be immobilized on a spinal (back) board, with head and neck in a neutral position, to prevent an incomplete injury from becoming complete.
- One member of the team must assume control of the patient's head to prevent flexion, rotation, or extension.
- The hands are placed on both sides of the head at about the ear to maintain traction and alignment while a spinal board or cervical immobilizing device is applied.
- At least four persons should slide the victim carefully onto a board for transfer to the hospital. Any twisting movement may irreversibly damage the spinal cord by causing a bony fragment of the vertebra to cut into, crush, or sever the cord completely.

It is desirable that the patient be referred to a regional spinal injury or trauma center because of the multidisciplinary personnel and support services required to counteract destructive changes that occur in the first few hours after injury.

Transferring the Patient. During treatment in the emergency and radiology departments, the patient is kept on the transfer board. The transfer of the patient to a bed presents a definite nursing problem.

- The patient must always be maintained in an extended position. No part of the body should be twisted or turned, nor should the patient be allowed to assume a sitting position.

The patient should be placed on a Stryker or other turning frame when transfer to a bed is planned. Later, if it has been proved that there is no cord injury, the patient can always be moved to a conventional bed without harm; the reverse, however, is not true. If a Stryker or other turning frame is not available, the patient should be placed on a firm mattress with a bedboard under it.

Clinical Manifestations

If conscious, the patient usually complains of acute pain in the back or neck, which may radiate along the involved nerve. Often the patient speaks of fear that the neck or back is broken. Severe spinal cord injury can result in paraplegia or quadriplegia as described in Chart 60-7. The consequences of spinal cord injury depend on the level of injury of the cord and the type of injury (Chart 60-8).

Neurologic level refers to that lowest level at which sensory and motor functions are normal. Below the neurologic level, there is total sensory and motor paralysis, loss of bladder and bowel control (usually with urinary retention and bladder distention), loss of sweating and vasomotor tone, and marked reduction of blood pressure from loss of peripheral vascular resistance.

Type of injury refers to the extent of injury to the spinal cord itself.

Respiratory problems are related to compromised respiratory function, the severity of which depends on the level of injury. The muscles contributing to respiration are the

CHART 60-7

Selected Terms Related to Spinal Cord Injury

- *Quadriplegia* (tetraplegia) results from a lesion involving one of the cervical segments of the spinal cord with dysfunction of both arms, both legs, bowel, and bladder.
- *Paraplegia* results from a lesion involving the thoracic lumbar, or sacral regions of the spinal cord with dysfunction of the lower extremities, bowel, and bladder.
- *Complete lesion* (*e.g.,* complete quadriplegia or complete paraplegia) implies total loss of sensation and voluntary muscle control below the injury.
- *Incomplete lesion* implies preservation of the sensory or motor fibers, or both, below the lesion. Incomplete lesions are classified according to the area of spinal cord damage: *central, lateral, anterior,* or *peripheral* (see Chart 60-8).

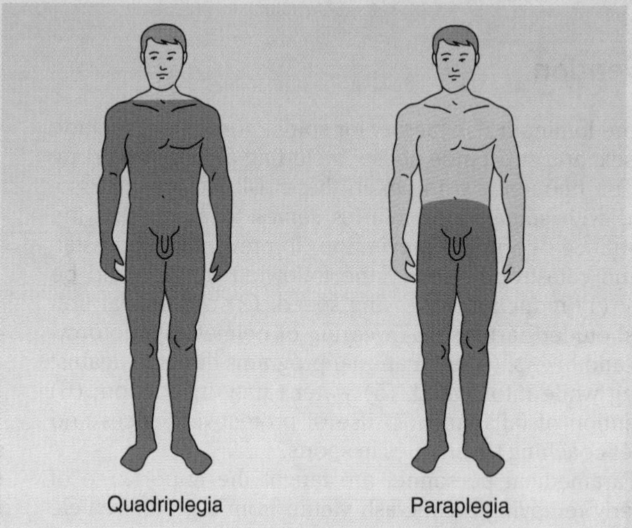

The shaded area shows the extent of motor and sensory loss.

(Adapted from Hickey JV. Clinical Practice of Neurological and Neurosurgical Nursing, 3rd ed. Philadelphia, JB Lippincott, 1992.)

abdominals, intercostals (T1–T11), and the diaphragm. In high cervical cord injury, acute respiratory failure is the leading cause of death.

Diagnostic Evaluation

A detailed neurologic examination is performed. Diagnostic x-rays (lateral cervical spine x-rays and CT scanning) are performed. A search is made for other injuries because spinal trauma often is accompanied by other injuries, commonly to the head and chest. Continuous ECG monitoring may be indicated because *bradycardia* (slow heart rate) and *asystole* (cardiac standstill) are common in acute cervical injuries.

Management of Spinal Cord Injuries (Acute Phase)

The goals of management are to prevent further spinal cord injury and to observe for symptoms of progressive neurologic deficits. The patient is resuscitated as necessary, and oxygenation and cardiovascular stability are maintained.

Pharmacotherapy. The administration of high dose corticosteroids, specifically methylprednisolone, has been found to improve prognosis and reduce disability if given within 8 hours of injury. A loading dose followed by a continuous infusion has been associated with significant clinical improvement for patients with acute spinal cord injury. Under investigation is treatment with high dose steroids, mannitol (given to decrease edema) and dextran (given to prevent the blood pressure from dropping and to improve capillary blood flow), given in combination. Naloxone, a drug that has shown promise in treating animals with spinal cord injury, has minimal side effects and may promote neurologic improvement in humans.

Hypothermia. The effectiveness of cooling techniques or hypothermia perfusion of the injured area of the spinal cord to counteract the autodestructive forces that follow this type of injury is being investigated.

Respiratory Measures. Oxygen is administered to maintain a high arterial PO_2, because anoxemia can create or worsen a neurologic deficit of the spinal cord. If endotracheal intubation is necessary, extreme care is taken to avoid flexing or extending the neck, which can result in an extension of cervical injury. **Diaphragm pacing** (electrical stimulation of the phrenic nerve) may be considered for the patient with a high cervical lesion but is usually carried out after the acute phase.

Skeletal Reduction and Traction. Management of spinal cord injury requires *immobilization* and *reduction* of dislocations (restoration of normal position) and *stabilization* of the vertebral column.

Cervical fractures are reduced and the cervical spine aligned with some form of skeletal traction, such as skeletal tongs or calipers, or with use of the halo device. A variety of skeletal tongs are available, all of which involve fixation in the skull in some manner (Fig. 60-9). The Gardner-Wells tongs require no predrilled holes in

CHART 60-8
Effects of Cord Injuries

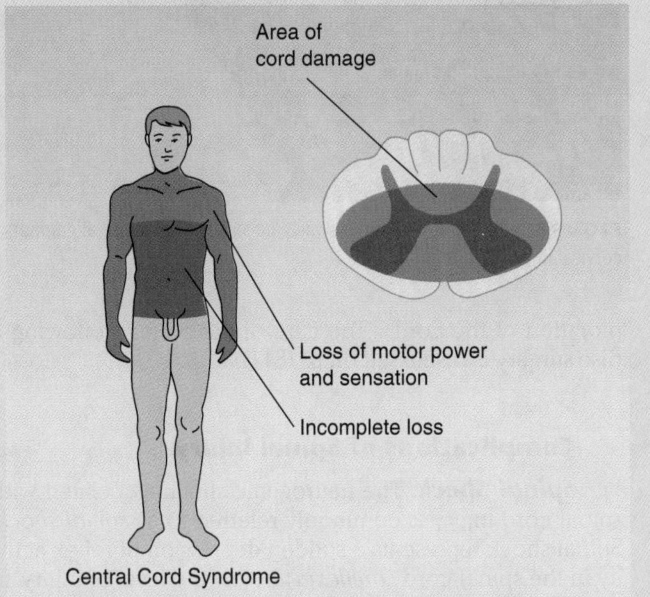

Central Cord Syndrome

- *Characteristics:* Motor deficits (in the upper extremities as compared to the lower extremities; sensory loss varies, but is more pronounced in the upper extremities); bowel/bladder dysfunction is variable, or function may be completely preserved.
- *Cause:* Injury or edema of the central cord, usually of the cervical area.

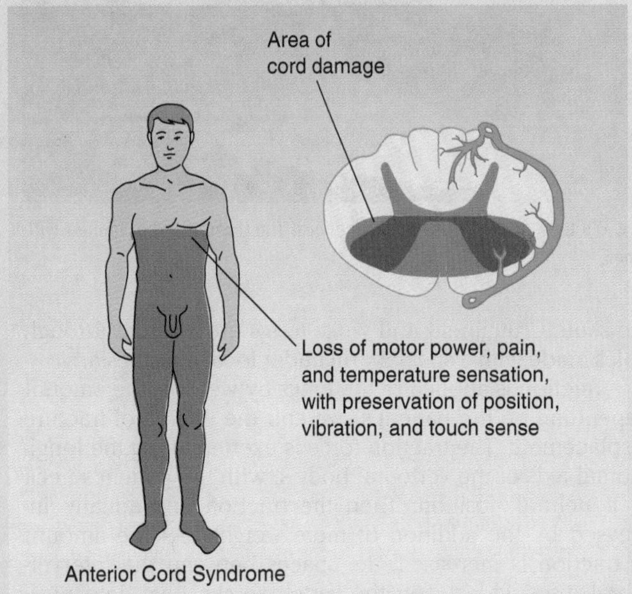

Anterior Cord Syndrome

- *Characteristics:* Loss of pain, temperature, and motor function is noted below the level of the lesion; light touch, position, and vibration sensation remain intact.
- *Cause:* The syndrome may be caused by acute disk herniation or hyperflexion injuries associated with fracture-dislocation of a vertebra. It also may occur as a result of injury to the anterior spinal artery, which supplies the anterior two-thirds of the spinal cord.

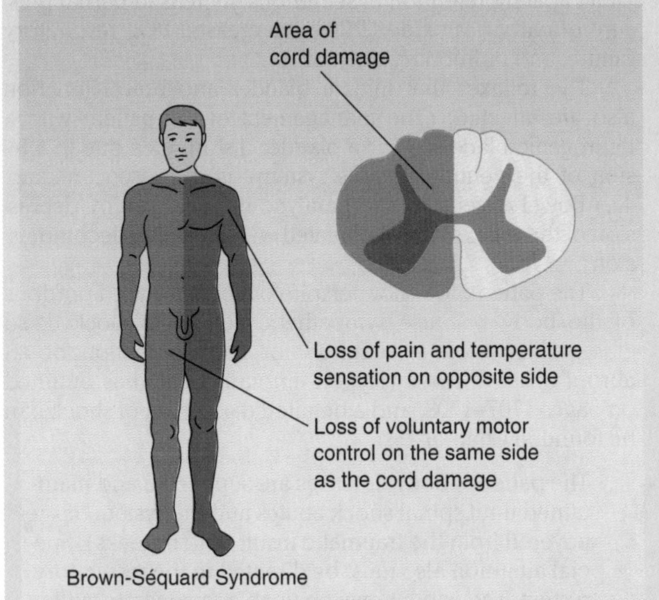

Brown-Séquard Syndrome (Lateral Cord Syndrome)

- *Characteristics:* Ipsilateral paralysis or paresis is noted, together with ipsilateral loss of touch, pressure, and vibration and contralateral loss of pain and temperature.
- *Cause:* The lesion is caused by a transverse hemisection of the cord (half of the cord is transected from north to south), usually as a result of a knife or missile injury, fracture–dislocation of a unilateral articular process, or possibly, an acute ruptured disk.

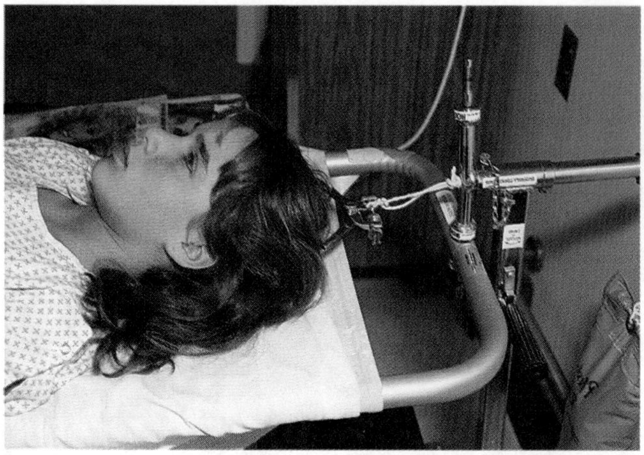

FIGURE 60-9. Traction for cervical fractures may be applied with tongs.

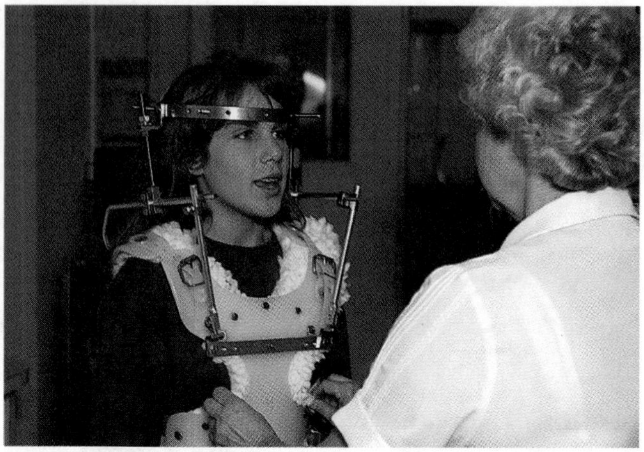

FIGURE 60-10. A halo vest may be used to maintain alignment in cervical injuries.

the skull. Crutchfield and Vinke tongs are inserted through holes made with a special drill under local anesthesia.

Traction is applied to the tongs by weights, the amount depending on the patient's size and the degree of fracture displacement. The traction force is exerted along the longitudinal axis of the vertebral bodies, with the patient's neck in a neutral position. Then the traction is gradually increased by the addition of more weights. As the amount of traction is increased, the spaces between the intervertebral discs widen, and the vertebrae slip back into position. Reduction usually takes place after correct alignment has been restored. Once reduction is achieved, as verified by cervical spine films and neurologic examination, the weights are gradually removed until the amount of weight needed to maintain the alignment is obtained. The weights should hang freely so as not to interfere with the traction. The patient is placed on a Stryker or other turning frame if one is available. (See p. 1797 for a method of transfer to the turning frame.)

A halo device may be used initially with traction or may be applied after removal of the tongs (Fig. 60-10). It consists of a stainless steel halo ring that is fixed to the skull by four pins. The ring is attached to a removable halo vest, which suspends the weight of the unit circumferentially around the chest. A metal frame connects the ring to the chest. Halo devices provide immobilization of the cervical spine while allowing early ambulation.

Thoracic and lumbar injuries are preferentially treated through surgical intervention followed by immobilization with a fitted brace. Traction is not indicated either pre- or postoperatively.

Surgical Intervention. Surgery is indicated when (1) the patient's deformities cannot be reduced by traction, (2) there is significant instability of the cervical spine, (3) the injury is in the thoracic or lumbar regions, or (4) the patient's neurologic status is deteriorating. Surgery is performed to reduce the spinal fracture or dislocation or decompress the cord.

A **laminectomy** (excision of the posterior arches and spinous processes of a vertebra) may be indicated in the presence of progressive neurologic deficit, suspected epidural hematoma, or penetrating injuries that require surgical debridement, or to permit direct visualization and exploration of the cord. (The care of the patient following a disc surgery is discussed on p. 1811.)

Complications of Spinal Injury

Spinal Shock. The neurogenic shock associated with spinal cord injury is commonly referred to as *spinal shock*. Spinal shock represents a sudden depression of reflex activity in the spinal cord (*areflexia*) below the level of injury. In this condition, the muscles innervated by the part of the cord segment situated below the level of the lesion become completely paralyzed and flaccid, and the reflexes are absent. The blood pressure falls, and the parts of the body below the level of the cord lesion are paralyzed and without sensation.

With injuries to the cervical and upper thoracic spinal cord, innervation to the major accessory muscles of respiration is lost and respiratory problems develop: decreased vital capacity, retention of secretions, increased partial pressure of carbon dioxide (PCO_2), decreased PO_2, respiratory failure, and pulmonary edema.

The reflexes that initiate bladder and bowel function also are affected. (The management of the patient with a neurogenic bladder—*i.e.*, a bladder disturbance due to a lesion of the central nervous system—is discussed in Chap. 42.) Bowel distention and paralytic ileus caused by depression of the reflexes may be treated with intestinal decompression.

The patient does not perspire on the paralyzed portions of the body, because sympathetic activity is blocked, so close observation is required for early detection of an abrupt onset of fever. (Hyperthermia is treated as outlined on pages 1707–1708, and a detailed discussion of shock can be found in Chapter 15.)

- The patient's body defenses are supported and maintained until spinal shock abates and the system has recovered from the traumatic insult (3 to 6 weeks). Special attention also must be directed to the respiratory system. The patient may be unable to generate sufficient intrathoracic pressure to cough effectively. Chest physical therapy and suctioning may assist in clearance of pulmonary secretions.

Deep Vein Thrombosis. Deep Vein Thrombosis (DVT) is a common complication of immobility and is common in spinal cord–injury patients. Those patients who develop DVT are at risk for developing a pulmonary embolism (PE), a life-threatening complication. Manifestations of PE include pleuritic chest pain, anxiety, shortness of breath, and abnormal blood gas values (increased PCO_2 and decreased PO_2). Thigh and calf measurements are made daily. The patient will be evaluated for the presence of DVT if there is a significant increase in the circumference of one extremity. Low-dose anticoagulation therapy usually is initiated to prevent DVT and pulmonary embolism along with thigh-high elastic stockings or pneumatic compression devices.

Other Complications. In addition to respiratory complications (respiratory failure; pneumonia) and autonomic hyperreflexia (characterized by pounding headache, profuse sweating, nasal congestion, piloerection [gooseflesh], bradycardia, and hypertension [see p. 1804]), other complications that may occur include pressure ulcers and infection (urinary, respiratory, and local infection at the pin sites).

❑ NURSING PROCESS
The Patient With Acute Spinal Cord Injury

Assessment

The breathing pattern is observed, the strength of the patient's cough is assessed, and the lungs are auscultated because paralysis of abdominal and respiratory muscles diminishes coughing and makes it difficult to clear bronchial and pharyngeal secretions. Reduced excursion of the chest also results.

The patient is monitored closely for any changes in motor or sensory function and symptoms of progressive neurologic damage. It may be impossible in the early stages of spinal cord injury to determine whether the cord has been severed because signs and symptoms of cord edema are indistinguishable from those of cord transection. Edema of the spinal cord may occur with any severe cord injury and may further compromise spinal cord function.

Motor and sensory function is assessed through careful neurologic examination. These findings are recorded so that changes in or progression from the baseline neurologic status can be evaluated accurately.

- ❑ Motor ability is tested by asking the patient to spread the fingers, squeeze the examiner's hand, and move the toes or turn the feet.
- ❑ Sensation is evaluated by pinching the skin or pricking it with the broken end of a cotton swab, starting at the shoulder level and working down both sides of the extremities. The patient is asked where the sensation is felt.
- ❑ Any decrease in neurologic function is reported immediately.

The patient is also assessed for the presence of spinal shock, in which there is complete loss of all reflex, motor, sensory, and autonomic activity below the level of the lesion, which causes bladder paralysis and distention. The patient's lower abdomen is palpated for signs of urinary retention and overdistention of the bladder. Further assessment is made for gastric dilation and ileus due to an atonic bowel, a result of autonomic disruption.

Temperature is monitored because the patient may have periods of hyperthermia as a result of alteration in temperature control due to autonomic disruption.

Diagnosis

Nursing Diagnoses

Based on all the assessment data, the patient's major nursing diagnoses may include the following:

- ❑ Ineffective breathing patterns related to weakness or paralysis of abdominal and intercostal muscles and inability to clear secretions
- ❑ Impaired physical mobility related to motor and sensory impairment
- ❑ Risk for impaired skin integrity related to immobility, sensory loss
- ❑ Urinary retention related to inability to void spontaneously
- ❑ Constipation related to presence of atonic bowel as a result of autonomic disruption
- ❑ Pain and discomfort related to treatment and prolonged immobility

Collaborative Problems/ Potential Complications

Based on the assessment data, potential complications that may develop include:

- ❑ Deep vein thrombosis
- ❑ Orthostatic hypotension
- ❑ Autonomic hyperreflexia

Planning and Implementation

Goals. The goals for the patient may include improvement of breathing pattern, improvement of mobility, maintenance of skin integrity, relief of urinary retention, improvement of bowel function, promotion of comfort, and absence of complications.

Nursing Interventions

Promoting Adequate Breathing. Possible impending respiratory failure is detected by observing the patient, measuring vital capacity, and monitoring arterial blood gas values. Early and vigorous attention to clearing bronchial and pharyngeal secretions can prevent retention of secretions and resultant atelectasis. Suctioning may be indicated, but caution must be used during suctioning because this procedure can stimulate the vagus nerve, producing bradycardia, which can result in cardiac arrest.

If the patient cannot cough effectively because of decreased inspiratory volume and inability to develop sufficient expiratory pressure, chest physical therapy and quad-assisted coughing may be indicated. Specific breathing exercises are supervised by the nurse to increase strength and endurance of inspiratory muscles, particularly the diaphragm. Assisted coughing provides an opportunity for the patient to clear the upper respiratory tract of secretions. It is important to ensure proper humidification and hydration to prevent secretions from becoming thick and difficult to remove even with coughing. The patient is assessed for signs of respiratory infection: cough, fever, and dyspnea. Smoking is discouraged because it increases bronchial and pulmonary secretions and impairs ciliary action.

- Ascending edema of the spinal cord in the acute phase may cause respiratory difficulty that requires immediate intervention. Therefore, the patient's respiratory status must be monitored frequently.

Improving Mobility. Proper body alignment is maintained at all times. The patient is placed in the dorsal or supine position as follows:

- The feet are positioned against a padded footboard to prevent footdrop. There should be a space between the end of the mattress and the footboard to allow free suspension of the heels. A wooden block on either end of the mattress prevents the mattress from pushing against the footboard.
- Trochanter rolls are applied from the crest of the ilium to the midthigh of both legs to prevent external rotation of the hip joints.

Patients with lesions above the midthoracic level have loss of sympathetic control of peripheral vasoconstrictor activity, leading to hypotension. These patients may tolerate changes in position poorly and require monitoring of blood pressure when positions are changed. Usually the patient is turned every 2 hours (Fig. 60-11). If not on a turning frame, the patient should not be turned unless the physician has indicated that it is safe to do so. Guidelines for turning a patient not on a turning frame are found in Guideline 60-2. Adequate preparation and time must be made for turning the patient, maintaining a gentle, firm, and steady touch.

Contractures develop rapidly in association with immobility and muscle paralysis. Atrophy of the extremities results from disuse. To avoid these complications, passive range-of-motion exercises may be prescribed within 48 to 72 hours after injury. These exercises preserve joint motion and stimulate circulation. A joint that is immobilized too long becomes fixed as a result of contractures of the tendon and joint capsule. Toes, metatarsals, ankles, knees, and hips should be put through a full range of motion at least four, and ideally five, times daily. Range-of-motion exercises can prevent many complications.

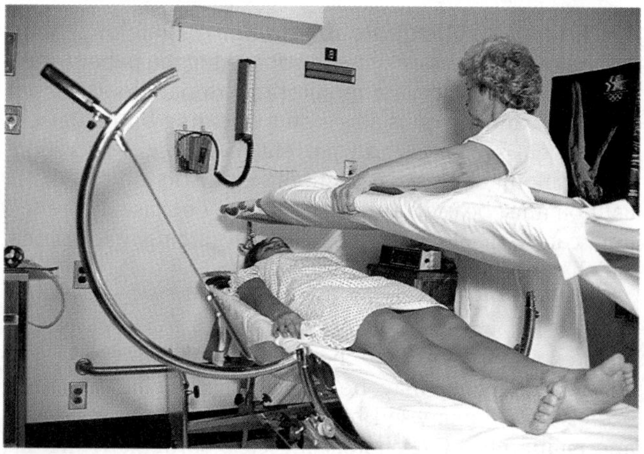

FIGURE 60-11. A patient on the Stryker frame is turned frequently to relieve pressure.

For patients with a cervical fracture without neurologic deficit, reduction in traction followed by rigid immobilization for about 16 weeks restores skeletal integrity in most patients. These patients are allowed to move gradually to an erect position. A four-poster neck brace or molded collar is applied when the patient is mobilized after traction is removed.

Maintaining Skin Integrity. Because the patient with a spinal cord injury is immobilized and has loss of feeling, there is an ever-present, life-endangering threat of pressure ulcers. In areas of local tissue ischemia where there is continuous pressure and where the peripheral circulation is inadequate as a result of the spinal shock and recumbency, pressure ulcers have developed within 6 hours. Prolonged immobilization of the patient on a transfer board increases the risk of pressure ulcers. The most common sites are over the ischial tuberosity, the greater trochanter, and the sacrum.

- The patient's position is changed at least every 2 hours. Turning not only aids in the prevention of pressure ulcers but also prevents the pooling of blood and tissue fluid in the dependent areas.
- Careful inspection of the skin is made each time the patient is turned. The skin over the pressure points is assessed for redness or breaks in the skin; the perineum is checked for soilage, and the catheter is observed for adequate drainage. The patient's general body alignment and comfort are assessed. Special attention should be given to pressure areas in contact with the transfer board.
- Every few hours the patient's skin should be washed with a mild soap, rinsed well, and *blotted* dry. Pressure-sensitive areas should be kept well lubricated and soft with bland cream or lotion. Massage should be performed gently with a circular motion.
- The patient is informed about the danger of pressure ulcers and encouraged to participate in preventive measures. (See Chapter 18 for other aspects of the prevention of pressure ulcers.)

Maintaining Urinary Elimination. Immediately after a spinal cord injury, the urinary bladder becomes atonic and cannot contract by reflex activity. Urinary retention is the immediate result of spinal cord injury. Because the patient has no sensation of bladder distention, overstretching of the bladder and detrusor muscle may occur and delay the return of bladder function.

Intermittent catheterization is carried out to avoid overstretching the bladder and urinary tract infection. If this is not feasible, an indwelling catheter is inserted temporarily. At an early stage, family members are shown how to carry out intermittant catheterization and are encouraged to participate in this facet of care, because they will be involved in long-term follow-up and must be able to recognize complications so that treatment can be instituted.

The patient is taught to record fluid intake, voiding pattern, amounts of residual urine after catheterization, quality of urine, and any unusual feelings that may be occurring.

GUIDELINE 60-2
Turning the Patient With Crutchfield Tongs

If Crutchfield tongs are used and the patient is not on a turning frame, a directive from the physician must be obtained before the patient is turned. The patient's head *should never be flexed,* either forward or laterally, and at all times must be kept in a direct line with the axis of the cervical spine.

To Turn the Patient

- Three persons should turn the patient in a logrolling fashion, making sure that the shoulder turns with the head and the neck. One nurse should support the head; the second nurse or assistant, the shoulders; and the third person, the hips and the legs.
- The nurse supporting the head gives the commands for turning.
- A pillow is placed between the legs of the patient to prevent the upper leg from slipping forward and jarring the patient's head.
- A pillow is placed longitudinally on the chest, with the patient's upper arm resting on it. The pillow prevents the shoulder from sagging and pulling on the neck as the patient is turned.
- As the patient is turned in a logrolling fashion, the traction should be moved carefully to keep it in a direct line with the cervical spine. The patient's position should be adjusted so that the traction, the patient's head, and the cervical spine are in correct alignment.
- While the nurse still supports the head in the lateral position, a small pillow is placed under the head to maintain cervical alignment.

The management of a neurogenic bladder is discussed in detail in Chapter 42.

Improving Bowel Function. Immediately after spinal cord injury, the patient usually develops a paralytic ileus due to neurogenic paralysis of the bowel and often necessitates a nasogastric tube to relieve distention and prevent aspiration.

Bowel activity usually returns within the first week. As soon as bowel sounds are heard by auscultation, the patient is given a high-calorie, high-protein, high-fiber diet, with the amount of food gradually increased. The nurse administers the prescribed stool softener to counteract the effects of immobility and pain medications. A bowel program is instituted as early as possible.

Providing Comfort Measures. Following cervical injury when tongs or calipers are in place, the patient's skull is assessed for signs of infection, including drainage around the tongs. The back of the head is checked periodically for signs of pressure and is massaged at intervals, with care taken not to move the neck. The hair around the tongs usually is shaved to facilitate inspection. Probing under encrusted areas is avoided.

The Patient in Halo Traction. Patients who have been placed in a halo device following cervical stabilization may experience a slight headache or discomfort around the skull pins for several days after the pins are inserted. The patient initially may not appreciate the rather startling appearance of this apparatus but can readily adapt to it because the device provides comfort for the unstable neck. The patient may complain of being caged in and of noise created by any object coming in contact with the steel frame but can be reassured that adaptation to such annoyances will occur.

The areas around the pin sites are cleansed daily and observed for redness, drainage, and pain. The pins are observed for loosening, which may contribute to infection. If one of the pins becomes detached, the patient's head is stabilized in a neutral position while another person notifies the neurosurgeon. A torque screwdriver should be readily available should the screws on the frame need tightening.

The skin under the halo vest is inspected for excessive perspiration, redness, and skin blistering, especially on the bony prominences. The vest is opened at the sides to allow the patient's torso to be washed. The liner of the vest is not allowed to become wet, because dampness causes skin problems. Powder is not used inside the vest, because it may contribute to the development of pressure ulcers.

Monitoring and Managing Potential Complications

Thrombophlebitis. Thrombophlebitis is a relatively common complication in patients following spinal cord injury. Over 20% of cord-injured patients develop deep vein thrombosis and thus are at risk for the development of pulmonary embolism. The patient must be assessed for symptoms of thrombophlebitis and pulmonary embolism; the occurrence of chest pain, shortness of breath, and changes in arterial blood gas values must be reported promptly to the physician. The circumferance of the thighs and calfs is measured and recorded daily; further diagnostic studies will be conducted if a significant increase in the circumference of one or both of the extremities is noted. Patients remain at risk for thrombophlebitis for up to 3 months following the initial injury. Immobilization and the associated venous stasis as well as varying degrees of autonomic disruption contribute to the high risk and susceptibility for DVT. Anticoagulation will be initiated once head and other injuries have been ruled out. Low-dose heparin may be followed by long-term oral anticoagulation (*i.e.*, Coumadin). Additional measures such as range-of-motion exercise, thigh-high elastic stockings, and adequate hydration are all important preventive measures. Pneumatic compression devices may also be used to reduce venous pooling and promote venous return. It is also important to avoid external pressure on the lower extremities that may result with flexion of the knees while the patient is in bed.

Orthostatic Hypotension. For the first 2 weeks following spinal cord injury blood pressure tends to to unstable and quite low. There is a gradual return to preinjury levels but periodic episodes of severe orthostatic hypotension frequently interfere with efforts to mobilize patients. Interruption in reflex arcs that normally produce vasoconstriction in the upright position coupled with dilation and pooling in abdominal and lower extremity vessels can result in blood pressure readings of 40 mm Hg systolic and 0 mm Hg diastolic. Orthostatic hypotension is a particularly common problem for patients with lesions above T7. It has been found that in some quadraplegic patients even slight elevations of the head can result in dramatic changes in blood pressure.

A number of techniques can be used to reduce the frequency of hypotensive episodes. Close monitoring of vital signs before and during position change is essential. Vasopressor medication can be used to treat the profound vasodilation. Thigh-high elastic stockings should be worn and will improve venous return from the lower extremities. Activity should be planned in advance and adequate time given for a slow progression of position change from recumbant to sitting and upright. Tilt tables frequently are helpful in assisting patients to make this transition.

Autonomic Hypereflexia. Autonomic hyperreflexia (autonomic dysreflexia) is an acute emergency that occurs as a result of exaggerated autonomic responses to stimuli that are innocuous in normal individuals. It will occur only after spinal shock has resolved. This syndrome is characterized by severe, pounding headache with paroxysmal hypertension, profuse diaphoresis (most often of the forehead), nasal congestion, and bradycardia. It occurs among patients with cord lesions above T6 level (the sympathetic visceral outflow level), generally after spinal shock has subsided. The sudden rise in blood pressure may cause a rupture of one or more cerebral blood vessels or lead to an increase in ICP. A number of stimuli may trigger this reflex: distended bladder (the most common cause), distended bowel, stimulation of the skin (tactile, pain, thermal stimuli), or distention or contraction of the viseral organs, especially the bowel (from constipation, impaction). Because this is an emergency situation, the objective is to remove the triggering stimulus and to avoid the possibly serious complications.

The following measures are carried out:

- ❑ The patient is placed immediately in a sitting position to lower blood pressure.
- ❑ The bladder is emptied immediately via a urinary catheter. If the catheter is not patent, it is irrigated or replaced with another catheter.
- ❑ After the symptoms subside, the rectum is examined for a fecal mass. If one is present, dibucaine ointment is inserted 10 to 15 minutes before the mass is removed, because viseral distention or contraction can cause autonomic dysreflexia.
- ❑ Any other stimulus that can be the triggering event, such as an object on the skin or a draft of cold air, must be removed.
- ❑ If these measures do not relieve the patient's hypertension and excruciating headache, a ganglionic blocking agent (hydralazine hydrochloride [Apresoline]) is prescribed and given slowly intravenously.
- ❑ The patient's medical record should be labeled with a clearly visible note about the risk for autonomic hyperreflexia.
- ❑ The patient is instructed in prevention and management measures.
- ❑ Any patient with a lesion above the T6 segment is informed that such an episode is possible and may even occur many years after the initial injury.

The rehabilitation of the patient with a permanent spinal cord injury (*i.e.*, the quadraplegic or paraplegic patient) is discussed in the next section.

Patient Education and Home Care Considerations. In most cases, patients will need long-term rehabilatation. The process begins during hospitalization as acute symptoms begin to abate or come under better control and the overall deficits and long-term effects become more clear. The goals begin to shift from merely surviving the injury to strategies necessary to cope with the alterations that injury imposes on the activities of daily living. The emphasis must now shift from ensuring that the patient is stable and free of complications to specific assessment and planning designed to meet particular patient and rehabilatation needs. Although maintaining function and preventing complications will remain important, goals regarding the skills necessary to carry out the tasks of daily living and preparation for discharge will assist in a smooth transition to rehabilatation and eventually the community. The ultimate goal of the rehabilitation process is independence. The nurse becomes a support to both the patient and the family, assisting them to accept responsibility for gaining the necessary skills.

Care for the patient with spinal cord injury must involve members from all the health care disciplines; these may include nursing, medicine, rehabilitation, respiratory therapy, physical therapy, social services, and so forth. The nurse is often in a key position to serve as coordinator of the management team and to serve as liaison with rehabilitation centers and home care agencies. The patient and family often require assistance in dealing with the psychological impact of the spinal cord injury and its consequences; referral to a psychiatric clinical nurse specialist or other mental health care professional often is helpful.

Evaluation

Expected Outcomes

1. Demonstrates improvement in gas exchange and clearance of secretions as evidenced by normal breath sounds on auscultation
   a. Breathe easily without shortness of breath
   b. Performs hourly deep breathing exercises, coughs effectively, and clears pulmonary secretions
   c. Is free of respiratory infection (*i.e.*, has normal temperature, respiratory rate and pulse, normal breath sounds, absence of purulent sputum)
2. Moves within limits of the dysfunction and demonstrates completion of exercises within functional limitations
3. Demonstrates optimal skin integrity
   a. Exhibits normal skin turgor and skin is free of reddened areas or breaks
   b. Participates in skin care and monitoring procedures within functional limitations
4. Regains urinary bladder function

a. Exhibits no signs of urinary tract infection (*i.e.*, has normal temperature, voids clear, dilute urine)
b. Consumes an adequate fluid intake
c. Participates in bladder training program within functional limitations

5. Regains bowel function
a. Reports regular pattern of bowel movement
b. Consumes adequate dietary fiber and oral fluids
c. Participates in bowel training program with functional limitations
6. Reports absence of pain and discomfort
7. Is free of complications
a. Demonstrates no signs of thrombophlebitis, deep vein thrombosis, or pulmonary embolus
b. Exhibits no manifestations of pulmonary embolism (*e.g.*, no chest pain or shortness of breath; arterial blood gases are normal)
c. Maintains blood pressure within normal limits
d. Experiences no lightheadedness with position changes
e. Exhibits no manifestations of autonomic hyperreflexia (*i.e.*, no headache, diaphoresis, nasal congestion, or bradycardia diaphoresis)

The Quadriplegic or Paraplegic Patient

Quadriplegia refers to the loss of movement and sensation in all four extremities and the trunk associated with injury to the cervical spinal cord. Paraplegia refers to loss of motion and sensation in the lower extremities and all or part of the trunk as a result of damage to the thoracic or lumbar spinal cord or to the sacral root. Both conditions most frequently follow trauma due to accidents and gunshot wounds but may also be the result of spinal cord lesions (intervertebral disc, tumor, vascular lesions), multiple sclerosis, infections and abscesses of the spinal cord, and congenital defects.

Management

The patient faces a lifetime of great disability, requiring ongoing follow-up and care and the expertise of a number of health professionals, including physicians (specifically a physiatrist), rehabilitation nurses, occupational therapist, physical therapist, psychologist, social worker, rehabilitation engineer, and vocational counselor at different times as the need arises.

As the years go by, these patients also have the same medical problems as others in the aging population. In addition, they face the threat of complications associated with their respective disability. Usually the patient is encouraged to attend a spinal clinic when problems arise. Lifetime care includes assessment of the urinary tract at prescribed intervals, because there is likelihood of continuing alteration in detrusor and sphincter function and the patient is prone to urinary tract infections.

Management includes observing and caring for any alteration in physiologic status and psychological outlook, and the prevention and management of long-term complications.

Long-term problems and complications of spinal cord injury include autonomic dysreflexia (discussed earlier), bladder and kidney infections (discussed in Chapter 42), spasticity, pressure ulcers with complications of sepsis, osteomyelitis, fistulas, and depression. Flexor muscle spasms may be particularly disabling. **Heterotopic ossification** (overgrowth of bone) in the hips, knees, shoulders, and elbows occurs in 20% to 40% of spinal cord injury patients. This complication is quite painful and can produce a loss of range of motion. The nursing role is that of emphasizing the need for vigilance in self-assessment and care.

❑ *NURSING PROCESS* *The Patient With Quadriplegia or Paraplegia*

Assessment

Assessment focuses on the patient's general condition, the presence of complications, and how the patient is managing at the particular point in time. A head-to-toe assessment and review of systems should be part of the data base, with particular emphasis on the areas prone to problems in this population. Specifically, a thorough inspection of all areas of the skin for redness or breakdown is critical. It is also important to review with the patient the established bowel and bladder program as the program must continue uninterrupted. Patients with quadriplegia or paraplegia have experienced varying degrees of loss of motor power, deep and superficial sensation, vasomotor control, bladder and bowel control, and sexual function. They are faced with potential problems related to immobility, skin breakdown and pressure ulcers, recurring urinary infection, contractures, and psychosocial disruptions. Knowledge regarding these particular problems can further guide the assessment in any setting. Nurses in all settings, including the home, must be cognizant of these potential problems in the lifetime management of these persons.

Psychosocial Assessment

An understanding of the emotional and psychological responses to quadriplegia or paraplegia is achieved by observing the responses and behaviors of the patient and family and by listening to expressed concerns. Documenting these assessments and reviewing the plan with the entire team on a regular basis provides insight into how both the patient and the family are coping with the changes in lifestyle and body functioning. Additional information frequently can be gathered from the social or psychiatric worker.

It usually takes time for the patient and the family to comprehend the magnitude of the resulting disability. They may go through stages of adjustment, including shock, disbelief, denial, depression, grief, and acceptance. During the acute phase of the injury, denial can be a protective mechanism to shield patients from the overwhelming reality of what has happened. As they realize the finality of paraplegia or quadriplegia, the grieving process may be prolonged and all-encompassing because of the recognition that long-held plans and expectations may be interrupted or permanently altered. A period of depression often follows as the patient experiences a loss of self-esteem in areas of self-identity, sexual functioning, and social and emotional roles. Self-esteem is related to being strong, loved, and lovable—all of which are threatened. Exploration and assessment of these issues can assist in developing a meaningful plan of care.

Diagnosis

Nursing Diagnoses

Based on all the assessment data, the major nursing diagnoses of the patient with quadriplegia or paraplegia may include the following:

- Immobility related to inability to walk
- Impairment of skin integrity related to permanent sensory loss and immobility
- Urinary retention related to level of spinal cord injury
- Constipation related to effects of spinal cord disruption
- Sexual dysfunction related to neurologic dysfunction
- Ineffective individual coping related to impact of dysfunction on daily living
- Knowledge deficit about requirements for long-term management

Collaborative Problems: Potential Complications

Based on all the assessment data, potential complications of quadriplegia or paraplegia that may develop include:

- Spasticity
- Infection and sepsis

Planning and Implementation

Goals. The goals for the patient may include attainment of some form of mobility, maintenance of healthy, intact skin, achievement of bladder management without infection, achievement of bowel control, achievement of sexual expression, strengthening of coping mechanisms, and absence of potential complictions.

Nursing Interventions

The patient requires extensive rehabilitation, which is less difficult if appropriate nursing management has been carried out during the acute phase of the injury or illness. (See Management of Spinal Cord Injuries [Acute Phase], p. 1798.) The nursing care is one of the determining factors in the success of the rehabilitation program. The main objective is for the patient to live as independently as possible in the home and community.

Increasing Mobility

Weight-Bearing Activities. A patient whose paralysis is due to complete severance of the cord can begin weight-bearing early, because no further damage can be incurred. The sooner muscles are strengthened, the less is the chance of disuse atrophy. The earlier the patient is brought to a standing position, the less opportunity there is for osteoporotic changes to take place in the long bones. Weight-bearing also reduces the possibility of renal calculi and enhances many other metabolic processes.

Exercise Program. The unaffected parts of the body are built up to optimal strength to promote maximal self-care. The muscles of the hands, arms, shoulders, chest, spine, abdomen, and neck must be strengthened in the paraplegic patient, because the patient must bear full weight on these muscles to ambulate. The triceps and the latissimus dorsi are important muscles used in crutch walking. The muscles of the abdomen and the back also are necessary for the balance and the maintenance of the upright position.

To strengthen these muscles, the patient can do push-ups when in a prone position and sit-ups when in a sitting position. Extending the arms while holding weights (traction weights can be used) also develops muscle strength. Squeezing rubber balls or crumbling newspaper promotes hand strength.

Through the encouragement of all of the members of the rehabilitation team, the patient develops the increased exercise tolerance needed for gait training and ambulation activities.

Mobilization. When the spine is stable enough to allow the patient to assume an upright posture, mobilization activities are initiated. A brace or vest may be used, depending on the level of the lesion. Braces and crutches enable some paraplegic patients to ambulate for short distances and even to drive manually operated automobiles. Crutch ambulation in paraplegics requires high energy expenditure. Modern technological developments, such as motorized wheelchairs and specially equipped vans, are contributing to the greater independence and mobility of patients with high-level spinal cord injuries or other lesions.

A major goal of nursing management is to help these patients overcome their sense of futility and to encourage them in the emotional adjustment that must be made before they are willing to venture into the outside world. To achieve this goal, it is important to realize that an excessively sympathetic attitude may cause patients to develop an overdependence that defeats the purpose of the entire rehabilitation program.

The patient is taught and assisted when necessary, but effort is made not to take over activities that patients can do for themselves with a little effort. This type of nursing care more than repays itself in the satisfaction of seeing a completely demoralized and helpless patient begin to find meaning in a newly emerging lifestyle.

Promoting Skin Integrity. Because these patients spend a great portion of their lives in a wheelchair, pressure ulcers are an ever-present threat. Contributing factors are permanent sensory loss over pressure areas, immobility that makes relief of pressure difficult, trauma from bumps (against the wheelchair, toilet) that cause unperceived abrasions and wounds, loss of protective function of the skin from excoriation and maceration due to excessive perspiration and possible urine and fecal incontinence, and poor general health (anemia, edema, malnutrition) leading to poor tissue perfusion.

The prevention and management of pressure ulcers are discussed in detail in Chapter 18 and under the care of the patient with a spinal cord injury (p. 1802).

The person with quadriplegia or paraplegia must take responsibility to personally monitor skin status. This involves relieving pressure and avoiding holding any position for longer than 2 hours, in addition to seeing that the skin receives meticulous attention and cleansing. The patient is taught that ulcers develop over bony prominences exposed to unrelieved pressure in the lying and sitting positions. The most vulnerable areas are identified. The paraplegic patient is instructed to use mirrors to inspect these areas morning and night, observing for redness, slight edema, or any abrasions. While in bed the patient should turn at 2-hour intervals and then inspect the skin again for redness that does not fade on pressure. The bottom sheet should be checked for wetness and for creases. The quadraplegic patient who is unable to perform these activities is encouraged to inform others of the need to check these problems and prevent them from developing.

The patient is taught to relieve pressure while in the wheelchair by doing push-ups, leaning from side to side to relieve ischial pressure, and tilting forward while leaning on a table. The caregiver for the quadriplegic patient will need to perform these activities if the patient cannot do so independently. Each person requires a wheelchair cushion prescribed to meet individual needs, which may change in time with alterations in posture, weight, and skin tolerance. A referral can be made to a rehabilitation engineer, who can measure pressure levels while the patient is sitting and then tailor the cushion and other necessary aids and assistive devices to the individual patient's needs.

The diet for the quadriplegic or paraplegic patient should be high in protein, vitamins, and calories to ensure minimal wasting of muscle, well-functioning kidneys, and the maintenance of healthy skin.

Improving Bladder Management. The effect of the spinal lesion on the bladder depends on the level of the cord injury, degree of cord damage, and length of time after injury. A patient with quadriplegia or paraplegia usually has either a reflex or a nonreflex bladder, which are discussed in Chapter 42. Both problems increase the risk of urinary tract infection.

The nurse emphasizes the importance of maintaining an adequate flow of urine by encouraging a fluid intake of about 2.5 L daily, emptying the bladder frequently so there is minimal residual urine, and giving attention to personal hygiene because infection of the bladder and kidneys almost always occurs by the ascending route. The perineum must be kept clean and dry and attention given to perianal skin after defecation. Underwear should be cotton (more absorbent) and changed at least daily.

If an external catheter (condom catheter) is used, the sheath is removed nightly; the penis is cleansed to remove urine and dried carefully because warm urine on the periurethral skin promotes growth of bacteria. Attention also is given to the collection bag. The nurse emphasizes the importance of monitoring for indications of urinary tract infection: cloudy, foul-smelling urine or *hematuria* (blood in the urine), fever, or chills.

The female patient who cannot achieve reflex bladder control or self-catheterization may need to wear pads or waterproof undergarments. Surgical intervention may be necessary to perform a urinary diversion procedure.

Establishing Bowel Control. The objective of a bowel training program is to establish bowel evacuation through reflex conditioning. This technique is described in Chapter 18. If a cord injury occurs above the sacral segments or nerve roots and there is reflex activity, the anal sphincter may be massaged to stimulate defecation. (If the cord lesion involves the sacral segment or nerve roots, anal massage is not performed because the anus may be relaxed and lack tone. Massage is also contraindicated if there is spasticity of the anal sphincter.) The anal sphincter is massaged by inserting a gloved finger (which has been adequately lubricated) 2.5 to 3.7 cm (1 to 1.5 in) into the rectum and moving it in a circular motion or from side to side. It soon becomes apparent which area triggers the defecation response. This procedure should be performed at the same time (usually every 48 hours), after a meal, and at a time that will be convenient for the patient on returning home. The patient also is taught the symptoms of impaction (frequent loose stools; constipation) and cautioned to watch for the development of hemorrhoids. A diet with sufficient fluids and fiber is essential to a successful bowel training program.

Counseling on Sexual Expression. Many paraplegic and quadriplegic patients can have some form of meaningful sexual relationship, although some modifications will have to be made. The patient and partner benefit from counseling on the range of sexual expression possible, special techniques, positions, exploration of body sensations offering sensual feelings, and urinary and bowel hygiene as related to sexual activity. Penile prostheses are available for men with erectile failure. Sexual education and counseling services are included in the rehabilitation services at spinal centers. Small group meetings in which the patients can share their feelings, receive information, and discuss sexual concerns and practical aspects are helpful in producing effective attitudes and adjustments.

Coping Mechanisms. The impact of the full realization of their disability and loss becomes marked when patients return home. Each time something new enters their life (*e.g.*, a new relationship, going to work), they are reminded anew of their limitations. Grief reactions and depression frequently are encountered.

To be able to work through this depression, patients must have some hope for relief in the future. Thus, they are guided toward a sense of confidence in their ability to achieve self-care and relative independence. The role of the nurse ranges from caretaker during the acute phase to teacher, counselor, and facilitator, as patients gain mobility and independence.

Adjustment to the disability leads to the development of realistic goals for the future, making the best of those abilities that are left intact, and reinvesting in other activities and relationships. Rejection of the disability causes self-destructive neglect and noncompliance with the therapeutic program, which leads to more frustration and depression. Crises for which interventions may be sought include social, psychologic, marital, sexual, and psychiatric problems. The family usually requires counseling, social services, and other support systems to help them cope with the changes in their lifestyle and socioeconomic status. (The psychologic implications of a disability are discussed also in Chapter 18.)

Patient Education and Home Care Considerations. Patients with quadriplegia or paraplegia are at risk for complications for the rest of their lives. Urinary tract infections and deconditioning resulting in contractures may appear and necessitate rehospitalization. For the rest of their lives, patients are at risk of developing pressure ulcers that pose a serious threat to life. To avoid these complications, the patient and a family member are taught skin care, catheter care, range-of-motion exercises, and other care techniques while the patient is still in the hospital and rehabilitation center. The teaching is reinforced during home visits by the home care nurse. Environmental modifications are made and specialized equipment is obtained before the patient goes home. Other complications during the extended care period may include lower extremity edema, joint contractures, pain, and alcohol abuse.

The home care nurse provides continuing follow-up evaluation to reinforce previous teaching and to determine if further physical help is needed. The patient's self-esteem and body-image may be very poor at this time.

Persons with high levels of social support who are satisfied with their social contacts and perceive that they have high levels of control generally report feelings of well-being despite major physical disability. Thus, it is beneficial for the nurse to assess and promote further development of the support system of each patient.

The local counselor for the Division of Vocational Rehabilitation works with the patient with respect to job placement or additional educational or vocational training.

The patient requires continuing, life-long follow-up by the physician, physical therapist, and other rehabilitation team members, because the neurologic deficit is usually permanent and new problems can erupt that require prompt attention before they take their toll in additional physical impairment, time, morale, and financial costs.

Monitoring and Managing Complications

Spasticity. Muscle spasticity is one of the most problematic complications of quadriplegia and paraplegia. These incapacitating flexor or extensor spasms, which occur below the level of the spinal cord lesion, interefere with both the rehabilatation process and activities of daily living. Spasticity results from an imbalance between the facilatory and inhibitory effects on neurons that exist normally. The area of the cord distal to the site of injury or lesion becomes disconnected from the higher inhibitory centers located in the brain. Facilatory impulses, which originate from muscles, skin, and ligaments, will thus predominate.

Spasticity is defined as a condition of increased muscle tone in a muscle that is weak. Initial resistance to stretching is quickly followed by sudden relaxation. The stimulus that precipatates spasm can be either obvious, such as movement or position change, or subtle such as slight jarring of the wheelchair. The majority of patients with quadriplegia or paraplegia experience some degree of spasticity. With SCI, the onset of spasticity usually occurs from a few weeks to 6 months following injury. The same muscles that are flaccid during the period of spinal shock will develop spasticity during recovery. The intensity of spasticity tends to peak around 2 years postinjury at which time the symptoms tend to regress.

Management of spasticity is complex and will be determined based on the severity of symptoms and the degree of incapacitation. Antispamodic medication such as Valium, Baclofen, and Dantrium are frequently effective in controlling spasm but can cause drowsiness, weakness, and vertigo in some patients. Passive range-of-motion exercises and frequent turning and repositioning are helpful as stiffness tends to increase spasticity. These activities also are essential in the prevention of contractures, pressure ulcers, and bowel and bladder dysfunction. The major problems that complicate day-to-day care are the difficulty with positioning and the lack of mobility. There are a number of surgical procedures that have been tried with varying degrees of success. These techniques are used if more conservative approaches fail.

Infection and Sepsis. Quadriplegic and paraplegic patients are at increased risk of infection and sepsis from a variety of sources: urinary tract, respiratory tract, and pressure ulcers. Sepsis remains a major cause of morbidity and mortality in these patients. Prevention of infection and sepsis is essential to reduce morbidity and mortality through maintenance of skin integrity, complete emptying of the bladder at regular intervals, and prevention of urinary and fecal incontinence. Risk of respiratory infection can be decreased by avoiding contact with persons with symptoms of respiratory infection, coughing and deep breathing exercises to prevent pooling of respiratory secretions, yearly administration of prophylactic influenza vaccines, and cessation of smoking. A high- protein diet is important in maintaining an adequate immune system as is avoidance of factors that may negatively affect immune system function; these include excessive stress, and use of illicit drugs and excessive alcohol.

If infection occurs, the quadriplegic or paraplegic patient requires thorough assessment and prompt treatment. Antibiotic therapy and adequate hydration in addition to local measures (depending on the site of infection) are initiated immediately. Urinary tract infections are minimized or prevented by:

- Aseptic technique in catheter management
- Adequate hydration
- Bladder training program
- Prevention of over distension of the bladder and stasis

Skin breakdown and infection are prevented by:

- Maintenance of a turning schedule
- Frequent back care
- Regular assessment of all skin areas
- Regular cleansing and lubrication of the skin
- Pressure relief, particularly over broken skin areas, bony prominances, and heels
- Wrinkle-free bed linen

Pulmonary infections are managed and prevented by:

- Frequent coughing, turning, and deep breathing exercises and chest physiotherapy
- Aggressive respiratory care and suctioning of the airway if a tracheostomy is present
- Assisted coughing
- Adequate hydration

Infections of any kind can be life-threatening. Therefore, aggressive nursing interventions are key to their prevention and management.

Evaluation

Expected Outcomes

See p. 1804 for other expected outcomes.

1. Attains some form of mobility
2. Maintains healthy, intact skin
3. Achieves bladder control, absence of urinary tract infection

4. Achieves bowel control
5. Reports sexual satisfaction
6. Shows improved adaptation to environment and others
7. Exhibits reduction is spasticity
8. Reports understanding of the precipitating factors
9. Reports understanding of measures to reduce spasticity
10. Describes long-term management required
11. Exhibits absence of complications (spasticity, infection, and sepsis)

Intraspinal Tumors

Tumors within the spine are classified according to their anatomic relation to the spinal cord. They include *intramedullary* lesions (within the spinal cord), *extramedullary-intradural* lesions (within the subarachnoid space), and *extradural* lesions (outside the dural membrane). Tumors that occur within the spinal cord or exert pressure on it cause symptoms ranging from weakness and loss of reflexes above the tumor level and localized or shooting pains, to progressive loss of motor function and paralysis. Usually sharp pain occurs in the area that is innervated by the spinal roots that arise from the cord in the region of the tumor. In addition, increasing paralysis develops below the level of the lesion.

The diagnosis is made by neurologic examination and myelography in combination with CT scanning and MRI.

Preoperative Management

The patient is assessed for weakness, muscle wasting, spasticity, and sensory or sphincter disorders. The patient is assessed for potential pulmonary problems, especially if a cervical tumor is present. The patient also is evaluated for coagulation deficiencies. A history of aspirin intake is obtained and reported because the use of aspirin may create problems with hemostasis postoperatively. Breathing exercises are taught and demonstrated preoperatively.

Surgical Management

The removal of the tumor is desirable but not always possible. The goal is to remove as much tumor as possible while sparing uninvolved portions of the spinal cord. Microsurgical techniques have improved the prognosis for surgical treatment of intramedullary tumors. The prognosis is related to the degree of neurologic impairment at the time of surgery, the speed with which symptoms occurred, and the tumor's origin. Patients with large neurologic deficits before surgery usually do not make significant functional recovery even after successful tumor removal.

Other treatment modalities include partial removal of the tumor, decompression of the spinal cord, chemotherapy, and radiation therapy.

If the patient has epidural spinal cord compression resulting from metastatic cancer (from breast, prostate, or lung), high-dose dexamethasone combined with radiation therapy is effective in relieving pain. (Spinal cord compression by tumor is discussed in Chapter 16).

Postoperative Nursing Interventions

The nursing management is similar to that after disc surgery (see p. 1811). The patient is monitored for deterioration in neurologic status. A sudden onset of neurologic deficit is an ominous sign. It may be due to vertebral collapse associated with spinal cord infarction. Neurologic checks are made, with emphasis on evaluating arm and leg movement, strength, and sensation. Sensory function is assessed by pinching the skin of the arms, legs, and trunk to determine if there is loss of feeling and, if so, at what level. Vital signs are monitored at intervals.

If the tumor was in the cervical area, there is always the possibility of postoperative respiratory compromise. Chest movement is observed for symmetry and abdominal breathing, and the chest is auscultated for abnormal breath sounds. In the instance of a high cervical lesion, the endotracheal tube is left in place until adequate respiratory function is assured. Deep breathing and coughing are encouraged.

The area over the patient's bladder is palpated for urinary retention. Incontinence may be present. Urinary dysfunction usually implies significant decompensation of spinal cord function. An intake and output record is maintained. Additionally, the abdomen is auscultated for bowel sounds.

The prescribed pain medication should be given in adequate amounts and at appropriate intervals to relieve pain and prevent its recurrence. Pain is the hallmark of spinal metastasis. Patients with sensory root involvement or vertebral collapse may suffer excruciating pain and require effective pain management.

The bed is usually kept flat. The patient is turned as a unit, keeping shoulders and hips aligned. The back is kept straight. The side-lying position usually is the most comfortable because it avoids pressure on the wound. A pillow is placed between the knees of the patient in a side-lying position, and extreme knee flexion is avoided.

Staining of the dressing may indicate leakage of CSF. Any CSF leakage from the surgical site may lead to serious infection or to an inflammatory reaction in the surrounding tissues that can cause severe pain in the postoperative period.

Patient Education

Patients with residual sensory involvement are cautioned about the dangers of extremes in temperature. They should be alert to the dangers of heating devices (*e.g.*, hot water bottles, heating pads, space heaters). The patient is taught to check skin integrity daily.

A patient who has impaired motor function related to motor weakness or paralysis may require training in activities of daily living and an assistive device such as a cane or walker.

Herniation of an Intervertebral Disc

The intervertebral disc is a cartilaginous plate that forms a cushion between the vertebral bodies. This tough, fibrous material is incorporated in a capsule. A ball-like cushion in the center of the disc is called the *nucleus pulposus*. In

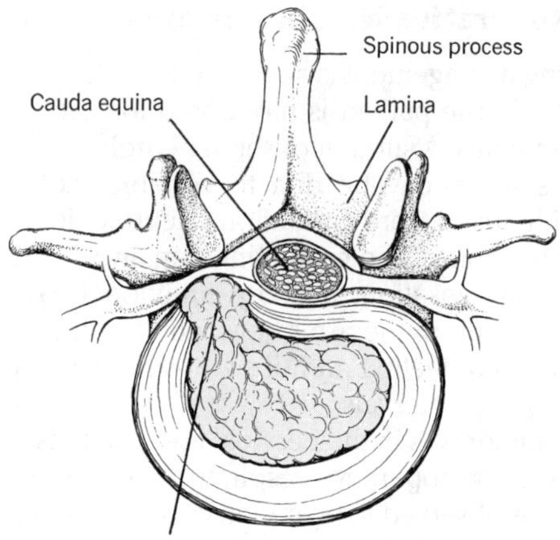

FIGURE 60-12. Ruptured vertebral disc.

herniation of the intervertebral disc (ruptured disc), the nucleus of the disc protrudes into the annulus (the fibrous ring around the disc), with subsequent nerve compression. Protrusion or rupture of the nucleus pulposus usually is preceded by degenerative changes that occur with aging. Loss of protein polysaccharides in the disc decreases the water content of the nucleus pulposus. The development of radiating cracks in the annulus weakens resistance to nucleus herniation. After trauma (falls, accidents, and repeated minor stresses, such as lifting), the cartilage may be injured.

In most patients, the immediate symptoms of trauma are short lived, and those resulting from injury to the disc do not appear for months or years. Then, with degeneration in the disc, the capsule pushes back into the spinal canal, or it may rupture and allow the nucleus pulposus to be pushed back against the dural sac or against a spinal nerve as it emerges from the spinal column (Fig. 60-12). This sequence produces pain due to pressure in the area of distribution of the involved nerve endings. Continued pressure may produce degenerative changes in the involved nerve, such as changes in sensation and reflex action.

Clinical Manifestations

A herniated disc with accompanying pain may occur in any portion of the spine: cervical, thoracic (rare), or lumbar. The clinical manifestations depend on the location, the rate of development (acute or chronic), and the effect on the surrounding structures.

Diagnostic Evaluation

Where available, MRI has become the diagnostic tool of choice for localizing even small disc protrusions, particularly for lumbar spine disease. In patients where clinical symptoms and the pathology seen on MRI are discrepant, CT and myelogram will then be performed. A neurologic examination is carried out to determine if there is reflex, sensory, or motor impairment from root compression and to provide a baseline for future assessment. Electromyography (EMG) may be used to localize the specific spinal nerve roots involved.

Management

Herniations of the cervical and the lumbar discs occur most commonly and usually are managed conservatively with bedrest and medication. The specific conservative management, along with surgical interventions for each form of herniation, are discussed below.

Disc Surgery. In general, surgical excision of a herniated disc is performed when there is evidence of a progressing neurologic deficit (muscle weakness and atrophy, loss of sensory and motor function, loss of sphincter control), and continuing pain and sciatica that are unresponsive to conservative management. The goal of surgical treatment is to lessen the pressure on the nerve root to relieve pain and reverse neurologic deficits. Microsurgical techniques are making it possible to remove precisely that amount of tissue that is absolutely necessary. This approach better preserves the integrity of normal tissue and imposes less trauma on the body. During these procedures, spinal cord function can be monitored electrophysiologically.

To achieve the goal of pain relief, several surgical techniques are used, depending on the type of disc herniation, surgical morbidity, and overall results of surgery:

Discectomy—removal of herniated or extruded fragments of intervertebral disc

Laminectomy—removal of the lamina to expose the neural elements in the spinal canal; allows the surgeon to inspect the spinal canal, identify and remove pathology, and relieve compression of the cord and roots

Laminotomy—division of the lamina of a vertebra

Discectomy with fusion—a bone graft (from iliac crest or bone bank) is used to fuse the vertebral spinous process; the object of spinal fusion is to bridge over the defective disc to stabilize the spine and reduce the rate of recurrence

Surgeries for herniated cervical disc and lumbar disc are discussed in detail in the sections that follow.

Herniation of a Cervical Intervertebral Disc

The cervical spine is subjected to stresses that result from disc degeneration (from aging, occupational stresses) and *spondylosis* (degenerative changes occurring in disc and adjacent vertebral bodies). Cervical disc degeneration may lead to lesions that can cause damage to the spinal cord and its roots.

A cervical disc herniation usually occurs at the C5–C6 and C6–C7 interspaces. Pain and stiffness may occur in the neck, the top of the shoulders, and the region of the scapulae. Sometimes patients interpret these signs as symptoms of heart trouble or bursitis. Pain may also occur in the upper extremities and head, accompanied by paresthesia and numbness of the upper extremities. The diagnosis is usually confirmed by cervical MRI.

Management

The goals of treatment are (1) to rest and immobilize the cervical spine to give the soft tissues time to heal, and (2) to reduce inflammation in the supporting tissues and the affected nerve roots in the cervical spine. Bed rest (usually 2 weeks) is important, because it eliminates the stress of gravity and frees the cervical spine from having to support the weight of the head. It also reduces inflammation and edema in soft tissues around the disc, relieving pressure on the nerve roots. Proper positioning on a firm mattress may bring dramatic relief from pain.

Immobilization. The cervical spine may be rested and immobilized by a cervical collar, cervical traction, or a brace. A collar allows maximal opening of the intervertebral foramina and holds the head in a neutral or slightly flexed position. The patient may have to wear the collar 24 hours a day during the acute phase. The skin under the collar is inspected for irritation. When the patient is free of pain, cervical isometric exercises are started to strengthen the muscles in the neck.

Traction. Cervical traction is accomplished by means of a head halter attached to a pulley and weight. It increases vertebral separation and thus relieves pressure on the nerve roots. The head of the bed is elevated to provide counteraction. If the skin becomes irritated, the halter can be padded. Experience has shown that a male patient may suffer more skin irritation if he shaves; the beard offers a natural form of padding.

Pain Relief. Hot, moist compresses (for 10 to 20 minutes) applied to the back of the neck several times daily increase blood flow to the muscles and help to relax the spastic muscles as well as the patient. Analgesics are given during the acute phase to relieve pain, and sedatives may be administered to control the anxiety often associated with cervical disc disease. Muscle relaxants are administered to interrupt the cycle of muscle spasm and to promote patient comfort. Anti-inflammatory drugs (aspirin, phenylbutazone [Butazolidin]) or corticosteroids are given to treat the inflammatory response that usually occurs in the supporting tissues and affected nerve roots. Occasionally an injection of a corticosteroid drug into the epidural space may be tried as a means of relieving radicular (spinal nerve root) pain. Anti-inflammatory agents are given with food and antacids to prevent gastrointestinal irritation. Periodic complete blood counts are indicated to detect the development of blood dyscrasias because hematologic toxicity to phenylbutazone can occur.

Surgical Management

Surgical excision of the herniated disc may be necessary when there is a significant neurologic deficit, progression of a neurologic deficit, evidence of cord compression, or pain that either fails to improve or worsens. A cervical discectomy, with or without fusion, may be performed to alleviate symptoms. In the cervical area, an anterior approach may be used through a transverse incision in the neck to remove disc material that has herniated into the spinal canal and foramina, or a posterior approach may be used at the appropriate level of the cervical spine.

Microsurgery may be performed in selected patients through a small incision and using magnification techniques. The patient who undergoes microsurgery usually has less tissue trauma and pain and consequently a shorter hospital stay than following conventional surgical approaches.

Postoperative Complications

Potential complications for the anterior approach include carotid or vertebral artery injury, recurrent laryngeal nerve dysfunction, esophageal perforation, and airway obstruction. Complications of the posterior approach include damage to the nerve root or to the spinal cord due to retraction or contusion of either of these structures, resulting in weakness of muscles supplied by the nerve root or cord.

❑ NURSING PROCESS
The Patient Undergoing a Cervical Discectomy

Assessment

The patient is asked about past injuries to the neck (whiplash), because unresolved trauma may cause persistent discomfort, pain and tenderness, and symptoms of arthritis in the injured joint of the cervical spine. Assessment of the patient's problems includes determining the onset, location and radiation of pain, paresthesias, limited movement, and diminished function of the neck, shoulders, and upper extremities. It is important to determine whether or not the symptoms are bilateral, because with large herniations bilateral symptoms may be due to cord compression. Examination of the area around the cervical spine includes palpation to assess muscle tone and tenderness.

Range of motion in the neck and shoulders is evaluated. The patient also is asked about any health problems that may influence the postoperative course. The nurse determines the patient's need for information about the surgical procedure and reinforces what has been explained by the physician. Strategies for pain management are discussed with the patient.

Postoperative Assessment

Assessment includes monitoring the blood pressure and pulse for evaluation of the cardiovascular status. The patient is evaluated for bleeding that is manifested by the complaint of excessive pressure in the neck or severe pain in the incisional area. The dressing is inspected for serosanguineous drainage, which suggests a dural leak. In this event, meningitis is a threat. A complaint of headache requires careful evaluation. Neurologic checks are made for upper and lower extremity weakness because cord compression may produce rapid or delayed onset of paralysis.

Throughout the postoperative course, the patient is monitored frequently to detect any signs of respiratory difficulty. Occasionally, during surgery, the recurrent laryngeal nerve may be injured by retractors, resulting in hoarseness and inability to cough effectively. The elimination of pulmonary secretions then becomes a problem requiring chest physical therapy.

One sign to observe for after an anterior cervical discectomy is a sudden return of radicular (spinal nerve root) pain, which may indicate that the spine is unstable.

Diagnosis

Nursing Diagnoses

Based on all the assessment data, the patient's major nursing diagnoses may include the following:

- Pain related to the surgical procedure
- Impaired physical mobility related to postoperative surgical regimen
- Knowledge deficit relative to the postoperative course and home care management

Other nursing diagnoses may include preoperative anxiety, postoperative constipation, urinary retention related to surgical procedure and dehydration, and self-care deficits related to neck orthosis; and sleep pattern disturbance related to disruption in lifestyle.

Collaborative Problems/ Potential Complications

Based on all the assessment data, the potential complications may include the following:

- Hematoma at the surgical site
- Recurrent or persistent pain following surgery

Planning and Implementation

Goals. The goals for the patient may include relief of pain, improved mobility, increased knowledge and self-care ability, and prevention of complications.

Nursing Interventions

Relieving Pain. The patient may be kept flat in bed for 12 to 24 hours. If the patient has had a bone fusion with bone removed from the iliac crest, considerable pain may be experienced. Interventions consist of monitoring the donor site for hematoma formation, administering the prescribed postoperative analgesic, positioning for comfort, and reassuring the patient that the pain can be relieved. If the patient experiences a sudden reappearance of pain, extrusion of the graft may have occurred, requiring reoperation and surgical repositioning of the graft. It should be promptly reported.

Usually the major complaints of the patient are a sore throat, hoarseness, and dysphagia due to temporary edema. These symptoms are relieved by throat lozenges, voice rest, and humidification. A blenderized diet may be given if the patient has dysphagia.

Monitoring and Managing Potential Complications. Bleeding at the surgical site and subsequent hematoma formation may occur. Severe localized pain not relieved by pain medication should be reported to the surgeon. Change in neurologic status (motor or sensory function) further suggests hematoma necessitating surgery to prevent irreversible motor and sensory deficits.

Improving Mobility. Postoperatively a cervical collar (neck orthosis) usually is worn, which contributes to limited neck motion and altered mobility. Patients are taught to turn the body instead of the neck when looking from side to side. The neck should be kept in a neutral (midline) position. Patients are assisted during position changes, making sure that head, shoulders, and thorax are kept aligned. When assisting a patient to a sitting position, the nurse supports the patient's neck and shoulders. Patients should wear shoes when ambulating to increase stability.

Patient Education and Home Care Considerations. The patient's hospital stay is likely to be short; therefore, the patient and family should understand the care that is important for a smooth recovery. Patients and family members are instructed to monitor for infection; if fever, wound drainage, or increased pain occurs, medical attention should be sought.

The cervical collar usually is worn for about 6 weeks. Patients are cautioned against flexing, extending, or rotating the neck in any extreme manner. The prone position should be avoided while sleeping. The head is to be kept in a neutral position. Patients should not prop themselves up in bed with pillows to minimize neck flexion.

The patient is instructed in care and use of the cervical collar as follows: Wear the collar at all times until directed otherwise by the physician. Wash the neck twice a day with mild soap. Keep the neck still while the collar is open. With the assistance of a helper, wash your neck in steps: (1) Lie flat on your back. Open the Velcro tabs on each side of the collar and remove its front portion. Gently wash and dry your neck. (2) Replace the front part of the collar and refasten the tabs. (3) Turn to one side with a thin pillow under your head. Open one tab. Gently wash and dry the back of the neck. Refasten the tab. (4) Turn to the other side and wash and dry this side. Refasten the tab. Place a wrinkle-free silk scarf under the collar to increase comfort. Men are instructed to shave without moving or twisting the neck. This may be done *with help* while lying flat or sitting. Only the front part of the collar is removed for shaving.

Sitting or standing for more than 30 minutes can cause neck strain. Patients are advised to alternate tasks in which the body does not move (*e.g.*, reading) with tasks that require greater body movement. Long automobile rides are avoided, because vibration is detrimental to the spine. Patients are instructed to see their physician prescribed intervals to document the disappearance of old symptoms and for examination of range of motion of the neck. The nurse assesses the patient's understanding of these limitations and recommendations. Additionally, the nurse assists the patient in identifying strategies to cope with activities of daily living (*i.e.*, self-care and child care) and minimize risks to the surgical site.

Recurrent or persistent pain may occur despite removal of the offending disc or disc fragments. Patients who undergo discectomy usually have consented to surgery after prolonged pain; they have often undergone repeated courses of ineffective conservative management and previous surgeries to relieve the pain. Therefore, the recurrence or persistence of symptoms, including pain and sensory deficits, postoperatively is often discouraging for the patient and family. The patient who experiences recurrence of symptoms requires emotional support and understanding. Additionally, the patient is assisted in modifying activities and in considering options for subsequent treatment.

Evaluation

Expected Outcomes

1. Achieves increasing comfort
2. Attains improved mobility
3. Acquires knowledge for self-care
   a. Lists the signs and symptoms to be reported
   b. Identifies prescribed activity limitations and restrictions
4. Is free of complications
   a. Reports no increase in incisional pain or sensory symptoms
   b. Demonstrates normal findings on neurologic assessment

Herniation of a Lumbar Disc

Most lumbar disc herniations occur at the L4–L5 or the L5–S1 interspaces. A lumbar disc produces low back pain accompanied by varying degrees of sensory and motor impairment. The patient complains of low back pain with muscle spasms, which is followed by radiation of the pain into one hip and down into the leg (*sciatica*). Pain is aggravated by actions that increase intraspinal fluid pressure (bending, lifting, straining, as in sneezing and coughing) and usually is relieved by bed rest. Usually there is some type of postural deformity because pain causes an alteration of the normal spinal mechanics. If the patient lies on the back and attempts to raise a leg in a straight position, pain radiates into the leg because this maneuver (*straight leg raising test*) stretches the sciatic nerve. Additional signs include muscle weakness, alterations in tendon reflexes, and sensory loss.

Diagnostic Evaluation

The diagnosis of lumbar disc disease is based on the history and physical findings and the use of imaging techniques such as MRI, CT, and myelogram.

Management

The objectives of treatment are to relieve the pain, slow the progression of the disease, and to increase the functional ability of the patient. Bed rest on a firm mattress (to limit spinal flexion) is encouraged to reduce the weight load and gravitational forces, thereby freeing the disc from stress. The patient is allowed to assume a comfortable position; usually, a semi-Fowler's position with moderate hip and knee flexion to relax the back muscles is most satisfactory. While in the side-lying position, a pillow is placed between the legs. To get out of bed, the patient lies on one side while pushing up to a sitting position.

Because muscle spasm is prominent during the acute phase, muscle relaxants are used. Anti-inflammatory agents and systemic corticosteroids may be administered to counter the inflammation that usually occurs in the supporting tissues and the affected nerve roots. Moist heat and massage help to relax spastic muscles and produce a sedative effect on the patient. See also Nursing Process: The Patient With Low Back Pain in Chapter 63 for nursing interventions.

Surgical Management

In the lumbar region, surgical treatment includes lumbar disc excision through a posterolateral **laminotomy** and the newer techniques of microdiscectomy and percutaneous **discectomy.**

Microdiscectomy incorporates the use of the operating microscope to visualize the offending disc and compressed nerve roots; it permits a smaller incision (2.5 cm [1 in]) and minimal blood loss, and takes about 30 minutes of operating time. Generally it involves a shorter hospital stay and the patient makes a more rapid recovery.

Percutaneous discectomy is an alternative treatment for herniated intervertebral discs of the lumbar spine at the L4–L5 level. One approach in current use is through a 2.5-cm (1-in) incision just above the iliac crest. A tube, trocar, or cannula is inserted under x-ray guidance through the retroperitoneal space to the involved disc space. Specially lengthened instruments are used to remove the disc. The operating time is about 15 minutes. Blood loss and postoperative pain are minimal, and the patient is generally discharged within 2 days after surgery. An example of a critical pathway for laminectomy is found on p. 1814.

The disadvantage of this procedure involves the possibility of damage to structures located in the surgical pathway.

Preoperative Nursing Management

Most patients fear surgery on any part of the spine, and therefore need assurance (that surgery will not weaken the back) and explanations all along the way. When data are being collected for the health history, any complaints of pain, paresthesia, and muscle spasm are recorded to provide a baseline for comparison after surgery. Preoperative assessment should also include an evaluation of movement in the extremities as well as bladder and bowel function. To facilitate the postoperative turning procedure, the patient is taught to turn as a unit (logroll), as part of the preoperative preparation (Fig. 60-13). Other facets of the postoperative regimen that should be practiced before surgery are deep-breathing, coughing, and muscle-setting exercises, which will help maintain muscle tone.

Postoperative Nursing Management

After lumbar disc excision, the vital signs are checked frequently and the wound is inspected for evidence of hemorrhage, because vascular injury is a complication of disc surgery. Because postoperative neurologic deficits may occur from nerve root injury, the sensation and motor power of the lower extremities are evaluated at specified intervals, along with the color and temperature of the legs and sensation of the toes. It is also important to assess for possible urinary retention, another sign of possible neurologic deterioration.

Most patients walk to the bathroom the same day as surgery, and all but a few are home by the second postoperative day. They are instructed in how to turn in bed (see

CRITICAL PATHWAY
Laminectomy

Outcome Criteria

Discharge to rehab POD #4 ☐ Ambulates independently ☐ Demonstrates knowledge of back precautions

	PAT Date:	OR Date:	POD #1 Date:	POD #2 Date:	POD #3 Date:
Assessments	History and physical NSG assessment* Evaluation social services/ home care	Post-op assessment*	Review of systems assessment*	Review of systems assessment*	Review of systems assessment*
Consults		PT/OT consult as needed			
Labs and Diagnostics	CBC PT/PTT EKG CXR CHEM7	Type & screen	H & H		
Interventions		Temptek*, Hemovac, Teds/Kendalls*, incentive spirometry*, obtain binder and elevated toilet seat*, straight cath PRN*, routine postop vital signs neurovascular checks with V.S. and q20*	Temptek*, DC Hemovac, Teds/Kendalls*, incentive spirometry*, Tegaderm / 4 × 4 / tape for PT DC*, V S W/ N.V. checks Q4*	Temptek*, incentive spirometry*, Teds/Kendalls*, change post op DSG*, vs W/N.V. checks TID*	D.C. Temptek*, incentive spirometry*, Teds*, apply Tegaderm for shower and replace w/dsg after shower*, VS W/N.V. checks*
IV's		IVF's*	DC IVF's if TOL diet; maintain HL or KVO IV on PCA*	DC H.L.*	
Medication	D/C ASA NSAIDS	Preop ABX*, PCA/IM analgesia*, IV ABX's*, stool softener*	DC PCA / IM analgesia*, begin PO analgesia*, IV ABX's*	PO analgesia*	PO analgesics*
Diet/GI		Clear; ADV as TOL	House MOM HS PRN*	MOM/SUPP PRN*	Supp/Fleets PRN*
Activity		Bedrest*, HOB <45°, logrolling*, bed exercises 1 hr. W/A*	Ambulate 1/2 hall BID w/binder in AM/PM/W/ assist*, OOB-BRP with elevated toilet seat*, no sitting or limited to <20 mins. w/meals*, bed exercises*	Ambulate 1/2 hall TID am, afternoon, eve independently/demonstrates safe transfer technique*/min. assist. W/ADLS/apply binder independently*, bed exercise 1 hour W/A*	OOB AD LIB independently w/binder*, independent W/ADL's*, bed exercises 1 hour W/A
Teaching	Review patient critical path*, give written itinerary*, review back basics booklet, C + DB exercises*, incentive spirometry*, bed exercises*, Teds and Kendalls*, activity limits*, logrolling*, PCA*	Review logrolling and proper positioning*	Teach transfer technique*, review back precautions*, give patient low back surgery discharge instructions*	Review back precautions PRN*, review written DC instructions*, teach wound care to patient and family, teach proper positioning for transportation via car*	Review all previous instructions*
D/C, Planning & Follow-Up	D/C planning, Rx for elevated toilet seat, arrangements for transportation or bed if needed		Social service if transportation is needed, home care if hospital bed is needed	Review all DC needs*, check that elevated toilet seat is available for home use*	Provide Rx's w/phone number, DC to home
*NSG Activities					
V = Variance	V V V	V V V	V V V	V V V	V V V
N = No Var.	N N N	N N N	N N N	N N N	N N N
NSG Care Performed:	☐ ☐ ☐	☐ ☐ ☐	☐ ☐ ☐	☐ ☐ ☐	☐ ☐ ☐
→	1. ________	1. ________	1. ________	1. ________	1. ________
Signatures: →	2. ________	2. ________	2. ________	2. ________	2. ________
→	3. ________	3. ________	3. ________	3. ________	3. ________

Legend: ABS or ABX = antibiotics; ADL's = activities of daily living; ADV = advance; ASA = salicylic acid; CHEM–7 = electrolyte screen; CXR = chest x-ray; D/C = discontinue or discharge; F/U = follow-up; H&H = hemoglobin and hematocrit; HL = heparin lock; HOB = head of bed; IVF's = intravenous fluids; KVO = keep vein open; N.V. = neurovascular; NSG = nursing; OT = occupational therapy; PCA = patient controlled analgesia; PT = physical therapy; PTT = prothrombin time; PTT = partial thromboplastin time; SOC SVCS = social services; SUPP = suppository; W/ = with; WA = while awake.

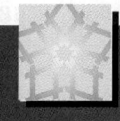

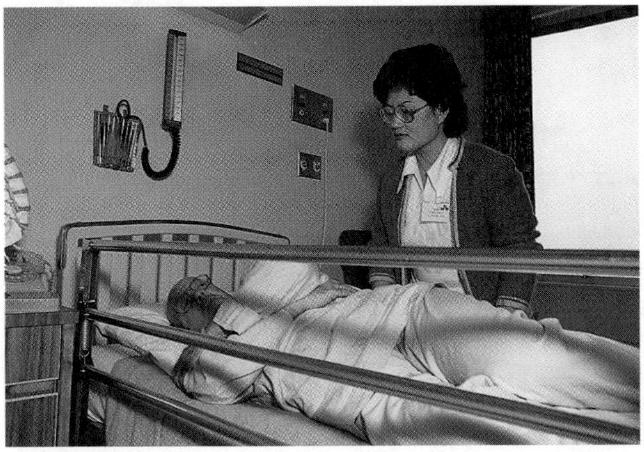

FIGURE 60-13. Logrolling technique for turning is taught to the laminectomy patient in the preoperative period.

below) and taught an exercise routine. Sitting is discouraged except for defecation.

To position the patient, a pillow is placed under the head, and the knee rest is elevated slightly, because slight knee flexion relaxes the muscles of the back. When the patient is lying on one side, however, extreme knee flexion must be avoided. The patient is encouraged to move from side to side to relieve pressure, but is first reassured that no injury will result from moving. When the patient is ready to turn, the bed is placed in a flat position and a pillow is placed between the legs. Turning is performed with the body as a unit (logrolling), without twisting the back.

To get out of bed, the patient lies on one side while pushing up to a sitting position. At the same time, the nurse eases the patient's legs over the side of the bed. Coming to a sitting or standing posture is accomplished by one long, smooth motion.

In cases requiring discectomy with fusion, the patient has an additional surgical wound if bone fragments are taken from the iliac crest or fibula to serve as wedges in the spine. The recovery period is somewhat longer than for those patients who have undergone removal of the ruptured portion of the disc without a spinal fusion, because bony union must take place.

Complications of Disc Surgery

A person having a disc procedure at one level may have degenerative process at other levels of the vertebral column. A herniation relapse may occur at the same level or elsewhere, so that the patient may become a candidate for another disc procedure. Arachnoiditis, (inflammation of the arachnoid membrane) may occur after surgery (and after myelography); it involves an insidious onset of diffuse, frequently burning pain in the lower back, radiating into the buttocks. Disc excision can leave adhesions and scarring around the spinal nerves and dura, which then produce inflammatory changes that create chronic neuritis and neurofibrosis. Disc surgery may relieve pressure on the spinal nerves, but it does not reverse the effects of neural injury and scarring and the pain that ensues. *Failed disc syndrome* (recurrence of sciatica after lumbar discectomy) remains a common cause of disability.

Patient Education

The patient is advised that activity is to be gradually increased up to the point of tolerance because it takes up to 6 weeks for the ligaments of the muscles to heal. Excessive activity may result in spasm of the paraspinal muscles.

Activities that produce flexion strain on the spine (*e.g.*, driving a car) should be avoided until healing has taken place. Heat may be applied to the back to soothe and relax muscle spasms and help absorb exudates in the tissues. Scheduled rest periods are important. Usually the patient is advised to avoid heavy work for 2 to 3 months after surgery. Exercises are prescribed to strengthen the abdominal and erector spinal muscles. A back brace or corset may be necessary if back pain persists (see also Patient Education for Low Back Pain in Chapter 63).

Cranial Nerve Disorders

There are 12 pairs of cranial nerves that emerge from the lower surface of the brain and pass through the *foramina* (openings) in the skull (Fig. 60-14). They are classified as motor, sensory, and mixed nerves. The cranial nerves are numbered in the order in which they arise from the brain. The names of the cranial nerves suggest their primary function or some anatomic characteristic. Most cranial nerves originate in the brain stem and innervate the head, neck, and structures associated with special senses.

The cranial nerves are examined separately and in sequence (see Chap. 58). Some cranial nerve deficits can be detected by observing the patient's face, eye movements, speech, and swallowing. Electromyography is used to investigate motor and sensory dysfunction. MRI produces excellent images of the cranial nerves and brain stem.

Because the brain stem and cranial nerves involve vital motor, sensory, or autonomic functions of the body, these nerves may be affected by conditions arising primarily within these structures or in secondary extension from adjacent disease processes. An overview of disorders that may affect each of the cranial nerves, including clinical manifestations and nursing interventions, is presented in Table 60-2. The following discussions center on trigeminal neuralgia, a condition affecting the fifth cranial nerve, and on Bell's palsy, caused by involvement of the seventh cranial nerve.

Trigeminal Neuralgia (Tic Douloureux)

Trigeminal neuralgia is a condition of the fifth cranial nerve characterized by paroxysms of pain similar to an electric shock or a lancinating burning sensation in the area innervated by one or more branches of the trigeminal nerve. The pain ends as abruptly as it starts. Each pain episode can be described as stabbing, lasting from a few seconds to minutes and produces contraction of some of the facial muscles, such as a sudden closing of the eye or a twitch of the mouth; hence the name *tic douloureux* (painful twitch). The cause is not certain, but chronic compression or irritation of the trigeminal nerve or degenerative changes in the gasserian ganglion are suggested causes. Some investigators believe that the condition may be due to vascular pressure

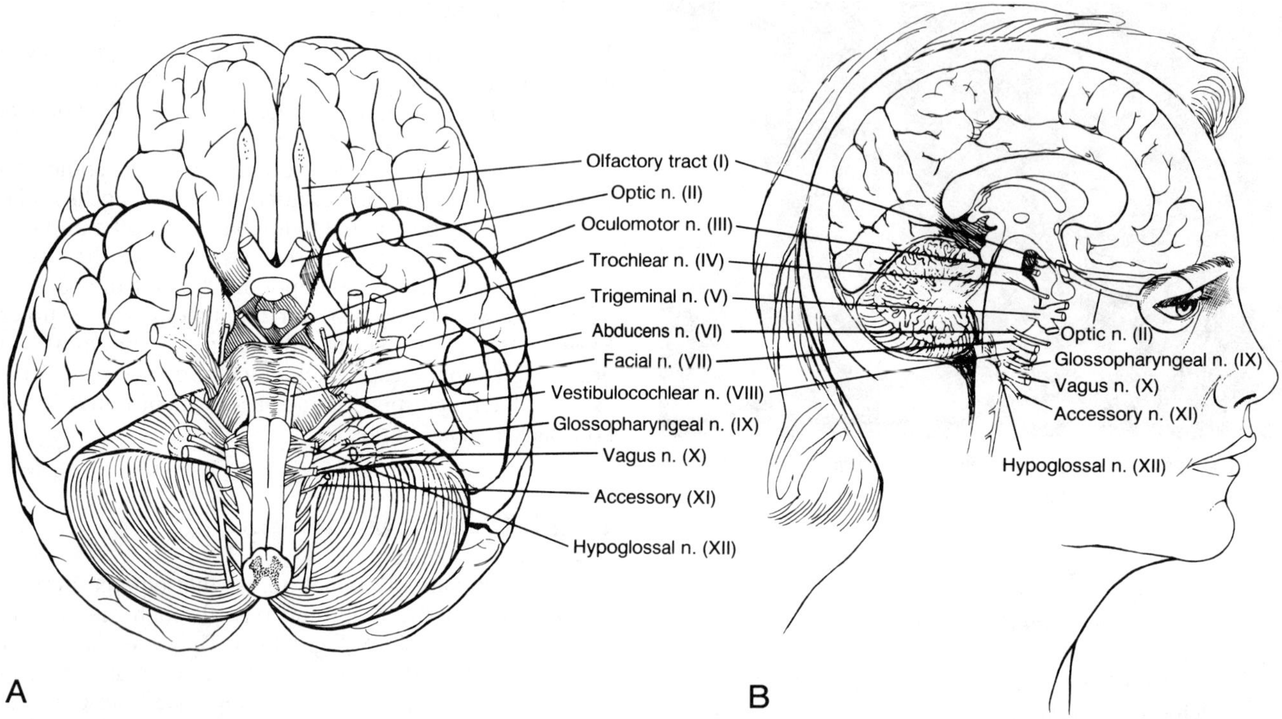

FIGURE 60-14. The cranial nerves. (**A**) inferior view of the brain showing the cranial nerves. (**B**) Lateral view showing a schematic version of the cranial nerves.

from structural abnormalities (loop of an artery) encroaching on the trigeminal nerve, gasserian ganglion, or root entry zone.

Early attacks, appearing most often in the fifth decade of life, are usually mild and brief. Pain-free intervals may be measured in terms of minutes, hours, days, or longer. With advancing years, the painful episodes tend to become more and more frequent and agonizing. The patient lives in constant fear of attacks.

The pain of this neuralgia is felt in the skin, not in the deeper structures, but it is more severe at the peripheral areas of distribution of the affected nerve, notably over the lip, the chin, the nostrils, and in the teeth. Paroxysms are aroused by any stimulation of the terminals of the affected nerve branches, such as washing the face, shaving, brushing the teeth, eating, and drinking. A draft of cold air and direct pressure against the nerve trunk may also cause pain. Certain areas are called *trigger points,* because the slightest touch immediately starts a paroxysm. To avoid stimulating these areas, patients with trigeminal neuralgia try not to touch or wash their faces, shave, chew, or do anything else that might cause an attack. Behavior of this type is a clue to diagnosis.

Management

The anticonvulsant agents carbamazepine (Tegretol) and phenytoin (Dilantin) relieve pain in most patients by reducing the transmission of impulses at certain nerve terminals. Carbamazepine is taken with meals, in dosages gradually increased until relief is obtained. Side effects include nausea, dizziness, drowsiness, and hepatic dysfunction. The patient is monitored for bone marrow depression during long-term drug therapy. Phenytoin also produces such side effects as nausea, dizziness, somnolence, ataxia, and skin allergies.

When medication fails to provide pain relief, a number of surgical options are available, as described in the following paragraphs. Patients should participate in choosing the procedure that best suits their health status.

Alcohol or phenol injection of the gasserian ganglion and peripheral branches of the trigeminal nerve relieves pain for several months. However, the pain returns after the nerve regenerates.

Percutaneous Radiofrequency Trigeminal Gangliolysis. Percutaneous radiofrequency interruption of the gasserian ganglion, whereby the small unmyelinated and thinly myelinated fibers that conduct the pain are thermally destroyed, is becoming the surgical procedure of choice for trigeminal neuralgia.

Under local anesthesia, the needle is introduced through the cheek on the affected side. Under fluoroscopic control, the needle electrode is guided through the foramen magnum into the gasserian ganglion. The divisions of the gasserian ganglion (mandibular, maxillary, and ophthalmic) are encountered sequentially. The nerve is stimulated with a small current while the patient is awake. The patient then reports when a tingling sensation is felt. When the electrode needle is in the desired position, the patient is anesthetized briefly and a radiofrequency current (heating current to destroy the nerve) is passed in a controlled manner to thermally injure the trigeminal ganglion and rootlets. The patient is then awakened from the anesthetic and examined for sensory deficits. Repeated lesions may be produced until the desired effect is achieved. The operative procedure takes less than 1 hour and gives permanent pain relief in

TABLE 60-2 Disorders of Cranial Nerves

Disorder	Clinical Manifestations	Nursing Interventions
Olfactory Nerve—I		
Head trauma Intracranial tumor Intracranial surgery	Unilateral or bilateral anosmia (temporary or persistent) Diminished taste for food	Assess for CSF rhinorrhea if patient has sustained head trauma.
Optic Nerve—II		
Optic neuritis Increased intracranial pressure Pituitary tumor	Lesions of optic tract produce homonymous hemianopsia.	Assess level of visual acuity. Restructure environment to prevent accidents. Teach patient to accommodate for visual loss.
Oculomotor Nerve—III **Trochlear Nerve—IV** **Abducens Nerve—VI**		
Vascular Brain stem ischemia Hemorrhage/infarction Neoplasm Trauma Infection	Dilation of pupil with loss of light reflex on one side Impairment of ocular movement Diplopia Gaze palsies Ptosis of eyelid	Assess extraocular movement and for nonreactive pupil.
Trigeminal Nerve—V		
Trigeminal neuraliga Head trauma Cerebellopontine lesion Sinus tract tumor/metastatic disease Compression of trigeminal root by tumor	Pain in face Diminished/loss of corneal reflex Chewing dysfunction	Assess for pain and triggering mechanisms for pain. Assess for difficulty in chewing. Discuss trigger zones and pain precipitants with patient. Protect cornea from abrasion. Ensure good oral hygiene. Educate patient about medication regimen.
Facial Nerve—VII		
Bell's palsy Facial nerve tumor Intracranial lesion Herpes zoster	Facial dysfunction; weakness and paralysis Hemifacial spasm Diminished/absent taste	Recognize facial paralysis as emergency; refer for treatment as soon as possible. Teach protective care for eyes. Select easily chewed foods; patient should eat and drink from unaffected side of mouth. Emphasize importance of oral hygiene. Provide emotional support for changed appearance of face.
Vestibulocochlear Nerve—VIII		
Tumors/acoustic neuroma Vascular compression of nerve Ménière's syndrome	Tinnitus Vertigo Hearing difficulties	Assess pattern of vertigo Provide for safety measures to prevent falls. Patient should obtain balance before ambulating. Caution patient to change positions slowly. Assist with ambulation. Encourage use of ADL aids.

(continued)

TABLE 60-2 *(continued)*

Disorder	Clinical Manifestations	Nursing Interventions
Glossopharyngeal Nerve—IX		
Glossopharyngeal neuralgia from neurovascular compression of IXth and Xth nerves Trauma Inflammatory conditions Tumor Vertebral artery aneurysms	Pain at base of tongue Difficulty in swallowing Loss of gag reflex Palatal, pharyngeal, and laryngeal paralysis	Assess for paroxysmal pain in throat, decreased or absent swallowing, gag and cough reflexes. Monitor for dysphagia, aspiration, nasal dysarthric speech. Position patient upright for eating or tube feeding.
Vagus Nerve—X		
Spastic palsy of larynx; bulbar paralysis; high vagal paralysis Guillain-Barré syndrome Carotid endarterectomy Vagal body tumors Nerve paralysis from malignancy, surgical trauma	Voice changes (temporary or permanent hoarseness) Vocal paralysis Dysphagia	Assess for airway obstruction/provide airway management. Prevent aspiration. Support patient having voice reconstruction procedures.
Spinal Accessory Nerve—XI		
Spinal cord disorder Amyotrophic lateral sclerosis Trauma Guillain-Barré syndrome	Drooping of affected shoulder with limited shoulder movement Weakness/paralysis of head rotation, flexion, extension; shoulder elevation	Support patient undergoing diagnostic tests.
Hypoglossal Nerve—XII		
Medullary lesions Amyotrophic lateral sclerosis Polio and motor system disease may destroy hypoglossal nuclei. Multiple sclerosis Trauma	Abnormal movements of tongue Weakness/paralysis of tongue muscles Difficulty in talking, chewing, and swallowing	Observe swallowing ability. Observe speech pattern. Be aware of attendant swallowing/vocal difficulties. Prepare for alternate feeding methods (tube feeding) to maintain nutrition.

most patients. Touch and proprioceptive functions are left intact.

Microvascular Decompression of the Trigeminal Nerve. An intracranial approach can be used to decompress the trigeminal nerve, because the pain may be caused by vascular compression of the entry zone of the trigeminal root by an arterial loop and occasionally by a vein. With the aid of an operating microscope, the artery loop is lifted from the nerve to relieve the pressure, and a small prosthetic device is inserted to prevent recurrence of impingement on the nerve. This procedure relieves facial pain while preserving normal sensation. It is a major procedure, involving a craniotomy. The postoperative management is the same as for other intracranial surgeries (see Chapter 59).

Nursing Interventions

Preoperative management of a patient with trigeminal neuralgia includes recognizing that certain factors may aggravate excruciating facial pain, such as food that is too hot or too cold or jarring the patient's bed or chair. Even washing the face, combing the hair, or brushing the teeth may produce acute bouts of pain. The nurse can prevent or reduce this pain in a variety of ways, such as providing cotton pads and room-temperature water for washing the patient's face, instructing the patient to rinse his or her mouth after eating when tooth brushing causes pain, and performing personal hygiene during pain-free intervals. The patient is advised to take food and fluids at room temperature, to chew on the unaffected side, and to ingest soft foods. The nurse must recognize that anxiety, depression, and insomnia often accompany chronic painful conditions and use appropriate interventions and referrals.

Bell's Palsy

Bell's palsy (facial paralysis) is due to peripheral involvement of the seventh cranial nerve on one side, which results in weakness or paralysis of the facial muscles. The cause is unknown, although possible causes may include vascular ischemia, viral disease (herpes simplex, herpes zoster), autoimmune disease, or a combination of all of these factors.

Pathophysiology

Bell's palsy is considered by some to represent a type of pressure paralysis. The inflamed, edematous nerve becomes compressed to the point of damage, or its nutrient vessel is occluded to the point of producing ischemic necrosis of the nerve within its long canal—a channel in which the fit at best is very snug. There is distortion of the face from paralysis of the facial muscles; increased lacrimation (tearing); and painful sensations in the face, behind the ear, and in the eye. The patient may experience speech difficulties and may be unable to eat on the affected side because of weakness or paralysis of the facial muscles.

Management

The objectives of treatment are to maintain the muscle tone of the face and to prevent or minimize denervation. The patient should be reassured that no stroke has occurred and that spontaneous recovery occurs within 3 to 5 weeks in most patients.

Corticosteroid therapy (prednisone) may be given to reduce inflammation and edema, which in turn reduces vascular compression and permits restoration of blood circulation to the nerve. Early administration of corticosteroid therapy appears to diminish the severity of the disease, relieve the pain, and help prevent or minimize denervation.

Facial pain is controlled with analgesics. Heat may be applied to the involved side of the face to promote comfort and blood flow through the muscles.

Electrical stimulation may be applied to the face to prevent muscle atrophy. Although most patients recover with conservative treatment, surgical exploration of the facial nerve may be undertaken in patients who are suspected of having a tumor or for surgical decompression of the facial nerve and for surgical rehabilitation of a paralyzed face.

Patient Education

While the paralysis lasts, the involved eye must be protected. Frequently, the patient's eye does not close completely, and the blink reflex is diminished so that the eye is vulnerable to dust and foreign particles. Corneal irritation and ulceration are potential complications in these patients. Sometimes there is an overflow of tears down the cheek (*epiphora*) from keratitis caused by drying of the cornea and absence of the blink reflex. The laxity of the lower lid alters the proper drainage of tears. To manage these problems, the eye should be covered with a protective shield at night. The eye patch may abrade the cornea, however, because there is some difficulty in keeping the partially paralyzed eyelids closed. The application of eye ointment at bedtime causes the eyelids to adhere to one another and remain closed during sleep. The patient can be taught to close the paralyzed eyelid manually before going to sleep. Wrap-around sunglasses or goggles are worn to decrease normal evaporation from the eye.

If the nerve is not too sensitive, the face may be massaged several times daily to maintain muscle tone. The technique is to massage the face with a gentle upward motion. Facial exercises, such as wrinkling the forehead, blowing out the cheeks, and whistling, may be performed with the aid of a mirror and are intended to prevent muscle atrophy. Exposure of the face to cold and drafts is avoided.

Disorders of the Peripheral Nervous System

Peripheral Neuropathies

A peripheral neuropathy is a disorder affecting the peripheral motor, sensory, or autonomic nerves. Peripheral nerves, by connecting the spinal cord and brain to all other organs, transmit motor impulses outward and relay sensory impulses to encode sensation in the brain.

A *mononeuropathy* affects a single peripheral nerve, whereas the involvement of multiple single peripheral nerves or their branches is termed *multiple mononeuropathy or mononeuritis multiplex*.

Polyneuropathies are characterized by bilaterally symmetric disturbance of function, usually beginning in the feet and hands. (Most nutritional, metabolic, and toxic neuropathies take this form.)

Causes. The most common causes of peripheral neuropathy are diabetes, alcoholism, and occlusive vascular disease. Many bacterial and metabolic toxins and exogenous poisons also affect the structure and function of the peripheral nerves. Because of the growing use of chemicals in industry, agriculture, and medicine, the number of substances known to cause peripheral neuropathies is increasing. In the developing countries, leprosy is a major cause of severe nerve disease because *Mycobacterium leprae* invade the peripheral nervous system.

Clinical Manifestations. The major symptoms of peripheral nerve disorders are loss of sensation, muscle atrophy, weakness, diminished reflexes, pain, and paresthesia (numbness, tingling) of the extremities. The patient frequently describes some part of the extremity as numb. Autonomic features include decreased or absent sweating, orthostatic hypotension, nocturnal diarrhea, tachycardia, impotence, and atrophic skin and nail changes.

Peripheral nerve disorders are diagnosed by EMG and the recording of the nerve and muscle responses evoked when electrical stimulation is applied to a nerve (somatosensory evoked potentials).

Mononeuropathy

Mononeuropathy is limited to a single peripheral nerve and its branches. It arises when the trunk of the nerve is compressed or entrapped (as by carpal tunnel syndrome, Chap. 63); traumatized, as when bruised by a blow, or overstretched, as in cases of dislocation of a joint; punctured by a needle used to inject a drug, or damaged by the drugs thus injected; or inflamed because an adjacent infectious process extends to the nerve's trunk. Mononeuropathy frequently is seen in the patient with diabetes.

Clinical Manifestations. Pain is seldom a major symptom of mononeuropathy when the condition is due to trauma, but in patients with complicating inflammatory conditions, such as arthritis, this feature is prominent. Such pain is increased by all body movements that tend to stretch, strain, or cause pressure on the injured nerve, and by sudden jarring of the body, such as that associated with coughing and sneezing. The skin in the areas supplied by nerves that are injured or diseased may become reddened and glossy; the subcutaneous tissue may become edematous, and the nutrition of the nails and the hair in this area defective. Chemical injuries to a nerve trunk, such as those caused by drugs injected into or near it, often are permanent.

Management. The objective of treatment of mononeuropathy is to remove the cause, if possible, such as by freeing the compressed nerve. Local corticosteroid injections may lessen inflammation and reduce pressure on the nerve. Pain may be relieved by aspirin or codeine.

Guillain-Barré Syndrome (Polyradiculoneuritis)

Guillain-Barré syndrome is a clinical syndrome of unknown cause involving the peripheral and cranial nerves. In most patients, the syndrome is preceded by an infection (respiratory or gastrointestinal) 1 to 4 weeks before the onset of neurologic deficits. In some instances, it has occurred after vaccination or surgery. It may be due to a primary viral infection, an immune reaction, some other process, or a combination of processes. One hypothesis is that a viral infection induces an autoimmune reaction that attacks the myelin of the peripheral nerves. (*Myelin* is a substance that surrounds or ensheaths the axons of certain nerves and plays an important role in the transmission of nerve impulses.)

Proximal portions of the nerves tend to be affected most often, and the nerve roots within the subarachnoid space are commonly involved. Autopsy findings have shown inflammatory edema and demyelination with some lymphocytic infiltration that is especially prominent in the spinal nerve roots.

Clinical Manifestations

There is variation in the mode of onset. The initial neurologic symptoms are *paresthesia* (tingling and numbness) and muscle weakness of the legs, which may progress to the upper extremities, trunk, and facial muscles. Muscle weakness may be followed quickly by complete paralysis. The cranial nerves frequently are affected, leading to paralysis of the ocular, facial, and oropharyngeal muscles and thus causing marked difficulty in talking, chewing, and swallowing. Autonomic dysfunction frequently occurs and takes the form of over-reactivity or under-reactivity of the sympathetic or parasympathetic nervous systems, as manifested by disturbances of heart rate and rhythm, blood pressure changes (transient hypertension, orthostatic hypotension), and a variety of other vasomotor disturbances. There may be severe and persistent pain in the back and calves of the legs. Frequently the patient exhibits loss of position sense as well as diminished or absent tendon reflexes. Sensory changes are manifested by paresthesias.

Most patients make a full recovery over several months to a year, but about 10% are left with a residual disability.

Diagnostic Evaluation

The spinal fluid shows an increased protein concentration with a normal cell count. Electrophysiologic testing demonstrates marked slowing of nerve conduction velocity.

Management

Guillain-Barré syndrome is considered a medical emergency and the patient is managed in an intensive care unit. A patient with respiratory problems requires mechanical ventilation, sometimes for prolonged periods. **Plasmapheresis** (plasma exchange), which produces a temporary reduction in circulating antibodies, may be used in the severely affected and deteriorating patient to limit the deterioration and demyelination. Continuous ECG monitoring may be required because of possible alteration in cardiac rate or rhythm. Cardiac dysrhythmias associated with autonomic abnormalities are treated with propranolol to prevent tachycardia and hypertension. Atropine may be administered to avoid episodes of bradycardia during endotracheal suctioning and physical therapy.

❑ NURSING PROCESS
The Patient With Guillain-Barré Syndrome

Assessment

Assessment for complications of Guillain-Barré syndrome involves constant monitoring for the life-threatening problem of acute respiratory failure. Other complications include cardiac dysrhythmias, which necessitate ECG monitoring and observing the patient for signs of deep vein thrombosis and pulmonary embolism, ever-present threats to any immobilized and paralyzed patient.

Diagnosis

Nursing Diagnoses

Based on the assessment data, the patient's major diagnoses may include the following:

- ❑ Ineffective breathing pattern and gas exchange related to rapidly progressive weakness and impending respiratory failure
- ❑ Impaired physical mobility related to paralysis
- ❑ Altered nutrition, less than body requirements, related to inability to swallow, which is secondary to cranial nerve dysfunction
- ❑ Impaired verbal communication related to cranial nerve dysfunction
- ❑ Fear and anxiety related to loss of control and paralysis

Collaborative Problems/ Potential Complications

Based on the assessment data, potential complications that may develop include:

- ❑ Respiratory failure

Planning and Implementation

Goals. The major goals of the patient may include maintenance of respiratory function, achievement of mobility, accomplishment of normal nutrition, achievement of communication, reduction of fear and anxiety, and absence of complications.

Nursing Interventions

Maintaining Respiratory Function. The patient with Guillain-Barré syndrome is dependent on nursing surveillance and care for recovery. Mechanical ventilation is likely if serial measurements of the patient's vital capacity show progressive deterioration, indicating worsening of respiratory muscle strength. The nursing management of the patient requiring mechanical ventilation is discussed in Chapter 25. The patient is at particularly high risk if unable to cough effectively to clear the airway and has difficulty in swallowing, which may cause aspiration of saliva and precipitate acute respiratory failure. Chest physical therapy and elevation of the head of the bed facilitate respirations and promote more effective coughing. Suctioning may be needed to maintain a clear airway.

Monitoring and Managing Potential Complications. Thorough assessment of respiratory function at regular intervals is essential because respiratory insufficiency and subsequent failure due to weakness or paralysis of the intercostal muscles and diaphragm may develop quickly. Respiratory failure is the major cause of mortality, which is reported to be as high as 10% to 20%. The patient's vital capacity is monitored frequently and at regular intervals in addition to respiratory rate and the quality of respirations so that respiratory insufficiency can be anticipated. Decreasing vital capacity associated with weakness of the muscles used in swallowing, which causes difficulty in both coughing and swallowing, indicates deterioration of respiratory function. Signs and symptoms include breathlessness while speaking, shallow and irregular breathing, use of accessory muscles, tachycardia, and changes in respiratory pattern.

Parameters for determining the onset of respiratory failure are established on admission. Intubation and the initiation of mechanical ventilation can be accomplished on a non-emergent basis. Patient preparation for this procedure may be possible in these circumstances and the procedure itself can take place in a controlled manner that reduces anxiety and complications.

Other complications for which the patient is assessed and monitored include **cardiac dysrhythmias,** which necessitate ECG monitoring, **deep vein thrombosis,** and **pulmonary embolism,** ever-present threats to any immobilized and paralyzed patient.

Reducing Effects of Immobility. The paralyzed extremities are supported in functional positions and given passive range-of-motion exercises at least twice daily. The nurse collaborates with the physical therapist to prevent contracture deformities by using careful positioning and range-of-motion exercises. Deep vein thrombosis and pulmonary embolism are threats to the paralyzed patient, who is unable to move the extremities. Nursing interventions include ensuring adequate hydration, assisting with physical therapy, the use of antiembolism stockings, and administering the prescribed anticoagulant regimen.

A paralyzed person has the potential to develop compression neuropathies, most often of the ulnar and peroneal nerves. Padding may be placed over the elbows and head of the fibula to prevent this problem. The prevention of pressure ulcers is a major nursing challenge. For paralyzed patients, the principles of nursing management of the unconscious patient (see Chap. 59) may be applied, although cognitive function is unaffected.

When recovery begins to take place, these patients may experience orthostatic hypotension (from autonomic dysfunction) and probably require the use of a tilt table to help them assume an upright posture.

Providing Adequate Nutrition. Attention is paid to adequate nutrition and prevention of muscle wasting. Paralytic ileus may result from insufficient parasympathetic activity. In this event, intravenous feedings are prescribed by the physician and administered and monitored by the nurse until bowel sounds are heard. If the patient is unable to swallow, nasogastric tube feedings may be prescribed. When the patient can swallow normally, oral feeding is gradually and carefully resumed.

Improving Communication. Because of paralysis, tracheostomy, and intubation, the patient is unable to talk, laugh, or cry, and thus has no outlet for emotional expression. These problems are compounded by boredom, dependency, isolation, and frustration. To establish some form of communication, lipreading and the use of picture cards, combined with a system of blinking the eyes to indicate yes or no, may be tried. If the patient remains on the ventilator for a prolonged period, a referral to a speech-language therapist may be made. Diversional therapy (television, cassette tapes, visits from the family) can alleviate some of the frustrations that are encountered.

Relieving Fear and Anxiety. Involving the family and friends with selected patient care activities and diversions (*e.g.,* reading aloud) will reduce the sense of isolation of the patient. Nursing interventions that are helpful in increasing the patient's sense of control (and hence reduction of fear) include providing information about the patient's condition, emphasizing a positive appraisal of coping resources, encouraging relaxation exercises and distraction techniques, and giving positive feedback. The attitude and atmosphere created by the nurse, physical therapist, and occupational therapist are important. Giving expert nursing care, explanations, and reassurance helps the patient gain some control over the situation.

Patient Education and Home Care Considerations. Most patients with Guillain-Barré Syndrome will experience complete recovery within weeks or months. Those patients who have experienced total or prolonged paralysis will likely require some type of rehabilitation following discharge from the hospital. The extent of such a program will depend on the assessment of need made by the health team members. Alternatives include a comprehensive inpatient program if deficits are significant and social support is limited to a home program of physical and occupational therapies.

The recovery phase may be long and will require patience as well as involvement on the part of the patient and family for return of former abilities. The acute onset and dramatic progression of symptoms may not allow time for the patient to adjust to the sudden change in function. A Guillain-Barré support group offers both information and

CRITICAL THINKING EXERCISES

1. Your patient has been informed that she has multiple sclerosis (MS). She is distraught and believes that MS is the same as ALS, which caused rapid deterioration and death in a family friend. How would you explain the differences between MS and ALS to her, and how would you devise a positive program to help her adjust to the diagnosis? Describe the patient behaviors that would indicate a successful outcome.
2. A patient who is experiencing frequent migraine headaches is being treated at a local clinic. She does not understand the relationship between her headaches and the recommended dietary restrictions. How would you explain this relationship and the reasons for the dietary restrictions? What assessment parameters would you expect were explored to determine other factors that would precipitate her headaches?
3. While you are in the grocery store, another shopper experiences a grand mal seizure. How would you respond to this event, and why would you take these actions? If the shopper had a 3-year-old child with her, how might you address this additional consideration?
4. You have a patient with epilepsy who develops status epilepticus. Based on your knowledge of this disorder, describe the medical management you would anticipate to control the seizures and the nursing measures that are indicated. Identify the patient outcomes that would indicate that the goals have been achieved.
5. A patient assigned to your care has been admitted to the hospital for control of myasthenic crisis. Describe the differences between myasthenic crisis (too little cholinergic activity or undermedication) and cholinergic crisis (excessive cholinergic activity or overmedication). Explain how your nursing actions would differ for myasthenic and cholinergic crisis and what the underlying rationale would be for these interventions.
6. You are assigned to care for one patient with a cervical spinal cord injury and another with a thoracic spinal cord injury. How would your assessment and care differ for these two patients?

group interaction, which may be helpful during the recovery phase.

Evaluation

Expected Outcomes

1. Maintains effective respirations and airway clearance
   a. Breath sounds normal on auscultation
   b. Demonstrates gradual improvement in respiratory function
2. Shows increasing mobility
   a. Regains use of extremities
   b. Participates in rehabilitation program
3. Demonstrates ability to swallow
4. Demonstrates recovery of speech
5. Shows lessening fear and anxiety
6. Is free of complications
   a. Breathes spontaneously
   b. Has vital capacity within normal range
   c. Exhibits normal arterial blood gases and oximetry

BIBLIOGRAPHY

Books

Adams R and Victor M. Principles of Neurology, 5th ed. New York, McGraw-Hill, 1993.

American Spinal Injury Association. Standards for Neurological and Functional Classification of Spinal Cord Injury, Revised 1992. Chicago, American Spinal Injury Association, 1992.

Asbury A, McKhann G, and McDonald I (ed). Diseases of the Nervous System: Clinical Neurobiology, 2nd ed. Philadelphia, WB Saunders, 1992.

Cailliet R. Head and Face Pain Syndromes. Philadelphia, FA Davis, 1992.

Cardona V. Trauma nursing: From Resuscitation Through Rehabilitation. Philadelphia, WB Saunders, 1994.

Chipps E, Clanin N, and Cambell V. Neurologic Disorders. St Louis, Mosby–Year Book, 1992.

Cook SD (ed). Handbook of Multiple Sclerosis. New York, Marcel Dekker, 1990.

Diamond S. Migraine Headache Prevention and Management. New York, Marcel Dekker, 1990.

Finlayson MAJ and Garner SH. Brain Injury Rehabilitation: Clinical Considerations. Baltimore, Williams & Wilkins, 1994.

Greenberg D, Ainoff M, and Simon R. Clinical Neurology, 2nd ed. Norwalk, CT, Appleton and Lange, 1993.

Gunderson C. Essentials of Clinical Neurology. New York, Raven Press, 1990.

Haerer AF. DeJong's The Neurologic Examination. Philadelphia, JB Lippincott, 1994.

Hanak M. Rehabilitation Nursing for the Neurological Patient. New York, Springer, 1992.

Hickey JV. The Clinical Practice of Neurological and Neurosurgical Nursing, 3rd ed. Philadelphia, JB Lippincott, 1992.

Johnson R (ed). Current Therapy in Neurologic Disease. Philadelphia, BC Decker, 1991.

Lechtenberg R. Seizure Diagnosis and Management. Philadelphia, FA Davis, 1990.

Marshall S et al. Neuroscience Critical Care: Pathophysiology and Patient Management. Philadelphia, WB Saunders, 1990.

Richardson T and McKinlay W. Clinical and Neuropsychological Aspects of Closed Head Injury. New York, Taylor & Francis, 1990.

Rosenthal M et al (eds). Rehabilitation of the Adult and Child with Traumatic Brain Injury, 2nd ed. Philadelphia, FA Davis, 1990.

Strub RL and Black FW. The Mental Status Examination in Neurology. Philadelphia, FA Davis, 1993.

Wesolowski MD and Zencius AH. A Practical Guide to Head Injury Rehabilitation: A Focus on Postacute Residential Treatment. New York, Plenum Press, 1994.

Westmoreland BF et al. Medical Neurosciences: An Approach to Anatomy, Pathology and Physiology by Systems and Levels. Boston, Little, Brown, 1994.

Yarkony GM (ed). Spinal Cord Injury: Medical Management and Rehabilitation. Gaithersburg, MD, Aspen, 1994.

Journals

Asterisks indicate nursing research articles.

General

Beck CK and Shue VM. Interventions for treating disruptive behavior in demented elderly people. Nurs Clin North Am 1994 Dec; 29(1):143–155.

Currie DM, Gershkoff AM and Cifu DX. Geriatric rehabilitation. 3. Mid- and late-life effects of early-life disabilities. Arch Phys Med Rehabil 1993 May; 74(5-S):S413–S416.

Davis M and Lucatorto M. Mannitol revisited. J Neurosci Nurs 1994 Jun; 26(3):170–174.

*Galindo-Clocon D et al. Functional impairment among elderly women with osteoporotic vertebral fractures. Rehabil Nurs 1995 Mar–Apr; 20(2):79–83, 130.

Guin PR and Freudenberger K. The elderly neuroscience patient: Implications for the critical care nurse. AACN Clin Iss Crit Care Nurs 1992 Feb; 3(1):98–105.

Hamilton MG, Hull RD and Pineo GF. Venous thromboembolism in neurosurgery and neurology patients: A review. Neurosurgery 1994 Feb; 34(2):280–296.

Held JL. Identifying spinal cord compression. Nursing 1994 May; 24(5):28.

Held JL et al. Nursing care of the patient with spinal cord compression. Oncol Nurs Forum 1993 Nov–Dec; 20(10):1507–1516.

Keller C and Williams A. Cardiac dysrhythmias associated with central nervous system dysfunction. J Neurosci Nurs 1993 Dec; 25(6):349–355.

Rose BA. Neurologic therapies in critical care. Crit Care Nurs Clin North Am 1993 Jun; 5(2):237–246.

St. George CL. Spasticity. Mechanisms and nursing care. Nurs Clin North Am 1993 Dec; 28(4):819–827.

Wall BM, Philips JP, and Howard JC. Validation of increased intracranial pressure and high risk for increased intracranial pressure. Nurs Diagn 1994 Apr–Jun; 5(2):74–81.

*Way C and Segatore M. Development and preliminary testing of the neurological assessment instrument. J Neurosci Nurs 1994 Oct; 26(5):278–287.

Yarkony GM. Pressure ulcers: A review. Arch Phys Med Rehabil 1994 Aug; 75(8):908–917.

Young RR. Spasticity: A review. Neurology 1994 Nov; 44(11 Suppl 9):S12–S20.

Zietlow SP et al. Multisystem geriatric trauma. J Trauma 1994 Dec; 37(6):985–988.

Amyotrophic Lateral Sclerosis

Bauman A. ALS—decision making under uncertainty: A positive approach. AXON 1991 Dec; 13(2):41–43.

Kaplan LM and Hollander D. Respiratory dysfunction in amotrophic lateral sclerosis. Clin Chest Med 1994 Dec; 15(4): 675–681.

Murphy P. Helping Joanne die with dignity: A nursing profile in courage. Nursing 1990 Sep; 20(9):44–49.

Sherman MS and Paz HL. Review of respiratory care of the patient with amotrophic lateral sclerosis. Respiration 1994; 61(2): 61–67.

Tidwell J. Pulmonary management of the ALS patient. J Neurosci Nurs 1993 Dec; 25(6):337–342.

Brain Tumors

Alexander E III and Loeffler JS. Radiosurgery using a modified linear accelerator. Neurosurg Clin North Am 1992 Jan; 3(1): 167–190.

Foote AW and Holcombe J. Acoustic neuroma: Suggestions for helping the patient adapt after translabyrinthine surgery. J Neurosci Nurs 1994 Jun; 26(3):162–165.

Furlong TG. Neurologic complications of immunosuppressive cancer therapy. Oncol Nurs Forum 1993 Oct. 20(9):1337–1352.

Laperriere NJ and Bernstein M. Radiotherapy for brain tumors. CA Cancer J Clin 1994 Mar–Apr; 44(2):96–108.

Newton C and Mateo MA. Uncertainty: Strategies for patients with brain tumor and their family. Cancer Nurs 1994 Apr; 17(2): 137–140.

Newton HB. Primary brain tumors: Review of etiology, diagnosis and treatment. Am Fam Physician 1994 Mar; 49(4):787–797.

Sarkissian S. Length of hospital stay and contributing variables in supratentorial craniotomy patients with brain tumor: A precare map study. AXON 1994 Jun; 15(4):86–89.

Stephanian E et al. Gamma knife surgery for sellar and suprasellar tumors. Neurosurg Clin North Am 1992 Jan; 3(1):207–218.

Cerebral Aneurysms and Intracranial Hemorrhage

Armstrong SL. Cerebral vasospasm: Early detection and intervention. Crit Care Nurs 1994 Aug; 14(4):33–37.

Coleman R et al. Treatment of posterior circulation aneurysms using platinum coils. J Neurosci Nurs 1994 Dec; 26(6):367–370.

Counsell C, Gilbert M, and Snively C. Nimodipine: A drug therapy for treatment of vasospasm. J Neurosci Nurs 1995 Feb; 27(1): 53–55.

Diringer MN. Intracerebral hemorrhage: Pathophysiology and management. Crot Care Med 1993 Oct; 21(10):1591–1603.

Ferguson R et al. Guarding against cerebral vasospasm. Am J Nurs 1994 Mar; 94(3):56A, 56D, 56F.

Nichols DA et al. Endovascular treatment of intracranial aneurysms. Mayo Clin Proc 1994 Mar; 69(3):272–285.

Parker CD. Fast action for subarachnoid hemorrhage. Am J Nurs 1995 Jan; 95(1):47.

Guillain-Barré Syndrome

Anderson SB. Guillain-Barré syndrome: Giving the patient control. J Neurosci Nurs 1992 Jun; 24(3):158–162.

*Farkkila M et al. Plasma exchange therapy reduces the nursing care needed in Guillain-Barré syndrome. J Adv Nurs 1992 Jun; 17(6):672–675.

Graves G et al. Therapeutic plasma exchange for Guillian-Barré syndrome during pregnancy. ANNA J 1994 Aug; 21(5):277–278.

Parobeck V et al. An unusual nursing challenge: Guillain Barré syndrome following cranial surgery. J Neurosci Nurs 1992 Oct; 24(5):251–255.

Penrose NJ. Guillain-Barré syndrome: A case study. Rehabil Nurs 1993 Mar–Apr; 18(2):88–90,94.

Ross AP. Nursing interventions for persons receiving immunosuppressive therapies for demyelinating pathology. Nurs Clin North Am 1993 Dec; 28(4):829–838.

Headache

Allen TG. Evaluating and treating headaches. Am J Nurs 1994 Apr; 94(4):16B–D, 16F, 16H.

*Basolo-Kunzer M et al. Chronic headache patients' marital and family adjustment. Issues Ment Health Nurs 1991 Apr–Jun; 12(2):133–148.

Buring JE et al. Migraine and subsequent risk of stroke in the Physicians' Health Study. Arch Neurol 1995 Feb; 52(2):129–134.

Dunajcik L. Biofeedback for headaches. Am J Nurs 1994 Oct; 94(10):17–18.

Gallagher RM. Headache diagnosis and treatment. J Am Acad Nurse Pract 1991 Jan–Mar; 3(1):3–10.

Gasser PA. Creating a headache diary. J Am Acad Nurse Pract 1991 Jan–Mar; 3(1):53–55.

Kennedy D and Barter R. Outpatient care of the headache client: A challenging specialty. J Neurosci Nurs 1994 Apr; 26(2):73–77.

Walling AD. Cluster headache. Am Fam Physician 1993 May 1; 47(6):1457–1465.

Head Injury

Acorn S et al. Head injury—impact on the wives. J Neurosci Nurs 1992 Dec; 24(6):324–326.

*Brown B et al. The effects of hyperventlation and lidocaine on intracranial pressure response to endotracheal suctioning. Heart Lung 1992 May; 21(3):286.

Brucia JJ et al. The effects of lidocaine on intracranial hypertension. J Neurosci Nurs 1992 Aug; 24(4):205–214.

*Crosby LJ et al. Cerebrovascular response of closed head injured patients to a standardized endotracheal tube suctioning and manual hyperventilation procedure. J Neurosci Nurs 1992 Feb; 24(1):40–49.

Dempsey DR. Nutritional support of the patient with head trauma. Trauma Q 1991 Jan; 7(2):71–77.

Gennarelli TA. Mechanisms of brain injury. J Emerg Med 1993; 11(Suppl 1):5–11.

Ghajar J et al. Survey of critical care management of comatose head-injured patients in the United States. Crit Care Med 1995 Mar; 23(3):560–567.

Godbole KB et al. A head-injured patient: Caloric needs, clinical progress and nursing care priorities. J Neurosci Nurs 1991 Oct; 23(5):290–294.

Hall M et al. Multidisciplinary approaches to management of acute head injury. J Neurosci Nurs 1992 Aug; 24(4):199–204.

Hammell KR. Psychosocial outcome following severe closed head injury. Int J Rehabil Res 1994 Dec; 17(4):319–332.

Hilton G. Secondary brain injury and the role of neuroprotective agents. J Neurosci Nurs 1994 Aug; 26(4):251–255.

Jackson S. Action STAT! Assessing a head injury: What to do until help arrives. Nursing 1992 Sep; 22(9):49.

Kerr ME et al. Hyperventilation in the head-injured patient: An effective treatment modality? Heart Lung 1993 Nov-Dec; 22(6): 516–522.

Martin KM. Loss without death: A dilemma for the head-injured patient's family. J Neurosci Nurs 1994 Jun; 26(3):134–139.

Ogg P et al. Connections and meanings . . . bringing patients back following head injury. J Neurosci Nurs 1993 Feb; 25(1):59–61.

*Reeber BJ. Evaluating the effects of a family education intervention. Rehabil Nurs 1992 Nov–Dec; 17(6):332–336.

Rice MJ. Minor head injury: Is anybody listening? J Neurosci Nurs 1992 Jun; 24(3):173–175.

Rosenwasser RH et al. Critical care management of head injury. Trauma Q 1992 Jan; 8(2):30–57.

*Ross AM et al. Prognosticators of outcome after major head injury in the elderly. J Neurosci Nurs 1992 Apr; 24(2):88–93.

Slazinski T and Johnson MC. Severe diffuse axonal injury in adults and children. J Neurosci Nurs 1994 Jun; 26(3):151–154.

Wald SL. Advances in the early management of patients with head injury. Surg Clin North Am 1995 Apr; 75(2):225–242.

Ward JD et al. Penetrating head injury. Crit Care Nurs Q 1994 May; 17(1):79–89.

Huntington's Disease

Cummings JL. Behavioral and psychiatric symptoms associated with Huntington's disease. Adv Neurol 1995; 65:179–186.

Hayden MR, Bloch M, and Wiggins S. Psychological effects of predictive testing for Huntington's disease. Adv Neurol 1995; 65: 201–210.

Mendez MF. Huntington's disease: Update and review of neuropsychiatric aspects. Int J Psychiatry Med. 1994 24(3):189–208.

Purdon SE et al. Huntington's disease: Pathogenesis, diagnosis and treatment. J Psychiatr Neurosci 1994 Nov; 19(5):359–367.

Kovach CR et al. Understanding Huntington's disease: An overview of symptomatology and nursing care. Geriatr Nurs 1993 Sep–Oct; 14(5):268–271.

Van der Weyden RS. Caring for a patient with Huntington's disease. Nurs Times 1994 Dec; 90(49):33–35.

Van der Weyden RS. Living at risk: Huntington's disease. J Psychosoc Nurs Ment Health Serv 1994 Jun; 32(6):63–64.

Meningitis and Brain Abscess

Adjunctive dexamethasone in bacterial meningitis. Nurses Drug Alert 1991 Jul; 15(7):50.

Mickles LI et al. Listeria meningitis: A case study. Crit Care Nurse 1994 Aug; 14(4):220, 225–232.

Mitrani-Schwartz A et al. Pseudomeningitis caused by pseudomonas paucimobilis. Heart Lung 1991 May; 20(3):305–307.

Mocsny N. Cryptococcal meningitis in patients with AIDS. J Neurosci Nurs 1992 Oct; 24(5):265–268.

Quagliarello VJ and Scheld WM. New perspectives on bacterial meningitis. Clin Infect Dis 1993 Oct; 17(4):603–608.

Singla S. Cryptococcal meningitis and the role of nutritional support. AIDS Patient Care 1992 Aug; 6(4):159.

Tunkel AR and Scheld WM. Pathogenesis and pathophysiology of bacterial meningitis. Ann Rev Med 1993 44; 103–120.

Multiple Sclerosis

*Dewis MEM et al. Nurturing a valuable resource: Family caregivers in multiple sclerosis. AXON 1992 Mar; 13(3):87–91.

*Gulick EE. Social support among persons with multiple sclerosis. Res Nurs Health 1994 Jun; 17(3):195–206.

*Gulick EE et al. Holistic health patterning in multiple sclerosis. Res Nurs Health 1992 Jan; 15(3):175–185.

*Hainsworth MA. Living with multiple sclerosis: The experience of chronic sorrow. J Neurosci Nurs 1994 Aug 26(4):237–140.

Hubsky EP et al. Fatigue in multiple sclerosis: Guidelines for nursing care. Rehabil Nurs 1992 Jul–Aug; 17(4):176–181.

Kelley CL and Smeltzer SC. Beta-interferon: The new MS treatment. J Neurosci Nurs 1994; 26(1):52–56.

*Long KA. Descriptions and perceptions of health among rural and urban adults with multiple sclerosis. Res Nurs Health 1992 Oct; 15(5):335–342.

Miller CM. Trajectory and empowerment theory applied to care of patients with multiple sclerosis. J Neurosci Nurs 1993 Dec; 25(6):343–348.

Miller CM and Hens M. Multiple sclerosis: A literature review. J Neurosci Nurs 1993 Jun; 25(3):174–179.

*O'Brian MT. Multiple sclerosis: The role of social support and disability. Clin Nurs Res 1993 Feb; 2(1):67–85.

Schapiro RT. Symptomatic management in multiple sclerosis. Ann Neurol 1994 36 Suppl: S123–S129.

*Smeltzer SC. Concerns of pregnant women with multiple sclerosis. Qual Health Res 1994 Nov; 4(4):480–502.

*Smeltzer SC et al. Respiratory function in multiple sclerosis: Utility of clinical assessment of respiratory muscle function. Chest 1992 Feb; 101(2):479–484.

Smeltzer SC. Use of the trajectory model of nursing in multiple sclerosis. Scholar Inq Nurs Pract 1991 Fall; 5(3):219–234.

*Stuifbergen AK. Meeting the demands of illness: Types and services of support for individuals with multiple sclerosis and their partners. Rehabil Nurs Res 1992 1(1):14–23.

*Wassem R. Self-efficacy as a predictor of adjustment to multiple sclerosis. J Neurosci Nurs 1992 Aug; 24(4):224–229.

*Weinert C et al. Challenging assumptions about multiple sclerosis. Rehabil Nurs Res 1994 Winter; 3(4):122–129.

Weiss J. Multiple sclerosis: will it come between us? Sexual concerns of clients and their partners. J Neurosci Nurs 1992 Aug; 24(4):190–193.

*Wineman NM et al. A comparative analysis of coping behaviors in persons with multiple sclerosis or a spinal cord injury. Res Nurs Health 1994 Jun; 17(3):185–194.

*Wineman NM et al. Congruence in uncertainty between individuals with multiple sclerosis and their spouses. J Neurosci Nurs 1993 Dec; 25(6):356–361.

Woolf K. Intravenous methylprednisolone for exacerbations in multiple sclerosis. Med surg Nurs 1995 Jun; 4(3):207–210.

Myasthenia Gravis

Burke ME. Myasthenia gravis and pregnancy. J Perinat Neonatal Nurs 1993 Jun; 7(1):11–21.
Donohoe KM. Nursing care of the patient with myasthenia gravis. Neurol Clin 1994 May; 12(2):369–385.
Hagen NA. Action STAT! Myasthenic crisis. Nursing 1991 June; 21(6):33.
Hardy EM and Rittenberry K. Myasthenia gravis: An overview. Orthop Nurs 1994 Nov–Dec; 13(6):37–42.
Hopkins LC. Clinical features of myasthenia gravis. Neurol Clin 1994 May; 12(2):243–261.
O'Donnell L. Caring for patients with myasthenia gravis . . . find out your role in assessing and managing this debilitating disorder. Nursing 1995 Mar; 25(3):60–61.
Phillips LH II. The epidemiology of myasthenia gravis. Neurol Clin 1994 May; 12(2):263–271.
Richman DP and Agius MA. Myasthenia gravia: Pathogenesis and treatment. Semin Neurol 1994 Jun; 14(2):106–110.
Sanders DB et al. The treatment of patients with myasthenia gravis. Neurol Clin 1994 May; 12(2):343–368.
Zulueta JJ and Fanburg BL. Respiratory dysfunction in myasthenia gravis. Clin Chest Med 1994 Dec; 15(4):683–691.

Parkinson's Disease

Ahlskog JE. Treatment of Parkinson's disease. From theory to practice. Postgrad Med 1994 Apr; 95(5):52–54, 57–58, 61–64.
Aminoff MJ. Treatment of Parkinson's disease. West J Med 1994 Sep; 161(3):303–308.
Calne S. Examining causes and care of idiopathic parkinsonism. Nurs Times 1994 Apr 20–26; 90(16):38–40.
Fitzsimmons B and Bunting LK. Parkinson's disease. Quality of life issues. Nurs Clin North Am 1993 Dec. 28(4):807–818.
Fowler SB et al. Continuous duodenal infusion of levodopa. J Neurosci Nurs 1993 Oct; 25(5):317–320.
Jenner P. The rationale for the use of dopamine agonists in Parkinson's disease. Neurology 1995 Mar; 45(3 Suppl 3):S6–S12.
Taira F. Facilitating self care in clients with Parkinson's disease. Home HealthCare Nurse 1992 Jul–Aug; 10(4):23–27.
Toledo LW. The postanesthesia patient with Parkinson's disease. J Post Anesth Nurs 1992 Feb; 7(1):32–37.

Seizures

Benbadis SR et al. Psychogenic seizures: A guide for patients and families. J Neurosci Nurs 1994 Oct; 26(5):306–308.
Cloyd JC et al. Antiepileptics in the elderly. Pharmacoepidemiology and pharmacokinetics. Arch Fam Med 1994 Jul; 3(7):589–598.
*DiIorio C. The development and testing of an instrument to measure self-efficacy in individuals with epilepsy. J Neurosci Nurs 1992 Feb; 24(1):9–13.
*DiIorio C. Self-efficacy and social support in self-management of epilepsy. West J Nurs Res 1992 Jun; 14(3):292–307.
*DiIorio C et al. Epilepsy self-management: Partial replication and extension. Res Nurs Health 1994 Jun; 17(3):167–174.
*DiIorio C and Manteuffel B. Preferences concerning epilepsy education: Opinions of nurses, physicians, and persons with epilepsy. J Neurosci Nurs 1995 Feb; 27(1):29–34.
*DiIorio C, Faherty B, and Manteuffel B. Learning needs of persons with epilepsy: A comparison of perceptions of persons with epilepsy, nurses and physicians. J Neurosci Nurs 1993 Feb; 25(1):22–29.
Ellis CR. Chronobiological aspects of epileptic phenomena: A literature review, implications for nursing and suggestions for research. J Neurosci Nurs 1992 Dec; 24(6):335–339.
Hanna DR. Purple glove syndrome: A complication of intravenous phenyotion. J Neurosci Nurs 1992 Dec; 24(6):340–345.
Hartshorn JC et al. Impact of epilepsy on quality of life. J Neurosci Nurs 1992 Feb; 24(1):24–29.
Hartshorn JC and Byers VL. Importance of health and family variables related to quality of life in individuals with uncontrolled seizures. J Neurosci Nurs 1994 Oct; 26(5):288–297.
Jordan KG. Status epilepticus: A perspective from the neuroscience intensive care unit. Neurosurg Clin North Am 1994 Oct; 5(4): 671–686.
Lannon SL. Epilepsy in the elderly. J Neurosci Nurs 1993 Oct; 25(5):273–285.
*Michael JE. Vagal nerve stimulation in treatment of intractable partial seizures: Nursing implications. J Neurosci Nurs 1992 Feb; 24(1):19–23.
Ziemba SK. Seizures. Am J Nurs 1995 Feb; 95(2):32–33.

Spinal Cord Injury

*Basta SM. Pressure sore prevention and outcome expectations: A study of people with spinal cord injury. Rehabil Nurs Res 1994 Spring; 3(1):11–17.
Boss BJ. The neurophysiological basis of learning. Part 2: Concept formation/abstraction, reason and executive functions. Implications for SCI nurses. SCI Nurs 1994 Mar; 11(1):3–6.
Cardenas DD and Hooton TM. Urinary tract infection in persons with spinal cord injury. Arch Phys Med Rehabil 1995 Mar; 76(3):272–280.
Casady L et al. Time period of immobility and pressure development in spinal cord-injured patients. J Neurosci Nurs 1992 Dec; 24(6):308.
*Charbonneau-Smith R. No touch catheterization and infection rates in a select spinal cord injured population. Rehabil Nurs 1993 Sep–Oct; 18(5):296–305, 355–356.
Coen SD. Spinal cord injury: preventing secondary injury. AACN Clin Issues Crit Care Nurs 1992 Feb; 3(1):44–54.
*Curry K et al. The relationship between extended periods of immobility and decubitus ulcer formation in the acutely spinal cord-injured individual. J Neurosci Nurs 1992 Aug; 24(4):185–189.
DiTunno JF Jr and Formal CS. Chronic spinal cord injury. N Engl J Med 1994 Feb 24; 330(8):550–556.
Donovan WH. Operative and nonoperative management of spinal cord injury. A review. Paraplegia 1994 Jun; 32(6):375–388.
Ducker TB and Zeidman SM. Spinal cord injury. Role of steroid therapy. Spine 1994 Oct 15; 19(20):2281–2287.
Hilton G et al. Methylprednisolone for acute spinal cord injury. J Neurosci Nurs 1992 Aug; 24(4):234–237.
Hixon AK et al. Improving continuity of care by evaluation of postdischarge outcomes. SCI Nurs 1992 Jun; 9(2):42–45.
Kim SW et al. Prevalence of deep venous thrombosis in patients with chronic spinal cord injury. Arch Phys Med Rehabil 1994 Sep; 75(9):965–968.
McBride DQ and Rodts GE. Intensive care of patients with spinal trauma. Neurosurg Clin North Am 1994 Oct; 5(4):755–766.
Montgomery JL and Montgomery ML. Radiographic evaluation of cervical spine trauma. Procedures to avoid catastrophe. Postgrad Med 1994 Mar; 95(4):173–174, 182–184.
Moore AD et al. Coping and emotional attributions following spinal cord injury. Int J Rehabil Res 1994 Mar; 17(1):39–48.
Peppers MP. Spinal Cord injury and methyprednisolone. Emergency 1992 Jun; 24(6):56–59.
*Radwanski M. Self-medicating practices for managing chronic pain after spinal cord injury. Rehabil Nurs 1992 Nov–Dec; 17(6):312–318.
*Richmond T et al. Cost of nursing care in acute spinal cord injury. Heart Lung 1992 May; 21(3):293.
*Richmond T et al. Powerlessness in acute spinal cord injury patients: a descriptive study. J. Neurosci Nurs 1992 Jun; 24(3):146–152.
*Richmond TS, Metcalf J and Daly M. Requirement for nursing care services and associated costs in acute spinal cord injury. J Neurosci Nurs 1995 Feb; 27(1):47–52.

Rinehart ME. Early mobilization in acute spinal cord injury: A collaborative approach. Crit Care Nurs Clin North Am 1990 Sep; 2(3):399–405.
Sauer PM and Harvey CJ. Spinal cord injury and pregnancy. J Perinat Neonatal Nurs 1993 Jun; 7(1):22–34.
Savoy SM et al. Intrathecal vaclofen infusion: An innovative approach for controlling spinal spasticity. Rehabil Nurs 1993 Mar–Apr; 18(2):105–113, 135–136.
Segatore M. Deafferentation pain after spinal cord injury. Part I. Theoretical aspects. SCI Nurs 1992 Jun; 9(2):46–50.
Segatore M. Deafferentation pain after spinal cord injury. Part II. Management. SCI Nurs 1992 Aug; 9(3):92–98.
Segatore M. Understanding chronic pain after spinal cord injury. J Neurosci Nurs 1994 Aug; 26(4):230–236.
Segatore M and Way C. Methylprednisolone after spinal cord injury. SCI Nurs 1993 Mar; 10(1):8–14.
Slack RS and Shucart W. Respiratory dysfunction associated with traumatic injury in the central nervous system. Clin Chest Med 1994 Dec; 15(4):739–749.
Smith EM and Bodner DR. Sexual dysfunction after spinal cord injury. Urol Clin North Am 1993 Aug; 20(3):535–542.
Stenger KM. Surveillance of spinal cord motor and sensory function. Nurs Clin North Am 1993 Dec; 18(4):783–792.
Waters RL, Sie IH and Adkins RH. Rehabilitation of the patient with a spinal cord injury. Orthop Clin North Am 1995 Jan; 26(1): 117–122.
*White MJ et al. A comparison of sexual concerns of men and women with spinal cord injuries. Rehabil Nurs Res 1994 Summer; 3(2):55–61.
Winkelman C. Neurologic trauma. AACN Clin Issues Crit Care Nurs 1992 Feb; 3(1):overall 7–54.

Cervical and Lumbar Disc Herniation

Bryant GA. When your patient needs back surgery. RN 1992 Jul; 55(7):46–52.
Feingold DJ et al. Complications of lumbar spine surgery. Orthop Nurs 1991 Jul–Aug; 10(4):39–58.
Hallal JC. Back pain with post-menopausal osteoporosis and vertebral fractures. Geriatr Nurs 1991 Nov–Dec; 12(6):285–287.
Partyka MB. Practical points in the care of the post-lumbar spine surgery patient. J Post Anesth Nurs 1991 Jun; 6(3):185–187.
Quigley MR et al. Lumbar surgery in the elderly. Neurosurgery 1992 May; 30(5):672–674.
Rizzolo SJ. Vaccaro AR and Cotler JM. Cervical spine trauma. Spine 1994 Oct 15; 19(20):2288–2298.

Trigeminal Neuralagia and Neuropathies

Blake GJ. Carbamazepine for trigeminal neuralagia and pain. Nursing 1991 Mar; 21(3):102.
Dyck Pj et al. When you suspect Bell's Palsy. Patient Care 1992 Jan 15; 26(1):151–154, 160–163.
Feinmann C and Peatfield R. Orofacial neuralgia. Diagnosis and treatment guidelines. Drugs 1993 Aug; 46(2):263–268.
McConaghy DJ. Trigeminal neuralgia: A personal review and nursing implications. J Neurosci Nurs 1994 Apr; 26(2):85–90.

INFORMATION/RESOURCES

Voluntary Agencies

American Cancer Society
1599 Clifton Road NE,
Atlanta, GA 30329

American Parkinson's Disease Association
60 Bay Street, Ste 401,
Staten Island, NY 10301

Amyotrophic Lateral Sclerosis Association
21021 Ventura Blvd. Ste 321,
Woodland Hills, CA 91364

Epilepsy Foundation of America
4351 Garden City Drive,
Landover, MD 20785

Guillain-Barrè Syndrome Foundation International
P.O. Box 262,
Wynnewood, PA 19096

Huntington's Disease Society of America
140 W 22nd Street, 6th Floor,
New York, NY 10011

Muscular Dystrophy Association
810 7th Avenue,
New York, NY 10019

Myasthenia Gravis Foundation
53 W Jackson Blvd, Ste 1352,
Chicago, IL 60604

National Head Injury Foundation
333 Turnpike Road,
Southborough, MA 01772

National Headache Foundation
5252 N Western Avenue,
Chicago, IL 60625

National Multiple Sclerosis Society
733 Third Avenue,
New York, NY 10017

National Parkinson's Foundation
1501 NW 9th Avenue,
Miami, FL 33136

National Spinal Cord Injury Association
600 W Cummings Park, Ste 2000,
Woburn, MA 01801

Paralyzed Veterans of America
801 18th Street NW,
Washington, DC 20006

Nursing Research Profile for Unit 15

Neuroscience Nursing

Overview

Research in neuroscience nursing reviewed here focuses on the nursing considerations, management, and implications for patients with head injuries and stroke. Such conditions are catastrophic for both patient and family; they require intensive nursing management and deserve the attention of nurse researchers.

Ross AM, Pitts LH, and Kobayasli S. Prognosticators of outcome after major head injury in the elderly. J Neurosci Nurs 1992 Apr; 24(2):88–93.

Although elderly patients who experience head injury are generally considered to have poorer outcomes than younger patients who experience similar injuries, few studies have systematically examined these outcomes in head-injured elderly patients. The purpose of the study was to determine whether outcomes following major head injury are poorer in older patients, as has been suggested.

The researchers prospectively reviewed clinical data of 195 head-injured patients over the age of 65 years of age. Data included Glasgow Coma Scale (GCS) scores at admission and 72 hours after injury, cause of injury, type of concurrent injuries, the presence of shock or apnea, type and results of surgical procedures, and Glasgow Outcome Scale (GOS) scores at 6 months. At the time of GCS determination an assessment of the degree of recovery was made and categorized as good recovery, moderately disabled, severely disabled, or vegetative. In addition, intracranial pressure (ICP) values of the 132 patients whose ICPs were monitored were used to categorize patients into two groups: Group I had values greater than 20 mm Hg at some time during monitoring, and Group II had ICP values that remained below 20 mm Hg throughout monitoring.

The mean age of the 195 patients in the sample was 75.5 years (range 65–99 years). Patients with elevated ICP (Group I) had greater mortality and morbidity than patients with normal ICP (Group II). In addition, all of the 79 patients who were in coma (GCS ≤ 8) on admission and remained in coma after 72 hours died within 6 months of their head injury. Of those 16 who were in coma at admission but not in coma at 72 hours, 9 (56%) were alive at 6 months. Of these 9 patients, 4 had moderate disability or a good recovery at 6 months, and the remaining 5 were severely disabled.

The findings revealed that patients over the age of 65 years had only a 25% chance of survival following a major head injury and a 13% chance of recovery with an independent lifestyle. Patients who were in a coma on admission tended to remain so and had a less than 10% chance of survival and a 4% chance of functioning independently once recovered. Patients in this study had an overall mortality rate of 75% at the 6-month follow-up, confirming previous reports of a higher mortality in the elderly head-injured patient when compared with younger patients.

Nursing Implications. When counseling family members regarding prognosis and outcome following major head injury in the elderly patient, particular attention should be given to the patient's hospital course during the first 72 hours as it is a strong predictor of later morbidity and mortality. Families should be given the opportunity to discuss the likelihood for meaningful survival and the anticipated degree of disability. The results of this study indicate that this opportunity for discussion with the family exists as early as 72 hours following head injury. Families and caregivers can then plan together for appropriate clinical care. The findings of this study have implications for end-of-life decision making in families and for future instutitional discussion about utilization of resources.

Rising C. The relationship of selected nursing activities to ICP. J Neurosci Nurs 1993 Oct; 25(5):302–308.

Intracranial pressure monitoring is frequently used in patients who have sustained some type of brain injury, surgery, or pathologic process. This study examined the effect that nursing activities (*e.g.*, turning, bathing, and suctioning) had on the ICP of five patients with brain injury due to trauma.

The five patients served as their own controls. Their mean ICPs were assessed with fiberoptic catheters and a continuous ICP monitoring system; ICP data were recorded 2 minutes before, during, and after each nursing activity was routinely performed throughout the time the ICP monitoring systems were in place. The study was completed by the nurse caring for the patient while another nurse was assigned to monitor that the nursing care acitivities were performed as outlined.

Turning was carried out by two nurses, keeping the head of the bed (HOB) elevated 30 degrees and maintaining body alignment. Suctioning involved inserting a suctioning catheter into the tracheostomy or endotracheal tube for a maximum period of 15 seconds and withdrawing the catheter at 80 to 100 mm Hg, followed by hyperventilation with 100% oxygen for 20 to 30 seconds. Bathing was completed with the patient in a supine position, using warm water at 48.9°C and covering the patient with a bath blanket to prevent chilling; the HOB was elevated 30 degrees.

The sample consisted of three males and two females ranging in age from 30 to 89 years. The ICP monitor was placed in the subdural space, with an initial mean opening ICP of 23.4 mm Hg (range 7–45 mm Hg). The mean Glasgow Coma Score of the five subjects was 9.4 (range 5–13).

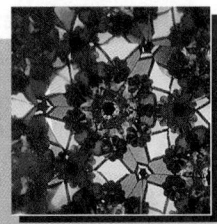

All patients were noted to have increases in ICP when turned and suctioned; however, there was no prolonged elevation of ICP. Bathing produced the least increase in ICP with only two baths (out of 22 baths given) resulting in ICP greater than 20 mm Hg in one of the five patients. This patient's ICP before bathing was 13.8 mm Hg, whereas other patients' ICP before bathing ranged from 2 to 8.55 mm Hg. Other subjects did not have an increase in ICP over 20 mm Hg when bathed.

Nursing Implications. Although this study is limited by the small sample size, it does provide important information about the effects of routine nursing activities on ICP in head-injured patients. It is important for the nurse, when providing nursing care activities to the patient, to keep in mind those activities that may cause an increase in ICP and the patient's baseline ICP value. Delaying routine activities may be warranted in those patients at risk for increased ICP.

Crosby L and Parsons LC. Cerebrovascular response of closed head injured patients to a standardized endotracheal tube suctioning and manual hyperventilation procedure. J Neurosci Nurs 1992 Feb; 24(1):40–51.

The purposes of this study were (1) to evaluate the cerebrovascular response to a standardized endotracheal tube suctioning and manual hyperventilation procedure and (2) to determine if a 5-minute rest period was adequate to allow the cerebrovascular parameters to return to pre-suctioning levels. The cerebrovascular parameters addressed in this study included mean arterial pressure (MAP), mean intracranial pressure (MICP), cerebral perfusion pressure (CPP), heart rate (HR), and the end tidal CO_2 ($PetCO_2$).

A sample of 49 patients with closed-head injury with ICP monitoring were enrolled in the study, with a total of 145 endotracheal suctioning and hyperventilation procedures performed. The suctioning procedure consisted of allowing the patient to rest undisturbed for 5 minutes before the procedure was initiated, removing the patient from the ventilator, and providing manual hyperventilation with 100% oxygen, using two hands. After the hyperventilation, the patient was suctioned through the endotracheal tube for 15 seconds and hyperventilated again. The procedure was repeated until the patient was suctioned three times and four periods of hyperventilation were given. The patient's endotracheal tube was then reattached to the ventilator and a 5-minute recovery phase initiated. The protocol was initiated as indicated based on results of assessment of the patient. Data were collected during the last 30 seconds of the 5-minute pre-procedure rest period, every 15 seconds during the procedure, and at the end of each minute of the 5-minute recovery period.

Analysis revealed significant differences ($p < .001$) among the 15-second data points during the suctioning/hyperventilation procedure and during the 5-minute recovery period on all cerebrovascular parameters. Stepwise increases in MICP associated with the first and second passes of the suctioning catheter were demonstrated. However, extension of hyperventilation from 30 to 60 seconds after the third suction procedure reversed this stair-step increase in MICP. It was also demonstrated that 2 full minutes of recovery time were needed for the cerebrovascular parameters examined in this study to return to baseline. Specific data points during the suctioning/hyperventilation procedure differed significantly compared with baseline.

Nursing Implications. Patients with head injuries are frequently intubated and require suctioning for the removal of retained secretions. This study highlights the important finding that suctioning alters the MICP, CPP, MAP, HR, and $PetCO_2$. Some critically injured patients with increased ICP may not tolerate the changes in the cerebrovascular parameters, which may lead to cerebral hypoxia. It is imperative that the nurse adequately oxygenate the patient before and after suctioning and plan nursing care so that adequate time is permitted for patients at risk for increased ICP to return to their baseline cerebrovascular parameters.

Nyswonger GD and Helmchen RH. Early enteral nutrition and length of stay in stroke patients. J Neurosci Nurs 1992 Aug; 24(4):220–223.

There is an extensive body of research demonstrating that early feeding of hospitalized patients can have an impact on the length of stay. Patients who have sustained a stroke have associated factors such as dysphagia, hemiplegia, and cognitive deficits that may impair their ability to receive adequate nutrition. The purpose of this study was to examine the effect of early enteral nutrition on length of hospital stay (LOS) of patients admitted to one hospital with the diagnosis of stroke.

A retrospective chart review of nonsurgical stroke patients admitted to a 750-bed community hospital during a 3-year period was conducted. There were 222 nonsurgical patients with a diagnosis of stroke admitted to this hospital during this period; 52 patients required enteral tube feedings during the course of hospitalization. Information collected from hospital records of the 52 patients included Glasgow Coma Scale score, age, sex, diagnosis, nutritional status at admission, time from hospital admission to initiation of enteral feeding, type of formula, date and time of admission and discharge, and discharge status.

The mean length of stay for the group was 26.06 days (SD = 18.12). There was a significant difference ($p = 0.036$) in length of stay of patients who received feedings within 72 hours of admission and those whose feedings were initiated after 72 hours. The mean LOS of those who received feedings early was 20.14 days (SD = 12.87), whereas those who were fed later had a mean LOS of 29.76 (SD = 20.05) days. The Glasgow Coma Scores (GCS) for the patients were also evaluated, showing no difference in LOS between the two groups. There were no statistical differences in LOS by discharge status (*i.e.*, home versus rehabilitation program versus extended care facility). LOS also did not differ by GCS score, admission nutritional status, gender, or age. Some patients had their hospital course complicated by congestive heart failure, preexisting malnutrition, borderline malnutrition, and development of complications (*e.g.*, pneumonia). Overall, the implementation of early feedings of stroke patients was associated with shorter LOS. Further study would include a larger sample size and concurrent rather than retrospective review.

Nursing Implications. Attention to nutritional status of patients admitted to the hospital with a stroke is warranted as many problems associated with stroke (*i.e.*, hemiplegia, dysphagia, and cognitive deficits) may affect their ability to swallow or eat adequately. Adequate nutritional status and shorter hospital stays may result from early nutritional assessment and intervention.

UNIT 16
Musculoskeletal Function

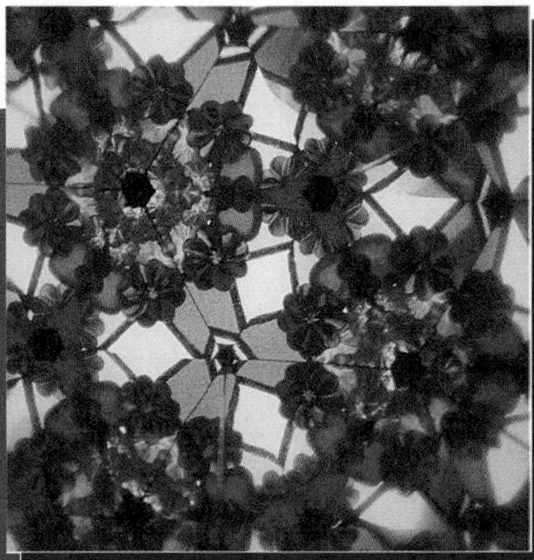

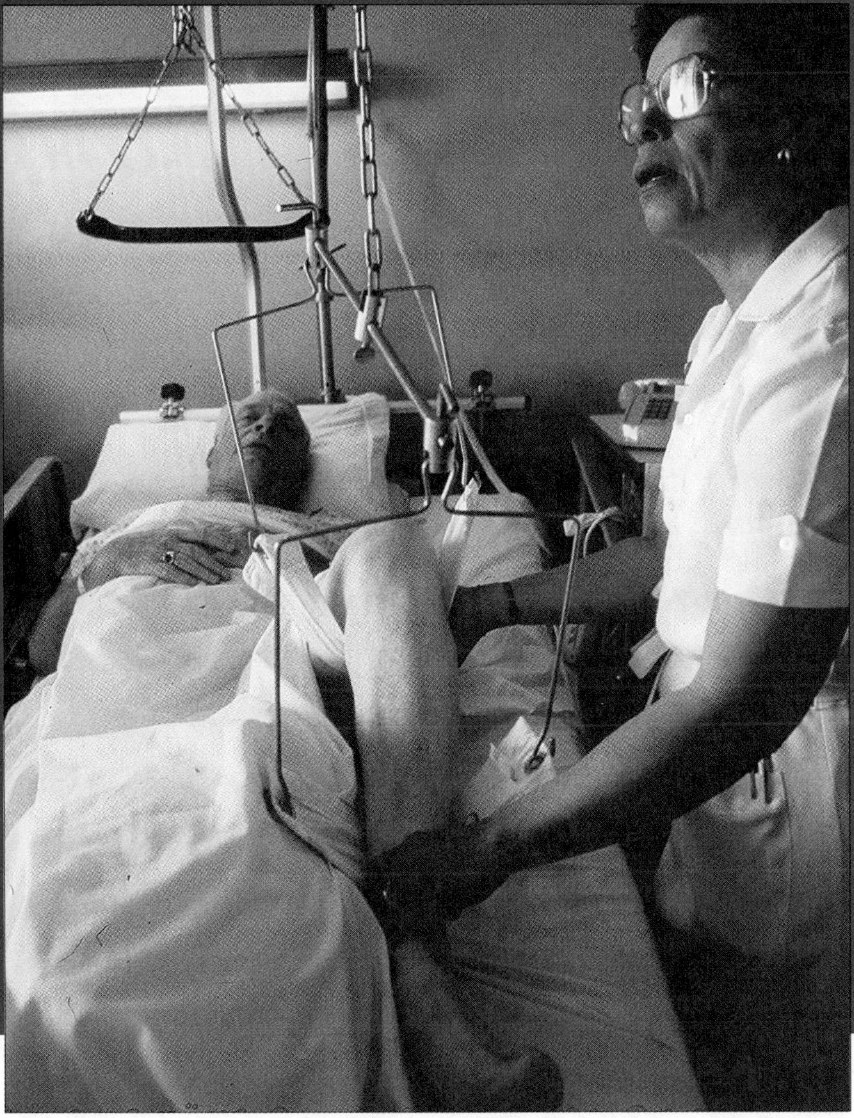

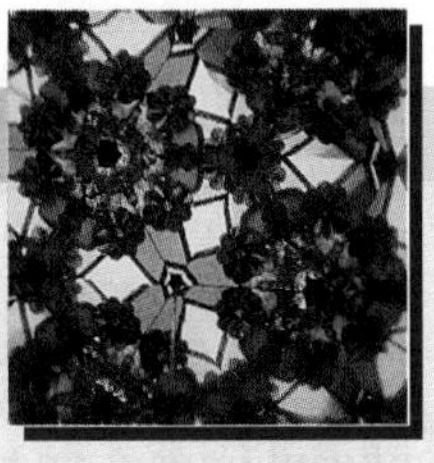

61

Assessment of Musculoskeletal Function

CHAPTER OUTLINE

LEARNING OBJECTIVES

On completion of this chapter, the learner will be able to:

1. Describe the physiology of the skeletal, articular, and skeletal muscle systems
2. Describe the physiology of bone healing
3. Describe the significance of physical assessment to the diagnosis of musculoskeletal dysfunction
4. Specify the diagnostic tests used for assessment of musculoskeletal function
5. Identify nursing diagnoses common to patients with musculoskeletal disorders

The musculoskeletal system includes the bones, joints, muscles, tendons, ligaments, and bursae of the body (see Chart 61-1 for a glossary of terms used in this chapter). The problems associated with these structures are very common and affect all age groups. Problems with the musculoskeletal system are generally not life threatening, but they have a significant impact on one's normal activities and productivity. Such problems may be encountered in any area of nursing practice, as well as during daily living experiences.

Physiologic Overview

Bony structures and connective tissue account for approximately 25% of the body weight, and muscle accounts for approximately 50%. The health and proper functioning of the musculoskeletal system are interdependent with those of the other body systems.

The bony structure provides protection for vital organs, including the brain, heart, and lungs. The bony skeleton provides a sturdy framework to support body structures. The muscles attached to the skeleton allow the body to move. The **bone matrix** stores calcium, phosphorus, magnesium, and fluoride. More than 99% of the total body calcium is present in bone. The red bone marrow located within bone cavities produces red and white blood cells in a process called **hematopoiesis.** Muscle contraction results in mechanical action for movement as well as heat production to maintain body temperature.

The Skeletal System

Anatomy of the Skeletal System. There are 206 bones in the human body, divided into four categories: **long bones** (*e.g.*, the femur), **short bones** (*e.g.*, the tarsals), **flat bones** (*e.g.*, the sternum), and **irregular bones** (*e.g.*, the vertebrae). The shape and construction of a specific bone are determined by its function and the forces exerted on it.

Bones are constructed of cancellous (trabecular or spongy) or cortical (compact) bone tissue. Long bones (*e.g.*, femur) are shaped like rods or shafts with rounded ends (Fig. 61-1). The shaft, or diaphysis, is primarily cortical bone. The ends of the long bones are called epiphyses and are primarily cancellous bone. The epiphyseal plate separates the epiphyses from the diaphysis and is the center for longitudinal growth in children. In the adult, it is calcified. The ends of long bones are covered by articular cartilage at

CHART 61-1
Glossary of Musculoskeletal Terms

Aponeurosis broad band of fibrous tissue connecting muscle to bone, connective tissue, other muscles, soft tissue, or skin

Bursa fluid-filled sac found in connective tissue usually in the area of joints

Callus fibrous tissue at fracture site

Cancellous bone spongy, lattice-like bone structure; trabecular bone

Cartilage special tissue at ends of bone

Clonus rhythmic contraction of muscle

Contracture abnormal shortening of muscle and/or joint fibrosis

Cortical bone compact bone

Crepitus grating sound; may be heard with movement of ends of a broke bone

Diaphysis shaft of long bone

Effusion excess fluid in joint

Endosteum marrow cavity lining of hollow bone

Epiphysis ends of long bone

Fascia (epimysium) fibrous tissue that covers, supports, and separates muscles

Fasciculation involuntary twitch of muscle fibers

Fasciculi parallel groups of muscle cells (myofibrils)

Flaccid absence of muscle tone

Isometric contraction muscle tension increased, length unchanged, no joint motion

Isotonic contraction muscle tension unchanged, muscle shortened, joint motion

Lamellar bone mature bone exhibiting concentric rings of bone matrix

Ligament fibrous band connecting bones

Myofibril muscle cell; contains sarcomeres

Ossification process in which minerals (calcium) are deposited in bone matrix

Osteoblast bone-forming cell

Osteocyte mature bone cell

Osteoclast bone resorption cell

Osteogenesis bone formation

Osteoid bone matrix tissue; prebone

Osteon microscopic functional bone unit

Periosteum fibrous connective tissue covering bone

Remodeling process of reorganizing new bone structure according to function

Resorption removal, destruction of bone

Sarcomere contractile unit of muscle cell

Spastic greater than normal muscle tone

Synovium membrane in joint which secretes lubricating fluid

Tendon cord of fibrous tissue connecting muscle to bone

Tone normal tension (resistance to stretch) in resting muscle

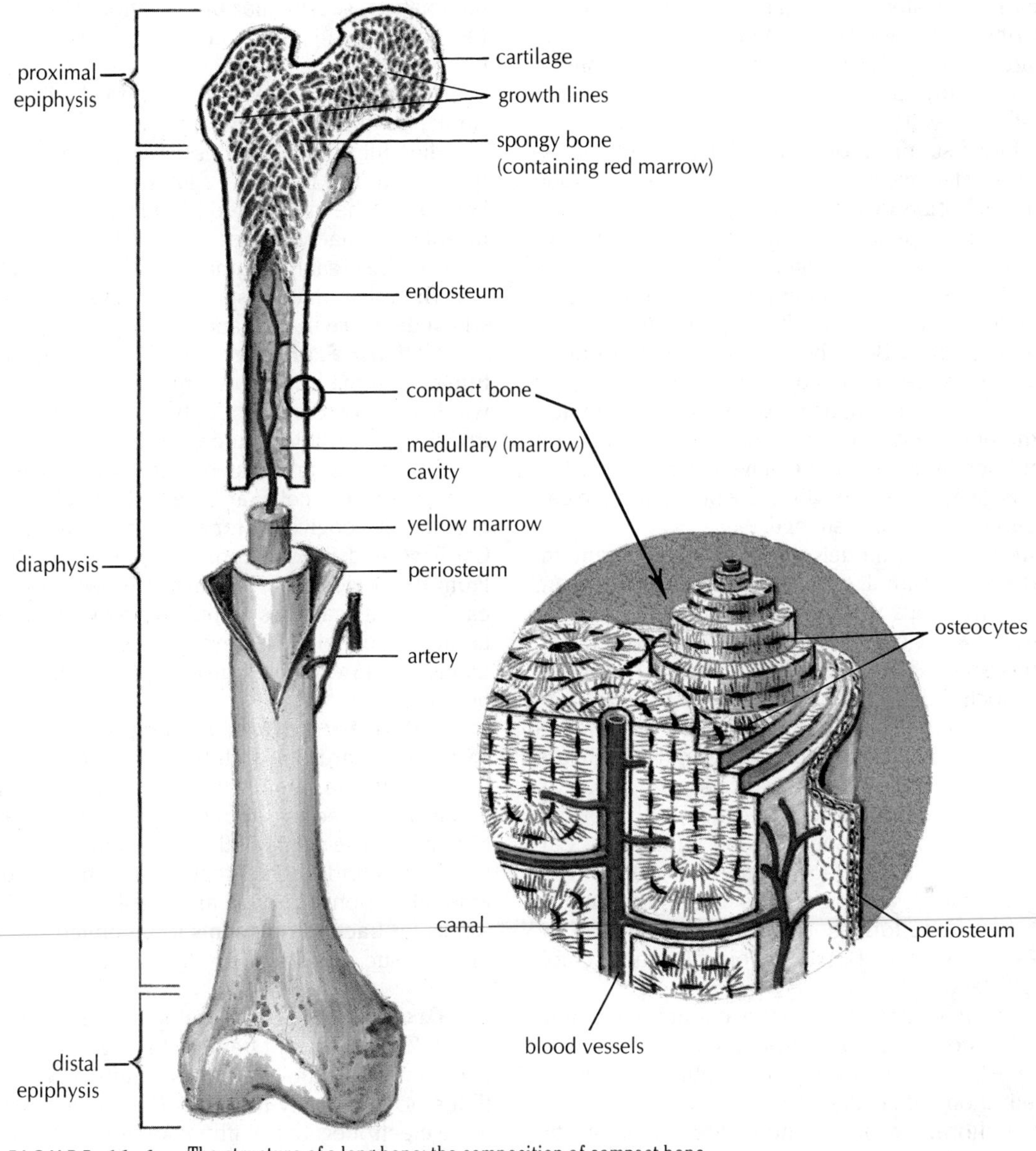

FIGURE 61-1. The structure of a long bone; the composition of compact bone.

the joints. Long bones are constructed for weight-bearing and movement. Short bones (*e.g.*, metacarpals) consist of cancellous bone covered by a layer of compact bone. Flat bones (*e.g.*, sternum) are important sites for hematopoiesis and frequently provide vital organ protection. They are made of cancellous bone layered between compact bone. Irregular bones (*e.g.*, vertebrae) have unique shapes related to their functions. Generally, irregular bone structure is similar to that of flat bones.

Bone is composed of cells, protein matrix, and mineral deposits. The cells are of three basic types—osteoblasts, osteocytes, and osteoclasts. Osteoblasts function in bone formation by secreting bone matrix. The matrix is 98% collagen and 2% foundation substances (glucosamine glycans [acid polysaccharides] and proteoglycans). The matrix is a framework in which inorganic mineral salts are deposited. Osteocytes are mature bone cells involved in bone-maintenance functions and are located in osteons (bone matrix units). Osteoclasts are multinuclear cells involved in destroying, resorbing, and remodeling bone.

The osteon is the microscopic functioning unit of mature bone. The center of the osteon contains a capillary. Around the capillary are circles of bone matrix called lamellae. Within the lamellae are osteocytes, which are nourished through processes that extend into tiny **canaliculi** (canals that communicate with blood vessels less than 0.1 mm away).

Covering the bone is a dense, fibrous membrane known as the periosteum. The periosteum nourishes bone and allows for its growth, as well as provides for the attachment of tendons and ligaments. The periosteum contains nerves, blood vessels, and lymphatics. The layer closest to the bone contains osteoblasts, which are bone-forming cells.

Endosteum is a thin, vascular membrane covering the marrow cavity of long bones and the spaces in cancellous bone. Osteoclasts, which dissolve bone to maintain the marrow cavity, are located near the endosteum and in Howship's lacunae (indentations on bone surfaces).

Bone marrow is a vascular tissue located in the medullary (shaft) cavity of long bones and in flat bones.

Red bone marrow, located mainly in the sternum, ilium, vertebrae, and ribs in the adult, is responsible for producing red and white blood cells. In the adult, the long bone is filled with fatty, yellow marrow.

Bone tissue is well vascularized. Cancellous bone receives a rich blood supply through metaphyseal and epiphyseal vessels. Periosteal vessels carry blood to compact bone through minute **Volkmann canals.** In addition, nutrient arteries penetrate the periosteum and enter the medullary cavity through **foramina** (small openings). Nutrient arteries supply blood to the marrow and bone. The venous system may accompany arteries or may exit independently.

Bone Formation. Bone begins to form long before birth. Ossification is the process by which the bone matrix (*e.g.*, collagen fibers and ground substance) is formed and hardening minerals (*e.g.*, calcium salts) are deposited on the collagen fibers in an electronegative environment. The collagen fibers give tensile strength to the bone, and the calcium provides compressional strength.

There are two basic models of ossification: intramembranous and endochondral. Intramembranous ossification, in which bone develops within membrane, occurs in the bones of the face and skull. Therefore, when the skull heals, it is by fibrous union. The other kind of bone formation is known as endochondral ossification, in which a cartilage model exists. Cartilage-like (osteoid) tissue is formed, resorbed, and replaced by bone. Most bones in the body are formed and heal by endochondral ossification.

Bone Maintenance. Bone is a dynamic tissue in a constant state of turnover (resorption and reforming). Calcium in bone in an adult is replaced at the rate of about 18% a year. The important regulating factors that determine the balance between bone formation and bone resorption include local stress, vitamin D, parathyroid hormone, calcitonin, and circulation.

Vitamin D functions to increase the amount of calcium in the blood by promoting absorption of calcium from the gastrointestinal tract. A deficiency of vitamin D results in bone mineralization deficit, deformity, and fracture.

Parathyroid hormone and calcitonin are the major hormonal regulators of calcium homeostasis. Parathyroid hormone regulates the concentration of calcium in the blood, in part by promoting movement of calcium from the bone. In response to low calcium levels in the blood, increased levels of parathyroid hormone prompt the mobilization of calcium, the demineralization of bone, and the formation of bone cysts. Calcitonin, from the thyroid gland, increases the deposit of calcium in bone.

Blood supply to the bone also affects bone formation. With diminished blood supply or **hyperemia** (congestion), osteogenesis is reduced and the bone becomes osteoporotic (less dense). Bone necrosis occurs when the bone is deprived of blood.

Bone Healing

Most fractures heal through endochondral ossification. When the bone is injured, the bone fragments are not merely patched together with scar tissue. The bone regenerates itself. There are several stages in fracture healing: (1) inflammation, (2) cellular proliferation, (3) callus formation, (4) callus ossification, and (5) remodeling into mature bone (Fig. 61-2).

Inflammation. With a fracture, the body's response is similar to that of injury elsewhere in the body. There is bleeding into the injured tissue and formation of a fracture hematoma. The fracture fragment ends become devitalized because of the interrupted blood supply. The injured area is invaded by macrophages (large white blood cells), which debride the area. Inflammation, swelling, and pain are present. The inflammatory stage lasts several days and resolves with a decrease in pain and swelling.

Cellular Proliferation. Within about 5 days, the fracture hematoma undergoes organization. Fibrin strands form within the clot, creating a network for revascularization and invasion by fibroblasts and osteoblasts.

Fibroblasts and osteoblasts (developed from osteocytes, endosteal cells, and periosteal cells) produce collagen and proteoglycans for a collagen matrix at the fracture. Cartilage and fibrous connective (osteoid) tissue develop. From the periosteum, a collar of growth is detectable. This cartilaginous callus is stimulated by minimal micromotion at the fracture site. However, excessive motion disrupts the callus structure. Actively growing bone exhibits electronegative potentials.

Callus Formation. Tissue growth continues and the cartilage collar from each bone fragment grows toward the others until the fracture gap is bridged. The fracture fragments are joined by fibrous tissue, cartilage, and immature fiber bone. The shape of the callus and the volume of tissue required to bridge the defect are directly proportional to the amount of bone damage and displacement. It takes 3 to 4 weeks for fracture fragments to be united by cartilage or fibrous tissue. Clinically, the fragments are no longer easily moved.

Ossification. The developed callus begins to ossify within 2 to 3 weeks of fracture through the process of endochondral ossification. Minerals continue to be deposited until the bone is firmly reunited. The callus surface continues to be electronegative. With major adult long bone fractures, ossification takes 3 to 4 months.

Remodeling. The final stage of fracture repair consists of removing any remaining devitalized tissue and reorganizing the new bone into its former structural arrangement. Remodeling may take months to years depending on the extent of bone modification needed, the function of the bone, and—in cases involving compact and cancellous bone—the functional stresses on the bone. Cancellous bone heals and remodels more rapidly than compact cortical bone, especially at points of direct contact. When remodeling is complete, the fracture surface charge is no longer negative.

The progress of bone healing is monitored by serial x-rays. Adequate immobilization is essential until there is evidence of callus formation on x-ray. Progression of the therapeutic regimen (*e.g.*, applying a cast brace to a patient who has had a femur fracture reduced and immobilized by skeletal traction) is determined by evidence of healing of the fracture.

Bone Healing With Fragments Firmly Approximated. When fractures are treated with open rigid fixation techniques, the bony fragments can be placed in direct con-

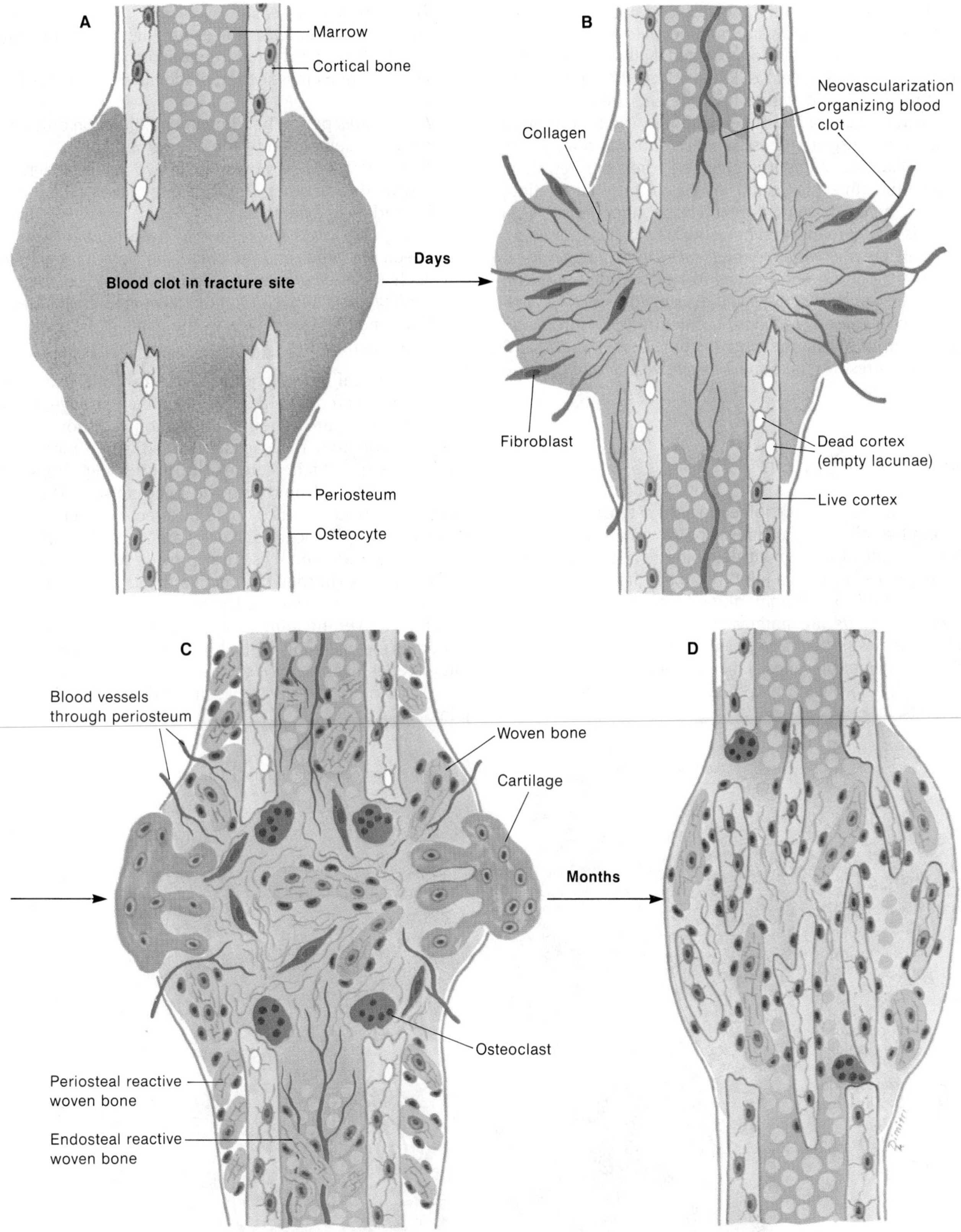

FIGURE 61-2. Healing of a fracture. (**A**) Soon after a fracture, an extensive blood clot forms in the subperiosteal and soft tissue. (**B**) Inflammatory phase: neovascularization and beginning organization of the blood clot. (**C**) Reparative phase: formation of a callus of cartilage and woven bone near the fracture site. (**D**) Remodeling phase: the cortex is revitalized. (Rubin E and Farber JL. Pathology, 2nd ed. Philadelphia, JB Lippincott, 1994.)

tact. Motion at the fracture is eliminated. In this situation, the stages of bone healing are modified. Hematoma formation is not essential and is not observed. Little or no external cartilaginous callus develops. Primary bone healing occurs.

Immature bone develops from the endosteum. There is an intensive regeneration of new osteons, which develop in the fracture line by a process similar to normal bone maintenance. Fracture strength is obtained when the new osteons have become established. With rigid internal fixation, the bone heals through cortical bone remodeling. This process is slower than when bone heals by callus formation.

Local stress (weight-bearing) acts to stimulate local bone formation and remodeling. Weight-bearing bones are thick and strong. When weight-bearing or stress is prevented, as in prolonged bedrest, calcium is lost from the bone (resorption) and the bone becomes osteoporotic and weak. If the stress on the bone is excessive, fracture or bone necrosis occurs.

The Articular System

The bones of the body are joined together at **joints** or **articulations** that allow for a variety of movements. Regardless of the amount of movement possible, the junction of two or more bones is called a joint. There are three basic kinds of joints: synarthrosis, amphiarthrosis, and diarthrosis joints. *Synarthrosis joints* are immovable, as exemplified by the skull sutures. *Amphiarthroses,* such as the vertebral joints and symphysis pubis, allow limited motion. The bones are separated by fibrous cartilage. *Diarthroses* are freely movable joints.

Types of Diarthrosis Joints

- *Ball and socket joints,* best exemplified by the hip and the shoulder, permit full freedom of movement (see Fig. 61-3 for a cross-section of the moveable joint of a hip).
- *Hinge joints* permit bending in one direction only and are best exemplified by the elbows and knees.
- *Saddle joints* allow movement in two planes at right angles to each other. The joint at the base of the thumb is a saddle, biaxial joint.
- *Pivot joints* are characterized by the articulation between the radius and the ulna. They permit rotation for such activities as turning a doorknob.
- *Gliding joints* allow for limited movement in all directions and are represented by the joints of the carpal bones in the wrist.

At a typical movable joint, the ends of the articulating bones are covered with a smooth hyaline cartilage. The articulating bones are surrounded by a tough, fibrous sheath, the **joint capsule.** The capsule is lined with a membrane, the synovium, which secretes the lubricating and shock-absorbing synovial fluid into the joint capsule. Therefore, the bone surfaces do not come in direct contact. In some synovial joints, fibrocartilage discs are located between the articular cartilage surfaces. They provide shock absorption.

Ligaments (fibrous connective tissue bands) bind the articulating bones together. Ligaments and muscle tendons, which pass over the joint, provide joint stability. Figure 61-3 illustrates the ligaments of the hip and pelvis. In some joints, interosseous ligaments (*e.g.,* the cruciate ligaments of the knee) are found within the capsule and add stability to the joint.

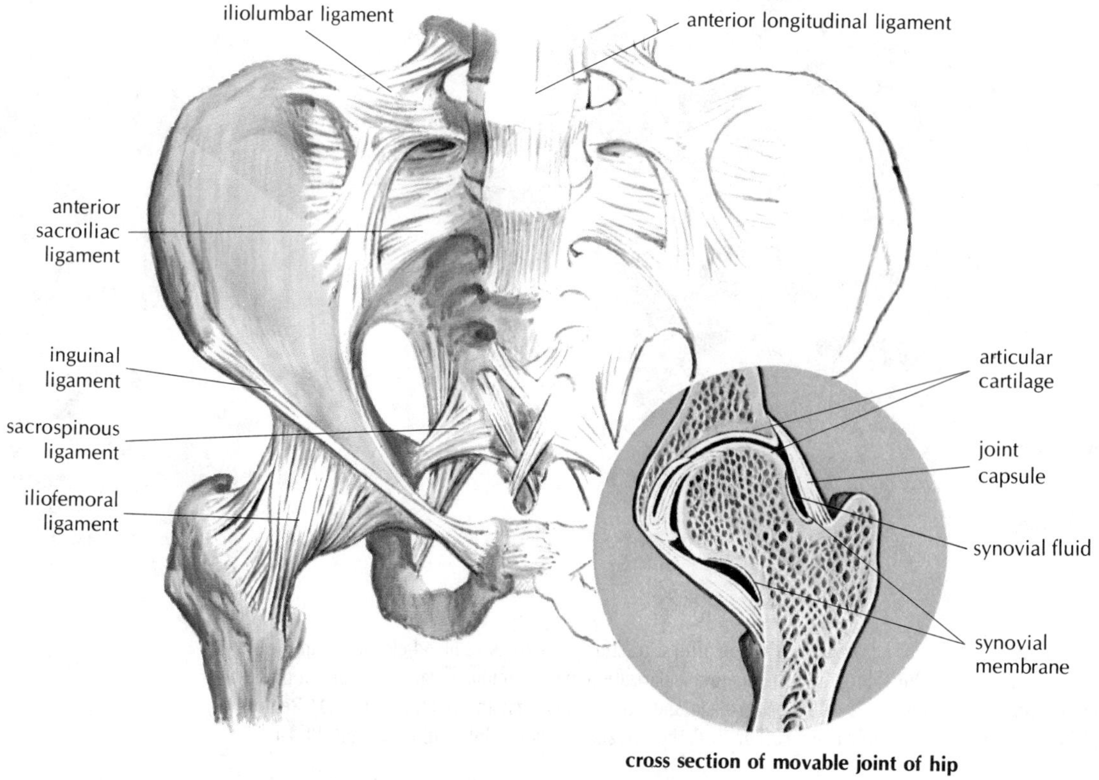

FIGURE 61-3. Ligaments of the hip and pelvis.

A bursa is a sac filled with synovial fluid that is located at a point of friction. Bursae are generally found cushioning the movement of tendons, ligaments, and bones at the elbow, shoulder, knee, and some other joints.

The Skeletal Muscle System

Anatomy of Skeletal Muscles. Skeletal (striated) muscles are involved in body movement, posture, and heat-production functions. Muscles are attached by tendons (cords of fibrous connective tissue) or **aponeuroses** (broad, flat sheets of connective tissue) to bones, connective tissue, other muscles, soft tissue, or skin. Muscles contract to bring the two points of attachment closer together. Muscles vary in shape and size according to the activity for which they are responsible. Muscles develop and are maintained when actively used. Age and disuse cause loss of muscular function as fibrotic tissue replaces the contractile muscle tissue.

The muscles of the body are composed of parallel groups of muscle cells (fasciculi) encased in fibrous tissue called epimysium or fascia. The more fasciculi contained in a muscle, the more precise the movements.

The speed of the muscle contraction is variable. **Myoglobulin** is a hemoglobin-like protein pigment that is present in striated muscle cells. It transports oxygen for the cell's metabolic needs from the blood capillaries to the mitochondria of the muscle cell. Muscles containing large quantities of myoglobulin **(red muscles)** have been observed to contract slowly and powerfully (*e.g.*, respiratory and postural muscles). Muscles containing little myoglobulin **(white muscles)** contract quickly and for extended periods of time (*e.g.*, extraocular eye muscles). Most body muscles contain both red and white muscle fibers.

Each muscle cell (also referred to as a muscle fiber) contains **myofibrils,** which in turn are composed of a series of **sarcomeres,** the actual contractile units of skeletal muscle. The components of the sarcomeres are known as thick and thin filaments. The thin filaments are composed mainly of a protein known as actin. The thick filaments are composed mainly of the protein myosin.

Skeletal Muscle Contraction. Contraction of a muscle is due to the contraction of each of its component sarcomeres. The contraction of a sarcomere is due to interactions between the myosin in the thick filaments and the actin in the thin filaments, brought about by a local increase in the calcium ion concentration. The thick and thin filaments slide across one another. When calcium concentration in the sarcomere subsequently falls, the myosin and actin filaments cease to interact and the sarcomere returns to its original resting length (relaxation). Actin and myosin do not interact in the absence of calcium.

Muscle fibers contract in response to electrical stimulation. When stimulated, muscle cells generate an action potential in a manner similar to that described for nerve cells. These action potentials propagate along the muscle cell membrane and lead to the release in the muscle cell of calcium ions that are stored in specialized organelles called the **sarcoplasmic reticulum.** It is the calcium that allows the interaction of actin and myosin in the sarcomere. Very shortly after the muscle cell membrane is depolarized, it recovers its resting membrane voltage. Calcium is rapidly removed from the sarcomeres by active reaccumulation in the sarcoplasmic reticulum, and the muscle relaxes.

Depolarization of the muscle cells normally occurs in response to a stimulus delivered by a nerve cell. The communication between the nerve cell and the muscle cell takes place at the **motor end plate.** The neurons that control the activity of skeletal muscle cells are called lower motor neurons. These neurons originate in the anterior horn of the spinal cord.

Energy is consumed during muscle contraction and relaxation. The rate of energy used by skeletal muscle varies; it increases markedly during exercise. The source of energy for the muscle cells is adenosine triphosphate (ATP) that is generated through cellular oxidative metabolism. Creatine phosphate, also present in muscle cells, functions as a second reservoir of metabolic energy; it can be converted to ATP when necessary. At low levels of activity, the skeletal muscle synthesizes ATP from the oxidation of glucose to water and carbon dioxide. During periods of high activity, when sufficient oxygen may not be available, glucose is metabolized primarily to lactic acid. Although ATP is generated during the production of lactic acid, the process is inefficient compared with that of oxidative pathways. Therefore, increased amounts of glucose are required and are supplied by muscle glycogen. Glycogen is a starch that is produced from glucose, stored in the cells during periods of rest, and utilized during periods of activity. Muscle fatigue is thought to be caused by depletion of glycogen and energy stores and accumulation of lactic acid. As a result, the cycle of muscle contraction and relaxation cannot continue.

During muscle contraction, the energy released from ATP is not completely used by the contractile apparatus. This excess energy is dissipated in the form of heat. During isometric contraction, almost all the energy is released in the form of heat; during isotonic contraction, some of the energy is expended in mechanical work. In some situations, such as shivering because of cold, the need to generate heat is the primary stimulus for muscle contraction.

Types of Muscle Contractions. The contraction of muscle fibers can result in either isotonic or isometric contraction of the muscle. In isometric contraction, the length of the muscles remains constant but the force generated by the muscles is increased; an example of this is when one pushes against an immovable wall. Isotonic contraction, on the other hand, is characterized by shortening of the muscle with no increase in tension within the muscle; an example of this is flexion of the forearm. In normal activities, many muscle movements are a combination of isometric and isotonic contraction. For example, during walking, isotonic contraction results in shortening of the leg, and during isometric contraction, the stiff leg pushes against the floor.

Muscle Tone. Relaxed muscles demonstrate a state of readiness to respond to contraction stimuli. This state of readiness is known as muscle tone (tonus) and is due to the maintenance of some of the muscle fibers in a contracted state. Sense organs in the muscles **(muscle spindles)** monitor muscle tone. Muscle tone is found to be minimal during sleep and increased when the person is anxious. A muscle that has less than normal tone is known as flaccid; a muscle with greater than normal tone is spastic. In lower motor neuron destruction (*e.g.*, polio), denervated muscle becomes atonic (soft and flabby) and atrophies.

Muscle Actions. Muscles accomplish movement only by contraction. Through the coordination of muscle groups, the body is able to perform a wide variety of movement. The **prime mover** is the muscle that causes a particular motion. The muscles assisting the prime mover are known as **synergists.** The muscle causing movement opposite to that of the primary mover is known as the **antagonist.** The antagonist must relax to allow the prime mover to contract, producing motion. For example, when contraction of the biceps causes flexion of the elbow joint, the biceps is the prime mover and the triceps is the antagonist. With muscle paralysis, a person may be able to retrain functioning muscles within a synergistic group to coordinate in such a way as to produce the needed movement. Secondary movers then become the primary mover.

The body movements that muscle contractions can produce are many. Flexion is characterized by bending at a joint (*e.g.*, elbow). The opposite movement is extension, or straightening at a joint. Abduction is the action of moving away from the midline of the body. To move toward the midline is adduction. Rotation describes turning around a specific axis (*e.g.*, shoulder joint). Circumduction is the cone-like movement of the thumb. Special body movements include supination (turning the palm up), pronation (turning the palm down), inversion (turning the sole of the foot inward), eversion (the opposite of inversion), protraction (pulling the jaw forward), and retraction (pulling the jaw backward).

Exercise, Disuse, and Repair. Muscles need to be exercised to maintain function and strength. When a muscle repeatedly develops maximum or close to maximum tension over a long period of time, as in regular exercise with weights, the cross-sectional area of the muscle increases **(hypertrophies)**. This is due to an increase in the size of individual muscle fibers without an increase in the number of muscle fibers. Hypertrophy will persist only if the exercise is continued.

The opposite phenomenon occurs with disuse of muscle over a long period of time. The decrease in the size of a muscle is called **atrophy.** Bedrest and immobility will cause loss of muscle mass and strength. When immobility is due to a treatment mode (*e.g.*, casting or traction), the patient can decrease the effects of immobility by isometric exercise of the muscles of the immobilized part. Quadriceps setting exercises (tightening the muscles of the thigh) and gluteal setting exercises (tightening of the muscles of the buttocks) help maintain the larger muscle groups that are important in ambulation. Active and weight-resistant exercises of uninjured parts of the body prevent muscle atrophy.

When muscles are injured, they need rest and immobilization until tissue repair occurs. The healed muscle then needs progressive exercise to resume its preinjury strength and functional ability.

Gerontologic Considerations

Multiple changes in the musculoskeletal system, including osteoporotic bones, enlarged joints, sclerosed tendons, limited range of motion, thinned intervertebral discs, and weakened muscles, occur with aging. Bone mass peaks at about age 35, after which there is a universal gradual loss of bone. Numerous metabolic changes, including menopausal withdrawal of estrogen and decreased activity, contribute to the loss of bone mass **(osteoporosis)**. Women lose more bone mass than men. By the age of 75, the average woman has lost 25% of her cortical (compact) bone and 40% of her trabecular (cancellous) bone. Additionally, bones change in shape and have reduced strength. If a fracture occurs, fibrous tissue develops more slowly in the aged.

In the elderly, collagen structures are less able to absorb energy. The articular cartilage degenerates in weight-bearing areas and heals less readily. This contributes to the development of osteoarthritis. Muscle mass and strength are similarly diminished. There is an actual loss in the number of muscle fibers due to myofibril atrophy with fibrous tissue replacement, which begins in the fourth decade of life.

In addition, remote musculoskeletal problems for which the patient has compensated may become new problems with age-related changes. For example, patients who have recovered from polio and who have been able to function normally by using synergistic muscle groups may discover increasing incapacity. They have a reduced compensatory ability.

Many of the effects of aging can be overcome if the body is kept healthy and active.

Physical Assessment

An examination of the musculoskeletal system ranges from a basic assessment of functional capabilities to sophisticated physical examination maneuvers that facilitate diagnosis of specific bone, muscle, and joint disorders. The nursing assessment is primarily a functional evaluation. Techniques of inspection and palpation are employed to evaluate the patient's bone integrity, posture, joint function, muscle strength, gait, and ability to perform activities of daily living.

The musculoskeletal assessment is commonly integrated into the routine progression of the physical examination. This system relates closely to the neurologic and cardiovascular systems; thus, assessments of all three systems are often carried out together. The basis of the assessment is a comparison of symmetric regions of the body. The extent of the assessment depends on the patient's physical complaints and health history and any physical clues detected by the examiner that warrant further exploration.

When specific symptoms or physical findings of musculoskeletal dysfunction are apparent, the examination findings are carefully documented and the information is shared with the physician, who may decide that a more extensive examination and diagnostic workup are necessary.

Assessing the Bony Skeleton. The bony skeleton is assessed for deformities and alignment. Abnormal bony growths due to bone tumors may be observed. Shortened extremities, amputations, and body parts that are not in anatomic alignment are noted. Abnormal angulation of long bones or motion at points other than joints is frequently indicative of fracture. Crepitus (a grating sound) at the point of abnormal motion may be detected. Movement of bony fragments must be minimized to avoid additional injury.

Assessing the Spine. The normal curvature of the spine is convex through the thoracic portion and concave through the cervical and lumbar portions. Common deformities of the spine that may be noted include **scoliosis** (a lateral curving deviation of the spine), **kyphosis** (an increased roundness of the thoracic spine curve), and **lordosis** (swayback; exaggeration of the lumbar spine curve) (Fig. 61-4). Kyphosis is frequently seen in the elderly patient with osteoporosis and in some patients with neuromuscular diseases. Scoliosis may be congenital, idiopathic (without an identifiable cause), or a result of damage to the paraspinal muscles, as in poliomyelitis. Lordosis is frequently seen during pregnancy as the woman adjusts her posture for changes in her center of gravity.

During inspection of the spine the patient's gown is open to expose the entire back, buttocks, and legs. The examiner inspects the spinal curves and trunk symmetry from anterior, posterior, and lateral views. Standing behind the patient, the examiner notes any differences in the height of the shoulders or iliac crests. The gluteal folds are normally symmetric. Shoulder and hip symmetry, as well as the straight line of the vertebral column, are inspected with the patient erect and bending forward (flexion). (Scoliosis is evidenced by abnormal lateral curve in the spine, unlevel shoulders, asymmetric waistline, and a prominent scapula, accentuated by the bending forward test.) In addition, older adults experience a loss in height due to loss of vertebral cartilage.

Assessing the Articular System. The articular system is evaluated by noting range of motion, deformity, stability, and nodular formation. Range of motion is evaluated both actively (joint is moved by the muscles surrounding the joint) and passively (joint is moved by the examiner). The examiner is familiar with the normal range of motion of major joints as defined by the American Academy of Orthopedic Surgeons. Precise measurement of range of motion can be made by a **goniometer** (a protractor designed for evaluating joint motion). If maximum extension of a joint reveals residual flexion, the range of motion is said to be limited. Limited range of motion may be due to skeletal deformity, joint pathology, or contracture of surrounding muscles and tendons. In elderly persons, limitations of range of motion associated with degenerative joint pathology may reduce their ability to perform activities of daily living.

If joint motion is compromised or the joint is painful, the joint is examined for the presence of excessive fluid within its capsule (effusion), swelling, and increased temperature that might reflect active inflammation. An effusion is suspected when the joint is swollen in size and the normal bony landmarks are obscured. The most common site for joint effusion is the knee. If a small amount of fluid is present in the joint spaces beneath the patella, it may be identified by the following maneuver: the medial and lateral aspects of the extended knee are milked firmly in a downward motion. This displaces any fluid downward. As pressure is exerted against the medial or lateral side, the examiner observes the opposite side for a bulge below the patella. When larger amounts of fluid are present, the patella becomes elevated from the femur during knee extension. When inflammation or fluid is suspected in a joint, physician consultation is indicated.

Joint deformity may be due to **contracture** (shortening of surrounding joint structures), **dislocation** (complete separation of joint surfaces), **subluxation** (partial separation of articular surfaces), or **disruption of structures** surrounding the joint. Weakness or disruption of joint-supporting structures may result in a joint that is too weak to function as designed, and it may therefore require an external supporting appliance (*e.g.*, brace).

Palpation of the joint while it is passively moved provides information about the integrity of the joint. Normally, the joint moves smoothly. A snap or a crack may indicate that a ligament is slipping over a bony prominence. Slightly roughened surfaces, as in arthritic conditions, will result in crepitus as the irregular surfaces of the joint are moved across one another.

The tissues surrounding joints are examined for nodule formation. Rheumatoid arthritis, gout, and osteoarthritis

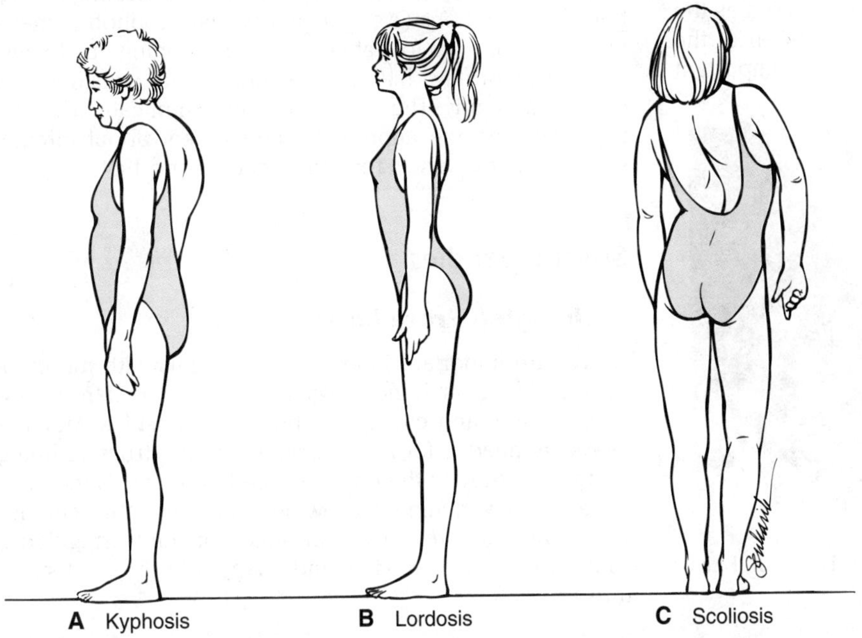

FIGURE 61-4. (**A**) Kyphosis: an increased convexity or roundness of the spine's thoracic curve. (**B**) Lordosis: swayback; exaggeration of the lumbar spine curve. (**C**) Scoliosis: a lateral curvature of the spine.

produce characteristic nodules. The subcutaneous nodules of rheumatoid arthritis are soft and occur within and along tendons that provide extensor function to the joints. Usually, involvement of the joints assumes a symmetric pattern (Fig. 61-5). The nodules of gout are hard and lie within and immediately adjacent to the joint capsule itself. Frequently they rupture, exuding white uric acid crystals onto the skin surface. Osteoarthritic nodules are hard and painless and represent bony overgrowth that has resulted from destruction of the cartilaginous surface of bone within the joint capsule. They are frequently seen in older adults.

Often the size of the joint is exaggerated by the atrophy of muscles proximal and distal to that joint. This is seen in rheumatoid arthritis of the knees, in which the quadriceps muscle may atrophy dramatically. The joint is kept immobile to avoid the pain, and the muscles that provide function for the joint atrophy from disuse (see Chapter 52.)

Assessing the Muscular System. The muscular system is assessed by noting the patient's ability to change position, muscular strength and coordination, and the size of individual muscles. Muscular weakness of a group of muscles might indicate a variety of conditions, such as polyneuropathy, electrolyte disturbances (particularly potassium and calcium), myasthenia gravis, poliomyelitis, and muscular dystrophy. By palpating the muscle while passively moving the relaxed extremity, the nurse can determine the muscle tone. Muscle strength can be estimated by having the patient perform certain tasks with and without added resistance. For example, the biceps can be tested by requesting the patient to fully extend the arm and then flex it against resistance applied by the nurse. A simple handshake provides an indication of grasp strength.

Muscle clonus (rhythmic contractions of a muscle) may be elicited in the ankle or wrist by sudden, forceful, sustained dorsiflexion of the foot or extension of the wrist. Fasciculations (involuntary twitching of muscle fiber groups) may be observed.

The girth of an extremity may be measured to monitor increased size due to edema or bleeding into the muscle; also, it may be used to detect a decrease in size due to atrophy. The unaffected extremity is measured and used as the reference standard. Measurements are to be taken at the maximum circumference of the extremity. It is important that the measurements be at the same location on the extremity and with the extremity in the same position with the muscle at rest. Distance from a specific anatomic landmark (*e.g.*, 10 cm below the medial aspect of the knee for measurement of the calf muscle) should be indicated in the patient's record so that subsequent measurements are made at the same point. For ease of serial assessment, the point of measurement can be indicated by marking the skin. Variations in size greater than 1 cm are considered significant.

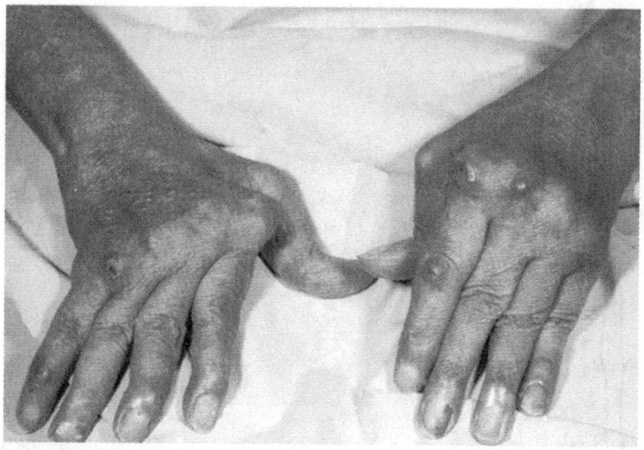

FIGURE 61-5. Rheumatoid arthritis. (Rubin E and Farber JL. Pathology, 2nd ed. Philadelphia, JB Lippincott, 1994.)

Assessing Gait. Gait is assessed by having the patient walk away from the examiner for a short distance. The examiner observes the gait for smoothness and rhythm. Any unsteadiness or irregular movements (frequently noted in elderly patients) are considered abnormal. When a limping motion is noted, it is most likely due to painful weight-bearing. In such instances, the patient can usually pinpoint the area of discomfort, thus guiding further examination. When one extremity is shorter than another, a limp may also be observed as the patient's pelvis drops downward on the affected side with each step. Limited joint motion may affect gait. A variety of neurologic conditions are associated with abnormal gaits (*e.g.*, spastic hemiparesis gait—stroke; steppage gait—lower motor neuron disease; shuffling gait—Parkinson's disease).

Assessing Skin and Peripheral Circulation. In addition to assessing the musculoskeletal system, the nurse inspects the skin and assesses peripheral circulation. Palpation of the skin can reveal if any areas are warmer or cooler than others and if edema is present. Peripheral circulation is evaluated by assessing peripheral pulses, color, temperature, and capillary refill time. Cuts, bruises, skin color, and evidence of decreased circulation or infection can influence nursing management.

Diagnostic Evaluation

Nursing Implications

Preparation for diagnostic studies includes assessing the patient for conditions (*e.g.*, pregnancy, claustrophobia, metal implants, ability to tolerate required positioning due to age, debility, deformity) that may require special consideration during the study. The nurse must communicate with the physician and the appropriate department about circumstances that may affect the prescribed diagnostic test.

Specific Studies

Imaging Procedures

X-rays are important in evaluating patients with musculoskeletal disorders. Bone x-rays determine bone density, texture, erosion, and changes in bone relationships. Multiple x-rays are needed for full assessment of the structure being examined. X-ray of the cortex of the bone reveals the presence of any widening, narrowing, and signs of irregularity. Joint x-rays will reveal the presence of fluid, irregularity, spur formation, narrowing, and changes in the joint structure.

Computed tomography (CT scan) shows in detail a specific plane of involved bone and can reveal tumors of the soft tissue or injuries to the ligaments or tendons. It is used to identify the location and extent of fractures in areas difficult to evaluate (*e.g.*, the acetabulum). Studies may be performed with or without contrast agents and last about an hour.

Magnetic resonance imaging (MRI) is a noninvasive, special imaging technique that uses magnetic fields, radio waves, and computers to demonstrate abnormalities (*i.e.*, tumors or narrowing of tissue pathways through bone) of soft tissue such as muscle, tendon, and cartilage. Because an electromagnet is used, patients with any metal implants, braces, or pacemakers are not candidates for this procedure. Jewelry must be removed. Patients who experience claustrophobia may be unable to tolerate the confinement of some MRI equipment without sedation.

Angiography is the study of vascular structures. Arteriography is the study of the arterial system. A radiopaque contrast agent is injected into the selected artery, and serial x-rays are taken of the arterial system supplied by that artery. The procedure is useful for assessing arterial perfusion and may be used to determine the level at which an amputation is to be performed. After the procedure, the patient is kept on bedrest for 12 to 24 hours to prevent hemorrhage at the arterial puncture site. The nurse monitors vital signs; the puncture site for swelling, bleeding, and hematoma; and the distal extremity for adequate circulation.

Digital subtraction angiography (DSA) uses computer technology to demonstrate the arterial system from a venous catheter access.

Venogram is a study of the venous system frequently used to detect venous thrombosis.

Myelography, the injection of a contrast agent into the subarachnoid space of the lumbar spine, is carried out to determine disc herniation, spinal stenosis (narrowing of the spinal canal), or the site of a tumor. (This technique is discussed in Chapter 58.)

Discography is a study of the intervertebral discs; a contrast agent is injected into the disc and its distribution is noted.

Arthrography is the injection of a radiopaque substance or air into the joint cavity to outline soft-tissue structures and the contour of the joint. The joint is put through its range of motion while a series of x-rays are obtained. Arthrograms are useful in identifying acute or chronic tears of the joint capsule or supporting ligaments of the knee, shoulder, ankle, hip, or wrist. (If a tear is present, the contrast agent will leak out of the joint and will be evident on x-rays.) Following the arthrogram, the joint is usually immobilized for 12 to 24 hours and a compression elastic bandage is applied as prescribed. Comfort measures are provided as appropriate.

Other Studies

An **arthrocentesis** (joint aspiration) is carried out to obtain synovial fluid for purposes of examination or to relieve pain due to effusion. Using aseptic technique, the physician inserts a needle into the joint and aspirates fluid. A sterile dressing is applied following aspiration.

Normally, synovial fluid is clear, pale, straw-colored, and scanty in volume. The fluid is examined grossly for volume, color, clarity, viscosity, and formation of mucin clot. It is examined microscopically for cell count, cell identification, Gram's stain, and formed elements. Examination of synovial fluid is helpful in the diagnosis of rheumatoid arthritis and other inflammatory arthropathies and will reveal the presence of **hemarthrosis** (bleeding into the joint cavity), which suggests trauma or a tendency to bleed.

Arthroscopy is an endoscopic procedure that allows direct visualization of a joint. The procedure is carried out in the operating room under sterile conditions; injection of a local anesthetic into the joint or general anesthesia is used. A large-bore needle is inserted and the joint is distended with saline. The arthroscope is introduced and joint structures, synovium, and articular surfaces are visualized. Following the procedure, the puncture wound is covered with a sterile dressing. The joint is wrapped with a compression dressing to control swelling. In addition, ice may be applied to control edema and discomfort.

Generally, the joint is kept extended and elevated to reduce swelling. The patient is advised to limit activity following the procedure. Neurovascular function is monitored. Analgesics may be prescribed to control discomfort. Complications are rare but may include infection, hemarthrosis, thrombophlebitis, stiffness, and delayed wound healing.

A **bone scan** (bone scintigraphy) reflects the degree to which the matrix of bone "takes up" a bone-seeking radioactive isotope that is injected into the system. The scan is performed 4 to 6 hours after the isotope is injected. The degree of nuclide uptake is related to the metabolism of the bone. An increased uptake of isotope is seen in primary skeletal disease (osteosarcoma), metastatic bone disease, inflammatory skeletal disease (osteomyelitis), and certain types of fractures.

No activity restrictions related to the study are needed. To increase excretion of the isotope, the patient is encouraged to drink plenty of fluids. Other radionuclide tests are not scheduled for 1 to 2 days.

Thermography measures the degree of heat radiating from the skin surface. Inflammatory conditions such as arthritis and infections, as well as neoplasms, may be evaluated. Serial studies may be used to document inflammatory episodes and the patient's response to anti-inflammatory medication therapy.

Electromyography provides information about the electric potential of the muscles and the nerves leading to them. The purpose of the procedure is to determine any abnormality of function of the motor end unit. Needle electrodes are inserted into selected muscles, and responses to electrical stimuli are recorded on an oscilloscope. Warm compresses may relieve residual discomfort following the study.

Single and dual photon absorptiometry are noninvasive tests to determine bone mineral content at the wrist or vertebrae. Osteoporosis may be monitored with this type of densitometry.

Biopsy may be performed to determine the structure and composition of bone, muscle, and synovium to help determine specific diseases. The biopsy site must be monitored for edema, bleeding, and pain. Ice may be prescribed to control bleeding and edema and analgesics prescribed for comfort.

Laboratory Studies

Examination of the patient's blood and urine can provide information about a primary musculoskeletal problem (*e.g.*, Paget's disease) or a developing complication (*e.g.*, infection), a baseline for instituting therapy (*e.g.*, anticoagulant therapy), or information regarding response to therapy. The complete blood count includes the hemoglobin level (frequently lower after bleeding associated with trauma) and the white blood cell count. Prior to surgery, coagulation studies are performed to detect bleeding tendencies, because bone is very vascular tissue.

Blood chemistry studies provide data about a wide variety of musculoskeletal conditions. Serum calcium levels are altered in osteomalacia, parathyroid function, Paget's disease, metastatic bone tumors, and with prolonged immobilization. Serum phosphorus levels are inversely related to calcium levels and are diminished in rickets associated with malabsorption syndrome. Acid phosphatase is elevated in Paget's disease and metastatic cancer. Alkaline phosphatase is elevated during fracture healing and in diseases with increased osteoblastic activity (*e.g.*, metastatic bone tumors). Bone metabolism may be evaluated through thyroid studies and determination of calcitonin, parathyroid hormone (PTH), and vitamin D levels. Serum enzyme levels of creatine kinase (CK) and serum glutamic-oxaloacetic transaminase (SGOT, aspartate aminotransferase) become elevated with muscle damage. Aldolase is elevated in muscle diseases (*e.g.*, muscular dystrophy and skeletal muscle necrosis).

Urine calcium levels increase with bone destruction (*e.g.*, parathyroid dysfunction, metastatic bone tumors, multiple myeloma).

Nursing Assessment and Diagnostic Considerations

Determining the patient's functional status and health care needs is an integral part of the nursing assessment. Nursing diagnoses and the care plan are developed and modified according to the patient's needs.

Initially, the patient will require support and nursing care during the period of assessment, including physical and psychologic preparation for examinations and tests. Patient education prior to the tests (including what is to be done; why it is being done; what the patient can expect to experience, including tactile, visual, and auditory sensations; and what patient participation is expected) will reduce anxiety and enable the patient to be an active participant in care.

The resulting medical diagnosis and prescribed treatment regimen will affect the nursing management of the patient. The nursing plan of care will reflect nursing measures that will facilitate the resolution of the patient's health problems and promotion of health.

The nursing assessment will enable the nurse to identify the health problems that can be improved by nursing interventions. Actual and potential nursing diagnoses common to patients with musculoskeletal disorders include the following:

- Impaired physical mobility
- Pain
- Risk for impaired skin integrity
- Risk for disuse syndrome
- Risk for peripheral neurovascular dysfunction
- Altered peripheral tissue perfusion
- Self-care deficits
- Knowledge deficit about the disease process and treatment regimen
- Risk for injury
- Activity intolerance
- Fatigue
- Altered role performance
- Self-esteem disturbance
- Body image disturbance
- Ineffective individual coping
- Powerlessness
- Altered family processes
- Risk for infection
- Constipation
- Sleep pattern disturbance
- Diversional activity deficit
- Altered nutrition: less than body requirements

In collaboration with the patient, health goals and nursing strategies are formulated to resolve the identified nursing diagnoses.

CRITICAL THINKING EXERCISES

1. A young man who has a cast applied to his fractured arm expresses concern that he will lose muscle strength because he cannot exercise his arm. How would you respond to him and address his concern? If the patient were an elderly woman who had broken her arm in a fall and now was fearful of falling again, how would your approach differ in addressing this patient's concerns?
2. The son of an elderly patient asks why his mother is "so much shorter than she used to be." How would you explain this phenomenon to him? How might you incorporate preventive measures related to his mother's musculoskeletal condition into a teaching session?
3. Following an arthroscopy, a patient complains that the dressing on his knee is too tight. He begins to loosen it. How would you react to his actions and why? If the patient had removed the dressing during the night without being detected and you discovered the fact early the next morning, how would the patient's situation have changed and how would you respond to this different set of circumstances?

REFERENCES AND SELECTED READINGS

Books

Bullock BL. Pathophysiology: Adaptations and Alterations in Function, 4th ed. Philadelphia, JB Lippincott, 1996.

Carpenito LJ. Nursing Diagnosis: Application to Clinical Practice, 6th ed. Philadelphia, JB Lippincott, 1995.

Davis PS. Nursing the Orthopaedic Patient. Edinburgh, Churchill Livingstone, 1994.

Gerard JA and Kleinfield SL. Orthopaedic Testing: A Rational Approach to Diagnosis. New York: Churchill Livingstone, 1993.

Guyton A. Human Physiology and Mechanisms of Disease, 5th ed. Philadelphia, WB Saunders, 1992.

Lewis CB and Knortz KA. Orthopedic Assessment and Treatment of the Geriatric Patient. St. Louis, CV Mosby, 1993.

Magee DJ. Orthopedic Physical Assessment, 2nd ed. Philadelphia, WB Saunders, 1992.

Maher AB et al. Orthopaedic Nursing. Philadelphia, WB Saunders, 1994.

Memmler R et al. Structure and Function of the Human Body, 5th ed. Philadelphia, JB Lippincott, 1992.

Mennell J. The Musculoskeletal System. Gaithersburg MD, Aspen, 1991.

Mercier LR. Practical Orthopedics, 3rd ed. St. Louis, Mosby Year Book, 1991.

Mourad LA. Orthopedic Disorders. St. Louis, Mosby Year Book, 1991.

Mourad LA and Droste MM. The Nursing Process in the Care of Adults With Orthopaedic Conditions, 3rd ed. Albany NY, Delmar Publishers, 1993.

National Association of Orthopaedic Nurses. Guidelines for Orthopaedic Nursing. Pitman NJ, National Association of Orthopaedic Nurses, 1992.

Porth CM. Pathophysiology: Concepts of Altered Health States, 4th ed. Philadelphia, JB Lippincott, 1994.

Salmond SW et al (ed). Core Curriculum for Orthopaedic Nursing, 2nd ed. Pitman NJ, National Association of Orthopaedic Nurses, 1991.

Sly D and Theis L (eds). Introduction to Orthopaedic Nursing: An Orientation Module. Pitman NJ, National Association of Orthopaedic Nurses, 1991.

Turek SL (ed). Orthopaedics: Principles and Their Application, 5th ed. Philadelphia, JB Lippincott, 1994.

Journals

Asterisks indicate nursing research articles.

Childs S. Avascular necrosis of the bone: The causes and the cures. Orthop Nurs 1993 Jul/Aug; 12(4):29–34.

*Daltory LH et al. Does the musculoskeletal function deteriorate in a predictable sequence in the elderly? Arthritis Care and Res 1992 Sep; 5(3):146–150.

Dublin S. The physiologic changes of aging. Orthop Nurs 1992 May/Jun; 11(3):45–50.

Einhorn T. Mechanisms of fracture healing. Hosp Pract 1991 Suppl 1; 26:41–45.

Gates S and Brooks M. Imaging of the orthopaedic patient: Implications for primary care. Nure Pract Forum 1991 Dec; 2(4):225–230.

Mundy GR. New concepts in bone metabolism: Clinical implications. Hosp Pract 1991 Jan; 26(Suppl 1):7–12.

Pavlik M. Measuring bone mineral content. Orthop Nurs 1991 Mar/Apr; 10(2):33–37.

Schurman S and Williamson A. Bone density studies: Current technology. Nurs Pract Forum 1991; Dec 2(4):246–250.

AGENCIES

National Institute of Arthritis and Musculoskeletal and Skin Diseases
National Institutes of Health,
Bethesda, MD 20892

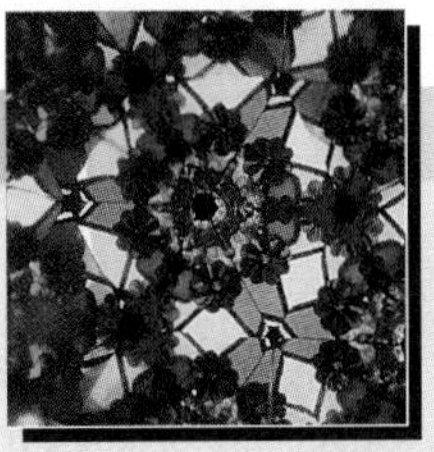

62

Management Modalities for Patients With Musculoskeletal Dysfunction

CHAPTER OUTLINE

LEARNING OBJECTIVES

On completion of this chapter, the learner will be able to:

1. Use the nursing process as a framework for care of the patient with musculoskeletal dysfunction
2. Use the nursing process as a framework for care of the patient with a cast
3. Describe the preventive and health teaching needs of the patient with a cast
4. Describe the various types of traction and the principles of effective traction
5. Specify the preventive nursing care needs of the patient in traction
6. Use the nursing process as a framework for care of the patient in traction
7. Use the nursing process as a framework for care of the patient undergoing orthopedic surgery
8. Compare the nursing needs of the patient undergoing total hip replacement with those of the patient undergoing total knee replacement

❑ NURSING PROCESS OVERVIEW

Assessment

The nursing assessment of the patient with musculoskeletal dysfunction includes an evaluation of the impact of the musculoskeletal problem on the patient. The nurse is concerned with assisting persons with musculoskeletal problems to maintain their general health, accomplish their activities of daily living (ADLs), and manage their treatment modalities. Systemic homeostasis is assured, optimal nutrition is encouraged, and problems related to immobility are prevented. Through an individualized plan of care the nurse helps the patient achieve maximum health.

Initial Interview

In the initial interview, the nurse obtains a general impression of the patient's health status. The nurse obtains subjective data from the patient concerning the onset of the problem and how it has been managed. The patient's perceptions and expectations related to the health problems may affect restoration of health. The existence of concurrent health problems (*e.g.*, diabetes, heart disease, upper respiratory infection) needs to be taken into consideration when developing the plan of care. A history of medication use and response to pain medication will aid in designing medication management regimens.

Allergies are noted and described in terms of the reactions they produce in the patient. The use of tobacco, alcohol, and other drugs is assessed to evaluate the effects of these agents on patient care. Information concerning the patient's ability to learn, economic status, and current occupation is needed for discharge planning and for rehabilitation. Additions to the initial interview data will be made as the nurse interacts with the patient. Such data allow for the nurse to adjust the individualized plan of care as needed.

Physical Assessment

The nurse is interested in identifying the functional abilities of the patient as well as in determining the effects that any disabilities and medical treatment have on the patient's ability to meet personal needs effectively and to perform ADLs. A general inspection of the body will disclose size, any significant deformity, asymmetry of contours, swelling, edema, bruising, or breaks in the skin. Observing the patient's posture, movement, and gait will provide information about alterations in the patient's mobility and the presence of pain and discomfort or involuntary movements (fasciculations or twitches) (see Chapter 61).

Any deviations from normal are noted. A baseline for noting and evaluating changes in the patient's abilities is established.

Subjective Assessment Data

During the interview and physical assessment, the patient may report the presence of pain, tenderness, tightness, and abnormal sensations. This information is assessed and documented.

Pain

Most patients with diseases and traumatic conditions of muscles, bones, and joints experience pain. Bone pain is characteristically described as a dull, deep ache that is boring in nature, whereas muscular pain is described as soreness or aching and is referred to as "muscle cramps." Fracture pain is sharp and piercing and is relieved by immobilization. Sharp pain may also result from bone infection with muscle spasm or pressure on a sensory nerve.

Most musculoskeletal pain is relieved by rest. Pain that increases with activity may indicate joint sprain or muscle strain, whereas steadily increasing pain points to a progression of an infectious process (osteomyelitis), a malignant tumor, or vascular complications. Radiating pain is seen in conditions in which pressure is exerted on a nerve root. Pain is variable, and its assessment and nursing management must be individualized.

- ❑ What was the patient doing before the pain occurred?
- ❑ Is the body in proper alignment?
- ❑ Is there pressure from traction, bed linens, a cast, or other appliances?
- ❑ Is there tension on the skin at the pin site?
- ❑ Is the pain localized?
- ❑ How does the patient describe it?
- ❑ How intense is the pain? (For example, have the patient rate the intensity of the pain on a scale of 0 to 10, with 10 being the worst possible pain.)
- ❑ What was the manner of onset?
- ❑ Does the pain radiate? If so, in what direction?
- ❑ Is there pain in any other part of the body?
- ❑ What is the character of the pain (sharp, dull, boring, shooting, throbbing, cramping)?
- ❑ Is it constant?
- ❑ What relieves it?
- ❑ What makes it worse?
- ❑ Does the patient experience increased discomfort when overly tired from lack of sleep, exciting stimuli, or too much activity?

It is important that the patient's pain and discomfort be managed successfully. Not only is pain exhausting, but if prolonged it can force the patient to become increasingly preoccupied and dependent.

Altered Sensations

Sensory disturbances are frequently associated with musculoskeletal problems. The patient may describe the presence of paresthesias (burning or tingling sensations) and numbness. These sensations may be due to pressure on nerves or circulatory impairment. Soft tissue swelling or direct trauma to these structures can impair their function. Loss of function can result from impaired nerves and circulatory structures located throughout the musculoskeletal system. The neurovascular status of the involved musculoskeletal area is assessed to provide information for planning interventions.

- ❑ Is the patient experiencing any abnormal sensations or numbness?
- ❑ When did this begin? Is it getting worse?
- ❑ Is the patient also experiencing pain?
- ❑ What is the color of the part distal to the affected area? Pale? Dusky? Cyanotic?
- ❑ Is there a pulse present distal to the affected area?
- ❑ Is there rapid capillary refill? (The nail is gently squeezed until it blanches; pressure is released and the

amount of time for color to return to normal is noted. Color normally returns quickly, within 3 seconds.)
- Is the motor component of the nerve intact? Is the patient able to move the innervated part?
- Is edema present?
- Is any constrictive device or clothing causing nerve or vascular compression?
- Are symptoms decreased by elevating the affected part or modifying its position?

Diagnosis

Nursing Diagnoses

Based on the nursing assessment data, the major nursing diagnoses for a patient with musculoskeletal dysfunction may include the following:

- Anxiety related to changes in body integrity
- Knowledge deficit about the treatment regimen
- Pain related to musculoskeletal disorder
- Altered peripheral tissue perfusion related to physiologic responses to injury, swelling, or increased pressure within a closed space (*i.e.*, muscle compartment, constrictive dressing, or cast)
- Impaired physical mobility related to musculoskeletal impairment

Planning and Implementation

Goals. The major goals of the patient with musculoskeletal dysfunction may include reduced anxiety, understanding of the treatment protocol, relief of pain, maintenance of adequate tissue perfusion, and improved physical mobility.

Nursing Interventions

Reducing Anxiety. Musculoskeletal problems may be due to an acute traumatic injury or may be of a persistent, recurrent, long-term nature. The problems take their toll on the psychologic and socioeconomic well-being of patients. The nurse assists the patient to cope with the problems associated with musculoskeletal dysfunction and its treatment.

Most patients with acute musculoskeletal problems are anxious and have pain. They experience fear and anticipation before definitive therapy begins. People who have long-term disabilities frequently undergo repeated reconstructive surgery. They are familiar with the routines of the hospital and are concerned with the ultimate outcome of the procedure. Their patience and hope may be limited. Such patients need an understanding, supportive nurse. (See Nursing Care Plan 10-1, Care of the Patient With Anxiety.)

Patient Education and Home Care Considerations. The patient who has been educated about the musculoskeletal disorder has an increased understanding of treatment alternatives. Information about what to expect, including sensations during and after the treatment, will encourage the patient to participate actively in developing and implementing the therapeutic regimen. When possible, specific information concerning anticipated equipment (*e.g.*, casts, traction), assistive devices (*e.g.*, trapeze, walker, crutches), exercise (*e.g.*, quadriceps setting, deep breathing), and medications (*e.g.*, analgesics, antibiotics) should be shared with the patient. At times patients can practice recuperative activities, such as crutch walking, before they have surgery and must use such devices.

Before discharge, patients should receive explicit instructions for continuing care at home. It is often helpful to provide these instructions in writing so that the patient can review them later. It is not enough to say "take it easy." Patients must be able to recognize any untoward signs and symptoms that should be reported to the physician. They must be aware of the importance of follow-up visits. If they have any difficulties, they should know where and how to get help. The nurse has a major responsibility for educating these patients before they leave the hospital (see Chapter 18).

Relieving Pain. Patients who have bone and joint problems frequently experience severe pain. Often the person who has undergone surgery to correct a foot condition is much more uncomfortable than one who has had extensive abdominal surgery. Opioids and other pain-relieving measures are administered as prescribed, taking into consideration the patient's age and body size as well as the type and the site of the musculoskeletal problem. Generally, elderly patients require close monitoring of their responses to pain medication because of age-related changes in pharmacokinetics and delayed excretion of medications.

Pain may result from either the primary musculoskeletal problem or associated problems (*e.g.*, pressure over bony prominences, muscle spasm, swelling). Prolonged pressure over bony prominences (*e.g.*, heel, head of fibula, tibial tuberosity) may cause a burning type of pain. Relieving the pressure is necessary to relieve the pain and prevent further tissue damage.

Muscle spasm is another associated cause of pain. When a muscle is injured, the natural response of that muscle is to contract, thereby splinting and protecting the injured area. Prolonged muscle contraction is painful. Relaxation techniques, traction, or medications may be used to reduce pain from muscle spasm.

Usually, swelling can be controlled and compartment syndrome (see p. 1852) avoided by elevating the injured part and intermittently applying an ice pack to the injury for 20 to 30 minutes.

Additional information and guidelines to nursing management of the patient with pain are presented in Chapter 13.

Improving Tissue Perfusion. Swelling usually accompanies musculoskeletal injury. The nurse monitors peripheral tissue perfusion frequently. The blood supply can be assessed by determining nailbed capillary refill. In addition, if the tissue perfusion is diminished, the skin will feel cool to the touch and will appear dusky, pale, or blue. Sensory and motor function may be altered or diminished. If the swelling occurs in a confined space (*e.g.*, cast, constrictive dressing, muscle fascia sheath), compartment syndrome may develop. Tissue pressure may be elevated and can be measured directly with a tissue pressure–monitoring device (Fig. 62-1). Excruciating pain and loss of motion and sensory function may result from tissue anoxia if compartment syndrome is undetected and untreated.

Swelling is controlled by elevating the affected area to the level of the heart and applying intermittent cold.

Improving Mobility. The immobility necessitated by some treatment modalities must not result in undue deterio-

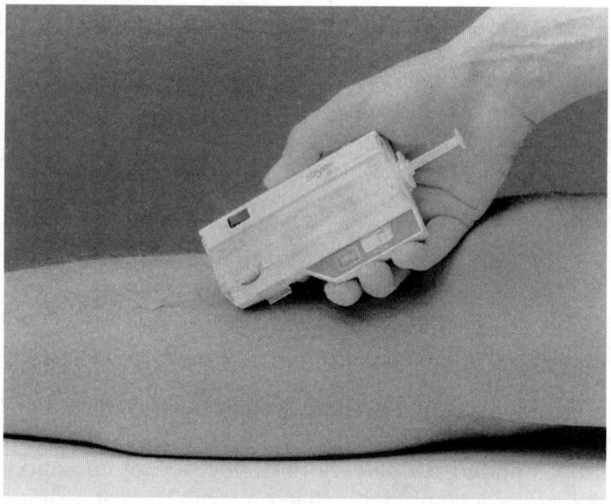

FIGURE 62-1. Tissue pressure–monitoring device. (Courtesy of Stryker Surgical.)

ration. Throughout the treatment period, the nurse is concerned with maintaining the patient's health and ultimately restoring function to the injured muscle and bone. Exercising nonimmobilized muscles and joints helps maintain their strength and function, minimizes cardiovascular deterioration, and prevents disuse osteoporosis. Isometric exercises of immobilized extremities help to maintain muscle strength.

Patients who are actively involved in performing ADLs (*e.g.*, hygiene, dressing, eating) typically feel a sense of independence and accomplishment. Coordinating nursing interventions with special therapy approaches (*e.g.*, physical therapy, occupational therapy) makes it easier for the patient to learn the therapeutic regimens. Emphasis is placed on what the patient is able to do within the limits of the treatment modalities.

Evaluation

Expected Outcomes

1. Exhibits minimal anxiety
   a. Appears relaxed and confident in abilities
   b. Uses effective coping strategies
   c. Participates in treatment plan
2. Relates plan for continued health management
   a. Describes planned treatment regimen
   b. States signs and symptoms to report to physician
   c. Makes appointment for follow-up care
3. Achieves pain relief
   a. Controls discomfort with occasional oral medications
   b. Moves with minimal discomfort
   c. Uses positioning to increase comfort
4. Maintains adequate tissue perfusion
   a. Controls swelling
   b. Demonstrates normal capillary refill
   c. Reports normal sensations
   d. Demonstrates motor function
5. Demonstrates improved physical mobility
   a. Transfers self independently or with minimal assistance
   b. Participates in activities of daily living
   c. Uses assistive devices safely

Managing the Patient in a Cast

A cast is a rigid external immobilizing device that is molded to the contours of the body to which it is applied. The purpose of a cast is to immobilize a body part in a specific position and to apply uniform pressure on encased soft tissue. It may be used to immobilize a reduced fracture, correct a deformity, apply uniform pressure to underlying soft tissue, or provide support and stability for weakened joints. Generally, casts permit mobilization of the patient while restricting movement of a body part.

Types of Casts

The condition being treated influences the type and thickness of the cast applied. Generally speaking, the joints proximal and distal to the area to be immobilized are included in the cast. With some fractures, however, cast construction and molding may allow movement of a joint while immobilizing a fracture (*e.g.*, three-point fixation in a patellar tendon weight-bearing cast).

Figure 62-2 illustrates some of the common types of cylindrical casts and areas in which pressure problems commonly occur.

Short arm cast—extends from below the elbow to the palmar crease, secured around the base of the thumb. If the thumb is included, it is known as a thumb spica or gauntlet cast.

Long arm cast—extends from the upper level of the axillary fold to the proximal palmar crease; the elbow usually is immobilized at a right angle

Short leg cast—extends from below the knee to the base of the toes. The foot is at a right angle in a neutral position.

Long leg cast—extends from the junction of the upper and middle third of the thigh to the base of the toes. The knee may be slightly flexed.

Walking cast—a short- or long-leg cast reinforced for strength. It might incorporate a walking heel.

Body cast—encircles the trunk

Spica cast—incorporates a portion of the trunk and one or two extremities (single or double spica cast)

Shoulder spica cast—a body jacket that encloses the trunk and the shoulder and elbow

Hip spica cast—encloses the trunk and a lower extremity; may be a single or double hip spica cast

Casting Materials

Plaster. The traditional cast is made of plaster. Plaster bandages mold very smoothly to the body contours. Rolls of crinoline are impregnated with powdered, anhydrous calcium sulfate (gypsum crystals). When wet, a crystallizing reaction occurs and heat is given off (an exothermic reaction).

- The heat given off during this reaction can be uncomfortable. Therefore, the water used should be cool.

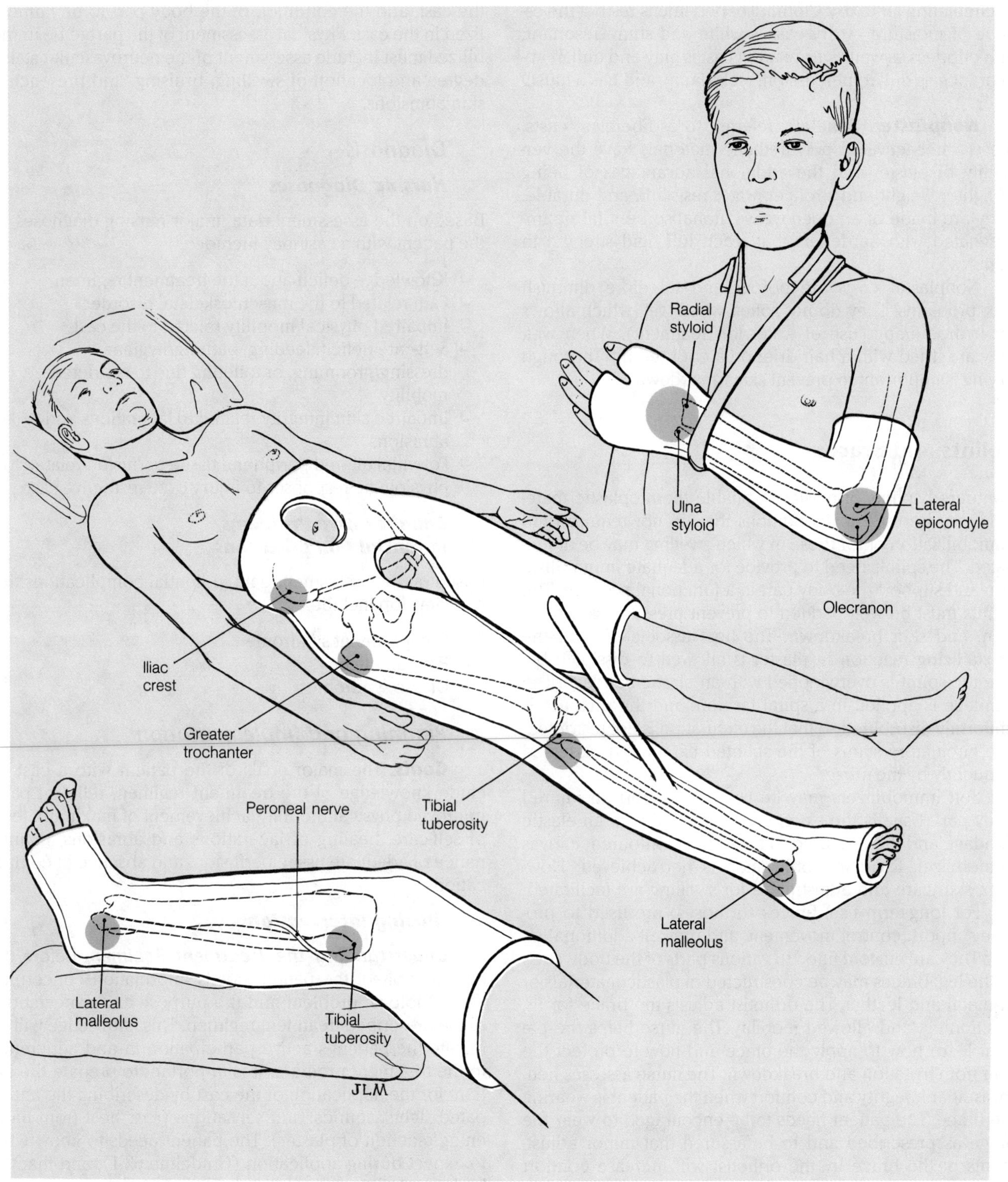

FIGURE 62-2. Pressure areas in different types of casts. (Suddarth DS. The Lippincott Manual of Nursing Practice, 5th ed. Philadelphia, JB Lippincott, 1991.)

- The cast needs to be exposed to allow maximum dissipation of the heat. Most casts are cool after about 15 minutes.

The crystallization produces a rigid dressing. The speed at which the reaction occurs varies from a few minutes to 15 to 20 minutes. The orthopedist will determine the plaster setting speed appropriate for the cast being applied.

After the plaster has set, the cast is still wet and somewhat soft. It does not have its full strength until dry. While damp, it can be dented if handled with the fingertips instead of the palms of the hand or if allowed to rest on hard surfaces or sharp edges. These dents produce pressure areas on the skin under the cast. The cast requires 24 to 72 hours to dry, depending on its thickness and the environmental drying conditions. A freshly applied cast should be exposed to circulating air to dry. Clothing or bed linens restrict the escape of moisture. A dry cast is white and shiny, resonant, and odorless as well as firm; a wet cast is gray and dull in appearance, is dull to percussion, feels damp, and has a musty odor.

Nonplaster. Generally referred to as fiberglass casts, these water-activated polyurethane materials have the versatility of plaster and the additional advantages of being of lighter weight and stronger, water resistant, and durable. They are made of an open-weave, nonabsorbent fabric impregnated with hardeners that reach full rigid strength in minutes.

Nonplaster casts are porous and therefore diminish skin problems. They do not soften when wet, which allows for hydrotherapy (use of water for treatment). When wet, they are dried with a hair drier on a cool setting. Thorough drying is important to prevent skin breakdown.

Splints and Braces

Contoured splints of plaster or pliable thermoplastic materials may be used for conditions that do not require rigid immobilization or for those in which swelling may be anticipated. The splints need to provide for adequate immobilization and support the body part in a functional position. The splints must be well padded to prevent pressure, skin abrasion, and skin breakdown. The heat associated with the crystallizing reaction in plaster is allowed to dissipate before the splint is overwrapped with an elastic bandage. The bandage is applied in a spiral fashion, and the pressure is uniformly distributed so that the circulation is not restricted. The circulatory status of the splinted extremity is assessed frequently by the nurse.

Soft immobilizers may be used to support an injured body part. Usually the extremity is wrapped with an elastic bandage and then secured to a padded, contoured, canvas immobilizer. Rigid immobilization is not achieved. However, skin care and adjustments for swelling are facilitated.

For long-term use, braces (orthoses) are used to provide support, control movement, and prevent additional injury. They are custom fitted to various parts of the body, such as the leg. Braces may be constructed of plastic materials or of metal and leather. The orthotist adjusts the brace for fit, positioning, and allowed mobility. The nurse helps the patient learn how to apply the brace and how to protect the skin from irritation and breakdown. The nurse assesses neurovascular integrity and comfort when the patient is wearing the brace. The patient needs to be encouraged to wear the brace as prescribed and to be assured that minor adjustments of the brace by the orthotist will increase comfort and minimize problems associated with its long-term use.

❑ *NURSING PROCESS*
The Patient in a Cast

Assessment

Before the cast is applied the nurse completes an assessment of the patient's general health, presenting signs and symptoms, emotional status, understanding of the need for the cast, and the condition of the body part to be immobilized in the cast. Physical assessment of the part to be immobilized must include assessment of the neurovascular status, degree and location of swelling, bruising, and presence of skin abrasions.

Diagnosis

Nursing Diagnoses

Based on the assessment data, major nursing diagnoses for the patient with a cast may include:

- ❑ Knowledge deficit about the treatment regimen
- ❑ Pain related to the musculoskeletal disorder
- ❑ Impaired physical mobility related to the cast
- ❑ Self-care deficit: feeding, bathing/hygiene, dressing/grooming, or toileting due to restricted mobility
- ❑ Impaired skin integrity related to lacerations and abrasions
- ❑ Potential altered peripheral tissue perfusion related to physiologic responses to injury or to restrictive cast

Collaborative Problems/ Potential Complications

Based on the assessment data, potential complications that may develop include:

- ❑ Compartment syndrome
- ❑ Pressure ulcer
- ❑ Disuse syndrome

Planning and Implementation

Goals. The major goals of the patient with a cast include knowledge of the treatment regimen, relief of pain, improved physical mobility, achievement of maximum level of self-care, healing of lacerations and abrasions, maintenance of adequate tissue perfusion, and absence of complications.

Nursing Interventions

Understanding the Treatment Regimen. Before the cast is applied, the patient needs information concerning the pathologic problem and the purpose and expectations of the prescribed treatment regimen. This knowledge will facilitate the patient's active participation in and adherence to the treatment program. It is important to prepare the patient for the application of the cast by describing the anticipated sights, sounds, and sensations (*e.g.*, heat from hardening reaction of plaster). The patient needs to know what to expect during application (Guideline 62-1), and that the body part will be immobilized after casting.

Relieving Pain. Pain associated with musculoskeletal problems must be evaluated carefully. The patient is asked to indicate the exact site and to describe the character and intensity of the pain to help determine its cause.

Pain may be indicative of complications: skin breakdown due to pressure on the tissues or bony prominences, or compartment syndrome due to impaired circulation. Severe pain over a bony prominence warns of an impending pressure ulcer. Pain decreases when ulceration occurs. Discomfort due to pressure on the skin may be relieved by ele-

GUIDELINE 62–1
Application of a Cast

Procedure	Rationale
1. Support extremity or body part to be casted.	1. Minimizes movement; maintains reduction and alignment; increases comfort
2. Position and maintain part to be casted in position indicated by physician during casting procedure.	2. Facilitates casting; reduces incidence of complications (*e.g.*, malunion, nonunion, contracture)
3. Drape patient.	3. Avoids undue exposure; protects other body parts from contact with casting materials.
4. Wash and dry part to be casted.	4. Reduces incidence of skin breakdown.
5. Place knitted material* (*e.g.*, stockinette) over part to be casted.	5. Protects skin from casting materials.
Apply in smooth and nonconstrictive manner.	Protects skin from pressure.
Allow additional material.	Folds over edges of cast when finishing application; creates smooth, padded edge; protects skin from abrasion.
6. Wrap soft, nonwoven roll padding* smoothly and evenly around part.	6. Protects skin from pressure of cast.
Use additional padding around bony prominences (see Fig. 62-2) and at nerve grooves (*e.g.*, head of fibula, olecranon process).	Protects skin at bony prominences. Protects superficial nerves.
7. Apply plaster or nonplaster casting material evenly on body part.	7. Creates smooth, solid, well-contoured cast.
Choose appropriate width bandage.	Facilitates smooth application.
Overlap preceding turn by half the width of the bandage.	Creates smooth, solid, immobilizing cast.
Use continuous motion, maintaining constant contact with body part.	Shapes cast properly for adequate support.
Use additional casting material (splints) at joints and at points of anticipated cast stress.	Strengthens cast.
8. "Finish" cast: • Edges smooth	8. Protects skin from abrasion.
• Trim and reshape with cast knife or cutter.	Assures full range of motion of adjacent joints.
9. Remove particles of casting materials from skin.	9. Prevents particles from loosening and sliding underneath cast.
10. Support cast during hardening and drying.	10. Casting materials harden in minutes. Maximum hardness of nonplaster cast occurs in minutes. Maximum hardness of plaster cast occurs with drying (24 to 72 hours, depending on thick ness of cast and environment).
Handle hardening casts with palms of hands; do not rest on hard surfaces or on sharp edges; avoid pressure on cast.	Avoids denting of cast and pressure areas.

**Nonabsorbent materials are used with nonplaster casts.*

vation that controls edema and positioning that alters pressure, or it may require modification of the cast or recasting. Pain associated with compartment syndrome is relentless and not controlled by modalities such as elevation, application of cold, and usual dosages of analgesics. Because of the risk of complications, complaints of discomfort must not go unheeded.

Pain associated with the disease process (*e.g.*, fracture) is frequently controlled by immobilization. Pain due to edema that is associated with trauma, surgery, or bleeding into the tissues can frequently be controlled by elevation and, if prescribed, intermittent application of cold. Ice bags (one-third to one-half full) or cold application devices are placed on each side of the cast, if prescribed, making sure not to indent the cast.

- Most pain can be relieved by elevating the involved part, applying cold as prescribed, and administering usual dosages of analgesics.
- The complaints of pain from the patient in a cast must never be ignored; potential problems including pressure ulcer formation or impaired tissue perfusion must be suspected.
- Unrelieved pain must be reported immediately to the physician to avoid possible necrosis and paralysis.

Improving Mobility. Every joint that is not immobilized should be exercised and moved through its range of motion to maintain function. If the patient has a leg cast, toe exercise is encouraged. If the patient has an arm cast, finger exercise is encouraged. The patient is encouraged to actively participate in personal care and to use assistive devices safely.

Achieving Maximum Level of Self-Care. Self-care deficits occur when a portion of the body is immobilized, resulting in reduced self-care abilities. The nurse must assist the patient in identifying areas of self-care deficit and develop strategies to best assist the patient to achieve independence in activities of daily living (ADLs). The patient's participation in planning and accomplishing ADLs is important in promotion of self-care, independence, maintenance of control, and avoidance of untoward psychological reaction such as depression.

Healing of Skin Abrasions. Before the cast is applied, skin lacerations and abrasions must be treated to enhance healing. The skin is cleansed thoroughly and treated as prescribed. Sterile dressings are used to cover the injured skin. If the skin wounds are extensive, an alternative method (*e.g.*, external fixator) may be chosen to immobilize the body part.

While the cast is on, the patient is observed for systemic signs of infection, odors from the cast, and purulent drainage staining the cast. The physician is notified if these occur.

Maintaining Adequate Tissue Perfusion. Swelling and edema are natural responses of the tissue to trauma and surgery. The patient may complain that the cast is too tight. Vascular insufficiency and nerve compression due to unrelieved swelling can reduce blood supply to an extremity and result in peripheral nerve damage. Generally, the extent of swelling can be controlled by elevating the injured area. If not controlled, the swelling can result in increased tissue pressure, ultimate occlusion of the blood supply, and subsequent anoxia resulting in loss of both nerve and muscle tissue. If this complication occurs, it is known as compartment syndrome.

In promoting tissue perfusion, the nurse monitors the affected extremity for pain, swelling, discoloration (paleness or blueness), paresthesia (tingling or numbness), diminished or absent pulses, paralysis, and coldness of the extremity. Fingers or toes of the casted extremity are assessed and compared with those of the opposite extremity. Normal findings include minimal discomfort, pink color, warm to touch, rapid capillary refill response, ability to move fingers or toes, and normal sensations. The patient is encouraged to move fingers and toes hourly to stimulate circulation.

Swelling (edema) reduces tissue perfusion. Cyanotic (blue-tinged) nail beds suggest venous congestion. White and cold fingers or toes suggest arterial obstruction. Reduced pulse indicates arterial insufficiency. Reduced motor abilities and occurrence of paresthesia (*e.g.*, abnormal sensations such as tingling) indicate nerve ischemia due to tissue pressure or nerve injury. Sensations in the fingers and toes and the ability to move them provide indications of specific sensory and motor function. Normal sensation in the thumb and index finger indicates function of the sensory branch of the musculocutaneous nerve—cervical nerve root 6. The patient is asked to dorsiflex the great toe to assess the function of the motor component of the peroneal nerve.

Tissue pressure can be measured directly by tissue pressure-monitoring devices when the muscle is accessible (see Fig. 62-1). Generally, indirect measures must be used to determine tissue perfusion.

Early recognition of diminished circulation and nerve function is essential to prevent loss of function and possible amputation. Frequent, regular assessments of neurovascular status must be done. When data indicate potential compartment syndrome (*e.g.*, progressive unrelieved pain, pain on passive stretch, paresthesia, motor loss, sensory loss, coolness, paleness, slow capillary refill, sensation of tightness), the nurse adjusts the extremity so that it is no higher than heart level to enhance arterial perfusion, notifies the physician at once, and anticipates treatment to include release of restrictive dressings (*e.g.*, bivalving cast) and possible fasciotomy.

Monitoring and Managing Potential Complications

Compartment Syndrome. **Compartment syndrome** occurs when there is an increase of tissue pressure within a limited space (*e.g.*, cast, muscle compartment) that compromises the circulation and the function of the tissue within the confined area.

- ❑ Unrelieved pain, excessive swelling, poor capillary refill response, inability to move toes or fingers, and elevated tissue pressure indicate compartment syndrome and must be reported to the physician at once.

To relieve the pressure, the cast must be bivalved (cut in half while maintaining alignment) and the extremity elevated (no higher than heart level). If pressure is not relieved and circulation is not restored, a fasciotomy may be necessary to relieve the pressure within the muscle compartment. The nurse closely monitors the patient's response to conservative and surgical management of compartment syndrome. Neurovascular responses are recorded and changes are reported to the physician promptly.

Pressure Ulcers. Pressure of the cast on soft tissues causes tissue anoxia and pressure ulcers. Lower extremity sites most susceptible to pressure are the heel, malleoli, dorsum of the foot, head of the fibula, and anterior surface of the patella. On the upper extremity, the main pressure sites are located at the medial epicondyle of the humerus and the ulnar styloid (see Fig. 62-2).

Generally, the patient with a pressure ulcer reports pain and tightness in the area. If the pressure is not relieved, the necrotic area may drain, stain the cast, and emit an odor. Discomfort may not be present when a pressure ulcer develops. Extensive loss of tissue may occur if signs and symptoms of pressure ulcer development are not monitored and reported.

To visually inspect the area in question, the physician may bivalve the cast or cut an opening (window) in the cast.

The procedure for bivalving a cast is as follows:

1. A longitudinal cut is made in the cast, dividing it into two halves.
2. The underlying padding is also cut.
3. The cast is spread apart to relieve pressure and to inspect and treat the pressure ulcer.
4. The anterior and posterior parts of the cast are secured together with an elastic compression bandage to maintain immobilization.
5. After the cast is bivalved, the extremity is elevated (no higher than heart level) to control swelling and promote circulation.

If the physician elects to create a window in the cast to inspect the pressure site, a portion of the cast is cut out. The affected area is inspected and possibly treated; the portion of the cast is replaced and held in place by an elastic compression dressing or tape. This prevents the underlying tissue from swelling through the window creating pressure areas around its margins.

Disuse Syndrome. While in a cast, the patient is taught to tense or contract muscles (*e.g.*, isometric muscle contraction) without moving the part; this helps to reduce muscle atrophy and maintain muscle strength. The patient with a leg cast, is instructed to "push down" the knee. The patient in an arm cast is encouraged to "make a fist." Muscle setting exercises (*e.g.*, quadriceps setting and gluteal setting exercises) are important in maintaining muscles essential for walking (Chart 62-1). Isometric exercises should be performed at least hourly while the patient is awake.

At times, portable electrical muscle stimulators may be attached to the skin over large muscles before cast application. Muscle contractions are electrically stimulated for about 8 hours a day to prevent the development of disuse atrophy.

Patient Education and Home Care Considerations. When the cast is dry, the patient is instructed as follows:

1. Move about as normally as possible. Avoid excessive use of the injured extremity.
2. Perform the prescribed exercises regularly, as scheduled.
3. Elevate the casted extremity to heart level frequently to prevent swelling.
4. Keep the cast dry.
   a. Wetness destroys the hardness of plaster casts.
      (1) Do not cover the cast with plastic or rubber, as this causes condensation and wetting of the cast.
      (2) Avoid walking on wet, slippery floors or sidewalks.
   b. Fiberglass casts, after being wet, must be dried thoroughly with a hair dryer on a cool setting to avoid skin problems.
5. Cushion rough edges of the cast with tape.
6. Report to the physician if the cast breaks; do not attempt to fix it yourself.
7. To clean a cast:
   a. Remove surface soil with a damp cloth.
   b. Stained areas may be touched up with a thin layer of white shoe polish.
8. Do not attempt to scratch the skin under the cast. This may cause a break in the skin and result in the formation of a skin ulcer. Cool air from a hair dryer may alleviate an itch.
9. Note odors about the cast, stained areas, warm spots, and pressure spots. Report them to the physician.
10. Also report the following to the physician: persistent pain, swelling that does not respond to elevation, changes in sensation, decreased ability to move exposed fingers or toes, and changes in skin color and temperature.

CHART 62-1
Muscle Setting Exercises

Isometric contraction of the muscle maintains muscle mass and strength and prevents atrophy.

Quadriceps-Setting Exercises

- Position patient supine with leg extended.
- Instruct patient to push knee back onto the mattress by contracting the anterior thigh muscles.
- Encourage patient to hold the position for 5 to 10 seconds.
- Let patient relax.
- Repeat exercise 10 times each hour when patient is awake.

Gluteal-Setting Exercises

- Position patient supine with legs extended, if possible.
- Instruct patient to contract muscles of buttocks and abdomen.
- Encourage patient to hold the contraction for 5 to 10 seconds.
- Let patient relax.
- Repeat exercise 10 times each hour when patient is awake.

Prepare the patient for cast removal or cast changes (Guideline 62-2) by explaining what to expect. The cast is cut using a cast cutter, which achieves its effect by oscillation. The patient will feel the vibration and pressure applied during its use. The cutter will not hurt the patient's skin. The cast padding is then cut with scissors.

The body part that has been casted will be weak from disuse, stiff, and may appear atrophied. Therefore, it requires support when the cast is removed. The skin is usually dry and scaling because of the accumulated dead skin and is vulnerable to injury from scratching. The skin needs to be washed gently and lubricated with an emollient lotion.

The patient is taught to gradually resume activities within the prescribed therapeutic regimen. Because the muscles are weak from disuse, the body part that has been casted is not able to withstand normal stresses immediately. In addition, the patient who has noticeable swelling of the affected extremity after the cast is removed is taught to continue to elevate the extremity to control swelling until normal muscle tone and use are reestablished.

Evaluation

Expected Outcomes

1. Patient actively participates in therapeutic regimen
   a. Elevates affected extremity
   b. Exercises according to instructions
   c. Keeps cast dry
   d. Reports any problems that develop
   e. Keeps follow-up clinic or physician appointments
2. Reports less pain
   a. Elevates extremity that is in the cast
   b. Repositions self
   c. Uses occasional oral analgesic
3. Demonstrates increased mobility
   a. Uses assistive devices safely
   b. Exercises to increase strength
   c. Changes position frequently

GUIDELINE 62-2
Cast Removal

Procedure	Rationale
1. Inform the patient about the procedure.	1. Facilitates cooperation and reduces fear about the procedure.
2. Assure patient that the electric saw or cast cutter will not cut skin.	2. Reduces anxiety. (Blade oscillates to cut cast.)
3. The cast is bivalved using a series of alternating pressures and linear movements of blade along the line to be cut.	3. Cuts cast in halves. Avoids burning sensation from prolonged contact of oscillating blade with padding.
4. Wear eye protection (patient and cast cutter operator).	4. Protects eyes from flying cast particles.
5. Cut padding with scissors.	5. Releases all of the casting materials.
6. Support body part as it is removed from the cast.	6. Reduces stresses on body part that has been immobilized.
7. Gently wash and dry area that has been immobilized.* Apply emollient lotion.	7. Removes dead skin that has accumulated during immobilization. Keeps skin supple.
8. Teach patient to avoid rubbing and scratching skin.	8. Prevents skin breakdown.
9. Teach patient to gradually resume active use of body part within the guidelines of prescribed therapeutic regimen.	9. Protects weakened part from excessive stress. Progressive exercises reduce stiffness, restore muscle strength and function.
10. Teach patient to control swelling by elevating the extremity or using elastic bandage if prescribed.	10. Facilitates circulation (*i.e.*, venous return) and controls fluid pooling.

**If a new cast is to be applied, follow guidelines for application of a cast and associated nursing care.*

   d. Performs range-of-motion exercises of joints not in the cast
4. Participates in self-care activities
   a. Performs hygiene and grooming activities independently or with minimal assistance
   b. Feeds self independently or with minimal assistance
5. Exhibits healing of abrasions and lacerations
   a. Demonstrates no systemic signs or symptoms of infection
   b. Demonstrates no local signs of infection (*i.e.*, local discomfort, purulent drainage, staining, odor)
   c. Demonstrates intact skin when cast is removed
6. Maintains adequate circulation to affected extremity
   a. Exhibits normal skin color and temperature
   b. Experiences minimal swelling
   c. Achieves satisfactory capillary refill on testing
   d. Demonstrates active movement of fingers or toes
   e. Reports normal sensations in casted body part
   f. Reports pain is controllable
7. Exhibits absence of complications
   a. Demonstrates normal neurovascular status of casted extremity
   b. Develops no pressure ulcers
   c. Exhibits minimal muscle wasting

Arm Casts

The patient whose arm is immobilized in a cast must readjust to many routine tasks. The unaffected arm must assume all the upper extremity activities. The patient may experience fatigue due to modification activities and the weight of the cast. Frequent rest periods are necessary.

To diminish and control swelling, the immobilized arm should be elevated. When the patient is lying down, the arm is elevated, with each joint positioned higher than the preceding proximal joint (*e.g.*, elbow higher than the shoulder, hand higher than the elbow). When the patient is sitting, the arm needs to be elevated also.

A sling may be used when the patient ambulates. To prevent pressure on the cervical spinal nerves, the sling should distribute the supported weight over a large area and not on the back of the neck. The patient is encouraged to remove the arm from the sling frequently and elevate it.

Circulatory disturbances in the hand may become apparent with signs of cyanosis, swelling, and an inability to move the fingers. One serious effect of circulatory constriction in an arm cast is Volkmann's contracture, a compartment syndrome. Contracture of the fingers and wrist occurs as the result of ischemia due to the obstruction of arterial flow to the forearm and hand. The patient is unable to extend the fingers, describes abnormal sensation (*e.g.*, unrelenting pain, pain on passive stretch), and exhibits signs of diminished circulation to the hand.

This serious complication can be prevented with nursing surveillance and proper care. Neurovascular checks need to be made frequently. Tissue pressure within muscle compartments may be measured directly, using pressure-monitoring devices (see Fig. 62-1). Compartment syndrome is managed in part by bivalving the cast to remove constricting cast and dressings. A fasciotomy may be necessary to improve vascular status. Permanent damage develops within a few hours if action is not taken.

Leg Casts

The application of a leg cast imposes a degree of immobility on the patient. The cast may be a short leg cast, extending to the knee, or a long leg cast, extending to the groin. The fresh cast must be handled in a manner that will not cause denting or disruption. The leg is supported on soft pillows to heart level to control swelling. Ice packs as prescribed may be applied over the fracture site for the first day or two.

As with other cast applications, the leg must be assessed for adequate circulation and normal nerve function. The circulation is assessed by observing the color, temperature, and capillary refill of the exposed toes. Nerve function is assessed by observing the patient's ability to move the toes and by asking about the sensations in the foot. Numbness, tingling, and burning may be due to peroneal nerve injury from pressure at the head of the fibula.

- Injury to the peroneal nerve as a result of pressure is a common cause of footdrop.

When the cast is dry, the patient is taught how to transfer and ambulate safely with assistive devices (*e.g.*, crutches, walker). The gait to be used depends on whether or not the patient's problem allows weight-bearing. If weight-bearing is allowed, the cast will be reinforced to withstand the body weight. A cast boot to wear over the casted foot (Fig. 62-3) provides a broad, anti-skid walking surface.

When seated, the patient is encouraged to elevate the casted leg. The patient should lie down several times a day with the casted leg elevated to further promote venous return.

Body or Spica Casts

Casts that encase the trunk (body cast) and portions of the trunk and one or two extremities (spica cast) require special nursing techniques. Body casts may be used in situations requiring spinal immobility. Hip spicas are used for patients after femoral fractures and some hip joint surgeries. Shoulder spica casts are used for some humeral neck fractures. Patient preparation, turning, and skin and hygienic care and monitoring for cast syndrome are nursing responsibilities.

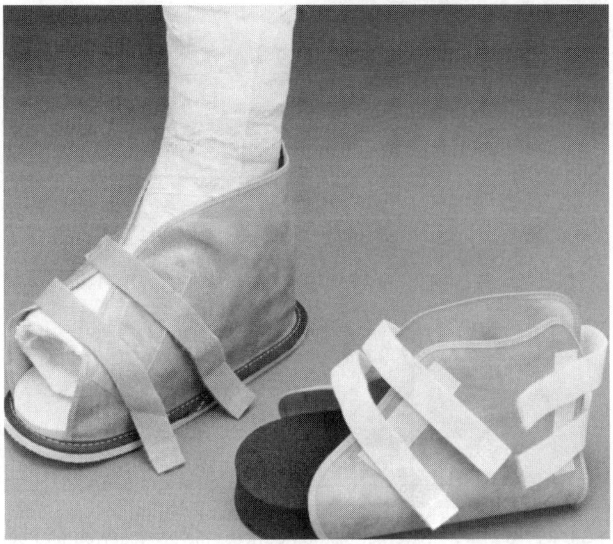

FIGURE 62-3. Cast boots. (Courtesy of Srouse Manufacturing, Inc., Ligonier, IN.)

Explaining the procedure will help reduce the patient's apprehension about being encased in a large cast. Often the patient has been immobilized in traction for weeks and anticipates recurrence of pain while being moved for casting. Also, the fracture table used for large cast application looks like a torture device. Saying that the patient will be cared for by several people during the application and that support for the injured body will be adequate and as gentle as possible may help to allay fear. Medications for pain and relaxation administered before the procedure will enable the patient to cooperate during the procedure by reducing discomfort and related anxiety.

After cast application, the patient needs to be supported by flexible, waterproof pillows until the cast is dry to prevent it from being dented. Inadequate cast support will cause a soft cast to crack or become dented, resulting in subsequent pressure points. The bed must have firm mattress support. Three pillows placed crosswise on the bed will suffice for the body cast; for a hip spica, one pillow placed crosswise at the waist and two pillows placed lengthwise for the affected leg are necessary. If both legs are involved, two additional pillows are necessary. It is important that the pillows be next to each other, because any spaces between the pillows will allow the damp cast to sag, become weak, and possibly break. It is also important to make sure that a pillow is not placed under the head and shoulders (of a patient in a body cast) while the cast is drying, as this causes pressure on the chest.

Patients are turned every 2 hours to relieve pressure and to allow the cast to dry (Guideline 62-3). The patient is turned as a unit toward the uninjured side. Twisting the patient's body within the cast is avoided. Sufficient personnel (at least three people) are needed when the patient is turned so that the fresh cast can be adequately supported with the palms of the hands at vulnerable points (*i.e.*, body joints) to prevent the cast from cracking. The patient is encouraged to assist in the repositioning by using the trapeze or bedrail. A stabilizing abduction bar incorporated into a spica cast should not be used as a turning device. Pillows are readjusted to provide support without creating areas of pressure.

The patient is turned to a prone position, twice daily if tolerated, to provide postural drainage of the bronchial tree and relieve pressure on the back. A small pillow under the abdomen enhances comfort, and a pillow placed lengthwise under the dorsa of the feet prevents the toes from being forced into the mattress. The toes are allowed to hang over the edge of the mattress.

The skin around the edges of the cast must be inspected frequently for signs of irritation. Some of the area under the cast can be inspected by pulling the skin taut and using a flashlight. Reaching under the cast edges with the fingers allows for removal of cast crumbs and massage of the skin. Accessible skin should be bathed carefully and massaged with an emollient.

The perineal opening must be large enough for hygienic care. If it is not, the cast must be adjusted. To make the cast resistant to soiling, the nurse protects the perineum with a towel and sprays the dry cast around the perineum with a protective plastic spray. To protect the cast from excreta soiling, clean dry plastic sheeting can be inserted under the cast and brought over the cast edge before each

GUIDELINE 62–3
Turning the Patient in a Hip Spica Cast

1. The patient is moved with a steady, even, pulling motion to the side of the bed.
2. Pillows are placed along the other side of the bed for cast support.
3. Instruct the patient to assist by using the arm on the involved side to pull the shoulder over when turning.
4. Two nurses are on the side to which the patient is being turned to provide support for the cast while rolling the patient toward them.
5. The third nurse assists in rolling the patient from behind, adjusts the patient's shoulder, and adjusts the pillows.
6. The patient's body should be turned as a unit and positioned comfortably in good alignment.

elimination. Generally, fracture bed pans are easier for hip spica patients to use than regular bed pans.

Cast Syndrome

Patients immobilized in large casts may develop psychologic and physiologic responses to the confinement. The psychologic component of cast syndrome is similar to a claustrophobic reaction. The patient exhibits an acute anxiety reaction characterized by behavioral changes and autonomic responses (*e.g.*, increased respiratory rate, diaphoresis, dilated pupils, increased heart rate, elevated blood pressure). The nurse needs to recognize the anxiety reaction and provide an environment in which the patient feels secure.

The physiologic responses to large casts are associated with the imposed immobility. With decreased physical activity, gastrointestinal motility decreases. With accumulation of intestinal gases, pressure increases and ileus occurs. The patient has distention, abdominal discomfort, nausea, and vomiting. As with other adynamic ileus situations, the patient is treated conservatively with decompression (nasogastric intubation connected to suction) and intravenous fluid therapy until gastrointestinal motility is restored. If the cast restricts the abdominal distention, a window must be cut in the cast over the abdominal area. The distention may place traction on the superior mesenteric artery, reducing the blood supply to the bowel. The bowel may become gangrenous, requiring surgical intervention.

The nurse needs to be aware of the possible development of cast syndrome in patients with large body casts and plan interventions for its prevention or resolution.

External Fixators

External fixation devices are used to manage open fractures with soft-tissue damage. They provide stable support for severe comminuted (crushed or splintered) fractures while permitting active treatment of damaged soft tissue (Fig. 62-4). Complicated fractures of the humerus, forearm, femur, tibia, and pelvis are managed with external skeletal fixators. The fracture is reduced, aligned, and immobilized by a series of pins inserted in the bone fragments. The pins are maintained in position through attachment to a portable frame. The fixators facilitate patient comfort, early mobility, and active exercise of adjacent uninvolved joints. Complications related to disuse and immobility are minimized.

It is important to prepare the patient psychologically for application of the external fixator. The apparatus looks clumsy and foreign to the patient. Reassurance that the discomfort associated with the device is mild and that early mobility is anticipated promotes acceptance of the device, as does involvement of the patient in the care associated with the fixator.

After the external fixator is applied, sharp points on the fixator or pins are covered to prevent device-induced injuries. The extremity is elevated to reduce swelling. The neurovascular status of the extremity is monitored every 2 hours. Each pin site is assessed for redness, drainage, ten-

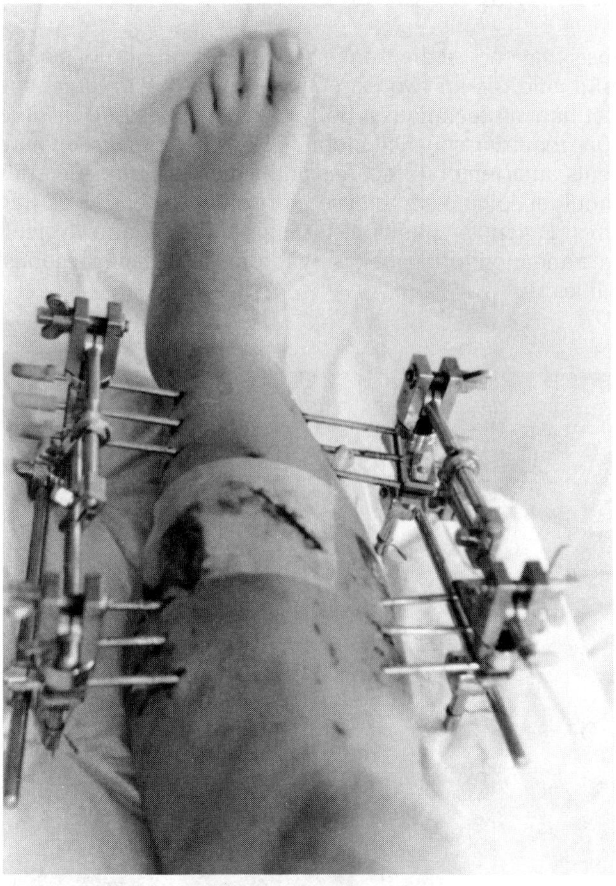

FIGURE 62-4. External fixation device. Pins are inserted into bone fragments. The fracture is reduced and aligned. The reduction is stabilized by attaching the pins to a rigid portable frame. The device facilitates treatment of soft tissue damaged in complex fracture situations.

derness, pain, and loosening of the pin. Some serous drainage from the pin sites is to be expected. The nurse must be alert for potential problems due to pressure by the device on the skin, nerves, or blood vessels.

Pin care to prevent pin tract infection is carried out according to the prescribed routine. Crusts should not form at the pin site, and the fixator must be kept clean. If pins or clamps loosen, the physician is notified.

- The clamps on the external fixator frame are never adjusted.

Isometric and active exercises are encouraged within the limits of tissue damage. When the swelling has subsided, the patient is mobilized within the limits of any other injuries. Weight-bearing limits are prescribed to minimize the chance of the pins loosening when stress is applied at the bone–pin interface.

The fixator is removed when the soft tissue has healed. The fracture may require additional stabilization by cast or molded orthosis for healing.

The **Ilizarov** external fixator is a special device using tension wires to attach fixator rings, which are joined by telescoping rods. The device is used to correct angulation and rotational defects, to treat nonunion, and to lengthen limbs. Callus and bone formation is stimulated by prescribed daily adjustment of the telescoping rods. The patient is taught how to adjust the telescoping rods and perform skin care. Weight-bearing is generally encouraged. When the desired correction has been achieved, no additional adjustments are made and the fixator is left in place until the bone heals.

Managing the Patient in Traction

Traction is the application of a pulling force to a part of the body. Traction is used to minimize muscle spasms; to reduce, align, and immobilize fractures; to reduce deformity; and to increase space between opposing surfaces. Traction must be applied in the desired direction and magnitude to obtain its therapeutic effects. Factors that reduce the effective pull of the traction must be eliminated.

At times, the traction needs to be applied in more than one direction to achieve the desired line of pull. When this is done, part of one of the lines of pull counteracts the other line of pull. These lines of pull are known as the vectors of force. The actual resultant pulling force is somewhere between the two lines of pull (Fig. 62-5). The effects of applied traction are evaluated with x-ray, and adjustments may be necessary. As the muscle and soft tissue relax, the amount of weight used may be changed to obtain the desired pulling force.

Types of Traction

Straight or running traction applies the pulling force in a straight line with the body part resting on the bed. Buck's extension traction (Fig. 62-6) and pelvic traction (see Fig. 63-1) are examples of straight traction.

Balanced suspension traction (Fig. 62-7) supports the affected extremity off the bed and allows for some patient mobility without disruption of the line of pull.

Traction may be applied to the skin (**skin traction**) or directly to the bony skeleton (**skeletal traction**). The mode of application is determined by the purpose of the traction.

Traction can be applied with the hands (**manual traction**). This is a very temporary traction that may be used when applying a cast, giving skin care under a Buck's extension foam boot, or adjusting traction apparatus.

Principles of Effective Traction

Whenever traction is applied, the **countertraction** must be considered. Countertraction is the force acting in the opposite direction. (Newton's third law of motion states that for every action there is an equal and opposite reaction.)

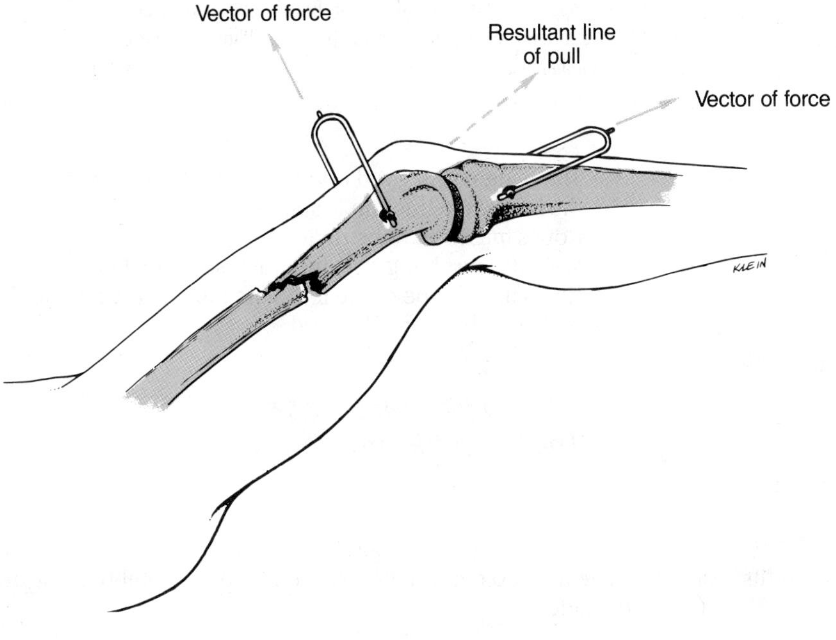

FIGURE 62-5. Traction may be applied in different directions to achieve the desired therapeutic line of pull. Adjustments in applied forces may be prescribed over the treatment period.

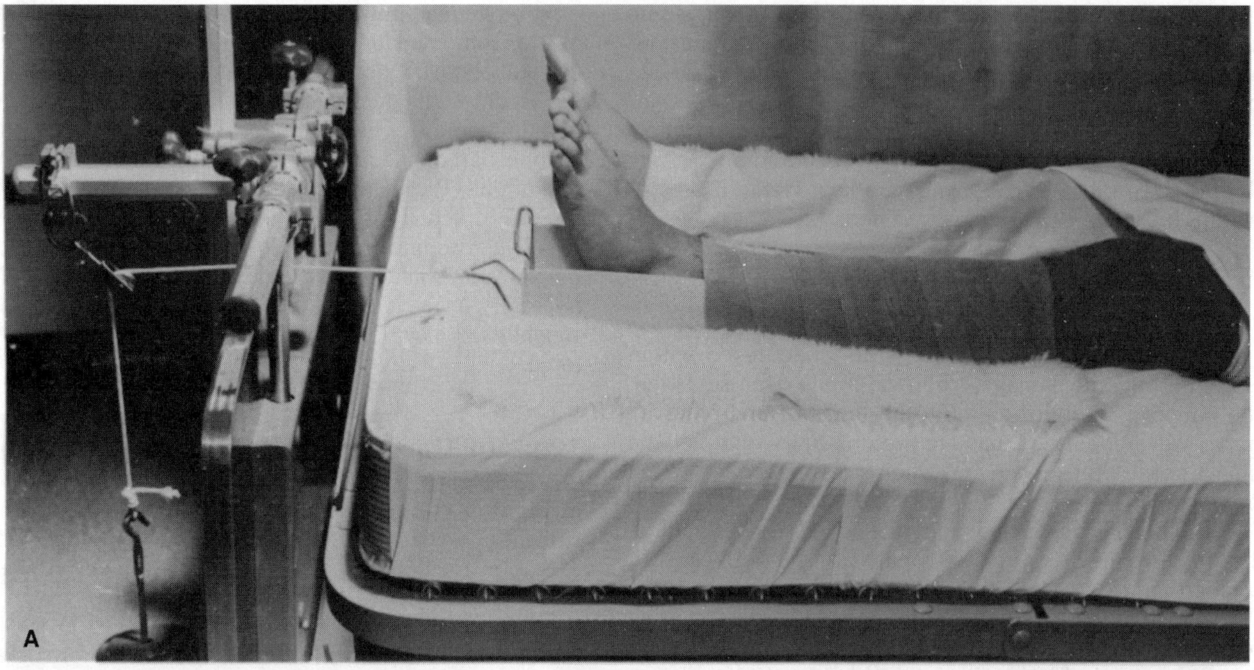

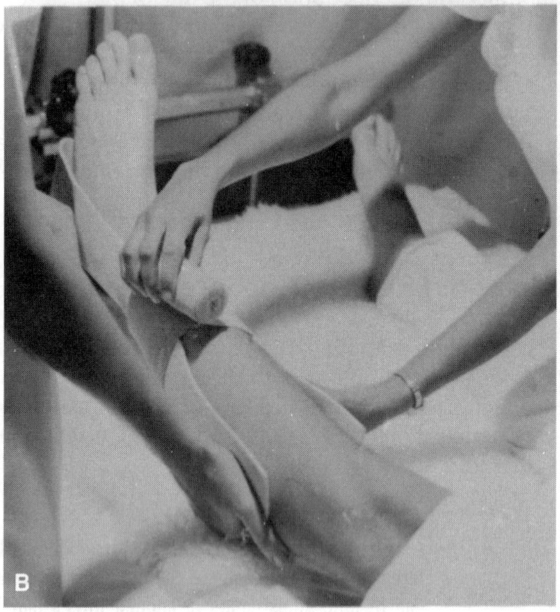

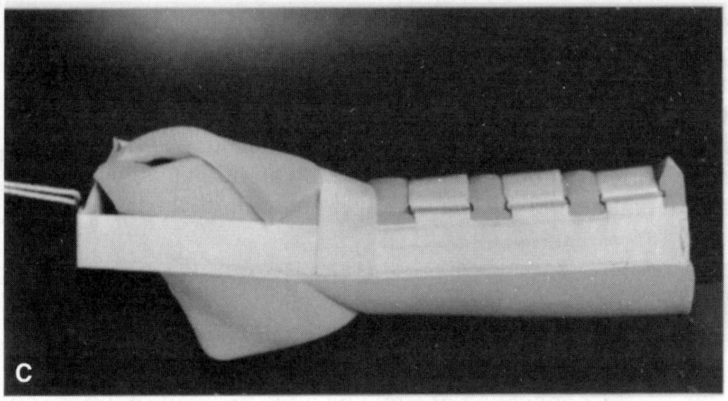

FIGURE 62-6. Buck's extension. (**A**) Lower extremity in Buck's extension traction. (**B**) Applying elastic bandage for Buck's extension traction. (**C**) Prepadded boot that may be used in Buck's extension. (Photo of boot courtesy of All Orthopedic Appliances.)

Generally, the patient's body weight and bed position adjustments supply the needed countertraction.

- Countertraction must be maintained for effective traction.

Traction must be continuous to be effective in reducing and immobilizing fractures. Pelvic and cervical skin tractions are frequently used to reduce muscle spasm and are usually prescribed as intermittent traction.

- Skeletal traction is *never* interrupted.
- Weights are not removed unless the traction is prescribed intermittently.

Any factor that might reduce the pull or alter its resultant line of pull must be eliminated.

- The patient is in good body alignment in the center of the bed when traction is applied.
- Ropes must be unobstructed.
- Weights must hang free and not rest on the bed or floor.
- Knots in the rope or the footplate must not touch the pulley or the foot of the bed.

❑ NURSING PROCESS
The Patient in Traction

Assessment

The psychologic and physiologic impact of the musculoskeletal problem, traction device, and immobility must be considered.

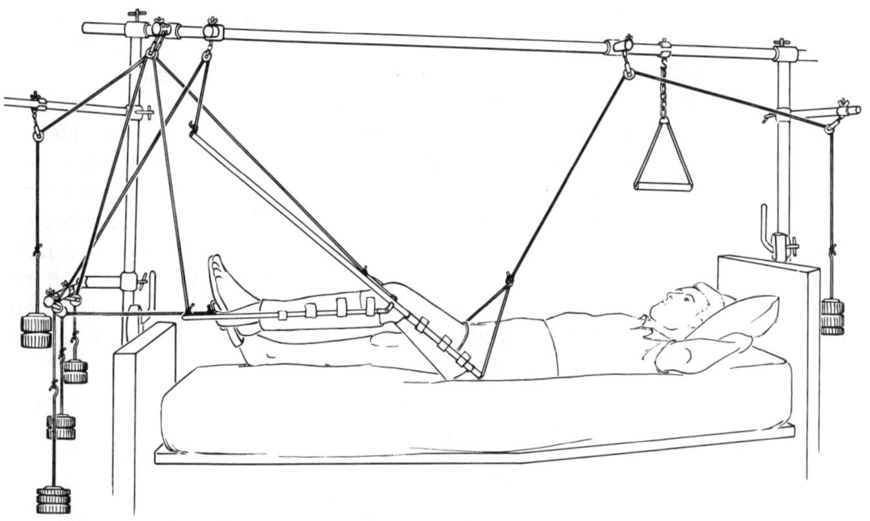

FIGURE 62-7. Balanced suspension traction with Thomas leg splint. Vertical movement of the patient is permitted as long as resultant line of pull is maintained.

Traction restricts one's mobility and independence. The equipment often looks threatening, and its application can be frightening. Confusion, disorientation, and behavioral problems may develop in patients who are confined in a limited space for an extended time. Therefore, the patient's anxiety level and psychologic responses to traction must be assessed and monitored.

The body part to be placed in traction must be assessed. The neurovascular status (*i.e.*, color, temperature, capillary refill, edema, pulses, sensations, ability to move) is evaluated and compared with the unaffected extremity. Skin integrity is noted.

Assessment of body system functioning is completed for baseline data, and ongoing assessment is indicated. Immobility may contribute to the development of integumentary, respiratory, gastrointestinal, urinary, and cardiovascular system problems. These may include pressure ulcers, lung congestion, stasis pneumonia, constipation, loss of appetite, urinary stasis, and urinary tract infections. Reports of calf tenderness, warmth, redness, or swelling, or a positive Homans' sign (discomfort in the calf when the foot is forcibly dorsiflexed) suggest the development of deep vein thrombosis. Early identification of preexisting or developing problems facilitates prompt interventions to resolve the problems.

Diagnosis

Nursing Diagnoses

Based on the nursing assessment, the patient's major nursing diagnoses related to traction may include the following:

- Knowledge deficit about the treatment regimen
- Anxiety related to health status and traction device
- Pain and discomfort related to traction and immobility
- Self-care deficit: feeding, hygiene, or toileting related to traction
- Impaired physical mobility related to disease process and traction

Collaborative Problems/ Potential Complications

Based on the assessment data, potential complications that may develop include:

- Pressure ulcer
- Lung congestion and pneumonia
- Constipation
- Anorexia
- Urinary stasis and infection
- Deep vein thrombosis

Planning and Implementation

Goals. The major goals of the patient in traction may include understanding of the treatment regimen, reduced anxiety, maximum comfort, maximum level of self-care, achieving maximum mobility within therapeutic limits of traction, and absence of complications.

Understanding the Treatment Regimen. The patient must understand the pathologic problem being treated and the rationale for the traction therapy. The information may need to be repeated and reinforced frequently. With increased understanding of the therapy, the patient will become an active participant in his health care.

Reducing Anxiety. Before any traction is applied, the patient needs to be informed about the procedure, its purpose, and its implications. Talking to the patient about what is being done, and why, helps to allay apprehension. After being in traction for a while the patient may react to being confined to a limited space. Frequent visits by the nurse will reduce feelings of isolation and confinement. Family and friends should be encouraged to visit frequently for the same reason. Diversional activities that can be performed within the limits of the traction are encouraged.

Achieving Maximum Level of Comfort. Because the patient will be immobilized in bed, the mattress needs to be firm and supported with a bed board. Special mattress pads designed to minimize the development of pressure ulcers should be placed on the bed before applying the traction.

- Pressure on dependent body parts can be relieved by turning and by positioning the patient for comfort within the limits of the traction.
- The bed linens are kept wrinkle-free and dry.
- Every complaint of the patient in traction is investigated immediately.

Achieving the Maximum Level of Self-Care. Initially, the patient may require assistance with self-care activities.

The nurse helps the patient learn to meet needs such as eating, bathing, dressing, and toileting while immobilized in the traction device. Assistive devices such as reachers and an overbed trapeze may facilitate self-care. With resumption of self-care activities the patient will feel less dependent and less frustrated and will experience improved self-esteem.

Some assistance will be required throughout the period of immobility; however, the nurse and the patient can creatively develop routines that will maximize the patient's independence.

Attaining Maximum Mobility Within the Limits of Traction. During traction therapy, the patient needs to exercise nonimmobilized muscles and joints to diminish their deterioration due to immobilization. Active motion of all unaffected joints is encouraged. The physical therapist can be consulted to design bed exercises that minimize loss of muscle strength. The nurse needs to encourage the patient to exercise. During exercising, the nurse must ensure that traction forces are maintained and that the patient is properly positioned to prevent complications resulting from poor alignment.

Monitoring and Managing Potential Complications

Pressure Ulcers. The patient's skin is examined frequently for evidence of pressure or friction. Special attention is given to bony prominences. Early intervention is necessary to relieve pressure. Frequent patient repositioning and use of skin protective devices (*e.g.*, elbow protectors) are helpful. If the risk of skin breakdown is high, such as with a multi-trauma patient or with a debilitated elderly patient, the nurse may consult with the physician concerning the use of a specialized bed to assist in prevention of skin breakdown. If a pressure ulcer develops, the nurse consults with the physician (and enterostomal therapist if one is available) concerning treatment.

Lung Congestion/Pneumonia. The patient's lungs are auscultated to determine respiratory status. The patient is taught deep breathing and coughing exercises to aid in full expansion of the lungs and to move pulmonary secretions. If patient history and baseline assessment indicate that the patient is at high risk for developing respiratory complications, the nurse should consult with the physician concerning use of specific therapies (*e.g.*, incentive spirometer). If a respiratory problem develops, prompt institution of prescribed therapy is needed.

Constipation and Anorexia. Reduced gastrointestinal motility results in constipation and anorexia. A diet high in fiber and fluids may help to stimulate gastric motility. If constipation does develop, the nurse consults with the physician concerning therapeutic measures, which might include stool softeners, laxatives, suppositories, and enemas. To improve the patient's appetite, the patient's food preferences are identified and included, as appropriate, within the prescribed therapeutic diet.

Urinary Stasis and Infection. Incomplete emptying of the bladder related to positioning in bed can result in urinary stasis and infection. In addition, the patient may find use of the bedpan uncomfortable and restrict fluids to minimize frequency of urination. The nurse must monitor the fluid intake and the character of the urine. The nurse teaches the patient to consume adequate amounts of fluid and to void every 2 to 3 hours. If the patient exhibits signs or symptoms of urinary tract infection, the nurse consults with the physician concerning treatment of the problem.

Deep Vein Thrombosis. Venous stasis occurs with immobility. The nurse teaches the patient to perform ankle and foot exercises within the limits of the traction therapy on a regular basis throughout the day to prevent the development of deep vein thrombosis (DVT). The patient is encouraged to drink fluids to prevent dehydration and associated hemoconcentration, which contribute to stasis. The nurse monitors the patient for development of signs of DVT and reports findings promptly to the physician for definitive evaluation and therapy.

Evaluation

Expected Outcomes

1. Demonstrates understanding of traction regimen
   a. Describes purpose of traction
   b. Participates in plan of care
2. Exhibits reduced anxiety
   a. Appears relaxed
   b. Uses effective coping mechanisms
   c. Expresses concerns and feelings
3. States increased level of comfort
   a. Requests occasional oral analgesia
   b. Repositions self frequently
4. Performs self-care activities
   a. Requires minimal assistance with feeding, bathing, dressing, and toileting
5. Demonstrates increased mobility
   a. Performs prescribed exercises
   b. Uses assistive devices safely
6. Exhibits absence of complications
   a. Intact skin
   b. Clear lungs
   c. No reports of shortness of breath
   d. No productive cough
   e. Regular bowel evacuation pattern
   f. Appetite normal
   g. Clear, yellow, nonconcentrated urine of adequate amount
   h. No signs or symptoms of deep vein thrombosis

Specific Traction Applications

Skin Traction

Skin traction is accomplished by a weight pulling on tape, sponge rubber, or canvas materials that have been attached to the skin. Traction on the skin transmits traction to the musculoskeletal structures. The amount of weight applied is limited: it must not exceed the tolerance of the skin. No more than 2 to 3 kg (4.5 to 7 lb) of traction can be used on an extremity. Pelvic traction is generally 4.5 to 9 kg (10 to 20 lb), depending on the weight of the patient. Skin traction is used to control muscle spasm and provide immobilization. When prolonged or heavy traction weight is necessary, skeletal traction is used rather than skin traction.

Appendicular (pertaining to the extremities) skin tractions used for adults include **Buck's extension traction,**

Russell's traction, and **Dunlop's traction.** Axial (involving the head and trunk) skin tractions, cervical and pelvic, are used to treat back pain (see Chapter 63).

Buck's Traction. Buck's extension (unilateral or bilateral) is a form of skin traction in which the pull is exerted in one plane when partial or temporary immobilization is desired (see Fig. 62-6*A*). It is used to provide comfort following injuries to the hip prior to surgical fixation.

Before the traction is applied, the skin is inspected for abrasions and circulatory disturbances. The skin and circulation must be in healthy condition to tolerate the traction. The extremity should be clean and dry before the foam boot or the traction tape is applied (see Fig. 62-6*B,C*).

To apply Buck's traction with tape, foam rubber—padded straps are applied with the foam surface against the skin on each side of the affected leg. A loop of tape about 10 to 15 cm (4 to 6 inches) long is extended beyond the sole of the foot. A spreader is applied to the distal end of the tape to prevent pressure along the side of the foot. The malleolus and proximal fibula are protected with cast padding to prevent pressure ulcers and skin necrosis. While one person elevates and supports the extremity under the patient's heel and knee, another person wraps the elastic bandage spiral fashion over the traction tape, beginning at the ankle and ending at the tibial tubercle. The elastic bandage helps the tape to adhere to the skin and prevents slipping. A sheepskin pad is placed under the leg to reduce the friction of the heel against the bed. When Buck's traction with a foam boot is applied, the patient's heel must be placed well into the heel of the boot. Velcro straps are secured around the leg and excessive pressure over the malleolus and proximal fibula is avoided. The weights are attached to the rope affixed to the spreader or footplate and passed over a pulley fastened to the end of the bed. The weight is attached to the rope.

Russell's Traction. Russell's traction, which may be used for fractures of the tibial plateau, supports the flexed knee in a sling and applies the horizontal pulling force via traction tape and elastic bandage to the lower leg. If prescribed, the leg may be supported by a pillow to assure proper knee flexion and to prevent pressure on the heel.

Dunlop's Traction. Dunlop's traction is skin traction applied to the upper extremity. Horizontal traction is applied to the abducted humerus, and vertical traction is applied to the flexed forearm.

Ensuring Effective Traction

To ensure effective traction, wrinkling and slipping of the traction bandage are avoided and countertraction is maintained. Proper positioning must be maintained to keep the leg or arm in a neutral position. To prevent bony fragments from moving against one another, the patient should not turn from side to side but can shift position slightly.

Potential Complications

Skin Breakdown. Skin traction can irritate the skin. Sensitive, fragile skin frequently seen in older adults must be identified during the initial assessment. Reaction of the skin to contact with tape and foam must be monitored closely. The skin traction must be applied firmly enough to ensure contact of the tapes or foam device with the skin. Shearing forces on the skin must be avoided. Traction tapes should be palpated daily to detect underlying tenderness. With the lower extremity, the ankle and the Achilles tendon should be inspected several times a day.

- The foam boots are removed to inspect the skin three times a day. A second nurse is needed to support the extremity during the inspection.
- Special back care is given to the patient at least every 2 hours to prevent pressure ulcers. Since the patient must remain in a supine position, the chance of developing a pressure ulcer is increased.
- Special mattresses (*e.g.*, air filled, high-density foam) may be indicated to minimize development of skin ulcers.

Nerve Pressure. Skin traction can place pressure on peripheral nerves. When applying traction to the lower extremity, care must be taken to avoid pressure on the peroneal nerve at the point at which it passes around the neck of the fibula just below the knee. Pressure at this point can cause footdrop (see Fig. 62-2). The patient is questioned about sensation and asked to move the toes and foot. Dorsiflexion of the foot demonstrates function of the peroneal nerve. Weakness of dorsiflexion or foot movement and inversion of the foot might indicate pressure on the common peroneal nerve. Plantar flexion demonstrates function of the tibial nerve.

When skin traction is applied to the arm, the area around the elbow where the ulnar nerve is located should not be wrapped tightly. Ulnar nerve function can be assessed by active abduction of the little finger and sensation on the ulnar side of the little finger.

- Sensation and motion must be assessed regularly.
- Any complaint of burning sensation under the traction bandage or boot must be investigated immediately.
- Altered sensation and motor function must be reported to the physician promptly.

Circulatory Impairment. After skin traction is applied, the foot or hand is inspected for circulatory difficulties within a few minutes and then every 1 to 2 hours.

- Peripheral pulses and the color, capillary refill, and temperature of the fingers or toes are assessed.
- The patient is assessed for calf tenderness and for a positive Homans' sign for indications of deep vein thrombosis.
- Active foot or hand exercise is encouraged hourly.

Skeletal Traction

Skeletal traction is applied directly to the bone. This method of traction is used most frequently to treat fractures of the femur, the tibia, the humerus, and the cervical spine. The traction is applied directly to the bone by use of a metal pin or wire (*e.g.*, Steinmann's pin; Kirschner wire) that is inserted through the bone distal to the fracture, avoiding nerves, blood vessels, muscles, tendons, and joints. Tongs applied to the head (*e.g.*, Gardner–Wells tongs) are fixed in the skull to apply traction that immobilizes cervical fractures.

Patient preparation is important and contributes to the patient's comfort and cooperation. Local or general anesthesia may be used.

Skeletal traction is applied under surgical asepsis. The insertion site is prepared with a surgical scrub such as povidone-iodine. A local anesthetic is administered at the insertion site and periosteum. A small skin incision is made and the sterile pin or wire is drilled through the bone. The patient feels pressure during this procedure and possibly some discomfort when the periosteum is penetrated.

After insertion, the pin or wire is attached to the traction bow or caliper. The ends of the wire are covered with corks or tape to prevent injury to the patient or personnel. The weights are attached to the pin or wire bow by a rope–pulley system that exerts the appropriate amount and direction of pull for effective traction. Skeletal traction frequently uses 7 to 12 kg (15 to 25 lb) to achieve the therapeutic effect. The weights applied initially must overcome the shortening spasms of the affected muscles. As the muscles relax, the traction weight is reduced to prevent fracture dislocation and to promote fracture healing.

Often skeletal traction is balanced traction, which supports the affected extremity, allows some movement of the patient, and facilitates patient independence and nursing care while maintaining effective traction.

The **Thomas splint with the Pearson attachment** is frequently used with skeletal traction in fractures of the femur (see Fig. 62-7). It may be used with skin traction and other balanced suspension apparatus. Because upward traction is required, an overbed frame is used. Figure 62-8 shows suspension traction using slings.

Maintaining Effective Traction. When traction is used, the apparatus is checked to see that the ropes are in the wheel grooves of the pulleys; that the ropes are not frayed; that the weights hang freely; and that the knots in the rope are tied securely. The patient's positioning is evaluated. Slipping down in bed results in ineffective traction.

- Weights should never be removed from skeletal traction unless a life-threatening situation occurs. If the weights are removed, the whole purpose of their use has been defeated and injury may result.

Positioning. The alignment of the patient's body in traction must be maintained as prescribed to promote an effective line of pull. The foot is positioned to avoid footdrop (plantar flexion), inward rotation (inversion), or outward rotation (eversion). The patient's foot may be supported in a neutral position by orthopedic devices (*e.g.*, foot supports).

Skin Care. When traction frames are used, a trapeze may be suspended overhead within easy reach of the patient. This apparatus is of great help in assisting the patient to move about in bed and on and off the bedpan.

The patient's elbows frequently become sore, and nerve injury may occur if most repositioning is done by pushing on the elbows. Often patients use the heel of the good leg to act as a brace when they raise themselves. This digging of the heel into the mattress may cause injury to the tissues; hence the heel must be protected and inspected for pressure areas.

Specific pressure points need to be checked for redness and skin breakdown. Areas that are particularly vulnerable to pressure caused by traction apparatus applied to the lower extremity include the ischial tuberosity, popliteal space, Achilles tendon, and heel.

When a patient is not permitted to turn on one side or the other, the nurse must make a special effort to provide back care and to keep the bed dry and free of crumbs and wrinkles. The patient can assist by holding onto the overhead trapeze and raising the hips off the bed. If the patient cannot raise himself or herself off the bed, the nurse can push down on the mattress with one hand to relieve pressure on the back and bony prominences and to provide for some shifting of weight.

Neurovascular Status. Neurovascular assessment of the immobilized extremity is conducted at least every hour initially and then several times a day. The patient is in-

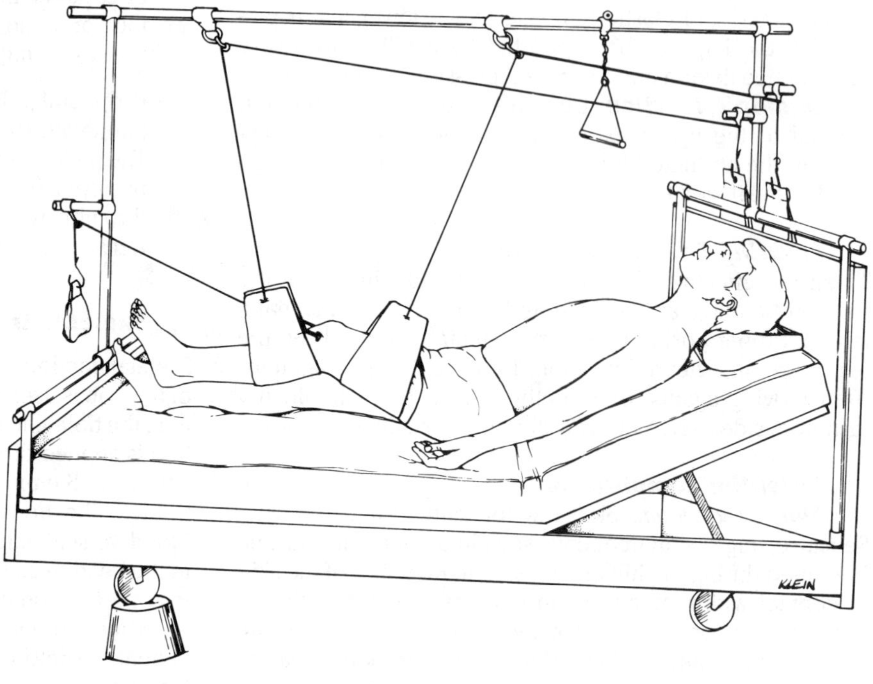

FIGURE 62-8. Balanced suspension traction using slings. Skeletal traction is applied to the patient's injured leg, which is supported in slings.

structed to report immediately any changes in sensation or movement so that they can be promptly evaluated. Prompt recognition of a developing neurovascular problem is essential so that corrective measures can be instituted promptly.

Pin Site. The wound at the insertion site requires attention. Initially, the site is covered with a sterile dressing. Subsequent care of the pin site is individually prescribed. The area must be kept clean. Slight serous oozing at the pin site is to be expected. Crusting should be prevented. The drainage and pin site are assessed for signs of infection such as purulent drainage, inflammation, and pain. The goal is to avoid infection and development of osteomyelitis. The patient may experience discomfort at the pin site due to traction on the skin caused by an unsupported muscle.

- The pin site is inspected at least every 8 hours for signs of inflammation and evidence of infection.

Exercise. Patient exercises are valuable in maintaining muscle strength and tone and in promoting circulation. Exercises are planned within the therapeutic limits of the traction. Active exercises include pulling up on the trapeze, flexing and extending the feet, and range-of-motion and weight-resistance exercises for noninvolved joints. The immobilized extremity benefits from isometric exercises. Quadriceps- and gluteal-setting exercises (see Chart 62-1) are important to maintain strength in major ambulatory muscles. Without bed exercises, the patient will lose muscle mass and strength, and rehabilitation time will be greatly prolonged.

Development of deep vein thrombosis is a significant risk for the immobilized patient. The patient is encouraged to do active flexion–extension ankle exercises and isometric contraction of the calf muscles (calf pumping exercises) 10 times an hour while awake to decrease venous stasis. In addition, elastic stockings, compression devices, and anticoagulant therapy may be prescribed to help prevent thrombus formation.

Pin Removal. When x-ray studies demonstrate the presence of callus, skeletal traction is discontinued. The extremity is gently supported while the weights are removed. The pin is cut close to the skin and removed by the physician. Casts or splints are then used to support the healing bone (see Chart 62-2 for nursing interventions for the patient in traction).

Managing the Patient Undergoing Orthopedic Surgery

Many patients who have musculoskeletal dysfunction need to undergo surgery to correct the problem. Problems that may be corrected by surgery include unstabilized fracture, deformity, joint disease, necrotic or infected tissue, impaired circulation (*e.g.*, compartment syndrome), and tumors or growths. Frequent surgical procedures include open reduction with internal fixation (ORIF) for fractures; arthroplasty, meniscectomy, and joint replacement for joint problems; amputation for severe extremity problems (*e.g.*, gangrene, massive trauma); bone graft for joint stabilization, defect-filling, or stimulation of healing; and tendon transplants for improving motion. The goals of most orthopedic surgery include improving function by restoring motion and stability and relieving pain and disability.

CHART 62-2
Nursing Interventions for the Patient in Traction

1. Assess the patient's neurovascular status.
2. Ensure that effective traction is maintained (*e.g.*, ropes and pulleys are freely moveable; prescribed weight hangs free; patient positioning is correct).
3. Maintain continuous traction unless otherwise prescribed.
4. Reposition within therapeutic limits of traction.
5. Involve the patient in care to reduce depression and boredom that frequently accompany weeks of traction therapy.
6. Encourage active foot exercises; use foot supporters as needed.
7. Encourage exercises to minimize deconditioning.
8. Observe for skin irritation and breakdown.
9. Observe for pressure under the sling and equipment and at common pressure points (*e.g.*, ischial tuberosity, popliteal space, heel).
10. Monitor pin sites and perform skin care.
11. Assess the patient for signs or symptoms of complications (*e.g.*, pin tract infection, deep vein thrombosis).

Types of Surgery

Orthopedic surgery generally falls into the following categories:

Open reduction—the reduction and alignment of the fracture after surgical dissection and exposure of the fracture

Internal fixation—the stabilization of the reduced fracture by the use of metal screws, plates, nails, and pins

Bone graft—the placement of bone tissue (autologous or homologous grafts) to promote healing, to stabilize, or to replace diseased bone

Amputation—the removal of a body part

Arthroplasty—the repair of joint problems through the operating arthroscope (an instrument that allows the surgeon to operate within a joint without a large incision) or through open joint surgery

Meniscectomy—the excision of damaged joint fibrocartilage

Joint replacement—the substitution of joint surfaces with metal or synthetic materials

Total joint replacement—the replacement of both articular surfaces within a joint with metal or synthetic materials

Tendon transfer—the movement of tendon insertion to improve function

Fasciotomy—the cutting of the muscle fascia to relieve muscle constriction or to reduce fascia contracture

❑ NURSING PROCESS
Preoperative Care of the Patient Undergoing Orthopedic Surgery

Assessment

Assessment of the patient is focused on hydration, current medication history, and possible infection.

Adequate hydration is an important goal for orthopedic patients. Immobilization and bed rest contribute to deep vein thrombosis, to urinary stasis and associated bladder infections, and to stone formation. Adequate hydration decreases blood viscosity and assures adequate urine flow and helps to prevent the occurrence of thrombophlebitis and urinary tract problems. To determine preoperative hydration, the nurse assesses the skin, vital signs, urinary output, and laboratory values for evidence of dehydration.

The medication history provides information for perioperative management. Corticosteroid therapy, whether current or in the recent past, may adversely affect the body's ability to withstand the stress of surgery. The person with chronic illness (*e.g.*, rheumatoid arthritis, chronic pulmonary disease) frequently has received corticosteroid medications to control symptoms. The corticosteroid should be administered preoperatively, intraoperatively, and postoperatively as prescribed to assure adequate corticosteroid levels and prevent occurrence of adrenal insufficiency because of suppressed adrenal function. The use of other medications, such as anticoagulants, cardiovascular agents, or insulin, needs to be documented and discussed with the surgeon and anesthesiologist to assure adequate management.

The patient is asked specifically about the presence of colds, dental problems, urinary tract infections, and other infections within the 2 weeks before surgery. Osteomyelitis could develop through hematologous spread. Permanent disability can result if infection occurs within a bone or joint. Preexisting infections must be resolved before elective orthopedic surgery.

Other areas of preoperative assessment are similar to those for any patient undergoing surgery. If the patient receives "on-call" preoperative medications, they are injected into an uninvolved area because tissue absorption is better in nontraumatized areas.

Diagnosis

Nursing Diagnoses

Based on the nursing assessment data, the patient's major preoperative nursing diagnoses related to orthopedic status may include the following:

- ❑ Pain related to fracture, orthopedic problem, swelling, or inflammation
- ❑ Altered peripheral tissue perfusion related to swelling, constricting devices, or impaired venous return
- ❑ Impaired health maintenance management related to loss of independence
- ❑ Impaired physical mobility related to pain, swelling, and possibly an immobilization device
- ❑ Disturbance in body image, self-esteem, or role performance related to impact of musculoskeletal problem

Planning and Implementation

Goals. The major goals of the patient before orthopedic surgery may include relief of pain, adequate tissue perfusion, health maintenance, improved mobility, and improved self-concept.

Relieving Pain. Physical, pharmacologic, and psychologic management techniques to control pain are useful in the preoperative period. Specific methods selected are tailored to the individual patient. Immobilization of a fractured bone or injured, inflamed joint will decrease discomfort. Elevation of a swollen extremity will promote venous return and reduce associated discomfort. Ice, if prescribed, will relieve swelling and directly reduce discomfort by diminishing nerve stimulation. Analgesics are frequently prescribed to control the acute pain of musculoskeletal injury and associated muscle spasm. During the immediate preoperative period, the nurse needs to discuss and coordinate administration of analgesic medications with the anesthesiologist and surgeon. Alternative methods of pain control (*e.g.*, distraction, focusing, guided imagery, quiet environment, back rubs) may be used to decrease pain perception.

Maintaining Adequate Tissue Perfusion. Trauma, swelling, or immobilization devices may interrupt tissue perfusion. The neurovascular status (*i.e.*, color, temperature, capillary refill, pulses, pain, edema, paresthesia, motion) of the extremity must be assessed frequently. If circulation is compromised, measures to restore adequate circulation are instituted. The physician is notified promptly, the extremity is elevated, and constricting wraps and casts are released as prescribed.

Maintaining Health. The nurse assists the patient in activities that will promote health during the perioperative and rehabilitative periods. Nutritional needs and hydration are assessed. Generally, nutrition for orthopedic patients is a reflection of their normal eating patterns. The preoperative fasting regimen is usually tolerated well. If the patient is diabetic, elderly and frail, or the victim of multiple trauma, special provisions may be necessary.

Abnormal urinalysis findings and complaints of burning on urination require further investigation before surgery. At times patients will decide to limit their fluid intake to minimize the use of a bedpan. A small fracture pan may be more comfortable for the patient to use. The nurse monitors fluid intake and urinary output. The use of an indwelling catheter should be avoided to reduce the risk of urinary tract infection.

Smoking should be stopped during the preoperative period to facilitate optimum respiratory function. Coughing, deep breathing, and use of the incentive spirometer are practiced preoperatively for improved respiratory function during the postoperative period. Preoperative teaching facilitates postoperative compliance.

Exercises are taught during the preoperative period. Gluteal-setting and quadriceps-setting isometric exercises are taught to maintain the muscles needed for ambulation (see p. 1853). Unless contraindicted, isometric contraction of the calf muscles and ankle exercises are practiced to minimize venous stasis and prevent deep vein thrombosis. Active range-of-motion exercises of uninvolved joints are encouraged. The patient who will be using assistive devices may exercise to strengthen the upper extremities and shoulders. If possible, assistive devices (*e.g.*, trapeze) are used and transfer techniques are practiced before surgery.

Skin care is provided, with special attention to pressure points. The use of pressure-reducing surfaces (*e.g.*, convoluted foam or air mattress) needs to be instituted before surgery for those at risk for skin breakdown.

To minimize the risk of infection, the skin is meticulously and gently cleaned with soap and water the day before surgery. If the operation is elective, the orthopedic surgeon may advise the patient to begin the skin cleansing with a germicidal soap several days before hospitalization.

Improving Mobility. Preoperatively, the patient's mobility may be impaired by pain, swelling, and immobilizing devices (*e.g.*, splints, casts, traction). The nurse must gently assist the patient in moving the injured part while providing adequate support. Swollen extremities are elevated and adequately supported with hands and pillows. Pain is controlled before an injured part is moved by splinting it and by administering medication in time to take effect before the injured part is moved. Movement within the limits of therapeutic immobility is encouraged. If assistive devices (*e.g.*, crutches, walker, wheelchair) are to be used postoperatively, the patient is encouraged to practice with them preoperatively, to facilitate their safe use and promote earlier independent mobility.

Improving Self-Concept. Preoperative orthopedic patients may need assistance in accepting changes in body image, diminished self-esteem, or inability to perform the responsibilities of their life roles. The degree of assistance required in this area varies greatly, depending on the events preceding hospitalization, the surgery and rehabilitation planned, the temporary or permanent nature of the altered body image, and the changes in role performance. The nurse promotes a trusting relationship for patients to express concerns and anxieties and helps them examine their feelings about changes in self-concept. The nurse can clarify any misconceptions patients may have and help them work through modifications that may be necessary because of alterations in physical capacity and self-concept.

Evaluation

Expected Outcomes

1. Reports controlled pain
   a. Uses multiple approaches to reduce pain
   b. States that medication is effective in controlling pain
   c. Moves with increasing comfort
2. Exhibits adequate tissue perfusion
   a. Skin color normal
   b. Skin warm
   c. Capillary refill response normal
   d. Sensation and motion normal
   e. Demonstrates reduced swelling
3. Promotes health
   a. Eats balanced diet appropriate to meet nutritional needs
   b. Maintains adequate hydration
   c. Abstains from smoking
   d. Practices respiratory exercises
   e. Repositions self to relieve skin pressure
   f. Engages in strengthening and preventive exercises
4. Maximizes mobility within the therapeutic limits
   a. Requests assistance when moving
   b. Elevates swollen extremity after transfer
   c. Uses immobilizing devices and assistive devices as prescribed
5. Expresses positive self-concept
   a. Acknowledges temporary or permanent changes in body image
   b. Discusses role performance changes
   c. Participates in care planning decisions

❑ *NURSING PROCESS*
Postoperative Care of the Patient Undergoing Orthopedic Surgery

Assessment

After orthopedic surgery, the nurse continues the preoperative care plan, modifying it to the current postoperative status. The nurse reassesses the patient's needs in relation to pain, tissue perfusion, health promotion, mobility, and self-concept.

Skeletal trauma and surgery performed on bones, muscles, and joints can produce significant pain, especially during the first several postoperative days.

Tissue perfusion must be monitored closely because edema and bleeding into the tissues may compromise circulation and result in compartment syndrome.

Assessment of respiratory, gastrointestinal, and urinary function provides data for promoting function of these systems. General anesthesia, analgesia, and immobility can result in altered functioning of these systems.

Prescribed limits on mobility are noted. The nurse assesses the patient's understanding of the mobility restrictions. Reassessing the patient's self-concept allows the nurse to modify the preoperative plan of care more easily.

In addition, the nurse is concerned with assessing and monitoring the patient for potential problems related to the surgery. Frequent assessment of vital signs, level of consciousness, wound drainage, breath sounds, bowel sounds, fluid balance, and pain will provide the nurse with data that may suggest the possible development of complications. Abnormal findings are reported to the physician promptly.

With major orthopedic surgery, there is a risk of hypovolemic shock because of blood loss. Muscle dissection frequently produces wounds in which hemostasis is poor. Wounds that are closed under tourniquet control may bleed during the postoperative period. The nurse must be alert for signs of hypovolemic shock (*e.g.*, rising pulse rate, falling blood pressure, confusion, restlessness) (see Chapter 15.)

Changes in the patient's pulse rate, respiratory rate, or color may indicate pulmonary or cardiac complications. The pulmonary complications of atelectasis and pneumonia are frequently seen and may be related to preexisting pulmonary disease, deep anesthesia, decreased activity, analgesics, and reduced respiratory reserve due to advanced age or an underlying musculoskeletal disorder (*e.g.*, restrictive lung expansion secondary to kyphosis and osteoporosis).

Voiding in unnatural positions may contribute to urinary retention. In addition, elderly men usually have some degree of prostate enlargement and may already have difficulty in voiding. Therefore it is important to monitor urinary output.

Temperature elevations within the first 48 hours are frequently related to atelectasis or other respiratory problems. Temperature elevations during the next few days are frequently associated with urinary tract infections. Superficial wound infections take about 5 to 9 days to develop. Phlebitis-associated fever generally occurs during the second week.

Thromboembolic disease (see Deep Vein Thrombosis, Chapter 31, and Pulmonary Embolism, Chapter 24) is one of the most common and most dangerous of all complications occurring in the postoperative orthopedic patient. Advancing age, hemostasis, lower extremity orthopedic surgery, and immobilization are significant risk factors. The nurse assesses the patient's legs daily for calf tenderness, warmth, redness, and edema, and a positive Homans' sign. Abnormal findings are reported to the physician promptly.

In addition, **fat embolus** (p. 1917) may occur with orthopedic surgery. The nurse must be alert to changes in respiration, behavior, and level of consciousness that might indicate the development of fat embolus.

Diagnosis

Nursing Diagnoses

Based on all assessment data, the patient's major nursing diagnoses after orthopedic surgery may include the following:

- Pain related to the surgical procedure, swelling, and immobilization
- Potential for altered peripheral tissue perfusion related to swelling, constricting devices, impaired circulation
- Altered health maintenance related to loss of independence
- Impaired physical mobility related to pain, swelling, surgical procedure, presence of immobilizing device (*e.g.*, splint, traction, cast)
- Altered body image, self-esteem, or role performance related to impact of musculoskeletal problems.

Collaborative Problems/ Potential Complications

Based on the assessment data, potential complications may include:

- Hypovolemic shock
- Atelectasis; pneumonia
- Urinary retention
- Infection
- Deep vein thrombosis

Planning and Implementation

Goals. The major goals of the patient after orthopedic surgery may include relief of pain, adequate tissue perfusion, health maintenance, improved mobility, improved self-concept, and absence of complications.

Nursing Interventions

Relieving Pain. After orthopedic surgery, pain can be intense. Edema, hematomas, and muscle spasms contribute to the pain experienced. Some patients will indicate that the pain is less than that experienced preoperatively, and only moderate amounts of analgesics are needed. The patient's pain level and response to therapeutic measures are monitored closely. Every effort is made to relieve the pain and discomfort.

Multiple pharmacologic approaches to pain management exist. Patient-controlled analgesia (PCA) and epidural analgesia may be prescribed to control the pain. If intramuscular and oral analgesics are prescribed on an as needed (PRN) basis, the patient is instructed to request the pain medication before the pain becomes severe. The medication should be administered promptly, within the prescribed intervals. Intramuscular injection sites should be rotated, avoiding the operative hip and thigh. Medications may be administered on a preventative basis within the prescribed intervals if the onset of pain can be predicted (*e.g.*, a half hour before planned activity such as transfer or exercise).

In addition to pharmacologic approaches to controlling pain, elevation of the operative extremity and application of cold, if prescribed, help to control edema and resulting pain. Portable suction of the wound decreases fluid accumulation and hematoma formation. The nurse may find that repositioning, relaxation, distraction, and guided imagery techniques are helpful in reducing and controlling the patient's pain.

Increasing and uncontrollable pain needs to be reported to the orthopedic surgeon for evaluation. Pain should diminish rapidly after the initial postoperative period. After 3 to 4 days, most patients require only occasional oral analgesia for residual muscle soreness and spasm.

Maintaining Adequate Tissue Perfusion. The preoperative plan of care is continued. The nurse monitors the neurovascular status of the involved body part and notifies the physician promptly of findings indicative of diminished tissue perfusion. The patient is reminded to perform muscle-setting, ankle, and calf-pumping exercises hourly while awake to enhance circulation.

Maintaining Health. The preoperative plan of care is continued. The patient is encouraged to participate in the postoperative treatment regimen.

A well-balanced diet with adequate protein and vitamins is needed for healthy tissue and wound healing. The patient is placed on a full balanced diet as soon as possible. Large amounts of milk should not be given to orthopedic patients who are on bed rest, however, because this only adds to the calcium pool in the body and requires that more calcium be excreted by the kidneys, which can lead to formation of urinary calculi.

The nurse monitors the patient for evidence of pressure ulcers, which are a constant threat to any patient who must spend an extended period in bed or who is elderly, malnourished, or unable to move without assistance. Turning, washing, and drying the skin, and minimizing pressure over bony prominences are necessary to avoid skin breakdown.

Improving Physical Mobility. Patients are frequently afraid to move after orthopedic surgery. A therapeutic relationship encourages the patient to participate in therapeutic activities designed to improve the level of physical mobility. Patients are usually receptive to increasing their mobility once they have been assured that movement within therapeutic limits is beneficial, that assistance will be provided by the nurse, that discomfort can be controlled, and that activity goals are attainable.

Soft tissue heals more rapidly than bone. The incision may appear healed; however, the underlying bone requires more time to repair and regain normal strength. This is especially important to remember in surgeries of the lower extremity.

Metal pins, screws, rods, and plates used for internal fixation are designed to maintain the position of the bone until ossification occurs. They are not designed to support the body's weight and can bend, loosen, or break if stressed. The estimated strength of the bone, the stability of the fracture, reduction and fixation, and the amount of bone healing are important considerations in determining the stress the bone can withstand after surgery. Some orthopedic procedures require prolonged protection from excessive stress, which is accomplished through weight-bearing restrictions. The orthopedic surgeon will prescribe the weight-bearing limits and use of protective devices (orthoses), if necessary, after surgery.

- ❑ Weight-bearing limits and use of protective devices are determined by the orthopedic surgeon before the patient begins transfer and ambulation.

The exercise program is tailored to the individual's needs. The goal is to return the patient to the highest level of function in the shortest time consistent with the surgical procedure. Rehabilitation involves progressively increasing the patient's activities and instituting progressive exercises as prescribed. Frequently some form of assistive device (crutches, walker) is used for postoperative mobility. Preoperative practice with assistive devices helps the patient use them postoperatively. Within the weight-bearing limits prescribed by the surgeon, the nurse monitors the patient's gait, making sure that it is safe. (Crutch walking and using a walker are discussed in Chapter 18.)

Improving Self-Concept. The preoperative plan of care is continued. The nurse and the patient set realistic goals. Increasing self-care activities within the limits of the therapeutic regimen and resumption of roles facilitate recognition of abilities and promote self-esteem, personal identity, and role performance. Acceptance of altered body image is facilitated by support provided by the nurse, family, and others.

Monitoring and Managing Potential Complications

Hypovolemic Shock. The nurse monitors the patient after surgery for the development of hypovolemic shock. Excessive loss of blood during or after surgery can result in shock. The nurse identifies early signs and symptoms of shock (*e.g.*, increased pulse rate, decreased blood pressure, urine output less than 30 ml per hour, restlessness, change in mentation, thirst, decreased hemoglobin and hematocrit) and reports the findings to the orthopedic surgeon for appropriate management. (See Chapter 15 for management of the patient with shock.)

Atelectasis and Pneumonia. The nurse monitors the patient's lung sounds and encourages deep breathing and coughing exercises. Full expansion of the lungs prevents accumulation of respiratory secretions and development of atelectasis and pneumonia. Incentive spirometry, if prescribed, is encouraged. If signs of respiratory problems develop (*e.g.*, increased respiratory rate, productive cough, diminished or adventitious breath sounds, fever), the nurse reports the findings to the surgeon for appropriate management.

Urinary Retention. The urinary output is monitored hourly after surgery. The patient is encouraged to void every 3 to 4 hours to prevent urinary retention and bladder distention. Privacy is provided during toileting. Because the patient may need to void in an unusual position, the nurse assists the patient with positioning. Fracture bedpans may be more comfortable than other bedpans. Voiding in the side-lying position may be helpful to the male patient. Some male patients can void only if standing, and clarification with the surgeon of the activity prescription may be needed before assisting the patient to a standing position. If the patient is unable to void, intermittent catheterizations may be prescribed until the patient is able to void independently.

Infection. Infection is a risk after any surgery. It is of particular concern for the postoperative orthopedic patient because of the high risk for osteomyelitis. Osteomyelitis often requires prolonged courses of intravenous antibiotics. At times the infected bone, prosthesis, and internal fixation devices must be surgically removed. Therefore, prophylactic systemic antibiotics are frequently prescribed during the perioperative and immediate postoperative period. The nurse assesses the patient's response to these antibiotics. When changing dressings and emptying wound drainage devices, aseptic technique is essential. The nurse monitors the patient's vital signs, inspects the wound, and notes the character of drainage. Because urinary retention is common after orthopedic surgery, the character of the urine is monitored for signs of urinary tract infection. Prompt recognition and reporting to the physician of an apparent infective process is essential.

Deep Vein Thrombosis. Prevention of deep vein thrombosis requires use of preventive measures (*e.g.*, ankle and calf pumping exercises; use of elastic stockings or sequential compression devices; adequate hydration; early mobilization). Prophylactic warfarin or adjusted-dose heparin may be prescribed. Aspirin has no apparent venous thromboembolism prophylactic effect in the orthopedic patient. The nurse monitors the patient for signs of deep vein thrombosis and promptly reports findings to the physician for management.

Evaluation

Expected Outcomes

1. Reports decreased level of pain
   a. Uses multiple approaches to reduce pain
   b. Uses occasional oral medication to control discomfort
   c. Elevates extremity to control swelling and discomfort
   d. Moves with greater comfort
2. Exhibits adequate tissue perfusion
   a. Skin color normal
   b. Skin warm
   c. Capillary refill response normal
   d. Sensation and motion normal
   e. Demonstrates reduced swelling

3. Promotes health
   a. Eats balanced diet appropriate to meet nutritional needs
   b. Maintains adequate hydration
   c. Abstains from smoking
   d. Practices respiratory exercises
   e. Repositions self to relieve skin pressure
   f. Engages in strengthening and preventive exercises
4. Maximizes mobility within the therapeutic limits
   a. Requests assistance when moving
   b. Elevates swollen extremity after transfer
   c. Uses immobilizing devices as prescribed
   d. Complies with prescribed weight-bearing limitation
5. Expresses positive self-concept
   a. Discusses temporary or permanent changes in body image
   b. Discusses role performances
   c. Views self as capable of assuming responsibilities
   d. Actively participates in planning care and in the therapeutic regimen
6. Exhibits absence of complications
   a. Does not experience shock
   b. Maintains normal vital signs and blood pressure
   c. Lung sounds clear
   d. Wound heals without signs of infection
   e. Wound drainage is not purulent
   f. Does not experience urinary retention
   g. Urine clear
   h. Exhibits no signs of deep vein thrombosis

Reconstructive Joint Surgery

At times, joint disease or deformity will necessitate surgical intervention to relieve pain, improve stability, and improve function. Surgical therapies used for joint disease include excision of damaged and diseased tissue, repair of damaged structures (*e.g.*, ruptured tendon), removal of loose bodies (debridement), immobilizing fusion of a joint (**arthrodesis**), and replacement of all or part of the joint surfaces (*e.g.*, arthroplasty, prosthesis, total joint).

Total joint replacement is the replacement of both articular surfaces within a joint capsule (*e.g.*, total hip replacement refers to implantation of both femoral and acetabular prostheses). Hemiarthroplasty refers to the replacement of one of the articular surfaces (*e.g.*, in a hip hemiarthroplasty the femoral head and neck are replaced with a femoral prosthesis—the acetabulum is not replaced).

The procedure is selected according to the patient's underlying orthopedic condition, general physical health, impact of joint disability on life, and age. Timing of these procedures is important to assure maximum function. Surgery should be performed before surrounding muscles become contracted and atrophied and serious structural abnormalities occur. The patient is carefully evaluated by the physician so that the most appropriate procedure is performed.

Joint Replacement

Patients with severe joint pain and disability may be selected for joint replacement. Conditions contributing to joint degeneration include rheumatoid arthritis, osteoarthritis (degenerative joint disease), trauma, and congenital deformity. Joint replacement may also be required in cases of disruption of the blood supply and subsequent avascular necrosis. Joints frequently replaced include the knee, hip (Fig. 62-9), shoulder, and finger joints. Less frequently, more complex joints (elbow, wrist, ankle) are replaced. The procedure is usually an elective one.

Most joint replacements consist of metal and high-density polyethylene components. Finger prostheses are generally Silastic. The joint implants may be cemented in the prepared bone with polymethyl methacrylate (PMMA; a bone-bonding agent), which has properties similar to bone. Loosening of the prosthesis due to cement—bone interface failure is a common reason for prosthesis failure. Ingrowth prostheses (porous-coated, cementless, artificial joint components) that allow the patient's bone to grow into and securely fix the prosthesis in the bone are being used more frequently. Accurate fitting and the presence of healthy bone with adequate blood supply are important in the use of cementless components. Efforts to reduce prosthesis failure rate through modification of techniques, improved materials, and use of bone grafts continue.

With joint replacement, excellent pain relief is obtained in 85% to 90% of patients. Return of motion and function de-

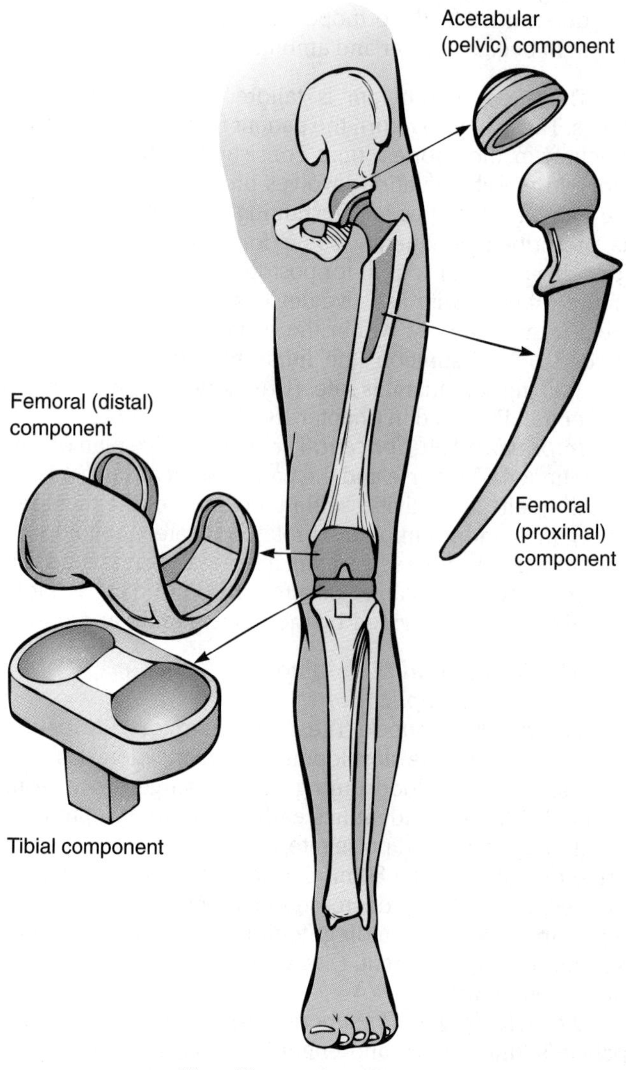

FIGURE 62-9. Hip and knee replacement.

pends on preoperative soft tissue condition, soft tissue reactions, and general muscle strength. Early failure of joint replacement is associated with high levels of activity and preoperative joint pathology.

Preoperative Assessment. Assessment of the patient and preoperative management are aimed at having the patient in optimal health at the time of surgery. A complete preoperative evaluation is directed toward cardiovascular, respiratory, renal, and hepatic function. Age, obesity, preoperative leg edema, history of deep vein thrombosis, and varicose veins increase the risk of postoperative deep vein thrombosis and pulmonary embolism. Every effort is made to prevent deep vein thrombosis and resulting pulmonary embolism, the most common cause of postoperative mortality in patients over 60 years of age undergoing total hip replacement.

Preoperatively, the neurovascular status of the extremity undergoing joint replacement is assessed. Postoperative assessment data are compared with preoperative assessment data to identify changes and deficits. Nerve palsy can occur during surgery. An absent pulse postoperatively is of concern unless the pulse was also absent preoperatively.

Preventing Infection. Careful preoperative assessment of the patient for sites of infection is necessary because of the risk of postoperative infection. Any infection 2 to 4 weeks before planned surgery may result in postponement of surgery. Preoperative urine cultures may be obtained because urinary tract infection is a frequent portal of entry for bacteria. It has been observed that infection occurs nearly twice as often in patients with rheumatoid arthritis as in those with osteoarthritis.

Preoperative skin preparation frequently begins a day or two before the surgery. The majority of deep infections are caused by bacteria, mostly from airborne sources, that are implanted into the wound at the time of surgery. Therefore, during surgery there is strict adherence to aseptic principles and the operating area is controlled and made as nearly bacteria free as possible.

Prophylactic antibiotics may be administered just before surgery or intraoperatively. Culture of the joint during surgery, before intraoperative antibiotic therapy is begun, may be important in identifying and treating subsequent infections.

Osteomyelitis is difficult to treat. Infection of the prosthesis generally requires removal of the implant and joint revision, a complex procedure. Also, it is not always possible to achieve a functional joint when the reconstruction procedure has to be repeated.

Ambulation After Surgery. Ambulation with a walker or crutches is usually started within a day or two after surgery. The goal is independent ambulation. At first the patient may only be able to stand for a brief period because of orthostatic hypotension. As the patient is able to tolerate more activity, transferring to a chair several times a day for short periods is encouraged.

Specific weight-bearing limits on the prosthesis are determined by the physician based on the patient's condition, the procedure, and the fixation method. Generally, cemented prostheses can have weight-bearing as tolerated by patient comfort. If the patient has an ingrowth prosthesis, weight-bearing may be limited after surgery to minimize micromotion of the prosthesis in the bone, in an attempt to prevent disruption of bone ingrowth.

Total Hip Replacement

Total hip replacement is the replacement of a severely damaged hip with an artificial joint. Indications for this surgery include arthritis (degenerative joint disease, rheumatoid arthritis), femoral neck fractures, failure of previous reconstructive surgeries (failed prosthesis, osteotomy, femoral head replacement), and problems resulting from congenital hip disease. A variety of total hip prostheses are available. Most consist of a metal femoral component topped by a spherical ball fitted into a plastic acetabular socket (see Fig. 62-9). The surgeon selects the prosthesis most suited to the individual, considering various factors including skeletal structure and activity level.

The patient is usually over age 60 with unremitting pain or irreversibly damaged hip joints. With the advent of improved prosthetic materials and operative techniques, the life of the prosthesis is extended, and younger patients with severely damaged painful hip joints are undergoing total hip replacement.

Nursing Interventions

The nurse must be aware of specific potential complications associated with total hip replacement and include them in the nursing care plan. These include dislocation of the hip prosthesis, excessive wound drainage, thromboembolism, and infection.

Dislocation of the Hip Prosthesis. Maintaining the femoral head component in the acetabular cup is essential. The patient is taught about positioning the leg in **abduction,** which helps to prevent dislocation of the prosthesis. The use of abduction splints, wedge pillows (Fig. 62-10), or two or three pillows between the legs keep the hip in abduction. When the patient in bed is turned, the operative hip must be kept in abduction and the entire length of the leg supported by pillows.

The hip is not flexed more than 45 to 60 degrees. Therefore the head of the bed should not be elevated more than 45 degrees to prevent acute hip flexion. When using the fracture bedpan, the patient is instructed to flex the unoperated hip and use the trapeze to lift the pelvis onto the pan; the patient is also reminded not to flex the operated hip.

Limited flexion is maintained during transfers and when sitting. When the patient is initially assisted out of bed, an abduction splint or pillows are kept between the legs. The patient is encouraged to keep the operative hip in extension. The patient is instructed to pivot on the unoperated leg while assisted by the nurse, who protects the operative leg from adduction, flexion, and excessive weight-bearing.

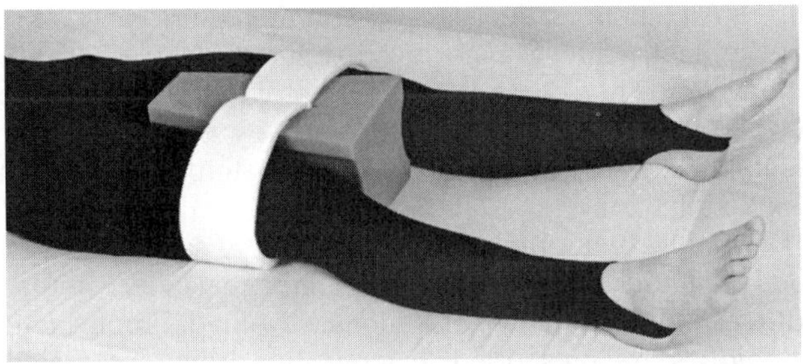

FIGURE 62-10. An abduction pillow may be used after a total hip replacement to prevent dislocation of the prosthesis.

Semi-reclining wheelchairs and toilet seat extenders may be used to minimize hip joint flexion.

The patient is taught protective positioning: maintain abduction, avoid internal and external rotation, hyperextension, and acute flexion. The patient should use a pillow between the legs when lying in a supine or side-lying position and when turning. The patient is instructed not to sleep on the operated side until this position is cleared with the surgeon. At no time should the patient cross the legs. Acute flexion of the hip is to be avoided.

Dislocation may occur with positioning that exceeds the limits of the prosthesis. Dislocation of the prosthesis must be recognized and reduced promptly so that circulatory and nerve damage to the leg does not occur.

- The indicators of dislocation are shortening of the leg, inability to move it, malalignment, abnormal rotation, and increased discomfort.

If a prosthesis becomes dislocated, the surgeon must be notified so that the hip can be reduced and stabilized. As the muscles and joint capsule heal, the chance of dislocation diminishes. Stresses to the new hip joint should be minimal for the first 3 to 6 months.

Wound Drainage. Fluid and blood accumulating at the surgical site are generally drained with a portable suction device. This prevents accumulation of fluid, which could contribute to discomfort and could provide a site for infection. Drainage of 200 to 500 ml in the first 24 hours is expected; by 48 hours postoperatively, the total drainage in 8 hours usually decreases to 30 ml or less, and the suction device is then removed. Drainage volumes greater than anticipated must be reported to the physician promptly.

When extensive blood loss is anticipated following total joint replacement surgery, an autotransfusion drainage system (*i.e.*, the drained blood is filtered and reinfused into the patient during the immediate postoperative period) may be used to decrease homologus blood transfusions.

Deep Vein Thrombosis. The risk for thromboembolism is particularly great after reconstructive hip surgery. The incidence of deep vein thrombosis is 45% to 70%. Of these patients, 20% develop pulmonary emboli, with 1% to 3% being fatal. Therefore the nurse must institute preventive measures and monitor the patient closely for the development of deep vein thrombosis and pulmonary emboli. Measures to promote circulation and decrease venous stasis are priorities for the patient having hip reconstruction. Low-dose heparin or enoxaparin (Lovenox), a low-molecular-weight heparin that requires no routine monitoring of coagulation times, may be used as prophylaxis for deep vein thrombosis following hip replacement surgery.

Infection. Infection is a serious complication after total hip replacement as deep infection may require removal of the implant. Patients who are diabetic, elderly, obese, or poorly nourished, who have rheumatoid arthritis, or who have concurrent infections (*e.g.*, urinary tract infections, dental abscesses) or develop large hematomas are at high risk for infection.

Because total joint infections are so disastrous, all efforts are undertaken to minimize their occurrence. Potential sources of infection are scrupulously avoided. Prophylactic antibiotics are prescribed. If indwelling urinary catheters and portable wound suction devices are used, they are removed as soon as possible to avoid infection. Prophylactic antibiotics may be prescribed if the patient needs any future surgical instrumentation, such as tooth extraction or cystoscopic examination.

Classic signs of infection may be present, or the patient may at some time months to years after the surgery experience return of discomfort in the hip, which could mean a late infection. Acute infections may occur within 3 months of surgery and are associated with progressive superficial infections or draining hematomas. Delayed surgical infections may appear 4 to 24 months after surgery. Infections occurring more than 2 years after surgery are attributed to the spread of infection through the bloodstream from another site in the body.

If an infection occurs, antibiotics are prescribed. Severe infections may require surgical débridement or removal of the prosthesis.

Other Complications. Other complications of total hip replacement include those associated with immobility, loosening of the prosthesis, **heterotrophic ossification** (formation of bone in the periprosthetic space) and **avascular necrosis** (bone death caused by loss of blood supply). Methods for improved cement fixation, ingrowth prosthesis, and bone grafts are aimed at reducing the chance of prosthesis loosening.

Patient Education and Home Care Considerations

Before the patient prepares to leave the acute care setting, a thorough teaching program is provided to promote continuity of the therapeutic regimen and full rehabilitation. The patient is expected to be an active participant in the rehabilitation process.

The patient is advised of the importance of the daily exercise program in maintaining the functional motion of the hip joint and strengthening the abductor muscles of the hip. It will take time to strengthen and reeducate the muscles.

Assistive devices (crutches, walker, or cane) are used for a time. When sufficient muscle tone has developed to permit a normal gait without discomfort, the cane may be abandoned. Walking efficiency after total hip replacement is improved because of the acquired painless normal gait. In general, by 3 months the patient is able to resume routine ADLs. Generally, stair climbing is avoided during the first 3 months after surgery and kept to a minimum for the next 3 months. Frequent walks, swimming, and use of a high rocking chair are excellent for hip exercises. Sexual activities should be carried out with the patient in the dependent position for 3 to 6 months to avoid excessive adduction and flexion of the new hip.

At no time should the patient cross the legs or flex the hip more than 90 degrees. Assistance in putting on shoes and socks may be needed. Low chairs are avoided, as well as sitting for more than 30 minutes at a time, to minimize hip flexion and the risk of prosthetic dislocation and to prevent hip stiffness and flexion contracture. Traveling long distances is to be avoided unless frequent changes in position are possible. Other activities to avoid include overexertion, lifting heavy loads, and excessive bending and twisting (lifting, shoveling snow, forceful turning). See Chart 62-3 for home care following hip replacement.

CHART 62-3
Home Care Management for Hip Replacement

Home Care Considerations	Nursing Intervention
Pain management	Discuss with patient methods to reduce pain: Periodic rest Distraction, relaxation Medications (*e.g.*, NSAIDs, opioid analgesics): actions, administration, side effects
Wound care	Instruct patient in the following: Keep incision clean and dry Wound care/dressing change Signs of wound infection (*e.g.*, pain, swelling, drainage, fever) Explain that sutures/staples will be removed 10 to 14 days following surgery.
Mobility	Instruct patient in the following: Safe use of assistive devices Weight bearing limits How to change positions frequently Limitations on hip flexion and adduction (*e.g.*, avoid acute flexion and crossing legs) How to stand without acutely flexing hip To avoid sitting in low chairs To sleep with pillow between legs to prevent adduction Gradual increase in activities and participation in prescribed exercise regimen Assess home environment for physical barriers.
Self-care (ADLs)	Instruct patient to use elevated toilet seat and to use reachers to aid in dressing. Encourage patient to accept assistance with ADLs during early convalescence until mobility and strength improve.
Potential problems	Instruct patient to report signs of potential problems: Dislocation of prosthesis (*e.g.*, increased pain, shortening of leg, inability to move leg, malalignment, abnormal rotation) Deep vein thrombosis (*e.g.*, calf pain, swelling) Wound infection (*e.g.*, swelling, purulent drainage, pain, fever, difficulty in ambulation) Assess patient for development of potential problems.

After successful surgery and rehabilitation, the patient can expect a hip joint that is free or nearly free of pain, has good motion, is stable, and that usually permits normal or near normal ambulation.

Nursing Care Planning

Based on the nursing assessment of the patient's needs and knowledge of care of the patient undergoing orthopedic surgery, specifically total hip replacement, the nurse develops with the patient an individualized plan of care that monitors for potential problems. A nursing care plan for the patient having a total hip replacement is presented in Nursing Care Plan 62-1.

Total Knee Replacement

Total knee replacement surgery is considered for patients who have severe pain and functional disabilities related to joint surfaces destroyed by arthritis (rheumatoid arthritis, osteoarthritis, posttraumatic arthritis), and bleeding into the joint, such as may result from hemophilia. Metal and acrylic prostheses designed to provide the patient with a functional, painless, stable joint may be used. If the patient's ligaments have weakened, a fully constrained (hinged) or semiconstrained prosthesis may be used to provide joint stability. A nonconstrained prosthesis depends on the patient's ligaments for joint stability.

Postoperative Management. Postoperatively, the knee is dressed with a compression bandage. Ice may be applied to control edema and bleeding. The neurovascular status of the leg is assessed. Active flexion of the foot is encouraged. Efforts are directed at preventing complications (thromboembolism, peroneal nerve palsy, infection).

A wound suction drain removes fluid accumulating in the joint. Drainage during the first 8 hours after surgery is

(text continues on page 1877)

NURSING CARE PLAN 62-1
Care of the Patient With a Total Hip Replacement

Nursing Interventions	Rationale	Expected Outcomes
NURSING DIAGNOSIS: Pain related to total hip replacement **GOAL:** Relief of pain		
1. Assess patient for pain.	1. Pain is expected after a surgical procedure because of the surgical trauma and tissue-response. Muscle spasms occur after total hip replacements. Immobility causes discomfort at pressure points.	• Patient describes discomfort. • Expresses confidence in efforts to control pain • States pain is reduced • Appears comfortable and relaxed • Uses physical, psychologic, and pharmacologic measures to reduce discomfort
2. Ask patient to describe discomfort.	2. Pain characteristics may help to determine cause of discomfort. Pain may be due to complication (hematoma, infection, flatus). Pain is an individual experience—it means different things to different people.	
3. Acknowledge existence of pain; inform patient of available analgesics or muscle relaxants.	3. Reduces the stress experienced by patient by communicating concern and availability of assistance to help patient deal with the pain	
4. Use pain-modifying techniques. a. Use analgesics.	a. Patient will require parenteral opioids during the first 24–48 hours, and then will progress to oral analgesics.	
b. Change position within prescribed limits.	b. Use pillows to provide adequate support; relieve pressure on bony prominences.	
c. Modify environment.	c. Interactions with others, distractions, and sensory overload or deprivation may affect pain experience.	
d. Notify surgeon if necessary.	d. Surgical intervention may be necessary if pain is due to hematoma or excessive edema.	
5. Evaluate and record discomfort and effectiveness of pain-modifying techniques.	5. Effectiveness of action is based on experience; notations provide data concerning pain experiences, management, and pain relief.	
NURSING DIAGNOSIS: Impaired physical mobility related to enforced bed rest after hip replacement **GOAL:** Achieves pain-free, functional, stable hip joint.		
1. Maintain proper positioning of hip joint (abduction, neutral rotation, limited flexion).	1. Prevents dislocation of hip prosthesis.	• Prescribed position maintained • Patient assists in position changes. • Shows increased independence in transfers • Exercises hourly • Participates in progressive ambulation program • Actively participates in exercise regimen • Uses ambulatory aids correctly and safely
2. Instruct and assist in position changes and transfers.	2. Encourage patient's active participation while preventing dislocation.	
3. Instruct and supervise isometric quadriceps and gluteal setting exercises.	3. Strengthens muscles needed for walking	
4. In consultation with physical therapist, instruct and supervise progressive safe ambulation within limitations of weight-bearing prescription.	4. Amount of weight-bearing depends on patient's condition and prosthesis; ambulatory aids are used to assist the patient with nonweight-bearing and partial weight-bearing ambulation.	

(continued)

NURSING CARE PLAN 62-1 *(continued)*
Care of the Patient With a Total Hip Replacement

Nursing Interventions	Rationale	Expected Outcomes
5. Offer encouragement and support exercise regimen.	5. Reconditioning exercises can be uncomfortable and fatiguing; encouragement helps patient comply with exercise program.	
6. Instruct and supervise safe use of ambulatory aids.	6. Prevents injury from unsafe use.	

COLLABORATIVE PROBLEMS: Hemorrhage; neurovascular compromise; dislocation of prosthesis; deep vein thrombosis; infection related to surgery

GOAL: Absence of complications

Hemorrhage

Nursing Interventions	Rationale	Expected Outcomes
1. Monitor vital signs, observing for shock.	1. Changes in pulse, blood pressure, and respirations may indicate development of shock. Blood loss and stress of surgery may contribute to development of shock.	• Vital signs stabilize within normal limits. • Amount of drainage decreases • No bright red bloody drainage • Hematology values are within normal limits.
2. Note character and amount of drainage.	2. Within 48 hours, bloody drainage collected in portable suction device decreases to 25–30 ml per 8 hours. Excessive drainage (more than 250 ml in first 8 hours after surgery) and bright red drainage may indicate active bleeding.	
3. Notify surgeon if patient develops shock or excessive bleeding and prepare for administration of fluids, blood component therapy, and medications.	3. Corrective measures need to be instituted.	
4. Note hemoglobin and hematocrit values.	4. Anemia due to blood loss may develop. Blood replacement therapy may be needed.	

Neurovascular Compromise

Nursing Interventions	Rationale	Expected Outcomes
1. Assess affected extremity for color and temperature.	1. The skin becomes pale and feels cool with decreased tissue perfusion. Venous congestion may produce cyanosis.	• Color normal • Extremity warm • Normal capillary refill • Moderate edema and swelling; tissue not palpably tense • Pain is controllable • No pain with passive dorsiflexion • Normal sensations • No paresthesia • Normal motor abilities • No paresis or paralysis • Pulses strong and equal
2. Assess toes for capillary refill response.	2. After compression of the nail, rapid return of pink color indicates good capillary perfusion.	
3. Assess extremity for edema and swelling. Listen to patient complaints of leg tightness.	3. The trauma of surgery will cause edema. Excessive swelling and hematoma formation can compromise circulation and function.	
4. Elevate extremity (keep lower than hip when in chair).	4. Minimizes dependent edema.	
5. Assess for deep, throbbing, unrelenting pain.	5. Surgical pain can be controlled; pain due to neurovascular compromise is refractory to treatment.	

(continued)

NURSING CARE PLAN 62-1 *(continued)*
Care of the Patient With a Total Hip Replacement

Nursing Interventions	Rationale	Expected Outcomes
6. Assess for pain on passive flexion of foot.	6. With nerve ischemia, there will be pain on passive stretch. Additionally, pain may indicate deep vein thrombosis—positive Homan's sign.	
7. Assess for sensations and numbness.	7. Diminished pain and paresthesia may indicate nerve damage. Sensation in web between great and second toe—peroneal nerve; sensation on sole of foot—tibial nerve.	
8. Assess ability to move foot and toes.	8. Dorsiflexion of ankle and extension of toes indicate function of peroneal nerve. Plantar flexion of ankle and flexion of toes indicate function of tibial nerve.	
9. Assess pedal pulses in both feet. Notify surgeon if diminished neurovascular status is noted.	9. Indicator of extremity circulation. Function of extremity needs to be preserved.	
Dislocation of Prosthesis		
1. Position patient as prescribed.	1. Hip component positioning (femoral component in acetabular component) needs to be maintained.	• Prosthesis not dislocated
2. Use abductor splint or pillows to maintain position and to support extremity.	2. Keep hip in abduction and in a neutral rotation to prevent dislocation.	
3. Support leg and place pillows between legs when patient is turning and side-lying; turn to the unaffected side.		
4. Avoid acute flexion of hip (head of bed at 45° or less).		
5. Avoid crossing legs.		
6. Assess for dislocation of prosthesis (extremity shortens, internally or externally rotated, severe hip pain, patient unable to move extremity)	6. Findings may indicate dislocation of prosthesis.	
7. Notify surgeon of possible dislocation.	7. Joint dislocations compromise neurovascular status and future function of extremity.	
Deep Vein Thrombosis		
1. Use elastic stocking or sequential compression device as prescribed.	1. Aid in venous blood return and prevent stasis.	• Wears elastic stockings/uses compression device
2. Remove stockings for 20 minutes twice a day and provide skin care.	2. Skin care is necessary to avoid breakdown. Extended removal of stockings defeats purpose of stockings.	• No skin breakdown • Pulses equal and strong • Skin temperature normal
3. Assess popliteal, dorsalis pedis, and posterior tibial pulses.	3. Pulses indicate arterial perfusion of extremity.	• Negative Homans' sign • Changes position with assistance and supervision.
4. Assess skin temperature of legs.	4. Local inflammation will increase local skin temperature.	• Participates in exercise regimen
5. Assess for Homans' sign every 8 hours.	5. Pain on dorsiflexion of ankle may indicate deep vein thrombosis.	• No chest pain; lungs clear to auscultation; no evidence of pulmonary emboli

(continued)

NURSING CARE PLAN 62–1 *(continued)*
Care of the Patient With a Total Hip Replacement

Nursing Interventions	Rationale	Expected Outcomes
6. Avoid pressure on popliteal blood vessels from applicances or pillows.	6. Compression of blood vessels diminishes blood flow.	
7. Change position and increase activity as prescribed.	7. Activity promotes circulation and diminishes venous stasis.	
8. Supervise ankle exercises hourly.	8. Muscle exercise promotes circulation.	
9. Monitor body temperature.	9. Body temperature increases with inflammation.	
Wound Infection		
1. Monitor vital signs.	1. Temperature, pulse, and respirations increase in response to infection. (Magnitude of response may be minimal in an elderly patient.)	• Vital signs normal • Well-approximated incision without drainage or excessive inflammatory response • Minimal discomfort; no hematoma • Patient tolerates antibiotics.
2. Use aseptic technique for dressing changes and emptying of portable drainage.	2. Avoid introducing organisms.	
3. Assess wound appearance and character of drainage.	3. Red, swollen, draining incision is indicative of infection.	
4. Assess complaints of pain.	4. Pain may be due to wound hematoma—a possible locus of infection—that needs to be surgically evacuated.	
5. Administer prophylactic antibiotics if prescribed, and observe for side effects.	5. Infected prosthesis is to be avoided.	

NURSING DIAGNOSIS: Potential impaired home maintenance management related to total hip replacement

GOAL: Cares for self at home.

Nursing Interventions	Rationale	Expected Outcomes
1. Assess home environment for discharge planning.	1. Physical barriers (especially stairs, bathrooms) may limit patient's ability to ambulate and care for self at home.	• Home is accessible for patient at time of discharge. • Patient appears relaxed and develops strategies to deal with identified problems. • Personal assistance is available. • Patient demonstrates ability to provide necessary assistance within therapeutic prescription. • Complies with home care program • Keeps follow-up health care appointments
2. Encourage patient to express concerns about care at home; explore together possible solutions to the problem.	2. Patient may have special problems that need to be identified and resolved.	
3. Assess availability of physical assistance for health care activities.	3. Because of limitation of mobility and limited hip range of motion, patient may require some assistance in routine health care.	
4. Teach caregiver home health care regimen.	4. Understanding of rehabilitative regimen is necessary for compliance.	
5. Instruct patient on posthospital care: a. Activity limitations (avoid stressing prosthesis) b. Reinforce exercise instructions. c. Safe use of ambulatory aids d. Wound care e. Measures to promote healing f. Medications, if any g. Potential problems h. Continuing health care supervision and management	5. Lack of knowledge and poor preparation for care at home contribute to patient anxiety, insecurity, and nonadherence to therapeutic regimen.	

CRITICAL PATHWAY
Total Knee Arthroplasty

Outcome Criteria

1. Discharge to rehab POD #4
   - □ Demonstrated rehab potential per P.T.
   - □ afeb vss | -Hg > 8
2. Discharge to home POD #5
   - □ independent with ambulation on level surfaces, stairs, and functional distances per individual needs
   - □ [I] with active knee exercises & use of immobilizer as needed
   - □ active knee flexion 80° or more

	PAT Date:	OR DAY Date:	POD #1 Date:	POD #5 Date:
Assessments/ Consults	History and physical (include dental status & BOO symptoms) PT, SS (V#1) + NSG assessment Risk assessment	Post-op assessment*	Rosa* Skin assessment*	Rosa*
Lab Tests and Diagnostics	CBC PT/PTT CHEM 7 CXR EKG	T&C	HG/HCT PT	PT
Interventions		Knee immobilizer*, elevation (pillow under heel)*, TEDS/Kendalls*, incentive spirometry q 1° W/A*, hemovac, orthoevac*, straight cath/foley prn*, don't gatch bed*, post-op routine VS*, NV checks q 2°*	Knee immobilizer*, elevation (pillow under heel)*, no pillow under knee*, TEDS/Kendalls*, incentive spirometry q 1° W/A*, D/C hemovac/foley, don't gatch bed*, VS q 4°*, NV checks q 4°*	Knee immobilizer PRN*, TEDS/ Kendalls*, incentive spirometry q 1° W/A*, DSG change/Ace, don't gatch bed*, VS q shift*, NV checks q shift*
Diet/GI	Nothing by mouth after MN	Clears → house as tolerated	House or per order	
IV's		IVF's*	IVF's → H.L. or KVO if using PCA*	
Meds	NSAIDS discontinued	ABX × 48 hrs*, PCA or IM analgesic*, heparin or coumadin*	PCA or IM analgesic*, heparin or coumadin*, antibiotics*, Revw meds; home meds, vitamins DVT prophylaxis, analgesics	P.O. analgesic*, heparin or coumadin*, home meds/vitamins*
Activity		Bedrest* Bed exercises q 1° W/A*	OOB → chair 2–3 hrs bid am & pm*, bed exercises*, to PT WBAT/PWB, gait training with walker, AROM 0–40°, initiate knee strengthening exercises	OOB → chair/amb with walker bid*, bed exercises q 1° W/A*, review of home exercise program by PT, review all previous gains, CPM as days 4 & 5*
Teaching	Review critical path*, review bed exercises*, review knee booklet*, review incentive spirometry*	Review bed exercises q shift*, review incentive spirometry, C + DB exercises q shift*	Review previous teaching PRN*	Family teaching by PT if needed, review D/C instructions*, wound care/reportable signs and symptoms, and F/U visit*
D/C Planning and Follow-up	Initial D/C planning with patient & family		SS Visit #2	Review D/C plans* | D/C to home, give written instructions*, give card w/phone number*
KEY: *NSG Care Activities				
V = Variance	V V V	V V V	V V V	V V V
N = No Variance	N N N	N N N	N N N	N N N
Nursing Care Performed	□ □ □	□ □ □	□ □ □	□ □ □
→	1. ______	1. ______	1. ______	1. ______
Signatures: →	2. ______	2. ______	2. ______	2. ______
→	3. ______	3. ______	3. ______	3. ______

Legend: ABX = antibiotics; BOO = bladder outlet obstruction; C+DB = cough and deep breathing; D/C = Discharge or continue; H.L. = heparin lock; IVF = intravenous fluids; KVO = keep vein open; OOB = out of bed; PCA = patient controlled analgesia; PT = physical therapy; PT (in Lab Tests and Diagnostics) = prothromin time; ROSA = review of systems assessment; SS = social service; V#1 = visit number one; W/A = while awake.

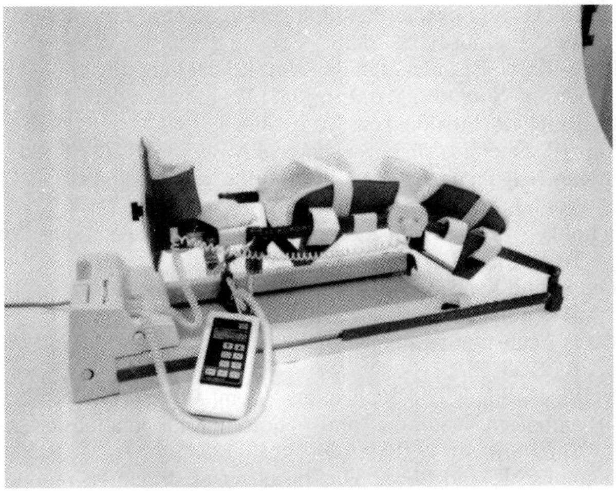

FIGURE 62-11. Continuous passive motion (CPM) device used for postoperative total knee arthroplasty patients to facilitate joint range of motion. (Courtesy of Sutter Biomedical Inc.)

about 200 ml; it diminishes to less than 25 ml by 48 hours postoperatively. The drains are then removed by the surgeon. If extensive bleeding is anticipated, an autotransfusion drainage system may be used during the immediate postoperative period.

Frequently the patient's leg is placed on a continuous passive motion (CPM) device (Fig. 62-11) in the postanesthesia area. This device promotes healing by increasing circulation and movement of the knee joint. The rate and amount of extension and flexion are prescribed. Usually 10 degrees of extension and 50 degrees of flexion are initiated, increasing to 90 degrees of flexion by discharge. The patient is encouraged to use the device most of the time. The physical therapist supervises exercises for strength and range of motion. If satisfactory flexion is not achieved, gentle manipulation of the knee joint under general anesthesia may be necessary about 2 weeks after surgery.

The patient is assisted with transfers out of bed the day after surgery. The knee is usually protected with a knee immobilizer and is elevated when the patient sits in a chair. Weight-bearing limits are prescribed by the physician. Progressive ambulation, using assistive devices and within the prescribed weight-bearing limits, begins a day or two after the surgery.

After discharge from the hospital, the patient may continue to use the CPM at home as well as to do physical therapy on an outpatient basis. Late complications that may occur include infection and loosening and wear of prosthetic components. Generally, the patient is able to achieve a pain-free, functional joint and participate more fully in life activities. Critical Path 62-1 is an example of a critical path for this type of surgery. (Note: This is a 5-day critical path; days 2 through 4 are not shown.)

CRITICAL THINKING EXERCISES

1. You are caring for two patients in the same room. One patient has had a knee replacement. The other patient has had a hip replacement. Both patients are experiencing pain. Compare and contrast the pain management strategies for each patient, and describe the differences in general care related to their respective mobility limitations.
2. A patient who was in a motor vehicle crash has a cast on his leg. He complains that the cast feels tight and that the pain medication is not relieving his pain. Analyze these data, explain what you think is happening, and describe the actions you would take and why.
3. A patient who has had internal fixation of the hip complains about his elastic stockings and requests that they be removed. How would you respond to this request, and how would you explain the purpose of the stockings? If the patient does not understand English and keeps trying to remove the stockings, describe two different strategies you could follow in this circumstance and the pros and cons of each intervention.
4. You are caring for two patients in the same room. One patient has skeletal traction applied to his leg, and the other has skin (pelvic) traction. The patients ask you why their traction setups are different. How would you explain the differences to them? Describe the different priorities of care for each of these patients.

REFERENCES AND SELECTED READINGS

Books

Carpenito LJ. Nursing Diagnosis: Application to Clinical Practice, 6th ed. Philadelphia, JB Lippincott, 1995.
Chapman MW and Madison M. Operative Orthopaedics, 2nd ed. Philadelphia, JB Lippincott, 1993.
Crenshaw A (ed). Campbell's Operative Orthopaedics, 8th ed. St. Louis, Mosby Year Book, 1992.
Davis PS. Nursing the Orthopaedic Patient. Edinburgh, Churchill Livingstone, 1994.
Goldstein TS. Geriatric Orthopaedics: Rehabilitative Management of Common Problems. Gaithersburg MD, Aspen Publishers, 1991.
Gregory B. Orthopaedic Surgery. St. Louis, Mosby, 1994.
Hogstel MO. Clinical Manual of Gerontological Nursing. St. Louis, Mosby Year Book, 1992.
Lewis CB and Knortz KA. Orthopedic Assessment and Treatment of the Geriatric Patient. St. Louis, Mosby, 1993.
Lotke PA and Ecker ML. Postoperative Infections in Orthopedic Surgery: Prevention and Treatment. Rosemont IL, American Academy of Orthopedic Surgeons, 1992.
Maher AB et al. Orthopaedic Nursing. Philadelphia, WB Saunders, 1994.
Mercier LR. Practical Orthopedics, 3rd ed. St. Louis, Mosby Year Book, 1991.
Mourad LA. Orthopedic Disorders. St. Louis, Mosby Year Book, 1991.

Mourad LA and Droste MM. The Nursing Process in the Care of Adults with Orthopaedic Conditions, 3rd ed. Albany NY, Delmar Publishers, 1993.
National Association of Orthopaedic Nurses. Guidelines for Orthopaedic Nursing. Pitman NJ, National Association of Orthopaedic Nurses, 1992.
Newman RJ. Orthogeriatrics: Comprehensive Orthopaedic Care for the Elderly Patient. Oxford, Butterworth-Heinemann, 1992.
Nickel VL and Botte MJ. Orthopaedic Rehabilitation, 2nd ed. New York, Churchill Livingstone, 1992.
Petty W. Total Joint Replacement. Philadelphia. WB Saunders, 1991.
Salmond SW et al (eds). Core Curriculum for Orthopaedic Nursing, 2nd ed. Pitman NJ, National Association of Orthopaedic Nurses, 1991.
Sly D and Theis L (eds). Introduction to Orthopaedic Nursing: An Orientation Module. Pitman NJ, National Association of Orthopaedic Nurses, 1991.
Steinberg G, Akins C, and Baran D (eds). Ramamurti's Orthopaedics in Primary Care, 2nd ed. Baltimore, Williams and Wilkins, 1992.
Turek SL (ed). Orthopaedics: Principles and Their Application, 5th ed. Philadelphia, JB Lippincott, 1994.
Wiesel SW, Delahany JN, and Connell MC. Essentials of Orthopaedic Surgery. Philadelphia, WB Saunders, 1993.

Journals

Asterisks indicate nursing research articles.

Arrlington RG et al. Postoperative orthopaedic blood salvage and reinfusion. Orthop Nurs 1992 May/Jun; 11(3):30–38.
Connolly ML. Ambulatory surgery and prepared discharges: Effects on orthopaedic patients and nursing practice. Nurs Clin North Am 1991 Mar; 26(1):105–112.
Carroll P. Deep venous thrombosis: Implications for orthopaedic nursing. Orthop Nurs 1993 May/Jun; 12(3):33–43.
Dykes PC. Minding the five Ps of neurovascular assessment. Am J Nurs 1993 Jun; 93(6):38–39.
Fecht-Gramley ME. Recognizing compartment syndrome. Am J Nurs 1994 Oct; 94(10):41.
Guanche C and Keenan MAE. Principles of orthopaedic rehabilitation. Phys Med Rehab Clin North Am 1992 May; 3(2):417–425.
Guinan JK. Early detection of pulmonary embolism. Rehabil Nurs 1992 Jul/Aug; 17(4):199–201.
Haines N. Same day surgery: Coordinating the educational process. AORN-J 1992 Feb; 55(2):573–576.
Is your patient complaining of "pain" or "burning"? Regan Rep Nurs Law 1992 Oct; 33(5):4.
Johnson G and Bowman R. Autologous blood transfusion. AORN J 1992 Aug; 56(2):282–292.
*Jones-Walton P. Clinical standards in skeletal traction pin site care. Orthop Nurs 1991 Mar/Apr; 10(2):12–16.
McConnell EA. Providing cast care. Nursing 1993 Jan; 23(1):19.
Monk HL. Fractures are never simple. RN 1993 Apr; 56(4):30–36.
Mooney N. Pain management in the orthopaedic patient. Nurs Clin North Am 1991 Mar; 26(1):73–87.
Nichol D. Preventing infection . . . patients with skeletal pins. Nurs Times 1993 Mar 31–Apr 6;89(13):78–80.
Reed LJ and Keegan MJ. Fat embolism syndrome: A complication of trauma. Crit Care Nurse 1993 Jun; 13(3):33–38.
Ross D. Acute compartment syndrome. Orthop Nurs 1991 Mar/Apr; 10(2):33–38.
Sly DA. Orthopedic complications: Compartment syndrome, fat embolism syndrome, and venous thromboembolism. Nurs Clin North Am 1991 Mar; 26(1):113–132.
*Timmons ME and Bower FL. The effect of structured preoperative teaching on patients' use of patient-controlled analgesia (PCA) and their management of pain. Orthop Nurs 1993 Jan/Feb; 12(1):23–31.
Weber N. The Ilizarov technique. CON J ACIIO 1991 Summer; 13(2):22–25.
Wells M and Ominsky-Mozenter L. From Russia with love: The Ilizarov technique. Point of View 1993 Apr; 30(1):2–6.

Joint Replacement

Carsten VL and Earnshaw PH. Postoperative orthopedic autotransfusion: Successful management for the total knee arthroplasty patient. AORN J 1992 Aug; 56(2):272–275.
Dale KG et al. Total elbow replacement. Orthop Nurs 1992 Sep/Oct; 11(5):23–29.
Dubin S. The physiologic changes of aging. Orthop Nurs 1992; 11(3):45–50.
*Evans et al. The efficacy of postoperative autotransfusion on total joint arthroplasty. Orthop Nurs 1993 May/Jun; 12(3):11–18.
Gannon D et al. An evaluation of the efficacy of postoperative blood salvage after total joint arthroplasty. J Arthroplasty 1991 Jun; 6(2):109–114.
*Giuffre M et al. Postoperative joint replacement pain: Description and opioid requirement. J Post Anesth Nurs 1991 Aug; 6(4):239–245.
Green K et al. Preoperative nutritional status of total joint patients: Relationship to postoperative wound complications. J Arthroplasty 1991 Dec; 6(4):321–325.

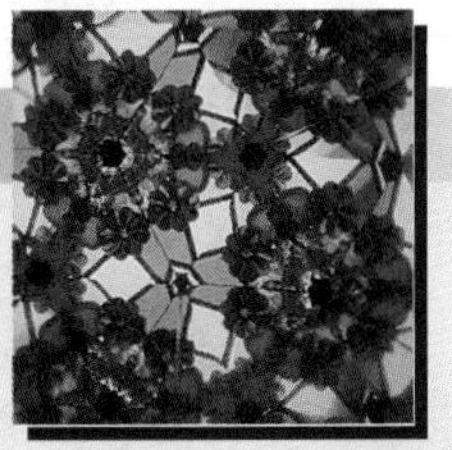

63 Management of Patients With Musculoskeletal Disorders

CHAPTER OUTLINE

LEARNING OBJECTIVES

On completion of this chapter, the learner will be able to:

1. Use the nursing process as a framework for care of the patient with low back pain
2. Describe the rehabilitation and health education needs of the patient with low back pain
3. Use the nursing process as a framework for care of the patient undergoing surgery of the hand or wrist
4. Use the nursing process as a framework for care of the patient undergoing foot surgery
5. Use the nursing process as a framework for care of the patient with spontaneous vertebral fracture related to osteoporosis
6. Use the nursing process as a framework for care of the patient with osteomalacia
7. Describe the medication therapy program for the patient with Paget's disease
8. Use the nursing process as a framework for care of the patient with osteomyelitis
9. Use the nursing process as a framework for care of the patient with a bone tumor

Common Musculoskeletal Problems

Low Back Pain

An estimated 80% of the population will experience low back pain sometime during their lifetime. Impairment of the back and spine, a major health problem, is the third leading cause of disability of people in their employment years. The limitations imposed on the individual by low back pain are severe. The economic cost, in terms of loss of productivity, is in the billions of dollars. The number of medical visits resulting from low back pain is second only to those for upper respiratory illnesses.

Most low back pain is caused by any one of a large number of musculoskeletal problems (*e.g.*, acute lumbosacral strain, unstable lumbosacral ligaments and weak muscles, osteoarthritis of the spine, spinal stenosis, intervertebral disc problems, inequality of leg length). Older patients may have back pain associated with osteoporotic vertebral fractures or bone metastasis. Other causes include kidney disorders, pelvic problems, retroperitoneal tumors, abdominal aneurysms, and psychosomatic problems. Most back pain due to musculoskeletal disturbances is aggravated by activity, whereas pain due to other conditions is not influenced by activity.

Obesity, stress, and occasionally depression may contribute to low back pain. Patients with chronic low back pain may develop a dependence on alcohol or analgesics.

Pathophysiology

The spinal column can be considered as an elastic rod constructed of rigid units (vertebrae) and flexible units (intervertebral discs) that are held together by complex facet joints, multiple ligaments, and paravertebral muscles.

The unique construction of the back allows for flexibility while providing maximum protection for the spinal cord. The spinal curves absorb vertical shocks from running and jumping. The trunk helps to stabilize the spine. The abdominal and thoracic muscles are important in lifting activities. Disuse weakens these supporting structures. Obesity, postural problems, structural problems, and overstretching of the spinal supports may result in back pain.

The intervertebral discs change in character as the person ages. In the young, the disc is mainly fibrocartilage with a gelatinous matrix. It becomes dense, irregular fibrocartilage in the elderly. Disc degeneration is a common cause of back pain. The lower lumbar discs, L4–L5 and L5–S1, are subject to the greatest mechanical stress and the greatest degenerative changes. Disc protrusion (herniated nucleus pulposa) or facet joint changes can cause pressure on nerve roots as they leave the spinal canal, which results in pain that radiates along the nerve. About 12% of people with low back pain have herniated nucleus pulposa. (Management of intervertebral disc disease is discussed in Chapter 60.)

Clinical Manifestations

The patient complains of either acute back pain or chronic back pain (lasting more than 2 months without improvement) and fatigue. During the initial interview, the location of the pain, its character, and whether it radiates along a nerve root (**sciatica**) are assessed. Pain that is musculoskeletal in origin usually is accentuated by movement.

The patient's gait, spinal mobility, reflexes, leg length, motor strength, and sensory perception are evaluated, along with the degree of discomfort experienced. Straight leg raising that causes pain indicates spinal root irritation.

Physical examination may disclose **paravertebral muscle spasm** (greatly increased muscle tone of the back postural muscles) with a loss of the normal lumbar lordotic curve and possible spinal deformity. When the patient is examined in a prone position, the paraspinal muscles relax and any deformity caused by spasm disappears.

If the patient has **radiculopathy** (nerve root problem) or chronic back pain, multiple diagnostic studies may be necessary.

At times, an organic basis for the back pain cannot be identified. Anxiety and stress may evoke muscle spasms and pain. Chronic low back pain may be a manifestation of depression or mental conflict or a reaction to environmental and life stressors.

When working with individuals with chronic low back pain, the nurse needs insight into family relationships, environmental variables, and work situations. In addition, the impact of chronic pain on the emotional well-being of the patient is assessed. The nursing care plan for the patient with chronic back pain may include psychiatric interventions to help the patient deal effectively with depression and psychosocial stressors that contribute to the chronic pain.

Diagnostic Evaluation

Multiple diagnostic tests may be performed to accurately diagnose the cause of back pain and nerve root compression and pain. The nurse must prepare the patient for these studies, provide the necessary support during the testing period, and monitor the patient for any adverse responses to the procedures.

The following diagnostic procedures may be prescribed for the patient with low back pain. An x-ray of the spine may demonstrate the presence of fracture, dislocation, infection, osteoarthritis, or scoliosis. Computed tomography (CT) is useful in identifying underlying problems such as obscure soft-tissue lesions adjacent to the vertebral column and problems of vertebral discs. Ultrasound helps to diagnose narrow spinal canals. Magnetic resonance imaging (MRI) permits visualization of the nature and location of spinal pathology. Myelogram and **discogram** (in which a small amount of contrast medium is injected into the intervertebral disc to allow x-ray visualization) may be performed to demonstrate degenerative disc or disc protrusions. Epidural venograms are used to assess lumbar disc disease by demonstrating displacement of epidural veins. Electromyogram (EMG) and nerve conduction studies are used to evaluate diseases of the spinal nerve root (radiculopathies).

Management

Most back pain is self-limiting and resolves within 6 weeks with bedrest, stress reduction, and relaxation. The patient is confined to bed on a firm, nonsagging mattress for 2 to 3 days. (A bedboard may be used.) Bathroom privileges may be permitted, but all other out-of-bed activities (*e.g.*, answering the phone, child care, general activity due to restlessness) are avoided. The patient is positioned to increase lumbar flexion, which reduces compression of the lumbar nerve roots. The head of the bed is elevated 30 degrees and the patient slightly flexes the knees (Fig. 63-1) or assumes a lateral position with knees and hips flexed (curled position) with a pillow between the knees and legs and a pillow under the head. A prone position is avoided because it accentuates lordosis.

Occasionally, the patient is hospitalized for "active conservative" treatment and physical therapy. Intermittent pelvic traction with 15 to 30 pounds of traction is usually prescribed. Traction promotes additional lumbar flexion and relaxation of the affected muscles (see Fig. 63-1).

Physical therapy may be prescribed to decrease pain and muscle spasm. Therapy may include use of therapeutic cold (*e.g.*, ice), infrared radiant heat, hot moist packs, ultrasound, diathermy, whirlpool, and traction. Appropriate treatment modes are determined by the patient's condition. Impaired circulation, diminished sensation, and trauma are contraindications for hot packs.

Whirlpool therapy may be contraindicated for patients with cardiovascular problems because they are not able to tolerate the associated massive peripheral vasodilation. Ultrasound produces deep heat, which may increase discomfort because of swelling in the acute stages. It is contraindicated if the patient has cancer or a bleeding disorder.

The treatment modality is continued as long as it provides the desired degree of pain relief.

Medications may be prescribed to treat acute pain. Narcotic analgesics are used to interrupt the pain cycle; muscle relaxants and tranquilizers are used to relax the patient and muscles in spasm, thereby providing pain relief. Anti-inflammatory agents, including aspirin and nonsteroidal anti-inflammatory drugs (NSAIDs), are helpful in reducing pain. Short-term corticosteroids decrease the inflammatory response and prevent the development of neurofibrosis, which results from ischemic changes.

The physician may use epidural corticosteroid injections, infiltrate paraspinal muscles with local anesthetics, or inject facet joints with steroids to achieve pain relief.

Transcutaneous electrical nerve stimulation (TENS) is a portable, noninvasive pain reduction modality that may allow the patient to participate in activities comfortably without medication. The TENS unit is thought to afford pain relief by overriding pain input (gate theory of pain) and stimulating endorphins.

As the patient achieves comfort at rest, activities can be gradually resumed and an exercise program initiated as prescribed. Exercises are begun gradually and increased as the patient recovers. The goal is to increase mobility, muscle strength, and flexibility. Hyperextension exercises strengthen the paravertebral muscles; flexion exercises increase back movement and strength; and isometric flexion exercises strengthen trunk muscles.

The exercise program is carried out under the direction of the physical therapist and is adapted to the individual patient. Each exercise period begins with relaxation.

Low back supports and braces may be prescribed to limit spinal motion, to correct posture, and to diminish stress on the lower lumbar spine. (Long-term use of these devices may result in disuse muscle atrophy and weakness and decreased muscle elasticity.)

❑ *NURSING PROCESS* *The Patient With Low Back Pain*

Assessment

The patient with low back pain is encouraged to describe the discomfort (*e.g.*, location, severity, duration, characteristics, radiation, associated weakness in the legs). Descriptions of how the pain occurred—with a specific action (*e.g.*, opening a garage door) or with an activity in which weak muscles were overused (*e.g.*, weekend gardening)—and how the patient has dealt with it often suggest areas for intervention and patient teaching. If back pain is a recurrent problem, information about previous successful pain control helps in planning current management. Additionally, the nurse may ask for evidence of how this back pain is affecting the patient's life-style. Information about job and recreational activities helps to identify areas for back health education.

During the interview, the nurse observes the patient's posture, position changes, and gait. Generally, the patient's movements are guarded, the back is kept as still as possible, and the chair selected for support tends to have arms and be of standard seat height. The patient may sit and stand in

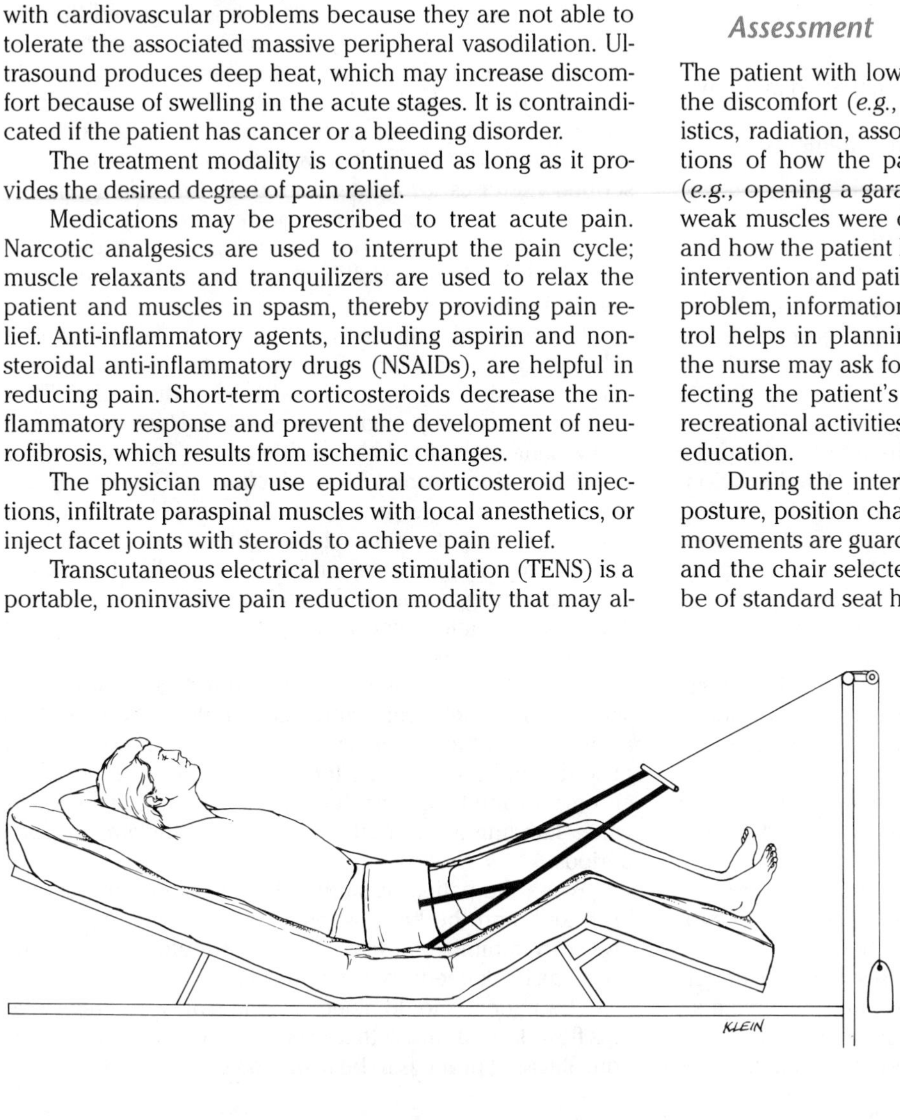

FIGURE 63-1. Positioning to promote lumbar flexion. Pelvic traction helps to alleviate low back pain.

an unusual position, leaning away from the most painful side, and may ask for assistance when undressing because back movements are uncomfortable.

On physical examination the spinal curves, pelvic crest, and shoulder symmetry are assessed. The paraspinal muscles are palpated, and spasm and tenderness are noted. The patient is asked to bend forward and laterally; discomfort and limitations in movement are noted. The effect of these limitations in movement on activities of daily living is determined. The patient is evaluated for nerve involvement by assessing for abnormal sensations (*e.g.*, paresthesia), muscle weakness or paralysis, and back and leg pain with straight leg raises (*e.g.*, with the patient supine, the patient's leg is lifted upward with the knee extended).

The patient is assessed for obesity as it can contribute to low back pain. A nutritional assessment is completed.

Diagnosis

Nursing Diagnoses

Based on the assessment data, the patient's major nursing diagnoses may include the following:

- Pain related to musculoskeletal problems
- Impaired physical mobility related to pain, muscle spasms, and decreased flexibility
- Knowledge deficit related to back-conserving body mechanics techniques
- Altered role performance related to impaired mobility and chronic pain
- Altered nutrition: More than body requirements, related to obesity

Planning and Implementation

Goals. The major goals of the patient may include relief of pain, improved physical mobility, use of back-conserving body mechanics techniques, improved role performance, and weight reduction.

Nursing Interventions

Relieving Pain. To relieve pain, the nurse encourages the patient to comply with prescribed bedrest and positioning to increase lumbar flexion. Patients are taught to control and modify the perceived pain through behavioral therapies that reduce muscular and psychologic tension. Diaphragmatic breathing and relaxation help reduce muscle tension contributing to low back pain. Diverting the patient's attention from the pain to another activity (*e.g.*, reading, conversation, watching TV) may be helpful in some instances. Guided imagery, in which the relaxed patient learns to focus on a pleasant event, may be used along with other pain relief strategies.

Gentle soft-tissue massage is useful to decrease muscle spasm, increase circulation, relieve congestion, and reduce pain.

If medication is prescribed, the nurse assesses the patient's response to each medication. As the acute pain subsides, medications are reduced as prescribed.

If TENS therapy is prescribed, nurses need to understand the device and its pain relief potential. The nurse may assist the patient in placing the electrodes over areas of the body where the patient is able to achieve maximum pain relief. The patient adjusts the stimulator's wavelength and intensity to achieve comfort (see Chapter 13). Patients who use cardiac pacemakers should *not* use TENS because of the risk of causing dysrhythmias. Those who operate machinery need to be aware of the potential for accidental shocks. Generally, the patient uses the device for 1 to 2 months, gradually decreasing its use as pain subsides and the back muscles are strengthened through graduated exercises.

Patient responses to various pain management modalities are evaluated and noted.

Improving Physical Mobility. Physical mobility is monitored through continuing assessments. The nurse assesses how the patient moves and stands. As the back pain subsides, self-care activities are resumed with minimal strain on the injured structures. Position changes should be made slowly and carried out with assistance as required. The patient should be taught to get out of bed with the least possible amount of discomfort. Twisting and jarring motions are avoided. The patient is encouraged to alternate lying, sitting, and walking activities and advised to avoid sitting, standing, and walking for long periods. Planning for recumbent rest periods several times throughout the day is important in minimizing stress on the back.

The nurse needs to encourage the patient to adhere to the prescribed exercise program; erratic exercising is ineffective. For most exercise programs it is suggested that the person exercise twice a day, increasing the number of exercises gradually. Prescribed exercises are designed to strengthen abdominal and trunk muscles, reduce lordosis, increase flexibility, and reduce strain on the back. Some patients may find it difficult to adhere to a program of prescribed exercises for a long period. These patients are encouraged to improve their posture, use good body mechanics on a regular basis, and engage in regular exercise activities such as walking or swimming to maintain a healthy back.

Recreational activities that the patient enjoys can be substituted for specific exercises. Activities should not cause excessive lumbar strain, twisting, or discomfort. They may be increased gradually as tolerated. Horseback riding and weight-lifting should be avoided.

Promoting Proper Body Mechanics. Good body mechanics and posture are essential to avoid recurrence of back pain. The patient must be taught how to stand, sit, lie, and lift properly (Figs. 63-2 and 63-3). Providing the patient with a list of suggestions will help in making these long-term changes. The patient who wears high heels is encouraged to switch to low heels.

The patient who is required to stand for long periods should shift weight frequently and should rest one foot on a low stool, which decreases lumbar lordosis. The proper posture can be verified by looking in a mirror to see if the chest is up and the stomach is tucked in. Locking the knees when standing is avoided, as is bending forward for long periods.

When the patient is sitting, the knees and hips should be flexed, and the knees should be level with the hips or higher to minimize lordosis. The feet should be flat on the floor. The back needs to be supported.

The patient should sleep on one side with knees and hips flexed, or supine with knees supported in a flexed position. Sleeping prone is to be avoided.

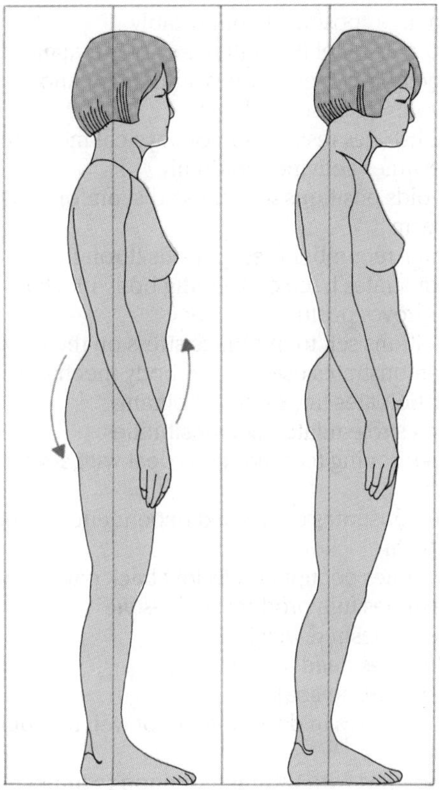

FIGURE 63-2. Proper and improper standing postures. (**Left**) Abdominal muscles contracted, giving a feeling of upward pull, and gluteal muscles contracted, giving a downward pull. (**Right**) Slouch position, showing abdominal muscles relaxed and body out of proper alignment.

The patient is instructed in the correct way to lift objects—using the strong quadriceps muscles of the thighs and with minimal use of weak back muscles. With feet placed to provide a wide base of support, the patient should bend the knees, tighten the abdominal muscles, and lift the object close to the body with a smooth motion, avoiding twisting and jerking. The patient should be instructed to wear a corset to support the back when repeated lifting is required and to avoid lifting more than one third of his weight without help. People with jobs that require heavy lifting may wear wide leather belts (trochanter belts) to decrease the strain on their backs.

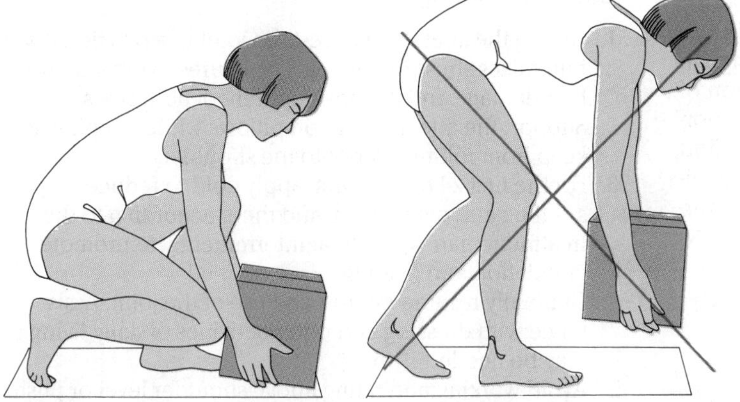

Patient Education and Home Care Considerations. It takes about 6 months for a person to readjust postural habits. Practicing these protective and defensive postures, positions, and body mechanics results in natural strengthening of the back and diminishes the chance that back pain will recur.

Standing:
- Avoid prolonged standing and walking.
- When standing for any length of time, rest one foot on a small stool or box to relieve lumbar lordosis.
- Avoid forward flexion work positions.

Sitting:
- Stress on the back may be greater in the sitting position than in the standing position.
- Avoid sitting for prolonged periods.
- Sit in a straight-back chair with back well supported.
- Use a foot stool to position knees higher than hips if necessary.
- Eradicate the hollow of the back by sitting with the buttocks "tucked under."
- Avoid knee and hip extension. When driving a car, have the seat pushed forward as far as possible for comfort.
- Maintain back support.
- Guard against extension strains—reaching, pushing, sitting with legs straight out.
- Alternate periods of sitting with walking.

Lying:
- Rest at intervals, because fatigue contributes to spasm of the back muscle.
- Place a firm bedboard under the mattress.
- Avoid sleeping in a prone position.
- When lying on the side, place a pillow under the head and one between the legs, which should be flexed at the hips and knees.
- When supine, use a pillow under the knees to decrease lordosis.

Lifting:
- When lifting, keep the back straight and hold the load as close to the body as possible. Lift with the large leg muscles, not the back muscles.
- Protect back with back-supporting corset when lifting.
- Squat while keeping the back straight when it is necessary to pick something off the floor.

FIGURE 63-3. Proper and improper lifting techniques. (**Left**) A good position for lifting is illustrated. This person is using the long and strong muscles of the arms and legs and holding the object so that the line of gravity falls within the base of support. (**Right**) This is an incorrect position for lifting because pull is exerted on the back muscles and leaning causes the line of gravity to fall outside the base.

Avoid twisting the trunk of the body, lifting above waist level, and reaching up for any length of time.

Exercise:

Daily exercise is important in the prevention of back problems.

Walking outdoors and gradually increasing the distance and pace of walking is recommended.

Do prescribed back exercises twice daily, increasing exercises gradually.

Avoid jumping.

Improving Role Performance. Role-related responsibilities may have been modified with the onset of low back pain. As recovery from acute low back pain and immobility progresses, the patient may resume former role-related responsibilities. If these activities contributed to the development of low back pain, however, it may be difficult to resume such responsibilities without risking chronic low back pain syndrome with associated disability and depression. The patient may need help in coping with specific stressors and in learning how to control stressful situations. Once people successfully deal with stress, they develop confidence in their abilities to manage other stressful situations.

Dependency is another problem associated with low back pain. Because of the immobility associated with low back pain, the patient will need to depend on others to do various tasks. Dependency may continue beyond physiologic needs and become a way to fulfill psychosocial needs. Assisting both the patient and support persons in recognizing extended dependency needs helps the patient to identify and cope with the underlying reason for continued dependency.

Referral to a back clinic or a pain clinic may be needed. These clinics use multidisciplinary approaches to help the patient with the pain and with resumption of role-related responsibilities. Working with these patients is a challenge because major adjustments are coupled with the cure. If the patient experiences secondary gains associated with the low back disability (*e.g.*, workman's compensation, easier life-style or work load, increased emotional support), a "low back neurosis" may develop. Psychotherapy or counseling will be needed to assist the person in resuming a full, productive life.

Modifying Nutrition for Weight Reduction. Weight reduction through diet modification may prevent recurrence of back pain. Obesity contributes to back strain by stressing the relatively weak back muscles. Exercises are less effective and more difficult to perform when the patient is overweight. With low back pain there may be a need to undertake a weight reduction program to decrease body weight and stress on the low back. Weight reduction is based on a sound nutritional plan that includes a change in eating habits to maintain desirable weight. Incorporation of weight reduction into the overall supervised plan is important. Monitoring weight reduction, noting achievement, and providing encouragement and positive reinforcement facilitate adherence. Frequently back problems resolve as normal weight is achieved.

Evaluation

Expected Outcomes

1. Experiences pain relief
   a. Rests comfortably
   b. Changes positions comfortably
   c. Obtains relief through use of physical modalities, psychologic techniques, and medications
   d. Avoids drug dependency
2. Demonstrates resumption of physical mobility
   a. Resumes activities gradually
   b. Avoids positions that cause discomfort and muscle spasm
   c. Plans recumbent rest periods throughout day
3. Demonstrates back-conserving body mechanics
   a. Improves posture
   b. Positions self to minimize stress on the back
   c. Demonstrates use of good body mechanics
   d. Participates in exercise program
4. Assumes role-related responsibilities
   a. Uses coping techniques to deal with stressful situations
   b. Demonstrates decreased dependence on others for self-care
   c. Resumes occupation as low back pain resolves
   d. Resumes full, productive life-style
5. Achieves desired weight
   a. Identifies need to lose weight
   b. Sets realistic goals
   c. Participates in development of weight-reduction plan
   d. Complies with weight reduction regimen

See Chart 63-1 for home care management for the patient with low back pain.

Common Problems of the Upper Extremity

Painful Shoulder Syndrome. The structures in and near the shoulder are frequently the sites of painful syndromes. With aging, degenerative alterations occur in all joints, including the articulations that make up the shoulder joint (glenohumeral, sternoclavicular, and acromioclavicular). Pain may arise from supraspinatus tendonitis or bicipital tendonitis, with the inflammation spreading to the tendon sheaths, other tendons and their sheaths (**tenosynovitis**), and the bursa, capsule, synovium, cartilage, bone, and surrounding muscles. Syndromes frequently encountered are listed in Table 63-1.

Patient Education. The nurse provides guidelines for general care and instructs the patient in how to carry out measures that will promote healing. Patient education includes the following:

1. During the acute phase, rest the joint in a position that minimizes stress on the joint structures to prevent further damage and the development of adhesions.
2. Support the affected arm on pillows while sleeping, to keep from rolling over onto the shoulder.
3. For the first 24 to 48 hours, apply cold to reduce swelling and discomfort, and then, according to the treatment plan, apply heat intermittently to promote circulation and healing.
4. Gradually resume motion and use of the joint. Assistance with dressing and other activities of daily living may be needed.
5. Avoid working and lifting above shoulder level or pushing an object against a "locked" shoulder.

CHART 63-1
Home Care Management for Low Back Pain

Home Care Considerations	Nursing Intervention
Pain management	Discuss with patient methods to reduce pain: Limited bedrest with knees flexed to decrease strain on back Nonpharmalogic approaches: Distraction, relaxation, imagery, thermal interventions (*e.g.*, ice or heat), stress reduction, TENS (transcutaneous electrical nerve stimulation) Pharmacologic approaches: Nonsteroidal anti-inflammatory agents, analgesics, muscle relaxants.
Exercise	Encourage patient to perform back exercises to increase function, emphasizing gradual increases in time and repetitions: Stretching, flexibility, strengthening.
Body mechanics	Instruct patient to: Practice good posture Avoid twisting body When lifting: Keep load close to body Bend knees and tighten abdominal muscles Avoid overreaching Use wide base of support Use back brace to protect back
Work modification	Encourage patient to: Adjust work area to avoid stress on back Adjust height of chair or work table Use lumbar support in chair Avoid prolonged standing and repetitive tasks Avoid bending, twisting, lifting heavy objects Avoid work involving continuous vibrations
Stress reduction	Discuss with patient the interdependence of stress and anxiety on muscle tension and pain Explore effective coping mechanisms Teach stress reduction techniques Refer patient to back clinic

6. Perform the prescribed daily range-of-motion and strengthening exercises.

Epicondylitis ("Tennis Elbow"). Epicondylitis is a chronic painful condition that is due to excessive pronation and supination activities of the forearm that result in damage to the tendons of the medial or lateral radial and ulnar epicondyles (*e.g.*, tennis, pitching, sculling, using a screwdriver). The pain characteristically radiates down the extensor (dorsal) surface of the forearm. The patient has a weakened grasp. Most often, relief is obtained by resting the arm in a molded splint, applying ice, and taking NSAIDs. In some instances, local injection of a corticosteroid or procaine is prescribed. Gentle daily exercises help to prevent elbow stiffness. A splint to limit extension of the elbow may be prescribed when activity is resumed.

Ganglion. A ganglion, a collection of gelatinous material near the tendon sheaths and joints, appears as a round, firm, cystic swelling, usually near the wrist. Ganglions develop through defects in the tendon sheath or capsule. They occur most frequently in women under the age of 50. The ganglion is tender and may cause an aching pain. When a tendon sheath is involved, weakness of the finger occurs. Treatment may include corticosteroid injection or surgical excision.

Carpal Tunnel Syndrome. Carpal tunnel syndrome is an entrapment neuropathy that occurs when the median nerve at the wrist is compressed by a thickened flexor tendon sheath, skeletal encroachment, edema, or soft-tissue mass. The patient experiences pain, numbness, paresthesia, and possibly weakness along the median nerve (thumb, first and second fingers). Night pain is common. Rest splints to prevent hyperextension and prolonged flexion of the wrist, avoidance of work that requires flexion of the wrist, and cortisone injections may relieve the symptoms. Diuretics may be helpful to control edema. Surgical release of the transverse carpal ligament may be necessary.

Dupuytren's Contracture. Dupuytren's deformity is a slowly progressive contracture of the palmar fascia that causes flexion of the fourth and fifth fingers and frequently

TABLE 63-1 Painful Shoulder Syndromes

Syndromes	Clinical Features	Clinical Manifestations	Management
Supraspinatus tendonitis and tenosynovitis	Reaction to mechanical stress and strain plus a degenerative process with traumatic inflammation	Pain in shoulder; "catching" sensation Patient grabs affected shoulder with opposite hand Night pain; inability to lie on affected side Painful arc beyond 60-degree abduction (as tendons and cuff impinge under coracoacromial arch)	Intermittent cold/heat applications Pendulum exercises Anti-inflammatory medications—salicylates (aspirin); NSAIDs Local injection of corticosteroid or anesthetic agent into shoulder joint
Calcific tendonitis	Calcium deposits develop in tendons; cause reaction in overlying bursa. Calcium tendonitis and bursitis often coexist.	Occurs in younger and more active persons Abrupt onset of severe aching pain, 1 to 4 days All shoulder and arm movement is painful. Acute phase followed by pain relief	Infiltration of subacromial area and aspiration of deposit Analgesics for pain Anti-inflammatory agents (aspirin, phenylbutazone, indomethacin) Applications of cold/heat Injection with local anesthetic agent and corticosteroid Operative treatment may be necessary for excision of calcified deposits.
Tears and rupture of rotator cuff	Tears occur at the insertion of rotator cuff into the bone, probably from overuse and degenerative changes.	Sports-related injury Occurs commonly after age 50 Abrupt shoulder pain in deltoid area Weakness/inability to abduct shoulder "Clicking" sensation felt in shoulder on abduction/rotation	Confirmation of defect by MRI or arthrogram Partial rupture usually responds to conservative management—rest, anti-inflammatory medications Infiltration with local anesthetic to relieve pain Surgical repair for complete rupture
Bicipital syndromes (lesions on the long head of biceps muscle); tendonitis and tenosynovitis	Long head of biceps is affected by arm and shoulder movement.	Chronic pain in anterolateral area of shoulder associated with muscle spasm and pain in trapezius, scalenus, deltoid	Rest of the extremity Salicylates; NSAIDs Intermittent cold/heat Gentle exercises within tolerance Avoid movements that stretch biceps tendon.
Bursitis	Almost all cases of subacromial bursitis have preceding tendonitis and tenosynovitis in the rotator cuff, biceps tendon, and sheath or an inflammatory process in bone or joint; the spread of inflammation to bursa is a secondary event.	Deep-seated ache in shoulder Pain on rotation of arm	Treatment consists of locating and treating the primary process causing the bursitis.

(Adapted from Bateman JE. The Shoulder and Neck. Philadelphia, WB Saunders.)

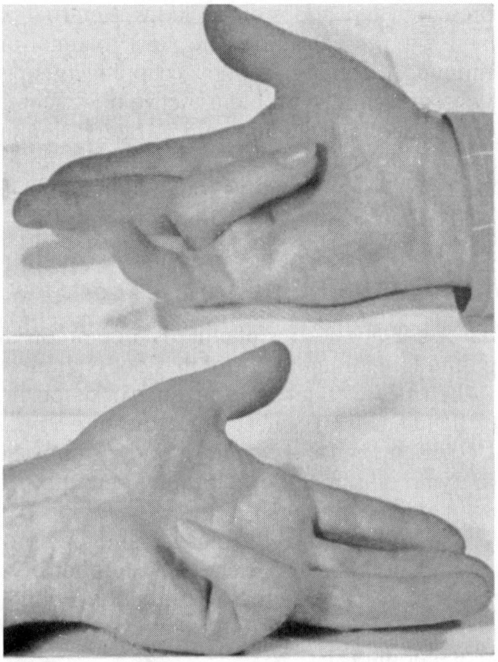

FIGURE 63-4. Dupuytren's contracture. (Boyes JH. Bunnell's Surgery of the Hand, 5th ed. Philadelphia, JB Lippincott.)

the middle finger, which renders them more or less useless (Fig. 63-4). It is a fairly common abnormality caused by an inherited autosomal dominant trait, occurring most frequently in men over the age of 50 who are of Scandinavian or Celtic origin. It starts as a tender nodule of the palmar fascia. The tenderness resolves, and the nodule may not change or it may progress so that the fibrous thickening extends to involve the skin in the distal palm and produces a contracture of the fingers. This condition always starts in one hand, but eventually both hands become deformed symmetrically. Surgery consists of limited palmar and digital fasciectomies that improve function. The recurrence and extension rate is 45% to 80%.

❑ NURSING PROCESS
The Patient Undergoing Surgery of the Hand or Wrist

Assessment

Surgery of the hand or wrist, unless related to major trauma, is generally an ambulatory surgery procedure. Before surgery, the nurse assesses the patient's level and type of discomfort and limitations in function caused by the ganglion, carpal tunnel syndrome, Dupuytren's contracture, or other condition of the hand. After surgery, the nurse assesses the patient for swelling, neurovascular status (circulation, sensation, motion), pain, and function. Pain may be related to edema, restrictive bandages, hematoma formation, or surgery.

Diagnosis

Nursing Diagnoses

Based on the assessment data, the nursing diagnoses for the patient with surgery of the hand or wrist may include the following:

- ❑ Pain related to inflammation and swelling
- ❑ Self-care deficit related to bandaged hands
- ❑ Risk for infection related to surgical procedure

Planning and Implementation

Goals. The goals of the patient may include relief of pain, improved self-care, and absence of infection.

Nursing Interventions

Relieving Pain. To control swelling that may increase the patient's pain and discomfort, the hand is elevated to heart level with pillows. When higher elevation is prescribed, an elevating sling may be attached to an IV pole or overhead frame. If the patient is ambulatory, the arm is elevated in a conventional sling.

Intermittent ice packs to the surgical area during the first 24 to 48 hours may be prescribed to control swelling. Active extension and flexion of the fingers promote circulation and are encouraged, even though movement is limited by the bulky dressing.

Neurovascular assessment of the exposed fingers every hour for the first 24 hours is essential for monitoring function of the nerves and perfusion of the hand. The patient is asked to describe the sensations in the hands and to demonstrate finger mobility. The patient's nerve function is observed carefully preoperatively because this information is needed for interpreting function after surgery. Compromised neurovascular functioning can contribute to pain.

Generally, the discomfort can be controlled by oral analgesics. The nurse evaluates the patient's response to analgesics and to other pain-control measures. Patient education concerning analgesics is important.

Improving Self-Care. During the first few days after surgery, the patient will need assistance with activities of daily living because one hand is bandaged and independent self-care is impaired. The patient may need to arrange for assistance with feeding, bathing/hygiene, dressing, grooming, and toileting. Within a few days the patient develops skills in one-handed activities of daily living and is usually able to function with minimal assistance. Use of the involved hand within the limits of discomfort is encouraged. As rehabilitation progresses, the patient will resume use of the injured hand. Physical therapy–directed exercises may be prescribed. Adherence to the therapeutic regimen is emphasized.

Preventing Infection. As with all surgery, there is a potential for infection. The patient is taught to monitor temperature and pulse for elevations that may indicate a possible infection. The patient also is instructed to keep the dressing clean and dry. Any drainage, foul odor associated with the dressing, or increased pain and swelling are reported. The wound is inspected for signs of infection. Patient education includes aseptic wound care as well as education related to prescribed prophylactic antibiotics.

Evaluation

Expected Outcomes

1. Achieves pain relief
   a. Reports increased comfort
   b. Controls edema through elevation of the hand
   c. Experiences no discomfort with movement

2. Demonstrates independent self-care
   a. Secures assistance with activities of daily living during first few days postoperatively
   b. Adapts to one-handed activities of daily living
   c. Uses injured hand functionally
3. Demonstrates absence of wound infection
   a. Complies with treatment protocol and prevention strategies
   b. Temperature and pulse within normal limits
   c. Experiences no purulent wound drainage
   d. Experiences no wound inflammation

Common Foot Problems

Disabilities of the human foot not only develop from poorly fitting shoes but may also be the result of hereditary influence. Probably the foot would cause little pain or disability on its own account if it were not for modern civilization, which disregards the physiology of the foot. Fashion, vanity, and eye appeal, rather than function, are for the most part the determining factors in the design of footwear. The restriction of ill-fitting shoes distorts normal anatomy while inducing deformity and pain.

The discomfort of foot strain can be treated by rest, elevation, physiotherapy, supportive strappings, and orthotic devices. Foot exercises in which active motion occurs will benefit the circulation and help strengthen the feet. Walking in properly fitting shoes is considered the best form of exercise.

Common Foot Ailments

A **corn** is an area of **hyperkeratosis** (overgrowth of a horny layer of epidermis) produced by internal pressure (the underlying bone is prominent because of congenital or acquired abnormality, commonly arthritis) or external pressure (shoes). The usual sites are the lesser toes, mainly the fifth toe, but all toes may be involved.

Corns are treated by soaking and scraping off the horny layer with an instrument by a podiatrist, by applying a protective shield or pad, or by surgical removal of the underlying offending osseous structure.

Soft corns are located between the toes and are kept soft by moisture and maceration. Treatment consists of drying the affected spaces and separating the affected toes. Usually, a podiatrist will be needed to treat the underlying cause.

A **callus** is a discretely thickened area of the skin that has been exposed to persistent pressure or friction. Faulty foot mechanics usually precede the formation of a callus. Treatment consists of eliminating the underlying causes and having the callus pared by a podiatrist if it is painful. A keratolytic ointment may be applied and a thin plastic cup worn over the heel if the callus is on this area. Felt padding with adhesive backing is also used to prevent and relieve pressure. Orthotic devices can be made to remove the pressure from the bony protuberance. The protuberance may be excised.

An **ingrown toenail** (onychocryptosis) is a condition in which the free edge of a nail plate penetrates the surrounding skin, either laterally or anteriorly. It may be accompanied by secondary infection or granulation tissue. This painful condition is caused by improper self-treatment, external pressure (tight shoes or stockings), internal pressure (deformed toes, growth under the nail), trauma, or infection. Trimming the nails properly (clipping them straight across) can prevent this problem. Active treatment consists of antibiotics and relieving the pain by decreasing the pressure on the surrounding soft tissue by the nail plate. Warm, wet soaks help to drain an infection. A toenail may need to be excised if there is severe infection.

Common Deformities of the Foot

Flatfoot. Flatfoot (pes planus) is a common disorder in which the longitudinal arch of the foot is diminished. It may be due to congenital abnormalities or associated with bone or ligament injury, muscle and posture imbalances, excessive weight, muscle fatigue, poorly fitting shoes, or arthritis. Symptoms include a burning sensation, fatigue, clumsy gait, edema, and pain.

Exercises to strengthen the muscles and to improve posture and walking habits are helpful. A number of foot devices are available to give the foot additional support. Severe flatfoot problems are usually treated by an orthopedic surgeon or a podiatrist.

Hammer Toe. Hammer toe is a flexion deformity of the interphalangeal joint and may involve several toes (Fig. 63-5). The condition is usually an acquired deformity. Tight socks or shoes may push an overlying toe back into the line of the other toes. The toes usually are pulled upward, forcing the metatarsal joints (ball of the foot) downward. Corns develop on top of the toes, and tender calluses develop under the metatarsal area. The treatment consists of conservative measures: carrying out manipulative exercises, wearing open-toed sandals or shoes that conform to the shape of the foot, and protecting the protruding joints with pads. Surgical correction is necessary for an established deformity.

Hallux Valgus. Hallux valgus (bunion) is a progressive deformity in which the great toe deviates laterally (see Fig. 63-5).

Associated with this is a marked prominence of the medial aspect of the first metatarsal–phalangeal joint. There is also osseous enlargement (exotosis) of the medial side of the first metatarsal head, over which a bursa may form (secondary to pressure and inflammation). Acute bursitis symptoms include a reddened area, edema, and tenderness. Factors contributing to bunion development include heredity, narrow shoes, and gradual lengthening and widening of the foot associated with aging. Osteoarthritis is frequently associated with hallux valgus.

Treatment depends on the patient's age, the degree of deformity, and the severity of symptoms. If a bunion deformity is uncomplicated, wearing a shoe that conforms to the shape of the foot or that is molded to the foot to prevent pressure on the protruding portions may be all the treatment that is needed. Corticosteroid injections to control acute inflammation and orthosis may be helpful; if not, surgical removal of the bunion (exotosis) and realignment of the toe may be required to improve function and appearance. Complications related to bunionectomy include limited range of motion, parethesias, tendon injury, and recurrence of deformity.

Postoperatively the patient may have intense throbbing pain at the operative site requiring rather liberal doses of

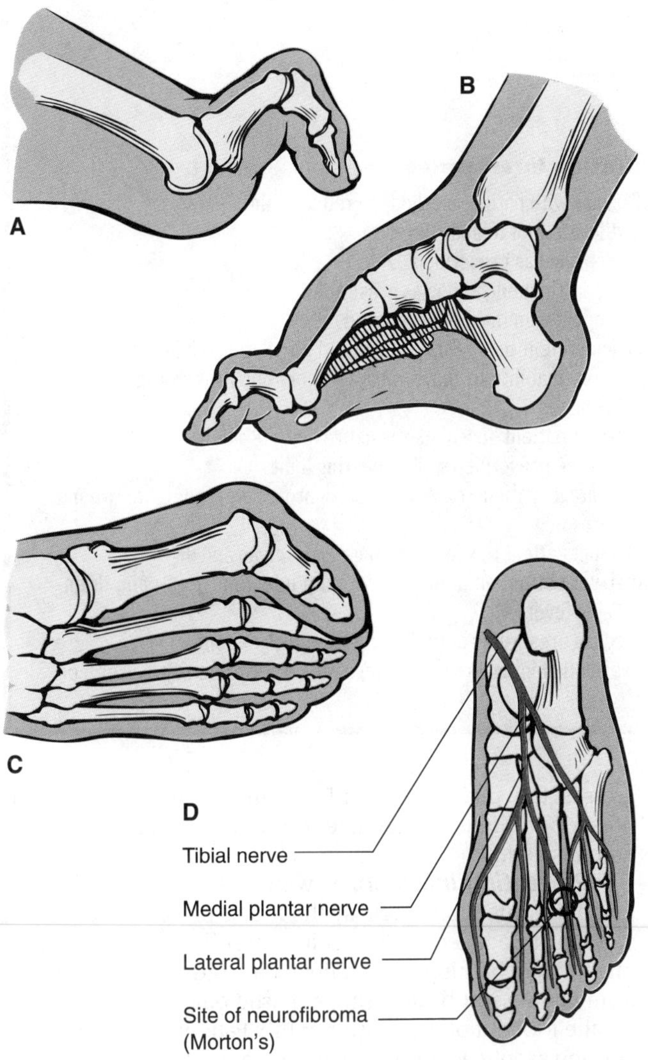

FIGURE 63-5. Common foot deformities. (**A**) Hammer toe. (**B**) Pes cavus (clawfoot). (**C**) Bunion (hallux valgus). (**D**) Site for Morton's neuroma.

analgesic medication. The foot is elevated to the level of the heart to decrease edema and pain. The neurovascular status of the toes is assessed. The duration of immobility and initiation of ambulation depend on the procedure used. Toe flexion and extension exercises are initiated to facilitate walking. Shoes that do not stress the foot are recommended.

Pes Cavus. Pes cavus (clawfoot) refers to a foot with an abnormally high arch, a fixed equinus deformity of the forefoot (see Fig. 63-5). There is shortening of the foot and increased pressure that produces calluses on the metatarsal area and on the dorsum (bottom) of the foot. Charcot-Marie-Tooth disease, a peripheral neuromuscular disorder associated with a familial degenerative disorder, diabetes mellitus, and tertiary syphilis are common causes of pes cavus. Exercises are prescribed to manipulate the forefoot into dorsiflexion and relax the toes. Bracing to protect the foot may be used. In severe cases, arthrodesis (fusion) is done to reshape and stabilize the foot.

Morton's Neuroma. Morton's neuroma (plantar digital neuroma, neurofibroma) is a swelling of the third (lateral) branch of the median plantar nerve (see Fig. 63-5). The third digital nerve, which is located in the third intermetatarsal space, is most commonly involved. Microscopically, digital artery changes cause an ischemia of the nerve.

The result is a throbbing, burning pain in the foot that is usually relieved when the patient rests. Pain sometimes radiates up the leg. Conservative treatment consists of inserting innersoles, metatarsal bars, and pads designed to spread the metatarsal heads and balance the foot posture. Local injections of hydrocortisone and a local anesthetic may provide relief. If these fail, surgical excision of the neuroma is necessary. Pain relief is immediate and permanent.

Other Foot Problems

Several systemic diseases affect the feet. In the case of rheumatoid arthritis, deformities result. Persons with diabetes are prone to develop corns and peripheral neuropathies with diminishing sensation, leading to ulcers over pressure points of the foot. Persons with peripheral vascular disease and arteriosclerosis complain of burning and itching feet with attendant scratching and excoriations. Dermatologic problems commonly affect the feet in the form of fungal infections and plantar warts.

❑ *NURSING PROCESS*
The Patient Undergoing Foot Surgery

Assessment

Surgery on the foot may be necessary because of a variety of conditions, including neuromas and foot deformities (bunion, hammer toe, clawfoot). Generally, foot surgery is performed on an outpatient basis. The nurse assesses the patient's ambulatory ability and balance and the neurovascular status of the foot before surgery. Additionally, the availability of assistance at home after surgery and the structural characteristics of the home are considered in planning for care during the first few days after surgery. These data, in addition to knowledge of the usual medical management of the problem, are used to formulate appropriate nursing diagnoses. Patient teaching for home care is planned (Chart 63-2). After surgery, the patient is assessed for swelling, neurovascular status (circulation, motion, sensation), pain, wound status, and mobility.

Diagnosis

Nursing Diagnoses

Based on the assessment data, the nursing diagnoses for the patient undergoing foot surgery may include the following:

- Pain related to inflammation and swelling
- Impaired physical mobility related to the foot-immobilizing device
- Risk for infection related to surgical procedure/break in skin

Planning and Implementation

Goals. The goals of the patient may include relief of pain, improved mobility, and absence of infection.

CHART 63-2
Home Care Management Following Foot Surgery

Home Care Considerations	Nursing Intervention
Pain management	Discuss with patient methods to reduce pain: Elevate foot to heart level Apply ice as prescribed Use pain medications as prescribed Report pain that is not relieved Teach patient indicators of impaired circulation: change in sensation, inability to move toes, toes or foot cool to touch, color changes
Mobility	Instruct patient how to use assistive devices safely Reinforce prescribed weight-bearing limits Encourage patient to wear special protective shoe over wound dressing
Wound care	Instruct patient to keep dressing or cast clean and dry Instruct patient about signs of wound infection (*e.g.*, pain, drainage, fever) Discuss prescribed antibiotic regimen with patient Explain that initial dressing change will be performed by the surgeon

Nursing Interventions

Relieving Pain. Pain experienced by patients who have had foot surgery is related to inflammation and edema. Formation of a hematoma may contribute to the discomfort. To control the swelling, the foot should be elevated on several pillows when the patient is sitting or lying.

Intermittent ice packs to the surgical area during the first 24 to 48 hours may be prescribed to control swelling and provide some pain relief. As activity increases, the patient may find that dependent positioning of the foot may be uncomfortable. Simply elevating the foot relieves the discomfort.

Neurovascular assessment of the exposed toes every 1 to 2 hours for the first 24 hours is essential to monitor the function of the nerves and the perfusion of the tissues. If the patient is discharged within several hours of the surgery, the patient and family are taught how to assess for swelling and neurovascular status. Compromised neurovascular function can increase the patient's pain. Oral analgesics may be used to control the pain, The patient and family are instructed about appropriate use of these medications.

Improving Mobility. After surgery, the patient will have a bulky dressing on the foot, protected by a light cast or a special protective boot. Weight-bearing on the foot will be prescribed by the surgeon. Some patients are allowed to walk on the heel and progress to weight-bearing as tolerated; other patients are restricted to non–weight-bearing. Assistive devices may be needed. Choice of the devices depends on the patient's general condition and balance and on the weight-bearing prescription. Safe use of the assistive devices must be ensured through adequate patient education and practice before discharge. Problems of moving around the house safely while using assistive devices are discussed with the patient. As healing progresses the patient gradually resumes ambulation within prescribed limits. Adherence to the therapeutic regimen is emphasized.

Preventing Infection. As with all surgery, there is a potential for infection. Because the foot is on or near the floor, care must be taken to protect it from soiling, dirt, and moisture. When bathing, the patient can prevent the dressing from getting wet by securing a plastic bag over it and keeping the foot out of the shower or tub. Patient instruction concerning aseptic wound care may be necessary.

The patient is taught to monitor temperature and pulse for elevations that could indicate a possible infection. Additionally, drainage on the dressing, foul odor, or increased pain and swelling could indicate infection and should be reported promptly to the physician.

If prophylactic antibiotics are prescribed, instruction about their correct use is indicated.

Evaluation

Expected Outcome

1. Achieves pain relief
   a. Elevates foot to control edema
   b. Applies ice to foot as prescribed
   c. Uses oral pain medications as needed and prescribed
   d. Reports decreased pain and increased comfort
2. Demonstrates increased mobility
   a. Uses assistive devices safely
   b. Resumes weight-bearing gradually as prescribed
   c. Exhibits diminished disability associated with preoperative condition
3. Develops no infection
   a. Temperature and pulse within normal limits

b. Reports no purulent drainage or signs of wound inflammation
c. Dressing is clean and dry
d. Takes prophylactic antibiotics as prescribed

Metabolic Bone Disorders

Osteoporosis

Osteoporosis is a disorder in which there is a reduction of total bone mass. There is a change in the normal homeostatic bone turnover; the rate of bone resorption is greater than the rate of bone formation, resulting in a reduced total bone mass. The bones become progressively porous, brittle, and fragile; they fracture easily under stresses that would not break normal bone. Osteoporosis frequently results in compression fractures (Fig. 63-6) of the thoracic and lumbar spine, fractures of the neck and intertrochanteric region of the femur, and Colles's fractures of the wrist. Multiple compression fractures of the vertebrae result in skeletal deformity.

Kyphosis

A gradual collapse of a vertebra may be asymptomatic; it is observed as progressive kyphosis. With the development of kyphosis ("dowager's hump"), there is an associated loss of height (Fig. 63-7). Some postmenopausal women may lose 2.5 to 15 cm (1 to 6 inches) in height from vertebral collapse. The postural changes result in relaxation of the abdominal muscles and hence a protruding abdomen. The deformity may also produce pulmonary insufficiency. Many patients complain of fatigue.

Loss of bone mass is a universal phenomenon associated with aging. Calcitonin, which inhibits bone resorption and promotes bone formation, is decreased. Estrogen, which inhibits bone breakdown, is also decreased with aging. Parathyroid hormone, on the other hand, increases with aging and increases bone resorption. The consequence of these changes is net bone mass loss over time. Women develop osteoporosis more frequently and more extensively than men owing to lower peak bone mass and the effect of estrogen loss during menopause. African-American women, who have a greater bone mass than Caucasian women, are less susceptible to osteoporosis. Small-framed, non-obese Caucasian women are at greatest risk for osteoporosis. More than half of all women over the age of 45 show evidence on x-ray of osteoporosis.

Early identification of at-risk teenage and young adult women and education to increase calcium intake, participate in regular weight-bearing exercise, and modify lifestyle (*e.g.*, reduce use of caffeine, cigarettes, and alcohol) will decrease the risk for developing osteoporosis, fractures, and associated disability later in life.

Gerontologic Considerations

The prevalence of osteoporosis in women over age 75 is 90%. The average 75-year-old woman has lost 25% of her cortical bone and 40% of her trabecular bone. With the aging of the

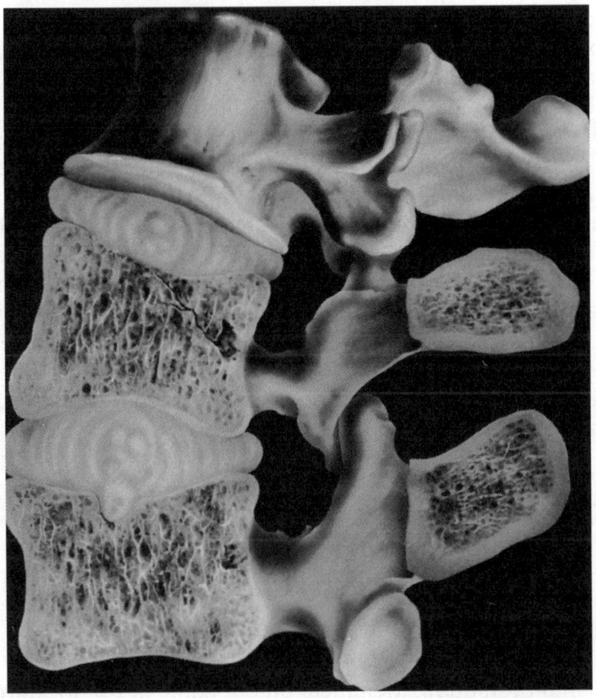

FIGURE 63-6. Diagram of progressive osteoporotic bone loss and compression fractures. (Courtesy of Ayerst Laboratories, New York, NY.)

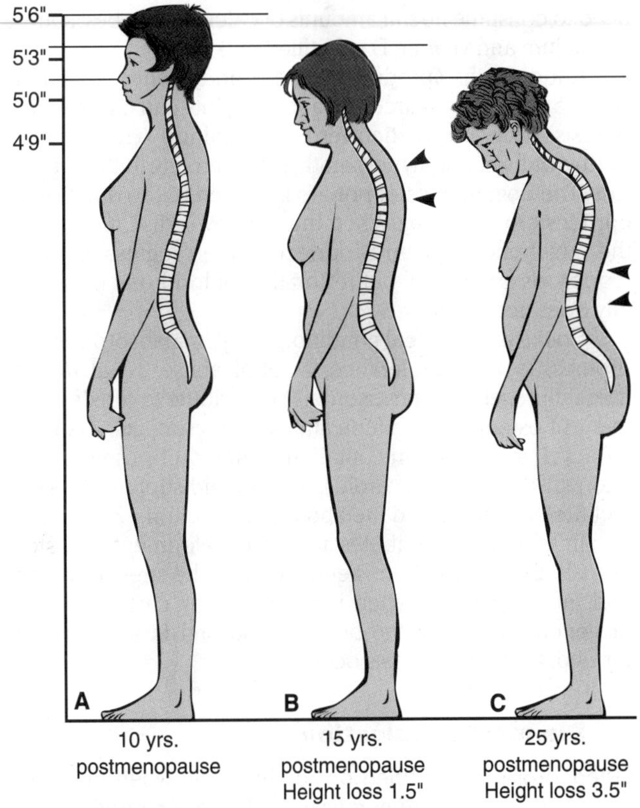

FIGURE 63-7. Typical loss of height associated with osteoporosis and aging. (Courtesy of Wilson Research Foundation.)

population, the incidence of fractures (1.3 million per year), pain, and disability associated with osteoporosis is rising.

Pathogenesis

Normal bone remodeling in the adult results in increased bone mass until about age 35. Genetics, nutrition, life-style choices (*e.g.*, smoking, caffeine and alcohol consumption), and physical activity influence the peak bone mass. Age-related loss begins soon after the peak bone mass is achieved. The withdrawal of estrogens at menopause and with oophorectomy causes an accelerated bone resorption that continues during the postmenopause years. Men have a greater peak bone mass and do not experience sudden hormonal changes. As a result, the incidence of osteoporosis is lower in men.

Nutritional factors contribute to the development of osteoporosis. Vitamin D is necessary for calcium absorption and for normal bone mineralization. Dietary calcium and vitamin D must be adequate to maintain bone remodeling and body functions. Inadequate intake of calcium or vitamin D over a period of years results in decreased bone mass and the development of osteoporosis. The recommended daily allowance (RDA) of calcium has been increased for adolescents and young adults (age 11 to 24) to 1200 mg to maximize peak bone mass. The RDA for an adult remains at 800 mg. However, 1000 to 1500 mg daily for postmenopausal women is usually recommended. The actual estimated average daily intake is 300 to 500 mg. Elderly persons absorb dietary calcium less efficiently and excrete it more readily through their kidneys; therefore, postmenopausal women and the elderly actually need to consume liberal amounts of calcium. The best source of calcium and vitamin D is fortified milk.

Endogenous (produced by the body) and exogenous (from an external source) catabolic agents can cause osteoporosis. Excessive corticosteroids, Cushing's syndrome, hyperthyroidism, and hyperparathyroidism contribute to bone loss. The degree of osteoporosis is related to the duration of corticosteroid therapy. When the therapy is discontinued or the metabolic problem is corrected, the progression of osteoporosis is stopped, but restoration of lost bone mass usually does not occur.

Coexisting medical conditions (*e.g.*, malabsorption syndromes, lactose intolerance, alcohol abuse, renal failure, liver failure, endocrine disorders) contribute to the development of osteoporosis. Medications (*e.g.*, isoniazid, heparin, tetracycline, aluminum-containing antacids, furosemide, anticonvulsants, corticosteroids, and thyroid supplements) affect the body's use and metabolism of calcium.

Immobility contributes to the development of osteoporosis. Bone formation is enhanced by the stress of weight and muscle activity. When immobilized by casts, paralysis, or general inactivity, the bone is resorbed faster than it is formed, and osteoporosis occurs.

Diagnostic Evaluation

Osteoporosis is identified on routine x-ray when there has been 25% to 40% demineralization. There is a radiolucency to the bone. When the vertebrae collapse the thoracic vertebrae become wedge shaped and the lumbar vertebrae become biconcave.

Laboratory studies (*e.g.*, serum calcium, serum phosphate, alkaline phosphatase, urine calcium excretion, urinary hydroxyproline excretion, hematocrit, erythrocyte sedimentation rate) and x-rays are used to exclude other possible medical diagnoses (*e.g.*, multiple myeloma, osteomalacia, hyperparathyroidism, malignancy) that contribute to bone loss.

Single-photon absorptiometry is used to monitor bone mass of the cortical bone in the wrist. Dual-photon absorptiometry, dual energy x-ray absorptiometry (DEXA), and CT provide information on bone mass at the spine and hip. They are useful in identifying osteoporotic bone and assessing response to therapy.

Management

An adequate, balanced diet rich in calcium and vitamin D throughout life, with an increased calcium intake beginning in the middle years, protects against skeletal demineralization. This would include three glasses of skim or whole vitamin D milk or other foods high in calcium (*e.g.*, Swiss cheese, steamed broccoli, canned salmon with bones) daily. To assure adequate calcium intake, a calcium preparation (calcium carbonate) may be prescribed.

At menopause, hormone replacement therapy (HRT) with estrogen and progesterone may be prescribed to retard bone loss and prevent occurrence of additional fractures. A woman who has had her ovaries removed or has undergone premature menopause may develop osteoporosis at a fairly young age; hormone replacement is considered for this patient. Estrogens decrease bone resorption but do not increase bone mass. The use of hormones for long-term therapy is being evaluated. Estrogens may not diminish the rate of bone loss indefinitely. Estrogen therapy has been associated with a slightly increased incidence of breast and endometrial cancers. Therefore, during HRT the patient must examine her breasts monthly and have a pelvic examination, including a Papanicolaou smear and endometrial biopsy (if indicated), one or two times a year.

Other medications that may be prescribed to manage osteoporosis include calcitonin, sodium fluoride, and etidronate sodium. Calcitonin primarily suppresses bone loss and is administered by subcutaneous or intramuscular injection. Side effects (*e.g.*, gastrointestinal disturbances, flushing, urinary frequency) are mild and experienced occasionally. Sodium fluoride promotes osteoblastic activity and bone formation; however, the quality of the new bone is being assessed. Etidronate sodium, which inhibits osteoclastic bone resorption, is being investigated for efficacy in the treatment of osteoporosis.

❑ *NURSING PROCESS*
The Patient With a Spontaneous Vertebral Fracture Related to Osteoporosis

Assessment

Health promotion, identification of people at risk for developing osteoporosis, and recognition of problems associated with osteoporosis form the basis for nursing assessment. The interview includes questions concerning the occurrence of osteoporosis in the family, previous fractures, dietary consumption of calcium, exercise patterns, onset of menopause, and use of corticosteroids as well as alcohol, smoking, and caffeine intake. Any symptoms the patient is experiencing, such as back pain, constipation, or altered body image, are explored.

Physical examination may disclose a fracture, kyphosis of the thoracic spine, or shortened stature. Problems in mobility and breathing may exist as a result of changes in posture and weakened muscles. Constipation may be present because of inactivity.

Diagnosis

Nursing Diagnoses

Based on the assessment data, the major nursing diagnoses for the patient who experiences a spontaneous vertebral fracture related to osteoporosis may include the following:

- Knowledge deficit about the osteoporotic process and treatment regimen
- Pain related to fracture and muscle spasm
- Constipation related to immobility or development of ileus (intestinal obstruction)
- Risk for injury: fracture, related to osteoporotic bone

Planning and Implementation

Goals. The major goals of the patient may include knowledge about osteoporosis and the treatment regimen, relief of pain, improved bowel elimination, and absence of additional fracture.

Nursing Interventions

Understanding Osteoporosis and the Treatment Regimen. Patient teaching focuses on factors influencing the development of osteoporosis, interventions to arrest or slow the process, and measures to relieve symptoms. Adequate dietary or supplemental calcium, regular weight-bearing exercise, and modification of life-style, if necessary (*e.g.*, reduced use of caffeine, cigarettes, and alcohol), help to maintain bone mass. Exercise and physical activity are the primary keys to developing high-density bones that are resistant to developing osteoporosis. It is emphasized that elderly persons continue to need sufficient calcium, vitamin D, sunshine, and exercise to minimize the osteoporotic effects.

Patient education related to medication therapy is important. Since gastric upsets and abdominal distention are frequent side effects of calcium supplements, the patient may find that taking calcium supplements with meals may reduce their occurrence. In addition, adequate fluid intake will reduce the risk of formation of renal calculi. If HRT is prescribed, the patient must be taught about the importance of periodic screening for breast and endometrial cancer.

Relieving Pain. Relief of back pain may be accomplished by resting in bed in a supine or side-lying position for several days. The mattress should be firm and nonsagging. Knee flexion increases comfort by relaxing muscles. Intermittent local heat and back rubs promote muscle relaxation. The patient is instructed to move the trunk as a unit, avoiding twisting. Good posture is encouraged and body mechanics are taught. When the patient is assisted out of bed, a lumbosacral corset may be worn for temporary support and immobilization, although such a device is frequently uncomfortable and poorly tolerated by many elderly persons. As the patient spends more time out of bed, intermittent recumbent rest periods are encouraged to relieve discomfort and reduce the stress of abnormal posture on weakened muscles.

Oral opioids may be needed for the first few days after the onset of back pain. After a few days, non-opioid analgesics afford relief.

Improving Bowel Elimination. Constipation is a problem related to immobility, medications, and age. Early institution of a high-fiber diet, increased fluids, and the use of prescribed stool softeners helps to prevent or minimize constipation. If the vertebral collapse involves a T10–L2 vertebra, the patient may develop an ileus. The nurse therefore monitors the patient's intake, bowel sounds, and bowel activity.

Preventing Injury. Physical activity is essential to strengthen muscles, prevent disuse atrophy, and retard progressive bone demineralization. Isometric exercises can be used to strengthen trunk muscles. Walking, good body mechanics, and good posture are encouraged. Sudden bending, jarring, and strenuous lifting are to be avoided. Daily weight-bearing activity, preferably outdoors in the sunshine, is necessary to enhance the body's ability to produce vitamin D.

Gerontologic Considerations. Elderly people fall frequently as a result of environmental hazards, neuromuscular disorders, diminished senses and cardiovascular responses, and responses to medications. Hazards must be identified and eliminated. Supervision and assistance should be readily available.

The patient and family need to be included in planning for continued care and preventive management regimens. The home environment is assessed for potential hazards (*e.g.*, scatter rugs, cluttered rooms, toys on the floor, pets underfoot) and a safe environment is created (*e.g.*, well-lighted staircases with secure hand rails, grab-bars in the bathroom, properly fitting footwear).

Evaluation

Expected Outcomes

1. Acquires knowledge about osteoporosis and the treatment regimen
   a. States relationship of calcium intake and exercise to bone mass
   b. Consumes adequate amounts of dietary calcium
   c. Increases level of exercise
   d. Takes prescribed hormonal therapy
   e. Undergoes prescribed screening procedures
2. Achieves pain relief
   a. Experiences pain relief at rest
   b. Experiences minimal discomfort during activities of daily living
   c. Demonstrates diminished tenderness at fracture site
3. Demonstrates normal bowel elimination
   a. Bowel sounds active
   b. Bowel movements regular
4. Experiences no new fractures
   a. Maintains good posture

b. Uses good body mechanics
c. Consumes balanced diet high in calcium and vitamin D
d. Engages in weight-bearing exercises (walks daily)
e. Rests by lying down several times a day
f. Participates in outdoor activities
g. Creates a safe home environment
h. Accepts assistance and supervision as needed

Osteomalacia

Osteomalacia is a metabolic bone disease characterized by inadequate mineralization of bone. (A similar condition in children is called **rickets**.) In adults the osteomalacia is chronic, and skeletal deformities are not as severe as in children because skeletal growth has been completed. In these patients, a large amount of osteoid or remolded bone does not calcify. It is thought that the primary defect is a deficiency in activated vitamin D (calcitrol), which promotes calcium absorption from the gastrointestinal tract and facilitates mineralization of bone. The supply of calcium and phosphate in the extracellular fluid is low. Without adequate vitamin D, calcium and phosphate are not moved to calcification sites in bones. As a result of this faulty mineralization, there is softening and weakening of the skeleton, causing pain, tenderness to touch, bowing of the bones, and pathologic fractures.

Pathophysiology

There are a variety of causes of osteomalacia resulting from a generalized disturbance in mineral metabolism. Risk factors for the development of osteomalacia include dietary deficiencies, malabsorption, gastrectomy, chronic renal failure, prolonged anticonvulsant therapy (phenytoin, phenobarbital), and insufficient vitamin D (dietary, sunlight).

The malnutrition type (deficiency in vitamin D often associated with poor intake of calcium) is mainly due to poverty, but food faddism and lack of knowledge of nutrition may also be factors. It occurs most frequently in parts of the world where vitamin D is not added to food and where dietary deficiencies exist and sunlight is rare.

Osteomalacia may occur as a result of failure of calcium absorption or excessive loss of calcium from the body. Gastrointestinal disorders in which fats are inadequately absorbed are likely to produce osteomalacia through loss of vitamin D (along with other fat-soluble vitamins) and calcium, the latter being excreted in the feces in combination with fatty acids. Such disorders include celiac disease, chronic biliary tract obstruction, chronic pancreatitis, and small bowel resections.

Severe renal insufficiency results in acidosis. Available calcium is used to combat the acidosis, and the parathyroid hormone continues to cause a release of skeletal calcium in an attempt to reestablish a physiologic *p*H. During this continual drain of skeletal calcium, bony fibrosis occurs and bony cysts form. Chronic glomerulonephritis, obstructive uropathies, and heavy metal poisoning result in a reduced serum phosphate level and demineralization of bone.

In addition, liver and kidney diseases can produce a lack of vitamin D, as these are the organs that convert vitamin D to its active form. Finally, hyperparathyroidism leads to skeletal decalcification, and thus to osteomalacia, by increasing phosphate excretion in the urine.

Gerontologic Considerations. A nutritious diet is particularly important in elderly persons. Adequate intake of calcium and vitamin D is promoted. Because sunlight is necessary, older people should be encouraged to spend some time in the sun.

Prevention, identification, and management of osteomalacia in the elderly are essential to reduce the incidence of fractures. When osteomalacia is combined with osteoporosis, the incidence of fracture increases.

Clinical Manifestations

The most common and distressing symptoms of osteomalacia are bone pain and tenderness. As a result of calcium deficiency, there is usually muscle weakness. The patient develops a waddling or limping gait. In the more advanced disease, the legs become bowed (because of body weight and muscle pull). The softened vertebrae become compressed, thus shortening the patient's trunk and deforming the thorax (**kyphosis**). The sacrum is forced down and forward, and the pelvis is compressed laterally. These two deformities explain the characteristic shape of the pelvis that often necessitates cesarean section in pregnant women affected with this disease. Weakness and unsteadiness increase the risk for falls and fractures.

Diagnostic Evaluation

On x-ray generalized demineralization of bone is evident. Studies of the vertebrae may show a compression fracture with indistinct vertebral end-plates. Laboratory studies show low serum calcium and phosphorus levels and a moderately elevated alkaline phosphatase level. Urine calcium and creatinine excretion is low. Bone biopsy demonstrates an increased amount of osteoid.

Management

The underlying cause of osteomalacia is corrected when possible. If osteomalacia is dietary in origin, a diet with adequate protein and increased calcium and vitamin D is provided.

Supplements of vitamin D may be prescribed. Vitamin D raises the concentration of calcium and phosphorus in the extracellular fluid and thus makes these ions available for mineralization of bone.

If osteomalacia is due to malabsorption, increased doses of vitamin D as well as supplemental calcium are usually prescribed. Exposure to sunlight for ultraviolet radiation to transform a cholesterol substance (7-dehydrocholesterol) present in the skin into vitamin D may be recommended.

Frequently, skeletal problems associated with osteomalacia resolve themselves when the underlying nutritional deficiency or pathologic process is adequately treated. Long-term monitoring of the patient is appropriate to ensure stabilization or reversal of osteomalacia. Some persistent orthopedic deformities may need to be treated with braces or surgery (osteotomy may be performed to correct long bone deformity).

❑ NURSING PROCESS
The Patient With Osteomalacia

Assessment

Patients with osteomalacia usually complain of generalized bone pain in the low back and extremities with an associated tenderness. The description of the discomfort may be vague. The patient may present with a fracture. During the interview, information concerning coexisting diseases (*e.g.*, malabsorption syndrome) and dietary habits is obtained.

On physical examination, skeletal deformities are noted. Spinal deformities and bending deformities of the long bones may give patients an unusual appearance and a waddling gait. Muscular weakness may be present. These patients may be uncomfortable with their appearance.

Diagnosis

Nursing Diagnoses

Based on the assessment data, the patient's major nursing diagnoses may include the following:

- Knowledge deficit about the disease process and the treatment regimen
- Pain related to bone tenderness and possible fracture
- Self-concept disturbance related to bowing legs, waddling gait, spinal deformities

Planning and Implementation

Goals. The major goals of the patient with osteomalacia may include knowledge of the disease process and treatment regimen, relief of pain, and improved self-concept.

Nursing Interventions

Understanding the Disease Process and Treatment Regimen. Patient education focuses on the cause of osteomalacia and approaches to controlling it. The patient is instructed about dietary sources of calcium and vitamin D (*e.g.*, fortified milk and cereals, eggs, chicken livers). The safe use of supplements is reviewed. Since high doses of vitamin D are toxic and enhance the risk of hypercalcemia, the importance of monitoring serum calcium levels is stressed.

The nurse encourages outdoor activities to expose the skin to the ultraviolet rays of the sun, which is necessary for the production of vitamin D within the body.

Relieving Pain. Physical, psychologic, and pharmaceutical measures are used to reduce the patient's discomfort and pain. Because the patient has both skeletal pain and tenderness, gentle handling is used when assisting the patient to change positions. Frequent position changes will decrease discomfort associated with immobility. A convoluted foam mattress and soft pillows will support the body and conform to existing deformities. Diversional activities and focusing attention on conversation, television, and other distractions will decrease the patient's perception of pain. At times, analgesics will be needed as prescribed to decrease the discomfort. The patient's response to the medications is monitored. As the condition responds to the therapy, the skeletal discomforts will diminish.

Improving Self-Concept. In an established, trusting relationship with the attending nurse, the patient is encouraged to discuss any changes in body image and methods for coping with the changes. The patient is encouraged to recognize and use existing strengths and is included in planning of care; being an active participant promotes self-control and improves feelings of self-worth. Interactions with family and friends are encouraged. Social interactions help provide a feeling of being accepted regardless of physical changes.

Evaluation

Expected Outcomes

1. Describes disease process and treatment regimen
   a. Describes specific factors contributing to disease process
   b. Consumes therapeutic amounts of calcium and vitamin D
   c. Exposes self to sunlight
   d. Has serum calcium level monitored throughout therapy
   e. Keeps follow-up health care appointments
2. Achieves relief of pain
   a. Reports feeling comfortable
   b. Reports less bone tenderness
3. Demonstrates improved self-concept
   a. Demonstrates confidence in abilities
   b. Increases level of activity
   c. Increases social interactions

Paget's Disease

Paget's disease (osteitis deformans) is a disorder of localized increased bone remodeling, most commonly affecting the skull, femur, tibia, pelvic bones, and vertebrae. There is a primary proliferation of osteoclasts, which produces bone resorption. This is followed by a compensatory increase in osteoblastic activity that repairs the bone. As bone turnover continues, a classic mosaic pattern of bone matrix develops. The bone formed is high in mineral content but poorly constructed. The bones are structurally weak and pathologic fractures occur. Frequently the legs bow; this causes malalignment of the hip, knee, and ankle joints, which contributes to the development of arthritis and pain.

Paget's disease occurs in approximately 3% of the population over age 50. The incidence is slightly greater in men than women and increases with aging. A family history has been noted, with siblings developing the disease. The cause of Paget's disease is not known. A viral cause is being actively researched.

Clinical Manifestations

Paget's disease is insidious; most patients never know they have it. Some patients are asymptomatic but have skeletal deformity. A few patients have symptomatic deformity and pain. The condition is most frequently identified on x-rays during a routine physical examination or in the course of workup for another problem. Sclerotic changes, skeletal deformities (*e.g.*, bowing of femur and tibia, enlargement of the skull) and cortical thickening of the long bones are seen. Bone scans may detect the disease quite early.

In the majority of patients, skeletal deformity involves the skull or long bones. The skull may be thickened and the patient may complain that a hat no longer fits. In some cases of Paget's disease, the cranium is much enlarged but not the face, which therefore appears small and triangular in shape. Most patients with skull involvement have impaired hearing due to cranial nerve compression and dysfunction. Other cranial nerves may be compressed also. Occasionally, obstructive hydrocephalus occurs.

The femurs and tibiae tend to bow, producing a waddling gait. The spine is bent forward and is rigid; the chin rests on the chest. The thorax is compressed and immobile on respiration. The trunk is flexed on the legs to maintain equilibrium; the arms are bent outward and forward and appear long in relation to the shortened trunk, giving the patient an apelike appearance. As a result of the kyphosis and the bowing of the legs, the patient's height may be reduced as much as 30 cm (12 in).

Pain and tenderness may be noted in the bones. The pain is mild to moderate, deep, and aching and increases with weight-bearing if the lower extremities are involved. Pain and discomfort may precede the skeletal changes of Paget's disease by years and are often wrongly attributed by the patient to old age or arthritis.

There is an increase in skin temperature overlying the affected bone because of increased vascularity of the bone. Patients with very large, highly vascular lesions may develop high-output cardiac failure because of the increased vascular bed and metabolic demands.

Malignant degeneration and osteosarcomas are seen in some patients with Paget's disease.

Diagnostic Evaluation

The serum alkaline phosphatase and the level of urinary hydroxyproline excretion are usually increased, reflecting increased osteoblastic activity; the higher these values, the more active the disease. Patients with Paget's disease have normal blood calcium levels.

X-rays confirm the diagnosis of Paget's disease. Local areas of demineralization and bone overgrowth produce characteristic mosaic patterns and irregularities. Bone scans and bone biopsy may aid in differential diagnosis.

Management

Usually, no treatment is recommended for the patient without symptoms. Pain usually responds to administration of NSAIDs.

Patients with a moderate to severe form of the disease may benefit from suppressive therapy. These patients have severe pain, neurologic deficits, extensive skeletal involvement, or high-output heart failure. At present, there are several agents that are potent inhibitors of bone resorption and under certain conditions may permit replacement of diseased bone with normal lamellar bone.

Calcitonin, a polypeptide hormone, retards bone resorption by decreasing the number and availability of osteoclasts. Calcitonin therapy facilitates remodeling of abnormal pagetic bone into normal lamellar bone, relieves bone pain, and helps alleviate neurologic and biochemical complications. Calcitonin is administered subcutaneously. Side effects of flushing of the face and nausea can be managed by taking the medication before bedtime or concurrently with an antihistamine; these effects tend to decrease with time. Calcitonin therapy is continued for about 3 months.

Disodium etidronate (EHDP), a diphosphonate compound, produces rapid reduction in bone turnover and relief of pain. It also reduces elevated serum alkaline phosphatase and urinary hydroxyproline levels. Food inhibits absorption. Side effects of nausea, cramping, and diarrhea may occur and can be alleviated by spacing the doses. Large doses may inhibit fracture healing and may contribute to osteomalacia. Calcitonin and EHDP may be combined and given to patients with very active disease.

Plicamycin (Mithracin), a cytotoxic antibiotic, may be used to control the disease. This drug is reserved for severely affected patients with neurologic compromise or for those who are resistant to other therapy. This medication has dramatic effects on pain reduction and on serum calcium, alkaline phosphatase, and urinary hydroxyproline levels. It is given by intravenous infusion and requires that hepatic, renal, and bone marrow function be monitored during therapy. Clinical remissions may continue for months after the medication is discontinued.

Fractures are managed according to location. Healing does occur if reduction, immobilization, and stability are adequate. Nonunion of a femoral neck fracture requires treatment with an endoprosthesis.

Loss of hearing is managed with hearing aids and communication techniques used with the hearing-impaired person (*e.g.*, lip reading, body language).

Gerontologic Considerations

Careful assessment of the patient's pain and discomfort is necessary. Frequently, elderly persons have discomfort associated with arthritis that may be accentuated by the bone deformities. Pain may indicate fracture. Patient education is important to help the patient compensate for altered neurologic functioning. The home environment needs to be assessed for safety to prevent falls and to reduce the incidence of fracture.

Musculoskeletal Infections

Osteomyelitis

Osteomyelitis is an infection of the bone. Bone infections are more difficult to cure than soft-tissue infections because of limited blood supply, inflammatory tissue response, increased tissue pressure, and involucrum formation (new bone around devitalized bone tissue). Osteomyelitis may become a chronic problem that affects quality of life or may result in loss of an extremity.

The infection may be due to **hematogenous** (blood-borne) spread from other foci of infection (*e.g.*, infected tonsils, boils, infected teeth, upper respiratory infections). Osteomyelitis due to hematogenous spread frequently occurs in a bone area where there has been trauma or where there is lowered resistance, possibly due to subclinical (non-apparent) trauma.

Osteomyelitis may be associated with extension of soft-tissue infection (*e.g.*, infected pressure or vascular ulcer, middle ear infection) or direct bone contamination (*e.g.*, open fracture, traumatic injury such as gunshot wound, bone surgery).

Patients who are at risk for developing osteomyelitis include those who are poorly nourished, elderly, obese, or diabetic. In addition, patients who have rheumatoid arthritis, have been hospitalized for a long time, have required long-term corticosteroid therapy, have had surgery on a joint previously operated on, or have a concurrent sepsis are susceptible, as are those who have undergone lengthy orthopedic surgery, have prolonged wound drainage, have marginal incisional necrosis or wound dehiscence, or require evacuation of postoperative hematomas.

Prevention

Prevention of osteomyelitis is the goal. Treatment of focal infections diminishes hematogenous spread. Management of soft-tissue infections controls erosion to the bone. Careful patient selection and attention to the surgical environment and technique can reduce the incidence of postoperative osteomyelitis.

Prophylactic antibiotics, administered to achieve adequate tissue levels at the time of surgery and for 24 to 48 hours after surgery, are helpful. Aseptic postoperative wound care techniques reduce the incidence of superficial infections and the potential development of an associated osteomyelitis.

Pathophysiology

Staphylococcus aureus causes 70% to 80% of bone infections. Other pathogenic organisms frequently found in osteomyelitis include *Proteus, Pseudomonas,* and *Escherichia coli.* There has been an increasing incidence of penicillin-resistant, nosocomial, gram-negative, and anaerobic infections.

The onset of osteomyelitis after orthopedic surgery may occur during the first 3 months (**acute fulminating—stage 1**) and is frequently associated with hematoma drainage or superficial infection. **Delayed onset (stage 2)** infections occur between 4 and 24 months after surgery. **Late onset (stage 3)** osteomyelitis is generally due to hematogenous spread and occurs 2 or more years after surgery.

The initial response to infection is one of inflammation, increased vascularity, and edema. After 2 or 3 days, thrombosis of the blood vessels occurs in the area, resulting in ischemia with bone necrosis due to increasing tissue and medullary pressure. The infection extends into the medullary cavity and under the periosteum and may spread into adjacent soft tissues and joints. Unless the infective process is controlled early, a bone abscess forms.

In the natural course of events, the abscess may spontaneously drain; more often, incision and drainage are performed by the surgeon. The resulting abscess cavity has in its walls areas of dead tissue, as in any abscess cavity; however, dead bone tissue (the **sequestrum**) does not easily liquefy and drain. The cavity cannot collapse and heal, as occurs in soft-tissue abscesses. New bone growth (the **involucrum**) forms and surrounds the sequestrum. Thus, although healing appears to take place, a chronically infected sequestrum remains that is prone to producing recurring abscesses throughout the patient's life. This is the so-called **chronic** type of osteomyelitis.

Clinical Manifestations

When the infection is carried by the blood, the onset is usually sudden, occurring often with the clinical manifestations of septicemia (*e.g.*, chills, high fever, rapid pulse, and general malaise). The systemic symptoms at first may overshadow the local signs completely. As the infection extends from the marrow cavity through the cortex of the bone, it involves the periosteum and the soft tissues, with the infected area becoming painful, swollen, and extremely tender. The patient may describe a constant, pulsating pain that intensifies with movement and is due to the pressure of the collecting pus.

When osteomyelitis occurs from spread of adjacent infection or direct contamination, there are no symptoms of septicemia. The area is swollen, warm, painful, and tender to touch.

The patient with chronic osteomyelitis presents with a continuously draining sinus or experiences recurrent periods of pain, inflammation, swelling, and drainage. The low-grade infection thrives in the scar tissue with its reduced blood supply.

Diagnostic Evaluation

With acute osteomyelitis, early x-rays demonstrate only soft-tissue swelling. In about 2 weeks areas of irregular decalcification, bone necrosis, periosteal elevation, and new bone formation are evident. Bone scans and MRI help with early definitive diagnosis. Blood studies reveal elevated leukocytes and an elevated sedimentation rate. Blood cultures and cultures of the abscess are needed for proper antibiotic therapy.

With chronic osteomyelitis, large, irregular cavities, raised periosteum, sequestra, or dense bone formations are seen on x-ray. Bone scans may be performed to identify areas of infection. The sedimentation rate and white blood cell count are usually normal. Anemia, associated with chronic infection, may be evident. The abscess is cultured to determine the infective organism and appropriate antibiotic therapy.

Management

The affected area is immobilized to decrease discomfort and to prevent fracture. Warm saline soaks for 20 minutes several times a day may be prescribed to increase circulation.

The initial goal of therapy is to control and arrest the infective process. Blood cultures and abscess fluid smears and cultures are performed to identify the organism and select the best antibiotic. Frequently, the infection is caused by more than one pathogen.

As soon as the culture specimens have been obtained, intravenous antibiotic therapy is begun, assuming the presence of a *Staphylococcus* infection that is sensitive to a semisynthetic penicillin or cephalosporin. The aim is to control the infection before the blood supply to the area diminishes as a result of thrombosis. Around-the-clock dosage administration is necessary to achieve a sustained high therapeutic blood level of the antibiotic. An antibiotic to which the causative organism is more sensitive is prescribed when the culture and sensitivity reports are known. When the infection appears to be controlled, the antibiotic may be administered orally and continued for up to 3 months. To enhance absorption of oral antibiotics, they should not be administered with food.

If the patient does not respond to antibiotic therapy, the involved bone is surgically exposed, the purulent and necrotic material removed, and the area irrigated directly with sterile physiologic saline solution. Antibiotic therapy is continued.

In chronic osteomyelitis, antibiotics are adjunctive therapy to surgical debridement. A **sequestrectomy** (removal of enough involucrum to enable the surgeon to remove the sequestrum) is performed. Often, sufficient bone is removed to convert a deep cavity into a shallow saucer (**saucerization**). All dead, infected bone and cartilage must be removed before permanent healing occurs.

The wound is either closed tightly to obliterate the dead space or packed, to be closed later by granulation or possibly by grafting. A closed suction irrigation system may be used to control the hematoma and remove debris. Physiologic saline solution is usually used for irrigation for 7 to 8 days. The development of superimposed infection may occur with prolonged irrigation.

The debrided cavity may be packed with cancellous bone graft to stimulate healing. With a very large defect, the cavity may be filled with a vascularized bone transfer or **muscle flap** (in which a muscle is moved from an adjacent area with blood supply intact). These microsurgery techniques enhance the blood supply; improved blood supply facilitates bone healing and eradication of the infection. These surgical procedures may be staged over time to ensure healing. Surgical debridement weakens the bone, which then may need stabilization or support from internal fixation or external supportive devices to prevent fracture.

❑ NURSING PROCESS
The Patient With Osteomyelitis

Assessment

The patient presents with an acute onset of symptoms (*e.g.*, localized pain, swelling, erythema, fever) or recurrent draining of an infected sinus with associated pain, swelling, and low-grade fever. The patient is assessed for risk factors (*e.g.*, older age, diabetes, or long-term corticosteroid therapy) and for previous injury, infection, or orthopedic surgery. The patient avoids pressure on the area and guards movement. In acute osteomyelitis, the patient will have generalized weakness due to the systemic reaction to the infection.

Physical examination reveals an inflamed, markedly swollen, warm area that is tender. Purulent drainage may be noted. The patient will have an elevated temperature. With chronic osteomyelitis the temperature elevation may be minimal, occurring in the afternoon or evening.

Diagnosis

Nursing Diagnoses

Based on the nursing assessment data, nursing diagnoses for the patient with osteomyelitis may include the following:

- Pain related to inflammation and swelling
- Impaired physical mobility associated with pain, immobilization devices, and weight-bearing limitations
- Risk for extension of infection: bone abscess formation
- Knowledge deficit about the treatment regimen

Planning and Implementation

Goals. The goals of the patient may include relief of pain, improved physical mobility within therapeutic limitations, control and eradication of infection, and knowledge of treatment regimen.

Nursing Interventions

Relieving Pain. The affected part may be immobilized with a splint to decrease pain and muscle spasm. The joints above and below the affected part should be gently placed through the range of motion. The wounds themselves are frequently very painful and must be handled with great care and gentleness.

Elevation reduces swelling and associated discomfort. The neurovascular status of the affected extremity is monitored. Techniques for reducing pain perception and prescribed analgesics may be useful.

Improving Physical Mobility. Treatment regimens restrict activity. The bone is weakened by the infective process and must be protected by immobilization devices and avoidance of stress on the bone. The patient must understand the rationale for the activity restrictions. Full participation in activities of daily living within the physical limitations is encouraged to promote general well-being.

Controlling the Infectious Process. The nurse monitors the patient's response to antibiotic therapy and observes the intravenous site for evidence of phlebitis or infiltration.

If surgery was necessary, measures are taken to ensure adequate circulation (wound suction to prevent fluid accumulation, elevation of the area to promote venous drainage, avoidance of pressure on grafted area), to maintain needed immobility, and to comply with weight-bearing restrictions.

The general health and nutrition of the patient are monitored. A balanced diet high in protein, vitamin C, and vitamin D is desired to ensure a positive nitrogen balance and to promote healing.

Patient Education and Home Care Considerations. Management of osteomyelitis, including wound care and intravenous antibiotic therapy, may be performed at home. The patient must be medically stable and motivated, and the family must be supportive. The home environment needs to be conducive to promotion of health and compliance with the therapeutic regimen.

It is important that the patient and family understand the antibiotic protocol. In addition, aseptic dressing changes and warm compress techniques are taught. Patient education before discharge from the hospital and adequate supervision and support from the home care nurse are important for successful home management of osteomyelitis.

These patients need to be monitored carefully for development of additional painful areas or sudden increases in temperature. The patient is instructed to observe and report elevated temperature, drainage, odor, and increased inflammation.

Evaluation

Expected Outcomes

1. Experiences pain relief
   a. Reports decreased pain
   b. Experiences no tenderness at site of previous infection
   c. Experiences no discomfort with movement
2. Increases physical mobility
   a. Participates in self-care activities
   b. Maintains full function of unimpaired extremities
   c. Demonstrates safe use of immobilizing device and assistive device
3. Absence of infection
   a. Takes antibiotic as prescribed
   b. Temperature normal
   c. Absence of swelling
   d. Absence of drainage
   e. WBC and sedimentation rate return to normal
   f. Wound cultures negative
4. Complies with therapeutic plan
   a. Takes medications as prescribed
   b. Protects weakened bones
   c. Demonstrates proper wound care
   d. Reports problems promptly
   e. Eats a balanced diet that is high in protein and vitamins C and D
   f. Keeps follow-up health appointments
   g. Reports increased strength
   h. Reports no elevation of temperature or recurrence of pain, swelling, or other symptoms at the site

Septic (Infectious) Arthritis

Joints can become infected by spread of infection from other parts of the body (hematogenous spread) or directly by trauma or surgical instrumentation. Previous trauma to joints, coexisting arthritis, and diminished host resistance contribute to the development of an infected joint. *Gonococci* and *Staphylococci* cause most adult joint infections. Prompt recognition and treatment of an infected joint are important because accumulating pus results in **chondrolysis** (destruction of hyaline cartilage), which heals poorly.

Clinical Manifestations. The patient with an acute septic arthritis usually presents with a warm, painful, swollen joint with decreased range of motion. Systemic chills, fever, and leukocytosis are present. Assessment for a primary locus of infection (*e.g.*, a carbuncle) is performed. Elderly patients and persons taking corticosteroids or immunosuppressive drugs may not exhibit typical clinical manifestations of infection.

Diagnostic Evaluation. Diagnostic studies include aspiration, examination, and culture of the synovial fluid. CT and MRI may disclose damage to the joint lining. Radioisotope scanning may be useful in localizing the process.

Management. Prompt treatment is essential. Antibiotics, such as nafcillin, cefoperazone, and gentamicin, should be started promptly by intravenous infusion. Penicillin G is used for gonococcal septic arthritis. The parenteral antibiotics are continued until symptoms disappear. The synovial fluid is monitored for sterility and decrease in white blood cells.

In addition to prescribing antibiotics, the physician may aspirate the joint with a needle to remove excessive joint fluid, exudate, and debris. This promotes comfort as well as decreases joint destruction due to the action of the proteolytic enzymes in the purulent fluid. Occasionally, arthrotomy or arthroscopy is used to drain the joint and remove dead tissue.

The inflamed joint is supported and immobilized in a functional position by a splint that increases the patient's comfort. Codeine may be prescribed to control pain. After the infection has responded to antibiotic therapy, NSAIDs may be prescribed.

The patient's nutrition and fluids are monitored to promote healing. Progressive range-of-motion exercises are prescribed when the infection subsides.

If septic joints are treated promptly, recovery of normal function should occur. The patient is assessed periodically for recurrence. If the articular cartilage was damaged during the inflammatory reaction, joint fibrosis and diminished function may result.

Bone Tumors

Neoplasms of the musculoskeletal system are of a variety of types, including osteogenic, chondrogenic, fibrogenic, muscle (rhabdomyogenic), and marrow (reticulum) cell tumors as well as nerve, vascular, and fatty cell tumors. They may be primary tumors or metastatic tumors from primary cancers elsewhere in the body (*e.g.*, breast, lung, prostate, kidney). Metastatic bone tumors are more common than primary bone tumors.

Benign Bone Tumors

Benign bone tumors generally are slow growing and well circumscribed, present few symptoms, and are not a cause of death. Benign primary neoplasms of the musculoskeletal system include osteoid osteoma, osteochondroma, enchondroma, bone cyst (*e.g.*, aneurysmal bone cyst), rhabdomyoma, and fibroma. Benign tumors of the bone and soft tissue are more common than malignant tumors. Some benign tumors, such as giant cell tumors, have the potential of undergoing malignant transformation.

Bone cysts are expanding lesions within the bone. *Aneurysmal bone cysts* are seen in young adults and present with a painful, palpable mass of the long bones, vertebrae, or flat bone. *Unicameral bone cysts* occur in children and cause mild discomfort and possible pathologic fractures of the upper humerus and femur. These may heal spontaneously. **Osteochondroma** is the most common benign bone tumor, usually occurring as a large projection of bone at the end of long bones (at the knee or shoulder). It develops during growth and then becomes a static bony mass. The cartilage cap of the osteochondroma may undergo malignant transformation after trauma, and a chondrosarcoma may develop. **Enchondroma** is a common tumor of the hyaline cartilage that develops in the hand, ribs, femur, tibia, humerus, or pelvis. Generally, the only symptom is a mild ache. Pathologic fractures may occur.

A painful tumor that occurs in children and young adults is the **osteoid osteoma.** The neoplastic tissue is surrounded by reactive bone formation that assists in its radiologic identification. **Giant cell tumors** (osteoclastoma) are benign for long periods but may invade local tissue and cause destruction. They occur in young adults and are soft and hemorrhagic. Eventually giant cell tumors may undergo malignant transformation and metastasize.

Malignant Bone Tumors

Primary malignant musculoskeletal tumors are relatively rare and arise from connective and supportive tissue cells (**sarcomas**) or bone marrow elements (**myelomas**). Malignant primary musculoskeletal tumors include osteosarcoma, chondrosarcoma, Ewing's sarcoma, and fibrosarcoma. Soft-tissue sarcomas include liposarcoma, fibrosarcoma of soft tissue, and rhabdomyosarcoma. Bone tumor metastasis to the lungs is common. *Osteogenic sarcoma* (osteosarcoma) is the most common and most often fatal primary malignant bone tumor. It is characterized by early hematogenous metastasis to the lungs. The tumor carries a high mortality rate because the sarcoma often has spread to the lungs by the time the patient seeks help. Osteogenic sarcoma appears most frequently in males in the age group between 10 and 25 years of age (in bones that grow rapidly) and in older persons with Paget's disease or as a result of radiation exposure. It is manifested by pain, swelling, limitation of motion, and weight loss (which is considered an ominous finding). The bony mass may be palpable, tender, and fixed, with an increase in skin temperature over the mass and venous distention. The primary lesion may involve any bone; the most common sites are the distal femur, the proximal tibia, and the proximal humerus.

Malignant tumors of the hyaline cartilage are called *chondrosarcomas* and are the second most common primary malignant bone tumor. They are large, bulky, slow-growing tumors that affect adults (men more frequently than women). The usual tumor sites include the pelvis, ribs, femur, humerus, spine, scapula, and tibia. Metastasis to the lungs occurs in fewer than half of patients. If these tumors are well differentiated, large block excision or amputation of the affected extremity results in increased survival rate. These tumors may recur.

Metastatic Bone Cancer

Metastatic bone carcinoma (secondary bone tumor) is more common than any primary malignant bone tumor. Tumors arising from tissues elsewhere in the body may invade the bone and produce localized bone destruction, with symptoms similar to those occurring in primary bone tumors. Tumors that metastasize to bone most frequently include carcinomas of the kidney, prostate, lung, breast, ovary, and thyroid. Metastatic tumors most frequently attack the skull, spine, pelvis, femur, and humerus.

Pathophysiology

The presence of a tumor in the bone causes the normal bone tissue to react by **osteolytic** response (bone destruction) or **osteoblastic** response (bone formation). Some of the bone tumors are common, and some are very rare. Some present no problem, whereas others rapidly become life threatening.

Clinical Manifestations

Patients with bone tumor present with a wide range of associated problems. They may be asymptomatic or may have pain (mild and occasional to constant and severe), varying degrees of disability, and, at times, obvious bone growth. Weight loss, malaise, and fever may be present. The tumor may be diagnosed only after pathologic fracture has occurred.

If spinal cord compression occurs it can progress rapidly or slowly. Neurologic deficits (*e.g.*, progressive pain, weakness, paresthesia, paraplegia, urinary retention) must be identified early and treated with decompressive laminectomy to prevent permanent spinal cord injury.

Diagnostic Evaluation

Differential diagnosis is based on the history, physical examination, and diagnostic studies including CT, bone scans (Fig. 63-8), myelograms, arteriography, MRI, biopsy, and biochemical assays of the blood and urine. Alkaline phosphatase is frequently elevated with osteogenic sarcoma. With metastatic carcinoma of the prostate, serum acid phosphatase is elevated. Hypercalcemia is present with breast, lung, and kidney cancer bone metastasis. Symptoms of hypercalcemia include muscle weakness, fatigue, anorexia, nausea, vomiting, polyuria, cardiac dysrhythmias, seizures, and coma. Hypercalcemia must be identified and treated promptly. Surgical biopsy is performed for histologic identification. Extreme care is taken during biopsy to prevent seeding and resulting recurrence after excision of the tumor.

Chest x-rays are performed to determine the presence of lung metastasis. Surgical staging of musculoskeletal tumors is based on tumor grade and site (intracompartmental or extracompartmental) as well as on metastasis. Staging is used for planning treatment.

During the diagnostic period, the nurse explains the diagnostic tests and provides psychologic and emotional support to the patient and family. Coping behaviors are assessed and use of support systems is encouraged.

Management

The goal of treatment is to destroy or remove the tumor. This may be accomplished by surgical excision (ranging from local excision to amputation and disarticulation), radiation when the tumor is radiosensitive, and chemotherapy (preoperative, postoperative, and adjunctive for possible mi-

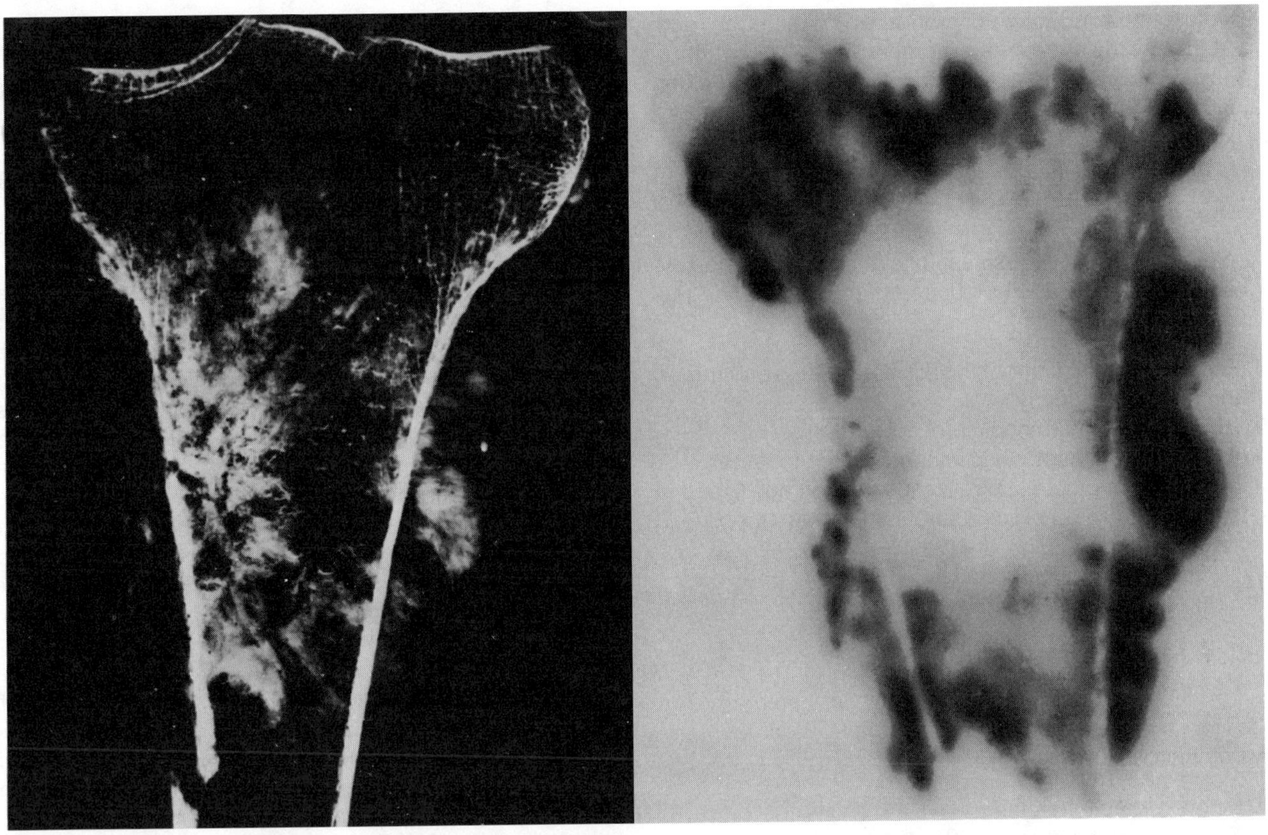

FIGURE 63-8. Bone scan of a patient with osteosarcoma. (**Left**) X-ray showing osteosarcoma at the proximal end of the tibia with destruction of the normal anatomy of the bone. (**Right**) The patient has received ^{85}Sr (strontium) intravenously for bone scanning. Note the high uptake (*black areas*) in the peripheral growing margin and the relative lack of uptake centrally. (Armed Forces Institute of Pathology; negatives 67-4-8, 67-4-9.)

crometastasis). Major gains are being made in using wide block excision with restorative grafting technique. Survival and quality of life are important considerations in procedures that attempt to save the involved extremity.

Surgical removal of the tumor frequently requires amputation of the affected extremity, with the amputation extending well above the tumor to achieve local control of the primary lesion. (See Nursing Process: The Patient Undergoing an Amputation in Chapter 64.)

Limb-sparing (salvage) procedures remove the tumor and adjacent tissue. The resected portion is replaced by a customized prosthesis, total joint arthroplasty, or bone tissue from the patient (autograft) or a cadaver donor (allograft). Soft tissue and blood vessels may need grafting because of the extent of the excision. Complications that may develop include infection, loosening or dislocation of the prosthesis, allograft nonunion, fracture, devitalization of the skin and soft tissues, joint fibrosis, and recurrence of the tumor. Function and rehabilitation after limb salvage depend on reducing the risk of complications and positive encouragement.

Because of the danger of metastasis with malignant tumors, combined chemotherapy is started before and continued after surgery in an effort to eradicate micrometastatic lesions. The hope is that combined chemotherapy will have a greater effect at a lower toxicity rate while reducing resistance to the drugs. There is an improved long-term survival rate (60%) when a localized osteosarcoma is removed and chemotherapy (doxorubicin hydrochloride and cisplatin or methotrexate) is initiated.

Soft-tissue sarcomas are treated with radiation, limb-sparing excision, and adjuvant chemotherapy.

The treatment of metastatic bone cancer is palliative, and the therapeutic goal is to relieve the patient's pain and discomfort as much as possible. Additional therapies are consistent with methods used to treat the original cancer. Internal fixation of pathologic fractures minimizes associated disability and pain. At times, large bones with metastatic lesions are strengthened by prophylactic internal fixation. Surgery may be indicated for fractures of long bones.

If hypercalcemia is present, treatment includes hydration with intravenous administration of normal saline solution, diuresis, mobilization, and medications such as phosphates, mithramycin, calcitonin, or corticosteroids.

❑ *NURSING PROCESS*
The Patient With a Bone Tumor

Assessment

The patient is encouraged to discuss the onset and course of symptoms. During the interview, the nurse notes the patient's understanding of the disease process, how the patient and the family have been coping, and how the patient has managed the pain. On physical examination the mass is palpated gently; its size and associated soft tissue swelling, pain, and tenderness are noted. Assessment of the neurovascular status and range of motion of the extremity provides baseline data for future comparisons. The patient's mobility and ability to perform activities of daily living are evaluated.

Diagnosis

Nursing Diagnoses

Based on the nursing assessment data, the major nursing diagnoses for the patient with a bone tumor may include the following:

- Knowledge deficit about the disease process and the therapeutic regimen
- Pain related to pathologic process and surgery
- Risk for injury: pathologic fracture related to tumor
- Ineffective coping related to fear of the unknown, perception of disease process, and inadequate support system
- Disturbance in self-esteem related to loss of body part or alteration in role performance

Collaborative Problems/ Potential Complications

Based on assessment data, potential complications that may develop include:

- Delayed wound healing
- Nutritional deficiency
- Infection

Planning and Implementation

Goals. The major goals of the patient include knowledge of the disease process and treatment regimen, control of pain, absence of pathologic fractures, effective patterns of coping, improved self-esteem, and absence of complications.

The nursing care of a patient who has undergone excision of a bone tumor is similar in many respects to that for other patients who have had skeletal surgery. Vital signs are monitored; blood loss is assessed; observations are made to assess for the development of complications such as deep vein thrombosis, pulmonary emboli, infection, contracture, and disuse atrophy. The operative part should be elevated to control swelling; the neurovascular status of the extremity should be assessed. Generally the area is immobilized by splints, casts, or elastic bandages until the bone heals.

Nursing Interventions

Understanding the Disease Process and Treatment Regimen. Patient and family education about the disease process and diagnostic and management regimens is essential. Explanation of diagnostic tests, treatments (*e.g.*, wound care), and expected results (*e.g.*, decreased range of motion, numbness, change of body contours) helps the patient deal with the procedures and changes. Cooperation and adherence to the therapeutic regimen are enhanced through understanding. The nurse can most effectively reinforce and clarify information provided by the physician by being present during these physician–patient discussions.

The patient is encouraged to be as independent as possible.

Controlling Pain. Psychologic and pharmacologic pain management techniques are used to control pain and increase the patient's comfort level. The nurse works with the patient in designing the most effective pain management regimen, thereby increasing the patient's control over the pain. The nurse prepares the patient and gives support during painful procedures.

After surgery the patient experiences pain at both the surgical and graft donor sites. Prescribed opioid analgesics are used during the early postoperative period. Later, oral, non-opioid analgesics are usually adequate to relieve pain.

Preventing Pathologic Fracture. Bone tumors weaken the bone to a point at which normal activities or position changes can result in fracture. During nursing care the affected bones must be supported and handled gently. External supports (*e.g.*, splints) may be used for additional protection. Prescribed weight-bearing restrictions must be followed. The patient is taught how to use assistive devices safely and how to strengthen unaffected extremities.

Coping Effectively. The patient and family are encouraged to verbalize their fears, concerns, and feelings. They need to be supported and to feel accepted as they deal with the impact of the malignant bone tumor. Feelings of shock, despair, and grief are expected. Referral to a psychiatric nurse liaison, psychologist, counselor, or clergy may be indicated for specific psychologic help.

Improving Self-Esteem. Independence versus dependence is an issue with the patient who has a malignancy. Life-style is dramatically changed, at least temporarily. The family is supported in working through the adjustments that must be made. Changes in body image due to surgery and possibly amputation need to be recognized. Realistic reassurance about the future and resumption of role-related activities is provided. Self-care and socialization are encouraged. The patient participates in planning daily activities. Involvement of the patient and family throughout treatment encourages confidence, restoration of self-concept, and a sense of being in control of one's life.

Monitoring and Managing Potential Complications

Wound Healing. Wound healing may be delayed because of tissue trauma from surgery or previous radiation. Pressure on the wound site is minimized to promote circulation to the tissues. An aseptic, nontraumatic wound dressing promotes healing. Monitoring and reporting of laboratory findings facilitate prescription of interventions to promote homeostasis and wound healing.

Repositioning the patient at frequent intervals reduces the incidence of skin breakdown due to pressure. Pain and avoidance of movement contribute to the potential for skin breakdown. Special therapeutic beds may be needed to prevent skin breakdown and to promote wound healing following extensive plastic surgery reconstruction and grafting.

Adequate Nutrition. Because loss of appetite, nausea, and vomiting are frequent side effects of chemotherapy and radiation therapy, it is necessary to provide adequate nutrition for healing and health promotion. Antiemetics and relaxation techniques reduce the gastrointestinal reaction.

Stomatitis is controlled with anesthetic or antifungal mouthwash. Adequate hydration is essential. Nutritional supplements or total parenteral nutrition may be prescribed to achieve adequate nutrition.

Osteomyelitis and Wound Infections. Prophylactic antibiotics and strict aseptic dressing techniques are used to diminish the occurrence of osteomyelitis and wound infections. During healing, other infections (*e.g.*, upper respiratory infections) need to be avoided so that hematogenous spread does not result in an osteomyelitis.

If the patient is receiving chemotherapy, the white blood cell count is monitored and he or she is instructed to avoid persons with colds and infections.

Patient Education and Home Care Considerations. Preparation for and coordination of continuing health care are begun early as a multidisciplinary effort. Patient education is directed at medication, dressing, and treatment regimens, as well as physical and occupational therapy programs. The safe use of special equipment is explained. The patient and family learn the signs and symptoms of possible complications. The patient is advised to have the phone numbers of persons to contact readily available in case problems arise. Frequently, arrangements are made with a home health care agency for home care supervision and follow-up. The need for long-term health supervision is emphasized to ensure cure or to detect tumor recurrence or metastasis.

Evaluation

Expected Outcomes

1. Describes disease process and treatment regimen
   a. Describes pathologic problem
   b. States goals of the therapeutic regimen
   c. Seeks clarification of information
2. Achieves control of pain
   a. Uses multiple pain control techniques, including prescribed medications
   b. Experiences no pain or decreased pain at rest, during activities of daily living, or at surgical sites
3. Experiences no pathologic fracture
   a. Avoids stress to weakened bones
   b. Uses assistive devices safely
   c. Strengthens uninvolved extremities
4. Demonstrates effective coping patterns
   a. Verbalizes feelings
   b. Identifies strengths and abilities
   c. Makes decisions
   d. Requests assistance as needed
5. Demonstrates positive self-concept
   a. Identifies home and family responsibilities that he or she is able to accomplish
   b. Exhibits confidence in own abilities
   c. Demonstrates acceptance of altered body image
   d. Demonstrates independence in activities of daily living
6. Exhibits absence of complications
   a. Demonstrates wound healing
   b. Experiences no skin breakdown
   c. Maintains or increases body weight
   d. Experiences no infections
   e. Manages side effects of therapies
   f. Reports symptoms of drug toxicity or complications of surgery
7. Participates in continuing health care at home
   a. Complies with prescribed regimen (*i.e.* takes prescribed medications, continues physical and occupational therapy programs)
   b. Acknowledges need for long-term health supervision
   c. Keeps follow-up health care appointments
   d. Reports occurrence of symptoms or complications

CRITICAL THINKING EXERCISES

1. A classmate who has a small child states that she has been having low back pain for several months. She asks for your advice. Describe how you would assess this situation, indicate the questions you would ask, and explain the kind of information you are seeking and why. How would your thinking redirect your asseessment if the woman (1) is overweight, (2) jogs regularly, and (3) is expecting another child?
2. You volunteer to help with a health fair in your community. You are asked to participate in the booth that will offer information about osteoporosis. How would your advice differ when you are talking to (1) teenagers, (2) young adults, and (3) elderly persons? Explain the reasons for your modifciations.
3. You are visiting with a patient in an extended-care facility. The patient's daughter states that her mother has osteoarthritis and her aunt has osteoporosis. She asks if these conditions are the same since her mother and aunt got them late in life and both are debilitated. What explanations do you feel would be helpful to her? How would the care of persons with these two disorders differ? How would the care be similar?

REFERENCES AND SELECTED READINGS

Books

Agency for Health Care Policy and Research. Acute Low Back Problems in Adults. Clinical Practice Guideline, Publication No. 95-0642. U.S. Department of Health and Human Services, Public Health Service, May 1995.

Baird S et al. Cancer Nursing. Philadelphia, WB Saunders, 1991.

Bullock BL and Philbrook P. Pathophysiology: Adaptations and Alterations in Function, 3rd ed. Philadelphia, JB Lippincott, 1992.

Carpenito LJ. Nursing Diagnosis: Application to Clinical Practice, 6th ed. Philadelphia, JB Lippincott, 1995.

Chapman M and Madison M. Operative Orthopaedics, 2nd ed. Philadelphia, JB Lippincott, 1993.

Conn R (ed). Current Diagnosis. Philadelphia, WB Saunders, 1991.

Crenshaw A (ed). Campbell's Operative Orthopaedics, 8th ed. St. Louis, Mosby Year Book, 1992.
Davis PS. Nursing the Orthopaedic Patient. Edinburgh, Churchill Livingstone, 1994.
Goldie B and Dunn D. Orthopaedic Diagnosis and Management: A Guide to the Care of Orthopaedic Patients. Oxford, Blackwell Scientific Publications, 1992.
Guyton A. Human Physiology and Mechanisms of Disease, 5th ed. Philadelphia, WB Saunders, 1992.
Hooper PD. Preventing Low Back Pain. Baltimore, Williams & Wilkins, 1992.
Hogstel MD (ed). Clinical Manual of Gerontological Nursing. St. Louis, CV Mosby, 1992.
Huvos A. Bone Tumors: Diagnosis, Treatment, and Prognosis, 2nd ed. Philadelphia, WB Saunders, 1991.
Lewis CB and Knortz KA. Orthopedic Assessment and Treatment of the Geriatric Patient. St. Louis, CV Mosby, 1993.
Lewis M (ed). Musculoskeletal Oncology: A Multidisciplinary Approach. Philadelphia, WB Saunders, 1992.
Maher AB et al. Orthopaedic Nursing. Philadelphia, WB Saunders, 1994.
Memmler R et al. Structure and Function of the Human Body, 5th ed. Philadelphia, JB Lippincott, 1992.
Mercier LR. Practical Orthopedics, 3rd ed. St. Louis, Mosby Year Book, 1991.
Mourad LA. Orthopedic Disorders. St. Louis, Mosby Year Book, 1991.
Mourad LA and Droste MM. The Nursing Process in the Care of Adults with Orthopaedic Conditions, 3rd ed. Albany, NY, Delmar Publishers, 1993.
National Association of Orthopaedic Nurses. Guidelines for Orthopaedic Nursing. Pitman, NJ, National Association of Orthopaedic Nurses, 1992.
Porth CM. Pathophysiology: Concepts of Altered Health States, 4th ed. Philadelphia, JB Lippincott, 1994.
Rakel RE (ed). Conn's Current Therapy. Philadelphia, WB Saunders, 1993.
Salmond SW et al (ed). Core Curriculum for Orthopaedic Nursing, 2nd ed. Pitman, NJ. National Association of Orthopaedic Nurses, 1991.
Sly D and Theis L (ed). Introduction to Orthopaedic Nursing: An Orientation Module. Pitman, NJ, National Association of Orthopaedic Nurses, 1991.
Turek SL (ed). Orthopaedics. Principles and Their Application, 5th ed. Philadelphia, JB Lippincott, 1994.
Watt-Watson J and Donovan M. Pain Management: Nursing Perspective. St. Louis, Mosby Year Book, 1992.
Wilson J and Foster D (ed). Williams Textbook of Endocrinology. Philadelphia, WB Saunders, 1992.
Wyngaarden J (ed). Cecil Textbook of Medicine, 19th ed. Philadelphia, WB Saunders, 1992.

Journals

Asterisks indicate nursing research articles.

Low Back Pain

Bowman JM. The meaning of chronic low back pain. AAOHN-J 1991 Aug; 39(8):381–384.
Chase JA. Outpatient management of low back pain. Orthop Nurs 1992 Jan/Feb; 11(1):11–21.
Deyo RA. Back pain revisted: Newer thinking on diagnosis and therapy. Consultant 1993 Feb; 33(2):88–90, 93–4, 97–8.
*Koku RV. Severity of low back pain: A comparison between participants who did and did not receive counseling. AAOHN-J 1992 Feb; 40(2):84–89.
Mayer T. Management of the patient with chronic low back pain: The functional restoration approach. Phys Med Rehabil Clin North Am 1991 Feb; 2(1):233–247.
Pedinoff S et al. Motion and progress in low-back pain. Patient Care 1991 May 15; 25(9):71–4, 76, 79–82.
*Pellino TA and Oberst MT. Perception of control and appraisal of illness in chronic low back pain. Orthop Nurs 1992 Jan/Feb; 11(1):22–26.
Popkess-Vawter S. and Patzel B. Compound problem: Chronic low back pain and overweight in adult females. Orthop Nurs 1992 Nov/Dec; 11(6):31–35.
Shelton JL and Robinson JP. Psychological aspects of chronic back pain. Phys Med Rehabil Clin North Am 1991 Feb; 2(1):127–144.
Wipf JE and Deyo RA. Low back pain. Med Clin North Am 1995 Mar; 79(2):247–260.

Arthroplasty

Johnson R. Total shoulder arthroplasty. Orthop Nurs 1993 Jan/Feb; 12(1):14–22.
*Kelley HK. Patient Perceptions of Pain and Disability after Joint Arthroplasty. Orthop Nurs 1991 Nov/Dec; 10(6):43–50.
*Lichtenstein R. et. al. Development and impact of a hospital-based preoperative patient education program in a joint replacement center. Orthop Nurs 1993 Nov/Dec; 12(6):17–25, 46.
Maskell M and Wright J. Preoperative preparation of patients undergoing total joint replacement. CONA J ACIIO 1993 Spring; 15(1):12–15.
Mather C. Total joint pre-admission clinic—Improve patient outcome and cost effectiveness. CONA J ACIIO 1992 Fall; 14(3): 9–12.
Mac HL et al. Comparison of autoreinfusion and standard drainage systems in total joint arthroplasty patients. Orthop Nurs 1993 May/Jun; 12(3):19–25.
Morrey B. Orthopedics. JAMA 1991 Jun 19; 265(23):3151.
*Selman SW and Mistretta EF. Perioperative concerns of the older adult undergoing total joint replacement. AORN 1992 Feb; 55(2):618–622.
Stranks GJ et al. The A-V impulse system reduces deep-vein thrombosis and swelling after hemiarthroplasty for hip fracture. J Bone Joint Surg [Br] 1992 Sep; 74-B(5):775–778.
*Tibbles L et al. Computer assisted instruction for preoperative and postoperative patient education in joint replacement surgery. Comput Nurs 1992 Sep/Oct; 10(5):208–212.

Osteoporosis

*Ali NS and Bennett SJ. Postmenopausal women. Factors in osteoporosis preventive behaviors. J Gerontol Nurs 1992 Dec; 18(12):23–32.
Bush TL. Feminine forever revisted: Menopausal hormone therapy in the 1990's. J Womens Health 1992 Spring; 1(1):1–4.
Bilezikian JP and Silverberg SH. Osteoporosis: A practical approach to the perimenopausal woman. J Womens Health 1992 Spring; 1(1):21–27.
Dubin S. The physiological changes of aging. Orthop Nurs 1992 May/Jun; 11(3):45–50.
Erickson GP. Osteoporosis risk assessment of mature working women: Primary and secondary prevention strategies. AAOHN-J 1992 Sept; 40(9):423–438, 453–455.
Gold DT et al. Psychosocial functioning and osteoporosis in late life: Results of a multidisciplinary intervention. J Womens Health 1993 Summer; 2(2):149–155.
Holm K et al. Bone loss in mid-life women. J Womens Health 1992 Summer; 1(2):131–136.
Kim K et al. Development and evaluation of the osteoporosis health belief scale. Resear Nurs & Heal 1991 Apr; 14(2):155–163.
Liscum B. Osteoporosis: The silent disease. Orthop Nurs 1992 Jul/Aug; 11(4):21–25.
Licata AA. Therapies of symptomatic primary osteoporosis. Geriatrics 1991 Nov; 46(11):62–63; 66–67.
Maddox MA. Women at midlife: Hormone replacement therapy. Nurs Clin North Am 1992 Dec; 27(4):959–969.

Marten SK. Complications of menopause and the risks and benefits of estrogen replacement therapy. J Am Acad Nurse Pract 1993 Mar–Apr; 5(2):55–61.
McMahon MA et al. Osteoporosis: Identifying high-risk persons. J Gerontol Nurs 1992 Oct; 18(10):19–26.
Mundy GR. New concepts in bone metabolism: Clinical implications. Hosp Pract 1991; 26(Suppl 1):7–12.
Optimal calcium intake. NIH Consensus Statement 1994 Jun 6–8; 12(4):1–31.
Orr P. Salmon calcitonin. Orthop Nurs 1993 Sep/Oct; 12(5):45–47.
Pavlik M. Measuring bone mineral content. Orthop Nurs 1991 Mar/Apr; 10(2):39–43.
Payling KJ. A safe way to reduce the symptoms? Advising women on hormone replacement therapy. Prof Nurse 1992 Oct; 8(1):37–41.
Rickert B. Estrogen replacement: Making informed choices. RN 1992 Sep; 55(9):26–33.
Sardana R. Nutritional management of osteoporosis. Geriatr Nurs 1992 Nov–Dec; 13(6):315–319.
Schurman S and Williamson A. Bone density studies: Current technology. Nurs Pract Forum 1991 Dec; 2(4):246–250.
Tollison CD et al. Etiology and diagnosis of osteoporosis. Physician Assist 1992 Apr; 16(4):57–8, 63–5, 153–5.

Paget's Disease

Freeman DA. Drug treatments for Paget's disease of bone. Physician Assist 1992 Mar; 16(3):125–6, 135–7, 162–4.
Hamdy RC et al. Clinical presentation of Paget's disease of the bone in older patients. South Med J 1993 Oct; 86(10):1097–1100.

Osteomyelitis

Cheatle MD. The effect of chronic orthopedic infection on quality of life. Orthop Clin North Am 1991 Jul; 22(3):539–547.
Mosher CM. The Papineau bone graft: A limb salvage technique. Orthop Nurs 1991 May/Jun; 10(3):27–32.
Tice A. Osteomyelitis. Hosp Pract 1991; 26(Suppl 5):31–36.

Bone Tumors

Frieden RA et al. Assessment of patient function after limb-sparing surgery. Arch Phys Med Rehabil 1993 Jan; 74(1):38–43.
Homa DM et al. Incidence and survival rates of children and young adults with osteogenic sarcoma. Cancer 1991 Apr 15; 67:2219–2223.
Petrilli AS et al. Increased surviv, limb preservation, and prognostic factors for osteosarcoma. Cancer 1991 Aug 15; 68:733–737.
Piasecki P. Update in orthopaedic oncology. Orthop Nurs 1992 Nov/Dec; 11(6):36, 38–43.
Piasecki PA. The nursing role in limb salvage surgery. Nurs Clin North Am 1991 Mar; 26(1):33–41.
Thatcher P. A young adult with chronic knee pain. J Am Acad Physician Assist 1993 Jul/Aug; 6(7):515–516.

INFORMATION/RESOURCES

Agencies

American Chronic Pain Association
P.O.Box 850,
Rocklin, CA 95677

Arthritis Foundation
1314 Spring Street NW,
Atlanta, GA 30309

National Easter Seals Society
70 East Lake Street,
Chicago, IL 60601

National Institute of Arthritis and Musculoskeletal and Skin Diseases
National Institutes of Health,
Bethesda, MD 20892

National Osteoporosis Foundation
2100 M Street NW, Suite 602,
Washington, DC 2003

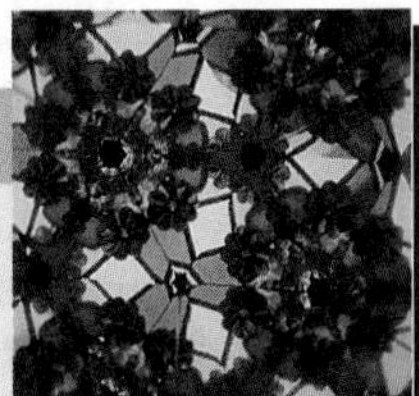

64

Management of Patients With Musculoskeletal Trauma

CHAPTER OUTLINE

LEARNING OBJECTIVES

On completion of this chapter, the learner will be able to:

1. Differentiate between contusions, strains, sprains, and dislocations
2. Specify the clinical manifestations of a fracture and the emergency management of the patient with a fracture
3. Describe the principles and methods of fracture reduction, fracture immobilization, and management of open fractures
4. Use the nursing process as a framework for care of the patient with a simple fracture
5. Describe the prevention and management of immediate and delayed complications of fractures
6. Describe the rehabilitative needs of patients with fractures of the clavicle, upper and lower extremities, pelvis, hips, ribs, and thoracolumbar spine
7. Use the nursing process as a framework for care of the elderly patient with fracture of the hip
8. Describe the rehabilitative and health education needs of the patient who has had an amputation
9. Use the nursing process as a framework for care of the patient with an amputation

Injury to one part of the musculoskeletal system usually produces injury or dysfunction of adjacent structures and of structures enclosed or supported by them. If the bones are broken, the muscles cannot function; if the nerves do not send impulses to the muscles, as in paralysis, the bones cannot move; if the joint surfaces do not articulate normally, neither the bones nor the muscles can function properly. Thus, although a fracture primarily affects the bone, it may also produce injury to the muscles, the blood vessels, and the nerves in the vicinity of the fracture.

Treatment of injury of the musculoskeletal system involves providing support for the injured part until healing is complete. Support may be provided by externally applied bandages, adhesive strapping, splints, or casts. Alternatively, support may be applied directly to the bone in the form of pins or plates. At times, traction must be applied to correct deformity or shortening.

After the immediate and the painful effects of the injury have passed, treatment efforts are focused on preventing fibrosis and the resulting stiffness in the injured muscles and joint structures. Proper exercise guards against this disability. In some cases, the support applied may permit early activity. The healing process and recovery of function may be hastened by various forms of physical therapy.

Contusions, Strains, and Sprains

A **contusion** is an injury of the soft tissues, produced by blunt force (*e.g.*, a blow, kick, or fall). The resultant rupture of many small vessels leads to bleeding into soft tissues (**ecchymosis,** bruising). A hematoma develops when the bleeding is sufficient to cause an appreciable collection of blood. The local symptoms (pain, swelling, and discoloration) are easily controlled with intermittent application of cold. Most contusions resolve in 1 to 2 weeks.

A **strain** is a "muscle pull" due to overuse, overstretching, or excessive stress. Strains are microscopic, incomplete muscle tears with some bleeding into the tissue. The patient experiences soreness or sudden pain with local tenderness upon muscle use and isometric contraction.

A **sprain** is an injury to the ligamentous structures surrounding a joint, caused by a wrenching or twisting motion. The function of a ligament is to maintain stability while permitting mobility. A torn ligament loses its stabilizing ability. Blood vessels are ruptured and significant edema occurs; the joint is tender and movement of the joint becomes painful. The degree of disability and pain increases during the first 2 to 3 hours after the injury because of the associated swelling and bleeding. The patient should have an x-ray examination to evaluate for bone injury. **Avulsion fracture** (a bone fragment is pulled away by a ligament or tendon) may be associated with a sprain.

Management. Treatment of contusions, strains, and sprains consists of resting and elevating the affected part, applying cold, and using a compression bandage. Rest prevents additional injury and promotes healing. Elevation controls the swelling. Moist or dry cold applied intermittently for 20 to 30 minutes during the first 24 to 48 hours after injury produces vasoconstriction, which decreases bleeding, edema, and discomfort. Care must be taken to avoid skin and tissue damage due to excessive cold. An elastic compression bandage controls bleeding, reduces edema, and provides support for the injured tissues. The neurovascular status of the injured extremity is monitored frequently. If the sprain is severe (torn muscle fibers and disrupted ligaments), surgical repair or cast immobilization may be necessary so that the joint will not lose its stability.

During the recovery phase, the injured muscles, ligaments, or tendons must be allowed to rest and repair themselves. After the acute inflammatory stage (*e.g.*, after 24 to 48 hours after injury) heat may be applied intermittently (for 15 to 30 minutes, 4 times a day) to relieve muscle spasm and to promote vasodilation, absorption, and repair. Depending on the severity of injury, progressive passive and active exercises may be begun in 3 to 5 days. Severe sprains may require 1 to 3 weeks of immobilization before protected exercises are initiated. Excessive exercise early in the course of treatment will delay recovery. Strains and sprains take weeks or months to heal. Splinting may be used to prevent reinjury.

Joint Dislocations

A dislocation of a joint is a condition in which the articular surfaces of the bones forming the joint are no longer in anatomic contact. The bones are literally "out of joint." A **subluxation** is a partial dislocation of the articulating surfaces. Traumatic dislocations are orthopedic emergencies, because the associated joint structures, blood supply, and nerves are distorted and severely stressed. If the dislocation is not treated promptly, **avascular necrosis** (tissue death due to anoxia and diminished blood supply) and nerve palsy may occur.

Dislocations may be (1) **congenital** (present at birth, due to some maldevelopment, most often noted at the hip); (2) spontaneous or **pathologic,** due to disease of the articular or the periarticular structures; or (3) **traumatic,** due to injury in which the joint is disrupted by force.

The signs and symptoms of a traumatic dislocation are (1) pain, (2) change in contour of the joint, (3) change in the length of the extremity, (4) loss of normal mobility, and (5) change in the axis of the dislocated bones.

X-ray studies confirm the diagnosis and demonstrate possible associated fracture.

Management. The affected joint needs to be immobilized while the patient is transported. The dislocation is reduced (*i.e.*, displaced parts brought into normal position), usually under anesthesia. The head of the dislocated bone is manipulated back into the joint cavity. The joint is immobilized by bandages, splints, casts, or traction and is maintained in a stable position. Several days to weeks after reduction, gentle active movement three or four times a day is begun to preserve range of motion. The joint is supported between exercise sessions.

Nursing concerns are directed at providing comfort, evaluating the neurovascular status, and protecting the joint during healing. The patient needs to learn how to manage the immobilizing devices and how to protect the joint from reinjury.

Sports Injuries

More and more people are participating in recreational sports. These recreational athletes may push themselves beyond the level of their physical conditioning and incur sports injuries. Injuries to the musculoskeletal system may be of an acute nature (sprains, strains, dislocations, fractures) or may result from gradual overuse (chondromalacia patella, tendinitis, stress fractures). Professional athletes are also susceptible to injury, even though their training is supervised closely to minimize the occurrence of injury and to enhance the development of athletic performance.

Musculoskeletal contusions result from direct falls or blows. The initial dull pain becomes greater, with edema and stiffness occurring by the next day. Sprains commonly occur in fingers, ankles, and knees. If the ligament damage is major, the joint becomes unstable and surgical repair may be required. An avulsion fracture may exist.

Strains present with a sharp, stabbing pain from bleeding and immediate protective muscle contraction. Tennis players often suffer calf muscle strains; soccer players often experience quadriceps strains; and swimmers, weight lifters, and tennis players often suffer shoulder strains. Tendinitis (inflammation of a tendon) is due to overuse and is seen in tennis players (epicondylar tendinitis or "tennis elbow"), runners and gymnasts (Achilles tendinitis), and runners and basketball players (infrapatellar tendinitis). Meniscal injuries of the knee occur with excessive rotational stress. Dislocations are seen with throwing and lifting sports. Fractures occur with falls. Skaters and bikers frequently suffer Colles's fractures of the wrist when they fall on outstretched arms; ballet dancers and track and field athletes may experience metatarsal fractures. Stress fractures occur with repeated bone trauma from activities such as jogging, gymnastics, basketball, and aerobics. The tibias, fibulas, and metatarsals are most vulnerable.

Management. Generally, musculoskeletal injuries need to be recognized and managed early to facilitate healing and to minimize residual disabilities. Most soft-tissue injuries are managed by RICE (*r*est, *i*ce, *c*ompression, *e*levation). The ice is applied for 20 to 30 minutes intermittently during the first 24 hours to control swelling and relieve pain. The area is wrapped with an elastic compression bandage to minimize effusion, support the area, and provide comfort. The wrap must not be constricting. Monitoring the neurovascular status of the extremity becomes an important nursing function. The injured extremity is elevated to the level of the heart to control swelling and to promote rest. Depending on the site and severity of injury, the extremity may be immobilized or treated by surgical intervention. Arthroscopic surgery may be required for meniscus tears and other joint injuries that limit joint function and contribute to articular cartilage wear.

Patients who have experienced a sports-related injury are often highly motivated to return to their previous level of activity. Compliance with restriction of activities and gradual resumption of activities may be a real problem for these patients. They need to be taught how to avoid further injury or new injury. With recurrence of symptoms, they need to learn to diminish the level and intensity of activity to a comfortable level and to treat the symptoms with RICE. Recovery from sports-related injury can take a few days or 6 or more weeks.

Sports-related injuries can be prevented by use of proper equipment (*e.g.*, running shoes) and by effectively training and conditioning the body. Changes in activities and stresses should occur gradually. The athlete needs to be taught to "tune in" to body symptoms indicating stress and to modify activities to minimize injury and to promote healing.

Internal Derangement of the Knee

Injury to most joints consists of a tear of the supporting ligaments. In the knee joint, however, there may also be a displacement or tear of the semilunar cartilages, which are two crescent-shaped cartilages attached to the edge of the shallow articulating surface of the head of the tibia. They normally move slightly backward and forward to accommodate the condyles of the femur when the leg is flexed or extended.

Normally, little torsion movement is permitted in the knee joint. In sports or accidents, twisting of the knee with the foot fixed may result in either tearing the cartilage or tearing the cartilage from its attachment to the head of the tibia.

These injuries leave loose cartilage in the knee joint that may slip between the femur and the tibia, preventing full extension of the leg. If this happens during walking or running, patients often describe their leg as "giving way" under them. Patients may hear or feel a click in the knee when they walk, especially when they extend the leg that is bearing weight, as in going upstairs. When the cartilage is attached front and back but torn loose laterally (bucket-handle tear), it may slide between the bones to lie between the condyles and prevent full flexion or extension. As a result, the knee "locks."

Internal derangements of the knee joint produce disturbing disabilities because the patients never know when their knee will malfunction. Usually, the damaged cartilage is surgically removed through an operating arthroscope.

After surgery, a pressure dressing is applied; a knee-immobilizing splint may be required. The leg is elevated on pillows to minimize edema. The most common complication is an effusion into the knee joint, which produces marked pain. If this occurs, the physician should be notified. Relief can be obtained by loosening the pressure dressing. The physician may need to aspirate the joint to remove fluid and relieve the pressure.

To prevent atrophy of the thigh muscles, these patients are taught quadriceps setting exercises. Additional exercises help to restore full function, stability, and strength.

Arthroscopic surgery is usually an outpatient procedure. The patient resumes activities in 1 to 2 days and sports can be resumed in several weeks, as prescribed by the physician.

Rupture of the Achilles Tendon

Traumatic rupture of the Achilles tendon, generally within the tendon sheath, occurs during activities when there is a sudden contraction of the calf muscle with the foot fixed firmly to the floor. The patient experiences sharp pain and is unable to plantar flex the foot. Immediate surgical repair of complete Achilles tendon ruptures is usually recommended to obtain satisfactory results. In some situations, conservative management with a plantar-flexed cast for 6 to 8 weeks may be used.

Fractures

A **fracture** is a break in the continuity of bone and is defined according to type and extent (Figs. 64-1 and 64-2). Fractures occur when the bone is subjected to stress greater than it can absorb. Fractures can be caused by a direct blow, crushing force, sudden twisting motion, and even extreme muscle contraction. Although the bone is broken, adjacent structures are also affected, resulting in soft-tissue edema, hemorrhage into the muscles and joints, joint dislocations, ruptured tendons, severed nerves, and damaged blood vessels. Body organs may be injured by the force that caused the fracture or by the fracture fragments.

Types of Fractures

A *complete fracture* involves a break across the entire cross section of the bone and is frequently displaced (removed from normal position). In an *incomplete fracture,* the break occurs through only part of the cross section of the bone.

A *closed fracture* (simple fracture) does not produce a break in the skin. An *open fracture* (compound/complex fracture) is one in which the skin or mucous membrane wound extends to the fractured bone. Open fractures are graded: Grade I is a clean wound less than 1 cm long; Grade II is a larger wound without extensive soft-tissue damage; and Grade III, which is highly contaminated and has extensive soft-tissue damage, is the most severe.

Fractures may also be described according to anatomic placement of fragments—*displaced/nondisplaced fracture.*

The following are specific types of fractures (see Figs. 64-1 and 64-2):

Greenstick—a fracture in which one side of a bone is broken and the other side is bent
Transverse—a fracture that is straight across the bone
Oblique—a fracture occurring at an angle across the bone (less stable than transverse)
Spiral—a fracture twisting around the shaft of the bone
Comminuted—a fracture in which bone has splintered into several fragments
Depressed—a fracture in which fragments are driven inward (seen frequently in fractures of skull and facial bones)
Compression—a fracture in which bone has been compressed (seen in vertebral fractures)
Pathologic—a fracture that occurs through an area of diseased bone (bone cyst, Paget's disease, bony metastasis, tumor)
Avulsion—a pulling away of a fragment of bone by a ligament or tendon and its attachment
Epiphyseal—a fracture through the epiphysis
Impacted—a fracture in which a bone fragment is driven into another bone fragment

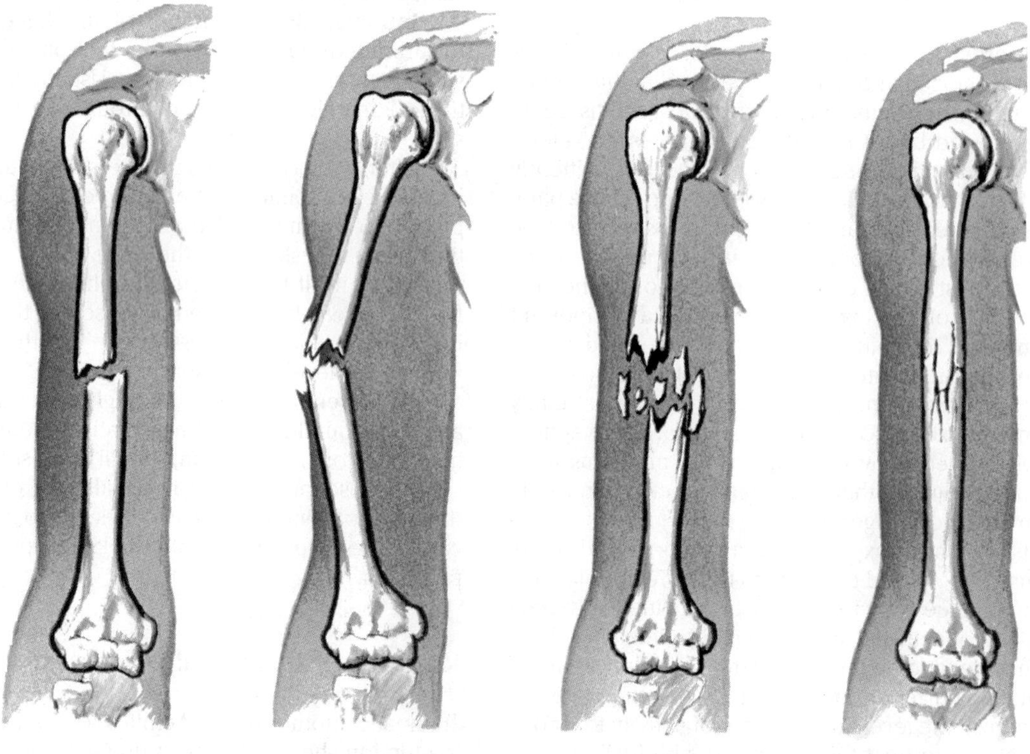

FIGURE 64-1. Types of fractures (simple, compound, comminuted, and greenstick).

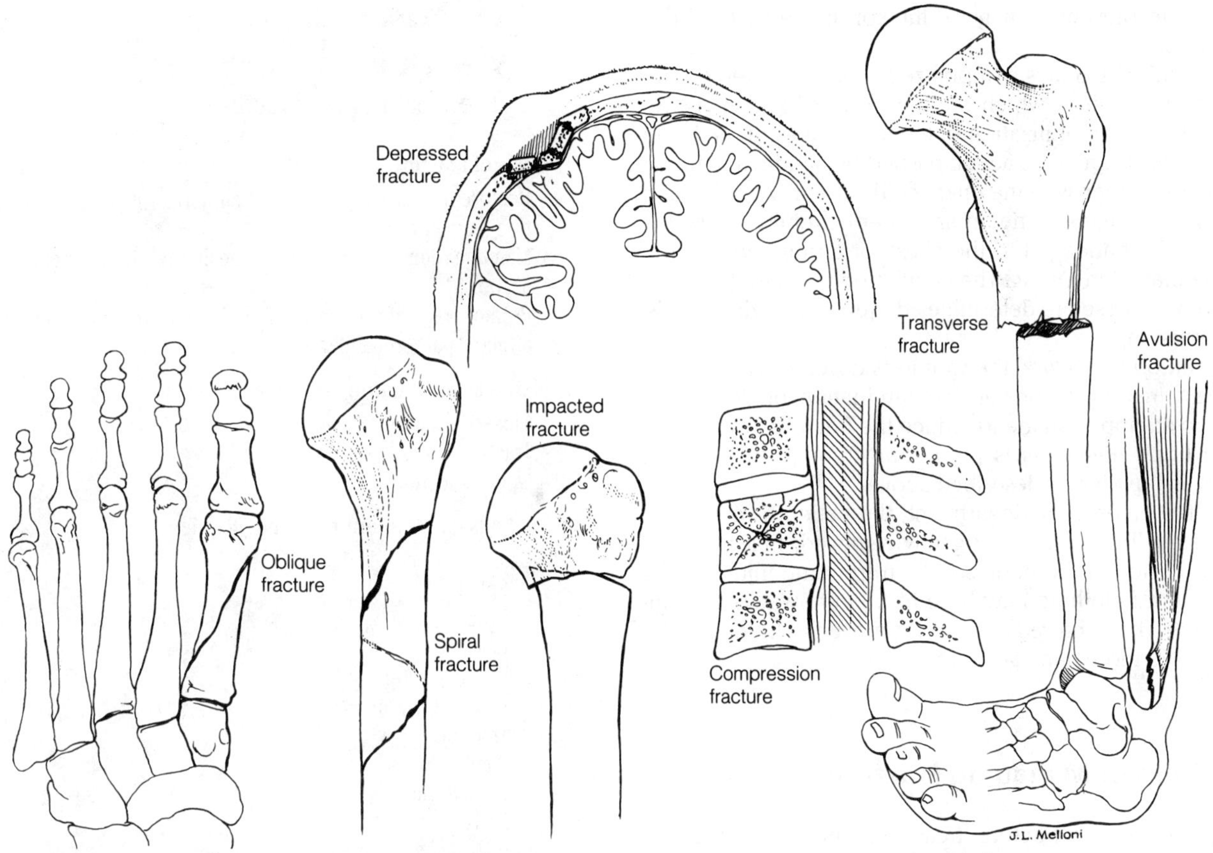

FIGURE 64-2. Types of fractures (transverse, oblique, spiral, impacted, depressed, compression, and avulsion).

Clinical Manifestations

The clinical manifestations of a fracture are pain, loss of function, deformity, shortening of the extremity, crepitus, local swelling, and discoloration.

1. The **pain** is continuous and increases in severity until the bone fragments are immobilized. The muscle spasm that accompanies fracture is a type of natural splinting designed to minimize further movement of the fracture fragments.
2. After a fracture, the part cannot be used and tends to move unnaturally (**false motion**) instead of remaining rigid as it normally would. Displacement of the fragments in a fracture of the arm or leg causes a **deformity** (either visible or palpable) of the extremity detectable when compared with the normal extremity. The extremity cannot function properly because normal function of the muscles depends on the integrity of the bones to which they are attached.
3. In fractures of long bones, there is actually **shortening** of the extremity because of the contraction of the muscles that are attached above and below the site of the fracture. The fragments may often overlap by as much as 2.5 to 5 cm (1 to 2 in).
4. When the extremity is examined with the hands, a grating sensation called **crepitus** can be felt because of the rubbing of the fragments against each other. (Testing for crepitus can produce further tissue damage.)
5. Localized **swelling** and **discoloration** of the skin occur as a result of trauma and hemorrhage that follow a fracture. These signs may not develop for several hours or days after the injury.

Not all of these signs and symptoms are present in every fracture. Many are not present with linear or fissure fractures or with impacted fractures (fractured surfaces are driven together). The diagnosis of a fracture depends on the patient's symptoms, the physical signs, and x-ray examination. Usually, the patient reports having sustained an injury to the area.

Emergency Management

Immediately after injury, a person may be in a state of confusion, be unaware of a fracture, and attempt to walk on a fractured leg. Therefore, when a fracture is suspected, it is important to immobilize that body part immediately before the patient is moved. If an injured patient must be removed from a vehicle before splints can be applied, the extremity is supported above and below the fracture site to prevent rotation as well as angular motion. Movement of fracture fragments will cause additional pain, soft-tissue damage, and bleeding.

The pain associated with a fracture is severe and can be reduced by preventing movement of the bone fragments and joints adjacent to the fracture. Adequate splinting is essential to prevent damage to the soft tissue by the bony fragments.

The injured area is immobilized by applying temporary, well-padded splints, which are then firmly bandaged over the clothing. Immobilization of the long bones of the lower extremities also may be accomplished by bandaging the extremities together, with the unaffected extremity serving as a splint for the injured one. In an upper extremity injury, the arm may be bandaged to the chest, or an injured forearm may be placed in a sling. The circulation distal to the injury should be assessed to determine adequacy of peripheral tissue perfusion.

In an *open fracture,* the wound is covered with a clean (sterile) dressing to prevent contamination of deeper tissues. No attempt is made to reduce the fracture, even if one of the bone fragments is protruding through the wound. Splints are applied as described above.

In the emergency department, the patient is evaluated completely. The clothes are gently removed, first from the uninjured side of the body and then from the injured side. The patient's clothing may have to be cut away on the injured side. The fractured extremity is moved as little as possible to avoid more damage.

CHART 64-1
The Treatment of Fractures

Goals of Fracture Treatment

- Restore fracture fragments to their normal anatomic position (reduction).
- Maintain reduction in place until healing occurs (immobilization).
- Promote regaining of normal function and strength of the affected part (rehabilitation).

Methods for Obtaining Fracture Reduction

- Closed reduction
- Traction
- Open reduction

Methods for Maintaining Immobilization

- External devices
  - Splint
  - Brace
  - Case
  - Pins in plaster
  - External fixator
  - Traction
  - Bandage
- Internal devices
  - Nails
  - Plates
  - Screws
  - Wires
  - Rods

Maintaining and Restoring Function

- Maintain reduction and immobilization
- Elevate to minimize swelling
- Monitor neurovascular status
- Control anxiety and pain
- Isometric and muscle-setting exercises
- Participation in activities of daily living
- Gradual resumption of activities

Principles of Managing Fracture

The principles of fracture treatment include reduction, immobilization, and regaining of normal function and strength through rehabilitation (Chart 64-1).

Fracture Reduction. Reduction of a fracture ("setting" the bone) refers to restoration of the fracture fragments into anatomic alignment and rotation.

Closed reduction, traction, or open reduction may be used to reduce a fracture. The specific method selected depends on the nature of the fracture; however, the underlying principles are the same. Usually the physician reduces fractures as soon as possible to prevent tissues from losing their elasticity from infiltration by edema or hemorrhage. In most cases, fracture reduction becomes more difficult as the injury begins healing.

Before fracture reduction and immobilization, the patient is prepared for the procedure; permission for the procedure is obtained, and an analgesic is administered as prescribed. Anesthesia may be administered. The extremity that is to be manipulated must be handled gently to avoid additional damage.

Closed Reduction. In most instances, closed reduction is accomplished by bringing the bone fragments into apposition (ends in contact) by **manipulation** and **manual traction.**

The extremity is held in the desired position while a cast, splint, or other device is applied by the physician. The immobilizing device maintains the reduction and stabilizes the extremity for bone healing. X-rays are obtained to determine that the bone fragments are correctly aligned.

Traction. Traction may be used to effect fracture reduction and immobilization. The amount of traction is modified as muscle spasm is overcome. X-rays are used to monitor the fracture reduction and approximation of the bony fragments. As the fracture heals, evidence of callus formation is noted on x-ray. When the callus is well established, a cast or splint may be used for continued immobilization. Use of traction and the nursing management of a patient in traction are discussed more fully in Chapter 62.

Open Reduction. Some fractures require open reduction. Through a surgical approach the fracture fragments are reduced. Internal fixation devices in the form of metallic pins, wires, screws, plates, nails, or rods may be used to hold the bone fragments in position until solid bone healing occurs. These devices may be attached to the sides of bone or inserted through the bony fragments or directly into the medullary cavity of the bone (Fig. 64-3); they ensure firm approximation and fixation of the bony fragments.

Fracture Immobilization. After the fracture has been reduced, bone fragments must be immobilized, or held in correct position and alignment until union has had

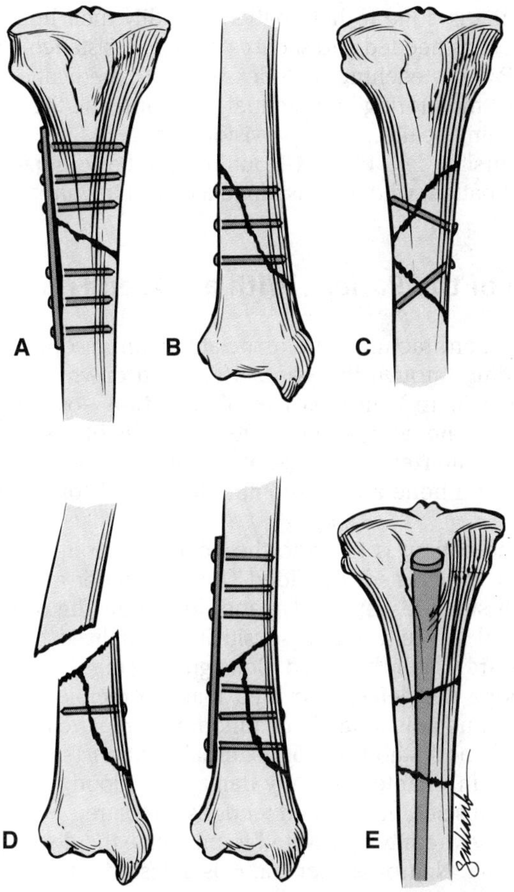

FIGURE 64-3. Techniques of internal fixation. (**A**) Plate and six screws for a transverse or short oblique fracture. (**B**) Screws for a long oblique or spiral fracture. (**C**) Screws for a long butterfly fragment. (**D**) Plate and six screws for a short butterfly fragment. (**E**) Medullary nail for a segmental fracture.

time to take place. Immobilization may be accomplished by external or internal fixation. Methods of external fixation include bandages, casts, splints, continuous traction, pin and plaster technique, or external fixators. Metal implants used for internal fixation serve as internal splints to immobilize the fracture.

Maintaining and Restoring Function. Efforts are directed toward facilitating bone and soft tissue healing. Reduction and immobilization are maintained as prescribed. Swelling is controlled by elevating the injured extremity and applying ice as prescribed. Neurovascular status (*i.e.*, assessment of circulation, pain, sensation, movement) is monitored, and the orthopedic surgeon is notified immediately if signs of neurovascular compromise are identified. Restlessness, anxiety, and discomfort are controlled with a variety of approaches (*i.e.*, reassurance; position changes; pain relief strategies, including analgesics). Isometric and muscle setting exercises are encouraged to minimize disuse atrophy and to promote circulation. Participation in activities of daily living is encouraged to promote independent functioning and self-esteem. Gradual resumption of activities is promoted within the therapeutic prescription. Usually, internal fixation allows for early mobilization. The surgeon estimates the stability of the fracture fixation, determines the amount of movement and stress the extremity can withstand, and prescribes the level of activity and weight-bearing. (See Chapter 62 for Nursing Process: The Patient in a Cast; The Patient in Traction; The Patient Undergoing Orthopedic Surgery.)

Factors Affecting Healing of Fracture. Weeks to months are required for most fractures to heal. Many factors influence the speed with which fractures heal (Chart 64-2). The reduction of the displaced fracture fragments must be accurate and successfully maintained to ensure healing. The affected bone must have an adequate blood supply. The age of the patient and the type of fracture also affect healing time. In general, fractures of flat bones (pelvis, scapula) heal quite rapidly. Fractures at the ends of long bones, where the bone is more vascular and cancellous, heal more quickly than do fractures in areas where the bone is dense and less vascular (midshaft). Weight-bearing will stimulate healing of stabilized fractures of the long bones in the lower extremities. In addition, activity minimizes the development of immobility-related **osteoporosis** (a reduction of total bone mass, producing porous and fragile bones because of imbalance in homeostatic bone turnover). Table 64-1 shows the approximate immobilization times necessary for union of the most common types of fractures.

If fracture healing is disrupted, the bone union time may be delayed or stopped completely. Factors that may interrupt fracture healing include inadequate blood supply

CHART 64-2
Factors Affecting Fracture Healing

Factors Enhancing Fracture Healing

- Immobilization of fracture fragments
- Maximum bone fragment contact
- Sufficient blood supply
- Proper nutrition
- Exercise—weight-bearing for long bones
- Hormones—growth hormone, thyroid, calcitonin, vitamin D, anabolic steroids
- Electric potential across fracture

Factors Inhibiting Fracture Healing

- Extensive local trauma
- Bone loss
- Inadequate immobilization
- Space/tissue between bone fragments
- Infection
- Local malignancy
- Metabolic bone diseases (*e.g.*, Paget's disease)
- Irradiated bone (radiation necrosis)
- Avascular necrosis
- Intra-articular fracture (synovial fluid contains fibrolysins, which lyse the initial clot and retard clot formation)
- Age (elderly persons heal more slowly)
- Corticosteroids (inhibit the repair rate)

TABLE 64-1 Approximate Immobilization Time Necessary for Union

Fracture	Number of Weeks
Phalanx (finger)	3–5
Metacarpal	6
Carpal	6
Scaphoid	10 (or until x-ray shows union)
Radius and ulna	10–12
Humerus:	
Supracondylar	8
Midshaft	8–12
Proximal (impacted)	3
Proximal (displaced)	6–8
Clavicle	6–10
Vertebra	16
Pelvis	6
Femur:	
Intracapsular	24
Intratrochanteric	10–12
Shaft	18
Supracondylar	12–15
Tibia:	
Proximal	8–10
Shaft	14–20
Malleolus	6
Calcaneus	12–16
Metatarsal	6
Phalanx (toe)	3

(Compare EL et al. Pictorial Handbook of Fracture Treatment, 5th ed. Chicago, Year Book Medical Publishers.)

to the fracture site or adjacent tissue, extensive space between bone fragments, interposition of soft tissue between bone ends, inadequate fracture immobilization, infection, complications from the treatment, and metabolic problems.

Care of the Patient With a Closed Fracture

Patients with closed (simple) fractures are encouraged to return to their usual activities as rapidly as possible. Fracture healing and restoration of full strength and mobility may take months. Patients are taught how to control swelling and pain associated with the fracture and soft-tissue trauma. They are encouraged to be active within the limits of the fracture immobilization. Bed rest is kept to a minimum. Exercises are begun to maintain the health of unaffected muscles and to increase strength of muscles needed for transferring and for using assistive devices (*e.g.*, crutches, walker). Patients are taught how to use these devices safely. Planning is done to help patients modify their home environment as needed and secure personal assistance if necessary. Patient teaching includes self-care, medication information, monitoring for potential problems, and the need for continuing health care supervision.

Nursing Care Plan 64-1 outlines the basic nursing care for the patient who has sustained a closed fracture.

Care of the Patient With an Open Fracture

In an open fracture (one associated with an open wound extending through the skin surface and down to the area of bone injury) there is risk of **infection**—osteomyelitis, gas gangrene, and tetanus. The objectives of management are to minimize the chance of infection of the wound, soft tissue, and bone and to promote healing of soft tissue and bone.

The patient is taken to the operating room, where the wound is cleansed, debrided (foreign matter and devitalized tissue are removed), and irrigated. The wound is swabbed for culture and sensitivity. Devitalized bone fragments are usually removed. Bone grafting may be necessary to bridge the defect, provided that the recipient tissue is healthy and able to facilitate union. The fracture is carefully reduced and stabilized by external fixation (see External Fixators in Chapter 62). Any damage to blood vessels, soft tissue, muscles, nerves, and tendons is repaired.

The extremity is elevated to minimize the development of edema. Neurovascular status is assessed frequently. The patient's temperature is taken at regular intervals, and the patient is monitored for signs of infection.

Primary closure may not be accomplished because of edema and potential ischemia, restricted wound drainage, and anaerobic infection. A heavily contaminated wound may be left unsutured, dressed with sterile gauze, and not closed until it is determined that the area is not infected. Tetanus prophylaxis is administered. Usually, intravenous antibiotics are prescribed to prevent or treat serious infection. The wound is closed by suture or by autogenous skin or flap graft in 5 to 7 days.

Complications of Fractures

Early Complications

The early complications after fracture are shock, which may be fatal within a few hours after injury; fat embolism, which may occur within 48 hours or later; and compartment syndrome, which may result in permanent loss of extremity function if not treated promptly. Other early complications associated with fracture are infection; thromboembolism (pulmonary embolism), which may cause death several weeks after injury; and disseminated intravascular coagulopathy (DIC).

Shock. Hypovolemic or traumatic shock, resulting from hemorrhage (both external and nonvisible blood loss) and loss of extracellular fluid into damaged tissues, may occur in fractures of the extremities, thorax, pelvis, and spine. Because the bone is very vascular, large quantities of blood

NURSING CARE PLAN 64–1
Care of the Patient With a Closed Fracture

NURSING DIAGNOSIS: Pain related to fracture

GOAL: Relief of pain

Nursing Interventions	Rationale	Expected Outcomes
1. Assess type and location of patient's pain and discomfort.	1. Pain and tenderness are expected with fracture and tissue damage; muscle spasms occur in response to injury and immobilization.	• Patient describes discomfort • Keeps injured extremity elevated • Uses ice during first 24 hours • Controls edema; neurovascular status intact • Uses relaxation techniques. • Demonstrates methods to control pain and swelling • Performs active and passive range-of-motion exercises on nonimmobilized joints; changes position frequently • Obtains pain relief
2. Assess patient's discomfort.	2. Pain assessment provides basis for planning nursing interventions.	
3. Use measures to control pain:	3.	
a. Splint and support injured area.	a. Prevents additional injury; minimizes movement of fracture fragments.	
b. Perform position changes gently.	b. Decreases muscle spasms.	
c. Elevate injured extremity to heart level.	c. Controls edema by promoting drainage.	
d. Apply ice, if prescribed.	d. Ice decreases pain and controls bleeding and edema.	
e. Monitor swelling and neurovascular status.	e. Edema and bleeding into the traumatized tissues cause discomfort; unrelenting pain may indicate compartment syndrome.	
f. Administer analgesics as prescribed early in pain experience.	f. Oral analgesics provide pain relief after fracture; control techniques are more effective early in pain cycle.	
g. Suggest relaxation techniques.	g. Modifies pain experience.	
4. Offer explanation of nursing measures to control pain, swelling, and additional tissue damage.	4. Damaged tissues cause pain; immobilization decreases discomfort from movement of fracture fragments; understanding of cause of pain reduces patient's perception of pain.	
5. Encourage active and passive range-of-motion exercises for nonimmobilized joints; encourage position changes as permitted within limits of immobilizing device.	5. Pressure on bony prominences and disuse contribute to discomfort.	
6. Minimize the time the injured extremity is in dependent position.	6. Swelling will occur in injured tissues when dependent; swelling contributes to discomfort.	

NURSING DIAGNOSIS: Risk for injury related to neurovascular compromise, pressure, and disuse

GOAL: Achievement of uncomplicated healing

Nursing Interventions	Rationale	Expected Outcomes
1. Assess for the development of neurovascular compromise: a. Increasing pain b. Cool skin temperature c. Increasing swelling d. Decreased motor abilities e. Abnormal sensations f. Diminished capillary refill	1. Early recognition of circulation and nerve problems due to compartment syndrome is needed to prevent loss of function.	• Neurovascular status distal to fracture is intact • Describes signs and symptoms of neurovascular compromise • Shows no evidence of skin breakdown • Describes signs and symptoms of skin breakdown • Reports problems to physician promptly
2. Teach the signs and symptoms of neurovascular compromise.	2. Patient education is needed for participation in care.	

(continued)

NURSING CARE PLAN 64–1 *(continued)*
Care of the Patient With a Closed Fracture

Nursing Interventions	Rationale	Expected Outcomes
3. Assess for the development of skin breakdown: a. Skin abrasion b. Cast "hot spots" c. Drainage d. Irritation sensations	3. Pressure of casts and appliances can cause skin breakdown.	• Participates in activities that will minimize diminished muscle function and loss of joint motion
4. Teach the signs and symptoms of skin breakdown.	4. Patient education is needed for self-care.	
5. Encourage active exercise and range-of-motion exercise of body parts not immobilized.	5. Disuse results in atrophy of muscles and loss of joint motion.	
6. Encourage isometric exercises of immobilized muscles.	6. Maintains muscle function and promotes self-care.	

NURSING DIAGNOSIS: Self-care deficit related to disruption of ability to perform activities of daily living

GOAL: Patient demonstrates satisfactory adjustment to altered performance of activities of daily living.

Nursing Interventions	Rationale	Expected Outcomes
1. Encourage patient to express concerns and to discuss injury and problems associated with injury. Listen actively.	1. Fractures result from accidents and affect one's ability to perform activities of daily living. Life-style is interrupted. Time loss from employment occurs.	• Patient discusses injury and its impact on life • Uses available resources and coping mechanisms to modify emotional stress
2. Support use of coping mechanisms.	2. Sudden disruption of routines and plans requires use of coping mechanisms.	• Participates in development of health care plan
3. Involve significant others and support services as needed and appropriate.	3. Others can assist patient with activities of daily living.	• Participates in activities of daily living • Demonstrates safe use of treatment modalities and mobilization aids
4. Modify home environment as necessary.	4. Accommodations for home management of fracture may be necessary to promote self-care and safety.	• Achieves appropriate level of self-care at home
5. Encourage patient participation in development of treatment regimen.	5. Patient regains independence by active participation in treatment plan decisions.	
6. Explain various facets of treatment regimen.	6. Patient education and understanding of rationale increase compliance.	
7. Encourage active participation in activities of daily living within therapeutic limits.	7. Self-esteem is enhanced through self-care activities.	
8. Teach safe use of treatment modalities and mobilization aids. Supervise use to assure safety.	8. Injury from unsafe use of modalities or mobilization aids can be prevented through education.	
9. Evaluate patient's ability to care for self at home: a. Planned treatment regimen b. Recognition of potential problems c. Recognition of unsafe situations d. Continued health supervision	9. Ensures patient's ability to manage fracture at home. Lack of knowledge and poor preparation for self-care at home contribute to anxiety and nonadherence to therapeutic regimen.	

may be lost as a result of trauma, especially in fractures of the femur and pelvis.

Treatment consists of restoring blood volume, relieving the patient's pain, providing adequate splinting, and protecting the patient from further injury (see Chapter 15).

Fat Embolism Syndrome. After fracture of long bones or pelvis, multiple fractures, or crush injuries, fat emboli may develop, especially in the young adult (20 to 30 years old) male. At the time of fracture, fat globules may move into the blood because the marrow pressure is greater than the capillary pressure or because catecholamines elevated by the patient's stress reaction mobilize fatty acids and promote the development of fat globules in the bloodstream. The fat globules combine with platelets to form emboli, which then block the small blood vessels that supply the brain, lungs, kidneys, and other organs. The onset of symptoms, which is rapid, may occur from a few hours to up to a week after injury, but usually occurs within 24 to 72 hours.

The presenting features include hypoxia, tachypnea, tachycardia, and pyrexia. Cerebral disturbances are manifested by mental status changes varying from mild agitation and confusion to delirium and coma that occur in response to hypoxia, due to the lodging of fat emboli in the brain.

The respiratory response includes tachypnea, dyspnea, crackles, wheezes, large amounts of thick white sputum, and tachycardia. Blood gases show PO_2 below 60 mm Hg, with an early respiratory alkalosis and later respiratory acidosis. The chest x-ray exhibits a typical "snow storm" infiltrate. Adult respiratory distress syndrome and heart failure develop.

With systemic embolization the patient appears pale. Petechiae are noted in the buccal membranes and conjunctival sacs, on the hard palate, on the fundus of the eye, and over the chest and anterior axillary folds. Free fat may be found in the urine when emboli reach the kidneys. Kidney failure may develop.

- Subtle personality changes, restlessness, irritability, or confusion in a patient who has sustained a fracture is an indication for immediate blood gas studies. Occlusion of a large number of small vessels causes the pulmonary pressure to rise, possibly resulting in acute right ventricular heart failure. Edema and hemorrhages in the alveoli impair oxygen transport, leading to hypoxia. There is an increase in respiratory rate, precordial chest pain, cough, dyspnea, and acute pulmonary edema.

Prevention and Management. Immediate immobilization of fractures, minimal fracture manipulation, and adequate support for fractured bones during turning and positioning are measures that may reduce the incidence of fat emboli. Monitoring high-risk patients (*e.g.*, adult males between 20 and 30 years of age, those with altered mental status) assists in the early identification of this problem. Prompt initiation of respiratory support is essential.

The objectives of management are to support the respiratory system and to correct homeostatic disturbances. Arterial blood gas analysis is performed to determine the degree of respiratory impairment, as respiratory failure is the most common cause of death. Respiratory support is provided with oxygen given in high concentrations. Controlled volume ventilation with positive end-expiratory pressure (PEEP) may be employed to prevent or treat pulmonary edema. Corticosteroids may be given to treat the inflammatory lung reaction and to control cerebral edema. Vasoactive medications to support cardiovascular function are given to prevent hypotension, shock, and interstitial pulmonary edema. Accurate intake and output records facilitate adequate fluid replacement therapy. Morphine may be prescribed for pain and anxiety for the patient on a ventilator. In addition, to allay apprehension, calm reassurance is provided. The patient's response to therapy is closely monitored.

Because fat emboli are a major cause of death in patients with fractures, respiratory support must be instituted early. The nurse must recognize early indications of fat embolism syndrome and report them to the physician for medical management.

Compartment Syndrome. Compartment syndrome is a problem that develops when tissue perfusion in the muscles is less than that required for tissue viability. This can be due to (1) reduction of the muscle compartment size because the enclosing muscle fascia is too tight or a cast or dressing is constrictive, or (2) an increase in muscle compartment contents because of edema or hemorrhage associated with a variety of problems (*e.g.*, ischemia, crush injuries, injection of tissue-destroying [toxic] substances, fractures). The forearm and the leg muscle compartments are involved most frequently. Permanent function can be lost if the situation continues for more than 6 to 8 hours and myoneural (muscle and nerve) ischemia and necrosis occur. Volkmann's contracture is an example of this complication.

The patient complains of deep, throbbing, unrelenting pain, which is not controlled by opioids. Palpation of the muscle, if possible, will reveal it to be swollen and hard. The actual tissue pressure can be monitored by inserting a fluid-filled needle or wick catheter into the compartment and determining the pressure with a pressure transducer monitoring setup (see Fig. 62-1). (Normal pressure is 8 mm Hg or less.) Nerve and muscle tissues deteriorate as compartment pressure increases. Prolonged pressure of 30 to 40 mm Hg can result in compromised microcirculation. Nerve tissue is more sensitive to elevated tissue pressures than muscle. Paresthesias generally occur before paralysis.

Passive stretching movement of the muscle will cause acute pain. If it does not, the patient's pain may be due to nerve ischemia.

Major arteries are not occluded by compartment syndrome. Tissue pressure would need to be above the systolic blood pressure to occlude arteries. Therefore, peripheral pulses are present with compartment syndrome but may be obscured by edema. Pulselessness is a sign of arterial occlusion and not compartment syndrome.

Prevention and Management. Compartment syndrome can be prevented by controlling edema, which is achieved by elevating the injured extremity to heart level and applying ice after injury as prescribed. If compartment syndrome occurs, restrictive dressings must be loosened. A fasciotomy (surgical excision of the fibrous membrane covering and separating muscles) may be needed if conservative measures do not restore tissue perfusion and relieve pain within 1 hour. Elevated tissue pressure warranting fasciotomy depends on multiple factors, including systolic blood pressure and hemodynamic status. After fasciotomy, the wound is not sutured but rather is left open and covered with moist sterile saline dressings. The limb is splinted in a functional position and passive range-of-motion exercises are usually prescribed every 4 to 6 hours. In 3 to 5 days, when the edema has resolved and tissue perfusion has been restored, the wound is debrided and closed.

Other Early Complications. Thromboembolism, infection (all open fractures are considered to be contaminated), and disseminated intravascular coagulopathy (DIC) are other possible complications of fractures. DIC includes a group of bleeding disorders with diverse causes, including massive tissue trauma. Manifestations of DIC include ecchymoses, unexpected bleeding after surgery, and bleeding from the mucous membranes, venipuncture sites, and gastrointestinal and urinary tracts. The treatment of DIC is discussed in Chapter 32.

Delayed Complications

Delayed Union and Nonunion. Delayed union occurs when healing does not advance at a normal rate for the location and type of fracture. Delayed union may be associated with systemic infection and distraction (pulling apart) of bone fragments. Eventually, the fracture heals.

Nonunion results from failure of the ends of a fractured bone to unite. The patient complains of persistent discomfort and movement at the fracture site. Factors contributing to union problems include infection at the fracture site; interposition of tissue between the bone ends; inadequate immobilization or manipulation, which disrupts callus formation; excessive space between bone fragments (bone gap); limited bone contact; and impaired blood supply resulting in avascular necrosis.

In nonunion, fibrocartilage or fibrous tissue exists between the bone fragments; no bone salts have been deposited. A false joint (**pseudarthrosis**) often develops at the site of the fracture. Fractures of the middle third of the humerus, the neck of the femur in elderly people, and the lower third of the tibia most frequently result in nonunion.

Nonunion may be managed by bone grafting. Surgically, the fractured bone fragments are trimmed, infection (if present) is removed, and a bone graft, frequently from the iliac crest, is placed in the bony defect. The bone graft provides a lattice work for invasion by bone cells. After grafting, rigid immobilization is required.

Electrical Stimulation of Osteogenesis. Osteogenesis in nonunion may be stimulated by electrical impulses; its effectiveness is similar to that of bone grafting. It is not effective with large bone gaps or synovial pseudarthrosis. The electrical stimulation modifies the tissue environment, making it electronegative, which enhances mineral deposition and bone formation.

In some situations, pins that act as cathodes are inserted percutaneously directly into the fracture site, and electrical impulses are directed to the fracture continuously. Direct current methods cannot be used when infection is present.

Another method is noninvasive inductive coupling. Pulsing electromagnetic fields (PEMFs) are delivered to the fracture for 3 to 10 hours a day by an electromagnetic coil implanted in the dressing over the nonunion site (Fig. 64-4). During the electrical stimulation treatment period, which takes about 3 to 6 months, rigid fracture fixation with adequate support is needed.

Avascular Necrosis of Bone. Avascular necrosis occurs when the bone loses its blood supply and dies. It may follow a fracture (especially of the femoral neck), dislocations, prolonged high-dosage corticosteroid therapy, chronic renal disease, sickle cell anemia, and other diseases. The devitalized bone may collapse or reabsorb and be replaced by new bone. The patient develops pain and experiences limited movement. X-rays reveal calcium loss and structural collapse. Treatment generally consists of attempts to revitalize the bone with bone grafts, prosthetic replacement, or **arthrodesis** (joint fusion).

Reaction to Internal Fixation Devices. Internal fixation devices may be removed after bony union has taken place, but for the majority of patients a device is not removed unless it produces symptoms. Pain and decreased function are the prime indicators that a problem has developed. Such problems may include mechanical failure

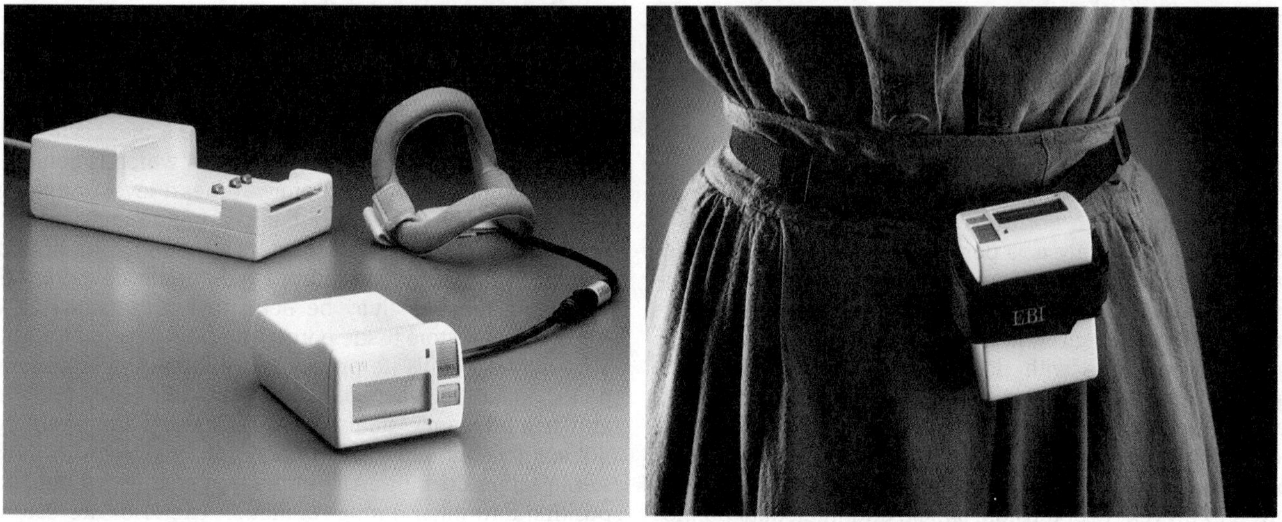

FIGURE 64-4. Electromagnetic bone-healing stimulator (**left**). Pulsed electromagnetic fields generated through the coils produce bone growth (osteogenesis) at the fracture site. The system is portable and battery powered (**right**). The therapy is used for 3 to 10 hours a day. (Courtesy of EBI Medical Systems, Inc., Parsippany, NJ.)

(inadequate insertion and stabilization); material failure (faulty or damaged devices); corrosion of the device, causing local inflammation; allergic response to the metallic alloy used; and osteoporotic remodeling adjacent to the fixation device (stress needed for bone strength is carried by the device, causing a disuse osteoporosis). If the device is removed, the bone needs to be protected from refracture related to osteoporosis, altered bone structure, and trauma. Bone remodeling reestablishes the bone's structural strength.

Fractures of Specific Sites

An injury to the skeletal structure may vary from a simple linear fracture to a severe crushing injury. Therapeutic management is determined by the type and location of the fracture and the extent of damage to surrounding structures. Maximum functional recovery is the goal of management.

Appendicular Skeletal Fractures

Clavicle Fractures

Fracture of the clavicle (collar bone) is a common injury that results from a fall or a direct blow to the shoulder. Associated head or cervical spinal cord injuries are often seen with these fractures.

The clavicle helps to hold the shoulder upward, outward, and backward from the thorax. Therefore, when the clavicle is fractured, the patient assumes a protective position—slumping the shoulders and immobilizing the arm to prevent shoulder movements. The treatment goal is to hold the shoulder in its normal position by means of closed reduction and immobilization.

More than 80% of these fractures occur in the middle or inner two-thirds of the clavicle. A modified shoulder spica (clavicular cast) or a figure-of-eight bandage or a commercially available clavicular strap (Fig. 64-5) may be used to reduce the fracture, pull the shoulders back, and hold them in this position. When a clavicular strap is used, the axillae are well padded to prevent a compression injury to the brachial plexus and axillary artery. Circulation and nerve function of both arms are monitored.

Fracture of the distal third of the clavicle without displacement and ligament disruption is treated with a sling and restricted motion of the arm. When a fracture in the distal third is accompanied by a disrupted coracoclavicular ligament, there is displacement, which may be treated by open reduction and internal fixation.

Complications of clavicular fractures include trauma to the nerves of the brachial plexus, injury to the subclavian vein or artery from a bony fragment, and malunion. Malunion may be a cosmetic problem when low-neckline clothing is worn.

Patient Education and Home Care Considerations. The patient is cautioned not to elevate the arm above shoulder level until the ends of the bone have united (about 6 weeks) but is encouraged to exercise the elbow, wrist, and fingers as soon as possible. When prescribed, shoulder exercises (Fig. 64-6) are performed to obtain full shoulder motion. Vigorous activity is limited for 3 months.

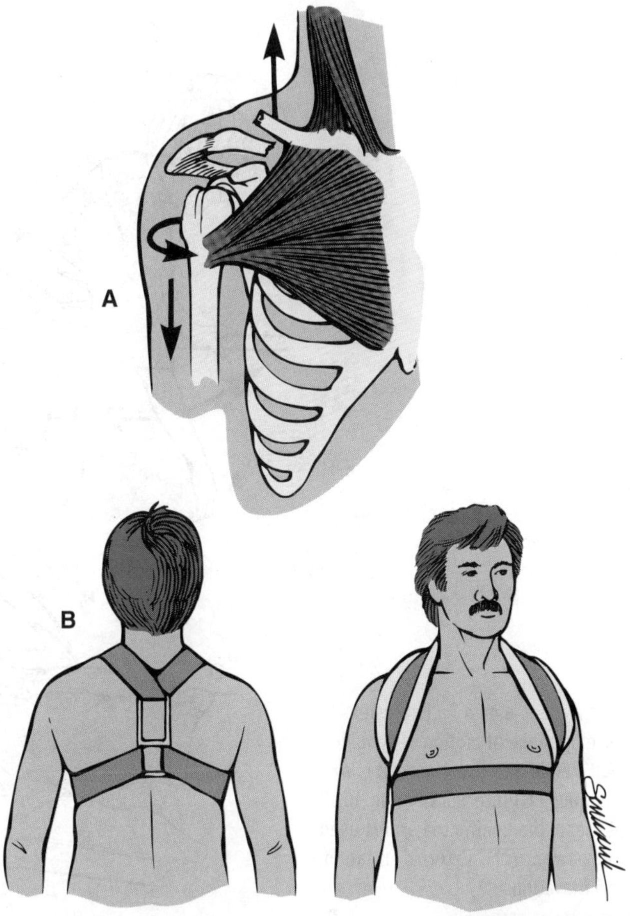

FIGURE 64-5. Fracture of the clavicle. (**A**) Anteroposterior view, showing typical displacement of midclavicle fracture. (**B**) Method of immobilization with a clavicular strap.

Upper Extremity Fractures

Fractures of the Humeral Neck

Fractures of the proximal humerus may occur through either the anatomic or the surgical neck of the humerus. The anatomic neck is located just below the humeral head. The surgical neck is the region below the tubercles. Impacted fractures of the surgical neck of the humerus are seen most frequently in older women after a fall on an outstretched arm. These are essentially nondisplaced fractures. Active middle-aged patients may suffer severely displaced humeral neck fractures with associated rotator cuff damage.

The patient presents with the affected arm hanging limp at the side and supported by the uninjured hand. Neurovascular assessment of the involved extremity is essential to fully evaluate the extent of injury and possible involvement of the neurovascular bundle (nerves and blood vessels) of the arm.

Many impacted fractures of the surgical neck of the humerus are not displaced and do not require reduction. The arm is supported and immobilized by a sling and swathe that secure the supported arm to the trunk (Fig. 64-7). A soft pad is placed in the axilla to absorb moisture and avoid skin breakdown. Limitation of motion and stiffness of the shoulder occur from disuse; therefore,

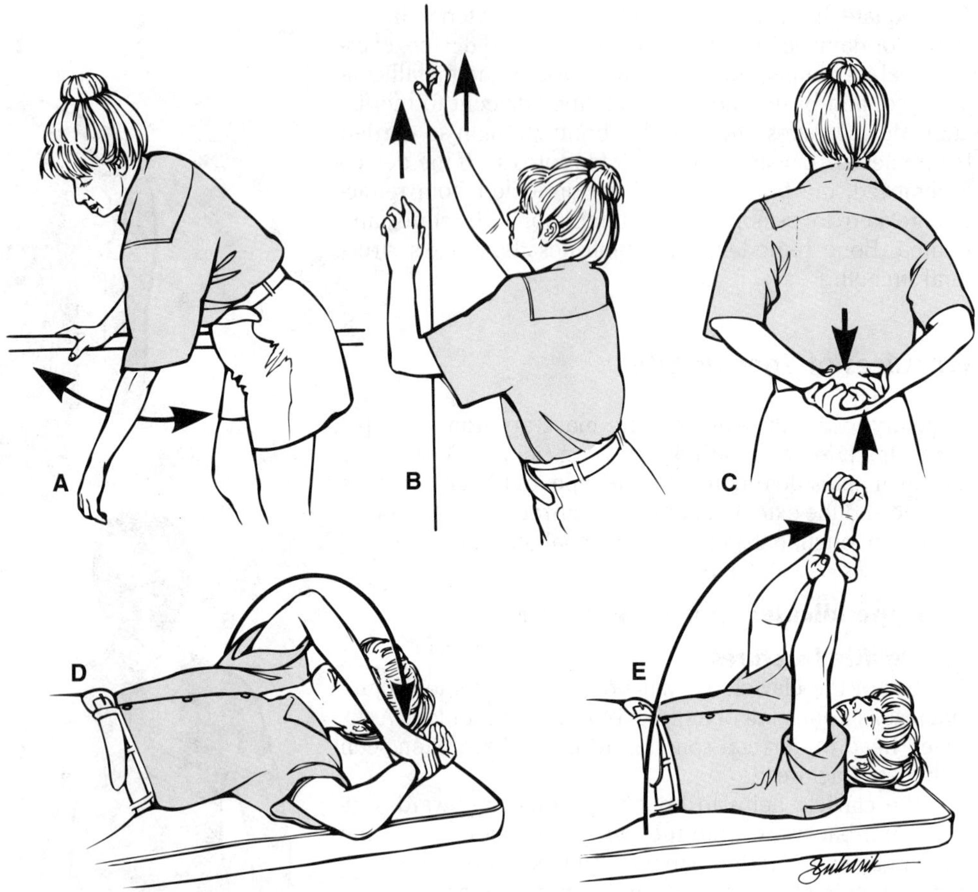

FIGURE 64-6. Exercises to develop range of motion of shoulder. (**A**) Pendulum exercise. (**B**) Wall climbing. (**C**) Internal rotation. In all of these, the unaffected arm is used for power. (**D**) External rotation. (**E**) Elevation.

pendulum exercises are begun as soon as tolerated by the patient. (In pendulum or circumduction exercises, the patient is instructed to lean forward and allow the affected arm to abduct and rotate [see Fig. 64-6].) Early motion of the joint does not displace the fragments if motion is carried out within the limits imposed by pain.

These fractures require 6 to 10 weeks to heal, and the patient should avoid vigorous activity, such as tennis, for an additional 4 weeks. Residual stiffness, aching, and some limitation of range of motion may persist for 6 or more months.

When a humeral neck fracture is displaced, treatment consists of closed reduction with x-ray visualization, open reduction, or replacement of the humeral head with a prosthesis. In this type of fracture, exercises are started only after a prescribed period of immobilization.

Fractures of the Shaft of the Humerus

Fractures of the shaft of the humerus are most frequently caused by (1) direct trauma that results in a transverse, oblique, or comminuted fracture, or (2) an indirect twisting force that results in a spiral fracture. The nerves and brachial blood vessels may be injured with these fractures. Wrist drop is indicative of radial nerve injury. Initial neurovascular assessment is essential to differentiate between trauma from the injury and complications from treatment.

Frequently, the weight of the arm helps to correct any displacement so that surgery is not required. With an oblique, spiral, or displaced fracture that has resulted in shortening of the humeral shaft, a hanging cast may be used. This cast is designed so that its weight provides traction to the arm when the patient is upright, thereby reducing and immobilizing the fracture. The hanging cast must be dependent (allowed to hang free without support) because the weight of the cast is the means by which continuous traction is applied to the long axis of the arm. The patient is advised to sleep in an upright position so that traction from the weight of the cast is maintained constantly. Complications encountered with this mode of therapy are fracture distraction (pulling fracture fragments too far apart) due to the weight of the cast and fracture angulation due to excessive fracture motion.

Finger exercises are started as soon as the cast is applied, and pendulum-shoulder exercises are performed as prescribed to provide active movement of the shoulder, thereby preventing adhesions of the shoulder joint capsule. Isometric exercises may be prescribed to prevent muscle atrophy.

After the cast is removed, a sling is applied and exercises of the shoulder, elbow, and wrist are begun. Humeral fractures require about 10 weeks to heal when treated with hanging casts.

Elderly patients may not tolerate a cast. A sling and swathe (see Fig. 64-7) may provide adequate comfort and immobilization. Shoulder exercises are begun in about 3 weeks.

Functional bracing is another form of treatment being used for these fractures. A hanging cast is applied for about

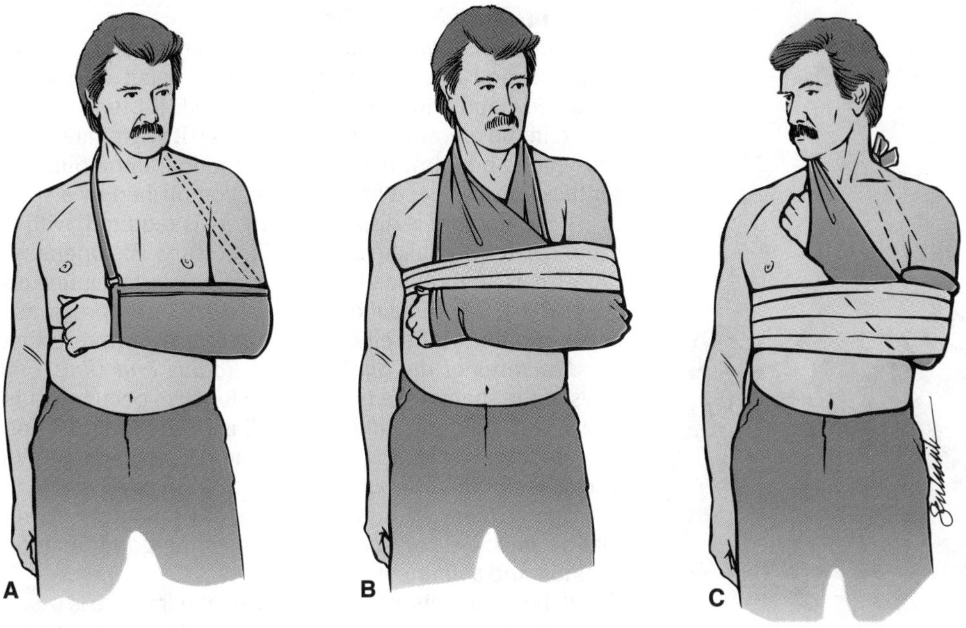

FIGURE 64-7. The types of immobilizing dressings used for proximal humeral fractures. (**A**) A commercial sling and swathe that permits easy removal of the arm for hygiene and is comfortable on the neck. (**B**) A conventional sling and swathe. (**C**) A stockinette Velpeau and swathe are used when there is an unstable surgical neck component, because this position relaxes the pectoralis major.

1 week, and then a contoured thermoplastic sleeve is secured in place with Velcro closures around the upper arm. As swelling decreases the Velcro is tightened, applying uniform pressure and stability to the fracture. Functional bracing allows active use of muscles, shoulder and elbow motion, and good approximation of fracture fragments. The callus that develops is substantial, and the sleeve can be discontinued in about 9 weeks.

Shoulder spica casts may be used during early treatment of unstable humerus fractures. Generally, the patient is uncomfortable and feels quite awkward.

Skeletal traction may be appropriate for patients who must remain in bed because of other injuries (Figs. 64-8 and 64-9). The patient is encouraged to perform active exercises of the hand and wrist.

Open fractures of the humeral shaft are frequently treated by external fixators (see Chapter 62). Open reduction of a humerus fracture is necessary with nerve palsy, pathologic fractures, or when other systemic or neurologic disease (*e.g.*, Parkinson's disease) would make management with a hanging cast inappropriate.

Fractures at the Elbow

Fractures of the distal humerus result from motor vehicle crashes, falls on the elbow (in the extended or flexed position), or a direct blow. These fractures may result in nerve damage from injury to the median, radial, or ulnar nerves. The patient is evaluated for paresthesias and signs of compromised circulation in the forearm and hand. The most serious complication of a supracondylar fracture of the humerus is Volkmann's ischemic contracture, which results from antecubital swelling or damage to the brachial artery.

The nurse must:

- Observe the hand for swelling, skin color, nailbed capillary refill, and temperature. The affected and unaffected hands are compared.
- Assess radial pulse.
- Assess for paresthesias (tingling and burning sensations) in the hand, because they may indicate nerve injury or impending ischemia.
- Assess for ability to move fingers.
- Assess intensity and character of pain.
- Directly measure tissue pressure as prescribed.
- Report indications of diminished nerve function or diminished circulatory perfusion promptly before

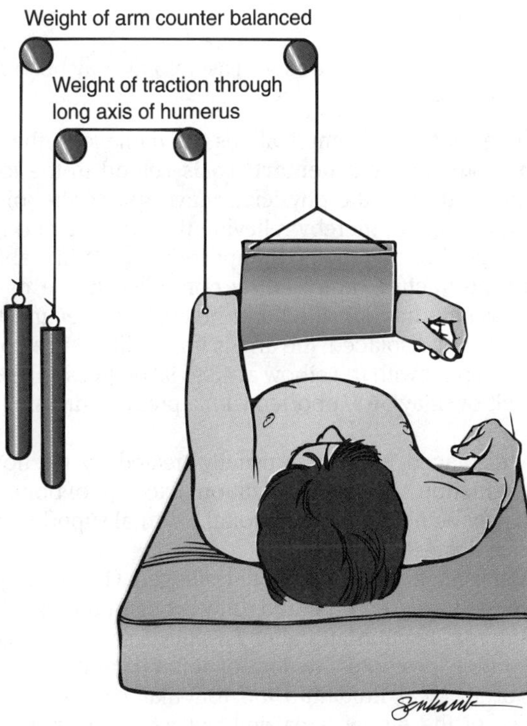

FIGURE 64-8. Over-the-face traction for supracondylar fracture reduces swelling by creating a very effective elevation of the extremity.

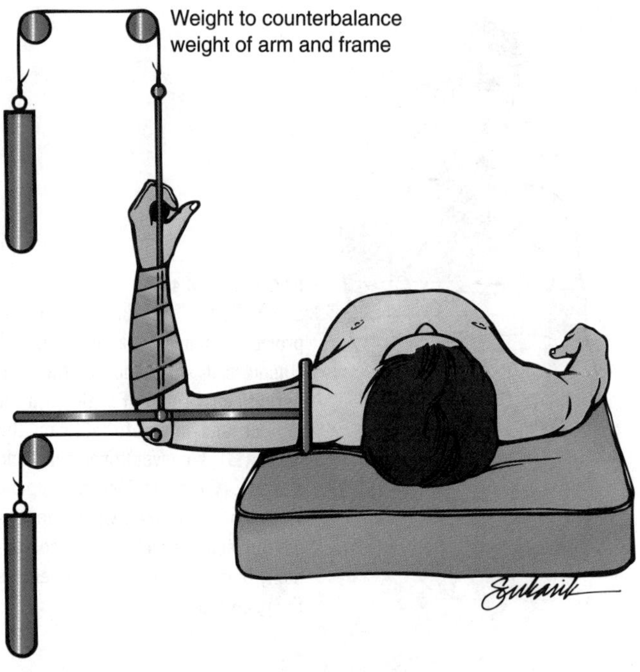

FIGURE 64-9. Balanced side-arm traction. The arm is passed through the ring, so that it encompasses the shoulder. The upright attachment for the forearm may be moved to accommodate the length of the humerus. A cloth sling is placed on the horizontal segment to provide a surface on which the arm may rest. The forearm is placed between the two upright supports and is usually held there with a circumferentially applied elastic bandage. A rope is attached to the vertical section and is passed through pulleys. A weight is attached to exactly counterbalance the weight of the arm and the frame. Skeletal traction is then applied in the desired amount through the pin in the olecranon. The entire extremity is counterbalanced so that a balanced traction system is created.

irreparable damage occurs. Fasciotomy may become necessary.

Other potential complications are damage to the joint articular surfaces and **hemarthrosis** (blood in the joint). With hemarthrosis, the physician may aspirate the joint to remove the blood, thereby relieving the pressure and pain.

The goal of therapy is prompt reduction and stabilization of the fracture, followed by controlled active motion when swelling has subsided and healing has begun. If the fracture is not displaced, the arm is immobilized in a cast or posterior splint with the elbow at 45 to 90 degrees of flexion, or the elbow may be supported with a pressure dressing and a sling.

A displaced fracture is usually treated by traction or open reduction and internal fixation. Excision of bone fragments may be necessary. Additional external support with a plaster splint is then applied.

Active finger exercises are encouraged. Gentle range-of-motion exercise of the injured joint is begun about 1 week after internal fixation and after 2 weeks with closed reduction. Motion promotes healing of injured joints by movement of synovial fluid into the articular cartilage. Active exercise of the elbow is carried out when prescribed, as residual limitation of motion may result without an intensive rehabilitation program.

Radial and Ulnar Fractures

Fractures of the Radial Head. Radial head fractures are common and are usually produced by a fall on the outstretched hand with the elbow extended. If blood has collected in the elbow joint (hemarthrosis), it is aspirated to relieve pain and allow early range of motion. Immobilization for these undisplaced fractures is accomplished by a splint.

If the fracture is displaced, surgery is required, with excision of the radial head when necessary. Postoperatively the arm is immobilized in a posterior plaster splint and sling. The patient is encouraged to carry out a program of active motion of the elbow and forearm when prescribed.

Fractures of the Shafts of the Radius and Ulna. Fractures of the shaft of the bones of the forearm occur most frequently in children. Either the radius or the ulna, or both, may be fractured at any level. Frequently, displacement occurs when both bones are broken.

The forearm's unique functions of pronation and supination must be preserved by maintaining good anatomic position and alignment.

If the fragments are not displaced, the fracture is treated by closed reduction with a long arm cast applied from the upper arm to the proximal palmar crease. A loop may be incorporated in the cast near the elbow and a sling pulled through it to prevent the cast from sagging against the forearm.

The circulation, motion, and sensation of the hand are assessed after the cast is applied. The arm is elevated to control edema. Frequent finger flexion and extension are encouraged to reduce edema. Active motion of the involved shoulder is essential. The reduction and alignment are monitored closely by x-ray to ensure adequate immobilization.

The fracture is immobilized for about 12 weeks; during the last 6 weeks the arm may be in a functional forearm brace that allows exercise of the wrist and elbow.

Displaced fractures are managed by open reduction with internal fixation, using a compression plate with screws, intramedullary nails, or rods. The arm is usually immobilized in a plaster splint, cast, or pressure dressing. Open fractures may be managed with external fixation devices. The arm is elevated to control swelling. Neurovascular status is monitored. Elbow, wrist, and hand exercises are begun as permitted by the immobilization device.

Fractures of the Wrist

Fractures of the distal radius (Colles's fracture) are common and are usually the result of a fall on an open dorsiflexed hand. This fracture is frequently seen in children and in elderly women with osteoporotic bones and weak soft tissues that do not dissipate the energy of the fall. The patient presents with a deformed wrist, radial deviation, pain, swelling, weakness, limited finger range of motion, and numbness.

Treatment usually consists of closed reduction and immobilization with a cast. For more severe fractures, a Kirschner wire may be inserted to maintain reduction. The wrist and forearm are elevated for 48 hours after reduction to control swelling.

Active motion of the fingers and shoulder is begun promptly. The patient is taught to do the following finger exercises to reduce swelling and prevent stiffness:

1. Hold the hand at the level of the heart.

2. Move the fingers from full extension to flexion. Hold and release. (Repeat at least 10 times every half hour when awake.)
3. Use the hand in functional activities.
4. Actively exercise the shoulder and elbow.

Fingers may swell from diminished venous and lymphatic return. The sensory function of the median nerve is assessed by pricking the distal aspect of the index finger, and the motor function is assessed by testing the ability to touch the thumb to the little finger. Diminished circulation and nerve function must be treated promptly by release of constricting casts and bandages.

Fracture of the Hand

Trauma to the hand often requires extensive reconstructive surgery. The objective of treatment is always to regain maximum function of the hand.

For an undisplaced fracture of the distal phalanx (finger bone), the finger is splinted for 3 to 4 weeks to relieve pain and protect the fingertip from further trauma. Displaced fractures and open fractures may require open reduction with internal fixation, using wires or pins.

The neurovascular status of the injured hand is evaluated. Swelling is controlled by elevation of the hand. Functional use of the uninvolved portions of the hand is encouraged.

Pelvic Fractures

The sacrum, ilium, pubis, and ischium bones form the pelvic bone, a fused, stable, bony ring in adults (Fig. 64-10). Pelvic fractures may be caused by falls, motor vehicle crashes, or crush injuries. General symptoms include ecchymosis; tenderness over the symphysis pubis, anterior iliac spines, iliac crest, sacrum, or coccyx; local swelling; and inability to bear weight without discomfort.

Pelvic fractures are serious because at least two-thirds of these patients have significant and multiple injuries. Management of severe, life-threatening pelvic fractures is coordinated with the trauma team. (The care of the patient with multiple injuries is discussed in Chapter 66.) A high mortality rate accompanies these fractures.

Hemorrhage and shock are two of the most serious consequences that may occur. Bleeding arises from the cancellous surfaces of the fracture fragments, from laceration of veins and arteries by bone spicules, and possibly from a torn iliac artery. The peripheral pulses of both lower extremities are palpated; absence of pulses may indicate a torn iliac artery or one of its branches. Peritoneal lavage may be performed to detect intra-abdominal hemorrhage. The patient is handled gently to minimize further bleeding and shock.

In addition to hemorrhage, the bladder, the urethra, or the intestines may be lacerated, resulting in conditions that can prove to be more serious than the fracture itself. To assess for urinary tract injury, the patient's urine is examined for blood. A voiding cystourethrogram and an intravenous urogram may be performed. Laceration of the urethra is suspected in males with anterior fracture of the pelvis and blood at the urethral meatus. (Females rarely experience lacerated urethra.) A catheter should not be inserted until the status of the urethra is known.

Hemorrhage, thoracic, intra-abdominal, and cranial injuries have priority over treatment of fractures. The nurse continues to assess for injuries to the bladder, rectum, intestines, other abdominal organs, and pelvic vessels and nerves. Paralytic ileus may accompany pelvic fractures and immobility. In addition, the patient is at risk for thrombophlebitis when immobilized or on bed rest. There is a high mortality rate associated with pelvic fractures from hemorrhage, pulmonary complications, fat emboli, intravascular coagulation, thromboembolic complications, and infection.

Numerous classification systems have been used to describe the pelvic fracture in relation to the anatomy, stability, and mechanism of injury. Some fractures of the pelvis do not disrupt the pelvic ring, whereas others disrupt the ring and may be rotationally and/or vertically unstable. The severity of pelvic fractures varies.

Stable fractures of the pelvis (Fig. 64-11) may include fracture of a single pubic or ischial ramus, fracture of ipsilateral pubic and ischial rami, fracture of the pelvic wing of ilium (*i.e.*, Duverney's fracture), or fracture of the sacrum or coccyx. Most fractures of the pelvis heal rapidly because the innominate bone (hip bone) is made up mostly of cancellous bone, which has a rich blood supply.

Stable pelvic fractures are treated with bed rest, using a bedboard under the mattress for additional firmness until the pain and discomfort resolve. Pelvic sling traction is rarely used because it is poorly tolerated by the patient. The patient in a pelvic sling complains of discomfort associated with the sling and is subject to developing skin breakdown.

The patient on bed rest is at risk for complications from immobility, including constipation, venous stasis, and pulmonary complications. Fluids, dietary fiber, ankle and leg exercises, log rolling, coughing and deep breathing, and skin care reduce the risk of complications and increase the patient's comfort. The patient with a fractured sacrum is at risk for paralytic ileus and bowel sounds should be monitored. The patient with fracture of the coccyx experiences pain on sitting and with defecation. Sitz baths may be prescribed to relieve pain, and stool softeners may be given to prevent the need to strain on defecation. As pain resolves, activity is gradually resumed.

Unstable fractures of the pelvis (Fig. 64-12) may be rotationally unstable (*e.g.*, the open book type in which separation occurs at the symphysis pubis) or vertically unstable (*e.g.*, vertical shear type with superior-inferior displacement of the sides of the pelvis) or a combination of both. Lateral or anterior-posterior compression of the pelvis produces rotationally unstable pelvic fractures. Vertically unstable pelvic fractures occur when force is exerted on the pelvis vertically, such as happens to those falling from a height onto extended legs or those struck from above by a falling object.

When an injury results in only a slight widening of the pubic symphysis and/or the anterior sacroiliac joint and the pelvic ligaments are intact and the patient is hemodynamically stable, the patient will be treated with bed rest. However, for rotationally unstable fractures, such as open book type fractures with symphysis pubis separation greater than 2 cm and some sacral ligament disruption, treatment generally involves external fixation or anterior open reduction

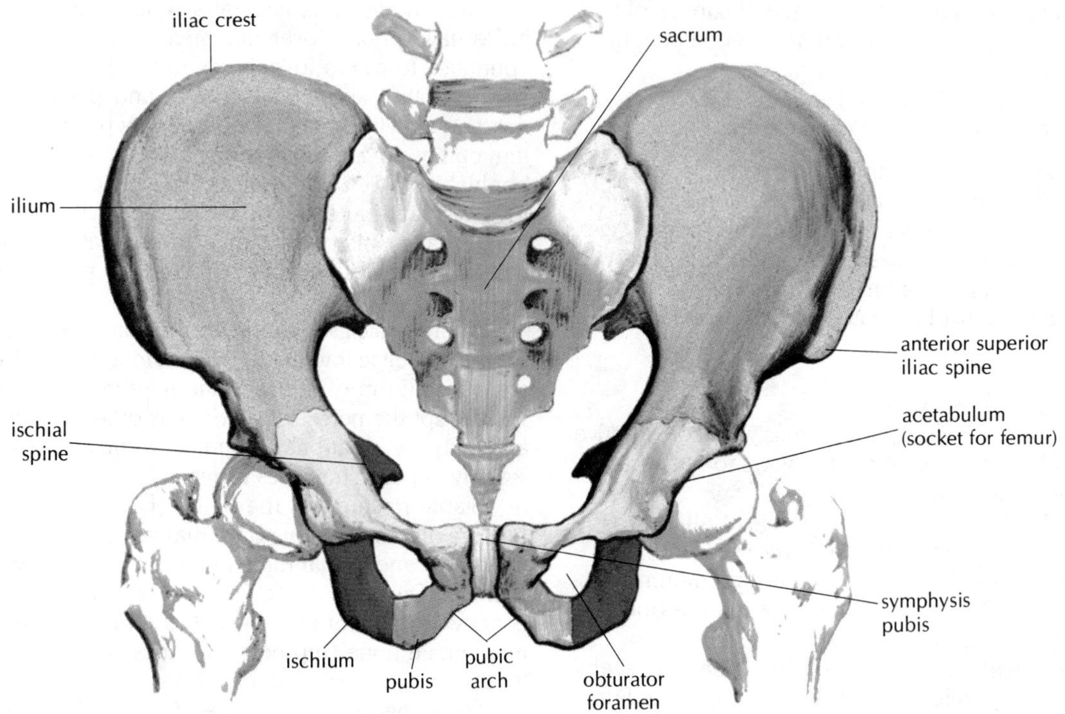

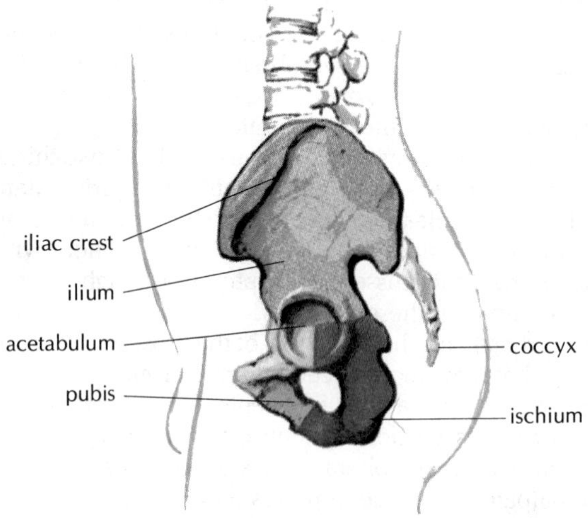

side view of male pelvis

FIGURE 64-10. Pelvic bones.

internal fixation. This promotes hemostasis, hemodynamic stability, comfort, and early mobilization.

Vertical shear pelvic fractures involve the anterior and posterior pelvic ring with vertical displacement, usually through the sacroiliac joint. There is generally complete disruption of posterior sacroiliac, sacrospinous, and sacrotuberous ligaments. Vertical displacement of the hemipelvis is usually evident. Treatment modalities may include external fixation with or without skeletal traction and open reduction internal fixation.

Undisplaced fractures of the acetabulum (Fig. 64-13) are seen after motor vehicle crashes in which the femur is jammed into the dashboard. Open reduction and fixation with multiple screws, arthroplasty, or direct lateral skeletal traction by insertion of a large trochanter screw into the femoral head is usually necessary. Traction is maintained for 6 weeks, followed by non–weight-bearing for another 6 weeks. Internal fixation permits earlier motion and function.

During the period of immobility associated with pelvic fractures, exercises (leg, respiratory, range-of-motion, and

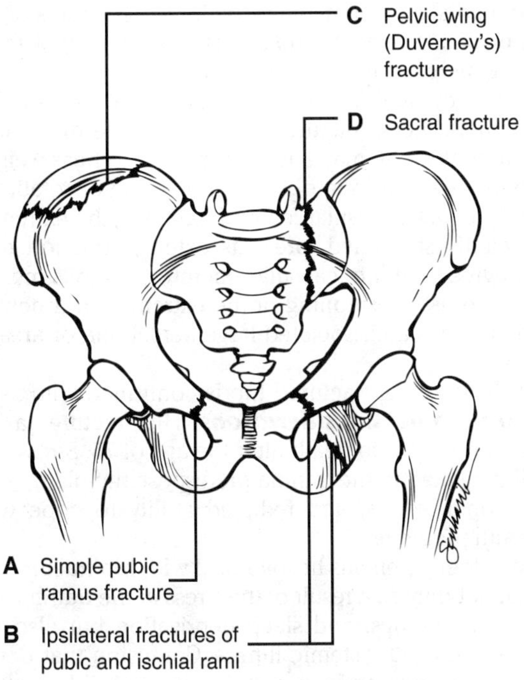

FIGURE 64-11. Stable pelvic fractures. (**A**) Single pubic ramus fracture. (**B**) Ipsilateral fractures of pubic and ischial rami. (**C**) Pelvic wing (Duverney's) fracture. (**D**) Sacral fracture.

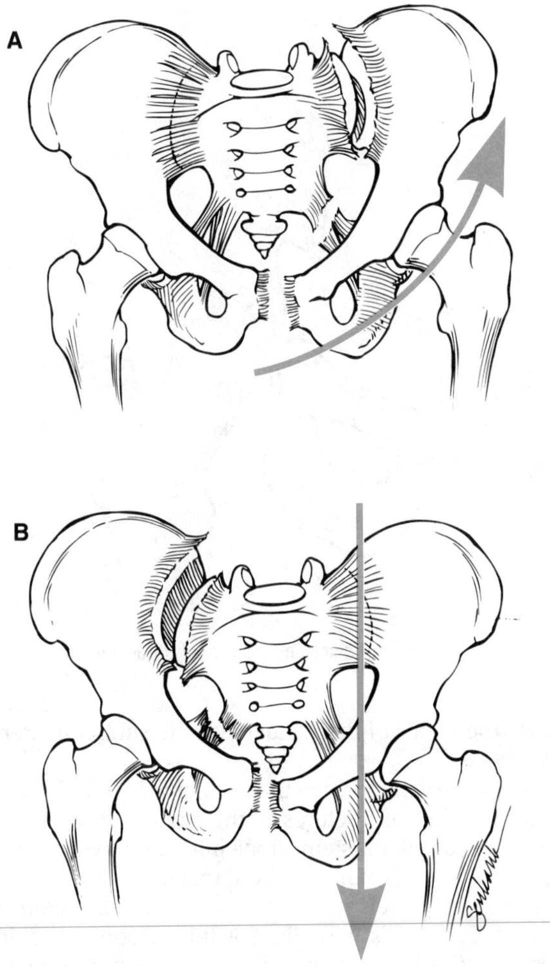

FIGURE 64-12. Unstable pelvic fracture. (**A**) Rotationally unstable fracture. Symphysis pubis separated and anterior sacroiliac, sacrotuberous, and sacrospinous ligaments disrupted. (**B**) Vertically unstable fracture. Displacement of hemipelvis anteriorly and posteriorly through symphysis pubis, and sacroiliac joint ligaments disrupted.

strengthening), elastic stockings, and elevation of the foot of the bed to aid venous return are appropriate measures to help diminish the effects of prolonged bed rest. When bone healing occurs, the patient is mobilized with progressive weight-bearing, usually with crutches. Long-term complications of pelvic fractures include malunion, nonunion, residual gait disturbances, and back pain from ligament injury.

Lower Extremity Fractures

The objectives of management of a fracture of the lower extremity are (1) to obtain adequate bony union with full length and normal alignment and without rotational or angular deformity, (2) to restore muscle power and joint motion, and (3) to restore the preinjury ambulatory status of the patient.

Practically all fractures of the lower extremity necessitate the use of crutches, walker, or cane during convalescence. The safe use of these assistive devices is discussed in Chapter 18.

Edema is common. Therefore, a fractured lower extremity is not placed in a dependent position for prolonged periods. The patient is encouraged to exercise regularly all joints that do not cause movement of the bone fragments. When the patient becomes ambulatory, the extremity is elevated for intervals to minimize recurrence of edema. It is best for the patient to lie down when elevating the healing leg. After the immobilizing device is removed, elastic stockings can be worn to support venous circulation, thus reducing the severity of edema.

Femur Fractures

Fractures of the femur can occur at several sites (Fig. 64-14). When the head, neck, or trochanteric region of the femur is involved, a hip fracture results. Fractures also occur in the femoral shaft and in the region of the knee (supracondylar and condylar fractures).

Hip Fractures

There is a high incidence of hip fractures among elderly people, whose bones are frequently brittle from osteoporosis (particularly women) and who tend to fall frequently. Weak quadriceps muscles, general frailty due to age, and conditions that produce decreased cerebral arterial perfusion (transient ischemic attacks, anemia, emboli, cardiovascular disease, effects of medications) contribute to the incidence of falls. The patient who has sustained a hip fracture frequently has associated medical (*i.e.*, cardiovascular, pulmonary, renal, endocrine) disorders. A hip fracture is viewed by the patient and the family as a catastrophic event that will have a negative impact on the patient's life-style and quality of life.

Classification. There are two major types of hip fractures. **Intracapsular fractures** are fractures of the neck of the femur. **Extracapsular fractures** are fractures of the trochanteric region (between the base of the neck and the

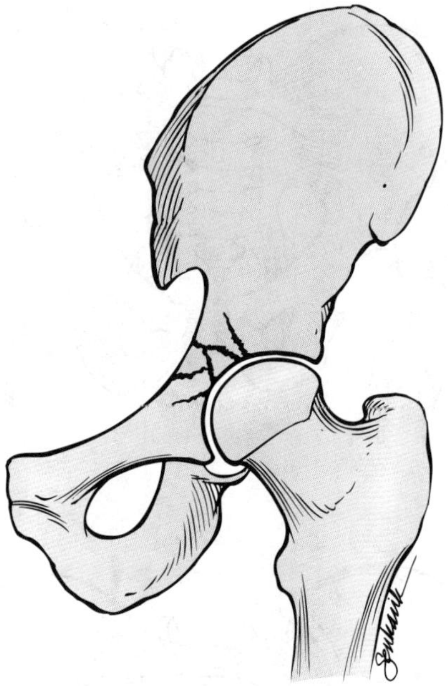

FIGURE 64-13. Undisplaced fracture of the acetabulum.

lesser trochanter of the femur) and the subtrochanteric region.

Healing of fractures of the neck of the femur is more difficult than that of fractures of the trochanteric region, because the vascular system supplying blood to the head and the neck of the femur may be damaged with the fracture. The nutrient vessels within the bone may be interrupted, and the bone cells may die. For this reason, nonunion or aseptic necrosis is common in patients with these types of fractures.

Extracapsular intertrochanteric fractures have an excellent blood supply and heal readily. There is, however, a fairly high mortality rate after intertrochanteric hip fractures, mainly because the patients are elderly (ages 70 to 85) and are not good surgical candidates. In addition, extensive soft tissue damage may occur at the time of injury, and it is not uncommon for the fracture to be comminuted and unstable.

Clinical Manifestations. With fractures of the femoral neck, the leg is shortened, adducted, and externally rotated. The patient may complain of slight pain in the groin

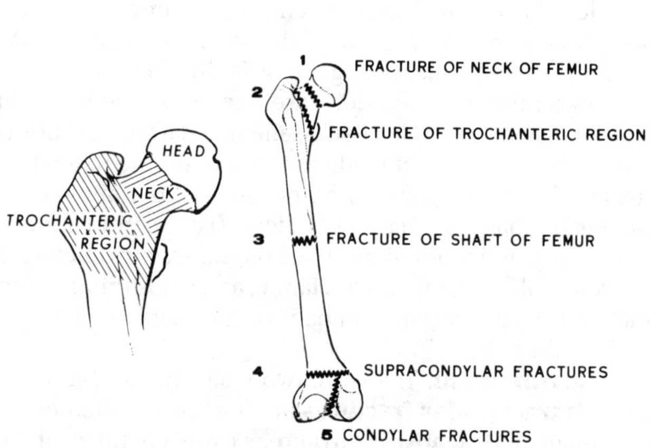

FIGURE 64-14. Sites of fracture of the femur.

or in the medial side of the knee. With most fractures of the femoral neck, the patient is unable to move the leg without significant increase in pain and is able to achieve some comfort with the leg slightly flexed in external rotation. Impacted femoral neck fractures cause moderate discomfort even with movement, may allow the patient to bear weight, and may not demonstrate obvious shortening or rotational changes. With extracapsular femoral fractures, the extremity is significantly shortened, presents external rotation to a greater degree than intracapsular fractures, exhibits muscle spasm that resists positioning of the extremity in a neutral position, and has an associated large hematoma or area of ecchymosis.

The diagnosis of fractured hip is confirmed with x-ray.

Gerontologic Considerations. Hip fractures are a frequent contributor to death after the age of 75. Stress and immobility related to the trauma predispose the older adult to pneumonia, sepsis, and reduced ability to cope with other health problems.

Many elderly persons hospitalized with hip fracture are confused, not only as a result of the stress of the trauma, unfamiliar surroundings, and sleep deprivation but also because of underlying systemic illness. Confusion that develops in some elderly patients may be due to mild cerebral ischemia. Other factors that may be associated with confusion include responses to medications and anesthesia, malnutrition, dehydration, infectious processes, mood disturbances, and blood loss.

To avoid complications, the nurse must assess the elderly patient for chronic conditions that require close monitoring. Examination of the legs may reveal edema due to congestive heart failure and absent peripheral pulses due to arteriosclerotic vascular disease. Similarly, chronic respiratory problems may be present and contribute to the possible development of inadequate pulmonary ventilation. Coughing and deep-breathing exercises are encouraged. Frequently, the elderly are taking cardiac, antihypertensive, or respiratory medications that need to be continued, requiring that their responses be monitored.

Dehydration and poor nutrition may be present. At times elderly persons who live alone are unable to summon help at the time of injury. A day or two may pass before assistance is provided, and as a result dehydration occurs. Dehydration contributes to hemoconcentration and predisposes to thromboembolism problems. Therefore the patient needs to be encouraged to consume adequate fluids and a balanced diet.

Muscle weakness and wasting may have contributed to the fall and fracture in the first place. Bed rest and immobility will cause an additional loss of muscle strength unless the nurse encourages the patient to move all joints except the involved hip and knee. Patients are encouraged to use their arms and the overhead trapeze to reposition themselves, thereby improving arm and shoulder strength, which will facilitate walking with assistive devices.

Management. Temporary skin traction, Buck's extension, may be applied to reduce muscle spasm, to immobilize the extremity, and to relieve pain. Sandbags or a trochanter roll may be used to control the external rotation.

The goal of surgical treatment of hip fractures is to obtain a satisfactory fixation so that the patient can be mobi-

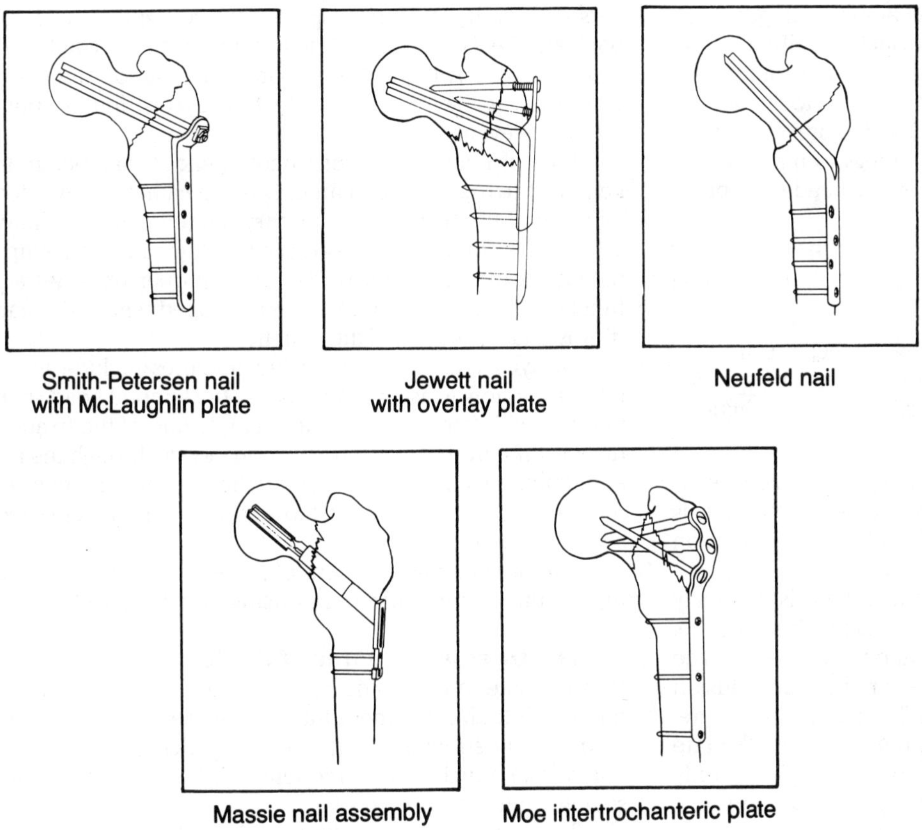

FIGURE 64-15. Examples of internal fixation for hip fractures. In fractures of the femoral neck and trochanteric region, internal fixation is achieved through the use of nails and plates specifically designed for stability and fixation. (Courtesy of Zimmer-USA, Warsaw, IN.)

lized quickly and thereby avoid secondary medical complications. Surgical treatment consists of (1) open reduction of the fracture and internal fixation or (2) replacement of the femoral head with a prosthesis (**hemiarthroplasty**). Surgical intervention is carried out as soon as possible after injury. The preoperative objective is to ensure that the patient is in as favorable a condition as possible for the surgery. Displaced femoral neck fractures may be treated as emergencies, and reduction and internal fixation are performed within 12 to 24 hours after fracture. This minimizes the effects of diminished blood supply and the development of avascular necrosis.

After general or spinal anesthesia, the hip fracture is reduced under x-ray visualization using an image intensifier. A stable fracture is usually fixed with nails, a nail-and-plate combination, multiple pins, or compression screw devices (Figs. 64-15 and 64-16). The choice of fixation device is determined by the fracture site and the preference of the orthopedic surgeon. Adequate reduction is important for fracture healing (the better the reduction, the better the healing).

Replacement of the head of the femur with a prosthesis is usually reserved for a fracture that cannot be satisfactorily reduced or securely nailed. Some orthopedic surgeons prefer this method because nonunion and avascular necrosis of the head of the femur are common complications of internal fixation techniques. Total hip replacement (see Chapter 62) may be used in selected patients with acetabular defects.

Postoperative Interventions. The immediate postoperative care of a patient with a hip fracture is similar to that for other patients undergoing major surgery (see Care of the Patient Undergoing Orthopedic Surgery in Chapter 62). Attention is given to preventing secondary medical problems, however, and to early mobilization of the patient so that independent functioning can be restored.

During the first 24 to 48 hours, attention is given to relief of pain and prevention of complications. Deep breathing,

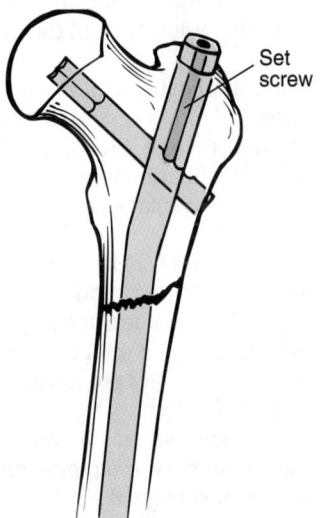

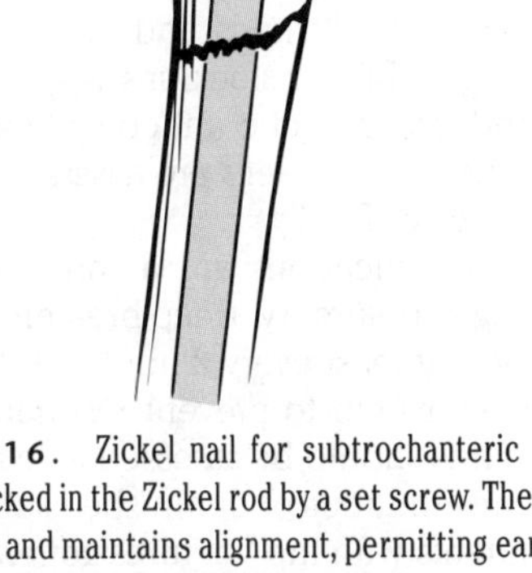

FIGURE 64-16. Zickel nail for subtrochanteric fractures. The triflanged nail is locked in the Zickel rod by a set screw. The Zickel nail fixation controls rotation and maintains alignment, permitting early active hip movement and early progressive weight-bearing ambulation.

coughing, and foot flexion exercises are encouraged each hour. Prescribed intravenous prophylactic antibiotics are administered. Hydration, nutritional status, and output are monitored. Thigh-high elastic compression stockings and pneumatic compression devices are used to prevent venous stasis. A pillow is placed between the legs to maintain abduction and alignment and to provide needed support when turning.

Turning. The patient may be turned on the affected or unaffected extremity as prescribed by the physician using the following method:

- A pillow is placed between the legs to keep the affected leg in an abducted position. The patient is then turned onto the side while maintaining proper alignment and supported abduction.

Exercise. It is important that the patient exercise as much as possible by means of the overbed trapeze. This helps strengthen the triceps and shoulders in preparation for ambulation.

On the first postoperative day, the patient is generally fairly comfortable and can transfer to a chair with assistance. The following day, assisted ambulation can begin. The amount of weight-bearing that can be permitted depends on the stability of the fracture reduction. The physician will prescribe the amount of weight-bearing permitted and the rate at which the patient can progress to full weight-bearing. Physical therapists will work with the patient on transfers, ambulation, and the safe use of walker and crutches.

The patient who has experienced a fractured hip can anticipate discharge with the use of an assistive device. Some modifications in the home may be needed to permit safe use of walkers and crutches and for the patient's continuing care.

Potential Complications. Elderly persons who suffer hip fractures are particularly prone to developing complications that may require more vigorous treatment than the fracture itself. In some instances, shock may prove fatal. Achievement of homeostasis after injury and surgery is accomplished through careful monitoring and collaborative management, including adjustment of therapeutic interventions as indicated.

Neurovascular complications may occur because of direct injury of nerves and blood vessels or from increased tissue pressure. With hip fracture, bleeding into the tissues is expected. Excessive swelling may be observed. Therefore, monitoring of the neurovascular status of the affected leg is essential.

Deep vein thrombosis (DVT) is the most common complication. To prevent DVT, fluids and ankle and foot exercises are encouraged. Elastic stockings, sequential compression devices, and prophylactic anticoagulant therapy may be prescribed. The patient's legs are assessed at least every 4 hours for evidence of DVT.

Pulmonary complications are a threat to elderly patients undergoing hip surgery. Deep-breathing exercises, a change of position at least every 2 hours, and the use of an incentive spirometer help to prevent respiratory complications. Breath sounds should be assessed at least every 4 to 8 hours to detect adventitious or diminished sounds.

Because patients with hip fractures generally have poor circulation and tend to remain in one position, pressure ulcers frequently develop. Proper skin care, especially to the back and heels and under the hips and shoulders, helps relieve pressure. A high-density foam, static air, or other special mattress may provide protection by distributing pressure more evenly.

Loss of bladder control (incontinence) may occur. In general, the routine use of an indwelling catheter is avoided because of the high risk for urinary tract infection. Urinary retention is common after surgery, and the patient's voiding patterns must be assessed. To assure proper urinary tract function, liberal fluid intake is encouraged within the cardiovascular tolerance of the patient.

Delayed complications of hip fractures include infection, nonunion, avascular necrosis of the femoral head (particularly with femoral neck fractures), failure of the fixation device, and protrusion of the fixation device through the acetabulum. Infection is suspected if the patient complains of moderate discomfort in the hip and has a mildly elevated sedimentation rate.

The nursing management of the elderly patient with a hip fracture is summarized in Nursing Care Plan 64-2.

Fractures of the Shaft of the Femur

Considerable force is required to break the shaft of the femur in adults. Most of these fractures are seen in young men who have been involved in a motor vehicle crash or have fallen from a high place. Frequently, these patients have associated multiple trauma.

The patient presents with an enlarged, deformed, painful thigh and cannot move the hip or the knee. The fracture may be transverse, oblique, spiral, or comminuted. Frequently, the patient develops shock, as the loss of 2 to 3 units of blood into the tissues is common with this fracture. The expanding diameter of the thigh may indicate continued bleeding.

Assessment includes checking the neurovascular status of the extremity, especially circulatory perfusion of the foot. (Popliteal and pedal pulses and toe capillary refill are assessed.) A Doppler ultrasound monitoring device may be needed to assess blood flow.

Dislocation of the hip and knee may accompany these fractures. Knee effusion suggests ligament damage and possible instability of the knee joint.

Management. Continued neurovascular monitoring is needed. Treatment is begun with skin traction for comfort and to immobilize the fracture so that additional soft-tissue damage does not occur. Generally, skeletal traction (Fig. 64-17) (suspension traction with Thomas splint and Pearson attachment or with slings; see Figs. 62-7 and 62-8) is used initially to achieve separation of the fracture fragments (which facilitates the operative procedure) for internal fixation or to achieve reduction and immobilization of the fracture site for subsequent cast bracing.

An external fixator may be used if the patient has experienced a Grade III fracture, has extensive soft-tissue trauma, has lost bone, has an infection, or has hip and tibial fractures.

Internal fixation is generally carried out a few days after injury. Intramedullary nailing devices or interlocking nail, plate, and screws provide adequate internal fixation, which allows for early mobilization. Active muscle movement is

(text continues on page 1935)

NURSING CARE PLAN 64–2
Care of the Elderly Patient With a Fractured Hip

Nursing Interventions	Rationale	Expected Outcomes
NURSING DIAGNOSIS: Pain related to fracture, soft-tissue damage, muscle spasm, and surgery		
GOAL: Relief of pain		
1. Assess type and location of patient's pain.	1. Pain is expected after fracture; soft-tissue damage and muscle spasm contribute to discomfort; pain is subjective and is evaluated through description of characteristics and location, which are important for determining cause of discomfort and for proposing interventions. Continuing pain may indicate development of neurovascular problems.	• Patient describes discomfort • Expresses confidence in efforts to control pain • Expresses little discomfort with position changes • Expresses comfort when fracture is positioned and immobilized • Minimizes movement of extremity before reduction and fixation • Uses physical, psychological, and pharmacologic measures to reduce discomfort • Relates a decrease in pain in 24–48 hours after surgery • Requests pain medications and uses pain relief measures early in pain cycle • States that positioning provides comfort • Appears comfortable and relaxed • Moves with increasing comfort as healing progresses
2. Acknowledge existence of pain; inform patient of available analgesics; record patient's baseline discomfort.	2. Reduces stress experienced by the patient by communicating concern and availability of help in dealing with pain. Documentation provides baseline data.	
3. Handle the affected extremity gently, supporting it with hands or pillow.	3. Movement of bone fragments is painful; muscle spasms occur with movement; adequate support diminishes soft-tissue tension.	
4. Apply Buck's traction as prescribed. Use trochanter roll.	4. Immobilizes fracture to decrease pain and additional tissue trauma; decreases muscle spasm and external rotation of hip.	
5. Use pain-modifying strategies.	5. Pain perception can be diminished by distraction and refocusing of attention.	
a. Modify the environment.	a. Interaction with others, distraction, and environmental stimuli may modify pain experiences.	
b. Administer prescribed analgesics as needed.	b. Analgesics reduce the pain; muscle relaxants may be prescribed to decrease discomfort associated with muscle spasm.	
c. Encourage patient to use pain relief measures before pain is "unbearable."	c. Mild pain is easier to control.	
d. Evaluate patient's response to medications and other pain-reduction techniques.	d. Assessment of effectiveness of measures provides basis for future management interventions; early identification of adverse reactions is necessary for corrective measures and care plan modifications.	
e. Consult with physician if relief of pain is not obtained.	e. Change in treatment plan may be necessary.	
6. Position for comfort and function.	6. Alignment of body facilitates comfort; positioning for function diminishes stress on musculoskeletal system.	
7. Assist with frequent changes in position.	7. Change of position relieves pressure and associated discomfort.	

(*continued*)

NURSING CARE PLAN 64–2 *(continued)*
Care of the Elderly Patient With a Fractured Hip

Nursing Interventions	Rationale	Expected Outcomes
NURSING DIAGNOSIS: Potential alteration in thought process related to age, stress of trauma, unfamiliar surroundings, and medication therapy		
GOAL: Remains oriented and participates in decision making		
1. Assess orientation status.	1. Evaluate presenting orientation of patient; confusion may result from stress of fracture, unfamiliar surroundings, coexisting systemic disease, cerebral ischemia, or other factors. Baseline data are important for determining change.	• Patient establishes effective communication • Demonstrates orientation to time, place, and person • Participates in self-care activities • Remains mentally alert • Avoids episodes of confusion
2. Interview family regarding patient's orientation and cognitive abilities before injury.	2. Provides data for evaluation of current findings.	
3. Assess patient for auditory and visual deficits.	3. Diminished vision and auditory acuity frequently occur with aging; glasses and hearing aid may increase patient's ability to interact with environment.	
a. Assist patient with use of sensory aids	a. Aids must be in good working order and available for use	
b. Control environmental distractors	b. Facilitates communication.	
4. Orient to and stabilize environment	4.	
a. Use orientation activities and aids (*e.g.,* clock, calendar, pictures, introduction of self).	a. Short-term memory may be faulty in the elderly; frequent reorientation helps.	
b. Minimize number of staff working with patient.	b. Consistency of caregivers promotes trust.	
5. Give simple explanations of procedures and plan of care.	5. Promotes understanding and active participation.	
6. Encourage participation in hygiene and nutritional activities.	6. Participation in routine activities promotes orientation; increases awareness of self.	
7. Provide for safety a. Keep side rails up when patient in bed b. Keep light on at night. c. Have call bell available d. Provide prompt response to requests for assistance.	7. Side rails decrease chance for additional injury from falls; mechanism for securing assistance is available to patient; independent activities based on faulty judgment may result in injury.	
8. Assess mental responses to medications, especially sedatives and analgesics.	8. Elderly persons tend to be more sensitive to medications; abnormal responses (*e.g.,* hallucinations, depression) may occur.	
NURSING DIAGNOSIS: Potential ineffective individual coping related to injury, anticipated surgery, and dependence		
GOAL: Uses effective coping mechanisms to modify stress		
1. Encourage patient to express concerns and to discuss the possible impact of fractured hip.	1. Verbalization helps patient deal with problems and feelings. Clarification of thoughts and feelings promotes problem-solving.	• Patient describes feelings concerning fractured hip and implications for lifestyle • Uses available resources and coping mechanisms; develops health promotion strategies • Uses community resources as needed
2. Support use of coping mechanisms. Involve significant others and support services as needed.	2. Coping mechanisms modify disabling effects of stress; sharing concerns lessens the burden and facilitates necessary modification.	

(continued)

NURSING CARE PLAN 64–2 *(continued)*
Care of the Elderly Patient With a Fractured Hip

Nursing Interventions	Rationale	Expected Outcomes
3. Contact social services, if needed.	3. Anxiety may be related to financial or social problems; facilitates management of problems associated with continuing care.	• Participates in development of health care plan
4. Explain anticipated treatment regimen and routines to facilitate positive attitude in relation to rehabilitation.	4. Understanding of plan of care helps to diminish fears of the unknown.	
5. Encourage patient to participate in planning.	5. Participating in care provides for some control of self and environment.	
COLLABORATIVE PROBLEMS: Hemorrhage; neurovascular compromise; deep vein thrombosis; pulmonary complications; pressure ulcers related to surgery and immobility		
GOAL: Patient experiences an absence of complications		
Hemorrhage		
1. Monitor vital signs, observing for shock.	1. Changes in pulse, blood pressure, and respirations may indicate development of shock; blood loss and stress may contribute to development of shock.	• Vital signs stabilized within normal limits • Experiences no excessive or bright red drainage • Exhibits hemoglobin and hematocrit values within normal limits
2. Consider preinjury blood pressure values and management of coexisting hypertension, if present.	2. Necessary for interpretation of current blood pressure determinations.	
3. Note character and amount of drainage.	3. Excessive drainage and bright red drainage may indicate active bleeding.	
4. Notify surgeon if patient develops shock or excessive bleeding.	4. Corrective measures need to be instituted.	
5. Note hemoglobin and hematocrit values and report decreases in values.	5. Anemia due to blood loss may develop; bleeding into tissues after hip fracture may be extensive; blood replacement may be needed.	
Neurovascular Compromise		
1. Assess affected extremity for color and temperature.	1. The skin becomes pale and feels cool with decreased tissue perfusion. Venous congestion may cause cyanosis.	• Patient has normal color and the extremity is warm • Demonstrates normal capillary refill response • Exhibits moderate swelling; tissue not palpably tense • States pain is controllable • Reports no pain with passive dorsiflexion • Reports normal sensations and no paresthesia • Demonstrates normal motor abilities and no paresis or paralysis • Has strong and equal pulses
2. Assess toes for capillary refill response.	2. After compression of the nail, rapid return of pink color indicates good capillary perfusion.	
3. Assess affected extremity for edema and swelling.	3. The trauma of surgery will cause swelling; excessive swelling and hematoma formation can compromise circulation and function; edema may be due to coexisting cardiovascular disease.	
4. Elevate affected extremity.	4. Minimizes dependent edema.	
5. Assess for deep, throbbing, unrelenting pain.	5. Surgical pain can be controlled; pain due to neurovascular compromise is refractory to treatment with analgesics.	
6. Assess for pain on passive flexion of foot.	6. With nerve ischemia, there will be pain on passive stretch. Additionally, pain	

(continued)

NURSING CARE PLAN 64–2 *(continued)*
Care of the Elderly Patient With a Fractured Hip

Nursing Interventions	Rationale	Expected Outcomes
	may indicate deep vein thrombosis (positive Homans' sign).	
7. Assess for sensations and numbness.	7. Diminished pain and paresthesia may indicate nerve damage. Sensation in web between great and second toe—peroneal nerve; sensation on sole of foot—tibial nerve.	
8. Assess ability to move foot and toes.	8. Dorsiflexion of ankle and extension of toes indicate function of peroneal nerve. Plantar flexion of ankle and flexion of toes indicate functioning of tibial nerve.	
9. Assess pedal pulses in both feet.	9. Indicator of circulatory status of extremities.	
10. Notify surgeon if diminished neurovascular status occurs.	10. Function of extremity needs to be preserved.	
Deep Vein Thrombosis		
1. Apply thigh-high elastic stockings or sequential compression device as prescribed.	1. Compression aids venous blood return and prevents stasis.	• Wears thigh-high elastic stockings. Uses sequential compression device • Experiences no skin breakdown • Experiences no more warmth than usual in skin areas • Demonstrates a negative Homans' sign • Changes position with assistance and supervision • Participates in exercise regimen • Experiences no chest pain; has lungs clear to auscultation; presents no evidence of pulmonary emboli • Exhibits no signs of dehydration; has normal hematocrit • Maintains normal body temperature
2. Remove stockings for 20 minutes twice a day and provide skin care.	2. Skin care is necessary to avoid skin breakdown. Extended removal of stocking or device defeats purpose.	
3. Assess popliteal, dorsalis pedis, and posterior tibial pulses.	3. Pulses indicate arterial perfusion of extremity. With coexisting arteriosclerotic vascular disease, pulses may be diminished or absent.	
4. Assess skin temperature of legs.	4. Local inflammation will increase local skin temperature.	
5. Assess for Homans' sign every 4 hours.	5. Pain in calf on dorsiflexion of ankle may indicate deep vein thrombosis.	
6. Avoid pressure on popliteal blood vessels from appliances or pillows.	6. Compression of blood vessels diminishes blood flow.	
7. Change position and increase activity as prescribed.	7. Activity promotes circulation and diminishes venous stasis.	
8. Supervise ankle exercises hourly.	8. Muscle exercise promotes circulation.	
9. Ensure adequate hydration.	9. Elderly persons may become dehydrated because of low fluid intake, resulting in hemoconcentration.	
10. Monitor body temperature.	10. Body temperature increases with inflammation (magnitude of response minimal in elderly).	
Pulmonary Complications		
1. Assess lung status: respiratory rate, depth, and duration, breath sounds, sputum. Monitor temperature.	1. Anesthesia and bedrest diminish respiratory effort and cause pooling of respiratory secretions. Adventitious breath sounds, respiratory pain, shortness of breath, blood tinged sputum, cough, etc., indicate possible pulmonary emboli.	• Patient has clear breath sounds • Breath sounds present in all fields

(continued)

NURSING CARE PLAN 64–2 *(continued)*
Care of the Elderly Patient With a Fractured Hip

Nursing Interventions	Rationale	Expected Outcomes
2. Report adventitious and diminished breath sounds and elevated temperature. 3. Supervise deep breathing and coughing exercises. Encourage use of incentive spirometer if prescribed. 4. Administer oxygen as prescribed. 5. Turn and reposition patient at least every 2 hours. Mobilize patient (assist patient out of bed) as soon as possible. 6. Ensure adequate hydration.	2. Elevated temperature in the early postoperative period may be due to a respiratory problem. 3. Promote optimal ventilation. Coexisting respiratory conditions diminish lung expansion. 4. Reduced ventilatory efforts may diminish PO_2 when patient is on room air. 5. Promotes optimal ventilation. Diminishes pooling of respiratory secretions. 6. Liquefies respiratory secretions. Facilitates expectoration.	• Exhibits no shortness of breath, chest pain, or elevated temperature • PO_2 on room air within normal limits • Performs respiratory exercises; uses incentive spirometer as instructed. • Changes position frequently • Consumes adequate fluids
Pressure Ulcers		
1. Monitor condition of skin at pressure points (*e.g.,* heels, sacrum, shoulders). 2. Reposition patient at least every 2 hours. Avoid skin shearing. 3. Administer skin care, especially to pressure points. 4. Use special care mattress and other protective devices (*e.g.,* heel protectors). 5. Institute care according to protocol at first indication of potential skin breakdown.	1. Elderly patients are subject to skin breakdown at points of pressure because of diminished subcutaneous tissue. 2. Avoids prolonged pressure and trauma to the skin. 3. Immobility causes pressure at bony prominences; position changes relieve pressure. 4. Devices minimize pressure on skin at bony prominences. 5. Early interventions prevent tissue destruction and prolonged rehabilitation.	• Patient exhibits no signs of skin breakdown • Skin remains intact • Repositions self frequently • Uses protective devices
NURSING DIAGNOSIS: Actual impairment of skin integrity related to surgical incision		
GOAL: Achieves wound healing		
1. Monitor vital signs. 2. Use aseptic dressing changes. 3. Assess wound appearance and character of drainage. 4. Assess complaint of pain. 5. Administer prophylactic antibiotic if prescribed, and observe for side effects.	1. Temperature, pulse, and respiration increase in response to infection. (Magnitude of response may be minimal in elderly patients.) 2. Avoids introducing infectious organisms. 3. Red, swollen, draining incision is indicative of infection. 4. Pain may be due to wound hematoma, a possible locus of infection, which needs to be surgically evacuated. 5. Osteomyelitis is to be avoided.	• Patient maintains vital signs within normal range • Exhibits well-approximated incision without drainage or excessive inflammatory response • Relates minimal discomfort; demonstrates no hematoma • Tolerates antibiotics; exhibits no evidence of osteomyelitis
NURSING DIAGNOSIS: Potential alteration in patterns of urinary elimination related to immobility		
GOAL: Maintains normal urinary elimination patterns		
1. Monitor intake and output.	1. Adequate fluid intake ensures hydration; adequate urinary output minimizes urinary stasis.	• Intake and output are adequate; patient exhibits normal voiding patterns

(continued)

NURSING CARE PLAN 64–2 *(continued)*

Care of the Elderly Patient With a Fractured Hip

Nursing Interventions	Rationale	Expected Outcomes
2. Avoid/minimize use of indwelling catheter.	2. Source of bladder infection.	• Demonstrates no evidence of urinary tract infection

NURSING DIAGNOSIS: Impaired physical mobility related to fractured hip

GOAL: Achieves pain-free, functional, stable hip

Nursing Interventions	Rationale	Expected Outcomes
1. Maintain neutral positioning of hip.	1. Prevents stress on fixation.	• Patient engages in therapeutic positioning
2. Use trochanter roll.	2. Minimizes external rotation.	• Uses pillow between legs when turning
3. Place pillow between legs when turning.	3. Supports leg; prevents adduction.	• Assists in position changes; shows increased independence in transfers
4. Instruct and assist in position changes and transfers.	4. Encourages patient's active participation while preventing stress on hip fixation.	• Exercises hourly
5. Instruct in and supervise isometric, quadriceps- and gluteal-setting exercises.	5. Strengthens muscles needed for walking.	• Uses trapeze
6. Encourage use of trapeze.	6. Strengthens shoulder and arm muscles necessary for use of ambulatory aids.	• Participates in progressive ambulation program
7. In consultation with physical therapist, instruct in and supervise progressive safe ambulation within limitations of weight-bearing prescription.	7. Amount of weight-bearing depends on the patient's condition, fracture stability, and fixation device; ambulatory aids are used to assist the patient with non–weight-bearing and partial-weight-bearing ambulation.	• Actively participates in exercise regimen
8. Offer encouragement and support exercise regimen.	8. Reconditioning exercises can be uncomfortable and fatiguing; encouragement helps patient comply with the program.	• Uses ambulatory aids correctly and safely
9. Instruct in and supervise safe use of ambulatory aids.	9. Prevents injury from unsafe use.	

NURSING DIAGNOSIS: Potential impaired home maintenance related to fractured hip and impaired mobility

GOAL: Cares for self at home

Nursing Interventions	Rationale	Expected Outcomes
1. Assess home environment for discharge planning.	1. Physical barriers (especially stairs, bathrooms) may limit patient's ability to ambulate and care for self at home.	• Home is accessible for patient at time of discharge
2. Encourage patient to express concerns about care at home; explore with patient possible solutions to problems.	2. Patient may have special problems that need to be identified and dealt with.	• Patient appears relaxed and develops strategies to deal with identified problems
3. Assess availability of physical assistance for health care activities.	3. Because of limitation of mobility, patient may require some assistance in routine health care.	• Has personal assistance available • Demonstrates ability to use necessary assistance within therapeutic prescription
4. Teach caregiver the home health care regimen.	4. Understanding of rehabilitative regimen is necessary for compliance.	• Complies with home care program; keeps follow-up health care appointments
5. Instruct patient in posthospital care. a. Activity limitations b. Reinforce exercise instructions. c. Safe use of ambulatory aids d. Wound care e. Measures to promote healing (nutrition, wound care) f. Medications, if any g. Potential problems h. Continuing health care supervision	5. Lack of knowledge and poor preparation for care at home contribute to patient anxiety, insecurity, and nonadherence to therapeutic regimen.	

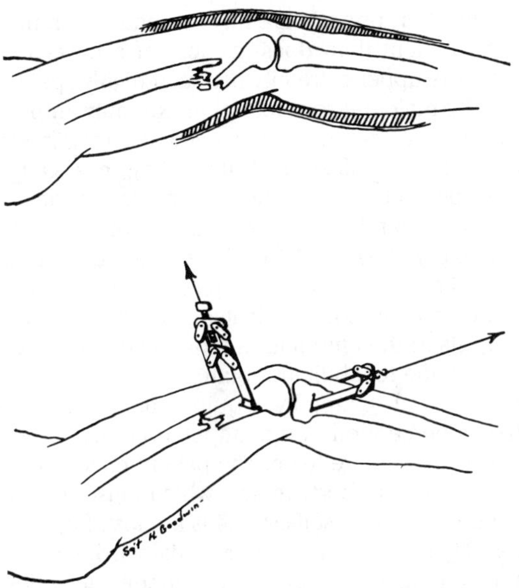

FIGURE 64-17. Two-wire skeletal traction for fracture of the femur in distal third. (**Top**) Deformity on admission to hospital. (**Bottom**) Adequate reduction when additional wire is inserted in lower femoral fragment and vertical lift is secured. (Hampton OP Jr. Wounds of the Extremities in Military Surgery. St. Louis, CV Mosby.)

important for increasing blood supply and electrical potentials at the fracture site, which enhances healing. A thigh cuff may be used for external support. Intramedullary implant and compression plates may be removed after 18 months. When plates are being removed, the resultant osteoporosis needs to be considered. A thigh cuff orthosis is used for several months after the removal of plates to provide support while bone remodeling occurs.

A cast brace may be used for fractures of the mid- and distal shaft (**supracondylar**). Two to four weeks after the injury, when pain and swelling have subsided, the patient is removed from skeletal traction and placed in a cast brace. The cast (fracture) brace is a total contact device that holds the reduced fracture. The muscle, through hydrodynamic compression, stabilizes the bone and stimulates healing. Minimal partial weight-bearing is begun and is progressed to full weight-bearing as tolerated. Functional ambulation stimulates fracture healing. The cast brace is worn for 12 to 14 weeks. In management of femoral shaft fractures, a major goal is rapid functional healing with sufficient strength to support the multiple stresses placed on the femur.

To preserve muscle strength, the patient should exercise the lower leg, foot, and toes on a regular basis. A common complication after fracture of the femoral shaft is restriction of knee motion. Active and passive knee exercises are performed as soon as possible, depending on the stability of the fracture and knee ligaments. Progressive strengthening exercises for the upper extremities are needed to prepare for ambulation.

Fractures of the Tibia and Fibula

The most common fracture below the knee is one of the tibia (and fibula) that results from a direct blow, falls with the foot in a flexed position, or a violent twisting motion. Fractures of the tibia and fibula often occur in association with each other. The patient presents with pain, deformity, obvious hematoma, and considerable edema. Frequently these fractures involve severe soft-tissue damage because there is little subcutaneous tissue in the area.

Peroneal nerve functioning is assessed to provide baseline data. If nerve function is impaired, the patient is unable to dorsiflex the great toe and has diminished sensation in the first web space. Tibial artery damage is assessed by testing the capillary refill response. The patient is monitored for an anterior compartment syndrome. Symptoms include pain unrelieved by medications and increasing with plantar flexion, tense and tender muscle lateral to tibial crest, and paresthesia. Fracture near the joint may be complicated by hemarthroses or ligament damage.

Most closed tibial fractures are treated with closed reduction and initial immobilization in a long leg-walking or patellar-tendon–bearing cast. Reduction must be relatively accurate in relation to angulation and rotation. At times it is difficult to maintain reduction, and percutaneous pins may be placed in the bone and held in position by a plaster cast (*i.e.*, pins-in-plaster technique) or an external fixator may be used. Partial weight-bearing is usually prescribed in 7 to 10 days. Activity decreases edema and increases circulation. The cast is changed to a short leg cast or brace in 3 to 4 weeks, which allows for knee motion. Fracture healing takes 6 to 10 weeks.

Open or comminuted fractures may be treated with skeletal traction, internal fixation with rods, plates, or nails, or external fixation. External plaster support may be used with internal fixation. Foot and knee exercises are encouraged within the limits of the immobilizing device. Weight-bearing is begun when prescribed, usually in about 4 to 6 weeks.

As with other lower-extremity fractures, the leg should be elevated to control edema. Continued neurovascular evaluation is needed. The development of compartment syndrome requires prompt recognition and resolution to prevent permanent functional deficit.

Axial Skeletal Fractures

Fractures of the skull and cervical spine have been described in Chapter 60. Fracture of the mandible is discussed in Chapter 34.

Rib Fractures

Uncomplicated fractures of the ribs occur frequently in adults and usually result in no impairment of function. Because these fractures produce painful respirations, the patient tends to decrease respiratory excursions and refrains from coughing. As a result, tracheobronchial secretions are not coughed up, aeration of the lung is diminished, and a predisposition to pneumonia and atelectasis results. To help the patient cough and take deep breaths, the nurse may splint the chest with her hands. Intercostal nerve blocks may be performed by the physician to relieve pain and permit productive coughing.

Chest strapping to immobilize the rib fracture is not usually used, because decreased chest expansion may result in pneumonia and atelectasis. The pain associated with rib fracture diminishes significantly in 3 or 4 days, and the fracture heals within 6 weeks.

Other serious complications may include a flail chest, **pneumothorax,** and **hemothorax.** The management of these patients is discussed in Chapter 24.

Fractures of the Thoracolumbar Spine

Fractures of the thoracolumbar spine may involve (1) the vertebral body, (2) the lamina and articulating processes, and (3) the spinous processes or transverse processes. The T12 to L2 area of the spine is most vulnerable to fracture. Fractures are generally due to indirect trauma caused by excessive loading, sudden muscle contraction, or excessive motion beyond physiologic limits. Osteoporosis contributes to vertebral body collapse.

The patient with a spinal fracture presents with acute tenderness, swelling, paravertebral muscle spasm, and change in normal curves or gap between spinous processes. Pain is greater when moving, coughing, or weight-bearing.

Immobilization is essential until initial assessments have determined if there is any spinal cord injury and if the fracture is stable or unstable. Few spinal fractures are associated with neurologic deficits. However, if spinal cord injury with neurologic deficit does occur, it usually requires immediate surgery (laminectomy with spinal fusion) to decompress the spinal cord.

Stable spinal fractures are due to flexion, extension, lateral bending, or vertical loading. The anterior structural column (vertebral bodies and discs) or the posterior structural column (neural arch, articular processes, ligaments) has been disrupted. Stable spinal fractures are treated conservatively with bed rest, with the head of bed elevated less than 30 degrees until the acute pain subsides (several days to 1 to 2 weeks). Analgesics are prescribed for pain relief. The patient is monitored for a transient ileus due to associated retroperitoneal hemorrhage. Sitting is avoided until the pain subsides. A spinal brace or plastic thoracolumbar orthosis may be applied for support during progressive ambulation and resumption of activities.

Unstable fractures occur with fracture-dislocations and exhibit disruption of both anterior and posterior structural columns. The potential for neural damage exists. The patient with an unstable fracture is placed on a side-to-side turning frame (*e.g.,* Stryker). Neurologic status is monitored closely during the preoperative and postoperative periods. Within 24 hours of fracture, open reduction and fixation with spinal fusion and Harrington or Luque rod stabilization are usually accomplished. Postoperatively, the patient continues to be cared for on the turning frame. Progressive ambulation is begun about 2 weeks after surgery, with the patient using a body jacket cast or brace.

Patient education emphasizes good posture, good body mechanics, and, when healing is sufficient, back-strengthening exercises.

Amputation

Amputation of a lower extremity is often necessary as a result of progressive peripheral vascular disease (often a sequela of diabetes mellitus), gangrene, trauma (crushing injuries, burns, frostbite, electrical burns), congenital deformities, or malignant tumor. Of all these causes, peripheral vascular disease accounts for the majority of amputations of lower extremities.

The loss of an upper extremity presents different problems to the patient than does the loss of a lower extremity, because the upper extremity has such highly specialized functions. The major reasons for upper-extremity amputation are severe trauma (acute injury, electrical burns, frostbite), malignant tumors, infection (fulminating gas gangrene, chronic osteomyelitis), and congenital malformations.

Amputation can be considered a type of drastic reconstructive surgery. It is used to relieve symptoms, improve function, and save or improve the patient's quality of life. If the health care team communicates a positive attitude, the patient adjusts to the amputation more readily and actively participates in the rehabilitative plan.

The loss of an extremity requires major adjustments. The patient's perception of the amputation must be understood by the health care team. The patient must adjust to a permanent change in body image, which must be incorporated in such a way that self-esteem is not lost. Physical mobility or ability to perform activities of daily living is altered, and the patient needs to learn how to modify activities and the environment to accommodate the use of mobility aids and assistive devices. The rehabilitation team is multidisciplinary (patient, nurse, physician, social worker, psychologist, prosthetist, vocational rehabilitation worker) and helps the patient achieve the highest possible level of function and participation in life activities.

Factors Affecting Amputation

Patients who require amputation are usually either young with severe extremity trauma or tumor or elderly with peripheral vascular disease. The young are generally healthy, heal rapidly, and participate in a vigorous rehabilitation program. Because the amputation is often the result of an injury, the patient needs much psychologic support in accepting the sudden change in body image and in dealing with the stresses of hospitalization, long-term rehabilitation, and modification of life-style. These patients need time to work through their feelings about their permanent loss. Their reactions are unpredictable and can include open bitterness and hostility.

Conversely, the elderly with peripheral vascular disease frequently have concurrent health problems, including diabetes mellitus and arteriosclerosis. Therapeutic amputations for long-standing conditions may relieve a patient of pain, disability, and dependency. These patients may have had time to work through some feelings and come to terms with the amputation. Planning for psychologic and physiologic rehabilitation begins before the amputation is performed. However, cardiovascular, respiratory, or neurologic disorders may limit their rehabilitation progress.

Management

Levels of Amputation

Amputation is performed at the most distal point that will heal successfully. The site of amputation is determined by two factors: circulation in the part and functional usefulness (*i.e.,* meets the requirements of the prosthesis).

The circulatory status of the extremity is evaluated through physical examination and specific studies. Muscle and skin perfusion is important for healing. Doppler flowmetry, segmental blood pressure determinations, and transcutaneous partial pressure of oxygen (PaO_2) are valuable studies. Angiography is performed if revascularization is considered to be an option.

The objective of surgery is to conserve as much extremity length as possible consistent with eradicating the disease process. Preservation of knee and elbow joints is desired. Figure 64-18 shows the different levels at which an extremity may be amputated. Almost any level of amputation can be fitted with a prosthesis.

Energy requirements and resultant cardiovascular demands increase as the patient progresses from using a wheelchair to a prosthesis or to crutch-walking without a prosthesis. Therefore, careful cardiovascular and nutritional monitoring is essential so that physiologic limits and demands can be met.

The amputation of toes and portions of the foot causes minor changes in gait and balance. A Syme's amputation (modified ankle disarticulation amputation) is performed most frequently for extensive foot trauma and produces a painless, durable extremity end that can withstand full weight-bearing. Below-knee amputations are preferred to above-knee amputations because of the importance of the knee joint and the energy requirements for walking. Preserving the knee joint of an elderly patient can mean the difference between walking with assistive devices and being confined to a wheelchair. Knee disarticulations are most successful with young, active patients who are able to develop precise control of the prosthesis. When above-knee amputations are performed, all possible length is preserved, muscles are stabilized and shaped, and hip contractures are prevented for maximum ambulatory potential. If a hip disarticulation amputation is performed, most people must rely on a wheelchair for mobility.

Upper-extremity amputations are performed to preserve the maximum functional length. The prosthesis is fitted early for maximum function.

Residual Limb Management

The major surgical objective is to achieve healing of the amputation wound, resulting in a nontender residual limb (stump) with healthy skin for prosthesis use. The elderly may have slower healing because of preexisting poor nutrition and other health problems. Healing is enhanced by gentle handling of the residual limb, controlling residual limb edema through rigid or soft compression dressings, and using aseptic technique in wound care to avoid infection.

Closed Rigid Dressings. A **closed rigid cast dressing** is frequently used to provide uniform compression, to support soft tissues and thereby control pain, and to prevent contractures. Immediately after surgery a rigid plaster dressing is applied and is equipped to attach a temporary prosthetic extension (pylon) and an artificial foot (Fig. 64-19). A

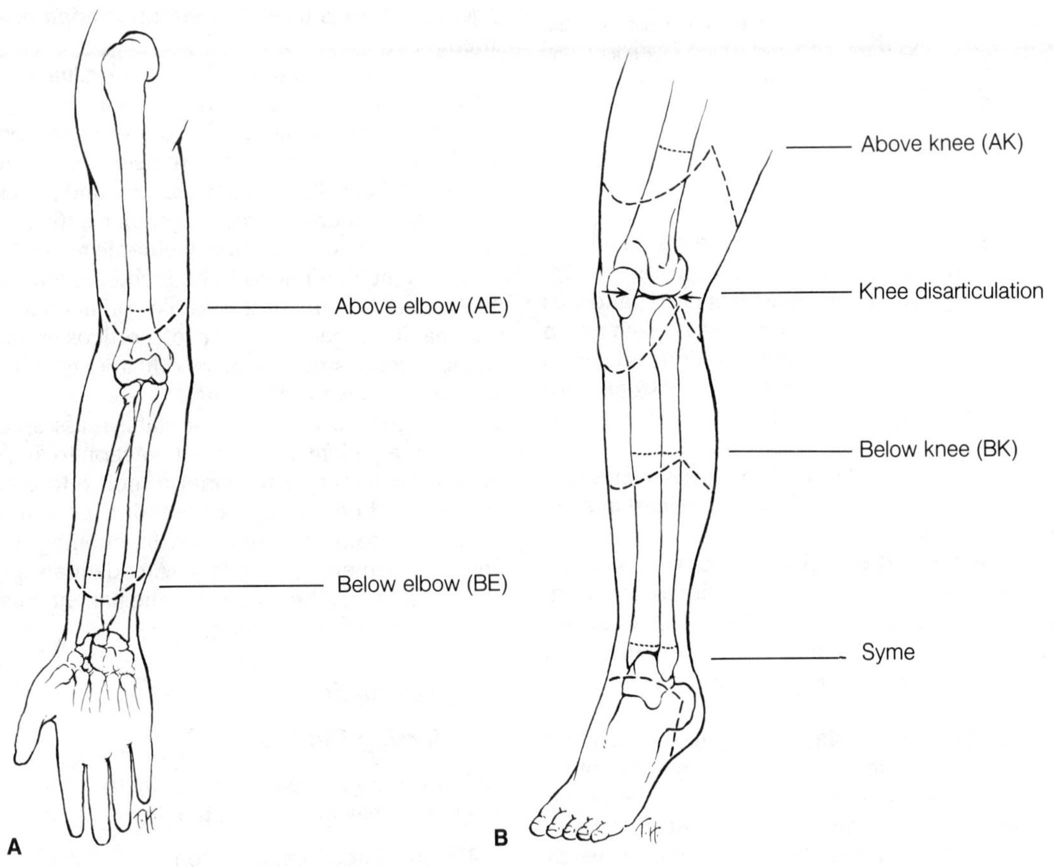

FIGURE 64-18. Levels of amputation are determined by circulatory adequacy, type of prosthesis, function of the part, and muscle balance. (**A**) Levels of amputation of upper extremity. (**B**) Levels of amputation of lower extremity.

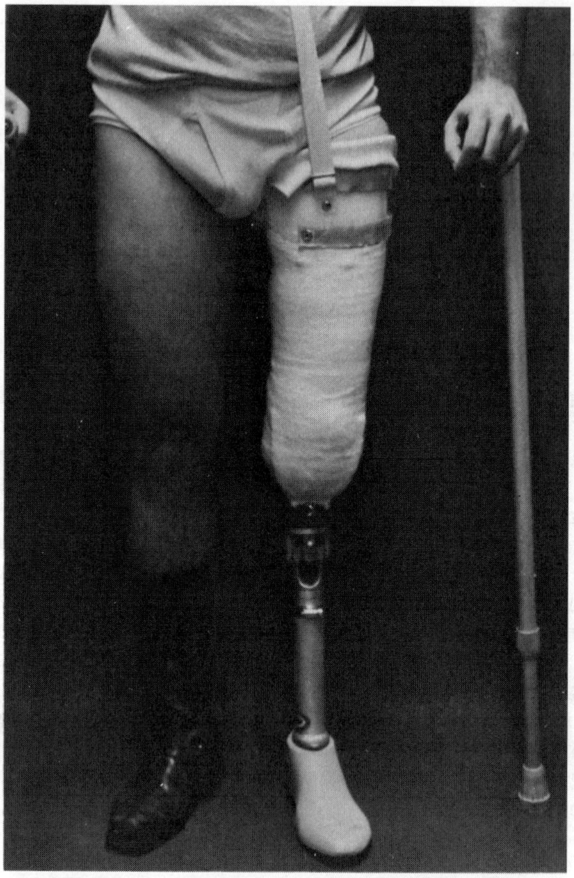

FIGURE 64-19. Immediate prosthetic fitting after amputation. Ambulation with temporary prosthetic extension (pylon) and an artificial foot. (Courtesy of the Prosthetics Research Study, Veterans Administration Contract V663P-784.)

sterilized residual limb sock is applied to the residual limb. Felt pads are placed over pressure-sensitive areas. The residual limb is wrapped with elastic plaster-of-paris bandages while firm, even pressure is maintained. Care is taken not to constrict circulation. This rigid dressing technique is used as a means of creating a socket for immediate postoperative prosthetic fitting. The length of the prosthesis is tailored to the individual patient.

The cast is changed in about 10 to 14 days. Elevated body temperature, severe pain, or a loose-fitting cast may require earlier replacement.

Soft Dressings. A **soft dressing** with or without compression may be used when frequent inspection of the residual limb (stump) is desired. An immobilizing splint may be incorporated in the dressing. Stump (wound) hematomas are controlled with wound drainage devices to minimize infection.

Staged Amputation. A **staged amputation** may be used when gangrene and infection exist. Initially, a guillotine amputation is performed to remove the necrotic and septic tissue. The wound is debrided and allowed to drain. The sepsis is treated with systemic antibiotics. In a few days, when the infection has been controlled and the patient has stabilized, a definitive amputation with skin closure is performed.

Complications

Complications of amputation include hemorrhage, infection, and skin breakdown. Since major blood vessels have been severed, massive bleeding could occur. Infection is a risk of all surgery; with poor circulation or contaminated wounds following traumatic amputation, the risk of infection increases. Poor wound healing and irritation caused by the prosthesis may result in skin breakdown.

❑ *NURSING PROCESS*
The Patient Undergoing an Amputation

Assessment

Before surgery, the neurovascular and functional status of the extremity must be evaluated through history and physical assessment (*e.g.*, color, temperature, palpable pulses, hair distribution, condition of skin, responses to positioning, sensations, pain, function). A Doppler (a hand-held ultrasonic instrument) may be used to evaluate arterial blood flow. Limitation of range of motion and presence of hip and knee flexion contractures are noted, since they may affect the function and fit of the prosthesis. If the patient has experienced a traumatic amputation, the function and condition of the residual limb are assessed. The circulatory status and function of the unaffected extremity also are assessed.

If infection or gangrene has set in, the patient may have associated enlarged lymph nodes, fever, and purulent drainage. A culture is taken to determine appropriate antibiotic therapy.

The patient's nutritional status is evaluated and a plan for nutritional care is made when necessary. Frequently, elderly persons are poorly nourished, obese, or on special diets because of concurrent health problems. For wound healing, a balanced diet with adequate vitamins and protein is essential.

Any concurrent health problems (*e.g.*, dehydration, anemia, cardiac insufficiency, chronic respiratory problems, diabetes mellitus) need to be identified and treated so that the patient is in the best possible condition to withstand the trauma of surgery. The use of corticosteroids, anticoagulants, vasoconstrictors, or vasodilators may influence management and wound healing.

The patient's psychologic status is assessed. Determination of the patient's emotional reaction to amputation is essential for nursing care. Grief response to a permanent alteration in body image is normal. Even if the amputation decreases pain and increases functioning, major psychologic adjustments are needed. An adequate support system and professional help can help the patient cope in the aftermath of amputation surgery.

Diagnosis

Nursing Diagnoses

Based on the assessment data, the patient's major nursing diagnoses may include the following:

- ❑ Pain related to amputation
- ❑ Sensory/perceptual alteration: phantom limb pain related to amputation

- Impaired skin integrity related to surgical amputation
- Body image disturbance related to amputation of body part
- Dysfunctional grieving related to loss of body part
- Self-care deficit: feeding, bathing, dressing, grooming, and toileting, related to loss of body part
- Impaired physical mobility related to loss of extremity

Collaborative Problems/ Potential Complications

Based on the assessment data, potential complications that may develop include:

- Postoperative hemorrhage
- Infection
- Skin breakdown

Planning and Implementation

Goals. The major goals of the patient may include relief of pain, absence of altered sensory perceptions, wound healing, acceptance of altered body image, resolution of the grieving process, independence in self-care, restoration of physical mobility, and absence of complications.

Nursing Interventions

Relieving Pain. Surgical pain can be readily controlled with opioid analgesics or evacuation of the hematoma or accumulated fluid.

If the patient has experienced much discomfort before surgery, the postoperative pain may be interpreted as minimal and may be controlled effectively by minimal doses of analgesics. Conversely, the pain may be combined with the expression of grief and alteration of body image and not relieved adequately by analgesics. Severe pain may be due to excessive pressure on a bony prominence or hematoma. The surgeon must be notified and the cause of the discomfort determined. Evaluation of the patient's pain and responses to interventions is an important part of the nurse's role in pain management.

Patients who are managed with a cast dressing generally experience less pain than those with soft dressings. Surgical pain is generally controlled effectively with oral analgesics and pain-modifying techniques within a few days. Early minimal weight-bearing on the residual limb with the pylon (a temporary prosthesis) attached produces little discomfort.

Muscle spasms may add to the patient's discomfort during convalescence. Changing the patient's position, applying heat, or placing a light sandbag on the residual limb to counteract the muscle spasm may improve the patient's level of comfort.

Absence of Altered Sensory Perceptions. Amputees usually experience **phantom limb pain** soon after surgery or 2 to 3 months after amputation. It occurs more frequently in above-knee amputations. The patient describes pain or unusual sensation in the part that has been amputated. The sensation creates a feeling that the extremity is present and possibly crushed, cramped, or twisted in an abnormal position. When a patient describes phantom pains or sensations, the nurse needs to acknowledge these feelings and help patients modify their perception of them.

Phantom sensation will eventually disappear. The pathogenesis of the phantom limb phenomenon is unknown. Keeping the patient active helps decrease the occurrence of phantom limb pain. Early intensive rehabilitation and stump desensitization with kneading massage affords relief. Distraction techniques and activity are helpful. Transcutaneous electrical nerve stimulation (TENS), ultrasound, or local anesthetics may provide relief for some patients. Multiple medications have been useful in controlling phantom limb pain. Beta blockers may relieve dull, burning discomfort; anticonvulsants control stabbing and cramping pain; and tricyclic antidepressants are used to improve mood and coping ability.

Promoting Wound Healing. Skin integrity has been altered by the surgical amputation. Potential healing problems may exist in relation to associated peripheral vascular, nutritional, or other concurrent health conditions such as diabetes mellitus. The residual limb must be handled gently. Whenever the dressing is changed, aseptic technique is required to prevent wound infections and possible osteomyelitis. When amputations of the leg are performed on elderly, debilitated patients, especially those with diabetes and arteriosclerosis, incontinence of urine and feces may occur. Plastic material secured by an adhesive strip above the dressing protects the residual limb from becoming soiled.

To promote healing, edema is controlled by a cast or compression dressing that promotes circulation and lymph drainage.

- If the cast or elastic dressing inadvertently comes off, the residual limb must immediately be wrapped with an elastic compression bandage. Excessive edema will develop in a very short time and will result in a delay in rehabilitation. The surgeon is notified if a cast dressing comes off so that another cast can be applied.

Residual limb shaping is important for prosthesis fitting. The patient is instructed in wrapping the residual limb with elastic dressings (Figs. 64-20 and 64-21). When the incision is healed, the patient is taught to care for the residual limb.

Enhancing Body Image. Amputation is a reconstructive procedure that alters the patient's body image. The nurse who has established a trusting relationship with the patient is better able to communicate acceptance of the patient who has experienced an amputation. The patient is encouraged to look at, feel, and then care for the residual limb. The patient's strength and resources are identified to facilitate rehabilitation. The patient is carefully assisted to regain the previous level of independent functioning. The patient who is accepted as a whole person is more readily able to resume responsibility for self-care; self-concept improves and body image changes are accepted. Even with highly motivated patients, this process may take months.

Resolving Grieving. The loss of an extremity, or part of one, may come as a shock even though the patient had been prepared preoperatively. The patient's behavior (*e.g.*, crying, withdrawal, apathy, anger) and expressed feelings (*e.g.*, depression, fear, helplessness) will demonstrate how the patient is coping with the loss and working through the grieving process. The nurse acknowledges the loss by listening and providing support.

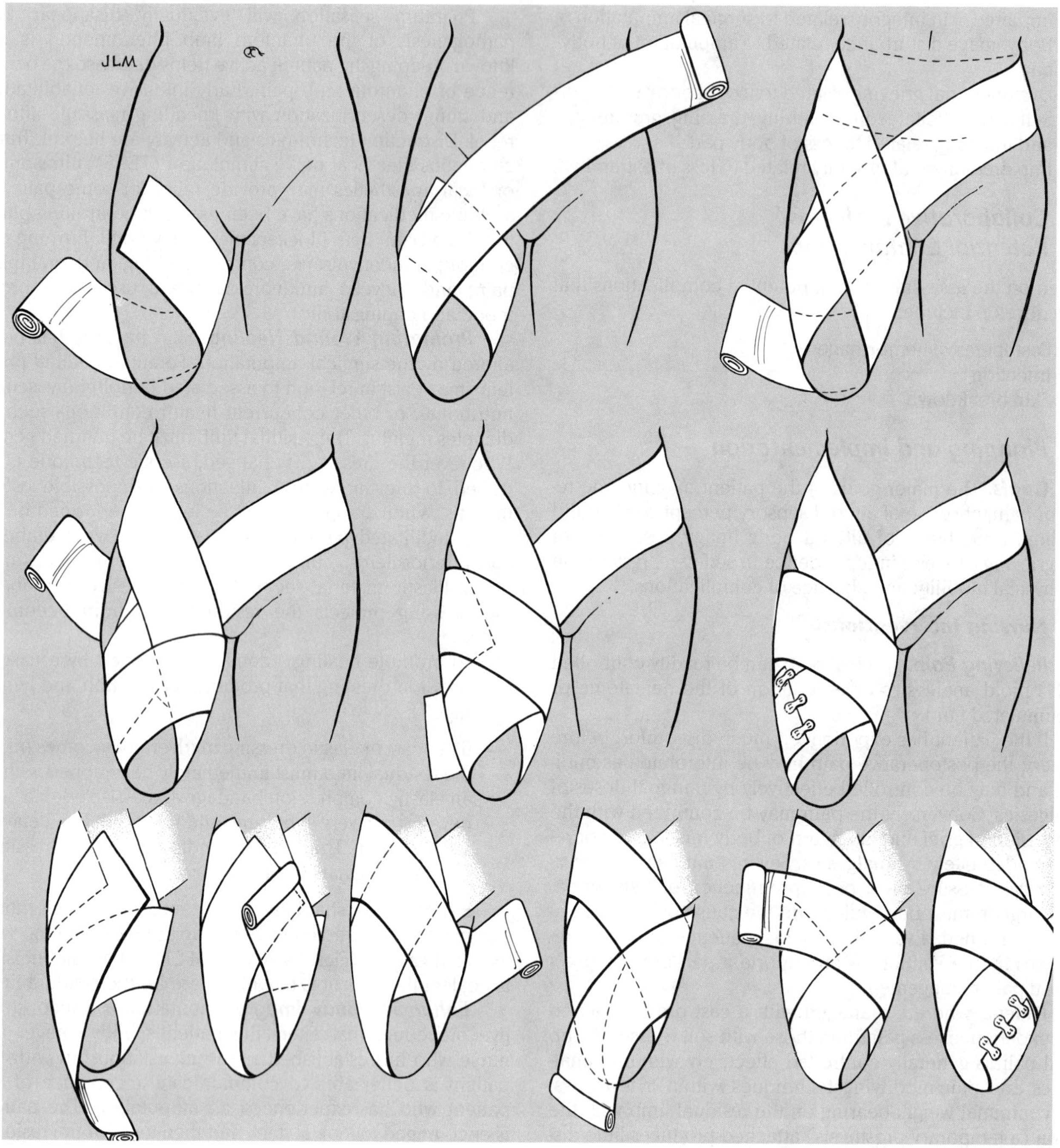

FIGURE 64-20. Wrapping above-knee residual limb. Elastic bandaging reduces edema and shapes the residual limb in a firm conical form for the prosthesis. (Suddarth DS. The Lippincott Manual of Nursing Practice, 5th ed. Philadelphia, JB Lippincott, 1991.)

The nurse creates an accepting and supportive atmosphere in which the patient and family are encouraged to express and share their feelings and work through the grief process. Support from family and friends promotes acceptance of the loss. The nurse helps the patient deal with immediate needs and become oriented to realistic rehabilitation goals and future independent functioning. Referrals to a mental health specialist and support groups may be appropriate.

Independent Self-Care. Amputation of an extremity affects the patient's ability to provide adequate self-care. The patient is encouraged to be an active participant in self-care. The patient needs time to accomplish these tasks and must not be rushed. Practicing an activity with consistent, supportive supervision in a relaxed environment will enable the person to learn self-care skills. The patient and nurse need to maintain positive attitudes and minimize fatigue and frustration during the learning process.

Independence in dressing, toileting, and bathing (shower or tub) depends on balance, transfer abilities, and physiologic tolerance of the activities. The nurse works with the physical therapist and occupational therapist in

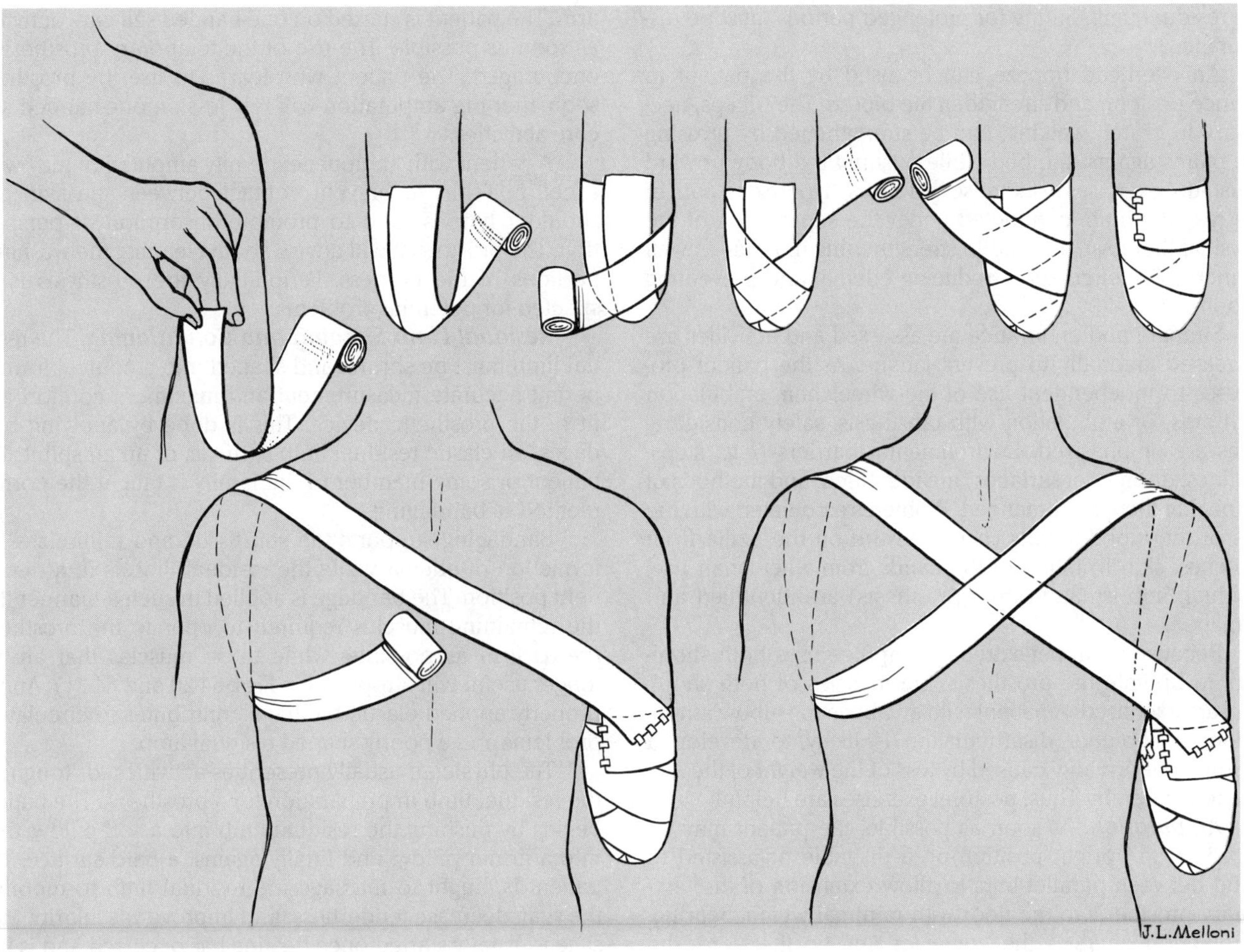

FIGURE 64-21. Wrapping above-elbow residual limb. An elastic bandage wrapping for an above-elbow residual limb minimizes edema and shapes it for a prosthesis. The bandage may need to be secured by wrapping across the back and shoulders. (Suddarth DS. The Lippincott Manual of Nursing Practice, 5th ed. Philadelphia, JB Lippincott, 1991.)

teaching and supervising the patient in these self-care activities.

The patient with an upper-extremity amputation will have self-care deficits in feeding, bathing, and dressing. Assistance is provided only as needed; the patient is encouraged to learn to do the task using feeding and dressing aids. The nurse, therapists, and prosthetist work with the patient to achieve maximum independence.

Restoring Physical Mobility. If the amputation is not an emergency procedure, efforts should be made preoperatively to strengthen the upper extremities as well as the trunk and the abdominal muscles. The extensor muscles in the arm and the depressor muscles in the shoulder especially need to be strengthened, as these muscle groups play an important part in crutch walking. The patient may flex and extend the arms while holding weights. Doing push-ups while in a prone position and sit-ups while seated will strengthen the triceps muscles. In addition, the patient should be taught to crutch walk before the surgical procedure to prepare for postoperative mobility.

Postoperative positioning to prevent the development of a hip or knee contracture is important. Abduction, external rotation, and flexion of the lower extremity are avoided. Depending on the surgeon's preference, the residual limb may be placed in an extended position or elevated for a brief period after surgery. If the residual limb is to be elevated, this should be done by raising the foot of the bed.

- The residual limb should not be placed on a pillow because a flexion contracture of the hip may result. A contracture of the joint above the amputation is a frequent complication.

In a lower-extremity amputation, the patient should be encouraged to turn from side to side and to assume a prone position to stretch the flexor muscles and to prevent flexion contracture of the hip. A pillow may be placed under the abdomen and the residual limb, with the foot resting over the edge of the mattress. The legs should remain close together to prevent an abduction deformity.

Postoperative Exercises. Postoperatively, range-of-motion exercises are started early because contracture deformities develop rapidly. Range-of-motion exercises include hip and knee exercises for below-the-knee amputations and hip exercises for above-the-knee amputations. It is important that the patient recognize the value of exercising the residual limb. Sitting for prolonged periods must be discouraged.

An overhead trapeze can be used by the patient to change position and strengthen the biceps. The triceps, necessary in crutch walking, can be strengthened by pressing the palms against the bed while pushing the body upward (push-up exercises). Exercises such as hyperextension of the residual limb, conducted under the supervision of the physical therapist, also aid in strengthening muscles as well as increasing circulation, reducing edema, and preventing atrophy.

Strength and endurance are assessed and activities are increased gradually to prevent fatigue. As the patient progresses to independent use of the wheelchair, ambulation with aids, or ambulation with prosthesis, safety considerations are emphasized. Environmental barriers (*e.g.*, steps, inclines, doors, wet surfaces) are identified, and methods of managing them are practiced. Problems associated with the use of the mobility aids (*e.g.*, pressure on the axilla from crutches, skin irritation of the hands from wheelchair use, residual limb irritation from prosthesis) are identified and managed.

Because an upper-extremity amputee uses both shoulders to operate the prosthesis, the muscles of both shoulders are exercised. A patient with an above-the-elbow amputation or shoulder disarticulation is likely to develop a postural abnormality caused by loss of the weight of the amputated extremity. Thus, postural exercises are helpful.

Ambulation. As soon as possible, the patient may be raised to an upright position on a tilt table or assisted to stand between parallel bars to allow extension of the temporary prosthesis to the floor with minimal weight-bearing. Amputation changes the center of gravity; therefore, the patient may need to practice position changes (*e.g.*, standing from sitting and standing on one foot). A well-fitting shoe with a nonslip sole should be worn. During position changes, the patient should be guarded and possibly stabilized with a transfer belt at the waist to prevent falling.

The patient is taught transfer techniques early and is reminded to maintain good posture upon getting out of bed.

- ❑ Excessive pressure on the residual limb is to be avoided because it may compromise wound healing.

How soon after surgery the patient is allowed to "touch down" the artificial foot depends on such factors as the patient's age and physical status and the condition of the other foot. Patients who are debilitated or have severe diabetes or peripheral vascular disease may not be able to tolerate the degree of pressure required to "touch down" the foot and thus must wait for a longer period before starting this activity.

The patient usually stands between parallel bars twice daily. As endurance increases, ambulation is started within the parallel bars, but full weight-bearing is not permitted on the amputated side. Crutch walking is started when stable balance is achieved. The patient should learn to use a normal gait. The residual limb should move back and forth while the patient is walking with the crutches. To prevent a permanent flexion deformity from occurring, the residual limb should *not* be held up in a flexed position.

The patient with an upper-extremity amputation is taught how to carry out the activities of daily living with one arm. The patient is started on one-handed self-care activities as soon as possible. The use of the temporary prosthesis is encouraged. The patient who learns to use the prosthesis soon after the amputation will rely less on one-handed self-care activities.

A patient with an upper-extremity amputation may wear a cotton T-shirt to prevent contact between the skin and shoulder harness and to promote absorption of perspiration. The prosthetist will advise about cleaning the washable portions of the harness. Periodically the prosthesis is inspected for potential problems.

Residual Limb Shaping and Conditioning. The residual limb must be shrunk and shaped into a conical form to permit accurate measurement and maximum comfort and fit of the prosthetic device. This is done by applying bandages, an elastic residual limb shrinker, or an air splint. The patient or some member of the family is taught the correct method of bandaging.

Bandaging supports the soft tissue and minimizes the formation of edema while the residual limb is in a dependent position. The bandage is applied in such a manner that the remaining muscles required to operate the prosthesis are as firm as possible, while those muscles that are no longer useful will atrophy (see Figs. 64-20 and 64-21). An improperly applied elastic bandage contributes to circulatory problems and a poorly shaped residual limb.

The physician usually prescribes activities to "toughen" the residual limb in preparation for a prosthesis. The patient begins by pushing the residual limb into a soft pillow, then into a firmer pillow, and finally against a hard surface. The patient is taught to massage the residual limb to mobilize the scar, decrease tenderness, and improve vascularity. Massage is usually started once healing has occurred and is first done by the physical therapist. Skin inspection and preventive care are taught.

Preparing for a Prosthesis. Patients who are candidates for a prosthesis will be seen by the prosthetist. Effective preprosthetic care is important to ensure proper fitting of the prosthesis. The major problems that can delay the prosthetic fitting during this period are (1) flexion deformities, (2) nonshrinkage of the residual limb, and (3) abduction deformities of the hip. These deformities must be avoided.

The prosthesis socket is custom-molded to the residual limb. Prostheses are designed for specific activity levels and patient abilities. Types of prostheses include hydraulic, pneumatic, biofeedback-controlled, myoelectrically controlled, and synchronized prostheses.

Gait training is continued under the supervision of a physical therapist until optimal gait is achieved. Adjustments of the prosthetic socket are made by the prosthetist to accommodate the residual limb changes that occur during the first 6 months to 1 year after surgery. A light plaster cast, an elastic bandage, or a shrinking sock is used to limit edema during the times the patient is not wearing the permanent prosthesis.

Monitoring and Managing Potential Complications. After any surgery, efforts are made to reestablish homeostasis and prevent problems related to surgery, anesthesia, and immobility.

Assessment of body systems (*e.g.*, respiratory, gastrointestinal, genitourinary) for problems associated with immobility (*e.g.*, pneumonia, anorexia, constipation, urinary stasis) is needed, and corrective management is instituted. Avoiding problems associated with immobility and restoring physical activity are necessary for maintenance of health.

Massive **hemorrhage** due to a loosened suture is the most threatening problem. The patient is monitored carefully for any signs or symptoms of bleeding. The patient's vital signs are monitored, and suction drainage is observed frequently.

- Immediate postoperative bleeding may develop slowly or take the form of a massive hemorrhage resulting from a loosened suture.
- A large tourniquet should be in plain sight at the patient's bedside so that if severe bleeding occurs, it can be applied to the residual limb to control the hemorrhage.
- The surgeon is notified immediately in the event of excessive bleeding.

Infection is a frequent complication of amputation. Patients who have undergone amputation frequently have poor circulation, a contaminated wound, or concurrent health problems that may contribute to infection. The incision, dressing, and drainage are monitored for indications of infection (*e.g.*, change in color, odor, consistency of drainage, increasing discomfort). Systemic indicators of infection (*e.g.*, elevated temperature) are monitored. Indications of infection are reported to the surgeon promptly.

Skin breakdown may result from immobilization and pressure from various sources. The prosthesis may cause pressure areas to develop. The nurse and the patient assess the skin for breaks.

Careful skin hygiene is essential to prevent skin irritation, infection, and breakdown. The residual limb is washed and dried (gently) at least twice daily. The skin is inspected for pressure areas, dermatitis, and blisters; if present, they must be treated before further skin breakdown occurs. Usually, a residual limb sock is worn to absorb perspiration and prevent direct contact between the skin and the prosthetic socket. The sock is changed daily and must fit smoothly to prevent irritation caused by wrinkles. The socket of the prosthesis is washed with a mild detergent, rinsed, and dried thoroughly with a clean cloth. The patient is advised that the socket must be thoroughly dry before the prosthesis is applied.

Rehabilitation. The complete rehabilitation of a patient who has had an amputation requires the concerted efforts of the entire rehabilitation team. The orthopedic surgeon, nurse, physiatrist, prosthetist, physical therapist, and occupational therapist work together to assist the patient to make a satisfactory adjustment to the prosthesis. Prosthetic clinics and amputee support groups facilitate this process. Vocational counseling and job retraining may be necessary to help patients return to work.

Psychologic problems (*e.g.*, denial, withdrawal) may be influenced by the type of support the patient receives from the rehabilitation team and by how quickly one-handed activities and use of the prosthesis are learned. Knowing the full options and capabilities available with the various prosthetic devices can give the patient a sense of control over the disability. The patient is not fully rehabilitated until a prosthesis has been fitted and the patient has learned how to use it. This is best accomplished in a specialized rehabilitation unit or center.

Nonambulatory Amputees. Some patients may not be candidates for a prosthesis. Conditions that may limit a patient's ability to walk with a prosthesis include heart disease, stroke, hypertension, circulatory insufficiency, advancing age, blindness, obesity, infections, delayed healing of the residual limb (amputation stump), and peripheral vascular disease. If use of a prosthesis is not possible, the patient is instructed in the use of a wheelchair to achieve independence.

A special wheelchair designed for patients who have had amputations is recommended. Because of the decreased weight in the front, a regular wheelchair may tip backward when the patient sits in it. In an amputee wheelchair, the rear axle is set back about 5 cm (2 in) to compensate for the change in weight distribution.

Patient Education and Home Care Considerations. When the patient has achieved physiologic homeostasis and has demonstrated achievement of major health care goals, rehabilitation will continue either in a rehabilitation facility or at home. Continued support and supervision by the community health nurse are essential.

Before the patient's discharge from the acute care facility, the home should be assessed. Modifications are made to assure the patient's continuing care, safety, and mobility. An overnight or weekend experience at home may be tried to identify problems that were not identified on the assessment visit. Physical therapy and occupational therapy may continue in the home or on an outpatient basis. Transportation to continuing health care appointments must be arranged. The social service department of the hospital or community agency managing continued health care may be of great assistance in securing personal assistance and transportation services.

During follow-up health visits, the nurse evaluates the patient's physical and psychosocial adjustment. Periodic preventive health assessments are necessary. Frequently an elderly spouse is unable to provide the assistance required, and additional help at home is needed. Modifications in the care plan are made on the basis of such findings. Often, the patient and family find involvement in an amputee support group to be of value; here they are able to share problems, solutions, and resources. Talking with those who have successfully dealt with a similar problem may help the patient develop a satisfactory solution.

Evaluation

Expected Outcomes

1. Experiences absence of pain
   a. Appears relaxed
   b. Verbalizes comfort
   c. Uses measures to increase comfort
   d. Participates in self-care and rehabilitative activities
2. Experiences absence of phantom limb pain
   a. Reports not perceiving sensations from amputated part
   b. Verbalizes absence of abnormal sensation in residual limb
3. Achieves wound healing
   a. Controls residual limb edema

   b. Achieves healed, nontender, nonadherent scar
   c. Demonstrates residual limb care
4. Demonstrates improved body image
   a. Acknowledges change in body image
   b. Participates in self-care activities
   c. Demonstrates increasing independence
   d. Projects self as a whole person
   e. Resumes role-related responsibilities
   f. Reestablishes social contacts
   g. Demonstrates confidence in abilities
5. Exhibits resolution of grieving
   a. Expresses grief
   b. Uses family and friends to work through feelings
   c. Focuses on future functioning
6. Achieves independent self-care
   a. Asks for assistance when needed
   b. Uses aids and assistive devices to facilitate self-care
   c. Verbalizes satisfaction with abilities to perform activities of daily living
7. Achieves maximum independent mobility
   a. Avoids positions contributing to contracture development
   b. Demonstrates full active range of motion
   c. Maintains balance when sitting and transferring
   d. Increases strength and endurance
   e. Demonstrates safe transferring technique
   f. Achieves functional use of prosthesis
   g. Overcomes environmental barriers to mobility
   h. Uses community services and resources as needed
8. Exhibits absence of complications of hemorrhage, infection, skin breakdown
   a. Does not experience excessive bleeding
   b. Maintains normal blood values
   c. Is free of local systemic signs of infection
   d. Repositions self frequently
   e. Is free of pressure-related problems
   f. Reports any skin discomfort and irritations promptly

CRITICAL THINKING EXERCISES

1. A classmate tells you that she is going to start jogging and that her goal is to run in a marathon in several months. Explain the kind of advice you would give her and your rationale for making these suggestions.
2. A middle-aged patient who has been hospitalized for 4 days with a fractured pelvis is making plans for discharge. His wife approaches you and expresses concern that he has become very irritable and that he "just doesn't seem to be himself." Analyze this information and speculate as to the possible causes for this behavior. Describe the additional kinds of information you would seek in a further assessment of the situation. What findings would confirm your initial speculation? What findings would lead to a different conclusion?
3. You witness a person falling on a patch of ice and you offer assistance. She does not seem to be seriously injured, but she complains that her left elbow is sore and her left hand feels weak. She indicates that she thinks she can drive herself home and will then decide if she needs to seek medical attention. What conclusions would you draw from the complaints she described? Based on that conclusion, how would you advise her and why?
4. You are visiting an elderly gentleman who is in an extended-care facility recovering from a below-the-knee amputation. He expresses satisfaction that he has progressed to the point that he has the stamina to sit in his wheelchair from breakfast time until after dinner. How would you advise him to modify his daily routine and why? Describe the plan of care you would devise for him and the outcomes you hope to have him achieve through this plan.

REFERENCES AND SELECTED READINGS

Books

Apley AG. Apley's System of Orthopaedics and Fractures, 7th ed. Oxford, Butterworth Heinemann, 1993.
Brooks M et al. Sports Injuries, 2nd ed. London, Gower Medical Pub., 1992.
Browner B et al (ed). Skeletal Trauma: Fractures, Dislocations, Ligamentous Injury. Philadelphia, WB Saunders, 1992.
Bullock BL and Philbrook P. Pathophysiology: Adaptations and Alterations in Function, 3rd ed. Philadelphia, JB Lippincott, 1992.
Carpenito LJ. Nursing Diagnosis: Application to Clinical Practice, 6th ed. Philadelphia, JB Lippincott, 1995.
Chapman M and Madison M. Operative Orthopaedics, 2nd ed. Philadelphia, JB Lippincott, 1993.
Crenshaw AH and Daugherty K (eds). Campbell's Operative Orthopaedics, 8th ed. St. Louis, Mosby Year Book, 1992.
Davis PS. Nursing the Orthopaedic Patient. Edinburgh, Churchill Livingstone, 1994.
Dolan JT. Critical Care Nursing: Clinical Management Through the Nursing Process. Philadelphia, FA Davis, 1991.
Goldie BS and Dunn Dc. Orthopaedic Diagnosis and Management. Oxford, Blackwell Scientific Publications, 1992.
Grana W and Kalenak A (eds). Clinical Sports Medicine. Philadelphia, WB Saunders, 1991.
Gustilo Rb, Kyle RF, and Templeman DC. Fractures and Dislocations, St. Louis, CV Mosby, 1993.
Hogstel MO. Clinical Manual of Gerontological Nursing. St. Louis, Mosby Year Book, 1992.
Lewis CB and Knortz KA. Orthopedic Assessment and Treatment of the Geriatric Patient. St. Louis, CV Mosby, 1993.
Karacoloff L, Hammersley C, and Schneider F. Lower Extremity Amputation, 2nd ed. Gaithersburg, MD, Aspen, 1992.
Maher AB et al. Orthopaedic Nursing. Philadelphia, WB Saunders, 1994.
Mercier LR. Practical Orthopedics, 3rd ed. St.Louis, Mosby Year Book, 1991.
Mourad LA. Orthopedic Disorders. St. Louis, Mosby Year Book, 1991.

Mourad LA and Droste MM. The Nursing Process in the Care of Adults with Orthopaedic Conditions, 3rd ed. Albany, NY, Delmar Publishers, 1993.
National Association of Orthopaedic Nurses. Guidelines for Orthopaedic Nursing. Pitman, NJ, National Association of Orthopaedic Nurses, 1992.
Nickel VL and Botte MJ. Orthopaedic Rehabilitation, 2nd ed. New York, Churchill Livingstone, 1992.
Porth CM. Pathophysiology: Concepts of Altered Health States, 4th ed. Philadelphia, JB Lippincott, 1994.
Rakel RE (ed). Conn's Current Therapy. Philadelphia, WB Saunders, 1993.
Rockwood C Jr, Green D, and Bucholz R (eds). Rockwood and Green's Fractures in Adults, 3rd ed. Philadelphia, JB Lippincott, 1991.
Salmond SW et al (eds). Core Curriculum for Orthopaedic Nursing, 2nd ed. Pitman, NJ. National Association of Orthopaedic Nurses, 1991.
Sly D and Theis L (eds). Introduction to Orthopaedic Nursing: An Orientation Module. Pitman, NJ, National Association of Orthopaedic Nurses, 1991.
Turek SL (ed). Orthopaedics: Principles and Their Application, 5th ed. Philadelphia, JB Lippincott, 1994.

Journals

Asterisks indicate nursing research articles.

Musculoskeletal Injury

Bailey M. and Michalski J. Close-up on clavicle fracture. Nursing 1992 Aug; 22(8):41.
Bailey M. and Michalski J. Close-up on Colles' fracture. Nursing 1992 Oct; 22(10):47.
Bailey M. and Michalski J. Close-up on scaphoid fracture. Nursing 1993 Mar; 23(3):49.
Bailey M. and Michalski J. Close-up on radial head fracture. Nursing 1993 Sep; 23(9):43.
Barden RM. and Sinkora GL. Bone stimulators of fusions and fractures. Nurs Clin North Am 1991 Mar; 26(1):89–103.
Belinsky JD. Acetabular fracture: ORIF . . . open reduction internal fixation. Orthop Nurs 1993 Jan/Feb; 12(1):42–45, 48–50.
Connolly M. Ambulatory surgery and prepared discharges. Nurs Clin North Am 1991 Mar; 26(1):89–104.
Cutts S. and Hood N. A role for nurses in sports injuries. Nurs Stan 1991 Jun 19–25; 5(39):25–27.
Dunwoody CJ. Pelvic fracture patient care: Reflections on the past, implications for the future. Nurs Clin North Am 1991 Mar; 26(1):65–72.
Edwards KP. Orthopedic trauma: Pelvic fracture. Today's OR Nurse 1993 Jul/Aug; 15(4):24–28.
Einhorn T. Mechanisms of fracture healing. Hosp Pract 1991 Jan; 26; Suppl 1:41–45.
Folcik M. Meniscal injuries. Nurs Clin North Am 1991 Mar; 26(1); 181–198.
Grisso J et al. Risk factors for falls as a cause of hip fracture in women. N Engl J Med 1991 May 9; 324(19):1326–1331.
Gruen G and Engle C. Verticle shear fractures of the pelvis. Orthop. Nurs 1993 Sep/Oct; 12(5):55–59.
Hip dislocation. Am J Nurs 1993 Aug; 93(8):46.
*Lerner RK et.al. Psychosocial, functional, and quality of life assessment of patients with posttraumatic fracture nonunion, chronic refractory osteomyelitis, and lower extremity amputation. Arch Phys Med Rehabil 1991 Feb; 72(2):122–126.
Miller K. Trauma to the extremities. Emergency 1991 Dec; 23(12): 28–31.
Mooney N. Pain management in the orthopaedic patient. Nurs Clin North Am 1991 Mar; 26(1):73–87.
Myerson M and Henderson M. Clinical applications of a pneumatic intermittent impulse compression device after trauma and major surgery to the foot and ankle. Foot and Ankle 1993; 14(4):198–203.
Nussman DS and Poole RC. Rescue and recovery in traumatic hip dislocation. Am J Nurs 1991 Nov; 91(11):34–38.
*O'Brien LA et. el. Hospitalized elders: Risk of confusion with hip fracture. J Gerontol Nurs 1993 Feb; 19(2):25–33.
Pellino TA. How to manage hip fractures Am J Nurs 1994 April; 94(4):46–50.
Rettig AC. and Kraft DE. Treat ankle sprains fast—it pays. Your Patient and Fitness 1991 Jul/Aug; 4(4):6–9.
Ross D. Acute compartment syndrome. Orthop Nurs 1991 Mar/Apr; 10(2):33–38.
Rothenberg JR. Innovations in treating anterior cruciate ligament deficiency. Orthop Nurs 1991 Mar/Apr; 10(2):17–25.
Ruda S. Common ankle injuries in the athlete. Nurs Clin North Am 1991 Mar; 26(1):167–180.
Ruhl JM. Pelvic trauma. RN 1991 Jul; 54(7):50–55.
Sly D. Orthopedic complications. Nurs Clin North Am 1991 Mar; 26(1):113–132.
Smrcina C. Stress fractures in athletes. Nurs Clin North Am 1991 Mar; 26(1):159–166.
Whittington CF and Carlson CA. Anterior cruciate ligament injuries: Evaluation, arthroscopic reconstruction, and rehabilitation. Nurs Clin North Am 1991 Mar; 26(1):149–158.

Amputation

Agne RAC. Rehabilitating a loved one: A personal story. Rehabil Nurs 1993 Jan/Feb; 18(1):23–25.
Casillas J et al. Transcutaneous oxygen presssure: An effective measure for prosthesis fitting on below-knee amputations. Am J Phys Med Rehabil 1993 Feb; 72(1):29–32.
Datta D, Nair P, and Payne J. Outcome of prosthetic management of bilateral lower-limb amputees. Disabil Rhabil 1992 Apr/Jun; 14(2):98–102.
Davis RW. Phantom sensation, phantom pain, and stump pain. Arch Phys Med Rehabil 1993 Jan; 74(1):79–91.
Evans J and Carlin P. Surgical approach to amputation. Phys Med Rehabil Clin North Am 1991 May; 2(2):263–277.
Fletcher E. Foot problems in people with diabetes. Nurs Stand 1992 Jun 3–9; 6(37):25–28.
Helt J. Foot care and footwear to prevent amputation. J Vasc Nurs 1991 Dec; 9(4):2–8.
Mikulaninec CE. An amputee critical path. J Vasc Nurs 1992 Jun; 10(2):6–9.
Mulvey MA and Sharma PK. Traumatic amputation. RN 1991 Sep; 54(6):26–30, 34.
Novotny MP. Psychosocial issues affecting rehabilitation. Phys Med Rehabil Clin North Am 1991 May; 2(2):373–393.
Rounseville C. Phantom limb pain: The ghost that haunts the amputee. Orthop Nurs 1992 Mar/Apr; 11(2):67–71.
Rudolphi D. Limb loss in the elderly peripheral vascular disease patient. J Vasc Nurs 1992 Sep; 10(3):8–13.
Stern P. The epidemiology of amputation. Phys Med Rehabil Clin North Am 1991 May; 2(2):253–261.
Vaida G and Friedmann LW. Postamputation phantoms: A review. Phys Med Rehabil Clin North Am 1991 May; 2(2):325–353.
Williamson VC. Amputation of the lower extremity: An overview. Orthop Nurs 1992 Mar/Apr; 11(2):55–65.

INFORMATION/RESOURCES

Agencies

Amputee Shoe and Glove Exchange
P.O. Box 27067,
Houston, TX 77227

National Amputation Foundation
12–45 150th Street,
Whitestone, NY 11357

National Easter Seal Society
70 E. Lake Street,
Chicago, IL 60601

National Handicap Housing Institute, Inc
4556 Lake Drive,
Robbinsdale, MN 55422

National Institute of Arthritis and Musculoskeletal and Skin Diseases
National Institutes of Health,
Bethesda, MD 20892

National Odd Shoe Exchange
P.O. Box 56845,
Phoenix, AZ 85079

Nursing Research Profile for Unit 16

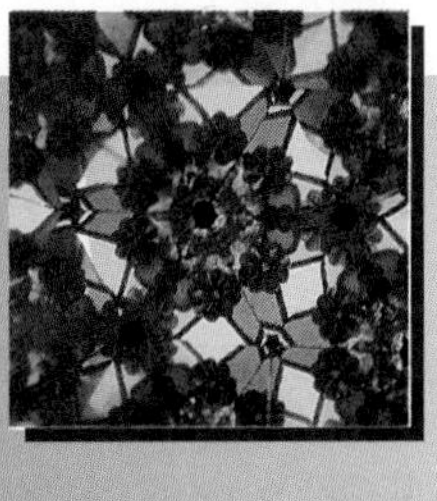

Musculoskeletal Function

Overview

The following nursing research studies focus on issues related to nursing management of individuals with orthopedic conditions and physical and psychosocial factors related to musculoskeletal disorders.

Daltroy LH et al. Does musculoskeletal function deteriorate in a predictable sequence in the elderly? Arthritis Care Res 1992 Sept; 5(3):146–150.

The aging process results in a loss of function that has been thought to reflect a reverse in sequence of abilities gained in youth. This study attempted to determine if functioning in areas requiring strength, skill, and endurance (*e.g.*, running errands or doing chores) would be lost before self-care activities (*e.g.*, rising from a chair, walking, picking up clothes, feeding oneself).

The study was part of a larger study of community-dwelling elderly persons in New England. Two hundred and eighty-nine subjects over 65 years of age participated in the study. Subjects were stratified by sex and age.

The 20-item Health Assessment Questionnaire (HAQ) was used to determine the subjects' self-reported difficulty with functional tasks. A Guttman scale was applied to the HAQ to allow for evaluation of patterns of decline in ability to perform tasks; in turn, the scale was used to predict functional loss and signal the need for professional intervention to prevent further loss. Based on analysis of ergonomics and strength required, activities were ranked as most difficult to least difficult as follows: doing chores, rising from a chair with no arms, walking on level ground, picking up clothes, rising from bed, and lifting a cup to the mouth.

The HAQ was administered by health professionals in the homes of the subjects. Subjects were asked if they were able to perform certain tasks independently or with assistance. The presence of arthritis was also determined.

Using a goodness-of-fit analysis, the order of activities was as expected except for the reversal of picking up clothes and walking on level ground. Persons with arthritis had greater difficulty in performing all of these activities than did persons without arthritis. The findings suggest that decline of function occurs in a predictable sequence except for patients with arthritis, whose hand function deterioration affects overall functioning.

Nursing Implications. Elderly patients generally lose functional ability in a predictable pattern. Awareness of this pattern could assist the professional nurse to determine whether functional losses are in an expected or unexpected pattern or rate and to determine needed nursing care. In addition, elderly patients with arthritis may have greater difficulty with fine motor activities, exhibit losses in an unpredictable pattern, and require greater assistance than those without arthritis. With early recognition of loss of functional ability, interventions can be more effectively planned and implemented.

Pellino TA and Oberst MT. Perception of control and appraisal of illness in chronic low back pain. Orthop Nurs 1992 Jan/Feb; 11(1):22–26, 106.

Chronic low back pain is a major health problem. How a person perceives the pain and illness situation and control over the pain may affect the outcomes (*i.e.*, pain and mood disturbance). This study developed a model of appraisal and perception of control for patients with chronic low back pain. Locus of control and demographic characteristics were viewed as causal antecedents; perception of pain control, emotional support, and appraisal of illness were viewed as mediating factors; and mood and pain rating were identified as the outcomes.

Patients, 20 males and 20 females, who had back pain for at least 6 months were included in this study. The subjects were middle aged and well educated. Most had a diagnosis of herniated disc, had had at least one surgical procedure, had a work-related injury, and were unemployed owing to the pain.

The subjects completed several questionnaires: the Appraisal of Illness Scale, which assessed types of appraisal (*i.e.*, harm/loss, threat, challenge, positive, benign), the Levensen Locus of Control Scales (*i.e.*, internal, external powerful others, and external chance), Perception of Control of Pain (adapted from the Headache Locus of Control Scale and Medical Cure and Pain Control subscales of the Pain Attitude Scale), Perceived Emotional Support (using items from the Solicitude subscale of the Survey of Pain Attitudes), Profile of Mood States (*i.e.*, anxiety, depression, anger, fatigue, vigor, and confusion), and a pain analogue scale for rating pain experienced over the past week. Variables entered in stepwise multiple regressions were selected on the basis of Pearson correlations.

Pain was positively correlated with negative appraisal and was negatively correlated with perceived internal locus of control and challenge appraisal. Perception of internal control of pain accounted for 29% of the variance in reported pain. Educational level of subjects affected perception of locus of control, with more highly educated subjects perceiving that they had more control over their pain. Perception of internal control of pain and challenge appraisal and negative appraisal accounted for 61% of the variance in mood disturbance. Perceived lack of social support and general ``powerful others'' locus of control accounted for 28% of the variance in challenge appraisal.

Nursing Implications. When working with patients with chronic back pain, the nurse needs to recognize that those who appraise their pain as harmful or threatening experience more pain and mood disturbance, whereas those who perceive themselves as having control over their pain experience less pain and mood disturbance. By using nursing interventions that assist the patient with low back pain to develop internal mechanisms for control over the pain and by promoting emotional support, the nurse can help the patient to successfully adapt to the pain situation.

Lichtenstein R et al. Development and impact of a hospital-based perioperative patient education program in a joint replacement center. Orthop Nurs 1993 Nov/Dec; 12(6):17–25, 46.

A hospital-based perioperative patient education program was developed and implemented in a tertiary care urban hospital in the Northeast. A 5-year retrospective evaluation study was completed using a one-group post-test–only research design to determine patients' perceptions of the education program and their perceptions of the outcome of surgery.

All patients scheduled for hip and knee joint replacements and their families were invited to participate in the educational program. The program consisted of a formal educational session presented by a nurse practitioner, covering the hospitalization experience, pathophysiology of arthritic joints, details of joint replacement, exercise, medications, potential complications, and postoperative discharge needs including life-style modification. An opportunity was provided for patients and their families to discuss individual concerns. Patient education materials were given to the patient to reinforce information presented orally. Volunteers who had had previous joint replacement talked with patients before and after surgery to help reduce anxieties and fears. All patients were invited to participate in the arthritis club, a self-help support group, 3 to 6 months after joint replacement surgery.

The characteristics of the patients participating in the program were as follows: 215 had total hip replacement surgery, 320 had total knee replacement surgery; osteoarthritis was present for 64% of the hip surgery patients and for 83% of the knee surgery patients; the mean age was 65 years for hip surgery patients and 69 years for knee surgery patients; 60% of the hip surgery patients were female versus 78% for knee surgery patients; two-thirds of all the patients were Caucasian.

Questionnaires were mailed to all participants 2 months following surgery; phone interviews were conducted with the participants 6 months and 1 year following surgery. The questionnaire gathered data on the patient's perceptions of the educational program, including problems encountered at home not addressed in the program; ability to function as expected; functional level (independent versus uses assistive devices); perception of health status; participation in prescribed exercises; and compliance with follow-up with a surgeon, as suggested. Most of these items were dichotomous so that negative responses could be studied for program modification.

Study findings indicated that the patients perceived the educational program to be helpful and that it covered most of the problems encountered at home. At 2 months, more than half the patients indicated they were able to function as expected, but about one-third indicated they had not yet recovered. Independent functional level was reported by about 70% of the patients by 1 year. More than three-fourths of the patients perceived themselves to be in good health by 6 months. Approximately 80% of the patients were back to their expected normal functioning by 1 year, and more than 80% performed exercises as recommended by the therapist at 6 months and at 1 year. Virtually all patients had had their follow-up visits with their surgeon as suggested.

Nursing Implications. This study supports the value of patient education to patients' compliance with exercise and follow-up care. The patients' perceptions of health status and functioning level may be seen as positive outcomes of patient education. Structured educational programs ensure that essential information is provided to the patient and provide an opportunity for clarifying questions and allaying anxieties.

O'Brien LA et al. Hospitalized elders: Risk of confusion with hip fracture. J Gerontol Nurs 1993 Feb; 19(2):25–33.

More than half of all patients admitted to the hospital for treatment of hip fracture experience confusion at some time during the course of their hospitalization. This study focused on identifying the characteristics of patients with hip fractures who experienced confusion, nurses' and physicians' documentation of the confusion, the risk of complications while hospitalized, and the length of hospitalization.

Subjects were drawn from a larger study population investigating risk factors for hip fracture. Profoundly cognitively impaired patients were excluded from participating. A total of 101 patients who had experienced hip fracture were included in the study.

Cognitive functioning was determined with the Kahn Goldfard Mental Status Questionnaire, administered by a trained nurse interviewer about 6 days following admission. Subjects were classified as experiencing severe confusion ($n = 45$), moderate confusion ($n = 26$), and no confusion or minimal confusion ($n = 30$).

An extensive chart review was performed to abstract demographic data, pre-admission clinical characteristics (*e.g.*, mental status, psychiatric history, sensory impairment, urinary incontinence), in-hospital characteristics (*e.g.*, length of stay, psychiatric and neurologic consultations, disruptive behaviors, documentation of mental status, medical complications), and discharge information (*e.g.*, discharge destination, orientation at discharge, ambulatory status, urinary incontinence).

Patients over 75 years of age were more likely to experience moderate to severe confusion. Also, education of no more than elementary-grade level was related to severe confusion. Patients with pre-hospitalization histories of psychiatric illness or urinary incontinence were more likely to experience severe confusion. Patients who experienced severe confusion were significantly more likely to experience medical complications (*e.g.*, urinary tract infections, heart failure, renal failure, pressure ulcers, sepsis) during hospitalization. However, cognitive status did not affect length of hospitalization even though severely confused patients experienced more medical complications. The likelihood of being discharged to a nursing home increased as a function of the level of confusion. Frequently, evidence of altered mental status was not noted in the medical record. However, nurses were more likely to document observations than physicians, who rarely documented the presence of confusion.

Nursing Implications. Patients over 75 years of age who have experienced hip fracture are vulnerable to confusion during hospitalization, and with confusion there is an increased incidence of medical complications. Multiple factors contributing to confusional states (*e.g.*, drug response, dehydration, infections, blood loss, environmental factors) have been identified in other research. The nurse must monitor for these factors and minimize their impact on the patient. Active nursing interventions can promote orientation and cognitive functioning of the older adult patient who has experienced a hip fracture.

UNIT 17

Other Acute Problems

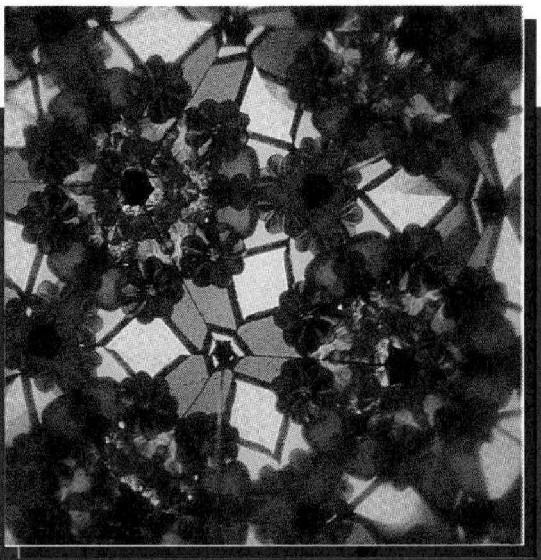

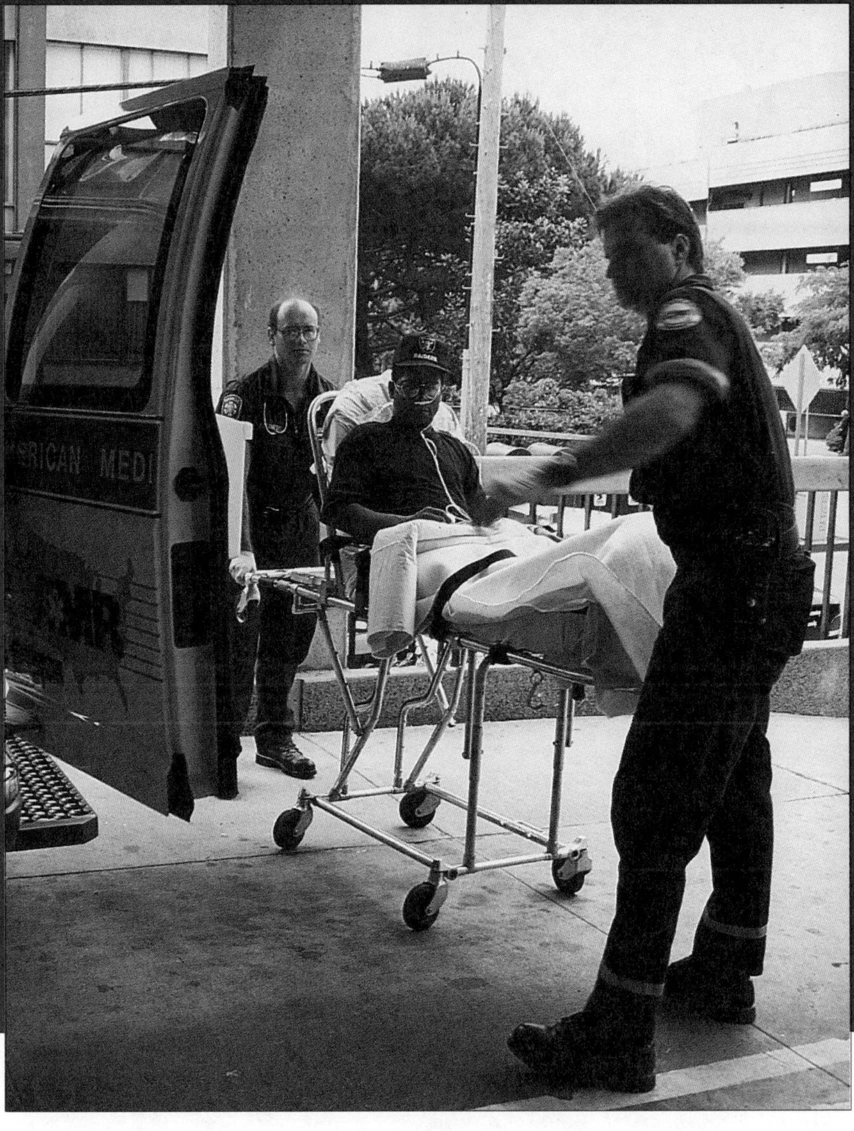

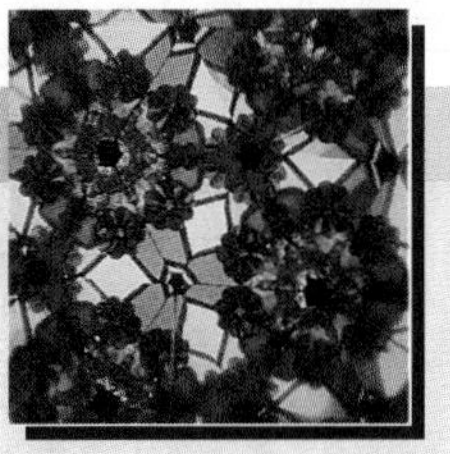

65

Management of Patients With Infectious Diseases

CHAPTER OUTLINE

LEARNING OBJECTIVES

On completion of this chapter, the learner will be able to:

1. Identify federal and local resources available to the nurse when seeking information about infectious diseases
2. Differentiate between colonization, infection, and disease
3. Use information obtained from the microbiology report to interpret infectious disease evidence
4. Identify the reasons for universal precautions and discuss recommended behaviors
5. Determine the nursing behaviors that decrease the risk of nosocomial infections
6. Contrast the various community-acquired infectious entities with particular emphasis on preventive aspects, management, and nursing and home health care implications
7. Identify the merit of vaccines recommended for health care workers
8. Describe home health care measures important in reducing the risk of infection
9. Use the nursing process as a framework for care of patients with infectious disease

Overview of Infectious Diseases

An infectious disease is any disease caused by growth of pathogenic organisms in the body. It may or may not be communicable (contagious). Within the last 2 decades, there has been a dramatic increase in the incidence of infectious diseases. HIV and AIDs, tuberculosis, hepatitis B, and all types of sexually transmitted diseases have become major concerns in health care today. In addition, there is a growing problem of antibiotic-resistant organisms that tend to thrive in health care facilities.

Therefore, it is important to understand general principles of infection and specific information about infectious diseases. In addition, it is important to understand the general patterns of infection in the human host and to be able to distinguish between those infectious diseases that are easily spread, are very serious, or are very common. Table 65-1 presents an overview of infectious diseases, their causative organisms, mode of transmission, and usual incubation periods. Chart 65-1 presents a glosssary of terms used in this chapter.

Transmission and control issues are important elements in dealing with infectious disease. The work of Ignaz Semmelweis, Florence Nightingale, and other early researchers in the area of contagion and its prevention is historically important for the findings that they made, and for the methods they used in the study of infectious disease transmission patterns.

Certainly, the role of the nurse has always been important in infection control as it is the nurse who provides consistent, around-the-clock care for most hospitalized patients. Handwashing, aseptic wound care, and promoting patient activity and nutrition have been viewed as important infection-reduction strategies.

The Infectious Process

A complete chain of events is necessary for infection to occur. Figure 65-1 illustrates the elements of the chain and points to weak links where health care workers' interventions can interrupt the chain. The necessary elements include:

- A causative organism
- A reservoir of available organisms
- A portal or mode of exit from the reservoir
- A mode of transmission from reservoir to host
- A susceptible host
- A mode of entry to host

Causative Organism. Any class of microorganism can serve as a *causative organism.* Infections can be caused by bacteria, rickettsiae, viruses, protozoa, fungi, or helminths.

Reservoir. *Reservoir* is the term used for any person, plant, animal, substance, or location that both provides nourishment for microorganisms and enables further dispersal of the organism. The causative organism and the reservoir represent the source for infection.

Means to Exit. The organism must have a *means to exit* from the reservoir. The infected host must shed the organisms to another host or to the environment for transmission to occur. Organisms exit through the respiratory tract, the gastrointestinal tract, or the genitourinary tract.

Route of Transmission. *Route of transmission* is necessary to connect the infectious source with its new host. Organisms may be transmitted through sexual or parenteral fluids; direct skin-to-skin, close contact or exposure; or through infectious particles in the air. It is important to recognize that different organisms require specific routes of transmission for infection to occur. For example, tuberculosis almost always is transmitted by the airborne route. Droplets present on the hands of health care workers would not present risk to other patients.

In contrast, bacteria such as *Staphylococcus aureus* are easily transmitted from patient to patient on the hands of health care workers. It is important for the nurse to understand and explain routes of disease transmission to patients with infectious diseases. For example, many patients question sharing a room with a patient with HIV infection. Concern should be reduced when the patient understands that transmission of HIV through recognized routes (sexual, perinatal, or parenteral exposure) is not likely to occur.

Susceptible Host. In order for infection to occur, the host must be *susceptible.* Previous infection or vaccine may render the host immune (not susceptible) to further infection with an agent. Many infections are prevented because of the powerful human immune defense. Although exposed to many organisms on a daily basis, relatively few individuals are actually infected.

Portal of Entry. If the host is susceptible to infection, a *portal of entry* is needed. The organism must gain access to the host through an entry point that allows organism interaction. For example, airborne tuberculosis does not cause disease when it settles on the skin of an exposed host. The only entry route of concern is through the respiratory system. Together susceptibility and point of entry represent the attack on the new host.

Colonization, Infection, and Disease

The brain, heart, and vascular system, and fluids from those sites (blood and cerebral spinal) are normally sterile. Most other human tissues have microorganisms in or on them. The majority of bacteria and other organisms introduce neither risk nor benefit. Others provide beneficial "normal flora" to compete with potential pathogens or to facilitate digestion.

Colonization. The term *colonization* is used to describe microorganisms present without host interference or interaction. Understanding the principle of colonization facilitates interpretation of microbiologic reports. Many reported results will reflect colonization rather than infection.

Infection. Infection indicates a host resistance to the organism. The host does not passively let the organism reside, but instead interacts and sets up a defense. A patient may have *Staphylococcus aureus* on the skin without any skin interruption or irritation (colonization). A culture of this area would show the presence of *S. aureus*, but would not distinguish infection from colonization. If the same patient were to have a cut and *S. aureus* entered the wound, the immune system would react with local inflammation and a routing of white cells to the site. The clinical evidence

TABLE 65-1 Infectious Diseases, Causative Organisms, Modes of Transmission, and Usual Incubation Period

Disease or Condition	Organism	Usual Mode of Transmission	Usual Incubation Period (Infection to First Symptom)
Acquired immunodeficiency syndrome (AIDS)	Human immunodeficiency virus	Sexual Percutaneous Perinatal	Median of 10 years
Amebiasis	*Entamoeba histolytica*	Contaminated water Through contact with raw vegetables	2–4 weeks
Chancroid	*Haemophilus ducreyi*	Sexual	3–5 days
Chickenpox	*Varicella zoster*	Airborne	Around 14 days
Cholera	*Vibrio cholera*	Ingestion of water contaminated with human waste	A few hours–5 days
Cryptococcosis	*Cryptococcus neoformans*	Probably by inhalation No person-to-person spread	Unknown
Cryptosporidiosis	*Cryptosporidium* species	Ingestion of contaminated water; direct contact with carrier	Probably 1–12 days
Cytomegalovirus (CMV) infection	Cytomegalovirus	Transfusion and transplant Sexual Perinatal Contact with mucous membranes	Highly variable; 3–8 weeks after transfusion 3–12 weeks after delivery of newborn
Diarrheal disease (Common causes)	*Campylobacter* species	Ingestion of contaminated food	3–5 days
	Clostridium difficile	Fecal-oral Efficient transfer by health care workers to patients	Variable; in part related to the influence of antibiotics
	Salmonella species	Ingestion of contaminated food or drink	12–36 hours
	Shigella species	Ingestion of contaminated food or drink; direct contact with carrier	1–3 days
	Yersinia species	Ingestion of contaminated food or drink; direct contact with carrier	3–7 days
Gonorrhea	*Neisseria gonorrhea*	Sexual	2–7 days
Hand, foot, and mouth disease	Coxsackie virus	Direct contact with nose and throat secretions, and with feces of infected persons	3–5 days
Foodborne hepatitis	Hepatitis A Hepatitis E	Ingestion of contaminated food or drink; direct contact with carrier	A: 15–50 days E: Unclear
Bloodborne hepatitis	Hepatitis B Hepatitis C Hepatitis D	Sexual Perinatal Percutaneous	B: 45–160 days C: 6–9 months D: Unclear
Herpangina	Coxsackie virus	Direct contact with nose and throat secretions and feces of infected persons	3–5 days
Herpes simplex	Human herpesvirus 1 and 2	Contact with mucous membrane secretions	2–12 days
Histoplasmosis	*Histoplasma capsulatum*	Inhalation of airborne spores	5–18 days
Hookworm disease	*Necator americanus* *Ancyclostoma duodenale*	Contact with soil contaminated with human feces	A few weeks to many months
Impetigo	*Staphylococcus aureus*	Contact with *S. aureus* carrier	4–10 days
Influenza	Influenza virus A, B, or C	Droplet spread	24–72 hours
Legionnaires' disease	*Legionella pneumophila*	Airborne from water source	2–10 days

(continued)

TABLE 65-1 *(continued)*

Disease or Condition	Organism	Usual Mode of Transmission	Usual Incubation Period (Infection to First Symptom)
Listeriosis	*Listeria monocytogenes*	Perinatal Sexual	Unclear; probably 3–70 days
Lyme disease	*Borrelia burgdorferi*	Tick bite	14–23 days
Lymphogranuloma venereum	*Chlamydia inguinale*	Sexual	Weeks to years
Malaria	*Plasmodium vivax* *Plasmodium malariae* *Plasmodium falciparum* *Plasmodium ovale*	Bite from *Anopheles* mosquito	12–30 days
Measles	Measles virus	Droplet spread	8–13 days
Meningococcal meningitis or bacteremia	*Neisseria meningitidis*	Contact with pharyngeal secretions; perhaps airborne	2–10 days
Mononucleosis	Epstein Barr virus	Contact with pharyngeal secretions	4–6 weeks
Mycobacterial diseases (non-tuberculosis *Mycobacterium* species)	*Mycobacterium avium* *Mycobacterium kansasii* *Mycobacterium fortuitum* *Mycobacterium gordonae* Other *Mycobacterium* species	Variable; probably contact with soil, water, or other environmental source. None are transmissible person to person	Variable
Mycoplasmal pneumonia	*Mycoplasma pneumonia*	Droplet inhalation	14–21 days
Pediculosis	*Pediculus humanus capitus* (head louse) *Pediculus humanus corporis* (body louse)	Direct contact	1–2 weeks
	Phthirus pubis (crab louse)	Sexual	
Pinworm disease	*Enterobius vermicularis*	Direct contact with egg-contaminated articles	4- to 6-week life cycle Often months of infection before recognition
Pneumocystis pneumonia	*Pneumocystis carinii*	Unknown Not transmitted person to person	Infants: 1–2 months; Adults: unclear
Pneumococcal pneumonia	*Streptococcus pneumoniae*	Droplet spread	Probably 1–3 days
Rabies	Rabies virus	Bite from rabid animal	2–8 weeks
Respiratory syncytial disease	Respiratory syncytial virus	Self inoculation by touching mouth or nose after contact with infectious respiratory secretions	3–7 days
Ringworm	*Microsporum* species *Trychophton* species *Epidermophyton floccosum*	Direct and indirect contact with lesions	4–10 days
Rocky Mountain Spotted fever	*Rickettsia ricketsii*	Bite from infected tick	3–14 days
Rotavirus gastroenteritis	Rota virus	Fecal–oral	Approximately 48 hours
Rubella	Rubella virus	Droplet spread Direct contact	14–21 days
Scabies	*Sarcoptes scabiei*	Direct skin contact	2–6 weeks
Syphilis	*Treponema pallidum*	Sexual	10 days–10 weeks
Tetanus	*Clostridium tetani*	Puncture wound	4–21 days
Trichinosis	*Trichinella spiralis*	Ingestion of insufficiently cooked foods, especially pork and beef	10–14 days
Tuberculosis	*Mycobacterium* tuberculosis	Airborne	4–12 weeks to the formation of primary lesion

CHART 65-1
Glossary

Bacteremia Laboratory-proven presence of bacteria in the bloodstream

Carrier A person who carries an organism without apparent symptomatology; able to transmit to others

Centers for Disease Control and Prevention (CDC) The federal agency with responsibility for conducting surveillance to measure endemic and epidemic disease; for recommending strategies to decrease infectious disease and other disease incidence; and for publishing guidelines to reduce risk to patients and health care workers

Colonization Microorganisms present in or on a host, without host interference or interaction, and without symptoms to the host

Disease The state in which the infected host displays a decline in wellness due to the infection.

Fungemia A bloodstream infection caused by a fungal organism

High-level disinfection The removal of all microorganisms with the possible exception of spores; this level of disinfection is appropriate for instruments that come in contact with mucous membranes but which cannot be sterilized because of mechanical difficulties

Host The person who provides living conditions to support a microorganism

Immune A person with protection in the form of antibodies or sensitized T cells from a previous infection or immunization, and who, as a result, is able to avoid reinfection when exposed to the same agent again

Incubation period The time between contact and development of the first symptomatology is recognized

Infection The condition in which the host interacts physiologically and immunologically with a microorganism

Latency The time interval after primary infection in which a microorganism dwells within the host without producing clinical evidence

Methicillin-Resistant Staphylococcus Aureus (MRSA) The bacterium *Staphylococcus aureus* that is not susceptible to extended-penicillin antibiotic formulas such as methicillin, oxacillin, or nafcillin

Normal flora Colonization with an organism or organisms that persists for long periods of time. In the skin, these organisms reside in low levels in the dermis layer

Nosocomial infection An infection acquired in the hospital that was not present nor incubating at the time of hospital admission

Primary bloodstream infection Bacteremia or fungemia, which occurs without infection, identified at another anatomic site

Reservoir Any person, plant, animal, substance, or location that provides living conditions for microorganisms and which enables further dispersal of the organism

Secondary bloodstream infection Bacteremia or fungemia infection of another anatomic site serves as a source for bloodstream contamination

Septicemia The presence of bacterial toxins in the bloodstream

Sterilization The complete removal of all microorganisms

Susceptible Not possessing immunity to a particular pathogen

Transient flora Organisms that recently have been acquired and are likely to be shed from skin or other site in a relatively short period of time

Universal precautions The strategy of considering all patients as though they may carry bloodborne infection and of using appropriate barrier precautions for all health care worker–patient interactions

Virulence The degree of pathogenicity of an organism

of redness, heat, and pain, and the presence of white cells on the blood smear would suggest infection. In this example, the host identifies the staphylococcus as "foreign." Infection is determined by host reaction as well as organism identification.

Disease. It is also important to recognize the difference between infection and disease. Infectious disease is the state in which the infected host displays a decline in wellness due to the infection. Often an infection will be present in which the host interacts immunologically with the organism, but remains well. Tuberculosis (TB) is an example of infection without disease. The host may become infected after exposure to the tubercle bacillus. The definition of infection is met when bacteria are first detected by nonspecific recognition, and later as newly sensitized immune system T cells propagate daughter lines of TB-specific T cells. After this initial infection, the untreated host has a low probability of actually becoming ill. Approximately 90% of infected hosts will not develop the disease of tuberculosis. Figure 65-2 depicts response to bacterial infection at the cellular level and at the host level.

The Microbiologic Report

The primary source of information about most bacterial infections is the microbiology report. The microbiology report should be viewed as a tool to be used along with clinical indicators to determine if a patient is colonized, infected, or diseased.

When specimens are sent to the laboratory for culture, results usually show three components: the smear and stain, the culture and organism identification, and the antimicrobial susceptibility (or sensitivity). As a marker for the

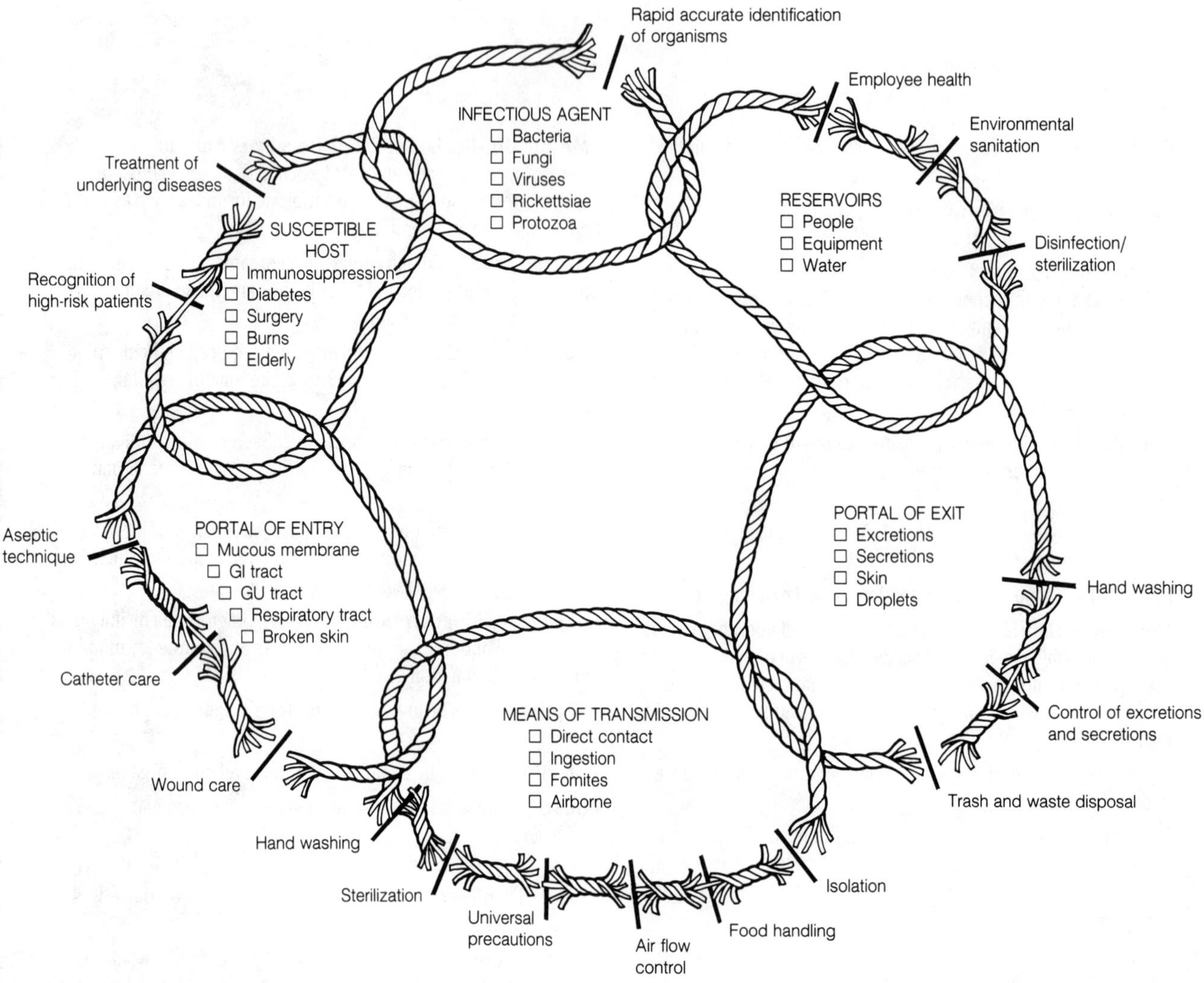

FIGURE 65-1. Health care workers' interventions used to break the chain of infection transmission.

likelihood of infection, the smear and stain generally provides the most helpful information as it most closely represents the mix of cells present at the site at the time of specimen collection. In contrast, culture and sensitivity processes refine and broaden information obtained on the smear, but may reflect distortion induced by laboratory manipulation rather than host reactions.

Infection Control and Prevention

Nurses specializing in infection control are responsible for agency-wide policy development and program direction. Staff nurses play an important role in risk reduction by careful attention to hand washing and by following guidelines to reduce technical risks associated with patient care.

Technological equipment issues become a focus of infection control as there is increased infection risk accompanying technical progress. In developing technically advanced outpatient services, such as clinics and home care programs, careful attention to risk reduction also becomes important.

Handwashing and Glove Use

Handwashing. Many outbreaks of infections in health care facilities are preventable with proper, consistent handwashing. **Normal skin flora** usually consist of coagulase-negative staphylococcus or diphtheroids. Only with host immune suppression or use of indwelling devices does the low quantity of colonization from these relatively nonpathogenic organisms have infectious potential.

In the health care setting, it is common for employees to carry **transient flora** such as *S. aureus*, *Pseudomonas aeruginosa*, and other organisms with strong pathogenic potential. Generally, these organisms are weakly attached and are shed with skin regeneration.

Handwashing is very important in the health care setting because transient organisms can be easily removed before transfer to other patients. Effective handwashing calls for at least 10 seconds of vigorous scrubbing with special attention to the area around nail beds and between fingers where there is generally an increased number of organisms present. Hands should be thoroughly rinsed after this step (Fig. 65-3).

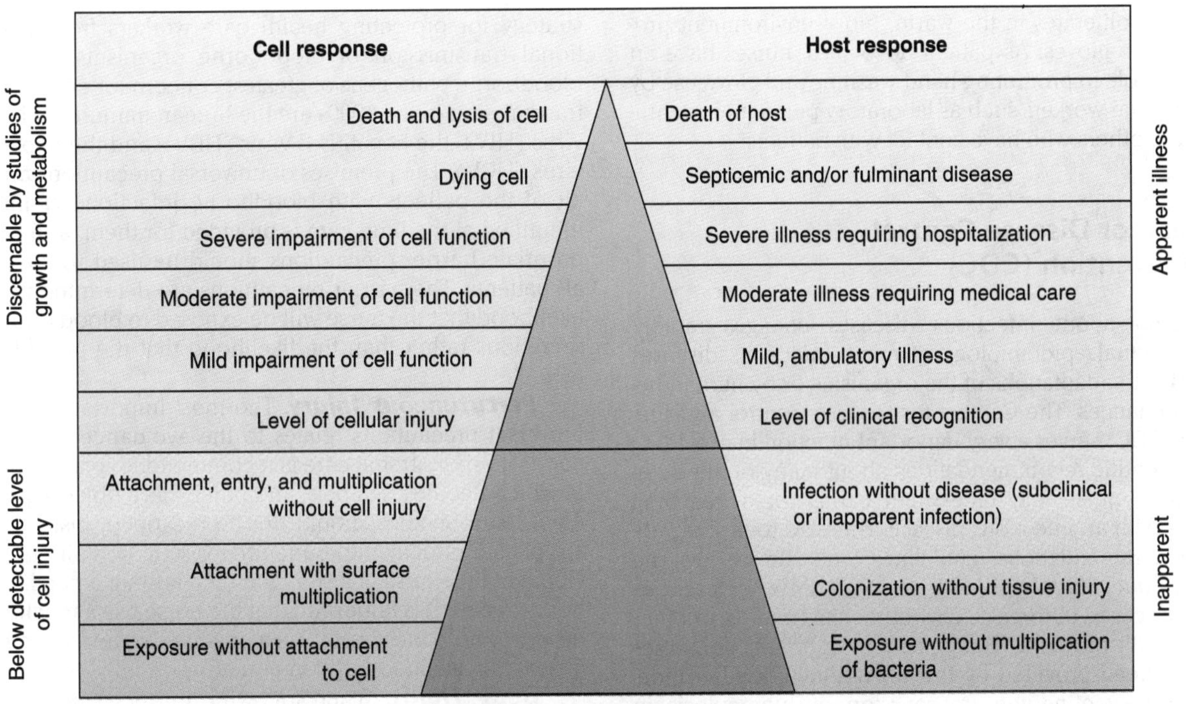

FIGURE 65-2. Biological spectrum of response to bacterial infection at the cellular level (*left*) and of the intact host (*right*). (Redrawn from Evans AS and Brachman PS. Bacterial Infections in Humans. New York, Plenum, 1991.)

When resistant organisms have been identified, or in intensive care units where there is likely to be a larger quantity of organisms present, antimicrobial handwashing agents are commonly used. Products appropriate for health care situations include solutions using chlorhexidine gluconate, alcohol, iodophors, chloroxylenol, or triclosan.

Glove Use. Gloves have been an important barrier protection in health care for a long time. Since the introduction of universal precautions and with increased awareness of barrier precautions for other types of infections, the use of gloves as protection for the health care worker has intensified significantly.

Gloves provide an effective skin barrier from the microflora associated with patient care. Infection control programs recommend the use of gloves whenever a health care worker has contact with secretions or excretions of any patient. Latex gloves are often preferred over vinyl gloves for comfort and better fit. Recent studies suggest that latex gloves may afford better protection than vinyl gloves.

To offer full protection, gloves must fit well, not tear, and not produce skin irritation. Irritation or allergy associated with glove use should be investigated by an occupational health specialist or dermatologist. When irritation or allergy to gloves occurs, decisions about the advisability of using an approved skin lotion, alternative types of gloves, or temporary relief from patient care activities should be made by occupational health specialists.

Because contaminated gloves can be the source of microorganism spread, it is important that gloves be discarded and hands washed thoroughly after every patient care exposure. Colonization of hospital organisms (some of which may be more virulent or more resistant than community or-

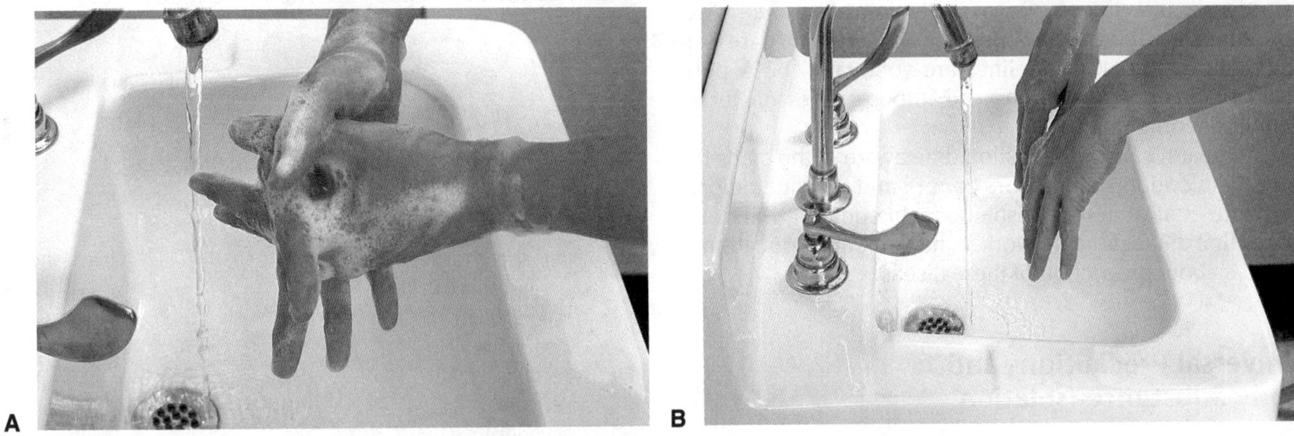

FIGURE 65-3. Effective handwashing. (**A**) Washing hands and forearms with firm rubbing and circular motions. (**B**) Rinsing thoroughly.

ganisms) proliferates in the warm, moist environment provided by the gloves. As patient advocates, nurses have an important role in promoting hand washing and glove use by other hospital workers such as laboratory personnel, technicians, and others who have contact with patients.

Centers for Disease Control and Prevention (CDC)

Information about infectious diseases changes rapidly, and the actual epidemiology of many infectious diseases changes with adaptations of the organisms or by human behavioral changes. The Centers for Disease Control and Prevention (CDC) serves a very important function in providing timely scientific recommendations about many of the questions that a nurse may face when caring for or teaching a patient with an infectious disease. The CDC routinely publishes recommendations, guidelines, and summaries. The *Morbidity and Mortality Weekly Report* (MMWR) describes significant cases, outbreaks, environmental hazards, or other public health problems. Examples of important summaries that have been provided by the MMWR include (1) Guidelines for Preventing the Transmission of Tuberculosis in Health Care Facilities, (2) Recommendations for Prevention of HIV Transmission in Health Care Settings, (3) Sexually Transmitted Diseases Treatment Guidelines, and (4) Standards for Pediatric Immunization Practices. In addition, the incidence of significant infectious diseases in the United States is summarized weekly.

The CDC itself can serve as an important resource if questions about a specific infectious disease or risk-reduction strategy arise. By contacting the CDC, nurses, epidemiologists, or other specialists often can obtain needed information or guidance.

Occupational Safety and Health Administration (OSHA)

Whereas the goal of the CDC is *disease reduction,* the goal for OSHA is the reduction of risk *exposure.* By law, OSHA has the duty to protect health care workers from hazards recognized in particular industries. OSHA has expanded its focus in infectious disease protection to enforce CDC Guidelines for Tuberculosis Prevention in Health Care Settings. Although CDC Guidelines are voluntary, OSHA publishes mandatory regulations and imposes fines on those found noncompliant.

All health care workers should be aware of the plans for both the bloodborne exposure control and the tuberculosis exposure control in their institutions. In addition, OSHA requires that all health care workers have routine educational updates about prevention of these diseases.

Universal Precautions and Body Substance Isolation

Universal Precautions. Universal precautions were first described in 1987 by the CDC. These precautions are a strategy for protecting health care workers from occupational transmission of bloodborne organisms. The three bloodborne pathogens of greatest concern for occupational transmission in the 1990s are the human immunodeficiency virus (HIV), the hepatitis B virus (HBV), and the hepatitis C virus (HCV). The premises of universal precautions are: (1) all of the patients with bloodborne infections cannot be identified at the time care is provided for them, and (2) appropriate barrier precautions should be used routinely for all patients. The barrier precautions are determined by the likelihood that the nurse will be exposed to blood or bloody secretions rather than the likelihood that the patient is infected.

Percutaneous Injury. The most important aspect of universal precautions relates to the avoidance of percutaneous injury. Extreme care is recommended in all situations in which needles, scalpels, and other sharp objects are handled. Used needles should not be recapped. Instead, they are placed directly into puncture-resistant containers in the vicinity of their use. If a situation dictates that a needle must be recapped, it is important that the nurse use a mechanical device to hold the cap, or use a one-handed approach to decrease the likelihood of skin puncture.

Body Fluids. When following universal precautions, the nurse recognizes that blood is the most important potential source of bloodborne pathogens such as HIV, HBV, and HCV. Other fluids are considered to present less risk of bloodborne infection, and still others are considered to represent no risk of transmission (unless visibly bloody). See Charts 65-2 and 65-3 for a list of fluids associated with the transmission of bloodborne pathogens and a list of fluids not considered to present risk (unless visibly bloody).

Barrier Precautions. Because of concern about transmission of diseases *other than* bloodborne diseases, gloves are recommended when touching feces, nasal secretions, sputum, urine, vomitus, and saliva.

Hands should be washed before and after contact with each patient and after the removal of gloves.

The eyes and mouth should be covered whenever there is reasonable anticipation of splashes, spray, splatter, or droplets of blood or other potentially infectious material to the face.

Although recognizing the very low risk of bloodborne infection as a result of contaminated clothes, it is still important to reduce this exposure. The nurse reduces the risk of

CHART 65-2
Fluids Associated With Transmission of Bloodborne Pathogens

- Semen and vaginal secretions
- Cerebrospinal fluid (CSF)
- Synovial fluid
- Pleural fluid
- Peritoneal fluid
- Pericardial fluid
- Amniotic fluid

CHART 65-3

Fluids Not Considered to Offer Risk of Transmission of Bloodborne Pathogens (Unless Visibly Bloody):

- Feces
- Nasal secretions
- Sputum
- Sweat
- Tears
- Urine
- Vomitus
- Saliva

contact of the skin with blood (minute breaks in skin theoretically could lead to transmission) by wearing appropriate protective clothing such as gowns, aprons, and laboratory coats. Nurses and other health care workers who have open lesions or weepy dermatitis should not have contact with patients or their secretions. Covering the head or shoes when there is a wide spray of blood is a wise and aestheticly sensitive practice.

Although saliva has not been implicated in HIV transmission, mouthpieces, resuscitation bags, or other ventilation devices should be available for use in areas in which the need for resuscitation is anticipated.

Pregnancy. Pregnant health care workers are not known to be at greater risk of contracting bloodborne infections than nonpregnant health care workers. However, if a health care worker develops a bloodborne infection during pregnancy, the infant bears a risk of perinatal transmission. Health care workers who are contemplating pregnancy are strongly advised to complete hepatitis B vaccine series and to be familiar with and adhere to universal precautions.

Body Substance Isolation. Some institutions have adopted a system of infection control and prevention called *body substance isolation* (BSI) rather than universal precautions (UP). BSI was devised because of the argument that UP is designed strictly for bloodborne disease risk reduction. UP may require the nurse or other health care worker to use one preventive strategy for bloodborne risk and another strategy for other infectious risks. Whereas UP focuses on bloodborne disease, BSI focuses on all moist and potentially infectious body substances. Glove use is emphasized as the most important aspect of control, and gloves are worn for exposure to any moist or wet substances. When patients have airborne transmitted diseases, such as tuberculosis, signs recommending the use of a mask are posted on the door.

The systems seem identical when caring for patients with recognized bloodborne infection or airborne infection. The difference between the systems is evident when caring for patients with other infectious diseases. For example, in a setting that uses UP, patients with *Salmonella* species would require enteric isolation and patients with antibiotic-resistant organisms would require contact isolation. In health care facilities that use BSI, isolation procedures would be identical in both instances.

The premise that supports BSI is that we cannot identify all of the pre-existing patient infections (not limited to bloodborne infections). Therefore, barrier precautions should be used routinely to protect from all sources of potential infection. Arguments against BSI are based on the concern that greater prevention attention should be directed at organisms that can have particularly serious outcomes or at infections that are easily transmitted in the health care setting.

Both UP and BSI demand the understanding that many infections are not easily recognizable in the patient population. Therefore, recommended precautions are based on nursing tasks rather than patient diagnosis.

Nosocomial Infections

Each year an estimated 2 million patients acquire infections while hospitalized. These infections, referred to as **nosocomial,** are estimated to cost more than $4.5 billion per year and cause more than 19,000 deaths per year in the United States. In addition, nosocomial infections are a contributing factor in over 55,000 deaths.

In the 1970s, the Centers for Disease Control conducted a massive investigation about the effectiveness of nosocomial infection reduction programs. That study, known as SENIC (Study of Nosocomial Infection Control) found that approximately one third of all nosocomial infections could be prevented when effective infection control programs are in place. An effective program was found to include the following four components: (1) a program of surveillance for nosocomial infections and vigorous control efforts, (2) at least one infection control practitioner for every 250 hospital beds, (3) a trained hospital epidemiologist, and (4) feedback to surgeons about individual surgical site infections. Unfortunately, the majority of hospitals have not yet introduced all four required aspects, and thus prevent only an estimated 9% of expected infections.

Nosocomial Bloodstream Infections (Bacteremia and Fungemia)

Bacteremia is defined as laboratory-proven presence of bacteria in the bloodstream. The term is often confused with septicemia, which is defined as the presence of bacterial toxins in the bloodstream.

Sepsis is a generalized host reaction to these toxins. Bacteremia is diagnosed with microbiologic data; septicemia is diagnosed with both microbiologic and clinical data.

Fungemia is a bloodstream infection caused by a fungal organism. Bloodstream infections are serious and require early recognition. The therapeutic goal is to prevent dissemination to other organs and other consequences including risk of mortality.

Pathophysiology

Normally the bloodstream is sterile. However, there are many opportunities for the introduction of organisms into the bloodstream. Common activities such as brushing or flossing teeth may produce a transient (temporary) bacteremia. In the immune competent host, the immune system usually is able to eradicate transient bacteria without producing symptoms. Without a strong immune system or when the source of organism overwhelms the immune system because of its virulence, number, or both, the bloodstream itself becomes infected.

The study of nosocomial bloodstream infections is usually divided into two categories: primary bacteremia and secondary bacteremia.

Primary Bloodstream Infections. **Primary bloodstream infections** are those in which the host has no preexisting infection, but through mechanical manipulation, (most frequently with intravascular devices) the bloodstream becomes contaminated.

Secondary Bloodstream Infection. **Secondary bloodstream infection** occurs when a host has another site of infection that can serve as a source of contamination to the bloodstream. For example, organisms present in a localized abscess can enter the bloodstream to cause disseminated bacteremia. Over the last decade, the rate of secondary nosocomial bacteremia has remained stable, while the rate of primary bacteremia has more than doubled. This increase represents largely preventable infections associated with advanced technology for diagnosis and therapy.

Vascular Access Devices. Any vascular access device (VAD) can serve as the source for bloodstream infection. Contamination can occur from the patient's own flora traversing the exterior of a catheter or by contamination of internal tubing during manipulation. The intravenous (IV) fluid itself can become contaminated and serve as a source of infection.

VADs are now used extensively for both hospitalized patients and outpatients receiving care in a clinic or home setting. In all instances, the nurse must consider the infectious potential of the VAD. Chart 65-4 identifies conditions that suggest the presence of nosocomial line-related bacteremia or fungemia.

CHART 65-4

Conditions That Suggest the Presence of Nosocomial Line-Related Bacteremia or Fungemia

- The patient has catheter in place, appears septic, but has no obvious reason to suggest predisposition to sepsis.
- There is no infection at another body site to indicate probable source of sepsis.
- The site of vascular line insertion is red, swollen, or draining (especially purulent drainage).
- The patient has a central vascular line in place at the onset of sepsis.
- The bloodstream infection is caused by *Candida* species or by common skin organisms such as coagulase-negative staphylococci, bacillus species, or corynebacterium.
- The patient remains septic after appropriate therapy without removal of the vascular access device.

Prevention

Disinfection. During the insertion of all vascular access devices, there must be strict attention to aseptic technique. Those inserting VADs must vigorously wash hands before insertion. Sterile gloves are worn for the placement of all central and arterial lines. Because the rate of bloodstream infection associated with central VADs is greater than with those peripherally placed, barrier methods such as gowns with long sleeves, masks, and a large drape over the patient are used in many settings for the insertion of such lines.

The site of insertion is disinfected with chlorhexidine gluconate, povidone iodine, or alcohol. The relative benefit of topical antimicrobial ointment use at the site has not yet been conclusively studied and its use varies among institutions.

Although there are inconclusive data about whether gauze or polyurethane transparent dressings confer greater benefit, the intended benefits of either type of dressing at the insertion site are to protect the catheter from contamination and to protect the site from trauma (Conley, Grieves and Peters, 1989; Maki and Ringer, 1987).

Guidewires. **Guidewires** generally are used to insert central lines. They offer decreased risk of vascular injury, less manipulation (with the goal of less contamination), and less risk of pneumothorax for subclavian and internal jugular catheters. As with many strategies for bacteremia risk reduction, it is not clear if guidewires offer infectious risk or benefit. In general, guidewires are helpful when there are limited alternative insertion sites available and when the central line requires removal because it has been in place for an extended period of time or when the catheter is cracked or leaking. However, if the patient has sepsis that may be linked to catheterization or if the insertion site is red or has purulent drainage, a new site should be chosen for catheter insertion.

Infusion Sets and Solutions. **Infusion sets and solutions** should be changed approximately every 72 hours unless an infusion set is used for the delivery of blood or lipid solutions, for arterial pressure monitoring, or when an infusion-related bacteremia is suspected. In these cases, the infusion set should be changed on completion of the solution or if infection is suspected. Policies to limit the duration of line insertion time for peripheral and central catheters must be followed. Signs of sepsis in patients with indwelling vascular lines should be promptly assessed and treated.

Nurses have an important role in the prevention of bloodstream infections as they assess patients for evidence of infection, make daily VAD site inspections, and monitor the interval of line changes.

Septic Shock

Invasion of the bloodstream by any microorganism has the potential to cause a generalized host reaction to these toxins. The result is a potentially life-threatening state of inadequate tissue perfusion called *septic shock*. Some organisms are more powerful in eliciting this response than others. In hospitalized patients, gram- negative organisms (*e.g., Escherichia coli, Klebsiella, Enterobacter,* and *Serratia* species, *Pseudomonas aeruginosa*, *Proteus* species, *Neisseria menin-*

gitidis, *Bacteroides fragilis*) are more frequently associated with septic shock than are gram-positive organisms (*e.g.*, *S. aureus*, *Streptococcus pneumoniae*). Scrutiny for early signs of shock and immediate treatment are crucial in reducing shock- related fatalities.

The organisms that invade the bloodstream are either endotoxins (a component of the cell wall of gram-negative organisms) or exotoxins (a toxin produced by *S. aureus* and other organisms). The immune system reaction to the recognition of these toxins is complex and variable with different organisms.

Clinical Manifestations

The clinical signs of septic shock may vary significantly among patients. Patients with recognized infections and severely immune suppressed patients at risk for shock should have vital signs monitored routinely and as warranted. In particular, the nurse must be alert for signs of:

- Fever
- Tachycardia (>90 beats/min)
- Tachypnea (>20 breaths/min)
- Evidence of lack of organ perfusion or dysfunction in the form of
  - Change of mental status
  - Hypoxemia as measured by arterial blood gas
  - Elevated lactate levels
  - Urine output (<30 ml/h)

Although the course of septic shock may be very rapid, especially when associated with a gram-negative organism, early administration of intravenous antibiotics, fluid replacement, vasopressors, and oxygen are essential components in the management of such a patient.

Gerontologic Considerations. In the elderly patient, septic shock may be manifested in atypical or confusing clinical signs. Septic shock should be suspected in any elderly person who develops an unexplained acute confused state, tachypnea, or hypotension.

Chapter 15 provides greater detail about the pathophysiology and nursing actions associated with septic shock.

Nosocomial Surgical Site Infections

Surgical site infections (SSI) are wound infections evident at the site of incision or in the anatomic pathway of a procedure following surgery.

The patient who develops a surgical wound infection may require a prolonged hospital stay with antibiotic therapy, wound care, and sometimes surgical repair. These consequences can cause depression, discomfort, and increased risk of other infections such as pneumonia or blood stream infection. Additionally, the patient may have increased concerns because of postponing a return to normal activities and employment. Financial concerns may become extreme as the length of stay exceeds that anticipated by the patient and the insurance company. The nurse who cares for such a patient can be very instrumental in orchestrating needed support from physicians, social workers, utilization management professionals, financial counselors, and others. Sensitivity to the unique problems caused by surgical site infection for each patient is crucial.

Pathophysiology

The probability of surgical site infection is directly related to the likelihood and volume of bacterial entry into the incision during surgery. Surgeries in which the incision is made through intact skin into sterile tissue represent lower infection risk than surgeries with entry into a contaminated site (such as following trauma) or into infected tissue (*e.g.*, a ruptured abdominal organ site such as the appendix). Because of the differences in risk of infection, surgical procedures are traditionally categorized by risk probability. The categories, their determinants, and their anticipated rates of postsurgical infection are summarized in Table 65-2.

Prevention

Because almost all surgical site infections originate at the time of surgery, preventive strategies for this type of infection must be aimed at reducing risk of introduction of organisms in the operating room.

The most likely source of organisms is the patient's own flora, either introduced from the surgical site or from other anatomic sites. Organisms also can gain wound entry by contamination from the surgical team members, from contaminated instruments or solutions, or from airborne introduction, especially in a heavily trafficked operating room setting.

Disinfection. In preparing the patient for surgery, instructions for showering and skin preparation must be carefully followed. Several studies have demonstrated that decreasing bacterial flora by shower or bathing with antimicrobial agent before surgery is associated with a lower infection risk (Cruse and Foord, 1973; Hayek, Emerson, and Gardner, 1987; Wihlborg, 1987). When procedures require removal of hair from the surgical site, clippers or depilatories are recommended rather than shaving. This tends to reduce the incidence of small cuts in the skin, thereby decreasing the potential for later wound infection (Seropian and Reynolds, 1971).

To reduce bacterial flora significantly in the surgical setting, the skin must be thoroughly cleaned and an antiseptic solution applied to the site just before incision is made. Operating room nurses are frequently responsible for this aspect of surgical preparation.

Antibiotics. Antibiotic prophylaxis should be used for procedures that have a high risk of infection or in which the risk of infection is associated with disastrous results. Antibiotic prophylaxis should be administered just prior to surgery to allow the drug concentration to be high enough to suppress growth of organisms that may enter the wound at the time of surgery.

Although the risk of introduction of organisms after surgery is very low, aseptic technique must be used when performing dressing changes.

Nosocomial Pneumonia

Pneumonia comprises approximately 15% of all nosocomial infections, and mortality rates have been calculated to be as

TABLE 65-2 Surgical Site Infection

Surgical Category	Determinants of Category	Expected Risk of Post Surgical Infection (%)
Clean	Nontraumatic site Uninfected site No inflammation No break in aseptic technique No entry into respiratory, alimentary, genitourinary or oropharyngeal tracts	1–3
Clean-contaminated	Entry into respiratory, alimentary, genitourinary or oropharyngeal tracts without unusual contamination Appendectomy Minor break in aseptic technique Mechanical drainage	3–7
Contaminated	Open, newly experienced traumatic wounds Gross spillage from gastrointestinal tract Major break in aseptic technique Entry into genitourinary or biliary tracts when urine or bile is infected	7–16
Dirty	Traumatic wound with delayed repair, devitalized tissue, foreign bodies, or fecal contamination Acute inflammation and purulent drainage encountered during procedure	16–29

high as 50%. The risk of infection is greatest for the postoperative patient, especially for those who have had thoracic or abdominal surgery. Other risk factors for pneumonia associated with **hospitalization** include: endotracheal intubation, mechanical ventilation, use of cimetidine for prevention of stress ulcer, the presence of a nasogastric tube, and recent bronchoscopy. High risk **patient-related** variables include: depressed level of consciousness, underlying chronic lung disease, old age, immune suppression, prior large volume aspiration, and severe trauma.

Pathophysiology

Bacteria can invade the lung after aspiration of oral and pharyngeal secretions or inhalation of contaminated aerosol, or through the hematogenous spread of organisms to the lung from another infected site. Another mechanism for contamination that is currently being investigated is the route of migration of organisms from the gastrointestinal tract to the lung (Fiddian-Green and Baaker, 1991).

Aspiration. **Aspiration** of organisms, which is the most frequent mode of transmission, is common in healthy individuals during sleep. However, it is particularly likely to occur in patients who have had recent surgery, those who have had mechanical instrumentation of the respiratory or gastrointestinal tract, those being mechanically ventilated, and those with depressed consciousness (CDC Guideline for Prevention of Nosocomial Pneumonia, 1994).

Transmission. Risk of pneumonia is heightened in hospitalized patients, as there is frequent colonization of the oropharynx with potentially pathogenic organisms soon after admission. Pathogenic organisms are frequently spread on the hands of health care workers. Increased transmission opportunity is seen in the ventilator- dependent patient who requires increased health care worker contact to manipulate ventilator equipment and suction. Organisms also can be acquired by contact with contaminated respiratory equipment or by inhaling aerosolized organisms from water sources used with this equipment.

Prevention

The behaviors listed in Chart 65-5 are those that are supported by epidemiologic studies and are recommended in the care of patients at risk for developing nosocomial bacterial pneumonia.

Sterilization. Further prevention strategies necessitate that all equipment that requires sterilization should be thoroughly cleaned with a detergent and mechanical cleaner prior to sterilizing. This is especially important for many pieces of respiratory equipment because small internal lumens can harbor mucus and other debris. Sterilization methods cannot reach surfaces that have not been first made accessible by cleaning.

Disinfection. If sterilization procedures are not feasible, *high level disinfection* must be used. High level disinfection is a process that removes all microorganisms except some spore-producing bacteria. Directions accompanying chemical disinfectant products must be carefully followed to determine appropriate methods for rinsing, drying, and

CHART 65-5
Prevention: Nosocomial Pneumonia

- Staff should be educated about infection control methods to prevent pneumonia.
- Gloves should be worn when handling mucous membrane or respiratory secretions.
- Gloves must be changed between patients and after handling respiratory secretions of a patient.
- Hands must be washed after each of these contacts even though gloves have been worn.
- Postoperatively, active efforts to reduce the risk of pneumonia include instructing the patient to regularly cough, take deep breaths, and to ambulate as soon as medically indicated. These methods are most important for the patient who has undergone abdominal, thoracic, or head and neck surgery, or for those with underlying decreased pulmonary function.
- Judicious control of pain during this time period may allow the patient to participate more effectively in the activities listed above.
- Incentive spirometry, intermittent positive pressure breathing, and chest physiotherapy are used as prescribed

storing. Sterile water is used for rinsing components that have been chemically disinfected.

The nurse should leave ventilator breathing circuits in place at least 48 hours between routine changes. Although the maximal safe interval between changes has not yet been well established, most experts advise changing circuits within 1 week. Condensate within the ventilator tubing or anesthesia machine should be drained periodically. Sterile water is used to fill bubbling humidifiers. It is not necessary to disinfect or sterilize internal components of mechanical ventilators and anesthesia breathing machines.

Suctioning. When suctioning a patient, it is important to use only sterile water for flushing the tube. If an open suction system is used, a sterile catheter must be used each time the patient is suctioned. In many settings, multi-use closed systems are used in an effort to decrease contamination and maintain oxygenation efficiency. The success of these instruments in decreasing contamination and maintaining oxygenation has not yet been demonstrated. When using such systems, nurses should carefully adhere to the manufacturer's recommendations for changing the catheter.

Feeding Tubes. Because endotracheal and enteral feeding tubes offer the opportunity for introduction of organisms, they should be removed at the earliest clinically acceptable time. Correct placement of feeding tubes should always be verified before initiation of feeding. Assessment of the patient's intestinal motility should include routinely listening for bowel sounds, measuring and recording the patient's girth for daily comparison, and measuring residual gastric volume. Decisions concerning the lumen size of the feeding tube, the timing, and quantity of tube feeding vary by institution and by patient condition. The risks or benefits of different enteral feeding options have not been verified scientifically at this time.

Nosocomial Urinary Tract Infections

Urinary tract infection (UTI) is a common nosocomial infectious disease that usually results when organisms ascend through the urethra into the bladder. Once organisms reach the bladder, they can multiply and ascend higher anatomically to cause infection of the ureters and kidneys.

Symptoms

Diagnosis of urinary tract infections should differentiate between lower urinary tract infections in which the bladder or urethra is infected, and upper urinary tract infection which includes infection of the ureter and kidney. Symptoms of lower UTI usually include dysuria, urgency, frequency, nocturia, or pelvic or suprapubic pain. Patients with upper UTI often exhibit more systemic signs including fever, nausea and vomiting, headache, and malaise along with specific site complaints of pain in the flank, low back, and abdomen. Complications of UTI can include perinephric abscesses and gram- negative sepsis.

Diagnosis

Diagnosis of UTI generally depends on identification of organisms as well as white blood cells in a specimen of voided or catheter- obtained urine. Because voided specimens are difficult to obtain without contamination, the quantification of organisms used to reflect likelihood of infection is usually set at 100,000 colony-forming units per milliliter (cfu/ml). Generally, the presence of white cells (usually >10 wbc/mm^3) in the urine specimen adds diagnostic strength, as these cells indicate host inflammatory response to organisms. The presence of organisms without accompanying white cells is considered *bacteriuria* rather than infection. Bacteriuria is a frequent finding in persons with catheters in place, in the elderly, and in pregnant women.

Pathogenesis

A frequent cause of nosocomial bacteriuria is the urinary catheter. Although urinary catheterization is an important component of care for the acutely ill, surgical patients, patients with neurogenic bladders, or elderly patients in extended care facilities, infection is a common outcome of catheter use. The risk of bacteriuria in the presence of catheter use has been calculated to be approximately 5% to 10% a day. Thus, virtually all patients will acquire bacteriuria after 10 days of catheter use.

Prevention

Intraluminal Contamination. In the catheterized patient, contamination of the bladder is increased by the presence of the catheter because organisms are able to ascend from contaminated urine in the collection bag to the bladder. Methods used to minimize this intraluminal approach include decontamination of the urine in the bag and attempts to decrease contamination while emptying urine. Vigorous efforts to maintain the closed system are important to reduce risk of intraluminal contamination.

Extraluminal Contamination. *Extraluminal contamination* can occur as organisms present in the perineal area ascend to the bladder via the space created along the area of the catheter and the mucosal lining of the urethra.

The tenets of keeping the collection system closed and keeping the collection bag lower than the patient appear to reduce the likelihood of infection, but do not eliminate risk when a catheter is used. Unfortunately, studies of all other strategies including decontamination methods and different types of catheters have not convincingly demonstrated reduced risk of catheter-related infection (Garibaldi et al, 1982; Wong and Hooten, 1983; Thompson et al, 1984).

Long-Term Catheterization. For the patient who requires long-term catheterization, such as the paralyzed patient with neurogenic bladder or the elderly patient with persistent incontinence (sometimes associated with pressure ulcer formation), the catheter virtually ensures bacteriuria. When assessing the need for long-term catheterization, potential complications of stone formation, renal infection, and systemic infection complicate the risk-to-benefit equation.

Specific Organisms With Nosocomial Infection Potential

Clostridium Difficile

Clostridium difficile is a bacterium with great potential as a nosocomial pathogen. The organism is a gram-positive spore-forming bacterium. Spore formation of this organism facilitates the organism's ability to be spread by environmental sources and personnel.

Pathophysiology. After antibiotic treatment, a person's normal intestinal flora is frequently interrupted. *C. difficile*, with its protective spore, is often resistant to antimicrobial therapy, and thus is able to proliferate relatively unimpeded in this setting.

The organism works as a pathogen by releasing toxins into the lumen of the bowel. The toxins cause destruction at the site, rather than actual invasion by the organism. In pseudomembranous colitis, the most extreme form of *C. difficile* infection, debris from the invaded lumen and white blood cells accumulate in the form of pseudomembranes or studded areas of the colon. The destruction of such a large anatomic area can produce profound sepsis.

Because many people receive antibiotics to treat infection, the risk for *C. difficile* pathology is widely distributed. This factor represents part of the nosocomial potential of this organism. To compound the problem, the spore is relatively resistant to cleaning and hand washing agents, and can be spread on the hands of health care workers and by contact with equipment that has been previously contaminated with *C. difficile*. Even in environments that have been cleaned, complete assurance that *C. difficile* has been eliminated is often unrealistic.

Diagnosis and Management. Diagnostic tools for this infection are culture and toxin assays. Because early diagnosis is important, stool specimens should be obtained and sent to the laboratory as soon as possible when the diagnosis of *C. difficile* infection is being explored.

C. difficile infection usually is treated with oral vancomycin or metronidazole. The patient who has been treated with one of these antibiotics and has apparent relief of symptoms should be taught that recurrence is a common problem. If there is recurrence of diarrhea after discharge from an acute care setting, patients need to relate the *C. difficile* diagnosis to their health care provider. Most experts discourage the use of antiperistaltic agents for treatment of diarrhea caused by *C. difficile*.

Prevention. It is important that nurses regularly wear gloves when caring for patients with *C. difficile* infection. Gloves provide a barrier protection to be removed between contact with other patients. Hands should be washed after gloves are removed. To decrease the risk of contaminated equipment being shared between patients, most infection control programs recommend the use of private rooms for patients with *C. difficile* infections.

Methicillin-Resistant *Staphylococcus Aureus* (MRSA)

Methicillin-resistant *Staphylococcus aureus* (MRSA) is a common nosocomial infection in hospitals and extended care facilities. MRSA is the term used to describe *S. aureus* that is resistant to Methicillin or its comparable pharmaceutical agents, oxacillin and nafcillin. Since the introduction of antibiotics in the 1940s, there has been concern about antibiotic-resistant *S. aureus*. At the time that penicillin was first made available almost all isolates of *S. aureus* were sensitive to the drug. Once resistance to penicillin was first seen, organisms rapidly became resistant. Fortunately alternative therapies in the forms of cephalosporins, and more importantly, synthetic penicillin solutions such as methicillin, oxacillin, or nafcillin were introduced.

Late in the 1970s MRSA was seen infrequently. The prevalence of this organism was originally linked epidemiologically to the intravenous drug abuse community. Since that time transmission within hospitals and nursing homes has become well documented. In fact, once found within a hospital, it is rare that control efforts are successful in eliminating this organism.

Despite the relative failure of eradication programs, there are several reasons for vigorous attempts to decrease the incidence of MRSA in hospitals. *S. aureus* remains the most frequently identified nosocomial pathogen and is a very common source of community-acquired infections as well. Therefore, *S. aureus* must initially be considered as a potential cause of infection in many patients.

Management. In a setting with increased prevalence of MRSA, initial therapy choices are severely limited. To assure antibiotic coverage for possible MRSA, patients may first require potentially less effective, more toxic, and more expensive alternative therapies. Many strains of *S. aureus* resistant to methicillin are also resistant to most other antibiotics. With this lack of antibiotic sensitivity, vancomycin may be the *only* appropriate antibiotic choice available.

There is a concern that MRSA may become resistant to vancomycin, which would make it an untreatable infection. The threat of vancomycin-resistant *S. aureus* suggests a return to health care in the preantibiotic era when patients died from common infections. Along with this concern, the need for vancomycin for those infected with MRSA, may induce vancomycin resistance in other organisms such as enterococcus.

Transmission. Transmission of MRSA from health care worker to patient appears very efficient because *S. aureus* is an organism that colonizes skin easily. Colonization is seldom recognized, so the health care worker must assume that *every* patient contact offers the possibility of MRSA exposure.

For patients who have alteration of normal flora with hospitalization, MRSA acquired in the hospital may persist as normal flora in the future. Although there is no evidence that MRSA is more virulent than other strains of staphylococcus, once colonized, the patient faces the likelihood of infection with MRSA when invasive procedures, such as intravenous therapy, respiratory therapy, or surgery are performed. If infected, very few antibiotics offer effective treatment options for MRSA. In addition, the patient colonized with MRSA serves as a reservoir of resistant organisms to be transmitted to others.

Prevention

Contact Isolation. Most hospitals use contact isolation, as designed by the CDC to control transmission of MRSA. Because MRSA easily colonizes skin, contact isolation emphasis is on hand washing and glove use before and after contact with the patient. In addition, in many hospitals, masks are recommended when caring for patients with MRSA pneumonia, although the value of this practice has not been well demonstrated.

Antimicrobial Agents. Decolonization of MRSA with antimicrobial agents has often been attempted. However, institutions that have used this strategy have frequently been unsuccessful in eradicating MRSA in the long run, and some may have induced resistance to the decolonizing agent. During clusters of MRSA infections, health care facilities may elect to treat colonized health care workers. A topical antimicrobial agent called mupirocin (Bactroban) has been shown to be one of the most effective agents used for eradication of the carrier state. It is important to recognize that identification of the carrier state among health care workers can be difficult. One negative culture does not eliminate the possibility that the health care worker is colonized or carries the organism from time to time. Similarly, one positive culture does not distinguish between transient or persistent colonization.

The American Hospital Association Technical Panel on Infections in Hospitals has recommended that nursing home facilities *should not* require that hospitalized patients have confirmed absence of MRSA before acceptance to a nursing home.

Vancomycin-Resistant Enterococcus (VRE)

Enterococcus is a gram-positive bacterium that is part of the normal flora of the gastrointestinal tract. However, it has the capability of producing significant infections in certain situations. Enterococcus is now the third most frequently isolated cause of nosocomial infection in the United States.

As a relatively resistant organism at baseline, therapy for enterococcus has been essentially limited to penicillin formulations (such as ampicillin), or vancomycin in combination with aminoglycoside (such as gentamicin). In the 1980s, initial recognition of resistance to all of these agents was reported. Between 1989 and 1993, the CDC recorded a 20-fold increase in the percentage of cases of infection with enterococcus resistant to vancomycin.

This rapidly growing problem has serious implications. Patients with vancomycin-resistant enterococcus are frequently resistant to all other antimicrobial therapies, leaving them with bacterial infections for which there is no pharmaceutical treatment available. Additionally, there is great theoretical concern that VRE may serve as a reservoir of genes coded for vancomycin resistance that can be transferred to the even more prevalent and virulent *S. aureus*.

Transmission. Enterococcus has the following traits that make it an ideal nosocomial organism: (1) the host carries an abundance of the organism even in a noninfected state, (2) it is bile resistant and can withstand harsh anatomic sites such as the intestine, (3) enterococcus has the potential for resistance to many antibiotics so that therapeutic agents reducing local bacterial competition may leave it to freely replicate, and (4) the enterococcus endures well on the hands of health care workers and on environmental objects.

Prevention. The best strategies for decreasing the prevalence of resistant enterococcus are not entirely clear. To reduce antibiotic induction of resistance, hospitals should have systems in place to determine that vancomycin is judiciously prescribed. Infection control efforts, such as isolating the patient with diagnosed VRE, may help to contain the organism. Unfortunately, it is not clear which control behaviors will prove the most successful. Extreme attention to hand washing and appropriate glove use are important parts of the risk-reduction strategy. In addition, equipment used for such patients must be appropriately disinfected before being used for other patients.

Sexually Transmitted Diseases

A sexually transmitted disease (STD) is a disease acquired through sexual contact with an infected person. Table 65-3 identifies diseases that can be classified as STDs and includes some that have other routes of transmission as well as. There are other organisms that can be transmitted during sexual contact although they are generally not considered STDs. For example *Giardia lamblia*, usually associated with contaminated water, can be transmitted through sexual exposure.

STDs are the most common infections in the United States and are epidemic in most parts of the world. Portals of entry of STD microorganisms and sites of infection include the skin and mucosal linings of the urethra, cervix, vagina, rectum, and oropharynx.

Risk Factors

Those at risk for acquiring STDs are sexual partners of infected persons. One's risk of infection increases proportionately with the number of sexual partners. Sexual activity in adolescence accounts for an increased incidence of STD

TABLE 65-3 Conditions Classified as Sexually Transmitted Diseases (STDs) and Their Routes of Transmission

Disease	Route(s) of Transmission
HIV infection/AIDS	*Sexual, Percutaneous, Perinatal*
Hepatitis B (HBV)	*Sexual, Percutaneous, Perinatal*
Hepatitis C (HCV)	*Percutaneous, Probably Sexual, Probably Perinatal*
Syphilis	*Sexual, Perinatal*
Gonorrhea	*Sexual, Perinatal*
Chlamydia	*Sexual*
Herpes simplex	*Sexual*
Human papillomavirus (HPV)	*Sexual*
Cytomegalovirus	*Sexual, Less intimate contact*
Chancroid, *Lymphogranuloma venereum,* and *Granuloma inguinale*	*Sexual*

cases in that age group. An increase in illicit drug use and homelessness promotes prostitution, which in turn influences a wide transmission of STDs. Oral and anal sexual practice exposes one to a potentially greater bacterial and viral load of organisms.

The use of the condom to provide a protective barrier from transmission of STD-related organisms has been broadly promoted especially since the recognition of AIDS. At first referred to as a method to assure *safe sex*, the use of condoms has been shown to reduce but not eliminate the risk of transmission of HIV and other venereal diseases. The term *safer sex* more appropriately connotes the public health message to be used when promoting the use of condoms.

Significance of Sexually Transmitted Diseases

Sexually transmitted diseases provide a unique set of challenges for the nurse, the physician, and public health official. Because of perceived stigma and possible threat to emotional relationships, those with symptoms of STDs often are reluctant to seek health care in a timely fashion. Similar to many other infectious diseases, STDs may progress without symptomatology. A delay in diagnosis and treatment is potentially harmful as the risk of complications for the infected individual and the risk of transmission to others increases over time.

Infection with one STD suggests the possibility of infection with other organisms as well. Therefore, once one STD is identified, diagnostic evaluation for others should be performed. The possibility of HIV infection should be pursued whenever any STD is diagnosed.

Complications for Women. STDs are of particular concern to women for several reasons. For most STDs, heterosexual transmission to women appears to occur more easily than heterosexual transmission to men. This may be because the vagina provides a location for prolonged contact with the infectious source. Women tend to have fewer symptoms and the aftereffect of infection is more likely to lead to sterility or neoplasm than infections in men. One of the greatest difficulties of STDs in women is that most infections can be transmitted to the fetus in utero or at the time of delivery. HIV, syphilis, cytomegalovirus, and herpes simplex cause some of the most catastrophic congenital infections in infants.

Human Immunodeficiency Virus (HIV)

HIV has been well established as the causative agent of acquired immunodeficiency syndrome (AIDS). AIDS is a syndrome of diseases that may occur when the immune system has been significantly weakened by the HIV virus. The definition of AIDS, as determined by the Centers for Disease Control, has changed several times since the syndrome was first recognized in 1981. In general, the definition sets a point in the continuum of HIV deterioration in which the host has clinically demonstrated profound immune dysfunction. A large number of opportunistic infections and neoplasms serve as markers for immune suppression severity. Since 1993, the AIDS definition has also included a $CD4^+$ count of less than 200 as a threshold criterion. The $CD4^+$ cell is a subset of the lymphocyte and is one of the target cells of HIV infection.

Types. HIV has two viral types identified. Almost all cases of recognized HIV infection in the United States are attributed to HIV-1. However, HIV-2, a similar virus with identical transmission routes and clinical course, also has the ability to cause AIDS. Since 1992, all donated blood and blood components or products have been screened for this rare virus. Serologic testing can distinguish between HIV-1 and HIV-2. Throughout the remainder of this section "HIV" will refer to HIV-1.

Pathophysiology

HIV is transmitted through sexual contact, percutaneous injection of contaminated blood, or perinatally from infected mother to fetus. The majority of those infected by the percutaneous route are intravenous drug users who share contaminated needles, but transmission is also remotely possible through contaminated blood transfusion. Since 1985, all blood transfusions have been screened and transfusion-related transmission of HIV is now extremely unlikely.

Risk to Health Care Workers. Health care workers can be infected through the percutaneous route if needlestick or other injury from sharp object introduces contaminated blood. Prospective studies of this risk demonstrate that fewer than 1% of such occupational exposures (in which the source patient is infected with HIV) lead to transmission. Despite the rarity of transmission, universal precautions are recommended by the CDC and enforced by OSHA as a strategy to decrease this risk. Health care workers are advised to take extreme care to avoid needlestick or mucous membrane exposure to blood of all patients.

STDs and HIV. There is strong evidence that other STDs, especially those characterized by ulceration, increase the risk of sexual transmission of HIV. Because of a failing immune system, persons with HIV infection may also be more susceptible to other STDs. Other related factors associated with increased risk of sexual transmission are failure to use condoms, frequency of sexual contact, anal intercourse, and sexual activity during menstruation.

Management

To date, there is no cure for AIDS, although antiviral therapy (using zidovudine or other therapies) may prolong the period of time that a patient with HIV is well. In addition, specific therapies to treat the different opportunistic infections and cancers associated with AIDS serve to increase life expectancy after diagnosis.

The impact of HIV is felt in all aspects of health care planning and delivery, as well as socially and financially throughout the world. HIV and AIDS are discussed in detail in Chapter 50.

Syphilis

Syphilis is an acute and chronic infectious disease caused by the spirochete, *Treponema pallidum*. It is acquired through sexual contact or may be congenital in origin.

Stages of Syphilis

In the untreated person, the course of syphilis can be divided into three stages: primary, secondary, and tertiary. These stages reflect the time from infection and the clinical manifestations observed in that period, and are the basis for treatment decisions.

Primary Syphilis. **Primary syphilis** occurs 2 to 3 weeks after initial inoculation with the organism. A painless lesion at the site of infection is called a *chancre*. Untreated, these lesions usually resolve spontaneously within about 2 months.

Secondary Syphilis. **Secondary syphilis** occurs when the hematogenous spread of organisms from the original chancre leads to generalized infection. The rash of secondary syphilis generally occurs approximately 2 to 8 weeks after the chancre, and involves the trunk, and the extremities, including the palms of the hands and the soles of the feet. Transmission of the organism can occur through contact with these lesions. Generalized signs of infection may include lymphadenopathy, arthritis, meningitis, hair loss, fever, malaise, and weight loss.

After the secondary stage, there is a period of *latency* in which the infected person is without signs or symptoms of syphilis. Latency can be interrupted by a recurrence of secondary syphilis.

Tertiary Syphilis. **Tertiary syphilis** is the final stage in the natural history of the disease. It is estimated that between 20% and 40% of those infected will not exhibit this final level of clinical findings. In this stage, syphilis presents as a slowly progressive inflammatory disease with the potential to affect multiple organs. The most common manifestations at this level are aortitis and neurosyphilis, as evidenced by dementia, psychosis, paresis, stroke, or meningitis.

Diagnostic Evaluation

Because syphilis shares symptoms with many diseases, clinical history and laboratory evaluation are important. The conclusive diagnosis of syphilis can be made by direct identification of the spirochete obtained from the chancre lesions of primary syphilis. Serologic tests used in the diagnosis of secondary and tertiary syphilis require clinical correlation in interpretation. The serologic tests are summarized below:

- *Nontreponemal or reagin tests* such as the Venereal Disease Research Laboratory (VDRL) or the rapid plasma reagin circle card test (RPR-CT) are generally used for screening and diagnosis. After adequate therapy, the test is expected to quantitatively decrease until it is read as negative, approximately 2 years after therapy.
- *Treponemal tests* such as the fluorescent treponemal antibody absorption test (FTA-ABS) and the microhemagglutination test (MHA-TP) are used to verify that the screening test did not represent a false- positive result. Positive results will usually be positive for life, and so are not appropriate to determine therapeutic effectiveness.

Management

The current treatment of all stages of syphilis is administration of antibiotics. Penicillin G benzathine is the medication of choice for early syphilis or latent syphilis of less than 1 year duration. It is given by intramuscular (IM) injection at a single session. The same therapy is recommended for patients with early latent syphilis. However, those with late latent or latent syphilis of unknown duration should receive three injections at 1-week intervals. Patients who are allergic to penicillin are usually treated with doxycycline. The patient treated with penicillin is monitored for 30 minutes after the injection to watch for a possible allergic reaction.

Treatment guidelines established by the CDC are updated on a regular basis. Recommendations provide special guidelines for treatment in the setting of pregnancy, allergy, HIV infection, pediatric infection, congenital infection, and neurosyphilis.

Nursing Interventions

Syphilis is a reportable communicable disease. In any health care facility, a mechanism should be in place to ensure that all patients who are diagnosed are reported to the state or local public health department to ensure follow-up. The public health department is responsible for interviewing the patient to determine sexual contacts, so that contact notification and screening can be initiated.

Lesions of primary and secondary syphilis may be highly infective. Gloves are worn when having direct contact with lesions, and hands are washed after gloves are

CHART 65-6
Patient Education: Treating and Preventing the Spread of Syphilis

- The patient is instructed to complete the full course of therapy if multiple penicillin injections are required.
- The patient with primary or secondary syphilis is assured that with proper treatment skin lesions and other sequelae of infection will improve, and serology eventually will reflect cure.
- The patient is instructed to refrain from sexual contact with previous or current partners until they have been treated.

removed. Isolation in a private room is not required. (See Chart 65-6 for patient education.)

Gonorrhea

Neisseria gonorrhea is a gram-negative bacterium, which is transmitted primarily through sexual contact. Infection also can occur in neonates as a result of contact during birth. *N. gonorrhea* can cause mucosal, local, or disseminated infection. Asymptomatic infection is somewhat common.

Clinical Manifestations

Gonorrhea most frequently presents with local manifestations. In men, urethritis and epididymitis are the most common symptoms. Gonorrhea is more likely to be asymptomatic in women than in men. The uterine cervix is the primary site of local infection, and symptoms often include urinary tract infection, increased vaginal discharge, and itching. The most common complication of localized gonococcal infection in women is pelvic inflammatory disease (PID) in which the organism infects the uterus, fallopian tubes, or peritoneal fluid. A complication of gonococcal PID is increased risk for ectopic pregnancy and bilateral tubal occlusion, which results in infertility.

In rare circumstances, the organism may disseminate in untreated, infected persons. Bacteremia can be accompanied by other systemic signs, such as arthritis or dermatitis. In rare instances, valves of the heart can be infected with *N. gonorrhea* or gonococcal meningitis can develop.

Diagnostic Evaluation

The patient is assessed for fever, urethral, vaginal, and rectal discharges, and for signs of arthritis. Culture and sensitivity studies are the usual and preferred methods of diagnosing and verifying effectiveness of therapy. In the male patient, specimens are obtained from the urethra, anal canal, and pharynx. In the female patient, cultures from the endocervix, pharynx, and anal canal are obtained. When obtaining these cultures, the nurse should wear disposable gloves and wash thoroughly after removing them. Lubricating jelly is not used for the vaginal examination because it may contain substances that inhibit growth or kill some pathogens. Instead, water is used as the lubricant. Because *N. gonococci* are susceptible to environmental changes, specimens must be delivered to the laboratory immediately after they are obtained.

Management

The CDC-recommended treatment for gonococcal infections is ceftriaxone (or cefixime, ciprofloxacin, or ofloxacin) along with doxycycline. Doxycycline is added to first line therapy to treat presumptive *Chlamydia trachomatis*, which commonly causes coinfection in patients with gonorrhea. Patients with uncomplicated gonorrhea who are treated with CDC-recommended therapy do not routinely need to return for a proof-of-cure visit. If the patient reports a new episode of symptoms or tests reveal gonorrhea again, the most likely explanation is reinfection rather than treatment failure.

Serologic testing for syphilis and HIV should be offered to patients with gonorrhea because any STD represents increased risk for other STD infections.

Nursing Interventions

Gonorrhea is a reportable communicable disease. In any health care facility, a mechanism should be in place to ensure that all patients diagnosed with gonorrhea are reported to the local public health department so that follow-up of the patient can be assured. In addition, the public health department is responsible for interviewing the patient to determine sexual contacts so that contact notification and screening can be initiated.

Chlamydia trachomatis Infections

Chlamydia trachomatis is a bacterium that requires attachment to the host cell, invasion, intracellular growth, and replication. This requirement for intracellular growth, which is similar to viruses, has made the identification and laboratory study more difficult than for organisms that grow and replicate independently. Recent advances have made diagnosis and screening much more available.

Clinical Manifestations in Women. In women, sexual intercourse is the usual route of transmission. The most frequent clinical manifestation is pelvic inflammatory disease, but many times symptoms are so subtle that pathologic progression can occur without detection. As with other causes of PID, diagnosis and treatment are not systematically applied. Long-term effects may include chronic pain, increased risk of ectopic pregnancy, postpartum endometritis, and infertility.

Clinical Manifestations in Infants. Transmission of infection from an infected pregnant woman to her vaginally born infant is very common. Approximately 15% to 20% of infected infants will develop chlamydia conjunctivitis and approximately 10% will develop chlamydia pneumonia.

Clinical Manifestations in Men. Although men infected with chlamydia are frequently nonsymptomatic, they easily transmit the infection to their sexual partners. Urethritis is the most common illness associated with infection in the symptomatic heterosexual man. Among homosexual men, the rectum is the common site of infection.

Diagnostic Evaluation and Management

Chlamydia should be suspected in cases of gonorrhea, nongonorreal urethritis, pelvic inflammatory disease, and epididymitis. Diagnostic tools include cell culture techniques and a relatively wide range of nonculture techniques including immunologic assays, DNA probes, and enzyme-sensitive tests.

Regimens for treating chlamydia usually are either doxycycline or azithromycin. Neither of these antibiotics is recommended in pregnancy. Guidelines published by the CDC should be used to determine alternative therapy for the patient who is pregnant or allergic or who has complicated chlamydial infection. It is important that both the patient and the sexual partner be treated.

Patient Education and Prevention

The target group for preventive patient education of *C. trachomatis* is the adolescent and young adult population. Abstinence, postponing the age of initial sexual exposure, limiting the number of sexual partners, and use of condoms for barrier protection should be promoted. It should also be stressed that screening for chlamydia and treating infection at an early stage are important methods to decrease disease progression common to women and to decrease the likelihood of infection in infants.

❑ NURSING PROCESS
The Patient With a Sexually Transmitted Disease

Assessment

History

The patient should be asked to describe the onset and progression of symptoms, and to characterize any lesions by location and description of drainage if present. Protecting confidentiality is important when discussing sexual issues. When a detailed sexual history is necessary, it is important to respect the patient's right to privacy. Brief explanations of why the information is asked and how confidentiality is maintained are often helpful. Clarification of terms may be necessary if the patient or nurse use language unfamiliar to the other. Asking specific information about sexual contacts should generally be done only when the nurse is part of a team that will contact the partners for follow-up. However, in the history-taking process, discussion about the patient's understanding of responsibility to inform sexual partners may be helpful in determining patient educational goals.

Physical Examination

During physical examination, the presence of rashes, lesions, drainage, discharge, or swelling are noted. Inguinal nodes are palpated to elicit tenderness and to note swelling. Women are examined for abdominal or uterine tenderness. The mouth and throat are examined for signs of inflammation or exudate.

The nurse wears gloves while examining the mucous membranes, and gloves are changed and replaced after vaginal or rectal examination.

Diagnosis

Nursing Diagnoses

Based on assessment data, the patient's major nursing diagnoses may include the following:

- ❑ Knowledge deficit about the disease and risk for spread of infection and reinfection
- ❑ Noncompliance with treatment
- ❑ Fear related to anticipated stigmatization and to prognosis and complications

Collaborative Problems/ Potential Complications

Based on assessment data, potential complications that may develop include:

- ❑ Increased risk of ectopic pregnancy
- ❑ Infertility
- ❑ Transmission of infection to fetus resulting in congenital abnormalities and other outcomes
- ❑ Neurosyphilis
- ❑ Gonococcal meningitis
- ❑ Gonococcal arthritis
- ❑ Syphilitic aortitis
- ❑ HIV-related complications

Planning and Implementation

Goals. Major goals are increased patient understanding of the natural history and treatment of the infection, increased compliance with therapeutic and preventive goals, reduction in fear, and absence of complications.

Nursing Interventions

Increasing Knowledge and Preventing Spread of Disease. Education and prevention of the spread of STDs to others often are simultaneous activities. Discussion concerning risk factors should be handled in the context that the same behaviors that led to infection with one STD may introduce risk for any other STD including HIV. Methods used to contact sexual partners should be discussed. The patient should understand that until the partner has been treated, continued sexual exposure to the same individual may lead to reinfection with STDs. Patients may need help in planning discussion with partners. If the patient is especially apprehensive about this aspect, a referral to a social worker or other specialist may be appropriate. Such support is especially important when the patient has newly recognized HIV infection.

The relative value of condoms in reducing the risk of infection with STDs should be addressed. When appropriate, the patient should be encouraged to discuss any reasons for resistance to condom use, so that decision making about this preventive method can be facilitated.

Increasing Compliance. In group settings (such as may be offered in an outpatient obstetric setting), or in a one-on-one setting, open sharing of information about STDs facilitates understanding. Socially driven discomfort can be lessened when factual representation of causes, consequences, treatments, prevention, and responsibilities are addressed. Because most communities have expanded STD prevention resources, referrals to appropriate agencies can complement individual educational efforts assuring that later questions or uncertainties can be addressed by experts. [The CDC-maintained STD National Hotline (1-800-227-8922) provides toll-free information and confidential referral services for STDs.]

The infected patient should be told what the causative organism is, and should receive an explanation of the usual course of the infection (including interval of potential communicability to others) and possible complications. The nurse should stress the importance of following therapy as prescribed and the need to report any therapeutic side effects or symptom progression.

Reducing Fear. When appropriate, the patient is encouraged to discuss anxieties and fear caused by the diagnosis, therapy, or prognosis. By individualizing education efforts, factual information applied to specific needs may offer reassurance. For example, patients with HIV should be encouraged to participate in well-coordinated programs in which support, education, counselling, and therapeutic goals are combined. Such programs are designed to offer coordinated care throughout the course of disease progression.

Monitoring and Managing Potential Complications

Infertility and Increased Risk of Ectopic Pregnancy. Pathology from these diseases may lead to pelvic inflammatory disease and with it the potential for increased ectopic pregnancy risk and infertility.

Congenital infections. All STDs can be transmitted to infants in utero or at the time of birth. Complications of congenital infection can range from localized infection (*e.g.*, throat infection with *N. gonorrhea*) to congenital abnormalities (*e.g.*, stunting of growth or deafness from congenital syphilis), to life-threatening disease (*e.g.*, congenital HSV).

Neurosyphilis, Gonococcal Meningitis, Gonococcal Arthritis, Syphilitic Aortitis. STDs can cause disseminated infection. The central nervous system may be infected as seen with neurosyphilis or gonococcal meningitis. Gonorrhea that infects the skeletal system may result in gonococcal arthritis. Syphilis can infect the cardiovascular system by forming vegetative lesions on the mitral or aortic valves.

HIV-Related Complications. HIV, which is primarily spread as an STD, leads to the profound immune suppression of AIDS. Complications of HIV infection include a long list of opportunistic infections including *Pneumocystis carinii*, *Cryptococcus neoformans*, cytomegalovirus, and *Mycobacterium avium*.

Evaluation

Expected Outcomes

1. Acquires knowledge and understanding of STDs
2. Complies with treatment
   a. Achieves effective treatment
   b. Reports for follow-up examination if necessary
3. Demonstrates a less anxious demeanor
   a. Recalls signs and symptoms of the most common STDs
   b. Inspects self for lesions, rashes, and discharge
   c. Assists with sharing information about infection to sexual partners
   d. Chooses a form of risk-reduction behavior through monogamy, reduction in sexual partners, and through the use of condoms
4. Experiences absence of complications
   a. When possible, infections are treated before opportunity for transmission to fetus
   b. Infection is treated before pelvic inflammatory disease or sterility develop
   c. Patients with syphilis are treated in primary stage so that progression to later stages or complications are avoided
   d. Patients with gonorrhea are treated in early stage before dissemination occurs

Community Infections

Tuberculosis

Tuberculosis (TB) is an infectious disease caused by the bacteria, *Mycobacterium tuberculosis*. It is the one of the oldest recognized infectious diseases and remains one of the greatest causes of infection-related deaths throughout the world. Since 1800, TB has been responsible for the deaths of approximately 100 million people around the world. Currently, TB causes approximately 2 to 3 million worldwide annual deaths, with developing countries most affected.

Incidence. In the United States TB incidence showed a steady decline from the 1940s through 1985. This decline was due to the effectiveness of antituberculosis chemotherapy and to a reduction in crowding and improvement of other standards of life in the United States. In the early 1980s elimination of TB in the United States (defined as annual case rate of <1/1,000,000 population) was considered an achievable goal and was included in the Public Health Service goals for the year 2010. However, between 1985 and 1993, there were approximately 60,000 more cases of TB than would have been predicted by previous trends. HIV infection, homelessness, and intravenous drug abuse are three of the major variables that have led to this rise in the number of cases.

Multidrug-Resistant TB. In recent years, clusters of multidrug-resistant TB (MDR-TB) cases have occurred in several US cities. Poor compliance or incomplete therapy regimens are factors leading to resistance in an individual. The resistant organisms can then be spread to others, whose initial therapy may not be effective against the resistant organism. The reservoir of resistant organisms grows in such a setting.

Intravenous Drug Use Community. The intravenous drug use (IVDU) community is one of the epicenters of the epidemic of multidrug resistance in the United States. The difficulty in assuring compliance, along with a growing proportion of persons who are HIV infected in the IVDU community, has led to epidemics of large numbers of exposed people becoming infected, and large numbers of newly infected people developing rapid and sometimes fatal disease.

Pathophysiology

The course of infection with *M. tuberculosis* varies in different hosts. Pulmonary disease is the usual presentation, but infection can occur at any site, including the meninges, kidneys, bones, and lymph nodes. Virtually all transmission of TB occurs from pulmonary infection with expression of the organism facilitated by sneezing, coughing, laughing, or any other vigorous expulsion of air. When a patient with TB coughs, droplet nuclei can remain suspended in the air to be inhaled by others. As droplet nuclei, the organisms can evade the protective mechanisms of the airway and reach the alveoli.

At this point, the patient is said to be "primarily infected." The organism is surrounded by nonspecific macrophages and is spread from the lungs via the hematogenous and lymphatic systems throughout the rest of the body. After time, the organisms are *recognized* by the T cells and a specific immune reaction develops. Frequently this immunity does not kill all organisms, but allows a latency period of months to years. During latency the organism is alive but not reproducing and, although not ill, the host remains infected.

Course of Infection. Although the usual course of infection is asymptomatic latency throughout life, approximately 10% of those infected eventually become ill with TB. With immune integrity interrupted by malnutrition, HIV infection, chemotherapeutic immune suppression, or advanced age, the immunologic barrier can become ineffective and a pathologic lesion can form. With renewed growth of the organism, the lesion may grow and cavitation is possible at the site of involvement. In the lung (where greater than 80% of disease is found), the cavity becomes a deposit site for enormous numbers of tuberculosis bacteria along with debris from cellular destruction and other immunologic cells. (See Chapter 24 for a detailed presentation of tuberculosis.)

Legionnaires' Disease

Legionnaires' disease is a multisystem illness that frequently includes pneumonia and is caused by the gram-negative bacteria, *Legionella pneumophila.* Named after an outbreak of the disease among persons attending a convention of the American Legion, its potential to cause outbreaks has been demonstrated numerous times in hospitals and other settings. *Legionella* organisms are found in many man-made and naturally occurring water sources. Although the organisms may initially be introduced in low numbers, growth is enhanced by water storage, scaling on the inside of water towers, temperatures ranging from 25° to 42°C, and certain amoebae frequently present in water that can support intracellular growth of legionellae.

Pathophysiology. *L. pneumophila* is transmitted by an aerosolized route from an environmental source to the respiratory tract of a person. There is no evidence that the organism can be transmitted from person to person. In hospitals, patients may be exposed to aerosols created by cooling towers, water sources from plumbing, and from respiratory therapy equipment. Because underlying medical conditions can increase host susceptibility and subsequent severity of disease, it is understandable that outbreaks in hospitals are recognized with greater frequency than at other community centers. Mortality rates among hospitalized patients are approximately twofold greater than for persons infected in the community.

Risk factors strongly associated with *Legionella* infection include diseases that lead to severe immune suppression such as AIDS, hematologic malignancy, end stage renal disease, or use of immunosuppressive agents. Other factors associated with increased risk include advanced age, diabetes, alcohol abuse, smoking, and other pulmonary disease.

Clinical Manifestations. The lungs are the principal organs of infection. However, other organs may be involved and disease without pulmonary involvement has been reported. The incubation period appears to range from 2 to 10 days. Early symptoms may include malaise, myalgias, headache, and dry cough. With disease progression, the patient develops increased pulmonary symptoms including productive cough, dyspnea, and chest pain. Patients are usually febrile, and fever curves may reach 103°F (39.4°C) and higher. Diarrhea, and other gastrointestinal complaints commonly accompany the pulmonary array of symptoms. In severe cases, multiorgan involvement and failure may follow.

Diagnosis. Laboratory diagnostic tests available for diagnosis of *Legionella* include culture (using special microbiologic methods and media), immunofluorescent microscopy, and antibody titer interpretation. Diagnosis of *Legionella* by antibody titer requires evidence that titers have increased at least fourfold over time. A single elevated titer is not sufficient to determine current disease. Frequently more than one laboratory test is used in the diagnosis of *Legionella*, as no one test is 100% sensitive. The diagnostic approach generally involves accumulation of information obtained from history, physical, radiologic, and laboratory findings, and assessment of therapeutic effectiveness. Chest x-ray abnormalities may vary in extensiveness and in location of diseased site.

Management. Erythromycin is considered the antibiotic of choice. Secondary choices include the use of rifampin, azithromycin, clarithromycin, and trimethoprim sulfa.

The nursing management described for the patient with any pneumonia (see Chapter 24) should form the basis of care for the patient with Legionnaire's pneumonia. Special isolation techniques should not be used for these patients as there is no evidence of transmission between humans.

Diarrheal Diseases

In developing countries of the world, infectious diarrhea kills about 4 million people per year. In the United States, it is estimated that children under the age of 5 experience over 20 million episodes of diarrheal diseases each year, with approximately 400 deaths per year attributed to such episodes. Dehydration associated with diarrheal diseases is the most important determinant of both morbidity and mortality. Dehydration is largely controllable by using rehydration therapy.

Transmission. The portal of entry of all diarrheal pathogens is oral ingestion. Although the food we eat is far from sterile, the high acidity of the stomach and the antibody-producing cells of the small bowel generally serve to decrease the potential of pathogens accumulating to the extent that they cause illness. However, if the number of organisms is large enough or if the food serves as a neutralized carrier to protect the organism in the acidic environment, pathogenic reactions can occur. Decreased gastric acidity with disruption of normal bowel flora, as is seen after surgery, use of antimicrobial agents, and the immune dysfunction of AIDS all lower intestinal defenses.

Specific Causes of Diarrheal Diseases. There are many viral, bacterial, and parasitic causes for diarrheal diseases. Rotavirus is the most important viral cause of diarrhea in young children. Common causes of bacterial infection include *Escherichia coli*, *Salmonella*, *Shigella*, *Campylobacter*, and *Yersinia* species. Parasitic infections of importance include *Giardia* and *Cryptosporidium* species, and *Entamoeba histolytica*.

Escherichia coli. *Escherichia coli* is the most common aerobic organism colonizing the large bowel. Most bacteriologic isolation of *E. coli* from fecal cultures does not represent pathologic habitation of the organism, but rather reflects normal flora. However, certain strains of *E. coli* with increased virulence have been responsible for significant morbidity and even a number of deaths in recent outbreaks. These stronger pathologic strains share the basic biologic properties of all *E. coli*, but can be subgrouped as "Enterotoxigenic *E. coli*" (ETEC). ETEC strains are distinguished by the enterotoxins they produce. ETEC strains are the most frequent cause of acute diarrhea throughout the world. Choleralike disease with rapid severe dehydration can follow infection with one of these strains.

During the 1980s, in the United States, outbreaks of an *E. coli* species, 0157:H7, were recognized as an important cause of bloody diarrhea, usually traced to undercooked hamburgers. This bacterium lives in the intestines of cattle and can be introduced into meat at the time of slaughter. Preventing disease from this strain of *E. coli* is aimed at teaching the public to thoroughly cook ground beef (until the meat is no longer pink and the juices run clear).

Salmonella. *Salmonella* is a gram-negative bacillus of which there are many species, including the very pathogenic *Salmonella typhi* (typhoid fever). Of the nontyphi species, most organisms are prevalent in animals that serve as food sources. It is estimated that *Salmonella* contaminates over 50% of commercially available chicken products and is frequently found in eggs (whether or not shells are broken), raw milk, and occasionally in beef. Along with contamination from food and water, person-to-person transmission can occur. Hospitals, long-term care facilities, and other institutions account for nearly one third of all reported epidemics of *Salmonella*. Routes of transmission in these settings are probably both through contaminated food and person-to-person transmission.

There is great variability of symptoms associated with *Salmonella* species infection, including asymptomatic carrier state, gastroenteritis, and systemic infection. Diarrhea with gastroenteritis is common. Less frequently disseminated disease and bacteremia will be accompanied by diarrhea.

The person with *Salmonella*-caused diarrhea can be a source for transmission to others. The importance of good hygiene should be emphasized and health care workers should use special care when handling bedpans, stool specimens, or other objects that may have fecal contamination. Handwashing is imperative after any contact with a person with *Salmonella* diarrhea.

Patients with gastroenteritis generally are not treated. Antibiotic use may increase the period of time that the patient carries the bacteria, while not improving the clinical outcome of the patient. However, those with systemic salmonellosis require antimicrobial therapy.

Shigella. The *Shigella* species is a gram-negative organism that invades the lumen of the intestine and causes disease and severe watery (possibly bloody) diarrhea.

Shigella species spread through the fecal-oral route, with easy transmission from one person to another. Small numbers of organisms are needed to cause disease.

Because of the ease of transmission with improper hygiene, it is not surprising that *Shigella* organisms disproportionately affect pediatric populations. Disease in the very young may infrequently be complicated by pulmonary or neurologic symptoms.

Antimicrobial therapy should be instituted early. Frequently, initial therapy choices must be altered when final microbiologic testing reveals the organism's sensitivity.

Campylobacter Infections. In the United States, diarrheal disease attributed to *Campylobacter* species surpasses that recorded for *Salmonella* and *Shigella* species. The organism is found abundantly in animal food sources. It is especially common in poultry, but also can be found in beef and pork. Cooking and storing food at appropriate temperatures protects against serving *Campylobacter*-contaminated food. In addition, keeping kitchen utensils used in meat preparation away from other food is important in the prevention of new infection with this organism.

Transmission appears to be almost entirely from a fecal-oral route with food sources serving as the reservoir of infection. Direct person-to-person transmission appears to be less common than for other enteric pathogens such as *Shigella*.

Once a person is infected, it is believed that the organism directly attacks the lumen of the intestine and may cause disease through enterotoxin release. Symptoms can range from mild abdominal cramping and minimal diarrhea to severe disease with profuse watery (sometimes bloody) diarrhea and debilitating abdominal cramping. Antimicrobial therapy is recommended only for those who are seriously ill.

Giardia lamblia. *Giardia lamblia* is a protozoan. Transmission occurs when food or drink is contaminated with viable cysts of the organism. People often become infected while traveling to endemic areas in both industrialized and nonindustrialized countries of the world, or by drinking contaminated water from mountain streams within the United States. The organism can be transmitted by close contact as seen in day care settings; transmission by sexual contact has also been documented.

Frequently, the infection goes unnoticed. Infection is generally recognized more clearly in children than in adults. In extreme cases, the patient may experience abdominal pain and chronic diarrhea, usually described as containing mucus and fat, but not blood. Microscopic examination of stool specimens will reveal the trophozoite or cyst stages of the parasitic life cycle.

The infection can be treated with quinacrine or metronidazole. Patients with *Giardia* infections should be instructed that the organism can be easily transmitted in family or group settings. Personal hygiene measures should be reinforced, and those who travel or camp where water is not treated and filtered should be advised to avoid local water supplies unless water is purified before drinking or used in cooking.

Vibrio cholera. Although in recent decades reported cases of cholera are rare in the United States, no discussion of infectious diarrhea is complete without mention of this very serious infectious disease. Historically, epidemics of cholera have influenced all aspects of life–from medical to political–and infection rates have been significant enough to destroy governments and armies.

The *Vibrio cholera* organism is a gram-negative organism with several different serotypes. The type usually associated with epidemics is toxigenic *V. cholera* 01. The organism is transmitted by contaminated food or water. In recent years, most cases in the United States have been from contaminated shellfish found in the Gulf of Mexico.

Cholera causes a disease with very rapid onset of copious diarrhea in which up to 1 L of fluid per hour can be lost. Dehydration, with cardiopulmonary collapse that follows, causes rapid progression from newly recognized disease to death. The principal therapy is rehydration. Rehydration efforts should be vigorous and sustained. If oral rehydration cannot be accomplished, the patient should be hospitalized for intravenous therapy support.

In the United States, cholera should be suspected in patients who have watery diarrhea after eating shellfish that have been harvested from the Gulf of Mexico. Confirmation of the causative organism can be made by stool culture. It is imperative that all cases are reported to local and state public health authorities.

❑ NURSING PROCESS
The Patient With Infectious Diarrhea

Assessment

The most important element of assessment in the patient with diarrhea is the determination of hydration status. The goal of rehydration is to correct the degree of dehydration. Assessment includes evaluation for thirst, oral mucous membrane dryness, sunken eyes, a weakened pulse, and loss of skin turgor. Careful observation for these signs is especially important in rapidly dehydrating diseases (most notably cholera) and in younger children.

Intake and output measurements are crucial in determining fluid balance. Liquid stool should be measured and recorded along with a record of the frequency of stools. It is important to note the consistency and appearance of stool as important indicators of the type and severity of the diarrheal disease. The presence of mucus or blood should also be noted.

When conducting a health history, it is important to determine if the patient has recently traveled, whether the patient is currently being treated with antibiotics, if the patient has been in contact with anyone who has recently had diarrheal disease, and what the patient has eaten recently. Frequently, patients will attribute the most recent meals eaten as the cause of symptoms. However, the incubation period for most diarrheal conditions is longer than the time interval between meals. Therefore, it is important to get detailed information, not only about the meal preceding the illness, but about all food intake in the previous 3 to 4 days. When eliciting this kind of history, it is helpful to ask the patient to list every food tasted and eaten completely. In addition, it is important to ask patients if they are employed in a food preparation service.

Diagnosis

Nursing Diagnoses

Based on the assessment data, the patient's major nursing diagnoses may include:

- Fluid volume deficit related to fluid lost through diarrhea
- Knowledge deficit about the infection, and the risk of transmission to others

Collaborative Problems/ Potential Complications

Based on the assessment data, potential complications that may develop include:

- Bacteremia
- Shock

Planning and Implementation

Goals. The most important goals are maintainence of fluid and electrolyte balance, knowledge about the disease and risk of transmission, and the absence of complications.

Nursing Interventions

Providing Rehydration Therapy for Diarrhea. The patient is assessed to determine the degree of dehydration. This assessment helps determine the amount and route of rehydration needed. Most patients can be rehydrated by using oral therapy. Oral rehydration therapy (ORT) is a strategy used to reduce the severe complications of diarrheal disease regardless of causative agent. It is inexpensive and effective, but is often underused because of sustained cultural beliefs discouraging oral intake during episodes of diarrhea. After much refinement of the formula, the World Health Organization (WHO) and the United Nation's International Children's Emergency Fund (UNICEF) agreed on the make-up of a single solution for treatment of dehydration and electrolyte imbalance associated with cholera and other forms of diarrheal disease. The solution contains (in mmol/l) sodium, 90; potassium, 20; chloride, 80; base, 30; and glucose 111.

Mild Dehydration. The patient exhibits dry mucous membranes of the mouth and increased thirst. The rehydration goal at this level is to deliver approximately 50 ml/kg oral rehydration solution (ORS) over a 4-hour interval.

Moderate Dehydration. Sunken eyes, loss of skin turgor, and dry oral mucous membranes are frequent manifestations. An infant may have a sunken fontanelle. The rehydration goal is approximately 100 ml/kg over 4 hours for the patient with moderate dehydration.

Severe Dehydration. The patient will show signs of shock (rapid thready pulse, cyanosis, cold extremities, rapid breathing, lethargy, or coma) and should receive intravenous replacement until hemodynamic and mental status return to normal. Once improvement is evident, the patient can be treated with ORS.

Administering Rehydration Therapy. Commercially available preparations in the United States such as Pedialyte and Ricelyte provide lower concentrations of sodium. They have been effective replacements for children with most of the viral diarrheal entities common in this country. However, when diarrheal losses are very high (>10 ml/kg/hr), concentrations of sodium such as those available through the WHO formulation are more appropriate.

In the hospitalized child, diarrheal fluid loss should be weighed and ORS should be administered at a rate of 1 ml for each gram of diarrheal stool. Stool losses can be approximated so that the patient receives approximately 10 ml/kg ORS for each diarrheal stool.

It is important for children and adults who are suffering from acute diarrheal symptoms to maintain caloric intake. Infants who are breast fed should continue to feed on demand; those who are receiving formula should receive full strength lactose-free or lactose-reduced formulas immediately following rehydration. Children who normally eat semisolid or solid food should have that food offered. Recommended foods include starches, cereals, yogurt, fruits, and vegetables. Foods that are high in simple sugars such as undiluted apple juice or Jello should be avoided.

Because diarrheal episodes often are accompanied by vomiting, rehydration and refeeding can be difficult. Oral rehydration therapy should be delivered in small, frequent amounts. When vomiting is persistent, small children often require administration of fluids by frequent spoonfuls rather than by drinking from a bottle or a cup. Intravenous therapy is necessary for the patient who is in shock or severely dehydrated.

Increasing Knowledge and Preventing Spread of Infection. Public health nurses, school nurses, and others who are involved in the education of families, new parents, and others should emphasize principles of safe food preparation. There should be great emphasis on meat preparation and cooking. Ground beef should be cooked until no longer pink, and all meat should be kept at temperatures below 45°F or over 140°F. In planning events for groups of people, adequate provision for storage and reheating to meet temperature thresholds is important. When preparing foods and meat, it is important to use different surfaces, knives, and other equipment.

Diarrheal diseases discussed in this section require reporting to local or state health departments. The goal of reporting is to provide information that will be used to assess disease incidence trends and to identify at the earliest point if there is a restaurant or other food preparation establishment that is serving contaminated food.

Necessity of rehydration and refeeding should be taught to parents of children with diarrheal disease. Beliefs about illness and food patterns may have a traditional or cultural basis and any teaching of health facts requires sensitivity.

Good hygiene in the health care delivery and home settings must be a focus when caring for patients with infectious diarrheal diseases. Diarrheal agents such as *Salmonella*, *Shigella*, and *Campylobacter* call for enteric precautions in most hospitals. The patient with recognized enteric infection would not be isolated in hospitals that use body substance isolation. However, principles of hand washing, glove use, and cleanliness are stressed.

Monitoring and Managing Potential Complications

Bacteremia. *E. coli*, *Salmonella*, and *Shigella* species are all organisms that can be introduced into the bloodstream and cause dissemination to other organs and systemic infection. It is important that the acutely febrile patient with diarrhea have blood cultures performed. If initial smear results reveal gram-negative organisms, antibiotic therapy is instituted.

Shock. Control of shock associated with diarrheal diseases demands accurate intake and output assessment and vigorous fluid replacement. In rare instances, patients with severe fluid imbalance will require intensive care unit support with aggressive hemodynamic monitoring.

Evaluation

Expected Outcomes

1. Attains fluid balance
   a. Output approximates intake
   b. Mucous membranes appear moist
   c. Normal skin turgor
   d. Ingests adequate amounts of fluids and calories
   e. Absence of vomiting
   f. Stools of normal color and consistency
2. Acquires knowledge and understanding about infectious diarrhea and transmission potential
   a. Takes proper precautions to prevent spread of infection to others
   b. Describes principles and techniques of safe food storage, preparation, and cooking
3. Absence of complications
   a. Temperature within normal range
   b. Negative blood culture reports
   c. Achieves fluid balance

Hepatitis Viruses

Hepatitis refers to any inflammation of the liver. Pathology can be caused by chemical or infectious means. Infectious causes include many agents that can cause damage and inflammation. The group of viruses known as hepatitis viruses are named alphabetically in the chronologic order of their discovery.

Parenterally and Sexually Transmitted Hepatitis Viruses

Hepatitis B, hepatitis C, and hepatitis D (known as delta hepatitis) are transmitted through parenteral, perinatal, or sexual routes.

Hepatitis B

Hepatitis B has been the virus most frequently studied because of availability of testing, prevalence of the disease, and morbidity and mortality associated with the disease. Hepatitis B infections, seen around the world, cause over 250,000 deaths per year. Since 1982, an effective vaccine for hepatitis B has become available and aggressive disease reduction campaigns will probably reduce the impact of this disease in the near future.

Transmission. In regions where the disease is endemic, (the Arctic, Africa, China, Southeast Asia, and the Amazon) the most frequent mode of transmission is perinatally from infected mother to infant. In developed countries with a lower prevalence of disease, primary routes of transmission are sexual and parenteral. In the United States, high-risk populations have included homosexual men, intravenous drug users, health care workers, and those who have had frequent blood transfusions.

Pathophysiology. The virus must gain access to the blood stream by direct inoculation, passage through mucous membranes, or breaks in skin in order to reach the liver. In the liver, replication takes place with an incubation of 6 weeks to 6 months before the host becomes symptomatic. Many infections are not apparent. For those with symptoms, the degree of liver destruction and associated manifestations varies greatly. Symptoms range from mild malaise to fever accompanied by rash, jaundice, arthritis, abdominal pain, and nausea. In extreme cases, liver failure with accompanying encephalopathy can occur. The mortality associated with this severe outcome approaches 50%.

Whether or not primary infection was clinically apparent, self resolution occurs within 1 to 2 weeks for the majority of patients. For fewer than 10% of cases, infection can persist for decades or for life. Hepatitis B is considered a chronic infection when the patient remains infectious for at least 6 months. Complications associated with chronic hepatitis B can be severe, with liver cancer, cirrhosis, and ascites occurring in years to decades after original infection.

Diagnosis. The serologic tests for hepatitis B give diagnostic information and information about degree of contagion and probable stage of disease. The available tests are directly related to the proteins of the virus and to the antibodies the host produces in response to those proteins. The virus has a central core and an outer surface or envelop. The proteins associated with these parts are the core antigen and the surface antigen. A laboratory test for core antigen is not available, but surface antigen, frequently expressed HB_sag, is detectable within weeks of initial infection. It rises in titer for several weeks and eventually drops to an undetectable level. The presence of HB_sag connotes recent infection and a relatively high degree of contagiousness. Another antigen that is part of the virus is called the *e antigen* (notated HB_eag). HB_eag is a very sensitive marker of acuity because it is detectable in close proximity to the time of clinical illness and at the point where there appears to be the greatest risk of contagion.

These antigens elicit human antibodies. Core antibody (notated HB_cab) is the first to be detected. It usually appears shortly after the appearance of HB_sag, during the acute phase of infection. Core antibody measured as IgM connotes a recent infection and is a laboratory value that should wane with recovery. Total core antibody (a measure of both IgM and IgG antibodies) will remain for decades or for life. It indicates that the host has at one time been infected. In this way, the HB_cab test serves as a helpful epidemiologic marker in comparing risk in various communities. An early marker of resolution of infection is the appearance of antibody to HB_eab. HB_eab usually appears while HB_sag is present and the patient is still considered infectious. Along with clinical evidence of improvement, the development of antibody to surface antigen (HB_sab) is seen. The presence of surface antibody indicates immunity and resolution. At that point, the patient is not considered infectious to others.

A patient who develops chronic hepatitis B continues to have surface antigen for prolonged periods of time without the anticipated development of surface antibody.

Vaccine. The hepatitis B vaccine, produced by using Hepatitis B antigen to stimulate antibody production and to provide protection from infection, is very safe and is effective in approximately 90% of those vaccinated. Because hepatitis B virus is easily transmitted by needlestick in a health care setting, vaccine is now recommended for all health care workers. To reduce both perinatal infection and risks of transmission occurring after infancy, hepatitis B vaccine is given routinely to infants at birth. The vaccinated individual (not previously infected) will have hepatitis B serology that is positive only for HB_sab. This assures that immunity produced by vaccine is distinguishable from that produced naturally, when antibody to core would also be present.

Hepatitis C

Until recently, *hepatitis Non-A, Non-B* was the designation used to describe viral hepatitis that was not hepatitis A, B, or any other causative agent. Most of hepatitis Non-A Non-B appeared to be parenterally transmitted. This previously unknown and unnamed virus is now identified and named *hepatitis C*. Furthermore, an antibody test to screen patients for this agent is available.

Pathophysiology. Hepatitis C is now estimated to infect approximately 150,000 people per year in the United States. It was once thought to be a disease transmitted almost exclusively by blood transfusion. However, there is a growing body of evidence that the virus is transmitted through other parenteral means as well (sharing of contaminated needles by intravenous drug users and accidental needlestick and other injury in health care workers). There is further evidence that this virus may be transmitted through sexual contact.

Diagnosis. Serologic tests currently available for hepatitis C detect only antibody and are therefore limited in interpretation. Most patients who have clinical evidence of a viral hepatitis will be followed to assure medical stability. Liver function tests are used as markers of hepatitis status. Typical disease course is not well understood at this time, but a repeated waxing and waning of liver enzymes appears to be a common finding. With this information and other clinical markers, it is believed that as many as half of all patients with hepatitis C infection develop chronic infection. It has been shown to be the leading cause of chronic liver disease and cirrhosis in the United States.

Management. At this time, there is no recognized therapy, vaccine, or accepted postexposure prophylactic agent for hepatitis C. Health care workers should follow the principles of universal precautions to minimize risk of occupational transmission. The principles are based on an understanding that there is no recognized population of infected carriers. Care with needles and appropriate barrier precautions must be used with all patients.

Hepatitis D (Delta Hepatitis)

Hepatitis D is a virus that is dependent on the more complex hepatitis B virus for survival. In this parasitic arrangement, hepatitis D is only a risk for those who are hepatitis B surface antigen positive.

Hepatitis D is suspected when a patient becomes acutely ill with new or renewed symptoms and has previously been ill with hepatitis B or has been a carrier of hepatitis B.

There is no specific treatment for hepatitis D. Prevention for this virus is achieved as a secondary benefit of the hepatitis B vaccine. Bloodborne preventive behaviors (not sharing needles and using condoms for sexual exposure) should be reinforced for those persons with hepatitis B infection who have not been infected with hepatitis D.

Hepatitis Viruses Transmitted by the Fecal–Oral Route

Hepatitis A

Hepatitis A is a virus almost always transmitted by the fecal-oral route. It leads to acute hepatitis with no chronic or persistent state such as is evident with the bloodborne hepatitis viruses.

In children, the disease is often unrecognized or is evident with benign complaints. Symptoms are more likely in adults, and can range from malaise to fever, jaundice, nausea, and vomiting. The disease is usually self-limiting within 1 to 3 weeks. Patients seldom require hospitalization and, when symptomatic, are rarely contagious to others.

Because it can be transmitted in contaminated food and water, hepatitis A has epidemic potential in countries with poor water treatment facilities. Infected food preparation workers have the potential of transmitting the disease to others unless personal hygiene measures are used.

Available hepatitis A antibody tests detect either IgM, which indicates acute, current infection, or IgG, which indicates resolved infection.

In February 1995, the US Food and Drug Administration approved the world's first vaccine against hepatitis A. The vaccine, called Havrix, is made from inactivated hepatitis virus. According to the manufacturer of the vaccine, one dose is 96% effective.

Hepatitis E

Hepatitis E is a viral infection spread by contaminated food or water through the fecal-oral route. Until recently, the infection has been designated as *enteric Non-A Non-B hepatitis*. Diagnosis had been made by excluding hepatitis A, B, and C, and determining that transmission was most likely from a contaminated food or water source. Now that a test for antibody for hepatitis E is available, epidemiologic studies will be greatly facilitated.

Hepatitis E has rarely been seen in the United States, but has been associated with epidemics from contaminated water in Asia, Africa, and the republics of the former Soviet Union. In the United States, hepatitis E should be considered in any person who has traveled abroad and has symptoms of viral hepatitis but has negative serology for other hepatitis viruses.

Herpes Family of Viruses

Viruses linked together as **herpesviridae** are grouped by biochemical properties but show substantial similarities in activity in the infected host. Six of the viruses in this family cause human infection: herpes simplex virus, type 1; herpes simplex virus, type 2; cytomegalovirus; varicella-zoster virus; Epstein Barr virus; and B-lymphotropic virus. All six produce life-long latent infection and can reactivate after initial infection and latency.

Herpes Simplex

Herpes simplex infections are among the most prevalent of viral infections. The range of presentations is broad and includes asymptomatic infections, cold sores, and genital herpes. Herpes simplex follows a pattern common to members of the herpes family of viruses: primary infection; incubation (latency); and reactivation (secondary infection). Person-to-person contact is the route of transmission for these viruses, usually from the mucous membrane of the infected person to the mucous membrane of the susceptible person.

Herpes simplex is divided into two serogroups: **herpes simplex 1 (HSV-1)** and **herpes simplex 2 (HSV-2)**. In general, HSV-1 causes oral, ocular, or facial infection; HSV-2 causes genital infection. However, either type of infection can cause disease at either body site.

Herpes simplex infections may be occupationally transmitted to health care workers. *Herpes whitlow* is a cutaneous manifestation of HSV that is seen most frequently in nurses, physicians, and dentists whose hands have had contact with pharyngeal secretions of patients. Whitlow, like other forms of HSV infection, is painful and recurrent. Health care workers with herpetic whitlow on their hands should not be allowed to participate in patient care while lesions are present. With increased use of gloves as advocated by universal precautions, it has been theorized that the incidence of herpes whitlow will probably decrease with time. It is important for health care workers to routinely use gloves when in contact with pharyngeal secretions of any patient because viral shedding may occur without visible lesions.

Primary Infection. Most newly infected people do not recognize the first episode of infection with herpes simplex. In symptomatic individuals, primary infection is the stage more likely to produce painful and prolonged symptoms than in any subsequent stages.

Symptoms. Symptoms can be discrete lesions of the mouth, pharynx, eyelids, or genitalia. Sometimes lesions in these areas will cluster. The infected host also may experience generalized signs of fever, sore throat, malaise, and lymphadenopathy. The severity of symptoms experienced by the immune suppressed host may include broadly disseminated disease with lesions appearing in a wide area including mucous membranes and skin. Primary infection symptoms may last for days.

Latency. The virus, which initially infects epithelial cells of mucous membranes and skin, will progress to sensory nerve cells during the period of latency. It does not actively replicate but remains alive. In this state, any physiologic or emotional stressor can induce the virus to reactivate.

Reactivation of Infection. The virus replicates either asymptomatically or symptomatically on reactivation of infection. In either case, viral shedding to others can occur. In general, symptomatic reinfection is substantially less severe and of shorter duration than primary infection. Recurrent symptomatic infections typically have a prodromal period that can be recognized by itching, burning, or tingling sensations.

Complications. The most significant complication of HSV is encephalitis which, although rare, has a case fatality rate of approximately 60% to 80%. HSV can present as a disseminated disease such as pneumonia, colitis, or esophagitis in AIDS patients. It has sometimes been widely disseminated in the patient with severe burns.

Primary or recurrent infections during pregnancy can lead to congenital infection of the fetus and newborn. Complications can range from mild localized infection to serious birth defects and even fatality.

Diagnosis. Diagnosis of herpes simplex virus can be made by viral culture or serologic testing. The frequently used Tzanck smear test uses a scraping of the lesion and adds special staining to directly observe giant multinucleated cells which indicate either HSV or herpes zoster infection.

Management. Herpes simplex encephalitis and neonatal infections are generally treated with acyclovir. Acyclovir also has been shown to be effective treatment for limiting the morbidity of initial episodes of genital herpes and for recurrent or severe herpes manifestations.

Cytomegalovirus

As a member of the herpes family, cytomegalovirus (CMV) shares traits of latency, persistence, and reactivation with other viral members of that family. The prevalence of cytomegalovirus is very wide and most people become infected at some point during their lifetime. Infection seldom has accompanying symptoms. Clinical disease from CMV is most frequent in transplant patients, in whom it is the most significant of all viral infections, and in AIDS patients, in whom CMV retinitis is the principal cause of blindness.

Primary Infection. Primary infection occurs when the host is first infected with the virus. Route of transmission is usually contact with mucous membranes, oral secretions, or sexual secretions. Thus, activities associated with the transmission of the virus include kissing, sexual contact, and childbirth. Medical interventions such as transfusion of blood and transplantation of organs may lead to transmission because the virus can be carried in any body fluid.

The host rarely has recognizable symptoms when first infected. When symptoms do occur, they frequently are suggestive of a common viral infection such as a cold or mononucleosis. Rarely in the immune competent host but frequently in the immune suppressed host, the initial infection is accompanied by localized symptomatic infection in the form of pneumonia, meningitis, hepatitis or other organ infection, or a generalized systemic infection.

Latency. After initial infection, which most frequently is benign, the host generally carries the virus asymptomatically throughout life. Despite absence of symptoms, the host may frequently shed the virus in urine, saliva, and other secretions. This unrecognized shedding of live virus facilitates the wide prevalence of the organism and exposure is probably extremely common.

Reactivation. Symptomatic reactivation can occur when immune defenses are weakened by emotional, physiologic, or chemical stressors. In HIV-infected and organ transplant populations, severe localized infections with CMV can cause devastating disease. CMV infections are a major complication of organ transplantation and a significant cause of transplant-related death.

Transmission. As routes of transmission would suggest, the risk of acquiring infection with cytomegalovirus is greatest in infancy, early childhood, and early adulthood. However, some risk persists throughout life, so that by the time a person advances in age the likelihood of having been infected approaches 100% (Cheeseman, 1992).

Infants may be born with cytomegalovirus that is acquired from the mother either in utero or perinatally at the time of birth. The pregnant woman with primary infection has a substantially greater likelihood of transmitting the virus to the fetus than does the previously infected woman who may intermittently shed virus throughout pregnancy. Breast milk may serve as a vehicle for transmission of virus from mother to baby. Kissing may also offer risk as the virus can be spread from parents and others to the baby.

Children with poor control of saliva, urine, and feces have an increased risk of primary infection with cytomegalovirus. In addition, the closeness often experienced in daycare settings puts children at increased risk. For the adolescent or adult who has not been infected with the virus, sexual activity provides risk of infection.

Complications. In the immune competent population acquisition of CMV generally poses no health risk. However, there is concern about CMV acquisition in pregnant woman and the fetus or infant. In fact, congenital CMV is the most common serious viral infection of newborns in the United States. Approximately 1% of all newborns are infected; and approximately 20% of those infected show symptomatology either initially, or within the first few months of life. When present, symptomatology varies widely in severity and organ system involvement. The most common clinical manifestations of infection are hematogenous with petechiae, hepatomegaly, and splenomegaly occuring in those affected. Severe, permanent neurologic complications can be associated with hematogenous complications. Although spontaneous abortion and congenital abnormalities associated with cytomegalovirus are relatively rare, primary infection during pregnancy represents an obstetric and public health concern. Opportunities for new infection during pregnancy are probably greatest for women who have other children in daycare settings because there is the opportunity for close exposure with newly infected children. Although there is concern for the pregnant health care or day care worker routinely exposed to secretions and excretions of patients and children, epidemiologic studies about these occupations do not consistently indicate increased risk of acquisition. However, pregnant workers in both occupations should be cautioned about the *potential* risk of acquisition in these settings.

Prevention. Handwashing and the use of gloves has been shown to greatly reduce the risk of transmission from patient to health care worker. Many patients (especially transplant patients and those with AIDS) will excrete cytomegalovirus in almost all body fluids. If pregnancy is used as a determinant for patient assignments, it is important that the pregnant nurse understand that exposure to CMV cannot be avoided by patient selection, but instead by consistent use of hand washing and glove use.

Transmission of cytomegalovirus also occurs with the transfusion of blood and the transplantation of organs. Fortunately, increased screening of blood for other viruses (hepatitis B, hepatitis C, and human immunodeficiency virus) also has decreased the risk of transfusion-associated cases of CMV. Reinfection of a previously infected organ transplant recipient with a new source of CMV (from the donor) can lead to severe illness in the immune suppressed patient.

Treatment. Ganciclovir is the therapy of choice for treatment of retinitis, pneumonitis, hepatitis, and other common CMV manifestations. Recently, Foscarnet has been used as an alternative therapy for CMV retinitis.

Varicella

Chickenpox

Varicella zoster is the causative viral agent of chickenpox and herpes zoster. The varicella virus attacks most individuals as children, causing disseminated disease in the form of chickenpox. Approximately 3 million cases of chickenpox occur in the United States each year. Varicella is quite contagious and humans serve as the reservoir. Transmission apparently occurs by the airborne and contact routes. With rare exception, varicella infects an individual only once. At the time of first infection (primary disease manifested as chickenpox) most hosts will experience a generalized illness with rash, fever, and malaise. The incubation period is about 2 weeks (with a range from 10 to 21 days). During a prodrome with general malaise (often noted about 2 days before the rash develops), the newly infected host is capable of transmitting the virus to other susceptible contacts. Typically, the rash is vesicular and pustular and spreads rapidly from few to many lesions in a matter of hours. New lesion formation continues for 2 to 3 days with lesions appearing at different stages throughout this time. By the fourth symptomatic day, the lesions begin to dry and new lesions usually do not develop. Fever is common during the 4 to 6 days of rash progression. When the lesions have crusted, the patient is no longer contagious to others.

Herpes Zoster

After recovery from chickenpox, the varicella virus exists in a latent stage throughout the remainder of life. As a latent virus, varicella is asymptomatic, but has the potential for reactivation. In its reactivated stage, varicella presents as herpes zoster, often referred to as *shingles*. Usually initiated by physiologic or emotional stress, the virus, which had been present in the dorsal spinal ganglion, follows a nerve branch to be expressed as a patch of erupted skin. Herpes zoster is typically very painful, as the nerve branch is severely inflamed. Rarely, herpes zoster disseminates with a broadly distributed rash extending beyond a single dermatome and crossing the midline of the body. Disseminated Herpes zoster is seen most frequently in immune compromised patients.

Herpes zoster is only infectious to those who do not have immunity to varicella (*i.e.*, those who have not previously been infected with varicella in the form of chickenpox). Localized herpes zoster is estimated to be approximately 25% less contagious than chickenpox with a much shorter period of contagion. In its disseminated presentation, the potential for transmission to others is increased.

The nurse who is uncertain of past varicella infection should be tested for immunity before caring for any patient with varicella infection or an undiagnosed rash. Attention must also be paid to home or community contacts who may have chickenpox or herpes zoster. This is most serious in settings where there are patients with immune suppression.

Control. Because varicella, especially chickenpox, is transmitted through the airborne route, it is important to isolate the patient from others in the acute care setting. A private room should be provided and other recommendations of respiratory isolation should be followed: the room should be maintained under negative pressure relative to hallway air, the air should be exhausted directly to the outside of the building, and the door should be kept closed at all times. Every effort to reduce contact of susceptible personnel should be made. For those who have a documented history of chickenpox or who have had serology verifying immunity, exposure to the infected patient should pose no risk.

Management. Acyclovir has been shown to be effective in reducing the severity of varicella infections (both as chickenpox and as herpes zoster) in the immunosuppressed patients. It is also recommended in the immune competent host with varicella pneumonia seen with chickenpox. Recently, immune competent children and adults with milder forms of chickenpox have been treated with oral acyclovir with notable decrease in symptomatology. At this point, the benefits of acyclovir treatment for herpes zoster manifestations in the immune competent patient are under study.

Varicella-specific immune globulin (V-zig) is available for the immunosuppressed or susceptible adult who has had recent exposure. V-zig has been shown to reduce the severity of varicella infection in these persons. Acyclovir is the antiviral therapy of choice for varicella. Because of toxicity associated with acyclovir, risk-benefit decisions about its use must be made on a case-by-case basis.

Vaccination. Vaccination for varicella is not currently part of the recommended routine childhood immunization schedule. A vaccine has been developed and is being actively evaluated. Immunosuppressed children are often given varicella vaccine, while chemotherapy is withheld in the immediate immunization period.

Epstein-Barr Virus

Epstein-Barr Virus (EBV) is a virus that causes the most cases of infectious mononucleosis (IM). Although all organs can be affected, IM is usually characterized by an intense proliferative response of the lymphoid tissue and organs (lymph nodes, spleen, tonsils). IM is usually self-limited, but there have been rare reports of complications including death. EBV is also associated with Burkitt's lymphoma and nasopharyngeal carcinoma.

Primary infection often is asymptomatic in younger children, although the more typical IM course may also occur. IM is most frequently diagnosed in the 15 to 25 year age group. Transmission of infectious mononucleosis is usually by oral contact, thus the name the *kissing disease*. The virus may persist in the pharynx for weeks or months so that recently ill persons probably serve as convalescent carriers of this disease.

Clinical Manifestations. Early clinical manifestations usually include fever, lymphadenopathy, and pharyngitis. In addition, a faint erythematous or maculopapular eruption may appear on the trunk and proximal extremities in the early stage of the disease. Hepatosplenomegaly is a common complication. Symptoms may persist for 2 to 3 weeks.

EBV can produce a chronic condition characterized by persistent lymphadenopathy, hepatosplenomegaly, and pneumonitis. There is a question of whether EBV can lead to another entity—chronic fatigue syndrome.

Diagnostic Evaluation. Diagnosis is made on the basis of the typical picture of clinical illness as well as laboratory findings such as lymphocytosis with atypical lymphocytes, detection of heterophile antibodies, and positive EBV-specific antibody test results.

Management. Treatment is symptomatic and supportive. Aspirin or acetaminophen is given for headache and muscle pains. Corticosteroids may be used when severe or life-threatening complications develop, such as marked hepatic dysfunction, neurologic manifestations, thrombocytopenia, hemolytic anemia, and airway obstruction.

Patient Education. The patient is encouraged to remain on bed rest while fever is present and to rest at intervals during recovery. Strenuous physical activity and competitive sports are discouraged until recovery is complete because the enlarged spleen of the patient with infectious mononucleosis is vulnerable to injury and may rupture if subjected to relatively mild trauma.

Meningitis

Meningitis is defined as inflammation of the arachnoid, the pia mater, or the cerebrospinal fluid (CSF). Causes include bacteria or viruses (frequently), fungal or rickettsial organisms (sometimes), and protozoa or helminths (rarely).

Severity ranges from benign, self-limited viral infectious disease, to slowly progressive fungal disease, to potentially rapidly fatal bacterial meningitis. Despite greater understanding of meningitis and a greater array of antibiotic choices, mortality associated with bacterial meningitis has not changed significantly in the last 30 years.

Bacterial meningitis is most frequently diagnosed in the very young or the very old, whereas viral meningitis is most common in children and young adults. Cryptococcal meningitis, the most common fungal meningitis, is now an important opportunistic infection associated with AIDS. It follows the same age distribution as other HIV-related manifestations.

Bacterial Meningitis

The most frequent bacterial species that cause meningitis are *Haemophilus influenza*, *Streptococcus pneumoniae* (also referred to as the *Pneumococcus*), and *Neisseria meningitidis* (also referred to as the *Meningococcus*). Onset of symptoms can be very rapid for any of these organisms. Meningococcus is especially noted for the rapidity of symptomatic onset and disease progression. The path of CSF penetration usually begins with oropharyngeal colonization and progresses to bloodstream invasion, and finally penetrates the bloodbrain barrier.

The risk for different bacterial causes varies by age group. Most *H. influenza* meningitis occurs in babies under age 2 with peak occurrence between 6 to 12 months. Risk is increased in babies with underlying immune globulin deficiency, sickle cell disease, or a history of splenectomy. *S. pnemoniae* is the most frequent source of meningitis among adults. Many patients who develop pneumococcal meningitis have concomitant *S. pneumoniae* bacteremia or pneumonia. Meningococcal meningitis is most frequently seen in young adults. The organism may seem mysterious because it often causes severe, rapidly progressive illness in previously healthy hosts.

Aseptic Meningitis

Aseptic meningitis is the term used for symptomatic meningitis in which no organism is identified and the CSF white cell count does not suggest a bacterial cause. The cause is usually viral, but can also be due to tuberculosis, insect-borne viruses such as Lyme disease and Rocky Mounted Spotted Fever. It can also be caused by noninfectious agents (such as medications or tumors) that may lead to irritation of the meninges.

Although laboratory tests for viral identification are seldom available in the diagnostic setting, researchers have identified that most aseptic meningitis is caused by the enterovirus. The virus is transmitted by the fecal-hand-oral route. Meningitis symptoms are often accompanied by those of gastrointestinal infection with nausea, vomiting, and malaise.

Cryptococcal Meningitis

Cryptococcal meningitis is one of the major causes of opportunistic infection associated with HIV and is seen most frequently in that setting. However, it can be a complication of any severe immune-suppressing disease. The meningitis it produces is usually mild, but persistent and slowly progressive.

Clinical Manifestations. Symptoms result from increased intracranial pressure and altered cerebral blood flow. The patient usually experiences severe headache, which may be accompanied by nausea, vomiting, photophobia, neck stiffness, and behavioral signs of cerebral dysfunction. Symptoms may vary due to the causative organism. *S. pneumonia* frequently leads to altered mental status; approximately 50% of patients with meningococcal meningitis have a rapidly progressive rash, whereas the patient with cryptococcal meningitis may report only headache and relatively subtle personality changes.

Physical examination reveals nuchal rigidity and the following signs of meningeal irritation which suggest meningitis:

- Positive Kernig's sign: when lying with the thigh flexed on the abdomen, the patient cannot completely extend the leg.
- Positive Brudzinski's sign: when the patient's neck is flexed, flexion of the knees and hips is produced; when passive flexion of the lower extremity of one side is made, a similar movement is seen for the opposite extremity.

Diagnosis. Diagnosis of meningitis and determination of the cause both depend on interpretation of the CSF white blood cell count. Normally CSF is clear, with a glucose count of approximately two thirds the value of peripheral blood, a protein of approximately 4.5 g/l, and fewer than 5 white cells. Meningitis usually produces significant changes in the CSF. White cell counts often are elevated above 1000/ml with bacterial meningitis. These white cells are predominately neutrophils. Glucose and protein are markedly decreased. Ultimate diagnosis is made by culture.

With viral or fungal meningitis (including cryptococcal), there is usually an increase in white cells, with a predominance of lymphocytes, relatively unchanged glucose, and a somewhat elevated protein count. Culture and other methods of direct identification of the causative agent are often unavailable. The CSF white cell count interpretation may also be helpful in monitoring the effectiveness of antibiotic therapy.

Management. Successful management depends on rapid administration of an antibiotic that crosses the blood-brain barrier into the subarachnoid space in sufficient concentration to halt the multiplication of bacteria. Antibiotics should be administered promptly after being prescribed.

Cerebral edema, shock, seizures, or coagulopathies that may accompany meningitis should be treated with standard methods. In addition to antibiotics, the patient may receive corticosteroids, mannitol, diazepam, or phenytoin. Fluid and electrolyte balance should be carefully monitored for all patients with meningitis.

Nursing Interventions

Vital signs are frequently assessed.

Hemodynamic stability may be monitored with central venous pressure or Swan-Ganz catheters to assess for incipient shock, which precedes cardiac or respiratory failure.

Generalized vasoconstriction, circumoral cyanosis, and cold extremities may be noted.

Rapid IV fluid replacement may be prescribed, but care is taken not to over hydrate the patient because of the risk of cerebral edema.

Body weight, serum electrolytes, and urine output are closely monitored.

Ongoing assessment of the patient's clinical status with attention to skin and oral hygiene, promotion of comfort, and protection during seizures and while comatose are important.

Prevention. *Haemophilus influenzae* type B (Hib) vaccine is now recommended as part of the routine childhood vaccination series. Meningococcal vaccine is recommended in outbreak situations, for travelers to countries with endemic or epidemic disease, and to individuals with immunologic deficiencies, including those who have had splenectomy performed. In addition, public health officials generally prescribe prophylactic antibiotics for household members of patients with either *H. influenza* or meningococcal meningitis. The goal of this prophylaxis is to eradicate oropharyngeal carriage of these organisms to decrease the risk of meningitis development. Pneumococcal vaccine is recommended for immunocompromised patients, adults with chronic diseases such as diabetes, those over 65 years of age, and those with HIV infection.

Clostridial Myonecrosis (Gas Gangrene)

Gas gangrene is a severe infection of skeletal muscle usually caused by one of several *Clostridium* species. Gas gangrene can complicate traumatic injuries, compound fractures, and postoperative wounds. The anaerobic organisms (*e.g.*, *Clostridium perfringens*, *Clostridium novyi*, *Clostridium septicum*) grow easily in wounds with low oxidation potential. Toxins within the clostridia are released in the wound and destroy affected tissue.

Although *Clostridium* species are found abundantly in nature, the patient's own intestinal tract flora usually presents the source for this wound infection.

Clinical Manifestations. Onset of gas gangrene is usually manifested by sudden severe pain occurring 1 to 4 days following injury. Pain is caused by gas and edema in the injured tissues. The surrounding skin initially appears normal or light colored and tense, but later becomes darkened. Vesicles filled with serous fluid appear and crepitus (crackling) produced by gas in the tissue may be felt. Frothy, foul smelling fluid may leak from the wound. Gas and retained fluid increase local pressure and impair blood supply and drainage. The involved muscles become discolored and necrotic.

In general, outcome associated with gas gangrene is poor. Amputation of the affected extremity is necessary in approximately 50% of cases. Risk of mortality is increased in patients with underlying immune suppressing diseases such as cancer, diabetes, or renal failure.

Management. Surgical debridement is the best treatment for gas gangrene. The surgical goal is to remove all devitalized tissue, dirt, and hematoma formation. Antibiotic treatment is also used. Use of hyperbaric oxygen (oxygen administered under pressure greater than atmospheric pressure) may add additional curative benefit.

Nursing Interventions. Because the patient is critically ill, intensive care unit support is usually warranted. The nurse should monitor pulmonary capillary wedge pressure, central venous pressure, and fluid and electrolyte balance. Nutritional demands may require enteral or parenteral support.

Rickettsial Infection

Rickettsias are microorganisms that have a cell wall similar to gram-negative bacteria. However, their parasitic dependence on other cells for survival is similar to viruses. With the exception of Q fever, all rickettsial infections are transmitted to humans through insects. Examples of rickettsial disease include Rocky Mountain Spotted fever, Lyme disease, and typhus. The microorganisms attack small blood vessels and cause a peripheral vasculitis, rash, and fever.

Rocky Mountain Spotted Fever

Rocky Mountain Spotted Fever (RMSF) is caused by *Rickettsia rickettsii.* There are approximately 1000 cases of this tick bite- transmitted disease reported in the United States each year. Currently, the greatest prevalence of disease is in the southeastern and southwestern regions of the United States. Incidence of infections increase in April and reach the highest level in May and June.

Pathophysiology. *R. rickettsii* organisms invade both the endothelial and smooth muscle cells of blood vessels, causing a generalized vasculitis. Cell damage may lead to alterations in capillary permeability, thrombosis, and hemorrhage. This generalized vasculitis may lead to cutaneous lesions and vascular injury of virtually every organ.

Clinical Manifestations. Several days after a bite by an infected tick early symptoms appear. They include severe headache, malaise, anorexia, photophobia, slight fever, and muscle and joint pain. Within a few days, fever, rash, and edema are pronounced.

The rash is the most specific manifestation of the infection and consists of rose-colored macules (nonelevated discolorations) of variable size that appear on the wrists, ankles, soles of the feet, and palms, gradually spreading over the entire body.

The rash becomes papular (consisting of solid elevated lesions), darker red, and slightly dusky; after a few days it develops a petechial or purpuric character. In some cases the rash appears in the terminal stages of illness or not at all. Evidence of extensive subcutaneous hemorrhages may appear, sometimes with necrosis of distal sites such as fingers, toes, or earlobes. The increase in vascular permeability may lead to generalized edema, hypovolemia, and hypotension. Renal failure, pulmonary edema, and pneumonia are potential complications of severe RMSF.

Diagnostic Evaluation. Early diagnosis is an important determinant of outcome. Therefore, inclusion of RMSF in a diagnostic work-up for the patient with headache and febrile illness is important, especially so during tick season. Laboratory confirmation of RMSF usually is made by serologic tests.

Management. Tetracycline and doxycycline are the medications of choice for rickettsial diseases. Severely ill patients should be cared for in an intensive care unit. Pulmonary artery catheter measurements are used to guide fluid and electrolyte replacement. The patient may require blood product transfusion.

Nursing Interventions. Nursing measures are used to decrease fever, restlessness, and pain. The patient is positioned carefully owing to the possibility of severe edema and necrosis from vasculitis. The circumferences of the abdomen, arms, and leg are measured at prescribed intervals to determine the extent of edema. Because the patient may develop renal failure, intake and output are monitored.

Prevention and Patient Education. RMSF prevention campaigns should be aimed at teaching people to avoid tick bite by wearing protective clothing, using tick repellent, and conscientiously searching for and removing ticks. Disease transmission usually occurs after an infected tick has been feeding several hours. Frequent examination of skin, scalp, and clothing will aid in finding and removing the tick before infection has occurred. Household pets also should be examined for ticks on a regular basis.

Ticks may be removed with tweezers. Another way to remove a tick is to cover it with a thick ointment to lessen the tick's hold on the skin. Care should be taken to avoid crushing the tick, contaminating the broken skin with infectious tick secretions, or leaving part of the tick in the skin. Immediately after tick removal, the tick bite is disinfected and the hands are washed.

Vaccine-Preventable Diseases

Vaccinations

Vaccination programs have greatly reduced morbidity and mortality associated with a number of infectious diseases. The goal of vaccination programs is to use wide-scale efforts to prevent specific infectious diseases from occurring in a population. Public health decisions about vaccine campaign implementation efforts are complex. Risks and benefits for the individual and the community must be evaluated in terms of morbidity, mortality, and financial benefit.

The most successful vaccine programs are those for the prevention of smallpox, measles, mumps, rubella, polio, diphtheria, pertussis, and tetanus. The eradication of smallpox (certified in 1979) and discontinuation of the smallpox vaccination program serve as a model for other vaccination and eradication planning endeavors.

There are currently 27 vaccines licensed in the United States. Vaccines are made of antigen preparations in a suspension and are intended to produce a human antibody response to protect the host from future encounters with the organism. No vaccine is completely safe for all recipients. Some persons are allergic to the antigen or the carrier substance. When live organisms are used as antigen, the actual disease (often with a modified course) may follow. It is very important that contraindications on package inserts of vaccine are heeded. These guidelines detail general experience with allergy and other complications, as well as provide critical information about refrigeration, storage, dosage, and administration.

Variations to the recommended vaccination schedule should be made on a case-by-case basis depending on the patient's risk factors and ability to return for follow-up vaccinations at the appointed time. For example, although the first dose of measles vaccine is recommended at the age of 12 to 15 months, babies in developing countries (where measles contributes significantly to childhood morbidity and mortality) should be vaccinated at 9 months.

The standard recommended vaccination schedule for infants and children as developed by the Centers for Disease Control is shown in Table 65-4. The schedule is revised as epidemiologic evidence warrants, and nurses are advised

TABLE 65-4 Centers for Disease Control, Advisory Committee on Immunization Practices 1994 Recommended Schedule for Routine Active Vaccination of Infants and Children

Vaccine	At birth (before hospital discharge)	1–2 months	6 weeks–2 months	4 months	6 months	6–18 months	12–15 months	15 months	4–6 years (before school entry)
Diphtheria-tetanus-pertussis (DTP)			DTP	DTP	DTP			DTP	DTP
Polio; live oral (OPV)			OPV	OPV	OPV				OPV
Measles-mumps-rubella (MMR)							MMR		MMR
Haemophilus influenzae; type B (Hib)*			Hib	Hib	Hib		Hib		
Hepatitis B (HepB)†	HepB	HepB				HepB			

*There are several different formulations of Hib vaccine available. Two of these formulations combine DTP vaccine in one dosage.

†Hepatitis B vaccine can be administered at the same time as DTP, OPV, Hib, and MMR vaccine. Hepatitis B vaccine should be offered to all infants in the newborn period; for those infants born to mothers known to have current infection with hepatitis B (surface antigen positive findings by serology), hepatitis B specific immune globulin should be given as soon as possible after birth.

to consult the CDC to determine when the most recent schedule has been published.

Vaccine recommendations for adults are designed to protect those with underlying diseases that increase their risks of infectious disease, those with potential for occupational exposure, and those who may be exposed to infectious agents during travel. Immunosuppressed adults (including those who have had splenectomy) should be vaccinated for pneumococcus, meningococcus, and *H. influenza*. Health care workers should have completed vaccination for measles, mumps, and rubella. It is recommended that all of the above adult groups and those with asthma or other chronic respiratory conditions receive annual influenza vaccine.

The CDC provides a 24-hour telephone hot-line for information about routine pediatric or adult vaccine advice (404-332-4553), and a 24-hour travelers' hotline for information about preventing specific communicable diseases while traveling abroad (404-332-4559).

Contraindications

There are certain conditions and circumstances which should alter routine vaccination schedules. Patients who have experienced previous anaphylaxis or anaphylactic-like reactions, patients who have developed an encephalopathy within 7 days of a previous diphtheria, tetanus, and pertussis (DTP) dose, or those who have developed other moderate or severe sequelae after a previous dose should not receive further doses. In addition, DTP is often deferred for the child who previously developed a fever of greater than 104°F (40°C) within 48 hours of vaccination, or who had seizure or developed a shocklike state within 3 days of previous vaccination. Live vaccines usually are not indicated for patients with severe immunosuppression such as is seen with HIV infection, leukemia, lymphoma, generalized malignancy, significant corticosteroid use, or in those receiving immunosuppressive medications to prevent transplant rejection.

Measles

Measles is also referred to as *rubeola*, *red measles*, or *hard measles*. Worldwide, measles causes approximately 1 million deaths (mostly in infants and children) annually.

After measles vaccine was licensed in 1963, there was a dramatic and steady decrease in the incidence of measles in the United States. However, in 1989 the trend temporarily reversed, with a dramatic increase observed in the preschool age group and in some ethnic minority communities. Reinvigorated vaccination campaigns have initiated a downward progression.

Pathogenesis and Clinical Manifestations. Measles is a highly contagious organism that is transmitted through the airborne route from an infected person to a susceptible person. The clinical course of measles generally begins with fever and malaise about 10 to 14 days after exposure. Within 24 hours of these initial symptoms, the patient usually develops nasal drainage, a cough, and conjunctivitis. At the end of this period Koplik spots, tiny raised specks appearing on the mucous membranes of the mouth and throat, frequently appear. After 2 to 3 days these symptoms worsen and a rash becomes apparent. The fine, red rash is first evident around the face and neck and then extends to the trunk and extremities.

Complications. The course of measles can vary greatly. Most complications involve the respiratory tract. Pneumonia following the onset of measles has been attributed either to the direct infection by the rubeola virus or to bacterial infections following the weakened host. Pneumonia is seen as a complication for preschool children, more than for older children or adults. In Africa, complications of diarrhea and malnutrition are responsible for many measles-related deaths.

Encephalitis is an unusual complication, usually associated with the older child or adult who has measles infection. When encephalitis does occur, it is most often seen when the rash stage diminishes.

Diagnosis and Managment. Diagnosis of measles is generally made by clinical findings and may be confirmed by serologic testing. Although there is no specific treatment for measles, antipyretic agents are generally indicated to control fever. The nurse should be alert for signs of subsequent bacterial respiratory infection as the initial infection resolves.

Mumps

Mumps is caused by an acute viral infection usually affecting children or young adults. Unilateral or bilateral parotitis is the most frequently observed manifestation of mumps, although the virus can infect many organs. The incidence of mumps has decreased significantly since mumps vaccine was licensed in 1968.

Pathophysiology. Mumps is transmitted through the airborne route. It appears to be somewhat less contagious than chickenpox and significantly less contagious than measles. The incubation period is 16 to 18 days. After incubation, the virus is contagious for about 3 to 5 days.

Clinical Manifestations. Up to a third of those newly infected will remain asymptomatic. For others the symptomatology is quite varied. In general, initial symptoms include fever, malaise, and anorexia. When present, parotitis usually is evident within a day of the earlier symptoms. Swelling and tenderness of the parotid gland usually progresses for 2 to 3 days, and then decreases within a week.

Complications. Complications include pancreatitis, orchitis, oophoritis, myocarditis, and meningoencephalitis. Central nervous system involvement is most common in children but is rarely associated with permanent sequelae. Deafness may occur in approximately 1 of 20,000 cases. In adult and adolescent men, orchitis is the most frequent complication. Studies have suggested that orchitis has not led to sterility or impotence (Feldman, 1991).

Diagnosis and Management. Diagnosis of mumps is based on symptoms, and diagnostic accuracy is greatly improved during an epidemic. Viral culture and serologic testing are used to confirm initial diagnosis.

There is no therapy that effectively shortens the course of the disease. Patients usually are confined to bed and given foods that are easy to chew and digest.

Influenza

Influenza is an acute viral disease that predictably and periodically causes worldwide epidemics. Epidemics occur every 2 to 3 years, with a highly variable degree of severity. During epidemics, an increase in the general mortality rate is seen as directly attributable to influenza and its accompanying pneumonia and other chronic cardiopulmonary sequelae. It is estimated that in excess of 70,000 deaths between 1977 and 1988 were attributed to influenza or its sequelae in vulnerable groups.

Pathophysiology. The virus is easily spread from host to host. The infected source typically sheds over 1 million infectious viral particles per milliliter of secretions. A small number of viral particles is necessary for transmission to occur. These factors lead to the epidemic potential of this disease. In addition, the virus is highly variable from viral generation to generation. Previous infection with influenza does not guarantee protection from future exposure to different subtypes or the same subtype following antigenic alteration.

Generally, epidemics are sudden and have high attack rates. Peak activity for influenza outbreaks is 6 to 8 weeks in winter months. During community epidemics, outbreaks in hospitals and extended care facilities are common, with pediatric, chronic care, and medical areas most effected.

The influenza virus is transmitted from person to person by spread of droplets to the upper respiratory tract of the person exposed. Transmission is most likely to occur in the first 3 days of illness, but viral shedding can occur in the period before symptoms appear.

Clinical Manifestations. Symptoms of influenza vary markedly between hosts. Generally there is an abrupt onset of multiple symptoms including fever, chills, headache, muscle aches, anorexia, and cough. Within a short time fever and upper respiratory symptoms progress. The patient usually begins to recover around the fourth day, but cough and some degree of debilitation may persist for a prolonged period of time.

Complications. Severe influenza can lead to viral pneumonia or superimposed bacterial pneumonia. Those at risk for progression of disease include the elderly and those with immunosuppression, diabetes, chronic renal failure, or chronic pulmonary disease.

Management. Goals of management are to relieve symptoms, treat complications, and prevent transmission to others.

The patient is encouraged to rest at home for greater comfort and reduction of transmission. Cough can be controlled with an expectorant-antitussive combination. Acetaminophen is frequently used for headache and myalgias. Aspirin is not given to children because of its association with Reye's syndrome. As with most febrile disease, the patient is encouraged to drink plenty of fluids.

Amantadine hydrochloride and rimantadine hydrochloride have been shown to be effective against influenza-A, but not against influenza-B. Amantadine is most effective when it is given before exposure, and may be given to groups of patients in a hospital or other health care facility when there is a recognition of influenza in the community. For those with symptomatic influenza, amantadine's effectiveness is increased when administered within the first 2 days of symptoms.

Prevention

Vaccination. The Immunization Practices Advisory Committee of the Public Health Service recommends annual influenza vaccinations for those at high risk for complications of influenza and for health care workers. Each year a new vaccine, composed of the three virus strains (usually two type A influenza and one type B influenza) considered most likely to be present in the coming season, is available. When the presumed influenza agents have been correctly anticipated and included in that year's vaccine, vaccine effectiveness reaches 70% protection for healthy children and young adults. Although less effective in the elderly (as low as 30% to 40% in the frail elderly), it decreases the severity of illness in those who do get infected, is 50% to 70% effective in preventing pneumonia and hospitalization, and is 80% effective in preventing death. In extended care facilities, risk of transmission is greatly reduced by vaccination of all residents.

The vaccine is recommended for the following groups who have increased risk of complications from influenza: those over 65 years of age, residents of extended care facilities, those with chronic pulmonary or cardiovascular diseases, and those with diabetes, immunosuppression, or renal dysfunction. Vaccination is also advised for children who require long-term aspirin therapy to reduce the likelihood of developing Reye's syndrome. Health care workers and household members of those in high-risk groups are advised to become vaccinated to reduce the risk of transmission to those vulnerable to influenza sequelae. Vaccine campaigns among health care workers and patients should be intensified when there is evidence of community influenza disease.

Isolation. Hospitalized patients with presumed or proven influenza should be kept in private rooms or in rooms with other patients with proven influenza. To the extent possible, rooms should be chosen that provide negative air pressure relative to the hallway. Employees who care for these patients should wear masks. During epidemics, institutions should establish policies to restrict visitation of those who may have febrile illness and screen elective admissions to decrease the likelihood of admitting those who are ill or are incubating influenza.

Infectious Diseases: Travel and Immigration

There is a well-founded concern that infectious diseases may be imported through travel or the influx of refugees. Historically, migration of populations often led to epidemics of disease in immunologically naive new lands. Because of trade, immigration, and wars, the Western Hemisphere has been brought yellow fever, malaria, hookworm, leprosy, smallpox, measles, mumps, syphilis, and many other infectious diseases.

Despite rapid travel, most of the diseases carried by immigrants and travelers to the United States do not efficiently spread in our environment. This is because of the infrastructure of public health with enforced vaccination, clean water, and insect and rodent control in the United States.

However, the potential for disease outbreaks linked to global travel persists. The CDC maintains an active surveillance system to prospectively monitor the incidence of many diseases that are now rare in the United States. This vigilance has proved to be effective in halting transmission of many diseases.

The most significant infectious disease transmission impact associated with immigration is from sexually transmitted diseases, vaccine preventable diseases, and tuberculosis. There is a growing concern that vector-borne diseases such as dengue may be transmitted by mosquitos if a reservoir of infected humans is established.

Immigration and Sexually Transmitted Diseases

HIV and AIDS. The fact that AIDS reached pandemic proportions in less than a decade after its recognition attests to the efficiency of world travel in spreading disease. The significance of such rapid transmission rates is especially dramatic in that HIV essentially requires intimate contact between two people either through sexual activity or sharing blood through needles.

Although the reservoir of HIV-1 in the United States is currently estimated to be greater than 1 million people, it was probably first introduced in the 1970s when asymptomatically infected travelers returned to the United States after having acquired the virus in other countries. The only cases of HIV-2 that have been identified in the United States are from people who have spent time in West Africa. Because of the long asymptomatic period associated with either HIV virus, carriers of HIV-2 may be unrecognized and introduce a chain of infection similar to that which we have witnessed with HIV-1. Control methods to prevent this occurrence involve routine seroprevalence studies to establish any introduction of the virus and routine screening of donated blood for the virus.

Hepatitis B. Similarly, hepatitis B is highly endemic in many parts of the world. Transmission is facilitated by the large proportion of asymptomatic carriers among infected persons. In the United States, travel and immigration are significant factors of disease transmission.

Immigration and Vaccine-Preventable Diseases

The incidence of vaccine-preventable diseases such as measles, mumps, rubella, and diphtheria is also affected by immigration from developing countries. Vaccine campaigns in developing countries are often financially and logistically constrained. Therefore, immigrants from such areas may increase the population of those susceptible to the disease, which in turn increases disease incidence.

It is important to increase vaccine programs in all locations, to include immigrants in such programs to reduce their direct health risks, and to reduce epidemic risk to other susceptible individuals.

Immigration and Tuberculosis

Immigration has always been an important influence in the dynamic epidemiology of TB in the United States. Tuberculosis is a major cause of death in developing nations. Immigration to the United States from such countries adds to the total number of U.S. inhabitants with latent and active disease.

Transmission potential is made greater because many tourists and immigrants visit and live in large cities, which are the epicenter of the HIV epidemic. Screening efforts are hampered as purified protein derivative (PPD) does not provide information about the infectivity of the host. The complexity of PPD interpretation is increased because of the common use of the vaccine BCG (bacille Calmette-Guérin) in many foreign countries. BCG is a vaccine designed to protect against TB, but its effectiveness is extremely variable. After receiving BCG, individuals are often PPD positive for a prolonged time, which affects the ability to interprete screening for TB infection.

Immigration and Vector-Borne Diseases

Malaria, yellow-fever, and dengue are diseases that cause significant morbidity and mortality throughout the developing world. These diseases are spread by infected mosquitos. Many other vector-borne parasitic diseases in developing countries rely on mosquitos and other organisms to complete their life cycles and transmit disease.

Dengue Fever. Dengue fever is an example of the risk of imported vector-borne disease. The disease is caused by a virus that is spread through human populations by the *Aedes aegypti* mosquitos. The mosquitos thrive in tropical zones and breed in stagnant water sources.

Infection from dengue produces flulike symptoms of fever, chills, eye pain, and back pain. Muscle and joint pain, along with nausea and vomiting may be present and patients may exhibit a hyperpigmented rash that blanches on touch. Symptoms often wax and wane and are generally self-limited. A small proportion of patients may develop hemorrhagic disease, which can be life-threatening in extreme forms.

Travelers, immigrants, and returning military personnel can serve as reservoirs of infection. There has been a recent increase in the incidence of dengue virus isolated in the Caribbean, which has caused concern about waves of infection in the United States in areas where vector mosquitos are present. There is no specific treatment for this infection. Control efforts rely on local effective mosquito control.

Immigration and Leprosy

Leprosy is an infectious disease caused by the bacterium, *Mycobacterium leprae*, an acid-fast bacillus, sharing many characteristics with *Mycobacterium tuberculosis*. Because of the long history of social ostracism associated with leprosy, it continues to be an emotional symbol of the risks of contagion.

Although nearly 12 million people worldwide are infected, the disease shows a wide variation of clinical presentation. In many people, the infection may be subclinical with no apparent disease. On the other hand, it can be a progressively disfiguring disease. It is rarely fatal. The organism is spread primarily through the airborne route, but may also be transmitted (rarely) through breaks in the skin.

In the United States, most diagnosed cases represent infection acquired abroad. However, a small but expanding focus of disease can be found in Louisiana, Texas, and Hawaii.

Diagnosis and Management. Diagnosis is made on the basis of the appearance of lesions and by finding acid-fast bacillus on slit skin smears. First-line therapy for leprosy is a combination of rifampin and dapsone. If the patient has extensive disease, clofazamine is frequently added.

Patient Education. Patients are educated to continue therapy to prevent progression of disease. After 1 week of therapy the patient is encouraged to return to work, social, and family activities. Because of peripheral neuropathy, patients are taught to use extreme caution to avoid injuring hands and feet. Those with advanced deformities may require plastic surgery and physical therapy to return to a maximal degree of functioning.

Care of the Patient in the Home

Reducing Risk

The nurse who cares for the patient in the home will need to provide infection risk prevention for the patient, the family, and the care giver.

Reducing Risk to the Patient

Patients requiring home care are often those with immune suppression either from underlying conditions such as HIV or cancer, or those who have therapy-induced immune suppression as may be seen with antineoplastic agents. Careful assessment for signs of infection are important.

Handwashing. Handwashing in the home is an important preventive strategy. Whether a treatment is performed by the nurse, the family, or the patient, handwashing will reduce the risk of transient flora.

Equipment Care. Health care equipment increases infection risk because it is complex and invasive. All care givers must be taught to pay careful attention to disinfection, asepsis, and appropriate usage intervals.

The nurse should maintain a record of the time intervals of vascular catheter insertion. Tunnelled catheters such as the Groshong should not be routinely changed. However, patients or family members who administer IV fluid or medication should be taught how to use aseptic technique during these procedures. The predetermined changing schedule of other vascular access devices should be followed. The nurse and the family members should be alert for any redness, swelling, or drainage around the catheter insertion site. Catheter-related sepsis should be highly suspected in any patient who has unexplained fever.

There is no recommended interval for the changing of urinary catheters. However, the nurse should promptly report to the patient's physician signs of urinary tract infection or of generalized sepsis.

Patient Education. When assessing the immune suppressed patient in the home environment for infectious risk, it is important to realize that intrinsic colonizing bacteria and latent viral infections present a greater risk than do extrinsic environmental contaminants. The patient and the family need reassurance that their home does not need to be sterile. Common sense approaches to cleanliness and risk reduction are helpful. The severely neutropenic patient should refrain from eating uncooked fruits and vegetables. For patients with neutropenia or with T-cell dysfunction (*e.g*, the AIDS patient) it is wise to restrict visits of persons with potentially contagious illnesses.

Reducing Risk to Household Members

Establishing Barriers and Precautions. Establishing careful barriers to infection transmission in the household is an important part of home care. The route of transmission of the organism in question must first be determined. Then the nurse can educate household members to reduce their risk of becoming infected.

If the patient has active pulmonary tuberculosis, the public health department should be contacted to provide screening and treatment for family members. Decisions about prevention of other airborne diseases, such as chickenpox, need to be made based on the family situation. For example, precautions are not usually recommended to prevent healthy siblings from being exposed to a child with chickenpox. However, if one of the household members is pregnant and has no previous history of chickenpox, avoiding contact during the infectious period is wise.

Food Preparation and Personal Hygiene. Organisms transmitted by the fecal-hand-oral route may be readily spread in a household setting unless very careful attention to food preparation and personal hygiene is maintained. Family care givers are vulnerable to acquiring organisms such as *Shigella* and *C. difficile* when assisting in personal care. Hands should be washed carefully after such contact. The family should be reassured that common household disinfectants are effective in killing environmental sources of such organisms.

Bloodborne Infection Risk. Family members who assist in the care of a patient with a bloodborne infection such as HIV should be alert for the potential of transmission if sharp objects contaminated with blood are handled. Family education may be designed to discuss the need for caution when shaving the patient, performing dressing changes, or administering any intravenous, intramuscular, or subcutaneous medication. It is important to set up an impenetrable container for the collection of needles, syringes, and vascular access equipment.

The nurse should also educate the family about infections that do not pose a risk. With the exception of tuberculosis, the opportunistic infections associated with AIDS do not pose a risk to the healthy family member. Family members should be reassured that dishes are safe to use after being washed with hot water, and linens and clothing also are safe to use after being washed in a hot water cycle.

Reducing Risk to the Caregiver

Recognizing that a health history may not identify all active or latent infections, the caregiver should follow careful infection control practices (including universal precautions) in all homes. Setting up a work environment in which hand washing and aseptic technique can be accomplished as carefully as they are in a hospital setting is important.

Receiving hepatitis B vaccination and yearly vaccination with the influenza vaccine is a wise preventative strategy. Having a purified protein derivative (PPD) test annually is an important method to verify that new infection with tuberculosis has not occurred.

❑ *NURSING PROCESS*
The Patient With an Infectious Disease

Assessment

Symptoms of infectious diseases vary significantly both between and within diseases. For some infections, such as chickenpox (varicella), widely disseminated rash represents the first suggestion of infection and is present in most newly infected people. In other infections, such as tuberculosis or HIV, latency is prolonged and the majority of those infected will not be symptomatic; instead, infection will be determined through diagnostic procedures.

History taking, physical examination, and the use of diagnostic tests are important determinants of infection and infectious diseases.

The goals of eliciting history are to establish the likelihood and probable source of infection and degree of associated pathology or pain. The patient's previous medical record is reviewed when possible. In obtaining a health history some of the following questions may be asked.

- ❑ Does the patient have a history of previous or recurrent infections? Is the patient aware of infection with an organism associated with prolonged latency such as HIV, herpes, or TB?
- ❑ Has there been fever? How high has the fever been? What is the fever pattern? Is the fever constant or does it rise and fall? Has fever been associated with chills? Has the patient taken medication to relieve fever?
- ❑ Is there cough? Is the cough chronic or acute? Is it associated with shortness of breath? Does the cough produce sputum? Is the sputum bloody? Has the patient had a PPD test performed recently? If so, what were the results? Has the patient been given isoniazid (INH) prophylaxis for TB infection? Has the patient been treated for TB in the past?
- ❑ Is there pain? Where is the pain? What is the nature of the pain? Are there sore throat, headache, myalgias, arthralgias? Is there pain on urination or other activity?
- ❑ Is there swelling? Is there drainage associated with the swelling? Is the swollen area warm to touch?
- ❑ Is there a draining site? Is the drainage associated with trauma or a previous procedure? Is the drainage purulent or clear?
- ❑ Does the patient have diarrhea, vomiting, or abdominal pain?
- ❑ Is there rash? What is the nature of the rash: flat, raised, red, crusted, purulent, lacelike?
- ❑ What is the vaccination history?
- ❑ Has the patient taken medications that could induce rash?
- ❑ Has there been exposure to another person who has an identified infectious disease or rash?
- ❑ Has there been an insect or animal bite? Has there been an animal scratch, or other exposure to pets, farm animals, or experimental animals?
- ❑ What medications are used? Have antibiotics been taken recently or chronically? Is the patient being treated with corticosteroids, immunosuppressing drugs, or chemotherapy?
- ❑ Is there a history of substance abuse?
- ❑ Has the patient been treated in the past for other infectious diseases? Has the patient been hospitalized for infectious diseases?
- ❑ If sexual history is pertinent, has there been sexual exposure to another person with a known sexually transmitted disease? Has the patient been treated for sexually transmitted diseases in the past? Is the patient

pregnant or has she recently been pregnant? Has the patient been tested for HIV?
- ❑ Has the patient traveled to or from a developing country or abroad? What was the immunization or antimicrobial prophylaxis used for protection while traveling?
- ❑ What is the patient's occupation?

Because infection may occur in any body system, physical examination may reveal signs of infection at any body site. Generalized signs of chronic infection may include significant weight loss or pallor associated with anemia of chronic diseases. Acute infection may present with fever, chills, lymphadenopathy, or rash. Localized signs vary significantly according to the source of infection. Purulence, pain, swelling, and redness are strongly associated with localized infection. Cough and shortness of breath may be due to influenza, pneumonia, or tuberculosis as well as to many noninfectious causes.

Diagnosis

Nursing Diagnoses

Infection may cause an interruption in normal function of any affected body system. For alteration in each system the reader should review nursing diagnoses for body systems listed in the appropriate chapter.

Based on assessment data, the patient's major nursing diagnoses which relate specifically to infection may include:

- ❑ Risk for infection transmission
- ❑ Knowledge deficit about the disease, cause of infection, treatment, and prevention measures
- ❑ Altered body temperature (fever) related to the presence of infection

Collaborative Problems/ Potential Complications

Based on the assessment data, potential complications that may develop include:

- ❑ Secondary bloodstream infection
- ❑ Septic shock
- ❑ Dehydration
- ❑ Abscess formation
- ❑ Endocarditis
- ❑ Infectious disease-related cancers
- ❑ Infertility
- ❑ Congenital abnormalities

Planning and Implementation

Goals. Major goals for the patient may include prevention of spread of infection, knowledge about the infection and its treatment, control of fever and related discomforts, and absence of complications.

Nursing Interventions

Preventing Infection Transmission. Preventing the spread of infection requires an understanding of the usual routes of transmission for the organism. The hospitalized patient may serve as a risk for transmission to other patients if the patient's disease was spread by the airborne route, or if infected by an organism such as *C. difficile*, which can be spread directly to others by persistence of spores in the environment. In these situations strict adherence to isolation measures is important in reducing the opportunity for spread. Risk of transmission of organisms from patient to patient usually requires participation of the health care team. Transmission of organisms on the hands and gloves of health care workers remains a common source of cross infection in the hospital or clinic setting.

Nurses serve an important function in prevention of transfer of organisms in two ways. First, as the health professional who often spends the greatest amount of time with patients, the opportunity for spreading organisms is great. It is imperative that nurses wash hands before and after contact with patients, and after performing a potentially hand contaminating activity. Hands must be washed each time gloves are removed. For example, the nurse who has performed endotracheal suctioning should remove gloves and wash hands before performing wound care on the same patient.

The second way that nurses reduce hand-to-hand spread is to serve as patient advocate. With the number of health care workers involved in patient care each day, there is a large opportunity for breaks in handwashing technique. To the degree feasible, the nurse should observe the hand washing activities of other professionals and discuss them when lapses in technique are observed.

Acquiring Knowledge About the Infectious Process. For infectious diseases, interruption of transmission requires infection recognition, as well as patient understanding of the significance of the infection and a commitment to prevention. The nurse's role in this situation is to educate, and in some settings, to report the case to public health officials for contact tracing and verification of follow-up.

In educational efforts it is also necessary to stress the importance of immunization to parents of young children and to others for whom certain vaccines are recommended. Nurses should assess their personal responsibility to receive hepatitis B and annual influenza vaccine to reduce potential transmission to self and vulnerable patient groups.

Infectious diseases often seem mysterious and frequently carry socially stigmatizing effects. Patient education efforts require empathy and sensitivity. For example, patients who are to receive INH prophylaxis for 6 months may be confused by the information that they are infected, but not diseased, and yet need to adhere to prolonged therapy. In the past, tuberculosis was a very stigmatized disease. Some still feel shame when learning of this infection. Patient education must be directed at the details and advantages of INH prophylaxis. It should be clarified that infection is not a guilt-associated issue.

Controlling Fever and Accompanying Discomforts. Whereas infectious diseases usually cause fever, there are other noninfectious causes of fever as well. Therefore, a new fever requires investigation of its source. There is evidence that fever, as mediated by the hypothalamus, is a part of a syndrome of reactions known as *acute phase reaction*. These reactions include changes in liver protein synthesis; alterations in serum metals, such as iron; increased production of certain classes of both white cells and other immune system cells. Fever may potentiate some beneficial functions of this acute phase reaction. Severe fever such as seen with

(text continues on page 1996)

NURSING CARE PLAN 65–1
Care of the Patient With an Infectious Disease

Nursing Interventions	Rationale	Expected Outcomes
NURSING DIAGNOSIS: Risk for infection transmission		
GOAL: Preventing transmission of infectious agents		
1. Prevent patient-to-patient infection spread	1. Organisms that are spread through an airborne route or are very contagious through direct contact can be transmitted in a health care setting from patient to patient	• No evidence of patient-to-patient transmission of infection • No evidence of transmission via health care workers • No occupationally acquired infections in nurses and other health care workers. • No evidence of transmission due to contaminated equipment • Absence of primary bloodstream infections • Absence of urinary tract infection • Absence of pneumonia
a. Provide isolation according to CDC, use of body substance isolation, or individual institution adaptation of isolation	a. CDC-adapted isolation strategies are developed to reduce the likelihood of transmission from patient to patient	
b. Ensure that patients with airborne infections remain in private rooms during their stay. If they must leave their rooms, arrangements should be made to decrease the likelihood of contact with other patients. Rooms should be ventilated according to CDC criteria. Personal protective equipment in the form of masks or respirators should be worn according to institution policy. In nursing homes and other locations where patients have increased risk of sequelae from influenza, annual influenza vaccination should be encouraged.	b. Engineering controls with ventilation focus are important in the prevention of transmission of airborne diseases. Influenza vaccine safely reduces risk of illness associated with this highly communicable, and frequently virulent organism.	
c. Ensure that patients with highly transmissible non-airborne organisms, such as *Clostridium difficile* and *Shigella* are physically separated from other patients if hygiene or institutional policy dictates	c. Increased preventive strategy is necessary when the organism has high epidemic potential	
2. Prevent health care worker's transfer of organisms from patient to patient	2. Transfer of organisms on the hands of health care workers is a common route of transmission. Hospital organisms which transiently colonize the hands of health care workers are frequently virulent	
a. Handwashing should be performed consistently and thoroughly—washing hands before and after each patient contact, and following procedures which offer contamination risk while caring for a single patient	a. Handwashing technique is important in reducing transient flora on outer epidermal layers of skin.	
b. Gloves must be used when handling any body fluid from any patient. Gloves must be changed between patient care activities and hands must be washed after gloves are removed.	b. Gloves provide an effective barrier protection. It must be recognized that gloves quickly become contaminated and then become a potential vehicle for transfer of organisms. Microflora of hands while gloves are worn is likely to proliferate.	

(continued)

NURSING CARE PLAN 65–1 *(continued)*
Care of the Patient With an Infectious Disease

Nursing Interventions	Rationale	Expected Outcomes
c. Nurses should monitor the hand washing and glove use behaviors of other health care professionals caring for patient	c. Poor compliance with handwashing among health care workers has been well documented, and should be expected. As the patient's advocate this protective communication is important to reduce infectious risk.	
3. Prevent patient-to-health care worker transmission of infection	3. Health care workers may occupationally acquire infections due to close contact with patients.	
a. Risk of infection with tuberculosis will be avoided by: (1) Participation in early identification of patients with active disease. Patients will be asked about risk factors, symptoms, previous exposure and PPD status. Diagnostic work-up with chest x-ray, sputum analysis for organisms, and PPD administration as appropriate are expedited.	a. The most important element in the reduction of transmission of tuberculosis is early identification. Many of the symptoms of tuberculosis are subtle, and may be first observed by the nurse who has prolonged contact with the patient.	
(2) Maintain engineering controls. Keep the patient in a private room with a closed door.	(2) Confining air flow to the immediate vicinity of the patient and exhausting air to the outside reduce the likelihood of transmission to health care workers in areas outside of the patient room.	
(3) Use protection in isolation room or when participating in procedures that are likely to generate cough such as suctioning, intubation, or administering nebulized medications.	(3) The benefit of masks and respirators is still under scientific study. However, it is theorized that such devices may reduce risk to the health care worker.	
b. Risk of transmission of bloodborne diseases such as hepatitis B, hepatitis C, and the human immunodeficiency virus will be avoided by:	b. Health care workers can contract bloodborne diseases via percutaneous injury such as needlestick or by contact with blood or bloody body fluids to mucous membranes such as eyes or mouth.	
(1) Vaccination with hepatitis B vaccine	(1) Without vaccine, health care workers with significant exposure such as needlestick face a relatively high risk of transmission of hepatitis B. The vaccine has been determined to be safe and effective.	
(2) Use universal precautions as outlined by the Centers for Disease Control and Prevention c. Avoid risk of infection with airborne diseases.	(2) Universal precautions are based on the recognition that most patients with bloodborne infections cannot be identified by physical assessment or history taking. Health care workers must assume that all patients may be infected and use appropriate barrier precautions routinely for *all* patients.	

(continued)

Care of the Patient With an Infectious Disease

Nursing Interventions	Rationale	Expected Outcomes
(1) Vaccination with influenza vaccine on an annual basis	(1) Influenza vaccine is recommended for health care workers to reduce the likelihood of transmission in health care agencies.	
(2) Vaccination or proof of immunity for measles, mumps and rubella	(2) Susceptible healthcare workers can become occupationally exposed, and can expose immunocompromised patients	
4. Prevent patient exposure to contaminated medical equipment	4. Technologic advances offer increased opportunity for invasive procedures, often using complex, difficult to clean equipment	
a. Equipment that enters through intact skin must be sterilized between patient uses	a. Sterilization renders equipment free of all microorganisms	
b. Equipment that has contact with mucous membranes must be sterilized or "high level" disinfected between patient uses	b. High-level disinfection with a product such as a glutaraldehyde renders an object free of all microorganisms with the possible exception of spore producing organisms	
c. Equipment used against intact skin should be thoroughly cleaned and "low level" disinfected between patient uses	c. The disinfection goal with this degree of contact is to reduce the load of microorganisms to be within a range that is not threatening to the host with intact skin.	
5. Follow established guidelines for the routine removal and replacement of intravenous equipment	5. Indwelling intravascular devices can serve as a conduit for organisms to migrate into the bloodstream to establish bacteremia	
6. Remove urinary catheters at the earliest time possible	6. The risk of urinary tract infection is directly proportional to the length of time that a urinary catheter remains in place, with the risk increasing until it reaches 100%	
7. Remove endotracheal and nasogastric tubes at earliest reasonable time	7. The risk of pneumonia is increased as the duration of the use of such equipment increases	

NURSING DIAGNOSIS: Knowledge deficit about disease, cause of infection, and preventive measures

GOAL: Acquisition of knowledge about the infectious process

Nursing Interventions	Rationale	Expected Outcomes
1. Listen carefully to what the patient says about the illness and treatment	1. Listening allows for detection and correction of misunderstanding and misinformation.	• Patient actively participates in treatment • Patient complies with infection control measures
2. Provide brief pertinent explanations about: a. Organism and route of transmission b. Treatment goals c. Follow-up schedule d. Prevention of transmission to others	2. Knowledge about specific diagnoses and treatments may promote compliance	
3. Allow opportunities for questions and discussions	3. The patient's questions indicate issues that need clarification	

(continued)

NURSING CARE PLAN 65–1 *(continued)*

Care of the Patient With an Infectious Disease

Nursing Interventions	Rationale	Expected Outcomes
4. Teach the patient and family about: a. Prophylaxis or immunization if recommended b. Community resources if necessary c. Means of preventing transmission within the home	4. Understanding of the risks and precautions associated with an infectious disease may reduce the opportunity for further spread	
NURSING DIAGNOSIS: Altered body temperature (fever) related to the presence of infection		
GOAL: Patient comfort and return of temperature to normal		
1. Monitor temperature, pulse, and respirations at regular intervals	1. Trends in fever can be classified as continuous, remittent, intermittent, and so forth, and provide diagnostic clues. Additionally, fever curves provide a measurement of severity and duration of infectious process.	• Body temperature within normal limits • Maintenance of fluid and electrolyte balance • Patient comfortable
2. Assess fever in elderly patients carefully	2. Elderly patients often are unable to generate fever effectively. Minimal fever or hypothermia may be indicative of infection. Fever increases metabolic demands and thus cardiac demands and workload. For many elderly patients cardiac function is already compromised; increase in cardiac workload can precipitate congestive heart failure.	
3. Encourage increased intake of fluids	3. Fluid replacement is important for replacement of losses due to increased respiration and diaphoresis	
4. Initiate cool baths or tepid sponge baths	4. Wetting the skin facilitates body cooling as evaporation occurs and promotes comfort	
5. Change linen when patient is diaphoretic	5. Dry linen may improve patient comfort	
COLLABORATIVE PROBLEMS: Different infectious agents have different potential for producing complications. Among potential complications are secondary bloodstream infection; septic shock; dehydration; abscess formation, endocarditis, infectious disease related cancers; obstructive pathology; infertility; congenital abnormalities		
GOAL: Absence of complications		
Secondary Bloodstream Infection		
1. Monitor patient for evidence of infection at any location	1. Vigilance for bacterial or fungal infection at any site promotes early recognition, treatment, and reduces the likelihood of secondary bloodstream infection	• No episodes of secondary bloodstream infection • Effective treatment of identified bacterial and fungal infections without progression to secondary bloodstream infection • Early improvement in septic course
2. Assess effectiveness of treatment for all identified infections	2. Effective control of localized infections reduces the risk of secondary bloodstream infection	
3. Administer antibiotics as prescribed with first dose given at earliest time possible.	3. Secondary infections are often from gram negative organisms which can very rapidly cause a septic course.	

(continued)

NURSING CARE PLAN 65–1 *(continued)*
Care of the Patient With an Infectious Disease

Nursing Interventions	Rationale	Expected Outcomes
Septic Shock		
1. Routinely, and as warranted, monitor vital signs for patients with recognized infections and severely immune suppressed patients at risk for shock. In particular be alert for signs of a. Fever b. Tachycardia (over 90 beats/min) c. Tachypnea (over 20 breaths/min) d. Evidence of decreased perfusion or dysfunction of vital organs in the form of (1) Change of mental status (2) Hypoxemia as measured by arterial blood gases (3) Elevated lactate levels (4) Urine output (less than 30 ml/h)	1. Early recognition of the signs of impending shock may reduce the associated severity or mortality.	• Absence of symptoms of septic shock • Hemodynamic and respiratory control
2. Administer antibiotics, fluid replacement, vasopressors, and oxygen as prescribed	2. Therapeutic maintenance of hemodynamic and respiratory status is necessary until infection is effectively treated with antimicrobial regimen	
Dehydration		
1. Assess for dehydration (thirst, dryness of mucous membranes, loss of skin turgor, reduced peripheral pulses, urine output less than 30 ml/hour)	1. Signs of dehydration provide basis for fluid replacement and suggest possible further complications of circulatory collapse	• Attains fluid balance (output approximates intake; body weight unchanged) • Mucous membranes appear moist; normal skin turgor • Serum electrolytes are within normal limits
2. Monitor weight	2. Rapid changes in weight indicate fluid volume changes	
3. Monitor intake and output, and serum electrolyte levels	3. Dehydration produces a deficit in some electrolytes. Decreased urine production may indicate a lack of systemic hydration	
4. Replace fluids as needed; If the patient can tolerate oral fluids, offer fluids every 2–4 hours. Administer intravenous fluids as prescribed.	4. When possible oral hydration is preferable, because the patient can select the beverage, control the rate and interval of replacement, and care for himself at home; in addition, the risks of vascular access devices are avoided. If intravenous fluid is required, intravenous solutions are formulated to facilitate intestinal reabsorption of fluid and electrolytes	
Abscess Formation		
1. Assess vascular access sites, wound sites, pressure ulcers, and other appropriate sites for apparent collections of purulent material	1. Collections of purulent material often require drainage before antimicrobial therapy is effective	• Absence of abscess • Early identification of signs of intra-abdominal sepsis to expedite procedural correction.

(continued)

NURSING CARE PLAN 65–1 *(continued)*
Care of the Patient With an Infectious Disease

Nursing Interventions	Rationale	Expected Outcomes
2. Assess the patient who has had abdominal surgery or trauma to abdominal area for localized signs of intra-abdominal abscess. These signs include: a. Low grade fever b. Elevated peripheral white blood cell count c. Localized pain d. Abdominal tenderness e. Visible or palpable mass f. Postoperative diarrhea g. GI bleeding	2. Intra-abdominal abscess formation is most common following traumatic or surgical disruption of the GI tract. Signs are often initially subtle.	
3. Assess patient who has had percutaneous abscess drainage to assess if drainage has been successful. Be alert for all of the above signs and symptoms.	3. After percutaneous drainage, recurrent or persistent signs of abscess may indicate the need for surgical treatment	
4. Administer antibiotics as prescribed.	4. Antibiotics, along with drainage, are the most important elements of intra-abdominal abscess management	
Endocarditis		
Prevention		
1. Patients with the following conditions should be taught about the value of antibiotic prophylaxis for events and procedures that may introduce risk of endocarditis: a. Valvular disease b. Congenital heart disease c. Intracardiac prostheses d. Previous endocarditis	1. Persons with underlying valvular disease and other cardiac entities are at increased risk for "seeding" of cardiac valves during procedures recognized to cause bacteremia	• Informs health care professionals of cardiac conditions that require antibiotic prophylaxis before procedures that can cause bacteremia • Takes prophylactic antibiotics as prescribed
Management		
1. Blood cultures should be obtained as ordered; results should be carefully recorded. Persistent bloodstream infection with an organism should be noted.	1. A definitive diagnosis of endocarditis requires blood culture confirmation	• When present endocarditis is diagnosed, treated, and cured.
2. Obtain detailed history about duration of fever in the absence of well-recognized cause.	2. Endocarditis should be suspected in patients who report an unexplained fever for over 1 week duration	
3. Administer intravenous antibiotic therapy at ordered time schedule.	3. Intravenous therapy is usually required for cure. The goal of therapy is complete eradication of all organisms. Careful adherence to following the scheduled regimen is therefore essential.	

Infectious disease-related cancers, infertility, congenital abnormalities: These potential complications of infectious diseases are prevented by primary avoidance of infection. Management of them is directed toward treating each of them as a non-infectious entity. For example, the management of cancer secondary to hepatitis B infection will be handled as an oncology issue, not as an infectious disease issue. Similarly, the care of the child with deafness will be managed from the otolaryngology and behavioral aspects of deafness rather than the treatment of CMV.

meningococcal meningitis may cause other complications in the form of heat stroke. However, this is very uncommon because most fevers are physiologically self-controlled to stay below 105.8°F (41°C). However, even with this control, fever and its accompanying fatigue, chills, and diaphoresis can be very uncomfortable for the patient. Decisions regarding fever control are made by the physician. Whether or not fever is treated, adequate fluid intake is very important during febrile episodes.

Because fever offers clues about infection severity and success of antibiotic therapy, outpatients with fever should be advised to obtain accurate readings. Frequently, parents will know that a child has warm skin, but will not trouble the child by taking a temperature reading. Body temperature information can be very helpful in adjusting therapy or in revaluating a preliminary diagnosis.

Monitoring and Managing Potential Complications. The patient with a rapidly progressive infectious disease should have vital signs and level of consciousness closely monitored for signs of sepsis. Laboratory values from microbiology, immunology, hematology, cytology, and parasitology along with x-ray findings must be interpreted in the context of other clinical findings to assess the infectious disease course. Antibiotic therapy is frequently complex with modifications necessary owing to sensitivity test results and disease progression. It is important to initiate antibiotic therapy as soon as it is prescribed, rather than waiting until routine medication scheduling times. This ensures that therapeutic blood levels can be attained as quickly as possible. See Nursing Care Plan 65-1 for nursing interventions for specific complications of infection.

Evaluation

Expected Outcomes

1. Uses appropriate methods to prevent the spread of infection
2. Acquires knowledge about the infectious process
3. Absence of elevated body temperature
4. Attains fluid balance

CRITICAL THINKING EXERCISES

1. A nurse who is returning to nursing after 10 years is being oriented to your nursing unit. She is assigned to take care of a patient with AIDS. She questions why the patient is not isolated. What conclusions might you draw from her comment? To ensure appropriate care for this patient, how would you explain to the nurse the best way to approach AIDS patients when giving care?
2. You are supervising a patient care technician who is changing the bed of a postoperative patient. There is fresh blood on the patient's sheet from a venipuncture that was just performed. The technician is not wearing gloves as she disposes of the linen. How would you evaluate this situation, and what action would you take? Explain the rationale for your decision.
3. You are caring for patients in an extended-care facility. A patient who has had a stroke is admitted, and the admission data indicate that the patient is incontinent of urine. A staff nurse indicates that she will obtain an order for an indwelling catheter. Evaluate the effectiveness of this approach, and describe the plan of care you would devise for this patient.
4. An elderly patient with cardiac disease questions you about why her physician suggested that she receive an influenza vaccination. She states that she received the vaccination years ago and then "got the flu from the vaccine." How would you respond to her and explain the situation? Describe the line of reasoning you would follow to convince her to get the vaccine. If she rejects your explanation, examine the different courses of action you could take and the pros and cons of each strategy.

BIBLIOGRAPHY

Books

Beaver PC, Jung RC, and Cupp EW. Clinical Parasitology. Philadelphia, Lea & Febiger, 1984.

Benenson A. Control of Communicable Diseases in Man; 1990. Washington, American Public Health Association, 1990.

Bennett JV and Brachman PS. Hospital Infections, 3rd ed. Boston, Little, Brown, 1992.

Cheeseman SH. Cytomegalovirus. In Gorbach JL, Bartlett JG, and Blacklow NR (eds). Infectious Diseases. Philadelphia, WB Saunders, 1992.

Evans S. Viral Infections of Humans: Epidemiology and Control, 2nd ed. New York, Plenum Medical Book, 1991.

Evans S and Brachman P. Bacterial Infections of Humans: Epidemiology and Control, 2nd ed. New York, Plenum Publishing, New York, 1991.

Feldman HA. Mumps. In Evans S (ed). Viral Infections of Humans: Epidemiology and Control. New York, Plenum Publishing, 1991.

Gorbach SL, Bartlett J, and Blacklow NR. Infectious Diseases. Philadelphia, WB Saunders, 1992.

Larson E. Clinical Microbiology and Infection Control. Boston, Blackwell Scientific Publications, 1984.

Mandell GL, Douglas RG, and Bennett JE. Principles and Practice of Infectious Diseases, 3rd ed. New York, Churchill Livingstone, 1990.

Remington JS and Klein JD. Infectious Diseases of the Fetus and Newborn Infant, 3rd ed. Philadelphia, WB Saunders, 1990.

Ryan F. The Forgotten Plague: How the Battle Against Tuberculosis Was Won—and Lost. Boston, Little, Brown, 1992.

Sandford J. Guide to Antimicrobial Therapy 1992. Dallas, Antimicrobial Therapy, 1992.

Stumacher RJ. Clinical Infectious Diseases. Philadelphia, WB Saunders, 1987.

Wenzel R. Prevention and Control of Nosocomial Infections. Baltimore, Williams and Wilkins, 1987.

Journals

Asterisks indicate nursing research articles.

Diarrheal Diseases

Centers for Disease Control. The management of acute diarrhea in children: Oral rehydration, maintenance, and nutritional therapy. MMWR 1992; 41:(RR16),1–20.

Lowry PW, Pavia AT, et al. Cholera in Louisiana: Widening spectrum of seafood vehicles. Arch Intern Med 1989 Sep; 149(9): 2079–2084.

Perez-Perez GI, Guerrant RL, et al. Clinical and immunologic significance of cholera-like toxin and cytotoxin production by Campylobacter species in patients with acute inflammatory diarrhea in the USA. J Infect Dis 1989 Sep; 160(3):460–468.

White KE, Hedeberg CW, et al. An outbreak of Giardiasis in a nursing home with evidence for multiple modes of transmission. J Infect Dis 1989 Aug; 160(2):298–304.

Federal Agencies

Centers for Disease Control. CDC: The nation's prevention agency. MMWR 1992; 41(44):833.

Decker M. OSHA enforcement policy for occupational exposure to tuberculosis. Infect Control Hosp Epidemiol 1993 Dec; 14(12): 689–693.

Gerberding JL. Occupational infectious diseases of infectious occupational diseases? Bridging the views of tuberculosis control. Infect Control Hosp Epidemiol 1993 Dec; 14(12):686–688.

Hepatitis

Alter MJ, Coleman PJ, et al. Importance of heterosexual activity in the transmission of hepatitis B and non-A, non-B hepatitis. JAMA 1989 Sep; 262(9):1201–1205.

Centers for Disease Control. Hepatitis E among US travelers, 1989–1992. MMWR 1993; 42(1):1–4.

Centers for Disease Control. Addressing emerging infectious disease threats: A prevention strategy for the United States; Executive summary. MMWR 1994; 43(RR-5):1–18.

Herpes Family of Viruses

Centers for Disease Control. Surveillance of congenital cytomegalovirus disease, 1990–1991. MMWR 1992; 41(SS-2):35–44.

Gerberding JL. Risks to health care workers from occupational exposure to hepatitis B virus, human immunodeficiency virus, and cytomegalovirus. Infect Dis Clin North Am 1989 Dec; 3(4):735–745.

Goldman DA. Prevention and management of neonatal infections. Infect Dis Clin North Am 1989 Dec; 3(4):779–813.

Meningitis

Tunkel A, Wispelwey B, et al. Pathogenesis and pathophysiology of meningitis. Infect Dis Clin North Am 1990 Dec; 4(4):555–575.

Saez-Llorens ET and McCracken GH. Bacterial meningitis in neonates and children. Infect Dis Clin North Am 1990 Dec; 4(4): 623–641.

Wispelwey B, Tunkel A, et al. Bacterial meningitis in adults. Infect Dis Clin North Am 1990 Dec; 4(4):645–659.

Methicillin-Resistant Staphylococcus Aureus

Boyce JM, et al. Methicillin-resistant *Staphylococcus aureus* (MRSA): A briefing for acute care hospitals and nursing facilities. Infect Control Hosp Epidemiol 1994 Feb; 15(2):105–115.

Nosocomial Infections and Care of Patients With Infections

Centers for Disease Control. Guideline for prevention of nosocomial pneumonia. Infect Control Hosp Epidemiol 1994 Sep; 15(9):588–627.

Centers for Disease Control. Public health focus: Surveillance, prevention, and control of nosocomial infections. MMWR 1992; 41(42):783–787.

Conly JM, Grieves K, and Peters B. Randomized study comparing transparent and dry dressings for central venous catheters. J Infect Dis 1989 Oct; 159:310–319.

*Craney JM, Hart EK,and Munro BH. A comparison of two techniques of care for indwelling arterial introducers after coronary angioplasty. J Cardiovasc Nurs 1992 Oct; 7(1):50–55.

Cruse PJE and Foord R. A five year prospective study of 23,649 surgical wounds. Arch Surg 1973 Aug; 107:206–210.

Fiddian-Green RG and Baaker S. Nosocomial pneumonia in the critically ill: Product of aspiration or translocation? Crit Care Med 1991 Jun; 19:763–769.

*Fitchie C. Central venous catheter-related infection and dressing type. Intensive Critical Care Nursing 1992 Dec; 8(4):199–202.

Hayek LJ, Emerson JM, and Gardner AMN. A placebo-controlled trial of the effects of two preoperative baths or showers with chlorhexidine detergent on postoperative wound infection rates. J Hosp Infect 1987 Feb; 10:165–172.

*Knowles HE. The experience of infectious patients in isolation. Nursing Times 1993 July 28–Aug 3; 89(30):53–56.

Maki DG and Ringer M. Evaluation of dressing regimens for prevention of infection with peripheral intravenous catheters: Gauze, a transparent polyurethane dressing, and a transparent iodophor dressing. JAMA 1987 Nov; 258:2396–2403.

*Robertson J. Changing central venous catheter lines: Evaluation of a modification to clinical practice. J Pediatr Oncol Nurs 1991 October; 8(4):173–179.

Seropian R and Reynolds BM. Wound infections after preoperative depilatory versus razor preparation. Am J Surg 1971 Mar; 121:251–254.

*White MC. Infections and infection risks in home settings. Department of Mental Health, Community and Administrative Nursing, University of California San Francisco 94143-0608. Infect Control Hosp Epidemiol 1992 Sept; 13(9):535–539.

Wihlborg O. The effect of washing with chlorhexidine soap on wound infection rates in general surgery. Ann Gynecol 1987 Apr; 76:263–265.

Resistant Enterococcus

Centers for Disease Control. Nosocomial Enterococci resistant to vancomycin—United States, 1989–1993. MMWR 1993; 42(30): 597–599.

Goldmann DA. Vancomycin-resistant *Enterococcus faecium:* Headline news [editorial]. Infect Control Hosp Epidemiol 1992 Jul; 13(7):695–699.

Karanfil LV and Murphy M. A cluster of vancomycin-resistant *Enterococcus faecium* in an intensive care unit. Infect Control Hosp Epidemiol 1992 Apr; 13(4):195–200.

Livornese LL, Dias S, et al. Hospital-acquired infection with vancomycin-resistant *Enterococcus faecium* transmitted by electronic thermometers. Ann Intern Med 1992 Jul; 117(2):112–116.

Sexually Transmitted Diseases

Centers for Disease Control. 1993 sexually transmitted diseases treatment guidelines. MMWR 1993; 42(RR-14):1–102.

Centers for Disease Control. Testing for antibodies to human immunodeficiency virus type 2 in the United States. MMWR 1992; 41(RR-12):1–9.

Centers for Disease Control. Special focus: Surveillance for sexually transmitted diseases. MMWR 1993; 42(SS-3):1–42.

Centers for Disease Control. Recommendations for the prevention and management of *Chlamydia trachomatis* infections, 1993. MMWR 1993; 42(RR-12):1–39.

Clottey C and Dallabetta G. Sexually transmitted diseases and human immunodeficiency virus. Infect Dis Clin North Am 1993 Dec; 7(4):753–770.

Tuberculosis

Pfaller M. Application of new technology to the detection, identification, and antimicrobial susceptibility testing of Mycobacteria. Am J Clin Pathol 1994 Mar; 101(3):329–337.

Urinary Tract Infections

Garibaldi RA, et al. An evaluation of daily bacteriologic monitoring to identify preventable episodes of catheter-associated urinary tract infection. Infection Control 1982 May–Jun; 3:466–470.

Johnson JR and Stamm WE. Diagnosis and treatment of acute urinary tract infections. Infect Dis Clin North Am 1987 Dec; 1(4):773–791.

Sobel J. Pathogenesis of urinary tract infections, host defenses. Infect Dis Clin North Am 1987 Dec; 1(4):751–772.

Thompson RL, et al. Catheter associated bacteriuria. Failure to reduce attack rates using periodic installation of a disinfectant into urinary drainage systems. JAMA 1984 Feb; 251(6):747–751.

Warren JW. Catheter-associated urinary tract infections. Infect Dis Clin North Am 1987 Dec; 1(4):823–854.

Wong ES and Hooten TM. Guidelines for prevention of catheter-associated urinary tract infections. Am J Infect Control 1983 Feb; 11(1):28–36.

Vaccine Issues

Centers for Disease Control. Prevention and control of influenza, Part I, vaccines. Recommendations of the Advisory Committee on Immunization Practices. MMWR 1993; 42(RR-6) 1–14.

Centers for Disease Control. Measles surveillance - United States 1991. MMWR 1992; 41(SS-6):1–12.

Centers for Disease Control. Immunization Practices Advisory Committee: General recommendations on immunization. MMWR 1989;38:223.

Centers for Disease Control. Immunization Practices Advisory Committee: Hepatitis B virus: A comprehensive strategy for eliminating transmission in the United States through universal childhood vaccination. Recommendations of the Immunization Practices Advisory Committee. MMWR 1991; 40(RR-13): 1–25.

Centers for Disease Control. Recommendations of the International Task Force for Disease Eradication. MMWR 1993; 42(RR-16): 1–38P.

INFORMATION/RESOURCES

International Agencies

World Health Organization
Avenue Appia, CH1211
Geneva 27, Switzerland

World Health Organization Collaborating Center on AIDS
c/o Centers for Disease Control,
1600 Clifton Road, NE,
Atlanta, GA 30333.

Governmental Agencies

Centers for Disease Control and Prevention
(Center for Prevention Services Center for Environmental Health, Center for Health Promotion and Education, Center for Infectious Diseases)
1600 Clifton Road NE,
Atlanta, GA 30333

National Institute of Allergy and Infectious Diseases
National Institutes of Health
9000 Rockville Pike,
Bethesda, Md 20205

US Department of Health and Human Services
Public Health Service
5600 Fishers Lane
Washington, DC 20201

Department of Infectious and Parasitic Disease Pathology
Armed Forces Institute of Pathology.
Washington DC 20306.

Voluntary Agencies

American Lung Association
1740 Broadway,
New York, New York 10019

American Public Health Association
1015 Fifteenth Street NW,
Washington DC 20005

Association for Professionals in Infection Control and Epidemiology, Inc.
1016 16th St. NW
Washington, DC 20036

National Foundation for Infectious Diseases
P.O. Box 42022,
Washington, DC 20015

Society for Healthcare Epidemiology of America
875 Kings Highway, Suite 200,
Woodbury, NJ 08096

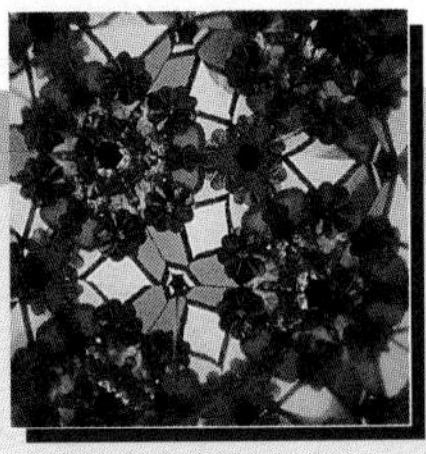

66 Emergency Nursing

CHAPTER OUTLINE

LEARNING OBJECTIVES

On completion of this chapter, the learner will be able to:

1. Describe emergency care as a holistic concept that includes the patient,the family, and significant others
2. Describe emergency resuscitation measures
3. Describe the emergency management of patients with hemorrhage due to trauma and hypovolemic shock
4. Describe the emergency management of patients with intra-abdominal injuries
5. Compare the immediate management of patients with fractures to long-term management
6. Describe the emergency management of patients with heat stroke, cold injuries, and anaphylactic reaction
7. Specify the emergency management of patients with swallowed, inhaled, and injected poisons, snakebites, and food poisoning
8. Describe the emergency management of patients with drug abuse and those with alcohol abuse
9. Differentiate between the emergency care of patients who are overactive, violent or depressed, and suicidal
10. Describe the significance of crisis intervention in the care of the rape victim

Suzanne C. Smeltzer and Brenda G. Bare: Brunner and Suddarth's Textbook of Medical-Surgical Nursing, 8th Edition. © 1996 Lippincott-Raven Publishers.

Nursing in Emergency Conditions

The term *emergency management* traditionally refers to care given to patients with urgent and critical needs. However, hospital emergency departments (ED) and emergency clinics are increasingly used for nonurgent problems. Thus, the philosophy of emergency care has broadened to include the concept that an emergency is whatever the patient or the family considers it to be. Emergency health care workers have an obligation to treat the patient with understanding and to respect any feelings of anxiety. Failure to do this may threaten the therapeutic process.

Large numbers of people seek emergency help for serious life-threatening cardiac conditions, such as myocardial infarction, acute congestive heart failure, pulmonary edema, and cardiac dysrhythmias. Priorities of management for cardiac conditions, as well as electrocardiographic (ECG) patterns evoked by dysrhythmias, are discussed in Unit 7. This chapter deals with emergency management of trauma and other conditions not found elsewhere in this book. *It is assumed that treatment is provided under the direction of a physician.*

The Nursing Process in the Emergency Department

The nursing process provides a logical framework for problem solving in the time-limited, pressurized environment of the emergency department. The emergency department nurse has had specialized education, training, and experience to gain expertise in assessing and identifying patients' health care problems in crisis situations. In addition, the emergency nurse establishes priorities, monitors acutely ill and injured patients, supports and attends to families, supervises allied health personnel, and teaches patients and families. Nursing interventions are accomplished interdependently in consultation with or with direction from the physician. The strengths of nursing and medicine are complementary in an emergency situation. Appropriate nursing and medical interventions are anticipated based on assessment data. The emergency health care staff members work as a team in performing the highly technical, high-touch skills necessary in the care of emergency patients.

Patients in the emergency department have a wide variety of actual or potential problems. The patient's condition may change constantly, therefore nursing assessment must be continuous. Nursing diagnoses must change with the patient's condition. Although a patient may have several diagnoses at a given time, the following discussions focus on the most immediate ones and assume both independent and interdependent nursing interventions.

Gerontologic Considerations

The elderly make up 12% of the U.S. population and are major consumers of emergency health care. In fact, this population accounts for 20% to 35% of visits to urban emergency facilities. Many of these visits are nonurgent, with skin, cardiovascular, and abdominal problems predominating. Elderly clients often arrive in the emergency department with one or more presenting conditions that, although not considered urgent in a younger person, can readily become life-threatening if untreated. The role of the ED in the care of the elderly is an expanding one. Acute illness may be manifested in the elderly person by nonspecific symptoms such as weakness and fatigue, episodes of falling, incontinence, and change in mental status.

Social service support may need to be initiated during the visit to the emergency department. The elderly client may perceive the emergency as a crisis signaling the end of an independent lifestyle or even resulting in death.

Infection Control Considerations

Because of the increasing numbers of people infected with human immunodeficiency virus (HIV), there is an increased risk that health care providers will be exposed to HIV-infected blood or other body fluids. It is essential that all care givers in the emergency department consider all patients as potentially infected with blood-borne pathogens and strictly adhere to universal infection control precautions for minimizing exposure. The re-emergence of tuberculosis is a major health problem of the 1990s and is complicated by multi-drug resistant tuberculosis and tuberculosis concomitant with HIV. Early identification and isolation of potentially infected patients are critical.

Discharge Planning Considerations

A large majority of patients who receive emergency care are discharged directly from the emergency department to their homes. Prior to discharge, instructions for continuing care are given to the patient and the family or significant others. All instructions should be both verbal and written so that the patient can refer to them later. Many EDs have preprinted standard instruction sheets for more common conditions. These instructions are then individualized for each patient. In many cases, these instructions are available in a variety of different languages. If instructions are not available in the language that the patient needs, an interpreter should be used. Instructions should include information about prescribed medications, treatments, diet, activity, when to contact a health care provider, and follow-up appointments.

Community Services. Prior to discharge, some patients require the services of a social worker to help them plan for meeting continuing health care needs. For patients unable to meet health care needs at home, it is critical that the services of community agencies (*e.g.*, Visiting Nurse Services) be arranged prior to discharge. This is particularly important for elderly patients who will need assistance when they return home. Identifying continuing health care needs and making arrangements for meeting these needs can prevent re-admission to the emergency department.

For patients returning to extended care facilities or for those who already rely on community agencies for continuing health care, it is important to make sure that communication is provided to these facilities or agencies about the patient's condition and any changes that have occurred in health care needs. This communication is essential in promoting continuity of care and in assuring ongoing care that meets the patient's changing health care needs.

Psychologic Management of Patients and Families in Emergency and Crisis Situations

Approaching the Patient

Sudden illness or trauma is an insult to physiologic and psychologic homeostasis that requires physiologic and psychologic healing.

Assessment of the patient's psychologic functioning includes evaluation of emotional expression, degree of anxiety, and cognitive functioning (orientation to time, place, and person). A brief physical examination is also performed, which focuses on the clinical problem that caused the patient to seek help. Nursing diagnoses may include anxiety related to uncertain potential outcomes of the illness or trauma and ineffective individual coping related to acute situational crisis. The first major goal is reduction of anxiety, which is a prerequisite to recovering the ability to cope.

Interventions

Patients experiencing sudden injury or illness often are overwhelmed by anxiety because they have not had time to mobilize their resources to adapt to the crisis. They experience real and terrifying fear of death, mutilation, immobilization, and other assaults on their personal identity and body integrity. Those caring for the patient should act confidently and competently to relieve anxiety. Reacting and responding to the patient in a warm manner promotes a sense of security. Explanations should be given on a level that the patient can grasp; an informed patient is able to cope more positively with psychologic and physical stress. Human contact and reassuring words reduce the panic of the severely injured person and aid in dispelling fear of the unknown.

The unconscious patient should be treated as if conscious. The patient should be touched, called by name, and given an explanation of every procedure that is performed. A primary concern as soon as the patient regains consciousness is to orient that person by stating his or her name, the date, and the location. This basic information should be repeated over and over in a calm, reassuring way if necessary.

Approaching the Family

The family is kept informed of where the patient is and that expert care is being given. When confronted with trauma, severe disfigurement, and sudden death, the family experiences several stages of feelings. The stages begin with anxiety and progress through denial, remorse, grief, anger, and reconciliation. In addition to anxiety, nursing diagnoses may include grieving and alterations in family processes related to acute situational crises.

Anxiety and Denial. Family members are encouraged to recognize and talk about their feelings of anxiety. Although denial is an ego-defense mechanism that protects one from recognizing painful and disturbing aspects of reality, prolonged denial is not encouraged or supported. The family must be prepared for the reality of what has happened and what may come.

Remorse and Guilt. Expressions of remorse and guilt are frequently heard and family members accuse themselves (or each other) of negligence or minor omissions. The nursing approach is to allow family members to verbalize expressions of remorse until they realize that there was probably little that they could have done to prevent the accident or illness.

Anger. Expressions of anger are common in crisis situations; they are a way of handling the anxiety. Anger is frequently directed at the patient, but it is also often expressed toward the physician, the nurse, or admitting personnel. The therapeutic approach is to allow the anger to be ventilated to help the family identify their feelings of frustration.

Grief. Grief is a complex emotional response to anticipated or actual loss. The nursing intervention is to help family members work through their grief and to support their coping mechanisms, letting them know that it is normal and acceptable for them to cry and feel pain and loss (see Guideline 66-1).

Post-traumatic Stress Disorder

Post-traumatic stress disorder is the development of characteristic symptoms after a psychologically stressful event that is considered outside the range of normal human experience (rape, combat, motor vehicle crash, natural catastrophe). Symptoms of this disorder include intrusive thoughts and dreams, phobic avoidance reaction (avoidance of activities that arouse recollection of the traumatic event), heightened vigilance, exaggerated startle reaction, generalized anxiety, and societal withdrawal. Post-traumatic stress disorder may be acute, chronic, or delayed.

Assessment includes an evaluation of the patient's pretrauma history, the trauma itself, and post-trauma functioning.

Interventions

The patient's goal is to organize and begin to integrate the experience in order to return to the pretrauma level of functioning as soon as possible. The nurse carries out a wide range of interventions including crisis intervention strategies, establishing a trusting and sharing relationship, and educating the patient and family about stress management and support services available in the community.

Priorities and Principles of Emergency Management

Priorities of Emergency Management

When care is given to a patient in an emergency situation, many crucial decisions must be made. These decisions require sound judgment based on an understanding of the condition that produced the emergency and its effect on the person.

GUIDELINE 66-1
Crisis Intervention Strategies for Helping a Family Deal With Sudden Death in the Emergency Department

- Take the family to a private place.
- Talk to the family together, so that they can mourn together.
- Assure the family that everything possible was done; inform them of the treatment rendered.
- Avoid using euphemisms such as "passed on." Show the family that you care by touching, offering coffee, and offering the services of a chaplain.
- Encourage family members to support each other and to express emotions freely (grief, loss, anger, helplessness, tears, disbelief).
- Avoid giving sedation to family members; this may mask or delay the grieving process, which is necessary to achieve emotional equilibrium and to prevent prolonged depression.
- Encourage the family to view the body if they wish; this action helps to integrate the loss. Cover mutilated areas before the family sees the body. Go with the family to see the body. Show acceptance by touching the body to give the family "permission" to touch.
- Spend a few minutes with the family, listening to them and identifying any needs that they may have for which the nursing staff can be helpful.
- Allow the family members to talk about the deceased and what he or she meant to them; this permits ventilation of feelings of loss. Encourage the family to talk about events preceding admission to the emergency department. Do not challenge initial feelings of anger or denial.
- Avoid volunteering unnecessary information (*e.g.*, patient was drinking).

Major goals of emergency medical treatment are to preserve life, to prevent deterioration before more definitive treatment can be given, and to restore the patient to useful living.

When the patient enters the emergency department, the primary goals are to determine the extent of injury or illness and to establish priorities for the initiation of treatment. These priorities are determined by any threat to the person's life. Injuries or conditions interfering with vital physiologic function (obstructed airway, massive bleeding) take precedence. Injuries of the face, neck, and chest that impair respiration usually are the highest priorities. Members of the emergency team work together to provide comprehensive, individualized patient care.

Principles of Emergency Management

The following principles are applicable to the emergency management of any patient:

1. Maintain a patent airway and provide adequate ventilation, employing resuscitation measures when necessary. Assess for chest injuries with subsequent airway obstruction.
2. Control hemorrhage and its consequences.
3. Evaluate and restore cardiac output.
4. Prevent and treat shock; maintain or restore effective circulation.
5. Carry out a rapid initial and ongoing physical examination; the clinical course of the injured or seriously ill patient is not static.
6. Determine if the patient can follow commands; evaluate the size and reactivity of the pupils and motor responses.
7. Start ECG monitoring if appropriate.
8. Splint suspected fractures, including fractures of the cervical spine in patients with head injuries.
9. Protect wounds with sterile dressings.
10. Check to see if the patient has a Medic Alert tag or similar identification designating allergies and other health problems.
11. Start a flow sheet of the patient's vital signs, blood pressure, and neurologic status, to guide decision making.

Obtaining Data From the Patient

If possible, a brief history of the injury or illness is obtained from the patient or the person accompanying the patient to the emergency department. The following questions should be asked and the answers documented:

1. What were the circumstances, precipitating events, location, and time of the injury or illness?
2. When did the symptoms appear?
3. Was the patient unconscious after the injury?
4. How did the patient get to the hospital?
5. What was the health status of the patient before the injury or illness?
6. Is there a history of illness? of admissions to the hospital?
7. Is the patient currently taking any medications, especially hormones, insulin, digitalis, anticoagulants?
8. Does the patient have any allergies?
9. Does the patient have any bleeding tendencies?
10. When was the last meal eaten? (Important if general anesthesia is to be given.)
11. Is the patient under a physician's care? What is the name of the physician?
12. What was the date of the patient's most recent tetanus immunization?

Recording of Data

Consent to examine and treat the patient is part of the emergency department record. The patient must consent to invasive procedures (*e.g.*, angiography, lumbar puncture). If the patient is unconscious and brought to the emergency department without family or friends, this fact should be documented. Monitoring of the patient's condition and all instituted treatment modalities must be documented. After treatment, a notation is made on the record about the patient's condition on discharge or transfer and instructions given to the patient and family for follow-up care.

Emergency Resuscitation Measures

Establishing an Airway

The first priority in the treatment of any emergency condition is establishing the airway. If the airway is obstructed, resulting hypoxia produces permanent brain damage or death within 3 to 5 minutes.

- *Complete airway obstruction* is recognized immediately: the patient suddenly stops breathing, becomes cyanotic, and loses consciousness for no apparent reason.
- *Partial airway obstruction* that interferes with air flow produces an apprehensive appearance, inspiratory and expiratory stridor, labored use of accessory muscles (suprasternal and intercostal retraction), flaring nostrils, increasing anxiety, restlessness, and confusion. Cyanosis of the earlobes and nail beds may be a late sign. Partial obstruction of the airway can lead to progressive hypoxia, hypercarbia, and respiratory and cardiac arrest.

Emergency Management of Airway Obstruction

1. Gently shake the victim and shout, "Are you okay?" to prevent injury from attempted resuscitation of a person who is not truly unconscious.
2. Place the patient supine on a firm, flat surface; if the patient is lying face down, turn the body as a unit so that the head, shoulders, and torso move simultaneously with no twisting.
3. Open the airway using one of two methods:
   a. Head-tilt–chin-lift maneuver.
      (1) Place one hand on the victim's forehead and apply firm backward pressure with the palm to tilt the head back.
      (2) Place the fingers of the other hand under the bony part of the lower jaw near the chin and lift. Bring the chin forward and the teeth almost to occlusion in order to support the jaw and help to tilt the head back.
   b. Jaw-thrust maneuver:
      (1) Grasp the angles of the victim's lower jaw and lift with both hands (one on each side), displacing the mandible forward while tilting the head backward. (This is a safe approach to opening the airway of a victim with suspected neck injury, because it can usually be accomplished without extending the neck.)
4. Remove any foreign body obstructing the airway.
5. Start cardiopulmonary resuscitation (CPR) immediately (see Chap. 28) to provide oxygen to the brain, heart, and other vital organs until definitive medical treatment can restore normal heart and ventilatory action. (CPR consists of establishing an effective airway and providing artificial ventilation and external cardiac compression.)

Airway management is discussed in detail in Chapter 25.

Management of Foreign Body Upper Airway Obstruction

Obstruction of the upper airway by food (café coronary) causes unconsciousness and cardiopulmonary arrest. Foreign bodies may cause either partial or complete airway obstruction. In adults, a piece of meat is the most common cause of obstruction. Factors associated with choking on food include large, poorly chewed pieces of food, alcohol consumption, and the presence of upper or lower dentures.

Assessment reveals that the victim is unable to speak, breathe, or cough. The patient may clutch the neck between the thumb and fingers (universal distress signal). The first response is to ask this person if he or she is choking.

Emergency Management. For partial obstruction (if patient is breathing and able to cough spontaneously):

1. Encourage the victim to cough forcefully; there may be some wheezing between coughs.
2. Continue to encourage the victim to persist with spontaneous coughing and breathing efforts as long as good air exchange persists.
3. If demonstrating a weak, ineffective cough, high-pitched noise while inhaling, increased respiratory difficulty, and possibly cyanosis, the patient is managed as if there were complete airway obstruction.

For complete obstruction, see Guideline 66-2.

Gerontologic Considerations. In extended care facilities, sedatives and hypnotic drugs as well as diseases affecting motor coordination (*e.g.*, Parkinson's disease) and mental functioning (*e.g.*, senility, mental retardation) are risk factors for asphyxiation by food. Nursing staff involved in the care of elderly patients must be aware of the symptoms of upper airway obstruction; skill in performing the Heimlich maneuver is essential.

Methods for Obtaining a Patent Airway

Insertion of an Oropharyngeal Airway. An oropharyngeal airway is a semicircular-shaped tube or tubelike device of plastic or rubber that is inserted over the back of the tongue into the lower posterior pharynx in a spontaneously breathing, unconscious patient; it prevents the tongue from falling back against the posterior pharynx and obstructing the airway, and allows for suctioning of secretions (see Guideline 66-3).

Insertion of an Esophageal Obturator Airway. The esophageal obturator airway (EOA) is a ventilatory device used in respiratory emergencies for resuscitation. Its primary use is in prehospital care. It consists of (1) a face mask to seal off the nose and mouth and anchor the airway, (2) a cuffed, blind-ended flexible tube with openings at the level of the pharynx to permit ventilation of the lungs, and

GUIDELINE 66–2
Management of Foreign Body Airway Obstruction

Action	Rationale/Amplification
Assess for Indications of Airway Obstruction Victim may clutch his neck between his thumb and fingers. Weak, ineffective cough; high-pitched noises on inspiration. Increased respiratory distress. Inability to speak, breathe, or cough. Collapse.	Air movement is absent in the presence of *complete airway obstruction.* Oxygen saturation in the blood decreases rapidly because the obstructed airway prevents entry of air into the lungs. Thus, oxygen deficit occurs in the brain, resulting in unconsciousness, with death following rapidly.
Heimlich Maneuver (subdiaphragmatic abdominal thrusts):	The term *Heimlich maneuver* is used for the sake of uniformity. The terms *subdiaphragmatic abdominal thrusts* and *abdominal thrusts* are used interchangeably, depending on the circumstances.
For Standing or Sitting Conscious Patient 1. Stand behind the patient; wrap your arms around his waist and proceed as follows: 2. Make a fist with one hand, placing the thumb side of the fist against the patient's abdomen, in the midline slightly above the naval and well below the xiphoid process. Grasp the fist with the other hand. 3. Press your fist into the patient's abdomen with a quick upward thrust. Each new thrust should be a separate and distinct maneuver. *With Patient Lying (Unconscious)* 1. Position patient on his back. 2. Kneel astride the patient's thigh, facing his head. 3. Place the heel of one hand against the patient's abdomen, in the midline slightly above the navel and well below the tip of the xiphoid; place the second hand directly on top of the first. 4. Press into the abdomen with a quick upward thrust.	A subdiaphragmatic abdominal thrust, by elevating the diaphragm, can force air from the lungs to create an artificial cough intended to move and expel an obstructing foreign body in the airway.
Finger Sweep 1. Open patient's mouth by grasping both the tongue and lower jaw between the thumb and fingers and lifting the mandible (tongue–jaw lift). 2. Insert the index finger of the other hand down along the inside of the cheek and deeply into the throat to the base of the tongue.	This maneuver is to be used *only in the unconscious patient.* This action draws the tongue away from the back of the throat and away from the foreign body that may be lodged there.
3. Use a hooking action to dislodge the foreign body and maneuver it into the mouth for removal.	Use care not to force the object deeper into the throat.
Chest Thrusts With Conscious Patient Standing or Sitting 1. Stand behind patient with arms under patient's axillae to encircle patient's chest. 2. Place thumb side of your fist on middle of patient's sternum, taking care to avoid xiphoid process and margins of rib cage.	This technique is to be used *only in the advanced stages of pregnancy or in the markedly obese person.*
3. Grasp your fist with the other hand and perform backward thrusts until the foreign body is expelled or patient becomes unconscious.	Each thrust should be administered with the intent of relieving the obstruction.
Chest Thrust With Patient Lying (Unconscious) 1. Place the patient on his back and kneel close to the side of his body. 2. Place the heel of your hand on the lower half of the sternum. 3. Deliver each chest thrust slowly and distinctly with the intent of relieving the obstruction.	This maneuver is used *only in the advanced stages of pregnancy or when the rescuer cannot apply the Heimlich maneuver effectively to the unconscious, markedly obese person.*

(Adapted from Cardiopulmonary Resuscitation [CPR]. Tulsa, CPR Publishers, 1993.)

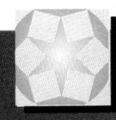

GUIDELINE 66-3
Insertion of an Oropharyngeal Airway

1. Extend the patient's head by placing one hand beneath the neck close to the occiput. Gently lift the neck; simultaneously, with other hand, tilt the head backward by applying pressure to the forehead.

2. Open the patient's mouth.

3. (A). Insert the oropharyngeal airway with the tip facing up toward the roof of the mouth until it passes the uvula. (B). Rotate the tip 180 degrees so that the tip is pointed down toward the pharynx. This displaces tongue anteriorly, and the patient then breathes through and around the airway.

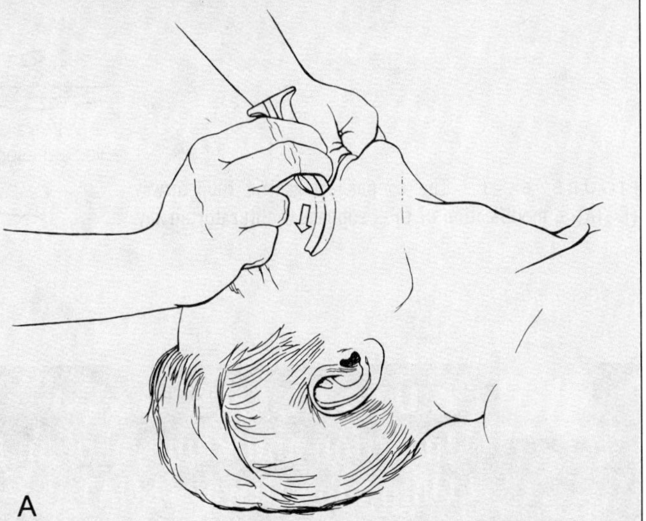

A

4. The distal end of the oropharyngeal airway is in the hypopharynx and the flange is approximately at the patient's lips. Make sure that the tongue has not been pushed into the airway.

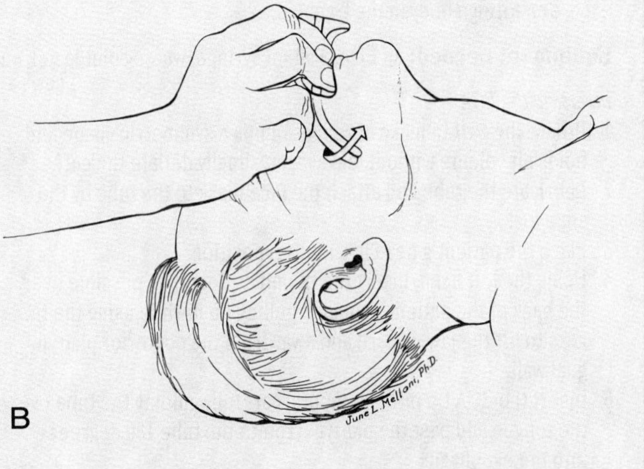

B

(3) a balloon on the distal end of the tube to block the esophagus, thus reducing the possibility of aspirating gastric contents. The purpose of the EOA is to ventilate the apneic, unconscious patient when endotracheal intubation is not possible. Use of a laryngoscope is not needed.

The tube is inserted through the mouth and advanced into the esophagus just below the bifurcation of the trachea. The proximal part of the tube has air holes at the level of the pharynx through which air or oxygen is blown into the lungs (see Guideline 66-4).

The esophageal gastric tube airway (EGTA) (Fig. 66-1) is a modification of the EOA. It has a central lumen that permits passage of a nasogastric tube so that suctioning of the stomach can be accomplished without interfering with ventilation.

Emergency Endotracheal Procedures

Endotracheal Intubation. The purpose of endotracheal intubation is to establish and maintain the airway in patients with respiratory insufficiency or hypoxia. Endotracheal intubation is indicated for the following reasons: (1) to establish an airway for patients who cannot be adequately ventilated with an oropharyngeal airway, (2) to bypass an upper airway obstruction, (3) to prevent aspiration, (4) to permit connection of the patient to a resuscitation bag or mechanical ventilator, and (5) to facilitate the removal of tracheobronchial secretions.

Because the procedure requires skill, endotracheal intubation may be performed only by those who have had intensive training in which they have practiced the technique on a mannequin. It should be performed under expert clinical supervision.

Details for emergency endotracheal intubation are outlined in Guideline 66-5 and Figure 66-2.

Cricothyroidotomy (Cricothyroid Membrane Puncture). Cricothyroidotomy is the puncture or incision of the cricothyroid membrane to establish an airway. This procedure is used in certain emergency situations in which

(text continues on page 2008)

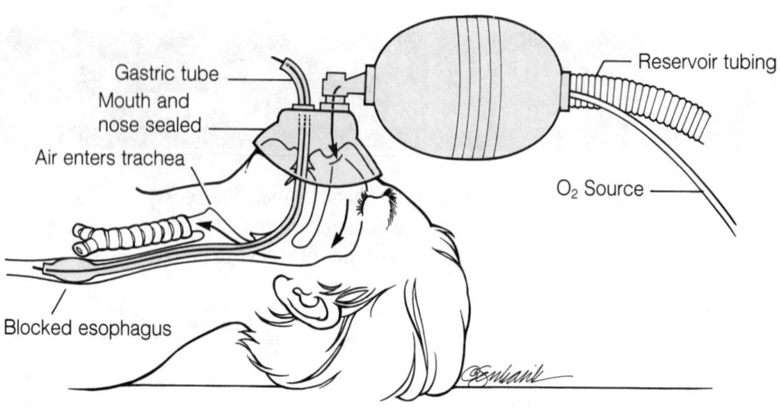

FIGURE 66-1. The esophageal gastric tube airway (EGTA), a modification of the esophageal obturator airway.

GUIDELINE 66–4
Insertion and Removal of an Esophageal Obturator Airway (EOA)

Warning: This procedure is contraindicated in conscious or semiconscious patients and in those with corrosive poisoning, esophageal disease, or a foreign body in the trachea.

Equipment needed: An EOA, a 50-ml syringe, water-soluble gel, and a manual resuscitation bag with mask.

Inserting the EOA

1. Inflate the cuff to make sure it assumes a symmetric shape and holds air volume without leakage; maximally deflate the cuff.
2. Lubricate the tube and attach the face mask to the tube by the snap lock.
3. Place the patient's head in a neutral position.
4. Using the left hand, insert the thumb as deeply as possible over the back of the patient's tongue, pulling on it while using the fingers to lift the jaw upward and away from the posterior pharyngeal wall.
5. Insert the EOA tip into the mouth, carefully guiding the tube over the tongue and past the pharynx; rotate the tube 180 degrees into the esophagus.
6. Stop advancing the tube when the mask reaches the face; press the mask firmly against the face.
7. Ventilate the patient by using manual resuscitation. If the tube is correctly positioned in the esophagus, the chest will rise.
8. If the chest does not rise or no breath sounds are heard, the airway is possibly blocking the trachea; remove the airway. Continue ventilating the patient (by bag-mask ventilation) and prepare for and proceed with second attempt at insertion.
9. Auscultate over *both* lung fields to check that *both* lungs are receiving adequate ventilation and that the EOA is in the esophagus and not in the trachea.
10. Inflate the cuff (balloon) with about 20 ml. of air. Inflating the cuff results in occlusion of the esophagus, minimizes the incidence of regurgitation, and prevents air leakage.
11. Connect the end of the EOA to a bag-mask or mechanical ventilator, and continue ventilating the patient.

Removing the EOA

1. The EOA must be removed when patient regains consciousness, begins to breath spontaneously, and has a gag reflex.
2. Explain to the patient where he is, why he cannot speak, and what is to be done.
3. Turn the patient's head to the side to prevent aspiration if vomiting occurs.
4. Maintain head and neck alignment until cervical spine injury is ruled out.
5. Remove the mask from the tube to prevent aspiration.
6. Attach a large syringe to the cuff inflation port and withdraw all the air. Inspect and palpate the test bulb to ensure that the esophageal balloon is deflated.
7. The EOA tube *must* be deflated before it is removed. If the tube is taken out prematurely, regurgitation and aspiration are almost inevitable.
8. Remove the tube following the curvature of the patient's airway. Have suction available. Turn the patient's head to the side; deflate the cuff and remove the tube.
9. Expect vomiting to occur. Carefully suction secretions and vomitus from the mouth and oropharynx.

GUIDELINE 66–5
Assisting With Emergency Endotracheal Intubation

Clinical Indications for Intubation

1. Respiratory arrest
2. Respiratory insufficiency—marked respiratory effort, substernal retraction, nostril flaring, increasing or decreasing pulse rate, increasing or decreasing respiratory rate, changing color (*cyanosis is a late sign*)
3. Airway obstruction (asphyxia)

Equipment

1. Laryngoscope with curved and straight blades and working light source (check batteries and bulb regularly)
2. Endotracheal tubes with low-pressure cuffs (to seal airway) and adapter (to connect tube to ventilator or bag)
3. Stylet to guide endotracheal tube
4. Oral airway (assorted sizes) or bite block (to keep patient from biting into and occluding endotracheal tube)
5. Adhesive tape or tube fixation system
6. Sterile anesthetic lubricant jelly (water-soluble)
7. Syringe
8. Suction source
9. Resuscitation bag and mask connected to oxygen source
10. Anesthetic spray
11. Sterile towel
12. Gloves
13. Goggles or other eye protection

Action	*Rationale/Amplification*
1. Remove the patient's dental bridgework and plates.	1. May interfere with insertion; will not be able to remove dentures easily once patient is intubated.
2. Remove headboard of bed (optional).	2. Provides easy access to the head.
3. Prepare equipment.	3.
a. Ensure function of resuscitation bag and mask, and suction.	a. Patient may require ventilatory assistance prior to and/or during procedure. Suction apparatus must be readily available, because gagging and emesis may occur during procedure.
b. Assemble the laryngoscope; make sure the lightbulb is tightly attached and functional.	
c. Select an endotracheal tube of the appropriate size (6–9 mm for average adult).	
d. Place the endotracheal tube on a sterile towel.	d. Although the tube will pass through the contaminated mouth or nose, the airway below the vocal cords is sterile, and efforts must be made to prevent iatrogenic contamination of the distal end of the tube and cuff. The proximal end of the tube may be handled, because it will reside in the upper airway.
e. Inflate the cuff to make sure it assumes a symmetric shape and holds air without leakage. Then deflate maximally.	e. Malfunction of the cuff must be ascertained *before* tube placement occurs.
f. Lubricate the distal end of tube liberally with the sterile anesthetic water-soluble jelly.	f. Aids in insertion.
g. Insert the stylet into the tube (if oral intubation is planned; nasal intubation does not employ use of the stylet).	g. Stiffens the soft tube, allowing it to be more easily directed into the trachea.
4. Assist the physician as he performs the following:	4.
a. If cervical spine is not injured, for oral intubation place head in a "sniffing" position: extended at the junction of the neck and thorax and flexed at the junction of the spine and skull.	a. Upper airway is open maximally in this position and mouth of the unconscious patient will often open.
b. Spray the back of the patient's throat with an anesthetic spray if time is available.	b. This will decrease gagging.
c. Ventilate and oxygenate the patient with the resuscitation bag and mask before intubation.	c. This decreases the likelihood of cardiac dysrhythmias or respiratory distress secondary to hypoxemia.
d. Hold the handle of the laryngoscope in the left hand and hold the patient's mouth open with the right hand by placing crossed fingers on the teeth.	d. Leverage is improved by crossing the thumb and index fingers when opening the patient's mouth (scissor-twist technique).

(continued)

GUIDELINE 66-5 *(continued)*
Assisting With Emergency Endotracheal Intubation

Action	*Rationale/Amplification*
e. Insert the curved blade of the laryngoscope along the right side of the tongue, push the tongue to the left, and use right thumb and index finger to pull patient's lower lip away from lower teeth.	e. Rolling the lip away from teeth prevents injury from the lips being caught between teeth and blade.
f. Lift laryngoscope forward (toward ceiling) to expose the epiglottis.	f. Do not use teeth as a fulcrum; this could lead to dental damage.
g. Lift laryngoscope upward and forward at a 45-degree angle to expose glottis and visualize vocal cords.	g. This stretches the hypoepiglottis ligament, folding the epiglottis upward and exposing the glottis.
h. As the epiglottis is lifted forward (toward ceiling), the vertical opening of the larynx between the vocal cords will come into view.	h. Do not use wrist; use shoulder and arm to lift epiglottis.
i. Once vocal cords are visualized, insert tube into the right corner of the mouth and pass the tube—guided by blade, but keeping vocal cords in constant view.	i. Make sure you do not insert tube into esophagus; the esophageal mucosa is pink and the opening is horizontal rather than vertical.
j. Gently push the tube through the triangular space formed by the vocal cords and back wall of trachea.	j. If the vocal cords are in spasm (closed), wait a few seconds before passing tube.
k. Stop insertion just after the tube cuff has disappeared from view beyond the cords.	k. Advancing tube further may lead to its entry into a main-stem bronchus (usually the right bronchus), causing collapse of the unventilated lung.
l. Withdraw laryngoscope while holding endotracheal tube in place. Disassemble mask from resuscitation bag and ventilate the patient.	l. Provides for resumption of oxygenation of the patient.
m. Inflate cuff with the minimal amount of air required to occlude the trachea.	m. The amount of air used for cuff inflation depends on the size of the cuff and the diameter of the patient's trachea. Occlusion occurs when no air is felt or heard passing through the patient's nose or mouth.
n. Insert oral airway or bite block if necessary.	n. This keeps patient from biting down on the tube and obstructing the airway.
o. Ascertain expansion of both sides of the chest by observation and auscultation of breath sounds.	o. Observation and auscultation help in determining that tube remains in position and has not slipped into the right main-stem bronchus.
p. Mark proximal end of tube with marking pen or tape at the point where the tube reaches the corner of the patient's mouth.	p. This allows for detection of any later change in tube position.
q. Secure tube to the patient's face with adhesive tape or apply a commercially available endotracheal tube stabilization device.	q. The tube must be fixed securely to ensure that it will not be dislodged. Dislodgement of a tube with an inflated cuff may result in damage to the vocal cords.
r. Obtain chest x-ray.	r. Verifies correct position of tube.
s. Measure cuff pressure with manometer, adjust pressure. Make adjustment in tube placement on the basis of chest x-ray results.	s. The tube may be advanced or withdrawn several centimeters for proper placement on the basis of the chest x-ray findings.
t. Record tube type and size, cuff pressure, and patient tolerance of the procedure. Auscultate breath sounds every 1 to 2 hours or if signs and symptoms of respiratory distress occur. Assess arterial blood gases after intubation if requested by physician.	t. Arterial blood gases may be prescribed to ensure adequacy of ventilation and respiration. Tube displacement outward may result in extubation (cuff above vocal cords). Tube displacement forward may result in tube touching carina (causing paroxysmal coughing) or intubation of a main-stem bronchus (resulting in collapse of the unventilated lung).

endotracheal intubation and tracheostomy are either not possible or contraindicated, as in airway obstruction from extensive maxillofacial trauma, cervical spine injuries, laryngospasm, laryngeal edema (after an allergic reaction), hemorrhage into neck tissue, or obstruction of the larynx (see Guideline 66-6).

Special Resuscitation Situation: Near-Drowning

Near-drowning is survival for at least some period of time under water without ventilation. The most common consequence is hypoxemia.

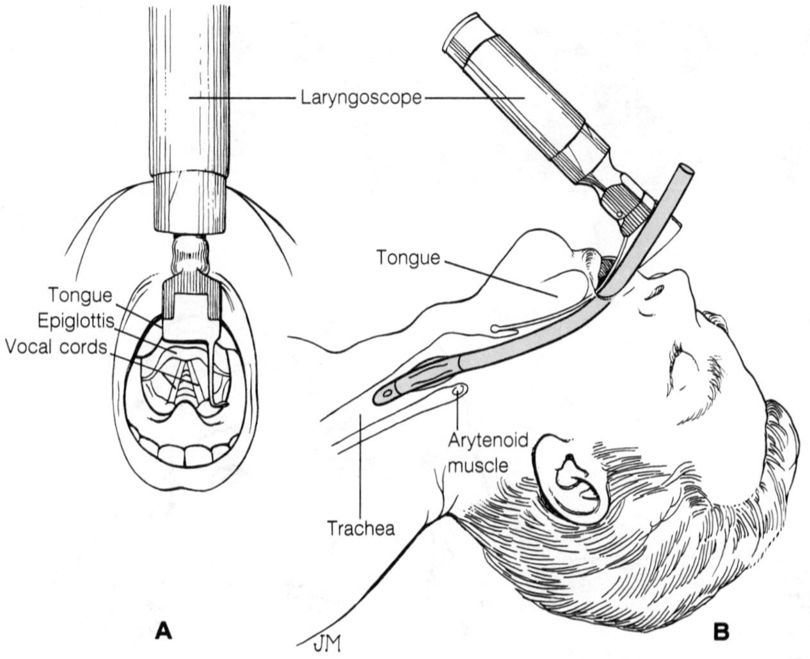

FIGURE 66-2. Endotracheal intubation. (**A**) The primary glottic landmarks for tracheal intubation as visualized with proper placement of the laryngoscope. (**B**) Positioning the endotracheal tube.

Drowning is the fourth leading cause of accidental death; an estimated 9000 fatalities from drowning and 80,000 near-drownings occur yearly in the United States. Children under 4 years of age account for 40% of drownings. Factors associated with drowning and near-drowning include alcohol ingestion, inability to swim, diving injuries, hypothermia, and exhaustion. Efforts to save the victim should not be abandoned prematurely; successful resuscitation with full neurologic recovery has occurred in near-drowning victims with prolonged submersion in cold water. This is possible owing to a decrease in metabolic demands or the diving reflex.

After resuscitation, hypoxia and acidosis are the primary problems of a victim who has nearly drowned and they require immediate intervention in the emergency department. Resultant pathophysiologic changes and pulmonary injury depend on the type of fluid (fresh water or salt water) and the volume of aspiration. When water has been aspirated, pulmonary function alterations may be anticipated. After a person has survived immersion, acute adult respiratory distress syndrome with hypoxia, hypercarbia, and respiratory or metabolic acidosis can occur.

Management in the Emergency Department. Therapy is aimed at maintaining cerebral perfusion and adequate oxygenation to prevent further damage to vital organs. Immediate cardiopulmonary resuscitation is the factor with the greatest influence on survival. The treatment goal is prevention of hypoxia.

1. Ensure adequacy of airway, respiration, and peripheral perfusion.
   a. Use a rectal probe to determine the degree of hypothermia if the patient has been submerged in cold water.
   b. Start rewarming procedures during resuscitation as prescribed (extracorporeal warming, warmed peritoneal dialysis, inhalation of warm aerosolized oxygen, surface warming); the choice is determined by the severity and duration of hypothermia and available resources.
2. Draw arterial blood to evaluate oxygen and carbon dioxide tensions and *p*H and bicarbonate levels; these parameters determine the type of ventilatory support required and the subsequent dosage of sodium bicarbonate to be given.
   a. Hypotension and impaired tissue perfusion are managed by intravascular volume expansion and inotropic agents.
3. Improve ventilation and oxygenation. Assist with endotracheal intubation with positive pressure ventilation (with positive end expiratory pressure [PEEP]) to improve oxygenation, prevent aspiration, and correct intrapulmonary shunting and ventilation–perfusion abnormalities (caused by aspiration of water). Continue with supplemental oxygen using a mask (if patient is breathing spontaneously) or an endotracheal tube (if patient is not breathing spontaneously).
   a. Respiratory acidosis is managed by improving ventilation.
4. Initiate ECG monitoring, because dysrhythmias frequently occur.
5. Assist with nasogastric intubation to empty the stomach and to prevent the patient from regurgitating gastric contents.
6. Continue to monitor the patient closely: vital signs, serial arterial blood gas values, *p*H, ECG, intracranial pressure, serum electrolytes, and serial chest x-rays.
7. Insert an indwelling catheter to determine urinary output; metabolic acidosis may compromise renal function.
8. Admit the patient to an intensive care unit. The appearance of the patient may be deceptive and the following complications of near-drowning that can lead to death include:
   a. Hypoxic or ischemic cerebral injury

GUIDELINE 66-6
Emergency Medical Management: Performing a Cricothyroidotomy

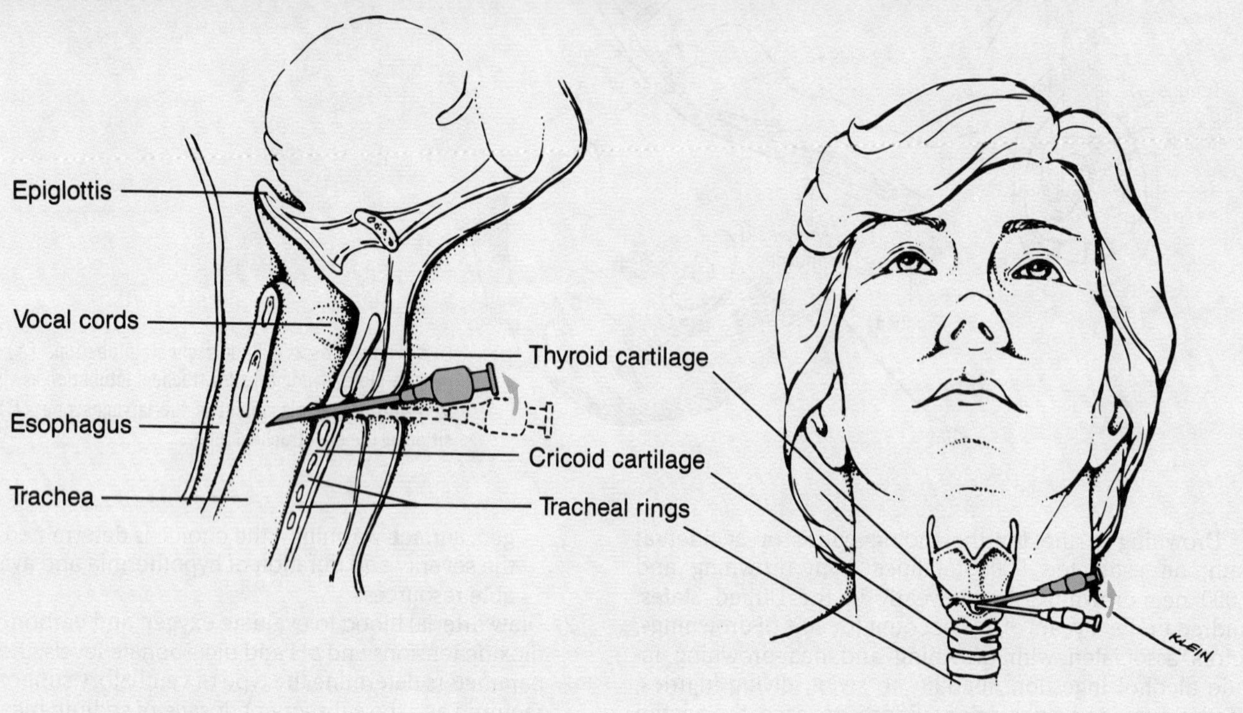

1. With the patient in a supine position, extend the neck so that the cricothyroid membrane can be palpated readily. Place a towel roll beneath the shoulders.
2. Identify the prominent thyroid cartilage (Adam's apple) and allow your finger to descend in the midline to the depression between the lower border of the thyroid cartilage and the upper border of the cricoid cartilage. This depression represents the cricothyroid membrane.
3. Insert a needle or any sharp instrument at a 10- to 20-degree angle, caudal direction in the midline just above the upper part of the cricoid cartilage.
   a. Listen for air passing back and forth through the needle synchronously with the patient's respiration.
   b. Direct the needle downward and posteriorly.
   c. Tape the needle with adhesive for stability.
4. After the patient is stabilized, a more permanent means of ventilatory support is implemented; prepare for endotracheal intubation or tracheostomy.
5. Monitor for potential complications: vocal cord injury, subcutaneous emphysema, bleeding, aspiration.

b. Acute respiratory distress syndrome and pulmonary damage secondary to aspiration
c. Cardiac arrest

Control of Hemorrhage

A primary cause of shock is the reduction in circulating blood volume. Only a few conditions, such as obstructed airway or a sucking wound of the chest, take precedence over the immediate control of hemorrhage. Stopping the bleeding is essential to the care and survival of patients in an emergency or disaster situation. Minor bleeding, which is usually venous, generally stops spontaneously unless the patient has a bleeding disorder.

The patient is assessed for cool, moist skin (resulting from poor peripheral perfusion), falling blood pressure, increasing heart rate, and decreasing urine volume. The nursing diagnoses may include fluid volume deficit, decreased cardiac output, and altered tissue perfusion. Goals of emergency management are to control the bleeding, maintain an adequately circulating blood volume for tissue oxygenation, and prevent shock. Nursing interventions are carried out collaboratively with other members of the health care team.

Emergency Management

1. Cut the patient's clothing away to identify the area of hemorrhage and perform a rapid physical assessment.

2. Apply direct, firm pressure over the bleeding area or the involved artery (Fig. 66-3). Most bleeding can be stopped by applying direct pressure (except when a major artery has been severed). Unchecked arterial bleeding produces death.
3. Apply a firm pressure dressing. Elevate the injured part to stop venous and capillary bleeding. Immobilize an injured extremity to control blood loss.
4. Insert a large-bore needle or IV cannula to provide a means for fluid and blood replacement.
   a. Withdraw blood samples for analysis, typing, and cross-matching.
   b. Administer replacement fluids as prescribed, including isotonic electrolyte solutions, plasma or plasma protein fractions, or blood component therapy (depending on clinical estimates of the type and volume of fluid lost).
      (1) Fresh blood is infused when there is massive blood loss.
      (2) Additional platelets and clotting factors are given when large amounts of blood are needed because replacement blood is deficient in clotting factors.
      (3) Blood may be warmed using a commercial warmer or basin of warm water (massive blood replacement has a cooling effect that can cause cardiac arrest).
      (4) Rate of infusion depends on the severity of blood loss and clinical evidence of hypovolemia.
5. Take the following steps for internal bleeding:
   a. Suspect internal bleeding in patients with hypovolemic shock but no external signs of bleeding: tachycardia; falling blood pressure; thirst; apprehension; cool, moist skin.
   b. Administer whole blood or plasma expanders as prescribed at the rate of blood loss.
   c. Apply an antishock garment (pneumatic counterpressure device), if available, to control internal bleeding and to facilitate the blood flow to vital areas. (The primary use is for hypovolemic shock secondary to bleeding in the lower part of the body.) Deflate the device in the emergency department after sufficient volume expansion in a controlled environment.
   d. Prepare the patient for surgical intervention.
   e. Monitor the patient's hemodynamic responses.
   f. Obtain arterial blood for blood gas determination and establish hemodynamic pressure monitoring as an index of the amount of fluid the patient can tolerate.

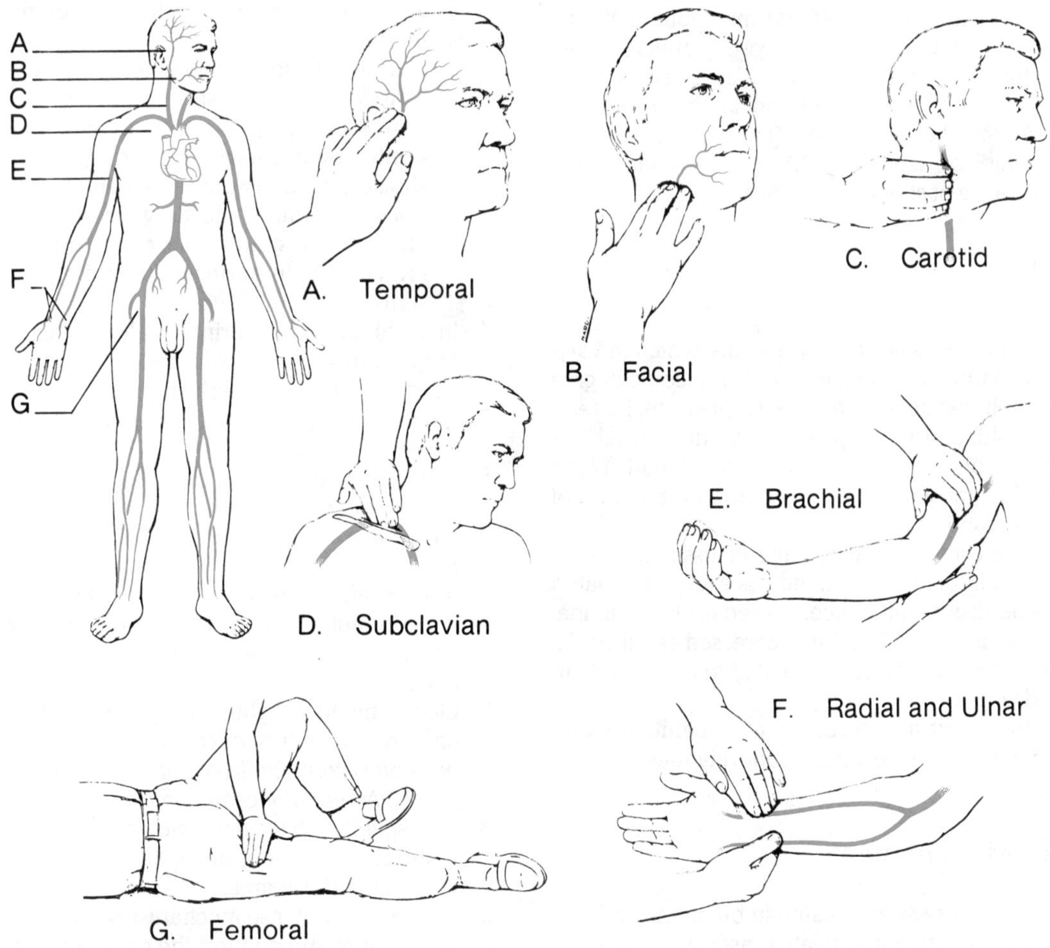

FIGURE 66-3. Pressure points for control of hemorrhage.

g. Maintain patient in supine position until hemodynamic or circulatory parameters improve.

6. Apply a tourniquet on an extremity only as a *last resort* when the hemorrhage cannot be controlled by any other method. Anticipate loss of an extremity if a tourniquet is applied.
   a. Apply the tourniquet just proximal to the wound; tie it tightly enough to control arterial blood flow.
   b. Tag the patient with a skin-marking pencil or on adhesive tape on the forehead with a T, stating the location of the tourniquet and the time applied.
   c. Loosen the tourniquet as directed to prevent irreparable vascular or neurologic damage if the patient is in an emergency facility. If there is no arterial bleeding, remove the tourniquet and again try a pressure dressing.
   d. In the event of a traumatic amputation, leave the tourniquet applied until the patient is in the operating room.
7. Observe for cardiac arrest; patients who hemorrhage are candidates for cardiac arrest caused by hypovolemia with secondary anoxia.

Control of Hypovolemic Shock

Shock is a condition in which there is loss of effective circulating blood volume. Inadequate organ and tissue perfusion follows, resulting ultimately in cellular metabolic derangements. In any emergency situation it is wise to anticipate onset of shock. Injured persons should be assessed immediately to determine the presence of shock. The underlying cause of shock must be determined (hypovolemic, cardiogenic, neurogenic, or septic shock). Hypovolemia is the most common cause of shock (see Chapter 15).

Assessment

Assess for the following signs and symptoms, which in varying combinations indicate that the patient is in some degree of hypovolemic shock: decreasing arterial pressure; increasing pulse rate; cold, moist skin; pallor; thirst; diaphoresis; altered sensorium; oliguria; metabolic acidosis; and hyperpnea. Of these, the most dependable criterion is the level of arterial blood pressure.

Nursing diagnoses may include altered tissue perfusion related to failing circulation; impaired gas exchange related to ventilation–perfusion imbalance; altered urinary elimination (oliguria or anuria) related to decreased renal perfusion; and decreased cardiac output related to decreased circulating blood volume.

Goals of treatment are to restore and maintain tissue perfusion and to correct physiologic abnormalities.

Emergency Management

1. Ensure a patent airway and maintain breathing and circulation. Give additional ventilatory assistance as required.
2. Restore the circulating blood volume with rapid fluid and blood replacement as prescribed to optimize cardiac preload, correct hypotension, and maintain tissue perfusion.
   a. A central venous pressure catheter is inserted in or near the right atrium to serve as a guide for fluid replacement. Continuous central venous pressure (CVP) readings give the direction and degree of change from baseline readings; the catheter is also a vehicle for emergency fluid volume replacement.
   b. Large-gauge IV needles or catheters are inserted into peripheral veins. Two or more catheters may be necessary for rapid fluid replacement and reversal of hemodynamic instability; emphasis is on volume replacement.
      (1) Establish IV lines in both upper and lower extremities if it is suspected that a major vessel in the chest or abdomen has been disrupted.
      (2) Withdraw blood for the following specimens: arterial blood gases, chemistry studies, typing and cross matching, and hematocrit.
3. Start IV infusion at a rapid rate until CVP rises to a satisfactory level above the baseline measurement or until there is improvement in the patient's clinical condition.
   a. Infusion of lactated Ringer's solution is useful initially because it approximates plasma electrolyte composition and osmolality, allows time for blood typing and cross matching, restores circulation, and serves as an adjunct to blood component therapy.
   b. Start transfusion of blood component therapy as prescribed, especially when blood loss has been severe or when the patient continues to hemorrhage.
   c. Control hemorrhage; hemorrhage compounds the shock state. Carry out serial hematocrit examinations if continued bleeding is suspected.
   d. Maintain the systolic blood pressure at a satisfactory level by administering fluids and blood as prescribed.
4. Insert an indwelling urinary catheter; record urinary output every 15 to 30 minutes. Urinary volume reveals adequacy of kidney perfusion.
5. Carry out a rapid physical assessment to determine the cause of shock.
6. Maintain ongoing nursing surveillance of the *total patient*—blood pressure, heart and respiratory rates, skin temperature, color, CVP, arterial blood gases, ECG, hematocrit, hemoglobin, coagulation profile, electrolytes, and urinary output—to assess patient response to treatment. Maintain a flow sheet of these parameters; trend analysis reveals improvement or deterioration of patient.
7. Elevate the feet slightly to improve cerebral circulation and promote return of venous blood to the heart. (*This position is contraindicated in patients with head injuries.*) Avoid unnecessary movement.
8. Give specific pharmacologic agents as prescribed (*e.g.*, inotropic drugs such as dopamine) to improve cardiovascular performance.
9. Support the defense mechanisms of the body.
   a. Reassure and comfort the patient; sedation may be necessary to relieve apprehension.

b. Relieve pain by *cautious* use of analgesics or narcotics.
c. Maintain body temperature.
   (1) Too much heat produces vasodilation, which counteracts the body's compensatory mechanisms of vasoconstriction and increases fluid loss by perspiration.
   (2) A patient who is in septic shock should be kept cool; high fever increases the cellular metabolic effects of shock.

Wounds

Wounds (injury to tissues) vary from minor lacerations to severe crushing injuries. Life-threatening problems, such as airway obstruction, hemorrhage, and shock, must be dealt with before the wound is treated.

Assessment

1. Determine *when* as well as *how* the wound occurred; a delay in treatment of more than 3 hours increases infection risk.
2. Inspect the wound, using aseptic technique, to determine the extent of damage to underlying structures.
3. Assess for sensory, motor, or vascular complications.

Nursing diagnoses may include impaired skin integrity (puncture wound, laceration) related to injury and risk for infection.

The patient's goal is restoration of the physical integrity and function of the injured tissue without the development of infection and with minimal scarring.

Emergency Management

1. Clip hairs or shave around the wound (with the exception of eyebrows) only if directed (this is done when it is anticipated that hairs will interfere with wound closure).
2. Cleanse around the wound with prescribed agent. Do not allow the cleansing solution to get into the wound; it may injure exposed tissues.
3. The area is infiltrated with a local intradermal anesthetic through the wound margins or by regional block. (Patients with soft tissue injuries usually have pain localized at the site of injury.)
4. Assist the physician in cleansing and débrideing the wound.
   a. Irrigate gently and copiously with isotonic sterile saline to remove surface dirt.
   b. Remove devitalized tissue and foreign matter. These impair the wound's ability to resist infection.
   c. Clamp and tie small bleeding vessels, or achieve hemostasis with cautery.
5. Suture the wound (usually done by the physician) if primary closure is indicated. Suturing depends on the nature of the wound, the time since the injury was sustained, the degree of contamination, and the vascularity of tissues.
   a. Subcutaneous fat is brought together loosely with a few sutures to close off the dead space.
   b. The subcuticular layer is then closed.
   c. The epidermis is closed; sutures are placed close to the wound edge with the skin edges leveled carefully to promote optimal healing.
   d. Sterile strips of reinforced microporous tape may be used to close clean, superficial wounds.
6. Apply nonadherent dressing to protect the wound. (The dressing may serve as a splint and as a reminder to the patient that an injury has been sustained.)
7. Delaying primary closure:
   a. A thin layer of gauze (to ensure drainage and prevent pooling of exudate) covered by an occlusive dressing may be used. Other options include split-thickness cadaver or porcine xenografts because they simulate the function of epithelium.
   b. Splint the wound in a position of rest to prevent motion.
   c. The wound is closed (using local anesthesia) when there are no signs of suppuration.
8. Administer antimicrobial treatment as prescribed. (Use of antibiotics depends on factors such as how the injury occurred, the age of the wound, and the presence of soil-infection potential.)
9. Immobilize the site if the wound is contaminated; elevate the site to limit accumulation of fluid in wound interstitial spaces.
10. Give tetanus prophylaxis as prescribed, based on the condition of the wound and the patient's immunization status.
11. Inform the patient to contact the physician or clinic if there is sudden or persistent pain, fever or chills, bleeding, rapid swelling, foul odor, drainage, or redness surrounding the wound.

Trauma

Trauma is the third leading cause of death in the United States following atherosclerosis and cancer. Trauma is the leading cause of death in children and in adults under the age of 44. Alcohol and drug abuse have been implicated as factors in blunt and penetrating trauma as well as intentional and unintentional trauma.

Intra-abdominal Injuries

Penetrating Abdominal Injuries

Penetrating abdominal injuries (gunshot wounds, stab wounds) are serious and usually require surgery. In penetrating injuries, the most important factor is the velocity with which the missile entered the body. High-velocity missiles (bullets) create extensive tissue damage. Almost all gunshot wounds require surgical exploration. Stab wounds may be more conservatively managed. Penetrating trauma of the abdomen results in a high incidence of injury to hollow organs, particularly the small bowel. The liver is the most frequently injured solid organ.

Assessment for Abdominal Injuries

- Obtain a history of the mechanism of the injury: penetrating force (gunshot, stab); blunt force (blow).
- Inspect the abdomen for obvious signs of injury: penetrating injuries, bruises, and exit sites.
- Auscultate for the presence or absence of bowel sounds and record baseline data so changes can be noted. Absence of bowel sounds is an early sign of intraperitoneal involvement; if signs of peritoneal irritation are present, an exploratory laparotomy (surgical incision into the abdominal cavity) is usually performed.
- Assess the patient for progression of abdominal distention, involuntary guarding, tenderness, pain, muscular rigidity or rebound tenderness, diminished bowel sounds, hypotension, and shock.
- Assess for chest injuries that frequently accompany intra-abdominal injuries; observe for associated injuries.
- Record all physical signs during patient examination.

Nursing Diagnoses. Nursing diagnoses may include impaired skin integrity related to penetrating injuries and high risk for infection related to disruption of skin integrity. Goals of the patient may include control of bleeding, maintenance of blood volume, and prevention of wound infection.

Emergency Management

1. Initiate resuscitation procedures (restoration of airway, breathing, circulation) as indicated.
2. Keep the patient on the stretcher or backboard; movement may cause fragmentation of a clot in a large vessel and produce massive hemorrhage.
   a. Ensure patency of the airway and stability of the respiratory, circulatory, and nervous systems.
   b. If the patient is comatose, splint the neck until after cervical neck x-rays are taken.
   c. Cut clothing away from the wound.
   d. Count the number of wounds.
   e. Locate entrance and exit wounds.
3. Assess for signs and symptoms of hemorrhage. *Hemorrhage frequently accompanies abdominal injury,* especially if the liver and spleen have been traumatized.
4. Control bleeding and maintain blood volume until surgery is performed.
   a. Apply compression to external bleeding wounds and occlusion of chest wounds.
   b. Insert indwelling large-bore IV catheter for rapid fluid replacement to restore circulatory dynamics.
   c. Watch for occurrence of shock after an initial response to transfusion therapy; this is often the first sign of internal hemorrhage.
   d. The physician may perform a paracentesis to identify the site of bleeding.
5. Aspirate the stomach contents with a nasogastric tube. This procedure helps detect gastric wounds, lessens contamination of the peritoneal cavity, and prevents lung complications due to aspiration.
6. Cover protruding abdominal viscera with sterile, moist saline dressings to prevent drying of the viscera.
   a. Flex the patient's knees; this position prevents further protrusion.
   b. Withhold oral fluids to prevent increased peristalsis and vomiting.
7. Insert an indwelling urethral catheter to ascertain the presence of hematuria and to monitor urinary output.
8. Maintain an ongoing flow sheet of the patient's vital signs, urinary output, central venous pressure readings (when indicated), hematocrit values, and neurologic status.
9. Prepare for paracentesis or peritoneal lavage when there is uncertainty about intraperitoneal bleeding.
10. Prepare for sinography to determine whether there is peritoneal penetration in the case of stab wounds.
    a. A purse string suture is placed around the wound.
    b. A small catheter is introduced through the wound.
    c. A contrast agent is introduced through the catheter; x-rays reveal whether peritoneal penetration has taken place.
11. Administer tetanus prophylaxis as prescribed.
12. Administer a broad-spectrum antibiotic as prescribed to prevent infection. Trauma predisposes to infection by disruption of mechanical barriers, exogenous bacteria from the environment at the time of injury, and diagnostic and therapeutic maneuvers (nosocomial infection).
13. Prepare the patient for surgery if there is continuing evidence of shock, blood loss, free air under the diaphragm, evisceration, or hematuria.

Blunt Abdominal Trauma

Blunt trauma to the abdomen may result from motor vehicle crashes, falls, and blows. Patients with blunt trauma are a challenge because of potential hidden injuries that may be difficult to detect. The incidence of delayed trauma-related complications is greater than that associated with penetrating injuries. This is especially true of blunt injuries involving the liver, kidneys, spleen, or blood vessels, which can lead to substantial blood loss into the peritoneal cavity. Blunt abdominal trauma frequently is associated with extra-abdominal injuries to the chest, head, or extremities. Evaluation and treatment of these injuries may take precedence over the abdominal injury.

Assessment

1. Obtain a detailed history when possible (this is frequently unobtainable, inaccurate, or misleading). Obtain all possible data about the following:
   a. Method of injury.
   b. Time of symptom onset.
   c. Passenger location if in a motor vehicle crash (driver frequently sustains rupture of the spleen or liver.) Seat belts on or off, type of restraint used.
   d. Time of last food or fluid intake.
   e. Bleeding tendencies.
   f. Concurrent diseases and medications.
   g. Immunization history, with attention to tetanus.
   h. Allergies.
2. Perform a rapid examination of the entire patient to detect life-threatening problems.

Clinical Manifestations

Clinical manifestations of blunt abdominal trauma include pain (especially on movement), rebound and maximal point tenderness (may indicate peritoneal irritation from blood or gastrointestinal fluid), muscle guarding, and diminishing or absent bowel sounds.

Emergency Management

1. Begin resuscitation procedures (as indicated) and evaluation of the patient simultaneously.
2. Carry out ongoing physical assessment: inspection, palpation, auscultation, and percussion of the abdomen. Changes noted in subsequent examinations may reveal an undetected abdominal injury.
   a. Avoid moving the patient until the initial assessment has been completed. Movement may fragment a clot in a large vessel and produce massive hemorrhage.
   b. Expect a wide variety of signs and symptoms resulting from blood loss, bruising and tearing of solid organs, and leaking of secretions from hollow abdominal viscera.
   c. Observe for chest injuries, especially fractures of the lower ribs.
   d. Inspect the front of the body, flanks, and back for bluish discoloration, asymmetry, abrasion, and contusion.
   e. Evaluate for signs and symptoms of hemorrhage, which frequently accompany abdominal injury, especially if the liver and spleen have been traumatized. Massive intraperitoneal bleeding is associated with shock.
   f. Note tenderness, rebound tenderness, guarding, rigidity, and spasm. Rebound tenderness is assessed as follows:
      (1) Press the area of maximal tenderness (have the patient point to the area).
      (2) Lift the fingers quickly; pain at the suspected point indicates peritoneal irritation.
   g. Observe for increased abdominal distention. Measure abdominal girth at the umbilical level on admission; this serves as a baseline from which changes can be determined.
   h. Ask about referred pain. This is helpful in detecting intraperitoneal injury. Pain in the left shoulder may be encountered in a patient bleeding from a ruptured spleen; pain in the right shoulder can result from laceration of the liver.
   i. Auscultate for bowel sounds. (Silent abdomen accompanies peritoneal irritation.)
   j. Note loss of dullness over the solid organs (liver or spleen), which indicates presence of free air. (Dullness over regions normally containing gas indicates presence of blood.)
3. Assist with rectal or vaginal examination for diagnosis of injury to the pelvis, bladder, and intestinal wall.
4. Avoid giving narcotics during the observation period because they may mask the clinical picture.
5. Monitor vital signs frequently and carefully. This may be the only clue to intra-abdominal bleeding.
6. Prepare the patient for diagnostic procedures.
   a. Laboratory studies include:
      (1) Urinalysis: as a guide to possible urinary tract injury (hematuria).
      (2) Serial hematocrit levels: trend reflects presence or absence of bleeding.
      (3) Complete blood count (CBC): white blood cell count is elevated with trauma in general.
      (4) Serum amylase determinations: rising level may indicate pancreatic injury or perforations of gastrointestinal tract.
   b X-ray studies:
      (1) Computed tomography (CT) scans: permit detailed evaluation of abdominal contents and retroperitoneal examination.
      (2) Abdominal and chest x-rays: may reveal free air beneath diaphragm, indicating a ruptured hollow viscus (a large interior organ).
7. Prepare for diagnostic peritoneal lavage to test for intraperitoneal bleeding; organ laceration or bleeding may be diagnosed by gross and microscopic examination of fluid returned after peritoneal lavage.
8. Assist with insertion of a nasogastric tube to prevent vomiting and subsequent aspiration. It is also helpful in removing fluid and air from the gastrointestinal tract.
9. Complications
   a. Immediate: hemorrhage, shock, and associated injuries
   b. Delayed: infection

Crush Injuries

Crush injuries occur when a person is crushed beneath debris, run over by a moving vehicle, or compressed by machinery.

Assessment

Observe for the following:

- Oligemic shock due to extravasation of blood and plasma into injured tissues after compression has been released.
- Paralysis of a body part.
- Erythema and blistering of skin.
- Damaged body part (usually an extremity) becomes swollen, tense, and hard.
- Renal dysfunction (prolonged hypotension causes kidney damage and acute renal insufficiency; myoglobinuria secondary to muscle damage can cause acute renal failure).

Emergency Management

1. Control shock.
2. Observe for acute renal insufficiency. Injury to the back may cause severe kidney damage.
3. Splint major soft tissue injuries early to control bleeding and pain.

4. Elevate the extremity. To relieve pressure of extravasated fluid it may be necessary for the physician to incise the fascia.
5. Administer medication for pain and anxiety as prescribed.

Multiple Injuries

The patient with multiple injuries requires a team approach, with one person responsible for coordinating the treatment. Multiple trauma potentially affects every body system. The nursing staff assumes responsibility for IV access, medications, recording data, and laboratory specimen collection.

Assessment. Evidence of gross trauma may be slight or absent. The injury regarded as the least significant may be the most lethal. Following trauma, there may be general depression of body functions, which leads to complications such as reduced blood pressure, oxygen deficiency in the blood and primary organ systems, dysrhythmias, and respiratory and cardiac failure. It is thought that the defense mechanisms of the body become depressed, contributing to total organ failure. Mortality in patients with multiple injuries is related to the severity of the injuries and the number of systems and organs involved.

Emergency Management. The goals of treatment are to determine the extent of injuries and to establish priorities of treatment. Any injury interfering with a vital physiologic function (*e.g.*, airway, breathing, circulation) is an immediate threat to life and has the highest priority for immediate treatment. *Imperative lifesaving procedures are performed simultaneously by the emergency team.* As soon as the patient is resuscitated, clothes are usually cut off and a rapid physical assessment is performed. Critically traumatized patients should not be moved from the stretcher or backboard until they are stable. Transfer from field management to ED must be orderly and controlled. Treatment in a level I trauma center is appropriate for major trauma patients.

Treatment priorities are as follows (Fig. 66-4):

1. Carry out a *rapid* physical examination to determine if the patient is breathing, bleeding, or in shock; determine the status of responsiveness and if there are severe wounds or fracture deformities.
2. Start resuscitation procedures (*i.e.*, airway, breathing, circulation) simultaneously while another team member is conducting a physical assessment.
   a. Note the character and symmetry of chest wall motion and the pattern of breathing. Auscultate the chest.
   b. Ask the conscious patient whether he or she is having difficulty breathing. Ask if there is chest pain.
   c. Suction to clear the trachea and bronchial tree of secretions.
   d. Insert an oropharyngeal airway to prevent occlusion by the tongue.
   e. Ventilate the patient (bag-mask system) to alleviate hypoxia.
   f. Prepare for endotracheal intubation if an adequate airway cannot be maintained.
   g. Suspect serious intrathoracic injuries if respiratory distress continues after an adequate airway has been established. (See Chapter 24 for management of chest injuries.)
3. Assess cardiac function and treat cardiac arrest; hypoxia, metabolic acidosis, and chest trauma may precipitate cardiac arrest.
   a. In the event of cardiac arrest, start closed chest compression and ventilation (see Chapter 28).
   b. If the chest wall is unstable (flail chest), emergency thoracostomy and manual compression may be necessary.
4. Control hemorrhage.
   a. Apply pressure over bleeding points if there is overt hemorrhage.
   b. Expect significant blood loss in the patient with a fracture of the shaft of the femur, with multiple fractures, or with major pelvic trauma.
   c. Use caution in applying tourniquets to extremities for massive arterial bleeding that cannot be halted with pressure.
   d. Prepare for immediate surgical intervention if the patient is bleeding internally.
5. Prevent and treat hypovolemic shock.
   a. Insert at least two (sometimes four) large-bore peripheral IV lines as prescribed. Central venous line insertion may be necessary. As shock progresses, the number of IV acesses needed increases.
   b. Draw blood for laboratory studies as directed (typing and cross matching, baseline CBC, electrolytes, blood urea nitrogen [BUN], glucose, prothrombin time).
   c. The physician may introduce a central venous catheter (multilumen catheter preferred) to monitor the patient's response to fluid infusion, to prevent fluid overload, and as a route for fluid infusion.
   d. Start IV infusions.
      (1) Lactated Ringer's solution is usually indicated for volume replacement until blood is available.
      (2) Give IV infusions rapidly to keep central venous pressure readings at or between 5 to 15 cm H_2O; monitor the rate and direction of change (important parameters).
   e. Administer blood component therapy as prescribed. Blood may be warmed to counteract the cooling effect of massive transfusions that can cause cardiac irritability and arrest.
   f. Insert an indwelling urinary catheter and monitor urinary output to aid in diagnosis of shock and to monitor therapy effectiveness and renal function. Do not force the catheter because the patient may have a ruptured urethra.
   g. Monitor the ECG to detect changes.
   h. Continue clinical evaluation to observe for improvement or deterioration. Improvement in the level of responsiveness, skin warmth, speed of capillary filling, and so forth, shows a reversal of the shock state.
   i. Prepare for surgical intervention if the patient does not respond to fluids or blood. Inability to restore blood pressure and circulatory volume in the patient usually indicates major internal bleeding.

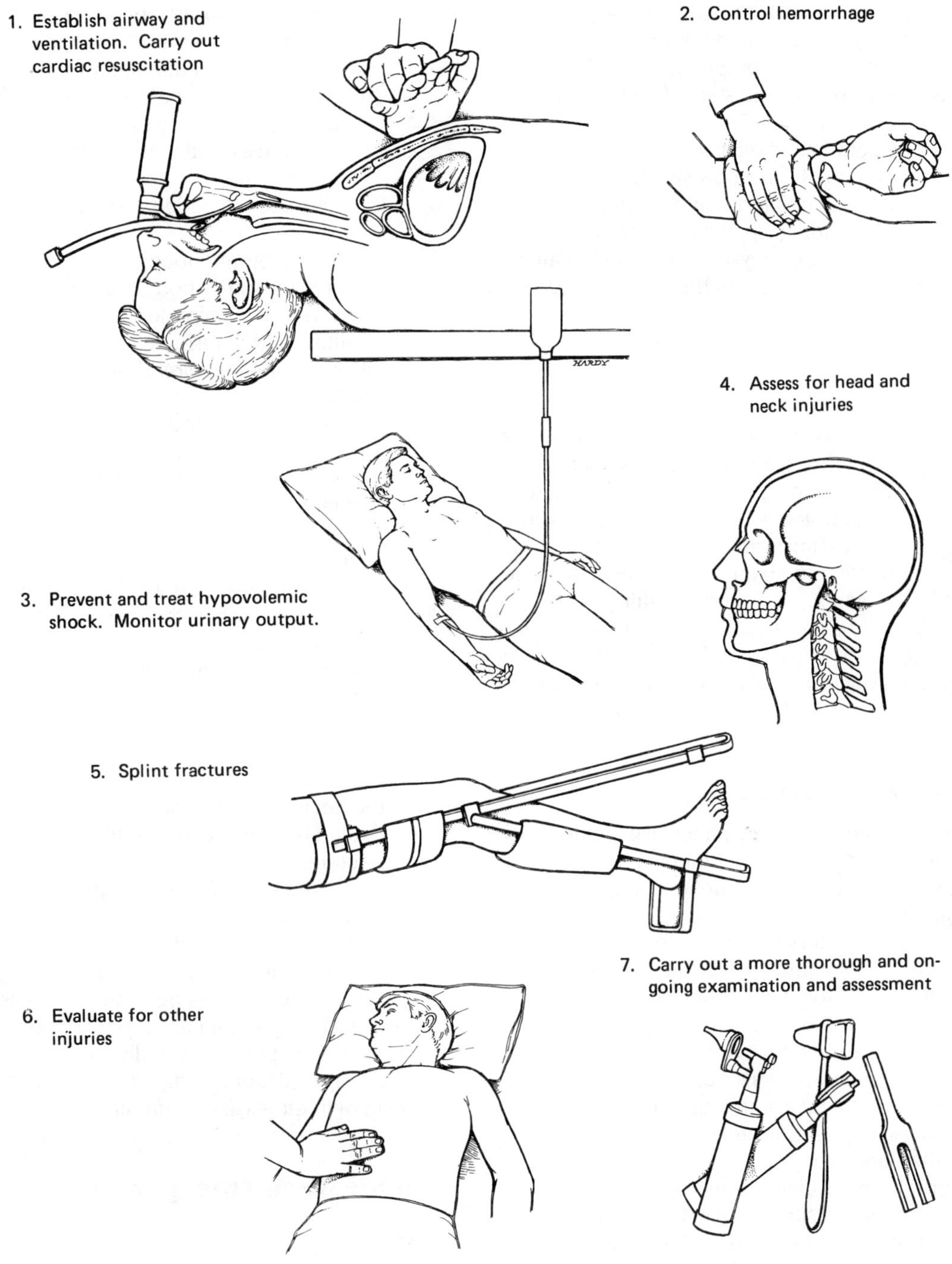
1. Establish airway and ventilation. Carry out cardiac resuscitation
2. Control hemorrhage
HARDY
4. Assess for head and neck injuries
3. Prevent and treat hypovolemic shock. Monitor urinary output.
5. Splint fractures
7. Carry out a more thorough and ongoing examination and assessment
6. Evaluate for other injuries

FIGURE 66-4. Management of the patient with multiple injuries.

6. Assess for head and neck injuries.
   a. Determine the baseline neurologic status of the patient: level of responsiveness, size and reactivity of pupils, motor power, and reflexes.
   b. Neck (and chest) x-rays may be taken; apply rigid cervical collar until the possibility of cervical spine injury is ruled out.
   c. Intracranial pressure monitoring may be instituted.
7. Administer dexamethasone as directed; corticosteroids appear to protect pulmonary function in patients with multiple injuries and help prevent posttraumatic pulmonary insufficiency. (However, this therapy is considered controversial.)
8. Splint fractures to prevent further trauma to soft tissues and blood vessels and to relieve pain; note the presence or absence of pulses in fractured extremities.
9. Assess the patient for gastrointestinal injuries.
   a. Examine the patient repeatedly for abdominal pain, muscular rigidity, tenderness, rebound tenderness, diminished bowel sounds, hypotension, and shock.
   b. Prepare for diagnostic peritoneal lavage to assess for intraperitoneal bleeding.
   c. Assist with insertion of a nasogastric tube if upper gastrointestinal bleeding is suspected or if gaseous distention of the stomach develops; this decreases the incidence of vomiting and aspiration.

d. Prepare for laparotomy if the patient shows continuing signs of hemorrhage and deterioration.
10. Continue to monitor urinary output hourly; urinary output reflects cardiac output and state of perfusion of visceral organs.
    a. Assess for hematuria and oliguria.
    b. Record measurements on a flow sheet.
11. Evaluate patient for other injuries and institute appropriate treatment, including tetanus immunization.
12. Carry out a more thorough physical examination after resuscitation and management of the above priorities.

Fractures

Immediate management of a fracture may determine the patient's outcome and make the difference between recovery and disability. When examining the patient for fracture, the body part is handled gently and as little as possible. Clothing is cut off to minimize trauma to the body part. Assessment is conducted for pain over or near a bone, swelling (from blood, lymph, and exudate infiltrating the tissue), and circulatory disturbance. The patient is assessed for ecchymosis, tenderness, and crepitation. *It must be remembered that the patient may have multiple fractures accompanied by head, chest, and other serious injuries.*

Emergency Management

1. Give immediate attention to the patient's general condition. If there is any question of multiple injury, the patient needs to be completely undressed, draped, and continuously monitored.
    a. Evaluate for respiratory difficulties from edema due to facial and neck injuries, accumulation of secretions in the respiratory tract; follow the ABCs of resuscitation.
        (1) Examine the chest for evidence of sucking chest wounds, pneumothorax, flail chest, and so forth.
        (2) Prepare for tracheal intubation or emergency tracheostomy as indicated.
    b. Control hemorrhage.
        (1) Control venous bleeding by applying direct pressure on the site along with digital pressure over the artery nearest to the bleeding area.
        (2) Suspect internal hemorrhage (pleural, pericardial, or abdominal) in the event of continuing shock and in the presence of injuries to the chest and abdomen.
    c. Treat for shock, which in patients with fractures is usually the result of blood loss.
        (1) Assess for falling blood pressure; cold, clammy skin; and rapid, thready pulse.
        (2) Keep in mind that a large amount of blood loss may accompany fractures of the femur and pelvis.
        (3) Maintain blood pressure with IV infusions, plasma, or plasma expanders as prescribed.
        (4) Administer blood transfusion or blood component therapy as prescribed as soon as blood is available.
        (5) Administer oxygen because cardiopulmonary obstruction causes decreased oxygen supply to the tissues and ultimately circulatory collapse.
        (6) Administer an analgesic as prescribed to control pain. Splinting the extremity and controlling pain are essential in treating shock accompanying fractures.
        (7) Observe for evidence of head, chest, and other injuries.
2. Inspect the fractured body part.
    a. Observe the entire body using a systematic head-to-toe physical examination; inspect for lacerations, swelling, and deformities.
    b. Observe for *angulation* (bending), *shortening*, and *rotation*.
    c. Palpate the pulse distal to the extremity fracture and all peripheral pulses.
    d. Assess for coolness, blanching, decreased sensation and motor function, and diminished or absent pulses; these indicate injury to nerves or blood supply.
    e. Handle the body part gently and as little as possible.
3. Apply the splint before the patient is moved; splinting relieves pain, improves circulation, prevents further tissue injury, and prevents a closed fracture from becoming an open one.
    a. Immobilize the joint above and below the fracture. Place one hand distal to the fracture and apply some traction while placing the other hand beneath the fracture for support.
    b. Extend the splints beyond the joints adjacent to the fracture.
    c. Check the vascular status of the extremity after splinting; check color, temperature, pulse, and blanching of nail bed.
    d. Assess for neurologic deficits caused by the fracture.
    e. Apply a sterile dressing if the fracture is open.
4. Investigate any complaint of pain or pressure.
5. Transport the patient carefully and gently.
6. See Chapter 64 for a complete discussion of the treatment of fractures at specific sites.

Temperature Emergencies

Heat Stroke

Heat stroke is an acute medical emergency caused by failure of the heat-regulating mechanisms of the body. It usually occurs during extended heat waves, especially when accompanied by high humidity. Persons at risk are those not acclimatized to heat, the elderly, those unable to care for themselves, those with chronic and debilitating diseases, and those taking certain medications (major tranquilizers, anticholinergics, diuretics, beta-adrenergic blocking agents). *Exertional heat stroke*, or exercise in extreme heat and humidity, can also cause death. This type of heat stroke occurs in healthy individuals during sports or work activities when hyperthermia results because of inadequate heat loss.

Gerontologic Considerations. Most heat-related deaths occur in the aged because their circulatory systems are unable to compensate for stress imposed by heat.

Assessment. Heat stroke causes thermal injury at the cellular level and resulting widespread damage to the heart, liver, kidney, and blood coagulation. Recent patient history reveals exposure to elevated ambient temperature or excessive exercise during extreme heat. When assessing the patient, the following symptoms are noted: profound central nervous system dysfunction (manifested by confusion, delirium, bizarre behavior, coma); elevated body temperature (40.6°C [105°F] or more); hot, dry skin; usually anhidrosis (absence of sweating), tachypnea, and tachycardia.

Nursing diagnoses may include ineffective thermoregulation related to inability of the body's homeostatic mechanisms to maintain normal body temperature. The goal is reduction of the high temperature as quickly as possible, because mortality is directly related to the duration of hyperthermia. Simultaneous treatment focuses on stabilization of oxygenation via the ABCs of basic life support.

Emergency Management

1. Remove the patient's clothing.
2. Reduce the core (internal) temperature to 39°C (102°F) as rapidly as possible. Use one or more of the following as directed:
   a. Use cool sheets and towels or continuous sponging with cool water.
   b. Apply ice to the skin while spraying with tepid water.
   c. Use cooling blankets.
   d. Iced saline lavage of stomach or colon may be prescribed if the temperature does not decrease.
3. Massage the patient to promote circulation and maintain cutaneous vasodilation during the cooling procedure.
4. Position an electric fan so that it blows on the patient to augment heat dissipation by convection and evaporation.
5. Constantly monitor the patient's temperature using a thermistor probe in the rectum or esophagus (monitors core temperature); avoid hypothermia; hyperthermia may recur spontaneously within 3 to 4 hours.
6. Monitor the patient carefully; vital signs, ECG, CVP, and level of responsiveness change with rapid alterations in body temperature; a seizure may be followed by recurrence of hyperthermia.
7. Administer oxygen to supply tissue needs exaggerated by the hypermetabolic condition. Assist in intubating the patient with a cuffed endotracheal tube and attach to a ventilator if necessary to support failing cardiorespiratory systems.
8. Start IV infusion as directed to replace fluid losses and maintain adequate circulation; administer slowly because of the dangers of myocardial injury from high body temperature and poor renal function. Cooling will redistribute fluid volume from the periphery to the core.
9. Measure urinary output; acute tubular necrosis is a complication of heat stroke.
10. Give supportive care as prescribed:
    a. Dialysis for renal failure.
    b. Anticonvulsant agents to control seizures.
    c. Potassium for hypokalemia and sodium bicarbonate to correct metabolic acidosis.
11. Continue to monitor ECG for possible myocardial ischemia, myocardial infarction, and dysrhythmias.
12. Perform serial testing for bleeding disorders (disseminated intravascular coagulopathy) and serum enzymes to estimate thermal hypoxic injury to the liver and muscle tissue.
13. Admit the patient to the intensive care unit. There may be permanent liver, cardiac, and central nervous system damage.

Patient Education and Home Care Considerations

1. Advise the patient to avoid immediate re-exposure to high temperatures; hypersensitivity to high temperatures may remain for a considerable length of time.
2. Emphasize the importance of maintaining adequate fluid intake, wearing loose clothing, and reducing activity in hot weather.
3. Advise athletes to monitor fluid losses, replace fluids, and use a gradual approach to physical conditioning, allowing sufficient time for acclimatization.
4. Direct the frail elderly living in urban settings with high environmental temperatures to places where air conditioning is available (shopping mall, library, church).

Cold Injuries

Frostbite

Frostbite is trauma from exposure to freezing temperatures and actual freezing of the tissue fluids in the cell and intercellular spaces. It results in vascular damage. Body parts most frequently affected by frostbite are the feet, hands, nose, and ears. A frozen extremity may be hard, cold, insensitive to touch, and appear white or mottled blue-white. The extent of injury from exposure to cold is not always initially known.

Nursing diagnoses may include hypothermia, risk for infection, altered tissue perfusion, and sensory alteration: tactile.

Emergency Management. The goal of management is to restore normal body temperature.

1. Do not allow the patient to walk if lower extremities are involved.
2. Remove all constricting clothing and jewelry that can impair circulation.
3. Rewarm the extremity by controlled and rapid rewarming. The extremity is usually placed in a 37° to 40°C (98.6° to 104°F) whirlpool until the tips of the injured part flush (about 30 to 45 minutes). Flush indicates that circulatory flow is re-established. Early rewarming appears to decrease the amount of tissue loss.
   a. Administer an analgesic for pain as prescribed; the rewarming process may be very painful.
   b. Handle the part gently to avoid further mechanical injury. *Do not massage.*
   c. Protect the rewarmed part; do not rupture blebs, which develop 1 hour to a few days after rewarming.
   d. Place sterile gauze or cotton between affected fingers or toes to prevent maceration.

e. Elevate the body part to help control swelling.
f. Use a foot cradle to prevent contact with bedclothes if the feet are involved.
4. Conduct physical assessment to observe for concomitant injury (soft tissue injury, dehydration, alcohol coma, fat embolism).
5. Restore electrolyte balance; dehydration and hypovolemia occur frequently in frostbite victims.
6. Use strict aseptic technique during dressing changes; frostbite injuries make the patient susceptible to infection.
7. Give tetanus prophylaxis as prescribed if there is associated trauma.
8. The following may be carried out when appropriate:
   a. Whirlpool bath for the affected extremity to aid circulation, débride necrotic tissue, and help prevent infection.
   b. Escharotomy (incision through the eschar) to prevent further tissue damage, to allow for normal circulation, and to permit joint motion.
   c. Fasciotomy (incision in fascia to release pressure on the muscles, nerves, and blood vessels) to treat compartment syndrome.
9. Encourage hourly active motion of the affected digits to promote maximal restoration of function and to prevent contractures.
10. Advise patient not to use tobacco because of the vasoconstrictive effects of nicotine that further reduce the already deficient blood supply to injured tissues.

Accidental Hypothermia

Accidental hypothermia is a condition in which the core (internal) temperature is 35°C (95°F) or below as a result of exposure to cold. Hypothermia occurs when a patient looses the ability to maintain body temperature. Urban hypothermia (extreme exposure to cold in an urban setting) is associated with a high mortality rate; elderly people, infants, persons with concurrent illnesses, and the homeless are particularly susceptible. Alcohol ingestion increases susceptibility. Trauma victims are at risk for hypothermia due to treatment with cold fluids and unwarmed oxygen.

Assessment. The following factors are kept in mind when assessing the patient. Hypothermia leads to physiologic changes in all organ systems. There is progressive deterioration with apathy, poor judgment, ataxia, dysarthria, drowsiness, and eventual coma. Shivering may be suppressed below a temperature of 32.2°C (90°F) because the body's self-warming mechanisms become ineffective. The heartbeat and blood pressure may be so weak that peripheral pulsation becomes undetectable. Cardiac irregularities may also occur. Other physiologic abnormalities include hypoxemia and acidosis.

Emergency Management. Management consists of continual monitoring, rewarming, and supportive care.

1. Monitor the patient: vital signs, CVP, urinary output, arterial blood gases, blood chemistry determinations (BUN, creatinine, glucose, electrolytes), chest x-ray. The ABCs of basic life support are a priority.
   a. Monitor body temperature with an esophageal or rectal thermistor probe.
   b. Employ continuous ECG monitoring; cold-induced myocardial irritability leads to conduction disturbances, especially ventricular fibrillation.
   c. Maintain an arterial line for recording blood pressure and to facilitate blood sampling.
2. Rewarm the patient. Rewarming methods include active core (internal) rewarming, active external rewarming, and passive or spontaneous rewarming. The optimal method has not been determined.
3. Supportive care during rewarming includes the following as directed:
   a. External cardiac compression.
   b. Electrical cardioversion of ventricular fibrillation.
   c. Mechanical ventillation with PEEP and heated humidified oxygen to maintain tissue oxygenation.
   d. IV fluids (warmed) to correct hypotension and maintain urinary output.
   e. Sodium bicarbonate to correct metabolic acidosis.
   f. Antidysrhythmic drugs.
   g. Indwelling urethral catheter to monitor fluid status.
   h. Prophylactic antibiotics. (A large percentage of hypothermic patients develop serious infections.)

Anaphylactic Reaction

An anaphylactic reaction is an acute systemic hypersensitivity reaction that occurs within seconds to minutes after exposure to a variety of foreign substances such as medications (*e.g.*, penicillin, iodinated contrast material) and stinging insects (*Hymenoptera* [bee, wasp, yellow jacket, hornet]). Repeated administration of parenteral or oral therapeutic agents may also precipitate an anaphylactic reaction.

An anaphylactic reaction is the result of an antigen—antibody interaction in a sensitized individual who, as a consequence of previous exposure, has developed a special type of antibody (immunoglobulin) that is specific for this particular allergen. The antibody immunoglobulin IgE is responsible for most of the immediate type of human allergic responses. The individual becomes sensitive to a particular antigen after production of IgE to this antigen.

Clinical Manifestations. Anaphylactic reaction produces a wide range of clinical manifestations.

Respiratory Signs. Respiratory signs include nasal congestion, itching, sneezing and coughing; possible respiratory distress that progresses rapidly and is caused by bronchospasm or edema of the larynx; tightness of the chest; and other respiratory difficulties, such as wheezing, dyspnea, and cyanosis.

Skin Manifestations. Skin manifestations appear in the form of flushing with a sense of warmth and diffuse erythema. *Generalized itching over the entire body indicates that a general systemic reaction is developing.* Urticaria (hives) may also appear. When massive facial angioedema develops, upper respiratory edema may occur.

Cardiovascular Manifestations. Cardiovascular manifestations include tachycardia or bradycardia and peripheral vascular collapse as indicated by pallor, imperceptible pulse, decreasing blood pressure, and circulatory failure, leading to coma and death.

Gastrointestinal Problems. Gastrointestinal problems may include nausea, vomiting, and colicky abdominal pains or diarrhea.

Nursing diagnoses may include decreased cardiac output, impaired gas exchange, risk for fluid volume deficit, and anxiety.

Emergency Management

1. Establish an airway. (This is performed while another person administers epinephrine.)
   a. Turn the face to one side; support the angles of the mandible.
   b. An oropharyngeal or endotracheal tube is inserted; apply oropharyngeal suction for excessive secretions.
   c. Employ resuscitative measures (especially for patients with stridor and progressive pulmonary edema).
   d. If glottal edema is present, an incision through the cricothyroid membrane provides an airway.
   e. Administer positive pressure oxygen therapy by mask and resuscitation bag.
   f. Closed chest cardiac massage is administered if necessary.
2. Administer aqueous epinephrine as prescribed to provide rapid relief of hypersensitivity reaction. (This should be done simultaneously as another person is establishing the airway.) Epinephrine may be repeated if necessary as prescribed. Judgment is used in choosing the route for administration of epinephrine:
   a. Subcutaneous injection for mild, generalized symptoms.
   b. Intramuscular injection when the reaction is more severe and progressive, and when there is concern that vascular collapse will inhibit absorption.
   c. IV route (aqueous epinephrine diluted in saline and given *slowly*), used in rare instances in which there is complete loss of consciousness and severe cardiovascular collapse. This method may precipitate cardiac dysrhythmias; *monitor ECG and have defibrillator available.*
3. To retard antigen absorption apply a tourniquet above the injection site if an anaphylactic reaction followed an injection (medication to which the patient is allergic) or insect sting.
   a. Infiltrate the injection site with epinephrine as directed.
   b. Loosen the tourniquet at regular intervals to allow adequate circulation to the extremity.
4. Start an IV infusion of saline for emergency access to a vein and for hypotension.

Additional Treatments as Indicated

1. Give antihistamine medications as prescribed. For example, diphenhydramine hydrochloride (Benadryl, IM) is given to block further histamine binding at target cells.
2. Give aminophylline IV *slowly* as prescribed over a period of time for patients with severe bronchospasm and wheezing that is refractory to other treatment. Monitor vital signs.
3. Treat prolonged hypotension as prescribed with crystalloids or colloids and possibly vasopressors; monitor blood pressure. A patient with reduced cardiac output may respond to an infusion of isoproterenol or dopamine.
4. Administer oxygen if significant respiratory or cardiovascular deficits are present.
5. Observe for dysrhythmias and cardiorespiratory arrest.
6. If the patient is having seizures, administer short-acting barbiturate or diazepam IV as prescribed over a period of several minutes.
7. Administer corticosteroids as prescribed if the patient is having a prolonged reaction with persistent hypotension or bronchospasm.
8. The patient usually is admitted to the hospital after symptoms abate.

Preventive Measures and Patient Education

1. Be aware of the danger of anaphylactic reactions and the early signs of anaphylaxis.
2. Ask about the patient's previous allergies to medications.
3. Question the patient before giving a foreign serum or other type of antigenic agent to determine whether it had been received at some earlier time.
4. Question the patient about previous allergic reactions to food or pollen.
5. Avoid giving medications to patients with hay fever, asthma, and other allergic disorders unless absolutely necessary.
6. Avoid giving parenteral medications unless absolutely necessary. Anaphylactic reactions are more likely to occur when the agent is given parenterally.
7. Perform a skin test before administration of certain materials known to produce anaphylactic reactions, such as horse serum. It must be remembered that skin testing can precipitate anaphylaxis in highly sensitive individuals.
   a. A negative skin test does not always indicate safety.
   b. Have epinephrine, IV infusions, and intubation and tracheostomy equipment available as precautionary measures.
8. If being treated as an outpatient, keep the patient in the office, hospital, or clinic for at least 30 minutes after injection of any agent. Caution the patient to return if symptoms develop.
9. Caution patients who are sensitive to insect bites to carry kits equipped to treat insect stings (tourniquet, epinephrine); instruct the patient, the family, and significant others in the use of the emergency supplies.
10. Encourage persons with allergies to wear identification tags or bracelets.

Poisoning

A poison is any substance that when ingested, inhaled, absorbed, applied to the skin, or produced within the body in relatively small amounts causes injury to the body by its chemical action. Poisoning from inhalation and ingestion of toxic materials, both accidental and by design, constitutes a major health hazard. About 7% of all emergency department visits are a result of toxic problems.

Ingested (Swallowed) Poisons

Goals of emergency treatment are to remove or inactivate the poison before it is absorbed, to give supportive care to maintain vital organ systems, to use the specific antidote to neutralize the poison, and to give treatment to hasten the elimination of the absorbed poison.

General Management

1. Attain control of the airway, ventilation, and oxygenation. In the absence of cerebral or renal damage, the patient's prognosis depends largely on successful management of respiratory and circulatory systems.
   a. Assess adequacy of ventilation by observing ventilatory effort through blood gas analysis or spirometry.
   b. Assess cardiovascular function by measurement of pulse, blood pressure, central venous pressure, and temperature (core and peripheral).
   c. Prepare for mechanical ventilation if respirations are depressed. Positive expiratory pressure applied to the airway (bag-mask) may help keep the alveoli inflated.
   d. Administer oxygen for respiratory depression, unconsciousness, cyanosis, and shock.
   e. Prevent aspiration of gastric contents by positioning patient on side with head down, using an oropharyngeal airway, and suctioning.
   f. Stabilize cardiovascular function and monitor ECG.
   g. Insert an indwelling urinary catheter to monitor renal function.
   h. Obtain blood specimen to test for concentration of drug or poison.
   i. Monitor neurologic status (including cognitive function); monitor the course of vital signs and neurologic status over time.
   j. Conduct a rapid physical examination.
2. Try to determine what product was taken, the amount, time since ingestion, symptoms, age and weight of the patient, and pertinent health history. Call the poison control center in the area if an unknown toxic agent has been taken or if it is necessary to identify an antidote for a known toxic agent.
3. Treat shock appropriately. It may be due to the cardiodepressant action of the drug ingested, venous pooling in lower extremities, or a reduction in circulating blood volume due to increased capillary permeability.
4. Remove the toxin or decrease its absorption. Use gastric emptying procedures as prescribed; the following may be used:
   a. Syrup of ipecac to induce vomiting in the alert patient. (Do not induce vomiting after ingestion of caustic substances or petroleum distillates).
   b. Gastric lavage (Fig. 66-5 and Guideline 66-7 for the obtunded patient). Save gastric aspirate for toxicology screens.
   c. Activated charcoal administration if poison is one that is absorbed by charcoal.
   d. Cathartic, when appropriate.
5. Give specific therapy. Administer the specific chemical antagonist or physiologic antagonist as early as possible to reverse or diminish effects of the toxin.
6. Support the patient having seizures. Poisons may excite the central nervous system or the patient may have seizures from oxygen deprivation.
7. Assist in carrying out procedures to promote the removal of the ingested substance if the above are not effective:
   a. Diuresis for agents excreted by the renal route.
   b. Dialysis.
   c. Hemoperfusion (process of passing blood through an extracorporeal circuit and a cartridge containing an adsorbent [such as charcoal or resins], after which the detoxified blood is returned to the patient).
   d. Multiple doses of charcoal.
8. Monitor central venous pressure as indicated.
9. Monitor for fluid and electrolyte imbalance.
10. Reduce elevated temperature.

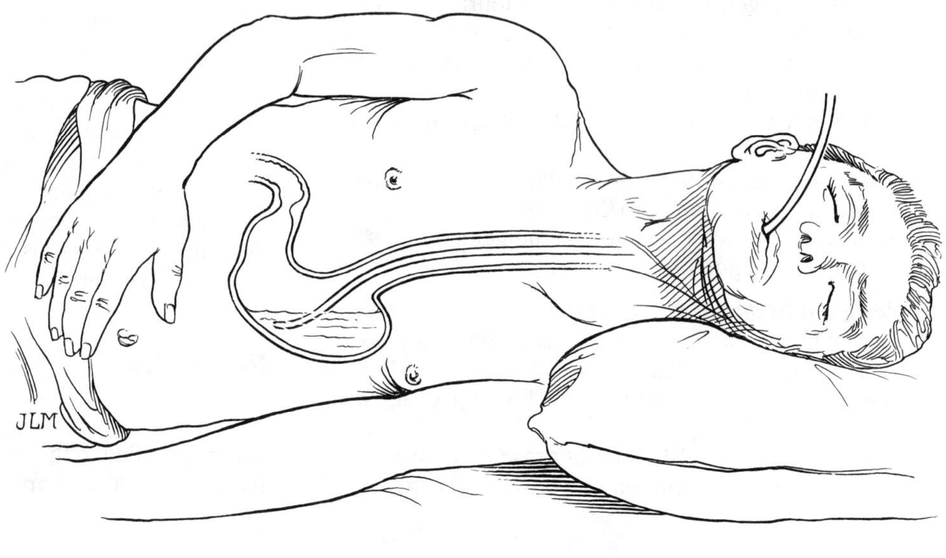

FIGURE 66-5. Gastric lavage. During gastric lavage the patient is positioned on his left side to allow pooling of the gastric contents and decrease the passage of fluid into the duodenum during lavage.

GUIDELINE 66–7
Assisting With Gastric Lavage

Gastric lavage is the aspiration of the stomach contents and washing out of the stomach by means of a gastric tube. Gastric lavage is contraindicated after acid or alkali ingestion, in the presence of seizures, or after ingestion of hydrocarbons or petroleum distillates. It is particularly dangerous after ingestion of strong corrosive agents.

Purposes

1. For urgent removal of ingested substance in order to decrease systemic absorption
2. To empty the stomach before endoscopic procedures
3. To diagnose gastric hemorrhage and to arrest hemorrhage

Equipment

Large-bore/nasogastric tubes or large-bore Ewald tube
Large irrigating syringe with adapter
Large plastic funnel with adapter to fit tube
Water-soluble lubricant
Tap water or appropriate antidote (milk, saline solution, sodium bicarbonate solution, fruit juice, activated charcoal)
Container for aspirate
Mouth gag, nasotracheal or endotracheal tubes with inflatable cuffs
Containers for specimens

Procedure

Action	Rationale/Amplification
1. Remove dentures and inspect the oral cavity for loose teeth.	1. This will prevent accidental aspiration of teeth.
2. Measure the distance between the bridge of the nose and the xiphoid process. Mark the tube with indelible pencil or tape.	2. This distance is a rule-of-thumb measurement of the distance the tube is passed to reach the stomach. This avoids curling and kinking of excess tubing in the stomach.
3. Lubricate the tube with water-soluble lubricant.	3. Lubrication eases insertion of the tube.
4. If comatose, the patient is intubated with a cuffed nasotracheal or endotracheal tube.	4. A cuffed nasotracheal or endotracheal tube prevents aspiration of gastric contents.
5. Place the patient in a left lateral position with the head lowered about 15 degrees downward.	5. This position decreases passage of gastric contents into the duodenum during lavage and minimizes the possibility of aspiration into the lungs.
6. Pass the tube by the oral route while keeping the head in a neutral position. Pass the tube to the adhesive marking or about 50 cm (20 in). After the lavage tube is passed, the head of the table is lowered. Have standby suction available.	6. The depth of insertion of the tube will vary with the size of the patient. If the tube enters the trachea instead of the esophagus, the patient will experience coughing, dyspnea, stridor, and cyanosis. Positive confirmation of tube placement can be accomplished with an x-ray.
7. Aspirate the stomach contents with the syringe attached to the tube before instilling water or an antidote. Save the specimen for analysis.	7. Aspiration is carried out to determine that the tube is in the stomach and to remove the stomach contents. Positive confirmation of tube placement can be accomplished with x-ray.
8. Remove the syringe. Attach the funnel to the end of the tube, or use a 50-ml syringe to inject lavage solution in the gastric tube. The volume of fluid placed in the stomach should be small.	8. Overfilling the stomach may cause regurgitation and aspiration or force the stomach contents through the pylorus.
9. Elevate the funnel above the patient's head and pour approximately 150 to 200 ml of solution into the funnel.	
10. Lower the funnel and siphon the gastric contents into the bucket.	10. The fluid should flow in freely and drain by gravity.
11. Save samples of the first two washings.	11. Keep the first washing sample isolated from other washings for toxicologic analysis.
12. Repeat the lavage procedure until the returns are relatively clear and no particulate matter is seen.	12. This usually requires a total volume of at least 2 liters; some clinicians advocate the use of 5 to 20 liters.
13. At the completion of lavage:	13.
a. The stomach may be left empty.	
b. An adsorbent (powder form of activated charcoal mixed with water to form slurry, the consistency of thick soup) may be instilled in the tube and allowed to remain in the stomach.	b. Activated charcoal reduces absorption by adsorbing (attaching to its surface) a wide range of substances; it renders the poison inaccessible to the circulation, thereby reducing its toxicity.

(continued)

GUIDELINE 66-7 (continued)
Assisting With Gastric Lavage

Procedure

Action	Rationale/Amplification
c. A saline cathartic may be instilled in the tube.	c. A cathartic may be given to hasten the elimination of remaining ingested material.
14. Pinch off the tube during removal or maintain suction while the tube is being withdrawn.	14. Pinching off the tube prevents aspiration and the initiation of the gag reflex. Keeping the patient's head lower than the body also helps to prevent initiation of the gag reflex.
15. Warn the patient that his stools will turn black from the charcoal.	

11. Cautiously give analgesics as prescribed for pain; severe pain causes vasomotor collapse and reflex inhibition of normal physiologic functions.
12. Assist in obtaining specimens of blood, urine, stomach contents, and vomitus.
13. Provide constant nursing surveillance and attention to the patient in a coma; coma from poisoning results from interference with brain cell function or metabolism.
14. Monitor and treat for complications such as hypotension, cardiac dysrhythmias, and seizures.
15. If the patient is discharged, give written material indicating signs and symptoms of potential problems and procedures for call-back or return.
    a. Request a psychiatric consultation if poisoning was a suicide attempt.
    b. In cases of accidental poison ingestion provide poison prevention and home poison-proofing instructions to the patient or family.

Corrosive Poisons

Corrosive poisons include alkaline and acid agents that can cause tissue destruction after coming in contact with mucous membranes.

- *Alkaline products:* Lye, drain cleaners, toilet bowl cleaners, bleach, nonphosphate detergents, oven cleaners, button batteries (batteries used to power watches, calculators, cameras), Clinitest tablets.
- *Acid products:* Toilet bowl cleaners, pool cleaners, metal cleaners, rust removers, battery acid.

Assessment

1. Note type and quantity of ingested agent.
2. Assess for pain and burning sensations in the mouth and throat, pain on swallowing, inability to swallow, vomiting, drooling, and hematuria.

Nursing diagnoses may include altered oral mucous membranes related to swallowing corrosive poison and risk for self-directed violence.

Emergency Management

1. Give water (or milk) to drink for dilution.
    a. Dilution is *not* attempted if patient has acute airway edema or obstruction or if there is clinical evidence of esophageal, gastric, or intestinal perforation.
    b. *Do not induce vomiting if the patient has consumed a strong acid, alkali, or other corrosive substance.*
2. The patient is usually admitted to the hospital for observation and elective endoscopy to evaluate for the presence of burns and deep ulceration.
3. Request a psychiatric evaluation if poisoning was a suicide attempt.

Inhaled Poisons

General Management

1. Carry the patient to fresh air immediately; open all doors and windows.
2. Loosen all tight clothing.
3. Initiate cardiopulmonary resuscitation (CPR) if required.
4. Prevent chilling; wrap the patient in blankets.
5. Keep the patient as quiet as possible.
6. Do not give alcohol in any form.

Carbon Monoxide Poisoning

Carbon monoxide poisoning may occur as a result of industrial or household accident, or attempted suicide. It is implicated in more deaths than any other toxic agent except alcohol. Carbon monoxide exerts its toxic effect by binding to circulating hemoglobin, which reduces the oxygen-carrying capacity of the blood. Hemoglobin absorbs carbon monoxide more than 200 times more readily than it absorbs oxygen. Carbon monoxide–bound hemoglobin, called *carboxyhemoglobin,* does not transport oxygen.

Clinical Manifestations and Assessment. Because the central nervous system has a critical need for oxygen it shows signs of carbon monoxide toxicity. A person suffering from carbon monoxide poisoning appears intoxicated (from cerebral hypoxia). Other signs and symptoms include headache, muscular weakness, palpitation, dizziness, and mental confusion, which can progress rapidly to coma. Skin color is not a reliable sign; it can range from pink or cherry red to cyanotic or pale. Exposure to carbon monoxide requires immediate treatment.

Nursing diagnoses may include impaired gas exchange and risk for self-directed violence.

Emergency Management. Goals of management are to reverse cerebral and myocardial hypoxia and to hasten carbon monoxide elimination.

1. Administer 100% oxygen at atmospheric or hyperbaric pressures to reverse hypoxia and accelerate the elimination of carbon monoxide.
2. Draw blood for carboxyhemoglobin levels; oxygen is administered until the carboxyhemoglobin level is less than 5%.
3. Observe the patient constantly. Psychoses, spastic paralysis, ataxia, visual disturbances, and deterioration of personality may persist after resuscitation and may be symptoms of permanent central nervous system damage.
4. When unintentional carbon monoxide poisoning occurs, contact the health department. The dwelling or building in question should also be inspected.
5. Request a psychiatric consultation if poisoning was a suicide attempt.

Skin Contamination Poisoning (Chemical Burns)

Injuries from exposure to chemicals are challenging because of the large number of offending agents with diverse actions and metabolic effects. The severity of a chemical burn is determined by the mechanism of action, penetrating strength and concentration, and amount and duration of exposure of the chemical to the skin.

Emergency Management

1. Drench the skin with running water from a shower, hose, or faucet.
2. Continue to apply a stream of water to the skin while removing the clothing; the skin of health care personnel should be appropriately protected if the burn is extensive or the agent significantly toxic.
3. Apply *prolonged* lavage with generous amounts of tepid water.
4. Attempt to determine the identity and characteristics of the chemical agent for future treatment.
5. Provide the standard burn treatment appropriate for the size and location of the wound (antimicrobial treatment, tetanus prophylaxis as prescribed).
6. Instruct the patient to have the affected area reexamined at 24 and 72 hours and 7 days. There is a risk of underestimating these types of injuries.

Injected Poisons: Stinging Insects

A person may have an extreme sensitivity to the venoms of the *Hymenoptera* (the stings of bees, hornets, yellow jackets, and wasps). Venom allergy is thought to be an IgE-mediated reaction, which constitutes an acute emergency. Stings of the head and neck are especially serious, although stings in any area of the body can result in anaphylaxis.

Clinical manifestations range from generalized urticaria, itching, malaise, and anxiety to laryngeal edema, severe bronchospasm, shock, and death. Generally, the shorter the time between the sting and the onset of severe symptoms, the worse the prognosis.

Emergency Management

1. Administer epinephrine (aqueous) as directed. Massage the site to hasten absorption.
2. If the sting is on an extremity, apply a tourniquet with sufficient compression to occlude venous and lymphatic flow.
3. See Chapter 15 for treatment of anaphylactic shock.
4. Counsel all persons sensitive to *Hymenoptera* venom to carry a prescription-available self-treatment kit containing a tourniquet, injectable and inhalant forms of epinephrine, an oral antihistamine, and written instructions. Instruct the patient to do the following if stung:
   a. Inject self immediately with epinephrine.
   b. Remove the stinger with one quick scrape of the fingernail. *Do not* squeeze the venom sac as this may cause injection of additional venom.
   c. Cleanse the area with soapy water and apply ice.
   d. Apply a tourniquet proximal to the sting.
   e. Report to the nearest health care facility for further examination.
5. All allergic individuals should wear medical warning bracelets indicating hypersensitivity.
6. Hyposensitization therapy should be given to persons who have had systemic or large local reactions.

Patient Education and Home Care Considerations. Instruct the patient, family, and significant others to limit exposure to stinging insects by the following measures:

- Avoid places where stinging insects congregate (camp and picnic sites).
- Avoid insect feeding areas (flower beds, ripe fruit orchards, garbage, fields of clover).
- Avoid going barefoot outdoors (yellow jackets may nest and pollinate on the ground).
- Avoid perfumes, scented soaps, and bright colors, which attract bees.
- Keep car windows closed.
- Spray garbage cans with quick-acting insecticide.
- Secure a professional exterminator to dispose of wasp and hornet nests or beehives in the home area.
- Remain motionless if an insect is buzzing around. (Motion, especially running, increases the likelihood of being stung.)
- Learn self-injection of epinephrine.

Snakebites

Venomous (poisonous) snakes cause approximately 8000 of the 45,000 snakebites that occur each year in the United States and result in 9 to 15 deaths. Children between the ages of 1 and 9 years are the most likely victims. The greatest number of bites occur during daylight hours in summer months. Venomous snakebites are medical emergencies.

Venomous snakes are found in every part of the United States. Different parts of the country and the world have different types of snakes. Because snakebites are medical emergencies, the nurse should be familiar with the types of snakes that are common to the geographic region.

Snake venom consists primarily of proteins that have a broad range of physiologic effects. Multiple organ systems, especially the neurologic, cardiovascular, and respiratory systems, may be affected.

Initial first aid at the site of the snakebite includes having the victim rest, removing constrictive items such as rings, providing warmth, cleansing the wound, covering the wound with a light sterile dressing, and immobilizing the injured body part below the level of the heart. Ice or a tourniquet *is not* applied. Initial evaluation in the emergency department is performed quickly and includes:

- Determining whether the snake was venomous or nonvenomous.
- Determining where and when the bite occurred and the circumstances of the bite.
- Establishing the sequence of events, signs and symptoms (fang puncture(s), pain, edema, and erythema of the bite and nearby tissues).
- Determining the severity of poisonous effects.
- Monitoring vital signs.
- Measuring and recording the circumference of the bitten extremity or area at several points.
- Obtaining appropriate laboratory data (*i.e.*, CBC, urinalysis, and clotting studies).

The course and prognosis of snakebites depend on the kind and amount of venom injected, where on the body the bite occurred, and the general health, age, and size of the victim. There is no one specific protocol for treatment of snakebites. General guidelines include the following:

1. Obtain baseline laboratory data.
2. *Do not* use ice, tourniquets, heparin, or corticosteroids during the acute stage. Corticosteroids are contraindicated in the first 6 to 8 hours after the bite because they may depress antibody production and hinder the action of antivenin (antitoxin for the snake venom).
3. Parenteral fluids may be used to treat hypotension. If vasopressors are used to treat hypotension, their use should be short-term.
4. Surgical exploration of the bite is rarely indicated.
5. Observe the patient closely for at least 6 hours; the patient is *never* left unattended.

Administration of Antivenin (Antitoxin). Antivenin is most effective if administered within 12 hours of the snakebite. The dosage depends on the type of snake and the estimated severity of the bite. Children may require more antivenin than adults because smaller bodies are more susceptible to toxic effects of venom. A skin or eye test should be performed prior to the initial dose to detect allergy to the antivenin.

Before administering antivenin and every 15 minutes thereafter, the circumference of the affected part is measured proximally. Antivenin is administered as an IV drip whenever possible, although intramuscular administration can be used. Depending on the severity of the bite, the antivenin is diluted in 500 to 1000 ml of normal saline; the fluid volume may be reduced for children. The infusion is started slowly and the rate is increased after 10 minutes if there is no reaction. The total dose should be infused during the first 4 to 6 hours after poisoning. The initial dose is repeated until symptoms decrease. After the symptoms decrease, the circumference of the affected part should be measured every 30 to 60 minutes for the next 48 hours.

The most common cause of serum reaction is too rapid infusion of antivenin, although approximately 3% of patients with negative skin tests develop reactions not related to infusion rate. Reactions may consist of a feeling of fullness in the face, urticaria, pruritus, malaise, and apprehension. These symptoms may be followed by tachycardia, shortness of breath, hypotension, and shock. In this situation, infusion should be stopped immediately and IV diphenhydramine administered. Vasopressors are used in the presence of shock. Emergency resuscitation equipment must be on standby while antivenin is infusing.

Food Poisoning

Food poisoning is a sudden, explosive illness that may occur after ingestion of contaminated food or drink. Botulism is a serious form of food poisoning that requires continual surveillance.

Emergency Management

1. Determine the source and type of food poisoning.
   a. Have suspected food brought to the medical facility.
   b. Obtain the history:
      (1) How soon after eating did the symptoms occur? (Immediate onset suggests chemical, plant, or animal poisoning.)
      (2) What was eaten in the previous meal? Did the food have an unusual odor or taste? (Most foods causing bacterial poisoning *do not* have unusual odor or taste.)
      (3) Did anyone else become ill from eating the same food?
      (4) Did vomiting occur? What was the appearance of the vomitus?
      (5) Did diarrhea occur? (Diarrhea is usually absent with botulism and with shellfish or other fish poisoning.)
      (6) Are any neurologic symptoms present? (These occur in botulism and in chemical, plant, and animal poisoning.)
      (7) Does the patient have a fever? (Fever is seen in salmonella, favism [ingestion of fava beans], and some fish poisoning.)
      (8) What is the patient's appearance?
2. Collect food, gastric contents, vomitus, serum, and feces for examination.
3. Monitor vital signs on a continuing basis.
   a. Assess respiration, blood pressure, sensorium, CVP (if indicated), and muscular activity.

b. Weigh the patient for future comparisons.
4. Support the respiratory system. Death from respiratory paralysis can occur with botulism, fish poisoning, and so forth.
5. Maintain fluid and electrolyte balance. Severe vomiting produces alkalosis, and severe diarrhea produces acidosis; large amounts of electrolytes and water are lost by vomiting and diarrhea.
   a. Observe for hypovolemic shock from severe fluid and electrolyte losses.
   b. Evaluate for lethargy, rapid pulse, fever, oliguria, anuria, hypotension, and delirium.
   c. Carry out blood electrolyte studies.
6. Correct and control hypoglycemia.
7. Control nausea.
   a. Administer an antiemetic medication parenterally as prescribed if the patient cannot tolerate fluids or medications by mouth.
   b. Give sips of weak tea, carbonated drinks, or tap water for mild nausea.
   c. Give clear liquids 12 to 24 hours after nausea and vomiting subside.
   d. Gradually progress to a low-residue, bland diet.

Substance Abuse

Substance abuse is the misuse of specific substances to alter mood or behavior; drug and alcohol abuse are two examples of substance abuse.

Drug Abuse

Drug abuse is the use of drugs for other than legitimate medical purposes. Clinical manifestations vary with the drug used, but underlying principles of management are essentially the same. Table 66-1 notes commonly abused drugs, listing their clinical manifestations and therapeutic management.

Drug users tend to take a variety of drugs simultaneously (*e.g.*, alcohol, barbiturates, narcotics, and tranquilizers), which may have additive effects. IV drug users are at increased risk for HIV infection, AIDS, hepatitis B, and are the most frequent victims of tetanus in the United States.

Treatment goals for a patient suffering from drug overdose are to support the respiratory and cardiovascular functions and to enhance clearance of the agent.

Emergency Management of Acute Drug Reaction

1. Assess the presence and adequacy of respirations. Attain control of the airway, ventilation, and oxygenation.
   a. Use a cuffed endotracheal tube and provide assisted ventilation in a severely depressed patient with absent gag or cough reflexes.
   b. Measure arterial blood gases for hypoxia due to hypoventilation and acid–base abnormalities.
   c. Administer oxygen.
2. Stabilize the cardiovascular system. (This is done simultaneously with airway management.)
   a. Begin external cardiac compression and ventilation in the absence of heartbeat.
   b. Start ECG monitoring.
   c. Draw blood samples for testing glucose, electrolytes, BUN, creatinine, and appropriate toxicologic screen.
   d. Start IV fluids.
3. Give a specific drug antagonist as prescribed if the drug is known. Naloxone hydrochloride (Narcan) is frequently used; 50% dextrose in water is also used (for hypoglycemia).
4. Remove the drug from the stomach as soon as possible.
   a. Induce vomiting if the patient is seen early after ingestion; save the vomitus for toxicologic study.
   b. Use gastric lavage if the patient is unconscious or if there is no way to determine when the drug was ingested. (In patients with absent gag or cough reflexes, carry out this procedure *only* after intubation with a cuffed endotracheal tube to prevent aspiration of the stomach contents.)
   c. Activated charcoal may be a useful adjunct to therapy and is used after vomiting or lavage.
   d. Save gastric aspirate for toxicologic analysis.
5. Provide supportive care.
   a. Take rectal temperature; extremes of thermoregulation (hyperthermia and hypothermia) must be recognized and treated.
   b. Treat seizures as directed; initiate seizure precautions.
   c. Assist with hemodialysis and peritoneal dialysis for potentially lethal poisoning.
   d. Insert a urinary catheter to maintain a free urine flow because the drug or metabolites are excreted by the urine.
6. Perform a thorough physical examination to rule out insulin shock, meningitis, subdural hematoma, stroke, and other possible causes.
   a. Assess for needle marks and external evidence of trauma.
   b. Carry out a rapid neurologic assessment (level of responsiveness, pupil size and reaction, reflexes, focal neurologic findings).
   c. Keep in mind that many drug users take multiple drugs simultaneously.
   d. Be aware that there is a high incidence of HIV infection and hepatitis B among IV drug users, which is the result of communal use of unsterile needles and syringes.
   e. Examine the patient's breath for the characteristic odor of alcohol, acetone, and so forth.
7. Try to obtain the drug experience history (from either the person accompanying the patient or the patient).
   a. Adopt a supportive and realistic relationship with the patient.
   b. Do not leave the patient alone; there is the potential for self-directed harm or harm to emergency department staff.
8. Admit the patient to intensive care unit (ICU) if unconscious; if the patient has deliberately overdosed, psychiatric consultation is necessary.
9. Make every effort to enroll the patient in a drug treatment program (detoxification *and* rehabilitation).

(text continues on page 2031)

TABLE 66-1 Emergency Management of Drug Abuse Patients and Patients with Drug Overdose

Drug	Clinical Manifestations	Therapeutic Management
Narcotics (Opioids)		
Cocaine Intranasally ("snorting"): inhaled into nostrils through straws By smoking ("freebasing"): cocaine hydrochloride dissolved in ether to yield a pure cocaine alkaloid base (called "crack"); smoking in a small pipe delivers large quantities of cocaine to lungs Intravenously	Cocaine is a CNS stimulant that can increase heart rate and blood pressure and cause hyperpyrexia, seizures, and ventricular dysrhythmias. It produces intense euphoria, then anxiety, sadness, insomnia, and sexual indifference; cocaine hallucinosis with delusions; psychosis with extreme paranoia with ideas of persecution; and hypervigilance. Chronic psychotic symptoms may persist.	1. Ensure airway and ventilation. 2. Control seizures. 3. Monitor cardiovascular effects; have lidocaine and defibrillator available. 4. Treat for hyperthermia. 5. Refer for psychiatric evaluation and treatment in an inpatient unit that eliminates access to the drug.
Heroin Opium or paregoric Morphine, codeine, synthetic derivatives (methadone, meperidine) Fentanyl (Sublimaze)	Acute intoxication (overdose) Pinpoint pupils (may be dilated with severe hypoxia); decreased blood pressure Marked respiratory depression Stupor → coma Fresh needle marks along course of any superficial vein; skin abscesses	1. Support respiratory and cardiovascular functions. 2. Establish an IV line; withdraw blood for chemical and toxicologic analysis. Patient may be given bolus of glucose to eliminate possibility of hypoglycemia 3. Give narcotic antagonist (naloxone hydrochloride [Narcan]) as prescribed to reverse severe respiratory depression and coma. 4. Continue to monitor level of responsiveness and respirations, pulse, and BP. Duration of action of naloxone hydrochloride is shorter than that of heroin; repeated dosages may be necessary. 5. Send urine for analysis; opiates can be detected in urine. 6. Obtain an ECG. 7. Do not leave patient unattended; he may lapse back into coma rapidly. Clinical status may change from minute to minute. Hemodialysis may be indicated for severe drug intoxication. 8. Monitor for pulmonary edema, which is frequently seen in patients who abuse/overdose on narcotics. 9. Refer patient for psychiatric evaluation prior to discharge.
Barbiturates		
Pentobarbital (Nembutal) Secobarbital (Seconal) Amobarbital (Amytal)	Acute intoxication (may mimic alcohol intoxication): Respiratory depression Flushed face Decreased pulse rate; decreased blood pressure Increasing nystagmus Depressed tendon reflexes Decreasing mental alertness	1. Maintain airway and give respiratory support. 2. Endotracheal intubation or tracheostomy is considered if there is any doubt about the adequacy of airway exchange. a. Check airway frequently. b. Perform suctioning as necessary. 3. Support cardiovascular and respiratory functions; most deaths result from respiratory depression or shock.

(continued)

TABLE 66-1 *(continued)*

Drug	Clinical Manifestations	Therapeutic Management
	Difficulty in speaking Poor motor coordination Coma, death	4. Start intravenous infusion through large-gauge needle or intravenous catheter to support blood pressure; coma and dehydration result in hypotension and respond to infusion of intravenous fluids with elevation of blood pressure. Sodium bicarbonate may be prescribed to alkalinize urine; it promotes excretion of barbiturates. 5. Evacuate stomach contents or lavage as soon as possible to prevent absorption; repeated doses of activated charcoal may be administered. 6. Assist with hemodialysis for severely overdosed patient. 7. Maintain neurologic and vital sign flow sheet. 8. Patient awakening from overdose may demonstrate combative behavior; this can stimulate automatic angry response by health care personnel. 9. Refer for psychiatric consultation to evaluate suicide potential and drug abuse.
Amphetamine-Type Drugs (Pep Pills, "Uppers," "Speed," "Crystal," "Meth")		
Amphetamine (Benzedrine) Dextroamphetamine (Dexedrine) Methamphetamine (Desoxyn) MDMA ("Ecstasy," "Adam") MDEA ("Eve") MDA	Nausea, vomiting, anorexia, palpitations, tachycardia, increased blood pressure, tachypnea, anxiety, nervousness, diaphoresis, mydriasis Repetitive or stereotyped behavior Irritability, insomnia, agitation Visual misperceptions, auditory hallucinations Fearful anxiety/depression, cold, distant hostility, paranoia Hyperactivity, rapid speech, euphoria Seizures, coma, hyperthermia, cardiovascular collapse	1. Provide airway support, ventilation, cardiac monitoring; insert IV line. 2. Employ gastrointestinal decontamination in cases of oral overdose; activated charcoal, gastric lavage. 3. Keep in calm, quiet environment; elevated temperature potentiates amphetamine toxicity. 4. Use small doses of diazepam (IV) as prescribed for CNS and muscular hyperactivity. 5. Administer appropriate pharmacologic therapy as prescribed for severe hypertension and ventricular dysrhythmias. 6. Try to communicate with patient if delusions, hallucinations, are present 7. Place in a protective environment (preferably psychiatric security room with video monitoring) to observe for suicide attempt. 8. Refer for psychiatric evaluation.
Hallucinogens or Psychedelic-Type Drugs		
Lysergic acid diethylamide (LSD) Phencyclidine HCI (PCP, "angel dust") Mescaline, psilocybin	Nystagmus, mild hypertension Marked confusion bordering on panic Incoherence, hyperactivity	*Emergency Management* 1. Evaluate and maintain patient's airway, breathing, and circulation. 2. Determine whether the patient has ingested hallucinogenic drug or has a toxic psychosis.

(continued)

TABLE 66-1 *(continued)*

Drug	Clinical Manifestations	Therapeutic Management
	Combative behavior; delirium, mania, self-injury Hallucinations, body image distortion Hypertension, hyperthermia, renal failure *Flashback:* recurrence of LSD-like state without having taken the drug; may occur weeks or months after drug was taken Seizures, coma, circulatory collapse, death	3. Try to communicate with the patient; reassure him. a. "Talking down" involves understanding the process through which the patient is proceeding and helping him overcome his fears while establishing contact with reality. b. Remind the patient that fear is common with this problem. c. Reassure the patient that he is not losing his mind—that he is experiencing effect of drugs and that this will wear off. d. Instruct the patient to keep his eyes open; this reduces intensity of reaction. e. Reduce sensory stimuli: minimize noise, lights, movement, tactile stimulation. 4. Sedate the patient as prescribed if his hyperactivity cannot be controlled; diazepam (Valium) or a barbiturate may be prescribed. 5. Search for evidences of trauma; hallucinogen users have a tendency to "act out" their hallucinations. 6. Manage seizures. 7. Observe patient closely; his behavior may become hazardous. 8. Monitor for hypertensive crisis if patient has prolonged psychosis due to drug ingestion. 9. Place patient in a protected environment under proper medical supervision to prevent self-inflicted bodily harm. *Management for Phencyclidine Abusers* 1. Place patient in a calm, supportive environment to minimize stimuli; protect from self-injury. 2. Avoid talking down. 3. Do not leave patient unobserved. Treat symptoms as they occur. a. Drug effects are unpredictable and prolonged. b. Symptoms are likely to exacerbate; patient becomes out of control. 4. Refer patient for psychiatric evaluation.
Drugs Producing Sedation, Intoxication, or Psychologic and Physical Dependence (Nonbarbiturate Sedatives)		
Diazepam (Valium) Chlordiazepoxide (Librium) Oxazepam (Serax) Lorazepam (Ativan)	Acute intoxication: Respiratory depression Decreasing mental alertness Confusion Slurred speech, decreased blood pressure	*Management* 1. Endotracheal tube is inserted as a precaution; use assisted ventilation to stabilize and correct respiratory depression. Observe for sudden apnea and laryngeal spasm (especially in patients dependent on glutethimide [Doriden]).

(continued)

TABLE 66-1 (continued)

Drug	Clinical Manifestations	Therapeutic Management
	Ataxia Pulmonary edema Coma, death	2. Assess for hypotension. a. Insert indwelling catheter for comatose patient; decreased urinary volume is an index of reduced renal flow associated with reduced intravascular volume or vascular collapse. b. Start volume expansion with saline or dextrose as prescribed. 3. Evacuate stomach contents; emesis; lavage; activated charcoal; cathartic. 4. Start ECG monitoring. Observe for dysrhythmias.
Salicylate Poisoning		
Aspirin (present in compound analgesic tablets)	Restlessness, tinnitus, deafness, blurring of vision Hyperpnea, hyperpyrexia, sweating Epigastric pain, vomiting, dehydration Respiratory and metabolic acidosis Disorientation, coma, cardiovascular collapse	1. Treat respiratory depression. 2. Induce gastric emptying: emesis or lavage. 3. Give activated charcoal to adsorb aspirin; a cathartic may be administered with charcoal to help assure intestinal cleansing. 4. Support patient with intravenous infusions as prescribed to establish hydration and correct electrolyte imbalances. 5. Enhance elimination of salicylates as directed by forced diuresis, alkalinization of urine, peritoneal dialysis, or hemodialysis, according to severity of intoxication. 6. Monitor serum salicylate level for efficacy of treatment. 7. Administer specific prescribed pharmacologic agent for bleeding and other problems.

Alcohol Abuse

Acute Alcohol Intoxication

Alcohol is a psychotropic drug affecting mood, judgment, behavior, concentration, and consciousness. Many heavy drinkers are young adults as well as people over 60 years of age. There is a high prevalence of alcoholism in emergency department patients. Because alcoholic patients return frequently to the ED, they often are exasperating and tax the patience of health professionals caring for them. Their management requires increased patience as well as thoughtful and accurate treatment.

Assessment. *Ethanol* (alcohol) is a direct multisystem toxin and central nervous system depressant that causes drowsiness, incoordination, slurring of speech, sudden mood changes, aggression, belligerency, grandiosity, and uninhibited behavior. It can cause stupor, coma, and death if taken excessively.

The patient is assessed for head injury, hypoglycemia (which mimics intoxication), and other health problems. Nursing diagnoses may include ineffective breathing pattern related to central nervous system depression and risk for violence (self-directed or directed at others) related to severe intoxication from alcohol.

Emergency Management of the Acutely Intoxicated Patient. Treatment involves detoxification of the acute poisoning, recovery, or "drying out," and rehabilitation.

1. Approach the patient with a nonjudgmental manner.
   a. Expect the patient to use mechanisms of denial and defensiveness.
   b. Adopt a firm, consistent, accepting, and reasonable attitude.
   c. Speak calmly and slowly; alcohol interferes with thought processes.
   d. If appearing intoxicated, the patient probably is intoxicated even though he or she denies alcohol intake.
2. Obtain a sample for a blood alcohol test as directed.
3. Allow the drowsy patient to sleep off the state of alcoholic intoxication.
   a. Observe for symptoms of central nervous system depression.
   b. Maintain a patent airway.

c. Undress the patient and cover with a blanket.
4. Sedate the noisy, belligerent patient as directed.
   a. *Monitor the patient carefully;* observe for hypotension and decreased level of consciousness.
   b. Monitor cardiac and respiratory rates and blood pressure.
5. Examine the patient for injuries and organic disease, which can be masked by alcoholic intoxication. Persons with alcoholism suffer more injuries than the general population. Also, acute alcohol intoxication is the cause of trauma for many nonalcoholics.
   a. Assess neurologic status; observe for symptoms of head injury.
   b. *Assess for alcoholic coma, which is a medical emergency.*
   c. Monitor carefully for seizures.
   d. Evaluate for pulmonary infection.
      (1) Pulmonary infections are more common in patients with alcoholism, resulting from respiratory depression, an impaired defense system, and a tendency toward gastric aspiration.
      (2) The patient may show little increase in temperature or white blood cell count.
   e. Observe for hypoglycemia.
6. Hospitalize the patient if necessary or admit to a detoxification center; an effort should be made to examine problems underlying substance abuse.

Alcohol Withdrawal Delirium (Delirium Tremens)

Alcohol withdrawal delirium is an acute toxic state that occurs as a result of sudden withdrawal following a bout of heavy drinking or, more usually, prolonged intake of alcohol. Severity of symptoms depends on how much alcohol was ingested and for how long. It may be precipitated by acute injury or infection (pneumonia, pancreatitis, hepatitis).

Clinical Manifestations. Patients suspected of alcohol withdrawal delirium show signs of anxiety, uncontrollable fear, tremor, irritability, agitation, insomnia, and incontinence. They are talkative and preoccupied, and experience visual, tactile, olfactory, and auditory hallucinations that often are terrifying. Autonomic overactivity occurs and is evidenced by tachycardia, dilated pupils, and profuse perspiration. Usually, all vital signs are elevated in the alcoholic toxic state. Alcohol withdrawal delirium is life-threatening and carries a high mortality rate.

Emergency Management. Goals of management are to give proper sedation and support to allow the patient to rest and recover without danger of injury or peripheral vascular collapse.

1. Monitor blood pressure because the patient's subsequent treatment may depend on blood pressure readings.
2. Perform a physical examination to identify pre-existing or contributing illnesses or injuries (*e.g.*, head injury, pneumonia).
3. Obtain a drug history to elicit information that may facilitate adjustment of sedative requirement.
4. Sedate the patient as directed with a sufficient dosage of medication to establish and maintain sedation, which reduces agitation, prevents exhaustion, and promotes sleep.
   a. A variety of medications and combinations of medications are used; for example, chlordiazepoxide, diazepam, and paraldehyde. Haloperidol may be given for severe acute alcohol withdrawal delirium.
   b. Dosages are adjusted according to the patient's symptoms (agitation, anxiety) and blood pressure response.
5. Place the patient in a private room and observe closely.
   a. Keep the room lighted to minimize potential for illusions and hallucinations.
   b. Close closet and bathroom doors to eliminate shadows.
   c. Keep the environment calm and nonstressful.
   d. Observe the patient closely; homicidal or suicidal responses may result from hallucinations.
   e. Have someone stay with the patient as much as possible; the presence of another person has a reassuring and calming effect, which helps the patient maintain contact with reality.
   f. Explain visual misrepresentations (illusions) to strengthen the link with reality.
   g. Explain every procedure being performed.
   h. Eliminate loud noises.
   i. Call the patient by name.
   j. Use protective devices and restraints as prescribed if necessary or if the patient is not under direct and constant observation. (Precaution: The least restrictive device that will prevent the patient from injuring self and others is used. Caution is taken to ensure that restraints are applied properly and that they are not applied in such a way that they impair circulation to any part of the body or interfere with respirations. Physical observation (*e.g.*, skin integrity, circulatory status, respiratory status) is ongoing and the patient's response is documented.
6. Maintain electrolyte balance and hydration by way of oral or IV route as prescribed. Fluid losses may be present from gastrointestinal losses (diarrhea) profuse perspiration, and from the respiratory tract (hyperventilation). Or the patient may be overhydrated as a result of the effect of alcohol on antidiuretic hormone.
7. Record temperature, pulse, respiration, and blood pressure frequently (every 30 minutes in severe forms of delirium) in anticipation of peripheral circulatory collapse or hyperthermia (the two most lethal complications).
8. Administer phenytoin (Dilantin) or other anticonvulsant medications as prescribed to prevent or control repeated withdrawal seizures.
9. Assess the respiratory, hepatic, and cardiovascular status. Frequent complications are infections (pneumonia), trauma, hepatic failure, hypoglycemia, and cardiovascular problems.
   a. Hypoglycemia may accompany alcohol withdrawal because alcohol depletes liver glycogen stores and impairs gluconeogenesis; many patients with alcoholism suffer from malnutrition.
   b. Administer parenteral dextrose as prescribed if liver glycogen is depleted. Give orange juice, Gatorade, or other carbohydrates to stabilize the blood sugar and counteract tremulousness.

10. Provide supplemental vitamin therapy and a high-protein diet as prescribed to counteract vitamin deficiency.
11. Refer the patient to an alcoholic treatment center for follow-up and rehabilitation.

Psychiatric Emergencies

A psychiatric emergency is an urgent, serious disturbance of behavior, affect, or thought that makes the patient unable to cope with life situations and interpersonal relationships. A patient presenting with a psychiatric emergency may be overactive or violent, underactive or depressed, or suicidal.

The most important concern of the emergency department personnel is whether the patient is likely to inflict personal harm or cause injury to others. The aim is to try to maintain the patient's self-esteem (and life, if necessary) while carrying out assessment and management procedures. The patient is asked whether he or she is currently under psychiatric treatment.

Overactive Patients

Patients display disturbed, uncooperative, and paranoid behavior and have anxiety and panic-like feelings. They may be prone to assaultive and destructive impulses and abnormal social behavior. Intense nervousness, depression, and crying are evident in some patients. Disturbed and noisy behavior may be compounded by alcohol or drug intoxication.

Emergency Management

1. Determine from a reliable source the events that led to the crisis; whether the patient has had past mental illness, hospitalizations, injuries, or serious illnesses; whether the patient uses alcohol or drugs or has experienced crises in interpersonal relationships or intrapsychic conflicts.
   a. Be aware that abnormal thoughts and behavior may be manifestations of an underlying physical disorder, such as hypoglycemia, stroke, epilepsy, and drug or alcohol toxicity.
   b. Perform a physical assessment when possible.
2. Attempt to gain control of the situation.
   a. Approach the patient with a calm, confident, and firm manner; this attitude is therapeutic and has a calming effect.
   b. Introduce yourself by name.
   c. Tell the patient: "I am here to help you."
   d. Repeat the patient's name from time to time.
   e. Speak in one-thought sentences. Be consistent.
   f. Give the patient space. Let the patient slow him- or herself down and become compliant.
   g. Be interested in and listen to the patient; encourage the patient to talk about personal thoughts and feelings.
   h. Offer appropriate explanations. Tell the truth.
3. Administer a psychotropic agent for emergency management of functional psychosis as prescribed. Chlorpromazine (Thorazine) or haloperidol (Haldol) acts specifically against psychotic symptoms of thought fragmentation and perceptual and behavioral aberrations.
   a. The initial dosage depends on the patient's body weight and the severity of the symptoms.
   b. Observe the patient for 1 hour after the initial dose to determine the degree of change in psychotic behavior.
   c. Subsequent dosages depend on the patient's reaction.
   d. If the behavior is caused by hallucinogens (*e.g.*, LSD), psychotropic medications (exerting an effect on the mind) are not used.
4. Use restraints only as a last resort and as prescribed.
5. The patient is admitted to a psychiatric unit, or psychiatric outpatient treatment is arranged.

Violent Behavior

Violent and aggressive behavior is usually episodic and is a means of expressing feelings of anger, fear, or hopelessness about a situation. Usually, the patient has a history of outbursts of rage, temper tantrums, or impulsive behavior. Persons with a tendency for violence frequently lose control when intoxicated with alcohol or drugs. Family members are the most frequent victims of their aggression. Patients with a propensity for violence include those intoxicated by drugs or alcohol; those going through drug or alcohol withdrawal; and those with acute paranoid schizophrenic state, acute organic brain syndrome, acute psychosis, a paranoid character, a borderline personality, or an antisocial personality.

A specially designated room with at least two exits should be used for the interview. No objects that could be used as weapons should be in sight. If the interviewer feels anxious or uneasy about the patient's response, security staff, a family member, or another health care worker should be asked to remain in the hall nearby in the event that additional help is needed.

Nursing diagnoses could include risk for violence (self-directed or directed at others) related to out-of-control behavior. The goal is to bring the violence under control.

Emergency Management

1. Keep the door of the room open and remain in clear view of the staff. Stay between the patient and the door. However, do not block the patient's exit to the door because the patient may feel closed in and threatened.
2. Help the patient bring violence under control.
   a. Give the patient space. Do not make any sudden movement.
   b. If the patient is carrying a weapon, ask that it be surrendered.
   c. If the patient is unwilling to surrender the weapon, call the security staff; they may seek assistance from the local police department.
3. Do not leave the patient alone; this may be interpreted as rejection or provide an opportunity for self-harm.
4. Adopt a calm, noncritical approach and remain in control of the situation. External calm and structure may help the patient gain control.

5. Talk and listen to the patient.
   a. Crisis intervention is best done with an attitude of interest in the patient's well-being and with an attempt to tune in to the patient while remaining firm.
   b. Acknowledge the patient's state of agitation; for example, "I want to work with you to relieve your distress."
   c. Give the patient the opportunity to ventilate anger verbally; avoid challenging the delusional patient.
   d. Try to hear what the patient is saying.
   e. Convey an expectation of appropriate behavior and make the patient aware that help is available to gain control.
      (1) Let the patient know that the violent behavior may be frightening others and that violence is not acceptable.
      (2) Describe the help available in crisis situations: clinic, emergency department, mental health facility.
6. Allow security personnel or police to intervene if the patient does not become calm.
   a. Offer protection of hospitalization; this is usually welcomed by the patient who fears losing control or harming self or others.
   b. If the above fails to alleviate the patient's tension, administer medication as prescribed (rapid tranquilization with haloperidol, diazepam, or chlorpromazine) to reduce tension, anxiety, and hyperactivity.
   c. Use restraints when necessary but with a minimum of force. Obtain a physician's order for the restraints.
      (1) Use restraints with verbal intervention to calm and make the patient more compliant.
      (2) Have appropriate personnel available when applying restraints. (Precaution: The least restrictive device that will prevent the patient from injuring self and others is used. Caution is taken to ensure that restraints are applied properly and that they are not applied in such a way that they impair circulation to any part of the body or interfere with respirations. Physical observation (*e.g.*, skin integrity, circulatory status, respiratory status) is ongoing, and the patient's response is documented.)
7. Refer the patient for further mental health treatment after combativeness, agitation, and fear have decreased.

Depressed Patients

In the emergency department, depression may be seen as the primary condition bringing the patient to the health care facility, or depression may be masked by anxiety and somatic complaints.

The depressed person has some sort of mood disturbance. Assessment includes observing for sadness, apathy, feelings of worthlessness, self-blame, suicidal thoughts, desire to escape, avoidance of simple problems, anorexia and weight loss, lessened interest in sex; sleeplessness and ceaseless activity or reduction in activity.

The agitated depressed individual may exhibit motor restlessness and severe anxiety.

Emergency Management

1. Listen to the patient in a calm, unhurried manner.
   a. The patient benefits from ventilating personal feelings.
   b. Give the patient an opportunity to talk about personal problems.
   c. Anticipate that the patient may be suicidal.
   d. Attempt to find out if the patient has thought about or attempted suicide: "Have you ever thought about taking your own life?" The patient is generally relieved because of the opportunity to discuss personal feelings.
   e. Find out if there is an illness, perceived or real.
   f. Assess whether there has been sudden worsening of depression.
   g. Notify relatives about a seriously depressed patient. Do not leave the patient alone, because suicide usually is committed in solitude.
2. Give antidepressant and antianxiety agents as prescribed.
3. Emphasize to the patient that depression is treatable.
4. Be aware of crisis and supportive services in the community: mental health center, telephone counseling and referral, suicide prevention centers, group therapy, martial and family counseling, befriending programs.
5. Refer the patient for psychiatric consultation or to a psychiatric unit.

Suicidal Patients

Attempted suicide is an act that stems from depression (the loss of a loved one, the loss of body integrity or status, poor self-image) and can be viewed as a cry for help and intervention. Those at risk include elderly people; males; young adults; people who are enduring unusual loss or stress; those who are unemployed, divorced, widowed, or living alone; those who are showing significant depression (weight loss, sleep disturbances, somatic complaints, suicidal preoccupation); and those who have a history of previous suicidal attempt or completed suicide in the family, or who have a psychiatric illness.

Prevention

1. Be aware of persons at risk.
2. Determine whether a person has communicated *suicidal intent,* such as preoccupation with death or talking of someone else's suicide:
   "I'm tired of living."
   "I've put my affairs in order."
   "I'm better off dead."
   "I'm a burden to my family."
3. Determine whether there has been a previous suicide attempt as the risk is much greater in these cases.
4. Is there a family history of suicide?
5. Was there loss of a parent at an early age?

6. Is there a specific plan for suicide? A means to carry out the plan?

Emergency Management

1. Treat the consequences of the suicide attempt (*e.g.*, gunshot wound, drug overdose).
2. Prevent further self-injury; a patient who has made a suicidal gesture may do so again.
3. Employ crisis intervention (a form of brief psychotherapy) to determine suicidal potential; discover areas of depression and conflict; find out about the patient's support system; and determine whether hospitalization or psychiatric referral is necessary.
4. Arrange for admission to ICU if condition warrants; arrange for follow-up care or admission to the psychiatric unit depending on the suicide potential.

Family Violence, Abuse, and Neglect

Emergency departments are often the first place where victims of family violence, abuse, or neglect go to seek help. Statistics show that each year 3 to 4 million women are battered, 1.5 million children are seriously abused, an additional 5 million children are maltreated, and 2.5 million elders are abused or neglected (Tilden VP, et al, 1994). However, these figures are likely to underestimate the true extent of abuse and neglect.

Clinical Manifestations. When victims of abuse seek treatment, they may present with physical injuries or health problems such as anxiety, insomnia, or gastrointestinal symptoms that are related to stress. They usually do not disclose their abuser.

The possibility of abuse should be investigated whenever a person presents with multiple injuries that are in various stages of evolution or when injuries are unexplained or the explanation does not fit the physical picture. The possibility of neglect should be investigated whenever a dependent person with adequate resources and a designated care provider shows evidence of inattention to hygiene, nutrition, or to known medical needs such as unfilled medication prescriptions or missed appointments with health care providers. In EDs the most common physical injuries seen are unexplained bruises, lacerations, abrasions, head injuries, or fractures. The most common clinical manifestations of neglect are malnutrition and dehydration (Lachs & Pillemer, 1995).

Whenever evidence leads one to suspect abuse or neglect, an evaluation with careful documentation of descriptions of events and drawings of injuries is critical because the medical record may be used as part of a legal document. The patient's general appearance, interactions with significant others, an examination of the entire surface area of the body, and a mental status examination are crucial.

Detection. Nurses in EDs are in a unique position to provide early detection and interventions for victims of domestic violence. This requires an acute awareness of the signs of possible abuse, maltreatment, and neglect. They must be skilled in interviewing techniques that are likely to elicit accurate information. A careful history is crucial in the screening process. The following questions, asked and discussed in privacy from others, may be helpful in eliciting information about abuse, maltreatment, and neglect:

I noticed that you have a number of bruises. Can you tell me how they happened? Has anyone at home hurt you?
You seem frightened. Has anyone at home ever hurt you?
Sometimes patients tell me that they have been hurt by someone at home. Could this be happening to you?
Are you afraid of anyone at home? Or of anyone with whom you come in contact?
Has anyone failed to help you to take care of yourself when you needed help?
Has anyone prevented you from seeing friends or other people whom you wish to see?
Have you signed any papers that you did not understand?
Has anyone forced you to sign papers against your will?

Management. Whenever abuse, maltreatment, or neglect are suspected, the health care worker's primary concern should be the safety and welfare of the patient. Protocols of most emergency departments indicate that a multidisciplinary approach be used. Nurses, physicians, social workers, and community agencies work collaboratively to develop and implement a plan for meeting the patient's needs.

If in immediate danger, the patient should be separated from the abusing or neglecting person whenever possible. On the basis of this danger, or on the basis of injuries or neglected medical conditions, hospitalization is justified until alternative plans are made. However, it must be remembered that third-party payers may not approve hospitalization that is based solely on abuse or neglect.

When abuse or neglect is considered to be the result of stress experienced by a care giver who is no longer able to cope with the burden of caring for an elderly person or a person with chronic disease, respite services may be necessary. Support groups may be helpful to these care givers. When pathologic mental factors in the person who is abusing or neglecting are responsible for the situation, alternative living arrangements may be required.

It must be remembered that competent adults are free to accept or refuse the help that is offered to them. Some patients will insist on remaining in the home environment where the abuse or neglect is occurring. For patients who are competent and not cognitively impaired, their wishes should be respected. However, all possible alternatives and available resources should be explored with the patient.

Mandatory reporting laws that require health care workers to report suspected abuse to an official agency, usually Adult (or Child) Protective Services, exist in 42 states. In most of these states suspected abuse is all that is required for reporting and the health care worker is not required to prove anything. Likewise, health care workers who report suspected abuse are immune to civil or criminal liability if the report is made in good faith. The subsequent home visit that results from the reporting of suspected abuse is part of the process of gathering further information about the patient in the home environment. In addition, many states have resource hotlines that can be used by health care workers and patients who seek answers to questions about abuse and neglect.

Sexual Assault

The legal definition of *rape* is carnal knowledge of a female by force or the threat of force against her will. However, rape is not only a female crime. It happens to males, especially young males. It is one of the fastest growing violent crimes. The feminist movement has focused on the rights and care of rape victims, and law enforcement agencies are becoming increasingly sensitive and aggressive in managing these crimes. Rape crisis centers offer extensive support, educate victims, and help them through the subsequent courtroom experience.

The manner in which the patient is received and treated in the emergency department is important to his or her future psychologic well-being. Crisis intervention should begin when the patient enters the health facility. The patient should be seen immediately on entry into the emergency department. Most hospitals have a written protocol that reflects consideration for the victim's physical and emotional needs as well as concern for meeting requirements for subsequent legal proceedings.

Phases of Psychologic Reaction to Rape

The patient's reaction to rape has been termed *rape trauma syndrome* and is seen as an acute stress reaction to a life-threatening situation. The nurse performing the assessment is aware that the patient may go through several phases of psychologic reactions:

1. Acute disorganization phase that may be manifested in two ways:
   a. Expressed state, in which shock, disbelief, fear, guilt, humiliation, anger, and other such emotions are encountered.
   b. Controlled state, in which feelings are masked or hidden and the victim appears composed.
2. Phase of denial and unwillingness to talk about the incident, followed by a phase of heightened anxiety, fear, flashbacks, sleep disturbances, hyperalertness, and psychosomatic reactions.
3. Phase of reorganization, in which the incident is put into perspective. Some victims never fully recover and develop chronic stress disorders and phobias.

Nursing diagnoses may include rape trauma syndrome related to a life-threatening situation. The patient's goal is to regain control over his or her life.

Emergency Management. Goals of management are to give sympathetic support, to reduce the emotional trauma of the patient, and to gather available evidence for possible legal proceedings.

1. Respect the privacy and sensitivity of the patient; be kind and supportive.
   a. Reassure the patient that anxiety is natural and that appropriate support is available from professional and community resources. Contact Rape Victim Companion Program, if available in the community, and request services of a volunteer.
   b. Accept the emotional reactions of the patient (*e.g.*, hysteria, stoicism, overwhelmed feeling).
   c. Do not leave the patient alone.
2. Assist with the physical examination.
   a. Secure written, witnessed informed consent from the patient (or parent or guardian if the patient is a minor) for examination, for taking photographs if necessary, and for release of findings to police.
   b. Take history only if the patient has not already talked to a police officer, social worker, or crisis intervention worker. Do not ask the patient to repeat the history. Record the history of the event in the patient's own words.
   c. Ask if the patient has bathed, douched, brushed teeth, changed clothes, urinated, or defecated since the attack; this may alter interpretation of subsequent findings.
   d. Record the time of admission, time of examination, date and time of alleged rape, and general appearance of the patient.
      (1) Document any evidence of trauma: discoloration, bruises, lacerations, secretions, torn and bloody clothing.
      (2) Document emotional state.
   e. Assist the patient to undress; drape properly.
      (1) Ask the patient to place each item of clothing in a separate paper bag. (Plastic bags promote moisture retention, which may lead to the formation of mold and mildew which can destroy evidence.)
      (2) Label bags appropriately; give to appropriate law enforcement authorities.
   f. Examine the patient (from head to toe) for injuries, especially to the head, neck, breast, thighs, back, and buttocks.
      (1) Assess for external evidence of trauma (bruises, contusions, lacerations, stab wounds).
      (2) Assess for dried semen stains (appearing as crusted, flaking areas) on the patient's body or clothes.
      (3) Inspect fingers for broken nails and tissue and foreign materials under nails.
      (4) Assist in conducting oral examination. Secure a specimen of saliva; take prescribed cultures of gum and tooth areas.
      (5) Document evidence of trauma with body diagrams and photographs.
3. Assist with pelvic and rectal examinations.
   a. Advise the patient of the nature and necessity of each procedure; give the rationale for each question asked.
      (1) Examine perineum (and other areas) with a Woods lamp or other filtered ultraviolet light; areas that are found fluorescent may indicate semen stains.
      (2) Note color and consistency of any discharge present.

(3) Use a water-moistened vaginal speculum for examination; do not use lubricant, which contains chemicals that may interfere with later forensic testing of specimens and acid phosphatase determinations.

b. Assist with securing laboratory specimens.

(1) Collect vaginal aspirate, which is examined for presence or absence of motile and nonmotile sperm.

(2) Use a sterile swab to draw secretions from the vaginal pool for acid phosphatase, blood group antigen of semen, and precipitin test against human sperm and blood.

(3) Obtain separate smears from the oral, vaginal, and anal areas.

(4) Obtain culture of body orifices for gonorrhea.

(5) Obtain blood serum for syphilis; a sample of serum may be frozen and saved for future testing.

(6) Conduct a pregnancy test if there is a possibility that the patient may be pregnant.

(7) Collect foreign material (leaves, grass, dirt) and place in a clean envelope.

(8) Comb the pubic hairs with a prepackaged clean comb. Trim areas of pubic hair suspected of containing semen. Obtain several pubic hairs with follicles; place in separate containers and identify these as patient's pubic hairs.

(9) Examine rectum for signs of trauma, blood, semen stains.

(10) Label each specimen with name of patient, date, time of collection, body area from which specimen was obtained, and names of personnel collecting specimens to preserve chain of evidence; give to designated person (*e.g.*, crime laboratory technician) and obtain an itemized receipt.

(11) Photographs are taken by designated person.

4. Treat associated injuries as indicated. Give the patient the option of prophylaxis against sexually transmitted disease.
   a. Intramuscular ceftriaxone (Rocephin) administered with 1% xylocaine may be prescribed as prophylaxis for gonorrhea.
   b. Doxycycline (Vibramycin) taken for 10 days may be prescribed as prophylaxis for syphilis and chlamydia.
5. Antipregnancy measures may be considered if the patient is of childbearing age, is not using contraceptives, and is at high risk in her menstrual cycle.
   a. A postcoital contraceptive drug may be prescribed after a pregnancy test: Ovral contains estrogen ethinyl estradiol and progestin norgestrel.
   b. To promote effectiveness, it is preferable that Ovral be administered within 12 to 24 hours and no later than 72 hours after intercourse; the 21-day package rather than the 28-day package is prescribed so that the patient does not take the inert tablets by mistake.
   c. An antiemetic may be given as prescribed to decrease discomfort from side effects.
6. Offer cleansing douche, mouthwash, and fresh clothing.
7. Provide for follow-up services:
   a. Make an appointment for follow-up surveillance for pregnancy, sexually transmitted disease, and HIV testing.
   b. Inform the patient of counseling services to prevent long-term psychologic effects; counseling services should be made available to both the patient and the family; referral is made to the Rape Victim Companion Program if available.
   c. Encourage the patient to return to the previous level of functioning as soon as possible.

CRITICAL THINKING EXERCISES

1. You are assigned to the triage area of an emergency department. A middle-aged man walks up to you and says that he drove himself to the hospital after experiencing indigestion at a local restaurant. He states, "It's probably nothing, but I thought I should be checked." Describe how you would proceed to assess this patient; what possible findings are you checking for? What is the range of possibilities, and what findings would indicate a serious situation or confirm the patient's feeling that it is nothing serious?
2. A homeless man comes to the emergency department for treatment of frostbite of his feet. He insists that his feet be placed in a pan of hot water. Describe how you would respond and the explanation you would give to this patient. How would you proceed with discharge planning for a homeless person?
3. A young woman with a toddler in her arms waits her turn in line at the triage desk of the emergency department. The child is crying and rubbing her eyes and face. You overhear the mother telling another patient that the child has had an allergic reaction to her first soft-cooked egg, which the child smeared on her face. Analyze this information and explain the conclusion you would draw and why; then describe the action you would take and the rationale for your decision.
4. An elderly patient is brought to the emergency department by her son. She is complaining of pain in her hip, and the son says that she tripped over a child's toy and fell. Upon initial assessment you notice that the patient has many bruises on her body in varying stages of resolution. What conclusions might you draw from these findings, and how might you proceed to evaluate the situation to determine what your course of action will be?

d. The patient should be accompanied by a family member or friend when leaving the health care facility.

BIBLIOGRAPHY

Books

Roberts JR and Hedges J. Clinical Procedures in Emergency Medicine, 2nd ed. Philadelphia, WB Saunders, 1991.

Wright JE and Shelton BK. Desk Reference for Critical Care Nursing. Boston, Jones and Bartlett, 1993.

Journals

Arendt DL and Arendt DB. Rescue operations for Snakebite. Am J Nurs 1992 Jul; 92(7):26–30.

Bauer J et al. Evaluation of behavioral and cognitive changes: The mental status examination. Emerg Med Clin North Am 1991 Feb; 9(1):1–12.

Beachley M. Abdominal trauma: Putting the pieces together. Am J Nurs 1993 Nov; 11:93(11):26–33.

Birrer RB. Heat stroke: Don't wait for the classic signs. Emerg Med 1994 Jul; 26(9):43–50.

Blackwell TH. Prehospital care. Emerg Med Clin North Am 1993 Feb;11(1):1–14.

Bonilla J et al. Hemorrhagic shock: Contemporary and future therapy. Trauma Q 1992 Aug; 8(4):38–53.

Buzan RD and Weissberg MP. Suicide: Risk factors and therapeutic considerations in the Emergency Department. J Emerg Med 1992 May/Jun; 10(3):335–343.

Chez N. Helping the victim of domestic violence. Am J Nurs 1994 July; 94(7):32-37.

Chisholm CD. Wound evaluation and cleansing. Emerg Med Clin North Am 1992 Sep; 10(4):665–672.

Colucciello SA. Blunt abdominal trauma. Emerg Med Clin North Am 1993 Feb; 11(1):107–123.

Coniglio K. Cocaine-induced acute myocardial infarction. Crit Care Nurse 1991 Feb; 11(2):16–22.

Denis DM. Acquired immunodeficiency syndrome: Ten years later. J Emerg Nurs 1991 Dec; 17(6):419-423.

Denis DM. ED response to the increased incidence of tuberculosis. J Emerg Nursing 1991 Aug; 17(4):244–245.

Edlich RF and Kubler-Ross E. On death and dying in the Emergency Department. J Emerg Med 1992 Mar/Apr; 10(2):225–229.

Glankler DM. Caring for the victim of near drowning. Crit Care Nurse 1993 Aug; 13(4):25–32.

Gold BS and Barish RA. Venomous snakebites. Emerg Med Clin North Am 1992 May; 10(2):249–267.

Goldman B. Facing up to violent patients. Emerg Med 1994 Jun; 26(8):121–126.

Green E. Charting the future of emergency drug protocols. Nursing 1992 Jun; 22(6):55–57.

Griffiths SE. Removing an esophogeal obturator airway. Nursing 1992 Oct; 22(10):33.

Harrahil M. Patterns of sharp force injury. J Emerg Nurs 1992 Aug; 18(4):355-356.

Hoffman DP and Dubovsky SL. Depression and suicide assessment. Emerg Med Clin North Am 1991 Feb; 9(1):107–121.

Hopkins AG. The trauma nurse's role with families in crisis. Crit Care Nurse 1994 Apr; 14(2):35–43.

Hurlbut K. Drug-induced psychoses. Emerg Med Clin North Am 1991 Feb; 9(1):31–52.

Jackimczyk K. Blunt chest trauma. Emerg Med Clin North Am 1993 Feb; 11(1):81–96.

Jackson L. Quick responses to hypothermia and frostbite. Am J Nurs 1995 Mar; 95(3):52-53.

Jolly T and Ghezzi KT. Accidental hypothermia. Emerg Med Clin North Am 1992 May; 10(2):311–327.

Jordan RC. Penetrating chest trauma. Emerg Med Clin North Am 1993 Feb; 11(1):97–206.

Kercher EE. Crisis intervention in the Emergency Department. Emerg Med Clin North Am 1991 Feb; 9(1):219–232.

Kinkle SL. Violence in the ED: How to stop it before it starts. Am J Nurs 1993 Jul; 93(7):22-24.

Kuhn MM. Colloids vs. crystalloids. Crit Care Nurse 1991 May; 11(5):37–51.

Kulig K. Initial management of ingestions of toxic substances. N Engl J Med 1992 Jun; 326(25):1677–1681.

Lachs MS and Pillemer K. Abuse and neglect of elderly persons. New Engl J Med 1995 Feb; 332(7):437–443.

Marx JA. Penetrating abdominal trauna. Emerg Med Clin North Am 1993 Feb; 11(1):125–135

Messerve KL. Preserving medicolegal evidence: A guide for emergency care providers. J Emerg Nurs 1992 Apr; 18(2):120–123.

Mathews PJ. Artificial airways. Nursing 1992 Jan; 22(1):53–59.

Olshaker JS and Whye DW. Head trauma. Emerg Med Clin North Am 1993 Feb; 11(1):165–186.

Olshaker JS. Near drowning. Emerg Med Clin North Am 1992 May; 10(2):339–350.

Rice MM and Moore GP. Management of the violent patient. Emerg Med Clin North Am 1991 Feb; 9(1):13–30.

Rice V. Shock, a clinical syndrome: An update. Part 1. Crit Care Nurse 1991 Apr; 11(4):20–27.

Rice V. Shock, a clinical syndrome: An update. Part 2. Crit Care Nurse 1991 May; 11(5):74–85.

Rice V. Shock, a clinical syndrome: An update. Part 3. Crit Care Nurse 1991 Jun; 11(6):34–39.

Rice V. Shock, a clinical syndrome: An update. Part 4. Crit Care Nurse 1991; 11(6):28–40.

Rogers B and Travers P. Overview of work-related hazards in nursing: Health and safety issues. Heart Lung 1991 Sep; 20(5): 486–495.

Rorison DG and McPherson SJ. Acute toxic inhalations. Emerg Med Clin North Am 1992 May; 10(2):409–435.

Russel S. Septic shock. Can you recognize the clues? Nursing 1994 Apr; 24(4):40–46.

Russel S. Septic shock. Is your patient at risk? Nursing 1994 Apr; 24(4):34–39.

Ruth-Sahd L. Pulmonary contusion: The hidden danger in blunt chest trauma. Crit Care Nurse 1991 Jun; 11(6):46–57.

Ruth-Sahd L. Treating carbon monoxide poisoning. Nursing 1992 Jan; 22(1):33.

Schmidt J and Moore GP. Management of multiple trauma. Emerg Med Clin North Am 1993 Feb; 11(1):29–51.

Schmidt TA et al. Sudden death in the ED: Educating residents to compassionately inform families. J Emerg Med 1992 Sep/Oct; 10(5):643–647.

Snyder JA. Emergency department protocols for domestic violence. J Emerg Nurs 1994 Feb; 20(1):65–68.

Soloway RA. Street smart advice on treating drug overdoses. Am J Nurs 1993 Sep; 93(9):65–68.

Sommers MS. The near-death experience following multiple trauma. Crit Care Nurse 1994 Apr; 14(2):62–66.

Stoloff R et al. Emergency medical recognition and management of idiopathic anaphylaxis. J Emerg Med 1992 Nov/Dec; 10(6): 693–698.

Tek D and Olshaker JS. Heat illness. Emerg Med Clin North Am 1992 May; 10(2):299–310.

Tilden VP et al. Factors that influence clinicians' assessment and management of family violence. Am J Pub Health 1994 April; 84(4):628-633.

Trunkey D. Initial treatment of patients extensive trauma. Current Concepts 1991 May; 324(18):1259–1263.

Utecht MJ et al. Heroin body packers. J Emerg Med 1993 Jan/Feb; 11(1):33–40.
Walls RM. Airway management. Emerg Med Clin North Am 1993 Feb; 11(1):53–60.
Walters DT and Tupin JP. Family grief in the Emergency Department. Emerg Med Clin North Am 1991 Feb; 9(1):189–206.
Weinman SA. Emergency management of drug overdose. Crit Care Nurse 1993 Dec; 13(6):45–51.
Willens JS. Strengthen your life support skills. Nursing 1993 Apr; 23(4):54–58.
Wofford JL et al. The role of emergency services in health care for the elderly: A review. J Emerg Med 1993 May/Jun; 11(3):317–326.

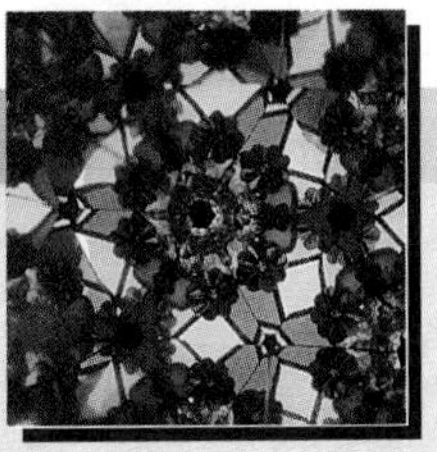

OUTLINE

Abbreviations
Reference Ranges—Hematology
Reference Ranges—Serum, Plasma, and Whole Blood Chemistries
Reference Ranges—Urine Chemistry
Reference Ranges—Cerebrospinal Fluid (CSF)
Miscellaneous Values
Reference Ranges—Immunodiagnostic Tests

Appendix: Diagnostic Studies and Their Meaning

Abbreviations

Conventional Units

kg = kilogram
gm = gram
mg = milligram
μg = microgram
μμg = micromicrogram
ng = nanogram
pg = picogram
dl = 100 milliliters
ml = milliliter
mm^3 = cubic millimeter
fL = femtoliter
mM = millimole
nM = nanomole
mOsm = milliosmole
mm = millimeter
μ = micron or micrometer
mmHg = millimeters of mercury
U = unit
mU = milliunit
μU = microunit
mEq = milliequivalent
IU = International Unit
mIU = milliInternational Unit

SI Units

g = gram
L = liter
d = day
h = hour
mol = mole
mmol = millimole
μmol = micromole
nmol = nanomole
pmol = picomole

Reference Ranges—Hematology*

	Reference Range		
Determination	**Conventional Units**	**SI Units**	**Clinical Significance**
A_2 hemoglobin	1.5%–3.5% of total hemoglobin	Mass fraction: 0.015–0.035 of total hemoglobin	Increased in certain types of thalassemia
Bleeding time	1–9 min	2–8 min	Prolonged in thrombocytopenia, defective platelet function, and aspirin therapy
Factor V assay (proaccelerin factor)	60%–140%		
Factor VIII assay (antihemophiliac factor)	50%–200%		Deficient in classical hemophilia
Factor IX assay (plasma thromboplastin component)	75%–125%		Deficient in Christmas disease (pseudohemophilia)
Factor X (Stuart factor)	60%–140%		Deficient in Stuart clotting defect
Fibrinogen	200–400 mg/dl	2–4 g/dl	Increased in pregnancy, infections accompanied by leukocytosis, nephrosis Decreased in severe liver disease, abruptio placenta
Fibrin split products	< 10 mg/L	Less than 10 mg/L	Increased in disseminated intravascular coagulation
Fibrinolysins (whole blood clot lysis time)	No lysis in 24 hr		Increased activity associated with massive hemorrhage, extensive surgery, transfusion reactions
Partial thromboplastin time (activated)	20–45 sec		Prolonged in deficiency of fibrinogen, factors II, V, VIII, IX, X, XI, and XII, and in heparin therapy
Prothrombin consumption	> 20 sec		Impaired in deficiency of factors VIII, IX, and X
Prothrombin time INR	9.5–12 sec 1.0		Prolonged by deficiency of factors, I, II, V, VII, and X, fat malabsorption, severe liver disease, coumarin-anticoagulant therapy. INR used to standardize the prothrombin time and anticoagulation therapy.
Erythrocyte count	Males: 4,6000,000–6,200,000/ mm^3	4.6–6.2 × 10^{12}/L	Increased in severe diarrhea and dehydration, polycythemia, acute poisoning, pulmonary fibrosis
	Females: 4,200,000–5,400,000/ mm^3	4.2–5.4 × 10^{12}/L	Decreased in all anemias, in leukemia, and after hemorrhage, when blood volume has been restored
Erythrocyte indices			
Mean corpuscular volume (MCV)	80–94 (cu μ)	80–94 fL	Increased in macrocytic anemias; decreased in microcytic anemia
Mean corpuscular hemoglobin (MCH)	27–32 μμg/cell	27–32 pg	Increased in macrocytic anemias; decreased in microcytic anemia
Mean corpuscular hemoglobin concentration (MCHC)	33%–38%	Concentration fraction: 0.33–0.38	Decreased in severe hypochromic anemia

(continued)

Reference Ranges—Hematology* *(continued)*

Determination	Reference Range: Conventional Units	Reference Range: SI Units	Clinical Significance
Reticulocytes	0.5%–1.5% of red cells	Number fraction: 0.005–0.015	Increased with any condition stimulating increase in bone marrow activity (*i.e.,* infection, blood loss [acute and chronic]); following iron therapy in iron deficiency anemia, polycythemia rubra vera Decreased with any condition depressing bone marrow activity, acute leukemia, late stage of severe anemias
Erythrocyte sedimentation rate (ESR)—Westergren method	Males under 50 yr: <15 mm./hr Males over 50 yr: <20 mm/hr Females under 50 yr: <20 mm/hr Females over 50 yr: <30 mm/hr	<15 mm/hr <20 mm/hr <20 mm/hr <30 mm/hr	Increased in tissue destruction, whether inflammatory or degenerative; during menstruation and pregnancy; and in acute febrile diseases
Erythrocyte sedimentation ratio—Zeta centrifuge	41%–54% in both sexes	Fraction: 0.41–0.54	Significance similar to ESR
Hematocrit	Males: 42%–50% Females: 40%–48%	Volume fraction: 0.42–0.5 Volume fraction: 0.4–0.48	Decreased in severe anemias, anemia of pregnancy, acute massive blood loss Increased in erythrocytosis of any cause, and in dehydration or hemoconcentration associated with shock
Hemoglobin	Males:13–18 gm/dl Females: 12–15 gm/dl	2.02–2.79 mmol/L 1.86–2.48 mmol/L	Decreased in various anemias, pregnancy, severe or prolonged hemorrhage, and with excessive fluid intake Increased in polycythemia, chronic obstructive pulmonary diseases, failure of oxygenation because of congestive heart failure, and normally in people living at high altitudes
Hemoglobin F	Less than 2% of total hemoglobin	Mass fraction: <0.02	Increased in infants and children, and in thalassemia and many anemias
Leukocyte alkaline phosphatase	Score of 40–100		Increased in polycythemia vera, myelofibrosis, and infections Decreased in chronic granulocytic leukemia, paroxysmal nocturnal hemoglobinuria, hypoplastic marrow, and viral infections, particularly infectious mononucleosis

(continued)

Reference Ranges—Hematology* *(continued)*

	Reference Range		
Determination	**Conventional Units**	**SI Units**	**Clinical Significance**
Leukocyte count Neutrophils Eosinophils Basophils Lymphocytes Monocytes	Total: 5,000–10,000/mm^3 60%–70% 1%–4% 0%–0.5% 20%–30% 2%–6%	5–10 × 10^9/L Number fraction: 0.6–0.7 Number fraction: 0.01–0.04 Number fraction: 0.00–0.05 Number fraction: 0.2–0.3 Number fraction: 0.02–0.06	Elevated in acute infectious diseases, predominantly in the neutrophilic fraction with bacterial diseases, and in the lymphocytic and monocytic fractions in viral diseases Elevated in acute leukemia, following menstruation, and following surgery or trauma Depressed in aplastic anemia, agranulocytosis, and by toxic agents such as chemotherapeutic agents used in treating malignancy Eosinophils elevated in collagen disease, allergy, intestinal parasitosis
Osmotic fragility of red cells	Increased if hemolysis occurs in over 0.5% NaCl Decreased if hemolysis is incomplete in 0.3% NaCl		Increased in congenital spherocytosis, idiopathic acquired hemolytic anemia, isoimmune hemolytic disease, ABO hemolytic disease of newborn Decreased in sickle cell anemia, thalassemia
Platelet count	100,000–400,000/mm^3	0.1–0.4 × 10^{12}/L	Increased in malignancy, myeloproliferative disease, rheumatoid arthritis, and postoperatively; about 50% of patients with unexpected increase of platelet count will be found to have a malignancy Decreased in thrombocytopenic purpura, acute leukemia, aplastic anemia, and during cancer chemotherapy, infections, and drug reactions

*Laboratory values vary according to the techniques used in different laboratories.

Reference Ranges—Serum, Plasma, and Whole Blood Chemistries

	Normal Adult Reference Range		Clinical Significance	
Determination	**Conventional Units**	**SI Units**	**Increased**	**Decreased**
Acetoacetate	0.2–1.0 mg/dl	19.6–98 μmol/L	Diabetic acidosis Fasting	
Acetone	0.3–2.0 mg/dl	51.6–344.0 μmol/L	Toxemia of pregnancy Carbohydrate-free diet High-fat diet	

(continued)

Reference Ranges—Serum, Plasma, and Whole Blood Chemistries *(continued)*

Determination	Normal Adult Reference Range: Conventional Units	Normal Adult Reference Range: SI Units	Clinical Significance: Increased	Clinical Significance: Decreased
Adrenocorticotropic hormone (ACTH) (plasma)—RIA*	Less than 50 pg/ml	Less than 50 mg/L	Pituitary-dependent Cushing's syndrome Ectopic ACTH syndrome Primary adrenal atrophy	Adrenocortical tumor Adrenal insufficiency secondary to hypopituitarism
Aldolase	3–8 Sibley-Lehninger U/dl at 37°C	22–59 mU/L at 37°C	Hepatic necrosis Granulocytic leukemia Myocardial infarction Skeletal muscle disease	
Aldosterone (plasma)—RIA	Supine: 3–10 ng/dl Upright: 5–30 ng/dl Adrenal vein: 200–800 ng/dl	0.08–0.30 nmol/L 0.14–0.90 nmol/L 5.54–22.16 nmol/L	Primary aldosteronism (Conn's syndrome) Secondary aldosteronism	Addison's disease
Alpha-1-antitrypsin	200–400 mg/dl	2–4 g/L		Certain forms of chronic lung and liver disease in young adults
Alpha-1-fetoprotein	None detected		Hepatocarcinoma Metastatic carcinoma of liver Germinal cell carcinoma of the testis or ovary Fetal neural tube defects—elevation in maternal serum	
Alpha-hydroxybutyric dehydrogenase	Up to 140 U/ml	Up to 140 U/L	Myocardial infarction Granulocytic leukemia Hemolytic anemias Muscular dystrophy	
Ammonia (plasma)	40–80 µg/dl (enzymatic method); varies considerably with method	22.2–44.3 µmol/L	Severe liver disease Hepatic decompensation	
Amylase	60–160 Somogyi U/dl	111–296 U/L	Acute pancreatitis Mumps Duodenal ulcer Carcinoma of head of pancreas Prolonged elevation with pseudocyst of pancreas Increased by drugs that constrict pancreatic duct sphincters: morphine, codeine, cholinergics	Chronic pancreatitis Pancreatic fibrosis and atrophy Cirrhosis of liver Pregnancy (2nd and 3rd trimesters)
Arsenic	6–20 µg/dl; if 50 µg/dl, suspect toxicity	0.78–2.6 µmol/L	Accidental or intentional poisoning Excessive occupational exposure	
Ascorbic acid (vitamin C)	0.4–1.5 mg/dl	23–85 µmol/L	Large doses of ascorbic acid as a prophylactic against the common cold	
Bilirubin	Total: 0.1–1.2 mg/dl	1.7–20.5 µmol/L	Hemolytic anemia (indirect)	

*By radioimmunoassay

(continued)

Reference Ranges—Serum, Plasma, and Whole Blood Chemistries *(continued)*

	Normal Adult Reference Range		**Clinical Significance**	
Determination	**Conventional Units**	**SI Units**	**Increased**	**Decreased**
	Direct: 0.1–0.2 mg/dl	17–3.4 μmol/L	Biliary obstruction and disease	
	Indirect: 0.1–1 mg/dl	1.7–17.1 μmol/L	Hepatocellular damage (hepatitis) Pernicious anemia Hemolytic disease of newborn	
Blood gases				
Oxygen, arterial (whole blood):				
Partial pressure (PaO_2)	95–100 mm Hg	12.64–13.30 kPa	Polycythemia	Anemia
Saturation (SaO_2)	94%–100%	Volume fraction: 0.94–1	Anhydremia	Cardiac decompensation Chronic obstructive pulmonary disease
Carbon dioxide, arterial (whole blood): partial pressure ($PaCO_2$)	35–45 mm Hg	4.66–5.99 kPa	Respiratory acidosis Metabolic alkalosis	Respiratory alkalosis Metabolic acidosis
*p*H (whole blood, arterial)	7.35–7.45	7.35–7.45	Vomiting Hyperpnea Fever Intestinal obstruction	Uremia Diabetic acidosis Hemorrhage Nephritis
Calcitonin	Basal: nondetectable 400 pg/ml	400 ng/L	Medullary carcinoma of the thyroid Some nonthyroid tumors Zollinger-Ellison syndrome	
Calcium	8.5–10.5 mg/dl	2.125–2.625 mmol/L	Tumor or hyperplasia of parathyroid Hypervitaminosis D Multiple myeloma Nephritis with uremia Malignant tumors Sarcoidosis Hyperthyroidism Skeletal immobilization Excess calcium intake: milk-alkali syndrome	Hypoparathyroidism Diarrhea Celiac disease Vitamin D deficiency Acute pancreatitis Nephrosis After parathyroidectomy
CO_2, venous	Adults: 24–32 mEq/L Infants: 18–24 mEq/L	24–32 mmol/L 18–24 mmol/L	Tetany Respiratory disease Intestinal obstruction Vomiting	Acidosis Nephritis Eclampsia Diarrhea Anesthesia
Carcinoembryonic antigen (CEA)—RIA	0–2.5 ng/ml (nonsmoker) 0–5 ng/ml (smoker)	0–2.5 μg/L (nonsmoker) 0–5 μg/L (smoker)	The repeatedly high incidence of this antigen in cancers of the colon, rectum, pancreas, and stomach suggests that CEA levels may be useful in the therapeutic monitoring of these conditions.	

(continued)

Reference Ranges—Serum, Plasma, and Whole Blood Chemistries *(continued)*

	Normal Adult Reference Range		Clinical Significance	
Determination	**Conventional Units**	**SI Units**	**Increased**	**Decreased**
Catecholamines (plasma)—RIA	Epinephrine, random: up to 90 pg/ml Norepinephrine, random 100–550 pg/ml Dopamine, random up to 130 pg/ml	Up to 490 pmol/L 590–3240 pmol/L Up to 850 pmol/L	Pheochromocytoma	
Ceruloplasmin	30–80 mg/dl	300–800 mg/L		Wilson's disease (hepatolenticular degeneration)
Chloride	95–105 mEq/L	95–105 mmol/L	Nephrosis Nephritis Urinary obstruction Cardiac decompensation Anemia	Diabetes Diarrhea Vomiting Pneumonia Heavy metal poisoning Cushing's syndrome Burns Intestinal obstruction Febrile conditions
Cholesterol	150–200 mg/dl	3.9–5.2 mmol/L	Lipemia Obstructive jaundice Diabetes Hypothyroidism	Pernicious anemia Hemolytic anemia Hyperthyroidism Severe infection Terminal states of debilitating disease
Cholesterol esters	60%–70% of total	Fraction of total cholesterol 0.6–0.7		The esterified fraction decreases in liver diseases
Cholinesterase	Serum: 0.6–1.6 delta pH Red cells: 0.6–1 delta pH	0.6–1.6 U 0.6–1 U	Nephrosis Exercise	Nerve gas intoxication (greater effect on red cell activity) Insecticides, organic phosphates (greater effect on plasma activity)
Chorionic gonadotropin, beta subunit—RIA	0–5 IU/L	0–5 IU/L	Pregnancy Hydatidiform mole Choriocarcinoma	
Complement, human C_3	70–150 mg/dl	880–2520 mg/L	Some inflammatory diseases, acute myocardial infarction, cancer	Acute glomerulonephritis Disseminated lupus erythematosus with renal involvement
Complement C_4	16–45 mg/dl	140–510 mg/L	Some inflammatory diseases, acute myocardial infarction, cancer	Often decreased in immunologic disease, especially with active systemic lupus erythematosus Hereditary angioneurotic edema
Complement, total (hemolytic)	90%–94% complement	25–70 U/ml	Some inflammatory diseases	Acute glomerulonephritis Epidemic meningitis Subacute bacterial endocarditis

(continued)

Reference Ranges—Serum, Plasma, and Whole Blood Chemistries *(continued)*

	Normal Adult Reference Range		Clinical Significance	
Determination	**Conventional Units**	**SI Units**	**Increased**	**Decreased**
Copper	70–165 µg/dl	11–25.9 µmol/L	Cirrhosis of liver Pregnancy	Wilson's disease
Cortisol—RIA	8 AM: 7–25 µg/dl 4 PM: 2–9 µg/dl	193–690 nmol/L 55–248 nmol/L	Stress: infectious disease, surgery, burns, etc. Pregnancy Cushing's syndrome Pancreatitis Eclampsia	Addison's disease Anterior pituitary hypofunction
C-peptide reactivity	1.5–10 ng/ml	1.5–10 µg/L	Insulinoma	Diabetes
Creatine	0.2–0.8 mg/ml	15.3–61 µmol/L	Pregnancy Skeletal muscle necrosis or atrophy Starvation Hyperthyroidism	
Creatine phosphokinase (CPK)	Males: 50–325 mU/ml Females: 50–250 mU/ml	50–325 U/L 50–250 U/L	Myocardial infarction Skeletal muscle diseases Intramuscular injections Crush syndrome Hypothyroidism Alcohol withdrawal delirium Alcoholic myopathy Cerebrovascular disease	
Creatine phosphokinase isoenzymes	MM: 100% MB: 0% BB: 0%		MB increased in myocardial infarction, ischemia	
Creatinine	0.7–1.4 mg/dl	62–124 µmol/L	Nephritis Chronic renal disease	Kidney diseases
Creatinine clearance	100–150 ml of blood cleared of creatinine per min	1.67–2.5 ml/sec		
Cryoglobulins, qualitative	Negative		Multiple myeloma Chronic lymphocytic leukemia Lymphosarcoma Systemic lupus erythematosus Rheumatoid arthritis Infective subacute endocarditis Some malignancies Scleroderma	
11-Deoxycortisol	1 µg/dl	<0.029 µmol/L	Hypertensive form of virilizing adrenal hyperplasia due to an 11-β-hydroxylase defect	
Dibucaine number	Normal: 70%–85% inhibition Heterozygote: 50%–65% inhibition Homozygote: 16%–25% inhibition			Important in detecting carriers of abnormal cholinesterase activity who are susceptible to succinylcholine anesthetic shock

(continued)

Reference Ranges—Serum, Plasma, and Whole Blood Chemistries *(continued)*

	Normal Adult Reference Range		Clinical Significance	
Determination	**Conventional Units**	**SI Units**	**Increased**	**Decreased**
Dihydrotestosterone	Males: 50–210 ng/dl Females: none detectable	1.72–7.22 nmol/L		Testicular feminization syndrome
Estradiol—RIA	Females: Follicular: 10–90 pg/ml Midcycle: 100–500 pg/ml Luteal: 50–240 pg/ml Follicular phase: 2–20 ng/dl Midcycle: 12–40 ng/dl Luteal phase: 10–30 ng/dl Postmenopausal: 1–5 ng/dl Males: 0.5–5 ng/dl	 37–370 pmol/L 367–1835 pmol/L 184–881 pmol/L	Pregnancy	Depressed or failure to peak—ovarian failure
Estriol—RIA	Nonpregnant females: <0.5 ng/ml Pregnant females: 1st trimester: up to 1 ng/ml 2nd trimester: 0.8–7 ng/ml 3rd trimester: 5–25 ng/ml	<1.75 nmol/L Up to 3.5 nmol/L 2.8–24.3 nmol/L 17.4–86.8 nmol/L	Pregnancy	Depressed or failure to peak—ovarian failure
Estrogens, total—RIA	Females: cycle days: Day 1–10: 61–394 pg/ml Day 11–20: 122–437 pg/ml Day 21–30: 156–350 pg/ml Males: 40–115 pg/ml	 61–394 ng/L 122–437 ng/L 156–350 ng/L 40–115 ng/L	Pregnancy Measured on a daily basis, can be used to evaluate response of hypogonadotrophic, hypoestrogenic women to human menopausal or pituitary gonadotropin	Fetal distress Ovarian failure
Estrone—RIA	Females: Day 1–10: 4.3–18 ng/dl Day 11–20: 7.5–19.6 ng/dl Day 21–30: 13–20 ng/dl Males: 2.5–7.5 ng/dl	 15.9–66.6 pmol/L 27.8–72.5 pmol/L 48.1–74 pmol/L 9.3–27.8 pmol/L	Pregnancy	Depressed or failure to peak—ovarian failure
Ferritin—RIA	Males: 29–438 ng/ml Females: 9–219 ng/ml	29–438 μg/L 9–219 μg/L	Nephritis Hemochromatosis Certain neoplastic diseases Acute myelogenous leukemia Multiple myeloma	Iron deficiency
Folic acid—RIA	2.5–20 ng/ml	6–46 nmol/L		Megaloblastic anemias of infancy and pregnancy Inadequate diet Liver disease Malabsorption syndrome Severe hemolytic anemia

(continued)

Reference Ranges—Serum, Plasma, and Whole Blood Chemistries *(continued)*

	Normal Adult Reference Range		Clinical Significance	
Determination	**Conventional Units**	**SI Units**	**Increased**	**Decreased**
Follicle stimulating hormone (FSH)—RIA	Males: 2–10 mIU/ml Females: Follicular phase: 5–20 mIU/ml Peak of middle cycle: 12–30 mIU/ml Luteinic phase: 5–15 mIU/ml Menopausal females: 40–200 mIU/ml	 5–20 IU/L 12–30 IU/L 5–15 IU/L 40–200 IU/L	Menopause and primary ovarian failure	Pituitary failure
Galactose	<5 mg/dl	<0.28 mmol/L		Galactosemia
Gamma glutamyl transpeptidase	Males: <45 IU/L Females: <30 IU/L	45 U/L 30 U/L	Hepatobiliary disease Anicteric alcoholism Drug therapy damage Myocardial infarction Renal infarction	
Gastrin—RIA	Fasting: 50–155 pg/ml Postprandial: 80–170 pg/ml Zollinger-Ellison syndrome: 200–over 2000 pg/ml Pernicious anemia: 130–2260 pg/ml (mean 912)	50–155 ng/L 80–170 ng/L 200–over 2000 ng/L 130–2260 ng/L (mean 912)	Zollinger-Ellison syndrome Peptic ulceration of the duodenum Pernicious anemia	
Glucose	Fasting: 60–110 mg/dl Postprandial (2 h.): 65–140 mg/dl	3.3–6.05 mmol/L 3.58–7.7 mmol/L	Diabetes Nephritis Hyperthyroidism Early hyperpituitarism Cerebral lesions Infections Pregnancy Uremia	Hyperinsulinism Hypothyroidism Late hyperpituitarism Pernicious vomiting Addison's disease Extensive hepatic damage
Glucose tolerance (oral)	Features of a normal response: 1. Normal fasting between 60–110 mg/dl 2. No sugar in urine 3. Upper limits of normal: Fasting = 125 1 hour = 190 2 hours = 140 3 hours = 125	 3.3–6.05 mmol/L 6.88 mmol/L 10.45 mmol/L 7.70 mmol/L 6.88 mmol/L	(Flat or inverted curve) Hyperinsulinism Adrenal cortical insufficiency (Addison's disease) Anterior pituitary hypofunction Hypothyroidism Sprue and celiac diseases	(High or prolonged curve) Diabetes Hyperthyroidism Primary adrenal cortical tumor or hyperplasia Severe anemia Certain central nervous system disorders
Glucose-6 phosphate dehydrogenase (red cells)	Screening: Decolorization in 20–100 min Quantitative: 1.86–2.5 IU/ml RBC	 1860–2500 U/L		Drug-induced hemolytic anemia Hemolytic disease of newborn
Glycoprotein (alpha-1-acid)	40–110 mg/dl	400–1100 mg/L	Neoplasm Tuberculosis Diabetes complicated by degenerative vascular disease	

(continued)

Reference Ranges—Serum, Plasma, and Whole Blood Chemistries *(continued)*

Determination	Normal Adult Reference Range: Conventional Units	Normal Adult Reference Range: SI Units	Clinical Significance: Increased	Clinical Significance: Decreased
			Pregnancy Rheumatoid arthritis Rheumatic fever Infectious liver disease Lupus erythematosus	
Growth hormone—RIA	<10 ng/ml	<10 mg/L	Acromegaly	Failure to stimulate with arginine or insulin—hypopituitarism
Haptoglobin	50–250 mg/dl	0.5–2.5 g/L	Pregnancy Estrogen therapy Chronic infections Various inflammatory conditions	Hemolytic anemia Hemolytic blood transfusion reaction
Hemoglobin (plasma)	0.5–5 mg/dl	5–50 mg/L	Transfusion reactions Paroxysmal nocturnal hemoglobinuria Intravascular hemolysis	
Hemoglobin A1 (Glycohemoglobin)	Nondiabetics & diabetics whose control of glucose is: Good: 4.4%–8.2% Fair: 8.3%–9.2% Poor: >9.2%			
Hexosaminidase, total	Controls: 333–375 nM/ml/hr Heterozygotes: 288–644 nM/ml/hr Tay-Sachs disease: 284–1232 nM/ml/hr Diabetics: 567–3560 nM/ml/hr	333–375 µmol/L/hr 288–644 µmol/L/hr 284–1232 µmol/L/hr 567–3560 µmol/L/hr	Diabetes Tay-Sachs disease	
Hexosaminidase A	Controls: 49%–68% of total Heterozygotes: 26%–45% of total Tay-Sachs disease: 0%–4% of total Diabetics: 39%–59% of total	Fraction of total: 0.49–0.68 0.26–0.45 0–0.04 0.39–0.59		Tay-Sachs disease and heterozygotes
High-density lipoprotein cholesterol (HDL cholesterol)				HDL cholesterol is lower in patients with increased risk for coronary heart disease

Age *(yr)*	**Males** *(mg/dl)*	**Females** *(mg/dl)*	**Males** *(mmol/L)*	**Females** *(mmol/L)*
0–19	30–65	30–70	0.78–1.68	0.78–1.81
20–29	35–70	35–75	0.91–1.81	0.91–1.94
30–39	30–65	35–80	0.78–1.68	0.91–2.07
40–49	30–65	40–85	0.78–1.68	1.04–2.2
50–59	30–65	35–85	0.78–1.68	0.91–2.2
60–69	30–65	35–85	0.78–1.68	0.91–2.2

(continued)

Reference Ranges—Serum, Plasma, and Whole Blood Chemistries *(continued)*

	Normal Adult Reference Range		Clinical Significance	
Determination	**Conventional Units**	**SI Units**	**Increased**	**Decreased**
17-Hydroxy-progesterone—RIA	Males: 0.4–4 ng/ml Females: 0.1–3.3 ng/ml Children: 0.1–0.5 ng/ml	1.2–12 nmol/L 0.3–10 nmol/L 0.3–1.5 nmol/L	Congenital adrenal hyperplasia Pregnancy Some cases of adrenal or ovarian adenomas	
Immunoglobulin A	Adults: 50–300 mg/dl (in children the normals are lower and vary with age)	0.5–3 g/L	Gamma A myeloma Wiskott-Aldrich syndrome Autoimmune disease Hepatic cirrhosis	Ataxia telangiectasis Agammaglobulinemia Hypogammaglobulinemia, transient Dysgammaglobulinemia Protein-losing enteropathies
Immunoglobulin D	0–30 mg/dl	0–300 mg/L	IgD multiple myeloma Some patients with chronic infectious diseases	
Immunoglobulin E	20–740 ng/ml	20–740 µg/L	Allergic patients and those with parasitic infestations	
Immunoglobulin G	Adults: 565–1765 mg/dl	6.35–14 g/L	IgG myeloma Following hyperimmunization Autoimmune disease states Chronic infections	Congenital and acquired hypogammaglobulinemia IgA myelomas, Waldenstrom's (IgM) macroglobulinemia Some malabsorption syndromes Extensive protein loss
Immunoglobulin M	Adults: 55–375 mg/dl	0.4–28 g/L	Waldenstrom's macroglobulinemia Parasitic infections Hepatitis	Agammaglobulinemias Some IgG and IgA myelomas Chronic lymphatic leukemia
Insulin—RIA	5–25 µU/ml	0.2–1 µg/L	Insulinoma Acromegaly	Diabetes mellitus
Iron	50–160 µg/dl	9–29 µmol/L	Pernicious anemia Aplastic anemia Hemolytic anemia Hepatitis Hemochromatosis	Iron deficiency anemia
Iron-binding capacity	IBC: 150–235 µg/dl TIBC: 230–410 µg/dl % Saturation: 20–50	26.9–42.1 µmol/L 41–73 µmol/L Fraction of total iron-binding capacity: 0.2–0.5	Iron deficiency anemia Acute and chronic blood loss Hepatitis	Chronic infectious diseases Cirrhosis
Isocitric dehydrogenase	50–180 U	0.83–3 U/L	Hepatitis; cirrhosis Obstructive jaundice Metastatic carcinoma of the liver Megaloblastic anemia	

(continued)

Reference Ranges—Serum, Plasma, and Whole Blood Chemistries *(continued)*

Determination	Normal Adult Reference Range: Conventional Units	Normal Adult Reference Range: SI Units	Clinical Significance: Increased	Clinical Significance: Decreased
Lactic acid (whole blood)	Venous: 5–20 mg/dl Arterial: 3–7 mg/dl	0.6–2.2 mmol/L 0.3–0.8 mmol/L	Increased muscular activity Congestive heart failure Hemorrhage Shock Some varieties of metabolic acidosis Some febrile infections May be increased in severe liver disease	
Lactic dehydrogenase (LDH)	100–225 mU/ml	100–225 U/L	Untreated pernicious anemia Myocardial infarction Pulmonary infarction Liver disease	
Lactic dehydrogenase isoenzymes Total lactic dehydrogenase LDH-1 LDH-2 LDH-3 LDH-4 LDH-5	 100–225 mU/ml 20%–35% 25%–40% 20%–30% 0–20% 0–25%	 100–225 U/L Fraction of total LDH: 0.2–0.35 0.25–0.4 0.2–0.3 0–0.2 0–0.25	LDH-1 and LDH-2 are increased in myocardial infarction, megaloblastic anemia, and hemolytic anemia LDH-4 and LDH-5 are increased in pulmonary infarction, congestive heart failure, and liver disease	
Lead (whole blood)	Up to 40 μg/dl	Up to 2 μmol/L	Lead poisoning	
Leucine aminopeptidase	80–200 U/ml	19.2–48 U/L	Liver or biliary tract diseases Pancreatic disease Metastatic carcinoma of liver and pancreas Biliary obstruction	
Lipase	0.2–1.5 U/ml	55–417 U/L	Acute and chronic pancreatitis Biliary obstruction Cirrhosis Hepatitis Peptic ulcer	
Lipids, total	400–1000 mg/dl	4–10 g/L	Hypothyroidism Diabetes Nephrosis Glomerulonephritis Hyperlipoproteinemias	Hyperthyroidism

Lipoprotein Phenotype: Summary of Findings in the Primary Hyperlipoproteinemias

					Lipoprotein Staining				
Type	**Frequency**	**Appearance**	**Triglyceride**	**Cholesterol**	*Beta*	*Pre-Beta*	*Alpha*	*Chylomicrons*	**Secondary Causes**
Normal		Clear	Normal	Normal	Moderate	Zero to moderate	Moderate	Weak	
I	Vary rare	Creamy	Markedly increased	Normal to moderately increased	Weak	Weak	Weak	Markedly increased	Dysglobulinemia

(continued)

Reference Ranges—Serum, Plasma, and Whole Blood Chemistries *(continued)*

Lipoprotein Phenotype: Summary of Findings in the Primary Hyperlipoproteinemias

Type	Frequency	Appearance	Triglyceride	Cholesterol	Lipoprotein Staining: *Beta*	*Pre-Beta*	*Alpha*	*Chylomicrons*	Secondary Causes
II	Common	Clear	Normal to slightly increased	Slightly to markedly increased	Strong	Zero to strong	Moderate	Weak	Hypothyroidism, myeloma, hepatic syndrome, macroglobulinemia, and high dietary cholesterol
III	Uncommon	Clear, cloudy, or milky	Increased	Increased	Broad intense band	Extends into beta	Moderate	Weak	
IV	Very common	Clear, cloudy, or milky	Slightly to markedly increased	Normal to slightly increased	Weak to moderate	Moderate to strong	Weak to moderate	Weak	Hypothyroidism, diabetes mellitus, pancreatitis, glycogen storage diseases, nephrotic syndrome, myeloma, pregnancy, and oral contraceptives
V	Rare	Cloudy to creamy	Markedly increased	Increased	Weak	Moderate	Weak	Strong	Diabetes mellitus, pancreatitis, and alcoholism

Types I and II are fat induced; types III and IV are carbohydrate induced; type V is fat and carbohydrate induced.

Determination	Normal Adult Reference Range: Conventional Units	SI Units	Clinical Significance: Increased	Decreased
Low-density lipoprotein cholesterol (LDL cholesterol)	Age (yr.) mg/dl 0–19 50–170 20–29 60–170 30–39 70–190 40–49 80–190 50–59 80–210	mmol/L 1.30–4.40 1.55–4.40 1.80–4.92 2.07–4.92 2.07–5.44	LDL cholesterol is higher in patients with increased risk for coronary heart disease	
Luteinizing hormone—RIA	Males: 4.9–15 mIU/ml Females: Follicular phase: 2–3 mIU/ml Ovulatory peak: 40–200 mIU/ml Luteal phase: 0–20 mIU/ml Postmenopausal: 35–120 mIU/ml	4.9–15 0.5–6.9 mg/L 9.2–46 mg/L 0–5 mg/L 8–27.5 mg/L	Pituitary tumor Ovarian failure	Depressed or failure to peak—pituitary failure
Lysozyme (muramidase)	2.8–8 µg/ml	2.8–8 mg	Certain types of leukemia (acute monocytic leukemia) Inflammatory states and infections	Acute lymphocytic leukemia
Magnesium	1.3–2.4 mEq/L	0.7–1.2 mmol/L	Excess ingestion of magnesium-containing antacids	Chronic alcoholism Severe renal disease Diarrhea Defective growth
Manganese	0.04–1.4 µg/dl	72.9–255 nmol/L		
Mercury	Up to 10 µg/dl	Up to 0.5 µmol/L	Mercury poisoning	
Myoglobin—RIA	Up to 85 ng/ml	Up to 85 µg/ml	Myocardial infarction Muscle necrosis	

(continued)

Reference Ranges—Serum, Plasma, and Whole Blood Chemistries *(continued)*

	Normal Adult Reference Range		Clinical Significance	
Determination	**Conventional Units**	**SI Units**	**Increased**	**Decreased**
5′ Nucleotidase	3.2–11.6 IU/L	3.2–11.6 U/L	Hepatobiliary disease	
Osmolality	280–300 mOsm/kg	280–300 mmol/L	Useful in the study of electrolyte and water balance	Inappropriate secretion of antidiuretic hormone
Parathyroid hormone	160–350 pg/ml	160–350 ng/L	Hyperparathyroidism	
Phenylalanine	1.2–3.5 mg/dl 1st week 0.7–3.5 mg/dl thereafter	0.07–0.21 mmol/L 0.04–0.21 mmol/L	Phenylketonuria	
Phosphatase, acid, total	0–11 UL	0–11 UL	Carcinoma of prostate Advanced Paget's disease Hyperparathyroidism Gaucher's disease	
Phosphatase, acid, prostatic—RIA	0–10 ng/ml Borderline: 2.5–3.3 IU/L	0–10 µg/L	Carcinoma of prostate	
Phosphatase, alkaline	Adults: 30–115 mU/ml	30–115 µ/L	Conditions reflecting increased osteoblastic activity of bone Rickets Hyperparathyroidism Liver disease	
Phosphatase, alkaline, thermostable fraction	Thermostable fraction >35%: hepatic disease and combined disease with predominant hepatic component Thermostable fraction between 25% and 35%: combined hepatic and skeletal disease Thermostable fraction <25%: skeletal disease with increased osteoblastic activity		Hepatic disease	
Phosphohexose isomerase	20–90 IU/L	20–90 U/L	Malignancy Disease of heart, liver, and skeletal muscles	
Phospholipids	125–300 mg/dl	1.25–3 g/L	Diabetes Nephritis	
Phosphorus, inorganic	2.5–4.5 mg/dl	0.8–1.45 mmol/L	Chronic nephritis Hypoparathyroidism	Hyperparathyroidism Vitamin D deficiency
Potassium	3.8–5 mEq/L	3.8–5 mmol/L	Addison's disease Oliguria Anuria Tissue breakdown or hemolysis	Diabetic acidosis Diarrhea Vomiting
Progesterone—RIA	Follicular phase: up to 0.8 ng/ml Luteal phase: 10–20 ng/ml End of cycle: <1 ng/ml Pregnant: up to 50 ng/ml in 20th week	2.5 nmol/L 31.8–63.6 nmol/L <3 nmol/L Up to 160 nmol/L	Useful in evaluation of menstrual disorders and infertility and in the evaluation of placental function during pregnancies complicated by toxemia, diabetes mellitus, or threatened miscarriage	

(continued)

Reference Ranges—Serum, Plasma, and Whole Blood Chemistries *(continued)*

	Normal Adult Reference Range		Clinical Significance	
Determination	**Conventional Units**	**SI Units**	**Increased**	**Decreased**
Prolactin—RIA	6–24 ng/ml	6–24 µg/L	Pregnancy Functional or structural disorders of the hypothalamus Pituitary stalk section Pituitary tumors	
Prostate-specific antigen	<4 ng/ml		Prostatic cancer, benign prostatic hyperplasia, prostatitis	
Protein, total Albumin Globulin	6–8 gm/dl 3.5–5 gm/dl 1.5–3 gm/dl	60–80 g/L 35–50 g/L 15–30 g/L	Hemoconcentration Shock Multiple myeloma (globulin fraction) Chronic infections (globulin fraction) Liver disease (globulin)	Malnutrition Hemorrhage Loss of plasma from burns Proteinuria
Electrophoresis (cellulose acetate)				
Albumin	3.5–5 gm/dl	35–50 g/L		
Alpha-1 globulin	0.2–0.4 gm/dl	2–4 g/L		
Alpha-2 globulin	0.6–1 gm/dl	6–10 g/L		
Beta globulin	0.6–1.2 gm/dl	6–12 g/L		
Gamma globulin	0.7–1.5 gm/dl	7–15 g/L		
Protoporphyrin erythrocyte (whole blood)	15–100 µg/dl	0.27–1.80 µmol/L	Lead toxicity Erythropoietic porphyria	
Pyridoxine	3.6–18 ng/ml			A wide spectrum of clinical conditions such as mental depression, peripheral neuropathy, anemia, neonatal seizures, and reactions to certain drug therapies
Pyruvic acid (whole blood)	0.3–0.7 mg/dl	34–80 µmol/L	Diabetes Severe thiamine deficiency Acute phase of some infections, possibly secondary to increased glycogenolysis and glycolysis	
Renin (plasma)—RIA	Normal diet: Supine: 0.3–1.9 ng/ml/h Upright: 0.6–3.6 ng/ml/h Low salt diet: Supine: 0.9–4.5 ng/ml/h Upright: 4.1–9.1 ng/ml/h	 0.08–0.52 ng/L/S 0.16–1.00 µg/L/S 0.25–1.25 µg/L/S 1.13–2.53 µg/L/S	Renovascular hypertension Malignant hypertension Untreated Addison's disease Primary salt-losing nephropathy Low-salt diet Diuretic therapy Hemorrhage	Frank primary aldosteronism Increased salt intake Salt-retaining steroid therapy Antidiuretic hormone therapy Blood transfusion
Sodium	135–145 mEq/L	135–145 mmol/L	Hemoconcentration Nephritis Pyloric obstruction	Alkali deficit Addison's disease Myxedema

(continued)

Reference Ranges—Serum, Plasma, and Whole Blood Chemistries *(continued)*

Determination	Normal Adult Reference Range: Conventional Units	SI Units	Clinical Significance: Increased	Decreased
Sulfate (inorganic)	0.5–1.5 mg/dl	0.05–0.15 mmol/L	Nephritis Nitrogen retention	
Testosterone—RIA	Females: 25–100 ng/dl Males: 300–800 ng/dl	0.9–3.5 nmol/L 10.5–28 nmol/L	Females: Polycystic ovary Virilizing tumors	Males: Orchidectomy for neoplastic disease of the prostate or breast Estrogen therapy Klinefelter's syndrome Hypopituitarism Hypogonadism Hepatic cirrhosis
T_3 (triiodothyronine) uptake	25%–35%	Relative uptake fraction: 0.25–0.35	Hyperthyroidism TBG deficiency Androgens and anabolic steroids	Hypothyroidism Pregnancy TBG excess Estrogens and antiovulatory drugs
T_3, total circulating—RIA	75–200 ng/dl	1.15–3.1 nmol/L	Pregnancy Hyperthyroidism	Hypothyroidism
T_4 (thyroxine)—RIA	4.5–11.5 μg/dl	58.5–150 nmol/L	Hyperthyroidism Thyroiditis Elevated thyroxine-binding proteins caused by oral contraceptives Pregnancy	Primary and pituitary hypothyroidism Idiopathic involvement Cases of diminished thyroxine-binding proteins caused by androgenic and anabolic steroids Hypoproteinemia Nephrotic syndrome
T_4, free	1–2.2 ng/dl	13–30 pmol/L	Euthyroid patients with normal free thyroxine levels may have abnormal T_3 and T_4 levels caused by drug preparations	
Thyroid-stimulating hormone (TSH)—RIA		0.3–5 m/IU/L	Hypothyroidism	Hyperthyroidism
Thyroid-binding globulin	10–26 μg/dl	100–260 μg/L	Hypothyroidism Pregnancy Estrogen therapy Oral contraceptives Genetic and idiopathic	Androgens and anabolic steroids Nephrotic syndrome Marked hypoproteinemia Hepatic disease
Transaminase, serum glutamic-oxaloacetate (SGOT, also called aspartate aminotransferase or AST)	7–40 U/ml	4–20 U/L	Myocardial infarction Skeletal muscle disease Liver disease	
Transaminase, serum glutamic-oxaloacetate (SGPT, also called alanine aminotransferase or ALT)	10–40 U/ml	5–20 U/L	Same conditions as SGOT, but increase is more marked in liver disease than SGOT	
Transferrin	230–320 mg/dl	2.3–3.2 g/L	Pregnancy Iron-deficiency anemia due to hemorrhaging Acute hepatitis	Pernicious anemia in relapse Thalassemic and sickle cell anemia

(continued)

Reference Ranges—Serum, Plasma, and Whole Blood Chemistries *(continued)*

	Normal Adult Reference Range		Clinical Significance	
Determination	**Conventional Units**	**SI Units**	**Increased**	**Decreased**
			Polycythemia Oral contraceptives	Chromatosis Neoplastic and hepatic diseases
Triglycerides	10–150 mg/dl	0.10–1.65 mmol/L	See *Lipoprotein Phenotype*	
Tryptophan	1.4–3 mg/dl	68.6–147 nmol/L		Tryptophan-specific malabsorption syndrome
Tyrosine	0.5–4 mg/dl	27.6–220.8 mmol/L	Tyrosinosis	
Urea nitrogen (BUN)	10–20 mg/dl	3.6–7.2 mmol/L	Acute glomerulonephritis Obstructive uropathy Mercury poisoning Nephrotic syndrome	Severe hepatic failure Pregnancy
Uric acid	2.5–8 mg/dl	0.15–0.5 mmol/L	Gouty arthritis Acute leukemia Lymphomas treated by chemotherapy Toxemia of pregnancy	Xanthinuria Defective tubular reabsorption
Viscosity	1.4–1.8 relative to water at 37°C. (98.6°F.)		Patients with marked increases of the gamma globulins	
Vitamin A	50–220 μg/dl	1.75–7.7 μmol/L	Hypervitaminosis A	Vitamin A deficiency Celiac disease Sprue Obstructive jaundice Giardiasis Parenchymal hepatic disease
Vitamin B_1 (thiamine)	1.6–4 μg/dl	47.4–135.7 nmol/L		Anorexia Beriberi Polyneuropathy Cardiomyopathies
Vitamin B_6 (pyridoxal phosphate)	3.6–18 ng/ml	14.6–72.8 nmol/L		Chronic alcoholism Malnutrition Uremia Neonatal seizures Malabsorption, such as celiac syndrome
Vitamin B_{12}—RIA	130–785 pg/ml	100–580 pmol/L	Hepatic cell damage and in association with the myeloproliferative disorders (the highest levels are encountered in myeloid leukemia)	Strict vegetarianism Alcoholism Pernicious anemia Total or partial gastrectomy Ileal resection Sprue and celiac disease Fish tapeworm infestation
Vitamin E	0.5–2 mg/dl	11.6–46.4 μmol/L		Vitamin E deficiency
Xylose absorption test	2 hr., 30–50 mg/dl	2–3.35 mmol/L		Malabsorption syndrome
Zinc	55–150 μg/dl	7.65–22.95 μmol/L	Zinc is essential for the growth and propagation of cell cultures and the functioning of several enzymes	

Reference Ranges—Urine Chemistry

	Normal Adult Reference Range		Clinical Significance	
Determination	**Conventional Units**	**SI Units**	**Increased**	**Decreased**
Acetone and acetoacetate	Zero		Uncontrolled diabetes Starvation	
Acid mucopolysaccharides	Negative		Hurler's syndrome Marfan's syndrome Morquio-Ulrich disease	
Aldosterone	Normal salt: Normal: 4–20 μg/24 hr Renovascular: 10–40 μg/24 hr Tumor: 20–100 μg/24 hr	 11.1–55.5 nmol/24 hr 27.7–111 nmol/24 hr 55.4–277 nmol/24 hr	Primary aldosteronism (adrenocortical tumor) Secondary aldosteronism Salt depletion Potassium loading ACTH in large doses Cardiac failure Cirrhosis with ascites formation Nephrosis Pregnancy	
Alpha amino nitrogen	50–200 mg/24 hr	3.6–14.3 mmol/24 hr	Leukemia Diabetes Phenylketonuria Other metabolic diseases	
Amylase	35–260 units excreted per hr	6.5–48.1 U/hr	Acute pancreatitis	
Arylsulfatase A	>2.4 U/ml			Metachromatic leuko-dystrophy
Bence-Jones protein	None detected		Myeloma	
Calcium	<150 mg/24 hr	<3.75 mmol/24 hr	Hyperparathyroidism Vitamin D intoxication Fanconi syndrome	Hypoparathyroidism Vitamin D deficiency
Catecholamines	Total: 0–275 μg/24 hr Epinephrine: 10%–40% Norepinephrine: 60%–90%	0–275 μg/24 hr. Fraction total: 0.10–8.4 Fraction total: 0.60–0.90	Pheochromocytoma Neuroblastoma	
Chorionic gonadotrophin, qualitative (pregnancy test)	Negative		Pregnancy Chorionepithelioma Hydatidiform mole	
Copper	20–70 μg/24 hr	0.32–1.12 μmol/24 hr	Wilson's disease Cirrhosis Nephrosis	
Coproporphyrin	50–300 μg/24 hr	0.075–0.45 μmol/24 hr	Poliomyelitis Lead poisoning Porphyria hepatica Porphyria erythropoietica Porphyria cutanea tarda	
Cortisol, free	20–90 μg/24 hr	55.2–248.4 nmol/d	Cushing's syndrome	
Creatine	0–200 mg/24 hr	0–1.52 mmol/24 hr	Muscular dystrophy Fever Carcinoma of liver Pregnancy Hyperthyroidism Myositis	

(continued)

Reference Ranges—Urine Chemistry *(continued)*

Determination	Normal Adult Reference Range: Conventional Units	SI Units	Clinical Significance: Increased	Decreased
Creatinine	0.8–2 gm/24 hr	7–17.6 mmol/24 hr	Typhoid fever Salmonella infections Tetanus	Muscular atrophy Anemia Advanced degeneration of kidneys Leukemia
Creatinine clearance	100–150 ml of blood cleared of creatinine per min	1.67–2.5 ml/sec		Measures glomerular filtration rate Renal diseases
Cystine and cysteine	10–100 mg/24 hr	0.08–0.83 mmol/24 hr	Cystinuria	
Delta aminolevulinic acid	0–0.54 mg/dl	0–40 µmol/L	Lead poisoning Porphyria hepatica Hepatitis Hepatic carcinoma	
11-Desoxycortisol	20–100 µg/24 hr	0.6–2.9 µmol/day	Hypertensive form of virilizing adrenal hyperplasia due to an 11-beta hydroxylase defect	
Estriol (placental)	**Weeks of pregnancy** — **µm./24 h.** — **nmol./24 h.** 12 — <1 — <3.5 16 — 2–7 — 7–24.5 20 — 4–9 — 14–32 24 — 6–13 — 21–45.5 28 — 8–22 — 28–77 32 — 12–43 — 42–150 36 — 14–45 — 49–158 40 — 19–46 — 66.5–160			Decreased values occur with fetal distress of many conditions, including preeclampsia, placental insufficiency, and poorly controlled diabetes mellitus
Estrogens, total (fluorometric)	Females: Onset of menstruation: 4–25 µg/24 hr Ovulation peak: 28 µg/24 hr Luteal peak: 22–105 µg/24 hr Menopausal: 14–19.6 µg/24 hr Males: 5–18 µg/24 hr	 4–25 µg/24 hr 28 µg/24 hr 22–105 µg/24 hr 1.4–19.6 µg/24 hr 5–18 µg/24 hr	Hyperestrogenism due to gonadal or adrenal neoplasm	Primary or secondary amenorrhea
Etiocholanolone	Males: 1.9–6 mg/24 hr Females: 0.5–4 mg/24 hr	6.5–20.6 µmol/24 hr 1.7–13.8 µmol/24 hr	Adrenogenital syndrome Idiopathic hirsutism	
Follicle-stimulating hormone—RIA	Females: Follicular: 5–20 IU/24 hr Luteal: 5–15 IU/24 hr Midcycle: 15–60 IU/24 hr Menopausal: 50–100 IU/24 hr Males: 5–25 IU/24 hr	 5–20 IU/day 5–15 IU/day 15–60 IU/day 50–100 IU/day 5–25 IU/day	Menopause and primary ovarian failure	Pituitary failure
Glucose	Negative		Diabetes mellitus Pituitary disorders Intracranial pressure Lesion in floor of 4th ventricle	

(continued)

Reference Ranges—Urine Chemistry *(continued)*

Determination	Normal Adult Reference Range: Conventional Units	Normal Adult Reference Range: SI Units	Clinical Significance: Increased	Clinical Significance: Decreased
Hemoglobin and myoglobin	Negative		Extensive burns Transfusion of incompatible blood Myoglobin increased in severe crushing injuries to muscles	
Homogentisic acid, qualitative	Negative		Alkaptonuria Ochronosis	
Homovanillic acid	Up to 15 mg/24 hr	Up to 82 μmol/day	Neuroblastoma	
17-hydroxycorticosteroids	2–20 mg/24 hr	5.5–27.5 μmol/day	Cushing's disease	Addison's disease Anterior pituitary hypofunction
5-Hydroxyindoleacetic acid, qualitative	Negative		Malignant carcinoid tumors	
Hydroxyproline	15–43 mg/24 hr	0.11–0.33 μmol/day	Paget's disease Fibrous dysplasia Osteomalacia Neoplastic bone disease Hyperparathyroidism	
17-ketosteroids, total	Males: 10–22 mg/24 hr Females: 6–16 mg/24 hr	35–76 μmol/day 21–55 μmol/day	Interstitial cell tumor of testes Simple hirsutism, occasionally Adrenal hyperplasia Cushing's syndrome Adrenal cancer, virilism Arrhenoblastoma	Thyrotoxicosis Female hypogonadism Diabetes mellitus Hypertension Debilitating disease of mild to moderate severity Eunuchoidism Addison's disease Panhypopituitarism Myxedema Nephrosis
Lead	Up to 150 μg/24 hr	Up to 60 μmol/24 hr	Lead poisoning	
Luteinizing hormone	Males: 5–18 IU/24 hr Females: Follicular phase: 2–25 IU/24 hr Ovulatory peak: 30–95 IU/24 hr Luteal phase: 2–20 IU/24 hr Postmenopausal: 40–110 IU/24 hr	 2–25 IU/day 30–95 IU/day 2–20 IU/day 40–110 IU/day	Pituitary tumor Ovarian failure	Depressed or failure to peak—pituitary failure
Metanephrines, total	Less than 1.3 mg/24 hr	Less than 6.5 μmol/day	Pheochromocytoma; a few patients with pheochromocytoma may have elevated urinary metanephrines but normal catecholamines and VMA	
Osmolality	Males: 390–1090 mM/kg Females: 300–1090 mM/kg	390–1090 mmol/kg 300–1090 mmol/kg	Useful in the study of electrolyte and water balance	

(continued)

Reference Ranges—Urine Chemistry *(continued)*

	Normal Adult Reference Range		Clinical Significance	
Determination	**Conventional Units**	**SI Units**	**Increased**	**Decreased**
Oxalate	Up to 40 mg/24 hr	Up to 456 μmol/day	Primary hyperoxaluria	
Phenylpyruvic acid qualitative	Negative		Phenylketonuria	
Phosphorus, inorganic	0.8–1.3 gm/24 hr	26–42 mmol/24 hr	Hyperparathyroidism Vitamin D intoxication Paget's disease Metastatic neoplasm to bone	Hypoparathyroidism Vitamin D. deficiency
Porphobilinogen, qualitative	Negative		Chronic lead poisoning Acute porphyria Liver disease	
Porphobilinogen, quantitative	0–1 mg/24 hr	0–4.4 μmol/24 hr	Acute porphyria Liver disease	
Porphyrins, qualitative	Negative		See porphyrins, quantitative	
Porphyrins, quantitative (coproporphyrin and uroporphyrin)	Coproporphyrin: 50–160 μg/24 hr Uroporphyrin: up to 50 μg/24 hr	 0.075–0.24 μmol/24 hr Up to 0.06 μmol/24 hr	Porphyria hepatica Porphyria erythropoietica Porphyria cutanea tarda Lead poisoning (only coproporphyrin increased)	
Potassium	40–65 mEq/24 hr	40–65 mmol/24 hr	Hemolysis	
Pregnanediol	Females: Proliferative phase: 0.5–1.5 mg/24 hr Luteal phase: 2–7 mg/24 hr Menopause: 0.2–1 mg/24 hr Pregnancy:	 1.6–4.8 μmol/24 hr 6–22 μmol/24 hr 0.6–3.1 μmol/24 hr	Corpus luteum cysts When placental tissue remains in the uterus following parturition Somes cases of adrenocortical tumors	Placental dysfunction Threatened abortion Intrauterine death
	Weeks of gestation — **mg/24 hr**	**μmol/24 hr**		
	10–12 — 5–15	15.6–47		
	12–18 — 5–25	15.6–78.0		
	18–24 — 15–33	47.0–103.0		
	24–28 — 20–42	62.4–131.0		
	28–32 — 27–47	84.2–146.6		
	Males: 0.1–2 mg/24 hr	0.3–6.2 μmol/24 hr		
Pregnanetriol	0.4–2.4 mg/24 hr	1.2–7.1 μmol/24 hr	Congenital adrenal androgenic hyperplasia	
Protein	Up to 100 mg/24 hr	Up to 100 mg/24 hr	Nephritis Cardiac failure Mercury poisoning Bence-Jones protein in multiple myeloma Febrile states Hematuria	
Sodium	130–200 mEq/24 hr	130–200 mmol/24 hr	Useful in detecting gross changes in water and salt balance	
Titratable acidity	20–40 mEq/24 hr	20–40 mmol/24 hr	Metabolic acidosis	Metabolic alkalosis
Urea nitrogen	9–16 gm/24 hr	0.32–0.57 mol/L	Excessive protein catabolism	Impaired kidney function

(continued)

Reference Ranges—Urine Chemistry *(continued)*

	Normal Adult Reference Range		Clinical Significance	
Determination	**Conventional Units**	**SI Units**	**Increased**	**Decreased**
Uric acid	250–750 mg/24 hr	1.48–4.43 mmol/24 hr	Gout	Nephritis
Urobilinogen	Random urine: <0.25 mg/dl 24-hour urine: up to 4 mg/24 hr	<0.42 mol/24 hr Up to 6.76 μmol/24 hr	Liver and biliary tract disease Hemolytic anemias	Complete or nearly complete biliary obstruction Diarrhea Renal insufficiency
Uroporphyrins	Up to 50 μg/24 hr	Up to 0.06 μmol/24 hr	Porphyria	
Vanillylmandelic acid (VMA)	0.7–6.8 mg/24 hr	3.5–34.3 μmol/24 hr	Pheochromocytoma Neuroblastoma Coffee, tea, aspirin, bananas, and several different drugs	
Xylose absorption test (5 hour)	16%–33% of ingested xylose	Fraction absorbed: 0.16–0.33		Malabsorption syndromes
Zinc	0.15–1.2 mg/24 hr	2.3–18.4 μmol/24 hr	Zinc is an essential nutritional element	

Reference Ranges—Cerebrospinal Fluid (CSF)

	Normal Adult Reference Range		Clinical Significance	
Determination	**Conventional Units**	**SI Units**	**Increased**	**Decreased**
Albumin	15–30 mg/dl	150–300 mg/L	Certain neurologic disorders Lesion in the choroid plexus or blockage of the flow of CSF Damage to the blood–CNS barrier	
Cell count	0–5 mononuclear cells per mm^3	0–5 $\times$ 10^6/L	Bacterial meningitis Neurosyphilis Anterior poliomyelitis Encephalitis lethargica	
Chloride	100–130 mEq/L	100–300 mmol/L	Uremia	Acute generalized meningitis Tuberculous meningitis
Glucose	50–75 mg/dl	2.75–4.13 mmol/L	Diabetes mellitus Diabetic coma Epidemic encephalitis Uremia	Acute meningitides Tuberculous meningitis Insulin shock
Glutamine	6–15 mg/dl	0.41–1 mmol/L	Hepatic encephalopathies, including Reye's syndrome Hepatic coma Cirrhosis	
IgG	0–6.6 mg/dl	0–66 mg/L	Damage to the blood–CNS barrier Multiple sclerosis Neurosyphilis Subacute sclerosing panencephalitis Chronic phases of CNS infections	

(continued)

Reference Ranges—Cerebrospinal Fluid (CSF) *(continued)*

	Normal Adult Reference Range		Clinical Significance	
Determination	**Conventional Units**	**SI Units**	**Increased**	**Decreased**
Lactic acid	<24 mg/dl	<2.7 mmol/L	Bacterial meningitis Hypocapnia Hydrocephalus Brain abscesses Cerebral ischemia	
Lactic dehydrogenase	1/10 that of serum	Activity fraction: 0.1 of serum	CNS disease	
Protein:			Acute meningitides Tubercular meningitis Neurosyphilis Poliomyelitis Guillain-Barré syndrome	
Lumbar	15–45 mg/dl	150–450 mg/L		
Cisternal	15–25 mg/dl	150–250 mg/L		
Ventricular	5–15 mg/dl	50–150 mg/L		
Protein electrophoresis (cellulose acetate)	% of total:	Fraction:	An increase in the level of albumin alone can be the result of a lesion in the choroid plexus or a blockage of the flow of CSF. An elevated gamma globulin value with a normal albumin level has been reported in multiple sclerosis, neurosyphilis, subacute sclerosing panencephalitis, and the chronic phase of CNS infections. If the blood–CNS barrier has been damaged severely during the course of these diseases, the CSF albumin level may also be elevated.	
Prealbumin	3–7	0.03–0.07		
Albumin	56–74	0.56–0.74		
$Alpha_1$ globulin	2–6.5	0.02–0.065		
$Alpha_2$ globulin	3–12	0.03–0.12		
Beta globulin	8–18.5	0.08–0.185		
Gamma globulin	4–14	0.04–0.14		

Gastric Analysis

	Normal Adult Reference Range		Clinical Significance	
Determination	**Conventional Units**	**SI Units**	**Increased**	**Decreased**
*p*H	<2	<2		Pernicious anemia
Basal acid output	0–6 mEq/hr	0–6 mmol/hr	Peptic ulcer	Gastric carcinoma
Maximum acid	5–40 mEq/hr	5–40 mmol/hr	Zollinger-Ellison syndrome	Chronic atrophic gastritis Decreased normally with age

Miscellaneous Values

		Clinical Significance	
Determinations	**Normal Value**	**Conventional Units**	**SI Units**
Acetaminophen	0	Therapeutic level = 10–20 μg/ml	10–20 mg/L
Aminophylline (theophylline)	0	Therapeutic level = 10–20 μg/ml	10–20 mg/L

(continued)

Miscellaneous Values *(continued)*

Determinations	Normal Value	Clinical Significance: Conventional Units	Clinical Significance: SI Units
Bromide	0	Therapeutic level = 5–50 mg/dl	50–500 mg/L
Carbamazepine	0	Therapeutic level = 8–12 μg/ml	34–51 μmol/L
Carbon monoxide	0%–2%	Symptoms with >20% saturation	
Chlordiazepoxide	0	Therapeutic level = 1–3 μg/ml	1–3 mg/L
Diazepam	0	Therapeutic level = 0.5–2.5 μg/dl	5–25 μg/L
Digitoxin	0	Therapeutic level = 5–30 ng/ml	5–30 μg/L
Digoxin	0	Therapeutic level = 0.5–2 ng/ml	0.5–2 μg/L
Ethanol	0%–0.01%	Legal intoxication level = 0.10% or above 0.3%–0.4% = marked intoxication 0.4%–0.5% = alcoholic stupor	
Gentamicin	0	Therapeutic level = 4–10 μg/ml	4–10 mg/L
Lithium	0	Therapeutic level = 0.6–1.2 mEq/ml	0.6–1.2 mmol/L
Methanol	0	May be fatal in concentration as low as 10 mg/dl	100 mg/L
Phenobarbital	0	Therapeutic level = 15–40 μg/ml	10–20 mg/L
Phenytoin	0	Therapeutic level = 10–20 μg/ml	10–20 mg/L
Primidone	0	Therapeutic level = 5–12 μg/ml	5–12 mg/L
Quinidine	0	Therapeutic level = 0.2–0.5 mg/dl	2–5 mg/L
Salicylate	0	Therapeutic level = 2–25 mg/dl Toxic level = >30 mg/dl	20–250 mg/L 300 mg/L

Reference Ranges—Immunodiagnostic Tests

Determination	Normal Value	Clinical Significance
Acetylcholine receptor binding antibody	Negative or <0.03 nmol/L	Considered to be diagnostic for myasthenia gravis in patients with symptoms.
Anti-ds-DNA antibody	<70 units by ELISA <1:20 by indirect fluorescence	Valuable in supporting diagnosis or monitoring disease activity and prognosis of systemic lupus erythematosus (SLE).
Anti-glomerular basement membrane antibody	Negative or less than 10 units	Primarily used in the differential diagnosis of glomerular nephritis induced by antiglomerular basement membrane antibodies from other types of glomerular nephritis.
Anti-insulin antibody	<3% binding of labelled beef and pork insulin by patient's serum, or <9 MIU/L	Helpful in determining the best therapeutic agent in diabetics and the cause of allergic manifestations. Also used to identify insulin resistance.
Anti-mitochondrial antibody and anti–smooth muscle antibody	<1:5 and <1:20, respectively	Increased in cirrhosis, autoimmune disease, thyroiditis, pernicious anemia.
Anti-nuclear antibody	Negative, <1:20	Increased in SLE, chronic hepatitis, scleroderma, leukemia, and mononucleosis.
Anti–parietal cell antibody	Negative, <1:20	Helpful in diagnosing chronic gastric disease and differentiating autoimmune pernicious anemia from other megaloblastic anemias.
Anti-ribonucleoprotein antibody	Negative	Helpful in differential diagnosis of systemic rheumatic disease.
Anti-scleroderma antibody	Negative	Highly diagnostic for scleroderma.
Anti-Smith antibody	Negative	Highly diagnostic of SLE.

(continued)

Reference Ranges—Immunodiagnostic Tests *(continued)*

Determination	Normal Value	Clinical Significance
Anti-SS-A anti-SS-B antibody	Negative	SS-A antibodies are found in Sjögren's syndrome alone or associated with lupus. SS-B antibodies are associated with primary Sjögren's syndrome.
Antithyroglobulin and antimicrosomal antibodies	<1:100 titer by gelatin or hemagglutination	Presence and concentration is important in evaluation and treatment of various thyroid disorders such as Hashimoto's thyroiditis and Graves' disease. May also be indicative of previous autoimmune disorders.
Ca 15-3 tumor marker	<22 IU/ml	Increased in metastatic breast cancer.
Ca 19-9 tumor marker	<37 IU/ml	Increased in pancreatic, hepatobiliary, gastric, and colorectal cancer; gallstones; cirrhosis.
Ca 125	0–35 IU/ml	Increased in colon, upper GI, ovarian, and other gynecologic cancers; pregnancy, peritonitis.
Cold agglutinins	<1:16	Increased in mycoplasma pneumonia, viral illness, mononucleosis, multiple myeloma, scleroderma
C-reactive protein	<0.8 mg/dl	Increase indicates presence of active inflammation
Hepatitis A virus antibodies, IgM (HAV-Ab/IgM)	Negative	Positive in acute stage hepatitis A; develops early in disease.
Hepatitis A virus antibodies, IgG (HAV-Ab/IgG)	Negative	Positive if previous exposure and immunity to hepatitis A.
Hepatitis B surface antigen (HBsAg)	Negative	Positive in acute stage hepatitis B.
Hepatitis B surface antibody (HBsAb)	Negative	Positive if previous exposure and immunity to hepatitis B.
Infectious mononucleosis tests (monospot, mono-test, heterophile antigen test, EBV antiviral capsid antigen IgM and IgG)	Negative, <1:80	Positive monospot and monotest are presumptive; positive Epstein-Barr virus (EBV) IgM and IgG indicate acute and recent or past infection, respectively.
Lyme disease titer	Negative, <1:256 by indirect fluorescent antibody method <0.8 by ELISA	Positive results help diagnose Lyme disease. False positive may occur with high rheumatoid factor titers or syphilis. Positive ELISA confirmed by Western blot test.
Pyroglobulin test	Negative	These abnormal proteins may be associated with myeloma, lymphoma, polycythemia vera, and SLE.
Rheumatoid factor	Negative or less than 60 IU/ml	Elevated in rheumatoid arthritis, lupus, endocarditis, tuberculosis, syphilis, sarcoidosis, cancer.
T and B cell lymphocyte surface markers T-helper/T-suppressor ratio	T and B surface markers: Percent T cells (CD2) 60%–88% Percent helper cells (CD4) 34%–67% Percent suppressor cells (CD8) 10%–42% Percent B cells (CD19) 3%–21% Absolute counts: Lymphocytes 0.66–4.60 thou/ml T cells 644–2201 cells/ml Helper cells 493–1191 cells/ml Suppressor T cells 182–785 cells/ml B cells 92–392 cells/ml Lymphocyte ratio: T/T ratio >1	Done to evaluate immune system by identifying the specific cells involved in the immune response. Valuable in diagnosis of lymphocytic leukemia, lymphoma, and immunodeficiency diseases including AIDS, and in the assessment of patient response to chemotherapy and radiation.

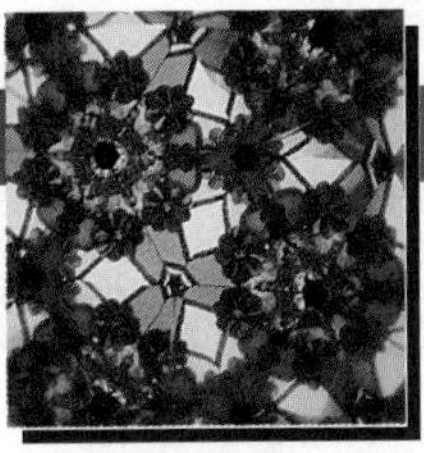

Index

Letters following page numbers indicate chart (*c*), figure (*f*), guideline (*g*), and table (*t*).

H

Self-Study Program Instructions

This electronic self-study program has been designed for use with an IBM or IBM-compatible computer and requires DOS version 3.0 or higher, 512KB RAM, a 3.5-inch disk drive, and a CGA graphics card or better.

To start the program, insert the diskette in your disk drive and type "a:" (or the appropriate letter for your disk drive—usually a or b), and press the <Enter> key. At the prompt (A:\>or B:\>), type "go" and press the <Enter> key to start the program.

This self-study program enables you to answer approximately 350 questions in a manner similar to the way you will take the NCLEX examination. As in the NCLEX, all questions in this program are multiple choice. To answer the questions, you will need to use only the up and down arrow keys and the <Enter> key. Use the arrow keys to highlight the answer you wish to select, and press <Enter> to make the selection. Instructions are provided at the bottom of the screen.

The Main Menu of the program looks like this:

1. Instructions
2. Choose a Test
3. Review Results
4. Quit

Highlight your choice using the arrow keys, and press <Enter>to select it.

Selecting the **Instructions** option will display an instructions screen.

Selecting the **Choose a Test** option will provide you with a list of 15 tests, each corresponding to a unit in *Brunner and Suddarth's Textbook of Medical-Surgical Nursing* (Units 1 and 2 do not have corresponding tests). To begin taking a test, use the arrow keys to highlight the name of the test you wish to take, and press the <Enter> key.

After you have selected a topic, you will be asked if you wish to take the test in *Study Mode* or *Test Mode.* To select a mode, press the <Alt> key at the same time as the underlined letter in your choice (<Alt>S for *Study Mode,* <Alt>T for *Test Mode*).

Study Mode lets you know immediately if the answer you select is correct and provides you with feedback for correct and incorrect choices. If you select an incorrect answer, try again until you find the correct answer.

If you select *Test Mode,* you will be given the option of having the test timed (press <Alt>I), having the screen display the time remaining (press <Alt>R), and having the screen display the number of questions remaining in the test (press <Alt>Q). While in *Test Mode* you will not receive immediate feedback on your answers. When you have answered all the questions or when time has expired, you will be shown how many questions you have answered correctly.

After seeing your test results in *Test Mode,* you will have the option of printing the results of the test (press <Alt>P), reviewing the questions again in *Study Mode* (press <Alt>S), or returning to the main menu (press <Alt>M).

If you choose to review the questions in *Study Mode,* you will see all the questions in that particular test again. The questions you answered correctly will be indicated with a check mark in front of the question number. All questions without a check mark were either answered incorrectly or not answered. In this mode you will receive instant feedback on the answers you select.

The results for each test taken in a single session are temporarily stored in memory. Choosing the **Review Results** option from the Main Menu will show you the results for any test you have taken during this session.

Selecting the **Quit** option from the Main Menu will end the session and return you to DOS.